# Textbook of Respiratory Medicine

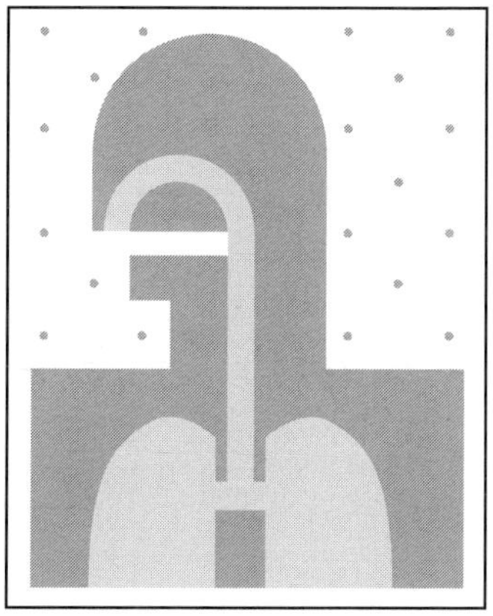

# Textbook of Respiratory Medicine

*Third Edition*


**Editors:**

**JOHN F. MURRAY,** M.D., D.Sc. (Hon), FRCP
Professor Emeritus of Medicine
University of California, San Francisco
Senior Staff, Pulmonary and Critical Care Division
San Francisco General Hospital
Senior Staff, Cardiovascular Research Institute
San Francisco, California

**JAY A. NADEL,** M.D., D.Sc. (Hon)
Professor of Medicine
Physiology and Radiology
University of California, San Francisco
Chief, Division of Pulmonary and Critical Care Medicine
Senior Staff, Cardiovascular Research Institute
San Francisco, California

**Associate Editors:**

**ROBERT J. MASON,** M.D.
Professor of Medicine
University of Colorado Health Sciences Center
Senior Faculty Member
National Jewish Medical and Research Center
Denver, Colorado

**HOMER A. BOUSHEY, JR.,** M.D.
Professor of Medicine
Department of Medicine
University of California, San Francisco
Director, Asthma Clinical Research Center
Chief, Division of Allergy and Immunology
San Francisco, California



**W.B. SAUNDERS COMPANY**
*A Harcourt Health Sciences Company*
Philadelphia • London • New York • St. Louis • Sydney • Toronto

**W.B. SAUNDERS COMPANY**
*A Harcourt Health Sciences Company*

The Curtis Center
Independence Square West
Philadelphia, Pennsylvania 19106



**Library of Congress Cataloging-in-Publication Data**

Textbook of respiratory medicine / [edited by] John F. Murray, Jay A. Nadel, Robert J. Mason, Homer A. Boushey, Jr.—3rd ed.

p. cm.

Includes bibliographical references and index.

ISBN 0-7216-7711-8 (set)

1. Respiratory organs—Diseases. I. Murray, John F. (John Frederic) II. Nadel, Jay A. Mason, Robert J. Boushey, Homer A., Jr. [DNLM: 1. Respiratory Tract Diseases. WF 140 T355 2000]

RC731.T48 2000 616.2—dc21

DNLM/DLC 99-045310

*Acquisitions Editor:* Richard Zorab
*Senior Developmental Editor:* Dolores Meloni
*Manuscript Editor:* Anne Ostroff
*Production Manager:* Natalie Ware
*Illustration Specialist:* Walter Verbitski

Set ISBN 0-7216-7711-8
Vol. 1 ISBN 0-7216-7712-6
Vol. 2 ISBN 0-7216-7713-4

TEXTBOOK OF RESPIRATORY MEDICINE



Printed in the United States of America.

Last digit is the print number: 9 8 7 6 5 4 3 2 1

*We dedicate this textbook to Dr. Julius H. Comroe, Jr., who was our mentor during the formative years of our professional development. Dr. Comroe was one of the truly great academicians of his generation. He was an investigator of exceptional merit, an educator whose influence was worldwide, and a medical statesman of exemplary integrity and vision. In dedicating this book, we acknowledge especially Dr. Comroe's scholarly contributions and his commitment to the importance of basic science in the solution of clinical problems.*

J.F.M.

J.A.N.

# Contributors

**Lewis Adams, Ph.D.**
National Heart and Lung Institute, Imperial College School of Medicine, London, United Kingdom
*Dyspnea*

**Richard K. Albert, M.D.**
Professor and Vice-Chair for Education, University of Colorado Health Sciences Center; Chief of Medicine, Denver Health Medical Center, Denver, Colorado
*Preoperative Evaluation*

**Kurt H. Albertine, Ph.D.**
Course Director—Gross Anatomy, Department of Neurobiology and Anatomy, and Professor, Departments of Pediatrics, Medicine, and Neurobiology and Anatomy, University of Utah, School of Medicine, Salt Lake City, Utah
*Anatomy of the Lungs*

**Thomas K. Aldrich, M.D.**
Professor of Medicine and Director, Pulmonary Medicine Division, Albert Einstein College of Medicine and Montefiore Medical Center, Bronx, New York
*The Lungs and Neuromuscular Disease*

**John R. Balmes, M.D., M.P.H.**
Professor of Medicine, University of California, San Francisco; Chief, Division of Occupational and Environmental Medicine, San Francisco General Hospital, San Francisco, California
*Evaluation of Respiratory Impairment/Disability; Occupational Asthma and Byssinosis; Air Pollution*

**Joan Albert Barberà, M.D.**
Senior Specialist, Servei de Pneumologia i Allèrgia Respiratòria, Hospital Clinic, Barcelona, Spain
*Pulmonary Complications of Abdominal Disease*

**Peter J. Barnes, D.M., D.Sc., FRCP**
Professor of Thoracic Medicine, National Heart and Lung Institute, and Chairman of Respiratory Medicine, Imperial College, London, United Kingdom
*General Pharmacologic Principles; Airway Pharmacology*

**Scott Barnhart, M.D., M.P.H.**
Associate Professor, Department of Medicine and Environmental Health, University of Washington; Medical Director/Associate Dean, Harborview Medical Center, University of Washington, Seattle, Washington
*Evaluation of Respiratory Impairment/Disability*

**Carol Basbaum, Ph.D.**
Professor of Anatomy, University of California, San Francisco, California
*Mucus Secretion and Ion Transport in Airways*

**Robert P. Baughman, M.D.**
Professor of Medicine, Division of Pulmonary and Critical Care Medicine, Department of Internal Medicine, University of Cincinnati Medical Center, Cincinnati, Ohio
*Bronchoscopy, Lung Biopsy, and Other Diagnostic Procedures*

**Margaret R. Becklake, M.B., B.Ch., M.D., FRCP, FRS(C)**
Professor Emeritus, Departments of Medicine and of Epidemiology, Biostatistics and Occupational Health, McGill University; Honorary Physician, McGill University Health Center, Royal Victoria Hospital Pavilion, Montréal, Québec, Canada
*Pneumoconioses*

**Albert J. Berger, Ph.D.**
Professor of Physiology and Biophysics, School of Medicine, University of Washington, Seattle, Washington
*Control of Breathing*

**Paul D. Blanc, M.D., M.S.P.H.**
Associate Professor of Medicine, University of California, San Francisco, California
*General Principles and Diagnostic Approach; Acute Pulmonary Responses to Toxic Exposures*

**Barry R. Bloom, Ph.D.**
Dean of the Faculty and Professor of Immunology and Infectious Diseases, Harvard School of Public Health, Boston, Massachusetts
*Tuberculosis and Other Myobacterial Diseases*

**R. C. Boucher, M.D.**
Kenan Professor of Medicine, University of North Carolina at Chapel Hill; Director, Cystic Fibrosis/Pulmonary Research and Treatment Center, University of North Carolina Hospitals, Chapel Hill, North Carolina
*Cystic Fibrosis*

**Homer A. Boushey, Jr., M.D.**
Professor of Medicine, Department of Medicine, University of California, San Francisco; Director, Asthma Clinical Research Center, Chief, Division of Allergy and Immunology, San Francisco, California
*Asthma*

**Alfred A. Bove, M.D., Ph.D.**
Professor of Medicine and Associate Dean for Practice Plan Affairs, Temple University School of Medicine, Philadelphia, Pennsylvania
*Diving Medicine*

**T. Douglas Bradley, M.D.**
Professor of Medicine, University of Toronto; Director, Sleep Research Laboratory, Toronto Rehabilitation Institute, Toronto, Ontario, Canada
*Sleep Disorders*

**V. Courtney Broaddus, M.D.**
Associate Professor of Medicine, University of California, San Francisco; Chief, Division of Pulmonary and Critical Care Medicine, San Francisco General Hospital, San Francisco, California
*General Principles and Diagnostic Approach; Pleural Effusion; Pneumothorax, Chylothorax, Hemothorax, and Fibrothorax; Tumors of the Pleura*

**Philip Bromberg, M.D.**
Bonner Professor of Medicine and Director, Center for Environmental Medicine and Lung Biology, University of North Carolina School of Medicine, Chapel Hill, North Carolina
*Pulmonary Complications of Hematologic Disease*

**Robert Cameron, M.D.**
Assistant Professor, Cardiothoracic Surgery and Surgical Oncology, and Director, Thoracic Oncology, University of California, Los Angeles, School of Medicine, Los Angeles, California
*Bronchogenic Carcinoma*

**Bartolome R. Celli, M.D.**
Professor of Medicine, Tufts University; Chief, Pulmonary and Critical Care, St. Elizabeth's Medical Center, Boston, Massachusetts
*Pulmonary Rehabilitation*

**Reuben M. Cherniack, M.D.**
Professor of Medicine, University of Colorado Health Sciences Center, National Jewish Medical and Research Center, Denver, Colorado
*Principles of and Approach to the Patient with Interstitial Lung Disease; Diffuse Alveolar Hemorrhage and Other Rare Infiltrative Disorders*

**Noreen M. Clark, Ph.D.**
Dean and Marshall H. Becker Professor of Public Health, University of Michigan School of Public Health, Ann Arbor, Michigan
*Individual Measures: Social and Behavioral Aspects*

**Franklin R. Cockerill III, M.D.**
Professor of Microbiology and Laboratory Medicine and Professor of Medicine, Mayo Medical School; Chairman of Microbiology, Director of Bacteriology and Molecular Microbiology, and Consultant in Microbiology and Infectious Diseases, Mayo Clinic and Mayo Foundation, Rochester, Minnesota
*Microbiologic Diagnosis of Lower Respiratory Tract Infection*

**David B. Corry, M.D.**
Assistant Professor of Medicine, Baylor College of Medicine, Houston, Texas
*Asthma*

**Robert L. Cowie, M.D.**
Professor, Departments of Medicine and of Community Health Sciences, and Head, Division of Respiratory Medicine, University of Calgary; Physician, Foothills Medical Centre; Director, Tuberculosis Services, Calgary, Alberta, Canada
*Pneumoconioses*

**Stephen Crawford, M.D.**
Associate Clinical Professor of Medicine, Pulmonary and Critical Care Division, University of California, San Diego, California
*Pulmonary Complications of Hematologic Disease*

**Scott F. Davies, M.D.**
Professor of Medicine, University of Minnesota Medical School; Chief, Division of Pulmonary and Critical Care Medicine, Hennepin County Medical Center, Minneapolis, Minnesota
*Fungal Infections*

**R. M. du Bois, M.D.**
Professor, Imperial College School of Medicine, London, United Kingdom
*The Lungs and Connective Tissue Diseases*

**Steven R. Duncan, M.D.**
Assistant Professor, The Scripps Research Institute, Department of Immunology; Attending Physician, Chest and Critical Care Medicine, Scripps Hospital, La Jolla, California
*Pulmonary Complications of Organ Transplantation and Primary Immunodeficiencies*

**Richard M. Effros, M.D.**
Professor of Medicine, Medical College of Wisconsin; Chief, Pulmonary and Critical Care Medicine, Froedtert Lutheran Memorial Hospital, Milwaukee, Wisconsin
*Acid-Base Balance*

**Virginia L. Ernster, Ph.D.**
Professor and Vice-Chair, Department of Epidemiology and Biostatistics, School of Medicine, University of California, San Francisco, California
*Epidemiology of Lung Cancer*

**John V. Fahy, M.D.**
Associate Professor of Medicine, University of California, San Francisco; Investigator, Cardiovascular Research Institute; Attending Physician, Critical Care Medicine and Pulmonary Medicine, Moffitt-Long Hospital, University of California, San Francisco, California
*Asthma*

**Barry L. Fanburg, M.D.**
Professor of Medicine, Tufts University School of Medicine; Chief, Pulmonary and Critical Care Division, New England Medical Center, Boston, Massachusetts
*Sarcoidosis*

**Peter F. Fedullo, M.D.**
Professor of Medicine, University of California, San Diego, Medical Center, San Diego, California
*Pulmonary Thromboembolism*

**Robert A. Figlin, M.D., FACP**
Professor of Medicine, Division of Hematology/Oncology, University of California, Los Angeles, School of Medicine, Los Angeles, California
*Bronchogenic Carcinoma*

**Sydney M. Finegold, M.D.**
Professor of Medicine and Professor of Microbiology and Immunology, University of California, Los Angeles, School of Medicine; Staff Physician, Infectious Diseases Section, Veterans Affairs Greater Los Angeles Health Care System; West Los Angeles Health Care Center, Los Angeles, California
*Pyogenic Bacterial Pneumonia, Lung Abscess, and Empyema*

**Jeffrey R. Fineman, M.D.**
Associate Professor of Pediatrics (Critical Care Medicine), University of California, San Francisco, California
*Vascular Pharmacology*

**Walter E. Finkbeiner, M.D., Ph.D.**
Professor and Director, Anatomic Pathology, Department of Pathology, University of California, Davis, School of Medicine, Sacramento, California
*General Features of Respiratory Pathology*

**Michael R. Flick, M.D., J.D.**
Associate Clinical Professor of Medicine, University of California, San Francisco, San Francisco; Visiting Scholar, Center for the Study of Law and Society, University of California, Berkeley; Chest Service, San Francisco General Hospital, San Francisco, California
*Pulmonary Edema and Acute Lung Injury*

**Kwun M. Fong, M.D., Ph.D.**
Assistant Professor, Department of Thoracic Medicine, The Prince Charles Hospital, Chermside, Brisbane, Australia
*Biology of Lung Cancer*

**Andrew P. Fontenot, M.D.**
Assistant Professor of Medicine, University of Colorado Health Sciences Center; Staff Physician, National Jewish Medical and Research Center, Denver, Colorado
*Immune Recognition and Responses*

**Judith Ford, Ph.D., MRCP, FRCR**
Assistant Professor, Radiation Oncology, University of California, Los Angeles, California
*Bronchogenic Carcinoma*

**Robinson Fulwood, M.S.P.H.**
Senior Manager, Public Health Program Development, National Institutes of Health/National Heart, Lung, and Blood Institute, Office of Prevention, Education, and Control, Bethesda, Maryland
*Community Measures: Public Policy and Education*

**Adi F. Gazdar, M.D.**
Professor of Pathology and Deputy Director, Hamon Center for Therapeutic Oncology Research, University of Texas Southwestern Medical Center, Dallas, Texas
*Biology of Lung Cancer*

**Gerald F. Gebhart, Ph.D.**
Professor and Head, Department of Pharmacology, University of Iowa College of Medicine, Iowa City, Iowa
*Chest Pain*

**Julie Louise Gerberding, M.D., M.P.H.**
Associate Professor of Medicine (Infectious Diseases), University of California, San Francisco; Staff Physician, San Francisco General Hospital, San Francisco, California
*General Principles and Diagnostic Approach*

**Matthew Bidwell Goetz, M.D.**
Professor of Clinical Medicine, Department of Medicine, University of California, Los Angeles, School of Medicine; Chief, Infectious Diseases, Veterans Affairs Greater Los Angeles Healthcare System, Los Angeles, California
*Pyogenic Bacterial Pneumonia, Lung Abscess, and Empyema*

**Edward J. Goetzl, M.D.**
Professor of Medicine and Immunology and Director of Immunology and Allergy Research, University of California, San Francisco, Medical Center, San Francisco, California
*Eosinophilic Lung Diseases*

**Warren M. Gold, M.D.**
Professor of Medicine, University of California, San Francisco; Attending Physician, Moffitt-Long Hospitals; Associate Staff and Director, Adult Pulmonary Laboratories, Clinical Physiological Services, Cardiovascular Research Institute, University of California, San Francisco, California
*Pulmonary Function Testing*

**Jeffrey A. Golden, M.D.**
Professor of Clinical Medicine, Director of Bronchoscopy, and Medical Director, Lung Transplant Program, and Professor of Clinical Medicine, Department of Medicine, University of California, San Francisco, California
*Bronchoscopy, Lung Biopsy, and Other Diagnostic Procedures*

**Ramya Gopinath, M.B., B.S.**
Visiting Associate, Helminth Immunology Section, Laboratory of Parasitic Diseases, National Institutes of Health, Bethesda, Maryland
*Parasitic Diseases*

**Alexander Gottschalk, M.D.**
Professor, Department of Radiology, Michigan State University, East Lansing, Michigan
*Nuclear Medicine Techniques and Applications*

**Peter H. Hackett, M.D.**
Affiliate Associate Professor of Medicine, University of Washington, Seattle, Washington; Staff Physician, St. Mary's Hospital and Medical Center, Grand Junction, Colorado
*High Altitude*

**Jesse B. Hall, M.D.**
Professor of Medicine, Anesthesia, and Critical Care, University of Chicago; Director of Critical Care Services, University of Chicago Hospitals and Clinics, Chicago, Illinois
*Principles of Critical Care of Respiratory Failure; Acute Hypoxemic Respiratory Failure; Ventilatory Failure*

**Frederick G. Hayden, M.D.**
Professor of Internal Medicine and Pathology and Stuart S. Richardson Professor of Clinical Virology, University of Virginia School of Medicine; Professor of Internal Medicine and Pathology, Department of Internal Medicine, University of Virginia Health System, Charlottesville, Virginia
*Viral Infections*

**Peter M. Henson, B.V.M.S., Ph.D.**
Professor of Pathology, Medicine, and Immunology, University of Colorado School of Medicine; Senior Faculty Member, Department of Pediatrics, National Jewish Medical and Research Center, Denver, Colorado
*Inflammation, Injury, and Repair*

**Michael A. Heymann, M.D.**
Professor of Pediatrics (Cardiology), University of California, San Francisco, California
*Vascular Pharmacology*

**Michele Hindi-Alexander, Ph.D.**
Health Scientist Administrator, Division of Lung Diseases, National Heart, Lung, and Blood Institute, Bethesda, Maryland
*Community Measures: Public Policy and Education*

**Julien I. E. Hoffman, M.D.**
Professor of Pediatrics (Cardiology), University of California, San Francisco, California
*Vascular Pharmacology*

**Philip C. Hopewell, M.D.**
Professor of Medicine, University of California, San Francisco; Associate Dean, San Francisco General Hospital, San Francisco, California
*Tuberculosis and Other Myobacterial Diseases*

**Thomas F. Hornbein, M.D.**
Professor of Anesthesiology, University of Washington, Seattle, Washington
*High Altitude*

**Laurence Huang, M.D.**
Assistant Professor of Medicine, University of California, San Francisco; Medical Director, Inpatient AIDS Unit and Consultation Service, and Chief, AIDS Chest Clinic, San Francisco General Hospital, San Francisco, California
*Pulmonary Complications of Human Immunodeficiency Virus Infection*

**J. Michael B. Hughes, D.M., FRCP**
Professor of Thoracic Medicine, Imperial College School of Medicine, and Honorary Consultant Physician, Department of Respiratory Medicine, Hammersmith Hospital, London, United Kingdom
*Pulmonary Arteriovenous Malformations and Other Pulmonary Vascular Abnormalities; Pulmonary Complications of Heart Disease*

**Dallas M. Hyde, Ph.D.**
Veterinary Anatomy, Department of Anatomy, Physiology and Cell Biology, and Professor and Associate Dean of Research, University of California, Davis, School of Veterinary Medicine, Davis, California
*Anatomy of the Lungs*

**Michael C. Iannuzzi, M.D.**
Senior Staff Physician, Pulmonary and Critical Care Medicine, Henry Ford Health System, Detroit, Michigan
*Genetic Basis of Lung Disease*

**Richard S. Irwin, M.D.**
Professor of Medicine, University of Massachusetts Medical School; Director, Division of Pulmonary Allergy and Critical Care Medicine, University of Massachusetts Memorial Health Care, Worcester, Massachusetts
*Cough*

**Susan Janson, R.N., A.N.P., D.N.Sc.**
Professor, School of Nursing; Adjunct Professor, School of Medicine, University of California, San Francisco, California
*Individual Measures: Social and Behavioral Aspects*

**Kenneth G. Kalassian, M.D.**
Medical Director, Critical Care Services, White Memorial Medical Center, Los Angeles, California
*Lymphangioleiomyomatosis*

**Haskins K. Kashima, M.D.**
Professor of Otolaryngology and Professor of Oncology, Johns Hopkins University School of Medicine; Active Full-Time Staff, Johns Hopkins Hospital, Baltimore, Maryland
*Disorders of the Upper Airways*

**Michael P. Keane, M.D.**
Assistant Professor of Medicine, Division of Pulmonary and Critical Care Medicine, University of Michigan Medical School, Ann Arbor, Michigan
*Inflammation, Injury, and Repair*

**Fraser M. Keith, M.D.**
Associate Clinical Professor, University of California, San Francisco, California
*Bronchoscopy, Lung Biopsy, and Other Diagnostic Procedures*

**Talmadge E. King, Jr., M.D.**
Constance B. Wofsy Distinguished Professor, University of California; Chief of Medical Services, and Vice Chair, Department of Medicine, San Francisco; San Francisco General Hospital, San Francisco, California
*Principles of and Approach to the Patient with Interstitial Lung Disease; Idiopathic Interstitial Pneumonias; Diffuse Alveolar Hemorrhage and Other Rare Infiltrative Disorders*

**M. R. Knowles, M.D.**
Professor of Medicine, University of North Carolina at Chapel Hill; Co-Director, Adult Cystic Fibrosis Program, University of North Carolina Hospitals, Chapel Hill, North Carolina
*Cystic Fibrosis*

**Brian L. Kotzin, M.D.**
Professor of Medicine and Immunology, University of Colorado Health Sciences Center; Professor of Medicine, National Jewish Medical and Research Center, Denver, Colorado
*Immune Recognition and Responses*

**Stephen C. Lazarus, M.D.**
Professor of Medicine, Division of Pulmonary and Critical Care Medicine; Senior Investigator, Cardiovascular Research Institute; Director, Chest Faculty Practice; and Director, Medical Specialty Practices, University of California, San Francisco, California
*Disorders of the Intrathoracic Airways*

**Claude Lenfant, M.D.**
Director, National Heart, Lung, and Blood Institute, National Institutes of Health, Bethesda, Maryland
*Community Measures: Public Policy and Education*

**James Lewis, M.D., FRCPC**
Associate Professor of Medicine and Physiology, University of Western Ontario; Associate Professor of Medicine and Physiology, Lawson Research Institute, St. Joseph's Health Centre, London, Ontario, Canada
*Pulmonary Surfactant*

**Richard W. Light, M.D.**
Professor of Medicine, Vanderbilt University; Director of Pulmonary Diseases, Saint Thomas Hospital, Nashville, Tennessee
*General Principles and Diagnostic Approach; Pleural Effusion; Pneumothorax, Chylothorax, Hemothorax, and Fibrothorax; Tumors of the Pleura*

**Glen A. Lillington, M.D., FRCPC (Medicine)**
Clinical Professor of Medicine, Stanford University, Stanford; Ombudsman, Palo Alto Medical Foundation, Palo Alto, California
*Benign Tumors*

**Andrew H. Limper, M.D.**
Associate Professor of Medicine, Biochemistry and Molecular Biology, Mayo Graduate School of Medicine; Staff Physician, Mayo Clinic, St. Mary's Hospital, and Rochester Methodist Hospital, Rochester, Minnesota
*Drug-Induced Pulmonary Disease*

**John M. Luce, M.D.**
Professor of Medicine and Anesthesia, University of California, San Francisco; Associate Director, Medical-Surgical Intensive Care Unit, San Francisco General Hospital, San Francisco, California
*Bronchiectasis; Pulmonary Arteriovenous Malformations and Other Pulmonary Vascular Abnormalities; Eosinophilic Lung Diseases*

**Judith A. Luce, M.D.**
Clinical Professor of Medicine, University of California, San Francisco; Director, Oncology Services, San Francisco General Hospital, San Francisco, California
*Lymphoma, Lymphoproliferative Diseases, and Other Primary Malignant Tumors; Metastatic Malignant Tumors*

**Neil R. MacIntyre, M.D.**
Professor of Medicine, Duke University Medical Center, Durham, North Carolina
*Principles of Mechanical Ventilation*

**Asrar B. Malik, Ph.D.**
Professor and Head, Department of Pharmacology, University of Illinois College of Medicine, Chicago, Illinois
*Pulmonary Circulation and Regulation of Fluid Balance*

**Gregory R. Mason, M.D.**
Professor of Medicine, University of California, Los Angeles (UCLA), School of Medicine, Los Angeles; Director, Chest Services, Department of Medicine, Division of Respiratory and Critical Care Physiology and Medicine, Harbor-UCLA Medical Center, Torrance, California
*Pulmonary Alveolar Proteinosis*

**Robert J. Mason, M.D.**
Professor of Medicine, University of Colorado Health Sciences Center; Associate Vice President for Academic Affairs and Senior Faculty Member, National Jewish Medical and Research Center, Denver, Colorado
*Pulmonary Surfactant*

**Michael A. Matthay, M.D.**
Professor, Medicine and Anesthesia, University of California, San Francisco; Senior Associate, Cardiovascular Research Institute; Associate Director, Intensive Care Unit, Moffitt Hospital, San Francisco, California
*Pulmonary Edema and Acute Lung Injury*

**Janet R. Maurer, M.D., FCCP**
Head, Section of Lung Transplantation, Department of Pulmonary and Critical Care Medicine; Associate Medical Director, Transplant Center, Cleveland Clinic Foundation, Cleveland, Ohio
*Lung Transplantation*

**F. Dennis McCool, M.D.**
Associate Professor of Medicine, Brown University Medical School, Providence; Medical Director of Respiratory Care, Memorial Hospital of Rhode Island, Pawtucket, Rhode Island
*The Lungs and Chest Wall Disease*

**John A. McDonald, M.D., Ph.D.**
Professor of Internal Medicine, Biochemistry and Molecular Biology, Mayo Graduate School of Medicine, Rochester, Minnesota; Director for Research, Mayo Clinic, Scottsdale, Arizona
*Lung Growth and Development*

**John D. Minna, M.D.**
Professor, Internal Medicine and Pharmacology, and Director, Hamon Center for Therapeutic Oncology Research, University of Texas Southwestern Medical Center, Dallas, Texas
*Biology of Lung Cancer*

**Richard D. Minshall, Ph.D.**
Research Assistant Professor, University of Illinois College of Medicine, Chicago, Illinois
*Pulmonary Circulation and Regulation of Fluid Balance*

**Jann Mortensen, M.D., D.Sc.**
Associate Professor, Department of Clinical Physiology and Nuclear Medicine, The Center of Imaging, Informatics and Engineering in Medicine, The Rigshospital, Copenhagen University Hospital, Copenhagen, Denmark
*Deposition and Clearance*

**John F. Murray, M.D., D.Sc. (Hon), FRCP**
Professor Emeritus of Medicine, University of California, San Francisco; Chief, Chest Service, 1966–1989, San Francisco General Hospital, San Francisco, California
*Chest Pain; History and Physical Examination; General Principles and Diagnostic Approach*

**Piero Mustacchi, M.D.**
Clinical Professor of Medicine and of Epidemiology, School of Medicine, University of California, San Francisco; Attending Physician, University of California Hospitals and California Pacific Medical Center, San Francisco, California
*Epidemiology of Lung Cancer*

**Jay A. Nadel, M.D., D.Sc. (Hon)**
Professor of Medicine, Physiology and Radiology, University of California, San Francisco; Chief, Division of Pulmonary and Critical Care Medicine, Senior Staff, Cardiovascular Research Institute, San Francisco, California
*General Principles and Diagnostic Approach*

**Tom Neuman, M.D.**
Professor of Medicine and Surgery, University of California, San Diego, California
*Diving Medicine*

**Thomas B. Nutman, M.D.**
Head, Helminth Parasitology Immunology Section and Clinical Parasitology Unit, Laboratory of Parasitic Diseases, National Institutes of Health, Bethesda, Maryland
*Parasitic Diseases*

**Kathryn E. Osann, Ph.D.**
Associate Adjunct Professor, Department of Medicine, Division of Hematology/Oncology, College of Medicine, University of California, Irvine, California
*Epidemiology of Lung Cancer*

**David R. Park, M.D.**
Acting Assistant Professor of Medicine, Division of Pulmonary and Critical Care Medicine, University of Washington, Seattle, Washington
*General Principles and Diagnostic Approach; Pneumomediastinum and Mediastinitis; Tumors and Cysts of the Mediastinum*

**Thomas L. Petty, M.D.**
Professor of Medicine, University of Colorado, Denver, Colorado; Professor of Medicine, Rush University, Chicago, Illinois
*Pulmonary Rehabilitation*

**Eliot A. Phillipson, M.D.**
Sir John and Lady Eaton Professor and Chair, Department of Medicine, University of Toronto, Toronto, Ontario, Canada
*Hypoventilation and Hyperventilation Syndromes; Sleep Disorders*

**David J. Pierson, M.D.**
Professor of Medicine, Division of Pulmonary and Critical Care Medicine, University of Washington; Medical Director of Respiratory Care, Harborview Medical Center, Seattle, Washington
*General Principles and Diagnostic Approach; Pneumomediastinum and Mediastinitis; Tumors and Cysts of the Mediastinum*

**Craig A. Piquette, M.D.**
Assistant Professor of Medicine, Section of Pulmonary and Critical Care Medicine, Department of Internal Medicine, University of Nebraska Medical Center; Staff Physician, Pulmonary Section, Medical Service, Omaha Veterans Administration Medical Center, Omaha, Nebraska
*Chronic Bronchitis and Emphysema*

**Diane Prager, M.D.**
Assistant Professor of Medicine, University of California, Los Angeles, School of Medicine, Los Angeles, California
*Bronchogenic Carcinoma*

**Donald F. Proctor, M.D.**
Emeritus Professor, Environmental Health Science, Otolaryngology, and Anesthesiology, Johns Hopkins University School of Medicine; Active Staff, Johns Hopkins Hospital, Baltimore, Maryland
*Disorders of the Upper Airways*

**Thomas A. Raffin, M.D.**
Colleen and Robert Haas Professor of Medicine and Biomedical Ethics; Chief, Division of Pulmonary and Critical Care Medicine; and Co-Director, Stanford University Center for Biomedical Ethics, Stanford University Medical School, Stanford, California
*Lymphangioleiomyomatosis; Pulmonary Complications of Organ Transplantations and Primary Immunodeficiencies; Ethics and Withdrawal of Life Support*

**Elliot Rapaport, M.D.**
Professor of Medicine and William Watt Kerr Professor of Clinical Medicine, University of California, San Francisco; Attending Cardiologist, San Francisco General Hospital, San Francisco, California
*Cor Pulmonale*

**Stephen I. Rennard, M.D.**
Professor of Medicine, Pulmonary and Critical Care Medicine, Department of Internal Medicine, University of Nebraska Medical Center, Omaha, Nebraska
*Chronic Bronchitis and Emphysema*

**David W. H. Riches, Ph.D.**
Division of Pulmonary Sciences and Critical Care Medicine, University of Colorado Health Sciences Center; Senior Faculty Member, National Jewish Medical and Research Center, Denver, Colorado
*Monocytes, Macrophages, and Dendritic Cells of the Lungs*

**Norman W. Rizk, M.D.**
Professor of Medicine, Stanford University School of Medicine; Medical Director and Senior Associate Chair, Department of Medicine, Stanford University, Stanford, California
*Benign Tumors; The Lungs in Obstetric and Gynecologic Disease*

**Dudley F. Rochester, M.D.**
Professor Emeritus, University of Virginia Medical School, Charlottesville, Virginia
*The Lungs and Neuromuscular Disease; The Lungs and Chest Wall Disease*

**Joseph R. Rodarte, M.D.**
Professor of Medicine and Molecular Physiology and Biophysics, and Chief of Pulmonary and Critical Care Section, Department of Medicine, Baylor College of Medicine; Chief of Pulmonary and Critical Care Service, Methodist Hospital, Houston, Texas
*Respiratory System Mechanics*

**Robert Rodriguez-Roisin, M.D., FRCP(E)**
Professor and Chairman, Department of Medicine, School of Medicine, University of Barcelona; Chief of Service and Senior Consultant, Servei de Pneumologia i Allèrgia Respiratòria, Hospital Clinic, Barcelona, Spain
*Pulmonary Complications of Abdominal Disease*

**Cecile S. Rose, M.D., M.P.H.**
Associate Professor of Medicine, University of Colorado Health Sciences Center; Staff Physician, National Jewish Medical and Research Center, Denver, Colorado
*Hypersensitivity Pneumonitis*

**Edward C. Rosenow III, M.D.**
Professor Emeritus of Medicine, Mayo Graduate School of Medicine, Rochester, Minnesota
*Drug-Induced Pulmonary Disease*

**Lewis J. Rubin, M.D.**
Professor of Medicine and Director, Division of Pulmonary and Critical Care Medicine, University of California, San Diego, School of Medicine, San Diego, California
*Pulmonary Vasculitis and Primary Pulmonary Hypertension*

**George A. Sarosi, M.D.**
Professor of Medicine, Indiana University; Chief, Medical Service, Roudebush Veterans Affairs Medical Center, Indianapolis, Indiana
*Fungal Infections*

**Gregory A. Schmidt, M.D.**
Professor of Clinical Medicine and Clinical Anesthesia and Critical Care, University of Chicago, Pritzker School of Medicine, Chicago, Illinois
*Principles of Critical Care of Respiratory Failure; Acute Hypoxemic Respiratory Failure; Ventilatory Failure*

**Robert B. Schoene, M.D.**
Professor of Medicine, Division of Pulmonary and Critical Care Medicine, University of Washington; Director of Internal Medicine Education, Providence Seattle Medical Center, Seattle, Washington
*High Altitude*

**Alan R. Schwartz, M.D.**
Associate Professor of Medicine, Johns Hopkins University School of Medicine, Baltimore, Maryland
*Disorders of the Upper Airways*

**Marvin I. Schwarz, M.D.**
James C. Campbell Professor of Pulmonary Medicine and Head, Division of Pulmonary Sciences and Critical Care Medicine, University of Colorado Health Sciences Center, Denver, Colorado
*Principles of and Approach to the Patient with Interstitial Lung Disease; Idiopathic Interstitial Pneumonias; Diffuse Alveolar Hemorrhage and Other Rare Infiltrative Disorders*

**Yoshitaka Sekido, M.D., Ph.D.**
Assistant Professor, Department of Clinical Preventive Medicine, Nagoya University School of Medicine, Nagoya, Japan
*Biology of Lung Cancer*

**Felix R. Shardonofsky, M.D.**
Assistant Professor of Pediatrics, Baylor College of Medicine, Houston, Texas
*Respiratory System Mechanics*

**Arthur S. Slutsky, M.D.**
Professor and Director, Division of Respiratory Medicine, University of Toronto, Toronto, Ontario, Canada
*Hypoventilation and Hyperventilation Syndromes*

**Philip L. Smith, M.D.**
Professor of Medicine, Johns Hopkins University School of Medicine; Active Full-Time Staff, Johns Hopkins Hospital, Johns Hopkins Bayview Medical Center, Baltimore, Maryland
*Disorders of the Upper Airways*

**Gordon L. Snider, M.D.**
Maurice B. Strauss Professor of Medicine, Boston University School of Medicine; Chief, Medical Service, Veterans Affairs Boston Healthcare System, Boston, Massachusetts
*Chronic Bronchitis and Emphysema*

**H. Dirk Sostman, M.D.**
Professor of Radiology, Cornell Medical College; Radiologist in Chief, New York Hospital, New York, New York
*Radiographic Techniques*

**John D. Stansell, M.D.**
Associate Professor of Medicine, University of California, San Francisco; Medical Director, Positive Health Program, San Francisco General Hospital, San Francisco, California
*Pulmonary Complications of Human Immunodeficiency Virus Infection*

**Robert M. Strieter, M.D.**
Professor of Medicine and Vice-Chair of Medicine, Chief Division of Pulmonary and Critical Care Medicine, University of California, Los Angeles, School of Medicine, Los Angeles, California
*Inflammation, Injury, and Repair*

**Michael S. Stulbarg, M.D.**
Professor of Clinical Medicine, University of California, San Francisco, California
*Dyspnea*

**Ira B. Tager, M.D., M.P.H.**
Professor of Epidemiology, School of Public Health, University of California, Berkeley, California
*Air Pollution*

**Virginia S. Taggart, M.P.H.**
Health Science Administrator, Division of Lung Diseases, National Heart, Lung, and Blood Institute, Bethesda, Maryland
*Community Measures: Public Policy and Education*

**C. Tiruppathi, Ph.D.**
Assistant Professor, University of Illinois College of Medicine, Chicago, Illinois
*Pulmonary Circulation and Regulation of Fluid Balance*

**Alkis Togias, M.D.**
Associate Professor of Medicine, Johns Hopkins University, Baltimore, Maryland
*Disorders of the Upper Airways*

**John J. Treanor, M.D.**
Associate Professor of Medicine, Infectious Diseases Unit, University of Rochester Medical Center, Rochester, New York
*Viral Infections*

**Otto Villa, M.D., Ph.D.**
Fellow, Pulmonary and Critical Care Division, New England Medical Center, Boston, Massachusetts
*Sarcoidosis*

**Stephen M. Vogel, Ph.D.**
Research Assistant Professor, University of Illinois College of Medicine, Chicago, Illinois
*Pulmonary Circulation and Regulation of Fluid Balance*

**Peter D. Wagner, M.D.**
Professor of Medicine and Bioengineering, Division of Physiology, Department of Medicine, University of California, San Diego, School of Medicine, La Jolla, California
*Ventilation, Blood Flow, and Gas Exchange*

**John A. Washington II, M.D.**
Professor of Pathology, The Ohio State University, Columbus; Chairman Emeritus, Department of Clinical Pathology, and Section Head Emeritus, Clinical Microbiology, The Cleveland Clinic Foundation, Cleveland, Ohio
*Microbiologic Diagnosis of Lower Respiratory Tract Infection*

**Karlman Wasserman, M.D., Ph.D.**
Professor of Medicine, Department of Medicine, University of California, Los Angeles (UCLA), School of Medicine, Los Angeles; Attending Physician, Division of Respiratory and Critical Care Physiology and Medicine, Harbor-UCLA Medical Center, Torrance, California
*Exercise; Pulmonary Alveolar Proteinosis*

**W. Richard Webb, M.D.**
Professor of Radiology and Chief of Thoracic Imaging, University of California, San Francisco, California
*Radiographic Techniques*

**John V. Weil, M.D.**
Professor of Medicine, Cardiovascular Pulmonary Research Laboratory, University of Colorado Health Sciences Center, Denver, Colorado
*Pulmonary Complications of Hematologic Disease*

**A. U. Wells, M.D.**
Consultant Chest Physician, Royal Brompton Hospital, London, United Kingdom
*The Lungs and Connective Tissue Diseases*

**Michael J. Welsh, M.D.**
Professor of Medicine and of Physiology and Biophysics, University of Iowa College of Medicine; Investigator, Howard Hughes Medical Institute, Iowa City, Iowa
*Mucous Secretion and Ion Transport in Airways*

**John B. West, M.D., Ph.D., D.Sc.**
Professor of Medicine and Physiology, School of Medicine, University of California, San Diego, La Jolla, California
*Ventilation, Blood Flow, and Gas Exchange*

**Brian J. Whipp, Ph.D., D.Sc.**
Professor of Physiology, St. George's Hospital Medical School, London, United Kingdom
*Exercise*

**John Widdicombe, D.M., D.Phil., FRCP**
Emeritus Professor, Human Physiology and Aerospace Medicine, GKT School of Biomedical Sciences, London, United Kingdom
*Cough*

**Jeffrey L. Widell, M.D.**
Clinical Assistant Professor, Medical College of Wisconsin; Attending Physician (Pulmonary/Critical Care), St. Luke's Hospital, Milwaukee, Wisconsin
*Acid-Base Balance*

**Jeanine P. Wiener-Kronish, M.D.**
Professor of Anesthesia and Medicine; Vice-Chairman, Department of Anesthesia and Perioperative Care; Medical Director, Preoperative Program; and Investigator, Cardiovascular Research Institute, University of California, San Francisco, California
*Preoperative Evaluation*

**Mary C. Williams, Ph.D.**
Professor, Boston University School of Medicine, Pulmonary Program K–6, Boston, Massachusetts
*Anatomy of the Lungs*

**Lawrence D. H. Wood, M.D., Ph.D.**
Professor of Medicine and Anesthesia and Critical Care and Faculty Dean of Medical Education, University of Chicago, Pritzker School of Medicine, Chicago, Illinois
*Principles of Critical Care of Respiratory Failure; Acute Hypoxemic Respiratory Failure; Ventilatory Failure*

**Daniel Worsley, M.D.**
Assistant Professor, Department of Radiology, University of British Columbia, Vancouver, British Columbia, Canada
*Nuclear Medicine Techniques and Applications*

**J. R. Yankaskas, M.D.**
Professor of Medicine, University of North Carolina at Chapel Hill; Co-Director, Adult Cystic Fibrosis Program, and Director, Critical Care Medicine, University of North Carolina Hospitals, Chapel Hill, North Carolina
*Cystic Fibrosis*

**Donovan B. Yeates, Ph.D.**
Research Professor, Departments of Medicine and Bioengineering, University of Illinois at Chicago; Senior Research Career Scientist, Veterans Affairs Chicago Healthcare System, West Side Division, Chicago, Illinois
*Deposition and Clearance*

**Noe Zamel, M.D., FRCPC, FCCP**
Professor of Medicine, Faculty of Medicine, and Director, Trihospital Pulmonary Fn. Laboratories, University of Toronto, Toronto, Ontario, Canada
*Lung Transplantation*

**Leslie Zimmerman, M.D.**
Associate Professor of Clinical Medicine, University of California, San Francisco; Medical Director, Intensive Care Unit, San Francisco Veterans Administration Medical Center, San Francisco, California
*Pulmonary Complications of Endocrine Disease*

# Foreword

Medical texts often begin with a note of thanks to the authors' wives for their supportive forbearance. We are pleased that in this case the wives have been given the opportunity to add a few remarks of their own. We did forbear to confess a certain lack of sympathy for this project at the outset. To ordinary nonmedical readers like ourselves, such vast medical tomes are of little interest, except to be consulted surreptitiously when one has a symptom, and then they are seen to have something in common with horror and mystery literature, full of frightening events and magic.

In other respects, it first appeared, a medical book, unlike the books of fiction we are used to writing and reading, above all, is lacking in narrative interest and plot. As time went on, however, we came to see that what the editors were doing had much similarity to a work of fiction. Their idea was of course to bring order and reassurance to the turbulent field of pulmonary medicine, rather as a novelist attempts to bring meaningful order to the chaotic events of reality. But the editors had an even more difficult task. While the novelist contents herself with a modest slice of life, they have tried to assemble as much as is known to date about anatomy, physiology, pharmacology, and pathology—in short the scientific basis of pulmonary medicine—as well as all the clinical aspects of chest diseases. (And, from what they have told us, this is the only book of its kind in which this is done.)

There are difficulties spared the novelist but faced by the medical editor—the conflicting opinions of contributing authors, or the wish of several to speak of the same thing, or dilatory authors who are too busy to finish their observations on time. For work unfinished, the novelist has only herself to blame. But the biggest problem in this book, from the nonmedical point of view, is that, unlike a novel in which things can conveniently be wound up, a textbook of respiratory medicine seems to have no tidy endings. It shows, unquestionably, how very much progress has been made in understanding the basis of pulmonary disease, but one can't help but note that it also demonstrates that doctors neither prevent nor cure such horrible conditions as emphysema, asthma, lung cancer, or even the common cold. In fiction, illness can be related to wickedness or moral defect and given to the character that deserves it, while in life these afflictions seem arbitrary and unjust. We hope this book will prove inspiring to clinicians and researchers in their quest for causes, cures, and happy endings.

Diane Johnson Murray
Judy Nadel
San Francisco, 1988

In our foreword to the first edition we noted certain similarities between a medical book and a novel. The comparison remains true. The sequel to a novel introduces new events and characters, so does the second edition of Murray and Nadel, which has chapters on exciting new subjects and introduces 65 additional authors. All this while keeping, one hopes, the qualities that made the first edition a household word (or so we are told).

Diane Johnson Murray
Judy Nadel
San Francisco, 1993

The third edition is even longer, because the plot has thickened. New villains have emerged to threaten lung health, and new weapons to rout them must be deployed. But serious readers are always pleased when a favorite or useful volume grows fatter.

Diane Johnson Murray
Judy Nadel
San Francisco, 1999

# PREFACE TO THE THIRD EDITION

The science and practice of modern respiratory medicine got its start in the 1970s owing to an infusion of talented young men and women into this specialty, the availability of research and training funds from the newly inaugurated Lung Division of the National Heart and Lung Institute (now the National Heart, Lung, and Blood Institute), the development of new tools such as the fiberoptic bronchoscope and pulmonary function measurement techniques, and the emergence of critical care medicine as an allied discipline. Accompanying this rapid growth were numerous monographs and books that dealt with specific topics, but no single work tried to encompass all that was known about the entire subject. To satisfy this need, we coedited the *Textbook of Respiratory Medicine,* which was first published in 1988. Our goal was to integrate and consolidate the expanding base of essential knowledge that was available at the time and to provide the reader, whether practicing chest physician or internist, graduate physician in training or medical student, or someone who wanted to know, with an authoritative and thoroughly documented source of information in the field. These efforts were well received and led to the second edition of the *Textbook* in 1994. To accommodate the ongoing explosion of knowledge, we added additional chapters, reorganized some of the sections, and enlisted the help of many new authors. That updated version was also well received.

Now it is time for publication of the third edition, which includes descriptions of the many new and important scientific discoveries and their clinical applications that occurred during the six years after the second edition was published. Once again, to present this material in the most efficient and understandable fashion, we have reorganized several sections, added new chapters and consolidated others, and obtained the help of more than 50 new authors, all acknowledged authorities in their subjects. While doing this, we have tried to retain two of the elements that helped bring about the success of the first two editions: first, to continue our emphasis on integrating basic science with the practice of respiratory medicine; second, to include an extensive list of references both to classic works as well as to the most recent (1999) important articles.

There has been one major change that deserves special attention: we are pleased and proud to acknowledge the inclusion of two distinguished physician-scientists, Dr. Homer A. Boushey, Jr., and Dr. Robert J. Mason, as Associate Editors. These two friends and colleagues have made vital contributions to planning the text, recruiting new authors, writing certain chapters, and editing several manuscripts for this edition. With their help, we hope that this edition continues the tradition of scholarship, usefulness, and readability that the *Textbook* has brought to its readers in the past.

Time has brought changes to W.B. Saunders as well. At the beginning of this publication cycle, our editor in Philadelphia was Judith Fletcher, who was later promoted and replaced by Richard Zorab. From beginning to end, we received strong and much needed production help from Dolores Meloni; Anne Ostroff handled the copyediting.

We also want to thank all our contributors and readers. Preparing a textbook the size and scope of this one is a lot of work. But the continued interest and support of our authors, who generously share their expertise, and our readers, who want to enrich their education, has made it worthwhile. We take considerable pleasure in the belief that the outcome of this complex enterprise will improve the care of patients with respiratory disease.

JOHN F. MURRAY, M.D.
JAY A. NADEL, M.D.

# Preface to the Second Edition

*Textbook of Respiratory Medicine* was created to meet a perceived need for a comprehensive and fully documented book that integrates the scientific basis with the practice of respiratory medicine. With the publication of the first edition, we expressed concern about how our "offspring" would make its way in the real world. Now, however, its broad acceptance reassures us that this ambitious text fulfills an important informational need.

During the last five years, the field of respiratory medicine has continued its stupendous growth at both the basic science and clinical levels, and the second edition attempts to keep the reader informed about this explosion of information. Several approaches have been utilized to accomplish this. First, all the chapters have been revised and updated. New chapters have been added concerning the physiology of the pulmonary circulation, the pulmonary complications of acquired human immunodeficiency virus infection, and the respiratory problems found in gynecologic and obstetric diseases. Several sections have been completely reorganized: "Defense Mechanisms and Immunology," for example, now incorporates the many important recent discoveries in lung cell biology; "Respiratory Pathology" includes modern concepts of lung inflammation, injury, and repair; "Neoplasms" adds recent advances in the biology of carcinogenesis and the epidemiology and clinical manifestations of pulmonary tumors; and "Respiratory Failure" contains new chapters on "Ethics and Withdrawal of Support" and "Lung Transplantation." The section on Diagnostic Evaluation has also undergone extensive updating and rewriting to include the latest imaging, functional, and invasive procedures and to emphasize their applications to clinical disorders and the evaluation of impairment and disability, operability, and cardiac function.

To accomplish this ambitious undertaking, we have added 65 *new* authors, all recognized experts in their fields. In many instances, a basic scientist has been added as a coauthor of a chapter on a clinical subject to provide a thorough description of relevant basic scientific principles and their application to specific clinical disorders.

Despite the extensive changes that have been introduced in the second edition, the aims of the textbook remain the same: to present complete coverage of the broad field of respiratory medicine in an expert and understandable fashion, with a fully documented text, containing extensive references (more than 20,000) to both classic works as well as the most recent and important articles.

A textbook of this size is a demanding assignment, but we have had considerable help. The job has been made easier by the many expert authors who worked hard and skillfully on their assignments. The two editors in San Francisco had proficient and meticulous secretarial support from Natalie Holt, Dorothy Ladd, and Shauna McDonough. We give special thanks to our editorial associate, Aja Lipavsky, who labored diligently with proofing and computer transformation of the text and to Susan Nutter and Alvin Averbach for careful editing. At W.B. Saunders Company in Philadelphia, Judith Fletcher provided considerable editorial help and tireless devotion to excellence. We received superb production assistance from Dolores Meloni, Linda R. Garber, and Evelyn Weiman.

In the end, we are thankful for being able to participate in the science and art of a field in which new discoveries are daily being applied to the care and prevention of respiratory disease.

John F. Murray, M.D.
Jay A. Nadel, M.D.

# Contents


## PART 1 Scientific Principles of Respiratory Medicine 1

### *Section A.* Anatomy and Development of the Respiratory Tract 3

**1. Anatomy of the Lungs** 3
Kurt H. Albertine, Ph.D. •
Mary C. Williams, Ph.D. •
Dallas M. Hyde, Ph.D.

**2. Lung Growth and Development** 35
John A. McDonald, M.D., Ph.D.

**3. Genetic Basis of Lung Disease** 45
Michael C. Iannuzzi, M.D.

### *Section B.* Respiratory Physiology 55

**4. Ventilation, Blood Flow, and Gas Exchange** 55
John B. West, M.D., Ph.D., D.Sc. •
Peter D. Wagner, M.D.

**5. Respiratory System Mechanics** 91
Joseph R. Rodarte, M.D. •
Felix R. Shardonofsky, M.D.

**6. Pulmonary Circulation and Regulation of Fluid Balance** 119
Asrar B. Malik, Ph.D. •
Stephen M. Vogel, Ph.D. •
Richard D. Minshall, Ph.D. •
C. Tiruppathi, Ph.D.

**7. Acid-Base Balance** 155
Richard M. Effros, M.D. •
Jeffrey L. Widell, M.D.

**8. Control of Breathing** 179
Albert J. Berger, Ph.D.

**9. Exercise** 197
Brian J. Whipp, Ph.D., D.Sc. •
Karlman Wasserman, M.D., Ph.D.

### *Section C.* Respiratory Pharmacology 231

**10. General Pharmacologic Principles** 231
Peter J. Barnes, M.A., D.M., D.Sc., FRCP

**11. Airway Pharmacology** 267
Peter J. Barnes, M.A., D.M., D.Sc., FRCP

**12. Vascular Pharmacology** 297
Jeffrey R. Fineman, M.D. •
Michael A. Heymann, M.D. •
Julien I. E. Hoffman, M.D.

### *Section D.* Defense Mechanisms 307

**13. Pulmonary Surfactant** 307
Robert J. Mason, M.D. •
James Lewis, M.D.

**14. Mucus Secretion and Ion Transport in Airways** 327
Carol Basbaum, Ph.D. •
Michael J. Welsh, M.D.

**15. Deposition and Clearance** 349
Donovan B. Yeates, Ph.D. •
Jann Mortensen, M.D., D.Sc.

**16. Monocytes, Macrophages, and Dendritic Cells of the Lungs** 385
David W. H. Riches, Ph.D.

**17. Immune Recognition and Responses** 413
Andrew P. Fontenot, M.D. •
Brian L. Kotzin, M.D.

### *Section E.* Respiratory Pathology and Inflammation 443

**18. General Features of Respiratory Pathology** 443
Walter E. Finkbeiner, M.D., Ph.D.

**19. Inflammation, Injury, and Repair** 495
Michael P. Keane, M.D. •
Peter M. Henson, B.V.M.S., Ph.D. •
Robert M. Strieter, M.D.

## PART 2 Manifestations and Diagnosis of Respiratory Disease 539

### *Section F.* Manifestations of Respiratory Disease 541

**20. Dyspnea** 541
Michael S. Stulbarg, M.D. •
Lewis Adams, Ph.D.

**21. Cough** 553
Richard S. Irwin, M.D. •
John Widdicombe, D.PHIL.

**22. Chest Pain** 567
John F. Murray, M.D. •
Gerald F. Gebhart, PH.D.

*Section G.* Diagnostic Evaluation 585

**23. History and Physical Examination** 585
John F. Murray, M.D.

**24. Microbiologic Diagnosis of Lower Respiratory Tract Infection** 607
Franklin R. Cockerill III, M.D. •
John A. Washington II, M.D.

**25. Radiographic Techniques** 633
H. Dirk Sostman, M.D. •
W. Richard Webb, M.D.

**26. Nuclear Medicine Techniques and Applications** 697
Daniel Worsley, M.D. •
Alexander Gottschalk, M.D.

**27. Bronchoscopy, Lung Biopsy, and Other Diagnostic Procedures** 725
Robert P. Baughman, M.D. •
Jeffrey A. Golden, M.D. •
Fraser M. Keith, M.D.

**28. Pulmonary Function Testing** 781
Warren M. Gold, M.D.

**29. Preoperative Evaluation** 883
Jeanine P. Wiener-Kronish, M.D. •
Richard K. Albert, M.D.

**30. Evaluation of Respiratory Impairment/Disability** 895
John R. Balmes, M.D., M.P.H. •
Scott Barnhart, M.D., M.P.H.

PART 3 **Clinical Respiratory Medicine** 913

*Section H.* Infectious Diseases of the Lungs 915

**31. General Principles and Diagnostic Approach** 915
Julie Louise Gerberding, M.D., M.P.H

**32. Viral Infections** 929
John J. Treanor, M.D. •
Frederick G. Hayden, M.D.

**33. Pyogenic Bacterial Pneumonia, Lung Abscess, and Empyema** 985
Matthew Bidwell Goetz, M.D. •
Sydney M. Finegold, M.D.

**34. Tuberculosis and Other Mycobacterial Diseases** 1043
Philip C. Hopewell, M.D. •
Barry R. Bloom, PH.D.

**35. Fungal Infections** 1107
Scott F. Davies, M.D. •
George A. Sarosi, M.D.

**36 Parasitic Diseases** 1143
Ramya Gopinath, M.B., B.S. •
Thomas B. Nutman, M.D.

*Section I.* Obstructive Diseases 1173

**37. General Principles and Diagnostic Approach** 1173
Jay A. Nadel, M.D.

**38. Chronic Bronchitis and Emphysema** 1187
Craig A. Piquette, M.D. •
Stephen I. Rennard, M.D. •
Gordon L. Snider, M.D.

**39. Asthma** 1247
Homer A. Boushey, Jr., M.D. •
David B. Corry, M.D. •
John V. Fahy, M.D.

**40. Cystic Fibrosis** 1291
R. C. Boucher, M.D. •
M. R. Knowles, M.D. •
J. R. Yankaskas, M.D.

**41. Bronchiectasis** 1325
John M. Luce, M.D.

**42. Disorders of the Upper Airways** 1343
Alan R. Schwartz, M.D. •
Philip L. Smith, M.D. •
Haskins K. Kashima, M.D. •
Donald F. Proctor, M.D. •
Alkis Togias, M.D.

**43. Disorders of the Intrathoracic Airways** 1361
Stephen C. Lazarus, M.D.

*Section J.* Neoplasms of the Lungs 1375

**44. Biology of Lung Cancer** 1375
Yoshitaka Sekido, M.D., PH.D. •
Kwun M. Fong, M.D., PH.D. •
Adi F. Gazdar, M.D. •
John D. Minna, M.D.

**45. Epidemiology of Lung Cancer** 1395
Kathryn E. Osann, Ph.D. •
Virginia L. Ernster, Ph.D. •
Piero Mustacchi, M.D.

**46. Bronchogenic Carcinoma** 1415
Diane Prager, M.D. •
Robert Cameron, M.D. •
Judith Ford, Ph.D. •
Robert A. Figlin, M.D., F.A.C.P.

**47. Lymphoma, Lymphoproliferative Diseases, and Other Primary Malignant Tumors** 1453
Judith A. Luce, M.D.

**48. Metastatic Malignant Tumors** 1469
Judith A. Luce, M.D.

**49. Benign Tumors** 1477
Glen A. Lillington, M.D. •
Norman W. Rizk, M.D.

*Section K.* Disorders of the Pulmonary Circulation 1485

**50. General Principles and Diagnostic Approach** 1485
John F. Murray, M.D.

**51. Pulmonary Thromboembolism** 1503
Peter F. Fedullo, M.D.

**52. Pulmonary Vasculitis and Primary Pulmonary Hypertension** 1533
Lewis J. Rubin, M.D.

**53. Pulmonary Arteriovenous Malformations and Other Pulmonary Vascular Abnormalities** 1557
J. Michael B. Hughes, D.M., F.R.C.P. •
John M. Luce, M.D.

**54. Pulmonary Edema and Acute Lung Injury** 1575
Michael R. Flick, M.D., J.D. •
Michael A. Matthay, M.D.

**55. Cor Pulmonale** 1631
Elliot Rapaport, M.D.

*Section L.* Infiltrative and Interstitial Lung Diseases 1649

**56. Principles of and Approach to the Patient with Interstitial Lung Disease** 1649
Marvin I. Schwarz, M.D. •
Talmadge E. King, Jr., M.D. •
Reuben M. Cherniack, M.D.

**57. Idiopathic Interstitial Pneumonias** 1671
Talmadge E. King, Jr., M.D. •
Marvin I. Schwarz, M.D.

**58. The Lungs and Connective Tissue Diseases** 1691
R. M. du Bois, M.D. •
A. U. Wells, M.D.

**59. Sarcoidosis** 1717
Barry L. Fanburg, M.D. •
Otto Villa, M.D., Ph.D.

**60. Diffuse Alveolar Hemorrhage and Other Rare Infiltrative Disorders** 1733
Marvin I. Schwarz, M.D. •
Reuben M. Cherniack, M.D. •
Talmadge E. King, Jr., M.D.

**61. Eosinophilic Lung Diseases** 1757
Edward J. Goetzl, M.D. •
John M. Luce, M.D.

**62. Lymphangioleiomyomatosis** 1775
Kenneth G. Kalassian, M.D. •
Thomas A. Raffin, M.D.

**63. Pulmonary Alveolar Proteinosis** 1789
Karlman Wasserman, M.D., Ph.D. •
Gregory R. Mason, M.D.

*Section M.* Environmental and Occupational Disorders 1803

**64. General Principles and Diagnostic Approach** 1803
Paul D. Blanc, M.D., M.S.P.H.

**65. Pneumoconioses** 1811
Margaret R. Becklake, M.D. •
Robert L. Cowie, M.D.

**66. Occupational Asthma and Byssinosis** 1853
John R. Balmes, M.D., M.P.H.

**67. Hypersensitivity Pneumonitis** 1867
Cecile S. Rose, M.D., M.P.H

**68. Air Pollution** 1885
John R. Balmes, M.D., M.P.H. •
Ira Tager, M.D.

**69. Acute Pulmonary Responses to Toxic Exposures** 1903
Paul D. Blanc, M.D., M.S.P.H.

**70. High Altitude** 1915
Robert B. Schoene, M.D. •
Peter H. Hackett, M.D. •
Thomas F. Hornbein, M.D.

**71. Diving Medicine** 1951
Alfred A. Bove, M.D., Ph.D. •
Tom Neuman, M.D.

**72. Drug-Induced Pulmonary Disease** 1971
Andrew H. Limper, M.D. • Edward C. Rosenow, III, M.D.

*Section N.* Disorders of the Pleura 1995

**73. General Principles and Diagnostic Approach** 1995
V. Courtney Broaddus, M.D. • Richard W. Light, M.D.

**74. Pleural Effusion** 2013
Richard W. Light, M.D. • V. Courtney Broaddus, M.D.

**75. Pneumothorax, Chylothorax, Hemothorax, and Fibrothorax** 2043
Richard W. Light, M.D. • V. Courtney Broaddus, M.D.

**76. Tumors of the Pleura** 2067
Richard W. Light, M.D. • V. Courtney Broaddus, M.D.

*Section O.* Disorders of the Mediastinum 2079

**77. General Principles and Diagnostic Approach** 2079
David R. Park, M.D. • David J. Pierson, M.D.

**78. Pneumomediastinum and Mediastinitis** 2095
David R. Park, M.D. • David J. Pierson, M.D.

**79. Tumors and Cysts of the Mediastinum** 2123
David R. Park, M.D. • David J. Pierson, M.D.

*Section P.* Disorders in the Control of Breathing 2139

**80. Hypoventilation and Hyperventilation Syndromes** 2139
Eliot A. Phillipson, M.D. • Arthur S. Slutsky, M.D.

**81. Sleep Disorders** 2153
T. Douglas Bradley, M.D. • Eliot A. Phillipson, M.D.

*Section Q.* Respiratory Manifestations of Extrapulmonary Disorders 2171

**82. Pulmonary Complications of Human Immunodeficiency Virus Infection** 2171
Laurence Huang, M.D. • John D. Stansell, M.D.

**83. Pulmonary Complications of Organ Transplantation and Primary Immunodeficiencies** 2223
Steven R. Duncan, M.D. • Thomas A. Raffin, M.D.

**84. Pulmonary Complications of Heart Disease** 2247
J. Michael B. Hughes, D.M., F.R.C.P.

**85. Pulmonary Complications of Abdominal Disease** 2267
Robert Rodriguez-Roisin, M.D. • Joan Albert Barberà, M.D.

**86. Pulmonary Complications of Hematologic Disease** 2285
John V. Weil, M.D. • Stephen Crawford, M.D. • Philip Bromberg, M.D.

**87. Pulmonary Complications of Endocrine Disease** 2309
Leslie Zimmerman, M.D.

**88. The Lungs in Obstetric and Gynecologic Disease** 2317
Norman W. Rizk, M.D.

**89. The Lungs and Neuromuscular Disease** 2329
Thomas K. Aldrich, M.D. • Dudley F. Rochester, M.D.

**90. The Lungs and Chest Wall Disease** 2357
F. Dennis McCool, M.D. • Dudley F. Rochester, M.D.

*Section R.* Respiratory Failure 2377

**91. Principles of Critical Care of Respiratory Failure** 2377
Lawrence D. H. Wood, M.D., Ph.D. • Gregory A. Schmidt, M.D. • Jesse B. Hall, M.D.

**92. Acute Hypoxemic Respiratory Failure** 2413
Jesse B. Hall, M.D. • Gregory A. Schmidt, M.D. • Lawrence D. H. Wood, M.D., Ph.D.

**93. Ventilatory Failure** 2443
Gregory A. Schmidt, M.D. • Jesse B. Hall, M.D. • Lawrence D. H. Wood, M.D., Ph.D.

**94. Principles of Mechanical Ventilation** 2471
Neil R. MacIntyre, M.D.

**95. Ethics and Withdrawal of Life Support** 2487
Thomas A. Raffin, M.D.

**96. Pulmonary Rehabilitation** 2505
Bartolome R. Celli, M.D. • Thomas L. Petty, M.D.

**97. Lung Transplantation** 2517
Janet R. Maurer, M.D., FCCP • Noe Zamel, M.D., FRCPC, FCCP

*Section S.* Prevention and Control 2531

**98. Individual Measures: Social and Behavioral Aspects** 2531
Noreen M. Clark, Ph.D. • Susan Janson, R.N., A.N.P., D.N.Sc.

**99. Community Measures: Public Policy and Education** 2543
Virginia S. Taggart, M.P.H. • Robinson Fulwood, M.S.P.H. • Michele Hindi-Alexander, Ph.D. • Claude Lenfant, M.D.

**Appendix** i

**Index** v

SECTION I

# Obstructive Diseases

# 37 General Principles and Diagnostic Approach

JAY A. NADEL, M.D.

Introduction
Etiology and Pathogenesis of Obstructive Diseases
- Asthma
- Chronic Obstructive Pulmonary Diseases (Emphysema and Chronic Bronchitis)
- Bronchiectasis
- Cystic Fibrosis
- Disorders of the Upper Airways
- Other Disorders of the Intrathoracic Airways

Differential Diagnosis of Obstructive Diseases
- Clinical Features
- Tests of Pulmonary Function and Other Diagnostic Procedures

Summary

## INTRODUCTION

As animals moved from sea to land, the ability to breathe air required a shift from the exchange of gases between exposed gills and water to a gas-liquid interface in the lungs. The lungs developed within the thoracic cavity in close proximity to the heart so that gas exchange could occur efficiently between the pulmonary capillaries and the alveoli. The airways developed as the "plumbing" that was required to connect the gas exchange area with the outside gaseous environment. During respiration, foreign particles and gases, bacteria, and viruses deposit on the airway surface and threaten the lungs and airways. The body has developed a series of defense mechanisms to protect itself. Because the lungs are an important port of entry into the body, complicated pulmonary defense mechanisms have evolved to protect the body; these are discussed in detail in Chapters 14 to 17. Abnormal stimulation by inflammatory stimuli (e.g., cigarette smoke) and abnormal or prolonged inflammatory responses by the person (e.g., in asthma) play important roles in airway diseases.

The subsequent chapters in this section review in detail the various obstructive diseases. Obstructive diseases include asthma (Chapter 39), chronic bronchitis and emphysema (Chapter 38), bronchiectasis (Chapter 41), cystic fibrosis (Chapter 40), diseases of the extrathoracic airways (Chapter 42), and other disorders of the intrathoracic airways (Chapter 43).

In the case of obstructive diseases, understanding the pathogenesis depends on knowledge of the structures involved; these are discussed in detail in Chapters 1 and 18. Knowledge of the changes in the mechanical properties of the lungs (Chapter 5) and of the changes in ventilation, blood flow, and gas exchange (Chapter 4) is essential to the understanding of the pathophysiology of obstructive diseases, for differentiating them from one another, for following the course of disease, and for evaluating therapeutic interventions. The pharmacologic principles of treatment of obstruction diseases are covered in Chapters 10 to 12. Prevention of obstructive diseases (especially those associated with cigarette smoking) require education and behavioral modification (Chapters 98, 99).

The external environment contains important stimuli that cause airway inflammation and disease. The impact of the environment is discussed in Chapter 64. Damaging exposures occur because of air pollution (Chapter 68) and occupation (Chapters 65 to 69).

Obstructive diseases of the airways are a diverse group. In general, they have in common airway narrowing, with the consequent increase in the work of breathing. The sites of obstruction vary from the upper airways to the most peripheral bronchioles. In obstructive lung diseases, the mechanisms of airway obstruction may be quite varied. For example, the decrease in maximal expiratory air flow in emphysema is due, at least in part, to the loss of lung elastic recoil secondary to the breakdown of lung tissue and the enlargement of the alveolar spaces. In chronic bronchitis, an inflammatory disease of the airways, the narrowing occurs in the airways themselves. Nevertheless, these two diseases are difficult to differentiate clinically. Thus, in the past, some clinicians pooled these diseases and gave them the common name "chronic obstructive pulmonary disease" (COPD). Intraluminal airway obstruction has multiple causes. Airway smooth muscle contraction, a classic mechanism in asthma, is the most commonly considered cause of airway narrowing because its presence can be evaluated (and reversed) by treatment with airway smooth muscle relaxants. Infiltration with inflammatory cells, scarring, edema, and intraluminal narrowing by secretions are also common causes of airway obstruction. Their presence and extent are, however, difficult to evaluate.

Another point of confusion relates to the definition of different diseases. Chronic bronchitis is defined *clinically* by the chronic presence of cough and sputum production. Emphysema, on the other hand, is defined *anatomically* on the basis of the breakdown of lung tissue and the enlargement of the alveolar spaces.

Because of anatomic differences, airway obstruction may vary with the breathing cycle. Thus, extrathoracic lesions such as laryngeal narrowing, extrathoracic tracheal stenosis, and tracheomalacia cause symptoms predominantly during inspiration. Some other diseases, such as intrathoracic tracheomalacia, cause symptoms of airway obstruction mainly during expiration.

Nevertheless, classifying the various obstructive diseases has important advantages in terms of treatment and prognosis. The combination of differences in signs and symptoms, utilization of various tests of structure and function, and response to different treatment modalities enables the physician to deal effectively with the different obstructive diseases.

The exact cause of most diseases of airways is not well understood. We know that cigarette smoking is associated with both chronic bronchitis and emphysema. We do not, however, know why cigarette smoke causes lung tissue destruction in some people, predominantly chronic bronchitis in others, and no detectable illness in many people. Similarly, the exact causes and pathophysiologic mechanisms underlying asthma still elude us. We believe that allergic mechanisms are often involved. In many people with asthma that starts in adulthood, however, no allergic mechanisms may be identifiable, and these patients often have severe asthma. Recently, the concept has evolved that asthma, like many of the other airway diseases, is inflammatory in nature, and research has focused on the cellular basis of the inflammatory responses. Cystic fibrosis is an example of a disease for which there are many clues and many tools but still few clinically relevant answers.

Because the precise pathophysiologic mechanisms of chronic airway diseases still elude us, it is not surprising that the symptoms of the diseases are mostly treated empirically and, in the case of some symptoms, often ineffectively. For example, the mainstay of therapy of mild asthma is bronchodilator therapy (i.e., the use of beta-adrenergic agonists that relax airway smooth muscle regardless of the cause of contraction). In more severe asthma, therapy with the anti-inflammatory corticosteroids is usually efficacious, even though we do not know the mechanisms responsible for the improvement. There is limited treatment for two common symptoms of airway disease, hypersecretion (Chapter 14) and cough (Chapter 21). It is hoped that the intense research activities that aim to elucidate the inflammatory cascades and cell-to-cell interactions that cause the various manifestations of airway diseases will soon produce insights that will enable more precise therapy and eventually prevention of the diseases.

Airway hypersecretion is an important manifestation of many chronic airway diseases, including chronic bronchitis,[1] bronchiectasis,[2] cystic fibrosis,[3] and acute asthma.[4] No known therapies are effective, and there is evidence that hypersecretion may lead to deterioration and death. In acute asthma, there is postmortem evidence that incriminates mucous plugging of peripheral airways as an important cause of death.[4]

Mucous secretion is derived from airway submucosal glands (located in large conducting airways) and from goblet cells in the airway epithelium (located throughout the airways). In healthy humans and in pathogen-free animals, peripheral airways contain few goblet cells,[5] but goblet cell metaplasia occurs in COPD,[1] cystic fibrosis,[2] and acute asthma.[4]

Submucosal glands are located adjacent to cough receptors, so clearance of these secretions may therefore be associated with cough. Chronic bronchitis (*defined* by cough and sputum production) causes disturbing symptoms (e.g., cough) but does not appear to be an important cause of deterioration or death in COPD.[6–8] Peripheral airways normally have low cuboidal epithelium, with few goblet cells,[5] but in hypersecretory diseases epithelial goblet cell metaplasia occurs.[1, 2, 4] Although symptoms of hypersecretion derived from large conducting airways draws major attention because of the associated symptom of cough, plugging of peripheral airways by secreted mucins derived from peripherally located goblet cells may cause no symptoms early, but extensive plugging may lead to deterioration and death. Furthermore, tests of pulmonary function are relatively insensitive to obstruction in peripheral airways (discussed in Chapter 28).

Goblet cell secretion can be divided into two steps: First, epithelial cells are converted to mucus-containing goblet cells. Second, goblet cell degranulation of the peripheral airways may be induced, leading to obstruction by plugging. Mucous secretion is reviewed in detail elsewhere (Chapter 14). The discussion here is limited to a few recently described mechanisms that appear likely to have therapeutic implications.

Stimulation of epidermal growth factor receptors (EGF-R) by its ligands (e.g., EGF, transforming growth factor-α) causes mucin expression in airway epithelial cells that can be inhibited by a selective EGF-R tyrosine kinase inhibitor in animals.[5] Furthermore, in an experimental model of asthma, ovalbumin sensitization in rats resulted in goblet cell metaplasia, an effect that was also prevented with a selective EGF-R tyrosine kinase inhibitor. In addition to allergic stimuli, other stimuli reported to cause the growth of goblet cells may also act via the EGF-R cascade. Further studies show that mechanical irritation of airways also stimulates goblet cell growth by activating the EGF-R cascade.[8a] By preventing EGF-R activation and the consequent mucous cell growth, selective inhibitors may provide effective therapy for hypersecretory diseases.

Another approach to treatment of hypersecretion is the inhibition of secretory cell *degranulation*. Neutrophils are recruited into the airways in hypersecretory diseases,[9] and neutrophil elastase is a very potent secretagogue in airway secretory cells.[10] Chemoattractants cause neutrophil-dependent goblet cell degranulation by a novel adhesive interaction between goblet cells and neutrophils in animals and in human airways, with the resultant release of elastase, which causes secretory cell degranulation.[10] Neutrophil recruitment that occurs in acute asthma, COPD exacerbations, and cystic fibrosis may thus cause serious clinical deterioration by obstructing peripheral airways. These results suggest several potential strategies of therapeutic intervention.

The pathogenesis, physiologic consequences, and differential diagnosis of the various obstructive diseases are reviewed in brief in this chapter. Detailed descriptions are given in individual chapters of this section.

## ETIOLOGY AND PATHOGENESIS OF OBSTRUCTIVE DISEASES

### Asthma

Asthma is a disease of the airways characterized by airway narrowing with spontaneous and pharmacologic reversibility. For many years, reversibility of obstruction was the only point of agreement among various clinicians and investigators to define asthma.[11]

A second important feature of asthma is the increased responsiveness of the airways to various physiologic stimuli (e.g., inhalation of cold air, exercise,[12] and pharmacologic stimulation with inhaled aerosols of bronchoconstrictor substances).[13] A third, recently recognized feature of asthma is the presence of inflammation in the airways.

The morphologic changes in patients who die of severe asthma (status asthmaticus) are well known and are summarized in Table 37.1. The airways are edematous and swollen, the blood vessels are congested, and cellular infiltrates (especially eosinophils) are conspicuous.[14, 15] Mucous plugs fill peripheral airways,[16] and epithelial cells are desquamated.[17] Clumps of these cells can be found in the sputum[18] and are known as Creola bodies[18] or Curschmann's spirals.[19]

A quantitative analysis of the peripheral airway changes has recently been published.[20] Permanent changes in the structure of the airways are also reported.[21]

Abnormalities in airway cell growth and differentiation occur in patients with asthma and are similar to those in other diseases that are associated with chronic inflammation (e.g., chronic bronchitis and cystic fibrosis). These abnormalities include metaplasia of the lining epithelium from ciliated cells to squamous and goblet cells. The basement membrane is thickened, a condition also seen in other diseases associated with increased cell turnover.[22] Airway submucosal glands and smooth muscle are increased in amount,[23] and this increased bulk may account, at least in part, for the hyperresponsive muscle responses that are characteristic of asthma. Anatomic studies in patients with asthma who have not died of status asthmaticus also demonstrate inflammatory changes. Thus, airway biopsy material shows epithelial cell desquamation, squamous cell transformation, leukocyte infiltration,[24, 25] an increase in goblet cells, and thickening of the basement membrane. Bronchoalveolar lavage has recently been used to obtain pathologic information (Chapter 27).[26]

In asthmatic subjects, local airway challenge with antigen caused an increase in neutrophils and eosinophils in lavage fluid[27, 28] associated with an immediate onset of mucosal edema and narrowing of the airway.[29] In another study of asthmatic patients with delayed bronchoconstriction after antigen challenge, lavage showed predominantly eosinophils, providing evidence that eosinophils

**Table 37.1 AIRWAY TISSUE RESPONSES IN ASTHMA**

| | |
|---|---|
| Vascular effects | Vascular dilation<br>Increased vascular permeability<br>Edema formation<br>Inflammatory cell infiltration |
| Cell growth and differentiation | Epithelial desquamation<br>Epithelial metaplasia (squamous and goblet cell proliferation)<br>Increase in submucosal gland and airway smooth muscle bulk |
| Specific cellular effects | Smooth muscle contraction<br>Hypersecretion |

might be involved in late asthmatic reactions.[30] The numbers of mast cells in lavage fluid are reported to be increased in asthmatic subjects, and there is indirect evidence that the mast cells have increased releasability.[31] In studies of repeated bronchial biopsies, the number of eosinophils in the airway wall is reported to decrease rapidly between attacks.

All of these morphologic studies provide evidence that people with asthma have chronic inflammatory changes in the walls of their airways and that stimuli such as antigen cause further responses characterized by infiltration with neutrophils and eosinophils and by airway edema. These inflammatory processes are exaggerated in patients who die of status asthmaticus.

Asthma is a disease with a clinical course that has long been recognized for which symptomatic treatment is reasonably satisfactory. The causes of asthma are still, however, only partially understood. The disease is discussed in detail in Chapter 39, so only selected issues of etiology are discussed here.

It has long been recognized that the clinical pattern of asthma varies markedly among populations, and on this basis two types of asthma have been recognized (Table 37.2). One group of patients ("extrinsic" asthmatics) develop asthma at a young age, have a family history of atopic predisposition, may have other atopic manifestations (e.g., skin and nasal allergies), and have evidence of IgE-mediated responses and allergic "triggers" to some attacks. Another group of patients ("intrinsic" asthmatics) develop asthma later in life, have a negative family history of asthma or atopy, have no evidence of IgE-mediated mechanisms, but often have severe asthma that is difficult to treat. Still another group includes patients whose asthma is clearly related to specific occupational exposures (Chapter 66). These clinical differences suggest that multiple mechanisms (and perhaps multiple cells) are involved in the pathogenesis of asthma in different subjects.

With two discoveries—the IgE antibody and the fact that IgE antigen binds to mast cells and activates them to release inflammatory mediators—it was tempting to develop a unifying concept of asthma: Introduction of an antigen produces IgE antibody, which attaches to mast cells. When the antigen is reintroduced into the airway, it binds to mast cells, creating an IgE-mediated antigen-antibody response with subsequent release of mast cell mediators and asthma. (These immunologic responses are important in allergic asthmatic people and are discussed in Chapter 17.[32, 33])

**Table 37.2 CLASSIFICATION OF ASTHMA**

| | |
|---|---|
| Extrinsic asthma | Strong family history of allergies<br>Onset usually at young age<br>Other allergic manifestations in patient<br>History of childhood allergies<br>Evidence of allergic association<br>History of specific allergic trigger (e.g., pollen, animal dander)<br>Correlation with skin and inhalation responses to specific antigens<br>Specific IgE levels |
| Intrinsic asthma | No allergic (personal or family) history<br>Onset usually in adulthood<br>Often follows severe respiratory illness<br>Symptoms usually perennial<br>More refractory to treatment |

Despite intensive investigation, asthma rates are increasing in developed western countries,[34–36] and the causes are unclear. Asthma has long been suspected of having a strong genetic component, and recent studies confirm this.[37, 38] Viral infections, especially early in life, may also play a role.[39–41] Considerable advances have been made in the understanding of immune responses in allergic asthma,[42–44] and these discoveries are likely to affect therapy in the future. It is hoped that future research will discover the causes of asthma and that this will lead to more definitive treatment and prevention. Epidemiologic studies have provided evidence for the important role of allergens in causing asthma.[45–47] House dust mites probably represent the most potent allergen in asthma.[48]

Mast cells can also be activated to release mediators by non-IgE mechanisms, so these inflammatory cells may be involved in responses to stimuli other than specific antigens. Because allergy could not explain many of the manifestations of asthma, investigators sought other mechanisms. Two phenomena were important in the next discoveries relevant to asthma: hyperresponsiveness and inflammation.

Airway smooth muscle hyperresponsiveness has been shown to play an important role in asthma. The concept evolved that the clinical airway response depends on both the strength of the stimulus and the degree of responsiveness of the smooth muscle. Thus, stimuli that normally produce no clinical response can produce clinical symptoms in the presence of increased responsiveness. Stated differently, in asthmatics, the "gain" of the airway system is increased, causing magnified and clinically significant responses. This concept is illustrated in Figure 37.1.

It was debated whether the hyperresponsiveness that is characteristic of asthma is due to hereditary predisposition, so studies were performed to determine whether otherwise healthy persons could develop hyperresponsive airways. The first demonstration of induced hyperresponsiveness occurred with respiratory viral infections. Viral infections were recognized as triggers to asthma attacks,[49] so it was questioned whether the mechanism was an induced increase in responsiveness. Spontaneous respiratory viral infections[50] and experimental infections with attenuated influenza virus[51] cause transient airway hyperresponsiveness in otherwise healthy individuals. The mechanism by which virus infections cause transient increases in airway responsiveness is still unknown. Respiratory viruses grow in airway epithelium and cause epithelial inflammation,[52] and Empey and colleagues[50] suggested that inflammation of epithelium could be important in the hyperresponsiveness that occurs with viral infections.

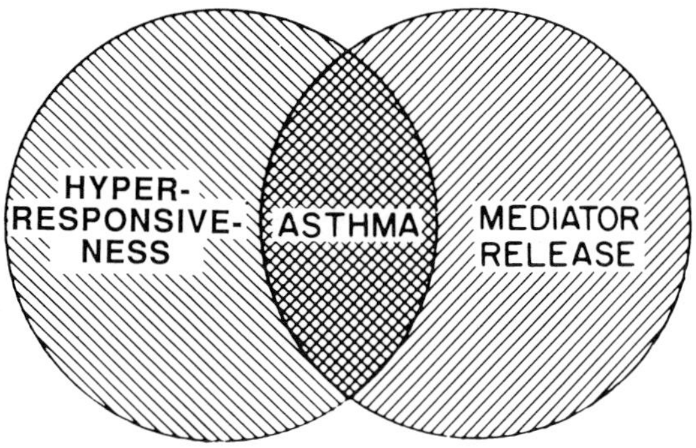


**Figure 37.1** The diagram shows the proposed mechanisms of asthma. Each circle represents a group of individuals. Inflammation of various etiologies causes airway hyperresponsiveness *(left circle)*. Alone, this does not result in asthma. Likewise, release of bronchoactive mediators from various cells (e.g., mast cells; *right circle*) does not result in asthma in the absence of hyperresponsiveness. When the hyperresponsive state and mediator release coexist (*cross-hatched area* where circles superimpose), clinical asthma results.

This evidence that hyperresponsiveness could be produced in otherwise healthy persons stimulated investigators to search for cells and mediators that might induce hyperresponsiveness. Studies in various laboratories have produced evidence that inflammation and inflammatory cells play an important role in the increased responsiveness of the airways that occurs in asthma.[50, 53–64]

Although airway hyperresponsiveness occurs in patients with asthma, it is not specific for the presence of asthma in individual patients, because symptoms of asthma may occur in the absence of hyperresponsiveness,[65] and airway hyperresponsiveness has been reported in patients with other chronic inflammatory diseases of the airways.[66, 67] Disappointingly, the relationship between the degree of hyperresponsiveness and the severity of asthma is not always consistent.[68, 69] Presumably, this is due to the fact that the degree of the airway narrowing that occurs in a person depends on both the degree of hyperresponsiveness and the amount of bronchoactive mediators released (see Fig. 37.1).

The concept that asthma is basically an inflammatory disease led to intense investigation of the contributions of various cells to the inflammatory cascades that may be responsible for the pathophysiology of asthma.[63, 64] Because animal models of asthma have only limited similarities to human asthma, investigators have moved increasingly to the study of asthmatic people. Utilization of techniques such as endobronchial biopsy and bronchoalveolar lavage have provided new information.[63]

One concept that has evolved is that the resident cells in the airways (e.g., epithelial cells, mast cells, and nerves) must play the principal roles in the induction of asthma and that other cells (e.g., leukocytes, lymphocytes) recruited into the airways may play important roles in the secondary cascades that lead to manifest disease.

Because the airway epithelium exists as an interface between the body and the external environment, the airway epithelium must contain mechanisms to protect the internal milieu from potentially damaging organisms and irritants. Therefore, it seems reasonable to assume that the superficial cells have important protective functions in airways. Figure 37.2 shows a diagram of the epithelium and some of its component cells. I suggest that various "sentinel" cells in the epithelium respond to foreign materials. These cells modify their own activities and produce mediators that signal other airway cells to act and call in inflammatory cells from the bloodstream.

In summary, the superficial tissues of the epithelium contain multiple cells. Each cell has specialized functions that protect against the deleterious effects of irritants and infectious agents. Their actions, via the release of such materials as cytokines, lipid mediators (e.g., arachidonic acid metabolites), enzymes (e.g., neutrophil and mast cell proteases), and peptide mediators (e.g., neuropeptides), may be exerted upon the same cell that released them (autocrine actions) or on neighboring cells (paracrine ac-

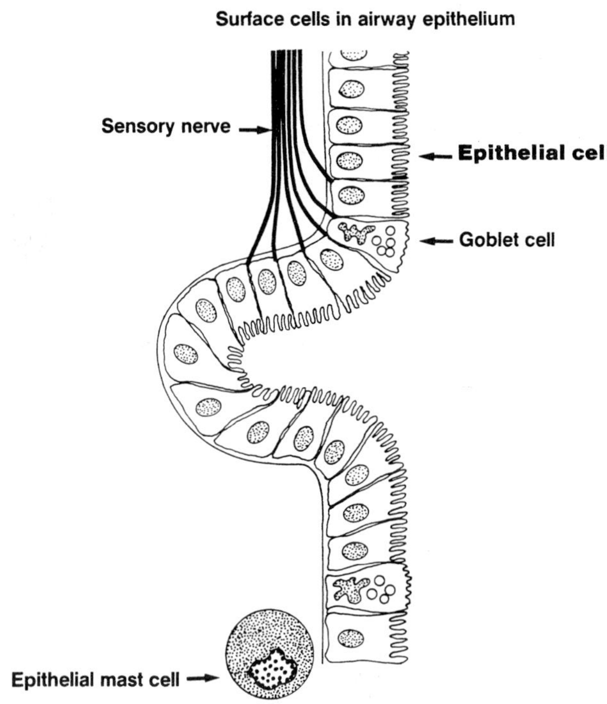


**Figure 37.2** The diagram shows the airway epithelium and some of its "sentinel" cell systems. The epithelium uses its cilia to clear foreign materials and (perhaps) its glycocalyx to prevent viral and bacterial entry. When "activated," it releases arachidonic acid metabolites that modulate smooth muscle tone, mast cell activation, and leukoycte chemotaxis. Superficial mast cells in the epithelium are posed to respond to antigenic and other stimuli by releasing inflammatory, bronchoactive, and secretagogue mediators. The sensory nerves receive irritating signals and respond in two ways: (1) via reflexes, whose pathways include the central nervous system; these reflexes cause cough, bronchospasm, and increased mucous secretion; and (2) via release of neuropeptides (e.g., substance P), with resultant inflammatory and other tissue-specific responses.

tions). Abnormal or excessive release of these mediators or the inability to break them down or inactivate them may result in excessive activities and lead to symptomatic disease.

## Chronic Obstructive Pulmonary Diseases (Emphysema and Chronic Bronchitis)

Cigarette smoking is the primary risk factor for COPD.[70] This subject is discussed in detail in Chapter 38. The most significant factor in the connection, however, is the individual variation in susceptibility. Thus, long-continued cigarette smoking is believed to be an important cause of lung cancer in one patient, of emphysema in another, and of bronchitis in a third; moreover, many heavy smokers have no pulmonary disability. Clearly, the defense mechanisms of the individual smoker must play an important role in determining whether he or she develops serious pulmonary disease or none at all. The fact that we have few insights into the causes of these differences among people is evidence of our ignorance of the basic biology of the lung. It is interesting that most cigarette smokers show a rate of decline of lung function only slightly greater than the rate of decline in nonsmokers. If we understood how most smokers defend the lungs successfully against the deleterious effects of cigarette smoke, we could identify those at risk. For those at risk who are unable to stop smoking, therapeutic intervention might then become feasible.

Because of the important association between cigarette smoking and COPD, investigators have worked intensively at discovering the mechanism(s) of smoke effects. The mechanisms by which cigarette smoke causes emphysema and chronic bronchitis are still not obvious. Although other environmental risk factors may also play a role in the pathogenesis of COPD, cigarette smoking stands far above all others. This is the most compelling reason to encourage people to stop smoking, to educate (especially the young) about the risks of smoking, and to modify behavior to achieve these ends (Chapters 98, 99).

### Emphysema

Emphysema is defined as a lung condition characterized by permanent enlargement of the alveolar spaces that is accompanied by destruction of their walls.[71–73] In any discussion of the mechanisms of lung disease it is useful to remember that lung tissue has a limited number of ways to respond to injury. First, there may be an acute inflammatory response followed by complete resolution. Second, the lungs may respond by generating scar tissue (fibrosis). Third, the response to lung injury may not permit healing to occur, but instead tissue breakdown occurs with subsequent destruction (emphysema). Thus, emphysema may simply be a stereotyped response (destruction of tissue) to many different types of injury. Emphysema, a destructive disease involving alveolar tissue, and chronic bronchitis, an inflammatory disease involving the airways, are separate disorders, but they usually occur together.[74]

Until relatively recently, the mechanisms responsible for emphysema remained entirely unknown. Although the exact molecular events involved in the production of this disease still escape us, two sets of observations have produced insights that are being pursued productively. In 1963, Laurell and Eriksson[75] discovered that homozygous deficiency in alpha$_1$-protease inhibitor (alpha$_1$-PI) is associated with premature development of severe emphysema.[76, 77] Studies of augmentation therapy in patients with alpha$_1$-PI deficiency are underway.[78–80]

Alpha$_1$-PI inhibits many proteolytic enzymes, including pancreatic elastase, trypsin, and chymotrypsin granulocyte elastase and collagenase, proteases from microorganisms, and collagenases from skin and synovia.[81] This knowledge led to the proposal that emphysema is caused by an imbalance between lung proteases and antiproteases. The proposal was given credence by experimental studies in animals in which administration of pancreatic elastase produced lung lesions similar to those of human emphysema.[82] Although leukocyte elastase has been particularly incriminated in the pathogenesis of emphysema, it is likely that other cells such as macrophages[83] and inhaled industrial intoxicants such as cadmium[84] may play a role.

Overwhelming evidence implicates cigarette smoking as an etiologic factor, but the mechanisms of the effect remain obscure. Even among persons with hereditary predisposition to the development of emphysema (i.e., persons with homozygous alpha$_1$-PI deficiency), smokers have a significantly lower life expectancy than nonsmokers.[85] Because cigarette smoking causes neutrophil chemotaxis into the lungs, purified human neutrophil elastase was delivered into the lungs of experimental animals; it resulted in the production of emphysema in exposed animals.[86, 87]

Could alpha$_1$-PI be involved in the pathogenesis of emphysema in persons with a normal complement of this inhibitor? It is known that oxidation of this molecule functionally inactivates it. Furthermore, cigarette smoke generates oxidants that also inactivate alpha$_1$-PI. Thus, cigarette smoke could create a deficiency of active alpha$_1$-PI and thereby promote emphysema. This possibility is being pursued, but results are controversial.[88–90]

In summary, enzymatic breakdown of lung tissue can be produced by various proteases, perhaps the most interesting of which is neutrophil elastase. Protective mechanisms, including antiproteases, defend the lungs against this destructive process. Therapeutic approaches might include supplying supplemental antiproteases. If neutrophils do play a role in pathogenesis and if we knew what ingredient in cigarette smoke caused neutrophils to move into lung tissue and release their toxic substances, we could develop the means to prevent the neutrophil effects. Thus, new insights into the pathogenesis of emphysema have recently been generated, but insufficient knowledge exists to produce sure therapeutic or preventive strategies (except for abstinence from smoking).

### Chronic Bronchitis

Chronic bronchitis is characterized pathologically by inflammatory changes in the airways.[71] Thus, neutrophils and chronic inflammatory cells are found in the epithelium in chronic bronchitis. Major additional pathophysiologic features of chronic bronchitis include the effects on cell growth and differentiation in the airways: Ciliated epithelial cells undergo squamous metaplasia and goblet cell proliferation, and smooth muscle and glands are increased in volume.[91–95] In addition, varying degrees of scarring and airway plugging with mucus are found. Thus, the pathology of chronic bronchitis is a combination of inflammation and altered cell proliferation.

As in emphysema, the exact cellular mechanisms underlying most of the changes found in patients with chronic bronchitis remain to be elucidated, but one thing is certain: The evidence is overwhelming that cigarette smoke is causally related to COPD (see Chapter 38 for documentation). Other agents suspected of causing chronic airway inflammation include air pollution (Chapter 68) and respiratory viruses. Major determinants are host factors, including genetic determinants. Why so many people exposed to cigarette smoke do not develop clinically evident disease raises the question of how the body's defenses cope with the respiratory insult and how failures in response result in the development of inflammatory disease of the airways.

Disappointingly, there is little specific therapy. Smoking cessation is important[96] but not immensely successful.

## Bronchiectasis

Bronchiectasis is a condition characterized by an abnormal dilation of bronchi due to the destruction of the elastic and muscular elements of their walls.[97] In developed countries, bronchiectasis was a devastating and relatively common disease before the antibiotic era, and it is still a public health problem in developing countries. In the United States today, bronchiectasis usually occurs in people with underlying systemic diseases in whom airway infection is superimposed (e.g., cystic fibrosis, allergic bronchopulmonary aspergillosis, primary ciliary dyskinesia, and immune deficiency). The major cause of the airway damage is inflammation, which may be produced by a combination of mediators, including neutrophil and monocyte products.[98–100]

## Cystic Fibrosis

Cystic fibrosis (CF) is a genetic disorder that is transmitted as an autosomal recessive trait. It is the most common genetic disease in Caucasian children, occurring in approximately 1:2500 live births,[101] and 1 in 20 Caucasians carries the CF gene. The progressive improvement in projected age of survival suggests that, although the disease is genetic in origin, a better understanding of the pathogenesis will allow further improvements in survival and in quality of life for CF patients. The disease affects exocrine glands and produces protean abnormalities, including sinusitis, nasal polyposis, hyperglycemia, and biliary cirrhosis. The most severe manifestations are, however, generally in two organs, the pancreas and the lung. In the pancreas, thick secretions are found early and lead to obstruction and later to gland tissue destruction and scarring.[102] Airway infection is probably a secondary complication, although it is the major cause of clinical deterioration and ultimate death. With progression of disease, the airways show evidence of inflammation, gland and goblet cell hypertrophy, and obstruction by secretions. At death, scarring and dilation of airways are common; lung tissue is less affected than airways, but alveolar damage, organizing pneumonia, and fibrosis can occur, especially in older persons.[103] Secondary cardiac involvement occurs in patients with severe hypoxemia, with resultant pulmonary vasoconstriction, pulmonary hypertension, and right ventricular overload (Chapter 55), but this complication usually occurs late in the course of the disease.[104]

CF has been known for many years to be a genetic disorder, but the molecular defects have only been discovered in the past 15 years: The responsible gene is located on the long arm of chromosome 7.[105–107] The gene encodes for an integral protein of epithelial cells called *CF transmembrane conductance regulator* (CFTR).[108] This protein is a chloride channel, but it may also have regulatory functions. Knockout of the CFTR gene in transgenic mice results in some characteristics similar to human CF.[109–111] Genotype analysis provides confirmation of the diagnosis and also has predictive implications concerning the course of disease.[112, 113]

The airways are a major site of disturbed function in CF, and their obstruction is a prevalent cause of premature death of patients with this lethal disease. Airway obstruction occurs owing to accumulated secretions and secondary bacterial infection. In fact, hypersecretion, neutrophil influx into the airways, and chronic bacterial infection are three of the conspicuous and unusual findings in patients with CF and are responsible for the progressive airway obstruction and death. The cause of hypersecretion in CF (and in all other diseases) is not known for certain. The sputum from these patients, however, contains large numbers of neutrophils and a high concentration of neutrophil proteases.[114, 115] Neutrophil elastase is an extremely potent secretagogue of airway submucosal glands and goblet cells.[10, 98, 99] Furthermore, CF sputum induces a secretory response from tracheal gland serous cells in vitro, and this secretion has been shown to be due to neutrophil proteases present in CF sputum.[115] These studies suggest that proteases released from neutrophils in airways may play an important role in causing airway hypersecretion in these patients. Clinical studies with inhibitors of neutrophil proteases are required to determine the clinical significance of these observations.

If neutrophil infiltration is important to the airway hypersecretion and other deleterious effects in the airways, what causes the neutrophils to accumulate in CF airways? In 1993, Richman-Eisenstat and associates[116] reported that CF sputum has significant neutrophil chemotactic activity and that this activity is inhibited by a blocking antibody to interleukin-8 (IL-8), a cytokine known to be potently chemotactic for neutrophils. The sputum contained high concentrations of IL-8.[116] Thus IL-8, possibly produced by airway epithelial cells or monocytes, or both, or by other airway cells, may be a major mechanism for recruitment of neutrophils in CF airways.

Can bacterial infection be involved in the "neutrophil cascade" just described? Recently, Massion and coworkers[117] discovered an exoproduct from *Pseudomonas aeru-*

*ginosa* (the predominant organism in CF airways) that potently induces IL-8 expression and activity in human airway epithelial cells and monocytes.[117]

These findings led to the following hypothesis: Bacterial infection (e.g., with *P. aeruginosa*) causes the release of a bacterial exotoxin that induces IL-8 production in airway cells, which in turn causes the influx of neutrophils into the airways where the neutrophil enzymes are released, causing hypersecretion. On their death, the neutrophils release large amounts of deoxyribonucleic acid (DNA), which causes the secretions to increase their viscosity. If this cascade plays a role in the pathogenesis of the deterioration of airway function in CF patients, it provides several strategies for potential therapeutic intervention.

The major clues to the cause of CF have derived from the clinical observations that secretions in various exocrine glands are inadequately cleared and that these secretions contain abnormal concentrations of electrolytes. The discovery that excessive loss of salt occurs in patients with CF via sweat was an important landmark in diagnosing the disease and, in retrospect, in developing a unifying concept of its pathogenesis.[118] A series of studies of active ion transport in sweat gland ducts[119, 120] and in placental trophoblast microvillus membrane vesicles[121] have provided powerful evidence that epithelial cells in these organs are impermeable to chloride. The chloride channels are located on the luminal membranes. When they open, chloride ions may move into the airway lumen; an osmotic gradient is produced, which draws water into the lumen. In patients with CF, the epithelium is impermeable to chloride and does not respond to normal stimuli. This lack of chloride permeability could lead to a lack of water movement into the airway lumen and thus cause relative dehydration of the airway lumen. The cilia lining the airway cells are normally bathed in a watery sol (Fig. 37.3). The tips of the cilia contact the mucous gel that floats on the sol, transporting the gel and entrapped foreign materials mouthward and thus clearing the airways.[122] In patients with CF, the ineffective chloride transport could limit water movement into the airways and thus contribute to mucous inspissation and impaired ciliary transport (Chapter 14) and impaired cough clearance of secretions (Chapter 15).

There have been multiple important new approaches to treatment, including lung transplantation,[123, 124] gene transfer,[125] and novel pharmacologic interventions (see Chapter 40).

## Disorders of the Upper Airways

Strictly speaking, diseases of the upper airways (nose, oropharynx, and larynx) are not treated as respiratory diseases (which are normally limited to the lungs). The upper airways are, however, directly "attached" to the lower airways and are important to normal respiration and to the understanding of the pathophysiology of some respiratory diseases (e.g., sleep disorders). In addition, diseases of the upper airways may masquerade as respiratory disorders because they limit breathing or cause dyspnea, cough, or wheezing. The physiology of the upper airways and the pathophysiologic features of diseases of these structures are reviewed in Chapter 42.

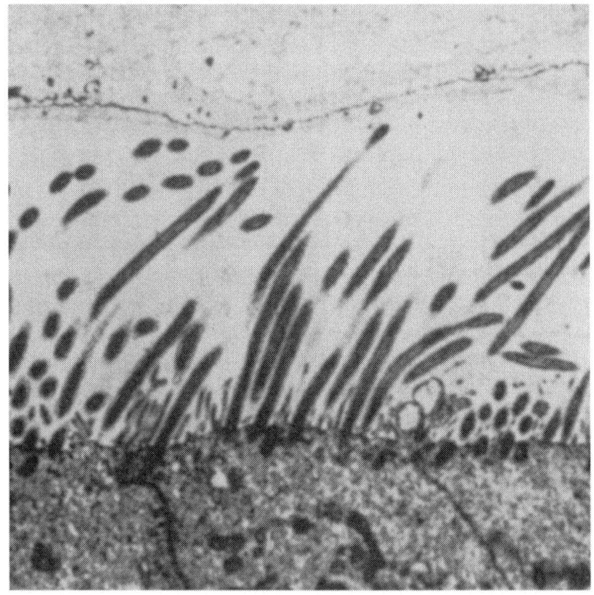

**Figure 37.3** The electron micrograph shows three airway epithelial cells. Cilia project from epithelial cells into the airway lumen. Cilia are surrounded by a watery sol layer (clear area between cilia) through which they can move easily. The tips of the cilia contact the gel (granular material at the top of photomicrograph). During the forward stroke, the cilia move the gel layer forward.

## Other Disorders of the Intrathoracic Airways

In addition to the common diseases of the airways, there also exist two other groups of airway diseases: diffuse diseases of the peripheral airways and localized diseases of the bronchi. The peripheral airways, bronchioles, do not normally contain cartilage, glands, or goblet cells.[126, 127] In various diseases usually thought of primarily as diseases of the large conducting airways (e.g., asthma, chronic bronchitis, and CF), increased numbers of goblet cells exist in bronchioles.[128] Secretion of the mucous contents of these cells could obstruct the peripheral airways and play a significant role in the pathogenesis of these diseases.

Inflammatory narrowing of the bronchioles (bronchiolitis) occurs especially in early childhood. This condition is rare in adults, but inhalation of relatively insoluble corrosive gases (e.g., nitrogen dioxide) is an example of a cause in adults (Chapter 69). Obliterative bronchiolitis may also occur as a result of respiratory infection, after bone marrow or heart-lung transplantation, or in association with connective tissue disorders. Pathologically, the bronchioles may be partially or totally filled with organizing connective tissue.[129–131] The pathologic changes may extend into the alveoli, and the process is then called *bronchiolitis obliterans with organizing pneumonia*.[132]

Bronchopulmonary dysplasia occurs in newborn infants

as a complication of the respiratory distress syndrome after oxygen therapy[133] and was reported in adults as a complication of adult respiratory distress syndrome.[134] Histologically, the bronchioles show obliterative changes with the formation of cysts.

Localized abnormalities of bronchi (discussed in Chapter 43) include common conditions (e.g., airway compression by infectious or malignant processes) and many rarer diseases (e.g., granulomatous disease, malacic lesions, broncholithiasis, amyloidosis, and traumatic injury). The manifestations of localized airway disease generally relate to the primary disease. These localized lesions do, however, cause symptoms and have physiologic effects on the respiratory system. Their detection usually also depends on clues presented by the causative disease.

Diseases in peripheral airways are difficult to diagnose early. With diffuse involvement, airway obstruction is not difficult to determine, but differentiation from diseases of large airways can be difficult.

## DIFFERENTIAL DIAGNOSIS OF OBSTRUCTIVE DISEASES

### Clinical Features

Clinical features of the obstructive diseases are discussed in detail in individual chapters on each disease. Here, only a few points are discussed. In "classic" cases, differential diagnosis may not cause problems, but in other cases there may be considerable overlap. Thus, in patients with previous attacks of reversible bronchospasm, especially young persons with a family history of asthma, atopic symptoms in childhood, evidence of allergic manifestations (so-called extrinsic asthma), and attacks triggered by specific antigen exposure, the diagnosis is apparent. Certain occupational exposures are known to precipitate asthma. In some cases, the connection between occupation and symptoms and disease is obvious, but in others, the connection is made only with a meticulous history and evaluation of the specific exposure. In persons who have no allergic or occupational background and whose symptoms occur later in life (so-called intrinsic asthma), however, the diagnosis is sometimes not obvious, and occupational asthma may easily be confused with chronic bronchitis. For clinical purposes, establishing the presence of reversibility of the obstruction and of airway smooth muscle hyperresponsiveness is useful in developing a therapeutic strategy for such patients. Therefore, in patients with chronic cough, part of the clinical workup is the evaluation of airway smooth muscle.

Localized disease of the airways may be difficult to establish. Localized physical findings may or may not be obvious, and pulmonary function tests play a limited role in the diagnosis (see later section). Specialized tests such as roentgenography, radioisotope scanning, and bronchoscopy can be useful.

CF presents a special challenge in diagnosis. Previously, CF patients rarely survived to adulthood, and CF problems were relegated to textbooks of pediatric medicine. With modern medical care, however, the age of survival has increased progressively, and now 50% of patients survive to age 25 years. This prolonged survival makes it mandatory to consider CF in the differential diagnosis of chronic airway obstruction in adults. Present evidence suggests that airway disease occurs after birth in patients with CF and is caused by abnormalities of secretion.[134] The chronic airway obstruction itself has no specific distinguishing features. Patients may have increased airway smooth muscle responsiveness that may simulate asthma. Chronic airway infection plays a major role in the deterioration of CF patients. The airways of many of the patients are colonized with *P. aeruginosa.*

### Tests of Pulmonary Function and Other Diagnostic Procedures

During the 1950s and 1960s, tests of pulmonary function were developed, and together with correlative studies of lung pathology they led to improved understanding of the pathophysiology of various diseases of the lungs and airways. These tests now play an important role in the diagnosis of diseases of the airways and in following the course of disease and the effects of various interventions. The alveoli act as an elastic element (e.g., like a balloon), and these properties are evaluated by studying lung compliance. The airways act as conducting tubes. Narrowing of the airways may lead to an increase in airflow resistance, which can be measured in a pulmonary function laboratory with a body plethysmograph. This measurement is not practical for day-to-day evaluation of most patients, but it is useful for laboratory evaluation (e.g., acute experimental exposures, studies of airway responsiveness). The plethysmograph has certain advantages: The measurement can be repeated easily, with little effort by the patient, and no deep breathing or forced exhalation is required.

The standard test for evaluating airway narrowing is spirometry. The test is based on the fact that, during exhalation, increasing effort does not continue to increase expiratory air flow; maximal flow occurs without great effort, and airway narrowing due to disease can be detected as a decrease in expiratory air flow. The patient inhales to total lung capacity and then exhales completely with a forceful effort. The standard reported value relates the volume exhaled in 1 second ($FEV_1$) to the total exhaled forced vital capacity (FVC). A decrease in this ratio implicates airway obstruction. On the basis of theoretic considerations, measurements of different portions of the exhaled curve have been made, and these have been shown to increase the sensitivity of the test (for discussion, see Chapter 28). In patients with irritable airways (e.g., those with asthma), deep inspiration or forced exhalation can trigger bronchospasm,[136] which can confound the evaluation. Nevertheless, spirometry is an excellent objective method for diagnosing obstructive airway disease and for evaluating the efficacy of therapeutic interventions.

Patients can evaluate therapy themselves using a peak flowmeter. This apparatus is small and portable. It measures the peak value for expiratory flow; when the airways are narrowed, peak flow decreases. This value is influenced more by the patient's effort, but it nonetheless gives useful information about the patient's status.

Other tests have been devised to better localize the

disease process and to increase the sensitivity (Chapter 28). For example, narrowing of the intrathoracic or extrathoracic trachea or larynx produces a characteristic pattern of air flow obstruction.[137–140] Investigators have attempted to devise tests to detect narrowing of peripheral airways, the so-called silent zone of the lungs. Various tests, including closing volume, frequency dependence of compliance,[141] and frequency dependence of resistance[142] and density dependence,[143, 144] have been evaluated. In general, these tests have not been successful because of various confounding problems (discussed in Chapters 5 and 28).

In general, tests of airway obstruction are more successful in diagnosing airway obstruction than in differentiating among diseases. Thus, spirometric abnormalities are often similar when the obstruction is due to bronchospasm (e.g., in asthma), mucus (e.g., CF), or luminal narrowing by edema and inflammation or scarring (e.g., some cases of chronic bronchitis) and when the "tethering" of the airways by the lungs is faulty because of lung tissue destruction (e.g., bullae and emphysema).

To differentiate smooth muscle contraction from other causes of airway narrowing, the response to the inhalation of bronchodilator aerosols is helpful. However, it is not uncommon for a patient to show little improvement after use of a bronchodilator on a single occasion in the laboratory, but to show improvement after treatment with bronchodilators for 7 to 10 days. This may be due at least in part to the fact that aerosolized bronchodilators are delivered mostly to the airways with the best ventilation (i.e., the least obstructed airways). Prolonged bronchodilator therapy may gradually improve access to the obstructed airways. Similarly, a 2 week trial of steroids occasionally shows striking reversibility of airway obstruction in patients in whom a bronchodilator has no acute salutary effect.

Sometimes, specific diseases can be distinguished by a combination of pulmonary function tests. For example, patients with emphysema have decreased air flow. Because alveolar-capillary membrane destruction is an integral part of their disease, they also tend to have a decrease in the measured diffusing capacity, whereas patients with bronchitis or asthma have normal values for diffusing capacity.[145]

Blood gas abnormalities in patients with obstructive airway diseases give important clues to cause. Regardless of etiology, patients with obstructive diseases tend to develop some degree of hypoxemia. Characteristically, however, patients with asthma show chronic respiratory alkalosis.[146] When the arterial $P_{CO_2}$ level begins to rise in patients with asthma, there is cause for alarm. Curiously, however, many patients with chronic bronchitis have dissimilar findings: With a similar degree of hypoxemia, they develop alveolar hypoventilation, with a raised arterial $P_{CO_2}$ level (Chapter 38). Despite much research, the exact cause of these differences in respiratory drive remains enigmatic. Single samples of arterial blood give only limited information in an individual patient. The discomfort associated with the procedure may cause acute hyperventilation. Furthermore, nocturnal blood gas levels often show marked depression during sleep. The blood bicarbonate level, therefore, often gives important information about the status of ventilatory control.

Most pulmonary function tests are performed at rest, but most patients complain of symptoms during or after exercise. Evaluation of exercise performance is therefore an important diagnostic strategy. It provides information on the level of the patient's performance and provides clues about underlying disease mechanisms. For example, in asthmatic subjects, exercise is a potent stimulus to bronchospasm. Therefore, measurement of spirometry before and after exercise may provide important diagnostic information. Similarly, in various diseases, exercise may exaggerate subtle abnormalities that are undetectable at rest.[116] Estimations of severity of airway obstruction by both the patient (based on symptoms) and the clinician (based on physical findings) leave much to be desired. Spirometry provides a simple inexpensive method for documenting the presence and degree of airway obstruction.

In localized diseases of the lungs (Chapter 43), the usefulness of pulmonary function tests is limited. In a patient with symptoms but without other objective evidence of lung disease, however, an abnormal test for distribution of ventilation (Chapter 28) may be the first evidence that lung disease exists, although it does not locate the lesion. Other tests are more useful, and these are discussed in Chapter 43.

## SUMMARY

Airway obstruction may result from contraction of airway smooth muscle (typified by asthma), edema, and mucous hypersecretion (e.g., chronic bronchitis) or loss of the elastic tethering of the airways by lung tissue (e.g., emphysema). Clinical manifestations of the airway obstruction and screening pulmonary function test abnormalities are similar, regardless of the pathologic cause. Thus, simple tests of pulmonary function (i.e., spirometry) are diagnostic of obstruction and are reliable means of studying the effects of therapy, but they usually do not differentiate among the causes of airway obstruction. In asthma, the degree of reversibility and evidence of airway smooth muscle responsiveness are important diagnostic features. Diseases of peripheral airways (bronchioles) and localized obstruction may be difficult diagnostic challenges.

Mucous hypersecretion is a major manifestation of many chronic inflammatory diseases of the airways. Presently, there is no effective therapy, but recent discoveries provide opportunities for novel therapeutic approaches.

A great deal is now known about the pathophysiology of the various obstructive diseases, but the cellular and molecular mechanisms are still understood only to a limited extent. New insights into the basic mechanisms of these diseases promise to provide new strategies for treatment and prevention. Regardless of the exact mechanisms causing chronic bronchitis and emphysema, cigarette smoking looms as the overwhelming cause. Prevention of smoking is the best method to avoid COPD.

## References

1. Snider GL, Faling LJ, Rennard SI: Chronic bronchitis and emphysema. *In* Murray JF, Nadel JA (eds): Textbook of Respiratory Medicine (Vol 2, 2nd ed). New York: WB Saunders, 1994, pp 1331–1397.

2. Fahy JF, Schuster A, Ueki I, et al: Mucus hypersecretion in bronchiectasis. The role of neutrophil proteases. Am Rev Respir Dis 146:1430–1433, 1992.
3. Boat TF, Boucher RD: Cystic fibrosis. *In* Murray JF, Nadel JA (eds): Textbook of Respiratory Medicine (Vol 2, 2nd ed). New York: WB Saunders, 1994, pp 1418–1450.
4. Shimura S, Andoh Y, Haraguchi M, et al: Continuity of airway goblet cells and intraluminal mucus in the airways of patients with bronchial asthma. Eur Respir J 9:1395–1401, 1996.
5. Takeyama K, Dabbagh K, Lee H-M, et al: Epidermal growth factor system regulates mucin production in airways. Proc Natl Acad Sci USA 96:3081–3086, 1999.
6. Speizer RF, Fay MD, Dockery DS, et al: Chronic obstructive pulmonary disease mortality in six U.S. cities. Am Rev Respir Dis 140:S49–S55, 1989.
7. Lang P, Nyboe J, Appleyard M, et al: Relation of ventilatory impairment and of chronic mucus hypersecretion to mortality from obstructive lung disease and from all causes. Thorax 45:579–585, 1990.
8. Annesi I, Kauffman F: Is respiratory mucus hypersecretion really an innocent disorder? Am Rev Respir Dis 134:688–693, 1986.
8a. Lee HM, Takeyama K, Ueki IF, et al: Agarose plugs in airways induce goblet cell metaplasia by activating epidermal growth factor receptors. Am J Respir Crit Care Med 159:A472, 1999.
9. Hill AT, Bayley D, Stockley RA: The interrelationship of sputum inflammatory markers in patients with chronic bronchitis. Am J Respir Crit Care Med 160:893–898, 1999.
10. Takeyama K, Agusti C, Ueki I, et al: Neutrophil-dependent goblet cell degranulation: Role of membrane-bound elastase and adhesion molecules. Am J Physiol 275 (Lung Cell Mol Physiol 19): L294–302, 1998.
11. Ciba Guest Symposium: Terminology, definitions and classifications of chronic pulmonary emphysema and related conditions. Thorax 14:286–299, 1959.
12. Anderson S: Asthma provoked by exercise, hyperventilation and the inhalation of non-isotonic aerosols. *In* Barnes P, Rodger I, Thomson N (eds): Asthma: Basic Mechanisms and Clinical Management (2nd ed). London: Academic Press, 1992, pp 473–490.
13. Hargreave FE, Juniper EF, Ryan G, et al: Clinical significance of nonspecific airway hyperreactivity. *In* Hargreave FE (ed): Airway Reactivity. Hamilton, Ontario: Astra Pharmaceuticals, 1980, pp 216–221.
14. Cardell BS, Pearson RSB: Death in asthmatics. Thorax 14:341–352, 1959.
15. Dunnill MS: The pathology of asthma. *In* Middleton E, Reed CE, Ellis EE (eds): Allergies, Principles and Practice. St. Louis: CV Mosby, 1978, pp 678–686.
16. Rigler L, Koucky R: Roentgen studies of the pathological physiology of bronchial asthma. Am J Roentgenol 39:353–362, 1938.
17. Houston JC, deNavasquez S, Trounce JR: A clinical and pathologic study of fatal cases of status asthmaticus. Thorax 8:207–213, 1953.
18. Naylor B: The shedding of the mucosa of the bronchial tree in asthma. Thorax 17:69–72, 1962.
19. Curschmann H: Ueber Bronchiolitis exudativa und ihr Verhaltniss zum Asthma nervosum. Dtsch Arch Klin Med 32:1–34, 1883.
20. Saetta M, Stefano AD, Rosina C, et al: Quantitative structural analysis of peripheral airways and arteries in sudden fatal asthma. Am Rev Respir Dis 143:138–143, 1991.
21. Bousquet J, Chanez P, Lacoste JY, et al: Asthma: A disease remodelling of the airways. Allergy 47:3–11, 1992.
22. Vracko R., Benditt EP: Manifestations of diabetes mellitus—Their possible relationship to an underlying cell defect. Am J Pathol 75:204–221, 1974.
23. Hossain S: Quantitative measurement of bronchial muscle in man with asthma [abstract]. Am Rev Respir Dis 107:99, 1973.
24. Glynn AA, Michaels L: Bronchial biopsy in chronic bronchitis and asthma. Thorax 15:142–153, 1960.
25. Laitinen LA, Heino M, Laitinen A, et al: Damage of the airway epithelium and bronchial reactivity in patients with asthma. Am Rev Respir Dis 131:599–606, 1985.
26. Reynolds HY: Bronchoalveolar lavage. State of the art. Am Rev Respir Dis 135:250–263, 1987.
27. Metzger WJ, Hunninghake GW, Richerson HB: Late asthmatic responses: Inquiry into mechanisms and significance. Clin Rev Allergy 3:145–165, 1985.
28. Metzger WJ, Richerson HB, Worden K, et al: Bronchoalveolar lavage of allergic asthmatic patients following allergen bronchoprovocation. Chest 89:477–483, 1986.
29. Metzger WJ, Zavala D, Richerson HB, et al: Local allergen challenge and bronchoalveolar lavage of allergic asthmatic lungs. Am Rev Respir Dis 135:433–440, 1987.
30. DeMonchy JGR, Kauffman HF, Venge, P, et al: Bronchoalveolar eosinophilia during allergen-induced late asthmatic reactions. Am Rev Respir Dis 131:373–376, 1985.
31. Tomioka M, Ida S, Shindoh Y, et al: Mast cells in bronchoalveolar lumen of patients with bronchial asthma. Am Rev Respir Dis 129:1000–1005, 1984.
32. Schleimer RP, MacGlashan DW, Jr, Peters SP, et al: Characterization of inflammatory mediator release from purified human lung mast cells. Am Rev Respir Dis 133:614–617, 1986.
33. Wasserman SI: Mediators of immediate hypersensitivity. J Allergy Clin Immunol 72:101–115, 1983.
34. Beasley R, Pearce N, Crane J: International trends in asthma mortality. *In* Chadwick DJ, Cardew G (eds): The Rising Trends in Asthma/Ciba Foundation Symposium 206. West Sussex, England: John Wiley & Sons 1997, pp 140–156.
35. Jackson RT, Sears MR, Beaglehole R, et al: International trends in asthma mortality: 1970–1985. Chest 94:914–918, 1988.
36. Evans R, Mullally DI, Wilson RW, et al: National trends in the morbidity and mortality of asthma in the U.S.: Prevalence, hospitalization and death from asthma over two decades: 1965–1984. Chest 91 (6): 65S–74S, 1987.
37. Duffy DL, Martin NG, Battistutta D, et al: Genetics of asthma and hay fever in Australian twins. Am Rev Respir Dis 142:1351–1358, 1990.
38. Ober C: Do genetics play a role in the pathogenesis of asthma? J Allergy Clin Immunol 101 (2, part 2):S417–S420, 1998.
39. Pattermore PK, Johnston SL, Bardin PG: Viruses as precipitants of asthma symptoms. I. Epidemiol Clin Exp Allergy 22:325–336, 1992.
40. Nicholson KG, Kent J, Ireland DC: Respiratory viruses and exacerbations of asthma in adults. BMJ 307:982–996, 1993.
41. Frick OL, German DF, Mills J: Development of allergy in children. I. Association with virus infections. J Allergy Clin Immunol 63(4):228–241, 1979.
42. McWilliam AS, Nelson D, Thomas JA, et al: Rapid dendritic cell recruitment is a hallmark of the acute inflammatory response at mucosal surfaces. J Exp Med 179(4):1331–1336, 1994.
43. Schon-Hegrad MA, Oliver J, McMenamin PG, et al: Studies on the density, distribution, and surface phenotype of intraepithelial class II major histocompatibility complex antigen 1(a)–bearing dendritic cells (DC) in the conducting airways. J Exp Med 173:1345–1356, 1991.
44. Dupuis M, McDonald DM: Dendritic-cell regulation of lung immunity. Am J Respir Cell Mol Biol 17(3):284–286, 1997.
45. Cockcroft DW, Murdock KY, Berscheid BA: Relationship between atopy and bronchial responsiveness to histamine in a random population. Ann Allergy 53:26–29, 1984.
46. Burrows B, Martinez FD, Halonen M, et al: Association of asthma with serum IgE levels and skin-test reactivity to allergens. N Engl J Med 320:271–277, 1989.
47. Sears MR, Burrows B, Flannery EM, et al: Relation between airway responsiveness and serum IgE in children with asthma and in apparently normal children. N Engl J Med 325:1067–1071, 1991.
48. Platts-Mills TAE, Chapman MD: Dust mites: Immunology, allergic disease, and environmental control. J Allergy Clin Immunol 80:755–775, 1987.
49. Lambert HP, Stern H: Infective factors in exacerbations of bronchitis and asthma. BMJ 3:323–326, 1972.
50. Empey DW, Laitinen LA, Jacobs L, et al: Mechanisms of bronchial hyperreactivity in normal subjects following upper respiratory tract infection. Am Rev Respir Dis 113:131–139, 1976.
51. Laitinen LA, Elkin RB, Empey DW, et al: Bronchial hyperresponsiveness in normal subjects during attenuated influenza virus infection. Am Rev Respir Dis 143:358–361, 1991.
52. Walsh JJ, Dietlein LF, Low FN, et al: Bronchotracheal response in human influenza. Arch Intern Med 108:376–382, 1961.

53. Behrens BL, Clark RAF, Marsh W, et al: Modulation of the late asthmatic response by antigen-specific immunoglobulin G in an animal model. Am Rev Respir Dis 130:1134–1139, 1984.
54. Chung KF, Becker AB, Lazarus SC, et al: Antigen-induced airway hyperresponsiveness and pulmonary inflammation in allergic dogs. J Appl Physiol 58:1347–1353, 1985.
55. Fabbri LM, Aizawa H, Alpert SE, et al: Airway hyperresponsiveness and changes in cell counts in bronchoalveolar lavage after ozone exposure in dogs. Am Rev Respir Dis 129:288–291, 1984.
56. Golden JA, Nadel JA, Boushey HA: Bronchial hyperirritability in healthy subjects after exposure to ozone. Am Rev Respir Dis 118:287–294, 1978.
57. Holtzman MJ, Fabbri LM, O'Byrne PM, et al: Importance of airway inflammation for hyperresponsiveness induced by ozone in dogs. Am Rev Respir Dis 127:686–690, 1983.
58. Holtzman MJ, Fabbri LM, Skoogh BE, et al: Time course of airway hyperresponsiveness induced by ozone in dogs. J Appl Physiol 55:1232–1236, 1983.
59. Lee L-Y, Bleecker ER, Nadel JA: Effect of ozone on bronchomotor response to inhaled histamine aerosol in dogs. J Appl Physiol 43:626–631, 1977.
60. Marsh WR, Irvin CG, Murphy KR, et al: Increases in airway reactivity to histamine and inflammatory cells in bronchoalveolar lavage after the late asthmatic response in an animal model. Am Rev Respir Dis 131:875–879, 1985.
61. Nadel JA, Holtzman MJ: Regulation of airway responsiveness and secretion: Role of inflammation. *In* Kay AB, Austen KF, Lichtenstein LM (eds): Asthma: Physiology, Immunopharmacology, and Treatment. London: Academic Press, 1984, pp 129–155.
62. Snapper JR, Brigham KL: Inflammation and airway reactivity. Exp Lung Res 6:83–89, 1984.
63. Djukanovic R, Roche WR, Wilson JW, et al: State of the art: Mucosal inflammation in asthma. Am Rev Respir Dis 142:434–457, 1990.
64. Bigby TD, Nadel JA: Asthma. *In* Gallin JI, Goldstein IM, Snyderman R (eds): Inflammation: Basic Principles and Clinical Correlates (2nd ed). New York: Raven Press, 1992, pp 889–906.
65. Stanescu DC, Frans A: Bronchial asthma without increased airway reactivity. Eur J Respir Dis 63:5–12, 1982.
66. Varpela E, Laitinen LA, Keskinen H, et al: Asthma, allergy and bronchial hyper-reactivity to histamine in patients with bronchiectasis. Clin Allergy 8:273–280, 1978.
67. Laitinen LA, Haahtela T, Kava T, et al: Nonspecific bronchial reactivity and ultrastructure of the airway epithelium in patients with sarcoidosis and allergic alveolitis. Eur J Respir Dis 64:267–284, 1983.
68. Brand P, Postma DS, Kerstjens HAM, et al: The Dutch CNSLD Study Group: Relationship of airway hyperresponsiveness to respiratory symptoms and diurnal peak flow variation in patients with obstructive lung disease. Am Rev Respir Dis 143:916–921, 1991.
69. Josephs LK, Gregg I, Mullee MA, et al: Nonspecific bronchial reactivity and its relationship to the clinical expression of asthma. A longitudinal study. Am Rev Respir Dis 140:350–357, 1989.
70. US Department of Health, Education, and Welfare: The Health Consequences of Smoking. Chronic Obstructive Lung Disease. Rockville: US Department of Health and Human Services Office of Smoking, DHHS (PHS) 84-50205, 1984.
71. Thurlbeck WM: Pathology of chronic airflow obstruction. *In* Cherniack NS (ed): Chronic Obstructive Pulmonary Disease. Philadelphia: WB Saunders, 1991, pp 3–20.
72. Thurlbeck WM: Chronic Airflow Obstruction in Lung Disease. Vol 5: Major Problems in Pathology. Philadelphia: WB Saunders, 1976.
73. Snider GL, Kleinerman J, Thurlbeck WM, et al: The definition of emphysema: Report of a National Heart, Lung and Blood Institute, Division of Lung Diseases, Workshop. Am Rev Respir Dis 132:182–185, 1985.
74. Burrows B, Bloom JW, Traver GA, et al: The course and prognosis of different forms of chronic airways obstruction in a sample from the general population. N Engl J Med 317:1309–1314, 1987.
75. Laurell CB, Eriksson S: The electrophoretic alpha-1-globulin pattern of serum in alpha-1 antitrypsin deficiency. Scand J Clin Lab Invest 15:132–140, 1963.
76. Larsson C: Natural history and life expectancy in severe alpha$_1$-antitrypsin deficiency, PiZ. Acta Med Scand 204:345–351, 1978.
77. Tobin MJ, Cook PJL, Hutchison DCS: Alpha$_1$-antitrypsin deficiency: The clinical features and physiological features of pulmonary emphysema in subjects homozygous for Pi type Z. A survey by the British Thoracic Association. Br J Dis Chest 77:14–27, 1983.
78. Hubbard RC, Sellers SE, and Czerski D: Biochemical efficacy and safety of monthly augmentation therapy for alpha-1-antitrypsin deficiency. JAMA 260:1259–1264, 1992.
79. Hubbard RC, Brantly ML, Sellers SE, et al: Antineutrophil-elastase defenses of the lower respiratory tract in alpha-1-antitrypsin deficiency directly augmented with an aerosol of alpha-1-antitrypsin. Ann Intern Med 111:206–212, 1988.
80. Hubbard RC, et al: Recombinant DNA-produced alpha 1-antitrypsin administered by aerosol augments lower respiratory tract antineutrophil elastase defenses in individuals with alpha 1-antitrypsin deficiency. J Clin Invest 84:1349–1354, 1989.
81. Idell S, Cohen HB: Alpha-1-antitrypsin deficiency. Clin Chest Med 4:359–376, 1983.
82. Snider GL, Lucey EC, Stone PJ: State of the art: Animal models of emphysema. Am Rev Respir Dis 133:149–169, 1986.
83. Senior RM, Connolly NL, Cury JD, et al: Elastin degradation by human alveolar macrophages: A prominent role of metalloproteinase activity. Am Rev Respir Dis 139:1251–1256, 1989.
84. Snider GL, Lucey EC, Faris B, et al: Cadmium chloride-induced airspace enlargement with interstitial pulmonary fibrosis is not associated with destruction of lung elastin. Implications for the pathogenesis of human emphysema. Am Rev Respir Dis 137:918–923, 1988.
85. Black LF, Kueppers F: Alpha$_1$-antitrypsin deficiency in nonsmokers. Am Rev Respir Dis 117:421–428, 1978.
86. Senior RM, Tegner H, Kuhn C, et al: The induction of pulmonary emphysema with human leukocyte elastase. Am Rev Respir Dis 116:469–475, 1977.
87. Snider GL, Lucey EC, Christensen TG, et al: Emphysema and bronchial secretory cell metaplasia induced in hamsters by human neutrophil products. Am Rev Respir Dis 129:155–160, 1984.
88. Stone PJ, Calore JD, McGowan SE, et al: Functional alpha-1-protease inhibitor in the lower respiratory tract of cigarette smokers is not decreased. Science 221:1187–1189, 1983.
89. Boudier C, Pelletier A, Pauli G, et al: The functional activity of alpha-1-proteinase inhibitor in bronchoalveolar lavage fluids from healthy human smokers and nonsmokers. Clin Chim Acta 132:309–315, 1983.
90. Abboud RT, Fera T, Richter A, et al: Acute effect of smoking on the functional activity of alpha-1-proteinase inhibitor in bronchoalveolar lavage fluid. Am Rev Respir Dis 131:79–85, 1985.
91. Reid L: Measurement of the bronchial mucous gland layer. A diagnostic yardstick in chronic bronchitis. Thorax 15:132–141, 1960.
92. Thurlbeck WM, Angus GE: A distribution curve for chronic bronchitis. Thorax 19:436–442, 1964.
93. Mitchell RS, Ryan SF, Petty TL, et al: The significance of morphologic chronic hyperplastic bronchitis. Am Rev Respir Dis 93:720–729, 1966.
94. Scott KWM: An autopsy study of bronchial mucous gland hypertrophy in Glasgow. Am Rev Respir Dis 97:54–61, 1968.
95. Mitchell RS, Silvers GW, Dart GA, et al: Morphologic correlations in chronic airway obstruction. Am Rev Respir Dis 97:54–61, 1968.
96. Fisher EB Jr, Rose K: Smoking cessation: A practical guide for physicians. Clin Chest Med 7:551–566, 1986.
97. Heard BE, Khatchatourov V, Otto H, et al: The morphology of emphysema, chronic bronchitis, and bronchiectasis: Definition, nomenclature, and classification. J Clin Pathol 32:882–892, 1979.
98. Schuster A, Ueki I, Nadel JA: Neutrophil elastase stimulates tracheal submucosal gland secretion that is inhibited by ICI 200, 355. Am J Physiol 262: L86–L91, 1992.
99. Sommerhoff CP, Nadel JA, Basbaum CB, et al: Neutrophil elastase and cathepsin G stimulate secretion from cultured bovine airway gland serous cells. J Clin Invest 85:682–689, 1990.
100. Owen CA, Campbell EJ, Hill SL, et al: Increased adherence of monocytes to fibronectin in bronchiectasis. Am Rev Respir Dis 145:626–631, 1992.

101. Hammond KB, Reardon MC, Accurso FJ, et al: Early detection and followup of cystic fibrosis in newborns: The Colorado experience. *In* Carter TP, Willey AM (eds): Genetic Disease: Screening and Management. New York: Alan R. Liss, 1986, pp 81–101.
102. di Sant'Agnese PA, Hubbard VS: The pancreas. *In* Taussig LM (ed): Cystic Fibrosis. New York: Thieme-Stratton, 1984, pp 230–295.
103. Tomashefski JF Jr, Konstan MW, Bruce M: The pathology of interstitial pneumonia in cystic fibrosis [abstract]. Am Rev Respir Dis 133:A365, 1986.
104. Stern RC, Borkat G, Hirschfield SS, et al: Heart failure in cystic fibrosis. Am J Dis Child 134:267–272, 1980.
105. Tsui LC, Buchwaid M, Baker D, et al: Cystic fibrosis locus defined by a genetically linked polymorphic DNA marker. Science 230:1054–1057, 1985.
106. White R, Woodward W, Leppert M, et al: A closely linked genetic marker for cystic fibrosis. Nature 318:382–384, 1985.
107. Wainwright BJ, Scambler PJ, Schmidtke J, et al: Localization of the cystic fibrosis locus to human chromosome 7 cenq22. Nature 318:384–385, 1985.
108. Riordan J, Rommens JM, Kerem BS, et al: Identification of the cystic fibrosis gene: Cloning and characterization of the complementary DNA. Science 245:1066–1073, 1989.
109. Egan M, Flotte T, Afione S, et al: Defective regulation of outwardly rectifying $Cl^-$ channels by protein kinase A corrected by insertion of CFTR. Nature 358:581–584, 1992.
110. Snouwaert JN, Brigman KK, Latour AM, et al: An animal model for cystic fibrosis made by gene targeting. Science 257:1083–1088, 1992.
111. Clarke LL, Grubb BR, Sherif GE, et al: Defective epithelial chloride transport in a gene-targeted mouse model of cystic fibrosis. Science 257:1125–1128, 1992.
112. Kerem E, Corey M, Kerem B-S, et al: The relation between genotype and phenotype in cystic fibrosis—Analysis of the most common mutation ($DF_{508}$). N Engl J Med 323:1517–1522, 1990.
113. Liechti-Gallati S, Bonsall I, Malik N, et al: Genotype/phenotype association in cystic fibrosis: Analyses of the delta F508, R553X, and 3905insT mutations. Pediatr Res 32:175–178, 1992.
114. Jackson AH, Hill SL, Afford SC: Studies of sputum sol phase proteins and elastase activity of patients with cystic fibrosis. Eur J Respir Dis 65:114–124, 1984.
115. Schuster A, Ueki I, Fahy JV, et al: CF sputum induces a secretory response from tracheal gland serous cells that can be inhibited by antiproteases [abstract]. Pediatr Pulmonol (Suppl 6):299, 1991.
116. Richman-Eisenstat JBY, Jorens PG, Hébert CA, et al: Interleukin-8: An important chemoattractant in sputum of patients with chronic inflammatory airway diseases. Am J Physiol: Lung Cell Mol Physiol 264:L413–418, 1993.
117. Massion PP, Inoue H, Grunberger D, et al: A *Pseudomonas aeruginosa* exoproduct induces interleukin-8 expression by human airway epithelial cells: Partial characterization. Am Rev Respir Dis 147:A29, 1993.
118. di Sant'Agnese PA, Darling RC, Perera GA, et al: Abnormal electrolytic composition of sweat in cystic fibrosis of the pancreas. Clinical significance and relationship of the disease. Pediatrics 12:549–563, 1953.
119. Quinton PM: Chloride impermeability in cystic fibrosis. Nature 301:421–422, 1983.
120. Quinton PM: Missing Cl conductance in cystic fibrosis. Am J Physiol 251:C649–C652, 1986.
121. Davis B, Shennan DB, Boyd CAR: Chloride transport in cystic fibrosis placenta. Lancet 1:392–393, 1985.
122. Nadel JA, Widdicombe JH, Peatfield AC: Regulation of airway secretions, ion transport, and water movement. *In* Fishman AP, Fisher AB (eds): Handbook of Physiology, Section 3: The Respiratory System (Vol 3, Part 1). Bethesda, MD: The American Physiological Society, 1985, pp 419–445.
123. Yankaskas JR, Mallory GB Jr: Lung transplantation in cystic fibrosis: Consensus Conference Statement. Chest 113:217–226, 1998.
124. Barr ML, Schenkel FA, Cohen RG, et al: Recipient and donor outcomes in living related and unrelated lobar transplantation. Transplant Proc 30:2261–2263, 1998.
125. Johnson LG, Knowles MR: New therapeutic strategies for cystic fibrosis lung disease. In Yankaskas JR, Knowles MR (eds): Cystic Fibrosis in Adults. Philadelphia: Lippincott-Raven, 1999, pp 233–258.
126. Hayek H: The Human Lung. New York: Hafner, 1960, pp 298–314.
127. Miller WS: The Lung (2nd ed). Springfield, IL: Charles C Thomas, 1947.
128. Thurlbeck WM: Chronic Airflow Obstruction in Lung Disease. Philadelphia: WB Saunders, 1976, pp 45–46.
129. Gosink BB, Friedman PJ, Liebow AA: Bronchiolitis obliterans. Roentgenologic-pathologic correlation. Am J Roentgenol 117:816–832, 1973.
130. Wright JL, Cagle P, Churg A, et al: Diseases of the small airways. Am Rev Respir Dis 146:240–262, 1992.
131. Epler GR, Colby TV: The spectrum of bronchiolitis obliterans. Chest 83:161–162, 1983.
132. Epler GR, Colby TV, McLoud TC, et al: Bronchiolitis obliterans organizing pneumonia. N Engl J Med 312:152–158, 1985.
133. Northway WH, Rosen RC, Porter DY: Pulmonary disease following respiratory therapy of hyaline-membrane disease. N Engl J Med 276:357–368, 1967.
134. Churg A, Golden J, Fligiel S, et al: Bronchopulmonary dysplasia in the adult. Am Rev Respir Dis 127:117–120, 1983.
135. Zuelzer WW, Newton WA Jr: The pathogenesis of fibrocystic disease of the pancreas. A study of 36 cases with special reference to the pulmonary lesions. Pediatrics 4:53–69, 1949.
136. Simonsson BG, Jacobs FM, Nadel JA: Role of autonomic nervous system and the cough reflex in the increased responsiveness of airways in patients with obstructive airway disease. J Clin Invest 46:1812–1818, 1967.
137. Gamsu G, Borson DB, Webb WR, et al: Structure and function in tracheal stenosis. Am Rev Respir Dis 120:519–531, 1980.
138. Hyatt RE, Black LF: The flow-volume curve: A current perspective. Am Rev Respir Dis 107:191–199, 1973.
139. Kryger M, Bode F, Antic R: Diagnosis of obstruction of the upper and central airways. Am J Med 61:85–93, 1976.
140. Miller RD, Hyatt RE: Evaluation of obstructing lesions of the trachea and larynx by flow-volume loops. Am Rev Respir Dis 108:475–481, 1973.
141. Woolcock AJ, Vincent NJ, Macklem PT: Frequency dependence of compliance as a test for obstruction in the small airways. J Clin Invest 48:1097–1106, 1969.
142. Grimby G, Takashima T, Graham W, et al: Frequency dependence of flow resistance in patients with obstructive lung disease. J Clin Invest 47:1455–1465, 1968.
143. Schilder DP, Roberts A, Fry DL: Effect of gas density and viscosity on the maximal expiratory flow-volume relationships. J Clin Invest 42:1705–1713, 1963.
144. Staats BA, Wilson TA, Lai-Fook SJ, et al: Viscosity and density dependence during maximal flow in man. J Appl Physiol 48:313–319, 1980.
145. Gelb AF, Gold WM, Wright, RR, et al: Physiologic diagnosis of subclinical emphysema. Am Rev Respir Dis 107:50–63, 1973.
146. McFadden ER Jr, Lyons HA: Arterial-blood gas tension in asthma. N Engl J Med 278:1027–1032, 1968.

# 38 Chronic Bronchitis and Emphysema

CRAIG A. PIQUETTE, M.D. • STEPHEN I. RENNARD, M.D.*
GORDON L. SNIDER, M.D.

Introduction
Definitions
Chronic Obstructive Pulmonary Disease
Chronic Bronchitis
Emphysema
Historical Background
Clinical Features of Chronic Obstructive Pulmonary Disease
History
Physical Examination
Laboratory Findings
Complications of Chronic Obstructive Pulmonary Disease
Differential Diagnosis of Chronic Obstructive Pulmonary Disease
Unilateral Hyperlucent Lung
Unilateral Bronchiolitis Obliterans
Further Considerations
Epidemiology
Magnitude of the Problem in the United States
Risk Factors for Chronic Obstructive Pulmonary Disease
Natural History
Prognosis and Course of Chronic Obstructive Pulmonary Disease
Pathology
Chronic Bronchitis
Simple Air-Space Enlargement
Emphysema
Structure-Function Correlations
Mucous Gland Size and Sputum Production
The Cause of Airflow Limitation in Chronic Obstructive Pulmonary Disease
Compliance and Lung Volumes in Emphysema
Carbon Monoxide Diffusing Capacity
Pathogenesis of Chronic Obstructive Pulmonary Disease
Introduction
Alpha$_1$-Protease Inhibitor Deficiency
The Elastase-Antielastase Hypothesis
Chronic Bronchitis
Treatment
Specific Therapy
Symptomatic Therapy
Secondary Therapy
Overall Therapeutic Strategy
Summary

## INTRODUCTION

Earlier in the 20th century, tuberculosis was the major disease occupying the professional efforts of physicians devoted to caring for patients with pulmonary diseases. Its place as the leading pulmonary cause of disability and death has been taken in the latter half of the 20th century by two diseases: carcinoma of the lung and chronic obstructive pulmonary disease (COPD). The number of deaths from these two conditions are similar. However, COPD, including both chronic bronchitis and emphysema, with their cardinal symptoms of cough, expectoration, wheezing, and labored breathing, runs an indolent course and is much more prevalent.

## DEFINITIONS

### Chronic Obstructive Pulmonary Disease

Chronic bronchitis and emphysema (see below) may occur with or without airflow limitation, whereas asthma, by definition[1] (Chapter 39), is always associated with discernible airflow limitation, although tests of bronchial provocation may be necessary to diagnose variant asthma. Chronic bronchitis and emphysema, because both are frequent results of the same etiologic factors (i.e., exposure to cigarette smoke), often occur together.[2] Asthma, a disease whose hallmark is reversible airflow limitation, may also lead to fixed airflow limitation.[3, 4] The clinical

*Corresponding author.

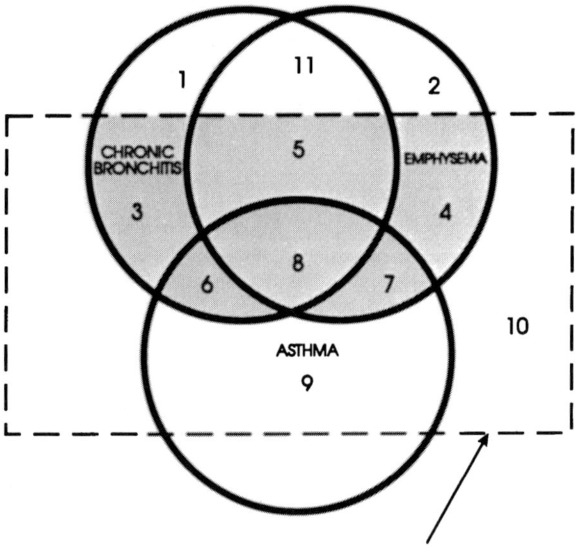


**Figure 38.1** Schema of chronic obstructive pulmonary disease. A nonproportional Venn diagram shows subsets of patients with chronic bronchitis, emphysema, and asthma in three overlapping circles; the subsets comprising COPD are shaded. The areas of the subsets are not proportional to the size of the subset. Most patients with severe disease have features of both chronic bronchitis and emphysema and fall into subset 5; some patients have features of asthma as well and fall into subset 8. Patients with features of asthma and chronic bronchitis (asthmatic bronchitis or the asthmatic form of COPD) fall into subset 6. Patients with asthma whose airflow obstruction is completely reversible (subset 9) and patients with chronic bronchitis or emphysema without airflow obstruction (subsets 1, 2, and 11) are not classed as COPD. See text for discussion.

and physiologic features of asthma, emphysema, and chronic bronchitis are often similar. Accordingly, precise classification of a patient's disease state can become difficult. To deal with this problem, a variety of terms have come into common usage to identify patients who have evidence of one or more of the diseases of chronic bronchitis, emphysema, and asthma. These terms are used synonymously: chronic obstructive lung disease, chronic obstructive airway disease, and chronic obstructive pulmonary disease (COPD); the last is used in this chapter.

A generally agreed on definition of COPD has been difficult to obtain. It has been argued that the term COPD should be used only for patients who have airflow limitation determined objectively. Chronic bronchitis and emphysema may, however, occur with little evidence of airflow limitation.[5] The term COPD (or one of its synonyms) can be used to record a diagnosis that does not imply a scientifically indefensible degree of precision. In contrast, the term asthma, rather than COPD, should be used for patients who have completely reversible airflow limitation without the symptoms of chronic bronchitis or the findings of emphysema (Fig. 38.1). This terminology is adequate when therapy is largely supportive and is not specific. Attempts to elucidate the underlying mechanisms of disease as well as efforts both to develop more specific interventions and to prevent the progression of disease have, however, created a need for a more detailed categorization.

## Chronic Bronchitis

Chronic bronchitis is defined for epidemiologic purposes as the presence of chronic productive cough for 3 months in each of 2 successive years in a patient in whom other causes of chronic cough, such as infection with *Mycobacterium tuberculosis,* carcinoma of the lung, bronchiectasis, cystic fibrosis, and chronic congestive heart failure, have been excluded.[1, 6] It is practical for clinical purposes to define chronic bronchitis more simply as chronic productive cough without a medically discernible cause that is present for more than half the time for 2 years. This broad, symptom-based definition has been useful despite including a number of conditions that share an etiology based on chronic irritation induced by inhaled substances.

## Emphysema

Respiratory air-space enlargement has been divided[7] into three categories (Table 38.1). Simple *air-space enlargement* is defined as enlargement of the respiratory air spaces without destruction, and it may be congenital, as in Down's syndrome, or acquired, as in the overdistention of the remaining lung that follows pneumonectomy. *Emphysema* is defined as a condition of the lung characterized by abnormal permanent enlargement of the air spaces distal to the terminal bronchioles accompanied by destruction of their walls and without obvious fibrosis. Destruction is defined as nonuniformity in the pattern of respiratory air-space enlargement; the orderly appearance of the acinus and its components is disturbed and may be lost. The third category of air-space enlargement occurs with obvious *fibrosis.* This form of the disease may be associated with infectious granulomatous disease such as tuberculosis, noninfectious granulomatous disease such as sar-

**Table 38.1** CLASSIFICATION OF RESPIRATORY AIR-SPACE ENLARGEMENT

| |
|---|
| **Simple Air-Space Enlargement** |
| Congenital |
| Congenital lobar overinflation |
| Down's syndrome |
| Acquired |
| Secondary to loss of lung volume |
| **Emphysema** |
| Proximal acinar emphysema |
| Focal emphysema |
| Centrilobular emphysema |
| Panacinar emphysema |
| Distal acinar emphysema |
| **Air-Space Enlargement with Fibrosis** |

coidosis, or fibrosis of undetermined cause. Air-space enlargement with fibrosis was formerly termed *irregular* or *paracicatricial emphysema.*

## HISTORICAL BACKGROUND

Although obstructive airway disorders have been known since antiquity, the appearance of enlarged respiratory air spaces on the surface of human lungs was not illustrated until 1691, by Ruysch.[8] Late in the 18th century, Matthew Baillie provided the earliest illustration[9] and a brief description[10] of emphysema. In the early 19th century, Laennec,[11, 12] using air-dried inflated lung specimens, gave us a description of emphysema that stood in its essentials for 125 years. He thought that the peripheral airways were the primary site of obstruction in emphysema and speculated that loss of elastic recoil was a likely contributor to diminished airflow from the enlarged alveoli. Orsos,[13] in the early 20th century, provided comprehensive descriptions of parenchymal elastic fibers and their extensive destruction in emphysema. He distinguished between emphysema and the simple overdistention of alveoli and the atrophy of elastic fibers that occur with aging.

In the 1950s, Gough and collaborators,[14–16] using sections of whole inflation-fixed lungs mounted on paper, ushered in the modern era of pathologic study of emphysema. They described centriacinar emphysema and distinguished it from panacinar emphysema. There followed a period of rapid expansion in our knowledge of the pathology, epidemiology, and pathophysiology of emphysema. Attempts to understand the pathogenesis of emphysema and bronchitis began in the early 1960s. The association of homozygous alpha$_1$-protease inhibitor deficiency with emphysema[17] and animal models of emphysema induced by the protease papain[18] led to the concept of proteolytic destruction of lung as a major factor. In ensuing decades the key role of inflammatory cells that can activate several potentially destructive mechanisms has been developed. The concept that the lung has some capacity to repair has emerged, with emphysema representing an imbalance between destruction and repair. Therapy has largely focused on supportive care based on the physiologic abnormalities associated with these disorders. In parallel with advancing understanding, however, attempts to correct the underlying mechanisms and thus improve the natural history are now being undertaken.

## CLINICAL FEATURES OF CHRONIC OBSTRUCTIVE PULMONARY DISEASE

### History

Cough is the most frequent symptom reported by patients with COPD. Cough precedes the onset of dyspnea or occurs at the same time in most patients. Most patients with COPD manifest cough, expectoration, and dyspnea, but it is usually the dyspnea that causes them to seek medical attention. Cough usually does not interfere with daily activities, and often the patient is unaware of cough frequency. Use of cough suppressants for a chronic productive cough is believed to lead to retention of secretions. A chronic daily cough is predictive of frequent exacerbations.[19]

Sputum production is insidious in its onset, and in most patients it is "scanty," defined as less than several tablespoons per day. Sputum production is much greater in smokers. The sputum is usually mucoid but becomes purulent during infective episodes and may take 2 to 3 weeks to clear. Following smoking cessation, sputum may become transiently more difficult to expectorate due to decreased cough clearability, but symptoms generally improve.[20]

Chronic bronchitis is the most common cause of hemoptysis in the United States and usually occurs in association with an infective episode.[21] Other etiologies of hemoptysis must, however, be kept in mind in this susceptible population.[22]

Dyspnea during exertion is usually the presenting symptom, and as the disease progresses it occurs with less and less effort. Measurement of dyspnea correlates weakly with FEV$_1$ and can be used to study these patients objectively. Dyspnea is not closely correlated with arterial blood gases, as the typical "blue bloater" with peripheral edema, hypoxemia, and hypercapnia generally has less dyspnea, in contrast to the "pink puffer," who generally does not have these blood gas abnormalities but is much more dyspneic. Dyspnea may also contribute to disturbed sleep and decreased caloric intake.

The hallmarks of an exacerbation of COPD include increased cough, purulent sputum, increased dyspnea, and on occasion perceptible wheezing. The presence of new onset or increased wheezing may indicate increased obstruction, as can its absence in a patient who frequently wheezes.

### Physical Examination

Physical examination of many patients with COPD reveals little abnormality, especially during quiet breathing. Coarse crackles early in inspiration have been associated with obstructive lung disease, although other adventitious sounds may be present. Rhonchi are more prevalent in patients complaining of dyspnea and are usually present during both inspiration and expiration. Wheezing is not a consistent finding and does not relate to the severity of obstruction. The most consistent finding in patients with symptomatic COPD is the prolonged expiratory time, which is best determined by listening over the larynx during a forced expiratory maneuver. Prolongation of the expiratory phase longer than the normal 4 seconds is indicative of significant obstruction.

As COPD becomes more severe, patients demonstrate more apparent physical signs. These include the barrel-shaped chest, pursed lip breathing, emaciation, and, frequently, inguinal hernias. Patients may be observed sitting forward and leaning on their elbows, or supporting their upper body with extended arms, in a position known as tripodding. This position stabilizes the shoulder girdle and helps to maximize intrathoracic volume.

Pulmonary hypertension may be suspected with a loud pulmonary component of the second heart sound. Heart sounds maybe displaced to the midline due to hyperinflation.

## Laboratory Findings

### Chest Radiography

COPD is a functional diagnosis, and, as such, only chest radiographs can suggest this diagnosis. Chronic bronchitis can never be diagnosed by chest radiographs, but there are radiographic signs that can suggest the diagnosis. Analysis of bronchial wall thickness viewed end-on was of some value in discrimination between patients with and without chronic bronchitis. Tubular shadows, or "tramlines," were not as discriminatory. The presence of prominent lung markings may also suggest the diagnosis of chronic bronchitis among others.

Chest radiographs from patients with emphysema generally do not show evidence of this disease until it is moderately advanced. There are two patterns recognized as being associated with emphysema. These are arterial deficiency and increased markings. The triad of overinflation, oligemia (deficiency in the volume of the blood), and bullae constitutes the arterial deficiency pattern, most often associated with emphysema, and the increased markings pattern is characterized by the "dirty chest" appearance seen in chronic bronchitis. The best evidence of overinflation is flattening of the diaphragm with a concavity of its superior surface (Fig. 38.2). Another sign is an increase in the width of the retrosternal air space, but this is less sensitive. Clinical correlation is important when overdistention is present on the chest radiograph, as these findings may also be seen with severe asthma. This sign, however, resolves in asthma, with clinical improvement in airflow limitation.

### Computed Tomography

Computed tomography (CT) can delineate the pulmonary parenchyma much better than the standard radiograph (Fig. 38.3).[23] Collimation is 1.0 to 2.0 mm in high-resolution CT rather than the standard 10 mm in conventional CT. CT may also be used to quantitate the amount of air trapping by a comparison of images during inspiration and full expiration.[24]

### Pulmonary Function Tests

Pulmonary function measurements serve to assess the severity of airflow limitation, to quantify the presence of the various abnormalities, and to identify and quantify reversible airflow limitation. The tests are also helpful in documenting the progress of disease and making a prognosis. (See Chapter 28 for a detailed discussion of this topic.) Airflow limitation accompanies the development of systemic dysfunction and impairment of gas exchange and is the most important functional defect in chronic bronchitis and emphysema. Loss of elastic recoil in emphysema allows collapse of distal, poorly supported airways at much higher lung volumes than normal. Increasing pleural pressure during active expiration by the patient

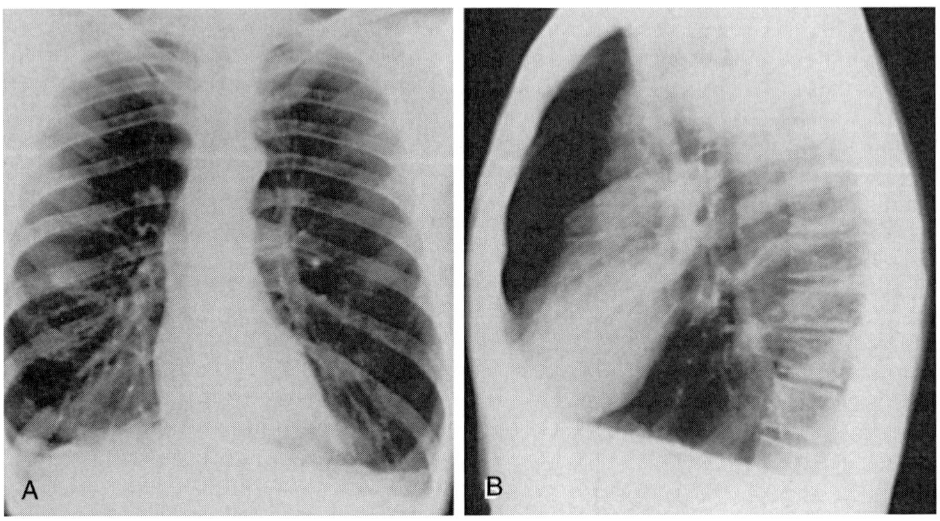


**Figure 38.2** Chest radiograph showing severe emphysema in a 40-year-old man with homozygous alpha$_1$-antiprotease deficiency. There was onset of dyspnea on effort at age 32 years with marked worsening after bouts of pneumonia at ages 36 and 39 years. Patient smoked 20 cigarettes daily from age 18 to 36 years. At the time of these films, patient was living a chair-and-bed existence. The frontal radiograph *(A)* shows marked flattening and depression of the diaphragm, which is located at the 7th anterior rib and 11th posterior rib shadow. There is marked attenuation of the pulmonary vascular shadows. The lateral projection *(B)* shows flattening of the diaphragm with an obtuse angle between the sternum and the diaphragm. The retrosternal air space is increased from front to back and extends lower than usual. The radiographic appearance is indistinguishable from that of a person of Pi MM phenotype with emphysema. (Reproduced with permission from Snider GL: Clinical Pulmonary Medicine. Boston: Little, Brown & Company, 1981.)

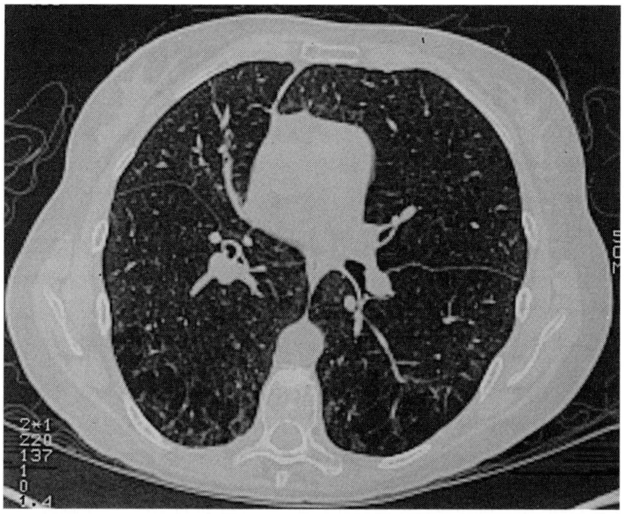

**Figure 38.3** High-resolution computed tomographic scan of the chest of a 65-year-old woman shows enlarged respiratory air spaces posteriorly in both lung fields, representing emphysema. The posterior location of the lesions in the upper portions of both lower lobes suggests that the emphysema is centrilobular in type. (Reproduced by courtesy of Dr. Robert Pugatch.)

worsens the collapse of distal airways and may give rise to dynamic narrowing of the trachea and large bronchi as the gradient between extraluminal and intraluminal pressures invaginates their soft posterior walls.[25, 26] Peripheral airway narrowing from luminal mucus, fibrosis, and inflammation of the walls and from increased smooth muscle is related to airflow limitation.[27] The $FEV_1$ cannot distinguish among these lesions. It has also become clear that none of the sensitive parameters of airflow obstruction, derived from the single-breath nitrogen curve, the frequency dependence of compliance, or the density dependence of maximum expiratory flow, is specific for peripheral airway disease. The results of all these tests are affected by loss of elastic recoil of the lung.[28]

**Forced Expiratory Spirometry.** The forced expiratory spirogram is the most useful test of airflow dynamics. Various indices can be determined from the volume-time record.[29] A few of these are the volume expired in the first second ($FEV_1$), the flow in the first one fourth of the FVC ($FEF_{0-25}$) or the middle half of the FVC ($FEF_{25-75}$), and the peak expiratory flow (PEF). The PEF and $FEF_{0-25}$ are largely effort dependent; the $FEF_{25-75}$ is relatively effort independent. Above a relatively modest expiratory effort, maximal flow is strongly volume dependent; accordingly, when flow limitation is severe, ventilation can be maintained only by prolonging expiratory time or increasing lung volume. Both of these adaptations are characteristic of COPD. The PEF is heavily effort dependent but can be measured with relatively inexpensive peak flow meters, which patients can be taught to use. Portable pneumotachograph-based spirometers are now available and may be used to monitor $FEV_1$, FVC, and PEF rate. During an exacerbation, the PEF rate and $FEV_1$ may not be accurately determined by portable equipment, and such values cannot be used interchangeably with those obtained by a volume displacement spirometer.[30, 31]

The $FEV_1$ has less variation and is more accurately predictable from age, sex, and height than the $FEF_{0-25}$ and $FEF_{25-75}$. The $FEV_1/FVC$ ratio is diminished in patients with obstructive lung disease but is maintained or increased in those with restrictive lung disease, making it an important differential point.

The $FEV_1$ and the $FEV_1/FVC$ ratio fall progressively, and plethysmographically measured airway resistance rises progressively with advances in the severity of emphysema. Many patients with COPD may have limited improvement in airflow in response to a bronchodilator, although airflow usually does not normalize. The percentage of individuals improving at least 15% increases with increasing severity of disease.[32] Repeated testing increases the number of individuals with reversibility. The absence of a response to a bronchodilator in a single study in the laboratory should never be a reason to withhold bronchodilator drug therapy.

**Lung Volumes.** The total lung capacity is increased in emphysema because the loss of elastic recoil permits the inspiratory muscles to stretch the lungs to a greater maximal volume. The residual volume is increased because of airway closure at a higher lung volume, which is due to a combination of loss of elastic recoil and bronchiolitis. The functional residual capacity is increased because of loss of elastic recoil. With severe airflow limitation, expiration may be interrupted by the next inspiration; in this circumstance, a dynamic component is added to the normal static determinants of functional residual capacity.[33] The vital capacity is decreased because of the increase in residual volume.

Variation in the pattern of lung volume abnormality is observed. Some patients tend to have a markedly increased total lung capacity with a relatively well-maintained vital capacity, as well as marked increases in residual volume. Others tend to have a near-normal total lung capacity with a greater decrease in vital capacity and a modest increase in residual volume.[34, 35] These differences tend to disappear as the disease becomes more severe.

**Volume-Pressure Relations.** With severe emphysema, lung compliance is increased and transpulmonary pressure at total lung capacity is reduced, reflecting the disruption of the elastic tissue network of the lungs.[36] All published studies have, however, failed to find a relationship between indices of lung elasticity and grade of emphysema.[37] The discrepancy has been particularly great with mild emphysema,[38] raising the question whether in mild emphysema elastic fiber degeneration is occurring between foci of emphysema. Measurement of the volume-pressure curve of the lung is a research procedure not generally used in routine clinical practice.

**Diffusing Capacity.** The single-breath diffusing capacity is decreased in proportion to the severity of emphysema because of the destruction of the alveoli and the loss of alveolar capillary bed.[36] However, the measurement is not sensitive to low grades of emphysema.[39] Furthermore, $DL_{CO}$ values are lower in smokers than in nonsmokers, even in young smokers who are not likely to have much emphysema.[40]

**Arterial Blood Gases.** Arterial blood gases reveal mild or moderate hypoxemia without hypercapnia in the early stages of COPD. In the later stages of the disease, hypoxemia tends to become more severe and may be accompanied by hypercapnia with increased serum bicarbonate levels.[36] Blood gas abnormalities worsen during acute exacerbations and may also worsen during exercise[41] and sleep.[42] The relationship between impaired spirometric values and blood gas abnormalities is weak; hypercapnia is observed with increasing frequency with values of the $FEV_1$ of less than 1 L. (Acid-base balance is discussed in Chapter 7.)

**Erythrocytosis.** In normal persons living at different altitudes, the development of erythrocytosis is proportional to arterial $PO_2$ values. Concerning patients with COPD, the literature is controversial, with various studies reporting that the response to $PO_2$ is normal, diminished, or even excessive.[43] The controversy in the literature may stem from differences in the methods used to study erythrocytosis. First, isolated hemoglobin and hematocrit values are poor indicators of the erythroid response to hypoxemia because of the wide variations of plasma volume in COPD patients.[44] Second, single measures of blood oxygenation are not representative of a patient's daily mean saturation. In a case-control study, hypoxemic patients with erythrocytosis had levels of renin and aldosterone that were threefold higher than those of controls.[45] It appears that the renin-angiotensin system is associated with the development of secondary erythrocytosis.

Intermittent hypoxemia is a potent stimulus for erythropoietin production, and both sleep and exercise can produce episodic desaturation in COPD. A relationship between arterial oxygen saturation of less than 80% in sleep and development of erythrocytosis has been shown.[46] Persistently elevated levels of blood carboxyhemoglobin contribute to the development of polycythemia in smokers.[47] Given the many factors that influence oxygen delivery to the tissues (hemoglobin concentration, red blood cell 2,3-diphosphoglycerate concentration, blood carboxyhemoglobin concentration, cardiac output, blood pH, and $PCO_2$, and local tissue blood flow), a varying relationship between blood oxygen level and red blood cell mass should be expected in patients with COPD.[43]

**Sputum Examination.** In stable bronchitis, sputum is mucoid, and microscopic examination reveals a predominance of macrophages; bacteria are few. During an exacerbation, the sputum becomes grossly purulent, and microscopy of a wet preparation or an appropriately stained smear shows the purulence to be due to an influx of neutrophils. The number of organisms seen on Gram's stain usually increases. A predominance of gram-positive diplococci or of fine gram-negative pleomorphic rods may be seen. The pathogens most often cultured from the sputum are *Streptococcus pneumoniae* and *Haemophilus influenzae*. Other oropharyngeal commensal flora such as *Moraxella catarrhalis* can be recovered. The cultures provide only qualitative data, and because these organisms are regularly found in the upper respiratory tract, their significance is uncertain. The number of organisms observed in the stained smear provides semiquantitative information that is helpful in suggesting whether bacterial infection is playing an important role and in guiding the physician in instituting antibiotic therapy and selecting the most appropriate drug.[48] Development of purulent sputum is not, however, correlated with the presence of one or another of these bacteria in quantitative cultures. It may be that a subtype of the nontypeable bacteria may be associated with increased pathogenicity.[49, 50] Cultures and even Gram's stain, however, are rarely necessary for institution of antimicrobial therapy unless the patient has sustained an exacerbation during or soon after receiving a course of antibiotic therapy.[51]

## Complications of Chronic Obstructive Pulmonary Disease

### Pneumothorax

The occurrence of a spontaneous pneumothorax in a person with normal lungs produces minor symptoms and disruption of lung function (Chapter 75). Pneumothorax complicating COPD often precipitates severe dyspnea and acute respiratory failure and may be life-threatening. Even a small pneumothorax can cause severe respiratory impairment in COPD patients who have only a marginal pulmonary reserve, and, because it is often accompanied by a persistent air leak between the involved lung and pleural space (bronchopleural fistula), it may be difficult to treat.

Pneumothorax should be suspected in any COPD patient who experiences sudden worsening of dyspnea. Depressed or absent breath sounds on auscultation is the most important clinical sign but may be difficult to detect because breath sounds are often already diminished in severe emphysema. The diagnosis is made from the chest radiograph; films taken on expiration have greater diagnostic sensitivity. Occasionally, large bullae may mimic pneumothorax, but prior chest radiographs resolve this dilemma.

Asymptomatic or mildly symptomatic patients with a small pneumothorax can be managed by serial observation, but, in the presence of emphysema, it is more conservative to place a chest tube attached to a one-way valve. The presence of a large or tension pneumothorax requires the prompt insertion of an intercostal chest tube with water seal drainage. Most bronchopleural fistulas will close after several days of treatment by tube thoracostomy, although a negative pressure of up to 30 cm $H_2O$ or more applied to the water seal system may be needed to expand the lung fully. If spontaneous sealing fails to occur within 48 to 72 hours, surgical closure of the air leak together with pleurodesis or parietal pleurectomy is often justified because failure to heal spontaneously is more frequent after this interval.[52] New techniques employing thoracoscopy are rapidly replacing standard open thoracotomy because these methods substantially reduce length of hospitalization and postoperative morbidity.[53, 54]

When pulmonary function impairment is severe, thus increasing the risk of surgical treatment, a longer period of closed chest tube drainage is often employed. An attempt to obliterate the pleural space by instilling a sclerosing agent may be a successful alternative approach to surgery if closure of the air leak fails to occur.[55, 56] This method often fails, however, even after repeated attempts in patients with large bronchopleural fistulas.

## Cor Pulmonale

Chronic cor pulmonale is defined as enlargement of the right ventricle (hypertrophy or dilatation) due to increased right ventricular afterload from diseases of the lungs or pulmonary circulation (see Chapters 50 and 55). Resting mean pulmonary arterial pressures may rise to 30 to 40 mm Hg in patients with advanced COPD as opposed to the normal value of 10 to 18 mm Hg. With exercise, mean pressures may rise as high as 50 to 60 mm Hg or greater. The causes of the pulmonary hypertension in COPD are several.[57, 58]

**Pathophysiology.** Emphysema results in a loss of pulmonary vascular bed. The major cause of increased pulmonary vascular resistance in patients with COPD is, however, vasoconstriction due to alveolar hypoxia. There is subsequent remodeling of the pulmonary vasculature with medial hypertrophy of muscular pulmonary arteries along with the appearance of smooth muscle in normally nonmuscular vessels of the pulmonary circulation. Sleep-related hypoxemia was shown not to favor the development of pulmonary hypertension in patients with moderate COPD.[58a] Although it is not clear how alveolar hypoxia gives rise to vasoconstriction, evidence is accumulating that an imbalance between endothelial cell–generated vasoconstrictor and vasodilator agents promotes vascular smooth muscle constriction and hyperplasia.[59]

Acidemia augments hypoxic vasoconstriction and can play a role in transient rises in pulmonary blood pressure during acute exacerbations of COPD. Increased intrathoracic pressures as a result of airflow limitation with air trapping can also increase pulmonary vascular resistance by compressing pulmonary vessels. Greater viscosity of blood occurring with erythrocytosis secondary to hypoxemia may play a role in the genesis of pulmonary hypertension, although this factor is far less important than hypoxic pulmonary vasoconstriction. Blood volume may be increased in patients with cor pulmonale, in part from impaired sodium and water excretion,[60] and, with increases in cardiac output occurring in response to hypoxemia, may contribute to higher mean pulmonary arterial pressure in the presence of a restricted pulmonary vascular bed.

Although left ventricular dysfunction is relatively uncommon in patients with cor pulmonale due to COPD, when such dysfunction is present, the occurrence of left ventricular failure and raised pulmonary venous pressure may also contribute to pulmonary hypertension. In addition, COPD patients are prone to develop chronic pulmonary thromboembolic disease, and emboli should always be considered when the magnitude of pulmonary hypertension is out of proportion to a patient's underlying lung disease and arterial hypoxemia.

**Diagnosis.** The detection of pulmonary hypertension and right ventricular enlargement by noninvasive means is difficult, but an R or R′ greater than or equal to the S wave in $V_1$, an R wave less than the amplitude of the S wave in $V_6$, and right axis deviation greater than 110 degrees without right bundle branch block are all supportive of the diagnosis of cor pulmonale.[58] Physical findings of a prominent systolic impulse along the lower left sternal border, accentuation of the pulmonic component of the second heart sound, murmurs of pulmonic or tricuspid insufficiency, and a right ventricular gallop are difficult to detect in patients with emphysema because the overdistended lungs are interposed between the heart and the sternum. Two-dimensional echocardiography, especially with an esophageal transducer, and pulsed Doppler techniques with echocardiography to estimate mean pulmonary arterial pressure can assess pulmonary hypertension and right ventricular function.[61–63] Left ventricular size and performance are generally normal in patients with COPD in the absence of other associated cardiac abnormalities. Esophageal electrocardiography appears to be more sensitive and correctly diagnosed cor pulmonale in 24 of 25 COPD patients in one study.[64] This technique is, however, impractical for routine use.

Increasing width of the cardiac shadow in serial chest radiographs, especially if accompanied by encroachment of the cardiac shadow on the retrosternal space, strongly suggests cor pulmonale. A width of the descending branch of the right pulmonary artery of 20 mm or more and measurement of the hilar cardiothoracic ratio are useful screens for pulmonary hypertension.[57]

First-pass and gated radionuclide angiographic methods, employing technetium ($^{99m}Tc$), can provide estimates of right ventricular size and function, with gated equilibrium studies providing acceptable measurements of right ventricular ejection fraction.[57] Right ventricular ejection fraction is frequently abnormal in patients with COPD who go on to develop right ventricular failure associated with cor pulmonale. Abnormalities of right ventricular ejection fraction are more frequently noted during exercise than at rest. Myocardial scintigraphy with thallium ($^{201}Tl$) to measure ventricular blood flow may be employed as an early indicator of right ventricular hypertrophy and abnormalities of right ventricular performance. Resting right ventricular blood flow in normal persons is insufficient to be visualized by this test.

**Treatment.** Successful treatment of cor pulmonale in patients with COPD begins with optimal management of the underlying airflow limitation. Correction of hypoxemia with long-term oxygen therapy is of the greatest importance. Although pulmonary hemodynamics with long-term oxygen therapy improves only modestly,[65, 66] patient survival is substantially increased. Phlebotomy is rarely required to reduce blood viscosity and elevated blood volume after patients employ supplemental oxygen for 1 or 2 months, but it can be used in acutely decompensated COPD patients when the hematocrit exceeds 60%. Diuretic therapy is useful to reduce intravascular volume and to control edema. The possibility of diuretic-induced hypokalemia and hypochloremic metabolic alkalosis should be kept in mind.

Use of pulmonary vasodilators employing a wide range of agents has thus far been disappointing, with no sustained improvement in hemodynamics or enhanced survival with these medications. Nifedipine taken for 8 weeks was shown to blunt the pulmonary vasodilator response to acute oxygen therapy, and it failed to reduce mean pulmonary arterial pressure in patients with COPD.[67] Theophylline, which both promotes pulmonary vasodilation and has a positive inotropic effect on the right ventricle, may provide sustained improvement in pulmonary hemodynamics.[68, 69] Beta agonists have an inotropic effect, and, although short-term therapy with pirbuterol decreased pulmonary artery pressure, the effect was not sustained. Studies with the angiotensin-converting enzyme inhibitor captopril have yielded conflicting results, possibly indicating a need for long-term studies.[70] Digoxin is generally used only when needed to control heart rate.

## Pneumonia

COPD is generally considered to be an important predisposing condition for pneumonia, although data confirming that the risk of pneumonia for COPD patients is higher than for the general population are lacking.[71] The presence of airflow limitation and colonization of the lower respiratory tract with bacteria (described earlier in this chapter) are considered risk factors for pneumonia. Precise figures for the frequencies of the organisms causing pneumonia are unavailable. Pneumococcal disease, aerobic gram-negative rods, *H. influenzae, M. catarrhalis,* and *Legionella pneumophila* have been implicated. *Pseudomonas aeruginosa* is an occasional cause of pneumonia, especially in patients who have been recently hospitalized; *Staphylococcus aureus* is rarely implicated. As with other community-acquired pneumonias, the cause remains uncertain in about 50% of cases.[72]

Mortality data are not available for pneumonia in patients with COPD, but clinical experience indicates that pneumonia is an important contributing cause of death (see discussion of prognosis of COPD, later in this chapter). Broad-spectrum antibiotic empirical coverage is generally recommended for pneumonia in COPD patients because of both their respiratory compromise and their common history of frequent antibiotic use, which increases the likelihood of resistant organisms.

## Sleep Abnormalities

A slight decrease in alveolar ventilation with an accompanying modest rise in arterial $P_{CO_2}$ and fall in arterial $P_{O_2}$ is normal during sleep.[73] (Sleep disorders are discussed in detail in Chapter 81.) Because of their daytime hypoxemia, with an arterial $P_{O_2}$–arterial oxygen saturation point that is close to the steep part of the oxygen-hemoglobin dissociation curve, the degree of fall in arterial oxygen saturation for a given fall in arterial $P_{O_2}$ is greater in patients with COPD than it is in normal persons. The major cause of sleep-induced hypoxemia in COPD patients is thought to be hypoventilation during rapid eye movement (REM) sleep related to rapid shallow breathing. An additional factor is reduction in functional residual capacity, accompanied by increased ventilation-perfusion mismatch.[74]

The blood gas abnormalities are greater during REM sleep than during non-REM sleep.[75] The severity of decrease in arterial $P_{O_2}$ tends to become greater as the night wears on, perhaps as a result of widening of the alveolar arterial $P_{O_2}$ difference due to suppression of the cough reflex during sleep and subsequent retained secretions. Even patients with awake arterial $P_{O_2}$ values of 60 mm Hg or greater may experience periods of major nocturnal desaturation, which are of uncertain clinical significance.[76] Although patients with COPD may have long episodes of hypopnea during sleep, true sleep apnea is no more common than in the general population.[77] When sleep apnea does complicate COPD, however, nocturnal hypoxemia tends to be more severe than in the general population because of baseline hypoxemia.

Patients with COPD have impaired sleep quality, with arousals often noted during periods of desaturation[78] and with less REM sleep. Increased hypoxemia during sleep is associated with a modest increment in clinically unimportant premature ventricular contractions,[79] as well as transient worsening of existing pulmonary hypertension. It remains uncertain whether repetitive nocturnal desaturations alone can result in chronic pulmonary hypertension, although findings supporting this concept have been reported.[80, 81] Erythrocytosis is enhanced by nocturnal desaturation in patients with significant daytime hypoxemia, but not in those whose daytime hypoxemia is mild (resting arterial $P_{O_2} > 60$ mm Hg).[81]

It is not thought appropriate to monitor routinely for nocturnal desaturation. Such a study should be done only in COPD patients who do not meet the criteria for long-term oxygen therapy but whose clinical assessment suggests the effects of intermittent hypoxemia, such as pulmonary hypertension, erythrocytosis, or mental status changes. This approach is supported by the finding that nocturnal hypoxemia alone does not impair survival in COPD patients[82] and that administering supplemental nocturnal oxygen for sleep desaturation in patients with a daytime arterial $P_{O_2}$ above 60 mm Hg does not reduce mortality.[81] Patients who manifest the ill effects of hypoxemia, who have nonqualifying daytime blood oxygen measurements, but who desaturate while asleep should have nighttime oxygen.

## Giant Bullae

**Clinical Features.** Bullae occupying one third to one half of one or both hemithoraces may occasionally produce a dramatic chest radiograph (Fig. 38.4). Such bullae may occur with airflow limitation and other loss of lung function ranging from minimal to severe. The extent of loss depends on the size of the bullae, the amount of normal or mildly diseased lung tissue the bullae are compressing (Fig. 38.5), and whether the bullae represent a locally severe region of generalized emphysema. Patients with bullae filling up to one half of both hemithor-

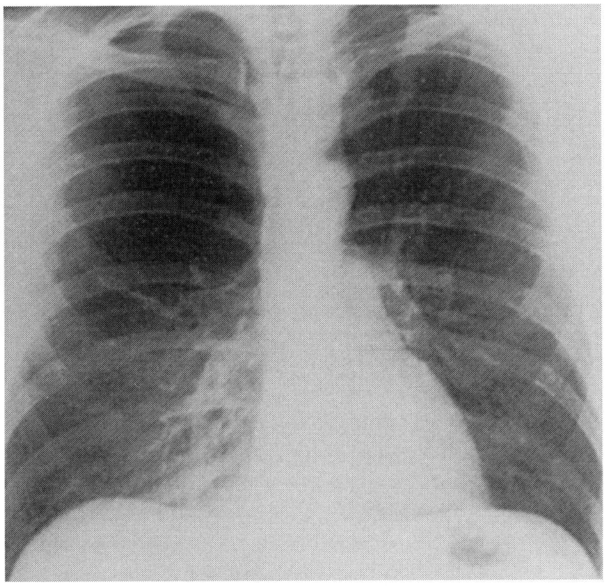

**Figure 38.4** Chest radiograph showing bullous disease with mild airflow obstruction. A 36-year-old man with a 10-year history of bullae smoked an average of 25 cigarettes per day since age 18 years. For 5 years he has had morning cough productive of sputum. Despite intensive efforts to do so, he has not been able to stop smoking. Dyspnea was not present. The chest radiograph shows marked radiolucency in both upper lung fields, extending lower on the right than on the left. An arcuate hairline shadow delimits the radiolucency below on the right. Pulmonary function studies at the time showed $FEV_1$ 5.05 L, 90% of predicted and 64% of FVC; TLC 7.78 L or 104% predicted; VC 5.29 L, 94% predicted; FRC 4.48 L or 104% predicted; RV 2.49 L, 120% predicted; arterial blood studies showed $Po_2$ 84 mm Hg, $Pco_2$ 40 mm Hg, pH 7.41.

aces may, however, have little abnormality of lung function.

The bullae may enlarge progressively over time, trapping a large volume of air. The difference in values of functional residual capacity as determined by body plethysmography and the gas dilution method indicates the amount of gas that is "trapped" in the bulla, which may approach several liters.[83] It is not clear whether this is because of a check-valve mechanism that allows air to enter the bulla more readily than it can leave or whether the enlargement occurs because severely emphysematous areas fill preferentially during breathing because of their increased compliance owing to extensive destruction of parenchymal connective tissue.[84] Both mechanisms are probably operative.

Bullae are seen most frequently in smokers. They occur most often in the upper lung zones (see Fig. 38.4 and Fig. 38.5). The selective involvement is attributed to the combination of the relatively lower blood flow to the upper lung in upright humans and to the pleural pressure gradient from apex to base, which augments stress in the upper lung zones. A striking 2:1 right-sided preponderance is generally attributed to the larger size of the right lung.[85] Basilar bullae in elderly nonsmokers should prompt investigation for $alpha_1$-protease inhibitor deficiency.[86] In patients without generalized emphysema, bullae are almost always associated with subpleural or paraseptal emphysema,[87] a finding that is best appreciated in CT scans.[88, 89]

**Complications of Bullous Disease.** Bullae may be complicated by infection with ordinary pyogenic organisms or with an *Aspergillus* species or another mycotic organism that gives rise to a mycetoma. Antibiotics should be used for pyogenic organisms. In many instances, fluid within the bulla may be sterile with active infection in the adjacent lung tissue.[90] Subsidence of the process is the rule, and a marked decrease in the size of the bulla is occasionally observed.[91] Excisional therapy should be reserved for an infected bulla that fails to respond to antibiotics; this is almost always due to failure of the bulla to drain properly. Percutaneous pneumonostomy can be helpful in a patient with large, persistently infected bulla whose lung function or general condition does not permit resection.[92, 93] Mycetomas rarely require therapy unless they are associated with life-threatening hemoptysis. In that event, bronchial arterial embolization should be considered.[94] Systemic antifungal therapy is not indicated for mycetomas unless there is clear evidence of tissue invasion by fungus.

There is an increased frequency of association of carcinoma of the lung with large bullae.[95, 96] Three major patterns of radiographic appearance have been reported: a nodular opacity within or adjacent to the bulla, partial or diffuse thickening of the bulla wall, and alteration in the bulla's appearance, change in diameter or air-fluid level, or presence of a pneumothorax.[97] The latter two appearances are nonspecific. Thickening of the wall occurs because of growth of tumor along the bulla wall. Tumors may occur in young men with bullae,[96] but the highest frequency is in the sixth decade of life.[97] The possibility of carcinoma complicating giant bullae warrants radiographic monitoring of these patients.

## DIFFERENTIAL DIAGNOSIS OF CHRONIC OBSTRUCTIVE PULMONARY DISEASE

The differential diagnosis of chronic airflow limitation relates back to the Venn diagram shown in Figure 38.1. The diagnosis of chronic bronchitis is made on the basis of symptoms, that of asthma is made on the basis of nearly complete reversibility spontaneously or with bronchodilators, and that of emphysema is made on the basis of pathologic changes best seen on CT scans of the chest. History and physical examination provide an initial data base. The chest radiograph is essential both for its value in excluding other pulmonary disorders that may produce the same respiratory symptoms and for showing overdistention of the lungs or the specific findings of emphysema. Forced expiratory spirometry and arterial blood gas measurements with the patient breathing room air provide the physiologic assessment that is necessary to establish the diagnosis, document the course of the disease, and establish a prognosis. The response of a spirometric index such as the $FEV_1$ to a bronchodilator regimen helps to differentiate COPD from asthma.

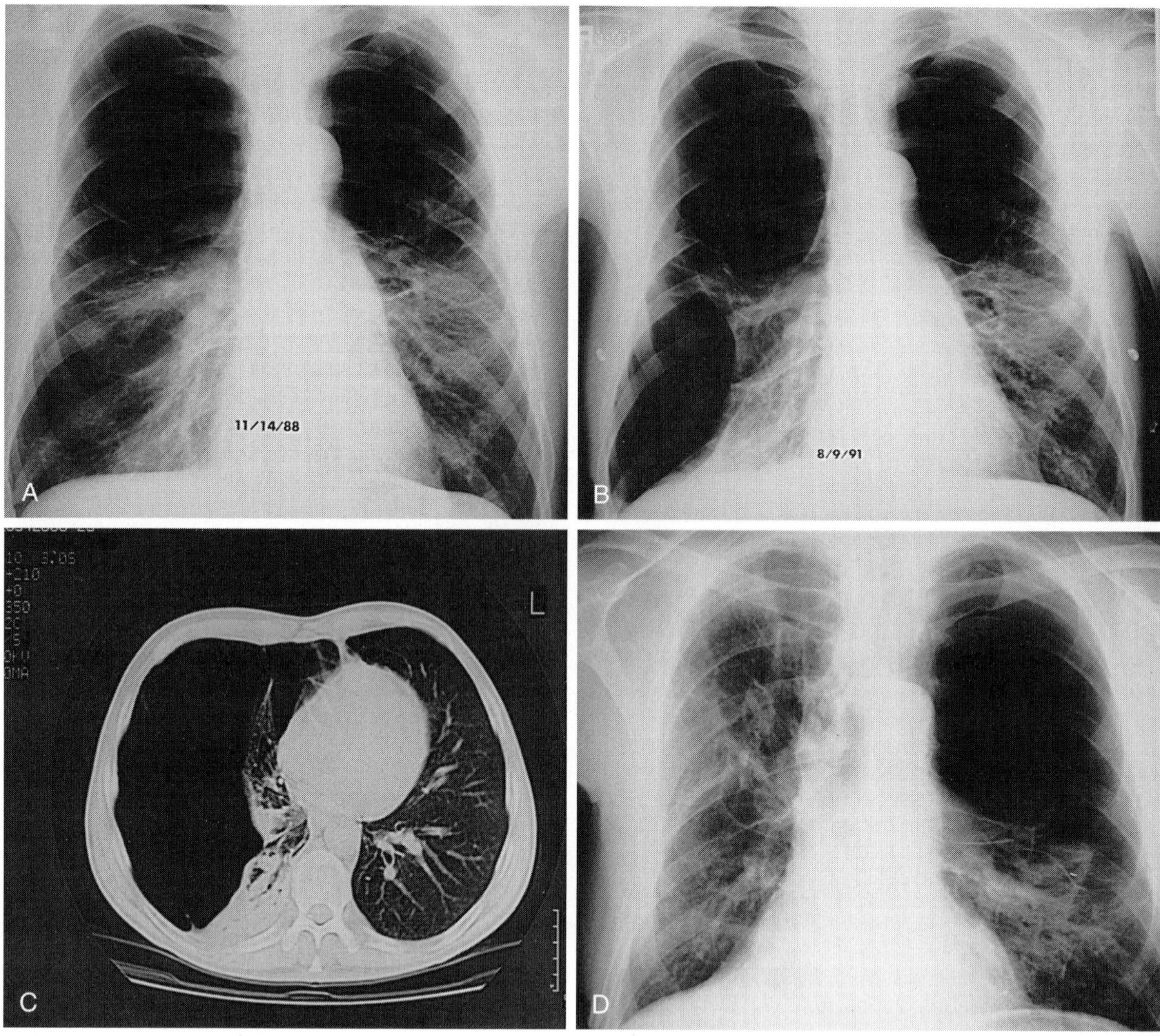


**Figure 38.5** Radiographs are shown of a 46-year-old man who had smoked an average of two packs of cigarettes daily from age 18 years and who presented in the summer of 1991 with dyspnea after walking 20 yards on the level. He was known to have giant bullous lung disease and had had multiple episodes of bronchitis and pneumonia. His serum $alpha_1$-antitrypsin level was normal. Pulmonary function studies revealed a FVC of 2.22 L (44% predicted), $FEV_1$ 1.28 L (34% predicted), $FEV_1/FVC$ 0.58, and carbon monoxide diffusing capacity of 9.09 mL/min per mm Hg. Arterial blood gases while breathing air were pH 7.43, arterial $Pco_2$ 38 mm Hg, and arterial $Po_2$ 58 mm Hg. Hematocrit was 51%. Lung perfusion scintiscan showed that virtually all of the perfusion went to the lower half of the left lung. Chest radiograph of November 14, 1988 *(A)*, reveals giant bullae occupying the upper half of both lung fields, with crowding of vascular shadows in the lower lung fields. In the radiograph of August 9, 1991 *(B)*, an additional giant bulla is seen in the right lower lung field, and a small bulla is noted at the left base. CT scan on October 16, 1991 *(C)*, shows atelectasis of the right lower lobe due to compression by giant bullae. The patient stopped smoking. Right thoracotomy with bullectomy was performed on January 14, 1992. The chest radiograph of February 24, 1992 *(D)*, shows expansion of the left lower lobe and residual small bullae in the right upper lung field. On November 3, 1992, the forced vital capacity was 2.81 L, $FEV_1$ 1.80 L, $FEV_1/FVC$ 0.64, and the carbon monoxide diffusing capacity was 19.7 mL/min per mm Hg. Arterial blood gases breathing room air were pH 7.43, arterial $Pco_2$ 40 mm Hg, and arterial $Po_2$ 71 mm Hg. The hematocrit was 42%. Dyspnea was markedly improved, and the patient had returned to clerical work.

Important actions by the physician rarely depend on the measurement of either lung volumes or the single-breath $DL_{CO}$. These studies, as well as measurements of cardiopulmonary function during exercise, may be necessary in complex cases when chronic airflow limitation represents only part of the physiologic picture and some other disease is suspected or in which dyspnea appears to be out of proportion to the impairment in lung function. Measurements of arterial oxygen saturation may be made during exercise with acceptable reliability using pulse oximetry; arterial blood gas measurements made with an indwelling arterial cannula provide more complete information. If the history suggests that sleep apnea is present, screening oximetry or complete polysomnography should be carried out. (See Chapter 81 for a discussion of sleep disorders.)

## Unilateral Hyperlucent Lung

The most common radiographic presentation of emphysema is that of increased lung volume and vascular shadow attenuation and, therefore, of increased transradiancy of the involved lung compared with nonemphysematous lung tissue. A number of conditions presenting as unilateral or lobar hyperlucency in the chest radiograph are different in pathogenesis and natural history from those of emphysema.[98] These conditions may need to be differentiated from unilaterally preponderant emphysema (Table 38.2). Greater transradiancy in the chest radiograph may also have a chest wall origin, such as from congenital absence of the pectoralis major muscle or absence of the female breast and pectoral muscles after radical mastectomy.

## Unilateral Bronchiolitis Obliterans

In the 1950s, Swyer and James[99] and Macleod,[100] giving much more detail, described patients with unilateral hyperlucent lungs. Subsequent study showed this entity to be due to patchy bronchitis and bronchiolitis obliterans (discussed in Chapter 43), sometimes with bronchiectasis and generally with respiratory air-space enlargement. This condition is best called *unilateral bronchiolitis obliterans with hyperinflation* but it is referred to by many other terms in the literature, including Swyer-James or Macleod's syndrome, unilateral hyperlucent lung, or unilateral emphysema.[101]

Unilateral bronchiolitis obliterans with hyperinflation is quite rare, with one case being seen only once every 2 to 4 years in a large chest service and occurring with a prevalence of 0.01% in 17,450 survey chest radiographs.[98] The condition is usually asymptomatic and is discovered accidentally by chest radiography. Mild productive cough may be present. If there is bronchiectasis, purulent expectoration may be present. Dyspnea during effort is uncommon, and severe pulmonary insufficiency is distinctly uncommon. In about half the cases there is a history of measles, a viral or mycoplasma respiratory infection, or, rarely, tuberculosis in childhood.[98, 102–105] Depressed breath sounds and coarse crackles may be found on physical examination. A decrease in the size of the affected hemithorax may be evident.

**Table 38.2 CLASSIFICATION OF CAUSES OF UNILATERAL HYPERLUCENT LUNG***

| |
|---|
| **Increased Transradiancy of Chest Wall Origin (Spurious)** |
| Congenital absence of pectoralis major muscle |
| Mastectomy |
| **Patent Airways** |
| Congenital anomalies |
|   Absence or hypoplasia of one pulmonary artery |
|   Pulmonary agenesis |
|   Extrapulmonary sequestration |
| Intrinsic obstruction of one pulmonary artery |
|   Embolus |
|   Tumor |
| Extrinsic compression of one pulmonary artery |
|   Tumor |
|   Nodes |
| Compensatory hyperinflation |
|   Atelectasis |
|   Status after lobectomy |
| **Partially Obstructed Airways** |
| Intrinsic obstruction of major bronchus |
|   Tumor, benign or malignant |
|   Postinflammatory stricture |
|   Foreign body |
|   Amyloid |
| Extrinsic obstruction |
|   Congenital |
|     Aberrant vessel |
|     Extrapulmonary sequestration |
|   Tumor |
|   Nodes |
| Congenital malformation of bronchus (defective cartilage or mucosal fold) causing "congenital emphysema" |
| Unilateral acquired bronchitis and bronchiolitis obliterans |
|   Swyer-James-Macleod syndrome |
| Unilateral preponderance of emphysema |

*The list includes samples; all possible conditions are not mentioned.

Modified from Gaensler, EA: Unilateral hyperlucent lungs. *In* Simon M, Potchen EJ, LeMay M (eds): Frontiers of Pulmonary Radiology. New York: Grune & Stratton, 1969, pp. 312–359.

Pathologic study, mostly of resected specimens, shows a normal or small lung that nevertheless remains inflated after removal and when the chest is first opened at thoracotomy.[85, 106, 107] In city dwellers, pigment is irregularly distributed over the surface, with pink and black areas alternating. Microscopically, there is evidence of patchy obliterative bronchitis and bronchiolitis. The bronchi appear to have the normal number of orders of branching, suggesting normal development of the bronchial tree. The respiratory air spaces may be normal or may be uniformly enlarged and simpler in outline than normal (panacinar emphysema). Large air spaces are unusual. Although there is thickening of pulmonary arteriolar walls and some apparent decrease in the number of branches, specimen angiograms and microscopic examination show much better preservation of the arterial tree than would be expected from the in vivo pulmonary arteriogram. Much of the poor in vivo vascular filling may occur because of increased resistance to flow through the affected lung.

Chest radiography shows a normal or small lung with increased transradiancy owing to small hilar vessels that arborize sparsely and are attenuated.[85, 98, 101] Fluoroscopy and inspiration-expiration radiographs show delayed and incomplete emptying of the affected lung with impaired opacification on expiration and shift of the mediastinum to the contralateral side. On angiography, the main pulmonary artery and its immediate branches are small, and there is poor filling and arborization of vessels in the periphery. Bronchograms show poor peripheral filling of airways; the contrast may end suddenly, or there may be irregular tapering or small bulbous expansions. Lack of normal tapering or frank dilation of bronchi, which may be focal, is observed in some cases; in other cases distinct bronchiectasis is found. CT scanning is useful for determining bronchial patency, lung parenchymal changes such as subpleural infiltrates, atelectasis or cavities, and the extent and degree of bronchiectasis.[108]

Pulmonary function studies show little to mild airflow limitation.[98, 109, 110] The residual volume is generally increased. Hypoxemia is usually not present at rest or during exercise. Ventilation-perfusion lung scintiscans show virtually no blood flow to the affected side and, in contrast to pulmonary embolism, also show impaired ventilation of the hyperlucent lung. Distribution of the equilibrium ventilation scan is normal, but washout is markedly delayed.[110, 111]

For most patients, and certainly for those without symptoms, the outlook is excellent. There is no need for intervention other than careful prevention and management of intercurrent respiratory infections. Occasionally, secondary infection of ectatic bronchi that cannot be adequately controlled with antibiotic therapy justifies lung resection.

Unilateral bronchiolitis obliterans is believed to originate from a destructive bronchitis and bronchiolitis. Both inhalation of corrosive gases and infections, especially by adenovirus, have been implicated. This usually occurs in childhood, but cases have been documented in adults who were previously normal. Air-space enlargement may be due to failure of increase in alveolar number after 8 years of age, with distention as the thorax grows.

### Further Considerations

Emphysema predominant in one lung usually causes a marked increase in lung size with a shift of the mediastinum to the contralateral side even on full inspiration. The presence of bullae or complicating spontaneous pneumothorax virtually excludes unilateral obliterative bronchiolitis. Pulmonary function studies and perfusion and ventilation scintigrams are not helpful in differentiating the two conditions.

Congenital hypoplasia or absence of a pulmonary artery may also give rise to a small transradiant lung[98, 101, 112, 113]; the amount of transradiancy varies, depending on the extent of bronchial artery hyperplasia. Unlike unilateral hyperlucent lung with bronchiolitis obliterans, the affected lung empties at a normal rate.

Atelectasis of a lobe, especially the left lower lobe, may occasionally occur with impressive transradiance of the overdistended upper lobe. The atelectasis and normal emptying of the overdistended lobe enable easy diagnosis.

Extrinsic compression of a main bronchus by bronchogenic carcinoma with distal air trapping usually presents no diagnostic problem. An intrabronchial neoplasm or postinflammatory stricture of a main bronchus may complicate the differential diagnosis if transradiancy of the affected lung results. Emptying of the diseased lung will be delayed and incomplete with contralateral mediastinal shift on expiration. A localized wheeze may be heard. A CT scan or bronchoscopy can yield definitive results.

Marked overdistention of a lobe, usually the upper lobe, may give rise to severe respiratory distress in infancy. The condition may also occur later in life and is usually referred to as *congenital lobar emphysema.* Its cause is unclear. Bronchial cartilage abnormalities and mucosal folds have been identified in some cases.[85, 114–116] Occasionally, a hyperlucent lung or lobe is seen as part of bronchial atresia or pulmonary agenesis.[85, 98, 117, 118] Both of these conditions are usually manifested in childhood, but bronchial atresia may not manifest until adulthood. In infancy and childhood, resection is indicated if normal lung tissue is severely compressed, with resultant pulmonary insufficiency. Most adults are asymptomatic, and differentiation from unilateral obliterative bronchiolitis may not be possible short of pathologic examination of the resected tissue. Such resection is usually not indicated.

## EPIDEMIOLOGY

### Magnitude of the Problem in the United States

**Morbidity.** The 1993 National Health Interview Survey provided estimates that about 13.8 million American men and women have chronic bronchitis and about 2 million have emphysema.[119] The overall prevalence of COPD cannot be estimated from these data because the number of persons reporting more than one condition is not given. The Tecumseh Community Health Study of over 9000 men and women of all ages showed that about 14% of adult men and 8% of adult women have chronic bronchitis, obstructive airway disease, or both.[120] Estimates of a physician's diagnosis of emphysema or chronic airflow obstruction in the majority of population-based studies in the United States were 4% to 6% of adult white men and 1% to 3% of adult white women.[121] The number of days per year of restricted activity due to chronic bronchitis and emphysema was 114 million, ranking these conditions among the highest in terms of morbidity.[122]

**Mortality.** In 1993, there were 95,900 deaths certified as due to COPD and allied conditions; this category ranked as the fourth leading cause of death in the United States.[123] In an examination of all causes of mortality between 1979 and 1993, obstructive lung disease was the underlying cause of death in 3.5% but was the underlying cause of death on 43.3% of death certificates that listed the presence of obstructive lung disease.[124] COPD takes its toll primarily at the older ages; more than 95% of all deaths from COPD in 1985 occurred in persons over the age of 55 years. Men and women have similar mortality rates for COPD before age 55 years, but men have appreciably higher rates thereafter. Thus, mortality for men is more than double that for women at age 70 years and is more than 3.5 times that for women at age 85 years and over.[125] The age-adjusted death rate continues to increase for a large segment of the population.[126]

**Trends Over Time.** The age-adjusted death rate for COPD rose 71% between 1966 and 1986, during which time the death rate from all causes declined by 22% and the rates for heart disease and cerebrovascular disease declined by 45% and 58%, respectively.[121] The age-adjusted death rate increased 22% between 1983 and 1993 and is higher in African-American males until around 60 years of age, when it becomes higher in white males. The rate in both white and African-American females is increasing markedly.[127] Age-adjusted prevalence rates for men rose only slightly over the period from 1979 to 1985, with a prevalence of 110/1,000 in 1985. Among women, however, prevalence rates increased by more than one third between 1979 and 1985, with a prevalence of 119/1,000 in 1985.[125]

The observed increases in mortality and morbidity cannot be explained by a change in diagnostic methods. Much of the trend of increasing morbidity and mortality from COPD appears to be due to past temporal trends in cigarette smoking. The current data are explainable by the effects of cigarette smoking on members of birth cohorts now reaching an advanced age. In contrast to cardiovascular mortality rates, COPD mortality rates are relatively insensitive to intermittent or short-term smoking cessation. Part of the continued rise in morbidity and mortality may be due to the increasing numbers of people living to an advanced age; the increases are particularly striking in those who continue to smoke. Because smoking frequency has fallen sharply in the United States over the past three decades, there may eventually be a decrease in COPD mortality,[128] although trends are expected to increase for several decades.[129]

## Risk Factors for Chronic Obstructive Pulmonary Disease

**Gender, Race, and Socioeconomic Status.** Most population studies have reported a higher prevalence of respiratory symptoms in men than in women, even when the data are controlled for smoking.[130] Additional data became available with the publication of the Third National Health and Nutrition Examination Survey.[131] Mortality rates for COPD are higher in whites than in nonwhites, but the difference is becoming less among men.[121] Morbidity and mortality rates are inversely related to socioeconomic status as measured by level of education and income and, generally, are higher for blue-collar workers than for white-collar workers.[121, 130, 132] Apart from homozygous alpha$_1$-protease inhibitor deficiency, COPD may aggregate in families.[133]

**Tobacco Smoking.** Cigarette smoking is firmly established as the most important risk factor for COPD. Data from longitudinal, cross-sectional, and case-control studies show that, compared with nonsmokers, cigarette smokers have higher death rates from chronic bronchitis and emphysema. They have a higher prevalence for, and incidence of, chronic bronchitis (Fig. 38.6), emphysema, and obstructive airway disease and higher frequencies of respiratory symptoms and lung function abnormalities than nonsmokers. Cigarette smokers also have a greater average annual rate of decline in FEV$_1$. Differences between cigarette smokers and nonsmokers increase as cigarette consumption increases. Pipe and cigar smokers have higher morbidity and mortality rates for COPD than nonsmokers, although their rates are lower than those of cigarette smokers. Only a minority, or about 10% to 15%, of smokers develop clinically significant COPD (Fig. 38.7); the reasons for the increased susceptibility in this subgroup of smokers is not known.[121, 130, 132, 134–138]

In the United States, tobacco smoking accounts for 80% to 90% of the risk of developing COPD.[132] The smoking-attributable fraction of COPD mortality in the United States during the 1980s was 0.850 for men and 0.694 for women.[139] The only other risk factor of comparable importance for the individual person is homozygous alpha$_1$-protease inhibitor deficiency, which is discussed subsequently, but this accounts for less than 0.1% of people with COPD in the United States. High levels of environmental air pollution have been established to be harmful to persons with heart or lung disease. The role of environmental air pollution in producing COPD is unclear; its role is small compared with that of cigarette smoking (see Chapter 68). In the developing world, exposure to smoke generated from the use of biomass fuels may be of comparable importance in some settings.

Passive or involuntary smoking is the exposure of nonsmokers to cigarette smoke in the indoor environment. Cigarette smoke in the air can irritate the eyes. The children of smoking parents have a higher prevalence of respiratory symptoms and respiratory disease and appear to have a small but measurable difference in tests of pulmonary function compared with children of nonsmoking parents. The significance of these findings in relation to the future development of lung disease is unknown.

**Asthma and Atopy.** In 1961, Oric and colleagues[140] from the Netherlands proposed that an "asthmatic constitution" underlies the development of chronic airflow limitation. Smoking was only one extrinsic factor that could lead to chronic airflow limitation. This asthmatic constitution consisted of a predisposition to atopic disease, airway hyperresponsiveness, and sometimes eosinophilia.[140] This formulation has come to be known as the "Dutch hypothesis." In contrast, Burrrows and colleagues[141] identified a group of patients with chronic airflow limitation and features of asthma who have a better prognosis than patients with usual COPD. Asthma itself can progress to severe chronic airflow limitation, so persistent forms of the disease are inseparable from COPD. There is also the likelihood that asthma is made worse by smoking, with development of chronic sputum production and the overlap condition often referred to as "asthmatic bronchitis." In contrast to asthma, the diagnosis of chronic bronchitis or emphysema or the presence of ventilatory impairment in the absence of asthma is not related to age- or sex-

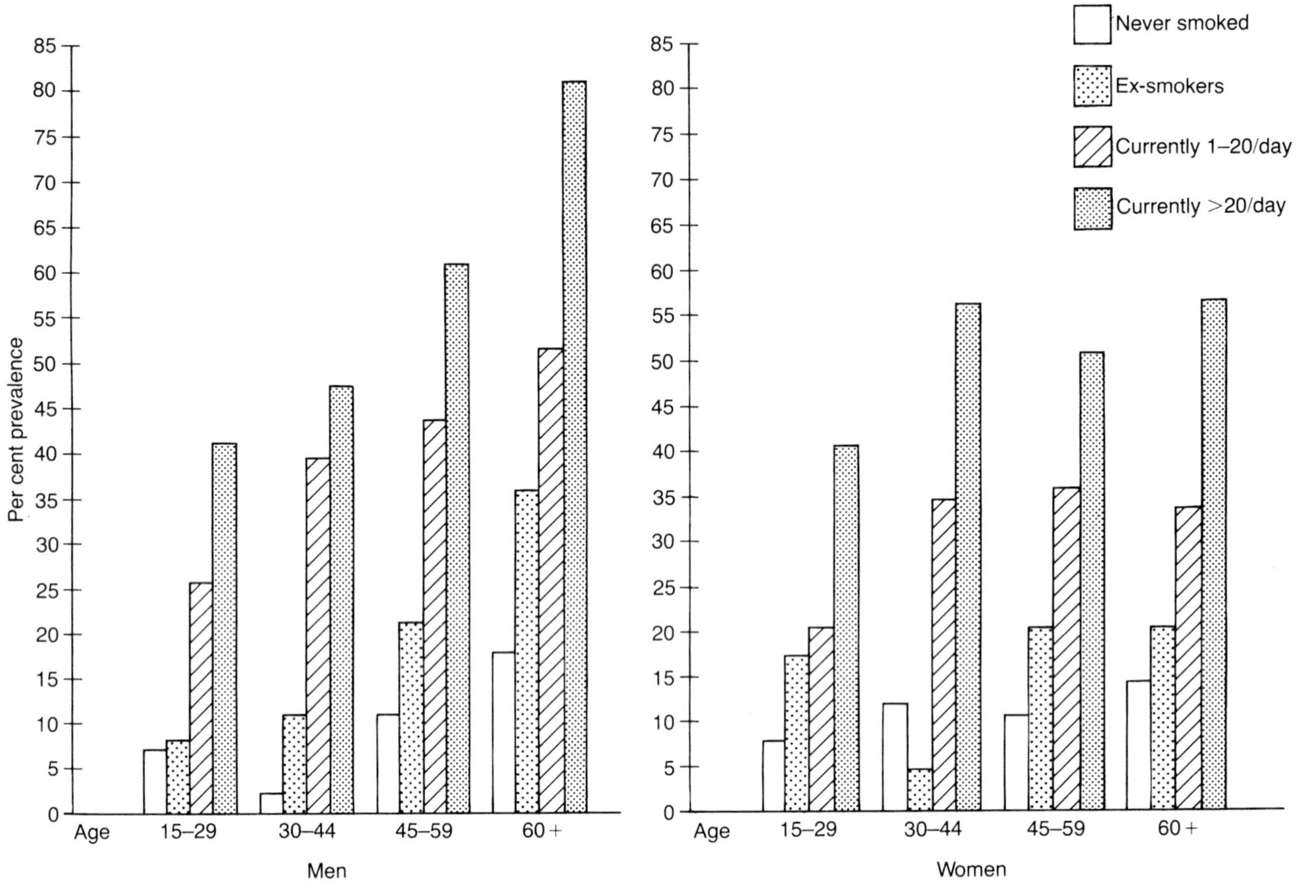


**Figure 38.6** Prevalence of chronic cough with or without chronic sputum production in samples of men and women in Tucson, Arizona, is depicted by age and smoking history. The prevalence of the symptoms increases with age even in nonsmokers, but the increase is greater in ex-smokers and current smokers. The prevalence is greater in 20+/cigarettes/day than in 1–20 cigarettes/day smokers. (Reproduced with permission from Liebowitz MD, Burrows B: Quantitative relationships between cigarette smoking and chronic productive cough. Int J Epidemiol 6:107–113, 1977.)

standardized serum immunoglobulin E (IgE) levels.[143] Thus, American investigators generally formulate the pathogenesis of COPD quite differently than do Dutch investigators.[141]

**Nonspecific Airway Hyperresponsiveness.** The possibility that nonspecific airway hyperresponsiveness (AHR) might be a risk factor for COPD was first raised as a part of the Dutch hypothesis.[140] In brief, studies based on histamine or methacholine challenge as a measure of AHR show mild increases in AHR in smokers similar to that in never-smoking workers exposed to grain dust. This change may be a result of irritation, and there is some evidence of reversibility of AHR with smoking cessation. There is no difference in responsiveness between COPD patients with and without high sputum production, and the observed alterations appear to be a function of airway caliber. In epidemiologic studies, the possible inclusion of asthmatics with their marked increase in AHR may have biased the results. There may be a relationship between the presence of AHR and the rate of decline of lung function.[144] AHR is related to airway caliber; those with smaller airways are more likely to demonstrate AHR.[145] The relationship between increased airway responsiveness and risk for the development of cigarette smoke–induced COPD, however, remains controversial.[146, 147]

**Occupation.** Population-based studies based on measures of either morbidity or mortality suggest that having an occupation in which the atmosphere is polluted with chemical fumes or nonhazardous dust gives rise to an increased prevalence of chronic airflow obstruction, increased rates of decline of $FEV_1$, and greater mortality from COPD. Farming or work in dusty occupations increases the risk of developing chronic bronchitis twofold to threefold, and in combination with smoking the risk increases to sixfold.[148, 149] Interaction between cigarette smoking and exposure to hazardous dusts such as cotton dust and crystalline silica results in higher rates of COPD. In all of these studies, however, smoking effects are

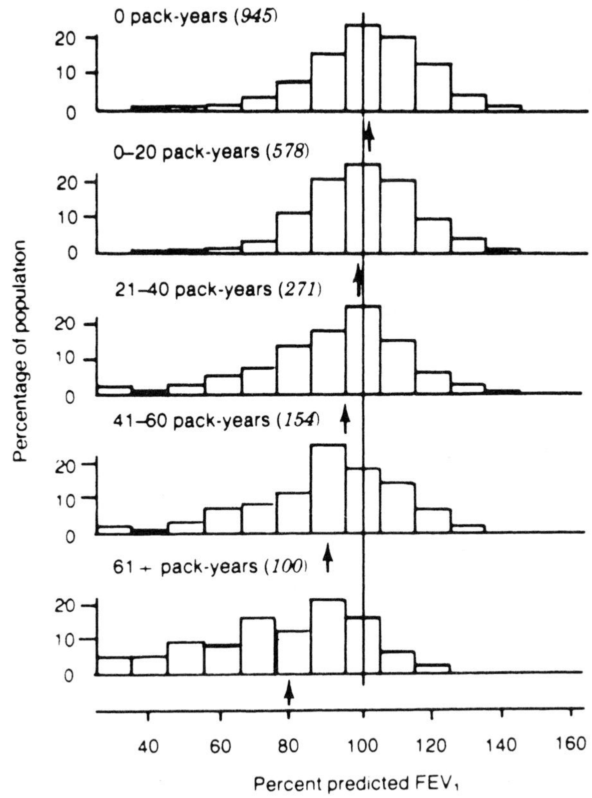


**Figure 38.7** Percentage distribution of predicted $FEV_1$ values in subjects with varying pack-years of smoking is depicted. Subjects with "respiratory trouble" before age 16 years were excluded. Medians *(arrows)* SD are shown for each group in the abscissae. Note that among the 425 persons with 20+ pack-years of smoking, only 15% have an $FEV_1$ of 60% predicted or less. (Reproduced with permission from Burrows B, Knudson RJ, Cline MG, et al: Quantitative relationships between cigarette smoking and ventilatory function. Am Rev Respir Dis 115:751–760, 1979.)

generally much greater than the occupational effects.[150] Occupational asthma is discussed in Chapter 66.

**Perinatal and Childhood Effects.** Maternal smoking has been associated with an increased incidence of respiratory illnesses, including asthma, in children[151, 152] and with lower birth weights. There is contradictory evidence that low birth weight in itself may be predictive of the development of asthma.[153, 154] It has been suggested that low birth weight and childhood respiratory infections may lead to the development of COPD.[152] There is a strong correlation between childhood respiratory infections and the development of COPD.[155, 156] Studies of the effects of low birth weight on development of chronic airflow limitation later in life have, however, been contradictory.[156, 157]

## NATURAL HISTORY

The natural history of airflow obstruction is still only partially characterized. Longitudinal studies, however, as well as much less satisfactory cross-sectional studies of persons of various ages, show that ventilatory function as measured by the $FEV_1$ in nonsmokers without respiratory disease declines by 25 to 30 mL/year beginning at about age 25 to 30 years (Fig. 38.8). The rate of decline of $FEV_1$ with age is steeper for smokers than for nonsmokers. It is also steeper for heavy smokers than for light smokers. The decline in function occurs along a slowly accelerating curvilinear path. In most persons, the loss is assumed to occur uniformly, although, in general, not enough measures have be obtained to ascertain the course of disease. In some individuals, the diseases appears to develop in stages with relatively steep declines.

A direct relationship between initial $FEV_1$ level and the slope of $FEV_1$ decline is known as the "horse race effect"; this term describes the observation that the horse leading in the middle of the race is most likely to win the race.[158] An association between initial $FEV_1$ and the slope of $FEV_1$ decline and a somewhat stronger association between a low $FEV_1/FVC$ on entry into the study and subsequent decline in $FEV_1$ were noted in men but not in women.[158] Thus, middle-aged male smokers who are likely to develop disabling COPD as they grow older can be identified on the basis of their demonstrated loss of $FEV_1$ or a low $FEV_1/FVC$ ratio ($<70\%$). This prediction

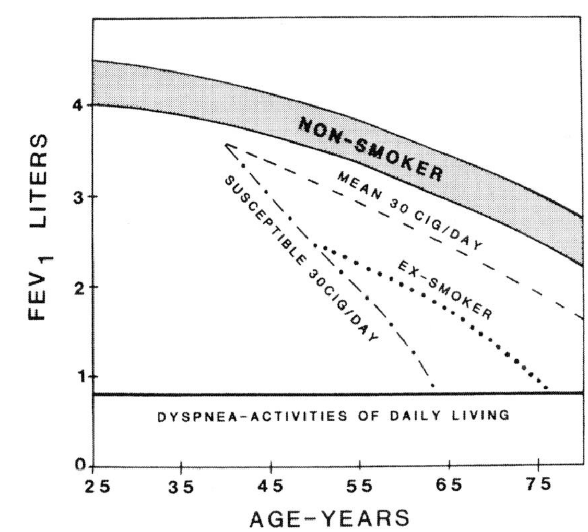


**Figure 38.8** Schema showing effect of age on $FEV_1$ in chronic obstructive pulmonary disease (COPD). Nonsmokers lose $FEV_1$ at an accelerating rate with age; the average loss is about 30 mL/year. Smokers of 30 cigarettes/day average a slightly greater rate of decline and have $FEV_1$ values slightly below average when first studied at age 40 years. A small proportion of susceptible smokers (10% to 15% of the smoking population) lose function much more rapidly, 150 mL/year, and have an $FEV_1$ of 0.8 L at age 65 years, a level that is so low that they experience dyspnea during activities of daily living. A susceptible smoker who stops smoking at age 50 years does not regain any lost function but subsequently loses function at the rate for nonsmokers. Dyspnea on activities of daily living will develop on average at age 76 years, 11 years later than if the person had continued to smoke.

becomes stronger if several years of study show an excessively rapid decline in the spirometric indices. Age, which cannot be separated from the number of years of cigarette smoking, is clearly a risk factor for more rapid decline of lung function; so are lifetime smoking history and the number of cigarettes currently smoked (Fig. 38.9).

Longitudinal studies have taught us a great deal about the natural history of COPD. Lung Health Study I suggested that treatment with anticholinergic drugs did not alter the natural history of COPD.[159] This does not discount the usefulness of the therapy as a bronchodilator. Data from the EUROSCOP Study, the Copenhagen City Lung Study, and the ISOLDE trial have demonstrated that use of inhaled steroids does not alter the rate of decline in airflow limitation.[160] To date, only smoking cessation has altered the natural history of lung function loss in COPD. Oxygen therapy for hypoxemic COPD patients increases survival, but the survival is no better than that of nonhypoxemic COPD patients with comparable airflow limitation. This expensive therapy does not impact the natural history of COPD in terms of decline in airflow limitation.

Individuals with COPD have more frequent acute chest illnesses than do those without COPD. Transient decreases of lung function occur with most episodes; after about 90 days, there is usually restoration of function to the level at the beginning of the acute chest illness.[158] Cough and mucus hypersecretion in smokers are not strongly associated with rate of decline of lung function or with mortality from COPD,[161] although there may be an association.[162] Only airflow limitation, best measured as the postbronchodilator $FEV_1$, relates to the development of disability and death from the disease. The relative contribution of peripheral airway disease and loss of elastic recoil remains unclear. Indices such as the closing capacity, whether expressed as a ratio to the vital capacity or to the total lung capacity, and the slope of the alveolar plateau derived from a single-breath nitrogen test are unable to identify persons who are highly susceptible to the development of chronic airflow limitation early in the course of their cigarette smoke exposure.[163] Tests reflecting emphysema such as carbon monoxide diffusing capacity, functional residual capacity, and total lung capacity predict survival in a relatively minor way.[164]

After the cessation of smoking, lung function lost as a result of smoking is, for the most part, not regained; the rate of decline of lung function with increasing age in former smokers slows to that seen in nonsmokers of the same age (see Figs. 38.8 and 38.9).[132, 165] As already noted, data from several studies strongly suggest that the susceptible subgroup of smokers with more rapid decline of lung function in the midyears of life can be defined by their greater loss of $FEV_1$[138] or their $FEV_1$/FVC ratio.[165] For example, it has been suggested that a smoker of 20 to 30 cigarettes per day for 20 years with an $FEV_1$ that is more than 1 L below the predicted value for age and height or an $FEV_1$/FVC ratio less than 70% is in the susceptible group. The goal of smoking cessation is to delay the rate of decline of ventilatory function and, therefore, the onset of dyspnea and disability; persons shown by spirometry to be at risk of developing disabling COPD should be specially targeted for antismoking interventions.

## PROGNOSIS AND COURSE OF CHRONIC OBSTRUCTIVE PULMONARY DISEASE

The prognosis of patients with COPD who have mild airflow limitation is favorable; survival in a group with

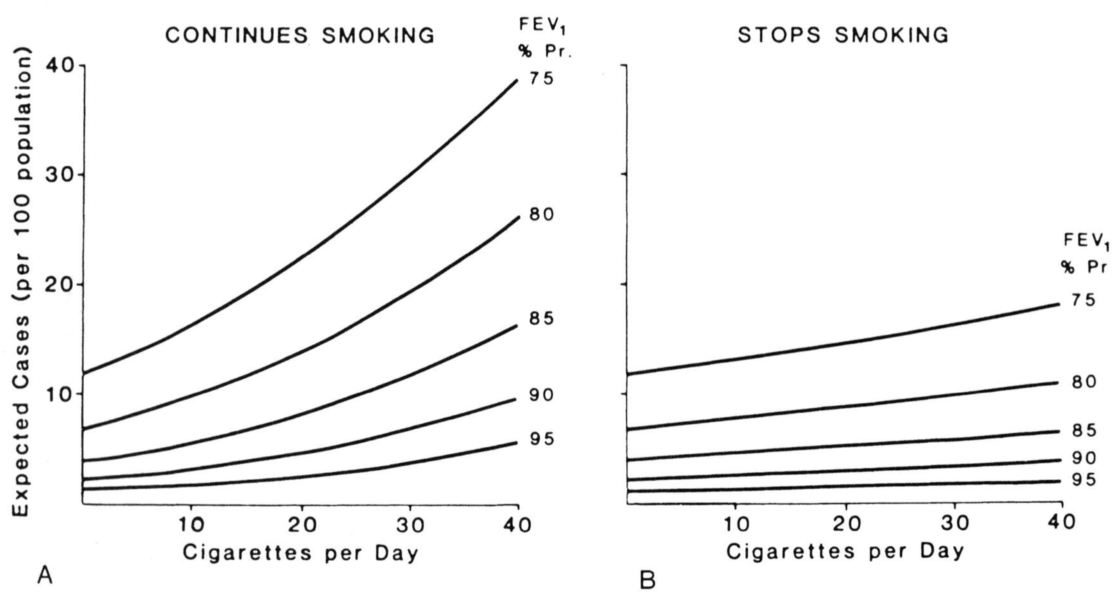


**Figure 38.9** Probabilities are shown of developing chronic obstructive pulmonary disease (COPD) within 10 years for 45-year-old men by cigarette smoking habit *(A)* and with decreased risk from smoking cessation *(B)*. (Reproduced with permission from Higgins MW: An index of risk for obstructive airways disease. Am Rev Respir Dis 125:144–151, 1982.)

initial postbronchodilator $FEV_1$ of 50% of predicted or greater was only slightly worse than in a group of smokers without airflow obstruction.[164] The prognosis is generally poor in patients with severe airflow limitation, especially if it is accompanied by hypercapnia. In patients presenting with values of $FEV_1$ less than 0.75 L, the approximate mortality rate at 1 year is 30% and at 10 years is 95%. Patients with electrocardiographic evidence of cor pulmonale have a shorter median survival rate than do those without electrocardiographic evidence of cor pulmonale.[166] Advanced age, an $FEV_1$ less than 50% predicted, and comorbidities such as chronic renal failure and cor pulmonale are associated with poor prognosis.[167] Median survival in a Finnish population after the first hospital admission for COPD was 5.7 years.[168] The 2-year mortality rate for patients admitted for acute exacerbation of COPD in the SUPPORT trial was 49%.[169]

Death generally occurs as a result of some medical complication, such as an overwhelming infection, retained secretions with atelectasis and pneumonia, pneumothorax, cardiac arrhythmia, or pulmonary embolism. Severe hypoxemia relates adversely to survival, and its correction by domiciliary oxygen therapy improves survival.[170–172] Patients surviving a bout of heart failure due to cor pulmonale or to an episode of acute respiratory failure, however, may live for many more years. Follow-up studies in several medical centers have shown that some patients with severe obstructive airway disease may survive for periods as long as 15 years.[164, 173–175] Assiduous and thoughtful management and facilitation of their entry into the medical care system when they are acutely ill are important in giving these patients the maximum possible length of life.

## PATHOLOGY

### Chronic Bronchitis

**Bronchi.** A number of morphologic changes in the bronchi have been described in chronic bronchitis.[132, 176] The submucosal glands reveal dilated ducts and hypertrophy and hyperplasia of their glandular elements (Fig. 38.10).[177–180] The most common way of measuring glandular enlargement is the Reid index, which is the ratio of gland to bronchial wall thickness.[181] Goblet cell frequency is also increased. Patchy areas of squamous metaplasia may replace normal ciliated epithelium.[182] The airway wall contains an infiltrate of inflammatory cells in which monocytes and lymphocytes[183] and $CD8^+$ lymphocytes are prominent.[184] This contrasts with the $CD4^+$ Th2 cells, which are prominent in asthma. Eosinophils may be present, but much less commonly than in asthma.[185] Neutrophils are more prominent in the airway lumen[186, 187] and in the glands[188] than in the airway wall. The amount of airway smooth muscle is increased.[189, 190]

**Bronchioles.** The respiratory bronchioles of smokers reveal a predominantly mononuclear inflammatory process.[191] Membranous airways less than 2 mm in diameter, the bronchioles, show varying degrees of plugging with mucus, goblet cell metaplasia, inflammation, increased smooth muscle, and distortion due to fibrosis and loss of alveolar attachments,[27, 192] which is related to concurrent emphysema.[193–195] Bronchiolar deformity is related to airflow obstruction.[196, 197]

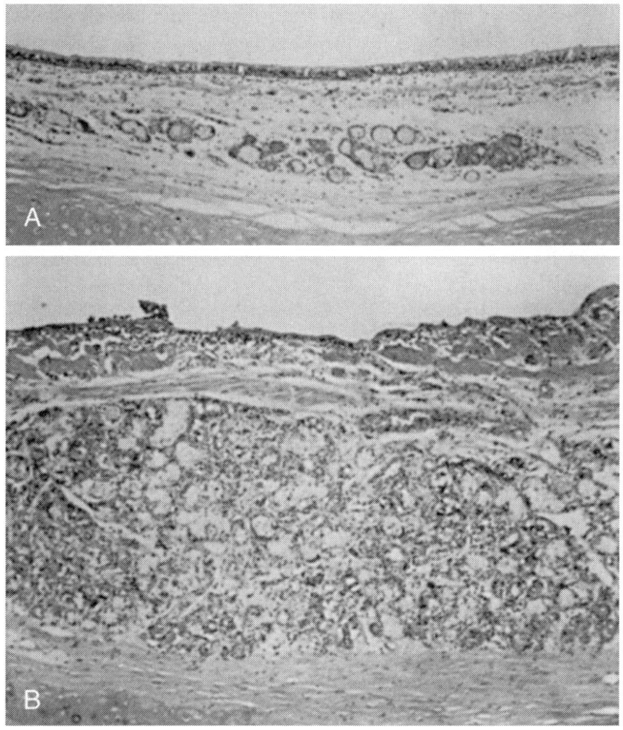


**Figure 38.10** Photomicrographs showing left main bronchus from a patient without respiratory symptoms *(A)* and from a patient with many years of productive cough and airflow obstruction *(B)*. Both serous acini (dark staining) and mucous acini (light staining) are seen to constitute the submucosal gland in *A*; the average gland thickness represents about one third the distance between the epithelial basement membrane and the perichondrium. The submucosal gland in *B* is markedly thickened, is made up mostly of mucous acini, and constitutes most of the wall thickness between the epithelial basement membrane and the perichondrium; note also that the epithelium has desquamated. (Reproduced with permission from Snider GL: Clinical Pulmonary Medicine. Boston: Little, Brown & Company, 1981.)

**Airway Pathology as a Defining Characteristic for Chronic Bronchitis.** The pathologic changes in the airways are not adequately specific for use as a basis for defining chronic bronchitis. The distribution of bronchial gland size is unimodal, so there is a gradual transition from normal glands to the enlarged glands of chronic bronchitis; there is considerable overlap of gland size between persons with and without clinically evident mucous hypersecretion.[176, 177, 198] Mucous gland enlargement is also a feature of other pulmonary diseases such as pneumoconiosis and cystic fibrosis.[199–201]

### Simple Air-Space Enlargement

The term *simple air-space enlargement* is applied to forms of air-space enlargement in which there is no loss of the orderly appearance of the lung acinus and evidence of destruction is wanting. In Down's syndrome, the number of alveoli is decreased, and alveoli are enlarged.[202] Air-space enlargement occurs with chronic overinflation, as in the contralateral lung after pneumonectomy, with air trapping in acute asthma, or in lung tissue adjacent to atelectasis. The air spaces also enlarge with advancing age, associated with a loss of elastic recoil.[203]

## Emphysema

Localization of the lesions of mild emphysema in the acinus serves as the basis for classification into several types of emphysema (see Table 38.1).[106, 176] The acinus or secondary lung lobule is the unit of lung structure distal to the terminal bronchiole. The acinus is composed of three to five orders of respiratory bronchioles, which have alveoli originating directly from their walls (Fig. 38.11). All of the structures distal to the terminal bronchiole participate in gas exchange and constitute the respiratory tissues of the lungs. The description of subtypes of emphysema based on location and distribution has been useful. For most patients, however, the process within the lung is heterogeneous to varying degrees.

**Centriacinar Emphysema.** As the term suggests, *centriacinar emphysema* begins in the respiratory bronchioles.[16, 176] Scarring and focal dilation of the bronchioles and of the adjacent alveoli result in the development of an enlarged air space or microbulla in the center of the secondary lung lobule. Air-space enlargement spreads peripherally from the centriacinar region.

***Focal Emphysema.*** A widespread form of centriacinar emphysema, occurring in persons who have had heavy exposure to a relatively inert dust such as coal dust,[204] is called *focal emphysema.* Large numbers of pigment-laden macrophages are noted in association with focal emphysema, which is uniformly distributed throughout the lungs.

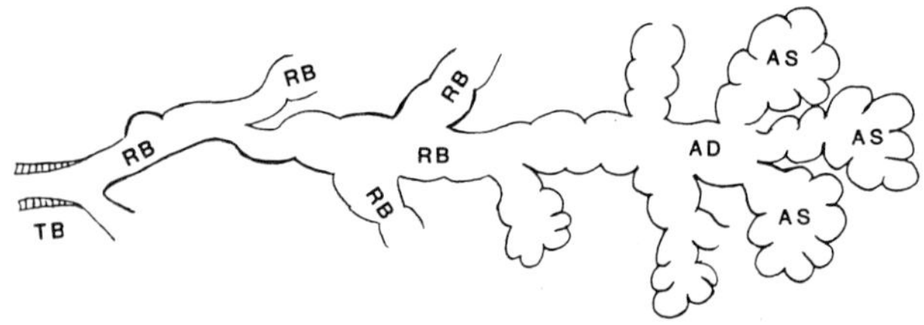


**Figure 38.11** Schematic diagram depicting normal respiratory air spaces. The terminal bronchiole (TB) leads into several orders of respiratory bronchioles (RB), which in turn open into alveolar ducts (AD) and alveolar sacs (AS). The respiratory air spaces arising from a single terminal bronchiole constitute the secondary lung lobule. Centrilobular emphysema begins in first-order respiratory bronchioles, hence its central localization in the secondary lung lobule. Panlobular emphysema involves all the respiratory spaces. (Reproduced with permission from Snider GL: Clinical Pulmonary Medicine. Boston: Little, Brown & Company, 1981.)

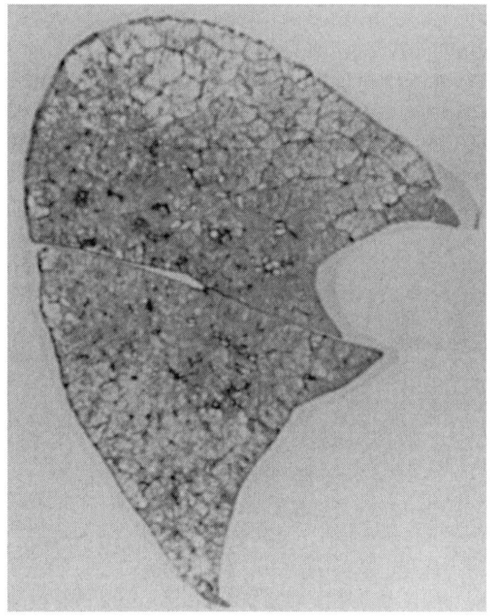

**Figure 38.12** Centrilobular emphysema is shown in this mounted section of inflation-fixed left lung. The disruption of respiratory air spaces is present in the basilar segments of the left lower lobe and lingula but is locally most severe in the apicoposterior segment of the upper lobe and superior segment of lower lobe. (Reproduced with permission from Snider GL: Clinical Pulmonary Medicine. Boston: Little, Brown & Company, 1981.)

***Centrilobular Emphysema.*** Centrilobular emphysema is the form of centriacinar emphysema most frequently associated with prolonged cigarette smoking in persons who have had no unusual dust exposure.[106, 132] This lesion involves the upper and posterior portions of the lungs more than the lower portions (Fig. 38.12).[106, 205, 206]

**Panacinar Emphysema.** The term *panacinar emphysema* refers to dilation of all of the respiratory air spaces of the secondary lung lobule (Fig. 38.13). This form of emphysema may be either focal or diffuse; in the focal form, lesions are more common at the lung bases than at the apices and are often seen in older persons.[205, 206] Panacinar emphysema also commonly occurs in the lung bases of smokers with normal serum proteins in association with centrilobular emphysema in the lung apices. As the disease process becomes more severe, the lesion becomes indistinguishable from panacinar emphysema.[176, 207]

Diffuse panacinar emphysema is the lesion most often associated with alpha$_1$-protease inhibitor deficiency; the emphysema is usually worse at the bases than at the apices.[106] Congenital lobar overinflation or emphysema results in infancy from bronchial atresia, most often in the apicoposterior segmental bronchus of the left upper lobe; available information suggests that the accompanying emphysema is panacinar in type.[85] A group of young (average age about 35 years) intravenous Ritalin (methylphenidate tablet) abusers with severe airflow obstruction and severe panacinar emphysema has been described.[208]

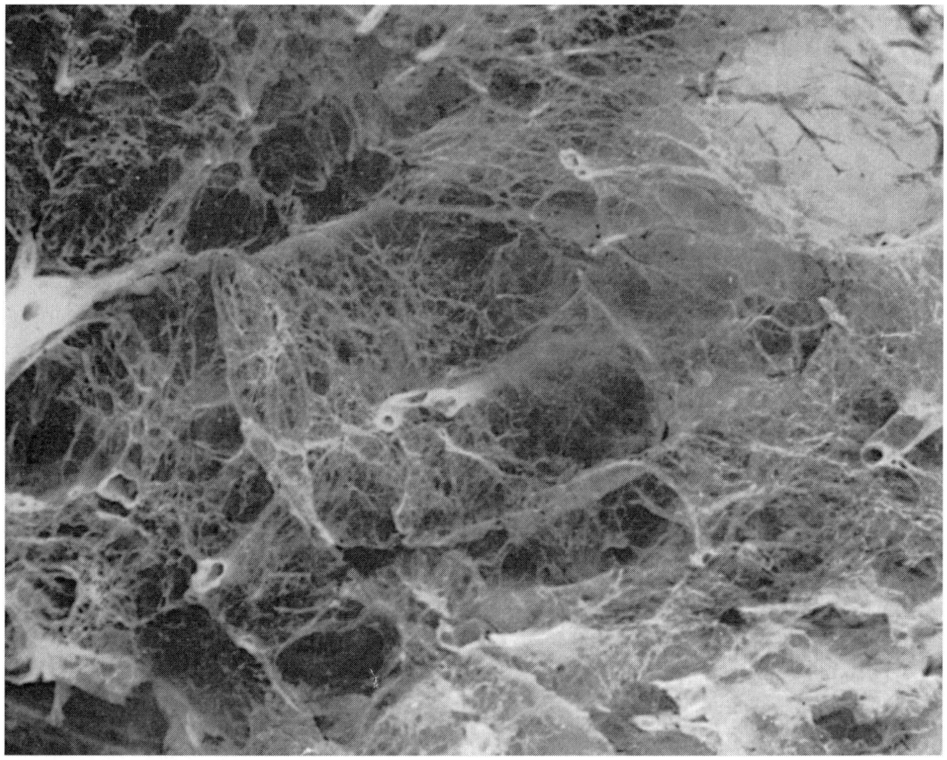

**Figure 38.13** Panlobular emphysema is shown. Close-up view of cut surface of inflation-fixed lung of patient with severe generalized panlobular emphysema. Note the extensive enlargement, distortion, and coalescence of the respiratory air spaces. (Reproduced with permission from Snider GL: Clinical Pulmonary Medicine. Boston: Little, Brown & Company, 1981.)

**Distal Acinar Emphysema.** In contrast to other forms of emphysema that tend to be generalized, distal acinar emphysema, which is also known as *paraseptal* or *subpleural emphysema,* is localized along fibrous interlobular septa or beneath the pleura. The remainder of the lung is often spared, so pulmonary function may be normal or nearly so despite the presence of many superficial areas of locally severe emphysema.[85, 209, 210] This is the type of emphysema that produces the apical bullae giving rise to simple spontaneous pneumothorax in young persons, as described in Chapter 75.

**Air-Space Enlargement with Pulmonary Fibrosis.** Another type of localized emphysema, air-space enlargement with pulmonary fibrosis, is commonly seen as an inconsequential lesion adjacent to scars. At times the air-space enlargement may be quite extensive and may be important clinically, occurring as a complication of fibrosing diseases such as tuberculosis, silicosis, and sarcoidosis.[106, 176] The underlying disease is usually evident radiographically, with extensive linear or nodular shadows evident along with the enlarged air spaces. Air-space enlargement with fibrosis is the anatomic lesion underlying emphysema associated with the pulmonary apical cap.[211] Honeycombing or the end stage of interstitial lung disease is different from air-space enlargement with fibrosis. Cystic spaces 0.5 to 2 cm in diameter are located mainly in the periphery of the lung, although they can sometimes be widespread. The spaces have dense fibrous walls and are mostly lined by bronchiolar epithelium.[212]

**Bullae.** Bullae are areas of marked focal dilation of respiratory air spaces that may result from coalescence of adjacent areas of emphysema, from locally severe panacinar emphysema, or from a ball-valve effect in the bronchi supplying an emphysematous area.[85, 106, 176] The bullae may be simple air spaces or may retain the trabeculae of the emphysema that led to them. Most frequently, bullae occur as a part of widespread emphysema. Although locally severe emphysema of any type can give rise to bullae, giant bullae are particularly likely to complicate distal acinar emphysema. The amount of emphysema in adjacent lung without bullae varies. In distal acinar emphysema, the emphysematous changes may be confined to the bullous areas; however, if these bullae become large and compress adjacent lung tissue, they may have important physiologic consequences.

**Blebs and Cysts.** Blebs are intrapleural collections of air and are, therefore, a form of interstitial emphysema. They may be a complication of interstitial emphysema in the neonatal period or a complication of pulmonary barotrauma complicating mechanical ventilation. They may also be a part of the spontaneous pneumomediastinum of adults. Ruptured blebs are a cause of spontaneous pneumothorax.[85, 106, 176]

Cysts in the lung are air spaces lined by epithelium, which usually have the characteristics of bronchial epithelium.[213] They are classically known as *intrapulmonary bronchogenic cysts* and usually occur near the tracheal bifurcation,[214, 215] but they may be seen more peripherally in the lung parenchyma. Air spaces with fibrous walls, as seen in fibrosing disorders such as sarcoidosis and open healing of tuberculous cavities, are sometimes referred to as *cysts.* They are better referred to as *air-space enlargements with fibrosis.*

**The Heterogeneity of Emphysema—Pathogenetic and Clinical Implications.** The anatomic patterns and age and sex distributions of the various types of emphysema suggest the presence of specific pathogenetic mechanisms. Unfortunately, the various types of emphysema cannot be identified with certainty by the clinician. Centrilobular emphysema can be identified on bronchograms as flower-like air-space dilations or pools in the distal airways.[216–218] Distal acinar emphysema may be suspected in patients with bullae and normal or near-normal lung function. A predominance of emphysema at the lung bases suggests the presence of panacinar emphysema. Noninvasive imaging techniques, however, particularly high-resolution CT, have permitted description of the anatomic distribution of emphysema. They also provide a method to grade relative severity within the lungs of an individual.[219–221] These methods have been very important in guiding lung volume reduction surgery (see below).

## STRUCTURE-FUNCTION CORRELATIONS

### Mucous Gland Size and Sputum Production

The tracheobronchial mucous glands constitute the major volume of mucus-secreting cells, the other source being the goblet cells, and are thought to be the major source of mucus in sputum. Studies have, however, shown only a weak or absent correlation between mucous gland enlargement and sputum production[178, 196, 222] in patients with COPD. The relationship between gland size and mucous production remains to be elucidated. Similarly, whether anatomic changes in the secretory apparatus are associated with alterations in mucus composition are also unknown.

### The Cause of Airflow Limitation in Chronic Obstructive Pulmonary Disease

The mechanical principles underlying airflow limitation are presented in Chapter 5, and the pulmonary function tests used to evaluate airflow limitation are discussed in Chapter 28. Bronchial gland enlargement is not related to airflow limitation,[196, 222–225] perhaps because the process gives rise to only slight thickening of the mucosa, and encroachment on the lumen of the cartilaginous airways is minimal.

Studies in elastase-treated animals show that emphysema causes airflow limitation in the absence of bronchiolitis. Because emphysema and bronchiolitis occur together in moderate or severe COPD, it is no simple matter to determine the relative roles of these two lesions in causing airflow limitation. It is only possible to clearly evaluate the role of bronchiolar changes in the absence of emphysema. In a study of subjects with varying smoking histories and with an $FEV_1$ greater than 75% of predicted and mild or no emphysema,[226] the internal diameter of respiratory and membranous bronchioles correlated strongly with $FEV_1$ values predicted ($r = .79$ and $.82$, respectively). Weaker correlations were noted between $FEV_1$ values and goblet cell metaplasia in membranous bronchioles ($r = .52$) and fibrosis ($r = .41$) and in intraluminal macrophages of respiratory bronchioles ($r = .41$).

The relationship between airflow limitation and bronchiolar pathology persists as airflow limitation and emphysema become moderate in severity, but the strength of the association is less. Cosio and coworkers[27] studied 36 smokers or ex-smokers who had lung resection for solitary nodules. A semiquantitative scoring system was applied to the airways less than 2 mm in diameter. The severity of the pathologic changes in the bronchioles was related to the ratio of $FEV_1/FVC$, the maximum midexpiratory flow, the closing capacity, the volume at which air and helium flows were equal, and the slope of phase III of the single-breath nitrogen washout curve. In this study, however, the severity of bronchiolar pathology was also related to the severity of emphysema.[227] In subjects with severe airflow limitation, there is no relationship between $FEV_1$ and the membranous bronchiolar score or any of its components.[196]

Another approach to evaluating the relative roles of emphysema and airway pathology in causing airflow limitation is to analyze findings in patients in whom observations on bronchi, bronchioles, parenchyma, and airflow obstruction are all available. A postmortem study was performed on the lungs of 48 subjects who had been entered into the National Institutes of Health Intermittent Positive-Pressure Breathing Trial[190, 196] in whom pulmonary function measurements had been made at regular intervals during life. The subjects had a mean emphysema panel grade of 62.5, but with a wide range, from 5 to 95. Emphysema scores showed modest correlations with tests of impaired expiratory flow such as the $FEV_1/FVC$. There was no relationship between scores of bronchial gland size or the membranous bronchiolar pathology scores and indices of airflow obstruction. The exceptions to this were weak correlations between tests of airflow limitation and the proportion of bronchioles less than 400 $\mu m$ in diameter and an index of distortion of respiratory bronchioles.

Similar conclusions were drawn in an earlier study by Mitchell and associates[228] of lungs in 242 subjects. The diagnosis of chronic airflow limitation in that study was based on clinical features. The authors concluded that the severity of emphysema was overwhelmingly the most important correlate of the clinical state of chronic airflow limitation. Pathologic changes in bronchi or bronchioles correlated weakly with chronic airflow limitation; they were seldom associated with chronic airflow limitation in the absence of emphysema. Hale and coworkers[229] compared the involvement of bronchial gland enlargement, bronchiolar pathology, and emphysema in three populations: a group of nonsmokers, a group of smokers who died outside the hospital without known pulmonary disease, and a group of smokers who died with severe airflow limitation. Two thirds of the last group had emphysema with a panel grade of 30 or more compared with 12% of smokers without airflow obstruction and 7% of nonsmokers. Although mean bronchiolar inflammation, smooth muscle, and fibrosis scores were lowest in nonsmokers, intermediate in smokers without airflow obstruction, and highest in smokers with airflow limitation, there was marked overlap among the three groups. Premortem $FEV_1$ measurements correlated with emphysema ($r = .74$, $P < .01$), with average bronchiole diameter ($r = .54$, $P < .05$), and with percentage of bronchioles less than 400 μm (r = .51, $P < .05$) but not with bronchiolar pathology scores. In a multiple regression analysis, with percentage predicted $FEV_1$ as the dependent variable and morphologic indices as independent variables, only emphysema entered at a significant level. The authors concluded that, among smokers with airflow obstruction, no feature of bronchiolar pathology was an independent predictor of ventilatory function beyond that of emphysema alone.

These data, taken together, suggest that when emphysema is mild or moderate in severity, bronchiolar inflammation and accompanying pathologic changes play an important role in causing airflow limitation. As emphysema becomes more severe, the emphysema becomes the predominant cause of airflow limitation. This is consistent with the various processes that often coexist in lungs of the COPD patient progressing with somewhat independent natural histories. Airway disease may be manifest earlier and may be a more important cause of airflow limitation in mild disease. Emphysema, in contrast, may become more important later in more severe disease.

## Compliance and Lung Volumes in Emphysema

Increased compliance of the lungs was first described in severe emphysema more than 50 years ago.[230] More recent studies show that in mild emphysema, quantified by the panel grade method, elastic recoil pressures are consistently decreased.[38, 231] There is increased lung distensibility with an accompanying increase in total lung capacity, functional residual capacity, and residual volume and a decrease in vital capacity. The volume-pressure curve of the lungs is usefully described by an exponential function, $V = A - Be^{-KP}$, where V is lung volume, P is static recoil pressure, and A, B, and K are constants. The constant K is an index of lung distensibility that describes the shape of the volume-pressure curve over the upper half of the lung volume; it is inversely related to the bulk elastic modulus of the lungs. The constant K is a better predictor of emphysema than other measures of elastic recoil or lung volumes.[232]

The correlations of all measures of the volume-pressure relationship with pathologic severity of emphysema are, however, relatively weak.[233] The reason for this weak relationship may be that the volume-pressure relationship of the whole lung is a net measurement reflecting the contributions of regions with varying degrees of alteration in lung compliance. The air spaces of centrilobular emphysema have been shown to be less compliant than normal and less compliant than the overall compliance of the lungs that contain them[234]; compliance may also be increased in some areas of destruction with little air-space enlargement.[235]

## Carbon Monoxide Diffusing Capacity

The carbon monoxide diffusing capacity, whether measured by the single-breath or steady-state method and whether values are expressed in absolute terms, as percentage predicted, as a function of alveolar volume, or as fractional uptake of carbon monoxide, has consistently been the best functional predictor of the severity of emphysema.[106] The correlation coefficients have ranged between 0.60 and 0.87. This relationship probably reflects the loss of internal surface area and of capillary bed of the lung that occurs in emphysema. The diffusing capacity is decreased in young smokers within a few years of starting smoking.[40] Because of the large test-to-test variation and the fact that other conditions can affect the diffusion capacity, however, this test is neither a specific nor a sensitive test of mild emphysema.

# PATHOGENESIS OF CHRONIC OBSTRUCTIVE PULMONARY DISEASE

## Introduction

Current concepts of the pathogenesis of COPD stem from several lines of evidence. Epidemiologic studies suggest that exposures, particularly to particulates and fumes, play a major role. Without doubt, the most important exposure in the developed world is cigarette smoke. In addition, studies of genetic disorders provide important insights. The first of these concerns the congenital deficiency of $alpha_1$-protease inhibitor (API), which led to the concept of a protease-antiprotease imbalance in emphysema. Finally, experimental studies in animals and in vitro support these general concepts and also indicate that disordered repair likely also plays an important role. The overall concept suggests that exposures may directly or indirectly damage the lung through the inflammatory processes that they initiate. If the inflammatory processes that include proteases and oxidants are not adequately balanced by control mechanisms, excessive damage may result. If the damage is not adequately balanced by repair mechanisms, tissue dysfunction may result.

Only 15% of smokers develop clinically symptomatic COPD, and, although there is a clear relationship to the amount smoked, there is considerable individual variation in susceptibility.[137] Probably there are both genetic and environmental reasons for this varying susceptibility. A number of genetic factors have been associated with the development of emphysema. The best characterized of these is API deficiency, which is discussed in detail below because it may be considered a syndrome in its own right and it serves as a paradigm for current concepts of mechanism in COPD. Individuals with API, however, also demonstrate variable susceptibility for the development of emphysema, and it is likely that other factors also play a role in individuals with this genetic predisposition.[236, 237] Polymorphisms in several other genes have been described to have associations with risk for COPD, although the functional relationships with pathogenesis are not entirely clear. These include microsomal epoxide hydrolase,[238] glutathione S-transferase,[239] $alpha_1$-antichymotrypsin,[240] the complement component GcG,[241] and the cytokine tumor necrosis factor-alpha.[242]

Childhood viral infections are also a risk factor for the development of COPD in later life. Hogg and colleagues[243] advanced the hypothesis that these infections can lead to a chronic state predisposing to the development of excessive inflammation. Consistent with this, most adults express adenoviral DNA within their lung, presumably due to incorporation of viral DNA into the host genome during childhood. Patients with COPD manifest increased expression of viral DNA compared with control subjects.[244] The product of the adenoviral E1A gene is capable of interacting with host transcription factors, thus exacerbating inflammatory responses.[245, 246] Chronic adenoviral infection in an animal model has been associated with inflammation and can potentiate inflammation induced by cigarette smoke.[247] Taken together, this series of studies suggests that acquired susceptibility to COPD may result from viral infections. It seems likely that viruses other than adenovirus function similarly.

These various mechanisms support the idea that individuals differ with respect to inflammation in the lung. These differences probably include varying susceptibility to develop inflammation, to produce inflammatory mediators capable of damaging the lung, to repair the lung following damage, and to protect the lung against inflammatory cell-mediated damage. The last of these is, at present, the best characterized, particularly the syndrome of API deficiency, which is presented in detail below.

## Alpha$_1$-Protease Inhibitor Deficiency

### Physiologic Role of Alpha$_1$-Protease Inhibitor

API is a serum protein that is capable of inhibiting several types of proteolytic enzymes. (API inhibitor is also known as *alpha$_1$-antitrypsin,* a term used in many references on this subject and elsewhere in this book.) Its molecular weight is 52 kd. The protein is present in the bronchoalveolar lavage fluid of normal humans.[248] API appears to play an important role in inflammatory states. It is an acute phase reactant, with its serum concentration rising during pregnancy, during infections, after severe burns, and in the presence of malignant tumors. Smoking elevates serum API concentration by about 20%. Proteolytic enzymes whose activities are inhibited by API include pancreatic trypsin, chymotrypsin and elastase, granulocytic elastase and collagenase, collagenases from synovia and skin, and proteases from some microorganisms.[248] Its main substrate in vivo is, however, believed to be neutrophil elastase.[249]

### Genetic Variations

API is a glycoprotein composed of 394 amino acids, and it is coded for by a single gene on chromosome 14. The serum protease inhibitor phenotype (Pi type) is determined by the independent expression of the two parental alleles. The API gene is highly pleomorphic. More than 75 alleles are known, and they have been classified into normal (associated with normal serum levels of normally functioning API), deficient (associated with serum API levels lower than normal), null (associated with undetectable API in the serum), and dysfunctional (API is present in normal amount but does not function normally).[250]

Most variants of API occur because of point mutations that result in a single amino acid substitution. The Z variant results from the substitution of a lysine for a glutamic acid in the M protein.[251] The substitution changes the charge of the molecule and therefore its electrophoretic mobility. Granules in the hepatocytes of affected persons stain with the periodic acid-Schiff reaction and probably represent the unsecreted protein. The Z protein is also incompletely glycosylated, and it has been suggested that this defect may interfere with the protein's excretion from the liver into body fluids.[252]

The normal M alleles (the alleles are assigned a letter code) occur in about 90% of persons of European descent with normal serum API levels; their phenotype is designated Pi MM. Normal values of serum API are 150 to 350 mg/dL or 20 to 48 μmol. More than 95% of persons in the severely deficient category are homozygous for the Z allele, designated Pi ZZ, and have serum API levels of 2.5 to 7 μmol (mean, 16% of normal). Almost all of these persons are Caucasians of northern European descent, because the Z allele is rare in Asians and African Americans. Rarely observed phenotypes that are associated with these low levels of serum API include the following: Pi SZ in persons with nonexpressing alleles; Pi-null, occurring in homozygous form; Pi null-null; and Pi Z null, occurring in heterozygous form with a deficient allele. Persons with phenotype Pi SS have API values ranging from 15 to 33 μmol (mean, 52% of normal). The threshold protective level of 11 μmol or 80 mg/dL (35% of normal) is based on the knowledge that Pi SZ heterozygotes, with serum API values of 8 to 19 μmol (mean, 37% of normal), rarely develop emphysema. Pi MZ heterozygotes have serum API levels that are intermediate between Pi MM normals and Pi ZZ homozygotes (12 to 35 μmol; mean, 57% of normal) and may be at increased risk for emphysema, although this is controversial.[253]

### Lung Disease in Alpha$_1$-Protease Inhibitor–Deficient Phenotypes

The premature development of severe emphysema is the hallmark of homozygous API deficiency.[254] The onset of dyspnea occurs at a median age of 40 years in Pi Z smokers compared with 53 years in Pi Z nonsmokers. Chronic cough and sputum production sufficient to meet the definition of chronic bronchitis is present in about half of the symptomatic persons.[255] Bronchiectasis has been reported in association with API deficiency.[256, 257] More than half of subjects who are type Pi Z die from pulmonary disease.[258]

Symptoms or signs of pulmonary disease rarely develop before age 25 years.[255, 258–260] Of 22 subjects 12 to 18 years of age with API deficiency discovered through neonatal screening,[261] all had normal spirometric values after bronchodilator aerosol inhalation, as well as normal lung volumes and carbon monoxide diffusing capacity values.

Tobacco smoking and the development of pulmonary disease are strongly associated. Dyspnea begins at an earlier age in smokers than in nonsmokers; smokers who are type Pi Z have a significantly lower life expectancy than nonsmokers who are type Pi Z, although male and female nonsmokers also have a reduced life expectancy.[255, 258, 259] Annual decline of $FEV_1$ is greater than normal in nonsmokers who are type Pi Z but is much greater in smokers who are type Pi Z than in nonsmokers.[259]

Severity of lung disease varies markedly; lung function is well preserved in some smokers who are type Pi Z and severely impaired in some nonsmokers.[255, 258–260] Nonindex cases tend to have better lung function, whether they smoke or not, than do index cases,[255] and the annual decline of $FEV_1$ in nonindex cases tends to be only moderately greater than normal.[260] Pi ZZ persons who are nonsmokers may live into their eighth or ninth decade; however, they usually develop some airflow obstruction as they age.[258, 259, 262] In addition to cigarette smoking, asthma, recurrent respiratory infections, and unidentified familial factors were identified as possible risk factors for chronic airflow limitation.[263] AHR is a common accompaniment of chronic bronchitis and emphysema, and therefore it is difficult to assess the significance of asthma as a risk factor.

Radiographically, Pi Z patients characteristically have much more definite evidence of emphysema than Pi M patients with COPD. The finding of basilar emphysema is not constant in Pi Z patients, but when present it is strongly suggestive of the diagnosis (Fig. 38.14).[264, 265] It is common with advanced disease to see hairline arcuate shadows separating markedly radiolucent areas in the lung bases from the less severely involved upper portions of the lungs.

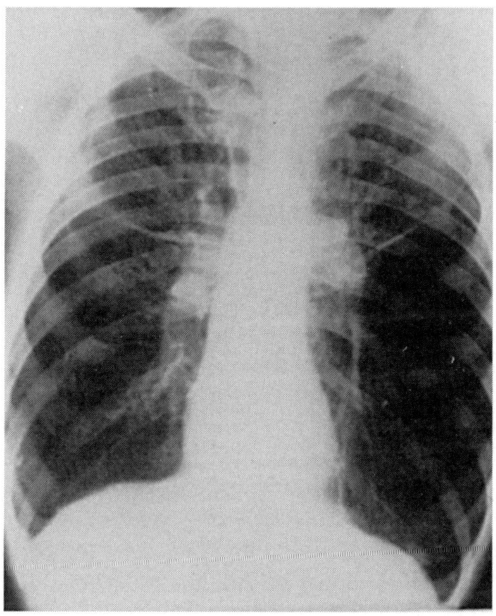

**Figure 38.14** Frontal chest radiograph of a 42-year-old man with homozygous alpha₁-protease inhibitor deficiency is shown. He began smoking 25 cigarettes daily at age 19 years. By age 31 years he was unable to continue working as a professional baseball player because of dyspnea during exertion. At the time of this examination, his $FEV_1$ was 0.6 L, his arterial $P_{O_2}$ was 49 mm Hg, and his arterial $P_{CO_2}$ was 50 mm Hg breathing air. Note the marked transradiancy in the lower half of both hemithoraces limited above by hairline shadows. Vascular markings are evident in the upper lung fields but not in the mid-lung and lower lung zones. The heart shadow is narrow, and the pulmonary artery shadows are enlarged. At autopsy the basilar areas were zones of very severe panacinar emphysema similar to those shown in Figure 38.5.

## Lung Disease in Other Alpha$_1$-Protease Inhibitor Phenotypes

Persons who are heterozygous for the Pi allele (Pi MZ) constitute 2% to 3% of the white population of the United States compared with 0.02% for those who are homozygous. The results of studies of heterozygotes are controversial.[253] Subjects with the Pi MZ phenotype who are studied because they are relatives of persons known to be Pi ZZ may have a slightly higher frequency of COPD than control subjects.[266] In studies in which Pi MZ patients have been identified as part of population surveys, however, their lung functions appear not to differ from those of control subjects.[267, 268]

Several reports suggest that DNA polymorphisms in the flanking regions of the alpha$_1$-antitrypsin gene may be associated with an increased frequency of development of emphysema in persons with normal serum protein.[269–271] This polymorphism does not appear to be associated with altered baseline levels of API.[270, 272–274] The mutation appears, however, to be located in a region that may serve as an interleukin-6 regulatory sequence. This raises the possibility that the polymorphism may be associated with a defective upregulation of API during stress. This could result in a relative API deficiency and increased risk for emphysema in the face of environmental or infectious exposures.

## Liver Disease in Alpha$_1$-Protease Inhibitor–Deficient Phenotypes

Homozygous API deficiency is often associated in infancy with hepatomegaly or hepatosplenomegaly and evidence of cholestasis and elevation of hepatocellular enzymes. Some patients with this abnormality may go on to develop cirrhosis. Cirrhosis, often with hepatoma, is second in frequency to emphysema as a cause of death.[255, 258, 275] Hepatic failure due to API deficiency can be treated with liver transplantation. Because the transplanted liver produces normal API, the disorder is effectively cured.[276] The development of liver disease may be related to a second genetic defect that impairs the hepatic degradation of the unsecreted API.[277]

## Diagnosis of Alpha$_1$-Protease Inhibitor Deficiency

The diagnosis of API deficiency is made by measuring the serum API level, followed by Pi typing for confirmation. These tests should be performed in patients with premature onset of chronic bronchitis, emphysema, and dyspnea and in COPD occurring in nonsmokers. A predominance of basilar emphysema should raise the possibility of the genetic defect.

Estimates of the frequency of the Pi ZZ phenotype in North America and Europe range from about 1 in 1600 to 1 in 4000,[278] a prevalence approximating that of cystic fibrosis and suggesting that severe API deficiency is among the most common potentially serious genetic conditions. Nevertheless, in large studies in both Sweden[258] and Great Britain,[278] rigorous attempts to identify all available cases have garnered 10% of estimated cases at most. This suggests that most subjects who are type Pi Z are either asymptomatic or masquerading under other diagnoses such as asthma.

## Alpha$_1$-Protease Inhibitor Augmentation Therapy

Augmentation therapy with purified human API for patients with severe API deficiency is based on the concept that a deficient protein is being restored to protective levels.[279] The American Thoracic Society has published guidelines for augmentation therapy.[280] It should be reserved for patients whose serum concentration of API is less than 11 μmol; it is not indicated for patients with cigarette smoking–related emphysema who have normal or heterozygous phenotypes. It is also not indicated for patients who have liver disease associated with API deficiency unless they also have lung disease.

Persons with normal lung function should be monitored but not treated; augmentation therapy should be considered when lung function is abnormal and especially if serial studies show deterioration. The American Thoracic Society[280] guidelines make the point that it is inappropriate to define a lower limit of lung function or an upper limit of age for administration of augmentation therapy, because it is unethical to withhold treatment that may have benefit even in severe end-stage disease. However, it seems reasonable to weigh carefully the advantages and disadvantages of augmentation therapy and to reach jointly a decision with elderly persons or those with severe impairment of lung function ($FEV_1$ values less than 0.8 L). For the severely impaired person less than 50 years of age, lung transplantation[281] may be a reasonable consideration.

Augmentation therapy may become less expensive and less unpleasant in the future. Monthly augmentation therapy[282] and the aerosol route of administration[283] are currently being explored and, perhaps, recombinant instead of human API can be inhaled as an aerosol.[284] Synthetic elastase inhibitors are also being evaluated. Whether these highly selective inhibitors will prevent emphysema or whether inhibition of enzymes in addition to elastase will also be required remains to be determined.

## The Elastase-Antielastase Hypothesis

The elastase-antielastase hypothesis of emphysema (Fig. 38.15) can be summarized briefly as follows. The lung is protected from elastolytic damage by antiproteases, including API. Of these, alpha$_2$-macroglobulin enters the lungs if capillary permeability is increased. Secretory leukoprotease inhibitor is secreted by bronchial glands and goblet cells. Elastase is a major product of neutrophils and other cells. Macrophages elaborate an elastaselike metalloprotease and may ingest, and later release, neutrophil elastase; macrophage-derived cysteine proteinases cathepsin B and cathepsin L may also play a role. Oxidants derived from neutrophils and macrophages or from cigarette smoke may inactivate API and may interfere with lung matrix repair. Endogenous antioxidants such as superoxide dismutase, glutathione, and catalase protect the lungs against oxidant injury.[227, 285] Toxic substances such as defensins[286] may also contribute to tissue damage.

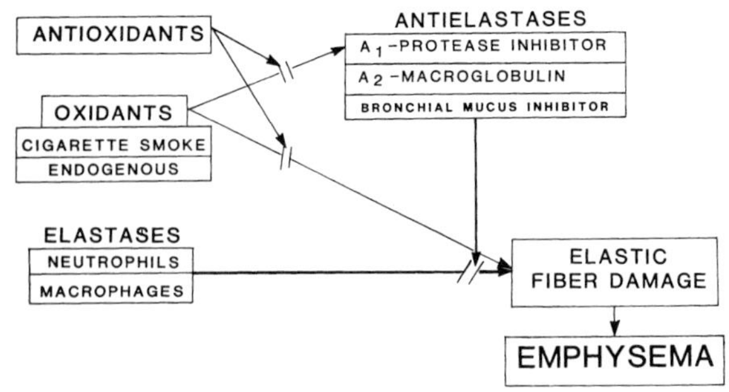


**Figure 38.15** Schema of elastase-antielastase hypothesis of emphysema is depicted. The lung is protected from elastolytic damage by alpha$_1$-protease inhibitor and alpha$_2$-macroglobulin. Bronchial mucous inhibitor protects the airways. Elastase is derived primarily from neutrophils, but macrophages secrete an elastaselike metalloprotease and may ingest and later release neutrophil elastase. Oxidants derived from neutrophils and macrophages or from cigarette smoke may inactivate alpha$_1$-protease inhibitor and may interfere with lung matrix repair. Endogenous antioxidants such as superoxide dismutase, glutathione, and catalase protect the lung against oxidant injury. (Reproduced with permission from Snider GL: Experimental studies on emphysema and chronic bronchial injury. Eur J Respir Dis 69(Suppl 146):17–35, 1986.)

## Animal Models of Emphysema with Elastin Damage

**Elastase-Induced Emphysema.** Elastolytic enzymes can induce experimental emphysema; proteolytic but nonelastolytic enzymes administered exogenously do not do so. Although early investigators reported a correlation between in vitro measures of elastolytic potency and in vivo emphysema-inducing ability,[18, 287] there are notable exceptions. Treatment with human neutrophil elastase causes increased air-space size and lung volumes,[288–290] but the changes are considerably less severe than those induced by doses of pancreatic elastase with comparable in vitro elastolytic effects (Fig. 38.16). Different susceptibilities of various lung tissues to the two enzymes and different accessibilities of the enzymes to alveolar elastic tissue may contribute to the differing severities of induced emphysema.[291] Alternatively, the enzymes may differ in their abilities to activate proteolytic and inflammatory cascades that amplify the initial proteolytic insult.[292] Emphysema induced by these models persists indefinitely but without progression.[293]

Studies of lung function performed on excised lungs and in anesthetized animals with elastase-induced emphysema have shown increases in lung compliance, functional residual capacity, residual volume, and total lung

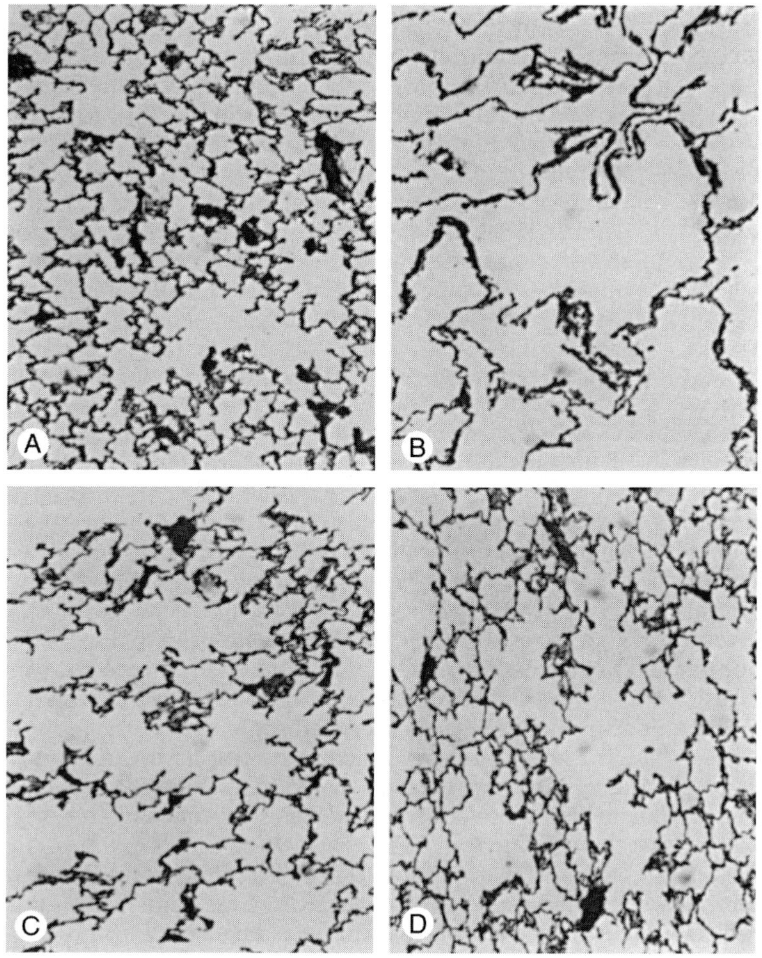

**Figure 38.16** Photomicrographs of hamster lungs are shown. (Hematoxylin and eosin stain; original magnification ×100.) *A,* Normal saline control. *B,* Severe emphysema with marked enlargement of respiratory air spaces 21 days after a single intratracheal instillation of 200 μg of porcine pancreatic elastase. *C,* Mild emphysema 56 days after a single intratracheal instillation of 350 μg of human neutrophil elastase. *D,* Mild emphysema 28 days after 20 instillations of endotoxin of 10 μg each over 8 weeks. (Reproduced with permission from Snider GL: Protease-antiprotease imbalance in the pathogenesis of emphysema and chronic bronchial injury: A potential target for drug development. Drug Dev Res 10:235–254, 1987. © by Wiley-Liss, a division of John Wiley & Sons, Inc.)

capacity.[294] Airflow limitation occurs during forced expiration due to loss of elastic recoil, because bronchiolitis is not present. The diffusing capacity for carbon monoxide is decreased in proportion to the severity of the emphysematous lesion induced. Arterial blood gas studies show hypoxemia without carbon dioxide retention. Right ventricular hypertrophy occurs in hamsters with elastase-induced emphysema and is only partially preventable by treatment of the animals with 35% oxygen.[295]

Treatment with elastase results in a diminution of lung elastin content at 24 hours, followed by rapid restoration of total lung elastin to normal levels.[289, 296] The anatomic arrangement of the elastic fibers, however, remains grossly disordered. The marked increase in total lung capacity that occurs in experimental (and human) emphysema is not likely to occur without disruption of the collagen network of the lungs. There is biochemical evidence of damage and subsequent repair of collagen in experimental elastase-induced emphysema.[297]

**Emphysema Induced by Pulmonary Neutrophilia.** Intravenous administration of endotoxin causes intravascular pulmonary leukocyte sequestration. Mild emphysema has been induced by multiple intravenous injections of endotoxin in rhesus monkeys[298] and in dogs.[299] Emphysema has also been induced by multiple intratracheal instillations of endotoxin in hamsters.[300] Combined treatment of rats with D-galactosamine and repeated injections of endotoxin over 10 weeks resulted in emphysema.[301] The D-galactosamine produces liver disease, which decreases plasma API levels; treatment with endotoxin alone produced milder changes. It was postulated that the emphysema in these experiments is induced by release of enzymes from sequestered leukocytes. Consistent with this concept, neutrophil transit through the lungs is reduced following exposure to cigarette smoke, partly because of changes in neutrophil deformability.[302–304] Transit is also decreased in COPD, raising the possibility of intravascular damage leading to tissue destruction.[305] Taken together, these studies suggest that the tissue destruction of emphysema may originate with an intravascular lesion.

**Emphysema and Impaired Cross-Linking of Elastin.** In the blotchy mouse (a model of genetically occurring emphysema) and in young animals fed lathyrogens, which prevent collagen and elastin cross-linking, emphysema results.[306] Elastase-induced emphysema is worse in lathyritic animals. These observations support the importance of elastic fiber damage in the pathogenesis of emphysema. They also raise the possibility that defective elastic fiber repair contributes to the development of emphysema.

## Evidence from Humans of Elastin Degradation in the Genesis of Emphysema

Investigators have sought direct evidence for involvement of elastin degradation in human emphysema in a number of ways.

**Blood Leukocyte Elastase Levels.** Some investigators report an association between blood leukocyte elastase concentration and airflow obstruction in homozygous or heterozygous API deficiency,[307–310] whereas others do not.[311, 312] Similarly, in persons with normal levels of API, some studies report increased serum leukocyte elastase concentration,[311, 312] and others do not.[313] The possibility remains that elevated leukocyte elastase is a risk factor for emphysema in both normal and API-deficient individuals.

**Proteases in Blood.** Serum immunoreactive leukocyte elastase concentration in patients with chronic obstructive bronchitis has been found to be double that in age-matched control subjects. Patients with other active lung diseases, however, have similarly increased leukocyte elastase concentrations in serum.[314]

**Inflammatory Cells.** Inflammatory cells are present in normal alveoli, but are present in increased numbers in smokers.[191] It is likely that smoke leads to increased alveolar inflammation by a variety of mechanisms. Smoke can activate the alternate complement pathway leading to the generation of the chemotactic factor C5a.[315, 316] Similarly, smoke can inactivate chemotactic factor inhibitor, a molecule that modulated the activity of the cochemotaxin GcG.[317] By both mechanisms, smoke could lead to inflammatory cell recruitment. Smoke can also directly activate cells, including both macrophages[318] and epithelial cells,[319, 320] to release chemotactic factors, including both lipid and chemokine mediators. The absolute number of neutrophils recovered in the bronchoalveolar lavage fluid of smokers is increased fourfold to fivefold in parallel with the increase in the total number of cells.[318] Neutrophils are rich in elastolytic proteinases, including neutrophil elastase, cathepsin-G,[291] and proteinase-3.[321] Increased bronchoalveolar lavage neutrophil elastase levels (measured as a complex with API) and decreased functional antielastase activity were found to correlate with emphysema as measured from CT scan and $DL_{CO}$ measurement.[322] The decrease in antielastase activity may result from oxidation of the API either directly by cigarette smoke[323] or by oxidants released by inflammatory cells.[324] By such mechanisms, cigarette smoke may lead to a functional API deficiency.

Macrophages are the major inflammatory cells recovered in the bronchoalveolar lavage fluid of smokers with and without emphysema, and recovery is increased fourfold to fivefold compared with nonsmokers. Macrophages may play a key role in elaborating cytokines that can recruit and activate other inflammatory cells, including neutrophils, but epithelial cells may also mediate these functions. Macrophages can also produce metalloelastase[325] and human alveolar macrophages and are capable of degrading elastin. This elastin degradation is inhibited by the tissue inhibitor of metalloproteases and is inhibited minimally or not at all by inhibitors of cysteine proteases or by the serine protease inhibitor eglin-c. Consistent with a role for metalloelastase in human emphysema, smaller amounts of elastase-like esterase activity have been shown in the bronchoalveolar lavage fluid of nonsmokers than smokers.[326, 327] Much of this activity appears to be due to a metalloprotease.

Consistent with these observations, transgenic mice deficient in metalloelastase (MMP-12) did not develop either emphysema or increased alveolar macrophage populations when exposed to cigarette smoke.[292] Macrophage recruitment to the lung, but not the development of emphysema, could be initiated by exogenous monocyte chemotactic peptide-1 (MCP-1), suggesting that the metalloelastase deficiency led to both defective macrophage recruitment and decreased tissue destruction. This is consistent with the concept that macrophage-generated matrix fragments may play a role in the development of emphysema by mediating the recruitment of inflammatory cells.[328, 329]

Macrophages also synthesize and express cathepsin B,[330, 331] and levels of the enzyme are approximately three times higher in the macrophages of healthy cigarette smokers than in nonsmokers and approximately 10 times higher in the bronchoalveolar lavage fluid of smokers.[332] Cathepsin B induces emphysema on instillation into hamster lungs.[333] Cathepsins D and L may also play a role in elastin degradation by macrophages.[334, 335] Finally, transgenic mice overexpressing collagenase develop emphysema.[336] As most of the matrix-degrading enzymes are released as inactive precursors,[292] it seems likely that complex interactions among these enzymes are likely, including mutual activation and augmented secretion due to cellular recruitment and activation.

**Elastin Degradation Products in Blood and Urine.** Whether increased elastin degradation products can be used as a marker of disease activity in emphysema is controversial. Early studies did not find elevated levels of the elastin-specific cross-link desmosine in the urine of smokers with COPD compared with normal smokers or nonsmokers.[337, 338] Urinary desmosine values are also similar in normal persons, Pi ZZ subjects with emphysema, and subjects with interstitial lung diseases, and these markers also were not elevated in children with Pi ZZ.[339] Stone and associates,[340] however, using a high-pressure liquid chromatographic technique and isotope dilution, found ratios of urinary desmosine to creatinine that were 10% to 20% of previously reported values, perhaps because of the presence of interfering substances in the urine. Studies with an enzyme-linked immunosorbent assay[341] showed that patients with COPD have higher plasma elastin peptide levels than normal nonsmokers, and normal smokers had intermediate values; however, the three groups overlapped. Decreased urinary excretion of desmosine has been reported in API-deficient subjects receiving replacement.[342] Similarly, smoking subjects with COPD and rapid decline in lung function had greater desmosine excretion than subjects with COPD and less rapid loss of function.[343] Although methodologic issues remain to be resolved, these results are consistent with a potential role for elastin fragments as markers of disease activity in emphysema.

**Immunocytochemical Localization of Elastase in Lung.** Controversy surrounds a report that provides direct evidence of the protease-antiprotease hypothesis of emphysema in smokers. One investigative group[344] showed that neutrophil elastase is bound to elastic fibers in the lungs of smokers and that the amount of elastase is proportional to the amount of emphysema present. Another group reports an inability to reproduce these findings,[345] while another group reports confirmation.[346]

***Lung Elastin in Emphysema.*** Early attempts to confirm by biochemical analysis the involvement of elastin damage in patients with emphysema failed to show a decrease in lung elastin compared with normal control subjects.[347–349] In one study,[350] five of eight patients showed a decrease in lung elastin, expressed as a proportion of crude connective tissue, compared with control subjects. The significance of this result is not clear, as the ratio of elastin to crude connective tissue could have been decreased because the crude connective tissue was elevated. In this regard, the collagen content of the lungs in early emphysema and the total lung weight may be increased,[347, 351] consistent with the activation of repair processes. Similarly, in experimental elastase-induced emphysema, after an initial decrease in lung elastin, normal lung elastin values are restored after the third to sixth week.[296, 297] The amount of connective tissue in the lungs therefore represents a balance between destruction and new production.

***Emphysema Without Elastin Damage.*** A number of animal models of emphysema have been developed that do not depend directly on elastin damage. Emphysema was caused by the following agents or conditions.

*Cadmium.* Some patients who survive severe lung injury with vaporized cadmium salts develop air-space enlargement with fibrosis.[352] Administration of cadmium chloride by multiple aerosol treatments to rats resulted in a lesion resembling human centrilobular emphysema.[353] The addition of the lathyritic agent beta-aminopropionitrile (BAPN) to the intratracheal cadmium chloride treatment resulted in marked air-space enlargement.[354] In a study[354] in which lung elastin was radiolabeled in the neonatal period, it was demonstrated that neonatally formed lung elastin is not destroyed in the model of cadmium chloride air-space enlargement with fibrosis in hamsters. Hoidal and coworkers[355] also showed that rendering hamsters neutropenic with antineutrophil globulin did not inhibit the air-space enlargement produced by combined cadmium chloride–BAPN treatment. Thus, it seems likely that cadmium chloride–induced air-space enlargement with fibrosis is not caused by neutrophil elastase.

A number of observations suggest that this finding may be important in relation to centrilobular emphysema in smokers. Fibrosis is a part of the microbullae of centrilobular emphysema.[16] Cigarette smoke is an important source of cadmium accumulation in humans,[356] and cadmium is found in emphysematous lungs in direct proportion to the severity of emphysema.[357] Finally, the compliance of the microbullae of centrilobular emphysema is less than that of normal lungs and much less than that of the lungs that contain them.[234] The centrilobular lesions, therefore, may represent focal air-space enlargement with fibrosis.

*Hyperoxia.* Exposure of rats to hyperoxia has been shown to give rise to air-space enlargement and increased lung volumes without alteration of compliance or alveolar number. There was an almost 50% increase in collagen content of the lungs. Treatment of the oxygen-exposed rats with an analogue of proline that prevents synthesis of cross-linked collagen prevented the development of these changes.[358] The mechanism of air-space enlargement in this model is not known. Because rats grow throughout their life spans and the number of alveoli did not change in this model, however, abnormal growth of alveoli related to an imbalance in their connective tissue elements may be the cause of the enlargement.

*Other Oxidants.* Workers in a number of laboratories have observed air-space enlargement with exposure of rats,[359–361] hamsters,[362–364] mice,[365] rabbits,[366] and dogs[177] to nitrogen dioxide. Hamsters exposed to 30 ppm nitrogen dioxide showed decreased lung elastin and collagen content 4 and 10 days (respectively) after starting exposure. The collagen content returned to control levels by day 14 of exposure. Total elastin did not return to control levels until after exposure to nitrogen dioxide was stopped.[367] During exposure, neutrophils accumulated rapidly in the lungs. There is suggestive but not definitive evidence that the neutrophils released elastase during their migration through the lung interstitium.[360] Air-space enlargement has also been shown with ozone.[368]

*Starvation.* Severe starvation induced air-space enlargement and reduced alveolar number in rats[369–372] and hamsters.[373] Saline-filled volume-pressure relations corrected for lung volume were consistent with increased compliance in one study.[374] Saline-filled volume-pressure curves were, however, found to be unaltered by two other groups of investigators.[372, 373] Lung DNA content was unchanged,[375] suggesting no increase in lung cells, such as neutrophils, in this model. Lung collagen and elastin were decreased compared with fed control rats but not compared with baseline values[372, 373]; this observation does not exclude increased turnover of connective tissues. This form of emphysema may be related to disordered growth of the rodent lungs, with an imbalance between lung and chest wall growth. It does not appear to be related to neutrophil elastase.

*Tobacco Smoke.* Prolonged exposure of rats and hamsters to cigarette smoke has failed to produce emphysema consistently, although cigarette smoke exposure did potentiate the emphysema induced by pancreatic elastase in hamsters.[376] Air-space enlargement and alveolar wall fibrosis have been induced in tracheotomized beagles by exposure to smoke.[377] Mice exposed to cigarette smoke also develop emphysema.[378] This may be a particularly important model, as the ability to create mice with defined genetic alterations promises to provide important insights into the pathogenesis of emphysema.

### Beyond the Protease-Antiprotease Hypothesis: Emphysema Is a Stereotyped Response of the Lungs to Injury

The production of experimental emphysema by diverse agents[379] suggests that air-space enlargement is a stereotyped response of the lungs to a wide variety of injuries (Fig. 38.17). It seems quite clear from the experimental data that not all air-space enlargement occurs with a background of elastin destruction, although elastin damage results in emphysema. The balance between injury and repair of connective tissue (collagen, elastin, and proteoglycans) plays a central role leading to air-space enlargement.

## Chronic Bronchitis

Many of the pathogenetic mechanisms discussed above with regard to emphysema are likely relevant to the development of chronic bronchitis. Specifically, inflammatory processes and host defense mechanisms in the airways are, at the cellular and biochemical levels, quite similar. This probably accounts for the marked clinical concurrence of disease in the airways with disease in the alveolar structures.

As noted earlier, neither the symptoms that define the syndrome of chronic bronchitis, chronic cough, and sputum production nor the characteristic pathologic features, inflammation, and enlargement of the secretory apparatus are specific for the condition. Other airway diseases such as cystic fibrosis and asthma have clinical and histologic features similar to those of chronic bronchitis. There is probably overlap among the pathogenetic mechanisms that give rise to the pathologic changes of these chronic airway conditions. The major distinction between chronic bronchitis and other airway disorders is, at present, etiologic. For example, in chronic bronchitis, the etiologic stimulus is presumed to be airway injury in response to cigarette smoke, air pollutants, or occupational exposures. Abnormalities in host defense and mucociliary clearance can lead to bronchiectasis. Alterations in salt and water transport due to mutations in the cystic fibrosis transmembrane regulator gene and a special spectrum of infecting bacteria are present in cystic fibrosis. It seems reasonable to expect that advances in understanding of the precise nature of and the host responses to these various stimuli will lead to an improved nosology of chronic bronchitis.

### Alterations in the Secretory Apparatus

A number of stimuli, considered from epidemiologic or clinical data to be potentially injurious, produce enlargement of the secretory apparatus in exposed animals. These

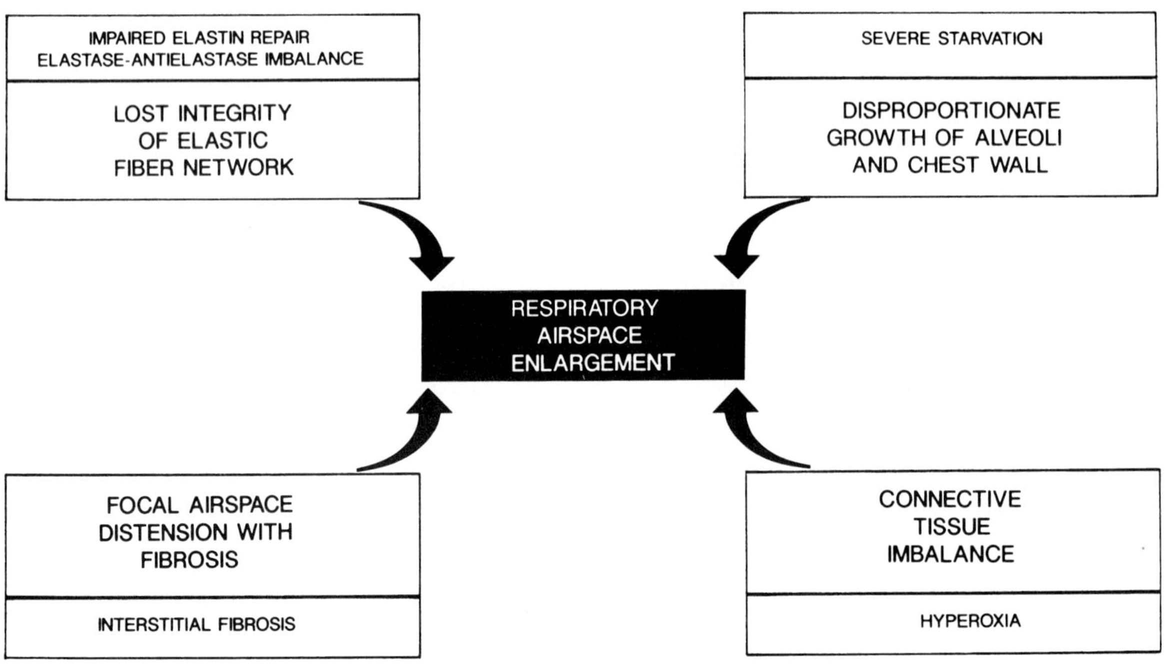


**Figure 38.17** Schema suggesting that respiratory air-space enlargement is a stereotyped response of the lungs to a variety of injuries is shown. Different injuries may give rise to air-space enlargement by different mechanisms: as a result of lost integrity of the elastic fiber network of the lungs, by focal air-space enlargement accompanying loss of alveoli and interstitial fibrosis, by the development of connective tissue imbalance, and by altering lung growth. (Reproduced with permission from Snider GL: Emphysema: The first two centuries and beyond; a historical overview, with suggestions for future research: Part 2. Am Rev Respir Dis 146:1615–1622, 1992.)

changes are considered analogous to the changes observed in chronic bronchitis. Included are irritant gases, endotoxin, acids, and proteases (Fig. 38.18).

Experimental chronic bronchial injury has been produced in rodents and dogs by sulfur dioxide[380–384] and tobacco smoke.[385, 386] The precise nature of the injury depends on the agent, its concentration, and the duration of the exposure. Chronic exposure of rats to sulfur dioxide induces predominantly central airway lesions, a finding generally attributed to the high solubility of the gas. There is a marked increase in the size of submucous glands in appropriate species and an increase in the proportion of goblet cells.[381] Exposing specific pathogen–free rats to cigarette smoke from 25 cigarettes daily for 14 days produces an increase in secretory cell proportion throughout the airways that is most marked in the peripheral airways.[386]

Secretory cell metaplasia also occurs in the central intrapulmonary airways of hamsters treated with 20 intratracheal instillations of endotoxin given over an 8-week period.[387] Similarly, dilute nitric, sulfuric, and hydrochloric acids instilled into the lungs of hamsters give rise to secretory cell metaplasia in the central airways.[388] The lesions appear to be related to the pH and persist for more than 4 months. (Regulation of airway secretion is reviewed in Chapter 14.)

## Experimental Bronchiolitis

Prolonged exposure of experimental animals to ozone[389–392] and nitrogen dioxide,[359, 389] at concentrations less than 1.0 and 10.0 ppm, respectively, produces damage focused on the junction of the conducting airways and the adjacent respiratory bronchioles in the centriacinar region; there is little injury to central airways. The lower the concentration of the oxidant gas, the more precise is this localization. The cells most susceptible to injury include the ciliated and secretory cells of the membranous bronchioles and the type I alveolar epithelial cells of the alveolated regions of the respiratory bronchioles; in contrast, type II alveolar epithelial cells are highly resistant. Following injury, bronchiolar secretory cell metaplasia becomes evident. The epithelium in adjacent alveolated airways changes from flat to cuboidal. Inflammatory cells are observed in the bronchiolar walls and lumens. With return of the animal to air breathing for extended periods, the bronchiolar and alveolated airway epithelium tends to return to normal. After 3 weeks of exposure of hamsters to ozone, for example, airflow limitation is present, but this disappears after 1 week of recovery.[387]

## Airway Inflammation

A variety of stimuli that can injure the airways are also capable of inducing airway neutrophilia. This has been demonstrated in animal models and in limited human exposures.[393–395] As noted earlier, the neutrophil is a potent source of both proteases and toxic oxidant species.[396] These substances, which can be released during inflammation, are capable of injuring airway epithelial cells in vitro[397–399] and in vivo. Instillation of neutrophil elastase and other serine proteases in hamster induces secretory cell metaplasia that is persistent (see Fig. 38.18).[290, 400] The human airways secrete a 12-kd protein, a secretory leukocyte protease inhibitor, that is capable of inactivating human neutrophil elastase[401] and preventing the induction of secretory cell metaplasia in hamsters.[402]

Intraluminal neutrophilia is a feature of chronic bronchitis,[186, 403] and infiltration of the airway wall with acute inflammatory cells including neutrophils is present during exacerbations.[404, 405] In chronic disease, neutrophils are present in the vicinity of glands.[188] Neutrophil elastase is a potent secretogogue, so it is likely that airway inflammation plays a key role in regulation of secretions.[406] In chronic disease, the airway wall is infiltrated with mononuclear cells, including monocytes and $CD8^+$ lymphocytes.[184, 407] These inflammatory cells appear to be one feature that may differentiate the inflammation of

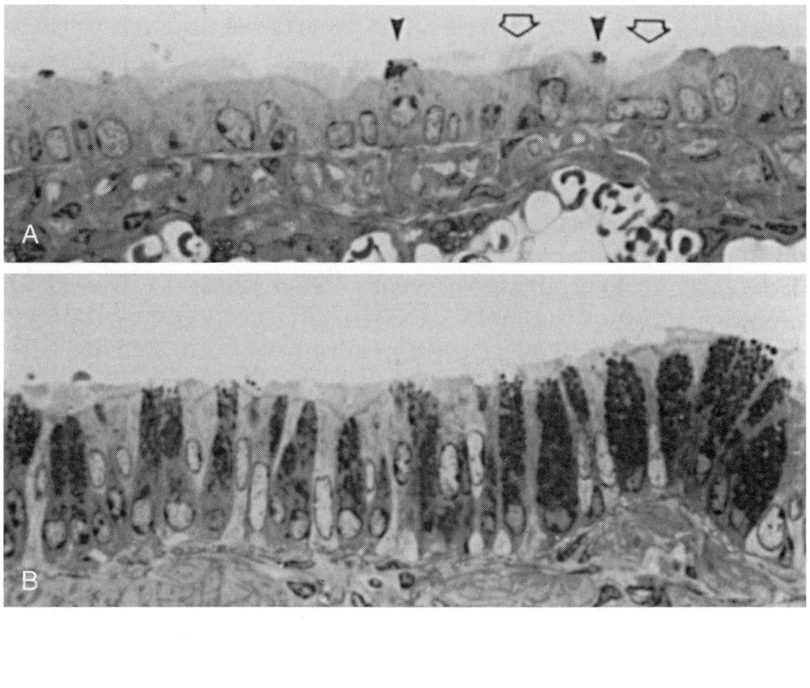


**Figure 38.18** Photomicrographs of plastic-embedded 1-μm section of main intrapulmonary bronchi of hamsters are shown. *A,* Saline-treated control. *B,* Hamster treated 16 days previously with 300 μg of human neutrophil elastase given intratracheally. In the saline-treated control only a few cells with black secretory granules are seen *(solid arrow),* many ungranulated secretory cells are present, as well as a few ciliated cells *(open arrows).* In the elastase-treated specimen, there has been a marked increase in the number of granulated secretory cells. Most cells are stuffed with large numbers of granules with a resultant increase in the height of the bronchial epithelium. This process is persistent. (Toluidine blue stain; original magnification ×620.) (Courtesy of Dr. Thomas Christensen, Boston, MA.)

chronic bronchitis from that of asthma. The presence of these chronic inflammatory cells is consistent with the concept that injuries that lead to altered airway anatomy in chronic bronchitis result not only from the direct effects of a toxic exposure but also from the secondary effects of the inflammatory response. In this regard, it is now clear that inflammatory mediators can alter the behavior of airway epithelial cells in many ways, including the induction of mucin gene expression.[408, 409]

The mechanisms by which various injuries lead to the development of inflammation and architectural changes in the airway are incompletely defined. Airway epithelial cells are capable of releasing a number of cytokines that can modulate the activity of inflammatory cells,[410–414] fibroblasts,[415–420] and other epithelial cells.[420, 421] Inflammatory cells are also capable not only of injuring parenchymal cells but also releasing cytokines that stimulate both epithelial cell[422, 423] and fibroblast[424] recruitment and proliferation. The processes that mediate airway repair under normal and pathologic conditions probably depend on complex quantitative, temporal, and spatial relationships among mediators produced by many cells present in the airways.

## Injury and Repair of Epithelial Cells

Injury of the airway epithelium from a variety of insults may lead to desquamation of cells.[397] Neighboring epithelial cells replicate rapidly and migrate to cover the wound.[405, 425, 426] These cells subsequently proliferate and differentiate, thus restoring epithelial integrity.[425–427] As with other migrating cell populations, however, the epithelial cells of the airways express attachment factors for extracellular matrix[398, 428, 429] and migrate in response to specific chemotactic stimuli.[421, 430, 431] Similarly, airway epithelial cells proliferate in response to a complex set of potential growth factors that might be involved in repair following injury.[432] Finally, differentiation of airway epithelial cells appears to involve a number of features, including the interactions with extracellular matrix and the presence of specific mediators.[433] This suggests that the repair process involves interactions between epithelial cells, mediators present within the local milieu, and the composition of the local extracellular matrix.

Repair of the airways involves not only the epithelial cells that line the airways but also the epithelial cells of the airway glands, the mesenchymal cells (fibroblasts and smooth muscle) present within the subepithelium, and the blood vessels that supply the airway structures. Undoubtedly, all these cells are also involved in the repair processes following injury. It seems likely that the processes that lead to smooth muscle[189] and glandular[181, 434] hypertrophy, peribronchiolar fibrosis,[27] and neovascularization,[404, 405, 435] which also characterize chronic bronchitis, are also initiated as part of the repair response.

Of these features, peribronchial fibrosis may be particularly important in contributing to expiratory airflow limitation.[27, 436] In this regard, a general property of fibrotic tissues is contraction. In the skin, this may serve to limit wound size and to maintain structural integrity. In a parenchymal organ, this contraction may lead to tissue distortion. This process may be responsible for the airway narrowing that characterizes airflow limitation in mild to moderate COPD. The mechanisms by which airway narrowing results are not delineated. Fibroblasts can, however, contract three-dimensional collagenous matrices, and this process can be modulated by exogenous mediators. Interestingly, epithelial cells can both regulate fibroblast contraction of collagenous matrices[437] and contract the matrices themselves.[438] This suggests that interactions between the epithelium and the mesenchyme in the airway may be important in regulating airway luminal diameter.

## Other Mediators of Airway Alteration

Some of the features of chronic bronchitis can develop without gross "injury." For example, the cells of the airway epithelium apparently undergo secretory cell metaplasia in response to protease treatment without the occurrence of a marked inflammatory cell recruitment and apparently without epithelial cell proliferation.[290] In this regard, features of glandular hypertrophy and secretory cell metaplasia can be produced in animal models by the administration of pilocarpine, isoproterenol, and methacholine.[380, 439] This suggests that the same mediators that regulate airway secretion and smooth muscle tone might also be able to regulate airway epithelial cell populations.

Data also support a role for other mediators to operate at several levels within the airway. Neuropeptides, for example, can acutely alter vascular[440, 441] and bronchial tone[442] and vascular permeability.[441, 443] Moreover, they can alter the ability of the epithelium to recruit inflammatory cells.[444] Similarly, inflammatory cell proteases may also function at several levels. As noted earlier, neutrophil elastase causes airway injury when administered at high doses.[290] At low concentrations, neutrophil elastase is a potent secretagogue.[406] Proteases, including neutrophil elastase, have been demonstrated to interact with cells through specific receptors regulating a variety of functions, including proliferation.[445, 446] Thus, it seems likely that a single mediator might have varying effects depending on its local concentration, the chronicity of its presence, and its interactions with other factors.

Finally, it is likely that many airway functions can be altered in an inflammatory environment. The airway epithelium, for example, produces a complex mixture of secretions that are responsible for mucociliary clearance and host defense.[447] Inflammatory mediators can alter not only cilia beating[448] but also the secretion of ions and water[449] as well as the secretion of macromolecules.[450, 451] The production of altered secretions and their altered handling appear to be important features of chronic airway injury. It is likely that factors present in the inflammatory milieu contribute to these alterations.

## Infection

The causal role of infection in chronic bronchitis remains unclear. Four potential scenarios are commonly considered, as pointed out in a critical review[452]: recurrent acute infectious exacerbations accelerate airway and parenchymal damage; bacteria cause acute exacerbations; chronic colonization and infection contribute to progressive airway and parenchymal damage; and childhood respiratory tract infection predisposes to development of COPD in adult life.

### Summary

There are a number of species differences in the growth and differentiation properties of cultured airway epithelial cells.[453, 454] Similarly, there are species differences in the responses of airways in animal models. Caution is therefore needed in generalizing from the animal models of chronic bronchitis to the human syndrome. An understanding of the human disorders requires studies performed on human cells and tissues to confirm concepts derived from animal studies.

The similarities of responses to a variety of injuries, however, suggest that a limited number of cellular processes are involved. The variations in the clinical syndrome, however, from some persons relentlessly developing airflow limitation to others remaining stable and yet others improving, implies that the processes are not fixed. Through better definition of these processes, it is likely that new therapeutic strategies for this syndrome can be developed.

## TREATMENT

Patients with COPD can be managed in an ambulatory setting, except when an exacerbation gives rise to the development of acute respiratory failure. Ambulatory therapy may be divided into three categories: specific, symptomatic, and secondary (therapy that improves the whole person without affecting lung function).

### Specific Therapy

Unfortunately, there is little available in the way of specific therapy. Occupational and other environmental inhaled irritants should be evaluated carefully and dealt with as circumstances dictate. Influenza vaccine should be given annually, and the pneumococcal vaccine should be given with a booster, currently recommended after 5 years for persons older than 65 years and for those with compromised host defense.[455] Both can be administered safely at the same time. The efficacy of the pneumococcal vaccine in preventing serious pneumococcal infections in COPD patients remains controversial,[456, 457] but its routine use is supported.[458]

### Smoking Cessation

Cigarette smoking is the most important cofactor in the cause of COPD, and every effort should be made to help the patient stop smoking, especially if the airflow limitation is only mild or moderate. (The many strategies that have been used to help patients stop smoking are reviewed in Chapters 98 and 99.) Unfortunately, no regimen can readily help all patients. Physicians should have a plan for assisting with smoking cessation. It has been shown that even a 1- to 2-minute delivery of advice to quit smoking has an important impact. As many as 5% of patients stop smoking in response to such advice.[459] The cessation rate is higher if this advice is supplemented by a self-help pamphlet such as the American Lung Association's *Freedom from Smoking* manual.

Nicotine replacement therapy is available with four formulations, all of which about double quit rates compared with a placebo.[460] Nicotine gum[461, 462] and transdermal nicotine,[463] when used in combination with behavior modification techniques, enhance smoking cessation rates. Nicotine transdermal systems are more convenient and without the oral side effects of nicotine gum. Bupropion is an antidepressant whose effectiveness as an aid to smoking cessation was demonstrated in two large trials.[464, 465] It can be used in combination with nicotine replacement. Smoking cessation rates in the best programs, however, rarely exceed 25% to 30% a year after a program is begun.[466]

The physician's greatest responsibility in counseling smoking cessation is to cigarette smokers who are found in the course of other examinations to have mild airflow limitation. In contrast to moderate airflow obstruction (which does not remit), mild pulmonary function abnormalities in persons who have been smoking for a relatively few years have been shown to be completely reversible.[467, 468]

### Development of New Therapeutic Initiatives

Efforts are going forward to develop and test artificial antiproteases that are administered by aerosol or by mouth to persons with normal serum protein levels. Similar efforts with other agents have been directed at other aspects of the inflammatory process. Antioxidants and agents that modulate inflammatory cell recruitment and activation have been suggested as potential therapeutic strategies.

The concept that lung function may be restored after its loss is also undergoing assessment. In this context, the observation that retinoids can induce accelerated alveolar development in neonatal animals[469] has been extended to animals with emphysema. In rats exposed to elastase, retinoic acid is able to induce an increase in alveolar surface area even if given after the emphysematous lesion has developed.[470] Studies extending these observations at both the mechanistic and clinical levels are underway or planned.

All studies designed to improve the natural history of COPD face a common problem. Because the disease progresses slowly, a relatively long time is needed to demonstrate a slowing of progression.[135] In addition, the changes likely to be observed are small, particularly when compared with the variation in the physiologic measures classically assessed in COPD (e.g., spirometry). As a result, studies of more than 1000 subjects for a period of years are needed in order to have adequate statistical power.[471] This is a function of the means of assessment and is independent of the intervention. More responsive measures of outcome in COPD are, therefore, urgently needed. A number have been suggested, including high-resolution CT, quality of life assessment, and measures of surrogate markers, particularly assessment of inflammation by histology, bronchoalveolar lavage, induced sputum, measures of elastin turnover, and exhaled air analysis. The hope is that it will be possible to prevent the progression of emphysema in persons who have the beginnings of this disease but are unable to stop smoking.[51, 472]

## Surgical Treatment for Emphysema

**Lung Volume Reduction Surgery.** Dr. Otto Brantigan pioneered resectional surgery for diffuse emphysema in the late 1950s. He hypothesized that removal of 20% to 30% of the most diseased-appearing sections of lung would increase traction on the distal airways and restore the dome shape of the diaphragm, thereby reducing airflow obstruction and improving the efficiency of the respiratory muscles. No physiologic measures were taken, but there was subjective improvement in 75% of survivors. A mortality rate of 16% soon caused the procedure to fall out of favor.[473]

Advances in technology and in surgical techniques resulting from experience with lung transplantation led to a revival of surgical treatment of emphysema. Wakabayashi and coworkers[474] and Brenner and coworkers[475] reported successful treatment of bullous emphysema with video-assisted thoracoscopy with carbon dioxide or yttrium-argon-gadolinium (YAG) laser. In 1993, Barth and colleagues[476] presented results from 20 patients who had undergone a resection of between 20% and 30% of each lung via median sternotomy. The improvements in physical measures were remarkable, as were the improvements in functional and quality of life measures. This report attracted considerable attention from the media, which led to an increased demand from the public for a surgical treatment of their debilitating disease. In December 1995, Medicare ceased payment for lung volume reduction surgery, justifying the decision by stating that no proof of efficacy had been established. The National Institutes of Health and the Health Care Financing Administration then decided to sponsor a randomized, controlled trial at a number of medical centers to evaluate the short-term effects of lung volume reduction surgery on pulmonary function, the mortality rate of the procedure, and the effect of resection on the rate of change in lung function.

A number of indications for lung volume reduction surgery have been published.[477, 478] Patients generally have severe fixed expiratory obstruction that has not improved with maximal medical therapy and who are markedly symptomatic with severe dyspnea. Patients with CT scans showing a prominent distribution of emphysema in the upper lobes, with a heterogeneous distribution confirmed by ventilation-perfusion scans, appear to be the best candidates for surgery.

Changes in multiple physiologic parameters have been reported for lung volume reduction surgery. Improvements in $FEV_1$ measured 3 to 6 months after bilateral surgery demonstrate mean increases of 25% to 58%, with a range between 16% and 96%. Changes in FVC range from 12% to 40%. Changes in total lung capacity have ranged from an increase of 7% to a decrease of 20%. Residual volume is reduced by 10% to 33%.[477] Despite these remarkable improvements, evidence is now emerging that they may be short-lived.

As discussed earlier, the natural history of COPD results in a loss of 20 to 40 mL per year in measurements of $FEV_1$. In Lung Health Study I, $FEV_1$ declined 34 mL per year in those patients who successfully quit smoking. Brenner and colleagues[479] reported an average loss in $FEV_1$ of 163 mL per year in a number of patients who had undergone a variety of lung volume reduction surgery procedures. Cooper and colleagues[480] reported a decline in $FEV_1$, estimated at 120 mL per year. In a recent report on a smaller group of patients from Boston, Ingenito and colleagues[481] reported an annualized decline in $FEV_1$ of 93 to 140 mL per year. The data suggest that the procedures that result in the greatest change in $FEV_1$ also result in the most rapid decline in $FEV_1$ postoperatively. An extrapolation of this more rapid decline would suggest that the majority of those patients undergoing lung volume reduction surgery derive a benefit in lung function that lasts only 3 to 4 years. This natural history following the surgical procedure may become more clear when the results of the National Emphysema Treatment Trial are released.[482]

Multiple reports demonstrate improvements in functional capacity as measured by exercise testing or a 6-minute walk test. Health-related quality of life is another measure that has been used in studies of lung volume reduction surgery. There are two types of health-related quality of life measures: general health measures such as the Sickness Impact Profile, the Quality of Well-Being Scale, and the Medical Outcomes Survey Short Form 36 (MOS SF-36); and disease-specific measures such as the Chronic Respiratory Disease Questionnaire or the St. Georges Respiratory Questionnaire. Disease-specific questionnaires are more sensitive to therapeutic interventions in COPD, and one study has demonstrated significant improvements in all four domains of the Chronic Respiratory Disease Questionnaire, while another has demonstrated significant improvements in patients undergoing lung volume reduction surgery as measured by the St. Georges Respiratory Questionnaire.[483, 484] Follow-up on the health-related quality of life questionnaires has been reported for only 6 months after lung volume reduction surgery. With regard to the MOS SF-36, significant improvements have been reported in the domains of physical functioning, social functioning, and vitality, with social functioning appearing to have the best correlation with improvement in $FEV_1$ and improvements in physical functioning correlating best with improvement in the 6-minute walk.[485]

The 16% mortality rate reported by Brantigan reduced acceptance of the procedure. More recent published operative mortality rates for lung volume reduction surgery range from 0% to 19%. The variability in these rates is probably due to a number of factors, including different definitions of surgical mortality, patient selection, surgical technique, experience with the procedure, and perioperative management. As a recent review suggests, comparison of surgical and nonsurgical treatments is not easily done.[482] In a recent study comparing patients denied lung volume reduction surgery with a similar group of patients who underwent the procedure, the survival rate for the surgical group was 82% and for the medical group, 64%.[486] In recent data on 722 patients released by the Health Care Financing Administration,[482] mortality was 23% at 12 months after surgery and 28% at 18 months postoperatively. Morbidity also increased in terms of acute hospitalization from 197 to 304 in the year following surgery, increasing from an average of 11.8 days a year before surgery to 18.7 days in the year after surgery.[482]

The future of lung volume reduction surgery as a viable treatment option for emphysema remains unclear. The National Emphysema Treatment Trial will provide some indication of where surgery might fit into the armamentarium of therapy for emphysema, but the results of that trial lie many years hence. For now, those patients who are willing to travel to a center in the National Emphysema Treatment Trial should be aware that it is a randomized, controlled trial. Other trials are either underway or are planned in both the United States and other countries. Some medical centers will allow surgery for individuals with financial resources.

**Lung Transplantation.** Transplantation of the lung has proved more difficult than transplantation of other solid organs such as kidney, heart, or liver. It is the only organ in constant communication with the atmosphere, it is prone to infection as well as rejection, and there are special problems related to its preservation before transplantation.[487] Nevertheless, there has been considerable progress in lung transplantation over the past 15 years. Most initial operations were heart-lung or double-lung transplantations, but currently single-lung transplantation is the more prevalent procedure. Since the early 1980s, when the first successful lung transplantations were performed, there have been more than 6400 lung transplantation procedures performed worldwide.[488]

The experience with single-lung transplantation in the 1970s was unsatisfactory.[489] The problem was thought to be preferential inflation and ventilation of the native lung because of its greater compliance. As a result, there was mediastinal shift and compression of the transplanted lung. Perfusion of the transplanted lung without proportional ventilation resulted in ventilation-perfusion mismatch.[281, 489–491] Consequently, as lung transplantation came of age during the 1980s, surgeons developed single-lung transplantation for use in patients with interstitial pulmonary fibrosis.[492] Only heart-lung and double-lung transplantation were used for patients with end-stage chronic obstructive airway diseases. Most of the patients receiving transplants had emphysema, frequently with API deficiency; other patients suffered from cystic fibrosis, bronchiectasis, bronchiolitis obliterans, eosinophilic granuloma, and lymphangioleiomyomatosis.[281, 491, 493]

In 1989, Mal and colleagues[494] reported two successful single-lung transplants for end-stage emphysema, and the procedure was then quickly revived by transplant surgeons.[491, 495] Single-lung transplantation is a much easier operation to perform than double-lung transplantation, and cardiac bypass is usually not necessary. The operative early and late morbidity and mortality rates are lower than for double-lung transplantation. Provided that the predicted vital capacity of the donor is larger than the recipient's by an average of 1.4, mediastinal shift has not been a problem.[496] Postoperative follow-up is still brief.

The FVC and $FEV_1$ are lower for single-lung than for double-lung transplantation. There is an excess of ventilation over perfusion in the transplanted lung, but this has little effect on improvement in exercise performance in single-lung compared with double-lung transplantation. Arterial blood gases are similarly improved in the two procedures.[491]

Single-lung transplantation is more applicable to an older population (50 to 60 years) than double-lung transplantation; despite its relative ease, the procedure still requires the full expertise of a lung transplant group. The limiting factor in the performance of single-lung transplantation for emphysema at this time is the paucity of donor lungs. COPD is the most common reason for lung transplantation worldwide. Lung transplantation is discussed in detail in Chapter 97.

**Surgery for Bullous Lung Disease.** In the presence of a giant radiolucent air space in the chest in a patient with compromised lung function, surgical excision may be considered. If lung function is not improved by the surgery, however, the morbidity and mortality rates of the procedure are high. It is not easy to know when to undertake surgery.

The determinants of the outcome of surgery are the size of the bulla and the impairment of function of the nonbullous lung tissue. Two mechanisms have been invoked for impairment of function by a giant bulla. There may be compression of nonbullous lung by a giant bulla whose intrapleural pressure is high and whose volume does not change during respiration, or there may be impairment of ventilation because of the large amount of space occupied in the thorax by the bulla, with resultant loss of linkage between the chest wall and the nonbullous lung tissue.[21, 84] There is little improvement in function after excision when bullae occupy less than one third of the hemithorax and lung function is normal or minimally impaired. The presence of generalized emphysema is also a predictor of a poor result.

As already noted, surgery in the presence of a low $FEV_1$, hypercapnia, or cor pulmonale is fraught with danger unless compressed, relatively normal lung can be released by the operation.[83, 497] Study of serial chest radiographs and pulmonary function data are helpful in judging whether compression of normal lung by bullae is responsible for the patient's current functional state or whether this represents progression of generalized emphysema. The presence of emphysema in nonbullous lung and the amount of compression can, however, be best assessed by CT, performed if possible at both full inspiration and full expiration.[84, 89] Bronchography, angiography, and studies of regional pulmonary function add little to CT data. In general, patients do best who have large bullae occupying at least 30% to 50% of the hemithorax and an $FEV_1$ of about half the predicted normal value.[21, 497] Other physiologic parameters predictive of successful surgery include plethysmographic lung volumes substantially larger than those measured by helium dilution, indicating sequestered gas, and a reasonably well-preserved diffusing capacity and normocapnia.[498]

The amount of uninvolved lung tissue resected should be kept to a minimum. Follow-up reveals that resection of giant bullae does not affect the size of remaining bullae.[497, 499]

## Symptomatic Therapy

Symptomatic relief is directed against the four reversible elements of airflow limitation: mucosal congestion and edema, increased secretions, bronchial smooth muscle contraction, and cellular infiltration and inflammation. The airways may be hyperresponsive, with excessive narrowing occurring in response to various stimuli.[500] The relative proportions of the mechanisms that cause airflow limitation vary markedly from patient to patient and in the same patient at different times. Careful clinical assessment, coupled with sputum examination, provides insights into which mechanisms are most important in a particular patient at a particular time.

### Bronchodilators

Bronchodilator agents, including beta-agonists, anticholinergic agents, and theophylline, remain mainstays in the treatment of COPD. Theophylline and to a lesser extent beta-agonists demonstrate many physiologic effects other than bronchodilation that may benefit patients with COPD. (Airway pharmacology is discussed in Chapter 11, and the drugs used in asthma are discussed in Chapter 39.)

**Sympathomimetic Drugs (Beta-Agonists).** Beta$_2$-adrenergic agonists have less effect on cardiac acceleration for a given degree of bronchodilation than do beta$_1$-agonists and are the sympathomimetic drugs of choice for treating COPD. In this chapter, the term *beta-agonist* used without further specification refers to a beta$_2$-agonist.

There is substantial evidence supporting the usefulness of beta-agonists in treating patients with COPD. First, many COPD patients demonstrate a significant bronchodilator response to these agents[501]; initial spirometry in the intermittent positive pressure breathing trial with approximately 900 patients showed an average bronchodilator response to 250 μg of inhaled isoproterenol of 15% of baseline FEV$_1$, with more than 30% of patients showing responses of 20% or greater.[32, 502] Of importance, failure to achieve a significant bronchodilator response at the outset of this study did not necessarily signify fixed airflow limitation. Approximately 70% of the patients who were initially unresponsive showed at least one response of more than 15% of baseline during the seven follow-up spirometry tests.

Beta-agonists enhance mucous clearance in COPD patients by accelerating mucociliary transport[503] and perhaps by inducing a chloride transport–mediated water shift into the bronchial lumen.[504] They do not appear to inhibit mucous gland secretion.[505] Beta-agonists may improve the endurance of fatigued respiratory muscles, but do not alter respiratory muscle strength.[506] It has been suggested but not proven that either regularly scheduled[507] or as-needed[508] beta-agonist therapy can delay deterioration of lung function in COPD patients with reversible airflow limitation. The long-acting beta-agonist salmeterol is effective in COPD[509] and is associated with improvement in quality of life using a validated health status instrument.[510]

The preferred mode for administering beta-agonists is by inhalation with a metered-dose inhaler (MDI) or a dry powder inhaler (DPI). These methods are superior to oral administration in improving FEV$_1$ and produce fewer side effects.[511] A large number of studies have also shown convincingly that a properly used MDI is as effective as and less expensive than nebulized aqueous solutions of beta-agonist. The ease of use of DPIs and the lack of necessity for a propellant suggest that they will become the standard. There is a place for beta-agonist solution administered by electrically powered nebulizers in patients too weak to use an inhaler device, in those with altered mental status,[512] or in those whose inspiratory capacity is too limited to permit effective inhalation[512]; intermittent positive pressure breathing is not indicated for this purpose.[501]

Careful and repeated instruction is often necessary if patients are to derive maximum benefit from an MDI (Table 38.3).[513] Modest dose increases beyond the usually recommended 2 puffs every 4 to 6 hours may be necessary for maximum bronchodilation.[514] Such dosing is generally safe because even with five or six actuations of an MDI only a few milligrams of a beta-agonist are inhaled. By this route, side effects are usually limited to a modest increase in heart rate and mild skeletal muscle tremor.[515] These symptoms usually diminish after long-term drug use. Small falls in serum potassium level are generally of no consequence.[515] The technique of sequential inhalation, taking 2 to 5 inhalations from an MDI separated by 1 to 2 minutes, may maximize pulmonary function by facilitating penetration of inhaled beta-agonist through previously obstructed airways.

MDI extension devices or spacers are another means of improving beta-agonist delivery to the lungs. The actual deposition in the lungs of a beta-agonist using the most popular spacers (Aerochamber, Monoghan; Inspirease, Schering) is only marginally improved over deposition by a properly used MDI alone.[516] Spacers improve beta-agonist inhalation by minimizing problems of hand-to-

**Table 38.3** STEPS FOR APPROPRIATE USE OF METERED DOSE INHALER

| |
|---|
| Remove cap |
| Shake inhaler |
| Hold inhaler upright |
| Tilt head back 10 to 15 degrees |
| Position inhaler 2–4 cm in front of open mouth* |
| Begin inhalation and then activate inhaler |
| Inhale slowly and deeply to total lung capacity |
| Hold breath for 5–10 seconds |
| Exhale slowly through nose† |
| Inhale on puff; wait 3–5 minutes between inhalation of subsequent puff |

*Patients with poor hand-to-breath coordination should seal lips around mouthpiece.
†May deliver medication to nose and sinuses with improvement of coexisting rhinitis and sinusitis.

breath coordination because aerosolized particles remain in suspension for 5 seconds or longer. They may be used by stable patients who display poor MDI technique and by all COPD patients during acute exacerbations of their disease, when a slow inspiratory maneuver and a 5- to 10-second inspiratory breath-hold are difficult to accomplish. The prevailing opinion is that an MDI without a spacer suffices for most COPD patients.[517] Use of a spacer not specifically designed for use with an inhaler may result in unpredictable administration and, if used, should be guided by empirical clinical results.

Because they require substantially higher dosing with enhanced risk of toxicity, oral beta-agonists should be reserved for COPD patients who fail to respond satisfactorily to a regimen of inhaled bronchodilators and used together with a modest dose of oral theophylline or for patients who consistently refuse to employ an MDI, a DPI, or a compressor nebulizer. If used, they should be prescribed in low doses (5 to 10 mg of metaproterenol, 2 mg of albuterol, or 2.5 mg of terbutaline) every 6 to 8 hours. Oral albuterol and metaproterenol both produce less skeletal muscle tremor than does oral terbutaline.[518, 519] Mild tachycardia and an increase in premature ventricular contractions have been noted with these agents.[520]

**Anticholinergics.** Anticholinergic bronchodilators have been used in Western medicine since the early 1800s[521] and have recently regained importance in the management of patients with COPD. Unlike atropine, ipratropium bromide given as an inhaled aerosol is not absorbed and is essentially free of anticholinergic side effects. It has become the prototypic anticholinergic agent in modern use. Glycopyrrolate, which, like ipratropium, is a quaternary ammonium compound, is available as a solution for nebulizer use, although it is not approved by the US Food and Drug Administration for this purpose. Oxitropium bromide is not available in the United States. Tiotropium is an anticholinergic agent with a markedly prolonged duration of action, lasting at least 36 hours.[522] It is currently in clinical trials.

Like all current anticholinergic agents, ipratropium acts by competing with acetylcholine for postganglionic muscarinic receptors on airway smooth muscle cells. Bronchodilation by ipratropium is thought to be due to inhibition of cholinergically mediated bronchomotor tone[523, 524]; greater relative bronchodilation by anticholinergic agents seems to occur as the severity of airflow limitation worsens.[525] The main bronchodilator effect has been reported to be within the larger airways,[526] but muscarinic receptors have been shown to be present in all human airways, suggesting the potential for a more generalized bronchodilator response.[527] Ipratropium can also block the efferent limb of vagally mediated reflex arcs, thereby preventing bronchoconstriction triggered by a wide range of nonspecific agents such as dusts, fumes, and cigarette smoke that act on sensory receptors within the respiratory tract.

Ipratropium for bronchodilation is currently available as an MDI, as a nebulized solution in the United States, and as an MDI combined with albuterol. The MDI delivers 18 μg of ipratropium/puff and can be employed with a spacer. The usual dose is 36 μg (2 puffs) on a fixed schedule every 4 to 6 hours, although doses up to 72 μg (4 puffs) or 108 μg (6 puffs) may provide further benefit to some COPD patients.[528–530] Tachyphylaxis does not occur even after long-term use.[531] Side effects are limited to occasional mild xerostomia, short paroxysms of cough, and mydriasis with blurred vision if the aerosol is accidentally sprayed into the eyes. Ipratropium does not affect airway mucociliary clearance adversely[532] and, unlike beta-agonists, does not worsen hypoxemia[533] or cause tachycardia or skeletal muscle tremor.[534]

Ipratropium can increase the $FEV_1$ and FVC significantly in COPD patients, generally in the range of 200 to 400 mL.[525, 528, 529] Major improvement in airway conductance has also been noted, with reductions in functional residual capacity and residual volume, indicating diminished air trapping.[528] Ipratropium can further improve pulmonary function in COPD patients receiving maintenance corticosteroids,[531, 532] as well as in patients who have therapeutic blood levels of theophylline.[528, 531] A recent report suggests that ipratropium may decrease exacerbation frequency and decreased total medical costs compared with the beta-agonist albuterol.[535] If this analysis is subsequently confirmed, it will represent a significant new clinical goal of ipratropium therapy.

**Inhaled Anticholinergics vs. Beta-Agonists.** It is not clear from the literature whether ipratropium or a beta-agonist is preferable for initial management of COPD. Ipratropium produces fewer side effects than inhaled beta-agonists. On the other hand, beta-agonists reduce bronchial hyperactivity to a greater extent than ipratropium,[536] and this may be advantageous. Patients often prefer an inhaled beta-agonist to ipratropium because of the agonist's more rapid onset of action and relief of dyspnea.[521] Because the newer anticholinergic drugs are poorly absorbed when delivered by aerosol, because they have been reported to produce greater bronchodilation than normally prescribed doses of beta-agonists,[528] and because they decrease sputum volume without altering its viscosity,[537] anticholinergics drugs have been recommended as first-line therapy.[538]

The result of controlled trials in COPD are controversial. In studies that compared the usual doses of both agents, the bronchodilator efficacy of ipratropium has been reported to be comparable with,[539] superior to,[531, 540, 541] or inferior to[542] that of beta-agonists. In studies in which the agents were given sequentially in large doses, the ipratropium was sometimes superior to the beta-agonists,[524] but it has more often been equipotent.[528, 536, 543–545] The problem is that, when planning comparisons, it is not clear how to determine equipotent doses of the two agents.

To date bronchodilators are used for symptom relief, and their use is empirical. It is reasonable to give them a clinical trial. If little benefit is obtained, it may be reasonable to forego therapy. A repeated clinical trial, however, may be warranted over time, as, with disease progression, responsiveness may increase. The following seems a reasonable approach at this time. Because of lower cost and more rapid onset of action, bronchodilator therapy can be initiated with an inhaled beta-agonist, particularly if symptoms are episodic, and continued in patients whose airflow limitation is well controlled. A trial of a fixed schedule of inhaled ipratropium can be performed for COPD patients who are not doing well with the beta-agonist, whether because of severe side effects or poor bronchodilator response. For patients who fail to improve sufficiently after standard dose therapy with ipratropium or a beta-agonist, a trial of high-dose ipratropium, 4 to 6 puffs (72 to 108 μg) four to six times daily, may provide further benefit with no increase in side effects, as would likely be the case if higher doses of inhaled beta-agonist were employed,[528, 529] but this has not been proven.[543] A combination of inhaled ipratropium and a beta-agonist may be more effective than monotherapy.

During an acute exacerbation of COPD requiring emergency room treatment, ipratropium appeared to be only equally effective as inhaled beta-agonists, with no further benefit from combination therapy.[546, 547] Ipratropium did not provide additional improvement when added to an emergency room regimen of inhaled beta-agonists and corticosteroids.[547] There is one report, however, that addition of ipratropium to beta-agonist therapy accelerated the improvement of COPD exacerbations and shortened the duration of emergency room treatment.[548]

**Theophylline.** Theophylline has been employed by physicians in the United States for about 70 years. Some disillusionment with theophylline, however, stems from a high frequency of toxicity[549–551] and from difficulties in dosing owing to substantial variation in hepatic metabolism of the drug. Furthermore, several double-blind crossover studies[552–554] demonstrated little or no improvement in patients' symptoms of dyspnea, wheezing, and cough, even though increases of 10% to 15% were observed in patients' baseline $FEV_1$ and FVC values.

This assault on theophylline has been countered by reports that document improved maximal exercise performance of patients taking theophylline,[555] a 16% decrease in pulmonary work during walking, and a preference by patients for theophylline over placebo.[556] A significant reduction in dyspnea based on an elaborate three-component dyspnea scoring system has also been reported.[557] Moreover, investigators in a well-conducted trial have shown that theophylline in COPD significantly improves arterial partial pressures of oxygen and carbon dioxide through increases in tidal volume and minute ventilation.[558] On the basis of these findings, many authorities believe that theophylline, when used judiciously, continues to have a useful role in the ambulatory management of COPD. The development of more selective phosphodiesterase inhibitors[559] may provide the benefits of theophylline without its difficulties.

***Physiologic Benefits.*** Although theophylline functions as a bronchodilator with minimal, if any, tachyphylaxis even after long-term use, its bronchodilator activity in COPD patients is less than that produced by ipratropium bromide[560] or an inhaled beta-agonist.[561, 562] Theophylline has many other physiologic effects that might benefit patients with COPD, and these generally occur at theophylline blood levels around 10 μg/mL. These benefits include enhancement of mucociliary clearance,[563] stimulation of central respiratory drive,[564] reduction in pulmonary vascular resistance together with improved cardiac contractility manifested by increases in right and left ventricular ejection fractions,[565] and improved lung function during sleep without impairment of sleep quality.[566] Theophylline has also been shown to augment diaphragmatic strength and endurance in COPD patients,[558, 567] although such benefit has not been found consistently.[568]

***Toxicity.*** The minor side effects of theophylline in patients with COPD consist of tremor, insomnia, irritability, and upper gastrointestinal upset with nausea and heartburn, as well as lower intestinal tract upset such as flatulence and bloating. These symptoms may occur at blood levels well below 20 μg/mL, generally subside after several weeks of treatment, and can often be avoided by starting the drug at a low dose followed by a gradual increase until a therapeutic level is attained.

Major side effects include vomiting and more importantly supraventricular arrhythmias (especially multifocal atrial tachycardia), ventricular arrhythmias, hypotension, and seizures. The latter may be fatal or result in serious impairment of cerebral function. Major toxicity generally occurs at blood levels that are quite high, above 30 to 35 μg/mL.[569] It is important to note, however, that life-threatening consequences may occur with serum theophylline concentrations close to 20 μg/mL, a level at which only minor toxicity is usually thought to occur. Patients older than 60 years are especially prone to serious theophylline toxicity at these relatively low levels[570]; major toxicity can occur without prior warning by minor toxicity.

***Metabolism.*** Approximately 85% to 90% of orally administered theophylline is metabolized into relatively inactive compounds in the liver, probably by the cytochrome P-450 system.[569, 571] Many factors can influence theophylline metabolism (Table 38.4).[572] Theophylline metabolism is increased by tobacco and marijuana smoking, hyperthyroidism, cystic fibrosis, and ingestion of some drugs such as phenytoin. Metabolism is higher in children and adolescents than in adults and decreases as adults grow older. There are genetically programmed slow and rapid metabolizers.[573] Occasional patients display nonlinear dose-dependent kinetics of the Michaelis-Menten type; under these circumstances, a small dose increase in theophylline can cause a disproportionately large increase in serum level.[574] Theophylline metabolism is decreased in patients with hepatic dysfunction due to hepatitis, cirrhosis, or congestive heart failure; the daily theophylline dose required to maintain a particular blood level may fall by 25% to 50%. Metabolism of the drug is decreased by a high carbohydrate diet and severe acute illnesses. Many drugs may slow theophylline excretion and require a major reduction in standard theophylline dosing to avoid possible toxicity.[575] In summary, many factors can result in enormous variations in the theophylline blood levels of patients receiving similar daily theophylline doses.

***Preparations.*** Slow-release anhydrous theophylline preparations were a major advance in ambulatory theophylline therapy. These are well absorbed after oral inges-

**Table 38.4 FACTORS AFFECTING THEOPHYLLINE METABOLISM IN CHRONIC OBSTRUCTIVE PULMONARY DISEASE (COPD)**

| Increase Metabolism | Decrease Metabolism |
|---|---|
| Cigarette smoking | Age > 60 years |
| High-protein diet | COPD with severe hypoxemia (arterial $Po_2$ < 45 mm Hg) |
| Hyperthyroidism | Congestive heart failure |
| Marijuana smoking | Hepatic dysfunction |
| Drugs | High-carbohydrate diet |
| Barbiturates | Severe acute illness |
| Carbamazepine | Viral infections (influenza) |
| Phenytoin | Drugs |
| Rifampin | Allopurinol |
| | Cimetidine |
| | Ciprofloxacin |
| | Erythromycin |
| | Oral contraceptives |
| | Propranolol |
| | Ticlopidine |
| | Thiabendazole |
| | Troleandomycin |
| | Verapamil |

tion and improve patient compliance. Preparations are available for once-daily (every 24 hours) or twice-daily (every 12 hours) dosing. It is often necessary for rapid theophylline metabolizers, however, to prescribe the every-12-hour preparations every 8 hours and the every-24-hour preparations twice daily to avoid wide fluctuations in theophylline blood concentrations.[576]

***Dosing.*** The problems of theophylline toxicity and its highly varied metabolism, together with the recognition that most if not all of the physiologic benefits of theophylline, including improvement in airflow obstruction, occur at theophylline blood levels around 10 μg/mL,[572, 577] have led to a recommendation that the ideal target level for theophylline should be 10 ± 3 μg/mL. A reasonable initial dose for an average-sized adult without heart failure or liver disease is 200 mg of a slowly absorbed theophylline preparation every 12 hours. If the therapeutic response is not satisfactory, the dose may be increased by 100 or 200 mg daily at 4- to 7-day intervals to a dose of 800 to 1000 mg/day. If the response is still not satisfactory, a blood level should be measured at a time midway between doses, before proceeding with further increases of the drug dose.[549, 575] The availability of dipstick theophylline kits that can use a drop of blood has made routine office monitoring of theophylline levels practical.

***Combination Therapy with Inhaled Agents.*** Several studies of patients with COPD have convincingly shown that combination therapy with oral theophylline and an inhaled beta-agonist produces more bronchodilation than either drug alone.[561, 578–580] The benefit seems to be additive, with improvement in breathlessness as well as spirometric indices; the response is less in patients who respond poorly to an inhaled beta-agonist (<15% to 20% increase in $FEV_1$). Dosing may be the same as when each drug is taken alone, but lower doses of each may provide satisfactory bronchodilation without toxicity.

## Corticosteroids

Corticosteroids objectively benefit only 15% to 20% of stable COPD patients with significant airflow limitation as determined by a 20% or greater improvement in baseline $FEV_1$.[581, 582] A far larger proportion of COPD patients feel subjectively better while taking these agents, with some patients also showing $FEV_1$ increases greater than 20% after placebo.[583] In a meta-analysis of 16 well-designed corticosteroid trials, patients with stable COPD treated with oral corticosteroids experienced a 20% or better improvement in their baseline $FEV_1$ only about 10% more often than similar patients receiving a placebo.[583] Long-term corticosteroid use is known to produce a myriad of side effects, including osteoporosis with disabling fractures,[584] difficult-to-control diabetes mellitus, systemic hypertension, peptic ulcer disease, and enhanced susceptibility to serious infections.[585] Patients with COPD may be particularly susceptible to steroid-induced bone disease.[586]

Unfortunately, a trial of therapy is the only way of identifying corticosteroid responders. A trial of corticosteroids based on morning doses of prednisone in the range of 0.25 to 0.5 mg/kg per day or its equivalent has been recommended for COPD patients who are doing poorly with an otherwise optimal bronchodilator regimen. Baseline spirometry values should be obtained and the test repeated after 2 to 3 weeks of corticosteroids. If the postcorticosteroid $FEV_1$ value has not increased by at least 20% to 25% over the baseline $FEV_1$ value, the drug should be rapidly tapered and stopped. If corticosteroids prove helpful, the daily dose should be tapered to the smallest amount that will sustain improvement. Substitution with an inhaled corticosteroid is common practice. Periodic COPD flare-ups can be managed with short-term high-dose oral corticosteroids with rapid tapering over 10 to 14 days[587]; intravenous and oral steroids also reduce further relapses after emergency room treatment of COPD exacerbations.[588] Another approach, designed to decrease side effects, is to institute alternative-day prednisone in doses that are twice the daily dose.[589]

Corticosteroid aerosols are safer than oral corticosteroids and are often used to avoid the toxicity of oral steroids. Inhaled corticosteroids have clear benefits in COPD, both improving airflow and reducing exacerbation frequency and severity,[590] although some studies suggest that they are less beneficial than oral corticosteroid therapy in relieving airflow limitation and in improving symptoms.[591–594] Nevertheless, patients often experience partial clinical benefit, and some patients respond to inhaled but not oral corticosteroids.[593, 595] When high-dose steroids are used, the steroid MDI should be attached to a spacer to minimize oropharyngeal deposition of the drug with the intent of decreasing the risk of oral candidiasis and hoarseness due to laryngeal myopathy.[596] Rinsing the mouth after inhaler use is usually sufficient to prevent these side effects when small steroid doses are used.

Adrenal suppression may occur at inhaled doses greater than 1500 μg of beclomethasone dipropionate per day.[597] Inhaled corticosteroids may also be associated with increased risk of fracture in COPD patients.[586]

Because of their reduced systemic delivery of drug, inhaled corticosteroids have a significant therapeutic advantage for chronic use in COPD patients. As a result, many clinicians have initiated therapeutic trials with inhaled corticosteroids. There are as yet no clear guidelines for this practice, but some evidence suggests that it is very reasonable. This is supported by the idea that oral clinical challenges of several weeks may be of insufficient duration to provide clinical benefit.

Inhaled corticosteroids have also been evaluated as agents to alter the relentless loss of function that characterizes COPD. Four large trials have been initiated, and three are completed. The results, as presented at international meetings, suggest that glucocorticoids do not slow decline in function. In contrast, the benefits in airflow noted above were generally confirmed, particularly in more severe patients. In addition, the reduction in exacerbations was confirmed in one study along with an improvement in health status compared with the results with a placebo. When these studies are published, the data will help to guide the use of inhaled corticosteroids for COPD.

## Cromolyn Sodium and Nedocromil

There are no data establishing that either cromolyn or nedocromil is effective in the treatment of COPD. Nevertheless, a clinical trial may be warranted, particularly with patients with evidence of hyperreactive airways.[598]

## Thinning and Mobilization of Airway Secretions

Increased mucous production by hypertrophied and hyperplastic airway submucosal glands and goblet cells together with impaired mucociliary clearance and cough are the rule in COPD patients. Sputum expectoration may range from only a few milliliters on awakening in the morning to frank bronchorrhea, with day-long production of sputum exceeding 100 mL/day.

The most successful means of controlling excessive airway mucous secretion is avoidance of inhaled irritants. Smoking cessation usually reduces sputum expectoration dramatically over several months[20]; the early period of smoking cessation is often associated with more difficult cough and expectoration, especially in the morning. Patients should avoid smoke-filled rooms and stay indoors when air pollution reaches dangerous levels. Air conditioners and electrostatic precipitators can reduce indoor air pollution.

Mucolytic agents are not used in the United States, but some agents are used widely elsewhere. *N*-acetylcysteine, in particular, is popular in Europe. This agent has been evaluated in large well-designed trials and is associated with an improvement in symptoms and in exacerbation frequency.[599] The agent is an active antioxidant, and this may be its means of action rather than its properties as a mucolytic. Because it can also reverse epithelial metaplasia in an animal model,[386] it continues to attract interest. Iodinated glycerol was previously available in the United States and may have some symptomatic benefits,[600] but this drug has been removed from the marketplace because of toxicity concerns. SSKI (potassium iodide) may be an alternative. Recombinant human DNAse, currently used for cystic fibrosis, has not proved useful for chronic bronchitis despite initial favorable reports in acute exacerbations of bronchitis.[601]

**Expectorants.** Therapy with beta-agonists and theophylline enhances mucociliary clearance. Bronchorrhea may be controlled by oral corticosteroids[505] and by inhaled indomethacin[602] and atropine.[603] Ipratropium bromide is not used to influence airway mucous production or clearance. The role of oral expectorants in promoting mucous clearance in COPD patients remains controversial; the consensus is that agents such as guaifenesin and glyceryl guaiacolate provide little or no benefit for most patients.[604]

Although patients can be encouraged to drink several glasses of water per day, aggressive hydration in COPD patients has not been shown to affect sputum volume, the physical properties of sputum, or the ease of expectoration favorably.[605] Bland aerosols of water or saline are also of limited value in clearing airway secretions in COPD, and such aerosols can precipitate bronchospasm.[606] Some patients expectorate thick secretions more readily after inhaling steam from hot water in a sink.

**Controlled Coughing.** Cough is usually impaired in COPD patients, with frequent uncontrolled coughing inducing fatigue, chest wall pain, and dyspnea. An effective cough is the best means of expelling airway mucus. Controlled cough and the forced expiratory technique, or huffing, have been advocated as safe, useful alternatives.[607] With controlled cough, patients are taught to inspire deeply, hold their breath for a few seconds, and then cough two or three times with the mouth open and without taking another breath. After repeating this sequence several times, patients should rest before beginning the procedure again if this is necessary. Controlled cough is believed to work because the cleansing action of cough in large airways takes place primarily during the first one or two coughs of a cough sequence.[608] The forced expiratory technique consists of one or two forced exhalations without glottic closure, starting at mid-lung volume. This is followed by a forced expectoration or a controlled cough at high lung volume to clear mucus from the central airways.

**Physical Therapy.** It is appropriate to try postural drainage with patients who are major sputum producers (>30 mL/day) and who have difficulty coughing up their secretions. This technique is safe for COPD patients who have negligible changes in lung volumes and in arterial oxygen saturation after being positioned in up to a 25-degree head-down tilt for 20 to 30 minutes.[609] An inhaled bronchodilator should be administered 20 to 30 minutes before postural drainage.[610] If difficulty in clearing airway secretions persists, family members can be taught cupped-hand chest wall percussion or the use of an electromechanical percussor. The routine use of postural drainage and chest percussion and vibration in all COPD patients is not indicated. Patients who produce only small quantities of sputum, either when stable or during an acute COPD exacerbation, benefit minimally or not at all.[572]

### Antibiotics

Less than half of acute exacerbations of chronic bronchitis are due to bacterial infection by pathogens that commonly colonize the respiratory tract: *H. influenzae, S. pneumoniae,* and *M. catarrhalis.*[452, 611] Infected patients generally have larger numbers of bacteria in their sputum than when they are clinically stable.[452, 612] The sputum Gram's stain provides semiquantitative information on the number of bacteria in the sputum; the culture provides information only on the identity of the organisms[613] and cannot separate colonization from infection. Clinical criteria alone are sufficient to justify a course of antibiotic therapy for a COPD exacerbation in the ambulatory setting. Patients having at least two of the triad of increased dyspnea, increased sputum volume, and sputum purulence are more likely to have their exacerbation shortened by an antibiotic than are patients with only one of these symptoms.[614]

A large number of oral antimicrobial agents have been approved for treatment of acute COPD exacerbations. Treatment is usually empirical and not based on sputum cultures.[615] Because response is generally good even without treatment,[614] a low-cost antibiotic such as trimethoprim-sulfamethoxasole, ampicillin, or a tetracycline is often used for mild exacerbations in relatively uncompromised patients. A 7- to 10-day course is most often prescribed. Providing patients with a prescription to fill if needed for an increase in symptoms is a commonly accepted practice. As baseline disease and exacerbation severity increase, broader spectrum antibiotics that are effective against resistant strains of *H. influenzae* and *S. pneumoniae* becomes increasingly recommended. If systemic symptoms such as fever are prominent, the patient should be regarded as having pneumonia and treated with broad-spectrum antibiotic coverage, as recommended.[616]

For the patient with frequent purulent exacerbations, a treatment approach similar to that used for bronchiectasis with the regular use of prophyllactic antibiotics may be beneficial. High-resolution CT of such patients may reveal bronchiectasis not apparent on routine chest roentgenography.[617]

## Secondary Therapy

Secondary therapy improves the functioning of the afflicted person without altering the status of the lungs.

### Long-Term Oxygen Therapy

Two studies, the British Medical Research Council trial[170] that evaluated oxygen for 15 hours/day vs. no oxygen and the NIH Nocturnal Oxygen Therapy Trial[171] that compared 12 vs. 24 hours of oxygen/day, have firmly established a place for prolonged long-term oxygen therapy in the management of severe COPD. The cardinal message from these studies is that long-term oxygen therapy extends life in hypoxemic COPD patients and that the 24-hour regimen is more beneficial than the 12-hour regimen.[171]

Other benefits of continuous oxygen therapy are a reduction in hematocrit,[171] modest neuropsychologic improvement,[618] and some improvement in pulmonary hemodynamics[65] (see discussion of cor pulmonale in Chapter 55). Oxygen therapy may also improve dyspnea and the work of breathing by reducing airway resistance[619] and decreasing minute ventilation needs.[620] Domiciliary oxygen therapy causes only small increases in arterial $P_{CO_2}$ in patients with hypercapnia[621] and does not result in pulmonary oxygen toxicity.[622] Although patients must be taught the dangers of smoking during oxygen use and some other simple precautions, there is no appreciable increase in fire hazard.[623]

**Indications.** Long-term oxygen therapy should be prescribed for patients who have a resting arterial $P_{O_2}$ level of 55 mm Hg or less while breathing air. For those whose resting arterial $P_{O_2}$ level is between 56 and 59 mm Hg, long-term oxygen therapy is indicated if they demonstrate erythrocytosis (hematocrit 55% or more) or evidence of cor pulmonale (Table 38.5). Stable ambulatory patients should meet these criteria after being on an optimal treatment regimen for at least 30 days.[624–626] Patients recovering from a bout of acute respiratory failure may be given ambulatory oxygen treatment, even though they have not been observed for sufficiently long periods. They must be reevaluated after 30 days at home, however, to ascertain that they meet the necessary criteria. This is a cost-effective decision, because 1 day of hospital care costs more than 1 month of ambulatory oxygen therapy.

**Oxygen During Exercise.** Patients with an arterial $P_{O_2}$ level of 60 mm Hg or higher while breathing room

**Table 38.5 MEDICARE INDICATIONS AND REQUIREMENTS FOR LONG-TERM OXYGEN THERAPY**

| |
|---|
| Indications |
| Arterial $P_{O_2} < 55$ mm Hg or saturated $O_2 < 88\%$ breathing ambient air |
| Arterial $P_{O_2}$ 56–59 mm Hg or saturated $O_2$ 89% with either of the following: |
| Evidence of cor pulmonale by electrocardiogram |
| Erythrocytosis (hematocrit > 56%) |
| or |
| Arterial $PO_2 > 60$ mm Hg or $SaO_2$ $O_2 > 90\%$ with compelling medical justification |
| Requirements |
| Optimal medical management before certification for long-term oxygen therapy |
| Measurement of arterial blood gases or arterial oxygen saturation by qualified laboratory |
| Completion of form HCFA-484 by the physician or an employee of the physician with physician's signature |

HCFA = Health Care Financing Administration.
Reproduced with permission from O'Donohue WJ Jr: Prescribing home oxygen therapy. Arch Intern Med 152:746–748, 1992.

air may develop worsening hypoxemia with exercise. In addition, oxygen therapy has been shown to improve exercise endurance in many studies,[627, 628] in part because of greater oxygen transport and improved oxygen utilization by exercising muscles.[629, 630] Oxygen has also been found to delay fatigue in exercising ventilatory muscle, as shown by the late appearance of paradoxic inward abdominal movement during inspiration due to diaphragmatic fatigue and a delayed fall in the high-to-low frequency components of the diaphragm electromyogram (a marker of fatigue).[631] It makes little sense, however, to perform exercise testing or to prescribe oxygen for patients who undertake little or no exercise. It is also likely that falls in arterial $Po_2$ level during brief exercise are of little physiologic significance unless the patient has significant underlying ischemic heart disease.

The diffusing capacity for carbon monoxide accurately predicts desaturation with exercise in patients with COPD; desaturation generally occurs only when the single-breath diffusing capacity is below 55% of predicted.[632, 633] It seems reasonable to limit exercise testing to COPD patients with limited exercise tolerance who have a diffusing capacity less than 55% predicted, whose room air $Po_2$ level is 60 mm Hg or higher, and who are highly motivated to work or perform major exercise. Prescription guidelines for oxygen therapy require patients with an arterial $Po_2$ level greater than 60 mm Hg to desaturate on low-level exercise to an arterial $Po_2$ level of 55 mm Hg or less.[626] (For additional information about the indications for and benefits of oxygen therapy, see Chapter 96.)

**Modes of Administration**

***Nasal Cannulas.*** The most frequently used oxygen delivery system at rest is the nasal cannula at a flow rate sufficient to achieve an arterial $Po_2$ level of 60 to 75 mm Hg (saturation > 90%). It is unusual to require a flow rate greater than 3 L/min to achieve this oxygen level. For patients using continuous oxygen, it is common practice to increase the resting oxygen flow rate by 1 L/min during sleep and exercise to prevent falls in arterial $Po_2$ level during these periods. For patients who qualify for oxygen only during sleep or exercise, the oxygen flow rate should be set to maintain a saturation of 90% or greater.

***Ambulatory Systems.*** A primary goal of oxygen therapy is to allow all patients to be as active as possible both in the home and, where appropriate, outside. Attaining this goal requires prescription of special equipment permitting ambulation. Liquid oxygen systems with refillable portable units are the most flexible but are also the most expensive ambulatory system.[624, 634, 635] Electrically driven concentrators with a 50-ft length of tubing along with small tanks of compressed oxygen for portable use in a stroller may be used for patients who spend only brief periods outside the home. Nevertheless, concentrators, because of their low equipment and service costs, are often provided to patients who should be using a liquid system. Vendors are motivated to do this because home oxygen is reimbursed under a fixed schedule, keyed to the prescribed oxygen flow rate, regardless of the oxygen system used or the needs of the patients.[634] Market forces seem, however, to be driving a change in this practice.

*Oxygen-Conserving Devices.* Several oxygen-conserving devices are now available that improve the efficiency of oxygen delivery by collecting oxygen flowing during expiration or by demand systems that permit oxygen flow only during inspiration. These systems result in oxygen savings of 50% or more, thereby prolonging the time of use of ambulatory reservoirs. The two systems that have gained widest acceptance are a reservoir pendant leading to a two-pronged nasal cannula (Oxymizer; Chad Therapeutics, Inc., Chatsworth, CA) and several demand oxygen delivery systems.[626]

*Transtracheal Catheters.* Transtracheal catheters are permanently sited in the trachea. The respiratory dead space is filled with undiluted oxygen flowing from the catheter, thus providing high-concentration oxygen early in inspiration. Several transtracheal catheter systems are available.[636] These systems are invasive and are associated with a wide range of complications, including occasional life-threatening tracheal obstruction by mucous balls.[637, 638] They may, however, correct severe hypoxemia in COPD patients who are refractory to high-flow oxygen by nasal cannula.[639] They can be almost completely concealed by clothing and result in increased compliance by some patients who will not accept the visibility of a nasal cannula.

**Oxygen Therapy During Commercial Air Travel.** The cabins of commercial airliners flying in the stratosphere are pressurized to an altitude between 5000 and 10,000 ft. Accordingly, patients with COPD in these cabins are subject to the added stress of a reduced inspired oxygen partial pressure. The arterial $Po_2$ level may fall below 40 mm Hg in some patients with COPD.[640] Fortunately, extensive experience has proved that flying without supplemental oxygen is safe for most subjects with COPD.[641] Hypercapnic COPD patients should employ supplemental oxygen while flying. Normocapnic patients with a sea level arterial $Po_2$ level above 68 mm Hg generally have a flight arterial $Po_2$ level above 50 mm Hg and do not require supplemental oxygen.[640, 642] One hundred per cent oxygen at a flow rate of 1 to 3 L/min by nasal cannula should provide a safe arterial $Po_2$ level.

To arrange for in-flight oxygen, patients should contact the airline more than 48 hours in advance. The patient's physician may be contacted by the airline for an oxygen prescription as well as for medical clearance to fly.[643] Patients are not permitted to use their own oxygen equipment on domestic (US) flights; airlines provide supplemental oxygen for in-flight use at a cost to the passenger of about $50.00 for each flight segment.[644] Because some airlines provide only face masks for oxygen delivery, patients should bring their own nasal cannulas. The patient should also know that the airline companies are not responsible for providing oxygen at stopover points or at the final destination.[643, 645]

Compact modern respirators can be brought into airplanes by patients, although this usually requires the purchase of an additional seat. Only gel-cell batteries are approved for air travel. Some airlines provide inverters that convert cabin power to a usable form of electricity for respirators.[644]

Finally, if the patient has major bullous disease, the physician should always warn the patient that ascent to a high altitude can precipitate life-threatening pneumothorax. Such a patient should probably not fly.

## Pulmonary Rehabilitation

Pulmonary rehabilitation, which attempts to return patients to their highest possible functional capacity, has become an essential component in comprehensive care of patients with severe COPD.[615] Successful rehabilitation requires an approach that draws on the expertise of respiratory therapists, respiratory nurse specialists, and physical and occupational therapists, all working under the direction of a pulmonary physician. Although such a program often begins in a hospital setting, continuation of rehabilitation in the home is essential, with family members often assisting.[646] This topic is covered separately in Chapter 96 and is outlined here only briefly; some critical components of rehabilitation, such as smoking cessation and oxygen therapy, are discussed elsewhere. Numerous studies have confirmed the overall value of such a program for COPD patients.[647] The benefits are improved independence and quality of life, decreased hospital days, and improved exercise capacity. Lung function usually is not improved.

**Patient Selection.** Any patient with severe symptomatic COPD should be considered; even patients with hypercapnia can benefit.[648] Patients' enthusiasm and ability to cooperate are critical factors for success. Confounding illness such as severe cardiac disease, arthritis, and major neurologic impairment may limit participation, especially for exercise conditioning.

### Methods of Improving Patient Performance

***Exercise.*** Exercise conditioning is the single most important aspect of rehabilitation and has been repeatedly shown to improve exercise capacity and endurance in COPD patients, albeit only modestly. Patients should undertake both general exercises and specific muscle training. As with any exercise program, gains in conditioning are quickly lost if the exercise program is stopped. For general reconditioning, graded leg exercises by stationary cycling, stair climbing, and walking are safe and well tolerated. Possible mechanisms of improved exercise tolerance include improved aerobic capacity, increased motivation, and better tolerance of dyspnea. Oxygen during exercise is recommended for patients who both have significant exercise desaturation ($<88\%$) and show improved exercise tolerance while using oxygen.[649] (Exercise is discussed in Chapter 9, and evaluation of exercise performance in patients is discussed in Chapter 28.)

Upper extremity exercises with light weights should be instituted. This approach is based on the observation that unsupported arm exercise results in dyspnea and fatigue at a much lower oxygen uptake than exercise performed by the lower extremities.[650] As accessory muscles of respiration, the shoulder girdle muscles are involved in breathing in COPD patients, and arm work quickly overloads them.[651] Such training improves upper extremity performance and reduces fatigue.[652]

Respiratory muscle training is controversial. The simplest, most reliable method for home use is a pressure-threshold breathing device for endurance training. The inspiratory pressure needed to achieve training has to be at least 30% of the maximum inspiratory pressure that the patient can generate, and the training duration should eventually reach 30 min/day.[653] An analysis of nine controlled trials of ventilatory-muscle resistive training in COPD patients[654] concluded that such training increases the endurance time that these muscles can tolerate a given load and may improve respiratory muscle strength, diminish dyspnea to the inspired load, and modestly increase walking distance. Up to 50% of patients, however, fail to complete training, and some develop respiratory muscle fatigue and even acute respiratory failure during training. It is unclear whether this method provides sufficient clinical advantage to justify its incorporation into a rehabilitation program.[655]

***Controlled Breathing.*** Controlled breathing techniques include pursed-lip breathing, deliberately slow and prolonged expiration, which may be coupled with manual upper abdominal compression, and the standing bent-forward position, with the outstretched arms and hands supporting the body. The benefits of these methods include control of resting dyspnea, anxiety, and panic attacks.[656] Some patients adopt breathing with pursed lips and the bending-forward posture intuitively during bouts of dyspnea; others adopt them only after instruction. The goal of these methods is a reduced respiratory rate and enhanced expiratory tidal volume, thus decreasing air trapping. Pursed-lip breathing may also stent the airways and thus prevent dynamic airway collapse[657] and may transiently improve arterial $Po_2$ level.[658] The bending-forward posture improves diaphragmatic function by increasing abdominal pressure, thus placing the diaphragm in a better position for contraction.[659]

## Nutrition

Patients with advanced COPD and a predominance of emphysema often experience progressive weight loss, with some becoming frankly cachectic.[660] Such patients have marked somatic depletion, including a significant reduction in triceps skinfold thickness. They show no evidence of protein malnutrition, however, as indicated by normal serum albumin levels and blood lymphocyte counts. The cause of this excessive weight loss is mainly a 15% to 25% increase in resting energy expenditure,[661, 662] perhaps the result of a markedly elevated work of breathing. A higher energy cost of daily activities, a reduced caloric intake relative to need, and an increase in circulating inflammatory cytokines[663, 664] may be other important factors. The main consequence of this excessive weight loss is reduced muscle strength, including weakness of both the inspiratory and expiratory muscles.[665]

Improved nutrition can restore respiratory and general muscle strength and endurance, but such improvement occurs only after clear-cut weight gain.[666, 667] Unfortunately, this has been consistently accomplished only within a controlled hospital environment with little success in patients living at home. Patients tolerate concentrated nutritional supplements poorly,[668] and feeding by nasogastric tube or parenterally is impractical and too invasive for long-term use. Better refeeding approaches are required, and new strategies need to be further evaluated.

The opposite approach appears necessary for chronically hypercapnic COPD patients with or without cor pulmonale who are overweight. Weight loss often improves breathlessness as well as hypoxemia and hypercapnia and reduces lower extremity edema.[669] The concern that large, mainly carbohydrate meals might acutely worsen arterial blood gas values in stable COPD patients with or without baseline hypercapnia because of an increase in the respiratory quotient, or might significantly limit exercise tolerance, has not been borne out in studies.[670, 671]

## Therapy for Dyspnea

**Pharmacologic.** Many COPD patients, especially those with severe emphysema, experience intolerable dyspnea, especially during exertion, that is poorly responsive to standard bronchodilator therapy. The data regarding the use of nebulized or oral narcotics in the treatment of dyspnea are conflicting. In five studies of oral narcotics and in three studies of nebulized morphine, most patients derived no significant benefit.[628, 672–678]

**Carotid Body Resection.** Bilateral but not unilateral carotid body resection has been reported to relieve dyspnea in patients with severe COPD, during both rest and exercise, mainly because of a large fall in respiratory rate and minute ventilation. In most patients, hypoxemia and hypercapnia worsen, and death may be hastened by such surgery.[679]

## Therapy for Respiratory or Ventilatory Failure

**Chronic Ventilatory Failure: Noninvasive Mechanical Ventilation.** The use of noninvasive mechanical ventilators in an attempt to rest the respiratory muscles is based on the concept that in patients with severe COPD the respiratory muscles are at the fatigue threshold, with small increases in respiratory requirements having the potential of precipitating fatigue and perhaps acute respiratory failure. Some studies, however, cast doubt on the existence of chronic fatigue of the diaphragm and the possibility that overt respiratory muscle fatigue causes ventilatory failure.[680, 681] Two forms of noninvasive ventilatory support have been used to rest the respiratory muscles, negative pressure ventilation by cuirass or poncho wrap, and intermittent positive-pressure ventilation by nasal mask.

Although some studies of negative-pressure ventilation show benefit, other long-term trials do not demonstrate improved gas exchange or respiratory muscle function, and many patients did not tolerate the treatment. Studies of long-term nocturnal nasal intermittent positive-pressure ventilation show mixed results. Strumpf and associates[682] found that the treatment was poorly tolerated and failed to improve pulmonary or respiratory muscle function, exercise endurance, or sleep efficiency. On the other hand, several investigators believe that the technique showed promise.[683, 684] Elliott and colleagues[684] studied eight hypercapnic COPD patients after 6 months of nocturnal nasal intermittent positive-pressure ventilation. Six patients showed a decrease and two showed an increase in arterial $P_{CO_2}$ level. These authors found no evidence of relief of muscle fatigue; there was evidence of decreased gas trapping and improved ventilatory drive. Other groups report improvements in total sleep time and sleep efficiency and a decrease in dyspnea.[685, 686] These methods are being widely adapted due to aggressive marketing, without substantial evidence of benefit.

### Altering Ventilatory Control

***Almitrine.*** Almitrine bismesylate, a peripheral chemoreceptor agonist not currently available in the United States, significantly improves resting room air arterial $P_{O_2}$ levels in about 80% of stable COPD patients in a dose-dependent fashion; a maximal increase of about 10 to 11 mm Hg is seen after 100 mg of the drug.[687] This increase results mainly from improved ventilation-perfusion relationships as almitrine enhances hypoxic pulmonary vasoconstriction by way of sympathetic efferent pathways.[688] Improvement in arterial blood gases persists during exercise[689] and with sleep.[690] The concern that almitrine might significantly increase pulmonary vascular resistance and pulmonary artery pressures has not been borne out in long-term studies.[691] Blood levels of almitrine steadily increase beyond a therapeutic level of 150 to 300 μg/mL if the drug is given continuously. An intermittent dosing schedule with 100 mg of almitrine daily given for 2 consecutive months followed by a 1-month washout period maintains therapeutic efficacy while avoiding serious complications such as progressive weight loss and peripheral neuropathy.[691]

***Analeptic Agents.*** The benefit of the true analeptic agents in COPD, like acetazolamide, which stimulates respiration by acidifying plasma and cerebrospinal fluid, and medroxyprogesterone acetate, which directly acts on brain-stem respiratory neurons, is far less certain. Acetazolamide does not effectively sustain increased ventilation in most COPD patients with chronic hypercapnia,[692] whereas medroxyprogesterone in a dose of 20 to 40 mg thrice daily mainly helps COPD patients whose hypoventilation is clearly out of proportion to their abnormal lung mechanics. Patients with severe ventilatory limitation ($FEV_1 < 0.5$ to 0.75 L) who are unable to reduce their arterial $P_{CO_2}$ with voluntary hyperventilation do not respond to this medication.[692]

### Acute Respiratory Failure

***Clinical Features.*** Acute respiratory failure in COPD is defined as the development of an arterial $P_{CO_2}$ level above 50 mm Hg or an arterial $P_{O_2}$ level below 50 mm Hg in association with recent clinical worsening. In patients with COPD, acute or chronic ventilatory failure is more common, but hypoxemic respiratory failure may contribute. Most episodes are caused by a superimposed acute chest illness, usually acute bronchitis, although other reversible causes such as pneumothorax, congestive heart failure, pulmonary embolus, and metabolic derangements such as hypophosphatemia or hypokalemia should be looked for.[693, 694] Detailed discussions of respiratory failure are given in Chapters 91 to 94, and the topic as it relates to COPD is only summarized here.

Patients with acute respiratory failure due to COPD usually arrive at the hospital awake and with an arterial $P_{CO_2}$ level of less than 80 mm Hg, provided that they have not received supplemental oxygen. Rapid rises in arterial $P_{CO_2}$ level may occur after administration of unnecessarily high amounts of oxygen. The rising arterial $P_{CO_2}$ level occurs because of the suppression of hypoxic peripheral chemoreceptor ventilatory drive, the Haldane effect in which oxygenated hemoglobin transports less carbon dioxide than deoxygenated hemoglobin, and the worsening of ventilation-perfusion matching.[695] A reduced hypoxic ventilatory drive does not usually occur until an arterial $P_{O_2}$ level of 60 mm Hg or higher has been reached.

***Conservative Therapy.*** The primary requirements for treatment of acute respiratory failure in patients with COPD are to improve hypoxemia and to prevent the development of tissue hypoxia with its potentially disastrous effects. These are best accomplished over the short term by administration of controlled low-dose oxygen with a Venturi mask with a concentration of 24% to 28% oxygen or by nasal cannula with an oxygen flow of 1 to 2 L/min. The intent is to achieve an arterial $P_{O_2}$ level in the range of 60 mm Hg, which allows an arterial oxygen saturation of 90% or more, thus preventing the development of tissue hypoxia. Some patients require higher concentrations or flows of inspired oxygen to attain this level of oxygenation. Although the increase in arterial $P_{O_2}$ level may be modest, it occurs on the steep portion of the oxygen-hemoglobin dissociation curve, thus resulting in a large increase in arterial saturation and oxygen content. It is hoped that keeping the arterial $P_{O_2}$ level of about 60 mm Hg will avoid significant abolition of hypoxic ventilatory drive. Slight increases in arterial $P_{CO_2}$ level may develop, but, because bicarbonate levels in blood will have risen in patients who have chronic hypercapnia, a further increase in arterial $P_{CO_2}$ level usually does not give rise to much worsening of acidemia. Unless the pH falls below 7.25, the consequences of this oxygen-induced rise in arterial $P_{CO_2}$ level are tolerable.

Once severe hypoxemia has been relieved, attention can be turned to relieving airflow limitation. The clinical presentation dictates the intensity of the therapy.

***Noninvasive Mechanical Ventilation.*** A number of review articles regarding the use of noninvasive ventilation in the treatment of acute respiratory failure have appeared.[696, 697] These alternative methods for ventilating acutely decompensated COPD patients, including negative-pressure ventilation[698] as well as nasal[699, 700] and face mask[701] intermittent positive-pressure ventilation, have been shown to reduce the need for intubation, decrease the length of stay in the intensive care unit, and may reduce mortality but require more careful monitoring than for ventilation through an endotracheal tube.[702] A ventilator system that provides inspiratory and expiratory (bilevel) pressure support ventilation through a nasal or facial mask is the most common means of noninvasive positive-pressure ventilation. The use of these systems should probably be limited to COPD patients who are thought to have quickly correctable causes of respiratory failure, such as excessive sedation or left ventricular failure. The use of continuous positive airway pressure by mask to counter intrinsic positive end-expiratory pressure appears to reduce the work of breathing and hyperinflation,[703, 704] but this approach carries the risk of further worsening intrinsic positive end-expiratory pressure if excessive levels of continuous positive airway pressure are employed.[705]

***Invasive Mechanical Ventilation.*** Most patients with acute respiratory failure due to COPD can be managed by a conservative regimen. A trend toward worsening hypercapnia and hypoxemia coupled with clinical deterioration, as indicated by progressive fatigue and difficulty in cooperation, guides the physician in deciding when to intubate and begin mechanical ventilation.

If the decision is made to intubate and ventilate the patient, it is important that ventilation not be so vigorous as to decrease the arterial $P_{CO_2}$ level rapidly; with the increased arterial blood bicarbonate level that is generally present, severe alkalemia with convulsions, coma, cardiac arrhythmias, and death may result. Levels of intrinsic positive end-expiratory pressure should be monitored closely during mechanical ventilation because excessive intrinsic positive end-expiratory pressure can promote diminished venous return, a reduced cardiac output, and hypotension. This phenomenon results from worsened airflow limitation during acute respiratory failure with increased air trapping and elevation of end-expiratory alveolar and intrapleural pressures; resetting the ventilator with a reduced rate, higher inspiratory flows, and an increased expiratory time helps to minimize this problem.[706]

Patients may be managed with an endotracheal tube and mechanical ventilator for up to 3 weeks without having to undergo a tracheostomy[707]; however, a much shorter period of mechanical ventilation is all that is needed for most patients to allow the factors that precipitated the acute respiratory failure to subside and to allow the respiratory muscles to rest adequately before extubation can be accomplished.

## Tracheal Stenosis

Severe tracheal stenosis after intubation for acute respiratory failure may contribute to respiratory disability in COPD patients.[708] Inspiratory stridor is rarely audible. The characteristic flow limitation seen on maximal inspiratory and expiratory flow volume curves with tracheal stenosis may be modified in COPD patients. A high degree of clinical suspicion followed by diagnostic bronchoscopy should lead to standard or laser surgery to remedy the condition.

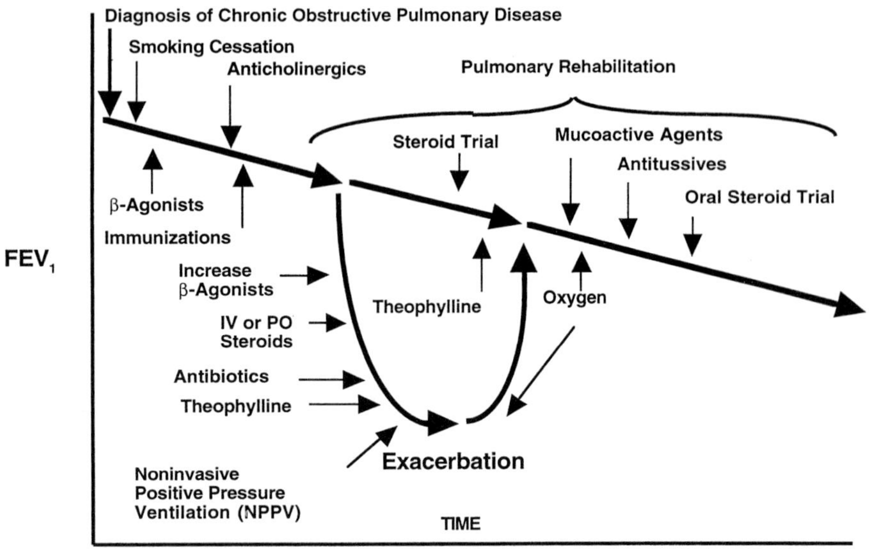


**Figure 38.19** Displayed against a background of the natural history of COPD showing the decline in pulmonary function over time is a schematic of various therapies that are used to treat this disease. The *arrows* are not meant to indicate specific time points when these therapies are to be applied but only represent the therapies in relation to the overall natural history. With exacerbations, lung function may deteriorate acutely, and temporary interventions may be required.

## Overall Therapeutic Strategy

The treatment techniques discussed here need to be applied to patients with COPD in a graded manner depending on the severity and reversibility of their airflow limitation, their symptoms, and the individual patient responses to and tolerance for the medications (Fig. 38.19). In mild disease, a beta-agonist or ipratropium bromide administered by an MDI or DPI may be all that is necessary. An alternative for patients who refuse to use an inhaler is a long-acting oral theophylline preparation. A long-acting beta-agonist or oral theophylline should be used if nocturnal symptoms dominate the clinical picture. For more troublesome complaints, various combinations of these medications can be given in low doses, thereby minimizing the toxicity of higher doses of beta-agonists and theophylline. For patients with severe disease, higher doses may be used at the cost of additional toxicity. A beta-agonist MDI should be prescribed for as-needed use, and patients need to be taught to carry such inhalers at all times, although the episodes requiring "rescue" are markedly fewer than in asthma.

With severe COPD, a short course of high-dose (0.5 to 1 mg/kg oral corticosteroids should be considered for patients with acute exacerbations of their disease. With severe chronic disease, a trial of inhaled corticosteroids should be undertaken. Every-other-day or daily prednisone by mouth, especially in high doses, should be employed only by the sickest patients who fail to respond to other treatments. Oral corticosteroids should be given over long periods only if they are shown objectively to be effective. Patients should be taught to inspect their sputum and to distinguish between mucoid and purulent secretions. They should begin a course of antibiotics at home for an established bronchial infection. If cough alone is inadequate to mobilize excessive secretions, chest physical therapy measures may be instituted. Long-term oxygen therapy should be administered to relieve hypoxemia and the effects of tissue hypoxia. A rehabilitation program should be instituted, especially for patients who have required a period of hospitalization for an acute incident.

Patients should be instructed on how they may intensify their therapy during an exacerbation of their disease and then diminish it to a maintenance level as the exacerbation subsides. Life-long medical supervision and support is an essential part of effective care for these patients.

## SUMMARY

Chronic obstructive pulmonary disease is a heterogeneous collection of disorders characterized by decreased expiratory airflow. The two major component syndromes, emphysema and chronic bronchitis, both commonly result from cigarette smoking and frequently coexist in an individual patient. Control of cigarette smoking is a key to disease prevention and management. Other exogenous and endogenous factors also contribute to the development of COPD, and coexistent infections probably result in the varied clinical presentations typical of COPD. Aggressive specific and supportive management can improve both patient well-being and survival.

## References

1. American Thoracic Society: Chronic bronchitis, asthma and pulmonary emphysema. A statement by the committee on diagnostic standards for nontuberculous respiratory diseases. Am Rev Respir Dis 85:762–768, 1962.
2. Burrows B, Bloom JW, Traver GA, et al: The course and prognosis of different forms of chronic airways obstruction in a sample from the general population. N Engl J Med 317:1309–1314, 1987.
3. Peat JK, Woolcock AJ, Cullen K: Rate of decline of lung function in subjects with asthma. Eur J Respir Dis 70:171–179, 1987.
4. Lange P, Parner J, Vestbo J, et al: A 15-year follow-up study of ventilatory function in adults with asthma. N Engl J Med 339:1194–1200, 1998.
5. Higgins M: Risk factors associated with chronic obstructive lung disease. Ann NY Acad Sci 624:7–17, 1991.
6. Ciba Foundation Guest Symposium: Terminology, definitions and classification of chronic pulmonary emphysema and related conditions. Thorax 14:286–299, 1959.

7. Snider GL, Kleinerman J, Thurlbeck WM, et al: The definition of emphysema. Report of a National Heart, Lung and Blood Institute, Division of Lung Diseases Workshop. Am Rev Respir Dis 132:182–185, 1985.
8. Ruysch F: Observationem Anatomico-Chirurgicarum. Amsterdam: Henricum Boom, 1691, pp 25–27.
9. Baillie M: A Series of Engravings, Accompanied with Explanations Which are Intended to Illustrate the Morbid Anatomy of Some of the Most Important Parts of the Human Body, Divided into 10 Fasciculi. London: W. Bulmer and Co, 1799.
10. Baillie M: The Morbid Anatomy of Some of the Most Important Parts of the Human Body. Brattleborough: W. Fessenden, 1808, pp 52–53.
11. Laennec RTH: De L'Auscultation Mediate, ou traite du diagnostic des maladies des poumons et du coeur. Tome Premier: Paris, 1819.
12. Laennec RTH: A Treatise on the Diseases of the Chest and on Mediate Auscultation. [Translated by John Forbes.] Philadelphia: Thomas & Co, 1835, pp 135–163.
13. Orsos F: Au Uber das elastische Gerauust der normalen und der emphysematosen Lunge. Pathol Anat 41:95–121, 1907.
14. Gough J, Wentworth JW: The use of thin sections of entire organs in morbid anatomical studies. J R Microsc Soc 69:231–235, 1949.
15. Gough J: Discussion on the diagnosis of pulmonary emphysema. The pathological diagnosis of emphysema. Proc R Soc Med 45:576–577, 1952.
16. Leopold JG, Gough J: The centrilobular form of hypertrophic emphysema and its relation to chronic bronchitis. Thorax 12:219–235, 1957.
17. Laurell CB, Eriksson S: The electrophoretic alpha 1-globulin pattern of serum in alpha 1-antitrypsin deficiency. Scand J Clin Lab Invest 15:132–140, 1963.
18. Snider GL, Hayes JA, Franzblau C, et al: Relationship between elastolytic activity and experimental emphysema-inducing properties of papain preparations. Am Rev Respir Dis 110:254–262, 1974.
19. Seemungal TA, Donaldson GC, Paul EA, et al: Effect of exacerbation on quality of life in patients with chronic obstructive pulmonary disease. Am J Respir Crit Care Med 157:1418–1422, 1998.
20. Buist AS, Sexton GJ, Nagy JM, et al: The effect of smoking cessation and modification on lung function. Am Rev Respir Dis 114:115–122, 1976.
21. Kinnear WJM, Tattersfield AE: Emphysematous bullae: Surgery is best for large bullae and moderately impaired lung function. BMJ 300:208–209, 1990.
22. Thompson AB, Teschler H, Rennard SI: Pathogenesis, evaluation, and therapy for massive hemoptysis. Clin Chest Med 13:69–82, 1992.
23. Bergin C, Muller N, Nichols DM, et al: The diagnosis of emphysema: A computed tomographic-pathologic correlation. Am Rev Respir Dis 133:541–546, 1988.
24. Knudson RJ, Standen JR, Kaltenborn WT, et al: Expiratory computed tomography for assessment of suspected pulmonary emphysema. Chest 99:1357–1366, 1991.
25. Stevens PM, Orman BF, Graves G: Contribution of lung recoil and airway resistance to forced expiratory flow limitation. Am Rev Respir Dis 100:54–62, 1969.
26. Beck CS, Heiner DC: Selective immunoglobulin G4 deficiency and recurrent infections of the respiratory tract. Am Rev Respir Dis 124:94–96, 1981.
27. Cosio M, Ghezzo H, Hogg JC, et al: The relations between structural changes in small airways and pulmonary function tests. N Engl J Med 298:1277–1281, 1978.
28. Buist AS, Ducic S: Smoking. Evaluation of studies which have demonstrated pulmonary function changes. *In* Macklem PT, Permutt S (eds): The Lung in Transition Between Health and Disease. New York: Marcel Dekker, 1978, pp 271–286.
29. West JB: Pulmonary Pathophysiology: The Essentials (5th ed). Baltimore: Williams & Wilkins, 1998.
30. Emerman CL, Cydulka RK: Use of peak expiratory flow rate in emergency department evaluation of acute exacerbation of chronic obstructive pulmonary disease. Ann Emerg Med 27(2):159–163, 1996.
31. Rebuck DA, Hanania NA, D'Urzo AD, et al: The accuracy of a handheld portable spirometer. Chest 109:152–157, 1996.
32. Anthonisen NR, Wright E, Group IT: Bronchodilator response in chronic obstructive pulmonary disease. Am Rev Respir Dis 133:814–819, 1986.
33. Hoppin FG: Pulmonary function tests for diagnosis and evaluation of COPD. *In* Cherniack NS (ed): Chronic Obstructive Pulmonary Disease. Philadelphia: WB Saunders, 1991, pp 363–372.
34. Burrows B, Niden AH, Fletcher CM, et al: Clinical types of chronic obstructive lung disease in London and in Chicago. Am Rev Respir Dis 90:14–20, 1964.
35. Burrows B, Fletcher CM, Heard BE: The emphysematous and bronchial types of chronic airways obstruction: A clinicopathological study of patients in London and Chicago. Lancet 1:830–836, 1966.
36. Bates DV: Respiratory Function in Disease (3rd ed). Philadelphia: WB Saunders, 1989, pp 172–187.
37. Thurlbeck WM: Overview of the pathology of pulmonary emphysema in the human. Clin Chest Med 4:337–350, 1983.
38. Silvers GW, Petty TL: Elastic recoil changes in early emphysema. J Clin Invest 35:490–495, 1980.
39. Symonds G, Rensetti AD, Mitchell MM: The diffusing capacity in pulmonary emphysema. Am Rev Respir Dis 109:391–394, 1974.
40. Miller A, Thornton JC, Warshaw R: Single breath diffusing capacity in a representative sample of the population of Michigan, a large industrial state. Predictive values, lower limits of normal, and frequencies of abnormality of smoking history. Am Rev Respir Dis 127:270–277, 1983.
41. Belman MJ: Exercise in patients with chronic obstructive pulmonary disease. Thorax 48:936–946, 1993.
42. Mulloy E, McNicholas WT: Ventilation and gas exchange during sleep and exercise in severe COPD. Chest 109:387–394, 1996.
43. Donahoe M, Rogers RM: Laboratory evaluation of the patient with chronic obstructive pulmonary disease. *In* Cherniack NS (ed): Chronic Obstructive Pulmonary Disease. WB Saunders, Philadelphia: 1991, pp 373–386.
44. Stradling JR, Lane DJ: Development of secondary polycythemia in chronic airways obstruction. Thorax 34:777–782, 1981.
45. Vlahakos DV, Kosmas EN, Dimopoulou I, et al: Association between activation of the renin-angiotensin system and secondary erythrocytosis in patients with chronic obstructive pulmonary disease. Am J Med 106:158–164, 1999.
46. Wedzicha JA, Cotes PM, Empey DW, et al: Serum immunoreactive erythropoietin in hypoxic lung disease with and without polycythemia. Clin Sci 69:413–422, 1985.
47. Smith JR, Landau SA, Smokers' polycythemia. N Engl J Med 298:6–10, 1978.
48. Chodosh S: Why, when, how and by whom. *In* Brody JS, Snider GL (eds): Current Topics in the Management of Respiratory Diseases. New York: Churchill Livingstone, 1985, pp 123–145.
49. Sethi S: Infectious exacerbations of chronic bronchitis: Diagnosis and management. J Antimicrob Chemother 43(Suppl A):97–105, 1999.
50. Yi K, Sethi S, Murphy TF: Human immune response to nontypeable *Haemophilus influenzae* in chronic bronchitis. J Infect Dis 176:1247–1252, 1997.
51. Snider GL, Stone PJ, Lucey EC: Development and evaluation of antiproteases as drugs for preventing emphysema. *In* Grassi C, Travis J, Casali L, et al. (eds): Biochemistry of Pulmonary Emphysema. Verona: Bi and Gi Publishers, 1992, pp 143–158.
52. Schoenenberger RA, Haefli WE, Weiss P, et al: Timing of invasive procedures in therapy for primary and secondary spontaneous pneumothorax. Arch Surg 126:764–766, 1991.
53. Wakabayashi A: Expanded applications of diagnostic and therapeutic thoracoscopy. J Thorac Cardiovasc Surg 102:721–723, 1991.
54. Yim AP, Ho JK, Chung SS, et al: Video-assisted thoracoscopic surgery for primary spontaneous pneumothorax. Aust NZ J Surg 64:667–670, 1994.
55. Rodriguez-Panadero F, Antony VB: Pleurodesis: State of the art. Eur Respir J 10:1648–1654, 1997.
56. Light RW, Vargas FS: Pleural sclerosis for the treatment of pneumothorax and pleural effusion. Lung 175:213–223, 1997.
57. Matthay RA, Niederman MS, Wiedemann HP: Cardiovascular

pulmonary interaction in chronic obstructive pulmonary disease with special reference to the pathogenesis and management of cor pulmonale. Med Clin North Am 74:571–618, 1990.

58. Klinger JR, Hill NS: Right ventricular dysfunction in chronic obstructive pulmonary disease. Chest 99:715–723, 1991.

58a. Chaouat A, Weitzenblum E, Kessler R, et al: Sleep-related $O_2$ desaturation and daytime pulmonary haemodynamics in COPD patients with mild hypoxaemia. Eur Resp J 10:1730–1735, 1997.

59. Dinh-Xuan AT, Higgenbottam TW, Clelland CA, et al: Impairment of endothelium-dependent pulmonary-artery relaxation in chronic obstructive lung disease. N Engl J Med 324:1539–1547, 1991.

60. Farber MO, Roberts LR, Weinberger MH, et al: Abnormalities of sodium and $H_2O$ handling in chronic obstructive lung disease. Arch Intern Med 142:1326–1330, 1982.

61. Dabestani A, Mahan G, Gardin JM, et al: Evaluation of pulmonary artery pressure and resistance by pulsed Doppler echocardiography. Am J Cardiol 59:662–668, 1987.

62. Tramarin R, Torbicki A, Marchandise B, et al: Doppler echocardiographic evaluation of pulmonary artery pressure in chronic obstructive pulmonary disease. A European multicentre study. Working group on noninvasive evaluation of pulmonary artery pressure. European office of the World Health Organization. Eur Heart J 12:103–111, 1991.

63. Sajkov D, Cowie RJ, Bradley JA, et al: Validation of new pulsed Doppler echocardiographic techniques for assessment of pulmonary hemodynamics. Chest 103:1348–1353, 1993.

64. Mittal SR, Jain SC, Sharma SK, et al: The role of electrocardiographic criteria for the diagnosis of right ventricular hypotherapy in chronic obstructive pulmonary disease. Int J Cardiol 11:165–173, 1986.

65. Timms RM, Khaja FU, Williams GW, et al: Hemodynamic response to oxygen therapy in chronic obstructive pulmonary disease. Arch Intern Med 102:29–36, 1985.

66. Weitzenblum E, Sautegeau A, Ehrahart M, et al: Long-term oxygen therapy can reverse the progression of pulmonary hypertension in patients with chronic obstructive pulmonary disease. Am Rev Respir Dis 131:493–498, 1985.

67. Agostoni P, Doria E, Galli C, et al: Nifedipine reduces pulmonary pressure and vascular tone during short- but not long-term treatment of pulmonary hypertension in patients with chronic obstructive lung disease. Am Rev Respir Dis 139:120–126, 1989.

68. Matthay RA: Favorable cardiovascular effects of theophylline in COPD. Chest 92:22S–26S, 1987.

69. Winter RJD, Langford JA, George RJD, et al: The effects of theophylline and salbutamol on right and left ventricular function in chronic bronchitis. Chest 78:358–362, 1984.

70. MacNee W: Pathophysiology of cor pulmonale in chronic obstructive pulmonary disease. Part two. Am J Respir Crit Care Med 150:1158–1168, 1994.

71. Griffith DE, Mazurek GH: Pneumonia and chronic obstructive lung disease. Infect Dis Clin North Am 5:467–484, 1991.

72. Fang GD, Fine M, Orloff J, et al: New and emerging etiologies for community-acquired pneumonia with implications for therapy: A prospective multicenter study of 359 cases. Medicine (Baltimore) 69:307–316, 1990.

73. Midgren B, Hansson L: Changes in the transcutaneous $P_{CO_2}$ with sleep in normal subjects and in patients with chronic respiratory diseases. Eur J Respir Dis 71:384–387, 1987.

74. Catterol JR, Calverley PMA, MacNee W: Mechanism of transient nocturnal hypoxemia in hypoxic chronic bronchitis and emphysema. J Appl Physiol 59:1698–1703, 1985.

75. Douglas NJ, Flenley DC: Breathing during sleep in patients with obstructive lung disease. Am Rev Respir Dis 141:1055–1070, 1990.

76. Fletcher EC, Miller J, Divine GW, et al: Nocturnal oxyhemoglobin desaturation in COPD patients with arterial oxygen tensions above 60 mmHg. Chest 92:604–608, 1987.

77. Catteral JR, Douglas NJ, Calverly PMA: Transient hypoxemia during sleep in chronic obstructive pulmonary disease is not a sleep apnea syndrome. Am Rev Respir Dis 128:24–29, 1983.

78. Fleetham J, West P, Mezan B, et al: Sleep arousals and oxygen desaturation in chronic obstructive pulmonary disease. Am Rev Respir Dis 126:429–433, 1982.

79. Shepard JW, Jr, Garrison MW, Grither DA, et al: Relationship of ventricular ectopy to nocturnal oxygen desaturation in patients with chronic obstructive pulmonary disease. Am J Med 78:28–34, 1985.

80. Fletcher EC, Luckett RA, Miller T, et al: Pulmonary vascular hemodynamics in chronic lung disease patients with and without oxyhemoglobin desaturation during sleep. Chest 95:157–166, 1989.

81. Fletcher EC, Luckett RA, Goodnight-White S, et al: A double-blind trial of nocturnal supplemental oxygen for sleep desaturation in patients with chronic obstructive pulmonary disease and a daytime $P_{aO_2}$ above 60 mm Hg. Am Rev Respir Dis 145:1070–1076, 1992.

82. Connaughton JJ, Catterall JR, Elton RA, et al: Do sleep studies contribute to the management of patients with severe chronic obstructive pulmonary disease? Am Rev Respir Dis 138:341–344, 1988.

83. Gaensler EA, Angell DW, Knudson RJ, et al: Surgical management of emphysema. Clin Chest Med 4:443–463, 1983.

84. Morgan MDL, Denison DM: The value of computed tomography for selecting patients with bullous lung disease for surgery. Thorax 41:855–862, 1986.

85. Reid L: The Pathology of Emphysema. Chicago: Year Book Medical Publishers, 1967.

86. Jack CI, Evans CC: Three cases of alpha-1 antitrypsin deficiency in the elderly. Postgrad Med J 67:840–842, 1991.

87. Viola AR Zuffardi EA: Physiologic and clinical aspects of pulmonary bullous disease. Am Rev Respir Dis 94:574–578, 1966.

88. Sanders C: The radiographic diagnosis of emphysema. Radiol Clin North Am 29:1019–1030, 1991.

89. Morgan MDL: Computed tomography in the assessment of bullous lung disease. Chest 78:10–25, 1984.

90. Peters JI, Kubitschek KR, Gotlieb MS, et al: Lung bullae with air-fluid levels. Am J Med 82:759–763, 1987.

91. Khan MA, Dulfano MJ: Disappearance of a giant bulla following acute pneumonitis. Chest 68:746–747, 1975.

92. Head JR, Avery EE: Intracavitary suction (Monaldi) in the treatment of emphysematous bullae and blebs. J Thorac Surg 18:761–767, 1949.

93. Verma RK, Nishiki M, Mukai M, et al: Intracavitary drainage procedure for giant bullae in compromised patients. Hiroshima J Med Sci 40:115–118, 1991.

94. Hayakawa K, Tanaka F, Mitsumori M, et al: Bronchial artery embolization for hemoptysis: Immediate and long term results. Cardiovasc Intervent Radiol 15:154–158, 1992.

95. Goldstein MJ, Snider GL, Liberson M, et al: Bronchogenic carcinoma and giant bullous disease. Am Rev Respir Dis 97:1062–1070, 1968.

96. Aronberg DJ, Sagel SS, LeFrak S, et al: Lung carcinoma associated with bullous lung disease in young men. AJR 134:249–252, 1980.

97. Tsutsui M, Araki Y, Shirakusa T, et al: Characteristic radiographic features of pulmonary carcinoma associated with large bulla. Ann Thorac Surg 46:679–683, 1988.

98. Gaensler EA: Unilateral hyperlucent lung. *In* Simon M, Potchen EJ, LeMay M. (eds): Frontiers of Pulmonary Radiology. New York: Grune & Stratton, 1969, pp 312–359.

99. Swyer P, James G: A case of unilateral pulmonary emphysema. Thorax 8:133–136, 1953.

100. Macleod WM: Abnormal transradiancy of one lung. Thorax 9:147–153, 1954.

101. Fraser RG, Pare JAP, Pare PS: Diagnosis of diseases of the chest. Philadelphia: WB Saunders, 1990, pp 2116–2144.

102. MacPherson RI, Cumming GR, Chernick V: Unilateral hyperlucent lung: A complication of viral pneumonia. J Can Assoc Radiol 20:225–232, 1969.

103. Stokes D, Sigler A, Khouri NE, et al: Unilateral hyperlucent lung (Swyer-James syndrome) after severe *Mycoplasma pneumoniae* infection. Am Rev Respir Dis 117:145–152, 1978.

104. Llames R, Schwartz RA, Gupta SK, et al: Unilateral hyperlucent lung with polycythemia and cor pulmonale. Chest 59:690–694, 1971.

105. Avital A, Shulman DL, Bar-Yishay E, et al: Differential lung function in an infant with the Swyer-James syndrome. Thorax 44:298–302, 1989.

106. Thurlbeck WM: Chronic airflow obstruction in lung disease. *In* Major Problems in Pathology. Philadelphia: WB Saunders, 1976.

107. Reid L, Simon G: Unilateral lung transradiancy. Thorax 17:230–239, 1962.
108. Marti-Bonmati L, Ruiz-Perales F, Catala F, et al: CT findings in Swyer-James syndrome. Radiology 172:477–480, 1989.
109. Weg JG, Krumholz RA, Hadderoad LE: Unilateral hyperlucent lung: A physiologic syndrome. Ann Intern Med 62:675–684, 1965.
110. Gottlieb LS, Turner FA: Swyer-James (Macleod's) syndrome: Variations in pulmonary-bronchial arterial blood flow. Chest 69:62–66, 1976.
111. O'Dell CW Jr, Taylor R, Higgins CB, et al: Ventilation perfusion lung images in the Swyer-James syndrome. Radiology 121:423–426, 1976.
112. Gluck MC, Moser KM: Pulmonary artery agenesis. Diagnosis with ventilation and perfusion scintiphotography. Circulation 41:859–867, 1970.
113. Isawa T, Taplin GV: Unilateral pulmonary artery agenesis, stenosis and hypoplasia. Radiology 99:605–614, 1971.
114. Raynor AL, Capp ML, Sealy WC: Lobar emphysema of infancy. Diagnosis, treatment and etiologic aspects. Ann Thorac Surg 4:374–385, 1967.
115. Murray GF: Congenital lobar emphysema. Surg Gynecol Obstet 124:611–625, 1967.
116. Lincoln JCR, Stark J: Congenital lobar emphysema. Ann Surg 173:55–62, 1971.
117. Waddell WR, Simon G, Reid L: Bronchial atresia of the left upper lobe. Thorax 20:214–221, 1965.
118. Thurlbeck WM: Chronic airflow obstruction. *In* Thurlbeck WM (ed): Pathology of the Lung. New York: Thieme Medical Publishers, 1988, pp 519–575.
119. Sears MR, Holdaway MD, Flannery EM, et al: Parental and neonatal risk factors for atopy, airway hyper-responsiveness, and asthma. Arch Dis Child 75:392–398, 1996.
120. Higgins MW, Keller JB, Metzner HL: Smoking, socioeconomic status, and chronic respiratory disease. Am Rev Respir Dis 116:403–410, 1977.
121. Higgins MW: Incidence, prevalence, and mortality: Intra- and intercountry differences. *In* Hensley MJ, Saunders NA (eds): Clinical Epidemiology of Chronic Obstructive Pulmonary Disease. New York: Marcel Dekker, 1990.
122. Collins JG, National Center for Health Statistics (US): Prevalence of Selected Chronic Conditions: United States, 1986–88. Vital and Health Statistics Series 10. Data from the National Health Survey, No. 182. Hyattsville, MD: US Dept. of Health and Human Services, Public Health Service, Centers for Disease Control, National Center for Health Statistics, pp iv, 87, 1993.
123. Singh G, Matthews TJ, Clarke SC, et al: Annual Summary of Births, Marriages, Divorces and Deaths: United States, 1994: Monthly Vital Statistics Report (Vol 43, No. 13). Hyattsville, MD: National Center for Health Statistics, 1994.
124. Mannino DM, Brown C, Giovino GA: Obstructive lung disease deaths in the United States from 1979 through 1993. An analysis using multiple-cause mortality data. Am J Respir Crit Care Med 156:814–818, 1997.
125. Feinlieb M, Rosenberg HM, Collins JG: Trends in COPD morbidity and mortality in the United States. Am Rev Respir Dis 140:S9–S18, 1989.
126. Morbidity and Mortality Chartbook on Cardiovascular, Lung, and Blood Diseases. Bethesda, MD: National Heart, Lung and Blood Institute, 1994.
127. National Lung Health Education Program Executive Committee: Strategies in preserving lung health and preventing COPD and associated diseases. Chest 113:123S–163S, 1998.
128. Speizer FE: The rise in chronic obstructive pulmonary disease mortality: Overview and summary. Am Rev Respir Dis 140:S106–S107, 1989.
129. Murray CJ, Lopez AD: Alternative projection of mortality by cause 1990–2020: Global burden of disease study. Lancet 349:1498–1504, 1997.
130. Sherrill D, Lebowitz M, Burrows B: Epidemiology of chronic obstructive pulmonary disease. Clin Chest Med 11:375–387, 1990.
131. Burt VL, Harris T: The third National Health and Nutrition Examination Survey: Contributing data on aging and health. Gerontologist 34:486–490, 1994.
132. US Surgeon General: The Health Consequences of Smoking: Chronic Obstructive Lung Disease. US Dept. of Health and Human Research, 84-50205, 1984.
133. Faling LJ: Genetic influences in the development of emphysema in persons with normal serum proteins. Clin Chest Med 4:377–387, 1983.
134. Auerbach O, Hammond EC, Garfinkel L, et al: Relation of smoking and age to emphysema. Whole-lung section study. N Engl J Med 286:853–857, 1972.
135. Fletcher C, Peto R, Tinker C, et al: The Natural History of Chronic Bronchitis and Emphysema. New York: Oxford University Press, pp 1–272, 1976.
136. Lebowitz MD, Burrows B: Quantitative relationships between cigarette smoking and chronic productive cough. Int J Epidemiol 6:107–113, 1977.
137. Burrows B, Knudson RJ, Cline MG, et al: Quantitative relationships between cigarette smoking and ventilatory function. Am Rev Respir Dis 115:195–205, 1977.
138. Higgins MW, Keller JB, Becker M: An index of risk for obstructive airways disease. Am Rev Respir Dis 125:144–151, 1982.
139. Davis RM, Novotny TE: The epidemiology of cigarette smoking and its impact on chronic obstructive pulmonary disease. Am Rev Respir Dis 140:S82–S84, 1989.
140. Orie NG, Sluiter HJ, DeVries K, et al: The host factor in bronchitis. *In* Orie NGM, Sluiter HJ (eds): Bronchitis, An International Symposium. Netherlands: Assen, 1961, pp 43–59.
141. Burrows B: Airways obstructive diseases: Pathogenetic mechanisms and natural histories of the disorders. Med Clin North Am 74:547–560, 1990.
142. Burnett D, Chamba A, Hill SL, et al: Neutrophils from subjects with chronic obstructive lung disease show enhanced chemotaxis and extracellular proteolysis. Lancet 2:1043–1046, 1987.
143. Burrows B, Martinez FD, Halonen M: Association of asthma with serum IgE levels and skin-test reactivity to allergens. N Engl J Med 320:271–277, 1989.
144. Tashkin DP, Altose MD, Connett JE, et al: Methacholine reactivity predicts changes in lung function over time in smokers with early chronic obstructive pulmonary disease. Am J Respir Crit Care Med 153:1802–1811, 1996.
145. Kanner RE, Connett JE, Altose MD, et al: Gender difference in airway hyperresponsiveness in smokers with mild COPD: The Lung Health Study. Am J Respir Crit Care Med 150:956–961, 1994.
146. Dosman JA, Gomez SR, Zhou C: Relationship between airways responsiveness and the development of chronic obstructive pulmonary disease. Med Clin North Am 74:561–569, 1990.
147. Burrows B, Martinez FD: Bronchial responsiveness, atopy, smoking and chronic obstructive pulmonary disease. Am Rev Respir Dis 140:1515–1517, 1989.
148. Frost F, Tollestrup K, Starzyk P: History of smoking from the Washington State death certificate. Am J Prev Med 10:335–339, 1994.
149. Melbostad E, Eduard W, Magnus P: Chronic bronchitis in farmers. Scand J Work Environ Health 23:271–280, 1997.
150. Becklake MR: Occupational exposures: Evidence for a causal association with chronic obstructive pulmonary disease. Am Rev Respir Dis 140:S85–S91, 1989.
151. Oliveti JF, Kercsmar CM, Redline S: Pre- and perinatal risk factors for asthma in inner city African-American children. Am J Epidemiol 143:570–577, 1996.
152. Shaheen S: The beginnings of chronic airflow obstruction. BMJ Bull 53:58–70, 1997.
153. Hagstrom B, Nyberg P, Nilsson PM: Asthma in adult life—Is there an association with birth weight? Scand J Prim Health Care 16:117–120, 1998.
154. Svanes C, Omenaas E, Heuch JM, et al: Birth characteristics and asthma symptoms in young adults: Results from a population-based cohort study in Norway. Eur Respir J 12:1366–1370, 1998.
155. Shaheen SO, Barker DJ, Shiell AW, et al: The relationship between pneumonia in early childhood and impaired lung function in late adult life. Am J Respir Crit Care Med 149:616–619, 1994.
156. Shaheen SO, Sterne JA, Florey CD: Birth weight, childhood lower respiratory tract infection, and adult lung function. Thorax 53:549–553, 1998.
157. Barker DJP, et al: Relation of birthweight and childhood respira-

tory infection to adult lung function and death from chronic obstructive airways disease. BMJ 303:671–675, 1991.
158. Burrows B, Knudson RJ, Camilli AE, et al: The "horse-racing effect" and predicting decline in forced expiratory volume in one second from screening spirometry. Am Rev Respir Dis 135:788–793, 1987.
159. Anthonisen NR, Connett JE, Kiley JP, et al: Effects of smoking intervention and the use of an inhaled anticholinergic bronchodilator on the rate of decline of $FEV_1$. JAMA 272:1497–1505, 1994.
160. Pauwels RA, Lofdahl CG, Laitinen LA, et al: Long-term treatment with inhaled budesonide in persons with mild chronic obstructive pulmonary disease who continue to smoke. N Engl J Med 340:1948–1953, 1999.
161. Peto R, Speizer FE, Cochrane AL, et al: The relevance in adults of airflow obstruction, but not of mucus hypersecretion, to mortality from chronic lung disease. Results from 20 years of prospective observation. Am Rev Respir Dis 128:491–500, 1983.
162. Vestbo J, Prescott E, Lange P: Association of chronic mucus hypersecretion with $FEV_1$ decline and chronic obstructive pulmonary disease morbidity. Am J Respir Crit Care Med 153:1530–1535, 1996.
163. Buist AS, Vollmer WM, Johnson LR: Does the single breath $N_2$ test identify the susceptible individual? Am Rev Respir Dis 128:491–500, 1983.
164. Anthonisen NR: Prognosis in chronic obstructive pulmonary disease: Results from multicenter clinical trials. Am Rev Respir Dis 133:S95–S99, 1989.
165. Camilli AE, Burrows B, Knudson RJ, et al: Longitudinal changes in forced expiratory volume in one second in adults. Am Rev Respir Dis 135:794–799, 1987.
166. Incalzi RA, Fuso L, De Rosa M, et al: Electrocardiographic signs of chronic cor pulmonale: A negative prognostic finding in chronic obstructive pulmonary disease. Circulation 99:1600–1605, 1999.
167. Antonelli A, Incalzi R, Fuso L, et al: Co-morbidity contributes to predict mortality of patients with chronic obstructive pulmonary disease. Eur Respir J 10:2794–2800, 1997.
168. Vilkman S, Keistinen T, Tuuponen T, et al: Survival and cause of death among elderly chronic obstructive pulmonary disease patients after first admission to hospital. Respiration 64:281–284, 1997.
169. Connors AF Jr, Dawson NV, Thomas C, et al: Outcomes following acute exacerbation of severe chronic obstructive lung disease. The SUPPORT investigators (Study to Understand Prognoses and Preferences for Outcomes and Risks of Treatments) [published erratum appears in Am J Respir Crit Care Med 155:386, 1997]. Am J Respir Crit Care Med 154:959–967, 1996.
170. Medical Research Council Working Party: Long-term domiciliary oxygen therapy in chronic hypoxic cor pulmonale complicating chronic bronchitis and emphysema. Lancet 1:681–686, 1981.
171. Nocturnal Oxygen Therapy Trial Group: Continuous or nocturnal oxygen therapy in hypoxemic chronic obstructive lung disease. Ann Int Med 93:391–398, 1980.
172. Cooper CB, Waterhouse J, Howard P: Twelve year clinical study of patients with hypoxic cor pulmonale. Thorax 42:105–110, 1987.
173. Traver GA, Cline MG, Burrows B: Predictions of mortality in COPD: A 15 year follow-up study. Am Rev Respir Dis 119:895–902, 1979.
174. Kanner RE, Renzetti AD Jr, Stanish WM, et al: Predictions of survival in subjects with chronic airflow limitation. Am J Med 174:249–255, 1983.
175. Kanner RE, Renzetti AD Jr: Predictions of spirometric changes and mortality in the obstructive airway disorders. Chest 85:15S–17S, 1984.
176. Thurlbeck WM: Pathology of chronic airflow obstruction. *In* Cherniack NS (ed): Chronic Obstructive Pulmonary Disease. Philadelphia: WB Saunders, 1991, pp 3–20.
177. Thurlbeck WM, Angus GE: A distribution curve for chronic bronchitis. Thorax 19:436–442, 1964.
178. Mitchell RS, et al: The significance of morphologic chronic hyperplastic bronchitis. Am Rev Respir Dis 93:720–729, 1966.
179. Scott KWM: An autopsy study of bronchial mucous gland hypertrophy in Glasgow. Am Rev Respir Dis 97:54–61, 1968.
180. Mitchell RS, Silvers GW, Dart GA, et al: Clinical and morphologic correlations in chronic airway obstruction. Am Rev Respir Dis 97:54–61, 1968.
181. Reid LM: Measurement of bronchial mucous gland layer. A diagnostic yardstick in chronic bronchitis. Thorax 15:132–141, 1960.
182. Auerbach O, Stout AP, Hammond EC, et al: Changes in bronchial epithelium in relation to cigarette smoking and in relation to lung cancer. N Engl J Med 265:253–258, 1961.
183. Saetta M: Activated T-lymphocytes and macrophages in bronchial mucosa of subjects with chronic bronchitis. Am Rev Respir Dis 147:301–306, 1993.
184. Saetta M, et al: CD8+ T-lymphocytes in peripheral airways of smokers with chronic obstructive pulmonary disease. Am J Respir Crit Care Med 157:822–826, 1998.
185. Saetta M, et al: Airway eosinophilia and expression of interleukin-5 protein in asthma and in exacerbations of chronic bronchitis. Clin Exp Allergy 26:766–774, 1996.
186. Thompson AB, et al: Intraluminal airway inflammation in chronic bronchitis: Characterization and correlation with clinical parameters. Am Rev Respir Dis 140:1527–1537, 1989.
187. Thompson AB, et al: Aerosolized beclamethasone in chronic bronchitis: Improved pulmonary function and diminished airway inflammation. Am Rev Respir Dis 146:389–395, 1992.
188. Saetta M, et al: Macrophage and neutrophil infiltration in the bronchial glands of subjects with chronic obstructive pulmonary disease. Am J Respir Crit Care Med 155:A595, 1997.
189. Hossain S, Heard BE: Hyperplasia of bronchial muscle in chronic bronchitis. J Pathol 101:171–184, 1970.
190. Nagai A, West WW, Paul JL, et al: The National Institutes of Health intermittent positive pressure breathing trial: Pathology studies. I. Interrelationships between morphologic lesions. Am Rev Respir Dis 132:937–945, 1985.
191. Niewoehner DE, Kleinerman J, Rice DB, et al: Pathologic changes in the peripheral airways of young cigarette smokers. N Engl J Med 291:755–758, 1974.
192. Wright JL, Cagle P, Churg A, et al: Disease of the small airways. Am Rev Respir Dis 146:240–262, 1992.
193. Linhartova A, Anderson AE, Foraker AG: Radial traction and bronchiolar obstruction in pulmonary emphysema. Arch Pathol 92:384–391, 1974.
194. Linhartova A, Anderson AE, Foraker AG: Further observations on luminal deformity and stenosis of nonrespiratory bronchioles in pulmonary emphysema. Thorax 32:53–59, 1977.
195. Saetta M, Ghezzo H, Kim WD, et al: Loss of alveolar attachments in smokers. Am Rev Respir Dis 132:894–900, 1985.
196. Nagai A, West WW, Thurlbeck WM: The National Institutes of Health intermitent positive-pressure breathing trial: Pathology studies II. Correlation between morphologic findings, clinical findings, and evidence of expiratory airflow obstruction. Am Rev Respir Dis 132:946–953, 1985.
197. Nagsai A, Yamawaki I, Takizawa T, et al: Alveolar attachments in emphysema of human lungs. Am Rev Respir Dis 144:888–891, 1991.
198. Hayes JA: Distribution of bronchial gland measurements in a Jamaican population. Thorax 24:619–622, 1969.
199. McKenzie HI, Glick N, Outhred KJ: Chronic bronchitis in coal miners. Ante-mortem/post-mortem comparisons. Thorax 24:527–535, 1969.
200. Ryder RC, Lyons JP, Campbell H: Bronchial mucous gland status in coal-workers' pneumoconiosis. Ann NY Acad Sci 200:370–380, 1972.
201. Bedrossian CWM, Greenberg SD, Singer DB: The lung in cystic fibrosis. Hum Pathol 7:195–204, 1976.
202. Cooney TP, Thurlbeck WM: Pulmonary hypoplasia in Down's syndrome. N Engl J Med 307:1170–1173, 1982.
203. Brody JS, Thurlbeck WM: Development, growth and aging of the lung. Handbk Physiol (Sec 3) 1:335–386, 1986.
204. Morgan WKC, Seaton A: Occupational Lung Diseases. *In* Occupational Lung Diseases. Philadelphia: WB Saunders, 1984.
205. Snider GL, Brody JS, Doctor L: Subclinical pulmonary emphysema. Am Rev Respir Dis 85:666–683, 1962.
206. Thurlbeck WM: The incidence of pulmonary emphysema: With observations on the relative incidence and spatial distribution of various types of emphysema. Am Rev Respir Dis 87:206–215, 1963.

207. Kim WD, Eidelman DH, Izquierdo JL: Centrilobular and panlobular emphysema in smokers: Two distinct morphologic and functional entities. Am Rev Respir Dis 144:1385–1390, 1991.
208. Schmidt RA, Glenny RW: Panlobular emphysema in young intravenous Ritalin abusers. Am Rev Respir Dis 143:649–656, 1991.
209. Heard BE: Further observations on the pathology of pulmonary emphysema in chronic bronchitis. Thorax 14:58–70, 1959.
210. Edge J, Simon G, Reid L: Peri-acinar (paraseptal) emphysema—its clinical, radiological and physiological features. Br J Dis Chest 60:10–18, 1966.
211. Butler C, Kleinerman J: Pathology of chronic obstructive pulmonary disease. Am J Pathol 60:205–216, 1970.
212. Thurlbeck WM: Pathology of chronic obstructive pulmonary disease. Clin Chest Med 11:389–404, 1990.
213. Spencer H: Pathology of the Lung. New York: Pergamon Press, 1985, pp 98–108.
214. Rogers LF, Osmer JC: Bronchogenic cyst: A review of 46 cases. AJR 91:273–283, 1964.
215. Reed JC, Sobonya RE: Morphologic analysis of foregut cysts in the thorax. AJR 120:851–860, 1974.
216. Simon G, Galbraith JJB: Radiology of chronic bronchitis. Lancet 265:850–853, 1953.
217. Reid LM: Correlations of certain bronchographic abnormalities seen in chronic bronchitis with the pathological changes. Thorax 10:199–204, 1955.
218. Duinker AVW, Huizinga E: The "flowers" in bronchography. Thorax 17:175–180, 1962.
219. Webb WR, Stein MG, Finkbeiner WE, et al: Normal and diseased isolated lungs: High resolution CT. Radiology 166:81–87, 1988.
220. Klein JS, Gamsu G, Webb WR: High-resolution CT diagnosis of emphysema in symptomatic patients with normal chest radiographs and isolated low diffusing capacity. Radiology 182:817–821, 1992.
221. Hruban RH, Meziane MA, Zerhouni EA, et al: High resolution computed tomography of inflation-fixed lungs: Pathologic-radiologic correlation of centrilobular emphysema. Am Rev Respir Dis 136:935–940, 1987.
222. Jamal K, Cooney TP, Fleetham JA, et al: Chronic bronchitis: Correlation of morphological findings to sputum production and flow rates. Am Rev Respir Dis 129:719–722, 1984.
223. Mullen JBM, Wright JL, Wiggs BR, et al: Reassessment of inflammation of airways in chronic bronchitis. BMJ 281:1235–1239, 1985.
224. West WW, et al: The National Institutes of Health intermittent positive-pressure breathing trial: Pathology studies. III. The diagnosis of emphysema. Am Rev Respir Dis 135:123–129, 1987.
225. Matsuba K, Ikeda T, Nagai A, et al: The National Institutes of Health intermittent positive-pressure breathing trial: Pathology studies. Am Rev Respir Dis 139:1439–1445, 1989.
226. Matsuba K, Takayuki S, Kuwano K: Small airways disease in patients without chronic airflow limitation. Am Rev Respir Dis 136:1105–1111, 1987.
227. Snider GL: Chronic obstructive pulmonary disease: Risk factors, pathophysiology and pathogenesis. Annu Rev Med 40:411–429, 1989.
228. Mitchell RS, Stanford RE, Johnson JM, et al: The morphologic features of the bronchi, bronchioles and alveoli in chronic airway obstruction: A clinicopathologic study. Am Rev Respir Dis 114:137–145, 1976.
229. Hale KA, Ewing SL, Gosnell BA, et al: Lung disease in long-term smokers with and without chronic airflow obstruction. Am Rev Respir Dis 130:716–721, 1984.
230. Christie RV, McIntosh CA: The measurement of the intrapleural pressure in man. J Clin Invest 13:279–294, 1934.
231. Petty TL, Silvers W, Stanford RE: Mild emphysema is associated with reduced elastic recoil and increased lung size, but not with airflow limitation. Am Rev Respir Dis 136:867–876, 1980.
232. Pare PD, Brooks LA, Bates J, et al: Exponential analysis of the pressure-volume curve as a predictor of emphysema. Am Rev Respir Dis 126:54–61, 1982.
233. Clausen JL: The diagnosis of emphysema, chronic bronchitis and asthma. Am Rev Respir Dis 126:405–416, 1990.
234. Hogg JC, Nepszy SJ, Macklem PT: Elastic properties of the centrilobular emphysematous space. J Clin Invest 48:1306–1312, 1969.
235. Saetta M: Destructive index: A measurement of lung parenchymal destruction in smokers. Am Rev Respir Dis 131:764–769, 1985.
236. Silverman EK, Chapman HA, Dreazen JM, et al: Genetic epidemiology of severe, early-onset chronic obstructive pulmonary disease. Risk to relatives for airflow obstruction and chronic bronchitis. Am J Respir Crit Care Med 157:1770–1778, 1998.
237. Luisetti M, Pignatti PF: The search for susceptibility genes of COPD. Monaldi Arch Chest Dis 50:28–32, 1995.
238. Smith CA, Harrison DJ: Association between polymorphism in gene for microsomal epoxide hydrolase and susceptibility to emphysema. Lancet 350:630–633, 1997.
239. Harrison DJ, Cantlay AM, Rae F, et al: Frequency of glutathione S-transferase M1 deletion in smokers with emphysema and lung cancer. Hum Exp Toxicol 16:356–360, 1997.
240. Faber J, Poller W, Olek K, et al: The molecular basis of alpha 1-antichymotrypsin deficiency in a heterozygote with liver and lung disease. J Hepatol 18:313–321, 1993.
241. Schellenberg D, Pare PD, Weir TD, et al: Vitamin D binding protein variants and the risk of COPD. Am J Respir Crit Care Med 157:957–961, 1998.
242. Huang SL, Su CH, Chang SC: Tumor necrosis factor-α gene polymorphism in chronic-bronchitis. Am J Respir Crit Care Med 156:1436–1439, 1997.
243. Elliott WM, Hayashi S, Hogg JC: Immunodetection of adenoviral E1A proteins in human lung tissue. Am J Respir Cell Mol Biol 12:642–648, 1995.
244. Matsuse T, Hayashi S, Kuwano K, et al: Latent adenoviral infection in the pathogenesis of chronic airways obstruction. Am Rev Respir Dis 146:177–184, 1992.
245. Keicho N, et al: Adenovirus E1A upregulates interleukin-8 expression induced by endotoxin in pulmonary epithelial cells. Am J Physiol 272:L1046–1052, 1997.
246. Keicho N, Elliott WM, Hogg JC, et al: Adenovirus E1A gene dysregulates ICAM-1 expression in transformed pulmonary epithelial cells. Am J Respir Cell Mol Biol 16:23–30, 1997.
247. Vitalis TZ, Kern I, Croome A, et al: The effect of latent adenovirus 5 infection on cigarette smoke-induced lung inflammation. Eur Respir J 11:664–669, 1998.
248. Idell S, Cohen HB: Alpha-1-antitrypsin deficiency. Clin Chest Med 4:359–376, 1983.
249. Travis J: Alpha 1-proteinase inhibitor deficiency. *In* Massaro M (ed): Lung Cell Biology. New York: Marcel Dekker, 1989, pp 1227–1246.
250. Brantly M, Nukiwa T, Crystal RG: Molecular basis of alpha-1-antitrypsin deficiency. Am J Med 84:13–31, 1988.
251. Yoshida L, Lieberman L, Gaidulis L: Molecular abnormality of human alpha-1-antitrypsin variant (piZ) associated with plasma activity deficiency. Proc Natl Acad Sci USA 73:1324–1330, 1976.
252. Jeppson JO, Larsson C, Eriksson C: Characterization of α-1-antitrypsin deficiency. N Engl J Med 293:576–581, 1975.
253. Sanford AJ, Weir TD, Spinelli JJ, et al: Z and S mutations of the alpha 1-antitrypsin gene and the risk of chronic obstructive pulmonary disease. Am J Respir Cell Mol Biol 20:287–291, 1999.
254. Eriksson S: Studies in α-1-antitrypsin deficiency. Acta Med Scand 432:1–85, 1965.
255. Tobin MJ, Cook PJL, Hutchinson DCS: α1-antitrypsin deficiency: The clinical features and physiological features of pulmonary emphysema in subjects homozygous for Pi type Z. A survey by the British Thoracic Association. Br J Dis Chest 77:14–27, 1983.
256. Ericksson S: Pulmonary emphysema and alpha-1 antitrypsin deficiency. Acta Med Scand 175:197–205, 1964.
257. Jones DK, Godden D, Cavanagh P: Alpha-1-antitrypsin deficiency presenting as bronchiectasis. Br J Dis Chest 79:301–304, 1985.
258. Larsson C: Natural history and life expectancy in severe alpha 1-antitrypsin deficiency, PiZ. Acta Med Scand 204:345–351, 1978.
259. Janus ED, Phillips NT, Carrell RW: Smoking, lung function, and alpha-1-antitrypsin deficiency. Lancet 1:152–154, 1985.
260. Brantly ML, Paul LD, Miller BH: Clinical features and history of the destructive lung disease associated with alpha-1-antitrypsin deficiency of adults with pulmonary symptoms. Am Rev Respir Dis 138:327–336, 1988.

261. Wall M, Moe E, Eisenberg J: Long term follow-up of a cohort of children with alpha-1-antitrypsin deficiency in nonsmokers. J Pediatr 116:248–251, 1990.
262. Black LF, Kueppers F: Alpha-1-antitrypsin deficiency in nonsmokers. Am Rev Respir Dis 117:421–428, 1990.
263. Silverman EK, Pierce JA, Province MA, et al: Variability of pulmonary function in alpha-1-antitrypsin deficiency: Clinical correlates. Ann Intern Med 111:982–991, 1989.
264. Hepper NG, Mulm JR, Sheehan WC: Roentgenographic study of chronic obstructive pulmonary disease by alpha-1-antitrypsin phenotype. Mayo Clin Proc 53:166–172, 1978.
265. Gishen P, Saunders AJS, Tobin MJ: Alpha-1-antitrypsin deficiency: The radiologic features of pulmonary emphysema in subjects of pi type Z and SZ: A survey by the British Thoracic Association. Clin Radiol 33:371–380, 1982.
266. Mittman C: The PiMZ phenotype: Is it a significant risk factor for the development of chronic obstructive lung disease? Am Rev Respir Dis 118:649–652, 1978.
267. Morse LO, Lebowitz MD, Knudson RA, et al: Relation of protease inhibitor phenotypes to obstructive lung disease in a community. N Engl J Med 296:190–194, 1977.
268. Bruce RM, Cohen BH, Diamond EL, et al: Collaborative study to assess risk of lung disease in PiMZ phenotype subjects. Am Rev Respir Dis 130:386–390, 1984.
269. Poller W, Meisen C, Olek K: DNA polymorphisms of the alpha 1-antitrypsin gene region in patients with chronic obstructive pulmonary disease. Eur J Clin Invest 20:1–7, 1990.
270. Kalsheker NA, Watkins GL, Hill S: Independent mutations in the flanking sequence of the alpha-1-antitrypsin gene are associated with chronic obstructive airways disease. Dis Markers 8:151–157, 1990.
271. Kalsheker N: Serine proteinase inhibitors on chromosome 14 and the genetics of familial chronic obstructive lung disease. Med Hypotheses 31:67–70, 1990.
272. Hodgson I, Kalsheker N: RFLP for a gene-related sequence of alpha 1-antitrypsin (AAT). Nucleic Acids Res 14:6779, 1986.
273. Morgan K, Scobie G, Kalsheker N: The characterization of a mutation of the 3′ flanking sequence of the alpha 1-antitrypsin gene commonly associated with chronic obstructive airways disease. Eur J Clin Invest 22:134–137, 1992.
274. Morgan K, Scobie G, Kalsheker NA: Point mutation in a 3′ flanking sequence of the alpha-1-antitrypsin gene associated with chronic respiratory disease occurs in a regulatory sequence. Hum Mol Genet 2:253–257, 1993.
275. Eriksson RM, Carlson J, Velez R: Risk of cirrhosis and primary liver cancer in alpha-1-antitrypsin deficiency. N Engl J Med 314:736–739, 1986.
276. Pratschke J, Steinmuller T, Bechstein WO, et al: Orthotopic liver transplantation for hepatic-associated metabolic disorders. Transplant Proc 31:382–384, 1999.
277. Wu Y, Whitman I, Molmenti E, et al: A lag in intracellular degradation of mutant $\alpha_1$-antitrypsin correlates with the liver disease phenotype in homozygous piZZ $\alpha_1$-antitrypsin deficiency. Proc Natl Acad Sci USA 91:9014–9018, 1994.
278. Hutchison DC: Natural history of alpha-1-protease inhibitor deficiency. Am J Med 84:3–12, 1988.
279. Wewers MD, Casolaro MA: Replacement therapy for alpha-antitrypsin deficiency associated with emphysema. N Engl J Med 316:1055–1062, 1987.
280. Buist AS, Burrows B, Cohen A, et al: Guidelines for the approach to the individual with severe hereditary alpha-1-antitrypsin deficiency. An official statement of the American Thoracic Society. Am Rev Respir Dis 140:1494–1497, 1989.
281. Low DE, Trulock EP, Kaiser LR: Morbidity, mortality, and early results of single versus double lung transplantation for emphysema. J Thorac Cardiovasc 103:1119–1126, 1992.
282. Hubbard RC, Sellers S, Czerski D: Biochemical efficacy and safety of monthly augmentation therapy for alpha-1-antitrypsin deficiency. JAMA 260:1259–1264, 1992.
283. Hubbard RC, Brantly ML, Sellers SE, et al: Anti-neutrophil-elastase defenses of the lower respiratory tract in alpha-1-antitrypsin deficiency directly augmented with an aerosol of alpha-1-antitrypsin. Ann Intern Med 111:206–212, 1988.
284. Hubbard RC, Brantly ML, Sellers SE, et al: Recombinant DNA-produced alpha 1-antitrypsin administered by aerosol augments lower respiratory tract antineutrophil elastase defenses in individuals with alpha 1-antitrypsin deficiency. J Clin Invest 84:1349–1354, 1989.
285. Janoff A: Elastases and emphysema. Current assessment of the protease-antiprotease hypothesis. Am Rev Respir Dis 132:417–433, 1985.
286. Ganz T, Lehrer RI: Defensins. Curr Opin Immunol 6:584–589, 1994.
287. Blackwood CE, Hosannah Y, Perman E: Experimental emphysema in rats: Elastolytic titer of inducing enzyme as determinant of the response. Proc Soc Exp Med 144:450–454, 1973.
288. Janoff A, Sloan B, Weinbaum G, et al: Experimental emphysema induced with purified human neutrophil elastase: Tissue localization of the instilled protease. Am Rev Resp Dis 115:461–478, 1977.
289. Senior RM, Tegner H, Kuhn C, et al: The induction of pulmonary emphysema with human leukocyte elastase. Am Rev Resp Dis 116:469–475, 1977.
290. Snider GL, Lucey EC, Christensen TG, et al: Emphysema and bronchial secretory cell metaplasia induced in hamsters by human neutrophil products. Am Rev Respir Dis 129:155–160, 1984.
291. Lucey EC, Stone PJ, Snider GL: Consequences of proteolytic injury. *In* Crystal RG (ed): The Lung: Scientific Foundations. New York: Raven Press, 1991, pp. 1789–1801.
292. Shapiro SD: Matrix metalloproteinase degradation of extracellular matrix: Biological consequences. Curr Opin Cell Biol 10:602–608, 1998.
293. Lucey EC, Stone PJ, Christensen TG: An 18 month study of the effects on hamster lungs of intratracheally administered human neutrophil elastase. Exp Lung Res 14:671–686, 1988.
294. Snider GL, Sherter CB, Koo KW, et al: Respiratory mechanics in hamsters following treatment with endotracheal elastase or collagenase. J Appl Physiol 42:206–215, 1977.
295. Icochea A, Cooper BS, Kuhn C: The effect of oxygen on cor pulmonale in experimental emphysema induced by elastase or elastase and beta-aminopropionitrile in hamsters. Am Rev Respir Dis 126:792–796, 1982.
296. Karlinsky JB, Fredette J, Davidovits G: The balance of lung connective tissue elements in elastase-induced emphysema. J Lab Clin Med 102:151–162, 1983.
297. Kuhn C, Yu SY, Chraplyvy M: The induction of emphysema with elastase: II. Changes in connective tissue. Lab Invest 34:372–380, 1976.
298. Wittels EH, Coalson JJ, Jacques J: Pulmonary intravascular leukocyte sequestration: A potential mechanism of lung injury. Am Rev Respir Dis 109:502–509, 1974.
299. Guenter CA Coalson JJ, Jacques J: Emphysema associated with intravascular leukocyte sequestration. Comparison with papain-induced emphysema. Am Rev Respir Dis 123:79–84, 1981.
300. Rudolphus A, Kramps JA, Dijkman JH: Effect of human antileucoprotease on experimental emphysema. Eur Respir J 4:103–108, 1991.
301. Blackwood RA, Moret J, Mandl I: Emphysema induced by intravenously administered endotoxin in an alpha-1-antitrypsin-deficient rat model. Am Rev Respir Dis 130:231–236, 1984.
302. Selby C, Drost E, Wraith PK, et al: In vivo neutrophil sequestration within lungs of humans is determined by in vitro "filterability." J Appl Physiol 71:1996–2003, 1991.
303. MacNee W, Wiggs B, Belzberg AS, et al: The effect of cigarette smoking on neutrophil kinetics in human lungs. N Engl J Med 321:924–928, 1989.
304. Drost EM, Selby C, Lannan S, et al: Changes in neutrophil deformability following in vitro smoke exposure: Mechanism and protection. Am J Respir Cell Mol Biol 6:287–295, 1992.
305. Selby C, Drost E, Lannan S, et al: Neutrophil retention in the lungs of patients with chronic obstructive pulmonary disease. Am Rev Respir Dis 143:1259–1264, 1991.
306. Snider G, Lucey E, Stone P: Animal models of emphysema. Am Rev Respir Dis 133:149–169, 1986.
307. Galdston M, Melnick EL, Goldring RM: Interactions of neutrophil elastase, serum trypsin inhibitory activity, and smoking history as risk factors for chronic obstructive pulmonary disease in patients with MM, MZ and ZZ phenotypes for $alpha_1$-antitrypsin. Am Rev Respir Dis 116:837–846, 1977.

308. Kidokoro Y, Kravis TC, Moser KME: Relationship of leukocyte elastase concentration to severity of emphysema in homozygous $alpha_1$-antitrypsin-deficient persons. Am Rev Respir Dis 115:793–803, 1977.
309. Abboud RT, Rushton JM, Grzybowski S: Interrelationships between neutrophil elastase, serum $alpha_1$-antitrypsin, lung function and chest radiography in patients with chronic airflow obstruction. Am Rev Respir Dis 120:31–40, 1979.
310. Lam S, Abboud RT, Chan-Yeung M: Neutrophil elastase and pulmonary function in subjects with intermediate $alpha_1$-antitrypsin deficiency (MZ phenotype). Am Rev Respir Dis 119:941–951, 1979.
311. Rodriguez JR, Seal JE, Radin AEA: Neutrophil lysosomal elastase activity in normal subjects and in patients with chronic obstructive pulmonary disease. Am Rev Respir Dis 119:409–417, 1979.
312. Kramps JA, Bakker W, Dijkman JH: A matched-pair study of the leukocyte elastase-like activity in normal persons and in emphysematous patients with and without $alpha_1$-antitrypsin deficiency. Am Rev Respir Dis 121:253–261, 1980.
313. Binder R: Serum antielastase and neutrophil elastase levels in PiM phenotype cigarette smokers with airflow obstruction. Respiration 47:267–267, 1985.
314. Stockley RA, Ohlsson K: Serum studies of leucocyte elastase in acute and chronic lung disease. Thorax 37:114–117, 1982.
315. Perricone R, et al: Complement activation by cigarette smoke condensate and tobacco infusion. Arch Environ Health 38:176–179, 1983.
316. Kew RR, Ghebrehiwet B, Janoff A: The fifth component of complement (C5) is necessary for maximal pulmonary leukocytosis in mice chronically exposed to cigarette smoke. Clin Immunol Immunopathol 43:73–81, 1987.
317. Robbins RA, Gossman GL, Nelson KJ, et al: Inactivation of chemotactic factor inactivator by cigarette smoke. A potential mechanism of modulating neutrophil recruitment to the lung. Am Rev Respir Dis 142:763–768, 1990.
318. Hunninghake GW, Crystal RG: Cigarette smoking and lung destruction: Accumulation of neutrophils in the lungs of cigarette smokers. Am Rev Respir Dis 128:833–838, 1983.
319. Shoji S, Ertl RF, Koyama S, et al: Cigarette smoke stimulates release of neutrophil chemotactic activity from cultured bovine bronchial epithelial cells. Clin Sci 88:337–344, 1995.
320. Mio T, Romberger DJ, Thompson AB, et al: Cigarette smoke induces interleukin-8 release from human bronchial epithelial cells. Am J Respir Crit Care Med 155:1770–1776, 1997.
321. Rao NV, Wehner NG, Marshall BC: Proteinase-3 (Pr-3): A polymorphonuclear leukocyte serine proteinase. Ann NY Acad Sci 624:60–68, 1991.
322. Fujita J, Nelson NL, Daughton DM, et al: Evaluation of elastase and antielastase balance in patients with bronchitis and pulmonary emphysema. Am Rev Respir Dis 142:57–62, 1990.
323. Carp H, Miller F, Hoidal JR, et al: Potential mechanism of emphysema: Alpha-1-proteinase inhibitor recovered from lungs of cigarette smokers contains oxidized methionine and has decreased elastase inhibitory capacity. Proc Natl Acad Sci USA 79:2041–2045, 1979.
324. Hubbard RC, Ogushi F, Fells GA, et al: Oxidants spontaneously released by alveolar macrophages of cigarette smokers can inactivate the active site of alpha-1 antitrypsin, rendering it ineffective as an inhibitor of neutrophil elastase. J Clin Invest 80:1289–1295, 1987.
325. Shapiro SD: Elastolytic metalloproteinases produced by human mononuclear phagocytes. Am J Respir Crit Care Med 150:S160–S164, 1994.
326. Janoff A: Levels of elastase activity in bronchoalveolar lavage fluids of healthy smokers and nonsmokers. Am Rev Respir Dis 127:540–544, 1983.
327. Niewoehner DE, Leatherman JW: Bronchodilator therapy in chronic airflow obstruction. Chest 86:161–162, 1984.
328. Hunninghake GW, Davidson JM, Rennard SI, et al: Elastin fragments attract macrophage precursors to diseased sites in pulmonary emphysema. Science 212:925–927, 1981.
329. Senior RM, Griffin GL, Meacham RP: Chemotactic activity of elastin-derived peptides. J Clin Invest 66:859–862, 1980.
330. Kominami E, Tsukahara T, Katunuma N: Biosynthesis and processing of lysosomal cysteine proteinases in rat macrophages. FEBS Lett 231:225–228, 1988.
331. Gariola CG, Galicki NI, Cardozo C: Cigarette smoke stimulates cathepsin B activity in alveolar macrophages of rats. Lab Clin Med 114:419–425, 1989.
332. Chang JC, Lesser M, Yoo OH, et al: Increased cathepsin B-like activity in alveolar macrophages and bronchoalveolar lavage fluid from smokers. Am Rev Respir Dis 134:538–541, 1986.
333. Lesser M, Padilla ML, Cardozo D: Induction of emphysema in hamsters by intratracheal instillation of cathepsin B. Am Rev Respir Dis 145:661–668, 1992.
334. Chang J, Yoo OH, Lesser M: Cathepsin D activity is increased in alveolar macrophages and bronchoalveolar lavage fluid of smokers. Am Rev Respir Dis 140:958–960, 1989.
335. Lesser M, Galicki N, Cardozo C: Cathepsin L activity in alveolar macrophages of rats: Response to cigarette smoke. Am J Respir Cell Mol Biol 1:371–376, 1989.
336. D'Armiento J, Dalal SS, Okada Y, et al: Collagenase expression in the lungs of transgenic mice causes pulmonary emphysema. Cell 71:955–961, 1992.
337. Davies SF, Offord KP, Brown MG, et al: Urine desmosine is unrelated to cigarette smoking or to spirometric function. Am Rev Respir Dis 128:473–475, 1983.
338. Harel S, Janoff A, Yu SY, et al: Desmosine radioimmunoassay for measuring elastin degradation in vitro. Am Rev Respir Dis 122:769–773, 1980.
339. Pelham F, Wewers M, Crystal R, et al: Urinary excretion of desmosine (elastase cross-links) in subjects with PiZZ alpha-1-antitrypsin deficiency, a phenotype associated with hereditary predisposition to pulmonary emphysema. Am Rev Respir Dis 132:821–823, 1985.
340. Stone PJ, Bryan-Rhadfi J, Lucey EC, et al: Measurement of urinary desmosine by isotope dilution and high performance liquid chromatography. Correlation between elastase-induced air-space enlargement in the hamster and elevation of urinary desmosine. Am Rev Respir Dis 144:284–290, 1991.
341. Kucich U, Christner P, Lippmann M, et al: Utilization of a peroxidase antiperoxidase complex in an enzyme-linked immunosorbent assay of elastin-derived peptides in human plasma. Am Rev Respir Dis 131:709–713, 1985.
342. Stone PJ, Morris TA, Franzblau C, et al: Preliminary evidence that augmentation therapy diminishes degradation of cross-linked elastin in alpha-1-antitrypsin-deficient humans. Respiration 62:76–79, 1995.
343. Grove A, Lipworth BJ, Reid P, et al: Effects of regular salmeterol on lung function and exercise capacity in patients with chronic obstructive airways disease. Thorax 51:689–693, 1996.
344. Damiano VV, Tsang A, Kucich U, et al: Immunolocalization of elastase in human emphysematous lungs. J Clin Invest 78, 1986.
345. Fox B, Bull TB, Guz A, et al: Is neutrophil elastase associated with elastic tissue in emphysema? J Clin Pathol 41:435–440, 1988.
346. Ge YM, Zhu YJ, Lou WC: Damaging role of neutrophil elastase in the elastic fiber and basement membrane in human emphysematous lung. Chin Med J 103:588–594, 1990.
347. Pierce JA, Hocott JB, Ebert RV: The collagen and elastin content of the lung in emphysema. Ann Intern Med 55:210–221, 1961.
348. Pecora LJ, Manne WR, Feldman DP: Biochemical study of ground substances in normal and emphysematous lungs. Am Rev Respir Dis 95:623–630, 1967.
349. Fitzpatrick M: Studies of human pulmonary conncective tissue III. Am Rev Respir Dis 96:254–265, 1967.
350. Chrzanowski P, Keller S, Cerreta J: Elastin content of normal and emphysematous lung parenchyma. Am J Med 69:351–359, 1988.
351. Lang MR, Fiaux GW, Gillooly M, et al: Collagen content of alveolar wall tissue in emphysematous and non-emphysematous lungs. Thorax 49:319–326, 1994.
352. Lane RE, Campbell ACP: Fatal emphysema in two men making a copper cadmium alloy. Br J Ind Med 11:118–122, 1954.
353. Snider GL, Hayes JA, Korthy AL, et al: Centrilobular emphysema experimentally induced by cadmium chloride aerosol. Am Rev Respir Dis 108:40–48, 1973.
354. Niewoehner DE, Hoidal JR: Lung fibrosis and emphysema: Divergent responses to a common injury? Science 217:359–360, 1982.

355. Hoidal JR, Niewoehner DE, Rao NV, et al: The role of neutrophils in the development of cadmium chloride-induced emphysema in lathyrogen-fed hamsters. Am J Pathol 120:22–29, 1985.
356. Lewis GP, Jusko WJ, Coughlin LL, et al: Contribution of cigarette smoking to cadmium accumulation in man. Lancet 1:291–292, 1972.
357. Hirst RN, Perry HM, Cruz MG, et al: Elevated cadmium concentration in emphysematous lungs. Am Rev Respir Dis 108:30–39, 1973.
358. Riley D: Prevention of collagen deposition following pulmonary oxygen toxicity in the rat by cis-4-hydroxy-L-proline. J Clin Invest 65:643–651, 1980.
359. Freeman G, Stephens RJ, Crane SC: Lesion of the lung in rats continuously exposed to two parts per million of nitrogen dioxide. Arch Environ Health 17:181–190, 1968.
360. Glasgow JE, Pietra GG, Abrams WR, et al: Neutrophil recruitment and degranulation during induction of emphysema in the rat by nitrogen dioxide. Am Rev Respir Dis 135:1129–1136, 1987.
361. Blank J, Glasgow JE, Pietra GG, et al: Nitrogen-dioxide–induced emphysema in rats: Lack of worsening by beta-aminopropionitrile treatment. Am Rev Respir Dis 135:376–379, 1988.
362. Lam C, Kattan M, Collins A: Long-term sequelae of bronchiolitis induced by nitrogen dioxide in hamsters. Am Rev Respir Dis 128:1020–1023, 1983.
363. Kleinerman J, Ip MPC, Gordon RE: The reaction of the respiratory tract to chronic $NO_2$ exposure. *In* Scarpelli DG, Craighead JE, Kaufman N (eds): The Pathologist and the Environment—International Academy of Pathology Monograph. Baltimore: Williams & Wilkins, 1995, pp 200–210.
364. Lafuma C, Harf A, Lange F, et al: Effect of low level $NO_2$ chronic exposure on elastase-induced emphysema. Environ Res 43:75–84, 1987.
365. Blair WH, Henry MC, Ehrlich R: Chronic toxicity of nitrogen dioxide: Effect on histopathology of lung tissue. Arch Environ Health 18:186–192, 1969.
366. Haydon GB, Davidson JT, Lillington GA: Nitrogen dioxide–induced emphysema in rabbits. Am Rev Respir Dis 95:797–805, 1967.
367. Kleinerman J, Ip MPC: Effect of nitrogen dioxide on elastin and collagen contents of lung. Arch Environ Health 34:228–232, 1979.
368. Lucey EC, Stone PJ, Christensen TG, et al: Human neutrophil elastase-induced and ozone-induced emphysema in hamsters are additive (abstract). Am Rev Respir Dis 141:A736, 1990.
369. Sahebjami H, Vassallo CL: Effects of starvation and refeeding on lung mechanics and morphometry. Am Rev Respir Dis 119:443–451, 1979.
370. Sahebjami H, Wirman JA: Emphysema-like changes in the lungs of starved rats. Am Rev Respir Dis 124:619–624, 1981.
371. Harkema JR, Mauderly JL, Gregory RE, et al: A comparison of starvation and elastase models of emphysema in the rat. Am Rev Respir Dis 129:584–591, 1984.
372. Kerr JS, Riley DJ, Lanza-Jacoby S, et al: Nutrition emphysema in the rat: Influence of protein depletion and impaired lung growth. Am Rev Respir Dis 131:644–650, 1985.
373. Karlinsky JB, Goldstein RH, Ojserkis B, et al: Lung mechanics and connective tissue levels in starvation-induced emphysema in hamsters. Am J Physiol 251:R282–R288, 1986.
374. Sahebjami H, MacGee J: Effects of starvation on lung mechanics and biochemistry in young and old rats. J Appl Physiol 58:778–784, 1985.
375. Sahebjami H, MacGee J: Effects of starvation and refeeding on lung biochemistry in rats. Am Rev Respir Dis 126:483–487, 1982.
376. Hoidal JR, Niewoehner DE: Cigarette smoke inhalation potentiates elastase-induced emphysema in hamsters. Am Rev Respir Dis 127:478–481, 1983.
377. Frasca JM, Auerbach O, Carter HW: Morphologic alterations induced by short-term cigarette smoking. Am J Pathol 111:11–20, 1983.
378. Hautamaki RD, Kobayashi DK, Senior RM, et al: Requirement for macrophage elastase for cigarette smoke–induced emphysema in mice. Science 277:2002–2004, 1997.
379. Snider GL: Chronic obstructive pulmonary disease—A continuing challenge. Am Rev Respir Dis 133:942–944, 1986.
380. Reid L, Jones R: Experimental chronic bronchitis. Int Rev Pathol 24:335–382, 1983.
381. Lamb D, Reid L: Mitotic rates, goblet cell increase and histochemical changes in mucus in rat bronchial epithelium during exposure to sulphur dioxide. J Pathol Bacteriol 96:97–111, 1968.
382. Lightowler NM, Williams JRB: Tracheal mucous flow rates in experimental bronchitis in rats. Br J Exp Pathol 50:139–145, 1969.
383. Charkin LW, Saunders LZ: Experimental chronic bronchitis, pathology in dog. Lab Invest 30:145–150, 1974.
384. Scanlon PD, Seltzer J, Ingram RM Jr, et al: Chronic exposure to sulfur dioxide. Physiologic and histologic exposure of dogs exposed to 50 or 15 ppm. Am Rev Respir Dis 135:831–839, 1987.
385. Lamb D, Reid L: Goblet cell increase in rat bronchial epithelium after exposure to cigarette and cigar tobacco smoke. BMJ 1:33–35, 1969.
386. Rogers DF, Jeffery PK: Inhibition by oral *N*-acetylcysteine of cigarette smoke–induced "bronchitis" in the rat. Exp Lung Res 10:267–283, 1986.
387. Snider GL: Animal models of chronic airways injury. Chest 101:74S–79S, 1992.
388. Christensen TG, Lucey EC, Breuer R, et al: Acid-induced secretory cell metaplasia in hamster bronchi. Environ Res 45:78–90, 1988.
389. Evans MJ, Johnson LV, Stephens RJ, et al: Renewal of the terminal bronchial epithelium in the rat following exposure to $NO_2$ or $O_3$. Lab Invest 35:246–257, 1976.
390. Evans MJ, Johnson LV, Stephens RJ, et al: Cell renewal in the lungs of rats exposed to low levels of ozone. J Exp Mol Pathol 24:70–76, 1976.
391. Lum H, Schwartz LW, Dungworth DL, et al: A comparative study of cell renewal after exposure to ozone or oxygen. Am Rev Respir Dis 118:335–345, 1978.
392. Mellick PW, Dungworth DL, Schwartz LW, et al: Short term morphologic effects of high ambient levels of ozone on lungs of rhesus monkeys. Lab Invest 36:82–90, 1977.
393. Davis WG, Rennard SI, Bittermann P, et al: Pulmonary oxygen toxicity: Early reversible changes in human alveolar structures induced by hyperoxia. N Engl J Med 309:878–883, 1983.
394. Koren HS, Devlin RB, Graham DE, et al: Ozone-induced inflammation in the lower airways of human subjects. Am Rev Respir Dis 139:407–415, 1989.
395. Von Essen SG, McGranaghan S, Cirian D, et al: Inhalation of grain sorghum dust extract causes respiratory tract inflammation in human volunteers. Am Rev Respir Dis 143:A105, 1991.
396. Abramson SL, Malech HL, Gallin JI: Neutrophils. *In* Crystal RG, West JB (eds): The Lung: Scientific Foundations. New York: Raven Press, 1991, pp 553–564.
397. Boucher RC, Van Scott MR, Willumsen N, et al: Epithelial cell injury. Mechanisms and cell biology of airway epithelial cell injury. Am Rev Respir Dis 138:S41–44, 1988.
398. Venaille TJ, Mendis AH, Warton A, et al: Study of human epithelial cell detachment and damage: Development of a model. Immunol Cell Biol 67:359–369, 1989.
399. Rickard KA, Taylor J, Rennard SI: Observations on development of resistance to detachment of cultured bovine epithelial cells in response to protease treatment. Am J Respir Cell Mol Biol 6:414–420, 1992.
400. Breuer RN, Lucey EC, Stone PJ: Proteolytic activity of human neutrophil elastase and porcine pancreatic trypsin causes bronchial secretory cell metaplasia in hamsters. Exp Lung Res 9:167–175, 1985.
401. DeWater R, Willems LNA, Van Muijen NP, et al: Ultrastructural localization of bronchial antileukoprotease in central and peripheral human airways by a gold-labelling technique using monoclonal antibodies. Am Rev Respir Dis 133:882–890, 1985.
402. Lucey EC, Stone PJ, Ciccolella DE, et al: Recombinant human secretory leukocyte-protease inhibitor: In vitro properties, and amelioration of human neutrophil elastase-induced emphysema and secretory cell metaplasia in the hamster. J Lab Clin Med 115:224–232, 1990.
403. Martin TR, Raghu G, Maunder RJ, et al: The effects of chronic bronchitis and chronic airflow obstruction on lung cell populations recovered by bronchoalveolar lavage. Am Rev Respir Dis 132:254–260, 1985.
404. Spencer H: Chronic bronchitis and bronchiolitis. *In* Pathology of the Lung. Oxford: Pergamon Press, 1968, pp 121–131.

405. McDowell EM, Beals TF: Biopsy Pathology of the Bronchi. Philadelphia: WB Saunders, 1987, pp 140–191.
406. Sommerhoff CP, Nadel JA, Basbaum CB, et al: Neutrophil elastase and cathepsin G stimulate secretion from cultured bovine airway gland serous cells. J Clin Invest 85:682–689, 1990.
407. Saetta M, Di Stefano A, Maestrelli P, et al: Activated mononuclear cells in the airway mucosa of subjects with chronic bronchitis. Eur Respir J 5:125S, 1992.
408. Teamann UA, Prasad B, Gallup MW, et al: A novel role for murine IL-4 in vivo: Induction of MUC5AC gene expression and mucin hypersecretion. Am J Respir Cell Mol Biol 16:471–478, 1997.
409. Adler KB, Fischer BM, Wright DT, et al: Interactions between respiratory epithelial cells and cytokines: Relationships to lung inflammation. Ann NY Acad Sci 725:128–145, 1994.
410. Von Essen SG, Robbins RA, Thompson AB, et al: Mechanisms of neutrophil recruitment to the lung by grain dust exposure. Am Rev Respir Dis 138:921–927, 1988.
411. Koyama S, Rennard SI, Leikauf G, et al: Endotoxin stimulates bronchial epithelial cells to release chemotactic factors for neutrophils. J Immunol 147:4293–4301, 1991.
412. Mattoli S, Colotta F, Fincato G, et al: Time course of IL1 and IL6 synthesis and release in human bronchial epithelial cell cultures exposed to toluene diisocyanate. J Cell Physiol 149:260–268, 1991.
413. Hamid Q, Azzawa M, Ying S, et al: Expression of mRNA for interleukin-5 in mucosal bronchial biopsies from asthma. J Clin Invest 87:1541–1546, 1991.
414. Marini M, Vittori E, Hollemborg J, et al: Expression of the potent inflammatory cytokines, granulocyte-macrophage colony stimulating factor and interleukin 6 and interleukin 8, in bronchial epithelial cells of patients with asthma. J Allergy Clin Immunol 89:1001–1009, 1992.
415. Shoji S, Rickard KA, Ertl RF, et al: Bronchial epithelial cells produce lung fibroblast chemotactic factor: Fibronectin. Am J Respir Cell Mol Biol 1:13–20, 1989.
416. Wang A, Cohen DS, Palmer E, et al: Polarized regulation of fibronectin secretion and alternative splicing by transforming growth factor. J Biol Chem 266:15558–15560, 1991.
417. Han RN, Mawdsley C, Souza P, et al: Platelet-derived growth factors and growth-related genes in rat lung III. Immunolocalization during fetal development. Pediatr Res 31:323–329, 1992.
418. Nakamura Y, Ertl RF, Kawamoto M, et al: Bronchial epithelial cells modulate fibroblast proliferation: Role of prostaglandin E2. Am Rev Respir Dis 145:A827, 1992.
419. Romberger DJ, Beckmann JD, Claassen L, et al: Modulation of fibronectin production of bovine bronchial epithelial cells by transforming growth factor-beta. Am J Respir Cell Mol Biol 7:149–155, 1992.
420. Sacco O, Romberger D, Rizzino A, et al: Spontaneous production of transforming growth factor beta 2 by primary cultures of bronchial epithelial cells: Effects on cell behavior in vitro. J Clin Invest 90:1379–1385, 1992.
421. Shoji S, Ertl RF, Linder J, et al: Bronchial epithelial cells produce chemotactic activity for bronchial epithelial cells: Possible role for fibronectin in airway repair. Am Rev Respir Dis 141:218–225, 1990.
422. Takizawa H, Beckmann J, Shoji S, et al: Pulmonary macrophages can stimulate cell growth of bovine bronchial epithelial cells. Am J Respir Cell Mol Biol 2:245–255, 1990.
423. Crystal RG: Alveolar macrophages. *In* Crystal RG, West JB (eds): The Lung: Scientific Foundations. New York: Raven Press, 1991, pp 527–538.
424. Crystal RG, Ferrans VJ, Basset F: Biologic basis of pulmonary fibrosis. *In* Crystal RG, West JB (eds): The Lung: Scientific Foundations. New York: Raven Press, 1991, pp 2031–2046.
425. Lane BP, Gordon R: Regeneration of rat tracheal epithelium after mechanical injury. I. Proc Soc Exp Biol Med 145:1139–1144, 1974.
426. Keenan KP, Combs JW, McDowell EM: Regeneration of hamster tracheal epithelium after mechanical injury. Virchows Arch (Cell Pathol) 41:193–214, 1982.
427. McDowell EM, et al: Differentiation of tracheal mucociliary epithelium in primary cell culture recapitulates normal fetal development and regeneration following injury in hamsters. Am J Pathol 129:511–522, 1987.
428. Rickard KA, et al: Attachment characteristics of bovine bronchial epithelial cells to extracellular matrix components. Am J Respir Cell Mol Biol 4:440–448, 1991.
429. Damjanovich L, et al: Distribution of integrin cell adhesion receptors in normal and malignant lung tissue. Am J Respir Cell Mol Biol 6:197–206, 1992.
430. Rickard KA, et al: Extracellular matrix and bronchial epithelial cell migration. Chest 101:17S–18S, 1992.
431. Shoji S, et al: Bronchial epithelial cells respond to insulin and insulin-like growth factor-I as a chemoattractant. Am J Respir Cell Mol Biol 2:553–557, 1990.
432. Jetten AM, Vollberg TM, Nervi C, et al: Positive and negative regulation of proliferation and differentiation in tracheobronchial epithelial cells. Am Rev Respir Dis 142:S36–S39, 1990.
433. Rearick JI, Jetten AM: Effect of substratum and retinoids upon the mucosecretory differentiation of airway epithelial cells in vitro. Environ Health Perspect 80:229–237, 1989.
434. Reid LM: Pathology of chronic bronchitis. Lancet 1:275–281, 1954.
435. Wright JL, Lawson L, Pare PD, et al: The structure and function of the pulmonary vasculature in mild chronic obstructive pulmonary disease. Am Rev Respir Dis 128:702–707, 1983.
436. Kuwano K, Bosken CH, Pare PD, et al: Small airways dimensions in asthma and in chronic obstructive pulmonary disease. Am Rev Respir Dis 148:1220–1225, 1993.
437. Mio T, Adachi Y, Romberger DJ, et al: Human bronchial epithelial cells modulate collagen gel contraction by fibroblasts. Am J Respir Crit Care Med 151:A561, 1995.
438. Liu X, Umino T, Cano M, et al: Human bronchial epithelial cells can contract type I collagen gels. Am J Phys 274:L58–L65, 1998.
439. Sturgess J, Reid L: The effect of isoprenaline and pilocarpine on (a) bronchial mucous secreting tissue and (b) pancreas, salivary glands, heart, thymus, liver and spleen. Br J Exp Pathol 54:388–399, 1973.
440. Salonen RO, Webber SE, Widdicombe JG: Effects of neurotransmitters on tracheobronchial blood flow. Eur Respir J Suppl 12:630s–636s, 1990.
441. Widdicombe JG: Neural control of airway vasculature and edema. Am Rev Respir Dis 143:S18–S21, 1991.
442. Solway J, Leff AR: Sensory neuropeptides and airway function. J Appl Physiol 71:2077–2087, 1991.
443. Barnes PJ: Regulatory peptides in the respiratory system. Experientia (Suppl) 56:317–333, 1989.
444. Von Essen SG, O'Neill D, Wisecarver J, et al: Grain sorghum dust extract causes lymphocyte chemotaxis directly and by stimulating bronchial epithelial cells to secrete chemotactic activity. Am Rev Respir Dis 143:A47, 1991.
445. Nadel JA: Role of mast cell and neutrophil proteases in airway secretion. Am Rev Respir Dis 144:S48–S51, 1991.
446. Bar-Shavit R, Benezra M, Sabbah V, et al: Thrombin as a multifunctional protein: Induction of cell adhesion and proliferation. Am J Respir Cell Mol Biol 6:123–130, 1992.
447. Reynolds HY, Chretien J: Respiratory tract fluids: Analysis of content and contemporary use of understanding lung diseases. Disease-A-Month 30:1–103, 1984.
448. Kobayashi K, Salathe M, Pratt MM, et al: Mechanism of hydrogen peroxide–induced inhibition of sheep airway cilia. Am J Respir Cell Mol Biol 6:667–673, 1992.
449. Widdicombe JH: Ion transport by airway epithelia, *In* Crystal RG, West JB (eds): The Lung: Scientific Foundations. New York: Raven Press, 1991, pp 263–272.
450. Marom Z, Shelhamer J, Berger M, et al: Anaphylatoxin C3a enhances mucous glycoprotein release from human airways in vitro. J Exp Med 161:657–668, 1985.
451. Marom Z, Shelhamer JH, Kaliner M: Human monocyte-derived mucus secretagogue. J Clin Invest 75:191–198, 1985.
452. Murphy T, Sethi S: Bacterial infection in chronic obstructive pulmonary disease. Am Rev Respir Dis 146:1067–1083, 1992.
453. Van Scott MR, Yankaskas JR, Boucher RC: Culture of airway epithelial cells: Research techniques. Exp Lung Res 11:75–94, 1986.
454. Rennard SI, Beckmann JD, Robbins RA: Biology of airway epithelial cells. In Crystal RG, West JB (eds): The Lung: Scientific Foundations. Vol 1. New York: Raven Press, 1991, pp 157–167.

455. Prevention of Pneumococcal Disease: Recommendations of the Advisory Committee on Immunization Practices (ACIP): MMWR Morbid Mortal Weekly Rep 46(RR-8):1–24, 1997.
456. Slmberkoff M: Efficacy of pneumococcal vaccine in high-risk patients. N Engl J Med 315:1318–1327, 1986.
457. Shapiro ED, Berg AT, Austrian R, et al: The protective efficacy of polyvalent pneumococcal polysaccharide vaccine. N Engl J Med 325:1453–1460, 1991.
458. Centers for Disease Control and Prevention: Prevention of pneumococcal diseases. Recommendations of the Advisory Committee on Immunization Practices (ACIP). MMWR 46(RR–8):1–24, 1997
459. Fisher EB Jr, Rose K: Smoking cessation: A practical guide for physicians. Clin Chest Med 7:551–566, 1986.
460. Rennard SI, Daughton DM: Nicotine replacement therapy: What are the options today? J Respir Dis 19:S20–S25, 1998.
461. Hall SM, Tunstall C, Rugg D, et al: Nicotine gum and behavioral treatment in smoking cessation. J Consult Clin Pathol 53:256–258, 1985.
462. Russell MAH, Merriman R, Stapleton J, et al: Effect of nicotine chewing gum as an adjunct to general practitioners' advice against smoking. BMJ 287:1782–1785, 1983.
463. The Transdermal Nicotine Study Group: Transdermal nicotine for smoking cessation. Six-month results from two multicenter controlled clinical trials. JAMA, 266:3133–3138, 1991.
464. Hurt RD, Sachs DP, Glover ED, et al: A comparison of sustained-release bupropion and placebo for smoking cessation. N Engl J Med 337:1195–1202, 1997.
465. Jorenby DE, Leischow SJ, Nides MA, et al: A controlled trial of sustained-release bupropion, a nicotine patch, or both for smoking cessation. N Engl J Med 340:685–691, 1999.
466. Ockene JK, Kuller LH, Svendsen KH, et al: The relationship of smoking cessation to coronary heart disease and lung cancer in the multiple risk factor intervention trial (MRFIT). Am J Public Health 80:954–958, 1990.
467. Ingram RH, O'Cain CF: Frequency dependence of compliance in apparently healthy smokers versus nonsmokers. Bull Physiopathol Respir 7:195–210, 1971.
468. McCarthy DS, Craig DB, Cherniack RM: Effect of modification of the smoking habit on lung function. Am Rev Respir Dis 114:103–113, 1976.
469. Massaro GD, Massaro D: Postnatal treatment with retinoic acid increases the number of pulmonary alveoli in rats. Am J Physiol 270:L305–L310, 1996.
470. Massaro G, Massaro D: Retinoic acid treatment abrogates elastase-induced pulmonary emphysema in rats. Nat Med 3:675–677, 1997.
471. Anthonisen N, Connett J, Friedman B, et al: Design of a clinical trial to test a treatment of the underlying cause of emphysema. Ann NY Acad Sci 624:31–34, 1991.
472. Snider GL, Stone PJ, Lucey EC: The specific treatment of emphysema. Eur Respir J 3(Suppl 9):23S–28S, 1990.
473. Fein AM: Lung volume reduction surgery: Answering the crucial questions. Chest 113:277S–282S, 1998.
474. Wakabayashi A, Brenner M, Kayaleh RA, et al: Thoracoscopic carbon dioxide laser treatment of bullous emphysema. Lancet 337:881–883, 1991.
475. Brenner M, Kayaleh RA, Milne EN, et al: Thoracoscopic laser ablation of pulmonary bullae. Radiographic selection and treatment response. J Thorac Cardiovasc Surg 107:883–890, 1994.
476. Barth J, Mollmann HW, Armbruster B, et al: Analysis of shape, particle size distribution and aggregation of the crystals of sodium cromoglycate and nedocromil sodium. Eur J Hosp Pharm 3:20–28, 1993.
477. Benditt JO, Albert RK: Surgical options for patients with advanced emphysema. Clin Chest Med 18:577–593, 1997.
478. Gelb AF, Zamel N, McKenna RJ Jr, et al: Mechanism of short-term improvement in lung function after emphysema resection. Am J Respir Crit Care Med 154:945–951, 1996.
479. Brenner M, McKenna RJ, Gelb AF, et al: Rate of FEV change following lung volume reduction surgery. Chest 113:652–659, 1998.
480. Cooper JD, Patterson GA, Sundaresean RS, et al: Results of 150 consecutive bilateral lung volume reduction procedures in patients with severe emphysema. J Thorac Cardiovasc Surg 112:1319–1330, 1996.
481. Ingenito EP, Evans RB, Loring SH, et al: Relation between preoperative inspiratory lung resistance and the outcome of lung-volume-reduction surgery for emphysema. N Engl J Med 338:1181–1185, 1998.
482. Fessler HE, Wise RA: Lung volume reduction surgery: Is less really more? Am J Respir Crit Care Med 159:1031–1035, 1999.
483. Bagley PH, Davis SM, O'Shea M, et al: Lung volume reduction surgery at a community hospital: Program development and outcomes. Chest 111:1552–1559, 1997.
484. Norman M, Hillerdal G, Orre L, et al: Improved lung function and quality of life following increased elastic recoil after lung volume reduction surgery in emphysema. Respir Med 92:653–658, 1998.
485. Moy ML, Ingenito EP, Mentzer SJ, et al: Health-related quality of life improves following pulmonary rehabilitation and lung volume reduction surgery. Chest 115:383–389, 1999.
486. Meyers BF, Yusen RD, Lefrak SS, et al: Outcome of Medicare patients with emphysema selected for, but denied, a lung volume reduction operation. Ann Thorac Surg 66:331–336, 1998.
487. Cooper JD, Vreim CE: Biology of lung preservation for lung transplantation. Am Rev Respir Dis 146:803–807, 1992.
488. Hosenpud JD, Bennett LE, Keck BM, et al: The Registry of the International Society for Heart and Lung Transplantation: Fourteenth official report—1997. J Heart Lung Transplant 16:691–712, 1997.
489. Egan TM, Kaiser LR, Cooper JD: Lung transplantation. Curr Probl Surg 26:675–751, 1989.
490. Cooper JD, Patterson GA, Grossman R, et al: Double-lung transplant for advanced chronic obstructive lung disease. Am Rev Respir Dis 139:303–307, 1989.
491. Patterson GA, Maurer JR, Williams TJ, et al: Comparison of outcomes of single and double lung transplantation for obstructive lung disease. The Toronto Lung Transplant Group. J Thorac Cardiovasc Surg 101:623–631, 1991.
492. Toronto Lung Transplant Group: Unilateral lung transplantation for pulmonary fibrosis. N Engl J Med 314:1140–1145, 1986.
493. Khaghani A, Banner N, Ozdogan E, et al: Medium-term results of combined heart and lung transplantation for emphysema. J Heart Lung Transplant 10:15–21, 1991.
494. Mal H, Andreassian B, Pamela F: Unilateral lung transplantation in end stage pulmonary emphysema. Am Rev Respir Dis 140:797–802, 1989.
495. Editorial: Single lung transplantation for pulmonary emphysema. Lancet 339:216–217, 1991.
496. Kaiser LR, Cooper JD, Trulock EP, et al: The evolution of single lung transplantation for emphysema. The Washington University Lung Transplant Group. J Thorac Cardiovasc Surg 102:333–339, 1991.
497. Nickoladze GD: Functional results of surgery for bullous emphysema. Chest 101:119–122, 1992.
498. Ohta M, Nakahara K, Yasumitsu T, et al: Prediction of postoperative performance status in patients with giant bullae. Chest 101:668–673, 1992.
499. Fitzgerald MX, Keelan PJ, Cugell DW, et al: Long term results of surgery for bullous emphysema. J Thorac Cardiovasc Surg 68:566–587, 1974.
500. Brand PLP, Postma DS, Kerstjens HAM: Relationship of airway hyperresponsiveness to respiratory symptoms and diurnal peak flow variation in patients with obstructive lung disease. Am Rev Respir Dis 143:916–921, 1991.
501. Intermittent Positive Pressure Breathing Trial Group: Intermittent positive pressure breathing therapy of chronic obstructive pulmonary disease: A clinical trial. Ann Intern Med 99:612–620, 1983.
502. Anthonisen RN, Wright EC, IPPB Trial Group: Response to inhaled bronchodilators in COPD. Chest 91:37S–39S, 1987.
503. Santa Cruz R, Landa J, Hirsch J, et al: Tracheal mucous velocity in normal man and patients with obstructive lung disease: Effects of terbutaline. Am Rev Respir Dis 109:458–463, 1974.
504. Davis B, Marin MG, Yee JW, et al: Effect of terbutaline on movement of $Cl^-$ and $Na^+$ across the trachea of the dog in vitro. Am Rev Respir Dis 120:547–552, 1979.
505. Kaliner M, Shelhamer JH, Borson B, et al: Human respiratory mucus. Am Rev Respir Dis 134:612–621, 1986.
506. Nava S, Crotti P, Gurrieri G, et al: Effect of a B2-agonist (broxaterol) on respiratory muscle strength and endurance in patients

with COPD with irreversible airway obstruction. Chest 101:133–140, 1992.

507. Postma D, De Vries K, Koeter GH, et al: Independent influence of reversibility of airflow obstruction and non-specific hyperreactivity on the long-term course of lung function in chronic airflow obstruction. Am Rev Respir Dis 134:276–280, 1986.
508. van Schayck CP, Dompeling E, van Herwaarden CLA, et al: Bronchodilator treatment in moderate asthma or chronic bronchitis: Continuous or on demand? A randomized controlled study. BMJ 303:1426–1431, 1991.
509. Boyd G, Morice AH, Pousford JC, et al: An evaluation of salmeterol in the treatment of chronic obstructive pulmonary disease (COPD). Eur Respir J 10:815–821, 1997.
510. Jones PW, Bosh TK: Quality of life changes in COPD patients treated with salmeterol. Am J Respir Crit Care Med 155:1283–1289, 1997.
511. Shim CS, Williams MH Jr: Bronchodilator response to oral aminophylline and terbutaline versus aerosol albuterol in patients with chronic obstructive pulmonary disease. Am J Med 75:697–701, 1983.
512. Tenholder MG, Bryson MJ, Waller RF, et al: Can MDIs be used effectively by extubated ICU patients? Am J Med 77:834–838, 1992.
513. DeBlaquiere P, Christensen DB, Carter WB, et al: Use and misuse of metered-dose inhalers by patients with chronic lung disease. Annu Rev Respir Dis 140:910–916, 1989.
514. Teale C, Morrison JFJ, Page RL, et al: Dose response to inhaled salbutamol in chronic obstructive airways disease. Postgrad Med J 67:754–756, 1991.
515. Lipworth BJ, Clark RA, Dhillon DP: Comparison of the effects of prolonged treatment with low and high doses of inhaled terbutaline on beta-adrenoceptor responsiveness in patients with chronic obstructive pulmonary disease. Am Rev Respir Dis 142:338–342, 1990.
516. Kim CS, Eldridge MA, Sackner MA: Oropharyngeal deposition and delivery aspects of metered-dose inhaler aerosols. Am Rev Respir Dis 135:157–164, 1987.
517. American Thoracic Society: Standards for the diagnosis and care of patients with chronic obstructive pulmonary disease (COPD) and asthma. Am Rev Respir Dis 136:225–244, 1987.
518. Jenne JW, Valcarenghi G, Druz WS, et al: Comparison of tremor responses to orally administered albuterol and terbutaline. Am Rev Respir Dis 134:708–713, 1986.
519. Jenne JW, Ridley DJ, Marcucci RA, et al: Objective and subjective tremor responses to oral beta 2 agents on first exposure. Am Rev Respir Dis 126:607–610, 1982.
520. Conradson TB, Eklundh G, Olofsson B, et al: Arrhythmogenicity from combined bronchodilator therapy in patients with obstructive lung disease and concomitant ischemic heart disease. Chest 91:5–9, 1987.
521. Gross NJ: Ipratropium bromide. N Engl J Med 319:486–494, 1988.
522. Maesen FPV, Smeets JJ, Sledsens TJH, et al: Tiotropium bromide, a new long-acting antimuscarinic bronchodilator: A pharmacodynamic study in patients with chronic obstructive pulmonary disease (COPD). Eur Respir J 8:1506–1513, 1995.
523. Gross NJ, Skorodin MS: Anticholinergic, antimuscarinic bronchodilators. Am Rev Respir Dis 129:856–870, 1984.
524. Gross NJ, Skorodin MS: Role of the parasympathetic system in airway obstruction due to emphysema. N Engl J Med 311:421–425, 1984.
525. Gross NJ, Co E, Skorodin MS: Cholinergic bronchomotor tone in COPD. Chest 96:984–987, 1989.
526. Ohrui T, Yanai M, Sekizawa K, et al: Effective site of bronchodilation by beta-adrenergic and anticholinergic agents in patients with chronic obstructive pulmonary disease: Direct measurement of intrabronchial pressure with a new catheter. Am Rev Respir Dis 146:88–91, 1992.
527. Mak JCW, Barnes PJ: Autoradiographic visualization of muscarinic receptor subtypes in human and guinea pig lung. Am Rev Respir Dis 141:1559–1568, 1990.
528. Easton PA, Jadue C, Dhingra S, et al: A comparison of the bronchodilating effects of a beta-2 adrenergic agent (albuterol) and an anticholinergic agent (ipratropium bromide), given by aerosol alone or in sequence. N Engl J Med 315:735–739, 1986.
529. Baigelman W, Chodosh S: Bronchodilator action of the anticholinergic drug, ipratropium bromide (Sch 1000), as an aerosol in chronic bronchitis and asthma. Chest 71:324–328, 1977.
530. Hunt D, MacDonald GF, Reilly P, et al: Bronchodilator response to several doses of ipratropium bromide in asthmatics and bronchitics. Curr Ther Res 33:651–659, 1983.
531. Tashkin DP, Ashutosh K, Bleecker ER, et al: Comparison of the anticholinergic bronchodilator ipratropium bromide with metaproterenol in chronic obstructive pulmonary disease. Am J Med 81:81–89, 1986.
532. Wanner A: Effect of ipratropium bromide on airway mucociliary function. Am J Med 81:23–27, 1986.
533. Gross NJ, Bankwala Z: Effects of anticholinergic bronchodilator on arterial blood gases of hypoxemic patients with chronic obstructive pulmonary disease. Am Rev Respir Dis 136:1091–1094, 1987.
534. Chapman KR, Smith DL, Rebuck AS, et al: Hemodynamic effects of inhaled ipratropium bromide alone and combined with an inhaled beta2-agonist. Am Rev Respir Dis 132:845–847, 1985.
535. Friedman M, Serby CE, Menjoge SS, et al: Pharmacoeconomic evaluation of a combination of ipratropium plus albuterol compared with ipratropium alone and albuterol alone in COPD. Chest 115:635–641, 1999.
536. Higgins BG, Powell RM, Cooper S, et al: Effect of salbutamol and ipratropium bromide on airway calibre and bronchial reactivity in asthma and chronic bronchitis. Eur Respir J 4:415–420, 1991.
537. Ghafouri MA, Patil K, Kass I: Sputum changes associated with the use of ipratropium bromide. Chest 86:387–393, 1984.
538. Ferguson GT, Cherniack RM: Management of chronic obstructive pulmonary disease. N Engl J Med 328:1017–1022, 1993.
539. Poppius H, Salorinne Y: Comparative trial of a new anticholinergic bronchodilator, Sch 1000, and salbutamol in chronic bronchitis. BMJ 4:134–136, 1973.
540. Marlin GE, Bush DE, Berend N: Comparison of ipratropium bromide and fenoterol in asthma and chronic bronchitis. Br J Clin Pharmacol 6:547–549, 1978.
541. Braun SR, Levy SF: Comparison of ipratropium bromide and albuterol in chronic obstructive pulmonary disease: A three-center study. Am J Med 21:28S–32S, 1991.
542. Wesseling G, Mostert R, Wouters EFM: A comparison of the effects of anticholinergic and beta-2 agonist and combination therapy on respiratory impedance in COPD. Chest 101:166–173, 1992.
543. LeDoux EJ, Morris JF, Temple WP, et al: Standard and double dose ipratropium bromide and combined ipratropium bromide and inhaled metaproterenol in COPD. Chest 95:1013–1016, 1989.
544. Karpel JP: Bronchodilator responses to anticholinergic and beta-adrenergic agents in acute and stable COPD. Chest 99:871–876, 1991.
545. Heimer D, Brami JL, Liberman D, et al: Comparison of a beta2 adrenergic agonist and an anticholinergic agent given by sequential inhalation in patients with severe chronic obstructive pulmonary disease. Isr J Med 27:307–310, 1991.
546. Karpel JP, Pesin J, Greenberg D, et al: A comparison of the effects of ipratropium bromide and metaproterenol sulfate in acute exacerbations of COPD. Chest 98:835–839, 1990.
547. Patrick DM, Dales RE, Stark RM, et al: Severe exacerbations of COPD and asthma. Chest 98:295–297, 1990.
548. Shrestha M, O'Brien T, Haddox R, et al: Decreased duration of emergency department treatment of chronic obstructive pulmonary disease exacerbations with the addition of ipratropium bromide to beta-agonist therapy. Ann Emerg Med 20:1206–1209, 1991.
549. Sessler CN, Brady W: Theophylline toxicity: How to minimize the potential risk factors that complicate use: Manifestations of overdose. J Crit Illness 6:1045–1054, 1990.
550. Sessler CN: Theophylline toxicity: Clinical features of 116 consecutive cases. Am J Med 88:567–576, 1990.
551. Schuff CN, Hegde HK, LaCloche L, et al: Inpatient theophylline toxicity: Preventable factors. Ann Intern Med 114:748–753, 1991.
552. Alexander MR, Dull WL, Kasik JE: Treatment of chronic ob-

structive pulmonary disease with orally administered theophylline: A double blind, controlled study. JAMA 244:2286–2290, 1980.
553. Eaton ML, Green BA, Church TR, et al: Efficacy of theophylline in "irreversible" airflow obstruction. Ann Intern Med 92:758–761, 1980.
554. Eaton ML, McDonald FM, Church TR: Effects of theophylline on breathlessness and exercise tolerance in patients with chronic airflow obstruction. Chest 82:538–542, 1982.
555. Nietrzeba RM, Elliott CG, Adams TD, et al: Effects of aminophylline upon the exercise performance of patients with stable chronic airflow obstruction. Bull Eur Physiopathol Respir 20:361–367, 1984.
556. Jenne JW, Siever JR, Druz WS, et al: The effect of maintenance theophylline on lung work in severe chronic obstructive pulmonary disease while standing and walking. Am Rev Respir Dis 130:600–605, 1984.
557. Mahler DA: Sustained-released theophylline reduces dyspnea in nonreversible obstructive airway disease. Am Rev Respir Dis 131:22–25, 1985.
558. Murciano D: A randomized, controlled trial of theophylline in patients with severe chronic obstructive pulmonary disease. N Engl J Med 320:1521–1525, 1989.
559. Torphy TJ, Undem BJ: Phosphodiesterase inhibitors: New opportunities for the treatment of asthma. Thorax 46:512–523, 1991.
560. Bleecker ER, Britt EJ: Acute bronchodilating effects of ipratropium bromide and theophylline in chronic obstructive pulmonary disease. Am J Med 91:24S–27S, 1991.
561. Filuk RB, Easton PA, Anthonisen NR: Responses to large doses of salbutamol and theophylline in patients with chronic obstructive pulmonary disease. Am Rev Respir Dis 132:871–874, 1985.
562. Dullinger D, Kronenberg R, Niewoehner DE: Efficacy of inhaled metaproterenol and orally-administered theophylline in patients with chronic airflow obstruction. Chest 89:171–173, 1986.
563. Wanner A: Effects of methylxanthines on airway mucociliary function. Am J Med 79:16–21, 1985.
564. Dowell AR, Heyman A, Sieker HU, et al: Effect of aminophylline on respiratory center sensitivity in Cheyne-Stokes respiration and in pulmonary emphysema. N Engl J Med 273:1447–1453, 1965.
565. Matthay RA, Berger HJ, Davies R, et al: Improvement in cardiac performance by oral long-acting theophylline in chronic obstructive pulmonary disease. Am Heart J 104:1022–1026, 1982.
566. Martin RJ, Pak J, Moore EG: Overnight theophylline concentrations and effects on sleep and lung function in chronic obstructive pulmonary disease. Am Rev Respir Dis 145:540–544, 1992.
567. Murciano D: Effects of theophylline on diaphragmatic strength and fatigue in patients with chronic obstructive pulmonary disease. N Engl J Med 311:349–353, 1984.
568. Foxworth JW, Reisz GR, Knudson SM, et al: Theophylline and diaphragmatic contractility. Am Rev Respir Dis 138:1532–1534, 1988.
569. Weinberger M, Hendeles L, Ahrens R: Pharmacologic management of reversible obstructive airways disease. Med Clin North Am 65:579–614, 1981.
570. Shannon MN, Lovejoy FH Jr: The influence of age vs peak serum concentration in life-threatening events after chronic theophylline intoxication. Arch Intern Med 150:2045–2048, 1990.
571. Jenne J, Nagasawa HT, Thompson RD: Relationship of urinary metabolites of theophylline to serum theophylline levels. Clin Pharmacol Ther 19:375–381, 1976.
572. Faling LJ, Snider GL: Treatment of chronic obstructive pulmonary disease. *In* Simmons D (ed): Current Pulmonology. Chicago: Year Book Medical Publishers, 1989, pp 209–263.
573. Miller CA, Slusher LB, Vesell ES: Polymorphism of theophylline metabolism in man. J Clin Invest 75:1415–1425, 1985.
574. Butts JD, Secrest B, Berger R: Nonlinear theophylline pharmacokinetics: A preventable cause of iatrogenic theophylline toxic reactions. Arch Intern Med 151:2073–2077, 1991.
575. Hill N: The use of theophylline in irreversible chronic obstructive pulmonary disease. Arch Intern Med 148:2579–2584, 1988.
576. Weinberger M, Hendeles L: Slow-release theophylline: Rationale and basis for product selection. N Engl J Med 308:760–764, 1983.
577. Rogers RM, Owens GR, Pennock BE: The pendulum swings again toward a rational use of theophylline. Chest 87:280–282, 1985.
578. Taylor DR, Buick B, Kinney C, et al: The efficacy of orally administered theophylline, inhaled salbutamol, and a combination of the two as chronic therapy in the management of chronic bronchitis with reversible air-flow obstruction. Am Rev Respir Dis 131:747–751, 1985.
579. Guyatt GH, Townsend M, Pugsley SO, et al: Bronchodilators in chronic air-flow limitation. Am Rev Respir Dis 135:1069–1074, 1987.
580. Thomas P, Pugsley JA, Stewart JH: Theophylline and salbutamol improve pulmonary function in patients with irreversible chronic obstructive pulmonary disease. Chest 101:160–165, 1992.
581. Mendella LA, Manfreda J, Warren CPW, et al: Steroid response in stable chronic obstructive pulmonary disease. Ann Intern Med 96:17–21, 1982.
582. Shim C, Stover DE, Williams MH Jr: Response to corticosteroids in chronic bronchitis. J Allergy Clin Immunol 62:363–367, 1978.
583. Callahan CM, Dittus RS, Katz BP: Oral corticosteroid therapy for patients with stable chronic obstructive pulmonary disease. Ann Intern Med 114:216–223, 1991.
584. Adinoff AD, Hollister JR: Steroid-induced fractures and bone loss in patients with asthma. N Engl J Med 309:265–268, 1983.
585. Wiest PM, Flanigan T, Salata RA, et al: Serious infectious complications of corticosteroid therapy for COPD. Chest 95:1180–1184, 1989.
586. McEvoy C, Ensrud KE, Bender E, et al: Association between corticosteroid use and vertebral fractures in older men with chronic obstructive pulmonary disease. Am J Respir Crit Care Med 157:704–709, 1998.
587. Thompson WH, Nielson CP, Carvalho P, et al: Controlled trial of oral prednisone in outpatients with acute COPD exacerbation. Am J Respir Crit Care Med 154:407–412, 1996.
588. Murata GH, Gorby MS, Chick TW, et al: Intravenous and oral corticosteroids for the prevention of relapse after treatment of decompensated COPD. Chest 98:845–849, 1990.
589. Blair GP, Light RW: Treatment of chronic obstructive pulmonary disease with corticosteroids. Chest 86:524–528, 1984.
590. Paggiaro PL, Dahle R, Bakran I, et al: Multicentre randomised placebo-controlled trial of inhaled fluticasone propionate in patients with chronic obstructive pulmonary disease. Lancet 351:773–780, 1998.
591. Harding SM, Freedman S: A comparison of oral and inhaled steroids in patients with chronic airways obstruction. Thorax 33:214–217, 1978.
592. Shim CS, Williams MHJ: Aerosol beclomethasone in patients with steroid-responsive chronic obstructive pulmonary disease. Am J Med 78:655–658, 1985.
593. Weir D: Corticosteroid trials in non-asthmatic chronic airflow obstruction: A comparison of oral prednisolone and inhaled beclomethasone dipropionate. Thorax 45:112–117, 1990.
594. Wesseling GJ, Guaedvlieg M, Wouters EFM: Inhaled budesonide in chronic bronchitis. Effects on respiratory impedance. Eur Respir J 4:1101–1105, 1991.
595. Robertson AS, Gove RI, Wieland GA, et al: A double-blind comparison of oral prednisolone, 40 mg/day with inhaled beclomethasone dipropionate, 1500-g/day in patients with adult onset chronic obstructive airways disease. Eur J Respir Dis 69:565–569, 1986.
596. Newhouse MT, Dolovich M: Aerosol therapy of reversible airflow obstruction. Chest 91:58S–64S, 1987.
597. Smith MI, Hodson ME: Effects of long term inhaled high dose beclomethasone dipropionate on adrenal function. Thorax 38:676–681, 1983.
598. deJong JW, Postma DS, van der Mark TW, et al: Effects of nedocromil sodium in the treatment of non-allergic subjects with chronic obstructive pulmonary disease. Thorax 49:1022–1024, 1994.
599. Multicenter Study Group: Long-term oral acetylcysteine in chronic bronchitis, a double-blind controlled study. Eur J Respir Dis 61:93–108, 1980.
600. Petty TL: The National Mucolytic Study. Results of a randomized, double-blind, placebo-controlled study of iodinated glycerol in chronic obstructive bronchitis. Chest 97:75–83, 1990.
601. Fick RB, Ansueto A, Mahutte K: Recombinant DNase mortality

reduction in acute exacerbations of chronic bronchitis. Clin Res 42:294A, 1994.
602. Tamaoki J, Chiyotani A, Kobayashi K, et al: Effect of indomethacin on bronchorrhea in patient with chronic bronchitis, diffuse panbrochitis, or bronchiectasis. Am Rev Respir Dis 145:548–552, 1992.
603. Wick MM, Ingram RH: Bronchorrhea responsive to aerosolized atropine. JAMA 235:1356, 1976.
604. Hirsch SR, Viernes PF, Kory RC: The expectorant effect of glyceryl guaiacolate in patients with chronic bronchitis. Chest 63:9–14, 1973.
605. Shim C, King M, Williams MR Jr: Lack of effect of hydration on sputum production in chronic bronchitis. Chest 92:679–682, 1987.
606. Sheppard D, Rizk N, Boushey HA, et al: Mechanism of cough and bronchoconstriction induced by distilled water aerosol. Am Rev Respir Dis 127:691–694, 1983.
607. Sutton PP, Parker RA, Webber BA, et al: Assessment of the forced expiration technique, postural drainage and directed coughing in chest physiotherapy. Eur J Respir Dis 64:62–68, 1983.
608. Harris RS, Lawson TV: The relative mechanical effectiveness and efficiency of successive voluntary coughs in healthy young adults. Clin Sci 34:569–577, 1968.
609. Marini JJ, Tyler ML, Hudson LD, et al: Influence of head-dependent positions on lung volumes and oxygen saturation in chronic airflow obstruction. Am Rev Respir Dis 129:101–105, 1984.
610. Sutton PP, Gemmell HG, Innes N, et al: Use of nebulized saline and nebulized terbutaline as an adjunct to chest physiotherapy. Thorax 43:57–60, 1988.
611. Fagon JY, Chastre J, Trouillet JL, et al: Characterization of distal bronchial microflora during acute exacerbation of chronic bronchitis. Am Rev Respir Dis 142:1004–1008, 1990.
612. Chodosh S: Treatment of acute exacerbations of chronic bronchitis: State of the art. Am J Med 91(Suppl):87–92, 1991.
613. Murray PR, Washington JA: Microscopic and bacteriologic analysis of expectorated sputum. Mayo Clin Proc 50:339–344, 1975.
614. Anthonisen NR, Manfreda J, Warren CPW, et al: Antibiotic therapy in exacerbations of chronic obstructive pulmonary disease. Ann Intern Med 106:196–204, 1987.
615. American Thoracic Society: Standards for the Diagnosis and Care of Patients with Chronic Obstructive Pulmonary Disease. Am J Respir Crit Care Med 152:S78–S121, 1995.
616. Guidelines for the initial management of adults with community-acquired pneumonia: Diagnosis, assessment of severity and initial antimicrobial therapy. Am Rev Respir Dis 148:1418–1426, 1993.
617. Lee PH, Carr DH, Rubens MB et al: Accuracy of CT in predicting the cause of bronchiectasis. Clin Radiol 50:839–841, 1995.
618. Heaton RK, Grant I, McSweeny J, et al: Psychologic effects of continuous and nocturnal oxygen therapy in hypoxemic chronic obstructive pulmonary disease. Arch Intern Med 143:1941–1947, 1983.
619. Astin TW, Penman RWB: Airways obstruction due to hypoxemia in patients with chronic lung disease. Am Rev Respir Dis 95:567–575, 1967.
620. Couser JI, Make BJ: Transtracheal oxygen decreases inspired minute ventilation. Am Rev Respir Dis 139:627–631, 1989.
621. Goldstein R: Effect of supplemental nocturnal oxygen on gas exchange in patients with severe obstructive lung disease. N Engl J Med 310:425–429, 1984.
622. Petty TL, Standford RE, Neff TA: Continuous oxygen therapy in chronic airway obstruction: Observations on possible oxygen toxicity and survival. Ann Intern Med 75:361–367, 1971.
623. Petty TL, Neff TA, Creagh CE, et al: Outpatient oxygen therapy in chronic obstructive pulmonary disease. Arch Intern Med 139:28–32, 1979.
624. Petty TL, Snider GL: Second Oxygen Consensus Conference report: Further recommendations for prescribing and supplying long-term oxygen therapy. Am Rev Respir Dis 138:745–747, 1988.
625. Petty TL: Home oxygen—A revolution in the care of advanced COPD. Med Clin North Am 74:715–729, 1990.
626. Tiep B: Long-term home oxygen therapy. Clin Chest Med 11:505–521, 1990.
627. Cotes JE, Gilson JC: Effect of oxygen on exercise ability in chronic respiratory insufficiency. Lancet 1:872–876, 1956.
628. Woodcock AA, Gross ER, Gellert AA, et al: Effects of dihydrocodeine, alcohol, and caffeine on breathlessness and exercise tolerance in patients with chronic obstructive lung disease and normal blood gases. N Engl J Med 305:1611–1616, 1981.
629. Vyas MN, Banister EW, Morton JW, et al: Response to exercise in patients with chronic airway obstruction: II. Effects of breathing 40 percent oxygen. Am Rev Respir Dis 103:401–412, 1971.
630. Stanek KA, Nagle FJ, Bisgard GE, et al: Effect of hyperoxia in oxygen consumption in exercising ponies. J Appl Physiol 46:1115–1118, 1979.
631. Bye PTP, Esau SA, Levy RD, et al: Ventilatory muscle function during exercise in air and oxygen in patients with chronic airflow limitation. Am Rev Respir Dis 132:236–240, 1985.
632. Owens GR, Rogers RM, Pennock BE, et al: The diffusing capacity as a predictor of arterial oxygen desaturation during exercise in patients with chronic obstructive pulmonary disease. N Engl J Med 310:1218–1221, 1984.
633. Kelley MA, Panettieri RA, Krupinski AV: Resting single-breath diffusing capacity as a screening test for exercise-induced hypoxemia. Am J Med 80:807–812, 1986.
634. Report C: New problems in supply, reimbursement, and certification of medical necessity for long-term oxygen therapy. Am Rev Respir Dis 142:721–724, 1990.
635. O'Donohue WJ Jr: Prescribing home oxygen therapy: What the primary care physician needs to know. Arch Intern Med 152:746–748, 1992.
636. Barker AF, Burgher LW, Plummer AL: Oxygen conserving methods for adults. Chest 105:248–252, 1994.
637. Adamo JP, Mehta AC, Stelmach K, et al: The Cleveland Clinic's initial experience with transtracheal oxygen therapy. Respir Care 35:153–160, 1990.
638. Harrow EM, Oldenburg FA, Lingenfelter MS, et al: Respiratory failure and cor pulmonale associated with tracheal mucoid accumulation from SCOOP transtracheal oxygen catheter. Chest 101:580–581, 1992.
639. Christopher KL, Spofford BT, Brannin PKEA: Transtracheal oxygen therapy for refractory hypoxemia. JAMA 256:494–497, 1986.
640. Schwartz JS, Bencowitz HZ, Moser KM: Air travel hypoxemia with chronic obstructive pulmonary disease. Ann Intern Med 100:473–477, 1984.
641. Dillard TA, Berg BW, Rajagopal KR, et al: Hypoxemia during air travel in patients with chronic obstructive pulmonary disease. Ann Intern Med 111:362–367, 1989.
642. Gong HJ, Tashkin DP, Lee EY, et al: Hypoxia-altitude simulation test. Am Rev Respir Dis 130:980–986, 1984.
643. Gong H, Jr: Air travel and patients with pulmonary and allergic conditions. J Allergy Clin Immunol 87:879–885, 1991.
644. Poundstone W: Air travel and supplemental oxygen. Respir Ther Jan:79–82, 1983.
645. Stoller JK, Hoisington E, Auger G: A comparative analysis of arranging in-flight oxygen aboard commercial air carriers. Chest 115:991–995, 1999.
646. Alkalay I, Kaplan AS, Sharma R, et al: Chronic obstructive pulmonary disease: Rehabilitation program with continuation on an outpatient basis. J Am Geriatr Soc 28:88–92, 1980.
647. American Association of Cardiovascular and Pulmonary Rehabilitation. Pulmonary rehabilitation: Joint ACCP/AACVPR evidence-based guidelines. ACCP/AACVPR Pulmonary Rehabilitation Guidelines Panel. American College of Chest Physicians. Chest 112:1363–1396, 1997.
648. Foster S, Lopez D, Thomas HM, et al: Pulmonary rehabilitation in COPD patients with elevated $P_{CO_2}$. Am Rev Respir Dis 138:1519–1523, 1988.
649. American Thoracic Society: Standards for the diagnosis and care of patients with chronic obstructive pulmonary disease (COPD) and asthma. Am Rev Respir Dis 136:225–244, 1987.
650. Celli BR, Rassulo J, Make B: Dyssynchronous breathing associated with arm but not leg exercises in patients with COPD. N Engl J Med 314:1485–1490, 1986.
651. Martinez FJ, Couser JI, Celli BR: Respiratory response to arm elevation in patients with chronic airflow obstruction. Am Rev Respir Dis 143:476–480, 1991.

652. Ries A, Ellis B, Hawkins R: Upper extremity exercise training in chronic obstructive pulmonary disease. Chest 93:688–692, 1988.
653. Larson JL, Kim MJ, Sharp JT, et al: Inspiratory muscle training with a pressure threshold breathing device in patients with chronic obstructive pulmonary disease. Am Rev Respir Dis 138:689–696, 1988.
654. Celli B: Training and the respiratory muscles. *In* Marini JJ, Roussos C (eds): Ventilatory Failure Update in Intensive Care and Emergency Medicine. Berlin: Springer-Verlag, 1991.
655. Smith K, Cook D, Guyatt GH, et al: Respiratory muscle training in chronic airflow limitation: A meta-analysis. Am Rev Respir Dis 145:533–539, 1992.
656. Faling LJ: Pulmonary rehabilitation—Physical modalities. Clin Chest Med 7:599–618, 1986.
657. Ingram RH Jr, Schilder DP: Effect of pursed lips expiration on the pulmonary pressure-flow relationship in obstructive lung disease. Am Rev Respir Dis 96:381–388, 1967.
658. Tiep BL, Burns M, Kao D, et al: Pursed lips breathing training using ear oximetry. Chest 90:218–221, 1986.
659. Sharp JT, Drutz WS, Moisan T, et al: Postural relief of dyspnea in severe chronic obstructive pulmonary disease. Am Rev Respir Dis 122:201–211, 1980.
660. Openbrier DR, Irwin MM, Rogers RM, et al: Nutritional status and lung function in patients with emphysema and chronic bronchitis. Chest 83:17–22, 1983.
661. Donahoe M, Rogers RM, Wilson DO, et al: Oxygen consumption of the respiratory muscles in normal and in malnourished patients with chronic obstructive pulmonary disease. Am Rev Respir Dis 140:385–391, 1989.
662. Goldstein S: Nitrogen and energy relationships in malnourished patients with emphysema. Am Rev Respir Dis 138:636–644, 1988.
663. de Godoy I, Donahoe M, Calhoun WJ, et al: Elevated TNF-alpha production by peripheral blood monocytes of weight-losing COPD patients. Am J Respir Crit Care Med 153:633–637, 1996.
664. Di Francia M, Barbier D, Mege JL, et al: Tumor necrosis factor-alpha levels and weight loss in chronic obstructive pulmonary disease. Am J Respir Crit Care Med 150:1453–1455, 1994.
665. Rochester DF, Esau SA: Malnutrition and the respiratory system. Chest 85:411–415, 1984.
666. Wilson D: Nutritional intervention in malnourished patients with emphysema. Am Rev Respir Dis 134:672–677, 1986.
667. Whittaker JS, Ryan CF, Buckley PA, et al: The effects of refeeding on peripheral and respiratory muscle function in malnourished chronic obstructive pulmonary disease patients. Am Rev Respir Dis 142:283–288, 1990.
668. Lewis MI, Belman MJ, Dorr-Uyemura L: Nutritional supplementation in ambulatory patients with chronic obstructive pulmonary disease. Am Rev Respir Dis 135:1062–1068, 1987.
669. Tirlapur VB, Mir MA: Effect of low calorie intake on abnormal pulmonary physiology in patients with chronic hypercapnic respiratory failure. Am J Med 77:987–994, 1984.
670. Gieseke T, Gurushanthaiah G, Glauser FL: Effects of carbohydrates on carbon dioxide excretion in patients with airway disease. Chest 71:55–58, 1977.
671. Brown SE, Nagendran RC, McHugh JW, et al: Effects of a large carbohydrate load on walking performance in chronic air-flow obstruction. Am Rev Respir Dis 132:960–962, 1985.
672. Eiser N, Denman WT, West C, et al: Oral diamorphine: Lack of effect on dyspnoea and exercise tolerance in the "pink puffer" syndrome. Eur Respir J 4:926–931, 1991.
673. Young IH, Daviskas E, Keena VA: Effect of low dose nebulised morphine on exercise endurance in patients with chronic lung disease. Thorax 44:387–390, 1989.
674. Light RW, Muro JR, Sato R: Effects of oral morphine on breathlessness and exercise tolerance in patients with chronic obstructive pulmonary disease. Am Rev Respir Dis 139:126–133, 1989.
675. Rice KL, Kronenberg RS, Hedemark LL, et al: Effects of chronic administration of codeine and promethazine on breathlessness and exercise tolerance in patients with chronic airflow obstruction. Br J Dis Chest 81:287–292, 1987.
676. Poole PJ, Veale AG, Black PN: The effect of sustained-release morphine on breathlessness and quality of life in severe chronic obstructive pulmonary disease. Am J Respir Crit Care Med 157:1877–1880, 1998.
677. Leung R, Hill P, Burdon J: Effect of inhaled morphine on the development of breathlessness during exercise in patients with chronic lung disease. Thorax 51:596–600, 1996.
678. Masood AR, Reed JW, Thomas SHL: Lack of effect of inhaled morphine on exercise-induced breathlessness in chronic obstructive pulmonary disease. Thorax 50:629–634, 1995.
679. Stulbarg MS, Winn WR: Bilateral carotid body resection for the relief of dyspnea in severe chronic obstructive pulmonary disease. Chest 96:1123–1128, 1989.
680. Similowski T, Yan S, Gauthier APEA: Contractile properties of the human diaphragm during chronic hyperinflation. N Engl J Med 325:917–923, 1991.
681. Efthimou J, Fleming J, Spiro SG: Sternomastoid muscle function and fatigue in breathless patients with severe respiratory disease. Am Rev Respir Dis 136:1099–1105, 1987.
682. Strumpf DA, Millmam RP, Carlisle CC, et al: Nocturnal positive-pressure ventilation via nasal mask in patients with severe chronic obstructive pulmonary disease. Am Rev Respir Dis 144:1234–1239, 1991.
683. Petrof BJ, Kimoff RJ, Levy RD, et al: Nasal continuous positive airway pressure facilitates respiratory muscle function during sleep in severe chronic obstructive pulmonary disease. Am Rev Respir Dis 143:928–935, 1991.
684. Elliott MW, Mulvey DA, Moxham J, et al: Domiciliary nocturnal nasal intermittent positive pressure ventilation in COPD: Mechanisms underlying changes in arterial blood gas tensions. Eur Respir J 4:1044–1052, 1991.
685. Krachman SL, Quaranta AJ, Berger TJ, et al: Effects of noninvasive positive pressure ventilation on gas exchange and sleep in COPD patients. Chest 112:623–628, 1997.
686. Renston JP, DiMarco AF, Supinski GS: Respiratory muscle rest using nasal BiPAP ventilation in patients with stable severe COPD. Chest 105:1053–1060, 1994.
687. Bury T, Jeannot JP, Ansquer JC, et al: Dose-response and pharmacokinetic study with almitrine bismesylate after single oral administrations in COPD patients. Eur Respir J 2:49–55, 1989.
688. Romaldini H, Rodriguez-Roisin R, Wagner PD, et al: Enhancement of hypoxic pulmonary vasoconstriction by almitrine in the dog. Am Rev Respir Dis 128:288–293, 1983.
689. Simmonneau G, Meignan M, Denjean A, et al: Cardiopulmonary effects of a single oral dose of almitrine at rest and on exercise in patients with hypoxic chronic airflow obstruction. Chest 89:174–179, 1986.
690. Connaughton JJ, Douglas NJ, Morgan AD, et al: Almitrine improves oxygenation when both awake and asleep in patients with hypoxia and carbon dioxide retention caused by chronic bronchitis and emphysema. Am Rev Respir Dis 132:206–210, 1985.
691. Weitzenblum E, Schrijen F, Apprill M, et al: One year treatment with almitrine improves hypoxaemia but does not increase pulmonary artery pressure in COPD patients. Eur Respir J 4:1215–1222, 1991.
692. Skatruc JB, Dempsey JA: Relative effectiveness of acetazolamide versus medroxyprogesterone acetate in correction of chronic carbon dioxide retention. Am Rev Respir Dis 127:405–412, 1983.
693. Derenne J, Fleury B, Pariente R: Acute respiratory failure of chronic obstructive pulmonary disease. Am Rev Respir Dis 138:1006–1033, 1988.
694. Schmidt GA, Hall JB: Acute or chronic respiratory failure. Assessment and management of patients with COPD in the emergent setting. JAMA 261:3444–3453, 1989.
695. Dunn WF, Nelson SB, Hubmayr RD: Oxygen-induced hypercarbia in obstructive pulmonary disease. Am Rev Respir Dis 144:526–530, 1991.
696. Mehta S, Hill NS: Noninvasive ventilation in acute respiratory failure. Respir Care Clin North Am 2:267–292, 1996.
697. Hillberg RE, Johnson DC: Noninvasive ventilation. N Engl J Med 337:1746–1752, 1997.
698. Corrado A, Bruscoli G, Messori A, et al: Iron lung treatment of subjects with COPD in acute respiratory failure. Chest 101:692–696, 1992.
699. Carrey Z, Gottfried SB, Levy RD: Ventilatory muscle support in respiratory failure with nasal positive pressure ventilation. Chest 97:150–158, 1990.
700. Marino W: Intermittent volume cycled mechanical ventilation via nasal mask in patients with respiratory failure due to COPD. Chest 99:681–684, 1991.

701. Brochard L, Isabey D, Piquet JEA: Reversal of acute exacerbations of chronic obstructive lung disease by inspiratory assistance with a face mask. N Engl J Med 323:1523–1530, 1990.
702. Chevrolet JC, Jolliet P, Abajo B, et al: Nasal positive pressure ventilation in patients with acute respiratory failure. Chest 100:775–782, 1991.
703. Fessler HE, Brower RG, Permutt S: CPAP reduces inspiratory work more than dyspnea during hyperinflation with intrinsic PEEP. Chest 108:432–440, 1995.
704. Kacmarek RM, Kirmse M, Nishimura M, et al: The effects of applied vs auto-PEEP on local lung unit pressure and volume in a four-unit lung model. Chest 108:1073–1079, 1995.
705. Petroff B: Continuous positive airway pressure reduces work of breathing and dyspnea during weaning from mechanical ventilation in severe chronic obstructive pulmonary disease. Am Rev Respir Dis 141:281–289, 1990.
706. Pepe PE, Marini JJ: Occult positive and end-expiratory pressure in mechanically ventilated patients with airflow obstruction. The auto-PEEP effect. Am Rev Respir Dis 126:166–170, 1982.
707. Atauffer JL, Olson DE, Petty TL: Complications and consequences of endotracheal intubation and tracheotomy. Am J Med 70:65–76, 1981.
708. Gelb AF, Tashkin DP, Epstein JD, et al: Nd-YAG laser surgery for severe tracheal stenosis physiologically and clinically masked by severe diffuse obstructive pulmonary disease. Chest 91:166–170, 1987.

# 39 Asthma

Homer A. Boushey, Jr., M.D. • David B. Corry, M.D.
John V. Fahy, M.D.

Introduction
Definition
Epidemiology and Risk Factors
- Population Trends
- Risk Factors
- Infection as a Risk Factor

Genetics
- Segregation Analysis
- Gene Association Studies

Pathology
- Structural Changes in the Airway
- Changes in Airway Mucus
- Large vs. Small Airway Pathology
- Airway Pathology in Allergic and Nonallergic Asthma
- Fatal Asthma
- Relationship Between Airway Pathology and Asthma Severity
- Specificity of Airway Inflammation

Pathophysiology
- Origin and Evolution
- Cellular and Mediator Basis
- Airway Remodeling

Physiology
- Physiologic Disturbances
- Pulmonary Function Testing
- Tests of Bronchial Responsiveness

Clinical Features
- History
- Physical Examination
- Laboratory Studies
- Differential Diagnosis
- Special Considerations
- Clinical Forms of Asthma

Natural History
- Remission
- Mortality
- Morbidity
- Progressive Airflow Obstruction
- Effects of Treatments on the Natural History of Asthma

Management
- General Principles
- Pharmacologic Therapy
- Acute Severe Asthma
- Chronic Asthma

Summary

## INTRODUCTION

Although asthma is one of the diseases longest recognized as a distinct entity, it has moved to center stage as a public health problem only in the last 30 years. Asthma is now recognized as a common cause of disability, of great economic cost, and of preventable deaths. The disease has engaged the full spectrum of biomedical investigation, from studies of the prevalence of asthmatic symptoms in various populations to studies of the effects of substitution of single base pairs in genes suspected to be important in asthma. These studies have stimulated rapid evolution in the scientific conception of asthma, followed by changes in the approach to its diagnosis and treatment. The breadth and vigor of current scientific study of asthma presents two insurmountable problems to its review. One problem is the sheer volume of scientific literature on asthma; the other is the rapidity of the advance in knowledge. Therefore, this review is necessarily idiosyncratic, a reflection of the perspectives of the authors, and represents a "snapshot" of a body of knowledge expanding at an explosive pace.

## DEFINITION

Although most physicians seem comfortable with their ability to recognize the clinical entity of asthma, agreement on a definition of the disease has proved elusive.[1] The difficulty probably arose from overreliance on description of the characteristic physiologic abnormality (airflow obstruction that reverses spontaneously or as a result of treatment) in early definitions of the disease. Definitions of diseases seem to be most satisfactory when they are derived from identification of a discrete single causative agent or from detection of a characteristic pathologic abnormality.

Because no single agent has been identified as causing asthma and because no pathologic feature is unique to asthma, the disease has been more described than defined.

The earliest feature described was presumably the labored, rapid breathing that is typical of asthmatic attacks, for the word "asthma" is derived from the ancient Greek word for "panting."[2] As knowledge about asthma has grown, the features described as characteristic have grown as well. Measurement of maximal expiratory flow led to recognition of reversible airflow obstruction as a characteristic feature; measurement of changes in airflow after inhalation of chemical or physical irritants led to the addition of bronchial hyperresponsiveness. And more recent studies of bronchial biopsies added descriptions of certain pathologic features.[3] This evolution in the understanding of asthma is summarized in the definition offered in the National Heart, Lung, and Blood Institute's 1995 Global Initiative for Asthma:

> Asthma is a chronic inflammatory disorder of the airways in which many cells and cellular elements play a role, in particular, mast cells, eosinophils, T lymphocytes, macrophages, neutrophils, and epithelial cells. In susceptible individuals, this inflammation causes recurrent episodes of wheezing, breathlessness, chest tightness, and coughing, particularly at night or in the early morning. These episodes are usually associated with widespread but variable airflow obstruction that is often reversible either spontaneously or with treatment. The inflammation also causes an associated increase in the existing bronchial hyperresponsiveness to a variety of stimuli.

This summary of the features of asthma serves well as a description of the major features of the disease, but it does not hold up as a definition. No feature is unique to asthma, and no feature is universal in those with the condition. For example, all tests of airway caliber may be normal between attacks, even in patients whose attacks are sudden and severe.[4, 5] Bronchial responsiveness may be normal over most of the year in patients with seasonal asthma,[6] and bronchial hyperresponsiveness is often found in people with allergic rhinitis but without asthma.[7] Even the association of eosinophilic bronchial inflammation and asthma is inconstant. Some patients with recurrent episodes of wheezing and dyspnea associated with reversible airflow obstruction and bronchial hyperresponsiveness have no evidence of eosinophilic inflammation in bronchial biopsies.[8] Other patients have eosinophilic inflammation of the bronchial mucosa and chronic cough that is responsive to treatment with an inhaled corticosteroid but have neither airflow obstruction nor bronchial hyperresponsiveness.[9] And some patients with severe asthma have a predominance of neutrophils, not eosinophils, in their bronchial mucosa.[10]

In practical terms, the limitations of the descriptive definitions of asthma have not proved crippling. The features of asthma requiring treatment are, for the most part, easy to recognize, so "working definitions" have sufficed. The lack of firm, universally agreed-upon criteria for defining asthma still complicates epidemiologic studies of the prevalence of asthma in various populations or of changes in prevalence in the same population over time, but the agreement on "working definitions" has enabled many informative studies.[11]

Logically, studies of the genetic basis of asthma should be most retarded by the lack of definitive diagnostic criteria, but the approach developed by genetic researchers is actually refining the general conception of the disease. Geneticists recognized early that asthma probably reflects the results of variations in many genes and is also the expression of an interaction between a genetic predisposition and some factor in the environment. So genetic researchers have examined the genetic determinants of well-defined phenotypes, rather than those of "asthma." This approach has clarified the role of genes as determinants of atopy, bronchial responsiveness, and responsiveness to asthma therapies (e.g., beta-agonists).[12] In other words, recognition of asthma as a complex, multifactorial disorder has led to greater focus on the individual, varied disturbances in function that contribute to a more or less common clinical expression. It is not so much that recent advances in science have enabled more precise definition of asthma as it is that advances have made the need for agreement on a definition seem less urgent.

## EPIDEMIOLOGY AND RISK FACTORS

### Population Trends

For studies of the epidemiology of asthma, agreement on a definition of the disease remains as necessary as ever. Few long-term, prospective, population-based studies have been done, so assessments of changes in the prevalence of asthma over time depend on the use of historical data. Because changes in diagnostic criteria have followed changes in the definition of asthma, and the latter have followed advances in the scientific conception of the disease, even medical records cannot be assumed to be reliable as a source of data. By the same reasoning, studies of differences in asthma prevalence among various populations require close similarity in the definitions of asthma used by physicians treating the populations being compared.

One approach to dealing with the first problem, possible inconsistency in diagnostic criteria over time, has been to analyze the frequency of dramatic events, such as death or hospitalization from asthma. The rationale for this approach is that recognition and classification of these events is unlikely to be affected by subtle differences in diagnostic criteria. To further sharpen accuracy, the analysis is often limited to those patients between 5 and 34 years of age, in whom other confounding diseases are uncommon.

Death from asthma was once thought to be so uncommon as to prompt Osler's adage that "the asthmatic pants into old age."[13] In retrospect, it can now be seen that in most Western countries asthma mortality has increased gradually since the 1940s,[14] but the event that attracted attention was a dramatic, abrupt increase in asthma deaths in the 1960s, especially in the British Isles, Australia, New Zealand, and Norway.[15] In these countries, asthma mortality increased 2- to 10-fold in less than 5 years. This increase was attributed to use of a high-dose preparation of a highly potent, nonselective inhaled beta-agonist, isoproterenol, and mortality fell after withdrawal of the preparation. A second, even more dramatic increase in asthma mortality in New Zealand in the 1970s was again attributed to sales of a particular beta-agonist, fenoterol.[16]

The New Zealand epidemic prompted reviews of asthma deaths in other Western countries, where fenoterol had not been marketed, almost all of which noted a gradual, 1.5- to 2-fold increase in the asthma mortality rate between the mid-1970s and the mid-1980s.[17] This increase occurred also in the United States, where the asthma mortality rate had historically been low, but disproportionately affected African-Americans, particularly those living in urban centers.[18]

The increase in deaths from asthma was mirrored by an increase in hospitalizations. The increases in asthma-related hospitalizations in the United States between 1965 and 1984, 50% in adults and more than 200% in children,[19] resembled similar but usually greater rates of increase in other Western countries.[20] The numbers continued to increase between 1979 and 1993 in the United States, from 386,000 to 466,000 cases per year,[21] but a slowing of the rate of increase was later noted in some countries, such as Sweden. This "leveling off" in hospitalization rates has been attributed to greater use of inhaled corticosteroids.[22]

The increases in asthma deaths and asthma hospitalizations probably reflect increases in asthma's prevalence. Surveys of asthma-like symptoms in a population are highly sensitive to the symptoms selected,[23] but surveys of constant constellations of symptoms within populations over time have been consistent in showing steady increases in their prevalence. Typical of the annual rates of increase reported are 3.4% in Melbourne, Australia[24]; 7.9% in Finland[25]; 3.5% in France[26]; and 4.8% in the United States.[27] Increase in asthma prevalence is by no means limited to Western countries. In Taiwanese children, prevalence rose from 1.3% in 1974 to 5.8% in 1985.[28] The most striking, even abrupt, increases observed have been in populations migrating from a rural to an urban environment[29–31] or from a nonindustrialized to a Westernized region.[32]

The changes in prevalence of symptoms suggestive of asthma are echoed by changes in the prevalence of "harder" end points, such as bronchial hyperresponsiveness to histamine.[33] Changes in the prevalence of physician-diagnosed asthma over long periods are harder to assess, because of varying diagnostic customs, but investigators in Olmsted County, Minnesota, were able to take advantage of a unique system of medical record-keeping.[34] This county, whose demographic makeup roughly mirrors that of the United States as a whole, has had a system in place to store all diagnoses recorded by all medical practitioners. The original, complete medical records are available for review. This enabled the application of explicit predetermined criteria to all encounters linked to a diagnosis of asthma over the 20 years surveyed. With this strict method, the annual incidence of asthma was found to have increased from 183 per 100,000 population in 1964 to 284 per 100,000 in 1983. The biggest increase occurred among children aged 1 to 14 years. This last finding, that increases in children account for most of the increase in prevalence in the population, suggests that the changes accounting for the rise in asthma are a "cohort effect" taking place early in life.

Evidence is now accumulating that the increase in the prevalence of asthma is probably an expression of a general increase in the prevalence of allergic disease. This is best established for eczema, which has been well documented as increasing over time in Denmark and in the United Kingdom.[35, 36] The prevalence of cutaneous sensitivity to inhaled allergens (aeroallergens) and of specific immunoglobulin E (IgE) antibodies against common aeroallergens also appears to be increasing.[37, 38] Again, the increases have been greatest in children, suggesting a cohort effect. Increases in the prevalence in allergic rhinitis appear to parallel the increases in asthma over the same period. For example, during a single decade asthma prevalence doubled (from 1% to 2% in 1971 to 2% to 5% in 1981) and allergic rhinitis also increased (from 3% to 6% in 1971 to 6% to 12% in 1981) among Swedish conscripts.[39] Over roughly the same period, the prevalence of rhinitis among Finnish adolescents increased from 5% to 15%.[40] In England and Wales, annual visits to general practitioners for grass pollen seasonal allergic rhinitis increased fourfold between 1955–1956 and 1981–1982.[41]

The general picture that has emerged from study of the trends in asthma in Western countries over the past 30 or more years is that the increases in the mortality and morbidity are real, widespread, and sustained. These increases in the dramatic expressions of asthma appear to reflect an increase in the overall prevalence of the disease, and this in turn appears to reflect an increase in the prevalence of all allergic diseases. The rates of increase have been much greater in children than in adults.[42, 43] This "cohort effect" is consistent with the interaction of some environmental agent with susceptible persons during an early "window" of development, during which allergic sensitization occurs. This general picture has properly alerted public health authorities, but, before effective preventive measures can be initiated, a far better understanding of the determinants of the risk for allergic disease and for asthma is required. Although all determinants have by no means been identified, epidemiologic studies comparing the incidence and prevalence of allergies and asthma in different populations, or in different subgroups within the same population, have provided important clues.[44]

## Risk Factors

The main requirement for investigating differences among populations is a valid and standard method for detecting the conditions of interest. Accordingly, the lack of uniformity of survey methods has complicated comparisons among the hundreds of asthma-prevalence studies done in various parts of the world. This accounts for the extraordinary importance of the International Study of Asthma and Allergies in Childhood (ISAAC),[45] which involved investigators at 155 centers in 56 countries around the world. To ensure consistency in their surveys of disparate populations, the investigators developed simple, 1-page questionnaires regarding the symptoms of asthma, allergic rhinoconjunctivitis, and atopic eczema. Recognizing that the words for asthma symptoms used in various languages correspond imperfectly, the surveys in some countries were complemented by an asthma video questionnaire that showed clinical signs and symptoms followed by questions. These tools were used to survey almost half a million children aged 13 to 14 years.

The results of this monumental study were dramatic, showing differences of 20- to 60-fold among centers in the prevalence of symptoms of asthma, allergic rhinoconjunctivitis, and atopic eczema (Fig. 39.1). For asthma symptoms, prevalences were highest (up to 20% of children) in the United Kingdom, Australia, New Zealand, and Ireland; they were lowest (as low as 2% to 3%) in Eastern European countries, Indonesia, Greece, Uzbekistan, India, and Ethiopia. For allergic rhinitis, the centers with the highest prevalences were scattered geographically, but the lowest prevalences were found in the same centers where asthma prevalence was low. For atopic eczema, some of the centers with the highest prevalences, such as those in Scandinavia and in Africa, were not among the centers with the highest prevalences of asthma.

Even the simplest interpretation of these findings is important: that factors in addition to atopic sensitization are important in the development of asthma, allergic rhinoconjunctivitis, and eczema, and that the factors responsible for asthma are more common in wealthy, Westernized countries. The findings further suggest that outdoor air pollution is not a major risk factor for the development of asthma in populations. Some centers with the lowest levels of air pollution (e.g., New Zealand) had the highest rates of asthma. Regions with high levels of particulate matter and sulfur dioxide (e.g., China, Eastern Europe) had low rates of asthma. A comparison of children raised in West and East Germany found significantly lower rates of current asthma and hay fever in East German children[46] despite the severe pollution due to heavy industrialization and private coal burning in the East German cities.[47]

The further findings of ISAAC and of other large international studies[48] will undoubtedly lead to new hypotheses regarding the causation of asthma.[49] But much has already been learned from studies of variations in the rates of asthma, rhinitis, and eczema among subunits of the same population. These subunits range in size from cities or regions of a state to families or even pairs of siblings. Studies of relationships in these smaller units have established some of the major risk factors.[41] The strongest is a family history of atopic disease.[50, 51] A positive family history increases the risk of developing allergic rhinitis by fivefold and that of asthma by threefold to fourfold.[52] Atopy greatly increases the risk of asthma. In children 3 to 14 years old, both positive skin tests and increases in total serum IgE are strongly associated with the presence of asthma.[53, 54] Serum IgE concentration also correlates strongly with bronchial hyperresponsiveness to a methacholine challenge.[55]

The nature of the sensitizing allergen seems to be an independent determinant of the risk for development of asthma. This has been best established for the house dust mite. The level of this antigen in the home environment has been linked to the likelihood, first, of cutaneous reactivity, and then of asthma itself, in a dose-dependent manner.[56–58] Other allergen exposures linked to a heightened risk of asthma are cat dander, cockroach, and *Alternaria,* but not, at least in a New Zealand study, grass pollen, a common cause of allergic rhinitis.[59–62] The conditions optimal for growth of house dust mites (warm temperatures, relatively high atmospheric humidity, and a ready food supply of shed human skin) may account for the greater prevalence of asthma in warm, coastal regions and in Westernized societies, in which mattresses, layers of bedding, and carpeted bedrooms are favored.

The diet favored by Westernized societies (or perhaps the balance of diet and activity that is favored) may also increase the risk for asthma.[63] In Britain and the United States, the rise in asthma among children has been accompanied by an almost epidemic increase in the prevalence of obesity.[64–66] Among Taiwanese girls (13 to 16 years old), the prevalence of symptoms of allergic rhinitis, positive skin test responses, bronchial hyperresponsiveness, and wheezing increased stepwise among quintiles for body mass index.[67] The large Nurses' Health Study in the United States is the first longitudinal study to demonstrate a strongly positive association between body mass index and risk of incident asthma.[68]

Other factors that are associated with asthma, but less strongly so, are male gender, low birth weight, prematurity, maternal smoking in pregnancy, parental smoking, and high intake of salt.[41, 69] Some protective factors are large family size,[70, 71] consumption of oily fish,[72] and, perhaps, breast feeding to the age of 3 months.[73] So far, no primary prevention study has shown that reduction of any risk factor, even house dust mite, significantly reduces asthma prevalence, but large trials are now under way.[73]

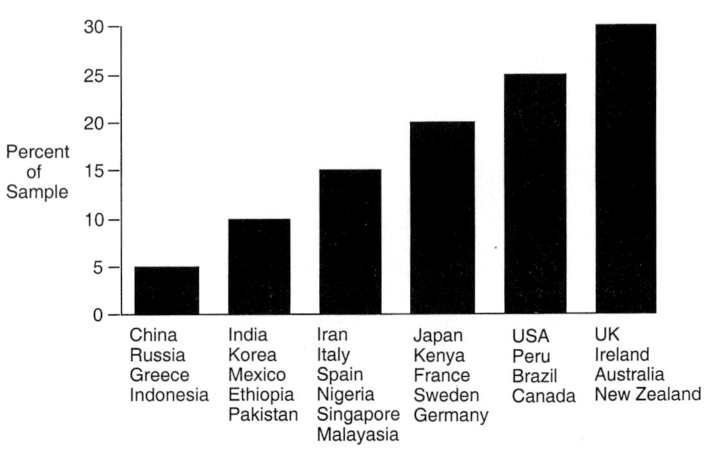


**Figure 39.1** The graph shows prevalence of wheeze in the last 12 months among 13- to 14-year old children, as measured in the International Study of Asthma and Allergies in Childhood (ISAAC) studies.[45] Only a selection of the 56 participating countries is shown. (Redrawn from Peat JK, Li J: Reversing the trend: Reducing the prevalence of asthma. J Allergy Clin Immunol 103:1–10, 1999, with permission.)

## Infection as a Risk Factor

Symptoms typical of ordinary "colds" often precede asthma exacerbations, but involvement of viral infections could not be proven until the highly sensitive method of polymerase chain reaction (PCR) was added to conventional methods of culture to detect viruses in respiratory secretions. The addition of PCR enabled detection of viruses in 80% of the episodes of worsening asthma in children and in 44% of the exacerbations in adults.[74, 75] The virus most frequently isolated was rhinovirus, the most common cause of the common cold.

That viral infection of the airways might also have a role in the induction of asthma has also long been suspected. A population-based study reported that a history of bronchiolitis or croup in early childhood was a predictor of increased bronchial responsiveness and of atopy in later years.[76] And in a prospective, longitudinal study of children born to allergic parents, upper respiratory infections were noted to occur 1 to 2 months before the onset of allergic sensitization.[77] The rise in virus-specific IgE in nasal secretions after respiratory syncytial virus infection in children suggests a possible mechanism by which viral infections might induce asthma.[78]

Only one third of infants who have wheezing with a lower respiratory tract illness have persistent episodes of wheezing at the age of 6 years. The strongest correlate of wheezing before age 3 is small airway caliber, whereas wheezing after 3 years of age correlates with elevated serum IgE and a maternal history of asthma.[79] The reduction in production of interferon-γ, the prototypic type 1 helper T-lymphocyte (Th1) cytokine, by monocytes in the cord blood of neonates with atopic parents[80] prompted speculation that viral infection does not so much induce asthma as unmask a predisposition to predominant Th2-like responses that is already present at the time of the infection.[81]

This predisposition to Th2-like responses is not necessarily fixed. The immunologic milieu at the fetal-maternal interface is naturally skewed toward a Th2 phenotype, and this immune bias is carried into neonatal life. Unless the pattern of immune response in the airways is "reprogrammed" toward a Th1 pattern, the infant will have a prolonged high-risk "window" for allergic sensitization to aeroallergens.[80] The principal impetus to this reprogramming of the mechanisms of immune response toward a normal Th1/Th2 balance is hypothesized to be contact with pathogenic and commensal microorganisms at the body's mucosal surfaces.[82, 83] In essence, this hypothesis proposes that recurrent infections of the airways may be protective against the development of asthma and suggests that the rising trends of asthma may be a result of medical and social changes that have reduced the frequency of respiratory infections in childhood, such as smaller family size, vaccination against respiratory pathogens, and widespread use of antibiotics (Fig. 39.2).

This theory also has some support from epidemiologic studies. It could account, for example, for the inverse relationship between sibling number and atopy,[46, 84] by the rationale that the frequency of respiratory infections is related to the number of children in a household. It could account also for the findings of a historical cohort study

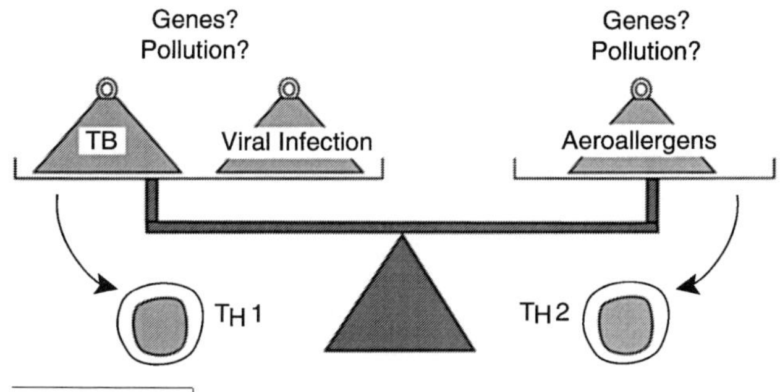


**Figure 39.2** Determinants of the direction of differentiation of precursor T cells in neonatal life are shown. Repeated infections of the respiratory tract favor differentiation toward the type 1 helper T-lymphocyte (Th1) phenotype; exposure to aeroallergens favors differentiation toward the Th2 phenotype. Various genes and air pollutants may have opposing effects on the direction of T-cell differentiation. Abbreviation: TB = tuberculosis. (Redrawn from Cookson WOCM, Moffatt MF: Asthma: An epidemic in the absence of infection. Science 275:41–42, 1997, with permission.)

in Guinea-Bissau, which showed that a history of measles was associated with a reduction in skin test reactivity to common allergens.[85] And this theory was cited as an explanation for the finding of an inverse association between tuberculin responses and markers of atopy in Japanese schoolchildren.[86]

It is possible that viral infections in early childhood may either protect against or induce asthma depending on the nature of the virus. Some viruses, for example, appear to have evolved to activate Th2 responses, which are less effective in containing or eliminating viral infection.[87] All that can be confidently stated at present is that viral infections of the airways are a common cause of exacerbations in people who have asthma and that the pattern of immune response that viral respiratory tract infections elicit in infants and young children may influence their risk of acquiring asthma in later years.

Although bacterial infections are not thought to worsen asthma, increasing attention is being focused on two of the bacterial causes of "atypical" pneumonia, *Chlamydia pneumoniae* and *Mycoplasma pneumoniae*. A prospective study of 365 adults with acute community-acquired pneumonia found that almost half of those with acute *C. pneumoniae* infection had bronchospasm during the illness, and a matched comparison study showed that those with high titers of *C. pneumoniae* antibody were more likely to be diagnosed as having "asthmatic bronchitis" after the respiratory illness.[88] A study of children similarly concluded that infection with *C. pneumoniae* can trigger acute episodes of wheezing,[89] and a study of 108 asthmatic children who were observed for 13 months found that nasal titers of *C. pneumoniae* secretory IgA antibodies were seven times higher among children who reported more than four exacerbations of asthma, compared with those who reported one or fewer attacks.[90]

The proposal that chronic infection with *M. pneumoniae* might be important in chronic severe asthma drew support from the application of PCR to detect infection in bronchial mucosal biopsies. *M. pneumoniae* was detected in more than half of the biopsies from asthmatics but in fewer than 1 in 10 of those from control subjects.[91]

Both *C. pneumoniae* and *M. pneumoniae* commonly infect the airway epithelium, and both are known to stimulate local inflammatory reactions.[92] The idea that they may worsen asthma in persons who have the disease or trigger it in those with atopy or some other predisposing condition fits well with current concepts of asthma as an inflammatory disease of the airways. Both organisms are sensitive to macrolide antibiotics, so it is tempting to speculate that infection with these organisms may account for the favorable response to prolonged courses of treatment with troleandomycin, a macrolide antibiotic once used for its "steroid-sparing" effects.[93]

## GENETICS

Asthma has been suspected of having a strong genetic component at least since 1860, when Henry Salter stated that he found "distinct traces of inheritance . . . in two cases out of every five."[94] Salter's certainty appears to have been confirmed by studies demonstrating increased prevalence of asthma among first-degree relatives of asthmatic subjects (20% to 25%, compared with a general population prevalence of 4%)[12, 95, 96] and greater concordance rates among monozygotic than dizygotic twins (50% vs. 33%, respectively).[97–99] But members of families share common environments, so familial "clustering" of a disease may reflect the effects of a common environmental exposure, rather than a genetic cause.[100] One such comparison showed no differences in the concordance for seasonal rhinitis (about 60%), positive skin tests, or serum IgE levels,[101] suggesting that the genetic contribution to these traits is much greater than the environmental contribution.[12] Twin studies have also revealed a genetic predisposition to the organ-specific manifestations of allergic disease: monozygotic and dizygotic twins who are concordant for an allergic disorder (asthma, eczema, or allergic rhinitis) are most likely to be concordant for the same disorder.[99] This may even be true of the particular manifestations of a specific disorder. The symptoms of cough and wheeze track separately in asthmatic families.[102]

### Segregation Analysis

Formal study of the pattern of inheritance of a disorder is done by segregation analysis. In this method, the distribution of disease in multiple families or in single large families is analyzed, and the frequency of the disorder among offspring and siblings is compared with the distribution to be expected from various modes of inheritance (e.g., autosomal dominant, autosomal recessive). Studies of the distribution of asthma have been complicated by the lack of an agreed definition of the disease (see previous discussion), but its distribution does not seem to follow any simple Mendelian pattern. Asthma is therefore thought to be both multifactorial and complex.[12, 100] The term *multifactorial* refers to the probable involvement of genetic and environmental components; *complex* refers to the involvement of many genes that interact to determine susceptibility. In other words, what is genetically determined in a multifactorial disease is not the condition itself but instead the susceptibility to acquiring the condition on encountering the causative stimuli in the environment. Differences in the probability of encountering the causative stimuli complicate studies of the genetic basis of a multifactorial disease. For example, the finding of a bimodal distribution of serum levels of specific IgE for house dust mite among residents in a single area may reflect differences in housing, not in genetic makeup. The finding of a bimodal distribution of specific IgE for an aeroallergen ubiquitous for the region more strongly suggests the presence of a susceptible subgroup in the population.[12, 103]

Because of the difficulties in defining asthma, segregation analysis has been used to determine the mode of inheritance of discrete, quantifiable traits that characterize asthma: total and specific IgE levels, skin test reactivity, and bronchial responsiveness. Studies of total IgE should be limited to populations with a low rate of parasitic infestation and should be controlled for other factors that also influence IgE levels, such as age, gender, and smoking habits. Most studies show total serum IgE levels to be distributed continuously and unimodally, a pattern most consistent with complex or polygenic determination.[12, 104] In contrast, skin test responses and serum IgE levels to specific allergens are often found to be distributed bimodally,[103] a pattern suggesting the presence of a uniquely susceptible subgroup in the population. It therefore appears that "basal" IgE levels and specific IgE responses to aeroallergens may be under different genetic controls.

Segregation analyses of bronchial responsiveness also suggest a mixed pattern of regulation. Atopy and bronchial hyperresponsiveness are strongly associated.[55, 105] However, because some people with atopy do not have bronchial hyperresponsiveness and some with bronchial hyperresponsiveness do not have atopy, it may be that bronchial responsiveness is under its own, separate genetic influence. As with total serum IgE levels, bronchial responsiveness is unimodally distributed in populations,[105] so its genetic determinants appear to be complex. But studies of bronchial responsiveness among atopic asthmatic children and their relatives show a different pattern of distribution.[106, 107] These findings are interpreted as demonstrating two components to the development of hyperresponsiveness: one genetic and the other acquired. That the mechanism for the acquired component is allergic inflammation of the airways[12] is supported by a study of monozygotic twin pairs discordant for allergic rhinitis. The allergic twins had greater bronchial responsiveness, and this hyperresponsiveness increased further during the relevant pollen season.[108]

### Gene Association Studies

Two major strategies have been used to identify genetic variants that contribute to the development of asthma: positional cloning and the candidate gene approach. *Positional cloning* takes advantage of the identification of more than 2000 "markers" scattered throughout the human genome. These markers are used in family or population studies to examine the concordance of inheritance of a trait with the transmission of a genetic marker. The underlying idea is that when a genetic marker and the gene for the trait are located close to each other on the same chromosome, the marker and the trait will tend to appear together, or to be "linked" in succeeding generations. Once linkage of the trait to a particular marker is established, then additional studies can refine the location of the gene for the trait.

Genome-wide searches have provided evidence for linkage of several chromosomal regions with various atopic phenotypes (eosinophil count, skin test responsiveness, atopy, and asthma).[109–111] Because of the great number of genes in the human genome (60,000 to 100,000), the statistical risk for false-negative findings is high, and many of the linkages found in one study have not been found in others. Some linkages have nonetheless attracted attention because of their biologic plausibility. For example, Young and colleagues reported linkages of a broadly defined allergic phenotype to an area of chromosome 11q[112] and also reported variations (polymorphisms) in the gene for the high-affinity IgE receptor in this region.[113] Similarly, reports of linkage between the 5q31–33 region and asthma attracted attention because the region is known to contain the genes encoding many of the cytokines that are thought to be important in the pathogenesis of atopic diseases (e.g., interleukin 3 [IL-3], IL-4, IL-5, IL-9, and IL-13).[114, 115]

The *candidate gene* approach starts with selection of a gene whose function is thought likely to influence a disease's pathogenesis, perhaps from studies of animal models.[116] The next step is to identify variants or polymorphisms within or close to the gene that could affect its function, as in the promoter locus. Once the gene has been selected and the polymorphism identified, the next step is to conduct *association studies* to determine whether the polymorphism occurs more frequently in persons who have the disease than in individuals from a control population, most often by studies of a *prospective cohort* or by a retrospective *case-control design.*

Association studies need not be limited to study of well-characterized candidate genes believed to regulate a function that is important in a disease's pathogenesis. They can be used to examine association with markers in a chromosomal region, the genes for which might be poorly known, but which emerged from a genome-wide search as strongly linked to the disease (a so-called hot spot). Several reports have been published of linkages of asthma or atopy to regions on chromosomes where potentially important "candidate genes" are located (Table 39.1). However, confirmation of linkages with these regions by various studies has been inconsistent.[100] A promising application of the candidate gene approach is the study of the genetic basis of responsiveness to particular therapies. This reduces the number of genes of potential importance. An example of the power of this approach is the identification of polymorphisms in the gene for the beta-adrenergic receptor and their possible influence on responsiveness to regular or intermittent beta-agonist treatment.[117]

Fulfillment of the promise of genetic studies of asthma still lies well in the future. A big step will be taken with completion of the Human Genome Project, when all genes at all chromosomal locations will be known. At present, it is clear that the susceptibility to asthma is inherited, but the specific genes responsible have yet to be identified. Most data suggest that asthma susceptibility is transmitted by multiple genes, with the various features of the disease under independent genetic regulation. There is strong reason to believe that other genes modify asthma's severity and its responsiveness to various treatments even though they may not contribute to its causation.[118] Identification of the genes that are primarily responsible is certain to lead to further revisions in scientific conceptions of the disease and ultimately to the development of far more effective strategies for prevention and treatment.

## PATHOLOGY

Chronic stable asthma is characterized by inflammation of the airway wall, with abnormal accumulation of eosinophils, lymphocytes, mast cells, macrophages, dendritic cells, and myofibroblasts. Inflammatory mediators and proteins secreted by these and other cells contribute directly and indirectly to changes in airway structure and function. The structural changes are found in both the epithelium and the submucosa and include abnormal deposition of collagen in the subepithelium and hyperplasia and/or hypertrophy of goblet cells, submucosal gland cells, smooth muscle cells, and blood vessel cells.

### Structural Changes in the Airway

#### Epithelial Changes

Whether epithelial desquamation or denudation is a pathologic feature of asthma or an artifact of tissue sampling and processing is controversial. Early descriptive autopsy reports emphasized epithelial desquamation in the airways of asthmatic patients but did not quantify the abnormality and included few controls. In the 1980s there were several reports of epithelial damage and epithelial denudation in endobronchial biopsies from asthmatic subjects.[3, 119] Again, these studies did not include many control subjects and were not always quantitative. More recently, the potential for artifactual disruption of the airway epithelium during the biopsy procedures or during fixation and embedding procedures has been emphasized,[120] and several quantitative studies have failed to show any difference between asthmatic and nonasthmatic subjects in the degree of epithelial desquamation in the airways.[121–124]

In areas of intact epithelium, squamous metaplasia has been described as a pathologic feature of asthma,[125] but it is not consistently mentioned in all pathologic studies. In contrast, goblet cell hyperplasia or hypertrophy is a consistent feature of case reports or case series of patients with fatal asthma.[126, 127] These goblet cell abnormalities result in a threefold increase, on average, in the amount of mucin stored in the airway epithelium.[128]

#### Eosinophilic Inflammation

A pathologic hallmark of asthma is an increase in the numbers of activated eosinophils in the airway epithelium

**Table 39.1 SUMMARY OF GENETIC LINKAGE ANALYSES RELEVANT TO HUMAN AND EXPERIMENTAL ASTHMA**

| Human Chromosome No. | Candidate Genes | Trait | References |
|---|---|---|---|
| ***Human*** | | | |
| 1 | IL-10 | Asthma | Borish et al, 1996[520] |
| 5 | IL-4, IL-5, IL-9, IL-13, GM-CSF, β2AdR, GCR, LTC4 synthase | Total serum IgE, BHR | Marsh et al, 1994[114]; Meyers et al, 1994[115]; Postma et al, 1995[521]; Douli et al, 1996[522]; Hopes et al, 1998[523] |
| 6 | TNF locus, HLA | Asthma, specific serum IgE titers | Moffatt et al, 1997[524]; Daniels et al, 1996[109]; Young et al, 1994[525] |
| 7 | TCR-α | Specific serum IgE titers | Young et al, 1994[525] |
| 11 | FcεRI-β chain | Atopy, asthma | Cookson et al, 1989[526]; Young et al, 1992[112]; Shirakawa et al, 1994[527]; Van Herwerden et al, 1995[528]; Doull et al, 1996[522] |
| 12 | IFN-γ, NOS, LTA4 hydrolase | Asthma, total IgE | Barnes et al, 1996[529] |
| 13 | Esterase D | Atopy, asthma | Daniels et al, 1996[109]; CSGA, 1997[110] |
| 14 | TCR β, NFκB-1 | Atopy | Moffatt et al, 1994[530] |
| 16 | IL-4Rα | Atopy, asthma | Mitsuyasu et al, 1998[531] Hershey et al, 1997[532] |
| ***Mouse*** | | | |
| 2 | IL-1 β, AchR, Gsα | Native airway hyperresponsiveness | De Sanctis et al, 1995[533] |
| 6 | IL-5R, CD4, CD8 (α and β), G β 3, Ly-36, Ly-49 | Native airway hyperresponsiveness | Ewart et al, 1996[534] |
| 15 | IL-2R β, IL-3R β 1, IL-3R β 2, PDGF β | Native airway hyperresponsiveness | De Sanctis et al, 1995[533] |
| 17 | HLA, TNF, MCP 6-7 | Native airway hyperresponsiveness | De Sanctis et al, 1995[533] |

IL, interleukin, GM-CSF = granulocyte-macrophage colony stimulating factor; β2AdR = beta 2 adrenergic receptor; GCR = glucocorticoid receptor; LTC4 synthase = leukotriene C4 synthase; TNF locus = tumor necrosis factor gene locus; HLA = human leukocyte antigen gene locus; TCR = T cell receptor; FcεRI-β chain = beta chain of the Fc epsilon receptor; IFN-γ = interferon gamma; NOS = nitric oxide synthase: LTA4 hydrolase = leukotriene A4 hydrolase; NFκB-1 = nuclear factor kappa B-1; IL-4Rα = alpha chain of the interleukin 4 receptor, IL-1 β = interleukin 1 beta; AchR = acetylcholine receptor; Gsα = G protein S alpha; IL-5R = interleukin 5 receptor; Gβ3 = G protein beta 3; PDGFb = platelet-derived growth factor beta; MCP = mast cell protease; IgE = immunoglobulin E; BHR = bronchial hyperreactivity.

and submucosa[129–132] (Fig. 39.3). The degree of eosinophilia is highly variable, however, and relatively few eosinophils are identifiable in the airway tissue of a sizable subgroup of asthmatic subjects.[131] Eosinophil numbers are often increased in the peripheral blood, but peripheral blood eosinophilia is not as sensitive as sputum eosinophilia as an indicator of asthma.[133]

### Subepithelial Changes

Increased amounts of collagen type III and type V, as well as fibronectin and tenascin, are deposited immediately beneath the bronchial epithelium in the asthmatic airway[134, 135] (see Fig. 39.3). These structural proteins differ from typical basement membrane proteins such as collagen IV and laminin; therefore, the subepithelial fibrosis of asthma is not a thickening of the true basement membrane but rather a deposition of a layer of interstitial collagens immediately beneath it. The likely source of these structural proteins is myofibroblasts, which are increased in number in asthma.[136]

The number and size of bronchial blood vessels are increased in asthma.[137] These vessels may have an important role in regulating airway caliber, because an increase in vascular volume can swell the mucosa and narrow the airway lumen.[138] Many inflammatory mediators cause vasodilation, a response that may be accompanied by increased permeability at the postcapillary venule, plasma extravasation, and airway mucosal edema.[139, 140]

Airway smooth muscle is hypertrophied and hyperplastic in asthma,[123, 141, 142] although the extent of these changes varies widely among patients, especially in the peripheral airways.[123, 143] Hyperplasia seems to dominate over hypertrophy as the dominant abnormality of airway smooth muscle in asthma,[144] with the number of smooth muscle cells increased twofold to threefold above normal.[141, 145, 146]

Studies have also found abnormalities in the structure of airway cartilage in asthma. Specifically, degeneration of cartilage with pericartilaginous fibrosis has been described.[147]

## Changes in Airway Mucus

In asthma, airway mucus is qualitatively and quantitatively abnormal, reflecting interactions between the inflammatory cells infiltrating the airway wall and the pathologic changes in secretory cells and blood vessels

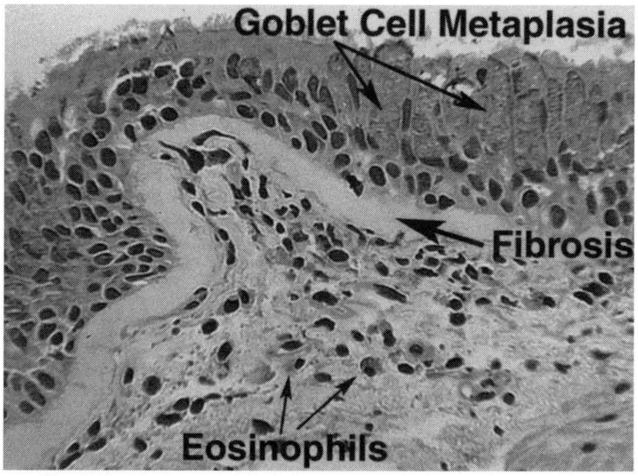


**Figure 39.3** Airway pathology in asthma is depicted in this photomicrograph of a hematoxylin and eosin-stained section from an endobronchial biopsy taken during bronchoscopy from a subject with mild chronic asthma. Goblet cell hyperplasia, subepithelial fibrosis, and eosinophilic infiltration of the submucosa are shown. (Hematoxylin and eosin stain; original magnification ×1200.)

in the airway epithelium and submucosa. These changes result in abnormalities in the viscoelastic and rheologic characteristics of airway mucus and in abnormalities in mucociliary clearance. The cellular and biochemical composition of airway secretions in asthma is abnormal in several respects. Eosinophil numbers are increased and account for the presence of bipyramidal crystals (Charcot-Leyden crystals), which are composed of eosinophil lysophospholipase.[148, 149] In addition, mucin concentrations in airway secretions are higher than normal in asthma[150]; this accounts for the occasional finding of corkscrew-shaped twists of inspissated mucus (Curschmann's spirals) in sputum from asthmatic patients.[148] Clumps of sloughed epithelial cells (Creola bodies) are occasionally seen in sputum, as well.[151] Furthermore, albumin and DNA concentrations are increased in sputum from asthmatic subjects,[150, 152] reflecting abnormal bronchovascular permeability and increased cellular inflammation, respectively. Finally, airway secretions in asthma are characterized by increases in a variety of plasma-derived proteins, cytokines, and chemokines,[153] reflecting the complex inflammation that is characteristic of asthma. The accumulation of abnormal mucus in the airways worsens airflow obstruction and provokes the symptoms of cough and sputum production. In addition, mucus accumulation contributes importantly to airway obstruction in fatal attacks of asthma.[154–156]

## Large vs. Small Airway Pathology

In general, studies comparing pathologic changes at various sites in the tracheobronchial tree have found that the changes of asthma are qualitatively similar in large and small airways.[119, 123, 143, 157] For example, the degree of subepithelial fibrosis in proximal airways is representative of its thickness in distal airways.[119] A 1996 report that eosinophilic inflammation extends into the alveolar septa in asthmatic subjects[158] challenges the notion that asthma is a disease whose pathology is limited to the airway wall. Goblet cell metaplasia may be particularly important as the source of mucus that occludes many small airways, because small, noncartilaginous airways do not have submucosal glands.

## Airway Pathology in Allergic and Nonallergic Asthma

The pathology of "extrinsic" or allergic asthma and that of "intrinsic" or nonallergic asthma (as judged by skin test reactivity and IgE levels) does not differ.[159, 160] Both forms of asthma are characterized by increases in eosinophils, mast cells, and CD4-positive T lymphocytes expressing cytokine profiles typical of the Th2 lymphocyte subgroup.[159, 161–164]

## Fatal Asthma

Extensive mucus plugging of the airways is typically found in autopsies of asthma fatalities and is considered a major cause of the asphyxiation of the lethal attack.[123, 154–156, 165, 166] It is only in a small minority of asthma deaths that mucus impaction of the airways is not found.[167] In addition, autopsy studies show that the degrees of airway wall thickening, smooth muscle hypertrophy, and submucosal gland hypertrophy are greater in patients who die from an asthmatic attack than in patients with asthma who die from other causes.[123] Eosinophils are prominent in the airways in fatal asthma,[155, 156, 165] but neutrophils are also prominent in the airways of asthmatic patients who die very quickly after the onset of the lethal attack.[168, 169]

## Relationship Between Airway Pathology and Asthma Severity

All of the characteristic findings of asthma are at least qualitatively similar in mild, moderate, and severe asthma.[119, 125, 170–174] There is some evidence that eosinophil numbers in airway tissue or airway secretions are higher in asthmatic patients with more severe disease, as assessed by the $FEV_1$ percent predicted, bronchial reactivity to methacholine, or composite asthma severity scores.[131, 175–178] The correlation between extent of subepithelial fibrosis and asthma severity is less certain.[122, 134, 179, 180] The pathologic features of the airway that result in difficult-to-control disease or risk for near-fatal or fatal asthma are not completely understood.

## Specificity of Airway Inflammation

Other airway diseases, such as chronic bronchitis or chronic obstructive pulmonary disease, may have an element of eosinophilic inflammation, but to a lesser degree than is found in asthma.[181, 182] Similarly, modest increases in airway eosinophilia are found in subjects with allergic rhinitis but no history of asthma.[178, 183] Smooth muscle hypertrophy is a feature of chronic bronchitis as well as of asthma.[184] Mononuclear cell infiltrates of the airway wall are characteristic of both asthma and chronic bronchitis, but the nature of the infiltrate differs: in asthma, the cells consist predominantly of CD4$^+$ lymphocytes; in chronic bronchitis, they consist predominantly of CD8$^+$ lymphocytes.[185] Also, subepithelial fibrosis can be observed in chronic bronchitis and in allergic rhinitis, but the degree of subepithelial fibrosis is much lower than in asthma.[122]

## PATHOPHYSIOLOGY

### Origin and Evolution

Asthma is a complex disease characterized physiologically by variable airflow obstruction and pathologically by multiple abnormalities in the airway epithelium, lamina propria, and submucosa. The clinical symptoms of wheeze, dyspnea, and sputum production reflect these physiologic and pathologic abnormalities and cannot be explained by simple abnormalities in airway smooth muscle responsiveness. Any explanation for the abnormal pathology and physiology of asthma must account for the facts that asthma is heritable, is strongly associated with atopy, and is currently increasing rapidly in prevalence.

Because of increasing recognition that airway inflammation is a key component of asthma and represents a complex interaction of inflammatory cells and resident airway cells, hypotheses have been proposed for various cells that might "orchestrate" this complex airway inflammation. The mast cell, the eosinophil, the airway epithelial cell, and the CD4$^+$ lymphocyte have been proposed as candidate "conductors" of the "inflammation orchestra" in the airway. Of the cases made for each of these cells as the key orchestrator of airway inflammation in asthma, the most compelling is that made for the CD4$^+$ lymphocyte. Consensus is building for a theory that proposes that persons with appropriate susceptibility genes for atopy and asthma, when placed in a specific early life environment, develop a particular type of lymphocytic airway inflammation that results in asthma (see Fig. 39.2). In utero fetal programming by the mother, coupled with a relative absence of early childhood infections, may create a biologic environment whereby naive T cells in the neonate are encouraged to differentiate toward a Th2 subtype. Secretion of typical Th2 cytokines such as IL-4, IL-5, and IL-13 in the airway might then promote eosinophilic and mast cell inflammation and structural airway changes typical of the asthma phenotype. Chronic airway inflammation originating in this way might be exacerbated by episodes of acute inflammation caused by viral or allergen exposures, resulting in further cycles of inflammation that contribute to airway remodeling and abnormal airway responses (Fig. 39.4).

This theory for the origin and evolution of asthma has some support from epidemiologic and experimental studies. If it is proven true, it will have profound consequences on strategies for treatment and prevention. Meanwhile, consistent incremental increases in understanding of the pathophysiology of asthma have been made from detailed studies of individual cells and mediators in asthma, from the development of murine models of allergic asthma, and from clinical studies in asthmatic subjects, including studies of airway secretions and airway tissue. These studies have largely validated the hypothesis that the CD4$^+$ cell is an important orchestrator of airway inflammation in asthma and that eosinophils, mast cells, basophils, and B cells are important effector cells. However, these studies also demonstrate that inflammatory events in the airway are dynamic and that cells such as airway epithelial cells, smooth muscle cells, fibroblasts and cartilage cells (previously considered helpless "target" cells) actually "fire back" mediators when stimulated and have influences of their own on asthmatic inflammatory cascades.

### Cellular and Mediator Basis

#### Overview of Immune Mechanisms in Asthma

Intensive investigation over the past 10 years has shown that the airway immune response in allergic asthma is coupled to, and probably responsible for, the clinical manifestations of disease. Although much remains to be learned regarding the genetic and environmental elements that conspire to elicit an "asthmatic" immune response, many of the key effector cells and molecules have been identified through work in humans and experimental models. Allergic airway inflammation begins with the uptake and processing of aeroallergens by antigen-presenting cells such as dendritic cells and macrophages. The context in which antigen is processed and presented to T cells critically influences the nature of the subsequent inflammation. Depending on the cytokines acting on precursor T cells at the time of antigen presentation, different classes of effector T cells (i.e., Th1 and Th2 cells) are produced (Fig. 39.5). The sources of these critical cytokines affecting T-cell differentiation are many, including T cells themselves, antigen-presenting cells, airway epi-

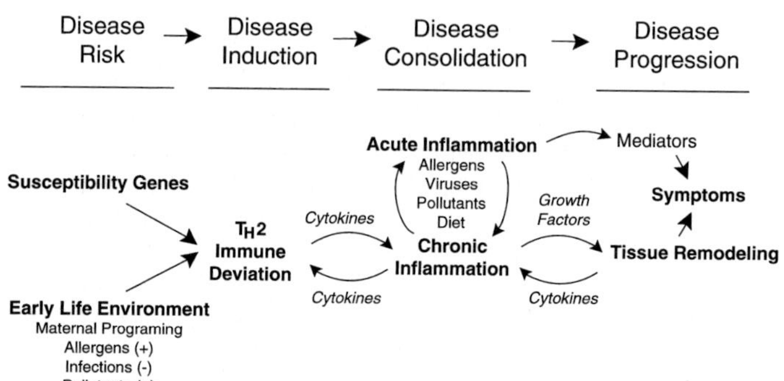


**Figure 39.4** A summary of current hypotheses for the evolution of asthma is shown. (Redrawn from Holgate ST: The cellular and mediator basis of asthma in relation to natural history. Lancet 350(Suppl II):5–9, 1997, with permission.)

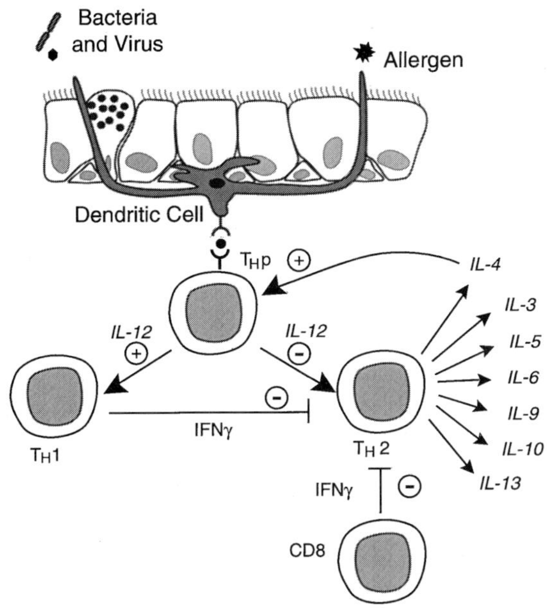


**Figure 39.5** A schematic representation of the key events in the asthmatic immune response is shown. Aeroallergens are ingested by airway antigen-presenting cells, particularly dendritic cells, and presented to CD4+ precursor T-helper cells (ThP). Depending on the context in which antigen is presented, ThP cells differentiate into either Th1 or Th2 cells, each with distinct patterns of secreted cytokines. Concomitant infections, particularly from certain bacteria and viruses, may promote the local release of interleukin-12 (IL-12), which favors Th1 cell development. Other infectious agents may promote Th2 cell development and chronic inflammation. The cytokines secreted by Th2 cells are largely responsible for the signs and symptoms of asthma. Interferon-gamma (IFNγ), released by Th1 and CD8+ T cells, down-regulates Th2 cell effector function. Airway epithelial cells may be an important additional source of cytokines that modulate airway immunity.

thelial cells, eosinophils, mast cells, macrophages, and perhaps airway smooth muscle cells and fibroblasts. The types of cytokines released during antigen presentation, and therefore the type of effector T cell produced, may be determined in part by concomitant infections and the nature of the allergens, with important implications for asthma (see Fig. 39.2). The cytokine secretion patterns of Th1 and Th2 cells are entirely distinct. Only the type 2 pattern of Th2 cells (IL-3, IL-4, IL-5, IL-6, IL-9, IL-10, and IL-13) is associated with asthma; type 1 cytokines (interferon-gamma [IFN-γ] and IL-12) counteract type 2 cytokines and attenuate allergic inflammation.

Research is ongoing to establish the mechanism by which the Th2 cell mediates airway hyperresponsiveness and other phenotypic characteristics of asthma. One possibility is that cytokine products of Th2 cells such as IL-4 and IL-5 act indirectly through effector cells, such as B cells, mast cells, and eosinophils, to mediate the asthma phenotype (Fig. 39.6). In this scenario, B cells, mast cells, and eosinophils play important roles in the disease expression of asthma. Another possibility is that cytokine products of Th2 cells such as IL-13 and IL-4 act directly to mediate the asthma phenotype (Fig. 39.7). In this scenario, B cells, mast cells, and eosinophils may have roles in potentiating asthma in some predisposed persons but are not required for disease expression.

## Dendritic Cells, Antigen Presentation, T Cells, and Cytokines

Although many cells (including airway epithelial cells and macrophages) can potentially present antigen, airway dendritic cells are thought to be the most important antigen-presenting cell and the most potent at initiating and sustaining airway inflammation (see Fig. 39.5). Dendritic cells (also referred to as Langerhans cells) are found within and below the epithelium and are ideally situated to receive, process, and present antigen.[186–189] These cells have a short half-life (less than 2 days), and their density in the airway can increase rapidly on airway stimulation.[188, 190] Their numbers are increased in asthma,[191] and they may initiate and sustain airway inflammation through enhanced expression of costimulatory molecules that facilitate T-cell activation and differentiation.[192, 193] Dendritic cells also secrete a number of mediators, including IL-12,[194] prostaglandin $E_2$, and IL-10,[195] that critically influence effector CD4+ T-cell development.

The immune response in asthma is characterized by the presence of CD4+ T cells in the epithelium and submucosa.[161, 196] These cells accumulate in the lungs in response to a variety of chemotactic stimuli, especially IL-16.[197] The presence of activated Th2 cells is revealed indirectly by the increased levels of Th2 cytokines such as IL-4, IL-5, and IL-13 in airway biopsies and bronchoalveolar lavage specimens from asthmatic subjects.[161, 196] CD4+ T cells, especially Th2 cells, appear to be absolutely required for induction of the asthma phenotype in murine models of asthma,[198] although other T cells, particularly γδ T cells[199] and CD8+ T cells,[200, 201] may have important regulatory roles.

Although all Th2 cytokines contribute to the asthma phenotype, IL-4 and IL-13 are particularly relevant. These cytokines are similar in structure, function, and chromosomal organization.[202] IL-4 functions primarily as a growth or differentiation factor for Th2 cells and promotes IgE secretion by B cells. Although IL-13 may also promote IgE secretion in humans, in experimental asthma this cytokine (and to a lesser extent IL-4) elicits disease through its proximal and perhaps direct mediation of airway hyperresponsiveness, goblet cell metaplasia, and airway eosinophilia[203, 204] (see Fig. 39.7). In murine models of asthma, the effects of IL-13 are mediated by the alpha subunit of the IL-4 receptor, but the relevant target tissues are unknown.[205]

IL-10 and IL-12 are also important cytokines in asthma. Originally described as a product of Th2 cells, IL-10 is synthesized by a wide variety of other cells, including airway epithelial cells and macrophages. IL-10 negatively regulates both Th1 and Th2 cytokines in vitro but may promote allergic responses in vivo through effects on dendritic cells.[206] Lack of IL-10 in antigen-challenged mice results in an exaggerated allergic phenotype.[207] IL-12 (together with IL-18[208, 209]) is required for

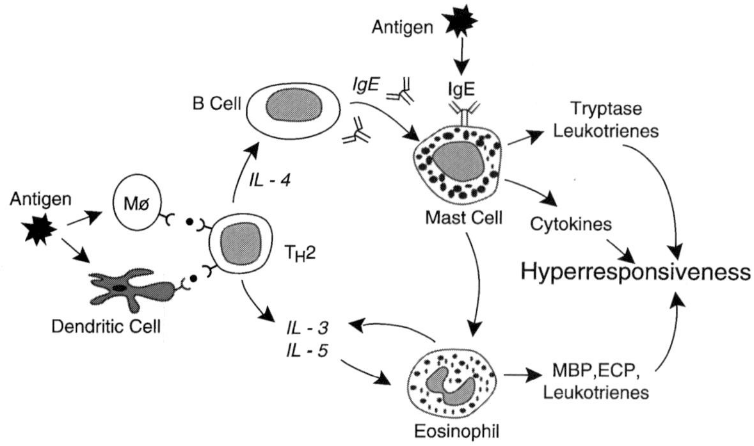


**Figure 39.6** The role of Th2 cells in the pathophysiology of asthma, in which cytokine products of Th2 cells act indirectly through effector cells to mediate the asthma phenotype, is depicted. Specifically, Th2 cells are activated to secrete type 2 cytokines (interleukin-3 (IL-3), IL-4, IL-5) after stimulation by antigen-presenting cells (dendritic cells and macrophages (Mϕ)) expressing cognate antigen. IL-4 induces B cells to synthesize and secrete immunoglobulin E (IgE); IL-3 and IL-5, together with granulocyte-macrophage colony-stimulating factor (GM-CSF) and other factors, mediate differentiation and recruitment of granulocytes, particularly eosinophils and mast cells. Secreted IgE is bound to surface IgE receptors present on mast cells and other cell types. After subsequent encounter with IgE-specific antigen, IgE receptors are cross-linked, leading to cellular activation and release of a wide variety of proinflammatory substances that together mediate eosinophil activation, airway hyperreactivity, and other elements of the asthma phenotype. In this scenario, B cells, mast cells, and eosinophils play important roles in the disease expression of asthma. Abbreviations: ECP = eosinophil cationic protein; MBP = major basic protein. (Redrawn from Drazen et al: Sorting out the cytokines of asthma. J Exp Med 183:1–5, 1996, with permission.)

maximal production of IFN-γ. IL-12 and IFN-γ antagonize many of the biologic effects of Th2 cytokines, and their administration to antigen-challenged mice abrogates the asthma phenotype.[210–213]

A number of cytokine-transgenic mice that demonstrate robust asthma phenotypes have been reported. This growing list includes mice overexpressing the cytokines IL-4, IL-5, IL-9, IL-11, IL-13, and granulocyte-macrophage colony-stimulating factor (GM-CSF) in the lung.[214–220] These data indicate that the lung is highly predisposed to an allergic phenotype after immune perturbation and confirm the existence of multiple pathways leading to the asthma phenotype.

## Role of the Airway Epithelium

Airway epithelial cells serve functions well beyond those of barrier protection, mucus secretion, and mucociliary clearance necessary for host defense.[221–223] More sophisticated host defense functions include modulation of local immune responses and limitation of inflammatory processes by degradation or inhibition of proinflammatory mediators and proteins. The epithelium can respond to a range of proinflammatory stimuli by producing biologically active mediators that influence airway inflammation. These mediators include cytokines and chemokines that can influence inflammatory cell trafficking and activation (Table 39.2), as well as lipid and peptide mediators (including arachidonic acid metabolites), endothelin-1, nitric oxide, and reactive oxygen species.[223] With an improved understanding of the biology of airway epithelial cells in health and disease, the classic concept of the epithelium as a physical barrier between the host and the environment has been replaced by a more complex concept in which epithelial cells also act as central modulators of the inflammatory response.[223]

The inflammatory mediators generated by the airway epithelium have multiple consequences, including recruitment of circulating leukocytes to the airway, regulation of airway tone, regulation of airway secretions, and promotion of antimicrobial and antiviral activity. The mechanisms responsible for epithelial cell activation are not well understood, but a number of stimuli, including air pollutants, respiratory viruses, aeroallergens, bacterial products, eosinophil and neutrophil granule products, and Th2 cytokines, may activate epithelial cells directly or indirectly.[221, 223, 224] It has been suggested that the activity of a protease-activated receptor (PAR-2) on epithelial cells represents a mechanism for prostanoid-dependent cytoprotection in the airways.[225] Other protective responses of the epithelium may include secretion of IL-10 and transforming growth factor-β, which may dampen airway inflammatory responses in certain circumstances.[226, 227]

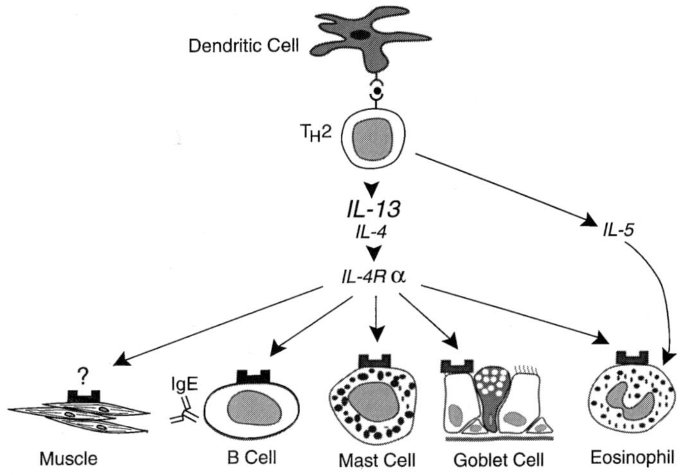


**Figure 39.7** The role of Th2 cells in the pathophysiology of asthma, in which cytokine products of Th2 cells act directly to mediate the asthma phenotype, is depicted. Specifically, Th2 cells, activated by dendritic cells, secrete type 2 cytokines that induce functional changes in many relevant tissues. Interleukin-13 (IL-13) and IL-4, signaling through the alpha chain of the IL-4 receptor (IL-4Rα), promote airway hyperresponsiveness through effects on smooth muscle, secretion of immunoglobulin E (IgE) from B cells, mast cell growth and differentiation, and goblet cell metaplasia with mucin overproduction. Together with IL-5, IL-4 and IL-13 also elicit airway eosinophilia. Although additional steps may be required, the cytokines may act directly on the target tissues: with the exception of airway smooth muscle and goblet cells, where expression has not been carefully examined, IL-4Rα is expressed on most of these target cells. In this scenario, B cells, mast cells, and eosinophils may have roles in potentiating asthma in some predisposed persons but may not be required for disease expression.

**Table 39.2** EPITHELIAL-DERIVED CYTOKINES

| Colony-Stimulating Factors (CSFs) | Pleiotropic Cytokines | Growth Factors | Receptor Antagonists | Chemoattractant Cytokines: Lymphocyte Chemoattractant Factor | Chemoattractant Cytokines: C-X-C/α Chemokines | Chemoattractant Cytokines: C-C/β Chemokines |
|---|---|---|---|---|---|---|
| GM-CSF | IL-6 | TGF-β | Type 1 TNFR | IL-16 | IL-6 | RANTES |
| G-CSF | IL-11 | TGF-α | icIL-1Ra Type 1 | | GRO-α | MCP-1 |
| M-CSF | IL-1 | SCF | | | GRO-γ | MCP-4 |
| CSF-1 | IL-10 | bFGF | | | | Eotaxin |
| | TNFα | | | | | |

GM = granulocyte-macrophage; G = granulocyte; CSF = colony stimulating factor; M = macrophage; IL = interleukin; TNF = tumor necrosis factor; TGF = transforming growth factor; SCF = stem cell factor; bFGF = basic fibroblast growth factor; TNFR = tumor necrosis factor receptor; icIL-1Ra = intracellular IL-1 receptor antagonist; GRO = growth-related oncogene; RANTES = regulated on activation, normal T-cell expressed and secreted; MCP = monocyte chemoattractant protein.

Adapted from Polito AJ, Proud D. Epithelial cells as regulators of airway inflammation. J Allergy Clin Immunol 102:714–718, 1998.

## B Cells, Mast Cells, Basophils, and Immunoglobulin E

Type I hypersensitivity reactions are considered to be an important cause of acute asthma exacerbations and may contribute to chronic airway inflammation in asthma. In these reactions, a cognate antigen cross-links IgE (and perhaps other antibody classes) bound to high affinity receptors on mast cells or basophils. This cross-linking activates the cells to release a variety of products, including histamine, tryptase, chymase, leukotrienes, platelet-activating factor, and various cytokines (IL-4, IL-5, TNF-α) that in turn promote airway hyperresponsiveness, mucus overproduction, fibroblast activation, and neuropeptide degradation. IgE-mediated activation of mast cells and basophils and IgE-facilitated antigen presentation to T cells are considered to be important mechanisms of the early and late phase responses to inhaled allergen[228] (Fig. 39.8), and inhibition of IgE attenuates both the early and late phase responses to inhaled allergen in asthmatic subjects.[229, 230]

Investigation of the relevance of type 1 hypersensitivity reactions in murine models of allergic asthma have yielded surprising results. Although passive transfer of antigen-specific IgE and IgE-bearing B cells induces airway hyperresponsiveness in mice,[231, 232] mice entirely deficient in antibodies and B cells develop a complete asthma phenotype,[198, 233, 234] indicating that type I hypersensitivity mechanisms are redundant in these models. These results are confined to the effects of acute antigen challenge; the role of antibodies in chronic disease is not well studied.

## Eosinophils

Eosinophils secrete an array of inflammatory mediators, including granule proteins, proteolytic enzymes, lipid mediators, oxygen metabolites, and cytokines.[235] These mediators are capable (directly or indirectly) of causing airway narrowing, airway hyperreactivity, and mucus hypersecretion, and the eosinophil has been considered the most important effector cell in asthma.[236] Support for this hypothesis comes from clinical studies and clinical observations. First, eosinophil numbers increase dramatically in the airways of asthmatic subjects 4 to 24 hours after an aerosolized allergen challenge,[173, 237–240] and their appearance coincides with the development of late phase asthmatic responses.[239, 241, 242] Second, eosinophil numbers increase in airway secretions in asthma exacerbations induced by corticosteroid withdrawal,[243, 244] and eosinophils are prominent both in secretions and in the airway

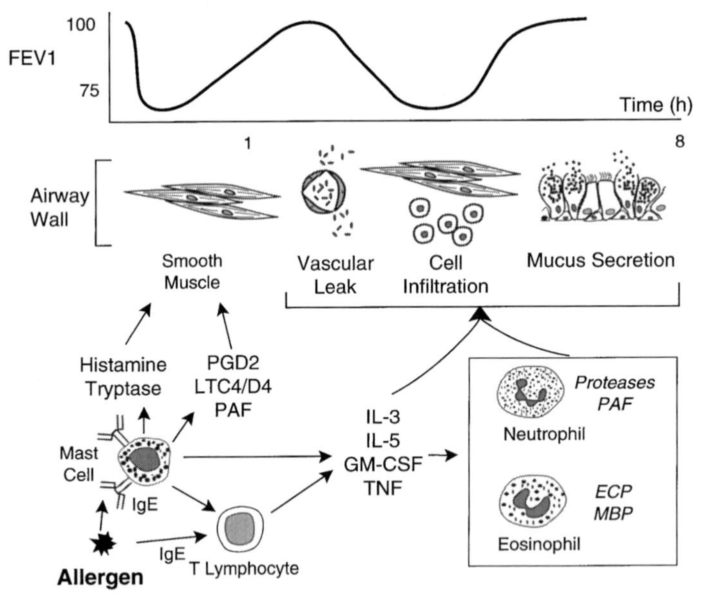


**Figure 39.8** Mechanisms of the early and late phase response to allergen. Allergic asthmatic subjects who inhale an aeroallergen to which they are sensitive develop immediate bronchoconstriction, which usually resolves spontaneously within 1 to 2 hours; in approximately 50% of subjects, this immediate response is followed 3 to 12 hours later by further bronchoconstriction and the development of airway inflammation and increased bronchial hyperresponsiveness. The mechanism of the early and late phase responses is thought to involve allergen-induced activation of mast cells (mediated by cross-linking of immunoglobulin E (IgE) molecules bound via the high-affinity IgE receptor) and T cells (perhaps mediated via a mechanism involving CD23 and IgE receptors[228]) that result in smooth muscle contraction, vascular leak, accumulation of activated eosinophils and mast cells, and degranulation of goblet cells. ECP = eosinophil cationic protein; LTC4/D4 = leukotriene $C_4/D_4$; MBP = major basic protein; PAF = platelet-activating factor; PGD2 = prostaglandin $D_2$.

wall in fatal cases of asthma.[141, 169] Finally, the beneficial effects of corticosteroids in asthma are hypothesized to result at least in part from the eosinophilopenic effects of these drugs.[245, 246]

Despite the compelling case for the eosinophil as an important effector cell in human asthma, attempts to show that the eosinophil is the key mediator of bronchial hyperresponsiveness in the murine model of asthma have not consistently succeeded. Although eosinophils accumulate in the airways of sensitized mice exposed to allergen, and although secreted products of eosinophils such as major basic protein, eosinophil cationic protein, and peroxidase can induce airway hyperresponsiveness under some conditions,[215, 234, 247–251] several studies showed no contribution of eosinophils to airway hyperresponsiveness or goblet cell metaplasia.[198, 252–255] Therefore, current data from the murine model of asthma can be interpreted as indicating that eosinophils may potentiate asthma but are not required for disease expression. A greater understanding of the role of the eosinophil in human asthma will be facilitated by therapies specifically targeting eosinophils (e.g., antibodies against IL-5) that are currently in clinical development.[256]

## Neutrophils

The role of the neutrophil in airway inflammation in asthma has been the subject of some debate. Neutrophil numbers are not increased in airway secretions or in airway tissue from asthmatic subjects with chronic, stable disease, except perhaps in subjects with severe steroid-dependent asthma.[10] In contrast, neutrophil numbers are increased in acute severe asthma, and particularly in fatal attacks.[168, 169, 257, 258]

Neutrophil elastase, cathepsin G, and proteinase 3 are secreted by neutrophils and are important mediators of goblet cell and submucosal gland cell degranulation.[259, 260] Therefore, neutrophils may potentiate asthma, particularly acute exacerbations, by inducing mucin hypersecretion and possibly by increasing bronchovascular permeability. The abnormal accumulation of neutrophils in the airways during acute exacerbations may be mediated by IL-8 secretion from airway epithelial cells activated by virus or antigen exposure.

## Mechanisms of Leukocyte Accumulation in the Airway

The recruitment of eosinophils, neutrophils, and other inflammatory cells from the vascular space to the airways requires the coordinated expression of a number of gene products that together mediate the essential steps of tethering and rolling, firm adhesion, and gradient-dependent chemotaxis. A series of receptor-ligand interactions must occur between leukocytes and endothelial cells during the initiation of transmigration. Selectins, expressed on leukocytes, bind to their ligands on endothelial cells to initiate tethering and rolling, the first step in endothelial transmigration. Tethering and rolling is followed by firm adhesion, mediated by integrins. The integrin gene family includes many members that generally pair as alpha and beta subunits on leukocytes. Integrin $\alpha_4\beta_1$ (formerly called *very late activation molecule 4* [VLAM-4]) interacts with its receptor on endothelial cells, CD106 (formerly called *vascular cell adhesion molecule 1* [VCAM-1]), to promote firm adhesion of most leukocytes except neutrophils. Neutrophils express integrin $\alpha_v\beta_2$ (formerly called *lymphocyte function antigen 1* [LFA-1]) which binds to CD54 (formerly called *intercellular adhesion molecule 1* [ICAM-1]) on vascular endothelium to mediate firm adhesion. Chemotaxis is the final step in inflammatory cell recruitment. Chemoattractants, typically chemokines secreted by resident and recruited airway cells, are bound to matrix molecules in the interstitium; recruited cells respond only to chemokine gradients and migrate in the direction of higher concentration. Under normal conditions, cellular recruitment occurs principally at sites of high endothelial venules present in secondary lymphoid organs such as lymph nodes. During inflammation, vascular adhesion molecules and chemokines are produced locally in response to TNF-α, GM-CSF, IL-8, and other soluble mediators. This allows recruitment of inflammatory cells through local bronchial blood vessels, not just through high endothelial venules in local lymphoid tissue.[261, 262]

The role of adhesion molecules in the airway is not restricted to leukocyte trafficking. Cell adhesion molecules facilitate T-lymphocyte adhesion to airway smooth muscle cells, resulting in smooth muscle hypertrophy and hyperplasia,[263] and CD54 (ICAM-1) facilitates neutrophil-mediated goblet cell degranulation, which requires adhesion of neutrophils and goblet cells.[260, 264]

## Macrophages

Macrophages may be involved in both the induction and the effector phases of immune responses in asthma. In the induction phase, macrophages could perform several functions, including uptake, processing, and presentation of antigens and secretion of immunostimulatory hormones.[265] In the effector phase, macrophages could function as cytotoxic cells and as effector cells capable of secreting a wide variety of proinflammatory mediators, including cytokines, arachidonic acid metabolites, and proteases.[266, 267] Alveolar macrophages from asthmatic subjects are phenotypically and functionally activated,[268, 269] but the consequences of this activation for acute and chronic airway inflammation in asthma are not well understood. Support for the relevance of activated macrophages in the airway is indirect and comes largely from studies demonstrating that the beneficial effects of corticosteroids in asthma may be mediated at least in part by downregulation of alveolar macrophages.[267, 270]

Although they normally are considered to be important in limiting the proliferative potential of T cells, macrophages from asthmatic subjects may be stimulated by specific allergens to augment T-cell proliferation[271] and enhance IL-5 secretion by peripheral blood $CD4^+$ cells.[272] Hypotheses have been advanced proposing that failure of macrophage-mediated T-cell regulation is an important factor in T-cell proliferation and activation in asthma.[273, 274] These hypotheses remain unproven, however, and the precise role of the macrophage in the immune dysregulation of human asthma remains uncertain.

## Airway Smooth Muscle Cells and Hyperreactivity

Measurements of isometric tension in airway smooth muscle tissue from asthmatic subjects have not shown consistent evidence for enhanced force generation, but the few isotonic measurements that have been made in these tissues show increased shortening.[275] Such increases in isotonic shortening could result from alterations in contractile apparatus,[276] tissue elastance, or extracellular matrix.[277] Also, some inflammatory mediators, such as tryptase, may increase force generation in response to subsequent application of others, such as histamine, in isolated human bronchi.[278] Changes in airway geometry may themselves contribute to bronchial hyperreactivity. For example, thickening of the airway wall, as occurs in asthmatic patients because of the changes described earlier (smooth muscle hyperplasia/hypertrophy and mucosal edema), result in larger increases in airway resistance from a given amount of smooth muscle shortening than would occur in a comparably sized airway with a normal wall thickness from the same degree of smooth muscle shortening.[279] Airway smooth muscle tissue from asthmatic patients has diminished relaxant responses to beta-adrenergic agonists,[280] which may relate to cytokine-induced up-regulation of a pertussis toxin–sensitive G protein.[281]

When dispersed and cultured in serum-containing media, airway smooth muscle cells undergo modulation from a contractile to a secretory-proliferative phenotype; once confluence is reached and serum is withdrawn, some of the cells revert to the contractile state.[276] In vivo, a similar sequence of changes occurs in vascular smooth muscle cells after arterial injury, but it is not yet known whether such changes occur in the airways of asthmatic patients. Studies of airway smooth muscle cells in culture have identified several potential mitogens, including growth factors whose receptors have intrinsic tyrosine kinase activity (platelet-derived growth factor, insulin-like growth factor-1, epidermal growth factor, fibroblast growth factor), inflammatory mediators (leukotriene $D_4$, thromboxane), cytokines (IL-1β), and serine proteases (thrombin, tryptase). Cultured airway smooth muscle cells of the secretory-proliferative phenotype secrete cytokines, including GM-CSF, and express adhesion molecules such as ICAM-1 and VCAM-1. These effects, to the extent which they occur in vivo, may contribute to the persistence of chronic inflammation in asthma.[282]

## Mechanisms of Mucus Hypersecretion

Hypersecretion of mucus in asthma represents the combined effects of hypersecretion of mucin glycoproteins from airway goblet cells and submucosal gland cells, excessive leakage of plasma proteins from the bronchial vasculature, and other abnormalities including leukocyte accumulation and abnormal mucociliary clearance in the airway.[283] In terms of mucin hypersecretion, there are two distinct pathophysiologic mechanisms that need to be considered. These are the mechanisms underlying secretory cell metaplasia and hyperplasia and the separate mechanisms underlying secretory cell degranulation. More is known about goblet cell metaplasia and hyperplasia than about submucosal gland hyperplasia. Important mediators of goblet cell metaplasia and hyperplasia include growth factors such as epidermal growth factor[284] and IL-4 and IL-13.[203, 204, 285] Important mediators of goblet cell degranulation include environmental stimuli (smoke, sulfur dioxide, chlorine, ammonia) and inflammatory mediators with secretagogue activity, including neutrophil elastase, leukotrienes, histamine, nonprotease neutrophil products, and tachykinins.[283, 286, 287] Many of these mediators have also been shown to degranulate submucosal gland serous cells. Neutrophil elastase may be an especially important secretagogue in acute exacerbations of asthma, because free elastase activity is detectable in sputum in this situation.[260, 288]

Increased concentrations of plasma proteins have been measured in airway secretions from patients with asthma.[152, 289] The relative importance of hypersecretion of mucin glycoproteins and excessive bronchovascular leakage of plasma proteins as causes of mucus hypersecretion is unknown. The mixture of albumin and mucin yields a very viscous material,[290] so the combination of mucin hypersecretion and plasma protein leak may be particularly dangerous in asthma. Mucociliary clearance is abnormally reduced in asthma,[291] and the cause is multifactorial.[292–295] The decline in clearance exacerbates the consequences of mucus hypersecretion.

## Nerves and Neurogenic Mediators

The lungs are highly innervated, and peptidergic, cholinergic, adrenergic, and other neurogenic mediators and their receptors may contribute to modulation of airway tone and even to airway inflammation.[296–298] Adrenergic receptor agonists and cholinergic receptor antagonists are mainstays of current bronchodilator therapy for asthma, but these agents are not thought to have antiinflammatory activity. Nerves themselves are not required for airway hyperresponsiveness and allergic inflammation, because lung transplant recipients with no intact neuronal connections can develop asthma.[299, 300]

In the airways, the term *neurogenic inflammation* refers to the inflammatory responses caused by tachykinins that activate specific receptors as part of the nonadrenergic noncholinergic (NANC) system. Excitatory NANC (eNANC) effects are mediated by release of tachykinins such as neurokinin A and substance P acting on natural killer (NK) 1 and 2 receptors.[301, 302] In general, NK-1 receptors mediate gland secretion, plasma extravasation, vasodilation, and leukocyte adhesion, whereas NK-2 receptors mediate contractions of airway smooth muscle.[303] Inhibitory NANC (iNANC) effects are thought to be mediated principally by vasoactive intestinal peptide and nitric oxide.[304]

Evidence for operation of the NANC system in asthma comes from studies showing that asthmatic subjects develop bronchoconstriction after inhaling neurokinin A or substance P.[305, 306] These tachykinins are degraded by neutral endopeptidase (NEP), which is active in the airway epithelium. An imbalance between tachykinin activity and NEP activity has been postulated as a pathophysiologic mechanism in asthma.[307] However, at present, the roles of tachykinins and NEP in asthma remain unproven. Although an NK-1/NK-2 receptor antagonist protected against bradykinin-induced bronchoconstriction in asthmatic subjects,[308] a selective NK-1 receptor antagonist did not protect against hypertonic saline-induced cough or bronchoconstriction.[303] In addition, inhaled thiorphan, an inhibitor of NEP, did not accentuate aeroallergen-induced bronchoconstriction in asthmatic subjects.[309]

## Airway Remodeling

The term *airway remodeling* in asthma refers to structural changes in the airway that are thought to occur as a consequence of chronic airway inflammation (Fig. 39.9). The net result of the alterations in the airway epithelium, lamina propria, and submucosa is thickening of the airway wall. The increase in wall area involves both cartilaginous (large) airways and membranous (small) airways. The thickening of the airway is evident both in pathologic studies (described previously) and in radiographic studies.[310, 311]

Airway remodeling in asthma may have at least three distinct consequences. First, moderate amounts of airway wall thickening, which have little effect on baseline airway resistance, can profoundly affect the airway narrowing caused by smooth muscle shortening and contribute to bronchial hyperresponsivenesss.[312] Second, airway wall thickening may explain the occurrence of persistent and incompletely reversible airway narrowing in a subgroup of asthmatic patients.[313] Third, increased vascularity of the airway wall coupled with hyperplasia of goblet cells and hypertrophy of submucosal gland cells may amplify the mucin secretion and plasma protein leakage that are responsible for formation of the mucus "plugs" that commonly obstruct airways in severe asthma exacerbations.[288, 314]

A wide range of mediators and growth factors have been implicated in the multiple pathologic abnormalities that result in airway remodeling in asthma[315] (Table 39.3). Interest is growing in a possible role for matrix metalloproteinases (MMPs), especially MMP-9 and MMP-2. However, apart from a possible role for these proteases in the transmigration of eosinophils and lymphocytes from the vascular space to the airway,[316] there is so far little firm data to suggest they have a direct role in airway fibrosis or cellular hyperplasia.

Programmed cell death, also called apoptosis, is a primary mechanism in the precise regulation of cell numbers in tissue homeostasis. Apoptosis is a genetically controlled, active cell process, and great progress has been made in identifying the genes responsible for its regulation.[317] For example, the Bcl-2 protein product of the *Bcl-2* gene enhances cell survival by blocking apoptotic cell death, and dysregulation of Bcl-2 is proposed as a mechanism of ozone-induced goblet cell metaplasia in the airway.[318] In experimental airway disease, apoptosis is believed to be a major mechanism for elimination of lymphocytes and consequent down-regulation of airway inflammatory responses.[319]

## PHYSIOLOGY

Unlike the other common obstructive lung diseases, emphysema (defined by pathologic criteria) and chronic bronchitis (defined by clinical criteria), asthma is defined by its characteristic disturbances in function: airflow obstruction that varies spontaneously or as a result of treatment and airway hyperresponsiveness. The diagnosis of asthma thus requires assessment of the physiology of the lungs and airways. This section will first review the nature of the disturbances in function and will then review their effects on standard tests of pulmonary function (see Chapter 28).

### Physiologic Disturbances

The disturbances in function caused by asthma are most clearly seen during severe attacks. Almost all physiologic

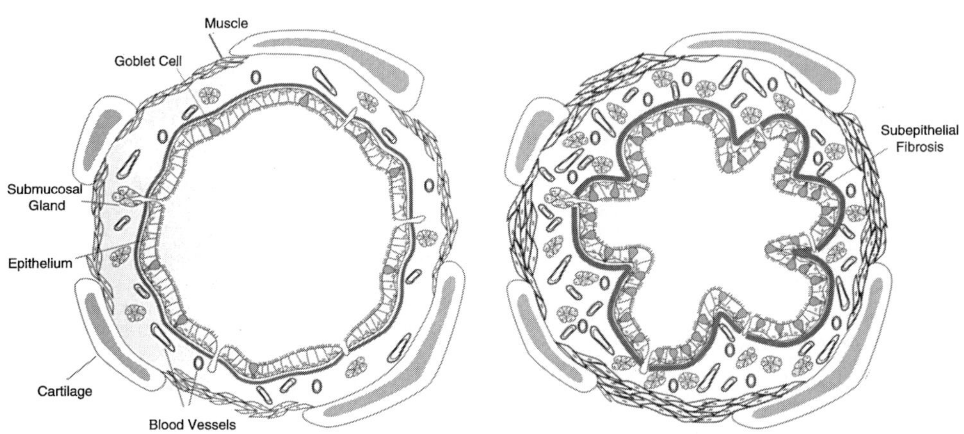


**Figure 39.9** Airway remodeling in asthma is depicted through schematic representations of the airway wall in health *(left)* and in asthma *(right)*. In asthma there is goblet cell hyperplasia/hypertrophy, subepithelial fibrosis, increased vascularity, and smooth muscle hypertrophy and hyperplasia. Not shown is increased collagen deposition throughout the airway wall, smooth muscle proliferation throughout the airway wall, degenerative changes in cartilage, and pericartilaginous fibrosis.

**Table 39.3** PUTATIVE MEDIATORS OF STRUCTURAL CHANGES IN THE AIRWAY IN ASTHMA

| Change | Mediators |
|---|---|
| Goblet cell metaplasia and hyperplasia | EGF, neutrophil elastase, leukotrienes, IL-13, IL-4, IL-11 |
| Increased vascularity/angiogenesis | bFGF, VEGF, TNFα, EGF |
| Airway smooth muscle hypertrophy and hyperplasia | EGF, tryptase, lysophosphatidic acid, endothelin-1, leukotriene D4, histamine, 5-hydroxytryptamine, thrombin, IL-1 |
| Subepithelial fibrosis | TGFβ1, TGFβ2, bFGF, PDGF, endothelin-1, IGF-1, IL-4, IL-11, IL-13, GM-CSF |

EGF, epidermal growth factor; IL = interleukin; bFGF = basic fibroblast growth factor; VEGF, vascular endothelial growth factor; TNF = tumor necrosis factor; TGF = transforming growth factor; PDGF = platelet-derived growth factor; IGF = insulin-like growth factor; GM-CSF = granulocyte-macrophage colony-stimulating factor.

For review, see references 144, 284, 315, 535, and 536.

consequences derive from narrowing of the airways. During attacks, this narrowing is diffuse, affecting all levels of the tracheobronchial tree, but is probably maximal in small bronchi 2 to 5 mm in diameter.[320] Tests of airway function are abnormal.[321] Airway resistance is increased and maximal expiratory flow is reduced at all lung volumes. Maximal inspiratory flow is also reduced, but less so. Narrowing of peripheral airways results in their premature closure, at higher lung volumes, causing marked increases in residual volume[322] (Fig. 39.10). Also contributing to thoracic hyperinflation is the tendency to breathe at a higher lung volume. Several mechanisms account for this increase in functional residual capacity. One is simply the inability of the lungs to empty during the expiratory phase of the respiratory cycle, because of the high resistance to expiratory flow[323]; another is a sustained increase in the activity of inspiratory muscles even during expiration.[324, 325] The adaptive advantages of breathing at higher lung volumes are an increase in the circumferential traction (tethering force) on intrapulmonary airways, which tends to hold them open, and an increase in the elastic recoil of the lungs, which increases the driving pressure for expiration. These adaptive gains are partially offset by a decrease in lung elastic recoil in severe asthma.[326]

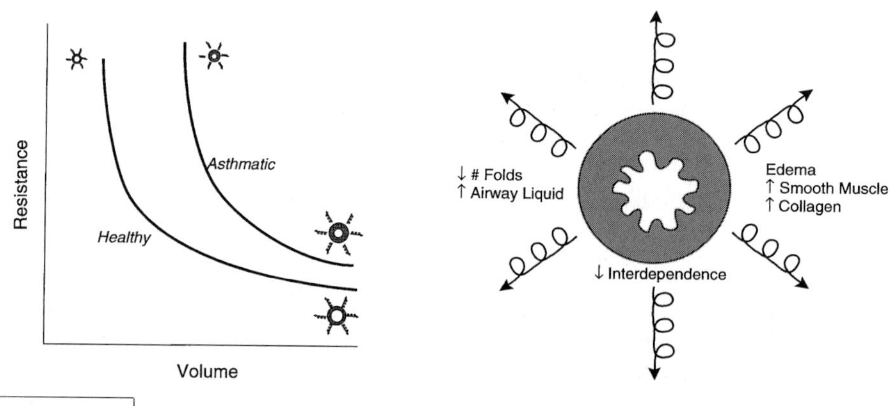


**Figure 39.10** The relationships between lung volume and airway caliber are shown. *Left,* the relationship in healthy and asthmatic subjects. At high lung volumes, the "tethering" action of elastic elements of the lung parenchyma opens the airways widely. As lung volume decreases, loss of this elastic force allows the airways to narrow; critical narrowing occurs at a higher lung volume when the airway wall is thickened. *Right,* the mechanism of interdependence between lung volume and airway caliber, which is thought to involve tethering attachments of the lung parenchyma to the airway wall. Interdependence may be attenuated by thickening of the airway wall, as from edema, smooth muscle proliferation, collagen deposition, or decreased numbers of mucosal folds. (Redrawn from Eidelman DH, Irvin CG: Air mechanics in asthma. *In* Holgate S, Busse W (eds): Rhinitis and Asthma. Boston: Blackwell Scientific Publications, 1995, pp 1033–1043, with permission.)

Together, these changes greatly increase the work of breathing, however, because resistive work is increased from narrowing of the airways and elastic work is increased from the flattening of the pressure-volume curve of the lungs at high volumes. This increased work must be performed by muscles of breathing placed at a mechanical disadvantage by overinflation of the thorax. At high thoracic volumes, the diaphragm and intercostal muscles must function over a suboptimal range of their length-tension curve, and accessory muscles (e.g., the sternocleidomastoids) are brought into play.[327] The increase in the work of breathing causes fatigue, and the inappropriateness of the length-tension relationship in the muscles of breathing is perceived as dyspnea.

The airway narrowing of asthma also affects gas exchange. The severity of obstruction is not uniformly distributed. Some airways are completely occluded, others are severely narrowed, and some are unobstructed. Shifts in pulmonary blood flow cannot completely compensate for the underventilation of the regions of lung subtended by the most obstructed airways. The resulting mismatch of ventilation to perfusion widens the alveolar-arterial oxygen difference $[(A-a)P_{O_2}]$, and the arterial $P_{O_2}$ in patients presenting with an acute attack of asthma is typically between 60 and 69 mm Hg.[328] The hypocapnia that also is typically found is only partly caused by overventilation of other lung units, because an increase in respiratory drive, possibly mediated by stimulation of neural receptors supplied by afferent fibers in the vagus nerves, is almost invariable in acute asthmatic attacks. An elevated or even normal $P_{CO_2}$ is therefore a sign that airflow obstruction is so severe that the muscles of respiration cannot maintain the ventilation demanded by the respiratory center. With any worsening of airflow obstruction, any loss in muscle performance (as from fatigue), or any decline in respiratory drive (as from administration of a narcotic or sedative drug), alveolar ventilation can fall precipitously. The rise in $P_{CO_2}$ further inhibits muscle performance and respiratory drive ("$CO_2$ narcosis"), putting the patient on a steep slope to respiratory failure and death.[329, 330] Hypercapnia therefore indicates an attack of extreme severity, requiring aggressive treatment with bronchodilators and preparation for intubation and mechanical ventilation should the treatment be ineffective.

Severe airflow obstruction usually improves quickly with treatment but resolves entirely much more slowly. When symptoms have resolved, $FEV_1$ and residual volume still average 50% and 200% of normal, respectively. Even when wheezing has resolved and the physical examination is entirely normal, maximal expiratory flow is still markedly reduced, especially at middle and low lung volumes, and residual volume remains increased.[327]

## Pulmonary Function Testing

Pulmonary function testing performed between attacks, or even after long periods of remission of asthmatic symptoms, usually shows characteristic changes. The easiest to detect are reductions in maximal expiratory flow. Peak flow is effort dependent, but it is reproducible when performed by a cooperative patient and can be measured repeatedly with any of several lightweight, portable, and inexpensive devices that meet American Thoracic Society criteria for accuracy.[331] The best use of peak flow measurements is probably in monitoring of ambulatory patients. Changes in peak flow can serve as a guide to patients for adjusting treatment.[332] Calculation of peak flow variability (the difference between the morning and afternoon values divided by the mean of the two) can also be used to detect abnormal airway lability, as an indirect measure of bronchial responsiveness.[333] Because peak flow is determined largely by the diameter of central airways, it is less sensitive to changes in peripheral airways than are measurements of flow at lower lung volumes. These flows contribute more importantly to the $FEV_1$, which may explain why peak flow underestimates $FEV_1$ by 10% to 20% in 30% to 50% of asthmatics.[334, 335]

$FEV_1$ (the volume of air expired in the first second of a forced expiratory maneuver from total lung capacity) is the best-standardized, most widely used test for airflow obstruction. An improvement in $FEV_1$ of more than 12% and more than 200 mL after administration of a bronchodilator is a hallmark of asthma.[336] Interpretation of the $FEV_1$ often requires simultaneous measurement of the forced vital capacity (FVC), which is the total volume exhaled from TLC to residual volume. Usually the reduction in $FEV_1$ exceeds the reduction in FVC, so the $FEV_1$/FVC ratio is typically low in asthma. An exception is severe asthma, in which residual volume may be so increased that the reduction in FVC is proportional to the reduction in $FEV_1$. Conversely, treatment may reverse the narrowing of peripheral airways, allowing exhalation of a greater volume before airway closure occurs, so the improvement in FVC can be proportionately greater than the improvement in $FEV_1$.[337] In some cases, improvement after treatment may be reflected only by reversal of pulmonary hyperinflation, without any apparent change in $FEV_1$.[326]

An index of flow derived from the FVC is the maximum midexpiratory flow ($FEF_{25-75\%}$), the average rate of flow over the middle half of the vital capacity. Flow over this lower lung volume was thought to be more specific for obstruction in small airways than the $FEV_1$,[338] and a normal value for $FEF_{25-75\%}$ indeed makes asthma unlikely,[339] although not impossible. Problems with measurement of $FEF_{25-75\%}$ are the wide range of normal values and the dependence of the measurement on correct measurement of vital capacity, which reduces its reproducibility.

Although the ease of measurement of derivatives of the FVC have made them standard in assessing the severity of airflow obstruction, their physiologic determinants are not straightforward. Maximal expiratory flow is not simply a reflection of airway narrowing. It is also a function of lung elastic recoil and of compressibility of central airways (see Chapter 28). Another problem with all measurements derived from the FVC is that the maneuver is necessarily preceded by inhalation to total lung capacity. This inhalation stretches intrapulmonary airways, transiently decreasing smooth muscle tone.[340] The bronchoconstriction caused by inhalation of methacholine, which can easily be demonstrated by measurement of airway resistance in a body plethysmograph, is reversed by inhalation to TLC in some asthmatic patients,[341] but not in others.[342] This effect, a function of the interdependence of the airways and the lung parenchyma, may be of great significance as a determinant of tests of bronchial responsiveness (see later discussion).

Residual volume and functional residual volume are increased in asthma but may be underestimated by methods that depend on dilution of a tracer gas (e.g., helium, neon) because of the poor ventilation of many lung units. More reliable estimates are obtained by body plethysmography. Total lung capacity can also be increased, possibly from a true increase in lung compliance,[343] but plethysmographically measured total lung capacity can be artifactually increased by intra-abdominal gas in patients with severe hyperinflation.[344]

Except in attacks so severe that hyperinflation results in expiratory intra-alveolar pressures that exceed pulmonary artery pressure, asthma does not reduce the volume of blood in alveolar capillaries, so the diffusing capacity for carbon monoxide ($DL_{CO}$) is usually normal or increased.[345] Reductions in $DL_{CO}$ should prompt a search for an alternate or additional diagnosis.

## Tests of Bronchial Responsiveness

Bronchial responsiveness is assessed by delivering progressively increasing doses of a provocative stimulus until a chosen index of airway caliber changes by a fixed amount. The stimulus used most often is methacholine or histamine, delivered as a nebulized aerosol in doubling concentrations at 10-minute intervals until $FEV_1$ falls by more than 20%. The concentration causing a 20% fall is calculated by interpolation and is expressed as the "$PC_{20}$": that is, the provocative concentration causing a 20% fall in $FEV_1$. Bronchial hyperresponsiveness, defined as a $PC_{20}$ of less than 8 mg/mL for either agent, is characteristic of asthma but may be found in other disorders, such as chronic obstructive pulmonary disease (COPD), cystic fibrosis, and allergic rhinitis. The degree of bronchial responsiveness roughly correlates with the severity of asthma.[7]

Other provocative stimuli can be used. Some—such as exercise; eucapnic hyperpnea of cold, dry air; and aerosols of hypertonic saline, distilled water, and adenosine—differ from histamine and methacholine in that they have no direct action on airway smooth muscle but stimulate release of mediators from cells resident in the airways (e.g., mast cells).[346, 347] Comparison of the changes in bronchial responsiveness to histamine and to adenosine has been used to infer whether down-regulation of beta-adrenergic responsiveness involves primarily beta receptors on airway smooth muscle or those on airway mast cells.[348]

It has been proposed that bronchial hyperresponsiveness results from loss of the normal interdependence of intrapulmonary airways and lung parenchyma. Normally, inhalation to a high lung volume dilates intrapulmonary airways through the tethering effect of the elastic elements of parenchymal attachments on the airway wall (see Fig. 39.10). This stretch of bronchial smooth muscle lowers its tone, at least transiently. Hyperinflation of the lungs can be regarded, in this sense, as a defense mechanism against airway closure.[349] If, however, some process in the airway wall, such as edema or inflammation, "uncouples" the mechanical linkage between the airway and lung parenchyma, then deep inhalation will no longer reverse bronchoconstriction. This may account for the finding that deep inspirations reverse the bronchoconstriction caused by methacholine or histamine challenge but do not reverse, or may even augment, the spontaneous bronchoconstriction associated with viral respiratory infection or allergic inflammation.[350] An extension of this line of reasoning is that prevention of deep inhalations might amplify bronchial responses to methacholine, and it was indeed found that when healthy subjects were kept from taking a deep breath during a methacholine challenge, they responded in a manner similar to asthmatic subjects.[351]

# CLINICAL FEATURES

## History

The cardinal symptoms of asthma are wheezing, chest tightness, and shortness of breath.[352] These symptoms are often precipitated by exercise, exposure to allergens, or viral respiratory infections. The symptoms of asthma characteristically vary over time. Variability from day to day is almost universal, but many patients note variations within a day, with symptoms worsening at night.[353, 354] Others report variations in symptoms over minutes, and a few have sudden severe attacks after long periods without symptoms.

The triad of wheezing, chest tightness, and shortness of breath is prototypic for asthma, and one or more of these symptoms are reported by more than 90% of patients,[355] but even this symptom complex is nonspecific. Wheezing is named as an important complaint by 76% of those with COPD and by 28% of those with heart disease. Shortness of breath and chest tightness discriminate even less well, being named by 60% to 80% of patients with COPD and 40% to 50% of patients with heart disease.[355] The choice of words used to describe asthmatic symptoms varies substantially among patients, and may vary further among different ethnic and cultural groups. "Throat tightness," "choking," "stuffed chest," and "chest congestion" are examples of terms sometimes volunteered by asthmatics to describe the sensation of bronchoconstriction.[356]

Forms of asthma have been recognized in which wheezing and chest tightness are absent and exertional dyspnea or cough is the sole presenting symptom,[357] as in "cough-variant asthma."[358] As many as 30% to 50% of patients with chronic cough have unrecognized asthma.[359, 360] This variant of asthma is more common in children,[361] but 13% of cases of cough-variant asthma occur in adults older than 50 years of age.[362] Up to 75% of the children with this form of asthma develop wheezing within 5 to 7 years.[363]

The cough associated with asthma is typically nonproductive, nocturnal, and chronic, sometimes persisting for several years. It is worsened by the same stimuli that worsen the classic symptoms of asthma: exercise, inhalation of cold air, allergen exposure, and upper respiratory infections.[361, 364] Relief is often prompt after initiation of appropriate bronchodilator and antiinflammatory therapy.

Sputum production, an expression of the goblet cell and submucosal gland cell hyperplasia consistently found in asthmatic airways,[141, 365] may be the dominant symptom of asthma.[366] Asthma is frequently misdiagnosed as "recurrent acute bronchitis," perhaps because asthmatic attacks, like acute bronchitis, are often preceded by viral upper respiratory infections. Clues to this error are youth, a family or personal history or atopy, a history of multiple previous bouts of bronchitis after viral respiratory infections (often treated with repeated courses of antibiotics), and associated symptoms of breathlessness and wheezing. The finding of a marked predominance of eosinophils on examination of the sputum virtually establishes the diagnosis.[367]

In distinguishing asthma from other causes of the symptoms of cough, chest tightness, wheezing, and sputum production, it is helpful to consider conditions often associated with asthma. For example, asthma clusters in families, and its genetic determinants appear to be linked to those of other allergic IgE-mediated diseases,[54, 368, 369] so a personal or family history of allergic rhinitis, atopic dermatitis, and eczema increases the likelihood of a diagnosis of asthma.

The symptoms described by people with asthma are often so characteristic that a strong likelihood of asthma can be established by the medical history alone. The next task is to obtain information about the condition's severity, because guidelines for asthma treatment propose a stepwise approach that matches the intensity of treatment to the severity of the disease.[370] Furthermore, morbidity and mortality from asthma are borne disproportionately by a subgroup of patients with identifiable features. The features of "fatality-prone asthma," for example, include a history of two or more emergency department visits or a hospitalization for asthma in the past year, the requirement for intubation and mechanical ventilation for any previous attack, a history of extremely rapid progression of symptoms,[5, 371] and a history of anaphylactic sensitivity to certain foods, such as nuts or shrimp.[372, 373] For all patients with asthma, but especially for those with adult-onset asthma and nasal polyps, specific questions should be asked about the effects of ingestion of aspirin or foods likely to contain sulfites (dried fruits, restaurant salads, some wines and beers). Both aspirin and sulfite ingestion can provoke severe, life-threatening attacks in patients who otherwise have features of mild or moderate asthma.[374–376]

The role of the history extends well beyond the assessment of severity. Information should be obtained about exposures to agents known to worsen asthma in the home or workplace, such as pets, cockroaches, house dust mites, and environmental tobacco smoke. Questions should be directed toward eliciting clues as to the presence of conditions that complicate or aggravate asthma, such as allergic rhinitis, chronic sinusitis, or gastroesophageal reflux. The medical interview also presents an opportunity to assess the patient's understanding of the causes and treatments of asthma and to learn how asthma has compromised the patient's full enjoyment of life. Finally, the manner in which the initial medical history is obtained is the first step in establishing the sense of partnership with the patient that is fundamental to the success of treatment.

## Physical Examination

The most characteristic finding of asthma is polyphonic expiratory wheezing, which is thought to reflect turbulence of airflow in peripheral airways. Wheezing is the first physical finding detected as airflow obstruction progresses, but its absence does not indicate the absence of airflow obstruction.[327] As a reflection of turbulence of airflow, wheeze clearly requires respiratory effort. Wheezing may be faint or inaudible in patients making little effort to move air, and the disappearance of wheezing in an infant has rarely, but tragically, been mistaken as indication that airflow obstruction was not present. At the other extreme, the wheeze produced with rapid, forced exhalation does not correlate with airflow obstruction or with bronchial hyperresponsiveness.[377, 378]

The other physical findings of asthma are also reflections of airflow obstruction. Overinflation of the thoracic cage may be obvious, resulting in part from the air trapping caused by narrowing of peripheral airways and in part from the adaptive response of breathing at high lung volumes, where airway caliber and lung recoil are greatest (see previous discussion).

Examination of nonthoracic organs often provides important diagnostic information. Swelling and pallor of the nasal mucosa suggest allergic rhinitis, and nasal polyps, especially in a patient with adult-onset asthma, suggest an increased risk of aspirin sensitivity.[379, 380] Sinus tenderness and purulent nasal discharge may indicate chronic sinusitis.[381] Obesity is an obvious but important finding, because obesity reduces functional residual volume, so that tidal breathing is done at low lung volumes, magnifying the effects of any intrinsic narrowing of the airways. Even modest airflow obstruction can cause severe dyspnea in an obese patient.

## Laboratory Studies

Tests of airway caliber are the only means of directly assessing two of the features central to the definition of asthma: widespread but reversible narrowing of the airways and increased bronchial responsiveness to inhaled stimuli. Tests of maximal expiratory flow, such as peak flow and $FEV_1$, are well standardized and easily performed.[382, 383] Many guidelines for the treatment of asthma recommend spirometry at the time the diagnosis is first made, again when there is a change in the severity of symptoms or in the intensity of treatment, and within 2 years in all cases.[384]

A reduction in maximal expiratory flow is a highly nonspecific finding. Clues to some of the other causes can be recognized easily from a simultaneous display of the flow-volume curve with the spirometry tracing. This greatly facilitates detection of submaximal effort and of upper airway (rather than intrapulmonary or bronchial) obstruction.[385, 386]

Measurement of maximal expiratory flow is also insensitive as a test for asthma, because asthma may cause only episodic airway narrowing. If expiratory flow is normal, support for the diagnosis requires demonstration of bronchial hyperresponsiveness (see previous discussion).

Measurement of bronchial responsiveness presents several advantages as a diagnostic test. Bronchial hyperresponsiveness is almost ubiquitous in patients with asthma, and its degree correlates with the severity of the disease.[7] The test therefore is highly sensitive; the absence of bronchial hyperresponsiveness should stimulate close reexamination of the grounds for suspecting asthma and consideration of other possible diagnoses. The major disadvantage of this test is that it is nonspecific. Bronchial hyperresponsiveness is found in some patients with chronic obstructive bronchitis[387] or allergic rhinitis.[388] As a practical matter, the detection of bronchial hyperresponsiveness in children with symptoms suggestive of asthma holds up well as a definition for asthma in epidemiologic studies.[11] Further, follow-up of students with bronchial hyperresponsiveness but without symptoms at the time of testing show that a high proportion go on to develop asthma as defined by clinical criteria.[389]

Other laboratory tests provide only supportive evidence of asthma. Elevation in serum IgE levels, positive skin prick tests to common antigens, and blood eosinophilia demonstrate the atopic diathesis associated with asthma[54, 369] but do not confirm the diagnosis. The routine chest radiograph may show overinflation of the lungs, bronchial wall thickening, and mucus plugs, but it may also be entirely normal (see Chapter 25). The association of eosinophilia, high serum levels of IgE, and changing pulmonary infiltrates in a patient with recurrent asthma, especially asthma associated with cough productive of plugs of mucus, should raise suspicion of allergic bronchopulmonary mycosis.[390]

A laboratory test that is now used in clinical research but has potential applicability for diagnostic purposes is analysis of induced sputum.[152, 391] Sputum induction, performed by gathering the material expectorated after inhalation of an aerosol of hypertonic saline, is well tolerated and safe, provided pretreatment with an inhaled beta-agonist is given and monitoring for bronchoconstriction is performed.[392] Analysis of the secretions expectorated may allow detection of eosinophilic inflammation of the airways, now considered a characteristic feature of even mild asthma.[130, 393] The cells and chemicals in induced sputum samples are more concentrated than in bronchial lavage samples.[257] Induced sputum from asthmatics contains a higher percentage of eosinophils and a higher concentration of eosinophilic cationic protein than do samples from healthy subjects, but the range of values overlap,[152, 391] with as many as 20% to 30% of asthmatics having no demonstrable increases. The diagnostic sensitivity of measurements of eosinophil percentages or eosinophil cationic protein concentrations therefore appears to be poor, but it is possible that sensitivity can be improved by the application of new methods for examination of inflammatory mediators, such as flow cytometry for detection of specific cells and activation markers[394] or the polymerase chain reaction for detection of specific cytokines.[395] The specificity of elevated values also appears to be imperfect, and it seems likely that further study of the sensitivity and specificity of markers of inflammation in induced sputum, or even in bronchial lavage or biopsy samples, will require a reappraisal of the definition of asthma. Examples at one extreme are patients with persistent cough but without bronchial hyperresponsiveness who are found to have increased eosinophils in induced sputum samples and to respond to corticosteroid treatment.[9, 396] At the other extreme are patients with asthma exacerbations who are found to have no detectable increase in sputum eosinophils.[257, 397]

The deficiencies of sputum induction (at least as it is currently performed) as a diagnostic test do not mean that it may not prove useful as a guide to treatment. Ongoing research is examining whether the number of eosinophils in induced sputum predicts responsiveness to increases in corticosteroid treatment[398] or deterioration in asthma if corticosteroid treatment is reduced or withdrawn.

## Differential Diagnosis

Because asthma is so common, it may too readily be assumed to be the cause of airflow obstruction or to account for complaints of dyspnea, cough, or wheezing. Other causes of dyspnea are legion (Table 39.4), and this is also true of cough. Particular care must be taken in diagnosing asthma in a patient with seasonal allergic rhinitis who complains of chronic or recurrent cough; although the patient's atopic predisposition does indicate an increased risk for the development of asthma, it also indicates that inflammatory disease of the upper airway may be the cause of cough. In this setting, documentation of reversible airflow obstruction or heightened bronchial responsiveness is mandatory for the diagnosis of asthma.

The third major symptom of asthma, wheezing, is more specific for asthma, but the adage that "all that wheezes is not asthma" is well founded. In infants younger than 3 years of age, wheezing is so commonly caused by viral bronchiolitis that it is not predictive of asthma at later ages.[79] In adults, wheezing can result from any cause of airflow obstruction (see Table 39.4).

Among adults, the diseases that most often overlap with asthma are chronic obstructive bronchitis and emphysema. These diseases and asthma are not mutually exclusive. A single patient with airflow obstruction can have destruction of alveolar tissue distal to the terminal bronchioles (emphysema), chronic production of sputum on most mornings for three or more consecutive months in two or more successive years (chronic bronchitis), chronic narrowing of the airways that does not reverse with maximal medical therapy (chronic airflow obstruction), and partially reversible airway narrowing associated with eosinophilic inflammation of the airway mucosa (asthma). Differentiation of asthma from chronic obstructive bronchitis has been made even more difficult with the recognition that unremitting airflow obstruction may develop in patients with asthma,[313, 399] especially in those who smoke.[400] For individual patients, the important question is whether the airflow obstruction is likely to reverse with therapy. Reversibility is made unlikely by a history of cigarette smoking and by the clinical features of emphysema.[401] At least partial reversibility of airflow obstruction and an increase in bronchial responsiveness may be found, however, in "pure" cases of chronic obstructive bronchitis: for example, in patients with a long history of cigarette smoking, without blood or sputum eosinophilia, and without a personal or family history of atopic dis-

Table 39.4 DIFFERENTIAL DIAGNOSIS

| CATEGORY | EXAMPLES |
|---|---|
| Diseases causing recurrent episodic dyspnea | Chronic obstructive pulmonary disease, coronary artery disease, congestive heart failure, pulmonary emboli, recurrent gastroesophageal reflux with aspiration, recurrent anaphylaxis, systemic mastocytosis, carcinoid syndrome |
| Common diseases causing cough | Rhinitis, sinusitis, otitis, bronchitis (chronic or postviral), bronchiectasis, cystic fibrosis, pneumonia, diffuse pulmonary fibrosis |
| Common diseases causing airflow obstruction | Chronic obstructive bronchitis and emphysema, bronchiolitis obliterans, cystic fibrosis, organic or functional laryngeal narrowing, extrinsic or intrinsic narrowing of trachea or major bronchus. |

From Boushey HA: Clinical diagnosis in adults. *In* Barnes PJ, Grunstein MM, Leff AR, et al (eds): Asthma. Philadelphia: Lippincott-Raven, 1997.

ease.[402] Reversibility therefore is best determined directly, with a trial of corticosteroid and bronchodilator therapy.[403]

A condition important to distinguish from asthma is upper airway obstruction, which can easily be missed if only the spirometry tracing is examined but is easily detected on a flow-volume curve.[385, 386, 404] "Organic" or mechanical obstruction of the larynx or trachea is infrequent but may result from vocal cord paralysis, arthritis of the cricoarytenoid joints, trauma, vocal cord polyps, or laryngeal tumors. A form of upper airway obstruction that is often confused with asthma is "vocal cord dysfunction," a functional disorder of the larynx that appears to be associated with somatiform-conversion, factitious, or other psychologic disorders.[405–407] The patient presents with recurrent, episodic dyspnea, sometimes with airflow obstruction so severe that carbon dioxide retention occurs.[408] Of the patients found to have this disorder on referral to National Jewish Medical Center, most were overweight, had required multiple emergency department visits or hospitalizations for asthma, and were receiving chronic oral corticosteroid therapy. Twenty-five percent had been intubated, some repeatedly. Stridor was reported by only 10% of the patients. Sputum production was uncommon, as was blood eosinophilia. Between attacks, the $FEV_1$ was normal or minimally reduced and did not improve after bronchodilator treatment. Analysis of the flow-volume curve was often helpful, however; it showed truncation of the inspiratory limb in 23%.

The diagnosis of vocal cord dysfunction requires visualization of the vocal cords. The diagnostic findings are inspiratory anterior vocal cord closure with airflow passage through a posterior glottic chink.[405, 409] This finding may be apparent only during attacks, whether spontaneous or provoked, as by histamine or methacholine challenge.[410]

Detection of vocal cord dysfunction arrests the medical and human costs of misdirected therapy and calls attention to important psychologic issues. Psychiatric disease is common; almost 40% of these patients give a history of sexual, physical, or emotional abuse in childhood.[408, 411] Psychiatric consultation and speech therapy, in which techniques for relaxed throat breathing are taught (as for functional voice disorders), are often effective.[412]

Disorders in the regulation of mast cell numbers or activity are also sometimes confused with asthma. These rare disorders include systemic mastocytosis[413] and recurrent anaphylaxis, in which the respiratory component is so dominant that the patient fails to mention, or the physician fails to appreciate, the significance of associated symptoms of hypotension, abdominal cramping, or skin rash.[373, 414] When these diagnoses are suspected, measurement of tryptase in a blood sample immediately after an attack may prove definitive.[415]

Another rare condition in which wheezing is associated with coincident systemic symptoms is the carcinoid syndrome, which is mediated by the release of serotonin, bradykinin, prostaglandin, and histamine from a carcinoid tumor. High urinary levels of the major metabolite of serotonin, 5-hydroxyindoleacetic acid, strongly suggest the diagnosis.[416]

The finding of parenchymal pulmonary infiltrates on chest radiographs in a wheezing patient with peripheral blood eosinophilia may reflect mucus plugs in the airways, with atelectasis of the subtended lung, but may also reflect parasitic infections, allergic bronchopulmonary mycosis, bronchocentric granulomatosis, or pulmonary vasculitides. Evaluation for these disorders should be pursued if the infiltrates recur despite the institution of effective antiasthmatic therapy with an inhaled corticosteroid and a bronchodilator.[417]

## Special Considerations

Asthma is often overlooked in the elderly,[418, 419] even though the morbidity and mortality of asthma are greater in older patients.[420] The failure to recognize asthma in elderly patients is more likely a result of failure to consider the diagnosis than of any difference in the clinical presentation of asthma, because the symptoms and signs of asthma in older patients do not differ from those in younger persons.[421] Other allergic diseases are slightly less common, serum levels of IgE are lower, and, although airflow obstruction is at least partially reversible, fixed airflow obstruction is more often found.[422, 423] One reason for the failure of physicians to consider asthma is that elderly patients themselves often attribute shortness of breathing and wheezing to aging. Another reason is the high prevalence of other diseases that cause cough and dyspnea, such as COPD, congestive heart failure, gastroesophageal reflux disease, and lung cancer.[424] Asthma responds well to treatment in these patients, so a high clinical index of suspicion should be maintained and objective measurement of airflow should be done routinely in elderly patients with pulmonary complaints.

Another special group are the so-called "poor perceivers": those with a blunted ability to detect airflow obstruction. These patients are thought to have an increased risk of fatal or near-fatal asthma, because they may be uncomfortable enough to seek treatment only when airflow obstruction is far advanced.[425, 426] Survivors of attacks that are so severe as to require intubation and mechanical ventilation are poor at detecting added external resistive loads and have weak ventilatory responses to hypercapnia and hypoxemia.[427] The prevalence of "poor perceivers" and their actual risk of morbidity or mortality are not known, perhaps because there is no simple test for perceptive ability.

At the other end of the spectrum from the "poor perceivers" are patients with the "hyperventilation syndrome." This condition, characterized by recurrent bouts of hyperventilation, sometime so severe as to result in syncope, is widely considered to be a form of anxiety neurosis or phobic response. The prevalence of bronchial hyperresponsiveness in patients with recurrent hyperventilation approaches 80%, however, and treatment with reassurance and bronchodilators is often curative.[428]

A category of asthma that is not reviewed here, because it is so important as to warrant its own chapter, is occupational asthma[429] (see Chapter 66).

## Clinical Forms of Asthma

All asthma is characterized by the coincidence of recurrent symptoms of wheezing, dyspnea, chest tightness, and/or cough, reversible airflow obstruction, and bronchial hyperresponsiveness, but the spectrum of clinical presentation is so wide that clinicians have found it useful to develop subcategories of asthma. Formal diagnostic criteria have been developed for very few of these subcategories. An exception is the classification of asthma according to severity (as a guide to therapy) by expert panels.[370] The categories of *mild intermittent, mild persistent, moderate persistent,* and *severe persistent* asthma are based on the frequency and severity of symptoms, especially nocturnal awakenings from asthma, the frequency of "as-needed" use of an inhaled beta-agonist, and the severity of airflow obstruction or liability (Table 39.5).

Some of the informally developed subcategories of asthma also evolved to recognize the importance of differences in the severity of the condition. At one extreme is *steroid-dependent asthma.* This category is intended to include patients who require continuous or frequent treatment with an oral glucocorticoid, usually prednisone or methylprednisolone. In informal use, this category does not include patients who require daily inhalation of an inhaled corticosteroid, even in high doses, but there are no guidelines as to frequency or duration of the need for treatment with an oral glucocorticoid that offer criteria for steroid-dependent asthma. This subcategory is at least partially a function of the quality of care, whether by the clinician or by the patient, because many patients referred to specialists for steroid-dependent asthma are weaned from oral glucocorticoid treatment after changes in their inhaled therapy, treatment of complicating conditions (especially chronic sinusitis and gastroesophageal reflux), and education in self-management (see Chapter 98). The patients who continue to do poorly despite expert management may include those with *steroid-resistant asthma,* as defined by failure of 2 weeks of treatment with 40 mg/day of methylprednisolone to cause a 15% improvement in $FEV_1$.[430]

Also at the extreme end of the spectrum of severity is *difficult asthma.*[431] This very loose classification includes patients with asthma prone to recurrent sudden attacks, or *brittle asthma,*[4, 5] as well as asthma that rarely causes severe exacerbations but that regularly interferes with sleep, exercise tolerance, or the ability to work, study, or play.[432]

At the other extreme of the spectrum of severity is asthma so mild that the clinician or patient resists application of the diagnosis from denial, fear of social stigma, or fear of loss of medical insurability. This may account for the inappropriate use of "reactive airways dysfunction" as a diagnosis. Historically, the term was developed to describe previously healthy patients who manifested symptoms of asthma, recurrent bouts of airflow obstruction, and bronchial hyperresponsiveness after brief exposure to high concentrations of an irritant or toxin in the workplace,[433] but it is now often (and inappropriately) applied to patients with mild or transient asthma.

Some of the informal subcategories of asthma arose from a need to classify the disease by its presumed pathogenesis. Apparent differences in the role of allergy among different people with asthma provided the underlying rationale for the classification of asthma as *extrinsic* or *intrinsic.*[434] Patients with extrinsic asthma had evidence of allergic sensitization, such as a history of allergic rhinitis, positive skin tests to aeroallergens, and high serum levels of IgE. Patients with intrinsic asthma, usually those with adult-onset asthma, lacked such features. Belief in the validity of the distinction has been eroded by reports that the values for serum IgE are actually elevated in patients with intrinsic asthma when the predicted value is corrected for age[54] and that the pathologic findings in bronchial biopsies from patients with extrinsic and intrinsic asthma do not differ.[159] A better accepted variant of extrinsic asthma is *seasonal asthma,* a category for patients who develop symptoms only during seasons in which they are exposed to high levels of a particular allergen, such as grass or birch pollen.

Other informal categories classify asthma according to the agents or events that trigger bronchoconstriction.

**Table 39.5 CLASSIFICATION OF ASTHMA SEVERITY**

| | Clinical Features Before Treatment* | | |
|---|---|---|---|
| Classification | Symptoms† | Nighttime Symptoms | Lung Function |
| STEP 4: Severe persistent | Continual symptoms<br>Limited physical activity<br>Frequent exacerbations | Frequent | $FEV_1$ or PEF ≤60% predicted<br>PEF variability >30% |
| STEP 3: Moderate persistent | Daily symptoms<br>Daily use of inhaled short-acting $beta_2$-agonist<br>Exacerbations affect activity<br>Exacerbations ≥2 times a week; may last days | >1 time a week | $FEV_1$ or PEF >60%–<80% predicted<br>PEF variability >30% |
| STEP 2: Mild persistent | Symptoms >2 times a week but <1 time a day<br>Exacerbations may affect activity | >2 times a month | $FEV_1$ or PEF ≥80% predicted<br>PEF variability 20–30% |
| STEP 1: Mild intermittent | Symptoms ≤2 times a week<br>Asymptomatic and normal PEF between exacerbations<br>Exacerbations brief (from a few hours to a few days): Intensity may vary | ≤2 times a month | $FEV_1$ or PEF ≥80% predicted<br>PEF variability <20% |

*The presence of one of the features of severity is sufficient to place a patient in that category. An individual should be assigned to the most severe grade in which any feature occurs. The characteristics noted are general and may overlap because asthma is highly variable. Furthermore, an individual's classification may change over time.

†Patients at any level of severity can have mild, moderate, or severe exacerbations. Some patients with intermittent asthma experience severe and life-threatening exacerbations separated by long periods of normal lung function and no symptoms.

From National Asthma Education and Prevention Program (NAEPP). Clinical Practice Guidelines. Expert Panel Report 2: Guidelines for the diagnosis and management of asthma. NIH Publication No. 91-4051. Bethesda, MD: National Institutes of Health/National Heart Lung and Blood Institutes, July, 1997.

*Exercise-induced asthma* is an example. A more correct description of the phenomenon is *exercise-induced bronchospasm,* because exercise provokes airway narrowing in most people with asthma. The pathways responsible are not entirely worked out, but the initial stimulus is thought to be the evaporative loss of water, and possibly also of heat, from the bronchial mucosa, caused by the inhalation of large volumes of unconditioned air.[435, 436] The resulting rise in osmolality is thought to stimulate activation of mast cells or afferent nerve endings, with the mediators released causing contraction of bronchial smooth muscle and vasodilation of the bronchial vasculature.[437] Exercise-induced asthma is therefore simply a reflection of the nonspecific bronchial hyperresponsiveness of asthma. The label is nonetheless applied to patients who develop symptoms only during or immediately after exercise.

*Nocturnal asthma,* or asthma causing awakenings from sleep, is so common that it should probably be regarded, like exercise-induced asthma, as simply an expression of asthma, not a discreet subcategory. In a survey of more than 7000 outpatients with asthma in the United Kingdom, 94% reported that asthmatic symptoms awaken them at least one night per month; 39% reported being awakened nightly.[353] That nocturnal awakenings may be a marker of severity or risk from asthma was suggested by a study of 168 deaths in Victoria, Australia, over a 1-year period; 53% of the deaths occurred during the 9 hours between 10 p.m. and 7 a.m.[438] Comparison of bronchoalveolar lavage fluid samples obtained at 4 p.m. and at 4 a.m. has shown remarkable nocturnal increases in eosinophils and neutrophils,[439] suggesting that asthmatic inflammation follows a circadian rhythm.

An important subcategory is *drug-induced asthma.* The drugs responsible include aspirin and other nonsteroidal antiinflammatory drugs, beta-blockers, and angiotensin-converting enzyme inhibitors. This form of asthma is discussed in Chapter 11.

The term *asthmatic bronchitis* is used in two senses. One sense refers to the coincidence of asthma and chronic obstructive bronchitis in a cigarette smoker. Again, there are no formal criteria for this subcategory of asthma, but the usual features are recurrent dyspnea and wheezing, chronic productive cough, and airflow obstruction that is partially, but not completely, reversible with treatment. Overlap between asthma and chronic obstructive disease is common. The so-called Dutch hypothesis has even proposed that the mechanisms responsible for asthma predispose to the development of COPD,[440] and the rate of decline in $FEV_1$ is indeed faster in smoking asthmatics than in nonsmoking asthmatics or healthy smokers.[400] The other sense of the term *asthmatic bronchitis* refers to episodes of prolonged production of cough and sputum purulence that often follow viral respiratory infections in asthmatic patients.

An important but rare form of asthma is *allergic bronchopulmonary mycosis.* This form of asthma is believed to reflect hypersensitivity to a fungus, usually *Aspergillus fumigatus,* that has colonized the bronchial mucosa. This form of asthma is characterized by eosinophilia, very high IgE levels, precipitating serum antibodies to *Aspergillus,* positive skin test response to *Aspergillus,* and recurrent localized infiltrates on chest radiography.[441] Unless diagnosed and treated, usually with an oral corticosteroid, central airway bronchiectasis can develop and progress.[442]

## NATURAL HISTORY

### Remission

In the definition of asthma as a "chronic inflammatory disease of the airways," the word *chronic* is meant to refer to the disease's tendency to last a long time or to recur often, as distinguished from "acute" diseases. For some patients, at least, the adjective is also true in its second sense, as "continuing indefinitely; perpetual; constant."[2] Whether the second sense will be true for a child with asthma is always high on the list of concerns of parents.

Some understanding of the determinants of the long-term outcomes of childhood asthma can be gleaned from the observations made in cohorts of asthmatic children observed prospectively for many years.[69, 443–445] These have shown that only 20% of children who had one or more attacks of wheezing before the age of 5 years had similar attacks at the age of 9 years. Of the children diagnosed as having asthma at age 5, only 50% still had the diagnosis at age 10.

Long-term studies have supported the notion that children can "outgrow" their asthma, and childhood asthma does appear sometimes to enter prolonged periods of clinical remission during the years of adolescence.[446–448] But true remissions may not occur as frequently as is commonly believed. A review of 15 studies of the natural history of asthma led Barbee and Murphy to conclude that about 50% of adults who recall having childhood asthma continue to have symptoms.[69] This figure could be suspected of being artifactually raised by recall bias, but follow-up studies of children who wheezed at 7 years of age showed that 25% to 50% had wheezing at least once a year at age 30.[444, 449] Overall, asthma improved and worsened in about the same number of people, and, in general, those with lower lung function and greater airway responsiveness as children were more likely to have asthma as adults.[450]

Spontaneous remissions can also occur in adults with asthma. Based on responses to simple questions about asthma symptoms, 60% of those identified as asthmatic on an initial survey were considered to be in remission 6 years later.[451] A more sophisticated longitudinal study of a general population sample showed that 22% of 136 asthmatics surveyed twice over a period of 9 years entered a sustained remission.[452] The rate of remission was highest in adolescents and fell off sharply in adults older than 30 years of age. Adults between the ages of 30 and 60 years with active asthmatic symptoms had only a 10% chance of losing their symptoms over 9 years. On the basis of a more rigorous definition of asthma remission (absence of pulmonary symptoms, normal bronchial responsiveness, and an $FEV_1$ greater than 90% of predicted), only 11% of adult asthmatics referred to a regional asthma clinic between 1962 and 1970 had remission of the disease when studied again 25 years later.[453] The features at the initial visit that correlated with remission at follow-up were younger age, less severe airflow obstruction, and a shorter period between the onset of asthma symptoms and specialized treatment of the disease.

### Mortality

Asthma rarely causes death. But because most deaths are considered preventable, because effective treatment is available, and because some of these deaths occur in children and young adults, the mortality rate from asthma is excessive. Retrospective study of asthma fatalities and follow-up study of survivors of near-fatal attacks has identified features of "potentially fatal asthma"[454, 455] (see earlier discussion). Other risk factors of importance include psychosocial problems, family dysfunction, low education, and unemployment. A risk factor pertinent to diverse populations is language barrier, which has been associated with a high (17.3) odds ratio for intubation, a surrogate marker for a potentially fatal attack.[456]

A disturbing but consistent finding of retrospective surveys is that 15% to 30% of asthma deaths occur in patients with only mild asthma.[438, 457, 458] Two explanations seem possible. One is that the information gathered retrospectively, largely relating to the severity of symptoms and medication requirements, underestimates the severity of the disease. The other possibility is that even patients with mild asthma are at some risk, albeit a very low one. Both possibilities seem likely. One group of investigators noted that "judgement of the severity of asthma prior to death was severely limited by the lack of objective measures of ventilatory function."[458] Other investigators found a relationship between asthma mortality and sudden extreme peaks of allergens in the environment as a result of industrial or climatologic activity.[459–461]

Few prospective studies of asthma mortality have been done. One study of more than 1000 patients with moderate or severe asthma identified associations between clinical features on entry and the subsequent risk of death.[462] Not surprisingly, age older than 70 years, a smoking history of more than 20 pack-years, and a reduced $FEV_1$ were factors associated with a high relative risk of death from asthma, but the relative risk was just as high for patients who had a greater than 50% improvement in $FEV_1$ after inhalation of a bronchodilator and for those with a blood eosinophil count higher than $0.45 \times 10^9$ cells/L. These findings invite speculation that the risk of dying from asthma may be related to the intensity of eosinophilic airway inflammation and of the resulting increase in airway liability.[463]

### Morbidity

Asthma causes substantial morbidity. The most visible morbid events are attacks requiring emergency care or hospitalization. One estimate put the annual cost of hospitalizations for asthma in the United States at $4.5 billion in 1985.[464] Emergency department visits were estimated to account for more than $200 million per year.

In any given year, 80% of the costs for these morbid events are attributable to 20% of patients with asthma.[465] The approach to reducing the morbidity of asthma seems to be obvious: to target measures of proven efficacy at the subpopulation of asthmatics who suffer most of the attacks. The key to this approach, of course, is identifying the right 20%.[432] To what extent does the natural history of asthma follow a predictable course in different individuals? Is it the same patients who suffer repeated attacks from year to year, and, if so, is their condition characterized by some identifiable markers of disease?

This question is analogous to the question about the distribution of risk for asthma mortality. There indeed appears to be a subgroup of patients with identifiable features indicating a heightened risk for severe attacks, but these patients make up a small proportion of the total population of asthmatics. Many, perhaps most, severe attacks of asthma occur in patients whose asthma had not previously been identified as severe. Again, two explanations seem possible. One is that these patients were at high risk but the markers for such risk were not assessed or are unknown. The other possibility is that some events, such as infection with a particularly "asthmogenic" virus or contact with an usually high level of an allergen, can precipitate severe attacks even in patients with truly mild asthma.

Again, few prospective studies of the determinants of asthma morbidity have been done. One study focused on adults who had made at least three physician visits for asthma during the previous year, were considered to have moderate or severe asthma, and were taking medications daily.[466] Prospectively, follow-up of these patients identified characteristics associated with a high (more than 50%), moderate (10% to 15%) and low (less than 5%) risk of hospitalization. The high-risk features included hospitalization within the previous year, moderate or severe reduction in $FEV_1$, a medication regimen consistent with severe asthma, a history of systemic corticosteroid use, overnight variability of peak flow greater than 40%, and a mean evening peak flow less than 60% predicted. Multivariate analysis showed that the first three risk factors listed provided most of the information needed. A single measurement of spirometry was more informative for risk stratification than was regular measurement of peak flow for 2 weeks.

## Progressive Airflow Obstruction

Acceptance of the idea that irreversible airflow obstruction as an outcome of the natural history of asthma may have been delayed by the emphasis on the reversibility of airway narrowing in the definitions of asthma. Some longitudinal studies have shown asthmatics to have greater rates of decline in pulmonary function than healthy nonsmokers,[400, 467] and many nonsmoking asthmatics have been found to have severe, irreversible airflow obstruction.[313, 399, 423] The progressive narrowing of the airways in chronic asthma is hypothesized to result from the deposition of collagen and growth of vessels, smooth muscle, and secretory cells and glands, presumably mediated by the products of inflammatory cells activated in the airways[134, 312] (see earlier discussion).

## Effects of Treatments on the Natural History of Asthma

The idea that inhaled corticosteroids may be a "disease-modifying" treatment led to the hope that their early, sustained use would increase the chance of remission of the disease after they were withdrawn. This hope was nurtured by a report of maintenance of improvements in airway responsiveness and clinical asthma when budesonide was discontinued in 8 adults with mild asthma who had taken 400 μg/day of the drug for 1 year.[468] More than 3 months after therapy was stopped, asthmatic symptoms had recurred in only three subjects, all of whom either had continued exposure to allergens or had contracted an upper respiratory infection.

The hopes raised by this study were diminished by subsequent studies. A follow-up study of adults with newly diagnosed asthma who had been treated with high-dose (1200 μg/day) budesonide for 2 years found that when the dose of budesonide was reduced most subjects continued to do well, but when the inhaled corticosteroid was discontinued, the subjects did poorly.[469] Again, the deteriorations in asthma control did not occur in all subjects. About a third of them continued to do as well as they had while taking budesonide.

Remission of asthma is not easily achieved, even when the definition of "remission" is eased to mean only the absence of symptoms while inhaled corticosteroid treatment is continued, not after its withdrawal. A 3-year study of asthmatic children treated with an inhaled corticosteroid found that, although two thirds of the children had a least one 8-month period free of asthma symptoms, most had a relapse of symptoms at some later stage, even though the inhaled corticosteroid was continued.[470] Therefore, 28 to 36 months of inhaled corticosteroid treatment may improve both symptoms and objective measures of lung function, but it does not cure asthma. This conclusion is underlined by a later report that withdrawal of inhaled corticosteroid from these patients was followed by rapid reappearance of symptoms and a deterioration in lung function.[471]

The idea that treatment might alter the clinical consequences of asthma is well supported by a large body of sound clinical research.[472] Although demonstration that treatment alters the risk of death in a classic, prospective study would require enrollment of so large a number of subjects as to be unfeasible, indirect evidence suggests strongly that treatment is protective. The markers of a heightened risk for death, such as one or more hospitalizations or emergency department visits for asthma,[473, 474] highly variable peak flow rates,[475, 476] and markedly increased bronchial reactivity,[477, 478] have all been shown to be altered favorably by inhaled corticosteroid treatment, even in survivors of near-fatal attacks.[479]

Hospitalization rates are also reduced by treatment. The decreased number of hospitalizations and number of days spent in hospital for asthma in Sweden that were recorded during a period when the prevalence of asthma doubled were attributed to greater use of inhaled corticosteroids.[22] A more persuasive study examined retrospectively a cohort of almost 17,000 asthmatics enrolled in a health maintenance organization in Massachusetts.[480] Filling of prescriptions for an inhaled corticosteroid reduced the risk of hospitalization by 50% overall, and by 70% among those who were dispensed more than eight canisters of an inhaled beta-agonist per year. Finally, a clinical study of classic design confirmed the association between use of an inhaled corticosteroid and reduction in the risk of exacerbations.[481] A similar association was also shown for regular treatment with a leukotriene-receptor antagonist.[482, 483]

Recognition that asthma can lead to irreversible airflow obstruction, attributed to pathologic changes in the airway wall, combined with the finding that even mild asthma is associated with fibrotic remodeling,[484] led to the attribution of great importance to differences in $FEV_1$ among patients chronically treated with placebo or with an inhaled corticosteroid. Two studies of patients with mild-to-moderate asthma, one in children[485] and one in adults,[486] showed greater declines in $FEV_1$ among those treated with an inhaled beta-agonist than among those treated with inhaled budesonide for 2 to 5 years. Among the patients for whom inhaled corticosteroid therapy was delayed, starting the treatment did not lead to a "catch-up" in $FEV_1$. Even after 1 year of treatment, the improvement in $FEV_1$ was only half as great as it had been in those in whom treatment had been started at the outset of the study.[469] These findings led to recommendations for early institution of treatment to modify the natural history of asthma. They led, for example, to emphasis on the importance of identifying young adults with asthma so that treatment can be started "to prevent the evolution of respiratory impairment."[487] They were also an important contributor to the recommendation for "chronic controller therapy" (e.g., with an inhaled corticosteroid) for patients with mild persistent asthma.[370]

Much remains to be learned about the natural history of asthma, but it is indisputable that regular treatment, especially with an inhaled corticosteroid, is effective in preventing some of the disease's short-term consequences. Treatment improves asthma symptoms, quality of life, airway caliber, and airway responsiveness. It further reduces the risks of need for emergency care and hospitalization, and it almost certainly reduces the risk of death from asthma. These are real and important benefits. Studies suggesting that treatment retards or prevents the development of irreversible airflow obstruction are few, however, and additional studies of large numbers of asthmatic subjects are needed. It may well be that the development of progressive airflow obstruction only occurs in a subgroup. As for the hope that treatment can alter the chances for sustained remission, new and better therapies must be awaited. Although current treatments are effective in altering the natural history of asthma, they appear to be effective only so long as they are taken.

## MANAGEMENT

### General Principles

Changes in the scientific conception of asthma have led national and international expert panels to propose guidelines for its diagnosis and management.[370, 488, 489] They emphasize the importance of long-term maintenance and control as a goal of therapy rather than simply treating symptomatic episodes. The recommendations for treatment are organized into four components: (1) use of objective measures of lung function to assess the severity of asthma and to monitor the efficacy of therapy; (2) identification and elimination of factors that worsen symptoms, precipitate exacerbations, or promote ongoing airway inflammation; (3) comprehensive pharmacologic therapy to reverse bronchoconstriction and to reverse and prevent airway inflammation; and (4) creation of a therapeutic partnership between the patient and the provider of care.[370] The process of developing guidelines and the elements of the patient-clinician partnership are reviewed elsewhere (see Chapters 98 and 99).

### Pharmacologic Therapy

Pharmacologic treatment of acute symptoms of dyspnea, chest tightness, and wheezing still focuses on reversing bronchoconstriction with "quick-relief" medications, such as short-acting beta$_2$-agonists and anticholinergics. Because asthma is now recognized as a chronic inflammatory disease of the airways, attention is additionally focused on regular, sustained use of "long-term control" medications, such as corticosteroids, leukotriene modifiers, cromolyn or nedocromil, or methylxanthines. The pharmacology of the drugs used in the treatment of asthma is reviewed in detail in Chapter 11.

### Acute Severe Asthma

Asthma is the most common respiratory emergency in clinical practice. In the United States, it accounts for 1.8 million visits to emergency departments each year, with costs exceeding $430 million.[464, 490] About 10% of asthmatics presenting for emergency care require hospitalization, further adding to the economic burden of asthma.

The most common precipitant of asthma exacerbations is infection with a respiratory viral pathogen.[74, 75, 491] Other precipitants include infection with *M. pneumoniae* or *C. pneumoniae*, exposure to allergens or irritants (e.g., sulfur dioxide, particulate pollutants), medication use (especially of aspirin-like or beta-blocking drugs), emotional crisis, and medication noncompliance. Knowledge of the cause of the attack is helpful in projecting the duration of treatment that is likely to be necessary, but it has no effect on initial management. Regardless of the cause of the attack, the first steps are to assess the severity of airflow obstruction and to initiate treatment.

Diagnosis usually presents little difficulty, so the purpose of clinical assessment is to determine the severity of the attack as a guide to the urgency of aggressive care. Except in those with life-threatening asthma, signs and symptoms correlate poorly with the severity of airflow obstruction, so $FEV_1$ or peak expiratory flow should be measured. Serial measurements provide valuable information about the response to therapy and help avoid both unnecessary admission and premature discharge.[492]

Clues that an attack of asthma is life-threatening include an altered sensorium, upright posture, diaphoresis, telegraphic speech, cyanosis, and fatigue. Other clues are an inspiratory fall in systolic blood pressure (pulsus paradoxus) of more than 15 mm Hg, intercostal retractions, poor air movement, peak flow less than 25% of predicted or less than 100 L/min, and $FEV_1$ less than 25% of predicted or less than 1.0 L.[493, 494] Pneumothorax is a life-threatening complication of asthma, because of the rapidity of progression to lung collapse or tension pneumothorax. When any of these signs are present, aggressive treatment should be given and early transfer to an intensive care unit arranged.

Except for the evaluation of suspected pneumothorax, chest radiography is usually unnecessary. Bacterial pneumonia rarely causes exacerbations, and the purulent sputum produced by asthmatics usually reflects inflammation of the airways caused by viral infection or by allergen inhalation, rather than bacterial bronchitis or pneumonia.

Except in mild attacks, oximetry should be done and supplemental oxygen given as necessary. Arterial blood gas measurement is rarely necessary. The typical profile of attacks is mild hypoxemia ($Pa_{O_2}$, 66 to 69 mm Hg), hypocapnia ($Pa_{CO_2}$, 33 to 36 mm Hg), and respiratory alkalosis. Respiratory drive is invariably increased, and even a normal value for $P_{CO_2}$ indicates extremely severe airflow obstruction and fatigue of the muscles of respiration (see earlier discussion). But patients with carbon dioxide retention often respond well to therapy, and the important goal of initial assessment is to recognize the attack as severe and to administer effective treatment. Peak flow measurement is sufficient for this purpose. The information from arterial blood gases becomes important when an attack does not respond to initial therapy, to guide decisions about the need for intubation and mechanical ventilation. In severe attacks, arterial blood gas analysis may also reveal acidosis, variably from metabolic and respiratory causes (lactic acidosis and alveolar hypoventilation); this rarely needs any treatment beyond effective oxygenation and relief from airflow obstruction.[495]

Treatment should be started as soon as an asthma exacerbation is recognized and its severity assessed. Measurements of lung function should be repeated periodically, at least at 2 hours after initial treatment.

For all patients, an inhaled $beta_2$-agonist should be given by nebulizer (2.5 to 5.0 mg of albuterol in isotonic saline) or by metered-dose inhaler (MDI) with a spacer (90 μg per puff; four to six puffs) every 20 to 30 minutes for 1 hour. Thereafter, the frequency of treatment should be adjusted to the improvement in airflow obstruction. For severe exacerbations, continuous administration of a nebulized $beta_2$-agonist may be given for up to 1 hour. Addition of an anticholinergic agent to the nebulized $beta_2$-agonist has been shown to cause additional bronchodilation.[496–498] Supplemental oxygen (by nasal cannulae or mask) should be administered to maintain an arterial blood oxygen saturation level higher than 90%.

For moderate to severe exacerbations, and for exacerbations that are incompletely responsive to initial $beta_2$-agonist therapy, treatment with an oral corticosteroid should be started and continued for 7 to 10 days (e.g., prednisone, 40 to 60 mg/day, given in a single or divided dose). Supplemental doses of an oral corticosteroid should be given to patients who take them regularly, even if the exacerbation is mild.[499–501]

Methylxanthines are no longer recommended for treatment of acute asthma, because they appear to add no benefit to optimal inhaled $beta_2$-agonist therapy and may increase adverse effects.[502–504] Antibiotics are also not routinely recommended, but they may be necessary for comorbid conditions (e.g., pneumonia, bacterial sinusitis) and should be considered for patients with fever and sputum purulence or pulmonary infiltrates on chest radiography. If an antibiotic is used, a macrolide antibiotic should be considered, because *M. pneumoniae* and *C. pneumoniae* are known to provoke asthma exacerbations.

Most attacks of asthma respond well to therapy, but for those that do not, hospitalization must be considered. A small subset of patients require monitoring in the intensive care unit, and some require intubation and mechanical ventilation. These are patients with severe airway obstruction that is unresponsive to treatment (status asthmaticus), especially if complicated by fatigue and increases in arterial $P_{CO_2}$, indicating impending respiratory arrest. With the institution of mechanical ventilation, pleural pressure abruptly becomes positive throughout the respiratory cycle. This impedes venous return, and a fall in cardiac output and hypotension should be anticipated. Hemodynamic instability can be further exacerbated by additional lung hyperinflation due to incomplete expiration of machine-delivered tidal volumes. Strategies to minimize hyperinflation during mechanical ventilation in acute severe asthma include relative hypoventilation with permissive hypercapnia, avoidance of ventilator-applied positive end-expiratory pressure, and adjustments in inspiratory airflow rates and patterns so as to maximize the duration of expiration. This strategy concomitantly helps limit barotrauma, especially pneumothorax, which is catastrophic in this setting. It is important to note that these ventilator strategies require the patient to be deeply sedated with narcotics, benzodiazepines, or anesthetic agents such as propofol or anesthetic gases.[505] Sometimes muscle relaxants are also required, but they should be avoided if possible because of the risk of prolonged muscle weakness when these agents are used in conjunction with corticosteroids in patients with severe asthma.[506]

The realization that the hemodynamic consequences of mechanical ventilation may contribute significantly to mortality from acute severe asthma has led to the widespread adoption of ventilator strategies designed to limit lung hyperinflation. At the same time, the mortality rates in published series of intubated asthmatic patients have decreased, often to zero.[505] Although these studies do not allow evaluation of the relative contribution of changes in ventilator practice, compared with other changes in clinical practice, to this decreased mortality, they do suggest a relationship.

To avoid the hazards of intubation, additional treatments are sometimes attempted. One of these is administration of heliox, a blend of helium and oxygen that has a lower gas density than air.[507, 508] This treatment seems most promising for patients with acute severe asthma with respiratory acidosis and a short duration of symptoms.[509] Another treatment is intravenous administration of magnesium sulfate.[510, 511] Although this may be effective among certain subgroups,[512] it has not proved consistently effective.

## Chronic Asthma

Guidelines for the management of asthma uniformly recommend adjusting the intensity of treatment to the clinical severity of asthma[370, 488, 489] (Table 39.6; see Table 39.5). For patients with occasional symptoms promptly relieved by a bronchodilator and with normal pulmonary function between episodes, no treatment other than an inhaled beta-agonist taken on an "as-needed" basis is necessary. But if symptoms occur more than twice a week, affect activity, or cause awakening from sleep more than twice a month, use of a long-term controller mediation is recommended. The treatment most strongly recommended is regular use of an inhaled corticosteroid, because this is predictably effective in improving control of asthma and has been shown to reduce airway mucosal inflammation. Cromolyn and nedocromil, the leukotriene modifiers, and theophylline are all regarded as acceptable alternatives but have not been proven to modify airway inflammation. For more severe asthma, higher doses of an inhaled corticosteroid are recommended, as is the combination of treatment with an inhaled corticosteroid and a long-acting beta-agonist.[481, 513, 514]

As for any chronic disease, successful treatment requires enlistment of the patient as a partner in his or her care. This in turn requires educating the patient about the nature of the disease, the purposes of the different treatments, and the actions to be taken when symptoms and signs worsen (i.e., an Action Plan). Simply providing information is not sufficient. Self-care requires mastery of certain skills, especially those of self-assessment (e.g., performance and interpretation of peak flow tests) and treatment (e.g., correct use of inhalers, correct dosing of an oral corticosteroid) (see Chapter 98).

The chronicity of asthma has other important implications for care. One is of the need to identify sources of exposure to allergens or irritants that can be reduced or eliminated. The most important allergens (house dust mite, cockroach, cat dander, and molds) are found in homes. Sensitivity to these allergens can be demonstrated by skin testing, and instructions can then be given regarding measures for reducing or avoiding exposure.

Another implication of chronicity is that care must be iterative. Assessments of the severity of symptoms, of airway caliber, of disruption of attendance at work or school, and of impairment of the quality of life must be made repeatedly. Review of the patient's knowledge and skills must be made regularly. And pharmacologic therapy must be adjusted periodically to maintain optimal control with minimal risk of toxicity.

A subgroup of asthmatic subjects with chronic asthma have "chronic severe asthma," as reflected by high medication requirements to maintain good disease control or by persistent symptoms, recurrent exacerbations, or continuing airflow obstruction despite high medication use. The term *chronic severe asthma* is meant to encompass other asthma subgroups, such as refractory asthma, steroid-dependent asthma, difficult-to-control asthma, poorly controlled asthma, brittle asthma, or irreversible asthma. This subgroup should logically include patients with steroid-resistant asthma, but this is customarily regarded as a specific and separate asthma phenotype.[515]

Because asthma severity is not defined consistently and is relatively difficult to measure, the size of this subgroup is unknown. Among the 6.4% of Israeli military recruits who were found to have asthma, fewer than 1% had severe asthma, defined narrowly as steroid dependence and an $FEV_1$ less than 50% of predicted.[516] Severe hyperreactivity to histamine ($PC_{20}$ histamine less than 0.1 mg/mL), a possible but indirect marker of severe asthma, was found in approximately 12% of asthmatic children and adults in Australia.[515] Both of these studies probably underestimated the prevalence of chronic severe asthma as defined earlier in this chapter.

Most recent studies of airway pathology in asthma have examined biopsies obtained from subjects with mild or moderate disease, but a study of patients with chronic severe asthma reported high numbers of neutrophils and high levels of thromboxane and leukotriene $B_4$, rather than the expected dramatic increases in numbers of eosinophils.[10]

The clinical approach to the assessment of patients with chronic severe asthma starts with review of the basics: confirmation of the diagnosis (see previous discussion) and evaluation of the patient's actual use of the medications prescribed. Once it has been confirmed that the patient indeed has asthma and that the medications prescribed are appropriate, attention should first be directed to confirming the patient's understanding of the disease, of the purposes and correct use of the medications prescribed, and of the importance of regular compliance with therapy. Noncompliance with the prescribed use of an inhaled corticosteroid may be the most important cause of inadequate control of asthma, and patients grossly overreport the regularity of their use of inhaled medication.[517] Another important cause of chronic severe asthma is the patient's failure to recognize, or reluctance to report, an irritant or allergen in the home or workplace, such as a beloved pet, or even a large number of pets. It is in the evaluation and treatment of chronic severe asthma that the creation of a therapeutic partnership in care may be most important (see Chapter 98). But even some patients whose understanding, skills, and compliance are ideal continue to have chronic severe asthma despite optimal use of inhaled medications. For these patients, computed tomographic scanning of the sinuses and esophageal pH monitoring should probably be undertaken, even in the absence of typical symptoms of sinusitis or gastroesophageal reflux, because a growing body of clinical observation suggests that treatment of these disorders can improve asthma control.[381, 518] Even the application of all of these measures is ineffective in a small proportion of patients, who are sometimes then offered aggressive immunosuppressive or other presumably immunomodulatory therapy.[519] This should be done in the context of a rigorously controlled clinical trial.

## SUMMARY

Asthma is an important cause of disability, death, and economic cost. Its incidence is increasing in developed

**Table 39.6** STEPWISE APPROACH FOR MANAGING ASTHMA IN ADULTS AND CHILDREN OLDER THAN 5 YEARS OF AGE*

| | TREATMENT† | | |
|---|---|---|---|
| CLASSIFICATION | **Long-Term Control** | **Quick Relief** | **Education** |
| STEP 4: Severe persistent | Daily medications:<br>**Anti-inflammatory: inhaled corticosteroid (high dose)**<br>AND<br>Long-acting bronchodilator: either **long-acting inhaled beta$_2$-agonist,** sustained-release theophylline, or long-acting beta$_2$-agonist tablets<br>AND<br>Corticosteroid tablets or syrup long term (2 mg/kg/day, generally do not exceed 60 mg/day). | Short-acting bronchodilator: **inhaled beta$_2$-agonists** as needed for symptoms<br>Intensity of treatment will depend on severity of exacerbation<br>Use of short-acting inhaled beta$_2$-agonists on a daily basis, or increasing use, indicates the need for additional long-term-control therapy | Steps 2 and 3 actions plus:<br>Refer to individual education/counseling |
| STEP 3: Moderate persistent | Daily medication:<br>Either<br>**Anti-inflammatory: inhaled corticosteroid (medium dose)**<br>OR<br>**Inhaled corticosteroid (low-medium dose)** and add a long-acting bronchodilator, especially for nighttime symptoms: either **long-acting inhaled beta$_2$-agonist,** sustained-release theophylline, or long-acting beta$_2$-agonist tablets<br>If needed:<br>Anti-inflammatory: **Inhaled corticosteroids (medium-high dose)**<br>AND<br>**Long-acting bronchodilator,** especially for nighttime symptoms; either **long-acting inhaled beta$_2$-agonist,** sustained-release theophylline, or long-acting beta$_2$-agonist tablets. | Short-acting bronchodilator: **inhaled beta$_2$-agonists** as needed for symptoms.<br>Intensity of treatment will depend on severity of exacerbation<br>Use of short-acting inhaled beta$_2$-agonists on a daily basis, or increasing use, indicates the need for additional long-term-control therapy | Step 1 actions plus:<br>Teach self-monitoring<br>Refer to group education if available<br>Review and update self-management plan |
| STEP 2: Mild persistent | One daily medication:<br>**Anti-inflammatory:** either **inhaled corticosteroid** (low doses) or **cromolyn or nedocromil** (children usually begin with a trial of cromolyn or nedocromil)<br>Sustained-release theophylline to serum concentration of 5–15 μg/mL is an alternative, but not preferred, therapy; Zafirlukast or zileuton may also be considered for patients ≥12 years of age, although their position in therapy is not fully established | Short-acting bronchodilator: **inhaled beta$_2$-agonists** as needed for symptoms.<br>Intensity of treatment will depend on severity of exacerbation<br>Use of short-acting inhaled beta$_2$-agonists on a daily basis, or increasing use, indicates the need for additional long-term-control therapy | Step 1 actions plus:<br>Teach self-monitoring<br>Refer to group education if available<br>Review and update self-management plan |

*Table continued on following page*

**Table 39.6** STEPWISE APPROACH FOR MANAGING ASTHMA IN ADULTS AND CHILDREN OLDER THAN 5 YEARS OF AGE* *Continued*

| | TREATMENT† | | |
|---|---|---|---|
| CLASSIFICATION | **Long-Term Control** | **Quick Relief** | **Education** |
| STEP 1: Mild intermittent | No daily medication needed. | Short-acting bronchodilator: **inhaled beta$_2$-agonists** as needed for symptoms.<br>Intensity of treatment will depend on severity of exacerbation<br>Use of short-acting inhaled beta$_2$-agonists more than 2 times a week may indicate the need to initiate long-term-control therapy | Teach basic facts about asthma<br>Teach inhaler/spacer/holding chamber technique<br>Discuss roles of medications<br>Develop self-management plan<br>Develop action plan for when and how to take rescue actions, especially for patients with a history of severe exacerbations<br>Discuss appropriate environmental control measures to avoid exposure to known allergens and irritants |

*The stepwise approach presents general guidelines to assist clinical decision making; it is not intended to be a specific prescription. Asthma is highly variable; clinicians should tailor specific medication plans to the needs and circumstances of individual patients.
†Preferred treatments are in bold print.

↓ Step down
Review treatment every 1 to 6 months; a gradual stepwise reduction in treatment may be possible.

↑ Step up
If control is not maintained, consider step up. First, review patient medication technique, adherence, and environmental control (avoidance of allergens or other factors that contribute to asthma severity).

From National Asthma Education and Prevention Program (NAEPP). Clinical Practice Guidelines. Expert Panel Report 2: Guidelines for the diagnosis and management of asthma. NIH Publication No. 91-4051. Bethesda, MD: National Institutes of Health/National Heart Lung and Blood Institutes, April, 1997.

Western countries and appears to be increasing epidemically in non-Western societies that have adopted some features of Western culture. On a fundamental level, it is a disease of misdirected immunity, with the direction of immune function being influenced by many genes, and probably also by airway infections, especially with viruses, but established in early neonatal life. The cells that are most important in orchestrating this "misdirected" immune response in the airways are the dendritic cell and the $CD4^+$ Th2 lymphocyte. The cytokines produced by this lymphocyte, especially IL-13, alter the functions of structural cells in the airways, either directly through activation of specific receptors on the cells or indirectly through their effects on other cells, such as B lymphocytes, mast cells, eosinophils, and polymorphonuclear leukocytes. Repeated release of these cytokines alters the function and structure of the airways. The structural changes, often referred to as "remodeling," are now recognized as potentially irreversible.

The approach to the diagnosis, assessment, and treatment of asthma has changed in response to its recognition as a chronic inflammatory disease punctuated by intermittent exacerbations. The therapies that are available are effective in controlling asthma, but their efficacy depends on engagement of the patient as a full partner in care.

Until a curative treatment is developed, only the combined use of antiinflammatory and bronchodilator therapies, coupled with measures to reduce environmental exposures, can reduce the costs of asthma for the individuals affected. Applied widely, these measures will also reduce the consequences and costs for society at large. Before the most economic and effective approach to prevention of asthma can be undertaken, more must be learned about the interplay of genotype and environment that is responsible for initiation and progression of the disease.

## References

1. A report of the conclusions of a Ciba Guest Symposium: Terminology, definitions and classifications of chronic pulmonary emphysema and related conditions. Thorax 14:286–299, 1959.
2. Webster's New World Dictionary of the American Language (2nd College ed). Englewood Cliffs, NJ: Prentice-Hall, 1986.
3. Laitinen LA, Heino M, Laitinen A, et al: Damage of the airway epithelium and bronchial reactivity in patients with asthma. Am Rev Respir Dis 131:599–606, 1985.
4. Ayres JG: Classification and management of brittle asthma. Br J Hosp Med 57:387–389, 1997.
5. Wasserfallen JB, Schaller MD, Feihl F, et al: Sudden asphyxic asthma: A distinct entity? Am Rev Respir Dis 142:108–111, 1990.
6. Hensley MJ, Scicchitano R, Saunders NA, et al: Seasonal variation in non-specific bronchial reactivity: A study of wheat workers with a history of wheat associated asthma. Thorax 43:103–107, 1988.
7. Cockcroft DW, Killian DN, Mellon JJ, et al: Bronchial reactivity to inhaled histamine: A method and clinical survey. Clin Allergy 7:235–243, 1977.
8. Crimi E, Spanevello A, Neri M, et al: Dissociation between air-

way inflammation and airway hyperresponsiveness in allergic asthma. Am J Respir Crit Care Med 157:4–9, 1998.
9. Gibson PG, Hargreave FE, Girgis-Gabardo A, et al: Chronic cough with eosinophilic bronchitis: Examination for variable airflow obstruction and response to corticosteroid. Clin Exp Allergy 25:127–132, 1995.
10. Wenzel SE, Szefler SJ, Leung DYM, et al: Bronchoscopic evaluation of severe asthma: Persistent inflammation associated with high dose glucocorticoids. Am J Respir Crit Care Med 156:737–743, 1997.
11. Toelle BG, Peat JK, Salome CM, et al: Toward a definition of asthma for epidemiology. Am Rev Respir Dis 146:633–637, 1992.
12. Sandford A, Weir T, Pare P: State of the art: The genetics of asthma. Am J Respir Crit Care Med 153:1749–1765, 1996.
13. Osler W: The Principles and Practice of Medicine (4th ed). Edinburgh: Pentland, 1901.
14. Beasley R, Pearce N, Crane J: International trends in asthma mortality. *In* Chadwick DJ, Cardew G (eds): The Rising Trends in Asthma/Ciba Foundation Symposium 206. West Sussex, UK: John Wiley, 1997, pp 140–156.
15. Stolley PD: Why the United States was spared an epidemic of death due to asthma. Am Rev Respir Dis 105:883–890, 1972.
16. Pearce N, Beasley R, Crane J, et al: End of the New Zealand asthma mortality epidemic. Lancet 345:41–44, 1995.
17. Jackson RT, Sears MR, Beaglehole R, et al: International trends in asthma mortality: 1970–1985. Chest 94:914–918, 1988.
18. Weiss KB, Wagener DK: Changing patterns of asthma mortality: Identifying target populations at high risk. JAMA 264:1683–1687, 1990.
19. Evans R, Mullally DI, Wilson RW, et al: National trends in the morbidity and mortality of asthma in the US: Prevalence, hospitalization and death from asthma over two decades, 1965–1984. Chest 91:65S–74S, 1987.
20. Mitchell EA: International trends in hospital admission rates for asthma. Arch Dis Child 60:376–378, 1985.
21. Mannino DM, Brown C, Giovino GA: Obstructive lung disease deaths in the United Sates from 1979 through 1993: An analysis using multiple-cause mortality data. Am J Respir Crit Care Med 156:814–818, 1997.
22. Wennergren G, Kristjainsson S, Strannegard I-L: Decrease in hospitalization for treatment of childhood asthma with increased use of antiinflammatory treatment, despite an increase in the prevalence of asthma. J Allergy Clin Immunol 97:742–748, 1996.
23. Jarvis D, Lai E, Luczynska C, et al: Prevalence of asthma and asthmalike symptoms in young adults living in three East Anglian towns. Br J General Practice 44:493–497, 1994.
24. Robertson CF, Heycock E, Bishop J, et al: Prevalence of asthma in Melbourne school children: Changes over 26 years. BMJ 302:1116–1118, 1991.
25. Haahtela T, Lindholm H, Bjorksten F, et al: Prevalence of asthma in Finnish young men. BMJ 301:266–268, 1990.
26. Perdrizet S, Neukirch F, Cooreman J, et al: Prevalence of asthma in adolescents in various parts of France and its relationship to respiratory allergic manifestations. Chest 91:104S–106S, 1987.
27. Weitzman G, Gortmaker SL, Sobol AM, et al: Recent trends in the prevalence and severity of childhood asthma. JAMA 268:2673–2677, 1992.
28. Hsieh KH, Shen JJ: Prevalence of childhood asthma in Taipei, Taiwan, and other Asian Pacific countries. J Asthma 25:73–82, 1988.
29. Godfrey RC: Asthma and IgE levels in rural and urban communities of The Gambia. Clin Allergy 5:201–207, 1975.
30. Odhiambo JA, Ng'ang'a LW, Mungai MW, et al: Urban-rural differences in questionnaire-derived markers of asthma in Kenyan school children. Eur Respir J 12:1105–1112, 1998.
31. Ng'ang'a LW, Odhiambo JA, Mungai MW, et al: Prevalence of exercise induced bronchospasm in Kenyan school children: An urban-rural comparison. Thorax 53:919–926, 1998.
32. Waite DA, Eyles EF, Tonkin SL, et al: Asthma prevalence in Tokelauan children in two environments. Clin Allergy 10:71–75, 1980.
33. Peat JK, Van Den Berg RH, Green WF, et al: Changing prevalence of asthma in Australian children. Br Med J 308:1591–1596, 1994.
34. Yunginger JW, Reed CE, O'Connell EJ, et al: A community-based study of the epidemiology of asthma: Incidence rates, 1964–1983. Am Rev Respir Dis 146:888–894, 1992.
35. Schultz LF, Holm N, Henningsen K: Atopic dermatitis: A genetic-epidemiologic study in a population based twin sample. J Am Acad Dermatol 15:487–494, 1986.
36. Taylor B, Wadsworth M, Wadsworth J, et al: Changes in the reported prevalence of childhood eczema since the 1939–1945 war. Lancet 2:1255–1257, 1984.
37. Barbee RA, Kaltenborn W, Lebowitz MD, et al: Longitudinal changes in allergen skin test reactivity in a community population sample. J Allergy Clin Immunol 79:16–24, 1987.
38. Gassner M: Immunologische-allergologische reactionen unter veranderten unweltbedungingen. Schweitz Rundsch Med Prax 81:426–430, 1992.
39. Aberg N: Asthma and allergic rhinitis in Swedish conscripts. Clin Exp Allergy 19:59–63, 1989.
40. Rimpela AH, Savonius B, Rimpela MK, et al: Asthma and allergic rhinitis among Finnish adolescents in 1977–1991. Scand J Soc Med 23:60–65, 1995.
41. Lundback B: Epidemiology of rhinitis and asthma. Clin Exp Allergy 28(Suppl 2):3–10, 1998.
42. Peat JK, Gray EJ, Mellis CM, et al: Differences in airway responsiveness between children and adults living in the same environment: An epidemiological study in two regions of New South Wales. Eur Respir J 7:1805–1813, 1994.
43. Sunyer J, Anto JM, Kogevinas M, et al: Risk factors for asthma in young adults: Spanish group of the European community respiratory health survey. Eur Respir J 10:2490–2494, 1997.
44. Holgate ST, Ciba Foundation: The Rising Trends in Asthma. Ciba Foundation Symposium 206. West Sussex: John Wiley & Sons, 1997.
45. The International Study of Asthma and Allergies in Childhood Steering Committee: Worldwide variation in prevalence of symptoms of asthma, allergic rhinoconjunctivitis, and atopic eczema: ISAAC. Lancet 351:1225–1232, 1998.
46. Von Mutius E, Martinez FD, Fritzsch C, et al: Prevalence of asthma and atopy in two areas of West and East Germany. Am J Respir Crit Care Med 149:358–364, 1994.
47. Nicolai T, Von Mutius E: Pollution and the development of allergy: The East and West Germany story. Arch Toxicol Suppl 19:201–206, 1997.
48. Burney P, Chinn S, Luczynska C, et al: Variations in the prevalence of respiratory symptoms, self-reported asthma attacks, and use of asthma medication in the European community respiratory health survey (ECRHS). Eur Respir J 9:687–695, 1996.
49. Lewis S: Commentary: ISAAC—A hypothesis generator for asthma? Lancet 351:1220–1221, 1998.
50. Aberg N: Familial occurrence of atopic disease: Genetic vs. environmental factors. Clin Exp Allergy 23:829–834, 1993.
51. Aberg N, Sundell J, Eriksson B, et al: Prevalence of allergic diseases in schoolchildren in relation to family history, upper respiratory infections, and residential characteristics. Allergy 51:232–237, 1996.
52. Ronmark E, Lundback B, Jonsson EA, et al: Incidence of asthma in adults: Report from the obstructive lung disease in Northern Sweden study. Allergy 52:1071–1081, 1997.
53. Burrows B, Halonen M, Lebowitz MD, et al: The relationship of serum immunoglobulin E, allergy skin tests, and smoking to respiratory disorders. J Allergy Clin Immunol 70:199–204, 1982.
54. Burrows B, Martinez FD, Halonen M, et al: Association of asthma with serum IgE levels and skin-test reactivity to allergens. N Engl J Med 320:271–277, 1989.
55. Sears MR, Burrows B, Flannery EM, et al: Relation between airway responsiveness and serum IgE in children with asthma and in apparently normal children. N Engl J Med 325:1067–1071, 1991.
56. Sporik R, Holgate ST, Platts-Mills TAE, et al: Exposure to house-dust mite allergen (Der p1) and the development of asthma in childhood. N Engl J Med 323:502–507, 1990.
57. Sporik R, Chapman MD, Platts-Mills TAE: House dust mite exposure as a cause of asthma. Clin Exp Allergy 22:897–906, 1992.
58. Peat JK, Tovey E, Toelle BG, et al: House dust mite allergens: A major risk factor for childhood asthma in Australia. Am J Respir Crit Care Med 153:141–146, 1996.

59. Peat JK, Tovey E, Mellis CM, et al: Importance of house dust mite and Alternaria allergens in childhood asthma: An epidemiological study in two climatic regions of Australia. Clin Exp Allergy 23:812–820, 1993.
60. Platts-Mills TAE, Sporic R, Ingram JM, et al: Dog and cat allergens and asthma among school children in Los Alamos, New Mexico, USA, Altitude 7200 feet. Int Arch Allergy Immunol 107:301–313, 1995.
61. Kmietowicz Z: Cockroaches blamed for high asthma rates. Br Med J 314:1437, 1997.
62. Sears MR, Herbison GP, Holdaway MD, et al: The relative risks of sensitivity to grass pollen, house dust mite and cat dander in the development of childhood asthma. Clin Exp Allergy 19:419–424, 1989.
63. Weiss ST: Diet as a risk factor for asthma. Ciba Found Symp 206:244–257, 1997.
64. Kuczmarski RJ, Flegal KM, Campbell SM, et al: Increasing prevalence of overweight among US adults: The National Health and Nutrition Examination Surveys, 1960–1991. JAMA 272:205–211, 1994.
65. Chinn S, Rona RJ: Trends in weight-for-height and triceps skinfold thickness for English and Scottish children, 1972–1982 and 1982–1990. Paediatr Perinat Epidemiol 8:90–106, 1994.
66. Troiano RP, Flegal KM, Kuczmarski RJ, et al: Overweight prevalence and trends for children and adolescents: The National Health and Nutrition Examination Surveys, 1963–1991. Arch Pediatr Adolesc Med 149:1085–1091, 1995.
67. Huang S-L, Shiao G-M, Chou P: Association between body mass index and allergy in teenage girls in Taiwan. Clin Exp Allergy 29:323–329, 1998.
68. Camargo CA, Weiss ST, Zhang S, et al: Prospective study of body mass index and risk of adult-onset asthma. Am J Respir Crit Care Med 157(Suppl):A47, 1998.
69. Barbee RA, Murphy S: The natural history of asthma. J Allergy Clin Immunol 102:S65–S72, 1998.
70. Von Mutius E, Martinez FD, Fritzsch C, et al: Skin test reactivity and number of siblings. Br Med J 308:692–695, 1994.
71. Jarvis D, Chinn S, Luczynska C, et al: The association of family size with atopy and atopic disease. Clin Exp Allergy 27:240–245, 1997.
72. Hodge L, Salome CM, Peat JK, et al: Consumption of oily fish and childhood asthma risk. Med J Aust 164:137–140, 1996.
73. Peat JK, Li J: Reversing the trend: Reducing the prevalence of asthma. J Allergy Clin Immunol 103:1–10, 1999.
74. Pattemore PK, Johnston SL, Bardin PG: Viruses as precipitants of asthma symptoms: I. Epidemiology. Clin Exp Allergy 22:325–336, 1992.
75. Nicholson KG, Kent J, Ireland DC: Respiratory viruses and exacerbations of asthma in adults. Br Med J 307:982–996, 1993.
76. Weiss ST, Tager IB, Munoz A, et al: The relationship of respiratory infections in early childhood to the occurrence of increased levels of bronchial responsiveness and atopy. Am Rev Respir Dis 131:573–578, 1985.
77. Frick OL, German DF, Mills J: Development of allergy in children: I. Association with virus infections. J Allergy Clin Immunol 63:228–241, 1979.
78. Welliver RC, Wong DT, Sun M, et al: The development of respiratory syncytial virus-specific IgE and the release of histamine in nasopharyngeal secretions after infection. N Engl J Med 305:841–847, 1981.
79. Martinez FD, Wright AL, Taussig LM, et al: Asthma and wheezing in the first six years of life. N Engl J Med 332:133–138, 1995.
80. Warner JA, Miles EA, Jones AC, et al: Is deficiency of interferon gamma production by allergen triggered cord blood cells a predictor of atopic eczema? Clin Exp Allergy 24:423–430, 1994.
81. Martinez FD, Stern DA, Wright AL, et al: Differential immune responses to acute lower respiratory illness in early life and subsequent development of persistent wheezing and asthma. J Allergy Clin Immunol 102:915–920, 1998.
82. Holt PG: Environmental factors and primary T-cell sensitisation to inhalant allergens in infancy: Reappraisal of the role of infections and air pollution. Pediatr Allergy Immunol 6:1–10, 1995.
83. Holt PG, Yabuhara A, Prescott S, et al: Allergen recognition in the origin of asthma. *In* Chadwick DJ, Cardew G (eds): The Rising Trends in Asthma. Ciba Foundation Symposium 206. West Sussex, UK: John Wiley, 1997, pp 35–55.
84. Strachan DP, Harkins LS, Johnston ID, et al: Childhood antecedents of allergic sensitization in young British adults. J Allergy Clin Immunol 99:6–12, 1997.
85. Shaheen SO, Aaby P, Hall AJ, et al: Measles and atopy in Guinea-Bissau. Lancet 347:1792–1796, 1996.
86. Shirakawa T, Enomoto T, Shimazu S, et al: The inverse association between tuberculin responses and atopic disorder. Science 275:77–79, 1997.
87. Openshaw PJM, O'Donnell DR: Asthma and the common cold: Can viruses imitate worms? Thorax 49:101–103, 1994.
88. Hahn DL, Dodge RW, Golubjatnikov R: Association of *Chlamydia pneumoniae* (strain TWAR) infection with wheezing, asthmatic bronchitis, and adult-onset asthma. JAMA 266:225–230, 1991.
89. Emre U, Roblin PM, Gelling M, et al: The association of *Chlamydia pneumoniae* infection and reactive airway disease in children. Arch Pediatr Adolesc Med 148:727–732, 1994.
90. Cunningham AF, Johnston SL, Julious SA, et al: Chronic *Chlamydia pneumoniae* infection and asthma exacerbations in children. Eur Respir J 11:345–349, 1998.
91. Kraft M, Cassell GH, Henson JE, et al: Detection of *Mycoplasma pneumoniae* in the airways of adults with chronic asthma. Am J Respir Crit Care Med 158:998–1001, 1998.
92. McDonald DM: Experimental models of bronchial reactivity: Effect of airway infections. *In* Ogra PL, Mestecky J, Lamm ME, et al (eds): Mucosal Immunology (2nd ed). New York: Academic Press, 1998, pp 1177–1185.
93. Spector SL, Katz FH, Farr RS: Troleandomycin: Effectiveness in steroid-dependent asthma and bronchitis. J Allergy Clin Immunol 54:367–379, 1974.
94. Salter HH: On asthma: Its pathology and treatment. Philadelphia: Blanchard & Lea, 1864.
95. Sibbald B, Turner-Warwick M: Factors influencing the prevalence of asthma among first degree relatives of extrinsic and intrinsic asthmatics. Thorax 34:332–337, 1979.
96. Hopp RJ, Bewtra AK, Biven R, et al: Bronchial reactivity pattern in nonasthmatic parents of asthmatics. Ann Allergy 61:184–186, 1988.
97. Hopp RJ, Bewtra AK, Watt GD, et al: Genetic analysis of allergic disease in twins. J Allergy Clin Immunol 73:265–270, 1984.
98. Edfors-Lubs M-L: Allergy in 7000 twin pairs. Acta Allergol 26:249–285, 1971.
99. Duffy DL, Martin NG, Battistutta D, et al: Genetics of asthma and hay fever in Australian twins. Am Rev Respir Dis 142:1351–1358, 1990.
100. Ober C: Do genetics play a role in the pathogenesis of asthma? J Allergy Clin Immunol 101:S417–S420, 1998.
101. Hanson B, McGue M, Roitman-Johnson B, et al: Atopic disease and immunoglobulin E in twins reared apart and together. Am J Hum Genet 48:873–879, 1991.
102. Duffy DL, Mitchell CA: Lower respiratory tract symptoms in Queensland schoolchildren: Risk factors for wheeze, cough and diminished ventilatory function. Thorax 48:1021–1024, 1993.
103. Barbee RA, Lebowitz MD, Thompson HC, et al: Immediate skin-test reactivity in a general population sample. Ann Intern Med 84:129–133, 1976.
104. Barbee RA, Halonen M, Lebowitz M, et al: Distribution of IgE in a community population sample: Correlations with age, sex, and allergen skin test reactivity. J Allergy Clin Immunol 68:106–111, 1981.
105. Burrows B, Sears MR, Flannery EM, et al: Relationships of bronchial responsiveness assessed by methacholine to serum IgE, lung function, symptoms, and diagnoses in 11 year old New Zealand children. J Allergy Clin Immunol 90:376–385, 1992.
106. Konig P, Godfrey S: Exercise-induced bronchial liability in monozygotic and dizygotic twins. J Allergy Clin Immunol 54:280, 1974.
107. Townley RG, Bewtra AK, Nair NM, et al: Methacholine inhalation challenge studies. J Allergy Clin Immunol 64:569–574, 1979.
108. Ericsson CH, Svartengren M, Mossberg B, et al: Bronchial reactivity and allergy-promoting factors in monozygotic twins discordant for allergic rhinitis. Ann Allergy 67:53–59, 1991.

109. Daniels SE, Bhattacharrya S, James A, et al: A genome-wide search for quantitative trait loci underlying asthma. Nature 383:247–250, 1996.
110. The Collaborative Study on the Genetics of Asthma: A genome-wide search for asthma susceptibility loci in ethnically diverse populations: The Collaborative Study on the Genetics of Asthma. Nat Genet 15:389–392, 1997.
111. Ober C, Cox NJ, Abney M, et al: Genome-wide search for asthma susceptibility loci in a found population: The Collaborative Study on the Genetics of Asthma. Hum Mol Genet 7:1393–1398, 1998.
112. Young RP, Sharp PA, Lynch JR, et al: Confirmation of genetic linkage between atopic IgE responses and chromosome 11q13. J Med Genet 29:236–238, 1992.
113. Shirakawa T, Li A, Dubowitz M, et al: Association between atopy and variants of the beta-subunit of the high-affinity immunoglobulin E receptor. Nat Genet 7:125–130, 1994.
114. Marsh DG, Neely JD, Breazeale DR, et al: Linkage analysis of IL4 and other chromosome 5q31.1 markers and total serum immunoglobulin E concentrations. Science 264:1152–1156, 1994.
115. Meyers DA, Postma DS, Panhuysen CIM, et al: Evidence for a locus regulating total serum IgE levels mapping to chromosome 5. Genomics 23:464–470, 1994.
116. Thomas NS, Wilkinson J, Holgate ST: The candidate region approach to the genetics of asthma and allergy. Am J Respir Crit Care Med 156:S144–S151, 1997.
117. Liggett SB: Polymorphisms of the beta2-adrenergic receptor and asthma. Am J Respir Crit Care Med 156:S156–S162, 1997.
118. Drazen JM, Silverman EK: Genetic of asthma: Conference summary. Am J Respir Crit Care Med 156:S69–S71, 1997.
119. Jeffery PK, Wardlaw AJ, Nelson FC, et al: Bronchial biopsies in asthma: An ultrastructural quantitative study and correlation with hyperreactivity. Am Rev Respir Dis 140:1745–1753, 1989.
120. Soderberg M, Hellstrom S, Sandstrom T, et al: Structural characterization of bronchial biopsies from healthy volunteers: A light and microscopical study. Eur Respir J 3:261–266, 1990.
121. Lozewicz S, Wells C, Gomez E, et al: Morphological integrity of the bronchial epithelium in mild asthma. Thorax 45:12–15, 1990.
122. Boulet LP, Laviolette M, Turcotte H, et al: Bronchial subepithelial fibrosis correlates with airway responsiveness to methacholine. Chest 112:45–52, 1997.
123. Carroll N, Elliot J, Morton A, et al: The structure of large and small airways in nonfatal and fatal asthma. Am Rev Respir Dis 147:405–410, 1993.
124. Ordõnez CL, Ferrando RE, Hyde DM, et al: Denudation of the bronchial epithelium in mild and moderate asthma: Artifact or pathology? Am J Respir Crit Care Med 157:A503, 1998.
125. Cutz E, Levison H, Cooper DM: Ultrastructure of airways in children with asthma. Histopathology 2:407–421, 1978.
126. Aikawa T, Shimura S, Sasaki H, et al: Marked goblet cell hyperplasia with mucus accumulation in the airways of patients who died of severe acute asthma attack. Chest 101:916–921, 1992.
127. Shimura S, Andoh Y, Haraguchi M, et al: Continuity of airway goblet cells and intraluminal mucus in the airways of patients with bronchial asthma. Eur Respir J 9:1395–1401, 1996.
128. Ordõnez CL, Khasayar R, Ferrando RE, et al: Increased goblet cell mucin content in mild and moderate asthma. Am J Respir Crit Care Med 157:A392, 1998.
129. Djukanovic R, Wilson JW, Britten KM, et al: Quantitation of mast cells and eosinophils in the bronchial mucosa of symptomatic atopic asthmatics and healthy control subjects using immunohistochemistry. Am Rev Respir Dis 142:863–871, 1990.
130. Laitinen LA, Laitinen A, Haahtela T: Airway mucosal inflammation even in patients with newly diagnosed asthma. Am Rev Respir Dis 147:697–704, 1993.
131. Bousquet J, Chanez P, Lacoste JY, et al: Eosinophilic inflammation in asthma. N Engl J Med 323:1033–1039, 1990.
132. Riise GC, Andersson B, Ahlstedt S, et al: Bronchial brush biopsies for studies of epithelial inflammation in stable asthma and nonobstructive chronic bronchitis. Eur Respir J 9:1665–1671, 1996.
133. Pizzichini E, Pizzichini MMM, Efthimiadis A, et al: Measuring airway inflammation in asthma: Eosinophilia and eosinophil cationic protein in induced sputum compared with peripheral blood. J Allergy Clin Immunol 99:539–544, 1997.
134. Roche WR, Beasley R, Williams JH, et al: Subepithelial fibrosis in the bronchi of asthmatics. Lancet 1989:520–524, 1989.
135. Laitinen A, Altraja A, Kampe M, et al: Tenascin is increased in airway basement membrane of asthmatics and decreased by an inhaled steroid. Am J Respir Crit Care Med 156:951–958, 1997.
136. Brewster CEP, Howarth PH, Djukanovic R, et al: Myofibroblasts and subepithelial fibrosis in bronchial asthma. Am J Respir Cell Mol Biol 3:507–511, 1990.
137. Li X, Wilson JW: Increased vascularity of the bronchial mucosa in mild asthma. Am J Respir Crit Care Med 156:229–233, 1997.
138. Mitzner W, Wagner E, Brown RH: Is asthma a vascular disorder? Chest 107:97S–102S, 1995.
139. Laitinen LA, Laitinen A, Widdicombe JG: Effects of inflammatory and other mediators on airway vascular beds. Am Rev Respir Dis 135:S67–S70, 1987.
140. McDonald DM: Neurogenic inflammation in the respiratory tract: Actions of sensory nerve mediators on blood vessels and epithelium in the airway mucosa. Am Rev Respir Dis 136:S65–S72, 1987.
141. Dunnill MS, Massarella GR, Anderson JA: A comparison of the quantitative anatomy of the bronchi in normal subjects, in status asthmaticus, in chronic bronchitis, and in emphysema. Thorax 24:176–179, 1969.
142. Ebina M, Takahashi T, Chiba T, et al: Cellular hypertrophy and hyperplasia of airway smooth muscles underlying bronchial asthma. Am Rev Respir Dis 148:720–726, 1993.
143. Roche WR: Inflammatory and structural changes in the small airways in bronchial asthma. Am J Respir Crit Care Med 157:S191–S194, 1998.
144. Knox AJ: Airway remodeling in asthma: Role of airway smooth muscle. Clin Sci 86:647–652, 1994.
145. Heard BE, Hossain S: Hyperplasia of bronchial muscle in asthma. J Pathol 110:319–331, 1973.
146. Hossain S: Quantitative measurement of bronchial muscle in men with asthma. Am Rev Respir Dis 107:99–109, 1973.
147. Haraguchi M, Shimura S, Shirato K: Morphometric analysis of bronchial cartilage in chronic obstructive pulmonary disease and bronchial asthma. Am J Respir Crit Care Med 159:1005–1013, 1999.
148. Sakula A: Charcot-Leyden crystals and Curschmann spirals in asthmatic sputum. Thorax 41:503–507, 1986.
149. Weller PF, Goetzyl EJ, Austen KF: Identification of human eosinophil lysophospholipase as the constituent of Charcot Leyden crystals. Proc Natl Acad Sci U S A 77:440–443, 1980.
150. Fahy JV, Steiger DJ, Liu J, et al: Markers of mucus secretion and DNA levels in induced sputum from asthmatic and from healthy subjects. Am Rev Respir Dis 147:1132–1137, 1993.
151. Naylor B: The shedding of the mucosa of the bronchial tree in asthma. Thorax 17:69–72, 1962.
152. Fahy JV, Liu J, Wong H, et al: Cellular and biochemical analysis of induced sputum from asthmatic and from healthy subjects. Am Rev Respir Dis 147:1126–1131, 1993.
153. Smith DL, Deshazo RD: Bronchoalveolar lavage in asthma. Am Rev Respir Dis 143:523–532, 1993.
154. Huber HC, Koessler KK: The pathology of bronchial asthma. Arch Intern Med 30:689–760, 1922.
155. Houston JC, De Navasquez S, Trounce JR: A clinical and pathological study of fatal cases of status asthmaticus. Thorax 8:207–213, 1953.
156. Dunnill MS: The pathology of asthma with special reference to changes in the bronchial mucosa. J Clin Pathol 13:27–33, 1960.
157. Hamid Q, Song Y, Kotsimbos TC, et al: Inflammation of small airways in asthma. J Allergy Clin Immunol 100:44–51, 1997.
158. Kraft M, Djukanovic R, Wilson S, et al: Alveolar tissue inflammation in asthma. Am J Respir Crit Care Med 154:1505–1510, 1996.
159. Humbert M, Durham SR, Ying S, et al: IL-4 and IL-5 mRNA and protein in bronchial biopsies from patients with atopic and nonatopic asthma: Evidence against "intrinsic" asthma being a distinct immunopathologic entity. Am J Respir Crit Care Med 154:1497–1504, 1996.
160. Mattoli S, Mattoso VL, Soloperto M, et al: Cellular and biochemical characteristics of bronchoalveolar lavage fluid in symptomatic nonallergic asthma. J Allergy Clin Immunol 87:794–802, 1991.

161. Humbert M, Durham SR, Kimmitt P, et al: Elevated expression of messenger ribonucleic acid encoding IL-13 in the bronchial mucosa of atopic and nonatopic subjects with asthma. J Allergy Clin Immunol 99:657–665, 1997.
162. Kotsimbos TC, Ghaffar O, Minshall EM, et al: Expression of the IL-4 receptor alpha-subunit is increased in bronchial biopsy specimens from atopic and nonatopic subjects. J Allergy Clin Immunol 102:859–866, 1998.
163. Yasruel Z, Humbert M, Kotsimbos TC, et al: Membrane-bound and soluble αIL-5 receptor mRNA in the bronchial mucosa of atopic and nonatopic asthmatics. Am J Respir Crit Care Med 155:1413–1418, 1997.
164. Ying S, Humbert M, Barkans J, et al: Expression of IL-4 and IL-5 mRNA and protein product by $CD4^+$ and $CD8^+$ T cells, eosinophils, and mast cells in bronchial biopsies obtained from atopic and nonatopic (intrinsic) asthmatics. J Immunol 158:3539–3544, 1997.
165. Earle BV: Fatal bronchial asthma. Thorax 8:195–206, 1953.
166. Cardell BS, Pearson RSB: Death in asthmatics. Thorax 14:341–352, 1959.
167. Reid LM: The presence or absence of bronchial mucus in fatal asthma. J Allergy Clin Immunol 80:415–416, 1987.
168. Sur S, Crotty TB, Kephart GM, et al: Sudden-onset fatal asthma: A distinct entity with few eosinophils and relatively more neutrophils in the airway submucosa? Am Rev Respir Dis 148:713–719, 1993.
169. Carroll N, Carello S, Cooke C, et al: Airway structure and inflammatory cells in fatal attacks of asthma. Eur Respir J 9:709–715, 1996.
170. Kirby JG, Hargreave FE, Gleich GJ, et al: Bronchoalveolar cell profiles of asthmatic and non-asthmatic subjects. Am Rev Respir Dis 136:379–383, 1987.
171. Wardlaw AJ, Dunnette S, Gleich GJ, et al: Eosinophils and mast cells in bronchoalveolar lavage in subjects with mild asthma. Am Rev Respir Dis 137:62–69, 1988.
172. Lozewicz S, Gomez E, Ferguson H, et al: Inflammatory cells in the airways in mild asthma. Br Med J 297:1515–1516, 1988.
173. Beasley R, Roche WR, Roberts JA, et al: Cellular events in the bronchi in mild asthma and after bronchial provocation. Am Rev Respir Dis 139:806–817, 1989.
174. Kay AB: Pathology of mild, severe, and fatal asthma. Am J Respir Crit Care Med 154:S66–S69, 1996.
175. Claman D, Boushey HA, Liu J, et al: Analysis of induced sputum to examine the effects of prednisone on airway inflammation in asthmatic subjects. J Allergy Clin Immunol 94:861–869, 1994.
176. Minshall EM, Leung DYM, Martin RJ, et al: Eosinophil-associated TGF-β1 mRNA expression and airways fibrosis in bronchial asthma. Am J Respir Cell Mol Biol 17:326–333, 1997.
177. Grootendorst DC, van den Bos J-W, Romeijn JJ, et al: Induced sputum in adolescents with severe stable asthma: Safety and the relationship of cell counts and eosinophil cationic protein to clinical severity. Eur Respir J 13:647–653, 1999.
178. Foresi A, Leone C, Pelucchi A, et al: Eosinophils, mast cells, and basophils in induced sputum from patients with seasonal allergic rhinitis and perennial asthma: Relationship to methacholine responsiveness. J Allergy Clin Immunol 100:58–64, 1997.
179. Chetta A, Foresi A, Del Donno M, et al: Airways remodeling is a distinctive feature of asthma and is related to severity of disease. Chest 111:852–857, 1997.
180. Ollerenshaw SL, Woolcock AJ: Characteristics of the inflammation in biopsies from large airways of subjects with asthma and subjects with chronic airflow limitation. Am Rev Respir Dis 1992:922–927, 1992.
181. Lacoste JY, Bousquet J, Chanez P, et al: Eosinophilic and neutrophilic inflammation in asthma, chronic bronchitis, and chronic obstructive pulmonary disease. J Allergy Clin Immunol 92:537–548, 1993.
182. Saetta M, DiStefano A, Maestrelli P, et al: Airway eosinophilia and expression of IL-5 protein in asthma and in exacerbations of chronic bronchitis. Clin Exp Allergy 26:766–774, 1996.
183. Bradley BL, Azzawi M, Jacobson M, et al: Eosinophils, T-lymphocytes, mast cells, neutrophils, and macrophages in bronchial biopsy specimens from atopic subjects with asthma: Comparison with biopsy specimens from atopic subjects without asthma and normal control subjects and relationship to bronchial hyperresponsiveness. J Allergy Clin Immunol 88:661–674, 1991.
184. Kuwano K, Bosken CH, Pare PD, et al: Small airways dimensions in asthma and in chronic obstructive pulmonary disease. Am Rev Respir Dis 148:1220–1225, 1993.
185. Saetta M, Di Stefano A, Turato G, et al: $CD8^+$ T-lymphocytes in peripheral airways of smokers with chronic obstructive pulmonary disease. Am J Respir Crit Care Med 157:822–826, 1998.
186. McWilliam AS, Nelson DJ, Holt PG: The biology of airway dendritic cells. Immunol Cell Biol 73:405–413, 1995.
187. Lawrence M, Wolfe J, Webb DR, et al: Efficacy of inhaled fluticasone propionate in asthma results from topical and not from systemic activity. Am J Respir Crit Care Med 156:744–751, 1997.
188. McWilliam AS, Nelson D, Thomas JA, et al: Rapid dendritic cell recruitment is a hallmark of the acute inflammatory response at mucosal surfaces. J Exp Med 179:1331–1336, 1994.
189. Gong JL, McCarthy KM, Rogers RA, et al: Interstitial lung macrophages interact with dendritic cells to present antigenic peptides derived from particulate antigens to T cells. Immunology 81:343–351, 1994.
190. Schon-Hegrad MA, Oliver J, McMenamin PG, et al: Studies on the density, distribution, and surface phenotype of intraepithelial class II major histocompatibility complex antigen I(a)-bearing dendritic cells (DC) in the conducting airways. J Exp Med 173:1345–1356, 1991.
191. Moller GM, Overbeek SE, Van Helden-Meeuswsen CG, et al: Increased numbers of dendritic cells in the bronchial mucosa of atopic asthmatic patients: Downregulation by inhaled corticosteroids. Clin Exp Allergy 26:517–524, 1996.
192. Lambrecht BN, Salomon B, Klatzmann D, et al: Dendritic cells are required for the development of chronic eosinophilic airway inflammation in response to inhaled antigen in sensitized mice. J Immunol 160:4090–4097, 1998.
193. Dupuis M, McDonald DM: Dendritic-cell regulation of lung immunity. Am J Respir Cell Mol Biol 17:284–286, 1997.
194. Sousa CR, Hieny S, Scharton-Kersten T, et al: In vivo microbial stimulation induces rapid CD40 ligand-independent production of interleukin 12 by dendritic cells and their redistribution to T cell areas [see comments]. J Exp Med 186:1819–1829, 1997.
195. Kalinski P, Schuitemaker JH, Hilkens CM, et al: Prostaglandin E2 induces the final maturation of IL-12-deficient $CD1a^+CD83^+$ dendritic cells: The levels of IL-12 are determined during the final dendritic cell maturation and are resistant to further modulation. J Immunol 161:2804–2809, 1998.
196. Robinson DS, Hamid Q, Ying S, et al: Predominant TH2-like bronchoalveolar T-lymphocyte population in atopic asthma. N Engl J Med 326:298–304, 1992.
197. Hessel EM, Cruikshank WW, Van Ark I, et al: Involvement of IL-16 in the induction of airway hyper-responsiveness and up-regulation of IgE in a murine model of allergic asthma. J Immunol 160:2998–3005, 1998.
198. Corry DB, Grunig G, Hadeiba H, et al: Requirements for allergen-induced airway hyperreactivity in T and B cell-deficient mice. Mol Med 4:344–355, 1998.
199. Zuany-Amorim C, Ruffié C, Hailé S, et al: Requirement for gammadelta T cells in allergic airway inflammation. Science 280:1265–1267, 1998.
200. Hamelmann E, Oshiba A, Paluh J, et al: Requirement for $CD8^+$ T cells in the development of airway hyperresponsiveness in a murine model of airway sensitization. J Exp Med 183:1719–1729, 1996.
201. Coyle AJ, Erard F, Bertrand C, et al: Virus-specific $CD8^+$ cells can switch to interleukin 5 production and induce airway eosinophilia. J Exp Med 181:1229–1233, 1995.
202. Zurawski G, De Vries JE: Interleukin 13, an interleukin 4-like cytokine that acts on monocytes and B cells, but not on T cells. Immunol Today 15:19–26, 1994.
203. Grunig G, Warnock M, Wakil AE, et al: Requirement for IL-13 independently of IL-4 in experimental asthma. Science 282:2261–2263, 1998.
204. Wills-Karp M, Luyimbazi J, Xu X, et al: Interleukin-13: Central mediator of allergic asthma. Science 282:2258–2261, 1998.
205. Zurawski SM, Chomarat P, Djossou O, et al: The primary binding subunit of the human interleukin-4 receptor is also a component of the interleukin-13 receptor. J Biol Chem 270:13869–13878, 1995.

206. De Smedt T, Van Mechelen M, De Becker G, et al: Effect of interleukin-10 on dendritic cell maturation and function. Eur J Immunol 27:1229–1235, 1997.
207. Grunig G, Corry DB, Leach MW, et al: Interleukin-10 is a natural suppressor of cytokine production and inflammation in a murine model of allergic bronchopulmonary aspergillosis. J Exp Med 185:1089–1099, 1997.
208. Okamura H, Tsutsi H, Komatsu T, et al: Cloning of a new cytokine that induces IFN-gamma production by T cells. Nature 378:88–91, 1995.
209. Robinson D, Shibuya K, Mui A, et al: IGIF does not drive Th1 development but synergizes with IL-12 for interferon-gamma production and activates IRAK and NFkappaB. Immunity 7:571–581, 1997.
210. Gavett SH, O'Hearn DJ, Li X, et al: Interleukin 12 inhibits antigen-induced airway hyperresponsiveness, inflammation, and Th2 cytokine expression in mice. J Exp Med 182:1527–1536, 1995.
211. Kips JC, Brusselle GJ, Joos GF, et al: Interleukin-12 inhibits antigen-induced airway hyperresponsiveness in mice. Am J Respir Crit Care Med 153:535–539, 1996.
212. Hofstra CL, Van Ark I, Hofman G, et al: Differential effects of endogenous and exogenous interferon-gamma on immunoglobulin E, cellular infiltration, and airway responsiveness in a murine model of allergic asthma. Am J Respir Cell Mol Biol 19:826–835, 1998.
213. Hofstra CL, Van Ark I, Hofman G, et al: Prevention of Th2-like cell responses by coadministration of IL-12 and IL-18 is associated with inhibition of antigen-induced airway hyperresponsiveness, eosinophilia, and serum IgE levels. J Immunol 161:5054–5060, 1998.
214. Tang W, Geba GP, Zheng T, et al: Targeted expression of IL-11 in the murine airway causes lymphocytic inflammation, bronchial remodeling, and airways obstruction. J Clin Invest 98:2845–2853, 1996.
215. Lee JJ, McGarry MP, Farmer SC, et al: Interleukin-5 expression in the lung epithelium of transgenic mice leads to pulmonary changes pathognomonic of asthma. J Exp Med 185:2143–2156, 1997.
216. Rankin JA, Picarella DE, Geba GP, et al: Phenotypic and physiologic characterization of transgenic mice expressing interleukin 4 in the lung: Lymphocytic and eosinophilic inflammation without airway hyperreactivity. Proc Natl Acad Sci U S A 93:7821–7825, 1996.
217. Temann UA, Geba GP, Rankin JA, et al: Expression of interleukin 9 in the lungs of transgenic mice causes airway inflammation, mast cell hyperplasia, and bronchial hyperresponsiveness. J Exp Med 188:1307–1320, 1998.
218. Lei XF, Ohkawara Y, Stampfli MR, et al: Compartmentalized transgene expression of granulocyte-macrophage colony-stimulating factor (GM-CSF) in mouse lung enhances allergic airways inflammation. Clin Exp Immunol 113:157–165, 1998.
219. Zhou Z, Homer RJ, Wang Z, et al: Pulmonary expression of interleukin-13 causes inflammation, mucus hypersecretion, subepithelial fibrosis, physiologic abnormalities, and eotaxin production. J Clin Invest 103:779–788, 1999.
220. Tang W, Geba GP, Zheng T, et al: Targeted expression of IL-11 in the murine airway causes lymphocytic inflammation, bronchial remodeling, and airway obstruction. J Clin Invest 98:2845–2853, 1999.
221. Davies RJ, Devalia JL: Epithelial cells. Br Med Bull 48:85–96, 1992.
222. Campbell AM: Bronchial epithelial cells in asthma. Allergy 52:483–489, 1997.
223. Polito AJ, Proud D: Epithelial cells as regulators of airway inflammation. J Allergy Clin Immunol 102:714–718, 1998.
224. Li L, Xia Y, Nguyen A, et al: Effects of Th2 cytokines on chemokine expression in the lung: IL-13 potently induces eotaxin expression by airway epithelial cells. J Immunol 162:2477–2487, 1999.
225. Cocks TM, Fong B, Chow JM, et al: A protective role for protease-activated receptors in the airways. Nature 398:156–160, 1999.
226. Aubert JD, Dalal BI, Bai TR, et al: Transforming growth factor beta 1 gene expression in human airways. Thorax 49:225–232, 1994.
227. Bonfield TL, Konstan MW, Burfeind P, et al: Normal bronchial epithelial cells constitutively produce the anti-inflammatory cytokine interleukin-10, which is downregulated in cystic fibrosis. Am J Respir Cell Mol Biol 13:257–261, 1995.
228. Coyle AJ, Wagner K, Bertrand C, et al: Central role of immunoglobulin (Ig) E in the induction of lung eosinophil infiltration and T helper 2 cell cytokine production: Inhibition by a non-anaphylactogenic anti-IgE antibody. J Exp Med 183:1303–1310, 1996.
229. Fahy JV, Fleming HE, Wong HH, et al: The effect of an anti-IgE monoclonal antibody on the early- and late-phase responses to allergen inhalation in asthmatic subjects. Am J Respir Crit Care Med 155:1828–1834, 1997.
230. Boulet L-P, Chapman KR, Cote J, et al: Inhibitory effects of an anti-IgE antibody E25 on allergen-induced early asthmatic response. Am J Respir Crit Care Med 155:1835–1840, 1997.
231. Lack G, Oshiba A, Bradley KL, et al: Transfer of immediate hypersensitivity and airway hyperresponsiveness by IgE-positive B cells. Am J Respir Crit Care Med 152:1765–1773, 1995.
232. Oshiba A, Hamelmann E, Takeda K, et al: Passive transfer of immediate hypersensitivity and airway hyperresponsiveness by allergen-specific immunoglobulin (Ig) E and IgG1 in mice. J Clin Invest 97:1398–1408, 1996.
233. Korsgren M, Erjefalt JS, Korsgren O, et al: Allergic eosinophil-rich inflammation develops in lungs and airways of B cell-deficient mice. J Exp Med 185:885–892, 1997.
234. Hogan SP, Mould A, Kikutani H, et al: Aeroallergen-induced eosinophilic inflammation, lung damage, and airways hyperreactivity in mice can occur independently of IL-4 and allergen-specific immunoglobulins. J Clin Invest 99:1329–1339, 1997.
235. Kita H, Adolphonson CR, Gleich GJ: Biology of eosinophils. *In* Middleton E, Reed CE, Ellis EF, et al (eds): Allergy Principles and Practice (5th ed). St. Louis: Mosby, 1998, pp 242–260.
236. Busse WW, Sedgwick JB: Eosinophils in asthma. Ann Allergy 68:286–290, 1992.
237. Montefort S, Gratziou C, Goulding D, et al: Bronchial biopsy evidence for leukocyte infiltration and upregulation of leukocyte-endothelial cell adhesion molecules 6 hours after local allergen challenge of sensitized asthmatic airways. J Clin Invest 93:1411–1421, 1994.
238. Fahy JV, Liu J, Wong H, et al: Analysis of cellular and biochemical constituents of induced sputum after allergen challenge: A method for studying allergic airway inflammation. J Allergy Clin Immunol 93:1031–1039, 1994.
239. Wooley KL, Adelroth E, Wooley MJ, et al: Effects of allergen challenge on eosinophils, eosinophil cationic protein, and granulocyte-macrophage colony stimulating factor in mild asthma. Am J Respir Crit Care Med 151:1915–1924, 1995.
240. Kroegel C, Julius P, Matthys H, et al: Endobronchial secretion of interleukin-13 following local allergen challenge in atopic asthma: Relationship to interleukin-4 and eosinophil counts. Eur Respir J 9:899–904, 1996.
241. Cookson WOCM, Craddock CF, Benson MK, et al: Falls in peripheral eosinophil counts parallel the late asthmatic response. Am Rev Respir Dis 139:458–462, 1989.
242. O'Byrne PM, Dolovich J, Hargreave FE: State of art: Late asthmatic responses. Am Rev Respir Dis 136:740–751, 1987.
243. Gibson PG, Wong BJO, Hepperle MJE, et al: A research method to induce and examine a mild exacerbation of asthma by withdrawal of inhaled corticosteroid. Clin Exp Allergy 22:525–532, 1992.
244. Pizzichini MMM, Pizzichini E, Clelland L, et al: Prednisone-dependent asthma: Inflammatory indices in induced sputum. Eur Respir J 13:15–21, 1999.
245. Schleimer RP: Mechanisms of glucocorticoid actions in asthma. Insights in Allergy 7:1–8, 1992.
246. Barnes PJ: Inhaled glucocorticoids for asthma. N Engl J Med 332:868–875, 1995.
247. Foster PS, Hogan SP, Ramsay AJ, et al: Interleukin 5 deficiency abolishes eosinophilia, airways hyperreactivity, and lung damage in a mouse asthma model [see comments]. J Exp Med 183:195–201, 1996.
248. Mauser PJ, Pitman AM, Fernandez X, et al: Effects of an antibody to interleukin-5 in a monkey model of asthma. Am J Respir Crit Care Med 152:467–472, 1995.

249. Eum SY, Haile S, Lefort J, et al: Eosinophil recruitment into the respiratory epithelium following antigenic challenge in hyper-IgE mice is accompanied by interleukin 5-dependent bronchial hyperresponsiveness. Proc Natl Acad Sci U S A 92:12290–12294, 1995.
250. Mauser PJ, Pitman A, Witt A, et al: Inhibitory effect of the TRFK-5 anti-IL-5 antibody in a guinea pig model of asthma. Am Rev Respir Dis 148:1623–1627, 1993.
251. Schwarze J, Hamelmann E, Bradley KL, et al: Respiratory syncytial virus infection results in airway hyperresponsiveness and enhanced airway sensitization to allergen. J Clin Invest 100:226–233, 1997.
252. Lilly CM, Chapman RW, Sehring SJ, et al: Effects of interleukin 5-induced pulmonary eosinophilia on airway reactivity in the guinea pig. Am J Physiol 270:L368–L375, 1996.
253. Henderson WR, Chi EY, Albert RK, et al: Blockade of CD49d (alpha4 integrin) on intrapulmonary but not circulating leukocytes inhibits airway inflammation and hyperresponsiveness in a mouse model of asthma. J Clin Invest 100:3083–3092, 1997.
254. Tanaka H, Nagai H, Maeda Y: Effect of anti-IL-4 and anti-IL-5 antibodies on allergic airway hyperresponsiveness in mice. Life Sci 62:L169–L174, 1998.
255. Corry DB, Folkesson HG, Warnock ML, et al: Interleukin 4, but not interleukin 5 or eosinophils, is required in a murine model of acute airway hyperreactivity. J Exp Med 183:109–117, 1996.
256. Cuss FM: Therapeutic effects of antibodies to IL-5. Allergy 53:S89–S92, 1998.
257. Fahy JV, Kim KW, Liu J, et al: Prominent neutrophilic inflammation in sputum from subjects with asthma exacerbation. J Allergy Clin Immunol 95:843–852, 1995.
258. Lamblin C, Gosset P, Tillie-Leblond I, et al: Bronchial neutrophilia in patients with non-infectious status asthmaticus. Am J Respir Crit Care Med 157:394–402, 1998.
259. Sommerhoff CP, Nadel JA, Basbaum CB, et al: Neutrophil elastase and cathepsin G stimulate secretion from cultured bovine airway gland serous cells. J Clin Invest 85:682–689, 1990.
260. Nadel JA, Takeyama K, Agusti C: Role of neutrophil elastase in hypersecretion in asthma. Eur Respir J 13:190–196, 1999.
261. Timens W: Cell adhesion molecule expression and homing of hematologic malignancies. Crit Rev Oncol Hematol 19:111–129, 1995.
262. Pilewski JM, Albelda SM: Cell adhesion molecules in asthma: Homing, activation, and airway remodeling. Am J Respir Cell Mol Biol 12:1–3, 1995.
263. Lazaar AL, Albelda SM, Pilewski JM, et al: T lymphocytes adhere to airway smooth muscle cells via integrins and CD44 and induce smooth muscle cell DNA synthesis. J Exp Med 180:807–816, 1994.
264. Takeyama K, Agusti C, Ueki I, et al: Neutrophil-dependent goblet cell degranulation: Role of membrane-bound elastase and adhesion molecules. Am J Physiol (Lung Cell Mol Physiol) 275:L294–L302, 1998.
265. Unanue ER, Allen PM: The basis for the immunoregulatory role of macrophages and other accessory cells. Science 236:551–554, 1987.
266. Nathan CF: Secretory products of macrophages. J Clin Invest 79:319–326, 1987.
267. John M, Lim S, Sebold J, et al: Inhaled corticosteroids increase interleukin-10 but reduce macrophage inflammatory protein-1α, granulocyte-macrophage colony stimulating factor, and interferon-γ release from alveolar macrophages in asthma. Am J Respir Crit Care Med 157:256–262, 1998.
268. Viksman MY, Liu MC, Bickel CA, et al: Phenotypic analysis of alveolar macrophages and monocytes in allergic airway inflammation. Am J Respir Crit Care Med 155:858–863, 1997.
269. Agea E, Forenza N, Piattoni S, et al: Expression of B7 co-stimulatory molecules and CD1a antigen by alveolar macrophages in allergic bronchial asthma. Clin Exp Allergy 28:1359–1367, 1998.
270. Wenzel SE, Trudeau JB, Westcott JY, et al: Single dose of prednisone decreases leukotriene B4 production by alveolar macrophages from patients with nocturnal asthma but not control subjects: Relationship to changes in cellular influx and FEV1. J Allergy Clin Immunol 94:870–881, 1994.
271. Spiteri M, Knight RA, Jeremy JR, et al: Alveolar macrophage-induced suppression of T-cell hyperresponsiveness in bronchial asthma is reversed by allergen exposure. Eur Respir J 7:1431–1438, 1994.
272. Tang C, Rolland JM, Ward C, et al: Differential regulation of allergen-specific TH2- but not TH1-type responses by alveolar macrophages in atopic asthma. J Allergy Clin Immunol 102:368–375, 1998.
273. Holt PJ: Downregulation of immune responses in the lower respiratory tract: Role of alveolar macrophages. Clin Exp Immunol 63:261–270, 1985.
274. Poulter LW, Janossy G, Power C, et al: Immunological/physiological relationships in asthma: Potential regulation by lung macrophages. Immunol Today 15:258–261, 1994.
275. Thompson R, Bramley A, Schellenberg R: Airway smooth muscle stereology: Implications for increased shortening in asthma. Am J Respir Crit Care Med 154:749–757, 1996.
276. Stephens N, Li W, Wang Y, et al: The contractile apparatus of airway smooth muscle: Biophysics and biochemistry. Am J Respir Crit Care Med 158:S80–S94, 1998.
277. Seow C, Schellenberg R, Pare P: Structural and functional changes in the airway smooth muscle of asthmatic patients. Am J Respir Crit Care Med 158:S179–S186, 1998.
278. Johnson PR, Ammit AJ, Carlin SM, et al: Mast cell tryptase potentiates histamine-induced contraction in human sensitized bronchus. Eur Respir J 10:38–43, 1997.
279. James AL, Pare PD, Hogg JC: The mechanics of airway narrowing in asthma. Am Rev Respir Dis 139:242–246, 1989.
280. Bai T, Mak J, Barnes P: A comparison of beta-adrenergic receptors and in vitro relaxant responses to isoproterenol in asthmatic airway smooth muscle. Am J Respir Cell Mol Biol 6:647–651, 1993.
281. Hakonarson H, Herrick D, Gonzalez P, et al: Mechanism of cytokine-induced modulation of beta-adrenoreceptor responsiveness in airway smooth muscle. J Clin Invest 97:2593–2600, 1996.
282. Pannettieri R: Cellular and molecular mechanisms regulating airway smooth muscle proliferation and adhesion molecular expression. Am J Respir Crit Care Med 158:S133–S140, 1998.
283. Fahy JV: Airway mucus and the mucociliary system. *In* Middleton E, Reed CE, Ellis EF, et al (eds): Allergy Principles and Practice (5th ed). St. Louis: Mosby, 1998, pp 520–531.
284. Takeyama K, Dabbagh K, Lee HM, et al: Epidermal growth factor system regulates mucin production in airways. Proc Natl Acad Sci U S A 96:3081–3086, 1999.
285. Temann UA, Prasad B, Gallup MW, et al: A novel role for murine IL-4 in vivo: Induction of MUC5AC gene expression and mucin hypersecretion. Am J Respir Cell Mol Biol 16:471–478, 1997.
286. Rogers DF: Airway goblet cells: Responsive and adaptable frontline defenders. Eur Respir J 7:1690–1706, 1994.
287. Wanner A, Salathe M, O'Riordan TG: Mucociliary clearance in the airways. Am J Respir Crit Care Med 154:1868–1902, 1996.
288. Fahy JV, Kim KW, Liu J, et al: Prominent neutrophilic inflammation in sputum from subjects with asthma exacerbation. J Allergy Clin Immunol 95:843–852, 1995.
289. Brogan TD, Ryley HC, Neale L, et al: Soluble proteins of bronchopulmonary secretions from patients with cystic fibrosis, asthma, and bronchitis. Thorax 30:72–79, 1975.
290. List SJ, Findlay BP, Fornster GG, et al: Enhancement of the viscosity of mucin by serum albumin. Biochem J 175:565–571, 1978.
291. O'Riordan TG, Zwang J, Smaldone GC: Mucociliary clearance in adult asthma. Am Rev Respir Dis 146:598–603, 1992.
292. Dulfano MJ, Luk CK: Sputum and ciliary inhibition in asthma. Thorax 37:646–651, 1982.
293. Di Benedetto G: Lung mucociliary clearance and arachidonic acid metabolites. Prostaglandins Leukot Essent Fatty Acids 37:235–239, 1989.
294. Hastie AT, Loegering DA, Gleich GJ, et al: The effect of purified human eosinophil major basic protein on mammalian ciliary activity. Am Rev Respir Dis 135:848–853, 1987.
295. Amitani R, Wilson R, Rutman A, et al: Effects of human neutrophil elastase and *Pseudomonas aeruginosa* proteinases on human respiratory epithelium. Am J Respir Cell Mol Biol 4:26–32, 1991.
296. Perrin LF, Laurent PE. Asthma and neuropeptides. Eur J Med 2:164–169, 1993.

297. Barnes PJ: Neural mechanisms in asthma. Br Med Bull 48:149–168, 1992.
298. Barnes PJ: Neuropeptides as modulators of airway function. Agents Actions Suppl 31:175–196, 1990.
299. Liakakos P, Snell GI, Ward C, et al: Bronchial hyperresponsiveness in lung transplant recipients: Lack of correlation with airway inflammation. Thorax 52:551–556, 1997.
300. Herve P, Picard N, Le Roy Ladurie M, et al: Lack of bronchial hyperresponsiveness to methacholine and to isocapnic dry air hyperventilation in heart/lung and double-lung transplant recipients with normal lung histology: The Paris-Sud Lung Transplant Group. Am Rev Respir Dis 145:1503–1505, 1992.
301. Barnes PJ: Asthma as an axon reflex. Lancet 1:242–243, 1986.
302. Chung KF: Airway neuropeptides and neutral endopeptidase in asthma. Clin Exp Allergy 26:491–493, 1996.
303. Fahy JV, Wong HH, Geppetti P, et al: Effect of an NK-1 receptor antagonist (CP-99,994) on hypertonic saline-induced bronchoconstriction and cough in male asthmatic subjects. Am J Respir Crit Care Med 152:879–884, 1995.
304. Belvisi MG, Stretton CD, Yacoub M, et al: Nitric oxide is the endogenous neurotransmitter of bronchodilator nerves in humans. Eur J Pharmacol 210:221–222, 1992.
305. Crimi N, Palermo F, Oliveri R: Effect of nedocromil on bronchospasm induced by inhalation of substance P in asthmatic subjects. Clin Allergy 18:375–382, 1988.
306. Joos G, Pauwels R, Van Der Straeten M: The effect of inhaled substance P and neurokinin A on the airways of normal and asthmatic subjects. Thorax 42:779–783, 1987.
307. Nadel JA: Neutral endopeptidase modulates neurogenic inflammation. Eur Respir J 4:745–754, 1991.
308. Ichinose M, Nakajima N, Takahashi T, et al: Protection against bradykinin-induced bronchoconstriction in asthmatic subjects by neurokinin receptor antagonist. Lancet 340:1248–1251, 1992.
309. Diamant Z, Van Der Veen H, Kuipjers AP, et al: The effect of inhaled thiorphan on allergen-induced airway responses in asthmatic subjects. Clin Exp Allergy 26:525–532, 1996.
310. Lynch DA, Newell JD, Tschomper BA, et al: Uncomplicated asthma in adults: Comparison of CT appearance of the lungs in asthmatic and healthy subjects. Radiology 188:829–833, 1993.
311. Paganin F, Seneterre E, Chanez P, et al: Computed tomography of the lungs in asthma: Influence of disease severity and etiology. Am J Respir Crit Care Med 153:110–114, 1996.
312. Wiggs BR, Bosken C, Pare PD, et al: A model of airway narrowing in asthma and in chronic obstructive pulmonary disease. Am Rev Respir Dis 145:1251–1258, 1992.
313. Brown PJ, Greville HW, Finucane KE: Asthma and irreversible airflow obstruction. Thorax 39:131–136, 1984.
314. Nadel JA, Takeyama K: Mechanisms of hypersecretion in acute asthma, proposed cause of death, and novel therapy. Pediatr Pulmonol Suppl 18:54–55, 1999.
315. Vignola AM, Chiappara G, Chanez P, et al: Growth factors in asthma. Monaldi Arch Chest Dis 52:159–169, 1997.
316. Kumagai K, Ohno I, Okada S, et al: Inhibition of matrix metalloproteinases prevents allergen-induced airway inflammation in a murine model of asthma. J Immunol 162:4212–4219, 1999.
317. White E: Life, death, and the pursuit of apoptosis. Genes Dev 10:1–15, 1996.
318. Tesfaigzi J, Hotchkiss JA, Harkema JR: Expression of the Bcl-2 protein in nasal epithelia of F344/N rats during mucous cell metaplasia and remodeling. Am J Respir Cell Mol Biol 18:794–799, 1998.
319. Milik AM, Buechner-Maxwell VA, Sonstein J, et al: Lung lymphocyte elimination by apoptosis in the murine response to intratracheal particulate antigen. J Clin Invest 99:1082–1091, 1997.
320. Kessler G-F, Austin JHM, Graf PD, et al: Airway constriction in experimental asthma in dogs: Tantalum bronchographic studies. J Appl Physiol 35:703–708, 1973.
321. Permutt S: Physiologic changes in the acute asthmatic attack. *In* Austen KF, Lichtenstein LM (eds): Asthma: Physiology, Immunopharmacology, and Treatment. New York: Academic Press, 1973, pp 15–27.
322. McFadden ER: Pulmonary structure, physiology, and clinical correlates in asthma. *In* Middleton E, Reed C, Ellis E, et al (eds): Allergy: Principles and Practice. St. Louis: Mosby, 1993, pp 672–693.
323. Eidelman DH, Irvin CG: Airway mechanics in asthma. *In* Busse WW, Holgate ST (eds): Rhinitis and Asthma. Oxford: Blackwell Scientific Publications, 1995, pp 1033–1043.
324. Martin J, Powell E, Shore S, et al: The role of respiratory muscles in the hyperinflation of bronchial asthma. Am Rev Respir Dis 121:441–447, 1980.
325. Muller N, Bryan AC, Zamel N: Tonic inspiratory muscle activity as a cause of hyperinflation in histamine-induced asthma. J Appl Physiol 49:869, 1980.
326. Woolcock AJ, Read J: Improvement in bronchial asthma not reflected in forced expiratory volume. Lancet 2:1323–1325, 1965.
327. McFadden ER, Kiser R, DeGroot WJ: Acute bronchial asthma: Relations between clinical and physiologic manifestations. N Engl J Med 288:221–225, 1973.
328. McFadden ER, Lyons HA: Arterial blood gas tension in asthma. N Engl J Med 278:1027–1032, 1968.
329. Stanescu DC, Teculescu DB: Pulmonary function in status asthmaticus: Effect of therapy. Thorax 25:581, 1975.
330. Ferrer A, Roca J, Wagner PD, et al: Airway obstruction and ventilation-perfusion relationships in acute severe asthma. Am Rev Respir Dis 147:579, 1993.
331. American Thoracic Society: Standardization of spirometry: 1994 update. Am J Respir Crit Care Med 152:1107–1136, 1995.
332. Lahdensuo A, Haahtela T, Herrala J, et al: Randomised comparison of guided self management and traditional treatment of asthma over one year. BMJ 312:748–752, 1996.
333. Ryan G, Latimer KM, Dolovich J, et al: Bronchial responsiveness to histamine: Relationship to diurnal variation of peak flow rate, improvement after bronchodilator, and airway calibre. Thorax 37:423–429, 1982.
334. Ritchie B: A comparison of forced expiratory volume and peak flow in clinical practice. Lancet 2:271–273, 1962.
335. Meltzer AA, Smolensky MH, D'Alonzo GE, et al: An assessment of peak expiratory flow as a surrogate measurement of $FEV_1$ in stable asthmatic children. Chest 96:329–333, 1989.
336. American Thoracic Society: Lung function testing: Selection of reference values and interpretative strategies. Am Rev Respir Dis 144:1202–1216, 1991.
337. McFadden ER, Lyons HA: Serial studies of factors influencing airway dynamics during recovery from acute asthma attacks. J Appl Physiol 452–459, 1969.
338. McFadden ER, Linden DA: A reduction in maximum mid-expiratory flow rate: A spirographic manifestation of small airways disease. Am J Med 52:725–737, 1972.
339. Alberts WM, Ferris MC, Brook SM, et al: The FEF25-75 and the clinical diagnosis of asthma. Ann Allergy 73:221–225, 1994.
340. Mead J, Takishima T, Leith D: Stress distribution in lungs: A model of pulmonary elasticity. J Appl Physiol 28:596–608, 1970.
341. Ding DG, Martin JG, Macklem PT: Effects of lung volume on maximal methacholine-induced bronchoconstriction in normal humans. J Appl Physiol 62:1324–1330, 1987.
342. Orehek J, Gayrard P, Smith AP, et al: Airway response to carbachol in normal and asthmatic subjects. Am Rev Respir Dis 115:937–943, 1977.
343. Gold WM, Kaufman HA, Nadel JA: Elastic recoil of the lungs in chronic asthmatic patients before and after therapy. J Appl Physiol 23:433–438, 1967.
344. Brown R, Hoppin FG, Ingram RH, et al: Influence of abdominal gas on the Boyle's law determination of thoracic gas volume. J Appl Physiol 44:469, 1978.
345. Keens TG, Mansell A, Krastins IRB: Evaluation of the single breath diffusing capacity in asthma and cystic fibrosis. Chest 76:41–44, 1979.
346. Smith CM, Anderson SD: Inhalation provocation tests using nonisotonic aerosols. J Allergy Clin Immunol 84:781–790, 1989.
347. Polosa R, Ng WH, Crimi N, et al: Release of mast-cell-derived mediators after endobronchial adenosine challenge in asthma. Am J Respir Crit Care Med 151:624–629, 1995.
348. Taylor DA, Jensen MW, Aikman SL, et al: Comparison of salmeterol and albuterol-induced bronchoprotection against adenosine monophosphate and histamine in mild asthma. Am J Respir Crit Care Med 156:1731–1737, 1997.
349. Macklem PT: Mechanical factors determining maximum bronchoconstriction. Eur Respir J 2(Suppl 6):516s–519s, 1989.
350. Pliss LB, Ingenito EP, Ingram RH: Responsiveness, inflammation

and effects of deep breaths on obstruction in mild asthma. J Appl Physiol 66:2298–2304, 1989.
351. Skloot G, Permutt S, Togias A: Airway hyperresponsiveness in asthma: A problem of limited smooth muscle relaxation with inspiration. J Clin Invest 96:2393–2403, 1995.
352. Li JTC, O'Connell EJ: Clinical evaluation of asthma. Ann Allergy Asthma Immunol 76:1–14, 1996.
353. Turner-Warwick M: Epidemiology of nocturnal asthma. Am J Med 85(Suppl 1B):6–8, 1988.
354. McFadden ER, Gilbert IA: Medical progress: Asthma. N Engl J Med 327:1928–1937, 1992.
355. Elliott MW, Adams L, Cockcroft A: The language of breathlessness: Use of verbal descriptors by patients with cardiopulmonary disease. Am Rev Respir Dis 144:826–832, 1991.
356. Hardie GE, Janson S, Boushey HA, et al: Ethnic differences in the language of breathlessness used by African American and Caucasian asthmatics. Am J Respir Crit Care Med 157:A631, 1999.
357. McFadden ER: Exertional dyspnea and cough as preludes to acute attacks of bronchial asthma. N Engl J Med 292:555–559, 1975.
358. Glauser FL: Variant asthma. Ann Allergy 30:457, 1972.
359. Irwin RS, Corrao WM, Pratter MR: Chronic persistent cough in the adult: The spectrum and frequency of causes and successful outcome of specific therapy. Am Rev Respir Dis 123:413, 1981.
360. Holinger LD: Chronic cough in infants and children. Laryngoscope 96:316, 1986.
361. Hannaway PJ, Hopper DK: Cough variant asthma in children. JAMA 247:206–208, 1982.
362. Ellul-Micallef R: Effect of terbutaline sulphate in chronic "allergic" cough. Br Med J 287:940, 1983.
363. Johnson D, Osborn LM: Cough variant asthma: A review of the clinical literature. J Asthma 28:85–90, 1991.
364. Konig P: Hidden asthma in childhood. Am J Dis Child 135:1053–1055, 1981.
365. Glynn AA, Michaels L: Bronchial biopsy in chronic bronchitis and asthma. Thorax 15:142–153, 1960.
366. Shimura S, Sasaki T, Sasaki H, et al: Chemical properties of bronchorrhea sputum in bronchial asthma. Chest 94:1211–1215, 1988.
367. Gibson PG, Girgis-Gabardo A, Morris MM, et al: Cellular characteristics of sputum from patients with asthma and chronic bronchitis. Thorax 44:689–692, 1989.
368. Burrows B: Allergy and the development of asthma and bronchial hyperresponsiveness. Clin Exp Allergy 25(Suppl 2):15–16, 1995.
369. Burrows B, Martinez FD, Cline MG, et al: The relationship between parental and children's serum IgE and asthma. Am J Respir Crit Care Med 152:1497–1500, 1995.
370. National Asthma Education and Prevention Program [NAEPP]. Clinical Practice Guidelines. Expert Panel Report 2: Guidelines for the diagnosis and management of asthma. NIH Publication No. 97-4051. Bethesda, MD: National Institutes of Health/National Heart Lung and Blood Institutes, July, 1997.
371. Benatar SR: Medical progress: Fatal asthma. N Engl J Med 314:423–429, 1986.
372. Sampson HA, Mendelson L, Rosen JP: Fatal and near-fatal anaphylactic reactions to food in children and adolescents. N Engl J Med 327:380–384, 1992.
373. Kemp SF, Lockey RF, Wolf BL, et al: Anaphylaxis: A review of 266 cases. Arch Intern Med 155:1749–1754, 1995.
374. Samter M, Beers RF: Intolerance to aspirin: Clinical studies and consideration of its pathogenesis. Ann Intern Med 68:975–983, 1968.
375. Stevenson DD, Mathison DA: Aspirin sensitivity in asthmatics: When may this drug be safe? Postgrad Med 78:111–117, 1985.
376. Baker GJ, Collette P, Allen DH: Bronchospasm induced by metabisulfite-containing foods and drugs. Med J Aust 2:614, 1981.
377. Marini JJ, Pierson DJ, Hudson LD, et al: The significance of wheezing in chronic airflow obstruction. Am Rev Respir Dis 120:1069–1072, 1979.
378. Holleman DR, Simel DL: Does the clinical examination predict airflow limitation? JAMA 273:313–319, 1995.
379. Bianco S, Robuschi M, Petrigni G: Aspirin sensitivity in asthmatics. Br Med J 282:146, 1981.
380. Lumry WR, Curd JG, Zeiger RS: Aspirin sensitive rhinosinusitis: The clinical syndrome and effects of aspirin administration. J Allergy Clin Immunol 71:588, 1983.
381. Slavin RG: Asthma and sinusitis. J Allergy Clin Immunol 90:534–537, 1992.
382. Gardner RM, Baker CD, Broennle AMJ, et al: ATS Statement—Snowbird workshop on standardization of spirometry. Am Rev Respir Dis 119:831–838, 1979.
383. Crapo RO, Morris AH, Gardner RM: Reference spirometric values using techniques and equipment that meet ATS recommendations. Am Rev Respir Dis 123:659–694, 1981.
384. National Asthma Education and Prevention Program [NAEPP]. Clinical Practice Guidelines: Expert Panel Report 2: Guidelines for the diagnosis and management of asthma. NIH Publication No. 91-4051. Bethesda, MD: National Institutes of Health/National Heart Lung and Blood Institutes, April, 1991.
385. Miller D, Hyatt E: Evaluation of obstructing lesions of the trachea and larynx by flow-volume loops. Am Rev Respir Dis 108:475–481, 1973.
386. Shim C, Corro P, Park SS, et al: Pulmonary function studies in patients with upper airway obstruction. Am Rev Respir Dis 106:233–238, 1972.
387. Ramsdale EH, Roberts RS, Morris MM, et al: Differences in responsiveness to hyperventilation and methacholine in asthma and chronic bronchitis. Thorax 40:422–426, 1985.
388. Townley RG, Ryo UY, Kolotkin BM, et al: Bronchial sensitivity to methacholine in current and former asthmatic and allergic rhinitis patients and control subjects. J Allergy Clin Immunol 56:429–442, 1975.
389. Zhong MS, Chen RC, Yang MO: Is asymptomatic bronchial hyperresponsiveness an indication of potential asthma? Chest 102:1104–1109, 1992.
390. Greenberger PA: Allergic bronchopulmonary aspergillosis. J Allergy Clin Immunol 74:645, 1984.
391. Pin I, Gibson PG, Kolendowicz R, et al: Use of induced sputum cell counts to investigate airway inflammation in asthma. Thorax 47:25–29, 1992.
392. Wong HH, Fahy JV: Safety of one method of sputum induction in asthmatic subjects. Am J Respir Crit Care Med 156:299–303, 1997.
393. Djukanovic R, Lai CKW, Wilson JW, et al: Bronchial mucosal manifestations of atopy: A comparison of markers of inflammation between atopic asthmatics, atopic nonasthmatics and healthy controls. Eur Respir J 5:538–544, 1992.
394. Hansel TT, Braunstein JB, Walker C, et al: Sputum eosinophils from asthmatics express ICAM-1 and HLA-DR. Clin Exp Immunol 86:271–277, 1991.
395. Gelder CM, Thomas PS, Yates DH, et al: Cytokine expression in normal, atopic, and asthmatic subjects using the combination of sputum induction and the polymerase chain reaction. Thorax 50:1033–1037, 1995.
396. Gibson PG, Dolovich J, Denburg J, et al: Chronic cough: Eosinophilic bronchitis without asthma. Lancet 1:1346–1348, 1989.
397. Turner MO, Hussack P, Sears MR, et al: Exacerbations of asthma without sputum eosinophilia. Thorax 50:1057–1061, 1995.
398. Pizzichini E, Pizzichini MM, Gibson P, et al: Sputum eosinophilia predicts benefit from prednisone in smokers with chronic obstructive bronchitis. Am J Respir Crit Care Med 158:1511–1517, 1998.
399. Backman KS, Greenberger PA, Patterson R: Airways obstruction in patients with long-term asthma consistent with "irreversible asthma." Chest 112:1234–1240, 1997.
400. Lange P, Parner J, Vestbo J, et al: A 15-year follow-up study of ventilatory function in adults with asthma. N Engl J Med 339:1194–1200, 1998.
401. Snider GL, Faling LJ, Rennard SI: Chronic bronchitis and emphysema. *In* Murray JF, Nadel JA (eds): Textbook of Respiratory Medicine (2nd ed). Philadelphia: WB Saunders, 1994, pp 1331–1397.
402. Dosman JA, Gomez SR, Zhou C: Relationship between airways responsiveness and the development of chronic obstructive pulmonary disease. Med Clin North Am 74:561–569, 1990.
403. Callahan CM, Dittus RS, Katz BP: Oral corticosteroid therapy for patients with stable chronic obstructive pulmonary disease: A meta-analaysis. Ann Intern Med 114:216–223, 1991.

404. Tenholder MF, Moser RJ, Koval JC: The flow volume loop in upper airway obstruction masquerading as asthma. Immunol Allergy Prac 9:33–43, 1987.
405. Christopher KL, Wood RP, Eckert RC, et al: Vocal cord dysfunction presenting as asthma. N Engl J Med 308:1566–1570, 1983.
406. Rodenstein DO, Francis C, Stanescu DC: Emotional laryngeal wheezing: A new syndrome. Am Rev Respir Dis 127:354–356, 1983.
407. Remirez RJ, Leon I, Rivera LM: Episodic laryngeal dyskinesia: Clinical and psychiatric characterization. Chest 90:716–721, 1986.
408. Newman KB, Mason UG, Schmaling KB: Clinical features of vocal cord dysfunction. Am J Respir Crit Care Med 152:1382–1386, 1995.
409. Wood RP, Jafek BW, Cherniack RM: Laryngeal dysfunction and pulmonary disorder. Otolaryngol Head Neck Surg 94:374–378, 1986.
410. Selner JC, Staudenmeyer H, Koepke JW, et al: Vocal cord dysfunction: The importance of psychologic factors and provocation challenge testing. J Allergy Clin Immunol 79:726–733, 1987.
411. Freedman MR, Rosenberg SJ, Schmaling KB: Childhood sexual abuse in patients with paradoxical vocal cord dysfunction. J Nerv Ment Dis 179:295–298, 1991.
412. Pitchenik AE: Functional laryngeal obstruction relieved by panting. Chest 100:1465–1467, 1991.
413. Horan RF, Austen KF: Systemic mastocytosis: Retrospective review of a decade's clinical experience at the Brigham and Women's Hospital. J Invest Dermatol 96:5S, 1991.
414. Sheffer AL, Soter NA, McFadden ER, et al: Exercise-induced anaphylaxis: A distinct form of physical allergy. J Allergy Clin Immunol 71:311–316, 1983.
415. Schwartz LB, Metcalfe DD, Miller JS: Tryptase levels as an indicator of mast-cell activation in systemic anaphylaxis and mastocytosis. N Engl J Med 316:1622, 1987.
416. Creutzfeldt W, Stockmann F: Carcinoids and carcinoid syndrome. Am J Med 82:4, 1987.
417. Lynch JP, Flint A: Sorting out the pulmonary eosinophilic syndromes. J Respir Dis 5:61, 1984.
418. Banerjee D, Lee G, Malik S: Underdiagnosis of asthma in the elderly. Br J Dis Chest 81:23–29, 1987.
419. Dow L: The diagnosis of asthma in older people. Clin Exp Allergy 24:156–159, 1994.
420. Weiss KB, Gergen PJ, Wagener DK: Breathing better or wheezing worse? The changing epidemiology of asthma morbidity and mortality. Annu Rev Public Health 14:491–513, 1993.
421. Burrows B, Lebowitz M, Barbee R: Findings before diagnoses of asthma among the elderly in a longitudinal study of a general population sample. J Allergy Clin Immunol 88:870–877, 1991.
422. Burrows B, Barbee R, Cline M: Characteristics of asthma among elderly adults in a sample of the general population. Chest 100:935–941, 1991.
423. Braman SS, Kaemmerlen JT, Davis SM: Asthma in the elderly: A comparison between patients with recently acquired and long-standing disease. Am Rev Respir Dis 143:336–340, 1991.
424. Sherman CB: Late-onset asthma: Making the diagnosis, choosing drug therapy. Geriatrics 50:24–33, 1995.
425. Barnes PJ: Poorly perceived asthma. Thorax 47:408–409, 1992.
426. Boulet L-P, Deschesnes F, Turcotte H, et al: Near fatal asthma: Clinical and physiologic features, perception of bronchoconstriction, and psychologic profile. J Allergy Clin Immunol 88:838–846, 1991.
427. Kikuchi Y, Okabe S, Tamura G, et al: Chemosensitivity and perception of dyspnea in patients with a history of near-fatal asthma. N Engl J Med 330:1329–1334, 1994.
428. Demeter SL, Cordasco EM: Hyperventilation syndrome and asthma. Am J Med 81:989–994, 1986.
429. Newman LS: Occupational asthma: Diagnosis, management, and prevention. Clin Chest Med 16:621–636, 1995.
430. Lane SJ, Lee TH: Mechanism and detection of glucocorticoid insensitivity in asthma. Allergy Clin Immunol Int 9:165–173, 1997.
431. Holgate ST, Boushey HA, Fabbri LM (eds): Difficult Asthma. London: England: Martin Dunitz, 1999.
432. Abisheganaden JA, Boushey HA: Difficult asthma: The dimensions of the problem. *In* Holgate ST, Boushey HA, Fabbri LM (eds): Difficult Asthma. London, UK: Martin Dunitz, 1999, pp 1–11.
433. Brooks SM, Weiss MA, Bernstein IL: Reactive airways dysfunction syndrome (RADS): Persistent asthma syndrome after high level irritant exposures. Chest 88:376–384, 1985.
434. Rackermann FM: A clinical study of one hundred and fifty cases of bronchial asthma. Arch Intern Med 22:517–552, 1918.
435. Deal EC, McFadden ER, Ingram RH, et al: Role of respiratory heat exchange in production of exercise-induced asthma. J Appl Physiol 46:467–475, 1979.
436. Anderson SD, Schoeffel RE, Black JL, et al: Airway cooling as the stimulus to exercise-induced asthma: Re-evaluation. Eur J Respir Dis 67:20–30, 1985.
437. Smith CM, Anderson SD: Hyperosmolarity as the stimulus to asthma induced by hyperventilation? J Allergy Clin Immunol 77:729–736, 1986.
438. Robertson CF, Rubinfeld AR, Bowes G: Deaths from asthma in Victoria: A 12-month survey. Med J Aust 152:511–517, 1990.
439. Martin RJ, Cicutto LC, Ballard RD, et al: Airways inflammation in nocturnal asthma. Am Rev Respir Dis 143:351–357, 1991.
440. Sluiter HJ, Koeter GH, De Monchy JGR, et al: The Dutch hypothesis (chronic non-specific lung disease) revisited. Eur Respir J 4:479–489, 1991.
441. Greenberger PA, Patterson R: Diagnosis and management of allergic bronchopulmonary aspergillosis. Ann Allergy 56:444–452, 1986.
442. Neeld DA, Goodman LR, Gurney JW, et al: Computerized tomography in the evaluation of ABPA. Am Rev Respir Dis 142:1200–1205, 1990.
443. Sporik R, Holgate ST, Cogswell JJ: Natural history of asthma in childhood: A birth cohort study. Arch Dis Child 66:1050–1053, 1991.
444. Strachan DP, Butland BK, Anderson HR: Incidence and prognosis of asthma and wheezing illness from early childhood to age 33 in a national British cohort. Br Med J 312:1195–1199, 1996.
445. Roorda RJ, Gerritsen J, Van Aalderen WMC, et al: Follow-up of asthma from childhood to adulthood: Influence of potential childhood risk factors on the outcome of pulmonary function and bronchial responsivness in adulthood. J Allergy Clin Immunol 93:575–584, 1994.
446. Blair H: Natural history of childhood asthma. Arch Dis Child 52:613–619, 1977.
447. Martin AJ, McLennan LA, Landau LI, et al: The natural history of childhood asthma to adult life. Br Med J 280:1397–1400, 1980.
448. Kelly WJW, Hudson I, Phelan PD, et al: Childhood asthma in adult life: A further study at 28 years of age. Br Med J 294:1059–1062, 1987.
449. McNicol KN, Williams HB: Spectrum of asthma in children: I. Clinical and physiological components. Br Med J 4:7–11, 1973.
450. Godden DJ, Ross S, Abdalla M, et al: Outcome of wheeze in childhood: Symptoms and pulmonary function 25 years later. Am J Respir Crit Care Med 149:106–112, 1994.
451. Schachter EN, Doyle CA, Beck GJ: A prospective study of asthma in a rural community. Chest 85:623–630, 1984.
452. Bronnimann S, Burrows B: A prospective study of the natural history of asthma: Remission and relapse rates. Chest 90:480–484, 1986.
453. Panhuysen CIM, Vonk JM, Koeter GH, et al: Adult patients may outgrow their asthma: A 25-year follow-up study. Am J Respir Crit Care Med 155:1267–1272, 1997.
454. Greenberger PA, Patterson R: The diagnosis of potentially fatal asthma. N Engl Reg Allergy Proc 9:147–152, 1988.
455. Miller TP, Greenberger PA, Patterson R: The diagnosis of potentially fatal asthma in hospitalized adults: Patient characteristics and increased severity of asthma. Chest 102:515–518, 1992.
456. LeSon S, Gershwin ME: Risk factors for asthmatic patients requiring intubation: III. Observations in young adults. J Asthma 33:27–35, 1996.
457. Sears MR, Rea HH, Beaglehole R, et al: Asthma mortality in New Zealand: A two year national study. N Z Med J 98:271–275, 1985.
458. Robertson CF, Rubinfeld AR, Bowes G: Pediatric asthma deaths in Victoria: The mild are at risk. Pediatr Pulmonol 13:95–100, 1992.
459. Ferrer A, Torres A, Roca J, et al: Characteristics of patients with soybean dust-induced acute severe asthma requiring mechanical ventilation. Eur Respir J 3:429–433, 1990.

460. Ordman D: An outbreak of bronchial asthma in South Africa, affecting more than 200 persons, caused by castor bean dust from an oil-processing factory. Int Arch Allergy 7:10–24, 1955.
461. Packe GE, Ayres JG: Asthma outbreak during a thunderstorm. Lancet 2:199–204, 1985.
462. Ulrik CS, Frederiksen J: Mortality and markers of risk of asthma death among 1075 outpatients with asthma. Chest 108:10–15, 1995.
463. Boushey HA. Relationship of asthma severity to fatalities. *In* Sheffer AL (ed): Fatal Asthma, Lung Biology in Health and Disease. New York: Marcel Dekker, 1998, pp 363–385.
464. Weiss KB, Gergen PJ, Hodgson TA: An economic evaluation of asthma in the United States. N Engl J Med 326:862–866, 1992.
465. Smith DH, Malone DC, Lawson KA, et al: A national estimate of the economic costs of asthma. Am J Respir Crit Care Med 156:787–793, 1997.
466. Li D, German D, Lulla S, et al: Prospective study of hospitalization for asthma: A preliminary risk factor model. Am J Respir Crit Care Med 151:647–655, 1995.
467. Peat JK, Woolcock AJ, Cullen K: Rate of decline of lung function in subjects with asthma. Eur J Respir Dis 70:171–179, 1987.
468. Juniper EF, Kline PA, Vanzieleghem MA, et al: Reduction of budesonide after a year of increased use: A randomized controlled trial to evaluate whether improvements in airway responsiveness and clinical asthma are maintained. J Allergy Clin Immunol 87:483–489, 1991.
469. Haahtela T, Jarvinen M, Kava T, et al: Effects of reducing or discontinuing inhaled budesonide in patients with mild asthma. N Engl J Med 331:700–705, 1994.
470. Van Essen-Zandvliet EE, Hughes MD, Waalkens HJ, et al: Remission of childhood asthma after long-term treatment with an inhaled corticosteroid (budesonide): Can it be achieved? Eur Respir J 7:63–68, 1994.
471. Waalkens HJ, Van Essen-Zandvliet EE, Hughes MD, et al: Cessation of long-term treatment with inhaled corticosteroid (budesonide) in children with asthma results in deterioration. Am Rev Respir Dis 148:1252–1257, 1993.
472. Boushey HA: Effects of inhaled corticosteroids on the consequences of asthma. J Allergy Clin Immunol 102:S5–S16, 1998.
473. Rea HH, Scragg R, Jackson R, et al: A case-control study of deaths from asthma. Thorax 41:833–839, 1986.
474. Crane J, Pearce N, Burgess C, et al: Markers of risk of asthma death or readmission in the 12 months following a hospital admission for asthma. Int J Epidemiol 21:737–744, 1992.
475. Hetzel MR, Clark TJH, Branthwaite MA: Asthma: Analysis of sudden deaths and ventilatory arrests in hospital. Br Med J 1:808–811, 1977.
476. Bateman JRM, Clarke SW: Sudden death in asthma. Thorax 34:40–44, 1979.
477. Drazen JM, Boushey HA, Holgate ST, et al: The pathogenesis of severe asthma: A consensus report from the workshop on pathogenesis. J Allergy Clin Immunol 80:428–437, 1987.
478. Matsuse H, Shimoda T, Kohno S, et al: A clinical study of mortality due to asthma. Ann Allergy Asthma Immunol 75:267–272, 1995.
479. Ruffin RE, Latimer KM, Schembri DA: Longitudinal study of near fatal asthma. Chest 99:77–83, 1991.
480. Donahue JG, Weiss ST, Livingston JM, et al: Inhaled corticosteroids and the risk of hospitalization for asthma. JAMA 277:887–891, 1997.
481. Pauwels RA, Lofdahl C-G, Postma DS, et al: Effect of inhaled formoterol and budesonide on exacerbations of asthma. N Engl J Med 337:1405–1411, 1997.
482. Malmstrom K, Rodriguez-Gomez G, Guerra J, et al: Oral montelukast, inhaled beclomethasone, and placebo for chronic asthma: A randomized, controlled trial. Montelukast/Beclomethasone Study Group. Ann Intern Med 130:487–495, 1999.
483. Suissa S, Dennis R, Ernst P, et al: Effectiveness of the leukotriene receptor antagonist zafirlukast for mild-to-moderate asthma: A randomized, double-blind, placebo-controlled trial. Ann Intern Med 126:177–183, 1997.
484. Vignola AM, Chanez P, Campbell AM, et al: Airway inflammation in mild intermittent and in persistent asthma. Am J Respir Crit Care Med 157:403–409, 1998.
485. Agertoft L, Pedersen S: Effects of long-term treatment with an inhaled corticosteroid on growth and pulmonary function in asthmatic children. Respir Med 88:373–381, 1994.
486. Haahtela T, Jarvinen M, Kava T, et al: Comparison of a $\beta_2$-agonist, terbutaline, with an inhaled corticosteroid, budesonide, in newly detected asthma. N Engl J Med 325:388–392, 1991.
487. Jaakkola MS, Jaakkola JJK, Ernst P, et al: Respiratory symptoms in young adults should not be overlooked. Am Rev Respir Dis 147:359–366, 1993.
488. WHO Workshop Report. National Heart Lung and Blood Institutes: Global initiative for asthma: Global strategy for asthma management and prevention NHLBI/WHO workshop report, March 1993. NIH Publication No. 95-3659. Bethesda, MD: National Institutes of Health/National Heart Lung and Blood Institutes, 1995.
489. British Guidelines on Asthma Management, 1995: Review and position statement. Thorax 52(Suppl 1):S1–S21, 1997.
490. US Dept. of Health and Human Services. Centers for Disease Control. Data from the National Health Survey, no. 193. DHHS no. (PHS) 96–1521.
491. Johnston SL, Pattemore PK, Sanderson G, et al: Community study of the role of viral infections in exacerbations of asthma in 9- to 11-year-old children. BMJ 310:1225–1229, 1995.
492. Taylor DR, Sears MR, Herbison GP, et al: Regular inhaled beta-agonists in asthma: Effects on exacerbations and lung function. Thorax 48:134–138, 1993.
493. Rebuck AS, Read J: Assessment and management of severe asthma. Am J Med 51:788–798, 1971.
494. Brenner BE, Abraham E, Simon RR: Position and diaphoresis in acute asthma. Am J Med 74:1005–1009, 1983.
495. Mountain RD, Heffner JE, Brackett NC, et al: Acid-base disturbances in acute asthma. Chest 98:651–655, 1990.
496. Schuh S, Johnson DW, Callahan S, et al: Efficacy of frequent nebulized ipratropium bromide added to frequent high-dose albuterol therapy in severe childhood asthma. J Pediatr 126:639–645, 1995.
497. Reisman J, Galdes-Sebalt M, Kazim F, et al: Frequent administration by inhalation of salbutamol and ipratropium bromide in the initial management of severe acute asthma in children. J Allergy Clin Immunol 81:16–20, 1988.
498. O'Driscoll BRC, Ruffles SP, Ayres JG, et al: Long term treatment of severe asthma with subcutaneous terbutaline. Br J Dis Chest 82:360–367, 1988.
499. Connett GJ, Warde C, Wooler E, et al: Prednisolone and salbutamol in the hospital treatment of acute asthma. Arch Dis Child 70:170–173, 1994.
500. Rowe BH, Keller JL, Oxman AD: Effectiveness of steroid therapy in acute exacerbations of asthma: A meta-analysis. Am J Emerg Med 10:301–310, 1992.
501. Singh NP, Despars JA, Stansbury DW, et al: Effects of buspirone on anxiety levels and exercise tolerance in patients with chronic airflow obstruction and mild anxiety. Chest 103:800–804, 1993.
502. Fanta CH, Rossing TH, McFadden ER: Treatment of acute asthma: Is combination therapy with sympathomimetics and methylxanthines indicated? Am J Med 80:5–10, 1986.
503. Rossing TH, Fanta CH, Goldstein DH, et al: Emergency therapy of asthma: Comparison of the acute effects of parenteral and inhaled sympathomimetics and infused aminophylline. Am Rev Respir Dis 122:365–371, 1980.
504. Murphy DG, McDermott MF, Rydman RJ, et al: Aminophylline in the treatment of acute asthma when $\beta_2$-adrenergics and steroids are provided. Arch Intern Med 153:1784–1788, 1993.
505. Corbridge TC, Hall JB: The assessment and management of adults with status asthmaticus. Am J Respir Crit Care Med 151:1296–1316, 1995.
506. Douglass JA, Tuxen DV, Horne M, et al: Myopathy in severe asthma. Am J Respir Dis 146:517–519, 1992.
507. Manthous CA, Hall JB, Caputo MA, et al: Heliox improves pulsus paradoxus and peak expiratory flow in nonintubated patients with severe asthma. Am J Respir Crit Care Med 151:310–314, 1995.
508. Gluck EH, Onorato DJ, Castriotta R: Helium-oxygen mixtures in intubated patients with status asthmaticus and respiratory acidosis. Chest 98:693–698, 1990.
509. Kass JE, Castriotta RJ: Heliox therapy in acute severe asthma. Chest 107:757–760, 1995.

510. Kuitert LM, Kletchko SL: Intravenous magnesium sulfate in acute, life-threatening asthma. Ann Emerg Med 20:1243–1245, 1991.
511. Skorodin MS, Tenholder MF, Yetter B, et al: Magnesium sulfate in exacerbations of chronic obstructive pulmonary disease. Arch Intern Med 155:496–500, 1995.
512. Bloch H, Silverman R, Mancherje N, et al: Intravenous magnesium sulfate as an adjunct in the treatment of acute asthma. Chest 107:1576–1581, 1995.
513. Greening AP, Ind PW, Northfield M, et al: Added salmeterol versus higher-dose corticosteroid in asthma patients with symptoms on existing inhaled corticosteroid. Lancet 344:219–224, 1994.
514. Woolcock A, Lundback B, Ringdal N, et al: Comparison of addition of salmeterol to inhaled steroids with doubling of the dose of inhaled steroids. Am J Respir Crit Care Med 153:1481–1488, 1996.
515. Woolcock AJ: Steroid resistant asthma: What is the clinical definition? Eur Respir J 6:743–747, 1993.
516. Auerbach I, Springer C, Godfrey S: Total population survey of the frequency and severity of asthma in 17 year old boys in an urban area in Israel. Thorax 48:139–141, 1993.
517. Rand CS, Wise RA, Nides M, et al: Metered-dose inhaler adherence in a clinical trial. Am Rev Respir Dis 146:1559–1564, 1992.
518. Harding SM, Richter JE: The role of gastroesophageal reflux in chronic cough and asthma. Chest 111:1389–1402, 1997.
519. Alexander AG, Barnes NC, Kay AB: Trial of cyclosporin A in corticosteroid-dependent chronic severe asthma [see comments]. Lancet 339:324–328, 1992.
520. Borish L, Aarons A, Rumbyrt J, et al: Interleukin-10 regulation in normal subjects and patients with asthma. J Allergy Clin Immunol 97:1288–1296, 1996.
521. Postma DS, Bleecker ER, Amelung PJ, et al: Genetic susceptibility to asthma: Bronchial hyperresponsiveness coinherited with a major gene for atopy. N Engl J Med 333:894–900, 1995.
522. Doull IJ, Lawrence S, Watson M, et al: Allelic association of gene markers on chromosomes 5q and 11q with atopy and bronchial hyperresponsiveness. Am J Respir Crit Care Med 153:1280–1284, 1996.
523. Hopes E, McDougall C, Christie G, et al: Association of glutamine 27 polymorphism of beta 2 adrenoceptor with reported childhood asthma: Population based study. BMJ 316:664, 1998.
524. Moffatt MF, Cookson WO: Tumour necrosis factor haplotypes and asthma. Hum Mol Genet 6:551–554, 1997.
525. Young RP, Dekker JW, Wordsworth BP, et al: HLA-DR and HLA-DP genotypes and immunoglobulin E responses to common major allergens. Clin Exp Allergy 24:431–439, 1994.
526. Cookson WOCM, Sharp PA, Faux JA, et al: Linkage between immunoglobulin E responses underlying asthma and rhinitis and chromosome 11q. Lancet 1:1292–1295, 1989.
527. Shirakawa T, Hashimoto T, Furuyama J, et al: Linkage between severe atopy and chromosome 11q13 in Japanese families. Clin Genet 46:228–232, 1994.
528. Van Herwerden L, Harrap SB, Wong ZYH, et al: Linkage of high-affinity IgE receptor gene with bronchial hyperreactivity, even in absence of atopy. Lancet 346:1262–1265, 1995.
529. Barnes KC, Neely JD, Duffy DL, et al: Linkage of asthma and total serum IgE concentration to markers on chromosome 12q: Evidence from Afro-Caribbean and Caucasian populations. Genomics 37:41–50, 1996.
530. Moffatt MF, Hill MR, Cornelis F, et al: Genetic linkage of T-cell receptor alpha/delta complex to specific IgE responses. Lancet 343:1597–1600, 1994.
531. Mitsuyasu H, Izuhara K, Mao XQ, et al: Ile50Val variant of IL4R alpha upregulates IgE synthesis and associates with atopic asthma. Nat Genet 19:119–120, 1998.
532. Hershey GK, Friedrich MF, Esswein LA, et al: The association of atopy with a gain-of-function mutation in the alpha subunit of the interleukin-4 receptor. N Engl J Med 337:1720–1725, 1997.
533. De Sanctis GT, Merchant M, Beier DR, et al: Quantitative locus analysis of airway hyperresponsiveness in A/J and C57BL/6J mice. Nat Genet 11:150–154, 1995.
534. Ewart SL, Mitzner W, DiSilvestre DA, et al: Airway hyperresponsiveness to acetylcholine: Segregation analysis and evidence for linkage to murine chromosome 6. Am J Respir Cell Mol Biol 14:487–495, 1996.
535. Redington AE, Howarth PH: Airway wall remodeling in asthma. Thorax 52:310–312, 1997.
536. Wilson JW: What causes airway remodeling in asthma? Clin Exp Allergy 28:534–536, 1998.

# 40 Cystic Fibrosis

R. C. BOUCHER, M.D. • M. R. KNOWLES, M.D.
J. R. YANKASKAS, M.D.

Introduction
Historical Perspectives
Epidemiology
Genetic Basis
Pathology
- Lung Pathology
- Other Respiratory Tract Pathology
- Nonrespiratory Pathologic Features

Pathophysiology
- CFTR Protein: Structure, Metabolism, and Function
- Abnormal Airway Mucosal Physiology
- Ion Transport
- Macromolecule Secretion
- Pathophysiology of Infection

Clinical Manifestations
- Lower Respiratory Tract Disease
- Upper Respiratory Tract Disease
- Complications of Respiratory Tract Disease
- Gastrointestinal Manifestations
- Pancreatic Disease
- Hepatobiliary Disease
- Genitourinary Tract Abnormalities
- Sweat Gland Dysfunction

Diagnosis
Treatment
- Ambulatory Care
- Hospital Therapy

Course of the Disease and Prognosis
Summary

## INTRODUCTION

Cystic fibrosis (CF) is a multisystem disorder affecting children and, increasingly, adults.[1] CF is characterized chiefly by chronic airway obstruction and infection and by exocrine pancreatic insufficiency with its effects on gastrointestinal function, nutrition, growth, and maturation. This condition is the most common life-threatening genetic trait in the white population.[2] Numerous mutations of a single gene are responsible for the CF syndrome and for variations in its severity. The gene encodes a membrane protein called the *cystic fibrosis transmembrane regulator* (CFTR). CFTR functions in many tissues as a kinase-regulated $Cl^-$ channel. In some tissues, CFTR also regulates the activity of other ion channels. Typically, mutations in CFTR affect both of these functions.

CF is an important medical problem for a number of reasons. It is the major source of severe chronic lung disease in children, and it has become an important cause of morbidity and mortality from chronic lung disease in young adults. CF is responsible for most cases of exocrine pancreatic insufficiency in childhood and early adulthood and for many cases of nasal polyposis, pansinusitis, rectal prolapse, nonketotic insulin-dependent hyperglycemia, and biliary cirrhosis in these age groups. Therefore, CF enters into the differential diagnosis for many pediatric and young adult patients. Finally, research advances have introduced the challenge of designing pharmacologic and gene transfer therapies to combat the broad range of manifestations and complications.

Central to CF diagnosis and care is a carefully integrated and closely monitored network of approximately 115 referral centers in the United States, sponsored by the Cystic Fibrosis Foundation. The Foundation also supports a smaller number of multidisciplinary research centers aimed at elucidating the molecular pathophysiology and improving the quality of life for patients with CF. Similar care and research centers are found in Canada and in many European countries.

## HISTORICAL PERSPECTIVES

CF was first described as a distinct clinical entity in the late 1930s. Numerous references to infants and children with meconium ileus and characteristic pancreatic and lung diseases are, however, sprinkled throughout the literature as early as 1650. Of interest are references in European folklore to the association of salty skin and early demise.[3] Dorothy Andersen, a pathologist at Babies Hospital in New York City, is usually credited with having written the first comprehensive description of CF in 1938.[4] She coined the term *cystic fibrosis of the pancreas.* In 1945, Farber[5] suggested that CF is a disease of exocrine glands, characterized largely by failure to clear their mucous secretory product. He introduced the term *mucoviscidosis,* which was used for a number of years.

Chronic infection of the lungs was recognized early as a major contributing factor, and antibiotics were first used for the treatment of CF in the 1940s. At the same time, an autosomal-recessive inheritance pattern for CF was suggested by Andersen and Hodges.[6] In 1953, di Sant'Agnese and colleagues[7] investigated salt depletion in children with CF during a summertime heat wave and concluded that excessive loss of salt occurred via the sweat. Subsequently, they documented that sodium and chloride levels in sweat are elevated in virtually all persons (more than 98%) with CF. This observation led to a description by Gibson and Cooke[8] of the pilocarpine iontophoresis method for sweat testing, a method that remains the diagnostic standard to this day. By the late 1950s, CF was reported occasionally in older children and in young adults. Soon thereafter, comprehensive and aggressive approaches to the care of patients were instituted in many treatment centers, and these approaches have been credited with the survival into adulthood of a steadily increasing number of patients with CF. In the past 40 years, a markedly refined description of the CF syndrome and the many related complications has emerged.

Several observations have resulted in a partial understanding of CF pathogenesis at the molecular level. In the early 1980s, epithelial physiologists described abnormalities of both sodium and chloride transport by CF respiratory epithelia[9] and chloride impermeability of sweat gland ducts from patients with CF.[10] These observations focused attention on a pathogenetic role for abnormal electrolyte and water movement across CF epithelia. From 1985 to 1987, geneticists, using restriction fragment-length polymorphism analysis, located the CFTR gene on the long arm of chromosome 7.[11–14] Shortly thereafter, the CFTR gene was isolated, cloned, sequenced,[15] and the major mutation of this gene was characterized.[16] Transfer of a wild-type (normal) gene into CF cells corrected the chloride transport defect.[17, 18] The product of the CF gene, CFTR, was studied and found to be both a $Cl^-$ channel[19–21] and a regulator of other channels.[22, 23] Studies of the metabolism of CFTR suggested that mutations could lead to abnormal folding and mislocation of the protein.[24–26] Knockout of the CFTR gene in transgenic mice has provided an animal model that possesses several physiologic and clinical similarities to human CF.[27–30] These observations provided a detailed understanding of CFTR structure and function and have laid the groundwork for development of more specific therapeutic interventions, including gene therapy.

## EPIDEMIOLOGY

CF is recognized in approximately 1:2500 and 1:17,000 live births in white[31] and black[32] populations, respectively, in the United States. The range of reported incidence figures worldwide varies from 1:569 in a confined Ohio Amish population[33] to 1:90,000 in an Asian population of Hawaii.[34]

Generally, mutations of the CF gene are most prevalent in northern and central Europeans and in persons who derive from these areas. An intermediate incidence is likely, although less well documented in non-European whites. CF is considered rare in Native Americans, Asian populations, and black natives of Africa. It has been suggested that the relatively low frequency in populations living in tropical and semitropical geographic locations is related to adverse consequences in the past from excessive salt loss in heterozygotes as well as homozygotes for the CF gene. In white populations, 2% to 5% are carriers of a CF gene mutation. These people have no clinical stigmas of CF. Although a number of chemical or physiologic alterations have been described in heterozygotes, these alterations can be identified only on a statistical basis.

## GENETIC BASIS

CF is an autosomal recessive trait, resulting from mutations at a single gene locus on the long arm of chromosome 7.[2, 31] This locus spans approximately 250 kb of DNA, contains at least 27 exons, and codes for a large protein that has several transmembrane domains, two cytoplasmic nucleotide (ATP)–binding folds, and numerous phosphorylation sites contained in a cytoplasmic regulatory (R) domain (Fig. 40.1). The primary and secondary structures of the protein product of the CF gene resemble those of other membrane proteins that act as pumps (e.g., the ATP-binding cassette transporters).[15]

The predominant CFTR mutation is a 3 basepair deletion that eliminates the phenylanine of CFTR at position 508, the so-called ΔF508 mutation.[16] This deletion has been detected in 66% of more than 20,000 CF patients' chromosomes analyzed worldwide,[2, 31, 35] but its prevalence varies considerably from population to population (Table 40.1). In general, ΔF508 is more prevalent in Northern than Southern European or Middle Eastern populations.[31] More than 850 other mutations of the CF gene have been reported but all at a relatively low frequency. The occurrence of known mutations accounts for only 90% of all CF gene abnormalities.[31] CFTR mutations include other deletions, missense mutations, nonsense mutations, frameshift mutations, and introductions of new splice sites.[31]

Correlations between genotype and phenotype are beginning to emerge. For example, homozygosity for the ΔF508 mutation almost always confers exocrine pancreatic insufficiency.[32] A severe phenotype, including meconium ileus and liver disease, is strongly associated with the presence of two "severe" (i.e., pancreatic exocrine insufficiency) alleles.[36–38] A region on human chromosome 19q13 has recently been identified as a modifier locus for meconium ileus.[39] Conflicting data exist on whether ΔF508 homozygosity versus other severe alleles is associated with a more severe form of chronic lung disease.[33] In contrast, "mild" mutations (i.e., preservation of pancreatic exocrine function) have been identified that are associated with normal concentrations of sweat chloride, exocrine pancreatic sufficiency, or both.[40] In summary, it is now clear that CF is indeed a syndrome caused by many combinations of mutations at a single gene locus, each of which may confer a slightly different phenotype. The ultimate phenotype of each person with CF is undoubtedly also influenced by genetic background

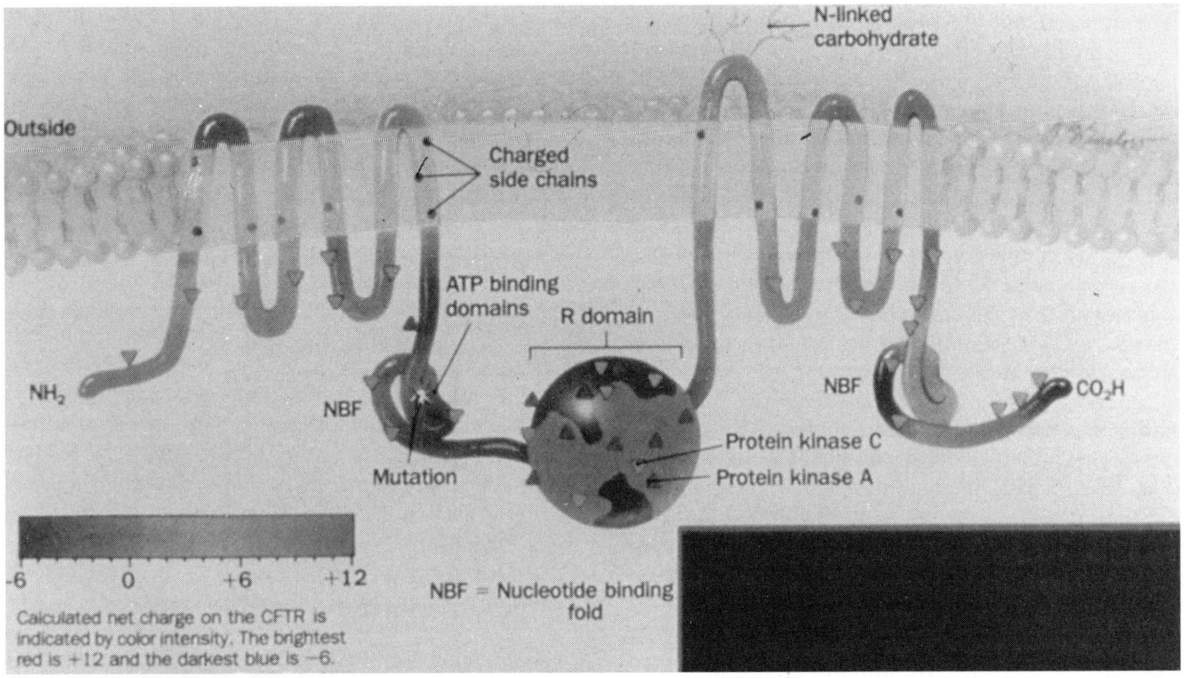


**Figure 40.1** A proposed structure for the cystic fibrosis transmembrane regulator (CFTR) protein is shown. Two repeat segments each consist of six transmembrane spans followed by a nucleotide-binding fold (NBF). The segments are joined by a highly charged region that contains multiple phosphorylation sites, the R domain. Much of the CFTR is intracytoplasmic. Glycosylation occurs on an extracellular loop of the second motif.

(i.e., "modifier genes") as well as by postnatal environmental factors.

Deoxyribonucleic acid (DNA) analysis can now be used to confirm the diagnosis, make prenatal diagnoses, and screen for carrier status in selected cases. For example, probes for 28 of the most common CF mutations in North Carolina provided definitive diagnostic information in less than 90% of persons with CF. Screening for CF carriers with the ΔF508 probe identifies only 50% to 60% of couples at risk of having a CF child.[41]

The high frequency of CF gene mutations in many populations has been ascribed to an unknown heterozygote advantage. Some evidence suggests a reproductive advantage for the carrier state.[42, 43] Others have postulated that reduced capacity to generate a secretory diarrhea in response to cholera infection, because of diminished intestinal chloride transport, may have provided an historical survival advantage to heterozygotes.[44–46]

**Table 40.1** FREQUENCY OF THE ΔF508 MUTATION*

| Population | Cystic Fibrosis Chromosomes (%) |
|---|---|
| North America, Caucasians | 76 |
| North America, Hispanics | 46 |
| United Kingdom | 74 |
| Spain | 49 |
| Italy | 43 |
| Ashkenazi Jews | 30 |

*Reproduced with permission from Leinna WK, Feldman GL, Kerem B, et al: Mutation analysis for heterozygote detection and the prenatal diagnosis of cystic fibrosis. N Engl J Med 322:291–296, 1990.

## PATHOLOGY

Soon after the original description of the CF syndrome, Farber[5] pointed out the prominent accumulation of mucus in the respiratory and gastrointestinal tracts. Subsequently, mucus stasis has been described in numerous sites, including the conducting airways of the lung,[47] paranasal sinuses, mucus-secreting salivary glands, apocrine sweat glands, small intestine, appendix, pancreas, biliary system, uterine cervix, and wolffian duct structures. The eccrine sweat gland, however, which figures prominently in the pathophysiology of CF, is morphologically normal at all ages. Pathologic changes in the lung, which is the primary site of organ dysfunction, also reflect chronic infection.

### Lung Pathology

It is clear that disease of the conducting airways in CF is acquired postnatally. The airways of children with CF who have died within the first days of life display only subtle abnormalities. The earliest macroscopic pathologic lesion is reported to be mucous obstruction of bronchioles.[47] The numbers and distribution of mucus-producing goblet cells and the numbers and sizes of submucosal glands, however, appear to be within normal ranges at birth. A careful morphometric analysis of CF airways early in life demonstrated dilation of submucosal gland acinar and ductal lumens before reaction to chronic infection would be expected.[48] This finding suggests that either hypersecretion or, more likely, failure to clear secretions at an early age accounts for mucus accumulation in bronchial regions, whereas the mucus retention in bronchioles presumably reflects the failure to clear mucus secreted by surface secretory (goblet) cells. Failure to clear secretions from the airway lumens probably initiates infection.

With the progression of lung disease, evidence for bronchiolitis and bronchitis becomes more prominent, the submucosal glands hypertrophy, and goblet cells not only become more numerous but also propagate into the bronchioles. Small airways may be completely obstructed by secretions (Fig. 40.2).[49] Bronchiolectasis and then bronchiectasis are consequences of persistent obstruction-infection cycles. Bronchiectasis had been thought to be manifest in the second decade of life, but now it is being detected earlier in life with increased use of computed tomographic (CT) scans. Pneumonia, when present, generally assumes a peribronchial pattern.

Detailed pathologic descriptions of lung disease are based on examination of lungs at autopsy and reflect advanced changes.[50, 51] Bronchiectatic cysts occupy as much as 50% of the cross-sectional area of the late-stage CF lung.[52] In general, bronchiectasis is more severe in upper than in lower lobes. In addition to dilatation of the small airways, bronchioles may be stenotic or even obliterated. The extent of obliterative bronchiolitis appears to be directly correlated with age at death.[51] Autopsied lungs also show extensive overinflation of air spaces. Small amounts of destructive emphysema are seen in many patients, especially those who have lived for two or three decades.[51] Absence of more extensive alveolar wall destruction can be explained by the confinement of chronic infection to conducting airways.

Several patterns of interstitial pneumonia have also been described in autopsied lungs, including usual interstitial pneumonitis, interstitial pneumonitis with organizing pneumonia, and diffuse alveolar damage.[53] Fibrosis is extensive in peribronchiolar and peribronchial regions and may contribute to the restrictive lung function pattern that is superimposed on obstruction in end-stage lung disease.[54] Subpleural cysts often occur on the mediastinal surfaces of the upper lobes and are thought to be related to the frequent occurrence of pneumothorax in patients with advanced lung disease.[55] The bronchial arteries become large and tortuous,[56] contributing to a propensity for hemoptysis in ectatic airways. The pulmonary arteries display varying degrees of change reflecting pulmonary hypertension.

## Other Respiratory Tract Pathology

Hypertrophy and hyperplasia of secretory elements, mucus accumulation, and chronic inflammatory changes are also features of the paranasal sinuses and the nasal passages. A common feature of nasal pathology is inflammatory edema of the mucosa with subsequent pedunculation and formation of polyps.[57]

## Nonrespiratory Pathologic Features

Most of the nonpulmonary pathology in CF occurs in the gastrointestinal tract and related organs. Striking changes are seen in the exocrine pancreas.[58] Obstruction of ducts by inspissated secretions is an early feature, followed by dilatation of the secretory ducts and acini and flattening

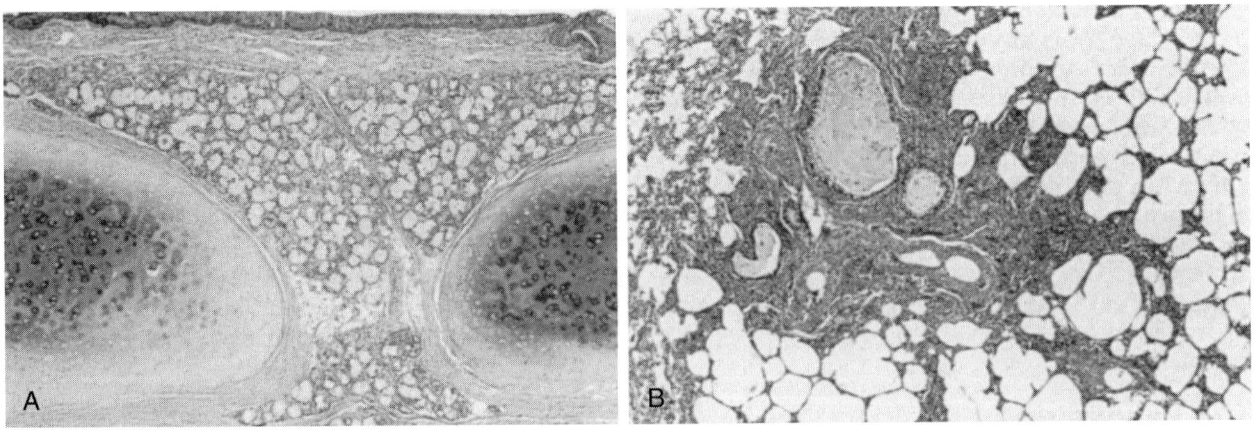


**Figure 40.2** *A,* hypertrophied submucosal gland in the trachea of an 18-year-old woman with cystic fibrosis is shown. Mucus-containing acini are distended. The gland occupies almost the entire thickness of the tracheal wall. (Hematoxylin and eosin stain; original magnification ×42.) *B,* The large and small bronchioles in the lungs of a 21-year-old man with cystic fibrosis are shown. These airways are completely obstructed with secretions and display chronic inflammation of the walls and surrounding tissues. Peribronchiolar fibrosis also can be demonstrated with appropriate stains. Air space enlargement is prominent *(right),* but more normal-appearing peripheral lung architecture is also present *(left).* (Hematoxylin and eosin stain; original magnification ×42.)

of the epithelium. Loss of acinar cells is widespread, and areas of destruction are replaced by fibrous tissue and fat. Intraluminal calcifications may occur and may be recognized roentgenographically. Small cysts are common and generally represent dilated ducts. Inflammatory changes are not prominent. The islets of Langerhans are spared until later periods of life. Changes in the islets include disruption by fibrous tissue bands that may provide a barrier between hormone-secreting cells and the vascular spaces.[59] Pathologic changes in the pancreas are used occasionally to make a postmortem diagnosis in atypical or missed cases of CF.

The pancreas is abnormal in almost all patients with CF and is virtually destroyed in approximately 90% of CF patients studied at autopsy. Liver changes are not as frequent or consistent.[60] In 25% or more of all autopsies, islands of relatively normal parenchymal cells are divided by fibrotic bands, creating a distinctive multilobular appearance. Microscopically, this focal biliary cirrhosis is characterized by inspissation of secretions within the bile ductules, bile duct proliferation, inflammatory reaction, and a paucity of evidence for bile stasis. Approximately 30% of patients also display fatty infiltration of the liver, which cannot always be ascribed to malnutrition. In approximately 25% of cases, the gallbladder is hypoplastic and contains a gelatinous mucus-like material. Cholelithiasis is an increasingly frequent observation.

Changes in the intestinal tract itself are less prominent.[61] Brunner's glands of the duodenum are hypertrophied, with dilated ducts and acinar lumens filled with mucus. There is little if any primary change in the small intestinal tract mucosa. The appendix frequently displays goblet cell hyperplasia of the epithelium and accumulation of secretions within crypts and in the lumen, changes that may be diagnostic of CF. A number of investigators have claimed the ability to diagnose CF by rectal biopsy, based on goblet cell hyperplasia and accumulation of mucus in the crypts. Subsequent studies have, however, demonstrated that these findings are not consistent in the rectal mucosa of patients with CF.[62]

Reproductive abnormalities are frequent and characteristic.[63] In most male patients with CF, the vas deferens, the tail and body of the epididymis, and the seminal vesicles are obliterated by fibrous tissue or are completely absent. Women with CF have mucus-distended uterine cervical glands and plugging of the cervical canal with tenacious mucous secretions. Endocervicitis is a frequent finding. Non–mucus-secreting glands such as the sweat glands and the parotid salivary glands have a normal gross and histologic appearance. Mucus-secreting salivary glands are usually somewhat enlarged, contain prominent mucus-secreting cells, and display a varied amount of mucous plugging in duct lumens.

## PATHOPHYSIOLOGY

### CFTR Protein: Structure, Metabolism, and Function

The CFTR is a single peptide chain containing 1480 amino acids and is *N*-glycosylated. The calculated molecular weight is 170 kd, but CFTR migrates in its mature form as a 180 kd glycoprotein.[31, 64] Figure 40.1 demonstrates the domain structure of CFTR, with two repeat motifs, each consisting of six transmembrane segments followed by a consensus nucleotide-binding fold (ATP-binding region). These two segments are linked by a highly charged region, the R (regulatory) domain, that contains multiple phosphorylation sites.[15] The CFTR structure closely resembles that of a number of other solute transport proteins and places the CF gene product in the ATP-binding cassette superfamily of proteins.[65]

CFTR mRNA transcripts are largely restricted to epithelial cells and are found at moderate levels in human pancreas, salivary glands, sweat glands, intestine, and the reproductive tract.[15, 64] In airways, CFTR mRNA may be more abundant in gland ducts than in surface epithelium.[66] These sites of CFTR mRNA expression are consistent with the locations of tissue dysfunction in patients with CF. Physiologic studies describe an apical membrane location for CFTR in most epithelia, although insertion into organelle membranes (e.g., endoplasmic reticulum,[67] endosomes,[68] and Golgi membranes[69]) may occur.

Most studies indicate that a central feature of the molecular pathophysiology of CF is that mutated CFTR (e.g., ΔF508) is not normally folded or processed and does not reach the Golgi or the apical membranes.[24, 70] The abnormal CFTR ΔF508 trafficking is temperature sensitive; normal processing and delivery to the plasma membrane can be achieved when temperatures are lowered.[71] More than 80% of the other identified CFTR mutations also produce a protein that is not completely processed.[72] An important caveat to the folding/processing theories of ΔF508 pathogenesis has been noted in recent studies,[73] suggesting that abnormal folding of ΔF508 may not occur in all affected tissues in vivo, including the airway epithelium.

Abnormal processing is not characteristic of all mutations.[72, 74] Dysfunctional CFTR may reach the plasma membrane but may be refractory to regulatory influences or exhibit conduction abnormalities as a consequence of several types of CFTR gene mutations.[75]

CFTR appears to have multiple functions (Fig. 40.3). It serves as a $Cl^-$ channel,[20, 21] modulates the activity of other plasma membrane channels,[22, 23] and perhaps regulates exocytotic and endocytotic events.[68, 76] Although CFTR resembles known solute pumps, as yet CFTR itself has not been shown to act as a pump. Its chloride conductance function is regulated through cyclic adenosine monophosphate(cAMP)–dependent kinase, C-kinase, and perhaps tyrosine kinase pathways.[77–79] Phosphorylation of R-domain serine residues and ATP binding and hydrolysis are necessary and independent steps in the activation of chloride conductance.[80, 81]

### Abnormal Airway Mucosal Physiology

CF is a disease that affects the epithelia lining various organs of the body. Because the native functions of affected epithelia in these organs vary widely, that is, some are salt absorbing but not volume absorbing (sweat duct), some are volume absorbing (airways), and others are volume secreting (pancreas), it is not surprising that the

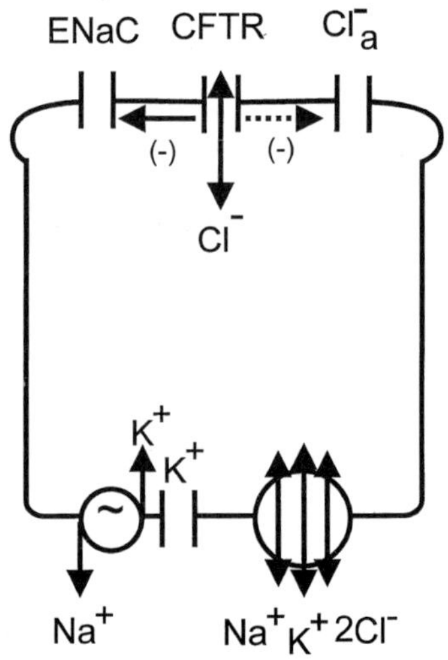


**Figure 40.3** Schematic describing the spectrum of activities and locations of the cystic fibrosis transmembrane (CFTR) protein in airway epithelia. The CFTR functions as a cyclic adenosine monophosphate (cAMP)–regulated $Cl^-$ channel in the plasma membrane. Other functions may include negative regulation of the activities of the epithelial sodium channel (ENaC) and possibly the alternative $Cl^-$ channel ($Cl^-_a$). At intracellular sites, CFTR may also act as a cAMP-regulated $Cl^-$ channel as well as act to direct vesicle trafficking (not shown).

physiologic consequences of the CF defect in these epithelia differ widely.

In the lung, airway but not alveolar epithelia are clinically affected. It is not yet clear whether the predominant pathophysiology of CF in the airway occurs in the superficial epithelium or in the glandular elements in the airway wall. The best-studied defects in CF airway epithelia are the $Na^+$ and $Cl^-$ transport defects in the superficial epithelia covering nasal polyp and bronchial surfaces. The likelihood that the superficial epithelium is the more important target epithelium in the lung is strengthened by data indicating that the earliest functional manifestation of CF in the lung is airflow obstruction in the bronchioles, a region that contains no glands. For discussion of the specificity of tests of function in the small airways, see Chapter 28.

A central premise of CF research has been that abnormalities of $Na^+$ and $Cl^-$ transport lead to a depletion of both salt and water (volume) on the airway surface. As a result of airway surface liquid (ASL) volume reduction, mucins are concentrated, the periciliary liquid depleted, and mucus clearance by ciliary and cough-dependent mechanisms diminished, which causes airflow obstruction and ultimately bacterial infection. Recently, a second hypothesis focusing on differences in salt concentration and perhaps tonicity of ASL has been proposed.[82, 83] This hypothesis rests on NaCl concentrations being low (less than 50 mmol/L) in the airway surface liquids of normal individuals and "high" in CF (more than 100 mmol/L). Table 40.2 describes the ASL composition in normal subjects and in CF subjects before infection. These data do not support a difference in ASL NaCl composition as central to the initiation of CF lung disease.

As discussed in Chapter 14, the role of active ion systems in the pulmonary epithelium can be reviewed on two levels: (1) the requirement of pulmonary epithelium to coordinate intrapulmonary surface liquid flow, that is, the so-called axial flow between different pulmonary regions such as alveolar and airway surfaces; and (2) the requirement to regulate surface-liquid volume and perhaps the composition relevant to the local microenvironment (i.e., to permit efficient mucus transport). Evidence that the CF defect leads to dysfunction at both levels is emerging. Confocal microscopy studies of well-differentiated cultures that exhibit rotational mucous transport have revealed that the mucus and periciliary liquid layers are both transported, imposing a requirement for volume absorption in airway epithelia.[84] Further studies with this system have revealed that net volume hyperabsorption is a feature of CF airway epithelia and abolishes mucous transport by both depletion of the periciliary liquid layer and concentration of mucins in the mucous layer[85] (Fig. 40.4). The depletion of periciliary liquid is predicted to hinder both cilial-dependent and cough-dependent mucous clearance. Consistent with this prediction is the mounting evidence that mucociliary and cough clearance

**Table 40.2** COMPOSITION OF AIRWAY SURFACE LIQUID IN NORMAL SUBJECTS AND UNINFECTED CYSTIC FIBROSIS PATIENTS

| Region/Phenotype | Study | N | $Na^+$ (mmol/L) | $Cl^-$ (mmol/L) | $K^+$ (mmol/L) |
|---|---|---|---|---|---|
| Normal nose | Knowles* | 8 | 109 ± 5 | 126 ± 5 | 29 ± 3 |
| | Hull† | 10 | 106 ± 4 | 115 ± 4 | ND |
| CF nose | Knowles | 8 | 110 ± 6 | 132 ± 5 | 28 ± 3 |
| | Hull | 10 | 116 ± 7 | 125 ± 4 | ND |
| Normal lower airway | Knowles | 11 | 91 ± 7 | 81 ± 6 | 17 ± 3 |
| | Hull | 7 | 85 ± 10 | 108 ± 5 | ND |
| CF lower airway | Knowles | 8 | 87 ± 4 | 77 ± 6 | 21 ± 2 |
| | Hull | 5 | 78 ± 16 | 77 ± 7 | ND |

*Knowles et al.[133]
†Hull et al.[388]

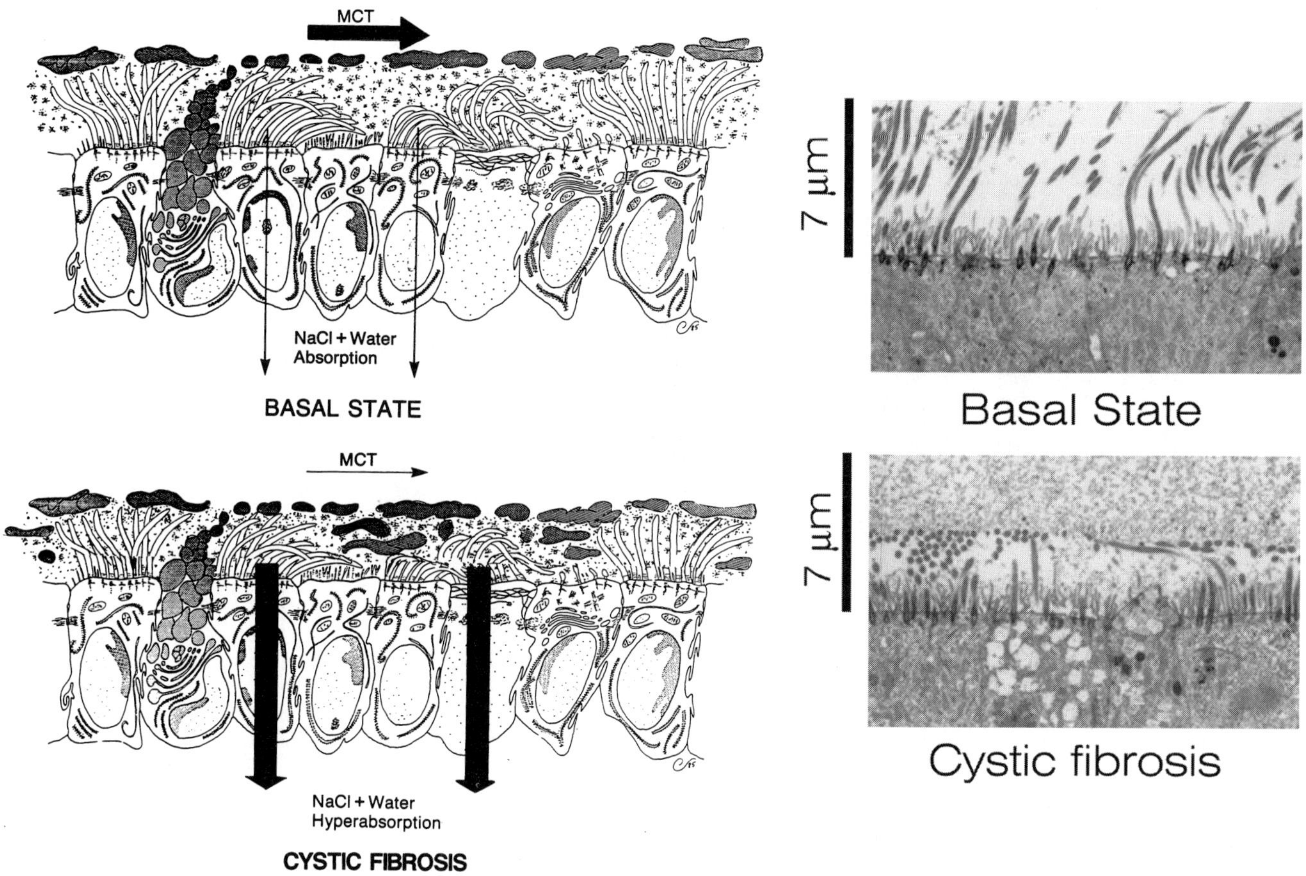


**Figure 40.4** Schema describing the mucociliary transport (MCT) apparatus in normal and CF airway epithelia. In normal airways *(upper left),* the volume and composition of airway surface liquids (''stars'' between cilia) are adjusted so that the extended cilium can transmit energy to the mucous layer that rests on the surface of the periciliary liquid layer. The height (volume) and the composition of this liquid layer are regulated by the superficial epithelial cells. The low-power electron micrograph *(upper right),* shows the 7 μm deep periciliary liquid layer on the surface of a cultured normal airway epithelium that exhibits mucous transport.[85] In CF airways *(lower left),* hyperabsorption of volume in response to excessive $Na^+$ transport depletes the height (volume) of the airway surface periciliary layer. It is postulated that this depletion of liquid contributes to slower airway clearance in CF by impacting mucus on cilial shafts and by altering cough clearance properties of mucus. The low-power electron micrograph *(lower right)* shows the depleted periciliary liquid layer on the surface of a CF airway epithelial culture that has lost the ability to perform mucous transport.[85] Other composition abnormalities of the periciliary secretory layer also may be important but are as yet unidentified.

are depressed in CF patients.[86, 87] It is possible, however, that CF-specific defects in addition to mucus retention contribute to lung disease.[88, 89]

## Ion Transport

The diagnostic biophysical hallmark of CF in airway epithelia is the raised transepithelial potential difference (PD).[9] The transepithelial PD can be analyzed simply as the product of the active ion transport rate (short-circuit current [$I_{sc}$]) and the ionic resistance of the epithelium ($R_t$). A series of in vivo ion substitution studies,[9] complemented by in vitro isotopic flux studies of excised tissues,[9, 90, 91] have revealed that the raised PD in CF airway epithelia reflects contributions of both increased transport ($Na^+$ absorption) and increased tissue resistance (due to decreased cellular $Cl^-$ permeability) (Fig. 40.5). Indirect evidence from studies measuring the effects of amiloride, an $Na^+$ channel blocker, in vivo indicates that the elevated $Na^+$ absorptive rate rather than the defective $Cl^-$ conductance dominates the resting electrical abnormalities of the superficial epithelium of CF airways.

### Abnormalities of Superficial Epithelial $Cl^-$ Transport

In vivo PD,[9] Ussing flux chamber,[90] and microelectrode studies[92–96] agree that CF airway epithelial cells exhibit an

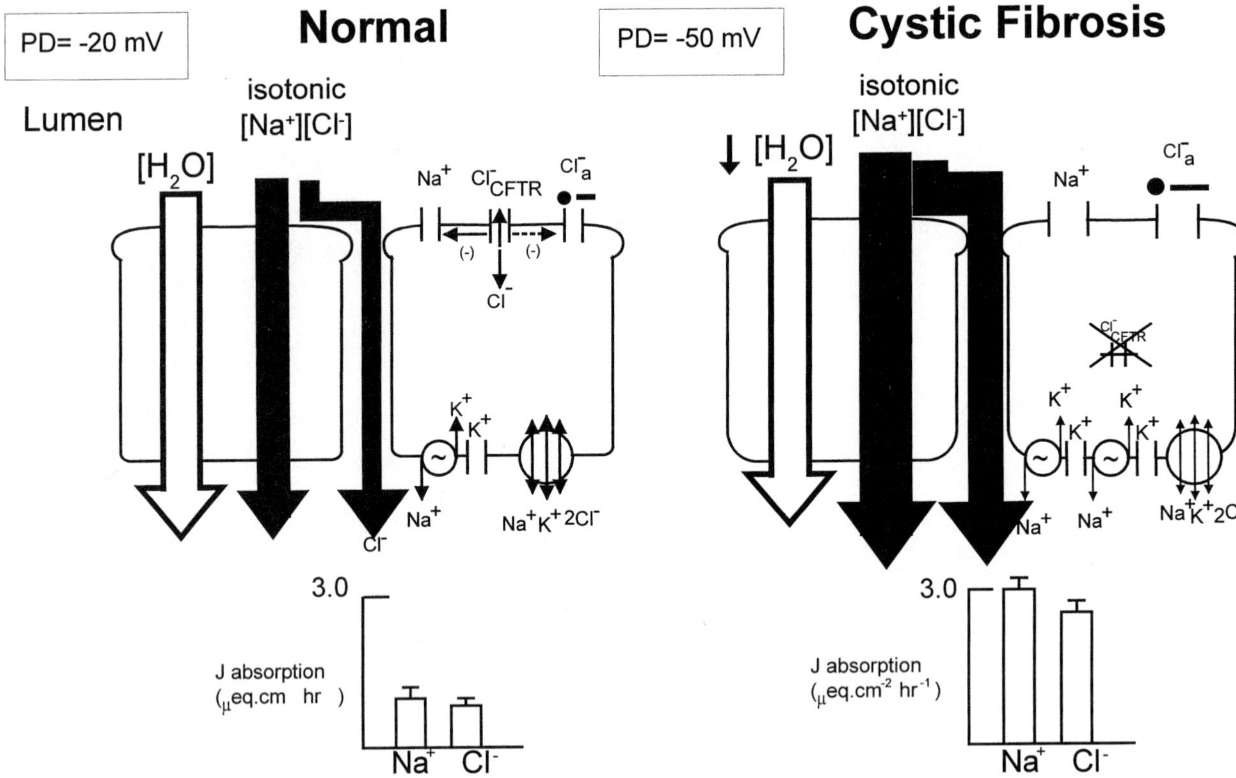


**Figure 40.5** Schema describing routes and magnitudes of ion transport across airway epithelia. In normal airway epithelia *(left)*, vectors describe routes and magnitudes of $Na^+$ (transcellular) and $Cl^-$ transport (paracellular). $H_2O$ is depicted as moving transcellularly. Bar graphs below describe absolute magnitude of $Na^+$ and $Cl^-$ absorption. In normal airway epithelia, the NaCl concentrations on the epithelial surface are depicted as isotonic. In CF, the NaCl concentrations are also depicted as isotonic, but the volume (↓ $H_2O$) is depicted as reduced. The reduction in volume in CF is depicted as reflecting a twofold to threefold greater rate of $Na^+$ absorption than for normal airway epithelia. $Cl^-$ hyperabsorption presumably accompanies $Na^+$ via the paracellular path (see bar graphs below). In addition, in CF, the capacity for induction of $Cl^-$ secretion is abolished by failure of cystic fibrosis transmembrane (CFTR) $Cl^-$ channel regulation. J = ion flux; PD = potential difference.

abnormal apical membrane conductive $Cl^-$ permeability. Studies utilizing double-barreled $Cl^-$-selective microelectrodes indicate that the basolateral membrane $Cl^-$ conductance and $Na^+,K^+,2Cl^-$ cotransport activities of CF cells are not different from those of normal cells.[94, 95, 97]

The abnormality in the apical membrane $Cl^-$ conductance of airway epithelia is one of selective defects in regulation of this pathway. The most extensively studied regulatory system in airway epithelia is the cAMP-dependent system. Like other affected epithelia, CF airway epithelia do not respond with $Cl^-$ secretion to agents that raise cellular cAMP (e.g., beta-agonists), whereas normal airway epithelia (amiloride-pretreated) do respond.[78, 91, 98–101] This abnormal response in CF airway epithelia does not reflect dysfunction of adenylyl cyclase or cAMP-dependent protein kinase activities. Rather, studies of expressed CFTR and purified CFTR proteins have demonstrated that wild-type CFTR functions as a cAMP-regulated $Cl^-$ channel[21] and have pinpointed the inability of CF airway epithelial cells to secrete $Cl^-$ to the defective CFTR protein itself.

CF airway epithelia, unlike normal airway epithelia, do not respond with $Cl^-$ secretion to activators of protein kinase C.[78, 100, 102, 103] The failure of the CF $Cl^-$ channel to respond to phosphorylation is, therefore, not selective for a specific kinase. Studies with the expressed CFTR protein have indicated that the CFTR $Cl^-$ channel can be directly regulated by protein kinase C activities.[104] Thus, the failure of CF airway epithelia to respond to protein kinase C also reflects dysfunction of the mutated CFTR $Cl^-$ channel itself. An area of intense interest at present is how CFTR is functionally and physically located in specialized domains (i.e., compartments), in epithelial cells.[105]

CF airway epithelial cells retain the capacity to secrete $Cl^-$ in response to elevations in intracellular $Ca^{2+}$.[106, 107] Data derived from studies of cultured monolayers impaled with double-barreled $Cl^-$-selective microelectrodes indicate that elevation of intracellular $Ca^{2+}$ with calcium ionophores (e.g., ionomycin) initiate $Cl^-$ secretion in both CF and normal cells. Two important issues need to be resolved to understand this phenomenon. First, there is the issue of which $Cl^-$ channel participates in this response. Because the CFTR $Cl^-$ channel does not respond to $Ca^{2+}$ calmodulin-dependent kinases and because the responses to $Ca^{2+}$ ionophores are preserved in mice whose CFTR gene has been disrupted by gene-targeting techniques,[28] the $Cl^-$ channel regulated by raised $Ca^{2+}$ in CF airway epithelial cells must be molecularly distinct from CFTR. This "alternative" $Cl^-$ channel, however, has still not been described biophysically with single-channel (patch electrode) techniques. Second, there is the issue of the second-messenger pathway that regulates this channel. It has not been resolved whether this $Cl^-$ channel responds to raised $Ca^{2+}$ itself or requires the participation of a kinase (e.g., a $Ca^{2+}$ calmodulin-dependent kinase).[106–109]

Regardless, these observations have potential therapeutic implications. In a search for compounds that interact with receptors on the lumen of airway epithelial cells that regulate intracellular $Ca^{2+}$ levels, it was discovered that the triphosphate nucleotides (ATP and uridine triphosphate [UTP]) are highly effective in initiating $Cl^-$ secretion in CF and normal airway epithelial cells.[110–113] Triphosphate nucleotides increase intracellular $Ca^{2+}$ via receptor-induced increases in inositol triphosphate levels. In vivo studies found that ATP and UTP were effective $Cl^-$ secretagogues in the nasal mucosa of CF subjects.[112] Indeed, an intriguing finding was that the triphosphate nucleotides were more effective in initiating $Cl^-$ secretion in CF than in normal subjects. These observations have led to the development of analogues of UTP that by virtue of being resistant to hydrolysis in CF airways may have longer duration of action.[114]

## Abnormalities of Superficial Epithelial $Na^+$ Transport

Abnormalities in $Na^+$ transport appear to be confined to epithelia that are involved in volume absorption. Thus, data have been reported that accelerated $Na^+$ absorption is a feature of the proximal tubule of the kidney,[115, 116] the jejunum and the ileum of the small intestine,[117–119] and the airways of CF patients.[91] Interestingly, the mechanisms of $Na^+$ hyperabsorption may differ in the three affected epithelia. $Na^+$-coupled solute movements may be the major affected pathways in the intestine, whereas the channel-mediated $Na^+$ absorption is the major abnormality in the lung (see subsequent discussion).

Studies of freshly excised airway specimens established that the raised PD that characterizes CF airway epithelia reflects in part an accelerated basal rate of active $Na^+$ absorption.[92] These studies also identified a defect in acute regulation of $Na^+$ transport rates in CF.[92] Beta-agonists and other reagents that raise intracellular cAMP levels paradoxically raise the already accelerated basal rate of $Na^+$ transport in CF tissues but do not affect $Na^+$ transport rates in normal tissues.[92]

Studies with microelectrodes in freshly excised tissues indicate that the principal abnormality in the $Na^+$ transport path in CF airway epithelia resides in the apical membrane $Na^+$ conductance.[92] Studies of cultured airway epithelia with double-barreled $Na^+$ selective microelectrodes show that the apical membrane $Na^+$ permeability in CF is twofold to threefold higher than in normal cells.[120, 121] Thus, these studies place a second ion permeability abnormality in the CF apical membrane and strongly suggest that the $Na^+$ transport abnormality is not secondary to the changes in the electrochemical driving forces for $Na^+$ entry consequent to absence of an apical membrane $Cl^-$ permeability.

The effects of the CF defect on the regulation of $Na^+$ transport rates at the single-channel level are not understood. The available evidence indicates that the fraction of time that the $Na^+$ channel is capable of conducting ions, the open probability ($P_o$), is approximately threefold greater in CF than in normal cells.[122–124] This finding suggests that the defect responsible for accelerated $Na^+$ transport in airway epithelia resides at the level of regulation of the $Na^+$ channel.

A major issue that is presently unresolved is the regulatory relationship between the CF gene product, CFTR, and the $Na^+$ transport defects. Clearly, the abnormalities in $Cl^-$ transport are expressed in all epithelia affected by CF and probably reflect the CFTR $Cl^-$ channel dysfunction. The $Na^+$ transport abnormalities are more restricted with regard to expression in particular epithelia, but the $Na^+$ transport abnormality appears to be unique to CF and therefore must be related to the abnormal gene product. The expression of the $Na^+$ transport defect in only one functional type of epithelium indicates that the abnormal $Na^+$ transport may be a direct consequence of an epithelium-specific CFTR function. Recent data indicate that CFTR negatively regulates the activity of $Na^+$ channels in the apical membrane.[125] Current efforts to understand the capacity for wild-type CFTR to exhibit cAMP-mediated "negative" feedback to the airway epithelia $Na^+$ channel have focused on protein-protein interactions that form microdomains or compartments. The cloning of the epithelial $Na^+$ channel expressed in airway epithelia has facilitated these efforts.[126, 127]

A key issue with respect to the $Na^+$ transport defect relates to its role in the pathogenesis of airway infection. Two studies have demonstrated increased $Na^+$-dependent volume absorption across CF airways.[85, 128] The more recent study has linked this defect to failure of mucous clearance.[85] Definitive evidence of this linkage, however, requires in vivo studies (e.g., producing similar abnormalities in mice or therapeutic trials in humans). The recent report that nucleotides also slow $Na^+$ transport in CF airways[129] suggest that data from therapeutic trials with these agents may be informative.

## Ion Transport Defects of Glandular Epithelium

CFTR may be expressed at high levels in certain regions of proximal airway glands. In situ hybridization studies indicate that lung CFTR is expressed at the highest level in serous cells contained in submucosal gland acini and a minor cell type in the ductal epithelium, the so-called oncocyte.[130]

CF airway gland acini, like superficial airway epithelia, do not respond to beta-agonists with $Cl^-$ secretion, whereas glands from normal subjects exhibit small responses.[131, 132] In vitro studies indicate that cultured CF gland cells, unlike the superficial airway epithelium of

CF subjects, do not respond to raised intracellular $Ca^{2+}$ with $Cl^-$ secretion, whereas normal glandular tissue does. Thus, the glands could have a $Cl^-$ transport phenotype that is more similar to gastrointestinal epithelia than to the superficial airway epithelium.[119, 131, 132] More recent in vivo studies of nasal gland secretion, however, have suggested a similar capacity for glands to secrete volume in CF and normal subjects.[133] Indeed, these studies raise the possibility that submucosal gland ducts modify the gland secretion so that it is hypotonic (i.e., it has a reduced NaCl concentration). Unlike the sweat duct, but similar to the parotid duct, the functions of the ductal epithelium in nasal glands of CF patients appear similar to those from normal subjects. Similar studies of lower airway glands are necessary to assess whether gland dysfunction contributes to CF airway pathogenesis.

## Macromolecule Secretion

Following Farber's report[5] of mucous obstruction in many exocrine glands, a search was initiated for abnormal macromolecules that might change the physical properties of CF exocrine secretions. Particular emphasis was placed on analysis of mucus glycoproteins (mucins), the high-molecular-weight glycoconjugates that are putative determinants of the viscoelastic properties of mucus.[134] One of the difficulties in comparing these substances sampled from CF and control airways is that they are susceptible to proteolytic and perhaps other degradative enzymes to which they are exposed in vivo. In addition, these glycoproteins display extensive microheterogeneity of carbohydrate constituents and therefore are difficult to compare from subject to subject or even from patient group to control group.

Overall, purified mucins from CF patients and control subjects show considerable similarity. Early suggestions that the fucose content of CF glycoproteins is elevated and the sialic acid content is decreased seem to been true for gastrointestinal mucins, but these phenomena are only observed postinfection in CF airways.[135] CF fibroblast membrane glycoproteins seem, however, to be excessively fucosylated. Sialylation of transferrin and the glycosphingolipid asialoganglioside GM1 (asialoGM1) by immortalized CF respiratory epithelial cells is reduced perhaps because of failure of these cells to acidify intracellular organelles secondary to reduced $Cl^-$ conductance.[69] Although this is an attractive hypothesis, further evidence is needed to link CFTR dysfunction to abnormal glycoprotein biosynthesis.

There is evidence that CF mucus glycoproteins are excessively glycosylated.[136] In addition, several investigators have reported that CF mucus glycoproteins from both respiratory and gastrointestinal sources contained increased numbers of sulfated sugars.[136–139] Goblet cells within the bronchial epithelium of patients with CF have an elevated sulfur content,[140] which, if present as sulfate, could promote sulfation of secretory glycoconjugates. Studies of CF fibroblasts and pancreatic cells suggest an increased influx capacity for the sulfate anion.[141, 142] Tracheal cells from CF subjects, however, transport sulfate normally via an $Na^+$-independent anion exchanger.[143] Theoretically, highly sulfated glycoproteins might be expected to have altered physical properties, which could lead to poor clearance of mucus. It is not yet certain, however, that alterations of sulfation play a primary pathophysiologic role. Attempts to document that CF respiratory tract mucous secretions differ rheologically from similar secretions of control subjects have met with mixed results.[144] This outcome may reflect difficulty in obtaining unaltered secretions and in developing highly sensitive methods for analysis of viscoelastic properties of mucus. Alternatively, surface characteristics of mucus such as adhesiveness may be more important determinants of clearance.[145]

There is no convincing evidence that CF epithelial cells hypersecrete macromolecules before the onset of airway injury. Hypersecretion in response to proteases, oxidative metabolites, and other products of inflammation undoubtedly, however, contributes to mucous obstruction in CF airways once infection has developed.[146]

Analyses of other macromolecular secretory products from patients with CF have failed to uncover substantial abnormalities. These macromolecules have included alpha-amylase, ribonuclease, and lysozyme from salivary secretions and pancreatic enzymes, including chymotrypsin, trypsin, carboxypeptidase, amylase, and lipase.

## Pathophysiology of Infection

Failure of the airways to clear mucus normally is likely to be the primary pathophysiologic event in CF. Adherent mucous plaques and plugs may form the surface for the biofilm growth of bacterial organisms.[147] The generation of immobile mucous surfaces thus constitutes the nidus for the chronic infection in the respiratory tract that is the major contributor to the loss of lung function and eventual demise of patients with CF.

The chronic airway infection of CF may be unique, particularly with respect to its endobronchial location and the organisms involved, particularly *Staphylococcus aureus* and *Pseudomonas aeruginosa*. Whether this predilection represents unique bacterial-mucous interactions[148, 149] or other factors is not known. Once established, infection of the lungs is rarely eradicated. Bacterial infection extending beyond the airways is, however, distinctly uncommon. Therefore, local airways rather than general host or pulmonary defense mechanisms must be impaired.

The old concept that a generalized failure of mucous clearance from airways is a central feature of CF airway infection has been supplemented with respect to mechanisms by recent clinical and laboratory data. Studies of airway mucous transport velocity have found that clearance from the central airways is usually reduced.[87] Clearance from the more peripheral airways, where mucus first accumulates, has recently been studied and found to be routinely reduced.[150] Studies to date suggest that ciliary morphology and beat frequency in CF airway epithelia are normal.[151, 152] In contrast, data from model systems indicate that the volume of liquid on CF airway surfaces is severely reduced.[85] The key concept is that volume depletion, by removing both the periciliary liquid and concentrating mucus, leads to a failure of both mucociliary and cough clearance. This virtually complete failure to clear mucus is probably responsible for the severe and unrelenting lung infections. In contrast, patients with pseudohypoaldosteronism due to loss-of-function mutations in the epithelial sodium channel gene have excess liquid on airway surfaces and increased rates of mucociliary transport and do not develop chronic airway infection.[85a]

*S. aureus* and *P. aeruginosa* are infrequent respiratory tract pathogens of children and adults, except in CF. The role played by these organisms in endobronchial infection has prompted the suggestion that surface properties of CF airway epithelia are altered in a fashion that promotes their adherence. *S. aureus* does not preferentially adhere to CF airway epithelial cells.[153] *P. aeruginosa* has been reported to adhere more avidly to buccal epithelial cells of patients with CF than to cells from control age-matched patients.[154] *P. aeruginosa* also adheres to upper and lower airway epithelial cells,[155, 156] but studies of respiratory cell interactions with *P. aeruginosa* do not demonstrate consistent differences between CF and normal cells.[157, 158] In contrast to studies reporting increased adherence of bacteria to CF airway epithelia, other studies have suggested that the wild-type CFTR expressed on normal epithelial cells binds to *Pseudomonas* and mediates bacterial internalization, which ultimately kills the microorganism. CF cells are reported to fail to perform this function.[88] A general experimental problem with most data examining bacterial-epithelial cell interactions is that they emanate from model systems that have not employed well-differentiated airway epithelia.

An emerging concept is that airway bacterial infections reflect initial binding, colonization, and infection of the mucous layer rather than the epithelial cell surface.[149, 159] Indeed, there is increasing evidence that CF airway infection reflects the infection of the mucous layer to form biofilms of bacteria that are resistant to host defense.[147] No differences in bacterial binding to CF versus normal mucins have been detected for *Staphylococcus* or *Pseudomonas*.[153] Rather, it is likely that increased bacterial adherence due to the increased concentration of mucins (reflecting volume depletion), which renders the surface of the mucous layer more adhesive or "tacky," coupled with the failure to clear mucus, produces these infections.[160] Once bacterial infection of mucus has occurred, the bacteria release products that can diffuse to the underlying epithelial cells and stimulate upregulation of mucin production[161, 162] and cytokine responses[163] and mediate cell damage. Once cell damage has occurred, the infection may be worsened by bacterial binding to the injured (but not uninjured) cells.[164]

Pulmonary immunology in CF has been investigated extensively. There is little reason to believe that a primary immunologic deficiency state exists. Although CF subjects tend to have a low level of serum immunoglobulin G (IgG) in the first decade of life, this level increases dramatically as chronic infection is established.[165] Secretory antibody levels appear to be normal or enhanced.[166] Antibody responses specific for infecting organisms in the respiratory tract are brisk.[167, 168] Numbers of B lymphocytes and plasma cells that differentiate into immunoglobulin-secreting cells are not depressed.[169] T-lymphocyte numbers are adequate, and these lymphocytes proliferate in response to nonspecific mitogens.[170] With advancing severity of pulmonary disease, lymphocytes of CF patients may proliferate less briskly in response to *P. aeruginosa* and other gram-negative organisms.[171] This acquired dysfunction can be reversed in some patients by intensive antibiotic treatment, but it may contribute to the resistance of end-stage lung disease to antimicrobial therapy.

Polymorphonuclear leukocytes and macrophages are plentiful in CF airways. CF pulmonary macrophages function normally when removed from their usual environment.[172] Polymorphonuclear cells also function normally outside of the host environment. These observations suggest that potential phagocytic defects in vivo could reflect infection-induced degradation of opsonins (e.g., IgG and complement) and possibly defective leukocyte migration through thickened, adhesive mucus.

Much recent work has focused on the magnitude of the inflammatory response to airway infection in CF and or the regulatory systems that modulate this response.[173] Studies from lung lavage fluid from CF neonates indicate that the magnitude of the neutrophil response normalized to bacterial counts in lavage fluid is higher in CF than in non-CF infants with lung infections.[174] Other workers have suggested that the cytokine interleukin-10, which normally serves to dampen epithelial cell interleukin-6 and interleukin-8 responses to luminal bacterial infection, is not produced at normal levels in CF airway epithelia.[175, 176] Because the enormous neutrophil influx into airway lumens produces a large amount of intraluminal DNA that is difficult to clear, it is important therapeutically to understand whether the neutrophil influx reflects persistent failure to kill bacteria growing in biofilms on thickened plaques or a failure of an epithelial regulatory mechanism for neutrophil influx.

The mechanisms by which progressive obstructive lung disease and destruction of airway walls occur in CF have been studied. The role of proteinases in this process has been intensively studied.[177] Leukocytes and bacteria produce large quantities of elastase that exceed the neutralization capacity of airway surface antiproteinases. Thus, elastases can work directly to destroy airway walls. Both leukocyte and bacterial elastases also generate C5a nonimmunologically in CF secretions.[178] High levels of this chemotactic factor may contribute to the brisk polymorphonuclear leukocyte response characteristic of infected CF airways, further exacerbating the burden of free elastase. *Pseudomonas*,[179] neutrophil,[180] and mast cell[181] proteases are potent stimulators of goblet cell and gland cell mucous secretion. Furthermore, proteolytic enzymes introduced into the airways of animals produce marked hyperplasia of mucus-secreting cells in the surface epithelium.[182] Proteinases also are capable of interfering with ciliary function[183] and damage epithelial cells.[184] Once damage to epithelial cells occurs, bacteria can adhere to cells and accelerate airway wall damage. Finally, proteolytic injury to airway walls probably contributes to their destruction with subsequent development of widespread bronchiolectasis and bronchiectasis.[185] The fact that destructive emphysema is not a prominent feature of CF lungs, especially early in the course of lung disease, can be attributed to confinement of infection to endobronchial spaces in mild to moderate lung disease. Other mechanisms of conducting airway tissue injury undoubtedly exist but have not yet been described in detail.

## CLINICAL MANIFESTATIONS

CF presents in many different ways and mimics a number of other clinical entities. Usual presentations include early onset of respiratory tract symptoms, particularly persistent cough and recurrent or refractory lung infiltrates. Usual gastrointestinal presentations include meconium ileus in approximately 10% of patients and failure to thrive with steatorrhea. A surprising number of people with CF escape detection in the first decade or two of life, often because symptoms are unusual, subtle, or even absent. Patients with "mild" mutations may present in childhood or later in life.[35] Unusual presentations are listed in Table 40.3, and presentations that may be expected at adolescence or early adulthood are highlighted. Recognition of the protean manifestations of CF and a high index of suspicion are required to detect all cases of CF, either in childhood or later in life.

### Lower Respiratory Tract Disease

The earliest manifestation of CF lung disease is generally cough. At first it is intermittent, coinciding with episodes of acute respiratory tract infection and persisting longer than expected. With time, the cough becomes a daily event. It is often worse at night and especially on arising in the morning. With progression of lung disease, the cough becomes productive and then paroxymal, with associated gagging and emesis. Sputum is usually tenacious, purulent, and often green, reflecting *P. aeruginosa* infection. Hyperinflation of the lungs is noted early in the progression of lung disease. In fact, it is unusual to see CF respiratory tract disease without at least a moderate increase in lung volume. Asthmatic or bronchiolitic-type wheezing is most common during the first 2 years of life but may be encountered at any age. Wheezing may occur with or without evidence of atopy, which is probably not more frequent in patients with CF.[186] Lung sounds are often unremarkable for extended periods of time, sometimes for years. Not infrequently, diminution in the intensity of breath sounds may be the only abnormality noted, correlating with the extent of hyperinflation. Adventitious lung sounds are usually heard first over the upper lobes and often are localized to the right side.

CF patients may have only mild bronchitic symptoms for long periods of time, in some cases for a decade or two, but eventually these periods of stability are punctuated with exacerbations of symptoms, including increased intensity of cough, tachypnea, shortness of breath, decreased activity and appetite, and weight loss. It has been assumed that these exacerbations are triggered by acute respiratory infections, perhaps of viral or mycoplasmal origin, although studies differ concerning evidence for these infections during periods of increased lung symptoms.[187–192] Environmental factors, including cigarette smoke,[193] also may evoke more respiratory symptoms. Intense antibiotic therapy and assistance with clearance of mucus are usually required to reduce lung symptoms and improve lung function. Exacerbations characteristically occur with increasing frequency. Frank limitation of activity or disability is associated with end-stage lung disease and heralds a sequence of terminal events, including substantial hypoxemia, pulmonary hypertension, cor pulmonale, and death.

#### Microbiology

The airways of patients with CF are colonized early with bacteria, and, once established, infection is rarely, if ever,

**Table 40.3 UNUSUAL PRESENTATIONS OF CYSTIC FIBROSIS***

| | |
|---|---|
| Respiratory | Bronchiolitis/asthma |
| | ***Pseudomonas aeruginosa* or *Staphylococcus aureus* colonization of the respiratory tract** |
| | Staphylococcal pneumonia |
| | **Nasal polyposis** |
| | **Nontuberculous mycobacterial infection** |
| Gastrointestinal | Meconium plug syndrome |
| | Rectal prolapse |
| | **Recurrent abdominal pain and/or right lower quadrant mass** |
| | Hypoproteinemic edema |
| | Prolonged neonatal jaundice |
| | **Biliary cirrhosis with portal hypertension** |
| | Vitamin deficiency states (A, D, E, K) |
| | Acrodermatitis enteropathica-like eruption with fatty acid and zinc deficiency |
| | **Recurrent pancreatitis** |
| Genitourinary | **Male infertility** |
| | **Female infertility** |
| Other | Hypochloremic, hyponatremic alkalosis |
| | **Mother of a child with cystic fibrosis** |

*Those in boldface may occur in adolescents or adults with CF.

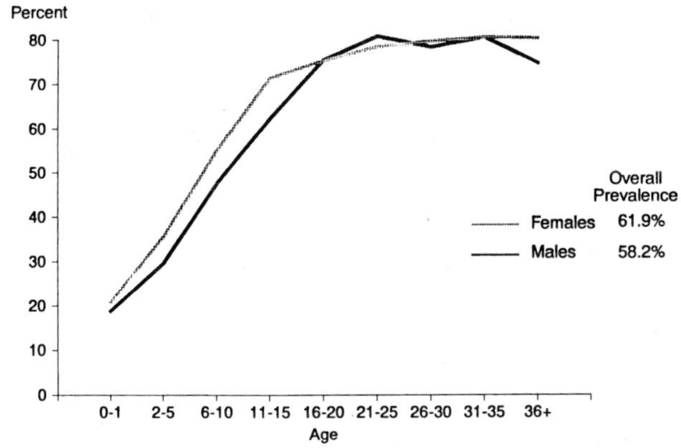


**Figure 40.6** Prevalence of *Pseudomonas aeruginosa* infection is shown by age and sex in CF patients enrolled in the US Cystic Fibrosis Foundation Registry, 1991, based on an analysis of 16,417 patients. (Courtesy of Dr. S. FitzSimmons, Cystic Fibrosis Foundation.)

eradicated. *S. aureus* and *Haemophilus influenzae* are often the first organisms detected.[194] *P. aeruginosa* characteristically is cultured from respiratory secretions months to years later, although this organism is present at diagnosis with increasing frequency. Age at acquisition of *P. aeruginosa* is graphed in Figure 40.6 and depends in part on genotype, with earlier acquisition occurring in persons homozygous for ΔF508.[33] The possibility of nosocomial acquisition of *P. aeruginosa* has been raised.[195] With progression of lung disease, *P. aeruginosa* is often the only organism recovered from sputum and may be present in several types of colonies, usually with different antibiotic sensitivity patterns. Typically, one of these types is mucoid, due to elaboration of large amounts of alginate. These mucoid organisms are found in microcolonies of pseudomonads embedded and growing in biofilms of alginate.[196] Mucoid properties are thought to inhibit opsonic and nonopsonic phagocytosis, enhance adherence properties, and decrease sensitivity to antibiotics and toxic, reactive intermediates produced by leukocytes.[147, 197–199] The recovery of *P. aeruginosa*, particularly the mucoid form, from the lower respiratory tract of a child or young adult with chronic lung symptoms is virtually diagnostic of CF.

Recently, other species have been recovered from CF lungs with increasing frequency, particularly *Burkholderia cepacia*. This organism has become prevalent in a few CF care centers and is particularly difficult to treat because it is usually resistant to most antimicrobial drugs. Evidence for patient to patient spread is strong and has led to recommendations for stringent infection control measures within CF care settings.[200] Colonization has been linked to the rapid demise of a small percentage of patients[201] with what is called the "cepacia syndrome." Recently, molecular techniques have allowed designation of different genetic groups of *B. cepacia*, which are called *genomovars*.[202–205] Genomovars II and III have been associated with the cepacia syndrome, and genomovar III includes the highly transmissible strain that may be linked to expression of the cable pilus.[204–206] Occasionally, other gram-negative rods are present in sputum, including mucoid *Escherichia coli, Stenotrophomonas maltophilia, Alcaligenes xylosoxidans*, *Klebsiella*, and *Proteus*. Anaerobes have been recovered from CF lung tissue; they may be undetected pathogens and are found in large abscess cavities on rare occasions.[207]

Sputum bacteriology correlates reasonably well with specimens obtained directly from the lower respiratory tract. Oropharyngeal swab cultures that yield *S. aureus* or *P. aeruginosa* are highly predictive of results from bronchoscopic specimens, but negative pharyngeal cultures do not rule out the presence of these organisms in lower airways.[208] Quantitative bacteriology may be particularly useful for determining the relative contributions of organisms isolated.

A large number of sputum specimens contain yeast and *Aspergillus fumigatus*. Neither organism has been considered a serious pathogen, although the latter causes the symptoms of allergic bronchopulmonary aspergillosis in a small percentage of patients.[209] Colonization of lungs with rapidly growing mycobacteria has been documented with increasing frequency. Up to 20% of adult patients in some clinics are colonized by nontuberculous mycobacteria, occasionally prompting treatment with agents directed against these organisms.[210–212] *Mycobacterium tuberculosis* infection has been seen in only very sporadic cases.

## Radiology

The earliest radiographic change is usually hyperinflation of the lungs, reflecting obstruction of small airways. The degree of hyperinflation generally increases with age. As bronchitis progresses, peribronchial cuffing becomes increasingly prominent. Mucous impaction in airways may be seen as branching fingerlike shadows. Evidence of bronchiectasis, such as enlarged ring shadows and cysts, is common by 5 to 10 years of age. Frequently, peripheral rounded densities are noted during acute exacerbations and may disappear with treatment, leaving residual cysts. Subpleural blebs often become evident during the second decade of life and are most prominent along the mediastinal border. For reasons that remain unexplained, the right upper lobe usually displays the earliest and most severe changes. With advancing disease, the pulmonary artery segments become more prominent. A relatively small and vertical cardiac shadow is typical, but the heart enlarges with onset of cor pulmonale. Hilar adenopathy is rarely prominent. Lobar or segmental atelectasis is uncommon, but is most often seen in infants or small children. Chest radiographic scoring systems have been introduced and may be useful for clinical studies and to chart the course of lung injury.[213]

Radiographic improvement with intensive treatment is not readily appreciated because of the fixed nature of airway changes. The most striking improvement often is reduced inflation of the lungs, a change that tends to make the fixed lung markings more prominent.

CT of the chest has not been used routinely for monitoring the course of CF lung changes. The cost is high, and the resolution for younger patients was initially poor. With rapid scanning, however, mild bronchiectasis and mucoid impaction can be observed at all ages.[214] CT scanning detects these lesions, even when the chest radiograph is nearly normal. The severity of bronchiectasis can be graded in older patients.[215] The indications for CT scanning in place of routine chest roentgenography are not established. One indication may be the evaluation of a patient considered for lobectomy. Magnetic resonance imaging (MRI) also defines peribronchial thickening, mucoid impaction, and bronchiectasis but has no well-documented advantage over CT scans in these areas of imaging.[216] MRI may be superior for distinguishing hilar adenopathy and prominent pulmonary vessels.[217]

## Lung Function

Newborns with CF are thought to have normal lung function. However, within weeks to months, many infants with CF show evidence of increased airway resistance, gas trapping, and diminished flow rates.[218] When children reach an age that makes cooperation possible, more complete testing first demonstrates airway obstruction, which presumably occurs in small airways as indicated by reduced maximum midexpiratory flow rates, reduced flows at low lung volumes, and elevated ratio of residual volume to total lung capacity (RV/TLC).[219–221] Other sensitive indicators of lung pathology include increased alveolar-arterial oxygen difference, frequency dependence of dynamic compliance, reduced response of flows to a helium-oxygen mixture, elevated slope of phase III of the single-breath nitrogen washout, and elevated wasted ventilation.[218] Tests that are used most often to follow the course of pulmonary function include spirometry, lung volume measurements, and measures of oxygenation. In general, patients progress from initial reductions in maximum midexpiratory flow rates to reductions in $FEV_1$/FVC and then to diminished vital capacity and total lung volumes. This progression from peripheral airway obstruction to more generalized obstruction and then to acquisition of a restrictive component is illustrated in Table 40.4. These tests are described and evaluated in Chapter 28.

**Table 40.4** REPRESENTATIVE PULMONARY FUNCTION TEST RESULTS FROM THREE YOUNG ADULT MALES WITH MILD (A), MODERATE (B), AND SEVERE (C) LUNG DISEASE*

| Test | Patient A | Patient B | Patient C |
|---|---|---|---|
| FVC | 98 | 72 | 48 |
| $FEV_1$ | 92 | 46 | 34 |
| $FEV_1$/FVC | (0.81) | (0.70) | (0.64) |
| MMEF | 83 | 15 | 6 |
| $\dot{V}max_{50}$ | 91 | 19 | 11 |
| $\dot{V}max_{25}$ | 52 | 10 | 5 |
| FRC | 162 | 112 | 75 |
| RV | 189 | 200 | 120 |
| TLC | 131 | 105 | 62 |
| RV/TLC | (0.29) | (0.45) | (0.50) |
| $Pa_{O_2}$ (room air) | [87] | [74] | [48] |

FRC = functional residual capacity; MMEF = maximal midexpiratory flow; RV = residual volume; TLC = total lung capacity.

*Values are per cent predicted, except those in parentheses, which are simple ratios, and those in brackets, which are mm Hg. Patient A coughs several times a day; the cough is occasionally productive. He shows no restriction of activity. Patient B coughs frequently, expectorates moderately large amounts of mucus, but is able to jog 3 miles daily and is a full-time student in a professional school. Patient C has chronic right heart failure, but is able to work daily as a hair stylist.

By the time a diagnosis is made, many children with CF show mild decrements of arterial $Po_2$. Oxygenation declines slowly throughout life. As a rule, patients who maintain satisfactory oxygenation do well, independent of the extent of the obstructive impairment. When arterial $Po_2$ values dip below 55 mm Hg on a sustained basis, symptomatic pulmonary hypertension can be expected.[222, 223] Exaggerated nocturnal desaturation experienced by patients with CF may be a contributing factor to pulmonary hypertension.[224] Hypoxemia generally is not accompanied by polycythemia, at least in part due to an expanded plasma volume and in some persons to suppressed erythropoiesis secondary to chronic infection. Elevation of arterial $Pco_2$ generally occurs with $FEV_1$ volumes less than 30% of those predicted and constitutes an end-stage event for most patients. Less than 50% of patients with $FEV_1$ below 30% of predicted, arterial $Pco_2$ more than 50 mm Hg, or arterial $Po_2$ below 55 mm Hg live for 24 additional months.[225]

Airway hyperreactivity is a frequent feature of CF lung disease and can be demonstrated by exercise testing, histamine challenge, or response to bronchodilators. Up to 68% of the CF population demonstrates decreased flows after histamine, and flows improve in as many as 40% with aerosolized bronchodilators.[226] In contrast to cross-sectional studies, repeated tests every 1 to 3 months for 1 year have demonstrated bronchodilator responsiveness at least once in 95% of subjects.[226] Responsiveness is unrelated to the severity of pulmonary disease or to indices of atopy, and it seems to be more prevalent during winter than during summer months. Responsiveness diminishes with exacerbations of lung disease, but returns as lung function improves over 2 weeks of intensive in-hospital therapy. Several investigators have noted that occasional patients with CF have a paradoxic response to bronchodilators, perhaps due to further loss of tone in bronchiectatic airways. The pathogenesis of bronchial hyperreactivity in CF is unclear. Airway hyperreactivity is discussed in Chapter 39.

Exercise tolerance is related to the severity of airway obstruction.[227, 228] Most patients with CF maintain adequate oxygen saturation, even with maximal exercise. In one study, however, 12 of 29 patients with an $FEV_1$ less than 50% of FVC had an arterial oxygen saturation below 90% at peak exercise compared with no drop for patients with higher $FEV_1$ values.[229] Persons with CF have higher than expected ventilatory muscle endurance, and this endurance can be further improved with inspiratory muscle training. Improved inspiratory muscle strength and endurance do not, however, augment exercise performance.[230] Exercise does improve cardiorespiratory fitness, but it does not improve standard pulmonary function test results. In one study, however, weight training increased weight and muscle size and in addition reduced RV/TLC by 12%.[231] Another study demonstrated that adults with CF and advanced lung disease increase but those with only moderate lung disease decrease end-expiratory lung volumes after graded exercise on a cycle ergometer.[232] Maximum oxygen consumption during exercise appears to be a better predictor of survival than routine pulmonary function testing.[233] (The physiology of exercise is discussed in Chapter 9, and exercise testing is discussed in Chapter 28.)

Resting energy expenditure is variably elevated in patients with CF. Although some have claimed that there are genetically determined increases in energy expenditure (e.g., increased ATP hydrolysis) related to certain CFTR mutations,[234] others have found increased work of breathing to be a more plausible explanation.[235]

## Upper Respiratory Tract Disease

Virtually all patients with CF have roentgenographic opacification of the paranasal sinuses[236] and intermittent symptoms of increased upper airway secretions and moderate airflow obstruction.[237] *Nasal polyps* occur in 15% to 20% of patients and are most common toward the end of the first decade and during the second decade of life.[57] Manifestations include severe or complete nasal airflow obstruction, rhinorrhea, and occasionally widening of the bridge of the nose. Despite the presence of roentgenographic abnormalities, acute or chronic symptoms of *sinusitis* occur in less than 10% of children[238] and in approximately 24% of adults.[239, 240]

## Complications of Respiratory Tract Disease

Lobar and segmental *atelectasis* occurs in about 5% of patients.[241] This complication is most prevalent in the first 5 years of life and thereafter has a diminishing frequency. The right lung is the site of atelectasis in most patients. Many episodes occur in conjunction with an exacerbation of clinical symptoms, but silent atelectasis is common. Occasionally, volume loss is associated with allergic aspergillosis and endobronchial mucus plugs. In most instances, however, a discrete plug is not evident on bronchoscopy.

*Pneumothorax* is a more frequent complication and is caused by rupture of subpleural blebs. The overall incidence is about 1% per year, and it increases with age and disease severity so that about 20% of CF adults will experience at least one pneumothorax.[242] Pneumothorax occurs equally in both sexes and is more frequent in the right chest. A small asymptomatic pneumothorax may be discovered at the time of routine chest roentgenographic examination. More commonly, patients develop acute onset of shortness of breath, chest pain, and/or hemoptysis. The incidence of tension pneumothorax is probably higher in patients with CF than in those with less severe or no lung disease, and, under these circumstances, the accumulation of pleural air may become a life-threatening event. Simultaneous bilateral pneumothoraces have been described and constitute an urgent situation. Recurrent pneumothoraces are very common.

*Hemoptysis* is a common event in older CF patients, correlates with clinical and radiologic evidence of bronchiectasis, and is usually due to airway inflammation rather than to vigorous activity or trauma to the chest. Blood streaking in the sputum ("minor hemoptysis") is common, whereas massive hemoptysis (more than 240 mL blood in 24 hours) occurs in approximately 5% of patients.[243] There is a strong correlation between the occurrence of both small and large volume hemoptysis and exacerbation of lung infection. Patients with relatively large-volume hemoptysis may be able to localize the site of bleeding by describing a bubbling or gurgling sensation in one area of the chest. Any lobe may be involved, and localization is difficult in most patients. Even emergent bronchoscopy often does not detect the location of blood in the airways. The immediate mortality rate with massive hemoptysis may be as high as 10%, but with proper treatment most patients with massive hemoptysis have a prognosis that is not much different from the remainder of the CF population.[244]

From 1% to 10% of patients develop *allergic bronchopulmonary aspergillosis* at some time in their lives.[245] In one study, more than 50% of patients with CF had precipitating antibodies to *A. fumigatus* in their serum, and this organism can be recovered from the sputum with a similar frequency.[246] New lung infiltrates, increased cough, respiratory distress, wheezing, and the expectoration of rusty brown plugs of sputum containing many eosinophils suggest this diagnosis. Atelectasis due to plugging of a lobar or segmental bronchus with hyphae-laden mucus may occur. Chronic airway colonization with *A. fumigatus* (or other species) is common, and diagnosis of allergic bronchopulmonary aspergillosis requires new clinical findings plus skin hypersensitivity and elevated levels of IgG and IgE antibodies against *A. fumigatus* or other fungi.[209]

*Pleural effusions* and *empyema* are uncommon in patients with CF, but pleuritic symptoms and signs may accompany exacerbations of lung disease. Staphylococcal and pseudomonal empyemas have been described, but respiratory tract infections usually spare the pleural space.[247]

Digital *clubbing* occurs in virtually all patients with cystic fibrosis and is usually present early in the course of symptomatic lung disease. The cause of clubbing is unknown, but its severity generally correlates with the severity of lung disease.[248] *Hypertrophic pulmonary osteoarthropathy* occurs in as many as 15% of older adolescents and adults.[170, 249] If roentgenographic evidence for periostitis is used as the definition, the incidence is 8%. The most common sites are the distal aspects of the tibia, fibula, radius, and ulna. Signs and symptoms include pain, bone tenderness, swelling, and warmth over the involved areas. Effusions in nearby joints may occur. There is often discomfort with ambulation. Hypertrophic pulmonary osteoarthropathy frequently becomes more symptomatic with pulmonary disease exacerbations and tends to subside when control of pulmonary symptoms is achieved. There are rare instances of cutaneous vasculitis due to CF, which causes a self-limited, painless, palpable purpura, typically involving the lower extremities.[249]

*Respiratory failure* leads to death in more than 90% of CF patients. *Hypoxemia* often develops during exertion[250] or sleep[251] and progresses over years. Hypercapnia reflects severe airway obstruction and increases with disease severity and acute exacerbations. Hepatic congestion and peripheral edema caused by pulmonary hypertension and cor pulmonale may develop in the last year of life,[252] particularly if hypoxemia is not treated adequately. Occasionally, infections such as respiratory syncytial virus or influenza cause acute respiratory failure that is fully reversible.[253]

## Gastrointestinal Manifestations

Meconium ileus occurs in 10% to 15% of newborns with CF and is virtually diagnostic for CF.[61] These infants fail to pass meconium in the first day or two of life, develop abdominal distention, and proceed to bilious emesis. Occasionally, perforation occurs, and peritonitis accompanied by shock intervenes. Flat and upright abdominal films reveal multiple dilated loops of intestine and air-fluid levels. The lower abdomen often takes on a granular appearance, representing accumulated meconium containing small air bubbles. A barium enema demonstrates a small colon, and, if contrast material can be refluxed into the ileum, the point of ileal obstruction can be identified. In utero, ileal perforation results in peritoneal and scrotal calcification. Occasionally, obstruction occurs lower in the intestinal tract and causes only delayed passage of meconium. This condition has been termed the *meconium plug syndrome* and is much less specific for CF.[254] Meconium ileus is also a prominent feature of transgenic mice with a disrupted CFTR gene.[27]

Beyond the newborn period, intestinal obstruction may occur for a variety of reasons. Perhaps the most common (occurring in 20% of patients) is called the *meconium ileus equivalent* or the *distal intestinal obstruction syndrome*.[36, 61, 255] As with meconium ileus of the newborn, obstruction occurs in the terminal ileum and is usually associated with voluminous, sticky, incompletely digested intestinal contents. In some instances, partial obstruction occurs, accompanied by intermittent abdominal pain. Complete obstruction is associated with failure to pass stools, abdominal distention, and vomiting. A mobile right lower quadrant mass may be palpable. Obstruction beyond the immediate newborn period is also characteristic of the CF mouse model. Other causes of abdominal pain associated with obstruction include intussusception, intestinal adhesions from previous abdominal surgery, which is a particular problem in patients with CF, and low-grade appendicitis, partially suppressed by antibiotic therapy, and periappendiceal abscess.[256] Nonfilling of the appendix with contrast enema is frequent in patients with CF, even in the absence of appendicitis.[257] Duodenal irritation, caused by failure to buffer gastric acid, may underlie radiographic changes in this area and recurrent epigastric pain.[258]

Rectal prolapse occurs in nearly 20% of children, but is an infrequent event for adults with CF.[259] In fact, CF is said to be the most common cause of rectal prolapse in the United States. Factors contributing to rectal prolapse include the presence of bulky sticky stools that adhere to rectal mucosa, loss of the perirectal fat that normally supports the rectum, and increased frequency of high intra-abdominal pressure due to paroxysmal coughing. *Pneumatosis coli* has been reported in association with rectal prolapse in an 18-year-old with CF.

## Pancreatic Disease

Pancreatic exocrine insufficiency is present from birth in most patients with CF.[260] It has been estimated that only 5% to 10% of patients have significant pancreatic enzyme release. Exocrine pancreatic sufficiency has been associated with several mutations, including 3789 + 10 kb C to T, R117H, R334W, R347H, R347P, A455E, P574H, and Y563N. Enzyme deficiency results in fat and protein maldigestion, producing a distended abdomen and frequent bulky, greasy, foul-smelling stools. Uncorrected maldigestion results in failure to gain weight and ultimately in a failure of linear growth. Poor growth may also, however, be associated with increased expenditure of energy to accomplish the work of breathing, a point that is often overlooked in the assessment of patients who are short or excessively thin.[261] Fat loss in stools may be as high as 50% to 70% of total intake. Nitrogen malabsorption is roughly comparable or perhaps somewhat less severe. In general, carbohydrates are adequately absorbed in CF. Deficient absorption of fat-soluble vitamins occasionally produces symptoms. Symptomatic vitamin A deficiency, initially a prominent part of the CF syndrome, is rare and occurs only in patients who do not take supplementary vitamins or pancreatic enzymes. Increased intracranial pressure, xerophthalmia, and night blindness may result. Vitamin D deficiency, rickets, is rarely seen. Bone demineralization is, however, common in CF patients.[262–265] Vitamin E deficiency is common in unsupplemented patients but only rarely causes symptoms, including increased red blood cell destruction and neuroaxonal dystrophy. Vitamin K–dependent coagulation factors may also be deficient, resulting in a hemorrhagic diathesis. Although severe hemorrhagic problems occur mostly in young children, associated symptoms such as hemoptysis are occasionally seen in older patients.

It is now recognized that symptoms of pancreatitis are encountered in less than 1% of identified adolescent or adult CF patients and are limited to those who have retained some exocrine pancreatic function.[266] Recurrent pancreatitis has, however, recently been reported as associated with mutations in CFTR and is becoming more frequently recognized as a presenting symptom in adults with CF.[267, 268] Pancreatic calcifications are occasionally seen roentgenographically, but do not seem to correlate with symptomatic pancreatitis.

## Hepatobiliary Disease

Focal biliary cirrhosis is characteristic of CF, but produces symptoms in less than 5% of CF patients and causes death in about 2%.[37, 269] Hepatic abnormalities can present as hepatosplenomegaly or as persistent elevation of hepatic enzymes (particularly alkaline phosphatase). Rarely, patients present with esophageal varices and hemorrhage due to portal hypertension. Fatty liver is more common and may improve with adequate nutrition. Gallbladder disease is common in adults with CF. From 10% to 30% of patients have dysfunctional gallbladders[270] or gallstones.[271] Common bile duct stenosis secondary to CF is rare.[272]

## Genitourinary Tract Abnormalities

More than 98% of male patients with CF have obstructive azoospermia due to obstruction of the vas deferens.[273] Relatively high incidences of inguinal hernia and hydrocele also have been noted. Failure of reproductive function does not become an issue until well into the second decade of life. Semen analysis may be required to identify the 1% to 2% of male CF patients who are fertile. The volume of ejaculate is usually one third to one half of normal. There usually is complete absence of spermatozoa, and a number of chemical abnormalities of semen that reflect absence of secretions from the seminal vesicles can be demonstrated.[274]

Female infertility in CF may be as high as 20%.[274] Some women with CF are anovulatory because of chronic lung disease and malnutrition. Another obstacle to conception may be the presence of thick tenacious cervical mucus, which is difficult to dislodge from the os. This mucus is dehydrated and has abnormal electrolyte concentrations, preventing the usual ferning at midcycle and perhaps impeding normal sperm migration.[275] Endocervicitis is commonly noted.

More than 600 pregnancies in CF females have been reported. A longitudinal study of 325 pregnant women with CF demonstrated 258 live births (79%) and 67 therapeutic abortions.[276] Compared with 1142 age-match and severity-matched controls, pregnancy in a woman with CF did not have an independent negative effect on pulmonary status or mortality over 2 years. It is essential, however, that CF females consider their own health and expected lifespan in the context of family planning. Women with CF can breastfeed successfully.[277]

## Sweat Gland Dysfunction

Sweat chloride level is elevated in most CF patients due to abnormal NaCl reabsorption in the sweat ducts.[278] Excessive loss of salt in the sweat predisposes young children to depletion episodes, especially at times when there is additional salt loss due to vomiting or diarrhea. These children present with lethargy, anorexia, and hypochloremic alkalosis, a presentation that is more common in warm arid zones. Such hypochloremic alkalosis is rare in older children and adults.[276]

## DIAGNOSIS

The diagnosis of CF is based on carefully defined clinical criteria and laboratory evidence of CFTR dysfunction, including abnormal sweat $Cl^-$ levels.[278, 280] Accepted diagnostic criteria are listed in Table 40.5. Any one of these clinical features, if accompanied by a sweat chloride level greater than 60 mEq/L, is sufficient to make the diagnosis.

**Table 40.5 CRITERIA FOR THE DIAGNOSIS OF CYSTIC FIBROSIS**

| |
|---|
| Phenotypic clinical features |
| Chronic sinopulmonary disease |
| Chronic cough and sputum production |
| Persistent infection with characteristic pathogens (*Staphylococcus aureus* and *Pseudomonas aeruginosa*) |
| Airflow obstruction |
| Chronic chest radiographic abnormalities |
| Sinus disease; nasal polyps |
| Gastrointestinal and nutritional abnormalities |
| Pancreatic exocrine insufficiency; recurrent pancreatitis |
| Meconium ileus; distal intestinal obstruction syndrome |
| Obstructive azoospermia in males |
| Laboratory evidence of CFTR dysfunction |
| Elevated sweat $Cl^-$ |
| Mutation in the CF gene on both alleles |
| Characteristic bioelectric abnormalities (potential difference) in nasal epithelium in vivo |

*Adapted from Rosenstein BJ, Cutting GR: The diagnosis of CF: A consensus statement. Cystic Fibrosis Foundation Consensus Panel. J Pediatr 132: 589–595, 1998.
CFTR = cystic fibrosis transmembrane conductance regulator.

Characteristic nasal epithelial bioelectric abnormalities can also serve as laboratory evidence of CFTR dysfunction and can be used to diagnose CF when phenotypic clinical features are present.[278, 281] Many diagnoses are verified by identifying a mutation in CFTR on both alleles. At this time, however, a substantial number of patients have unidentified mutations. A few persons with sweat chloride values persistently in the diagnostic range but without clinical features of CF or a family history have been identified. As long as they remain symptom free and mutations of both CFTR genes are not identified, the diagnosis of CF cannot be made. Other clinical entities may be accompanied by elevated sweat chloride concentrations; these are listed in Table 40.6. None of these disorders is easily confused with CF. It is now recognized that a small percentage of persons with CF have sweat values in an intermediate (40 to 60 mEq/L) or even normal range.[35, 282, 283]

For the 1% to 2% of patients with compatible clinical features but normal sweat chloride levels, several approaches to the diagnosis are available. Clinical criteria for making the diagnosis of CF in the presence of a normal sweat chloride value were proposed before modern diagnostic options.[282] The discovery that bioelectric potential differences across respiratory epithelia are abnormal in patients with CF[9, 281] offers a more quantitative diagnostic test that has been useful in the evaluation of atypical patients. Also, DNA analysis techniques are now available for detection of the CF gene, particularly in clinical variants. For example, a single mutation of the CFTR gene, 3789 + 10 kb C to T, is associated with many of the suspected cases of CF whose sweat chloride values are in the normal range.[35, 284]

Although DNA analysis is becoming a standard of care

**Table 40.6 CONDITIONS OTHER THAN CYSTIC FIBROSIS ASSOCIATED WITH ELEVATED SWEAT CHLORIDE LEVELS**

| |
|---|
| Adrenal insufficiency |
| Anorexia nervosa |
| Atopic dermatitis |
| Pseudohypoaldosteronism |
| Hypothyroidism |
| Hypoparathyroidism |
| Nephrogenic diabetes insipidus |
| Ectodermal dysplasia |
| Glycogen storage disease (type I) |
| Mucopolysaccharidosis |
| Fucosidosis |
| Malnutrition |
| Mauriac's syndrome |
| Familial cholestasis syndrome |
| Prostaglandin $E_1$ administration |
| Hypogammaglobulinemia |

in CF, the sweat test remains the diagnostic standard. Only one method is recognized by the Cystic Fibrosis Foundation as adequate for the definitive diagnosis of CF. This test involves collection of sweat by pilocarpine iontophoresis, coupled with chemical determination of the chloride concentration.[285, 286] The procedure must be carried out in a meticulous fashion to avoid errors that frequently contribute to misleading values. As many as 40% of patients referred to CF centers have been inaccurately diagnosed elsewhere because of false-positive or false-negative sweat test results. In addition to frequent laboratory errors, faulty values can be obtained if the sweat rate is not sufficiently high. At least 50 mg of sweat must be collected in a 30-minute period. Potential pitfalls in interpretation include the presence of hypoproteinemic edema, failure to consider age-related effects, and concurrent administration of corticosteroids. Although a threshold level of 60 mEq/L of chloride in sweat appears to discriminate nearly all adults with CF from those with other lung conditions,[287] normal values of sweat chloride do increase with age, and some investigators insist on documentation of sweat chloride levels in excess of 70 mEq/L for the diagnosis of CF in adults.

Newborn screening for CF is carried out on all infants in several US states. The test used is an assay of immunoreactive trypsin in dried blood spots collected on filter paper in the first several days of life. Experience thus far suggests that many, but not all, newborns with CF may be identified with this test.[288] This test has an acceptable rate of false-positive results. Screening for gene mutations is currently precluded by the large number of mutations. If screening were based on ΔF508 alone, less than half of all newborns with CF would be identified. If parents were to be screened by DNA analysis, only 70% of carriers or 50% of carrier couples would be detected. At present, routine newborn screening cannot be strongly recommended largely because there is not yet a specific highly efficacious therapy for this condition that demands early intervention. Studies of newborns with CF discovered by screening have, however, detected nutritional deficits, which suggests that early identification and treatment may be useful to protect against loss of lung function.[289–292] In addition, pharmacologic and gene transfer therapies currently at an experimental stage are theoretically most effective early in life, and, if their efficacy is documented, newborn screening will play an important role.

Antenatal diagnosis can now be carried out, especially when the genotype of the parents is established. A 1997 National Institutes of Health Consensus Statement recommended that genetic testing for CF be offered to couples currently planning a pregnancy.[293]

## TREATMENT

The primary objectives of CF treatment are to control infection, promote mucous clearance, and improve nutrition.[294] In addition, experience has repeatedly demonstrated that attention to preventive aspects of lung care and psychosocial factors are important. The efficacy of a number of currently used and new approaches is being tested in controlled multicenter clinical trials.

### Ambulatory Care

At diagnosis, most patients are introduced to a care program that includes postural drainage with chest percussion, administration of antibiotics as indicated, and a nutritional regimen including pancreatic enzymes and fat-soluble vitamins. Other therapeutic modalities are prescribed as indicated.

#### Airway Clearance

The use of postural drainage with chest percussion to clear mucus is based on the concept that cough clears mucus from large airways, but chest vibrations are necessary to move secretions from the small airways where expiratory flow rates are low. The most compelling argument for the use of this therapeutic modality comes from a study of older children with mild to moderate airflow limitation.[295] When patients were receiving chest physical therapy on a regular basis, the only immediate effect documented was an increase in peak expiratory flow rate 30 minutes after therapy. After 3 weeks without chest physical therapy, however, both forced vital capacity and flow rates were significantly reduced. The diminution in lung function could be reversed with renewal of regular chest physical therapy. A recent meta-analysis of 35 studies concluded that standard chest physical therapy increases sputum production and improves expiratory airflow ($FEV_1$).[296] Most care centers prescribe this therapy one to four times a day, depending on the severity of illness.

A variety of mechanical percussors are available to assist, especially for those patients who do their own therapy. Several studies suggest that repeated forced expiratory maneuvers,[297] use of positive expiratory pressure,[298] and vigorous exercise[299–301] may substitute for chest physical therapy. The advisability of chest physical therapy for patients who have minimal cough and no apparent sputum production is open to question. Study results are not available to answer this question. Theoretically, chest physical therapy might prevent or delay inspissation of mucus in small airways, which is the earliest lesion. In addition, caregivers have found that many patients who do not receive chest physical therapy on a regular basis are unlikely to initiate this therapy when pulmonary exacerbations arise.

## Antibiotics

Lung infection is the major source of morbidity and mortality in CF. Therefore, antibiotic therapy is a mainstay of therapy designed to control progression of disease. In general, antibiotic therapy should be predicated on the presence of symptoms and guided by the identification of organisms from the lower respiratory tract. There is evidence that early and vigorous use of antibiotics produces better results than delaying the administration of antibiotics until symptoms are well developed or advanced.[302] Similarly, *P. aeruginosa* infection has been treated by regularly scheduled courses of intravenous antibiotics.[303] Data justifying these approaches are lacking.

Another principle of antimicrobial therapy in CF is that dosages need to be higher than for non–CF-related chest infections. Both total body clearance and volume of distribution are considerably greater for CF than for other patients.[304] In addition, large doses are needed to achieve therapeutic levels in the infected and mucus-filled or pus-filled endobronchial space. Sputum levels achieved are highly varied but usually are less than half of the levels measured in serum.[305] Experience also has led many caregivers of CF patients to use longer than usual courses of antibiotics, continuing for at least 2 weeks and, frequently, 3 or 4 weeks.

The choice of antibiotics optimally should be based on the results of sputum culture and sensitivity tests. For patients with nonproductive cough, specimens are best obtained by harvesting secretions with a throat swab placed just above the glottis during repetitive coughing. Nasopharyngeal cultures are not useful as a guide for selection of antibiotics. If *S. aureus* is present or expected, the choice may include a semisynthetic penicillin, a combination of ampicillin and clavulanic acid, a cephalosporin, or clindamycin. Suggested drugs and doses are listed in Table 40.7. *Haemophilus* infections are best treated with ampicillin, trimethoprim-sulfamethoxazole, cefuroxime, or cefaclor. In most cases, these antibiotics eradicate *S. aureus* and *H. influenzae* from the airways on a temporary basis. In older children and adults, tetracyclines may provide useful empiric therapy. Ciprofloxacin appears to

**Table 40.7 ANTIMICROBIAL AGENTS USED TO TREAT CF LUNG INFECTION**

| | | | Dose | | |
|---|---|---|---|---|---|
| Route | Organism | Agent | Pediatric (mg/kg/day) | Adult (g/day) | Doses/Day |
| Oral | *S. aureus* | Dicloxacillin | 50–100 | 2–4 | 4 |
| | | Cefaclor | 40 | 0.75–1.5 | 3 |
| | | Clindamycin | 10–20 | 0.6–1.2 | 4 |
| | | Erythromycin | 50 | 2 | 4 |
| | | Amoxicillin/clavulanate | 50 | 1.5 | 3 |
| | | Azithromycin | — | 0.5 day 1, then 0.25 daily for 2–5 days | 1 |
| | *H. influenzae* | Amoxicillin | 50 | 1.5 | 3 |
| | | Trimethoprim-sulfamethoxazole | 20* | 0.32–0.64* | 2–4 |
| | *P. aeruginosa* | Ciprofloxacin | — | 1.5–2.25 | 3 |
| | | Ofloxacin | — | 0.8–1.2 | 2–3 |
| | Empirical | Tetracycline | 25–50 | 2 | 3–4 |
| Intravenous | *S. aureus* | Oxacillin | 150–200 | —† | 4 |
| | | Vancomycin | 40 | 2 | 2–4 |
| | *P. aeruginosa* | Gentamicin or tobramycin | 10 | —† | 2–3 |
| | | Amikacin | 30 | —† | 2–3 |
| | | Carbenicillin or ticarcillin | 400 | —† | 4–6 |
| | | Piperacillin, mezlocillin, or azlocillin | 400 | —† | 4–6 |
| | | Ticarcillin/clavulanate | 400 | —† | 4–6 |
| | | Imipenem/cilastatin | 100 | 4 | 3–4 |
| | *P. aeruginosa* and *B. cepacia* | Ceftazidime | 300 | 3–6 | 3 |
| Aerosol | *P. aeruginosa* | Gentamicin | 40–600† | 80–600† | 2–4 |
| | | Tobramycin | 40–600† | 80–600† | 2–4 |

*Quantity of trimethoprim.
†Usually dosed by mg/kg/day as with children.
‡Total dose in milligrams.

control symptoms and reduces numbers of *Pseudomonas* organisms in CF airways, but its usefulness is limited by rapid emergence of resistant organisms.[306]

Because of limited options for treatment of *Pseudomonas* with oral antibiotics, parenteral preparations of aminoglycosides or other antibiotics have been delivered to the lower respiratory tract by aerosol.[307, 308] Recent studies show clear short-term benefit of aerosolized tobramycin (300 mg in nebulizer) taken twice daily.[309] This treatment, taken in alternate months for three cycles, improved lung function, decreased bacterial burden, and decreased relative risk for hospitalization. The rate of acquired tobramycin resistance was about 7% over 24 weeks in the treated group.

### Aerosolized rhDNase

The lysis of viscous DNA with the recombinant enzyme DNase offers benefit to some patients with purulent airway secretions.[310] When taken once daily, aerosolized DNase reduced the relative risk of respiratory exacerbations by 28% and improved $FEV_1$ approximately 6% above baseline over 6 months. Not all patients had objective improvement in lung function, but symptomatic benefit occurred in many of the treated patients without improved lung function. The long-term effect of DNase on lung function is currently being evaluated in an open-label multinational study.

### Other Aerosol Therapy

Other solutions given by aerosol have the objective of providing volume of liquid to hydrate inspissated mucous secretions. One frequently used solution is normal saline, but the efficacy of this approach has not been substantiated. Studies from Australia in 1996 suggest that aerosolized hypertonic saline (3% to 12%) may offer short-term benefit with acute improvement in lung function and mucociliary clearance.[311, 312]

### Bronchodilators

As detailed in the discussion of clinical manifestations, many patients demonstrate bronchial lability, prompting frequent use of bronchodilators,[218] particularly beta-adrenoceptor agonists. Although their immediate effectiveness can be documented in the pulmonary function laboratory, overall improvement or long-term benefit has not been established. Indications for the use of bronchodilators include troublesome wheezing and a documented improvement in pulmonary function (e.g., at least a 15% improvement of $FEV_1$). Beta-agonists can be nebulized, administered by meter-dosed inhalers, or given orally. Caution should be exercised concerning long-term therapy with these agents because animal studies show that administration of large amounts of beta-adrenoceptor agonists cause submucosal gland hypertrophy and presumably a hypersecretory state.[313] Theophylline preparations also may be effective in selected cases. CF patients seem, however, to be less tolerant of theophylline because of frequent gastrointestinal irritation.[314] Ipratropium bromide is at least as effective as beta-agonists in CF,[315–317] although distal intestinal obstruction syndrome has been reported coincident with use of this agent.[318] Cromolyn sodium has also been used; a single study failed to demonstrate efficacy.[319]

### Corticosteroids

An initial double-blind controlled study of alternate-day oral corticosteroid administration demonstrated better maintenance of pulmonary function and fewer exacerbations of lung disease requiring hospitalization over a 4-year period.[320] A subsequent large multicenter study of corticosteroids administered in a dose of 1.0 or 2.0 mg/kg every other day, however, failed to confirm efficacy and was attended by an unacceptable rate of side effects, including growth suppression and hyperglycemia.[320a] Widespread use of corticosteroids cannot be advocated. They may be used for specific indications such as allergic bronchopulmonary aspergillosis.

### Anti-Inflammatory Therapy with Ibuprofen

A recent study of high-dose ibuprofen over 4 years indicates that young CF patients (younger than 13 years) with mild lung disease have remarkable slowing of decline of lung function (eightfold) compared with placebo-control subjects.[321] No effect was documented in patients older than 13 years, even among patients with the mildest lung disease. There were few side effects, but most of the patients were taking antacids or $H_2$-receptor blockers.

### Other Respiratory Therapies

Mucolytics, expectorants, and cough suppressants have been used for relief of chest symptoms. In general, cough is an important mucous clearance mechanism for patients with CF and should not be suppressed. Expectorants, which assist in the elimination of airway secretions during cough, probably do not achieve that objective. Rather than being helpful, long-term administration of iodides to patients with CF has been associated with a high incidence of goiter and hypothyroidism.[322] Mucolytics such as *N*-acetylcysteine are injurious to respiratory epithelium and promote bronchitis when used regularly. Therefore, aerosol inhalation of this substance should be used selectively and only for short periods. Another experimental approach, delivery of elastase inhibitors to airways by aerosol, is the subject of several clinical trials.

Other experimental drugs include $Na^+$ conductance inhibitors[323, 324] and triphosphate nucleotides.[112, 150] Both act to increase salt and water availability at the epithelial surface of the airway and may improve mucous clearance properties.

Exercise is generally considered beneficial for patients with CF and should be encouraged for all but those with the most severe lung disease and hypoxemia.[325] A 12-week exercise program consisting of three 1-hour sessions a week, during which jogging was used to produce a heart rate averaging 70% to 85% of peak heart rate, has been shown to increase exercise tolerance and cardiorespiratory fitness, probably by increasing respiratory muscle endurance.[231] This program did not, however, improve pulmonary function. Most caregivers of patients with CF believe that regular, vigorous exercise promotes a positive self-concept and increases the perception of wellness. In addition to cardiopulmonary conditioning exercises, isometric exercises such as weight lifting may build abdominal and upper body muscle strength and in this way promote deep breathing and effective coughing.

### Gene Transfer Technology

It is technically possible with genetically engineered viral vectors to transfer the wild-type CFTR gene to respiratory epithelial cells in vitro, where it can be expressed at least for days to weeks.[326] Systems for efficient targeted delivery and optimal integration in vivo are being studied and contribute to the hope that genetic reconstitution will be a feasible approach to lung therapy in the future.

### Nutrition

Approximately 90% of patients with CF require mealtime pancreatic enzymes, packaged as granules that are coated with acid-resistant material to promote delivery to the small intestine. Capsules containing 1000 to 20,000 U of lipase are available. Numbers of capsules taken should be adjusted based on weight gain, presence or absence of abdominal cramping, and the character of stools. Dosage should be limited to current guidelines (500 to 2500 lipase units per kg per meal) because a large total daily dose of enzyme activity has been associated with fibrosing colonopathy.[327–330] Vitamins A and D are generally supplied by a daily multiple-vitamin preparation. Also, 200 to 400 IU of vitamin E daily for patients older than 10 years are recommended because serum levels are generally low in unsupplemented patients. Vitamin K is given sporadically to treat bleeding complications or to correct prolonged prothrombin times. Other vitamins and trace minerals may be deficient and require supplementation on a selective basis.[261]

Many patients with CF have a higher than normal caloric need because of the increased work of breathing. In general, patients should be encouraged to eat a balanced diet, including at least a moderate amount of fat. When the anorexia of chronic infection supervenes, failure to gain weight or weight loss occurs. Further encouragement to eat high-calorie foods may be helpful. Supplementation with elemental dietary preparations by mouth is unlikely to be sustained over an extended period of time. Some CF care centers administer supplementary elemental feedings nocturnally by nasogastric tube or by percutaneous duodenostomy.[261, 331] Although short-term benefits such as increased weight gain can be achieved, long-term beneficial effects on pulmonary function have not been established.

Patients with CF who retain exocrine pancreatic function and maintain good nutrition experience a slower rate of decline of pulmonary function than do those with pancreatic dysfunction.[332] This observation has been used as a rationale for emphasizing nutritional interventions. Although this approach may have merit, it is generally more efficacious to maintain good nutrition by preventing progression of lung disease than to maintain good lung function by emphasizing nutritional therapy.

### Psychosocial Factors

As with any chronic disease, compliance with therapy and ability to function fully are highly dependent on the patient's attitude. Therefore, approaches that promote a positive self-concept and foster the ability of patients to take control of their medical management and that enable them to participate fully in life events are likely to promote well-being and perhaps longevity. Medical care that provides continuity and fosters trust may pay large dividends. Personnel who specifically provide psychosocial support are important contributors to CF care teams.

### Immunization for Lung Pathogens

Rubeola, pertussis, and influenza infections are particularly injurious to CF lungs and may trigger a downward spiral of lung function. Adequate immunization early in life for pertussis and measles is mandatory. In addition, patients of all ages should be adequately immunized for influenza virus infection on a yearly basis. The early use of amantadine for acute respiratory illnesses during epidemics of influenza A infections may further prevent adverse consequences of this infection. Other routine vaccines should be administered as for the general population. There is no evidence that administration of pneumococcal vaccine is useful.

## Hospital Therapy

Indications for hospitalization and intensive pulmonary therapy include increased cough or wheezing, respiratory distress with decreased activity tolerance, weight loss, sustained downward trend in pulmonary function, increasing hypoxemia, or one of the major pulmonary complications of CF. Although all the modalities of therapy can be intensified in the hospital, the major advantage of hospitalization is the ability to administer intravenous antimicrobial agents that control *Pseudomonas* infection and to intensify physical maneuvers to clear airway secretions.

Antibiotics for intravenous administration should be selected on the basis of respiratory tract cultures and susceptibility studies. Two-drug treatment of *Pseudomonas* infection is the rule. A third antibiotic may be added as necessary for control of *S. aureus* or other organisms. Drugs and dosages currently used for intravenous therapy are listed in Table 40.7. A clinical response is often not seen for 4 to 7 days after initiation of therapy. In general, a 2-week course provides good improvement in pulmonary function[333, 334] and more sustained benefit than shorter courses. With refractory infection, treatment for 3 weeks or more is not unusual. Some advocate intensive therapy until pulmonary function has returned to a previous baseline or until improvement has reached a plateau. Prolonged courses of antibiotic therapy should include periodic monitoring of respiratory tract organisms and their antibiotic sensitivities, as shifts in either are common.

Aminoglycosides have been the mainstay of anti-*Pseu-*

*domonas* therapy for many years. A major advantage is the ability to monitor and adjust blood levels. For gentamicin or tobramycin, two to three times a day dosage and achievement of peaks in the range of 10 to 12 μg/mL and troughs less than 2 μg/mL seem to be optimal. Patients should be monitored during aminoglycoside therapy for nephrotoxicity and ototoxicity. An aminoglycoside is usually paired with one of the penicillin derivatives or with ceftazidime.

Patients with CF, particularly those who are in school or working full-time jobs, may opt to administer intravenous antibiotics at home for all or a portion of the treatment course. This seems to work well for selected patients and may be as effective as hospital treatment.[335, 336] For patients requiring frequent courses or long-term home antibiotic therapy, central intravenous catheters have been surgically placed and used for prolonged periods.

One study suggested that the infusion of 100 mg/kg of intravenous immunoglobulin daily for three days during a course of intravenous antibiotics enhances the pulmonary function response.[337] Further studies are needed to confirm these observations.

Interest in bronchial lavage as a therapeutic modality has been tempered by the realization that long-term benefits are unlikely to accrue from this approach and that acute deterioration of lung function is a possible outcome.[338] In fact, there is no evidence that bronchoscopy and lavage, whether it be whole lung, lobar, or segmental, is superior to intensive antibiotic therapy and chest percussion.

## Treatment of Lung Complications

Hypercapnic and hypoxemic *respiratory failure* in CF are primarily due to progressive obstructive airway disease with alveolar hypoventilation and ventilation/perfusion mismatching. Treatment of airway infection and inflammation with antibiotics and the airway clearance measures summarized earlier is essential. Low flow oxygen is effective at relieving nocturnal, exertional, and resting hypoxemia and does not usually cause significant hypercapnia.[339] The use of supplemental oxygen in children has been discouraged[340] because nocturnal oxygen did not improve survival or prevent the development of cor pulmonale in one controlled trial.[341] A larger study demonstrated that the development of pulmonary hypertension in adults with CF is strongly correlated with hypoxemia and is associated with increased mortality.[342] Therefore, supplemental oxygen in accordance with the guidelines established for COPD[343] is recommended.[344] Diuretics, inotropic agents, and theophylline produce few benefits and are rarely used. Cor pulmonale is a late complication of airway obstruction, and no treatment options beyond those for the primary disease processes are effective.

Ventilatory assistance is effective in CF patients with acute respiratory failure caused by reversible insults,[253] but it produces few long-term benefits in patients with respiratory failure due to irreversible lung damage caused by bronchiectasis.[345] Assisted ventilation with nasal or face masks[346, 347] or endotracheal tubes[348] can effectively treat patients awaiting lung transplantation. The airway disease progresses, however, and long-term ventilatory support is rarely feasible.

*Atelectasis* is best treated by vigorous standard therapy, including airway clearance and antibiotics. Corticosteroids may be helpful in the presence of reactive airways or severe airway inflammation. There is no evidence that bronchoscopy and lavage are effective in expanding collapsed segments of lobes.[241] *Allergic bronchopulmonary aspergillosis* responds to standard doses of systemic corticosteroids.[349] Inhaled steroids[350] and the oral antifungal agent itraconazole[351] may prove to be useful.

*Pneumothorax* can be observed for spontaneous resolution if it is small and minimally symptomatic. A large pneumothorax (more than 20% of the hemithorax volume, compromising ventilation or causing hypotension) requires tube drainage.[223] Recurrences are very common and may require thoracoscopic talc poudrage or surgical pleural abrasion.[247]

*Hemoptysis* requires treatment of airway infection and supplemental vitamin K if the prothrombin time is prolonged due to inadequate absorption. Massive hemoptysis may resolve with such conservative therapy and modest cough suppression for 1 to 2 days,[243] but bronchial artery embolization[352] provides more definitive control, which usually persists for more than 6 months.

## Treatment of Gastrointestinal Complications

*Meconium ileus* can be relieved in a number of cases with enemas and meglumine diatrizoate (Gastrografin) or other contrast materials, which are refluxed into the terminal ileum under fluoroscopy. If this fails, or if there is evidence of perforation, surgical intervention is required. *Distal intestinal obstruction syndrome* also can be relieved with contrast enemas that reach the terminal ileum. This approach has, however, been largely supplanted by intestinal "flushes" with a balanced salt solution; 1 to 2 L rapidly instilled into the stomach is usually effective. Occasionally, surgical intervention is necessary. *Rectal prolapse* usually can be reduced voluntarily by older patients, using abdominal, perineal, and gluteal muscles, but in small children rectal prolapse must be reduced manually by continuous gentle pressure with the patient in the knee-chest position[259]; sedation may be helpful. Adequate pancreatic enzyme therapy, decreased fat in the diet, and control of pulmonary infection usually prevent recurrences. A few patients may require surgical stabilization of the rectum.

*Cirrhosis* is generally focal and usually does not require specific therapy. Localization of CFTR to bile ductule cells suggests that abnormal bile secretion may be germane to CF liver disease. Ursodeoxycholic acid is effective treatment for primary biliary cirrhosis.[353] Early trials of ursodeoxycholic acid in CF patients showed improved liver function tests, but the long-term effect on liver function is not known.[354, 355] The thresholds for initiating therapy and clinical outcomes are under investigation. Bleeding esophageal varices that complicate cirrhosis often can be managed with banding or sclerotherapy. In the past, significant bleeding has been treated successfully with portosystemic shunting.[356] Splenorenal anastomoses have been most effective, and hepatic encephalopathy has not been a problem. The transjugular intrahepatic portosystemic shunt procedure[357, 358] can relieve portal hypertension and reduce bleeding episodes. Liver failure and ascites are treated as in other patients. Liver transplantation has been successfully performed, with a 2-year survival rate exceeding 50%.[359, 360] Pancreatitis, when it occurs in adolescents or young adults with CF, is treated with standard measures.

Hyperglycemia as a complication of CF can occur at any age, but it is generally a problem of the second and third decades of life.[262] Ketoacidosis is rarely encountered. When blood glucose levels are only intermittently elevated and glycosuria is not present, no treatment is necessary. With the advent of sustained glycosuria, insulin treatment should be instituted. Oral hypoglycemic agents, considered ineffective in the past, may be helpful in selected patients.[361] The development of significant hyperglycemia may not affect longevity.[362, 363] Vascular disease affecting the retina and kidneys has, however, been documented in CF patients who have had prolonged hyperglycemia.[364, 365] Therefore, careful control of blood sugar levels is desirable.

### Surgical Therapy

Nasal polypectomy to relieve obstruction is the most common surgical procedure in CF, and most patients obtain symptomatic improvement.[366] Recurrence of polyps is common,[367] but the incidence of polyposis usually wanes after the second decade. Gallstones are common, and symptomatic disease may require elective cholecystectomy in as many as 5% of CF adults.[368] Lobectomy is occasionally indicated for massive hemoptysis that is refractory to bronchial artery embolization. Partial lung resection has been advocated for apparently localized disease and recurrent severe exacerbations.[369] The generalized lung disease, however, continues to progress; the limited probability of long-term benefits dictates caution in patient selection.

### Transplantation

Lung transplantation has become an accepted therapy for respiratory failure secondary to CF.[370] Heart-lung transplantation has been largely replaced by sequential double lung transplantation because of limited organ availability. Patients should be referred when their prognosis is about equal to the waiting time for donor lungs, currently about 2 years after acceptance as a lung transplant candidate. More than 1600 lung transplantations have been performed for CF around the world. The transplanted lungs remain free of CF but are subject to secondary infection, acute rejection, and chronic rejection (bronchiolitis obliterans syndrome). The 5-year survival rate is 48%, as good as that of lung transplant recipients with other causes of lung disease. Living lobar transplantation is an effective alternative to conventional cadaveric lung transplants.[371] The lobe donors must have sufficiently large lungs so that their lower lobe will fill the recipient's hemithorax. Survival appears to be similar to that following conventional lung transplantation.

## COURSE OF THE DISEASE AND PROGNOSIS

CF has a highly varied course, ranging from death due to complications of meconium ileus in the first days of life or death from severe respiratory tract problems within the first months of life to essentially asymptomatic existence for 10 to 20 years[372] and protracted survival. A few patients with CF do live into the sixth and seventh decades of life.[255] More than 7500 (36%) of the patients in the US CF registry are 18 years of age or older.[34] The changing age distribution is demonstrated in Figure 40.7.

At most CF care centers, patients are monitored by general clinical assessment, which often involves the use of a scoring system,[373, 374] periodic monitoring of respiratory tract pathogens, periodic chest roentgenograms, serial pulmonary function testing, and ongoing nutritional assessment. Initial intensive treatment is usually followed by improvement in pulmonary function tests, substantial improvement in weight-to-height ratios, and accelerated linear growth in children. After initial improvement or stabilization, there is often an extended period of stable lung function that may last 5, 10, or even 15 years. Progressive dysfunction inevitably supervenes. Longitudinal patterns of pulmonary function in older individuals with CF are highly variable.[375, 376]

The most recent statistics from the Cystic Fibrosis Foundation indicate that 50% of patients can now be expected to survive beyond age 30 years. These data were generated from all patients under care in Cystic Fibrosis Foundation–sponsored centers in 1997 (Fig. 40.8). Analyses of survival curves over the years suggest that longevity has increased steadily to the present time. Some of the improvement in survival may have resulted from the diagnosis of milder forms of the disease. There is, however, considerable opinion that improved symptomatic therapy has also contributed to better survival.

Multiple factors determine the prognosis for individuals with CF.[377] Data from all US CF centers suggest that survival is better for patients living in northern climates

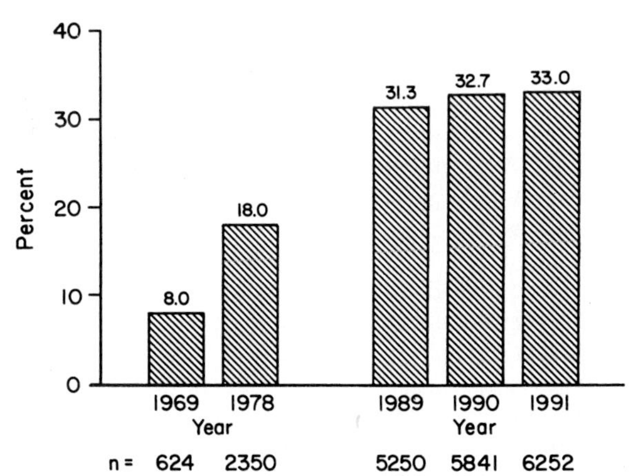


**Figure 40.7** Per cent of CF patients aged 18 or older are shown for 1969 to 1991. Data are from the Patient Registry, Cystic Fibrosis Foundation, Bethesda, MD. (Courtesy of Dr. S. FitzSimmons, Cystic Fibrosis Foundation.)

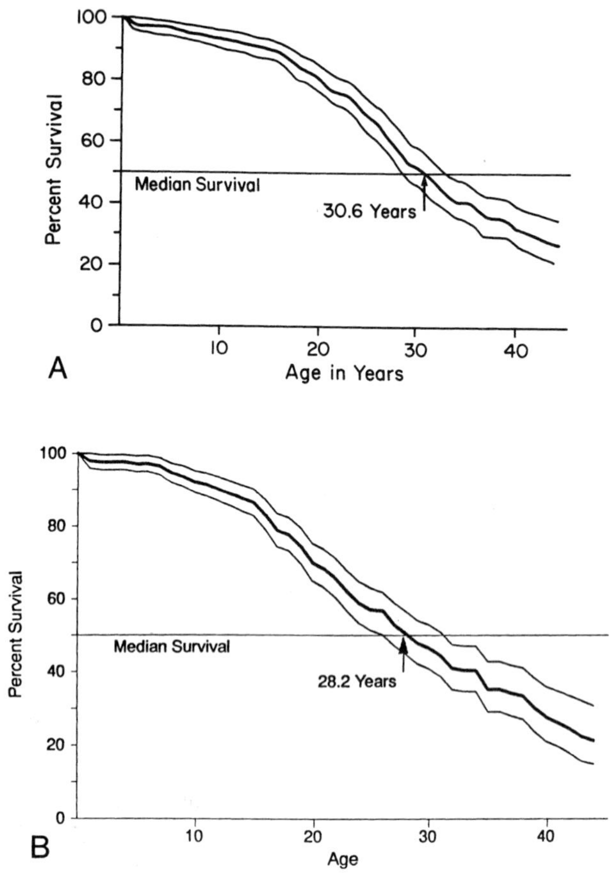


**Figure 40.8** Survival curves are shown for the male *(A)* and female *(B)* CF patients studied in all US CF Centers in 1991. The curves demonstrate that the median survival age, or age to which 50% of the patient population may be expected to survive, exceeds 30 years for males and 28 years for females. Aggregate median survival is 29.4 years. Data are from the Patient Registry, Cystic Fibrosis Foundation, Bethesda, MD. (Courtesy of Dr. S. FitzSimmons, Cystic Fibrosis Foundation.)

than for those in the South. On average, male patients live 3 years longer than do female patients. Blacks who survive the first several years of life may have a better prognosis than whites. Age at diagnosis has not emerged as a clear determinant of survival. A study of sibling pairs, however, suggests that the younger sibling who is diagnosed before 1 year of age, before the onset of symptoms, usually has better pulmonary function at 7 years of age than does the older sibling diagnosed at an older age because of symptoms.[378] Outcome analyses of patients who have been identified at birth by screening procedures and those who have been diagnosed after onset of symptoms should provide more definitive evidence for the efficacy of early diagnosis and treatment.

Several studies suggest that the clinical features present when the patient is first seen make a difference. Patients who initially have only steatorrhea and failure to thrive generally improve remarkably after institution of therapy and do well for extended periods. In contrasts, patients who have respiratory tract symptoms when first seen usually continue to have respiratory tract problems and have a less favorable prognosis.[379] When the entire CF population is considered, those patients who retain pancreatic exocrine function display a slower progression of pulmonary disease.[32, 380] Meconium ileus does not influence longevity if the patient survives the first months of life. Initial claims that CF patients with allergies have improved survival cannot be substantiated. There are numerous indicators of poor prognosis once airway disease has been established, including colonization with *P. aeruginosa* or *B. cepacia* and occurrence of pulmonary complications such as pneumothorax and massive hemoptysis.[381] Onset of insulin-dependent hyperglycemia has been considered a risk factor,[363] but some evidence suggests that survival rates of these patients parallel those of patients who have no overt problem of glucose metabolism.[382]

Little is known about the influence of medical care on longevity. Several studies suggest that patients studied at established care centers have a greater median survival rate than do those who receive care in nonspecialized settings.[383, 383a] In addition, evidence suggests that center to center variation in survival of patients is directly related to the intensity of the care rendered in each center, including frequency of monitoring, antibiotic use, and hospitalization for treatment of pulmonary exacerbations.[302]

Finally, psychosocial factors undoubtedly play a prominent role in outcome, although this is difficult to document.[384–386] The role of a supportive family is crucial. Suicide is uncommon. It is widely recognized, however, that a substantial number of adolescent and adult patients do not comply fully with therapy regimens because of denial, unresolved dependence-independence issues, and depression. Clearly, attitude and the ability to cope with a fatal illness during maturation and early adulthood do influence outcome.

Even though faced with a life-threatening illness and burdened with staggering demands on time, energy, and financial resources to comply with therapy, most adolescents and young adults cope admirably and are able to achieve a satisfactory quality of life. Successful relationships,[387] advanced education, and a full-time occupation are frequently achieved (Table 40.8), indicating that independent lifestyles and full participation in life events are attainable goals for many patients.

## SUMMARY

CF is a prevalent autosomal recessive syndrome that causes life-threatening chronic lung disease of childhood and adulthood. It is caused by one or two of more than 850 identified mutations occurring in a gene on chromosome 7 that codes for an integral membrane protein of epithelial cells (CFTR). This protein is a chloride channel and also regulates other ion channels in epithelial cells. Disturbed function results in alterations of electrolyte content, intraluminal volume, and diminished clearance of exocrine secretions. Lung pathophysiology reflects airway obstruction by accumulated mucus and secondary bacterial infection.

Diagnosis requires the identification of typical pulmo-

**Table 40.8** EDUCATIONAL AND EMPLOYMENT RECORDS OF ADULTS WITH CYSTIC FIBROSIS*

| RECORDS | PERCENT |
|---|---|
| Highest educational degree (n = 686) | |
| Associate | 10 |
| Bachelor's | 14 |
| Master's | 5 |
| Doctorate | 2 |
| Other | 4 |
| No advanced degree or no response | 65 |
| Employment (n = 679) | |
| Full time | 37 |
| Part time | 21 |
| Unemployed, seeking work | 12 |
| Unemployed, not seeking work | 30 |

*Data from a national survey by the Cystic Fibrosis Foundation. (Adapted from Lewiston NJ: Psychosocial impact of cystic fibrosis. Semin Respir Med 6:321-332, 1985, with permission.)

nary or pancreatic manifestations or a family history of CF, combined with documentation of elevated chloride concentrations in sweat. Genotype analyses confirm the diagnosis and have predictive implications for the clinical course.

Treatment currently focuses on control of mucus retention and chronic infection in the lungs, replacement of pancreatic enzymes, and nutritional therapy. Close monitoring, vigorous attempts to reverse deterioration of lung function and nutritional deficits, and psychosocial support offer additional benefits. The outcome is highly variable, but longevity has increased steadily and median survival now exceeds 29 years. Quality of life for patients with CF has also improved. New approaches to therapy, including lung transplantation, pharmacologic interventions targeted to epithelial cell pathophysiology, and gene transfer to airway epithelium offer hope for further substantial therapeutic advances.

## References


1. Davis PB, Drumm M, Konstan MW: Cystic fibrosis. Am J Respir Crit Care Med 154:1229–1256, 1996.
2. Zielenski J, Tsui LC: Cystic fibrosis: Genotypic and phenotypic variations. Annu Rev Genet 29:777–807, 1995.
3. Taussig LM: Cystic Fibrosis. New York: Thieme-Stratton, 1984.
4. Andersen DH: Cystic fibrosis of the pancreas and its relation to celiac disease: A clinical and pathologic study. Am J Dis Child 56:344–399, 1938.
5. Farber S: Some organic digestive disturbances in early life. J Mich Med Sci 44:587–594, 1945.
6. Andersen DH, Hodges RG: Celiac syndrome. V. Genetics of cystic fibrosis of the pancreas with a consideration of etiology. Am J Dis Child 72:62–80, 1946.
7. di Sant'Agnese PA, Darling RC, Perera GA, et al: Abnormal electrolyte composition of sweat in cystic fibrosis of the pancreas. Pediatrics 12:549–563, 1953.
8. Gibson LE, Cooke RE: A test for concentration of electrolytes in sweat in cystic fibrosis of the pancreas utilizing pilocarpine by iontophoresis. Pediatrics 23:545–549, 1959.
9. Knowles M, Gatzy J, Boucher R: Increased bioelectric potential difference across respiratory epithelia in cystic fibrosis. N Engl J Med 305:1489–1495, 1981.
10. Quinton PM, Bijman J: Higher bioelectric potentials due to decreased chloride absorption in the sweat glands of patients with cystic fibrosis. N Engl J Med 308:1185–1189, 1983.
11. Tsui LC, Buchwald M, Barker D, et al: Cystic fibrosis locus defined by a genetically linked polymorphic DNA marker. Science 230:1054–1057, 1985.
12. Zengerling S, Tsui LC, Grzeschik KH, et al: Mapping of DNA markers linked to the cystic fibrosis locus on the long arm of chromosome 7. Am J Hum Genet 40:228–236, 1987.
13. White R, Woodward S, Leppert M, et al: A closely linked genetic marker for cystic fibrosis. Nature 318:382–384, 1985.
14. Wainwright BJ, Scambler PJ, Schmidtke J, et al: Localization of cystic fibrosis locus to human chromosome 7cen-q22. Nature 318:384–385, 1985.
15. Riordan JR, Rommens JM, Kerem B-T, et al: Identification of the cystic fibrosis gene: Cloning and characterization of complementary DNA. Science 245:1066–1073, 1989.
16. Kerem B-T, Rommens JM, Buchanan JA, et al: Identification of the cystic fibrosis gene: Genetic analysis. Science 245:1073–1080, 1989.
17. Drumm ML, Pope HA, Cliff WH, et al: Correction of the cystic fibrosis defect in vitro by retrovirus-mediated gene transfer. Cell 62:1227–1233, 1990.
18. Rich DP, Anderson MP, Gregory RJ, et al: Expression of cystic fibrosis transmembrane conductance regulator corrects defective chloride channel regulation in cystic fibrosis airway epithelial cells. Nature 347:358–363, 1990.
19. Anderson MP, Rich DP, Gregory RJ, et al: Generation of cAMP-activated chloride currents by expression of CFTR. Science 251:679–682, 1991.
20. Anderson MP, Gregory RJ, Thompson S, et al: Demonstration that CFTR is a chloride channel by alteration of its anion selectivity. Science 253:202–205, 1991.
21. Bear CE, Li C, Kartner N, et al: Purification and functional reconstitution of the cystic fibrosis transmembrane conductance regulator (CFTR). Cell 68:809–818, 1992.
22. Egan M, Flotte T, Afione S, et al: Defective regulation of outwardly rectifying $Cl^-$ channels by protein kinase A corrected by insertion of CFTR. Nature 358:581–584, 1992.
23. Stutts MJ, Canessa CM, Olsen JC, et al: CFTR as a cAMP-dependent regulator of sodium channels. Science 269:847–850, 1995.
24. Cheng SH, Gregory RJ, Marshall J, et al: Defective intracellular transport and processing of CFTR is the molecular basis of most cystic fibrosis. Cell 63:827–834, 1990.
25. Jensen TJ, Loo MA, Pind S, et al: Multiple proteolytic systems, including the proteasome, contribute to CFTR processing. Cell 83:129–135, 1995.
26. Gunderson KL, Kopito RR: Conformational states of CFTR associated with channel gating: The role of ATP binding and hydrolysis. Cell 82:231–239, 1995.
27. Snouwaert JN, Brigman KK, Latour AM, et al: An animal model for cystic fibrosis made by gene targeting. Science 257:1083–1088, 1992.
28. Clarke LL, Grubb BR, Gabriel SE, et al: Defective epithelial chloride transport in a gene targeted mouse model of cystic fibrosis. Science 257:1125–1128, 1992.
29. Dorin JR, Dickinson P, Alton EWFW, et al: Cystic fibrosis in the mouse by targeted insertional mutagenesis. Nature 359:211–215, 1992.
30. Grubb BR, Boucher RC: Pathophysiology of gene-targeted mouse models for cystic fibrosis. Physiol Rev 79:S193–S214, 1999.
31. Tsui L-C, Buchwald M: Biochemical and molecular genetics of cystic fibrosis. Adv Hum Genet 20:153–266, 1991.
32. Kerem E, Corey M, Kerem B-S, et al: The relation between genotype and phenotype in cystic fibrosis–analysis of the most common mutation ($DF_{508}$). N Engl J Med 323:1517–1522, 1990.
33. Liechti-Gallati S, Bonsall I, Malik N, et al: Genotype/phenotype association in cystic fibrosis: Analyses of the delta F508, R553X, and 3905insT mutations. Pediatr Res 32:175–178, 1992.
34. FitzSimmons SC: CFF Patient Registry. 1997 Annual Data Report. Bethesda, MD: Cystic Fibrosis Foundation, 1998.
35. Knowles MR, Friedman KJ, Silverman L: Genetics, diagnosis, and clinical phenotype. *In* Yankaskas JR, Knowles MR (eds):

Cystic Fibrosis in Adults. Philadelphia: Lippincott-Raven, 1999, pp 27–42.
36. Gaskin KJ: Intestines. *In* Yankaskas JR, Knowles MR (eds): Cystic Fibrosis in Adults. Philadelphia: Lippincott-Raven, 1999, pp 325–342.
37. Colombo C, Crosignani A, Melzi ML, et al: Hepatobiliary system. *In* Yankaskas JR, Knowles MR (eds): Cystic Fibrosis in Adults. Philadelphia: Lippincott-Raven, 1999, pp 309–324.
38. Duthie A, Doherty DG, Williams C, et al: Genotype analysis for delta F508, G551D and R553X mutations in children and young adults with cystic fibrosis with and without chronic liver disease. Hepatology 15:660–664, 1992.
39. Zielenski J, Corey M, Rozmahel R, et al: Detection of a cystic fibrosis modifier locus for meconium ileus on human chromosome 19q13. Nat Genet 22:128–129, 1999.
40. Strong TV, Smit LS, Turpin SV, et al: Cystic fibrosis gene mutation in two sisters with mild disease and normal sweat electrolyte levels. N Engl J Med 325:1630–1634, 1991.
41. Wilfond BS, Fost N: The cystic fibrosis gene: Medical and social implications for heterozygote detection. JAMA 263:2777–2783, 1990.
42. Danks DM, Allan J, Anderson CM: A genetic study of fibrocystic disease of the pancreas. Ann Hum Genet 28:323–356, 1965.
43. Ten Kate LP: A method for analysing fertility of heterozygotes for autosomal recessive disorders, with special reference to cystic fibrosis, Tay-Sachs disease and phenylketonuria. Ann Hum Genet 40:287–297, 1977.
44. Romeo G, Devoto M, Galietta LJV: Why is the cystic fibrosis gene so frequent? Hum Genet 84:1–5, 1989.
45. Boat TE, Dearborn DG: Etiology and pathogenesis. *In* Taussig LI (ed): Cystic Fibrosis. New York: Thieme-Stratton, 1984, pp 25–84.
46. Gabriel SE, Brigman KN, Koller BH, et al: Cystic fibrosis heterozygote resistance to cholera toxin in the cystic fibrosis mouse model. Science 266:107–109, 1994.
47. Zuelzer WW, Newton WA Jr: The pathogenesis of fibrocystic disease of the pancreas. A study of 36 cases with special reference to the pulmonary lesions. Pediatrics 4:53–69, 1949.
48. Sturgess J, Imrie J: Quantitative evaluation of the development of tracheal submucosal glands in infants with cystic fibrosis and control infants. Am J Pathol 106:303–311, 1982.
49. Baker D, Kupke KG, Ingram P, et al: Microprobe analysis in human pathology. Scan Electron Microsc 1985:659–680, 1985.
50. Tomashefski JF Jr, Bruce M, Goldberg HI, et al: Regional distribution of macroscopic lung disease in cystic fibrosis. Am Rev Respir Dis 133:535–540, 1986.
51. Sobonya RE, Taussig LM: Quantitative aspects of lung pathology in cystic fibrosis. Am Rev Respir Dis 134:290–295, 1986.
52. Tomashefski JF Jr, Dahms BB, Abramowsky CR: The pathology of cystic fibrosis. *In* Davis PB (ed): Cystic Fibrosis (1st ed). New York: Marcel Dekker, 1993, pp 435–489.
53. Tomashefski JF Jr, Konstan MW, Bruce M: The pathology of interstitial pneumonia in cystic fibrosis. Am Rev Respir Dis 133:A365, 1986.
54. Tomashefski JF Jr, Bruce M, Stern RC, et al: Pulmonary air cysts in cystic fibrosis: Relation of pathologic features to radiologic findings and history of pneumothorax. Hum Pathol 16:253–261, 1985.
55. Boat TF, di Sant'Agnese PA, Warwick WJ, et al: Pneumothorax in cystic fibrosis. JAMA 209:1498–1504, 1969.
56. Mack JF, Moss AF, Harper WW, et al: The bronchial arteries in cystic fibrosis. JAMA 209:1498–1504, 1965.
57. Stern RC, Boat TF, Wood RE, et al: Treatment and prognosis of nasal polyps in cystic fibrosis. Am J Dis Child 136:1067–1070, 1982.
58. di Sant'Agnese PA, Hubbard VS: The pancreas. *In* Taussig LM (ed): Cystic Fibrosis. New York: Thieme-Stratton, 1984, pp 230–295.
59. Handwerger S, Roth J, Gorden P, et al: Glucose intolerance in cystic fibrosis. N Engl J Med 281:451–461, 1969.
60. di Sant'Agnese PA, Hubbard VS: The hepatobiliary system. *In* Taussig LM (ed): Cystic Fibrosis. New York, Thieme-Stratton, 1984, pp 296–322.
61. di Sant'Agnese PA, Hubbard VS: The gastrointestinal tract. *In* Taussig LM (ed): Cystic Fibrosis. New York: Thieme-Stratton, 1984, pp 212–229.
62. Neutra MR, Trier JS: Rectal mucosa in cystic fibrosis. Morphological features before and after short term organ culture. Gastroenterology 75:701–710, 1978.
63. Brugman SM, Taussig LM: The reproductive system. *In* Taussig LM (ed): Cystic Fibrosis. New York: Thieme-Stratton, 1984, pp 323–337.
64. Gregory RJ, Cheng SH, Rich DP, et al: Expression and characterization of the cystic fibrosis transmembrane conductance regulator. Nature 347:382–386, 1990.
65. Hyde SC, Emsley P, Hartshorn MJ, et al: Structural model of ATP-binding proteins associated with cystic fibrosis, multidrug resistance and bacterial transport. Nature 346:362–365, 1990.
66. Engelhardt JF, Yankaskas JR, Ernst SA, et al: Submucosal glands are the predominant site of CFTR expression in human bronchus. Nat Genet 2:240–247, 1992.
67. Hoogeveen AT, Keulemans J, Willemsen R, et al: Immunological localization of cystic fibrosis candidate gene products. Exp Cell Res 193:435–437, 1991.
68. Bradbury NA, Jilling T, Berta G, et al: Regulation of plasma membrane recycling by CFTR. Science 256:530–532, 1992.
69. Barasch J, Kiss B, Prince A, et al: Defective acidification of intracellular organelles in cystic fibrosis. Nature 352:70–73, 1991.
70. Riordan JR: Cystic fibrosis as a disease of misprocessing of the cystic fibrosis transmembrane conductance regulator glycoprotein. Am J Hum Genet 64:1499–1504, 1999.
71. Denning GM, Anderson MP, Amara JF, et al: Processing of mutant cystic fibrosis transmembrane conductance regulator is temperature-sensitive. Nature 358:761–764, 1992.
72. Gregory RJ, Rich DP, Cheng SH, et al: Maturation and function of cystic fibrosis transmembrane conductance regulator variants bearing mutations in putative nucleotide-binding domains 1 and 2. Mol Cell Biol 11:3886–3893, 1991.
73. Kalin N, Claabeta A, Sommer M, et al: DeltaF508 CFTR protein expression in tissues from patients with cystic fibrosis. J Clin Invest 103:1379–1389, 1999.
74. Anderson MP, Welsh MJ: Regulation by ATP and ADP of CFTR chloride channels that contain mutant nucleotide-binding domains. Science 257:1701–1704, 1992.
75. Drumm M: What happens to Delta F508 in vivo? J Clin Invest 103:1369–1370, 1999.
76. Bradbury NA, Cohn JA, Venglarik CJ, et al: Biochemical and biophysical identification of cystic fibrosis transmembrane conductance regulator chloride channels as components of endocytic clathrin-coated vesicles. J Biol Chem 269:8296–8302, 1994.
77. Berger HA, Anderson MP, Gregory RJ, et al: Identification and regulation of the cystic fibrosis transmembrane conductance regulator-generated chloride channel. J Clin Invest 88:1422–1431, 1991.
78. Hwang T-C, Lu L, Zeitlin PL, et al: $Cl^-$ channels in CF: Lack of activation by protein kinase C and cAMP-dependent protein kinase. Science 244:1351–1356, 1989.
79. Fischer H, Machen TE: CFTR displays voltage dependence and two gating modes during stimulation. J Gen Physiol 104:541–566, 1994.
80. Anderson MP, Berger HA, Rich DP, et al: Nucleoside triphosphates are required to open the CFTR chloride channel. Cell 67:775–784, 1991.
81. Cheng SH, Rich DP, Marshall J, et al: Phosphorylation of the R domain by cAMP-dependent protein kinase regulates the CFTR chloride channel. Cell 66:1027–1036, 1991.
82. Smith JJ, Travis SM, Greenberg EP, et al: Cystic fibrosis airway epithelia fail to kill bacteria because of abnormal airway surface fluid. Cell 85:229–236, 1996.
83. Zabner J, Smith JJ, Karp PH, et al: Loss of CFTR chloride channels alters salt absorption by cystic fibrosis airway epithelia in vitro. Mol Cell 2:397–403, 1998.
84. Matsui H, Randell SH, Peretti SW, et al: Coordinated clearance of periciliary liquid and mucus from airway surfaces. J Clin Invest 102:1125–1131, 1998.
85. Matsui H, Grubb BR, Tarran R, et al: Evidence for periciliary liquid layer depletion, not abnormal ion composition, in the pathogenesis of cystic fibrosis airways disease. Cell 95:1005–1015, 1998.
85a. Kerem E, Bistritzer T, Hanukoglu A, et al: Pulmonary epithelial sodium-channel dysfunction and excess airway liquid in pseudohypoaldosteronism. N Engl J Med 341:156–162, 1999.

86. Kohler D, App E, Schmitz-Schumann M, et al: Inhalation of amiloride improves the mucociliary and the cough clearance in patients with cystic fibroses. Eur J Respir Dis 69(Suppl 146):319–326, 1986.
87. Regnis JA, Robinson M, Bailey DL, et al: Mucociliary clearance in patients with cystic fibrosis and in normal subjects. Am J Respir Crit Care Med 150:66–71, 1994.
88. Pier GB, Grout M, Zaidi TS, et al: Role of mutant CFTR in hypersusceptibility of cystic fibrosis patients to lung infections. Science 271:64–67, 1996.
89. Imundo L, Barasch J, Prince A, et al: Cystic fibrosis epithelial cells have a receptor for pathogenic bacteria on their apical surface. Proc Natl Acad Sci USA 92:3019–3023, 1995.
90. Knowles M, Gatzy J, Boucher R: Relative ion permeability of normal and cystic fibrosis nasal epithelium. J Clin Invest 71:1410–1417, 1983.
91. Knowles MR, Stutts MJ, Spock A, et al: Abnormal ion permeation through cystic fibrosis respiratory epithelium. Science 221:1067–1070, 1983.
92. Boucher RC, Stutts MJ, Knowles MR, et al: $Na^+$ transport in cystic fibrosis respiratory epithelia. Abnormal basal rate and response to adenylate cyclase activation. J Clin Invest 78:1245–1252, 1986.
93. Cotton CU, Stutts MJ, Knowles MR, et al: Abnormal apical cell membrane in cystic fibrosis respiratory epithelium. An in vitro electrophysiologic analysis. J Clin Invest 79:80–85, 1987.
94. Widdicombe JH, Welsh MJ, Finkbeiner WE: Cystic fibrosis decreases the apical membrane chloride permeability of monolayers cultured from cells of tracheal epithelium. Proc Natl Acad Sci USA 82:6167–6171, 1985.
95. Willumsen NJ, Boucher RC: Shunt resistance and ion permeabilities in normal and cystic fibrosis airway epithelium. Am J Physiol 256:C1054–C1063, 1989.
96. Willumsen NJ, Davis CW, Boucher RC: Intracellular $Cl^-$ activity and cellular $Cl^-$ pathways in cultured human airway epithelium. Am J Physiol 256:C1033–C1044, 1989.
97. Willumsen NJ, Davis CW, Boucher RC: Cellular $Cl^-$ transport in cultured cystic fibrosis airway epithelium. Am J Physiol 256:C1045–C1053, 1989.
98. Frizzell RA, Rechkemmer G, Shoemaker RL: Altered regulation of airway epithelial cell chloride channels in cystic fibrosis. Science 233:558–560, 1986.
99. Welsh MJ: Abnormal regulation of ion channels in cystic fibrosis epithelia. FASEB J 4:2718–2725, 1990.
100. Welsh MJ, Liedtke CM: Chloride and potassium channels in cystic fibrosis airway epithelia. Nature 322:467–470, 1986.
101. Boucher RC, Cheng EHC, Paradiso AM, et al: Chloride secretory response of cystic fibrosis human airway epithelia: Preservation of calcium but not protein kinase C- and A-dependent mechanisms. J Clin Invest 84:1424–1431, 1989.
102. Schoumacher RA, Shoemaker RL, Halm DR, et al: Phosphorylation fails to activate chloride channels from cystic fibrosis airway cells. Nature 330:752–754, 1987.
103. Li M, McCann JD, Anderson MP, et al: Regulation of chloride channels by protein kinase C in normal and cystic fibrosis airway epithelia. Science 244:1353–1356, 1989.
104. Tabcharani JA, Chang XB, Riordan JR, et al: Phosphorylation-regulated $Cl^-$ channel in CHO cells stably expressing the cystic fibrosis gene. Nature 352:628–631, 1991.
105. Short DB, Trotter KW, Reczek D, et al: An apical PDZ protein anchors the cystic fibrosis transmembrane conductance regulator to the cytoskeleton. J Biol Chem 273:19797–19801, 1998.
106. Willumsen NJ, Boucher RC: Activation of an apical $Cl^-$ conductance by $Ca^{2+}$ ionophores in cystic fibrosis airway epithelia. Am J Physiol 256:C226–C233, 1989.
107. Wagner JA, McDonald TV, Nghiem PT, et al: Antisense oligodeoxynucleotides to the cystic fibrosis transmembrane conductance regulator inhibit cAMP-activated but not calcium-activated chloride currents. Proc Natl Acad Sci USA 89:6785–6789, 1992.
108. Anderson MP, Welsh MJ: Calcium and cAMP activate different chloride channels in the apical membrane of normal and cystic fibrosis epithelia. Proc Natl Acad Sci USA 88:6003–6007, 1991.
109. Worrell RT, Frizzell RA: CaMKII mediates stimulation of chloride conductance by calcium in T84 cells. Am J Physiol 260:C877–C882, 1991.
110. Brown HA, Lazarowski ER, Boucher RC, et al: Evidence that UTP and ATP regulate phospholipase C through a common extracellular 5′-nucleotide receptor in human airway epithelial cells. Mol Pharmacol 40:648–655, 1991.
111. Mason SJ, Paradiso AM, Boucher RC: Regulation of transepithelial ion transport and intracellular calcium by extracellular adenosine triphosphate in human normal and cystic fibrosis airway epithelium. Br J Pharmacol 103:1649–1656, 1991.
112. Knowles MR, Clarke LL, Boucher RC: Activation by extracellular nucleotides of chloride secretion in the airway epithelia of patients with cystic fibrosis. N Engl J Med 325:533–538, 1991.
113. Clarke LL, Boucher RC: Chloride secretory response to extracellular ATP in normal and cystic fibrosis nasal epithelia. Am J Physiol 263:C348–C356, 1992.
114. Noone PG, Accurso FJ, Aitken M, et al: Safety of aerosolized Ins365 in patients with mild to moderate CF: Results of a multicenter therapeutic development network study (abstract). Pediatr Pulmonol (Suppl 19):244–245, 1999.
115. Robson AM, Tateishi S, Ingelfinger JR, et al: Renal function in cystic fibrosis. J Pediatr 79:42–50, 1971.
116. Stenvinkel P, Hjelte L, Alvan G, et al: Decreased renal clearance of sodium in cystic fibrosis. Acta Paediatr Scand 80:194–198, 1991.
117. O'Loughlin EV, Hunt DM, Gaskin KJ, et al: Abnormal epithelial transport in cystic fibrosis jejunum. Am J Physiol 260:G758–G763, 1991.
118. Baxter P, Goldhill J, Hardcastle J, et al: Enhanced intestinal glucose and alanine transport in cystic fibrosis. Gut 31:817–820, 1990.
119. Berschneider HM, Knowles MR, Azizkhan RG, et al: Altered intestinal chloride transport in cystic fibrosis. FASEB J 2:2625–2629, 1988.
120. Willumsen NJ, Boucher RC: Sodium transport and intracellular sodium activity in cultured human nasal epithelium. Am J Physiol 261:C319–C331, 1991.
121. Willumsen NJ, Boucher RC: Transcellular sodium transport in cultured cystic fibrosis human nasal epithelium. Am J Physiol 261:C332–C341, 1991.
122. Chinet T, Fullton J, Yankaskas J, et al: Characterization of sodium channels in the apical membrane of nasal epithelial cells (abstract). Am Rev Respir Dis 141:A164, 1990.
123. Chinet T, Fullton J, Boucher R, et al: Sodium channels in the apical membrane of normal and CF nasal epithelial cells (abstract). Pediatr Pulmonol (Suppl 5):209, 1990.
124. Chinet T, Fullton J, Yankaskas J, et al: Characteristics of cation channels in cell-attached patches of normal and CF nasal epithelial cells (abstract). Am Rev Respir Dis 143:A148, 1991.
125. Stutts MJ, Rossier BC, Boucher RC: Cystic fibrosis transmembrane conductance regulator inverts protein kinase A–mediated regulation of epithelial sodium channel single channel kinetics. J Biol Chem 272:14037–14040, 1997.
126. Canessa CM, Horisberger J-D, Rossier BC: Epithelial sodium channel related to proteins involved in neurodegeration. Nature 361:467–470, 1993.
127. Canessa CM, Schild L, Buell G, et al: Amiloride-sensitive epithelial $Na^+$ channel is made of three homologous subunits. Nature 367:463–467, 1994.
128. Jiang C, Finkbeiner WE, Widdicombe JH, et al: Altered fluid transport across airway epithelium in cystic fibrosis. Science 262:424–427, 1993.
129. Devor DC, Pilewski JM: UTP inhibits $Na^+$ absorption in wild-type and DeltaF508 CFTR-expressing human bronchial epithelia. Am J Physiol 276:C827–C837, 1999.
130. Engelhardt JF, Stratford-Perricaudet LD, Yang Y, et al: Direct transfer of recombinant genes into human bronchial epithelia of xenografts with E1 deleted adenoviruses. Nat Genet 4:27–34, 1993.
131. Yamaya M, Finkbeiner WE, Widdicombe JH: Ion transport by cultures of human tracheobronchial submucosal glands. Am J Physiol 261:L485–L490, 1991.
132. Yamaya M, Finkbeiner WE, Widdicombe JH: Altered ion transport by tracheal glands in cystic fibrosis. Am J Physiol 261:L491–L494, 1991.
133. Knowles MR, Robinson JM, Wood RE, et al: Ion composition of airway surface liquid of patients with cystic fibrosis as compared

to normal and disease-control subjects. J Clin Invest 100:2588–2595, 1997.
134. Boat TF, Cheng PW: Biochemistry of airway mucus secretions. Fed Proc 39:3067–3074, 1980.
135. Davril M, Degroote S, Humbert P, et al: The sialylation of bronchial mucins secreted by patients suffering from cystic fibrosis or from chronic bronchitis is related to the severity of airway infection. Glycobiology 9:311–321, 1999.
136. Wesley A, Forstner J, Qureshi R, et al: Human intestinal mucin in cystic fibrosis. Pediatr Res 17:65–69, 1983.
137. Cheng P-W, Boat TF, Cranfill K, et al: Increased sulfation of glycoconjugates by cultured nasal epithelial cells from patients with cystic fibrosis. J Clin Invest 84:68–72, 1989.
138. Frates RC Jr, Kaizu TT, Last JA: Mucus glycoproteins secreted by respiratory epithelial tissue from cystic fibrosis patients. Pediatr Res 17:30–34, 1983.
139. Zhang Y, Jiang Q, Dudus L, et al: Vector-specific complementation profiles of two independent primary defects in cystic fibrosis airways. Hum Gene Ther 9:635–648, 1998.
140. Roomans GM, von Euler AM, Muller RM, et al: X-ray microanalysis of goblet cells in bronchial epithelium of patients with cystic fibrosis. J Submicrosc Cytol 18:613–615, 1986.
141. Elgavish A, Meezan E: Increased sulfate uptake in skin fibroblasts isolated from cystic fibrosis patients. Biochem Biophys Res Commun 152:99–106, 1988.
142. Elgavish A, Meezan E: Altered sulfate transport via anion exchange in CFPAC is corrected by retrovirus-mediated CFTR gene transfer. Am J Physiol 263:C176–C186, 1992.
143. Mohapatra NK, Cheng P-W, Parker JC, et al: Sulfate transport and concentrations are not altered in CF airway epithelial cells (abstract). Pediatr Pulmonol (Suppl 8):283, 1992.
144. Lethem MI, James SL, Marriott C: The role of mucous glycoproteins in the rheologic properties of cystic fibrosis sputum. Am Rev Respir Dis 142:1053–1058, 1990.
145. Pillai RS, Chandra T, Miller IF, et al: Work of adhesion of respiratory tract mucus. J Appl Physiol 72:1604–1610, 1992.
146. Leigh MW, Boat TF: Airway secretions. *In* Chernick V, Mellins RB (eds): Basic Mechanisms of Pediatric Respiratory Disease: Cellular and Integrative. Philadelphia: BC Decker, 1991, pp 328–345.
147. Lam J, Chan R, Lam K, et al: Production of mucoid microcolonies by *Pseudomonas aeruginosa* within infected lungs in cystic fibrosis. Infect Immun 28:546–556, 1980.
148. Vishwanath S, Ramphal R: Adherence of *Pseudomonas aeruginosa* to human tracheobronchial mucin. Infect Immun 45:197–202, 1984.
149. Nelson JW, Tredgett MW, Sheehan JK, et al: Mucinophilic and chemotactic properties of *Pseudomonas aeruginosa* in relation to pulmonary colonization in cystic fibrosis. Infect Immun 58:1489–1495, 1990.
150. Bennett WD, Olivier KN, Zeman KL, et al: Effect of uridine 5′-triphosphate plus amiloride on mucociliary clearance in adult cystic fibrosis. Am J Respir Crit Care Med 153:1796–1801, 1996.
151. Katz SM, Holsclaw DS Jr: Ultrastructural features of respiratory cilia in cystic fibrosis. Am J Clin Pathol 73:682–685, 1980.
152. Rutland J, Cole PJ: Nasal mucociliary clearance and ciliary beat frequency in cystic fibrosis compared with sinusitis and bronchiectasis. Thorax 36:654–658, 1981.
153. Ulrich M, Herbert S, Berger J, et al: Localization of *Staphylococcus aureus* in infected airways of patients with cystic fibrosis and in a cell culture model of *S. aureus* adherence. Am J Respir Cell Mol Biol 19:83–91, 1998.
154. Woods DE, Bass JA, Johanson WG Jr, et al: Role of adherence in the pathogenesis of *Pseudomonas aeruginosa* lung infection in cystic fibrosis patients. Infect Immun 30:694–699, 1980.
155. Saiman L, Ishimoto K, Lory S, et al: The effect of piliation and exoproduct expression on the adherence of *Pseudomonas aeruginosa* to respiratory epithelial monolayers. J Infect Dis 161:541–548, 1990.
156. Plotkowski MC, Chevillard M, Pierrot D, et al: Differential adhesion of *Pseudomonas aeruginosa* to human respiratory epithelial cells in primary culture. J Clin Invest 87:2018–2028, 1991.
157. Saiman L, Cacalano G, Gruenert D, et al: Comparison of adherence of *Pseudomonas aeruginosa* to respiratory epithelial cells from cystic fibrosis patients and healthy subjects. Infect Immun 60:2808–2814, 1992.
158. Plotkowski MC, Chevillard M, Pierrot D, et al: Epithelial respiratory cells from cystic fibrosis patients do not possess specific *Pseudomonas aeruginosa*–adhesive properties. J Med Microbiol 36:104–111, 1992.
159. Tsang KWT, Rutman A, Tanaka E, et al: Interaction of *Pseudomonas aeruginosa* with human respiratory mucosa in vitro. Eur Respir J 7:1746–1753, 1994.
160. Puchelle E, de Bentzmann S, Zahm JM: Physical and functional properties of airway secretions in cystic fibrosis—therapeutic approaches. Respiration 62(Suppl 1):2–12, 1995.
161. Li JD, Dohrman AF, Gallup M, et al: Transcriptional activation of mucin by *Pseudomonas aeruginosa* lipopolysaccharide in the pathogenesis of cystic fibrosis lung disease. Proc Natl Acad Sci USA 94:967–972, 1997.
162. Dohrman A, Miyata S, Gallup M, et al: Mucin gene (MUC 2 and MUC 5AC) upregulation by gram-positive and gram-negative bacteria. Biochim Biophys Acta 1406:251–259, 1998.
163. DiMango E, Zar HJ, Bryan R, et al: Diverse *Pseudomonas aeruginosa* gene products stimulate respiratory epithelial cells to produce interleukin-8. J Clin Invest 96:2204–2210, 1995.
164. Plotkowski MC, Zahm JM, Tournier JM, et al: *Pseudomonas aeruginosa* adhesion to normal and injured respiratory mucosa. Mem Inst Oswaldo Cruz 87(Suppl V):61–68, 1992.
165. Matthews WJ Jr, Williams M, Oliphint B, et al: Hypogammaglobulinemia in patients with cystic fibrosis. N Engl J Med 302:245–249, 1980.
166. Gugler E, Pallavicini JC, Swedlow H, et al: Immunological studies of submaxillary saliva from patients with cystic fibrosis and from normal children. J Pediatr 73:548–559, 1968.
167. Doring G, Obernesser HJ, Botzenhart K, et al: Proteases of *Pseudomonas aeruginosa* in patients with cystic fibrosis. J Infect Dis 147:744–750, 1983.
168. Baltimore RS, Fick RB Jr, Fino L: Antibody to multiple mucoid strains of *Pseudomonas aeruginosa* in patients with cystic fibrosis, measured by an enzyme-linked immunosorbent assay. Pediatr Res 20:1085–1090, 1986.
169. Sorensen RU, Ruuskanen O, Miller K, et al: B-lymphocyte function in cystic fibrosis. Eur J Respir Dis 64:524–533, 1983.
170. Sorensen RU, Stern RC, Polmar SH: Cellular immunity to bacteria: Impairment of in vitro lymphocyte responses to *Pseudomonas aeruginosa* in cystic fibrosis patients. Infect Immun 18:735–740, 1977.
171. Sorensen RU, Stern RC, Chase P, et al: Defective cellular immunity to gram-negative bacteria in cystic fibrosis patients. Infect Immun 23:398–402, 1979.
172. Thomassen MJ, Demko CA, Wood RE, et al: Ultrastructure and function of alveolar macrophages from cystic fibrosis patients. Pediatr Res 14:715–721, 1980.
173. Konstan MW, Berger M: Current understanding of the inflammatory process in cystic fibrosis: Onset and etiology. Pediatr Pulmonol 24:137–142, 1997.
174. Noah TL, Black HR, Cheng P-W, et al: Nasal and bronchoalveolar lavage fluid cytokines in early cystic fibrosis. J Infect Dis 175:638–647, 1997.
175. Bonfield TL, Konstan MW, Burfeind P, et al: Normal bronchial epithelial cells constitutively produce the anti-inflammatory cytokine interleukin-10, which is downregulated in cystic fibrosis. Am J Respir Cell Mol Biol 13:257–261, 1995.
176. Bonfleld TL, Panuska JR, Konstan MW, et al: Inflammatory cytokines in cystic fibrosis lungs. Am J Respir Crit Care Med 152:2111–2118, 1995.
177. Birrer P, McElvaney NG, Rudeberg A, et al: Protease-antiprotease imbalance in the lungs of children with cystic fibrosis. Am J Respir Crit Care Med 150:207–213, 1994.
178. Fick RB Jr, Robbins RA, Squier SU, et al: Complement activation in cystic fibrosis respiratory fluids: In vivo and in vitro generation of C5a and chemotactic activity. Pediatr Res 20:1258–1268, 1986.
179. Klinger JD, Tandler B, Liedtke CM, et al: Proteinases of *Pseudomonas aeruginosa* evoke mucin release by tracheal epithelium. J Clin Invest 74:1669–1678, 1984.
180. Sommerhoff CP, Nadel JA, Basbaum CB, et al: Neutrophil elastase and cathepsin G stimulate secretion from cultured bovine airway gland serous cells. J Clin Invest 85:682–689, 1990.
181. Sommerhoff CP, Caughey GH, Finkbeiner WE, et al: Mast cell

chymase. A potent secretagogue for airway gland serous cells. J Immunol 142:2450–2456, 1989.
182. Christensen TG, Korthy AL, Snider GL, et al: Irreversible bronchial goblet cell metaplasia in hamsters with elastase-induced panacinar emphysema. J Clin Invest 59:397–404, 1977.
183. Hingley ST, Hastie AT, Kueppers F, et al: Disruption of respiratory cilia by proteases including those of *Pseudomonas aeruginosa*. Infect Immun 54:379–385, 1986.
184. Niederman MS, Merrill WW, Polomski LM, et al: Influence of sputum IgA and elastase on tracheal cell bacterial adherence. Am Rev Respir Dis 133:255–260, 1986.
185. Bruce MC, Poncz L, Klinger JD, et al: Biochemical and pathologic evidence for proteolytic destruction of lung connective tissue in cystic fibrosis. Am Rev Respir Dis 132:529–535, 1985.
186. Davis PB: Clinical pathophysiology and manifestations of lung disease. *In* Yankaskas JR, Knowles MR (eds): Cystic Fibrosis in Adults. Philadelphia: Lippincott-Raven, 1999, pp 45–67.
187. Wang EEL, Prober CG, Manson B, et al: Association of respiratory viral infections with pulmonary deterioration in patients with cystic fibrosis. N Engl J Med 311:1653–1658, 1984.
188. Petersen NT, Hoiby N, Mordhorst CH, et al: Respiratory infections in cystic fibrosis patients caused by virus, *Chlamydia* and *Mycoplasma*—possible synergism with *Pseudomonas aeruginosa*. Acta Paediatr Scand 70:623–628, 1981.
189. Conway SP, Simmonds EJ, Littlewood JM: Acute severe deterioration in cystic fibrosis associated with influenza A virus infection. Thorax 47:112–114, 1992.
190. Winnie GB, Cowan RG: Association of Epstein-Barr virus infection and pulmonary exacerbations in patients with cystic fibrosis. Pediatr Infect Dis 11:722–726, 1992.
191. Abman SH, Ogle JW, Butler-Simon N, et al: Role of respiratory syncytial virus in early hospitalizations for respiratory distress of young infants with cystic fibrosis. J Pediatr 113:826–830, 1988.
192. Ramsey BW, Gore EJ, Smith AL, et al: The effect of respiratory viral infections on patients with cystic fibrosis. Am J Dis Child 143:662–668, 1989.
193. Campbell PW3d, Parker RA, Roberts BT, et al: Association of poor clinical status and heavy exposure to tobacco smoke in patients with cystic fibrosis who are homozygous for the F508 deletion. J Pediatr 120:261–264, 1992.
194. Gilligan PH: Microbiology of cystic fibrosis lung disease. *In* Yankaskas JR, Knowles MR (eds): Cystic Fibrosis in Adults. Philadelphia: Lippincott-Raven, 1999, pp 93–114.
195. Tummler B, Koopmann U, Grothues D, et al: Nosocomial acquisition of *Pseudomonas aeruginosa* by cystic fibrosis patients. J Clin Microbiol 29:1265–1267, 1991.
196. Costerton JW, Stewart PS, Greenberg EP: Bacterial biofilms: A common cause of persistent infections. Science 284:1318–1322, 1999.
197. May TB, Shinabarger D, Maharaj R, et al: Alginate synthesis by *Pseudomonas aeruginosa*: A key pathogenic factor in chronic pulmonary infections of cystic fibrosis patients. Clin Microbiol Rev 4:191–206, 1991
198. Blackwood LL, Pennington JE: Influence of mucoid coating on clearance of *Pseudomonas aeruginosa* from lungs. Infect Immun 32:443–448, 1981.
199. May TB, Chakrabarty AM: *Pseudomonas aeruginosa*: Genes and enzymes of alginate synthesis. Trends Microbiol 2:151–157, 1994.
200. LiPuma JJ, Dasen SE, Nielson DW, et al: Person-to-person transmission of *Pseudomonas cepacia* between patients with cystic fibrosis. Lancet 336:1094–1096, 1990.
201. Isles A, MacLusky I, Corey M, et al: *Pseudomonas cepacia* infection in cystic fibrosis: An emerging problem. J Pediatr 104:206–210, 1984.
202. Fisher MC, LiPuma JJ, Dasen SE, et al: Source of *Pseudomonas cepacia*: Ribotyping of isolates from patients and from the environment. J Pediatr 123:745–747, 1993.
203. Steinbach S, Sun L, Jiang RZ, et al: Transmissibility of *Pseudomonas cepacia* in clinic patients and lung-transplant recipients with cystic fibrosis. N Engl J Med 331:981–987, 1994.
204. Sun L, Jiang RZ, Steinbach S, et al: The emergence of a highly transmissible lineage of *cbl+Pseudomonas (Burkholderia) cepacia* causing CF centre epidemics in North America and Britain. Nat Med 1:661–666, 1995.
205. Kollberg H, Vandamme P: Analysis of genomovars of *Burkholderia cepacia*: A helpful epidemiologic and prognostic tool (abstract)? Pediatr Pulmonol (Suppl 13):297, 1996.
206. Goldstein R, Sun L, Jiang RZ, et al: Structurally variant classes of pilus appendage fibers coexpressed from *Burkholderia (Pseudomonas) cepacia*. J Bacteriol 177:1039–1052, 1995.
207. Lester LA, Egge A, Hubbard VS, et al: Aspiration and lung abscess in cystic fibrosis. Am Rev Respir Dis 127:786–787, 1983.
208. Ramsey BW, Wentz KR, Smith AL, et al: Predictive value of oropharyngeal cultures for identifying lower airway bacteria in cystic fibrosis patients. Am Rev Respir Dis 144:331–337, 1991.
209. Hutcheson PS, Rejent AJ, Slavin RG: Variability in parameters of allergic bronchopulmonary aspergillosis in patients with cystic fibrosis. J Allergy Clin Immunol 88:390–394, 1991.
210. Kilby JM, Gilligan PH, Yankaskas JR, et al: Nontuberculous mycobacteria in adult patients with cystic fibrosis. Chest 102:70–75, 1992.
211. Aitken ML, Burke W, McDonald G, et al: Nontuberculous mycobacterial disease in adult cystic fibrosis patients. Chest 103:1096–1099, 1993.
212. Olivier KN, Yankaskas JR, Knowles MR: Nontuberculous mycobacterial pulmonary disease in cystic fibrosis. Semin Respir Infect 11:272–284, 1996.
213. Brasfield D, Hicks G, Soong S, et al: The chest roentgenogram in cystic fibrosis: A new scoring system. Pediatrics 63:24–29, 1979.
214. Nathanson I, Conboy K, Murphy S, et al: Ultrafast computerized tomography of the chest in cystic fibrosis: A new scoring system. Pediatr Pulmonol 11:81–86, 1991.
215. Bhalla M, Turcios N, Aponte V, et al: Cystic fibrosis: Scoring system with thin-section CT. Radiology 179:783–788, 1991.
216. Kinsella D, Hamilton A, Goddard P, et al: The role of magnetic resonance imaging in cystic fibrosis. Clin Radiol 44:23–26, 1991.
217. Fiel SB, Friedman AC, Caroline DF, et al: Magnetic resonance imaging in young adults with cystic fibrosis. Chest 91:181–184, 1987.
218. Taussig LM, Landau LI, Marks MI: Respiratory system. *In* Taussig LI (ed): Cystic Fibrosis. New York: Thieme-Stratton, 1984, pp 115–174.
219. Levison H, Godfrey S: Pulmonary aspects of cystic fibrosis. *In* Mangos JA, Talamo RE (eds): Cystic Fibrosis: Projections into the Future. New York: Stratton Intercontinental, 1976, pp 3–24.
220. Hanrahan JP, Brown RW, Carey VJ, et al: Passive respiratory mechanics in healthy infants. Effects of growth, gender, and smoking. Am J Respir Crit Care Med 154:670–680, 1996.
221. Feher A, Castile R, Kisling J, et al: Flow limitation in normal infants: A new method for forced expiratory maneuvers from raised lung volumes. J Appl Physiol 80:2019–2025, 1996.
222. Siassi B, Moss AJ, Dooley RR: Clinical recognition of cor pulmonale in cystic fibrosis. J Pediatr 78:794–805, 1971.
223. Yankaskas JR, Egan TM, Mauro MA: Major complications. *In* Yankaskas JR, Knowles MR (eds): Cystic Fibrosis in Adults. Philadelphia: Lippincott-Raven, 1999, pp 175–193.
224. Francis PW, Muller NL, Gurwitz D, et al: Hemoglobin desaturation: Its occurrence during sleep in patients with cystic fibrosis. Am J Dis Child 134:734–740, 1980.
225. Boat T: Comparison of lung function and survival patterns between cystic fibrosis and emphysema or chronic bronchitis patients. *In* Sturgess JM (ed): Perspectives in Cystic Fibrosis. Mississanga, Ontario: Imperial Press, 1980, pp 236–245.
226. Hordvik NL, Koenig P, Morris D, et al: A longitudinal study of bronchodilator responsiveness in cystic fibrosis. Am Rev Respir Dis 131:889–893, 1985.
227. Godfrey S, Mearns M: Pulmonary function and response to exercise in cystic fibrosis. Arch Dis Child 46:144–152, 1971.
228. Lands LC, Coates AL: Cardiopulmonary and skeletal muscle function and their effects on exercise limitation. *In* Yankaskas JR, Knowles MR (eds): Cystic Fibrosis in Adults. Philadelphia: Lippincott-Raven, 1999, pp 365–382.
229. Henke KG, Orenstein DM: Oxygen saturation during exercise in cystic fibrosis. Am Rev Respir Dis 129:708–711, 1984.
230. Asher MI, Pardy RL, Coates AL, et al: The effects of inspiratory muscle training in patients with cystic fibrosis. Am Rev Respir Dis 126:855–859, 1982.
231. Orenstein DM, Franklin BA, Doershuk CF, et al: Exercise condi-

tioning and cardiopulmonary fitness in cystic fibrosis. Chest 80:392–398, 1981.
232. Regnis JA, Alison JA, Henke KG, et al: Changes in end-expiratory lung volume during exercise in cystic fibrosis relate to severity of lung disease. Am Rev Respir Dis 144:507–512, 1991.
233. Nixon PA, Orenstein DM, Kelsey SF, et al: The prognostic value of exercise testing in patients with cystic fibrosis. N Engl J Med 327:1785–1788, 1992.
234. O'Rawe A, McIntosh I, Dodge JA, et al: Increased energy expenditure in cystic fibrosis is associated with specific mutations. Clin Sci 82:71–76, 1992.
235. Davies PSW, Bronstein MN: Energy expenditures of infants with cystic fibrosis (abstract). Pediatr Pulmonol (Suppl 8):175–176, 1992.
236. Gharib R, Allen RP, Joos HA, et al: Paranasal sinuses in cystic fibrosis: Incidence of Roentgen abnormalities. Am J Dis Child 108:499–502, 1964.
237. Stern RC, Jones K: Nasal and sinus disease. *In* Yankaskas JR, Knowles MR (eds): Cystic Fibrosis in Adults. Philadelphia: Lippincott-Raven, 1999, pp 221–231.
238. Cepero R, Smith RJH, Catlin FI, et al: Cystic fibrosis—An otolaryngologic perspective. Otolaryngol Head Neck Surg 97:356–360, 1987.
239. Shwachman H, Kowalski M, Shaw K-T: Cystic fibrosis: A new outlook. Seventy patients above 25 years of age. Medicine (Baltimore) 56:129–149, 1977.
240. Jaffe BF, Strome M, Khaw K-T, et al: Nasal polypectomy and sinus surgery for cystic fibrosis—A 10-year review. Otolaryngol Clin North Am 10:81–90, 1977.
241. Stern RC, Boat TF, Orenstein DM, et al: Treatment and prognosis of lobar and segmental atelectasis in cystic fibrosis. Am Rev Respir Dis 118:821–826, 1978.
242. Spector ML, Stern RC: Pneumothorax in cystic fibrosis: A 26-year experience. Ann Thorac Surg 47:204–207, 1989.
243. Stern RC, Wood RE, Boat TF, et al: Treatment and prognosis of massive hemoptysis in cystic fibrosis. Am Rev Respir Dis 117:825–828, 1978.
244. Brinson GM, Noone PG, Mauro MA, et al: Bronchial artery embolization for the treatment of hemoptysis in patients with cystic fibrosis. Am J Respir Crit Care Med 157:1951–1958, 1998.
245. Becker JW, Burke W, McDonald G, et al: Prevalence of allergic bronchopulmonary aspergillosis and atopy in adult patients with cystic fibrosis. Chest 109:1536–1540, 1996.
246. Schonheyder H, Jensen T, Hoiby N, et al: Frequency of *Aspergillus fumigatus* isolates and antibodies to aspergillus antigens in cystic fibrosis. Acta Pathol Microbiol Scand 93:105–112, 1985.
247. Egan TM: Thoracic surgery for patients with cystic fibrosis. *In* Orenstein DM, Stern RC (eds): Treatment of the Hospitalized Patient with Cystic Fibrosis. New York: Marcel Dekker, 1998, pp 231–247.
248. Lemen RJ, Gates AJ, Mathe AA, et al: Relationships among digital clubbing, disease severity, and serum prostaglandins F2alpha and E concentrations in cystic fibrosis patients. Am Rev Respir Dis 117:639–646, 1978.
249. Noone PG, Bresnihan B: Rheumatic disease in cystic fibrosis. *In* Yankaskas JR, Knowles MR (eds): Cystic Fibrosis in Adults. Philadelphia: Lippincott-Raven, 1999, pp 439–447.
250. Nixon PA, Orenstein DM, Curtis SE, et al: Oxygen supplementation during exercise in cystic fibrosis. Am Rev Respir Dis 142:807–811, 1990.
251. Tepper RS, Skatrud JB, Dempsey JA: Ventilation and oxygenation changes during sleep in cystic fibrosis. Chest 84:388–393, 1983.
252. Stern RC, Borkat G, Hirschfeld SS, et al: Heart failure in cystic fibrosis. Treatment and prognosis of cor pulmonale with failure of the right side of the heart. Am J Dis Child 134:267–272, 1980.
253. Garland JS, Chan YM, Kelly KJ, et al: Outcome of infants with cystic fibrosis requiring mechanical ventilation for respiratory failure. Chest 96:136–138, 1989.
254. Rosenstein BJ, Langbaum TS: Incidence of meconium abnormalities in newborn infants with cystic fibrosis (abstract). Am J Dis Child 134:72–73, 1980.
255. di Sant'Agnese PA, Davis PB: Cystic fibrosis in adults: 75 cases and a review of 232 cases in the literature. Am J Med 66:121–132, 1979.
256. McCarthy VP, Mischler EH, Hubbard VS, et al: Appendiceal abscess in cystic fibrosis. A diagnostic challenge. Gastroenterology 86:564–568, 1984.
257. Fletcher BD, Abramowsky CR: Contrast enemas in cystic fibrosis: Implications of appendiceal nonfilling. AJR 137:323–326, 1981.
258. Taussig LM, Saldino RM, di Sant'Agnese PA: Radiographic abnormalities of the duodenum and small bowel in cystic fibrosis of the pancreas (mucoviscidosis). Radiology 106:369–376, 1973.
259. Stern RC, Izant RJ Jr, Boat TF, et al: Treatment and prognosis of rectal prolapse in cystic fibrosis. Gastroenterology 82:707–710, 1982.
260. Durie PR, Forstner GG: The exocrine pancreas. *In* Yankaskas JR, Knowles MR (eds): Cystic Fibrosis in Adults. Philadelphia: Lippincott-Raven, 1999, pp 261–287.
261. Kalnins D, Stewart C, Tullis E, et al: Nutrition. *In* Yankaskas JR, Knowles MR (eds): Cystic Fibrosis in Adults. Philadelphia: Lippincott-Raven, 1999, pp 289–307.
262. Robbins MK, Ontjes DA: Endocrine and renal disorders in cystic fibrosis. *In* Yankaskas JR, Knowles MR (eds): Cystic Fibrosis in Adults. Philadelphia: Lippincott-Raven, 1999, pp 383–418.
263. Henderson RC, Madsen CD: Bone density in children and adolescents with cystic fibrosis. J Pediatr 128:28–34, 1996.
264. Salamoni F, Roulet M, Gudinchet F, et al: Bone mineral content in cystic fibrosis patients: Correlation with fat-free mass. Arch Dis Child 74:314–318, 1996.
265. Aris RM, Neuringer IP, Weiner MA, et al: Severe osteoporosis before and after lung transplantation. Chest 109:1176–1183, 1996.
266. Shwachman H, Lebenthal E, Khaw KT: Recurrent acute pancreatitis in patients with cystic fibrosis with normal pancreatic enzymes. Pediatrics 55:86–95, 1975.
267. Cohn JA, Friedman KJ, Noone PG, et al: Relation between mutations of the cystic fibrosis gene and idiopathic pancreatitis. N Engl J Med 339:653–658, 1998.
268. Sharer N, Schwarz M, Malone G, et al: Mutations of the cystic fibrosis gene in patients with chronic pancreatitis. N Engl J Med 339:645–652, 1998.
269. Sokol RJ, Durie PR: Recommendations for management of liver and biliary tract disease in cystic fibrosis. Cystic Fibrosis Foundation Hepatobiliary Disease Consensus Group. J Pediatr Gastroenterol Nutr 28:S1–S13, 1999.
270. Jebbink MC, Heijerman HG, Masclee AA, et al: Gallbladder disease in cystic fibrosis. Neth J Med 41:123–126, 1992.
271. Nagel RA, Westaby D, Javaid A, et al: Liver disease and bile duct abnormalities in adults with cystic fibrosis. Lancet 2:1422–1425, 1989.
272. O'Brien S, Keogan M, Casey M, et al: Biliary complications of cystic fibrosis. Gut 33:387–391, 1992.
273. Wilschanski M, Corey M, Durie P, et al: Diversity of reproductive tract abnormalities in men with cystic fibrosis. JAMA 276:607–608, 1996.
274. Flume PA, Yankaskas JR: Reproductive issues. *In* Yankaskas JR, Knowles MR (eds): Cystic Fibrosis in Adults. Philadelphia: Lippincott-Raven, 1999, pp 449–464.
275. Kopito LE, Kosasky HJ, Shwachman H: Water and electrolytes in human cervical mucus from patients with cystic fibrosis. Fertil Steril 24:512–516, 1973.
276. FitzSimmons SC, Fitzpatrick S, Thompson B, et al: A longitudinal study of the effects of pregnancy on 325 women with cystic fibrosis (abstract). Pediatr Pulmonol 13(Suppl):99–101, 1996.
277. Michel SH, Mueller DH: Impact of lactation on women with cystic fibrosis and their infants: A review of five cases. J Am Diet Assoc 94:159–165, 1994.
278. Rosenstein BJ, Cutting GR: The diagnosis of CF: A consensus statement. Cystic Fibrosis Foundation Consensus Panel. J Pediatr 132:589–595, 1998.
279. Nussbaum E, Boat TF, Wood RE, et al: Cystic fibrosis with acute hypoelectrolytemia and metabolic alkalosis in infancy. Am J Dis Child 133:965–966, 1979.
280. Stern RC: The diagnosis of cystic fibrosis. N Engl J Med 336:487–491, 1997.
281. Knowles MR, Paradiso AM, Boucher RC: In vivo nasal potential difference: Techniques and protocols for assessing efficacy of gene transfer in cystic fibrosis. Hum Gene Ther 6:447–457, 1995.

282. Stern RC, Boat TF, Doershuk CF: Obstructive azoospermia as a diagnostic criterion for the cystic fibrosis syndrome. Lancet i:1401–1404, 1982.
283. Stern RC, Boat TF, Abramowsky CR, et al: Intermediate-range sweat chloride concentration and *Pseudomonas* bronchitis: A cystic fibrosis variant with preservation of exocrine pancreatic function. JAMA 239:2676–2680, 1978.
284. Highsmith WE, Burch LH, Zhou Z, et al: A novel mutation in the cystic fibrosis gene in patients with pulmonary disease but normal sweat chloride concentrations. N Engl J Med 331:974–980, 1994.
285. Anonymous: Sweat Testing: Sample Collection and Quantitative Analysis; Approved Guideline. Wayne, PA: National Committee for Clinical Laboratory Standards (Document C34-A), NCCLS 14:C34-A, 1994.
286. LeGrys VA: Sweat testing for the diagnosis of cystic fibrosis: Practical considerations. J Pediatr 129:892–897, 1996.
287. Davis PB, Del Rio S, Muntz JA, et al: Sweat chloride concentration in adults with pulmonary diseases. Am Rev Respir Dis 128:34–37, 1983.
288. Rock MJ, Mischler EH, Farrell PM, et al: Newborn screening for cystic fibrosis is complicated by age-related decline in immunoreactive trypsinogen levels. Pediatrics 85:1001–1007, 1990.
289. Reardon MC, Hammond KB, Accurso FJ, et al: Nutritional deficits exist before 2 months of age in some infants with cystic fibrosis identified by screening test. J Pediatr 105:271–274, 1984.
290. Ramsey BW, Farrell PM, Pencharz P: Nutritional assessment and management in cystic fibrosis: A consensus report. The Consensus Committee. Am J Clin Nutr 55:108–116, 1992.
291. Farrell PM, Kosorok MR, Laxova A, et al: Nutritional benefits of neonatal screening for cystic fibrosis. Wisconsin Cystic Fibrosis Neonatal Screening Study Group. N Engl J Med 337:963–969, 1997.
292. Waters DL, Wilcken B, Irwig L, et al: Clinical outcomes of newborn screening for cystic fibrosis. Arch Dis Child Fetal Neonatal Ed 80:F1–F7, 1999.
293. Anonymous: Genetic Testing for Cystic Fibrosis. April 14–16. NIH Consens Statement Online 15:1–20, 1997.
294. Noone PG, Knowles MR: Standard therapy of cystic fibrosis lung disease. *In* Yankaskas JR, Knowles MR (eds): Cystic Fibrosis in Adults. Philadelphia: Lippincott-Raven, 1999, pp 145–173.
295. Desmond KJ, Schwenk WF, Thomas E, et al: Immediate and long-term effects of chest physiotherapy in patients with cystic fibrosis. J Pediatr 103:538–542, 1983.
296. Thomas J, Cook DJ, Brooks D: Chest physical therapy management of patients with cystic fibrosis. A meta-analysis. Am J Respir Crit Care Med 151:846–850, 1995.
297. Mortensen J, Falk M, Groth S, et al: The effects of postural drainage and positive expiratory pressure physiotherapy on tracheobronchial clearance in cystic fibrosis. Chest 100:1350–1357, 1991.
298. Oberwaldner B, Evans JC, Zach MS: Forced expirations against a variable resistance: A new chest physiotherapy method in cystic fibrosis. Pediatr Pulmonol 2:358–367, 1986.
299. Blomquist M, Freyschuss U, Wiman L-G, et al: Physical activity and self treatment in cystic fibrosis. Arch Dis Child 61:362–367, 1986.
300. de Jong W, Grevink RG, Roorda RJ, et al: Effect of a home exercise training program in patients with cystic fibrosis. Chest 105:463–468, 1994.
301. Baldwin DR, Hill AL, Peckham DG, et al: Effect of addition of exercise to chest physiotherapy on sputum expectoration and lung function in adults with cystic fibrosis. Respir Med 88:49–53, 1994.
302. Wood RE: Determinants of survival in cystic fibrosis (abstract). Cystic Fibrosis Club Abstracts 26:69, 1985.
303. Pedersen SS, Jensen T, Hoiby N, et al: Management of *Pseudomonas aeruginosa* lung infection in Danish cystic fibrosis patients. Acta Paediatr Scand 76:955–961, 1987.
304. Smith A, Cohen M, Ramsey B: Pharmacotherapy. *In* Yankaskas JR, Knowles MR (eds): Cystic Fibrosis in Adults. Philadelphia: Lippincott-Raven, Publishers, 1999, pp 345–364.
305. Mendelman PM, Smith AL, Levy J, et al: Aminoglycoside penetration, inactivation, and efficacy in cystic fibrosis sputum. Am Rev Respir Dis 132:761–765, 1985.
306. LeBel M, Bergeron MG, Vallee F, et al: Pharmacokinetics and pharmacodynamics of ciprofloxacin in cystic fibrosis patients. Antimicrob Agents Chemother 30:260–266, 1986.
307. Hodson ME, Penketh ARL, Batten JC: Aerosol carbenicillin and gentamicin treatment of *Pseudomonas aeruginosa* infection in patients with cystic fibrosis. Lancet ii:1137–1139, 1981.
308. Wall MA, Terry AB, Eisenberg J, et al: Inhaled antibiotics in cystic fibrosis. Lancet i:1325, 1983.
309. Ramsey BW, Pepe MS, Quan JM, et al: Intermittent administration of inhaled tobramycin in patients with cystic fibrosis. The Cystic Fibrosis Inhaled Tobramycin Study Group. N Engl J Med 340:23–30, 1999.
310. Fuchs HJ, Borowitz DS, Christiansen DH, et al: Effect of aerosolized recombinant DNase on exacerbations of respiratory symptoms and on pulmonary function in patients with cystic fibrosis. The Pulmozyme Study Group. N Engl J Med 331:637–642, 1994.
311. Eng PA, Morton J, Douglass JA, et al: Short-term efficacy of ultrasonically nebulized hypertonic saline in cystic fibrosis. Pediatr Pulmonol 21:77–83, 1996.
312. Robinson M, Regnis JA, Bailey DL, et al: Effect of hypertonic saline, amiloride, and cough on mucociliary clearance in patients with cystic fibrosis. Am J Respir Crit Care Med 153:1503–1509, 1996.
313. Sturgess J, Reid L: The effect of isoprenaline and pilocarpine on (a) bronchial mucus-secreting tissue and (b) pancreas, salivary glands, heart, thymus, liver and spleen. Br J Exp Pathol 54:388–403, 1973.
314. Shapiro GG, Bamman J, Kanerek P, et al: The paradoxical effect of adrenergic and methylxanthine drugs in cystic fibrosis. Pediatrics 58:740–743, 1976.
315. Avital A, Sanchez I, Chernick V: Efficacy of salbutamol and ipratropium bromide in decreasing bronchial hyperreactivity in children with cystic fibrosis. Pediatr Pulmonol 13:34–37, 1992.
316. Sanchez I, Holbrow J, Chernick V: Acute bronchodilator response to a combination of beta-adrenergic and anticholinergic agents in patients with cystic fibrosis. J Pediatr 120:486–488, 1992.
317. Weintraub SJ, Eschenbacher WL: The inhaled bronchodilators ipratropium bromide and metaproterenol in adults with CF. Chest 95:861–864, 1989.
318. Mulherin D, FitzGerald MX: Meconium ileus equivalent in association with nebulized ipratropium bromide in cystic fibrosis. Lancet i:552, 1990.
319. Sivan Y, Arce P, Eigen H, et al: A double-blind, randomized study of sodium cromoglycate versus placebo in patients with cystic fibrosis and bronchial hyperreactivity. J Allergy Clin Immunol 85:649–654, 1990.
320. Auerbach HS, Williams M, Kirkpatrick JA, et al: Alternate-day prednisone reduces morbidity and improves pulmonary function in cystic fibrosis. Lancet ii:686–688, 1985.
320a. Eigen H, Rosenstein BJ, FitzSimmons S, et al: A multicenter study of alternate-day prednisone therapy in patients with cystic fibrosis. Cystic Fibrosis Foundation Prednisone Trial Group. J Pediatr 126:515–523, 1995.
321. Konstan MW, Byard PJ, Hoppel CL, et al: Effect of high-dose ibuprofen in patients with cystic fibrosis. N Engl J Med 332:848–854, 1995.
322. Dolan TF Jr, Gibson LE: Complications of iodide therapy in patients with cystic fibrosis. J Pediatr 79:684–687, 1971.
323. Knowles MR, Church NL, Waltner WE, et al: A pilot study of aerosolized amiloride for the treatment of lung disease in cystic fibrosis. N Engl J Med 322:1189–1194, 1990.
324. Hofmann T, Stutts MJ, Ziersch A, et al: Effects of topically delivered benzamil and amiloride on nasal potential difference in cystic fibrosis. Am J Respir Crit Care Med 157:1844–1849, 1998.
325. Sims DE, Westfall JA, Kiorpes AL, et al: Preservation of tracheal mucus by nonaqueous fixative. Biotech Histochem 66:173–180, 1991.
326. Johnson LG, Knowles MR: New therapeutic strategies for cystic fibrosis lung disease. *In* Yankaskas JR, Knowles MR (eds): Cystic Fibrosis in Adults. Philadelphia: Lippincott-Raven, 1999, pp 233–258.
327. Smyth RL, van Velzen D, Smyth AR, et al: Strictures of ascending colon in cystic fibrosis and high strength pancreatic enzymes. Lancet 343:85–86, 1994.

328. Borowitz DS, Grand RJ, Durie PR: Use of pancreatic enzyme supplements for patients with cystic fibrosis in the context of fibrosing colonopathy. Consensus Committee. J Pediatr 127:681–684, 1995.
329. Smyth RL, Ashby D, O'Hea U, et al: Fibrosing colonopathy in cystic fibrosis: Results of a case-control study. Lancet 346:1247–1251, 1995.
330. FitzSimmons SC, Burkhart GA, Borowitz D, et al: High-dose pancreatic-enzyme supplements and fibrosing colonopathy in children with cystic fibrosis. N Engl J Med 336:1283–1289, 1997.
331. Bertrand JM, Morin CL, Lasalle R, et al: Short-term clinical, nutritional, and functional effects of continuous elemental enteral alimentation in children with cystic fibrosis. J Pediatr 104:41–47, 1984.
332. Gaskin K, Gurevit D, Durie P, et al: Improved respiratory prognosis in patients with cystic fibrosis with normal fat absorption. J Pediatr 100:857–862, 1982.
333. Redding GJ, Restuccia R, Cotton EK, et al: Serial changes in pulmonary functions in children hospitalized with cystic fibrosis. Am Rev Respir Dis 126:31–36, 1982.
334. Regelmann WE, Elliott GR, Warwick WJ, et al: Reduction of sputum *Pseudomonas aeruginosa* density by antibiotics improves lung function in cystic fibrosis more than do bronchodilators and chest physiotherapy alone. Am Rev Respir Dis 141:914–921, 1990.
335. Donati MA, Guenette G, Auerbach H: Prospective controlled study of home and hospital therapy of cystic fibrosis pulmonary disease. J Pediatr 111:28–33, 1987.
336. Pond MN, Newport M, Joanes D, et al: Home versus hospital intravenous antibiotic therapy in the treatment of young adults with cystic fibrosis. Eur Respir J 7:1640–1644, 1994.
337. Winnie GB, Cowan RG, Wade NA: Intravenous immune globulin treatment of pulmonary exacerbations in cystic fibrosis. J Pediatr 114:309–314, 1989.
338. Braunstein MS, Fleet WF: Failure of bronchopulmonary lavage in cystic fibrosis. Chest 66:96–99, 1974.
339. Spier S, Rivlin J, Hughes D, et al: The effect of oxygen on sleep, blood gases, and ventilation in cystic fibrosis. Am Rev Respir Dis 129:712–718, 1984.
340. Coates AL: Oxygen therapy, exercise, and cystic fibrosis. Chest 101:2–4, 1992.
341. Zinman R, Corey M, Coates AL, et al: Nocturnal home oxygen in the treatment of hypoxemic cystic fibrosis patients. J Pediatr 114:368–377, 1989.
342. Fraser KL, Tullis DE, Sasson Z, et al: Pulmonary hypertension and cardiac function in adult cystic fibrosis: Role of hypoxemia. Chest 115:1321–1328, 1999.
343. Anonymous: Continuous or nocturnal oxygen therapy in hypoxemic chronic obstructive lung disease: A clinical trial. Nocturnal Oxygen Therapy Trial Group. Ann Intern Med 93:391–398, 1980.
344. Schidlow DV, Taussig LM, Knowles MR: Cystic Fibrosis Foundation Consensus Conference Report on pulmonary complications of cystic fibrosis. Pediatr Pulmonol 15:187–198, 1993.
345. Davis PB, di Sant'Agnese PA: Assisted ventilation for patients with cystic fibrosis. JAMA 239:1851–1854, 1978.
346. Hodson ME, Madden BP, Steven MH, et al: Non-invasive mechanical ventilation for cystic fibrosis patients—a potential bridge to transplantation. Eur Respir J 4:524–527, 1991.
347. Piper AJ, Parker S, Torzillo PJ, et al: Nocturnal nasal IPPV stabilizes patients with cystic fibrosis and hypercapnic respiratory failure. Chest 102:846–850, 1992.
348. Flume PA, Egan TM, Westerman JH, et al: Lung transplantation for mechanically ventilated patients. J Heart Lung Transplant 13:15–21, 1994.
349. Knutsen AP, Slavin RG: Allergic bronchopulmonary mycosis complicating cystic fibrosis. Semin Respir Infect 7:179–192, 1992.
350. Imbeault B, Cormier Y: Usefulness of inhaled high-dose corticosteroids in allergic bronchopulmonary aspergillosis. Chest 103:1614–1617, 1993.
351. Mannes GP, van der Heide S, van Aalderen WM, et al: Itraconazole and allergic bronchopulmonary aspergillosis in twin brothers with cystic fibrosis. Lancet 341:492, 1993.
352. Fellows KE, Taik Khaw K, Schuster S, et al: Bronchial artery embolization in cystic fibrosis: Technique and long-term results. J Pediatr 95:959–963, 1979.
353. Hofmann AF, Popper H: Ursodeoxycholic acid for primary biliary cirrhosis. Lancet ii:398–399, 1987.
354. Galabert C, Montet JC, Lengrand D, et al: Effects of ursodeoxycholic acid on liver function in patients with cystic fibrosis and chronic cholestasis. J Pediatr 121:138–141, 1992.
355. Colombo C, Battezzati PM, Podda M, et al: Ursodeoxycholic acid for liver disease associated with cystic fibrosis: A double-blind multicenter trial. The Italian Group for the Study of Ursodeoxycholic Acid in Cystic Fibrosis. Hepatology 23:1484–1490, 1996.
356. Stern RC, Stevens DP, Boat TF, et al: Symptomatic hepatic disease in cystic fibrosis: Incidence, course, and outcome of portal systemic shunting. Gastroenterology 70:645–649, 1976.
357. Rossle M, Haag K, Ochs A, et al: The transjugular intrahepatic portosystemic stent-shunt procedure for variceal bleeding. N Engl J Med 330:165–171, 1994.
358. Berger KJ, Schreiber RA, Tchervenkov J, et al: Decompression of portal hypertension in a child with cystic fibrosis after transjugular intrahepatic portosystemic shunt placement. J Pediatr Gastroenterol Nutr 19:322–325, 1994.
359. Mieles LA, Orenstein D, Teperman L, et al: Liver transplantation in cystic fibrosis. Lancet i:1073, 1989.
360. Noble-Jamieson G, Barnes N, Jamieson N, et al: Liver transplantation for hepatic cirrhosis in cystic fibrosis. J R Soc Med 27(Suppl):31–37, 1996.
361. Rosenbloom AL: Diabetes mellitus in cystic fibrosis (abstract). Pediatr Pulmonol (Suppl 6):209–210, 1991.
362. Rodman HM, Doershuk CF, Roland JM: The interaction of 2 diseases: Diabetes mellitus and cystic fibrosis. Medicine (Baltimore) 65:389–397, 1986.
363. Finkelstein SM, Wielinski CL, Elliot GR, et al: Diabetes mellitus associated with cystic fibrosis. J Pediatr 112:373–377, 1988.
364. Lass JH, Spurney RV, Dutt RM, et al: A morphologic and fluorophotometric analysis of the corneal endothelium in type I diabetes mellitus and cystic fibrosis. Am J Ophthalmol 100:783–788, 1985.
365. Allen JL: Progressive nephropathy in a patient with cystic fibrosis and diabetes. N Engl J Med 315:764, 1986.
366. Duplechain JK, White JA, Miller RH: Pediatric sinusitis. The role of endoscopic sinus surgery in cystic fibrosis and other forms of sinonasal disease. Arch Otolaryngol Head Neck Surg 117:422–426, 1991.
367. Cuyler JP: Follow-up of endoscopic sinus surgery on children with cystic fibrosis. Arch Otolaryngol Head Neck Surg 118:505–506, 1992.
368. Stern RC, Rothstein FC, Doershuk CF: Treatment and prognosis of symptomatic gallbladder disease in patients with cystic fibrosis. J Pediatr Gastroenterol Nutr 5:35–40, 1986.
369. Smith MB, Hardin WD Jr, Dressel DA, et al: Predicting outcome following pulmonary resection in cystic fibrosis patients. J Pediatr Surg 26:655–659, 1991.
370. Yankaskas JR, Mallory GB Jr: Lung transplantation in cystic fibrosis: Consensus Conference Statement. Chest 113:217–226, 1998.
371. Barr ML, Schenkel FA, Cohen RG, et al: Recipient and donor outcomes in living related and unrelated lobar transplantation. Transplant Proc 30:2261–2263, 1998.
372. Stern RC, Boat TF, Doershuk CF, et al: Cystic fibrosis diagnosed after age 13. Twenty-five teenage and adult patients including three asymptomatic men. Ann Intern Med 87:188–191, 1977.
373. Shwachman H, Kulczycki LL: Long-term study of one hundred five patients with cystic fibrosis. Study made over a five- to fourteen-year period. J Dis Child 96:6–15, 1958.
374. Taussig LM, Kattwinkel J, Friedewald WT, et al: A new prognostic score and clinical evaluation system for cystic fibrosis. J Pediatr 82:380–390, 1973.
375. Fink RJ, Doershuk CF, Tucker AS, et al: Pulmonary function and morbidity in 40 adult patients with cystic fibrosis. Chest 74:643–647, 1978.
376. Corey M, Levison H, Crozier D: Five- to seven-year course of pulmonary function in cystic fibrosis. Am Rev Respir Dis 114:1085–1092, 1976.
377. Wood RE: Prognosis. *In* Taussig LM (ed): Cystic Fibrosis. New York: Thieme-Stratton, 1984, pp 434–460.

378. Orenstein DM, Boat TF, Stern RC, et al: The effect of early diagnosis and treatment in cystic fibrosis: A seven-year study of 16 sibling pairs. Am J Dis Child 131:973–975, 1977.
379. Katz JN, Horwitz RI, Dolan TF, et al: Clinical features as predictors of functional status in children with cystic fibrosis. J Pediatr 108:352–358, 1986.
380. Hamosh A, Corey M: Correlation between genotype and phenotype in patients with cystic fibrosis. The Cystic Fibrosis Genotype-Phenotype Consortium. N Engl J Med 329:1308–1313, 1993.
381. Knoke JD, Stern RC, Doershuk CF, et al: Cystic fibrosis: The prognosis for five-year survival. Pediatr Res 12:676–679, 1978.
382. Reisman J, Corey M, Canny G, et al: Diabetes mellitus in patients with cystic fibrosis: Effect on survival. Pediatrics 86:374–377, 1990.
383. Hill DJ, Martin AJ, Davidson GP, et al: Survival of cystic fibrosis patients in South Australia. Evidence that cystic fibrosis centre care leads to better survival. Med J Aust 143:230–232, 1985.
383a. Mahadeva R, Webb K, Westerbeek RC, et al: Clinical outcome in relation to care in centres specialising in cystic fibrosis: Cross sectional study. BJM 316:1771–1775, 1998.
384. Denning CR, Gluckson MM: Psychosocial aspects of cystic fibrosis. *In* Taussig LM (ed): Cystic Fibrosis. New York: Thieme-Stratton, 1984, pp 461–492.
385. Lewiston NJ: Psychosocial impact of cystic fibrosis. Semin Respir Med 6:321–332, 1985.
386. Yankaskas JR, Fernald GW: Adult social issues. *In* Yankaskas JR, Knowles MR (eds): Cystic Fibrosis in Adults. Philadelphia: Lippincott-Raven, 1999, pp 465–476.
387. Levine SB, Stern RC: Sexual function in cystic fibrosis. Relationship to overall health status and pulmonary disease severity in 30 married patients. Chest 81:422–428, 1982.
388. Hull J, Skinner W, Robertson C, et al: Elemental content of airway surface liquid from infants with cystic fibrosis. Am J Respir Crit Care Med 157:10–14, 1998.

# 41 Bronchiectasis

John M. Luce, M.D.

Introduction
Classification
Pathogenesis and Pathology
Epidemiology
Pulmonary Function Abnormalities
Symptoms
Complications
Physical Findings
Diagnosis
Treatment
Prognosis
Prevention
Associated Conditions
- Allergic Bronchopulmonary Aspergillosis
- Alpha$_1$-Antitrypsin Deficiency
- Bronchial Obstruction
- Bronchopulmonary Sequestration
- Congenital Cartilage Deficiency
- Cystic Fibrosis
- Human Immunodeficiency Virus Infection
- Immunodeficiency
- Infection
- Inflammation
- Other Associated Conditions
- Primary Ciliary Dyskinesia
- Rheumatoid Arthritis
- Tracheobronchomegaly
- Unilateral Hyperlucent Lung
- Yellow Nail Syndrome

Summary

## INTRODUCTION

The term *bronchiectasis* is derived from the Greek words *bronkos*, "windpipe," and *ektasis*, "stretching" or "extension."[1] It refers to an abnormal dilation of the proximal medium-sized bronchi greater than 2 mm in diameter caused by destruction of the muscular and elastic components of their walls. This dilation commonly is associated with chronic bacterial infection and the production of large quantities of foul-smelling sputum. Bronchiectasis need not always be associated with purulent expectoration, however, especially when it involves areas of the lung with dependent drainage, such as the upper lobes, which frequently are involved in patients with pulmonary tuberculosis. In this circumstance, the bronchiectasis is called "dry" to distinguish it from the more common "wet" or productive variety.

Bronchial dilation may be temporary, as occurs in areas of atelectasis after acute pneumonia.[2] Complete reversal of bronchiectasis after several years has also been observed.[3] Nevertheless, bronchiectasis generally is thought of as a persistent, if not permanent, pathologic process. The word *process* is useful here because it stresses that bronchiectasis is not a discrete disease entity unless it is caused solely by bronchial obstruction or untreated infection. Rather, it is more commonly a pulmonary manifestation of systemic disorders, such as cystic fibrosis and primary ciliary dyskinesia, which are discussed at the end of this chapter.

Some investigators[4] have presumed bronchiectasis to be a focal process, in contrast to chronic bronchitis, which usually involves the entire lung. Bronchiectasis certainly can result from local airway obstruction and infection and therefore may be confined to one area. Focal bronchiectasis of this sort was particularly common before the advent of antibiotics. Even before antibiotics became available, however, bronchiectasis often was generalized. As a result, bronchiectasis cannot be distinguished from chronic bronchitis on the basis of distribution within the chest. Furthermore, patients with chronic bronchitis may demonstrate some degree of proximal bronchial dilation, whereas patients with bronchiectasis may demonstrate the pathologic changes associated with chronic bronchitis, especially if they smoke.[5] Thus, considerable clinical overlap between the two conditions commonly occurs.[5a]

## CLASSIFICATION

Several systems have been used to classify bronchiectasis, most of them based on anatomic abnormalities of the bronchi seen on bronchography or at autopsy.[6, 7] The classification system most commonly cited today was introduced in 1950 by Reid,[8] who correlated the pathologic and bronchographic findings in 45 bronchiectatic lobes removed during autopsy at the Royal Melbourne Hospital. The Reid classification consists of the following categories: (1) cylindrical bronchiectasis, in which sections of the bronchi are consistently widened; (2) varicose bronchiectasis, in which local constrictions in cylindrical bronchiectatic sections cause an irregularity resembling that of varicose veins; and (3) saccular or cystic bronchiectasis, in which dilation increases toward the lung periphery, so that the bronchi terminate in balloon-like structures. The Reid classification of bronchiectasis is helpful in roentgenographic descriptions of the process because it is based on a pathologic-bronchographic correlation. Nevertheless, little clinical, epidemiologic, or pathophysiologic difference has been demonstrated among cylindrical, varicose, and saccular bronchiectasis.

## PATHOGENESIS AND PATHOLOGY

In all forms of bronchiectasis, abnormal dilation is found in the proximal subdivisions of bronchi that contain cartilaginous walls. Its major cause is inflammation, which is mediated by elastase, collagenase, and other substances from neutrophils that are recruited into the lung and that stimulate hypersecretion.[9–14] Neutrophil recruitment results in large part from the release of cytokines such as interleukin-8 and leukotriene-$B_4$ from macrophages and airway epithelial cells.[15–16] The cytokine-mediated inflammation is reflected in a release of exhaled nitric oxide,[17] which may be localized or generalized.[18]

Although the initial cause of inflammation varies among patients depending on the origin of their bronchiectasis, the inflammation traditionally has been seen as a physiologic response to persistent infection. In support of this view, Konstan and associates[19] demonstrated that infection, as documented by the finding of *Pseudomonas aeruginosa, Staphylococcus aureus,* and/or *Haemophilus influenzae* in bronchoalveolar lavage fluid, was present in all of 18 patients with bronchiectasis related to cystic fibrosis who had stable, clinically mild lung disease. The same patients also had high concentrations of neutrophils and neutrophil elastase in their lavage specimens, indicating ongoing inflammation presumably caused by the bacteria. On the other hand, Khan and colleagues[20] showed that the lavage fluid of infants with cystic fibrosis (mean age, 6 months) also contained increased neutrophil counts, neutrophil elastase concentrations, and interleukin-8 levels despite negative cultures for bacteria, viruses, and fungi. This study suggests that, at least in patients with cystic fibrosis, inflammation occurs early in the course of disease and may precede infection. As Russell and associates[21] have speculated, defective regulation of the inflammatory response may play a role in the pathogenesis of cystic fibrosis and perhaps other disorders causing bronchiectasis.

The end result of inflammation of the bronchial walls is destruction of their elastic and muscular components; the surrounding undamaged lung tissue exerts a contractile force that expands the damaged bronchi and creates the characteristic dilation observed roentgenographically.[22] Chronic bronchial overdistention caused by the pull of surrounding lung tissue on the bronchial walls also provokes a contraction of the surrounding musculature, leading in turn to its hypertrophy and hyperplasia. In long-standing bronchiectasis, the peribronchial alveolar tissue is also damaged by inflammation. Diffuse peribronchial fibrosis frequently results from this process. Squamous metaplasia of the bronchial epithelium is assumed to stem from the same chronic inflammation. The inflammation is also associated with obliteration of the distal bronchi or bronchioles. This obliteration causes a reduction in the bronchial subdivisions between the hilum and the periphery of the lung, so that the usual airway arborization pattern appears to have been pruned.

In her original study, Reid[8] examined primarily the posterior basal segments of the left or right lower lobes, because these segments were most frequently involved in the bronchiectatic process, presumably because of their lack of gravitational drainage. Moll[6] and Perry and King[7] also found the lower lobes to be most commonly abnormal in patients with bronchiectasis. Bilateral lower lobe involvement occurs in one third of patients; unilateral involvement is seen in the left and the right lungs with equal frequency.[23]

Upper lobe bronchiectasis is usually seen in the posterior and apical segments and has been attributed to tuberculous endobronchitis, allergic bronchopulmonary aspergillosis, or cystic fibrosis.[24] Nevertheless, a study[25] using computed tomography (CT) demonstrated that bronchiectasis associated with systemic disorders can occur anywhere in the lungs and that the causes of bronchiectasis cannot be reliably diagnosed on the basis of CT appearance alone.

The most important functional result of the altered airway anatomy of bronchiectatic patients is impaired tracheobronchial clearance, which in time predisposes to airway colonization and infection with pathogenic organisms.[26] Such impaired clearance was first described in 1972 by Lourenco and colleagues.[27] In 1987, Currie and associates[28] confirmed these results using radiolabeled aerosols in bronchiectatic patients with presumably normal ciliary anatomy and function. These investigators also showed that tracheobronchial clearance was similarly impaired in smokers with chronic bronchiectasis but not in smokers who had negligible sputum production. More recently, Regnis and coworkers[29] demonstrated impaired mucociliary clearance in nonsmoking patients with cystic fibrosis. According to Deneuville and associates,[30] the impairment results in large part from decreased mucus hydration caused by infection with organisms such as *P. aeruginosa*.

Liebow and associates[31] first described enlargement of the bronchial arteries and extensive anastomoses between these vessels and the pulmonary arteries in the lungs of bronchiectatic patients. They attributed the increase in arterial size to augmented blood flow in the bronchial circulation and believed that it was related to the presence of chronic inflammation and the development of granulation in the bronchial walls and peribronchial tissues. The systemic-pulmonary anastomoses appeared to result both from new capillary channels and from the expansion of previously existing communications between the two circulations.

According to Spencer,[22] total pulmonary arterial flow may diminish because of obstructive endarteritis in patients with severe bronchiectasis. A functional decrease in the cross-sectional area of the pulmonary circulation also might be expected in the presence of alveolar hypoxia. The pulmonary hypertension resulting from this condition might worsen owing to the large volume of blood passing into the pulmonary artery through bronchial-pulmonary anastomoses until pressures in the two circulations equilibrate. The same mechanism might serve as a left-to-right shunt and increase the work of the right ventricle. Left-to-right intrapulmonary shunting was demonstrated in bronchiectatic patients by Tadavarthy and colleagues.[32]

## EPIDEMIOLOGY

Postinfectious bronchiectasis once was a common disease in the United States. However, it has become rare since the introduction of antibiotics and now occurs in very few Americans. Most affected persons have bronchiectasis in association with systemic disorders. Postinfectious bronchiectasis remains a public health problem today only in one segment of the U.S. population: Native Americans in Alaska, whose annual incidence of the condition was estimated to be 4 per 10,000 in 1968. This incidence was four times higher than any other reported in the United States but probably underestimated the problem in Alaska, because some asymptomatic persons and those living in isolated areas escaped diagnosis.[33] Despite its decline in the United States and in other industrialized nations, bronchiectasis persists in most resource-poor countries of the world.[34, 35]

## PULMONARY FUNCTION ABNORMALITIES

The pulmonary function abnormalities attributable to bronchiectasis are difficult to differentiate from those caused by the diseases that underlie or exist in concert with this condition. This difficulty limits the usefulness of early studies, in which bronchiectatic patients were not well characterized and concurrent chronic bronchitis and pulmonary emphysema were not accounted for. For example, in a study by Baum and associates[34] of Israelis with cystic lung disease, most of which was attributed to bronchiectasis, the forced vital capacity (FVC) and the ratio of $FEV_1$ to FVC were said to be normal or slightly reduced in patients 45 years of age or younger and invariably reduced in patients older than 45 years. These variables generally were not reversible and were thought by the investigators to be caused by concurrent infection. However, it was not clear what caused infections in these patients, whether the FVC or $FEV_1$/FVC ratio improved after their infections were treated, or whether their airflow obstruction was influenced by cigarette smoking.

Cherniack and colleagues[36] assessed pulmonary function in 50 patients with bronchiectasis, 41 of whom had bilateral disease on bronchography. Half of the patients were older than 50 years of age, 2 had hypogammaglobulinemia, 1 had situs inversus, and 20 had suspected chronic bronchitis or pulmonary emphysema in addition to bronchiectasis. None of the patients had active infection at the time of pulmonary function testing. Mean values for FVC, $FEV_1$, maximum breathing capacity, index of alveolar mixing, diffusing capacity, arterial $Po_2$, arterial $Pco_2$, and physiologic dead space all were minimally abnormal in this study. The investigators concluded that mild air flow obstruction and maldistribution of ventilation accounted for most of the abnormalities of pulmonary function in their patients.

A correlation between physiologic abnormalities and the extent of bronchiectasis was underscored by Bass and associates,[37] who performed bronchography, routine pulmonary function tests, and an assessment of regional lung function with inhaled and intravenous radiolabeled xenon in eight patients. In general, bronchographically abnormal areas were less well ventilated than normal areas, but some bronchiectatic areas were well ventilated. Although blood flow generally was diminished in the underventilated areas, some areas had increased blood flow, perhaps because of an increase in vascularity due to bronchial-pulmonary circulatory anastomoses in these regions.

Early studies such as these offer the only available information on pulmonary function in patients who were grouped together because of their common diagnosis of bronchiectasis. Newer work focuses on pulmonary function in subsets of bronchiectatic patients. For example, Nichols and associates[38] assessed pulmonary function in 16 patients with allergic bronchopulmonary aspergillosis during an acute episode and during a follow-up period of 49 months. Acute episodes of bronchopulmonary aspergillosis were associated with transient reductions in lung volumes and diffusing capacity in all 16 patients. However, functional loss was seen in only 3 of the 16 patients over time. These findings suggest that progressive deterioration is not inevitable in allergic bronchopulmonary aspergillosis, presumably because asthma is an integral part of the condition. On the other hand, worsening might be expected in cystic fibrosis and in other less reversible conditions.

Despite the heterogeneity of patients with bronchiectasis and their clinical variability, general patterns of pulmonary function abnormalities can be anticipated. Most patients with bronchiectasis demonstrate some degree of air flow obstruction. Mild restriction may also be present, especially if the bronchiectasis is associated with a disease that reduces lung volumes. The diffusing capacity for carbon monoxide also may be decreased. Most patients have mild hypoxemia owing to ventilation-perfusion mismatching and intrapulmonary shunt. Normocapnia or hypocapnia is observed in all but the most advanced cases. Cor pulmonale occurs in only a minority of patients with bronchiectasis, because hypoxemia usually is not severe in these patients.[39, 40]

## SYMPTOMS

Patients with bronchiectasis may have symptoms referable to the bronchiectatic process alone or to underlying disorders. Symptoms caused by bronchiectasis itself include chronic cough, purulent expectoration, fever, weakness, and weight loss. Sputum production often increases during acute respiratory infections. Using 24-hour sputum volume as an indicator of the severity of bronchiectasis, Ellis and associates[41] categorized patients who produced less than 10 mL, 10 to 150 mL, and more than 150 mL of sputum daily as having "mild," "moderate," and "severe" bronchiectasis, respectively.

Dyspnea is reported by some patients with bronchiectasis but is not a universal finding. As might be expected, breathlessness is especially common among patients with extensive bronchiectasis on the chest roentgenogram. As Ellis and associates[41] emphasized, however, marked dyspnea may relate more to concurrent illnesses such as chronic bronchitis and pulmonary emphysema than to pure bronchiectasis. As a result, the effect of cigarette smoking and the presence of severe airflow obstruction on pulmonary function testing may correlate better with subjective complaints than with the extent of bronchiectasis per se.

Hemoptysis is also common among patients with bronchiectasis, occurring in 44 of 48 Israelis in the series reported by Baum and colleagues.[34] Hemoptysis is said to be less common among patients with wet bronchiectasis than among those with dry bronchiectasis, including patients with pulmonary tuberculosis.[6] Hemoptysis is generally mild, most often consisting of the expectoration of purulent sputum flecked with blood. However, because the bleeding usually originates from bronchial arteries or bronchial-pulmonary anastomoses under systemic pressures, it may become massive, that is, more than 250 mL per day.[42–45]

## COMPLICATIONS

The complications most commonly associated with bronchiectasis are recurrent pneumonia, empyema, pneumothorax, and lung abscess.[6, 7, 42–45] Differentiating these conditions from bronchiectasis is difficult on clinical grounds alone, and their true prevalence is difficult to determine in most series. Brain abscess has also been reported in bronchiectatic patients. Amyloidosis once was frequently attributed to bronchiectasis[7] but is rarely seen today in developed countries. As noted earlier, cor pulmonale occurs in a minority of patients, but it nevertheless is a complication of grave concern.

## PHYSICAL FINDINGS

The physical signs of patients with bronchiectasis are neither sensitive nor specific for that process. The breath is fetid in some but not most patients. Digital clubbing also is an inconsistent finding, as are cyanosis and plethora reflective of polycythemia. Nasal polyps and signs of chronic sinusitis may be present. Crackles are often found at the lung bases; rhonchi may be encountered, especially if active infection is present; and scattered wheezes may be heard. Evidence of wasting and weight loss suggests advanced disease but is hardly diagnostic of bronchiectasis. The same is true for the physical stigmata of cor pulmonale.

## DIAGNOSIS

Bronchiectasis may be suspected on the basis of clinical presentation, especially if the process involves purulent expectoration and if disorders such as pneumonia, emphysema, and lung abscess have been ruled out. The onset of bronchiectasis may be traced to a clear-cut aspiration or febrile illness, especially in patients with postobstructive or infectious bronchiectasis. Field[42–44] found that childhood bronchiectasis in the preantibiotic era often followed an episode of pneumonia, pertussis, influenza, or measles; thereafter, the children suffered recurrent infections. Bronchiectasis that occurs in patients with underlying disorders such as cystic fibrosis or primary ciliary dyskinesia is more likely to have an insidious onset but may be associated with discrete infectious episodes as well.

Sputum analysis should reinforce the clinical impression of bronchiectasis. Such analysis might include visual inspection of expectorated sputum that has been allowed to settle into the characteristic three layers: an upper frothy and watery layer, a middle layer that is turbid and mucopurulent, and a bottom layer that is purulent and opaque.[12] The bottom layer may contain Dittrich's plugs, small white or yellow concretions. Bacteriologic studies of bronchiectatic sputum may reveal microorganisms such as *Streptococcus pneumoniae, H. influenzae,* and *S. aureus,* but these pathogens may also be present in the sputum of patients with chronic bronchitis. The finding of *Aspergillus* species is suggestive but not diagnostic of allergic bronchopulmonary aspergillosis. Mucoid strains of *Pseudomonas* and *Escherichia coli* are found in the respiratory secretions of not only patients with cystic fibrosis but also those with bronchiectasis due to other causes.[46, 47] Infection with *Pseudomonas cepacia* is associated with poor outcomes in patients with cystic fibrosis.[48] *Branhamella catarrhalis* is increasingly recognized as a pathogen in patients with bronchiectasis and other forms of chronic lung disease.[49]

Roentgenographic studies have long been the means by which the diagnosis of bronchiectasis is firmly made. The plain chest roentgenogram is normal in some patients with bronchiectasis, but most often it shows characteristic patterns. When cylindrical bronchiectasis is present, these patterns involve linear radiolucencies and thin parallel markings that radiate from the hili and are called *tram tracks* or *tram lines* (Fig. 41.1 and Fig. 41.2). Varicose bronchiectasis is characterized by variable degrees of bronchial dilation. The dilated bronchi may appear as thick, parallel markings or so-called *toothpaste lines* (Fig. 41.3). The roentgenographic appearance of cystic bronchiectasis involves isolated or clustered cysts that may contain air-fluid levels (Fig. 41.4 and Fig. 41.5). Peribronchial haziness, atelectasis, and consolidation also have been described.[50] Chest roentgenograms have not been shown to be useful in distinguishing chronic bronchiectasis in patients with cystic fibrosis from acute exacerbations of disease.[51]

Bronchography once was commonly used for confirming the presence of bronchiectasis and determining the extent of its involvement, but this technique is now virtually obsolete. The procedure may be performed with the installation of contrast material via a catheter or bronchoscope. Although it provides adequate visualization with minimal discomfort, bronchography can be dangerous in patients with respiratory compromise. Therefore, bronchography should not be performed during exacerbations of bronchiectasis or when significant bronchospasm is present, including that associated with allergic bronchopulmonary aspergillosis.[15]

CT of the chest, which involves little discomfort and few adverse complications, has for practical purposes

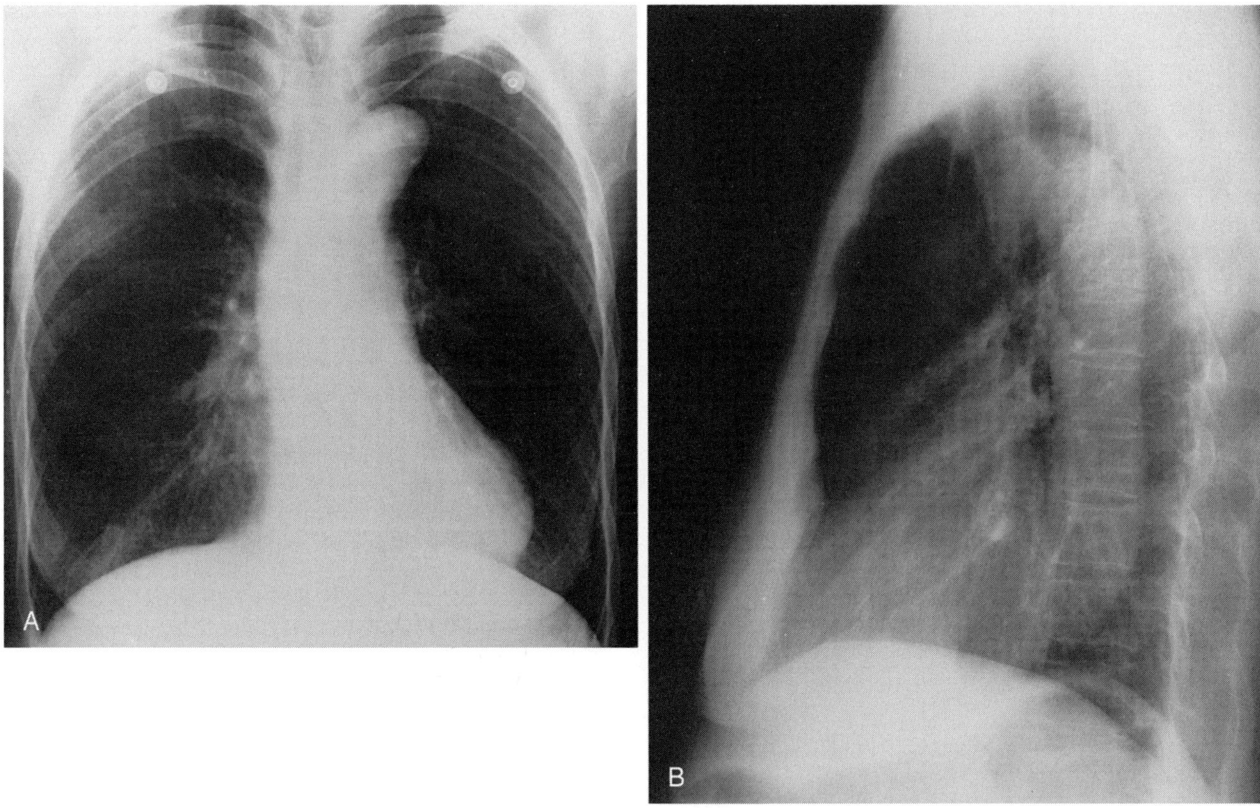

**Figure 41.1** Plain posterior-anterior *(A)* and lateral *(B)* roentgenograms showing thin parallel markings (tram lines) characteristic of cylindrical bronchiectasis in the left lower lobe. Bronchogram not available. (Courtesy of Philip C. Goodman, M.D., Duke University, Durham, North Carolina.)

replaced bronchography in the diagnosis of bronchiectasis, especially among patients with generalized disease.[51a] Early studies showed that routine, thick-section chest CT studies missed cylindrical and varicose bronchiectasis in a significant number of patients,[52] and the sensitivity and specificity of CT at a segmental level, compared with bronchography, were found to be 66% and 92%, respectively.[53] These deficiencies were all but overcome by the introduction of high-resolution, thin-section chest computed tomography (HRCT), which has a sensitivity and a specificity of more than 90% for the detection of bronchiectasis at a segmental level[54] (Fig. 41.6).

Bronchiectasis results in six characteristic HRCT findings, as originally described by Naidich and coworkers[55]: bronchial dilation, bronchial wall thickening, lack of normal bronchial tapering, gross irregularities in airway contact, and air-fluid levels in distended bronchi. According to Webb,[56] bronchiectasis generally can be diagnosed when the internal diameter of a bronchus is greater than that of an adjacent branch of the pulmonary artery. Exacerbations of cystic fibrosis are marked by the appearance of air-fluid levels in bronchiectatic cavities.[57] Patients infected with *P. aeruginosa* have more extensive and severe bronchiectasis on HRCT than those without *Pseudomonas* infection.[58] Although HRCT can distinguish among cylindrical, varicose, and saccular or cystic lesions, this distinction is of uncertain clinical significance, as it is when made by other methods. At the same time, HRCT findings in individual patients are of limited value for discriminating among the various causes of bronchiectasis.[59, 59a]

Helical or spiral CT scanning has been demonstrated to improve CT resolution of bronchiectasis, but this technique is not widely available and increases radiation exposure. As a result, helical scanning is recommended primarily for use in patients in whom HRCT is difficult to interpret.[60] Magnetic resonance scanning requires no radiation exposure and is increasingly available in developed countries. However, the resolution of magnetic resonance scanning at present does not compare well with that of HRCT in terms of accuracy.[61]

Bronchoscopy is less helpful than bronchography or HRCT for visualization of entire bronchiectatic segments. However, bronchoscopy may be useful for detection of aspirated foreign bodies and other obstructing lesions, and it is indicated when such lesions are suspected. Bronchoscopy also may be indicated in patients with hemoptysis to localize the bleeding site or to determine from which lung or lobe blood is coming. Bronchoscopy also can be used to collect bronchoalveolar lavage specimens for culture and sensitivity studies, as has been described in patients with cystic fibrosis.[62] Nevertheless, bronchoscopy cannot be recommended for the routine evaluation of bronchiectasis.

In countries where postinfectious bronchiectasis is common and medical resources are limited, the work-up

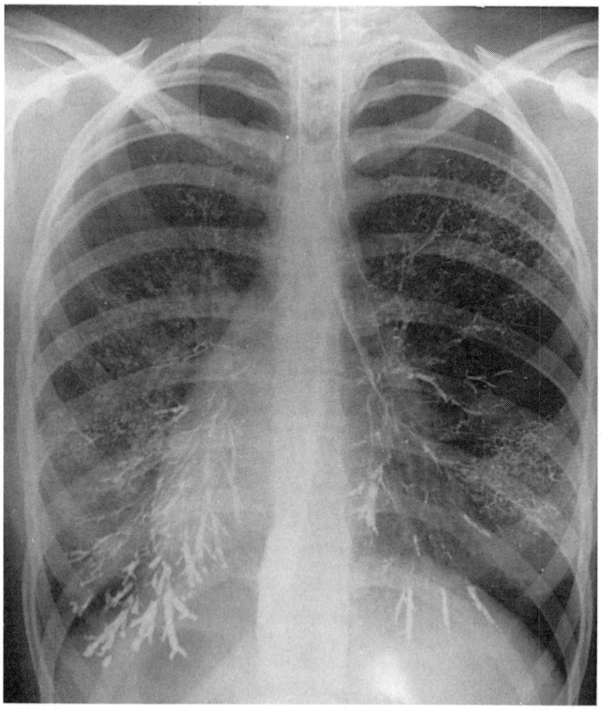

**Figure 41.2** Bronchogram showing cylindrical bronchiectasis in the right lower lobe of a patient with situs inversus from Kartagener's syndrome. (Reprinted with permission from Hinshaw HC, Murray JF: Diseases of the Chest (4th ed). Philadelphia: WB Saunders, 1980, p 594.)

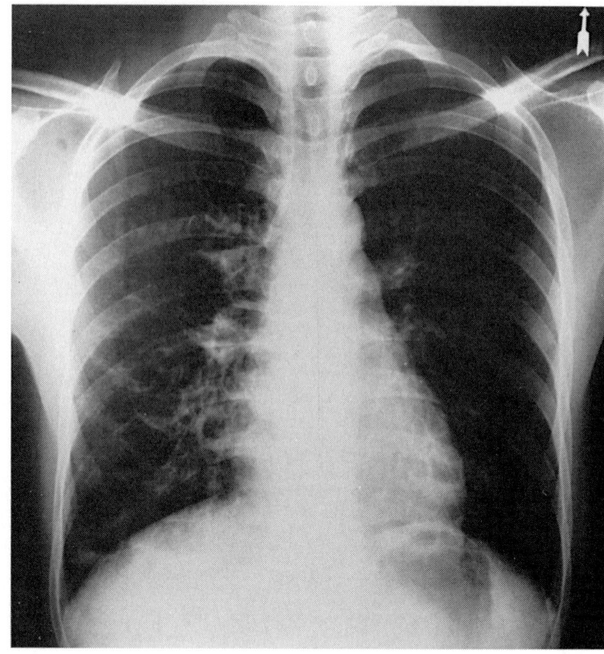

**Figure 41.4** Plain roentgenogram showing cystic bronchiectasis in the right middle lobe of a patient with cystic fibrosis. (Courtesy of Philip C. Goodman, M.D., Duke University, Durham, North Carolina.)

for bronchiectasis may extend no further than history-taking and sputum examination with or without a plain chest roentgenogram. In the United States and other industrialized countries, however, the detection of *de novo* bronchiectasis should prompt a search for its underlying cause. Depending on the type of patient involved, this search might include some or all of the following: serum protein electrophoresis for $alpha_1$-antitrypsin deficiency; immunoglobulin levels, including immunoglobulin G (IgG) subclasses, for hypogammaglobulinemia; pilocarpine iontophoresis (sweat test) for cystic fibrosis; determination of immunoglobulins and *Aspergillus* precipitins for allergic bronchopulmonary aspergillosis; and electron

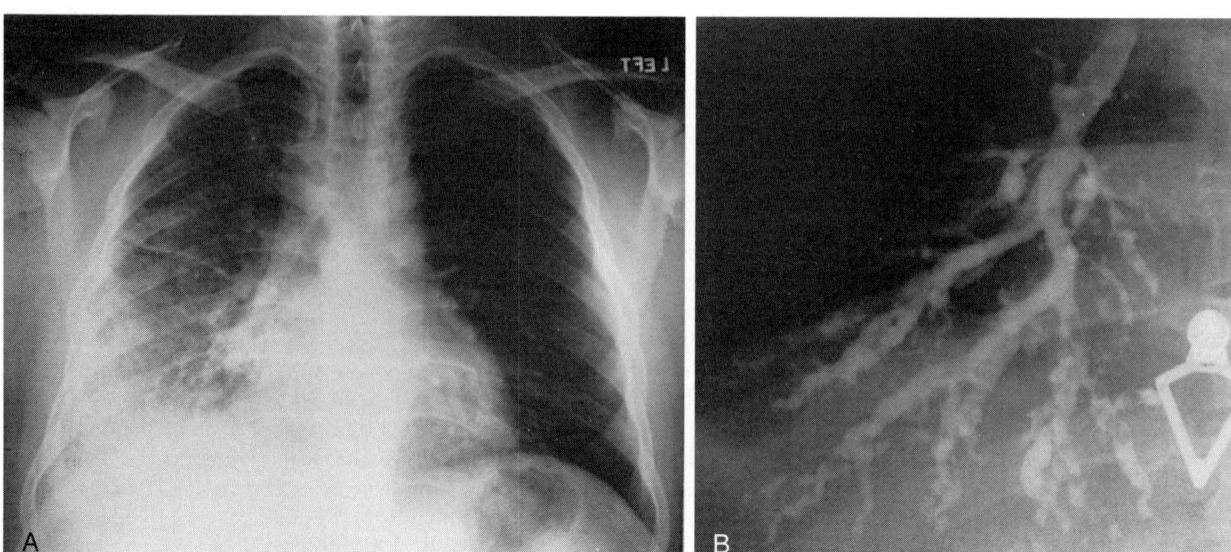


**Figure 41.3** Plain roentgenogram *(A)* and bronchographic detail *(B)* showing varicose bronchiectasis in the right lower lobe of a Polynesian patient. (Courtesy of Philip C. Goodman, M.D., Duke University, Durham, North Carolina.)

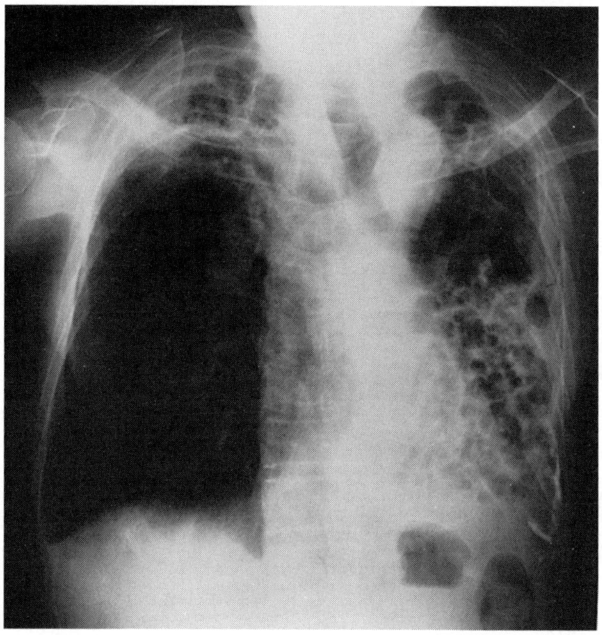

**Figure 41.5** Plain roentgenogram showing postinfectious cystic bronchiectasis in a patient from Central America. (Courtesy of Philip C. Goodman, M.D., Duke University, Durham, North Carolina.)

microscopic examination of sperm or respiratory epithelium for primary ciliary dyskinesia.[63]

## TREATMENT

Antimicrobial drugs have been the mainstay of treatment of bronchiectasis since their introduction more than 40 years ago. The choice of specific agents should be dictated by sputum or bronchoalveolar lavage fluid culture for aerobes, anaerobes, and mycobacteria whenever possible. If mixed flora are present, as is often the case, treatment consists of a broad-spectrum antibiotic such as amoxicillin, tetracycline, or trimethoprim-sulfamethoxazole. Antibiotics used to treat *Pseudomonas* infections include ticarcillin, gentamycin, tobramycin, ceftazidime, and ciprofloxacin.[64] Most clinicians prefer to give antimicrobial agents during acute exacerbations of bronchiectasis, but some prescribe them on a regular basis or during a given number of weeks each month, as is sometimes done for infectious chronic bronchitis. Aerosolized gentamycin and tobramycin have been shown to improve airway secretion and inflammation in patients with bronchiectasis related to cystic fibrosis and other conditions.[65, 66]

Chest physical therapy with postural drainage, chest clapping, humidification, the use of mucolytics, and other measures have also been recommended.[67] Techniques such as chest clapping can be administered by family members and certainly are of psychological benefit. Their physiologic utility has not been well demonstrated, although a meta-analysis by Thomas and colleagues[68] found that chest physical therapy resulted in significantly greater sputum expectoration than no treatment, whereas therapy and exercise were associated with a significant increase in expiratory flow rates. Aerosolized amiloride appears to increase mucociliary clearance in patients with cystic fibrosis,[69] as does the combination of amiloride, hypertonic saline, and cough.[70] The beta-adrenergic agonist terbutaline has been shown to increase tracheal mucus velocity in patients with cystic fibrosis,[71] as has albuterol.[72]

The most promising agent to facilitate secretion clearance in patients with cystic fibrosis is aerosolized recombinant human deoxyribonuclease (DNase). This substance appears to hydrolyze extracellular deoxyribonucleic acid (DNA) that accumulates, along with other neutrophil degradation products, in infected airways. Recombinant DNase was been shown to reduce the viscoelastic properties of sputum and to improve air flow rates in a small study of pediatric and adult patients with cystic fibrosis.[73] Also, the administration of recombinant DNase improved flow rates and reduced but did not eliminate exacerbations of respiratory symptoms in a large number of bronchiectatic patients with cystic fibrosis in a prospective, randomized trial.[74] Despite its beneficial effects in this group of patients, however, recombinant DNase has not been demonstrated to enhance sputum transportability or to improve symptoms in patients with bronchiectasis due to other causes.[75, 76]

A new approach to treating bronchiectasis is anti-inflammatory therapy. In this regard, inhaled indomethacin was shown to improve sputum viscosity and to relieve symptoms in patients with chronic bronchitis and bronchiectasis, although it did not affect pulmonary function.[77] Furthermore, in a group of patients with cystic fibrosis and mild lung disease monitored by Konstan and associates,[78] high-dose ibuprofen, given orally twice daily for 4 years, slowed the rate of decline in $FEV_1$ and FVC, the percentage of ideal body weight, and a chest roentgenogram score used to describe the severity of roentgenographic involvement.

Diuretics may be administered cautiously to bronchiectatic patients with cor pulmonale. These patients, as well as those with severe hypoxemia (arterial $Po_2$, 55 mm Hg or less) at rest despite intensive treatment, are candidates for continuous low-flow oxygen therapy, which is discussed further in Chapter 96. This approach improves hemodynamic performance and longevity in patients with chronic bronchitis and pulmonary emphysema[79, 80] and presumably should also benefit bronchiectatic patients. Supplemental oxygen has been demonstrated to improve exercise performance in patients with cystic fibrosis.[81] Long-term mechanical ventilation, including that administered by face mask, may be useful in patients with bronchiectasis and severe chronic respiratory failure.[82]

In addition to these general measures, specific therapies may be appropriate when the underlying cause of bronchiectasis has been identified. For example, the regular administration of immunoglobulin to patients with immunodeficiency may decrease their incidence of sinopulmonary infection.[83, 84] Replacement enzyme therapy is now available for patients with $alpha_1$-antitrypsin deficiency, and gene replacement therapy is being studied in patients with cystic fibrosis.[85] Other treatments are incidental to the lungs but of great overall importance; one example is the use of pancreatic enzymes to aid digestion in patients with cystic fibrosis.

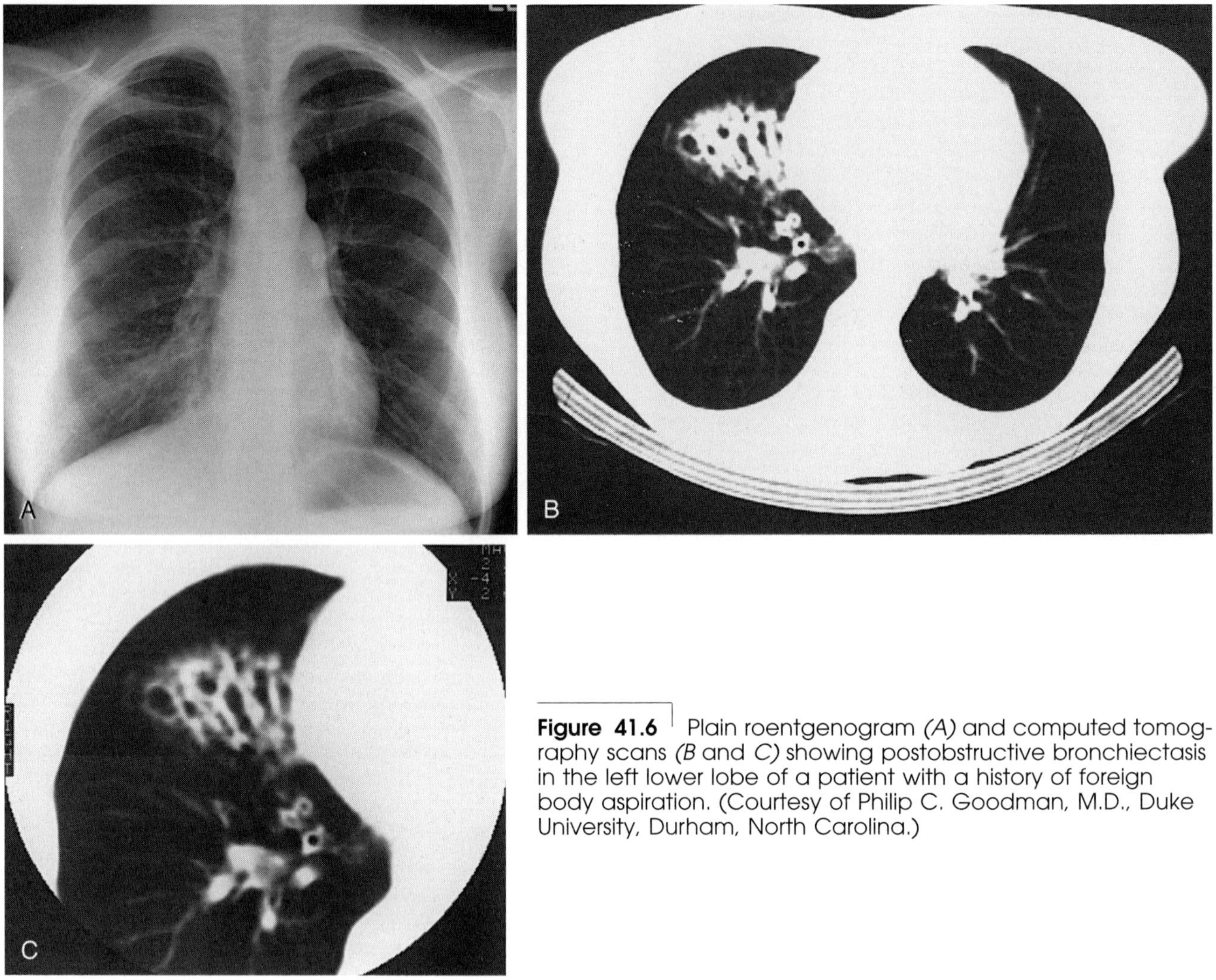


**Figure 41.6** Plain roentgenogram *(A)* and computed tomography scans *(B and C)* showing postobstructive bronchiectasis in the left lower lobe of a patient with a history of foreign body aspiration. (Courtesy of Philip C. Goodman, M.D., Duke University, Durham, North Carolina.)

The medical management of bronchiectasis should prove effective in the almost all patients. Nevertheless, consideration should be given to surgical resection in certain instances. The first successful resection for bronchiectasis was carried out in 1901, and segmentectomy, lobectomy, and even pneumonectomy became increasingly popular over subsequent years. Despite a mortality rate of 12% or more from these procedures in a series reported from Great Britain by Edwards[86] in 1939, surgery to be appeared justified because most investigators believed that the prognosis for bronchiectatic patients who did not undergo resection was grave.[6, 7] Subsequent reports by Field[42–44] and others cast doubt on this opinion, prompting surgeons to be more selective in their choice of patients for resection and to limit the amount of lung tissue removed. The operative mortality rate declined as a result, reaching 6% in 159 English patients reported by Helm and Thompson[87] in 1958.

More recent series[88–92] suggest that the operative mortality rate may be as low as 1% today in the surgical treatment of segmental and even multisegmental bronchiectasis. Although this reduction in mortality reflects better surgical techniques in some instances, the major reason for the improvement is that surgery is limited primarily to patients with local disease that has not responded to antibiotics. This limitation presumably accounts for reports of a greater reduction in symptoms in some patients managed surgically rather than medically. Nevertheless, a 1982 study by Annest and colleagues,[93] who compared groups of patients who met similar surgical criteria but did or did not undergo surgery because of physician preference or patient refusal of operation, suggested that the quality of life, as measured by the presence of persistent symptoms and the need for further medical attention, was superior in those patients treated with surgical resection; survival, however, was not improved.

A prospective, randomized trial comparing surgical and medical approaches to bronchiectasis never will be performed in the United States or other developed nations, where most patients have generalized bronchiectasis related to systemic disorders. Even in countries like Nigeria, where postinfectious bronchiectasis is more common, most bronchiectatic patients are managed medically rather than surgically.[35] Experience throughout the world justifies this approach and suggests that surgical resection should be reserved for patients who have focal abnormalities, are unwilling or unable to take antimicrobial agents, or present with life-threatening hemoptysis.

Although surgery remains the treatment of choice when hemoptysis is massive and a bleeding site has been identified or is strongly suspected, newer techniques provide a less invasive alternative in most cases. Such techniques include endobronchial bronchoscopic tamponade with a Fogarty balloon[94] and especially bronchial artery angiography and embolization with resorbable material.[95–97] Although inadvertent obstruction of the spinal arteries and subsequent neurologic deficits may occur with bronchial arteriography and embolization, this procedure is not unduly hazardous and has all but replaced surgery at some institutions.

In passing, it should be mentioned that double-lung and heart-lung transplantation has emerged as definitive treatment for patients with severe generalized bronchiectasis, most notably that related to cystic fibrosis.[98, 99] Generally, transplantation is considered about 2 years before operation in the United States, due to the scarcity of suitable donor organs and the need to prepare the potential recipient and start a rehabilitation program. Recognizing the usefulness of being able to predict the risk of death in patients with cystic fibrosis before transplantation, Kerem and colleagues[100] reviewed pulmonary function data and arterial blood gas levels in a cohort of 673 patients with cystic fibrosis monitored at their institution between 1977 and 1989. These investigators found that the relative risk of death of these patients within 2 years was 2.0 for each 10% decrement in the $FEV_1$ below the predicted value. They concluded that patients with cystic fibrosis should be considered for lung transplantation when the $FEV_1$ falls to less than 30% of the predicted value and that female and younger patients may need to be considered at an even earlier stage.

## PROGNOSIS

As noted previously, the prognosis for patients with bronchiectasis in the preantibiotic era was assumed to be dismal by most investigators. The 12-year study of 400 patients at the Massachusetts General Hospital, reported by Perry and King[7] in 1940, revealed a 26% mortality rate for patients treated nonsurgically. Only 15% of the patients lived 20 years or longer, and their lives were characterized by progressive decline in health and comfort punctuated by bleeding and acute infectious episodes. Perry and King[7] concluded that patients who developed bronchiectasis before the age of 10 years were unlikely to see their 40th birthday. By the 1960s, Field[43, 44] could report that deterioration was no longer inevitable and many patients stabilized, thanks to the advent of antibiotics. In 1981, Ellis and associates[101] described 116 patients whose bronchiectasis had been diagnosed at least 5 years previously, only 22 of whom had died. A full 77% of the survivors had missed less than 2 weeks of work annually from chest illness, and only 7% of the patients were considered disabled.

## PREVENTION

Of course, the prognosis for patients with bronchiectasis would not be a topic for discussion if the process could be prevented. Prevention involves the administration of vaccines against measles, pertussis, influenza, and other infections that may predispose to bronchiectasis. It includes prompt removal of foreign bodies and obstructing lesions in the airways and aggressive use of antibiotics for bacterial bronchopulmonary infections. And it requires further research into the systemic disorders associated with bronchiectasis in many patients.

## ASSOCIATED CONDITIONS

As stressed throughout this chapter, bronchiectasis often occurs in association with systemic diseases and other conditions (Table 41.1). These conditions are reviewed in the following section in alphabetic order. For further information on cystic fibrosis, see Chapter 40; for bronchopulmonary sequestration, see Chapter 53.

### Allergic Bronchopulmonary Aspergillosis

Allergic bronchopulmonary aspergillosis is characterized by bronchospasm, bronchiectasis, respiratory secretions containing *Aspergillus* species, and immunologic evidence of allergy to this antigen. The first three cases of allergic bronchopulmonary aspergillosis involving *Aspergillus fumigatus* were described in Great Britain by Hinson and coworkers[102] in 1952. Pepys and coworkers,[103] Campbell and Clayton,[104] Scadding,[105] and Henderson and associates[106] reported similar cases and noted the striking prevalence of this condition among asthmatic patients admitted to British hospitals.

Patterson and Golbert[107] in 1968, and Slavin and colleagues[108] 1 year later, described the first American patients with allergic bronchopulmonary aspergillosis. Today, the disease is still reported less often in the United States than in Great Britain, but it is far from rare.[109] It has also been associated with *Aspergillus* species other than *A. fumigatus* and with fungi other than *Aspergillus*.[110]

The pathophysiology of allergic bronchopulmonary aspergillosis involves a hypersensitivity reaction to the pres-

**Table 41.1 CONDITIONS ASSOCIATED WITH BRONCHIECTASIS**

| |
|---|
| Allergic bronchopulmonary aspergillosis |
| $Alpha_1$-antitrypsin deficiency |
| Bronchial obstruction (including middle lobe syndrome) |
| Bronchopulmonary sequestration |
| Congenital cartilage deficiency (Williams-Campbell syndrome) |
| Cystic fibrosis |
| Human immunodeficiency virus infection |
| Immunodeficiency |
| Infection |
| Inflammation |
| Other associated conditions |
| Primary ciliary dyskinesia |
| Rheumatoid arthritis |
| Tracheobronchomegaly (Mounier-Kuhn syndrome) |
| Unilateral hyperlucent lung (Swyer-James-MacLeod syndrome) |
| Yellow nail syndrome |

ence of inhaled antigen in the tracheobronchial tree. The bronchiectasis that occurs is assumed to result from airway plugging by viscid secretions containing *Aspergillus* hyphae. Tissue invasion is thought not to occur, differentiating this condition from the invasive form of aspergillosis that is encountered in severely immunocompromised hosts. The allergic process seems to include both type I (immediate) and type III (Arthus-type) reactions, as reflected in immediate and late skin reactivity and the presence of increased serum levels of IgG and IgE.[110a] Type IV (delayed) hypersensitivity has also been implicated.[111]

Elevated IgE concentrations, peripheral blood eosinophilia, precipitating antibodies against *Aspergillus* or other antigens, a history of asthma, central bronchiectasis, and characteristic chest roentgenographic patterns are required to confirm the diagnosis of allergic bronchopulmonary aspergillosis, according to Rosenberg and associates.[112, 113] Scadding[105] believed that the finding of saccular proximal bronchiectasis of the upper lobes was pathognomonic of allergic bronchopulmonary aspergillosis, but this pattern is not seen in all cases, and it exists in patients with bronchiectasis due to other causes. A variety of linear shadows, transient or peribronchial haziness, focal or platelike atelectasis, and patchy or massive consolidation also have been reported. In addition, the chest roentgenogram may be normal in some patients.[114] Further information about allergic bronchopulmonary aspergillosis, including its treatment, is available in Chapter 61.

Closely related to allergic bronchopulmonary aspergillosis are two other conditions also described in asthmatic patients: *mucoid impaction* of the bronchus and *bronchocentric granulomatosis*. Mucoid impaction is associated with proximal bronchial dilation and distention with thick secretions.[115] *Aspergillus* or other sporulating fungi frequently are present in these secretions, and a focal angiitis may be observed. Bronchocentric granulomatosis is characterized by necrotic granulomas consisting of lymphocytes, plasma cells, eosinophils, and epithelioid cells within the conducting airways. This process often extends into the surrounding lung parenchyma and pulmonary arteries, causing a vasculitis that is secondary to the bronchocentric lesion.[116] Peripheral blood eosinophilia is common among patients with bronchocentric granulomatosis; precipitins to *Aspergillus* may be identified, and fungi are frequently found in resected tissue.

Mucoid impaction may occur in patients without exposure to *Aspergillus.* Bronchocentric granulomatosis may also exist in patients without such exposure and has even been reported in nonasthmatics. Furthermore, neither mucoid impaction nor bronchocentric granulomatosis has been reported in a majority of patients with allergic bronchopulmonary aspergillosis. Nevertheless, the similarities among these three conditions and their coexistence in some patients has led Katzenstein and colleagues[117] to regard them as alternative expressions of hypersensitivity to *Aspergillus* and other fungi.

## Alpha$_1$-Antitrypsin Deficiency

Emphysema is the most widely appreciated pulmonary manifestation of deficiency of alpha$_1$-antitrypsin, the major protease inhibitor in serum. Nevertheless, bronchiectasis was present in two of the five patients with alpha$_1$-antitrypsin deficiency first described by Laurell and Eriksson[118] in 1963. Other investigators have noted a similar association,[119–122] and a CT study[123] of patients with this deficiency suggested that bronchiectasis may be more common among such patients than previously realized.

The pathogenesis of bronchiectasis in patients with protease inhibitor deficiency has not been resolved. Alpha$_1$-antitrypsin inhibits several proteolytic enzymes, any of which may injure the lungs. It is possible that the protease inhibitor capacity of serum protects the lungs during infection and other inflammatory states, when proteases are likely to be present, and that the parenchyma and airways become more susceptible to destruction when this protective capacity is lacking.

## Bronchial Obstruction

Granted that bronchiectasis is the end result of several diseases, investigators once assumed that a common pathogenic factor was proximal airway obstruction with distal infection of the bronchial walls and (in many cases) the surrounding lung parenchyma. Although this assumption proved to be incorrect, focal postobstructive bronchiectasis may indeed occur in patients with endobronchial tumors, broncholithiasis,[124] bronchial stenosis from inflammatory disorders such as tuberculosis, and aspirated foreign bodies such as coins, nuts, and timothy grass heads.[125, 126] It also may occur as part of the *middle lobe syndrome*.

Bronchiectasis and chronic bacterial pneumonia of the right middle lobe was first designated as a syndrome by Graham and coworkers[127] in 1948. This syndrome presumably results from the angulation of the lobar bronchus at its origin, impingement on the right middle lobe bronchus by enlarged lymph nodes, and a lack of collateral ventilation to that lobe.[127–129] Although some patients with the middle lobe syndrome are symptomatic, the condition is frequently detected on a plain chest roentgenogram taken for other purposes.

## Bronchopulmonary Sequestration

Sequestrations of the lung involve maldeveloped portions of lung tissue and abnormal arteries that usually arise from the aorta and supply the sequestered areas. The sequestrations presumably originate from accessory bronchial buds and are enveloped either within (intralobar) or without (extralobar) normally aerated lung tissue.[130] Sequestrations appear roentgenographically as masses or polycystic shadows, often in the posterior basal segments of the lower lobes.[131] They frequently contain dilated bronchial elements in addition to other normal or abnormal bronchoalveolar structures. Infection of these structures may lead to further bronchiectatic changes. The diagnosis and management of bronchopulmonary sequestration is described in Chapter 53.

## Congenital Cartilage Deficiency

Williams and Campbell[132] in 1960 first described five patients who developed recurrent bronchopulmonary infections, chronic cough and sputum production, fever, and failure to thrive in infancy. The segmental bronchi of these patients were normal on bronchoscopic examination, but bronchography revealed that the second and third bronchial divisions were dilated and either devoid of cartilage or invested only with discontinuous cartilaginous plaques. The involved areas expanded and narrowed with inspiration and expiration, and the distal bronchi resembled a series of elongated balloons that were being inflated and deflated.

Although concurrent infection frequently was present in the patients, Williams and Campbell[132] believed that their bronchiectasis was developmental because of the symmetry of the lesions and the lack of inflammation in adjacent noncartilaginous structures. This opinion was accepted by other investigators, who labeled this condition the Williams-Campbell syndrome.[133, 134] The congenital aspect of the syndrome is reflected in a more recent report of two siblings with similar roentgenographic findings who developed respiratory symptoms immediately after birth.[135]

## Cystic Fibrosis

Cystic fibrosis (see also Chapter 40) is the most common lethal genetic syndrome involving white children and a frequent cause of chronic pulmonary disease in childhood.[136] It occurs in approximately 2 of every 2000 Caucasians and 1 in 17,000 blacks in the United States. Cystic fibrosis is transmitted in an autosomal recessive pattern; approximately 5% of most white populations are carriers of the cystic fibrosis gene. The isolation of this gene, which is located on chromosome 7, was first reported in 1989 by Rommens and colleagues[137] and Riordan and associates.[138] The gene is predicted to encode a 1480-amino-acid protein termed the *cystic fibrosis conductance regulator.* The most common mutation of the gene, $\Delta F_{508}$, causes the omission of a phenylalinine residue as the regulator.[139] The variable clinical course in patients with cystic fibrosis can be attributed at least in part to specific genotypes at the locus of the cystic fibrosis gene.[140]

Patients with cystic fibrosis are thought to have morphologically normal lungs at birth. Nevertheless, as noted earlier, inflammation and infection soon appear. In childhood, patients with cystic fibrosis manifest dilation and hypertrophy of bronchial glands, goblet cell hyperplasia, excessive mucous secretions, and impaired mucus transport, all of which lead to plugging of the proximal airways and subsequent bronchiectasis.[141, 142]

Humoral immune function has been assumed to be normal in patients with cystic fibrosis. However, Matthews and colleagues[143] detected hypogammaglobulinemia in 22% of 157 patients younger than 10 years old. Elevated serum IgG concentrations were observed in 7% of these patients, in 25% of patients 10 to 20 years old, and in 47% of patients 20 years of age or older. In this study, the patients with hypogammaglobulinemia had less severe lung disease, as defined by clinical and roentgenographic criteria, than age-matched patients with cystic fibrosis and either normal or increased IgG levels. This finding suggests that the progression of lung disease in cystic fibrosis might be a hyperimmune response.

## Human Immunodeficiency Virus Infection

The most frequently diagnosed respiratory diseases in a large cohort of patients in the prospective Pulmonary Complications of Human Immunodeficiency Virus (HIV) Infection Study[144] were upper respiratory tract infection, acute bronchitis, acute sinusitis, bacterial pneumonia, and *Pneumocystis carinii* pneumonia. However, HIV-positive patients were not screened for bronchiectasis by CT scanning in this study, and the prevalence of that condition among such patients had not been appreciated before the study was begun. Holmes and colleagues[145] in 1992, and Verghese and associates[146] in 1994, reported small series of HIV-infected patients with bronchiectasis, raising the possibility that bronchiectasis was common among patients with HIV disease.

Sheikh and associates[147] subsequently diagnosed bronchiectasis by chest roentgenogram in as many as 26 of 164 children with the acquired immunodeficiency syndrome (AIDS) seen at the Children's Medical Center of Brooklyn between 1984 and 1996; most of these patients had CD4-positive T-lymphocyte counts of less than 100 cells/μL. King and coworkers[148] detected CT evidence of bronchiectasis in 18 of 50 HIV-positive subjects, all of whom had significantly higher bronchoalveolar lavage fluid neutrophil counts than did subjects with normal bronchi on CT. This study suggests that bronchiectasis in HIV-positive subjects may reflect ongoing infection with bacteria and other organisms, including possibly *P. carinii.* The many other pulmonary complications of HIV infection are described in Chapter 82.

## Immunodeficiency

Bronchiectasis and other chronic or recurrent sinopulmonary infections are common among patients with congenital or acquired immunodeficiency. Abnormalities of B-lymphocyte functions are most frequently associated with bronchiectasis. Congenital or acquired hypogammaglobulinemia characterized by a decrease or absence of circulating IgG has been described in several patients with bronchiectasis.[149–152] Perhaps even more commonly associated with bronchiectasis are immunodeficiency states involving one or more of the four IgG subclasses in the presence of normal total IgG levels. In this regard, Beck and Heiner[153] described five patients with isolated absence of immunoglobulin subclass $IgG_4$ and recurrent severe sinopulmonary infections. Similarly, Umetsu and coworkers[154] reported 20 patients with $IgG_2$, $IgG_3$, or combined $IgG_2$ and $IgG_3$ deficiency who manifested recurrent infections and impaired antibody response to bacterial capsular polysaccharide antigen.

De Gracia and associates[155] studied 65 patients with bronchiectasis of unknown origin and determined that 31 had low serum concentration of one or more IgG subclasses. This study indicated that IgG subclass deficiencies are a common cause of bronchiectasis and that serum subclass levels should be assessed whenever other causes of bronchiectasis have been ruled out. Although bronchiectasis previously has been reported in patients with selective IgA deficiency, some of whom had normal IgG subclass levels,[156, 157] it is possible that the sinopulmonary infections associated with selective IgA deficiency in some series were actually caused by undetected IgG subclass deficiencies.[158]

## Infection

Previously in the developed nations and currently in resource-poor countries, bronchiectasis may occur as a result of necrotizing pulmonary infections that are poorly treated or left untreated. Rosensweig and Stead[24] first drew attention to bronchiectasis occurring after bronchopulmonary necrosis due to *Klebsiella, S. aureus,* other aerobic bacteria, or *Mycobacterium tuberculosis.* Since that time, bronchiectasis has been reported in patients with pulmonary disease caused by nontuberculous mycobacteria[159] or by aerobic bacteria such as *Mycoplasma pneumoniae.*[160, 161] Bronchiectasis may also result from anaerobic lung infections, and it may be encountered as a complication of measles, pertussis, influenza, or adenovirus type 7 infection.[162] The potential importance of antecedent viral infection in the pathogenesis of bronchiectasis was underscored by the finding by Carson and associates[163] of acquired ciliary defects in the nasal epithelium of children with viral upper respiratory infections.

## Inflammation

Bronchiectasis has been reported in patients with ammonia burns of the respiratory tract[164] and after gastric acid aspiration in which bronchopulmonary infection probably occurred. Two such patients aspirated gastric acid as a result of heroin intoxication.[165, 166] Bronchiectasis also may occur after exposure to paraquat[167] or sulfur mustard gas.[168]

## Other Associated Conditions

In addition to its association with conditions previously discussed, bronchiectasis has been reported in patients with a wide range of diseases, including Ehlers-Danlos syndrome,[169] Marfan's syndrome,[170] peripheral neuropathy,[171] and ulcerative colitis.[172] Finally, bronchiectasis has been detected by HRCT in patients after heart-lung transplantation, in whom it may be a sign of chronic lung allograft rejection.[173]

## Primary Ciliary Dyskinesia

The triad of situs inversus totalis, bronchiectasis, and either nasal polyps or recurrent sinusitis has carried Kartagener's name since he reported on three patients with these findings in 1933[174] and seven more in 1935.[175] Other patients with Kartagener's triad were subsequently described,[176] as were patients without the complete syndrome.[177] Kartagener and Stucki[178] argued that the syndrome was congenital, noting that situs inversus was detected during mass roentgenographic screening in Norway in only 1 of every 10,000 persons; 25% of those with situs inversus also had bronchiectasis or all three components of the triad. Similarly, Katsuhara and coworkers[179] observed that bronchiectasis occurred in at least 25% of patients with situs inversus but in only about 0.5% of the general population throughout the world. In subsequent years, numerous investigators[180–183] offered various explanations for the association between the two conditions.

In 1975, Afzelius and colleagues[184] noted a lack of inner and outer dynein arms on electron microscopic examination of immotile human spermatozoa. This group subsequently reported the presence of nonfunctioning cilia and impaired mucociliary transport in the tracheobronchial tract of two patients with Kartagener's syndrome and speculated that the syndrome might be caused by ciliary dysfunction.[185] In 1976, Afzelius[186] noted a lack of dynein arms in the sperm and cilia of four subjects; three subjects had Kartagener's syndrome, and the fourth was a brother of one of them. In this report, Afzelius suggested that situs inversus is caused by a deficiency of motile cilia at a particular embryonic stage in which ciliary beating normally causes a rotation of presumptive organ tissue. In 1977, Eliasson and associates[187] proposed that what they called the "immotile cilia syndrome" is responsible for chronic airway infections and male sterility in a wide variety of persons.

Since these original reports, the term *immotile cilia syndrome* has been applied to many patients with or without Kartagener's syndrome.[188–193] In recent years, however, it has been replaced by the term *primary ciliary dyskinesia.* This replacement reflects the finding that the cilia of many patients do move, albeit in an uncoordinated fashion, and that ciliary disorientation alone can cause primary ciliary dyskinesia.[194, 195] Primary ciliary dyskinesia is believed to be an autosomal recessive disorder that affects between 1 in 15,000 and 1 in 30,000 persons. The genetic link between ciliary dyskinesia and situs inversus, which occurs in approximately 50% of patients with the disorder, still is not clear.

## Rheumatoid Arthritis

The most common pulmonary manifestations of rheumatoid arthritis are pleuritis with or without pleural effusions, rheumatoid nodules, obliterative bronchiolitis, diffuse interstitial pneumonitis, and pulmonary vasculitis.[196] Bronchiectasis also has been reported in patients with rheumatoid arthritis, but it has been thought to be rare. Nevertheless, Shadick and associates[197] identified 23 patients with rheumatoid arthritis and bronchiectasis among a cohort of 4000 patients with rheumatoid arthritis at the Brigham and Women's Hospital in Boston between 1984 and 1991, 18 of whom had arthritis preceding lung disease.

The prevalence of bronchiectasis of 0.6% among the patients with rheumatoid arthritis in Boston is even greater than the prevalence of 0.4% in the Native American population in Alaska, suggesting more than a chance association between the two diseases. Other studies[198–200] based on HRCT findings support this suggestion. Whether bronchiectasis results from subclinical infection or inflammation related to obstructive bronchiectasis in patients with rheumatoid arthritis is unclear.

### Tracheobronchomegaly

First described in 1932 by Mounier-Kuhn,[201] tracheobronchomegaly is characterized by a striking dilation of the intrathoracic trachea and major bronchi. Enlargement of the airways and the deep corrugations produced by redundant musculomembranous tissues between the cartilaginous rings gives a roentgenographic appearance of multiple diverticula. Katz and associates[202] found the mean tracheal diameter to be greater than 31 mm, the right main-stem bronchial diameter to be greater than 24 mm, and the left main-stem bronchial diameter to be greater than 23 mm in five patients with the Mounier-Kuhn syndrome, compared with mean diameters of 20, 16, and 15 mm, respectively, in normal adults.

The cause of tracheobronchomegaly is unknown; although it has been attributed to severe, chronic bronchopulmonary suppuration, the latter condition may be a result of tracheobronchomegaly rather than its cause. Enlargement of the cartilaginous tracheal rings as well as the membranous trachea supports a congenital cause, as does one report of familial occurrence.[203] A study by Roditi and Weir[204] using HRCT suggested that tracheomegaly is a frequent finding in patients with bronchiectasis, although it did not determine whether tracheomegaly was the result of bronchiectasis or the cause.

### Unilateral Hyperlucent Lung

Swyer and James[205] and later MacLeod[206] originally described "unilateral lung transradiancy" on the chest roentgenograms of 10 patients in the 1950s. Although these patients were initially thought to manifest emphysema secondary to bronchial obstruction, such obstruction was not demonstrated by bronchoscopy or bronchography. However, cystic abnormalities were noted in the proximal bronchi. These abnormalities presumably related to antecedent bronchopulmonary infections during infancy. Today, such infections are thought to cause hypoplasia of lung parenchyma and the pulmonary artery on the involved side.

### Yellow Nail Syndrome

Samman and White[207] coined the term *yellow nail syndrome* in 1964 to describe the association of yellow discoloration of the fingernails and lymphedema. Since then, some but not all patients with these findings have also been reported to have pleural effusions and bronchiectasis. The bronchiectasis has been attributed either to hypoplasia of the lymphatic system with altered lung drainage or to immunologic deficiencies that were demonstrated in certain patients.[208] Of the 12 patients with various manifestations of the yellow nail syndrome described by Hiller and colleagues,[209] three of the five with bronchographically confirmed bronchiectasis also had chronic sinusitis, suggesting the possibility of underlying mucociliary dysfunction.

## SUMMARY

In industrialized nations, bronchiectasis is neither as common nor as devastating a condition as it once was, although in low-income countries it remains an important public health problem. In countries such as the United States, the pathologic process called bronchiectasis usually occurs in patients with underlying systemic disorders on which airway infection is superimposed. Primary ciliary dyskinesia, cystic fibrosis, allergic bronchopulmonary aspergillosis, immunodeficiency, and HIV infection are the most important of these disorders. Further elucidation of their pathogenesis should help decrease the incidence of bronchiectasis even further in Western society.

Bronchiectasis in patients with underlying disorders can usually be diagnosed with little difficulty, particularly with the use of HRCT. Identification of bronchiectasis also may provide clues as to the presence of a systemic disease that has not yet been diagnosed. In such circumstances, and when bronchiectasis is related to obstruction or previously untreated infection, it usually improves with the administration of antibiotics in concert with therapy aimed at the underlying condition when appropriate. Surgery is rarely indicated for bronchiectasis; it should be limited to patients with massive hemoptysis who do not respond to bronchial artery embolization and patients with local disease that is unresponsive to antibiotics.

## References

1. Baum GL, Herschko EP: Bronchiectasis. *In* Baum GL, Wolinsky E (eds): Textbook of Pulmonary Medicine (3rd ed). Boston: Little Brown, 1983, pp 615–634.
2. Lander FPL: Bronchiectasis and atelectasis: Temporary and permanent changes. Thorax 1:198–210, 1946.
3. Pontius JR, Jacobs LG: The reversal of advanced bronchiectasis. Radiology 68:204–207, 1957.
4. Fraser RG, Macklem PT, Brown WG: Airway dynamics in bronchiectasis: A combined cinefluorographic-manometric study. AJR Am J Roentgenol 93:821–835, 1965.
5. Heard BE, Khatchatourov V, Otto H, et al: The morphology of emphysema, chronic bronchitis, and bronchiectasis: Definition, nomenclature, and classification. J Clin Pathol 32:882–892, 1979.

5a. Mysliwiec V, Pina JS: Bronchiectasis: The "other" obstructive lung disease. Postgrad Med 106:123–126, 1999.

6. Moll HH: A clinical and pathological study of bronchiectasis. Q J Med 25:457–469, 1932.
7. Perry K, King D: Bronchiectasis: A study of prognosis based on a follow-up of 400 patients. Am Rev Tuberc 41:531–548, 1940.
8. Reid LM: Reduction in bronchial subdivision in bronchiectasis. Thorax 5:233–247, 1950.
9. Schuster A, Ueki I, Nadel JA: Neutrophil elastase stimulates tracheal submucosal gland secretion that is inhibited by ICI 200,355. Am J Physiol 262:L86–L91, 1992.
10. Sommerhoff CP, Nadel JA, Basbaum CB, et al: Neutrophil elastase and cathepsin G stimulate secretion from cultured bovine airway gland serous cells. J Clin Invest 85:682–689, 1990.
11. Owen CA, Campbell EJ, Hill SL, et al: Increased adherence of monocytes to fibronectin in bronchiectasis. Am Rev Respir Dis 145:626–631, 1992.
12. Sepper R, Konttinen YT, Ding Y, et al: Human neutrophil collagenase (MMP-8), identified in bronchiectasis BAL fluid, correlates with severity of disease. Chest 107:1641–1647, 1995.
13. Power C, O'Connor CM, Macfarlane D, et al: Neutrophil collagenase in sputum from patients with cystic fibrosis. Am J Respir Crit Care Med 150:818–822, 1994.
14. Fahy JV, Schuster A, Ueki I, et al: Mucus hypersecretion in bronchiectasis: The role of neutrophil proteases. Am Rev Respir Dis 146:1430–1433, 1992.

15. Richman-Eisenstat JBY, Jorens PG, Hébert CA, et al: Interleukin-8: An important chemoattractant in sputum of patients with chronic inflammatory airway diseases. Am J Physiol 264:L413–L418, 1993.
16. Mikami M, Llewellyn-Jones CG, Bayley D, et al: The chemotactic activity of sputum from patients with bronchiectasis. Am J Respir Crit Care Med 157:723–728, 1998.
17. Kharitonov SA, Wells AU, O'Connor BJ, et al: Elevated levels of exhaled nitric oxide in bronchiectasis. Am J Respir Crit Care Med 151:1889–1893, 1995.
18. Meyer KC, Sharma A, Rosenthal NS, et al: Regional variability of lung inflammation in cystic fibrosis. Am J Respir Crit Care Med 156:1536–1540, 1997.
19. Konstan MW, Hilliard KA, Norvell TM, et al: Bronchoalveolar lavage findings in cystic fibrosis patients with stable, clinically mild lung disease suggest ongoing infection and inflammation. Am J Respir Crit Care Med 150:448–454, 1994.
20. Khan TZ, Wagener JS, Bost T, et al: Early pulmonary inflammation in infants with cystic fibrosis. Am J Respir Crit Care Med 151:1075–1082, 1995.
21. Russell KJ, McRedmond J, Mukherji N, et al: Neutrophil adhesion molecule surface expression and responsiveness in cystic fibrosis. Am J Respir Crit Care Med 157:756–761, 1998.
22. Spencer HP: Pathology of the Lung (2nd ed). Oxford: Pergamon Press, 1968, pp 132–151.
23. Jaffe HJ, Katz S: Current ideas about bronchiectasis. Am Fam Physician 7:69–76, 1973.
24. Rosenzweig DY, Stead WW: The role of tuberculosis and other forms of bronchopulmonary necrosis in the pathogenesis of bronchiectasis. Am Rev Respir Dis 93:769–785, 1966.
25. Lee PH, Carr DH, Rubens MB, et al: Accuracy of CT in predicting the cause of bronchiectasis. Clin Radiol 50:839–841, 1995.
26. Barker AF, Bardana EJ: Bronchiectasis: Update of an orphan disease. Am Rev Respir Dis 137:969–978, 1988.
27. Lourenco RV, Loddenkemper R, Carton RW: Patterns of distribution and clearance of aerosols in patients with bronchiectasis. Am Rev Respir Dis 106:857–866, 1972.
28. Currie DC, Pavia D, Agnew JE, et al: Impaired tracheobronchial clearance in bronchiectasis. Thorax 42:126–130, 1987.
29. Regnis JA, Robinson M, Bailey DL, et al: Mucociliary clearance in patients with cystic fibrosis and in normal subjects. Am J Respir Crit Care Med 150:66–71, 1994.
30. Deneuville E, Perrot-Minot C, Pennaforte F, et al: Revisited physicochemical and transport properties of respiratory mucus in genotyped cystic fibrosis patients. Am J Respir Crit Care Med 156:166–172, 1997.
31. Liebow AA, Hales MR, Lindskog GE: Enlargement of the bronchial arteries and their anastomoses with the pulmonary arteries in bronchiectasis. Am J Pathol 25:211–231, 1949.
32. Tadavarthy SM, Klugman J, Castaneda-Zuniga WR, et al: Systemic-to-pulmonary collaterals in pathological states. Radiology 144:55–59, 1982.
33. Fleshman MD, Wilson JF, Cohen JJ: Bronchiectasis in Alaska native children. Arch Environ Health 17:517–523, 1968.
34. Baum GL, Racz I, Bubis JJ, et al: Cystic disease of the lung: Report of eighty-eight cases, with an ethnologic relationship. Am J Med 40:578–602, 1966.
35. Adebonojo SA, Grillo IA, Osinowo O, et al: Suppurative diseases of the lung and pleura: A continuing challenge in developing countries. Ann Thorac Surg 33:40–47, 1982.
36. Cherniack N, Vosti KL, Saxton GA, et al: Pulmonary function tests in fifty patients with bronchiectasis. J Lab Clin Med 53:693–707, 1959.
37. Bass H, Henderson JAM, Heckscher T, et al: Regional structure and function in bronchiectasis: A correlative study using bronchography and Xe. Am Rev Respir Dis 97:598–609, 1968.
38. Nichols D, Dopico GA, Braun S, et al: Acute and chronic pulmonary function changes in allergic bronchopulmonary aspergillosis. Am J Med 67:631–637, 1979.
39. Fraser RG, Pare JAP: Diagnoses of Diseases of the Chest (2nd ed). Philadelphia: WB Saunders, 1979, pp 1443–1455.
40. Konietzko NFJ, Carton RW, Leroy EP: Causes of death in patients with bronchiectasis. Am Rev Respir Dis 100:852–858, 1969.
41. Ellis DA, Thornley PE, Wightman AJ, et al: Present outlook in bronchiectasis: Clinical and social study and review of factors influencing prognosis. Thorax 36:659–664, 1981.
42 Field CE: Bronchiectasis in childhood. Pediatrics 4:21–47, 231–254, 355–372, 1949.
43. Field CE: Bronchiectasis. A long-term follow-up of medical and surgical cases from childhood. Arch Dis Child 36:587–603, 1961.
44. Field CE: Bronchiectasis. Third report on a follow-up study of medical and surgical cases from childhood. Arch Dis Child 44:551–561, 1969.
45. Bradshaw HH, Putrey FJ, Clerf CH: The fate of patients with untreated bronchiectasis. JAMA 116:2561–2563, 1941.
46. Rivera M, Nicotra MB: *Pseudomonas aeruginosa*-mucoid strain: Its significance in adult chest diseases. Am Rev Respir Dis 126:833–836, 1982.
47. Pang JA, Cheng A, Chan HS, et al: The bacteriology of bronchiectasis in Hong Kong investigated by protected catheter brush and bronchoalveolar lavage. Am Rev Respir Dis 139:14–17, 1989.
48. Steinbach S, Sun L, Jiang R-Z, et al: Transmissibility of *Pseudomonas cepacia* infection in clinic patients and lung-transplant recipients with cystic fibrosis. N Engl J Med 331:981–987, 1994.
49. Klingman KL, Pye A, Murphy TF, et al: Dynamics of respiratory tract colonization by *Branhamella catarrhalis* in bronchiectasis. Am J Respir Crit Care Med 152:1072–1078, 1995.
50. McCarthy DS, Simon G, Hargreave FE: The radiological appearances in allergic broncho-pulmonary aspergillosis. Clin Radiol 21:366–375, 1970.
51. Greene KE, Takasugi JE, Godwin JD, et al: Radiographic changes in acute exacerbations of cystic fibrosis in adults: A pilot study. AJR Am J Roentgenol 163:557–562, 1994.
51a. Lynch DA, Newell J, Hale V, et al: Correlation of CT findings with clinical evaluations in 261 patients with symptomatic bronchiectasis. AJR Am J Roentgenol 173:53–58, 1999.
52. Muller NL, Bergin CJ, Ostrow DN, et al: Role of computed tomography in the recognition of bronchiectasis. AJR Am J Roentgenol 143:971–976, 1984.
53. Cooke JC, Currie DC, Morgan AD, et al: Role of computed tomography in diagnosis of bronchiectasis. Thorax 42:272–277, 1987.
54. Grenier P, Maurice F, Musset D, et al: Bronchiectasis: Assessment by thin-section CT. Radiology 161:95–99, 1986.
55. Naidich DP, McCauley DI, Khouri NF, et al: Computed tomography of bronchiectasis. J Comput Assist Tomogr 6:437–44, 1982.
56. Webb WR: Radiology of obstructive pulmonary disease. AJR Am J Roentgenol 169:637–647, 1997.
57. Shah RM, Sexauer W, Ostrum BJ, et al: High-resolution CT in the acute exacerbation of cystic fibrosis: Evaluation of acute findings, reversibility of those findings, and clinical correlation. AJR Am J Roentgenol 169:375–380, 1997.
58. Miszkiel K, Wells AU, Rubens MB, et al: Effects of airway infection by *Pseudomonas aeruginosa*: A computed tomographic study. Thorax 52:260–264, 1997.
59. Reiff DB, Wells AU, Carr DH, et al: CT findings in bronchiectasis: Limited value in distinguishing between idiopathic and specific types. AJR Am J Roentgenol 165:261–267, 1995.
59a. Cartier Y, Havanagh PV, Johkoh T, et al: Bronchiectasis: Accuracy of high-resolution CT in the differentiation of specific diseases. AJR Am J Roentgenol 173:47–52, 1999.
60. Lucidarme O, Grenier P, Coche E, et al: Bronchiectasis: Comparative assessment with thin-section CT and helical CT. Radiology 200:673–679, 1996.
61. Carr DH, Oades P, Trotman-Dickenson B, et al: Magnetic resonance scanning in cystic fibrosis: Comparison with computed tomography. Clin Radiol 50:84–89, 1995.
62. Baughman RP, Keeton DA, Perez C, et al: Use of bronchoalveolar lavage semiquantitative cultures in cystic fibrosis. Am J Respir Crit Care Med 156:286–291, 1997.
63. Stern RC: The diagnosis of cystic fibrosis. N Engl J Med 336:487–491, 1997.
64. Ramsey BW: Management of pulmonary disease in patients with cystic fibrosis. N Engl J Med 335:179–188, 1996.
65. Lin H-C, Cheng H-F, Wang C-H, et al: Inhaled gentamicin reduces airway neutrophil activity and mucus secretion in bronchiectasis. Am J Respir Crit Care Med 155:2024–2029, 1997.

66. Ramsey BW, Dorkin HL, Eisenberg JD, et al: Efficacy of aerosolized tobramycin in patients with cystic fibrosis. N Engl J Med 328:1740–1746, 1993.
67. Mortensen J, Falk M, Groth S, et al: The effects of postural drainage and positive expiratory pressure physiotherapy on tracheobronchial clearance in cystic fibrosis. Chest 100:1350–1357, 1991.
68. Thomas J, Cook DJ, Brooks D: Chest physical therapy management of patients with cystic fibrosis. Am J Respir Crit Care Med 151:846–850, 1995.
69. Knowles MR, Church NL, Waltner WE, et al: A pilot study of aerosolized amiloride for the treatment of lung disease in cystic fibrosis. N Engl J Med 322:1189–1194, 1990.
70. Robinson M, Regnis JA, Bailey DL, et al: Effect of hypertonic saline, amiloride, and cough on mucociliary clearance in patients with cystic fibrosis. Am J Respir Crit Care Med 153:1503–1509, 1996.
71. Wood RE, Wanner A, Hirsch J, et al: Tracheal mucociliary transport in patients with cystic fibrosis and its stimulation by terbutaline. Am Rev Respir Dis 111:733–738, 1975.
72. Hordvik NL, Sammut PH, Judy CG, et al: The effects of albuterol on the lung function of hospitalized patients with cystic fibrosis. Am J Respir Crit Care Med 154:156–160, 1996.
73. Ramsey BW, Astley SJ, Aitken ML, et al: Efficacy and safety of short-term administration of aerosolized recombinant human deoxyribonuclease in patients with cystic fibrosis. Am Rev Respir Dis 148:145–151, 1993.
74. Fuchs HJ, Borowitz DS, Christiansen DH, et al: Effect of aerosolized recombinant human DNase on exacerbations of respiratory symptoms and on pulmonary function in patients with cystic fibrosis. N Engl J Med 331:637–642, 1994.
75. Wills PJ, Wodehouse T, Corkery K, et al: Short-term recombinant human DNAse in bronchiectasis: Effect on clinical state and in vitro sputum transportability. Am J Respir Crit Care Med 154:413–417, 1996.
76. O'Donnell AE, Barker AF, Ilowite JS, et al: Treatment of idiopathic bronchiectasis with aerosolized recombinant human DNase I. Chest 113:1329–1334, 1998.
77. Tamaoki J, Chiyotani A, Kobayashi K, et al: Effect of indomethacin on bronchorrhea in patients with chronic bronchitis, diffuse panbronchiolitis, or bronchiectasis. Am Rev Respir Dis 145:548–552, 1992.
78. Konstan MW, Byard PJ, Hoppel CL, et al: Effect of high-dose ibuprofen in patients with cystic fibrosis. N Engl J Med 332:848–854, 1995.
79. Nocturnal Oxygen Therapy Trial Group: Continuous or nocturnal oxygen therapy in hypoxemic chronic obstructive lung disease. Ann Intern Med 93:391–394, 1980.
80. British Medical Research Council Working Party: Long term domiciliary oxygen therapy in chronic hypoxic cor pulmonale complicating chronic bronchiectasis and emphysema. Lancet 1:681–685, 1981.
81. Marcus CL, Bader D, Stabile MW, et al: Supplemental oxygen and exercise performance in patients with cystic fibrosis with severe pulmonary disease. Chest 101:52–57, 1992.
82. Benhamou D, Muir JF, Raspaud C, et al: Long-term efficiency of home nasal mask ventilation in patients with diffuse bronchiectasis and severe chronic respiratory failure: A case-control study. Chest 112:1259–1266, 1997.
83. Cunningham-Rundles C, Siegal FP, Smithwick EM, et al: Efficacy of intravenous immunoglobulin in primary humoral immunodeficiency disease. Ann Intern Med 101:435–439, 1984.
84. Roifman CM, Lederman HM, Lavi S, et al: Benefit of intravenous IgG replacement in hypogammaglobulinemic patients with chronic sinopulmonary disease. Am J Med 79:171–174, 1985.
85. Knowles MR, Hohneker KW, Zhou Z, et al: A controlled study of adenoviral-vector-mediated gene transfer in the nasal epithelium of patients with cystic fibrosis. N Engl J Med 333:823–831, 1995.
86. Edwards AT: Treatment of bronchiectasis. Med J 1:809–815, 1939.
87. Helm WH, Thompson VC: The long-term results of resection for bronchiectasis. Q J Med 107:353–367, 1958.
88. Sealy WC, Bradham RR, Young WG: The surgical treatment of multisegmental and localized bronchiectasis. Surg Gynecol Obstet 123:80–90, 1966.
89. Sanderson JM, Kennedy MCS, Johnson MF, et al: Bronchiectasis: Results of surgical and conservative management: A review of 393 cases. Thorax 29:407–416, 1974.
90. George SA, Leonardi HK, Overholt RH: Bilateral pulmonary resection for bronchiectasis: A 40-year experience. Ann Thorac Surg 28:48–53, 1979.
91. Wilson JF, Decker AM: The surgical management of childhood bronchiectasis: A review of 96 consecutive pulmonary resections in children with nontuberculous bronchiectasis. Ann Surg 195:354–363, 1982.
92. Smit HJM, Schreurs JM, Van den Bosch JMM, et al: Is resection of bronchiectasis beneficial in patients with primary ciliary dyskinesia? Chest 109:1541–1544, 1996.
93. Annest LS, Kratz JM, Crawford FA: Current results of treatment of bronchiectasis. J Thorac Cardiovasc Surg 83:546–550, 1982.
94. Swersky RB, Chang JB, Wisoff BG, et al: Endobronchial balloon tamponade of hemoptysis in patients with cystic fibrosis. Ann Thorac Surg 27:262–264, 1979.
95. Wholey MH, Chamorro HA, Rao G, et al: Bronchial artery embolization for massive hemoptysis. JAMA 236:2501–2504, 1976.
96. Remy J, Arnaud A, Fardou H, et al: Treatment of hemoptysis by embolization of bronchial arteries. Radiology 122:33–37, 1977.
97. Brinson GM, Noone PG, Mauro MA, et al: Bronchial artery embolization for the treatment of hemoptysis in patients with cystic fibrosis. Am J Respir Crit Care Med 157:1951–1958, 1998.
98. Scott J, Higenbottam T, Hutter J: Heart-lung transplantation for cystic fibrosis. Lancet 2:192–194, 1988.
99. Whitehead B, Helms P, Goodwin M: Heart-lung transplantation for cystic fibrosis: 2. Outcome. Arch Dis Child 66:1022–1026, 1991.
100. Kerem E, Reisman J, Corey M, et al: Prediction of mortality in patients with cystic fibrosis. N Engl J Med 326:1187–1191, 1992
101. Ellis DA, Thornley PE, Wightman AJ, et al: Present outlook in bronchiectasis: Clinical and social study and review of factors influencing prognosis. Thorax 36:659–664, 1981.
102. Hinson KFW, Moon AJ, Plummer NS: Broncho-pulmonary aspergillosis: A review and a report of eight new cases. Thorax 7:317–333, 1952.
103. Pepys J, Riddell RW, Citron KM, et al: Clinical and immunologic significance of *Aspergillus fumigatus* in the sputum. Am Rev Respir Dis 80:167–175, 1959.
104. Campbell MJ, Clayton YM: Bronchopulmonary aspergillosis: A correlation of the clinical and laboratory findings in 272 patients investigated for bronchopulmonary aspergillosis. Am Rev Respir Dis 89:186–196, 1964.
105. Scadding JG: The bronchi in allergic aspergillosis. Scand J Respir Dis 48:372–377, 1967.
106. Henderson AH, English MP, Vecht RJ: Pulmonary aspergillosis: A survey of its occurrence in patients with chronic lung disease and a discussion of the significance of diagnostic tests. Thorax 23:513–518, 1968.
107. Patterson R, Golbert TM: Hypersensitivity disease of the lung. Univ Mich Med Cent J 34:8–12, 1968
108. Slavin RG, Stanczyk DJ, Lonigro AJ, et al: Allergic bronchopulmonary aspergillosis: A North American rarity. Clinical and immunologic characteristics. Am J Med 47:306–313, 1969.
109. Hoehne JH, Reed CE, Dickie HA: Allergic bronchopulmonary aspergillosis is not rare: With a note on preparation of antigen for immunologic tests. Chest 63:177–181, 1973.
110. Ricketti AJ, Greenberger PA, Mintzer RA, et al: Allergic bronchopulmonary aspergillosis. Chest 86:773–778, 1984.
110a. Cockrill BA, Hales CA: Allergic bronchopulmonary aspergillosis. Annu Rev Med 50:303–316, 1999.
111. Wang JLF, Patterson R, Rosenberg M, et al: Serum IgE and IgG antibody activity against *Aspergillus fumigatus* as a diagnostic aid in allergic bronchopulmonary aspergillosis. Am Rev Respir Dis 117:917–927, 1978.
112. Yocum MW, Saltzman AR, Strong DM, et al: Extrinsic allergic alveolitis after *Aspergillus fumigatus* inhalation: Evidence of a type IV immunologic pathogenesis. Am J Med 61:939–944, 1976.
113. Rosenberg M, Patterson R, Mintzer R, et al: Clinical and immunologic criteria for the diagnosis of allergic bronchopulmonary aspergillosis. Ann Intern Med 86:405–414, 1977.
114. Rosenberg M, Mintzer R, Aaronson DW, et al: Allergic broncho-

pulmonary aspergillosis in three patients with normal chest x-ray films. Chest 72:597–600, 1977.
115. Irwin RS, Thomas HM, III: Mucoid impaction of the bronchus: Diagnosis and treatment. Am Rev Respir Dis 108:955–962, 1973.
116. Liebow AA: The J Burns Amberson lecture: Pulmonary angiitis and granulomatosis. Am Rev Respir Dis 108:1–18, 1973.
117. Katzenstein AL, Liebow AA, Friedman PJ: Bronchocentric granulomatosis, mucoid impaction, and hypersensitivity reactions to fungi. Am Rev Respir Dis 111:497–537, 1975.
118. Laurell CB, Eriksson S: The electrophoretic $\alpha$1-globulin pattern of serum in $\alpha$1-antitrypsin deficiency. Scand J Clin Lab Invest 15:132–140, 1963.
119. Longstreth GF, Weitzman SA, Browning RJ, et al: Bronchiectasis and homozygous alpha1-antitrypsin deficiency. Chest 67:233–235, 1975.
120. Scott JH, Anderson CL, Shankar PS, et al: Alpha1-antitrypsin deficiency with diffuse bronchiectasis and cirrhosis of the liver. Chest 71:535–538, 1977.
121. Jones DK, Godden D, Cavanagh P: Alpha-1-antitrypsin deficiency presenting as bronchiectasis. Br J Dis Chest 79:301–304, 1985.
122. Rodriguez-Cintron W, Guntupalli K, Fraire AE: Bronchiectasis and homozygous ($P_1ZZ$) $\alpha_1$-antitrypsin deficiency in a young man. Thorax 50:424–425, 1995.
123. King MA, Stone JA, Diaz PT, et al: $\alpha_1$-Antitrypsin deficiency: Evaluation of bronchiectasis with CT. Radiology 199:137–141, 1996.
124. Dixon GF, Donnerberg RL, Schonfeld SA, et al: Advances in the diagnosis and treatment of broncholithiasis. Am Rev Respir Dis 129:1028–1030, 1984.
125. Merriam JC, Storrs RC, Hoefnagel D: Lung disease caused by aspirated timothy-grass heads. Am Rev Respir Dis 90:947–952, 1964.
126. Dudgeon DL, Parker FB, Frittelli G, et al: Bronchiectasis in pediatric patients resulting from aspirated grass inflorescences. Arch Surg 115:979–983, 1980.
127. Graham EA, Burford TH, Mayer JH: Middle lobe syndrome. Postgrad Med 4:29–34, 1948.
128. Bradham RR, Sealy WC, Young WG Jr: Chronic middle lobe infection. Ann Thorac Surg 2:612–616, 1966.
129. Inners CR, Terry PB, Traystman RJ, et al: Collateral ventilation and the middle lobe syndrome. Am Rev Respir Dis 118:305–310, 1978.
130. Iwai K, Shindo G, Hajikano H, et al: Intralobar pulmonary sequestration, with special reference to developmental pathology. Am Rev Respir Dis 107:911–920, 1973.
131. Savic B, Birtel FJ, Tholen W, et al: Lung sequestration: Report of seven cases and review of 540 published cases. Thorax 34:96–101, 1979.
132. Williams H, Campbell P: Generalized bronchiectasis associated with deficiency of cartilage in the bronchial tree. Arch Dis Child 35:182–191, 1960.
133. Williams HE, Landau LI, Phelan PD: Generalized bronchiectasis due to extensive deficiency of bronchial cartilage. Arch Dis Child 47:423–428, 1972.
134. Mitchell RE, Bury RG: Congenital bronchiectasis due to deficiency of bronchial cartilage (Williams-Campbell syndrome). J Pediatr 87:230–234, 1975.
135. Wayne KS, Taussig LM: Probable familial congenital bronchiectasis due to cartilage deficiency (Williams-Campbell syndrome). Am Rev Respir Dis 114:15–22, 1976.
136. Wood RE, Boat TF, Doersuk CF: Cystic fibrosis. Am Rev Respir Dis 113:833–878, 1976.
137. Rommens JM, Iannuzzi MC, Kerem B: Identification of the cystic fibrosis gene: Chromosome walking and jumping. Science 245:1059–1065, 1989.
138. Riordan JR, Rommens JM, Kerem B: Identification of the cystic fibrosis gene: Cloning and characterization of complementary DNA. Science 245:1066–1073, 1989.
139. Kerem E, Corey M, Kerem B, et al: The relation between genotype and phenotype in cystic fibrosis: Analysis of the most common mutation ($DF_{508}$). N Engl J Med 323:1517–1522, 1990.
140. Shwachman H, Kowalski M, Khaw KT: Cystic fibrosis: A new outlook: 70 Patients above 25 years of age. Medicine (Baltimore) 56:129–149, 1977.
141. di Sant'agnese PA, Davis PB: Cystic fibrosis in adults: 75 Cases and a review of 232 cases in the literature. Am J Med 66:121–132, 1979.
142. Smith JJ, Travis SM, Greenberg EP, et al: Cystic fibrosis airway epithelia fail to kill bacteria because of abnormal airway surface fluid. Cell 85:229–236, 1996.
143. Matthews WJ Jr, Williams M, Oliphint B, et al: Hypogammaglobulinemia in patients with cystic fibrosis. N Engl J Med 302:245–250, 1980.
144. Wallace JM, Rao AV, Glassroth J, et al: Respiratory illness in persons with human immunodeficiency virus infection. Am Rev Respir Dis 148:1523–1529, 1993.
145. Holmes AH, Trotman-Dickenson B, Edwards A, et al: Bronchiectasis in HIV disease. J Med 85:307–308, 1992.
146. Verghese A, Al-Samman M, Nabhan D, et al: Bacterial bronchitis and bronchiectasis in human immunodeficiency virus infection. Arch Intern Med 154:2086–2091, 1994.
147. Sheikh S, Madiraju K, Steiner P, et al: Bronchiectasis in pediatric AIDS. Chest 112:1202–1207, 1997.
148. King MA, Neal DE, St. John R, et al: Bronchial dilatation in patients with HIV infection: CT assessment and correlation with pulmonary function tests and findings at bronchoalveolar lavage. AJR Am J Roentgenol 168:1535–1540, 1997.
149. Good RA, Mazzitello WF: Chest disease in patients with agammaglobulinemia. Dis Chest 29:9–35, 1956.
150. Hermans PE, Diaz-Buxo JA, Stobo JD: Idiopathic late-onset immunoglobulin deficiency: Clinical observations in 50 patients. Am J Med 61:221–237, 1976.
151. Knowles GK, Stanhope R, Green M: Bronchiectasis complicating chronic lymphatic leukaemia with hypogammaglobulinaemia. Thorax 35:217–228, 1980.
152. Suhs RH, Dowling HF, Jackson GG: Hypogammaglobulinemia with chronic bronchitis or bronchiectasis: Treatment of five patients with long-term antibiotic therapy. Arch Intern Med 116:29–38, 1965.
153. Beck CS, Heiner DC: Selective immunoglobulin $G_4$ deficiency and recurrent infections of the respiratory tract. Am Rev Respir Dis 124:94–96, 1981.
154. Umetsu DT, Ambrosino DM, Quinti I, et al: Recurrent sinopulmonary infection and impaired antibody response to bacterial capsular polysaccharide antigen in children with selective IgG-subclass deficiency. N Engl J Med 313:1247–1251, 1985.
155. De Gracia J, Rodrigo MJ, Morell F, et al: IgG subclass deficiencies associated with bronchiectasis. Am J Respir Crit Care Med 153:650–655, 1996.
156. Chipps BE, Talamo RC, Winkelstein JA: IgA deficiency, recurrent pneumonias, and bronchiectasis: Clinical conference in pulmonary disease from the Department of Pediatrics, the John Hopkins University School of Medicine. Chest 73:519–526, 1978.
157. Strober W, Krakauer R, Klaeveman HL, et al: Secretory component deficiency: A disorder of the IgA immune system. N Engl J Med 294:351–356, 1976.
158. Kagan E, Soskolne CL, Zwi S, et al: Immunologic studies in patients with recurrent bronchopulmonary infections. Am Rev Respir Dis 111:441–451, 1975.
159. Albelda SM, Kern JA, Marinelli DL, et al: Expanding spectrum of pulmonary disease caused by nontuberculous mycobacteria. Radiology 157:289–296, 1985.
160. Edwards C, Penny M, Newman J: Mycoplasma pneumonia, Stevens-Johnson syndrome, and chronic obliterative bronchitis. Thorax 38:867–869, 1983.
161. Whyte KF, Williams GR: Bronchiectasis after mycoplasma pneumonia. Thorax 39:390–391, 1984.
162. Simila S, Linna O, Lanning P, et al: Chronic lung damage caused by adenovirus type 7: A ten-year follow-up study. Chest 80:127–131, 1981.
163. Carson JL, Collier AM, Hu SCS: Acquired ciliary defects in nasal epithelium of children with acute viral upper respiratory infections. N Engl J Med 312:463–468, 1985.
164. Kass I, Zamel N, Dobry CA, et al: Bronchiectasis following ammonia burns of the respiratory tract: A review of two cases. Chest 62:282–285, 1972.
165. Warnock ML, Ghahremani GG, Rattenborg C, et al: Pulmonary complication of heroin intoxication: Aspiration pneumonia and diffuse bronchiectasis. JAMA 219:1051–1053, 1972.

166. Banner AS, Muthuswamy P, Shah RS, et al: Bronchiectasis following heroin-induced pulmonary edema: Rapid clearing of pulmonary infiltrates. Chest 69:552–555, 1976.
167. Lee SH, Lee KS, Ahn JM, et al: Paraquat poisoning of the lung: Thin-section CT findings. Radiology 195:271–274, 1995.
168. Emad A, Rezaian GR: The diversity of the effects of sulfur mustard gas inhalation on respiratory system 10 years after a single, heavy exposure: Analysis of 197 cases. Chest 112:734–738, 1997.
169. Robitaille G: Ehlers-Danlos syndrome and recurrent hemoptysis. Ann Intern Med 61:710–721, 1964.
170. Foster ME, Foster DR: Bronchiectasis and Marfan's syndrome. Postgrad Med J 56:718–719, 1980.
171. Caughey JE, Wilson RF, Borrie J: Peripheral neuropathy (peripheral neuritis) with bronchiectasis. Thorax 13:59–63, 1958.
172. Camus P, Piard F, Ashcroft T, et al: The lung in inflammatory bowel disease. Medicine (Baltimore) 72:151–183, 1993.
173. Loubeyre P, Revel D, Delignette A, et al: Bronchiectasis detected with thin-section CT as a predictor of chronic lung allograft rejection. Radiology 194:213–216, 1995.
174. Kartagener M: Zur pathogenese dir brmchiekrasien. Mitteilung: Bronchiektasien be situs viscerum inversus. Deitr Klin Erforsch Tuberk Lungenkr 83:489–501, 1933.
175. Kartagener M, Horlacher A: Bronchiektasiem bei situs viscerum inversus. Schweiz Med Wochenschr 65:782–784, 1935.
176. Mayo CW, Rice RG: Situs inversus totalis: A statistical review of data on seventy-six cases with special reference to disease of the biliary tract. Arch Surg 58:724–730, 1949.
177. Bergstrom WH, Cook CD, Scannell J, et al: Situs inversus, bronchiectasis and sinusitus: Report of a family with two cases of Kartagener's triad and two additional cases of bronchiectasis among six siblings. Pediatrics 6:573–582, 1950.
178. Kartagener M, Stucki P: Bronchiectasis with situs inversus. Arch Pediatr 79:193–207, 1962.
179. Katsuhara K, Kawamoto S, Wakabayashi T, et al: Situs inversus totalis and Kartagener's syndrome in a Japanese population. Chest 61:56–61, 1972.
180. Logan WD Jr, Abbott OA, Hatcher CR Jr: Kartagener's triad. Dis Chest 48:613–616, 1965.
181. Olsen AM: Bronchiectasis and dextrocardia: Observations on the aetiology of bronchiectasis. Am Rev Tuberc 47:435–439, 1943.
182. Overholt EL, Bauman DF: Variants of Kartagener's syndrome in the same family. Ann Intern Med 48:574–579, 1958.
183. Miller RD, Divertie MB: Kartagener's syndrome. Chest 62:130–135, 1972.
184. Afzelius BA, Eliasson R, Johnsen O, et al: Lack of dynein arms in immotile human spermatozoa. J Cell Biol 66:225–232, 1975.
185. Camner P, Mossberg B, Afzelius BA: Evidence for congenitally nonfunctioning cilia in the tracheobronchial tract in two subjects. Am Rev Respir Dis 112:807–809, 1975.
186. Afzelius BA: A human syndrome caused by immotile cilia. Science 193:317–319, 1976.
187. Eliasson R, Mossberg B, Camner P, et al: The immotile-cilia syndrome: A congenital ciliary abnormality as an etiologic factor in chronic airway infections and male sterility. N Engl J Med 297:1–6, 1977.
188. Rossman CM, Forrest JB, Ruffin RE, et al: Immotile cilia syndrome in persons with and without Kartagener's syndrome. Am Rev Respir Dis 121:1011–1016, 1980.
189. Corbeel L, Cornillie F, Lauweryns J, et al: Ultrastructural abnormalities of bronchial cilia in children with recurrent airway infections and bronchiectasis. Arch Dis Child 56:929–933, 1981.
190. Jahrsdoerfer R, Feldman PS, Rubel EW, et al: Otitis media and the immotile cilia syndrome. Laryngoscope 89:769–778, 1979.
191. Sturgess JM, Chao J, Turner JAP: Transposition of ciliary microtubules: Another cause of impaired ciliary motility. N Engl J Med 303:318–322, 1980.
192. Sturgess JM, Chao J, Wong J, et al: Cilia with defective radial spokes: A cause of human respiratory disease. N Engl J Med 300:53–56, 1979.
193. Neustein HB, Nickerson B, O'Neal M: Kartagener's syndrome with absence of inner dynein arms of respiratory cilia. Am Rev Respir Dis 2:979–981, 1980.
194. Rayner CFJ, Rutman A, Dewar A, et al: Ciliary disorientation alone as a cause of primary ciliary dyskinesia syndrome. Am J Respir Crit Care Med 153:1123–1129, 1996.
195. de Iongh RU, Rutland J: Ciliary defects in healthy subjects, bronchiectasis, and primary ciliary dyskinesia. Am J Respir Crit Care Med 151:1559–1167, 1995.
196. Hunninghake GW, Fauci AJ: Pulmonary involvement in the collagen vascular diseases. Am Rev Respir Dis 119:471–503, 1979.
197. Shadick NA, Fanta CH, Weinblatt ME, et al: A late feature of severe rheumatoid arthritis. Medicine (Baltimore) 73:161–170, 1994.
198. Hassan WU, Keaney NP, Holland CD, et al: High resolution computed tomography of the lung in lifelong non-smoking patients with rheumatoid arthritis. Ann Rheum Dis 54:308–310, 1995.
199. Cortet B, Flipo R-M, Rémy-Jardin M, et al: Use of high resolution computed tomography of the lungs in patients with rheumatoid arthritis. Ann Rheum Dis 54:815–819, 1995.
200. Remy-Jardin M, Remy J, Cortet B, et al: Lung changes in rheumatoid arthritis: CT findings. Radiology 193:375–382, 1994.
201. Mounier-Kuhn P: Dilatation de la trachea: Constatations radiographiques et bronchoscopiques. Lyon Med 150:106–109, 1932.
202. Katz I, LeVine M, Herman P: Tracheobronchiomegaly: The Mounier-Kuhn syndrome. AJR Am J Roentgenol 88:1084–1094, 1962.
203. Johnston RF, Green RA: Tracheobronchiomegaly: Report of five cases and demonstration of familial occurrence. Am Rev Respir Dis 91:35–50, 1965.
204. Roditi GH, Weir J: The association of tracheomegaly and bronchiectasis. Clin Radiol 49:608–611, 1994.
205. Swyer PR, James GCW: A case of unilateral pulmonary emphysema. Thorax 8:133–136, 1953.
206. MacLeod WM: Abnormal transradiancy of one lung. Thorax 9:147–153, 1954.
207. Samman PO, White WF: The "yellow-nail" syndrome. Br J Dermatol 76:153–157, 1964.
208. Dilley JJ, Kierland RR, Randall RV, et al: Primary lymphedema associated with yellow nails and pleural effusions. JAMA 204:670–125, 1968.
209. Hiller E, Rosenow EC, Olsen AM: Pulmonary manifestations of the yellow nail syndrome. Chest 61:452–458, 1972.

# 42 Disorders of the Upper Airways

ALAN R. SCHWARTZ, M.D. • PHILIP L. SMITH, M.D.
HASKINS K. KASHIMA, M.D. • DONALD F. PROCTOR, M.D.
ALKIS TOGIAS, M.D.

Introduction
Principles of Airflow Dynamics in the Upper Airways
The Nose
- Structure and Function
- Allergic and Nonallergic Rhinitis

The Pharynx
- Structure and Function
- Airflow Obstruction in Obstructive Sleep Apnea
- Other Clinical Disorders

The Larynx
- Structure and Function
- Laryngeal Disorders

## INTRODUCTION

The upper airways—anatomically complicated structures that extend from the airway openings at the nares and lips to the trachea—serve numerous physiologic functions. Their respiratory function includes filtering, conditioning, and conveying air to the lungs. The nasal airway also supports the sense of olfaction; the oral airway, pharynx, and larynx also support deglutition, phonation, and coughing. These processes have been studied extensively. This chapter focuses on the role of the upper airways in breathing and on disorders that impact this function. We also discuss some of the air-conditioning functions of the nasal mucosa because they have direct impact on the health of the lower airways.

The term *upper airways* includes several anatomically distinct regions (Figs. 42.1 and 42.2). The nose constitutes the upper segment, followed by the nasopharyngeal and oropharyngeal airways, which extend from the nasal choanae and oral cavity to the supraglottic space. The larynx divides the upper and lower airways, although some place it in the thoracic inlet.

We first lay the groundwork for considering the pathophysiologic mechanisms of airflow obstruction in these airways by outlining general principles of airflow dynamics. We then turn to a review of the functions of three relatively distinct anatomic regions (the nasal, oropharyngeal, and laryngeal airways) not only under resting conditions but also as shaped by the need for coordination with other vital functions, by sleep, and by increases in ventilatory demands (e.g., exercise). For each of these

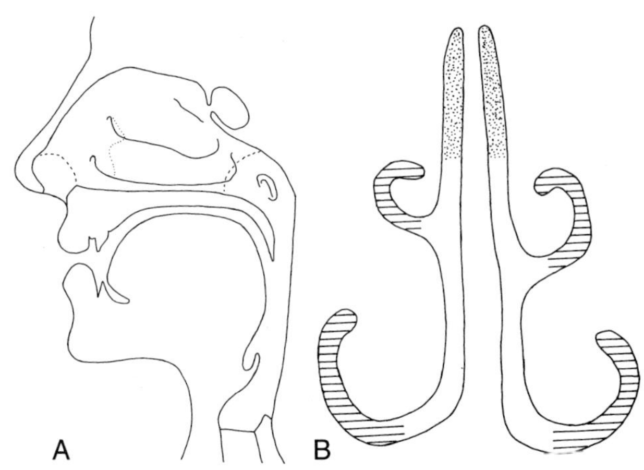


**Figure 42.1** The diagram show upper airways and nasal segments. *A,* Nasal and oropharyngeal airways are shown with the nasal septum omitted. The *dashed line on the left* marks the beginning of the nasal valve; the *dotted line* marks the approximate beginning of the ciliated mucosa; and *dashed line on the right* marks the termination of the nasal septum. Note the key position of the soft palate for control of the division between oral and nasal paths for airflow. *B,* This section through the main nasal passage shows the septum and folds of the turbinates. The *stippled areas* are the olfactory region, through which little inspiratory airflow passes. The *striped areas* are meatal spaces, through which there is little airflow. The *clear space* is a region of major inspiratory airflow (From Proctor DF, Anderson I (eds): The Nose: Upper Airway Physiology and the Atmospheric Environment. Amsterdam: Elsevier Biomedical Press, 1982.)

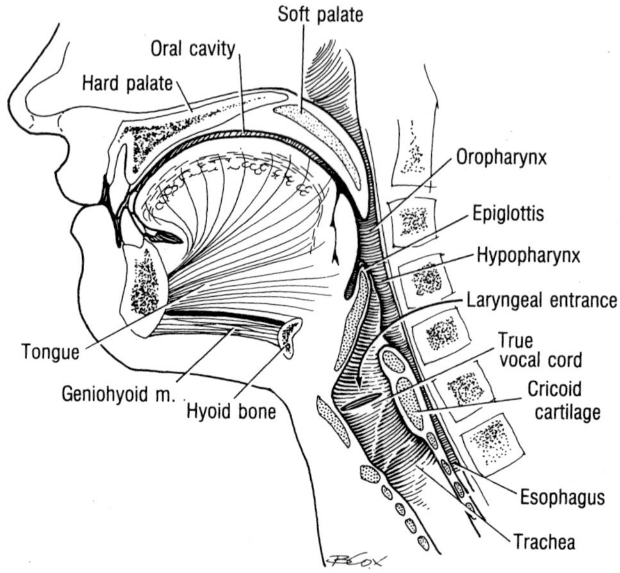


**Figure 42.2** The diagram illustrates the major structures comprising the oropharyngeal and laryngeal airway. (From Wiegand L, Zwillich CW: Pathogenesis of obstructive sleep apnea: Role of the pharynx. Semin Respir Med 9:540–546, 1988.)

anatomic regions, some common clinical disorders are discussed.

## PRINCIPLES OF AIRFLOW DYNAMICS IN THE UPPER AIRWAYS

The upper airways must permit the passage of air and food. This function requires exquisite neural control of numerous muscle groups. The actions of pharyngeal sphincters and glottic adductors enable complete occlusion of the airways at specific sites during deglutition. The action of dilators of several airway segments and the transition from solely nasal to oronasal breathing enables augmentation of airflow during exercise. When extreme increases in ventilation are required, airflow appears to be restricted only by the anatomic limits of the caliber of specific airway segments. These limits are approached as neuromuscular and non-neuromuscular mechanisms recruit airway dilators[1–9] and decongest the nasal and pharyngeal airways.[10–12]

The underlying mechanisms that modulate the flow-conducting properties in the airways have been elucidated by examining the effects of alterations in the properties of specific airway segments on airflow dynamics.[13–17] Narrowing can result from structural bony or soft-tissue abnormalities. When narrowing is fixed, airflow resistance increases. Narrowing can also result from dynamic collapse of upper airway segments.[18] When airway collapsibility is increased and inspiratory effort is sufficient, dynamic collapse results in airflow obstruction.[15, 19–21]

The effects of alterations in resistance or collapsibility on airflow through the upper airways can be clarified by consideration of airflow dynamics in a simple collapsible conduit (Fig. 42.3). In this mechanical analogue, the airway can be partitioned into three physiologically distinct segments.[21] In an absolutely compliant or collapsible segment, collapse occurs when the intraluminal pressure falls below the pressure in the surrounding tissue (the critical pressure or $P_{crit}$).[16, 17] Collapse is more likely to occur, of course, when the pressure in surrounding tissues is elevated[22, 23] and less likely when the segment has retained some rigidity. Because the cross-sectional areas of the segments upstream and downstream from the collapsible site change minimally with changes in intraluminal pressure, they can be modeled as resistances: upstream ($R_{US}$) and downstream ($R_{DS}$) resistance, respectively. If resistance upstream from a collapsible segment is increased, the pressure drop across it is also increased so that the intraluminal pressure within the collapsible segment is lower. Thus, changes in a "fixed" upstream resistance affect the flow at which limitation by a collapsible segment occurs.

Segmental resistances influence the initial parts of the inspiratory pressure-flow curves (Fig. 42.4). During single inspirations, increases in driving pressure are initially associated with progressive increases in airflow. For a given driving pressure, inspiratory airflow ($\dot{V}_I$) is determined by the combined resistances of the upstream and downstream airway segments, $R_{US}$ and $R_{DS}$. At low flows, below approximately 0.3 L/sec, airflow is laminar and can be approximated as follows:

$$\dot{V}_I = (P_{US} - P_{DS})/(R_{US} + R_{DS}) \quad (1)$$

At higher levels of flow, however, airflow becomes turbulent, and the relationship between airflow and driving pressure becomes curvilinear and follows the quadratic equation of Rohrer, as discussed by Sullivan and Chang.[24] Even under these circumstances, a detailed analysis can predict the effect of alterations in resistance on airflow.[25–27]

To determine how airway collapsibility influences airflow, consider the terminal segments of the pressure-flow relationships in Figure 42.4. As the driving pressure continues to rise, inspiratory airflow plateaus at a maxi-

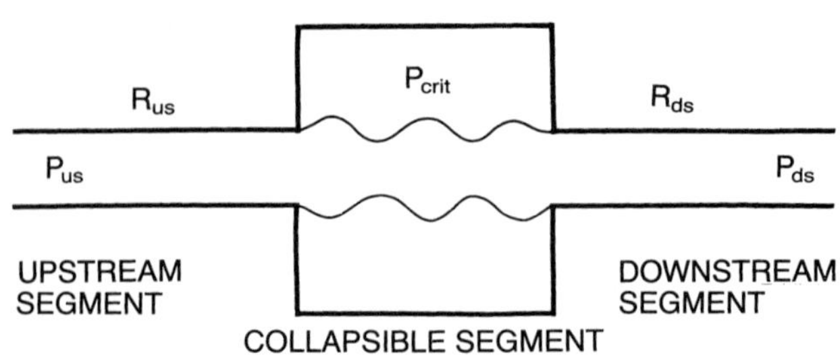


**Figure 42.3** A mechanical analogue of an upper airway region with a collapsible segment is illustrated. This segment is surrounded by a critical pressure, $P_{crit}$. Segments upstream and downstream are relatively rigid and have defined resistances, $R_{US}$ and $R_{DS}$, respectively. Pressures in these segments are represented by $P_{US}$ and $P_{DS}$. When intraluminal pressure immediately downstream from the collapsible segment falls below $P_{crit}$, pressure in the collapsible segment remains at $P_{crit}$, which becomes the effective downstream pressure to airflow (see Equation 2).

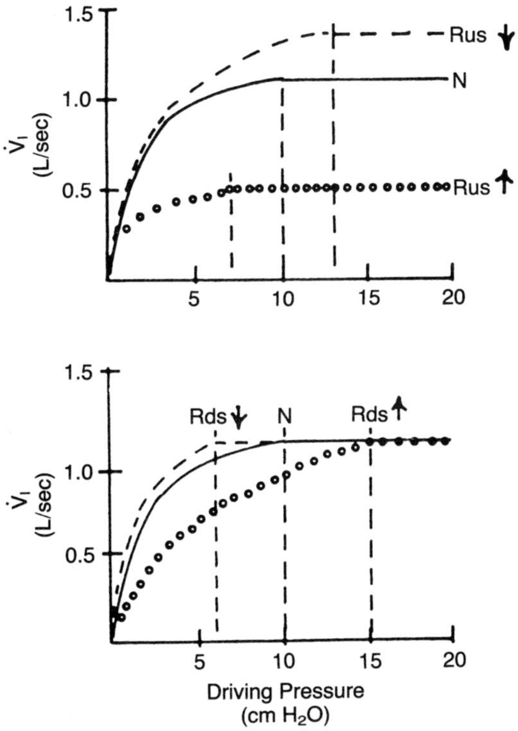


**Figure 42.4** Inspiratory airflow ($\dot{V}_I$ vertical axes) is plotted vs. driving pressure ($P_{US} - P_{DS}$, horizontal axes) across the nose during the initial portions of single inspirations. Note that each curve demonstrates a maximum (plateau) in inspiratory airflow as driving pressure exceeds a level shown by the *vertical dashed lines,* indicating the development of flow limitation. The effect of isolated changes in upstream resistance ($R_{US}$) and downstream resistance ($R_{DS}$) compared with baseline normal (N) conditions are illustrated in the *upper* and *lower* panels, respectively. Changes in maximal airflow are only related to changes in $R_{US}$ (and not $R_{DS}$). (From Brain, JD, Proctor, DF, Reid LM (eds): Respiratory Defense Mechanisms. New York: Marcel Dekker, 1977.)

mal level ($\dot{V}_I max$) and becomes independent of further increases in driving pressure. This finding, which is characteristic of flow limitation in collapsible biologic conduits, is due to dynamic collapse of the airway at a discrete locus.[16, 17, 28–32] Dynamic airway collapse, therefore, is characterized by the development of inspiratory airflow limitation at higher driving pressures.

When airflow limitation develops, maximal inspiratory airflow can be described as follows[15, 19, 29, 33, 34]:

$$\dot{V}_I max = (P_{US} - P_{crit})/R_{US} \qquad (2)$$

where $\dot{V}_I max$ is the plateau flow illustrated in Figure 42.4. In comparison with the relationship of Equation 1, $P_{crit}$ has replaced $P_{DS}$ as the effective downstream pressure. When airflow becomes limited, therefore, $V_I max$ is determined by airway collapsibility and by the upstream resistance. Furthermore, as this relationship suggests, airflow ceases whenever $P_{crit}$ rises above $P_{US}$.

The levels of driving pressure and airflow are low with resting tidal breathing. In this setting, airflow is not limited, but it varies directly with driving pressure. When driving pressure increases, however, airflow limitation may occur unless there are concomitant decreases in airway collapsibility or in the resistance upstream to the collapsible site (Fig. 42.4).

## THE NOSE

### Structure and Function

The nasal passage is divided by the nasal septum. Air enters the nose through the nasal vestibule, an approximately 1-cm channel in the cartilaginous portion of the nose. The nasal passages then become convoluted by the folds of the turbinates. This complex form alters airflow dynamics in the nose and is well suited for the specialized respiratory functions of humidification and warming or cooling of inspired air.

During nasal breathing in the erect position, air must enter the nose in an upward direction before turning horizontally just beyond the nasal valve to enter the main nasal passages. In contrast, the main nasal passage runs horizontally backward through the nasal passages. These passages run horizontally backward to the nasopharynx and have large cross-sectional and surface areas. As a result of the changes in direction, the inspiratory air stream undergoes two nearly 90° bends before entering the relatively straight pharyngolaryngotracheal path. The direction of the nasal air stream is more curvilinear during expiration.

The two bends in the airstream separate the nose into two anatomically and physiologically distinct segments (see Fig. 42.1). The passage of the nasal vestibule is narrow, and linear velocity becomes quite high.[35, 36] The combination of high linear velocities and the bend in the passage favors the deposition of most airborne particles in the anterior nose. Air velocities are lower in the main nasal passages where the cross-sectional area is greater. This reduction in air velocity allows prolonged contact of inspired air with the nasal mucosa, enabling the nose to modify the temperature and water vapor content[37–50] and to remove airborne pathogens and pollutants.[51–55]

Neuromuscular activity in the skeletal muscles that overlie the cartilaginous portion of the nose play a major role in the control of nasal vestibule patency.[1, 5, 11, 35, 36] Contraction of the transverse part of the alae nasi narrows this segment, whereas activation of the alar part of this muscle and of the depressor septi widens it. Dilators of the nasal vestibule are under voluntary control[1] and are recruited during inspiration when ventilatory drive is augmented (Table 42.1).[1, 56–59] Dilator activation typically precedes the onset of inspiration and peaks early in inspiration, when airflow is highest.[1] The activity of these muscles correlates with the level of nasal airflow and increases with the ventilatory response to hypercapnia, hypoxemia, and exercise.[11, 35, 56, 60–62] When ventilatory drive is elevated, the pressure difference from the nasal inlet to the pharynx increases as inspiratory effort increases. To avoid collapse of the alar cartilages and limitation of flow during inspiration, a rise in dilator activity at the nasal vestibule is thought to decrease both the resistance and the collapsibility of this nasal segment.[1, 15, 35, 56, 63]

**Table 42.1 MUSCLES SURROUNDING THE UPPER AIRWAYS**

| Region | Stabilizing or Widening | May Widen or Narrow | Narrowing or Closing |
|---|---|---|---|
| Nose | Dilator naris | Vascular smooth muscle | Compressor naris |
| | Alae nasi | | |
| Nasopharynx | | Tensor veli palatini | Levator veli palatini |
| | | | Palatopharyngeus |
| Mouth and pharynx | Lateral pterygoid | Salpingopharyngeus | Medial pterygoid |
| | Genioglossus | Muscles of the lips | Pharyngeal constrictors |
| | | Masseter | Pterygopharyngeus |
| | | Glossopalatinus | Buccopharyngeus |
| | | | Stylopharyngeus |
| | | | Mylopharyngeus |
| | | | Glossopharyngeus |
| | | | Chondropharyngeus |
| | | | Ceratopharyngeus |
| | | | Thyropharyngeus |
| | | | Cricopharyngeus |
| | | | Styloglossus |
| | | | Hyoglossus |
| | Digastric | | |
| | Mylohyoid | | |
| | Geniohyoid | | |
| | Stylohyoid | | |
| | | Omohyoid | |
| | | Thyrohyoid | |
| | | Sternohyoid | |
| | | Sternothyroid | |
| Larynx | Cricoarytenoid posterior | Cricothyroid | Aryepiglottic |
| | | | Interarytenoid |
| | | | Cricoarytenoid lateralis |
| | | | Thyroarytenoid |
| Trachea | | | Smooth muscle |

Congestion or obstruction in the nasal cavum leads to increases in the resistance downstream to the site of inspiratory airflow limitation in the nasal vestibule.[25, 62] These increases in downstream resistance reduce nasal airflow and increase the driving pressure required to reach maximal flow (see Fig. 42.4). To reduce the inspiratory effort required to generate a given level of flow, mouth breathing remains the only effective strategy when an elevated nasal resistance occurs.[64–66] Therefore, the individual with an elevated resistance must adopt a breathing strategy that balances the need to increase inspiratory effort for the sake of receiving the benefits of nasal airflow conditioning.

The specialized functions of the nose are of great importance to the lower airways. These functions are attributable to particular anatomic features of the nasal mucosa and are facilitated by the above-described airflow patterns. The nasal mucosa is characterized by an abundance of submucosal glands and goblet cells within the respiratory epithelium,[67] a dense subepithelial network of fenestrated capillaries,[68] an additional vascular network of capacitance vessels (venous sinusoids)[69] that can rapidly pool blood and engorge mucosal tissue,[70] and an abundance of sensory nerve endings that interdigitate between epithelial cells and act as nonspecialized nociceptors.[71] Production of mucus by seromucous glands and goblet cells provides the trapping material for particles entering the airways with inhaled air. The contents of nasal secretions, which include immunoglobulins (particularly secretory IgA),[72] antibacterial chemicals (lysozyme, lactoferrin),[73] or even antioxidants (uric acid),[74] offer innate and specific immune functions and chemical protection for the lower airways. The nasal and particularly the paranasal sinus epithelium are also rich in inducible nitric oxide synthase, which confers the ability to produce nitric oxide,[75–77] a substance with antibacterial,[78] antiviral,[79] and smooth muscle relaxant[80] properties. Indeed, under resting conditions, the concentrations of nitric oxide in the healthy sinus and nasal cavities are exceedingly high.[76, 77] Rapid passage of blood through the subepithelial capillaries acts as a heat exchanger with tremendous capacity for warming of inhaled air. By engorging the tissue, capacitance vessels increase the contact surface with inhaled air and facilitate heat and water exchange. The fenestrae of the subepithelial capillaries are thought to be important in allowing for rapid water transportation from the intravascular space to the epithelial layer. Water moves passively through the intraepithelial junctions and effectively humidifies inhaled air.[81] Finally, the nociceptors of the nasal mucosa generate several central reflexes such as the sneezing reflex, as well as nasonasal reflexes through which the glandular apparatus and the vasculature are activated. Neural reflexes act in concordance to protect the airways.

The functional role of the nasal airways as protectors of the lower airways becomes evident when we consider the impact of nasal breathing on exercise-induced asthma. The stimuli that induce bronchospasm in this condition are water loss leading to mucosal hypertonicity[82–84] and, possibly, mucosal cooling.[85, 86] Hypertonicity and cooling occur because, as a result of hyperventilation, breathing becomes oronasal, and a significant proportion of inhaled air reaches the lower airways without having been adequately conditioned by the nose. In experimental settings in which asthmatics were asked to exercise while breathing either through their mouth or through their nose at equal ventilatory rates, the reduction in lung function induced by exercise was markedly inhibited with nasal breathing.[87, 88]

## Allergic and Nonallergic Rhinitis

Nasal symptoms—sneezing, rhinorrhea, congestion, and posterior nasal drainage—are probably known to almost all humans because they typically occur in response to the most common infection affecting our species, the common cold. These symptoms can also occur in the absence of infection, as an expression of type I immunologic hypersensitivity to aeroallergens deposited in the nose (allergic rhinitis). In addition, such symptoms can be experienced as a result of a variety of other, less common, disorders of known etiology or without an identifiable mechanism (nonallergic rhinitis).

### Classification and Pathophysiology

Allergic rhinitis is classified into episodic, seasonal, and perennial on the basis of the duration of symptoms. Most patients with nonallergic rhinitis belong to the "unknown etiology" group. This group can be further classified into three conditions: nonallergic hyperplastic rhinosinusitis; nonallergic, noninflammatory rhinopathy (also referred to as "vasomotor rhinitis"); and nonallergic rhinitis with eosinophilia syndrome (NARES).[89] However, complete agreement on the classification of nonallergic rhinitis has not been achieved.[90]

The prevalence of allergic rhinitis ranges from 9% to 24% in most epidemiologic studies.[91–93] Because of such a high prevalence and because of the many comorbidities from the respiratory tract (sinus disease, otitis media, lower respiratory symptoms), the economic burden of allergic rhinitis is high.[94, 95] In fact, the annual direct cost in the United States has been estimated to lie between $1.23 and $3.4 billion.

Allergic rhinitis, very much like allergic asthma (Chapter 39), is characterized by mucosal inflammation and hyper-responsiveness. As in asthma, the allergens responsible are inhaled (aeroallergens). Outdoor allergens, such as plant pollens (especially from ragweed, grasses, and weeds) and molds (e.g., *Alternaria*) typically cause seasonal rhinitis, whereas indoor allergens such as house dust mite, cockroach, and pet danders cause perennial symptoms. In subtropical and tropical climates, where seasons are less distinct, the differentiation between seasonal and perennial patterns of disease is of less value.

As in allergic asthma, a basic cellular event is the interaction of antigen (allergen) with the Fab portion of specific IgE antibody molecules anchored on the surface of two types of cells, the mast cell (a stationary tissue cell) and the basophil (a peripheral blood leukocyte). The interaction between antigen and IgE bridges two nearby IgE molecules, leading to the activation of second-messenger pathways that cause the release of preformed inflammatory mediators, like histamine and tryptase, and the de novo synthesis and release of others, such as prostaglandin $D_2$ and sulfidopeptide leukotrienes.[96, 97] These substances cause acute symptoms such as intense local pruritus, sneezing, rhinorrhea, and nasal congestion with airflow limitation. Lacrimation is also part of this constellation. In this acute aspect of the clinical manifestation of allergic rhinitis, histamine is probably the most important mediator because it is the only one to generate the entire spectrum of rhinitic symptoms. In the human nasal mucosa, receptors for histamine (primarily the $H_1$ type) are found on sensory nerve endings and blood vessels.[98, 99] Blood vessels appear to bear $H_2$ receptors as well.[98, 100]

We emphasize that the allergic reaction does not end with the development of acute symptoms. As in asthma, exposure to allergen results not only in an early but also in a late reaction, which is marked by recrudescence of symptoms, especially of nasal congestion, a second wave of inflammatory mediator release, and an increase in the numbers of eosinophils, basophils, mononuclear cells, and neutrophils in nasal secretions.[101, 102] Although the late phase reaction has been studied as a laboratory phenomenon, it is thought to be important in the natural history of allergic rhinitis; the most effective treatment modalities, corticosteroids and immunotherapy, strongly suppress the clinical, biochemical, and cellular manifestations of this reaction.[103–107] Late phase reactions can be recognized in the natural course of allergic rhinitis as well. In general, they occur after exposure to high levels of allergen. In the laboratory setting, a good correlation between the magnitude of the symptomatology in the acute (early) and the late phase allergic reaction exists.[102]

Mucosal biopsies performed 24 hours after nasal provocation demonstrate an inflammatory infiltrate that is mostly lymphocytic.[108, 109] In addition, eosinophils, basophils, and neutrophils are found in increased numbers. Again, as in asthma, immunohistochemical staining and in situ hybridization studies reveal that most of the tissue lymphocytes are $CD4^+$ (helper) T cells primarily of the T helper type 2–like subclass (Chapter 39).[108] The histologic picture of chronic allergic rhinitis is in close resemblance.[109, 110] The exact role of the inflammatory infiltrate in the clinical presentation of the disease has not, however, been elucidated. Among the most important consequences of the presence and activation of leukocytes is the production of cytokines and chemokines (chemokines are also produced by resident epithelial and endothelial cells). These substances are thought to orchestrate the perpetuation of inflammation, which, as a result of the nature of these cytokines and chemokines, bears unique "allergic" characteristics. Some of the cytokines (including interleukin-4 [IL-4] and IL-13) drive the immune system toward an even more polarized "allergic" responsivity,[111, 112] others (such as IL-5) enhance the presence and activation of eosinophils,[113] while others (such as histamine-releasing factors) have the ability of activating basophils and possibly eosinophils to release symptom-producing mediators in the absence of direct allergen stimulation.[114, 115] The presence of increased numbers of mast cells and the accumulation of basophils and eosinophils at the site of allergic inflammation provides on the one hand more IgE targets for allergen and on the other hand more cells capable of releasing symptom-producing inflammatory mediators on activation. These complex interactions may explain additional clinical phenomena that characterize chronic allergic rhinitis, that is, nasal priming to allergens and nonspecific hyper-responsiveness.

Priming of the nasal mucosa to allergens is a phenomenon described in the 1960s by Connell,[116] detailing the observation that with increasing exposure to allergens, the symptoms progressively accentuate. This explains why, in the beginning of the pollen season, despite the fact that pollen counts rapidly increase, disease severity remains relatively mild. At the end of the season, despite very low pollen counts, patients with allergic rhinitis remain quite symptomatic. The presence of nonspecific nasal hyper-responsiveness explains the clinical observation that a large number of patients with allergic rhinitis specify not only allergens (pollen, pets, and so forth) but also various irritants (strong perfumes, smoke, cold, dry air) as triggers of their nasal symptoms.[117] In the laboratory setting, priming can be produced in the nose even after a single allergen provocation.[118] When a second provocation is performed a few hours after the first, in addition to the increased symptomatology, the level of symptom-producing mediators (e.g., histamine) is increased in nasal lavage fluids. This suggests either an increased number of cellular targets for allergen or an increased cellular releasability of mediators. In addition, following allergen provocation, the responsiveness of the nasal mucosa to histamine, an actual product of the allergic reaction, is increased,[119, 120] and this can also contribute to the priming phenomenon. Allergen-induced increased responsiveness to histamine is thought to reflect primarily hyper-responsiveness of the sensorineural apparatus.[121, 122] This type of hyper-responsiveness has been experimentally demonstrated in natural allergic rhinitis whether of seasonal or perennial nature.[123–125]

The pathophysiology of the most common nonallergic rhinitis syndromes is almost completely obscure. Hyperplastic nonallergic rhinosinusitis, similar to its allergic counterpart, is characterized by thickened nasal and paranasal sinus mucosa and excessive mucosal inflammation.[126–131] The cytokine pattern in the inflamed tissues, as assessed by immunhistochemistry, is, however, somewhat different between allergic and nonallergic disease.[132, 133] Also, compared with uncomplicated allergic rhinitis, hyperplastic rhinosinusitis, whether allergic or nonallergic, is characterized by increased neutrophilia in nasal secretions.[134] This raises the possibility of a chronic infectious process participating in this syndrome; yet most attempts to identify bacterial culprits have been unsuccessful.[135, 136] Also unknown is the etiology of the nonallergic rhinitis with eosinophilia syndrome,[137–140] the clinical presentation of which resembles that of allergic rhinitis. It is, therefore, possible that an as yet unknown allergen is responsible for this illness.[141]

Finally, in nonallergic, noninflammatory rhinopathy (vasomotor rhinitis), not only is nasal mucosal inflammation absent,[142–145] but very few functional alterations have been consistently described.[124, 146, 147] In contrast, many studies indicate that this syndrome benefits from treatment with repetitive nasal applications of capsaicin, which results in defunctionalization of mucosal nociceptors.[148–154] It is possible, therefore, that nonallergic, noninflammatory rhinopathy represents a state of sensorineural imbalance. The etiology is, however, unknown.

## Management

The management of allergic rhinitis is summarized in Table 42.2. As for allergic asthma, environmental control aiming at allergen avoidance together with pharmacotherapy and immunotherapy constitutes the backbone of our therapeutic strategies. Because the offending allergens are the same, environmental control for allergic rhinitis is identical to that recommended for the management of allergic asthma (Chapter 39). Perhaps, compared with asthma, pollen avoidance may be more beneficial for

**Table 42.2 MANAGEMENT OF ALLERGIC RHINITIS**

| Indication | Management |
|---|---|
| Mild disease | Allergen avoidance plus as-needed antihistamines/decongestants |
| Moderate disease | Allergen avoidance plus continuous cromolyn or topical steroids with or without as-needed antihistamines/decongestants |
| Severe disease | Allergen avoidance plus continuous topical steroids with or without immunotherapy and with or without as-needed antihistamines/decongestants |
| Difficult to control rhinorrhea | Ipratropium bromide |
| Thick secretions | High-dose guaifenesin |

allergic rhinitis because the size of pollen particles makes them more likely to deposit in the nasal mucosa. On the other hand, in patients with perennial allergic rhinitis, especially those lacking any evidence of seasonal, pollen-related exacerbations, indoor allergen exposure needs to be reduced as scrupulously as for patients with asthma.

The pharmacologic agents used to treat allergic rhinitis can be separated into two categories: those conferring symptom relief and those with anti-inflammatory properties. The first category includes three types of agents: antihistamines, decongestants, and ipratropium bromide, a locally active anticholinergic drug. Some also recommend the use of guaifenesin, at very high doses (1200 mg twice a day), to thin mucosal secretions, thus helping patients who complain of refractory posterior nasopharyngeal drainage. Antihistamines are $H_1$ receptor antagonists.[155, 156] They are effective in reducing pruritus, sneezing, tearing, and rhinorrhea, but less so nasal congestion. They can be used on an as-needed basis, although they have a better effect if taken either before symptom develop or continuously.

The use of the older compounds (first-generation or classic antihistamines) has been limited because of their significant side effects, primarily sedation and systemic anticholinergic activity. Newer agents, first introduced in the early 1980s, are essentially devoid of such adverse effects and can be used with great ease. Also, the newer antihistamines have longer half-lives and active metabolites, which prolong their action. This allows them to be taken once or twice daily, thus enhancing patient compliance. Currently, three of these agents, cetirizine, fexofenadine, and loratadine, are available in the United States. When the new-generation antihistamines are compared with each other, cetirizine appears to exert the strongest effects in studies involving skin testing with histamine as the outcome,[155] in trials involving relatively controlled provocations with allergen in large exposure rooms,[157] as well as in natural allergen exposure "park" studies.[158]

Because antihistamines do not have clinical potency against nasal congestion, oral and topical decongestants can be used in combination with antihistamines, or as single agents, to offer relief from this symptom.[159] These are alpha-adrenergic agonists (i.e., vasoconstrictors). Because vasodilation of the capacitance vessels of the nasal mucosa results in nasal congestion, constriction of the same vessels leads to tissue shrinking and decongestion. Oral agents (pseudephedrine, phenylpropanolamine) are, on the one hand, less potent than the topical ones (oxymetazoline, xylometazoline, phenylephrine) and, on the other hand, can cause significant sympathomimetic side effects, including insomnia, tachycardia, nervousness, and increased blood pressure.

Topical agents are quite potent, but they induce receptor down-regulation and pharmacologic tolerance, which results in a continuously increasing need for dosing and in rebound nasal congestion after discontinuation. Such agents should not be used for more than 4 to 5 consecutive days at a time. Ipratropium bromide, being an antagonist of acetylcholine on muscarinic receptors, can reduce the stimulation of the submucosal nasal glands by cholinergic neural pathways.[160] It is recommended when excessive rhinorrhea dominates the constellation of nasal symptoms. This agent will have no effects on the other symptoms of allergic rhinitis; therefore, rarely will it be sufficient, as a single agent, to control the disease. The two types of anti-inflammatory agents indicated for the treatment of allergic rhinitis, disodium cromoglycate (cromolyn) and topical nasal glucocorticosteroids, are thoroughly discussed in Chapter 11 in terms of their pharmacology and their use in asthma.

The strategic positioning of these agents in allergic rhinitis is very similar to that in asthma, as are their relative effectiveness and safety profiles. In moderate to severe rhinitis, topical glucocorticosteroids constitute the mainstay of treatment,[161, 162] benefiting all symptoms and reducing inflammation[103, 106, 163–166] and nasal hyper-responsiveness.[120, 167] Continuous use, as opposed to "as required," results in more effective symptoms control.[168] Safety profile is excellent, with most common side effects being local irritation, dryness, and headaches. In contrast to inhaled steroids, which can rather frequently result in oropharyngeal candidiasis, this adverse event is extremely rare with nasal agents. Several studies involving mucosal biopsies have ensured us that nasal steroids do not induce mucosal atrophy.[165, 169, 170] The systemic bioavailability of these agents with some metabolic effects have been documented.[171, 172] These effects, however, are of far less concern than those of systemically administered glucocorticosteroids.

The role of immunotherapy in allergic rhinitis is very well established.[107, 173–178] This treatment, during which increasing doses of allergenic extracts are progressively administered subcutaneously, once or twice per week, until a maintenance dose is reached, alters various aspects of the immune response to allergens,[179–184] leading to inhibition of many elements of the allergic reaction.[107, 176] The indications for immunotherapy include the presence of moderate to severe disease and either lack of effectiveness of conventional medical therapy, or intolerance to such therapy, or unavoidable allergen exposure.[185] The allergens used in immunotherapy are determined on the basis of a thorough diagnostic evaluation with immediate hypersensitivity skin tests or determination of the levels of specific IgE antibodies in the patient's serum. This evaluation has to be complemented by a meticulous exposure history and an assessment of the seasonality of the nasal symptoms so that the allergens that are *clinically* relevant are identified. Similar rules apply to the decision as to the doses of the allergenic extracts that will be used. Allergen immunotherapy is a safe form of treatment.[175, 186] Systemic anaphylactic reactions are infrequent and, most of the time, mild and easily manageable. Anaphylactic shock can, however, very rarely occur, and deaths from immunotherapy have been reported.[186] Therefore, health care providers who administer this treatment should be well trained in the management of anaphylaxis.[187, 188]

Because of the lack of any substantial understanding of the pathophysiology of any of the major nonallergic rhinitis syndromes, the management of this condition is poor.[89] In all of these syndromes, symptomatic treatment with antihistamines, decongestants, and ipratropium bromide could provide some help as long as the clinical presentation involves sneezing/pruritus, nasal congestion/

pressure, and excessive rhinorrhea, respectively.[189] In hyperplastic rhinosinusitis and in the nonallergic rhinitis with eosinophilia syndrome, nasal glucocorticosteroid treatment is indicated. The latter syndrome is highly responsive to nasal steroids, whereas a significant number of patients with hyperplastic inflammatory disease do not obtain adequate relief from these agents. In nonallergic, noninflammatory rhinopathy, nasal steroids are not indicated, and symptomatic treatment should be pursued. As mentioned earlier, defunctionalization of nasal nociceptors with the use of repetitive applications of capsaicin in the nasal mucosa may benefit patients with this syndrome.[148–154]

## THE PHARYNX

### Structure and Function

The pharyngeal airway extends caudally from the nasal choanae to the supraglottic space (see Fig. 42.2). Although it is surrounded by bony structures, (i.e., the cervical vertebrae, mandible, and hyoid bone), its caliber and function are modulated chiefly by the activity of the intrinsic muscles within the pharyngeal wall and the tongue and by the inframandibular and cervical strap muscles. The pharyngeal airway can be partitioned functionally into two segments: the nasopharyngeal segment, which ends at the rim of the soft palate, and the oropharyngeal and hypopharyngeal segment, which extends beyond this point to the aryepiglottic folds.

#### Nasopharynx

In the nasopharyngeal segment, the intrinsic muscles of the pharyngeal wall and the soft palate play major roles in deglutition, speech, and breathing.[190–194] Prescribed muscle recruitment patterns are required to perform each of these processes (see Table 42.1). An important function of these muscles is maintenance of palatal tension to prevent nasopharyngeal airflow obstruction during sleep.[9, 195, 196] Increases in tension also prevent prolapse of the tongue into the pharynx as it moves posteriorly against its ventral surface during sleep.[197, 198] A decline in the activity of the tensor veli palatini during sleep may predispose to the development of velopharyngeal obstruction in patients with sleep apnea. Another important function of the nasopharyngeal segment is its ability to adjust to allow high inspiratory and expiratory flows, particularly during exercise. This is achieved with changes in palatal and tongue position that take place when ventilation exceeds approximately 40 L/min during exercise. In this context, the nasopharynx also regulates partitioning of airflow during oronasal breathing.

#### Oropharynx

The oropharynx is composed of soft tissues and muscles (see Table 42.1), which permit a wide range of changes in its conformation and mechanical properties. This segment serves as a conduit for airflow into the lungs and for flow of liquids and solids into the esophagus. Despite similarities in the respiratory and digestive functions of the oropharynx, fundamentally different strategies have been adopted to facilitate flow into the respiratory and digestive systems. On the one hand, liquids and solids are actively propelled into the esophagus by constricting and foreshortening the oropharynx during the involuntary phase of swallowing. Constriction is due to localized increases in the pressure exerted by tissues surrounding the oropharynx. Air, on the other hand, flows passively through this segment as long as oropharyngeal patency is maintained by dilating muscles and supporting bony structures that reduce the pressures exerted by the surrounding tissues.[199–203] Thus, somewhat negative tissue pressures are required for air to flow to the lungs, whereas markedly positive tissue pressures are generated to propel food to the stomach.

Several reflexes are believed to play an important role in maintaining airway patency. Activity of the genioglossus and strap muscles begins just before the onset of inspiration.[1, 204] Moreover, recruitment of these muscles is augmented by chemical stimuli to ventilation, airway obstruction, negative intraluminal pressures, and the presence of flow in the upper airways.[6, 62, 205–213] Recruitment of these muscles ensures a patent pharyngeal airway when ventilatory drive is elevated.

Pharyngeal patency is modulated by the level of consciousness. Patency is poorly maintained, for example, during general anesthesia.[199, 200, 214, 215] Many centrally acting depressants, including anesthetic agents, sedatives, and alcohol, depress motor activity in these muscles.[216–225] During sleep, similar decreases in the activity of the genioglossus and strap muscles have been demonstrated, particularly during rapid eye movement sleep,[209, 226–236] which may be responsible for the development of airflow obstruction in obstructive sleep apnea. Regardless of the mechanism for this sleep-dependent decrease in neuromuscular activity, the resulting decreases in pharyngeal patency during anesthesia and sleep can have dramatic clinical consequences.[237]

### Airflow Obstruction in Obstructive Sleep Apnea

In patients with obstructive sleep apnea (see also Chapter 81), diminished pharyngeal patency during sleep leads to the development of airflow obstruction.[232, 238–241] Patients with this disorder exhibit recurrent periods of complete pharyngeal occlusion during sleep that often lead to oxyhemoglobin desaturation and arousals from sleep. In other patients, partial obstruction causes recurrent hypopnea often in association with oxyhemoglobin desaturations and arousals from sleep.[242–245] Less severe airflow obstruction may cause snoring without periodic apneas or hypopneas in otherwise asymptomatic individuals. Therefore, a spectrum of clinical disorders in pharyngeal function have been recognized that are associated with varying degrees of pharyngeal airflow obstruction during sleep.

Differences in the degree of airflow obstruction during sleep have been attributed to abnormalities in pharyngeal size,[197, 231, 246–248] compliance,[247, 249] collapsibility,[19, 21, 34, 198, 224, 225, 245, 250–255] and resistance.[232, 256–259] Although it is uncertain which of these mechanical properties accounts for the development of airflow obstruction, it is clear that the hypopneas and apneas are due to the development of inspiratory airflow limitation during sleep.[19, 21, 34, 198, 245, 250] A major finding is that airflow obstruction of increasing severity among these clinical groups is associated with progressively decreasing levels of maximal inspiratory airflow.

Previous studies have related these alterations in the level of $\dot{V}$Imax to changes in $P_{crit}$.[19, 34, 198, 245, 250] In patients with obstructive sleep apnea, a positive $P_{crit}$ accounts for the cessation of airflow (when $\dot{V}$Imax becomes zero, Equation 2). In contrast, reductions in $P_{crit}$ to subatmospheric levels of about $-5$ cm $H_2O$ increase $\dot{V}$Imax and resolve obstructive sleep apnea. Thus, current evidence indicates that the clinical manifestations of pharyngeal airflow obstruction are related to elevations in $P_{crit}$, which reflect increases in pharyngeal collapsibility.

As $P_{crit}$ rises toward the pressure upstream at the nares, maximal inspiratory airflow decreases (Equation 2). Conversely, when nasal pressure is lowered experimentally to subatmospheric levels, reductions in maximal inspiratory airflow have also been demonstrated.[19, 34] Reductions in upstream (nasal) pressure below $P_{crit}$ have been associated with periodic obstructive apneas, microarousals, and oxyhemoglobin desaturations, the hallmark polysomnographic features of the sleep apnea syndrome. These observations suggest that the level of $\dot{V}$Imax and the severity of pharyngeal airflow obstruction during sleep are related to the difference between the pressure at the nares and $P_{crit}$.

Based on these findings, two approaches can be adopted to treat patients with obstructive sleep apnea: First, nasal pressure can be increased and $\dot{V}$Imax restored by applying continuous positive airway pressure to the nose. As the level of nasal continuous positive airway pressure is increased, $\dot{V}$Imax progressively increases, which has been associated with diminished airflow obstruction and the amelioration of obstructive sleep apnea.[19, 224, 260–262] Second, steps can be undertaken to decrease $P_{crit}$. When $P_{crit}$ falls in patients with obstructive sleep apnea who lose weight[250] or undergo upper airway reconstructive surgery,[198] airflow ($\dot{V}$Imax) increases and sleep apnea remits. Decreases in $P_{crit}$ are also likely to account for improvements in airflow and apnea with changes in body posture[22, 254, 263–268] and with chemical stimulation of the pharyngeal and strap musculature.[196, 269–271] Thus, it is possible to treat obstructive sleep apnea by either raising the upstream pressure at the nares or by lowering $P_{crit}$. It is expected that new approaches to treating obstructive sleep apnea will result from specific structural[272] or neuromuscular maneuvers[196, 270, 273, 274] that decrease $P_{crit}$.

## Other Clinical Disorders

Only a few of the many causes of pharyngeal obstruction can be reviewed here, for illustrative purposes. Among the causes of gradually developing pharyngeal obstruction are pharyngeal stenosis from prior injury or inflammation and gross enlargement of the tonsils. A combination of enlarged tonsils and adenoids in childhood may result in severe airflow obstruction, particularly during sleep, with pulmonary edema or chronic alveolar hypoventilation, hypoxemia, and cor pulmonale.[275, 276] This syndrome rapidly reverses after tonsillectomy and adenoidectomy.

Infection in the tissues surrounding the pharynx may progress to severe obstruction with frightening speed. Patients with deep neck infections,[277] retropharyngeal abscess, or Ludwig's angina[278] need constant and careful observation. A fulminating course with progression to total airway obstruction may also occur in patients with trauma[279–281] from either external blows or intubation accidents. Foreign bodies in the pharynx or larynx are especially hazardous because these are so often overlooked.

# THE LARYNX

## Structure and Function

The larynx lies between the conducting airways of the lungs and the oronasal airway. In the hypopharynx, the air stream funnels into the larynx, where the cross-sectional area narrows. Skeletal support is principally provided by the thyroid and cricoid cartilages. Because the latter is the only ringed structure, the subglottis is particularly vulnerable to airway obstruction.

During inspiration, the cross-sectional area between the vocal cords widens.[282–286] This effect is augmented during deep inspiration.[287, 288] In contrast, the glottis narrows during expiration. This narrowing may retard expiratory airflow.[3, 4, 286, 289–301]

The movement of glottic structures is controlled by a number of muscles intrinsic to the larynx (Figs. 42.5 and 42.6).[286, 302] The thyroarytenoid, cricoarytenoid lateralis, interarytenoid, and aryepiglottic muscles close the glottis, whereas only the posterior cricoarytenoid is capable of abduction and glottic opening.[301] The cricothyroid muscles ordinarily stabilize the relative position of the thyroid and cricoid cartilages when the tracheobronchial tree lengthens during inspiration.[303] They are also capable of vocal fold elongation by approximating the anterior portions of the two cartilages. This occurs when singing high tones.

The laryngeal musculature is involved in the coordination of many important functions, including breathing, swallowing, coughing, phonating, and vomiting. To fulfill these roles, the central nervous system initiates and coordinates the neuromuscular control of glottic structures. In the glottis, the afferent pathway begins at numerous sensory nerve endings,[304–306] which return to the central nervous system primarily through the superior laryngeal nerves. Laryngeal feedback to the respiratory control centers modulates laryngeal function and the breathing pattern.[285, 307–309] Studies have demonstrated afferent fibers with single nerve recordings from the superior laryngeal nerve, which respond to alterations in intraluminal pressure, airflow, temperature, and laryngeal position.[310]

## Laryngeal Disorders

By virtue of the larynx's key role in breathing, swallowing, and speaking, a significant breakdown in any of its functions usually alters the performance of its other functions. The glottic aperture depends on vocal fold motion,[282–286] and the larynx is sheltered by supraglottic

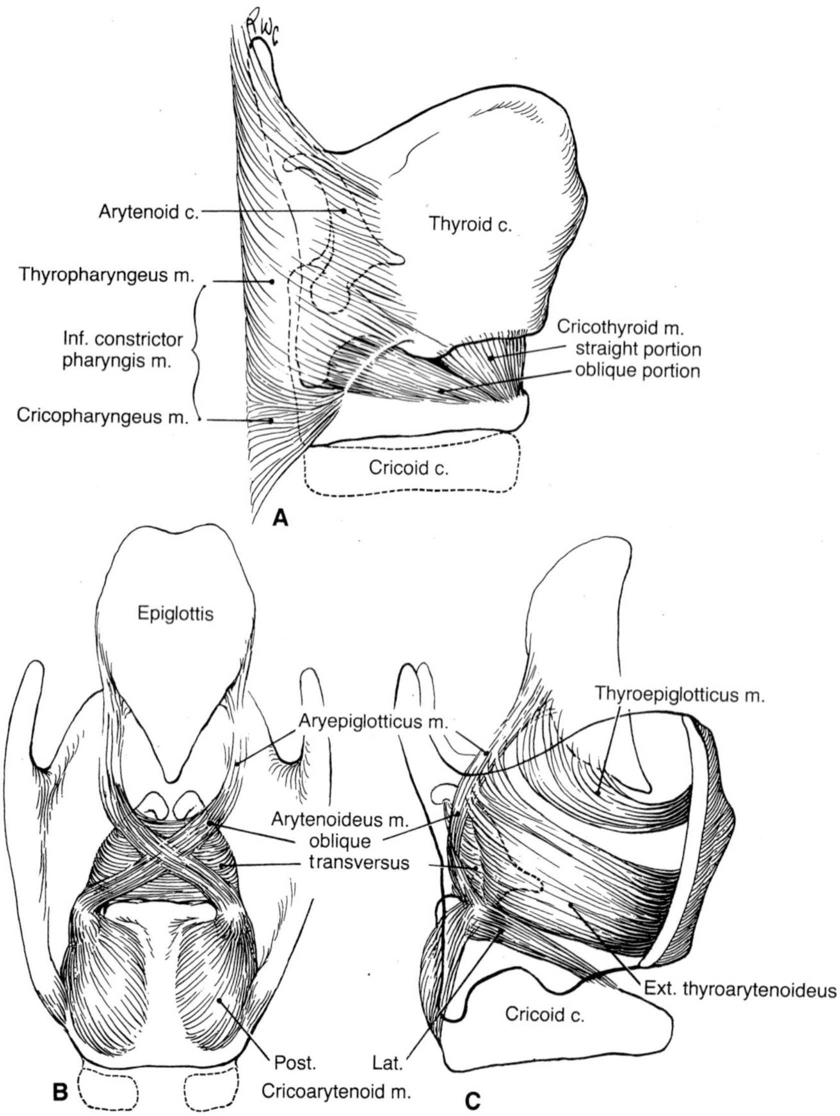


**Figure 42.5** Muscles of the larynx are shown from the right *(A)*, from behind *(B)*, and with the right side of the thyroid cartilage cut away *(C)*. Note in *A* that the cricothyroid muscle can act to draw the thyroid cartilage toward the cricoid and can draw the thyroid cartilage forward on the sliding cricothyroid joint. (From Proctor DF: Physiology of the upper airway. *In* Fenn WO, Rahn H (eds): Handbook of Physiology. Washington, DC: American Physiological Society, 1964.)

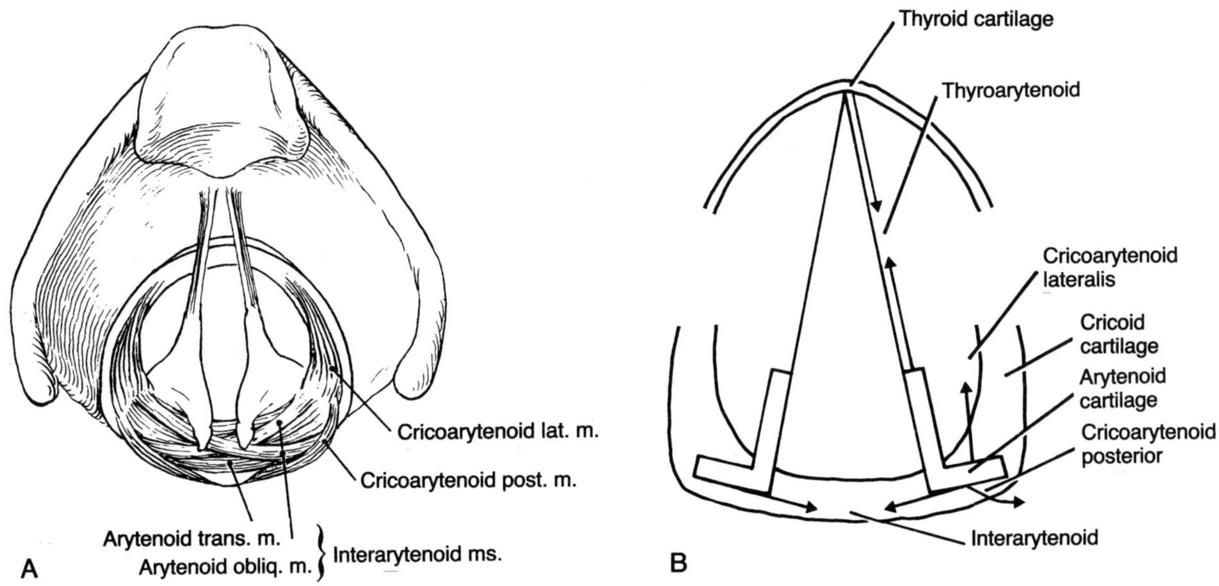


**Figure 42.6** The muscles involved in opening and closing the glottis are illustrated. *A*, The cricothyroid muscle is omitted. *B*, The action of these muscles is diagramed. (*B* from Proctor DF: Physiology of the upper airway. *In* Fenn WO, Rahn H (eds): Handbook of Physiology. Washington, DC: American Physiological Society, 1964.)

structures and supporting structures (false cords, epiglottis, the base of the tongue). Disorders of the larynx can result from dysfunction in any of its anatomic parts as well as of its sensorimotor coordination.

The history of a laryngeal disorder is often ambiguous because breathing difficulties often masquerade as a swallowing or voice disorder. Conversely, swallowing difficulties that result in failure to clear food particles from the throat may interfere with breathing. Airway obstruction is often marked by the complaint of shortened phrasing and excessively effortful speaking, singing, or both. Conversely, laryngeal complaints often reflect disorders of the pharynx or esophagus.

When airflow obstruction is confined to inspiration,[311] stridor may be present, and marked reductions in inspiratory airflow with well-preserved levels of expiratory airflow (extrathoracic airways obstruction) can be documented on flow-volume curves.[311–314] The plateau of inspiratory airflow over a wide range of inspiratory effort suggests that inspiratory airflow limitation is present.[315] In general, mid-vital capacity flow rates of 1.5 L/sec or greater on expiration and inspiration usually permits routine activities and moderate physical exertion.[311]

Fixed obstruction of the larynx or extrathoracic trachea produces roughly equal decrements in inspiratory and expiratory airflow. When the narrowing is severe, transmural pressures across the airways, upstream and downstream, fluctuate widely and can limit flow if airway collapsibility is increased. Spirometric findings in extrathoracic obstruction are discussed in Chapter 28.

Neuromuscular mechanisms appear to play an important role in the modulation of laryngeal patency in laryngeal disorders. Laryngeal airflow obstruction can result from either decreases in abductor activity or increases in adductor activity (see Table 42.1). Decreases in abductor activity account for the occurrence of inspiratory airflow obstruction in patients with unilateral and bilateral vocal cord paralysis, most often from damage to recurrent laryngeal nerves.[64, 316–319] When both recurrent laryngeal nerves are injured, the vocal cords move toward the midline (resulting from the action of the still active cricothyroid muscles). This may go unrecognized because hoarseness may be only slight, and the narrowed airway may still permit limited physical activity for years. Gradually, glottic airflow obstruction increases, and the diagnosis may be made 10 to 20 years later, at which point surgical intervention is necessary. Past history of a thyroidectomy is frequently elicited in these cases. Unilateral vocal cord paralysis[317] is diagnosed more frequently because, for unknown reasons, a patient with such a disorder is prone to aspiration and severe laryngospasm during sleep. In a significant percentage of patients, a search for the cause of this condition fails to uncover a specific etiology. Of course, the possibility of cervical or mediastinal malignancy or of aortic aneurysm encroaching on one recurrent laryngeal nerve (usually the left) must be considered.[64]

In other disorders, increases in vocal cord adductor activity can cause laryngeal airflow obstruction. this mechanism appears to account for the development of laryngospasm and of a curious disorder characterized by paradoxical movement of the vocal cords, also termed *vocal cord dysfunction* (see also Chapter 39).[320–326] In this disorder, active adduction of the vocal cords during inspiration occurs paroxysmally. Attacks are characterized by stridor, marked inspiratory effort, and dyspnea and are often mistaken for asthma. In contrast to asthma, however, these patients demonstrate paradoxical medial

**Table 42.3 DISORDERS ASSOCIATED WITH LARYNGEAL OBSTRUCTION**

| |
|---|
| May be associated with acute onset of obstruction |
| Anesthesia and other states of unconsciousness |
| Angioneurotic edema |
| Burns of the airway |
| Croup |
| Epiglottis |
| Foreign bodies |
| Infections involving surrounding structures |
| Deep neck infections |
| Ludwig's angina |
| Peritonsillar abscess |
| Retropharyngeal abscess |
| Intubation injury |
| Malfunction of muscles stabilizing the airways |
| Syphilitic gumma, tabes dorsalis |
| Laryngeal or tracheal trauma |
| Usually slowly developing obstruction |
| Arthritis cricoarytenoid joint |
| Enlarged tonsils and adenoids or laryngeal obstruction |
| Esophageal foreign body |
| Histiocytoma |
| Laryngeal carcinoma, papilloma, cartilaginous tumors, angioma, cystic hygroma, congenital malformations, polyp, granuloma |
| Malignant metastases to cervical glands |
| Neurologic disease |
| Relapsing polychondritis |
| Thyroid tumors, malignant and benign |
| Tracheal cyst, stenosis from cylindroma, tracheomalacia |
| Vocal cord paralysis |
| Unlikely to produce significant obstruction |
| Coccidiodomycosis |
| Cryptococcosis |
| Histiocytosis X |
| Histoplasmosis |
| Laryngeal cyst, granuloma, laryngocele, polyp |
| Lupus erythematosus |
| Rhabdomyosarcoma |
| Sarcoidosis |
| Tuberculosis |
| Unilateral vocal cord paralysis |

movement of the vocal cords during inspiration and a pattern of extrathoracic airway obstruction on flow-volume curves obtained during an attack.[327]

Laryngeal obstruction is also associated with many other conditions. These are listed in Table 42.3.

## References


1. Strohl K, Hensley M, Hallett M, et al: Activation of upper airway muscles before onset of inspiration in normal humans. J Appl Physiol 49:638–642, 1980.
2. Brancatisano T, Dodd D, Engel L: Responses of the posterior cricoarytenoid and alae nasi muscles to increased chemical drive in man. Respir Physiol 64:177–189, 1986.
3. Wyke B: Respiratory activity of intrinsic laryngeal muscles: An experimental study. *In* Wyke B.D. (ed): Ventilatory and Phonatory Control Systems. London: Oxford University Press, 1974, pp. 408–421.
4. Green J, Neil E: The respiratory function of the laryngeal muscles. J Physiol 129:134–141, 1955.
5. Mann D, Sasaki C, Suzuki M, et al: Dilator naris muscle. Ann Otol Rhinol Laryngol 86:362–372, 1977.
6. Brouillette R, Thach B: Control of genioglossus muscle inspiratory activity. J Appl Physiol 49:801–808, 1980.
7. Patrick G, Strohl K, Rubin S, et al: Upper airway diaphragm muscle responses to chemical stimulation and loading. J Appl Physiol 53:1133–1137, 1982.
8. Roberts J, Reed W, Thach B: Pharyngeal airway-stabilizing function of sternohyoid and sternothyroid muscles in the rabbit. J Appl Physiol 57:1790–1795, 1984.
9. Weiner D, Mitra J, Salamone J, et al: Effect of chemical stimuli on nerves supplying upper airway muscles. J Appl Physiol 52:530–536, 1982.
10. Cole P, Forsyth R, Haight J: Effects of cold air and exercise on nasal patency. Ann Otol Rhinol Laryngol 92:196–198, 1983.
11. Cole P, Haight J, Love L, et al: Dynamic components of nasal resistance. Am Rev Respir Dis 132:1229–1232, 1985.
12. Kirsten E, St John W: A feline decerebration technique with low mortality and long-term homeostasis. J Pharmacol Methods 1:263–268, 1978.
13. Van Lunteren E, Haxhiu M, Cherniack N: Relation between upper airway volume and hyoid muscle length. J Appl Physiol 63:1443–1449, 1987.
14. Pertuze J, Watson A, Pride N: Maximum airflow through the nose in humans. J Appl Physiol 70:1369–1376, 1991.
15. Bridger G, Proctor D: Maxium nasal inspiratory flow and nasal resistance. Ann Otol Rhinol Laryngol 79:481–488, 1970.
16. Permutt S, Riley R: Hemodynamics of collapsible vessels with tone. J Appl Physiol 18:924–932, 1963.
17. Permutt S, Bromberger-Barnea B, Bane B: Alveolar pressure, pulmonary venous pressure, and the vascular waterfall. Med Thorac 19:239–260, 1962.
18. Proctor D: The naso-oro-pharyngo-laryngeal airway. Eur J Respir Dis 64(Suppl 128):89–96, 1983.
19. Smith P, Wise R, Gold A, et al: Upper airway pressure-flow relationships in obstructive sleep apnea. J Appl Physiol 64:789–795, 1988.
20. Liistro G, Stanescu D, Veriter C, et al: Pattern of snoring in obstructive sleep apnea patients and in heavy snorers. Sleep 14:517–525, 1991.
21. Schwartz A, Smith P, Wise R, et al: Effects of nasal pressure on upper airway pressure flow relationships. J Appl Physiol 1989:1626–1634, 1989.
22. Liistro G, Stanescu D, Dooms G, et al: Head position modifies upper airway resistance in men. J Appl Physiol 64:1285–1288, 1988.
23. Koenig J, Thach B: Effects of mass loading on the upper airway. J Appl Physiol 64:2294–2299, 1988.
24. Sullivan K, Chang H: Steady and oscillatory transnasal pressure-flow relationships in healthy adults. J Appl Physiol 71:983–992, 1991.
25. Olson L, Fouke J, Hoekje P, et al: A biomedical view of upper airway function. *In* Mathew O. (ed): Respiratory Function of the Upper Airway. New York: Marcel Dekker, 1988, pp 359–389.
26. Wheatley J, Amis T, Engel L: Nasal and oral airway pressure-flow relationships. J Appl Physiol 71:2317–2324, 1991.
27. Tully A, Brancatisano A, Loring S, et al: Influence of posterior cricoarytenoid muscle activity on pressure-flow relationship of the larynx. J Appl Physiol 70:2252–2258, 1991.
28. Guyton A, Adkins Z: Quantitative aspects of the collapse factor in relationship to venous return. Am J Physiol 177:523–527, 1954.
29. Pride N, Permutt S, Riley R, et al: Determinants of maximal expiratory flow from the lungs. J Appl Physiol 23:646–662, 1967.
30. Schwartz A, Smith P, Wise R, et al: Effect of pressure loads on upper airway collapsibility in obstructive sleep apnea. Am Rev Respir Dis 135:A183, 1987.
31. Smaldone G, Bergofsky E: Delineation of flow-limiting segment and predicted airway resistance by moving catheter. J Appl Physiol 40:943–952, 1976.
32. Smaldone G, Smith P: Location of flow-limiting segments via air-

way catheters near RV in human subjects. J Appl Physiol 59:502–508, 1985.
33. Green J: Fundamental cardiovascular and pulmonary physiology. *In* Green J (ed): An Integrated Approach for Medicine. Philadelphia: Lea & Febiger, 1982, pp 10–13.
34. Schwartz A, Smith P, Wise R, et al: Induction of upper airway occlusion in sleeping individuals with subatmospheric nasal pressure. J Appl Physiol 64:535–542, 1988.
35. Haight J, Cole P: The site and function of the nasal valve. Laryngoscope 93:49–55, 1983.
36. Swift D, Proctor D: Access of air to the respiratory tract. *In* Brain J, Proctor D, Reid L (eds): Respiratory Defense Mechanisms, Part I. New York: Marcel Dekker, 1977, pp 63–93.
37. Morgan K, Monticello T: Airflow-gas deposition, and lesion distribution in the nasal passages. Environ Health Perspect 88:209–218, 1990.
38. Andersen I, Lundqvist G, Jensen P, et al: Human response to 78-hour exposure to dry air. Arch Environ Health 9:319–324, 1974.
39. Anggard A: Parasympathetic influence on the nasal mucosa. Acta Otolaryngol 83:22–24, 1977.
40. Anggard A, Strandberg K: Vascular effects of the slow reacting substance (SRS) in the cat nasal mucosa and the appearance of a SRS-like principle in cat nasal secretion on nerve stimulation. Acta Physiol Scand 111:329–333, 1981.
41. Anggard A, Lundberg JM, Lundblad L: Nasal autonomic innervation with special reference to peptidergic nerves. Eur J Respir Dis 64:143–149, 1983.
42. Batson O: The venous networks of the nasal mucosa. Ann Otol Rhinol Laryngol 63:571–580, 1954.
43. Bosma J, Showacre J: Development of upper respiratory anatomy and function. Washington, DC: National Institutes of Health, 1976.
44. Bosma J, Donner M: Physiology of the pharynx. *In* Paparella M, Shumrick D (eds): Otolaryngology (2nd ed.) Philadelphia: WB Saunders, 1980, pp 332–345.
45. Cauna N: Blood and nerve supply of the nasal lining. *In* Proctor DF, Andersen IB (eds): The Nose. Oxford: Elsevier Biomedical Press, 1982, pp 44–69.
46. Cole P: Upper respiratory airflow. *In* Proctor D, Andersen I (eds): The Nose: Upper Airway Physiology and the Atmospheric Environment. Amsterdam: Elsevier Biomedical Press, 1982, pp 163–190.
47. Cole P: Modification of inspired air. *In* Proctor DF, Andersen IB (eds): The Nose: Upper Airway Physiology and the Atmospheric Environment. Oxford: Elsevier Biomedical Press, 1982, pp 351–376.
48. Dawes J, Prichard M: Studies of the vascular arrangements of the nose. Am J Anat 87:311–325, 1953.
49. Eccles R: Neurological and pharmacological considerations. *In* Proctor DF, Andersen I (eds): The Nose: Upper Airway Physiology and the Atmospheric Environment. Oxford: Elsevier Biomedical Press, 1982, pp 191–214.
50. Ingelstedt S, Toremalm N: Airflow patterns and heat transfer within the respiratory tract. Acta Physiol Scand 51:204–217, 1960.
51. Proctor D: The upper airways I. Nasal physiology and defense of the lungs. Am Rev Respir Dis 115:97–130, 1977.
52. Proctor D, Andersen I: The fate and effects of inhaled materials. *In* Proctor D, Andersen I (eds): The Nose: Upper Airway Physiology and the Atmospheric Environment. Amsterdam: Elsevier Biomedical Press, 1982, pp 423–456.
53. Bau S, Aspin N, Wood D, et al: Measurement of fluid deposition in humans following mist tent therapy. Pediatrics 48:605–612, 1971.
54. Baumann A, Masing H: Uber den einfluss korperlicher arbeit auf den Nasenwiderstand. Laryngol Rhinol Otol 49:264–270, 1970.
55. Swindle P: The architecture of the blood vascular networks in the erectile and secretory lining of the nasal passages. Ann Otol Rhinol Laryngol 44:913–932, 1935.
56. Strohl K, O'Cain C, Slutsky A: Alae nasi activation and nasal resistance in healthy subjects. J Appl Physiol 52:1432–1437, 1982.
57. Suratt P, McTier R, Wilhoit S: Alae nasi electromyographic activity and timing in obstructive sleep apnea. J Appl Physiol 58:1252–1256, 1985.
58. Carlo W, Martin R, Abboud E, et al: Effect of sleep state and hypercapnia on alae nasi and diaphragm EMGs in preterm infants. J Appl Physiol 54:1590–1596, 1983.
59. Brancatisano A, Engel L: Role of the upper airway in the control of respiratory flow and lung volume in humans. *In* Mathew O, Sant'Ambrogio G (eds): Respiratory Function of the Upper Airway. New York: Marcel Dekker, 1988, pp 447–517.
60. Wheatley J, Amis T, Engel L: Relationship between alae nasi activation and breathing route during exercise in humans. J Appl Physiol 71:118–124, 1991.
61. Dallimore N, Eccles R: Changes in human nasal resistance associated with exercise, hyperventilation and rebreathing. Acta Otolaryngol 84:416–421, 1977.
62. Van Lunteren E, Van de Graff W, Parker D, et al: Nasal and laryngeal reflex responses to negative upper airway pressure. J Appl Physiol 56:746–752, 1984.
63. Forsyth R, Cole P, Shephard R: Exercise and nasal patency. J Appl Physiol 55:860–865, 1983.
64. Parnell F, Brandeburg J: Vocal cord paralysis: A review of 100 cases. Laryngoscope 80:1036–1045, 1970.
65. Bartlett D: Effects of hypercapnia and hypoxia on laryngeal resistance to airflow. Respir Physiol 37:293–302, 1979.
66. Miller R, Hyatt R: Obstructing lesions of the larynx and trachea: Clinical and physiologic characteristics. Proc Mayo Clin 44:145–161, 1969.
67. Tos M: Goblet cells and glands in the nose and paranasal sinuses. *In* Proctor DF, Andersen IB (eds): The Nose: Upper Airway Physiology and the Atmospheric Environment. Amsterdam: Elsevier Biomedical Press B.V., 1982, pp 99–144.
68. Watanabe K, Watanabe I: The ultrastructural characteristics of the capillary walls in human nasal mucosa. Rhinology 18:183–195, 1980.
69. Burnham HH: An anatomical investigation of blood vessels of the lateral nasal wall and their relation to turbinates and sinuses. J Laryngol Otol 50:569–593, 1935.
70. Cauna N: Fine structure of the arteriovenous anastomosis and its nerve supply in the human nasal respiratory mucosa. Anat Rec 168:9–22, 1970.
71. Cauna N, Hinderer K, Wentges R: Sensory receptor organs of the human nasal respiratory mucosa. Am J Anat 124:187–210, 1969.
72. Brandtzaeg P: Immunocompetent cells of the upper airway: Functions in normal and diseased mucosa. Eur Arch Oto-Rhino-Laryngol 252:S8–S21, 1995.
73. Raphael G, Jeney E, Baraniuk J, et al: Pathophysiology of rhinitis: Lactoferrin and lysozyme in nasal secretions. J Clin Invest 84:1528–1535, 1989.
74. Peden D, Swiersz M, Ohkubo K, et al: Nasal secretion of the ozone scavenger uric acid. Am Rev Respir Dis 148:455–461, 1993.
75. Lundberg J, Rinder J, Weitzberg E, et al: Nasally exhaled nitric oxide in humans originates mainly in the paranasal sinuses. Acta Physiol Scand 152:431–432, 1994.
76. Lundberg J, Farkas-Szallasi T, Wetzberg E, et al: High nitric oxide production in human paranasal sinuses. Nature Medicine 1:370–373, 1995.
77. Lundberg J, Lundberg J, Settergren G, et al: Nitric oxide, produced in the upper airways, may act in an "aerocrine" fashion to enhance pulmonary oxygen uptake in humans. Acta Physiol Scand 155:467–469, 1995.
78. Meng O, Springall D, Bishop A, et al: Lack of inducible nitric oxide synthase in bronchial epithelium: A possible mechanism of susceptibility to infection in cystic fibrosis. J Pathol 184:323–331, 1998.
79. Sanders SP, Siekierski ES, Porter JD, et al: Nitric oxide inhibits rhinovirus-induced cytokine production and viral replication in a human respiratory epithelial cell line. J Virol 72:934–942, 1998.
80. Hogman M, Frostell C, Hedenstrom H, et al: Inhalation of nitric oxide modulates adult human bronchial tone. Am Rev Respir Dis 148:1474–1478, 1993.
81. Anderson S, Togias A: Dry air and hyperosmolar challenge in asthma and rhinitis. *In* Busse W, Holgate S (eds): Asthma and Rhinitis. Boston: Blackwell, 1995, pp 1178–1195.
82. Anderson S: Is there a unifying hypothesis for exercise-induced asthma? J Allergy Clin Immunol 73:660–665, 1984.
83. Anderson S, Daviskas E, Smith C: Exercise-induced asthma: A difference in opinion regarding the stimulus. Allergy Proc 10:215–226, 1989.

84. Anderson S: Exercise-induced asthma. *In* O'Byrne P, Thompson N (eds): Manual of Asthma Management. Ca, Ltd.: WB Saunders Co., Ltd., 1995, pp 621–643.
85. McFadden E, Denison D, Waller J, et al: Direct recordings of the temperatures in the tracheobronchial tree in normal man. J Clin Invest 69:700–705, 1982.
86. McFadden E, Lenner K, Strohl K: Postexertional airway rewarming and thermally induced asthma. J Clin Invest 78:18–25, 1986.
87. Shturman-Ellstein R, Zeballos R, Buckley J, et al: The beneficial effect of nasal breathing on exercise-induced bronchoconstriction. Am Rev Respir Dis 118:65–73, 1978.
88. Griffin M, McFadden E, Ingram R: Airway cooling in asthmatic and nonasthmatic subjects during nasal and oral breathing. J Allergy Clin Immunol 69:354–359, 1982.
89. Togias A: Non-allergic rhinitis. *In* Mygind N, Naclerio R, Durham S (eds): Rhinitis. New York: Marcel Dekker, 1998, pp 383–399.
90. Zeiger RS: Allergic and nonallergic rhinitis: Classification and pathogenesis: Part II. nonallergic rhinitis. Am J Rhinol 3:113–139, 1989.
91. Sibbald B, Rink E: Epidemiology of seasonal and perennial rhinitis: Clinical presentation and medical history. Thorax 46:895–901, 1991.
92. Nathan R, Meltzer E, Selner J, et al: Prevalence of allergic rhinitis in the United States. J Allergy Clin Immunol 99:808–814, 1997.
93. Smith JM: Epidemiology. *In* Mygind N, Naclerio RM, Durham S (eds): Rhinitis. New York: Marcel Dekker, 1998, pp 29–44.
94. Malone D, Lawson K, Smith D, et al: A cost of illness study of allergic rhinitis in the United States. J Allergy Clin Immunol 99:22–27, 1997.
95. Storms W, Meltzer E, Nathan R, et al: The economic impact of allergic rhinitis. J Allergy Clin Immunol 99(Suppl):820–824, 1997.
96. Peebles R, Togias A: Role of mast cells and basophils in rhinitis. *In* Marone G (ed): Chemical Immunology, Human Basophils and Mast Cells—Clinical Aspects, Chemical Immunology. Switzerland; S. Karger AG, Basel Medical and Scientific Publishers, 1995, pp 60–83.
97. McNeil H, Austen KF: Biology of mast cell. *In* Frank MM, Austen KF, Claman HN, et al (eds): Samter's Immunologic Diseases (5th ed): Boston: Little Brown and Company, 1995, pp 185–204.
98. Ichimura K, Jackson R: H1 and H2 histamine receptors in the in vitro nasal mucosa. Acta Otolaryngol 99:610–619, 1985.
99. Okayama M, Baraniuk J, Hausfeld J, et al: Characterization and autoradiographic localization of histamine H1 receptors on human nasal turbinates. J Allergy Clin Immunol 89:1144–1150, 1992.
100. Secher C, Kirkegaard J, Borum P, et al: Significance of H1 and H2 receptors in the human nose: Rationale for topical use of combined antihistamine preparations. J Allergy Clin Immunol 70:211–218, 1982.
101. Naclerio R, Proud D, Togias A, et al: Inflammatory mediators in late antigen-induced rhinitis. N Engl J Med 313:65–70, 1985.
102. Peebles R, Togias A: Late-phase reactions in the nose. *In* Kay AB (ed): Allergy and Allergic Diseases. Oxford, England: Blackwell Science, 1997, pp 1139–1160.
103. Pipkorn U, Proud D, Lichtenstein L, et al: Inhibition of mediator release in allergic rhinitis by pretreatment with topical glucocorticoids. N Engl J Med 316:1506–1510, 1987.
104. Pipkorn U, Proud D, Lichtenstein L, et al: Effect of short-term systemic glucocorticoid treatment on human nasal mediator release after antigen challenge. J Clin Invest 80:957–961, 1987.
105. Bascom R, Pipkorn U, Lichtenstein L, et al: The influx of inflammatory cells into nasal washings during the late response to antigen challenge. Effect of steroid pretreatment. Am Rev Respir Dis 138:406–412, 1988.
106. Bascom R, Wachs M, Naclerio R, et al: Basophil influx occurs after nasal antigen challenge: Effects of topical corticosteroid pretreatment. J Allergy Clin Immunol 81:580–589, 1988.
107. Iliopoulos O, Proud D, Adkinson N, et al: Effects of immunotherapy on the early, late and rechallenge nasal reaction to provocation with allergen: Changes in inflammatory mediators and cells. J Allergy Clin Immunol 87:855–866, 1991.
108. Varney V, Jacobson M, Sudderick R, et al: Immunohistology of the nasal mucosa following allergen-induced rhinitis. Am Rev Respir Dis 146:170–176, 1992.
109. Lim M, Taylor R, Naclerio R: The histology of allergic rhinitis and its comparison to cellular changes in nasal lavages. Am J Respir Crit Care Med 151:136–144, 1995.
110. Igarashi Y, Goldrich M, Kaliner M, et al: Quantitation of inflammatory cells in the nasal mucosa of patients with allergic rhinitis and normal subjects. J Allergy Clin Immunol 95:716–725, 1995.
111. Ryan J: Interleukin-4 and its receptor: Essential mediators of the allergic response. J Allergy Clin Immunol 99:1–5, 1997.
112. de Vries J, Carballido J, Aversa G: Receptors and cytokines involved in allergic TH2 cell responses. J Allergy Clin Immunol 103:S492–S496, 1999.
113. Bagley C, Lopez A, Vadas M: New frontiers for IL-5. J Allergy Clin Immunol 99:725–718, 1997.
114. MacDonald S, Rafnar T, Langdon J, et al: Molecular identification of an IgE-dependent histamine-releasing factor. Science 269:688–690, 1995.
115. MacDonald S: Human recombinant histamine-releasing factor. Int Arch Allergy Immunol 113:187–189, 1997.
116. Connell J: Quantitative intranasal pollen challenges: III. The priming effect in allergic rhinitis. J Allergy 43:33–44, 1969.
117. Diemer FB, Sanico AM, Horowitz E, et al: Non-allergenic inhalant triggers in seasonal and perennial allergic rhinitis. J Allergy Clin Immunol 103:S2, 1999.
118. Wachs M, Proud D, Lichtenstein L, et al: Observations on the pathogenesis of nasal priming. J Allergy Clin Immunol 84:492–501, 1989.
119. Walden S, Proud D, Lichtenstein L, et al: Antigen-provoked increase in histamine reactivity: Observations on mechanisms. Am Rev Respir Dis 143:642–648, 1991.
120. Baroody F, Cruz A, Lichtenstein L, et al: Intranasal beclomethasone inhibits antigen-induced nasal hyperresponsivess to histamine. J Allergy Clin Immunol 90:373–376, 1992.
121. Sanico A, Togias A: Neuronal dysfunction and its role in rhinitis. *In* Oehling AK, Lopez JGH (eds): Proceedings of the ICACI XVI/EAACI 97. Seattle: Hogrefe and Huber, 1997, pp 185–190.
122. Sanico AM, Koliatsos VE, Stanisz AM, et al: Neural hyperresponsiveness and nerve growth factor in allergic rhinitis. Int Arch Allergy Immunol 118:153–158, 1999.
123. Riccio M, Proud D: Evidence that enhanced nasal reactivity to bradykinin in patients with symptomatic allergy is mediated by neural reflexes. J Allergy Clin Immunol 97:1252–1263, 1996.
124. Sanico A, Philip G, Proud D, et al: Comparison of nasal mucosal responsiveness to neuronal stimulation in nonallergic and allergic rhinitis: Effects of capsaicin nasal challenge. Clin Exp Allergy 28:92–100, 1998.
125. Sanico AM, Philip G, Lai G, et al: Hyperosmolar saline induces reflex nasal secretions, evincing neural hyperresponsiveness in allergic rhinitis. J Appl Physiol 86(4):1202–1210, 1999.
126. Harlin S, Ansel D, Lane S, et al: A clinical and pathologic study of chronic sinusitis: The role of the eosinophil. J Allergy Clin Immunol 81:867–875, 1988.
127. Hamilos D, Leung D, Wood R, et al: Chronic hyperplastic sinusitis: Association of tissue eosinophilia with mRNA expression of granulocyte-macrophage colony-stimulating factor and interleukin-3. J Allergy Clin Immunol 92:39–48, 1993.
128. Hamilos D, Leung D, Wood R, et al: Eosinophil infiltration in nonallergic chronic hyperplastic sinusitis with nasal polyposis (CHS/NP) is associated with endothelial VCAM-1 upregulation and expression of TNF-α. Am J Respir Cell Mol Biol 15:443–450, 1996.
129. Hamilos D, Plout M, Leung D, et al: GM-CSF, IL-5 and RANTES mRNA expression and protein levels in chronic hyperplastic sinusitis with nasal polyposis. J Allergy Clin Immunol 99:S130, 1997.
130. Ghaffar O, Durham S, Al-Ghamdi K, et al: Expression of IgE heavy chain transcripts in the sinus mucosa of atopic and nonatopic patients with chronic sinusitis. Am J Respir Cell Mol Biol 18:706–711, 1998.
131. Shimomura A, Ikeda K, Susuki H, et al: Expression of adhesion molecules in nonallergic chronic sinusitis. Laryngoscope 107:1519–1524, 1997.
132. Okuda M, Pawankar R: Characteristics of human nasal lympho-

cytes in perennial allergic rhinitis in comparison with chronic non-allergic hypertrophic rhinitis. J Allergy Clin Immunol 91:185, 1993.
133. Hamilos D, Leung D, Wood R, et al: Evidence for distinct cytokine expression in allergic versus nonallergic chromic sinusitis. J Allergy Clin Immunol 96:537–544, 1995.
134. Suzuki H, Takahashi Y, Wataya H, et al: Mechanisms of neutrophil recruitment induced by IL-8 in chronic sinusitis. J Allergy Clin Immunol 98:659–670, 1996.
135. Chester AC: Chronic sinusitis. Am Fam Physician 15:877–887, 1996.
136. Druce H, Rutledge J: Chronic sinusitis and rhinitis. Am J Rhinol 3:163–166, 1989.
137. Jacobs R, Freedman P, Boswell R: Nonallergic rhinitis with eosinphilia (NARES syndrome). J Allergy Clin Immunol 67:253–262, 1981.
138. Mullarkey M, Hill J, Webb D: Allergic and nonallergic rhinitis: Their characterization with attention to the meaning of nasal eosinophilia. J Allergy Clin Immunol 65:122–126, 1980.
139. Rupp G, Friedman P: Eosinophilic nonallergic rhinitis in children. Pediatrics 70:437–439, 1982.
140. Moneret-Vautrin D, Hsieh V, Wayoff M, et al: Nonallergic rhinitis with eosinophilia syndrome a precursor of the triad: Nasal polyposis, intrinsic asthma, and intolerance to aspirin. Ann Allergy 64:513–518, 1990.
141. Ward G, Rose G, Karlsson G, et al: Trichophyton asthma: Sensitisation of bronchi and upper airways to dermatophyte antigen. Lancet i:859–862, 1989.
142. Blom H, Godthelp T, Fokkens W, et al: Mast cells, eosinophils and IgE-positive cells in the nasal mucosa of patients with vasomotor rhinitis. Eur Arch Oto-Rhino-Laryngol 252:533–539, 1995.
143. Blom H, Godthelp T, Fokkens W, et al: The effect of nasal steroid aqueous spray on nasal complaint scores and cellular infiltrates in the nasal mucosa of patients with nonallergic, noninfectious perennial rhinitis. J Allergy Clin Immunol 100:739–747, 1997.
144. Ali M, Gaumond E, Yuta A, et al: Nonallergic rhinitis (NAR) of chronic fatigue syndrome (CFS). J Allergy Clin Immunol 99:S420, 1997.
145. Yuta A, Fujita K, Shimizu T, et al: Elastase in nasal lavage of cystic fibrosis and chronic fatigue syndrome (CFS) subjects with nonallergic rhinitis (NAR) J Allergy Clin Immunol 99:S420, 1997.
146. Borum P: Nasal methacholine challenge: A test for the measurement of nasal reactivity. J Allergy Clin Immunol 63:253–257, 1979.
147. Cook J, Hamilton J, Jones A: The diving reflex in non-eosinophilic non-allergic rhinitis. Clin Otolaryngol 21:226–227, 1996.
148. Wolf G, Andenhuber W, Hauser-Kronberger C, et al: Treatment of non-specific rhinopathy with capsaicin. Laryngorhinootologie 74:289–293, 1995.
149. Lacroix J, Buvelot J, Polla B, et al: Improvement of symptoms of non-allergic chronic rhinitis by local treatment with capsaicin. Clin Exp Allergy 21:595–700, 1991.
150. Rajakulasingam K, Howarth P: Topical capsaicin therapy in chronic rhinitis: A way forward? Clin and Exp Allergy 21:531–532, 1991.
151. Marabini S, Ciabatti P, Polli G, et al: Beneficial effects of intranasal applications of capsaicin in patients with vasomotor rhinitis. Eur Arch Otorhinolaryngol 248:191–194, 1991.
152. Stjarne P, Lundblad L, Anggard A, et al: Local capsaicin treatment of the nasal mucosa reduces symptoms in patients with nonallergic nasal hyperreactivity. Am J Rhinol 5:145–151, 1991.
153. Filiaci F, Zambetti G, Ciofalo A, et al: Local treatment of aspecific nasal hyperreactivity with capsaicin. Allergol Immunopathol 22:264–268, 1994.
154. Blom HM, Van Rijswijk JB, Garrelds IM, et al: Intranasal capsaicin is efficacious in non-allergic, non-infectious perennial rhinitis. A placebo-controlled study. Clin Exp Allergy 27:796–801, 1997.
155. Simons F, Simons K: The pharmacology and use of $H_1$-receptor-antagonist drugs. N Engl J Med 330:1663–1670, 1994.
156. Simons FE, Fraser TG, Maher J, et al: Central nervous system effects if $H_1$ receptor antagonists in the elderly. Ann Allergy Asthma Immunol 82:157–160, 1999.
157. Day J, Briscoe M, Widlitz M: Cetirizine, loratadine, or placebo in subjects with seasonal allergic rhinitis: Effects after controlled ragweed pollen challenge in an environmental exposure unit. J Allergy Clin Immunol 101:638–645, 1998.
158. Meltzer E, Weiler J, Widlitz M: Comparative outdoor study of the efficacy onset and duration of action, and safety of cetirizine, loratadine, and placebo for seasonal allergic rhinitis. J Allergy Clin Immunol 97:617–626, 1996.
159. Anggard A, Malm L: Orally administered decongestant drugs in disorders of the upper respiratory passages: A survey of clinical results. Clin Otolaryngol 9:43–49, 1984.
160. Kaiser H, Findlay S, Georgitis J, et al: Long-term treatment of perennial allergic rhinitis with ipratropium bromide nasal spray 0.06%. J Allergy Clin Immunol 95:1128–1132, 1995.
161. Naclerio R: Allergic rhinitis. N Engl J Med 325:860–869, 1991.
162. Mabry R: Uses and misuses of intranasal corticosteroids and cromolyn. Am J Rhinol 5:121–124, 1991.
163. Pipkorn U: Effect of topical glucocorticoid treatment on nasal mucosal mast cells in allergic rhinitis. J Allergy 38:125–129, 1983.
164. Pipkorn U, Hammarlund A, Enerback L: Prolonged treatment with topical glucocorticoids results in an inhibition of the allergen-induced weal-and-flare response and a reduction in skin mast cell numbers and histamine content. Clin & Exp Allergy 19:19–25, 1989.
165. Cheng C, Baroody F, Reed K, et al: Effects of one year treatment with fluticasone propionate aquenous nasal spray (FPANS) and terfenadine (TER) on the nasal mucosa: I. A safety study using electron and light microscopy. J Allergy Clin Immunol 99:S497, 1997.
166. Baroody F, Rouadi P, Driscoll P: Intranasal beclomethasone reduces allergen-induced symptoms and superficial mucosal eosinophilia without affecting submucosal inflammation. Am J Respir Crit Care Med 157:899–906, 1998.
167. Andersson M, Andersson P, Pipkorn U: Allergen-induced specific and non-specific nasal reactions. Reciprocal relationship and inhibition by topical glucocorticosteroids. Acta Otolaryngol 107:270–277, 1989.
168. Juniper E, Guyatt G, O'Bryne P, et al: Aqueous beclomethasone diproprionate nasal spray: Regular versus "as required" use in the treatment of seasonal allergic rhinitis. J Allergy Clin Immunol 86:380–386, 1990.
169. Holopainen E, Malmberg H, Binder E: Long-term follow-up intra-nasal beclomethasone treatment. A clinical and histologic study. Acta Otolaryngol 386:270–2273, 1982.
170. Knight A, Kolin A: Long term efficacy and safety of beclomethasone dipropionate aerosol in perennial rhinitis. Ann Allergy 50:81–84, 1983.
171. Knutsson U, Stierna P, Marcus C, et al: Effects of intranasal glucocorticoids on endogenous glucocorticoid peripheral and central function. J Endocrinol 144:301–310, 1995.
172. Wilson A, McFarlane L, Lipworth B: Effects of repeated once daily dosing of three intranasal corticosteroids on basal and dynamic measures of hypothalamic-pituitary-adrenal-axis activity. J Allergy Clin Immunol 101:470–474, 1998.
173. Lichtenstein L, Norman P, Winkenwerder W: A single year of immunotherapy for ragweed hay fever. Ann Intern Med 75:663–671, 1971.
174. Norman P: Immunotherapy for nasal allergy. J Allergy Clin Immunol 81:992–996, 1988.
175. Norman P: Safety of allergen immunotherapy. J Allergy Clin Immunol 84:439, 1989.
176. Furin M, Norman P, Creticos P, et al: Immunotherapy decreases antigen-induced eosinophil migration into the nasal cavity. J Allergy Clin Immunol 88:27–32, 1991.
177. Naclerio R, Proud D, Moylan B, et al: Clinical aspects of allergic diseases: A double-blind study of the discontinuation of ragweed immunotherapy. J Allergy Clin Immunol 100:293–300, 1997.
178. Bousquet J, Lockey R, Malling H-J: Allergen immunotherapy: Therapeutic vaccines for allergic diseases: A WHO position paper. J Allergy Clin Immunol 102:558–562, 1998.
179. Gleich J, Zimmermann B, Henderson L, et al: Effects of immunotherapy on immunoglobulin E and immunoglobulin G antibodies to ragweed antigens: A six year prospective study. J Allergy Clin Immunol 70:261–271, 1982.

180. Djurup R, Osterball O: IgG subclass antibody response in grass pollen-allergic patients undergoing specific immunotherapy. Allergy 39:433–441, 1984.
181. Varney V, Hamid Q, Gaga M, et al: Influence of grass pollen immunotherapy on cellular infiltration and cytokine mRNA expression during allergen-induced late phase-cutaneous responses. J Clin Invest 92:644–51, 1993.
182. Secrist H, Chelan C, Wen Y, et al: Allergen immunotherapy decreases interleukin 4 production in CD4+ Tells from allergic individuals. J Exp Med 178:2123–30, 1993.
183. Durham S, Ying S, Varney V, et al: Grass pollen immunotherapy inhibits allergen-induced infiltration of CDA4$^+$T lymphocytes and eosinophils in the nasal mucosa and increases the number of cells expressing messenger RNA for interferon-$\gamma$. J Allergy Clin Immunol 97:1356–1365, 1996.
184. Durham S, Till S: Immunologic changes associated with allergen immunotherapy. J Allergy Clin Immunol 102:157–164, 1998.
185. Malling H-J: Indications and contraindications for allergen-specific immunotherapy. Allergy Clin Immunol Int 10:76–80, 1998.
186. Editorial: Systemic reactions from allergen immunotherapy. J Allergy Clin Immunol 90:567–578, 1992.
187. Bochner B, Lichtenstein L: naphylaxis. N Engl J Med 324:1785–1790, 1991.
188. AAAI Board of Directors: The use of epinephrine in the treatment of anaphylaxis. J Allergy Clin Immunol 94:666–668, 1994.
189. Mygind N: Perennial rhinitis. Nasal Allergy (2nd Ed). Oxford: Blackwell Scientific Publications, 1979, pp 224–232.
190. Niinimaa V, Cole P, Mintz S, et al: The switching point from nasal to oronasal breathing. Respir Physiol 42:61–71, 1980.
191. Niinimaa V, Cole P, Mintz S, Shephard R: Oronasal distribution of respiratory airflow. Respir Physiol 43:69–75, 1981.
192. Rodenstein D, Stanescu D: The soft palate and breathing. Am Rev Respir Dis 134:311–325, 1986.
193. Schiratzki H: The oral and laryngeal components of the upper airway resistance during mouth breathing. Acta Otolaryngol 60:71–82, 1965.
194. Proctor D: Breathing Speech and Song. Vienna: Springer Verlag, 1980.
195. Tangel D, Mezzanotte M, White D: Influence of sleep on tensor palatini EMG and upper airway resistance in normal men. J Appl Physiol 70:2574–2581, 1991.
196. Remmers J, Anch A, deGroot W, et al: Oropharyngeal muscle tone in obstructive sleep apnea before and after strychnine. Sleep 3:447–453, 1980.
197. Suratt P, Dee P, Atkinson R, et al: Fluoroscopic and computed tomographic features of the pharyngeal airway in obstructive sleep apnea. Am Rev Respir Dis 127:487–492, 1983.
198. Schwartz A, Schubert N, Rothman W, et al: Effect of uvulopalatopharyngoplasty on upper airway collapsibility in obstructive sleep apnea. Am Rev Resp Dis 145:527–532, 1992.
199. Safar P, Escarraga L, Chang F: Upper airway obstruction in the unconscious patient. J Appl Physiol 14:760–764, 1968.
200. Safar P: Failure of manual respiration. J Appl Physiol 14:84–88, 1959.
201. Van de Graaff W, Gottfried S, Mitra J, et al: Respiratory function of hyoid muscles and hyoid arch. J Appl Physiol 57:197–204, 1984.
202. Van de Graaff W: Thoracic traction on the trachia: Mechanisms and magnitude. J Appl Physiol 70:1328–1336, 1991.
203. Cummiskey J, Williams T, Krumpe P, et al: The detection and quantification of sleep apnea by tracheal sound recordings. Am Rev Respir Dis 126:221–224, 1982.
204. Thach B, Brouillette R: The respiratory function of pharyngeal musculature: Relevance to clinical obstructive apnea. *In* Euler C, Lagercrantz H (eds): Central Nervous Control Mechanisms in Breathing. Oxford: Pergamon Press, 1979, pp 483–494.
205. Van Lunteren E, Strohl K, Parker D, et al: Phasic volume-related feedback on upper airway muscle activity. J Appl Physiol 56:730–736, 1984.
206. Mathew O, Abu-Osba Y, Thach B: Genioglossus muscle responses to upper airway pressure changes: Afferent pathways. J Appl Physiol 52:445–450, 1982.
207. Alex C, Aronson R, Onal E, Lopata M: Effects of continuous positive airway pressure on upper airway and respiratory muscle activity. J Appl Physiol 62:2026–2030, 1987.
208. Mathew O, Abu-Osba Y, Thach B: Influence of upper airway pressure changes on genioglossus muscle respiratory activity. J Appl Physiol 51:438–444, 1982.
209. Megirian D, Hinrichsen C, Sherrey J: Respiratory roles of genioglossus, sternothyroid, and sternohyoid muscles during sleep. Exp Neurol 90:118–128, 1985.
210. Onal E, Lopata M, O'Connor T: Diaphragmatic and genioglossal electromyogram responses to isocapnic hypoxia in humans. Am Rev Respir Dis 124:215–217, 1981.
211. Onal E, Lopata M, O'Connor T: Diaphragmatic and genioglossal electromyogram responses to CO2 rebreathing in humans. J Appl Physiol 50:1052–1055, 1981.
212. Parisi R, Neubauer J, Frank M, et al: Correlation between genioglossal and diaphragmatic responses to hypercapnia during sleep. Am Rev Respir Dis 135:378–382, 1987.
213. Basner R, Ringler J, Berkowitz S, et al: Effect of inspired air temperature on genioglossus activity during nose breathing in awake humans. J Appl Physiol 69:1098–1103, 1990.
214. Shelton R, Bosma J: Maintenance of the pharyngeal airway. J Appl Physiol 17:209–214, 1962.
215. Morikawa S, Safar P, DeCarlo J: Influence of the head-jaw position upon upper airway patency. Anesthesiology 22:265–270, 1961.
216. Hershenson M, Brouillette R, Olsen E, et al: The effect of chloral hydrate on genioglossus and diaphragmatic activity. Pediatr Res 18:516–519, 1984.
217. Nishino T, Shirahata M, Yonezawa T, et al: Comparison of changes in the hypoglossal and the phrenic nerve activity in response to increasing depth of anesthesia in cats. Anesthesiology 60:19–24, 1984.
218. Nishino T, Kohchi T, Yonezawa T, et al: Responses of recurrent laryngeal, hypoglossal, and phrenic nerves to increasing depths of anesthesia with halothane or enflurane in vagotomized cats. Anesthesiology 63:404–409, 1985.
219. Bonora M, Shields G, Knuth S, et al: Selective depression by ethanol of upper airway respieratory motor activity in cats. Am Rev Respir Dis 130:156–161, 1984.
220. Krol R, Knuth S, Bartlett D: Selective reduction in genioglossus muscle activity by alcohol in normal human subjects. Am Rev Respir Dis 129:247–250, 1984.
221. Remmers JE: Obstructive sleep apnea: A common disorder exacerbated by alcohol. Am Rev Respir Dis 130:153–155, 1984.
222. Bonora M, St. John W, Bledsoe T: Differential elevation by protriptyline and depression by diazepam of upper airway respiratory motor activity. Am Rev Respir Dis 31:41–45, 1985.
223. Wiegand L, Zwillich C, Wiegand D, et al: Changes in upper airway muscle activation and ventilation during phasic REM sleep in normal men. J Appl Physiol 71:488–497, 1991.
224. Issa F, Sullivan C: Upper airway closing pressures sin obstructive sleep apnea. J Appl Physiol 57:520–527, 1984.
225. Issa F, Sullivan C: Upper airway closing pressures in snores. J Appl Physiol 57:528–535, 1984.
226. Sauerland E, Orr W, Hairston L: EMG patterns of oropharyngeal muscles during respiration in wakefulness and sleep. Electroencephalogr Clin Neurophysiol 21:307–316, 1981.
227. Sauerland E, Harper R: The human tongue during sleep: Electromyographic activity of the genioglossus muscle. Exp Neurol 51:160–170, 1976.
228. Leiter J, Knuth S, Bartlett D: The effect of sleep deprivation on activity of the genioglossus muscle. Am Rev Respir Dis 132:1242–1245, 1985.
229. Wiegand D, Latz B, Zwillich C, et al: Geniohyoid muscle activity in normal men during wakefulness and sleep. J Appl Physiol 69:1262–1269, 1990.
230. Wiegand D, Latz B, Zwillich C, et al: Upper airway resistance and geniohyoid muscle activity in normal men during wakefulness and sleep. J Appl Physiol 69:1252–1262, 1990.
231. Rivlin J, Hoffstein V, Kalbfleisch J, et al: Upper airway morphology in patients with idiopathic obstructive sleep apnea. Am Rev Respir Dis 129:355–360, 1984.
232. Remmers J, deGroot W, Sauerland E, Anch A: Pathogenesis of upper airway occlusion during sleep. J Appl Physiol 44:931–938, 1978.
233. Jeffries B, Brouillette R, Hunt C: Electromyographic study of some accessory muscles of respiration in children with obstructive sleep apnea. Am Rev Respir Dis 129:696–702, 1984.

234. Hendricks J, Kline L, Kovalski R, et al: The English bulldog: a natural model of sleep-disordered breathing. J Appl Physiol 63:1344–1350, 1987.
235. Hudgel D, Chapman K, Faulks C, et al: Changes in inspiratory muscle electrical activity and upper airway resistance during periodic breathing induced by hypoxia during sleep. Am Rev Respir Dis 135:899–906, 1987.
236. Lopes J: Total airway resistance and respiratory muscle activity during sleep. J Appl Physiol 54:773–777, 1983.
237. Esclamado R, Glenn M, McCulloch T, et al: Perioperative complications and risk factors in the surgical treatment of obstructive sleep apnea syndrome. Laryngoscope 99:1125–1129, 1989.
238. Guilleminault C, Eldridge F, Tilkina A, et al: Sleep apnea syndrome due to upper airway obstruction. Arch Intern Med 137:296–300, 1977.
239. Mauer K, Staats B, Olsen K: Upper airway obstruction and disordered breathing in children. Mayo Clin Proc 58:349–353, 1983.
240. Gastaut H, Tassinari C, Duron B: Etude polygraphique des manifestations episodiques (hypniques et respiratoires) diurnes et nocturnes, du syndrome de Pickwick. Rev Neurol 112:568–579, 1965.
241. Onal E, Lopata M, O'Connor T: Pathogenesis of apneas in hypersomnia-sleep apnea syndrome. Am Rev Respir Dis 125:167–174, 1982.
242. Gould G, Whyte K, Rhind G, et al: The sleep hypopnea syndrome. Am Rev Respir Dis 137:895–898, 1988.
243. Block A, Boysen P, Wynne J, et al: Sleep apnea, hypopnea and oxygen desaturation in normal subjects. N Engl J Med 300:513–517, 1979.
244. Block A, Boysen P, Synne J, et al: Sleep apnea, hypopnea and oxygen desaturation in normal subjects: A strong male predominance. N Engl J Med 300:513–517, 1979.
245. Gleadhill IC, Schwartz AR, Schubert N, et al: Upper airway collapsibility in snorers and in patients with obstructive hypopnea and apnea. Am Rev Respir Dis 143:1300–1303, 1991.
246. Haponik E, Smith P, Bohlman M, et al: Computerized tomography in obstructive sleep apnea: Correlation of airway size with physiology during sleep and wakefulness. Am Rev Respir Dis 127:221–226, 1983.
247. Bradley T, Brown I, Grossman R, et al: Pharyngeal size of snorers, non-snorers, and patients with obstructive sleep apnea. N Engl J Med 315:1327–1331, 1986.
248. Brown J, Zamel N, Hoffstein V: Pharyngeal cross-sectional area in normal men and women. J Appl Physiol 61:890–895, 1986.
249. Brown I, Bradley T, Phillipson E, et al: Pharyngeal compliance in snoring subjects with and without obstructive sleep apnea. Am Rev Respir Dis 132:211–215, 1985.
250. Schwartz A, Gold A, Schubert N, et al: Effect of weight loss on upper airway collapsibility in obstructive sleep apnea. Am Rev Respir Dis 144:494–498, 1991.
251. Gleadhill I, Schwartz A, Smith P, et al: Measurement of upper airway critical pressure in patients with obstructive hypopnea. Am Rev Respir Dis 135:A185, 1987.
252. Smith P, Schwartz Z, Gauda E, et al: The modulation of upper airway critical pressures during sleep. *In* Issa F, Surratt P, Remmers J (eds): Sleep and Respiration. New York: Wiley-Liss, 1990 pp 253–260.
253. Issa F, Sullivan C: Arousal and breathing responses to airway occlusion in healthy sleeping adults. J Appl Physiol 55:1113–1119, 1983.
254. Wilson S, Thach B, Brouillette R, et al: Upper airway patency in the human infant: Influence of airway pressure and posture. J Appl Physiol 48:500–504, 1980.
255. Roberts J, Reed W, Mathew O, et al: Assessment of pharyngeal airway stability in normal and micrognathic infants. J Appl Physiol 58:290–299, 1985.
256. Anch A, Remmers J, Bunce H: Supraglottic airway resistance in normal subjects and patients with occlusive sleep apnea. J Appl Physiol 53:1158–1163, 1982.
257. Hudgel D: Mechanisms of obstructive sleep apnea. Chest 101:541–549, 1992.
258. Hudgel D, Harasick T: Physiologic effects of uvulopalatopharyngoplasty (UPP) in patients with transpalatal or hypopharyngeal upper airway obstruction during sleep. Am Rev Respir Dis 141:A865, 1990.
259. Skatrud J, Dempsey J: Airway resistance and respiratory muscle function in snorers during NREM sleep. J Appl Physiol 59:328–335, 1985.
260. Issa F, Sullivan C: The immediate effects of nasal continuous positive airway pressure treatment on sleep pattern in patients with obstructive sleep apnea syndrome. Electroencephalogr Clin Neurophysiol 63:10–17, 1986.
261. Sullivan C, Berthon-Jones M, Issa F, et al: Reversal of obstructive sleep apnea by continuous positive airway pressure applied through the nares. Lancet 1:862–865, 1981.
262. Strohl K, Redline S: Nasal CPAP therapy, upper airway muscle activation, and obstructive sleep apnea. Am Rev Respir Dis 134:555–558, 1986.
263. Cartwright R, Lloyd S, Lilie J, et al: Sleep position training as treatment for sleep apnea syndrome: A preliminary study. Sleep 8:87–94, 1985.
264. Kavey N, Blitzer A, Gidro-Frank S, et al: Sleeping position and sleep apnea syndrome. Am J Otolaryngol 6:373–377, 1985.
265. Bonora M, Bartlett D, Knuth S: Changes in upper airway muscle activity related to head position in awake cats. Respir Physiol 60:181–192, 1985.
266. McEvoy R, Sharp D, Thornton' A: The effects of posture on obstructive sleep apnea. Am Rev Respir Dis 133:662–666, 1986.
267. Cartwright R, Diaz F, Lloyd S: The effects of sleep posture and sleep stage on apnea frequency. Sleep 14:351–353, 1991.
268. Yildirim N, Fitzpatrick M, Whyte K, et al: The effect of posture on upper airway dimensions in normal subjects and in patients with the sleep apnea/hypopnea syndrome. Am Rev Respir Dis 144:845–847, 1991.
269. Smith P, Haponik E, Allen R, et al: The effects of protriptyline in sleep disordered breathing. Am Rev Respir Dis 127:8–13, 1983.
270. Oliven A, Odeh M, Gavriely N: Effect of salcylate on upper airway dilating muscles in anesthetized dogs. Am Rev Respir Dis 139:170–175, 1989.
271. Hudgel D, Hendricks C, Dadley A: Alteration in obstructive apnea pattern induced by changes in oxygen- and carbon-dioxide-inspired concentrations. Am Rev Respir Dis 138:16–19, 1988.
272. Riley R, Powell N, Guilleminault C: Maxillary, mandibular and hyoid advancement for treatment of obstructive sleep apnea: A review of 40 patients. J Oral Maxillofac Surg 48:20–26, 1990.
273. Miki H, Hida W, Shindoh, et al: Effects of electrical stimulation of the genioglossus on upper airway resistance in anesthetized dogs. Am Rev Respir Dis 140:1279–1284, 1989.
274. Miki H, Hida W, Chonan T, et al: Effects of submental electrical stimulation during sleep on upper airway patency in patients on obstructive sleep apnea. Am Rev Respir Dis 140:1285–1289, 1989.
275. Dijalilian M, Kern E, Brown H, et al: Hypoventilation secondary to chronic upper airway obstruction in childhood. Proc Mayo Clin 50:11–14, 1975.
276. Kanter R, Watchko J: Pulmonary edema associated with upper airway obstruction. Am J Dis Child 138:356–358, 1984.
277. Gates G: Deep neck infection. Am J Otolaryngol 4:420–421, 1983.
278. Patterson H, Kelly J, Strome M: Ludwig's angina: An update. Laryngoscope 92:370–378, 1982.
279. Cherry J, Hammond J: Transection of the cervical trachea resulting from closed trauma to the neck. J Laryngol Otol 948:97–100, 1984.
280. Dash H, Gode G: Blunt trauma to the cervical portion of the trachea. Br J Anaesth 55:1271–1272, 1983.
281. Schaefer S, Brown O: Selective application of CT in the management of laryngeal trauma. Laryngoscope 93:1473–1475, 1983.
282. Proctor D: The upper airways II. The larynx and trachea. Am Rev Respir Dis 115:315–342, 1977.
283. Proctor D: Form and function of the upper airways and the larynx. *In* Macklem P, Mead J (eds): Handbook of Physiology. Section 3. The Respiratory System. Mechanics of Breathing. Bethesda, MD: American Physiological Society, 1986, pp 63–74.
284. Ingelstedt S, Toremalm N: Aerodynamics within the larynx and trachea. Acta Otolaryngol 158:81–92, 1960.
285. Widdicombe J: Reflex control of the larynx. Bull Pathophysiol Respir 11:102–103, 1975.
286. Brancatisano T, Collett P, Engel L: Respiratory movements of the vocal cords. J Appl Physiology 54:1269–1276, 1983.

287. England S, Bartlett D: Changes in respiratory movements of the human vocal cords during hyperpnea. J Appl Physiol 52:780–785, 1982.
288. England S, Bartlett D: Influence of human vocal cord movements on airflow and resistance during eupnea. J Appl Physiol 52:773–779, 1982.
289. Baier H, Wanner A, Zarzecki S, et al: Relationships among glottis opening, respiratory flow, and upper airway resistance in humans. J Appl Physiol 43:603–611, 1977.
290. Bartlett D, Remmers J, Gautier H: Laryngeal regulation of respiratory airflow. Respir Physiol 18:196–204, 1973.
291. Bowden R: Innervation of intrinsic laryngeal muscles. *In* Wyke B (ed): Ventilatory and Phonatory Control Systems. London: Oxford University Press, 1974, pp 370–381.
292. Gautier H, Remmers J, Bartlett D: Control of the duration of expiration. Respir Physiol 18:205–221, 1973.
293. Jackson A, Gulesian P, Mead J: Glottal aperture panting with voluntary limitation of tidal volume. J Appl Physiol 39:834–836, 1975.
294. Kirchner J, Wyke B: Articular reflex mechanisms in the larynx. Ann Otol Rhinol Larygol 74:749–768, 1965.
295. Martensson A: The functional organization of the intrinsic laryngeal muscles. Ann NY Acad Sci 155:91–97, 1968.
296. Murakami Y, Kirchner J: Respiratory activity of the external laryngeal muscles. An electromyographic study in the cat. *In* Wyke BD (ed): Ventilatory and Phonatory Control Systems. London: Oxford University Press, 1974, pp 430–458.
297. Nakamura F, Uyeda Y, Sonoda Y: Electromyographic study of respiratory movements of the intrinsic laryngeal muscles. Laryngoscope 68:109–119, 1958.
298. Negus V: Comparative Anatomy and Physiology of the Larynx. New York: Hafner, 1962.
299. Rattenburg C: Laryngeal regulation of respiration. Acta Anaesthesiol Scand 5:129–140, 1961.
300. Remmers J, Bartlett D: Reflex control of expiratory airflow and duration. J Appl Physiol 42:80–87, 1977.
301. Wyke B, Kirchner J: Neurology of the larynx. *In* Hinchcliffe R, Harrison D (eds): Scientific Foundations of Otolaryngology. London: Wm. Heinemann, 1976, pp 546–574.
302. Widdicombe J: Studies on afferent airway innervation. Am Rev Respir Dis 115:88–106, 1977.
303. Freedman L: The role of the cricothyroid muscle in tension of the vocal cords. Arch Otolaryngol 62:347–353, 1955.
304. Adzaku F: The morphological and functional characteristics of the innervation of the subglottic mucosa of the larynx. Ann R Coll Surg Engl 62:426–431, 1980.
305. Adzaku F, Wyke B: Innervation of the subglottic mucosa of the larynx and its significance. Folia Phoniatr 31:271–283, 1979.
306. Sant'Ambrogio G, Mathew O, Fisher J, et al: Laryngeal receptors responding to tranmural pressure, airflow and local muscle activity. Respir Physiol 54:317–330, 1983.
307. McCaffrey T, Kern E: Laryngeal airway resistance 1. Chemoreceptor reflexes. Ann Otol Rhinol Laryngol 89:209–214, 1980.
308. McCaffrey T, Kern E: Laryngeal airway resistance. 2. Pulmonary receptor reflexes. Ann Otol Rhinol Laryngol 89:462–466, 1980.
309. Stransky A, Szereda-Przestaszewska M, Widdicombe J: The effects of lung reflexes on laryngeal resistance and motooneuron discharge. J Physiol 231:417–438, 1973.
310. Mathew O, Sant'Ambrogio F: Laryngeal reflexes. *In* Mathew O, Sant'Ambrogio G (eds): Respiratory Function of the Upper Airway. New York: Marcel Dekker, 1988, pp 259–302.
311. Kashima H: Documentation of upper airway obstruction vocal cord paralysis: flow-volume loop studies in 43 subjects. Laryngoscope 94:923–937, 1984.
312. Hyatt R: Evaluation of major airway lesions using the flow-volume loop. Ann Otol Rhinol Laryngol 84:635–642, 1975.
313. Miller R, Hyatt R: Evaluation of obstructing lesions of the trachea and larynx by flow-volume loops. Am Rev Respir Dis 18:475–481, 1973.
314. Owens G, Murphy D: Spirometric diagnosis of upper airway obstruction. Arch Intern Med 143:1331–1334, 1983.
315. Gibson G, Pride N, Empey D: The role of inspiratory dynamic compression in upper airway obstruction. Am Rev Respir Dis 108:1352–1360, 1973.
316. Smith R, Catlin F: Congenital anomalies of the larynx. Am J Dis Child 138:35–39, 1984.
317. Clerf L: Unilateral vocal cord paralysis. JAMA 161:900–903, 1953.
318. Cunning D: Unilateral vocal cord paralysis. Ann Otol Rhinol Laryngol 64:487–494, 1955.
319. New B, Childrey J: Paralysis of the vocal cords. Arch Otolaryngol 16:143–160, 1932.
320. Christopher K, Wood R, Eckert R, et al: Vocal cord dysfunction presenting as asthma. N Engl J Med 308:1566–1570, 1983.
321. Kellman R, Leopold D: Paradoxical vocal cord motion: An important cause of stridor. Laryngoscope 92:58–60, 1982.
322. Lisboa C, Jardin J, Angus E, et al: Is extrathoracic airway obstruction important in asthma? Am Rev Respir Dis 122:115–121, 1980.
323. Macklem P, Rector W, Wang K, et al: Upper airway obstruction in asthma. Johns Hopkins Med J 147:233–237, 1980.
324. Rogers J, Stell P: Paradoxical movement of the vocal cords as a cause of stridor. J Laryngol Otol 92:157–158, 1978.
325. Proctor DF: All that wheezes [editorial]. Am Rev Respir Dis 127:261–262, 1983.
326. Rodenstein D, Stanescu F: Emotional laryngeal wheezing. A new syndrome. Am Rev Respir Dis 127:354–356, 1983.
327. Cormier Y, Camus P, Desmeules M: Nonorganic acute upper airways obstruction and a diagnostic approach. Am Rev Resp Dis 121:147–150, 1981.

# 43 Disorders of the Intrathoracic Airways

STEPHEN C. LAZARUS, M.D.

Introduction
Disorders with Diffuse Involvement
- Anatomic and Physiologic Features
- Epidemiology
- Bronchiolitis
- Bronchiolitis Obliterans
- Respiratory Bronchiolitis
- Panbronchiolitis
- Bronchopulmonary Dysplasia

Localized Disorders
- Neoplasms
- Bronchial Compression
- Mediastinal Fibrosis
- Foreign Bodies
- Granulomatous Inflammation
- Broncholithiasis
- Amyloidosis
- Bronchomalacia
- Traumatic Injury
- Clinical Features
- Diagnosis
- Treatment
- Tracheobronchial Stents

Summary

## INTRODUCTION

Previous chapters in this section have described the major diseases that affect primarily intrathoracic airways: asthma, bronchitis, and bronchiectasis. In addition, a number of less common entities that involve these airways exist. Bronchiolitis, bronchiolitis obliterans, and bronchopulmonary dysplasia are diseases of the peripheral airways. Because they produce widespread involvement of small bronchi and bronchioles, their physiologic consequences may be major. Increasing awareness of these diseases has led to an increased frequency of diagnosis. In contrast to these generalized diseases of the peripheral airways, there are also a number of conditions whose effects are localized to more central airways. In this chapter, both the local and diffuse processes involving intrathoracic airways are discussed.

## DISORDERS WITH DIFFUSE INVOLVEMENT

### Anatomic and Physiologic Features

Intrapulmonary airways can be subclassified as bronchi, bronchioles, and gas-exchange ducts (Chapter 1). Although all the conducting airways contain smooth muscle, there are important differences that distinguish bronchi from bronchioles. *Bronchi* contain cartilage, submucosal glands, ciliated epithelial cells, and goblet cells.[1, 2] Bronchial smooth muscle is innervated by muscarinic output carried in the vagus nerves.[3] Nerve endings responsible for cough ("cough receptors") are found in the large bronchi, mostly at bifurcations.[4] Because of their limited total cross-sectional area, the bronchi are responsible for most of the resistance to airflow in the lung.[5, 6]

In contrast to bronchi, *bronchioles* normally do not contain cartilage, glands, or goblet cells.[1, 2] In many chronic diseases of the airways (e.g., chronic bronchitis, asthma, cystic fibrosis), increased numbers of goblet cells are found in peripheral airways, but the extent to which their secretions contribute to the pathophysiology of these diseases is uncertain.[7] Cilia are more sparse in bronchioles than in bronchi, and bronchiolar smooth muscle is not under vagal control. Repeated branching creates a large number of bronchioles arranged in parallel. This results in a large total cross-sectional area, such that bronchioles normally contribute little to total airflow resistance.[5, 6]

Because the walls of the airways are not rigid, their dimensions change with lung volume. The bronchioles are located within the connective tissue structure of the lung, and their walls are relatively thin.[8] Although the contribution of bronchioles to total airflow resistance is small at normal and high lung volumes, they narrow markedly at low lung volumes and their contribution to resistance increases as residual volume is approached. This increased collapsibility (high compliance) explains why normal peripheral bronchioles may close at low lung volumes.[9]

Narrowing of peripheral airways may have profound effects on lung function. For example, local peripheral narrowing may decrease ventilation to a diseased area, leading to hypoxemia, but this narrowing may not produce wheezing or striking increases in the total work of breathing. For these reasons, pathologic narrowing of peripheral airways is difficult to detect, and these airways may be considered a "silent zone" of the lung. Despite much effort to design tests to identify obstruction in peripheral airways, no method has been entirely successful (Chapter 28).

## Epidemiology

The frequency of disorders of the peripheral airways is unknown because of the difficulty of localizing abnormalities to these sites. Moreover, because of the continuity between bronchi and bronchioles, it is doubtful whether pure bronchitis or bronchiolitis ever exists. Indeed, some authors prefer to avoid making an anatomic distinction about the site of inflammation and collectively refer to these peripheral airways (< 2 mm in diameter) as "small airways."[10] Processes that obstruct small airways may result in severe functional disability.

## Bronchiolitis

Bronchiolitis, a cellular and mesenchymal reaction involving bronchioles, is relatively uncommon in adults. Although bronchiolitis may occur in response to various stimuli, identification may be delayed because of the difficulty in detecting this narrowing. A generalized inflammatory response of the peripheral airways may follow inhalation of a corrosive gas that penetrates deeply into the lungs. Highly soluble irritants such as sulfur dioxide and ammonia dissolve in the lining fluid of the upper airways, causing damage primarily there. Less soluble gases such as nitrogen dioxide and phosgene pass into peripheral airways, where they cause inflammatory changes in bronchioles and alveoli.[11, 12] Such toxic fume exposures are a significant industrial and environmental hazard. "Nitrous fumes," for example, may be found in silo gas, jet and missile fuel, metal pickling fumes, and certain fires. (This subject is discussed more fully in Chapter 69.)

After exposure to toxic fumes, three clinical patterns may develop (Fig. 43.1).[12–16] Acutely, patients may develop cough, dyspnea, cyanosis, hemoptysis, hypoxemia, and loss of consciousness. These symptoms and signs may disappear within hours, or they may persist for weeks before they eventually resolve. In patients exposed to higher concentrations, pulmonary edema and severe acute respiratory distress syndrome may develop immediately or after a latent period of 3 to 30 hours. Although most patients recover, death may occur. Finally, some patients develop irreversible airflow obstruction (bronchiolitis obliterans) 2 to 8 weeks after the initial exposure. Typically, this occurs after recovery from the acute symptoms of exposure or in patients who had no initial illness and is characterized by the gradual onset of dyspnea and a nonproductive cough.[16–18] Patients who develop bronchiolitis obliterans after toxic fume inhalation commonly experience progressive deterioration, often leading to death from respiratory failure.

In contrast to adults, in whom it is considered rare, infectious bronchiolitis is a common lower respiratory tract illness in infants and young children. The cause most commonly is a virus, especially respiratory syncytial virus.[19] In older children and adults, the disease has been associated with *Mycoplasma pneumoniae, Legionella pneumophila*, and several viruses.[20–22]

Bronchiolitis in children typically begins as an acute virus-like illness. Within several days, cough, dyspnea, and fever develop. Although wheezing, chest wall retractions, and cyanosis may be seen, respiratory failure is uncommon. Peribronchiolar inflammation with epithelial necrosis, when severe, causes airflow obstruction in the peripheral airways of infants, with resulting hyperinflation and severe gas exchange abnormalities.[23] Roentgenograms generally show overinflation of the lungs, and sometimes nodular shadows appear[24, 25] with areas of focal atelectasis and pneumonia.[26, 27] Bronchiolitis is usually self-limiting, and complete recovery usually occurs within days to weeks.[19, 28] Symptomatic treatment with supplementary oxygen and hydration is usually all that is necessary. Bronchiolitis in infancy has been associated with an increased risk of subsequent wheezing and bronchial hyperreactivity,[29–31a] but a direct link to chronic obstructive pulmonary disease has not been shown. Occasionally,

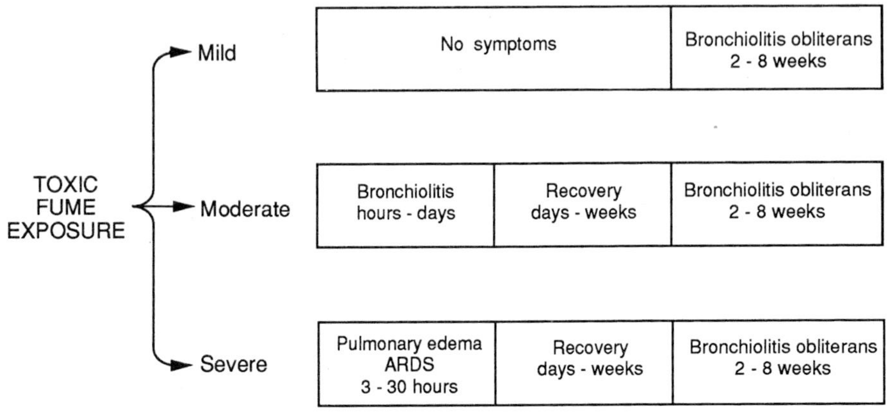


**Figure 43.1** The severity of bronchiolitis after inhalation of toxic fumes depends in part on the magnitude of the exposure. Most patients recover from the acute event, although some develop bronchiolitis obliterans 2 to 8 weeks after the initial insult. *Abbreviation:* ARDS = acute respiratory distress syndrome.

**Table 43.1 CONDITIONS ASSOCIATED WITH BRONCHIOLITIS OBLITERANS**

| |
|---|
| Toxic fume inhalation |
| Mineral dust exposure |
| Infection (viral, *Mycoplasma, Legionella*) |
| Bone marrow transplantation |
| Lung and heart-lung transplantation |
| Rheumatoid arthritis |
| Penicillamine |
| Systemic lupus erythematosus |
| Dermatomyositis, polymyositis |
| Hypersensitivity pneumonitis |

bronchiolitis obliterans, bronchiolectasis, and localized emphysema develop as sequelae to bronchiolitis.[32] No role has been proven for bronchodilators, antibiotics, or corticosteroids, although the latter often are used empirically in progressive disease in an attempt to reduce the severity of obliterative bronchiolitis.

Because of their anatomic features, diseases of peripheral airways are difficult to detect and to differentiate from diseases of large airways. In individual patients, the cause of acute bronchiolitis often is not established, and the disease in patients with progressive bronchiolitis obliterans frequently is classified as "idiopathic." Lung biopsy should be considered in those with chronic progressive disease.

## Bronchiolitis Obliterans

Obliterative bronchiolitis first was described by Reynaud in 1835.[33] In 1901, Lange[34] reported two young adults who died of rapidly progressive respiratory failure. At autopsy, their lungs revealed fibrous scarring of small airways with polypoid foci of exudate extending into the lumens. Since that time, bronchiolitis obliterans has been described after inhalation of toxic fumes, as a consequence of respiratory infections, in association with connective tissue disorders, and after bone marrow or heart-lung transplantation (Table 43.1). It appears that any damage to the bronchiolar epithelium may, during the repair phase, lead to excessive proliferation of granulation tissue. The reason this occurs in only a percentage of patients is unknown, but it probably reflects both differences in the magnitude of the provocative stimulus and abnormalities in the responses of host tissue. Bronchiolitis obliterans is classified clinically, based on etiology (see Table 43.1),[35] and histopathologically, based on tissue morphology.[36]

Bronchiolitis obliterans characteristically presents with the insidious onset of a nonproductive cough and dyspnea 2 to 8 weeks after an acute respiratory illness or toxic exposure. Physical examination is typically unremarkable but may reveal diffuse expiratory wheezing. Similarly, routine laboratory studies are not helpful. The roentgenographic pattern of bronchiolitis obliterans is variable and may show a miliary or diffuse nodular pattern or a reticulonodular pattern or may on occasion be normal. In some patients, narrowing of small bronchi and bronchioles may result in marked hyperinflation of the lungs, which is apparent on the chest roentgenogram. This postobstructive hyperinflation with associated roentgenographic hyperlucency may be generalized or confined to one lung. The unilateral hyperlucent lung syndrome first was described in children by Swyer and James,[37] and 1 year later, the same abnormality was reported in adults.[38] It currently is believed that these forms of hyperinflation with hyperlucency are postobstructive complications of bronchiolitis obliterans. (See Chapter 28 for more information about hyperinflation as a complication of airway obstruction.)

There are two distinct forms of bronchiolitis obliterans.[36, 39, 40] "Classic bronchiolitis obliterans," as described by Lange[34] and currently referred to as "proliferative bronchiolitis," is characterized by intraluminal polyps of organizing connective tissue. "Constrictive bronchiolitis," in contrast, is characterized by partial or complete obstruction of bronchiolar lumens that results from chronic bronchiolar inflammation, concentric submucosal or adventitial scarring, and smooth muscle hypertrophy.[39] These two forms show little clinical or histopathologic overlap.[41] Histologically, pure bronchiolitis obliterans is rare. When present, there is obliteration of bronchiolar lumens without spread of fibrosis to other air spaces or interstitium. Extension of the exudate and granulation tissue into alveoli is referred to as organizing pneumonia, and the entire process then is termed *bronchiolitis obliterans with organizing pneumonia*, or BOOP. Epler and Colby suggested the classification shown in Table 43.2 to describe the histologic effects, prognosis, and response to therapy of different clinical patterns of bronchiolitis obliterans.[35]

**Table 43.2 CLASSIFICATION, PROGNOSIS, AND THERAPY OF BRONCHIOLITIS OBLITERANS**

| Type | Organizing Pneumonia | Prognosis | Therapy |
|---|---|---|---|
| Toxic fume exposure | Rare | Poor-good | Steroids |
| Postinfectious | +/− | Fair-good | Steroids |
| Connective tissue disease | +/− | Poor-good | Steroids |
| Localized | Yes | Good | Resection |
| Idiopathic | Yes | Fair-good | Steroids |

Reproduced with permission from Epler GR, Colby TV: The spectrum of bronchiolitis obliterans. Chest 83:161–162, 1983.

## Bronchiolitis Obliterans and Connective Tissue Diseases

Bronchiolitis obliterans may occur as an uncommon manifestation of connective tissue or collagen vascular diseases. It has been reported in association with rheumatoid arthritis, where it affects primarily women with long-standing, seropositive rheumatoid arthritis in their fifth or sixth decade of life.[42–45] The onset and progression of dyspnea and nonproductive cough are rapid, as is the rate of progression of airflow obstruction. The chest roentgenogram usually shows no abnormalities. Unfortunately, no consistent response to corticosteroids has been documented, and the prognosis for these patients generally is poor.[46, 47] Penicillamine has been implicated as a potential cause of bronchiolitis obliterans,[48, 49] but confirmation of an etiologic relationship is lacking. Bronchiolitis obliterans also has been reported in systemic lupus erythematosus,[50] polymyositis, and dermatomyositis.[51]

## Bronchiolitis Obliterans After Bone Marrow Transplantation

Chronic graft-versus-host disease (GVHD) occurs in approximately one third of long-term survivors of allogeneic bone marrow transplantation. Bronchiolitis obliterans occurs in approximately 10% of bone marrow transplant patients who develop chronic GVHD. In this context, bronchiolitis obliterans is preceded, 2 to 3 months after transplantation, by typical findings of GVHD: mucositis, esophagitis, and skin rash. Four to 6 months later, the patients develop dry, nonproductive cough, and exertional dyspnea that may be severe and rapidly progressive. The physical examination reveals scattered wheezing, and bibasilar rales are often present. Hypoxemia is common. Of note, the chest roentgenogram usually shows no abnormalities or demonstrates hyperinflation.

Various mechanisms have been proposed to explain bronchiolitis obliterans after bone marrow transplantation. Chronic GVHD and prior methotrexate therapy appear to be risk factors for the development of airflow obstruction.[52] The GVHD may damage small airways directly. Lung epithelial cells can express Ia (class II major histocompatibility complex [MHC]) antigens that may activate T cells from the donor, thus making the airways a target for immunologically mediated injury.[52] Methotrexate, which alone does not cause bronchiolitis obliterans, may act as a "priming" agent in the presence of GVHD, perhaps by inducing antigen expression in the lungs. Finally, bronchiolitis obliterans may result from viral infection, and the increased immunosuppression given to treat GVHD may increase the risk of such opportunistic infections. A 25% to 30% incidence of viral infection has been reported in patients with bronchiolitis obliterans after bone marrow transplantation.[53–55]

## Bronchiolitis Obliterans After Lung or Heart-Lung Transplantation

Bronchiolitis obliterans is the major cause of death of long-term survivors of heart-lung transplantation, developing in 30% to 50% of transplant recipients (see Chapter 97).[56–61] Although various factors have been suggested as causes of bronchiolitis obliterans after heart-lung transplantation, including infections, altered mucociliary clearance, altered blood flow secondary to bronchial artery ligation, reaction to immunosuppressive drugs, and loss of the cough reflex with recurrent aspiration,[57] it appears that these entities may act mainly as "co-factors" and that the primary pathogenetic event is chronic transplant rejection.[57–65a] By multivariate analysis, human leukocyte antigen (HLA)–A locus mismatch stands out as a significant independent predictor of bronchiolitis obliterans.[66]

Bronchiolitis obliterans may present several months to several years after lung or heart-lung transplantation.[65] Clinical features include productive cough, dyspnea during exertion, progressive shortness of breath, and irreversible airflow obstruction with moderate reduction of diffusing capacity. Arterial hypoxemia and hypocapnia are almost always present.

Because bronchoscopy with bronchoalveolar lavage and transbronchial biopsy often are used as surveillance for rejection after lung transplantation, this model has provided much information on the immunologic processes involved in the development of bronchiolitis obliterans.[67] Enhanced expression of class II MHC antigens has been found in the epithelium of bronchioles and alveoli of patients with bronchiolitis obliterans after heart-lung transplantation.[68–70] T lymphocytes from the recipient may recognize these donor class II MHC antigens as foreign, resulting in a cascade of lymphocyte activation, proliferation, and differentiation.[71] This concept is supported further by the demonstration of activated T lymphocytes in the cellular infiltrates. Functional testing of bronchoalveolar lavage cells has been used to monitor patients for the development of bronchiolitis obliterans. Donor-specific activity (primed lymphocyte test, cell-mediated lympholysis) of cells removed from transplanted lung is strongly associated with bronchiolitis obliterans, and alloreactivity of bronchoalveolar lavage cells may be a significant risk factor for the subsequent development of bronchiolitis obliterans in clinically quiescent patients.[72, 72a] During rejection, there is marked lymphocytic infiltration of the transplanted organ,[73, 74] and infiltrating cells demonstrate $CD4^+$ and $CD8^+$ phenotypes.[75–77] A predominant $CD4^+$ cell population, mediating donor-specific class II antigen-directed reactivity, is associated with graft rejection; a predominant $CD8^+$ cell population, mediating donor-specific class I antigen-directed reactivity, is associated with bronchiolitis obliterans.[78]

The role of co-factors such as *Pneumocystis carinii* infection or cytomegalovirus pneumonia in the initiation of lung allograft rejection and development of bronchiolitis obliterans remains unclear. Pneumocystis infection is associated with an increased number and alloreactivity of bronchoalveolar lavage cells and a higher incidence of chronic rejection, leading to bronchiolitis obliterans.[79] It has been suggested that activated T cells, on presentation of antigen by macrophages, proliferate and produce cytokines such as interleukin-2 that lead to an expansion of the number of alloreactive T cells.[79] Similarly, cytomegalovirus infection may stimulate the release of cytokines such as interferon-gamma, which may lead to the increased expression of MHC antigens on epithelial and

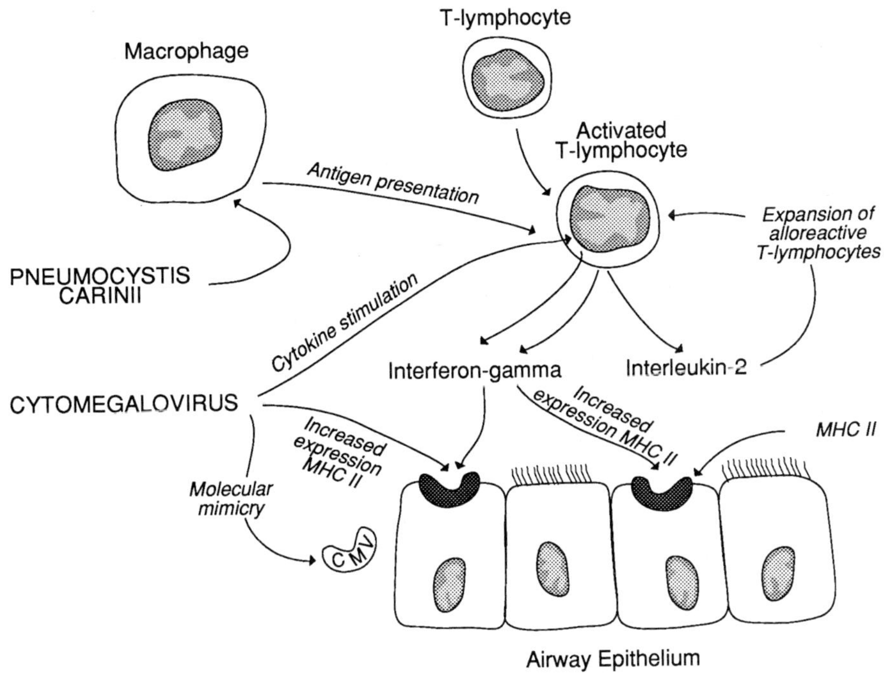


**Figure 43.2** Schematic diagram showing the potential interactions between infectious and immunologic stimuli that lead to bronchiolitis obliterans after transplantation of lung. Pneumocystis and cytomegalovirus (CMV) may act as "co-factors" to increase numbers of alloreactive T cells and increase expression of class II major histocompatibility complex (MHC) antigens on airway cells.

endothelial cells.[80–81a] Alternatively, cytomegalovirus may directly stimulate the up-regulation of MHC antigen expression on target cells. Finally, Fujinami and associates [82] have described a region of amino acid sequence homology between the immediate-early region of human cytomegalovirus and the HLA-DR beta-chain. By "mimicking" the molecular structure of HLAs in the lung, cytomegalovirus might induce a response directed against the graft (Fig. 43.2).

## Bronchiolitis Obliterans with Organizing Pneumonia

In 1985, Epler and associates[83] described 50 patients whose lung biopsy specimens showed patchy organizing pneumonia in association with bronchiolitis obliterans. They proposed that bronchiolitis obliterans with organizing pneumonia (BOOP) was a distinct component of the spectrum of infiltrative lung diseases. Clinically, most patients had a history suggesting a slowly resolving pneumonia spanning weeks or months. The most common symptom on presentation was a persistent, nonproductive cough, and approximately one third of patients reported a flu-like illness with fever, sore throat, and malaise. Dyspnea was a prominent feature in half the patients. On physical examination, crackles or "Velcro" rales were present in 68% of patients, and wheezes were rarely present.

Epler and associates[83] described an unusual radiographic pattern of bilateral patchy ground glass densities in 81% of their patients. Other radiographic patterns of BOOP include a miliary nodular pattern resembling miliary tuberculosis, bilateral symmetric lower lobe interstitial infiltrates, and, on rare occasions, a normal chest roentgenogram.

The physiologic abnormalities of BOOP are variable.[47, 83] In patients who are symptomatic, arterial hypoxemia is nearly always present. Pulmonary function tests demonstrate a restrictive pattern, with reduction in diffusing capacity in 72% of patients. Airflow obstruction is uncommon in patients who are not smokers.

The histologic pattern identified as BOOP is not specific for a single cause, but rather can occur in association with a large number of pulmonary conditions (Table 43.3). The idiopathic form of BOOP also is known as cryptogenic organizing pneumonitis (COP). Cordier and associates[84] have described three different clinical profiles. The first group had patchy migratory pneumonic foci. All patients recovered completely with corticosteroid therapy but relapsed when therapy was stopped rapidly. In a second group with diffuse interstitial lung disease, approximately half of the patients responded to corticosteroids. A third group had solitary foci of pneumonia that were resected because of concern over carcinoma. These patients recovered without relapse. Other studies have reported similar success with corticosteroid therapy, with an overall response rate of 60% to 70%, and similar rates of recurrence associated with early cessation of

**Table 43.3** ETIOLOGY OF BRONCHIOLITIS OBLITERANS WITH ORGANIZING PNEUMONIA (BOOP)

| |
|---|
| Infection |
| Acute respiratory distress syndrome |
| Bone marrow transplantation |
| Lung and heart-lung transplantation |
| Collagen vascular disease |
| Hypersensitivity pneumonitis |
| Toxic fume inhalation |
| Aspiration pneumonitis |
| Idiopathic |

corticosteroid therapy.[83, 85, 86] Because most patients with BOOP demonstrate complete clinical and physiologic recovery after therapy with corticosteroids, the diagnosis must be confirmed. Usually this requires an open-lung biopsy to distinguish BOOP from irreversible interstitial lung disease. BOOP should be considered whenever "community-acquired pneumonia" fails to respond to appropriate therapy.

### Treatment of Bronchiolitis Obliterans and Bronchiolitis Obliterans with Organizing Pneumonia

Early recognition and therapy of bronchiolitis obliterans is important because treatment is often ineffective when the disease has reached the late, fibrotic stage. Although there is little evidence that smooth muscle contraction plays a significant role, beta-adrenergic agonists usually are given in an attempt to provide symptomatic relief. Corticosteroids play an important role and, if administered early, may alter significantly the disease process. This is especially true of bronchiolitis obliterans after exposure to toxic fumes.[12, 16, 87, 88] Once instituted, corticosteroid therapy should be continued for at least 2 to 3 months, then reduced slowly, to minimize the likelihood of relapse.[48, 84–88] In some patients, it may be necessary to continue low-dose or alternate-day corticosteroid therapy for months or years.

In bronchiolitis obliterans after bone marrow transplantation, the response to therapy has been poor. Generally, by the time severe airflow obstruction has been established, there is minimal if any therapeutic response. Bronchodilators and corticosteroids have not improved airflow in most cases, and the use of immunosuppressive agents to treat chronic GVHD, although occasionally effective,[89, 90] has not consistently changed the course of bronchiolitis obliterans.[47] Better prophylaxis against GVHD and viral infection may reduce the incidence of bronchiolitis obliterans after bone marrow transplantation.

Bronchiolitis obliterans after lung or heart-lung transplantation has been treated by augmenting immunosuppression with high-dose corticosteroids, azathioprine, antithymocyte globulin (ATG), or OKT3 monoclonal antibody, or all, and the response has varied.[59, 60, 72, 91–93] If bronchiolitis obliterans is detected early and therapy is initiated immediately, the likelihood of reversal is enhanced.[59, 91, 94] Therapy begun late in the clinical course may stabilize the process or have no effect, although assessing this is difficult because the rate of progression of bronchiolitis obliterans tends to slow spontaneously with time.[61] The best therapy for bronchiolitis obliterans is prevention, and the addition of azathioprine to the post-transplant immunosuppression regimen has reduced significantly the incidence of bronchiolitis obliterans.[59, 95, 96] Rigorous surveillance for evidence of asymptomatic rejection makes it feasible to prevent the chronic rejection that is thought to lead to bronchiolitis obliterans.

BOOP represents a special situation. Corticosteroid therapy is effective in most cases, and clinical improvement is often dramatic, sometimes occurring within 1 to 2 days of starting therapy.[83, 97] In Epler's original study,[83] there was complete clinical and physiologic recovery in 65% of patients. Because this lesion is so "steroid-responsive," the diagnosis should be established early, so therapy can be initiated before irreversible changes in lung function occur.

## Respiratory Bronchiolitis

Respiratory bronchiolitis is characterized by the accumulation of pigmented alveolar macrophages in respiratory bronchioles and in the adjacent air spaces. It is a distinct pathologic entity commonly found in cigarette smokers and in patients with mineral dust exposure.[98–100] Previously considered an incidental finding at autopsy, respiratory bronchiolitis currently is thought to be a possible precursor to chronic lung disease in heavy smokers.[98, 101] Clinically, the disease resembles idiopathic pulmonary fibrosis. Patients present with cough, dyspnea, and rales, with diffuse interstitial infiltrates or reticulonodular opacities on chest roentgenogram and pulmonary function tests showing restrictive lung disease with decreased diffusing capacity. High-resolution computed tomography may be useful in differentiating respiratory bronchiolitis from interstitial lung disease, demonstrating diffuse or patchy ground glass densities or fine nodules in the former, and peripheral reticular opacities and honeycombing in the latter.[102] The duration of symptoms is considerably longer than for BOOP, with patients with respiratory bronchiolitis reporting an average of 37 months of symptoms.[101] Little is known about the natural history of respiratory bronchiolitis or about its therapy.

## Panbronchiolitis

Diffuse panbronchiolitis is an obscure inflammatory disease of the respiratory bronchioles and surrounding alveoli. Described originally in Japan, where more than 1000 cases have been identified,[103–107] it also has been reported in non-Japanese Asians[108] and in whites in the United States.[109]

Most individuals with diffuse panbronchiolitis are male[106, 107] and nonsmokers, and almost all have chronic sinusitis. Usual presenting symptoms are cough, dyspnea, and sputum production. The chest radiograph and high-resolution computed tomography are characteristic, showing diffuse small centrilobular nodular opacities and hyperinflation.[102, 110, 111] Pulmonary function tests typically reveal progressive airflow obstruction or a mixed obstructive-restrictive pattern, with reduced diffusing capacity.[109] Although the etiology of diffuse panbronchiolitis remains obscure, both genetic and environmental factors are believed to be important.[112–113a] Airway neutrophilia is a common feature, and chronic treatment with macrolide antibiotics has been shown to be beneficial,[114, 115] possibly by reducing levels of the neutrophil chemoattractant interleukin-8.[116, 116a]

## Bronchopulmonary Dysplasia

Bronchopulmonary dysplasia occurs in newborn babies with the infant respiratory distress syndrome (hyaline membrane disease) after prolonged treatment with high concentrations of inspired oxygen and positive pressure ventilation.[117, 118] Because these two therapeutic modalities are linked so closely in practice, it has not been possible to separate the pathogenetic contributions of each. In all likelihood, both oxygen and positive pressure play a role. Characteristic histologic features are unusual abnormalities of the bronchioles, including marked metaplasia, obliteration, and cystic changes. The disorder also has been described in adults after adult respiratory distress syndrome.[119] It is possible that this complication occurs more frequently in adults than currently is recognized. The pathologic findings may be misdiagnosed easily as "honeycombing," a nonspecific consequence of many different fibrosing disorders.

## LOCALIZED DISORDERS

Many of the specific causes of localized abnormalities of bronchi described pathologically also underlie abnormalities of the extrathoracic airways (Chapter 18). Examples are neoplasms, extrinsic compression, granulomatous disease, malacic lesions, and trauma. However, the manifestations, diagnosis, and therapy of localized bronchial disorders are substantially different from similar disorders in the larynx or trachea.

### Neoplasms

Because lung cancers are common, any endobronchial mass must be evaluated carefully for possible malignancy. All histopathologic types of primary lung cancer may protrude into a bronchus and narrow or occlude it. Malignant endobronchial tumors often have an irregular, rather than smooth, surface on bronchoscopic examination. Primary malignant tumors of the lung are described in detail in Chapter 46.

Of patients with extrapulmonary malignancies metastatic to the lungs, approximately 5% have predominantly endobronchial metastases.[120] The most common primary malignancies are renal cell, colonic, rectal, cervical, and breast carcinomas and malignant melanomas.[121] In most instances, the manifestations of the primary tumor are apparent before the endobronchial metastasis is discovered.[120] Metastatic malignancies of the lungs are discussed in detail in Chapter 48.

In patients with lymphomas or leukemia, malignant infiltrations of bronchial mucosa occur rarely. In Hodgkin's disease or non-Hodgkin's lymphoma, the endobronchial malignant cells may originate in bronchus-associated lymphoid tissue, may invade the bronchial mucosa by direct extension from hilar or peribronchial lymph nodes, or may seed the bronchial mucosa via lymphatic or blood vessels.[122] Leukemic infiltration of bronchial mucosa occurs as a rare, late manifestation of chronic lymphocytic leukemia.[123]

Involvement of the lungs occurs in one third to one half of patients with acquired immunodeficiency syndrome (AIDS) and Kaposi's sarcoma (Chapter 82).[124] Endobronchial lesions occur frequently, but they rarely cause bronchial obstruction or hemoptysis. The lesions are usually multiple, bright red or violaceous, and flat when visualized through the bronchoscope. The diagnosis of endobronchial Kaposi's sarcoma is established when a patient with AIDS has widespread extrapulmonary Kaposi's sarcoma and characteristic-appearing endobronchial lesions. Biopsy of the endobronchial lesions is seldom necessary and may be hazardous because of excessive bleeding.[125]

Benign lung tumors frequently originate from cells in the airways, including nerves (neurinomas, neurofibromas, neurolemmomas), smooth muscle (leiomyomas), cartilage (chondromas), blood vessels (hemangiomas), fat cells (lipomas), glands (cystoadenomas, oxyphilic adenomas), and epithelium (papillomas).[126, 127] These tumors often narrow or obstruct bronchi. By bronchoscopic examination, the tumors often are smooth, round, and well localized.[127] Benign tumors of the lung are described in detail in Chapter 49.

### Bronchial Compression

When peribronchial lymph nodes are enlarged by carcinoma, lymphoma, or granulomatous infection, narrowing of adjacent bronchi may occur. Although sarcoidosis frequently results in enlarged hilar and mediastinal lymph nodes, bronchial narrowing from compression by lymph nodes in sarcoidosis is rare. In infants with congenital heart defects such as tetralogy of Fallot and transposition of the great vessels with ventricular septal defect, bronchial compression by dilated pulmonary arteries is an occasional complication.[128]

### Mediastinal Fibrosis

In patients with pulmonary histoplasmosis or tuberculosis, an interesting and rare complication is mediastinal fibrosis.[129] In such patients, it appears that fungal or bacterial antigens from granulomatous foci in mediastinal lymph nodes stimulate fibrogenesis in surrounding tissue, perhaps because of unusual sensitivity to the antigens.[129] The fibrosis may result in narrowing or occlusion of vital mediastinal structures, and the structures affected depend on the specific lymph nodes involved by the original infection. Mediastinal fibrosis originating from subcarinal or hilar lymph nodes often results in occlusion of mainstem bronchi, pulmonary blood vessels, and the esophagus. Mediastinal fibrosis originating from right paratracheal lymph nodes commonly produces obstruction of the superior vena cava and azygos veins.[129]

### Foreign Bodies

Accidental inhalation of foreign bodies is a major cause of death in children: approximately 2000 children die annually in the United States of this cause.[130] The foreign bodies, which may be seeds, nuts, nails, or a variety of other objects, most frequently lodge in the right mainstem bronchus. Children with aspirated foreign bodies may present with immediate cyanosis, cough, and wheezing or with the delayed onset of pneumonia or bronchiectasis. Suspected aspiration of a foreign body is an indication for immediate fiberoptic bronchoscopy.[131]

### Granulomatous Inflammation

In patients with pulmonary tuberculosis, spillage of infected material into the middle and lower lobes occasionally causes localized endobronchial infection.[132] Endobronchial tuberculosis may present with hemoptysis, bronchorrhea, or localized bronchial obstruction, causing lobar collapse and persistent postobstructive pneumonitis. These findings may develop during active pulmonary infection by tuberculosis or many years after its treatment. The diagnosis is established most readily by fiberoptic bronchoscopy.[133] The typical finding is the presence of localized endobronchial gelatinous granulation tissue. The mucosa may be nodular, red, and ulcerated, and often the diagnosis of bronchogenic neoplasm is suggested until pathologic examination of biopsy material has been carried out.

In patients with pulmonary sarcoidosis, localized endobronchial granulomatous inflammation rarely may lead to stenosis of bronchi.[134] Pulmonary function tests often show airway obstruction, but the common causes of the obstruction are the structural distortion of bronchi and bronchioles that accompanies pulmonary fibrosis,[135] nonspecific bronchial hyperreactivity,[136] or laryngeal sarcoidosis.[137] Only rarely is bronchostenosis present.

*Bronchocentric granulomatosis* is an uncommon inflammatory lesion defined morphologically by the presence of necrotizing granulomas surrounding bronchi.[138] The entity occurs most commonly in asthmatic patients with allergic bronchopulmonary aspergillosis, and considerable evidence suggests that the granulomatous bronchitis is an immunologic response to endobronchial fungi. Narrowing or obliteration of bronchi may occur because of the inflammatory reaction itself or because of associated mucoid impaction.[138]

## Broncholithiasis

Broncholithiasis is defined as the presence of a calcified fragment of tissue within a bronchus.[139] Any disorder that leads to calcification of lung tissue or of lymph nodes may result in broncholithiasis. Most often, this occurs when hilar or peribronchial lymph nodes become calcified as a result of granulomatous infections, such as histoplasmosis or tuberculosis, or less commonly from actinomycosis, coccidioidomycosis, cryptococcosis, or silicosis.[139] Necrotizing pneumonias and bronchiectasis may lead to calcification of bronchial cartilage, which can fragment to produce broncholiths. Occasionally, retained foreign bodies may become calcified. Clinical manifestations of broncholithiasis occur when calcified stones erode or break loose into the airways (this is discussed in a subsequent section). These stones are composed of 85% to 90% calcium phosphate and 10% to 15% calcium carbonate and thus closely resemble bone.

## Amyloidosis

Amyloidosis (see also Chapter 86) is defined on the basis of the extracellular deposition of the fibrous protein amyloid.[140] In both the primary and secondary forms of the disease, these deposits can occur endobronchially, producing obstruction or incidental findings at the time of bronchoscopy.[141] As many as 30% of patients with primary amyloidosis are symptomatic. The definitive diagnosis of endobronchial amyloidosis requires biopsy and demonstration of amyloid deposits, as defined by their green birefringence when viewed with polarized light after staining with Congo red.[141]

## Bronchomalacia

Softening of the bronchial walls may contribute to expiratory narrowing of the airways in emphysema. Less commonly, bronchomalacia may be found in infants because of inadequate development of bronchial cartilage.[142] These infants generally present with dyspnea, atelectasis, or recurrent pneumonias.

## Traumatic Injury

Tears or complete ruptures of main-stem bronchi or the bronchus intermedius are occasional complications of blunt trauma to the chest. The diagnosis should be suspected in any post-traumatic patient with new onset of cough, respiratory distress, subcutaneous and mediastinal emphysema, or pneumothorax. The associated presence of hemoptysis or hemothorax indicates bronchial vascular damage. Occasionally, the development of manifestations of bronchial tears may be delayed for days or weeks after the traumatic injury.

## Clinical Features

Patients with localized endobronchial lesions generally present with symptomatic, physical, or radiographic manifestations of the lesion itself or of underlying conditions (e.g., malignancy, infection, AIDS, or sarcoidosis). Only the manifestations of the lesions themselves are described in this section.

The most common symptoms of localized endobronchial disease are cough, hemoptysis, wheeze, dyspnea, and fever and chills secondary to postobstructive pneumonia. If an endobronchial lesion only partially obstructs a bronchus, patients may show manifestations of chronic pulmonary infection, such as lung abscess (Chapter 33) or bronchiectasis (Chapter 41). A history of recurrent pneumonia in the same segment or lobe of the lung should prompt a careful evaluation for partial bronchial obstruction by an endobronchial lesion.[143] A similar caution should exist for any edentulous elderly patient with a history of a severe anaerobic pulmonary infection.[144]

Symptoms of broncholithiasis include cough, hemoptysis, fever associated with purulent sputum, and expectoration of stones. Often the cough in broncholithiasis is productive of a mixture of gritty, sandy particles and purulent or bloody sputum.

The physical examination in patients with localized endobronchial lesions may reveal fever and tachypnea. When a bronchus is narrowed but not completely obstructed, examination of the chest may reveal a unilateral palpable rhonchus, a prolonged forced inspiratory time on the affected side (the inspiratory "bagpipe" sign),[145] and a localized wheeze during a forced expiratory maneuver. Once the obstruction is complete, there is a loss of breath sounds and vocal fremitus during auscultation over the portion of the lung distal to the obstruction.

In patients with localized endobronchial disease, the

chest roentgenogram may show no abnormality. Radiographically, apparent lung collapse depends on the completeness of the obstruction and on the extent to which collateral ventilation from adjacent lung is present. In infants, the pores of Kohn, through which collateral ventilation normally occurs, are poorly developed.[146] Hence, the likelihood of complete collapse from localized bronchial disease is great in this age group. Other findings on the plain chest roentgenogram include mediastinal adenopathy with or without calcification, lung abscess, bronchiectasis, or pneumonia. The presence of air bronchograms in a consolidated region of the lung suggests that the bronchus supplying that region is at least partially patent.[147]

*Middle lobe syndrome* refers to chronic or recurrent radiographic evidence of collapse of the right middle lobe. Originally, it was postulated that the cause was tuberculous adenitis of lymph nodes in the right middle lobe, causing bronchial compression.[148] By bronchoscopic examination, however, most of these patients have completely normal right middle lobe bronchi. Therefore, in most instances, the collapse relates to the normal, relatively long length and narrow caliber of the right middle lobe bronchus or to the relatively ineffective collateral ventilation normally present in this lobe.[149]

## Diagnosis

In patients with only partial obstruction of a bronchus, comparing roentgenograms obtained at full inspiration with those obtained at full expiration may assist in establishing the diagnosis. On inspiration, the negative intrathoracic pressure distends the partially obstructed bronchus, and air enters the distal lung. On expiration, the obstruction becomes temporarily complete, and air is trapped behind it. The result is mediastinal shift away from the affected side on expiration. Computed tomography scans may identify hyperinflation, compressing lymph nodes or calcifications in patients with broncholithiasis, or subtle endobronchial abnormalities.[150, 151]

The definitive procedure for diagnosing localized bronchial abnormalities is direct bronchial examination via fiberoptic bronchoscopy. In general, any visualized abnormality should be biopsied, and the biopsied materials should be submitted for histologic examination as well as for culture. If the lesion is friable and bleeds easily during its examination and manipulation, rigid bronchoscopy may be required.

Routine pulmonary function tests in general do not distinguish between localized and widespread bronchial obstruction. In patients with bronchial compression or mediastinal fibrosis, skin tests for histoplasmosis or tuberculosis may be positive.[129] In bronchocentric granulomatosis, peripheral blood eosinophilia and serum precipitins for *Aspergillus* may be present.[138] In endobronchial amyloidosis, immunoelectrophoretic analysis of blood or urine shows evidence of monoclonal gammopathy in 90% of cases.[140]

## Treatment

The appropriate therapy of localized lesions of the bronchi depends on the specific underlying cause. Treatment of bronchial neoplasms is described in Chapters 44 to 49. In some patients with inoperable, obstructive neoplasms of the main-stem bronchi or bronchus intermedius, the use of the neodymium:yttrium-aluminum-garnet (Nd-YAG) laser has provided effective palliation of the obstructing lesions.[152] Bronchial obstruction from extrinsic compression or endobronchial granulomatous inflammation may be relieved by medical treatment of the underlying condition (e.g., lymphoma, tuberculosis), but irreversible fibrotic narrowing often requires surgical resection or stenting. Foreign bodies usually can be removed with specialized wire claws or baskets inserted through a bronchoscope.[131] When they are lodged in central airways, removal of foreign bodies is performed most effectively via a rigid bronchoscope. Broncholithiasis is often self-limited, requiring no further evaluation or treatment. However, if hemoptysis, persistent cough, atelectasis, or infection is present, bronchoscopic visualization is indicated. Stones sometimes can be removed bronchoscopically, and antibiotics should be administered to treat post-obstructive infection. Occasionally, surgical intervention is required to manage persistent or recurrent broncholithiasis.[139] In infants with bronchomalacia, effective treatment may require long-term ventilation of the lungs until normal cartilage is formed, which usually occurs by 6 months to 2 years of age.[142] Patients with suspected traumatic bronchial injury should undergo immediate endotracheal intubation and fiberoptic bronchoscopy, followed by thoracotomy.[153]

## Tracheobronchial Stents

Although prostheses have been used to relieve tracheal and bronchial obstruction for many years,[154] recent technical advances have made the procedure easier and more effective.[155] More than 20 kinds of tracheobronchial stents are now available, in metal, mesh, or silicone rubber, and insertion usually can be accomplished by fiberoptic bronchoscopy, without general anesthesia. Stents have been used effectively to relieve airway obstruction caused by malignancy, postinflammatory stenosis, and tracheobronchomalacia.[155–159] Fenestrated or mesh stents are more effective for benign lesions than for neoplasms, which tend to grow through the metal mesh.[160] Careful patient selection, choice of the correct stent, and an experienced bronchoscopist are important determinants of success.

## SUMMARY

This chapter includes discussion of a number of disorders that produce either diffuse or localized abnormalities of the intrathoracic bronchi and bronchioles. Bronchiolitis, bronchiolitis obliterans, and bronchiolitis obliterans with organizing pneumonia (BOOP) are being recognized increasingly in association with a wide range of respiratory insults and diseases. The clinical sequelae of these entities vary considerably, but in general, delayed diagnosis and therapy are associated with a poor prognosis. Because corticosteroid therapy may have a dramatic effect on the course of bronchiolitis obliterans and especially BOOP, early diagnosis is imperative. Diagnostic approaches include a high index of suspicion, careful physiologic testing, and histologic examination of involved lung. Localized dysfunction of intrathoracic airways may result from endobronchial neoplasms, compression of bronchi by lymph nodes, aneurysms, mediastinal fibrosis, foreign bodies, endobronchial granulomatous inflammation, endobronchial amyloidosis, bronchomalacia, or trauma. The clinical manifestations of these localized abnormalities include cough, hemoptysis, and complete or partial bronchial obstruction. Diagnosis depends primarily on direct visualization of the airways via fiberoptic bronchoscopy, and therapy is determined by the specific cause of the disorder.

## References


1. Hayek H: The Human Lung. New York: Hafner, 1960, pp. 298–314.
2. Miller WS: The Lung. Springfield, MI: Charles Thomas, 1947.
3. Richardson JB: Nerve supply to the lungs. Am Rev Respir Dis 119:785–802, 1979.
4. Widdicombe JG: Nervous receptors in the respiratory tract and lungs. *In* Hornbein TF (ed): Regulation of Breathing. New York: Marcel Dekker, 1981, pp. 429–472.
5. Hogg JC, Williams J, Richardson JB, et al: Age as a factor in the distribution of lower-airway conductance and in the pathologic anatomy of obstructive lung disease. N Engl J Med 282:1283–1287, 1970.
6. Wood LDH, Engel LA, Griffin P, et al: Effect of gas physical properties and flow on lower pulmonary resistance. J Appl Physiol 41:234–244, 1976.
7. Thurlbeck WM: Chronic Airflow Obstruction in Lung Disease. Philadelphia: WB Saunders, 1976, pp. 45–46.
8. Klingele TG, Staub NC: Terminal bronchiole diameter changes with volume in isolated, air-filled lobes of cat lung. J Appl Physiol 30:224–227, 1971.
9. Hughes JMB, Rosenzweig DY, Kivist PB: Site of airway closure in excised dog lungs: Histologic demonstration. J Appl Physiol 29:340–344, 1970.
10. Macklem PT, Thurlbeck WM, Fraser RG: Chronic obstructive disease of small airways. Ann Intern Med 74:167–177, 1971.
11. Milne JEH: Nitrogen dioxide inhalation and bronchiolitis obliterans. J Occup Med 11:538–547, 1969.
12. Horvath EP, doPico GA, Barbee RA, et al: Nitrogen dioxide–induced pulmonary disease. J Occup Med 20:103–110, 1978.
13. Von Oettingen WF: The toxicity and potential dangers of nitrous fumes. Public Health Bull 272:1–34, 1941.
14. Ramirez RJ, Dowell AR: Silo-filler's disease: nitrogen dioxide-induced lung injury: Long-term follow-up and review of the literature. Ann Intern Med 74:569–576, 1971.
15. Prowse K: Nitrous fume poisoning. Bull Europ Physiopathol Respir 13:191–202, 1977.
16. Milne JEH: Nitrogen dioxide inhalation and bronchiolitis obliterans. J Occup Med 11:538–547, 1980.
17. Darke CS, Warrack AJN: Bronchiolitis from nitrous fumes. Thorax 13:327–333, 1958.
18. Fleming GM, Chester EH, Montenegro HD: Dysfunction of small airways following pulmonary injury due to nitrogen dioxide. Chest 75:720–721, 1979.
19. Wohl MEB, Chernick V: Bronchiolitis. Am Rev Respir Dis 118:759–781, 1978.
20. Dines DE: Acute bronchiolitis as a cause of chronic obstructive lung disease in adults: Report of two cases. Lancet 87:281–282, 1967.
21. Sato P, Madtes DK, Thorning D, et al: Bronchiolitis obliterans caused by *Legionella pneumophila*. Chest 87:840–842, 1985.
22. Coultas DB, Samet JM, Butler C: Bronchiolitis obliterans due to *Mycoplasma pneumoniae*. West J Med 144:471–474, 1986.
23. Simpson H, Matthew DJ, Habel AH, et al: Acute respiratory failure in bronchiolitis and pneumonia in infancy. Br Med J 2:632–636, 1974.
24. Engel S: Bronchiolitis. Br J Dis Chest 53:125–127, 1959.
25. Koch DA: Roentgenologic considerations of capillary bronchiolitis. AJR Am J Roentgenol 82:433–436, 1959.
26. Sawazaki H, Watabe S, Onoki S, et al: Two cases of bronchiolitis obliterans. Jpn J Chest Dis 21:635–647, 1962.
27. Felson B, Felson H: Acute diffuse pneumonia of asthmatics. AJR Am J Roentgenol 74:235–241, 1955.
28. Green M: Bronchiolitis. *In* Sadul P, Milic-Emili J, Simonsson BG, Clark TJH (eds): Small Airways in Health and Disease. Amsterdam: Exerpta Medica, 1974, pp. 90–94.
29. Sims DG, Downham MAPS, Gardner PS, et al: Study of 8-year-old children with a history of respiratory syncytial virus bronchiolitis in infancy. Br Med J 1:11–14, 1978.
30. Hall CB, Hall WJ, Gala CL, et al: Long-term prospective study in children after respiratory syncytial virus infection. J Pediatr 105:358–364, 1984.
31. Weiss ST, Tager IB, Munoz A, et al: The relationship of respiratory infections in early childhood to the occurrence of increased levels of bronchial responsiveness and atopy. Am Rev Respir Dis 131:573–578, 1985.

31a. Kattan M: Epidemiologic evidence of increased airway reactivity in children with a history of bronchiolitis. J Pediatr 135:8–13, 1999.

32. Chang AB, Masel JP, Masters B: Post-infectious bronchiolitis obliterans: Clinical, radiological and pulmonary function sequelae. Pediatr Radiol 28:23–29, 1998.
33. Reynaud AC: Memoire sur l'obliteration des bronches. Mem Acad Med Paris 4:117–167, 1835.
34. Lange W: Ueber eine eigenthümliche Erkrankung der kleinen Bronchien und Bronchiolen (Bronchitis et Bronchiolitis obliterans). Deutsches Arch f klin Med 70:342–364, 1901.
35. Epler GR, Colby TV: The spectrum of bronchiolitis obliterans. Chest 83:161–162, 1983.
36. Meyers JL, Colby TV: Pathologic manifestations of bronchiolitis, constrictive bronchiolitis, cryptogenic organizing pneumonia, and diffuse panbronchiolitis. Clin Chest Med 14:611–621, 1993.
37. Swyer P, James G: Case of unilateral pulmonary emphysema. Thorax 8:133–136, 1953.
38. Macleod WM: Abnormal translucency of one lung. Thorax 9:147–153, 1954.
39. Gosink BB, Friedman PJ, Liebow AA: Bronchiolitis obliterans: Roentgenologic-pathologic correlation. AJR Am J Roentgenol 117:816–832, 1973.
40. Wright JL, Cagle P, Churg A, et al: Diseases of the Small Airways. Am Rev Respir Dis 146:240–262, 1992.
41. Colby TV: Bronchiolitis: Pathologic considerations. Am J Clin Pathol 109:101–109, 1998.
42. Collins RL, Turner RA, Johnson AM, et al: Obstructive pulmonary disease in rheumatoid arthritis. Arthritis Rheum 19:623–628, 1976.
43. Herzog CA, Miller R, Hoidal JA: Bronchiolitis and rheumatoid arthritis. Am Rev Respir Dis 124:636–639, 1981.
44. Bégin R, Massé S, Cantin A, et al: Airway disease in a subset of nonsmoking rheumatoid patients: Characterization of the disease and evidence for an autoimmune pathogenesis. Am J Med 72:743–750, 1982.
45. Yousem SA, Colby TV, Carrington CB: Lung biopsy in rheumatoid arthritis. Am Rev Respir Dis 131:770–777, 1985.
46. Geddes DM, Corrin B, Brewerton DA, et al: Progressive airway obliteration in adults and its association with rheumatoid disease. QJM 46:427–444, 1977.
47. King TE: Bronchiolitis obliterans. Lung 167:69–93, 1989.
48. Epler GR, Snider GL, Gaensler EA, et al: Bronchiolitis and bronchitis in connective tissue disease: A possible relationship to the use of penicillamine. JAMA 242:528–532, 1979.
49. Murphy KC, Atkins CJ, Offer RC, et al: Obliterative bronchiolitis in two rheumatoid arthritis patients treated with penicillamine. Arthritis Rheum 24:557–560, 1981.
50. Kinney WW, Angelillo VA: Bronchiolitis in systemic lupus erythematosis. Chest 82:646–649, 1982.
51. Schwartz MI, Matthay RA, Sahn SA, et al: Interstitial lung disease in polymyositis and dermatomyositis: Analysis of six cases and review of the literature. Medicine 55:89–104, 1976.
52. Clark JG, Schwartz DA, Flournoy N, et al: Risk factors for airflow obstruction in recipients of bone marrow transplants. Ann Intern Med 107:648–656, 1987.
53. Meyers JD, Flournoy N, Thomas ED: Nonbacterial pneumonia after allogenic bone marrow transplantation: A review of ten years' experience. Rev Infect Dis 4:1119–1132, 1982.

54. Winston DJ, Territo MC, Ho WG, et al: Alveolar macrophage dysfunction in human bone marrow transplant recipients. Am J Med 73:859–866, 1982.
55. Shields AF, Hackman RC, Fife KH, et al: Adenovirus infections in patients undergoing bone-marrow transplantation. N Engl J Med 312:529–533, 1985.
56. Burke CM, Theodore J, Dawkins KD, et al: Post-transplant obliterative bronchiolitis and other late lung sequelae in human heart-lung transplantation. Chest 86:824–829, 1984.
57. Yousem SA, Burke CM, Billingham ME: Pathologic pulmonary alterations in long-term human heart-lung transplantation. Hum Pathol 16:911–923, 1985.
58. Dawkins KD, Jamieson SW, Hunt SA, et al: Long-term results, hemodynamics, and complications after combined heart and lung transplantation. Circulation 71:919–926, 1985.
59. Glanville AR, Baldwin JC, Burke CM, et al: Obliterative bronchiolitis after heart-lung transplantation: Apparent arrest by augmented immunosuppression. Ann Intern Med 107:300–304, 1987.
60. Griffith BP, Paradis IL, Zeevi A, et al: Immunologically mediated disease of airways after pulmonary transplantation. Ann Surg 208:371–378, 1988.
61. Paradis I: Bronchiolitis obliterans: Pathogenesis, prevention, and management. Am J Med Sci 315:161–178, 1998.
62. Tazelaar HD, Prop J, Nieuwenhuis P, et al: Airway pathology in the transplanted rat lung. Transplantation 45:864–869, 1988.
63. Scott JP, Higenbottam TW, Sharples L, et al: Risk factors for obliterative bronchiolitis in heart-lung transplant recipients. Transplantation 51:813–817, 1991.
64. Ladowski JS, Hayhurst TE, Scheeringa RH, et al: Obliterative bronchiolitis following single-lung transplantation—Diagnosis by spirometry and transbronchial biopsy. Transplantation 55:207–209, 1993.
65. Kelly K, Hertz, MI: Obliterative bronchiolitis. Clin Chest Med 18:319–338, 1997.
65a. Husain AN, Siddiqui MT, Holmes EW, et al: Analysis of risk factors for the development of bronchiolitis obliterans syndrome. Am J Respir Crit Care Med 159:829–833, 1999.
66. Sundaresan S, Mohanakumar T, Smith MA, et al: HLA-A locus mismatches and development of antibodies to HLA after lung transplantation correlate with the development of bronchiolitis obliterans syndrome. Transplantation 65:648–653, 1998.
67. Duquesnoy RJ, Trager JDK, Zeevi A: Propagation and characterization of lymphocytes from transplant biopsies. Crit Rev Immunol 10:455–480, 1991.
68. Taylor PM, Rose ML, Yacoub MH: Expression of MHC antigens in normal human lungs and transplanted lungs with obliterative bronchiolitis. Transplantation 48:506–510, 1989.
69. Yousem SA, Curley JM, Dauber J, et al: HLA-class II antigen expression in human heart-lung allografts. Transplantation 49:991–995, 1990.
70. Romaniuk A, Prop J, Petersen AH, et al: Expression of class II major histocompatibility complex antigens by bronchial epithelium in rat lung allografts. Transplantation 44:209–214, 1987.
71. Lawrence EC, Holland VA, Young JB, et al: Dynamic changes in soluble interleukin-2 receptor levels after lung or heart-lung transplantation. Am Rev Respir Dis 140:789–796, 1989.
72. Rabinowich H, Zeevi A, Paradis IL, et al: Proliferative responses of bronchoalveolar lavage lymphocytes from heart-lung transplant patients. Transplantation 49:115–121, 1990.
72a. Jaramillo A, Smith MA, Phelan D, et al: Development of ELISA-detected anti-HLA antibodies precedes the development of bronchiolitis obliterans syndrome and correlates with progressive decline in pulmonary function after lung transplantation. Transplantation 67:1155–1161, 1999.
73. Veith FJ, Sinha SBP, Blümcke S, et al: Nature and evolution of lung allograft rejection with and without immunosuppression. J Thorac Cardiovasc Surg 63:509–520, 1972.
74. Prop J, Tazelaar HD, Billingham ME: Rejection of combined heart-lung transplants in rats: Function and pathology. Am J Pathol 127:97–105, 1987.
75. Platt JL, LeBien TW, Michael AF: Interstitial mononuclear cell populations in renal graft rejection: Identification by monoclonal antibodies in tissue sections. J Exp Med 155:17–30, 1982.
76. Marck K, Prop J, Wildevuur C, et al: Lung transplantation in the rat: histopathology of left lung iso- and allografts. Heart Transplant 4:263–265, 1985.
77. Bishop GA, Hall BM, Duggin GG, et al: Immunopathology of renal allograft rejection analyzed with monoclonal antibodies to mononuclear cell markers. Kidney Int 29:708–717, 1986.
78. Reinsmoen NL, Bolman RM, Savik K, et al: Differentiation of class I- and class II-directed donor-specific alloreactivity in bronchoalveolar lavage lymphocytes from lung transplant recipients. Transplantation 53:181–189, 1992.
79. Zeevi A, Fung JJ, Paradis IL: Bronchoalveolar macrophage lymphocyte reactivity in heart-lung transplant recipients. Transplant Proc 19:2537–2540, 1987.
80. Steinhoff G, Wonigeit K, Pichlmayr R: Analysis of sequential changes in major histocompatibility complex expression in human liver grafts after transplantation. Transplantation 45:394–401, 1988.
81. Grattan MT, Moreno-Cabral CE, Starnes VA, et al: Cytomegalovirus infection is associated with cardiac allograft rejection and atherosclerosis. JAMA 261:3561–3566, 1989.
81a. Ross DJ, Moudgil A, Bagga A, et al: Lung allograft dysfunction correlates with gamma-interferon gene expression in bronchoalveolar lavage. J Heart Lung Transplant 18:627–636, 1999.
82. Fujinami RS, Nelson JA, Walker L, et al: Sequence homology and immunologic cross-reactivity of human cytomegalovirus with HLA-DR β chain: A means for graft rejection and immunosuppression. J Virol 62:100–105, 1988.
83. Epler GR, Colby TV, McLoud TC, et al: Bronchiolitis obliterans organizing pneumonia. N Engl J Med 312:152–158, 1985.
84. Cordier J-F, Loire R, Brune J: Idiopathic bronchiolitis obliterans organizing pneumonia: Definition of characteristic clinical profiles in a series of 16 patients. Chest 96:999–1004, 1989.
85. Davison AG, Heard BE, McAllister WAC, et al: Steroid responsive relapsing cryptogenic organizing pneumonitis. Thorax 37:785–786, 1982.
86. Davison AG, Heard BE, McAllister WAC, et al: Cryptogenic organizing pneumonitis. QJM 52:382–394, 1983.
87. Tse RL, Bockman AA: Nitrogen dioxide toxicity: Reports of four cases in firemen. JAMA 212:1342–1344, 1970.
88. Jones GR, Proudfoot AT, Hall JI: Pulmonary effects of acute exposure to nitrous fumes. Thorax 28:61–65, 1973.
89. Wyatt SE, Nunn P, Hows JM, et al: Airways obstruction associated with graft versus host disease after bone marrow transplantation. Exp Hematol 12:17–18, 1984.
90. Ralph DD, Springmeyer SC, Sullivan KM, et al: Rapidly progressive air-flow obstruction in marrow transplant recipients: Possible association between obliterative bronchiolitis and chronic graft-versus-host disease. Am Rev Respir Dis 129:641–644, 1984.
91. Burke CM, Theodore J, Baldwin JC, et al: Twenty-eight cases of human heart-lung transplantation. Lancet 1:517–519, 1986.
92. Theodore J, Starnes VA, Lewiston NJ: Obliterative bronchiolitis. Clin Chest Med 11:309–321, 1990.
93. Ross DJ, Jordan SC, Nathan SD, et al: Delayed development of obliterative bronchiolitis syndrome with $OKT_3$ after unilateral lung transplantation: A plea for multi-center immunosuppressive trials. Chest 109:870–873, 1996.
94. Allen WE, Burke CM, McGregor CGA, et al: Steroid-responsive bronchiolitis after human heart-lung transplantation. J Thorac Cardiovasc Surg 92:449–451, 1986.
95. Hutter JA, Despins P, Higenbottam T, et al: Heart-lung transplantation: Better use of resources. Am J Med 85:4–11, 1988.
96. McCarthy PM, Starnes VA, Theodore J, et al: Improved survival after heart-lung transplantation. J Thorac Cardiovasc Surg 99:54–60, 1990.
97. Guerry-Force ML, Müller NL, Wright JL, et al: A comparison of bronchiolitis obliterans with organizing pneumonia, usual interstitial pneumonia, and small airways disease. Am Rev Respir Dis 135:705–712, 1987.
98. Niewoehner DE, Kleinerman J, Rice DB: Pathologic changes in the peripheral airways of young cigarette smokers. N Engl J Med 291:755–758, 1974.
99. Churg A, Wright JL: Small airways disease in persons exposed to nonasbestos mineral dusts. Hum Pathol 14:688–693, 1983.
100. Churg A, Wright JL: Small airway disease in mineral dust exposure. Pathol Annu 18(Part 2):233–251, 1983.
101. Bogin RM, Niccoli SA, Waldron JA, et al: Respiratory bronchiolitis: Clinical presentation and bronchoalveolar lavage findings. Chest 94:21S, 1988.

102. Lynch DA: Imaging of small airways diseases. Clin Chest Med 14:623–634, 1993.
103. Yamanaka A, Saeki S, Tamura S, et al: The problems of chronic obstructive pulmonary disease: Especially diffuse panbronchiolitis. Nakai-Inter Med 23:442–451, 1969.
104. Homma H: Diffuse panbronchiolitis. Jpn J Thorac Dis 13:383–395, 1975.
105. Homma H: Definition of diffuse panbronchiolitis. Jpn J Intern Med 65:645–659, 1976.
106. Homma H, Yamanaka A, Tanimoto S, et al: Diffuse panbronchiolitis: A disease of the transitional zone of the lung. Chest 83:63–69, 1983.
107. Izumi T: A nation-wide survey of diffuse panbronchiolitis in Japan. *In* Grassi C, Rizzato G, Pozzi E (eds): Sarcoidosis and Other Granulomatous Disorders. New York: Elsevier Science Publ, 1988.
108. Tsang KWT, Ooi CGC, Ip MSM, et al: Clinical profiles of Chinese patients with diffuse panbronchiolitis. Thorax 53:274–280, 1998.
109. Fitzgerald JE, King TE, Lynch DA, et al: Diffuse panbronchiolitis in the United States. Am J Respir Crit Care Med 154:497–503, 1996.
110. Akira M, Kitatani F, Yong-Sik L, et al: Diffuse panbronchiolitis: evaluation with high-resolution CT. Radiology 168:433–438, 1988.
111. Nishimura K, Kitaichi M, Izumi T, et al: Diffuse panbronchiolitis: High resolution CT and pathologic findings. Radiology 184:779–785, 1992.
112. Suzuki M, Usui K, Tamura N, et al: Familial cases of diffuse panbronchiolitis. Jpn J Thorac Dis 19:645–651, 1981.
113. Sugiyama Y, Kudoh S, Maeda H, et al: Analysis of HLA antigens in patients with diffuse panbronchiolitis. Am Rev Respir Dis 141:1459–1462, 1990.
113a. Emi M, Keicho N, Tokunaga K, et al: Association of diffuse panbronchiolitis with microsatellite polymorphism of the human interleukin 8 (IL-8) gene. J Hum Genet 44:169–172, 1999.
114. Kudoh S, Uetake T, Hagiwara K, et al: Clinical effect of low dose long term erythromycin chemotherapy of diffuse panbronchiolitis. Jpn J Thorac Dis 25:632–642, 1987.
115. Nagai H, Shishido H, Yoneda R, et al: Long-term low dose administration of erythromycin to patients with diffuse panbronchiolitis. Respiration 58:145–149, 1991.
116. Black PN: Anti-inflammatory effects of macrolide antibiotics. Eur Respir J 10:971–972, 1997.
116a. Nakamura H, Fujishima S, Inoue T, et al: Clinical and immunoregulatory effects of roxithromycin therapy for chronic respiratory tract infection. Eur Respir J 13:1371–1379, 1999.
117. Northway WH, Rosen RC, Porter DY: Pulmonary disease following respiratory therapy of hyaline-membrane disease. N Engl J Med 276:357–368, 1967.
118. Edwards DK, Dyer WM, Northway WH: Twelve years experience with bronchopulmonary dysplasia. Pediatrics 59:839–846, 1977.
119. Churg A, Golden J, Fligiel S, et al: Bronchopulmonary dysplasia in the adult. Am Rev Respir Dis 127:117–120, 1983.
120. Braman SS, Whitcomb ME: Endobronchial metastasis. Arch Intern Med 135:543–547, 1975.
121. Shepherd MP: Endobronchial metastatic disease. Thorax 37:362–365, 1982.
122. Rose RM, Grigas D, Strattemeir E, et al: Endobronchial involvement with non-Hodgkin's lymphoma: A clinical-radiologic analysis. Cancer 57:1750–1755, 1986.
123. Chernoff A, Rymuza J, Lippman ML: Endobronchial lymphocytic infiltration: Unusual manifestation of chronic lymphocytic leukemia. Am J Med 77:755–759, 1984.
124. Zibrak JD, Silvestri RC, Costello P, et al: Bronchoscopic and radiologic features of Kaposi's sarcoma involving the respiratory system. Chest 90:476–479, 1986.
125. Pitchenik AE, Fischl MA, Saldano MJ: Kaposi's sarcoma of the tracheobronchial tree: Clinical, bronchoscopic, and pathologic features. Chest 87:122–124, 1985.
126. Wang N, Morin J: Recurrent endobronchial soft tissue tumors. Chest 85:787–791, 1984.
127. Felson B: Neoplasms of the trachea and mainstem bronchi. Semin Roentgenol 20:23–37, 1983.
128. Corno A, Picardo S, Ballerini L, et al: Bronchial compression by dilated pulmonary artery: Surgical treatment. J Thorac Cardiovasc Surg 90:706–710, 1985.
129. Goodwin RA, Nickell JA, Des Prez RM: Mediastinal fibrosis complicating healed primary histoplasmosis and tuberculosis. Medicine 51:227–246, 1972.
130. Weissberg D, Schwartz I: Foreign bodies in the tracheobronchial tree. Chest 91:730–733, 1987.
131. Fieselman JF, Zavala DC, Keim LW: Removal of foreign bodies by fiberoptic bronchoscopy. Chest 72:241–244, 1977.
132. Ip MSM, So SY, Lam WK, et al: Endobronchial tuberculosis revisited. Chest 89:227–230, 1986.
133. Kim YH, Kim HT, Lee KS, et al: Serial fiberoptic bronchoscopic observations of endobronchial tuberculosis before and early after anti-tuberculosis chemotherapy. Chest 103:673–677, 1993.
134. Westcott JL, Noehren TH: Bronchial stenosis in chronic sarcoidosis. Chest 63:893–897, 1973.
135. Miller A, Tierstein AS, Jackler I, et al: Airway function in chronic pulmonary sarcoidosis with fibrosis. Am Rev Respir Dis 109:179–189, 1974.
136. Dines DE, Stubbs SE, McDougall JC: Obstructive disease of the airways associated with stage I sarcoidosis. Mayo Clin Proc 53:788–891, 1978.
137. James DG, Williams WJ: Sarcoidosis and Other Granulomatous Disorders. Philadelphia: WB Saunders, 1985, pp 58–59.
138. Katzenstein A, Liebow AA: State of the art: Bronchocentric granulomatosis, mucoid impaction, and hypersensitivity reactions to fungi. Am Rev Respir Dis 111:497–537, 1975.
139. Dixon GF, Donnerberg RL, Schonfeld SA, Whitcomb ME: Clinical commentary: Advances in the diagnosis and treatment of broncholithiasis. Am Rev Respir Dis 129:1023–1030, 1984.
140. Glenner GG: Amyloid deposits and amyloidosis. N Engl J Med 302:1283–1292, 1980.
141. Cordier JF, Loire R, Brune J: Amyloidosis of the lower respiratory tract: Clinical and pathologic features in 21 patients. Chest 90:827–831, 1986.
142. Denneny JC: Bronchomalacia in the neonate. Ann Otol Rhinol Laryngol 94:466–469, 1985.
143. Winterbauer RH, Bedon GA, Ball WC: Recurrent pneumonia: Predisposing illness and clinical patterns in 158 patients. Ann Intern Med 70:689–700, 1969.
144. Verghese A, Berk SL: Bacterial pneumonia in the elderly. Medicine 62:271–285, 1983.
145. Rabin CB: New or neglected signs in the diagnosis of chest diseases. *In* Fishman AP (ed): Pulmonary Diseases and Disorders. New York: McGraw-Hill, 1980, pp. 92–102.
146. Lakier JB, Stanger P, Heyman MA, et al: Tetralogy of Fallot with absent pulmonary valve: Natural history and hemodynamic considerations. Circulation 50:167–175, 1974.
147. Hinshaw HC, Murray JF: Diseases of the Chest. Philadelphia: WB Saunders, 1980, pp. 606–625.
148. Lindskog GE, Spear HC: Middle-lobe syndrome. N Engl J Med 253:489–495, 1955.
149. Inners CR, Terry PB, Traytsman RJ, et al: Collateral ventilation and the middle lobe syndrome. Am Rev Respir Dis 118:305–310, 1978.
150. Lau LSW, Simpson L, Murphy F: High resolution CT scanning of the bronchial tree. Australas Radiol 29:323–331, 1985.
151. Arakawa H, Webb WR: Air trapping on expiratory high-resolution CT scans in the absence of inspiratory scan abnormalities: Correlation with pulmonary function tests and differential diagnosis. Am J Radiol 170:1349–1353, 1998.
152. Brutinel WG, Cortese DA, McDougall JC, et al: A two year experience with the neodymium-YAG laser in endobronchial obstruction. Chest 91:159–165, 1987.
153. Kelley JP, Webb WR, Moulder PV, et al: Management of airway trauma. I. Tracheobronchial injuries. Ann Thor Surg 40:551–555, 1985.
154. Harkins WB: An endotracheal metallic prosthesis in the treatment of stenosis of the trachea. Ann Otol Rhinol Laryngol 61:932–935, 1952.
155. Phillips MJ: Stenting therapy for stenosing airway diseases. Respirology 3:215–219, 1998.
156. Wallace M, Charnsangavej C, Ogawa K, et al: Tracheobronchial tree: expandable metallic stents used in experimental and clinical applications. Radiology 158:309–312, 1986.

157. Simonds AK, Irving JD, Clarke SW, Dick R: Use of expandable metal stents in the treatment of bronchial obstruction. Thorax 44:680–681, 1989.
158. George PJ, Irving JD, Khaghani A, et al: Role of the Gianturco expandable metal stent in the management of tracheobronchial obstruction. Cardiovasc Intervent Radiol 15:375–381, 1992.
159. Monnier P, Mudry A, Stanzel F, et al: The use of the covered Wallstent for the palliative treatment of inoperable tracheobronchial cancers. Chest 110:1161–1168, 1996.
160. Sawada S, Tanigawa N, Kobayashi M, et al: Malignant tracheobronchial obstructive lesions: Treatment with Gianturco expandable metallic stents. Radiology 188:205–208, 1993.

SECTION J

# Neoplasms of the Lungs

# 44 Biology of Lung Cancer

Yoshitaka Sekido, M.D., Ph.D. • Kwun M. Fong, M.D., Ph.D.
Adi F. Gazdar, M.D. • John D. Minna, M.D.

Introduction
Lung Development, Differentiation, Preneoplasia, and Tumor Biology
- Lung Development
- Neuroendocrine Differentiation and Lung Cancer
- Preneoplasia: The Multistep Evolution of Lung Cancer
- Telomerase Activity
- Microsatellite Instability and Methylation Abnormalities
- Paraneoplastic Syndromes

Tumor Growth Stimulation and Dominant Oncogenes
- Transmembrane Receptors and Their Ligands
- *RAS* Family
- *MYC* Family

Tumor Suppressor Genes and Apoptosis
- P53 Pathway
- P16-Cyclin D1-CDK4-RB Pathway
- PTEN, FHIT, TGF-β, and Retinoids and Carotenoids
- Other Chromosome Loci for Candidate Tumor Suppressor Genes
- *BCL2* Family and Apoptosis

Host Response and Tumor Progression
- Host Immunity
- Tumor Angiogenesis
- Factors Influencing Metastases

Summary

## INTRODUCTION

Lung cancer is the most frequent cause of cancer death in the United States among both men and women, with an estimated 171,600 new cases and 158,800 deaths in 1999.[1] Despite many aggressive approaches to therapy and new chemotherapeutic agents, survival rates have changed little in the last decade. This has led to a major effort, aided by the rapid developments in molecular research, to increase the understanding of the processes leading to the development of lung cancer. The ultimate aim is to provide novel approaches to combat lung cancer by aiding in its early detection and prevention and devising new therapeutic strategies. This chapter reviews and summarizes some of these developments and attempts to provide some insight as to how these findings might affect future clinical work in lung cancer. Table 44.1 summarizes the major genetic alterations and biologic properties of lung cancer cells that are reviewed.

## LUNG DEVELOPMENT, DIFFERENTIATION, PRENEOPLASIA, AND TUMOR BIOLOGY

### Lung Development

Knowledge of the origin of the various cell types in the normal respiratory epithelium is essential to an understanding of the cells that give rise to the different types of lung cancer. Tracking cell lineages has hitherto been hampered by the lack of stem cell markers, but new molecular tools may help overcome this problem.

Specialized epithelial cells at all levels of the respiratory tract are thought to arise from the proliferation and subsequent differentiation of primordial undifferentiated cells from the foregut endoderm. The lungs develop from an evagination of a ventral groove in the endodermal tube at the level of the fourth visceral arch about 22 to 26 days after fertilization. This laryngotracheal diverticulum divides to form the trachea and primary bronchi, which branch further to give rise to the bronchial tree. Whereas basal, secretory, and ciliated cells are the major cell types constituting the pseudostratified portion of the tracheobronchial epithelium, the alveolar epithelium is composed of the morphologically distinct type I and type II alveolar cells.

Although stem cells must exist in the primitive embryonic lung, it is not known whether there are stem cells in the two epithelial-cell lineage compartments in the adult lung. In any case, both the airway and the alveolar compartments have a transiently dividing compartment of differentiated epithelial cells. These are the secretory cells and basal cells in the airway epithelium and the type II cells in alveolar epithelium. Conversely, ciliated airway cells and type I cells are considered to be terminally differentiated and do not appear to proliferate. It should be noted, however, that there is some plasticity in gene expression in the lung, and the role of stem cells in lung development has been reviewed.[2]

### Neuroendocrine Differentiation and Lung Cancer

**Neuroendocrine Phenotype.** A characteristic phenotype is common to the normal pulmonary neuroendocrine cells and a subset of lung malignancies, including small cell lung cancer (SCLC), carcinoids, and certain non–

**Table 44.1 MAJOR GENETIC ALTERATIONS AND BIOLOGIC PROPERTIES IN LUNG CANCER**

| | Small Cell Lung Cancer | Non–Small Cell Lung Cancer |
|---|---|---|
| Incidence | ~25% | ≈75% |
| Neuroendocrine phenotype | ~100% | LCNEs and carcinoids |
| Telomerase activity | ~100% | 80–85% |
| Microsatellite instabilities | ~35% | ≈22% |
| Paraneoplastic syndromes | Often | Occasional |
| Possible autocrine loop | GRP/GRP receptor<br>SCF/KIT | HGF/MET<br>NDF/ERBB |
| *RAS* mutation | <1% | 15–20% |
| *MYC* amplification* | 15–30% | 5–10% |
| *p53* mutation | 75–100% | ≈50% |
| *p53* abnormal expression (IHC) | 40–70% | 40–60% |
| RB absent protein expression | ≈90% | 15–30% |
| $p16^{INK4A}$ mutation | <1% | 10–40% |
| Absent $p16^{INK4A}$ expression (IHC) | 0–10% | 30–70% |
| BCL2 expression | 75–95% | 10–35% |
| Neuroendocrine phenotype | ≈100% | LCNEs and carcinoids |
| Radiation sensitivity | High | Low |
| Anti-tumor drug sensitivity | High | Low |

*Overexpression without amplification is observed in other cases; small cell lung cancer amplifications include *MYC, MYCN, MYCL*.

LCNE = large cell neuroendocrine carcinoma; IHC = immunohistochemical analysis; RB = retinoblastoma; GRP = gastrin-releasing peptide; HGF = hepatocyte growth factor; SCF = stem cell factor; NDF = neu differentiation factor.

small cell lung cancers (NSCLCs). In normal lung, pulmonary neuroendocrine cells show granular cytoplasmic staining with silver and may occur singly or in small clusters in the bronchi (neuroepithelial bodies). They are most numerous in late fetal and early postnatal life but are relatively scant in normal adult lung, suggesting that their secretions play a major role in pulmonary development and maturation. Many neuroendocrine properties are related to the synthesis, storage, and release of secretory products, which is thought to be the primary function of the neuroendocrine cells. Chromogranin A, synaptotagmin, and synaptophysin are proteins associated with secretory organelles (neurosecretory vesicles and dense-core granules) that store secreted products such as biogenic amines and regulatory peptides. L-Dopa decarboxylase, which is expressed by the neuroendocrine cells, is essential for biogenic amine formation.

SCLCs can express more than 30 different regulatory peptides and hormones that work in endocrine, autocrine, or paracrine fashions, as well as receptors for almost half of these factors. Certain peptides (gastrin-releasing peptide, calcitonin, neurotensin, arginine vasopressin, and corticotropin) are more frequently secreted than others (insulin, somatostatin, glucagon, gastrin, substance P, and parathyroid-like peptide). Neuroendocrine characteristics include expression of unique isozymes, such as neuron-specific enolase (NSE) and creatine kinase BB isozymes, or markers such as CD56 (or neural cell adhesion molecule [NCAM]) and CD57 (also known as Leu-7) and neuroendocrine-specific protein (NSP)—reticulons.[3] Expression of neuroendocrine markers in NSCLC tumors and cell lines has been associated with a poor prognosis and with in vitro chemoresistance.

Knowledge of the genetic program that induces neuroendocrine differentiation in lung cancer, and even normal lung, is limited. In *Drosophila* and in vertebrates, the achaete-scute family of basic helix-loop-helix transcription factors plays a critical developmental role in neuronal commitment and differentiation. A minority of normal bronchial epithelial cells and many lung cancers, especially SCLC, exhibit a neuroendocrine phenotype that may reflect a common precursor cell population. The transcription factor, human achaete-scute homologue-1 (hASH1), is selectively expressed in normal fetal pulmonary neuroendocrine cells, as well as in the diverse range of lung cancers with neuroendocrine features.[4] Newborn mice bearing a genetic disruption of the mouse homologue have no detectable pulmonary neuroendocrine cells. Further, hASH1 depletion from lung cancer cells by antisense oligonucleotides results in a significant decrease in the expression of neuroendocrine markers.[4]

**Transition Between SCLC and NSCLC.** Is there a common stem cell for all histologic types of lung cancer? Although lung cancers are classified into discrete histologic subtypes, individual tumors often display more than one histologic phenotype. For example, about 1% to 3% of cases of SCLC may be combined with adenocarcinoma or squamous cell carcinoma. One notion is that lung cancers represent a continuum of cell types and that transition among the cell types is possible within individual tumors. This phenotypic plasticity has been observed in cell lines and animal model system and in lung cancers in patients, raising the hypothesis that the four major lung cancer subtypes are related through a common differentiation pathway in the normal bronchial epithelium.

As described later, the finding of genetic abnormalities in lung cancer can be classified into two groups: those that are common to all lung cancers and those that segregate to some histologic subtypes of lung cancer. *RAS* mutation is limited to NSCLC, *RB* mutation relatively limited to SCLC, and *p16^INK4A^/CDKN2* mutation to NSCLC. Aberrant expression of CD44 is also considered to be a marker for NSCLC.[5, 6] In addition to *hASH1* and other differentiation genes, it is possible that some genetic changes of oncogenes or tumor suppressor genes (TSGs) affect the phenotypic commitment of lung cancers. Indeed, phenotypic transition has been demonstrated by the in vitro introduction of oncogenes or TSGs into lung cancer cell lines. For instance, *v-Ha-RAS* was shown to change SCLC cells into a NSCLC phenotype.[5, 7] In other words, RAS in combination with MYC may promote SCLC cell lines to lose SCLC markers and to gain phenotypic characteristics of NSCLC. Another in vitro study has suggested that transition form SCLC to NSCLC phenotype was accompanied by an increased binding activity of the phorbol 12-myristate 13-acetate (TPA)–responsive element (TRE) and recruitment of specific proteins of AP-1 transcription factor complex, which is one of four Fos family members.[8]

## Preneoplasia: The Multistep Evolution of Lung Cancer

A series of morphologically distinct preneoplastic changes (hyperplasia, metaplasia, dysplasia, and carcinoma in situ) can be observed in bronchial epithelium before the appearance of a clinically overt lung cancer, particularly squamous cell lung cancer. These preneoplastic cells and the bronchial epithelium adjacent to cancers contain a number of genetic abnormalities that are identical to some of the abnormalities found in overt cancer cells (discussed later), including *MYC* and *RAS* up-regulation, cyclin D1 expression, p53 immunoreactivity, BCL2 overexpression, and deoxyribonucleic acid (DNA) aneuploidy.[9–13] Immunohistochemical studies have shown p53 immunoreactivity (overexpression) in dysplasias,[9, 13] and a follow-up study confirmed a progression from p53-positive dysplasias to p53-positive squamous cell carcinomas in the bronchi of three former chromate workers.[11] BCL2 overexpression and BCL2-associated X protein (BAX) down-regulation occur in preinvasive lesions and are maintained during invasion.[13]

Allelotyping of precisely microdissected preneoplastic foci of cells shows that 3p allele loss is the earliest change, followed by 9p allele loss, 17p allele loss (and *p53* mutation), 5q allele loss, and *RAS* mutations.[14–16a] However, based on topographic analysis, others have speculated that *KRAS* activation occurs during the earliest stages of tumorigenesis.[12] Atypical alveolar hyperplasia, which might be a potential precursor lesion of adenocarcinomas, was also found to have *KRAS* mutations.[17, 18]

These observations are consistent with the multistep model of carcinogenesis and a "field cancerization" process, whereby the whole tissue region is repeatedly exposed to carcinogenic damage (e.g., tobacco smoke) and is at risk for development of multiple, separate foci of neoplasia.[19] The 3p, 9p, and 17p deletions often showed allele-specific loss (deletion of the same allele in preneoplastic tissues as in the primary tumor), consistent with either clonal evolution or another, unidentified mechanism specifically targeting the same allele, akin to imprinting.[14]

## Telomerase Activity

Human telomeres are specialized nucleoprotein structures located at the ends of chromosomes. They are composed of tandem hexameric repeats of the sequence 5′-TTAGGG-3′ bound to specific proteins. During normal cell division, the absence of telomerase activity is associated with progressive telomere shortening during replication. This progressive shortening is believed to represent an intrinsic "cellular clock," leading to cell senescence and normal cell "mortality." In contrast, germ cells, most stem cells, and most cancer cells have a telomerase activity that is able to compensate for telomere shortening by replacing the hexameric repeats onto the chromosomal ends, potentially leading to cellular "immortality." The telomerase holoenzyme is composed of both ribonucleic acid (RNA) and protein subunits. The human telomerase catalytic protein subunit, hTERT (telomerase reverse transcriptase), is expressed in human cancers and is able to restore telomerase activity if ectopically expressed. In almost all SCLCs and 80% to 85% of NSCLCs, the highly sensitive polymerase chain reaction (PCR)–based TRAP (telomeric repeat amplification protocol) assay demonstrates high levels of telomerase activity.[20, 21] High telomerase activity has also been associated with increased cell proliferation rates and advanced pathologic stage in primary NSCLCs.[21] However, telomerase activity and/or expression of the RNA component of human telomerase are frequently dysregulated in carcinoma *in situ* lesions, implicating its early involvement in the multistage development of lung cancer.[22]

## Microsatellite Instability and Methylation Abnormalities

**Microsatellite Instability.** Microsatellite repeats are highly polymorphic short tandem DNA repeat sequences, widely distributed throughout the genome. Studies of lung cancer have demonstrated abnormal sizes of these microsatellite repeats, referred to as microsatellite instability (MSI). The underlying mechanism generating these unstable sequences is not known, but it appears to be different from the related replication error repair phenotype caused by mutations in DNA mismatch repair genes that is seen in colon cancer.

There is a very wide range of reported MSI frequencies in lung cancer. Overall, 35% (37/106) of SCLCs and 22% (160/727) of NSCLCs showed some examples of MSI at individual loci.[23] In contrast, only 1% to 10% of all the samples showed MSI at multiple loci. The presence of MSI maybe related to reduced survival,[24] and it is controversial whether MSI is more frequently observed in advanced-stage tumors.[24, 25] The role of MSIs in lung cancer remains to be elucidated: does it play a causative role, resulting in disruption of specific genetic targets, or does it reflect nonspecific genome destabilization? In addition, the underlying defect affecting DNA synthesis and/or repair processes leading to MSI in lung cancer must be identified. Occasional mutations in the gene involved in the repair of oxidative DNA damage, the 8-oxoguanine DNA glycosylase *(OGGI)* gene, have been reported in lung cancer.[26]

**Aberrant Methylation in Lung Cancer.** The DNA of vertebrates contains tissue-specific patterns of methylated cytosine residues that have been transmitted by clonal inheritance through the strong preference of mammalian DNA (cytosine-5)-methyltransferase for hemimethylated DNA. Methylation patterns are established during early embryogenesis and gametogenesis. Appropriate methylation may help maintain genomic DNA stability, because hypomethylation in embryonic stem cells lacking a major enzyme responsible for methylation is associated with an elevation in mutation rates. Abnormalities of DNA methylation occur consistently in human neoplasia including lung cancer. Abnormal DNA methylation at cytosine residues in the CpG (C connected by a 3′,5′phosphodiester bond to a G) islands around the 5′ end of many genes may affect transcription, and it is believed that some TSGs may be epigenetically silenced by hypermethylation of the wild-type allele. Notably, hypermethylation in the 5′ region of the *RB, VHL,* $p16^{INK4A}$, *E-cadherin*, and *hMLH1* genes have been reported in human cancers. In a subset of NSCLCs, $p16^{INK4A}$ hypermethylation has been demonstrated.[27, 28] The methylated DNA sequences can be found in the tumor and patients' sera.[28a] Given the frequent absence of $p16^{INK4A}$ protein expression in primary NSCLCs and the lower frequency of structural gene mutations, it is likely that *p16* inactivation by methylation is a reasonably frequent event in lung cancer. Other regional sites of hypermethylation have been found in lung cancer, including 3p, 4q34, 10q26, and 17p13, although the precise gene targets are uncertain and the significance is not yet apparent.[29, 30]

Methylation also plays a role in mediating genomic imprinting that can be defined as a gamete-specific modification causing differential expression of the two alleles of a gene in somatic cells. Loss of genomic imprinting of the insulin-like growth factor 2 (*IGF2*) and *H19* genes, both mapped at 11p15, occurs in some lung cancers.[31, 32]

## Paraneoplastic Syndromes

Lung cancers, particularly SCLCs, are frequently associated with a number of clinical "paraneoplastic syndromes." The known underlying pathogenetic mechanisms can be grouped into two categories: hormonal and immunologic. In many cases, tumors retain their neuroendocrine phenotypes and produce hormones that are supraphysiologic and homeostatically inappropriate, resulting in endocrine manifestations. The production of such hormones may or may not be associated with overt clinical syndromes, depending on the functional activity and level of the ectopic hormone produced. Additionally, tumors not typically endocrine in nature, such as squamous cell carcinomas, can also produce factors with endocrine effects. The other paraneoplastic category involves an abnormal host immunologic response. Typically, an antibody or cellular cytotoxic response that has been generated against tumor-associated antigens cross-reacts against normal tissues, reminiscent of the autoimmune diseases.

**Syndrome of Inappropriate Antidiuretic Hormone.** Low serum sodium levels can occur in patients with lung cancer, most typically recognized as the syndrome of inappropriate antidiuretic hormone (SIADH). Approximately 14% (range, 7% to 35%) of patients with SCLC and far fewer of those with NSCLC have clinically evident hyponatremia or SIADH at the time of presentation. The mechanisms of SIADH include tumor cell expression of arginine vasopressin (AVP, also called antidiuretic hormone), and of atrial natriuretic factor (ANF) in the patients in whom AVP is not elevated. Most SCLC cell lines produce ANF, but a minority produce AVP. However this production, especially of ANF, does not necessarily cause clinical manifestations.[33, 34] Whether these two peptides account for all cases of hyponatremia in patients with SCLC is debatable.[33, 34]

**Humoral Hypercalcemia of Malignancy.** Hypercalcemia in cancer can be classified either as humoral hypercalcemia of malignancy (HHM), caused by circulating hormones, or local osteolytic hypercalcemia, caused by local paracrine factors secreted by cancers within bone. Parathyroid hormone-related protein (PTHrP), which is secreted by the tumor cells, causes most cases of HHM. PTHrP shares a significant homology with parathyroid hormone (PTH) in the critical amino terminus, which allows it bind to the PTH receptor. The clinical HHM syndrome and increased blood levels of PTHrP are more commonly found in patients with NSCLC, especially squamous cell carcinoma.[35]

**Paraneoplastic Cushing's Syndrome.** About half of patients with paraneoplastic Cushing's syndrome induced by ectopic production of corticotropin (ACTH) have lung cancer, predominantly SCLC. However, even in SCLC the clinical syndrome is rare, affecting fewer than 5% of SCLC patients. It is far more common to detect elevated serum and tissue levels of immunoreactive ACTH than to diagnose the clinical syndrome. Besides ACTH, other peptides processed from the precursor pro-opiomelanocortin (POMC), such as lipotropins, endorphins, and melanocyte-stimulating hormones, can be demonstrated at high levels in plasma and tissue extracts of patients with SCLC.

ACTH secretion by tumors of nonpituitary origin is characteristically resistant to negative feedback regulation by glucocorticoids. Although the general mechanism of the glucocorticoid-resistant state remains unclear, an ACTH-secreting SCLC cell line was reported to have both a structural defect in the intracellular glucocorticoid receptor and diminished glucocorticoid receptor–ligand binding activity.[36] Ectopic ACTH production may herald a poorer prognosis, because it has been associated with a low response to chemotherapy, short survival, and a high rate of complication to therapy.[37]

**Paraneoplastic Neuromuscular Syndromes.** A variety of the carcinoma-associated neuromyopathies (subacute cerebellar degeneration, optic neuritis and retinopathy, subacute necrotizing myelopathy, peripheral neuropathy, Lambert-Eaton syndrome, and polymyositis-dermatositis) have been reported in lung cancers. They are thought to result from immunologic cross-reactivity between tumor-associated antigens and normal host tissues. Unlike most other paraneoplastic disorders, the course of the neurologic abnormality is frequently independent of the clinical course of the underlying tumor.

The best studied of this group is the Lambert-Eaton syndrome, a disorder of neuromuscular transmission with diminished quantal release of acetylcholine. Acetylcholine is released from storage vesicles in the nerve ending in response to an action potential. This mechanism requires the regulated influx of calcium through voltage-gated channels in nerve terminals. In Lambert-Eaton syndrome, pathogenic autoantibodies are directed against the calcium channels that are present both on tumor cells and on distal motor nerve terminals. Autoantibodies found in the patients with this syndrome can react against the $\alpha 1$-subunits or beta subunits of the P/Q type or against the N- or L-types of calcium channels.[38, 38a]

SCLC patients with paraneoplastic encephalomyelitis/sensory neuropathy (PEN/SN) frequently have high titers in their serum and cerebrospinal fluid of antibodies called anti-Hu (or antineuronal nuclear autoantibody type 1 [ANNA-1]), which recognize 35- to 40-kd proteins. HuD, HuC, and Hel-N1 are anti-Hu antigens that consist of cytoplasmic RNA-binding proteins. Because only HuD is expressed in SCLC, it is thought to play a central role in the triggering of the anti-Hu immune response, although there is no direct evidence that these immune responses can induce the paraneoplastic syndrome.[39] Clinically, fewer than 1% of SCLC patients express high-titer anti-Hu antibodies and develop PEN/SN, but the presence of these antibodies at diagnosis may be a predictor of response to treatment.[40]

Recoverin, a photoreceptor-specific calcium-binding protein, is another autoantigen in cancer-associated degenerative retinopathy. Recoverin has been shown to be expressed in lung cancer,[41] but its clinical relevance has yet to be clarified.

## TUMOR GROWTH STIMULATION AND DOMINANT ONCOGENES

Many growth factors or regulatory peptides and their receptors are expressed by either the lung tumor or adjacent normal cells and thus provide a series of autocrine or paracrine growth stimulatory loops. Some components of these signaling pathways were initially identified as proto-oncogene products such as ERBB1, ERBB2, MET, and KIT. These can become abnormally activated in lung cancer by several different genetic mechanisms including point mutation, gene amplification/overexpression, and other, unidentified processes (Fig. 44.1).

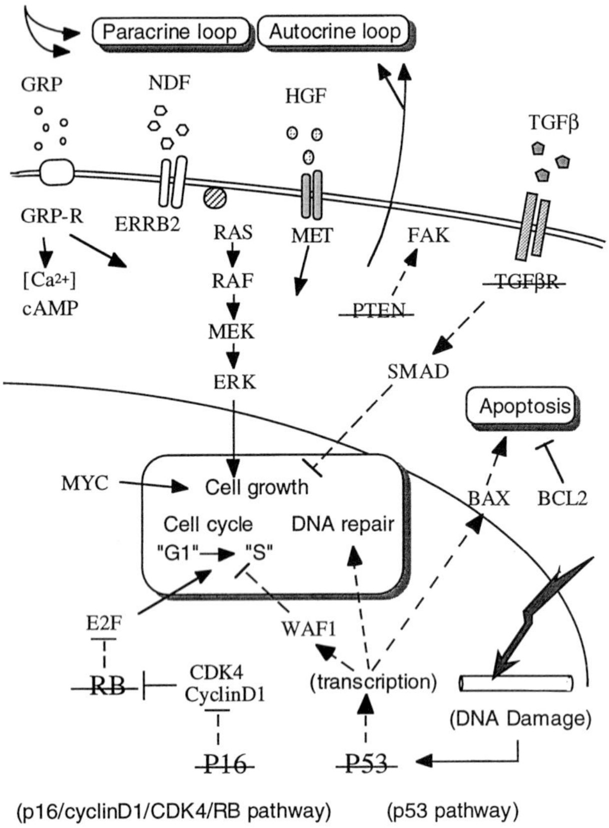


**Figure 44.1** A schematic representation of the major abnormalities involved in the regulation of growth control of lung cancer is presented. Frequent genetic mutations observed in lung cancer are gene amplification (MYC), activating mutations (RAS), and inactivating mutations (p53, p16, and RB, shown with line drawn through them to indicate mutation). GRP/GRP receptor, NDF/ERRB2, and hepatocyte growth factor (HGF)/Met oncogene (MET) consist of positive growth-stimulatory loops activating in autocrine or paracrine fashion. In contrast, TGFβ, TGFβR, and SMAD mediate a negative growth-stimulatory cascade.
Two major growth-regulatory pathways are inactivated in lung cancer, the p53 pathway and the p16$^{INK4A}$-cyclin D1-CDK4-RB pathway. Under stressed cellular conditions (DNA damage or hypoxia), p53 is activated by phosphorylation and can initiate downstream processes such as cell-cycle arrest, DNA repair, and apoptosis. CDK and cyclin D1 complex phosphorylate hypophosphorylated RB (active, growth-suppressing form) into hyperphosphorylated RB (inactive, non–growth-suppressing form). *Solid lines* and *dashed lines* indicate activated and inactivated signals in lung cancer, respectively. ERK = extracellular signal-regulated kinase; MEK = MAP kinase/ERK-activating kinase; NDF = neu differentiation factor; PTEN = phosphatase and tensin homologue deleted on chromosome 10; TGF = transforming growth factor; RB = retinoblastoma protein; GRP = gastrin-releasing peptide; CDK = cyclin dependent kinase.

## Transmembrane Receptors and Their Ligands

**Gastrin-Releasing Peptide.** The autocrine loop comprising gastrin-releasing peptide (GRP), other bombesin-like peptides (GRP/BN), and their receptors is the best characterized growth stimulatory loop in lung cancer. GRP is the 27-amino-acid mammalian homologue of the amphibian peptide bombesin. The human GRP/BN receptor subtypes, including GRP receptor (GRP-R), neuromedin B receptor (NMB-R), and bombesin receptor subtype-3 (BRS-3), belong to the G protein–coupled receptor superfamily with seven predicted transmembrane domains.[42] GRP/BN has been shown to be widely distributed in the central nervous system and gastrointestinal tract, but an important role of GRP/BN in lung development and repair also has been elucidated.[43] GRP/BN in embryonic pulmonary neuroendocrine cells augments epithelial growth and lung branching and stimulates migration of airway epithelial cells, a process thought to be essential for healing and restoration of function after airway injury.

Although no mutations in the genes encoding GRP/BN and the GRP/BN receptor subtypes have been found, the GRP/BN autocrine loop appears to be involved in the growth of SCLCs. It is possible that these embryogenic regulatory loops become reactivated during lung cancer development by unidentified mechanisms. Immunohistochemical studies showed that about 20% to 60% of SCLC cancers express GRP, and NSCLCs express GRP less frequently.[44] In comparison, expression of GRP/BN receptors has been shown to be widespread in both SCLC and NSCLC cell lines, with most tumors expressing at least one of the three receptors and many tumors expressing more than one.[42] The formation of soft agar clones in vitro and the in vivo growth of nude mouse xenografts of SCLC cell lines were inhibited by a neutralizing monoclonal antibody directed against the C-terminal domain of GRP/BN and by antagonists of bombesin.[45, 46] A clinical trial of the monoclonal antibody showed some antitumor activity among 12 patients with previously treated SCLC.[47]

**ERBB Family.** Neuregulins (also known as Neu differentiation factors [NDFs]) are peptide growth factors that interact with the ERBB family of transmembrane receptor tyrosine kinases (ERBB2, ERBB3, and ERBB4), which constitute other potential growth stimulatory loops in lung cancer. On binding neuregulin, the ERBB receptors homodimerize or heterodimerize, thereby inducing intrinsic kinase activities that initiate intracellular signal transduction cascades such as the mitogen-activated protein (MAP) kinase pathway. In lung cancer, *ERBB2* (also known as *HER2/neu*) is highly expressed in approximately 30% of NSCLCs, especially adenocarcinomas.[48, 49] *ERBB2* gene amplification as a mechanism of over-expression is rare in lung cancer. Experiments with transfected *ERBB2* in immortalized human bronchial epithelial cells suggests that *ERBB2* overexpression contributes to, but is not sufficient for, induction of tumorigenicity.[50] In any case, an anti-ERBB2 monoclonal antibody inhibited the in vitro growth of NSCLC cell lines expressing ERBB2.[51] Clinically, *ERBB2* overexpression correlates with a shorter survival time in some but not all studies of lung cancers.[52, 53] High levels of ERBB2 have also been associated with intrinsic multiple drug resistance in NSCLC cells[54] and increased metastatic potential in a NSCLC cell line,[55] which may help explain the poor outcome.

ERBB1 (also known as epidermal growth factor receptor [EGFR]) is homologous with ERBB2 and regulates epithelial proliferation and differentiation. Activation of *ERBB1* in lung cancer cells usually occurs by overexpression without amplification. More common in NSCLC than in SCLC, ERBB1 activation may be related to tumor stage and differentiation.[56, 57] Mice lacking *ERBB1/EGFR* have impaired epithelial development in several organs including the lung, with impaired branching, deficient alveolization, and septation.[58] Six characterized ligands bind to ERBB1, including epidermal growth factor (EGF) and transforming growth factor-α (TGF-α). Production of ERBB1/EGFR ligands, especially TGF-α, by lung cancer cells expressing cognate receptors suggests the existence of an autocrine loop.[49, 59] The JUN kinase/stress-activated protein kinase (JNK/SAPK) pathway is also required for EGF growth stimulation of A549 lung cancer cells.[60]

**Other Membrane Tyrosine Kinases.** The hepatocyte growth factor/scatter factor (HGF/SF) acts as a mesenchyme-derived morphogenic factor during fetal lung development.[61] HGF is also expressed in normal lung at very low levels, but these levels increase in response to lung injury.[62] HGF is a potent mitogen and/or motogen for human bronchial epithelial, alveolar type II, and SCLC cells in vitro. Whereas the *MET* proto-oncogene encoding the HGF receptor was expressed in normal lung, SCLC, and NSCLC, the HGF ligand was expressed in most NSCLCs but not in SCLCs; this suggests an autocrine loop specific for NSCLC.[63, 64] Elevated HGF was also strongly associated with poor outcome for patients with resectable NSCLC.[65]

The *KIT* proto-oncogene, which encodes yet another tyrosine kinase receptor, CD117, and its ligand, stem cell factor (SCF), are coexpressed in many SCLCs.[66, 67] Activation of this putative SCF/KIT autocrine loop may provide a growth advantage or mediate chemoattraction for SCLC. Insulin-like growth factors (IGF-1 and IGF-2) and the type I IGF receptor (IGF-R) are frequently coexpressed in both SCLC and NSCLC.[68] IGF-2 may be the predominant IGF involved in the autocrine growth stimulation of lung cancer. The proto-oncogene of *v-sis*, platelet-derived growth factor (PDGF), and its receptor (PDGFR, or CD140) were also found to be coexpressed in lung cancer, generating another potential autocrine loop.[69] Nerve growth factor (NGF) was shown to have antiproliferative effects on two SCLC cell lines expressing NGF receptors in vitro and in vivo.[70] In contrast, others reported that NGF stimulated clonal growth of three lung cancer cell lines.[71]

Finally, all histologic types of lung cancer express nicotine receptors, which have characteristics of acetylcholine receptors, and a variety of opioid receptors and are able to produce several opioid peptides. Opioids can inhibit lung cancer cell growth and cause apoptosis, leading to the apparent paradox whereby lung cancer cells express a negative opioid autocrine regulatory loop.[72] Although nicotine itself does not appear to stimulate growth of the majority of lung cancer cells, it can antagonize the apoptotic effect of opioids, and it is therefore possible that nicotine inhaled through cigarette smoking may play a direct role in lung cancer pathogenesis by inhibiting apoptosis.[72]

## *RAS* Family

The *RAS* gene family (*KRAS*, *HRAS*, and *NRAS)* represent oncogenes that are important in a subset of lung cancers. *RAS* genes are activated by point mutations at codons 12, 13, or 61 in approximately 20% to 30% of lung adenocarcinomas and 15% to 20% of all NSCLCs but very rarely in SCLCs.[44] Although the RAS protein usually works by binding to guanosine triphosphate transiently, owing to an intrinsic guanosine triphosphatase activity, mutations result in the protein's being locked in an "on" position, thus inappropriately signaling for continued cell division. Mutations in *KRAS* account for approximately 90% of *RAS* mutations in lung adenocarcinomas, with 85% of the *KRAS* mutations affecting codon 12. However, the finding of *KRAS* mutations in parenchymal but not in bronchial adenocarcinomas indicates genetic heterogeneity even within this subtype.[17] Furthermore, goblet-cell tumors appears to have the highest frequency of *KRAS* mutation among the adenocarcinoma subtypes.[73]

Most *KRAS* mutations (70%) are G-T transversions, with the substitution of either cysteine (TGT) or valine (GTT) for the normal glycine (GGT). Similar G-T transversions also affect the *p53* gene in lung cancer, and they represent the type of DNA damage to be expected from bulky DNA adducts caused by the polycyclic hydrocarbons and nitrosamines in tobacco smoke.[74] Further evidence for a causative role of tobacco smoke in these mutations is the correlation of *KRAS* mutations with a smoking history.[75] *KRAS* mutations portend a poor prognosis in both early- and late-stage NSCLC, and their presence may prove to be a clinically useful prognosticator,[76–78] although there have been some conflicting reports.[79] It has been suggested that *RAS* mutations induce resistance to chemotherapy and radiation, but no association between *RAS* mutation and resistance against a range of chemotherapeutic agents was found in a panel of NSCLC cell lines in vitro.[80] In addition, a prospective study showed that neither chemotherapy sensitivity nor survival correlated with *KRAS* mutation in patients with advanced (inoperable stage III or stage IV) lung adenocarcinoma.[81] There is much therapeutic optimism for attacking RAS malfunction with new agents such as farnesyltransferase and geranylgeranyltransferase I inhibitors. These agents, which inhibit posttanscriptional modification of KRAS, suppressed growth of lung cancer cells with mutant *KRAS* in nude mice.[82]

The major downstream factors to RAS include the RAF1/MEK/ERK pathway (ERK = extracellular signal-regulated kinase; MEK = MAP kinase/ERK-activating kinase; RAF1 = human homologue of v-*raf* oncogene). Although one copy of *RAF1* at chromosome region 3p25 is frequently deleted in human lung cancer, no *RAF1* mutations have been detected. Because allelic loss is more mechanistically consistent with a TSG rather than a dominant proto-oncogene role, it is intriguing that activated RAF1 causes growth arrest in SCLCs.[83] If activation of the RAF1/MEK/ERK pathway, perhaps accompanied by other genetic changes such as p27$^{KIP1}$ induction, suppresses SCLC growth, this could be the reason why *RAS* mutations are very infrequent in SCLCs.

## *MYC* Family

The RAS signal transduction cascade ultimately activates nuclear proto-oncogene products, such as MYC, that belong to the basic helix-loop-helix leucine-zipper (bHLHZ) class of transcription factors. Through heterodimerization with MAX, MYC-MAX heterodimers recognize specific DNA motifs with high affinity, which leads to transcriptional activation of downstream genes. MYC function has been implicated in normal cell-cycle progression, differentiation, and programmed cell death.

*MYC*, *MYCN*, and *MYCL* are the major members of the *MYC* family; *MYCL* was originally isolated from a lung cancer cell line.[84] *MYC* is the one most frequently activated in SCLC and NSCLC, whereas abnormalities of *MYCN* and *MYCL* usually occur only in SCLC. Activation of the *MYC* family of genes has been observed by gene amplification or by transcriptional dysregulation without amplification, both of which lead to protein overexpression. These genes are amplified to 20 to 115 copies per cell, but in most cases only one member of the *MYC* family is amplified. Richardson and Johnson[44] concluded from 17 studies that 36 (18%) of 200 SCLC tumors and 38 (31%) of 122 SCLC cell lines had gene amplification of one member of the *MYC* family. Conversely, only 25 (8%) of 320 NSCLC tumors and 3 (20%) of 15 NSCLC cell lines were amplified for the *MYC* gene family.[44] Although *MYC* translocations have not been reported in lung cancer, there are reports of *MYCL* amplification with *MYCL* fusion to the approximately 480-kb upstream *RLF* gene, causing a chimeric protein.[85]

*MYC* gene family amplification appears to occur more frequently in cell lines (often derived from metastases) than in primary tumors; in patients previously treated with chemotherapy; and in the "variant" subtype SCLC.[86] These findings may explain why *MYC* amplification correlates with adverse survival. In addition, *MYCL* expression may be associated with a high level of neuroendocrine differentiation in SCLC. The growth inhibition of an SCLC cell line by all-*trans*-retinoic acid (RA) was associated with increased neuroendocrine differentiation and increased *MYCL* but decreased *MYC* expression.[87] Finally, it is debatable whether an *Eco*RI restriction fragment length polymorphism (RFLP) in *MYCL* might be associated with lung cancer susceptibility, metastasis, and adverse survival.[88]

Although reports have implicated other nuclear proto-oncogenes such as *MYB, JUN,* and *FOS* in lung cancer, the biologic basis and significance of these genes in lung cancer are still being investigated.[89, 90] In addition, comparative genome hybridization studies have indicated the presence of several new amplified chromosome regions that probably contain new dominant oncogenes.[91, 92]

# TUMOR SUPPRESSOR GENES AND APOPTOSIS

## p53 Pathway

p53 maintains the integrity of the genome in the face of DNA damage by gamma-irradiation, ultraviolet irradiation, or carcinogens. In response to DNA damage or hypoxia, p53 activation results in a rapid increase of its protein, which acts as a sequence-specific transcription factor regulating downstream genes such as *p21, MDM2, GADD45,* and *BAX* (see Fig. 44.1). In general terms, these genes function to regulate either the G1/S phase transition or apoptosis. p53 also appears to participate in the DNA damage checkpoints of the cell cycle at the G2/M boundary.

Loss of p53 function allows the inappropriate survival of genetically damaged cells, setting the stage for the evolution of a cancer cell. *p53* gene plays a critical role in lung cancer[93] and other cancers, with thousands of mutations documented.[94] One copy of the chromosomal region 17p13, which houses *p53,* is frequently deleted in lung cancer, and mutational inactivation of the remaining allele occurs in 75% to 100% of SCLCs and approximately 50% of NSCLCs.[74] Somatic mutations are most common in the evolutionarily conserved *p53* exons 5 to 8, including missense and nonsense mutations, splicing abnormalities, and larger deletions. A causative role for tobacco carcinogens is suggested, because *p53* mutations in lung tumors correlate with cigarette smoking and are most commonly the G-T transversions expected from tobacco smoke carcinogens.[74] Furthermore, in bronchial epithelial cells, benzo(*a*)pyrene, a major cigarette smoke carcinogen, selectively forms adducts at nucleotides known to be the major *p53* mutational hot spots.[95] Most mutations are missense and prolong the half-life of the p53 protein to several hours, leading to increased protein levels that can be detected by immunohistochemistry.[96] Such studies have shown abnormal p53 expression in 40% to 70% of SCLCs and 40% to 60% of NSCLCs (higher in squamous cell carcinomas than in adenocarcinomas).[97, 98] Despite many studies the prognostic value of p53 mutations, determined by either immunohistochemical or molecular techniques, is controversial, and currently it appears that no prognostic significance should be placed on p53 abnormalities.[99]

The in vitro reintroduction of wild-type *p53* into lung cancer cells with various other genetic abnormalities besides *p53* blocked tumor cell growth by apoptosis but not G1 arrest.[100] Injection of wild-type p53 in a retroviral construct directly into tumors in nine patients with NSCLC for whom conventional treatment had failed led to tumor regression in a third and stabilized tumor growth in three others, with more frequent apoptosis in posttreatment compared with pretreatment biopsies.[101] A promising alternative strategy for early lesions involves the use of liposomal-p53 complexes delivered endobronchially.[102]

About 15% to 25% of lung cancer patients develop antibodies against the p53 protein, suggesting the possibility that mutant p53 protein overexpression can lead to a humoral immune response. Although p53 antibodies have been suggested as an early diagnostic marker,[103] the presence of antibodies does not appear to be a useful prognostic marker.[104] However, one study showed that p53 antibodies are rapidly reduced during chemotherapy.[105]

p73 and p51, proteins homologous to p53, have been isolated and mapped to 1p36 and 3q28, respectively. Both of these proteins can induce growth suppression and apoptosis. p73 mutations were not detected in lung cancers despite frequent loss of heterozygosity in this region (42%).[106] In contrast, others have suggested that p73 may play an important role in lung tumorigenesis through activation rather than as a TSG, because wild-type p73 was demonstrated to be highly expressed in lung tumors.[107] Similarly, p51 mutations were detected only infrequently in human tumors including lung cancer.[108]

*p21* (also known as *WAF1* or *CIP1*) is a p53-responsive gene that inhibits cyclin/cyclin-dependent kinase complexes at the G1 phase. Although it is not mutated in lung cancer, p21 overexpression is seen in 65% to 75% of NSCLCs, especially in well differentiated tumors. This high frequency suggests that p21 can be expressed independently of p53 alterations.[109] In one NSCLC study, p21 immunohistochemical expression was detected in almost 75% of tumors and was associated with favorable survival.[110] In another NSCLC study, concordant expression of p21 and TGF-$\beta_1$ predicted a better survival than did discordant p21 and TGF-$\beta_1$ expression.[111]

The *MDM2* oncogene product inhibits p53 by blocking the ability of p53 to regulate target genes and by reducing p53 levels through enhanced proteasome-dependent degradation. Conversely, p53 autoregulates the expression of the *MDM2* gene in a feedback loop. Although *MDM2* gene amplification was detected in 2/30 NSCLCs, the protein was expressed in 48/201 NSCLCs.[112] It has been suggested that several p53 mutants can still bind to the p53-responsive element of the *MDM2* gene, which may account for the overexpression of MDM2.[113] MDM2 expression without abnormal p53 expression was reported to be a favorable prognostic factor.

## p16$^{INK4A}$-Cyclin D1-CDK4-RB Pathway

**The Retinoblastoma Gene.** The p16$^{INK4A}$-cyclin D1-CDK4-RB pathway is central to controlling the G1/S phase transition of the cell cycle. One of the four genes that comprise this pathway is functionally altered or mutated in most lung cancers (see Fig. 44.1).

The retinoblastoma gene *(RB),* located in chromosomal region 13q14, encodes a nuclear phosphoprotein that was initially identified as a TSG in retinoblastomas. Hypophosphorylated RB (active growth-suppressing form) binds and controls a number of other cellular proteins, including the transcription factor E2F-1, which is essential for G1/S phase transition. RB has been shown to recruit histone diacetylase (HDAC1) to E2F; HDAC1 modifies chromatin architecture by deacetylation, thereby repressing E2F-mediated gene expression. Meanwhile, cyclin D1/cyclin-dependent kinase 4 (CDK4) and other cyclin/CDK complexes phosphorylate RB and inactivate the binding activity of RB to the transcription factors, thereby allowing entry into S phase. Thus, inhibition of G1/S progression is a major growth-suppressing function of RB.

Inactivation of both *RB* alleles is common in lung cancers,[114] with RB protein abnormalities present in approximately 90% of SCLCs and 15% to 30% of NSCLCs.[115–117] Underlying *RB* mutations include deletional truncation, nonsense mutations, and splicing abnormalities frequently leading to truncated RB protein. The few point mutation studies of the *RB* gene showed that most such mutations result in RB truncation.[118] The sensitivity of methods for detecting RB abnormalities in SCLCs varies: sensitivity is about 20% by Southern blot band loss; approximately 60% by Northern blot detection of absent or abnormal RNA; and almost 90% by protein or immunohistochemical analysis. Conversely, in NSCLCs, RB abnormalities were detected in 0.9% (2/219) by Southern analysis, 10% (22/219) by Northern analysis, and 32% (53/163) by immunohistochemistry.[115] Functionally, the in vitro reintroduction of a wild-type *RB* suppressed the growth of SCLC cells.[119]

Absence of RB expression was associated with poor prognosis in NSCLCs, particularly stage I and II disease,[120] in some but not all studies.[117, 121] Relatives of retinoblastoma patients who carry germline *RB* mutation are almost 15 times more likely to die from lung cancer than are persons in the general population.[122]

Two structurally and functionally related genes, *p107* and *pRB2/p130,* are other members of the *RB* gene family that have also been implicated in lung cancer. One SCLC cell line was shown to have a point mutation of *p130* in a splice acceptor site, leading to loss of exon 2 and expression of a truncated p130 protein.[123]

**Cyclin D1 and CDK4.** As cyclin D1 inhibits the activity of RB by stimulating its phosphorylation by CDK4, cyclin D1 over-expression seems to be an alternative way for disrupting the p16$^{INK4A}$-cyclin D1-CDK4-RB pathway in lung cancer. Overexpression of the CCND1 (also known as *PRAD1* or *BCL1*) proto-oncogene that encodes cyclin D1 can be induced by amplification or by chromosomal translocation in different tumors. Cyclin D1 was overexpressed at 4- to 100-fold higher levels in 11 of 12 NSCLC cell lines compared with an immortalized bronchoepithelial cell line.[124] In 53 primary resected NSCLCs, amplification of *CCND1* was detected in 8 samples (15%) and overexpression in 25 samples (47%).[125] Transfection of a cyclin D1 antisense construct into lung cancer cell lines induced destabilization of RB and retarded lung cancer cell growth.[126] Although amplification of *CDK4*, the other component of the cyclin D1 complex, has been reported in other human malignancies, its role in lung cancer has not yet been studied.

**The *p16$^{INK4A}$* Gene.** Chromosome 9p allele loss is observed in many lung cancers.[127] The *p16$^{INK4A}$* gene (also known as *CDKN2* or *MTS1*), situated at 9p21, undergoes allele loss and mutation in a variety of human cancers, including lung cancer.[23] Mutation of *p16$^{INK4A}$* represents another tumor strategy for disrupting the p16$^{INK4A}$-cyclin D1-CDK4-RB pathway in lung cancer. The p16$^{INK4A}$ protein is a cell-cycle modulator that appears to regulate RB function by inhibiting CDK4 and CDK6 kinase activity.

*$p16^{INK4A}$* abnormalities have been found frequently in NSCLC but rarely in SCLC. Homozygous deletion or point mutations have been observed in 10% to 40% of NSCLCs.[128, 129] Hypermethylation in the 5′ CpG island of the retained allele may also cause down-regulation of *$p16^{INK4A}$* in lung cancer.[27, 28] Early genetic assays underestimated the frequency of *$p16^{INK4A}$* inactivation because it often occurs by transcriptional silencing and hypermethylation in addition to allelic deletion and mutation. Each of these differing inactivation mechanisms contributes to the ultimate loss of *$p16^{INK4A}$* expression.[130] In NSCLC, the $p16^{INK4A}$-cyclin D1-CDK4-RB pathway is mostly inactivated through $p16^{INK4A}$ inactivation (30% to 70% of NSCLCs), whereas RB inactivation is the preferential mechanism in SCLC (90% of SCLCs and 15% to 30% of NSCLCs).[121, 131–134a] Inactivation of both *RB* and *$p16^{INK4A}$* is uncommon, but cyclin D1 overexpression can coexist with each of these changes.[135] Ten percent to 30% of NSCLCs appear to be normal for both *RB* and *$p16^{INK4A}$*, indicating the likely contribution from abnormalities of cyclin D1, CDK4, and other pathway members. It may well be that most, if not all, lung cancers have acquired abnormalities in this $p16^{INK4A}$-cyclinD1-CDK4-RB pathway.

It has been suggested that *$p16^{INK4A}$* mutations in lung cancer are associated with tumor progression,[136] and an immunohistochemical study of primary NSCLCs showed that the percentage of *$p16^{INK4A}$*-negative tumors increased correspondingly with clinical stage.[121] Although this finding was not confirmed in another study,[134] both studies showed that 30% to 40% of early-stage primary NSCLCs have absent *$p16^{INK4A}$* expression. Some studies have reported that the absence of *$p16^{INK4A}$* expression is a predictor of adverse survival in NSCLC.[121, 137] In addition, *$p16^{INK4A}$* expression was shown to be associated with the increased sensitivity of ectopic *$p16^{INK4A}$*-expressing NSCLC cells to DNA topoisomerase I inhibitors.[138]

The *$p16^{INK4A}$* locus encodes a second alternative reading frame (ARF) protein, $p14^{ARF}$ (the mouse homologue is called $p19^{ARF}$), which may be a TSG (possibly via direct binding to the MDM2-p53 complex) and prevents p53 degradation, resulting in p53 activation. An immunohistochemical analysis showed that $p19^{ARF}$ protein was more frequently lost in large cell neuroendocrine NSCLCs and SCLCs than in NSCLCs without neuroendocrine features.[139]

Although there are other CDK inhibitor genes, including *$p15^{INK4B}$*, *$p18^{INK4C}$*, *$p19^{INK4D}$*, *p21* (previously discussed), *$p27^{KIP1}$*, and *$p57^{KIP2}$*, mutational analyses of these genes have not detected significant genetic changes in lung cancer except for *$p15^{INK4B}$* (*CDKN2B* or *MTS2*). *$p15^{INK4B}$* shares about 70% amino acid similarity to *$p16^{INK4A}$*, and because it is immediately centromeric to *$p16^{INK4A}$*, codeletion of *$p15^{INK4B}$* with *$p16^{INK4A}$* has been frequently demonstrated in NSCLCs, whereas *$p15^{INK4B}$* point mutations are rare.

Similarly, *$p27^{KIP1}$* has not been found to be mutated in human lung cancers. However, reduced $p27^{KIP1}$ expression in NSCLC patients correlated with poor prognosis.[140, 141] In contrast, most SCLCs exhibited increased $p27^{KIP1}$ staining, suggesting a possible link between $p27^{KIP1}$ and neuronal differentiation.[141] Another CDK inhibitor, *$p57^{KIP2}$*, which mapped to 11p15, was found to be imprinted with maternal expression, and *$p57^{KIP2}$* expression was down-regulated by selective loss of the maternal alleles in some lung cancers.[142]

## *PTEN, FHIT,* TGF-β, and Retinoids and Carotenoids

**The *PTEN* Gene.** A large number of protein kinases, many of them oncogene products, have been implicated in carcinogenesis. This has led to the proposal that protein tyrosine phosphatases play a role in tumor suppression due to their ability to antagonize the growth-promoting protein kinases. A candidate is the phosphatase encoded by the *PTEN* (*MMAC1*) gene, which is located at chromosome region 10q23,[143] where lung cancer has also been shown to have frequent loss of heterozygosity.[144] PTEN has sequence similarity to the cytoskeletal protein tensin, and it dephosphorylates protein and peptide substrates phosphorylated on serine, threonine, and tyrosine residues, indicating a dual-specificity phosphatase activity. Moreover, PTEN interacts with the focal adhesion kinase (FAK) and regulates cell interactions with the extracellular matrix.[145]

Frequent somatic mutations of this gene have been found in various kinds of tumors, including glioblastoma, prostate, kidney, and breast cancers.[143] *PTEN* was also found to be mutated in a few primary lung cancers, and several lung cancer cell lines showed homozygous deletions of this gene.[146]

**The *FHIT* Gene.** Candidate TSGs are predicted at the chromosome 3p14.2 region on the basis of frequent hemizygous and occasional homozygous deletion in lung cancer cells. One such candidate is *FHIT*, which encodes a dinucleoside 5′,5‴-$P^1$,$P^3$-triphosphate ($Ap_3A$) hydrolase.

Forty percent to 80% of lung cancer cells express abnormal mRNA transcripts of *FHIT* and almost always also express wild-type *FHIT* transcripts.[147, 148] *FHIT* point mutations are very rare in lung cancers.[147, 148] In terms of these two characters, *FHIT* differs from classic TSGs. However, absent FHIT protein has been observed in primary lung tumors and cell lines, and this down-regulation has been associated with DNA and/or RNA abnormalities.[149] Also, more *FHIT* allele loss was observed in lung cancers from smokers (80%) than from nonsmokers (22%), suggesting that *FHIT* is a molecular target of tobacco smoke carcinogens.[150] Allelic deletion of the *FHIT* gene was associated with poorer survival in patients with NSCLC.[151] Furthermore, reintroduction of exogenous wild-type *FHIT* suppressed tumorigenicity of lung cancer cell lines in nude mice.[152, 152a] Unexpectedly, however, a *FHIT* mutant lacking wild-type hydrolase activity also showed tumor suppression. In contrast, others reported that *FHIT* transfection did not suppress tumor growth of human cancer cell lines but that absent FHIT protein expression was observed in 3 of 11 SCLCs and 15 of 28 NSCLCs.[153] Therefore, although the *FHIT* region is frequently altered in lung cancer, it is not yet clear whether *FHIT* is a target or merely a marker of alterations in the chromosomal inducible fragile site at 3p14.2.

**TGF-β Signaling Pathway.** The TGF-β family of signaling molecules regulate the proliferation of many cell types. TGF-β binds to transmembrane receptors with serine/threonine kinase activity, designated types I, II, and III. Despite being a growth factor for fibroblast cells, TGF-$\beta_1$ is a potent inhibitor of proliferation of most epithelial and hematopoietic cells. Indeed, many tumorigenic cell lines have been shown to lose responsiveness to the negative growth-regulatory effects of TGF-$\beta_1$. TGF-$\beta_1$ inhibits epithelial cell proliferation of developing lung, resulting in less branching.[154] TGF-$\beta_1$ also suppressed N-*myc* expression; this gene is known to be expressed during embryonic development in epithelial cells involved in branching morphogenesis, and homozygous null N-*myc* mice have defects in lung development.[154] In addition, the presence of mutant *p53* has been shown to diminish the growth inhibition by TGF-$\beta_1$ in human bronchial epithelial cells.[155]

In SCLC cell lines, resistance to growth inhibition by TGF-$\beta_1$ correlates with loss of messenger RNA (mRNA) expression of the type II receptor (TGFβ-RII).[156] Although mutations in TGFβ-RII situated at chromosome 3p22 (a site of frequent allele loss in lung cancer) have been reported in colon cancers with the MSI phenotype, this gene is rarely mutated in lung cancer.[157] However, transgenic mice overexpressing a dominant-negative mutant TGFβ-RII showed enhanced tumorigenesis in the mammary gland and lung in response to the carcinogen 7,12-dimethylbenz[*a*]anthracene.[158]

SMAD proteins, which comprise seven known members, are the downstream signaling mediators central to TGF-β ligand-receptor complexes. *SMAD4* was initially identified as a TSG and was mutated in some pancreatic and colon cancers. However, *SMAD* gene mutations (*SMAD4* and *SMAD2*) were infrequent in lung cancer.[159, 160]

**Retinoids and Carotenoids.** Retinoids have an important regulatory function in lung morphogenesis during development and in the control of proliferation and differentiation of tracheobronchial epithelial cells.[161] Vitamin A deficiency has been shown to result in hyperplasia and squamous metaplasia of the tracheobronchial epithelium. Many of the biologic effects of retinoids in cells involve nuclear retinoid receptors, comprising two subfamilies, retinoic acid receptors (RARs) and retinoid X receptors (RXRs), with each family containing α, β, and γ subtypes. Abnormalities of the signal transduction pathway mediated by RARs have been implicated in a variety of human malignancies, including lung cancer, and lung cancer cell lines usually exhibit resistance to retinoic acid.[162] RAR-β maps to chromosome region 3p24, a frequent site of allele loss in lung cancer, and RAR-β expression was found to be down-regulated in approximately 60% of primary NSCLCs.[163] Squamous cell lung cancers transfected with an RAR-β expression construct showed in vivo tumor suppression in xenograft studies.[164] In contrast, mice expressing an antisense RAR-$\beta_2$ transgene developed lung cancer at very high frequency.[165] Hundreds of retinoids have been synthesized, and current intensive efforts focus on the development of more active and less toxic retinoids for cancer prevention and therapy. Novel retinoid-related molecules have been demonstrated to be apoptosis inducers and effective inhibitors of lung cancer cells in vivo[166] and in vitro.[167, 168] For this reason, several retinoids are currently in lung cancer chemoprevention trials.

Carotenoids, such as beta-carotene (an antioxidant plant pigment that can be converted to vitamin A), share certain properties with retinoids. However, they also have distinct mechanisms of action and appear to have different biologic, pharmacologic, and clinical effects. Three large, randomized trials showed that beta-carotene has no chemopreventive benefit for lung cancer. The Alpha-Tocopherol, Beta-Carotene Cancer Prevention Study (ATBC study) tested 50 mg alpha-tocopherol (vitamin E), 20 mg beta-carotene, alpha-tocopherol and beta-carotene together, or a placebo daily in 29,133 men who smoked five or more cigarettes daily.[169] Although no overall effect was observed for lung cancer from alpha-tocopherol supplementation, beta-carotene supplementation was actually associated with increased lung cancer risk in heavy smokers. The Beta-Carotene and Retinol Efficacy Trial (CARET) tested the combination of 30 mg beta-carotene and 25,000 IU retinyl palmitate (vitamin A) taken daily against placebo in 18,314 men and women at high risk for development of lung cancer.[170] CARET participants receiving the combination of beta-carotene and vitamin A actually had excess lung cancer incidence and mortality. Finally, the Physicians' Health Study showed that 12-year supplementation with beta-carotene (50 mg on alternate days) did not have a significant effect on the incidence either of malignancies, including lung cancer, or of cardiovascular disease.[171] These studies have provoked a major reassessment of lung cancer chemoprevention trials. So far, the excess risk of lung cancer has been confined to continuous, heavy smokers, and similar adverse effects have not been seen in the retinoid trials.

## Other Chromosome Loci for Candidate Tumor Suppressor Genes

In addition to deletions targeting *p53* at 17p, *RB* at 13q, *p16*$^{INK4A}$ at 9p, *FHIT* at 3p14.2, and *PTEN* at 10q, cytogenetic and allelotyping studies have revealed many other tumor-specific hemizygous and some homozygous deletions in lung cancer at multiple chromosomal regions. In the classic TSG paradigm, such deletions suggest the presence of other underlying TSGs as the target of these genetic losses. The chromosomal regions showing frequent allelic deletions include 1p, 1q, 2q, 3p (multiple sites), 5q, 6p, 6q, 8p, 8q, 11p, 11q, 14q, 17q, 18q, and 22q.[172–178] Although several of these chromosomal arms contain known or candidate TSGs (e.g., *VHL* at 3p25, *APC* at 5q21, *WT1* at 11p13, *NF2* at 22q12), these genes were not found to be mutated in lung cancer.

**Chromosome Region 3p.** The very frequent hemizygous loss of one chromosome 3p in lung cancer provides strong evidence for the existence of TSGs.[179] At least four distinct 3p regions have been identified by allelotyping, including 3p25-26, 3p21.3-22, 3p14, and 3p12, which suggests that there are probably more than four different TSGs located on 3p.[180] In addition, five separate regions (including 3p21, 3p14.2, and 3p12-13) are homozygously deleted in several lung cancer cell lines.[23] The 3p21.3 region has been extensively examined for putative TSGs,[179] particularly at a 300-kb region homozygously deleted in three SCLC cell lines.[181, 182] Another approximately 800-kb deletion region at 3p21 was localized by the presence of overlapping homozygous deletions in five lung cancer cell lines.[183]

The presence of homozygous deletions resulting in two hits at chromosomal regions 2q33, 5p13-q14, 8, 21q, and X/Y in lung cancer further imply yet other unidentified TSGs.[184–186] Meanwhile, the molecular cytogenetic technique of comparative genomic hybridization (CGH) can survey a tumor genome for deletions or increased DNA copy number in lung cancer. CGH techniques have been used to detect lung cancer deletions at many chromosomes and to document some differences between SCLC and NSCLC, as well as between adenocarcinoma and squamous cell carcinoma subtypes.[91, 187]

Lung cancers also harbor many other structural cytogenetic abnormalities suggestive of allele loss, including nonreciprocal translocations and numeric abnormalities (aneuploidy). In yeast, chromosomal instability leading to aneuploidy has been consistently associated with the loss of function of a mitotic checkpoint. Therefore, the role of a family of genes controlling the G2/M checkpoint of the cell cycle needs to be studied in lung cancer.

## *BCL2* Family and Apoptosis

Unlike normal cells, tumor cells (including lung cancer) acquire the ability to escape programmed cell death (apoptosis) in response to certain conditions such as DNA damage. Proteins involved in apoptotic signaling that frequently show abnormality in lung cancer are BCL2 and p53. The BCL2 proto-oncogene product probably helps determine the chemotherapy response of cancer cells through repression of apoptosis. For instance, a BCL2-transfected human SCLC cell line exhibited higher chemoresistance by inhibiting apoptosis,[188] and SCLC cells transfected with BCL2 mRNA antisense oligodeoxynucleotides were less viable, with reduced BCL2 levels.[189]

BCL2 expression may be correlated with neuroendocrine differentiation of lung cancers.[190] BCL2 protein expression has been observed to be higher in SCLCs (75% to 95%) than in NSCLCs.[190, 191] Paradoxically, SCLCs are usually much more sensitive to chemotherapy, which usually occurs by apoptosis, than are NSCLCs. In addition, there was a trend toward longer survival in patients whose SCLC tumors expressed BCL2.[191] BCL2 expression is also relatively higher in squamous cell carcinoma (25% to 35%) than in adenocarcinoma (approximately 10%).[190, 192–194] Although the finding is controversial, better survival of BCL2-positive lung cancer cases also has been reported in NSCLC studies.[192–196]

Most SCLCs have both BCL2 and p53 overexpression, whereas some but not all NSCLC studies report an inverse relationship.[13, 195, 197] These results suggest the hypothesis that either *p53* mutation or up-regulation of BCL2 expression is sufficient to modify the apoptotic pathway in NSCLC and that BCL2-positive tumors may show less aggressive behavior.[195] Furthermore, *BAX*, which counteracts BCL2 and promotes apoptosis, is a direct downstream transcription target of p53. In certain human cancers with MSI, *BAX* may be a TSG, but mutations have not been reported in lung cancer. The expressions of BAX and BCL2 were inversely related in 121 neuroendocrine lung cancers; most carcinoids (both typical and atypical types) showed low BCL2 and high BAX expression, but this situation was reversed in most SCLCs and large cell neuroendocrine cancers.[97] These results would correlate with clinical behavior, with locally invasive and nonmetastatic carcinoids faring well in contrast to highly metastatic SCLCs.

# HOST RESPONSE AND TUMOR PROGRESSION

## Host Immunity

Tumor cells express a variety of novel epitopes that represent potential immune targets, and therefore clinically evident tumors are thought to have effectively avoided immune recognition and elimination. Several different mechanisms for this escape from immune surveillance have been elucidated in patients with lung cancer.

**Major Histocompatibility Complex Molecules.** The major histocompatibility complex (MHC) class I molecules mediate presentation of endogenous antigenic peptides to cytotoxic T lymphocytes. Class I MHC antigen expression is down-regulated in human cancers, including lung cancer.[198, 199] Mutations of the beta$_2$-microglobulin gene, whose product is a component of the class I molecules, occur rarely in lung cancer.[200] However, beta$_2$-microglobulin reintroduction into the mutated cells restores the MHC class I expression.[200] For the stable assembly of peptide-MHC class I complex, transporters associated with antigen presentation (TAP), TAP-1 and TAP-2, are necessary for conveying intracellular peptides into the endoplasmic reticulum for formation of a complex with class I MHC and subsequent recognition by cytotoxic T lymphocytes. The TAP-1 transporter has been shown to be down-regulated in lung cancer.[199, 201] Although *TAP-1* is not somatically mutated in lung cancer, one SCLC cell line was transcriptionally silent for its wild-type allele and expressed only a genetically defective TAP allele, leading to an acquired loss of antigen-presenting ability.[202]

**Fas and Fas Ligand.** Fas (CD95) and the Fas ligand (FasL) play key roles in the initiation of one apoptotic pathway. FasL can induce activated T cells to undergo apoptosis, and this mechanism is thought to contribute to immune privilege sites. FasL expressed on tumor cells counterattacks cytotoxic T lymphocytes and natural killer cells by causing apoptosis through binding of FAS on immune cells, a process that may account for the ability of tumor cells to evade host immune destruction. Lung cancer cell lines and primary tumors express FasL, and coculture of lung cancer cell lines with a Fas-sensitive human T-cell line induced apoptosis in the T cells.[203] Also, cell-surface Fas expression has been shown to be reduced in adenocarcinomas despite the existence of Fas protein in the cytoplasm, which potentially results from alterations in the posttranslational machinery and which may also account for their resistance to Fas-mediated apoptosis.[204]

## Tumor Angiogenesis

Like all solid cancers, primary and metastatic lung cancers recruit new blood vessels (induce angiogenesis) from the surrounding host vasculature. Without neovascularization or angiogenesis, a tumor mass is not capable of exceeding 1 or 2 mm in diameter. Tumor angiogenesis is a complex process, but the discovery and molecular characterization of a diverse family of inducers and inhibitors that govern angiogenesis and regulate endothelial cell proliferation and migration is very exciting. These molecules are released by both tumor cells and host cells, with their ultimate balance influencing tumor angiogenesis.

Vascular endothelial growth factor (VEGF) is perhaps the most important tumor angiogenesis inducer. VEGF expression is lower in NSCLCs that are poorly vascularized or that are wild-type for p53 (immunohistochemically negative).[205, 206] VEGF expression correlates with nodal metastasis.[207] In squamous cell carcinomas, the VEGF receptor, Flt-1, is frequently expressed and VEGF expression is associated with reduced survival.[208] Basic fibroblast growth factor (bFGF) is another angiogenesis inducer. Although bFGF expression was detected in approximately 70% of NSCLCs, the association between bFGF expression and its prognostic significance is controversial.[209, 210] In cocultures of NSCLC cell lines and normal pulmonary fibroblasts, NSCLC cells stimulated normal pulmonary fibroblasts to secrete stromelysin-3 and release bFGF.[211] In addition, the expression of platelet-derived endothelial cell growth factor (PD-ECGF), which is also angiogenic, correlated with tumor angiogenesis and with a worse prognosis, even in NSCLC patients without lymph node metastases (N0 stage).[212]

The role of angiogenic CXC chemokines containing the glutamic acid-leucine-arginine (ELR) motif, such as interleukin-8 (IL-8) and epithelial neutrophil activating peptide (ENA-78), and angiostatic non-ELR-CXC chemokines such as interferon-$\gamma$–inducible protein 10 (IP-10) is also becoming clearer in human lung cancer.[213] IL-8 has been suggested to act an angiogenic factor for SCLC, and its inhibition by passive immunization reduced tumorigenesis of human NSCLC xenografts in severe combined immunodeficiency (SCID) mice.[214] In contrast, IP-10 was shown to inhibit human NSCLC tumorigenesis and spontaneous metastases.[215]

Other angiogenesis inhibitors include angiostatin and endostatin. Endostatin administered to Lewis lung carcinoma–bearing mice was shown to cause tumor regression without inducing drug resistance.[216] The combined effects of angiostatin and ionizing radiation were shown to target the tumor vasculature in vivo.[217] Another inhibitor, thrombospondin-1 (TSP-1), is regulated by p53. Loss of p53 function leads to reduction in the levels of this angiogenesis inhibitor; restoration of p53 function up-regulates TSP-1 and impairs the angiogeneic capability of the tumor cells.

The number of microvessels in the tumor area, representing an index of angiogenesis, has been shown to correlate with an increased risk of metastatic disease and a worse overall survival rate for several human cancers. The higher the microvessel density, the poorer the clinical outcome of the patients with NSCLC,[218, 219] although conflicting data also have been reported.[220, 221] In addition, there appear to be distinct patterns of vascularization in primary stage I NSCLCs, one of which is characterized by lack of parenchymal destruction and absence of neovascularization, suggesting that a tumor can exploit an established vascular bed if one is available.[222] Tissue factor (TF) is a physiologic initiator of blood coagulation and has been suggested to regulate tumor growth and angiogenesis. Low expression of TF was associated with low microvessel density and poor prognosis in NSCLC.[223] Genes regulating apoptosis may also play a role in tumor angiogenesis; for instance, BCL2 expression was inversely related to microvessel density in NSCLC.[224]

## Factors Influencing Metastasis

Tumor metastasis is a complex, multistep process that depends on host factors as well as on tumor characteristics. To metastasize, tumor cells must detach from the primary tumor, invade the extracellular matrix, enter and survive the vasculature, arrest in a capillary bed, adhere to subendothelial basement membrane, enter the organ parenchyma, respond to paracrine growth factors, proliferate, and induce angiogenesis, all the while evading host defenses. Molecules involved in cell-cell and cell-matrix adhesion have been implicated in epithelial differentiation, carcinogenesis, and metastasis. Some tumor cells can down-regulate expression of cohesive molecules and have increased motility. Cell adhesion molecules (CAMs) can be grouped into four distinct families: integrins, selectins, the immunoglobulin superfamily, and cadherins.

**E-Cadherin.** E-cadherin is located at the epithelial junction complex and is responsible for the organization, maintenance, and morphogenesis of epithelial tissues. E-cadherin has been implicated in carcinogenesis because it frequently is lost in human epithelial cancers and is affected by germline mutations in familial gastric cancer.[225] Reduced E-cadherin expression has been shown to be associated with tumor dedifferentiation, increased lymphogenous metastasis, and poor survival in NSCLC patients.[226]

**Integrins.** Integrins ($\alpha_2$, $\alpha_3$, $\alpha_6$, $\beta_4$), which bind to collagen and laminin, the major basement membrane components, are down-regulated in NSCLCs.[227] Reduced integrin $\alpha_3$ expression has been associated with poor prognosis in patients with adenocarcinoma.[228]

**CD44.** CD44 is a surface adhesion molecule, known to be a lymphocyte homing receptor involved in cell-to-cell and cell-to-extracellular matrix interactions. Specific CD44 isoforms are associated with metastasis of a variety of tumors but not lung cancer.[229] However, the expression of CD44v6 (encoded by variant exon 6) isoform is correlated with adverse prognosis of patients with stage I NSCLC.[230]

**Type IV Collagen.** The degradation of the extracellular matrix and basement membrane components by tumor cells is an essential prerequisite for invasion and metastasis. Type IV collagen represents a major structural component of the basement membrane. Type IV collagen expression of adenocarcinomas is progressively lost with increasing tumor dedifferentiation.[231]

**Matrix Metalloproteinases.** Among the enzymes involved in stromal degradation are the matrix metalloproteinases (MMPs), a family of metal-dependent endopeptidases that are produced by connective tissue cells and by many tumor cells. Currently recognized families of MMPs include collagenases, gelatinases, stromelysins, membrane-type MMPs, and additional enzymes such as matrilysin and metalloelastase. These enzymes differ in substrate specificity regulation, tissue-specific expression, and potential interactions with additional MMP family members. It is increasingly recognized that lung tumors show changes in the expression of these degradative enzymes. Gelatinase A expression has been demonstrated in both SCLCs (approximately 50%) and NSCLCs (approximately 65%) by immunohistochemical analysis.[232] The activation of gelatinase A in lung cancer was correlated with membrane-type MMP mRNA expression, whose product is one of the progelatinase activators.[233] Stromelysin-3 was shown to be overexpressed by stromal elements in primary NSCLCs, in comparison with adjacent normal lung specimens.[234]

## SUMMARY

The understanding of the genes involved in molecular biologic changes in lung cancer pathogenesis is advancing rapidly. The proteins encoded by these genes appear to fall into key regulatory pathways of cell growth and differentiation, cell cycle processes, apoptosis, and tumor progression (metastasis and angiogenesis). Histologic types of lung cancers and even clinically relevant subsets within a histologic type can now be related to certain patterns of molecular lesions. Based on these findings, it is hoped that early detection, chemoprevention, and rationally derived therapies will begin to decrease mortality from this disease in the near future.

## References


1. Landis SH, Murray T, Bolden S, et al: Cancer statistics, 1999. CA Cancer J Clin 49:8–31, 1999.
2. Mason RJ, Williams MC, Moses HL, et al: Stem cells in lung development, disease, and therapy. Am J Respir Cell Mol Biol 16:355–363, 1997.
3. Senden NH, Timmer ED, de Bruine A, et al: A comparison of NSP-reticulons with conventional neuroendocrine markers in immunophenotyping of lung cancers. J Pathol 182:13–21, 1997.
4. Borges M, Linnoila RI, van de Velde HJ, et al: An *achaete-scute* homologue essential for neuroendocrine differentiation in the lung. Nature 386:852–855, 1997.
5. Penno MB, August JT, Baylin SB, et al: Expression of CD44 in human lung tumors. Cancer Res 54:1381–1387, 1994.
6. Tran TA, Kallakury BVS, Sheehan CE, et al: Expression of CD44 standard form and variant isoforms in non-small cell lung carcinomas. Hum Pathol 28:809–814, 1997.
7. Falco JP, Baylin SB, Lupu R, et al: v-rasH induces non-small cell phenotype, with associated growth factors and receptors, in a small cell lung cancer cell line. J Clin Invest 85:1740–1745, 1990.
8. Risse-Hackl G, Adamkiewics J, Wimmel A, et al: Transition from SCLC to NSCLC phenotype is accompanied by an increase TRE-binding activity and recruitment of specific AP-1 proteins. Oncogene 16:3057–3068, 1998.
9. Hirano T, Franzén B, Kato H, et al: Genesis of squamous cell lung carcinoma. Am J Pathol 144:296–302, 1994.
10. Betticher DC, Heighway J, Thatcher N, et al: Abnormal expression of *CCND1* and *RB1* in resection margin epithelia of lung cancer patients. Br J Cancer 75:1761–1768, 1997.
11. Satoh Y, Ishikawa Y, Nakagawa K, et al: A follow-up study of progression from dysplasia to squamous cell carcinoma with immunohistochemical examination of p53 protein overexpression in the bronchi of ex-chromate workers. Br J Cancer 75:678–683, 1997.
12. Li ZH, Zheng J, Weiss LM, et al: c-k-*ras* and p53 mutations occur very early in adenocarcinoma of the lung. Am J Pathol 144:303–309, 1994.
13. Brambilla E, Gazzeri S, Lantuejoul S, et al: p53 Mutant immunophenotype and deregulation of p53 transcription pathway (Bcl2, Bax, and Waf1) in precursor bronchial lesions of lung cancer. Clin Cancer Res 4:1609–1618, 1998.
14. Hung J, Kishimoto Y, Sugio K, et al: Allele-specific chromosome 3p deletions occur at an early stage in the pathogenesis of lung carcinoma. JAMA 273:558–563, 1995.
15. Kishimoto Y, Sugio K, Hung JY, et al: Allele-specific loss in chromosome 9p loci in preneoplastic lesions accompanying non-small-cell lung cancers. J Natl Cancer Inst 87:1224–1229, 1995.
16. Sugio K, Kishimoto Y, Virmani AK, et al: K-*ras* mutations are a relatively late event in the pathogenesis of lung carcinomas. Cancer Res 54:5811–5815, 1994.

16a. Wistuba II, Behrens C, Milchgrub S, et al: Sequential molecular abnormalities are involved in the multistage development of squamous lung cancer. Oncogene 18:643–650, 1999.

17. Cooper CA, Carey FA, Bubb VJ, et al: The pattern of K-*ras* mutation in pulmonary adenocarcinoma defines a new pathway of tumour development in the human lung. J Pathol 181:401–404, 1997.
18. Westra WH, Baas IO, Hruban RH, et al: K-*ras* oncogene activation in atypical alveolar hyperplasias of the human lung. Cancer Res 56:2224–2228, 1996.
19. Slaughter DP, Southvick HW, Smejkal W: "Field cancerization" in oral stratified squamous epithelium: Clinical implications of multicentric origin. Cancer 6:963–968, 1953.
20. Hiyama K, Hiyama E, Ishioka S, et al: Telomerase activity in small-cell and non-small-cell lung cancers. J Natl Cancer Inst 87:895–902, 1995.
21. Albanell J, Lonardo F, Rusch V, et al: High telomerase activity in primary lung cancers: Association with increased cell proliferation rates and advanced pathologic stage. J Natl Cancer Inst 89:1609–1615, 1997.
22. Yashima K, Litzky LA, Kaiser L, et al: Telomerase expression in respiratory epithelium during the multistage pathogenesis of lung carcinomas. Cancer Res 57:2373–2377, 1997.
23. Sekido Y, Fong KM, Minna JD: Progress in understanding the molecular pathogenesis. Biochim Biophys Acta 1378:F21–F59, 1998.
24. Rosell R, Pifarré A, Monzó M, et al: Reduced survival in patients with stage-I non-small-cell lung cancer associated with DNA-replication errors. Int J Cancer 74:330–334, 1997.
25. Adachi J, Shiseki M, Okazaki T, et al: Microsatellite instability in primary and metastatic lung carcinomas. Genes Chromosomes Cancer 14:301–306, 1995.
26. Chevillard S, Radicella JP, Levalois C, et al: Mutations in *OGG1*, a gene involved in the repair of oxidative DNA damage, are found in human lung and kidney tumours. Oncogene 16:3083–3086, 1998.
27. Merlo A, Herman JG, Mao L, et al: 5′ CpG island methylation is associated with transcriptional silencing of the tumour suppressor *p16/CDKN2/MTS1* in human cancers. Nature Med 1:686–692, 1995.

28. Otterson GA, Khleif SN, Chen W, et al: *CDKN2* gene silencing in lung cancer by DNA hypermethylation and kinetics of $p16^{INK4}$ protein induction by 5-aza 2′deoxycytidine. Oncogene 11:1211–1216, 1995.
28a. Esteller M, Sanchez-Cespedes M, Rosell R, et al: Detection of aberrant promoter hypermethylation of tumor suppressor genes in serum DNA from non-small cell lung cancer patients. Cancer Res 59:67–70, 1999.
29. Makos M, Nelkin BD, Lerman MI, et al: Distinct hypermethylation patterns occur at altered chromosome loci in human lung and colon cancer. Proc Natl Acad Sci USA 89:1929–1933, 1992.
30. Kohno T, Kawanishi M, Inazawa J, et al: Identification of CpG islands hypermethylated in human lung cancer by the arbitrarily primed-PCR method. Hum Genet 102:258–264, 1998.
31. Suzuki H, Ueda R, Takahashi T, et al: Altered imprinting in lung cancer. Nat Genet 6:332–333, 1994.
32. Kondo M, Suzuki H, Ueda R, et al: Frequent loss of imprinting of the *H19* gene is often associated with its overexpression in human lung cancers. Oncogene 10:1193–1198, 1995.
33. Gross AJ, Steinberg SM, Reilly JG, et al: Atrial natriuretic factor and arginine vasopressin production in tumor cell lines from patients with lung cancer and their relationship to serum sodium. Cancer Res 53:67–74, 1993.
34. Campling BG, Sarda IR, Baer KA, et al: Secretion of atrial natriuretic peptide and vasopressin by small cell lung cancer. Cancer 75:2442–2451, 1995.
35. Takai E, Yano T, Iguchi H, et al: Tumor-induced hypercalcemia and parathyroid hormone-related protein in lung carcinoma. Cancer 78:1384–1387, 1996.
36. Gaitan D, DeBold CR, Turney MK, et al: Glucocorticoid receptor structure and function in an adrenocorticotropin-secreting small cell lung cancer. Mol Endocrinol 9:1193–1201, 1995.
37. Shepherd FA, Laskey J, Evans WK, et al: Cushing's syndrome associated with ectopic corticotropin production and small-cell lung cancer. J Clin Oncol 10:21–27, 1992.
38. Lennon VA, Kryzer TJ, Griesmann GE, et al: Calcium-channel antibodies in the Lambert-Eaton syndrome and other paraneoplastic syndromes. N Engl J Med 332:1467–1474, 1995.
38a. Raymond C, Walker D, Bichet D, et al: Antibodies against the beta subunit of voltage-dependent calcium channels in Lambert-Eaton myasthenic syndrome. Neuroscience 90:269–277, 1999.
39. Manley GT, Smitt PS, Dalmau J, et al: Hu antigens: Reactivity with Hu antibodies, tumor expression, and major immunogenic sites. Ann Neurol 38:102–110, 1995.
40. Graus F, Dalmou J, Reñé R, et al: Anti-Hu antibodies in patients with small-cell lung cancer: Association with complete response to therapy and improved survival. J Clin Oncol 15:2866–2872, 1997.
41. Polans AS, Witkowska D, Haley TL, et al: Recoverin, a photoreceptor-specific calcium-binding protein, is expressed by the tumor of a patient with cancer-associated retinopathy. Proc Natl Acad Sci USA 92:9176–9180, 1995.
42. Fathi Z, Way JW, Corjay MH, et al: Bombesin receptor structure and expression in human lung carcinoma cell lines. J Cell Biochem Suppl 24:237–246, 1996.
43. Spurzem JR, Rennard SI, Romberger DJ: Bombesin-like peptides and airway repair: A recapitulation of lung development? Am J Respir Cell Mol Biol 16:209–211, 1997.
44. Richardson GE, Johnson BE: The biology of lung cancer. Semin Oncol 20:105–127, 1993.
45. Cuttitta F, Carney DN, Mulshine J, et al: Bombesin-like peptides can function as autocrine growth factors in human small-cell lung cancer. Nature 316:823–826, 1985.
46. Halmos G, Schally AV: Reduction in receptors for bombesin and epidermal growth factor in xenografts of human small-cell lung cancer after treatment with bombesin antagonist RC-3095. Proc Natl Acad Sci USA 94:956–960, 1997.
47. Kelley MJ, Linnoila RI, Avis IL, et al: Antitumor activity of a monoclonal antibody directed against gastrin-releasing peptide in patients with small cell lung cancer. Chest 112:256–261, 1997.
48. Weiner DB, Nordberg J, Robinson R, et al: Expression of the *neu* gene-encoded protein ($P185^{neu}$) in human non-small cell carcinomas of the lung. Cancer Res 50:421–425, 1990.
49. Rachwal WJ, Bongiorno PF, Orringer MB, et al: Expression and activation of erbB-2 and epidermal growth factor receptor in lung adenocarcinomas. Br J Cancer 72:56–64, 1995.
50. Noguchi M, Murakami M, Bennett W, et al: Biological consequences of overexpression of a transfected c-*erb*B-2 gene in immortalized human bronchial epithelial cells. Cancer Res 53:2035–2043, 1993.
51. Kern JA, Torney L, Weiner D, et al: Inhibition of human lung cancer cell line growth by an anti-p185HER2 antibody. Am J Respir Cell Mol Biol 9:448–454, 1993.
52. Kern JA, Slebos RJC, Top B, et al: C-*erb*B-2 expression and codon 12 K-*ras* mutations both predict shortened survival for patients with pulmonary adenocarcinomas. J Clin Invest 93:516–520, 1994.
53. Pfeiffer P, Clausen PP, Andersen K, et al: Lack of prognostic significance of epidermal growth factor receptor and the oncoprotein p185HER-2 in patients with systemically untreated non-small-cell lung cancer: An immunohistochemical study on cryosections. Br J Cancer 74:86–91, 1996.
54. Tsai C-M, Chang K-T, Wu L-H, et al: Correlations between intrinsic chemoresistance and *HER-2/neu* gene expression, *p53* gene mutations, and cell proliferation characteristics in non-small cell lung cancer cell lines. Cancer Res 56:206–209, 1996.
55. Yu D, Wang S-S, Dulski KM, et al: c-*erb*B-2/*neu* overexpression enhances metastatic potential of human lung cancer cells by induction of metastasis-associated properties. Cancer Res 54:3260–3266, 1994.
56. Tateishi M, Ishida T, Mitsudomi T, et al: Immunohistochemical evidence of autocrine growth factors in adenocarcinoma of the human lung. Cancer Res 50:7077–7080, 1990.
57. Damstrup L, Rygaard K, Spang-Thomsen M, et al: Expression of the epidermal growth factor receptor in human small cell lung cancer cell lines. Cancer Res 52:3089–3093, 1992.
58. Miettinen PJ, Warburton D, Bu D, et al: Impaired lung branching morphogenesis in the absence of functional EGF receptor. Dev Biol 186:224–236, 1997.
59. Rusch V, Baselga J, Cordon-Cardo C, et al: Differential expression of the epidermal growth factor receptor and its ligands in primary non-small cell lung cancers and adjacent benign lung. Cancer Res 53:2379–2385, 1993.
60. Bost F, McKay R, Dean N, et al: The JUN kinase/stress-activated protein kinase pathway is required for epidermal growth factor stimulation of growth of human A549 lung carcinoma cells. J Biol Chem 272:33422–33429, 1997.
61. Ohmichi H, Koshimizu U, Matsumoto K, et al: Hepatocyte growth factor (HGF) acts as a mesenchyme-derived morphogenic factor during fetal lung development. Development 125:1315–1324, 1998.
62. Yanagita K, Matsumoto K, Sekiguchi K, et al: Hepatocyte growth factor may act as a pulmotrophic factor on lung regeneration after acute lung injury. J Biol Chem 268:21212–21217, 1993.
63. Harvey P, Warn A, Newman P, et al: Immunoreactivity for hepatocyte growth factor/scatter factor and its receptor, met, in human lung carcinomas and malignant mesotheliomas. J Pathol 180:389–394, 1996.
64. Olivero M, Rizzo M, Madeddu R, et al: Overexpression and activation of hepatocyte growth factor/scatter factor in human non-small-cell lung carcinomas. Br J Cancer 74:1862–1868, 1996.
65. Siegfried JM, Weissfeld LA, Singh-Kaw P, et al: Association of immunoreactive hepatocyte growth factor with poor survival in resectable non-small cell lung cancer. Cancer Res 57:433–439, 1997.
66. Sekido Y, Takahashi T, Ueda R, et al: Recombinant human stem cell factor mediates chemotaxis of small-cell lung cancer cell lines aberrantly expressing the c-*kit* protooncogene. Cancer Res 53:1709–1714, 1993.
67. Krystal GW, Hines SJ, Organ CP: Autocrine growth of small cell lung cancer mediated by coexpression of c-*kit* and stem cell factor. Cancer Res 56:370–376, 1996.
68. Quinn KA, Treston AM, Unsworth EJ, et al: Insulin-like growth factor expression in human cancer cell lines. J Biol Chem 271:11477–11483, 1996.
69. Antoniades HN, Galanopoulos T, Neville-Golden J, et al: Malignant epithelial cells in primary human lung carcinomas coexpress in vivo platelet-derived growth factor (PDGF) and PDGF receptor mRNAs and their protein products. Proc Natl Acad Sci USA 89:3942–3946, 1992.

70. Missale C, Codignola A, Sigala S, et al: Nerve growth factor abrogates the tumorigenicity of human small cell lung cancer cell lines. Proc Natl Acad Sci USA 95:5366–5371, 1998.
71. Oelmann E, Sreter L, Schuller I, et al: Nerve growth factor stimulates clonal growth of human lung cancer cell lines and a human glioblastoma cell line expressing high-affinity nerve growth factor binding sites involving tyrosine kinase signaling. Cancer Res 55:2212–2219, 1995.
72. Maneckjee R, Minna JD: Opioids induce while nicotine suppresses apoptosis in human lung cancer cells. Cell Growth Differ 5:1033–1040, 1994.
73. Tsuchiya E, Furuta R, Wada N, et al: High K-*ras* mutation rates in goblet-cell-type adenocarcinomas of the lungs. J Cancer Res Clin Oncol 121:577–581, 1995.
74. Greenblatt MS, Bennett WP, Hollstein M, et al: Mutations in the *p53* tumor suppressor gene: Clues to cancer etiology and molecular pathogenesis. Cancer Res 54:4855–4878, 1994.
75. Slebos RJ, Hruban RH, Dalesio O, et al: Relationship between K-ras oncogene activation and smoking in adenocarcinoma of the human lung. J Natl Cancer Inst 83:1024–1027, 1991.
76. Slebos RJ, Kibbelaar RE, Dalesio O, et al: K-*ras* oncogene activation as a prognostic marker in adenocarcinoma of the lung. N Engl J Med 323:561–565, 1990.
77. Mitsudomi T, Steinberg SM, Oie HK, et al: *ras* Gene mutations in non-small cell lung cancers are associated with shortened survival irrespective of treatment intent. Cancer Res 51:4999–5002, 1991.
78. Rosell R, Li S, Skacel Z, et al: Prognostic impact of mutated K-ras gene in surgically resected non-small cell lung cancer patients. Oncogene 8:2407–2412, 1993.
79. Siegfried JM, Gillespie AT, Mera R, et al: Prognostic value of specific KRAS mutations in lung adenocarcinomas. Cancer Epidemiol Biomarkers Prev 6:841–847, 1997.
80. Tsai C-M, Chang K-T, Perng R-P, et al: Correlation of intrinsic chemoresistance of non-small-cell lung cancer cell lines with HER-2/neu gene expression but not with ras gene mutations. J Natl Cancer Inst 85:897–901, 1993.
81. Rodenhuis S, Boerrigter L, Top B, et al: Mutational activation of the K-*ras* oncogene and the effect of chemotherapy in advanced adenocarcinoma of the lung: A prospective study. J Clin Oncol 15:285–291, 1997.
82. Sun J, Qian Y, Hamilton AD, et al: Both farnesyltransferase and geranylgeranyltransferase I inhibitors are required for inhibition of oncogenic K-Ras prenylation but each alone is sufficient to suppress human tumor growth in nude mouse xenografts. Oncogene 16:1467–1473, 1998.
83. Ravi RK, Weber E, McMahon M, et al: Activated Raf-1 causes growth arrest in human small cell lung cancer cells. J Clin Invest 101:153–159, 1998.
84. Nau MM, Brooks BJ, Battey J, et al: L-myc, a new myc-related gene amplified and expressed in human small cell lung cancer. Nature 318:69–73, 1985.
85. Mäkela TP, Hellsten E, Vesa J, et al: The rearranged L-myc fusion gene (*RLF*) encodes a Zn-15 related zinc finger protein. Oncogene 11:2699–2704, 1995.
86. Johnson BE, Russell E, Simmons AM, et al: *MYC* family DNA amplification in 126 tumor cell lines from patients with small cell lung cancer. J Cell Biochem Suppl 24:210–217, 1996.
87. Ou X, Campau S, Slusher R, et al: Mechanism of all-*trans*-retinoic acid-mediated L-*myc* gene regulation in small cell lung cancer. Oncogene 13:1893–1899, 1996.
88. Fong KM, Kida Y, Zimmerman PV, et al: *MYCL* genotypes and loss of heterozygosity in non-small-cell lung cancer. Br J Cancer 74:1975–1978, 1996.
89. Levin WJ, Press MF, Gaynor RB, et al: Expression patterns of immediate early transcription factors in human non-small cell lung cancer. Oncogene 11:1261–1269, 1995.
90. Szabo E, Riffe ME, Steinberg SM, et al: Altered cJUN expression: An early event in human lung carcinogenesis. Cancer Res 56:305–315, 1996.
91. Levin NA, Brzoska PM, Warnock ML, et al: Identification of novel regions of altered DNA copy number in small cell lung tumors. Genes Chromosomes Cancer 13:175–185, 1995.
92. Schwendel A, Langreck H, Reichel M, et al: Primary small-cell lung carcinomas and their metastases are characterized by a recurrent pattern of genetic alterations. Int J Cancer 74:86–93, 1997.
93. Takahashi T, Nau MM, Chiba I, et al: p53: A frequent target for genetic abnormalities in lung cancer. Science 246:491–494, 1989.
94. Hainaut P, Hernandez T, Robinson A, et al: IARC Database of p53 gene mutations in human tumors and cell lines: Updated compilation, revised formats and new visualisation tools. Nucleic Acids Res 26:205–13, 1998.
95. Denissenko MF, Pao A, Tang M, et al: Preferential formation of benzo[*a*]pyrene adducts at lung cancer mutational hotspots in *P53*. Science 274:430–432, 1996.
96. Casey G, Lopez ME, Ramos JC, et al: DNA sequence analysis of exons 2 through 11 and immunohistochemical staining are required to detect all known p53 alterations in human malignancies. Oncogene 13:1971–1981, 1996.
97. Brambilla E, Negoescu A, Gazzeri S, et al: Apoptosis-related factors p53, Bcl2, and Bax in neuroendocrine lung tumors. Am J Pathol 149:1941–1952, 1996.
98. Nishio M, Koshikawa T, Kuroishi T, et al: Prognostic significance of abnormal p53 accumulation in primary, resected non-small-cell lung cancers. J Clin Oncol 14:497–502, 1996.
99. Graziano SL: Non-small cell lung cancer: Clinical value of new biological predictors. Lung Cancer 17:S37–S58, 1997.
100. Adachi J, Ookawa K, Shiseki M, et al: Induction of apoptosis but not G1 arrest by expression of the wild-type p53 gene in small cell lung carcinoma. Cell Growth Differ 7:879–886, 1996.
101. Roth JA, Nguyen D, Lawrence DD, et al: Retrovirus-mediated wild-type *p53* gene transfer to tumors of patients with lung cancer. Nature Med 2:985–991, 1996.
102. Zou Y, Zong G, Ling YH, et al: Effective treatment of early endobronchial cancer with regional administration of liposome-p53 complexes. J Natl Cancer Inst 90:1130–1137, 1998.
103. Lubin R, Zalcman G, Bouchet L, et al: Serum p53 antibodies as early markers of lung cancer. Nature Med 1:701–702, 1995.
104. Rosenfeld MR, Malats N, Schramm L, et al: Serum anti-p53 antibodies and prognosis of patients with small-cell lung cancer. J Natl Cancer Inst 89:381–385, 1997.
105. Zalcman G, Schlichtholz B, Trédaniel J, et al: Monitoring of p53 autoantibodies in lung cancer during therapy: Relationship to treatment. Clin Cancer Res 4:1359–1366, 1998.
106. Nomoto S, Haruki N, Kondo M, et al: Search for mutations and examination of allelic expression imbalance of the p73 gene at 1p36.33 in human lung cancers. Cancer Res 58:1380–1383, 1998.
107. Mai M, Yokomizo A, Qian C, et al: Activation of *p73* silent allele in lung cancer. Cancer Res 58:2347–2349, 1998.
108. Osada M, Ohba M, Kawahara C, et al: Cloning and functional analysis of human *p51*, which structurally and functionally resembles *p53*. Nature Med 4:839–843, 1998.
109. Marchetti A, Doglioni C, Barbareschi M, et al: p21 RNA and protein expression in non-small cell lung carcinomas: Evidence of p53-independent expression and association with tumoral differentiation. Oncogene 12:1319–1324, 1996.
110. Caputi M, Esposito V, Baldi A, et al: p21waf1/cip1mda-6 expression in non-small-cell lung cancer: Relationship to survival. Am J Respir Cell Mol Biol 18:213–217, 1998.
111. Bennett WP, El-Deiry WS, Rush WL, et al: $p21^{waf1/cip1}$ and transforming growth factor β1 protein expression correlate with survival in non-small cell lung cancer. Clin Cancer Res 4:1998.
112. Higashiyama M, Doi O, Kodama K, et al: *MDM2* gene amplification and expression in non-small-cell lung cancer: Immunohistochemical expression of its protein is a favourable prognostic marker in patients without p53 protein accumulation. Br J Cancer 75:1302–1308, 1997.
113. Gorgoulis VG, Zacharatos PV, Manolis E, et al: Effects of p53 mutants derived from lung carcinomas on the p53-responsive element (p53RE) of the MDM2 gene. Br J Cancer 77:374–384, 1998.
114. Harbour JW, Lai SL, Whang-Peng J, et al: Abnormalities in structure and expression of the human retinoblastoma gene in SCLC. Science 241:353–357, 1988.
115. Reissmann PT, Koga H, Takahashi R, et al: Inactivation of the retinoblastoma susceptibility gene in non-small-cell lung cancer. Oncogene 8:1913–1919, 1993.
116. Cagle PT, El-Naggar AK, Xu H-J, et al: Differential retinoblastoma protein expression in neuroendocrine tumors of the lung. Am J Pathol 150:393–400, 1997.

117. Dosaka-Akita H, Hu S-X, Fujino M, et al: Altered retinoblastoma protein expression in nonsmall cell lung cancer. Cancer 79:1329–1337, 1997.
118. Gouyer V, Gazzeri S, Bolon I, et al: Mechanism of retinoblastoma gene inactivation in the spectrum of neuroendocrine lung tumors. Am J Respir Cell Mol Biol 18:188–196, 1998.
119. Ookawa K, Shiseki M, Takahashi R, et al: Reconstitution of the *RB* gene suppresses the growth of small-cell lung carcinoma cells carrying multiple genetic alterations. Oncogene 8:2175–2181, 1993.
120. Xu H-J, Quinlan DC, Davidson AG, et al: Altered retinoblastoma protein expression and prognosis in early-stage non-small-cell lung carcinoma. J Natl Cancer Inst 86:695–699, 1994.
121. Kratzke RA, Greatens TM, Rubins JB, et al: *Rb* and $p16^{INK4a}$ expression in resected non-small cell lung tumors. Cancer Res 56:3415–3420, 1996.
122. Sanders BM, Jay M, Draper GJ, et al: Non-ocular cancer in relatives of retinoblastoma patients. Br J Cancer 60:358–365, 1989.
123. Helin K, Holm K, Niebuhr A, et al: Loss of the retinoblastoma protein-related p130 protein in small cell lung carcinoma. Proc Natl Acad Sci USA 94:6933–6938, 1997.
124. Schauer IE, Siriwardana S, Langan TA, et al: Cyclin D1 overexpression vs. retinoblastoma inactivation: Implications for growth control evasion in non-small cell and small cell lung cancer. Proc Natl Acad Sci USA 91:7827–7831, 1994.
125. Betticher DC, Heighway J, Hasleton PS, et al: Prognostic significance of *CCND1* (cyclin D1) overexpression in primary resected non-small-cell lung cancer. Br J Cancer 73:294–300, 1996.
126. Driscoll B, Wu L, Buckley S, et al: Cyclin D1 antisense RNA destabilizes pRb and retards lung cancer cell growth. Am J Physiol 273:L941–L949, 1997.
127. Merlo A, Gabrielson E, Askin F, et al: Frequent loss of chromosome 9 in human primary non-small cell lung cancer. Cancer Res 54:640–642, 1994.
128. Rusin MR, Okamoto A, Chorąży M, et al: Intragenic mutations of the $p16^{INK4}$, $p15^{INK4B}$ and *p18* genes in primary non-small-cell lung cancers. Int J Cancer 65:734–739, 1996.
129. Marchetti A, Buttitta F, Pellegrini S, et al: Alterations of *P16* (*MTS1*) in node-positive non-small cell lung carcinomas. J Pathol 181:178–182, 1997.
130. Shapiro GI, Park JE, Edwards CD, et al: Multiple mechanisms of $p16^{INK4A}$ inactivation in non-small cell lung cancer cell lines. Cancer Res 55:6200–6209, 1995.
131. Okamoto A, Demetrick DJ, Spillare EA, et al: Mutations and altered expression of $p16^{INK4}$ in human cancer. Proc Natl Acad Sci USA 91:11045–11049, 1994.
132. Nakagawa K, Conrad NK, Williams JP, et al: Mechanism of inactivation of *CDKN2* and *MTS2* in non-small cell lung cancer and association with advanced stage. Oncogene 11:1843–1851, 1995.
133. Kelley MJ, Nakagawa K, Steinberg SM, et al: Differential inactivation of CDKN2 and Rb protein in non-small-cell and small-cell lung cancer cell lines. J Natl Cancer Inst 87:756–761, 1995.
134. Kinoshita I, Dosaka-Akita H, Mishina T, et al: Altered $p16^{INK4}$ and retinoblastoma protein status in non-small cell lung cancer: Potential synergistic effect with altered p53 protein on proliferative activity. Cancer Res 56:5557–5562, 1996.
134a. Geradts J, Fong KM, Zimmerman PV, et al: Correlation of abnormal RB, $p16^{INK4A}$, and p53 expression with 3p loss of heterozygosity, other genetic abnormalities, and clinical features in 103 primary non-small cell lung cancers. Clin Cancer Res 5:791–800, 1999.
135. Shapiro GI, Edwards CD, Kobzik L, et al: Reciprocal Rb inactivation and $p16^{INK4}$ expression in primary lung cancers and cell lines. Cancer Res 55:505–509, 1995.
136. Okamoto A, Hussain SP, Hagiwara K, et al: Mutations in the $p16^{INK4}$/*MTS1*/*CDKN2*, $p15^{INK4B}$/*MTS2*, and *p18* genes in primary and metastatic lung cancer. Cancer Res 55:1448–1451, 1995.
137. Taga S, Osaki T, Ohgami A, et al: Prognostic value of the immunohistochemical detection of $p16^{INK4}$ expression in nonsmall cell lung carcinoma. Cancer 80:389–395, 1997.
138. Fukuoka K, Adachi J, Nishio K, et al: $p16^{INK4}$ expression is associated with the increased sensitivity of human non-small cell lung cancer cells to DNA topoisomerase I inhibitors. Jpn J Cancer Res 88:1009–1016, 1997.
139. Gazzeri S, Della Valle V, Chaussade L, et al: The human p19ARF protein encoded by the beta transcript of the p16INK4a is frequently lost in small cell lung cancer. Cancer Res 58:3926–3931, 1998.
140. Esposito V, Baldi A, De Luca A, et al: Prognostic role of the cyclin-dependent kinase inhibitor p27 in non-small cell lung cancer. Cancer Res 57:3381–3385, 1997.
141. Yatabe Y, Masuda A, Koshikawa T, et al: $p27^{KIP1}$ in human lung cancers: Differential changes in small cell and non-small cell carcinomas. Cancer Res 58:1042–1047, 1998.
142. Kondo M, Matsuoka S, Uchida K, et al: Selective maternal-allele loss in human lung cancers of the maternally expressed $p57^{KIP2}$ gene at 11p15.5. Oncogene 12:1365–1368, 1996.
143. Li J, Yen C, Liaw D, et al: *PTEN*, a putative protein tyrosine phosphatase gene mutated in human brain, breast, and prostate cancer. Science 275:1943–1947, 1997.
144. Petersen S, Wolf G, Bockmühl U, et al: Allelic loss on chromosome 10q in human lung cancer: Association with tumour progression and metastatic phenotype. Br J Cancer 77:270–276, 1998.
145. Tamura M, Gu J, Matsumoto K, et al: Inhibition of cell migration, spreading, and focal adhesions by tumor suppressor PTEN. Science 280:1614–1617, 1998.
146. Forgacs E, Biesterveld EJ, Sekido Y, et al: Mutation analysis of the *PTEN/MMAC1* gene in lung cancer. Oncogene 17:1557–1565, 1998.
147. Sozzi G, Veronese ML, Negrini M, et al: The *FHIT* gene at 3p14.2 is abnormal in lung cancer. Cell 85:17–26, 1996.
148. Fong KM, Biesterveld EJ, Virmani A, et al: *FHIT* and FRA3B 3p14.2 allele loss are common in lung cancer and preneoplastic bronchial lesions and are associated with cancer-related *FHIT* cDNA splicing aberrations. Cancer Res 57:2256–2267, 1997.
149. Sozzi G, Tornielli S, Tagliabue E, et al: Absence of Fhit protein in primary lung tumors and cell lines with *FHIT* gene abnormalities. Cancer Res 57:5207–5212, 1997.
150. Sozzi G, Sard L, De Gregorio L, et al: Association between cigarette smoking and FHIT gene alterations in lung cancer. Cancer Res 57:2121–2123, 1997.
151. Burke L, Khan MA, Freedma AN, et al: Allelic deletion analysis of the *FHIT* gene predicts poor survival in non-small cell lung cancer. Cancer Res 58:2533–2536, 1998.
152. Siprashvili Z, Sozzi G, Barnes LD, et al: Replacement of Fhit in cancer cells suppresses tumorigenicity. Proc Natl Acad Sci USA 94:13771–13776, 1997.
152a. Ji L, Fang B, Yen N, et al: Induction of apoptosis and inhibition of tumorigenicity and tumor growth by adenovirus vector-mediated fragile histidine triad (FHIT) gene overexpression. Cancer Res 14:3333–3339, 1999.
153. Otterson GA, Xiao GH, Geradts J, et al: Protein expression and functional analysis of the FHIT gene in human tumor cells. J Natl Cancer Inst 90:426–432, 1998.
154. Serra R, Pelton RW, Moses HL: TGFβ1 inhibits branching morphogenesis and N-*myc* expression in lung bud organ cultures. Development 120:2153–2161, 1994.
155. Gerwin BI, Spillare E, Forrester K, et al: Mutant p53 can induce tumorigenic conversion of human bronchial epithelial cells and reduce their responsiveness to a negative growth factor, transforming growth factor beta 1. Proc Natl Acad Sci USA 89:2759–2763, 1992.
156. Nørgaard P, Spang-Thomsen M, Poulsen HS: Expression and autoregulation of transforming growth factor β receptor mRNA in small-cell lung cancer cell lines. Br J Cancer 73:1037–1043, 1996.
157. Tani M, Takenoshita S, Kohno T, et al: Infrequent mutations of the transforming growth factor beta-type II receptor gene at chromosome 3p22 in human lung cancers with chromosome 3p deletions. Carcinogenesis 18:1119–1121, 1997.
158. Böttinger EP, Jakubczak JL, Haines DC, et al: Transgenic mice overexpressing a dominant-negative mutant type II transforming growth factor beta receptor show enhanced tumorigenesis in the mammary gland and lung in response to the carcinogen 7,12-dimethylbenz-[*a*]-anthracene. Cancer Res 57:5564–5570, 1997.
159. Nagatake M, Takagi Y, Osada H, et al: Somatic in vivo alterations of the *DPC4* gene at 18q21 in human lung cancers. Cancer Res 56:2718–2720, 1996.
160. Uchida K, Nagatake M, Osada H, et al: Somatic in vivo alter-

ations of the *JV18-1* gene at 18q21 in human lung cancers. Cancer Res 56:5583–5585, 1996.
161. Chytil F: Retinoids in lung development. FASEB J 10:986–992, 1996.
162. Minna JD, Mangelsdorf DJ: Retinoic acid receptor expression abnormalities in lung cancer: Important clues or major obstacles? J Natl Cancer Inst 89:602–604, 1997.
163. Xu XC, Sozzi G, Lee JS, et al: Suppression of retinoic acid receptor β in non-small-cell lung cancer in vivo: Implications for lung cancer development. J Natl Cancer Inst 89:624–629, 1997.
164. Houle B, Rochette-Egly C, Bradley WEC: Tumor-suppressive effect of the retinoic acid receptor β in human epidermoid lung cancer cells. Proc Natl Acad Sci USA 90:985–989, 1993.
165. Berard J, Laboune F, Mukuna M, et al: Lung tumors in mice expressing an antisense RARβ2 transgene. FASEB J 10:1091–1097, 1996.
166. Lu XP, Fanjul A, Picard N, et al: Novel retinoid-related molecules as apoptosis inducers and effective inhibitors of human lung cancer cells in vivo. Nat Med 3:686–690, 1997.
167. Sun SY, Yue P, Dawson MI, et al: Differential effects of synthetic nuclear retinoid receptor-selective retinoids on the growth of human non-small cell lung carcinoma cells. Cancer Res 57:4931–4939, 1997.
168. Adachi H, Preston G, Harvat B, et al: Inhibition of cell proliferation and induction of apoptosis by the retinoid AHPN in human lung carcinoma cells. Am J Respir Cell Mol Biol 18:323–333, 1998.
169. Albanes D, Heinonen OP, Taylor PR, et al: Alpha-tocopherol and beta-carotene supplements and lung cancer incidence in the alpha-tocopherol, beta-carotene cancer prevention study: Effects of base-line characteristics and study compliance. J Natl Cancer Inst 88:1560–1570, 1996.
170. Omenn GS, Goodman GE, Thornquist MD, et al: Risk factors for lung cancer and for intervention effects in CARET, the Beta-Carotene and Retinol Efficacy Trial. J Natl Cancer Inst 88:1550–1559, 1996.
171. Hennekens CH, Buring JE, Manson JE, et al: Lack of effect of long-term supplementation with beta carotene on the incidence of malignant neoplasms and cardiovascular disease. N Engl J Med 334:1145–1149, 1996.
172. Ohata H, Emi M, Fujiwara Y, et al: Deletion mapping of the short arm of chromosome 8 in non-small cell lung carcinoma. Genes Chromosomes Cancer 7:85–88, 1993.
173. Sato S, Nakamura Y, Tsuchiya E: Difference of allelotype between squamous cell carcinoma and adenocarcinoma of the lung. Cancer Res 54:5652–5655, 1994.
174. Shiseki M, Kohno T, Nishikawa R, et al: Frequent allelic losses on chromosomes 2q, 18q, and 22q in advanced non-small cell lung carcinoma. Cancer Res 54:5643–5648, 1994.
175. Otsuka T, Kohno T, Mori M, et al: Deletion mapping of chromosome 2 in human lung carcinoma. Genes Chromosomes Cancer 16:113–119, 1996.
176. O'Briant KC, Bepler G: Delineation of the centromeric and telomeric chromosome segment 11p15.5 lung cancer suppressor regions LOH11A and LOH11B. Genes Chromosomes Cancer 18:111–114, 1997.
177. Ueno K, Kumagai T, Kijima T, et al: Cloning and tissue expression of cDNAs from chromosome 5q21-22 which is frequently deleted in advanced lung cancer. Hum Genet 102:63–68, 1998.
178. Virmani AK, Fong KM, Kodagoda D, et al: Allelotyping demonstrates common and distinct patterns of chromosomal loss in human lung cancer types. Gene Chromosomes Cancer 21:308–319, 1998.
179. Kok K, Naylor SL, Buys CH: Deletions of the short arm of chromosome 3 in solid tumors and the search for suppressor genes. Adv Cancer Res 71:27–92, 1997.
180. Hibi K, Takahashi T, Yamakawa K, et al: Three distinct regions involved in 3p deletion in human lung cancer. Oncogene 7:445–449, 1992.
181. Kok K, van den Berg A, Veldhuis PMJF, et al: A homozygous deletion in a small cell lung cancer cell line involving a 3p21 region with a marked instability in yeast artificial chromosomes. Cancer Res 54:4183–4187, 1994.
182. Wei M-H, Latif F, Bader S, et al: Construction of a 600-kilobase cosmid clone contig and generation of a transcriptional map surrounding the lung cancer tumor suppressor gene (*TSG*) locus on human chromosome 3p21.3: Progress toward the isolation of a lung cancer TSG. Cancer Res 56:1487–1492, 1996.
183. Yamakawa K, Takahashi T, Horio Y, et al: Frequent homozygous deletions in lung cancer cell lines detected by a DNA marker located at 3p21.3-p22. Oncogene 8:327–330, 1993.
184. Kohno T, Morishita K, Takano H, et al: Homozygous deletion at chromosome 2q33 in human small-cell lung carcinoma identified by arbitrarily primed PCR genomic fingerprinting. Oncogene 9:103–108, 1994.
185. Wieland I, Böhm M, Bogatz S: Isolation of DNA sequences deleted in lung cancer by genomic difference cloning. Proc Natl Acad Sci USA 89:9705–9709, 1992.
186. Kohno T, Kawanishi M, Matsuda S, et al: Homozygous deletion and frequent allelic loss of the 21q11.1-q21.1 region including the ANA gene in human lung carcinoma. Genes Chromosomes Cancer 21:236–243, 1998.
187. Petersen I, Bujard M, Petersen S, et al: Patterns of chromosomal imbalances in adenocarcinoma and squamous cell carcinoma of the lung. Cancer Res 57:2331–2335, 1997.
188. Ohmori T, Podack ER, Nishio K, et al: Apoptosis of lung cancer cells caused by some anti-cancer agents (MMC, CPT-11, ADM) is inhibited by *bcl-2*. Biochem Biophys Res Commun 192:30–36, 1993.
189. Ziegler A, Luedke GH, Fabbro D, et al: Induction of apoptosis in small-cell lung cancer cells by an antisense oligodeoxynucleotide targeting the Bcl-2 coding sequence. J Natl Cancer Inst 89:1027–1036, 1997.
190. Jiang SX, Kameya T, Sato Y, et al: Bcl-2 protein expression in lung cancer and close correlation with neuroendocrine differentiation. Am J Pathol 148:837–846, 1996.
191. Kaiser U, Schilli M, Haag U, et al: Expression of bcl-2–protein in small cell lung cancer. Lung Cancer 15:31–40, 1996.
192. Pezzella F, Turley H, Kuzu I, et al: *bcl-2* protein in non-small-cell lung carcinoma. N Engl J Med 329:690–694, 1993.
193. Higashiyama M, Doi O, Kodama K, et al: *bcl-2* oncoprotein in surgically resected nonsmall cell lung cancer: Possibly favorable prognostic factor in association with low incidence of distant metastasis. J Surg Oncol 64:48–54, 1997.
194. Apolinario RM, van der Valk P, de Jong JS, et al: Prognostic value of the expression of p53, *bcl*-2, and *bax* oncoproteins, and neovascularization in patients with radically resected non-small-cell lung cancer. J Clin Oncol 15:2456–2466, 1997.
195. Fontanini G, Vignati S, Bigini D, et al: Bcl-2 protein: A prognostic factor inversely correlated to p53 in non-small-cell lung cancer. Br J Cancer 71:1003–1007, 1995.
196. Anton RC, Brown RW, Younes M, et al: Absence of prognostic significance of bcl-2 immunopositivity in non-small cell lung cancer: Analysis of 427 cases. Hum Pathol 28:1079–82, 1997.
197. Kitagawa Y, Wong F, Lo P, et al: Overexpression of Bcl-2 and mutations in p53 and K-*ras* in resected human non-small cell lung cancers. Am J Respir Cell Mol Biol 15:45–54, 1996.
198. Redondo M, Concha A, Oldiviela R, et al: Expression of HLA class I and II antigens in bronchogenic carcinomas: Its relationship to cellular DNA content and clinical-pathological parameters. Cancer Res 51:4948–4954, 1991.
199. Korkolopoulou P, Kaklamanis L, Pezzella F, et al: Loss of antigen-presenting molecules (MHC class I and TAP-1) in lung cancer. Br J Cancer 73:148–153, 1996.
200. Chen HL, Gabrilovich D, Virmani A, et al: Structural and functional analysis of $\beta_2$ microglobulin abnormalities in human lung and breast cancer. Int J Cancer 67:756–763, 1996.
201. Singal DP, Ye M, Qiu X: Molecular basis for lack of expression of HLA class I antigens in human small-cell lung carcinoma cell lines. Int J Cancer 68:629–636, 1996.
202. Chen HL, Gabrilovich D, Tampe R, et al: A functionally defective allele of TAP1 results in loss of MHC class I antigen presentation in a human lung cancer. Nat Genet 13:210–213, 1996.
203. Niehans GA, Brunner T, Frizelle SP, et al: Human lung carcinomas express Fas ligand. Cancer Res 57:1007–1012, 1997.
204. Nambu Y, Hughes SJ, Rehemtulla A, et al: Lack of cell surface Fas/APO-1 expression in pulmonary adenocarcinomas. J Clin Invest 101:1102–1110, 1998.
205. Mattern J, Koomägi R, Volm M: Association of vascular endothelial growth factor expression with intratumoral microvessel den-

sity and tumour cell proliferation in human epidermoid lung carcinoma. Br J Cancer 73:931–934, 1996.
206. Fontanini G, Vignati S, Lucchi M, et al: Neoangiogenesis and p53 protein in lung cancer: Their prognostic role and their relation with vascular endothelial growth factor (VEGF) expression. Br J Cancer 75:1295–1301, 1997.
207. Ohta Y, Watanabe Y, Murakami S, et al: Vascular endothelial growth factor and lymph node metastasis in primary lung cancer. Br J Cancer 76:1041–1045, 1997.
208. Volm M, Koomägi R, Mattern J: Prognostic value of vascular endothelial growth factor and its receptor Flt-1 in squamous cell lung cancer. Int J Cancer 74:64–68, 1997.
209. Takanami I, Imamura T, Hashizume T, et al: Immunohistochemical detection of basic fibroblast growth factor as a prognostic indicator in pulmonary adenocarcinoma. Jpn J Clin Oncol 26:293–297, 1996.
210. Volm M, Koomägi R, Mattern J, et al: Prognostic value of basic fibroblast growth factor and its receptor (FGFR-1) in patients with non-small cell lung carcinomas. Eur J Cancer 33:691–693, 1997.
211. Mari BP, Anderson IC, Mari SE, et al: Stromelysin-3 is induced in tumor/stroma cocultures and inactivated via a tumor-specific and basic fibroblast growth factor-dependent mechanism. J Biol Chem 273:618–626, 1998.
212. Koukourakis MI, Giatromanolaki A, O'Byrne KJ, et al: Platelet-derived endothelial cell growth factor expression correlates with tumour angiogenesis and prognosis in non-small-cell lung cancer. Br J Cancer 75:477–481, 1997.
213. Arenberg DA, Keane MP, DiGiovine B, et al: Epithelial-neutrophil activating peptide (ENA-78) is an important angiogenic factor in non-small cell lung cancer. J Clin Invest 102:465–472, 1998.
214. Arenberg DA, Kunkel SL, Polverini PJ, et al: Inhibition of interleukin-8 reduces tumorigenesis of human non-small cell lung cancer in SCID mice. J Clin Invest 97:2792–2802, 1996.
215. Arenberg DA, Kunkel SL, Polverini PJ, et al: Interferon-$\gamma$-inducible protein 10 (IP-10) is an angiostatic factor that inhibits human non-small cell lung cancer (NSCLC) tumorigenesis and spontaneous metastases. J Exp Med 184:981–992, 1996.
216. Boehm T, Folkman J, Browder T, et al: Antiangiogenic therapy of experimental cancer does not induce acquired drug resistance. Nature 390:404–407, 1997.
217. Mauceri HJ, Hanna NN, Beckett MA, et al: Combined effects of angiostatin and ionizing radiation in antitumor therapy. Nature 394:287–291, 1998.
218. Angeletti CA, Lucchi M, Fontanini G, et al: Prognostic significance of tumoral angiogenesis in completely resected late stage lung carcinoma (stage IIIA-N2): Impact of adjuvant therapies in a subset of patients at high risk of recurrence. Cancer 78:409–415, 1996.
219. Fontanini G, Lucchi M, Vignati S, et al: Angiogenesis as a prognostic indicator of survival in non-small-cell lung carcinoma: A prospective study. J Natl Cancer Inst 89:881–886, 1997.
220. Pastorino U, Andreola S, Tagliabue E, et al: Immunocytochemical markers in stage I lung cancer: Relevance to prognosis. J Clin Oncol 15:2858–2865, 1997.
221. Chandrachud LM, Pendleton N, Chisholm DM, et al: Relationship between vascularity, age and survival in non-small-cell lung cancer. Br J Cancer 76:1367–1375, 1997.
222. Pezzella F, Pastorino U, Tagliabue E, et al: Non-small-cell carcinoma tumor growth without morphological evidence of neo-angiogenesis. Am J Pathol 151:1417–1423, 1997.
223. Koomägi R, Volm M: Tissue-factor expression in human non-small-cell lung carcinoma measured by immunohistochemistry: Correlation between tissue factor and angiogenesis. Int J Cancer 79:19–22, 1998.
224. Koukourakis MI, Giatromanolaki A, O'Byrne KJ, et al: Potential role of bcl-2 as a suppressor of tumour angiogenesis in non-small-cell lung cancer. Int J Cancer 74:565–570, 1997.
225. Guilford P, Hopkins J, Harraway J, et al: E-cadherin germline mutations in familial gastric cancer. Nature 392:402–405, 1998.
226. Sulzer MA, Leers MP, van Noord JA, et al: Reduced E-cadherin expression is associated with increased lymph node metastasis and unfavorable prognosis in non-small cell lung cancer. Am J Respir Crit Care Med 157:1319–1323, 1998.
227. Smythe WR, LeBel E, Bavaria JE, et al: Integrin expression in non-small cell carcinoma of the lung. Cancer Metastasis Rev 14:229–239, 1995.
228. Adachi M, Taki T, Huang C, et al: Reduced integrin alpha3 expression as a factor of poor prognosis of patients with adenocarcinoma of the lung. J Clin Oncol 16:1060–1067, 1998.
229. Givehchian M, Woerner SM, Lacroix J, et al: Expression of CD44 splice variants in normal respiratory epithelium and bronchial carcinomas: No evidence for altered CD44 splicing in metastasis. Oncogene 12:1137–1144, 1996.
230. Hirata T, Fukuse T, Naiki H, et al: Expression of CD44 variant exon 6 in stage I non-small cell lung carcinoma as a prognostic factor. Cancer Res 58:1108–1110, 1998.
231. Clarke MR, Landreneau RJ, Finkelstein SD, et al: Extracellular matrix expression in metastasizing and nonmetastasizing adenocarcinomas of the lung. Hum Pathol 28:54–59, 1997.
232. Kawano N, Osawa H, Ito T, et al: Expression of gelatinase A, tissue inhibitor of metalloproteinases-2, matrilysin, and trypsin(ogen) in lung neoplasms: An immunohistochemical study. Hum Pathol 28:613–622, 1997.
233. Tokuraku M, Sato H, Murakami S, et al: Activation of the precursor of gelatinase A/72 kDa type IV collagenase/MMP-2 in lung carcinomas correlates with the expression of membrane-type matrix metalloproteinase (MT-MMP) and with lymph node metastasis. Int J Cancer 64:355–359, 1995.
234. Anderson IC, Sugarbaker DJ, Ganju RK, et al: Stromelysin-3 is overexpressed by stromal elements in primary non-small cell lung cancers and regulated by retinoic acid in pulmonary fibroblasts. Cancer Res 55:4120–4126, 1995.

# 45 Epidemiology of Lung Cancer

KATHRYN E. OSANN, PH.D. • VIRGINIA L. ERNSTER, PH.D.
PIERO MUSTACCHI, M.D.

Introduction
Patterns of Occurrence
- Mortality and Incidence in the United States
- Variations in Occurrence by Race or Ethnicity
- International Trends

Survival
Risk Factors
- Cigarette Smoking
- Occupational and Environmental Exposures
- Diet
- Host Factors

Summary

## INTRODUCTION

Lung cancer represents a true epidemic of the 20th century. Once rare, the disease is now the leading cause of cancer-related mortality in both men and women in the United States, accounting for 28% of all cancer deaths. This chapter reviews time trends in mortality and incidence in the United States, the influence of racial and ethnic differences, international patterns, and survival rates. In addition, the chapter discusses the major risk factors for lung cancer: smoking, environmental tobacco smoke, occupational and environmental exposures, diet, and host factors including biomarkers associated with susceptibility to the disease.

## PATTERNS OF OCCURRENCE

### Mortality and Incidence in the United States

In the 1930s lung cancer mortality rates in men began to rise steeply, and since the mid-1950s the disease has ranked first among causes of cancer death in men. Rates in women, initially low, have increased by more than 500% since 1950 (Fig. 45.1). In 1987, lung cancer surpassed breast cancer to become the leading cause of death from cancer among women in the United States. The disease now accounts for about 32% of all cancer deaths in men and 25% of cancer deaths in women. An estimated 90,900 men and 68,000 women died of lung cancer in the United States in 1999.[1] Lung cancer accounts for 15% of newly diagnosed cancers among men and 13% of new cases among women, ranking second in incidence in men to prostate cancer (29%) and in women to breast cancer (29%). An estimated 94,000 men and 77,600 women were diagnosed with the disease in the United States in 1999.[1]

In 1984, overall age-adjusted lung cancer incidence rates in men reached a peak and began to decline,[2] decreasing by 10% between 1992 and 1996.[3] Age-specific rates are declining for men aged 64 years and younger and are leveling off for older men. In women, recent incidence rates provide evidence of a plateau, with a 0.7% decline between 1992 and 1996.[3] Age-specific rates show downward trends among women younger than 45

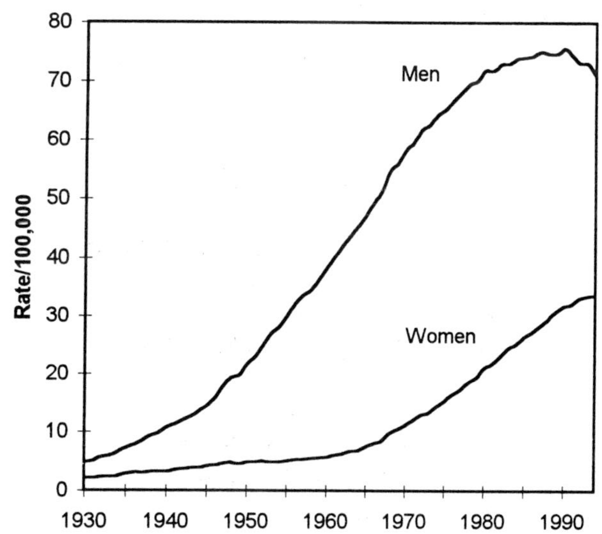


**Figure 45.1** Age-adjusted lung cancer death rates, United States, 1980–1994. Rates are age-adjusted to the 1970 U.S. standard population. (Data adapted from Landis SH, Murray T, Bolden, et al: Cancer Statistics, 1998. CA Cancer J Clin 48:6–29, 1998, Figs. 3 and 4.)

**Table 45.1 TRENDS IN AGE-SPECIFIC LUNG CANCER INCIDENCE RATES, 1973–1995, BY SEX AND RACE**

| Age Group (Yr) | Percent Change | | | |
|---|---|---|---|---|
| | Men | | Women | |
| | *White* | *Black* | *White* | *Black* |
| 15–34 | −9.2 | −46.4 | −23.4 | 110.9 |
| 35–44 | −53.6 | −13.3 | −29.2 | 2.2 |
| 45–54 | −32.9 | −27.9 | 28.6 | 28.6 |
| 55–64 | −12.9 | 3.7 | 102.2 | 118.2 |
| 65–74 | 6.5 | 21.9 | 232.4 | 216.2 |
| 75+ | 29.4 | 51.0 | 286.2 | 200.7 |

Data from Ries LAG, Kosary CL, Hankey BF, et al. (eds). SEER Cancer Statistics Review, 1973–1995. Bethesda, MD: National Cancer Institute, 1998.

years of age, though rates are still increasing sharply for older women (Table 45.1).[3a] These trends parallel changes in mortality rates and reflect declines in cigarette consumption and changes in the types of cigarettes smoked in more recent birth cohorts, with appropriate allowance for lag time between exposure changes and disease rates.

## Variations in Occurrence by Race or Ethnicity

There is marked variation in lung cancer mortality and incidence rates by race or ethnicity in the United States. In 1996, lung cancer mortality rates (age-adjusted to the 1970 population) were 66.8 and 94.4 per 100,000 population among white and African-American men and 35.0 and 33.5 per 100,000 among white and African-American women, respectively. Incidence rates were 50% higher in African-American than in white men (101.4 and 68.4 per 100,000, respectively) but similar in white and African-American women in 1996 (43.7 and 47.2, respectively).[3]

The downward trend in lung cancer incidence in younger age groups applies to both African-Americans and whites (see Table 45.1), consistent with recent declines in smoking among both African-Americans and whites.[4] After adjustment for smoking habits, racial differences between whites and African-Americans in Detroit mostly disappear.[5] However, in men and women aged 40 to 54 years, risks for some histologic types of lung cancer were two to four times higher in African-Americans than in whites after adjusting for smoking. These data and others support racial differences in the intake of cigarette smoke, its metabolism, and/or susceptibility to carcinogenic effects.[5a, 6]

Lung cancer incidence rates for 1988 to 1992 in the United States are lowest (about 14 per 100,000) in Native Americans and highest (117 per 100,000) in African-Americans. Rates for other ethnic groups fall between these extremes; incidence is low (42 to 53 per 100,000) among Hispanic, Japanese, Chinese, Filipino, and Korean men, whereas moderate rates (71 to 89 per 100,000) are observed among Vietnamese, non-Hispanic whites, Alaskan natives, and Hawaiians (Fig. 45.2).[6] Rates for women show less variation, ranging from 15 per 100,000 in Japanese women to 51 per 100,100 in Alaskan natives. Overall, groups with relatively low incidence rates (15 to 25.3 per 100,000) include Japanese, Korean, Filipino, Hispanic, and Chinese women, whereas higher rates (31.2 to 44.2) are observed in Vietnamese, Hawaiian, non-Hispanic white, and African-American women.[6]

## International Trends

Lung cancer has surpassed stomach cancer to become the most common cancer in the world.[7] The geographic distribution of lung cancer largely reflects the prevalence of tobacco smoking. Incidence and mortality rates have been high primarily among men in developed countries, reflecting smoking rates in the first half of the 20th century. In European countries, where the highest lung cancer rates were observed in the 1970s (England, Scotland, Germany, Scandinavia), a substantial reduction in

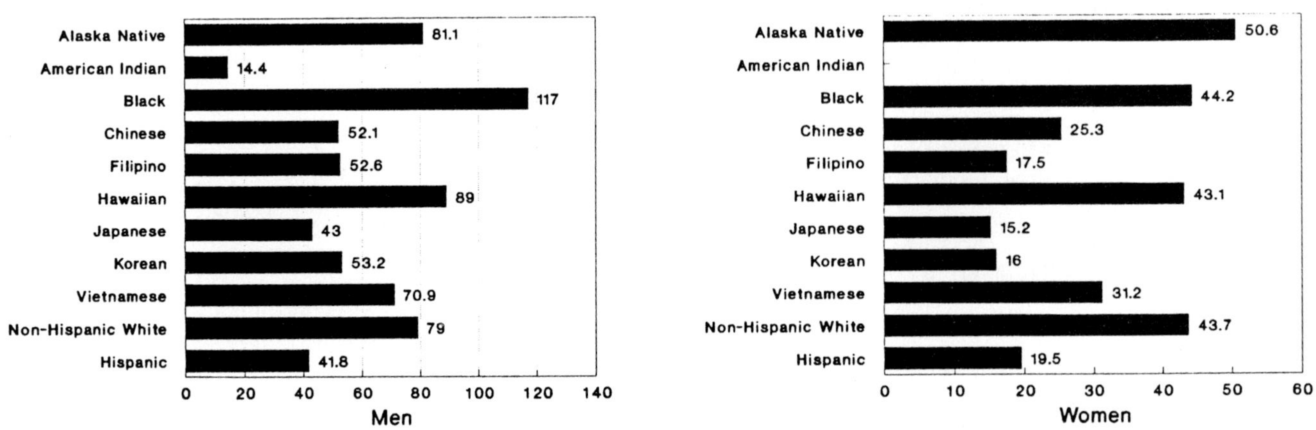


**Figure 45.2** Incidence rates by race or ethnicity: SEER, 1988–1992. (Data from Miller AB, Kolonel LN, Bernstein L, et al: Racial/Ethnic Patterns of Cancer Incidence in the United States 1988–1992 (NIH Publication No. 96-4104, 1996). Bethesda, MD: National Cancer Institute.)

smoking has resulted in a decline in lung cancer, particularly in the younger birth cohorts, similar to trends in the United States and Canada. Although still low, lung cancer rates have increased among men in Spain,[8] Portugal, and Italy.[7] A dramatic increase has been observed in Eastern European men, among whom death rates are now higher than ever observed in Western Europe.[9, 10] Trends for women are increasing in some Western and most Eastern European countries.[7–10]

Among Asians, risk of lung cancer is generally low in India, moderate but increasing in Japan, and high among Chinese men and women. A high prevalence of smoking among Chinese men, which exceeds 70% in Shanghai, is probably responsible[11]; however, lung cancer rates are also high among nonsmoking Chinese women.[12] The increase observed in the Japanese population can be explained by changes in per capita cigarette consumption, which increased from 360 to 3468 cigarettes annually between 1947 and 1980.[13] Despite the decline in smoking prevalence in the United States, total U.S. cigarette production has actually increased in recent years due to a dramatic increase in exports. Between 1984 and 1989, cigarette exports increased from 8.4% of U.S. tobacco production to 20.9%.[14] By the year 2000, it is projected that there will be 2 million cases of lung cancer diagnosed annually worldwide, of which 60% will be in developing countries.[15]

## SURVIVAL

Survival for lung cancer is poor compared with cancers of most other sites and has improved only slightly since 1960 (Table 45.2).[3] Among persons newly diagnosed with lung cancer between 1989 and 1995, the 5-year relative survival rate was 12.7% for white men, 9.9% for African-American men, 16.4% for white women, and 14.0% for African-American women. This rate was much higher for persons with localized disease at the time of diagnosis (50% overall); however, only 15% of all cases were in this category. The worst prognosis is for small cell (oat cell) carcinoma, with 5-year survival rates of 4.5% and 7.0% for white men and women, respectively, in 1989 to 1995.[3]

**Table 45.2** LUNG CANCER 5-YEAR RELATIVE SURVIVAL RATES (%), 1960–1994, BY SEX, RACE, AND YEAR OF DIAGNOSIS

| Year of Diagnosis | Men | | Women | |
|---|---|---|---|---|
| | White | Black | White | Black |
| 1960–1963 | 7 | 5 | 11 | 6 |
| 1970–1973 | 9 | 6 | 14 | 10 |
| 1974–1976 | 11.1 | 11.0 | 16.0 | 13.1 |
| 1977–1979 | 12.1 | 9.1 | 17.3 | 17.0 |
| 1980–1982 | 12.2 | 11.0 | 16.2 | 15.4 |
| 1983–1985 | 12.2 | 10.4 | 17.1 | 14.2 |
| 1986–1988 | 12.4 | 11.9 | 15.9 | 11.6 |
| 1989–1994 | 13.0 | 9.7 | 16.5 | 13.9 |

Data from Ries LAG, Kosary CL, Hankey BF, et al. (eds). SEER Cancer Statistics Review, 1973-1995. Bethesda, MD: National Cancer Institute, 1998.

**Table 45.3** LUNG CANCER 5-YEAR RELATIVE SURVIVAL RATES (%), 1960–1994, BY AGE, SEX, AND RACE

| Age at Diagnosis | Men | | Women | |
|---|---|---|---|---|
| | White | Black | White | Black |
| <45 | 18.3 | 12.8 | 29.2 | 22.8 |
| 45-54 | 15.7 | 11.4 | 20.1 | 15.2 |
| 55-64 | 14.4 | 9.5 | 17.9 | 17.4 |
| 65-74 | 12.8 | 10.2 | 16.1 | 10.8 |
| 75+ | 8.6 | 4.2 | 11.9 | 7.4 |

Data from Ries LAG, Kosary CL, Hankey BF, et al. (eds). SSER Cancer Statistics Review, 1973-1995. Bethesda, MD: National Cancer Institute, 1998.

Relative survival declines with age among whites; among African-Americans, the trend with age is less consistent, although relative survival tends to be worse among older persons (Table 45.3).[3] Women have consistently higher survival rates than men, and whites higher than African-Americans. Differences in stage at diagnosis and in histologic type do not entirely explain the differences in survival between whites and African-Americans.

## RISK FACTORS

The major established risk factors for lung cancer include smoking, which is responsible for about 85% of lung cancers in the United States, occupational and other environmental exposures, diet, and host or genetic factors.

### Cigarette Smoking

Lung cancer was a rare disease early in this century, and its epidemic occurrence, first in men and then in women, paralleled the widespread adoption of cigarette smoking, with a lag time of about 20 to 30 years. Early epidemiologic evidence for an association between cigarette smoking and lung cancer appeared in the medical literature in about 1950.[16–18] The growing body of case-control and cohort studies, along with other evidence, was summarized in the first report of the U.S. Surgeon General on smoking and health in 1964.[19] Subsequent reports from the Surgeon General and other reviews have contributed to the now overwhelming evidence.[20–24] Data supporting an association between exposure and disease have rarely, if ever, been as strong, as consistent, and as coherent as those linking smoking and lung cancer. Lung cancer rates remain low in populations with low smoking prevalence. Risk increases with number of years smoked, with number of cigarettes smoked daily, and with earlier age at smoking initiation. Unfiltered and high-tar cigarettes carry a higher risk than filtered and lower-tar cigarettes. Furthermore, risk decreases with time elapsed since smoking cessation. The primary contribution to risk of earlier age at initiation is the increased duration of smoking. However, there is some evidence of an independent effect of age that may alter biologic susceptibility, rendering smokers who begin earlier more susceptible to the carcinogenic effects of tobacco smoke.[25, 26] Duration of smoking is also important, because evidence suggests that smoking 1 pack per day for 40 years is more hazardous than smoking 2 packs per day for 20 years.[26]

**Variation in Smoking and Lung Cancer by Race/Ethnicity and Religion.** Differences in smoking account for much of the variation in lung cancer rates across ethnic and certain religious groups. Lung cancer remains relatively uncommon in religious groups in the United States that proscribe tobacco. Incidence is low in Utah, where residents are predominantly Mormon,[3] among Seventh Day Adventists in California,[27] and among Amish and Hutterite communities.[28] In the United States, Asian and Hispanic men and women, who are less likely to be current smokers and who smoke fewer cigarettes per day than whites, have lower incidence rates, whereas Alaskan natives, who have a high prevalence of smoking, experience high incidence rates.[3, 4]

The effect of smoking may be greater for some racial groups than for others. The relative risks associated with smoking among Hispanic and non-Hispanic whites in New Mexico are similar after amount smoked is taken into account.[29] However, higher rates among African-American and Hawaiian men may not entirely be explained by smoking history. African-Americans are 1.8 times more likely to develop lung cancer than whites after adjusting for smoking habits.[30] Although differences in smoking habits explain most of the difference in incidence at older ages, African-American men and women experience a two- to fourfold increase in lung cancer risk compared with whites at ages 40 to 54 years after controlling for cigarette smoking. At comparable smoking levels, native Hawaiians appear to have a substantially increased relative risk of lung cancer compared with Hawaiian whites, whereas Hawaiian Japanese have a substantially decreased risk.[31] The relatively high rates of lung cancer among nonsmoking Chinese women in Hawaii and in China[31, 32] also suggest that smoking is not entirely responsible for observed racial differences in lung cancer rates. Differences in occupational exposures, diet, or genetic susceptibility may be responsible for the residual differences in lung cancer incidence.

**Data on Women.** The 1980 Surgeon General's report on the health consequences of smoking for women eliminated any remaining doubt about the existence of a causal association between smoking and lung cancer in women.[21] Epidemiologic studies conducted since that time further document the association with smoking in women.[22–26] Because women started smoking in large numbers 20 to 30 years later and initially smoked fewer cigarettes than men, the epidemic occurred later in women and the relative risks reported in earlier studies were lower than in men.[21] Over time, the smoking habits of women have changed to resemble more closely those of men,[33] with a resulting increase in the relative risks associated with smoking for women. The relative risk for women smokers in the American Cancer Society's Cancer Prevention I (CPS-I) prospective study, begun in 1959, was approximately 2.7, one fifth the magnitude observed for men (11.9). By the time of the second Cancer Prevention Study (CPS-II), begun in 1982, the relative risk for women (12.8) had increased to approximately half the risk observed in men (23.2) and had equaled the level observed for men in CPS-I.[34, 35]

More recent data, reflecting earlier age at initiation and heavier smoking among later cohorts of women, show risk ratios for women smokers that are equal to or, in some studies, significantly exceed risk ratios in men.[36–40] Data from the American Health Foundation disclose a risk for lung cancer approximately 1.5 times higher for women smokers than for men even though men started to smoke earlier, inhaled more, and smoked more cigarettes per day.[40] A cohort mortality study found higher age-specific relative risks for women who were heavy smokers than for men.[39] Possible explanations for the higher risks observed in women smokers include inadequate adjustment for male-female differences in reported smoking habits, differences in exposure related to the types of cigarettes smoked, and higher susceptibility to the carcinogenic effects of cigarette smoke in women.

Current lung cancer mortality rates in women approximate those of men about 40 years ago.[20] Peak smoking prevalence in women (about 34% in 1965) was never as high as for men (more than 50% in the 1950s). However, because the smoking prevalence among women began to decline later than in men, lung cancer deaths among women will continue to rise until the years 2005 to 2010.[41]

**Smoking and Histologic Type.** Despite the many sources of variability in histologic typing of lung cancers, consistent differences have been observed between men and women and between smokers and nonsmokers. Squamous cell carcinoma has long been the most common histologic type among men, whereas adenocarcinoma predominates among women.[42, 43] Adenocarcinoma comprises 30% and 40% of lung cancers in men and women smokers, respectively, but 60% to 80% of lung cancers among nonsmokers.[44, 45] A significant association with smoking is noted for all major histologic types of lung cancer. In women, it is stronger for small cell carcinoma than for squamous cell carcinoma and is relatively weaker for adenocarcinoma; in men, smoking-associated risks are equally high for squamous and small cell carcinomas but lower for adenocarcinoma.[36–38, 40, 46]

Trends in incidence rates show a decline in most cell types for men but increases across all cell types for women. Rates for squamous, small cell, and large cell carcinomas in men reached a peak in the 1980s and have since declined. Rates for adenocarcinoma, however, continued to increase through the 1980s, showing evidence of a plateau in the early 1990s. A decline in rates of adenocarcinoma is now evident for white men younger than 65 years of age; among older men, rates continue to increase. Similar patterns are observed in African-American and in white men; peaks are reached 1 to 2 years later for squamous, small cell, and large cell carcinomas but several years earlier for adenocarcinoma. In African-American and white women, rates for all cell types exhibited a continuous increase through 1991, with the exception of a plateau in rates for large cell carcinoma in white women.[2, 43] More recent data suggest that rates for small cell and squamous cell carcinomas are beginning to decline for women younger than 65 years of age, although the incidence of adenocarcinoma in women continues to increase.[2, 3]

Trends in incidence rates by histologic type for age-, sex-, and race-specific groups largely reflect changes in smoking habits. However, not all of the observed trends and patterns of occurrence can be explained by what is known about the relationship between smoking and various histologic types of lung cancer. Long-term trends show that adenocarcinoma, which is less strongly associated with cigarette smoking, increases at a faster rate in men than do lung cancers of other cell types, and faster in women than squamous cell carcinoma.[47] Although men smoke more than women, women experience equal and sometimes higher relative risks associated with smoking for all three major histologic types.[36–38, 40] Changes in cigarette composition may contribute to the observed changes in lung cancer histology.[48]

**The Changing Cigarette.** Not only has the consumption of cigarettes changed over time, from a high of 3800 cigarettes per adult per year in the United States in 1965 to about 2800 cigarettes in 1993,[48] but also the composition of the average cigarette has changed. Today's cigarettes are lower in tar and nicotine and more likely to be filtered than in the 1950s. The sale-weighted average tar and nicotine yields of all cigarettes have decreased by approximately 60% over the last four decades, from 38 and 2.7 mg, respectively, to 12 and 0.9 mg.[49] Approximately 97% of cigarettes sold in the United States in 1992 were filtered, compared with 19% of those sold in 1955. Most epidemiologic studies have shown that lung cancer risk is lower in smokers of filtered and low-tar cigarettes. Risk decreases roughly in proportion to the tar yield and may be reduced by as much as half in lifelong smokers of filtered, compared with nonfiltered, cigarettes.[50–52]

Although changes in tar and nicotine content of cigarettes may explain some of the decline in lung cancer incidence rates, inconsistencies in case-control and cohort data suggest that use of low-tar cigarettes may involve additional risks. Some studies have failed to demonstrate lower risks with decreasing tar yield or increasing use of filtered cigarettes.[53, 54] Smokers of low-yield cigarettes are known to compensate for the lower nicotine levels by increasing puff volume, frequency, and retention, and they may receive two to three times the levels of tar and nicotine reported by the Federal Trade Commission.[55] When lung cancer death rates reported by the CPS-I and CPS-II studies are compared, those in CPS-II who smoked only filtered cigarettes had higher rates than smokers of nonfiltered cigarettes in the CPS-I, despite the lower tar and nicotine content of filtered cigarettes.

Possible explanations include differences in exposure (dose) not reflected by survey measures of dose, differences in other risk factors (e.g., diet, environment, occupation, host factors), and other changes in the constitution of cigarettes. The use of new tobacco blends, which has been responsible for the reduction in exposure to tar and polycyclic aromatic hydrocarbons (PAHs), has resulted in an increased exposure to carcinogenic tobacco-specific *N*-nitrosamines (TSNAs), including 4-(methylnitrosamino)-1-(3-pyridyl)-1-butanone (NNK), a systemic carcinogen that induces adenocarcinoma of the lung in laboratory animals.[49] Low-tar cigarettes, which contain higher concentrations of NNK and which are inhaled more deeply to compensate for their lower nicotine content, may be responsible for the increase in adenocarcinoma over time and may contribute to the higher smoking-associated risks in women, who are more likely to smoke low-tar cigarettes.

Mentholated cigarettes do not appear to convey a significantly greater adverse effect on lung cancer risk compared with nonmentholated brands. One study found no difference in the prevalence of use of mentholated cigarettes between smokers with and without lung cancer.[56] In another study, the increase in lung cancer among men who smoked menthol cigarettes was not explained by differences in amount smoked, and women who smoked mentholated brands experienced no increase in risk.[57] The fact that African-Americans are more likely to smoke mentholated cigarettes than whites[58] does not appear to explain the considerably greater lung cancer rate among African-American men compared with white men.

**Smoking Cessation.** Persons who quit smoking reduce their risk of lung cancer.[59] The relative risk for death is inversely related to the number of years since smoking cessation.[39, 60] Moreover, for a given duration of cessation, risk decreases with the number of cigarettes previously smoked per day.[60] Although some evidence suggests that lung cancer risk among persons who smoked for less than 20 years reverts to that of nonsmokers after 10 to 15 years of nonsmoking,[61] among U.S. veterans the risk of death from lung cancer remained 50% higher than in those who had never smoked even 40 or more years after cessation.[60] Higher lung cancer rates in the few years immediately after smoking cessation can be explained by the inclusion of persons who quit smoking because of illness. Consistent with other information on the critical contribution of duration of smoking to lifetime risk, at least one study showed that smokers who quit smoking for a reasonable period but later relapse have a reduced risk, compared with smokers who experience no nonsmoking interval.[62]

**Environmental Tobacco Smoke.** With some exceptions, most published studies on the link between passive smoking and lung cancer have reported a positive association. The evidence was deemed sufficient in 1986 for the Surgeon General to conclude, "Involuntary smoking is a cause of disease, including lung cancer, in healthy nonsmokers."[63] Comprehensive reviews by the National Research Council of the National Academy of Sciences[64] and the Environmental Protection Agency[65] reached similar conclusions and led to the classification of environmental tobacco smoke (ETS) as a group A carcinogen (along with radon, asbestos, and benzene).[65] Use of meta-analysis to combine data from the many case-control and four cohort studies resulted in estimates for the excess risk of lung cancer among nonsmokers married to smokers to be 1.2 in the United States[65] and 1.3 worldwide.[63] As many as 3000 to 4000 lung cancer deaths per year in the United States may be attributable to ETS exposure.[65]

More recent studies, designed to address many of the limitations of earlier ones (i.e., small sample size, inadequate adjustment for confounders, and possible selection and misclassification biases) are consistent with an excess risk of 1.2 to 1.3. Three population-based studies reported a statistically significant increase in lung cancer risk of 30% to 140% among women nonsmokers, associated with long-term exposure to ETS after adjustment for confounding factors.[66–68] A fourth, smaller study reported a consistent although nonsignificant excess risk for male nonsmokers married to smokers.[69] In the CPS-II cohort study, nonsmokers married to smokers experienced a 20% higher lung cancer death rate than those married to nonsmokers, and death rates increased with the number of cigarettes smoked by spouses.[70] Linear extrapolation from studies that used biochemical assessment to estimate tobacco exposure resulted in a predicted excess risk for nonsmokers of 19%, consistent with estimates from other studies of ETS exposure.[71] This was not verified in Chinese women,[72–73] possibly because of confounding from exposure to cooking fumes.

Most studies to date have been limited to the effect of household smoking, primarily by spouses. Exposure to ETS during childhood (parental smoking), in the workplace, or in social settings has been less frequently studied, and results are inconsistent. Despite the consistency of studies of exposure to ETS from spouses, some concern about the reliability of existing epidemiologic evidence for ETS has persisted, owing to the potential for poor accuracy in self-reporting of exposure levels and other methodologic problems.[74–76]

**Other Forms of Tobacco.** Compared with nonsmokers, risk of lung cancer is elevated in cigar and pipe smokers, increases with the number of cigars or pipes smoked daily, and is greater in persons who inhale smoke more deeply when they smoke.[21, 77] In the United States, relative risks of lung cancer for exclusive cigar or pipe smokers are generally much lower than for cigarette smokers[52, 78] because of the decreased frequency of smoking and depth of inhalation. However, in some areas of Europe where cigar and pipe smokers inhale more deeply, the risk of lung cancer is similar to that for cigarette smokers.[79] Use of cigars increased by 45% in the United States between 1993 and 1996; cigar consumption has increased particularly among teenagers, raising concern for the long-term consequences.[80] There are no reports of any associations of smokeless tobacco (chewing tobacco or snuff) and lung cancer.[81]

**Lung Cancer Deaths Attributable to Smoking.** It is estimated that about 90% of male and 76% of female lung cancer deaths are currently attributable to cigarette smoking—a total of approximately 132,470 lung cancers in the United States in 1995.[82] That figure does not include lung cancer deaths related to ETS or to pipe and cigar use. As noted, the decline in smoking prevalence and, to a lesser extent, the widespread adoption of filtered, lower-tar cigarettes in recent decades has led to a decline in lung cancer rates observed recently among young adults in the United States,[83] and presumably a decreasing fraction of lung cancers will be tobacco-related in the future. However, because changes in lung cancer mortality lag behind changes in smoking behavior by two to three decades, the great majority of lung cancers encountered by physicians at least through the first quarter of the 21st century will have been caused by cigarette smoking.

## Occupational and Environmental Exposures

**General Considerations.** The lung is both the portal of entry and the target organ for many respirable hazards, including known and suspected carcinogens. In the United States, an estimated 9000 to 10,000 men and 900 to 1900 women develop lung cancer annually as a result of occupational exposures.[84] Most of the current understanding of the occupational epidemiology of lung cancer is derived from studies of exposures sustained at least two decades ago, and data in many reports were not corrected for possible confounders (e.g., smoking history). Without minimizing the independent excess risks associated with specific occupational exposures, it is important to emphasize that the majority of lung cancers occurring in workers who smoke could be prevented if smoking were eliminated.[85]

Many occupational studies have attempted to identify differences in the distribution of histologic types of lung cancer associated with specific exposures. An overrepresentation of adenocarcinomas follows arsenic exposure; small cell carcinomas occur frequently after exposure to chloromethyl ethers[86] or to uranium[87]; and vinyl chloride has been linked to large cell cancers.[88] However, no study has unequivocally demonstrated any one lung cancer cell type to be uniquely associated with a specific physical or chemical exposure.[89]

### Established Human Carcinogens

***Aluminum Production.*** The aluminum reduction process, which involves exposure to condensed-pitch volatiles, is associated with a significant increase in mortality from lung cancer. In cohort data, risk is related to number of years of exposure and years since first exposure; risk develops after 21 or more years of exposure.[90]

***Arsenic.*** Occupational exposure to inorganic arsenic in copper smelting causes a 2- to 14-fold increase in respiratory cancer risk. After controlling for smoking, risk increases with cumulative exposure and time-weighted average, and it does not decline after cessation of exposure.[91] The relation between arsenic and smoking can be multiplicative.[92] Arsenic is considered a late-stage carcinogen, although an initial-stage effect is possible.[93, 94]

***Asbestos.*** Asbestos, the group of naturally occurring fibrous silicates, consists of two types: serpentine fibers (including chrysotile, the most common variety) and amphibole fibers (including crocidolite, amosite, anthophyllite, actinolite, and tremolite). Prolonged exposure, which occurs only after fibers are released during mining, manufacturing, or handling of finished products, is associated with a relative risk of lung cancer of 1.1 to 15.[95] Exposure to crocidolite or amosite may be more dangerous than exposure to chrysotile or anthophyllite alone.[96]

Asbestos-related lung cancer occurs more commonly in the lower lobes but may also occur in the upper lobe.[97] Lung cancer is accompanied by alveolitis and thickening of the alveolar walls and peribronchial regions. Although the presence of radiologic and autopsy evidence of asbestosis is associated with an increase in lung cancer risk,[98] it is uncertain whether asbestosis is a necessary precursor of lung cancer. Radiologic signs of asbestosis may be absent even in the presence of histologic evidence of fibrosis.[99] The precise role of asbestos in lung carcinogenesis remains to be defined, although it is probably a tumor promoter[100] affecting both proto-oncogenes and tumor suppressor genes.[101]

With some exceptions,[102] risk increases with cumulative exposure (duration times intensity)[103] and number of retained fibers.[104] The average latency period is 37 to 40 years, although risk can increase as early as 12.5 years after first exposure.[105, 106] Lung cancer risk declines after cessation of asbestos exposure, suggesting a late-stage carcinogenic effect.[107, 108] Smoking markedly intensifies the carcinogenic potential of occupational asbestos exposure.[109, 110] The interaction, which approximates a multiplicative model, is most evident with high levels of asbestos exposure.[110] The authors of a recent analysis of 12 previous studies of the combined risks of cigarette smoking and asbestos concluded that one third of lung cancer cases among smokers who were exposed to asbestos can be attributed to the synergistic behavior of the two carcinogens in excess of their independent effects or to other factors.[110a]

The question of whether there exists a threshold exposure below which lung cancer does not develop has not been answered satisfactorily. Although the linearity of the dose-response curve is impressive, there is some evidence of a threshold cumulative exposure below which the risk of lung cancer is not increased.[111] Amosite workers with a cumulative exposure of less than 6 fibers/mL-years did not experience increased lung cancer mortality until 25 years after first exposure.[112]

Information regarding mortality at the low levels characteristic of contemporary exposures is limited, and uncertainties exist in the extrapolation of risk to environmental exposures, which are likely to be two or three orders of magnitude lower than occupational exposures.[113] Exposure to 0.5 fibers/mL for 40 years beginning at age 25 is estimated to cause 82 lifetime excess lung cancers per 10,000 persons exposed. School children exposed to 0.001 fibers/mL for 6 years would experience an estimated risk of 5 excess lung cancers per 1,000,000 persons exposed.[114] Assuming a linear dose-response relationship, the risk for development of lung cancer from inhalation of a single asbestos fiber is estimated to be $0.4 \times 10^{-13}$.[115]

Exposure to asbestos resulted in an estimated 76,700 deaths from lung cancer for the 25-year period from 1985 to 2009.[116] Current projections regarding asbestos-related pathologic conditions relate to past industrial practices, and more stringent occupational and environmental controls will decrease asbestos-related lung cancer deaths in the future.

***Bis(chloromethyl)ether.*** BCME develops when hydrochloric acid and formaldehyde are mixed in the course of chloromethylation processes used in the textile, paint, and home insulation industries. Some 16 to 25 years after first exposure, or less if exposure is heavy, workers experience a 2.5- to more than 10-fold increased risk of lung cancer.[117–121] Risk increases with duration and cumulative exposure, is greatest for small cell lung cancer,[118, 121] and is reduced when production processes reduce exposure.[121] Exposure to BCME results in an earlier age at onset of lung cancer, with an average age at diagnosis 10.5 years younger than for persons with lung cancer who were not exposed to BCME.[122]

***Chromium.*** Hexavalent chromium compounds are established human carcinogens.[123] Elevated tissue chromium has been found in bronchial carcinomas.[124] Moreover, inhaled chromium remains in the lungs long after cessation of exposure.[125] Arc welders, chromium platers, and workers in bichromate production and chromate-pigment manufacturing are at increased risk for lung cancer. Among New Jersey chromium pigment workers monitored for more than 30 years, standardized mortality ratios (SMRs) for lung cancer were 81, 139, 201, and 321 for subjects with 0, less than 1, 1 to 9, and more than 10 years of exposure, respectively.[126] In England, chromate workers had a lung cancer SMR of 197 after adjustment for socioeconomic status.[127] The overall relative risk estimated from 10 large studies of workers exposed to chromium was 2.78 (95% confidence interval [CI], 2.47 to 3.52).[84]

***Coke Oven Emissions.*** Polycyclic aromatic hydrocarbons (PAHs) result from the incomplete combustion of organic material. PAHs include benzo(*a*)pyrene, a procarcinogen that can eventually react covalently with deoxyribonucleic acid (DNA) to form stable DNA adducts, and chrysene and benzo(*a*)anthracene, which react with DNA via diol epoxides to play a critical role in the initiation of the carcinogenic process.[128] The highest levels of human exposure to PAHs occur with industrial production of coke or with the use of coal tar and pitch in iron and steel foundries.[129] A number of epidemiologic studies have concluded that exposure to coal tar and pitch can lead to lung cancer.[129] Coke production was associated in one study with a lung cancer SMR of 251 after adjustment for smoking.[130] Levels of PAH-DNA adducts were detectable in the leukocytes of 47% of coke oven workers, compared with 30% of nonexposed controls, and were higher among smokers than among nonsmokers in both groups.[128] A tenfold higher average benzo(*a*)pyrene concentration at the oven top, compared with the side, is consistent with observed higher mortality rates among workers employed at topside jobs compared with those working at the side of the oven.[131–133] Lung cancer risk appears to be similar for coke oven workers with high and low levels of inhaled benzo(*a*)pyrene, suggesting that the effect of coke oven exposure may result in part from exposure to other carcinogens in the production process.[134]

***Iron and Steel Founding.*** PAHs are formed as a result of incomplete pyrolysis of organic binders and sand additives when molten metal is poured over sand molds and cores. Suggestive evidence for the carcinogenicity of foundry work has existed for more than half a century.[135] Epidemiologic studies of foundry workers have consistently reported an increased risk for lung cancer associated with exposure to hot metal fumes that is not attributable to smoking.[135–138] Risk estimates are remarkably consistent, ranging from 1.5 to 2.5 in more than ten studies.[137, 138] Steel workers exposed to acid mists have a smoking-corrected SMR of 150 (95% CI, 105 to 207).[139] In four out of six studies, risk increased with length of employment[137] but not with exposure to iron oxide fumes.[140]

***Mustard Gas.*** Significantly increased but widely varying risks of lung cancer were reported among Japanese and German workers engaged in the production of mustard gas during World War II.[141] The episodic exposure suffered by U.S. veterans of World War I was associated with a 50% increase in lung cancer risk, but no increased risk was reported among British veterans of the same war.[141]

***Nickel and Nickel Compounds.*** The increased lung cancer risk prevalent in nickel refinery workers was initially attributed to exposure to metallic nickel and nickel carbonyl, which are carcinogenic in animals.[142] However, subsequent epidemiologic evidence has suggested that exposure to combinations of nickel sulfides and oxides encountered in the refining industry increases lung cancer risk in humans, whereas evidence for the carcinogenicity of metallic nickel and nickel alloys is inconclusive.[142, 143] Ten cohort studies have reported increased risks for occupational exposure to nickel.[144] Excess mortality increases with length of exposure (SMR, 137 for less than 5 years and 489 for more than 5 years), and it takes at least 15 years from first exposure to diagnosis of lung cancer.[145] The association of nickel exposure and lung cancer may be confounded by the presence of asbestos in some nickel ores and the presence of chromium in stainless steel welding.[146]

***Radiation.*** Uranium, as found in nature, is normally at or near equilibrium with its decay products, which include the inert gas radon. The radioactive decay progeny of radon represent the major occupational radiation hazard to the lung. Significant lung cancer excesses have been observed in almost all of the 20 populations of underground miners studied thus far. Additional follow-up of the cohort of Colorado Plateau uranium miners confirmed the existence of significant trends between lung cancer mortality and increasing exposure (working-level months) and duration of employment.[147] Smoking and exposure to radon decay products interact in multiplicative or nearly multiplicative fashion to increase risk of lung cancer.[148, 149]

High radon levels have been detected in homes where uranium mill tailings were used in the construction process and in basements and structures made predominantly of concrete. There is considerable disagreement regarding the validity of extrapolating the risks experienced by miners to residential exposure to radon.[150] Exposure levels for indoor radon are much lower, and the exposed population includes women and children, who are not represented in the miner studies.

Some hold that there is no proven safe threshold for radiation exposure,[151] whereas others have challenged the linear, no-threshold theory of radiation carcinogenesis.[150]

The results from numerous case-control studies of indoor radon exposure, including two studies in Finland,[152, 153] have been equivocal. Inherent methodologic limitations, which include low risk ratios and difficulties with the measurement of exposure, may be responsible. When the data from eight case-control studies were combined using meta-analysis, results were consistent with risks predicted from miner data, showing a significant relative risk of 1.14 (95% CI, 1.0 to 1.3) for the exposure-response trend.[154] Combined analyses from cohort studies also support an increased risk with low-level exposure to radon consistent with the linear dose-response relationship observed in miners.[155] The existence of a smoking-radon interaction remains in question, however, because never-smokers experienced higher lung cancer risks than smokers in the cohort data.

Studies of exposure to ionizing radiation have failed to show an increase in lung cancer risk among plutonium workers[156] or among male employees at the Hanford nuclear site after adjusting for smoking habits.[157] However, in a follow-up study of residential exposure to a nuclear accident at Three Mile Island, exposure to the highest dose carried an increased risk for lung cancer of 3.92.[158] Studies of atomic bomb survivors support an interactive effect between radiation and smoking.[159] Persons undergoing radiation therapy have an increased relative risk for lung cancer,[160, 161] and there is a multiplicative effect for smoking and radiation therapy.[161] The radiation dose received by the lung under current radiotherapy procedures is substantially lower than in the past, lessening the potential for risk in the future.

***Vinyl Chloride.*** Although human exposure to vinyl chloride has been associated primarily with liver angiosarcoma, there is suggestive but inconsistent evidence that vinyl chloride is also a lung carcinogen.[162–164] An SMR of 149 that was not explained by smoking was observed in vinyl chloride workers who inhaled vinyl chloride dust.[88, 164]

### Suspected Human Carcinogens

***Beryllium.*** Two cohort mortality studies have reported a significant excess of lung cancer associated with exposure to beryllium.[165, 166] In follow-up of 689 men and women from the Beryllium Case Registry,[165] the SMR for lung cancer was 200, whereas an SMR of 124 not explained by smoking was observed in a cohort mortality study of workers from seven beryllium plants.[166] The highest lung cancer risk observed has been for workers who, during the 1940s and 1950s, developed acute berylliosis after intense exposure, although some of their excess risk may have been explained by repetitive diagnostic x-rays or sulfuric acid vapors.[167]

***Cadmium and Cadmium Compounds.*** Published SMRs for lung cancer among cadmium workers, principally exposed in electroplating industries, vary between 81 and 235, with a median value of 131 uncorrected for smoking.[168] Follow-up from a cohort study of cadmium smelter workers reported a relative risk of 1.49 not explainable by smoking.[169, 170] Swedish data also suggest that prolonged exposure to an ambient air level of 0.3 mg cadmium/m$^3$ or higher is associated with an increased risk for lung cancer in exposed workers.[171] The relative risk associated with cadmium exposure increases with cumulative duration of exposure.[170, 172]

***Crystalline Silica.*** Crystalline silica is genotoxic in vitro and is carcinogenic in the rat. The mechanism by which silica causes lung cancer in the rat is not clear; it possibly involves an initiating effect on DNA or promotion of growth in previously initiated cells.[173] Lung cancer risk increases with longer exposure to silica and "inert dusts"[174, 175] and with the presence of silicosis.[176, 177] Age- and smoking-adjusted SMRs were 3.9 times higher in silicotic than in nonsilicotic miners.[178]

Heavy smoking can impair pulmonary clearance, thereby prolonging silica's presence in the lungs and increasing the risk for silicosis. Heavy smokers developed significantly more silicosis after 20 or more years of silica exposure than did nonsmokers and moderate smokers combined.[179] Either the heavy doses of silica that result in silicosis also result in lung cancer, or some other aspect of the fibrotic process is responsible for the lung cancer excess.[84] Based on review of new evidence, the California Department of Toxic Substances Control recommended in 1995 that crystalline silica be classified a definite carcinogen.[179a] A causal association between silica exposure and lung cancer would be of considerable public health interest; in the United States alone, more than 3 million workers in 238,000 processing plants are potentially exposed to silica.[180] Of note, therefore, is the recent conclusion from a careful study of long-term exposure that "crystalline silica may well be a human carcinogen."[180a]

***Fibrous Glass.*** Studies of exposure to fibrous glass show increased SMRs for lung cancer ranging from 110 to 199. Many studies have not controlled for smoking and other confounders.[181, 182] Furthermore, SMRs were not influenced by duration of employment or increasing latency,[183] indicating the need for additional studies before concluding that fibrous glass is carcinogenic in humans.[184]

***Formaldehyde.*** Although one study noted a small excess of lung cancer in workers exposed to formaldehyde,[185] most have found no such association.[186–195] Two large cohort studies of American[196] and British exposed workers[197] also found no relationship between cumulative dose and lung cancer mortality. The absence of increased risk in "high-exposure" occupations and the possibility of confounding from unknown smoking habits argue against a causal association.[197]

***Welding Fumes.*** Exposure to welding fumes has been associated with a 30% to 50% increase in the risk for lung cancer.[198] Meta-analysis including 18 case-control and 31 cohort studies shows a combined relative risk for all types of welding of 1.38 (95% confidence interval, 1.29 to 1.48). No significant differences were observed between risks for shipyard and nonshipyard welders; nor did lung cancer risk differ significantly between stainless steel welders exposed to hexavalent chromium and nickel and mild steel welders.[199] An increased lung cancer risk among hard metal welders is attributed to simultaneous exposure to cobalt and tungsten carbide.[200]

### Other Environmental Exposures

***Air Pollution.*** Five major pollutants account for approximately 98% of air pollution: carbon monoxide (52%), sulfur oxides (18%), hydrocarbons (12%), particulate matter (10%), and nitrogen oxide (6%). The major sources of air pollution include transportation (60%), industry (18%), space heating (16%), electric power generation (13%), and refuse disposal (3%). The concentration of pollutants varies with the source. Downwind from a steel mill, particulate matter accounts for a greater percentage of the total pollution, whereas in areas where automobiles are the main source of pollution, carbon monoxide, hydrocarbons, and nitrogen oxides are higher and sulfur dioxide is lower. The adsorption of carcinogenic substances on inert particulate material could prolong residence time in the respiratory tract, further enhancing the carcinogenic potential of air pollution.

Although no lung cancer excess was found among residents living near any of ten nonferrous smelters located in five western states,[201] clusters of lung cancer cases have occurred downwind of foundries.[202, 203] In a community where smelter workers and miners had lung cancer relative risks greater than 3.0, a relative risk of 2.0 was calculated for men residing within 20 km of the smelter.[204] Indoor air pollution from "smoky" coal combustion was strongly related to lung cancer mortality in China.[205, 206] Air pollution is believed to interact multiplicatively with smoking and occupational exposure.[207] However, it is estimated that fewer than 5% of all lung cancers are attributable to pollution of ambient air.[208–210]

***Diesel Exhaust.*** Organic extracts of diesel particulates are carcinogenic in animals. Nine of 14 studies assessing lung cancer among truck drivers showed excess risks of 30% to 50% that persisted in the few studies that corrected for smoking.[211] Although several studies noted no increased risks for exposure to diesel exhaust,[212–214] significantly elevated risks were reported for railroad workers exposed to diesel fumes for at least 20 years,[215] for highly exposed Swedish bus garage workers,[216] and for long-haul diesel truck drivers.[217] In the United States, a 50% excess risk for lung cancer associated with employment in motor exhaust–related occupations was not explained by smoking habits or other occupational exposures.[218]

***Electromagnetic Fields.*** The association of pulsed electromagnetic fields (EMFs) and lung cancer has been attributed to the ability of the electric field component of power-frequency EMFs to attract and concentrate airborne radon progeny in their vicinity.[219, 220] Radar-exposed U.S. naval personnel experienced a twofold increase in lung cancer mortality in one study, although rates were not corrected for smoking.[221] Polish military personnel exposed to radiofrequency and microwave radiation experienced a relative risk for lung cancer of 1.41 compared with nonexposed personnel.[222] However, no lung cancer excess was identified among male and female employees of a large Swedish telecommunication company,[223] and the SMR for lung cancer among U.S. amateur radio operators was only 66.[224] In a study of electrical utility workers, lung cancer was not strongly associated with duration of employment in specific jobs involving high potential exposure to 60-Hz magnetic fields or to pulsed EMFs.[225]

***Miscellaneous.*** The lung cancer experiences of many other occupational groups have been examined, including agriculturalists exposed to fumes containing nickel and hexavalent chromium, meat cutters and slaughterhouse workers, firefighters, and others. The data regarding lung cancer risk in these occupational groups are often sparse, uncontrolled for confounders, inconsistent across studies, or lacking a persuasive dose effect. Estimates of exposure are often based on job classification rather than measurement of a relevant exposure. Use of biomarkers for exposure will improve the ability of future occupational studies to estimate past exposures and associated risks.

## Diet

A large body of experimental and epidemiologic evidence[226–230] supports the role of diet in modifying risk for lung cancer. Essential micronutrients, including vitamins A, C, and E and selenium, may be protective, whereas other dietary factors, including fats and cholesterol, may adversely affect risk.

**Vitamin A.** The term "vitamin A" refers to two dietary factors. *Preformed vitamin A,* the physiologically active form, occurs primarily as retinyl esters, retinal, and retinol. Dietary sources include animal products, supplements, and fortified foods. Vitamin A may exert a protective effect through its ability to control cellular differentiation and proliferation. The *provitamin A* carotenoids are found in plants, chiefly leafy green and yellow vegetables and fruits, and can be metabolized to retinol. Carotenoids may be active by way of conversion to retinol or through their ability to quench singlet oxygen.[231] Beta-carotene, the most common carotenoid, is also a potent scavenger of free radicals, a property not shared by retinol.

Since the 1970s, when the first studies suggested a lower risk for lung cancer in persons with high vitamin A intake, 8 prospective and more than 20 retrospective studies have investigated the role of vegetables and fruits, carotenoids, and related micronutrients in the etiology of lung cancer.[228–230, 232–234] The risk of developing lung cancer was reduced by approximately 30% to 60% in persons who had a higher intake of vegetables and/or fruits in all 8 cohort studies and all but 2 of 20 reviewed case-control studies.[228–230, 232–234] However, reduced risks were not always significant, and they sometimes were observed only in specific subgroups (e.g., whites but not African-Americans).[235] Small sample size and residual confounding due to inadequate adjustment for smoking or other behavioral correlates of smoking may be responsible for some of the inconsistencies.[229] The inverse trend in lung cancer risk with increasing consumption of fruits and vegetables was stronger than the trend with carotenoid intake in 13 of 15 studies examining both variables.[229] No association was observed with retinol intake.[236–240] Therefore, the protective effect of fruits and vegetables is not entirely explained by their carotenoid content and may be related to content of other phytochemicals, either alone or in combination with carotenoids.

A significant inverse association is consistently observed between serum levels of beta-carotene[241–243] and lung cancer risk. Although many studies have used stored samples of prediagnostic sera, data show that beta-carotene in stored blood degrades over time, casting some doubt on the validity of these associations.[229] Serum beta-carotene levels are inversely associated with current smoking, higher daily use of cigarettes, and increasing pack-years, and serum levels increase with increasing number of years since smoking cessation.[244] This suggests the existence of a biologic mechanism that lowers serum beta-carotene levels in smokers.

The consistency of inverse associations reported in observational studies led to several randomized, double-blind chemoprevention trials that used beta-carotene alone or in combination with other antioxidants. Results, however, did not confirm a protective effect for beta-carotene supplementation.[245–249] Lung cancer incidence was significantly increased by 18% in the Alpha-Tocopherol, Beta-Carotene Cancer Prevention Study (ATBC) of male heavy smokers in Finland who took beta-carotene with or without vitamin E[245] and by 36% in the Beta-Carotene and Retinol Efficacy Trial (CARET), a multicenter U.S. trial of heavy smokers and asbestos-exposed workers.[246, 247] Adverse effects occurred predominantly in heavier smokers and drinkers.[247, 248] A third study of U.S. physicians found no difference in lung cancer incidence between groups receiving beta-carotene versus placebo.[249]

Although observational studies continue to show a reduction in risk with increased consumption of carotenoid-rich fruits and vegetables, supplementation with a single carotenoid, beta-carotene, has not proved beneficial and, in some groups, may actually increase lung cancer risk. Even if beta-carotene supplementation has a beneficial effect in micronutrient-deficient populations, an adverse effect is possible in some subgroups if beta-carotene promotes tumor growth by inducing a pro-oxidant state in heavy smokers and drinkers.[230, 250] Fruits and vegetables contain a complex mixture of vitamins, minerals, fibers, and other phytochemicals. Persons consuming high levels of carotenoids also consume more of these substances and presumably less of other dietary components such as fats. Other antioxidants in fruits and vegetables, acting independently or together with beta-carotene, may be responsible for the observed protective effects. Though the exact dietary component responsible for the protective effect remains unknown, results of observational and intervention research indicate that significant public health benefits could be achieved by increasing consumption of fruits and vegetables. Supplementation with pharmacologic doses of beta-carotene, however, cannot be recommended for prevention of lung cancer.[250]

**Vitamin E.** Alpha-tocopherol, or vitamin E, is a lipid-soluble antioxidant that inhibits the formation of nitrosamines and *in vitro* carcinogenesis[251] and reduces the extent of oxidative damage to the lung epithelium in animals.[252] Although studies of vitamin E intake and lung cancer risk suggest a protective effect for vitamin E, inconsistencies have been noted.[229, 253, 254] In four reviewed studies assessing total vitamin E intake, results showed a significant inverse association in one,[255] differential effects for men and women in two,[236, 256] and no association in another.[257] Because of difficulty in estimating intake of vitamin E–rich fats and oils, blood levels of alpha-tocopherol are frequently studied. Only three of six prospective studies of prediagnostic serum levels reported an inverse association with lung cancer.[229] Observed associations could be explained by confounding due to the presence of beta-carotene or other dietary nutrients or by failure to adjust for other confounders. In the randomized ATBC Cancer Prevention Study,[245] supplementation with vitamin E did not result in any detectable beneficial effect on incidence or mortality from lung cancer. At present, evidence for a protective effect of vitamin E is not convincing.

**Vitamin C.** Vitamin C may exert a protective effect through its ability to scavenge free radicals and to protect against lipid peroxidation.[226] Vegetables and fruits, consistently associated with decreased risk for lung cancer,[228–230, 232–234] are the primary sources of vitamin C in the diet. Though early results showed weak protective effects for vitamin C intake,[236, 258–261] a review of more recent studies found conflicting results.[229] A significant protective effect for vitamin C was observed in several studies[238, 240, 262] but not in others.[236, 257, 263, 264] Inverse associations are often stronger and/or more consistent for intake of fruits and vegetables than for total vitamin C.[238, 265] Though data are suggestive of a protective effect for vitamin C, some other component of fruits and vegetables could be responsible for the observed decrease in risk.

**Other Dietary Factors.** Investigations of other dietary factors include possible protective effects for selenium,[229, 266–268] flavonoids,[269] glucosinolates in Brassica vegetables,[233] and black tea[270, 271] and adverse effects for alcohol[272, 273] and fats.[274–280] Significant supportive evidence exists only for the protective effect of selenium and the adverse effects of fats and alcohol. Selenium is present in the active site of glutathione peroxidase, an enzyme that prevents lipid peroxidation through the destruction of lipid hyperoxides and endogenous hydrogen peroxide.[226] A review of prospective studies of prediagnostic serum and toenail selenium produced discordant results describing positive, negative, and null associations.[229] However, the two largest studies reviewed showed significant inverse trends, with relative risks in the highest selenium quintile of 0.3[266] and 0.5,[267] compared with the lowest quintile. Moreover, a reduction in lung cancers was observed in a placebo-controlled prevention trial of selenium supplementation to prevent skin cancer.[268] Although the latter study was not designed to test hypotheses related to lung cancer, the results are promising and warrant further study.

Ecologic studies first supported an association between consumption of animal fats and lung cancer risk.[274, 275] Oxidation products of cholesterol are known mutagens and carcinogens. In addition, a high-fat diet may promote lung tumors through effects on the immune system, intercellular communication, endocrine processes, and cell proliferation.[226] Some analytic studies support a positive association between intake of dietary lipids and lung cancer risk,[257, 264, 275–278] one study noted no association,[279] and others reported inconsistencies in the excess risks for subgroups.[257, 276, 279] Because of the high correlation between saturated fat (or cholesterol or total fat) and total calories, it is difficult to estimate the effect of fat independent of total caloric intake.[280] Of the two studies that controlled for total energy intake, one reported a strong increasing trend in lung cancer risk with increased consumption of saturated fat[257] and the other reported no such increase.[279] Although the current evidence is suggestive, it is not sufficient to conclude that increased dietary intake of cholesterol and fats increases risks of lung cancer.

## Host Factors

**Familial Aggregation.** The fact that only one in ten smokers develops lung cancer emphasizes the importance of individual differences in susceptibility to the effects of tobacco smoke. Studies of family members support the notion that susceptibility is familial but not necessarily inherited; the relative contribution of heredity versus shared exposures is unclear. Lung cancer is known to aggregate in families and to cluster with other cancers.[281–285] In family studies, risk for lung and other cancers is higher in families of probands after adjusting for smoking and other risk factors.[286–289] Risk increases in direct proportion to the number of relatives with cancer[283, 290] and is greatest for squamous and small cell carcinomas.[291, 292] Smoking interacts synergistically with family history to increase lung cancer risk by 30 to 47 times the risk observed in nonsmokers with no family history.[281, 293]

Smoking is known to aggregate in families and, although analyses have attempted to adjust for smoking habits in family studies, some of the higher risks seen in family members may simply be attributable to inadequate statistical adjustment for smoking. Other aspects of shared environments may also contribute to familial clustering of lung cancer. Studies of twin pairs noted a familial effect possibly related to smoking but no evidence of a genetic mechanism.[294, 295] In segregation analysis of family data, the aggregation of lung cancer in families of nonsmokers was best explained by an environmental model rather than a heritable defect.[296] The clustering of cancers of both smoking-related and nonrelated sites in family members of lung cancer probands supports the existence of some heritable host factors that affect susceptibility or resistance to carcinogens.

**Biologic Markers.** Understanding of the multiple stages, diverse pathways, and gene alterations involved in carcinogenesis and susceptibility to carcinogens has increased substantially as a result of the research use of biologic markers.[297–299] Biomarkers may serve as indicators of internal exposure dose (e.g., serum cotinine or nicotine levels), or they may serve as measures of an individual's genetically determined predisposition to develop cancer.[300] For further discussion, see Chapter 44. Metabolism of absorbed compounds involves both the activation and deactivation of carcinogens. A shift in the balance between phase I procarcinogen-activating enzymes and phase II deactivating enzymes, resulting in genetic damage, is one way by which susceptibility can be conferred. Markers of early events in carcinogenesis, such as DNA adduction or somatic cell mutations, can also serve as intermediate markers for later events in the multistep process, including oncogene mutation, early neoplasia, and clinically apparent disease.

DNA and protein adducts constitute an early indication of biologic response to carcinogens and may lead to mutations that activate oncogenes or deactivate tumor suppressor genes.[301] Adduct levels are higher in smokers than in nonsmokers, increase in parallel with smoking dose,[302–304] and have been shown to correlate with the activity of aryl hydrocarbon hydroxylase (AHH), an enzyme involved in the metabolism of carcinogens.[305] Cytogenetic measures such as sister chromatid exchange (SCE) reflect the genotoxic effects of cigarette smoking[306] and may reflect defects in cellular repair mechanisms.[307] Although lung cancer patients do not differ from healthy smokers with respect to frequency of SCEs in peripheral blood lymphocytes,[307, 308] SCEs do reflect pack-years of exposure to cigarettes.[308] SCEs, however, are significantly elevated in patients with lung cancer in comparison with healthy subjects, because controls are less likely to smoke or they have smoked for fewer pack-years.[307] Mutagen sensitivity, measured by frequency of chromatid breaks, has been shown to be increased in lung cancer patients compared with controls, particularly in light smokers,[309] and may be greater in Hispanics than in non-Hispanic whites.[310] Consistent with the dysregulation of cell growth, cycling, and division, more frequent mutations in proto-oncogenes and tumor suppressor genes, including *KRAS* and *p53*, have been noted in lung cancer patients compared with controls.[311, 312] Deletions or translocations of chromosome 3 and loss of alleles on chromosomes 11 and 17 have been reported.[313, 314]

Genetic markers of susceptibility to lung cancer have focused on polymorphisms for enzymes involved in the metabolism of carcinogens, including AHH, cytochrome P-450, *N*-acetyltransferase (NAT), and glutathione-*S*-transferase (GSTM1). An increase in AHH enzyme activity occurs after exposure to PAHs in tobacco smoke and is associated with increased risk for lung cancer.[304, 315, 316] The high AHH-inducibility phenotype has been associated with a variant genotype of the polymorphic cytochrome P-450 (*CYP1A1* gene) involved in the metabolism of PAHs to reactive intermediate compounds capable of forming DNA adducts.[298] Studies using molecular methods have shown an association between the CYP1A1 *Msp1* polymorphism, first identified in Japanese populations, and lung cancer risk.[317, 318] Caucasians heterozygous or homozygous for the *Msp1* variant genotype carry a twofold increased risk for lung cancer after adjusting for confounders. The association is consistent for both genders, various smoking categories, and various histologic types.[319]

Another P-450 enzyme, CPY2D6, which is involved in the metabolism of the antihypertensive drug debrisoquine, has been linked to lung cancer risk through activation of the tobacco-specific carcinogen 4-methylnitrosamino-1-(3-pyridyl)-1-butanone (NNK). A strong interaction between CYP2D6 activity and smoking was observed in one study.[320] Smokers with the highest CYP2D6 activity experienced significantly increasing risk for lung cancer with increasing smoking; those with the heaviest smoking were at very high risk for lung cancer. At low or medium levels of CYP2D6 activity, however, a dose-response effect for smoking was not evident. An increase in the putative pathway for NNK detoxification has been reported in whites compared with African-Americans and could explain racial differences in lung cancer.[321] Consistent with this observation, slower clearance of the nicotine metabolite cotinine in blacks compared with whites has been reported.[5a] Studies of the CYP2D6 genotype and lung cancer, however, have been inconsistent.[322, 323] Any direct relationship between the CP2D6 genotype and lung cancer risk is not likely to be strong.

A third polymorphism involving the GSTs, a family of enzymes involved in conjugation and inactivation of toxic substances including PAHs, has been strongly implicated as a protective factor in lung cancer. GSTM1 (mu-class enzyme) deficiency is more common in lung cancer patients than in controls.[324] The null allele (*GSTM1*0* genotype) appears to produce no active enzyme owing to partial or total gene deletion. Deficiencies in the mu isoenzyme have also been associated with increased cytogenetic damage in smokers[325] and higher levels of PAH-DNA adducts in tissue.[326] Data strongly support a protective effect for GST.

Phase II metabolism (deactivation) of PAHs also involves reduced nicotinamide adenine dinucleotide (NADPH):quinone oxidoreductase (NQO), NAT, and other enzymes. The wild-type genotype of *NQO1* has been associated with lung cancer risk after controlling for age, gender, ethnicity, and smoking.[327] Carriers of the *NAT2*4/*4* genotype, with its high acetylation capacity, were noted to have a threefold increased risk for lung cancer after adjusting for age, gender, and smoking.[328]

No one single factor is likely to explain the increased susceptibility to lung cancer in a subset of smokers. The simultaneous presence of both the null *GSTM1* genotype and the mutant *CYP1A1* genotype, associated with a high relative risk for lung cancer of 41.0 (95% CI, 9 to 194),[329] conveys a higher risk than either marker alone.[330] Investigation of those who have multiple high-risk polymorphisms, including both phase I and phase II carcinogen-metabolizing enzymes, may eventually identify those smokers for whom lung cancer is probable.

## SUMMARY

Lung cancer is the leading cause of cancer mortality among both men and women in the United States, accounting for 28% of all cancer deaths in 1999. Mortality, which increased rapidly early in this century, leveled off for men in the mid-1980s and is now declining; rates for women continue to increase, although at a slower rate in recent years, and are decreasing in the younger age groups. The prognosis is poor, with only 12.6% of men and 16.2% of women surviving 5 years.

An estimated 85% of lung cancers are attributable to cigarette smoking. Risk increases with years of smoking, number of cigarettes smoked daily, earlier smoking initiation, deeper inhalation, and higher tar content, and it decreases with time after smoking cessation. Data suggest that women smokers may be at increased risk compared with men who smoke. Changes in the constitution of low-tar cigarettes may be responsible. Nonsmoking women married to smokers have a 20% to 30% increased risk of lung cancer.

Increased risk of lung cancer is well established for occupational exposures to aluminum production, arsenic, asbestos, bis(chloromethyl) ether, chromium, coke oven emissions, iron and steel founding, mustard gas, nickel and nickel compounds, radiation, and vinyl chloride. Suspected occupational carcinogens include beryllium, cadmium and cadmium compounds, crystalline silica, fibrous glass, formaldehyde, diesel exhaust, and electromagnetic fields, among others.

Although dietary intake of fruits and vegetables is consistently associated with a reduced risk of lung cancer, supplementation with beta-carotene has not proved beneficial for the prevention of lung cancer in smokers. Data are suggestive of a protective effect for vitamin C and for selenium and an adverse effect for cholesterol and for dietary fat intake. Evidence for a protective effect for vitamin E is not convincing.

The increase in risk associated with family history of lung and other cancers independent of smoking habits suggests the presence of heritable factors that influence susceptibility to lung cancer. Investigations of biologic markers of susceptibility include studies of inherited genetic polymorphisms that may identify increased susceptibility to lung cancer and studies of intermediate markers of carcinogenesis such as DNA adduction and somatic cell mutations. Research on the occurrence of multiple high-risk gene polymorphisms for enzymes involved in the metabolism of carcinogens in tobacco smoke may eventually lead to identification of those smokers who are most likely to develop lung cancer.

## References


1. Landis SH, Murray T, Bolden S, et al: Cancer statistics, 1999. CA Cancer J Clin 49:8–31, 1999.
2. Travis WD, Lubin J, Ries L, et al: United States lung carcinoma incidence trends: Declining for most histologic types among males, increasing for females. Cancer 77:2464–2470, 1996.
3. Ries L, Kosary CL, Hankey BF, et al (eds): SEER Cancer Statistics Review 1973–1996. Bethesda, MD: National Cancer Institute, 1999.

3a. Ries LAG, Kosary CL, Hankey BF, et al (eds): SEER Cancer Statistics Review 1973–1995. Bethesda, MD: National Cancer Institute, 1998.

4. US Department of Health and Human Services: Tobacco Use among US Racial/Ethnic Minority Groups: A Report of the Surgeon General. Rockville, MD: US Department of Health and Human Services, Public Health Service, Office on Smoking and Health, 1998.
5. Schwartz AG, Swanson GM: Lung carcinoma in African Americans and whites: A population-based study in metropolitan Detroit, Michigan. Cancer 79:45–52, 1997.

5a. Perez-Stable EJ, Herrera B, Jacob P, et al: Nicotine metabolism and intake in black and white smokers. JAMA 280:152–156, 1998.

6. Miller BA, Kolonel LN, Bernstein L, et al (eds): Racial/Ethnic Patterns of Cancer in the United States 1988–1992 (NIH Publication No. 96-4104). Bethesda, MD: National Cancer Institute, 1996.
7. Coleman MP, Esteve J, Damiecki P, et al: Trends in Cancer Incidence and Mortality. IARC Scientific Publications No. 21. Lyon: World Health Organization, International Agency for Research on Cancer, 1993.
8. Takkouche B, Gestal-Otero JJ: The epidemiology of lung cancer: Review of risk factors and Spanish data. Eur J Epidemiol 12:341–349, 1996.
9. Negri E, La Vecchia C, Franceschi S, et al: Patterns of mortality from major cancers in Europe. Cancer Epidemiol Biomarkers Prev 3:531–536, 1994.
10. Kubik A, Plesko I: Trends in cigarette sales and lung cancer mortality in four central European countries. Cent Eur J Public Health 6:37–41, 1998.
11. Gao YT, Zheng W, Gao RN, et al: Tobacco smoking and its effect on health in China. IARC Sci Publ 105:62–67, 1991.
12. Wang TJ, Zhou BS, Shi JP: Lung cancer in nonsmoking Chinese women: A case-control study. Lung Cancer 14(Suppl 1):S93–S98, 1996.
13. Kristein MM: Japanese lung cancer mortality rates, 1947–1980 and per capita cigarette consumption in Japan 5 (letter). Int J Epidemiol 15:140–141, 1986.
14. Garfinkel L, Silverberg E: Lung cancer and smoking trends in the United States over the past 25 years. Ann N Y Acad Sci 609:146–154, 1990.
15. Peto R, Lopez AD, Boreham J, et al: Mortality from tobacco in developed countries: Indirect estimation from national vital statistics. Lancet 339:1268–1278, 1992.
16. Wynder EL, Graham EA: Tobacco smoking as a possible etiologic factor in bronchogenic carcinoma. JAMA 143:329–336, 1950.
17. Levin ML, Goldstein H, Gerhardt PR: Cancer and tobacco smoking: A preliminary report. JAMA 143:336–338, 1950.
18. Hammond EC, Horn D: Smoking and death rates: Report on forty-four months of follow-up of 187,783 men. JAMA 251:2840–2853, 1958.
19. US Public Health Service: Smoking and Health: A Report of the Advisory Committee to the Surgeon General of the Public Health Service. Rockville, MD: US Department of Health, Education and Welfare, Center for Disease Control, 1964.
20. US Public Health Service: Smoking and Health: A Report of the Surgeon General. Rockville, MD: US Department of Health, Education, and Welfare, Public Health Service, Office on Smoking and Health, 1979.
21. US Public Health Service: The Health Consequences of Smoking for Women: A Report of the Surgeon General. Rockville, MD: US Department of Health and Human Services, Office on Smoking and Health, 1980.
22. US Department of Health and Human Services: The Health Consequences of Smoking: Cancer. A Report of the Surgeon General. DHHS Publication No. (PHS) 82–50179, 1982. Rockville, MD: US Department of Health and Human Services, Public Health Service, Office on Smoking and Health.
23. US Department of Health and Human Services: Reducing the Health Consequences of Smoking: 25 Years of Progress. A Report of the Surgeon General. DHHS Publication No. (CDC) 89–8411. Rockville, MD: US Department of Health and Human Services, Public Health Service, Centers for Disease Control, Center for Chronic Disease Prevention and Health Promotion, Office on Smoking and Health, 1989, pp. 43–55;249.
24. Loeb LA, Ernster VL, Warner KE, et al: Smoking and lung cancer: An overview. Cancer Res 44:5940–5958, 1984.
25. Burns DM, Shanks TG, Choi W, et al: The American Cancer Society Cancer Prevention Study I: 12-Year followup of 1 million men and women. *In* Shopland D (ed): Changes in Cigarette-Related Disease Risks and Their Implication for Prevention and

Control (Smoking and Tobacco Control Monograph No. 8). Bethesda, MD: US Department of Health and Human Services, Public Health Service, National Institutes of Health, National Cancer Institute, 1997.
26. Thun MJ, Myers DG, Day-Lally C, et al: Age and the exposure-response relationships between cigarette smoking and premature death in Cancer Prevention Study II. *In* Shopland D (ed): Changes in Cigarette-Related Disease Risks and Their Implication for Prevention and Control (Smoking and Tobacco Control Monograph No. 8). Bethesda, MD: US Department of Health and Human Services, Public Health Service, National Institutes of Health, National Cancer Institute, 1997.
27. Ullmann D, Phillips RL, Beeson WL, et al: Cause-specific mortality among physicians with differing life-styles. JAMA 265:2352–2359, 1991.
28. Troyer H: Review of cancer among 4 religious sects: Evidence that life-styles are distinctive sets of risk factors. Soc Sci Med 26:1007–1017, 1988.
29. Humble CG, Samet JM, Pathak DR, et al: Cigarette smoking and lung cancer in "Hispanic" whites and other whites in New Mexico. Am J Public Health 75:145–148, 1985.
30. Harris RE, Zang EA, Anderson JI, et al: Race and sex differences in lung cancer risk associated with cigarette smoking. Int J Epidemiol 22:592–599, 1993.
31. Le Marchand L, Wilkens LR, Kolonel LN: Ethnic differences in the lung cancer risk associated with smoking. Cancer Epidemiol Biomarkers Prev 1:103–107, 1992.
32. Gao YT, Blot WJ, Zheng W, et al: Lung cancer and smoking in Shanghai. Int J Epidemiol 17:277–280, 1988.
33. Burns DM, Lee L, Shen LZ, et al: Cigarette smoking behavior in the United States. *In* Shopland D (ed): Changes in Cigarette-Related Disease Risks and Their Implication for Prevention and Control (Smoking and Tobacco Control Monograph No. 8). Bethesda, MD: US Department of Health and Human Services, Public Health Service, National Institutes of Health, National Cancer Institute, 1997.
34. Thun MJ, Day-Lally C, Myers DG, et al: Trends in tobacco smoking and mortality from cigarette use in cancer prevention studies I (1959 through 1965) and II (1982 through 1988). *In* Shopland D (ed): Changes in Cigarette-Related Disease Risks and Their Implication for Prevention and Control (Smoking and Tobacco Control Monograph No. 8). Bethesda, MD: US Department of Health and Human Services, Public Health Service, National Institutes of Health, National Cancer Institute, 1997.
35. Garfinkel L, Stellman SD: Smoking and lung cancer in women: Findings in a prospective study. Cancer Res 48:6951–6955, 1988.
36. Osann KE, Anton-Culver HA, Kurosaki T, et al: Sex differences in lung cancer risk associated with cigarette smoking. Int J Cancer 54:44–48, 1993.
37. Risch HA, Howe GR, Jain M, et al: Are female smokers at higher risk for lung cancer than male smokers? Am J Epidemiol 138:281–293, 1993.
38. Brownson RC, Chang JC, Davis JR: Gender and histologic type variations in smoking-related risk of lung cancer. Epidemiology 3:61–64, 1992.
39. Friedman GD, Tekawa I, Sadler M, et al: Smoking and mortality: The Kaiser Permanente experience. *In* Shopland D (ed): Changes in Cigarette-Related Disease Risks and Their Implication for Prevention and Control (Smoking and Tobacco Control Monograph No. 8). Bethesda, MD: US Department of Health and Human Services, Public Health Service, National Institutes of Health, National Cancer Institute, 1997.
40. Zang EA, Wynder EL: Differences in lung cancer risk between men and women: Examination of the evidence. J Natl Cancer Inst 88:183–192, 1996.
41. Brown CC, Kessler LG: Projections of lung cancer mortality in the United States: 1985–2025. J Natl Cancer Inst 80:43–51, 1988.
42. Anton-Culver H, Culver BD, Kurosaki T, et al: Incidence of lung cancer by histological type from a population-based registry. Cancer Res 48:6580–6583, 1988.
43. Thun MJ, Lally CA, Flannery JT, et al: Cigarette smoking and changes in the histopathology of lung cancer. J Natl Cancer Inst 89:1580–1586, 1997.
44. Muscat JE, Wynder EL: Lung cancer pathology in smokers, ex-smokers and never smokers. Cancer Lett 88:1–5, 1995.
45. Brownson RC, Loy TS, Ingram E, et al: Lung cancer in non-smoking women. Cancer 75:29–33, 1995.
46. Schoenberg JB, Wilcox HB, Mason TJ, et al: Variation in smoking-related lung cancer risk among New Jersey women. Am J Epidemiol 130:688–695, 1989.
47. Thun MJ, Heath CW: Changes in mortality from smoking in two American Cancer Society prospective studies since 1959. Prev Med 26:422–426, 1997.
48. Wynder EL, Muscat JE: The changing epidemiology of smoking and lung cancer histology. Environ Health Perspect 103(Suppl 8):143–148, 1995.
49. Hoffman D, Djordjevic MV, Hoffman I: The changing cigarette. Prev Med 26:427–434, 1997.
50. Zang EA, Wynder EL: Cumulative tar exposure. Cancer 70:69–76, 1992.
51. Kaufman DW, Palmer JR, Rosenberg L, et al: Tar content of cigarettes in relation to lung cancer. Am J Epidemiol 129:703–711, 1989.
52. Lubin JH, Blot WJ, Berrino F, et al: Patterns of lung cancer risk according to type of cigarette smoked. Int J Cancer 33:569–576, 1984.
53. Pathak DR, Samet JM, Humble CG: Determinants of lung cancer risk in cigarette smokers in New Mexico. J Natl Cancer Inst 76:597–604, 1986.
54. Sidney S, Tekawa IS, Friedman GD: A prospective study of cigarette tar yield and lung cancer. Cancer Causes Control 4:3–10, 1993.
55. Djordjevic MV, Hoffman D, Hoffman I: Nicotine regulates smoking patterns. Prev Med 26:427–434, 1997.
56. Kabat GC, Hebert JR: Use of mentholated cigarettes and lung cancer risk. Cancer Res 51:6510–6513, 1991.
57. Sidney S, Tekawa IS, Friedman GD, et al: Mentholated cigarette use and lung cancer. Arch Intern Med 155:727–732, 1995.
58. Cummings KM, Giovino G, Mendicino AJ: Cigarette advertising and black-white differences in brand preference. Public Health Rep 102:698–701, 1987.
59. US Department of Health and Human Services: The Health Benefits of Smoking Cessation. Rockville, MD: US Department of Health and Human Services, Public Health Service, Centers for Disease Control, Center for Chronic Disease Prevention and Health Promotion, 1990.
60. Hrubec Z, McLaughlin JK: Former cigarette smoking and mortality among US veterans: A 26-year followup, 1954 to 1980. *In* Shopland D (ed): Changes in Cigarette-Related Disease Risks and Their Implication for Prevention and Control (Smoking and Tobacco Control Monograph No. 8). Bethesda, MD: US Department of Health and Human Services, Public Health Service, National Institutes of Health, National Cancer Institute, 1997.
61. Lubin JH, Blot WJ, Berrino F, et al: Modifying risk of developing lung cancer by changing habits of cigarette smoking. Br Med J 288:1953–1956, 1984.
62. Becher H, Jockel KH, Timm J, et al: Smoking cessation and non-smoking intervals: Effect of different smoking patterns on lung cancer risk. Cancer Causes Control 2:381–387, 1991.
63. US Department of Health and Human Services: The Health Consequences of Involuntary Smoking. A Report of the Surgeon General. Publication No. (CDC)87–8398. Rockville, MD: Department of Health and Human Services, Office on Smoking and Health, 1987.
64. Committee on Passive Smoking, Board on Environmental Studies and Toxicology, National Research Council: Environmental Tobacco Smoke: Measuring Exposures and Assessing Health Effects. Washington, DC: National Academy Press, 1986.
65. US Environmental Protection Agency: Health Effects of Passive Smoking: Assessment of Lung Cancer in Adults and Respiratory Disorders in Children. EPA Publication No. 600/6–90/006A. Washington, DC: EPA, 1990.
66. Brownson RC, Alavanja MCR, Hock ET, et al: Passive smoking and lung cancer in non-smoking women. Am J Public Health 82:1525–1530, 1992.
67. Stockwell HG, Goldman AL, Lyman GH, et al: Environmental tobacco smoke and lung cancer risk in nonsmoking women. J Natl Cancer Inst 84:1417–1422, 1992
68. Fontham ETH, Correa P, Reynolds P, et al: Environmental tobacco smoke and lung cancer in nonsmoking women: A multicenter study. JAMA 271:1752–1759, 1994.

69. Kabat GC, Stellman SD, Wynder EL: Relation between environmental tobacco smoke and lung cancer in lifetime nonsmokers. Am J Epidemiol 142:141–148, 1995.
70. Cardenas VM, Thun MJ, Austin H, et al: Environmental tobacco smoke and lung cancer mortality in the American Cancer Society's Cancer Prevention Study II. Cancer Causes Control 8:57–64, 1997.
71. Hackshaw AK, Law MR, Wald NJ: The accumulated evidence on lung cancer and environmental tobacco smoke. Br Med J 315:980–988, 1997.
72. Ko YC, Lee CH, Chen MJ, et al: Risk factors for primary lung cancer among non-smoking women in Taiwan. Int J Epidemiol 26:24–31, 1997.
73. Wang TJ, Zhou BS: Meta-analysis of the potential relationship between exposure to environmental tobacco smoke and lung cancer in nonsmoking Chinese women. Lung Cancer 16:145–150, 1997.
74. Gross AJ: The risk of lung cancer in nonsmokers in the United States and its reported association with environmental tobacco smoke. J Clin Epidemiol 48:587–598, 1995.
75. Koo LC, Kabat GC, Rylander R, et al: Dietary and lifestyle correlates of passive smoking in Hong Kong, Japan, Sweden, and the USA. Soc Sci Med 45:159–169, 1997.
76. Nilsson R. Environmental tobacco smoke and lung cancer: A reappraisal. Ecotoxicol Environ Saf 34:2–17, 1996.
77. Lubin JH, Richter BS, Blot WJ: Lung cancer risk with cigar and pipe use. J Natl Cancer Inst 73:377–381, 1984.
78. Higgins IT, Mahan CM, Wynder EL: Lung cancer among cigar and pipe smokers. Prev Med 17:116–128, 1988.
79. Damber LA, Larsson L-G: Smoking and lung cancer with special regard to type of smoking and type of cancer: A case-control study in north Sweden. Br J Cancer 53:673–681, 1986.
80. Cigar smoking among teenagers—United States, Massachusetts, and New York, 1996. MMWR Morb Mortal Wkly Rep 46:433-444, 1997.
81. US Department of Health and Human Services: The Health Consequences of Using Smokeless Tobacco. A Report of the Advisory Committee to the Surgeon General. NIH Publication No. (PHS) 86–2874. Rockville, MD: US Department of Health and Human Services, Public Health Service, Office on Smoking and Health, 1986.
82. Shopland DR: Tobacco use and its contribution to early cancer mortality with a special emphasis on cigarette smoking. Environ Health Perspect 103(Suppl 8):131–142, 1995.
83. Devesa SS, Blot WJ, Fraumeni JF Jr: Declining lung cancer rates among young men and women in the United States: A cohort analysis. J Natl Cancer Inst 81:1568–1571, 1989.
84. Steenland K, Loomis D, Shy C, Simonsen N: Review of occupational lung carcinogens. Am J Ind Med 29:474–490, 1996.
85. Kjuus H, Langard S, Skjaerven R: A case-referent study of lung cancer, occupational exposures and smoking: III. Etiologic fraction of occupational exposures. Scand J Work Environ Health 12:210–215, 1986.
86. Weiss W, Moser RL, Auerbach O: Lung cancer in chloromethyl ether workers. Am Rev Respir Dis 120:1031–1037, 1979.
87. Edling C: Lung cancer and smoking in a group of iron ore miners. Am J Ind Med 3:191–199, 1982.
88. Waxweiler RJ, Smith AH, Falk H, et al: Excess lung cancer risk in a synthetic chemicals plant. Environ Health Perspect 41:159–165, 1981.
89. Ives JC, Buffler PA, Greenberg SD: Environmental associations and histopathologic patterns of carcinoma of the lung: The challenge and dilemma in epidemiologic studies. Am Rev Respir Dis 128:195–209, 1983.
90. Gibbs GW: Mortality of aluminum reduction plant workers, 1950 through 1977. J Occup Med 27:761–770, 1985.
91. Sobel W, Bond GG, Baldwin CL, et al: An update of respiratory cancer and occupational exposure to arsenicals. Am J Ind Med 13:263–270, 1988.
92. Pershagen G, Wall S, Taube A, et al: On the interaction between occupational arsenic exposure and smoking and its relationship to lung cancer. Scand J Work Environ Health 7:302–309, 1981.
93. Brown CC, Chu KC: Implications of the multistage theory of carcinogenesis applied to occupational arsenic exposure. J Natl Cancer Inst 70:455–463, 1983.
94. Thomas DC, Whittemore AS: Methods for testing interactions, with applications to occupational exposures, smoking, and lung cancer. Am J Ind Med 13:131–147, 1988.
95. Muscat JE, Stellman SD, Wyner EL: Insulation, asbestos, smoking habits and lung cancer types. Am J Ind Med 27:257–269, 1995.
96. Health and Safety Commission: Asbestos. Vol 2: Papers Prepared for the Advisory Committee. London, Her Majesty's Stationery Office, 1979, pp. 8–55.
97. Weiss W: Lobe of origin in the attribution of lung cancer to asbestos. Br J Ind Med 45:544–547, 1988.
98. Craighead JE: Do silica and asbestos cause lung cancer? Arch Pathol Lab Med 116:16–20, 1992.
99. Hillerdal HG, Henderson DW: Asbestos, asbestosis, pleural plaques and cancer. Scand J Work Environ Health 23:93–103, 1997.
100. Topping DC, Nettesheim P: Two-stage carcinogenesis studies with asbestos in Fischer 344 rats. J Natl Cancer Inst 65:627–630, 1980.
101. Barrett JC, Lamb PW, Wiseman RW: Multiple mechanisms for the carcinogenic effects of asbestos and other mineral fibers. Environ Health Perspect 81:81–89, 1989.
102. Finkelstein MM: Mortality among long-term employees of an Ontario asbestos-cement factory. Br J Ind Med 40:138–144, 1983.
103. Lash TL, Crouch EAC, Green LG: A meta-analysis of the relation between cumulative exposure to asbestos and relative risk of lung cancer. Occup Environ Med 54:254–263, 1997.
104. Warnock ML: Lung asbestos burden in shipyard and construction workers with mesothelioma: Comparison with burdens in subjects with asbestosis or lung cancer. Environ Res 50:68–85, 1989.
105. Selikoff IJ, Hammond EC, Seidman H: Latency of asbestos disease among insulation workers in the United States and Canada. Cancer 46:2736–2740, 1980.
106. Liddell FDK: Latent periods in lung cancer mortality in relation to asbestos dose and smoking. *In* Wagner JD, Davis W (eds): Biological Effects of Mineral Fibres. Lyon: International Agency for Research on Cancer, 1980, pp. 661–665.
107. Walker AM: Declining relative risks for lung cancer after cessation of asbestos exposure. J Occup Med 26:422–426, 1984.
108. de Klerk NH, Musk AW, Armstrong BK, et al: Smoking, exposure to crocidolite, and the incidence of lung cancer and asbestosis. Br J Ind Med 48:412–417, 1991.
109. Kjuus H, Skjaerven R, Langård S, et al: A case-referent study of lung cancer, occupational exposures and smoking: II. Role of asbestos exposure. Scand J Work Environ Health 12:203–209, 1986.
110. Vainio H, Boffetta P: Mechanisms of the combined effects of asbestos and smoking in the etiology of lung cancer. Scand J Work Environ Health 20:235–242, 1994.
110a. Erren TC, Jacobsen M, Pierkarski C: Synergy between asbestosis and smoking on lung cancer risk. Epidemiology 10:405–411, 1999.
111. Browne K: A threshold for asbestos related lung cancer. Br J Ind Med 43:556–558, 1986.
112. Seidman H, Selikoff IJ, Gelb SK: Mortality experience of amosite asbestos factory workers: Dose-response relationships 5 to 40 years after onset of short-term work exposure. Am J Ind Med 10:479–514, 1986.
113. Omenn GS, Merchant J, Boatman E, et al: Contribution of environmental fibers to respiratory cancer. Environ Health Perspect 70:51–56, 1986.
114. Hughes JM, Weill H: Asbestos exposure: Quantitative assessment of risk. Am Rev Respir Dis 133:5–13, 1986.
115. Kelman GR: Can one fibre cause cancer? (letter). Med J Aust 143:92, 1985.
116. Lilienfeld DE, Mandel JS, Coin P, et al: Projection of asbestos related diseases in the United States, 1985–2009: I. Cancer. Br J Ind Med 45:283–291, 1988.
117. Weiss W: Epidemic curve of respiratory cancer due to chloromethyl ethers. J Natl Cancer Inst 69:1265–1270, 1982.
118. Weiss W, Figueroa WG: The characteristics of lung cancer due to chloromethyl ethers. J Occup Med 18:623–627, 1976.
119. Albert RE, Pasternack BS, Shore RE, et al: Mortality patterns among workers exposed to chloromethyl ethers: A preliminary report. Environ Health Perspect 11:209–214, 1975.

120. Pasternack BS, Shore RE, Albert RE: Occupational exposure to chloromethyl ethers. J Occup Med 19:741–746, 1977.
121. McCallum RI, Woolley V, Petrie A: Lung cancer associated with chloromethyl methyl ether manufacture: An investigation at two factories in the United Kingdom. Br J Ind Med 40:384–389, 1983.
122. Gowers DS, DeFonso LR, Schaffer P, et al: Incidence of respiratory cancer among workers exposed to chloromethyl-ethers. Am J Epidemiol 137:31–42, 1993.
123. Mancuso TF: Chromium as an industrial carcinogen: Part 1. Am J Ind Med 31:129–139, 1997.
124. Kollmeier H, Seemann J, Müller K-M, et al: Increased chromium and nickel content in lung tissue and bronchial carcinoma. Am J Ind Med 11:659–669, 1987.
125. Kishi R, Tarumi T, Uchino E, et al: Chromium content of organs of chromate workers with lung cancer. Am J Ind Med 11:67–74, 1987.
126. Hayes RB, Sheffet A, Spirtas R: Cancer mortality among a cohort of chromium pigment workers. Am J Ind Med 16:127–133, 1989.
127. Davies JM, Easton DF, Bidstrup PL: Mortality from respiratory cancer and other causes in United Kingdom chromate production workers. Br J Ind Med 48:299–313, 1991.
128. van Schooten FJ, van Leeuwen FE, Hillebrand MJX, et al: Determination of benzo[*a*]pyrene diol epoxide-DNA adducts in white blood cell DNA from coke-oven workers: The impact of smoking. J Natl Cancer Inst 82:927–933, 1990.
129. World Health Organization: Evaluation of the Carcinogenic Risk of Chemicals to Humans: Polynuclear Aromatic Compounds, Part 3, Industrial Exposures in Aluminium Production, Coal Gasification, Coke Production, and Iron and Steel Founding, vol 34. Lyon: International Agency for Research on Cancer, 1984, pp. 101–131.
130. Bertrand JP, Chau N, Patris A, et al: Mortality due to respiratory cancers in the coke oven plants of the Lorraine coalmining industry (Houilléres du Bassin de Lorraine). Br J Ind Med 44:559–565, 1987.
131. Mazumdar S, Redmond C, Sollecito W, et al: An epidemiological study of exposure to coal tar pitch volatiles among coke oven workers. J Air Pollut Control Assoc 25:382–389, 1975.
132. Redmond CK: Cancer mortality among coke oven workers. Environ Health Perspect 52:67–73, 1983.
133. Lloyd JW: Long-term mortality study of steelworkers: V. Respiratory cancer in coke plant workers. J Occup Med 13:53–68, 1971.
134. Pott F, Heinrich U: Relative significance of different hydrocarbons for the carcinogenic potency of emissions from various incomplete combustion processes. *In* Vainio H, Sorsa M, McMichael AJ (eds): Complex Mixtures and Cancer Risk. Lyon: International Agency for Research on Cancer, 1990, pp. 288–297.
135. Tola S: Epidemiology of lung cancer in foundries. J Toxicol Environ Health 6:1195–1200, 1980.
136. Breslow L, Hoaglin L, Rasmussen G, et al: Occupations and cigarette smoking as factors in lung cancer. Am J Public Health 44:171–181, 1954.
137. Simonato L: Definition of exposure in epidemiological studies on foundry workers. *In* Vainio H, Sorsa M, McMichael AJ (eds): Complex Mixtures and Cancer Risk. Lyon: International Agency for Research on Cancer, 1990, pp. 368–374.
138. Xu Z, Brown LM, Pam GW, et al: Cancer risks among iron and steel workers in Ashan, China. Part II: Case-control studies of lung and stomach cancer. Am J Ind Med 30:7–15, 1996.
139. Steenland K, Beaumont J: Further follow-up and adjustment for smoking in a study of lung cancer and acid mists. Am J Ind Med 16:347–354, 1989.
140. Steenland K, Beaumont J, Elliot L: Lung cancer in mild steel welders. Am J Epidemiol 133:220–229, 1991.
141. World Health Organization: Evaluation of Carcinogenic Risk of Chemicals to Man. IARC Monograph No. 9. Lyon: International Agency for Research on Cancer, 1975, pp. 181–192.
142. Doll R, Mathews JD, Morgan LG: Cancers of the lung and nasal sinuses in nickel workers: A reassessment of the period of risk. Br J Ind Med 34:102–105, 1977.
143. Kaldor J, Peto J, Easton D, et al: Models for respiratory cancer in nickel refinery workers. J Natl Cancer Inst 77:841–848, 1986.
144. Report of the International Committee on Nickel Carcinogenesis in Man. Scand J Work Environ Health 16:1–82, 1990.
145. Roberts RS, Julian JA, Muir DCF, et al: A study of mortality in workers engaged in the mining, smelting, and refining of nickel. II: Mortality from cancer of the respiratory tract and kidney. Toxicol Ind Health 5:975–993, 1989.
146. Langer AM, Rohl AN, Selikoff IJ, et al: Asbestos as a cofactor in carcinogenesis among nickel-processing workers. Science 209:420–422, 1980.
147. Roscoe RJ: An update of mortality from all causes among white uranium miners from the Colorado Plateau Study Group. Am J Ind Med 31:211–222, 1997.
148. Samet JM: Radon and lung cancer: Epidemiology and risk assessment. Fundam Appl Toxicol 13:632–634, 1989.
149. Lubin JH, Liang Z, Hrubec Z, et al: Radon exposure in residences and lung cancer risk among women: Combined analysis of three studies. Cancer Causes Control 5:114–128, 1994.
150. Cohen BL: Problems in the radon vs lung cancer test of the linear no-threshold theory and a procedure for resolving them. Health Phys 72:623–628, 1997.
151. Oge MT: Radon risk in the home. Science 255:1194, 1992.
152. Ruosteenoja E, Makelainen I, Rytomaa T, et al: Radon and lung cancer in Finland. Health Phys 71:185–189, 1996.
153. Auvinen A, Makelainen I, Hakama M, et al: Indoor radon exposure and risk of lung cancer: A nested case-control study in Finland. J Natl Cancer Inst 88:966–972, 1996.
154. Lubin JH, Boice JD: Lung cancer risk from residential radon: Meta-analysis of eight epidemiologic studies. J Natl Cancer Inst 89:49–57, 1997.
155. Lubin JH, Boice JD, Edling C, et al: Lung cancer in radon-exposed miners and estimation of risk from indoor exposure. J Natl Cancer Inst 87:817–827, 1995.
156. Voelz GL, Lawrence JNP: A 42-year medical follow-up of Manhattan Project plutonium workers. Health Phys 61:181–190, 1991.
157. Petersen GR, Gilbert ES, Buchanan JA, et al: A case-cohort study of lung cancer ionizing radiation, and tobacco smoking among males at the Hanford site. Health Phys 58:3–11, 1990.
158. Wing S, Richardson D, Armstrong D, et al: A reevaluation of cancer incidence near the Three Mile Island nuclear plant: The collision of evidence and assumptions. Environ Health Perspect 105:52–57, 1997.
159. Prentice RL, Yoshimoto Y, Mason MW: Relationship of cigarette smoking and radiation exposure to cancer mortality in Hiroshima and Nagasaki. J Natl Cancer Inst 70:611–622, 1983.
160. Inskip PD, Boice JD: Radiotherapy-induced lung cancer among women who smoke. Cancer 73:1541–1543, 1994.
161. Neugut AI, Murray T, Santos J, et al: Increased risk of lung cancer after breast cancer radiation therapy in cigarette smokers. Cancer 73:1615–1620, 1994.
162. Laplanche A, Clavel-Chapelon F, Contassot J-C, et al: Exposure to vinyl chloride monomer: Results of a cohort study after a seven year follow up. Br J Ind Med 49:134–137, 1992.
163. Simonato L, L'Abbé KA, Andersen A, et al: A collaborative study of cancer incidence and mortality among vinyl chloride workers. Scand J Work Environ Health 17:159–169, 1991.
164. Buffler PA, Wood S, Eifler C, et al: Mortality experience of workers in a vinyl chloride monomer production plant. J Occup Med 21:195–203, 1979.
165. Steenland K, Ward E: Lung cancer incidence among patients with beryllium disease: A cohort mortality study. J Natl Cancer Inst 83:1380–1385, 1991.
166. Ward E, Okun A, Ruder A, et al: A mortality study of workers at seven beryllium processing plants. Am J Ind Med 22:885–904, 1992.
167. Beryllium Industry Scientific Advisory Committee: Is beryllium carcinogenic to humans? J Occup Environ Med 39:205–208, 1997.
168. Warnock ML, Isenberg W: Asbestos burden and the pathology of lung cancer. Chest 89:20–26, 1986.
169. Thun MJ, Schnorr TM, Smith AB, et al: Mortality among a cohort of US cadmium production workers: An update. J Natl Cancer Inst 74:325–333, 1985.
170. Stayner L, Smith R, Thun M, et al: A dose-response analysis and quantitative assessment of lung cancer risk and occupational cadmium exposure. Ann Epidemiol 2:177–194, 1992.

171. Elinder C-G, Kjellström T, Hogstedt C, et al: Cancer mortality of cadmium workers. Br J Ind Med 42:651–655, 1985.
172. Sorahan T, Lancashire RJ: Lung cancer mortality in a cohort of workers employed at a cadmium recovery plant in the United Sates: An analysis with detailed job histories. Occup Environ Med 54:194–201, 1997.
173. Goldsmith DF, Guidotti TL, Johnston DR: Does occupational exposure to silica cause lung cancer? Am J Ind Med 3:423–440, 1982.
174. Rafnsson V, Gunnarsdottir H: Lung cancer incidence among an Icelandic cohort exposed to diatomaceous earth and cristobalite. Scand J Work Environ Health 23:187–192, 1997.
175. Neuberger M, Kundi M: Occupational dust exposure and cancer mortality: Results of a prospective cohort study. *In* Simonato L, Fletcher AC, Saracci R, et al (eds): Occupational Exposure to Silica and Cancer Risk. Lyon: International Agency for Research on Cancer, 1990, pp. 65–73.
176. Forastiere F, Lagorio S, Michelozzi P, et al: Silica, silicosis and lung cancer among ceramic workers. Am J Ind Med 12:221–222, 1987.
177. Mastrangelo G, Zambon P, Simonato L, et al: A case-referent study investigating the relationship between exposure to silica dust and lung cancer. Int Arch Occup Environ Health 60:299–302, 1988.
178. Forastiere F, Lagorio S, Michelozzi P, et al: Silica, silicosis and lung cancer among ceramic workers: A case-referent study (letter). Am J Ind Med 10:363–370, 1986.
179. Swaen GMH, Meijers JMM: Lung cancer risk among workers with silicosis: Potential confounding by smoking habits. Am J Ind Med 12:223–225, 1987.
179a. Klein AK, Christopher JP: Evaluation of crystalline silica as a threshold carcinogen. Scand J Work Environ Health 21(Suppl 2):95–98, 1995.
180. US Occupational Safety and Health Administration: Toxic and hazardous substances. US CFR 29, Part 1910–1000, 1983, pp. 603–604.
180a. Cherry NM, Burgess GL, Turner S, et al: Crystalline silica and risk of lung cancer in the potteries. Occup Environ Med 55:779–785, 1999.
181. Infante PF, Schuman LD, Huff J: Fibrous glass insulation and cancer: Response and rebuttal. Am J Ind Med 30:113–120, 1996.
182. Bender JR, Bunn W, Rossiter CE, et al: Epidemiologic studies of fiberglass: Methods, findings and implications. J Occup Environ Med 37:653–655, 1995.
183. Shannon HS, Jamieson E, Julian JE, et al: Mortality experience of glass fibre workers: Extended follow-up. Ann Occup Hyg 31:657–662, 1987.
184. Lee IM, Hennekens CH, Trichopoulos D, et al: Man-made vitreous fibers and risk of respiratory system cancer: A review of the epidemiologic evidence. J Occup Environ Med 37:725–738, 1995.
185. Bertazzi PA, Pesatori AC, Radice L, et al: Exposure to formaldehyde and cancer mortality in a cohort of workers producing resins. Scand J Work Environ Health 12:461–468, 1986.
186. Murdoch BS: Does formaldehyde cause cancer? Health Environ Digest 3:1–2, 1989.
187. Swenberg JA: Formaldehyde and cancer: Ten years of hindsight. Health Environ Digest 3:3–5, 1989.
188. Partanen T, Kauppinen T, Hernberg S, et al: Formaldehyde exposure and respiratory cancer among woodworkers: An update. Scand J Work Environ Health 16:394–400, 1990.
189. Bond GG, Flores GH, Shellenberger RJ, et al: Nested case-control study of lung cancer among chemical workers. Am J Epidemiol 124:53–66, 1986.
190. Walrath J, Fraumeni JF Jr: Cancer and other causes of death among embalmers. Cancer Res 44:4638–4641, 1984.
191. Jensen OM, Andersen SK: Lung cancer risk from formaldehyde. Lancet 1:913, 1982.
192. Hall A, Harrington JM, Aw T-C: Mortality study of British pathologists. Am J Ind Med 20:83–89, 1991.
193. Partanen T, Kauppinen T, Nurminen M, et al: Formaldehyde exposure and respiratory and related cancers. Scand J Work Environ Health 11:409–415, 1985.
194. Coggon D, Pannett B, Acheson ED: Use of job-exposure matrix in an occupational analysis of lung and bladder cancers on the basis of death certificates. J Natl Cancer Inst 72:61–65, 1984.
195. Callas PW, Pastides H, Hosmer DW: Lung cancer mortality among workers in formaldehyde industries. J Occup Env Med 38:747–748, 1996.
196. Marsh GM, Stone RA, Henderson VL: A reanalysis of the National Cancer Institute study on lung cancer mortality among industrial workers exposed to formaldehyde. J Occup Med 34:42–44, 1992.
197. Gardner MJ, Osmond C, Pannett B: Formaldehyde and lung cancer. Lancet 2:1366–1367, 1985.
198. International Agency for Research on Cancer: Chromium, Nickel, and Welding Fumes: Monographs on the Evaluation of Carcinogenic Risk of Chemical to Humans, vol. 49. Lyon: International Agency for Research on Cancer, 1990.
199. Moulin JJ: A meta-analysis of epidemiologic studies of lung cancer in welders. Scand J Work Environ Health 23:104–113, 1997.
200. Moulin JJ, Wild P, Romazini S, et al: Lung cancer in hard-metal workers. Am J Epidemiol 148:241–248, 1998.
201. Greaves WW, Rom WN, Lyon JL, et al: Relationship between lung cancer and distance of residence from nonferrous smelter stack effluent. Am J Ind Med 2:15–23, 1981.
202. Smith GH, Williams FLR, Lloyd OL: Respiratory cancer and air pollution from iron foundries in a Scottish town: An epidemiological and environmental study. Br J Ind Med 44:795–802, 1987.
203. Lloyd OL, Williams FLR, Gailey RAY: Is the Armadale epidemic over? Air pollution and mortality from lung cancer and other diseases, 1961–1982. Br J Ind Med 42:815–823, 1985.
204. Pershagen G: Lung cancer mortality among men living near an arsenic-emitting smelter. Am J Epidemiol 122:684–694, 1985.
205. Mumford JL, He XZ, Chapman RS, et al: Lung cancer and indoor air pollution in Xuan Wei, China. Science 235:217–220, 1987.
206. He X, Chen W, Liu Z, et al: An epidemiological study of lung cancer in Xuan Wei County, China: Current progress. Case-control study on lung cancer and cooking fuel. Environ Health Perspect 94:9–13, 1991.
207. Jedrychowski W, Becher H, Wahrendorf J, et al: A case-control study of lung cancer with special reference to the effect of air pollution in Poland. J Epidemiol Community Health 44:114–120, 1990.
208. Speizer FE: Overview of the risk of respiratory cancer from airborne contaminants. Environ Health Perspect 70:9–15, 1986.
209. Buffler PA, Cooper SP, Stinnett S, et al: Air pollution and lung cancer mortality in Harris County, Texas, 1979–1981. Am J Epidemiol 128:683–699, 1988.
210. Freeman DJ, Cattell FC: The risk of lung cancer from polycyclic aromatic hydrocarbons in Sydney air. Med J Aust 149:612–615, 1988.
211. Steenland K: Lung cancer and diesel exhaust: A review. Am J Ind Med 10:177–189, 1986.
212. Rushton L, Alderson MR, Nagarajah CR: Epidemiological survey of maintenance workers in London transport executive bus garages and Chiswick works. Br J Ind Med 40:340–345, 1983.
213. Paradis G, Theriault G, Tremblay C: Mortality in a historical cohort of bus drivers. Int J Epidemiol 18:397–402, 1989.
214. Hall NEL, Wynder EL: Diesel exhaust exposure and lung cancer: A case-control study. Environ Res 34:77–86, 1984.
215. Garshick E, Schenker MB, Mũnoz A, et al: A case-control study of lung cancer and diesel exhaust exposure in railroad workers. Am Rev Respir Dis 135:1242–1248, 1987.
216. Gustavsson P, Plato N, Lidström E-B, et al: Lung cancer and exposure to diesel exhaust among bus garage workers. Scand J Work Environ Health 16:348–354, 1990.
217. Steenland K, Silverman D, Hornung R: Case-control study of lung cancer and truck driving in the Teamsters Union. Am J Public Health 80:670–674, 1990.
218. Hayes RB, Thomas T, Silverman DT: Lung cancer in motor exhaust-related occupations. Am J Ind Med 16:685–695, 1989.
219. Erren T: Re: "Association between exposure to pulsed electromagnetic fields and cancer in electric utility workers in Quebec, Canada, and France." Am J Epidemiol 143:841, 1996.
220. Henshaw DL: Re: "Electromagnetic field exposure and cancer." Am J Epidemiol 146:366, 1997.
221. Robinette CD, Silverman C, Jablon S: Effects upon health of occupational exposure to microwave radiation (radar). Am J Epidemiol 112:39–53, 1980.

222. Szmigielski S, Bielec M, Lipski S, et al: Immunological and cancer-related aspects of exposure to low-level microwave and radiofrequency fields. *In* Marino A (ed): Modern Bioelectricity. New York: Marcel Dekker, 1988.
223. Vögerö D, Ahlbom A, Olin R, et al: Cancer morbidity among workers in the telecommunications industry. Br J Ind Med 42:191–195, 1985.
224. Milham S Jr: Increased mortality in amateur radio operators due to lymphatic and hematopoietic malignancies. Am J Epidemiol 127:50–54, 1988.
225. Savitz DA, Dufort V, Armstrong B, et al: Lung cancer in relation to employment in the electric utility industry and exposure to magnetic fields. Occup Environ Med 54:396–402, 1997.
226. Ames BN: Dietary carcinogens and anticarcinogens. Science 221:1256–1264, 1983.
227. Colditz GA, Stampfer MJ, Willett WC: Diet and lung cancer. Arch Intern Med 147:157–160, 1987.
228. Steinmetz KA, Potter JD: Vegetables, fruit, and cancer prevention: A review. J Am Diet Assoc 96:1027–1039, 1996.
229. Ziegler RG, Mayne ST, Swanson CA: Nutrition and lung cancer. Cancer Causes Control 7:157–177, 1996.
230. Mayne ST: Beta-carotene, carotenoids, and disease prevention in humans. FASEB J 10:690–701, 1996.
231. Peto R, Doll R, Buckley JD, et al: Can dietary beta-carotene materially reduce human cancer rates? Nature 290:201–208, 1981.
232. Riboli E: Nutrition and cancer of the respiratory and digestive tract: Results from observational and chemoprevention studies. Eur J Cancer Prev 1996;5(Suppl 2):9—17.
233. Verhoeven DT, Goldbohm A, van Poppel G, et al: Epidemiological studies on brassica vegetables and cancer risk. Cancer Epidemiol Biomarkers Prev 5:733–748, 1996.
234. Koo LC: Diet and lung cancer 20+ years later: More questions than answers? Int J Cancer 10(Suppl):22–29, 1997.
235. Dorgan JF, Ziegler RG, Schoenberg JB, et al: Race and sex differences in associations of vegetables, fruits, and carotenoids with lung cancer risk in New Jersey (United States). Cancer Causes Control 4:273–281, 1993.
236. Byers TE, Graham S, Haughey BP, et al: Diet and lung cancer risk: Findings from the western New York diet study. Am J Epidemiol 125:351–363, 1987.
237. Samet JM, Skipper BJ, Humble CG, et al: Lung cancer risk and vitamin A consumption in New Mexico. Am Rev Respir Dis 131:198–202, 1985.
238. Le Marchand L, Yoshizawa CN, Kolonel LN, et al: Vegetable consumption and lung cancer risk: A population based case-control study in Hawaii. J Natl Cancer Inst 81:1158–1164, 1989.
239. Ziegler RG, Mason TJ, Stemhagen A, et al: Carotenoid intake, vegetables, and the risk of lung cancer among white men in New Jersey. Am J Epidemiol 123:1080–1093, 1986.
240. Fontham ET, Pickle LW, Haenszel W, et al: Dietary vitamins A and C and lung cancer risk in Louisiana. Cancer 62:2267–2273, 1988.
241. Menkes MS, Comstock GW, Vuilleumeir JP, et al: Serum beta-carotene, vitamins A and E, selenium, and the risk of lung cancer. N Engl J Med 315:1250–1254, 1986.
242. Comstock GW, Helzlsouer KJ, Bush TL: Prediagnostic serum levels of carotenoids and vitamin E as related to subsequent cancer in Washington County, Maryland. Am J Clin Nutr 53:260S–264S, 1991.
243. Stahelin HB, Gey KF, Eichholzer M, et al: Beta-carotene and cancer prevention: The Basel study. Am J Clin Nutr 53:265S–269S, 1991.
244. Goodman GE, Thornquist M, Kestin M, et al: The association between participant characteristics and serum concentrations of beta-carotene, retinol, retinyl palmitate, and alpha-tocopherol among participants in the Beta-Carotene and Retinol Efficacy Trial (CARET) for prevention of lung cancer. Cancer Epidemiol Biomarkers Prev 5:815–821, 1996.
245. The Alpha-Tocopherol, Beta Carotene Cancer Prevention Study Group: The effect of vitamin E and beta carotene on the incidence of lung cancer and other cancers in male smokers. N Engl J Med 330:1029–1035, 1994.
246. Omenn GS, Goodman GE, Thornquist MD, et al: Effects of a combination of beta carotene and vitamin A on lung cancer and cardiovascular disease. N Engl J Med 334:1150–1155, 1996.
247. Omenn GS, Goodman GE, Thornquist MD, et al: Risk factors for lung cancer and for intervention effects in CARET, the Beta-Carotene and Retinol Efficacy Trial. J Natl Cancer Inst 88:1550–1559, 1996.
248. Albanes D, Heinonen OP, Taylor PR, et al: Alpha-tocopherol and beta-carotene supplements and lung cancer incidence in the Alpha-Tocopherol, Beta-Carotene Cancer Prevention Study: Effects of base-line characteristics and study compliance. J Natl Cancer Inst 88:1560–1570, 1996.
249. Hennekens CH, Buring JE, Manson JE, et al: Lack of effect of long-term supplementation with beta carotene on the incidence of malignant neoplasms and cardiovascular disease. N Engl J Med 334:1145–1149, 1996.
250. Mayne ST, Handelman GJ, Beecher G: Beta-carotene and lung cancer promotion in heavy smokers: A plausible relationship? J Natl Cancer Inst 88:1513–1515, 1996.
251. Chen LH, Boissonneault GA, Glauert HP: Vitamin C, vitamin E and cancer. Anticancer Res 8:739–748, 1988.
252. Chow CK: Dietary vitamin E and cellular susceptibility to cigarette smoke. Ann N Y Acad Sci 393:426–436, 1982.
253. Willett WC, Polk BF, Underwood BA, et al: Relation of serum vitamins A and E and carotenoids to the risk of cancer. N Engl J Med 310:430–434, 1984.
254. Knekt P, Aromaa A, Maatela J, et al: Vitamin E and cancer prevention. Am J Clin Nutr 53:283S–286S, 1991.
255. Mayne ST, Janerich DT, Greenwald P, et al: Dietary beta-carotene and lung cancer risk in US nonsmokers. J Natl Cancer Inst 86:33–38, 1994.
256. Shibata A, Paganini-Hill A, Ross RK, et al: Intake of vegetables, fruits, beta-carotene, vitamin C, and vitamin supplements and cancer incidence among the elderly: A prospective study. Br J Cancer 66:673–679, 1992.
257. Alavanja MCR, Brown CC, Swanson C, et al: Saturated fat intake and lung cancer risk among non-smoking women in Missouri. J Natl Cancer Inst 85:1906–1916, 1993.
258. Shekelle RB, Liu S, Raynor WJ, et al: Dietary vitamin A and risk of cancer in the Western Electric Study. Lancet 2:1185–1189, 1981.
259. Mettlin C, Graham S, Swanson M: Vitamin A and lung cancer. J Natl Cancer Inst 62:1435–1438, 1979.
260. Hinds MW, Kolonel LN, Hankin JH, et al: Dietary vitamin A, carotene, vitamin C, and risk of lung cancer in Hawaii. Am J Epidemiol 119:227–237, 1984.
261. Block G: Vitamin C and cancer prevention: The epidemiologic evidence. Am J Clin Nutr 53:270S–282S, 1991.
262. Candelora EC, Stockwell HG, Armstrong AW, et al: Dietary intake and risk of lung cancer in women who never smoked. Nutr Cancer 17:263–270, 1992.
263. Knekt P, Jarvinen R, Seppanen R, et al: Dietary antioxidants and the risk of lung cancer. Am J Epidemiol 134:471–479, 1991.
264. Jain M, Burch JD, Howe GR, et al: Dietary factors and risk of lung cancer: Results from a case-control study, Toronto, 1981–1985. Int J Cancer 45: 287–293, 1990.
265. Steinmetz KA, Potter JD, Folsom AR: Vegetables, fruit, and lung cancer in the Iowa Women's Health Study. Cancer Res 53:536–543, 1993.
266. Knekt P, Aromaa A, Maatela J, et al: Serum selenium and subsequent risk of cancer among Finnish men and women. J Natl Cancer Inst 82:864–868, 1990.
267. van den Brandt PA, Goldbohm A, van't Veer P, et al: A prospective cohort study on selenium status and the risk of lung cancer. Cancer Res 53:4860–4865, 1993.
268. Fleet JC: Dietary selenium repletion may reduce cancer incidence in people at high risk who live in areas with low soil selenium. Nutr Rev 55:277–279, 1997.
269. Knekt P, Jarvinen R, Seppanen R, et al: Dietary flavonoids and the risk of lung cancer and other malignant neoplasms. Am J Epidemiol 146:223–230, 1997.
270. Goldbohm RA, Hertog MG, Brants HA, et al: Consumption of black tea and cancer risk: A prospective cohort study. J Natl Cancer Inst 88:93–100, 1996.
271. Zheng W, Doyle T, Kushi LH, et al: Tea consumption and cancer incidence in a prospective cohort study of post-menopausal women. Am J Epidemiol 144:175–182, 1996.
272. Murata M, Takayama K, Choi BC, et al: A nested case-control

study of alcohol drinking, tobacco smoking, and cancer. Cancer Detect Prev 20:557–565, 1996.
273. Potter JD, Sellers TA, Folsom AR, et al: Alcohol, beer, and lung cancer in postmenopausal women: The Iowa Women's Health Study. Ann Epidemiol 2:587–595, 1992.
274. Taioli E, Nicolosi A, Wynder EL: Possible role of diet as a host factor in the aetiology of tobacco-induced lung cancer: An ecological study in southern and northern Italy. Int J Epidemiol 20:611–614, 1991.
275. Wynder EL, Hebert JR, Kabat GC: Association of dietary fat and lung cancer. J Natl Cancer Inst 79:631–637, 1987.
276. Goodman MT, Kolonel LN, Yoshizawa CN, et al: The effect of dietary cholesterol and fat on the risk of lung cancer in Hawaii. Am J Epidemiol 128:1241–1255, 1988.
277. Knekt P, Seppanen R, Jarvinen R, et al: Dietary cholesterol, fatty acids, and the risk of lung cancer among men. Nutr Cancer 16:267–275, 1991.
278. Shekelle RB, Rossof AH, Stamler J: Dietary cholesterol and incidence of lung cancer: The Western Electric Study. Am J Epidemiol 134:480–484, 1991.
279. Wu Y, Zheng W, Sellers TA, et al: Dietary cholesterol, fat, and lung cancer incidence among older women: The Iowa Women's Health Study (United States). Cancer Causes Control 5:395–400, 1994.
280. Swanson CA, Brown CC, Brownson RC, et al: Re: Dietary fat intake and lung cancer risk among nonsmoking women in Missouri. J Natl Cancer Inst 89:1724–1725, 1997.
281. Osann KE: Lung cancer in women: The importance of smoking, family history of cancer, and medical history of respiratory disease. Cancer Res 51:4893–4897, 1991.
282. Wu-Williams AH, Dai XD, Blot W, et al: Lung cancer among women in north-east China. Br J Cancer 62:982–987, 1990.
283. Shaw GL, Falk RT, Pickle LW, et al: Lung cancer risk associated with cancer in relatives. J Clin Epidemiol 44:429–437, 1991.
284. Wu AH, Yu MC, Thomas DC, et al: Personal and family history of lung disease as risk factors for adenocarcinoma of the lung. Cancer Res 48:7279–7284, 1988.
285. Wu AH, Fontham ET, Reynolds P, et al: Family history of cancer and risk of lung cancer among lifetime nonsmoking women in the United States. Am J Epidemiol 143:535–542, 1996.
286. Sellers TA, Ooi WL, Elston RC, et al: Increased familial risk for non-lung cancer among relatives of lung cancer patients. Am J Epidemiol 126:237–246, 1987.
287. Ooi WL, Elston RC, Chen VW, et al: Increased familial risk for lung cancer. J Natl Cancer Inst 76:217–222, 1986.
288. Lynch HT, Kimberling WJ, Markvicka SE, et al: Genetics and smoking-associated cancers. Cancer 57:1640–1646, 1986.
289. McDuffie HH: Clustering of cancer in families of patients with primary lung cancer. J Clin Epidemiol 44:69–76, 1991.
290. Brownson RC, Alavanja MC, Caporaso N, et al: Family history of cancer and risk of lung cancer in lifetime non-smokers and long-term ex-smokers. Int J Epidemiol 26:256–263, 1997.
291. Ambrosone CB, Rao U, Michalek AM, et al: Lung cancer histologic types and family history of cancer. Cancer 72:1192–1198, 1993.
292. Sellers TA, Elston RC, Atwood LD, et al: Lung cancer histologic type and family history of cancer. Cancer 69:86–91, 1992.
293. Horwitz RI, Smaldone LF, Voscoli CM: An ecogenetic hypothesis for lung cancer in women. Arch Intern Med 148:2609–2612, 1988.
294. Ahlbom A, Lichtenstein P, Malmstrom H, et al: Cancer in twins: Genetic and nongenetic familial risk factors. J Natl Cancer Inst 89:287–293, 1997.
295. Carmelli D, Page WF: Twenty-four year mortality in World War II male veteran twins discordant for cigarette smoking. Int J Epidemiol 25:554–559, 1996.
296. Yang P, Schwartz AG, McAllister AE, et al: Genetic analysis of families with nonsmoking lung cancer probands. Genet Epidemiol 14:181–197, 1997.
297. Spivack SD, Fasco MJ, Walker VE, et al: The molecular epidemiology of lung cancer. Crit Rev Toxicol 27:319–365, 1997.
298. Vineis P, Caporaso N: Tobacco and cancer: Epidemiology and the laboratory. Environ Health Perspect 103:156—160, 1995.
299. Devereux TR, Taylor JA, Barrett JC: Molecular mechanisms of lung cancer: Interaction of environmental and genetic factors. Chest 109(Suppl):14s–19s, 1996.
300. Ernster VL: The epidemiology of lung cancer in women. Ann Epidemiol 4:102–110, 1994.
301. Harris CG: Interindividual variation among humans in carcinogen metabolism, DNA adduct formation and DNA repair. Carcinogenesis 10:1563–1566, 1989.
302. Phillips DH, Hewer A, Martin CN, et al: Correlation of DNA adduct levels in human lung with cigarette smoking. Nature 336:790–792, 1988.
303. Randerath E, Miller RH, Mittal D, et al: Covalent DNA damage in tissue of smokers as determined by $^{32}$P-postlabeling assay. J Natl Cancer Inst 81:341–347, 1989.
304. Yoshikawa M, Arashidini K, Kawamoto T, et al: Aryl hydrocarbon hydroxylase activity in human lung tissue in relation to cigarette smoking and lung cancer. Environ Res 65:1–11, 1994.
305. Bartsch H, Petruzzelli S, De Flora S, et al: Carcinogen metabolism and DNA adducts in human lung tissues as affected by tobacco smoking or metabolic phenotype: A case-control study of lung cancer patients. Mutat Res 250:103–114, 1991.
306. Lambert B, Lindblad A, Holberg K, et al: The use of sister chromatid exchange to monitor human populations for exposure to toxicologically harmful agents. *In* Wolff S (ed): Sister Chromatid Exchange. New York: John Wiley & Sons, 1982, pp. 149–182.
307. Dosaka J, Abe S, Sasaki M, et al: Sister chromatid exchange induction by benzo(*a*)pyrene in cultured peripheral blood lymphocytes of lung cancer patients and healthy individuals with or without familial history of neoplasms. Int J Cancer 39:329–332, 1987.
308. Perera F, Mayer J, Jaretzki A, et al: Comparison of DNA adducts and sister chromatid exchange in lung cancer cases and controls. Cancer Res 49:4446–4451, 1989.
309. Spitz MR, Wu X, Jiang H, et al: Mutagen sensitivity as a marker of cancer susceptibility. J Cell Biochem 25S:80–84, 1996.
310. Wei Q, Gu J, Cheng L, et al: Benzo(a)pyrene diol epoxide-induced chromosomal aberrations and risk of lung cancer. Cancer Res 56:3975–3979, 1996.
311. Ronai A, Yabubovskaya MS, Zhang E, et al: K-ras mutation in sputum of patients with and without lung cancer. J Cell Biochem 25S:172–176, 1997.
312. Kondo K, Tsuzuki H, Sasa M, et al:. A dose-response relationship between the frequency of p53 mutations and tobacco consumption in lung cancer patients. J Surg Oncol 61:20–26, 1996.
313. Yamakawa K, Takahashi T, Horio Y, et al: Frequent homozygous deletions in lung cancer cell lines detected by a DNA marker located at 3p21.3-p22. Oncogene 8:327–330, 1993.
314. Minna JD, Battey JF, Brooks BJ, et al: Molecular genetic analysis reveals chromosomal deletion, gene amplification, and autocrine growth factor production in the pathogenesis of human lung cancer. Cold Spring Harbor Symp Quant Biol 51:843–853, 1986.
315. McLemore TL, Adelberg S, Liu MC, et al: Expression of CYP1A1 gene in patients with lung cancer: Evidence for cigarette smoke-induced gene expression in normal lung tissue and for altered gene regulation in primary pulmonary carcinomas. J Natl Cancer Inst 82:1333–1339, 1990.
316. Bartsch H, Petruzzelli S, De Flora S, et al: Carcinogen metabolism in human lung tissues and the effect of tobacco smoking: Results from a case-control multicenter study of lung cancer patients. Environ Health Perspect 98:119–124, 1992.
317. Kawajiri K, Nakachi K, Imai K, et al: Identification of genetically high-risk individuals to lung cancer by DNA polymorphism of the cytochrome P450 CYP1A1 gene. FEBS Lett 236:131–133, 1990.
318. Hayashi SI, Watanabe J, Nakachi K: Genetic linkage of lung cancer associated MspI polymorphisms with amino acid replacement in the heme binding region of the human cytochrome P450 1A1 gene. J Biochem 110:407–411, 1991.
319. Xu X, Kelsey KT, Wiencke JK, et al: Cytochrome p450 CYP1A1 mspI polymorphism and lung cancer susceptibility. Cancer Biomarkers Prev 5:687–692, 1996.
320. Bouchardy C, Benhamou S, Dayer P: The effect of tobacco on lung cancer risk depends on CYP2D6 activity. Cancer Res 56:251–253, 1996.

321. Richie JP, Carmella SG, Muscat JE, et al: Differences in the urinary metabolites of the tobacco-specific lung carcinogen 4-(methylnitrosamino)-1-(3-pyidyl)-1-butanone in black and white smokers. Cancer Epidemiol Biomarkers Prev 6:783–790, 1997.
322. Shaw GL, Falk RT, Deslauriers J, et al: Debrisoquine metabolism and lung cancer risk. Cancer Epidemiol Biomarkers Prev 4:41–48, 1995.
323. Caporaso N, Tucker MA, Hoover RN, et al: Lung cancer and the debrisoquine metabolic phenotype. J Natl Cancer Inst 82:1264–1272, 1990.
324. Sun GF, Shimojo N, Pi JB, et al: Gene deficiency of glutathione S-transferase mu isoform associated with susceptibility to lung cancer in a Chinese population. Cancer Lett 113:169–172, 1997.
325. van Poppel G, Verhagen H, van't Veer P, et al: Markers for cytogenetic damage in smokers: Associations with plasma antioxidants and glutathione S-transferase mu. Cancer Epidemiol Biomarkers Prev 2:441–447, 1993.
326. Ryberg D, Hewer A, Phillips DH, et al: Different susceptibility to smoking-induced DNA damage among male and female lung cancer patients. Cancer Res 54:5801–5803, 1994.
327. Wiencke JK, Spitz MR, McMillan A, et al: Lung cancer in Mexican-Americans and African Americans is associated with the wild-type genotype of the NAD(P)H:quinone oxidoreductase polymorphism. Cancer Epidemiol Biomarkers Prev 6:87–92, 1997.
328. Cascorbi I, Brockmoller J, Mrozikiewicz PM, et al: Homozygous rapid arylamine N-acetyltransferase (NAT2) genotype as a susceptibility factor for lung cancer. Cancer Res 56:3961–3966, 1996.
329. Nakachi K, Imai K, Hayashi S, et al: Polymorphisms of the CYP1A1 and glutathion-S-transferase genes associated with susceptibility to lung cancer in relation to cigarette dose in a Japanese population. Cancer Res 56:3961–3966, 1996.
330. Hayashi S, Watanabe J, Kawajiri K: High susceptibility to lung cancer analyzed in terms of combined genotypes of P4501A1 and mu-class glutathione-s-transferase genes. Jpn J Cancer Res 83:866–870, 1992.

# 46 Bronchogenic Carcinoma

DIANE PRAGER, M.D. • ROBERT CAMERON, M.D.
JUDITH FORD, M.D., PH.D. • ROBERT A. FIGLIN, M.D., F.A.C.P.

Introduction
Epidemiology
Molecular Biology
- *p53* Mutations
- *K-ras*
- Loss of Heterozygosity

Natural History
- Classification

Clinical Features and Diagnosis
- Screening
- Clinical Presentation
- Diagnostic Workup

Staging
Prognosis
Molecular Detection
- DNA-Based Techniques
- Polymerase Chain Reaction Assays for Oncogene Mutations
- Microsatellite Analysis

Surgical Management
- Non-Small Cell Lung Cancer
- Small Cell Lung Cancer

Radiation Therapy
- Radical Radiation Therapy for Non-Small Cell Lung Cancer
- Radiation Combined with Chemotherapy for Non-Small Cell Lung Cancer
- Superior Sulcus Tumors
- Small Cell Lung Cancer
- Palliative Radiation Therapy
- Complications of Radiation Therapy

Combined Modality Approaches
- Preoperative and Postoperative Chemotherapy for Resectable Non-Small Cell Lung Cancer
- Postoperative Adjuvant Chemotherapy or Chemoradiation
- Combined Modality Therapy for Stage IIIB Non-Small Cell Lung Cancer

Chemotherapy
- Chemotherapy for Advanced Disease
- Chemotherapy for Small Cell Lung Cancer

Guidelines
Solitary Pulmonary Nodules
Economic Issues
Summary

## INTRODUCTION

Lung cancer continues to be a major health problem in the United States accounting for 32% of all male cancer deaths and 25% of all female cancer deaths.[1] The estimated number of lung cancer cases in the United States for 1999 was 171,600 with 158,900 deaths.[2] Overall, the prognosis for patients with lung cancer is poor, with a 14% overall 5-year relative survival rate for whites and 11% for blacks.[2] Black men younger than 54 years of age appear to have an increased incidence of lung cancer, whereas black and white women appear to have equal incidence rates.[3]

### Epidemiology

The epidemiology of lung cancer is reviewed completely in Chapter 45; the key features are discussed here. The association between cigarette smoking and the development of lung cancer has been reviewed by Wynder and Hoffman,[4] Bartecchi,[5] and the Surgeon General.[6] More than 80% of lung cancers are attributed to tobacco exposure, with a 20-fold increase in the relative risk for lung cancer for current smokers versus nonsmokers.[7] Fewer than 20% of smokers develop lung cancer in their lifetime, which indicates an individual variation in susceptibility. At present, 46.3 million adults smoke, with the highest prevalence being the 25- to 44-year age group.[8] Quitting the use of tobacco has been shown to reduce the risk of subsequent lung cancer development, regardless of how long or how many cigarettes were smoked. However, the risk decreases slowly for 10 to 20 years, after which time it becomes almost the same as that for a person who never smoked.[9] Although total elimination does not seem possible, modification of U.S. smoking habits through education has resulted in a decreased smoking prevalence since the 1950s; however, the per capita cigarette consumption remains similar to that in 1952. Use of filters has not had a substantial effect on tobacco carcinogenicity.[10–13]

Denissenko and colleagues[14] recently mapped the distribution of benzo-[a]-pyrene diol-epoxide (BPDE) adducts along exons of p53 in BPDE-treated HeLa cells and bronchial epithelial cells noting selective adduct formation at codons 157, 248, and 273. These data provided the first direct link between tobacco smoke and lung cancer mutations. Studies suggest that nonsmokers exposed to second-hand smoke may have double the risk of getting lung cancer compared with unexposed nonsmokers.[15–18] It is estimated that 17% of lung cancer among nonsmokers may be attributed to high levels of exposure to cigarette smoke during childhood and adolescence.[19] Results of a case-control study of men with histologically confirmed lung cancer indicate that although quitting smoking resulted in a reduced risk of squamous cell and adenocarcinoma, the risk of small cell lung cancer (SCLC) was unaffected.[20] Whereas the number of cigarettes smoked per day was the strongest predictor of risk, early age at initiation of smoking significantly enhanced the risk of SCLC. The incidence of SCLC would be decreased by 80% if tobacco exposure were abolished.[21] Smokers with chronic obstructive pulmonary disease are at increased risk for developing SCLC. The risk of developing lung cancer for pipe smokers and cigar smokers is greater than that for nonsmokers but much less than that for cigarette smokers and appears to be related to inhalation practices.[22] The risk of lung cancer is not increased by chewing tobacco or using snuff; however, these practices are carcinogenic for the upper aerodigestive tract.[23]

Many occupational exposures to carcinogens have been shown to increase the risk of lung cancer; the proven and strongly suspected substances are listed in Table 46.1. Of special importance are the data on the risk of lung cancer when smokers also are exposed to occupational carcinogens. For example, smokers exposed to asbestos have almost 100 times the risk of lung cancer compared with nonsmokers without asbestos exposure. The combination of smoking and working as a uranium miner is almost as dangerous.[24] Radon gas, rising from the crust of the earth because of decay of uranium ($^{238}$Ur) may collect in homes, adding to the subsequent risk of lung cancer.[25–27]

Epidemiologic studies provide indirect evidence for genetic and familial predisposition to lung cancer.[28–30] Factors that influence carcinogen absorption, distribution, or accumulation in target tissues influence cancer susceptibility. The ultimate dose of tobacco carcinogen to which lung tissue is exposed may be modulated by metabolic polymorphisms in enzymes responsible for activation or detoxification of the substances present in tobacco smoke. Differences in these pathways may account for interindividual differences in susceptibility. The cytochrome P450 (CYP) 1Al gene encodes for aryl-hydrocarbon hydroxylase, which initiates a pathway that activates polycyclic hydrocarbons, including benzo-[a]-pyrene, to highly electrophilic metabolites. Numerous studies have shown an association between aryl-hydrocarbon hydroxylase activity or polymorphisms and lung cancer.[31, 32] Similarly, CYP2D6, which metabolizes tobacco-specific nitrosamine to mutagenic products, has a polymorphism that has been evaluated for lung cancer risk.[33, 34] Table 46.2 lists a variety of metabolic polymorphisms as markers of lung cancer susceptibility.

Certain systemic diseases also have been associated with lung cancer. Sarcoidosis is associated with a threefold increased risk of lung cancer.[35] Scleroderma is associated with an increased risk of bronchioloalveolar carcinoma (BAC)[36] Both these associations may be related to "scar carcinomas," in which lung cancers arise in pulmonary scars from sarcoidosis and scleroderma, as well as from tuberculosis, pneumonia, infection, and pneumoconiosis.[37, 38]

**Table 46.1 OCCUPATIONAL CARCINOGENS FOR LUNG CANCER**

| PROVEN | SUSPECTED |
|---|---|
| Arsenic | Acrylonitrile |
| Asbestos | Beryllium |
| Bis(chloromethyl)ether | Vinyl chloride |
| Chromium | Silica |
| Mustard gas | Iron ore |
| Nickel | Wood dust |
| Polycyclic aromatic hydrocarbons | |
| Ionizing radiation | |

Reproduced from Carr DT, Holaye PY, Kittong W: Bronchogenic carcinoma. *In* Murray JF, Nadel JA (eds): Textbook of Respiratory Medicine. Philadelphia: WB Saunders, 1994, with permission.

## MOLECULAR BIOLOGY

Many of the molecular genetic markers, which are reviewed in Chapter 44, are changes caused by cigarette smoking. These genetic changes may be useful for molecular screening.

### *p53* Mutations

Mutations in the *p53* tumor suppressor gene are the most common genetic alterations in human cancer and are clustered at several hot-spots, especially codons 157, 248, and 273 within the DNA-binding domain of *p53*.[14] Codon 157 is the lung cancer hot-spot. Tobacco-related mutations are transversions of GC base pairs, with a majority being G:C → T:A transversions.[39] *p53* mutations are associated with heavy tobacco use.[40, 41] Numerous studies show a linear increase in the occurrence of G:T transversion mutations with increasing tobacco use.[42–44] Conversely, lower tobacco exposure is associated with less frequent *p53* mutations.[45] Uranium miners and atomic bomb survivors with lung cancer do not show G:T transversions.

Table 46.2 MARKERS OF SUSCEPTIBILITY OF LUNG CANCER RISK

| Markers | Prevalence of Variant Allele or Phenotype in Controls | Ethnicity | Positive Association |
|---|---|---|---|
| **Metabolic Polymorphisms** | | | |
| *CYP1A1* | | | |
| MspI RFLP 3′ noncoding region | 0.30 | Japanese | 3 |
| A/G mutation in exon 7 | 0.37 | Japanese | 2.6 |
| Another MspI RFLP 3′ noncoding region | 0.15 | Black | 1.3 |
| *CYP2D6* | 0.09 | Not specified | 2.3 |
| *CYP2A6* | 0.15 | Finnish | NA |
| | 0.24 | English | NA |
| | 0.48 | Japanese | NA |
| | 0.17 | Taiwanese | NA |
| | 0.03 | Black | NA |
| *CYP2E1* | | | |
| *Dra* I polymorphism | 0.74 | Japanese | Yes |
| | 0.89 | Finnish | No |
| *pst* I polymorphism | 0.95 | Swedish | Yes |
| | 0.91 | White | No |
| | 0.95 | Black | No |
| | 0.69 | Japanese | No |
| *GSTM1* | 0.48 | Not specified | 3 |
| *GSTT1* | 0.53 | Not specified | No |
| *NAT2* | 0.40–0.70 | | |
| *EH* | | | |
| Exon 3 | 0.35 | Not specified | NA |
| Exon 4 | 0.23 | Not specified | NA |
| *p53* codon 72 | 0.35 | Japanese | 1.7 |
| | 0.34 | White | No |
| | 0.53 | Black | 1.6 |
| | 0.26 | Mexican-American | 2.0 |

Reproduced from Spitz MR, Wu X, Lippman SM: Markers of susceptibility. *In* Roth JA, Cox JD, Ki Hong W: Lung Cancer. Oxford, UK: Blackwell Science, 1998, pp. 1–24, with permission.

### *K-ras*

The *ras* family of oncogenes encodes genes for guanosine diphosphate (GDP)- and guanosine triphosphate (GTP)-binding proteins with GTPase activity important for signal transduction. *K-ras* mutations have been specifically associated with smoking and are mostly G → T transversions.[46, 47] *K-ras* mutations show specificity for adenocarcinomas.

### Loss of Heterozygosity

Loss of heterozygosity (LOH) on several chromosome loci containing candidate tumor suppressor genes has been reported for tobacco-related cancers. Specifically, LOH at 3p14, which includes the candidate tumor suppressor fragile and histidine triad, Fhit gene and 9p21 (p16 tumor suppressor gene) have been shown to be early specific genetic aberrations in lung cancer. Mao and associates[48] studied bronchial epithelium in 54 smokers with minimal histologic abnormalities by multiple biopsies. LOH at 3p14 was seen in 75% of 36 informative cases. LOH at 9p21 was seen in 24% of informative cases. The incidence of LOH at 17p13 was lower, suggesting that it is a later genetic event. Interestingly, LOH at 3p was more evident in current versus past smokers. Recently, Tomizawa and colleagues[49] analyzed the expression of Fhit protein in 105 cases of stage I non–small cell lung cancer (NSCLC). A marked reduction in Fhit expression was detected in squamous cell carcinomas compared with adenocarcinomas. This reduced expression was also correlated with a positive history of tobacco use.[49] Moreover, reduced Fhit expression was associated with a poorer prognosis, regardless of histologic cell type.

## NATURAL HISTORY

### Classification

Table 46.3 lists a modified version of the 1999 World Health Organizations Classification System developed for lung cancer. This classification is used by most pathologists and oncologists with minor modification. The overwhelming majority of cases are represented by the first four categories. Of the NSCLCs, 35% to 71% are squamous, 9% to 29% are adenocarcinomas, and 3% to 16 % are large cell carcinomas. SCLC represents 12% to 25%

**Table 46.3 THE 1999 PATHOLOGIC CLASSIFICATION OF LUNG CANCER**

**Epithelial Tumors**

- Squamous cell carcinoma
  - Variants
    - Papillary
    - Clear cell
    - Small cell
    - Basaloid
- Small cell carcinoma
  - Variants
    - Combined small cell carcinoma
- Adenocarcinoma
  - Acinar
  - Papillary
  - Bronchioloalveolar carcinoma
    - Nonmucinous (Clara cell/type II pneumocyte type)
    - Mucinous (Goblet cell type)
    - Mixed mucinous and nonmucinous or indeterminate
  - Solid adenocarcinoma with mucin formation
  - Adenocarcinoma with mixed subtypes
  - Variants
    - Well-differentiated fetal adenocarcinoma
    - Mucinous (colloid) adenocarcinoma
    - Mucinous cystadenocarcinoma
    - Signet ring adenocarcinoma
    - Clear cell adenocarcinoma
- Large cell carcinoma
  - Variants
    - Large cell neuroendocrine carcinoma
      - Combined large cell neuroendocrine carcinoma
    - Basaloid carcinoma
    - Lymphoepithelioma-like carcinoma
    - Clear cell carcinoma
    - Large cell carcinoma with rhabdoid phenotype
- Adenosquamous carcinoma
- Carcinomas with pleomorphic, sarcomatoid, or sarcomatous elements
  - Carcinomas with spindle or giant cells, or both
    - Pleomorphic carcinoma
    - Spindle cell carcinoma
    - Giant cell carcinoma
  - Carcinosarcoma
    - Pulmonary blastoma
  - Carcinoid tumor
    - Typical carcinoid
    - Atypical carcinoid
  - Carcinomas of salivary gland type
    - Mucoepidermoid carcinoma
    - Adenoid cystic carcinoma
    - Others
  - Unclassified carcinoma

**Soft-Tissue Tumors**

- Localized fibrous tumor
- Epithelioid hemangioendothelioma
- Pleuropulmonary blastoma
- Chondroma
- Calcifying fibrous pseudotumor of the pleura
- Congenital peribronchial myofibroblastic tumor
- Diffuse pulmonary lymphangiomatosis
- Desmoplastic round cell tumor
- Others

Reprinted with permission from Colby TV, Corrin B, Shimosato Y, et al: Histological typing of lung and pleural tumors. *In* Travis WD, Sobin LH (eds): WHO International Histological Classification of Tumors, 3rd ed, Berlin: Springer Verlag, 1999.

of cases.[50] The relative and absolute prevalence of adenocarcinoma is increasing, especially in women.[51, 52]

*Squamous cell carcinoma* arises from the bronchial epithelium.[53] The tumor usually develops as a polypoid or sessile mass in major bronchi, which often obstructs the lumen of the airway and causes obstructive pneumonitis; less often, squamous cell carcinoma develops as a peripheral mass. Because this tumor type is most likely to be resectable, it is associated with the most favorable prognosis. Squamous cell carcinomas account for nearly half of the superior sulcus tumors (Pancoast tumors).[54] Multiple karyotypic abnormalities have been detected.[55]

*Adenocarcinoma* of the lung develops most commonly as a peripheral parenchymal mass that usually remains asymptomatic until the mass becomes large. The tumors arise from the bronchioloalveolar epithelium or from mucous glands. Adenocarcinomas invade blood and lymph vessels early in their development and frequently give rise to metastases before the primary lesion causes any symptoms. They frequently involve the pleura and metastasize to the scalene lymph nodes. Although tobacco smoking is a risk factor for each of the subtypes of lung cancer, this is the histologic type that nonsmokers tend to have most. A subtype of adenocarcinoma, called bronchioloalveolar type (BAC) is believed to arise from Clara cells (nonciliated bronchiolar epithelial cells). Lesions are usually peripheral and may be related to pre-existing scars.[56, 57] Metastasis is by bronchogenic spread and results in multiple metastatic pulmonary nodules. An increase in this subtype appears to be responsible for the increase in adenocarcinomas.[58–60] A viral etiology for BAC is postulated. Jaagsiekte or pulmonary adenomatosis in sheep is similar to BAC in humans.[61–63] It is casually linked to a retrovirus, with documented sheep-to-sheep transmission. Reports of sheep farmers developing diffuse BAC have been published, but no sheep-to-human transmission is documented.[64] The role of tobacco in BAC is controversial.

*Large cell carcinoma* of the lung can be central or peripheral. Etiologic factors are similar to those for adenocarcinomas. A subset of large cell carcinomas with neuroendocrine features (chromogranin A, leu-7 antigen, high L-dopa carboxylase levels, and neuron-specific enolase positivity) has a more favorable response to chemotherapy than tumors without these markers.[65]

A small portion of cases are labeled adenosquamous, 1% to 3% at initial biopsy.[66] In fact, many bronchogenic carcinomas have evidence of two or even more cell types if enough areas of tumor are sampled.

*Small cell carcinoma* (SCLC) usually originates from a bronchus and causes narrowing of the lumen without producing a discrete intrabronchial mass. These tumors metastasize early to hilar and mediastinal lymph nodes and readily invade blood vessels. Tumors are classified into three groups: (1) pure small cell carcinoma, (2) small cell/large cell, and (3) combined tumors with SCLC components.[67] Pure small cell carcinoma accounts for 90% of cases, mixed small cell/large cell accounts for 4% to 6%, and less than 1% are combined SCLC and squamous or adenocarcinoma of the lung.

*Bronchial carcinoid tumors* are thought to derive from the Kulchitsky cell and make up approximately 2% of lung cancers.[68] These tumors are frequently invasive and metastasize. Histologic features do not predict behavior.[69, 70] Bronchial carcinoids occur in the main, lobar, or segmental bronchi and present with local obstructive symptoms. Peripheral lesions present with hemoptysis or are silent. Five hydroxy-indoleacetic acid may be elevated with or without carcinoid syndrome. The treatment of choice for resectable lesions is surgery, with a 5-year survival rate in the 60% to 80% range.[71] In the presence of distant metastases, 5-year survival rate is estimated at 11%.

*Bronchial gland tumors* occur less frequently than carcinoids but may behave malignantly.[72] Lesions are either infiltrative and locally invasive (adenoid cystic) or pedunculated (mucoepidermoid) and frequently cause bronchial obstruction. The treatment of choice is surgery.

## CLINICAL FEATURES AND DIAGNOSIS

### Screening

The concept of screening for lung cancer is based on the theory that there is a preclinical or asymptomatic but detectable phase in the life history of a lung cancer during which it may be discovered, diagnosed, and treated successfully by currently available methods. The routine use of tests (chest radiographs [CXRs] and sputum cytology) at appropriate intervals in a high-risk group might discover lung cancers while they are still localized enough to be surgically resectable. These theories led the National Cancer Institute to sponsor three large studies for lung cancer detection at the Mayo Clinic, Memorial Sloan-Kettering Hospital, and Johns Hopkins University Hospital (Table 46.4).

These studies showed that intensive screening results in the diagnosis being made at an earlier stage of the disease. The prevalence rates (5.5 to 8.3/1000 persons) and incidence rates (3 to 5.5/1000 persons/year) were similar.[73] The sputum and CXRs were complementary. These three studies did not show any improvement in decreasing lung cancer mortality.[73] Similarly, a case-control study from the German Democratic Republic and a randomized controlled trial of high-risk men in Czechoslovakia showed no benefit of screening on lung cancer mortality.[74, 75] A Swedish study that compared survival of lung cancer patients who had CXR screening showed a slight improvement in survival of patients with squamous cell carcinoma.[76]

Other possible screening modalities are being evaluated. The sensitivity and specificity of monoclonal antibodies to antigens present on SCLCs and NSCLCs in preserved sputum specimens also have been evaluated.[77] With 69 specimens with moderate or greater atypia, positive staining was present in 14 of 22 patients who progressed to lung cancer. Screening was nonreactive in 88% of specimens from patients who did not progress. Of note, all true positives were collected 24 months in advance of the diagnosis. When false-negative specimens that had been collected within this time frame were reanalyzed, the specimens did stain positively. Tockman and associates[78] recently demonstrated that hnRNP $A_2/B_1$, an RNA-binding protein, is up-regulated in pulmonary cancers. In archived preneoplastic sputum samples, hnRNP $A_2/B_1$

**Table 46.4 SCREENING OF LUNG CANCER**

| | Mayo Clinic | Memorial Sloan-Kettering | Johns Hopkins |
|---|---|---|---|
| Screening | CXR, sputum every 4 mo vs. control (optional yrly CXR) | CXR yrly ± sputum cytology every 4 mo | CXR yrly ± sputum cytology every 4 mo |
| Prevalence | 8.3/1000 | 5.5/1000 | 7/1000 |
| Incidence | 4.9/1000/yr overall<br>5.5/1000/yr screened<br>4.3/1000/yr control | 3/1000/yr | 4–5/1000/yr |
| Early disease | "Resectable" incidence cases 46% screened; 32% control | Overall results, stage I incidence and prevalence cases: 38% | 56% prevalence case and ≈45% incidence cases "resectable for cure" |
| Mortality | Incidence cases 5-yr survival 40% (3.2/1000/yr) screened<br>15% (3.0/1000/yr) control | 5-year survival (all cases) ≈90% stage I ≈5% stage II/III | Mortality rate 3.4/1000/yr with cytology 3.8/1000/yr without cytology |

Reproduced from Figlin R, Holmes EC, Turrisi, AT III: Neoplasms of the Lung, Pleura, and Mediastinum. *In* Haskell CM: Cancer Treatment (4th ed). Philadelphia: WB Saunders, 1995, pp. 385–413, with permission.

overexpression was detected. This test identified preclinical cancer more accurately than cytomorphology. In an ongoing prospective study of Yunnan tin miners at high risk for developing lung cancer, up-regulation of hnRNP $A_2/B_1$ in the sputum in 69 of 94 primary lung cancers was detected compared with 10 primary lung cancers detected cytologically. Sputum from resected stage I patients showed up-regulation of hnRNP $A_2/B_1$ in 32 of 42 specimens, compared with cytologic changes found in only one patient, and accurately predicted outcome. These studies predicted that 69% of the miners and 67% of resected stage I patients with elevated hnRNP $A_2/B_1$ would develop lung cancer as compared with background. The up-regulation of hnRNP $A_2/B_1$ is thus an early finding. The accuracy of this test appears similar to that of the prostate-specific antigen test used for prostate cancer screening.

The utility of mobile spiral computed tomography (CT) of the chest also has been assessed. In 1996, 5843 individuals in Japan aged 40 to 74 years underwent CXR, cytologic sputum assessment, and spiral CT of the chest.[79] Nineteen patients were diagnosed with lung cancer; 18 were surgically confirmed. In 4 of 19 patients, CT and CXR revealed an abnormality. Of these patients, 16 had stage I disease and the remainder had stage IV disease. The detection rate for CT screening was 0.48% (19 of 3967), compared with a 0.03% to 0.05% detection rate for CXR and sputum cytology screening previously performed in the same area. Therefore, the authors found a 10-fold increase in the detection rate for lung cancer, many of which were at an early stage. A recent reappraisal of detection failures in high-risk smokers after screening by spiral CT led to the recommendation to reexamine suspicious areas of old disease with thin-section CT and to perform follow-up examinations.[79a]

## Clinical Presentation

At presentation, about 90% of patients are symptomatic. Symptoms may be classified as local, distant, or systemic. Table 46.5 shows the local effects of lung cancer and an estimate of their frequency. Central lesions may cause cough, hemoptysis, dyspnea, hoarseness, dysphagia, wheezing, and symptoms compatible with superior vena caval or pericardial involvement. Peripheral lesions may present with pain, cough, or dyspnea secondary to pleural effusion. A new or increased chronic cough or expectoration in a middle-aged or older male smoker may mean the development of lung cancer.[80]

Lung cancer tends to metastasize to the bone, liver, lymph nodes, and brain. At presentation, up to 25% of patients may present with bone pain, 20% with hepatic involvement, 20% with lymphadenopathy, and 5% to 10% with neurologic manifestation of cranial involvement.

The systemic effects of lung cancer are numerous and are listed in Table 46.6. The most important of these are constitutional, which occur in virtually everyone with the disease. The paraneoplastic manifestations are described subsequently.

SCLC may present with the same signs and symptoms

**Table 46.5 LOCAL MANIFESTATIONS OF LUNG CANCER AT PRESENTATION**

| Symptom or Sign | Frequency (%) |
|---|---|
| Cough | 70 |
| Hemoptysis | 40 |
| Dyspnea | 40 |
| Chest pain | 35 |
| Hoarseness | 5 |
| Effects of superior vena caval obstruction | 5 |
| Wheezing | 2 |
| Pericardial effusion | Rare |
| Effects of brachial plexus compression or Horner's syndrome | Rare |

Reproduced from Figlin R, Holmes EC, Turrisi AT III: Neoplasms of the Lung, Pleura, and Mediastinum. *In* Haskell CM: Cancer Treatment (4th ed). Philadelphia: WB Saunders, 1995, pp. 385–413, with permission.

**Table 46.6 SYSTEMIC MANIFESTATIONS OF BRONCHOGENIC CARCINOMA**

| |
|---|
| **Constitutional** |
| Weight loss |
| Anorexia |
| Weakness |
| Fever |
| **Neurologic** |
| Autonomic overactivity (Horner's syndrome) |
| Corticocerebellar degeneration |
| Spinal-cerebellar degeneration |
| Carcinomatous myopathies (including Eaton-Lambert syndrome) |
| Carcinomatous neuropathy |
| Polymyositis |
| **Cutaneous** |
| Acanthosis nigricans |
| Dermatomyositis |
| Scleroderma |
| Tylosis |
| **Skeletal** |
| Clubbing |
| Hypertrophic pulmonary osteoarthopathy |
| **Vascular coagulation** |
| Thrombophlebitis |
| Disseminated intravascular coagulation |
| Nonbacterial thrombotic endocarditis |
| **Endocrine** |
| Antidiuretic hormone secretion |
| Hypercalcemia (parathyroid hormone-related protein) |
| Adrenocorticotropic hormone |
| Gynecomastia |
| Melanocyte-stimulating hormone |

Reproduced from Figlin R, Holmes EC, Turrisi AT III: Neoplasms of the Lung, Pleura, and Mediastinum. *In* Haskell CM: Cancer Treatment (4th ed). Philadelphia: WB Saunders, 1995, pp. 385–413, with permission.

as NSCLC. Because tumors are usually central and endobronchial in location, patients often present with cough, dyspnea, wheezing, chest pain, hemoptysis, or postobstructive pneumonia. Involvement of the mediastinum by tumor is not infrequent and may cause superior vena cava obstruction (10% of patients), hoarseness secondary to recurrent laryngeal nerve involvement, or dysphagia. About 4% of SCLCs have no detectable pulmonary or mediastinal primary tumor; these cases represent either an obvious extrapulmonary primary or nodal or disseminated metastases.[84, 85] These tumors resemble SCLC morphologically, may contain neurosecretory granules on electron microscopy, and may present with paraneoplastic manifestations. They are usually biologically aggressive and may arise from the uterine cervix, esophagus, larynx, pharynx, colon, rectum, prostate, or paranasal sinuses.

## Paraneoplastic Syndromes

There are several systemic paraneoplastic syndromes of lung cancer, many of which are nonspecific but which may be the presenting manifestation and thus attract attention to the underlying malignancy. The most important of those listed in Table 46.6 are the following:

**Neurologic.** Paraneoplastic syndromes can involve any part of the neuromuscular system: brain, spinal cord, peripheral nerves, and muscles; these have been associated with many types of malignancies, of which about half are lung cancer. They share the properties of rapid progression, severe disability, and the potential for improvement related to treatment of the underlying tumor.[81] The only one of the complications that is specific for malignancy is the *Eaton-Lambert syndrome*, a myasthenia gravis–like disorder linked to SCLC and, occasionally, to other cancers with a more favorable prognosis. The syndrome is caused by the formation of IgG antibodies directed at an omega conotoxin-sensitive voltage-gated calcium channel present both in the cancer and at the neuromuscular junction.[81a] More recently, a type 1 antineuronal nuclear autoantibody (ANNA-1, also known as "anti-Hu") has been identified as a marker of neurologic autoimmunity that is highly associated with SCLC (97%). ANNA-1 has been linked to many paraneoplastic neurologic abnormalities such as neuropathy (especially sensory), cerebellar ataxia, limbic encephalitis, and others, including Eaton-Lambert syndrome.[81b]

**Cutaneous.** All cutaneous manifestations of lung cancer are uncommon or rare. Sixty percent of cases of *acanthosis nigricans*, a symmetric verrucous and papillary dermatosis with hyperpigmentation located in the flexor areas such as the axilla and neck, are associated with malignancies, often bronchogenic in origin. According to Barnes,[82] a complicating lung or other visceral malignancy develops in 6% to 16% of patients with *dermatomyositis-polymyositis* and sometimes *scleroderma* (see also Chapter 58).

**Skeletal.** *Clubbing of the fingers*, with or without *hypertrophic pulmonary osteoarthropathy*, has many causes (see Chapter 23 for full discussion and references). Probably the most important of these associations is cancer of the lung, which may be announced or preceded by the onset of joint pains and digital abnormalities. The causal alliance between the cancer and the osteoarthropathy is dramatically demonstrated by the immediate relief of the disabling symptoms when the tumor is surgically removed.

**Vascular—Coagulation.** *Migratory thrombophlebitis*, also called *Trousseau's syndrome*, which was first associated with pancreatic and other gastrointestinal malignancies, is now more commonly caused by lung cancer. Its mechanism is unknown but presumably relates to the presence of excess circulating thromboplastin-like substances. Warfarin is often ineffective, and unfractionated or low-molecular-weight heparin is required to prevent recurrent thromboses.[82a]

**Endocrine.** The *syndrome of inappropriate antidiuretic hormone* (SIADH) secretion is found in 15% of patients with SCLC, 3% of patients with head and neck cancer, 0.7% of patients with NSCLC, and in many other conditions.[83] Excess release of arginine vasopressin by the tumor can be recognized by (1) hyponatremia, (2) continued renal excretion of sodium, (3) absence of signs of fluid volume depletion, (4) presence of urine osmolality higher than that appropriate for the concomitant plasma osmolality, and (5) normal function of the kidneys and adrenal and thyroid glands. *Hypercalcemia* occurs in about 10% of all lung cancer patients, of whom 10% to 15% do not have demonstrable bone metastases; most of these patients have squamous cell carcinomas (not SCLC) that elaborate a *parathyroid hormone–related peptide*, which shares considerable sequence homology with parathyroid hormone.[83a] The supraphysiologic production of *adrenocorticotropic hormone* is the most frequently detectable paraendocrine disorder of lung cancer and, since its description, has been classically linked to SCLC. Because of the short natural history of this cancer, however, patients do not usually manifest the classic clinical signs or symptoms of *Cushing's syndrome*; instead, the diagnosis is suggested by mild arterial hypertension, hypokalemia, and alkalosis. More recently, slower growing malignancies, pulmonary tumorlets and carcinoid tumors, have been reported to cause the full-blown syndrome.[83b, 83c]

## Diagnostic Workup

In a patient evaluated because of symptoms or an abnormal CXR, the diagnostic workup includes a thorough history and physical examination, CXR, blood chemistry, CT of the chest and upper abdomen, bronchoscopy, and selected pulmonary function tests. A positron-emission tomographic scan may also provide useful additional staging information. The minimum pulmonary function tests should include screening spirometry with or without bronchodilators (as needed), diffusing capacity, and resting oxygen saturation. Table 46.7 lists additional testing that may become necessary.

Positron-emission tomography (PET) scanning uses specialized radiation sensitive cameras to detect specific radioactive isotopes that decay by positron emission. Malignant tumors demonstrate enhanced cellular metabolism. $^{18}$F-fluorodeoxyglucose (FDG) is taken up by malignant cells and phosphorylated to FDG-6-$PO_4$, which remains trapped in the tumor cell and is therefore an excellent marker of cell metabolism. The persistence of this tracer in the tumor is essential for successful imaging.[86] Although PET scanning is not useful for determining size or adjacent structural invasion, the identification of pleural metastasis is useful. PET is also useful in determining nodal staging as well as metastatic disease status. PET scanning also may help to detect recurrent lung cancer and to assess response to therapy. Table 46.8 shows some of the conditions that may complicate PET interpretation.

**Table 46.7 ADDITIONAL PULMONARY FUNCTION TESTS FOR ASSESSMENT OF NON–SMALL CELL LUNG CANCER**

Patients with $FEV_1$ < 2.0 L (<70%), $D_{LCO}$ <70%, $O_2$ saturation <94%
May need:
- Resting and exercise arterial blood gas analysis
- Quantitative ventilation/perfusion scan
- Maximum oxygen consumption ($\dot{V}O_2$ max)

Reproduced from Cameron R, Finger J, Taylor C, et al: Practice guidelines for non-small cell lung cancer. Cancer J 562–567, 1996, with permission.

**Table 46.8 POSSIBLE CAUSES OF FALSE-POSITIVE OR FALSE-NEGATIVE $^{18}$F-FLUORODEOXYGLUCOSE POSITRON-EMISSION TOMOGRAPHY (PET) STUDIES**

| False-Positive PET | False-Negative PET |
|---|---|
| Infection | Low-grade malignancy |
| Acute inflammation | Microscopic/small focal malignancy |
| Recent surgery | Hyperglycemia |
| Muscle hypermetabolism | Adjacent highly metabolic focus |

Reproduced from Lowe VJ, Naunheim KS: Current role of positron emission tomography in thoracic oncology. Thorax 53:703–712, 1998, with permission.

Cytologic examination of early morning expectorated sputum is a noninvasive procedure that may be diagnostic. Optimal results usually are obtained from samples collected on 5 consecutive days.

Fiberoptic bronchoscopy is especially useful for central lesions. In addition to providing direct visualization of lesions, bronchoscopy permits biopsy of endobronchial lesions, brushings and washings of different areas and transbronchial biopsy of peribronchial lesions. A positive cytologic finding of malignancy from a sputum or bronchial washing is 98% reliable for a diagnosis of malignancy.[87–88] Rarely, a positive sputum cytology may be secondary to aspirated tumor cells shed from a head and neck cancer. For peripheral lesions not accessible by bronchoscopy, transthoracic aspiration or biopsy performed under fluoroscopy may provide a diagnosis[89, 90]; this technique is reported to have 74% to 94% diagnostic accuracy.[91, 92] In addition, pleural or pericardial fluid aspiration, mediastinoscopy, or supraclavicular lymph node biopsy may be helpful for diagnostic purposes. Video-assisted thoracoscopy may be useful for the identification and excision of peripheral nodules, pleural lesions, and pleural effusions. There remains a minority of patients in whom the diagnosis requires a thoracotomy. At the time of thoracotomy, the diagnosis can be confirmed by fine-needle aspiration, incisional or excisional biopsy, and frozen-section analysis. Further pathologic staging also may be performed.

A trial in the United States and Canada showed that the lung-imaging fluorescence endoscope improved the detection of intraepithelial lesions sixfold.[93] Lesions as small as 1 mm and only a few cell layers thick can be detected. There also appears to be a correlation between abnormal fluorescence and molecular changes. The technique clearly has the potential to enhance the detection of severe dysplasia and carcinoma in situ, although at present little is known about the natural history of these lesions, particularly their risk of progressing to invasive cancer.[93a] Fluorescence bronchoscopy also may be useful in detecting early versus late molecular changes and in monitoring the role of chemoprevention or other interventions.[93]

Tumor markers such as carcinoembryonic antigen may be elevated in patients with all histologic types of cancer. These markers are neither sensitive nor specific enough to be of generalized clinical use.

Diagnostic workup for SCLC routinely should include a magnetic resonance imaging (MRI) or CT scan of the brain (even if the patient is asymptomatic), an evaluation of the bone marrow by aspiration and biopsy or MRI of the vertebral column. Central nervous system metastasis is found in up to 30% of patients with SCLC. Patients with central nervous system disease as the sole site of metastasis may have a survival not dissimilar to that of limited stage disease; however, relapse in the brain after irradiation is frequent.

After the staging workup is completed, 30% to 40% of patients have limited-stage disease and 60% to 70% extensive stage disease.[94] Sites of distant metastases include the bone, liver, bone marrow, brain, lymph nodes, and soft tissues.

## STAGING

Accurate and reproducible staging information is key to lung cancer patient management, for clinical research and for communicating information regarding lung cancer worldwide. The majority of patients with lung cancer are not curable, with the 5-year survival rate less than 10%; therefore, until effective systemic therapy is available, development of new treatment strategies depends on results obtained for carefully staged groups of lung cancer patients. Variations in survival reported by different institutions likely reflect the extent of pretreatment evaluation, including the extent of mediastinal lymph node sampling and the accuracy of pathologic testing. Extensive pretreatment evaluation usually results in stage migration, with most patients classified as having more advanced disease, which results in better survival for each stage.[95] Estimates of percentages of patients suitable for resection at presentation are probably only 20% to 35%.[96–99] Table 46.9 shows the recommended staging workup.

About half the patients who are found to be unresectable at presentation have distant metastases. The most frequently involved sites are bone, brain, liver, lymph nodes, skin, and thorax. The presence of distant metastases varies according to histologic cell type.[100] One possible exception to the resection of a primary tumor in the presence of distant metastases is the scenario of a solitary resectable primary non–small cell lesion together with a solitary resectable brain metastasis. Uncontrolled studies show occasional long-term survival when both lesions are resected and the brain is radiated.[101, 102]

Whole-body PET scanning is now recognized as an important adjunct in the staging workup, with a sensitivity and specificity approaching 85%[102a]; in a recent comparison, PET was reported to be more accurate than thoracic CT, bone scintigraphy, and brain CT or MRI in staging patients with bronchogenic cancer.[102b] To compare the accuracy of CT scanning and PET scanning in locoregional lymph node staging, 68 patients underwent CT, PET, and surgical staging.[103] Surgical staging data were available for 690 lymph node samples. CT correctly identified nodal stage in 40 of 68 patients (59%), with understaging in 12 patients and overstaging in 16 patients. PET plus CT was accurate in 59 patients (87%), with understaging in 5 patients and overstaging in 4 patients. For N2/N3 disease, the sensitivity, specificity, and accuracy of CT were 75%, 63%, and 68%, respectively. For PET plus CT, they were 93%, 95%, and 94%. Therefore, CT plus PET appears to be significantly more accurate than CT alone. Thus, the high negative predictive value of mediastinal PET may reduce the need for mediastinoscopy.[103]

The revised international system for staging lung cancer is presented subsequently.[104, 105] Subsets of patients are combined according to TNM descriptors into stages, each having similar treatment options and survival expectations (Tables 46.10 and 46.11). Of note, stage I has been split into stages IA and IB. Stage II has been divided into IIA and IIB, with the patient group T3 N0 M0 being moved to the IIB category because of improved survival compared with other stage III patients. Fifty-five percent of patients with pT1 N1 M0 lesion (stage IIA) are expected to survive 5 years or more after complete resection versus a 39% survival rate for patients with pT2 N1 M0 and a 38% survival rate for patients with a pT3 N0 M0 lesion (stage IIB). Stage IIIA currently comprises T3 N1

**Table 46.9 RECOMMENDED STAGING WORKUP**

| |
|---|
| History, performance status, assessment of weight loss, and physical examination |
| Blood count, serum chemistries, urinalysis |
| Chest radiograph |
| CT oncology chest (chest plus upper abdomen) +/− positron-emission tomography scan |
| Bone scan with plain films of abnormal areas |
| Mediastinoscopy before surgery if tumor initially deemed resectable |

Reproduced from Figlin R, Holmes EC, Turrisi AT III: Neoplasms of the Lung, Pleura, and Mediastinum. *In* Haskell CM: Cancer Treatment (4th ed). Philadelphia: WB Saunders, 1995, pp. 385–413, with permission.

**Table 46.10 TNM DESCRIPTORS**

| | |
|---|---|
| **PRIMARY TUMOR (T)** | |
| TX | Primary tumor cannot be assessed, or tumor proved by the presence of malignant cells in sputum or bonchial washings but not visualized by imaging or bronchoscopy |
| T0 | No evidence of primary tumor |
| Tis | Carcinoma in situ |
| T1 | Tumor ≤ 3 cm in greatest dimension, surrounded by lung or visceral pleura, without bronchoscopic evidence of invasion more proximal than the lobar bronchus* (i.e., not in the main bronchus) |
| T2 | Tumor with any of the following features of size or extent:<br>> 3 cm in greatest dimension<br>Involves main bronchus, ≥ 2 cm distal to the carina<br>Invades the visceral pleura<br>Associated with atelectasis or obstructive pneumonitis that extends to the hilar region but does not involve the entire lung. |
| T3 | Tumor of any size that directly invades any of the following: chest wall (including superior sulcus tumors), diaphragm, mediastinal pleura, parietal pericardium; or tumor in the main bronchus < 2 cm distal to the carina, but without involvement of the carina; or associated atelectasis or obstructive pneumonitis of the entire lung |
| T4 | Tumor of any size that invades any of the following: mediastinum, heart, great vessels, trachea, esophagus, vertebral body, carina; or tumor with a malignant pleural or pericardial effusion,† or with satellite tumor nodules(s) within the ipsilateral primary-tumor lobe of the lung |
| **REGIONAL LYMPH NODES (N)** | |
| NX | Regional lymph nodes cannot be assessed |
| N0 | No regional lymph node metastasis |
| N1 | Metastasis to ipsilateral peribronchial or ipsilateral hilar lymph nodes, and intrapulmonary nodes involved by direct extension of the primary tumor |
| N2 | Metastasis to ipsilateral mediastinal or subcarinal lymph node(s) |
| N3 | Metastasis to contralateral mediastinal, contralateral hilar, ipsilateral, or contralateral scalene, or supraclavicular lymph node(s) |
| **DISTANT METASTASIS (M)** | |
| MX | Presence of distant metastasis cannot be assessed |
| M0 | No distant metastasis |
| M1 | Distant metastasis present‡ |

Reproduced from Mountain C: Revisions in the International System for Staging Lung Cancer. Chest 111:1710–1717, 1997, with permission.

*The uncommon superficial tumor of any size with its invasive component limited to the bronchial wall, which may extend proximal to the main bronchus, also is classified T1.

†Most pleural effusions associated with lung cancer are caused by tumor. However, there are a few patients in whom multiple cytopathologic examinations of pleural fluid show no tumor. In these cases, the fluid is nonbloody and is not an exudate. When these elements and clinical judgment dictate that the effusion is not related to the tumor, the effusion should be excluded as a staging element and the patient's disease should be staged T1, T2, or T3. Pericardial effusion is classified according to the same rules.

‡Separate metastatic tumor nodule(s) in the ipsilateral nonprimary-tumor lobe(s) of the lung also are classified M1.

M0, T1 N2 M0, T2 N2 M0, and T3 N2 M0. Clinically staged T3 N1 M0 tumors have a 9% 5-year survival rate compared with 13% for the remainder of the subsets in the group.[104] Of the N2 group, 72% are accounted for by the cT2 N2 M0 category, 22% by cT3 N2 M0, and 6% by T1 N2 M0. For stages IIIB and IV, the classification is unchanged. The presence of satellite tumor(s) in the primary tumor lobe should be classified as T4, whereas intrapulmonary ipsilateral metastasis in a nonprimary lobe is classified as M1. Of note, Urschel and colleagues[106] retrieved 11 articles from the literature in which 568 patients with satellite nodules underwent resection of the primary and satellite nodules; the 5-year actuarial survival rate was 20% with the 5-year survival being better if the satellite nodules were in the primary lobe. This survival is clearly better than that for T4 lesions, raising the question of whether the T4 designation is accurate. However, satellite nodules in ipsilateral nonprimary lobes share metastatic mechanisms and have survival results consistent with M1 stage disease. *Please note that all the studies described in the treatment section have used the old staging system.*

The international workshop on SCLC recommends the following staging system[94]:

Limited stage SCLC—to include patients with disease restricted to one hemithorax with regional lymph node metastases, including hilar, ipsi-, and contralateral mediastinal, or supraclavicular nodes. The inclusion of patients with contralateral mediastinal lymph nodes and supraclavicular lymph nodes was decided on because the prognostic influence of these metastatic sites is different from that of distant metastatic sites. The presence of an ipsilateral pleural effusion (benign or malignant) is included in this stage of disease.

**Table 46.11 STAGE GROUPING—TNM SUBSETS***

| STAGE | TNM SUBSET |
|---|---|
| 0 | Carcinoma in situ |
| IA | T1 N0 M0 |
| IB | T2 N0 M0 |
| IIA | T1 N1 M0 |
| IIB | T2 N1 M0 |
| | T3 N0 M0 |
| IIIA | T3 N1 M0 |
| | T1 N2 M0 |
| | T2 N2 M0 |
| | T3 N2 M0 |
| IIIB | T4 N0 M0 |
| | T4 N1 M0 |
| | T4 N2 M0 |
| | T1 N3 M0 |
| | T2 N3 M0 |
| | T3 N3 M0 |
| | T4 N3 M0 |
| IV | Any T Any N M1 |

Reproduced from Mountain C: Revisions in the International System for Staging Lung Cancer. Chest 111:1710–1717, 1997, with permission.

*Staging is not relevant for occult carcinoma, designated TX N0 M0.

Extensive stage disease—this classification includes all patients with disease who cannot be included in the limited stage.

## PROGNOSIS

Sixty-seven per cent of a collected series of patients with surgical-pathologic stage IA disease and 57% of those with stage IB disease are expected to survive 5 years or more after complete resection. Fifty-five per cent of patients with stage IIA disease are expected to survive 5 years or more, whereas 38% to 39% of stage IIB patients survive for this long. Five-year survival rates were 25% for surgically staged T3 N1 M0 tumors and 23% for T1–3 N2 M0 tumors. The T1 N2 M0 tumors represent 3% of the total surgical population. The expected 5-year survival rate of stage IIIB patients with T4 Nany M0 disease is 7%, Tany N3 M0 is 3%, and that for stage IV disease, Tany Nany M1 is 1%.[104] Figure 46.1 shows survival according to nodal involvement.

As a subgroup, patients with N2 disease who undergo resection have a varied outcome. Vansteenkiste and associates[107] reported an analysis of 18 series in the literature to determine whether any clinical prognostic factors could be identified. The absence of preoperative evidence of N2 disease was a favorable factor. The extent of surgery, lobectomy versus pneumonectomy, did not have a significant effect on outcome. The histopathologic tumor type favors squamous cell carcinoma with these patients generally doing better than those with other cell types. In all the series, the extent of the primary tumor, (lower T stage) was associated with a survival advantage. In addition, those patients with only one mediastinal lymph node station involved had a better prognosis, whereas metastasis to the subcarinal lymph nodes portended a poorer prognosis. These analyses all are hampered by the limited number of patients enrolled in the studies, therefore necessitating pooling of data.

Molecular analysis may be an important adjunct for accurate staging. A study of 244 stage I NSCLC patients treated at the Brigham and Women's Hospital investigated the effects of demographics, surgical extent, pathologic features, and molecular factors on cancer-free survival.[108] The molecular analysis consisted of immunohistochemical staining for *erb* B-2, *ras*-p21, p53, *rb, bcl*-2, blood group A antigen, and polymerase chain reaction and sequence analysis for *k-ras* codon 12. p53 positivity was associated with a decreased cancer free survival in univariate analysis ($P = .18$). Stepwise multivariate analysis identified solid mucin-producing adenocarcinoma tumor, lymphatic invasion, p53 expression, tumor dimension of

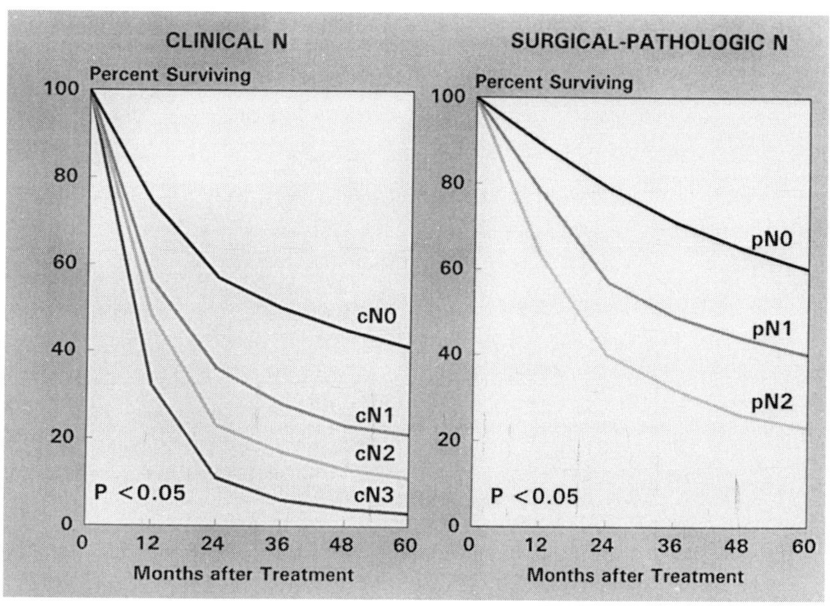


**Figure 46.1** Cumulative percent of patients surviving 5 years or more after treatment according to status by lymph nodes. (Reproduced from Mountain C, Dresler C: Regional lymph node classification for lung cancer staging. Chest 111:1718–1723, 1997.)

4 cm or larger, *k-ras* mutation, and *H-ras*–p21 negativity as influencing cancer-free survival. This study did not find any correlation with abnormalities of *rb, bcl*-2, *erb* B-2, which have been reported in other studies.

In general, for patients with inoperable disease, performance status is the strongest predictor of survival duration.[109, 110] Weight loss in the 6 months before diagnosis, brain metastases, advanced age (older than 70 years), and hepatic metastases are other poor prognostic factors.

The prognostic factors that help determine outcome for SCLC patients include stage (limited vs. extensive), performance status, sex (female gender is favorable), absence of mediastinal or supraclavicular lymph node involvement and pleural effusion (favorable limited stage disease), and few organs involved with absence of brain and liver lesions (favorable extensive stage). Elevated lactic dehydrogenase and alkaline phosphatase are unfavorable markers. Which factor is the most important is difficult to know because all the studies did not perform exactly the same pretreatment evaluation, and many of these factors are correlated.

## MOLECULAR DETECTION

### DNA-Based Testing

With the use of normal lymphocytes as germline control DNA, and DNA extracted from circulating plasma, microsatellite alterations (new alleles or loss of heterozygosity) were detected in 16 of 21 patients with SCLC.[111] Although the outcome for these patients is not available, tumor DNA is present in the circulation and accessible for analysis and may correlate with tumor burden.[112] It is feasible that a positive microsatellite test result in the serum might be predictive for patients predisposed to developing metastatic disease and those who would benefit from adjuvant systemic chemotherapy.

### Polymerase Chain Reaction Assays for Oncogene Mutations

With the use of the Johns Hopkins Lung Program repository of cytologic samples, samples that were nondiagnostic from patients who developed lung cancer were tested for p53 and *ras* mutations. Ten of 15 patients had either a p53 or *ras* mutation present. The assay amplifies sputum DNA, which then is subcloned into a phage vector, transferred to a nylon membrane, and hybridized with a panel of mutant-specific oligonucleotide probes (single stranded) for p53 and *k-ras*. Eight of 10 patients whose tumors harbored mutations were shown to have malignant cells in their previously normal cytologic specimen.[113] Sputum samples harboring clonal populations of cancer cells were detected from 1 to 13 months before clinical diagnosis of lung cancer. In a study using *k-ras* as a biomarker, healthy patients, smokers at high risk, and patients with NSCLC were tested.[114] *K-ras* codon 12 mutations were detected in 60% of patients with normal-appearing tissue but with a diagnosis of NSCLC compared with 10% of lung tissue obtained from healthy patients. Sputum from patients with NSCLC contained these mutations 47% of the time compared with only 12.5% of controls. In another study of 52 patients with lung cancer, more than half of them with adenocarcinoma were found to contain a *k-ras* mutation when bronchoalveolar fluid was examined versus no mutations if the histology was squamous cell carcinoma.[115] Tissue samples identified matching mutations. Interestingly, mutations were detected in samples from four patients with suspected but not histopathologically confirmed carcinoma.

### Microsatellite Analysis

Microsatellite alterations are rare in NSCLC but more prevalent in SCLC.[116] Alterations have been detected in corresponding sputum samples from lung cancer patients.[117, 118] In particular, tetranucleotide repeats (AAAG) appear to be altered in lung cancer. If well chosen, these repeats may identify a specific new allele in up to 50% of NSCLCs.[117] Table 46.12 lists some of the molecular and genetic alterations in lung cancer.

## SURGICAL MANAGEMENT

Although partial pulmonary resections for lung cancer were reported by Pean as early as 1895,[119] it was not

**Table 46.12 MOLECULAR ABNORMALITIES IN LUNG CANCER**

| Genes | Mutation | Abnormal Expression Frequency NSCLC (%) | SCLC (%) |
|---|---|---|---|
| Oncogenes | | | |
| *K-ras* | Point mutation (codon 12) | 30 | Not reported |
| *MYC* | DNA amplification overexpression | 10 | 10–40 |
| *c-erb B-2* | Increased expression | 25 | Not reported |
| *BCL-2* | Expression of protein | 25 | Not reported |
| Tumor-suppressor genes | | | |
| *3p* | Deletion | 50 | 90 |
| *RB* | Deletion, altered protein expression, and phosphorylation | 15 | > 90 |
| *p53* | Deletion, point mutation, and overexpression | 50 | 80 |
| *p16$^{INK4A}$* | Expression of protein | 60 | Not reported |

Reproduced from Salgia R, Skarin AT: Molecular Abnormalities in Lung Cancer. J Clin Oncol 6:1207–1217, 1998, with permission.

until after Graham and Singer[120] reported a successful pneumonectomy in 1933 that surgery for lung cancer became widespread. Since then, surgical removal has remained the primary curative therapy for lung cancers that are technically resectable.

## Non-Small Cell Lung Cancer

### General Considerations

To optimize the results of surgical treatment of NSCLC, it is necessary to examine the lymph nodes within the mediastinum (mediastinal staging) either by mediastinoscopy before or by dissecting and sampling during the operative procedure. In addition, the technical differences in the extent of resection and their impact on morbidity and mortality must be understood. Each of these considerations is discussed.

**Mediastinoscopy.** In this procedure, a small cervical incision is made, and a mediastinoscope is passed in front of the trachea into the superior mediastinum. Lymph nodes are sampled from multiple areas and are labeled according to the modified lymph node map originally designed by Naruke. For sampling of the aortopulmonary window lymph nodes, an extended mediastinoscopy can be performed by passing the mediastinoscope over the aortic arch at the base of the innominate artery or, alternatively, a left parasternal mediastinotomy incision (Chamberlain procedure) can be performed. Unfortunately, not all surgeons agree on the indications for mediastinoscopy. In locally advanced disease, there is general agreement that mediastinoscopy should be routine; yet, in earlier stage patients, there is not a uniform approach. Some believe that mediastinoscopy is indicated in all patients, but a more selective approach probably is warranted. Patients with T1 lesions, squamous histology, and no CT evidence of adenopathy probably do not require this procedure because the incidence of nodal involvement is probably less than 10%; however, in stage I patients with central lesions or adenocarcinoma histology and in patients with clinical stage II disease, it is worthwhile to exclude mediastinal metastases, particularly because there are numerous reports showing an 18% or greater false-negative rate based on CT scans and recent prospective trials have shown a significant benefit to preoperative induction chemotherapy in patients with N2 disease (discussed subsequently).[121]

**Intraoperative Lymph Node Dissection or Sampling.** The extent of intraoperative lymph node staging has been debated. Some surgeons perform a routine mediastinal lymph node dissection to remove all lymph nodes in the superior mediastinum and subcarinal space. Others prefer to simply sample a few lymph nodes from various areas. There has been some evidence that outcome is not affected by either method as long as lymph node sampling is combined with cervical mediastinoscopy.[122] This question, however, has not been subjected to a rigorous prospective randomized trial, although such a trial is planned by the American College of Surgeons Clinical Trials Group. Until more definitive evidence is published, both are thought to be equivalent in terms of survival, but complete lymph node dissection provides more accurate staging information.[122, 123]

**Limited Resection Versus Lobectomy/Pneumonectomy.** Uncontrolled studies have suggested that more limited resections might produce equivalent results to more radical procedures, such as lobectomy and pneumonectomy. This question was addressed by the Lung Cancer Study Group in a randomized trial in stage I patients. Patients were randomly assigned intraoperatively to a limited wedge or segmental resection versus standard lobectomy. Results showed that locoregional recurrence rates tripled with limited resection (0.022, 0.044, and 0.086 person/year for lobectomy, segmentectomy, and wedge resection, respectively). In addition, the overall cancer-related death rate was increased 50% with limited resections.[124] This has been confirmed by others.[125] Interestingly, there was no difference in postoperative pulmonary function between the two groups. Therefore, lobectomy and pneumonectomy currently are recommended, whenever possible. Limited resections, however, are still superior to other alternatives in patients with marginal pulmonary reserve.

**Advanced Resections (Sleeve Resections).** Some primary tumors involve the proximal right main-stem bronchus or the distal trachea at the level of the carina. If these tumors do not have lymph node metastases, sleeve resections can be performed. In the case of a right main-stem tumor, a sleeve resection removes the right upper lobe and a segment of proximal right main-stem bronchus. In the case of a carina tumor, the right (most often) lung and a segment of distal trachea are removed. Although sleeve lobectomy has been widely accepted because of its low complication and recurrence rates, both of which are equivalent to or better than pneumonectomy, sleeve pneumonectomy is performed only in highly selected cases in young patients because of its high mortality rate (15% to 30%) and overall limited prognosis (5-year survival rate, 20% to 40%).[126–128]

**Morbidity and Mortality.** The morbidity and mortality for both lobectomy and pneumonectomy have been well documented by the Lung Cancer Study Group in 2220 procedures. In experienced hands, the risk of death from lobectomy is 2.9% and 6.2% from pneumonectomy.[129] However, in centers with less experience, the mortality rate from pneumonectomy averages 11.6%.[130] The risk of major complications has been reported to be 10% in patients with stage I or II disease and 20% in patients with higher stage tumors.[131] Nearly 50% of all complications represent major complications.[132]

### Early-Stage Non-Small Cell Lung Cancer

Lung tumors that are confined completely to a single lung with or without intrapulmonary or hilar lymph node metastases are considered "early-stage" lung cancer (stages I and II). In the newly revised lung cancer staging system, tumors that invade the chest wall, diaphragm, mediastinal pleura, and proximal main-stem bronchi (within 2 cm of the carina) without any intrapulmonary, hilar or mediastinal lymph node metastases also are considered to be in this group (stage IIB).

**Occult Non–Small Cell Lung Cancer (TX N0 M0).** Lung cancer that is diagnosed by cytologic examination of sputa samples but associated with normal findings on chest imaging studies is considered "occult" lung cancer. The majority of these tumors are proximal squamous cell carcinomas. With widespread use of flexible bronchoscopy, the advent and increasing resolution of CT scans, and the introduction of new technologies (e.g., MRI and PET scans), the incidence of truly occult lung carcinoma has become rare. In addition, as many as one third of patients thought to have occult lung cancer are found to have a primary tumor in the head and neck region that explains the cytologic findings.[133] Therefore, a thorough upper aerodigestive tract examination is mandatory in these patients. Moreover, recent developments in lung cancer screening, including the generation of new monoclonal antibodies, which detect specific malignant changes on exfoliated cells in sputa, and the use of the lung-imaging fluorescence endoscope, which detects autofluorescence of malignant and premalignant cells through the use of a helium-cadmium (442 nm) laser, may increase the incidence of new occult lung cancers detected.[134, 135] In cases of true occult lung cancer, a systematic and meticulous sampling of cytologic specimens obtained by brushing and washing each individual segmental bronchus is necessary, taking great care to avoid cross-contamination of specimens from neighboring bronchi. Repeated positive findings (on at least two different occasions) from the same bronchus is enough evidence to warrant definitive treatment.

Treatment of occult lung carcinoma generally has been limited to surgical resection of the involved portion of the lung. This usually necessitates lobectomy or pneumonectomy, although segmentectomy is occasionally possible. However, other forms of therapy have been reported.[136] Successful treatment of occult and early lung cancers with a combination of external beam radiation and $^{192}$Ir endobronchial brachytherapy has been reported.[136] Japanese investigators also have produced impressive results with photodynamic therapy, using Photofrin as a photosensitizing agent and either an argon or excimer dye laser as the light source.[137] Finally, a study using transbronchoscopic electrocautery has shown some promise.[138] These latter treatments have been developed primarily as alternatives to surgical resection for those patients who are not surgical candidates, but if early success rates are substantiated, one or more of these therapies may replace surgery as the treatment of choice for these lesions.

Survival of patients treated for occult lung carcinoma is generally quite high. After surgical resection, recurrences are rare, but second primary lung cancers develop in many patients. Five-year survival rate in patients treated with external beam irradiation and endobronchial brachytherapy has been reported to exceed 85%.[136] Although photodynamic therapy also has a very high clinical complete response rate, with all 30 lesions in 26 patients responding in one report, only 5 of 15 lesions (33%) treated surgically after photodynamic therapy were confirmed to have a pathologically complete response.[139] Finally, electrocautery also has an impressive clinical complete response rate of 12 of 15 lesions (80%) in 10 of 13 patients (77%); however, histologic confirmation and long-term survival data are lacking.[138]

**Stage IA and IB Non–Small Cell Lung Cancer (T1 N0 M0 and T2 N0 M0).** Small (< 3 cm) T1 lung cancers are often peripheral, asymptomatic, and discovered only incidentally as solitary pulmonary nodules or "coin" lesions on radiographs obtained for unrelated reasons. Symptoms are more likely to occur with larger (> 3 cm) T2 tumors. The diagnosis may be confirmed in 90% of cases by either radiologically guided fine-needle aspiration cytology (peripheral lesions) or by bronchoscopic biopsy (central lesions). Because of the possibility of benign diseases, such as tuberculosis or hamartoma, and, in certain areas of the United States, fungal infections (coccidioidomycosis and histoplasmosis), attempts have been made to predict the nature of solitary pulmonary nodules through the use of CT and PET scans. However, because of a significant number of false-positive and false-negative findings, the results to date have shown that neither test can replace pathologic evaluation. Even without a diagnosis, new noncalcified solitary pulmonary nodules or enlarging nodules should be presumed to contain cancer until proven otherwise. Generally, this requires invasive excisional biopsy. For peripheral lesions, biopsy often may be accomplished with minimally invasive surgical techniques to minimize discomfort and disability. With T2 lesions, the diagnosis usually is less uncertain because few benign processes produce masses larger than 3 to 5 cm. Studies required in the evaluation of patients with stage IA and IB disease include a chest CT scan, including the upper abdomen (liver and adrenal glands), and pulmonary function tests. Quantitative lung perfusion scanning is optional, depending on the results of the pulmonary function tests. Bone scans and brain CT or MRI are not obtained without specific symptoms or other indications.

Treatment for stage IA and IB NSCLC is complete surgical resection whenever possible, preferably by lobectomy or pneumonectomy. Before resection, mediastinoscopy may be helpful to exclude the possibility of mediastinal lymph node metastases, particularly in stage IA patients with central lesions or histology showing adenocarcinoma and in all stage IB patients or patients with CT scans documenting enlarged hilar or mediastinal lymph nodes. At the time of surgery, a complete mediastinal lymph node dissection or at least a lymph node sampling (when mediastinoscopy also is performed) should be included as part of the procedure for accurate postresection staging. Patients with medical contraindications to surgery and those who refuse surgery can be treated with radical curative radiation therapy, albeit with less success than with surgical resection. However, radical curative radiation therapy requires inclusion and destruction of enough lung parenchyma that patients with poor pulmonary function often cannot tolerate such therapy, although newer techniques including three-dimensional conformal radiotherapy may help improve this situation.

The prognosis for patients who undergo complete surgical resection by lobectomy/pneumonectomy for T1 N0 M0 NSCLC is quite good, with more than 80% of patients surviving 5 years.[140] The prognosis for patients with T2 N0 M0 is only slightly worse, with 5-year survival rates exceeding 60% to 65%.[141] Stage I patients, however, do have an additional 20% to 33% risk of developing new primary tumors of the upper aerodigestive tract and need to be followed closely.[141] Those patients who do develop recurrence usually do so at distant systemic sites, with 20% of patients developing a solitary brain metastasis as their only site of disease. Postoperative adjuvant radiation therapy has not been shown to be of any benefit, and results with postresection chemotherapy have been inconclusive. Therefore, after resection, no further therapy is recommended other than an approved clinical trial. Neoadjuvant chemotherapy, which has been used successfully in more advanced (stage IIIA) disease, is showing promise in feasibility studies in stage IB patients.[142]

**Stage IIA Non–Small Cell Lung Cancer (T1 N1 M0).** Patients presenting with small (< 3 cm) NSCLCs that have metastasized to bronchopulmonary or hilar lymph nodes are more likely to report symptoms than patients with stage I disease. This group of patients usually is evaluated with a chest CT scan, including the upper abdomen to assess the liver and adrenal glands, pulmonary function tests, and, optionally, a quantitative lung perfusion scan. PET scans may be useful in staging the pulmonary hilum and mediastinum but so far have not replaced mediastinoscopy for definitive mediastinal lymph node staging.[103] In the absence of symptoms or an elevated serum alkaline phosphatase level, however, brain CT or MRI scan and bone scans are generally not of any utility. Many patients in this category have clinically staged IA disease, and it is only after surgical resection that the pathologic stage IIA is recognized.

Treatment for patients with stage IIA lesions remains complete surgical resection. In this subgroup of patients, nearly all patients require at least a lobectomy or pneumonectomy, with only a rare patient able to undergo a segmentectomy. Because of a significant incidence of mediastinal metastases, mediastinoscopy and, in some cases of left upper lobe tumors, left parasternal mediastinotomy before resection are mandatory for mediastinal staging. At the time of surgical resection, it is extremely important that accurate mediastinal staging be established, preferably with a complete mediastinal lymph node dissection or at least lymph node sampling. Intraoperative sampling of interlobar or "sump" lymph nodes also is performed to help determine the need for pneumonectomy. Patients who are not candidates for surgical resection because of medical contraindications or patient refusal should be palliated with radiation therapy or chemoradiotherapy.

The long-term survival of patients with stage IIA disease is significantly less than those patients with similar size lesions but without lymph node metastases (stage IA). In a review of data from Memorial Sloan-Kettering Cancer Center, Martini and coauthors[143] reported a 39% survival rate in stage II disease. There was no difference between T1 and T2 lesions, although patients with small (< 3 cm) tumors fared better than those with large (> 5 cm) ones. In this study, the best survival occurred in those patients with small (< 3 cm ) tumors and only a single lymph node metastasis (48% 5-year survival rate). In addition, local recurrence was more frequent with squamous cell histology, and systemic recurrence was more common with adenocarcinoma. Because of the high risk of postoperative recurrences, adjuvant radiation and chemoradiotherapy have been used in an attempt to improve survival. The Lung Cancer Study Group detected an increased disease-free survival in patients with adenocarcinoma treated with chemoradiotherapy.[144] A phase II trial of neoadjuvant chemotherapy with carboplatin and taxol in this high-risk patient population has begun, with encouraging early data.[142] The optimal adjuvant therapy, however, has yet to be determined.

**Stage IIB Non–Small Cell Lung Cancer (T2 N1 M0; T3 N0 M0).** Patients with larger (> 3 cm) NSCLCs that have metastasized to bronchopulmonary or hilar lymph nodes or with tumors that have invaded the parietal pleura of the chest wall, diaphragm, or mediastinum and beyond make up a small but significant subgroup of patients with NSCLC. In the 1993 revision of the Union Internationale Contre le Cancer (UICC) and the American Joint Committee on Cancer (AJCC) staging system for NSCLC, T3 N0 M0 tumors, which previously were classified as stage IIIA tumors, were changed to stage IIB along with T2 N1 M0 lesions. This was based on survival data. As with stage IIA disease, patients often present with clinical stage IB disease and are found only after surgical resection to have pathologic stage IIB disease. Furthermore, unless there is gross rib destruction, it is very difficult in most patients to determine without surgical exploration whether true involvement of the parietal pleura exists. Prospective studies evaluating the utility of CT scans and MRI in this area have shown that these modality are not as helpful in predicting this problem as was first hoped, although MRI may be of some benefit in specifically gauging mediastinal invasion.[145, 146] Although most of these patients ultimately develop systemic metastases, routine brain CT or MRI scans and bone scans still are not warranted, and preoperative radiologic evaluation consists primarily of a CT scan of the chest and upper abdomen.

Treatment for patients with known or suspected stage IIB NSCLC consists of standard complete surgical resection. As in stage IIA, nearly all patients require at least a lobectomy or pneumonectomy. In addition, for patients with parietal pleural involvement, all affected tissues must be removed en bloc. This may require chest wall resection, resection of a portion of the diaphragm, or removal of mediastinal tissues. Chest wall resection may require reconstruction, particularly if three or more ribs are affected and if the defect is anterior and not covered by the scapula. The techniques of reconstruction vary widely but include the use of Maarlex and Gortex mesh and, in some instances, methylmethacrylate for chest wall stability. A very small subset of patients may have tumors within 2 cm of the carina, and in some of these patients, a sleeve pneumonectomy may be required for complete resection. Surgical mediastinal staging (i.e., mediastinoscopy with or without a left parasternal mediastinotomy), again, is required before resection. At the time of surgery, complete mediastinal lymph node dissection is recommended for accurate pathologic staging. Intraoperative sampling of interlobar or "sump" lymph nodes is performed to help determine the need for pneumonectomy. Palliative radiation or radiochemotherapy are available for patients who are not candidates for surgical resection because of medical contraindications or who refuse surgery. The prognosis after complete surgical resection is similar to that in stage IIA disease (see previous discussion). Large (> 5 cm) tumors, however, have a particularly poor prognosis. In addition, patients with multiple lymph node metastases have decreased survival, with only 39% surviving 5 years.[143] The survival rate of patients with chest wall involvement, requiring chest wall resection, has been reported to be as high as 35% to 62% at 5 years.[147] Patients requiring sleeve pneumonectomy for primary tumors within 2 cm of the carina can have as high as a 40% 5-year survival rate; however, the surgical mortality also is substantial.[128] Survival of patients with Pancoast tumor and other superior sulcus tumors is discussed separately next. As in stage IIA disease, adjuvant therapy has yielded only an increase in locoregional control and disease-free survival but not increased overall survival. New approaches with neoadjuvant chemotherapy are currently under investigation.[142]

**Pancoast Tumor and Other Superior Sulcus Tumors.** T3 tumors that occur at the thoracic apex constitute an important subset of patients with NSCLC. Classically, Pancoast tumors involve the apex of the lung; invade the first and second ribs posteriorly; involve the lower brachial plexus nerve roots (T1 and C8), which produces pain that radiates down the inner aspect of the arm and forearm; often involve the stellate ganglion, causing Horner's syndrome; and frequently exhibit squamous histology. Anterior superior sulcus tumors involve the apex of the lung, invade the first and second ribs anteriorly, involve the subclavian vein and artery, and cause primarily chest wall pain. Radiologic evaluation includes a CT scan and often an MRI scan, particularly if involvement of the vascular structures is suspected. Although bone scans often are obtained to show local rib destruction, they usually do not demonstrate distant metastases and in most cases are unnecessary. Results from treatment of Pancoast and other superior sulcus tumors were dismal until Paulson and colleagues[148, 149] described the use of preoperative radiation therapy, resulting in a 5-year survival rate of 31%. These results have not changed up to the present time. It is imperative that patients initially undergo mediastinoscopy before therapy because a small group of these patients demonstrates mediastinal lymph node metastases that carry an extremely poor prognosis and are a contraindication to surgical resection. After this, radiation therapy is initiated either in 300-cGy fractions over 2 weeks or in 200-cGy fractions over 4 weeks.[150] Resection is then carried out 3 to 4 weeks later and includes en bloc removal of the upper lobe, involved ribs and transverse spinal processes, dorsal sympathetic chain, and lower trunk of the brachial plexus, if necessary. As in other stage II tumors, a complete mediastinal lymph node dissection is recommended. With this approach, from 21% to 90% of tumors can be completely resected.[151, 152]

The prognosis after preoperative radiation and complete surgical resection has not changed since Shaw and colleagues[149] first described this approach. Other reports have confirmed the 5-year survival rate of approximately 30%. Some variations on the delivery of radiation with a "sandwich" technique adding additional postoperative radiation may improve these results slightly, although this approach has not been widely adopted.[153] Recent trials are designed to assess the efficacy of the addition of chemotherapy to the preoperative treatment regimen. Results from these trials are still pending. Poor prognostic factors that have been identified include N2 disease, incomplete resection, and the use of wedge resection instead of lobectomy.[154]

## Locally Advanced Non-Small Cell Lung Cancer

**Stage IIIA Non–Small Cell Lung Cancer (T1–3 N2 M0; T3 N1 M0).** Patients with stage IIIA disease are probably the most heterogeneous group of patients within any stage of NSCLC. Patients may have a solitary microfocus of disease in a single mediastinal lymph node, many mediastinal lymph nodes with bulky extranodal tumor extension, or disease involving the mediastinum (T3) with one or more hilar lymph node metastases only. The radiographic evaluation of these patients includes a chest and upper abdominal CT scan and often may include a brain MRI scan, PET scan, and bone scan to exclude the possibility of distant metastases, particularly before any high-risk surgical procedure.

The treatment of patients with stage IIIA disease, and in particular N2 disease, has been very controversial. Historically, surgery first was used in these patients with poor results. Once radiation alone was shown to be equivalent to surgery, this modality became standard therapy. Surgery still is indicated in patients with "minimal" N2 disease that is detected only at the time of thoracotomy (after a negative mediastinoscopy) because of its more favorable prognosis (discussed later). Despite years of trials, which have documented only a modest increase in disease-free survival with postoperative adjuvant chemotherapy and chemoradiotherapy, more recent data with multimodality therapy, including neoadjuvant chemotherapy combined with surgery, neoadjuvant chemoradiotherapy combined with surgery, and chemoradiotherapy alone, have produced more encouraging results.[155] Based on preliminary phase II results and data from three randomized trials (discussed later) comparing surgery alone with neoadjuvant chemotherapy and surgery (with or without radiation), surgical resection after preoperative (induction) chemotherapy appears to offer a safe and reasonably effective treatment for patients with "resectable" N2 disease.

Before interpreting prognostic data, one must realize that N2 disease is quite variable and survival of patients with "N2" disease can vary substantially. For instance, 5-year survival rate with "minimal" microscopic disease in a single lymph node is nearly 41% after surgery alone.[156] In contrast, 5-year survival rates in bulky (visible on CXR) disease in multiple lymph nodes throughout the mediastinum may only be 5% to 10% after multimodality therapy.[155] Many phase II and phase III trials sponsored by the Lung Cancer Study Group, the Veterans Administration, and others have evaluated postoperative adjuvant treatment (radiation, chemotherapy, and radiochemotherapy) with only a modest increase in disease-free but not overall survival.[144] With this background, a multitude of phase II nonrandomized studies have suggested benefit to the addition of neoadjuvant (preoperative) chemotherapy to surgical resection in stage IIIA (N2) patients.[155] Based on these data, three randomized trials comparing surgery alone with neoadjuvant chemotherapy and surgery (with or without radiation) with a total of 147 patients have shown a definite survival advantage to the neoadjuvant chemotherapy group.[157–159] Median survivals have varied but have been reported to be as high as 64 months versus only 11 months for surgery alone.[157] Currently, the role of surgery is being evaluated in "resectable" N2 patients in an intergroup trial comparing neoadjuvant chemoradiotherapy to chemoradiotherapy alone. The results, however, are still unknown. Other stage IIIA patients (T3 N1) have a 5-year survival rate of approximately 37%.[160] These patients also are being included in trials of neoadjuvant chemotherapy in high-risk, early-stage patients.[142]

**Stage IIIB Non–Small Cell Lung Cancer (T4 N0–2 M0; T1–3 N3 M0).** NSCLCs with contralateral or supraclavicular lymph node metastases (N3), involvement of major mediastinal organs such as the heart, great vessels, esophagus, and vertebral body (T4), or associated with malignant pleural effusions (T4) are thought to be "unresectable." Japanese reports, however, have described radical resection of major thoracic organs, including the aorta, vertebral bodies, main pulmonary artery, and superior vena cava, sometimes with cardiopulmonary bypass in attempts to completely resect all disease. Even with these heroic attempts at removal, the 5-year survival rate is less than 13%, which is not significantly better than treatment with a more conservative regimen of chemotherapy and radiation.[161] However, there are some interesting data with regard to multimodality treatment. A Southwest Oncology Group Study (8805) treated both stage IIIA and stage IIIB patients with induction chemoradiotherapy followed by surgical resection. This was a phase II trial without a randomized control arm, but survival was noted to be identical in both arms.[162] Although these data are preliminary, further study with this aggressive multimodality treatment approach may be warranted.

## Metastatic (Stage IV) Non-Small Cell Lung Cancer (TX NX M1)

**Treatment with Curative Intent.** Although patients with stage IV NSCLC generally are thought to be incurable, certain distinct subsets of patients may be amenable to surgical therapy for possible cure.

Patients who present with either synchronous or metachronous *solitary brain metastases* may be treated by surgical resection of tumor at both the primary and metastatic sites. Wronski and associates[163] reviewed the experience with this approach at Memorial Sloan-Kettering Cancer Center. They noted 231 patients who had undergone up to four resections of solitary brain metastases with median survival rates of 46.3%, 14.7%, and 12.5% after 1, 3, and 5 years, respectively. Poor prognostic factors identified were male gender, incomplete resection of pulmonary disease, infratentorial location, age older than 60 years, and the presence of systemic metastases. In this experience, up to four resections were performed over time for metachronous recurrent solitary brain disease. Other reports have suggested a 21% or greater 5-year survival rate.[164] Phase II trials have been initiated to determine whether adjuvant chemotherapy (after resection of the brain metastases and before removal of the primary lung tumor) can impact on the modest survival advantage with this approach. Finally, the development of stereotactic radiation of brain metastases has demonstrated 94% growth control and may obviate the need for surgical resection of some metastases.[165]

Similar to brain metastases, *solitary adrenal metastases* seem to have a more favorable prognosis than the usual widespread metastatic disease when resected along with the primary lung cancer. In cases of synchronous adrenal lesions on the same side as the primary lung cancer, this can be done conveniently at the same time as the pulmonary resection through a transdiaphragmatic approach. Luketich and Burt[166] have reviewed the experience at Memorial Sloan-Kettering Cancer Center and reported a 3-year survival rate of 38%. In addition, patients who underwent resection had a median survival of 31 months compared with 8.5 months for patients receiving only chemotherapy. Others have confirmed a long-term survival rate of 17% at 15 years.[167] Solitary adrenal metastases also are being included in adjuvant chemotherapy protocols to determine whether systemic treatment increases the modest long-term survival afforded by surgical resection.

**Palliative Treatment.** Most patients with stage IV NSCLC are treated with nonoperative therapy. Surgery does, however, play an active role in the palliation of certain symptoms.

Direct surgical resection, usually with the aid of a neodymium:yttrium-aluminum-garnet (Nd-YAG) laser, can relieve dyspnea and symptoms of postobstructive pneumonia in patients with *bronchial obstruction* proximal to the segmental bronchi. The relief is immediate but only temporary unless other antitumor therapy is instituted. External beam radiation also can accomplish the same effect but is less reliable and often requires several weeks before the bronchus reopens. Brachytherapy is particularly useful in palliation of these residual endobronchial lesions and even has been reported to prolong survival in these patients.[168, 169] Some centers have described success with photodynamic therapy and radiofrequency resection combined with cryotherapy.[170, 171]

Rarely, surgeons are asked to perform a "toilet" lobectomy. This is frequently the case if proximal bronchial obstruction has not responded to treatment and a postobstructive pneumonia has evolved into a frank *pulmonary abscess* or if *massive hemoptysis* develops. Although it is tempting to perform such surgery to help the patient, this is almost never necessary. Pulmonary abscesses have been successfully, albeit not ideally, palliated with percutaneous drainage catheters if radiation fails to open obstructed bronchi. In addition, intravenous antibiotics have been fairly successful at suppression of postobstructive pneumonias. Furthermore, patients with massive hemoptysis may be treated quite successfully with bronchial artery embolization or with conservative endobronchial control measures (i.e., iced saline lavage, endobronchial balloon tamponade, Nd-YAG laser coagulation, etc.) with reasonable success. Therefore, it is extremely rare for patients to require this type of surgery, and the palliation afforded by this aggressive approach often is somewhat dubious.

## Small Cell Lung Cancer

Guidelines for the management of SCLC have recently been published.[171a] Although the disease is seldom amenable to surgical resection, SCLC equivalent to stage I NSCLC (e.g., solitary tumors without hilar, mediastinal, and distant metastases) can be treated quite successfully with surgical resection alone, with reported 5-year survival rates as high as 35% to 51%.[172, 173] Most often, suspected lung cancers are removed for diagnostic purposes and are found only postoperatively to represent SCLC. After resection, postoperative chemotherapy often has been given, and studies in this group of patients, including trials reported by the Veterans Administration Surgical Adjuvant Group, have demonstrated 5-year survival rates from 41% to 68%.[174, 175] Even if a known SCLC is detected that has no mediastinal or hilar lymph node involvement (requires mediastinoscopy), surgical resection should be strongly considered. Surgical treatment of patients with hilar lymph node metastases is more controversial, with many studies showing dramatically lower survival than in patients with clinical stage I disease. Other studies have evaluated patients with mediastinal lymph node metastases without distant metastases and found no benefit over standard chemotherapy and radiation. Finally, the role of surgical resection after induction chemotherapy as the best means for local control is still under investigation in an ongoing intergroup trial; however, data do indicate that surgical resection of residual disease after initial treatment in patients without distant spread occasionally is warranted because of the possibility of mixed tumors. In these patients, previous treatment eradicates the small cell component but leaves a non–small cell tumor that is amenable to surgical therapy.[176]

# RADIATION THERAPY

## Radical Radiation Therapy for Non–Small Cell Lung Cancer

### Medically Inoperable Non–Small Cell Lung Cancer

Radical radiation therapy may produce long-term survival for patients with stage I NSCLC (T1 or T2 N0) whose tumors are unresectable because of comorbid medical conditions or inadequate pulmonary function.[177–180] The reported 5-year survival rate is 10% to 32%, although some articles include patients with T3 or N1 disease. Overall survival may be considerably worse than cause-specific survival (e.g., 13% vs. 32% at 5 years) because of intercurrent deaths.[180, 181] Outcome depends on T stage, dose, and tumor size.[177, 178] The larger the tumor, the more clonogenic cells and the higher the radiation dose needed to eradicate them. Dose ultimately is limited by normal tissue tolerance, therefore larger tumors do less well. The corollary of this is that some small central tumors may be technically inoperable but still may be suitable for radical radiotherapy.

Isolated locoregional failure can account for up to 50% of relapses, but this number can be reduced with radiation doses greater than 60 Gy.[177, 178, 180–182] Overall outcome and local recurrence depends on the extent of the initial staging evaluation.[177] Most patients who receive radiation therapy have not had a mediastinoscopy. Kaskowitz and coauthors[181] reported on 53 patients with stage I NSCLC treated with radical radiotherapy and concluded that the results were inferior to those obtained with surgery; however, only 4 patients had been pathologically staged (with mediastinoscopy), and only 62% of patients received a minimum primary tumor dose of 60 Gy. Clinical staging almost always underestimates stage, therefore direct comparisons of surgery and radiation therapy may not be appropriate.

Many radiation therapists include the adjacent hilar and mediastinal nodes in the radiation field. However, treating the primary lesion alone still may achieve a good outcome while minimizing lung toxicity. This approach is appropriate for patients with poor lung function and a lower clinical stage of disease. Reasonable doses are 40 to 50 Gy to nodal areas (if treated) and a minimum of 60 Gy to the tumor bulk, given in 1.8- to 2-Gy fractions.

### Unresectable Non–Small Cell Lung Cancer

Unresectable NSCLC may be treated with palliative or curative intent depending on the extent of disease and the patient's overall physical condition. The most aggressive approach is to combine chemotherapy and radiation (either sequentially or concurrently). Radiation alone also may be used with curative intent. In clinical trials comparing radiation to chemoradiation therapy, median survival is 9 to 15 months and the long-term survival rate is 10% to 25% at 2 years and 5% at 5 years.[182–187] A recursive partitioning analysis of 1592 patients entered into Radiation Therapy Oncology Group (RTOG) trials showed that Karnofsky performance status (KPS) of 70% or less was associated with a median survival of only 5.9 months compared with 9.9 months for patients with KPS of 80% to 100%.[187] In general, clinical trials of radical radiation treatment often include only patients whose performance status is good (KPS $\geq$ 70%) and who present with less than a 5% weight loss. In normal clinical practice, a significant number of patients do not fall into this good prognostic group. The survival data show that most patients are palliated, not cured, therefore quality of life is an important consideration.[188]

**Conventional Radiation Therapy.** Nodal areas that are at risk for microscopic spread but negative on CT imaging receive a prophylactic dose of 40 to 50 Gy, and the bulk of disease receives a minimum of 60 Gy (in 1.8- to 2-Gy fractions). For upper lobe tumors, the nodal areas at risk include the supraclavicular nodes, but not the lower mediastinal nodes, and vice versa for lower lobe tumors. The mediastinal and bilateral hilar nodes generally are considered at risk in all cases.

**Dose Dependence.** The effect of dose on outcome was investigated in the RTOG trial 73-01, in which 500 patients were randomizely assigned to receive 40, 50, or 60 Gy.[183, 189] Local failure occurred within the radiation field in 58% of patients treated to 40 Gy compared with 35% of those receiving 60 Gy. There was a survival advantage for the 60-Gy dose group at 3 years (15% vs. 6% for 40 Gy), but this was not maintained beyond 3 years.

**Dose Escalation.** Most techniques of dose escalation increase acute side effects such as fatigue, dysphagia, and skin irritation, which must be managed symptomatically. Dose-limiting side effects are predominantly "late" radiation tissue damage (e.g., damage to lung, spinal cord, or bone), which occurs some months or years after the radiation is completed. These effects are irreversible.

*Hyperfractionation* is the use of smaller individual radiation doses (fractions) to reduce late tissue damage. By giving more than 1 dose per day, a higher total dose is given and the overall treatment time is not increased. Doses must be at least 6 hours apart, or sparing of late toxicity is incomplete.

RTOG trial 88-08 compared 69.6 Gy, given as 1.2 Gy twice a day over 6 weeks, with 60 Gy in 30 fractions of 2 Gy over 6 weeks.[189–191] Median survival was 12.3 months for the hyperfractionated group versus 11.4 months for the standard regimen. The 2-and 4-year survival rates were 24% and 9%, respectively, for the hyperfractionated regimen and 20% and 4%, respectively, for the standard regimen.[190] This trial included only patients with KPS greater than 70% and weight loss of less than 5%.

*Accelerated fractionation* is the reduction in the overall treatment time. The rationale is that there is evidence for accelerated growth of tumors after about 4 weeks. Accelerated treatment generally uses multiple doses per day.

Phase II studies by RTOG (83-12 and 84-07) investigated the effects of giving 70 to 75 Gy in 5 to 5.5 weeks.[189] With single daily doses, there was significant late toxicity, which was reduced by using divided doses, although acute toxicity remained high. Median survival was 9 to 10 months (no improvement), but 2-year survival rates appear improved, 22% to 25%, versus 15% to 19% for standard therapy.[187, 189]

Continuous hyperfractionated accelerated radiation therapy (CHART), a technique developed in the United Kingdom, uses small doses given 3 times per day, 6 hours apart, over a continuous period of 12 days (including weekends).[192] Full treatment therefore is given well before any accelerated tumor growth occurs, and the small fraction size reduces late toxicity. Treatment is completed before acute side effects become marked.

Acute toxicity with CHART is high because of the rapid accumulation of dose; however, toxicity occurs after treatment is completed. In a randomized trial of 563 patients, CHART, in 54 Gy in 36 fractions of 1.5 Gy over 12 days, was compared with 60 Gy in 30 fractions over 6 weeks.[191] Two-year survival rate was increased from 20% to 29% overall and from 19% to 33% for patients with squamous histology. Acute dysphagia was increased in the CHART group, but other side effects were comparable.

**Conformal Radiation Therapy.** Multiple shaped, noncoplanar radiation beams may be used to increase target dose while geometrically sparing normal tissue, particularly critical structures such as the spinal cord. Fixation of the target, however, remains a problem in treatment of the lung, although gating of the radiation beam with respiration is being investigated. Lung toxicity is also volume dependent and therefore paradoxically could be increased (i.e., a low dose to a large volume could be more toxic than a high dose to a small volume).

**Interruptions in Treatment.** Interruptions in radiation treatment reduce the chance of a favorable outcome. In a review of RTOG studies 83-21, 84-03 (conventional radiation), and 83-11 (hyperfractionated dose escalation), patients who completed treatment according to protocol had double the 2-year and 3 times the 5-year survival of those with treatment interruptions (24% vs. 13% and 10% vs. 3%).[189, 193] Overall, survival differences were statistically significant ($p = .016$). Interruptions occurred in up to 15% of patients receiving higher doses. For patients without unfavorable prognostic features, the 5-year survival rate was 15% if they completed 69.6 Gy or greater, 0% if treatment was interrupted, and 7% for conventional fractionation without interruption. Some patients may best be served by a conventional course of treatment that they can complete. Nonclinical interruptions during treatment caused by machine breakdown, patient transport, and other problems must be avoided.

**Endobronchial Brachytherapy.** Brachytherapy is a technique by which radioactive isotopes are inserted into or close to a tumor to give localized radiation therapy. Brachytherapy may be low-dose rate, given over several days, or high-dose rate, given over several minutes. High-dose rate brachytherapy generally is divided into a small number of fractions to avoid late toxicity to normal tissues but sometimes may be given as a single dose if in combination with external beam treatment. Brachytherapy can be applied to endobronchial tumors. Practical considerations mean that high-dose rate therapy is the most appropriate. The patient undergoes bronchoscopy, and a blind-ended nylon guide tube is passed through the bronchus at the level of the tumor. The radioactive wire then is passed into the tube until the radioactive part is at the level of the tumor and left for the amount of time required to give the specified dose.

Endobronchial brachytherapy may be used as a boost after radical or palliative external beam therapy, or as a palliative measure on its own.[194, 195] It sometimes is combined with laser surgery for a blocked bronchus or is used to prevent tumor regrowth and restenosis. The main limitation of endobronchial brachytherapy is that the radiation dose is only given to about a 1-cm radius. Therefore, tumor beyond this radius is relatively unaffected and will regrow. The wire also may sit asymmetrically in the bronchus, underdosing one side. Treatment is relatively well tolerated without systemic upset because of its localized nature. Rare but significant risks include hemorrhage or bronchial fistula if the tumor penetrates a vessel or bronchial wall.[194]

## Radiation Combined with Chemotherapy for Non-Small Cell Lung Cancer

### "Conventional" Chemoradiation

The current "gold standard" regimen of chemoradiation is cisplatin (100 mg/m$^2$ on days 1 and 29) and vinblastine, with radiation alone starting on day 50 (40 Gy in 20 fractions to nodal areas, 60 Gy in 30 fractions to primary tumor).[184] In a randomization of the same radiation versus chemoradiation for patients with stage III disease, median survival was 9.6 months for the radiation alone group versus 13.7 months for the chemoradiation group.[184] These differences were statistically significant, and there were no treatment-related deaths.

RTOG trial 88-08 compared 60 Gy alone to hyperfractionated radiation and to chemotherapy followed by 60 Gy as described previously.[190] Differences were small in absolute terms, but chemoradiation therapy improved both the median, 1-, and 2-year survivals. Those patients with squamous cell carcinoma had no overall survival benefit, whereas patients with adenocarcinoma did show a survival benefit.

### Concurrent Chemoradiation

The rationale for concurrent therapy is that those patients with chemotherapy insensitive tumors do not have their definitive radiation treatment delayed and that there may be sensitization of the tumor to the radiation by the chemotherapy. The risks include an increase in toxicity, making it difficult for either treatment to be completed on schedule.

The European Organization for Research and Treatment of Cancer (EORTC) demonstrated a significant survival advantage for low-dose cisplatin given daily during radiation versus radiation alone (2-year survival rate 26% vs. 13%), but the unusual split-course radiation regimen used in this trial complicates its interpretation.[196] Five other randomized trials have failed to show a benefit for concurrent chemoradiation versus radiation alone despite three trials including cisplatin.[197] RTOG trial 94-10 comparing preradiation chemotherapy (cisplatin and vinblastine) with the same chemotherapy given concurrently with radiation, and chemotherapy with hyperfractionated radiotherapy completed accrual in 1998. The Cancer and Leukemia Group B and the Eastern Cooperative Oncology Group reported the results of a phase III study that tested the effect of carboplatin radiosensitization in unresectable stage III patients with lung cancer. Two hundred eighty-three patients were entered. All patients received induction chemotherapy with cisplatin plus vindesine followed by 60 Gy over 6 weeks. One hundred forty-six patients were randomly assigned to receive carboplatin, 100 mg/m$^2$/wk concurrently with the radiation. The complete response rate was 18% for the carboplatin arm and 10% for the radiation alone arm, with a 13% 4-year survival rate for the carboplatin arm and a 10% 4-year survival rate for the radiotherapy arm. Thus, carboplatin did not impact on survival. Furthermore, the relapse rate within the chest remained greater than 50%.

## Superior Sulcus Tumors

Superior sulcus tumors erode the first rib and invade the lower brachial plexus so that they most commonly cause shoulder and arm pain. Symptoms may include paresthesias, numbness, and weakness. The pain is often unrelenting and severe. They may cause Horner's syndrome from involvement of the stellate ganglion. In unresectable patients with a poor prognosis, higher doses of radiation (60 Gy in 30 fractions rather than 30 Gy in 10 fractions) are recommended to provide optimum pain control. These tumors are challenging for the radiation oncologist because of their tendency to invade the upper thoracic vertebrae and to intrude through the vertebral foramina and encroach on the spinal cord.

## Small Cell Lung Cancer

### Chest Irradiation in Limited-Stage Disease

Several prospective randomized trials in which at least 80 patients with limited-stage SCLC disease were randomly assigned to chemotherapy or chemotherapy plus radiation have been published. Concurrent therapy is defined as combined modality treatment with chemotherapy and radiation being given together. In alternating therapy, radiation is given on days of the chemotherapy cycle in which no drug is given. Sequential therapy is defined as each modality being given separately, one after completion of the other, or delays in chemotherapy for delivery of radiation.

Four studies showed minimal to significantly improved survival for combined modality therapy (two utilizing concurrent therapy, one alternating and one sequential therapy).[199-203] Overall, the improvement in median survival was modest at 1 to 4 months, with an increase in the 2-year survival rate from 7% to 17%. For the studies with the longest follow-up, the advantage seen with the radiotherapy arms did not extend beyond 5 years because of intercurrent deaths and new primary tumors.[199, 203] A meta-analysis of 13 published and unpublished trials of more than 2100 limited-stage SCLC patients randomly assigned to chemotherapy or chemotherapy plus radiation showed a 14% decrease in the death rate and a 5.4% increase in the 3-year survival rate for the combination therapy arm.[204] Exactly how to integrate thoracic radiation with chemotherapy is not resolved; however, therapy combining radiation with chemotherapy in limited-stage SCLC improves survival, especially when radiation is given concurrently or in an alternating fashion. Results of sequential therapy are disappointing.

Combined modality therapy is associated with increased toxicity, such as pneumonitis, pulmonary fibrosis, esophagitis, and toxic cardiac effects. Thus, chest irradiation need not be offered to patients with poor pulmonary function or poor performance status. Results of randomized clinical trials show no role for chest irradiation in extensive stage SCLC other than for palliation.

### Prophylactic Cranial Irradiation

Cranial metastases are common in SCLC. Subclinical metastases are present in 10% of patients at diagnosis and develop in 20% of patients during treatment. Prophylactic cranial irradiation (PCI), although effective in reducing the frequency of clinically detectable brain metastases, does not improve survival.[205] Late neurologic sequelae include leukoencephalopathy and neuropsychological impairment. The recommended dose is 2000 to 4000 cGy in 200- to 250-cGy fractions.[206] Prophylactic cranial irradiation is recommended for complete respondents, although definitive recommendations await the results of several large ongoing clinical trials.

## Palliative Radiation Therapy

### Palliative Chest Radiation

A standard palliative radiation regimen is 30 Gy in 10 fractions of 3 Gy each, delivered over 2 weeks. Side effects are mild. Most patients experience some fatigue during the second week of treatment, lasting for 2 to 3 weeks, and transient esophagitis, usually lasting less than 1 week.

### Palliative Radiotherapy for Systemic Disease or Relapsed Disease

Patterns of relapse vary with histology. In particular, squamous cell carcinoma is more likely to show isolated locoregional relapse, whereas metastatic disease to the brain is more likely with adenocarcinoma.[182]

Patients with small-volume local relapses without evidence of systemic disease should be considered for aggressive chemoradiation therapy. Locoregional radiation may improve symptoms. Radiation therapy is more effective if given early, before collapse of a lung or lobe, and may prevent subsequent collapse.

**Bone Metastases.** Symptomatic bone metastases, being focal, are ideally treated by radiation.[194] Symptomatic relief is high (80% or more). Radiation therapy is particularly beneficial with bone pain, which is worse on movement and therefore difficult to control at all times with analgesics because of fluctuating pain levels with activity. Radiation of lytic lesions may prevent pathologic fractures, however, prophylactic surgical pinning may also be needed. A standard radiation regimen for bony lesions is 30 Gy in 10 fractions over 2 weeks. In general, pain relief occurs after radiation, but it starts to take effect about 2 weeks after the completion of treatment and may continue to improve over time. Adequate analgesia should be provided in the interim. Patients with a poor prognosis but in significant pain or at risk for fracture can be treated with a single fraction of 8 Gy. This is especially important for lesions in the proximal femur, which compromise the cortex of the bone. Such lesions should be irradiated prophylactically, even if asymptomatic.

**Spinal Cord Compression.** Spinal cord compression is an oncologic emergency.[194] Patients who receive treatment with either surgery or radiation therapy within a day of initial symptoms and before symptoms have progressed to complete paralysis have the best chance of maintaining or regaining function. Patients who have been paraplegic for some days seldom recover no matter what treatment is given, however, treatment always should be attempted. Urgent referral to specialists and workup with MRI scan is therefore mandatory whenever spinal cord compression is suspected. Symptoms may be minimal.

Initial treatment consists of steroids (dexamethasone loading dose, 8 to 10 mg, followed by dexamethasone, 4 mg every 6 hours) and surgical decompression or urgent radiation therapy. Response to dexamethasone is often indicative of overall response; no response to dexamethasone is a poor sign, suggesting nerve damage, not just compression. Radiation therapy is not helpful for compression due to fracture with bony displacement.

### Superior Vena Cava Obstruction

Radiation therapy can be therapeutic in superior vena cava obstruction provided that tumor shrinkage is reasonably rapid and no permanent blockage by thrombus has occurred. Standard treatment doses and techniques are used. For SCLC, chemotherapy may be equally as efficacious.

Symptomatic relief usually occurs after radiation therapy or chemotherapy for superior vena cava syndrome in patients with lung cancer; improvement, however, is partial in about 50%, and recurrence occurs in 10% to 32%.[206a] For patients with continued or recurrent venous obstruction following conventional treatment, stenting of the superior vena cava with various endovascular prostheses may offer relief.[206b]

### Brain Metastases

The outlook for patients with cerebral metastases has improved considerably because of advances in radiation therapy techniques. For NSCLC, surgical removal of a solitary metastasis followed by whole-brain irradiation results in a median survival of approximately 11 months.[207, 208] About 30% of patients relapse at the surgical site, despite radiation, and about 30% relapse elsewhere in the brain.[207] However, only about a third of patients die of their cerebral disease alone.[207] Standard therapy for brain metastases consists of 30 Gy in 10 fractions. The median survival for patients with inoperable or multiple cerebral metastases is 3 to 6 months.[209, 210] For patients with small numbers of metastases, including lesions in critical cortical areas, stereotactic radiosurgery offers median survival of 9 to 18 months in various series.[208, 211] A neurosurgical head frame is used for immobilization, and treatment is delivered with multiple arcs of radiation (Linac radiosurgery) or 201 beams (gamma knife). Single doses of 16 to 24 Gy are delivered providing 80% control of the treated site.[208, 211]

In SCLC, cerebral metastases are generally multiple, and stereotactic techniques or surgery are seldom appropriate. Treatment is with whole-brain irradiation, unless the patient already has received prophylactic cranial irradiation. In these patients, a response in the brain may be seen with systemic chemotherapy.

## Complications of Radiation Therapy

### Spinal Cord

Most lung radiation fields include the hilar and mediastinal nodes. Through the use of an anteroposterior/posteroanterior (AP/PA) parallel pair technique, the dose-limiting structure is the spinal cord. If multiple beams or an oblique AP/PA pair are used, the field arrangements tend to include larger regions of lung, thus increasing the risk of cord damage.

### Lung

Radiation pneumonitis is a subacute toxicity that presents about 6 weeks after the end of a course of radiation with a dry cough, fever, dyspnea, and pleuritic chest pain. The CXR shows patchy changes in the area of the radiation field. Extension outside the radiation field is extremely rare. Significant (grade 3) pneumonitis occurs in about 5% of patients treated with radiation alone.[191] It is more likely with large radiation fields, high total dose, and large daily doses.[191, 212] The incidence of this toxicity is higher with combined chemoradiation, and up to 50% of patients may have mild symptoms.[191, 212] Radiation pneumonitis responds well to steroids, but an abrupt taper can lead to a rebound worsening of symptoms. For patients receiving chemotherapy, infection must be excluded.

Long-term fibrosis is a late radiation effect, commencing months after treatment and occurring in areas of lung receiving above 20 to 25 Gy (fractionated treatment). Therefore, high doses should not be given to large volumes of lung, especially in patients with compromised lung function.

### Esophagus

The esophagus is usually encompassed in any radiation field that includes the mediastinal and hilar lymph nodes. Radiation esophagitis begins at about 3 weeks into a radical (6 to 7 week) course of treatment. Patients often report that their food seems to "stick," rather than report pain. The symptoms resolve 2 to 4 weeks after the end of therapy. Reduced oral intake and nutrition may occur, and patients are advised to avoid very hot or very cold foods, alcohol, spices, vinegar, and sharp toast. Some patients get relief from antacid liquids, which may be combined with viscous lidocaine. Most patients experience some esophagitis, but it is more marked with more aggressive regimens and with combined chemoradiation.[189]

### Other Toxicities

*Fatigue* is a significant side effect of radiation therapy. It is cumulative, often being inapparent for the first 2 to 3 weeks of treatment, and is most noticeable at the end of treatment and in the subsequent few weeks after completion of therapy. Recovery is gradual. Patients who are symptomatic from their disease conversely may improve during therapy. This is noted most often in patients with SCLC that responds rapidly to treatment.

The skin over the radiation beam entry and exit areas may become reddened with mild irritation. Because the targets of treatment are at a depth and at least two radiation fields are used, *skin changes* are generally mild. Hydrocortisone cream can be used to alleviate irritation. For patients with chest hair, hair loss may occur in the radiation port areas. Generally, it regrows.

## COMBINED MODALITY APPROACHES

### Preoperative and Postoperative Chemotherapy for Resectable Non-Small Cell Lung Cancer

A current phase II intergroup trial of combined chemoradiation (platinum-etoposide) before surgical resection for patients with N2-negative disease by mediastinoscopy is in progress. For patients with microscopic N2-positive disease, two phase II trials demonstrated a benefit for 2 to 3 cycles of preoperative chemotherapy. Rosell and colleagues[158] in Spain randomly assigned 60 patients to surgery versus 3 cycles of mitomycin, ifosfamide, and cisplatin followed by surgery. All patients received postoperative radiation. The median survival was 8 versus 26 months ($P < .001$) and the median disease-free survival was 5 versus 20 months.[158] Roth and colleagues[157] randomly assigned 60 patients with stage IIIA disease to 3 cycles of cisplatin (100 mg/m$^2$), VP-16, cyclophosphamide followed by surgery and then 3 cycles of the same chemotherapy postoperatively versus surgery alone. The estimated 1-, 2-, and 3-year survival rates were 75%, 60%, and 56% for the chemotherapy arm versus 45%, 25%, and 15% for the surgery arm alone. Pass and colleagues[159] also demonstrated benefit for neoadjuvant chemotherapy in a small study.

### Postoperative Adjuvant Chemotherapy or Chemoradiation

For resected stage I patients, a study in Helsinki, Finland, randomly assigned 110 patients to surgery versus surgery followed by cyclophosphamide (400 mg/m$^2$ ), doxorubicin (40 mg/m$^2$), cisplatin (40 mg/m$^2$) (CAP) every 4 weeks for 6 cycles. The recurrence rate was 48% for the control arm versus 31% for the postoperative CAP arm ($P = .01$) with a 56% 5-year survival rate for the control arm versus 67% for the CAP arm.[213] Of note, the clinical characteristics of the patients were disparate in favor of the CAP arm. A Lung Cancer Study Group phase III trial of 269 patients randomly assigned to CAP or no treatment with resected stage I disease, 4 cycles every 3 weeks, showed no difference in time to recurrence or overall survival at 3.8 years.[214]

A phase III trial in resected stage II and III patients by the Lung Cancer Study Group compared CAP with intrapleural bacille Calmette-Guérin (BCG) plus levamisole as an adjuvant to surgery. Although a significant increase in disease-free survival and overall survival was demonstrated, several phase III trials of levamisole in lung cancer have shown inferior survival compared with control arms without levamisole.[144]

A phase III study from Japan randomly assigned resected stage IIIA NSCLC patients to postoperative cisplatin (80 mg/m$^2$) and vindesine every 4 weeks for 3 courses or to no therapy. The 3-year survival rate was 37% for the chemotherapy arm versus 42% for the control arm.[215]

A multi-institutional French study randomly assigned 267 patients with resected NSCLC to either postoperative 60-Gy radiation or 3 cycles of cyclophosphamide, doxorubicin, CCN4, vincristine, and cisplatin every 4 weeks followed by radiation. Three percent had stage I, 27% had stage II, and 70% had stage IIIA disease. At follow-up (minimal 6 years), there was no difference in either disease-free survival ($P = .47$) or overall survival ($P = .68$).[216]

A phase III trial from Memorial Sloan-Kettering Cancer Center randomly assigned 72 patients with T1–3 N2 M0 to surgery plus postoperative radiation or postoperative radiation plus vindesine and cisplatin (120 mg/m$^2$ on days 1, 29, 71, and 113). Median survival of the chemotherapy arm was 17.5 months versus 24.5 months for the control arm.[217] The 1-, 2-, and 5-year survival rates were 72%, 31%, and 17% with chemotherapy versus 66%, 44%, and 30% for the control arm. Thus, although several large randomized trials have addressed the issue of postoperative adjuvant therapy, no survival benefit has emerged. Postoperative radiation therapy does reduce local recurrence.

## Combined Modality Therapy for Stage IIIB Non–Small Cell Lung Cancer

For patients with a good performance status, randomized trials and meta-analyses showed that chemotherapy improves survival in stage IIIB patients when added to radiotherapy. Combined modality therapy is associated with a 14- to 18-month median survival in both SCLC and NSCLC.

# CHEMOTHERAPY

## Chemotherapy for Advanced Disease

Over the past few years, newer active chemotherapeutic agents (vinorelbine, paclitaxel, docetaxel, and gemcitabine) have been shown to improve survival and symptoms in patients with stages IIIB and IV NSCLC.[218] Best supportive care regimens (including palliative radiotherapy) produce median survivals of 16 to 17 weeks, with only 10% to 15% of patients alive at 1 year.[219–221] Meta-analyses of multiple randomized trials conducted comparing best supportive care with cisplatin-based chemotherapy combinations demonstrated a modest improvement of 10 weeks in the median survival with a 10% increase in 1-year survival. Combination chemotherapy (cisplatin plus other drug) was superior to single-drug therapy. These combinations also were shown to improve quality of life.

A variety of new agents have been tested in multiple phase I and II trials. These drugs include two taxanes, paclitaxel and docetaxel; two topoisomerase I inhibitors, irinotecan and topotecan; one novel antimetabolite, gemcitabine; and a novel vinca alkaloid, vinorelbine. All agents produced response rates greater than 20% (with the exception of topotecan) with a median survival of 40 weeks. As a result of the activity of these new agents, a number of phase II trials were conducted with the combination of a new agent with cisplatin or carboplatin (Table 46.13). These studies all showed higher response rates for the combination than those reported for either agent alone.

### Randomized Phase III Studies

A phase III trial comparing gemcitabine plus cisplatin to etoposide plus cisplatin revealed a 40.6% response rate

**Table 46.13** PHASE II STUDIES OF NEW DRUGS + CISPLATIN OR CARBOPLATIN

| Agent | No. of Studies* | No. of Patients | Total CR + PR (%) | Median Survival (Weeks) | No. of Studies† | % 1-Year Survival | No. of Studies‡ |
|---|---|---|---|---|---|---|---|
| Vinorelbine + cisplatin | 7 | 328 | 135 (41) | 38 | 7 | 35–40§ | 1 |
| Paclitaxel + cisplatin | 8 | 286 | 121 (42) | 42 | 3 | 36 | 3 |
| Paclitaxel + carboplatin | 8 | 333 | 137 (46) | 38 | 4 | 40 | 4 |
| Docetaxel + cisplatin | 5 | 255 | 88 (35) | 35 | 3 | 58 | 1 |
| Gemcitabine + cisplatin | 6 | 245 | 114 (47) | 57 | 2 | 61 | 1 |
| Trinotecan + cisplatin | 7 | 185 | 81 (44) | 34 | 1 | NR | NR |
| Topotecan + cisplatin | 1 | 22 | 3 (22) | 32 | 1 | 26 | 1 |

Reproduced from Bunn P, Kelly K: New chemotherapeutic agents prolong survival and improve quality of life in non-small cell lung cancer: A review of the literature and future directions. Clin Cancer Res 5:1087–1100, 1998, with permission.
*Number of studies reporting results.
†Number of studies with median survival data.
‡Number of studies with 1-year survival data.
§Personal communication, Glaxo Wellcome.
CR = complete response; NR = not reported; PR = partial response.

for gemcitabine plus cisplatin versus a 21.9% response for the etoposide plus cisplatin combination, respectively.[222] Furthermore, the cisplatin plus gemcitabine combination had a significant delay in time to disease progression, 6.9 months versus 4.3 months for the cisplatin plus etoposide combination. There was no impairment of quality of life. Survival time was 8.7 months for the gemcitabine plus cisplatin arm and 7.2 months for the etoposide plus cisplatin arm, although the study was not sufficiently powered to show a difference in survival. Overall, the toxicity profiles for the drugs in each arm were similar.

In a randomized phase III study conducted by the Southwest Oncology Group comparing cisplatin to cisplatin plus vinorelbine, response rates of 12% and 26%, respectively, were observed.[223] The 1- and 2-year survival rates for the cisplatin arm were 20% and 6%, respectively, compared with 36% and 12% for the cisplatin plus vinorelbine arm, demonstrating the superiority of the combination. Similarly, a phase III trial comparing cisplatin to cisplatin plus gemcitabine revealed 31% versus 9.1% response rate in favor of the combination, with an interim survival analysis favoring the combination (8.7 vs. 7.6 months).[224]

Although there are few studies that specifically report on quality of life rather than objective response rates, all studies do show symptom relief for most patients. A randomized study conducted in the United Kingdom demonstrated an improved quality of life and prolonged survival for patients receiving a cisplatin-based combination regimen.[225] In the EORTC randomized study that compared paclitaxel plus cisplatin to teniposide plus cisplatin, the former combination was associated with a superior quality of life.[226]

Survival data with the newer chemotherapeutic agents are similar to those obtained in advanced SCLC (Table 46.14). In advanced NSCLC, the paclitaxel plus cisplatin combination produced median survivals of 40 to 43 weeks in phase III studies of EORTC and Eastern Cooperative Oncology Group, with a 40% 1-year survival rate.[226, 227] In contrast, a study in extensive-stage SCLC from the Southeast Cancer Study Group and Japanese Study Group comparing cisplatin plus etoposide to cyclophosphamide plus doxorubicin plus vincristine versus the alternation of the two combinations reported median survival of 37 and 36 weeks with a 1-year survival rate of 30%.[228, 229]

## Chemotherapy for Small Cell Lung Cancer

Combination chemotherapy for limited-stage disease usually produces overall response rates of 80% to 95%, with 50% to 60% complete responses and a median survival of 12 to 20 months. For patients with extensive-stage disease, overall response rates are 60% to 80% and complete response rates are 15% to 20%, with a median survival of 7 to 11 months. In 1974, patients with SCLC were treated with cyclophosphamide plus doxorubicin plus vincristine (CAV) combined with thoracic irradiation and PCI.[230] The remarkable chemosensitivity of SCLC was documented with significant improvement in quality of life and survival. Median survivals improved from 7 weeks to 6 to 10 months. Despite the routine response of this disease to chemotherapy, most patients relapse within 1 year, even those (10% to 20%) who achieved a complete response.

The combination of cisplatin plus etoposide (PE) is the most common drug regimen used and should be considered the standard of care. In studies that randomly assigned patients to PE versus CAV,[231, 232] patients receiving PE had improved response rates but similar survival to those receiving CAV. PE used as salvage, for those patients failing CAV, produced response rates twice as high as CAV given as salvage after PE. In patients with limited-stage disease who received 2 cycles of PE after 6 cycles of CAV with or without chest irradiation, a 30-

**Table 46.14 COMPARISON OF RESULTS OF PHASE III TRIALS WITH SMALL CELL LUNG CANCER (SCLC) AND NON–SMALL CELL LUNG CANCER (NSCLC)**

| | Extensive Stage | | | | Limited Stage | | | |
|---|---|---|---|---|---|---|---|---|
| | SCLC | | NSCLC | | SCLC | | NSCLC | |
| | *SECSG* | *JSG* | *ECOG* | *EORTC* | *SWOG* | *ECOG* | *SWOG* | *CALGB* |
| No. of patients | 140 | 51 | 198 | 168 | 215 | 186 | 126 | 78 |
| Median survival | 37 wk | 36 wk | 43 wk | 41 wk | 15.5 mo | 18.6 mo | 15 mo | 14 mo |
| % 1-year survival | 30 wk | 30 wk | 40 wk | NR | 35* | 43* | 25 mo | 25 mo |
| % 4-year survival | | | | | 20 | NR | 22 | 20 |

Reproduced from Bunn P Jr, Kelly K: New chemotherapeutic agents prolong survival and improve quality of life in non-small cell lung cancer: A review of the literature and future directions. Clin Cancer Res 5:1087–1100, 1998, with permission.

*2-year survival percentages.

CALGB = Cancer and Leukemia Group B; ECOG = Eastern Cooperative Oncology Group; EORTC = European Organization for Research and Treatment of Cancer; JSG = Japanese Study Group; NR = not reported; SECSG = Southeast Cancer Study Group.

week survival advantage for the PE arm was demonstrated.[233]

Substituting carboplatin or cisplatin reduces gastrointestinal toxicity but increases myelosuppression.[234] Addition of ifosfamide to PE improved median survival by 1 month in a single trial.[235] Oral etoposide has been shown to be inferior in numerous studies.[236–238]

### Dose Intensity

Numerous phase III studies have evaluated standard versus escalating doses of cyclophosphamide-based chemotherapy without any apparent benefit. Similarly, a National Cancer Institute (NCI) study that examined standard versus escalated doses of PE failed to demonstrate an advantage for the higher doses.[239]

### Second-Line Therapy

In two studies that used CAV as second-line therapy, response rates of 13% and 28% were noted.[240, 241] Topotecan, a topisomerase I inhibitor, as a single agent has shown response rates of 21.7%, 14%, and 19% in phase II trials.[242–244] A meta-analysis of these data produces an overall response rate of 18%, with a median survival of 30 weeks.[245] In a study of 211 patients comparing CAV with topotecan for relapsed SCLC, response rates were 24.3% (topotecan) versus 18.3% (CAV), with median survivals of 25.0 and 24.7 weeks, respectively. Control of symptoms appeared improved for the topotecan arm.[246] Therefore, topotecan is an acceptable second-line therapy for relapsed SCLC.

There have been numerous small trials testing newer chemotherapeutic agents such as vinorelbine, irinotecan, gemcitabine, taxol, and docetaxel for relapsed SCLC, but no randomized studies have been published.

### Maintenance Therapy

Maintenance therapy after induction chemotherapy for SCLC is controversial. Of 13 trials published since 1980, 1 trial shows a statistically significant survival advantage whereas 5 show some survival advantage for subsets of patients.[247] Six trials showed no difference and one trial showed reduced survival with maintenance.[247] Presently, the Eastern Cooperative Oncology Group is conducting a trial comparing observation to 4 cycles of topotecan after 4 cycles of PE therapy.

### Chemotherapy in Special Clinical Settings

For patients with superior vena cava syndrome, chemotherapy was shown to be as effective as chemotherapy plus chest irradiation in providing rapid palliation of symptoms.[248] Chemotherapy alone therefore may be appropriate for patients who otherwise would not receive radiation. Although cranial irradiation is administered to patients who develop brain metastases, chemotherapy also may induce regression.[249–251] Although the data would not support this as a routine approach outside of a clinical trial, it is reasonable in patients who progress or relapse in the brain after initial irradiation therapy. In general, most of the paraneoplastic syndromes associated with SCLC respond to chemotherapy, except Eaton-Lambert syndrome.

## GUIDELINES

The recommendations proposed in this chapter should be considered as guidelines for the care of lung cancer patients. Therapy, however, always should be individualized after taking into account the patient's age, comorbid conditions, performance status, and personal needs and wishes. The flow diagrams in Figures 46.2 to 46.6 outline strategies to be considered in the management of patients by stage of disease.

## SOLITARY PULMONARY NODULES

Approximately 150,000 new solitary pulmonary nodules (SPNs) are diagnosed each year in the United States. Of these, 45,000 require no additional workup other than a careful history and review of a prior CXR, whereas 105,000 cases require further evaluation.[252] The primary objective is to identify malignant nodules for surgical excision. Further testing almost always involves a CT scan followed by a biopsy or surgery if the scan is positive. Although CT technology continues to evolve, lack of specificity is an ongoing problem, with a significant number of false-positive results. Transthoracic needle aspiration biopsy is the method of choice for biopsy of an SPN together with fluoroscopy, CT, or ultrasonography. This procedure has a false-negative rate of 10% to 25%. Therefore, effective alternative diagnostic tests are required. Fiberoptic bronchoscopy is of limited value because most nodules are not accessible by bronchoscopy.[253, 254] Video-assisted thoracoscopy is performed under general anesthesia and involves inserting a small operating thoracoscope directly into the thorax. Malignant nodules can be resected immediately, however, malignant tissue may not be removed entirely. This procedure is 100% sensitive and specific. PET scanning for diagnostic workup of SPNs is growing. Specificity may be compromised by increased FDG uptake by active tuberculosis, histoplasmosis, or abscess, but the overall accuracy of PET warrants continued use. To model quantitatively the cost-effectiveness of various management strategies for SPNs, four decision trees were compared: watch and wait, surgery, CT, and CT plus PET.[252] Through the use of an incremental cost-effectiveness model, the CT plus PET strategy was the most cost-effective over a large pretest likelihood (probability of having a malignant nodule). This decision-making tree is illustrated in Figure 46.7.

## ECONOMIC ISSUES

Lung cancer represents 2% of all health-care costs and about 20% of all cancer care costs in the United States.[255] This constitutes about $8 billion to the U.S. health-care system.[256] Evans and colleagues,[256] using a lung cancer costing model, have reported that the total health-care costs to the Canadian system for an individual patient with NSCLC treated with radiation only was $14,110 versus $12,474 for surgery alone versus $17,889 for

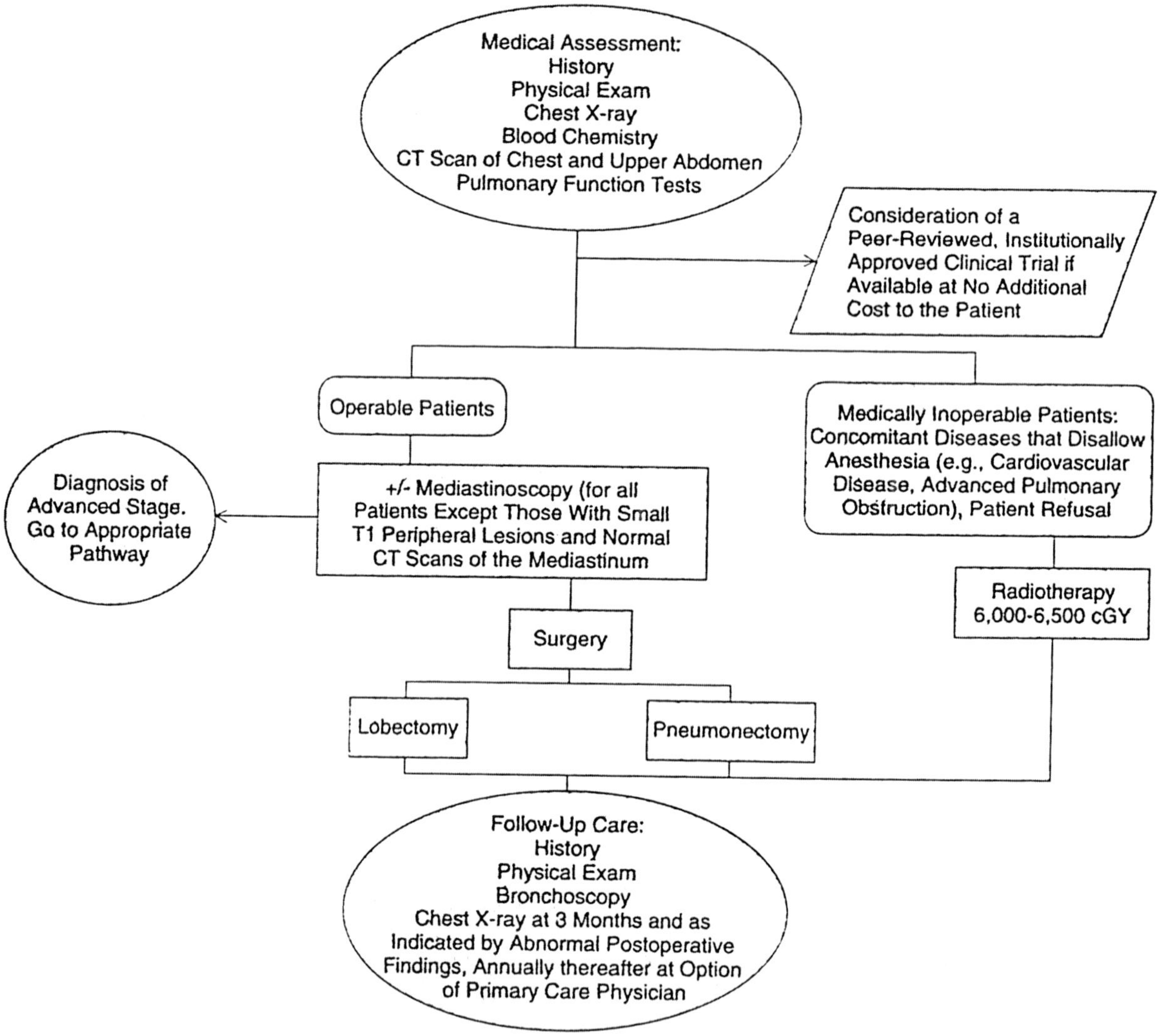


**Figure 46.2** Management of clinical stage I non-small cell lung cancer. (Reproduced from Cameron R, Fringer J, Taylor C, et al: Practice guidelines for non-small cell lung cancer. The Cancer J 2(3A suppl): S61–S68, 1996.)

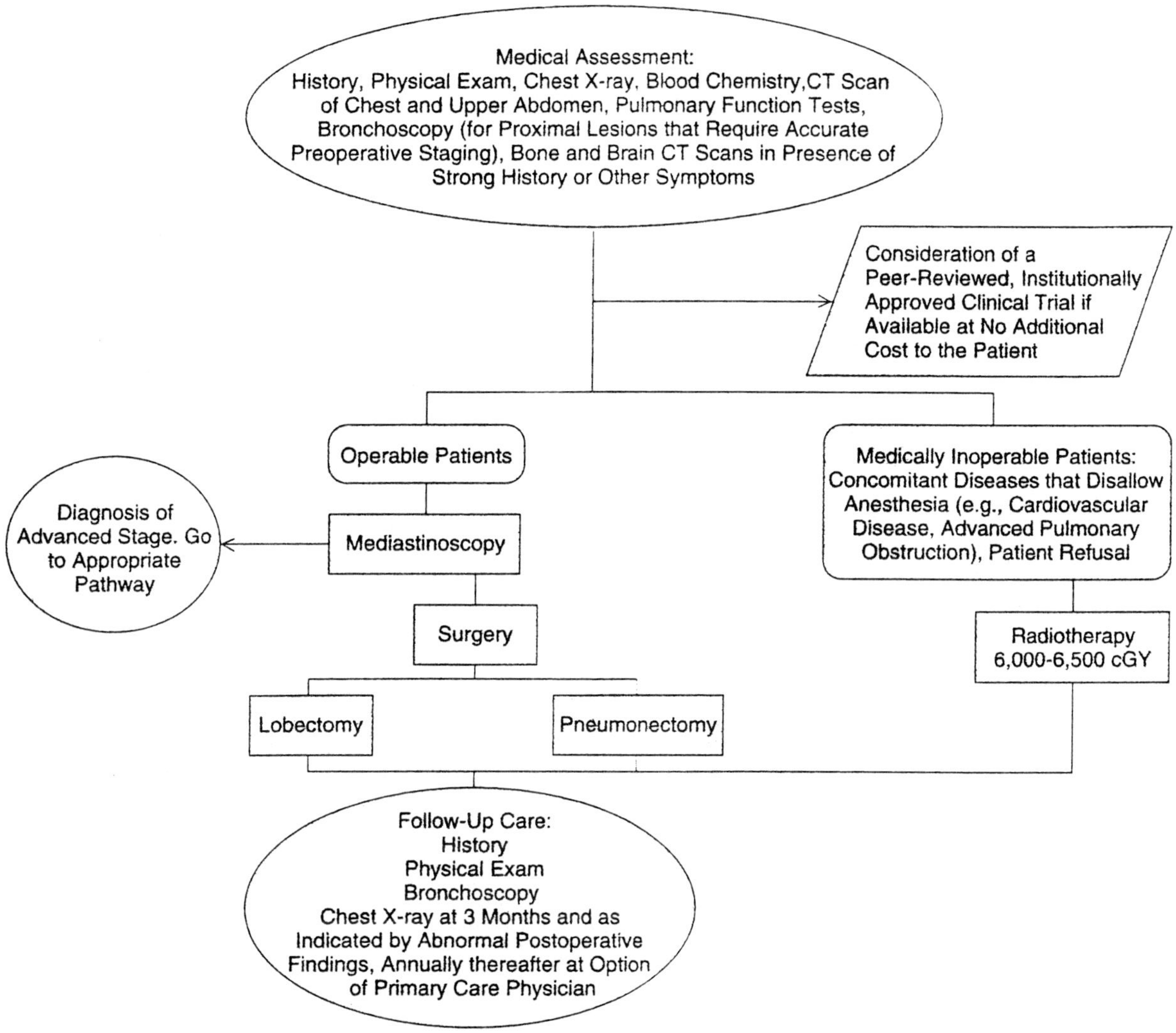


**Figure 46.3** Management of clinical stage II non-small cell lung cancer. (Reproduced from Cameron R, Fringer J, Taylor C, et al: Practice guidelines for non-small cell lung cancer. The Cancer J 2(3A suppl): S61–S68, 1996.)

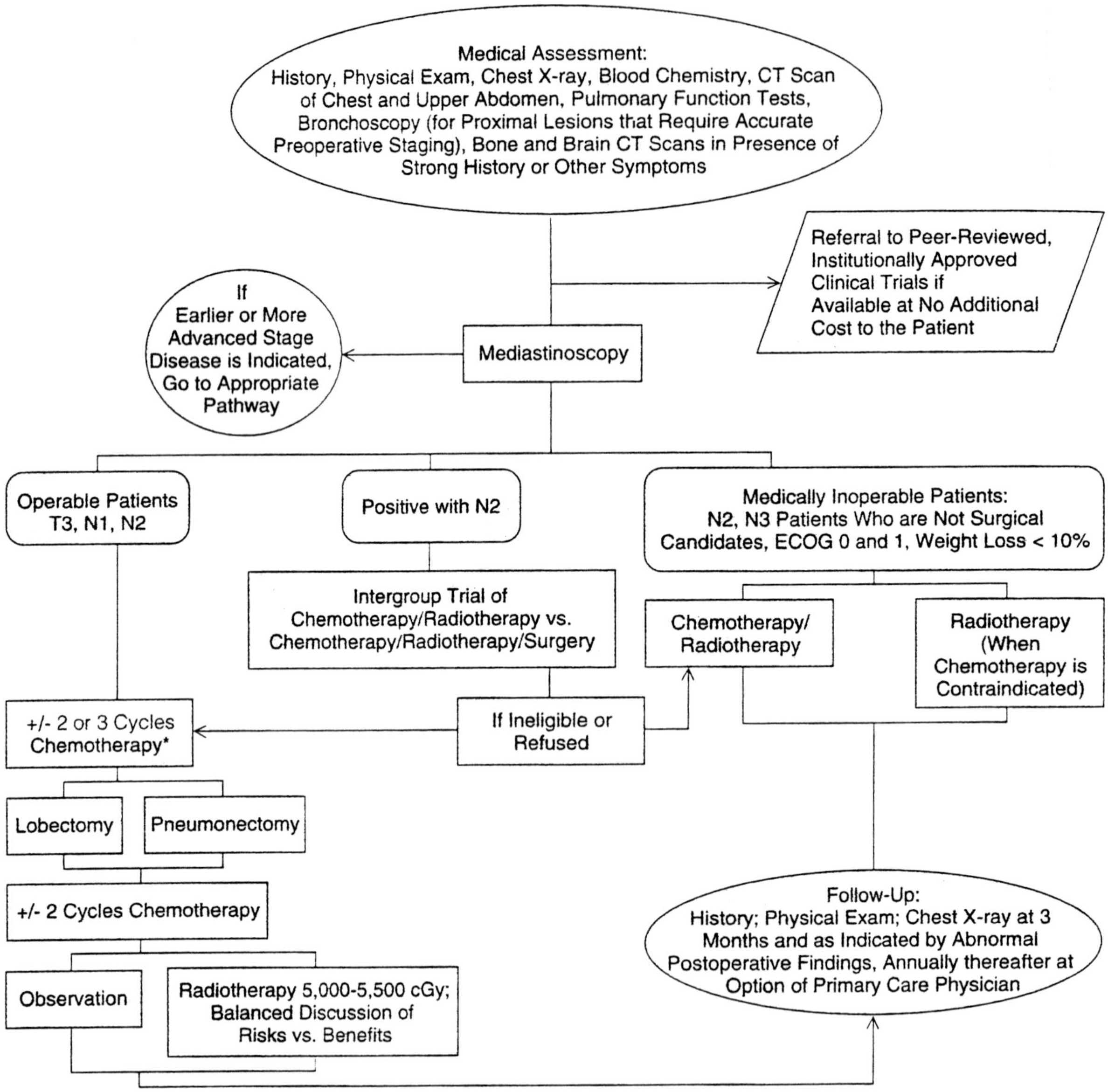


**Figure 46.4** Management of clinical stage IIIA non-small cell lung cancer. (Reproduced from Cameron R, Fringer J, Taylor C, et al: Practice guidelines for non-small cell lung cancer. The Cancer J 2(3A suppl): S61–S68, 1996.)

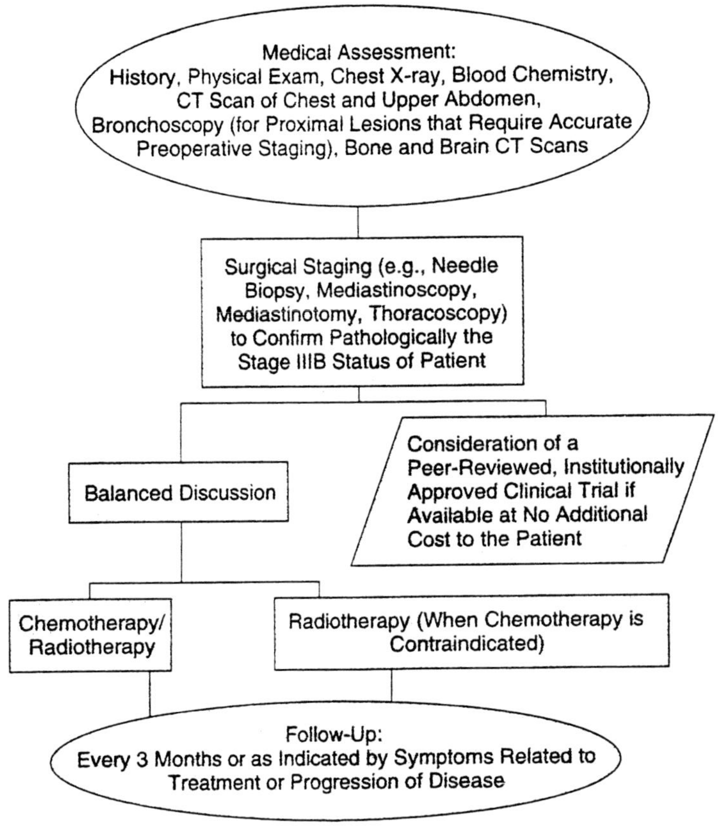


**Figure 46.5** Management of clinical stage IIIB non-small cell lung cancer. (Reproduced from Cameron R, Fringer J, Taylor C, et al: Practice guidelines for non-small cell lung cancer. The Cancer J 2(3A suppl): S61–S68, 1996.)

surgery plus radiation therapy (1988 Canadian dollars). Management of localized NSCLC cost $18,691 (Canadian dollars). For all stages of disease, hospitalization was the major cost. Despite growing evidence that combined modality therapy and combination chemotherapy induces remissions and prolongs survival, many patients with lung cancer do not have an opportunity to pursue these therapies. Although economic data demonstrate the cost-effectiveness of these strategies, the reluctance to offer these interventions to patients still remains. Evans and colleagues[256] showed that this may in part be the result of the absolute cost of introducing new treatments. Standard radiation therapy per patient for stages IIIA and IIIB disease is estimated to cost $16,086 and $13,391, respectively (Canadian dollars). When patients relapse, their diagnostic workup ($2,141 Canadian dollars) and supportive or palliative care ($17,575 Canadian dollars) increase costs significantly.[257] Thus, assuming that relapse will occur, the average cost to care for one patient with stage IIIA lung cancer is $34,595 (Canadian dollars) versus $31,928 (Canadian dollars) for stage IIIB lung cancer. Evaluating the cost-effectiveness of the combined modality strategies in patients with stage III disease, the costs associated with neoadjuvant therapy for stage IIIA and combined modality therapy for stage IIIB are acceptable.[257]

For advanced NSCLC, data on economic costs are again derived from Canadian studies that compared best supportive care with two cisplatin regimens.[258] Best supportive care costs ($8,595, 1984 Canadian dollars) were for a median survival of 17 weeks. Costs of the two chemotherapy arms were $7,645 and $12,232, respectively, with a median survival of 33 weeks for the higher costing arm. The extra costs were $3,637 for 16 additional weeks of life, which calculates into $11,820 per year of added life. For vinorelbine and cisplatin, the cost-effectiveness per year gained was $17,700.[259] In comparing the cost of treating patients with gemcitabine versus cisplatin plus etoposide, the gemcitabine therapy was less expensive, saving $1,500 to $7,000 per cycle.[260]

Although the costs of therapy for NSCLC are well within the range of other accepted medical therapies, efforts to reduce tobacco use should be vigorously pursued. Reducing tobacco consumption will likely be associated with enhanced quality of life and a net economic benefit.

## SUMMARY

This chapter reviews thc complex subject of bronchogenic carcinoma with emphasis on its clinical aspects, diagnosis, and treatment. Surgical therapy remains the treatment of choice, and considerable improvement has been made in selecting patients for operation and in determining their prognosis. New schedules of radiation therapy and new drugs for chemotherapy have extended survival and improved the quality of life. But much remains to be done, however, to improve overall 5-year survival rate from its present dismal 14%. Because bronchogenic carcinoma is, for the most part, a preventable disease, people must be persuaded to stop smoking cigarettes or, better yet, not to start at all. That is the fastest and most certain way of

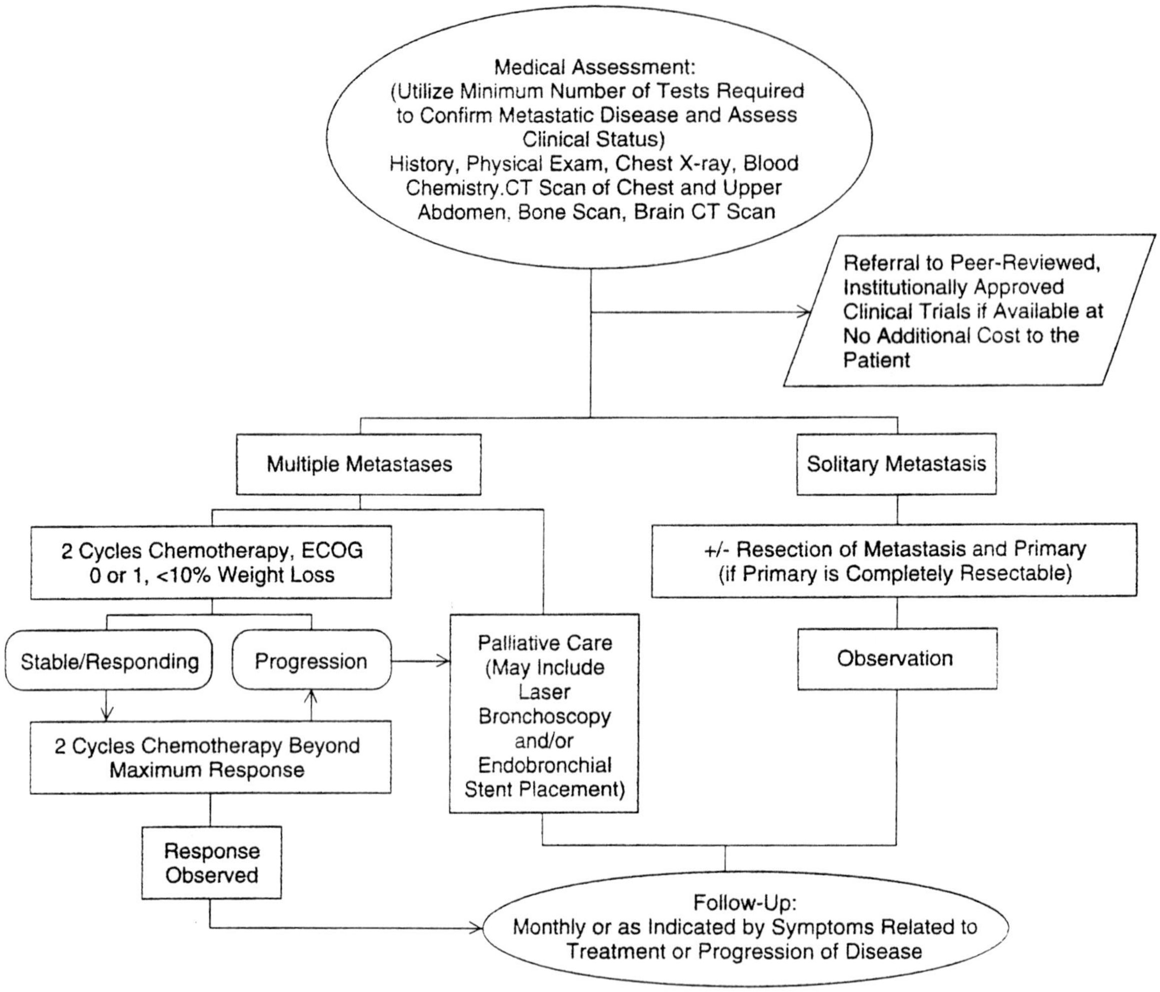


**Figure 46.6** Management of clinical stage IV non-small cell lung cancer. (Reproduced from Cameron R, Fringer J, Taylor C, et al: Practice guidelines for non-small cell lung cancer. The Cancer J 2(3A suppl): S61–S68, 1996.)

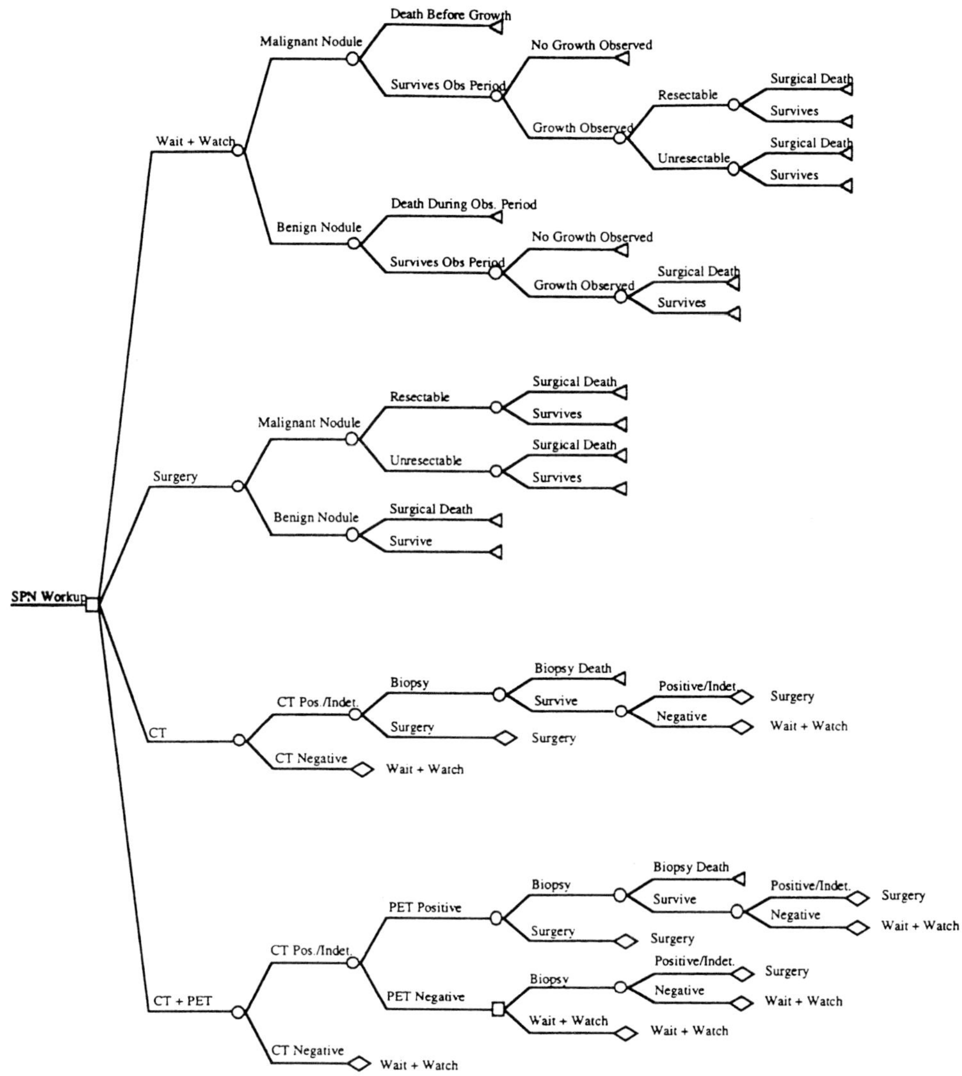


**Figure 46.7** Flow diagram of the four strategies analyzed. (Reproduced from Gambhir SS, Shepard JE, Shah BD, et al: Analytical decision model for the cost-effective management of solitary pulmonary nodules. J Clin Oncol 16:2113–2125, 1998.)

saving the lives of the more than 100,000 persons in the United States who will die each year in the foreseeable future from this prevalent cancer that kills more men and women than any other malignancy.

## References


1. Pierce JT, Frome MC, Novotny TE, et al: Trends in cigarette smoking in the United States: Projections to the year 2000. JAMA 261:61–65, 1989.
2. Landis SH, Murray T, Bolden S, et al: Cancer statistics, 1999. CA Cancer J Clin 49:8–31, 1999.
3. Satariano WA: Racial differences in cancer incidence: The significance of age-specific patterns. Cancer 62:2640–2653, 1988.
4. Wynder EL, Hoffman D: Tobacco and health: A societal challenge. N Engl J Med 300:894–903, 1979.
5. Bartecchi CE: The human costs of tobacco use (1). N Engl J Med 330:907–912, 1994.
6. Health Consequences of Smoking for Women: A Report of the Surgeon General. Rockville, MD: Dept of Health & Human Services, 1980.
7. Shopland DR, Eyre HJ, Pechacek TF: Smoking-attributable cancer mortality in 1991: Is lung cancer now the leading cause of death among smokers in the United States? J Natl Cancer Inst 83:1142–1148, 1991.
8. Update changes in notifiable disease surveillance data—United States 1992–1993. MMWR Morb Mortal Wkly Rep 42:824–836, 1993.
9. Wynder EL: The etiology, epidemiology, and prevention of lung cancer. Semin Respir Med 3:135–139, 1982.
10. Benowitz NL: Influence of smoking fewer cigarettes on exposure to tar, nicotine, and carbon monoxide. N Engl J Med 309:139–141, 1986.
11. Wynder EL: The effect of low-yield cigarette smoking on lung cancer risk. Cancer 62:1223–1230, 1988.
12. Lenfant C: Are "low-yield" cigarettes really safer? N Engl J Med 309:181–182, 1983.
13. Benowitz NL: Influence of smoking fewer cigarettes on exposure to tar, nicotine, and carbon monoxide. N Engl J Med 315:1310, 1986.
14. Denissenko MF, Pao A, Tang M et al: Preferential formation of benzo[a]pyrene adducts at lung cancer mutational hotspots in p53. Science 274:430–432, 1996.

15. Eriksen, MP, LeMaistre CA, Newell GR: Health hazards of passive smoking. Ann Rev Public Health 1998 9:47–70, 1988.
16. Janerich DT, Thompson WD, Varela LR: Lung cancer and exposure to tobacco smoke in the household. N Engl J Med 323:632–636, 1990.
17. Fleiss, JL, Gross AJ: Meta-analysis in epidemiology, with special reference to studies of the association between exposure to tobacco smoke and lung cancer: A critique. J Clin Epidemiol 44:127–139, 1991.
18. Fontham ETH, Correa P, Wu-Williams A, et al: Lung cancer in nonsmoking women: A multicenter case-control study. Cancer Epidemiol Biomarkers Prev 1:35–43, 1991.
19. Janerich DT: Lung cancer and exposure to tobacco smoke in the household. N Engl J Med 323:632, 1990.
20. Khuder S, Dayal H, Mutgi A, et al: Effect of cigarette smoking on major histological types of lung cancer in men. Lung Cancer 22:15–21, 1998.
21. Holoye PY, Shirinian M. Adjuvant surgery in the multimodality treatment of small-cell lung cancer: Department of Medical Oncology, University of Texas M.D. Anderson Cancer Center, Houston. Am J Clin Oncol 14:231–251, 1991.
22. Lubin JH: Lung cancer risk with cigar and pipe use. J Natl Cancer Inst 73:377, 1984.
23. Connolly GN: The reemergence of smokeless tobacco. N Engl J Med 314:1020, 1986.
24. Whittemore AS, McMillan A: Lung cancer mortality among U.S. uranium miners: A reappraisal. J Natl Cancer Inst 71:489–500, 1983.
25. Samet JM: Health effects and sources of indoor air pollution. Part II. Am Rev Respir Dis 137:221, 1988.
26. Logue J: Health hazards associated with elevated levels of indoor radon. MMWR Morbid Mortal Wkly Rep 34:657, 1985.
27. Samet JM: Indoor radon and lung cancer. N Engl J Med 320:591, 1989.
28. Tokuhata GK, Lilenfeld AM: Familial aggregation of lung cancer in humans. J Natl Cancer Inst 30:289–312, 1963.
29. Ooi WL, Elston RC, Chen VW, et al: Increased familiar risk for lung cancer. J Natl Cancer Inst 76:217–222, 1986.
30. Sellers TA, Elston RC, Rothschild H: Familial risk of cancer among randomly selected cancer probands. Genet Epidemiol 5:381–392, 1988.
31. Bartsch H, Petruzzelli S, De Flora S, et al: Carcinogen metabolism in human lung tissues and the effect of tobacco smoking: Results from a case-control multicenter study on lung cancer patients. Environ Health Perspect 98:119–124, 1992.
32. Bartsch H, Hietanen E, Petruzzelli S, et al: Possible prognostic value of pulmonary AH-locus-linked enzymes in patients with tobacco-related lung cancer. Int J Cancer 46:185–188, 1990.
33. Ayesh R, Idle SR, Ritchie JC, et al: Metabolic oxidation phenotypes as markers for susceptibility to lung cancer. Nature 312:169–170, 1984.
34. Crespi CL, Penman BW, Gelboin HV, et al: A tobacco smoke-derived nitrosamine, 4-(methylnitrosamino)-1-(3 pyridyl)-1-butanone, is activated by multiple human cytochrome P450s including the polymorphic human cytochrome P4502D6. Carcinogenesis 12:1197–1201, 1991.
35. Brincker H: The incidence of malignant tumors in patients with respiratory sarcoidosis. Br J Cancer 29:247, 1974.
36. Godeau P: Bronchioloalveolar carcinoma and scleroderma: Report of a case and review of the literature. Semin Hop Paris 50:1161, 1974.
37. Lee BY, Guerra J, Cagir B, et al: Pulmonary scar carcinoma: Report of three cases and review of the literature. Mil Med 160:537–541, 1995.
38. Bakris GL: Pulmonary scar carcinoma: A clinicopathologic analysis. Cancer 52:493, 1983.
39. Hollstein M, Shomer B, Greenblatt D, et al: Somatic point mutations in the p53 gene of human tumors and cell lines: Updated compilation. Nucleic Acid Res 24:141–146, 1996.
40. Ryberg D, Kure E, Lystad S, et al: p53 mutations in lung tumors: relationship to putative susceptibility markers for cancer. J Cancer Res 54:1551–1555, 1994.
41. Field JK, Spandidos DA, Malliri A, et al: Elevated p53 expression correlates with a history of heavy smoking in squamous cell carcinoma of the head and neck. Br J Cancer 64:573–577, 1991.
42. Wang X, Christiani DC, Wiencke JK, et al: Mutations in the p53 gene in lung cancer are associated with cigarette smoking and asbestos exposure. Cancer Epidemiol Biomarkers Prev 4:543–548, 1995.
43. Kawajiri K, Eguchi H, Nakachi K, et al: Association of CYP1A1 germline polymorphisms with mutations of the p53 gene in lung cancer. Cancer Res 56:72–76, 1996.
44. Kondo K, Tsuzuki H, Sasa M, et al: A dose-response relationship between the frequency of p53 mutations and tobacco consumption in lung cancer patients. J Surg Oncol 61:20–26, 1996.
45. Koch WM, Patel H, Brennan J, et al: Squamous cell carcinoma of the head and neck in the elderly. Arch Otoloaryngol Head Neck Surg 121:262–265, 1995.
46. Slebos RJC, Hruban RH, Dalesio O, et al: Relationship between *K-ras* oncogene activation and smoking in adenocarcinoma of the human lung. J Natl Cancer Inst 83:1024–1027, 1991.
47. Husgafvel-Pursianinen K, Kackman P, Ridanpaa M, et al: *K-ras* mutations in human adenocarcinoma of the lung: Association with smoking and occupational exposure to asbestos. Int J Cancer 53:250–256, 1993.
48. Mao L, Lee JS, Kurie JM, et al: Frequent genetic alterations in bronchial epithelium of smokers. Proc Am Assoc Cancer Res 38:246, 1997.
49. Tomizawa Y, Nakajima T, Kohno T, et al: Clinicopathological significance of Fhit protein expression in stage I non–small cell lung carcinoma. Cancer Res 58:5478–5483, 1998.
50. Mountain CF: A system for the clinical staging of lung cancer. Am J Roentgenol Radium Ther Nucl Med 120:130, 1974.
50. Barkley JE, Green MR: Bronchioloalveolar carcinoma. J Clin Oncol 14:2377–2386, 1996.
51. Linnoila I: Pathology of non–small cell lung cancer: New diagnostic approaches. Hematol Oncol Clin North Am 4:1027, 1990.
52. Wu A: Secular trends in histologic types of lung cancer. J Natl Cancer Inst 77:53, 1986.
53. McDowell EM: The respiratory epithelium. V. Histogenesis of lung carcinoma in the human. J Natl Cancer Inst 61:587–606, 1978.
54. Paulson DL: Superior sulcus tumors: Results of combined therapy. NY State J Med 71:2050, 1971.
55. Lee JS: Involvement of chromosome 7 in primary lung tumor. Cancer Res 47:6349, 1987.
56. Meyer EC, Liebow AA: Relationship of interstitial pneumonia, honeycombing and atypical proliferation to cancer of the lung. Cancer 18:322–349, 1965.
57. Fraire AE, Greenberg SD: Carcinoma and diffuse interstitial fibrosis of the lung. Cancer 31:1078–1086, 1973.
58. Auerbach O, Garfinkel L: The changing pattern of lung adenocarcinoma. Cancer 68:1973–1977, 1991.
59. Ikeda T, Kurita Y, Inutsuka S, et al: The changing pattern of lung cancer by histologic type: A review of 1151 cases from a university hospital in Japan. 1970–1989. Lung Cancer 7:157–164, 1991.
60. Barksy SH, Cameron R, Osann KE, et al: Rising incidence of bronchoioloalveolar lung carcinoma and its clinicopathologic features. Cancer 73:1163–1170, 1994.
61. Bonne C: Morphological resemblance of pulmonary adenomatosis (jaagsiekte) in sheep and certain cases of cancer of the lung in man. Am J Cancer 35:491–501, 1939.
62. Nobel TA, Perk K: Bronchioloalveolar cell carninoma. Animal model: Pulmonary adenomatosis of sheep, pulmonary carcinoma of sheep (jaagsiekte). Am J Pathol 90:783–786, 1978.
63. Perk K, Hod I: Sheep lung carcinoma: An endemic analogue of a sporadic human neoplasm. J Natl Cancer Inst 69:747–779, 1982.
64. Heiman HL, Samuel E: Pulmonary adenomatosis: Case report. S Afr Med J 29:934–935, 1953.
65. Graziano S: The use of neuroendocrine immunoperoxidase markers to predict chemotherapy response in patients with non–small-cell lung cancer. J Clin Oncol 7:1398, 1989.
66. Kreyberg L: Histologic typing of lung tumors. *In* Kreyberg L (ed): International Histologic Classification of Tumors, No. 1. Geneva: World Health Organization, 1987, p. 19.
67. Hirsch FR, Matthews MJ, Aisner S, et al: Histopathologic classification of small cell lung cancer: Changing concepts and terminology. Cancer 62:973–977, 1988.

68. Kulke MH, Mayer RJ: Carcinoid tumors. N Engl J Med 340: 858–868, 1999.
69. Smith RA: Bronchial carcinoid tumours. Thorax 24:43, 1969.
70. Hajdu SI: Carcinoid tumors. A study of 204 cases. Am J Clin Pathol 61:521, 1974.
71. Godwin JD II: Carcinoid tumors. An analysis of 2,837 cases. Cancer 36:560, 1975.
72. Yousem SA: Mucoepidermoid tumors of the lung. Cancer 60:1346, 1987.
73. Figlin R, Holmes EC, Turrisi AT III: Neoplasms of the lung, pleura, and mediastinum. *In* Haskell CM: Cancer Treatment. Philadelphia: WB Saunders, 1995, pp 385–413.
74. Ebeling K, Nischan P: Screening for lung cancer: Results from a case-control study. Int J Cancer 40:141–144, 1987.
75. Kubik A, Parkin DM, Khlat M, et al: Lack of benefit from semi-annual screening for cancer of the lung: Follow-up report of a randomized controlled trial on a population of high-risk males in Czechoslovakia. Int J Cancer 45:26–33, 1990.
76. Hillerdal G: Long-term survival of patients with lung cancer from a defined geographical area before and after radiological screening. Lung Cancer 15:21–30, 1996.
77. Tockman MS: Sensitive and specific monoclonal antibody recognition of human lung cancer antigen on preserved sputum cells: A new approach to early lung cancer detection. J Clin Oncol 6:1685, 1988.
78. Tockman MS, Mulshine JL, Piantadosi S, et al: Prospective detection of preclinical lung cancer: Results from two studies of heterogeneous nuclear ribonucleoprotein A2/B1 overexpression. Clin Cancer Res 3:2237–2246, 1997.
79. Sone S, Takashima S, Li F, et al: Mass screening for lung cancer with mobile spiral computed tomography scanner. Lancet 351:1242–1245, 1998.
80. Weiss W: The Philadelphia Pulmonary Neoplasm Research Project: Symptoms in occult lung cancer. Chest 73:57, 1978.
81. Levin KH: Paraneoplastic neuromuscular syndromes. Neurol Clin 15:597–614, 1997.
81a. Nakao YK, Motomura M, Suenaga A, et al: Specificity of omega-conotoxin MVIIC-binding and -blocking calcium channel antibodies in Lambert-Eaton myasthenic syndrome. J Neurol 246:38–44, 1999.
81b. Lucchinetti CF, Kimmel DW, Lennon VA: Paraneoplastic and oncologic profiles of patients seropositive for type I antineuronal nuclear antibodies. Neurology 50:652–657, 1998.
82. Barnes BE: Dermatomyositis and malignancy. Ann Intern Med 84:68–76, 1976.
82a. Zuger M, Demarmels-Biasiutti F, Wuillemin WA, et al: Subcutaneous low-molecular weight heparin for treatment of Trousseau's syndrome. Ann Hematol 75:165–167, 1997.
83. Sorensen JB, Andersen MK, Hansen HH: Syndrome of inappropriate secretion of antidiuretic hormone (SIADH) in malignant disease. J Intern Med 238:97–110, 1995.
83a. Takai E, Yano T, Iguchi H, et al: Tumor-induced hypercalcemia and parathyroid-related protein in lung carcinoma. Cancer 78:1384–1387, 1996.
83b. Arioglu E, Doppman J, Gomes M, et al: Cushing's syndrome caused by corticotropin secretion by pulmonary tumorlets. N Engl J Med 339:883–886, 1998.
83c. Matte J, Roufosse F, Rocmans P, et al: Ectopic Cushing's syndrome and pulmonary carcinoid tumour identified by [$^{111}$In-DTPA-D-Phe]octreotide. Postgrad Med J 74:108–110, 1998.
84. Levenson RM, Ihde DC, Matthews MJ, et al: Small cell carcinoma presenting as an extrapulmonary neoplasm: Sites of origin and response to chemotherapy. J Natl Cancer Inst 67:607, 1981.
85. Remick SC, Hafez GR, Carbone PP: Extrapulmonary small cell carcinoma: A review of the literature with emphasis on therapy and outcome. Medicine 110:707, 1984.
86. Lowe VJ, Naunheim KS: Current role of positron emission tomography in thoracic oncology. Thorax 53:703–712, 1998.
87. Kanhouwa SB: Reliability of cytologic typing of lung cancer. Acta Cytol (Baltimore) 20:229, 1976.
88. Gagneten CB: Diagnosis of bronchogenic carcinoma through the cytologic examination of sputum, with special reference to tumor typing. Acta Cytol (Baltimore) 20:530, 1976.
89. Pavy RD: Percutaneous aspiration biopsy of discrete lung lesions. Cancer 34:2109, 1974.
90. Lalli AF: Aspiration biopsies of chest lesions. Radiology 127:35, 1978.
91. Westcott JL: Percutaneous needle aspiration of hilar and mediastinal masses. Radiology 141:323, 1981.
92. Gibney RTN: Aspiration biopsy in the diagnosis of pulmonary disease. Chest 80:300, 1981.
93. Lam S, Kennedy T, Unger M, et al: Localization of bronchial intraepithelial neoplastic lesions by fluorescence bronchoscopy. Chest 113:696–702, 1998.
93a. George PJ: Fluorescence bronchoscopy for the early detection of lung cancer. Thorax 54:180–183, 1999.
94. Lassen U, Hansen HH: Small cell carcinoma of the Lung. *In* Haskells CM: Cancer Treatment. Philadelphia: WB Saunders, 1995, pp. 414–420.
95. Mountain CF: Lung cancer staging classification. Clin Chest Med 14:43–53, 1993.
96. Lince L: Carcinoma of the lung: A comparative series of 687 cases. Arch Surg 102:103, 1971.
97. Hyde L: Natural course of inoperable lung cancer. Chest 64:309, 1973.
98. Overholt RH: Primary cancer of the lung: A 42-year experience. Ann Thorac Surg 20:511, 1975.
99. Benfield JR: Current and future concepts of lung cancer. Ann Intern Med 83:93–106, 1975.
100. Cohen MH: Natural history of lung cancer. Clin Chest Med 3:229–241, 1982.
101. Deviri E: Carcinoma of lung with a solitary cerebral metastasis: Surgical management and review of the literature. Cancer 52:1507, 1983.
102. Sundaresan N: Surgical treatment of single brain metastasis from non–small cell lung cancer. Cancer Invest 3:107, 1985.
102a. Coleman RE: PET in lung cancer. J Nucl Med 40:814–820, 1999.
102b. Marom EM, McAdams HP, Erasmus JJ, et al: Staging non–small lung cancer with whole-body PET. Radiology 212:803–809, 1999.
103. Vansteenkiste JF, Stroobants SG, De Leyn PR, et al: Lymph node staging in non–small-cell lung cancer with FDG-PET scan: A prospective study on 690 lymph node stations from 68 patients. J Clin Oncol 16:2142–2149, 1998.
104. Mountain C: Revisions in the international system for staging lung cancer. Chest 111:1710–1717, 1997.
105. Mountain C, Dresler C: Regional lymph node classification for lung cancer staging. Chest 111:1718–1723, 1997.
106. Urschel JD, Urschel DM, Anderson TM, et al: Prognostic implications of pulmonary satellite nodules: Are the 1997 staging revisions appropriate? Lung Cancer 21:83–87, 1998.
107. Vansteenkiste JF, De Leyn PR, Deneffe GJ, et al: Clinical prognostic factors in surgically treated stage IIIA-N2 non–small cell lung cancer: Analysis of the literature. Lung Cancer 19:3–13, 1998.
108. Kwiatkowski DJ, Harpole DH Jr, Godleski J, et al: Molecular pathologic substaging in 244 stage I non–small-cell lung cancer patients: Clinical implications. J Clin Oncol 16:2468–2477, 1998.
109. Stanley KE: Prognostic factors for survival in patients with inoperable lung cancer. J Natl Cancer Inst 65:25, 1980.
110. Zelen M: Preliminary report on the treatment of nonresectable cancer of the lung. Cancer Chemother Rep 4(Suppl 3):31, 1973.
111. Chen XQ, Stroun M, Magnenat J-L, et al: Microsatellite alterations in plasma DNA of small cell lung cancer patients. Nature Med 2:1033–1035, 1996.
112. Nawroz H, Hoch W, Anker P, et al: Microsatellite alterations in serum DNA of head and neck cancer patients. Nature Med 2:1035–1037, 1996.
113. Mao L, Hruban RH, Boyle Jo, et al: Detection of oncogene mutations in sputum precedes diagnosis of lung cancer. Cancer Res 54:1634–1637, 1994.
114. Yakubovskaya MS, Speigelman V, Luo FC, et al: High frequency of *K-ras* mutations in normal appearing lung tissues and sputum of patients with lung cancer. Int J Cancer 63:810–814, 1995.
115. Mills NE, Fishman CL, Scholes J, et al: Detection of *K-ras* oncogene mutations in bronchoalveolar lavage fluid for lung cancer diagnosis. J Natl Cancer Inst 87:1056–1060, 1995.
116. Merlo A, Mabry M, Gabrielson E, et al: Frequent microsatellite instability in primary small cell lung cancer. Cancer Res 54:2098–2101, 1994.

117. Mao L, Lee DJ, Tockman MS, et al: Microsatellite alterations as clonal markers in the detection of human cancer. Proc Natl Acad Sci USA 91:9871–9875, 1994.
118. Miozzo M, Sozzi G, Musso K, et al: Microsatellite alterations in bronchial and sputum specimens of lung cancer patients. Cancer Res 56:2285–2288, 1996.
119. Pean J: Chirurgie des poumons. Discussion Ranc Chir Proc Verh Paris 9:72, 1895.
120. Graham EA, Singer JJ: Successful removal of the entire lung for carcinoma of the bronchus. JAMA 101:1371, 1933.
121. Kristensen S, Asaby C, Nielsen SM: Mediastinal staging of lung cancer. Is mediastinsoscopy still essential? Dan Med Bull 42:192–194, 1995.
122. Izbicki JR, Passlick B, Karg O. Impact of radical systematic mediastinal lymphadenectomy on tumor staging in lung cancer. Ann Thorac Surg 59:209–214, 1995.
123. Martini N. Mediastinal lymph node dissection for lung cancer: The Memorial experience. Chest Surg Clin North Am 5:189–203, 1995.
124. Ginsberg RJ, Rubinstein LV: Randomized trial of lobectomy versus limited resection for T1 N0 non–small cell lung cancer: Lung Cancer Study Group. Ann Thorac Surg 60:615–622, 1995.
125. Warren WH, Faber LP: Segmentectomy vs. lobectomy in patients with stage I pulmonary carcinoma: Five year survival and patterns of intrathoracic recurrence. J Thorac Cardiovasc Surg 107:1087, 1994.
126. Faber LP, Jensik RJ, Kittle CF: Results of sleeve lobectomy for bronchogenic carcinoma in 101 patients. Ann Thorac Surg 37:279, 1984.
127. Vogt-Moykopf I, Fritz TH, Meyer G, et al: Bronchoplastic and angioplastic operation in bronchial carcinoma: Long-term results of a retrospective analysis from 1973 to 1983. Int Surg 71:211, 1986.
128. Dartevelle P, Macchiarini P: Carinal resection for bronchogenic cancer. Semin Thorac Cardiovasc Surg 8:414–425, 1996.
129. Ginsberg RJ, Hill LD, Eagan RT: Modern thirty-day operative mortality for surgical resections in lung cancer. J Thorac Cardiovasc Surg 86:654–658, 1983.
130. Romano PS, Mark DH. Patient and hospital characteristics related to in-hospital mortality after lung cancer resection. Chest 101:1332–1337, 1992.
131. Deslauriers J, Ginsberg RJ, Dubois P, et al: Current operative morbidity associated with elective surgical resection for lung cancer. Can J Surg 32:335, 1989.
132. Nagasaki F, Flehinger BJ, Martini N: Complications of surgery in the treatment of carcinoma of the lung. Chest 82:25, 1982.
133. Martini N, Melamed MR. Occult carcinoma of the lung. Ann Thorac Surg 30:215, 1980.
134. Tockman MS, Erozan YS, Gupta PK, et al: The early detection of second primary lung cancers by sputum immunostaining. Chest 106(suppl):385S–390S, 1994.
135. Lam S, MacAulay C, Hung J, et al: Detection of dysplasia and carcinoma in situ with a lung imaging fluorescence endoscope device. J Thorac Cardiovasc Surg 105:1035–1040, 1993.
136. Morita K: Recent advances in radiation therapy for non–small cell lung cancer. Nippon Kyobu Shikkan Gakkai Zasshi 34(suppl):103–106, 1996.
137. Kawate KH, Kinoshita K, Yamamoto H, et al: Photodynamic therapy of early-stage lung cancer. Ciba Found Symp 146:183–194, 1989.
138. van Boxem TJ, Venmans BJ, Schramel FM, et al: Radiographically occult lung cancer treated with fibreoptic bronchoscopic electrocautery: A pilot study of a simple and inexpensive technique. Eur Respir J 11:169–172, 1998.
139. Kato H, Kawate N, Kinoshita K, et al: Photodynamic therapy of early-stage lung cancer. Ciba Found Symp 146:194–195, 1989.
140. McCormack P, Martini N: Primary lung cancer. NY State J Med 80:618, 1980.
141. Martini N, Bains MS, Burt ME, et al: Incidence of local recurrence and second primary tumors in resected stage I lung cancer. J Thorac Cardiovasc Surg 109:120–129, 1995.
142. Pisters KM, Ginsberg RJ: Phase II trial of induction paclitaxel and carboplatin (PC) in early stage (T2 N0, T1–2 N1, and selected T3 N0–1) non–small cell lung cancer (NSCLC). Proc ASCO 17:451a, 1998.
143. Martini N, Burt ME, Bains MS, et al: Survival after resection of stage II non–small cell lung cancer. Ann Thorac Surg 54:460–465, 1992.
144. Holmes EC, Gail M, the Lung Cancer Study Group: Surgical adjuvant therapy for stage II and III adenocarcinoma and large cell undifferentiated carcinoma. J Clin Oncol 4:710, 1986.
145. Menconi GF, Ambrogi MC, Melfi FM, et al: Endothoracic sonography with color Doppler availability during video assisted thoracic surgery (videothoracoscopic operative staging with ultrasound color Doppler) for lung cancer staging. Surg Endosc 12:816–819, 1998.
146. Webb WR, Gatsonis C, Zerhouni EA, et al: CT and MR imaging in staging non–small cell bronchogenic carcinoma: report of the Radiologic Diagnostic Oncology Group. Radiology 178:705–713, 1991.
147. McCaughan BC, Martini N, Bains MS, et al: Chest wall invasion of carcinoma of the lung: Therapeutic and prognostic implications. J Thorac Cardiovasc Surg 89:836, 1985.
148. Paulson DL: Combined preoperative irradiation and extended resection for carcinoma in the superior pulmonary sulcus. *In* Bonica JJ, Denise G, Albe-Fessard D (eds): Advances in Pain Research and Therapy. New York: Raven Press, 1982, p. 47.
149. Shaw RR, Paulson DL, Kee JL Jr: Treatment of the superior sulcus tumor by irradiation followed by resection. Ann Surg 154:29, 1961.
150. Hilaris BS, Martini N: Multimodality therapy of superior sulcus tumors. *In* Bonica JJ, Denise G, Albe-Fessard D (eds): Advances in Pain Research and Therapy. New York: Raven Press,1982, p. 113.
151. Hilaris BS, Martini N, Wong GY, et al: Treatment of superior sulcus tumor (Pancoast tumor). Surg Clin North Am 67:965–977, 1987.
152. Paulson DL. The "superior sulcus" lesion. *In* Delarue NC, Eschapasse H (eds): International Trends in General Thoracic Surgery. Philadelphia: WB Saunders, 1985, p. 121.
153. Shahian DM, Neptune WB, Ellis FH: Pancoast tumors: Improved survival with preoperative and postoperative radiotherapy. Ann Thorac Surg 43:32, 1987.
154. Dartevelle TG, Chapelier AR, Macchiarini P, et al: Anterior transcervical-thoracic approach for radical resection of lung tumors invading the thoracic inlet. J Thorac Cardiovasc Surg 105:1025, 1993.
155. Cameron R, Ginsberg RJ: Induction (pre-operative) therapy and surgery for locally advanced stage IIIa (N2) non–small cell lung cancer. *In* Carney DN (ed): Lung Cancer. London: Arnold, 1995, pp. 78–95.
156. Pearson FG, DeLarue NC, Ilves R: Significance of positive superior mediastinal nodes identified at mediastinoscopy in patients with resectable cancer of the lung. J Thorac Cardiovasc Surg 83:1–11, 1982.
157. Roth JA, Fossella F, Komaki R, et al: A randomized trial comparing perioperative chemotherapy and surgery with surgery alone in resectable stage IIIA non–small-cell lung cancer. J Natl Cancer Inst 86:673–680, 1994.
158. Rosell R, Maestre J, Font A, et al: A randomized trial of mitomycin/ifosfamide/cisplatin preoperative chemotherapy plus surgery versus surgery alone in stage IIIA non–small cell lung cancer. Semin Oncol 21(3, Suppl 4):28–33, 1994.
159. Pass HI, Pogrebniak HW, Steinberg SM, et al: Randomized trial of neoadjuvant therapy for lung cancer: Interim analysis. Ann Thorac Surg 53:992–998, 1992.
160. Pitz CC, Brutel de la Riviere A, Elbers HR, et al: Results of resection of T3 non–small cell lung cancer invading the mediastinum or main bronchus. Ann Thorac Surg 62:1016–1020, 1996.
161. Tsuchiya R, Asamura H, Kondo H, et al: Extended resection of the left atrium, great vessels, or both for lung cancer. Ann Thorac Surg 57:960–965, 1994.
162. Albain KS, Rusch VW, Crowley JJ, et al: Concurrent cisplatin/etoposide plus chest radiotherapy followed by surgery for stages IIIA (N2) and IIIB non–small-cell lung cancer: Mature results of Southwest Oncology Group phase II study 8805. J Clin Oncol 13:1880–1892, 1995.
163. Wronski M, Arbeit E, Burt M, et al: Survival after surgical treatment of brain metastases from lung cancer: A follow-up study of 231 patients treated between 1976 and 1991. J Neurosurg 83:605–616, 1995.

164. Magilligan DJ Jr, Duvernoy C, Malik G, et al: Surgical approach to lung cancer with solitary cerebral metastasis: Twenty-five years' exprerience. Ann Thorac Surg 42:360–364, 1986.
165. Kihlstrom L, Karlsson B, Lindquist C: Gamma knife surgery for cerebral metastases: Implications for survival based on 16 years expererience. Stereotact Funct Neurosurg 61(suppl 1):45–50, 1993.
166. Luketich JD, Burt ME: Does resection of adrenal metastases from non–small cell lung cancer improve survival? Ann Thorac Surg 62:1614–1616, 1996.
167. Kirsch AJ, Oz MC, Stoopler M, et al: Operative management of adrenal metastases from lung carcinoma. Urology 42:716–719, 1993.
168. Cavaliere S, Venuta F, Foccoli P, et al: Endoscopic treatment of malignant airway obstructions in 2,008 patients. Chest 110:1536–1542, 1996.
169. Tredaniel J, Hennequin C, Zalcman G, et al: Prolonged survival after high-dose rate endobronchial radiation for malignant airway obstruction. Chest 105:767–772, 1994.
170. LoCicero J 3d, Metzdorff M, Almgren C: Photodynamic therapy in the palliation of late stage obstructing non–small cell lung cancer. Chest 98:97–100, 1990.
171. Marasso A, Bernardi V, Gai R, et al: Radiofrequency resection of bronchial tumours in combination with cyrotherapy: Evaluation of a new technique. Thorax 53:106–109, 1998.
171a. Adjer AA, Marks RS, Bonner JA: Current guidelines for the management of small cell lung cancer. Mayo Clin Proc 74:809–816, 1999.
172. Shepherd FA, Ginsberg RJ, Feld R, et al: Surgical treatment for limited small-cell lung cancer: The University of Toronto Lung Oncology Group experience. J Thorac Cardiovasc Surg 101:385–393, 1991.
173. Prasad US, Naylor AR, Walker WS, et al: Long term survival after pulmonary resection for small cell carcinoma of the lung. Thorax 44:784–787, 1989.
174. Higgins GA: Use of chemotherapy as an adjuvant to surgery for bornchogenic carcinoma. Cancer 30:1383, 1972.
175. Ichinose Y, Hara N, Ohta M, et al: Comparison between resected and irradiated small cell lung cancer in patients in stages I through IIIa. Ann Thorac Surg 53:95–100, 1992.
176. Shepherd FA, Ginsberg RJ, Patterson GA, et al: Is there ever a role for salvage operations in limited small-cell lung cancer? J Thorac Cardiovasc Surg 101:196–200, 1991.
177. Sandler HM, Curran WJ Jr, Turrisi AT III: The influence of tumor size and pre-treatment staging on outcome following radiation therapy alone for stage I non–small cell lung cancer. Int J Radiat Oncol Biol Phys 19:9–13, 1990.
178. Dosoretz DE, Katin MJ, Blitzer PH, et al: Radiation therapy in the management of medically inoperable carcinoma of the lung: Results and implications for future treatment strategies. Int J Radiat Oncol Biol Phys 24:3–9, 1992.
179. Graham PH, Gebski VJ, Langlands AO: Radical radiotherapy for early nonsmall cell lung cancer. Int J Radiat Oncol Biol Phys 31:261–266, 1995.
180. Sibley GS, Jamieson TA, Marks LB, et al: Radiotherapy alone for medically inoperable stage I non–small cell lung cancer: The Duke experience. Int J Radiation Oncology Biol Phys 40:149–154, 1998.
181. Kaskowitz L, Graham MV, Emami B, et al: Radiation therapy alone for Stage I non–small cell lung cancer. Int J Radiat Oncol Biol Phys 27:517–523, 1993.
182. Perez CA, Pajak TF, Rubin P, et al: Long-term observations of the patterns of failure in patients with unresectable non-oat cell carcinoma of the lung treated with definitive radiotherapy. Cancer 59:1874–1881, 1987.
183. Van Houtte P: Induction or concomitant chemotherapy and radiotherapy for non–small-cell lung cancer: Myth or reality. Ann Oncol 6:S37–S40, 1995.
184. Dillman RO, Herndon J, Seagren SL, et al: Improved survival in stage III non–small-cell lung cancer: Seven-year follow-up of cancer and leukemia group B (CALGB) 8433 Trial. J Natl Cancer Inst 88:1210–1215, 1996.
185. Marino P, Preatoni A, Cantoni A: Randomized trials of radiotherapy alone versus combined chemotherapy and radiotherapy in stages IIIa and IIIb nonsmall cell lung cancer. Cancer 76:593–601, 1995.
186. Non–Small Cell Lung Cancer Collaborative Group: Chemotherapy in non–small cell lung cancer: A meta-analysis using updated data on individual patients from 52 randomised clinical trials. BMJ 3:899–909, 1995.
187. Scott C, Sause WT, Byhardt R, et al: Recursive partitioning analysis of 1592 patients on four Radiation Therapy Oncology Group studies in inoperable non–small cell lung cancer. Lung Cancer 17:S59–S74, 1997.
188. Lutz ST, Huang DT, Ferguson CL, et al: A retrospective quality of life analysis using the lung cancer symptom scale in patients treated with palliative radiotherapy for advanced nonsmall cell lung cancer. Int J Radiat Oncol Biol Phys 37:117–122, 1997.
189. Byhardt RW: The evolution of radiation therapy oncology group (RTOG) protocols for nonsmall cell lung cancer. Int J Radiat Oncol Biol Phys 32:1513–1525, 1995.
190. Komaki R, Scott CB, Sause WT, et al: Induction cisplatin/vinblastine and irradiation vs. irradiation in unresectable squamous cell lung cancer: Failure patterns by cell type in RTOG 88-08/ECOG 4588. Int J Radiat Oncol Biol Phys 39:537–544, 1997.
191. Komaki R, Scott C, Lee JS, et al: Impact of adding concurrent chemotherapy to hyperfractionated radiotherapy for locally advanced non–small cell lung cancer (NSCLC): Comparison of RTOG 83-11 and RTOG 91-06. Am J Clin Oncol 20:435–440, 1997.
192. Saunders M, Dische S, Barrett A, et al: Continuous hyperfractionated accelerated radioatherapy (CHART) versus conventional radiotherapy in non–small cell lung cancer: A randomized multicentre trial. Lancet 350:161–165, 1997.
193. Cox JD, Pajak TF, Asbell S, et al: Interruptions of high-dose radiation therapy decrease long-term survival of favorable patients with unresectable non–small small cell carcinoma of the lung: Analysis of 1244 cases from 3 radiation therapy oncology group (RTOG) trials. Int J Radiat Oncol Biol Phys 27:493–498, 1993.
194. Baldini EH: Palliative radiation therapy for non–small cell lung cancer. Hematol Oncol Clin North Am 11:303–319, 1997.
195. Huber RM, Fischer R, Hautmann H, et al: Does additional brachytherapy improve the effect of external irradiation? A prospective, randomized study in central lung tumors. Int J Radiat Oncol Biol Phys 38:533–540, 1997.
196. Schaake-Koning C, van den Bogaaert W, Dalesio O, et al: Effects of concomitant cisplatin and radiotherapy on inoperable non–small-cell lung cancer. N Engl J Med 326:524–530, 1992.
197. Arriagada R: Current strategies for radiation therapy in non–small cell lung cancer. Chest 112:209S–213S, 1997.
198. Clamon G, Herndon J, Cooper R, et al: Radiosensitization with carboplatin for patients with unresectable stage III non–small-cell lung cancer: A phase III trial of the Cancer and Leukemia Group B and the Eastern Cooperative Oncology Group. J Clin Oncol 17:4–11, 1999.
199. Bunn PA, Lichter AS, Makuch RW, et al: Chemotherapy alone or chemotherapy with chest radiation therapy in limited stage small cell lung cancer: A prospective randomized trial. Ann Intern Med 106:655, 1987.
200. Perry MC, Eaton WL, Propert KJ, et al: Chemotherapy with or without radiation therapy in limited small-cell carcinoma of the lung. N Engl J Med 316:912, 1987.
201. Perez CA, Einhorn L, Oldham RK, et al: Randomized trial of radiotherapy to the thorax in limited small-cell carcinoma of the lung treated with multi-agent chemotherapy and elective brain irradiation: A preliminary report. J Clin Oncol 2:1200, 1984.
202. Fox RM, Woods RL, Brodie GN, et al. A randomized study: Small cell anaplastic lung cancer treated by combination chemotherapy and adjuvant radiotherapy. Int J Radiat Oncol Biol Phys 6:1083, 1980.
203. Rosenthal MA, Tattersall MHN, Fox RM, et al: Adjuvant throracic radiotherapy in small cell lung cancer: Ten-year follow-up of a randomized study. Lung Cancer 7:235, 1991.
204. Pignon JP, Arriagada R, Ihde DC, et al: A meta-analysis of thoracic radiotherapy for small-cell lung cancer. N Engl J Med 327:1618, 1992.
205. Pedersen AG, Kristjansen PE, Hansen HH: Prophylactic cranial irradiation and small cell lung cancer. Cancer Treat Rev 15:85–103, 1988.
206. Turrisi AT: Brain irradiation and systemic chemotherapy for small cell lung cancer: Dangerous liaisons? J Clin Oncol 8:196, 1990.

206a. Brooks DM, Jackson JE: Stenting of superior vena caval obstruction. Thorax 50(Suppl 1):S31–S36, 1995.
206b. Gaines PA, Belli A-M, Anderson PB, et al: Superior vena caval obstruction managed by the Gianturco Z stent. Clin Radiol 49:202–208, 1994.
207. Wronski M, Arbit E, Burt M, et al: Survival after surgical treatment of brain metastases from lung cancer: A follow-up study of 231 patients treated between 1976 and 1991. J Neurosurg 83:605–616, 1995.
208. Flickinger JC, Kondziolka D, Lunsford LD, et al: A multi-institutional experience with stereotactic radiosurgery for solitary brain metastasis. Int J Radiat Oncol Biol Phys 28:797–801, 1994.
209. Coia L: The role of radiation therapy in the treatment of brain metastases. Int J Radiat Oncol Biol Phys 23:229–238, 1992.
210. Kurtz JM, Gelber R, Brady LW: The palliation of brain metastases in a favorable patient population: A randomized clinical trial by the radiation therapy oncology group. Int J Radiat Oncol Biol Phys 7:891–895, 1981.
211. Mehta MP, Rozental JM, Levin AB, et al: Defining the role of radiosurgery in the management of brain metastases. Int J Radiat Oncol Biol Phys 24:619–625, 1992.
212. Cox JD, Azarnia N, Byhardt RW, et al: A randomized phase I/II trial of hyperfractrionated radiation therapy with total doses of 60.0 Gy to 79.2 Gy: Possible survival benefit with ≥69.6 Gy in favorable patients with radiation therapy oncology group stage III non–small cell lung carcinoma: Report of radiation therapy oncoogy Group 83-11. J Clin Oncol 8:1543–1555, 1990.
213. Niiranen A, Niitamo-Korhonen S, Kouri M, et al: Adjuvant chemotherapy after radical surgery for non–small cell lung cancer: A randomized study. J Clin Oncol 10:1927–1932, 1992.
214. Feld R, Rubinstein L, Thomas PA: Adjuvant chemotherapy with CAP in patients with completely resected stage I non–small cell lung cancer. J Natl Cancer Inst 85:299–306, 1993.
215. Ohta M, Tsuchiya R, Shimoyama M, et al: Adjuvant chemotherapy for completely resected stage III NSCLC. J Thorac Cardiovasc Surg 106:703–708, 1993.
216. Dautzenberg B, Chastang C, Arriagada R, et al: Adjuvant radiotherapy versus combined chemotherapy followed by radiotherapy in the treatment of resected NSCLC. Cancer 76:779–786, 1995.
217. Pisters KMW, Kris MG, Gralla RJ, et al: Randomized trial of adjuvant vindesine plus cisplatin in patients with operable stage III non–small cell lung cancer. J Surg Oncol 56:236–241, 1994.
218. Bunn PA Jr, Kelly K: New chemotherapeutic agents prolong survival and improve quality of life in non–small cell lung cancer: A review of the literature and future directions. Clin Cancer Res 5:1087–1100, 1998.
219. Soquet PJ, Chauvin F, Boissel JP, et al: Polychemotherapy in non–small cell lung cancer: A meta-analysis. Lancet 342:19–21, 1993.
220. Non–small Cell Lung Cancer Collaborative Group: Chemotherapy in non–small cell lung cancer: Meta-analysis using updated data on individual patients from 52 randomized clinical trials. Br Med J 311:899–909, 1995.
221. Marino P, Pampallona S, Preatoni A: Chemotherapy *versus* supportive care in advandced non–small cell lung cancer: Results of a meta-analysis of the literature. Chest 106:861–865, 1994
222. Cardenal F, Lopez-Cabrerizo MP, Anton A, et al: Randomized phase III study of gemcitabine-cisplatin versus etopside-cisplatin in the treatment of locally advanced or metastatic non–small-cell lung cancer. J Clin Oncol 17:12–18, 1999.
223. Crowley JJ, Balcerzak SP, Weiss GR, et al: Randomized phase III trial of cisplatin (CDDP) vs. CDDP plus navelbine (NVB) in treatment of advanced non small cell lung cancer (NSCLC): An update of a Southwest Oncology Group Study (SWOG-9308). Proceedings of ASCO 17:1744, 1998.
224. Sandler J, Nemunaitis J, Dehnam C, et al: Phase III study of cisplatin (C) with or without gemcitabine (G) in patients with advanced nonsmall cell lung cancer (NSCLC). Proceedings of ASCO 17:1747, 1998.
225. Billingham LJ, Cullen MH, Woods J, et al: Mitomycin, ifosfamide and cisplatin in non–small cell lung cancer: Results of a randomized trial evaluating palliation and quality of life. Lung Cancer 18(Suppl 1):9, 1997.
226. Giaccone G, Ted AW, Splinter CD, et al: Randomized study of paclitaxel-cisplatin versus cisplatin-teniposide in patients with advanced non–small-cell lung cancer. J Clin Oncol 16:2133–2141, 1998.
227. Bonomi P, Kim K, Chang A, et al: Phase III trial comparing etoposide-cisplatin *versus* Taxol with cisplatin-G-CSF *versus* Taxol-cisplatin in advanced non–small cell lung cancer: An Eastern Cooperative Oncology Group trial. Proc Am Soc Clin Oncol 15:382, 1996.
228. Roth BJ, Johnson DH, Einhorn LH, et al: Randomized study of cyclophosphamide, doxorubicin, and vincristine *versus* etopside and cisplatin *versus* alternation of these two regimens in extensive small-cell lung cancer: A Phase III trial of the Southeastern Cancer Study Group. J Clin Oncol 10:282–291, 1992.
229. Fukuoka M, Furuse K, Saijo N, et al: Randomized trial of cyclophosphamide, doxorubicin and vincristine *versus* cisplatin and etopside *versus* alternation of these regimens in small cell lung cancer. J Natl Cancer Inst 83:855–861, 1991.
230. Einhorn LH, Bond WH, Horback IV, et al: Long-term results in combined modality treatment of SCLC. Semin Oncol 5:309–313, 1978.
231. Roth BJ, Johnson DH, Einhorn LH, et al: Randomized study of cyclophosphamide, doxorubicin, and vincristine versus etoposide and cisplatin versus alternation of these two regimens in extensive small-cell lung cancer: A phase III trial of the Southeastern Cancer Study Group. J Clin Oncol 10:282, 1992.
232. Fukuoka M, Furuse K, Saijo N, et al: Randomized trial of cyclophosphamide, doxorubicin, and vincristin versus cisplatin and etoposide versus alternation of these regimens in small-cell lung cancer. J Natl Cancer Inst 83:855, 1991.
233. Einhorn LH, Crawford J, Birch R, et al: Cisplatin plus etopside consolidation following cyclophosphamide, doxorubicin, and vincristine in limited small-cell lung cancer. J Clin Oncol 6:451, 1988.
234. Bishop JF, Raghavan D, Stuart-Harris R, et al: Carboplatin (CBDCA, JM-8) and VP-16-213 in previously untreated patients with small cell lung cancer. J Clin Oncol 5:1574, 1987.
235. Loehrer PJ, Ansari R, Gonin R, et al: Cisplatin plus etoposide with and without infosfamide in extensive small-cell lung cancer: A Hoosier Oncology Group study. J Clin Oncol 13:2594, 1995.
236. Johnson DH, Greco FA, Strupp J, et al: Prolonged administration of oral etoposide in patient with relapsed small-cell lung cancer: A phase II trial J Clin Oncol 8:1613–1617, 1990.
237. Comparison of oral etoposide and standard intravenous multidrug chemotherapy for small-cell lung cancer: A stopped multicentre randomized trial: Medical Research Council Lung Cancer Working Party. Lancet 348:563–566, 1996.
238. Souhami RL, Spiro SG, Rudd RM, et al: Five day etoposide treatment for advanced small-cell lung: Randomized comparison with intravenous chemotherapy. J Natl Cancer Inst 89:577–580, 1997.
239. Ihde D, Mulshine JL, Kramer BS, et al: Randomized trial of high versus standard $PVP_{16}$ in extensive SCLC. Proc ASCO 10:240, 1991.
240. Sculter JP, Klastersky J, Lipert P, et al: A phase II study evaluating CAVi (cyclophosphamide, adriamycin, vincristine) potentiated or not by amphotericin B entrapped into sonicated liposomes, as salvage therapy for small-cell lung cancer. Lung Cancer 6:110–118, 1990.
241. Shepard FA, Evans WK, MacCormick R, et al: Cyclophosphamide, doxorubicin and vincristine in etoposide and cisplatin-resistant small-cell lung cancer. Cancer Treat Rep 71:941–944, 1987.
242. Ardizzoni A, Hansen H, Dombernowksy P, et al: Topotecan, a new active drug in the second-line treatment of smal-cell lung cancer: A phase II study in patients with refractory and sensitive disease. J Clin Oncol 15:2090–2096, 1997.
243. Depierre A, von Pawel J, Hans K, et al: Evaluation of topotecan (Hycamtin) in relapsed small-cell lung cancer (SCLC): A multicenter phase II study. Lung Cancer 18 (abstr 126):35, 1997.
244. Eckardt J, Gralla R, Palmer MC, et al: Topotecan (T) as second-line therapy in patients pts. with small cell lung cancer (SCLC): A phase II study. Ann Oncol 7 (abs 513):107, 1996.
245. Eckardt J, Depierre A, Ardizzoni A, et al: Pooled analysis of topotecan (T) in the second-line treatment of patients (pts) with sensitive small cell lung cancer (SCLC). Proc Am Soc Clin Oncol 16 (abs 1624):452a, 1997.
246. von Pawel J, Schiller JH, Shepard FA, et al: Topotecan versus cy-

clophosphamide, doxorubicin, and vincristine for the treatment of recurrent small-cell lung cancer. J Clin Oncol 17:658–667, 1999.

247. Sculier JP, Berghmans T, Castaigne C, et al: Maintenance chemotherapy for small cell lung cancer: A critical review of the literature. Lung Cancer 19:141–151, 1998.
248. Spiro SG, Shah S, Harper PG, et al: Treatment of obstruction of the superior vena cava by combination chemotherapy with and without irradiation in small-cell carcinoma of the bronchus. Thorax 38:501, 1983.
249. Postmus PE, Smit EF, Haaxma-Reiche H, et al: Teniposide for brain metastases of small-cell lung cancer: A phase II study. J Clin Oncol 13:660, 1995.
250. Lee JS, Murphy WK, Glisson BS, et al: Primary chemotherapy of brain metastases in small-cell lung cancer. J Clin Oncol 7:916, 1989.
251. Twelves CJ, Souhami RL, Harper PG, et al: The response of cerebral metastases in small cell lung cancer to systemic chemotherapy. Br J Cancer 61:147, 1990.
252. Gambhir SS, Shepherd JE, Shah BD, et al: Analytical decision model for the cost-effective management of solitary pulmonary nodules. J Clin Oncol 16:2113–2125, 1998.
253. Goldberg S, Walkenstein M: The role of staging bronchoscopy in the preoperative assessment of a solitary pulmonary nodule. Chest 104:94–97, 1993.
254. Torrington K: The utility of fiberoptic bronchoscopy in the evaluation of pulmonary nodule. Chest 104:1021–1024, 1993.
255. Desch CE, Hillner BE, Smith TJ: Economic considerations in the care of lung cancer patients. Curr Opin Oncol 8:126–132, 1996.
256. Evans WK, Will BP, Berthelot J-M, et al: Estimating the cost of lung cancer diagnosis and treatment in Canada: The POHEM model. Can J Oncol 5:408–419, 1995.
257. Evans WK, Will BP, Berthelot JM, et al: Cost of Combined modality interventions for stage III non–small-cell lung cancer. J Clin Oncol 15:3038–3048, 1997.
258. Jaakinainen L, Goodwin PJ, Pater L, et al: Counting the costs of chemotherapy in a National Cancer Institute of Canada randomized trial in non–small cell lung cancer. J Clin Oncol 13:1301–1309, 1990.
259. Smith TJ, Hillner BE, Neighbors DM, et al: Economic evaluation of a randomized clinical trial comparing vinorelbine, vinorelbine plus cisplatin and vindesine plus cisplatin. J Clin Oncol 13:2166–2173, 1995.
260. Copley-Merriman C, Corral J, King K, et al: Economic value of gemcitabine compared to cisplatin and etoposide in non–small cell lung cancer. Lung Cancer 14:45–61, 1996.

# 47 Lymphoma, Lymphoproliferative Diseases, and Other Primary Malignant Tumors

JUDITH A. LUCE, M.D.

Introduction
Lymphomas
- Hodgkin's Disease
- Non-Hodgkin's Lymphoma

Lymphoproliferative Diseases
- Lymphomatoid Granulomatosis
- Angioimmunoblastic Lymphadenopathy
- Castleman's Disease

Other Primary Malignant Tumors
- Carcinoid and Neuroendocrine Carcinomas
- Mucoepithelial Malignancies
- Sarcomas
- Pulmonary Blastoma and Carcinosarcoma
- Pulmonary Tumorlets
- Other Tumors

Summary

## INTRODUCTION

Although most primary malignant pulmonary tumors are classified as bronchogenic carcinomas, other major types of neoplasms also occur in the lungs.[1] Lymphomas and sarcomas (cancers of presumptive mesenchymal origin) comprise the largest group of nonbronchogenic neoplasms. Carcinoid tumors, lymphoepithelial tumors, and mucoepithelial neoplasms of salivary gland origin are epithelial cancers that may occur in the lungs. The rarest of the nonbronchogenic carcinomas, melanoma, pulmonary blastoma, and pulmonary tumorlets, are of obscure origin. All of these diseases share no known epidemiologic associations with bronchogenic carcinoma and have no known preventive strategies. Correct diagnosis, often with special diagnostic techniques, may be necessary to appropriately manage these cancers. Treatment frequently differs from the approach to bronchogenic carcinoma, and curability may be greater for these cancers.

## LYMPHOMAS

### Hodgkin's Disease

#### Primary Pulmonary Hodgkin's Disease

Hodgkin's disease involving the lung alone is extremely rare, having been reported only in isolated cases.[2] The disease is thought to arise in lymphoid follicles or peribronchial lymph nodes that are scattered throughout the lung. Because histologic proof requires demonstration of the pathognomonic Reed-Sternberg cell, primary pulmonary Hodgkin's disease is usually diagnosed by open (or thoracoscopic) lung biopsy.[3] Fine-needle aspiration cytology, aided by the use of special immunohistochemical stains, may also provide the diagnosis.[4] Because Hodgkin's disease so rarely involves the lung alone, defining a case requires proof of the absence of hilar or mediastinal adenopathy as well as an undisputed histologic diagnosis of Hodgkin's disease.

Primary pulmonary Hodgkin's disease has been reported more frequently in older people and in women than has Hodgkin's disease. Systemic symptoms such as fever, night sweats, and weight loss are common. The radiologic pattern may include solitary pulmonary nodules, diffuse infiltration, and cavitation; the disease is rarely bilateral and most often involves the upper lobes.

Full staging evaluation is essential in making treatment decisions for such patients. In reported cases in which the lung was the only site of disease, patients were treated with surgery and radiotherapy with apparently excellent results. When other node involvement is documented, the treatment is stage dependent, and combinations of radiation therapy and chemotherapy are increasingly used. Current therapy for early stage extranodal Hodgkin's disease most often includes chemotherapy, although the issue remains controversial.[5]

## Hodgkin's Disease in Lymph Nodes with Lung Involvement

Hodgkin's disease involves the nodes of the mediastinum in approximately two thirds of all cases. Pulmonary involvement occurs in slightly more than 10% of patients and is virtually always an extension of mediastinal node involvement.[6, 7] Nodular sclerosing Hodgkin's disease is the presenting histologic type in 67% to 84% of patients having thoracic involvement. Extension of the disease to hilar nodes may result in contiguous spread to the lungs, which may take the form of interstitial linear infiltrates, or small nodules, or both (Fig. 47.1). Bulky mediastinal involvement, defined as a ratio of tumor mass to thoracic diameter of 0.30 or more, is associated with spread to the pleura, pericardium, and chest wall. In one prospective series, interstitial or nodular lung spread was never seen without hilar node involvement, and in virtually all cases of pleural, pericardial, and chest wall involvement bulky tumor was also found in the mediastinum.[4] There are insufficient data to demonstrate that magnetic resonance imaging, positron emission tomography, gallium, or other imaging methods are superior to computed tomography (CT) scanning in documenting the pulmonary extent of Hodgkin's disease.

Histologic confirmation of pulmonary extension by Hodgkin's disease may be necessary. When the disease is clearly a direct extension of known bulky involvement, such confirmation is usually not undertaken. However, patients with nodular or infiltrating pulmonary parenchymal lesions may require histologic proof before treatment is begun, especially because the differential diagnosis of such lesions includes many infectious processes.[8] The key Reed-Sternberg cell in the lung may be demonstrated in material from bronchial lavage,[9] endobronchial brushings,[10] sputum cytology,[11] fine-needle aspiration,[12] or more formal transbronchial biopsy or thoracoscopic or open lung biopsy. None of the reports compares techniques or provides adequate information to assess how frequently each of these methods is useful in making the proper diagnosis. The sole exception is diagnostic needle aspiration cytology: Its use in soft tissue extranodal sites, mostly pulmonary, resulted in a diagnosis of Hodgkin's disease in 15 of 18 cases.[11]

Treatment of individuals with pulmonary involvement due to Hodgkin's disease primarily depends on the stage of disease in each patient; therefore, careful staging is necessary for all such patients. Bulky mediastinal disease of any stage is most commonly treated with a combination of chemotherapy and radiation therapy. Extension of Hodgkin's disease into the lung in a nodular or interstitial infiltrate necessitates use of either chemotherapy or radiation therapy fields that adequately encompass the extension into the lung parenchyma; however, because radiation therapy permanently injures pulmonary parenchyma, chemotherapy is usually used first to diminish the size and extent of tumor to spare lung from radiation. Whether the prognosis of adequately treated patients having pulmonary extranodal extension of Hodgkin's disease is worse than for patients without extension is controversial.[13, 14]

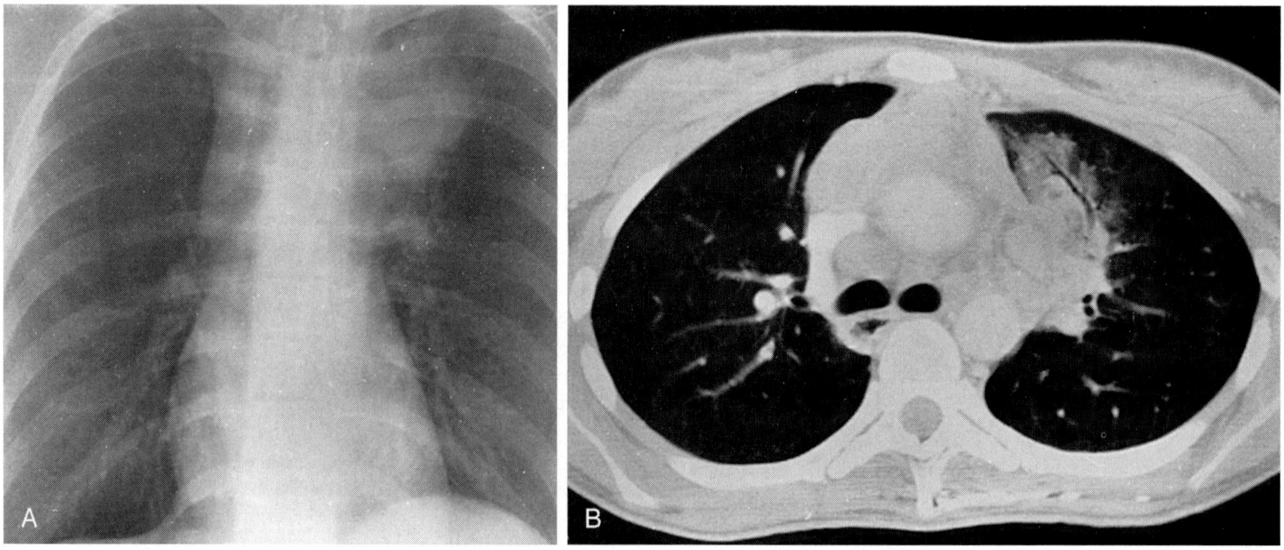


**Figure 47.1** Massive mediastinal involvement in a 35-year-old woman with nodular sclerosing Hodgkin's disease is shown. The diameter of the anterior mediastinal mass on posterior-anterior radiograph (*A*) is greater than 0.30 of the transverse diameter of the thorax. The computed tomographic scan (*B*) demonstrates an interstitial infiltrate involving the left upper lobe adjacent to the large mass, a typical feature of pulmonary involvement by Hodgkin's disease.

## Recurrent Hodgkin's Disease Involving the Lung

Because thoracic involvement is common in Hodgkin's disease, the lungs are a common site of disease recurrence. Factors predicting a high likelihood of pulmonary recurrence include advanced stage disease at the time of diagnosis, particularly if systemic symptoms are also present; bulky mediastinal node involvement[12–17]; and incomplete or inadequate initial staging and treatment.

The radiographic pattern of pulmonary recurrence and the radiographic differential diagnosis depend on the treatment used for the primary disease. Pulmonary recurrence in patients who have received mantle irradiation is most often seen as masses at the margins of the radiotherapy fields (Fig. 47.2) or diffusely in the pulmonary parenchyma adjacent to the field. Individuals who relapse after chemotherapy alone are likely to have recurrence in areas of prior nodal involvement, particularly if it was bulky, as well as extension into the lung.

The differential diagnosis of pulmonary recurrence in Hodgkin's disease includes infections, especially opportunistic infections, as well as pulmonary toxicity from treatment, including radiation pneumonitis and drug-induced interstitial pneumonitis.[18] Radiation pneumonitis may be present within the area of irradiated lung or diffusely throughout the lungs or may appear as a widening of the mediastinum.[19] The time of appearance of symptoms and abnormal radiographs may be helpful: Most radiation pneumonitis develops within 8 to 12 weeks after treatment, and it is unusual for Hodgkin's disease to relapse so quickly. New masses that appear on chest radiographs years after treatment for Hodgkin's disease may not be recurrent Hodgkin's disease; non-Hodgkin's lymphoma, solid tumors such as lung cancer, and radiation-induced tumors such as sarcomas are important causes of later mortality in both adult and pediatric patients.[20, 21] Other serious long-term cardiopulmonary complications of treatment are unusual.[22, 23]

## Non-Hodgkin's Lymphoma

Primary pulmonary non-Hodgkin's lymphoma is rare, comprising fewer than 5% of all primary extranodal lymphomas. *Non-Hodgkin's lymphoma* is a term applied to a variety of lymphoid malignancies that are usually classified according to the Revised European–American Lymphoma Classification,[24] shown in Table 47.1. This classification system sorts lymphomas into categories by histology, immunophenotyping, and certain other characteristics, including chromosomal translocations. The International Prognostic Index provides risk information based on the simple criteria shown in Table 47.2.[25]

Indolent follicular or diffuse B-cell lymphomas are the most common type among pulmonary lymphomas, and low-grade lymphoma of mucosa-associated lymphoid cells (MALT lymphomas) are the most common indolent subtype.[26, 27] Aggressive lymphomas, which may be composed of small, large, or mixed cell types, are more likely to be localized at diagnosis and are more commonly found in other extranodal sites.[28, 29] Indolent lymphomas have a long natural history with median survival times in excess of five years; in contrast, aggressive lymphomas are responsive to chemotherapy and radiation therapy but have a more rapid evolution and shorter median survival times. Only aggressive lymphomas are, however, considered curable with current therapies.[29]

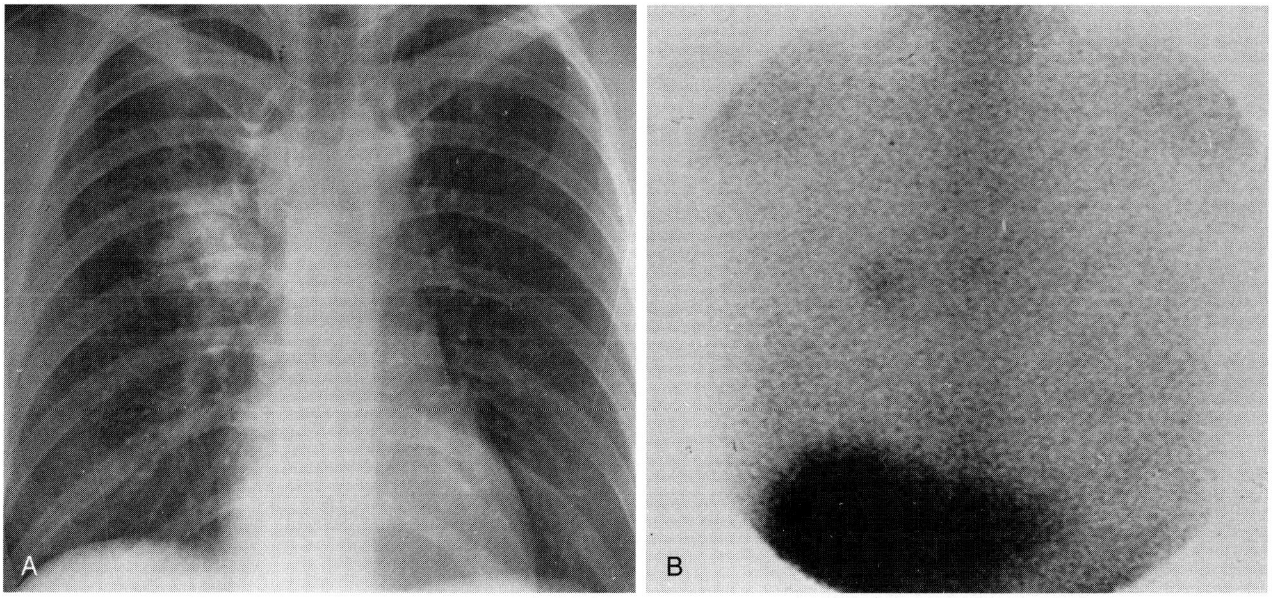


**Figure 47.2** This 34-year-old man had received "mantle" radiation therapy to the thorax for nodular-sclerosing Hodgkin's disease involving the anterior mediastinum 8 years before presenting with recurrent night sweats and the right hilar mass seen in *A*. The gallium scan shown in *B* reveals isolated uptake in the same area. The diagnosis of recurrent Hodgkin's disease was confirmed at thoracotomy, and the patient was treated with chemotherapy.

**Table 47.1 REVISED EUROPEAN-AMERICAN LYMPHOMA CLASSIFICATION**

| |
|---|
| **B-Cell Lymphoma** |
| Precursor B-lymphoblastic leukemia/lymphoma (B-ALL/LBL) |
| B-cell chronic lymphocytic leukemia/small lymphocytic lymphoma |
| B-cell prolymphocytic leukemia |
| Lymphoplasmacytic lymphoma |
| Splenic marginal zone B-cell lymphoma |
| Hairy cell leukemia |
| Plasma cell myeloma/plasmacytoma |
| Extranodal marginal zone B-cell lymphoma of MALT type |
| Mantle-cell lymphoma |
| Follicular lymphoma |
| Nodal marginal zone B-cell lymphoma |
| Diffuse large B-cell lymphoma |
| Burkitt's lymphoma |
| **T-Cell and NK-Cell Lymphomas** |
| Precursor T-lymphoblastic lymphoma/leukemia (T-ALL/LBL) |
| T-cell prolymphocytic leukemia |
| T-cell granular lymphocytic leukemia |
| Aggressive NK-cell leukemia |
| Adult T-cell lymphoma/leukemia (HTLV-I +) |
| Extranodal NK/T-cell lymphoma, nasal type |
| Enteropathy-type T-cell lymphoma |
| Hepatosplenic (γδ) T-cell lymphoma |
| Subcutaneous panniculitis-like T-cell lymphoma |
| Mycosis fungoides/Sezary's syndrome |
| Anaplastic large cell lymphoma, unspecified |
| Angioimmunoblastic T-cell lymphoma |
| Anaplastic large cell lymphoma, primary systemic type |

## Primary Pulmonary Lymphomas

The precise pathogenesis of primary pulmonary lymphomas is unknown. These tumors are thought to arise in either MALT or interbronchial nodes or lymphatic channels. In the lung, bronchus-associated lymphoid tissue is sparsely distributed and usually not associated with organized lymphoid follicles.[30] When indolent lymphomas develop, they are often multicentric or diffuse in distribution, and the monoclonal cells are most often small B lymphocytes with cleaved nuclei. Lymphoid proliferation may present as isolated masses, as peribronchial proliferation, or as interstitial infiltration,[31] and lymphoma may develop in any of those patterns. Aggressive lymphomas may present as extensions of mediastinal nodal disease or as isolated masses within the pulmonary parenchyma, bone, or pleura. Virtually all pulmonary lymphomas are of B-cell origin.[26]

Speculation about the pathogenesis of primary pulmonary MALT lymphomas is that they are related to immune responses within the lung. The pathogenesis of MALT lymphoma in the gastrointestinal tract has been shown to occur during *Helicobacter pylori* infection, and B cells responsive to *Helicobacter* antigens have been demonstrated. The presumption about the genesis of lymphoma is that during proliferation of the responding B-cell pool, mutations occur that result in immortalization of a clone of B cells. The similarity of MALT lymphomas at all sites suggests that chronic antigen stimulation is the cause; what is not known about pulmonary maltomas is what that antigen might be. Indolent, small B-cell lymphomas at all sites may evolve into large cell aggressive lymphomas late in their course; this transformation is presumed to be due to further mutation of the initial B-cell clone.

As is reflected in the most recent lymphoma classification system, a number of other techniques have been applied to diagnosing and classifying lymphoma. Immunohistochemical stains may be used to identify surface immunoglobulins and surface receptors that establish B- or T-cell lineage or other surface proteins unique to lymphoid lineage cells. Because these cancers are most often monoclonal proliferations of B cells, they display unique gene rearrangements of the immunoglobulin gene loci, unique surface immunoglobulin idiotypes, and other monoclonal markers. Cytologic studies have demonstrated several characteristic gene rearrangements such as the 14:18 translocation seen in follicular lymphomas,[32] and molecular probes have been designed for detecting these genetic characteristics in small samples of cells. Making a diagnosis of non-Hodgkin's lymphoma from an extremely small sample of tissue is now possible with immunohistochemical techniques or flow cytometry. Invasive techniques such as open lung biopsy, thoracoscopy, or transbronchial biopsy may be supplanted by transthoracic needle aspiration biopsy, bronchial lavage, or bronchial brushings.[33–35]

The signs and symptoms of non-Hodgkin's lymphoma involving the lung may be quite varied. Solitary masses may occur without symptoms. Patients with diffuse lung involvement may have cough, dyspnea, or chest pain. Lymphomas involving airways may produce cough, hemoptysis, and obstructive symptoms, including pneumonia. Systemic symptoms of lymphoma may be present: fever, night sweats, and weight loss. Patients with MALT lymphomas rarely have systemic symptoms. Patients may have other areas of extranodal lymphoma: in one series of MALT lymphomas, 25% had disease in other sites, including salivary glands, bone marrow, and orbit.[27] The

**Table 47.2 INTERNATIONAL PROGNOSTIC INDEX FOR AGGRESSIVE NON-HODGKIN'S LYMPHOMA**

| |
|---|
| **Risk Factors for Patients ≤60 Years** |
| Ann Arbor stage (I or II vs. III or IV) |
| Performance status (0 or 1 vs. 2–4) |
| Serum lactate dehydrogenase (LDH) level (≤normal vs. >normal) |
| **Risk Factors for All Patients** |
| Age (≤60 vs. >60 years) |
| Serum LDH level (≤normal vs. >normal) |
| Performance status (0 or 1 vs. 2–4) |
| Ann Arbor stage (I or II vs. III or IV) |
| Extranodal involvement (≤1 site vs. >1 site) |

chest radiographic appearance is nondiagnostic: diffuse infiltrates, reticulonodular infiltrates, small and large nodules, and effusions may be seen. The most common CT appearance in MALT lymphoma in one study was consolidation with air bronchograms, which correlated with cellular lymphocytic infiltration that expanded the interstitium and compressed adjacent alveoli.[35a] Paraneoplastic signs of lymphoma may include pruritus, erythema nodosum, autoimmune phenomena, coagulopathy, hypercalcemia, and central nervous system abnormalities.

Evaluation of individuals with non-Hodgkin's lymphoma involving the lung consists of defining the intrathoracic involvement carefully and staging the patient completely. Staging evaluation includes defining all areas of nodal and extranodal disease according to the Ann Arbor classification.[36] Staging may involve biopsies of liver, bone marrow, intra-abdominal nodes, and extranodal sites. Obtaining lymph node tissue is useful in making the distinction among the various kinds of lymphoma, provided nodal tissue is readily accessible. Laboratory evaluation should include performance of complete blood counts, liver function tests, and lactate dehydrogenase. As with Hodgkin's disease, the spectrum of opportunistic infections must be carefully considered in the differential diagnosis of pulmonary infiltrates in patients having non-Hodgkin's lymphoma.

## Treatment

Treatment of non-Hodgkin's lymphoma involving the lung, as with Hodgkin's disease, depends on the stage of disease; however, in non-Hodgkin's lymphoma the classification of disease is equally important. In contrast to Hodgkin's disease, patients having solitary extranodal non-Hodgkin's lymphoma are acknowledged to have the same prognosis as nodal disease of the same stage and histologic type. Indolent non-Hodgkin's lymphoma that does not produce significant symptoms may not be treated at all, because early intervention has not been shown to produce longer survival. Symptomatic patients with localized (stage I or II) low-grade non-Hodgkin's lymphoma may be treated with local radiotherapy or a combination of chemotherapy and radiotherapy.[37–39] Radiotherapy produces permanent pulmonary injury, so its use should be restricted to small volumes of lung. If the pulmonary involvement is diffuse, chemotherapy is the treatment of choice. Conventional dose chemotherapy treatment may produce prolonged remissions but will not cure indolent lymphomas, and whether a high-dose chemotherapy approach is clearly more efficacious is controversial. Patients with advanced stage (stage III or IV) indolent non-Hodgkin's lymphoma, such as MALT lymphoma, are candidates for chemotherapy: Treatment is usually started when patients are clearly symptomatic from their disease, and responses to therapy are quite common but relapse is the rule.[40]

Patients having aggressive non-Hodgkin's lymphoma are treated at the time of diagnosis, in keeping with the more rapid progression of these lymphomas and the potentially curative nature of therapy. Localized disease, if completely staged, may be treated successfully with radiation therapy to involved areas: 5-year survival rates of 65% were found in one study of patients with clinical stage I disease, including those with extranodal lymphoma,[41] but in a series in which all patients were totally staged, including laparotomy, the 5-year survival with local radiotherapy was 100%.[42] Incompletely staged patients and patients having stage II disease, however, fare poorly with only localized radiotherapy, with a survival rate of 25% or less at 5 years. Treatment with chemotherapy or combined chemotherapy and radiotherapy has clearly improved these rates: 5-year survival rates in excess of 80% are reported for patients with localized stage I or II intermediate-grade and high-grade disease.[43, 44] Advanced stage intermediate-grade and high-grade non-Hodgkin's lymphomas are treated with combination chemotherapy; local radiotherapy to bulky areas of disease may be appropriate for patients whose bulky masses do not resolve entirely with chemotherapy.

Pulmonary non-Hodgkin's lymphoma has a more unique clinical course in immunosuppressed patients. Epstein-Barr virus–driven lymphoproliferative syndromes, seen in transplant patients receiving immunosuppressive drugs, mimic lymphoma in their presentation, which is usually with widespread disease.[45, 46, 47] Withdrawal of immunosuppressive medication may result in diminution of the disease, but fatalities are common. Lymphoma associated with acquired immunodeficiency syndrome (AIDS) and congenital immunodeficiency often involves extranodal sites and is virtually always intermediate or high grade in histology and B cell in origin. AIDS-associated lymphoma displays both clinical and genetic heterogeneity.[48, 49] Whereas AIDS-associated lymphoma responds to radiotherapy and chemotherapy, poor tolerance of treatment and rapid relapse is the rule, and median survival is less than 1 year.[50, 51] A unique form of lymphoma, involving body cavity serosal surfaces, may present as lymphoma in the pleural space in patients having advanced AIDS. The causative agent is believed to be human herpesvirus 8, the virus associated with Kaposi's sarcoma.[52] Human herpesvirus 8–associated body cavity–based lymphomas respond to chemotherapy, but are usually associated with rapid relapse and short survival.[53]

Non-Hodgkin's lymphoma may recur after treatment in both nodal and extranodal sites. As with Hodgkin's disease, complications of therapy and opportunistic infections must be distinguished from tumor recurrence in the lung. Molecular studies of very small specimens obtained from lavage or fine-needle aspirate may be quite useful in making a diagnosis of recurrence. Recurrence is the rule in indolent lymphomas, although a long disease-free period may occur from initial treatment to recurrence, and the recurrence may be as an aggressive subtype of lymphoma. Aggressive lymphomas recur rapidly as a rule; most recurrence in diffuse large cell lymphoma, for example, occur within the first 3 years after initial remission.[29]

The development of pulmonary masses or infiltrates in patients who have been treated for non-Hodgkin's lymphoma may be a sign of recurrence, of opportunistic infection, of pulmonary injury due to therapy, or of new malignancy. Non-Hodgkin's lymphoma is itself a common second neoplasm following successful treatment of both childhood[54, 55] and adult neoplasms.[56] Second neoplasms are increased in incidence following treatment of non-Hodgkin's lymphoma and include leukemia, bladder cancer, carcinoma of the lung, and bone sarcomas.[57] Imaging techniques may be somewhat helpful in delineating the possibilities.[16, 17] Minimally invasive techniques such as fine-needle aspiration and lavage may also be useful.[32–34, 58] One series suggests that, when surgical exploration is necessary, most cases will prove to have recurrence of lymphoma rather than new primary cancers or infections.[59]

## LYMPHOPROLIFERATIVE DISEASES

Disorders that are characterized by lymphoid infiltration in the lungs are numerous and varied in their manifestations. Several of these lymphocyte-derived disorders, however, are without obvious infectious or inflammatory cause and are commonly associated with a progressive course that terminates in a lymphoma or lymphoma-like illness. These include lymphomatoid granulomatosis, angioimmunoblastic lymphadenopathy, and other lymphoproliferative diseases, which are given various names such as pseudolymphoma and angiocentric lymphoproliferative disease. This category excludes Wegener's granulomatosis, allergic granulomatoses, sarcoidosis, and lymphocytic interstitial pneumonitis, which are described in Section L.

Lymphoproliferative disorders of the lung have undergone reclassification because of the availability of new molecular techniques that show that many are clonal proliferations of a single lymphoid cell and are therefore really lymphomas. Revision of the concepts of how pulmonary lymphoproliferative diseases are classified has been the result of the efforts of many of the original describers of pulmonary lymphoproliferative syndromes.[60–63] Lymphoma-oriented treatment is useful in these diseases, and their termination in a therapy-resistant, often high-grade lymphoma resembles the clinical course of indolent lymphomas.

### Lymphomatoid Granulomatosis

First described by Liebow and colleagues[64] in 1972, this angiocentric lymphoproliferative disease has always been of unknown etiology and poorly understood. Because of skin and pulmonary parenchymal involvement, the disease usually presents in adults with cough, dyspnea, and occasionally sputum production, fevers, and malaise.[65–67] Central nervous system manifestations occur in one fourth of patients and are characterized by focal deficits in an asymmetric distribution, sometimes with seizures. Central nervous system features range from mild to very severe and have contributed to death of patients in all large series. Dermatologic involvement occurs in nearly half of patients, with patchy erythematous macular or papular areas, usually small and nonconfluent. Lesions occur most often on the extremities and may ulcerate; subcutaneous nodules can also occur.

Pulmonary involvement is almost invariably a feature of lymphomatoid granulomatosis, and the most common appearance is that of parenchymal masses, usually in the periphery and lower lobes. Extensive destruction of lung parenchyma sufficient to cause respiratory insufficiency has been reported in most series, as well as the occasional occurrence of massive hemoptysis or severe cavitary disease. Airway infiltration may also occur, usually in bronchioles, but lobar obstruction by endobronchial destructive lesions has been reported.

Other organ involvement by lymphomatoid granulomatosis is unusual. In contrast to Wegener's granulomatosis, renal involvement is rare as a clinical manifestation, but may be found at necropsy. Focal necrotic and proliferative lesions are seen, without glomerulonephritis. Hepatic involvement, although unusual, may carry a worse prognosis. Lymph node and splenic involvement is rare and does not appear to adversely affect prognosis. Also in contrast to Wegener's granulomatosis, lymphomatoid granulomatosis rarely involves the nasopharynx and upper airways.

The diagnosis of lymphomatoid granulomatosis is made histologically. This disease displays a destructive, inflammatory granulomatous angiitis, but, in contrast to Wegener's granulomatosis, the lymphoid infiltrate is composed of atypical and immature cells with abundant mitoses and a paucity of polymorphonuclear or eosinophilic leukocytes. These infiltrates have been shown to be composed of a population of B cells, usually with Epstein-Barr virus RNA within them, and surrounding reactive T cells.[68, 69] There are no characteristic laboratory values in lymphomatoid granulomatosis. In contrast to angioimmunoblastic lymphadenopathy, paraproteinemia, cytopenias, and autoimmune antibodies are uncommon.

The radiographic appearance of lymphomatoid granulomatosis is not unique: Multiple bilateral pulmonary nodules involving the lower and peripheral lung fields (Fig. 47.3) are also seen in metastases, other granulomatous diseases, and benign disorders such as eosinophilic granuloma. Cavitation, atelectasis or lobar obstruction, large mass-like lesions, and pneumothorax may be seen in lymphomatoid granulomatosis. The pulmonary lesions typically wax and wane, and some areas may regress while others are progressing. Hilar and mediastinal adenopathy is rare, as are normal chest radiographs.[70]

The pathogenesis of lymphomatoid granulomatosis is unknown. Although the disease may be associated with syndromes in which impaired immunity occurs, such as Sjögren's syndrome, chronic viral hepatitis, rheumatoid arthritis, AIDS, and renal transplant, there has been no clear association with a specific pathogen. Although Epstein-Barr virus is frequently found in the B cells in the granulomas,[65, 66] no investigator has demonstrated a causative relationship, and the virus may have infected the proliferating B cells coincidentally. Furthermore, reports that abnormal T-cell function occurs in lymphomatoid granulomatosis patients without other immune system disorders[71] suggest that lymphomatoid granulomatosis itself, or perhaps the high-grade lymphomas that frequently arise in the course of the disease, may be due to opportunistic pathogens or to an aberrant immune response to some pathogen. Both monoclonal T-cell proliferation and monoclonal B-cell proliferation have been identified in this disease, thereby confusing the issue of pathogenesis, but suggesting the possibility of evolution to lymphoma.[72–74] The identification of primary T-cell

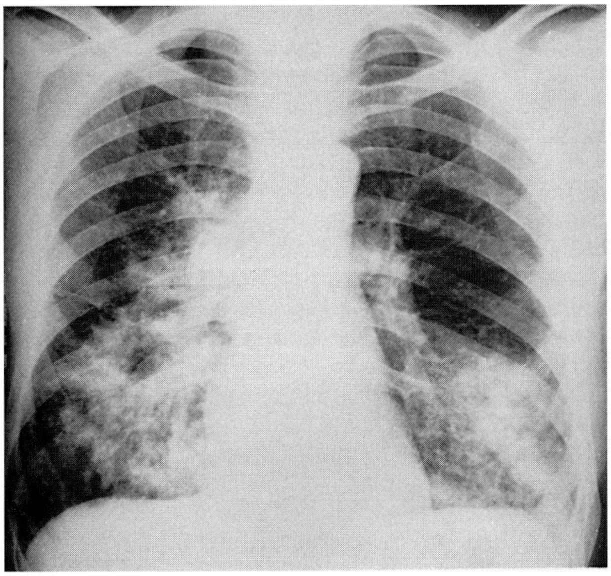

**Figure 47.3** Diffuse nodular pulmonary infiltrate in a 49-year-old man with pulmonary, renal, and central nervous system abnormalities is shown. The coalescing fluffy nodules were found to be lymphomatoid granulomatosis by biopsy. (Reproduced courtesy of Dr. G. Gamsu, University of California San Francisco, CA.)

lymphomas due to the human T-cell leukemia virus type I (HTLV-I) presenting with a syndrome much like lymphomatoid granulomatosis has further complicated the question of the pathogenesis of this disease.[75]

Treatment of lymphomatoid granulomatosis has been difficult. A significant fraction of patients have a benign disease course and may not require treatment for years or even longer. Individuals with symptomatic disease have been treated with steroids and antineoplastic drugs, predominantly low doses of cytotoxic drugs such as cyclophosphamide. Although the disease often responds to such measures, recurrence is frequent, and development of either refractory disease or high-grade lymphoma is common. Protracted responses to therapy may also occur, predominantly in patients having minimal disease with no central nervous system involvement. Radiotherapy works well for localized lesions,[76] but the optimum management of steroids, cytotoxic drugs, and radiotherapy remains unresolved. Lymphomatoid granulomatosis has a poor prognosis, with half or more of patients succumbing to the disease within 5 years. Its clinical course is quite heterogeneous, however, and long survivals and spontaneous remissions have been observed. The disease terminates in aggressive lymphoma in 15% to 25% of patients.

## Angioimmunoblastic Lymphadenopathy

Angioimmunoblastic lymphadenopathy was first described by Lukes and Tindle,[77] who noted that it resembled Hodgkin's disease but without the tell-tale Reed-Sternberg cell. Although known initially by a wide variety of names, this syndrome has ultimately been called either angioimmunoblastic lymphadenopathy or angioimmunoblastic lymphadenopathy with dysproteinemia (AILD).[78–80] Lymphadenopathy is a constant feature of the disease. Patients are virtually always adults and often have constitutional symptoms of fever, weight loss, and fatigue. Rash occurs in nearly half, and pruritus is a common symptom. Hepatosplenomegaly and splenomegaly are common findings, and the adenopathy may occur at any or all sites. Pulmonary involvement occurs as massive adenopathy, pleural effusion, pleural thickening, or diffuse interstitial pulmonary infiltrates. Patients with AILD have a 5% to 20% likelihood of developing aggressive lymphoma; the majority who die of the disease succumb to infection, including opportunistic infections. Approximately one third of patients have a benign course, with either mild disease or spontaneous remission. Overall, however, the median survival is poor: 1.5 years.

The characteristics of AILD that distinguish it from other lymphoproliferative diseases are the laboratory phenomena. Most patients are anemic, and 40% have both clinical and laboratory evidence of autoimmune hemolytic anemia. Dysproteinemia is another hallmark feature, with either nonspecific polyclonal hyperglobulinemia, which occurs in about 70% of cases, or late in the disease with hypoglobulinemia or monoclonal hyperglobulinemia. Leukocytosis, lymphopenia, thrombocytopenia, and eosinophilia have been reported in significant numbers of AILD patients. Autoantibodies abound: autoimmune thrombocytopenia, aplastic anemia, and serologic evidence of other autoimmune phenomena are common. Evidence of T-cell–mediated immune defects and dysregulation is also common.[81, 82]

The diagnosis of AILD may be suspected on clinical grounds, but the histologic features are necessary to finalize the diagnosis. The disease is characterized by proliferation and arborization of small blood vessels within the enlarged lymph nodes or lymphatic tissue; by effacement of normal lymph node architecture with a polymorphous inflammatory infiltrate and depletion of normal-appearing lymphocytes and germinal centers; and by the accumulation of amorphous eosinophilic material in intracellular spaces. It may resemble the histology of peripheral T-cell lymphomas, formerly called Lennert's lymphoma or Castleman's disease. Extranodal AILD may be found in bone marrow, skin, liver, lung, and rarely other internal organs. The infiltrate in such sites resembles the polymorphous appearance of Hodgkin's disease, although the Reed-Sternberg cell is absent. The appearance of the disease in human immunodeficiency virus (HIV)–infected patients is quite similar.[83] The differential diagnosis of pulmonary involvement by AILD includes infections, especially opportunistic infections. The lymphomas that occur in patients with AILD may be of any histologic type, though they are usually intermediate or high grade.[84, 85]

The pathogenesis of AILD is also unknown. The association of this disease with other immune dysfunction diseases such as Sjögren's syndrome and AIDS suggests that the primary problem may be immunodysregulation. The combination of B-cell–mediated overactivity and dysregulation with T-cell underfunction is similar to the immune defects in HIV-infected individuals, many of whom also develop lymphoma. Epstein-Barr virus has also been found in lymphatic tissue of AILD patients,[86, 87] but its etiologic relationship has not been established. The lymph node histology closely resembles that of patients with congenital rubella infections, and a rubella-like agent has been postulated; other infectious agents might include HTLV-III, HIV, and as yet unindentified retroviruses. Clonal populations of T cells have been identified in as many as 75% of cases of AILD,[88] leading to their inclusion in the current classification schemes (see Table 47.1). B-cell and T-cell proliferation unrestrained by a malfunctioning T-cell control mechanism has been proposed as the underlying problem, that permits the ultimate development of lymphoma in AILD patients.[89]

Treatment of AILD has followed the same pattern as lymphomatoid granulomatosis, with the early use of steroids and cytotoxic drugs, but the need to produce immunosuppression of the autoimmune phenomena has led to the use of other kinds of agents. Danazol, widely prescribed for autoimmune hemolytic anemia and thrombocytopenia, has been reported to have some efficacy in AILD patients.[90] Cyclosporine has also been used,[91] as has interferon alpha.[92, 93] Lymphoma arising in AILD patients has been treated with various types of combination chemotherapy. The prognosis of AILD remains poor despite treatment.

### Castleman's Disease

In 1956, Castleman and colleagues[94] described a lymphoproliferative disorder, sometimes called angiofollicular lymph node hyperplasia, of unknown etiology that now bears the senior author's name. Castleman's disease tends to present two different patterns of involvement: the first type is focal, localized or unicentric, whereas the second type includes diffuse multicentric disease with systemic manifestations.[94a] The lesions consist of large collections of lymphoid cells organized in loose follicles with interspersed vessels and small lymphoid cells. Unicentric Castleman's disease presents as one or more asymptomatic masses in the mediastinum or lungs in both children and adults. The masses are usually lobulated, are generally not calcified, mostly have smooth margins, and are found by CT scan to be very vascular.[94b, 94c] These solitary masses can be diagnosed as Castleman's disease only by wide, often excisional, biopsy; smaller specimens typically yield nonspecific results.

Multicentric Castleman's disease presents more clinical challenges. In addition to the lungs and mediastinum, lesions may occur in a variety of extrathoracic sites, including neck, retroperitoneum, pelvis, and axillary nodes. Patients often have systemic symptoms, including fever and night sweats, weight loss, fatigue, and neuropathy. Laboratory findings may include anemia, hyperglobulinemia, hypoalbuminemia, and autoimmune phenomena. Biopsies are more likely to show plasma cells than lymphocytes infiltrating among follicles. The multicentric variant has been described in patients with HIV infection and has been linked to the presence of human herpesvirus 8 (or Kaposi's sarcoma herpesvirus, KSHV); human herpesvirus has also been identified in pathologic lymph nodes from patients without HIV infection.[94d] The causal relationship between this virus and the disease has not been clearly defined, but the suspicion is that proliferation of B cells is actuated either by a host response to human herpesvirus infection or by genes in the virus itself. Investigators have shown that the stroma cells in Castleman's disease produce large quantities of interleukin-6 (IL-6)[94e] and that the B cells in the same masses have high levels of IL-6 receptors,[94f] suggesting an autocrine mechanism for growth in these masses. Excess levels of IL-6 may also be responsible for the systemic symptoms seen in multicentric Castleman's disease.

Treatment of Castleman's disease depends on the type of disease in a given patient. The nodules of unicentric Castleman's disease are usually resected surgically, with excellent long-term results. When these lymphoid nodules are located in areas difficult to resect, they may be treated with radiation therapy. Multicentric Castleman's disease has been treated with corticosteroids, immunosuppressive therapy, cytotoxic drugs, and radiation therapy. The results of these various therapies have not been systematically reported, but in general, the more symptomatic the patient, the poorer the response and the shorter the survival; optimal treatment is unknown.[95g] Anecdotal reports of patients with HIV-associated multicentric Castleman's disease suggest that highly active antiretroviral therapy for HIV may help, although there is a report of three patients with AIDS in whom symptoms of fulminant multicentric Castleman's disease developed after the initiation of highly active antiretroviral therapy.[94h] Neither unicentric nor multicentric Castleman's disease progresses to lymphoma, in contrast to the other lymphoproliferative syndromes discussed in this chapter.

## OTHER PRIMARY MALIGNANT TUMORS

### Carcinoid and Neuroendocrine Carcinomas

Carcinoid tumors arising in the lungs and bronchi were first described in 1937, when they were characterized as a neoplasm distinct from bronchial adenoma. In the 1960s their microscopic features were compared with carcinoids occurring in other components of the embryonic foregut: the stomach, duodenum, gallbladder, and pancreas. Later, the electron micrographic and immunohistochemical features of these tumors were expanded. Bronchial carcinoids share neuroendocrine properties with a family of tumors thought to be derived from primitive neural crest tissue, including the gut carcinoids, APUDomas, pheochromocytomas, medullary carcinoma of the thyroid, and other endocrine tumors. Typical bronchial carcinoid cells are small and uniform in appearance with acidophilic cytoplasm and finely stippled chromatin. They are argyrophilic and contain neurosecretory granules on electron microscopy. They stain positively with immunohistochemical stains for neuron-specific enolase, chromogranin A, synaptophysin, serotonin, and other neurosecretory cell markers. *Neuroendocrine carcinomas,* also referred to as *atypical bronchial carcinoids,* are characterized by larger cell size and fewer characteristic nuclear and cytoplasmic features, but they retain at least some immunohistochemical stain positivity and electron micrographic features of neuroendocrine neoplasms. Both must be distinguished from other bronchial tumors and from small cell carcinoma of the lung.[94–96]

## Incidence and Natural History

Bronchial carcinoids occur in a wide age range, with most clinical series showing a median age in the mid 40s. They are extremely rare in children but occur equally in both sexes. There are fewer than 2000 cases in the United States annually, and they represent about 2% of all primary lung tumors.[96a] Bronchial carcinoids represent about 25% of all carcinoid tumors and may be slightly more common in African-American males.[97] There is no known relationship to smoking or other environmental factors.

Carcinoid tumors may spread via either lymphatics or the bloodstream. The size and degree of differentiation of the primary tumor may be predictive of the likelihood of metastasis. Patterns of hematogenous spread show a predilection for the liver, bones, central nervous system, and adrenals. Serotonin-producing carcinoids are unusual in the lungs, and only about half of patients having elevated urinary serotonin metabolites also have the clinical carcinoid syndrome. Other endocrine syndromes such as Cushing's disease, antidiuretic hormone secretion; and fever have been reported, as have rare cases associated with multiple endocrine neoplasias.[98–101]

## Clinical Presentation

Central pulmonary carcinoid tumors that arise in the larger airways comprise about one half of all cases. Cough is the most common presenting symptom in such cases. Bronchial carcinoids are highly vascular tumors, and, although they originate submucosally, hemoptysis is a common presenting symptom, reported in 18% to 35% of series. Bronchial obstruction, causing stridor or wheezing, recurrent pneumonia, bronchiectasis, or lung abscess, is a common clinical feature, occurring in 15% to 25% of all patients. Weakness, weight loss, and fever are common accompanying symptoms in these patients. Systemic symptoms and local symptoms of metastasis, such as bone pain, are present in very few patients. Many patients (25% to 60%) are entirely asymptomatic, and the tumor is discovered on chest radiographs or CT scans taken for another purpose.

## Diagnosis

The radiographic features of bronchial carcinoid are few, although most patients with pulmonary carcinoids have abnormal chest radiographs, either due to the tumor itself or to airway obstruction and its consequences. The tumor masses are usually not necrotic or are variable in density on plain films, and fewer than 10% have visible calcifications. CT evaluation may be useful in establishing that a pulmonary parenchymal mass has an endobronchial component[102]; in general, however, both atypical and typical bronchial carcinoids are found to be very vascular, well-defined masses, some with detectable intratumoral calcification.[103, 104]

Adequate tissue for pathologic diagnosis of carcinoid or atypical carcinoid should be obtained, such as small samples from fine-needle aspiration or forceps biopsy at bronchoscopy, but this is not uniformly possible. Although these tumors are highly vascular, an increased risk of bleeding complications has not been reported in contemporary studies with flexible fiberoptic endoscopes and transbronchial biopsy. Bronchial brushings, sputum specimens, and lavage fluid are rarely worthwhile sources for tissue diagnosis. Thoracotomy and resection are frequently performed when the differential diagnosis includes a bronchogenic carcinoma.

Laboratory evaluation of patients with carcinoid tumors may include liver function tests, and 24-hour urine serotonin metabolites (5-hydroxyindoleacetic acid [5-HIAA]), which may be elevated in up to 25% of patients at diagnosis. Evaluation for metastatic disease may include a variety of sites: The central nervous system, adrenals, liver, and bones are the most common sites of hematogenous dissemination of bronchial carcinoid, both typical and atypical. Node metastases to the hila and mediastinum may occur in carcinoid tumors, but most patients with small typical carcinoids do not require metastatic evaluation at the time of diagnosis. If the tumor is less than 2 cm in diameter, resectable, and typical in histology, the prognosis is excellent, and metastatic evaluation not justified.[105] Persistent elevation of urinary 5-HIAA or other serum hormone level should, however, prompt an investigation for metastatic disease.

## Treatment

Surgical resection of carcinoid tumors is the only means of cure for these cancers. Because they are usually locally well defined, surgical margins may be extremely small and the risk of local recurrence low. Resection via bronchoscopy is technically possible for some tiny tumors, but the results from series with fulguration via bronchoscopy show that the recurrence rate is high.[93] If formal surgical salvage is also available, the prognosis may not be altered adversely,[106] and the procedure does offer palliation of symptoms. Tracheal carcinoids are amenable to tracheal resection or sleeve resection with good results.[107] When thoracotomy is performed and tumors are larger than 2 cm or are not well differentiated, staging by sampling the hilar and mediastinal nodes is appropriate.

Radiation therapy has a defined palliative role in the treatment of carcinoid tumors. The results from the largest reported series of patients with carcinoids of various sites suggest that, although 80% of treated patients have a partial or complete response to radiotherapy, curative therapy for gross disease is not a reasonable expectation.[108] Doses of 4500 to 5000 cGy are appropriate at sites where this is feasible. Prolonged symptomatic palliation may occur, especially with spinal cord metastases and osseous metastases. Hepatic and pulmonary metastases are not well treated by this therapy because of low tissue tolerance of radiation and the resulting low doses to tumor.

Chemotherapy has a limited role in the treatment of metastatic carcinoid tumors. The most effective regimens reported contain streptozotocin, 5-fluorouracil, cyclophosphamide, dacarbazine, or doxorubicin.[109] Objective response rates are less than 40%, and combination therapy has not been formally compared with the use of single drugs. Response durations, when reported, are usually short; no trial has demonstrated a prolongation of survival

tive bronchiolitis[143] and Cushing's syndrome[143a] have been reported.

Tumorlets are thought to be derived from normal neuroendocrine cells in the lungs. The tumorlets are argyrophilic and stain for neuron-specific enolase and other markers of neuroendocrine cells. What makes them proliferate is not understood, but they are thought to be part of the lung's inflammatory response.[144, 145] Pulmonary tumorlets were shown to have acquired novel neuroendocrine properties compared with normal pulmonary neuroendocrine cells, suggesting that the proliferation is associated with abnormal, perhaps even neoplastic features.[146] Pulmonary tumorlets remain a pathologic enigma.

## Other Tumors

### Multiple Myeloma and Waldenström's Macroglobulinemia

Multiple myeloma and Waldenström's macroglobulinemia derive from the immunoglobulin-producing B cells: plasma cells producing IgG, IgA, or IgE in myeloma and plasmacytoid lymphocytes producing IgM in Waldenström's macroglobulinemia. In rare cases, each of these diseases may present as either a pulmonary parenchymal mass or pleural effusion. In even rarer circumstances, these manifestations may be the first or only signs of the disease. Bone marrow involvement accompanies most cases of pulmonary involvement by these two diseases.[147, 148]

Primary pulmonary involvement is frequently asymptomatic. Dyspnea is usually the first symptom of large pleural effusions. Associated symptoms may reflect the underlying systemic disease and may include fatigue, bruisability, bone pain, fever, and weight loss. Clinical signs may include adenopathy or visceromegaly in Waldenström's macroglobulinemia, petechiae or purpura, and signs of hyperviscosity such as vascular plethora, edema, or congestive heart failure.

Radiographic signs are nonspecific. The parenchymal lesions are usually poorly circumscribed masses or nodules. Lytic bone lesions may be a useful sign of multiple myeloma, although diffuse osteopenia is common to both diseases. Diagnosis may be made by needle aspiration, especially if it includes immunohistochemical staining showing a monoclonal surface immunoglobulin. The differential diagnosis includes granulomatous diseases, infection, and benign lymphoproliferative diseases. Laboratory evaluation must include demonstration of the monoclonal immunoglobulin in the tumor as well as a diligent search for systemic disease, employing bone marrow biopsy, serum and urine immunoelectrophoresis, and skeletal radiographic survey.[149, 150]

True solitary plasmacytoma has a good prognosis if treated with excision or radiation therapy, but the tumor is very uncommon. It most often precedes the later development of clinically overt multiple myeloma. Patients having pleural effusion may be treated with intrapleural sclerotherapy and systemic chemotherapy. The median survival of patients with systemic disease is 3 to 4 years. Additional information about multiple myeloma and Waldenström's macroglobulinemia is provided in Chapter 86.

### Primary Pulmonary Melanoma

There are only 28 cases of primary pulmonary melanoma in the literature that are well enough documented to exclude a cutaneous or ocular primary site.[151, 152] The tumors in these cases were both bronchial and parenchymal, and all occurred in adults. Presenting signs are nonspecific, and an extremely careful search for a primary site or for other evidence of metastases is important before making the diagnosis of primary pulmonary melanoma,[153] and immunohistochemical staining and electron microscopy are useful confirmatory tests. The pathogenesis of primary pulmonary melanoma is not clear, but the similarity of melanoma to neuroendocrine carcinomas raises the possibility that these tumors may develop from pulmonary neuroendocrine cells. Primary pulmonary melanoma is more advanced locally at diagnosis than is cutaneous melanoma and thus more likely to recur after surgical excision. Standard treatment is surgical resection, and case reports suggest that prolonged remission of the disease is possible. Nonsurgical candidates may be palliated with radiation therapy. Newer biologic therapies and chemotherapy may be considered for individuals with recurrent or unresponsive disease.

## SUMMARY

The nonbronchogenic malignancies that involve the lung are a varied group of diseases with highly variable natural histories and outcomes. The non-Hodgkin's lymphomas range from highly aggressive but curable tumors to more indolent cancers that are incurable. Pulmonary Hodgkin's disease is most often seen as a direct extension of tumor involving the hilar and mediastinal nodes and is curable with aggressive therapy, usually a combination of chemotherapy and radiotherapy. Carcinoid tumors are surgically curable if small and not atypical in appearance; larger and less differentiated tumors, especially when metastatic, have no known curative treatment. Similarly, the better differentiated mucoepithelial cancers are curable when they can be completely removed surgically; sarcomas are likewise potentially curable. Neither class of tumor is curable when metastases occur, and both have a high rate of local recurrence, even when they are low grade and indolent in nature.

This group of cancers is becoming much better defined clinically in part due to advances in their molecular characterization. Indolent inflammatory diseases can be distinguished from low-grade lymphomas by means of newer technologies, allowing for more directed therapies for these patients. The same techniques may be used to define extranodal pulmonary involvement by other lymphomas, especially recurrent lymphomas, thereby making more appropriate treatment decisions possible with less invasive diagnostic procedures.

## References

1. Whimster WF: Lung tumors: Differentiation and classification. Pathol Annu 18:121–138, 1983.
2. Wood NL, Coltman CA: Localized primary extranodal Hodgkin's disease. Ann Intern Med 78:113–118, 1973.

3. Yousem SA, Weiss LM, Colby TV: Primary pulmonary Hodgkin's disease. Cancer 57:1217–1224, 1986.
4. Friedman M, Kim U, Shimaoka K, et al: Appraisal of aspiration cytology in management of Hodgkin's disease. Cancer 45:1653–1663, 1980.
5. Connors JM, Klimo P: Is it an E lesion or stage IV? An unsettled issue in Hodgkin's disease staging. J Clin Oncol 2:1421–1423, 1984.
6. Diehll LF, Hopper KD, Giguere J, et al: The pattern of intrathoracic Hodgkin's disease assessed by computed tomography. J Clin Oncol 9:438–443, 1991.
7. Lewis ER, Caskey CI, Fishman EK: Lymphoma of the lung: CT findings in 31 patients. AJR Am J Roentgenol 156:711–714, 1991.
8. McCloud TC, Naidich DP: Thoracic disease in the immunocompromised patient. Radiol Clin N Am 30:525–554, 1992.
9. Morales FM, Matthews JI: Diagnosis of parenchymal Hodgkin's disease using bronchoalveolar lavage. Chest 91:785–787, 1987.
10. Rubin A-HE, Ben-Shachar M, Malberger E: Cytologic diagnosis of pulmonary Hodgkin's disease via endobronchial brush preparation. Chest 96:948–949, 1989.
11. Reale FR, Varikojis D, Compton JC, et al: Cytodiagnosis of Hodgkin's disease in sputum specimens. Acta Cytol 27:258–261, 1983.
12. Friedman M, Kim U, Shimaoka K, et al: Appraisal of aspiration cytology in management of Hodgkin's disease. Cancer 45:1653–1663, 1980.
13. Torti FM, Portlock CS, Rosenberg SA, et al: Extralymphatic Hodgkin's disease: Prognosis and response to therapy. Am J Med 70:487–492, 1981.
14. Levi JA, Wiernik PH: Limited extranodal Hodgkin's disease: Unfavorable prognosis and therapeutic implications. Am J Med 63:365–372, 1977.
15. Lee CKK, Bloomfield CD, Goldman AI, et al: Prognostic significance of mediastinal involvement in Hodgkin's disease treated with curative radiotherapy. Cancer 46:2403–2409, 1980.
16. Mauch P, Goodman R, Hellman S: The significance of mediastinal involvement in early stage Hodgkin's disease. Cancer 42:1039–1045, 1978.
17. Prosnitz LR, Curtis AM, Knowlton AH: Supradiaphragmatic Hodgkin's disease: Significance of large mediastinal masses. Int J Radiat Oncol Biol Phys 6:809–813, 1980.
18. Jochelson MS: The treated thorax. Radiol Clin North Am 28:763–769, 1990.
19. Libshutz HI, Brosof AB, Southard ME: Radiographic appearance of the chest following extended field radiation therapy for Hodgkin's disease. Cancer 32:206–215, 1973.
20. Tucker MA, Coleman CN, Cox RS, et al: Risk of second malignancies following Hodgkin's disease after 15 years. N Engl J Med 318:76–81, 1988.
21. Meadows AT, Obringer AC, Marrero O, et al: Second malignant neoplasms following childhood Hodgkin's disease: Treatment and splenectomy as risk factors. Med Pediatr Oncol 17:477–484, 1989.
22. Putterman C, Polliack A: Late cardiovascular and pulmonary complications of therapy in Hodgkin's disease: Report of three unusual cases, with a review of relevant literature. Leuk Lymphoma 7:109–115, 1992.
23. Allavena C, Conreoy T., Aletti P, et al: Late cardiopulmonary toxicity after treatment for Hodgkin's disease. Br J Cancer 65:908–912, 1992.
24. Harris ML, Jaffe ES, Stein H, et al: A revised European-American classification of lymphoid neoplasms: A proposal from the International Lymphoma Study Group. Blood 84:1361–1392, 1994.
25. International Non-Hodgkin's Lymphoma Prognostic Factors Project: A predictive model for aggressive non-Hodgkin's lymphoma. N Engl J Med 329:987–994, 1993.
26. Cordier JF, Chailleux E, Lauque D, et al: Primary pulmonary lymphomas: A clinical study of 70 cases in non immunocompromised patients. Chest 103:201–208, 1993.
27. Fiche M, Capron F, Berger F, et al: Primary pulmonary non-Hodgkin's lymphomas. Histopathology 26:529–537, 1995.
28. Armitage JO, Weisenburger DD: New approach to classifying non-Hodgkin's lymphomas: Clinical features of the major histologic subtypes. J Clin Oncol 16:2780–2795, 1998.
29. A clinical evaluation of the International Lymphoma Study Group classification of non-Hodgkin's lymphoma. Blood 89:3909–3918, 1997.
30. Bienenstock J, Johnston N, Perey DYE: Bronchial lymphoid tissue. I. Morphologic characteristics. Lab Invest 28:686–692, 1973.
31. Kradin RL, Mark EJ: Benign lymphoid disorders of the lung, with a theory regarding their development. Hum Pathol 14:857–867, 1983.
32. Weiss LW, Warnke RA, Sklar J, et al: Molecular analysis of the t(14;18) chromosomal translocation in malignant lymphoma. N Engl J Med 317:1185–1189, 1987.
33. Pisani RJ, Witzig TE, Li C-Y, et al: Confirmation of lymphomatous pulmonary involvement by immunophenotypic and gene rearrangement analysis of bronchoalveolar lavage fluid. Mayo Clin Proc 65:651–656, 1990.
34. Nicholson AG, Wotherspoon AC, Diss TC, et al: Pulmonary B-cell non-Hodgkin's lymphomas. The value of immunohistochemistry and gene analysis in diagnosis. Histopathology 26:395–403, 1995.
35. Zaer F, Braylan M, Zander D, et al: Multiparametric flow cytometry in the diagnosis and characterization of low-grade pulmonary mucosa-associated lymphoid tissue lymphomas. Mod Pathol 11:525–532, 1998.
35a. Kinsely BL, Mastey LA, Mergo PJ, et al: Pulmonary mucosa-associated lymphoid tissue lymphoma: CT and pathologic findings. AJR Am J Roentgenol 172:1321–1326, 1999.
36. Chabner, BA, Johnson, RE, Young, RC, et al: Sequential nonsurgical and surgical staging of non-Hodgkin's lymphoma. Cancer 42:922–925, 1978.
37. McLaughlin P, Fuller LM, Velasquez WS, et al: Stage I-II follicular lymphoma. Treatment results for 76 patients. Cancer 58:1596–1602, 1986.
38. Monfardini S, Banfi A, Bonnadonna G, et al: Improved five year survival after combined radiotherapy-chemotherapy for stage I–II non-Hodgkin's lymphoma. Int J Radiat Oncol Biol Phys 6:125–134, 1980.
39. Gomez GA, Barcos M, Krishnomsetty RM, et al: Treatment of early—stages I and II—nodular, poorly differentiated lymphocytic lymphoma. Am J Clin Oncol 9:40, 1986.
40. Portlock CS, Rosenberg SA: No initial therapy for stage III and IV non-Hodgkin's lymphoma of favorable histologic types. Ann Intern Med 90:10–13, 1979.
41. Jones SE, Fuks A, Kaplan HS, et al: Non-Hodgkin's lymphomas. V. Results of radiotherapy. Cancer 32:682–691, 1973.
42. Vokes EE, Ultmann JE, Golomb HM, et al: Long-term survival of patients with localized diffuse histiocytic lymphoma. J Clin Oncol 3:1309–1313, 1985.
43. Cabanillas F, Bodey GP, Freireich EJ: Management with chemotherapy only of stage I and II malignant lymphoma of aggressive histologic types. Cancer 46:2356–2359, 1980.
44. Connors JM, Klimo P, Fairey RN, et al: Brief chemotherapy and involved field radiation therapy for limited-stage, histologically aggressive lymphoma. Ann Intern Med 107:25–30, 1987.
45. List AF, Greco FA, Vogler LB: Lymphoproliferative diseases in immunocompromised hosts: The role of Epstein-Barr virus. J Clin Oncol 5:1673–1689, 1987.
46. Young L, Alfieri C, Hennessy K, et al: Expression of Epstein-Barr virus transformation-associated genes in tissues of patients with EBV lymphoproliferative disease. N Engl J Med 321:1080–1085, 1989.
47. Purtilo DT, Strobach RS, Okano M, et al: Epstein-Barr virus-associated lymphoproliferative disorders. Lab Invest 67:5–23, 1992.
48. Northfelt DW, Kaplan LD Clinical aspects of AIDS-related non-Hodgkin's lymphoma. Curr Opin Oncol 3:872–880, 1991.
49. Shiramizu B, McGrath MS: Molecular pathogenesis of AIDS-associated non-Hodgkin's lymphoma. Hematol Oncol Clin North Am 5:323–330, 1991.
50. Northfelt DW, Kaplan, LD: Clinical manifestations and treatment of HIV related non-Hodgkin lymphoma. Cancer Surv 10:121–133, 1991.
51. Levine AM: Acquired immunodeficiency syndrome-related lymphoma. Blood 80:8–20, 1992.
52. Cesarman E, Chang Y, Moore, PS, et al: Kaposi's sarcoma-associated herpesvirus-like DNA sequences in AIDS-related body-cavity–based lymphomas. N Engl J Med 332:1186–1191, 1995.

53. Komanduri KV, Luce JA, McGrath MS, et al: The natural history and molecular heterogeneity of HIV-associated primary malignant lymphomatous effusions. J AIDS 13:215–226, 1996.
54. Eguiguren JM, Ribiero RC, Pui CH, et al: Secondary non-Hodgkin's lymphoma after treatment for childhood cancer. Leukemia 5:908–911, 1991.
55. Meadows AT, Baum E, Bellani-Fossati F, et al: Second malignant neoplasms in children: An update from the Late Effects Study Group. J Clin Oncol 3:532–538, 1985.
56. van Leeuwen FE: Second cancers. *In* DeVita VT Jr, Hellman S, Rosenberg SA (eds): Cancer: Principles and Practice of Oncology (5th ed). Philadelphia: Lippincott-Raven, 1997, pp 2773–2796.
57. Travis LB, Curtis RE, Boice JD Jr, et al: Second cancers following non-Hodgkin's lymphoma. Cancer 67:2002–2009, 1991.
58. Roggeri A, Prandi S, Iori I: Pulmonary involvement in non-Hodgkin's malignant lymphomas. Chest 99:527, 1991.
59. Yellin A, Pak HY, Burke JS, et al: Surgical management of lymphomas involving the chest. Ann Thorac Surg 44:363–369, 1987.
60. Colby TV, Carrington CB: Lymphoreticular tumors and infiltrates of the lung. Pathol Annu 18:27–70, 1983.
61. Churg A: Pulmonary angiitis and granulomatosis revisited. Hum Pathol 14:868–883, 1983.
62. Kennedy JL, Nathwani BN, Burke JS, et al: Pulmonary lymphomas and other pulmonary lymphoid lesions. Cancer 56:539–552, 1985.
63. Addis BJ, Hyjek E, Isaacson PG: Primary pulmonary lymphoma: A re-appraisal of its histogenesis and its relationship to pseudolymphoma and lymphoid interstitial pneumonitis. Histopathology 13:1–17, 1988.
64. Liebow AA, Carrington CRB, Friedman PJ: Lymphomatoid granulomatosis. Hum Pathol 3:457–558, 1972.
65. Katzenstein A-LA, Carrington CB, Liebow AA: Lymphomatoid granulomatosis. A clinicopathological study of 152 cases. Cancer 43:360–373, 1979.
66. Patton WF, Lynch JP III: Lymphomatoid granulomatosis. Clinicopathologic study of four cases and literature review. Medicine 61:1–12, 1982.
67. Fauci AS, Haynes BE, Costa J, et al: Lymphomatoid granulomatosis. Prospective clinical and therapeutic experience over 10 years. N Engl J Med 306:68–74, 1982.
68. Wilson WH, Kingma DW, Raffeld M, et al: Association of lymphomatoid granulomatosis with Epstein-Barr viral infection of B lymphocytes and response to interferon-alpha 2b. Blood 87:4531–4537, 1996.
69. Haque AK, Myers JL, Hudnall SD, et al: Pulmonary lymphomatoid granulomatosis in acquired immunodeficiency syndrome: Lesions with Epstein-Barr virus infection. Mod Pathol 11:347–356, 1998.
70. Frazier AA, Rosado-de-Christenson ML, Galvin JR, et al: Pulmonary angiitis and granulomatosis: Radiologic-pathologic correlation. Radiographics 18:687–710, 1998.
71. Sordillo PP, Epremian B, Koziner B, et al: Lymphomatoid granulomatosis: An analysis of clinical and immunologic characteristics. Cancer 49:2070–2076, 1982.
72. Gaulard P, Henni T, Marolleau JP, et al: Lethal midline granuloma (polymorphic reticulosis) and lymphomatoid granulomatosis. Evidence for a monoclonal T-cell lymphoproliferative disorder. Cancer 62:705–710, 1988.
73. Bleiweiss IJ, Strauchen JA: Lymphomatoid granulomatosis of the lung: Report of a case and gene rearrangement studies. Hum Pathol 19:1109–1112, 1988.
74. Jaffe ES, Wilson WH: Lymphomatoid granulomatosis: Pathogenesis, pathology, and clinical implications. Cancer Surv 30:233–248, 1997.
75. McNutt NS, Smoller BR, Kline M, et al: Angiocentric T-cell lymphoma associated with human T-cell lymphotropic virus type I infection. Arch Pathol Lab Med 114:170–175, 1990.
76. Nair BD, Joseph MG, Catton GE, et al: Radiation therapy in lymphomatoid granulomatosis. Cancer 64:821–824, 1989 [published erratum in Cancer 64:1795, 1989].
77. Lukes RJ, Tindle BH: Immunoblastic lymphadenopathy: A hyperimmune entity resembling Hodgkin's disease. N Engl J Med 292:1–8, 1975.
78. Frizzera G, Moran EM, Rappaport H: Angio-immunoblastic lymphadenopathy. Diagnosis and clinical course. Am J Med 59:803–818, 1975.
79. Aozasa K: Angioimmunoblastic lymphadenopathy: Review of 44 patients with emphasis on prognostic behavior. Cancer 63:1625–1629, 1989.
80. Knecht H: Angioblastic lymphadenopathy: Ten years' experience and state of current knowledge. Semin Hematol 26:208–215, 1989.
81. Neiman RS, Dervan P, Haudenschild C, et al: Angioimmunoblastic lymphadenopathy: An ultrastructural and immunologic study with review of the literature. Cancer 41:507–518, 1978.
82. Pizzolo G: Increased serum levels of soluble IL-2 receptor, CD30 and CD8 molecules, and gamma-interferon in angioimmunoblastic lymphadenopathy: Possible pathogenetic role of immunoactivation mechanisms. Br J Haematol 75:485–488, 1990.
83. Blumenfeld W: Angioimmunoblastic lymphadenopathy with dysproteinemia in homosexual men with acquired immune deficiency syndrome. Arch Pathol Lab Med 107:567–569, 1983.
84. Nathwani BN, Rappaport H, Moran EM, et al: Malignant lymphoma arising in angioimmunoblastic lymphadenopathy. Cancer 41:578–606, 1978.
85. Bluming AZ, Cohen HG, Saxon A: Angioimmunoblastic lymphadenopathy with dysproteinemia. A pathogenetic link between physiologic lymphoid proliferation and malignant lymphoma. Am J Med 67:421–428, 1979.
86. Lipford EH Jr, Margolick JB, Longo DL, et al: Angiocentric immunoproliferative lesions: A clinicopathologic spectrum of postthymic T cell proliferations. Blood 72:1674–1681, 1988.
87. Medeiros LJ, Jaffe ES, Chen YY, et al: Localization of Epstein-Barr viral genomes in angiocentric immunoproliferative lesions. Am J Surg Pathol 16:439–447, 1992.
88. Feller A, Griesser H, Schilling C, et al: Clonal gene rearrangement patterns correlate with immunophenotype and clinical parameters in patients with angioimmunoblastic lymphadenopathy. Am J Pathol 133:549–556, 1988.
89. Tindle B: The pathology of immunoblastic proliferations: Reaction, prelymphoma, lymphoma. Pathol Annu 26:145–186, 1991.
90. Banavali S: Danazol in treatment of angioimmunoblastic lymphadenopathy. Cancer 64:613–615, 1989.
91. Murayama T: Successful treatment of angioimmunoblastic lymphadenopathy with dysproteinemia with cyclosporin A. Cancer 69:1259–1267, 1992.
92. Schwarzmeier J: Interferon-alpha induces complete remission in angioimmunoblastic lymphadenopathy (AILD): Late development of aplastic anaemia with cytokine abnormalities. Br J Haematol 79:336–337, 1991.
93. Meuthen I: Lymphogranulomatosis X: Complete remission by low dose interferon-alpha. Br J Haematol 75:438–439, 1990.
94. Castleman B, Iverson L, Menedez VP: Localized mediastinal lymph node hyperplasia resembling thymoma. Cancer 9:822–839, 1956.
94a. McCarty JJ, Vukelja SJ, Banks PM, et al: Angiofollicular lymph node hyperplasia (Castleman's disease). Cancer Treat Rev 21:291–310, 1995.
94b. Onik G, Goodman P: CT of Castleman's disease. AJR Am J Roentgenol 140:691–692, 1983.
94c. Fiore D, Biondetti P, Calabro F, et al: CT demonstration of bilateral Castleman tumors in the mediastinum. J Comput Assist Tomogr 7:719–720, 1983.
94d. Cesarman E, Knowles DM: The role of Kaposi's sarcoma–associated herpesvirus (KSHV/HHV-8) in lymphoproliferative diseases. Semin Cancer Biol 9:165–174, 1999.
94e. Emilie D, Zou W, Fior R, et al: Production and roles of IL-6, IL-10, and IL-13 in B-lymphocyte malignancies and in B-lymphocyte hyperactivity of HIV infection and autoimmunity. Methods 11:133–142, 1997.
94f. Ishiyama T, Koike M, Nakamura S, et al: Interleukin-6 receptor expression in the peripheral B cells of patients with multicentric Castleman's disease. Ann Hematol 73:179–182, 1996.
94g. Bowne WB, Lewis JJ, Filippa DA, et al: The management of unicentric and multicentric Castleman's disease: A report of 16 cases and a review of the literature. Cancer 85:706–717, 1999.
94h. Zietz C, Bogner JR, Goebel F-D, et al: An unusual cluster of Castleman's disease during highly active antiretroviral therapy for AIDS. N Engl J Med 340:1923–1924, 1999.

95. Warren WH, Memoli VA, Gould VE: Well differentiated and small cell neuroendocrine carcinomas of the lung: Two related but distinct clinicopathologic entities. Virchows Arch Biol 55:299–310, 1988.
96. Paladugu RR, Benfield JR, Pak HY, et al: Broncho-pulmonary Kulchitsky cell carcinomas I and II—alias typical and atypical carcinoids. Cancer 55:1303–1311, 1985.
96a. Kulke MH, Mayer RJ: Carcinoid tumors. N Engl J Med 340:858–868, 1999.
97. Modlin IM, Sandor A: An analysis of 8305 cases of carcinoid tumors. Cancer 79:813–829, 1997.
98. Benfield JR: Neuroendocrine neoplasms of the lung. J Thorac Cardiovasc Surg 100:628–629, 1990.
99. Harpole DH, Feldman JM, Buchanan S, et al: Bronchial carcinoid tumor: A retrospective analysis of 126 patients. Ann Thorac Surg 54:50–55, 1992.
100. Okike N, Bernatz PE, Woolner LB: Carcinoid tumors of the lung. Ann Thorac Surg 22:270–277, 1976.
101. Stamatis G, Freitag L, Greschuchna D: Limited and radical resection for tracheal and broncho-pulmonary carcinoid tumor: Report on 227 cases. Eur J Cardiothorac Surg 4:527–533, 1990.
102. Davis SD, Zirn JR, Govoni AF, et al: Peripheral carcinoid tumor of the lung: CT diagnosis. AJR Am J Roentgenol 155:1185–1187, 1990.
103. Naidich DP, McCauley DI, Siegelman SS: Computed tomography of bronchial adenomas. J Comput Assist Tomogr 6:725–732, 1982.
104. Zweibel BR, Austin JHM, Grimes MM: Bronchial carcinoid tumors: Assessment with CT of location and intratumoral calcification in 31 patients. Radiology 179:483–486, 1991.
105. Ducrocq X, Thomas P, Massard G, et al: Operative risk and prognostic factors of typical bronchial carcinoid tumors. Ann Thorac Surg 65:1410–1414, 1998.
106. Van Boxem TJ, Venmans BJ, van Mourik JC, et al: Bronchoscopic treatment of intraluminal typical carcinoid: A pilot study. J Thorac Cardiovasc Surg 116:402–406, 1998.
107. Briselli M, Mark GJ, Grillo HC: Tracheal carcinoids. Cancer 42:2870–2879, 1978.
108. Schupak KD, Wallner KE: The role of radiation therapy in the treatment of locally unresectable or metastatic carcinoid tumors. Int J Radiatr Oncol Biol Phys 20:489–495, 1991.
109. Oberg K: The use of chemotherapy in the management of neuroendocrine tumors. Endocrinol Metab Clin North Am 22:941–952, 1993.
110. Moertel CG: An odyssey in the land of small tumors. J Clin Oncol 5:1503, 1987.
111. Janson ET, Oberg K: Long-term management of the carcinoid syndrome. Treatment with octreotide alone and in combination with alpha-interferon. Acta Oncol 32:225–229, 1993.
112. Kvols LK, Moertel CG, O'Connell MJ, et al: Treatment of the malignant carcinoid syndrome. Evaluation of a long-acting somatostatin analogue. N Engl J Med 315:663–666, 1986.
113. Mulvihill S, Pappas TN, Passaro E Jr, et al: The use of somatostatin and its analogs in the treatment of surgical disorders. Surgery 100:467–475, 1986.
114. Oberg K, Ericksson B: The role of interferon in the management of carcinoid tumors. Acta Oncol 30:519–522, 1991.
115. Grander D, Oberg K, Lundqvist M-L, et al: Interferon-induced enhancement of 2′,5′-oligoadenylate synthetase in mid-gut carcinoid tumors. Lancet 336:337–340, 1990.
116. Seifert G, Sobin LH: The World Health Organization's histological classification of salivary gland tumors. A commentary on the second edition. Cancer 70:379–385, 1992.
117. Aberle DR, Brown K, Young DA, et al: Imaging techniques in the evaluation of tracheobronchial neoplasms. Chest 99:211–215, 1991.
118. Chetty R, Forder MD, DeGroot M, et al: Muco-epidermoid and adenoid cystic carcinomas of the tracheobronchial tree. Aust NZ J Surg 61:360–362, 1991.
119. Wong MP, Chung LP, Yuen ST, et al: In situ detection of Epstein-Barr virus in non-small cell lung carcinomas. J Pathol 177:233–240, 1995.
120. Chan JK, Hui PK, Tsang WY, et al: Primary lymphoepithelioma-like carcinoma of the lung. A clinicopathological study of 11 cases. Cancer 76:413–422, 1995.
121. Chen FF, Yan JJ, Lai WW, et al: Epstein-Barr virus–associated nonsmall cell lung carcinoma: undifferentiated "lymphoepithelioma-like" carcinoma as a distinct entity with a better prognosis. Cancer 82:2334–2342, 1998.
122. Li W, Ellerbroek NA, Libshitz HI: Primary malignant tumors of the trachea. A radiologic and clinical study. Cancer 66:894–899, 1990.
123. Grillo HC, Mathisen DJ: Primary tracheal tumors: Treatment and results. Ann Thorac Surg 49:69–77, 1990.
124. Fields JN, Rigaud G, Emami BN: Primary tumors of the trachea. Results of radiation therapy. Cancer 63:2429–2433, 1989.
125. Chan AT, Teo PM, Lam KC, et al: Multimodality treatment of primary lymphoepithelioma-like carcinoma of the lung. Cancer 83:925–929, 1998.
125a. Bacha EA, Wright CD, Grillo HC, et al: Surgical treatment of primary pulmonary sarcomas. Eur J Cardiothorac Surg 15:456–460, 1999.
126. Gebauer C: The postoperative prognosis of primary pulmonary sarcomas: A review with a comparison between the histological forms and the other primary endothoracical sarcomas based on 474 cases. Scand J Thorac Cardiovasc Surg 18:251–254, 1984.
127. Wick MR, Ritter HH, Humphrey PA: Sarcomatoid carcinomas of the lung: A clinicopathologic review. Am J Clin Pathol 108:40–53, 1997.
128. Barson AJ, Jones AW, Lodge KV: Pulmonary blastoma. J Clin Pathol 21:480–485, 1968.
129. Jacobsen M, Francis D: Pulmonary blastoma. Acta Pathol Microbiol Immunol Scand [A] 88:151–160, 1980.
130. Kodama T, Koide T, Shimosato Y, et al: Six cases of well-differentiated adenocarcinoma simulating fetal lung tubules in pseudoglandular stage. Comparison with pulmonary blastoma. Am J Surg Pathol 8:735–744, 1984.
131. Nakatani Y, Dickersin R, Mark EJ: Pulmonary endodermal tumor resembling fetal lung: A clinicopathological study of five cases with immunohistochemical and ultrastructural characterization. Hum Pathol 21:1097–1107, 1990.
132. Kradin RL, Kirkham SE, Young RH, et al: Pulmonary blastoma with argyrophil cells and lacking sarcomatous features (pulmonary endodermal tumor resembling fetal lung). Am J Surg Pathol 6:165–172, 1982.
133. Priest JR, McDermott MB, Bhatia S, et al: Pleuropulmonary blastoma: A clinicopathologic study of 50 cases. Cancer 80:147–161, 1997.
134. Medbery CA III, Bibro MC, Phares JC, et al: Pulmonary blastoma: Case report and literature review of chemotherapy experience. Cancer 53:2413–2416, 1984.
135. Cutler CS, Michel RP, Yassa M, et al: Pulmonary blastoma: Case report of a patient with a 7-year remission and review of chemotherapy experience in the world literature. Cancer 82:462–467, 1998.
136. Cabarcos A, Dorronsoro MG, Beristain JL: Pulmonary carcinosarcoma: A case study and review of the literature. Br J Dis Chest 79:83–84, 1985.
137. Davis MP, Eagan, RT, Weiland LH, et al: Carcinosarcoma of the lung: Mayo Clinic experience and response to chemotherapy. Mayo Clin Proc 59:598–603, 1984.
138. Ishida T, Tateishi M, Kaneko S, et al: Carcinosarcoma and spindle cell carcinoma of the lung. Clinicopathologic and immunohistochemical studies. J Thorac Cardiovasc Surg 100:844–852, 1990.
139. Whitwell F: Tumourlets of the lung. J Pathol Bacteriol 70:529–541, 1955.
140. Bonikos DS, Archibald R, Bensch KG: On the origin of the so-called tumorlets of the lung. Hum Pathol 7:461–469, 1976.
141. Ranchod M. The histogenesis and development of pulmonary tumorlets. Cancer 39:1135–1145, 1977.
141a. Colby TV, Wistuba II, Gazdar A: Precursors to pulmonary neoplasia. Adv Anat Pathol 5:205–215, 1999.
142. D'Agati VD, Perzin KH: Carcinoid tumorlets of the lung with metastases to a peribronchial lymph node: Report of a case and review of the literature. Cancer 55:2472–2476, 1985.
143. Sheerin N, Harrison MK, Sheppard MN, et al: Obliterative bronchiolitis caused by multiple tumourlets and microcarcinoids suc-

cessfully treated by single lung transplantation. Thorax 50:207–209, 1995.

143a. Arioglu E, Doppman J, Gomes M, et al: Cushing's syndrome caused by corticotropin secretion by pulmonary tumorlets. N Engl J Med 339:883–886, 1999.

144. Gould VE, Linnoila C, Memoli VA, et al: Neuroendocrine components of the bronchopulmonary tract: Hyperplasias, dysplasias, and neoplasms. Lab Invest 49:519–537, 1983.

145. Gosney JR, Sissons MCJ, Allibone RO, et al: Pulmonary endocrine cells in chronic bronchitis and emphysema. J Pathol 157:127–133, 1989.

146. Gosney J, Green ART, Taylor W: Appropriate and inappropriate neuroendocrine products in pulmonary tumourlets. Thorax 45:679–683, 1990.

147. Kyle RA: Subject review: Multiple myeloma. Review of 869 cases. Mayo Clin Proc 50:29–40, 1975.

148. Fudenberg HH: Waldenstrom's macroglobulinemia. *In* Brodsky I, Kahn SB, Moyer JH (eds): Cancer Chemotherapy II. The Twenty-Second Hahnemann Symposium. New York: Grune & Stratton, 1972, pp 393–403.

149. Amin R: Extramedullary plasmacytoma of the lung. Cancer 56:152–156, 1985.

150. Hayes DW, Bennett WA, Heck FJ: Extramedullary lesions in multiple myeloma: Review of the literature and pathologic studies. Arch Pathol 53:262–272, 1982.

151. Jennings TA, Axiotis CA, Kress Y, et al: Primary malignant melanoma of the lower respiratory tract: Report of a case and literature review. Am J Clin Pathol 94:649–655, 1990.

152. Wilson RW, Moran CA: Primary melanoma of the lung: A clinicopathologic and immunohistochemical study of eight cases. Am J Surg Pathol 21:1196–1202, 1997.

153. Cagle P, Mace ML, Fudge DM, et al: Pulmonary melanoma: Primary vs. metastatic. Chest 85:125–126, 1984.

# 48 Metastatic Malignant Tumors

Judith A. Luce, M.D.

Introduction
Pathogenesis
- Hematogenous Dissemination
- Lymphogenous Dissemination
- Direct Invasion
- Intrabronchial Dissemination

Diagnosis
- Symptoms
- Physical Signs
- Radiographic Evaluation
- Tissue Diagnosis

Treatment
- Medical Therapy
- Surgical Therapy

Summary

## INTRODUCTION

The lungs are a common site of spread of malignancies, with pulmonary metastases occurring in 30% to 40% of all patients who have cancer. The frequency and number of these metastases are a function of both the time during the disease process when a patient is evaluated and the natural history of the particular malignancy. Autopsy studies may overestimate the clinical importance of metastatic disease to the lungs; the clinical relevance of pulmonary metastases is very much related to the natural history of various cancers. For example, although as many as 40% of pancreatic carcinoma patients may have pulmonary metastases at autopsy, the metastases are rarely a clinical problem or the cause of death. Table 48.1 summarizes the approximate autopsy incidences of pulmonary metastases and their relative clinical importance in common cancers.[1, 2]

## PATHOGENESIS

Malignancies originating within or outside of the thorax may spread to the lungs by several routes: hematogenous, or bloodborne, spread; lymphogenous dissemination; direct invasion; and perhaps intrabronchial dissemination. There is no current research that fully explains the precise mechanisms that cause pulmonary metastases. Tumor-specific factors may include the ability to form new vessels, to adhere to endothelium, to produce proteases capable of digesting matrix proteins, and to avoid host immune defenses. Organ-specific and host-specific factors may include either attractive or defensive features that preclude or permit tumor cell adhesion, invasion, and growth.

### Hematogenous Dissemination

Cancers are capable of inducing the formation of new blood vessels, and as a consequence of this complex process they are capable of invading the vascular space as either single cells or as small multicellular aggregates. Once in the venous circulation, malignant cells may passively come to rest in pulmonary capillaries as microemboli or actively attach to and invade through pulmonary capillary endothelium.[3] Animal studies with transplanted human tumors have demonstrated a broad range of capability for forming pulmonary metastases after venous injection of tumor cells.[4, 5] In addition, within a single human tumor cell line, individual clones may be identified that differ in their ability to form pulmonary metastases via the hematogenous route.[6] The balance between tumor-derived angiogenic factors and antiangiogenic factors may determine the ultimate fate of tumor cells that come to rest in the pulmonary circulation.[7] A combination of both tumor-related and pulmonary endothelial factors may also determine the predilection of particular cancers for formation of pulmonary metastases.[8] Human sarcomas, of both soft-tissue and bony origin, and certain carcinomas, such as renal cell, gestational trophoblastic neoplasms, thyroid carcinoma, and breast and lung carcinomas, show a high frequency of spread to the lungs via hematogenous dissemination.

### Lymphogenous Dissemination

Malignant cells may arrive in the lungs through two routes of lymphogenous dissemination. Extensive lymph node involvement in distant sites is believed to allow the spread of cancer cells into the larger lymphatic channels

**Table 48.1 FREQUENCY OF PULMONARY METASTASES IN CANCERS OF VARIOUS PRIMARY SITES**

| Primary Site | Autopsy Incidence (%) | Lung Only Site of Metastases (%) | Relative Risk as Major Site/ Cause of Death |
|---|---|---|---|
| Lung | 20–40 | >10 | + + |
| Colon/rectum | 20–40 | 9 | + |
| Breast | 60 | 21 | + + + |
| Prostate | 15–50 | 18 | + + |
| Pancreas | 25–40 | 3 | + |
| Stomach | 20–30 | 7 | + |
| Liver/bile ducts | 20 | * | + |
| Esophagus | 20–35 | 17 | + + |
| Melanoma | 60–80 | NA | + + + |
| Hodgkin's disease | 50–70 | * | + + |
| Non-Hodgkin's lymphoma | 30–40 | <10 | + + |
| Thyroid | 65 | N/A | + + + |
| Head/neck | 20–40 | N/A | + |
| Gynecologic | | | |
| Ovary | 10 | 0 | + |
| Uterus | 30–42 | 9 | + + |
| Cervix | 20–30 | 14 | + |
| Placenta, choriocarcinoma | 70–100 | † | + + + + |
| Renal | 50–75 | 27 | + + + |
| Bladder | 25–30 | 9 | + + |
| Testis (germ cell tumors) | 70–80 | 27 | + + + |
| Soft tissue sarcomas (adult) | 40–60 | N/A | + + + |
| Pediatric | | | |
| Ewing's sarcoma | 80–85 | † | + + + + |
| Wilms' tumor | 75–80 | † | + + + + |
| Neuroblastoma | 50–60 | * | + |
| Rhabdomyosarcoma | 55–60 | ‡ | + + + |
| Osteosarcoma | 80–100 | 75 | + + + + |

*Extremely uncommon, less than 2%.
†Very common, but consistent data not available.
‡Depends on the primary site; varies from rare (head and neck sites) to common (trunk sites).
+ = very low; + + = low; + + + = moderate; + + + + = high.
Data are from Weiss and Gilbert[1] and De Vita et al.[2]

and then to the thoracic duct, superior vena cava, and pulmonary vascular bed. Germ cell tumors, particularly testicular carcinoma, probably reach the lungs with characteristic high frequency via this route.

Alternatively, extensive mediastinal or hilar node involvement is thought to result in retrograde dissemination of malignant cells into pulmonary lymphatic channels, producing the clinical syndrome of lymphangitic metastases. This mechanism is seen most commonly in lymphomas, lung cancer, and breast cancer.

## Direct Invasion

The lungs may be directly invaded by malignancies originating in the chest wall (mainly soft-tissue sarcomas), mediastinum (mainly esophageal carcinomas or primary mediastinal tumors such as thymoma, lymphoma, and germ cell tumors), the abdominal viscera (especially carcinomas of the gastric cardia and liver), and retroperitoneal sarcomas.

## Intrabronchial Dissemination

It has long been believed that malignancies that originate in the upper aerodigestive tract (the head, neck, larynx, upper esophagus, and bronchi) could spread by direct implantation from one area of the airways to another. This theory has been invoked to explain the high frequency of second carcinomas, usually squamous cell carcinomas, in individuals treated for early cancers at another upper aerodigestive tract site. This theory has been difficult to prove for a number of reasons: Spread of cancer to bronchi via hematogenous dissemination has been documented; careful studies of individuals with early lung cancer have shown a high frequency of synchronous dysplastic or neoplastic lesions within the tracheobronchial epithelium; and techniques to show that second cancers were genetically related to the first primary tumors were lacking. New molecular techniques have, however, demonstrated the genetic relationship between primary tumors and subsequent recurrences in the same primary site[9]; thus, with careful analysis by molecular techniques, this theory may be either supported or contradicted.

## DIAGNOSIS

### Symptoms

Metastatic cancer may produce a variety of symptoms when pulmonary spread occurs. Involvement of airway mucosa may produce cough, hemoptysis, and airway obstruction with wheezing or stridor, obstructive pneumonitis, or lobar or segmental collapse and dyspnea. Bronchial metastasis is most common in breast cancer, melanoma, and other hematogenously disseminated cancers; bronchial spread without other pulmonary spread is rare.[10] Metastases to the pulmonary parenchyma, via either the lymphatic or hematogenous route, are most often asymptomatic. In their advanced state, they may be associated with dyspnea, tightness or fullness in the chest, cough, and, if the pleura is involved, pain or pleural effusion. When pulmonary metastases originate from mediastinal involvement, the presenting symptoms are most often related to the presence of mediastinal neoplasm. These symptoms include chest pressure or tightness; hoarseness due to recurrent laryngeal nerve invasion; facial and upper extremity edema and plethora due to superior vena cava compression; occasionally stridor or dysphagia due to compression of the esophagus or airways; and chest pain or pressure and other symptoms of pericardial tamponade.

### Physical Signs

The physical examination of a patient with suspected pulmonary metastases is most useful if it points to the primary site of a previously undiagnosed cancer or if it demonstrates a potential site, such as nodes or other masses, for obtaining tissue to make a diagnosis of cancer. Signs of pleural effusion, pericardial effusion, or partial or total airway obstruction are useful and should be sought. Superior vena cava syndrome is always a clinical diagnosis based on physical findings. Direct or indirect laryngoscopy may reveal or confirm vocal cord paralysis or a primary cancer in a hoarse patient with metastatic lung involvement. The physical examination of a patient with metastatic cancer in the lungs should include rectal examination, pelvic examination, and careful examination of the breasts.

### Radiographic Evaluation

The variety of clinical and physiologic manifestations of metastatic cancer in the lungs is mirrored in the variety of abnormalities shown by plain films of the thorax. Pleural effusions, parenchymal masses, obstructive pneumonia or lobar or segmental collapse, and hilar and mediastinal adenopathy may be seen. Lymphangitic spread is characterized by linear interstitial markings (Fig. 48.1), normally radiating outward from enlarged hilar or mediastinal nodes. Lymphomatous involvement most commonly consists of small nodules, a lymphangitic appearance, or a combination of the two findings. Parenchymal metastases may have any appearance, including both smooth and ill-defined nodules or masses, cavitary masses, and occasionally calcified masses (Figs. 48.2 and 48.3). Pneumothorax is a rare manifestation of pulmonary parenchymal metastases and must be distinguished from other benign causes of pulmonary nodules and pneumothorax such as eosinophilic granuloma.

Most patients with a new appearance of multiple pulmonary nodules or lymphangitic spread already have a diagnosis of cancer. In such patients the new finding is

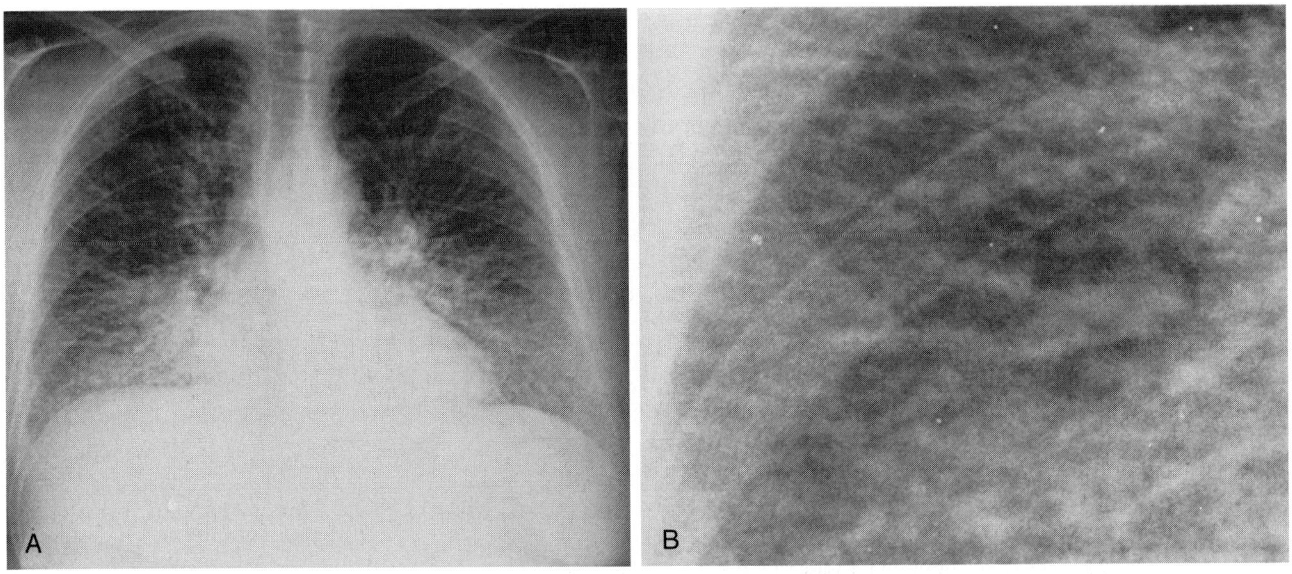


**Figure 48.1** Lymphangitic dissemination of breast carcinoma in a 59-year-old woman. The posteroanterior radiograph *(A)* shows widespread reticulonodular infiltrates, in addition to hilar and mediastinal adenopathy and a right mastectomy. The detail view of the right lower lobe *(B)* shows the fine interstitial pattern and small nodular densities typical of lymphangitic carcinomatosis.

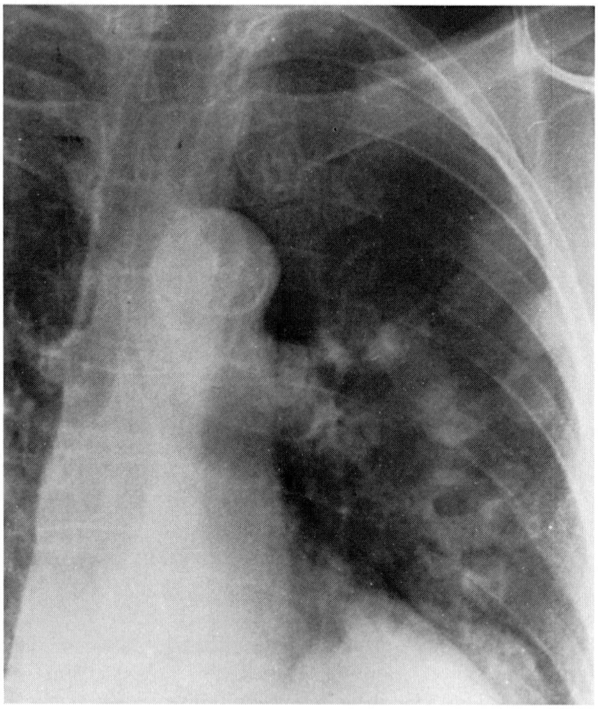

**Figure 48.2** Radiograph showing cavitation of hematogenous pulmonary metastases in a 79-year-old woman with metastatic colon carcinoma. The cavities are thick walled and occasionally eccentric. The differential diagnosis includes granulomatous diseases.

70% to 80% likely to represent metastatic cancer.[11] The differential diagnosis must, however, be carefully considered even in patients with known neoplasms, especially considering the clinical implications of their relative immunosuppression.[12] The differential diagnosis of lymphangitic spread includes congestive heart failure and interstitial inflammatory processes, especially those caused by cancer treatment (e.g., cytotoxic drugs, radiation). Tuberculosis, septic emboli, and other infectious processes must be considered in the differential diagnosis of multiple or single parenchymal masses (Table 48.2).

## Computed Tomography of the Thorax

Computed tomographic (CT) evaluation may play a role in the initial diagnosis of patients presenting with radiographic evidence of a thoracic neoplasm either in the search for a primary site outside of the thorax or in defining the intrathoracic extent of disease sufficiently to clarify its origin within the thorax. CT is of little help in further defining tumor in patients with known advanced cancer. CT is a necessary adjunct to radiation therapy treatment planning, if this mode of treatment is to be employed. Magnetic resonance imaging (MRI) offers no particular advantages over CT imaging of the thorax in the evaluation of metastatic disease.

CT imaging has been widely employed to screen for the presence of pulmonary parenchymal metastases, to evaluate patients with apparent solitary pulmonary metastasis, and to enumerate and evaluate pulmonary metastases when surgical resection is being considered. The use of CT in the evaluation of solitary pulmonary masses is discussed in Chapters 46 and 49. CT as a screening test for possible pulmonary metastases has been most widely used in the evaluation of patients with germ cell tumors, sarcomas, and melanoma, malignancies in which a high frequency of pulmonary metastases is found and in which their presence might dramatically alter the choice of therapy.[13] Helical CT is capable of near 100% sensitivity for masses of 6 mm or more, about half of which prove to be malignant at subsequent excision.[14, 15]

Despite its low specificity and because it is so much more sensitive than plain radiographs, the clinical usage of CT is unlikely to change until a better test is devised. Positron emission tomography scanning as a method for detecting pulmonary metastases is not well established and is not more sensitive than CT. As methods for evaluating patients for surgical resection, both CT and MRI are helpful in defining unresectable metastases, with 80% to 85% specificity. Careful surgical inspection remains the most important part of the evaluation of patients whose pulmonary metastases appear to be surgically resectable by imaging procedures.

## Tissue Diagnosis

The diagnosis of pulmonary metastases depends on a careful clinical strategy. If the patient is not known to have cancer, the search for a primary site relies primarily on a thorough history and physical examination. Laboratory tests that are abnormal require evaluation, and site-directed laboratory screening tests, such as biochemical tumor markers for germ cell tumors, gastrointestinal malignancy, ovarian cancer, or prostate cancer, may be indicated. Imaging procedures of the thorax or other sites are performed only as indicated by the results of the history, physical examination, and laboratory tests. The role of

**Table 48.2** DIFFERENTIAL DIAGNOSIS OF MULTIPLE PULMONARY NODULES IN CANCER PATIENTS

| |
|---|
| **Malignant Etiologies** |
| Metastatic disease from known primary site |
| New primary site, solid tumor |
| New primary site, lymphoma or lymphoproliferative disease |
| **Benign Etiologies** |
| Infectious granulomas—histoplasmosis, coccidioidomycosis, tuberculosis |
| Pyogenic abscesses—embolic, nonembolic |
| Parasitic disease—paragonimiasis, hydatid cyst, filariasis |
| Arteriovenous malformations |
| Wegener's granulomatosis |
| Rheumatoid nodules |
| Sarcoidosis |
| Benign tumors—hamartomas, papillomatosis |
| Opportunistic infections—aspergillosis, nocardiosis, cryptococcosis |

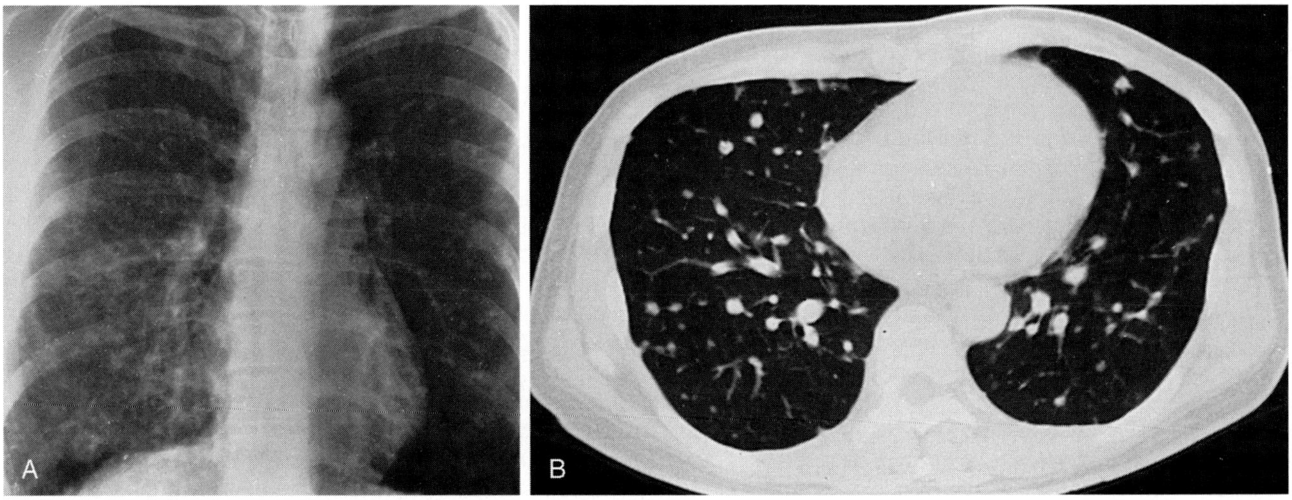


**Figure 48.3** Chest radiograph of a 47-year-old woman with metastatic breast cancer showing calcification of multiple hematogenous metastases. The postero-anterior chest film *(A)* shows the large number and variation of size of the metastases; the computed tomographic scan (*B*) more clearly shows the density of these metastases compared with soft tissues. The differential diagnosis includes tuberculosis, fungal infections, rheumatoid arthritis, multiple hamartomas, amyloidosis, and papillomatosis.

extensive radiographic evaluation of patients with metastatic carcinoma without an obvious primary site is controversial and ultimately of little benefit to patients.[16]

If the thorax is the best available site for making a tissue diagnosis, a variety of procedures may be employed, including sputum cytology (most useful for cavitary, endobronchial, and lymphangitic metastases); bronchoscopy with lavage (more sensitive than sputum cytology for the same type of metastases), brushings, or transbronchial biopsy; and transthoracic needle aspiration.[17] Immunohistochemical staining of such specimens may be extremely useful in defining occult primary cancers such as prostate cancer, melanoma, germ cell tumors, and breast and thyroid cancer. Thoracotomy is required infrequently but may be of therapeutic benefit.

Patients who have known cancers may require more individualized approaches to the diagnosis of pulmonary metastases. If the patient already has advanced neoplasm, the appearance of new lung findings is generally assumed to be due to metastatic disease if the radiographic or clinical differential diagnosis strongly favors metastases and the occurrence is consistent with the natural history of the cancer. For example, lymphangitic carcinomatosis is common in advanced breast cancer but rare in multiple myeloma; because patients with myeloma are also significantly immunosuppressed, a detailed evaluation is indicated. If the cancer diagnosis is distant from the appearance of new pulmonary findings, the clinical picture is inconsistent with the known primary disease, or the lungs are the only site of new onset of metastases, then biopsy proof of the diagnosis is indicated. Similarly, if there is any clinical evidence to suggest that the pulmonary findings represent a possible second primary cancer, then tissue diagnosis is also indicated.

# TREATMENT

## Medical Therapy

Patients who have pulmonary metastases from curable cancers should be treated with appropriate therapy. Testicular and ovarian germ cell tumors, neuroblastoma, gestational trophoblastic neoplasms, non-Hodgkin's lymphoma, Hodgkin's disease, and osteosarcoma are included in this category. One ongoing research issue with such patients is how to proceed when curative therapy has been delivered and residual masses remain in the mediastinum or lungs. Two strategies have emerged: aggressive resection of masses that have not resolved within some specific period of time from the completion of curative therapy and an observational strategy that allows the mass to resume growing before intervention occurs. Residual masses remain after the treatment of testicular carcinomas in approximately 40% of patients who have advanced disease and negative serum tumor markers at the conclusion of treatment. At surgical excision, these masses may be necrotic tissue (about half), residual carcinomas (about 25%), or mature teratoma (about 25%), which may continue to grow. Long-term follow-up studies suggest that about 90% of the patients with mature teratoma are cured by surgery, and perhaps as many as 50% of those with residual carcinoma are also cured surgically.[18, 19] Surgical guidelines are much less clear for patients with lymphoma, for whom treatment alternatives are more numerous and systemic therapy is necessary. Surgical biopsy rather than excision may be appropriate.

Unfortunately, most adults with pulmonary metastases do not have curable cancers, and palliative therapy is appropriate. For selected cancers, medical treatment may consist of chemotherapy, radiation therapy, hormonal therapy, or immunologic therapies. These may be employed with acceptable toxicity and temporary improvement, even with significant prolongation of survival in some cases. Symptom relief for untreatable patients may be aided by the selective use of radiation therapy,[20] perhaps endobronchial laser therapy,[21] and steroids. Opiates and oxygen therapy may relieve symptoms of end-stage dyspnea. Social, emotional, and physical rehabilitation support have important roles in the care of such patients.

## Surgical Therapy

The idea of curing pulmonary metastases surgically is an appealing one and has been widely practiced in the United States and Europe for more than 100 years.[21a] Despite the increasingly aggressive use of surgery for selected patients, there have been no prospective clinical trials comparing surgical with nonsurgical treatment, and most surgically treated patients still die of their malignancies.

The indications for pulmonary metastasectomy have evolved as surgery has become technically better and the understanding of individual diseases has expanded. Patient selection is better, and anesthetic and other supportive care has improved. The morbidity of surgery and the loss of lung parenchyma dictated that patients had to have few or solitary metastases; however, using current operative techniques, surgeons are now able to resect more than 50 pulmonary metastases at a single operation, and case reports of patients having had several thoracotomies for metastasectomy are not unusual. Current indications for pulmonary metastasectomy include the following situations[22]:

- Adequate control of the primary site has been or can be obtained.
- The patient can tolerate the planned procedure.
- There is no evidence of metastatic disease at another site.
- There is no definitive radiographic evidence of unresectable pulmonary metastases.

Knowledge of factors associated with poor outcome has evolved as the use of surgery has increased. Although it was once thought that the number of metastases was a prognostic indicator, there is no evidence in the current literature that this is, in fact, the case. It is, however, very clear that the metastases must be completely resected: In virtually all series with various primary sites, the presence of unresectable pulmonary metastases is associated with a survival rate comparable with no surgery. It was once thought that an indolent natural history was an important prognostic indicator. To some extent, this is still true: Breast cancer patients with less than a 1-year interval between the initial diagnosis and the onset of pulmonary metastases do not live long after surgical resection, for example. The largest series reveal that the disease-free interval is an important prognostic factor, but controversy remains.[23, 24] Cancers whose metastases commonly occur at sites other than the lungs are less likely to have favorable outcomes than are cancers such as sarcomas that metastasize almost exclusively to the lungs. Some authors have shown that the tumor doubling time predicts poor outcome if it is short, particularly shorter than 20 days; however, not all authors agree with that conclusion, particularly for osteosarcoma. Finally, a cancer that has responded well to chemotherapy is no more likely than a refractory cancer to have a good outcome after metastasectomy, especially osteosarcoma and soft-tissue sarcoma.[25]

Most adult solid tumor patients are not good candidates for metastasectomy; the surgical approach should be considered for individuals who meet the basic criteria and who have had a long interval between diagnosis and the appearance of pulmonary metastases. Such patients might include those having renal cell carcinoma, colorectal carcinomas, thyroid carcinomas, and soft-tissue sarcomas. Occasionally breast cancer, melanoma, and gynecologic cancer patients are eligible.[26–29] As Table 48.3 shows, overall outcome is poor: Most patients do not have prolonged survival. Whether a randomized trial might show benefit is not known. The judgment to perform metastasectomy remains a difficult one.[30, 31]

The approach to osteosarcoma has evolved differently, however. This disease rarely metastasizes to sites other than lung and adjacent bone. Based on some very long-term survival results[32] some individual investigators have advocated increased use of thoracotomy and resection of all pulmonary metastases[33, 34]; this procedure is repeated as often as is tolerable, and, because most of these patients are young, they tolerate multiple surgical procedures well. A striking number of them later develop second malignancies,[27] consonant with genetic evidence suggesting that osteosarcoma results from the deletion of an important tumor suppressor gene. This aggressive approach has been shown by a variety of investigators to result in 5-year survival rates of 25% to 50%, but these must be viewed with some caution because of the lack of prospective trials. A recent follow-up study reported a 3-year survival after excision of metastatic osteogenic sarcoma, which (surprisingly) was not influenced by the number of thoracotomies (up to four) that had to be performed.[34a]

Complications of pulmonary metastasectomy should be few. The procedure may be performed through a median sternotomy or via sequential lateral thoracotomies. Some surgeons prefer the latter approach because it allows more careful inspection of the posteroapical segments of lung. Most metastases are located subpleurally and may be

**Table 48.3** PER CENT FIVE-YEAR SURVIVAL RATES AFTER PULMONARY METASTASECTOMY (SERIES AFTER 1980)

| Primary Site | Five-Year Survival (%) |
|---|---|
| Soft tissue | 20–35 |
| Osteosarcoma | 25–50 |
| Melanoma | 5–33 |
| Colon/rectum | 13–40 |
| Testis (germ cell) | 50–80 |
| Renal | 15–20 |
| Breast | 25–50 |

excised with stapler, laser, electrocautery, or manual suture techniques; staplers require the removal of larger portions of lung. New laser technology is being evaluated and is said to offer advantages.[36] An effort must be made to locate all masses observed on a preoperative CT scan, as well as to carefully palpate and remove masses not visualized on the scan. More than 50 metastases may be removed during a single surgical procedure. Video-assisted thoracoscopy has been employed in metastasectomy, but its routine role has not been established.[35] Mortality in most series is less than 2%; morbid complications may occur in up to 10% of patients. The most common complications are persistent air leak and infection. Increased rates of infection have been reported in patients having had recent chemotherapy. Respiratory failure in thoracotomy patients having had extensive prior radiotherapy and chemotherapy has been reported, especially in those who received high fractional concentrations of oxygen postoperatively.

## SUMMARY

Regardless of their route of entry into the lungs, pulmonary metastases present a common clinical problem. Early signs and symptoms may be varied or absent. Most patients have an identified primary cancer, but for those who do not, careful history and physical examinations are useful to determine a possible primary site, and only a few laboratory tests contribute to the evaluation. Imaging studies may be very useful to find multiple pulmonary metastases not seen on conventional radiographs and to better define lymphagitic or locally invasive disease. When the thorax is the only available site for obtaining tissue, a variety of techniques may be used, aided by immunohistochemical stains, to help identify the site of origin of the cancer.

Treatment of pulmonary metastases is individualized and is highly dependent on the type of cancer. Patients having curable cancers are few. Treatment issues for these patients may include later resection of residual disease in the lungs for diagnostic and potentially therapeutic purposes. For most patients, palliative treatment is appropriate, employing both symptomatic and anticancer therapies. Surgical resection of metastases may be advisable for highly selected patients having isolated pulmonary metastases. Metastatic sarcomas are most often approached surgically, occasionally with long-term cure of patients. The lack of prospective data limits further application of surgical treatment.

## References

1. Weiss L, Gilbert HA: Pulmonary Metastasis. Boston: GK Hall & Co, 1978.
2. De Vita VT Jr, Hellman S, Rosenberg SA: Cancer: Principles and Practice of Oncology (3rd ed). Philadelphia: JB Lippincott, 1989.
3. Folkman J: The role of angiogenesis in tumor growth. Semin Cancer Biol 3:65–71, 1992.
4. Nicolson GL: Tumor and host molecules important in the organ preference of metastasis. Semin Cancer Biol 2:143–154, 1991.
5. Fidler IJ: Molecular biology of cancer: Invasion and metastasis. *In* DeVita VT Jr, Hellman S, Rosenberg SA (eds): Cancer: Principles and Practice of Oncology (5th ed): Philadelphia: Lippincott-Raven, 1997, pp 135–152.
6. Nicolson GL: Cancer metastasis: Tumor cell and host organ properties important in metastasis to specific secondary sites. Biochim Biophys Acta 948:175–224, 1988.
7. Folkman J: Angiogenesis inhibitors generated by tumors. Mol Med 1:120–122, 1995.
8. Cheng HC, Abdel-Ghany M, Elble RC, et al: Lung endothelial dipeptidyl peptidase IV promotes adhesion and metastasis of rat breast cancer cells via tumor cell surface-associated fibronectin. J Biol Chem 273:24207–24215, 1998.
9. Sidransky D, Frost P, Von Eschenbach A, et al: Clonal origin of bladder cancer. N Engl J Med 326:737–740, 1992.
10. Ikezoe J, Johkoh T, Takeuchi N, et al: CT findings of endobronchial metastasis. Acta Radiol 32:455–460, 1991.
11. Felson B: Pulmonary nodules and cysts. *In* Chest Roentgenology. Philadelphia: WB Saunders, 1973, pp 314–329.
12. Viggiano RW, Swensen SJ, Rosenow EC: Evaluation and management of solitary and multiple pulmonary nodules. Clin Chest Med 13:83–95, 1992.
13. Davis SD: CT evaluation for pulmonary metastases in patients with extrathoracic malignancy. Radiology 180:1–12, 1991.
14. Diederich S, Semik MN, Lentschig MG, et al: Helical CT of pulmonary nodules in patients with extrathoracic malignancy: CT-surgical correlation. AJR Am J Roentgenol 172:353–360, 1999.
15. Wright AR, Collie DA, Williams JR, et al: Pulmonary nodules: Effect on detection of spiral CT pitch. Radiology 199:837–841, 1996.
16. Levine MN, Drummond MF, Labelle RJ: Cost-effectiveness in the diagnosis and treatment of carcinoma of unknown primary origin. Can Med Assoc J 133:977–978, 1985.
17. Janzen DL, Adler BD, Padley SP, et al: Diagnostic success of bronchoscopic biopsy in immunocompromised patients with acute pulmonary disease: Predictive value of disease distribution as shown on CT. AJR Am J Roentgenol 160:21–24, 1993.
18. Jansen RL, Sylvester R, Sleyfer DT, et al: Long-term followup of nonseminomatous testicular cancer patients with mature teratoma or carcinoma at postchemotherapy surgery. EORTC Genitourinary Cancer Cooperative Group. Eur J Cancer 27:695–698, 1991.
19. Xiao H, Liu D, Bajorin DF, et al: Medical and surgical management of pulmonary metastases from germ cell tumors. Chest Surg Clin North Am 8:131–143, 1998.
20. Chetty KG, Moran EM, Sassoon CS, et al: Effect of radiation therapy on bronchial obstruction due to bronchogenic carcinoma. Chest 95:582–584, 1989.
21. Midthun DE: Endobronchial techniques in lung cancer. Options for nonsurgical care. Posgrad Med 101:169–172, 177–178, 1997.
21a. Downey RJ: Surgical treatment of pulmonary metastases. Surg Oncol Clin North Am 8:341, 1999.
22. Todd TR: The surgical treatment of pulmonary metastases. Chest 112(Suppl):287S–290S, 1997.
23. International Registry of Lung Metastases: Long-term results of lung metastasectomy: Prognostic analyses based on 5206 cases. J Thorac Cardiovasc Surg 113:37–49, 1997.
24. Robert JH, Ambrogi V, Mermillod B, et al: Factors influencing long-term survival after lung metastasectomy. Ann Thorac Surg 63:777–784, 1997.
25. Lanza LA, Putnam JB Jr, Benjamin RS, et al: Response to chemotherapy does not predict survival after resection of sarcomatous pulmonary metastases. Ann Thorac Surg 51:219–224, 1991.
26. Lanza LA, Natarajan G, Roth JA, et al: Long-term survival after resection of pulmonary metastases from carcinoma of the breast. Ann Thorac Surg 54:244–248, 1992.
27. Pogrebniak HW, Haas G, Linehan WM, et al: Renal cell carcinoma: Resection of solitary and multiple metastases. Ann Thorac Surg 54:33–38, 1992.
28. Harpole DH, Johnson LM, Wolfe WG, et al: Analysis of 945 cases of pulmonary metastatic melanoma. J Thorac Cardiovasc Surg 103:743–751, 1992.
29. Robinson BJ, Rice TW, Strong SA, et al: Is resection of pulmonary and hepatic metastases warranted in patients with colorectal cancer? J Thorac Cardiovasc Surg 117:66–75, 1999.
30. McIntosh R, Thatcher N: Management of the solitary metastasis. Thorax 45:909–911, 1990.
31. Moores DWO: Pulmonary metastases revisited. Ann Thorac Surg 52:178–179, 1991.
32. Beattie EJ, Harvey JC, Marcove R, et al: Results of multiple pul-

monary resections for metastatic osteogenic sarcoma after two decades. J Surg Oncol 46:154–155, 1991.
33. Snyder CL, Saltzman DA, Ferrell KL, et al: A new approach to the resection of pulmonary osteosarcoma metastases. Clin Orthop Rel Res 270:247–253, 1991.
34. Burk CD, Belasco JB, O'Neill JA Jr, et al: Pulmonary metastases and bone sarcomas: Surgical removal of lesions appearing after adjuvant chemotherapy. Clin Orthop Rel Res 262:88–92, 1991.
34a. Antunes M, Bernardo J, Salete M, et al: Excision of pulmonary metastases of osteogenic sarcoma of the limbs. Eur J Cardiothorac Surg 15:592–596, 1999.
35. Dowling RD, Landreneau RJ, Miller DL: Video-assisted thoracoscopic surgery for resection of lung metastases. Chest 113(Suppl):2S–5S, 1998.
36. Rolle A, Eulerich E: Extensive multiple and lobe-sparing pulmonary resections with the Nd:YAG laser and a new wavelength of 1318 nm. Acta Chir Hung 38:115–117, 1999.

# 49 Benign Tumors

GLEN A. LILLINGTON, M.D. • NORMAN W. RIZK, M.D.

Introduction
Clinical Manifestations
Classification
Tracheobronchial Benign Tumors
Solitary Parenchymal Tumors
Multiple Parenchymal Tumors
Pseudotumors
Summary

## INTRODUCTION

Benign tumors of the lung account for about 2% to 5% of primary lung tumors.[1–6] In general, the etiology and pathogenesis of these uncommon conditions are poorly understood. Some "benign" pulmonary tumors are really low-grade malignancies that may occasionally behave in a frankly malignant manner. Conversely, some pulmonary lesions, although not neoplastic in the pathologic sense, mimic the clinical and roentgenologic features of tumors; such "pseudotumors" should be included in the differential diagnosis of benign and malignant lung tumors.

## CLINICAL MANIFESTATIONS

The clinical picture depends primarily on the location of the lesion. Symptoms, signs, and roentgenologic features differ among benign tumors that arise in the trachea, the bronchi, and the lung parenchyma.

*Intratracheal benign tumors* may be asymptomatic but may manifest with pseudoasthmatic wheezing, cough, dyspnea, or hemoptysis. Careful examination of the tracheal air shadow by standard roentgenography may help detect the tumor, but confirmation by computed tomography (CT) is required.[7, 8] Bronchoscopy is usually diagnostic and may even permit adequate tumor removal by forceps or with the aid of laser technology. Surgical resection, however, is usually recommended.[8, 9]

*Endobronchial benign tumors* are frequently symptomatic, often causing partial or complete bronchial obstruction, which may result in recurrent pneumonias, bronchiectasis, unilateral wheezing, atelectasis, postobstructive pneumonitis, and postobstructive hyperinflation. Hemoptysis is occasionally noted. Standard roentgenography and CT may detect the obstructive consequences of the tumor rather than the tumor itself. Bronchoscopy usually reveals the location of the lesion. Because the tumor may be covered with normal mucosa, bronchial washings and brushings are often nondiagnostic, but forceps biopsy is usually successful in providing a suitable specimen. In some instances, the tumor can be completely removed endoscopically, but bronchotomy, sleeve resection, or even lobectomy/pneumonectomy may be required.[8–10]

*Parenchymal benign tumors* of the lung are typically asymptomatic, even when large, and are customarily an unexpected finding in a chest roentgenogram obtained for other purposes. A benign tumor in the lung parenchyma usually manifests radiologically as a *solitary pulmonary nodule* in an asymptomatic person. Because many solitary nodules are malignant and curable, resection may be required unless benignity can be established. Most benign nodules are granulomas, but about 10% to 20% are benign tumors.[10]

Certain patterns of calcification almost always indicate benignity. Even if the nodule is uncalcified, continued observation is justified if the lesion is "stable": that is, if there has been no increase in size during the previous 2 years.[10]

Examination of the nodule by CT is occasionally definitive. CT shows the pattern of calcification more clearly than plain roentgenograms, and CT densitometry may identify otherwise undetectable calcification.[11] More than 50% of hamartomas can be identified by high-resolution CT.[12] In indeterminate cases, an estimate of the probability that the nodule is malignant can be calculated by Bayesian techniques, and this information can be employed in the decision process.[10, 13] Magnetic resonance imaging has relatively little to offer in the evaluation of solitary nodules; positron emission tomography may be more useful, but further studies are needed to define its exact role.[14]

Transthoracic needle aspiration biopsy of pulmonary nodules is extremely sensitive for malignancy. In addition, this procedure often identifies benign lesions, including infectious processes and benign tumors. If the biopsy results are indeterminate, thoracotomy or thoracoscopy is usually indicated.[1, 15]

## CLASSIFICATION

Benign tumors are customarily classified in terms of their pathologic abnormalities. The classification used in this chapter mirrors the actual clinical presentation, being based on location and on whether single or multiple lesions are detectable. The clinical manifestations of benign tumors are largely dependent on whether the lesion is endobronchial or parenchymal in location.

## Tracheobronchial Benign Tumors

**Multiple Laryngeal Papillomatosis.** Laryngeal papillomatosis, a viral disease of the upper airways in young children, may spread to the intrapulmonary tracheobronchial tree in later years.[16–18] The lesions are sessile or stalked papillary growths lined with flattened squamous epithelium; they may cause hemoptysis, asthmatic wheezing, atelectasis, and obstructive pneumonitis. Standard roentgenograms may show multiple nodular lesions that are often cavitated. Some of these lesions may develop transformations in association with mutation of the p53 action gene.[19]

The diagnosis is suggested by the history of childhood laryngeal papillomatosis and is confirmed by bronchoscopic biopsy of the lesions. Resection is indicated where possible. Therapy with antiviral agents has been reported, but it is usually neither curative nor of long-term benefit.[20]

**Solitary Papilloma.** The solitary tracheobronchial papilloma, which is usually less than 1.5 cm in diameter, most commonly occurs in middle-aged men. The tumor is usually in a lobar or segmental bronchus, manifesting clinically with hemoptysis, atelectasis, or postobstructive pneumonitis.[16, 21, 22] The pathology is identical to that seen in viral papillomatosis. Endoscopic removal is usually feasible.

**Inflammatory Papilloma.** The inflammatory tracheobronchial papilloma, usually solitary, is a polypoid mass of exuberant granulation tissue secondary to chronic irritation, such as bronchiectasis, thermal injury, and indwelling foreign bodies.[16] The usual clinical manifestation is bronchial obstruction. Treatment is local excision plus efforts to control the underlying inflammation.

**Mucous Gland Adenoma.** This is the only lesion that truly deserves the appellation of *bronchial adenoma.* The latter term is often misapplied to malignant tracheobronchial tumors such as the carcinoid tumor, the cylindroma (adenoid cystic carcinoma), and the mucoepidermoid carcinoma, which are discussed in Chapter 46.

The mucous gland adenoma (bronchial cystadenoma) arises in main or lobar bronchi, often has a papillary appearance, and may cause obstructive symptoms.[23, 24] The cystic spaces within the tumor are lined by columnar cells. The tumor can often be removed endoscopically.

**Granular Cell Myoblastoma.** This tumor is composed of polygonal or spindle cells with granular eosinophilic cytoplasm; despite the name, it is now thought to have a neural origin, probably from Schwann cells. The tumor can arise in many organs, but fewer than 100 cases of bronchial origin have been reported. The respiratory tract lesions are usually in the larynx or main bronchi and are multiple in 10% of cases.[25–27] The disease, which is more common in men than in women, usually becomes clinically apparent between the ages of 30 to 50 years.

Clinical manifestations include cough, hemoptysis, recurrent infections, and wheezing. Bronchoscopic biopsy is usually diagnostic, and bronchoscopic removal is occasionally possible. Laser therapy is sometimes helpful, but complete surgical excision is usually advisable, particularly for lesions greater than 8 mm in diameter. These tumors show a propensity for local invasiveness and may recur after limited excision.[28, 29] In rare cases, a granular cell myoblastoma of the lung may present as a solitary pulmonary nodule.[30]

**Endobronchial Hamartoma.** The pathology and pathogenesis of intrapulmonary hamartomas are discussed subsequently. About 10% to 20% of all bronchopulmonary hamartomas are endobronchial in location; a literature review in 1972 listed 58 reported cases.[31] Although the endobronchial tumors may cause the usual obstructive complications, they are often asymptomatic.

Endobronchial hamartomas favor central bronchi and are usually polypoid. Cartilage is present in 82% of cases[32] but is often scanty. The epithelial clefts seen in the parenchymal tumors are often missing in the endobronchial form. Bronchoscopy is usually but not always diagnostic.[33] Resection is usually advisable for preventing or alleviating obstructive complications.

**Other Mesenchymal Tumors.** Several types of benign mesenchymal lung tumors that are usually parenchymal in location occasionally occur within the tracheobronchial tree, where they typically give rise to obstructive syndromes. Examples include *fibromas,*[34] which may recur after endoscopic removal; *myxomas*[35]; *chondromas*[36]; *neurofibromas*[37]; *glomus tumors*[38]; and *inflammatory pseudotumors.*[39, 40]

The intrapulmonary *lipoma,*[41, 42] in contrast, is almost always endobronchial in origin. About 50% of pulmonary *leiomyomas*[43, 44] are endobronchial in location and thus cause cough, expectoration, and symptoms of obstruction.

## Solitary Parenchymal Tumors

**Hamartoma.** Hamartomas[45, 46] are the most common form of benign lung tumors, occurring in 0.2% of routine autopsies and in 0.32% of 47,000 miners. They are twice as common in men as in women. About 5% to 10% of solitary pulmonary nodules are hamartomas.[10]

Although the name suggests that hamartomas are developmental abnormalities, the current belief is that they are true neoplasms; the term *benign mesenchymoma* has been suggested.[31, 47] Favoring tumoral status is the relatively late onset (from the late 30s, with a peak in the 60s) and a tendency to exhibit slow growth during prolonged observation. The results of cytogenetic studies[48, 49] indicate that only the mesenchymal component of the hamartoma is neoplastic; this led to the suggestion that the chondroid hamartoma should be renamed *pulmonary chondroma.* Malignant change is extremely rare,[6, 50] and some authorities doubt that it can occur.

Microscopic examination shows a central cartilaginous area in virtually all cases,[32] with calcification in some instances. Other areas of the tumor contain myxomatous and fibroblastic tissue, often accompanied by muscular and adipose tissue, bronchial glands, and chronic inflammatory cells. Slit-like spaces or clefts lined with epithelium are commonly present, usually near the periphery of the tumor.[5, 6]

The peripheral hamartoma is typically a well-circumscribed and asymptomatic nodule less than 3.0 cm in diameter, with a margin that is sharp and often lobulated. Slow growth may be detectable with serial roentgen examinations.[6] A variety of benign tumors and congenital anomalies may occur in association with pulmonary hamartomas.[51]

Calcification is detectable in 10% to 15% of cases on plain radiographs and may show a characteristic "popcorn" pattern.[6, 45, 46] The presence of calcification is better seen on standard tomograms or CT examination. High-resolution CT is diagnostic in more than 50% of hamartomas; the characteristic features (Fig. 49.1) are the combination of cartilage (with or without calcification) and focal areas of low attenuation due to fat deposits in the tumor.[12, 51a]

The diagnosis of peripheral hamartoma can be established by transthoracic needle aspiration biopsy in many cases[52, 53] and can sometimes be made by bronchoscopic transbronchial biopsy.[54] Although surgical excision is curative, it is not clear that resection is required in all or even most cases.[55, 56] Appropriate indications for surgery might include the presence of symptoms, growth of the tumor under roentgenographic observation, large size of the tumor, and impingement of the mass on a vital structure.

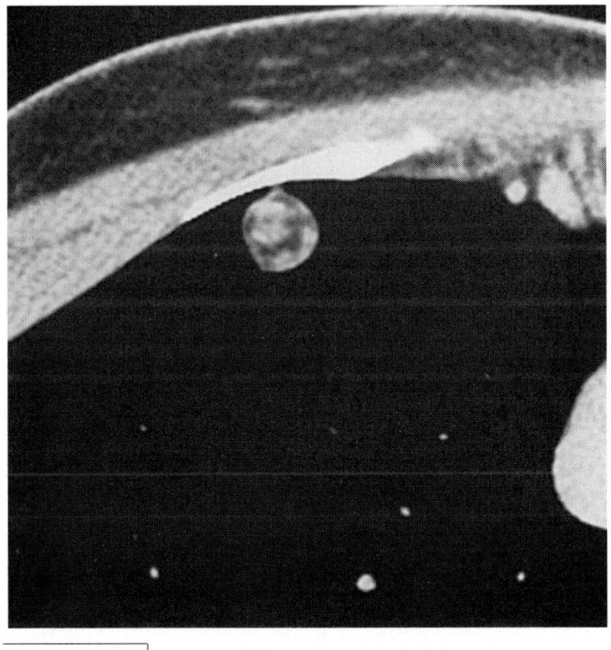

**Figure 49.1** High-resolution computed tomographic image of the right lung in an asymptomatic person, showing a well-circumscribed nodule with a diameter of 1.5 cm in the subpleural position anteriorly. The nodule shows areas of increased attenuation, representing cartilage. The intranodular areas of low attenuation are fat; note the similarity to the attenuation of the subcutaneous fat. The pathologic diagnosis was a chondroid hamartoma. (Courtesy of Dr. Nestor Müller.)

Mesenchymal cystic hamartomas[57] are rare tumors that may show malignant changes.[58] These lesions, however, should be differentiated from ordinary hamartomas.

**Sclerosing Hemangioma.** This uncommon tumor, originally considered vascular in origin, is now generally classified as an epithelial tumor derived from pneumocytes or terminal bronchiolar cells.[59] The name *sclerosing pneumocytoma* has been proposed.[60] The tumor usually contains several elements, including solid cellular areas, papillary structures, sclerotic regions, and dilated blood-filled spaces resembling hemangioma.[4, 5, 61–63]

The tumor is most common in middle-aged women and is usually asymptomatic.[4, 6] The roentgenographic appearance is a well-defined homogeneous nodule less than 4 cm in diameter. Slow growth has been noted in some cases. Diagnosis has usually been made by resection of the lesion at exploratory thoracotomy.[63]

**Other Mesenchymal Tumors of Lung Parenchyma.** Several types of benign tumors may arise from cells of mesenchymal origin within the lung parenchyma. Most are uncommon.

***Intrapulmonary Lipoma.*** These tumors are usually endobronchial, but parenchymal tumors have been described.[41, 42] The parenchymal tumor presents as a solitary nodule, and its fatty nature can be defined by the decreased attenuation noted on CT examination.

***Pulmonary Leiomyoma.*** This tumor appears as a sharply defined, lobulated, and asymptomatic parenchymal solitary nodule in 50% of cases, occurring most commonly in middle-aged adults.[43, 44] Some cases in women may actually be solitary examples of so-called *benign metastasizing leiomyoma*, which is discussed subsequently.

***Neural Tumors.*** The parenchymal nodule of neural origin is usually a *neurofibroma* and occasionally a *schwannoma*.[27] Some cases are part of the syndrome of neurofibromatosis.[64] Intrapulmonary *meningiomas* have been described.[65]

***Fibroma.*** The parenchymal fibroma is more common in men than in women[2] and is usually asymptomatic. Some cases diagnosed as fibroma may actually be fibrous histiocytomas[66] or leiomyomas.[4]

**Benign Clear Cell Tumor.** This rare tumor presents radiographically as a well-circumscribed pulmonary nodule. Symptoms are rarely present, and the tumors tend to first appear in adulthood. The lesion may be as large as 6 cm in diameter but is usually less than 3 cm.[67–69]

The cells are polygonal, with abundant clear or finely vacuolated cytoplasm. Multinucleated giant cells are often present. The richness of the cytoplasm in glycogen has prompted the term *sugar tumor.* The pathologic differential diagnosis includes metastatic hypernephroma and primary clear cell carcinoma of the lung[4]; the distinction can be made with special immunochemical studies.[68] On occasion, symptomatic necrotic clear cell tumors behave as though malignant.[69] In all reported cases, the diagnosis has been established by thoracotomy or autopsy.

**Teratoma.** Intrapulmonary teratomas are very rare (about 30 reported worldwide), often large, and only occasionally symptomatic. They are more often benign than malignant.[70] Calcification may be present, and radiologic evidence of an intratumoral tooth may be noted.

**Postinflammatory Pseudotumors.** These conditions are more inflammatory in nature than neoplastic. The specific name for each variant depends on the histology of the lesion.[4–6, 71] In most cases, the lesions have been diagnosed and treated at thoracotomy.[71, 71a] The diagnosis can sometimes be made by transthoracic needle aspiration biopsy; long-term follow-up with serial chest roentgenograms seems prudent in such cases.

***Plasma Cell Granuloma.*** The tumor is composed of fibrous tissue and polyclonal inflammatory cells, always with large numbers of plasma cells. Calcification and ossification are common, and amyloid degeneration may occur.[72–74] The lesion is usually a nodule between 2 and 5 cm in diameter, but large masses have been described. A relatively high proportion occur in children and adolescents. Slow growth or transformation to a lymphoma may occur, but in most cases there is no change over long observation periods.[6, 75] As noted previously, plasma cell granulomas may present in an endobronchial location.

Plasma cell granuloma should not be confused with *plasmacytoma,* which may appear in the trachea or the lung parenchyma[76] and is a highly malignant manifestation of multiple myeloma. The histopathology shows distinctive features of malignancy.

***Fibrous Histiocytoma, Histiocytoma, and Xanthoma.*** These tumors consist primarily of histiocytes with eosinophilic or foamy cytoplasm and of fibroblasts and fibrous tissue in varying proportions; plasma cells are scanty.[6] Their clinical characteristics are identical to those of plasma cell granulomas. Fibrous histiocytomas may be confused with fibromas.[66]

***Pulmonary Hyalinizing Granuloma.*** Approximately 50 cases of this rare tumor have been reported.[4, 77, 78] The tumor contains lamellae of homogeneous hyaline material, with interspersed plasma cells and giant cells.[5] The nodule is usually 2 to 4 cm in diameter, although large lesions have been reported, and some are cavitary.[79] In many cases, multiple lesions are present, simulating metastatic tumors.[80]

***Pulmonary Endometrioma.*** Catamenial hemoptysis (hemoptysis occurring at the time of menstruation) is a rare circumstance, which is presumed to be due to intrabronchial or parenchymal endometrial tissue deposits.[81] Pulmonary endometrioma may also present as an asymptomatic solitary pulmonary nodule; the diagnosis is usually established by exploratory thoracotomy. Intrapleural endometrial deposits are much more common than bronchopulmonary lesions and may be associated with catamenial pneumothorax[82] or catamenial hemothorax.[81]

***Pseudolymphoma.*** These large solitary nodular or irregular lung lesions are composed of a polymorphous mixture of lymphocytes, plasma cells, and histiocytes, which resembles the histologic changes in patients with lymphocytic interstitial pneumonitis. These are part of the spectrum of bronchus-associated lymphoid tissue proliferations, both benign and malignant.[83] Cough and sputum production are common. In many cases, such tumors are really low-grade lymphomas,[84] but in general, the prognosis is relatively good. (Further discussion about pulmonary lymphomas and lymphoproliferative diseases is available in Chapter 47.)

## Multiple Parenchymal Tumors

Many of the tumors already discussed as solitary intraparenchymal benign tumors occasionally present as multiple nodules in the lung. Such tumors include hamartomas,[85] hyalinizing granulomas,[6] leiomyomas, and sclerosing hemangiomas.[86]

**Benign Metastasizing Leiomyoma.** Multiple pulmonary leiomyomas occur predominantly in women and are associated in 80% of cases with a history of prior uterine surgery for fibroid tumors.[87] Some authorities have considered these lesions to be hamartomas or multiple primary lung tumors,[87] but the consensus favors metastatic deposits from a uterine tumor that appears benign histologically, hence the title.[87a] Current opinion is that the tumors, despite their relatively indolent behavior, are well-differentiated metastatic leiomyosarcomas.[6, 87, 88] There is often a response to hormonal manipulation.[89]

**Carney's Triad.** This bizarre syndrome consists of gastric epithelioid leiomyosarcoma, pulmonary chondromas, and extra-adrenal paragangliomas.[90, 90a] In some cases, only two of the three features are present. It occurs primarily in young women below the age of 30 years; less than 10% of the patients are men. The chondromas, which may be single or multiple, have been considered to be chondromatous hamartomas.[85] These tumors present as asymptomatic sharply circumscribed pulmonary nodules that may be calcified or even ossified (Fig. 49.2) and may show slow growth. Needle biopsy may be diagnostic.[91] In one patient with this syndrome, some of the lung nodules were metastases from the primary tumor and others were chondromas.[92]

**Pulmonary Tumorlets.** Tumorlets are minute collections of neuroendocrine cells scattered throughout the lungs that are usually discovered as an incidental finding in postmortem or surgical material. Most commonly they are found in elderly women[93, 94] and are not usually detectable by roentgenographic studies. Pulmonary tumorlets classically accompany inflammatory lesions in the airways but may also be multifocal and bilateral; when lesions exceed 0.5 cm in size, they are (arbitrarily) classi-

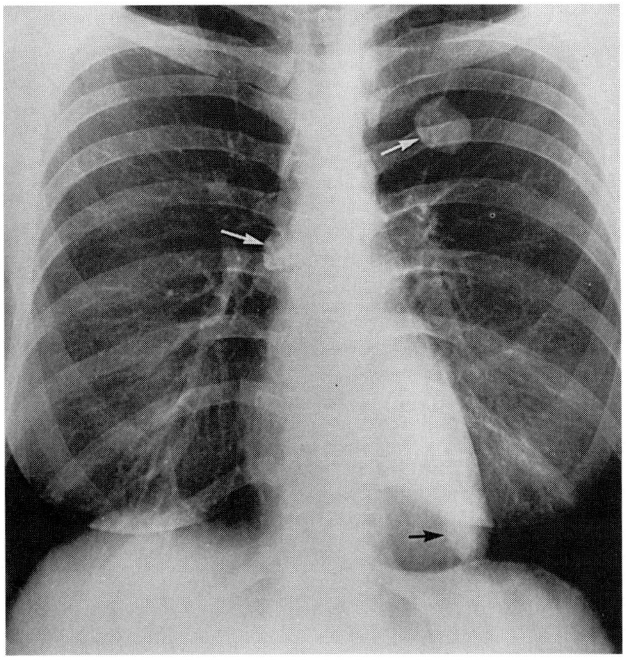

**Figure 49.2** Right lateral chest roentgenogram of a 21-year-old woman with recurrent gastric epithelioid leiomyosarcoma, showing several well-circumscribed intrapulmonary nodules bilaterally. Their roentgenographic densities were greater than those of soft tissue but less than that of calcium. The nodule shown *(top arrow)* was in the left upper lobe and had a lobulated but sharp margin. Transthoracic needle aspiration biopsy of this nodule yielded cartilage consistent with the diagnosis of chondroma. Mediastinal paragangliomas were discovered at a later thoracotomy. Diagnosis was pulmonary chondroma in a patient with Carney's triad.

fied as carcinoid tumors.[94a] Associated Cushing's syndrome has recently been reported.[94b]

**Pulmonary Chemodectoma.** Solitary intrapulmonary chemodectomas that are large enough to be detected by plain roentgenograms have been observed in the trachea[95] and in pulmonary parenchyma[96] in a handful of cases. They are apparently true paragangliomas and behave in a benign manner. Multiple minute pulmonary tumors, which are 1 to 3 mm in diameter and resemble chemodectomas, have been detected as asymptomatic incidental findings in a number of cases, almost all in women.[97, 98] These tumors appear to have no clinical significance and are probably not paragangliomas but resemble meningothelial cells.[98]

## Pseudotumors

Endobronchial pseudotumors include *tracheopathia osteochondroplastica,*[99, 99a] nodular *sarcoidosis,*[100] and tracheobronchial *amyloidosis,*[101] all of which may present as multiple plaques or as papillary lesions. An endobronchial *mucoid pseudotumor* may have the roentgenographic appearance of a solitary nodule.[102]

Parenchymal pseudotumors may be solitary or multi-

**Table 49.1** MANIFESTATIONS OF PULMONARY AMYLOIDOSIS

| MANIFESTATION | PATTERN | CLINICAL | PROGNOSIS |
|---|---|---|---|
| **Tracheobronchial** | | | |
| Plaques | Multiple | Wheezing | Fair |
| Papillary | Single | Asymptomatic airway obstruction | Good |
| **Parenchymal** | | | |
| Nodular | Single | Asymptomatic | Good |
| Diffuse | Interstitial | Dyspnea, respiratory failure | Poor |

ple. *Nodular amyloidosis* of the lung presents as asymptomatic well-defined nodules that are 2 to 4 cm in diameter.[103, 104] *Diffuse amyloidosis* complicating other diseases (e.g., multiple myeloma) may sometimes produce widespread infiltrates in the lung parenchyma (Table 49.1). (The various manifestations of bronchopulmonary amyloidosis are discussed in Chapter 86.) *Round atelectasis* is usually a solitary mass but occasionally is multiple; most cases are secondary to asbestos-induced pleural disease and are typically accompanied by distortion of blood vessels. The appearance on CT is characteristic, although not always diagnostic.[105] Intrapulmonary *hematomas* are recognized from the trauma history and the gradual shrinkage of the mass or masses with the passage of time.

Solitary pseudotumors that mimic bronchogenic carcinoma include *paraffinoma* (or *lipoid pneumonia*), which is due to recurrent aspiration of mineral oil (the presence of nonspecific areas of consolidation with low attenuation values and a "crazy-paving" pattern should strongly suggest the diagnosis)[106]; intrapulmonary *rheumatoid granuloma*[107]; and a solitary mass due to *Wegener's granulomatosis.*[108] The last condition can be diagnosed with a high degree of certainty by the combination of needle aspiration biopsy and a positive test for antineutrophilic cytoplasmic antibody.[109] Necrotizing granulomas that may simulate parenchymal tumors also include *infectious granulomas* and *bronchocentric granulomatosis.*[110]

A loculated *interlobar effusion* may simulate pulmonary tumor if seen in only one projection, but the roentgenographic appearances on multiple views are usually diagnostic. Serial films often show that the opacity shrinks with diuretic therapy. The terms *vanishing lung tumor* or *phantom tumor* have been applied to loculated effusions and hematomas that decrease in size.[111] A *pulmonary infarct* may be confused with pulmonary tumor[112, 113]; this has occasionally resulted in surgical resection of old infarcts.

## SUMMARY

Benign tumors of the lung are uncommon and often asymptomatic. Intratracheal and endobronchial tumors frequently give rise to symptoms of bronchial obstruction and are diagnosed (and often treated) by bronchoscopy.

Parenchymal benign tumors are usually asymptomatic and are discovered serendipitously on chest roentgenograms. In most cases, the diagnosis is made by thoracotomy or thoracostomy and resection, although the diagnostic usefulness of transthoracic needle biopsy is increasingly accepted. Pseudotumors may mimic benign and malignant lung tumors.

## References

1. Arrigoni MG, Woolner LB, Bernatz PE, et al: Benign tumors of the lung: A ten year surgical experience. J Thorac Cardiovasc Surg 60:589–599, 1970.
2. Miller DR: Benign tumors of the lung and tracheobronchial tree. Ann Thorac Surg 8:542–560, 1969.
3. Madewell JE, Feigin DS: Benign tumors of the lung. Semin Roentgenol 12:175–186, 1977.
4. Dail DH: Uncommon tumors. *In* Dail DH, Hammar SP (eds): Pulmonary Pathology (2nd ed). New York: Springer-Verlag, 1994, pp 1279–1461.
5. Churg A: Tumors of the lung. *In* Thurlbeck WM (ed): Pathology of the Lung. Stuttgart: Thieme, 1988, pp 311–423.
6. Fraser RG, Paré JAP, Paré PD, et al: Neoplastic diseases of the lungs. *In* Fraser RG, Paré JAP, Paré PD, et al (eds): Diagnosis of Diseases of the Chest (Vol 11, 3rd ed). Philadelphia: WB Saunders, 1989, pp 1327–1623.
7. McCarthy MJ, Rosado-de-Christenson ML: Tumors of the trachea. J Thorac Imaging 10:180–198, 1995.
8. Grillo HC, Mathisen DJ: Primary tracheal tumors: Treatment and results. Ann Thorac Surg 49:69–77, 1990.
9. Wang N-S, Morin J: Recurrent endobronchial soft tissue tumors. Chest 85:787–791, 1984.
10. Lillington GA: Management of solitary pulmonary nodules. Dis Mon 37:271–318, 1991.
11. Zwirewich CV, Vedal S, Miller RR, et al: Solitary pulmonary nodule: High resolution CT and radiographic-pathologic correlation. Radiology 179:469–476, 1991.
12. Siegelman SS, Khouri NF, Scott WW Jr, et al: Pulmonary hamartoma: CT findings. Radiology 160:313–317, 1986.
13. Swensen SJ, Silverstein MD, Ilstrup DM, et al: The probability of malignancy in solitary pulmonary nodules: Application to small, radiologically indeterminate nodules. Arch Intern Med 157:849–855, 1997.
14. Dewan NA, Shehan CJ, Reeb SD, et al: Likelihood of malignancy in a solitary pulmonary nodule: Comparison of Bayesian analysis and results of FDG-PET scan. Chest 112:416–422, 1997.
15. Khouri NF, Meziane MA, Zerhouni EA, et al: The solitary pulmonary nodule: Assessment, diagnosis and management. Chest 91:128–133, 1987.
16. Spencer H, Dail DH, Ameaud J: Noninvasive bronchial epithelial papillary tumors. Cancer 45:1486–1497, 1980.
17. Kramer SS, Wehaunt WD, Stocker JT, Kashima H: Pulmonary manifestations of juvenile laryngotracheal papillomatosis. AJR Am J Roentgenol 144:687–694, 1985.
18. Bauman NM, Smith RJ: Recurrent respiratory papillomatosis. Pediatr Clin North Am 43:1385–1401, 1996.
19. Rady PL, Schnadig VJ, Weiss RL, et al: Malignant transformation of recurrent respiratory papillomatosis associated with integrated human papillomavirus type 11 DNA and mutation of p53. Laryngoscope 108:735–740, 1998.
20. Healy GB, Gelber RD, Trowbridge AL, et al: Treatment of recurrent respiratory papillomatosis with human leukocyte interferon: Results of a multicenter randomized clinical trial. N Engl J Med 319:401–407, 1988.
21. Leventhal BG, Whisnant J, Kashima H, et al: Recurrent respiratory papillomatosis. J Biol Response Mod 4:525–530, 1985.
22. Maxwell RJ, Gibbons JR, O'Hara MD: Solitary squamous papilloma of the bronchus. Thorax 40:68–71, 1985.
23. Emory WB, Mitchell WT Jr, Hatch HG Jr: Mucous gland adenoma of the bronchus. Am Rev Respir Dis 108:1407–1410, 1973.
24. England DM, Hochholzer L: Truly benign "bronchial adenoma." Report of 10 cases of mucous gland adenoma with immunohistochemical and ultrastructural findings. Am J Surg Pathol 19:887–899, 1995.
25. Liu RC, McKenzie FN, Kim Y, Senderoff E: Primary endobronchial granular cell myoblastoma. Ann Thorac Surg 48:113–115, 1989.
26. Victoria LV, Hoffman HT, Robinson RA: Granular cell tumor of the larynx. J Laryngol Otol 112:373–376, 1998.
27. Young CD, Gay RM: Multiple endobronchial granular cell myoblastoma of the bronchus. Hum Pathol 15:193–194, 1984.
28. McLain WC, Olsen GN, Woolridge DB, et al: Endotracheal granular cell myoblastoma: A failure of laser therapy. Chest 86:136–137, 1984.
29. Montpreville T, Dulmet EM: Granular cell tumors of the lower respiratory tract. Histopathology 27(3):257–262, 1995.
30. Shulster PL, Khan FA, Azueta V: Asymptomatic granular cell tumor presenting as a coin lesion. Chest 68:256–258, 1975.
31. Sibala JL: Endobronchial hamartomas. Chest 62:631–634, 1972.
32. Tomashefski JF Jr: Benign endobronchial mesenchymal tumors: Their relationship to parenchymal pulmonary hamartomas. Am J Surg Pathol 6:531–540, 1982.
33. Borro JM, Moya J, Botella JA, et al: Endobronchial hamartoma: Report of 7 cases. Scand J Thorac Cardiovasc Surg 23:285–287, 1989.
34. Corona FE, Okeson GC: Endobronchial fibroma. Am Rev Respir Dis 110:350–353, 1974.
35. Littlefield JB, Drash EC: Myxoma of the lung. J Thorac Surg 37:745–749, 1959.
36. Walsh TJ, Healy TM: Chondroma of the bronchus. Thorax 24:327–329, 1969.
37. Bartley TD, Arean VM: Intrapulmonary neurogenic tumors. J Thorac Cardiovasc Surg 50:114–123, 1965.
38. Fabich DR, Hafez Z-R: Glomangioma of the trachea. Cancer 45:2337–2341, 1980.
39. Buell R, Wang NS, Seemayer TA, et al: Endobronchial plasma cell granuloma (xanthomatous pseudotumor): A light and electron microscopic study. Hum Pathol 7:411–426, 1976.
40. Duncan JD, Greenberg SD, Mattox KL, et al: Benign fibrous histiocytoma: A rare endobronchial neoplasm. Int Surg 71:110–111, 1986.
41. Schraufnagel DE, Morin JE, Wang NS: Endobronchial lipoma. Chest 75:97–99, 1979.
42. Politis J, Funahashi A, Gehlsen JA, et al: Intrathoracic lipomas: Report of 3 cases and review of the literature with emphasis on endobronchial lipoma. J Thorac Cardiovasc Surg 77:550–556, 1979.
43. Vera-Romn JM, Sobonya RE, Gomez-Garcia JL, et al: Leiomyoma of the lung: Literature review and case report. Cancer 52:936–941, 1983.
44. White SH, Ibrahim NBN, Forrester-Wood CP, et al: Leiomyomas of the lower respiratory tract. Thorax 40:306–311, 1985.
45. Murray J, Kielkowski D, Leiman G: The prevalence and age distribution of peripheral pulmonary hamartomas in adult males. South Afr Med J 79:247–249, 1991.
46. Gjavre JA, Myers JL, Prakash U: Pulmonary hamartomas. Mayo Clin Proc 71:14–20, 1996.
47. van den Bosch JMM, Wagenaar SS, Corrin B, et al: Mesenchymoma of the lung (so-called hamartoma): A review of 154 parenchymal and endobronchial cases. Thorax 42:790–793, 1987.
48. Fletcher JA, Pinkus GS, Weidner N, et al: Lineage-restricted clonality in biphasic solid tumors. Am J Pathol 138:1199–1207, 1991.
49. Johansson M, Dietrich C, Mandahl N, et al: Recombinations of chromosome bands 6p2l and 14q24 characterize pulmonary hamartomas. Br J Cancer 67:1236–1241, 1993.
50. Basile A, Gregoris A, Antoci B, et al: Malignant change in a benign pulmonary hamartoma. Thorax 44:232–233, 1989.
51. Gabrail NY, Zara RY: Pulmonary hamartoma syndrome. Chest 97:962–965, 1990.
51a. Potente G, Macori F, Caimi M, et al: Noncalcified pulmonary hamartomas: Computed tomography enhancement patterns with histologic correlation. J Thorac Imaging 14:101–104, 1999.
52. Hamper UM, Khouri NF, Stitik FP, et al: Pulmonary hamartoma: Diagnosis by transthoracic needle aspiration biopsy. Radiology 155:15–18, 1985.
53. Dunbar F, Leiman G: The aspiration cytology of pulmonary hamartomas. Diagn Cytopathol 5:174–180, 1989.

54. Panos RJ, Chang SW: Diagnosis of pulmonary hamartoma by bronchoscopic transbronchial biopsy. J Natl Med Assoc 81:460–463, 1989.
55. Hansen CP, Holtveg H, Francis D, et al: Pulmonary hamartoma. J Thorac Cardiovasc Surg 104:674–678, 1992.
56. de Rooij PD, Meijer S, Calame J, et al: Solitary hamartoma of the lung: Is thoracotomy still mandatory? Neth J Surg 40:145–148, 1988.
57. Mark EJ: Mesenchymal cystic hamartoma of the lung. N Engl J Med 315:1255–1259, 1986.
58. Hedlund GL, Bisset GS, Bove KE: Malignant neoplasms arising in cystic hamartomas of the lung in childhood. Radiology 173:77–79, 1989.
59. Yousem SA, Wick MR, Singh R, et al: So-called sclerosing hemangioma of the lung: An immunohistochemical study supporting a respiratory epithelial origin. Am J Surg Pathol 12:582–590, 1988.
60. Chan K-W, Gibbs AR, Lo WS, Newman GR: Benign sclerosing pneumocytoma of lung (sclerosing haemangioma). Thorax 37:404–412, 1982.
61. Leung AS, Chan KW, Sereviratne HS: A morphological and immunohistochemical study of 25 cases of so-called sclerosing hemangioma of the lung. Histopathology 27:121–128, 1995.
62. Katzenstein A-L, Fulling K, Weise DL, et al: So-called sclerosing hemangioma of the lung: Evidence for mesothelial origin. Am J Surg Pathol 7:3–14, 1983.
63. Sugio K, Yokoyama H, Kaneko S, et al: Sclerosing hemangioma of the lung: Radiographic and pathological study. Ann Thorac Surg 53:295–300, 1992.
64. Unger PD, Geller SA, Anderson PJ: Pulmonary lesion in a patient with neurofibromatosis. Arch Pathol Lab Med 108:654–657, 1984.
65. Flynn SD, Yousem SA: Pulmonary meningiomas: A report of 2 cases. Hum Pathol 22:469–474, 1991.
66. Viguera JL, Pujol JL, Reboiras SD, et al: Fibrous histiocytomas of the lung. Thorax 31:475–479, 1976.
67. Liebow AA, Castleman B: Benign clear cell tumors of the lung. Am J Pathol 43:13–14, 1963.
68. Andrion A, Mazzucco G, Gugliotta P, et al: Benign clear cell ("sugar") tumor of the lung. Cancer 56:2657–2663, 1985.
69. Gaffey MJ, Mills SE, Askin FB, et al: Clear cell tumor of the lung. A clinicopathologic, immunohistochemical and ultrastructural study of eight cases. Am J Surg Pathol 14:248–259, 1990.
70. Morgan DE, Sangers C, McElvein RB, et al: Intrapulmonary teratoma: A case report and review of the literature. J Thorac Imaging 7(3):70–77, 1992.
71. Spencer H: The pulmonary plasma cell/histiocytoma complex. Histopathology 8:903–916, 1984.
71a. Cerfolio RJ, Allen MS, Nascimento AG, et al: Inflammatory pseudotumors of the lung. Ann Thorac Surg 67:993–996, 1999.
72. Mandelbaum I, Brashear RE, Hull MT: Surgical treatment and course of pulmonary pseudotumor (plasma cell granuloma). J Thorac Cardiovasc Surg 82:77–82, 1981.
73. Bahadori M, Liebow AA: Plasma cell granulomas of the lung. Cancer 31:191–208, 1973.
74. Berardi RS, Lee SS, Chen HP, et al: Inflammatory pseudotumors of the lung. Surg Gynecol Obstet 156:89–96, 1983.
75. Copin MC, Gosselin BH, Ribet ME: Plasma cell granuloma of the lung: Difficulties in diagnosis and prognosis. Ann Thorac Surg 61:1477–1482, 1996.
76. Greene R, McLoud TC, Stark P: Other malignant tumors of the lung. Semin Roentgenol 12:225–237, 1977.
77. Engleman P, Liebow AA, Gmelich J, et al: Pulmonary hyalinizing granuloma. Am Rev Respir Dis 115:997–1008, 1977.
78. Yousem SA, Hochholzer L: Pulmonary hyalinizing granuloma. J Clin Pathol 87:1–6, 1987.
79. Gans SJ, Vander Elst AM, Straks W: Pulmonary hyalinizing granuloma. Eur Respir J 1:389–391, 1988.
80. Chalaoui J, Grégoire P, Sylvester P, et al: Pulmonary hyaline granuloma: A cause of pulmonary nodules. Radiology 152:23–26, 1984.
81. Joseph J, Sahn SA: Thoracic endometriosis syndrome: New observations from an analysis of 110 cases. Am J Med 100:164–170, 1996.
82. Lillington GA, Mitchell SM, Wood GA: Catamenial pneumothorax. JAMA 219:1328–1332, 1972.
83. Koss MN: Pulmonary lymphoid disorders. Semin Diagn Pathol 12:158–171, 1995.
84. Colby TV: Lymphoproliferative diseases. *In* Dail DH, Hammar SP (eds): Pulmonary Pathology (2nd ed). New York: Springer-Verlag, 1994, pp 1097–1122.
85. King TE Jr, Christopher KL, Scharwz MI: Multiple pulmonary chondromatous hamartomas. Hum Pathol 13:496–497, 1981.
86. Joshi K, Gopinath N, Shankar SK, et al: Multiple sclerosing hemangiomas of the lung. Postgrad Med J 56:50–53, 1980.
87. Wolff M, Gordon K, Silva F: Pulmonary metastases (with admixed epithelial elements) from smooth muscle neoplasms. Am J Surg Pathol 3:325–342, 1979.
87a. Esteban JM, Allen WM, Schaerf RH, et al: Benign metastasizing leiomyoma of the uterus. Arch Pathol Lab Med 123:960–962, 1999.
88. Parenti DJ, Morley TF, Giudice JC: Benign metastasizing leiomyoma. Respiration 56:347–350, 1992.
89. Clark DH, Weed JC: Metastasizing leiomyoma: A case report. Am J Obstet Gynecol 127:672–673, 1977.
90. Carney JA: The triad of gastric epithelioid leiomyosarcoma, pulmonary chondroma and functioning extra-adrenal paraganglioma: A five year review. Medicine 62:159–169, 1983.
90a. Carney JA: Gastric stromal sarcoma, pulmonary chondroma, and extra-adrenal paraganglioma (Carney triad): Natural history, adrenocortical component, and possible familial occurrence. Mayo Clin Proc 75:543–552, 1999.
91. Dajee A, Dajee H, Hinrichs S, et al: Pulmonary chondroma, extra-adrenal paraganglioma, and gastric leiomyosarcoma. J Thorac Cardiovasc Surg 84:377–391, 1982.
92. Chahinian AP, Kirschner PA, Dikman SH, et al: Pulmonary leiomyosarcoma coexisting with pulmonary chondroma in Carney's triad. Arch Intern Med 143:1462–1464, 1983.
93. Churg A, Warnock ML: Pulmonary tumorlet: A form of peripheral carcinoid. Cancer 37:1469–1477, 1976.
94. Miller MA, Mark GJ, Kanarek D: Multiple peripheral pulmonary carcinoids and tumorlets of carcinoid type, with restrictive and obstructive lung disease. Am J Med 65:373–378, 1978.
94a. Colby TV, Wistuba II, Gazdar A: Precursors to pulmonary neoplasia. Adv Anat Pathol 5:205–215, 1999.
94b. Arioglu E, Doppman J, Gomes M, et al: Cushing's syndrome caused by corticotropin secretion by pulmonary tumorlets. N Engl J Med 339:883–886, 1999.
95. Liew S-H, Leong A-Y, Tang HM: Tracheal paraganglioma: A case report with review of the literature. Cancer 47:1387–1393, 1981.
96. Singh G, Lee RE, Brooks DH: Primary pulmonary paraganglioma: Report of a case and review of the literature. Cancer 40:2286–2289, 1977.
97. Churg A, Warnock ML: So-called minute pulmonary chemodectoma: A tumor not related to paraganglioma. Cancer 37:1759–1769, 1976.
98. Gaffey MJ, Mills SE, Askin FB: Minute pulmonary meningothelial-like nodules: A clinicopathologic study of so-called minute pulmonary chemodectoma. Am J Surg Pathol 12:167–175, 1988.
99. Case 32-1999. Trachopathia osteoplastica. Case records of the Massachusetts General Hospital. N Engl J Med 341:1292–1299, 1999.
99a. Moore CE, Wiatrak BJ, McClatchey KD, et al: High-risk human papillomavirus types and squamous cell carcinoma in patients with respiratory papillomas. Otolaryngol Head Neck Surg 120:698–705, 1999.
100. Corsello BF, Lohaus GH, Funihashi A: Endobronchial mass lesion due to sarcoidosis: Complete resolution with corticosteroid. Thorax 38:157–158, 1983.
101. Chen KTK: Amyloidosis presenting in respiratory tract. Pathol Ann 24(Part 1):253–273, 1989.
102. Karasick D, Karasick S, Lally JF: Mucoid pseudotumor of the tracheobronchial tree in 2 cases. AJR Am J Roentgenol 132:459–461, 1979.
103. Cordier JF, Loire R, Brune J: Amyloidosis of the lower respiratory tract: Clinical and pathologic features in a series of 21 patients. Chest 90:827–833, 1986.
104. Scott PP, Scot WW Jr: Isolated nodular pulmonary amyloidosis: Diagnosis by percutaneous needle aspiration biopsy. South Med J 78:467–471, 1985.

105. O'Donavan PB, Schenk M, Lim K, et al: Evolution of the reliability of computed tomographic criteria used in the diagnosis of round atelectasis. J Thorac Imaging 12(l):54–58, 1997.
106. Laurent F, Philippe JC, Vergier B, et al: Exogenous lipoid pneumonia: HRCT, MR, and pathologic findings. Eur Radiol J 9:1190–1196, 1999.
107. Panetierre F, Chandler BF, Libcke JH: Pulmonary cavitation in rheumatoid disease. Am Rev Respir Dis 97:89–95, 1968.
108. Blennerhassett JB, Lichter BI, Taylor AJ: Localized Wegener's granulomatosis simulating lung cancer: Report of four cases. Thorax 31:576–584, 1976.
109. Pitman MB, Szyfelbein WM, Niles J, et al: Clinical utility of fine needle aspiration biopsy in the diagnosis of Wegener's granulomatosis. Acta Cytol 36:222–229, 1992.
110. Ulbright TM, Katzenstein A-L: Solitary necrotizing granulomas of the lung: Differentiating features and etiology. Am J Surg Pathol 4:13–28, 1980.
111. Meier MA, Helfrich GB, Levitsky S: Phantom tumor of the lung (letter). JAMA 218:1571, 1971.
112. Louie SM, Corbett MG, Lillington GA: Pseudo-pseudo-pseudotumor of the lung. Chest 88:470–471, 1985.
113. Miller JI, Harrison EG Jr, Bernatz PE: Surgically treated unsuspected pulmonary infarction. Ann Thorac Surg 14:181–188, 1972.

SECTION K

# Disorders of the Pulmonary Circulation

# 50 General Principles and Diagnostic Approach

JOHN F. MURRAY, M.D.

Introduction
- Anatomy
- Physiology
- Pulmonary Vascular Resistance

Pulmonary Hypertension
- Pathophysiology
- Clinical Findings
- Differential Diagnosis

Abnormal Vascular Communications
- Pathophysiology
- Clinical Findings
- Differential Diagnosis

Pulmonary Edema
- Pathophysiology
- Clinical Findings
- Differential Diagnosis

Summary

## INTRODUCTION

Disorders of the pulmonary circulation constitute a large group of diverse conditions, some arising primarily in the blood vessels of the lungs (e.g., primary pulmonary hypertension and pulmonary arteriovenous fistula) and others affecting the blood vessels as a consequence of a disease process originating in sites outside the lungs (e.g., pulmonary embolism, cardiogenic pulmonary edema). Because of this etiologic heterogeneity, there is no completely satisfactory classification of the clinical entities that involve the pulmonary circulation. The chapters in this section include the major categories of vascular disorders (pulmonary thromboembolism, pulmonary vasculitis, primary pulmonary hypertension, arteriovenous fistulas and other malformations, and acute lung injury) and the chief complications of these disorders (cor pulmonale and pulmonary edema).

The diagnostic approach to a suspected disorder of the pulmonary circulation varies widely and differs in each of the three disease categories shown in Table 50.1. At times, making a diagnosis is remarkably simple, as in a

Table 50.1 CLASSIFICATION OF DISORDERS OF THE PULMONARY CIRCULATION

| Type | Pulmonary Origin | Extrapulmonary Origin |
|---|---|---|
| Pulmonary hypertension | Primary pulmonary hypertension<br>Vasculitis | Pulmonary embolism<br>Drug-induced pulmonary hypertension |
| Abnormal vascular communications | Arteriovenous malformations<br>Sequestration of the lung | Cirrhosis of the liver<br>Acquired systemic-pulmonary communications |
| Pulmonary edema | Direct ARDS-type lung injury<br>Veno-occlusive disease | Indirect ARDS-type lung injury<br>Heart failure |

ARDS = Acute respiratory distress syndrome.

patient with acute pulmonary edema after inhalation of a known corrosive gas. At other times, however, the diagnosis can be elusive and, even when made, is always somewhat tenuous, as in a patient with acute respiratory distress syndrome. In this chapter the general principles of and the diagnostic approach to pulmonary vascular disorders are reviewed, including their pathophysiology, clinical and laboratory features, and differential diagnosis. Details concerning each of the many different conditions that may involve the pulmonary circulation are found in the subsequent chapters in this section and elsewhere in this book.

## Anatomy

The blood supply to the lungs comes from two different sources: the pulmonary circulation and the bronchial circulation. The general anatomic organization of the two circulations and their histologic components are described in Chapter 1. Additional information about the structure and function of the pulmonary and bronchial circulations and their interconnections are provided in Chapter 6, details about the factors that govern the distribution of pulmonary blood flow are described in Chapter 4, and the pharmacologic responses of the vasculature are reviewed in Chapter 12. Only the essential features that pertain to the pathophysiology of the principal pulmonary vascular disorders and their clinical consequences are considered here.

### Pulmonary Circulation

The pulmonary circulation extends from the pulmonary valve, which marks the vascular exit from the right side of the heart, to the orifices of the pulmonary veins in the wall of the left atrium, which marks the entrance into the left side of the heart. The pulmonary circulation includes the central pulmonary outflow tract; the right and left main pulmonary arteries and their lobar branches, intrapulmonary arteries, arterioles, capillaries, and venules; and the large pulmonary veins.[1] The anatomic relationships of the extrapulmonary and large intrapulmonary arteries and veins, down to about 2 mm in diameter, are well demonstrated on pulmonary angiograms (Fig. 50.1). The varying patterns of the lobar branches, which for the most part are unimportant clinically, have been catalogued.[2]

Because of differences in their physiologic behavior (described subsequently), the pulmonary circulation is sometimes subdivided into *extra-alveolar vessels* and *alveolar vessels*.[3] In addition, the small vessels that participate in liquid and solute exchange are often lumped together and called collectively the *pulmonary microcirculation*.[4] As later emphasized, however, the anatomic boundaries of the extra-alveolar and alveolar vessels and of the microcirculation are undefined and probably change, depending especially on the prevailing lung volume and vascular pressures.

The pulmonary capillaries form an extensive network in the interalveolar septa, the walls that separate adjacent alveoli from each other. The capillary endothelium is composed chiefly of the cytoplasmic extensions of the endothelial cells, which by their contiguous arrangement form a thin vascular tube; details about the anatomic and functional interrelationships of the pulmonary microcirculation are available elsewhere.[5, 6] Both the endothelium and the neighboring alveolar epithelium, chiefly types I and II pneumocytes, rest on separate basement membranes (Fig. 50.2). Over approximately half of the capillary perimeter, the two endothelial and epithelial basement membranes appear to be fused; this fusion forms the so-called thin portion of the alveolar-capillary membrane that, because of its narrowness, is the site of maximal gas diffusion. Over the other half of the capillary perimeter, the two basement membranes are separated to form an interstitial space; this is the so-called thick portion of the interalveolar septum and is the site of liquid and solute exchange. Pulmonary capillaries weave their way through the interstitial space of the interalveolar septum, first facing one alveolus and then the other. Thus, the interstitial space is perforated by capillaries and should be thought of as a communicating meshwork, not as a continuous sheet.[7]

The pulmonary arteries branch, and the veins converge continuously as they travel from the hilum to the periphery through the lungs, but their anatomic relations with each other and with the airways differ. Branches of both pulmonary arterial and bronchial systems travel together as close neighbors and supply the same terminal respiratory (gas exchange) units within a single lobule. In con-

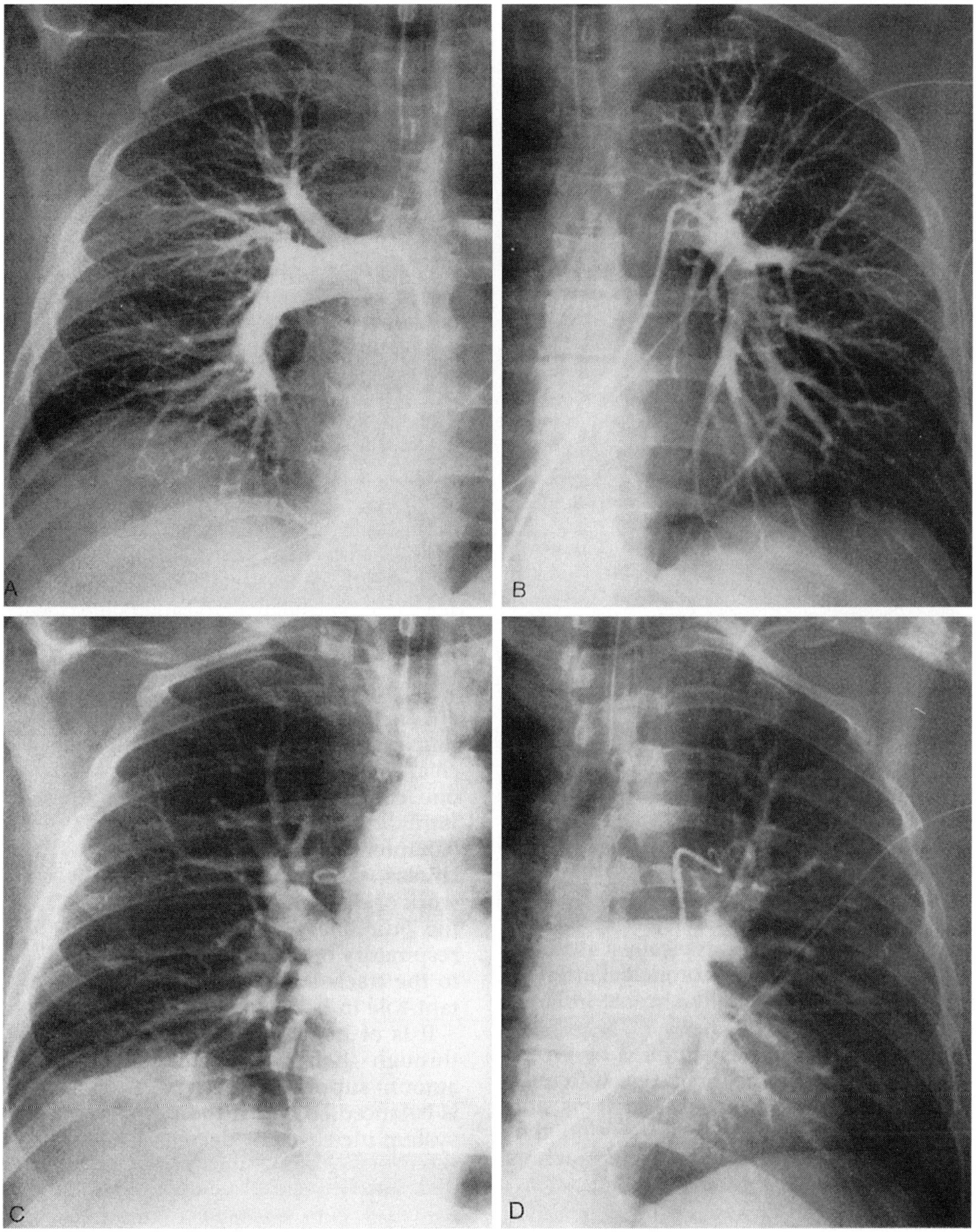


**Figure 50.1** Pulmonary angiogram showing normal anatomy of the arteries and veins. *A,* Arteries of the right lung after injection of contrast material into the right main pulmonary artery. *B,* Arteries of the left lung after injection into the left main pulmonary artery. *C,* Veins of the right lung and opacification of the left atrium, left ventricle, and aorta. *D,* Veins of the left lung and left atrium.

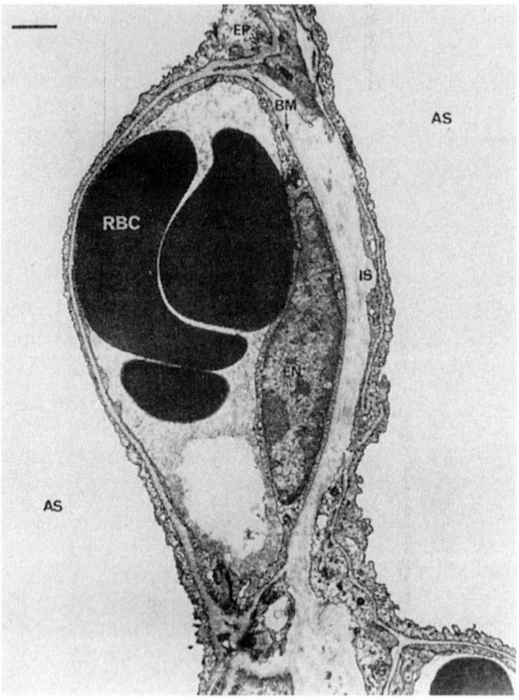


**Figure 50.2** Electron micrograph of a normal human lung. A capillary containing red blood cells (RBC) is suspended in the interalveolar septum between two alveolar spaces (AS). The basement membranes (BM) of the epithelium (EP) and endothelium (EN) appear to be fused over the thin portion of the septum and separated over the thick portion of the septum containing the interstitial space (IS). Horizontal bar = 1 μm. (Original photograph courtesy of Dr. Ewald R. Weibel, University of Berne.)

trast, pulmonary venules drain blood from several lobules, and as progressively larger veins form, they lie as far from the bronchial-arterial partners as is anatomically possible.[8] Both the veins and the paired bronchi and arteries are enclosed by the bronchovascular sheath. Within this surrounding membrane lies an interstitial space, the peribronchovascular space, which is filled with loose connective tissue, and the pulmonary lymphatic vessels, which use these conduits as exit pathways from the lungs; these structures play an important role in the formation and clearance of pulmonary edema.[4]

## Bronchial Circulation

There are substantial differences between the pulmonary circulation and the bronchial circulation in the amount of blood flow, composition of the blood, and functional importance, which have been comprehensively reviewed.[9] The pulmonary circulation consists of virtually the entire cardiac output; it contains venous blood, and the "arterialization" of this blood is essential for life. In contrast, the bronchial circulation consists of only 1% or 2% of the cardiac output; it contains systemic arterial blood, and the normal adult lung remains viable without it. However, this statement oversimplifies the role of the bronchial circulation, because it overlooks the importance of bronchial blood flow to development of the lungs in the fetus and its crucial contributions to gas exchange in many varieties of congenital cardiac anomalies. Furthermore, there is typically a striking increase in the size and number of bronchial arteries in certain lung diseases, especially chronic inflammation and neoplasms (Fig. 50.3).

Venous blood from capillaries supplied by bronchial arteries returns to the heart by two different pathways (see Fig. 6.2). True *bronchial veins* are formed from tributaries that originate around the lobar and segmental bronchi and from branches from the pleura in the neighborhood of the hilus. Bronchial venous blood flows into the azygos, hemiazygos, and intercostal veins and then into the right atrium. Veins that originate from bronchial capillaries within the lungs unite to form venous tributaries that join the pulmonary veins; these communicating vessels are sometimes called *bronchopulmonary veins*. Blood leaving the capillary bed around terminal bronchioles flows through anastomoses with the alveolar capillaries, and the mixture of blood returns to the left atrium through pulmonary veins.

## Physiology

The pulmonary circulation serves many important functions. Of these, the most vital is the maintenance of gas exchange through the constant flow of mixed venous (poorly oxygenated and carbon dioxide–rich) blood through the pulmonary arterial circulation to the pulmonary capillaries and the return of arterialized blood through the pulmonary venous circulation to the left atrium. But the pulmonary circulation has other important roles[10]: It provides substrates to satisfy the nutritional and metabolic needs of the lung parenchyma, including the synthesis of surfactant; it serves as the site for the synthesis, storage, and transformation of a variety of biochemical substances[11]; it furnishes a reservoir of blood for the left ventricle[12]; it filters the venous return from the entire body; and it provides a large surface for the absorption of lung liquid that must occur at the time of birth[13] or that may take place in unusual circumstances (e.g., bronchoalveolar lavage or near drowning).

The bronchial circulation is the principal source of nutrient blood and oxygen to virtually all intrapulmonary structures except the parenchyma; these structures include the bronchial tree from the main-stem bronchi to the terminal bronchioles, the pulmonary nerves and ganglia, the walls of elastic and some muscular pulmonary arteries and veins, the lymph nodes and lymph tissue, and the connective tissue septa in most mammals. The blood supply to the visceral pleura varies among different species[14]; in humans the visceral pleura is supplied by the bronchial circulation, a feature of some importance in view of the sites and magnitude of liquid formation and removal by the pleural surfaces (Chapter 73). Near the end of the terminal bronchioles, the bronchial arterioles terminate in a network of capillaries that anastomose extensively with the pulmonary capillaries supplying the adjoining respiratory bronchioles. The bronchial blood supply to the trachea and central airways plays an important role in heat and water exchange.[15]

It is of interest that the blood flow to the lungs through

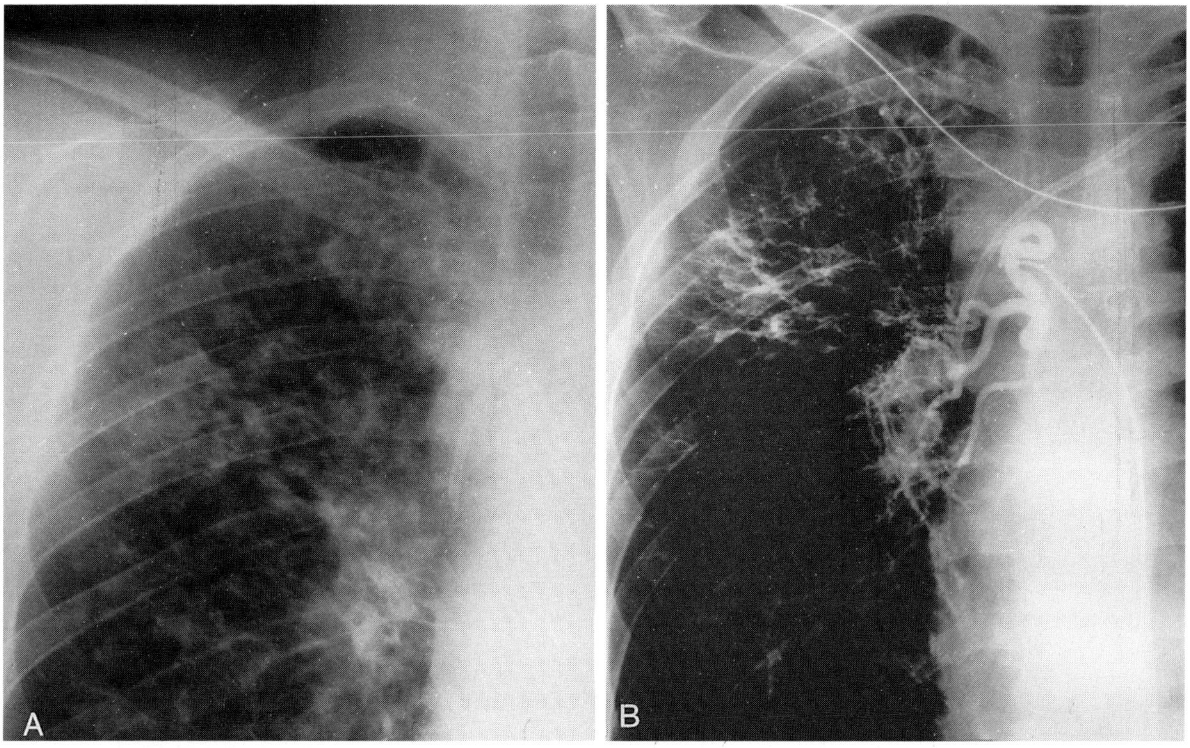

**Figure 50.3** *A,* Detailed view of the right upper lung field of a patient with cystic fibrosis after an episode of massive hemoptysis, showing a patchy infiltrate in the area. *B,* Selective right bronchial arteriogram demonstrating marked enlargement with hypervascularity in the right upper lobe and hilar lymph nodes. (Case courtesy of Dr. Jeffrey Dieden, Kaiser Permanente Medical Center. From Klein JS, Schultz S: Interventional chest radiology. Curr Prob Diagn Radiol 21:258–264, 1992.)

their two circulations, even though the amount supplied by each pathway differs markedly, is balanced so that if the perfusing pressure in one system increases or decreases, there is a change in the opposite direction in the amount of blood supplied by the other system.[16] This means that if pressure falls in part of the pulmonary arterial circulation (e.g., distal to the site of a pulmonary embolus), blood flow to the lung parenchyma through the bronchial circulation will increase; conversely, if pressure in the bronchial system falls (e.g., in lung transplantation, which deprives the lung of all its bronchial blood flow), blood flow in the pulmonary circulation will increase in an attempt to supply the tissues that formerly received blood through the bronchial circulation.

## Pulmonary Blood Flow

Not long after cardiac catheterization was introduced and direct measurements of pulmonary arterial pressures became available, Dock[17] suggested that the distribution of blood flow within the lungs must be nonuniform because the pulmonary circulation is a low-pressure system that is operating in a gravitational field. He also speculated that the presence of uneven blood flow would create important differences between regions of the lungs in their local defense capabilities and adequacy of gas exchange. Fifteen years later, the development of radioactive gas techniques for assessing the distribution of pulmonary blood flow confirmed Dock's theory.

On the basis of results of their original studies, West and coworkers[18] developed a model of the lung that accounts for the pattern of the regional distribution of blood flow (see Fig. 4.10 and accompanying discussion). They divided the lung into three zones according to the relationships among alveolar pressure ($P_{ALV}$), pulmonary arterial pressure ($P_{PA}$), and pulmonary venous ($P_{PV}$) or left atrial pressure. This model has provided important conceptual understanding of the behavior of the pulmonary circulation, but its application to the human lung is often misunderstood. As shown in Figure 50.4, in healthy persons in the upright position, most of the lung is in zone 3; there is usually a small zone 2 toward the apex and no zone 1. It is obvious that changing the hydrostatic pressures relative to the height of the lung must affect the distribution of blood flow. Accordingly, pulmonary blood flow is more uniform in the supine than in the upright position, because the vertical height of the lung is decreased and the pressures are relatively constant. Similarly, exercise in the upright position raises pulmonary arterial pressure and pulmonary venous pressure (Table 50.2), so that blood flow to the upper regions improves and overall perfusion becomes more uniform than at rest. Conversely, in patients with diseases that lower pulmonary arterial pressure (e.g., circulatory shock) or raise alveolar pressure (e.g.,

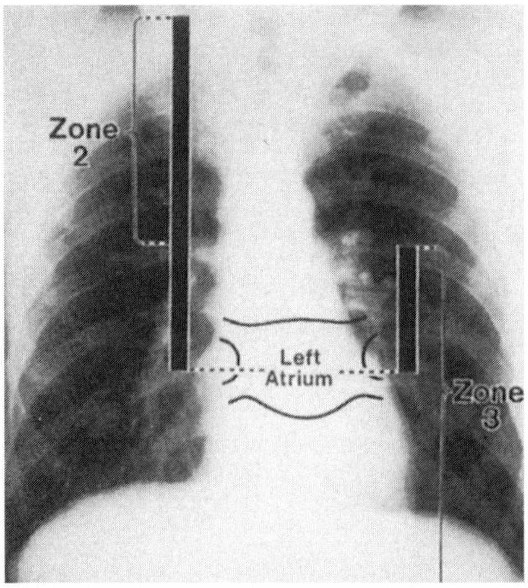


**Figure 50.4** Chest radiograph showing the distribution of zones in normal human lungs in the upright position. The solid bar on the left shows height "reached" by pulmonary arterial pressure, and the bar on the right shows height "reached" by pulmonary venous pressure; both pressures are referenced to the mid-left atrium. More of the lungs are in zone 3 than zone 2, and there is no zone 1.

use of end-expiratory pressure), the amount of lung in which zone 2 conditions prevail increases, and a zone 1 may develop.

## Pulmonary Vascular Resistance

The lungs normally "accept" the entire output of blood from the right ventricle, exchange oxygen and carbon dioxide between pulmonary capillary blood and alveolar gas, and return the arterialized blood to the left ventricle for distribution to the rest of the body. Although blood flow to the lungs is greater than that to any other organ, the pressure within the pulmonary circulation is low; normal mean pulmonary arterial pressure is less than one seventh of mean systemic arterial pressure. Not only is the pulmonary circulation a high-flow–low-pressure system at rest but it also can accommodate increases in cardiac output during exercise up to several times resting values with only a small increase in pulmonary arterial pressure. This means that pulmonary vascular resistance is low to begin with and decreases even further when pulmonary blood flow increases (see Table 50.2).

Resistance to blood flow through the lungs is computed from the same general equation used to calculate resistance in any system of flowing liquid: resistance = pressure difference ÷ flow. When this equation is applied to pulmonary vascular resistance (PVR), inflow and outflow pressures are mean pulmonary arterial pressure and pulmonary venous pressure, respectively, and flow through the system is total cardiac output ($\dot{Q}_T$):

$$\text{PVR} = \frac{P_{PA} - P_{PV}}{\dot{Q}_T} \qquad (1)$$

As discussed in detail in Chapter 6, an important advance in our knowledge concerning the distributions of pressures and vascular resistances in the pulmonary circulation was made by Bhattacharya and Staub,[19] who measured microvascular pressures with micropipets in an isolated perfused canine lung. The profile of the distribution of vascular resistance under zone 3 conditions (see Fig. 6.6) shows that the largest resistance (46%) lies in the capillaries of the alveolar septum, most of the remainder is in arterioles (20 to 50 μm in diameter), and there is negligible resistance from venules (20 μm in diameter) to pulmonary veins. Further analysis of these data suggests that they apply to the lungs as a whole and could be compatible with either network or sheet flow models of the microcirculation.[20]

### Regulation

Changes in pressures within or surrounding pulmonary blood vessels, shifts of blood into and out of the lungs, and alterations in whole blood viscosity all cause passive changes in pulmonary vascular resistance; the word *passive* is used to indicate that the change in caliber of the vessels is not caused by *active* contraction or relaxation of vascular smooth muscle. Originally, the pulmonary vascular bed was considered to respond chiefly in a passive manner, and these influences still appear to predominate. Abundant data, however, have established that the pulmonary vessels are capable of reacting actively, by contraction or relaxation of vascular smooth muscle, to neurogenic influences, humoral substances, or chemical stimuli, especially in response to alveolar hypoxia. (Additional information about neural and chemical regulation of the pulmonary circulation is available in Chapters 6 and 12.)

The most potent vasoconstrictor stimulus to the pulmonary circulation is *alveolar* hypoxia, as opposed to either arterial or mixed venous hypoxia. Alveolar hypoxia initiates an important adaptive response by redistributing blood flow from poorly ventilated to better ventilated regions of the lungs, thus improving gas exchange.[21] Perhaps for this reason, the response is unique to the lungs; exposure of systemic vessels to hypoxia causes vasodilation. The major site of hypoxia-induced pulmonary vasoconstriction lies in the small muscular pulmonary arteries (30 to 50 μm in diameter). Despite extensive investigation, the mechanism of hypoxia-induced pulmonary vasoconstriction remains unknown. In fact, it is still uncertain whether vasoconstriction is a direct effect of hypoxia on arterial smooth muscle or is actuated by a chemical mediator; neural stimulation is unlikely to be involved. Numerous candidate vasoconstrictor substances (for review, see Chapter 6 and reference 21) have failed to qualify, but new contenders continue to appear.[22] Cyclooxygenase inhibitors (e.g., indomethacin) augment hypoxia-induced vasoconstriction,[23] whereas nitric oxide (NO) inhibits it.[24] Because the far-reaching search for a chemical mediator has been so unsuccessful, there is renewed interest in mechanisms through which hypoxia may directly effect vascular smooth muscle cells; one possibility is by inhibiting the $K^+$ channel that provokes membrane depolarization, thereby opening a $Ca^{2+}$ chan-

**Table 50.2** COMPARISON OF PULMONARY AND SYSTEMIC HEMODYNAMIC VARIABLES DURING REST AND EXERCISE OF MODERATE SEVERITY IN A HEALTHY YOUNG MAN

| Condition | Rest (Sitting) | Exercise (Bicycling) |
|---|---|---|
| Oxygen consumption (mL/min) | 300 | 2000 |
| **Blood Flow** | | |
| Cardiac output (liters/min) | 6.3 | 16.2 |
| Heart rate (beats/min) | 70 | 135 |
| Stroke volume (mL/beat) | 90 | 120 |
| **Intravascular Pressures** | | |
| Pulmonary arterial pressure (mm Hg) | 20/10 | 30/11 |
| Mean (mm Hg) | 14 | 20 |
| Left atrial pressure (mean) (mm Hg) | 5 | 10 |
| Brachial arterial pressure (mm Hg) | 120/70 | 155/78 |
| Mean (mm Hg) | 88 | 122 |
| Right atrial pressure (mean) (mm Hg) | 3 | 1 |
| **Resistances** | | |
| Pulmonary vascular resistance (units*) | 1.43 | 0.62 |
| Systemic vascular resistance (units*) | 13.5 | 6.9 |

* Units = mm Hg/liter/min.
Reproduced with permission from Murray JF: The Normal Lung. Philadelphia: WB Saunders, 1986, p 140.

nel that permits calcium-mediated smooth muscle contraction.[25]

## PULMONARY HYPERTENSION

The low pulmonary arterial pressure in the lungs of healthy subjects while at rest depends on a pulmonary circulation with a large cross-sectional area and a low resistance to blood flow. As cardiac output increases during progressively heavy exercise, pulmonary arterial pressure increases, but only slightly; this means that resistance must decrease substantially because of an increase in the cross-sectional area of the vascular bed, both by dilation of vessels that were perfused at rest and by recruitment of previously unperfused vessels. Because the capillary network is the chief site of resistance to blood flow through the pulmonary circulation, much of the dilation and recruitment during exercise takes place in the capillaries. Pulmonary hypertension, an abnormal increase in pulmonary arterial pressure, is caused by an increase in pulmonary vascular resistance that in turn depends on a decrease in the cross-sectional area of the vascular bed. Narrowing of any segment of the pulmonary circulation—arteries, arterioles, capillaries, venules, and veins—if sufficient, will cause hypertension.

### Pathophysiology

The cross-sectional area of the pulmonary vascular bed may be decreased by vasoconstriction, by structural changes (e.g., obstruction or obliteration) of the blood vessels, or by both. As disorders associated with pulmonary hypertension increase in severity, vasoconstriction or structural narrowing or both progressively impair the capacity of pulmonary blood vessels to increase their caliber and to decrease their resistance during exercise. This behavior explains why the diagnosis of *early* vascular involvement can be established only by measuring pulmonary arterial pressure while the patient exercises (Fig. 50.5). By the time clinically recognizable pulmonary

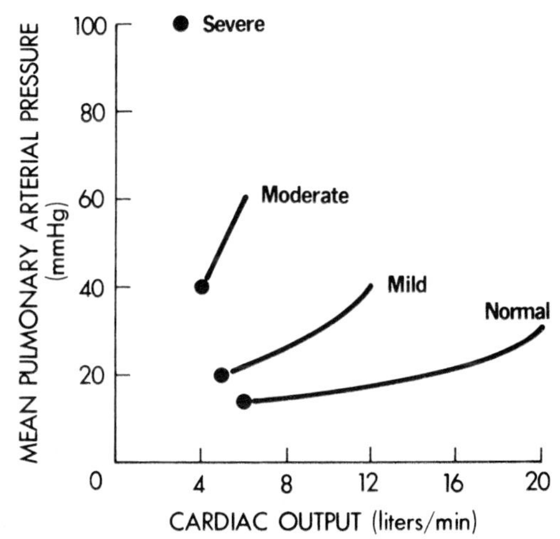


**Figure 50.5** Schematic representation of the relationship between mean pulmonary arterial pressure and cardiac output in normal subjects and in patients with mild, moderate, and severe pulmonary hypertension. *Solid circles* represent values at rest. Note that as the process worsens, resting pressure increases, resting output decreases, and an increase in output causes progressively steeper increases in pressure. (From Murray JF: Respiration. *In* Smith LH, Thier S (eds): Pathophysiology (2nd ed). Philadelphia: WB Saunders, 1985, p 835.)

hypertension is present at rest, the process is usually severe and inherently less reversible.

As with pulmonary vascular diseases in general, there is no completely satisfactory classification of the multiple causes of pulmonary hypertension. Wood's classification,[26] shown in Table 50.3, indicates that the quantity of blood flow and various intracardiac conditions as well as intrinsic pulmonary vascular diseases may increase pulmonary arterial pressure. Only the mechanisms directly related to abnormalities of respiration are considered in this chapter.

## Vasoconstriction

The pulmonary blood vessels are innervated and furnished with receptors that, in experimental animals, respond to neural and pharmacologic stimuli.[27, 28] These responses, however, are either impossible to demonstrate or weak in healthy human subjects. Although the widely used Wood classification (see Table 50.3) attempts to account for increased pulmonary artery hypertension strictly in hemodynamic terms, considerable evidence supports the likelihood that abnormal intrinsic responses of the pulmonary vasculature contribute to the development of pulmonary hypertension.[29] Many patients with pulmonary hypertension have an associated element of vasoconstriction, at times severe, that compounds whatever structural narrowing is present.[30] Prevailing pulmonary vasomotor tone seems to be determined by the interplay among locally produced or generated vasoactive substances, chiefly the vasodilators prostacyclin and NO, and the vasoconstrictors endothelin-1 (ET-1) and angiotensin II, but many other mediators are probably involved. Moreover, the vasodilators act generally to inhibit vascular smooth muscle growth, whereas the vasoconstrictors promote it,[21] thereby reinforcing the link between vasomotor structure and function.

From a clinical perspective, ET-1, which has both vasoconstrictor and growth-regulating cytokine activity, appears to be particularly important; patients with both primary pulmonary hypertension and a variety of secondary causes (thromboembolic, hypoxic, and associated with collagen vascular diseases and heart failure) have elevated levels of circulating ET-1 and increased expression of endothelin-converting enzyme-1 in the walls of diseased pulmonary arteries.[31, 32] Furthermore, patients with pulmonary hypertension have reduced amounts of endothelial NO synthase-III, the main enzyme responsible for generating the vasodilator NO, in their lungs,[33] and decreased amounts of NO in their expired air.[34] Thus, a plausible hypothesis is that a vasomotor imbalance in the pulmonary circulation, once established in favor of vasoconstriction and initiated or amplified by an excess of ET-1 and a deficiency of NO, triggers a complex series of reactions that promote smooth muscle and adventitial thickening and distort vascular morphology; attendant increased wall stresses and altered mechanical forces unleash other responses that exacerbate vascular remodeling. All of these responses are under genetic control, which is consistent with the familial clustering that has been observed in primary pulmonary hypertension.[35]

Acidemia exerts a direct pressor effect on the pulmonary circulation and, of more significance, compounds the vasomotor reaction to a given degree of hypoxia.[36] The synergistic vasoconstrictor response produced by hypoxia and acidosis combined may be important in the pathogenesis of pulmonary hypertension in patients in whom the two abnormalities coexist. Hypercapnia seems to have little or no effect on the human pulmonary circulation apart from the influence of increases in $P_{CO_2}$ on pH. Hypocapnia attenuates the vasoconstrictor effect of hypoxia, but it is not known whether this relates to a decrease in $P_{CO_2}$ or an increase in pH.

## Obliteration or Obstruction of Vessels

Obviously, one direct way of reducing the cross-sectional area of the pulmonary vascular bed is by obstructing or removing blood vessels in the lungs. Complete or partial occlusion of major pulmonary arteries is most often caused by recurrent pulmonary thromboembolism. Progressive narrowing of small pulmonary arteries is the

**Table 50.3 CLASSIFICATION OF PULMONARY HYPERTENSION: MODIFIED FROM WOOD WITH EXAMPLES OF EACH TYPE**

| Type | Mechanism | Examples |
|---|---|---|
| Passive | Impedance to pulmonary venous drainage | Mitral stenosis<br>Pulmonary veno-occlusive disease |
| Hyperkinetic | Increased pulmonary blood flow | Atrial septal defect<br>Ventricular septal defect |
| Obstructive | Impedance to flow through large pulmonary arteries | Pulmonary thromboembolism<br>Unilateral absence or stenosis of a pulmonary artery |
| Obliterative | Impedance to flow through small pulmonary blood vessels | Primary pulmonary hypertension<br>Collagen vascular diseases |
| Vasoconstrictive | Impedance to flow from hypoxia-induced vasoconstriction | Chronic mountain sickness<br>Sleep apnea syndrome |
| Polygenic | Two or more of the causes listed above | Chronic obstructive pulmonary disease (obliterative and vasoconstrictive)<br>Interstitial pulmonary fibrosis (obliterative and vasoconstrictive) |

outstanding feature of primary pulmonary hypertension and pulmonary vasculitis, and it occurs to some extent in patients with emphysema and interstitial fibrosis. Because the cross-sectional area of the pulmonary vascular system enlarges progressively from central pulmonary arteries to capillaries, the effect of an obstructive or obliterative process on pulmonary vascular resistance depends on the location of the abnormality. Millions of capillaries must be destroyed to equal the effect of occluding one lobar artery.

Once pulmonary hypertension occurs, regardless of its cause, secondary changes occur in the walls of pulmonary arteries that produce further narrowing. Early abnormalities are hypertrophy of smooth muscle in the media of small arteries and thickening of the adventitia. Later in the sequence, a cascade of reactions leads to increased deposition of elastin, intimal proliferation, and formation of atheromatous plaques. At times, fibrinoid necrosis develops, which predisposes to thrombosis in situ. Finally, aneurysmal and angiomatoid changes occur.[37] The effect of these reactions is to reduce an already restricted vascular bed. The progressively worsening vicious circle is shown in Figure 50.6. Once set in motion, the process is self-perpetuating and steadily accelerates, but it is not irreversible. Serial histologic studies of lungs from patients with primary pulmonary hypertension who responded to pharmacologic therapy with a reduction in pressure have shown improvement in the extent and severity of vascular remodeling.[38] The cellular and molecular mechanisms that underlie pulmonary vascular remodeling have been reviewed.[39]

### Cor Pulmonale

Cor pulmonale (see Chapter 55) is defined as hypertrophy and/or dilation of the right ventricle secondary to some form of respiratory disease; this condition is invariably associated with pulmonary hypertension. The term *respiratory disease,* rather than *pulmonary disease,* is used in this definition because abnormalities of organs other than the lungs cause or contribute to the pathogenesis of cor pulmonale. Implicit in both the definition and the clinical diagnosis of cor pulmonale is the exclusion of congenital and acquired forms of heart disease as causes of pulmonary arterial hypertension and right ventricular enlargement.

Although obviously parts of a continuum, the abnormal processes that cause cor pulmonale can be viewed as occurring in two stages: first, the onset of pulmonary hypertension as a result of narrowing of the vascular bed, and second, the development of right ventricular hypertrophy or dilation, or both, in response to the increased pulmonary arterial pressure. Cor pulmonale causes signs of right ventricular failure when pulmonary hypertension is severe and, usually, long lasting. Thus, patients with cor pulmonale always have pulmonary arterial hypertension but may or may not have right ventricular failure.

Pulmonary artery hypertension is clearly the most important determinant and is usually attributable to the effects of vascular obliteration or chronic alveolar hypoxia or both; however, other factors also contribute to the pathogenesis of cor pulmonale, especially in patients with chronic obstructive pulmonary disease (COPD), but exactly how these factors operate is poorly understood. In patients with COPD, the size of the right ventricle at postmortem examination does not correlate with the severity of emphysema as assessed morphometrically. Pulmonary hypertension and eventual cor pulmonale in these patients probably result from a complex interaction among such factors as hypoxic vasoconstriction, postinflammatory destruction of the pulmonary vascular bed, structural changes in the remaining vessels, increased blood viscosity, and abnormalities of lung mechanics, all of which probably vary from one patient to another.[40]

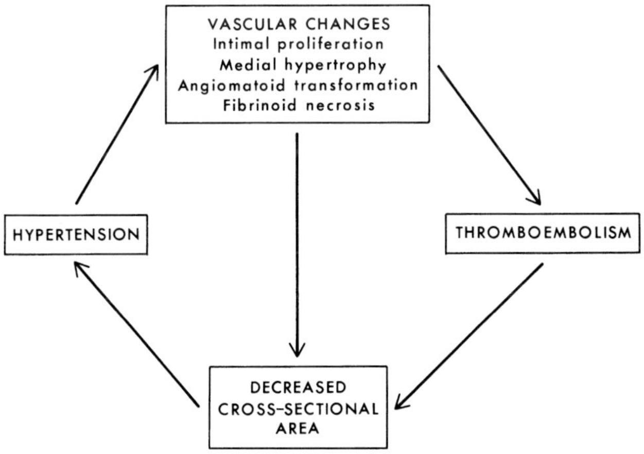


**Figure 50.6** Schematic diagram showing how pulmonary hypertension, once established from any cause, is compounded by secondary structural changes that predispose to thromboembolic narrowing, both of which further decrease the cross-sectional area of the pulmonary vascular pathways, which worsens the hypertension. (From Hinshaw HC, Murray JF: Diseases of the Chest (4th ed). Philadelphia: WB Saunders, 1979, p 687.)

## Clinical Findings

The signs and symptoms, radiographic features, and pulmonary function abnormalities associated with the pulmonary hypertensive diseases listed in Table 50.1 are extremely varied. Respiratory manifestations predominate mainly in the two intrinsic pulmonary diseases (primary pulmonary hypertension and veno-occlusive disease) and in two of the diseases of extrapulmonary origin (pulmonary embolism and drug-induced pulmonary hypertension). In patients with a generalized vasculitis that also involves the pulmonary circulation and in patients with pulmonary hypertension secondary to cirrhosis of the liver, the major abnormalities are apt to originate in organs other than the lungs.

### Symptoms and Signs

The chief symptom of pulmonary vascular occlusion is dyspnea. In early chronic occlusive diseases, dyspnea occurs first during exercise but, as the process worsens, may become severe during slight exertion and even at rest. In patients with acute thromboembolism, dyspnea is usually episodic and varies enormously from mild to incapacitating. Associated features of severe chronic vascular occlusion are syncope and peripheral edema. Symptoms that may accompany thromboembolism are hemoptysis and pleuritic pain.

There are often few or no detectable abnormalities on physical examination of the lungs in patients with chronic pulmonary vascular occlusive diseases. Crackles, a pleural friction rub, or signs of a pleural effusion may be found in patients with pulmonary embolism. More helpful, if present, are the signs of pulmonary hypertension on examination of the heart and circulatory system: a loud pulmonary second sound, which is often split and fixed with regard to the aortic second sound; a parasternal or subxyphoid heave, which is indicative of right ventricular enlargement; either a third or fourth heart sound, which may vary in intensity with respiration; distention of the neck veins, perhaps with an a-wave or a v-wave, which indicates high right-sided filling pressures; and hepatic enlargement and peripheral edema, which usually indicate right-sided heart failure.

### Radiographic Features

The radiographic abnormalities that accompany pulmonary vascular occlusive diseases are also varied. Several typical examples are shown in Chapter 51 (Pulmonary Thromboembolism) and Chapter 52 (Pulmonary Vasculitis and Primary Pulmonary Hypertension). In general, as with the physical examination, abnormalities are more likely to be found in the heart than in the lungs. The right ventricle may be enlarged, and the pulmonary trunk and central pulmonary arteries are often dilated with contrasting reduced vascular markings in the peripheral lung field. Irregular or marginated densities may be found in patients with pulmonary vasculitis, and a triad of elevated hemidiaphragm, unexplained parenchymal density, and small pleural effusion should raise the possibility of pulmonary embolism.

### Pulmonary Function Abnormalities

Because there is no pathophysiologic reason why intrinsic narrowing of the cross-sectional area of the pulmonary circulation should affect the results of tests of lung volumes or mechanics in any way, these results tend to be normal in patients with pure pulmonary vascular disorders. Theoretically, arterial hypoxia should not occur either, because a reduction in blood flow to gas exchange units means that ventilation-perfusion ratios should decrease and arterial $P_{O_2}$ values should increase; however, most studies, as reviewed by Voelkel and Reeves,[41] reveal a reduced arterial $P_{O_2}$ in patients with primary pulmonary hypertension. Of course, if pulmonary hypertension is secondary to airway, parenchymal, or neuromuscular disease, characteristic abnormalities of volumes and mechanics and severe disturbances of gas exchange are evident.

Pulmonary hypertension is associated with certain functional disturbances. First, arterial $P_{CO_2}$ is chronically decreased, presumably from reflex ventilatory drive; which receptors are stimulated is unclear, but distortion of mechanoreceptors in dilated pulmonary arteries may be involved. Second, wasted ventilation, which may be normal during rest, increases during exercise because the effects of taking deep breaths overcome the compensatory redistribution of ventilation away from poorly perfused regions.[42] Increased wasted ventilation was once thought to be the pathophysiologic hallmark of pulmonary vascular occlusive diseases, but similar findings have been reported in other (nonvascular) pulmonary diseases.[43] Diffusing capacity is reduced in these patients, probably because pulmonary capillaries are involved in the pathologic process.

Late in the evolution of pulmonary hypertension from vascular obliteration, arterial hypoxia may worsen as right-to-left shunting of blood supervenes. In some patients, the shunt occurs through a patent foramen ovale, which opens as right ventricular end-diastolic and right atrial pressures increase. In other patients, the shunt pathway is less evident but might be present through preexisting arteriovenous communications or newly formed angiomatoid malformations.

### Differential Diagnosis

The differential diagnosis of pulmonary vascular occlusive diseases can be difficult and frustrating for both patient and physician. In view of the poor prognosis of this entire group of disorders when untreated, every effort must be made to identify a condition for which treatment is available. All patients need a careful history and physical examination, posteroanterior and lateral chest radiographs, and an electrocardiogram. The possibility of underlying heart disease can usually be dealt with by thorough echocardiography; at times, cardiac catheterization is needed. Other causes of precapillary pulmonary hypertension such as connective tissue disease (particularly scleroderma and lupus erythematosus) and cirrhosis of the liver are typically evident on the initial examination. Underlying human immunodeficiency virus infection may be a cause of pulmonary hypertension[44]; if it is not already diagnosed, serologic studies are necessary. In addition, pulmonary hypertension may be associated with ingestion of appetite suppressants (most recently documented with fenfluramine and dexfenfluramine[45]) and the patient must be questioned specifically about their use.

One of the most important differential considerations is chronic pulmonary thromboembolism, which is easily confused with primary pulmonary hypertension unless suitable diagnostic studies are obtained. Important information about the risk factors that predispose to recurrent venous thromboembolism, especially heritable abnormalities of the clotting system, has become available.[46, 47] Usually the distinction between chronic pulmonary thromboembolism and primary pulmonary hypertension can be made by a perfusion lung scintigram, but in patients being evaluated for surgical thromboendarterectomy, which may be lifesaving,[48] pulmonary angiography is required.

## ABNORMAL VASCULAR COMMUNICATIONS

All the blood that enters the pulmonary arterial circulation should flow through pulmonary capillaries before leaving the lungs in the pulmonary veins. Pulmonary artery–to–pulmonary vein, or *arteriovenous,* communications do not occur in normal lungs. Vascular communications between the bronchial and pulmonary circulations have been identified in normal lungs, especially those of infants, but these anastomoses are so uncommon that they have no functional significance.

Clinically important pulmonary arteriovenous malformations are well known but, in general, are rare. Those of pulmonary origin (see Table 50.1) usually represent congenital or hereditary abnormalities. Abnormal vascular communications may also be found in several acquired conditions: most commonly in cirrhosis of the liver[49] and less often in schistosomiasis,[50] mitral stenosis,[51] actinomycosis,[51] trauma,[51] Fanconi's syndrome,[52] and malignancies.[53] A truly remarkable occurrence of acquired pulmonary arteriovenous malformations has been reported in infants with congenital heart disease after cavopulmonary anastomosis, a surgical procedure that prevents hepatic venous blood from flowing through the lungs; in several affected infants, redirection of hepatic flow to the pulmonary circulation has caused the malformations to disappear.[54] Vascular abnormalities involving the bronchial and other systemic arteries are also rare and may be either congenital or acquired.

## Pathophysiology

Abnormal vascular communications provide pathways for blood flow that either bypass the lung parenchyma, thus creating a right-to-left shunt that affects gas exchange, or connect the high-pressure systemic circulation with the low-pressure pulmonary circulation; usually, the latter types include a capillary bed and so are of little hemodynamic consequence, but in rare instances there may be a direct communication between the two circulations that is analogous to a peripheral arteriovenous fistula, thus creating a left-to-right shunt.

### Right-to-Left Shunts

A right-to-left shunt can be viewed as a pathway through which pulmonary arterial (mixed venous) blood is allowed to flow into the pulmonary venous circulation without having perfused *functioning* pulmonary capillaries and without having contributed to gas exchange. The concept of functioning is important, because most right-to-left shunts occur when blood flows through pulmonary capillaries that are normal but that supply nonventilated and thus functionless terminal respiratory units; this common type of shunt-induced hypoxia occurs when alveoli are closed (e.g., as a result of atelectasis) or when they are filled with liquid (e.g., as a result of pulmonary edema or with blood or pus).

In contrast to right-to-left shunts through normal vessels that are perfusing nonfunctioning regions of lung, pulmonary arteriovenous fistulas (Chapter 53) are abnormal vascular communications that bypass functioning lung. Obviously, however, the effect on gas exchange is exactly the same in both varieties. The admixture of poorly oxygenated blood from a right-to-left shunt with normally oxygenated blood from the remainder of the lungs decreases arterial $P_{O_2}$ and increases the alveolar-arterial $P_{O_2}$ difference. When flow through the shunt pathway or pathways is large, severe hypoxemia results. Pulmonary arteriovenous fistulas create a continuous right-to-left shunt, thereby causing unremitting hypoxemia with all of its pathophysiologic consequences: cyanosis, polycythemia, clubbing of the digits (but only rarely pulmonary hypertrophic osteoarthropathy), and a pathway for paradoxic embolism to systemic organs.[55]

### Left-to-Right Shunts

Most abnormal communications between the systemic arterial circulation, including the bronchial arteries, and the pulmonary circulation exist to perfuse the lungs themselves, such as in tetralogy of Fallot and other cyanotic congenital heart diseases, or because of a structural abnormality, such as a bronchopulmonary sequestration, neoplasm, tuberculosis, or bronchiectasis (see Fig. 50.3). In inflammatory disorders, the amount of bronchial blood flow may increase severalfold above normal.[56] But these abnormal pathways are not true left-to-right shunts because the vascular network includes arterioles that impose a vascular resistance between the high-pressure arterial inflow and low-pressure venous outflow and capillaries from which oxygen is extracted to sustain tissue metabolism. Bronchial blood flow is increased in patients with mitral stenosis[57] and probably contributes to the severe hemoptysis that may occur in this disorder.

When systemic arteries have direct access to a low-pressure system (in other words, when there is little or no interposed vascular resistance to cause a pressure drop), torrential blood flow results in a left-to-right shunt. Systemic arterial–pulmonary arterial or systemic arterial–pulmonary venous fistulas are extremely rare and usually result from some sort of penetrating traumatic injury to the chest wall and lungs[58] but may occur in inflammatory or neoplastic lesions. These communications create left-to-right shunts that may have adverse hemodynamic consequences, although high-output left ventricular failure is unusual.

## Clinical Findings

The symptoms, signs, radiographic features, and pulmonary function abnormalities associated with abnormal vascular communications vary considerably, from innocent to life-threatening. Manifestations depend on whether the aberrant channels are developmental or acquired, whether there are associated extrapulmonary disorders, and, most important, how much blood flows through the vascular pathway or pathways. Discriminating features are discussed in Chapter 53 and have been reviewed.[55]

### Symptoms and Signs

The symptoms of a large, or multiple, pulmonary arteriovenous fistula, the prototypical intrapulmonary right-to-left shunt, include dyspnea on exertion and chronic fatigue. The most serious complaint is probably hemoptysis, which is occasionally massive and life-threatening. Patients with multiple pulmonary and systemic arteriovenous malformations (hereditary hemorrhagic telangiectasia, or Rendu-Weber-Osler disease) often have a history of multiple bleeding episodes (hemoptysis, epistaxis, hematemesis, and melena). At times, presenting symptoms are related to paradoxic embolism, the most dangerous of which is a brain abscess.[59]

The peripheral signs of pulmonary arteriovenous fistula are indistinguishable from those of cyanotic congenital heart disease; they include cyanosis, plethora, and digital clubbing. In about half the patients, a continuous murmur can be heard over the chest wall near the intrapulmonary site of the fistula; typically, breathing maneuvers that increase systemic venous return (Müller's maneuver) or assuming the body position in which the fistula is gravitationally dependent augment the murmur, and conversely, decreasing venous return (Valsalva's maneuver) diminishes the intensity of the murmur. At times, the murmurs are audible only during systole and may even be absent. An important clue to the presence of pulmonary arteriovenous malformations is the finding of one or more peripheral telangiectases. These lesions are usually small (1 to 2 mm), red, and located under the fingernails, on the skin of the arms or trunk, or in the mucosa of the oropharynx.

### Radiographic Features

The abnormalities on routine chest radiographic examination in patients with one or more pulmonary arteriovenous malformations are likely to suggest the diagnosis, especially when viewed in conjunction with other clinical findings. One or more rounded densities of varying size can usually be seen in the peripheral lung fields. The vascular origin of the lesion is strongly suggested by the presence of incoming and outgoing blood vessels between the peripheral density and the hilum. Confirmation can be obtained with contrast-enhanced computed tomography (CT), three-dimensional helical CT, or magnetic resonance imaging, each of which is highly accurate. Nevertheless, pulmonary angiography remains the diagnostic gold standard (see Fig. 53.8), especially in patients being considered for resectional or obliterative therapy.[55]

### Pulmonary Function Abnormalities

Because most pulmonary arteriovenous malformations are small in relation to the total volume of the lungs, results of tests of vital capacity, total lung capacity, and maximal expiratory flow rates are likely to be normal unless coexisting lung disease is present. As might be expected, the most striking physiologic abnormalities are those of gas exchange. Of the various tests used to detect the presence and magnitude of right-to-left shunts, breathing 100% oxygen has been the most widely used. While patients with pulmonary arteriovenous malformations breathe 100% oxygen, the magnitude of the shunt typically increases when patients change from the supine to the erect position[60] and when breathing at a high lung volume, which enlarges the fistula.[61] Absolute diffusing capacity may be increased in the presence of polycythemia, but the observed value is usually normal when corrected for the patient's hemoglobin concentration. A decreased diffusing capacity suggests the possibility of coexisting diffuse pulmonary vascular disorder.[62]

## Differential Diagnosis

The differential diagnosis of pulmonary arteriovenous malformations is limited, and the workup is not difficult. The 100% oxygen breathing test is used first to document the presence and size of a right-to-left shunt; then, contrast echocardiography is performed to localize the shunt to either the heart or the lungs; saline with dissolved bubbles is a useful medium. Finally, an imaging study, especially pulmonary angiography, is conducted to establish the number and location of the lesions. Patients with cirrhosis of the liver occasionally have right-to-left shunts through abnormal pathways within the lungs.[49] Patients with this syndrome, like those with typical pulmonary arteriovenous fistulas, have cyanosis, clubbing, and polycythemia, unless there is coexisting bleeding from another source. The abnormal vascular communications have been demonstrated by casts made of postmortem lung specimens,[63] but they may be surprisingly difficult to demonstrate during life. Even the 100% oxygen breathing test may fail to document right-to-left shunting of blood, presumably because the arteriovenous communications involve many tiny blood vessels that are situated close to gas exchange units; thus, when 100% oxygen is breathed, oxygen can diffuse from the alveoli into the abnormal channels, thereby disguising their presence. The presence of right-to-left shunts in patients with cirrhosis can be demonstrated by intravenous injection of radiolabeled aggregates ($<50$ μm in diameter) of albumin or microspheres.[64] Ordinarily, all of the material is trapped in the lungs as it flows through the pulmonary circulation. In patients with cirrhosis and right-to-left shunts, the particles flow through the abnormal communications and can be identified as radioactivity deposited in systemic organs. This technique has largely been replaced by echocardiography during the injection of bubble-containing saline. (Further information about the pulmonary complications of chronic liver disease is presented in Chapter 85.)

### Systemic-Pulmonary Communications

Although pulmonary arteriovenous fistulas are uncommon, by 1963 they were well described and nearly 300 cases had been reported.[65] In contrast, fistulas between a systemic artery and a pulmonary artery or vein are so much rarer that in 1972, only 28 cases could be found in the world's literature.[66] The systemic vessel that penetrates the lung usually arises from the internal mammary artery, intercostal arteries, or an anomalous branch of the aorta; multiple fistulas between the coronary and pulmonary arteries have been reported.[67] Systemic-pulmonary vessel communications can be congenital, neoplastic, or traumatic in origin. Two cases have occurred as a complication of closed-tube thoracostomy.[58, 68] Probably the most common cause of an abnormality with a characteristic systemic-pulmonary vascular communication is *sequestration of the lung,* which is discussed fully in Chapter 53.

Most patients with systemic-pulmonary shunts are

asymptomatic, but massive hemoptysis can occur.[69] The communications are suggested by the presence of a continuous murmur heard on physical examination[66] or by radiographic abnormalities such as notching of the ribs, increased caliber of pulmonary vessels, pleural thickening, and cardiomegaly.[58] The diagnosis can be established by selective angiography of the relevant systemic vessel. Despite much uncertainty about the natural history of these vascular communications, surgery is frequently performed as definitive therapy.

The rare combination of *platypnea* (dyspnea induced by the upright position and relieved by recumbency) and *orthodeoxia* (arterial hypoxia accentuated by the upright position and improved during recumbency) has been observed in patients with intrapulmonary arteriovenous fistulas.[60] Similar abnormalities have been reported after pneumonectomy and pulmonary embolism and are associated with chronic lung disease.[70] In affected patients, dyspnea and desaturation in the upright position are usually related to substantial right-to-left shunting of blood through a patent foramen ovale. Careful studies of patients with platypnea and orthodeoxia after lung resection have demonstrated intra-atrial shunting, but the mechanism by which positional changes affect shunt flow is under speculation.[71] The diagnosis can be established by tilt-table two-dimensional echocardiography with peripheral venous contrast medium.[70] The presence of platypnea and orthodeoxia, especially after lung resection, warrants thorough investigation, because closure of the defect is curative.[72]

## PULMONARY EDEMA

One of the major advances since the 1960s has been the acquisition of important new knowledge concerning the physiology of liquid and solute exchange in normal and diseased lungs. This information has permitted better understanding and identification of various pathologic conditions in which pulmonary edema may develop. Pulmonary edema is not a disease, but rather a complication of some other abnormality, which may have its origin within the lungs or, more commonly, arises in extrapulmonary organs, particularly the heart (see Table 50.1).

### Pathophysiology

Pulmonary edema can be defined as a pathologic state in which there is abnormal accumulation of extravascular liquid in the lungs. The word *pathologic* is important for differentiating abnormal accumulation of liquid from the normal filling of the lungs with liquid that occurs during fetal development. This definition is not entirely satisfactory, however, because taken literally, it would include pneumonia, intrapulmonary hemorrhage, and other conditions in which various types of liquid accumulate in the lungs. The kind of pulmonary edema discussed here occurs when liquid is filtered into the lungs faster than it can be removed. Further information about the clinical features, diagnosis, and treatment of pulmonary edema is provided in Chapter 54, and a detailed discussion of normal liquid and solute exchange in healthy persons and of the pathophysiology of pulmonary edema is available in Chapter 6.

#### Normal Liquid and Solute Exchange

The factors that determine the rate of liquid and solute exchange across semipermeable membranes in the body were defined by Starling[73] more than 100 years ago and are included in the famous equation that bears his name:

$$Jv = LpS[(Pc - Pi) - \sigma d(\pi c - \pi i)] \qquad (2)$$

where Jv is the net transcapillary filtration rate, Lp is the hydraulic conductivity of the membrane (or "barrier" to fluid filtration), S is the surface area, Pc is the pulmonary capillary hydrostatic pressure, Pi is the interstitial hydrostatic pressure, $\pi c$ is the capillary plasma colloid osmotic (or oncotic) pressure, $\pi i$ is the interstitial fluid oncotic pressure, and $\sigma d$ is the osmotic reflection coefficient of the vessel wall ($\sigma d = 0$ if the membrane is freely permeable and $\sigma d = 1$ if the membrane "rejects" the molecule). The difference between intravascular and extravascular pressures is often referred to as the *transmural* or *transvascular pressure.* Collectively, the transmural hydrostatic and protein osmotic pressures are called the *Starling forces.* Normal values for intravascular pressures within the pulmonary circulation, for other variables in the Starling equation, and for the percentage of the total filtrate from the various segments of the microcirculation are shown in Table 50.4.[74] The derivation of these values in healthy persons, how they change in various disease states, and the protective roles of the several "safety factors" (see Table 54.1) are discussed in detail in Chapters 6 and 54.

#### Types of Pulmonary Edema

There are two fundamentally different pathophysiologic causes of pulmonary edema: an increase in net transmural filtration pressure from an imbalance of Starling forces, which leads to *increased pressure pulmonary edema* (sometimes called "hydrostatic" edema), and an increase in hydraulic conductivity and a decrease in reflection coefficient, which lead to *increased permeability pulmonary edema.* The physiologic basis for pulmonary edema formation has been the subject of several comprehensive reviews.[4, 74, 75]

**Increased Pressure Edema.** According to the Starling equation, an increase in the net transmural filtration pressure acting across the capillary endothelium could occur by appropriate directional changes in any or all of the four Starling forces: an increase in intravascular hydrostatic pressure, a decrease in perivascular (interstitial) hydrostatic pressure, a decrease in intravascular osmotic pressure, or an increase in perivascular osmotic pressure. The most common form of pulmonary edema clinically encountered occurs in patients with heart failure and is often called *cardiogenic edema;* when either left ventricular end-diastolic filling pressure increases (e.g., as in aortic valve disease, hypertensive or coronary arterial heart disease, and myocardiopathies) or left atrial

**Table 50.4** MEAN VALUES OF HYDROSTATIC PRESSURES (P), COLLOID OSMOTIC PRESSURES (π), AND REFLECTION COEFFICIENTS (σ) IN THE PULMONARY CIRCULATION AND IN THE PERIMICROVASCULAR INTERSTITIAL SPACE AND THE CONTRIBUTIONS OF ARTERIOLES, CAPILLARIES, AND VENULES TO OVERALL FILTRATION

| | Pulmonary Artery | Arterioles | Capillaries | Venules | Pulmonary Veins |
|---|---|---|---|---|---|
| Intravascular (mm Hg) | | | | | |
| P | 14.0 | 11.0 | 9.0 | 7.0 | 5.0 |
| π | 24.3 | 24.3 | 24.3 | 24.3 | 24.3 |
| Endothelium (mm Hg) | | | | | |
| σ | — | 0.9 | 0.85 | 0.8 | — |
| Interstitial (mm Hg) | | | | | |
| P | — | −5.0 | −2.0 | −5.0 | — |
| π | — | 10.0 | 14.6 | 15.6 | — |
| Percentage of total (%) filtrate | — | 7 | 66 | 27 | — |

Modified with permission from Staub NC: Pathophysiology of pulmonary edema. *In* Staub NC, Taylor AE (eds): Edema. New York: Raven Press, 1984, pp 719–746.

pressure increases (e.g., as in mitral valve disease and left atrial myxoma), intracapillary hydrostatic pressure in the lungs must also increase at least as much. When intravascular hydrostatic pressure rises sufficiently, the fluid that leaks becomes a low-protein ultrafiltrate of plasma; this liquid dilutes or washes out the proteins already present in the interstitial space, thereby decreasing the interstitial protein osmotic pressure and increasing the net transmural osmotic pressure. For every 2–mm Hg increase in intravascular hydrostatic pressure, there is approximately a 1–mm Hg decrease in interstitial protein osmotic pressure,[76] which nullifies 50% of the initial increase in hydrostatic pressure.

In patients with cardiogenic pulmonary edema, the changes in perivascular interstitial hydrostatic pressure are negligible because so little liquid accumulates in what is probably a high-compliance space. When surface tension at the alveolar air-liquid interface increases, however, interstitial pressure becomes more negative than usual, and this increases the transmural hydrostatic pressure, favoring fluid filtration. In experimental models, increased surface tension by itself causes pulmonary edema,[77] and in clinical disorders such as the acute (formerly adult) respiratory distress syndrome (ARDS)[78] or *Pneumocystis carinii* pneumonia,[79] in which surfactant dysfunction is well documented, increased surface tension must aggravate the forces that tend to cause pulmonary edema.

**Increased Permeability Pulmonary Edema.** This type of pulmonary edema is encountered clinically in the many forms of acute lung injury that are collectively lumped together under the generic term ARDS.[80] In an effort to further discriminate among the many types of acute lung injury, Murray and coworkers[80] added the terms "direct" and "indirect," to indicate whether the injury arose directly within the lungs themselves (e.g., as in pneumonia, acid aspiration, contusion) or whether the insult arose outside the lungs and they were injured indirectly (e.g., as in sepsis syndrome, pancreatitis, hemorrhagic shock). It was postulated that because there were unquestioned differences in etiology between these two broad categories of lung injury, they should be kept separate in clinical studies of mechanism, prognosis, and especially treatment. The same direct-indirect distinction was later incorporated into the American-European consensus conference definition of ARDS.[81] Subsequent reports concerning the physiologic consequences[82] and outcome[83] in patients with ARDS have substantiated the importance of differentiating rather than collectively categorizing the causes of acute lung injury.

The syndrome occurs most often in patients hospitalized for a serious medical or surgical problem that does not involve the lungs initially, especially sepsis and multiple traumatic injuries. The syndrome also develops in patients after the inhalation of smoke or corrosive chemicals or after aspiration of gastric contents; if patients are seen early, their lungs, although injured, may not yet show the full extent of damage. After a brief period in which manifestations of pulmonary parenchymal injury may be minimal or even absent, progressive physiologic abnormalities develop: arterial hypoxia from right-to-left shunting of blood and decreased lung compliance. Chest roentgenograms reveal extensive diffuse consolidation of air spaces without enlargement of the heart. Pathologic findings in the acute stage are marked hemorrhagic pulmonary edema and, often, hyaline membranes. Further information about the pathogenesis of direct and indirect parenchymal injury and ARDS is available in Chapter 54 and in reviews published during the 1990s.[84–86]

## Clinical Findings

The clinical findings in patients with pulmonary edema vary considerably, depending on the severity of the condition and its origin.

**Symptoms and Signs.** Patients with pulmonary edema nearly always complain of dyspnea. The only likely exception to this occurs when the patient is unable to give a history because of alterations in mental status due to drugs or causes of central nervous system depression. Even in these instances, although the patient may not complain of respiratory distress, it is evident on physical examination. Patients with cardiogenic pulmonary edema usually have recognizable symptoms of heart disease: a history of previous cardiac distress, recurrent pain of myocardial ischemia, exertional dyspnea, orthopnea, and paroxysmal nocturnal dyspnea. Patients with pulmonary edema from increased permeability are likely to have symptoms related both to the cause of the acute lung injury, when indirect, and to the pulmonary involvement. It is of interest that sepsis, one of the most common causes of ARDS, is often heralded by unexplained hyperventilation.[87]

Abnormal physical findings, especially crackles, are nearly always present on auscultation of the lungs of patients with pulmonary edema. In early cardiogenic edema, crackles are confined to the lung bases; when edema is generalized, so are the crackles. In patients with severe edema, particularly that caused by increased permeability, which often has a peripheral distribution, the lungs may appear consolidated, with dullness to percussion and increased transmission of breath sounds. Because the hydrostatic forces that cause or contribute to pulmonary edema are influenced by gravity, the physical findings associated with edema are apt to be most marked in the dependent regions of the lungs. Many patients with pulmonary edema from left-sided heart failure also have a detectable pleural effusion in one or both pleural cavities. When present, pleural effusion exaggerates the dullness to percussion and obscures the crackles and increased transmission of breath sounds over the dependent portions of the lungs. Coexisting signs of extrapulmonary involvement (e.g., heart failure, renal failure, and sepsis) are usually present and provide important clues to the origin of the pulmonary edema.

**Radiographic Features.** Because the symptoms and signs of pulmonary edema are hopelessly nonspecific, when present they serve as an indication for prompt roentgenographic examination of the chest to aid in the differential diagnosis. The chest radiograph is widely available, relatively inexpensive, and noninvasive. It is the best available means of determining the presence, assessing the severity, and monitoring the course of pulmonary edema. Obviously, the value of a particular chest roentgenogram depends on the quality of the product. This is often less than desirable, especially films taken in critical care units, because body position and depth of inspiration are often uncontrollable, and several important technical factors may vary from one examination to the next.

Using an indicator-dilution method developed and described by Pistolesi and Giuntini,[88] Pistolesi and associates[89] compared the measured values of extravascular lung water to a rigorous scoring system for evaluating chest roentgenograms of patients with heart disease. They found that the chest roentgenograms showed evidence of interstitial pulmonary edema when values of the indicator-dilution method were within normal limits. This means that the chest radiograph is the more sensitive method for detecting early pulmonary edema.

Subsequently, Milne and colleagues[90] developed a system for differentiating among the chest radiographic abnormalities caused by pulmonary edema associated with heart failure, renal failure-overhydration, and increased permeability. The roentgenographic features that they found discriminating are listed in Table 50.5. It is not entirely clear why they found such consistent differences between cardiogenic and renal failure pulmonary edema, both of which are caused by an increase in Starling forces; the effect of lung volume on the distribution of edema in the two conditions may be partly responsible.[91] In a later study, Milne and colleagues' criteria did not hold up well when applied to ordinary films taken under routine conditions in critical care units,[92] which led to controversy concerning whether it is possible to differentiate cardiogenic pulmonary edema from increased permeability pulmonary edema, especially in supine, mechanically ventilated patients in the intensive care unit. The consensus remains that making the distinction is difficult but, according to one publication, may be facilitated by using two readily assessed radiologic signs: the cardiothoracic ratio and the vascular pedicle width.[93]

**Pulmonary Function Abnormalities.** The continuum of pulmonary function abnormalities that result from pro-

**Table 50.5** RADIOGRAPHIC FEATURES OF INCREASED PRESSURE (CARDIAC), OVERHYDRATION (RENAL), AND INCREASED PERMEABILITY (INJURY) PULMONARY EDEMA*

| Feature | Cardiac | Renal | Injury |
|---|---|---|---|
| Heart size | Enlarged | Enlarged | Not enlarged |
| Vascular pedicle | Normal or enlarged | Enlarged | Normal or reduced |
| Pulmonary blood flow distribution | Inverted | Balanced | Normal or balanced |
| Pulmonary blood volume | Normal or increased | Increased | Normal |
| Septal lines | Not common | Not common | Absent |
| Peribronchial cuffs | Very common | Very common | Not common |
| Air bronchogram | Not common | Not common | Very common |
| Lung edema, regional distribution (horizontal axis) | Even | Central | Peripheral |
| Pleural effusions | Very common | Very common | Not common |

*Each factor listed has been shown to have statistical significance in determining which type of edema is present.

Reproduced with permission from Milne ENC, Pistolesi M, Miniati M, et al: The radiologic distinction of cardiogenic and noncardiogenic pulmonary edema. AJR Am J Roentgenol 144:879–894, 1985.

gressively worsening increased-pressure pulmonary edema has been thoroughly studied and well described (see Table 54.4). Less is known about the spectrum of abnormalities in increased-permeability pulmonary edema, particularly as it changes in degree from mild to severe and in structure from acute (edematous) to chronic (proliferative-fibrotic). The results of a comparison study of increased-pressure and increased-permeability pulmonary edemas on gas exchange and lung mechanics in sheep, at comparable amounts of edema, showed similar changes in the alveolar-arterial $Po_2$ difference and dynamic compliance; resistance to airflow, however, increased significantly when hydrostatic pressure was increased but did not change when permeability was increased.[94] These results suggest that other influences, perhaps mediated by reflexes, the presence of vascular engorgement, or the location and quantity of peribronchial edema, affect airway function in increased-pressure pulmonary edema.

Gattinoni and colleagues[82] described the abnormalities of lung and chest wall distensibilities that characterize direct and indirect types of ARDS. In patients with direct lung injury (chiefly bacterial pneumonia) and indirect lung injury (associated with, e.g., multiple trauma or peritonitis), overall distensibility, which was measured as respiratory system elastance, was similarly increased in the absence of end-expiratory pressure. (Because elastance is the reciprocal of compliance, this means that lung plus chest wall compliance was also decreased.) However, the mechanisms differed strikingly in the two groups: in the directly injured patients, lung elastance was increased, whereas chest wall elastance was normal; in the indirectly injured patients, the main abnormality was a marked increase in chest wall elastance. Moreover, as positive end-expiratory pressure was added in increments, total (respiratory system) elastance increased in the direct ARDS patients but decreased in the indirect ARDS patients; these findings are consistent with the belief that the prevailing abnormality in direct ARDS is consolidation, as opposed to interstitial and alveolar edema and alveolar collapse in indirect ARDS. Gattinoni and colleagues suggested that clinical management can be improved by taking into account the mechanical differences between pulmonary and extrapulmonary ARDS,[82] which underscores, again, the value of differentiating, not collectively categorizing, the causes of acute lung injury.

## Differential Diagnosis

There are two diagnostic steps to be taken in dealing with suspected pulmonary edema. The first step is to determine whether edema is indeed present, and the second is to establish the cause of the abnormality.

Usually, a chest radiograph suffices not only to document whether edema is present but also to provide some hints about its origin. At times, the roentgenographic findings are not diagnostic; this usually occurs when the distribution of densities is strikingly asymmetric or in the presence of coexisting lung diseases such as diffuse infiltrative disorders or emphysema. The availability of a previous radiograph is of great value in these circumstances. Coexisting bronchopneumonia, which may complicate underlying pulmonary edema or vice versa, is virtually impossible to rule in or out by chest x-ray examination. A variety of techniques have been used to assess the amount of edema present in the lungs[94]; suffice it to say here that, at least at present, no test other than the chest roentgenogram is suitable for routine clinical use.

Distinction between increased pressure and increased permeability pulmonary edemas can often be made on the basis of coexisting abnormalities. Heart disease is usually obvious in patients with cardiogenic pulmonary edema. The sudden onset of pulmonary edema in a patient with a severe medical or surgical disorder, such as the sepsis syndrome or multiple traumatic injuries, is likely to occur from increased permeability. The inclusion of widespread pneumonia from *P. carinii,* influenza virus, and other infectious agents within the ARDS family means that infectious diseases must always be considered and looked for. The value of measurements of pulmonary wedge pressure with a flotation catheter is debatable. In theory, the pressure should be high in cardiogenic or overhydration edema and normal in increased permeability pulmonary edema, but there are important exceptions to this in practice, and there are a number of potential pitfalls in the measurement and interpretation of pulmonary capillary pressure, which have been carefully reviewed.[95] Pulmonary artery catheterization has an appreciable incidence of complications,[96] and it is doubtful whether the measurements improve clinical outcome. More and more experts are questioning the value of the procedure, but favorable reports continue to appear.[97, 97a]

When florid pulmonary edema is present and it is possible to obtain a sample of the liquid through an endotracheal tube, differentiation between increased pressure and increased permeability types of edema can be made by measuring the protein (or albumin) concentration of the edema fluid and also of a simultaneously obtained specimen of plasma.[98] In increased-pressure pulmonary edema, the ratio of the protein concentration in the edema fluid to that in the plasma is less than 0.6, and in increased permeability pulmonary edema, the ratio is greater than 0.8. Intermediate values are occasionally observed and presumably are caused by reabsorption of alveolar fluid and concentration of protein, which in patients with ARDS implies an intact epithelium and is a favorable prognostic sign.[99] In certain disorders (near drowning), the edema fluid-plasma ratio is unusually low and is diagnostically and prognostically useful.[100]

## SUMMARY

This chapter has briefly reviewed the normal anatomy and physiology of the pulmonary circulation. Overviews of pulmonary vascular occlusive diseases, abnormal vascular communications in the lungs, and pulmonary edema emphasize the pathophysiology, clinical findings, and differential diagnosis of each of these groups of disorders. Detailed information about the principal disorders of the pulmonary circulation is available in the next five chapters: Chapter 51, "Pulmonary Thromboembolism"; Chapter 52, "Pulmonary Vasculitis and Primary Pulmonary Hypertension"; Chapter 53, "Pulmonary Arteriovenous Malformations and Other Pulmonary Vascular Abnormalities"; Chapter 54, "Pulmonary Edema and Acute Lung Injury"; and Chapter 55, "Cor Pulmonale."

## References


1. Harris P, Heath D: The Human Pulmonary Circulation. Its Form and Function in Health and Disease (3rd ed). Edinburgh, Churchill Livingston, 1986, pp 1–11.
2. Cory RAS, Valentine EJ: Varying patterns of the lobar branches of the pulmonary artery. A study of 524 lungs seen at operation on 426 patients. Thorax 14:267–280, 1959.
3. Mead J, Whittenberger JL: Lung inflation and hemodynamics. *In* Fenn WO, Rahn H (eds): Handbook of Physiology. Section 3: Respiration. Vol. 1. Washington, DC: American Physiological Society, 1964, pp 477–486.
4. Staub NC: Pulmonary edema. Physiol Rev 54:678–811, 1974.
5. Weibel ER: The Pathway for Oxygen. Structure and Function of the Mammalian Respiratory System. Cambridge, MA: Harvard University Press, 1984, pp 339–377.
6. Murray JF: The Normal Lung. The Basis of Diagnosis and Treatment of Pulmonary Disease (2nd ed). Philadelphia: WB Saunders, 1986, pp 23–59.
7. Weibel ER: Morphological basis of alveolar-capillary gas exchange. Physiol Rev 53:419–495, 1973.
8. Lauweryns JM: The blood and lymphatic microcirculation of the lung. *In* Sommers SC (ed): Pathology Annual 1971. New York: Appleton-Century-Crofts, 1971, pp 365–415.
9. Butler J (ed): The Bronchial Circulation. New York: Marcel Dekker, 1992, pp 45–100, 181–198.
10. Heinemann HO, Fishman AP: Nonrespiratory functions of mammalian lung. Physiol Rev 49:1–47, 1969.
11. Jenkinson SG (ed): Metabolic functions of the lungs. Clin Chest Med 10:1–128, 1989.
12. Hoffman JIE, Guz A, Charlier AA, et al: Stroke volume in conscious dogs: Effect of respiration, posture, and vascular occlusion. J Appl Physiol 20:865–877, 1965.
13. Bland RD: Dynamics of pulmonary water before and after birth. Acta Paediatr Scand Suppl 305:12–20, 1983.
14. McLaughlin RF Jr: Bronchial artery distribution in various mammals and in humans. Am Rev Respir Dis 128(Suppl):S557–S558, 1983.
15. McFadden ER Jr: Heat and water exchange in human airways. Am Rev Respir Dis 146(Suppl):S8–S10, 1992.
16. Auld PA, Rudolph AM, Golinko RJ: Factors affecting bronchial collateral flow in the dog. Am J Physiol 198:1166–1170, 1960.
17. Dock W: Apical localization of phthisis: Its significance in treatment by prolonged rest in bed. Am Rev Tuberc 53:297–305, 1946.
18. West JB, Dollery CT, Naimark A: Distribution of blood flow in isolated lung: Relation to vascular and alveolar pressures. J Appl Physiol 19:713–724, 1964.
19. Bhattacharya J, Staub NC: Direct measurements of microvascular pressures in the isolated perfused dog lung. Science 210:327–328, 1980.
20. Overholser KA, Bhattacharya J, Staub NC: Microvascular pressure in the isolated, perfused dog lung: Comparison between theory and measurement. Microvasc Res 23:67–76, 1982.
21. Reeves JT, Rubin LJ: The pulmonary circulation. Snapshots of progress. Am J Respir Crit Care Med 157:S101–S108, 1998.
22. Gaine SP, Hales MA, Flavahan NA: Hypoxic pulmonary endothelial cells release a diffusible contractile factor distinct from endothelin. Am J Physiol 274:L657–L664, 1998.
23. Garrett RC, Thomas HM III: Meclofenamate uniformly decreases shunt fraction in dogs with lobar atelectasis. J Appl Physiol 54:284–289, 1983.
24. Frostell CG, Blomqvist H, Hedenstierna G, et al: Inhaled nitric oxide selectively reverses human hypoxic pulmonary vasoconstriction without causing systemic vasodilation. Anesthesiology 78:427–435, 1993.
25. Barman SA: Potassium channels modulate hypoxic pulmonary vasocontriction. Am J Physiol 275:L64–L70, 1998.
26. Wood P: Pulmonary hypertension. Br Med Bull 8:348–353, 1952.
27. Hyman AL, Nandiwada P, Knight DS, et al: Pulmonary vasodilator responses to catecholamines and sympathetic nerve stimulation in the cat. Evidence that vascular b-2 adrenoreceptors are innervated. Circ Res 48:407–415, 1981.
28. Hyman AL, Kadowitz PJ: Evidence for existence of postjunctional $\alpha_1$- and $\alpha_2$-adrenoceptors in cat pulmonary vascular bed. Am J Physiol 249:H891–H898, 1985.
29. Loscalzo J: Endothelial dysfunction in pulmonary hypertension (editorial). N Engl J Med 327:117–119, 1992.
30. Wood P: Pulmonary hypertension with special reference to the vasoconstrictive factor. Br Heart J 20:557–570, 1958.
31. Michael JR, Markewitz BA: Endothelins and the lung. Am J Respir Crit Care Med 154:555–575, 1996.
32. Giaid A: Nitric oxide and endothelin-1 in pulmonary hypertension. Chest 114:208S–212S, 1998.
33. Giaid A, Saleh D: Reduced expression of endothelial nitric oxide synthase in the lungs of patients with pulmonary hypertension. N Engl J Med 333:214–221, 1995.
34. Kaneko FT, Arroliga AC, Dweik RA, et al: Biochemical reaction products of nitric acid as quantitative markers of primary pulmonary hypertension. Am J Respir Crit Care Med 158:917–923, 1998.
35. Barst RJ, Loyd JE: Genetics and immunogenetic aspects of primary pulmonary hypertension. Chest 114:231S–236S, 1998.
36. Rudolph AM, Yuan S: Response of the pulmonary vasculature to hypoxia and $H^+$ ion concentration changes. J Clin Invest 45:399–411, 1966.
37. Heath D, Edwards JE: The pathology of hypertensive pulmonary vascular disease: A description of six grades of structural changes in the pulmonary arteries with special reference to congenital cardiac septal defects. Circulation 18:533–547, 1958.
38. Rubin LJ: Primary pulmonary hypertension. N Engl J Med 336:111–117, 1997.
39. Stenmark KR, Mecham RP: Cellular and molecular mechanisms of pulmonary vascular remodeling. Annu Rev Physiol 59:89–144, 1997.
40. Macnee W: Pathophysiology of cor pulmonale in chronic obstructive pulmonary disease. Am J Respir Crit Care Med 150:833–852, 1158–1168, 1994.
41. Voelkel N, Reeves JT: Primary pulmonary hypertension. *In* Moser KM (ed): Pulmonary Vascular Diseases. New York: Marcel Dekker, 1979, pp 573–628.
42. Nadel JA, Gold WM, Burgess TH: Early diagnosis of chronic pulmonary vascular obstruction. Value of pulmonary function tests. Am J Med 44:16–25, 1968.
43. Mohsenifar Z, Brown HW, Koerner SK: Abnormal wasted ventilation fraction and normal pulmonary hemodynamics during exercise in patients with exertional dyspnea. Respiration 43:263–270, 1982.
44. Petitpretz P, Brenot F, Azarian R, et al: Pulmonary hypertension in patients with human immunodeficiency virus infection: Comparison with primary pulmonary hypertension. Circulation 89:2722–2726, 1994.
45. Simonneau G, Fartoukh M, Sitbon O, et al: Primary pulmonary hypertension associated with the use of fenfluramine derivatives. Chest 114:195S–199S, 1998.
46. Murin S, Marelich P, Arroliga AC, et al: Hereditary thrombophilia and venous thromboembolism. Am J Respir Crit Care Med 158:1369–1373, 1998.
47. Hyers TM: Venous thromboembolism. Am J Respir Crit Care Med 159:1–14, 1999.
48. Archibald CJ, Auger WR, Fedullo PF, et al: Long-term outcome after pulmonary thromboendarterectomy. Am J Respir Crit Care Med 160:523–528, 1999.
49. Rodriguez-Roisin R, Roca J: Hepatopulmonary syndrome: The paradigm of liver-induced hypoxaemia. Baillière's Clin Gastroenterol 11:387–406, 1997.
50. Bethlem EP, Schettino G de P, Carvalho CP: Pulmonary schistosomiasis. Curr Opin Pulm Med 3:361–365, 1997.
51. Prager RL, Laws KH, Bender HW Jr: Arteriovenous fistula of the lung. Ann Thorac Surg 36:231–239, 1983.
52. Taxman RM, Halloran MJ, Parker BM: Multiple pulmonary arteriovenous malformations in association with Fanconi's syndrome. Chest 64:118–120, 1973.
53. Caron F, Novati JP, Langlois D, et al: Metastatic pulmonary choriocarcinoma and pulmonary arteriovenous aneurysm. Rev Mal Respir 12:165–166, 1995.

54. Srivastava D, Preminger T, Lock JE, et al: Hepatic venous blood and the development of pulmonary arteriovenous malformation in congenital heart disease. Circulation 92:1217–1222, 1995.
55. Gossage JR, Kanj G: Pulmonary arteriovenous malformations. A state of the art review. Am J Respir Crit Care Med 158:643–661, 1998.
56. Butler J: Clinical aspects of the bronchial circulation. *In* Butler J (ed): The Bronchial Circulation. New York: Marcel Dekker, 1992, pp 477–492.
57. Agostini P, Agrifoglio M, Arena V, et al: Systemic to pulmonary bronchial blood flow in mitral stenosis. Chest 99:642–645, 1991.
58. Fein AB, Godwin JD, Moore AV, et al: Systemic artery-to-pulmonary vascular shunt: A complication of closed-tube thoracostomy. AJR Am J Roentgenol 140:917–919, 1983.
59. Finkelstein R, Engel A, Simri W, et al: Brain abscess: The lung connection. J Intern Med 240:33–36, 1996.
60. Robin ED, Laman D, Horn BR, et al: Platypnea related to orthodeoxia caused by true vascular lung shunts. N Engl J Med 294:941–943, 1976.
61. Huseby JS, Culver BH, Butler J: Pulmonary arteriovenous fistulas: Increase in shunt at high lung volume. Am Rev Respir Dis 115:229–232, 1977.
62. Pennington DW, Gold WM, Gordon RL, et al: Treatment of pulmonary arteriovenous malformations by therapeutic embolization. Rest and exercise physiology in eight patients. Am Rev Respir Dis 145:1047–1051, 1992.
63. Rydell R, Hoffbauer FW: Multiple pulmonary arteriovenous fistulas in juvenile cirrhosis. Am J Med 21:450–460, 1956.
64. Bank ER, Thrall JH, Dantzker DR: Radionuclide demonstration of intrapulmonary shunting in cirrhosis. AJR Am J Roentgenol 140:967–969, 1983.
65. Hodgson CH, Kaye RL: Pulmonary arteriovenous fistula and hereditary hemorrhagic telangiectasis: A review and report of 35 cases of fistula. Dis Chest 43:449–455, 1963.
66. Brundage BH, Gomez AC, Cheitlin MD, et al: Systemic artery to pulmonary vessel fistulas. Report of two cases and review of the literature. Chest 62:19–23, 1972.
67. Van Dam DW, Noyez L, Skotnicki SH, et al: Multiple fistulas between coronary and pulmonary arteries. Eur J Cardiovasc Surg 9:707–708, 1995.
68. Cox PA, Keshishian JM, Blades BB: Traumatic arteriovenous fistula of the chest wall and lung secondary to insertion of an intercostal catheter. J Thorac Cardiovasc Surg 54:109–112, 1967.
69. Sharifi M, Messersmith R, Newman B, et al: Bronchial arteriovenous malformation in a child with hemoptysis. A case report. Angiology 47:203–209, 1996.
70. Seward JB, Hayes DL, Smith HC, et al: Platypnea-orthodeoxia: Clinical profile, diagnostic workup, management, and report of seven cases. Mayo Clin Proc 59:221–231, 1984.
71. Franco DP, Kinasewitz GT, Markham RV, et al: Postural hypoxemia in the postpneumonectomy patient. Am Rev Respir Dis 129:1021–1022, 1984.
72. Begin R: Platypnea after pneumonectomy. N Engl J Med 293:342–343, 1975.
73. Starling EH: On the absorption of fluids from the connective tissue spaces. J Physiol (Lond) 19:312–326, 1896.
74. Staub NC: Pathophysiology of pulmonary edema. *In* Staub NC, Taylor AE (eds): Edema. New York: Raven Press, 1984, pp 719–746.
75. Bhattacharya J: Physiological basis of pulmonary edema. *In* Matthay MA, Ingbar DH (eds): Pulmonary Edema. New York: Marcel Dekker, 1998, pp 1–36.
76. Erdmann AJ, Vaughan TR, Brigham KL, et al: Effect of increased vascular pressure on lung fluid balance in unanesthetized sheep. Circ Res 37:271–284, 1975.
77. Albert RK, Lakshminarayan S, Hildebrandt J, et al: Increased surface tension favors pulmonary edema formation in anesthetized dogs' lungs. J Clin Invest 63:1015–1018, 1979.
78. Gregory TJ, Longmore WJ, Moxley MA, et al: Surfactant chemical composition and biophysical activity in acute respiratory distress syndrome. J Clin Invest 88:1976–1981, 1991.
79. Hoffman AGD, Lawrence MG, Ognibene FP, et al: Reduction of pulmonary surfactant in patients with human immunodeficiency virus infection and *Pneumocystis carinii* pneumonia. Chest 102:1730–1736, 1992.
80. Murray JF, Matthay MA, Luce JM, et al: An expanded definition of the adult respiratory distress syndrome. Am Rev Respir Dis 138:720–723, 1988.
81. Bernard GR, Artigas A, Brigham KL, et al: The American-European consensus conference on ARDS. Definition, mechanisms, relevant outcomes, and clinical trial coordination. Am J Respir Crit Care Med 149:818–824, 1994.
82. Gattinoni L, Pelosi P, Suter PM, et al: Acute respiratory distress syndrome caused by pulmonary and extrapulmonary disease: Different syndromes? Am J Respir Crit Care Med 158:3–11, 1998.
83. Milberg JA, Davis DR, Steinberg KP, et al: Improved survival of patients with acute respiratory distress syndrome (ARDS): 1983–1993. JAMA 273:306–309, 1995.
84. Kollef MH, Schuster DP: The acute respiratory distress syndrome. N Engl J Med 332:27–37, 1995.
85. Sachdeva RC, Guntupalli KK: Acute respiratory distress syndrome. Crit Care Clin 13:503–521, 1997.
86. Luce JM: Acute lung injury and the acute respiratory distress syndrome. Crit Care Med 26:369–376, 1998.
87. Simmons DH, Nicoloff J, Guze LB: Hyperventilation and respiratory alkalosis as signs of gram-negative bacteremia. JAMA 174:2196–2199, 1960.
88. Pistolesi M, Giuntini C: Assessment of extravascular lung water. Radiol Clin North Am 6:551–574, 1978.
89. Pistolesi M, Miniati M, Milne ENC, et al: The chest roentgenogram in pulmonary edema. Clin Chest Med 6:315–344, 1985.
90. Milne ENC, Pistolesi M, Miniati M, et al: The radiologic distinction of cardiogenic and noncardiogenic pulmonary edema. AJR Am J Roentgenol 144:879–894, 1985.
91. Staub NC: Only the shadow knows (editorial). AJR Am J Roentgenol 144:1086–1087, 1985.
92. Aberle DR, Wiener-Kronish JP, Webb WR, et al: Hydrostatic versus increased permeability pulmonary edema: Diagnosis based on radiographic criteria in critically ill patients. Radiology 168:73–79, 1988.
93. Thomason JWW, Ely EW, Chiles C, et al: Appraising pulmonary edema using supine chest roentgenograms in ventilated patients. Am J Respir Crit Care Med 157:1600–1608, 1998.
94. Staub NC, Hyde RW, Crandall E: Workshop on techniques to evaluate alveolar-microvascular injury. Am Rev Respir Dis 141:1071–1077, 1990.
95. Cope DK, Grimbert F, Downey JM, et al: Pulmonary capillary pressure: A review. Crit Care Med 20:1043–1056, 1992.
96. Altschule MD: A new branch of medicine: Complications of vascular catheters. Chest 89:446, 1986.
97. Dalen JE, Bone RC: Is it time to pull the pulmonary artery catheter? JAMA 276:916–918, 1996.
97a. Marinelli WA, Weinert CR, Gross CR, et al: Right heart catheterization in acute lung injury. An observational study. Am J Respir Crit Care Med 159:69–76, 1999.
98. Fein A, Grossman RF, Jones JG, et al: The value of edema fluid protein measurement in patients with pulmonary edema. Am J Med 67:32–38, 1979.
99. Matthay MA, Wiener-Kronish JP: Intact epithelial barrier function is critical for the resolution of alveolar edema in humans. Am Rev Respir Dis 142:1250–1257, 1990.
100. Cohen DS, Matthay MA, Cogan MG, et al: Pulmonary edema associated with salt water near-drowning: New insights. Am Rev Respir Dis 146:794–796, 1992.

# 51 Pulmonary Thromboembolism*

PETER F. FEDULLO, M.D.

Introduction
Pathogenesis and Risk Factors
Natural History: Deep Vein Thrombosis
Natural History: Pulmonary Embolism
Clinical Presentation
Diagnosis of Venous Thrombosis
- Contrast Venography
- Duplex Ultrasonography
- Impedance Plethysmography
- Magnetic Resonance Imaging

Diagnosis of Pulmonary Embolism
- Standard Laboratory Evaluation
- Echocardiography
- Hemostaseologic Assays
- Ventilation-Perfusion Scanning
- Spiral (Helical) Computed Tomography
- Pulmonary Angiography

Diagnostic Approach
Prevention of Venous Thromboembolism
- Low-Dose Unfractionated Heparin
- Low-Molecular-Weight Heparin
- Pneumatic Compression Devices
- Sodium Warfarin

Management of Venous Thromboembolism
- Heparin
- Inferior Vena Cava Filters

Massive Pulmonary Embolism
- Thrombolytic Therapy
- Pulmonary Embolectomy

Postembolic Prophylaxis
Chronic Thromboembolic Pulmonary Hypertension
- Diagnosis
- Treatment

Other Forms of Embolism
- Schistosomiasis
- Air Embolism
- Fat Embolism
- Amniotic Fluid Embolism
- Septic Embolism
- Other Emboli

Summary

## INTRODUCTION

The one generalization about venous thromboembolism that is free from controversy is that many aspects of this disorder remain controversial. There are multiple reasons why venous thromboembolism, despite extensive clinical and laboratory investigation, continues to engender lively debate. Perhaps the major reason, notwithstanding the substantial advances that have been made since 1990, is that a number of fundamental questions continue to exist regarding the pathogenesis, clinical presentation, diagnosis, and therapy of the disease.

Venous thromboembolism represents a potentially fatal disease process with a clinical presentation that is often silent or nonspecific and for which a wide range of diagnostic techniques is available, many with technical and interpretive limitations.[1] The best available information suggests that at least five million episodes of venous thrombosis occur annually in the United States; that at least 10% of these episodes lead to a pulmonary embolism; and that at least 10% of those who have an embolic event—50,000—die each year.[2,3] Despite vigorous debate regarding optimal therapeutic intervention, the overwhelming majority of these deaths are not the result of therapeutic failure. Instead, most deaths from embolism are a result of prophylactic oversight or diagnostic error. Furthermore, the incidence of venous thromboembolism and of a fatal pulmonary embolism does not appear to be decreasing, a finding that probably reflects the demographics of an aging population, that modern medicine has placed an increased population at risk for the disease, and that preventive measures are not being applied to this population in an appropriate manner.[4–6] The persistence of such incidence figures commands attention, particularly because many instances of venous thromboembolism are preventable and for this reason are an important cause of medical malpractice litigation in the United States.[6a]

Contributing to the debate surrounding venous thromboembolism is the involvement of a wide range of medical disciplines in its prevention, diagnosis, and management. Thrombosis is not a discrete subspecialty. The

*In memory of Dr. Kenneth M. Moser, original author of this chapter: clinician, educator, and scientist whose friendship and guidance were a source of inspiration and whose contributions to the fields of pulmonary medicine and pulmonary vascular disease enriched and gave hope to many.

problem of venous thromboembolism involves pulmonologists, cardiologists, internists, specialists in vascular disease, radiologists, a range of surgical subspecialists, obstetricians, and others. Because specific prophylactic, diagnostic, and therapeutic strategies within one discipline may not necessarily be applicable to another, a perception of coherence in the clinical approach to this disease process often appears to be lacking.

Fortunately, during the past decade, many of the longstanding controversies surrounding the natural history, diagnosis, and therapy of venous thromboembolism have been partially or completely reconciled. The persistence of a number of unresolved issues, therefore, should not be a cause for clinical cynicism. In the approach to the patient with suspected venous thromboembolism, an understanding of what is unknown can prove invaluable to the decision-making process.

## PATHOGENESIS AND RISK FACTORS

The triad of venous stasis, alterations in coagulation, and vascular injury identified by Virchow in 1845 as primary factors in the pathogenesis of venous thromboembolism has been supported by a considerable amount of clinical and experimental evidence. Inherited and acquired abnormalities of the coagulation and fibrinolytic system, including isolated deficiencies of antithrombin III, protein C, protein S, and plasminogen, as well as the presence of a lupus anticoagulant, had been described as etiologic factors in a minority of patients with venous thromboembolism.[7]

More recently, novel pathogenetic mechanisms capable of shifting the hemostatic balance toward thrombosis have been described in specific populations with an inherited predisposition to venous thromboembolic events. The term *thrombophilia* was conceived to describe recurrent venous thromboembolism from inherited causes.

In 1993, Dahlbeck and coworkers described an inherited resistance to activated protein C.[8] The defect responsible for this resistance, designated factor V Leiden mutation, was localized to a single point mutation on the factor V gene (adenine for guanine), resulting in factor $V_a$ with diminished sensitivity to the natural anticoagulant effect of activated protein C. Although initially detected in as many as 60% of *selected* patients with venous thromboembolism, subsequent studies have detected the mutation in 10% to 20% of unselected patients.[9–11] Among women having a thromboembolic event during pregnancy or during the postpartum period, as many as 60% carry this mutation.[10] Activated protein C resistance also is found in about one third of patients who develop venous thromboembolism while taking oral contraceptives. Approximately 5% of whites in Europe and North America are heterozygous for this genetic defect, although this figure varies among ethnic groups. The heterozygous state carries a 5- to 10-fold increase in lifetime risk for venous thromboembolism; the risk for venous thromboembolism among patients homozygous for this mutation is increased 80-fold.[11]

More recently, a sequence variation in the prothrombin gene (20210G $\rightarrow$ A) has been described that is estimated to occur in 1% to 2% of the population. This mutation is associated with higher plasma prothrombin levels as well as a three- to fourfold increased risk of lower extremity venous thrombosis.[12] The G20210A mutation also appears to increase the risk of cerebral vein thrombosis by a factor of 10. For women who are both carriers of the G20210A mutation and current users of oral contraceptives, the risk of cerebral vein thrombosis far exceeds the sum of the separate risks associated with these two factors.[13]

Hyperhomocysteinemia has also been identified as a predisposition to venous thromboembolism. Elevation of plasma homocysteine levels may be the result of genetic abnormalities, nutritional deficiencies of vitamins ($B_6$, $B_{12}$, folate), or a combination of the two. A number of studies have strongly suggested that hyperhomocysteinemia may contribute independently to the pathogenesis of venous thrombosis and that it may act in a synergistic manner with other inherited predisposing factors.[14, 15]

The identification of these risk factors, and the likelihood that others exist, raises the possibility that screening to determine relative thromboembolic risk may be feasible in the future. However, such an approach does not exist at the present time. Despite its high prevalence, screening for factor V Leiden mutation is not advised because most patients with this abnormality will never experience a thromboembolic event. Furthermore, the absence of this abnormality should not influence the decision to provide prophylaxis to patients at clinical risk. Currently, 70% to 80% of all patients with venous thromboembolism do not have an identifiable thrombophilic tendency. Thus, in most patients, even those with an identified thrombophilic state, some clinical state associated with venous stasis or intimal injury, or both, serves as the basis for the thromboembolic event.[16, 17] Along with these inherited thrombophilias, the medical and surgical risk factors associated with an increased likelihood of thromboembolism have been clearly identified (Table 51.1).

These risk factors should be regarded as cumulative, not independent. Thromboembolic risk in an otherwise healthy 45-year-old individual undergoing an elective cholecystectomy is considerably less than the risk experienced by an obese, 65-year-old with a history of venous thromboembolism undergoing the same procedure. Similarly, the patient with hip fracture or hip replacement has, by virtue of that condition alone, a 60% to 70% risk of deep venous thrombosis and a 2% to 4% risk of experiencing a fatal thromboembolic event. Add other risk factors, and the incidence of deep venous thrombosis, and the likelihood of a fatal complication, are even higher. These considerations allow for the development of a reasonable "risk profile" in an individual patient, a profile that should influence the intensity of prophylactic intervention.

## NATURAL HISTORY: DEEP VEIN THROMBOSIS

Extensive autopsy and clinical studies have established that some 90% of pulmonary emboli that achieve clinical

**Table 51.1 THROMBOEMBOLIC RISK FACTORS**

| |
|---|
| **Hereditary Thrombophilias** |
| Protein C deficiency |
| Protein S deficiency |
| Antithrombin III deficiency |
| Factor V Leiden mutation |
| Prothrombin 20210 G/A variation |
| Hyperhomocysteinemia |
| Dysfibrinogenemia |
| Familial plasminogen deficiency |
| **Acquired Surgical Predispositions** |
| Major thoracic, abdominal or neurosurgical procedures requiring general anesthesia and lasting > 30 minutes |
| Hip arthroplasty |
| Knee arthroplasty |
| Knee arthroscopy |
| Hip fracture |
| Major trauma |
| Open prostatectomy |
| Spinal cord injury |
| **Acquired Medical Predispositions** |
| Prior venous thromboembolism |
| Advanced age (particularly > 60 years) |
| Malignancy |
| Congestive heart failure |
| Cerebrovascular accident |
| Nephrotic syndrome |
| Estrogen therapy |
| Pregnancy and the postpartum period |
| Obesity |
| Prolonged immobilization |
| Antiphospholipid antibody syndrome |
| Lupus anticoagulant |
| Inflammatory bowel disease |
| Paroxysmal nocturnal hemoglobinuria |
| Behçet's syndrome |

attention arise from venous thrombosis in the deep veins of the lower extremities.[18] Venous thrombi capable of embolization can arise from other sites. Primary iliac or proximal femoral thrombi may develop in patients undergoing surgery involving the hip, whereas pelvic vein thrombosis can occur in patients undergoing pelvic or prostatic surgery. Axillosubclavian vein thrombosis may be spontaneous, resulting from congenital abnormalities of the thoracic outlet, or may be related to indwelling central venous catheters, pulmonary artery catheters, or transvenous pacing wires.[19] In patients with dilated right heart chambers or pulmonary arteries, thrombi can form at those sites and embolize distally into the branches of the pulmonary artery.

Available information also indicates that the likelihood of embolism is influenced by the location of thrombi in the veins of the lower extremity. Although most thrombi form at the site of venous valves in the veins of the calf, it has been demonstrated clearly that thrombi limited to the calf veins rarely are associated with embolism, whereas thrombi that extend proximally into the thigh (popliteal and ileofemoral systems) pose a risk of embolization that approaches 50%.[20, 21] This difference in natural history between calf-limited and proximal thrombi has several important diagnostic and therapeutic implications. First, because most emboli arise from veins in the lower extremity, diagnostic approaches to deep venous thrombosis can be focused on techniques that detect lower extremity thrombosis. Second, techniques that detect above-knee thrombi are of particular value, regardless of whether they can detect calf-limited thrombi. Finally, although it is true that calf-limited thrombi rarely embolize, many have concluded incorrectly from this information that *symptomatic*, calf-limited deep venous thrombosis represents a clinically unimportant condition. It must be emphasized that approximately 15% to 20% of calf-limited thrombi, if untreated, extend proximally, thereby posing an embolic risk. Furthermore, preliminary data suggest that untreated, symptomatic calf vein thrombosis may result in a higher risk of future recurrence. In view of the strong association between recurrent deep venous thrombosis and the development of the postphlebitic syndrome, anticoagulant therapy of *symptomatic* calf-limited thrombi appears to represent a prudent clinical approach.[22, 23]

Although most above-knee thrombi represent extensions from calf thrombi, some do arise in the larger, proximal veins de novo. This occurrence appears to be restricted principally to patients with hip fracture or replacement, pelvic surgery (including prostatic resection), and other high inguinal-pelvic trauma.

The natural history of deep venous thrombosis is reasonably well understood.[24] Venous thrombi appear to begin either in the vicinity of a venous valve, where eddy currents arise, or at the site of intimal injury. Platelet aggregation and release of mediators initiate the sequence. With local accumulation of such factors, the coagulation cascade is activated, and a red fibrin thrombus develops. As thrombus extension occurs, local fibrinolytic activity is enhanced. Thus, thrombus behavior becomes a dynamic process that may result in complete dissolution or an endothelialized remnant, resulting in a variable degree of intimal narrowing and valvular damage. If significant obstruction persists, collateral veins develop.

At any time during this process, a portion or all of the thrombus can detach as an embolus. This risk is highest early in thrombus development before significant fibrinolysis or organization occurs. Beyond this acute phase, the long-term outlook is influenced principally by the extent of residual venous obstruction and valvular damage. If significant obstruction persists, downstream stasis will be present, leading to a substantial risk of recurrent deep vein thrombosis.

## NATURAL HISTORY: PULMONARY EMBOLISM

As noted previously, pulmonary embolism is not a disease per se. It is merely a complication of venous thrombosis. Nonetheless, once it occurs, embolism can trigger a host of serious pulmonary and cardiac effects.[25]

The pulmonary effects of embolism can be numerous. First, if regional pulmonary vascular obstruction is total, alveolar dead space is created. Second, with total vascular occlusion, pneumoconstriction may occur in the lung distal to the area of obstruction as the result of alveolar hypocapnia.[26] This is probably uncommon in patients because they inhale some carbon dioxide ($CO_2$)–rich dead-space air into the unperfused lung regions at the beginning of each breath and because obstruction is rarely total. Third, hyperventilation almost always occurs, the mechanism for which remains uncertain. Fourth, some degree of arterial hypoxemia often occurs.[27] One common cause of arterial hypoxemia is widening of the arteriovenous oxygen difference resulting from an acute increase in right ventricular afterload and an ensuing decline in cardiac output.[28, 29] This lowering of the mixed venous oxygen content magnifies the effects of the normal venous admixture, thereby lowering the arterial $PO_2$. Another potential mechanism for hypoxemia is shunt, either on an intrapulmonary or intracardiac basis.[30] With embolic occlusion sufficient to increase pulmonary artery pressure, compensatory hypoxic vasoconstrictive mechanisms can be overcome, and perfusion to poorly ventilated or nonventilated lung regions may occur. On occasion, embolic events massive enough to increase right atrial pressure may result in the development of a patent foramen ovale and intracardiac right-to-left shunting.

The final mechanism for hypoxemia relates to the fifth pulmonary consequence of embolism, loss of pulmonary surfactant.[31] Unlike the first four consequences, loss of surfactant does not occur immediately. It requires approximately 24 hours of total occlusion to develop. At that time or later, surfactant depletion in the nonperfused alveolar zones may cause atelectasis and edema. If partial thrombus resolution and reperfusion to this atelectatic region develop, hypoxemia can result.

One uncommon pulmonary consequence of pulmonary embolism is pulmonary infarction (see Fig. 18.4). Infarction is uncommon because the pulmonary parenchyma has three potential sources of oxygen: the pulmonary arteries, the bronchial arteries, and the airways.[32] Two of these three sources apparently must be compromised before infarction develops. Therefore, in a patient with no coexisting cardiopulmonary disease, infarction is rare. Infarction occurs in approximately 20% of patients with significant cardiac or pulmonary disease that compromises either bronchial arterial flow or airway patency. In patients with left ventricular failure, increased pulmonary venous pressure may decrease bronchial flow, and infarction may occur.[33]

The cardiac and hemodynamic effects of embolism are related to two factors: reduction of the cross-sectional area of the pulmonary vascular bed and the preexisting status of the cardiopulmonary system.[34–36] Obstruction of the pulmonary vascular bed by embolism acutely increases the workload on the right ventricle, a chamber ill equipped to deal with a high pressure load. In patients without preexisting cardiopulmonary disease, obstruction of less than 20% of the pulmonary vascular bed results in a number of compensatory events that minimize adverse hemodynamic consequences. Recruitment and distension of pulmonary vessels occur, resulting in a normal or near-normal pulmonary artery pressure and pulmonary vascular resistance; cardiac output is maintained by increases in the right ventricular stroke volume and increases in the heart rate. As the degree of pulmonary vascular obstruction exceeds 30% to 40%, compensatory mechanisms are overcome and increases in pulmonary artery pressure and modest increases in right atrial pressure occur. The Frank-Starling mechanism maintains right ventricular stroke work and cardiac output. When the degree of pulmonary artery obstruction exceeds 50% to 60%, compensatory mechanisms are overcome, cardiac output begins to fall, and right atrial pressure increases dramatically. In patients without prior cardiopulmonary disease, a pulmonary artery mean pressure of 30 to 40 mm Hg (pulmonary artery systolic pressure of 50 to 60 mm Hg) represents severe pulmonary hypertension. With acute obstruction beyond 60% of the pulmonary vascular bed, the right heart dilates, cardiac output decreases, and systemic hypotension develops.

The hemodynamic response to acute pulmonary embolism in patients with preexisting cardiopulmonary disease may be considerably different.[34] Unlike patients without prior cardiopulmonary disease in whom there is a general relationship between the degree of pulmonary vascular obstruction and the level of the pulmonary artery pressure, patients with prior cardiopulmonary disease demonstrate degrees of pulmonary hypertension that are disproportionate to the degree of pulmonary vascular obstruction. As a result, severe pulmonary hypertension may develop in response to a relatively small reduction in pulmonary artery cross-sectional area. Thus, evidence of right ventricular hypertrophy (rather than ventricular dilation) associated with an estimated pulmonary artery systolic pressure in excess of 60 mm Hg in an embolic suspect should suggest an element of chronic pulmonary hypertension, which might result from a potentially diverse group of etiologic possibilities (e.g., chronic thromboembolic pulmonary hypertension, left ventricular failure, valvular disease, right-to-left cardiac shunts).

After the acute embolic event, the behavior of emboli parallels that previously described for venous thrombi; that is, they undergo resolution by fibrinolysis or organization and recanalization. The most rapid resolution of a large embolus that has been documented is 51 hours.[37] Other reports indicate that resolution is substantial during the first week and continues for 4 to 8 weeks.[38, 39] The term *resolution* is used here because it is uncertain, in humans, to what degree lysis (vs. organization) participates in embolic resolution. Most sequential data regarding resolution in humans are based on perfusion scans, not angiographic data. Reperfusion can occur with restoration of as little as 20% of the normal luminal diameter. Therefore, significant organized residuals may persist in patients whose scans return to normal. How often such residuals persist is not known. What is known is that residual obstruction sufficient to cause pulmonary hypertension is rare. The clinical course and management of this small group of patients is dealt with later in this chapter.

## CLINICAL PRESENTATION

The most common symptoms and physical findings of venous thrombosis include swelling, pain, erythema, and warmth. "Classic" findings such as Homans' sign (calf pain with flexion of the knee and dorsiflexion of the ankle), Moses' sign (pain with calf compression against the tibia), or a palpable cord occur infrequently and are nonspecific.

Multiple investigations have established that the clinical diagnosis of venous thrombosis is imprecise.[40–42] In patients with clinical signs and symptoms suggestive of venous thrombosis, the majority will not have the diagnosis established by venography. An algorithmic clinical model has been demonstrated to increase the sensitivity and specificity of clinical diagnosis in *symptomatic* patients, although not to a level in which clinical diagnosis, in the absence of objective testing, can be relied on exclusively to either confirm or exclude the diagnosis.[43] Furthermore, and even more disquieting, most high-risk patients who are monitored and who develop deep venous thrombosis do not have signs or symptoms suggesting that diagnosis.[18, 44]

Multiple investigations also have confirmed that the diagnosis of pulmonary embolism cannot be confirmed or excluded solely on clinical grounds.[20, 45, 46] The most comprehensive analysis of the presenting clinical findings in symptomatic patients with angiographically documented pulmonary embolism was provided by the PIOPED (Prospective Investigation of Pulmonary Embolism Diagnosis) trial.[47] In this trial, the clinical probability of embolism, based on history, physical examination, chest radiography, arterial blood gas analysis, and electrocardiographic findings, was estimated by the investigators before performing objective testing. Among 90 patients in whom the clinical probability of embolism was estimated to be 80% or greater, 32% did not have angiographic evidence of pulmonary emboli. Among the 228 patients in whom the clinical probability of pulmonary embolism was considered to be 19% or less, 9% had positive angiograms. Clinical probability, therefore, was much more useful in excluding the diagnosis than in confirming it. Unfortunately, most patients entered into the trial fell into a clinically indeterminate group in whom the incidence of angiographically confirmed embolism was 30%.

Despite their nonspecific nature, a review of the clinical signs and symptoms associated with embolism is worthwhile because clinical findings represent an essential first step in the diagnostic pathway. Although a somewhat arbitrary classification because presenting symptoms and signs of embolism frequently overlap, the presentation of pulmonary embolism can be categorized into one of three clinical syndromes: (1) isolated dyspnea; (2) pleuritic pain or hemoptysis; and (3) circulatory collapse.[48] Among patients without prior cardiopulmonary disease in the PIOPED study, the syndrome of pleuritic pain or hemoptysis was the most common mode of presentation, occurring in 65% of patients; isolated dyspnea occurred in 22%, and circulatory collapse occurred in 8%.

The most common presenting symptom of acute embolism in various studies is the sudden onset of dyspnea, which has occurred in most patients. It must be emphasized, however, that in PIOPED dyspnea was not present in 27% of patients ultimately proven to have embolism. A sense of impending doom also is reported, particularly with massive embolism. Angina also can occur with massive embolism; it is angina, but the cause is right ventricular ischemia. Syncope also may be a presenting complaint in major embolic occlusion.

The same factors influence the frequency and severity of clinical signs. The most common finding is unexplained tachypnea (respiratory rate $\geq$ 20 minute). In the PIOPED trial, however, tachypnea was not present in 30% of patients with embolism. Clinical findings found less frequently include crackles, tachycardia, a fourth heart sound, and an increased pulmonic component of the second heart sound. Fever may develop some hours after the event and often reaches but rarely exceeds 38.3°C. As noted previously, hemoptysis may be observed; it usually is quite modest in extent, although it persists for some days. Brisk hemoptysis is rare and almost never the initial finding. With massive embolism, there may be evidence of right ventricular overload or failure, such as a right ventricular tap along the left sternal border and an accentuated pulmonary valve closure sound. If right ventricular failure occurs, there may be fixed splitting of S2, the appearance of S3 or S4, or both, distended neck veins, and cyanosis. Careful examination of the legs may elicit evidence suggesting venous thrombosis. In the PIOPED trial, clinically apparent venous thrombosis was found in only 11% of patients.

Obviously, these symptoms and signs are nonspecific. In the PIOPED study, none of the presenting symptoms were capable of discriminating between those with positive angiograms and those in whom the angiographic findings were negative. Also, in terms of presenting signs, only the presence of crackles, a fourth heart sound, and an increased pulmonic component of the second heart sound could differentiate between those with positive and those with negative angiograms. Furthermore, in patients with underlying cardiopulmonary disease, the presenting symptoms and signs frequently are obscured by elements of the patient's underlying illness.[45] It is also important to recognize that the clinical presentation of embolism has been characterized in trials composed of symptomatic patients. Prospective studies of high-risk patients have established that asymptomatic emboli occur in some 40% or more of patients with proximal deep venous thrombosis.[1, 20, 49] It is likely that the frequency and severity of symptoms are influenced by the extent of embolic occlusion and the prior cardiopulmonary status of the patient. Small- or moderate-sized emboli may induce few or no symptoms in an otherwise healthy individual. In patients with preexisting cardiopulmonary disease, symptoms are more common and more severe.

Because of its nonspecific presentation, the differential diagnosis of pulmonary embolism is varied and extensive, especially in hospitalized patients with coexisting cardiac or pulmonary disease. Common considerations include congestive heart failure, exacerbation of chronic lung disease, postoperative atelectasis, and viral pleurisy. Emboli presenting with fever, dyspnea, and chest radiographic abnormalities easily can be confused with a bacterial pneumonia. The presence of fever and leukocytosis (rarely exceeding 15,000/μL) is uncommon, but they are well-described accompaniments of venous thromboembolism.[50, 51]

These precautionary statements regarding clinical diagnosis are not meant to suggest that the clinical presentation of pulmonary embolism cannot be used as a basis for clinical decision making. They are, however, meant as a reminder that the clinical presentation of pulmonary embolism may often be atypical or subtle and should serve only to generate a suspicion of that diagnosis. Most physicians would have little difficulty in considering the diagnosis of embolism in a patient presenting with the acute onset of dyspnea, pleuritic chest pain, and hemoptysis. Unfortunately, such a presentation is quite rare. A reliance on signs and symptoms that are considered "classic" before making the decision to proceed to confirmatory testing ultimately leads to underdiagnosis and unnecessary mortality.

## DIAGNOSIS OF VENOUS THROMBOSIS

The proper diagnostic approach to venous thromboembolism must take into account the central fact that venous thrombosis and pulmonary embolism are manifestations of the same disease process, venous thrombosis representing the source of pulmonary embolism and pulmonary embolism representing a complication of venous thrombosis. To regard venous thrombosis and pulmonary embolism as separate entities not only is inappropriate but also can lead to serious errors in management.

### Contrast Venography

In validating any test, there must be a gold standard. In the case of lower extremity venous thrombosis, that standard is contrast venography (Fig. 51.1). In investigative contexts, it is a good gold standard (as will be indicated, however, that is not always the case in clinical studies). The venogram is performed according to a specific protocol described by Rabinov and Paulin in 1972.[52] The most reliable criterion for the diagnosis of venous thrombosis is a constant intraluminal filling defect evident in two or more views. Other criteria such as nonvisualization of deep veins, finding collateral veins, or nonconstant filling defects are less reliable. Under circumstances in which the proper protocol and interpretative criteria are used, contrast venography has high sensitivity and specificity. The study, however, is not without shortcomings. As those who have seen many venograms recognize, the study is not easy to interpret, especially in patients with a history of venous thrombosis. Venous cannulation often may be difficult to define, especially in the presence of edema; expert interpretation is essential for accurate diagnosis; injection of contrast material with its associated risk is necessary; venous thrombosis may be induced by the procedure itself; and the cost, invasive nature, and discomfort of the study make sequential studies unfeasible.

Because of these limitations, a number of noninvasive studies capable of being performed on a sequential basis were introduced into clinical practice. Currently, two validated noninvasive techniques are available: impedance plethysmography and duplex ultrasonography. Magnetic resonance imaging (MRI), although less well validated, may play a valuable role in venous thrombosis diagnosis in the future.

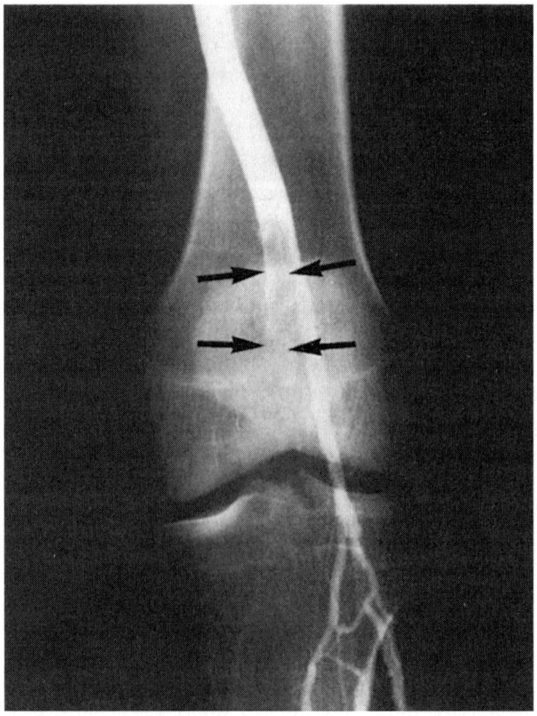

**Figure 51.1** Contrast venogram disclosing large filling defect *(arrows)* due to thrombus in popliteal and distal superficial femoral vein. Such thrombi pose substantial embolic risk.

### Duplex Ultrasonography

Since 1990, duplex ultrasonography, which refers to the combination of Doppler venous flow detection and real-time B-mode imaging, has assumed a central role in the noninvasive diagnosis of lower extremity deep venous thrombosis.[53–55] A number of criteria are used to diagnose venous thrombosis, the most reliable of which is noncompressibility of a venous segment (Fig. 51.2). Secondary, less reliable criteria include the presence of echogenic material within the venous lumen, venous distention, loss of phasicity, response to Valsalva maneuver, and augmentation of spontaneous flow. The absence of an echogenic luminal mass cannot be considered useful in excluding the diagnosis of venous thrombosis because acute thrombus may not demonstrate echogenicity. Multiple studies during the last decade have demonstrated sensitivity rates exceeding 90% and specificity rates exceeding 95% in symptomatic patients with proximal venous thrombosis. A clear advantage of real-time B-mode imaging alone, duplex ultrasonography, and color Doppler imaging has not been demonstrated because all rely on vein noncompressibility as the primary diagnostic endpoint. Although simplified compression examinations limited to the symptomatic leg or to the common femoral and popliteal veins (rather than the entire lower extremity venous system) have been suggested, the time saved with such approaches is limited.[56, 57] A more prudent approach appears to be a complete examination extending from the inguinal ligament to the popliteal vein.

Duplex ultrasonography is far less sensitive in the

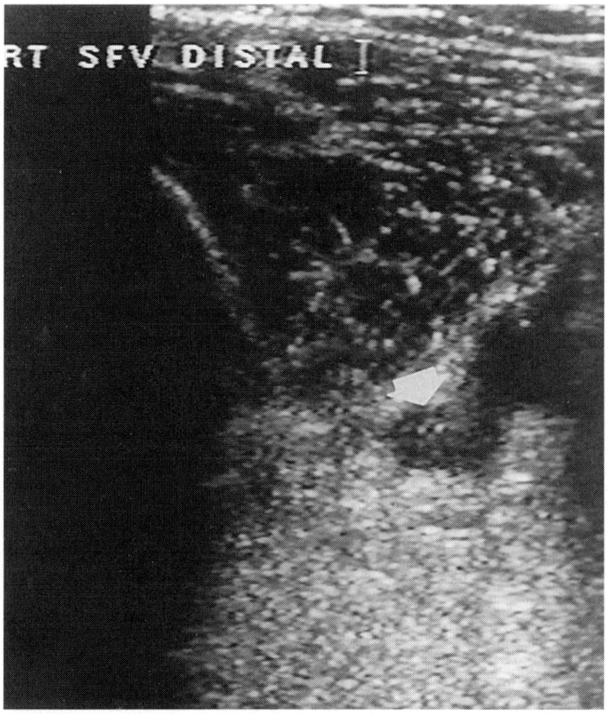


**Figure 51.2** Duplex ultrasonography demonstrating a noncompressible distal superficial femoral vein containing an echogenic mass *(arrow)*, consistent with venous thrombosis.

detection of symptomatic calf-limited thrombi (approximately 70%) and in asymptomatic proximal vein thrombi (approximately 50%), thereby limiting its utility as a screening study in high-risk populations.[58, 59] When ultrasonography is negative in patients with suspected venous thrombosis, a strategy of serial testing has proven to be effective in detecting proximal extension.

### Impedance Plethysmography

Impedance plethysmography (IPG), an indirect technique that measures the rate of venous outflow, has been well standardized and carefully validated against contrast venography.[60, 61] False-positive findings can result from conditions that diminish arterial inflow (congestive heart failure, shock, peripheral arterial disease) or that impede venous return (right ventricular failure, obstructive lung disease), thereby lowering the specificity of the technique. Early studies reported sensitivity rates of approximately 90% in symptomatic patients with proximal venous thrombosis.[60–62] Calf thrombi are detected in approximately 25%, a figure that reflects the lesser degree of venous obstruction in most (although not all) calf thrombi.

Studies of IPG accuracy have raised questions regarding the ability of IPG to detect even symptomatic, proximal vein thrombosis. Reported sensitivity rates in these studies have been in the range of 65% to 75%.[63, 64] The low sensitivity of IPG in these studies may result from its use in patients with less severe symptoms because these patients are more likely to have small, nonocclusive, or distal thrombi that IPG cannot readily detect. Supporting this premise is the fact that IPG sensitivity returns to 85% to 90% when more extensive thrombi and those that have extended into the distal superficial femoral vein are evaluated. These data support the current recommendation that a single negative IPG study result should not be used to exclude venous thrombosis in a symptomatic patient. A strategy of serial IPG testing, however, has been demonstrated to be useful in detecting proximal extension.[65–67] Although this strategy has proven effective, confirmatory testing with duplex ultrasonography or venography may be necessary when IPG results conflict with clinical impression, especially in patients with limited cardiopulmonary reserve in whom embolism would be tolerated poorly.

As is the case with duplex ultrasonography, the sensitivity rate of IPG is, at best, in the range of 40% in the detection of asymptomatic proximal vein thrombosis.[68] The low sensitivity of IPG in these patients may be attributed to the fact that thrombi in asymptomatic patients are less extensive and less likely to be occlusive.

The detection of possible recurrent venous thrombosis commonly represents a diagnostic challenge for which impedance plethysmography may play a valuable role.[69, 70] The resolution rate for IPG-documented venous thrombosis at 6 months has been found to be 85% and at 12 months to be 95%. Therefore, reversion of IPG results from normal to abnormal in a symptomatic patient with suspected recurrent venous thrombosis provides strong evidence that recurrence has occurred. The utility of such an approach, however, mandates that follow-up IPG be performed and that IPG normalization has been documented in an individual patient.

### Magnetic Resonance Imaging

MRI techniques for detecting venous thrombosis include spin-echo MRI, gradient-recalled-echo MRI, and magnetic resonance venography. Preliminary reports suggest that MRI is at least as sensitive and specific as duplex ultrasonography.[71, 72] A potential advantage of MRI is that the entire length of the venous system, including the pelvic veins, can be evaluated. Disadvantages associated with MRI include the cost and limited availability of scanner time as well as the expertise required to properly perform and interpret the studies.

## DIAGNOSIS OF PULMONARY EMBOLISM

There are certain parallels between the approaches to the diagnosis of pulmonary embolism and deep venous thrombosis. Perhaps the most important parallel is that clinical evidence cannot be relied on to confirm or exclude the diagnosis but merely can raise the suspicion of that diagnosis. Once that suspicion has been raised, however, diagnostic studies are required to confirm or deny the diagnosis.

### Standard Laboratory Evaluation

Routine laboratory studies, unfortunately, cannot make the diagnosis of pulmonary embolism. Although none has the discriminatory power to confirm the diagnosis of embolism, they do provide valuable adjunctive information, provide support for therapeutic interventions, and may confirm the presence of an alternative diagnosis.

Most patients with pulmonary embolism have abnormal chest radiographs.[73] These abnormalities, however, are usually subtle, nonspecific, and therefore nondiagnostic (Fig. 51.3). In the PIOPED study, the most common radiographic abnormalities were atelectasis or pulmonary infiltrates. There is some confusion about the diagnostic configuration of infiltrates due to embolism. These infiltrates, although usually abutting a pleural surface, can be of any shape, not necessarily wedge shaped. Although pleural effusions occur in almost half of the patients, most are small and involve only blunting of the costophrenic angle.[74] Findings once considered specific for embolism, such as Westermark's sign (focal areas of avascularity), Hampton's hump (pleural-based, wedge-shaped density), and Fleischner's sign (prominence of the central pulmonary artery), have not proven to have discriminatory value. A normal chest radiograph may be quite useful in raising the index of suspicion of embolism and by excluding confounding diagnostic options. The major role of chest radiography in suspected pulmonary embolism, therefore, is to exclude competing diagnoses and to evaluate the pulmonary parenchyma, which is essential for accurate interpretation of the ventilation-perfusion scan.

Likewise, electrocardiographic findings in pulmonary embolism, although occurring frequently, are diverse and nonspecific.[74, 75] The most common abnormalities include nonspecific T-wave inversion and abnormalities of the ST segment. With more extensive occlusion, the electrocardiogram may reveal an "$S_1Q_3T_3$" pattern, a pseudoinfarction pattern, right bundle-branch block, or right axis deviation. Rhythm disturbances other than sinus tachycardia are uncommon and usually are confined to patients with underlying cardiac disease.

Arterial blood gas analysis is helpful although not definitive.[75] Arterial hypoxemia may be present, and the more massive the obstruction, the more severe the hypoxemia is likely to be. However, many other conditions also cause hypoxemia, and embolism often does not cause hypoxemia or even a widening of the $(A-a)P_{O_2}$ gradient. Hypocapnia usually is present with embolism; hypercapnia, conversely, is rare. Hypercapnia appears with embolism only in patients with marked antecedent ventilatory limitation or when such limitation has been imposed because the patient is on controlled mechanical ventilation when embolism occurs.[78]

## Echocardiography

Echocardiography may serve a valuable role in the diagnostic approach to pulmonary embolism. Under appropriate clinical circumstances, the detection of unexplained right ventricular volume or pressure load should suggest the possibility of embolism and lead to confirmatory testing. A distinct echocardiographic pattern involving akinesia of the mid-free wall with apical sparing has been described.[78] Properly performed transesophageal echocardiography has demonstrated sensitivity and specificity rates exceeding 90% in the detection of emboli involving the pulmonary trunk and the right and left main pulmonary arteries.[79] Furthermore, transesophageal echocardiography has proven valuable in the evaluation of competing diagnostic possibilities such as right ventricular infarction, endocarditis, pericardial tamponade, and aortic dissection in patients with unexplained shock and evidence of elevated central venous pressure.[80] Although transesophageal echocardiography cannot be considered a primary diagnostic technique, strong consideration can be given to its use in that subset of patients with suspected massive pulmonary embolism who are too ill for transportation or too unstable to undergo angiography, or who have an absolute contraindication to the administration of a contrast agent.

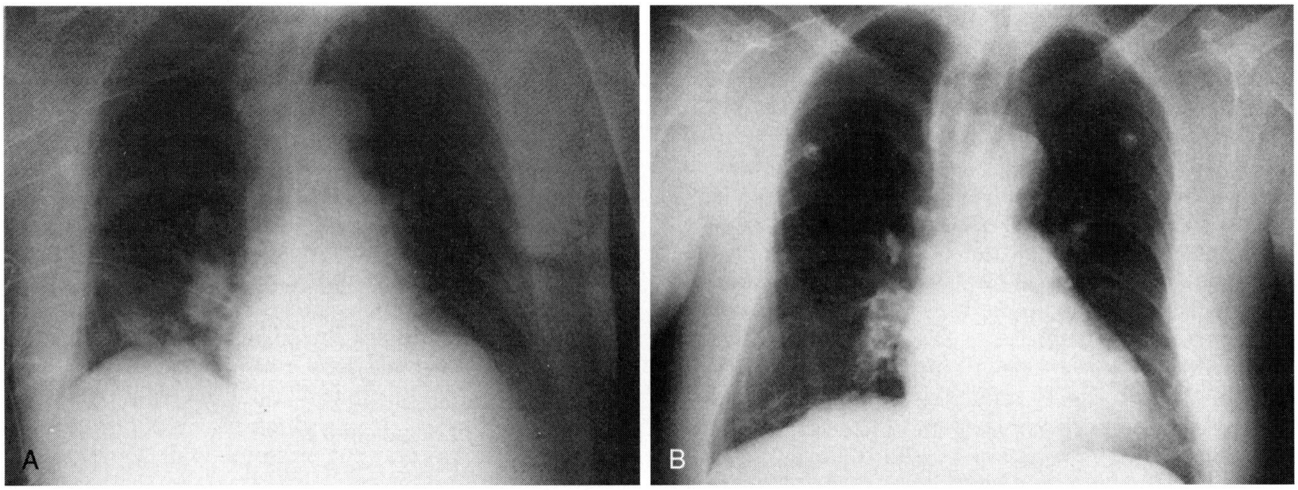


**Figure 51.3** Chest radiographs in a patient with pulmonary embolism. *A,* Infiltrates caused by atelectasis with edema in right lower lobe and in retrocardiac area in patient with angiographically confirmed pulmonary embolus. *B,* Two weeks later, the infiltrates have cleared.

## Hemostaseologic Assays

The development of a rapid and accurate blood test capable of diagnosing venous thromboembolism has held special appeal and has been the subject of considerable investigative interest. A number of different serologic markers have been investigated, including D-dimer, fibrin monomer, prothrombin fragment, thrombin-antithrombin III complex, and fibronectin. Of these, D-dimer, alone and in combination with other noninvasive studies such as IPG, duplex ultrasonography, or ventilation-perfusion scanning, has been subject to the most rigorous clinical evaluation.[81–83] Although preliminary results of D-dimer testing have been promising under a variety of clinical circumstances, two critical factors currently limit its diagnostic utility, especially for hospitalized patients.[84] A number of different assays (enzyme-linked immunosorbent assay [ELISA], latex agglutination, and more recently developed rapid methods) with different discriminatory values and with a wide range of sensitivities and specificities have been developed.[85] Furthermore, the low specificity of D-dimer testing (approximately 25% in hospitalized patients) excludes the possibility that it can be used as a confirmatory test for either venous thrombosis or pulmonary embolism. However, the reported high sensitivity but low specificity of elevated D-dimers suggests that the presence of normal values could be used to exclude the presence of pulmonary embolism, a hypothesis that was supported by finding a 100% negative predictive value in *selected* patients (no recent surgery, no malignancy, serum bilirubin level <2.0 mg/dL) suspected of having pulmonary embolism.[85a] Pending further investigation and establishment of a rapid, reproducible, standardized technique, D-dimer testing likely will play a valuable role in limiting the need for invasive testing in patients with indeterminate ventilation-perfusion scan results.

## Ventilation-Perfusion Scanning

Despite certain limitations, the perfusion lung scan is invaluable if interpreted appropriately. First, a negative perfusion scan rules out the diagnosis of pulmonary embolism with the same degree of certainty as a negative pulmonary angiogram (Fig. 51.4). Thus, in any patient in whom embolism is suspected, a perfusion scan is worth doing for its exclusionary value. Second, the PIOPED study demonstrated that a "high probability" scan (one characterized by multiple, segmental-sized, mismatched defects) is associated with embolism in approximately 87% of patients; when coupled with a high clinical probability of embolism, the positive predictive value increased to 96% (Fig. 51.5). However, the PIOPED data also provided several pieces of disquieting information: (1) the overwhelming majority of patients with suspected embolism did not have scan findings that fell into a high probability or normal category, the only categories that can be considered definitive; (2) most patients with embolism did not have a high probability scan finding; (3) the overwhelming majority of patients without embolism did not have a normal scan; and (4) a substantial and clinically significant percentage of patients with scan findings interpreted as intermediate probability (33%) and low probability (16%) subsequently were demonstrated to have angiographic evidence of embolism.[47] It is essential that clinicians recognize that the concept of a low-probability scan is misleading and potentially dangerous because of the frequency of pulmonary embolism in patients exhibiting this scan pattern.[86, 87]

To improve perfusion scan specificity, traditional inter-

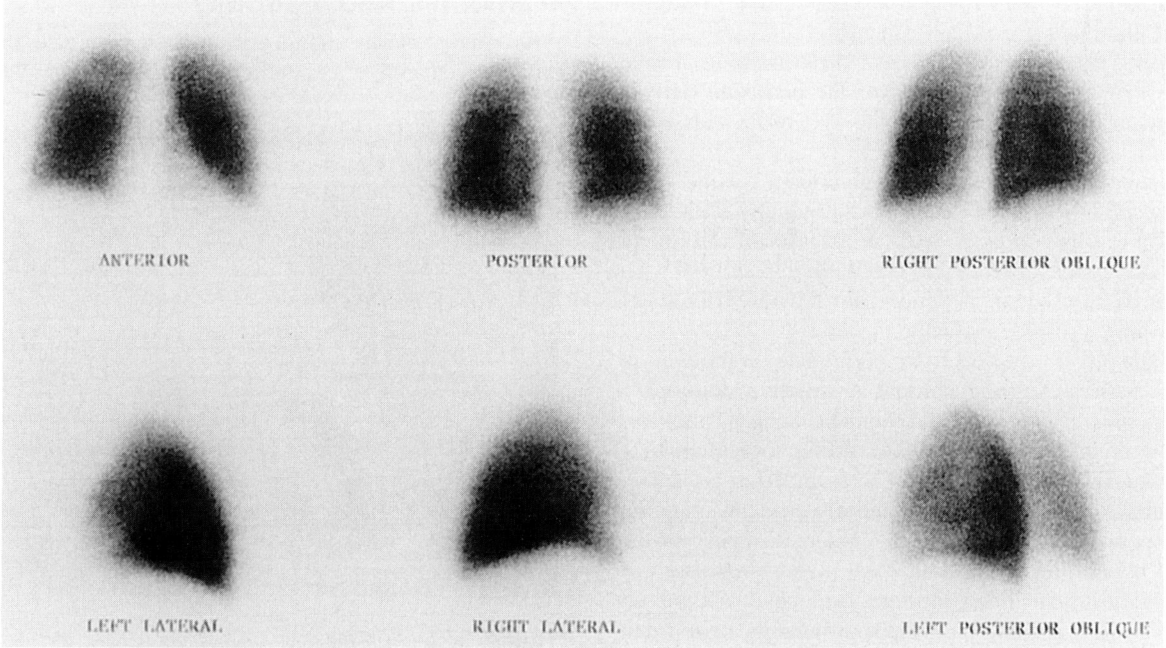


**Figure 51.4** Normal six-view perfusion scan. A normal finding is capable of excluding the diagnosis of embolism.

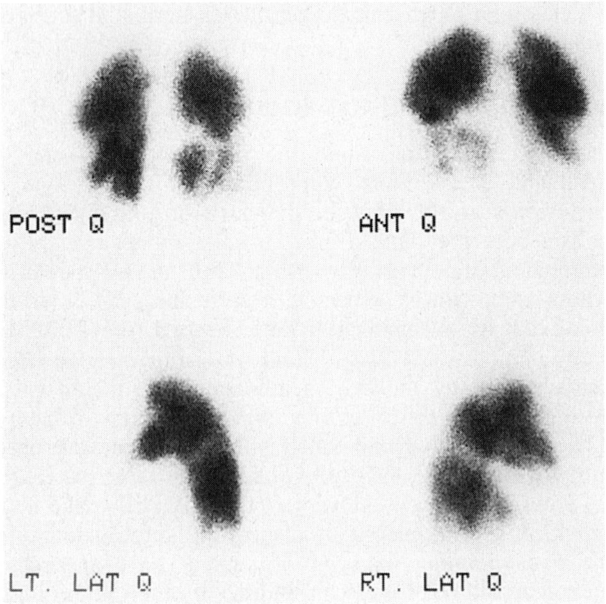


**Figure 51.5** Lung perfusion scan showing major segmental and lobar defects bilaterally. Ventilation scan and chest radiograph were normal. This "high probability" pattern is strongly associated with the presence of embolism.

pretive criteria, including the PIOPED criteria, rely on the number and size of the perfusion defects as well as on the results of a concurrent ventilation image. The intended basis for doing so is to differentiate pulmonary vascular obstruction ("mismatched" defects) from primary parenchymal disorders that result in compensatory pulmonary vasoconstriction ("matched" defects). In a more recent trial, the Prospective Investigative Study of Acute Pulmonary Embolism Diagnosis (PISA-PED) investigators used a fundamentally different interpretive scheme that relied on the shape of the perfusion defects alone, regardless of their number or size or their association with ventilation findings.[88] The results of this study and a later analysis suggest that embolism can be diagnosed accurately and the need for angiography limited by perfusion results combined with an assessment of clinical likelihood in the absence of ventilation imaging.[88a] An analysis of a subset of patients from the PIOPED study resulted in a similar conclusion.[89]

The diagnostic approach to pulmonary embolism in patients with underlying chronic obstructive pulmonary disease remains especially problematic because the presentation of pulmonary embolism in this population may closely mimic an exacerbation of their underlying disease. Unfortunately, the value of ventilation-perfusion scanning in this population is even more limited than that in the general population because an even higher proportion of scans fall into an indeterminate category.[90] However, among the few patients with high probability or normal/near-normal scan findings, both the positive predictive value and negative predictive value were equivalent to that in the general population.

## Spiral (Helical) Computed Tomography

The utility of spiral computed tomography (CT) scanning for diagnosing acute pulmonary embolism has been evaluated in a number of small studies.[91, 92] Its role in pulmonary embolism diagnosis remains undefined, although it does demonstrate promise. Several studies have demonstrated that spiral CT scanning is capable of visualizing central emboli (main, lobar, and segmental arteries) with a sensitivity rate exceeding 90% (Fig. 51.6). However, sensitivity appears to decline markedly when emboli are confined to the subsegmental arteries, not an uncommon finding in embolism.[93, 94] Accurate CT scan interpretation also requires considerable expertise and experience.

An advantage of spiral CT scanning includes the ability to define nonvascular structures such as lymphadenopathy, lung tumors, emphysema, and other parenchymal abnormalities. CT scanning requires patient transportation and a volume of contrast equivalent to that of a pulmonary angiogram. It is also unclear whether CT scanning will supplant ventilation-perfusion scanning, pulmonary angiography, or both, in the diagnostic sequence. Although some have strongly endorsed the incorporation of CT scanning into the diagnostic algorithm for pulmonary embolism, it is difficult to support this recommendation in the absence of a large, randomized trial comparing CT scanning (a CT "equivalent" of the PIOPED trial) with pulmonary angiography.[95] Of course, this recommendation may change as technical improvements occur and as additional data are accumulated regarding the sensitivity and specificity of CT scanning using an angiographic gold standard and outcome analysis for validation. At the present time, the only exception to this recommendation may be patients with severe chronic obstructive pulmonary disease (COPD) or extensive parenchymal infiltrates in whom the likelihood of a diagnostic ventilation-perfusion scan is exceedingly low.

## Pulmonary Angiography

The results of the diagnostic studies reviewed thus far often are capable of excluding or confirming the diagnosis

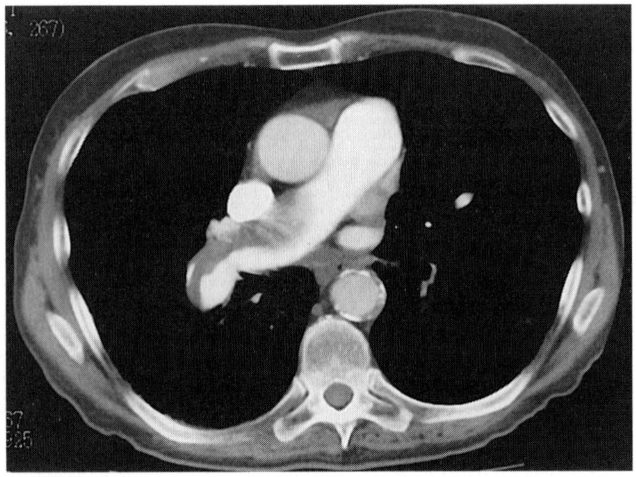

**Figure 51.6** Chest computed tomographic scan with contrast, demonstrating extensive embolization involving the right main, upper lobe, and lower lobe pulmonary arteries.

of embolism. But in a significant number of patients (20% to 80%, depending on the population studied), the diagnosis remains in doubt. At this juncture, pulmonary angiography may be required because it represents the ultimate diagnostic arbiter. Like contrast venography, however, pulmonary angiography has a number of limitations as a gold standard. First, the procedure is invasive and not without risk, especially in patients with acute right ventricular failure. Experience during the 1990s, however, has demonstrated that the perception of risk associated with angiography outweighs the actual risk.[96, 97] Pulmonary angiography can be performed quite safely if certain safeguards are observed and experienced personnel are involved.

Even though the risk of angiography should be nominal, the procedure has other, more subtle limitations. One is accessibility. Angiography must be performed in a special facility to which the patient must be transported. In some institutions, the logistic problems involved are modest; in others, they are substantial.

The other limitation is interpretation. Interpretation of pulmonary angiograms is influenced heavily by three factors: the location of the thromboembolic obstruction, the quality of the images, and the experience of the interpreters. Only two angiographic findings are diagnostic of acute embolism: the filling defect and abrupt cutoff of a vessel (Fig. 51.7). Technical adequacy of the angiogram is critical to accurate identification of both. Flow artifacts can suggest a filling defect. It is essential that good vessel opacification be obtained and that the filling defects be identified as real on a sequence of films.

Thus, although concern about risk should not deter pulmonary angiography, there are noteworthy limitations on its performance and value.[98] Still, it is a rather odd commentary on medical thinking that few, these days, would advise against performance of a coronary angiogram in a patient with coronary thrombosis or ischemia because of risk, yet the question of risk often deters pulmonary angiography in a patient in whom embolism is suspected. Inasmuch as the case fatality rate of undiagnosed and untreated embolism exceeds that of myocardial infarction, it is not clear why this disparity exists; and it should not exist, in view of equal competence in the performance and interpretation of these two procedures.

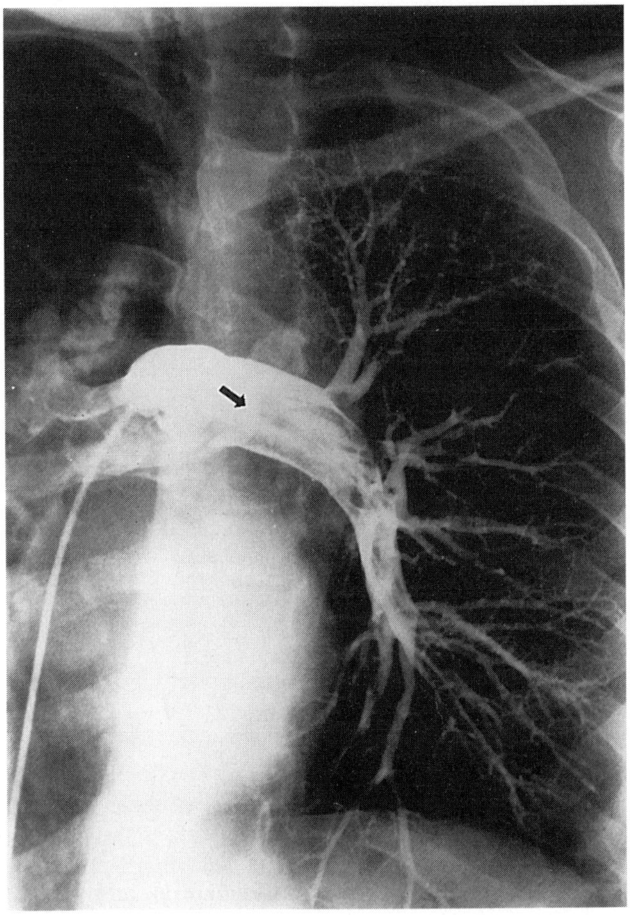

**Figure 51.7** Left-sided pulmonary angiogram showing extensive filling defects *(arrow)* within the left pulmonary artery and the upper lobe, lingula, and lower lobe arteries, which are consistent with the diagnosis of pulmonary embolism.

## DIAGNOSTIC APPROACH

In summary, an almost bewildering array of diagnostic possibilities are available for patients with suspected venous thromboembolism. What the clinician at the bedside must understand and accept is that a stepwise diagnostic strategy, rather than any single diagnostic technique, may be necessary to confirm or exclude the diagnosis (Fig. 51.8). Furthermore, the clinician must understand that these steps are essential and potentially lifesaving. Withholding anticoagulation in a patient who has experienced an embolic event places that patient at risk for recurrent, potentially lethal events; instituting empirical anticoagulant therapy in a patient who has not experienced an embolic event involves unnecessary hospitalization and therapy, places the patient at risk for hemorrhagic complications, and establishes a "preexisting" condition that may adversely affect future healthcare costs.

Ventilation-perfusion scanning, or perfusion scanning alone, should be the initial diagnostic study in embolic suspects. A normal perfusion scan is capable of excluding the diagnosis of embolism. A "high probability" scan can be used as the basis for therapy, with the exception of three circumstances: when a substantial discrepancy exists between the scan finding and the clinical probability of embolism; when the institution of anticoagulant therapy in an individual patient is associated with prohibitive risk; and when there is a history of embolism and no baseline perfusion scan for comparison. In these patients, as well as those with indeterminate lung scan findings (intermediate and low probability), lower extremity, noninvasive venous testing should be performed. The detection of lower extremity, proximal vein thrombosis, although not confirming that embolism has occurred, has the same therapeutic implications. It must be emphasized that a single, negative lower extremity test is not as useful. Therefore, in embolic suspects with preexisting cardiopulmonary compromise, an indeterminate lung scan finding, and negative lower extremity findings, pulmonary

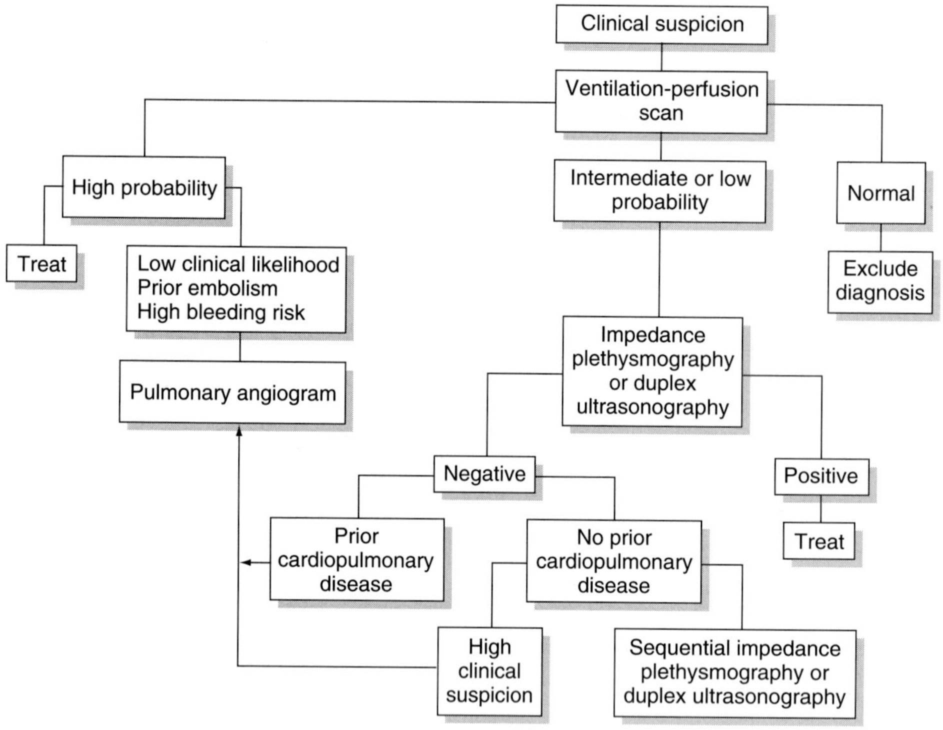


**Figure 51.8** Current algorithmic approach to venous thromboembolism. This approach is expected to change considerably as the roles of spiral computed tomographic scanning and D-dimer determination in embolism diagnosis and exclusion are resolved.

angiography should be pursued because of the mortal risk of a recurrent event. In embolic suspects with adequate cardiopulmonary reserve, indeterminate lung scan findings, a low clinical likelihood of embolism, and a negative lower extremity examination, a strategy of serial noninvasive leg studies may provide a practical alternative to pulmonary angiography. This strategy does not confirm that embolism has not occurred, only that recurrence is unlikely. It is also in this circumstance that D-dimer testing, once the methodologic difficulties have been overcome, may prove to be invaluable in the clinical decision-making process. As noted previously, spiral CT scanning should be considered in lieu of ventilation-perfusion scanning in those patients with severe underlying parenchymal lung disease or extensive radiographic abnormalities.

## PREVENTION OF VENOUS THROMBOEMBOLISM

One of the most striking changes in the field of venous thromboembolism during the last two decades has been emphasis on prevention. This emphasis is totally appropriate and, indeed, should be the cornerstone of modern management. It is clear that if the goal is to prevent pulmonary embolism, the only effective approach is to prevent deep venous thrombosis. The basic information and tools required for developing a prophylactic strategy are now available.

To develop such a strategy, three fundamentals must be in place: (1) the population at risk must be identified; (2) the duration of the increased thromboembolic risk should be ascertained; and (3) effective, low-risk prophylactic options must be available. Populations at risk for deep venous thrombosis and, therefore, for embolism, have been identified; and such risk can, to a considerable extent, be quantified as high, moderate, or low. Furthermore, there are a variety of effective and safe prophylactic approaches available. It should be emphasized that the trend toward earlier hospital discharge has been accompanied by an increased incidence of postdischarge venous thromboembolism. Thromboembolic risk does not necessarily end at the time of hospital discharge or transfer to a lower level of care.[99] In patients with an ongoing predisposition to thrombosis at the time of discharge from an acute inpatient setting, prophylaxis should be continued until the risk for venous thromboembolism has resolved.

The appropriate objective of this prophylactic strategy is to identify the degree of thromboembolic risk in the individual patient and to match the intensity of prophylaxis to that degree of risk. Although a variety of prophylactic approaches has been investigated and used, four approaches have proven effective: low-dose unfractionated heparin, low-molecular-weight heparin, intermittent pneumatic compression devices, and warfarin.

### Low-Dose Unfractionated Heparin

Low-dose heparin has been studied widely as a prophylactic modality. Heparin, given subcutaneously in a dose of 5000 units every 8 or 12 hours, is begun as soon as the risk of deep venous thrombosis is evident and is continued until that risk has abated. This regimen has been shown to be effective in reducing the incidence of deep venous thrombosis, pulmonary embolism, and fatal pulmonary embolism in patients at low to moderate risk, such as those undergoing surgical procedures requiring general anesthesia for 30 minutes or longer and those with medical conditions requiring bed rest for several days.[100] This form of prophylaxis, however, has not been optimally effective in patients whose thromboembolic risk is higher, such as those with hip fracture or hip replacement, those undergoing prostatic surgery, and patients with major traumatic injuries.[101, 102] Furthermore, although the bleeding risk of low-dose heparin is nominal in most patients, there are groups of patients in whom heparin administration is contraindicated, for example, those with active bleeding, hemorrhagic diathesis, hemorrhagic stroke, or neurologic surgery. Before being given prophylactic heparin, patients should be screened with an initial platelet count, partial thromboplastin time, and prothrombin time. During therapy, however, monitoring of coagulation tests is not useful because such tests do not reflect the safety or efficacy of the regimen.

### Low-Molecular-Weight Heparin

Low-molecular-weight heparin (LMWH) preparations represent another prophylactic option. When compared with unfractionated heparin, the ability of LMWH preparations to potentiate the inhibition of factor Xa relative to their inhibition of thrombin theoretically allows them to maintain an equivalent antithrombotic effect while minimizing their anticoagulant effect. In trials that have been performed comparing the prophylactic efficacy and bleeding risk of LMWH with unfractionated heparin in general surgical and medical populations, LMWH has not proven superior to unfractionated heparin.[103, 104] However, LMWH preparations appear more promising as prophylactic agents in several high-risk groups: patients undergoing hip or knee replacement, patients with spinal cord injury, patients with ischemic strokes, and patients with multiple trauma.[101–104]

### Pneumatic Compression Devices

Another extensively evaluated and effective prophylactic approach in low- to moderate-risk patients is the use of mechanical leg compressive devices.[105] These devices periodically (e.g., once or twice per minute) compress the leg by an air-inflatable bladder. A variety of devices are available: thigh length systems, which provide both thigh and calf compression; calf compressive devices; single-pulse systems; and sequential compressions systems. The various compressive devices do not appear to differ in efficacy. Instead, the major determinant of efficacy appears to be strict compliance with this intervention during the period of increased thromboembolic risk.[106]

### Sodium Warfarin

Warfarin and other prothrombinopenic drugs, administered as heparin at the onset of high risk (e.g., preoperatively), have also been shown to be effective and safe. Unfortunately, the use of prothrombinopenic agents has not gained wide favor as a prophylactic approach. There is a perception among physicians that bleeding risk is greater than that reported in the literature. This perception, warranted or not, has inhibited widespread application of these drugs in prophylaxis, even though they are widely used in long-term prophylaxis after acute venous thromboembolism. However, in patients at high risk undergoing hip replacement, warfarin has proven to be quite effective and has achieved general acceptance. Two regimens are widely used: small doses (1 to 2 mg) given for several days before surgery, with dose escalation to therapeutic range; or initiation after surgery.[107, 108] Although LMWH preparations appear equally effective in patients undergoing hip replacement, it has become evident that increased thromboembolic risk in this population can extend for 4 to 6 weeks after hospital discharge.[99] Although the use of warfarin requires monitoring, it is likely that compliance with a once-daily, orally administered drug is superior to that of a subcutaneously administered agent. In this population, a strategy of perioperative LMWH followed by 4 to 6 weeks of warfarin appears optimal.

There is one option available to prevent pulmonary embolism in patients at high risk who cannot be provided pharmacologic or mechanical prophylaxis. Patients with extensive trauma often fall into this category, particularly those with pelvic or lower extremity fractures and potential internal or intracranial bleeding. In such patients, prophylactic placement of an inferior vena cava (IVC) filter provides protection against otherwise nonpreventable emboli.[109]

In summary, in view of the effective options available, few patients at risk for venous thrombosis cannot be protected. Despite this awareness, however, surveys have demonstrated that prophylaxis is underused in populations at risk.[110, 111] A number of different rationales have been proposed to account for this lack of compliance. The overstated perception of bleeding complications associated with pharmacologic methods of prophylaxis appears to remain a deterrent. Furthermore, fatal pulmonary embolism is uncommon in any individual physician's experience, thereby diminishing the perception of risk. Finally, the issue of prophylaxis often is subordinated to the compelling demands of the patient's admitting diagnosis and therapy. Whatever the reason, however, increased use of prophylaxis must occur if significant impact is to be made on the substantial and often unnecessary morbidity and mortality of associated with pulmonary embolism. Not only must prophylaxis be administered, it must be applied in a manner proportionate to the patient's risk of thromboembolism. Such a stepwise approach to prophylaxis would involve low-dose subcutaneous heparin (5000 units every 12 hours) or intermittent compression devices alone in lower risk populations; higher dose of subcutaneous heparin (7500 units every 8 to 12 hours), LMWH, or the combination of low-dose subcutaneous unfractionated heparin plus pneumatic compression devices in those at intermediate risk; and warfarin, IVC filter placement, or sequential lower extremity monitoring, or all three, in those at highest risk.

## MANAGEMENT OF VENOUS THROMBOEMBOLISM

The basic approaches to management are defined chiefly by what we know, as already described, about the pathogenesis, pathophysiology, clinical presentation, and natural history of venous thrombosis and pulmonary embolism.

## Heparin

Heparin remains the mainstay of therapy for pulmonary embolism not associated with hemodynamic compromise or bleeding. Whenever there is a strong suspicion of embolism—based on clinical findings and laboratory tests—heparin therapy should be instituted immediately, without awaiting diagnostic confirmation, unless anticoagulation places the patient at significant risk. Although heparin can be administered by way of either intermittent intravenous injection or subcutaneous injection, the optimal heparin regimen consists of the continuous intravenous administration of a dose that maintains the activated partial thromboplastin time (APTT) between 1.5 and 2.5 times the control value.[112, 113]

Data suggest that physician practices in the administration of heparin often result in levels of anticoagulation that fall below those currently recommended in the literature.[114] To overcome these problems, standardized protocols for heparin administration and monitoring have been recommended. A number of different intravenous heparin dosing schemes have been published, all of which have demonstrated the potential to reach a therapeutic threshold more rapidly than a nonstandardized approach: (1) a weight-based system that includes an 80-unit/kg bolus of heparin followed by an 18-unit/kg/hr infusion; (2) a standard regimen involving a 5000-unit bolus followed by 1280 units/hr; and (3) a variable regimen involving a 5000-unit bolus followed by 40,000 units/day if the patient is at low risk for bleeding or 30,000 units/day if the patient is at high risk for bleeding.[115–117] More recently, an effective, algorithmic approach has been devised for the subcutaneous administration of unfractionated heparin.[118] Each regimen, whether intravenous or subcutaneous, includes standardized dose adjustments based on subsequent APTT values. Whatever regimen is used, an APTT should be obtained 6 hours after the bolus dose, 6 hours after each prescribed dose adjustment, and then on a daily basis for the duration of therapy. Because maintenance of the APTT within a rigidly defined range does not appear to increase the efficacy or safety of the drug, frequent dosage adjustments are not necessary once the dose has been stabilized within a therapeutic range of 1.5 to 2.5 times control. It should be recognized that heparin requirements tend to decrease during the course of therapy, resulting in an increase in the level of the APTT. For patients with heparin resistance (defined as the need for more than 40,000 units/day), monitoring heparin with an anti-factor Xa assay appears safe and effective and results in less escalation of the heparin dose than monitoring with the APTT.[119]

Supporting the importance of achieving a therapeutic threshold as early as possible are data that suggest that a *subtherapeutic* APTT is strongly correlated with thromboembolic recurrence whereas a *supratherapeutic* APTT is not associated with an increased risk of clinically important bleeding complications.[112, 120] There is no direct evidence that the absolute dose of heparin or the level of the APTT can predict the likelihood of bleeding. Instead, bleeding during heparin therapy appears to be related to the presence of concurrent illness, such as renal disease, a history of heavy alcohol consumption, aspirin use, and prior surgical procedures or peptic ulcer disease. Failure to reach a therapeutic range within 24 hours appears to have long-term as well as short-term implications for thromboembolic recurrence. Data strongly suggest that patients who fail to achieve a therapeutic threshold within 24 hours have a subsequent recurrence rate significantly higher than those who do.[121]

Many physicians, unaware of these relationships, initiate therapy with inadequate doses of heparin and then attempt to reach a therapeutic range by time-consuming, marginal increments in dose. In many instances, thrombus extension during this period of subtherapeutic anticoagulation serves to increase heparin requirements, thereby prolonging the process even further. Once a therapeutic range is reached, many "straddle" the lower therapeutic limit of APTT in an attempt to reduce hemorrhagic risk. It must be recognized that fluctuations in APTT levels can occur, and therefore, a single APTT value is not necessarily predictive of results over a 24-hour period.[122] Attempts to maintain the APTT in a low therapeutic range based on the results of a single daily APTT may result in periods of inadequate anticoagulation and an increased risk of thromboembolic recurrence. Furthermore, because commercial thromboplastin reagents differ in their sensitivity to heparin, an APTT ratio of 1.5 obtained with a highly responsive reagent may not represent a therapeutic range.[123] In view of these concerns, a more prudent target for the lower limit of the APTT ratio during heparin therapy may be 2.0 rather than 1.5, especially during the initial few days of therapy.

The complexities involved in heparin administration and APTT monitoring may be diminished by the introduction of LMWH preparations into clinical practice that require a once- or twice-daily subcutaneous dose without monitoring. Thus, as these agents are introduced into clinical practice, current controversies about dose regimens and monitoring strategies may become historical footnotes.

A growing body of evidence suggests that LMWH administered subcutaneously is as safe and effective as conventional heparin administered intravenously for both venous thrombosis and pulmonary embolism.[104, 124, 125] The advantage of LMWH preparations arises from their increased bioavailability and longer half-life as well as the simplicity of subcutaneous administration once or twice daily without need for APTT monitoring. Clinicians must recognize, however, that the administration of LMWH preparations also requires clinical judgment. Standardized dosing is not possible in patients at the extremes of body weight; dose adjustments are necessary in patients with renal insufficiency due to renal clearance of the drug; the anticoagulant effect of the drug cannot be monitored easily; populations exist (e.g., patients at high bleeding risk) in which a longer drug half-life is not a desirable effect; the ability of protamine sulfate to reverse the anticoagulant effect remains uncertain; and drug costs are substantially higher than unfractionated heparin. Neither can all patients with venous thromboembolism be treated with LMWH in the outpatient setting. In studies performed, approximately 50% of patients were ineligible for outpatient therapy because of such factors as major bleeding risk, compliance problems, renal failure, significant comorbid disease, inadequate cardiopulmonary reserve, and inaccessibility for follow-up. Furthermore, early embolic recurrence can and does occur in patients treated with both unfractionated and LMWH preparations. Although this recurrence rate would not be diminished in an inpatient setting, the potential consequences of recurrence, especially in patients with preexisting cardiopulmonary disease, would be detected and managed more promptly in this setting. Even in patients who require initial inpatient management, however, the duration of hospitalization may be decreased considerably by a transition to outpatient LMWH. Validation in ongoing clinical trials is necessary to determine the safety, efficacy, and cost-effectiveness of these agents, particularly in potential early discharge or outpatient treatment of venous thromboembolism.

Recommendations regarding the duration of heparin therapy remain undefined. Although 7 to 10 days of intravenous heparin therapy has been the usual practice, studies using a 5-day course of therapy in patients with proximal venous thrombosis is associated with a recurrence rate identical to that of a 10-day course.[126] This assumes, of course, that warfarin is started early and is in a therapeutic range for 2 consecutive days before heparin is discontinued, an often difficult target to achieve. It is likely that a short course of intravenous heparin therapy would be similarly effective in patients with uncomplicated pulmonary embolism. However, a longer course of therapy is advisable in patients with major pulmonary embolism or extensive iliofemoral venous thrombosis.

The major complications of heparin are bleeding and the development of thrombocytopenia.[127, 128] There are no predisposing factors to heparin-associated thrombocytopenia other than a history of a previous incident. The incidence of arterial thrombosis with heparin-associated thrombocytopenia appears to be low, but when it occurs it is associated with considerable morbidity and mortality. If heparin-associated thrombocytopenia develops, warfarin should be instituted and consideration given to placement of an IVC filter. If more rapid anticoagulation is necessary than that provided by warfarin, a number of options exist that include defibrinating agents (ancrod), antithrombin drugs (hirudin and analogs), or heparanoids (danaparoid).[128] Danaparoid has minimal cross reactivity (5% to 10%) with unfractionated heparin and, in view of its ease of administration, appears to be the drug of choice in patients with heparin-associated thrombocytopenia. Cross reactivity with LMWH is relatively common, and these drugs should be avoided.[129]

### Inferior Vena Cava Filters

The established indications for filter placement include: protection against pulmonary embolism in patients with acute venous thromboembolism in whom conventional anticoagulation is contraindicated (e.g., recent surgery, hemorrhagic cerebrovascular accident, active bleeding, heparin-associated thrombocytopenia); protection against pulmonary embolism in patients with acute venous thromboembolism in whom conventional anticoagulation has proven ineffective; and protection of an already compromised pulmonary vascular bed from further thromboembolic risk (massive pulmonary embolism, chronic thromboembolic pulmonary hypertension).

With the increased ease of percutaneous filter placement, however, those indications have been expanded to include prophylaxis for patients without acute venous thrombosis but who are at high risk of developing it. This expansion in the indications for filter placement has occurred before the risks and benefits of such a strategy have been evaluated in a controlled manner. As noted previously, established prophylactic options, both pharmacologic and nonpharmacologic (intermittent pneumatic compression devices), are available for most high-risk patients.

Mortality from filter placement appears to be quite low regardless of which filter is used.[130, 131] Nonfatal complications of IVC filters, which occur with increased frequency, include: (1) complications relating to the insertion process; (2) venous thrombosis at the site of insertion; (3) filter migration; (4) filter erosion through the IVC wall; and (5) IVC obstruction. Most clinically important complications appears to involve venous thrombosis at the insertion site and IVC obstruction.

Whether anticoagulant therapy should follow filter placement is not clear. Filter placement, although protecting the pulmonary vascular bed, does nothing to lessen the occurrence or the extension of venous thrombosis. Small thrombi can pass through patent filters or through collateral vessels around obstructed filters; furthermore, thrombus extension can occur through the filter itself. Data suggest that vena caval filters are capable of diminishing the incidence of early thromboembolic recurrence; however, this benefit is offset by an increased long-term risk of recurrent deep vein thrombosis.[132] Before filter placement, the physician must be aware that this intervention is an irrevocable one (Fig. 51.9). In view of these considerations, long-term anticoagulation should be used after filter placement if no contraindications exist.

## MASSIVE PULMONARY EMBOLISM

The significant mortality associated with massive pulmonary embolism justifies a separate consideration of the diagnostic and therapeutic approach to this problem.[133]

The definition of massive pulmonary embolism should be based on hemodynamic considerations rather than purely anatomic ones. This impression is supported by mortality statistics from the urokinase trials and others.[134, 135] Although anatomically massive emboli have a greater likelihood of being associated with hemodynamic compromise, not all anatomically massive emboli lead to hemodynamic compromise. Regardless of the degree of vascular obstruction, patients with pulmonary embolism who present with shock have a mortality that is at least three- to fourfold greater than those without shock.

The therapeutic approach to the patient with hemodynamically massive pulmonary embolism should be designed to counteract the adverse physiologic consequence

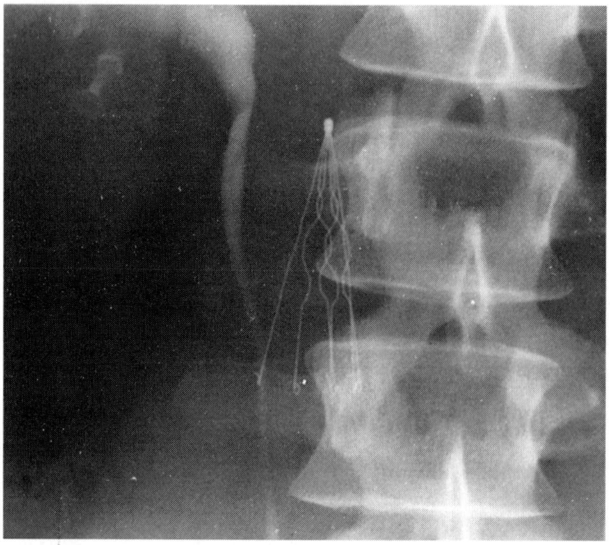

**Figure 51.9** Inferior vena cava filter in place below renal veins.

of pulmonary vascular obstruction, whether or not that obstruction is anatomically massive. Basic care of a critically ill patient should not be overlooked while specific diagnostic and therapeutic considerations are being implemented.[133] Oxygen should be administered to alleviate the hypoxic pulmonary vasoconstriction that might be contributing to the pulmonary hypertension. Intubation and mechanical ventilatory support might be required to improve oxygenation and decrease metabolic demands. Although volume resuscitation has been advised, excessive preload may further distend the right ventricle, resulting in decreased coronary perfusion and right ventricular ischemia. The judicious use of inotropic support also can prove useful in increasing blood pressure and supporting right ventricular function.[136] Although there is a tendency to use central hemodynamic monitoring in critically ill, hypotensive patients, this intervention should be considered carefully in the patient with massive pulmonary embolism. Inserting the catheter through the femoral vein poses the risk of dislodging residual ileofemoral thrombus. Furthermore, balloon flotation through the right ventricle poses the risk of dislodging embolic material that might be trapped within the atrial or ventricular cavities.

Although the central goal of therapy in massive pulmonary embolism should be to relieve pulmonary vascular obstruction, the severely compromised nature of the pulmonary vascular bed makes prevention of recurrence an important secondary consideration. Therefore, assuming the requisite expertise in filter placement is available and that placement of a filter will not interfere with the primary management of the patient, placement of a filter should be considered in all patients with hemodynamically massive embolism.

## Thrombolytic Therapy

The use of thrombolytic agents in acute pulmonary embolism remains controversial. Although thrombolytic therapy does appear to accelerate the rate of thrombolysis, there is no convincing evidence to suggest that it decreases mortality, increases the ultimate extent of resolution when measured at 7 days, reduces thromboembolic recurrence rates, improves symptomatic outcome, or decreases the incidence of thromboembolic pulmonary hypertension.[137] The one issue about which there can be little controversy is that the use of thrombolytic agents is associated with a substantially increased risk of bleeding, including intracranial hemorrhage. Intracranial hemorrhage has occurred in 0.5% to 2.0% of patients treated with thrombolytic agents in trials evaluating the use of these agents in both pulmonary embolism and myocardial infarction.

Based on these data, the role of thrombolytic therapy in pulmonary embolism should be limited to those circumstances in which an accelerated rate of thrombolysis may be considered lifesaving; that is, in those patients with pulmonary embolism associated with hemodynamic compromise. The finding of right ventricular dysfunction on echocardiography, a common accompaniment of embolism, in the absence of hemodynamic compromise should not serve as significant justification for thrombolytic therapy. There is little basis for exposing a patient to the considerable risk of hemorrhagic complications associated with thrombolytic therapy for a disease process whose outcome is excellent with the use of heparin therapy alone. This is especially true in view of the advances that have occurred in heparin administration strategies. Some have called for more widespread use of thrombolytic therapy based on the results of nonrandomized trials.[138] However, until it has been demonstrated in a randomized trial that the use of thrombolytic therapy results in improved mortality or long-term patient outcome, not short-term hemodynamic or angiographic improvement, when compared with heparin therapy alone, then such changes in the management philosophy remain unwarranted.

## Pulmonary Embolectomy

The role of pulmonary embolectomy in acute, hemodynamically massive pulmonary embolism also remains controversial.[139, 140] Patients with anatomically massive or submassive emboli who are hemodynamically compromised, who have not had a cardiac arrest, and who do not have an absolute contraindication to thrombolytic therapy should be managed initially with aggressive medical therapy: specifically, thrombolytic therapy plus heparin. Patients in whom acute embolectomy might be considered are those with hemodynamically massive pulmonary embolism who have an absolute contraindication to anticoagulant or thrombolytic therapy, those who have had a cardiopulmonary arrest (although the mortality associated with embolectomy in those who have is far greater than in those who have not), and those in whom aggressive medical therapy, including the use of thrombolytic agents, has proven ineffective. The concept of relieving the pulmonary vascular obstruction and decreasing right ventricular afterload with a percutaneous device designed to extract or fragment thrombi has been appealing. Several such devices have been tested, but their role in the treatment of massive pulmonary embolism remains investigative.[133, 141, 142]

## POSTEMBOLIC PROPHYLAXIS

The duration of outpatient anticoagulation for patients with pulmonary embolism remains a subject of controversy. Although the "standard" recommendation was for 3 months of outpatient therapy, durations of therapy as short as 4 weeks and as long as 6 months have been recommended. The most recent data suggest that a 6-month course of prophylactic oral anticoagulants after a first episode of venous thromboembolism leads to a lower recurrence rate than does treatment lasting 6 weeks. However, even beyond 6 months, recurrences continue.[143]

Much of the difficulty in making definitive recommendations regarding the duration of outpatient anticoagulation is the result of study design and the diverse populations studied. The presence of persistent venous outflow obstruction or postthrombotic venous valvular damage may represent continued risk factors for recurrence beyond those responsible for the initiating event. Patients with a clearly defined initial predisposition, whose initial thromboembolic risk factors have resolved and whose ventilation-perfusion scan and noninvasive lower extremity testing have normalized can likely be managed with a 3-month course of anticoagulation. Patients without a defined predisposition to thromboembolism and those with persistent ventilation-perfusion scan defects or abnormal lower extremity test results should be treated for 6 months or more. Patients with an ongoing risk factor should be treated until that risk factor resolves. Finally, patients with an irreversible acquired *or* genetic predisposition to venous thrombosis, major ventilation-perfusion scan defects, or a history of recurrent thromboembolic events should be treated with lifelong anticoagulation, even though such a strategy is associated with an increased risk of hemorrhagic complications.[144]

Such a strategy assumes that new "baseline" studies be performed when decisions whether outpatient anticoagulation can be stopped are first made. Although some may disagree with this approach for cost reasons, these studies provide useful information in guiding the duration of anticoagulation and may prove invaluable in the diagnostic and therapeutic sequence if recurrent venous thromboembolism is suspected after anticoagulation is discontinued.

Regarding postembolic anticoagulant "intensity," evidence suggests that maintaining the prothrombin time (PT) ratio at 1.3 to 1.5 times the control value is as effective in reducing recurrence rates as is maintaining the PT ratio at 2 times the control values, as previously recommended. However, as a result of considerable variability in the sensitivity of commercially available thromboplastins, the absolute PT or the PT ratio may understate or exaggerate the actual degree of warfarin effect, thereby leading to either excessive or inadequate anticoagulation.[145] To correct for these differences in thromboplastin sensitivity, the international normalized ratio (INR) as a means of reporting warfarin effect has been adopted.[146] The recommended therapeutic range for the INR in most patients with venous thromboembolism is 2.0 to 3.0. The exception to this rule are patients with antiphospholipid antibody syndrome in whom an INR of 3.0 to 4.0 appears more effective in reducing recurrence rates than an INR of less than 3.0.[147] In patients with a lupus anticoagulant, in whom the baseline INR may be elevated, the INR may not reliably reflect the level of anticoagulation. In these patients, the use of tests that are insensitive to the lupus anticoagulant, such as the prothrombin-proconvertin time or chromogenic factor X assay, have been recommended.[148]

## CHRONIC THROMBOEMBOLIC PULMONARY HYPERTENSION

As already discussed, most treated pulmonary emboli resolve over some weeks, which restores the pulmonary arterial bed to normal or near-normal status. In a very small percentage of patients, estimated to represent no more than 0.1% of the 450,000 patients who survive a pulmonary embolic event each year in the United States, such resolution does not occur and the residual obstruction is of sufficient extent to cause persistent pulmonary hypertension.[149]

There are, in fact, two forms of pulmonary hypertension that require consideration: one controversial and the other rather clearly defined. The controversial form consists of the obstruction of small, distal pulmonary arteries, the so-called thrombotic variant of primary pulmonary hypertension. The controversy centers on whether this entity ever is the result of recurrent, very small, unresolved emboli, or whether the thrombi seen are local consequences of endothelial injury. There is mounting evidence that embolism is not a cause but a consequence of primary pulmonary hypertension (see Chapter 52). All the small vessel lesions encountered in primary pulmonary hypertension, including the thrombotic lesions, also are found in other pulmonary hypertensive states. In terms of management options, however, this issue does not matter. Patients with small-vessel obstruction, with or without thrombotic lesions, are managed in the same fashion with vasodilator therapy, anticoagulation, and the potential consideration of transplantation.[150]

Quite different, however, is the other form of thromboembolic pulmonary hypertension that involves the central elastic vessels (main, lobar, and segmental arteries). Such patients should be considered separately because their thrombi are potentially accessible to pulmonary thromboendarterectomy.[151] The reasons that thromboembolic pulmonary hypertension develops are not clear; that is, it is not evident why this special minority of patients fails to resolve their emboli. It has been found that, in approximately half the patients, the initial diagnosis of pulmonary embolism was not made, and therefore, no treatment given.[151] Despite extensive investigation, the only identifiable thrombotic predisposition has been the presence of lupus anticoagulant in approximately 10% of patients.[152] The prevalence of antithrombin III or protein C or protein S deficiency does not appear to be higher than that encountered in the general population. Preliminary evidence also suggests that the factor V Leiden mutation is no more common in patients with chronic thromboembolic pulmonary hypertension than in the general population.

Neither has any consistent defect in fibrinolytic activity been identified.[153]

The diagnosis of thromboembolic pulmonary hypertension usually is not made until the degree of pulmonary hypertension is advanced. As a result, the exact hemodynamic evolution of the disease has not been fully established. The progressive nature of the pulmonary hypertension in most patients with chronic thromboembolic disease does not appear to be the result of recurrent embolic events or in situ thrombosis, as initially postulated. The majority of patients with sequential perfusion scans available for review experience symptomatic and hemodynamic decline in the absence of new perfusion defects. As experience with the diagnosis and surgical management of this disease process has grown, however, it has become increasingly apparent that the increase in pulmonary artery pressures arises from two different sources: a decrease in the cross-sectional area of the pulmonary vascular bed associated with the unresolved thromboembolic component of the disease and the development over time of a distal, small-vessel arteriopathy (see Fig. 50.6), which are pathologically indistinct from that seen in a wide range of pulmonary hypertensive disorders.[154] It appears that these secondary pulmonary hypertensive changes, perhaps induced by high pulmonary artery pressures or flows, result in an incremental increase in right ventricular afterload, progressive pulmonary hypertension, and, ultimately, right ventricular failure.

## Diagnosis

Perhaps the most important aspect of dealing with this patient group is the proper approach to its recognition. Progressive dyspnea is common to all patients with chronic thromboembolic pulmonary hypertension. Later in the course of the disease, exertional chest pain, near-syncope or syncope, or lower extremity edema may develop.

Although a history of documented thromboembolism may not be present, many patients can provide a history consistent with an acute embolic event. They may describe an episode of "pleurisy," lower extremity "muscle strain," or prolonged, atypical "pneumonia." They may describe a hospitalization or surgical procedure from which they never fully recovered. An episode of venous thromboembolism that was not diagnosed, or was misdiagnosed, is not surprising in view of data that confirm the high frequency with which venous thrombosis and pulmonary embolism are overlooked in the population at large.[20] Diagnostic delay, particularly in the absence of an acute history of venous thromboembolism, occurs commonly. Progressive dyspnea and exercise intolerance are often attributed to coronary artery disease, cardiomyopathy, interstitial lung disease, asthma, deconditioning, or psychogenic dyspnea. Unfortunately, the duration of diagnostic delay does not appear to have shortened substantially since the early 1990s, emphasizing that the status of the pulmonary vascular bed should be considered in any patient with persistent or progressive dyspnea in whom no compelling cause can be established.

Physical examination findings may be subtle early in the course of the illness, thereby contributing to this diagnostic delay. Before the development of significant right ventricular hypertrophy or overt right ventricular failure, physical examination abnormalities may be limited to a widening of the second heart sound or to a subtle accentuation of its pulmonic component. In time, obvious findings such as a right ventricular heave, jugular venous distension, prominent A and V wave venous pulsations, fixed splitting of S2, a right ventricular S3, murmurs of tricuspid regurgitation or pulmonic insufficiency, hepatomegaly, and ascites may develop. Peripheral edema, a result of chronic lower extremity venous outflow obstruction or right ventricular failure, may be present.

A unique physical finding in certain patients with chronic thromboembolic disease is the presence of flow murmurs over the lung fields.[155] These subtle bruits, which appear to originate from turbulent flow through partially obstructed or recanalized thrombi, are high pitched and blowing in quality, heard over the lung fields rather than the precordium, accentuated during inspiration, and frequently heard only during periods of breath-holding. Their importance arises in not having been described in primary pulmonary hypertension, which represents the most common competing diagnostic possibility.

The intent of the diagnostic evaluation is to establish the presence and degree of pulmonary hypertension, to define its etiology, and, if major vessel thromboembolic disease is present, to determine whether it is accessible to surgical intervention. Findings on standard laboratory tests are nonspecific, dependent on the point in the natural history of the disease at which they are obtained, and reflective of the hemodynamic and gas exchange consequences of the thromboembolic obstruction and the accompanying cardiac dysfunction.

Chest radiography, although often normal, may demonstrate findings that suggest the diagnosis. Enlargement of both main pulmonary arteries or asymmetry in the size of the central pulmonary arteries may be present (Fig. 51.10). Areas of hypoperfusion or hyperperfusion may be present. There may also be evidence of old pleural disease, unilaterally or bilaterally. The cardiac silhouette may reflect obvious right atrial or right ventricular enlargement; more often, right ventricular hypertrophy and enlargement are suggested only on the lateral film by encroachment on the normally empty retrosternal space.

Early in the course of the disease, electrocardiographic findings may be normal. Later in the course, electrocardiography demonstrates evidence of right ventricular hypertrophy. Pulmonary function testing, performed to evaluate the patient's dyspnea, is often within normal limits. Most patients have a reduction in the single breath diffusing capacity for carbon monoxide ($D_{LCO}$); a normal value, however, does not exclude the diagnosis. Approximately 20% of patients demonstrate a mild to moderate restrictive defect.[156] A mild obstructive defect also may be present as a result of mucosal hyperemia related to the large bronchial arterial collateral circulation that develops after pulmonary artery occlusion. The degree of spirometric defect, however, whether restrictive or obstructive, is almost always disproportionate to the patient's gas exchange abnormalities, symptomatic complaints, and degree of pulmonary hypertension.

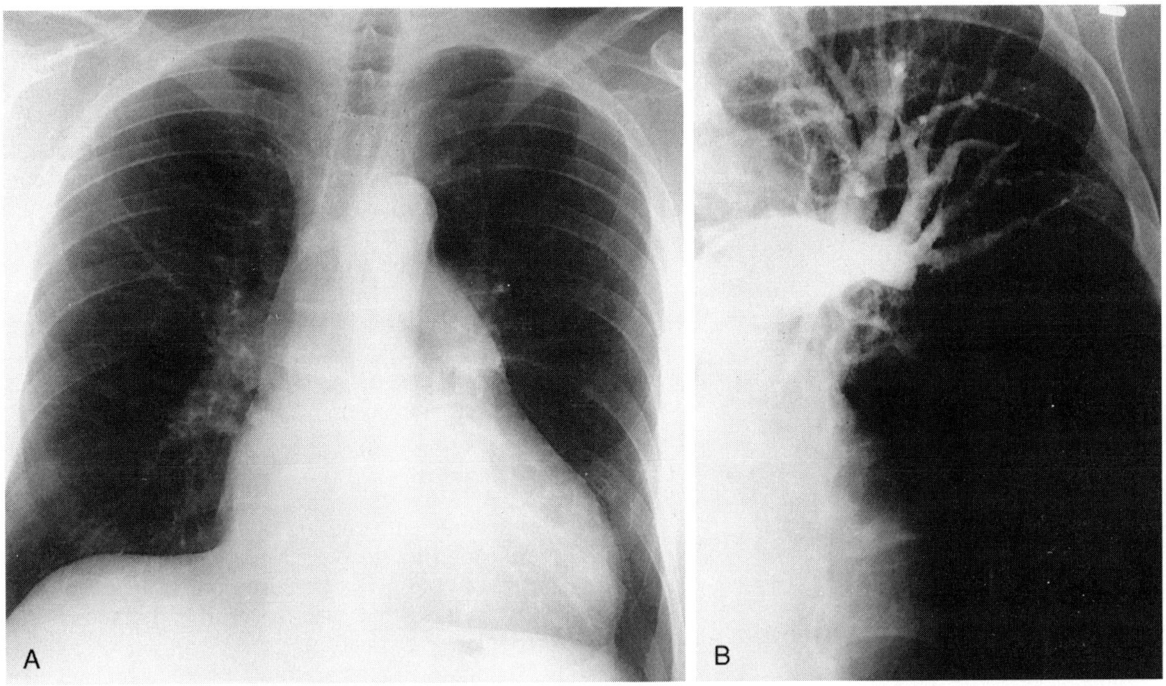


**Figure 51.10** Chest radiograph in a patient with chronic thromboembolic pulmonary hypertension. *A,* Note asymmetry of central pulmonary arteries, absence of descending left pulmonary artery, left lower lobe oligemia, and peripheral density representing prior infarct. *B,* Angiogram in same patient, demonstrating complete proximal occlusion of descending left pulmonary artery.

In terms of gas exchange findings, the arterial $P_{O_2}$ may be within normal limits. However, the alveolar-arterial oxygen gradient typically is widened, and most patients have a decline in the arterial $P_{O_2}$ with exercise. Wasted (dead-space) ventilation ($V_D/V_T$) often is increased at rest and worsens with exercise. Minute ventilation typically is elevated as a result of this increased dead-space ventilation.

Echocardiography commonly provides the initial objective evidence that pulmonary hypertension is present. Once the diagnosis of pulmonary hypertension has been established, determination of whether it originates from abnormalities of the small, resistance vessels or from central, chronic thromboembolic obstruction is essential. Ventilation-perfusion lung scanning appears to provide an excellent, noninvasive means of distinguishing between potentially operable major-vessel thromboembolic pulmonary hypertension and small-vessel pulmonary hypertension.[157] In chronic thromboembolic disease, at least one (and more commonly, several) segmental or larger mismatched ventilation-perfusion defects are present. In primary pulmonary hypertension, perfusion scans are either normal or exhibit a "mottled" appearance characterized by subsegmental defects.

The ventilation-perfusion scan often understates the actual extent of central pulmonary vascular obstruction.[158] Channels through—or partial flow around—central obstructing lesions, a result of the often complex patterns of recanalization and organization that occur after an embolic event, allow the radioisotopic agent to reach the periphery of the lung. Depending on the distribution of flow, these areas may appear normal or as relatively hypoperfused "gray zones." Ventilation-perfusion scanning, therefore, although capable of suggesting the potential presence of chronic thromboembolic obstruction, is incapable of determining the magnitude, location, or proximal extent of the disease, information critical to the question of surgical accessibility.

Right-heart catheterization and pulmonary angiography are essential to designate the degree of pulmonary hypertension, to exclude competing diagnoses, and to define the surgical accessibility of the obstructing thrombotic lesions. If hemodynamic measurements at rest demonstrate only modest degrees of pulmonary hypertension, measurements should be obtained after a short period of exercise.[159] In patients with chronic thromboembolic obstruction sufficient to abolish normal compensatory mechanisms, exercise-related increases in cardiac output are accompanied by an excessive elevation in pulmonary artery pressure.

The angiographic findings in chronic thromboembolic disease bear little resemblance to the sharply defined, intraluminal defects diagnostic of acute embolism.[160] Five distinct angiographic patterns have been described that correlate with the finding of organized thromboembolic material at the time of thromboendarterectomy (Fig. 51.11): (1) "pouch defects"; (2) pulmonary artery webs or bands; (3) intimal irregularities; (4) abrupt narrowing of the major pulmonary arteries; and (5) obstruction of lobar or segmental vessels at their point of origin, with complete absence of blood flow to pulmonary segments normally perfused by those vessels.

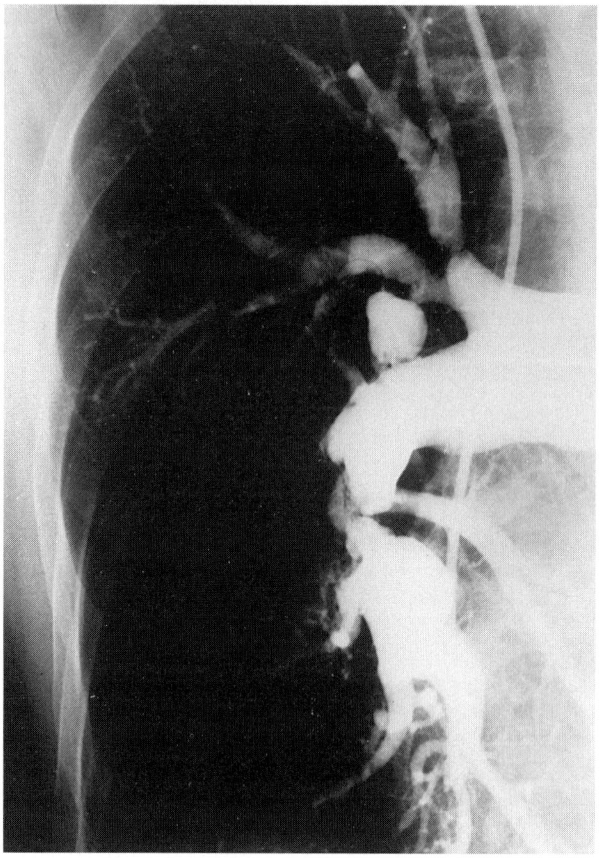

**Figure 51.11** Right-sided pulmonary angiogram in a patient with chronic thromboembolic pulmonary hypertension. Many of the classic angiographic findings associated with this disease are present, including pouch defects, intimal irregularity, pulmonary artery webs with poststenotic dilatation, and complete obstruction to flow of the right middle lobe and several lower lobe segmental arteries.

Pulmonary angioscopy has proven invaluable in confirming the presence of chronic thromboembolic obstruction and in determining whether it is accessible to surgical intervention.[161] The pulmonary angioscope is a fiberoptic device that allows visualization of the pulmonary arteries to the segmental level. The normal pulmonary artery has a round or oval contour with a smooth, pale, glistening appearance to the intima, and bright red blood filling the lumen (Fig. 51.12). The features of organized chronic emboli consist of roughening or pitting of the intimal surface, bands and webs across the lumen, pitted masses of chronic embolic material within the lumen, and partial recanalization.

Although pulmonary angiography/angioscopy usually completes the diagnostic sequence and confirms surgical accessibility, adjunctive studies may be necessary to exclude competing diagnoses. Computed tomography of the chest can be useful in determining whether a mediastinal process (e.g., fibrosing mediastinitis or malignancy) is responsible for the angiographic findings and, in selected cases, defining the extent and accessibility of the obstructing thrombi.[162] Arch aortography can be useful if an arteritis is being considered.[163]

The major conditions from which thromboembolic pulmonary hypertension must be distinguished are the following: primary pulmonary hypertension and other forms of secondary pulmonary hypertension, including fibrosing mediastinitis with pulmonary arterial or venous obstruction; pulmonary hypertension associated with congenital atrial or ventricular septal defects; congenital pulmonary artery branch stenoses; pulmonary artery agenesis; tumors arising in or obstructing the central pulmonary arteries; and Takayasu's arteritis. The standard diagnostic approaches previously discussed, preferably performed at a center experienced in the management of pulmonary hypertension, are capable of excluding most of these competing diagnoses.

## Treatment

For patients with chronic thromboembolic pulmonary hypertension, the decision to proceed to pulmonary thromboendarterectomy is based on both objective and subjective factors that are carefully defined during the preoperative evaluation.[151]

The first and most absolute criterion for potential surgical intervention is the accessibility of the thrombi as defined by angiography and angioscopy. Present surgical techniques allow removal of chronic thrombi whose proximal location extends to the main, lobar, and segmental arteries. Those that begin more distally are not subject to endarterectomy. The decision to recommend thromboendarterectomy is based on a complex decision-making process that includes pulmonary hemodynamic findings, pulmonary angiographic findings, and, when indicated, pulmonary angioscopic findings. The hemodynamic abnormality in chronic thromboembolic disease involves elements of the central, surgically accessible component of the disease; the distal, surgically inaccessible component of the disease; and the secondary, small-vessel arteriopathy resulting from the pulmonary hypertension itself. Operating on patients in the latter two categories is contraindicated. This determination is critical. Failure to remove sufficient chronic thromboembolic material to lower pulmonary vascular resistance, especially in patients with severe pulmonary hypertension and right ventricular dysfunction, is associated with an adverse long-term outcome and may result in an inability to wean the patient from cardiopulmonary bypass at the time of the thromboendarterectomy. Therefore, during the evaluative process, it is essential to partition the three elements of the patient's pulmonary hypertension. To do so successfully, considerable expertise is required in angiographic-angioscopic-surgical correlation, expertise that can be gained only through extensive clinical experience with this unique group of patients.

The second criterion involves the presence of hemodynamic or ventilatory impairment as a consequence of the chronic thromboembolic pulmonary vascular obstruction. The majority of operated patients have a pulmonary vascular resistance in excess of 300 dyne-sec•cm$^{-5}$, at rest or with exercise. Occasionally, patients, especially those with involvement of one main pulmonary artery, have a significant exercise impairment because of high minute ventilation demands without substantially altered pulmo-

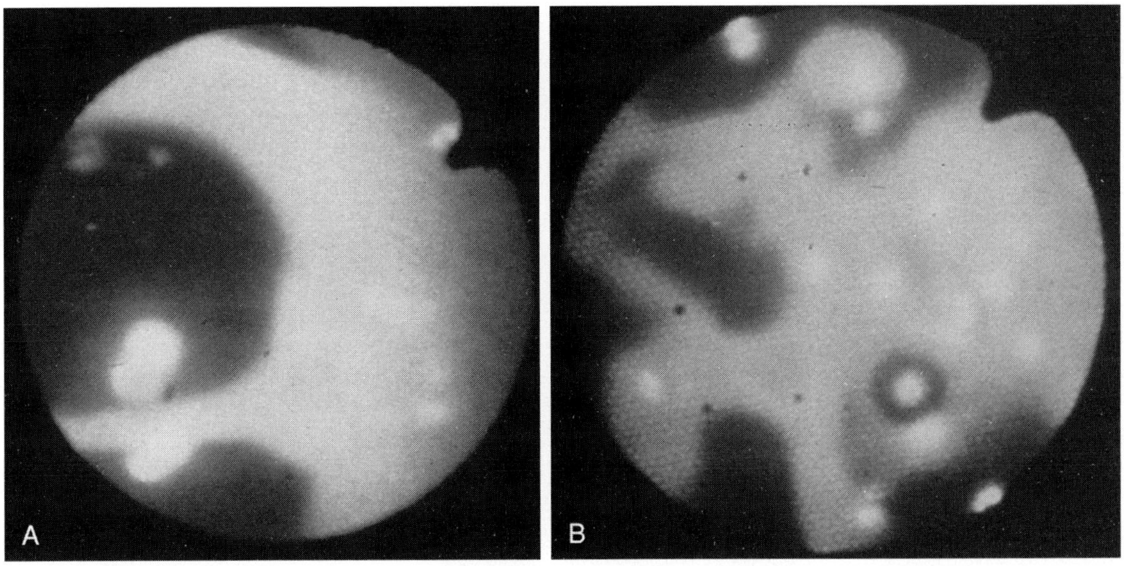


**Figure 51.12** Pulmonary angioscopy. *A*, Angioscopic appearance of normal pulmonary artery. *B*, Angioscopic appearance of chronic thromboembolic pulmonary artery obstruction demonstrating multiple, recannalized channels.

nary hemodynamics. The option of surgery also is considered in those patients with only moderate degrees of pulmonary hypertension at rest but who demonstrate significant increases in pulmonary artery pressure with exercise. Because this hemodynamic response reproduces events during the patient's activities of daily living, it may reflect the true workload of the right ventricle. Furthermore, in view of what now is known about the pathophysiologic mechanisms of the disease, it is likely that the exercise-related augmentation of pressure and flow over a sufficient period of time will result in progressive worsening of pulmonary hypertension.

The third criterion is the absence of comorbid conditions, such as severe parenchymal lung disease, which may adversely affect outcome. Although the presence of coexisting disease processes does not represent an absolute contraindication to the procedure, the risks imposed by the condition and its potential effect on long-term outcome are reviewed carefully with the patient before a surgical decision is made. Age in itself is not a contraindication to the procedure. Patients up to 80 years of age, if they are otherwise fit, have successfully undergone a pulmonary thromboendarterectomy.

Before surgery, several other essential issues must be considered. It is important that the patient be protected against embolic recurrence, both over the long term and during the high-risk perioperative period. Therefore, an IVC filter should be placed before surgery unless an obvious nonleg or nonpelvic source of embolism is present. For those at risk of coronary artery disease, coronary angiography is performed routinely before surgery, usually at the time of the right-heart catheterization and pulmonary angiogram. Coronary artery bypass grafting, if necessary, can be performed at the time of the thromboendarterectomy.

Although a thoracotomy approach to chronic thromboembolic pulmonary hypertension has been used in the past, sternotomy with cardiopulmonary bypass and periods of circulatory arrest represent the procedure of choice because sternotomy allows access to both pulmonary arteries, provides a bloodless operative field, and ensures more complete removal of the chronically obstructing material.[164, 165] Considerable experience is required by the surgical team to identify the correct operative plane and to remove the segmental-level extensions of the more proximal obstruction (Fig. 51.13). Failure to do so results in an inadequate hemodynamic outcome.

Although an immediate improvement in pulmonary hemodynamics occurs, the postoperative course can be complex. In addition to complications common to other forms of cardiac surgery (arrhythmias, atelectasis, wound infection, pericardial effusions, delirium), patients undergoing pulmonary thromboendarterectomy often experience two unique complications capable of significantly impairing gas exchange: reperfusion pulmonary edema and pulmonary artery "steal."[166–168]

Pulmonary artery "steal" (Fig. 51.14) represents a postoperative redistribution of pulmonary arterial blood flow away from previously well-perfused segments and into the newly endarterectomized segments.[166] Long-term follow-up has demonstrated that pulmonary vascular steal resolves in most patients.[167] Reperfusion pulmonary edema appears to represent a form of high-permeability lung injury, which is limited to those areas of lung from which proximal thromboembolic obstructions have been removed (Fig. 51.15). It may appear up to 72 hours after surgery and is highly variable in severity, ranging from a mild form of edema resulting in postoperative hypoxemia to an acute, hemorrhagic, and fatal complication.[168] When associated with pulmonary artery steal, reperfusion pulmonary edema can represent a significant challenge in terms of postoperative gas exchange. Pulmonary blood flow is directed toward edematous, noncompliant areas of lung, which contribute poorly to gas exchange. Manage-

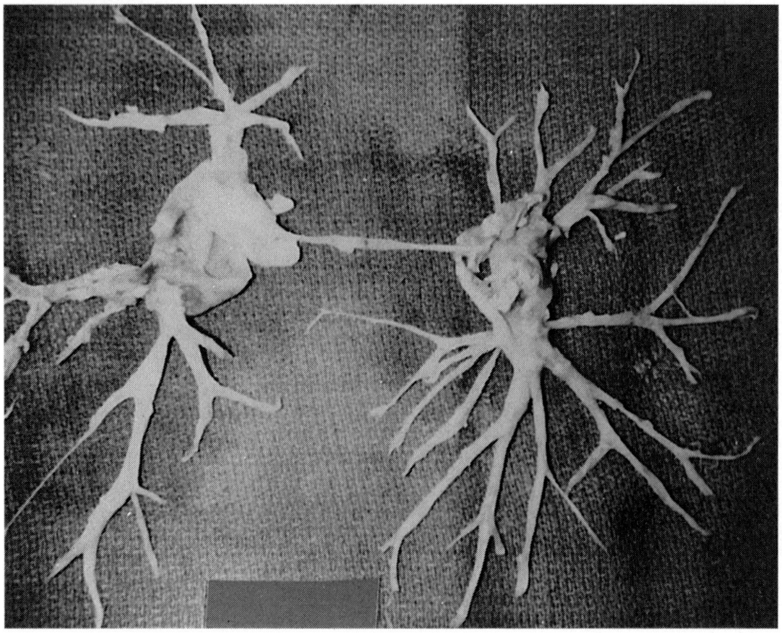

**Figure 51.13** Specimen obtained at the time of pulmonary thromboendarterectomy. In addition to central thromboembolic obstruction, note multiple segmental extensions. Failure to adequately remove these distal extensions results in an inadequate hemodynamic outcome.

ment of reperfusion edema, as with other forms of acute lung injury, is supportive until resolution occurs.

Among survivors of thromboendarterectomy, the immediate hemodynamic improvement observed has been dramatic, with marked reductions in pulmonary artery pressures and pulmonary vascular resistance (Fig. 51.16). At centers experienced with this procedure, the total operative and postoperative mortality rate has approximated 7%, with most deaths occurring in patients in New York Heart Association Class IV. At centers with less experience in the evaluation, surgical management, and postoperative care of these patients, the reported mortality has

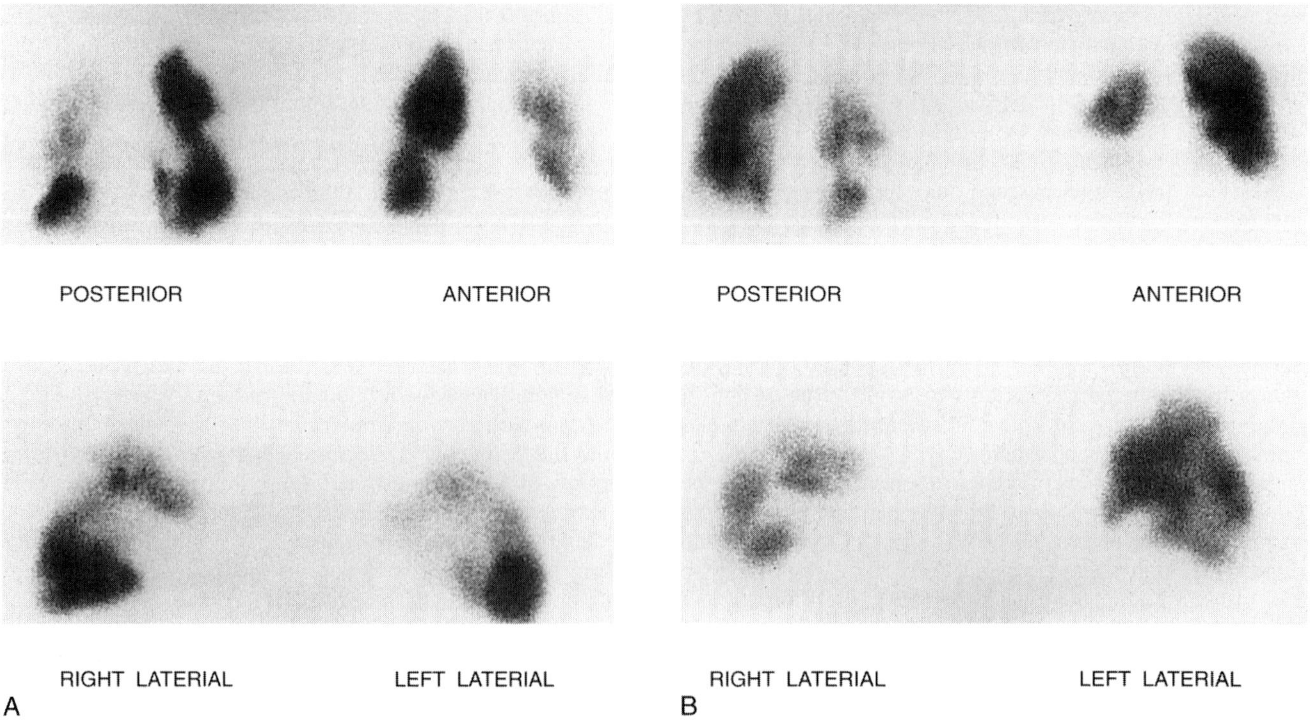


**Figure 51.14** Perfusion scans showing pulmonary artery steal. *A,* Preoperative perfusion scan demonstrating minimal flow to the left lung. *B,* Perfusion scan obtained in early postoperative period demonstrating dramatic reversal of flow with vascular "steal" from right lung. Equilibration and normalization of flow over time is the rule.

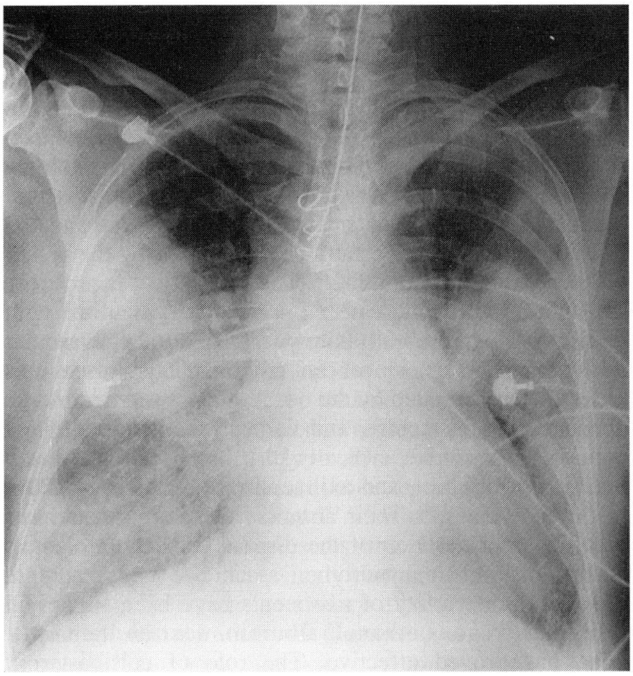

**Figure 51.15** Chest radiograph showing postoperative reperfusion pulmonary edema. Only the upper lobes are spared, from which no thromboembolic material was dissected.

been approximately threefold higher.[169–170] The long-term hemodynamic and symptomatic outcomes have been equally dramatic. Many patients are restored to normal activity, and essentially all have improved at least one grade in the classification of cardiac disability.[171] Long-term follow-up of 308 patients showed sustained benefit and greatly improved quality of life.[171a]

## OTHER FORMS OF EMBOLISM

Because the lungs receive all the blood flow returned from the venous system, the pulmonary vascular bed serves as a "sieve" for all particulates entering the venous blood and is the first vascular bed to be exposed to any toxic substance injected intravenously. As a result of its strategic position, the pulmonary vascular bed is, therefore, exposed to a wide variety of potentially obstructing and injurious agents.

### Schistosomiasis

Among such agents, the most common on a worldwide basis, although not within the United States, is schistosomiasis.[172] This parasitic disorder causes severe pulmonary vascular obstruction by two mechanisms: anatomic obstruction by the organism itself and an intense, inflammatory vasculitic response to the components of the organism. In endemic areas, schistosomal disease is the most common cause of cor pulmonale. Limited data suggest that cardiopulmonary schistosomiasis is seen most often in *Schistosoma mansoni* infection. This form of cor pulmonale does not occur in the absence of concomitant severe schistosomal liver disease because the liver always is involved, usually extensively, before pulmonary involvement occurs. The premortem diagnosis of cardiopulmonary schistosomiasis depends on the detection of viable schistosomal ova in stool or urine, along with evidence of hepatic fibrosis and pulmonary hypertension. Treatment options are discussed in Chapter 36. Several agents can effectively eradicate schistosomal infections

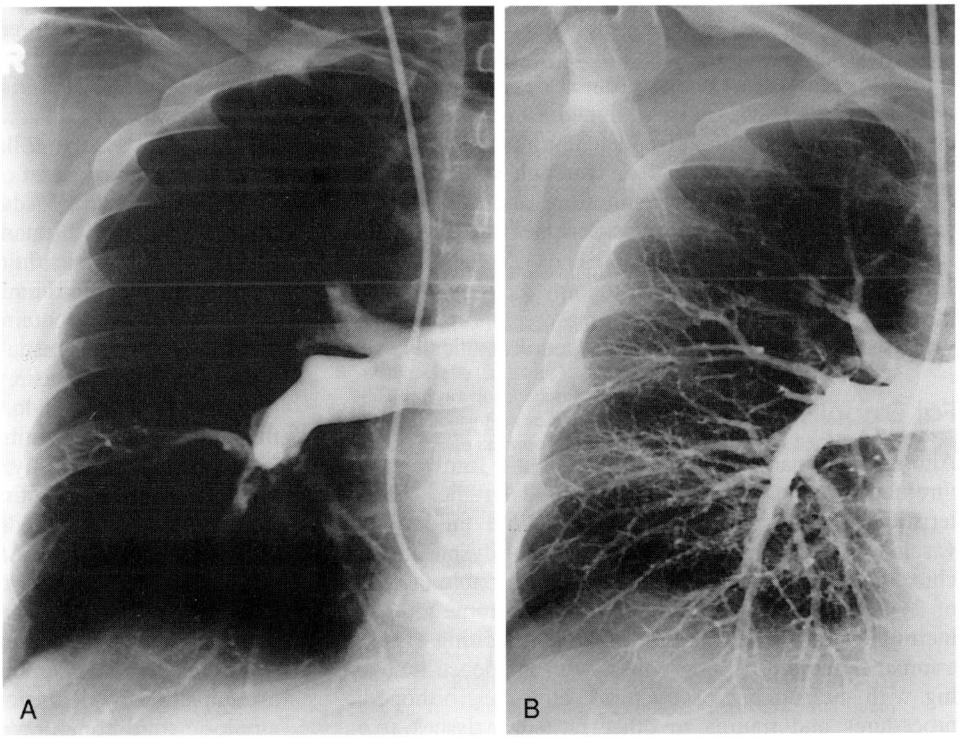


**Figure 51.16** *A,* Preoperative pulmonary angiogram showing thromboembolic obstruction involving left upper lobe, lingula, and lower lobe pulmonary arteries. *B,* Postoperative angiogram showing dramatic improvement of flow. This angiographic improvement was accompanied by a corresponding hemodynamic improvement.

12. Poort SR, Rosendaal FR, Reitsma PH, et al: A common genetic variation in the 3′-untranslated region of the prothrombin gene is associated with elevated plasma prothrombin levels and an increase in venous thrombosis. Blood 88:3698–3703, 1996.
13. Martinelli I, Sacchi E, Landi G, et al: High risk of cerebral-vein thrombosis in carriers of a prothrombin-gene mutation and in users of oral contraceptives. N Engl J Med 338:1793–1797, 1998.
14. Heijer M, Koster T, Blom HJ, et al: Hyperhomocysteinemia as a risk factor for deep-vein thrombosis. N Engl J Med 334:759–762, 1996.
15. Mandel H, Brenner B, Berant M, et al: Coexistence of hereditary homocystinuria and factor V Leiden—Effect on thrombosis. N Engl J Med 334:763–768, 1996.
16. Nachman RL, Silverstein R: Hypercoagulable states. Ann Intern Med 119:819–827, 1993.
17. Anderson FA, Wheeler HB: Venous thromboembolism: Risk factors and prophylaxis. Clin Chest Med 16:235–251, 1995.
18. Sevitt S, Gallagher N: Venous thrombosis and pulmonary embolism: A clinicopathological study in injured and burned patients. Br J Surg 48:475–489, 1961.
19. Haire D: Arm vein thrombosis. Clin Chest Med 16:341–352, 1995.
20. Ryu JH, Olson EJ, Pellikka PA: Clinical recognition of pulmonary embolism: Problem of unrecognized and asymptomatic cases. Mayo Clin Proc 73:873–879, 1998.
21. Moser KM, LeMoine JR: Is embolic risk conditioned by location of deep venous thrombosis? Ann Intern Med 94:439–434, 1981.
22. Lagerstedt CI, Olsson CG, Fagher B, et al: Need for long-term anticoagulant treatment in symptomatic calf-vein thrombosis. Lancet 2:515–518, 1985.
23. Stradness DE, Langlois Y, Cramer M, et al: Long-term sequelae of acute venous thrombosis. JAMA 250:1289–1292, 1983.
24. Hirsh J, Hull RD, Raskob GE: Epidemiology and pathogenesis of venous thrombosis. J Am Coll Cardiol 8:104B–113B, 1986.
25. Moser KM: Venous thromboembolism: State of the art. Am Rev Respir Dis 141:235–249, 1990.
26. Severinghaus JW, Swenson EW, Finley TN, et al: Unilateral hypoventilation produced by occlusion of one pulmonary artery. J Appl Physiol 16:53–57, 1961.
27. Sergysels R: Pulmonary gas exchange abnormalities in pulmonary embolism. *In* Morpurgo M (ed): Pulmonary Embolism: Lung Biology in Health and Disease. Vol 75. New York: Marcel Dekker, 1994, pp. 89–96.
28. Huet Y, Lemaire F, Brun-Buisson C, et al: Hypoxemia in acute pulmonary embolism. Chest 88:829–836, 1985.
29. Manier G, Castaing Y, Guenard H: Determinants of hypoxemia during the acute phase of pulmonary embolism in humans. Am Rev Respir Dis 132:332–338, 1985.
30. D'Alonzo GE, Bower JS, Dehart P, et al: The mechanisms of abnormal gas exchange in acute massive pulmonary embolism. Am Rev Respir Dis 128:170–172, 1983.
31. Cherniak V, Hodson WA, Greenfield LJ: Effect of chronic pulmonary artery ligation on pulmonary mechanics and surfactant. J Appl Physiol 21:1315–1319, 1966.
32. Shure D: The bronchial circulation in pulmonary vascular obstruction. *In* Butler J (ed): The Bronchial Circulation: Lung Biology in Health and Disease (Vol 57). New York: Marcel Dekker, 1992, pp. 579–597.
33. Jandik J, Endrys J, Rehulová E, et al: Bronchial arteries in experimental pulmonary infarction: Angiographic and morphometric study. Cardiovasc Res 27:1076–1083, 1993.
34. McIntyre KM, Sasahara AA: Hemodynamic and ventricular response to pulmonary embolism. Prog Cardiovasc Dis 17:175–190, 1974.
35. McIntyre KM, Sasahara AA: The hemodynamic response to pulmonary embolism in patients without prior cardiopulmonary disease. Am J Cardiol 17:288–294, 1971.
36. Elliott CG: Pulmonary physiology during pulmonary embolism. Chest 101:163S–171S, 1992.
37. James WS, Minh VD, Minteer MA, et al: Rapid resolution of pulmonary embolus in man. West J Med 128:60–64, 1978.
38. Dalen JE, Banas JS, Brooks HL: Resolution rate of acute pulmonary embolism in man. N Engl J Med 280:1194–1199, 1969.
39. Tow DE, Wagner HN Jr: Recovery of pulmonary arterial blood flow in patients with pulmonary embolism. N Engl J Med 275:1053–1059, 1967.
40. Cranley JJ, Canos AJ, Sull WJ: The diagnosis of deep venous thrombosis: Fallibility of clinical symptoms and signs. Arch Surg 111:34–36, 1976.
41. Kakkar VV, Howe CT, Flanc C, et al: Natural history of post-operative deep vein thrombosis. Lancet 2:230–232, 1969.
42. Landefeld CS, McGuire E, Cohen AM: Clinical findings associated with deep vein thrombosis: A basis for quantifying clinical judgement. Am J Med 88:382–388, 1990.
43. Wells PS, Hirsh J, Anderson DR, et al: Accuracy of clinical assessment of deep-vein thrombosis. Lancet 345:1326–1330, 1995.
44. Moser KM, Fedullo PF: Venous thromboembolism: Three simple decisions. Chest 83:117–121, 256–260, 1983.
45. Goldhaber SZ, Hennekens CH, Evans DA, et al: Factors associated with the correct antemortem diagnosis of major pulmonary embolism. Am J Med 73:822–826, 1982.
46. Stein PD, Terrin ML, Hales CA, et al: Clinical, laboratory, roentgenographic, and electrocardiographic findings in patients with acute pulmonary embolism and no pre-existing cardiac or pulmonary disease. Chest 100:598–603, 1991.
47. The PIOPED Investigators: Value of the ventilation/perfusion scan in acute pulmonary embolism: Results of the Prospective Investigation Of Pulmonary Embolism Diagnosis (PIOPED). JAMA 263:2753–2759, 1990.
48. Stein PD, Terrin ML, Hales CA, et al: Clinical, laboratory, roentgenographic, and electrocardiographic findings in patients with acute pulmonary embolism and no pre-existing cardiac or pulmonary disease. Chest 100:598–603, 1991.
49. Monroel M, Ruiz J, Olazabal A, et al: Deep venous thrombosis and the risk of pulmonary embolism: A systematic study. Chest 102:677–681, 1992.
50. Murray HW, Ellis GC, Blumenthal DS, Sos TA: Fever and pulmonary thromboembolism. Am J Med 67:232–235, 1979.
51. Aburahma AF, Saiedy S: Deep vein thrombosis as probable cause of fever of unknown origin. W V Med J 93:368–370, 1997.
52. Rabinov K, Paulin S: Roentgen diagnosis of venous thrombosis in the leg. Arch Surg 104:134–144, 1972.
53. Lensing AWA, Prandoni P, Brandjes D, et al: Detection of deep-vein thrombosis by real-time b-mode ultrasonography. N Engl J Med 320:342–345, 1989.
54. Cronan JJ, Dorfman GS, Scola FH, et al: Deep venous thrombosis: US assessment using vein compression. Radiology 162:191–194, 1987.
55. Pedersen OM, Aslaksen A, Vik-Mo H, et al: Compression ultrasonography in hospitalized patients with suspected deep venous thrombosis. Arch Intern Med 151:2217–2220, 1991.
56. Pezzulo JA, Perkins AB, Cronan JJ: Symptomatic deep vein thrombosis: Diagnosis with limited compression ultrasound. Radiology 198:67–70, 1996.
57. Naidich JB, Torre JR, Pellerito JS, et al: Suspected deep venous thrombosis: Is US of both legs necessary? Radiology 200:429–431, 1996.
58. Wells PS, Lensing AWA, Davidson BL, et al: Accuracy of ultrasound for the diagnosis of deep venous thrombosis in asymptomatic patients after orthopedic surgery: A meta-analysis. Ann Intern Med 122:47–53, 1995.
59. Habscheid W, Höhmann M, Wilhelm T, et al: Real-time ultrasound in the diagnosis of acute deep venous thrombosis of the lower extremity. Angiology 41:599–608, 1990.
60. Hull R, Hirsh J, Sackett DL, et al: Combined use of leg scanning and impedance plethysmography in suspected venous thrombosis: An alternative to venography. N Engl J Med 296:1497–1500, 1977.
61. Hull R, Hirsh J, Sackett DL, et al: Replacement of venography in suspected venous thrombosis by impedance plethysmography and 125-I-fibrinogen leg scanning: A less invasive approach. Ann Intern Med 94:12–15, 1981.
62. Heijboer H, Cogo A, Buller HR, et al: Detection of deep-vein thrombosis with impedance plethysmography and real-time compression ultrasonography in hospitalized patients. Arch Intern Med 152:1901–1903, 1992.
63. Ginsberg JS, Wells PS, Hirsh J, et al: Reevaluation of the sensitivity of impedance plethysmography for the detection of proximal deep vein thrombosis. Arch Intern Med 94:439–444, 1994.
64. Wells PS, Hirsh J, Anderson DR, et al: Comparison of the accu-

racy of impedance plethysmography and compression ultrasonography in outpatients with clinically suspected deep vein thrombosis: A two centre paired-design prospective trial. Thromb Haemost 74:1423–1427, 1995.
65. Huisman MV, Buller HR, ten Cate JW, et al: Serial impedance plethysmography for suspected deep venous thrombosis in outpatients. N Engl J Med 314:823–828, 1986.
66. Huisman MV, Buller HR, ten Cate JW, et al: Management of clinically suspected acute venous thrombosis in outpatients with serial impedance plethysmography in a community hospital setting. Arch Intern Med 149:511–513, 1989.
67. Heijboer H, Buller HR, Lensing AWA, et al: A comparison of real-time compression ultrasonography with impedance plethysmography for the diagnosis of deep-vein thrombosis in symptomatic outpatients. N Engl J Med 329:1365–1369, 1993.
68. Ginsberg JS, Caco CC, Brill-Edwards P, et al: Venous thrombosis in patients who have undergone major hip or knee replacement: Detection with compression ultrasound and impedance plethysmography. Radiology 181:651–654, 1991.
69. Hull RD, Carter CJ, Jay RM: The diagnosis of acute, recurrent deep vein thrombosis: A diagnostic challenge. Circulation 67:901–906, 1983.
70. Huisman MV, Buller HR, ten Cate JW: Utility of impedance plethysmography in the diagnosis of recurrent deep-vein thrombosis. Arch Intern Med 148:681–683, 1988.
71. Evans AJ, Sostman HD, Witty LA, et al: Detection of DVT: Prospective evaluation of MRI and sonography. J Magn Reson Imaging 1:44–51, 1996.
72. Carpenter JP, Holland GA, Baum RA, et al: Magnetic resonance venography for the detection of deep venous thrombosis: comparison with contrast venography and duplex Doppler ultrasonography. J Vasc Surg 18:734–741, 1993.
73. Worsley DF, Alavi A, Aronchick JTT, et al: Chest radiographic findings in patients with acute pulmonary embolism: Observations from the PIOPED study. Radiology 189:133–136, 1993.
74. Stein PD, Terrin ML, Hales CA, et al: Clinical, laboratory, roentgenographic, and electrocardiographic findings in patients with acute pulmonary embolism and no pre-existing cardiac or pulmonary disease. Chest 100:598–603, 1991.
75. Stein PD, Dalen JE, McIntyre KM, et al: The electrocardiogram in acute pulmonary embolism. Prog Cardiovasc Dis 17:247–257, 1975.
76. Stein PD, Goldhaber SZ, Henry JW, et al: Arterial blood gas analysis in the assessment of suspected acute pulmonary embolism. Chest 109:78–81, 1996.
77. Benotti JR, Dalen JE, Alpert JS: Pulmonary embolism. *In* Rippe JM, Irwin RS, Alpert JS, et al (eds): Intensive Care Medicine (2nd ed). Boston: Little Brown and Company, 1991, pp. 308–314.
78. McConnell MV, Solomon SD, Rayan ME: Regional right ventricular dysfunction detected by echocardiography in acute pulmonary embolism. Am J Cardiol 78:469–473, 1996.
79. Krivec B, Voga G, Zuran I, et al: Diagnosis and treatment of shock due to massive pulmonary embolism: Approach with transesophageal echocardiograpy and intrapulmonary thrombolysis. Chest 112:1310–1316, 1997.
80. Sohn DW, Shin GJ, Oh JK, et al: Role of transesophageal echocardiograpy in hemodynamically unstable patients. Mayo Clin Proc 70:925–931, 1995.
81. Ginsberg JS, Kearon C, Douketis J, et al: The use of D-dimer testing and impedance plethysmographic examinations in patients with clinical indications of deep venous thrombosis. Arch Intern Med 157:1077–1081, 1997.
82. Perrier A, Bounameaux H, Morabia A, et al: Diagnosis of pulmonary embolism by a decision analysis-based strategy including clinical probability, D-dimer levels, and ultrasonography: A management study. Arch Intern Med 156:531–536, 1996.
83. Perrier A, Desmarais S, Goehring C, et al: D-dimer testing for suspected pulmonary embolism in outpatients. Am J Respir Crit Care Med 156:492–496, 1997.
84. Moser KM: Diagnosing pulmonary embolism: D-dimer needs rigorous evaluation. BMJ 309:1525–1526, 1994.
85. Freyburger G, Trillaud H, Labrouche S, et al: D-dimer strategy in thrombosis exclusion—A gold standard study in 100 patients suspected of deep venous thrombosis or pulmonary embolism: 8 DD methods compared. Thromb Haemost 79:32–37, 1998.
85a. Quinn DA, Fogel RB, Smith CD, et al: D-Dimers in the diagnosis of pulmonary embolism. Am J Respir Crit Care Med 159:1445–1449, 1999.
86. Hull RD, Raskob GE, Pineo GF, et al: The low-probability lung scan: A need for change in nomenclature. Arch Intern Med 155:1845–1851, 1995.
87. Bone RC: The low-probability lung scan: A potentially lethal reading. Arch Intern Med 153:2621–2622, 1993.
88. Miniati M, Pistolesi M, Marini C, et al: Value of perfusion lung scan in the diagnosis of pulmonary embolism: Results of the Prospective Investigative Study of Acute Pulmonary Embolism Diagnosis (PISA-PED). Am J Respir Crit Care Med 154:1387–1393, 1996.
88a. Miniati M, Prediletto R, Formichi B, et al: Accuracy of clinical assessment in the diagnosis of pulmonary embolism. Am J Respir Crit Care Med 159:864–871, 1999.
89. Stein PD, Terrin ML, Gottschalk A, et al: Value of ventilation/perfusion scans versus perfusion scans alone in acute pulmonary embolism. Am J Cardiol 69:1239–1241, 1992.
90. Lesser BA, Leeper KV, Stein PD, et al: The diagnosis of acute pulmonary embolism in patients with chronic obstructive lung disease. Chest 102:17–22, 1992.
91. Remy-Jardin M, Remy J, Deschildre F, et al: Diagnosis of pulmonary embolism with spiral CT: Comparison with pulmonary angiography and scintigraphy. Radiology 200:699–706, 1996.
92. Remy-Jardin M, Remy J, Wattinne L, et al: Central pulmonary thromboembolism: Diagnosis with spiral volumetric CT with the single breath hold technique—Comparison with pulmonary angiography. Radiology 185:381–387, 1992.
93. Goodman LR, Curtin JJ, Mewissen MW, et al: Detection of pulmonary embolism in patients with unresolved clinical and scintigraphic diagnosis: Helical CT versus angiography. AJR Am J Roentgenol 164:1369–1374, 1995.
94. Oser RF, Zuckerman DA, Gutierrez FR, et al: Severity of pulmonary emboli at pulmonary arteriography: Implications for spiral and ultrafast CT (abstract). Radiology 193(P):352, 1994.
95. Goodman LR, Lipchik RJ: Diagnosis of acute pulmonary embolism: time for a new approach. Radiology 199: 25–27, 1996.
96. Stein PD, Athanasoulis C, Alavi A, et al: Complications and validity of pulmonary angiography in acute pulmonary embolism. Circulation 85:462–468, 1992.
97. Nicod P, Peterson K, Levine M, et al: Pulmonary angiography in severe chronic pulmonary hypertension. Ann Intern Med 107:565–568, 1987.
98. Newman GE: Pulmonary angiography in pulmonary embolic disease. J Thorac Imaging 4:29–39, 1989.
99. Planes A, Vochelle, Darmon JY, et al: Risk of deep-venous thrombosis after hospital discharge in patients having undergone total hip replacement: Double-blind randomised comparison of enoxaparin versus placebo. Lancet 348:224–228, 1996.
100. Prevention of fatal postoperative pulmonary embolism by low doses of subcutaneous heparin. An International Multicentre Trial. Lancet 2:45–51, 1975.
101. Mohr DN, Silverstein MD, Murtaugh PA, et al: Prophylactic agents for venous thrombosis in elective hip surgery. Arch Intern Med 153:2221–2228, 1993.
102. Geerts WH, Jay RM, Code KI, et al: A comparison of low-dose heparin with low-molecular weight heparin as prophylaxis against venous thromboembolism after major trauma. N Engl J Med 335:701–707, 1996.
103. Clagett GP, Anderson FA Jr, Heit J, et al: Prevention of venous thromboembolism. Chest 108:312S–334S, 1995.
104. Weitz JI: Low-molecular-weight heparins. N Engl J Med 337:688–698, 1997.
105. Clagett GP, Reisch JS: Prevention of venous thromboembolism in general surgical patients. Ann Surg 208:227–240, 1988.
106. Comerota AJ, Katz ML, White JV: Why does prophylaxis with external pneumatic compression for deep venous thrombosis fail? Am J Surg 164:265–269, 1992.
107. Francis CW, Marder VJ, McCollister EC, et al: Two step warfarin therapy: Prevention of postoperative venous thrombosis without excessive bleeding. JAMA 249:374–378, 1983.
108. Hirsh J: Oral anticoagulant drugs. N Engl J Med 324:1865–1875, 1991.
109. Becker DM, Philbrick JT, Selby JB: Inferior vena cava filters: In-

dications, safety, effectiveness. Arch Intern Med 152:1985–1994, 1992.
110. Anderson FA Jr, Wheeler HB, Goldberg RG, et al: Physician practices in the prevention of venous thromboembolism. Ann Intern Med 115:591–595, 1991.
111. Keane MC, Ingenito EP, Goldhaber SZ: Utilization of venous thromboembolism prophylaxis in the medical intensive care unit. Chest 106:13–22, 1994.
112. Hull RD, Pineo GF: Current concepts of anticoagulation therapy. Clin Chest Med 16:269–280, 1995.
113. Hull RD, Raskob GE, Hirsh J, et al: Continuous intravenous heparin compared with intermittent subcutaneous heparin in the initial treatment of proximal vein thrombosis. N Engl J Med 315:1109–1114, 1986.
114. Wheeler RH, Jaquiss RD, Newman JH: Physician practices in the treatment of pulmonary embolism and deep venous thrombosis. Arch Intern Med 148:1321–1325, 1988.
115. Cruikshank MK, Levine MN, Hirsh J, et al: A standard nomogram for the management of heparin therapy. Arch Intern Med 151:333–337, 1991.
116. Raschke RA, Reilly BM, Guidry JR, et al: The weight based heparin dosing nomogram compared with a "standard care" nomogram: A randomized controlled study. Ann Intern Med 119:874–881, 1993.
117. Hull RD, Raskob GE, Rosenbloom DR, et al: Optimal therapeutic level of heparin therapy in patients with venous thromboembolism. Arch Intern Med 152:1589–1595, 1992.
118. Prandoni P, Bagatella P, Bernardi E, et al: Use of an algorithm for administering subcutaneous heparin in the treatment of deep venous thrombosis. Ann Intern Med 129:299–302, 1998.
119. Levine MN, Hirsh J, Gent M, et al: A randomized trial comparing actived thromboplastin time with heparin assay in patients with acute venous thromboembolism requiring large daily doses of heparin. Arch Intern Med 154:49–56, 1994.
120. Hull RD, Raskob GE, Rosenbloom DR, et al: Optimal therapeutic level of heparin therapy in patients with venous thromboembolism. Arch Intern Med 152:1589–1595, 1992.
121. Hull RD, Raskob GE, Brant RF, et al: The importance of initial heparin threatment on long-term clinical outcomes of antithrombotic therapy: The emerging theme of delayed recurrence. Arch Intern Med 157:2317–2321, 1997.
122. Decousus HA, Croze M, Levi FA, et al: Circadian changes in anticoagulant effect of heparin infused at a constant rate. BMJ 200:341–344, 1985.
123. Baker BA, Adelman MD, Smith PA, Osborn JC: Inability of the activated partial thromboplastin time to predict heparin levels. Time to reassess guidelines for heparin assays. Arch Intern Med 157:2475–2479, 1997.
124. The Columbus Investigators: Low-molecular weight heparin in the treatment of patients with venous thromboembolism. N Engl J Med 337:657–662, 1997.
125. Simonneau G, Sors H, Charbonnier B, et al: A comparison of low-molecular weight heparin with unfractionated heparin for acute pulmonary embolism. N Engl J Med 337:663–669, 1997.
126. Hull RD, Raskob GE, Rosenbloom D, et al: Heparin for 5 days as compared with 10 days in the initial treatment of proximal venous thrombosis. N Engl J Med 322:1260–1264, 1990.
127. Landfeld CS, Beyth RJ: Anticoagulant-related bleeding: Clinical epidemiology, prediction and prevention. Am J Med 95:315–328, 1993.
128. Hirsh J, Raschke R, Warkentin TE, et al: Heparin: Mechanisms of action, pharmacokinetics, dosing considerations, monitoring, efficacy and safety. Chest 108:258S–275S, 1995.
129. Warkentin TE, Levine MN, Hirsh J, et al: Heparin-induced thrombocytopenia in patients treated with low molecular weight heparin or unfractionated heparin. N Engl J Med 332:1330–1335, 1995.
130. Becker DM, Philbrick JT, Selby JB: Inferior vena cava filters: Indications, safety, effectiveness. Arch Intern Med 152:1985–1994, 1992.
131. Ferris, EJ, McCowan TC, Carver DK, et al: Percutaneous inferior vena caval filters: Follow-up of seven designs in 320 patients. Radiology 188:851–856, 1993.
132. Decousus H, Leizorovicz A, Parent F, et al: A clinical trial of vena caval filters in the prevention of pulmonary embolism in patients with proximal deep-vein thrombosis. N Engl J Med 338:409–415, 1998.
133. Tapson VF, Witty LA: Massive pulmonary embolism: Diagnostic and therapeutic strategies. Clin Chest Med 16:329–340, 1995.
134. Blackmon JR, Sautter RD, Wagner HN, et al: Urokinase pulmonary embolism trial: Phase 1 results. JAMA 214:2163–2172, 1970.
135. Bell W, Blackmon JR, DeGroot W, et al: Urokinase-streptokinase embolism trial: Phase 2 results. JAMA 229:1606–1613, 1974.
136. Layish DT, Tapson VF: Pharmacologic hemodynamic support in massive pulmonary embolism. Chest 111:218–224, 1997.
137. Dalen JE, Alpert JS, Hirsch J: Thrombolytic therapy for pulmonary embolism: Is it effective? Is it safe? When is it indicated? Arch Intern Med 157:250–2556, 1997.
138. Konstantinides S, Geigel A, Olschewski M, et al: Association between thrombolytic treatment and the prognosis of hemodynamically stable patients with major pulmonary embolism: Results of a multicenter registry. Circulation 96:882–888, 1997.
139. Gray HH, Miller GAH, Paneth M: Pulmonary embolectomy: Its place in the management of pulmonary embolism. Lancet 1:1441–1445, 1988.
140. Gray HH, Morgan JM, Paneth M, et al: Pulmonary embolectomy for acute massive pulmonary embolism: An analysis of 71 cases. Br Heart J 60:196–200, 1988.
141. Greenfield LJ, Proctor MS: Role of catheter-embolectomy in treating pulmonary embolism. Semin Respir Crit Care Med 17:95–99, 1996.
142. Stein PD, Sabbah HN, Basha MA, et al: Mechanical disruption of pulmonary emboli in dogs with a flexible rotating-tip catheter (Kensey Catheter). Chest 98:994–998, 1990.
143. Schulman S, Sofie-Rhedin A, Lindmarker P, et al: A comparison of six weeks with six months of oral anticoagulant therapy after a first episode of venous thromboembolism. N Engl J Med 332:1661–1665, 1995.
144. Schulman S, Granqvist S, Holmstrom M, et al: The duration of oral anticoagulant therapy after a second episode of venous thromboembolism. N Engl J Med 336:393–398, 1997.
145. Bussey HI, Force RW, Bianco TM, et al: Reliance on prothrombin time ratios causes significant errors in anticoagulation therapy. Arch Intern Med 152:278–282, 1992.
146. Hirsh J, Poller L: The international normalized ratio: A guide to understanding and correcting its problems. Arch Intern Med 154:282–288, 1994.
147. Khamashta MA, Cuadrado MJ, Jujic F, et al: The management of thrombosis in the antiphospholipid-antibody syndrome. N Engl J Med 332:993–997, 1995.
148. Moll S, Ortel TL: Monitoring warfarin therapy in patients with lupus anticoagulants. Ann Intern Med 127:177–185, 1997.
149. Moser KM, Auger WR, Fedullo PF: Chronic major-vessel thromboembolic pulmonary hypertension. Circulation 81:1735–1743, 1990.
150. Rubin LJ: Primary pulmonary hypertension. Chest 104:236–250, 1993.
151. Fedullo PF, Auger WR, Channick RN, et al: Chronic thromboembolic pulmonary hypertension. Clin Chest Med 16:353–374, 1995.
152. Auger WR, Moser KM, Fedullo PF, et al: The association of heparin-induced thrombocytopenia and the lupus anticoagulant in patients with chronic thromboembolic pulmonary hypertension. Am Rev Respir Dis 143:A-803, 1991.
153. Olman MA, Marsh JJ, Lang IM, et al: Endogenous fibrinolytic system in chronic large-vessel thromboembolic pulmonary hypertension. Circulation 86:1241–1248, 1992.
154. Moser KM, Bloor CM: Pulmonary vascular lesions occurring in patients with chronic major vessel thromboembolic pulmonary hypertension. Chest 103:685–692, 1993.
155. Auger WR, Moser KM: Pulmonary flow murmurs; a distinctive physical sign found in chronic pulmonary thromboembolic disease (abstract). Clin Res 37:145A, 1989.
156. Morris TA, Auger WR, Ysrael MZ, et al: Parenchymal scarring is associated with restrictive defects in patients with chronic thromboembolic pulmonary hypertension. Chest 110:399–403, 1996.
157. Fishmann AJ, Moser KM, Fedullo PF: Perfusion lung scans vs pulmonary angiography in evaluation of suspected primary pulmonary hypertension. Chest 84:679–683, 1983.

158. Ryan KL, Fedullo PF, Davis GB, et al: Perfusion scan findings understate the severity of angiographic and hemodynamic compromise in chronic thromboembolic pulmonary hypertension. Chest 93:1180–1185, 1988.
159. Fedullo PF, Auger WR, Moser KM, et al: Hemodynamic response to exercise in patients with chronic, major vessel thromboembolic pulmonary hypertension (abstract). Am Rev Respir Dis 141:A-890, 1990.
160. Auger WR, Fedullo PF, Moser KM, et al: Chronic major-vessel thromboembolic pulmonary artery obstruction: Appearance at angiography. Radiology 182:393–398, 1992.
161. Shure D, Gregoratos G, Moser KM: Fiberoptic angioscopy: Role in the diagnosis of chronic pulmonary arterial obstruction. Ann Intern Med 103:844–850, 1995
162. Bergin CJ, Sirlin CB, Hauschildt JP, et al: Chronic thromboembolism: Diagnosis with helical CT and MR imaging with angiographic and surgical correlation. Radiology 204:695–702, 1997.
163. Kerr KM, Auger WR, Fedullo PF, et al: Large vessel pulmonary arteritis mimicking thromboembolic disease. Am J Respir Crit Care Med 152:367–373, 1995.
164. Chitwood WR, Sabiston DC, Wechsler AS, et al: Surgical treatment of chronic unresolved pulmonary embolism. Clin Chest Med 5:507–536, 1984.
165. Jamieson SW, Auger WR, Fedullo PF, et al: Experience and results with 150 pulmonary thromboendarterectomy operations over a 29-month period. J Thorac Cardiovasc Surg 106:116–127, 1993.
166. Olman MA, Auger WR, Fedullo PF, Moser KM: Pulmonary vascular steal in chronic thromboembolic pulmonary hypertension. Chest 98:1430–1434, 1990.
167. Moser KM, Metersky JL, Auger WR, Fedullo PF: Resolution of vascular steal after pulmonary thromboendarterectomy. Chest 104:1441–1444, 1993.
168. Levinson R, Shure D, Moser KM: Reperfusion pulmonary edema after pulmonary artery thromboendarterectomy. Am Rev Respir Dis 134:1241–1245, 1986.
169. Hartz R, Byrne JG, Levitsky S, et al: Predictors of mortality in pulmonary thromboendarterectomy. Ann Thorac Surg 62:1255–1260, 1996.
170. Mayer E, Dahm M, Hake U, et al: Mid-term results of pulmonary thromboendarterectomy for chronic thromboembolic pulmonary hypertension. Ann Thorac Surg 61:1788–1792, 1996.
171. Moser KM, Daily PO, Peterson K, et al: Thromboendarterectomy for chronic major-vessel thromboembolic pulmonary hypertension: Immediate and long-term results in 42 patients. Ann Intern Med 107:560–565, 1987.
171a. Archibald CJ, Auger WR, Fedullo PF, et al: Long-term outcome after pulmonary thromboendarterectomy. Am J Respir Crit Care Med 160:523–528, 1999.
172. Morris W, Knauer CM: Cardiopulmonary manifestations of schistosomiasis. Semin Respir Infect 12:159–170, 1997.
173. King MB, Harmon KR: Unusual forms of pulmonary embolism. Clin Chest Med 15:561–580, 1994.
174. Butler BD, Hills BA: The lung as a filter for microbubbles. J Appl Physiol 47:537–543, 1979.
175. Durant TM, Long J, Oppenheimer MJ: Pulmonary (venous) air embolism. Am Heart J 33:269–281, 1947.
176. Alvaran SB, Tuong JK, Graff TE, et al: Venous air embolism: Comparative merits of external cardiac massage, intracardiac aspiration, and left lateral decubitus position. Anesth Analg 57:166–170, 1978.
177. Armon C, Deschamps C, Adkinson C, et al: Hyperbaric treatment of cerebral air embolism sustained during an open-heart surgical procedure. Mayo Clin Proc 66:565–571, 1991.
178. Tibbles PM, Edelsberg JS: Hyperbaric-oxygen treatment. N Engl J Med 334:1642–1648, 1996.
179. Johnson MJ, Lucas GL: Fat embolism syndrome. Orthopedics 19:41–48, 1996.
180. Gossling H, Pellegrini V: Fat embolism syndrome: A review of the pathophysiology and physiological basis for treatment. Clin Orthop 165:68–82, 1982.
181. Bruecke P, Burke JF, Lam KW, et al: Pathophsiology of the pulmonary fat embolism. J Thorac Cardiovasc Surg 61:949–955, 1971.
182. Richards RR: Fat embolism syndrome. Can J Surg 40:334–349, 1997.
183. Martin RW: Amniotic fluid embolism. Clin Obstet Gynecol 39:101–106, 1996.
184. Hollingsworth HM, Irwin RS: Acute respiratory failure in pregnancy. Clin Chest Med 13:723–740, 1992.
185. Clark SL: Amniotic fluid embolism. Crit Care Clin 7:877–883, 1991.
186. Clark SL, Hankins GD, Dudley DA, et al: Amniotic fluid embolism: Analysis of the national registry. Am J Obstet Gynecol 172:1158–1167, 1995.
187. Collins CG: Suppurative pelvic thrombophlebitis: II. Symptomatology and diagnosis. Surgery 30:311–327, 1951.
188. Julander I. Staphylococcal septicaemia and endocarditis in 80 drug users. Scand J Infect Dis 41:49–54, 1983.
189. Pittet D, Hulliger S, Auckenthaler R: Intravascular device-related infections in critically ill patients. J Chemother 7(Suppl 3):55–66, 1995.
190. Clarke DE, Raffin TA: Infectious complications of indwelling long-term central venous catheters. Chest 97:966–972, 1990.
191. Robertson CH Jr, Reynolds RC, Wilson JE: Pulmonary hypertension and foreign body granulomas in intravenous drug abusers. Am J Med 61:657–662, 1976.

# 52 Pulmonary Vasculitis and Primary Pulmonary Hypertension

LEWIS J. RUBIN, M.D.

Introduction
Pulmonary Vasculitis
- Classification
- Epidemiology
- Pathology
- Pathogenesis and Etiology
- Symptoms
- Physical Findings
- Diagnosis
- Treatment
- Specific Disorders

Primary Pulmonary Hypertension
- Classification
- Epidemiology
- Pathology
- Pathogenesis and Etiology
- Symptoms
- Physical Findings
- Diagnosis
- Treatment and Prognosis

Summary

## INTRODUCTION

Disorders affecting the pulmonary circulation constitute a heterogeneous group without unifying or characteristic etiologic, physiologic, or pathologic features. Many of these diseases, however, share a variety of clinical manifestations that are the result of the disruption of the delicate interface between the ventilation and perfusion components of gas exchange and the impact of altered pulmonary vascular dynamics on the function of the right ventricle. This chapter addresses two forms of pulmonary vascular disease: the vasculitides and primary pulmonary hypertension. Other pulmonary vascular disorders or complications that are discussed in this section include thromboembolism in Chapter 51, arteriovenous fistulas and other malformations in Chapter 53, pulmonary edema and acute lung injury in Chapter 54, and cor pulmonale in Chapter 55.

## PULMONARY VASCULITIS

The vasculitides are a diverse group of disorders that are characterized by inflammation within and surrounding the blood vessel walls.[1] When the inflammation leads to destruction of the blood vessels, the process often is referred to as a necrotizing vasculitis.[2] Many investigators restrict application of the terms *vasculitis* and *angiitis* to only those disorders in which necrosis is evident. In this chapter, the terms *pulmonary vasculitis* and *pulmonary angiitis* are applied to inflammatory disorders of the pulmonary blood vessels with or without necrosis.[3]

### Classification

Vasculitis first was identified as a distinct clinicopathologic entity in 1837 by Schönlein[4] in describing the disease currently known as *anaphylactoid purpura*. Kussmaul and Maier[5] in 1866 described the syndrome of *polyarteritis nodosa* in a patient with fever, muscle weakness, gastrointestinal symptoms, and renal disease in whom a diffuse necrotizing vasculitis was found at autopsy. Over the subsequent years, this term has been used to describe patients with a variety of vasculitides attributed to hypersensitivity reactions to drugs, infectious antigens, rheumatic diseases, and other disorders.

A number of attempts have been made to classify and organize the pulmonary vasculitides.[8] However, these efforts have lacked consensus because these conditions overlap considerably in clinical manifestations and morphologic features and because their causes are unknown. The American College of Rheumatology has proposed diagnostic criteria for various vasculitides, based on a study of 807 patients who met specific criteria established for the diagnosis of several types of vasculitis.[9–17] Subjects with vasculitis secondary to underlying connective tissue diseases were excluded from this study. These criteria may prove useful to clinicians for both the diagnosis and the classification of vasculitic entities.

## Epidemiology

Pulmonary vasculitis is an uncommon condition despite the relative frequency of collagen vascular diseases and other conditions that may be associated with vasculitis in the general population. Even *Wegener's granulomatosis*, perhaps the best known pulmonary vasculitis, rarely is encountered in clinical practice; Fauci and Wolff[18] noted that only 200 cases of this disorder had been reported up to 1967, although the true incidence probably was higher. The incidence of other pulmonary vasculitides for the most part remains unknown.

Pulmonary vasculitis can occur in persons of all ages, although anaphylactoid purpura is more common among children, and the granulomatous vasculitides usually affect patients in their fifth and sixth decades.[8] Vasculitis associated with collagen vascular disease is described most often among women, as is *necrotizing sarcoid angiitis* and granulomatosis. Conversely, Wegener's granulomatosis, *lymphomatoid granulomatosis*, and *allergic granulomatosis* and angiitis are reported most frequently in men. Familial and racial predispositions are noted primarily in patients with the collagen vascular disorders and giant cell arteritis.

## Pathology

Inflammation, frequently extending through all layers of the blood vessel wall, is the hallmark of pulmonary vasculitis. With the exception of *bronchocentric granulomatosis*, this process is angiocentric because it appears to originate in the blood vessels, although surrounding tissues frequently are involved. Arteries and veins of all sizes may be involved, and capillaritis may accompany these pathologic changes in some conditions. Fibrinoid necrosis often accompanies the inflammation, as do intimal proliferation and perivascular fibrosis. Because these processes may cause obstruction of the blood vessels, pulmonary vasculitis often leads to obliterative pulmonary vascular disease. Secondary thrombosis also may contribute to vascular obstruction in this setting.

The inflammatory cells responsible for pulmonary vasculitis include neutrophils, normal and abnormal lymphocytes, eosinophils, monocytes, macrophages, histiocytes, plasma cells, multinucleated giant cells, and combinations thereof. Vasculitis is called leukocytoclastic if neutrophils predominate and granulomatous if lymphocytes predominate. However, lymphocytes may be abundant in areas of leukocytoclastic vasculitis if the process is more than 24 hours old, just as mononuclear cells, histiocytes, and multinucleated giant cells may outnumber lymphocytes in the later stages of granulomatous vasculitis.[2, 19]

## Pathogenesis and Etiology

Despite their differences, the pulmonary vasculitides appear to share a common immunopathogenesis. This concept is supported by several observations.[1–3] Leukocytoclastic vasculitis, polyarteritis nodosa, and essential mixed cryoglobulinemia may occur with illnesses such as hepatitis B infection, which are associated with immune complex deposition within blood vessel walls. Vasculitis may be a component of collagen vascular disorders, in which immunologic pathogenetic mechanisms are well accepted. Patients with vasculitis may manifest serologic abnormalities associated with immunodysfunction, including the presence of rheumatoid factor, cryoglobulinemia, hyperglobulinemia, hypocomplementemia, and circulating immune complexes. Vasculitis may be associated temporally with infections, drug ingestion, and other kinds of antigen exposure. The upper and lower airway involvement with granulomatous vasculitis in particular suggests that foreign antigens may enter the body via the respiratory tract. Finally, these and other vasculitides frequently respond to immunosuppressive or cytotoxic therapy.

Many investigators believe that pulmonary vasculitis is caused by a type III hypersensitivity reaction involving the deposition of immune complexes in blood vessels.[1] Although the antigens responsible for this process rarely have been identified, streptococcal M protein, hepatitis B surface antigen, and *Mycobacterium tuberculosis* have been found in or near the site of vascular inflammation. Immunoglobulins M, G, and A and complement breakdown products also have been localized in the blood vessels of patients with leukocytoclastic vasculitis, polyarteritis nodosa, and collagen vascular disorders.[2] How the antigens and antibodies come together is not certain; the antigens may bind to vascular basement membranes, diffuse into the blood vessels from surrounding tissues, or travel in the bloodstream. Whatever the mechanism, a significant excess of antigen over antibody is necessary to create immune complexes that are small enough to elude the reticuloendothelial system yet insoluble enough to deposit in blood vessel walls.[8]

The blood vessels also must be predisposed to accept immune complexes. Such acceptance probably involves local vasodilation and increased vascular permeability that are mediated by vasoactive amines released by platelets, mast cells, and basophils. After the immune complexes are deposited, complement activation is thought to occur by either the direct or the alternate pathway.[1] Certain complement components, such as C3a, cause further vasodilation and increased vascular permeability, whereas C5a and its breakdown product, C5a des arginine, attract neutrophils; circulating total complement and complement components are decreased. The neutrophils then are stimulated to ingest the immune complexes and to release toxic enzymes and oxygen radical species.[3]

Although this sequence can be implicated in leukocytoclastic vasculitis and polyarteritis nodosa, it may not apply to granulomatous vasculitis, in which immune complex deposition rarely is demonstrated and complement levels are increased. These facts and the characteristic histology of granulomatous vasculitis have prompted the hypothesis that cell-mediated immune events are involved in this condition. The involvement may be secondary because it follows immune complex deposition that cannot be detected. Whether such deposition occurs or not, sensitized T lymphocytes are assumed to contact antigens and either cause direct cytotoxicity or recruit mononuclear cells to the site. These mononuclear cells in turn become activated macrophages that release lysosomal enzymes. At the same time, some of the cells evolve into the histiocytes and multinucleated giant cells that participate in granuloma formation.[1]

## Symptoms

In general, systemic symptoms more commonly accompany the vasculitides that produce minimal pulmonary involvement, whereas respiratory complaints predominate among the vasculitides that primarily involve the lungs.[1–3, 8] For example, the initial manifestations of leukocytoclastic vasculitis include fever, malaise, arthralgias, and skin lesions. Symptoms referable to the skin and joints also are seen among patients with collagen vascular disorders and polyarteritis nodosa.[20] In contrast, dyspnea and cough frequently occur among patients with granulomatous vasculitis; symptoms related to the upper airways, including sinus pain and epistaxis, suggest Wegener's granulomatosis and lymphomatoid granulomatosis.[8] Hemoptysis also is reported in these disorders and may be massive in patients with pulmonary artery aneurysms[3] or diffuse capillaritis. Periodic dyspnea or a history of asthma is characteristic of allergic granulomatosis and angiitis (Churg-Strauss syndrome)[15, 21]; according to a recent review of 96 patients, asthma was the most frequent manifestation at presentation.[21a]

## Physical Findings

The physical findings generally parallel the symptoms of patients with pulmonary vasculitis. For example, purpura, bullae, and dermal ulcers may be evident in patients with leukocytoclastic vasculitis.[2] Joint deformity is suggestive of rheumatoid arthritis, whereas thickening of the skin and Raynaud's phenomenon may accompany progressive systemic sclerosis.[20] Erosions of the nose and upper airways are characteristic of Wegener's granulomatosis and lymphoid granulomatosis; proptosis caused by orbital pseudotumors and sclerouveitis also are seen in the former condition.[8] Iritis and oral and genital ulcers are hallmarks of Behçet's syndrome. Peripheral nerve lesions are especially common in polyarteritis nodosa. Central nervous system lesions are described in the giant cell arteritides and other conditions.[1] Patients with eosinophilia-myalgia syndrome frequently manifest many of the features of systemic sclerosis; in addition, they may have peripheral neuropathy, myositis, and fasciitis.[22, 23]

## Diagnosis

Despite certain characteristic presentations, the vasculitides rarely can be diagnosed solely on clinical grounds. Potentially helpful laboratory studies include the erythrocyte sedimentation rate, which usually is elevated in giant cell arteritis, and the differential white blood cell count, which is normal in most patients with vasculitis but may show an eosinophilia in patients with allergic granulomatosis and angiitis[13] or eosinophilia-myalgia syndrome.[22, 23] An elevation of immunoglobulins, a decrease in total complement and complement components, and the presence of circulating immune complexes may be present in leukocytoclastic vasculitis.[2] Determinations of rheumatoid factor levels, antinuclear antibody patterns, and antineutrophil cytoplasmic antibodies[24] are useful in the differential diagnosis of collagen vascular diseases and Wegener's granulomatosis, respectively.

Leukocytoclastic vasculitis and the vasculitis associated with collagen vascular disorders characteristically cause patchy infiltrates when they involve the lungs. Pleural effusions have been reported among patients with anaphylactoid purpura, collagen vascular disease,[8] and Churg-Strauss syndrome.[25] The angiocentric granulomatous vasculitides usually cause patchy infiltrates or pulmonary nodules; the latter often are bilateral and may cavitate.[8] Bronchocentric granulomatosis, conversely, is associated with fleeting infiltrates similar to those seen in allergic bronchopulmonary aspergillosis and mucoid impaction.[26] Visualization of the upper airways through plain roentgenograms or computerized tomography often is employed in the evaluation of Wegener's granulomatosis and lymphoid granulomatosis.[3] Angiographic studies frequently are undertaken in patients with polyarteritis nodosa, giant cell arteritis, and Takayasu's arteritis.

Hypoxemia, often in concert with hypocapnia and chronic respiratory alkalosis, is present in many patients whose lungs are involved with vasculitis.[3] Pulmonary function tests usually reveal normal or mildly reduced flow rates and lung volumes, unless obstructive or restrictive disorders coexist. Pulmonary vascular obstruction may be suggested by a decreased diffusing capacity for carbon monoxide, an increased dead space-to-tidal volume ratio, and an increased alveolar-to-arterial $PO_2$ difference at rest, which worsen during progressive exercise.[27]

Given the general lack of clinical experience with pulmonary vasculitis, a tissue biopsy may be needed for diagnosis. Skin biopsy is the preferred initial approach in patients with lesions attributable to granulomatous vasculitis, leukocytoclastic vasculitis, or polyarteritis nodosa.[2] If this approach is not helpful, upper airway biopsy may be revealing in patients suspected of having Wegener's granulomatosis or lymphomatoid granulomatosis. Renal biopsy is not recommended in patients with the former condition because granulomas usually are not present; the lungs are therefore a preferred biopsy site.[8] Transbronchial biopsy frequently is not helpful in the evaluation of pulmonary vasculitis because of the small amount of tissue obtained. As a result, many investigators recommend lung biopsy, which now can be performed thoracoscopically.[8] This recommendation needs to be reconsidered in light of the recent information that nearly all patients (>90%) with active Wegener's granulomatosis have a test result positive for cytoplasmic (as opposed to perinuclear) antineutrophil cytoplasmic antibodies (ANCAs).[28] Current opinion holds that ANCAs are a highly specific objective marker for the important group of vasculitides that includes Wegener's granulomatosis, polyarteritis nodosa, Churg-Strauss syndrome, and pauci-immune glomerulonephritis with or without pulmonary hemorrhage.[29] Temporal artery biopsy is employed in establishing the diagnosis of temporal arteritis.

## Treatment

Leukocytoclastic vasculitis often is self-limited and responds to removal of the offending antigen. A trial of corticosteroids may be used if extensive disease or pulmonary complications such as hypoxemia are present, although their general utility is unclear.[2] Corticosteroids also have been used for allergic granulomatosis and angiitis, necrotizing sarcoid granulomatosis, bronchocentric granulomatosis, eosinophilia-myalgia syndrome, and giant cell arteritis.[3, 8] Failure to respond to corticosteroids usually leads to cytotoxic therapy, especially when lung and renal involvement is severe. Wegener's granulomatosis, in particular, may respond dramatically to cyclophosphamide, as is discussed subsequently.[30] Cyclophosphamide and other cytotoxic agents have been used in patients with lymphomatoid granulomatosis, allergic granulomatosis and angiitis, polyarteritis nodosa, and vasculitis associated with collagen vascular disorders.[1–3, 8]

## Specific Disorders

Although there is considerable overlap among the various disorders that constitute the continuum of pulmonary vasculitides, numerous entities have been recognized as having certain clinical and pathologic specificity. In this section, each of the specific disorders listed in Table 52.1 is described briefly. Many of these diseases, particularly the connective tissue diseases (also known as collagen vascular disorders), also may present with manifestations of infiltrative and interstitial involvement of the lung parenchyma. For further information about these aspects of the disorders, the reader is referred to Chapter 58.

**Table 52.1 CLASSIFICATION OF PULMONARY VASCULITIDES**

| SPECIFIC DISORDERS |
|---|
| Granulomatous vasculitis |
| Wegener's granulomatosis |
| "Limited" Wegener's granulomatosis |
| Lymphomatoid granulomatosis |
| Allergic granulomatosis and angiitis (Churg-Strauss syndrome) |
| Necrotizing sarcoid granulomatosis |
| Bronchocentric granulomatosis |
| Leukocytoclastic vasculitis |
| Anaphylactoid purpura (Henoch-Schönlein purpura) |
| Essential mixed cryoglobulinemia |
| Vasculitis associated with collagen vascular disorders |
| Rheumatoid arthritis |
| Systemic lupus erythematosus |
| Progressive systemic sclerosis |
| Polymyositis and dermatomyositis |
| Mixed connective tissue disease |
| Classic polyarteritis nodosa |
| Giant cell (temporal) arteritis |
| Takayasu's disease |
| Behçet's syndrome |
| Hughes-Stovin syndrome |
| Eosinophilia-myalgia syndrome |

### Wegener's Granulomatosis

Wegener[31] in 1936 described the clinical syndrome that now bears his name and that consists chiefly of necrotizing granulomatous vasculitis of the upper and lower respiratory tract and glomerulonephritis. He considered the syndrome a variant of polyarteritis nodosa and called it rhinogenic granuloma, with reference to the prominent nasal and paranasal involvement.[32] Although clinical attention usually is focused on the respiratory and renal lesions of Wegener's granulomatosis, the disease also may involve the eyes, ears, heart, skin, joints, and peripheral and central nervous systems.[8, 32, 33] The cause of Wegener's granulomatosis is unknown. However, an immunopathogenesis is supported by the finding of hypergammaglobulinemia and circulating antibodies in patients with the disorder, in addition to their dramatic response to cytotoxic therapy.[31, 33–35]

Of the vasculitides that typically affect the lungs, Wegener's granulomatosis is the most common, comprising approximately 10% of all systemic vasculitides clinically diagnosed.[3] Wegener's granulomatosis may affect persons of all ages but is most common in middle-aged patients, predominantly men.[8, 11, 35] Sinusitis is the most frequent presenting symptom, followed by fever, arthralgias, cough, rhinitis, hemoptysis, otitis, and ocular inflammation.[35] Upper respiratory tract involvement may include destruction of tissue and bone and secondary bacterial infection; this may lead to confusion with midline granuloma, a necrotizing and ulcerating granulomatous process usually limited to the nose and face.[36] Pulmonary involvement ranges from minimal to life-threatening. The chest roentgenogram is abnormal in two thirds of patients, with infiltrates occurring most frequently (63%), followed by nodules (31%), infiltrates with cavitation (8% to 10%), and nodules with cavitation (10%).[11, 37, 38] Bilateral abnormalities occur with nearly equal frequency as unilateral abnormalities. Atelectasis due to endobronchial obstruction and pleural disease with thickening or effusions also have been reported.[39] Lung biopsy usually reveals parenchymal necrosis, granulomatous inflammation accompanied by an infiltrate consisting of a mixture of neutrophils, lymphocytes, plasma cells, eosinophils, and histiocytes, and vasculitis with blood vessel obstruction and bland infarcts (Fig. 52.1). Capillaritis can be seen in almost one third of patients and is a significant cause of hemoptysis.[40] Less commonly, interstitial fibrosis, acute and chronic bronchiolitis, bronchiolitis obliterans, lipoid pneumonia, and tissue eosinophilia can be seen.[41]

In 1985, van der Woude and associates[42] reported a high sensitivity of ANCAs for active Wegener's granulomatosis, and suggested that ANCAs may be useful as a marker of disease activity. Although ANCA activity may be detected in other vasculitides, its presence is associated most strongly with Wegener's granulomatosis, and the cytoplasmic staining pattern is reported to be present in more than 90% of patients with untreated active disease.[43–45] The rate of positivity declines substantially when the disease is in remission, but the test is not sufficiently sensitive to serve as a guide to therapy.[29]

In the past, patients with Wegener's granulomatosis died within months or a few years of diagnosis because of

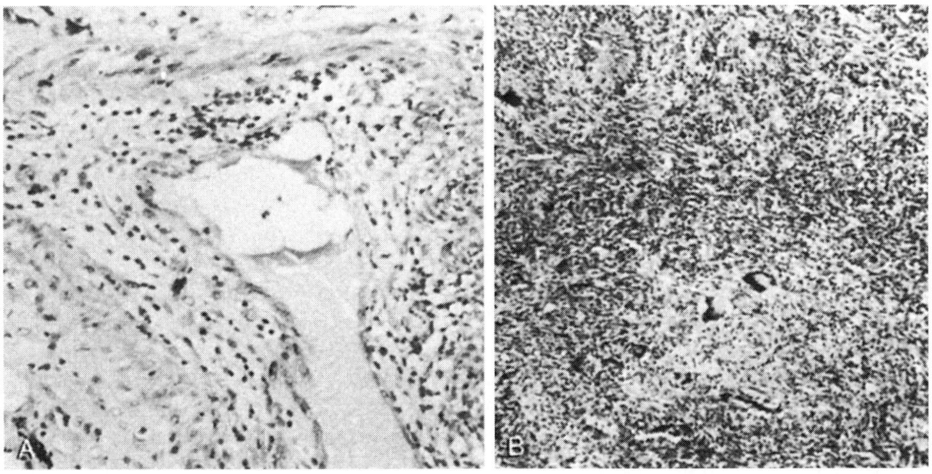

**Figure 52.1** Hematoxylin and eosin stains of autopsy specimens from a patient with Wegener's granulomatosis. *A,* Angiitis in wall of pulmonary blood vessel. *B,* At higher power, note granulomatous inflammation with histiocytes and giant cells. (Courtesy of Martha L. Warnock, M.D.; reproduced with permission from Luce JM: Vasculitis, primary pulmonary hypertension, and arteriovenous fistulas. *In* Murray JF, Nadel JA (eds): Textbook of Respiratory Medicine. Philadelphia: WB Saunders, 1988.)

disseminated vasculitis and renal failure.[31] Corticosteroids rarely affected this prognosis, but it was altered considerably after the advent of cytotoxic drugs. The current cytotoxic agent of choice is cyclophosphamide in a dosage of 1 to 2 mg/kg per day, either alone or in combination with lower doses of corticosteroids, continued for at least 1 year after a decline in disease activity.[46] From 75% to 90% of patients treated with this regimen experience a complete remission. Some investigators have advocated the use of intermittent, pulsed intravenous therapy with cyclophosphamide in an attempt to reduce the incidence of complications (neutropenia, infection, hemorrhagic cystitis) associated with daily oral therapy.[47] The antimicrobial agent trimethoprim-sulfamethoxazole also has been reported to produce improvement or reduce the incidence of relapse in several patients.[48]

## "Limited" Wegener's Granulomatosis

Carrington and Liebow[49] in 1966 described 16 patients with clinical and morphologic features of Wegener's granulomatosis but without glomerulonephritis. There was no evidence of asthma or eosinophilia to suggest allergic granulomatosis and angiitis in these patients. Six of them died of progressive pulmonary disease, but another six survived for 12 months or more without immunosuppressive or cytotoxic therapy. The favorable outcome subsequently was confirmed in other studies,[50] and "limited" Wegener's granulomatosis now is considered by some authors to represent a disease distinct from "classic" Wegener's granulomatosis. However, others believe that limited Wegener's granulomatosis represents an earlier form of the disease rather than a separate clinical entity and advocate aggressive treatment using the same strategy employed for classic Wegener's granulomatosis.

## Lymphomatoid Granulomatosis

In 1972, Liebow and associates[51] first described a unique form of pulmonary angiitis and granulomatosis that they called lymphomatoid granulomatosis. The disorder is characterized histologically by an angiocentric and angiodestructive infiltration of the upper and lower respiratory tracts, skin, central nervous system, and kidneys by lymphoblasts, plasma cells, histiocytes, and large atypical lymphocytes with abnormal mitotic activity.[51, 52] Although the histogenesis of the disease is uncertain, immunologic markers have indicated a predominance of T lymphocytes in one well-studied patient.[53]

Although the original report of lymphomatoid granulomatosis cited only 40 patients, Katzenstein and colleagues[52] in 1979 identified and reported on 157 patients in Liebow's consultation files. The 150 patients whose ages were known ranged from 7 to 85 years, with a mean age of 48 years. Men outnumbered women almost 2 to 1. In contrast to persons with Wegener's granulomatosis, the patients with lymphomatoid granulomatosis usually presented with lower respiratory tract symptoms, including chest pain, dyspnea, and cough. Their chest roentgenograms, however, were indistinguishable from those of patients with Wegener's granulomatosis. Central nervous system involvement also was common, but renal disease was uncommon despite autopsy evidence of glomerulonephritis.

Several of the patients with lymphomatoid granulomatosis in Katzenstein's series had preexisting lymphomas, and lymphomas eventually developed in another 16%.[52] The median survival of all patients was 17 months despite immunosuppressive or cytotoxic therapy, with death usually due to progressive pulmonary or central nervous system involvement. In a prospective series collected by Fauci and associates,[54] half the patients who received daily cyclophosphamide and every-other-day corticosteroids enjoyed remissions lasting an average of 4 years. However, virtually all the patients who did not achieve remissions eventually developed lymphomas. These findings and their own experience led DeRemee and coworkers[55] to classify lymphomatoid granulomatosis as a malignant lymphoproliferative disorder. Colby and Carrington[56] agreed with this hypothesis and speculated that lymphomatoid granulomatosis probably is a lymphoma whose malignant nature may be obscured by the accompanying polymorphous infiltration, as discussed in Chapter 47.

Israel and colleagues[57] and Saldana and associates[58] have argued that pulmonary angiitis and granulomatosis comprise three predominant types: a lymphocyte-depleted type (corresponding to classic and limited Wegener's granulomatoses), a malignant lymphoproliferative type (corresponding to lymphomatoid granulomatosis), and a benign lymphocytic type (a previously unnamed entity). Their patients with benign lymphocytic angiitis and granulomatosis manifested a polymorphous but histologically benign lymphocytic infiltrate with a mild to moderate vasculitis and little or no tissue necrosis. These patients also had consistent responses to chlorambucil. Nevertheless, two patients who appeared to have a benign process eventually developed fatal lymphomatoid granulomatosis. Because of this, benign lymphocytic angiitis and granulomatosis are best considered not as separate entities but rather as one end of a spectrum of disease.[59]

## Allergic Granulomatosis and Angiitis (Churg-Strauss Syndrome)

In 1951, Churg and Strauss[21] reported 13 cases of severe asthma associated with fever and hypereosinophilia. Pathologically, there were granulomatous extravascular lesions and inflammatory, granulomatous, and necrotizing vascular changes in the small arteries and veins of the lungs, heart, pancreas, spleen, kidneys, and skin. Although most of the patients had been assumed to have polyarteritis nodosa, Churg and Strauss[21] believed that the pathologic findings suggested the presence of a distinct clinical process. The cause of this disease remains unknown, but an immunologic basis is supported by the presence of elevations in immunoglobulins and circulating immune complexes in many patients.[13, 60]

Allergic granulomatosis and angiitis, or the Churg-Strauss syndrome, primarily affects middle-aged men with current or previous asthma.[21a] The lungs, peripheral nerves, skin, heart, and viscera are the most commonly injured organs.[13] Renal disease is infrequent, but the prostate and lower urinary tract may be involved.[61] Unlike Wegener's granulomatosis, Churg-Strauss syndrome is characterized by peripheral eosinophilia, which usually exceeds 10% of the peripheral white blood cell count.[13] Plain chest roentgenograms most often reveal patchy infiltrative or nodular densities. Treatment has included corticosteroids, azathioprine, or cyclophosphamide. Before the availability of corticosteroids, Churg-Strauss syndrome was frequently a rapidly progressive disease. However, recent studies suggest that most patients respond favorably to therapy: none of the 20 patients reported in the American College of Rheumatology registry died as a result of the syndrome.[15]

## Necrotizing Sarcoid Granulomatosis

Liebow[7] in 1973 introduced the term necrotizing sarcoid granulomatosis to describe 11 patients with (1) histologic evidence of confluent granulomas similar to those seen in sarcoidosis, in association with a minimally necrotic granulomatous vasculitis involving pulmonary arteries and veins; (2) pulmonary nodules or infiltrates, usually in the absence of bilateral hilar lymphadenopathy; and (3) a benign clinical course with or without the use of corticosteroids. These histologic and roentgenographic characteristics suggested that necrotizing sarcoid granulomatosis was a variant of angiocentric granulomatosis with sarcoid-like features. However, the clinical characteristics favored the concept that necrotizing sarcoid granulomatosis was a variant of sarcoidosis (see Chapter 59).

Subsequent studies[62–64] have supported the latter concept and have confirmed that necrotizing sarcoid granulomatosis is a comparatively benign condition. Indeed, Churg and colleagues[65] proposed that this entity is the same as or similar to nodular sarcoidosis as described by Sharma and coworkers[66] and Onal and associates.[67] Why necrotizing sarcoid granulomatosis includes a vasculitic component is not understood. Nevertheless, the relative lack of necrosis, the female preponderance, and the likelihood of spontaneous clinical and roentgenographic remission emphasize that this condition differs from the other granulomatous vasculitides.

## Bronchocentric Granulomatosis

Liebow[7] described bronchocentric granulomatosis as a disease in which the lower airways were invaded by lymphocytes and plasma cells and ultimately were ulcerated and destroyed. Although adjacent arteries and veins could be injured in the process, their involvement was more or less incidental, unlike that found in angiocentric disorders such as Wegener's granulomatosis. Bronchocentric granulomatosis appeared to affect primarily persons with asthma and produced infiltrates, nodules, or areas of atelectasis on the chest roentgenogram. However, despite its roentgenographic manifestations and disturbing histologic picture, the disease often caused few respiratory symptoms. Furthermore, it lacked the common extrapulmonary manifestations of other vasculitides.

Katzenstein and associates[26] subsequently updated Liebow's original cases and described other patients with bronchocentric granulomatosis. Approximately half the patients in their series had asthma along with eosinophilia and serologic evidence of exposure to *Aspergillus* species and other fungi. *Aspergillus* was recovered from the sputa of several patients, and eosinophils and degraded fungal hyphae were present within necrotizing granulomas in their lungs. These findings and the clinical and roentgenographic similarities among bronchocentric granulomatosis, allergic bronchopulmonary aspergillosis, and mucoid impaction of the bronchi led the investigators to suggest that all three disorders represented hypersensitivity reactions to fungi. However, bronchocentric granulomatosis occurred without serologic or histologic evidence of allergy in the other half of the patients that were reviewed as well as in patients from other series.[68, 69] Although immunopathogenic mechanisms are suspected in these patients, the antigen responsible for their illness has not been identified.

## Leukocytoclastic Vasculitis

This type of vasculitis is a systemic disease that involves arterioles, venules, and capillaries in the skin and other organs. It also has been called hypersensitivity vasculitis, allergic vasculitis, and necrotizing vasculitis.[2, 70] The term *leukocytoclastic* is preferred because it describes the neutrophilic infiltration characteristic of the disorder. Leukocytoclastic vasculitis is manifested clinically by palpable purpura of the lower extremities. Other cutaneous lesions include nodules and necrotic ulceration.[70] Eye, joint, gastrointestinal, peripheral and central nervous system, and pulmonary involvement also have been reported, and leukocytoclastic vasculitis may cause respiratory failure.[8]

Leukocytoclastic vasculitis has been observed after infections with streptococci, *M. tuberculosis*, and hepatitis B virus.[2, 71] It also is associated with several drugs, including sulfa compounds and penicillin, and may accompany malignancies such as chronic lymphocytic leukemia, lymphoma, and multiple myeloma.[3] Leukocytoclastic vasculitis presumably represents a response to a wide variety of antigens. This is supported by the finding in affected patients of immunoglobulins and complement components in vessel walls of cutaneous lesions and normal skin.[72]

## Anaphylactoid Purpura

Anaphylactoid purpura (Henoch-Schönlein syndrome) is a form of leukocytoclastic vasculitis that has been reported primarily in infants and young children.[14, 73] However, adults also may develop the disease.[74] It commonly follows an upper respiratory infection and manifests as a triad of purpura, arthritis, and abdominal pain. Renal involvement may range from hematuria and other abnormalities of the urinary sediment to severe glomerulonephritis and renal failure. Respiratory tract disease occurs only rarely[8, 14] and consists of alveolar hemorrhage and patchy perihilar infiltrates. Elevated serum immunoglobulin A (IgA)– and IgG-containing complexes often are observed in adults with this disease, and most patients have IgA deposition in the kidneys and skin detected by immunofluorescence microscopy. These findings suggest that the disease may represent an immunologic response to a previous infection.[1]

## Essential Mixed Cryoglobulinemia

This disease is characterized by recurrent episodes of purpura, weakness, arthralgias, and multiorgan involvement in persons with elevated serum cryoglobulins with rheumatoid factor activity. The histologic picture is that of a leukocytoclastic vasculitis; immunoglobulins and complement components may be found in blood vessels and along the glomerular basement membrane.[2] Bombardieri and associates[75] described lung involvement in 23 patients with essential mixed cryoglobulinemia, only half of whom had serologic evidence of exposure to hepatitis B virus. Most of the patients were hypoxemic, had decreased expiratory flows at low lung volume, and manifested mild inhomogeneity on regional lung perfusion scanning. Although the last test suggested vascular involvement, pathologic studies were not performed.

## Rheumatoid Arthritis

Rheumatoid arthritis is a systemic disease characterized by inflammation of the peripheral joints and other organs. The common pleuropulmonary manifestations (see also Chapter 58) include pleurisy with or without effusion, necrobiotic nodules (nonpneumoconiotic intrapulmonary nodules), Caplan's syndrome (rheumatoid pneumoconiosis), diffuse interstitial disease, and pulmonary vasculitis and hypertension.[20, 76] The last condition is extremely uncommon; patients alleged to have rheumatoid vasculitis of the lung[77] may well have had primary pulmonary hypertension. Indeed, angiitis was found in only 1 of 40 open lung biopsy specimens from patients with rheumatoid lung disease by Yousem and coworkers.[78]

## Systemic Lupus Erythematosus

This connective tissue disease is characterized by inflammatory changes in connective tissue, blood vessels, and solid organs. The pleuropulmonary manifestations of this disease (see also Chapter 58) include pleurisy with or without effusion, atelectasis, uremic pulmonary edema, acute pneumonitis, diffuse interstitial disease, diaphragmatic dysfunction, and vasculitis.[20] Pulmonary vascular changes consisting of leukocytoclastic vasculitis and fibrinoid necrosis were found in most autopsy specimens from systemic lupus erythematosus patients by Fayemi[79] and Gross and coworkers.[80] In contrast, such findings were rare in autopsy studies reported by Matthay and associates[81] and Miller and colleagues.[82] These and other investigators agree that whatever the true incidence of pulmonary vasculitis is in patients with systemic lupus erythematosus, few develop clinical manifestations of pulmonary hypertension and right-heart failure.

## Progressive Systemic Sclerosis

Another member of the connective tissue disease family that also is discussed in Chapter 58, progressive systemic sclerosis (scleroderma), is associated with Raynaud's phenomenon, distal vasculitis, and inflammation of the skin and internal organs. Pulmonary dysfunction is common among patients with progressive systemic sclerosis, and some degree of interstitial fibrosis is identified in almost all patients at autopsy.[20] Although severe fibrosis and, possibly, recurrent aspiration and pneumonitis may account for pulmonary hypertension and cor pulmonale in some persons, others primarily have pulmonary vascular disease.[83, 84] Pulmonary vascular involvement also may predominate in patients with the CREST syndrome (calcinosis, Raynaud's disease, esophageal dysmotility, sclerodactyly, and telangiectasia) (Fig. 52.2).[85]

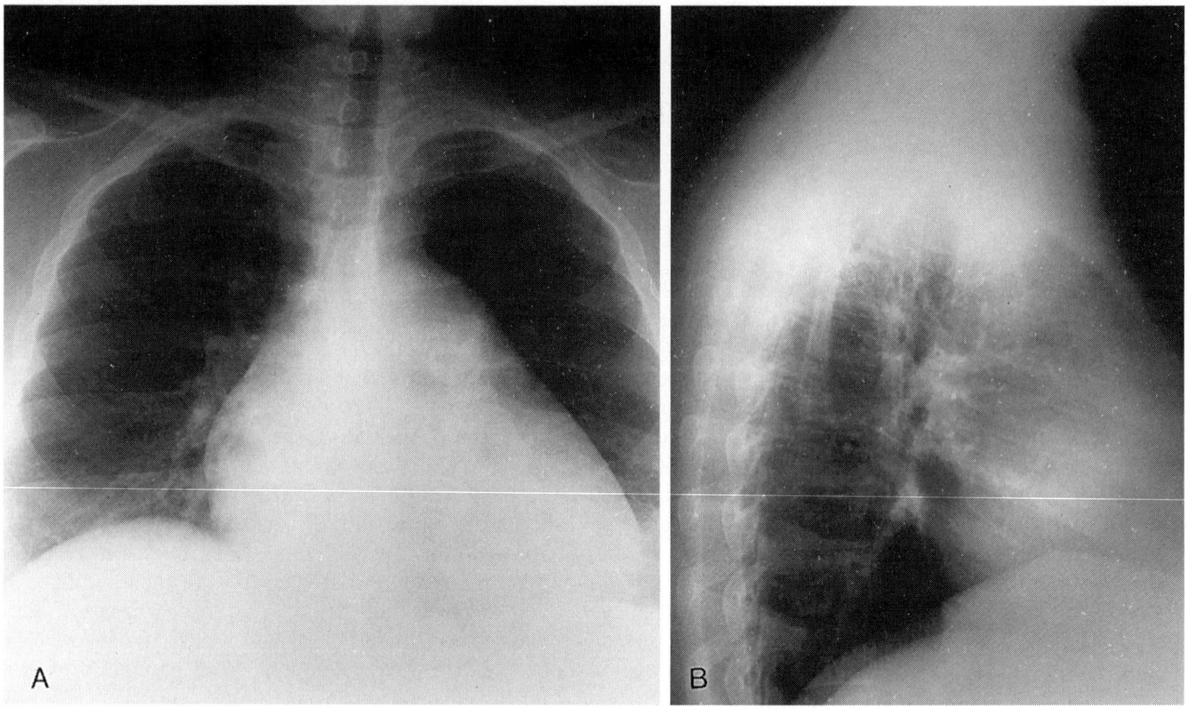

**Figure 52.2** Frontal and lateral chest roentgenograms of 24-year-old woman with pulmonary hypertension associated with the CREST syndrome, showing dilated pulmonary outflow tract and widened cardiac silhouette from right ventricular enlargement.

The pulmonary vascular lesions of progressive systemic sclerosis and the CREST syndrome variant are similar to vascular lesions seen in the kidneys and other organs. They consist of intimal proliferation and concentric fibrosis of the small arteries and arterioles, which frequently are narrowed or occluded. Necrotizing angiitis and fibrinoid necrosis are uncommon, indicating that the lesions lack a strong vasculitic component.[86–88] A vasoconstrictor component similar to that seen in primary pulmonary hypertension is suggested by the frequent finding of medial hypertrophy in biopsy specimens. Whatever its pathologic basis, the pulmonary vascular disease of progressive systemic sclerosis and the CREST syndrome should be suspected when low diffusing capacity for carbon monoxide is found by pulmonary function testing.[89]

## Polymyositis and Dermatomyositis

Polymyositis is an inflammatory disease of skeletal muscle that causes weakness and atrophy; the term dermatomyositis describes a characteristic skin rash.[20] Interstitial lung disease is the most common pulmonary manifestation of these two conditions.[90] Pulmonary vascular disease has been described in two patients, both of whom on further analysis were thought to have progressive systemic sclerosis.[91] It therefore appears that vasculitis occurs infrequently, if at all.

## Mixed Connective Tissue Disease

Patients with mixed connective tissue disease have clinical features characteristic of systemic lupus erythematosus, progressive systemic sclerosis, and polymyositis and dermatomyositis, in addition to antibodies to extractable nuclear antigen.[92] Although lung disease has been assumed to be absent or mild in most of these patients, abnormal pulmonary function tests, including a reduced diffusing capacity for carbon monoxide, have been reported.[93] In addition, severe pulmonary involvement has been described by Jones and coworkers[94] and by Wiener-Kronish and associates.[95] Some autopsies performed on patients with mixed connective tissue disease revealed vasculitic changes similar to those seen in systemic lupus erythematosus and other connective tissue disorders; other examinations disclosed lesions more characteristic of primary pulmonary hypertension (Fig. 52.3) and thromboembolic disease. Thus, the nature of the pulmonary vascular involvement in patients with mixed connective tissue disease is unresolved.

## Classic Polyarteritis Nodosa

As noted previously, Kussmaul and Maier[5] in 1866 introduced the term periarteritis nodosa to describe patients with a necrotizing vasculitis of the small- and medium-sized muscular arteries that was associated with subcutaneous skin nodules. Rose and Spencer[96] preferred the term polyarteritis nodosa, which rightfully drew attention away from perivascular phenomena and emphasized the multiorgan involvement so characteristic of this disease. Most current investigators use polyarteritis nodosa to describe a widespread vasculitis that involves a neutrophilic inflammation of the blood vessels and perivascular space associated with intimal proliferation, fibrinoid necrosis, vessel occlusion and aneurysmal dilatation, and tissue ischemia and infarction. Although the cause is uncertain, hepatitis B infection frequently is implicated.

Classic polyarteritis nodosa may occur in patients of all ages, most of whom do not have an allergic history. The clinical manifestations of this disease depend on the number of organs involved. Vasculitis frequently affects the joints, liver, abdominal viscera, and peripheral and central nervous systems.[12] Renal disease is caused by either vasculitis or glomerulonephritis. Polyarteritis nodosa also may involve the testes, epididymis, bladder, and ovaries. Coronary arteritis is especially common in younger patients. Despite the importance of subcutaneous nodules in the original description, skin involvement is far from universal in polyarteritis nodosa. In fact, the term *cutaneous periarteritis nodosa* has been introduced to describe patients with nodules, livedo reticularis, and ulcers but little evidence of systemic disease.[97]

Although polyarteritis nodosa may be distributed throughout the body, the lungs usually are spared. Sweeney and Baggenstoss[98] detected vasculitis in the bronchial and pulmonary arteries in 8 of 28 patients on whom autopsies were performed at the Mayo Clinic before 1950, but these patients had granulomatous lesions with eosinophilic, rather than neutrophilic, infiltration. In 1945, Wilson and Alexander[99] reported that asthma and peripheral eosinophilia were present in a large number of the 300 patients reported until then in the literature. Rose and Spencer,[96] who analyzed 104 cases from London hospitals from 1946 to 1953, found that only 14 patients with polyarteritis nodosa had lung involvement. Twelve of the 14 patients had asthma, 7 had peripheral eosinophilia, and 7 had granulomatous lesions in the lungs and other organs. In retrospect, it appears that most, if not all, of the patients once thought to have polyarteritis nodosa with pulmonary involvement actually had allergic granulomatosis and angiitis, as described by Churg and Strauss[21] in 1951.

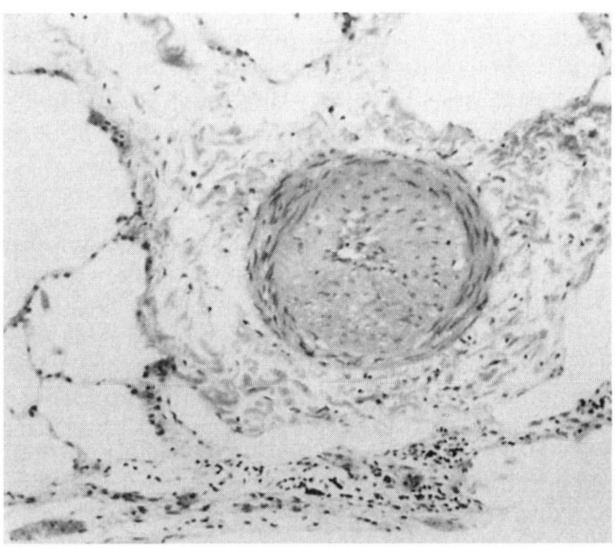

**Figure 52.3** Hematoxylin and eosin stain of autopsy specimen of lung from a patient with mixed connective tissue disease. Note marked endothelial proliferation and endarteritis obliterans in a small pulmonary artery. (Courtesy of Martha L. Warnock, M.D.; reproduced with permission from Luce JM: Vasculitis, primary pulmonary hypertension, and arteriovenous fistulas. *In* Murray JF, Nadel JA (eds): Textbook of Respiratory Medicine. Philadelphia: WB Saunders, 1988.)

## Giant Cell (Temporal) Arteritis

The symptoms of giant cell (temporal) arteritis include headache, tenderness of the temporal arteries, myalgias, and ocular abnormalities that may progress to blindness, vertigo, dementia, and cerebrovascular accidents.[15] These symptoms occur more frequently in women than in men, usually are associated with mild anemia and elevation of the erythrocyte sedimentation rate, and should respond to low doses of corticosteroids. Biopsy of the temporal artery (or other cranial arteries at autopsy) reveals an inflammatory infiltrate consisting of lymphocytes and giant cells, intimal proliferation, and destruction of elastic membranes. Immunofluorescent studies demonstrate immunoglobulin and complement deposition in the renal walls.

Temporal arteritis traditionally has been thought of as a local process, in contrast to *polymyalgia rheumatica*, a syndrome consisting of fever, weakness, weight loss, and pain and stiffness of the proximal limb muscles and back. Yet many patients with temporal arteritis also have symptoms of polymyalgia rheumatica; patients with polymyalgia rheumatica may develop temporal arteritis; and temporal artery biopsies in patients with polymyalgia rheumatica have revealed vasculitic changes. Most important, involvement of extracranial vessels, including the aorta and pulmonary arteries,[100, 101] has been reported in patients with temporal arteritis. These findings suggest that the underlying disorder in both temporal arteritis and polymyalgia rheumatica is a generalized vasculitis.

## Takayasu's Disease

In 1908, Takayasu[102] described a young woman with cataracts and arteriovenous anastomoses around the optic discs who subsequently was shown to lack pulses in her arms. Later investigators determined that the "pulseless disease" resulted from a granulomatous vasculitis involving primarily the aorta and its branches and that these lesions led to blood vessel narrowing and occlusion with aneurysm formation. These histologic changes have been reported predominantly in young Japanese women and are associated with an elevated erythrocyte sedimentation rate. Despite therapy with corticosteroids and anticoagulants, Takayasu's disease may cause blindness, cerebrovascular accidents, severe hypertension, left ventricular failure, and aortic aneurysm rupture.[17, 103] Pulmonary symptoms have been reported in patients with this disorder. Pulmonary artery involvement, with or without pulmonary hypertension, has been confirmed by angiographic and autopsy studies, and pulmonary arteritis probably occurs in most patients.[17, 103–105]

## Behçet's Syndrome

Behçet's syndrome was described in 1937 as a symptom complex of recurrent aphthous stomatitis, genital ulceration, and uveitis.[106] It subsequently has become recognized as a systemic inflammatory disorder that also may involve the gastrointestinal tract, cardiovascular system, brain, kidneys, and lungs.[107] The underlying pathologic process is a vasculitis involving neutrophils and mononuclear cells that usually affects veins, venules, and capillaries. Immunoglobulin staining of the lesions has revealed IgG and complement. Susceptibility to Behçet's disease has been strongly linked to the presence of the HLA-B51 allele.[107a]

Pulmonary involvement occurs in approximately 10% of patients with Behçet's syndrome and includes recurrent pneumonia and often fatal episodes of hemoptysis.[108–111] The latter problem has been attributed to vasculitis of small lung vessels and to rupture of bronchial veins when intraluminal pressure is increased by thrombosis of the superior vena cava.[112] However, hemoptysis also may result from rupture of large pulmonary artery aneurysms and arteriovenous fistulas.[111, 112]

### Hughes-Stovin Syndrome

Hughes and Stovin[113] in 1959 described two patients who died of massive hemoptysis due to rupture of segmented pulmonary artery aneurysms. Recurrent venous thrombosis also was detected in these patients, as was intracranial hypertension that probably was related to thrombosis of intracranial and extracranial vessels. That these abnormalities were caused by vasculitis was suggested by the finding of an inflammatory infiltrate consisting largely of lymphocytes and plasma cells in the walls of the elastic pulmonary arteries at autopsy. Neither these patients nor similar patients subsequently reported by Durieux and associates[112] and Meireles and coworkers[114] met the diagnostic criteria for Behçet's syndrome. The Hughes-Stovin syndrome therefore appears to be either a separate entity or a variant of Behçet's syndrome.

### Eosinophilia-Myalgia Syndrome

An epidemic of the eosinophilia-myalgia syndrome in the late 1980s has been linked to the dietary ingestion of contaminated L-tryptophan, with more than 1500 cases reported to the Centers for Disease Control and Prevention through 1990.[23, 115-119] This compound was used extensively as an over-the-counter remedy for insomnia, stress, and depression. Although the pathogenesis remains unclear, the disease appears to result from a reaction to a contaminant that was introduced during the manufacturing process.[120, 121] The clinical manifestations of eosinophilia-myalgia syndrome include myalgias, arthralgias, skin rashes, muscle pain, edema, fatigue, neuropathy, and marked peripheral eosinophilia.[121] More than half the patients with eosinophilia-myalgia syndrome have respiratory ailments, with dyspnea occurring most frequently (see also Chapter 61). Acute eosinophilic pneumonitis, pleural effusions, chronic interstitial lung disease, and chronic pulmonary hypertension have been reported.[122–124] Lung biopsies have demonstrated the presence of vasculitis with fibrointimal hyperplasia, often associated with varying degrees of interstitial infiltrate.[123, 124] Although some patients have improved with the discontinuation of L-tryptophan or corticosteroid therapy, the response is often incomplete and the disease may be chronic and progressive.[122]

## PRIMARY PULMONARY HYPERTENSION

Primary pulmonary hypertension is a disease in which there is a persistent elevation of pulmonary artery pressure without demonstrable cause.[125] Although there is no uniformly accepted hemodynamic definition for pulmonary hypertension, the primary pulmonary hypertension registry of the United States National Institutes of Health[125] required a resting mean pulmonary artery pressure greater than 25 mm Hg or a mean pressure in excess of 30 mm Hg during exercise. These criteria facilitate the inclusion of patients identified early in the course of their illness.

### Classification

Primary pulmonary hypertension by definition is a diagnosis of exclusion. It must be differentiated on clinical grounds from pulmonary hypertension related to chronic pulmonary thromboembolism, chronic airflow obstruction, parenchymal lung disease, severe hypoventilation, left ventricular failure, left-sided valvular heart disease, and congenital heart disease with intracardiac shunts.[125] A World Health Organization[126] conference in 1973 categorized chronic pulmonary thromboembolism, pulmonary veno-occlusive disease, and plexogenic pulmonary arteriopathy under the rubric pulmonary hypertension of unknown cause. However, the morphologic characteristics of these conditions are quite distinct despite their clinical similarities, and plexogenic pulmonary arteriopathy is the histologic lesion that most investigators associate with primary pulmonary hypertension.[127] Pulmonary veno-occlusive disease most likely represents a variant of plexogenic pulmonary arteriopathy.

### Epidemiology

Primary pulmonary hypertension first was described at autopsy by Romberg[128] in 1891. Patients with pulmonary hypertension of unknown cause were reported infrequently over the next 60 years, with only two cases identified from 10,000 consecutive autopsies at Massachusetts General Hospital.[129] However, the condition was recognized more commonly after the advent of cardiac catheterization. Wood[130] in 1950 detected six cases of what he called idiopathic pulmonary hypertension among 233 unselected British patients with presumed congenital heart disease, 152 of whom were catheterized. One year later, the term primary pulmonary hypertension was introduced by Dresdale and associates[131] in a detailed clinical and hemodynamic study of similar patients.

Since these original studies, primary pulmonary hypertension has been reported with increased frequency. Shephard and colleagues[132] and Chapman and coworkers[133] described 14 patients with the condition in 1957; in 1958, Yu[134] reviewed the findings in 55 persons older than 12 years of age reported previously in the literature. Wolcott and colleagues[135] selected 23 cases from among

Mayo Clinic patients seen from 1946 to 1965. A review of 17,901 autopsies performed on persons older than 1 year of age from 1944 to 1981 at the Johns Hopkins Hospital yielded 24 cases of primary pulmonary hypertension; this amounted to a prevalence of 0.13% of all patients.[136] The primary pulmonary hypertension registry included 187 cases collected from 32 centers between 1981 and 1985. In 1984, Rich and Brundage[137] noted that primary pulmonary hypertension was found at autopsy in approximately 1% of patients with cor pulmonale.

Primary pulmonary hypertension customarily has been considered a disease of young women. Indeed, all of Wood's[130] six patients were women between 20 and 45 years of age, as were the three patients described by Dresdale and associates.[131] An overall female:male ratio of 1.7:1 was found in the U.S. registry.[125] However, primary pulmonary hypertension has been reported in both sexes within a wide age range. For example, the mean age of patients in the registry series was 36 years, with a range of 1 to 81 years.[125] The disease appears to affect older men and women in equal numbers, although most younger patients continue to be female.[125]

## Pathology

Wood[138] in 1958 divided pulmonary hypertension into six types: *passive*, as seen with increased pulmonary venous pressure due to raised left atrial or ventricular pressure; *hyperkinetic*, caused by increased pulmonary blood flow; *obstructive*, resulting from pulmonary embolism or thrombosis; *obliterative*, manifested by a reduction of pulmonary vascular capacity; *vasoconstrictive*, brought about by functional and presumably reversible vasospasm; and *polygenic*, arising in two or more of the preceding ways (further details are provided in Table 50.3). Vasoconstrictive pulmonary hypertension occurred most characteristically in response to alveolar hypoxia and usually responded to the inhalation of oxygen or the injection of acetylcholine into the pulmonary artery. Reversible vasoconstriction also was seen as an added component of the passive hypertension of mitral stenosis and the hyperkinetic hypertension caused by congenital left-to-right intracardiac shunts before the onset of Eisenmenger's syndrome. The histologic lesions observed in these reversible kinds of pulmonary hypertension consisted of medial hypertrophy of the pulmonary artery and scant intimal hyperplasia.

Also in 1958, Heath and Edwards[139] documented the pathology of hypertensive pulmonary vascular disease in a study of 67 patients with congenital heart disease and 2 patients with primary pulmonary hypertension. These investigators argued that the progression of lesions in these patients was so stereotyped as to allow division of the structural effects of pulmonary hypertension into six grades as follows: grade 1, medial hypertrophy of the pulmonary arteries and arterioles without intimal changes; grade 2, medial hypertrophy with cellular intimal proliferation; grade 3, medial hypertrophy, intimal proliferation, and intimal fibrosis; grade 4, progressive generalized vascular dilation and occlusion by intimal fibrosis and fibroelastosis; grade 5, appearance of dilation lesions, including vein-like branches of occluded pulmonary arteries, plexiform lesions, angiomatoid lesions, and cavernous lesions; and grade 6, necrotizing arteritis.

Heath and Edwards' grading system focused on the muscular pulmonary arteries 100 to 1000 μm in size. Grades 1 and 2, which were characterized by medial thickening, were comparable to the reversible vasoconstrictive phase of Wood's scheme. In grades 3 and 4, intimal changes led to progressive obstruction of the vessels, which then dilated in the presence of high pressure. Some of the dilated areas evolved into microaneurysms in which there was endothelial proliferation and the formation of in situ thrombosis; these made up the characteristic plexiform lesions. In grade 5, the dilation became rigid, and hemosiderin was extruded from vessels that either burst or allowed the diapedesis of erythrocytes. Grade 6 was seen rarely and involved perivascular neutrophilic inflammation and fibrinoid necrosis.

Heath and Edwards[139] lumped the pathology of congenital heart disease and primary pulmonary hypertension together, and a large series of patients with the latter disorder was not available until 1970. In that year, Wagenvoort and Wagenvoort[140] described the morphology of the pulmonary vessels of 150 persons in whom the diagnosis of primary pulmonary hypertension had been made on clinical grounds. Despite their common diagnosis, the cases could be divided into several groups on histologic analysis: chronic pulmonary thromboembolism, chronic pulmonary venous hypertension, pulmonary veno-occlusive disease, sarcoidosis, chronic bronchitis and pulmonary emphysema, pulmonary schistosomiasis, and vasoconstrictive primary pulmonary hypertension. The patients with the last disorder were the largest group, consisting of 36 men and 74 women with a mean age of 23 years and an age range of 4 days to 69 years.

The lesions that Wagenvoort and Wagenvoort attributed to vasoconstrictive primary pulmonary hypertension were strikingly similar to those described earlier by Heath and Edwards[139] and Wood.[138] The earliest abnormalities were medial hypertrophy of the muscular pulmonary arteries and muscularization of the arterioles. These findings were especially prominent in children and were the only irregularities found in young infants. Although the medial thickening might be interpreted as a persistence of the high-resistance fetal circulation, it was considerably greater than that observed in infants of the same age. Less marked in children but apparent in all adults studied were intimal proliferation and laminar intimal fibrosis that gave an onionskin appearance to the pulmonary arteries. This pattern was not seen in any patients with initially unsuspected chronic pulmonary thromboembolism and also was absent from an additional 20 patients with known thromboembolic disease.

Dilation lesions, including the plexiform variety, were observed in 77 patients with vasoconstrictive primary pulmonary hypertension and one patient with schistosomiasis (who also had *Schistosoma mansoni* ova) but was not evident in persons with chronic pulmonary thromboembolism or other disorders. Necrotizing arteritis occurred in 34 patients with chronic pulmonary thromboembolism; it never involved the veins as it does in pulmonary veno-occlusive disease. Wagenvoort and Wagenvoort[140] noted that vasculitis occurred only in persons with advanced disease and probably was a result rather than a cause of pulmonary hypertension, in contrast to the true pulmonary vasculitides. They believed that the progression of lesions in primary pulmonary hypertension was entirely consistent with a vasoconstrictive mechanism.

Subsequent investigators[127] confirmed the findings of Wagenvoort and Wagenvoort,[140] including the histologic distinctions between primary pulmonary hypertension (Fig. 52.4), chronic pulmonary thromboembolism (Fig. 52.5), and pulmonary veno-occlusive disease (Fig. 52.6). Nevertheless, the vasoconstrictive nature of primary pulmonary hypertension has not been universally accepted; Anderson and coworkers,[141] for example, concluded from their autopsy experience that the essential lesion in this disorder is not medial hypertrophy but intimal proliferation of the pulmonary arteries. Because the pathogenesis of primary pulmonary hypertension is still open to debate, the term *vasoconstrictive primary pulmonary hypertension* has been superseded by the term *plexogenic pulmonary arteriopathy,*[127] despite the fact that plexiform lesions also may be seen in patients with congenital heart disease and pulmonary schistosomiasis.[140]

## Pathogenesis and Etiology

Although the pathogenesis of primary pulmonary hypertension is uncertain, the pathologic similarity between this disease and congenital intracardiac shunts strongly suggests an early vasoreactive phase. Functional vasoconstriction also is supported by the demonstration of immediate reductions in the pulmonary artery pressure of some patients during cardiac catheterization and reports of long-term sustained hemodynamic responses to therapy and spontaneous regression in a few patients, including an 11-year-old girl.[142] Presumably, such persons have a preponderance of medial hypertrophy rather than intimal proliferation and fibrosis. Whether their lesions are chronologically earlier than or pathogenetically different from those of patients with less reversible primary pulmonary hypertension is unclear.

The cause of vasoconstriction in primary pulmonary hypertension also has not been fully characterized; a variety of potential mediators have been suggested, including endothelin, thromboxane, or deficiencies in endothelial production of prostacyclin or nitric oxide.[143] Recently, a defect in pulmonary artery smooth muscle cell

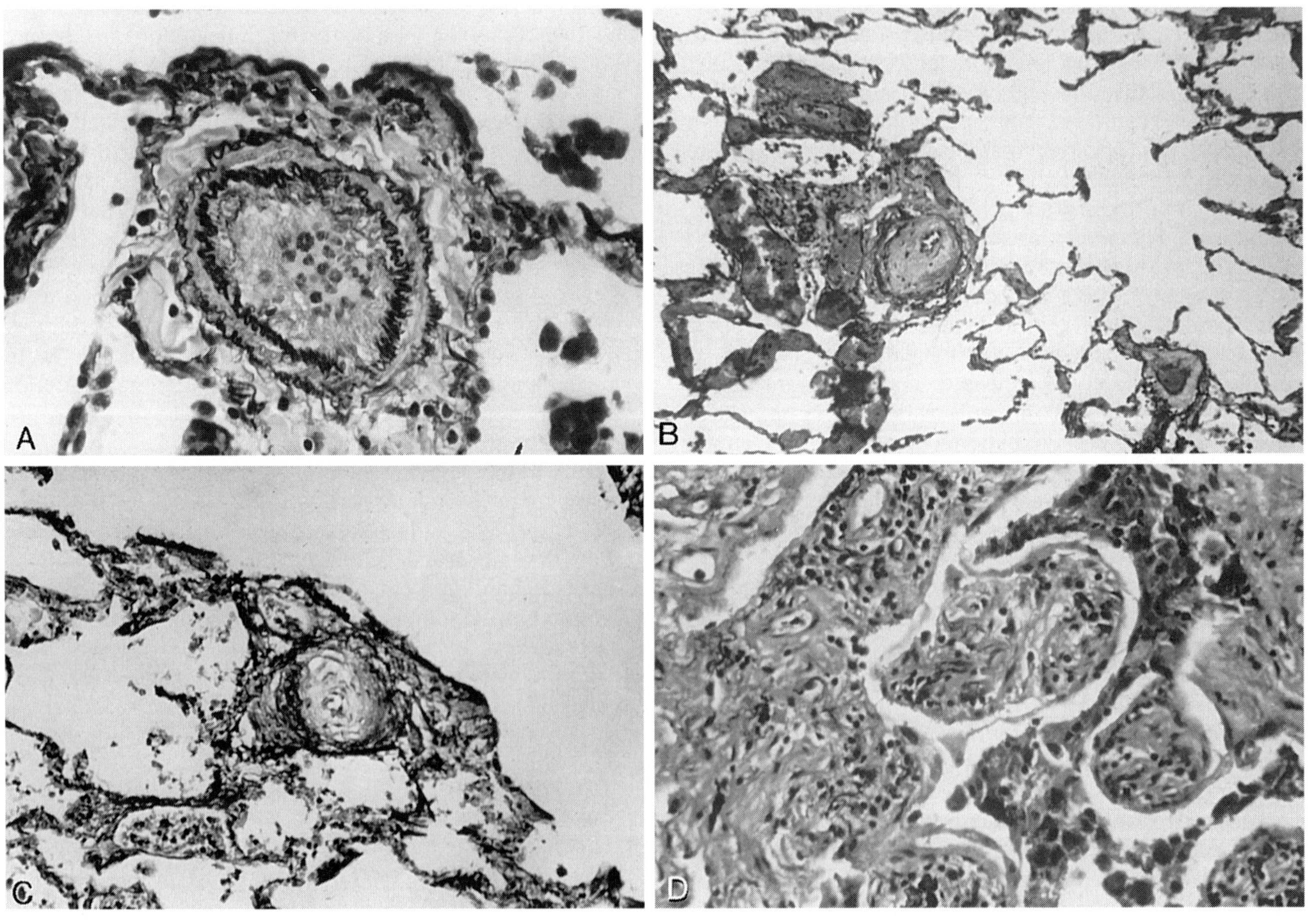


**Figure 52.4** Pathologic changes of primary pulmonary hypertension. *A,* Elastic stain demonstrating medial hypertrophy and intimal proliferation. *B,* Hematoxylin and eosin stain demonstrating eccentric intimal fibrosis. *C,* Hematoxylin and eosin stain demonstrating concentric intimal fibrosis (onion-skinning). *D,* Hematoxylin and eosin stain demonstrating a plexiform lesion.

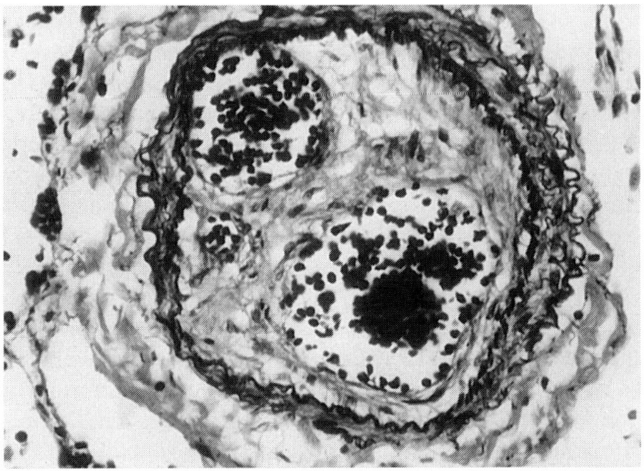

**Figure 52.5** Elastic stain of lung tissue from patient with chronic pulmonary thromboembolism showing that there is little medial hypertrophy and that the organized thrombus has recanalized.

membrane potassium channel activity in primary pulmonary hypertension has been reported.[144] Goodale and Thomas,[129] among others, argued that disease was the result of the persistence of the vasoreactive fetal circulation, but their argument was contradicted by the findings of Wagenvoort and Wagenvoort,[140] cited earlier. Dresdale and coworkers,[131] who named the condition, speculated that patients with primary pulmonary hypertension might be congenitally sensitive to sympathetic stimulation. Although its mechanism has not been fully elucidated, such sensitivity is supported by reports of primary pulmonary hypertension in identical twins,[145] two siblings and their father,[146] five members of one family across three generations,[147] and six members of the same family over two generations.[148] Genetic studies of some of these families suggests that the gene for pulmonary hypertension is transmitted in an autosomal-dominant pattern and that its locus resides on chromosome 2q31-32. [149] Familial disease was reported in 7% of patients in the U.S. registry.[125] Susceptibility to high-altitude pulmonary hypertension appears to have a genetic basis in animals[150] and humans,[151] and wide individual and species variation in vascular reactivity is well described.

The association of primary pulmonary hypertension and Raynaud's phenomenon[152–154] also supports the notion of a vasoconstrictive pathogenesis. Raynaud's phenomenon was either the initial complaint or an eventual symptom in 30% of patients with primary pulmonary hypertension seen at the Mayo Clinic,[135] and in 10% of patients in the U.S. registry.[125] Primary pulmonary hypertension has been linked with Raynaud's phenomenon, migraine, and variant angina as manifestations of a generalized vasospastic disorder.[154]

Raynaud's phenomenon also is common among patients with collagen vascular disorders. The concurrence of these two abnormalities and primary pulmonary hypertension first was noted in 1960 by Rawson and Woske,[155] who hypothesized that primary pulmonary hypertension actually might be a collagen vascular disease. Since that time, antinuclear antibodies have been detected in the sera of up to 30% of persons with primary pulmonary hypertension,[125, 156] and pulmonary hypertension has been described in an even larger number of persons with rheumatoid arthritis,[76–78] systemic lupus erythematosus,[79–81] progressive systemic sclerosis and the CREST syndrome,[83–88] polymyositis and dermatomyositis,[90, 91] and mixed connective tissue disease.[93–95]

Some patients with these diseases have been found at autopsy to have plexogenic pulmonary arteriopathy. Furthermore, medial hypertrophy and concentric intimal fibrosis are prominent in progressive systemic sclerosis, although plexiform lesions are not seen. The frequent finding of Raynaud's phenomenon and the occasional response to vasodilators in patients with progressive systemic sclerosis and pulmonary hypertension prompted Sackner and associates[83] to suggest the likely role of generalized vasospasm in progressive systemic sclerosis.

Raynaud's phenomenon, progressive systemic sclerosis, and primary pulmonary hypertension occur most commonly in women. Primary pulmonary hypertension also may be noted initially during pregnancy,[157, 158] when pulmonary vascular reactivity normally is blunted and pulmonary artery pressure should be low.[159] In addition, primary pulmonary hypertension has been reported with striking frequency in patients taking oral contraceptives.[160, 161] These observations suggest that estrogens and perhaps other vasoactive hormones play a role in primary pulmonary hypertension, although this role has never been well characterized.

Portal hypertension is another disease occasionally associated with pulmonary hypertension, although the expected structural alteration in the pulmonary vessels is diffuse dilation of the arteries and veins.[162] Mantz and Craige[163] first described simultaneous occurrence of portal

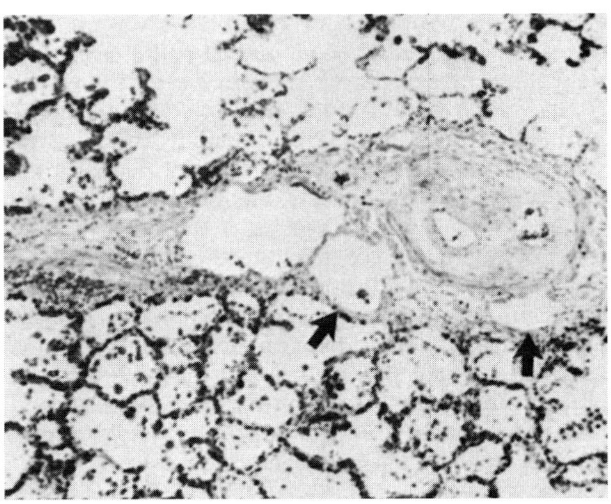

**Figure 52.6** Hematoxylin and eosin stain of lung tissue from patient with pulmonary veno-occlusive disease showing occluded vein and dilated perivenous lymphatics *(arrows)*. (Courtesy of Martha L. Warnock, M.D.; reproduced with permission from Luce JM: Vasculitis, primary pulmonary hypertension, and arteriovenous fistulas. *In* Murray JF, Nadel JA (eds): Textbook of Respiratory Medicine. Philadelphia: WB Saunders, 1988.)

and pulmonary hypertension in a patient with portal vein thrombosis and speculated that multiple emboli emanating from portacaval anastomoses were responsible for the pulmonary hypertension. Naeye[164] in 1960 reported six cases of coexisting portal and pulmonary hypertension and also implicated embolization from the portal vein. It also has been suggested that a vasoactive agent or a substance harmful to the pulmonary circulation might have been produced in the gut but escaped hepatic detoxifying mechanisms. This hypothesis is supported by reports of six patients who had been treated by portal-systemic shunting before the clinical onset of pulmonary hypertension[165, 166] and patients with plexogenic arteriopathy associated with congenital agenesis of the portal vein.[167] In addition, orthotopic liver transplantation in a patient with severe pulmonary hypertension from hepatitis C–associated cirrhosis resulted in striking hemodynamic improvement.[167a] (For further discussion, see Chapter 85.)

The possibility that the liver is not metabolizing a toxin or vasoconstrictive substance in patients with portal and pulmonary hypertension is strengthened by mounting evidence of dietary pulmonary hypertension.[168] In 1957, Bras and colleagues[169] described veno-occlusive disease of the liver in Jamaican patients who drank bush tea made from *Crotalaria spectabilis,* a plant containing the pyrrolidine alkaloid monocrotaline. Another alkaloid, fulvine, causes similar disease after the ingestion of *Crotalaria fulva.* Although these agents are hepatotoxic in humans, they do not produce pulmonary lesions. However, both monocrotaline and fulvine damage the pulmonary vessels in rats.[170, 171] Neither laminar intimal fibrosis nor plexiform lesions are part of the pulmonary toxicity of these agents, but these reports serve as reminders that substances taken by mouth can cause pulmonary vascular disease.

This possibility was dramatized vividly between 1967 and 1970 in Switzerland, Austria, and Germany, where a 20-fold increase in pulmonary hypertension was observed after the introduction of aminorex, an appetite suppressant resembling epinephrine and amphetamine.[172] The pulmonary lesions produced by this agent resembled plexogenic pulmonary arteriopathy in every respect. Although the case against aminorex was weakened by the facts that 20% of patients with idiopathic pulmonary hypertension in Central Europe did not take the drug, only 1 in 1000 persons taking the drug actually developed pulmonary hypertension, and an animal model could not be created,[173] the case was strengthened by the observation that the incidence of pulmonary hypertension decreased to its previous level after aminorex was withdrawn from the market. Pulmonary hypertension has been associated with another family of appetite suppressants with similar chemical structure, fenfluramine and dexfenfluramine.[174] In a case-controlled prospective study performed in Europe, the risk of developing pulmonary hypertension was increased by 20-fold in individuals who used these drugs for periods exceeding 3 months. Reversible pulmonary hypertension has been reported after discontinuation of a similar agent.[175] Interestingly, application of both aminorex and fenfluramine to pulmonary artery smooth muscle cells results in K channel function alterations that are similar to those observed in cells from patients with "spontaneous" primary pulmonary hypertension.[176]

In 1983, an epidemic of pulmonary hypertension was observed in Spain among people who ingested rapeseed oil contaminated with aniline and acetanilide dyes used to mark the oil as unfit for human consumption.[177] Most of the poisoned patients with pulmonary complications died of increased permeability pulmonary edema shortly after ingestion. However, several survivors manifested pulmonary hypertension during cardiac catheterization, and pathologic studies revealed medial thickening and intimal proliferation, early histologic findings of plexogenic pulmonary arteriopathy.[178] Strikingly similar findings have been observed in some patients who developed the eosinophilia-myalgia syndrome after the ingestion of contaminated L-tryptophan. Although the systemic manifestations predominated in most patients, several patients developed varying degrees of pulmonary hypertension, characterized by intimal proliferation and medial hypertrophy of small pulmonary arteries, in the absence of significant parenchymal lung disease.

Illicit drug use has been observed with increasing frequency as a cause of severe pulmonary hypertension; this may be the result of a combination of factors, including granulomatous pulmonary arteritis resulting from a reaction to talc, which commonly is used as an adulterant of parenteral drugs; obstruction of the vasculature due to other foreign material, such as cotton fibers; and the vasoconstrictive properties of some agents, such as cocaine.

## Symptoms

Dyspnea is the cardinal symptom of primary pulmonary hypertension, occurring in more than 95% of patients in the major clinical series.[125, 126, 133–135] Breathlessness is the presenting symptom in 60% of patients and usually is noted first on exertion, but eventually occurs at rest. Its mechanism is probably complex: the most likely cause for the dyspnea of pulmonary hypertension is the inadequacy of cardiac output relative to metabolic requirements.[179] Reeves and Groves[180] have postulated that stretch receptors on the main pulmonary arteries also may be involved. Regardless of its mechanism, Packer[181] stresses that the severity of dyspnea does not correlate with the elevation of pulmonary artery pressure in patients with primary pulmonary hypertension.

Closely related to dyspnea are sensations of fatigue and weakness, reported by a majority of patients with primary pulmonary hypertension.[125] These sensations usually are experienced before the general disability that is present with advanced disease. They presumably reflect impaired tissue oxygenation resulting from the depressed cardiac output in patients with primary pulmonary hypertension. This impairment is usually evident during cardiac catheterization as both a low cardiac output and a decreased mixed venous $P_{O_2}$.

Substernal chest pain also commonly is reported in patients with primary pulmonary hypertension.[133, 134] It frequently occurs on exertion, radiates to the left shoulder or axilla, and is relieved by rest. The pain has been likened to angina pectoris and has been attributed to coronary insufficiency in the presence of increased right ventricular work and hypoxemia[180]; this concept is supported by the occasional relief produced by nitroglycerin. However, pain may be present in young patients without coronary artery disease, prompting Viar and Harrison[182] to argue that the pain is caused by distention of the pulmonary artery, whose afferents enter the nervous system along the same pathways as afferents from the heart. Another plausible but unproved explanation is that the chest pain of primary pulmonary hypertension is variant angina in patients with generalized vasospastic disease.

Syncope occurs in some patients with primary pulmonary hypertension and may be its initial manifestation.[125] This symptom also is experienced first on exertion but may happen later at rest. The syncope probably is caused by a decrease in cerebral blood flow that follows an increase in pulmonary artery pressure and a decrease in cardiac output. Dresdale and associates[131] speculated that cardiac output would be especially depressed in patients with concurrent coronary insufficiency and right ventricular failure. Conversely, James[183] believed that depression of the cardiac output results primarily from bradycardia due to ischemia of the sinus node.

Another symptom associated with primary pulmonary hypertension is hemoptysis that presumably stems from microvascular aneurysms that rupture under the high pulmonary artery pressure. In addition, hoarseness may result from pressure of the enlarged main pulmonary artery on the recurrent laryngeal nerve.[184] Peripheral edema and ascites may develop after the onset of right ventricular failure.[143]

## Physical Findings

Patients with early primary pulmonary hypertension may manifest no physical abnormalities. However, signs of pulmonary hypertension and a decreased cardiac output should be evident with advanced disease. As Wood[185] observed, the hands and feet of a patient with severe pulmonary hypertension are cold, the peripheral pulse is diminished, the blood pressure is likely to be low, and the pulse pressure is reduced. Signs of systemic venous hypertension should be present, including a prominent jugular venous *a* wave, which is exaggerated by abdominal compression (hepatojugular reflux) and transmitted to the liver in a presystolic hepatic pulse, and prominent *c-v* waves, which are indicative of tricuspid regurgitation. Palpation of the chest should reveal a right ventricular lift at the left sternal border that is sustained throughout the pressure-overloaded cardiac contraction, in contrast to the unsustained parasternal impulse felt in pure volume overload.

On auscultation of the chest, the second heart sound is closely split, and the second (pulmonic) component is accentuated. The valvular closure sound should increase in intensity on inspiration and may become palpable as pulmonary artery pressure rises. A systolic ejection click reflecting sudden distention of the right ventricular wall also may be heard. A murmur of tricuspid regurgitation, heard best along the left sternal border and increasing in intensity with inspiration, is heard frequently. A pulmonary regurgitant murmur may become evident after dilation of the main pulmonary artery and its valve annulus. Diastolic vibration of the aortic valve leaflet (Graham Steell's murmur) may be present along with third and fourth heart sounds. In addition to these findings, patients with right-sided heart failure usually have peripheral edema and abdominal distention due to ascites. If tricuspid regurgitation is present, the liver may become pulsatile.

Cyanosis occurs with variable frequency in patients with primary pulmonary hypertension and is likely to be a late phenomenon.[96] It is most marked during exercise but also may be present at rest. Peripheral vasoconstriction and impaired oxygenation of arterial blood due to mixed venous hypoxemia resulting from the decreased cardiac output appear to be the most common mechanisms. Patients in whom right atrial pressure equals or exceeds left atrial pressure may develop severe hypoxemia and cyanosis because of opening of the foramen ovale with subsequent right-to-left shunting of blood. In addition to cyanosis, vascular plethora may be observed in hypoxemic patients with secondary polycythemia. With the exception of patients with cirrhosis and pulmonary hypertension, clubbing is not a usual manifestation of primary pulmonary hypertension. The presence of clubbing warrants a careful search for other causes of pulmonary vascular disease.

## Diagnosis

Although pulmonary hypertension may be appreciated on physical examination, primary pulmonary hypertension cannot be distinguished from the other causes of pulmonary hypertension by examination alone. The major entities in the differential diagnosis are chronic pulmonary thromboembolism (Chapter 51); cardiac disorders, such as congenital heart disease, mitral stenosis, and left atrial tumors (Chapter 84); and pulmonary veno-occlusive disease (discussed subsequently). Although the severity of pulmonary hypertension may be assessed by physical examination, laboratory evaluation is required for precise quantitation.

Blood studies are an important part of the laboratory evaluation. The complete blood count is particularly helpful in documenting polycythemia, which is present in hypoxemic patients with primary pulmonary hypertension.[125] An even smaller number are anemic, thrombocytopenic, or both. Two patients recently have been reported with microangiopathic hemolytic anemia and primary pulmonary hypertension, one of whom had portal hypertension as well. In both cases, intravascular fragmentation of erythrocytes and platelets was attributed to blood flow through plexiform lesions in the pulmonary circulation.[186, 187] Pulmonary hypertension also has been associated with a familial platelet storage pool disease, in which platelet function was impaired and plasma levels of serotonin were elevated.[188]

The plain chest roentgenogram is potentially useful in suggesting the presence of pulmonary hypertension and in providing clues of underlying conditions such as parenchymal lung disease (Fig. 52.7). In patients with primary pulmonary hypertension, the roentgenogram characteristically reveals protrusion of the main pulmonary artery, increased width of the descending branch of the right

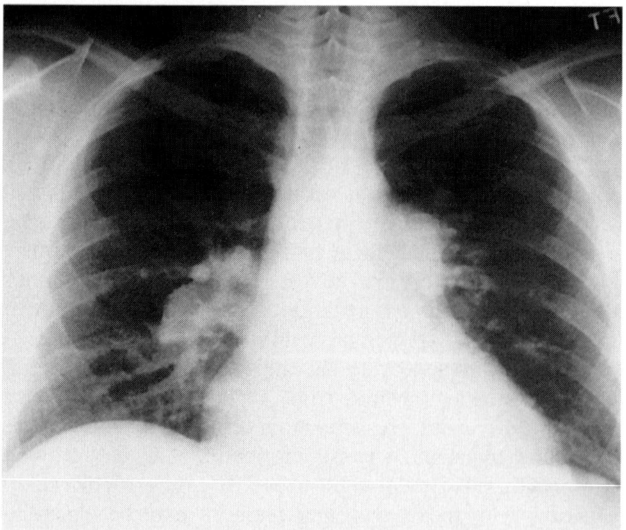

**Figure 52.7** Chest roentgenogram from a patient with primary pulmonary hypertension showing the marked dilation of the main pulmonary arteries and right ventricular enlargement.

pulmonary artery, peripheral oligemia, and an increase in the cardiothoracic ratio.[180]

Systemic arterial blood gas analysis in patients with primary pulmonary hypertension usually reveals a low $P_{CO_2}$ and a normal pH, reflecting chronic respiratory alkalosis. The systemic arterial $P_{O_2}$ may be normal or abnormal, but the alveolar-to-arterial $P_{O_2}$ difference usually is increased.[125] Several mechanisms have been proposed for the hypoxemia of patients with primary pulmonary hypertension, including diffusion impairment caused by a reduction in the number of pulmonary vessels coupled with the shortened time spent by erythrocytes in traversing the pulmonary circulation; ventilation-perfusion mismatching due to alterations in pulmonary blood flow and concomitant conditions such as bronchospasm; and right-to-left intracardiac shunting through a patent foramen ovale. Dantzker and Bower[189] demonstrated with the multiple inert gas elimination technique that the hypoxemia is caused by a combination of ventilation-perfusion mismatching, intrapulmonary shunt, and a low mixed venous $P_{O_2}$ resulting from a reduced cardiac output.

Pulmonary function tests performed in patients with primary pulmonary hypertension usually reveal normal expiratory flow rates with normal or mildly reduced lung volumes.[125] The modest restrictive defect has been attributed to diminished distensibility of the pulmonary vessels.[190] The diffusing capacity for carbon monoxide often is reduced to a mild or moderate degree.[125]

Exercise testing serves to bring out physiologic abnormalities in patients with primary pulmonary hypertension if these abnormalities are not present at rest. Characteristically, patients with pulmonary hypertension achieve their target heart rate and anaerobic threshold at low levels of exercise, often accompanied by a reduction in the systemic arterial $P_{O_2}$ or an increase in the alveolar-to-arterial $P_{O_2}$ difference. The dead space-to-tidal volume ratio either fails to decrease as it should in healthy persons or actually increases during graded exercise. Of course, exercise may be accompanied by an increase in pulmonary artery pressure and a demand for oxygen transport that cannot be met by a compromised circulation. Exercise testing may therefore be hazardous in patients with primary pulmonary hypertension, and a death has been reported during one such study.[152]

The electrocardiogram usually discloses right ventricular hypertrophy in patients with advanced primary pulmonary hypertension.[185] Electrocardiographic criteria for right ventricular hypertrophy include a QRS axis in the frontal plane that is greater than or equal to 110 degrees, an R wave in lead $V_1$ that is greater than 5 mm, an R-to-S ratio in $V_1$ that is greater than 1, and an R-to-S ratio in lead $V_6$ that is less than 1. Patients also may manifest right atrial enlargement with a symmetric and peaked P wave in lead II that is greater than 2.5 mm in amplitude. ST segment depression and T wave inversion may be seen in the anterior chest leads. These abnormalities may not be present if pulmonary hypertension is not pronounced or if patients are young.[180]

The echocardiogram may be helpful in documenting pulmonary hypertension and in ruling out conditions such as mitral stenosis and left ventricular dysfunction. Primary pulmonary hypertension has been associated in one-dimensional echocardiography with midsystolic notching, diminution of the *a* dip, prolongation of the right ventricular pre-ejection period, increased right ventricular systolic dimensions, and midsystolic fluttering of the pulmonary valve.[191–193] Two-dimensional echocardiography helps quantitate right atrial and right ventricular size and may identify systolic flattening or diastolic bulging of the interventricular septum due to increased pulmonary artery pressure.[194] Intracardiac shunting may be observed after the intravenous injection of microbubbles. In addition, Doppler techniques may allow estimation of pulmonary artery pressure.[195, 196]

Perfusion lung scanning has been used primarily to differentiate primary pulmonary hypertension from chronic pulmonary thromboembolism. Wilson and coworkers[197] scanned 21 patients with chronic obliterative pulmonary hypertension and observed three patterns: large multiple, segmental defects; multiple ill-defined defects; and no defects. The first pattern occurred exclusively among patients with documented thromboembolic disorders, whereas the third pattern was found exclusively among patients with primary pulmonary hypertension. The second pattern was attributed to disease of the small pulmonary arteries, although recurrent embolization or idiopathic hypertension could not be excluded. Later, D'Alonzo and associates[198] studied 25 patients; in all 8 patients with chronic pulmonary thromboembolism, lung scans indicated a high probability of embolic disease due to multiple segmental defects, whereas 17 patients with primary pulmonary hypertension had scans that were normal or indicated a low probability of embolism. This study suggests that lung scans are highly specific in differentiating the two conditions and might replace angiography, especially because of their relative safety. Not all investigators agree with this suggestion, however, and perfusion scanning was associated with sudden death in a patient with obliterative pulmonary vascular disease,[199] presumably because of transient obstruction of a critical number of small pulmonary vessels by the macroaggregates of radiolabeled albumin. Nevertheless, perfusion scanning generally is considered to be a safe procedure in patients with unexplained pulmonary hypertension; reduced doses of tracer material can be used for scanning if concern about patient safety exists. Scanning over the head or abdomen may yield images of the brain or kidneys, indicative of a right-to-left shunt (Fig. 52.8).

As indicated in the preceding discussion, pulmonary angiography remains the most accepted method of ruling out chronic pulmonary thromboembolism and other disorders in patients suspected of having primary pulmonary hypertension (Fig. 52.9). Arteriography is practical because it can be combined with pressure measurements in one session. However, death has been reported in patients with pulmonary hypertension undergoing arteriography, particularly when overt right ventricular failure is present.[200] The risk of compromising the pulmonary vascular bed during arteriography may be decreased by using smaller amounts of nonionic contrast material with selective injections or by digital subtraction angiography. Magnification arteriography through a catheter in the wedge position has been used in children to determine the nature and extent of pulmonary vascular disease.[201] Helical spiral computed tomography is also useful in excluding thrombotic disease of the proximal pulmonary vessels.

Right-heart catheterization traditionally has been employed to document severity of pulmonary hypertension, to help establish its cause, to determine the potential for acute pulmonary vasodilatation with oxygen and pharmacologic agents, and to assess the utility of chronic vasodilator therapy.[180] Cardiac chamber pressures are recorded, and the wedge pressure is measured to rule out disease at the level of the left ventricle, left atrium, or large pulmonary veins. Cardiac output is measured and from it and vascular pressures the pulmonary and systemic vascular resistances are calculated. Blood gas samples are taken to determine oxygen contents in the two circulations. These and other variables may be studied at rest or during exercise. Intracardiac shunts may be excluded by the measurements of blood oxygen contents in the various cardiac chambers and by indicator techniques.

Cardiac catheterization in patients with primary pulmonary hypertension usually reveals elevated right atrial pressure, pulmonary arterial pressures that are increased often to systemic levels, and depression of cardiac output. Pulmonary vascular resistance generally is increased, whereas systemic vascular resistance is in the normal range.[125, 202] In the US registry, mean values ($\pm 1$ SD) were as follows: right arterial pressure, $9.7 \pm 6$ mm Hg; pulmonary artery pressure, $60 \pm 18$ mm Hg; wedge pressure, $8.4 \pm 4$ mm Hg; cardiac index, $2.3 \pm 0.9$ L/min/m$^2$; and pulmonary vascular resistance index, $26 \pm 14$ mm Hg/L/min/m$^2$.[125] Mixed venous oxygen tensions usually are low, and the arterial-to-mixed venous oxygen content difference is increased. Approximately 20% of patients have a patent foramen ovale. Unless performed carefully, catheterization may increase pulmonary arterial pressure, worsen oxygen transport, and cause death.[203] Because of this possibility, cardiac catheterization should be performed only under controlled conditions, and its risks must be balanced against the information gained.

Virtually identical hemodynamic and clinical findings may be encountered in the extremely rare disease termed *pulmonary veno-occlusive* disease, which accounts for fewer than 10% of patients with unexplained pulmonary hypertension. Like primary pulmonary hypertension, pulmonary veno-occlusive disease appears to be a morphologic rather than an etiologic entity. In addition, pulmo-

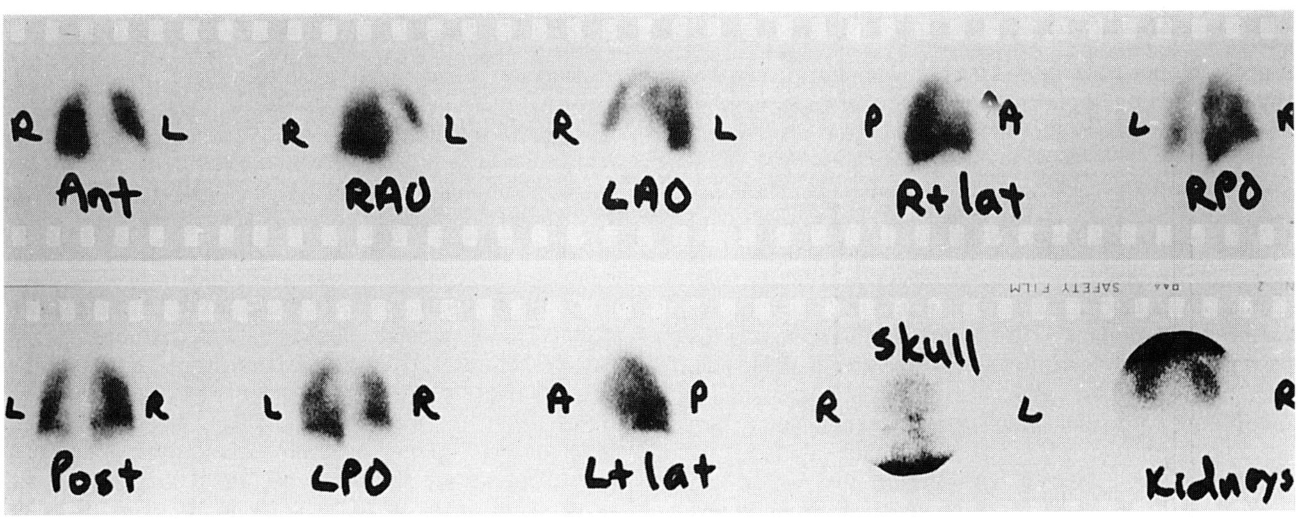


**Figure 52.8** Perfusion lung scan from a patient with primary pulmonary hypertension with a right-to-left shunt through a patent foramen ovale. The overall pattern of perfusion is normal; the presence of a shunt is demonstrated by the appearance of tracer when scanning over the skull and kidneys. Projections are as follows: Ant = anterior; LAO = left anterior oblique; Lt lat = left lateral; LPO = left posterior oblique; Post = posterior; RAO = right anterior oblique; Rt lat = right lateral; RPO = right posterior oblique.

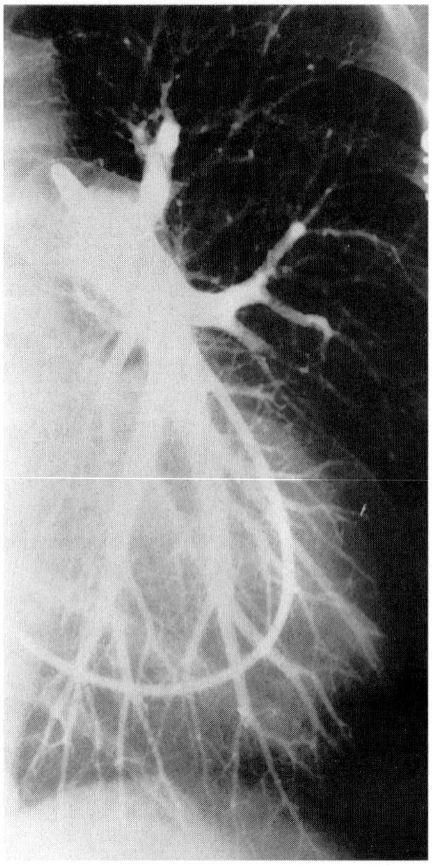

**Figure 52.9** Left pulmonary angiogram from a patient with primary pulmonary hypertension, showing the characteristic "pruning" of the peripheral vessels.

nary veno-occlusive disease tends to afflict infants, children, and young adults, although patients older than 60 years of age have been reported. However, in the adults with veno-occlusive disease who have been reported, there is a slight male preponderance. A familial occurrence of veno-occlusive disease also has been noted. Veno-occlusive disease has been associated with viral syndromes, toxin exposure, and chemotherapy. The characteristic histologic feature of pulmonary veno-occlusive disease is obstruction of pulmonary venules and veins by intimal fibrosis; intravascular fibrous septa, which usually are considered pathognomonic of recanalized thrombi, are nearly always present.[204] These findings have led to the speculation that thrombosis is an essential pathogenetic mechanism in most cases, but the factors causing or contributing to thrombus formation are completely unknown.

Of considerable interest is the recent observation that narrowing or obliteration of pulmonary arteries is found in approximately half the cases of pulmonary veno-occlusive disease.[204] The morphologic appearance of the arterial lesions indicates that they also were produced by organization of intravascular thrombi and that the abnormalities were not merely secondary to pulmonary venous obstruction with attendant medial hypertrophy and arterial hypertension. These observations raise the question whether there are two variations of the same basic disorder: the classic form of pulmonary veno-occlusive disease, in which the arteries are spared, and a generalized form, in which both arteries and veins are involved. It has even been suggested that the latter variety be called *pulmonary vascular occlusive disease*.[205]

Pulmonary veno-occlusive disease cannot be distinguished with certainty from primary pulmonary hypertension by right-heart catheterization unless the pulmonary capillary wedge pressure is elevated. Apart from the difficulties of successfully wedging a catheter in patients with pulmonary hypertension, whether the wedge pressure is elevated depends on whether the venous obstruction is in the venules or the large veins.[206] This is because the pressure actually measured at the tip of a catheter positioned in an obstructed pulmonary artery, by either wedging or inflating a balloon, is the pressure in the next freely communicating downstream vessel. Accordingly, if venules are occluded, as is often the case in pulmonary veno-occlusive disease, the next freely communicating vessel may be a vein in which the pressure is normal. In contrast, if (large) veins are the sites of occlusion, then the pulmonary venous pressure is likely to be elevated proximally and to be detectable at catheterization. Indeed, the wedge pressure may vary in different sites within the lung in patients with veno-occlusive disease. Some authors have suggested that a diffuse, patchy pattern on perfusion lung scanning in a patient with unexplained pulmonary hypertension is strongly suggestive of pulmonary veno-occlusive disease.[207] The chest radiograph may show signs of pulmonary hypertension with prominent Kerley B lines in the absence of other signs of left-sided heart failure, and this is often the most useful clue to the diagnosis in a patient with unexplained severe pulmonary hypertension. In addition, patients with veno-occlusive disease may develop acute pulmonary edema in response to pharmacologic agents that reduce upstream pulmonary vascular resistance and increase cardiac output, such as prostacyclin.[208] This phenomenon probably is caused by an increase in pulmonary blood volume in the face of downstream vascular obstruction.

The final diagnostic technique to be considered in patients suspected of having primary pulmonary hypertension or pulmonary veno-occlusive disease is lung biopsy. In their morphologic study of 156 patients in whom primary pulmonary hypertension was suspected, Wagenvoort and Wagenvoort[140] demonstrated that 45 persons had other disorders, some of which were treatable. More recently, Wagenvoort[209] showed that open-lung biopsy may be helpful not only in diagnosing patients but also in predicting their responses to therapy for pulmonary hypertension and congenital cardiac disorders. Despite these studies, open-lung biopsy remains a potentially harmful procedure that does not affect the clinical outcome of most patients. Its major value has been in documenting the heterogeneity of lesions in patients with pulmonary hypertension and elucidating the natural history of this condition.

## Treatment and Prognosis

A comprehensive medical approach is essential in managing patients with primary pulmonary hypertension. In particular, patients should be instructed to avoid circumstances that may increase pulmonary artery pressure and decrease cardiac output. The alveolar hypoxia of high altitude (e.g., flying in commercial aircraft) is one stimulus that may exacerbate pulmonary hypertension. Similarly, concurrent cardiopulmonary disease should be treated, oxygen should be given to hypoxemic patients, and cigarette smoking should be avoided. Indomethacin and related prostaglandin synthesis inhibitors and sympathomimetic drugs should be avoided because of their vasoconstrictive actions, as should barbiturates and other drugs that depress cardiac output.[210]

Another potentially adverse circumstance is pregnancy, which imposes an additional burden on the cardiovascular system.[157, 158] Conception probably should be prevented in women with primary pulmonary hypertension, preferably without oral contraceptives, and consideration should be given to terminating pregnancies that occur. If abortion is chosen, abortifacients such as prostaglandin $F_{2\alpha}$, which may increase pulmonary artery pressure, should not be used.[211]

Warfarin has been given to many patients with primary pulmonary hypertension because chronic pulmonary thromboembolism had not been ruled out, because in situ thrombosis was perceived as part of the pathogenesis of primary pulmonary hypertension, or because no other treatment was available. A retrospective review from the Mayo Clinic[212] suggested that anticoagulants actually may have improved survival in patients with pulmonary hypertension of unknown cause, although they often were initiated late in the course of the disease; another later study came to the same conclusion.[213] Whether the improvement was caused by alteration of the underlying lesion of plexogenic pulmonary arteriopathy, by treatment of patients who actually had chronic pulmonary thromboembolism or pulmonary veno-occlusive disease, or by preventing in situ thrombosis from becoming superimposed on these three disorders is not clear from these studies. Furthermore, the value of anticoagulation has yet to be established in a prospective randomized trial of patients with either pulmonary hypertension of unknown cause or plexogenic pulmonary arteriopathy in particular. Anticoagulation poses a potential risk, especially in persons prone to syncope or hemoptysis. If anticoagulation is contemplated in such patients, adjusted-dose subcutaneous heparin may be considered as an alternative to warfarin. Patients with intracardiac shunting through a patent foramen ovale are at additional risk for a paradoxic embolism.

Vasodilators have been used to treat patients with primary pulmonary hypertension for many years. Sublingual isoproterenol,[214] phentolamine,[215] hydralazine,[216, 217] diazoxide,[218] nifedipine,[219, 220] captopril,[221] nitrates,[222] and prostaglandin inhibitors[223] have been used on a long-term basis.

The studies of vasodilators in primary pulmonary hypertension are hampered by the lack of a meaningful physiologic end point. Most investigators focus on pulmonary vascular resistance, a variable that is calculated from pressure and flow data rather than measured directly. Pulmonary vascular resistance does indeed decline in some patients receiving vasodilators, but often this decline is not caused by a decrease in pulmonary artery pressure but by an increase in cardiac output related to tachycardia, the augmented venous return, and the recruitment of previously unused pulmonary vascular channels. Furthermore, the price paid for a decline in pulmonary vascular resistance may be a decrease in systemic vascular resistance associated with severe hypotension and an interference with hypoxic pulmonary vasoconstriction that worsens oxygenation.[224] Conversely, pulmonary vascular resistance may be a better variable to follow than pulmonary artery pressure. Survival in patients with primary pulmonary hypertension cannot be predicted by the severity of pulmonary hypertension per se and probably is related, as is symptom relief, to increases in transpulmonary blood flow.[180, 225]

Whatever the variable observed, sustained beneficial hemodynamic and symptomatic responses to vasodilators probably occur in 20% to 40% of patients with primary pulmonary hypertension.[226–228] Because syncope and sudden death may result from vasodilators, these agents should be used cautiously. Furthermore, because hemodynamic response cannot be predicted, the drugs should be administered initially in the catheterization laboratory or under carefully controlled conditions in an intensive care unit. Some investigators have advocated using potent titratable, short-acting intravenous agents, such as prostaglandin $I_2$ or adenosine, or nitric oxide by inhalation as screening agents with which pulmonary vasoreactivity can be assessed with relative safety.[143, 227–229] Patients receiving vasodilators should be followed closely, and responsiveness should be evaluated by repeat catheterization, as required.[230] The most widely used vasodilators are the calcium-channel blocking agents nifedipine and diltiazem.[213, 219, 220, 227] In responsive patients, these drugs produce improvement in pulmonary hemodynamics and right ventricular function, often accompanied by improved exercise tolerance. Recently, high doses of calcium-channel blockers in patients with primary pulmonary hypertension who responded with reductions in pulmonary artery pressure and pulmonary vascular resistance were shown to improve survival over a 5-year period.[213] Rich and Brundage[232] have advocated using a regimen consisting of large doses of these agents, which they believe may be required to elicit the sustained beneficial responses. Continuous intravenous infusions of prostacyclin (prostaglandin $I_2$, epoprostenol) have been used in patients who were refractory to conventional therapy, either as a primary mode of treatment or as a bridge to transplantation, and produce sustained improvement in hemodynamics and exercise tolerance as well as prolonged survival.[208]

Until recently, combined heart-lung transplantation was the only remaining therapy for patients who did not respond to vasodilators. First performed at Stanford University in 1981, this procedure was associated with both functional improvement and increased longevity in severely disabled persons who would have died without surgery.[233, 234] However, in addition to complications directly related to immunosuppression, such as opportunistic infections and graft rejection, obliterative bronchiolitis occurs with striking frequency in heart-lung transplant patients and can substantially compromise lung function.[234] In addition, organ availability has further limited the widespread application of this technique. (The benefits and complications of lung transplantation are discussed in detail in Chapter 97.)

The remarkable capacity of the right ventricle to revert to normal or near-normal function after pulmonary thromboendarterectomy in patients with chronic thrombotic pulmonary vascular obstruction,[235] which has now been associated with substantial long-term improvement in survival, function, and quality of life,[235a] led to the suggestion that single- or double-lung transplantation may be a viable option for patients with primary pulmonary hypertension who are refractory to medical management. Single-lung transplantation has been reported to result in a prompt decline in pulmonary artery pressure and normalization of right-sided heart function in several patients.[236] However, organ rejection may be associated with severe hypoxemia in this setting because of an inability to redistribute blood flow to the native hypertensive lung in the setting of impaired ventilation in the donor lung. In addition, obliterative bronchiolitis occurs in lung transplant recipients as well, although the incidence may be lower than in heart-lung transplant patients.

Survival of patients with primary pulmonary hypertension is generally poor, with a median survival in the U.S. registry of 2.8 years.[125] Variables associated with poor survival included a New York Heart Association functional class III or IV, presence of Raynaud's phenomenon, elevated right atrial and mean pulmonary artery pressures, decreased cardiac index and diffusing capacity for carbon monoxide, and exercise intolerance using the 6-minute walk test.[125, 208, 225] Sudden death occurs frequently and probably is caused by acute right ventricular decompensation, arrhythmia, or a thromboembolic event. Nevertheless, improvements in management have lengthened survival in the subgroup of patients with reversible pulmonary artery hypertension,[208, 213] and there is hope for other patients with the disease.[237]

## SUMMARY

Pulmonary vasculitis is a relatively rare condition despite its association with the collagen vascular disorders and other systemic processes. It is a major component of illnesses such as the granulomatous vasculitides that affect the lungs primarily; it also may be a part of diseases, such as the leukocytoclastic vasculitides, in which the lungs are minimally involved. Because of the considerable overlap among the various pulmonary vasculitides, it seems likely that they have a similar immunopathogenesis. The diagnosis of vasculitis usually is made by biopsy of involved tissues, such as the skin, upper airways, or lungs. Some but not all of these disorders respond to immunosuppressive or cytotoxic drugs. More specific treatment awaits an understanding of the etiology of the pulmonary vasculitides.

Primary pulmonary hypertension is a severely debilitating illness that too often is diagnosed only when it is far advanced. Mortality is related to impaired right ventricular function and is best predicted on the basis of relationships between stroke volume index and right atrial and pulmonary artery pressures. Iatrogenic insults also contribute to mortality, and clinicians frequently are frustrated both by their inability to treat primary pulmonary hypertension and by complicity in their patients' poor outcome. Despite this frustration, there is reason for cautious hope in the treatment of primary pulmonary hypertension. Some patients do benefit from vasodilators; others gain extra time with good medical management; still others appear so far to have been helped by combined heart-lung or lung transplantation. The future should bring better tools for the noninvasive assessment of pulmonary hemodynamics and thereby facilitate improved diagnosis and follow-up of patients. Further research also should help elucidate the cause(s) of this baffling disease.

## References


1. Fauci AS: The spectrum of vasculitis. Ann Intern Med 89:660–676, 1978.
2. Sams WM Jr: Necrotizing vasculitis. J Am Acad Dermatol 3:1–13, 1980.
3. Sullivan EJ, Hoffman GS: Pulmonary vasculitis. Clin Chest Med 19:759–776, 1998.
4. Schönlein JL: Allegemeine und spezielle Pathologie und Therapie (3rd ed, Vol 2). Freiberg: Hexisan, 1837.
5. Kussmaul A, Maier K: Uber eine bisher nicht beschriebene eigenthumliche Arterienerkrankung (periarteritis nodosa) die mit Morbus Brightii: und rapid fortschreitender allemeiner Muskellahmung einhergeht Dtsch. Arch Klin Med 1:484–517, 1866.
6. Zeek PM: Periarteritis nodosa and other forms of necrotizing angiitis. N Engl J Med 248:764–772, 1953.
7. Liebow AA: Pulmonary angiitis and granulomatosis. Am Rev Respir Dis 108:118, 1973.
8. Fulmer JD, Kaltreider B: The pulmonary vasculitides. Chest 82:615–624, 1982.
9. Bloch DA, Michel BA, Hunder GG, et al: The American College of Rheumatology 1990 criteria for the classification of vasculitis: Patients and methods. Arthritis Rheum 33:1068–1073, 1990.
10. Hunder GG, Arend WP, Bloch DA, et al: The American College of Rheumatology 1990 criteria for the classification of vasculitis: Introduction. Arthritis Rheum 33:1065–1067, 1990.
11. Leavitt RY, Fauci AS, Bloch DA, et al: The American College of Rheumatology 1990 criteria for the classification of Wegener's granulomatosis. Arthritis Rheum 33:1101–1107, 1990.
12. Lightfoot RW, Michel BA, Bloch DA, et al: The American College of Rheumatology 1990 criteria for the classification of polyarteritis nodosa. Arthitis Rheum 33:1088–1093, 1990.
13. Masi AT, Hunder GG, Lie JT, et al: The American College of Rheumatology 1990 criteria for the classification of Churg-Strauss syndrome (allergic granulomatosis and angiitis). Arthritis Rheum 33:1094–1100, 1990.
14. Mills JA, Michel BA, Bloch DA, et al: The American College of Rheumatology 1990 criteria for the classification of Henoch-Schönlein purpura. Arthritis Rheum 33:1114–1121, 1990.
15. Hunder GG, Bloch DA, Michel BA, et al: The American College of Rheumatology 1990 criteria for the classification of giant cell arteritis. Arthritis Rheum 33:1122–1128, 1990.
16. Calabrese LH, Michel BA, Bloch DA, et al: The American College of Rheumatology 1990 criteria for the classification of hypersensitivity vasculitis. Arthritis Rheum 33:1108–1113, 1990.
17. Arend WP, Michel BA, Bloch DA, et al: The American College of Rheumatology 1990 criteria for the classification of Takayasu arteritis. Arthritis Rheum 33:1129–1134, 1990.
18. Fauci AS, Wolff SM: Wegener's granulomatosis: Studies in eighteen patients with a review of the literature. Medicine 52:535–561, 1973.
19. Gilliam JN, Smiley JD: Cutaneous necrotizing vasculitis and related disorders. Ann Allergy 37:328–339, 1976.
20. Hunninghake GW, Fauci AS: Pulmonary involvement in the collagen vascular diseases. Am Rev Respir Dis 119:471–503, 1979.
21. Churg J, Strauss L: Allergic granulomatosis, allergic angiitis, and periarteritis nodosa. Am J Pathol 27:277–301, 1951.

21a. Guillevin L, Cohen P, Gayraud M, et al: Churg-Strauss syndrome:

Clinical study and long-term follow-up of 96 patients. Medicine 78:26–37, 1999.
22. Clauw DJ, Nashel DJ, Umhau A, et al: Tryptophan-associated eosinophilic connective tissue disease: A new clinical entity? JAMA 263:1502–1506, 1990.
23. Centers for Disease Control: Eosinophilia-myalgia syndrome: New Mexico. MMWR Morb Mortal Wkly Rep 38:756–767, 1989.
24. Rao JK, Weinberger M, Oddone EZ, et al: The role of antineutrophil cytoplasmic antibody (C-ANCA) testing in the diagnosis of Wegener's granulomatosis. Ann Intern Med 123:925–932, 1995.
25. Erzurum SC, Underwood GA, Hamilos DL, et al: Pleural effusion in Churg-Strauss syndrome. Chest 95:1357–1359, 1989.
26. Katzenstein A, Liebow AA, Friedman PJ: Bronchocentric granulomatosis, mucoid impaction, and hypersensitivity reactions to fungi. Am Rev Respir Dis 111:497–537, 1975.
27. Wasserman K, Whipp BJ: Exercise physiology in health and disease. Am Rev Respir Dis 112:219–249, 1975.
28. Hoffman GS, Kerr GS, Leavitt RY, et al: Wegener granulomatosis: An analysis of 158 patients. Ann Intern Med 116:488–498, 1992.
29. Niles JL: Value of tests for antineutrophil cytoplasmic autoantibodies in the diagnosis and treatment of vasculitis. Curr Opin Rheumatol 5:18–24, 1993.
30. Novack SN, Pearson CM: Cyclophosphamide therapy in Wegener's granulomatosis. N Engl J Med 17:938–942, 1971.
31. Wegener F: Über generalisierte, septische Gefässerkrankungen. Verh Dtsch Ges Pathol 29:202–210, 1936.
32. Godman GC, Churg J: Wegener's granulomatosis. Arch Pathol 58:533–553, 1954.
33. Howell SB, Epstein WV: Circulating immunoglobulin complexes in Wegener's granulomatosis. Am J Med 60:259–268, 1976.
34. Fahey JL, Leonard E, Churg J, et al: Wegener's granulomatosis. Am J Med 17:168–179, 1954.
35. Fauci AS, Haynes BF, Katz P, et al: Wegener's granulomatosis: Prospective clinical and therapeutic experience with patients for 21 years. Ann Intern Med 98:76–85, 1983.
36. Fauci AS, Johnson RE, Wolff SM: Radiation therapy of midline granuloma. Ann Intern Med 84:140–147, 1976.
37. Landman S, Burgener I: Pulmonary manifestations in Wegener's granulomatosis. AJR Am J Roentgenol 122:750–757, 1974.
38. Gohel VK, Dalinka MK, Israel HL, et al: The radiological manifestations of Wegener's granulomatosis. Br J Radiol 46:427–432, 1973.
39. Maguire R, Fauci AS, Doppman JL, et al: Unusual radiographic features of Wegener's granulomatosis. AJR Am J Roentgenol 130:233–238, 1978.
40. Travis WD, Colby TV, Lombard C, et al: A clinicopathologic study of 34 cases of diffuse pulmonary hemorrhage with lung biopsy confirmation. Am J Surg Pathol 14:1112–1125, 1990.
41. Travis WD, Hoffman GS, Leavitt RY, et al: Surgical pathology of the lung in Wegener's granulomatosis. Am J Surg Pathol 15:315–333, 1991.
42. van der Woude FJ, Rasmussen N, Lobatto S, et al: Autoantibodies against neutrophils and monocytes: Tool for diagnosis and marker of disease activity in Wegener's granulomatosis. Lancet 1:425–429, 1985.
43. Specks U, Wheatley CL, McDonald TJ, et al: Anticytoplasmic autoantibodies in the diagnosis and followup of Wegener's granulomatosis. Mayo Clin Proc 64:28–36, 1989.
44. Beer DJ: ANCAs aweigh. Am Rev Respir Dis 146:1128–1130, 1992.
45. Bosch X, Font J, Mirapeix E: Antimyeloperoxidase autoantibody associated necrotizing alveolar capillaritis. Am Rev Respir Dis 146:1326–1329, 1992.
46. Fauci AS, Wolff SM, Johnson JS: Effect of cyclophosphamide upon the immune response in Wegener's granulomatosis. N Engl J Med 285:1493–1496, 1971.
47. Haubitz M, Schellong S, Gobel U, et al: Intravenous pulse administration of cyclophosphamide versus daily oral treatment in patients with antineutrophil cytoplasmic antibody–associated vasculitis and renal involvement: A prospective, randomized study. Arthritis Rheum 41:1835–1844, 1998.
48. Stegeman CA, Tervaert JWC, de Jong PE, et al: Trimethoprim-sulfamethoxazole (co-trimoxazole) for the prevention of relapses of Wegener's granulomatosis. N Eng J Med 335:16–20, 1996.
49. Carrington CB, Liebow AA: Limited forms of angiitis and granulomatosis of Wegener's type. Am J Med 41:497–527, 1966.
50. Cassan SM, Coles DT, Harrison EG: The concept of limited forms of Wegener's granulomatosis. Am J Med 49:366–379, 1970.
51. Liebow A, Carrington C, Friedman P: Lymphomatoid granulomatosis. Hum Pathol 3:457–506, 1972.
52. Katzenstein A-L, Carrington CB, Liebow AA: Lymphomatoid granulomatosis. Cancer 43:360–373, 1979.
53. Nichols PW, Koss M, Levine AM, et al: Lymphomatoid granulomatosis: T-cell disorder? Am J Med 72:467–471, 1982.
54. Fauci AS, Haynes BF, Costa J, et al: Lymphomatoid granulomatosis: Prospective clinical and therapeutic experience over 10 years. N Engl J Med 306:68–74, 1982.
55. DeRemee RA, Weiland LH, McDonald TJ: Polymorphic reticulosis, lymphomatoid granulomatosis: Two diseases or one? Mayo Clin Proc 53:634–640, 1978.
56. Colby TV, Carrington CB: Pulmonary lymphomas simulating lymphomatoid granulomatosis. J Surg Pathol 6:19–32, 1982.
57. Israel HL, Patchefsky AS, Saldana MJ: Wegener's granulomatosis, lymphomatoid granulomatosis, and benign lymphocytic angiitis and granulomatosis of lung. Ann Intern Med 87:691–699, 1977.
58. Saldana MJ, Patchefsky AS, Israel HI, et al: Pulmonary angiitis and granulomatosis. Hum Pathol 8:391–409, 1977.
59. Fauci AS: Granulomatous vasculitides: Distinct but related. Ann Intern Med 87:782–783, 1977.
60. Kus J, Bergin C, Miller R, et al: Lymphocyte subpopulations in allergic granulomatosis and angiitis (Churg-Strauss syndrome). Chest 87:826–828, 1985.
61. Koss N, Monovych T, Hochholzer L: Allergic granulomatosis (Churg-Strauss syndrome): Pulmonary and renal morphologic findings. Am J Surg Pathol 5:21–28, 1981.
62. Bottcher E: Disseminated sarcoidosis with a marked granulomatous arteritis. Arch Pathol 68:419–423, 1959.
63. Rosen Y, Moon S, Huang C, et al: Granulomatous pulmonary angiitis in sarcoidosis. Arch Pathol Lab Med 101:170–174, 1977.
64. Stephen JG, Braimbridge MV, Corrin B, et al: Necrotizing "sarcoidal" angiitis and granulomatosis of the lung. Thorax 31:356–360, 1976.
65. Churg A, Carrington CB, Gupta R: Necrotizing sarcoid granulomatosis. Chest 76:406–413, 1979.
66. Sharma O, Hewlett R, Gordonson JC: Nodular sarcoidosis: An unusual radiographic appearance. Chest 64:189–192, 1973.
67. Onal E, Lopata M, Lourenco R: Nodular pulmonary sarcoidosis. Chest 72:296–300, 1977.
68. Koss MN, Robinson RG, Hochholzer L: Bronchocentric granulomatosis. Hum Pathol 12:632–638, 1981.
69. Robinson RG, Wehunt WD, Tsou E, et al: Bronchocentric granulomatosis: Roentgenographic manifestations. Am Rev Respir Dis 125:751–756, 1982.
70. Winkelmann RK, Ditto WB: Cutaneous and visceral syndromes of necrotizing or "allergic" angiitis: A study of 38 cases. Medicine 43:59–89, 1964.
71. Sergent JS, Lockshin MD, Christian CL, et al: Vasculitis with hepatitis B antigenemia: Long-term observation in nine patients. Medicine 55:1–18, 1976.
72. Sams WM Jr, Claman HN, Kohler PF, et al: Human necrotizing vasculitis: Immunoglobulins and complement in vessel walls of cutaneous lesions and normal skin. J Invest Dermatol 64:441–445, 1975.
73. Allen DM, Diamond LK, Howell DA: Anaphylactoid purpura in children (Schönlein-Henoch syndrome). Am J Dis Child 99:147–168, 1960.
74. Cream JJ, Gumpel JM, Peachey RD: Schönlein-Henoch purpura in the adult. QJM 34:461–487, 1970.
75. Bombardieri S, Paoletti P, Ferri C, et al: Lung involvement in essential mixed cryoglobulinemia. Am J Med 66:748–756, 1979.
76. Petty TL, Wilkins M: The five manifestations of rheumatoid lung. Dis Chest 49:75–82, 1966.
77. Kay JM, Banik S: Unexplained pulmonary hypertension with pulmonary arteritis in rheumatoid disease. Br J Dis Chest 71:53–59, 1977.
78. Yousem SA, Colby TV, Carrington CB: Lung biopsy in rheumatoid arthritis. Am Rev Respir Dis 131:770–777, 1985.

patterns of pulmonic valve motion with pulmonary hypertension. Circulation 50:905–910, 1974.
192. Nanda NC, Gramiak R, Robinson TI, et al: Echocardiograph evaluation of pulmonary hypertension. Circulation 50:575–581, 1974.
193. Lew W, Karliner JS: Assessment of pulmonary valve echogram in normal subjects and in patients with pulmonary arterial hypertension. Br Heart J 42:147–161, 1979.
194. Tanaka H, Tei C, Nakao S, et al: Diastolic bulging of the interventricular septum toward the left ventricle. Circulation 62:558–563, 1980.
195. Kitabatake A, Inoue M, Asao M, et el: Noninvasive evaluation of pulmonary hypertension by a pulsed Doppler technique. Circulation 68:302–309, 1983.
196. Hinterlitter AL, Willis PW, Barst RJ, et al: Effects of long-term infusion of prostacyclin (epoprostenol) on echocardiographic measures of right ventricular structure and function in primary pulmonary hypertension. Circulation 95:1479–1486, 1997.
197. Wilson AG, Harris CN, Lavender JP, et al: Perfusion lung scanning in obliterative pulmonary hypertension. Br Heart J 35:917–930, 1973.
198. D'Alonzo G, Bower JS, Dantzker DR: Differentiation of patients with primary and thromboembolic pulmonary hypertension. Chest 85:457–462, 1984.
199. Child JS, Wolfe JD, Tashkin D, et al: Fatal lung scan in a case of pulmonary hypertension due to obliterative pulmonary vascular disease. Chest 67:308–310, 1975.
200. Perlmutt LM, Braun SD, Newman GE, et al: Pulmonary arteriography in the high-risk patient. Radiology 162:187–189, 1987.
201. Nihill MR, McNamara DG: Magnification pulmonary wedge angiography in the evaluation of children with congenital heart disease and pulmonary hypertension. Circulation 58:1094–1106, 1978.
202. Sleeper JC, Orgain ES, McIntosh HD: Primary pulmonary hypertension: Review of clinical features and pathologic physiology with a report of pulmonary hemodynamics derived from repeated catheterization. Circulation 26:1358–1369, 1962.
203. Caldini P, Gensini GG, Hoffman MS: Primary pulmonary hypertension with death during right heart catheterization. Am J Cardiol 4:519–527, 1959.
204. Wagenvoort CA, Wagenvoort N, Takahashi T: Pulmonary veno-occlusive disease: Involvement of pulmonary arteries and review of the literature. Hum Pathol 16:1033–1041, 1985.
205. Päakkö, P, Sutinen S, Remes M, et al: A case of pulmonary vascular occlusive disease: Comparison of postmortem radiography and histology. Histopathology 9:253–262, 1985.
206. Rich S: Primary pulmonary hypertension. Prog Cardiovasc Dis 31:205–238, 1988.
207. Rich S, Pietra GG, Kieras K, et al: Primary pulmonary hypertension: Radiographic and scintigraphic patterns of histologic subtypes. Ann Intern Med 105:499–502, 1986.
208. Barst RJ, Rubin LJ, Long WA, et al: A comparison of continuous intravenous epoprostenol (prostacyclin) with conventional therapy for primary pulmonary hypertension. N Eng J Med 334: 296–302, 1996.
209. Wagenvoort CA: Lung biopsy specimens in the evaluation of pulmonary vascular disease. Chest 77:614–625, 1980.
210. Inkley SR, Gillespie L, Funkhouser RK: Two cases of primary pulmonary hypertension with sudden death associated with the administration of barbiturates. Ann Intern Med 43:396–406, 1955.
211. Weir EK, Greer BE, Smith SC, et al: Bronchoconstriction and pulmonary hypertension during abortion induced by 15-methyl-prostaglandin $F_2$. Am J Med 60:556–562, 1976.
212. Fuster V: Primary pulmonary hypertension: Natural history and the importance of thrombosis. Circulation 70:580–587, 1984.
213. Rich S, Kaufmann RN, Levy PS: The effect of high doses of calcium-channel blockers on survival in primary pulmonary hypertension. N Engl J Med 327:76–81, 1992.
214. Shettigar UR, Hultgren HN, Specter M, et al: Primary pulmonary hypertension: Favorable effect of isoproterenol. N Engl J Med 295:1414–1415, 1976.
215. Ruskin JN, Hutter AM: Primary pulmonary hypertension treated with oral phentolamine. Ann Intern Med 90:772–774, 1979.
216. Rubin LJ, Peter RH: Oral hydralazine therapy for primary pulmonary hypertension. N Engl J Med 302:69–74, 1980.
217. Lupi-Herrera E, Sandoval J, Sloane M, et al: The role of hydralazine therapy for pulmonary arterial hypertension of unknown cause. Circulation 65:645–650, 1982.
218. Klinke WP, Gilbert JAL: Diazoxide in primary pulmonary hypertension. N Engl J Med 302:91–92, 1980.
219. Rubin LJ, Nicod P, Hillis LD, et al: Treatment of primary pulmonary hypertension with nifedipine: A hemodynamic and scintigraphic evaluation. Ann Intern Med 99:433–438, 1983.
220. Feyter PJ, Kerkkamp HJJ, deJong JP: Sustained beneficial effect of nifedipine in primary pulmonary hypertension. Am Heart J 105:333–334, 1982.
221. Rich S, Martinez J, Lam K, et al: Captopril as treatment for patients with pulmonary hypertension: Problem of variability in assessing chronic drug treatment. Br Heart J 48:272–277, 1982.
222. Pearl RG, Rosenthal MH, Schroeder JS, et al: Acute hemodynamic effects of nitroglycerin in pulmonary hypertension. Ann Intern Med 99:9–13, 1983.
223. Hermiller JB, Bambach D, Thompson MJ, et al: Vasodilators and prostaglandin inhibitors in primary pulmonary hypertension. Ann Intern Med 97:480–489, 1982.
224. Rich S, Martinez J, Lam W, et al: Reassessment of the effects of vasodilator drugs in primary pulmonary hypertension: Guidelines for determining a pulmonary vasodilator response. Am Heart J 105:119–127, 1985.
225. D'Alonzo GE, Barst RJ, Ayres SM, et al: Survival in patients with primary pulmonary hypertension. Results from a national prospective registry. Ann Intern Med 115:343–349, 1991.
226. Weir EK, Rubin LJ, Ayres SM, et al: The acute administration of vasodilators in primary pulmonary hypertension. Am Rev Respir Dis 140:1623–1630, 1989.
227. Brown G: Pharmacologic treatment of primary and secondary pulmonary hypertension. Pharmacotherapy 11:137–156, 1991.
228. Rubin LJ, Groves BM, Reeves JT, et al: Prostacyclin-induced pulmonary vasodilation in primary pulmonary hypertension. Circulation 66:334–338, 1982.
229. Long W, Rubin LJ: Prostacyclin and prostaglandin $E_1$ treatment of pulmonary hypertension. Am Rev Respir Dis 136:773–776, 1987.
230. Rounds S, Hill NS: Pulmonary hypertensive diseases. Chest 85:397–405, 1984.
231. D'Alonzo GE, Gianotti L, Dantzker DR: Noninvasive assessment of hemodynamic improvement during chronic vasodilator therapy in obliterative pulmonary hypertension. Am Rev Respir Dis 133:380–384, 1986.
232. Rich S, Brundage BH: High-dose calcium channel-blocking therapy for primary pulmonary hypertension: Evidence for long-term reduction in pulmonary arterial pressure and regression in right ventricular hypertrophy. Circulation 76:135–141, 1987.
233. Reitz BA, Wallwork JL, Hernt SA, et al: Heart-lung transplantation. N Engl J Med 306:557–564, 1982.
234. Theodore J, Jamieson SW, Burke CM, et al: Physiologic aspects of human heartlung transplantation: Pulmonary function status of the posttransplanted lung. Chest 86:349–357, 1984.
235. Moser KM, Daily PO, Peterson K, et al: Thromboendarterectomy for chronic, major vessel thromboembolic pulmonary hypertension: Immediate and longterm results in 42 patients. Ann Intern Med 107:560–565, 1987.
235a. Archibald CJ, Auger WR, Fedullo PF, et al: Long-term outcome after pulmonary thromboendarterectomy. Am J Respir Crit Care Med 160:523–528, 1999.
236. Pasque MK, Trulock EP, Kaiser LR, et al: Single-lung transplantation for pulmonary hypertension. Circulation 84: 2275–2279, 1991.
237. Reeves JT, Groves BM, Turkevich D: The case for treatment of selected patients with primary pulmonary hypertension. Am Rev Respir Dis 134:342–346, 1986.

# 53 Pulmonary Arteriovenous Malformations and Other Pulmonary Vascular Abnormalities

J. MICHAEL B. HUGHES, D.M., F.R.C.P. • JOHN M. LUCE, M.D.

Introduction
Pulmonary Arteriovenous Malformations
- Classification
- Hereditary Hemorrhagic Telangiectasia
- Clinical Features of Pulmonary Arteriovenous Malformations
- Diagnosis
- Pathophysiology
- Treatment
- Idiopathic Pulmonary Arteriovenous Malformations

Systemic-Pulmonary Vascular Communication
- Classification
- Diagnosis and Treatment

Bronchopulmonary Sequestration
- Pathogenesis
- Epidemiology and Pathology
- Symptoms
- Diagnosis, Treatment, and Prognosis

Pulmonary Artery Aneurysms
- Classification
- Etiology and Pathogenesis
- Pathology
- Symptoms
- Diagnosis
- Treatment and Prognosis

Summary

## INTRODUCTION

Pulmonary vascular abnormalities occur in a variety of acquired and congenital conditions. These abnormalities include vascular communications that either are confined to the pulmonary circulation, as is the case with pulmonary arteriovenous malformations, or join the systemic and pulmonary circulations, as with bronchopulmonary sequestration. Aneurysmal dilations of the pulmonary artery also occur and are considered in this chapter. The vast array of congenital cardiac abnormalities and associated aberrant vascular communications, such as cor triatriatum[1] and total anomalous pulmonary venous connection,[2] are discussed elsewhere.[3]

## PULMONARY ARTERIOVENOUS MALFORMATIONS

### Classification

From a functional viewpoint, pulmonary arteriovenous malformations (PAVMs) behave as right-to-left intrapulmonary shunts. There is arterial hypoxemia and a predisposition to paradoxical embolism. A characteristic, and diagnostic, finding is that after intravenous injection, radiolabeled albumin macroaggregates pass through the lung (in proportion to the shunt) and into the systemic circulation and can be detected by a gamma camera placed over the head or the kidneys. Alternatively, contrast echocardiography will show microcavitations in the left atrium after intravenous injection of agitated saline (or other contrast media). Excluding right-to-left intracardiac shunts, intrapulmonary right-to-left shunting occurs either on a macroscopic basis, as in hereditary hemorrhagic telangiectasia and idiopathic and developmental arteriovenous malformations, or on a microscopic basis, as in the hepatopulmonary syndrome or portal hypertension with or without cirrhosis.

All three varieties of PAVMs have similar physiological features but differ in other characteristics (Table 53.1). The two macroscopic types of PAVM are indistinguishable except that hereditary hemorrhagic telangiectasia is accompanied by extrapulmonary manifestations and by a strong family history, and the developmental type is usually confined to the lungs. These malformations represent communications between the pulmonary arterial tree and the pulmonary venous system, and they are associated with pulmonary capillary dysgenesis; a large fraction of the microvascular bed (mostly capillaries and venules), corresponding to an acinus or secondary lobule, coalesces into a single vascular sac. These sacs vary from 3 to 50 mm in diameter and are readily seen on pulmonary angiograms (Fig. 53.1).

The PAVMs associated with the hepatopulmonary syndrome are not the result of genetic mutation but represent a remodeling of existing septal capillaries with dilation of individual vessels to a diameter of 80 to 100 μm, at least, as illustrated in Figure 2 in Davis and associates.[4] The dilated capillary vessels in hepatopulmonary syndrome are not true malformations; "acquired intrapulmonary vascular shunts" might be a better term. The pulmonary angiogram is usually normal but may have a diffuse, "spongy" appearance with spidery vascular abnormalities. These intrapulmonary shunts associated with liver disease are dealt with more fully in Chapter 85.

Other causes of PAVMs are very rare. Macroscopic PAVMs may develop over time in about 20% of patients with severe congenital heart disease who have undergone a Glenn shunt (superior vena cava to right pulmonary artery anastomosis).[5] Trauma or neoplastic infiltration can in theory establish a direct communication between pulmonary arteries and veins, termed *arteriovenous fistula*; however, the different anatomic locations of pulmonary arteries (centrilobular, accompanying the bronchi) and veins (in the interlobular septae) make this an unlikely occurrence. Schistosomiasis is considered a cause of PAVMs, but the lesions are probably microscopic and related to the associated portal hypertension and cirrhosis. Twenty per cent of PAVMs seen on angiography are not associated with hereditary hemorrhagic telangiectasia, although the angiographic appearances are identical. Such patients have no family history, no telangiectasia, and no chronic epistaxes. Because they do not bleed from their noses or gastrointestinal tracts, they are more likely to have polycythemia. They usually have less than five abnormal vascular channels, all of which are amenable to curative embolization.

## Hereditary Hemorrhagic Telangiectasia

Eighty per cent of macroscopic PAVMs are associated with hereditary hemorrhagic telangiectasia (HHT) (formerly called the Rendu-Osler-Weber syndrome). Hanes,[6] in an excellent review published in 1909, coined the term "hereditary hemorrhagic telangiectasia," and his paper gives a fascinating account of the early descriptions of HHT from 1865 to 1896, but the condition was generally considered to be a variant of hemophilia until 1896, when Rendu[7] described a man with persistent epistaxes and facial telangiectasia (his mother and brother had recurrent epistaxes) but without any symptoms or signs of hemophilia. This was followed by Osler's landmark paper in 1901.[8]

HHT is a disorder of vascular development that has an autosomal dominant inheritance pattern. The reported prevalences vary from 2.5 to 43 per 100,000 population,[9, 10] with particularly high frequencies in isolated communities in mountainous areas[10] or islands.[11, 12] HHT is characterized by frequent epistaxes, usually beginning in childhood, mucocutaneous telangiectasia, and a clear-

**Table 53.1 DISTINGUISHING FEATURES OF MACROSCOPIC AND MICROSCOPIC PULMONARY ARTERIOVENOUS MALFORMATIONS**

| | Macroscopic PAVMs | Microscopic PAVMs |
|---|---|---|
| Arterial $P_{O_2}$ | Low | Low |
| $^{99m}$Tc-MAA perfusion scan | Radioactivity appears in brain and kidneys | Radioactivity appears in brain and kidneys |
| Pulmonary diffusion ($D_{L_{CO}}$) | Normal or low | Low to very low |
| Chest radiograph | Circular opacities supplied by enlarged vessels | Normal |
| Pulmonary angiogram | Early filling and emptying of saclike lesions | Normal or "diffuse spongy" |
| Pulmonary arterial pressure and vascular resistance | Low | Low |
| Cardiac output | Increased *in proportion* to right-to-left shunt | Increased *out of proportion* to right-to-left shunt |
| Paradoxical embolism | Common | Rare |
| Treatment | Percutaneous catheter embolization | Liver transplantation |

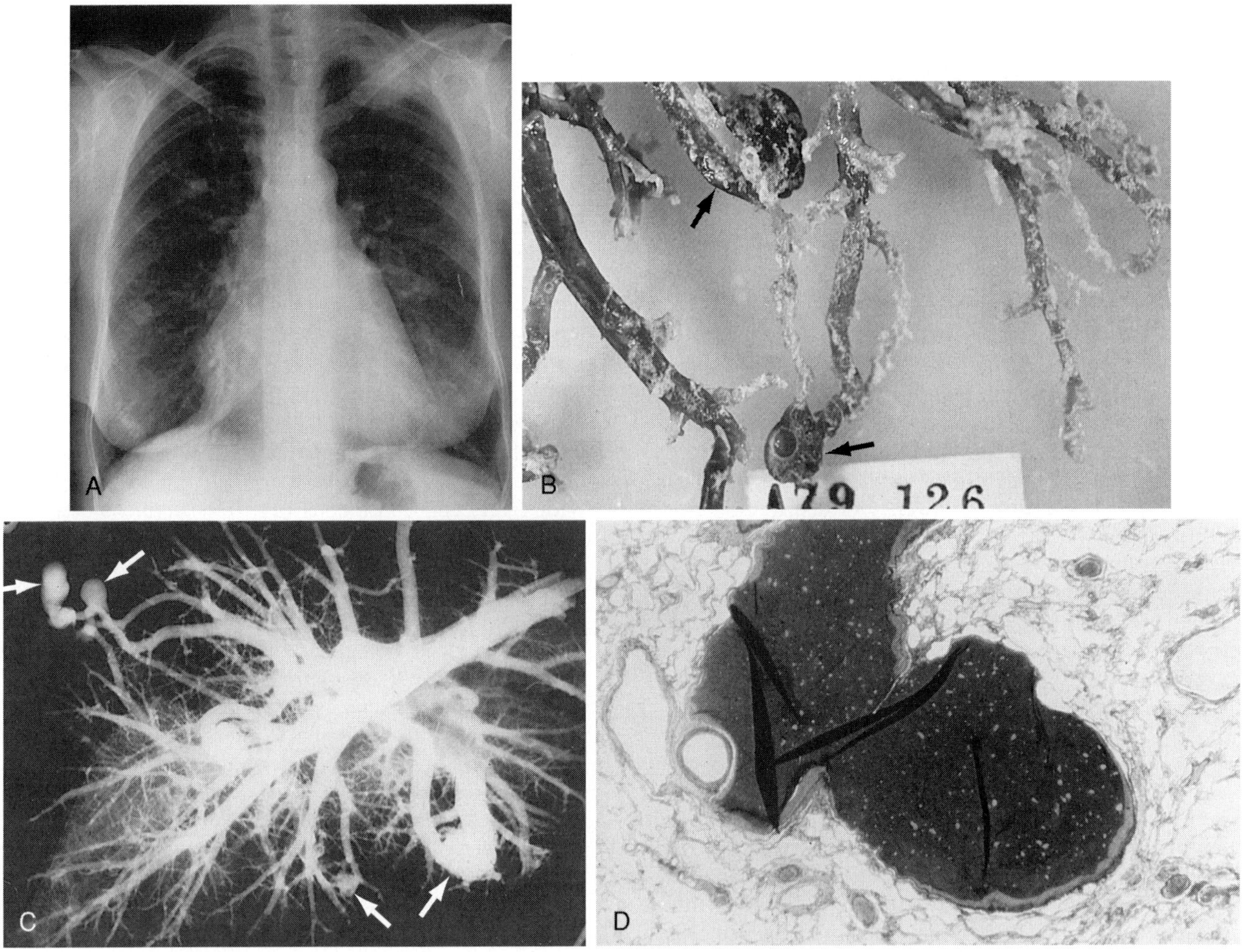


**Figure 53.1** Images are from a woman with hereditary hemorrhagic telangiectasia who died at 54 years of age. *A*, Premortem chest roentgenogram shows multiple pulmonary arteriovenous fistulas, cardiomegaly attributed to cor pulmonale, and incidental left superior sulcus tumor. *B*, Casts of fistulas *(arrows)* show feeding and draining vessels. *C*, Pulmonary angiogram from autopsy specimen shows multiple fistulas *(arrows)*. *D*, Microscopic view shows single fistula.

cut family history. For more information about HHT, some recent reviews should be consulted.[13–16a]

## Pathogenesis

The pathogenic mechanisms in HHT and PAVM have recently been reviewed.[16a] Mutations in two genes have been found in families with HHT. The first mutation to be described (HHT 1) was found on the long arm of chromosome 9[17, 18] in the gene encoding for the protein *endoglin*.[19] Endoglin is a homodimeric transmembrane glycoprotein, expressed most abundantly on endothelial cell surfaces.[20] It is part of the transforming growth factor-$\beta_1$ (TGF-$\beta_1$) complex and associates with TGF-β receptors (I and II). The precise way it binds to, interacts with, and regulates tissue levels of TGF-β is not known. TGF-β stimulates the production of extravascular matrix and is likely to be important in the formation of microvascular networks. More than 16 different mutations in the endoglin gene have been described, one common to two families but the rest unique to a particular family,[21] which in most cases predict a truncated protein. In a neonate with HHT parentage having mutant endoglin, *normal* endoglin was expressed on umbilical vein endothelial cell surfaces at 50% of control levels[22]; no mutated endoglin was found (only its metabolic products), presumably because it was transiently expressed intracellularly and then destroyed.[22] Therefore, HHT 1 would appear to be associated with a 50% reduction in endoglin levels per se rather than from an interaction of the abnormal with the normal protein (a so-called dominant-negative protein effect).

Production of a protein at half the normal level by one chromosomal allele (the other allele producing none) is called *haploinsufficiency*. An interesting feature of HHT is that the vascular abnormality is localized predominately in certain endothelial beds (i.e., nasal mucosa, oro-mucocutaneous surfaces, gastric mucosa, and the pulmonary circulation). Perhaps these vascular beds require especially high levels of endoglin (and possibly TGF-β) for normal development, whereas a level of 50% will suffice elsewhere.

In families with HHT and normal endoglin genes, mutations have been found on the long arm of chromosome 12 in the activinlike kinase 1 (ALK-1) gene.[23] Mutations in ALK-1 are considered to be functionally null alleles like the endoglin mutations. ALK-1 also binds to TGF-$\beta_1$. A single family, unusual for its high frequency of hepatic arteriovenous malformations, has been found not to have mutations in either endoglin or ALK-1[24]; the location of this mutation remains to be found.

Clinical observation commonly shows that disease severity and location in HHT varies widely among affected members of the same family who share the same mutation. In 30 individuals from families with seven different endoglin mutations, there was no statistically significant correlation between disease severity or distribution either within or between families.[21] This is consistent with haploinsufficiency in which a variety of factors (sex hormone levels being the most obvious) interact with low endoglin levels during the formation in utero or the repair process (after birth) of individual vascular beds. A milder phenotype with a lower incidence of PAVMs is a feature of the ALK-1 mutation (HHT 2).[25]

## Clinical Features

The lesions associated with HHT affect specific sites, and their appearance in affected individuals is related to age (Table 53.2). The vascular malformations and telangiectasia that affect the lungs, gastrointestinal (GI) tract, liver, and central nervous system may remain silent and unnoticed for many years; small lesions may never be detected unless specific screening is undertaken.

The earliest and most frequent symptom and sign is recurrent epistaxis, usually unprovoked by trauma. Epistaxes vary in frequency (1 per month to 4 per day) and severity (a trickle for 1 to 2 minutes to severe hemorrhage lasting 30 to 60 minutes). The telangiectasias appear later than the epistaxes; they are recognizable from about the age of 20 years as pinpoint cherry-red spots on the lips, palate, tongue, and buccal mucosa. With advancing years, the lesions enlarge (rarely to more than 5 mm diameter) and may appear on the face and pulps of the fingers. Histopathologically, the telangiectasias of HHT occur first as focal dilations of postcapillary venules[26] in the upper dermis. In the fully developed lesion, the venules are markedly dilated and convoluted, external to all layers of the dermis, and often connect directly to dilated arterioles.

The mucocutaneous telangiectasias do not in general cause any problem; bleeding from them is usually slight and infrequent. Bleeding from the telangiectasias involving the nasal mucosa is severe in 10% to 20% of patients with HHT, and continuous oral iron supplementation or multiple transfusions may be required. Estrogen therapy is effective in some, but a controlled trial did not show a significant benefit.[27] Cauterization with argon or yttrium-aluminum-garnet lasers, septodermoplasty, and embolization of the nasal vasculature give short-term to medium-term relief only (see Guttmacher and colleagues[28] for references). Superficial telangiectasias also occur in the GI tract, particularly in the stomach. Bleeding from the GI tract generally occurs after the age of 50 years, at an age when epistaxes may also worsen. This is probably related to hormonal changes, especially the menopause. A randomized double-blind study showed that a combination of estrogen and progesterone decreased transfusion requirements in patients with HHT and GI bleeding.[29] Treatment with antifibrinolytic agents such as ϵ-aminocaproic acid or tranexamic acid may be effective for a few patients, but not for most.[30] Endoscopic ablation of superficial gastric and duodenal telangiectasis with heat or laser is beneficial.[30a]

**Table 53.2 HEREDITARY HEMORRHAGIC TELANGIECTASIA: CLINICAL MANIFESTATIONS**

| Site | Frequency (%) | Age at Presentation (Years) | Consequences |
|---|---|---|---|
| Nose | 90–95 | 3–20 | Hemorrhage (epistaxes) |
| PAVMs | 15–30 | 3–20 | Hypoxemia<br>Paradoxical embolism |
| Telangiectasia (oral/mucocutaneous) | 50–80 | 15–30 | Cosmetic, may bleed |
| Telangiectasia (facial) | 30–50 | 30–50 | Cosmetic, may bleed |
| Gastrointestinal telangiectasia | 20–40 | 40–60 | Anemia |
| Central nervous system AVMs | 20–30 | ? | Epilepsy, paresis |
| Hepatic AVMs | ? | ? | High-output cardiac failure |

The other vascular lesions of HHT are arteriovenous malformations (AVMs), which are similar to superficial telangiectasias but are much larger, with direct communication between larger arteries and veins. A common site for these "macrotelangiectasias" or AVMs is the lung (see Table 53.2).

**Diagnosis of HHT.** A definite clinical diagnosis of HHT is based on the presence of three of four key features of HHT: spontaneous recurrent epistaxis, characteristic telangiectasia, visceral AVMs (pulmonary, cerebral, hepatic), and an affected first-degree relative.[30b] The presence of recurrent epistaxis alone, in the presence of a positive family history, is suggestive (absence of telangiectasia in subjects less than 20 years old is quite usual) and, although not diagnostic, warrants screening for PAVMs (see discussion of screening, later). Similarly, the diagnosis of HHT should always be considered in anyone presenting with a cerebral abscess or a cerebral, pulmonary, or hepatic AVM. In 95% of persons with a parent afflicted by HHT, epistaxis or telangiectasia or visceral AVMs will have declared themselves by age 35 years[10, 21]; nevertheless, the diagnosis can never be finally excluded and, from a young age, the phrase "has a parent affected by HHT" should be part of these persons' medical record.

**Frequency of PAVMs in HHT.** The incidence of small PAVMs will not be known until large numbers of HHT-affected persons are screened with sensitive and safe techniques. In earlier series, in which only the more obvious lesions would have been detected, the incidence ranges from 15% to 25%.[32] As mentioned earlier, there is a much lower incidence of reported PAVMs (about 3%) in families in whom the HHT mutation is linked to chromosome 12 rather than to chromosome 9.[25]

## Clinical Features of Pulmonary Arteriovenous Malformations

In the Hammersmith Hospital series (n = 53),[33] the average age was 43 years (range, 9 to 78 years). In more than half the patients, PAVMs were recognized in persons aged 20 to 50 years, with 28% presenting at older than 50 years and 19% at younger than 20 years. There is an interesting (and unexplained) female sex preponderance (F/M ratio, 1.6:1).[31] For HHT itself, there is no gender bias; in the 324 cases of HHT reported by Plauchu and coworkers,[10] the F/M ratio was 1.04. This suggests that female sex hormones have an important influence on the growth of PAVMs.

In an analysis of 53 patients with PAVMs,[33] only 26% presented because of respiratory symptoms, notably exertional dyspnea. Four patients were asymptomatic despite arterial oxygen saturation ($So_2$) values averaging 89%. Hemoptysis is a relatively uncommon symptom in PAVMs, with a frequency of 6% to 13%.[10, 33, 34] Polycythemia (Hb > 16 g/dL) occurs in 45%, but iron deficiency anemia (Hb < 12.5 g/dL) was seen in 13%.[33]

### Paradoxical Embolism

The seriousness of PAVMs lies not so much in the hypoxemia (except in the severest cases) but in the frequency of paradoxical embolization, leading to transient ischemic attacks, embolic stroke, and cerebral abscess. Our overall neurologic complication rate in patients with PAVMs was 40%.[33] In the largest series studied in North America,[34] ischemic lesions were present in 21 of 59 (36%) patients who had had brain computed tomography (CT) scans. The incidence of cerebral abscess in different series ranged from 6% to 20% (reviewed by Wirth and coworkers[35]). The organisms that are found in cerebral abscesses are usually anaerobes or *Actinomyces* species. This suggests an origin in the mouth and stresses the importance of antibiotic prophylaxis for all dental work in afflicted patients. The frequencies of ischemic attacks and cerebrovascular accidents range from about 15% to 36% for both diagnoses,[35] but this may reflect differences in nomenclature or definition. Migraine is also common.

### Pregnancy

There is evidence that PAVMs enlarge during pregnancy,[31, 36] and there is an increased risk of pulmonary hemorrhage and stroke in women with extensive PAVMs who become pregnant.[37] The larger the right-to-left shunt, the more hazardous the pregnancy for the mother. There does not seem to be any particular risk for the fetus. In women with extensive and multiple PAVMs, arterial oxygenation improves during pregnancy, only to deteriorate markedly afterward to a level lower than before pregnancy.[38] The influence of estrogens and progesterones would seem to be important modifiers of the clinical expression of HHT. PAVMs are more common in women than men[31]; hemorrhage from the nose or GI tract occurs more severely after the menopause and may be alleviated by hormonal therapy (see Shovlin and coworkers[31] for further discussion).

## Diagnosis

Many cases are diagnosed as a result of a chest radiograph obtained either routinely or for nonspecific respiratory symptoms. Sometimes the diagnosis of HHT will have been made and a chest radiograph (and other investigations; see later discussion of screening) ordered to confirm or refute the diagnosis of PAVMs. It is particularly important to think of the diagnosis of PAVMs (and to undertake the appropriate investigations such as a chest radiography and measurement of arterial $Po_2$) in patients who present with a cerebral abscess or, if under the age of 50 years, with recurrent ischemic attacks or an embolic stroke.

The chest radiograph is abnormal in 80% to 90% of patients, although careful scrutiny is required to detect the abnormalities, which are frequently subtle. One or more well-circumscribed peripheral noncalcified opacity, connected by prominent blood vessels to the hilum, may be seen (see Fig. 53.1). The enlargement of these feeding vessels is probably physiological due to the low vascular resistance of the PAVM and the higher than normal flow. PAVMs occur preferentially in the lower zones (in 95% of cases in one series[33]), and their caudal location means that they are often partially obscured by the diaphragm. PAVMs are commonly multiple, 72% of affected subjects having lesions in both lungs.[33] White and coworkers[34] maintain that 65% of PAVMs are in the lower lobes, with a further 24% in the right middle lobe or lingula; only 12% are located in the upper lobes.

Three-dimensional spiral (or helical) CT is a very elegant way of demonstrating the anatomy of PAVMs and their feeding vessels,[39] particularly if the latest reconstruction techniques are used.[40] No contrast medium is required because of the natural contrast of the gas in the lung.

Most HHT patients who screen positive for PAVMs will come to pulmonary angiography for consideration of therapy by transcatheter embolization. A superselective angiographic technique is necessary if the smaller lesions are not to be missed.[33] In terms of resolution, the best digital subtraction angiography is superior to helical CT. The advantage of CT is that it is noninvasive. Most PAVMs can, however, be diagnosed or suspected on clinical and physiological grounds. Therefore, a CT scan is not required if a decision has already been made to proceed to pulmonary angiography.

## Measurement of the Right-to-Left Shunt

Although the arterial $Po_2$ level (or arterial $So_2$ with pulse oximetry) is a very useful measure of PAVMs, it is not specific for the detection of an intrapulmonary shunt because $\dot{V}A/\dot{Q}$ mismatching from any cause will also lower the arterial $Po_2$. In the classic measurement of an anatomic shunt, the subject breathes 100% oxygen for 15 minutes; then, arterial blood is sampled for measurements of $Po_2$ and hemoglobin.

An alternative method makes use of the lung perfusion scan. The principle of the lung perfusion scan for the diagnosis of pulmonary embolism is that, after intravenous injection, small (20 to 50 μm diameter) radiolabeled ($^{99m}$Tc) human serum albumin particles impact in the pulmonary circulation wherever there is normal blood flow. In the presence of an anatomic shunt (in the heart or lungs), a fraction of the particles (proportional to the shunt flow) will escape into the systemic circulation, where they can be detected by a gamma camera placed over the kidneys. For macroscopic PAVMs, this method has been quantitated[41] and shown to be in good agreement with the 100% oxygen technique.[42] It has the advantage of being less invasive than pulmonary angiography, and it can be used during exercise[42] and in transient unsteady states such as breath-holding.[43]

Contrast echocardiography is an alternative method for demonstrating intrapulmonary shunts.[44] After intravenous injection of agitated saline solution (or galactose-based microbubbles), microcavitations will be observed in the left atrium in the presence of a right-to-left shunt; the appearance time will be more than 3 heartbeats slower (relative to appearance in the right atrium) for an intrapulmonary shunt than for an atrial septal defect, for example. The technique is simple, safe and noninvasive, but it is qualitative rather than quantitative,[44] and its sensitivity and specificity remain to be determined.

In patients with PAVMs, the right-to-left shunt (supine posture) varies widely, from 4% to 60% of the cardiac output with a mean (n = 53) of 23% ± 3.5%.[33]

## Screening

Many patients with PAVMs are asymptomatic from the respiratory point of view (20/53 [38%] in one study[33] and 17/32 [53%] in another[45]). Because of the serious consequences of paradoxical embolization, the hazards of pregnancy,[31] and the possibility of hemoptysis and hemothorax,[37] all patients with HHT should be screened for the presence of PAVMs. This involves a comprehensive family screening policy when a physician is dealing with an HHT patient. The proband must be reminded of the importance of his or her relatives' being screened for HHT and PAVMs, especially for women of childbearing age.

The question remains: What screening tests should be employed? With adults, it is usually possible to determine whether a relative has inherited HHT. It is not at all easy to be sure with children and teenagers. Cyanosis, clubbing, and pulmonary bruits are physical signs of large intrapulmonary shunts, but in many patients who have mild to moderate PAVMs these signs are absent. The chest radiograph (posteroanterior and lateral), carefully scrutinized, has a sensitivity and specificity of 83% and 92%, respectively.[45] Due to the shape of the oxygen dissociation curve, the measurement of arterial $Po_2$ is rather too sensitive and may be low in asymptomatic cigarette smokers, for example. Haitjema and associates[45] screened 98 HHT family members (36 had HHT, and 12 of these had PAVMs). An abnormal arterial $Po_2$ level was found in 8 of 12 of the PAVM subjects and in a further 33 subjects who were subsequently found not to have PAVMs, giving a positive predictive value of only 19.5% (8/[33 + 8]).

Pulse oximetry measures arterial $So_2$ with a simple photosensitive probe placed on the vasodilated ear lobe or finger. It is a simple and noninvasive method and the only technique that can be used at home. Because it is so simple to perform, meticulous attention to good technique (a good flow pulse, readings taken for 10 minutes) is sometimes neglected. With extensive PAVMs and a large right-to-left shunt, the low arterial $So_2$ signal on pulse oximetry will be obvious, and there will be a characteristic further fall in arterial $So_2$ when the patient stands upright from the supine posture. The difficulty comes when PAVMs are small and not readily indentifiable on a chest radiograph. Thompson and coworkers studied this situation in 66 patients whose PAVMs had been treated by coil embolization (see later discussion of treatment), 40 of whom had residual PAVMs too small to embolize as shown on selective digital subtraction pulmonary angiography, which served as the gold standard. Arterial $So_2$ of 96% or less in the erect posture detected by pulse oximetry correctly classified 60% of the patients, and pulse oximetry had a sensitivity of 73% and a specificity of 35% for detecting these small PAVMs. Measurement of right-to-left shunt with $^{99m}$Tc-MAA–labeled particles was more accurate (based on a threshold of ≥3.5% shunt), correctly classifying 78% of the patients, with a sensitivity of 87% and a specificity of 78%.

In a patient with HHT, once an abnormality has been found on a chest radiograph or with a measurement of arterial $Po_2$ or $So_2$, the next step is to confirm or refute the existence of a right-to-left shunt with a radionuclide perfusion scan[41, 42] or contrast echocardiography,[44] or by the measurement of arterial $Po_2$ during 100% oxygen breathing. Finally, helical CT scanning or pulmonary arteriography will constitute the definitive examination.

## Pathophysiology

### Pulmonary Hemodynamics

The main physiological features of PAVMs are pulmonary hypotension and a right-to-left intrapulmonary shunt. In a series of patients with PAVMs associated with HHT,[47] mean pulmonary artery pressure was $14 \pm 1.8$ mm Hg ($n = 6$) and pulmonary vascular resistance was $0.33 \pm 0.24$ mm $Hg \cdot L^{-1} \cdot min^{-1}$ (normal range, 0.5 to 1.0). The finding of a raised pulmonary artery pressure suggests another cause such as pulmonary thromboembolic disease or pulmonary hypertension secondary to left ventricular dysfunction or smoking-related lung disease. Sapru and colleagues[48] described three patients with pulmonary hypertension who also had HHT. The pulmonary wedge pressures were normal, and the angiograms in two of three cases showed some peripheral pruning but no evidence of pulmonary embolism. Interestingly, all patients had been taking estrogens for persistent epistaxes.

A raised pulmonary capillary pressure may be one of the factors, the other being pregnancy,[31] that promotes growth of PAVMs. Chow and coworkers[49] documented massive enlargement of a PAVM over 5 years in an elderly woman with mitral stenosis. There was a similar patient at Hammersmith Hospital in whom the onset of left ventricular dysfunction and secondary pulmonary hypertension led to enlargement of a previously small PAVM.

### Gas Exchange at Rest and on Exercise

There is wide variation in the arterial hypoxemia of patients with PAVM, with a mean arterial $So_2$ in 53 patients of $89\% \pm 1\%$ (SEM) in the supine posture and a minimum of 62%[33]; in 7 patients, arterial $So_2$ was greater than 95% (i.e., within the normal range). The shunt calculation while breathing air (venous admixture), obtained with pulse oximetry, predicts the anatomic right-to-left shunt quite accurately,[43] which suggests that the arterial hypoxemia is wholly caused by the intrapulmonary PAVM shunts (except when there is coexisting intrinsic lung disease). Arterial $Pco_2$ tends to be low.[50]

A 2% or greater fall in arterial $So_2$ in the erect posture (orthostatic hypoxemia or orthodeoxia) is a very characteristic finding in PAVMs. The average fall in arterial $So_2$ from the supine to the erect position in our series[33] was $6\% \pm 1\%$; eight patients had an arterial $\Delta So_2$ value of more than 10% absolute. On the other hand, 4 of 53 subjects had an arterial $So_2$ level higher than 95% in both the erect and the supine postures. PAVMs are much more common in the lower than upper zones, which accounts for the postural fall in arterial $So_2$. The low pulmonary vascular pressure in PAVMs means that the fraction of total pulmonary blood flow to the lung bases will be particularly high in the erect posture.

The fall in arterial $So_2$ in the erect posture is accompanied by an increase in the right-to-left shunt $\dot{Q}s/\dot{Q}_T$.[43] In eight subjects with HHT and PAVMs, $\dot{Q}s/\dot{Q}_T$ increased from $29\% \pm 10\%$ (supine) to $39\% \pm 14\%$ (erect).[47] An increase also occurred if the shunt measurement was made at a high lung volume. $\dot{Q}s/\dot{Q}_T$ was $17\% \pm 11\%$ at functional residual capacity compared with $23\% \pm 12\%$ at total lung capacity.[43]

The exercise capacity may be surprisingly well preserved despite severe hypoxemia. Maximum workloads exceeding 70% predicted were found in 11 of 15 patients.[51] Resting arterial $So_2$ was reduced (average, 86%), and in 13 of 15 patients it fell further on exercise (mean fall on maximum exercise, $8\% \pm 2\%$). There are two possible reasons for the fall in arterial $So_2$ on exercise: an increase in the shunt fraction and a fall in the mixed venous oxygen content. Both are important, and in one study of 12 patients with PAVMs, each mechanism accounted for about 50% of the observed fall in arterial $So_2$ during steady-state exercise.[42] Somewhat surprisingly, others[50] found no change in the ideal alveolar-arterial oxygen tension gradient on exercise in eight patients with HHT and PAVMs. This suggests that these patients had a decrease in their shunt fraction on exercise.

In a further study of seven patients with HHT and PAVMs,[47] total cardiac output on exercise exceeded the normal value (for a given oxygen consumption), remarkably, by an amount equal to the flow through the pulmonary arteriovenous shunts. The shunt flow on exercise (at an average of 33% of predicted maximum) averaged 5 L/min for a cardiac output of 15 L/min. Because of the high cardiac output and hemoglobin concentration from compensatory polycythemia, which mitigated to some extent the fall in arterial $So_2$, the delivery of oxygen to the tissues relative to the needs of the body (oxygen consumption) was actually increased.

What is driving the cardiac output to such high levels at rest and on exercise, resulting in "overcompensation" in terms of oxygen delivery? One mechanism might be the low right ventricular afterload, which is peculiar to patients with intrapulmonary shunts and in marked contrast to the pulmonary hypertension that accompanies normal subjects who exercise at high (or simulated) altitudes, and it is a feature of most respiratory conditions. In addition, the high oxygen delivery implies a higher than normal blood flow-to-work rate ratio in exercising muscle. This suggests a low systemic vascular resistance due either to hypoxemic vasodilation or to increased muscle vascularity (in response to chronic hypoxemia) or (rather unlikely) to microscopic AVMs in the muscles of patients with HHT.

### Pulmonary Function

Lung volumes are normal, and there is no airflow obstruction. Diffusion for carbon monoxide is reduced, $DL_{CO}$ being $78\% \pm 3.2\%$ (SEM) predicted and $DL/VA$ $85\% \pm 3.2\%$ ($n = 53$).[33] Those with the lowest $DL_{CO}$ and $DL/VA$ have the most widespread vascular malformations. Because of the low vascular resistance of PAVMs, a vascular steal might contribute to the low diffusion values. For two reasons this is unlikely: (1) there is only a small rise in DL/VA after macroscopic PAVMs have been eliminated by embolization techniques,[33, 50] and (2) pulmonary blood flow to nonshunting lung is normal.[47]

## Treatment

Successful excision of a PAVM was first reported in 1942, and surgery remained the treatment of choice until the 1980s. Surgery was never the ideal solution when PAVMs were multiple (as they frequently are in HHT). Percutaneous transcatheter embolization with detachable balloons was introduced in 1978.[52] Steel coils have largely replaced balloons.[33, 53] Considerable skill is required. In selective pulmonary arteriography with or without digital subtraction (Fig. 53.2), the tip of the catheter must be placed close to the neck of the AVM sac; too proximal a placement means sacrificing normal lung, and too peripheral risks loss of the coil into the sac and passage into the left atrium.[33]

Steel coil embolization is well tolerated. A general anesthetic is rarely required except for young children. Dutton and coworkers[33] reported on 102 procedures in 53 patients of whom 42 had associated HHT; there were 18 complications (18%) of which only 4 were classed as severe (systemic embolization requiring retrieval of a coil [2], myocardial puncture [1], and cerebrovascular accident [1]), but the final outcome was satisfactory in all cases. Haitjema and coworkers,[53] also using steel coils, treated 32 patients (31 had HHT) in 44 sessions; there was similarly an 18% complication rate, including systemic embolization of a coil (later retrieved) in two patients.

White and colleagues have been the pioneers and advocates of embolization with detachable balloons.[34, 52, 54, 55] Two hundred seventy-six PAVMs have been occluded in 76 patients.[55] There were only two instances of systemic embolization of a balloon, and the outcome was uneventful. In expert hands, embolization by either coils or balloons appears to be a safe procedure. Pulmonary hypertension developed in one case after embolization, and it was attributed to the hemodynamic consequences of a large left-to-right shunt caused by a large hepatic AVM.[56]

After occlusion of all PAVMs with feeding vessels of more than 3 mm diameter, mean arterial $S_{O_2}$ in the 53 patients reported by Dutton and associates[33] increased from 89% ± 1% (SEM) to 94% ± 1% (supine posture) and from 83% ± 1% to 92% ± 1% (erect posture). Mean

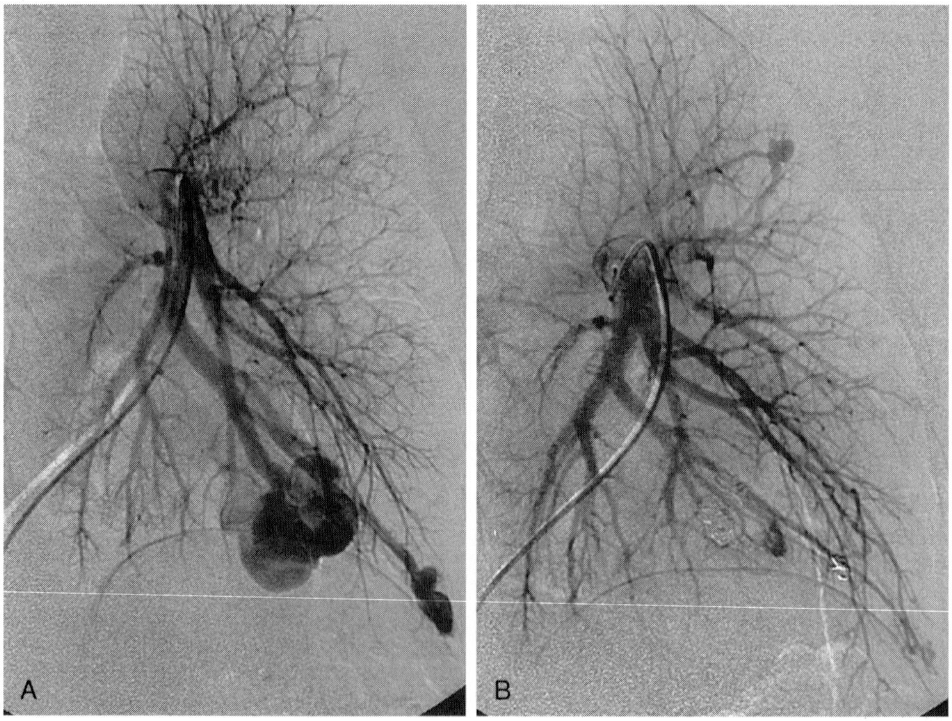


**Figure 53.2** *A,* Digital subtraction selective pulmonary angiogram (arterial phase) shows a very large and complex PAVM at the left base with two feeding vessels (7 and 5 mm diameter). A smaller PAVM with 4 mm feeding vessel lies at the costophrenic angle. Both PAVMs were embolized with steel coils. *B,* A follow-up angiogram was performed 3 months after the embolization (note that the coils appear as white or light gray). Part of the larger PAVM is still patent at the base. Another PAVM is now visible in the left upper zone (4 mm feeding vessel). Both PAVMs were subsequently embolized with coils. Very small PAVMs are visible at the lowermost costophrenic angle with 1 to 2 mm diameter feeding vessels, but they are too small to embolize.

arterial $SO_2$ on exercise at an equivalent workload increased from 81% ± 2% to 91% ± 1%. The right-to-left shunt decreased from 23% ± 2% to 9% ± 1%.[33] With an arterial $SO_2$ level above 95% and right-to-left shunt below 5% as criteria of "normality," supine arterial $SO_2$ had returned to normal in 64% of patients, erect arterial $SO_2$ in 53%, and right-to-left shunt in 40%. In HHT (most of the cases), there are often multiple small PAVM channels that cannot be embolized, in addition to the larger ones that have been treated. Changes in pulmonary function after embolization were small, only the increase in DL/VA (from 85% ± 3.2% to 90% ± 4%) being significant,[33] as previously observed.[51]

In the series from the Netherlands,[53] in 32 patients with PAVMs, mean right-to-left shunt (100% oxygen method) decreased from 16.6% to 7.4%, and the arterial $PO_2$ level increased from 72 to 86 mm Hg (equivalent to an arterial $SO_2$ increase from 92.5% to 95%). Using detachable balloons, White and coworkers[34] found arterial $PO_2$ increases of 58 to 75 mm Hg (supine) and 47 to 68 mm Hg (erect), implying the persistence of significant residual right-to-left shunts.

After all feeding vessels with diameters more than 3 mm had been embolized with steel coils, Dutton and coworkers[33] noted that residual shunts with smaller feeding vessels were present in two-thirds of treated patients. This explains the failure of arterial oxygenation and the right-to-left shunt to return to normal, as mentioned above. Somewhat surprisingly, a low value of $DL_{CO}$ ($TL_{CO}$) or DL/VA (KCO) at initial presentation, or at follow-up, did not predict the likelihood of there being residual shunts.

The clinical message is that, owing to the persistent shunt flow, antibiotic prophylaxis should continue indefinitely after embolization of PAVMs. Other salient features of pulmonary arteriovenous malformations are summarized in Table 53.3.

**Tabe 53.3 SALIENT POINTS ABOUT PULMONARY ARTERIOVENOUS MALFORMATIONS**

1. The diagnosis of HHT with PAVMs should be considered when there is a history of recurrent epistaxes from childhood and neurologic events or cyanosis in a young person.
2. If HHT is confirmed, screening for PAVMs should be undertaken in the index case and in all affected relatives because of the risk of paradoxical embolization to the brain.
3. An adequate screen consists of chest radiographs and measurements of oxygenation (arterial $PO_2$ or arterial $SO_2$) in the erect and supine postures. PAVMs themselves cause few symptoms. If there is doubt, a measurement of intrapulmonary right-to-left shunt should be undertaken with radioisotope scanning or contrast echocardiography.
4. Pulmonary angiography and CT scanning are the definitive investigations.
5. Embolization with steel coils or detachable balloons is an effective treatment.
6. Antibiotic prophylaxis should continue indefinitely because of persistence of PAVMs too small to treat or detect.

## Idiopathic Pulmonary Arteriovenous Malformations

Twenty per cent of PAVMs seen on angiography are not associated with HHT, although the angiographic appearances are identical. These patients have no family history, no telangiectasia, and no chronic epistaxes. They are more likely to have polycythemia, because they are not bleeding from the nose or the GI tract. Diagnosis and treatment are similar to HHT-associated PAVMs. Afflicted patients usually have less than five abnormal vascular channels, all of which are amenable to embolization. Typically, they are not left with any residual shunt. In retrospect, some of these patients may represent an atypical presentation of HHT, and a careful family history should be taken with this possibility in mind.

# SYSTEMIC-PULMONARY VASCULAR COMMUNICATION

## Classification

Direct communications between the systemic arterial circulation, including the bronchial arteries, and the pulmonary circulation are much less common than communications within the pulmonary circulation. Such communications are so uncommon, in fact, that only 28 could be found by Brundage and associates[57] in the world's literature in 1972. Most of these communications are traumatic in origin; several have resulted from placement of thoracostomy tubes.[58, 59] The systemic vessel that penetrates the lung usually arises from the coronary arteries,[60] the intercostal arteries,[61] or the internal mammary artery.[62] A left-to-right shunt is thereby created between the high-pressure systemic circulation and the low-pressure pulmonary circulation, and massive amounts of blood flow through the abnormal vascular channels. This may have adverse hemodynamic consequences, although high-output left ventricular failure is unusual.

A second type of "reactive" systemic-pulmonary vascular communication develops in patients with intrapulmonary neoplasms and inflammatory disorders, presumably in response to the angiogenic stimuli that cause new blood vessels to form in these conditions. Although large amounts of blood may flow through these channels, the abnormal pathways do not constitute true left-to-right shunts because the vascular network contains arterioles that impose a vascular resistance between the two circulations and capillaries from which oxygen is extracted to sustain tissue metabolism. In contrast to the direct, usually posttraumatic, variety, reactive systemic-pulmonary vascular communications are clinically much more important because they are more common and are the source of major episodes of bleeding.

## Diagnosis and Treatment

Most patients with direct left-to-right noncardiac systemic-pulmonary shunts are asymptomatic. The presence of the vascular abnormalities is suggested by detection of a continuous murmur during physical examination[57] or by roentgenographic findings such as notching of the ribs, increased caliber of the pulmonary vessels, pleural thickening, or cardiomegaly.[59] The diagnosis can be established by selective angiography of the relevant systemic vessel. Although there is little information about the natural history of these vascular communications, surgery is frequently performed as definitive therapy.

The clinical features in patients with the reactive type of systemic-pulmonary vascular communications are usually dominated by the underlying neoplastic or inflammatory disease, classically tuberculosis or bronchiectasis, sometimes primary or metastatic carcinoma or aspergilloma. The presence of the abnormal blood supply is usually heralded by the onset of *hemoptysis*, which may be mild or massive. Bleeding is apt to be more severe from a bronchial arterial source than from a pulmonary arterial communication because of the much higher pressure in systemic than in pulmonary vessels. At times the origin of the bleeding can be inferred from the color of the blood: bright red from the bronchial artery and dark red from the pulmonary artery. Systemic-pulmonary vascular communications are the chief source of brisk bleeding from the lung. In one large series of cases of massive hemoptysis, defined as more than 200 mL of blood in 24 hours, bleeding in 103 of the 120 patients (85%) was from inflammatory lung diseases,[63] typically either pulmonary tuberculosis or bronchiectasis, conditions in which abnormal bronchial arterial communications are well described.[63a]

Massive hemoptysis is a life-threatening emergency that requires urgent diagnosis and treatment. A careful history and physical examination are needed to establish that the lungs, rather than the gastrointestinal tract or upper air passages, are the source of bleeding. Chest radiography occasionally reveals the cause of hemoptysis but is more often nonlocalizing because the lungs usually show alveolar densities from blood that has been widely dispersed by aspiration through the bronchial tree.[63b] Bronchoscopy is recommended in an effort to lateralize which lung the blood is coming from and, if possible, to identify a more specific location; at times, the bleeding can be contained or controlled locally.[64] The role of CT and its new applications, which are considered complementary to bronchoscopy and of considerable value in ordinary hemoptysis,[63b] are not well established in massive bleeding.

Resectional surgery was once the only available treatment for massive hemoptysis, but the operative mortality was high and many patients could not be operated on because of poor pulmonary function from underlying generalized lung disease. In 1974, Remy and coworkers[64a] introduced a new interventional radiologic approach of selective bronchial artery embolization, which has now virtually replaced surgery as the initial treatment for hemoptysis.[64b, 64c] Not all patients, however, can be embolized, but new techniques of "superselective" catheterization and improvements in embolization materials should increase the rate of success.[65] Both acute (less than 30 days) and long-term recurrences have been reported,[65a] and the procedure should be considered palliative (or temporizing) rather than definitive.

## BRONCHOPULMONARY SEQUESTRATION

The most common developmental disorder characterized by an abnormal systemic-pulmonary vascular communication is bronchopulmonary sequestration, which was first described in 1861 by Rokitansky[66] and Rektorzik.[66a] The term *sequestration*, which is derived from the Latin verb *sequestrare*, "to separate," was coined in 1946.[66b] Most investigators now accept the definition proposed by Pryce and colleagues[67, 68]: Bronchopulmonary sequestration is a region of lung parenchyma that has an incomplete or no connection with the airways and is supplied by an aberrant artery arising from the aorta or one of its branches. A distinction is made between intralobar sequestrations, which share a common visceral pleural investment with the adjacent normal lung tissue, and extralobar sequestrations, which have their own pleural lining that separates them from the remaining lung tissue.

### Pathogenesis

Although the mechanism of formation of bronchopulmonary sequestrations has long been debated, there is an increasing tendency to regard them, along with bronchogenic cysts, as developmental abnormalities of the embryologic foregut.[69–72] For example, Heithoff and colleagues[71] proposed that an accessory lung bud forms caudad to the normal lung bud. If this occurs early in embryologic life, the accessory bud remains within the pleura and becomes an intralobar sequestration. If the accessory bud appears after the pleura has formed, the result is an extralobar sequestration with its own pleural investment.[73] The differential timing of this process explains why sequestrations in general, and extralobar sequestrations in particular, are associated with other congenital foregut anomalies.

### Epidemiology and Pathology

Extralobar sequestrations are quite rare and occur most commonly in men. Most patients with these sequestrations manifest other congenital abnormalities, the most common of which is diaphragmatic hernia, but associated cystic adenomatoid malformations are being described with increasing frequency.[73a, 73b] Extralobar sequestrations also may communicate with the lower esophagus and stomach.[69] They usually are located within the lower chest, twice as commonly on the left than on the right side, but a retroperitoneal location also has been described.[74] Because the sequestrations lack communication with the airways, they rarely contain air. The sequestrations resemble masses of rubbery tissue that on microscopic examination contain orderly and disorderly arrangements of normal lung tissue.[73] Their arterial supply usually is from the aorta.[75] Because venous drainage usually is through the azygous or hemiazygous system, extralobar sequestrations are not true systemic-pulmonary vascular communications.

Intralobar sequestrations are more common than extralobar sequestrations and are found equally among men and women. These sequestrations often occur in the absence of other congenital abnormalities. They tend to blend into the surrounding lung and usually are located in the medial or posterior basal segments of the lower lobes, again more often on the left. Because they either communicate directly with the airways or are aerated by adjacent lung, they often contain some air. They also tend to become secondarily infected. Pathologic examination reveals normal lung tissue with superimposed inflammation and cyst formation (Fig. 53.3). Arterial supply usually is from the aorta, with venous outflow via the pulmonary veins; because of this, intralobar sequestrations contain true systemic-pulmonary vascular communications.[73, 76] Arterial flow from the coronary arteries also has been described.[77, 78]

Of the 547 cases of bronchopulmonary sequestration analyzed by Savic and associates,[79] 400 were intralobar, 133 extralobar, and 14 of mixed origin. In intralobular sequestrations, the aberrant artery arose from the thoracic aorta in 74% of cases, and there was more than one anomalous artery in 15%; the venous drainage was nearly always (96%) via the pulmonary veins; and the lower lobes were the most common (98%) site of involvement. Extralobar sequestrations were usually (77%) located between the diaphragm and lower lobes. The aberrant artery arose from the thoracic aorta or, slightly less often, the abdominal aorta; and the venous drainage was more variable than in the intralobar variety.

## Symptoms

Extralobar sequestrations usually are asymptomatic and may be discovered accidentally during roentgenographic evaluation for other purposes or during repair of a congenital lesion such as a diaphragmatic hernia. Large sequestrations may, however, cause respiratory distress in the neonate.[76] The chief symptoms of intralobar sequestration are cough, fever, recurrent pneumonia, and hemoptysis, often occurring in adolescence.[80, 81] This clinical picture resembles bronchiectasis and also may be confused with lung abscess when a cystic mass is seen on the chest roentgenogram.[82] White and colleagues[83] also described infants with heart failure due to large right-to-left shunts

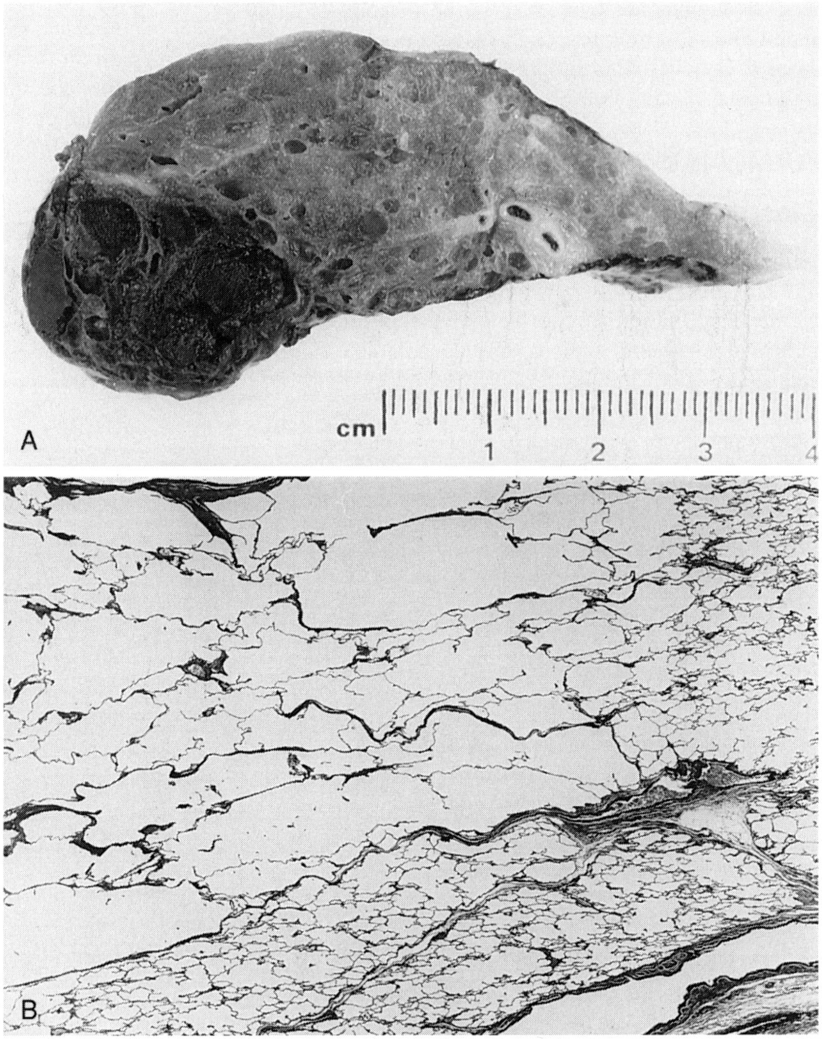


**Figure 53.3** *A*, The photograph of an autopsy specimen of intralobar sequestration reveals normal lung at the upper left, cysts in the middle of the sequestration, and an artery supplying sequestration below. *B*, High-power view of intralobar sequestration shows normal lung at the bottom separated from distorted cystic spaces of the sequestration by an ill-defined boundary. (Reproduced courtesy of Martha L. Warnock, M.D.; original magnification ×20.)

through intralobar sequestrations. Fabre and coworkers[84] have described the same condition in adults.

## Diagnosis, Treatment, and Prognosis

The diagnosis of bronchopulmonary sequestration can be suspected by the typical basilar location of the density on the chest roentgenogram (Fig. 53.4*A*). This is a relatively unusual location for pyogenic lung abscess, although bronchogenic cysts and other lesions may occur in this area. Although communication between sequestrations and the surrounding airways may exist, the sequestrations rarely fill during bronchography and cannot be visualized by bronchoscopy. Instead, the anatomy can be delineated by CT and the diagnosis confirmed by demonstrating the aberrant artery by angiography (Fig. 53.4*B*). Spiral CT scanning and magnetic resonance imaging also can be used.[85] Most surgeons believe that preoperative localization of the abnormal blood supply is desirable to avoid bleeding at the time of resection; spiral CT angiography seems ideal for the purpose because it allows simultaneous imaging of the anomalous vessels and the lung parenchyma in a single examination.[85a] Extralobar sequestrations often can be removed without disruption of surrounding normal lung tissue; lobectomy is the procedure of choice for intralobar sequestrations.[73] Video-assisted thoracoscopic resection may be possible in selected cases.[86] Patients who undergo resection have an excellent prognosis, barring complications at the time of surgery.

# PULMONARY ARTERY ANEURYSMS

## Classification

Pulmonary artery aneurysms have been defined by Bartter and coworkers[87] as roentgenographically visible sacs formed by dilation of the wall of the pulmonary artery. Other investigators have identified two shapes of these aneurysms: fusiform aneurysms, formed by localized dilation of the entire circumference of the vessel wall; and saccular aneurysms, formed by localized dilations involving only part of the circumference. Bartter and associates[87] do not use this distinction because it lacks diagnostic and prognostic significance. They do, however, distinguish between aneurysms that include abnormal arteriovenous communications and those that do not. Aneurysms with arteriovenous communications are covered earlier in this chapter; those lacking such communication are discussed here.

## Etiology and Pathogenesis

Pulmonary artery aneurysms are a rare vascular anomaly. This was suggested by Deterling and Clagett,[88] who in 1947 reported that only 8 cases of such aneurysms were documented in a study of 109,571 autopsies. From 40% to 50% of pulmonary artery aneurysms are associated with congenital cardiac defects such as patent ductus arteriosus, ventricular septal defect, tetralogy of Fallot, and pulmonic value stenosis.[88, 89] Infection is the other major cause of these aneurysms. Historically, infectious or mycotic aneurysms were seen for the most part in patients with syphilis and tuberculosis; in the latter group, they are called Rasmussen's aneurysms.[90] In developing countries today, mycotic aneurysms occur primarily in patients with bacterial[91] or fungal[92] infections involving either the lung or, more commonly, the heart valves.

Pulmonary artery aneurysms also occur in patients with underlying vascular disorders, including atherosclerosis and especially cystic medial necrosis. Cystic medial necrosis of the aorta and pulmonary arteries is well recognized, especially in the setting of severe pulmonary hypertension,[93, 94] and this process also may account for pulmonary artery aneurysms in patients with Marfan's syndrome.[87] In addition, systemic and pulmonary artery aneurysms have been reported in patients with giant cell arteritis,[95] Behçet's syndrome,[96, 96a] and Hughes-Stovin

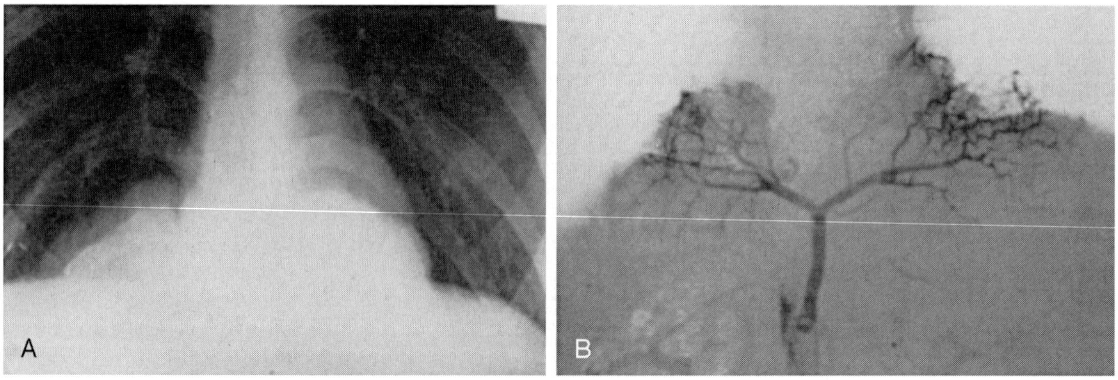


**Figure 53.4** *A,* A detailed view of a posteroanterior projection shows bilateral pulmonary sequestrations in typical basilar locations. *B,* Angiogram, with subtraction techniques, shows that the blood supply to both lesions comes from a large branch of abdominal aorta. (Reproduced courtesy of Gordon Gamsu, M.D.; reproduced with permission from Hinshaw HC, Murray JF: Diseases of the Chest (4th ed). Philadelphia: WB Saunders, 1979, p 191.)

syndrome.[97, 97a] The last three disorders are forms of pulmonary vasculitis and are discussed in Chapter 52.

Finally, pulmonary artery aneurysms may be traumatic in origin. Penetrating stab wounds have long been associated with aneurysms,[98] and aneurysms can occur after tube thoracostomy.[99] Several reports,[100–103] however, suggest that pulmonary artery catheterization is emerging as the most common traumatic cause. Catheterization can cause a pseudoaneurysm if the vessel wall is lacerated by the catheter tip and bleeding is contained, temporarily or permanently, by the surrounding tissues. Alternatively, a true aneurysm, with or without rupture, can develop if the catheter balloon is overinflated in a small branch of the pulmonary artery.

## Pathology

The histologic appearances of pulmonary artery aneurysms and pseudoaneurysms differ according to their etiology. With Rasmussen's aneurysms, the vessel wall is replaced by granulomatous inflammation in a centripetal fashion, leaving a thickened and weakened wall that has a tendency either to form an aneurysm, in which blood flow is contained within the intima of the vessel, or to rupture.[87, 90] Aneurysms secondary to necrotizing bacterial pneumonias probably develop in a similar fashion, but those related to endocarditis or septicemia show an angiocentric pattern that suggests endovascular seeding. As noted earlier, cystic medial necrosis is a common feature of aneurysms in patients with degenerative vascular disease and frequently is associated with intimal tears that allow blood to dissect between the wall layers.[93, 94] Vasculitic changes may be present in patients with noninfectious generalized vascular disorders, and trauma frequently causes pseudoaneurysm formation.

## Symptoms

Pulmonary artery aneurysms may be clinically silent and come to light only at autopsy, or they may be confused with central or peripheral neoplasms on the chest roentgenogram.[104–106] Alternatively, large lesions may cause dyspnea or chest pain[107] and may simulate pulmonary embolism.[108] Patients with severe pulmonary hypertension may manifest right-sided heart failure, whereas patients with underlying infectious or inflammatory disorders usually have fever and systemic complaints. The symptoms of greatest concern in these patients and in those with trauma is pulmonary artery rupture, which may be massive and uncontrollable.[109]

## Diagnosis

Pulmonary artery aneurysms and pseudoaneurysms may be suspected on routine chest roentgenography (Fig. 53.5*A* and *B*). They are better visualized by echocardiography[89] or CT.[98] Magnetic resonance imaging may prove to be superior to CT for these aneurysms and for abnormal vascular communications in the lung because flowing blood appears as an empty space on the scan, allowing clear differentiation between vascular and nonvascular lesions.[70] The best diagnostic procedure is angiography, however, which allows clear delineation of the aneurysms and may be combined with therapy at one session (Fig. 53.5*C*).

## Treatment and Prognosis

The exact prognosis of pulmonary artery aneurysms is unknown, and many of these lesions are neither detected nor cause symptoms during life. In autopsy series,[89, 94] only one third of the patients died because of aneurysm rupture, and two-thirds died of right heart failure, pulmonary embolism, or unrelated causes. Yet aneurysms are inherently unstable because any further dilatation greatly increases wall tension according to the law of Laplace. Because of this, many patients with these lesions, and especially those with hemoptysis, probably should be treated. At the very least, therapy should be directed toward underlying infection or inflammatory causes if they exist. Definitive removal or obliteration of the aneurysms may, however, be required.

The first surgical repair of an aneurysm was reported by Williams and associates[110] in 1971. Since then, pulmonary artery banding also has been shown to be successful.[111] As is the case with pulmonary arteriovenous malformations, however, percutaneous catheter embolization has emerged as the preferred approach to aneurysms that do not involve the proximal pulmonary arteries. After the first catheter-directed occlusion of a single pulmonary arteriovenous malformation was performed by Taylor and colleagues[112] in 1978, others[109, 113–115] reported excellent results in embolizing pulmonary artery aneurysms using both steel coils and inflatable balloons.

## SUMMARY

Pulmonary arteriovenous malformations (except the microscopic variety seen in the hepatopulmonary syndrome) are nearly always associated with *hereditary hemorrhagic telangiectasia*, an autosomal dominant disorder of microvascular development. Patients with pulmonary arteriovenous malformations are often asymptomatic, even when cyanosed. They are at risk of paradoxical embolization and may present with cerebrovascular events (paresis or transient ischemic attacks) or cerebral abscess. Modern treatment involves embolization with steel coils or detachable balloons. Therapy is very effective and has low morbidity, but malformations with small feeding vessels may remain; therefore, follow-up and antimicrobial prophylaxis (for dental procedures, etc.) should continue indefinitely.

Bronchopulmonary sequestrations are rare congenital anomalies that often are asymptomatic but that may produce symptoms that relate to underlying infection or that cause confusion on chest roentgenographic interpretation. They are diagnosed by their characteristic roentgenographic appearance and by arteriography. Treatment is surgical, and the results usually are excellent.

Pulmonary artery aneurysms with arteriovenous communications are rare but clinically significant vascular abnormalities. Their etiology is diverse, their clinical presentation varies, and they may be the source of life-threatening bleeding. These lesions can be definitively

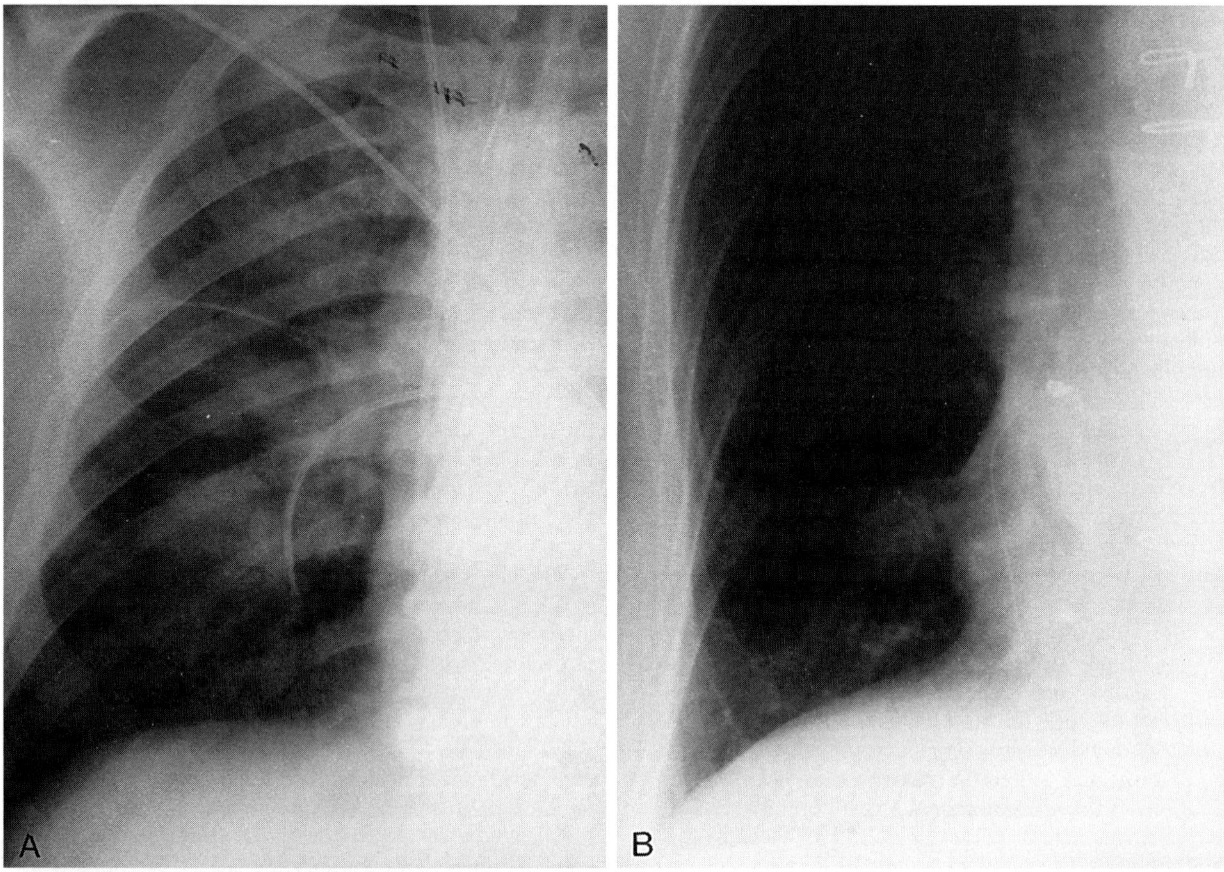

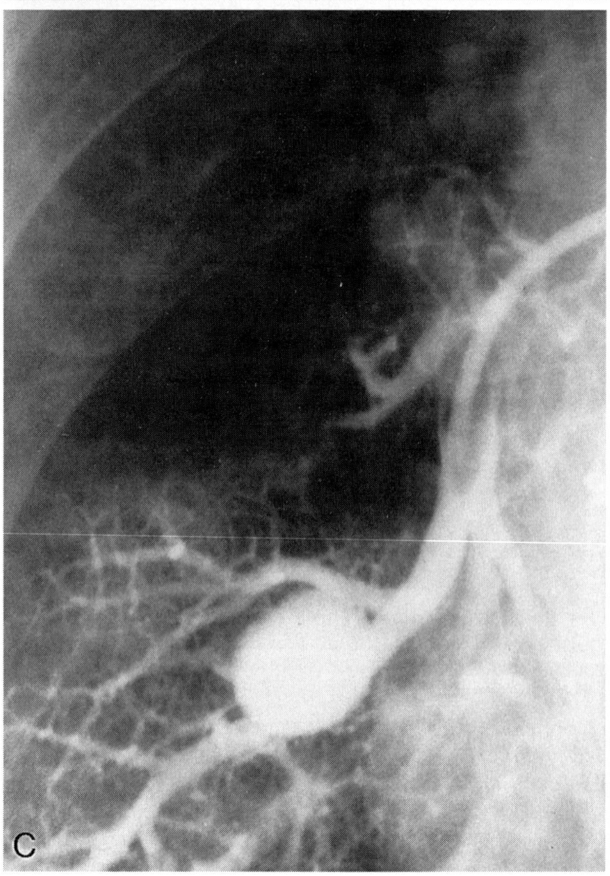

**Figure 53.5** *A,* A posteroanterior projection shows the pulmonary artery catheter in the distal branch of the right pulmonary artery, surrounded by ill-defined density. *B,* A similar projection shows a rounded lesion after the catheter is removed. *C,* A detailed view of the angiogram reveals the lesion to be a pulmonary arterial pseudoaneurysm presumably caused by laceration of the vessel by the catheter tip. (Reproduced courtesy of Jeffrey S. Klein, M.D.)

diagnosed by angiography and treated by several methods, of which transcutaneous catheterization with embolization is preferred.

## References


1. Niwayama G: Cor triatriatum. Am Heart J 59:291–317, 1960.
2. Burroughs JT, Edwards JE: Total anomalous pulmonary venous connection. Am Heart J 59:913–931, 1960.
3. Perloff JK, Child JS (eds): Congenital Heart Disease in Adults (2nd ed). Philadelphia: WB Saunders, 1998, pp 1–393.
4. Davis HA, Schwartz DJ, Lefrak SS, et al: Alveolar-capillary oxygen disequilibrium in hepatic cirrhosis. Chest 73:507–511, 1978.
5. Trusler GA, Williams WG, Cohen AJ, et al: William Glenn lecture. The cavopulmonary shunt. Evolution of a concept. Circulation 82:131–138, 1990.
6. Hanes FM: Multiple hereditary telangiectasis causing hemorrhage (hereditary hemorrhagic telangiectasia). Bull Johns Hopkins Hosp 20:63–73, 1909.
7. Rendu M: Epistaxis répétées: Chez un sujet porteur de petits angiomes cutanes et muqueux. Gaz des hôpitaux 49:1322–1323, 1896.
8. Osler W: On family form of recurring epistaxis, associated with multiple telangiectasis of skin and mucous membranes. Bull Johns Hopkins Hosp 12:333–337, 1901.
9. Porteous ME, Burn J, Proctor SJ: Hereditary haemorrhagic telangiectasia: A clinical analysis. J Med Genet 29:527–530, 1992.
10. Plauchu H, de Chadarevian J-P, Bideau A, et al: Age-related clinical profile of hereditary hemorrhagic telangiectasia in an epidemiologically recruited population. J Med Genet 32:291–297, 1989.
11. Vase P, Holm M, Arendrup H: Pulmonary arteriovenous fistulas in hereditary haemorrhagic telangiectasia. Acta Med Scand 218:105–109, 1985.
12. Jessurun GA, Kamphuis DJ, van dZF, et al: Cerebral arteriovenous malformations in the Netherlands Antilles. High prevalence of hereditary hemorrhagic telangiectasia–related single and multiple cerebral arteriovenous malformations. Clin Neurol Neurosurg 95:193–198, 1993.
13. Guttmacher AE, McKinnon WC, Upton MD: Hereditary hemorrhagic telangiectasia: A disorder in search of the genetics community [letter]. Am J Med Genet 52:252–253, 1994.
14. Haitjema T, Westermann CJ, Overtoom TT, et al: Hereditary hemorrhagic telangiectasia (Osler-Weber-Rendu disease): New insights in pathogenesis, complications, and treatment. Arch Intern Med 156:714–719, 1996.
15. Hughes JMB: Pulmonary arteriovenous malformations in hereditary hemorrhagic telangiectasia. Semin Respir Crit Care Med 19:79–89, 1998.
16. Shovlin CL: Molecular defects in rare bleeding disorders: Hereditary haemorrhagic telangiectasia. Thromb Haemost 78:145–150, 1997.
16a. Shovlin CL, Letarte M: Hereditary haemorrhagic telangiectasia and pulmonary arteriovenous malformations: Issues in clinical management and review of pathogenic mechanisms. Thorax 54:714–729, 1999.
17. McDonald MT, Papenberg KA, Ghosh S, et al: A disease locus for hereditary haemorrhagic telangiectasia maps to chromosome 9q33–34. Nat Genet 6:197–204, 1994.
18. Shovlin CL, Hughes JM, Tuddenham EG, et al: A gene for hereditary haemorrhagic telangiectasia maps to chromosome 9q3. Nat Genet 6:205–209, 1994.
19. McAllister KA, Lennon F, Bowles BB, et al: Genetic heterogeneity in hereditary haemorrhagic telangiectasia: Possible correlation with clinical phenotype. J Med Genet 31:927–932, 1994.
20. Gougos A, Letarte M: Primary structure of endogline, an RGD-containing glycoprotein of human endothelial cells. J Biol Chem 265:8361–8364, 1990.
21. Shovlin CL, Hughes JMB, Scott J, et al: Characterization and identification of novel mutations in hereditary hemorrhagic telangiectasia. Am J Hum Genet 61:68–79, 1997.
22. Pece N, Vera S, Cymerman U, et al: Mutant endoglin in hereditary hemorrhagic telangiectasia type 1 is transiently expressed intracellularly and is not a dominant negative. J Clin Invest 100:2568–2579, 1997.
23. Berg JN, Galline CJ, Stenzel TT, et al: The activin receptor-like kinase gene: Genomic structure and mutations in hereditary hemorrhagic telangiectasia type 2. Am J Hum Genet 61:60–67, 1997.
24. Piantinida M, Buscarini E, Dellavecchia C, et al: Hereditary haemorrhagic telangiectasia with extensive liver involvement is not caused by either HHT1 or HHT2. J Med Genet 31:441–443, 1996.
25. Berg JN, Guttmacher AE, Marchuk DA, et al: Clinical heterogeneity in hereditary haemorrhagic telangiectasia: Are pulmonary arteriovenous malformations more common in families linked to endoglin? J Med Genet 33:256–257, 1996.
26. Braverman IM, Keh A, Jacobsen BS: Ultrastructure and three-dimensional organization of the telangiectasias of hereditary hemorrhagic telangiectasia. J Invest Dermatol 95:422–427, 1990.
27. Vase P: Estrogen treatment of hereditary haemorrhagic telangiectasia. Acta Med Scand 209:393–396, 1981.
28. Guttmacher AE, Marchuk DA, White RJ: Hereditary hemorrhagic telangiectasia. N Engl J Med 333:918–924, 1995.
29. van Cutsem E, Rutgeerts P, Vantrappen G: Long-term effect of hormonal therapy for bleeding gastrointestinal malformations. Eur J Gatroenterol 5:439–443, 1993.
30. Korzenik JR, Topazian MD, White RI: Treatment of bleeding in hereditary hemorrhagic telangiectasia with aminocaproic acid [letter]. N Engl J Med 331:1326, 1994.
30a. Sargeant I, Loizon LR, Ramptar DA, et al: Laser ablation of upper gastrointestinal vascular ectasias: Long-term results. Gut 34:470–475, 1993.
30b. Shovlin CL, Guttmacher AE, Buscanni E, et al: Diagnostic criteria for hereditary hemorrhagic telangiectasia (Rendu-Osler-Weber syndrome). Am J Med Genet (in press).
31. Shovlin CL, Winstock AR, Peters AM, et al: Medical complications of pregnancy in hereditary haemorrhagic telangiectasia. Q J Med 88:879–887, 1995.
32. Dines DE, Seward JB, Bernatz PE: Pulmonary arteriovenous fistulas. Mayo Clin Proc 58:176–181, 1983.
33. Dutton JA, Jackson JE, Hughes JM, et al: Pulmonary arteriovenous malformations: Results of treatment with coil embolization in 53 patients. Am J Roentgenol 165:1119–1125, 1995.
34. White RJ, Lynch NA, Terry P, et al: Pulmonary arteriovenous malformations: Techniques and long-term outcome of embolotherapy. Radiology 169:663–669, 1988.
35. Wirth JA, Pollack JS, White RI: Pulmonary arteriovenous malformations. Curr Pulmonol Crit Care Med 17:261–298, 1996.
36. Swinburne AJ, Fedulla AJ, Gangemi R, et al: Hereditary hemorrhagic telangiectasia and multiple arteriovenous fistulas. Clinical deterioration during pregnancy. Chest 89:459–460, 1986.
37. Ference BA, Shannon TM, White RJ, et al: Life-threatening pulmonary hemorrhage with pulmonary arteriovenous malformations and hereditary hemorrhagic telangiectasia. Chest 106:1387–1390, 1994.
38. Hughes JMB, Shovlin CL, Simonds A: Pulmonary disease and cor pulmonale. *In* Oakley CM (ed): Heart Disease in Pregnancy. London: BMJ Publishing Group, 1997, pp 180–200.
39. Remy-Jardin M, Remy J: Spiral CT angiography of the pulmonary circulation. Radiology 212:615–636, 1999.
40. Remy J, Remy-Jardin M, Giraud F, et al: Angioarchitecture of pulmonary arteriovenous malformations: Clinical utility of three-dimensional helical CT. Radiology 191:657–664, 1994.
41. Chilvers ER, Peters AM, George P, et al: Quantification of right to left shunt through pulmonary arteriovenous malformations using $^{99}$Tcm albumin microspheres. Clin Radiol 39:611–614, 1988.
42. Whyte MK, Peters AM, Hughes JM, et al: Quantification of right to left shunt at rest and during exercise in patients with pulmonary arteriovenous malformations. Thorax 47:790–796, 1992.
43. Ueki J, Hughes JM, Peters AM, et al: Oxygen and $^{99}$mTc-MAA shunt estimations in patients with pulmonary arteriovenous malformations: Effects of changes in posture and lung volume. Thorax 49:327–331, 1994.
44. Barzilai B, Waggoner AD, Spessert C, et al: Two-dimensional contrast echocardiography in the detection and follow-up of congenital pulmonary arteriovenous malformations. Am J Cardiol 68:1507–1510, 1991.
45. Haitjema T, Disch F, Overtoom TT, et al: Screening family members of patients with hereditary hemorrhagic telangiectasia. Am J Med 99:519–524, 1995.

46. Thompson RD, Jackson JE, Peters AM, et al: Sensitivity and specificity of radioisotope right to left shunt measurements and pulse oximetry for the early detection of pulmonary arteriovenous malformations. Chest 115:109–113, 1999.
47. Whyte MK, Hughes JM, Jackson JE, et al: Cardiopulmonary response to exercise in patients with intrapulmonary vascular shunts. J Appl Physiol 75:321–328, 1993.
48. Sapru RP, Hutchison DCS, Hall JI: Pulmonary hypertension in patients with pulmonary arteriovenous fistulae. Br Heart J 31:559–569, 1969.
49. Chow LT, Chow W, Ma K: Pulmonary arteriovenous malformation. Progressive enlargement with replacement of the entire middle lobe in a patient with mitral stenosis. Med J Aust 158:632–634, 1992.
50. Pennington DW, Gold WM, Gordon RL, et al: Treatment of pulmonary arteriovenous malformations by therapeutic embolization. Rest and exercise physiology in eight patients. Am Rev Respir Dis 145:1047–1051, 1992.
51. Chilvers ER: Clinical and physiological aspects of pulmonary arteriovenous malformations. Br J Hosp Med 39:188–192, 1988.
52. Terry PB, White RJ, Barth KB, et al: Pulmonary arteriovenous malformations. Physiologic observations and results of therapeutic balloon embolization. N Engl J Med 308:1197–1200, 1983.
53. Haitjema TJ, Overtoom TT, Westermann CJ, et al: Embolisation of pulmonary arteriovenous malformations: Results and follow up in 32 patients. Thorax 50:719–723, 1995.
54. Barth KH, White RJ, Kaufman SL, et al: Embolotherapy of pulmonary arteriovenous malformations with detachable balloons. Radiology 142:599–606, 1982.
55. White RI, Pollack JS, Wirth JA: Pulmonary arteriovenous malformations: Diagnosis and transcatheter embolotherapy. J Vasc Intervent Radiol 7:787–804, 1996.
56. Haitjema T, Ten BJ, Overtoom TT, et al: Unusual complications after embolization of a pulmonary arteriovenous malformation. Chest 109:1401–1404, 1996.
57. Brundage BH, Gomez AC, Cheitlin MD, et al: Systemic artery to pulmonary vessel fistulas: Report of two cases and a review of the literature. Chest 62:19–23, 1972.
58. Cox PA, Keshishian JM, Blades SB: Traumatic arteriovenous fistula of the chest wall and lung: Secondary to insertion of an intercostal catheter. J Thorac Cardiovasc Surg 54:109–112, 1967.
59. Fein AB, Godwin JD, Moran JF, et al: Systemic artery-to-pulmonary vascular shunt: A complication of closed-tube thoracostomy. AJR 140:917–919, 1983.
60. Iskandrian AS, Kimbiris D, Bemis CE, et al: Coronary artery to pulmonary artery fistulas. Am Heart J 96:605–609, 1978.
61. Kiphart R, Mackenzie JW, Templeton AW, et al: Systemic-pulmonary arteriovenous fistula of the chest wall and lung: A report of a case and review of the literature. J Thorac Cardiovasc Surg 54:113–120, 1967.
62. Hearne SF, Burbank MK: Internal mammary artery-to-pulmonary artery fistulas: Case report and review of the literature. Circulation 62:1131–1135, 1980.
63. Knott-Craig CJ, Oostuized JG, Rossouw G, et al: Management and prognosis of massive hemoptysis. J Thorac Cardiovasc Surg 105:394–397, 1993.
63a. Liebow AA, Hales MR, Lindskog GE: Enlargement of the bronchial arteries, and their anastomoses with the pulmonary arteries in bronchiectasis. Am J Pathol 25:211–231, 1949.
63b. Marshall TJ, Flower CDR, Jackson JE: The role of radiology in the investigation and management of patients with haemoptysis. Clin Radiol 51:391–400, 1996.
64. Dweik RA, Stoller JK: Role of bronchoscopy in massive hemoptysis. Clin Chest Med 20:89–105, 1999.
64a. Rémy J, Voisin C, Dupuis C, et al: Traitement des hémoptysies par embolisation de la circulation bronchique. Ann Radiol (Paris) 17:5–16, 1974.
64b. Marshall TJ, Jackson JE: Vascular intervention in the thorax: Bronchial artery embolization for haemoptysis. Eur Radiol 7:1221–1227, 1997.
64c. Najarian KE, Morris CS: Arterial embolization in the chest. J Thorac Imaging 13:93–104, 1998.
65. White RI Jr: Bronchial artery embolotherapy for control of acute hemoptysis. Analysis of outcome. Chest 115:912–915, 1999.
65a. Mah H, Rullon I, Mellot F, et al: Immediate and long-term results of bronchial artery embolization for life-threatening hemoptysis. Chest 115:996–1001, 1999.
66. Rokitansky C: Lehrbuch der pathologiochen Anatomie (3rd ed). Wien, 1861, p 44.
66a. Rektorzik E: Über accessorische Lungenlappen. Wochenblatt der Zeitschrift der Kaiserlichen und Königlichen Gesellschaft der Ärzte in Wien. 17:4, 1861.
66b. Carter R: Pulmonary sequestration. Ann Thorac Surg 7:68–88, 1969.
67. Pryce DM: Lower accessory artery with intralobular sequestration of the lung. J Pathol Bacteriol 58:457–467, 1946.
68. Pryce DM, Sellors JH, Blair LG: Intralobar sequestration of the lung associated with an abnormal pulmonary artery. Br J Surg 35:18–19, 1947.
69. Gerle RD, Jaretzki A III, Ashley CA, et al: Congenital bronchopulmonary-foregut malformation: Pulmonary sequestration communicating with the gastrointestinal tract. N Engl J Med 278:1413–1419, 1968.
70. Heithoff KB, Sane SM, Williams HJ, et al: Bronchopulmonary foregut malformations: A unifying etiological concept. AJR 126:46–55, 1976.
71. Rodgers BM, Harman PK, Johnson AM: Bronchopulmonary foregut malformations: The spectrum of anomalies. Ann Surg 203:517–524, 1985.
72. Laurin S, Hagerstrand I: Intralobar bronchopulmonary sequestration in the newborn—a congenital malformation. Pediatr Radiol 29:174–178, 1999.
73. Ferguson TB: Congenital lesions of the lungs and emphysema. *In* Sabiston DC, Spencer FC (eds): Gibbon's Surgery of the Chest (4th ed). Philadelphia: WB Saunders, 1983, pp 668–709.
73a. Conran RM, Stocker JT: Extralobar sequestration with frequently associated congenital cystic adenomatoid malformation, type 2: Report of 50 cases. Pediatr Dev Pathol 2:454–463, 1999.
73b. Samuel M, Burge DM: Management of antenatally diagnosed pulmonary sequestration associated with congenital cystic adenomatoid malformation. Thorax 54:701–706, 1999.
74. Hernanz-Schulman M, Johnson JE, Holcomb GW, et al: Retroperitoneal pulmonary sequestration: Imaging findings, histopathologic correlation, and relationship to cystic adenomatoid malformation. AJR 168:1277–1281, 1997.
75. Rosado-de-Christenson ML, Frazier AA, Stocker JT: Extralobar sequestration: Radiologic-pathologic correlation. Radiographics 132:425–441, 1993.
76. Khalil KG, Kilman JW: Pulmonary sequestration. J Thorac Cardiovasc Surg 70:928–937, 1975.
77. Hilton TC, Keene WR, Blackshear JL: Intralobar pulmonary sequestration with nutrient systemic arterial flow from multiple coronary arteries. Am Heart J 129:823–826, 1995.
78. Temes RT, Talbot WA, Carrillo YM, et al: Sequestration of the lung arising from the circumflex coronary artery. Ann Thorac Surg 65:257–259, 1998.
79. Savic B, Birtel FJ, Tholen W, et al: Lung sequestration: Report of seven cases and review of 540 published cases. Thorax 34:96–101, 1979.
80. Rubin EM, Garcia H, Horowitz MD, et al: Fatal massive hemoptysis secondary to intralobar sequestration. Chest 106:954–955, 1994.
81. Avishai V, Dolev E, Weissberg D, et al: Extralobar sequestration presenting as massive hemothorax. Chest 109:843–845, 1996.
82. Sippel JM, Ravichandran PS, Antonovic R, et al: Extralobar pulmonary sequestration presenting as a mediastinal malignancy. Ann Thorac Surg 63:1169–1171, 1997.
83. White JJ, Donahoo JS, Ostrow PT, et al: Cardiovascular and respiratory manifestations of pulmonary sequestration in childhood. Ann Thorac Surg 18:286–294, 1974.
84. Fabre OH, Porte HL, Godart FR, et al: Long-term cardiovascular consequences of undiagnosed intralobar pulmonary sequestration. Ann Thorac Surg 65:1144–1146, 1998.
85. Frush DP, Donnelly LF: Pulmonary sequestration spectrum: A new spin with helical CT. AJR 169:679–682, 1997.
85a. Franco J, Aliaga FJ, Domingo ML, et al: Diagnosis of pulmonary sequestration by spiral CT angiography. Thorax 53:1089–1092, 1998.
86. Mezzetti M, Dell'Agnola CA, Bedoni M, et al: Video-assisted thoracoscopic resection of pulmonary sequestration in an infant. Ann Thorac Surg 61:1836–1838, 1996.

87. Bartter T, Irwin RS, Nash G: Aneurysms of the pulmonary arteries. Chest 94:1065–1075, 1988.
88. Deterling RA, Clagett DT: Aneurysms of the pulmonary artery: Review of the literature and report of a case. Am Heart J 34:471–498, 1947.
89. Bhandari AK, Nanda NC: Pulmonary artery aneurysms: Echocardiographic features in 5 patients. Am J Cardiol 53:1438–1441, 1984.
90. Auerbach O: Pathology and pathogenesis of pulmonary artery aneurysm in tuberculous cavities. Am Rev Tuberc 39:99–115, 1939.
91. Navarro C, Dickinson PCT, Kondlapoodi P, et al: Mycotic aneurysms of the pulmonary arteries in intravenous drug addicts. Am J Med 76:1124–1131, 1984.
92. Roush K, Scala-Barnett DM, Donabedian H, et al: Rupture of a pulmonary artery mycotic aneurysm associated with candidal endocarditis. Am J Med 84:142–144, 1988.
93. Natelson EA, Watts HD, Fred HL: Cystic medionecrosis of the pulmonary arteries. Chest 57:333–335, 1970.
94. Butto F, Lucas RV, Edwards JE: Pulmonary arterial aneurysm: A pathologic study of five cases. Chest 91:237–241, 1987.
95. Dennison AR, Watkins PM, Gunning AJ: Simultaneous aortic and pulmonary artery aneurysms due to giant cell arteritis. Thorax 40:156–157, 1985.
96. Durieux P, Bietry D, Huchon G, et al: Multiple pulmonary artery aneurysms in Behçet's disease and Hughes-Stovin syndrome. Am J Med 71:730–741, 1981.
96a. Tunaci M, Ozkorkmaz B, Tunaci A, et al: CT findings of pulmonary artery aneurysms during treatment for Behçet's disease. AJR Am J Roentgenol 172:729–733, 1999.
97. Hughes JP, Stovin PG: Segmental pulmonary artery aneurysms with peripheral venous thrombosis. Br J Dis Chest 53:19–27, 1959.
97a. Herb S, Hetzel M, Hetzel J, et al: An unusual case of Hughes-Stovin syndrome. Eur Respir J 11:1191–1193, 1998.
98. Daykin EL, Irwin GAL, Harrison DA: CT demonstration of a traumatic aneurysm of the pulmonary artery. J Comput Assist Tomogr 10:323–324, 1986.
99. Podbielski FJ, Wiesman IM, Yaghmai B, et al: Pulmonary artery pseudoaneurysm after tube thoracostomy. Ann Thorac Surg 64:1478–1480, 1997.
100. Bartter T, Irwin RS, Phillips DA, et al: Pulmonary artery pseudoaneurysm: A potential complication of pulmonary artery catheterization. Arch Intern Med 148:471–473, 1988.
101. Ray CE, Kaufman JA, Geller SC, et al: Embolization of pulmonary catheter-induced pulmonary artery pseudoaneurysms. Chest 110:1370–1373, 1996.
102. Ferretti GR, Thony F, Link KM, et al: False aneurysm of the pulmonary artery induced by a Swan-Ganz catheter: Clinical presentation and radiologic management. AJR 167:941–945, 1996.
103. Karak P, Dimick R, Hamrick KM, et al: Immediate transcatheter embolization of Swan-Ganz catheter-induced pulmonary artery pseudoaneurysm. Chest 111:1450–1452, 1997.
104. Buckingham WB, Sutton GC, Meszaros WT: Abnormalities of the pulmonary artery resembling intrathoracic neoplasms. Dis Chest 40:698–704, 1961.
105. Gibbs PM, Hami A: Pulmonary arterial aneurysm presenting as an endobronchial mass. Thorax 50:1013–1014, 1995.
106. Chung CW, Doherty JU, Kotler R, et al: Pulmonary artery aneurysm presenting as a lung mass. Chest 108:1164–1166, 1995.
107. Jaffin BW, Gundel WD, Capeless MA, et al: Aneurysm of the pulmonary artery as a cause of severe chest pain. Arch Intern Med 143:1484–1485, 1983.
108. Dillon WP, Taylor AT, Mineau DE, et al: Traumatic pulmonary artery pseudoaneurysm simulating pulmonary embolism. AJR 139:818–819, 1982.
109. Remy J, Lemaitre L, Lafitte JJ, et al: Massive hemoptysis of pulmonary arterial origin: Diagnosis and treatment. AJR 143:963–969, 1984.
110. Williams JE, Schiller M, Craenen J, et al: Pulmonary artery aneurysms. J Thorac Cardiovasc Surg 62:63–66, 1971.
111. Opie C, Sandor GGS, Ashmore PG, et al: Successful palliation by pulmonary artery banding in absent pulmonary valve syndrome with aneurysmal pulmonary arteries. J Thorac Cardiovasc Surg 85:125–128, 1983.
112. Taylor BG, Cockerill EM, Manfredi F, et al: Therapeutic embolization of the pulmonary artery in pulmonary arteriovenous fistula. Am J Med 64:360–366, 1978.
113. Remy L, Smith M, Lemaitre L, et al: Treatment of massive hemoptysis by occlusion of a Rasmussen aneurysm. AJR 135:605–606, 1980.
114. Renie WA, Rodeheffer RJ, Mitchell S, et al: Balloon embolization of a mycotic pulmonary artery aneurysm. Am Rev Respir Dis 126:1107–1110, 1982.
115. Santelli ED, Katz DB, Goldschmidt AM, et al: Embolization of multiple Rasmussen aneurysms as a treatment of hemoptysis. Radiology 193:396–398, 1994.

Fluid exchange in larger vessels in the lungs is probably limited by their thick walls and small surface area.

The essential factors that govern fluid exchange in the lungs are expressed in the Starling equation for the microvascular barrier:

$$Jv = LpS[(Pc - Pi) - \sigma d(\pi c - \pi i)]$$

where Jv is the net fluid-filtration rate (volume flow) across the microvascular barrier, Lp is the hydraulic conductivity ("permeability") of the microvascular barrier to fluid filtration (a measure of how easy it is for water to cross the barrier), S is the surface area of the barrier, Pc is the pulmonary capillary (microvascular) hydrostatic pressure, Pi is the interstitial ("perimicrovascular") hydrostatic pressure, $\pi c$ is the capillary (microvascular) plasma colloid osmotic (or oncotic) pressure, $\pi i$ is the interstitial (perimicrovascular) fluid osmotic pressure, and $\sigma d$ is the average osmotic reflection coefficient of the barrier (a measure of how effective the barrier is in hindering the passage of solutes from one side of the barrier to the other).

The osmotic forces oppose the hydrostatic forces at the fluid exchange sites. Because molecules smaller than plasma proteins pass unhindered and have nearly the same concentrations on both sides of the microvascular barrier, the osmotic forces across the barrier are generated by the plasma proteins and other macromolecules. The microvascular osmotic reflection coefficient ($\sigma d$) is a measure of how effective the barrier is in hindering the passage of solutes from one side of the barrier to the other. Solutes that pass freely across the microvascular barrier, such as the plasma electrolytes, have an osmotic reflection coefficient of 0 (because they are at equal concentrations on both sides of the barrier, they exert no osmotic pressure). A solute restricted entirely to the vascular lumen and not found in the perimicrovascular space has an osmotic reflection coefficient of 1. Because macromolecules pass across the microvascular barrier in relation to their size, the osmotically active solutes have reflection coefficients that are proportional to their radii and that vary from 0 to 1. The substantial protein concentration normally present in the perimicrovascular interstitium is important because if this were not the case, the high osmotic pressure relative to hydrostatic pressure within the bloodstream would result in a balance of forces favoring net fluid absorption rather than filtration, and the lungs would be dry rather than wet.

Because the normal microvascular barrier is leaky, the alveolar barrier must serve as the principal protection against the accumulation of alveolar edema. Fluid and protein do not normally move into alveoli, because the alveolar barrier has a low permeability even to small molecules (similar to cell-membrane permeability) and because the fluid that is filtered is continuously being pumped back into the interstitium by alveolar epithelial cells,[8, 9] drained away from the alveolar walls through the interstitium, and removed by lymphatic vessels.

The microvascular pressure is the principal force that causes fluid filtration in the lungs. If blood were not flowing through the lungs, the opposing hydrostatic and osmotic forces on either side of the microvascular barrier would be equal, their sum would be zero, and there would be no filtration. It is the pumping action of the heart that causes blood to flow through the lungs, and the microvascular hydrostatic pressure generated in the process establishes the steady-state values of the other driving pressures and causes fluid to filter.[1, 10]

According to the Starling equation, the balance between the prevailing transmural hydrostatic pressures (Pc − Pi) and the colloid osmotic pressures ($\pi c - \pi i$) provides the "driving force" for fluid filtration. The actual amount of filtrate that forms at any given driving force is determined by the integrity of the barrier to filtration, which is reflected in the conductivity (Lp) and reflection ($\sigma d$) coefficients. The equation predicts the development of two fundamentally different kinds of pulmonary edema: the first, *increased pressure pulmonary edema*, occurs when the balance of the driving forces increases, forcing fluid across the barrier at a rate that can no longer be accommodated by lymphatic drainage; the second, *increased permeability pulmonary edema*, occurs in the presence of acute lung injury that damages the normal barriers to fluid filtration and allows increased conductance of liquid and protein in the lungs. There also is a third type of pulmonary edema caused by impaired lymphatic drainage of filtered fluid, but this has less clinical relevance and is not discussed in detail. The lymphatic drainage of the lungs is an important means of removing filtered fluid and proteins from the perimicrovascular interstitial space, and pulmonary edema can occur when lymphatic ducts are interrupted (e.g., in transplanted lungs[11]) or obstructed (e.g., by fibrosis[12] or tumor[13]).

The several factors (Table 54.1) that normally protect the lungs against edema have been called *safety factors*. Under normal conditions, the lymphatic system pumps

**Table 54.1 SAFETY FACTORS PROTECTING THE LUNGS AGAINST ALVEOLAR EDEMA ACCUMULATION**

| |
|---|
| Alveolar barrier properties opposing edema |
| Extremely low alveolar epithelial barrier permeability |
| Low alveolar surface tension (surfactant) |
| Active transport by alveolar epithelial cells |
| Microvascular barrier properties opposing increased pressure filtration |
| Low permeability to protein |
| Washdown of perimicrovascular protein osmotic pressure |
| Plasma protein concentration |
| Interstitial exclusion volume |
| Alveolohilar interstitial pressure gradient |
| Perimicrovascular interstitial compliance |
| Coagulation of edema fluid |
| Liquid clearance pathways |
| Lung lymphatic system |
| Loose peribronchovascular connective tissue sumps |
| Resorption into blood vessels |
| Mediastinal drainage |
| Pleural space |
| Expectoration |

filtered fluid and protein out of the lungs as rapidly as they are formed, even when filtration of fluid and protein from the bloodstream into the interstitium is increased. Increases in fluid and protein filtration across the microvascular barrier also can be drained away from the alveolar walls down the prevailing pressure gradient into the loose peribronchovascular connective tissue or can be resorbed directly into blood vessels.[7] The lung lymphatics can increase their pumping capacity many fold, particularly when the microvascular wall has been injured.[14] When the balance of driving forces is upset by higher hydrostatic pressure, the increase in filtration of water across the microvascular barrier is much larger than that in protein flux because the microvascular barrier has a low protein conductance. This results in dilution ("washdown") of interstitial protein concentration and thereby an increase in the balance of the osmotic pressure opposing the higher hydrostatic pressure (because plasma protein concentration remains high). The interstitial gel is also hydrated. Exclusion volume for protein decreases, either because of swelling or because of alteration of composition as hyaluronan is washed out from the interstitium, reducing the concentration of protein by expanding the available volume.

The osmotic safety factors work only when the microvascular barrier is normal (increased pressure edema). If the endothelial barrier is injured and its functional integrity is compromised (increased permeability edema), barrier conductance increases and the osmotic reflection coefficient decreases, making this safety factor much less effective or virtually ineffective. The compliance of the interstitial space also protects the lungs against edema. Increases in interstitial volume result in only small elevations of interstitial pressure until the interstitial volume is large. This keeps the hydrostatic driving pressure across the alveolar barrier suitably low. When interstitial pressure is elevated to greater than pleural pressure, fluid flows across the visceral pleura into the pleural space, where its effects on lung function are relatively minor. Pleural fluid is drained by parietal pleural lymphatics and, even when pleural liquid accumulates, does not appear to flow back from the pleural space into the lungs. The extremely low alveolar barrier solute conductance provides an osmotic force that favors absorption of water out of the air space rather than filtration of water into the air space. Fluid that does accumulate in the alveoli is pumped out by alveolar epithelial cell active transport.[8] Alveolar type II cells can proliferate, thus increasing the removal of fluid from the air space. In addition, alveolar epithelial cell swelling in edema appears to decrease alveolar barrier fluid conductivity. The spread of lung injury and edema may be limited by coagulation in damaged microvascular beds, interstitium, and alveoli flooded with plasma proteins. Some fluid in the lungs' air spaces can be cleared by coughing and expectoration.

In summary, pulmonary edema results from increases in either driving pressures (increased pressure edema) or barrier conductance (increased permeability edema). What distinguishes the two types is barrier permeability, which is normal in increased pressure edema but abnormal in increased permeability edema. Fluid flow into the lungs is driven across the barrier in both types of edema by the balance of pressures; therefore, the fundamental therapeutic strategy is to lower it.

## Increased Pressure Edema

Increased pressure pulmonary edema (Fig. 54.1) is caused by an increase in the balance of driving forces for fluid filtration into the lungs. The essential feature of this edema is that the barriers to fluid and protein flow into the lungs are functionally intact. Increased pressure edema is often called *cardiogenic, high-pressure, hydrostatic*, or *secondary pulmonary edema* but more appropriately would be called *normal barrier pulmonary edema* because it is the barrier resistance to fluid and solute movement into the lungs that distinguishes the types of pulmonary edema. Increased pressure edema was the subject of two reviews.[15, 16]

### Pathophysiology

The flow of fluid and protein into the lungs increases when the sum of driving pressures is elevated. If the rate of fluid accumulation exceeds the rate at which it can be removed, increased pressure edema occurs. Because the barriers limiting fluid and protein flow into the lungs are intact, the lungs are protected against edema by the normal safety factors. Especially important is the ability to protect against increases in the principal driving pressure, lung microvascular hydrostatic pressure. Because of the microvascular barrier's low protein conductance, fluid flow increases much more than protein flow with an elevation in microvascular hydrostatic pressure. Interstitial protein concentration is diluted both by this higher fluid flow relative to protein flow and by a diminished exclusion volume for proteins as the interstitial gel is hydrated and swells. Lower interstitial protein concentra-

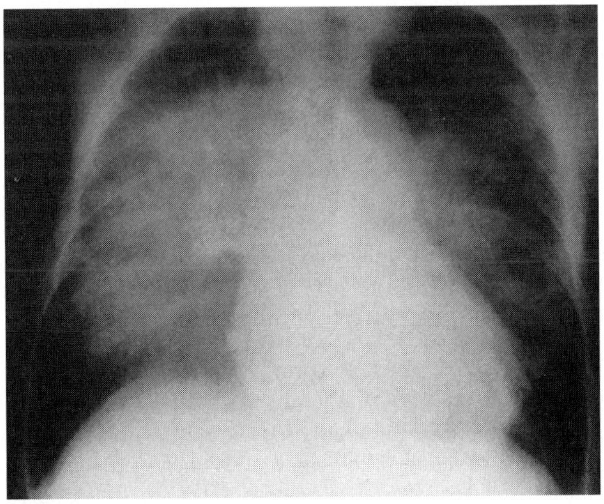

**Figure 54.1** Chest roentgenogram in a patient with increased pressure pulmonary edema. The heart is enlarged, and the vascular pedicle is widened. The "butterfly" pattern of edema (infiltrates centrally distributed, close to the heart and hila) is often seen with volume overload. The patient had chronic renal failure and overhydration.

tion (washdown or washout of interstitial proteins) results in lower perimicrovascular osmotic pressure and thereby a greater protein osmotic pressure difference across the barrier opposing any rise in hydrostatic pressure. In experimental animals, slightly less than 50% of an increase in hydrostatic pressure is offset by the increase in osmotic pressure difference.[17] Increased pressure edema may be slow and gradual in onset and progression because any elevation in microvascular hydrostatic pressure is attenuated by a rise in osmotic pressure difference across the microvascular barrier, owing to a decline in interstitial protein osmotic pressure.

There are, of course, limits to the ability of widening osmotic pressure difference to oppose increases in hydrostatic pressure at the microvascular barrier. Because the barrier is leaky, some protein is always carried into the interstitial space with water by convection, and washdown is limited by the barrier osmotic reflection coefficient. These impose limits to the decrease in interstitial protein concentration such that the maximum osmotic pressure difference able to oppose an increase in hydrostatic pressure can at most about double, from close to 10 mm Hg to just over 20 mm Hg. This effect is also limited by the concentration of proteins in the vascular space. At low plasma protein concentrations, the capacity to oppose hydrostatic pressure increases is reduced[18, 19] because the osmotic pressure difference across the barrier cannot be as large as normal. Lymphatic function is essential to this safety factor. Protein flow is greatly enhanced in increased pressure edema because proteins are swept into the lungs with water, and all the extravasated protein must be removed in lymph if washdown is to succeed. Lymphatic function may be compromised by an elevation in hydrostatic pressure at the outflow of the pulmonary lymphatic system into the large thoracic veins, which afford the back pressure that must be pumped against,[20, 21] and lymphatics in the lungs may be compressed by accumulating edema and rising pressure in the peribronchovascular connective tissue spaces. In long-standing or chronic high-pressure states (e.g., mitral stenosis), lymphatics have been said to proliferate and hypertrophy, improving the effectiveness of the lymphatic system for fluid and protein removal.[1, 22] Because osmotic pressure across the alveolar barrier is determined mainly by the concentration of molecules much smaller than protein that are present in the interstitial space at the same concentrations as in the blood, washdown of interstitial plasma protein concentration has little effect on the osmotic pressure across the alveolar barrier.

The consequences of increased pressure edema on lung mechanics and gas exchange (Table 54.2) depend on how much edema accumulates.[23] Dehydration of normal subjects increases lung volumes and improves tests of ventilatory function,[24] indicating that water in the lungs affects even the normal condition. Early in the progression of edema, increases in hydrostatic pressure result in greater intrapulmonary blood volume (as vessels are opened or distended by rising pressure), and the diffusing capacity of the lung for carbon monoxide ($DL_{CO}$) may actually be greater than normal because pulmonary capillary blood volume is increased. Similarly, arterial $Po_2$ may also rise because ventilated units are better perfused when vascular pressures are higher.[25] Whether lung compliance may be decreased by acute congestion of the lungs with blood is controversial.[1] Small, reversible changes in air flow resistance and dynamic compliance, unaffected by vagotomy, in congested lungs appear to be due to reflex bronchoconstrictor responses when baseline bronchial tone is normal.[26] When baseline tone is increased (e.g., by histamine), vagal reflexes appear to contribute to bronchial hyperreactivity.[27]

**Table 54.2 EFFECTS OF VASCULAR CONGESTION AND EDEMA ON PULMONARY FUNCTION AND LUNG MECHANICS**

| |
|---|
| Vascular congestion |
| Increased diffusing capacity |
| Increased arterial $Po_2$ |
| ± Decreased compliance |
| Bronchoconstriction |
| Interstitial edema |
| Increased closing volume |
| Decreased maximal expiratory flow |
| Increased ventilation-perfusion mismatching |
| Decreased arterial $Po_2$ |
| Alveolar flooding |
| Increased closing volume (air trapping) |
| Increased vascular resistance |
| Decreased lung volume (especially vital and inspiratory capacities) |
| Decreased compliance |
| Decreased diffusing capacity |
| Right-to-left shunting of blood (severely compromised gas exchange) |

When interstitial edema is present, closing volume may be increased[28] and maximum expiratory flows may be decreased. These changes were originally believed to be due to a decrease in caliber of small airways caused by compression by rising volume and pressure in the peribronchovascular connective tissue spaces. This effect would have to be in airways larger than bronchioles because bronchioles and smaller airways do not have loose connective tissue sheaths[1] and their diameter is a function of lung volume, not transpulmonary pressure.[29] Current evidence is that interstitial edema does not result in significant changes in airway diameter.[30] Lung compliance may be decreased in interstitial edema, but changes have been found not to be related closely to the amount of lung water[1, 31]; decreased lung compliance may be due to decreased lung volume, a reflex phenomenon, or to large-airway compression.[32] Chronic interstitial edema may provoke fibrotic changes in the lungs that can significantly decrease compliance.[1] Arterial $Po_2$ may fall as a result of ventilation-perfusion mismatching, but gas exchange is not seriously compromised until alveoli are flooded.

With alveolar flooding, lung volumes are diminished.[25] This is most marked in measurements of vital capacity, with inspiratory capacity affected more than expiratory capacity. Airways may close at higher than normal distending pressures, resulting in trapping of larger volumes of gas in the lungs.[33] Lung compliance is lessened when alveolar edema is present because lung volume is decreased.[25, 34] The elastic properties of edematous lungs were found to be not very different from those of normal lungs when surface forces were minimized, and edematous lungs had normal compliance when the number of ventilatable units was increased by elevated distending pressures.[34] Gas exchange is, of course, severely compromised when flooded alveoli are perfused (right-to-left shunt),[35] and there is an increase in wasted ventilation (ventilation of units where no gas exchange occurs).

Resistance to air flow across the lungs increases more with increased pressure edema than with increased permeability edema, perhaps due to effects on the bronchial circulation: bronchial veins drain into the right atrium, so increased systemic venous pressure would result in increased bronchial venous and capillary pressures.[36] In addition to changes in resistance of the lungs to air flow, the resistance of the lungs to blood flow increases as edema progresses.[37] Mild interstitial edema causes small arterioles to constrict, and capillaries are recruited, thus maintaining low lung microvascular pressure and acting as a safety factor to delay development of edema.[38] Vessels are not found to be compressed by interstitial edema,[30] and pulmonary blood flow is not much affected until alveolar flooding occurs.[37, 39] The cause of decreased pulmonary blood flow with edema is believed to be compression of alveolar wall vessels by the weight of the edema fluid. Greater resistance to blood flow in extra-alveolar vessels at low lung volumes[40, 41] and increases in hematocrit[42, 43] may add to this effect. Blood flow may also be redistributed: flow decreases at the bases as lung volume is diminished by edema.[44, 45]

Intact red blood cells are sometimes found in the edema fluid in increased pressure edema, especially if the edema is caused by increased hydrostatic pressure. Their presence may be due to rupture of a small number of tiny blood vessels with very high pressure, probably at the base of the lungs, where pressure is highest, and mixing of extravasated cells with edema fluid. Increased pressure edema fluid has low protein concentration, and there is no evidence that new pathways for leaking blood into the air spaces are opened up as the pressure climbs. If new pathways were created, the protein concentration of the edema fluid would increase along with the pressure. Protein concentrations in edema fluid decrease as pressure increases, indicating that proteins are sieved by the barrier (passing in proportion to their size) regardless of the pressure.

Light and electron microscopic examination of human and animal lung tissue in increased pressure edema shows alveolar edema and hemorrhage; thickened interstitial compartments (especially large peribronchovascular fluid cuffs) with separated, dispersed collagen fibrils; and increased capillary surface area and volume.[46–50] More intercellular vesicles can be seen, but otherwise no detectable changes in the ultrastructure of the vascular endothelium occur, and the gap widths at intracellular junctions are not different from those in normal lungs.[47] Electron-lucent zones (laminae rarae) may be seen in the basement membranes, particularly where the alveolar capillary barrier is thinnest.[46] Long-standing edema (e.g., in patients with mitral stenosis) can be associated with basement membrane thickening and increased distance between the alveoli and capillaries[48]; increases in fibroblasts, histiocytes, and bulky strands of collagenous fibers can be seen in the interstitium.[50] Permeability might be lowered across these widened barriers.[51, 52] Dogs with pacing-induced chronic congestive heart failure developed a significant increase in the threshold for high-vascular-pressure edema formation (about a 50% reduction in the amount of water and protein cleared across the lung microvascular endothelial barrier at high pulmonary vascular pressures as compared with controls).[53] Morphometric analysis of the alveolocapillary barrier showed endothelial, interstitial, and epithelial thickness were increased compared with controls, indicating that remodeling confers an increase in the resistance to development of high-pressure–induced alveolar edema. Alveolar type II cells may be more numerous than in normal lungs, and alveolar macrophages proliferate.[50] Chronic, severe increased pressure edema may also become organized and fibrotic, may calcify, and may even result in bone formation.[54]

A study[55, 56] of the morphology of experimental high-vascular-pressure pulmonary edema in excised, isolated, nonpulsatile-perfused, bloodless rabbit lungs held at a volume of 60% of total lung capacity showed marked inhomogeneity of interstitial and alveolar edema fluid distribution and albumin concentrations that were interpreted as indicating different sources of alveolar flooding (localized epithelial leaks resulting in direct filling of alveoli and distant leaks resulting in retrograde filling of alveoli via the airways) and local differences in the sieving properties of both the epithelial and the endothelial barriers. Unlike previous studies,[6, 7, 57, 58] alveolar flooding could not be characterized as an all-or-none phenomenon. Distinct and numerous lesions of the epithelial cell layer were observed, including formation of epithelial blebs and frank disruptions (epithelial discontinuities on the thin and thick sides of the blood-gas barrier). Epithelial lesions were absent in dry alveoli, which was interpreted as demonstrating direct association between barrier lesions and alveolar edema. In contrast to these epithelial lesions, endothelial lesions were rare. The authors and a commentator[59] suggested that formation of pulmonary edema cannot be explained by the classic, generally accepted membrane models for fluid exchange (i.e., fluid escape into alveoli cannot be described by the Starling equations) and that the difference between increased pressure and increased permeability edemas is not in barrier leaks, which are present in both, but rather in the severity and the extent of injury to the alveolar epithelial barrier and the associated inflammatory reaction.

There are serious problems, however, with the experimental preparation and with the interpretation of the morphologic findings. First, unlike clinical and most experimental increased pressure pulmonary edema, edema was induced by high vascular pressures very rapidly (in a few minutes), rather than with a latency of hours (as occurs clinically) and with more modest pressures (as occurs in most experimental preparations). Second, the lungs were perfused with hypertonic 6% albumin, which has been shown to cause barrier deterioration in rat lungs.[60] Already damaged barriers would be unmasked when vascular pressures are raised, even if no ultrastructural alterations could be seen at normal pressures.[61] Third, the perfusion pressure in these experiments was quite high, and small rodent lungs are known to be more fragile than the lungs of larger mammals (including humans). Fourth, no quantitative studies were reported, so it is not possible to know how extensive were the barrier injuries observed. Fifth, the edema fluid produced was not sampled for protein concentration, and no other measurements of barrier function were made, so it is impossible to know whether the authors were studying normal-barrier or abnormal-barrier pulmonary edema. The inhomogeneity of edema protein concentration they observed seems to indicate that they were studying a mixed type of pulmonary edema, one with both increased pressure and altered permeability mechanisms. Finally, their morphologic findings are inconsistent with those in all other studies of increased pressure pulmonary edema and with physiologic observations since 1950. On balance, these anomalous experiments likely represent an unmasking of already injured lungs by elevated microvascular pressure and do not demand any new concepts in the formation of pulmonary edema. The membrane damage hypothesis to explain alveolar flooding in increased pressure pulmonary edema remains unsubstantiated.

## Mechanisms

The most common cause of increased pressure edema is elevated microvascular hydrostatic pressure. The sum of driving pressures might also be greater if perimicrovascular hydrostatic pressure or the osmotic pressure difference across the microvascular barrier were decreased. At the alveolar barrier, an increase in interstitial hydrostatic pressure, a decrease in alveolar hydrostatic pressure, or a decrease in osmotic pressure difference across the barrier might result in a greater sum of driving pressures. The possibilities are listed in Table 54.3 and are discussed in the following paragraphs.

**Increased Microvascular Hydrostatic Pressure.** Congestive heart failure is the most common cause of increased pressure edema. That is why increased pressure edema is often called *cardiogenic* even though the heart is not always primarily involved. Elevated pressures in the pulmonary microvasculature are usually due to left-sided heart failure, with elevated left atrial pressures transmitted retrograde into the pulmonary circulation. Common causes are left ventricular dysfunction (e.g., caused by acute myocardial infarction, severe coronary insufficiency, tachyarrhythmias, bradyarrhythmias, cardiomyopathies, constrictive pericarditis, aortic stenosis or regurgitation, mitral regurgitation, coarctation of the aorta, rupture of chordae tendineae or intraventricular septum, systemic hypertension) or mechanical obstruction of the left atrial outflow tract (e.g., as in mitral stenosis, left atrial myxoma). An uncommon cause is impaired ventricular function secondary to scorpion envenomization.[62, 63] Left atrial pressure and subsequent pulmonary microvascular pressure can also be elevated by severe volume overloading in a patient with a normal or diseased heart. This is a cause of pulmonary edema in pregnant women who have preeclampsia or who are treated with tocolytic therapy, for example, as discussed in Chapter 88. A very rare cause of congestive heart failure and pulmonary edema is a pseudomineralocorticoid excess state caused by binge licorice consumption.[64]

An unusual cause of increased microvascular hydrostatic pressure is pulmonary venous hypertension in the absence of left ventricular or atrial disease, which can occur if the pulmonary veins are contracted (e.g., by possible muscular sphincters[65]), compressed, or obstructed (e.g., because of veno-occlusive disease or mediastinal fibrosis[66]). Bronchial venous hypertension does not appear to significantly increase fluid filtration in the lungs.[67]

Increases in fluid filtration can also be associated with increases in vascular pressure proximal to the filtration sites in the lungs. For example, pulmonary hypertension, in combination with depressed left ventricular function, has been implicated in the pathogenesis of cocaine-induced pulmonary edema.[68] Whether such increases lead to pulmonary edema depends on what happens to microvascular pressure. If high right-sided pressures are caused by increased resistance before the main site of filtration in the lungs (e.g., hypoxic pulmonary vasoconstriction of small arterial vessels,[69–71] primary pulmonary hypertension, pulmonary artery or valvular stenosis), edema does not occur. Conversely, if the lung vascular bed is only partially constricted or obstructed, or if the vascular surface area is greatly decreased (e.g., by lung resection), higher flow in perfused vessels leads to increased pressure edema[71] because microvascular pressures at the fluid exchange site are elevated in the overperfused lung. Pulmonary edema occurred in about 15% of patients after pneumonectomy and seemed to be exacerbated by administration of fresh frozen plasma,[72] probably because intravascular volume is increased by such transfusions. Any increase in blood flow through the lungs increases the pulmonary microvascular pressure at the fluid exchange sites even if the pulmonary venous pressure remains constant because pulmonary microvascular pressure is the sum of pulmonary venous pressure plus the product of pulmonary venous resistance and blood flow.[16] High systemic venous pressure might also promote edema forma-

**Table 54.3 MECHANISMS OF INCREASED PRESSURE PULMONARY EDEMA**

| |
|---|
| Increased lung microvascular hydrostatic pressure |
| Left ventricular dysfunction |
| Mechanical obstruction of left atrial outflow |
| Volume overload |
| Pulmonary venous hypertension |
| Overperfusion |
| Increased lymphatic outflow pressure |
| Decreased perimicrovascular hydrostatic pressure |
| Increased alveolar surface tension |
| ? Re-expansion of the lung |
| ? Pleural fluid evacuation |
| ? Pericardial fluid evacuation |
| ? Inspiratory airway obstruction |

tion by raising the outflow pressure and thereby reducing the flow of lymph.[20, 21]

The mechanisms of two exotic pulmonary edemas, those occurring at high altitude and during severe neurologic insults, may involve increased microvascular hydrostatic pressure. *High-altitude pulmonary edema,*[73, 74] which is also discussed in Chapters 6 and 70, appears to be caused by severe pulmonary hypertension that develops in susceptible individuals as a consequence of hypoxic vasoconstriction. Nonhomogeneous obstruction of the pulmonary vascular bed by exaggerated hypoxic vasoconstriction results in high blood flow and transmission of pressure to portions of the pulmonary vascular bed that are not protected by vasoconstriction, and the result is pulmonary edema. Patients who develop high-altitude pulmonary edema have been found to have very high pulmonary arterial pressure (sometimes at systemic levels), the excessive rise in pressure precedes the development of the edema, and agents that lower pulmonary arterial pressure (e.g., oxygen, nifedipine, hydralazine, phentolamine, and inhaled nitric oxide) are effective in prevention or treatment or both.

Postmortem edema fluid has been described as "proteinaceous" in high-altitude pulmonary edema, and measurements of edema fluid protein concentration have been made in two patients.[75] In one, edema fluid to plasma protein concentration ratio (0.6) was in the range predicted for increased pressure edema; in the other, the ratio (0.8 in one sample, 1.1 in another) was in the range typical of increased permeability pulmonary edema. Bronchoalveolar lavage fluid of six climbers with high-altitude pulmonary edema showed a marked increase in high-molecular-weight proteins (as well as many red blood cells and alveolar macrophages).[76] Because water is resorbed from edema fluid in the alveoli much faster than protein,[77, 78] the protein concentration of edema fluid increases progressively as edema resolves. The high protein concentration of postmortem high-altitude pulmonary edema and bronchoalveolar lavage fluids may be due to observations made during a time when fluid was being resorbed from, rather than added to, alveoli. Water loss from the alveoli by evaporation may be accentuated in these patients, but only if they are hyperventilating and the air at high altitude is extremely dry. More measurements of protein concentrations in edema fluid and plasma during the development of high-altitude pulmonary edema are needed to clarify the type of edema produced and its mechanism.

As noted earlier, overperfusion of a restricted pulmonary vascular bed, even in the presence of hypoxia, causes increased pressure edema, not increased permeability edema.[71] This can explain why some cases of high-altitude pulmonary edema are correctly classified as increased pressure pulmonary edema. Other cases likely are increased permeability pulmonary edemas, perhaps caused by physical damage to vascular walls (so-called stress failure), which has been shown to occur at extreme, but sometimes transient, increases in pulmonary vascular pressures in experimental animals.[79–80a] Such structural failures need not occur in large numbers to explain even severe increased permeability edema, because edema would form readily and in a quantity driven by the prevailing elevated vascular pressure.[81] The suggestion has been made that high-altitude pulmonary edema results from the stress failure of overdistended, relatively thin-walled pulmonary arteries rather than from microvascular rupture,[82] which might help explain why the prevailing vasoconstriction does not seem to offer much protection to downstream vessels, why there are no reports of gradual progression through an indolent prodrome of increased pressure edema before stress failure occurs, and why high-altitude pulmonary edema is first detected radiographically in the central lung fields surrounding large vessels rather than in the lung bases and periphery.

Plasma selectins have been measured in subjects at high altitude.[83] Levels of E-selectin were inversely related to arterial oxygen saturation in control subjects and in subjects with acute mountain sickness and with high-altitude pulmonary edema. Because endothelial cells are the only known source of E-selectin, increased plasma levels were considered to be a sign of activation or injury of endothelial cells. Plasma levels of P-selectin were not found to be elevated at high altitude. P-selectin is elevated in acute lung injuries and would be expected to be elevated if "stress failure" occurred, because exposure of subendothelial matrix would activate thrombin, which in turn elevates P-selectin.

Several alternative mechanisms for the increased permeability in high-altitude pulmonary edema have been proposed. Vulnerability to high-altitude pulmonary edema may be immunogenetically mediated, perhaps through an inherent human leukocyte antigen–associated susceptibility to pulmonary hypertension.[84] Some patients likely are infected and develop increased permeability pulmonary edema on that basis. High-altitude pulmonary edema could be a result of a noninfectious inflammatory response in the lungs: a preliminary communication claimed that increases in sheep lung lymph flow at simulated high altitude were caused by intravascular formation of air bubbles during decompression.[85] Air emboli–induced increased permeability edema in sheep is believed to be mediated by leukocytes.[86] Inflammatory responses in high-altitude pulmonary edema, however, are probably a consequence rather than a cause of the edema.[73, 87, 88] The ready reversibility of high-altitude pulmonary edema with descent to lower elevation, oxygen therapy, or pharmacologic reduction of pulmonary vascular pressure are not characteristics of acute lung injuries and increased permeability pulmonary edemas suspected to be caused by or related to inflammation, and high-altitude pulmonary edema patients do not experience clinical courses similar to those of patients with acute lung injuries. At this time, the precise mechanism of high-altitude pulmonary edema remains uncertain.

*Neurogenic pulmonary edema,*[89] which is also discussed in Chapter 6, may also be related to elevated pulmonary vascular pressures. Measurements of edema fluid protein concentration relative to plasma protein concentration in 12 patients with neurogenic pulmonary edema have been reported.[90] Seven of the patients had ratios typical of increased pressure pulmonary edema, and the other five had ratios consistent with either increased permeability pulmonary edema or with sampling during the resolution phase of increased pressure pulmonary edema (when edema fluid protein concentration rises as fluid is resorbed from the alveoli at a faster rate than protein). Measurements in eight patients had previously been reported; two of the measurements indicated increased pressure edema, and six indicated increased permeability edema or sampling during the resolution phase (as discussed earlier). Thus, half the cases of neurogenic pulmonary edema in which edema fluid protein concentration has been measured appear to be increased pressure edemas, and the fraction is perhaps even higher, depending on the timing of edema sampling.

Measurements of alveolar-to-plasma protein concentration ratios in dogs with intracisternal veratrine-induced neurogenic pulmonary edema showed a wide range of values, indicating that both increased pressure and increased permeability mechanisms may play roles to varying degrees in the development of that type of neurogenic pulmonary edema.[91] In other animal experiments, filtration increases in neurogenic edemas[92–96] and edema following transient pulmonary hypertension[94, 97] were attributable to increased pressure or increased vascular surface area, or both, perhaps in combination with acute lymphatic insufficiency.[97] Animal studies can be difficult to interpret. Some models have been complicated by primary lung injury that is separate from effects on the central nervous system[98] or by evidence that vascular permeability was abnormal in control experiments[97] performed in surgically traumatized, acutely prepared animals.[99]

Both human and experimental neurogenic pulmonary edema can be associated with massive discharge of the sympathetic nervous system, resulting in systemic vasoconstriction and translocation of blood from the systemic to the pulmonary circulation, producing marked increases in pulmonary blood flow and vascular pressures. Peak pulmonary arterial pressure can reach systemic levels. Hydrostatic pressure at the fluid exchange sites in the lungs can also be elevated by catecholamine-induced left ventricular dysfunction, increased pulmonary venous resistance, and mitral valve insufficiency secondary to left ventricular dilation. Thus, as in high-altitude pulmonary edema, high pulmonary vascular pressures could result in either increased pressure edema (from elevated microvascular hydrostatic pressure) or increased permeability edema (if pulmonary vascular pressures were high enough to cause stress failure of pulmonary vessels). Whether neurogenic pulmonary edema can occur by pressure-independent mechanisms remains controversial and unproven.[89] Some neurogenic edemas are increased pressure edemas; others appear to be increased permeability edemas. More information is needed to sort out the precise causes.

**Decreased Perimicrovascular Hydrostatic Pressure.** The sum of driving pressures would be greater if perimicrovascular hydrostatic pressure were diminished, thereby resulting in an increase in fluid and protein filtration at the microvascular barrier in the lungs. Pulmonary edema has been described in circumstances in which this might occur. The best clinical example is *postobstructive pulmonary edema* as a consequence of upper airway obstruction or its release, which can be caused, for example, by laryngospasm, endotracheal tube obstruction, foreign-body aspiration, epiglottitis, croup, severe acute asthma, airway compression by tumors, strangulation, or hanging. High negative intrathoracic pressures generated by inspiration attempts against the occluded airway are transmitted to the interstitium, thereby sucking fluid into the lungs. Mechanical effects on the cardiovascular system likely contribute to this kind of edema: high negative intrathoracic pressure causes increases in cardiac preload and afterload and in pulmonary blood flow, all of which increase the microvascular pressure that drives fluid out into the interstitium. Three patients with upper airway obstruction and pulmonary edema were reported, all with low edema fluid protein concentration relative to plasma protein concentration (ratios of 0.44, 0.31, and 0.52), indicating increased pressure pulmonary edema.[100] Pulmonary edema may also occur after evacuations of pericardial fluid,[101, 102] but measurements of edema fluid protein in humans have not been made to determine which type of edema is associated with pericardiocentesis.

Aspiration of air or fluid from the pleural space with consequent re-expansion of collapsed lung could result in a decrease in perimicrovascular hydrostatic pressure as the lung expands to fill the thorax. So-called *re-expansion pulmonary edema* has been reported in experimental animals[103, 104] and in patients[105–108] after lung re-expansion, but the high edema fluid protein concentration measured in three patients[109, 110] indicated that re-expansion may result in an increased permeability edema rather than an increased pressure edema. Support for this hypothesis was found in a dual isotope scintigraphic study in humans[111] and in studies of rabbits with experimental re-expansion edema.[112–116] Precisely why increased permeability edema might occur in re-expanded lung is not known. The hypothesis that this edema is due to vascular stretching seems untenable because blood flow to rapidly re-expanded lung has been shown to be significantly less than normal blood flow[117] and because vascular distention causes increased pressure edema, not increased permeability edema.[71]

An alternative hypothesis is that re-expansion pulmonary edema is a form of ischemia/reperfusion injury,[118] the increase in lung microvascular permeability being related to restoration of blood flow, formation of oxygen free radicals, release of proinflammatory mediators, and activation of neutrophils. On reperfusion, pulmonary vascular resistance shifts more toward postcapillary venules, which elevates pressure in the microvascular vessels at the fluid exchange sites in the lungs and would aggravate edema formation across the injured barrier.[119] A patient with apparent reperfusion pulmonary edema complicating thrombolytic therapy for pulmonary embolism has been reported,[120] and reperfusion injury is believed to be one of the causes of the pulmonary edema that occurs in transplanted lungs. Hemorrhagic and traumatic shock have also been conceived of as types of a "whole-body ischemia/reperfusion syndrome."[121] Reperfusion pulmonary edema is discussed in more detail in Chapter 6.

If high alveolar surface tension were transmitted to the interstitium, perimicrovascular hydrostatic pressure would also be lowered, thereby increasing filtration across the microvascular barrier. Such an effect has been suggested by experimental findings in dog lungs.[122, 123] The effect of alveolar surface tension on lung fluid balance is discussed later.

**Decreased Transmural Osmotic Pressure Difference.** The sum of driving pressures would be increased if the osmotic pressure difference opposing the hydrostatic pressure difference across the microvascular barrier were decreased (by lowering plasma protein concentration or by raising interstitial protein concentration), resulting in an increase in the sum of driving pressures for fluid and protein flow into the lungs. This theoretical mechanism of increased pressure edema has been the subject of study in experimental animals. Results are contradictory. In some studies, hypoproteinemia was not found to increase lung microvascular liquid conductance or protein permeability.[124, 125] Because the microvascular-perimicrovascular osmotic pressure gradient is generated by the microvascular hydrostatic pressure and by the barrier descriptors (conductivity and reflection coefficient), it is not possible to decrease the osmotic pressure gradient by depleting plasma proteins except transiently while a new steady state is being established. Although fluid flow would be increased temporarily, it would return to normal when a new steady state is reached, unless hydrostatic pressure or barrier characteristics were also changed. This is not to imply that protein concentrations are not important forces in lung fluid balance. Although isolated decreased osmotic pressure gradient across the microvascular barrier cannot be sustained or be an important mechanism for increased pressure edema, the absolute concentration of protein has a profound effect on lung fluid balance when hydrostatic driving pressure is increased.[18] When plasma osmotic pressure is low, the ability of the osmotic pressure gradient to widen in response to increased hydrostatic pressure is diminished, and edema accumulates at hydrostatic driving pressures lower than those needed to cause edema when protein concentration is normal.

In other studies, plasma protein depletion apparently increased calculated lung liquid conductance,[126] but problems in study design and in the calculations were noted.[127] The apparent increase in lung liquid conductance might have been an artifact of the method used in its calculation, which combined microvascular barrier, interstitial, and lymphatic conductances. An increase in interstitial or lymphatic conductance, rather than in microvascular barrier conductance, might explain the results. For example, were interstitial resistance decreased by edema, as when hyaluronan is washed out or the interstitium expands,[128–130] calculated lung liquid conductance would be increased, even if microvascular barrier conductance were unchanged. Similarly, a decrease in lymphatic resistance with edema[14] would cause the calculated lung liquid conductance to increase, even if microvascular barrier conductance were unchanged. The authors proposed an alternative filtration theory[131] to explain their results, but the possibility of increased lung microvascular liquid conductance or protein permeability caused by hypoproteinemia must be regarded as controversial and unproved.

**Alveolar Barrier Function.** The driving pressure for fluid and protein flow across the alveolar barrier would be elevated, resulting in increased pressure edema, if the interstitial hydrostatic pressure were raised or if the alveolar hydrostatic pressure or the osmotic pressure difference across the alveolar barrier were lowered. Because the osmotic pressure difference across the barrier is established by the relevant hydrostatic forces and barrier descriptors (as across the microvascular barrier), an isolated decrease in the osmotic difference could result in only a transiently increased pressure filtration until a new steady state is achieved. This transient phenomenon would not be an important mechanism for alveolar increased pressure edema.

Interstitial hydrostatic pressure rises as interstitial edema accumulates in the lungs.[5, 6, 132, 133] Increased interstitial hydrostatic pressure would raise the sum of driving pressures across the alveolar barrier and could drive edema formation across the alveolar or airway epithelium. The role of interstitial hydrostatic pressure in edema formation is not simple, however. Although increased interstitial hydrostatic pressure favors edema formation across the alveolar barrier, it opposes edema formation across the microvascular barrier. The relative contributions of these disparate effects have not been elaborated. The osmotic pressure difference across the intact alveolar barrier provides a powerful force that opposes filtration increases driven by hydrostatic pressure. Because the barrier is normally virtually impermeable even to small solutes, filtration of water would result in a decrease in alveolar osmotic pressure. A decrease of only 1 mOsm (<0.5% of the normal alveolar osmotic pressure) would balance a 19 mm Hg increase in interstitial hydrostatic pressure.

Greater pressure filtration across the alveolar barrier would also result from an increase in the sum of driving pressures if alveolar hydrostatic pressure were lowered. This is complicated by the interrelation between alveolar and interstitial hydrostatic pressures.[6, 133, 134] A drop in alveolar hydrostatic pressure, which increases the sum of driving pressures across the alveolar barrier, also results in a lowering of interstitial hydrostatic pressure, which decreases the sum of driving pressures across the alveolar barrier but increases the sum of driving pressures across the microvascular barrier. The influence of alveolar surface tension on lung fluid balance has been investigated in dogs. Administration of a detergent aerosol resulted in loss of surfactant activity, higher alveolar surface tension, lower static compliance, atelectasis, and pulmonary edema; low protein concentration in alveolar edema fluid and left-hilar afferent lymph relative to plasma protein concentration indicated that this was an increased pressure type of pulmonary edema.[135, 136] Higher alveolar surface tension has also been associated with lower isogravimetric pressure (i.e., fluid accumulated in the lungs at lower vascular pressures) in open-chested dogs,[122] with increased ratios of lung wet-to-dry weights[135] and altered mechanical properties and lung morphology[137] in rabbits, and detergent aerosol apparently disrupted the alveolar lining and increased microvascular permeability in sheep.[138] Because increased pressure edema has been shown to impair surface activity of dog lung extracts[139] and isolated rabbit lungs,[140] it is possible that changes in alveolar surface tension may accelerate edema formation. However, the notion that changes in alveolar surface tension in edema lead to a self-perpetuating vicious circle of edema formation is not borne out clinically, and in experimental animals, alveoli fill with edema fluid in a patchy, all-or-none fashion with no evidence that edema formation is self-perpetuating or spreads uncontrollably to adjacent alveoli.[57]

Surfactant could act as an antiwetting agent to antagonize edema formation if the alveoli were dry and the epithelial cells were covered with an adsorbed surfactant film. There has been controversy about whether the alveoli are normally dry or covered by a thin, continuous or discontinuous liquid hypophase. The present consensus is that a continuous layer is always present.[141]

The only kind of clinical pulmonary edema caused by transmural osmotic pressure differences is near drowning.[142, 143] Seawater is three times more hyperosmotic (1000 mOsm) than plasma, so the volume of fluid in the air spaces after salt water aspiration increases threefold to reach osmotic equilibrium, thus markedly increasing the alveolar edema already present because of the volume of seawater itself in the alveoli. Osmotic equilibrium is reached in minutes as water is sucked from the vasculature into the alveoli by osmotic pressure. Alveolar barrier function is not significantly compromised (unless perhaps the patient aspirates gastric contents or the seawater is contaminated or rich in particulate matter), and the alveolar edema is cleared very rapidly (50% to 60% of excess alveolar fluid is cleared in 4 hours). Transient, minimal disturbances in endothelial barrier function may occur, however, if cellular water loss causes cell shrinkage, thereby opening up paracellular pathways (junctions between cells) for fluid and solute movement. Fresh water near drowning proceeds in the opposite fashion: osmotic equilibrium is reached rapidly by flow of water out of the alveoli into the interstitium and bloodstream, causing interstitial rather than alveolar edema. Severe hemodilution, with hemolysis and fibrinolysis, also occurs, and the rapid water flux and hypotonicity cause severe distortion of pulmonary ultrastructure, including damage to type I and type II cells, endothelial cell swelling, basement membrane detachment, and cell disruption. Both alveolar epithelium and microvascular endothelium can thus be injured by the hypotonic fluid, leading to increased permeability pulmonary edema rather than a normal barrier type of pulmonary edema.

## Increased Permeability Edema and Acute Lung Injury

Increased permeability pulmonary edema (Fig. 54.2) is caused by an increase in liquid and protein conductance across the barriers in the lungs. The essential feature of this edema is that the integrity of the barrier to fluid and protein flow into the lungs is altered. Increased permeability edema is sometimes called *noncardiogenic* or *primary pulmonary edema*, and the resulting clinical syndromes in humans are commonly lumped together as the *acute* (formerly *adult*) *respiratory distress syndrome* (ARDS).[144] Introductory remarks in one text summarized the history of acute lung injury since the problem was first recognized in World War I and the progress made in defining and understanding acute lung injury since that time.[145] Epidemiology of acute lung injury was reviewed in the same text,[146] and new reviews appear regularly.[147–150]

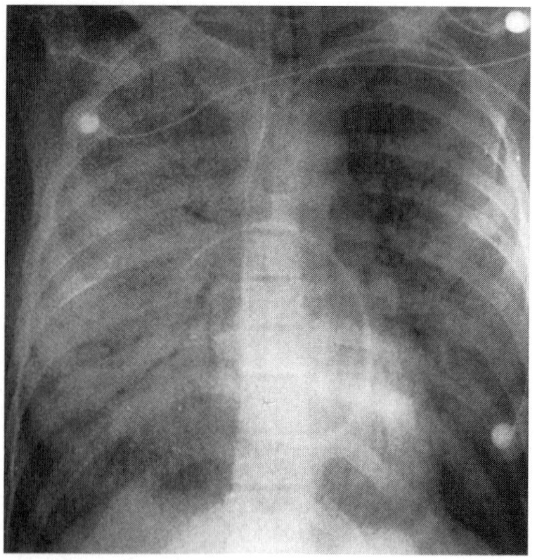

**Figure 54.2** Chest roentgenogram in a patient with increased permeability pulmonary edema. The heart is not enlarged, and the vascular pedicle is of normal size. Edema is peripheral and not gravitationally distributed. Air bronchograms are present, a finding more common in increased permeability edema than in increased pressure edema. The patient had drug overdose, coma, and hypotension.

### Pathophysiology

Flow of fluid and protein into the lungs increases when the lung parenchyma is injured. If the rate of fluid accumulation exceeds the rate at which it can be removed, increased permeability edema occurs. Because the barriers limiting fluid and protein flow into the lungs do not function normally when the lungs are injured, the lungs are not protected against edema by the usual safety factors. Although increases in fluid and protein filtration across the barriers are removed by lymphatics and drained away from the alveolar walls as in increased pressure edema, much more fluid and protein are filtered at any given sum of driving pressures because the barriers to their flow are much less restrictive than normal. Edema formation in injured lungs is very sensitive to driving pressures.[81] Driving pressures are often increased when the lungs are injured because of, for example, the vasoconstrictive effects of inflammatory mediators, which may shift the main site of resistance to postcapillary venules, thus increasing hydrostatic pressure at the microvascular fluid exchange sites,[151] or because of effects on the heart as well as on the circulation, for example, elevated left atrial pressure, pulmonary venoconstriction, and increased cardiac output in sepsis, all of which can increase hydrostatic pressure at the microvascular fluid exchange sites.[152] Microvascular hydrostatic pressure in injured lungs is not related simply to pulmonary artery occlusion ("wedge") pressure, and such measurements can be very misleading.

Because the barriers are inordinately leaky, protective osmotic pressure differences are lost across them; driving pressure is unopposed by osmotic pressure, and even normal hydrostatic pressure results in significant fluid and protein extravasation into the lungs. Lymphatic capability to pump the excess filtrate away is increased when the lungs are injured. Maximal lung lymph flow increases more when the microvascular wall has been injured than when hydrostatic pressure alone is increased (as a result of poorly understood "edema-dependent lymphatic factors"),[14] but even this augmented lymphatic-pumping capability is taxed at lower driving pressures. If the epithelial barrier is injured, edema may accumulate readily in the alveoli, even if the endothelial barrier is normal, because most of the resistance to fluid and protein flow into the alveoli is in the epithelial barrier.[153, 154] Increased permeability edema is often rapid in onset and progression because injured barriers offer much less resistance to flow and because hydrostatic driving pressure is unopposed by increases in osmotic pressure difference. Clinically, patients with increased permeability edema usually have a low sum of driving pressures, commonly measured as a low or normal pulmonary capillary wedge pressure. This is not an intrinsic feature of increased permeability edema but simply reflects the reduced likelihood of survival when fluid and protein are driven at higher pressures virtually unopposed across barriers into the lungs, or it reflects the low vascular pressures associated with underlying disease (e.g., sepsis).

The consequences of increased permeability edema on lung mechanics and gas exchange depend on how much edema accumulates and how severe the causative lung injury is.[23, 155] As with increased pressure edema, the major effects on pulmonary mechanics occur with alveolar flooding. In experimental lung injury, functional residual capacity was found to be decreased as a consequence of alveolar flooding, and this loss of ventilatable units accounted for virtually all the observed decrease in static lung compliance.[156, 157] Computed tomography has provided new insights into structure/function relationships in human acute lung injury.[158–161] In the early stage of lung injury, when alveolar edema predominates, the lungs are characterized by a homogeneous alteration of vascular permeability, and edema accumulates evenly in all lung regions with a nongravitational distribution. Increased lung weight due to edema causes collapse of lung regions along the vertical axis through the transmission of hydrostatic forces (compression atelectasis, caused by the weight of edema). Thus, collapse occurs mainly in the dependent lung, where the superimposed weight from above is greatest.

Measurements of pulmonary mechanics in mechanically ventilated patients with acute lung injuries[155] showed decreased static lung compliance as a consequence of this loss of ventilatable lung. In addition, lung resistance was found to be increased as a result of decreased lung volume. Bronchospasm adds to the increase in air flow resistance and can be substantially reversed with bronchodilator inhalation.[162] Chest wall compliance was reduced, probably because of alterations of intrinsic mechanical properties of the chest wall by abdominal distention, chest wall edema, and pleural effusion.[155] Different respiratory mechanics and response to positive end-expiratory pressure (PEEP) during mechanical ventilation were reported in patients with ARDS originating from pulmonary disease (pneumonia, which caused consolidation) or from extrapulmonary disease (which caused edema and subsequent alveolar collapse).[163] Lung elastance was higher in pneumonia, whereas chest wall elastance and intra-abdominal pressure were higher in patients with extrapulmonary causes of their lung injuries. PEEP appeared to primarily stretch alveoli in pneumonia, whereas in extrapulmonary causes of acute lung injury, it appeared to recruit previously collapsed alveoli.

Although the effects of surface forces on decreased lung compliance in acute lung injury were believed to be small, results of experiments in isolated rabbit lungs indicated that increased permeability edema may result in more severe mechanical changes than equivalent degrees of increased pressure edema.[140] In contrast, experiments in awake sheep showed that similar degrees of pulmonary edema, regardless of the mechanism, caused similar changes in compliance and gas exchange.[36] Other experiments showed that dynamic and static lung compliance decreased early in evolving lung injury.[164] Surfactant is strongly thromboplastic, and there may be a coagulative type of surfactant depletion when plasma proteins enter the air spaces.[165] Surfactant may also be inactivated by compression at the low lung volumes present in edema.[166, 167] The injured lung may release substances that can interfere with the normal low surface tension in the alveoli,[168] and activated polymorphonuclear leukocytes (PMNs) have been shown to impair surfactant function in vitro and to degrade the major surfactant apoprotein by a combination of proteolysis and oxidant-radical–mediated mechanisms.[169] Other in vitro studies have shown that phospholipases and the fatty acids they release both inactivate surfactant and, at lower concentrations, increase the sensitivity of surfactant to other inhibitory agents, such as albumin.[170] Human lung surfactant obtained by bronchoalveolar lavage of patients at risk for acute lung injury and patients with established acute lung injuries has been reported to be abnormal in chemical composition and functional activity.[171] Abnormalities also could be caused by interactions between surfactant and edema proteins because plasma proteins[165] (especially fibrin monomers but also fibrinogen and albumin[172]) interfere with surfactant function. Proteinaceous edema fluid has been associated with surfactant inhibition in various experimental models.[173–176] Surfactant depletion or abnormal function might also increase the resistance to flow in the lymphatic system, where surface-active material may be important in preventing proteins from acting as adhesives that could glue lymph vessels shut.[177] The role of surfactant in the development and treatment of acute lung injury was the subject of a review,[178] and the possibility of surfactant therapy is discussed in more detail later in this chapter.

As in increased pressure edema, gas exchange is severely compromised in increased permeability edema, owing both to intrapulmonary shunting of blood and to ventilation-perfusion inequalities.[179–181] The available evidence taken as a whole does not support the concept that tissue oxygenation may be further compromised by an abnormality in the regulation of oxygen extraction that has been hypothesized to occur in patients with acute lung injury (so-called pathologic dependency).[182, 183] Unlike in increased pressure edema, pulmonary blood volume is usually not expanded in increased permeability edema,[184] probably because intravascular pressures are lower at equivalent degrees of edema.

Mechanical and gas exchange abnormalities change with time through the course of acute lung injuries.[185] The early, exudative stage of injury, in which edema predominates, is characterized by small but not stiff ventilatable lungs (so-called baby lung) and true shunt; the later, proliferative stage of injury, in which fibrosis and remodeling predominate, is characterized by small and stiff ventilatable lungs, with superimposed emphysema-like alterations (bullous disease), decreased alveolar ventilation, and probable ventilation-perfusion maldistribution rather than true shunt.

Other consequences of acute lung injury (beyond those related to edema accumulation) probably depend on the cause and extent of injury. Bronchoconstriction, caused by injury and mediator release, may add to mechanical and gas exchange abnormalities.[162, 186, 187] Vascular reactivity to hypoxia and other stimuli may also be altered in the injured lung's vascular bed.[188–190] Perhaps because lung metabolic function is compromised, the injured lung may add or fail to extract vasoactive substances (e.g., biogenic amines, arachidonic acid metabolites, and drugs) from the blood, and angiotensin-converting enzyme (ACE) activity may be abnormal.[191] This could have effects on the heart and on the systemic as well as on the pulmonary circulation.[192, 193] Increases in microvascular permeability may lead to activation of the clotting cascade.[194] Disseminated intravascular coagulation, often associated with endotoxemia and gram-negative infections, is an ominous complication associated with thromboses, hemorrhage, and endothelial cell injury in the lungs and other organs.[195] Abnormalities of fibrin turnover[196] and lung fibrinogen uptake[197] have been reported in acute lung injuries. Pulmonary vascular resistance between arteries and veins also may increase as a result of morphologic alterations of the microvascular endothelium[43] or disruption and loss of the pulmonary vascular bed.[198] If the lungs have severe structural damage, mechanical and gas exchange abnormalities may be much greater than can be explained by edema accumulation alone.

The light and electron microscopic appearance of human[58, 198–210] and animal[45, 58, 206, 207, 211–215] lung tissue in acute lung injury is variable. Lung morphology depends on the severity and the duration of injury and on the treatments administered rather than on the cause of injury. Exudative, proliferative, and fibrotic changes usually appear in sequence. Death (or recovery) can occur at any stage.

The earliest changes are marked by widespread alveolar and interstitial edema and hemorrhage. Injury to alveolar ducts may be particularly severe.[202] Hyaline membranes, composed of precipitated plasma proteins, fibrin, and necrotic debris, can be seen. The alveolar epithelium may be more extensively damaged than the vascular endothelium, even if the underlying insult is bloodborne. Widespread, local areas of destruction of type I alveolar epithelial cells alternate with normal-appearing alveoli. The injured alveolar epithelium is swollen, disorganized, discontinuous, and often lifted off exposed, but usually intact, basement membranes, which are covered by hyaline membranes. Type I cells are more severely damaged than type II cells, and the thin cytoplasmic extensions of the cells far from the nucleus covering the thin side of the alveolar-capillary barrier may be most severely affected. The interstitium is widened by edema (especially in peribronchovascular cuffs) and may be choked with leukocytes, platelets, red blood cells, fibrin, and debris (especially near the alveolar walls). The thick portion of the alveolar interstitium is usually involved more than the thin portion. The microvascular endothelium is preserved, usually showing little other than irregular, focal thickening as a result of cytoplasmic swelling or vacuoles and greater numbers of luminal leukocytes. Intracapillary thrombi are rare in this and subsequent phases. Large endothelial gaps are not seen, probably because they would be incompatible with even brief survival because massive edema pours across even small, focal gaps. The alveolar capillary is the usual site of injury, but some insults involve other vessels (e.g., focal gaps in arterioles less than 1 mm in diameter in air-emboli–induced lung injury).[213]

The exudative phase can be followed, usually after 7 to 10 days, by a proliferative phase.[216] The relative contributions of the original insult, repair processes, and effects of therapies to this and subsequent phases are not known, but some of the abnormalities that occur after the initial exudative phase could be related to such factors as oxygen toxicity and mechanical ventilation as well as to the original lesion. In the proliferative phase, fluid has been resorbed from the air spaces. Fibrin may be prominent in alveoli and interstitium, and there is infiltration with inflammatory cells and fibroblasts (which may have been activated very early in the course of lung injury[217]). The alveolar epithelium is often cuboidal, made up largely of proliferating type II cells. The air-blood barrier can be greatly thickened by interstitial and epithelial enlargement. The pulmonary vascular bed may be partially or completely disrupted, and structural alterations may greatly reduce its surface area. The proliferative phase can present clinically as an inflammatory syndrome with fever, leukocytosis, low systemic vascular resistance, diffuse alveolar infiltrates, diffuse and intense pulmonary uptake of gallium, and neutrophilia on bronchoalveolar lavage, all in the absence of any infection.[218, 219]

A final stage may follow, often about 2 weeks after the initial insult, in which fibrotic changes of the alveolar ducts, alveoli, and interstitium predominate. Alveoli may be obliterated, alveolar walls coalesced, and functional lung units lost. The lungs may be emphysema-like, with extensive bullous disease.[185] Even severe changes at any stage may be reversible, with slow recovery toward normal lung function. Recovery may be related to the intensity of any fibrotic response and to the severity of the initial damage to the architecture of the lungs.

## Mechanisms

New causes of acute lung injury are continually being reported in humans and experimental animals. Table 54.4 lists most of the conditions that have been associated with acute lung injury in humans. The common causes, accounting for most of the cases, are pneumonia, sepsis, aspiration, and trauma. The insult can be via the airways or bloodborne. The exact mechanisms by which the lungs are injured have been the subject of intense investigation. Because information from humans is difficult to obtain and interpret, most of our knowledge about the mechanism of acute lung injuries comes from experimental animal models. Current reviews summarize most of what we have learned about the possible mechanisms of experimental acute lung injuries that result in pathophysiologic changes similar to those occurring in patients with ARDS,[149, 220, 221] and the mechanisms of various particular acute lung injuries are discussed in Chapter 6.

Major hypotheses of current research interest are discussed here. Although there are both considerable enthusiasm and experimental support for these hypotheses, significant problems still need to be resolved. Because support comes largely from in vitro and animal experiments and not from studies in humans, the relevance of the hypotheses being studied to the human disorder is unknown. This is especially true in studies of isolated cells and tissues, in which the complexity and redundancy of intact systems have been bypassed to provide more controlled conditions for the study of possible disease mechanisms. Intact animal models of acute lung injury often involve pathophysiologic responses that reverse quickly and completely, even if no therapy is given. Significant differences are seen between humans and experimental animals in the magnitude and the duration of response to the same lung injury (e.g., air embolization of the lungs[222]), and no animal model faithfully replicates human disease.

Studies in isolated organs and small animals in which hemodynamic variables are not measured are also difficult to evaluate because indices of lung injury, usually measured by appearance of markers in lungs or in lavage or perfusion fluids, are not determined solely by the barrier function of the microvasculature. Lavage fluid may be a nonspecific and potentially misleading indicator of lung injury.[223] For example, when the vascular endothelium is injured, fluid and protein movement from the vascular space into the lungs is extremely sensitive to hydrostatic driving pressures and surface area for filtration,[81] and the effects of experimental interventions may be caused by changes in these parameters and not by changes in microvascular barrier function. The effects of microvascular driving pressures and surface area can be difficult to evaluate even in large, instrumented animals. In sheep and goats, interpretation of lung lymph fluid and protein flow changes are further complicated by contributions from lymphatics outside the lungs,[224, 225] physical forces acting on lymphatics, [20, 21, 226] and possible intranodal modification of lymph.[227] These effects are probably more important when transport coefficients are being measured than when the animals' response to injury is being evaluated.

Investigators sometimes develop a kind of tunnel vision that distorts the importance of their areas of research into a comprehensive and sole explanation for the cause of acute lung injury. Investigative efforts are sometimes driven by fashion, technology, or quest for funding rather than oriented to problem solving.[228] Most experimental work purposely controls and excludes interactions of multiple components of causation and thereby turns the reality of complexity into the simplicity of a final common pathway. The concept that multiple and diverse insults lead to a stereotypical sequence of lung injury is attractive because it offers hope of specific intervention, but unfortunately, it is not consistent with the evidence.[221] In acute lung injury, as in all aspects of medicine, what is most important is that one must be imaginative and have an open mind. An important part of that process is to avoid fixation on theory and to concentrate on the evidence. Increased permeability pulmonary edema may be caused by some extent of interaction of all of the hypotheses at hand.[229]

From experimental animal models, we seem to have learned that there are at least two broad categories of mechanisms of acute lung injury: those that are *indirect* (i.e., requiring the participation of intermediary mechanisms, e.g., host defenses) and those that are *direct* (i.e., not requiring intermediary mechanisms, and injury probably occurs as a result of contact between an offending substance and lung tissue).[230] These categories overlap because once the lungs are injured, inflammatory responses occur, and, of course, inflammatory responses directly injure the lungs. The relevance of animal models to human disease is largely unknown,[231–233] and human disease is not well understood, but three major hypotheses about the mechanism of acute lung injury have emerged. Each is discussed separately, but they are interrelated.

**Role of Infection.** Acute lung injury develops in 10% to 45% of patients with the sepsis syndrome.[234–237] Increased microvascular permeability to albumin has been shown to accompany human sepsis,[238] and infection and the sepsis syndrome are the major causes of acute lung injury in humans.[239] Patients who develop shock in response to known or suspected infection have a particularly high incidence of acute lung injury, and the mortality of patients with acute lung injury associated with infection, the sepsis syndrome, or bacteremia is greatly increased.[240–242] Acute lung injury also appears to predispose the lungs to infection, and infection and/or host defense responses account for many of the deaths of patients who survive the initial lung insult.[219, 243–245]

The mechanism by which infection and the sepsis syndrome injure the lungs is not known with certainty.[246] It seems likely that lung injury may be related to factors other than direct damage by bacteria or other microorganisms because prognosis has not been found to be related to documented bacteremia or pneumonia.[247–249] In experimental animals, intravenous infusions of live *Pseudomonas aeruginosa,*[250] endotoxins from *Escherichia coli*[251–253] or *Salmonella typhimurium,*[252] the precursor (lipid X) of the biologically active lipid A portion of gram-negative endotoxin,[254] and surgically induced peritonitis[255] all resulted in increased permeability pulmonary edema in

**Table 54.4** CLINICAL DISORDERS ASSOCIATED WITH ACUTE LUNG INJURY

- Infectious causes
  - Gram-negative sepsis
  - Sepsis syndrome
  - Endotoxemia
  - Toxic shock syndrome
  - Bacterial pneumonia
  - Viral pneumonia
  - Mycoplasmal pneumonia
  - Fungal pneumonia
  - *Pneumocystis carinii* pneumonia
  - Mycobacterial disease
    - Miliary tuberculosis
    - Tuberculous pneumonia
    - Atypical mycobacteria
  - Rickettsial disease
    - Rocky Mountain spotted fever
    - Boutonneuse fever
  - Malaria
  - Strongyloidiasis
  - Herxheimer's reaction (treatment of syphilis, other infectious diseases)
- Aspiration
  - Gastric acid
  - Food and other particulate matter
  - Fresh water (near drowning)
  - Blood
    - Gastrointestinal bleeding
    - Nasopharyngeal bleeding
  - Hydrocarbon fluids
    - Gasoline
    - Kerosine
- Trauma
  - Lung contusion
  - Fat emboli
  - Nonthoracic trauma
  - Overdistention (mechanical ventilation)
  - Blast injury (explosion, lightning)
  - Thermal injury (burns)
  - Ruptured viscus (bowel, appendix, kidney, uterus)
- Hemodynamic disturbances
  - Shock of any etiology
  - Anaphylaxis
  - High-altitude pulmonary edema
  - Reperfusion
  - Embolization
    - Thromboembolism
    - Air embolism
    - Amniotic fluid embolism
  - Bowel infarction
- Drugs
  - Suicide gesture (aspiration)
  - Heroin
  - Methadone
  - Propoxyphene
  - Naloxone
  - Cocaine
  - Barbiturates
  - Colchicine
  - Salicylates
  - Ethchlorvynol
  - Interleukin-2
  - Protamine
  - Hydrochlorothiazide
  - Amiodarone
  - Paraldehyde
  - Kamisyoyo-san
  - Cancer chemotherapy
    - Cytosine arabinoside
    - Cyclosporine
    - Methotrexate
    - Vinca alkaloids
    - Mitomycin
    - Nitrosoureas
    - Alkylating agents
- Inhaled toxins
  - Oxygen (high concentrations)
  - Combustion products (smoke)
  - Lacrimators (tear gas)
  - Corrosive chemicals
    - Silo-filler's disease ($NO_2$)
    - Chlorine
    - Ammonia
    - Phosgene
    - Cadmium
    - Paraquat
    - Methylene chloride
    - Ozone
    - Nitric acid
- Hematologic disorders
  - Disseminated intravascular coagulation
  - Incompatible blood transfusion
    - ABO incompatibility
    - Rh incompatibility
    - Antileukocyte antibodies
  - Leukoagglutinin reactions
  - Postcardiopulmonary bypass, pump oxygenator
- Metabolic disorders
  - Pancreatitis
  - Uremia
  - Diabetic ketoacidosis
- Neurologic disorders
  - Head trauma
  - Grand mal seizures
  - Increased intracranial pressure (any cause)
  - Subarachnoid or intracerebral hemorrhage
  - Cerebrovascular accident
  - Spinal cord injury
  - Trigeminal nerve block
- Obstetric/gynecologic disorders
  - Tocolytic therapy
  - Preeclampsia
  - Eclampsia
  - Abruptio placentae
  - Retained placenta
  - Uterine hemorrhage or rupture
  - Trophoblastic disease
  - Hysteroscopy (anaphylaxis)

**Table 54.4 CLINICAL DISORDERS ASSOCIATED WITH ACUTE LUNG INJURY** *Continued*

| | |
|---|---|
| Miscellaneous | Goodpasture's syndrome |
| Obstruction or its release | Pustular and erythrodermic psoriasis |
| Lung re-expansion | Electrical injury |
| Thoracentesis | Electroconvulsive therapy |
| Upper airway obstruction | Electrocution |
| Epiglottitis | Lightning |
| Laryngotracheobronchitis | Envenomization |
| Laryngospasm after endotracheal intubation | Stonefish |
| Strangulation | Jellyfish |
| Interrupted hanging | Heat stroke |
| Tumors | Hypothermia |
| Foreign body aspiration | Postcardioversion |
| Nd:YAG phototherapy | Radiation pneumonitis |
| Lymphangitic carcinomatosis | Induction of anesthesia |
| Hematologic malignancy | Sudden infant death syndrome |
| Carcinomas | Psychologic stress (fright) |
| Hepatoma | |
| Esophagus | |
| Pheochromocytoma | |

Nd:YAG = neodymium:yttrium-aluminum-garnet.

sheep. Instillation of endotoxin into the airways of sheep also led to severe lung injury.[256] *P. aeruginosa* has also been reported to cause lung injury in pigs (but not dogs),[257] and *E. coli* endotoxin has been reported to injure the lungs of baboons[258] and dogs[259] and to result in neutrophilic alveolitis in rats.[260] Acute lung injury caused by endotoxin in sheep is believed to be an inflammatory response mediated at least in part by PMNs[261] and by tumor necrosis factor (TNF).[262] Endotoxin can also affect the clotting system[195] and metabolic functions of the lungs,[263] and it may dispose the lung to the development of pulmonary infections by increasing adherence of bacteria to endothelium.[264] However, acute lung injury in septic humans does not appear to be necessarily related to endotoxemia, because endotoxin may be undetectable or present only in low concentrations in septic patients. In one study, endotoxin was detected in plasma samples of 74% of patients believed to be at risk who subsequently developed acute lung injury, 64% of patients with acute lung injury, and 22% of patients believed to be at risk who did not develop acute lung injury.[265] Exoproducts of bacteria, such as elastase and exoenzyme S, also might injure the lungs.[246]

Both increased pressure edema and increased permeability edema are associated with impaired antibacterial defenses,[266, 267] and bacillary infections worsen acute lung injury in dogs,[268] baboons,[269] and hamsters.[270, 271] The cause of impaired bacterial defenses in acute lung injury is not known. Bactericidal properties of the alveolar lining material[272–274] might be altered in injured or flooded lungs, but alterations in surfactant concentration and function were not found to be a factor in one study.[275] Alveolar macrophage function has been reported to be compromised in pigs[276] but not in hamsters[270] with acute lung injury. Although PMNs may be present in large numbers in the bronchoalveolar lavage fluid of patients with acute lung injury, evidence indicates the function of these PMNs is compromised.[277, 278] Drugs (e.g., aspirin[279] and aminophylline[280]) used in the treatment of acute lung injury may also compromise antibacterial defenses. The reason for, and the significance of, impairment of bacterial defenses in acute lung injuries need to be worked out. The central role of inflammation hypothesized in the mechanism of many acute lung injuries (discussed later) focuses attention on its destructive potential and invites suppressive therapies. It is important, however, to keep in mind the protective functions of inflammation and increased permeability pulmonary edema, both of which are integral to host defenses against infection. Effort should concentrate on developing reversible and selective drugs that decrease the harmful, while retaining (or even enhancing) the beneficial, effects of host defenses.

**Role of Inflammation.** Substantial evidence has accumulated implicating host defenses and inflammatory responses in the underlying mechanism of many acute lung injuries. Neutrophils, complement, and other humoral mediators of inflammation, injury, and repair are discussed in detail in Chapter 19. Succinct reviews present the theory of acute lung injury mediated by inflammation.[221, 281, 282]

The main actor in this hypothesis is the PMN,[283, 284] which wears two hats. In one role, PMNs are a vital component of host defenses, crucial in the killing of invading microorganisms (and instrumental in defending against oxidants,[285] modifying the inflammatory response, and initiating repair processes). In their other role, PMNs are potent offensive weapons that can turn their armamentarium against the lungs. Other cellular actors include alveolar[283] and pulmonary intravascular[286] macrophages, circulating eosinophils,[287–290] and other leukocytes, each of which also can act both to protect and to destroy. The main humoral mediators of the inflammatory response are listed in Table 54.5. Normally, the pulmonary circulation contains a very large pool of marginated PMNs,[291, 292] and, of course, the circulating inflammatory cells pass through

**Table 54.6 EXPANDED DEFINITION OF ACUTE LUNG INJURY**

| |
|---|
| Phase (acute or chronic) |
| Lung injury score (see Table 54.7) |
| Etiology (underlying cause or association; see Table 54.4) |
| Nonpulmonary organ dysfunction |

vascular pressures, and other measurements must be before this syndrome can be diagnosed.[343] This is a serious problem that makes evaluation of the burgeoning acute lung injury literature difficult, if not impossible, and that hampers progress in understanding the incidence, risk, mechanism, clinical course, appropriate supportive and specific therapy, and prognosis of the many disorders amalgamated into ARDS.[344] Two definitions have gained some acceptance: the expanded definition of acute lung injury[345] (often only its component "lung injury score" is cited, which is sometimes called the "Murray score") and the American-European Consensus Conference definition.[346] Both of these definitions should be used whenever lung injury is diagnosed.

The expanded definition of acute lung injury has four elements (Table 54.6). The first element establishes the time at which the diagnosis is made and separates the group of patients suffering from the immediate consequences of acute lung injury from those who have progressed to more indolent, chronic disease. This is an important distinction because the causes of morbidity and mortality, appropriate supportive and specific therapy, and prognosis differ between the two phases. The second element is the actual Lung Injury Score (Table 54.7), which provides an assessment of the severity of lung injury, taking into account supportive therapy, such as mechanical ventilation with PEEP and oxygen supplementation. This score is important because not all lung injuries are of equal severity and severity changes over time. The term *acute respiratory distress syndrome* is applied only to the most severe injuries (those that yield a score of >2.5); milder lung injuries, termed mild to moderate, may have a better prognosis and may differ from ARDS in other important aspects. Pulmonary artery catheterization is not required for the diagnosis of acute

**Table 54.7 COMPONENTS AND INDIVIDUAL VALUES OF THE LUNG INJURY SCORE**

| | Value |
|---|---|
| 1. Chest roentgenogram score | |
| No alveolar consolidation | 0 |
| Alveolar consolidation confined to 1 quadrant | 1 |
| Alveolar consolidation confined to 2 quadrants | 2 |
| Alveolar consolidation confined to 3 quadrants | 3 |
| Alveolar consolidation in all 4 quadrants | 4 |
| 2. Hypoxemia score | |
| $Pa_{O_2}/FI_{O_2} \geq 300$ | 0 |
| $Pa_{O_2}/FI_{O_2}$ 225–299 | 1 |
| $Pa_{O_2}/FI_{O_2}$ 175–224 | 2 |
| $Pa_{O_2}/FI_{O_2}$ 100–174 | 3 |
| $Pa_{O_2}/FI_{O_2} < 100$ | 4 |
| 3. PEEP score (when ventilated) | |
| PEEP ≤5 cm $H_2O$ | 0 |
| PEEP 6–8 cm $H_2O$ | 1 |
| PEEP 9–11 cm $H_2O$ | 2 |
| PEEP 12–14 cm $H_2O$ | 3 |
| PEEP ≥15 cm $H_2O$ | 4 |
| 4. Respiratory system compliance score (when available) | |
| Compliance ≥80 mL/cm $H_2O$ | 0 |
| Compliance 60–79 mL/cm $H_2O$ | 1 |
| Compliance 40–59 mL/cm $H_2O$ | 2 |
| Compliance 20–39 mL/cm $H_2O$ | 3 |
| Compliance ≤19 mL/cm $H_2O$ | 4 |

The final value is obtained by dividing the aggregate sum by the number of components that were used

| | Score |
|---|---|
| No lung injury | 0 |
| Mild-to-moderate lung injury | 0.1–2.5 |
| Severe lung injury (ARDS) | >2.5 |

$Pa_{O_2}/FI_{O_2}$ = arterial oxygen tension to inspired oxygen concentration ratio; PEEP = positive end-expiratory pressure.

From Murray JF, Matthay MA, Luce JM, et al: An expanded definition of the adult respiratory distress syndrome. Am Rev Respir Dis 138:720–723, 1988.

lung injury and is used only as needed to aid in clinical management. The third element, etiology, separates out the many underlying disorders that can result in acute lung injury (see Table 54.4, which is not meant to be an exhaustive or exclusive list). Multiple etiologies may be present, which should be noted if that is the case. This element is important because the many disorders may differ in important particulars, such as suitable markers for early diagnosis, specific therapy, and prognosis. There are significant unresolved problems about diagnostic criteria for some of the underlying disorders, particularly sepsis and the sepsis syndrome. Because sepsis and the sepsis syndrome are the cause of many acute lung injuries and large-scale clinical trials are often based on or incorporate many patients suffering from them, uniform definitions would help with communication and understanding. However, defining these conditions is beyond the scope of this chapter. Standardized sepsis terminology has been proposed[347] and used, somewhat modified, in large clinical sepsis studies.[348] Finally, the fourth element, which was not parsed out when the expanded definition of acute lung injury was first proposed, recognizes the occurrence of injury of organs other than the lungs. This is important because injury is often not limited to the lungs. Dysfunction of other organs is common,[349, 350] and prognosis varies between isolated pulmonary and generalized systemic disorders.

The Glasgow Coma Scale is widely used to assess neurologic status. Criteria have been proposed to evaluate abnormalities in renal, cardiovascular, hepatic, gastrointestinal, and hematologic function, all of which can complicate or coexist with acute lung injury.[351] The APACHE II scoring system has been used to define the patient's overall severity of injury.[352, 353] Another stratification system of acute lung injury ("GOCA") has been proposed,[354] but it appears to add nothing to the expanded definition.

The American-European Consensus Conference Definition (Table 54.8) also has four elements: (1) timing (onset must be "acute"); (2) oxygenation (arterial $Po_2/FI_{O_2} \leq 300$ mm Hg, regardless of PEEP level, for the diagnosis of acute lung injury to be made, and arterial $Po_2/FI_{O_2} \leq 200$ mm Hg, regardless of PEEP level, for the diagnosis of ARDS to be made); (3) chest radiograph (bilateral infiltrates seen on frontal view); and (4) pulmonary artery wedge pressure ($\leq$18 mm Hg when measured or no clinical evidence of left atrial hypertension).

**Table 54.8** AMERICAN-EUROPEAN CONSENSUS CONFERENCE DEFINITION OF ACUTE LUNG INJURY AND ACUTE RESPIRATORY DISTRESS SYNDROME

| |
|---|
| Timing |
| Acute |
| Oxygenation (regardless of PEEP level) |
| $Pa_{O_2}/FI_{O_2} \leq 300$ mm Hg = acute lung injury |
| $Pa_{O_2}/FI_{O_2} \leq 200$ mm Hg = acute respiratory distress syndrome |
| Chest radiograph |
| Bilateral infiltrates on frontal view |
| Pulmonary artery wedge pressure |
| $\leq$18 mm Hg when measured, or |
| No clinical evidence of left atrial hypertension |

$Pa_{O_2}/FI_{O_2}$ = arterial oxygen tension to inspired oxygen concentration ratio; PEEP = positive end-expiratory pressure.

The two definitions differ in the exact (and arbitrary) criteria that must be met for a diagnosis to be established, but they identify similar patients[355] and are complimentary. The powers of the Consensus Conference definition are that it was reached by consensus and that it is easy to remember. The powers of the expanded definition are that it provides a grading system (the Lung Injury Score) whereby equally injured patients can be grouped and compared and the progress (or lack thereof) of any individual patient's course over time can be measured, that it recognizes the distinct phases of the progression of lung injuries (early vs. late disease), that it separates out the different underlying conditions that can become associated with acute lung injury (conditions in which the exact etiology and mechanism of acute lung injury may differ), and that it recognizes and requires identification of associated extrapulmonary disease (which has profound effects on mortality of patients with acute lung injuries).

All that being said, definition of acute lung injury and ARDS is not without its problems.[356] The most serious deficiency of both definitions is failure to link the underlying pathophysiology of acute lung injury to the functional abnormalities that are at the core of the definitions (i.e., data are lacking that link any particular arterial $Po_2/FI_{O_2}$ to any particular change in the structure or function of the relevant barriers in the lungs or to the degree of edema). What defines acute lung injury in a meaningful way is the altered barrier permeability of the lungs. What defines ARDS in a meaningful way (if anything can) is structural damage to the lung microvascular endothelial barrier or to the alveolar epithelial barrier or both. All other designations are arbitrary. Many respiratory disorders can reach the definitions' thresholds for "diagnosis," and many acute lung injuries, especially mild ones, fail to reach them at all. For example, bacterial pneumonia is not a different disease when it crosses some arbitrary threshold and meets criteria for acute lung injury or ARDS; venous-air-emboli–induced and heroin-induced pulmonary edemas are acute lung injuries, even if they fail to disturb oxygenation sufficiently to satisfy an arbitrary definition of acute lung injury or ARDS. In small numbers of patients, the Lung Injury Score has correlated with bedside measurements of lung vascular permeability[357–359] and with the extent of abnormalities on computed tomography.[360]

The Consensus Conference definition suffers from its own particular further problems. First, it requires that timing be acute, but it neither specifies the degree of acuity required nor accounts for the considerable heterogeneity in the course of patients with acute lung injuries, each progressing, or not progressing, at its own given pace, through exudative, proliferative, and recovery phases. Second, it requires an arbitrary pulmonary artery wedge pressure (or no clinical evidence of left atrial hypertension), but left atrial hypertension or the lack thereof is not part of the basic pathophysiology of acute lung injury. It is the pulmonary microvascular pressure that matters when the lungs are injured, and that pressure can be low, normal, or (often) elevated. The Consensus Conference definition is, however, simple to apply and has facilitated enrollment of patients in clinical trials.[150]

Both definitions have been faulted for failing to allow early diagnosis and for failing to accurately predict mortality.[361, 362] It is not necessary, however, that a definition should bear the burden of either task. Regarding early diagnosis, the interval between "at risk" and "diagnosis" for acute lung injuries is often painfully short, and patients who are appropriately "diagnosed" are never more than a small fraction of those who appear to be "at risk." No simple definition is ever going to solve the early detection problem (which is discussed in more detail later). Regarding mortality, the relevant question about any definition is not whether it can predict who will live and who will die, but rather can it correctly identify and quantify who has acute lung injury and who does not. Death is often not directly related to acute lung injury, but rather to nonpulmonary organ dysfunction, chronic liver disease, or sepsis.[362] The severity of oxygenation defect, which is what the definitions mainly measure, just does not have major prognostic value early in the course of clinical lung injury. Finally, putative assessment of the accuracy of definitions[355] is difficult because there is no "gold standard" against which the accuracy of any given definition can be measured.

**Chest Roentgenograms.** The plain chest radiograph is the most practical laboratory study available for the detection of pulmonary edema.[1, 363–367] Disadvantages are that chest radiographs are insensitive to small changes in lung water and are only semiquantitative.[1, 363, 368] They are also not specific: alveolar filling disorders (e.g., infections, alveolar proteinosis, Goodpasture's syndrome, bronchoalveolar carcinoma) and many parenchymal diseases (e.g., infections, extrinsic allergic alveolitis, immunologic disorders, hemosiderosis, inhalational pneumoconioses, chronic obstructive pulmonary disease) can produce the same patterns of radiographic density as edema. Conversely, edema can produce the same patterns of radiographic density as parenchymal diseases (e.g., lobar pneumonia, metastases, and embolic disease).[369] An additional limitation is that chest radiographs are not helpful in distinguishing increased pressure edema from increased permeability edema.[370–372] These disadvantages are balanced by the advantages that chest radiographs are noninvasive, have a cost appropriate to the value of the information that can be obtained, and are easily repeatable, readily available, and free of side effects.

Before alveolar flooding, the plain chest radiograph can show distended vascular shadows (particularly in the upper lung fields), enlargement and loss of definition of hilar structures, development of septal lines (Kerley's lines), loss of peribronchial and perivascular definition (cuffing), and perihilar haze indicating the presence of interstitial pulmonary edema. Acinar shadows, often confluent and creating irregular, patchy increases in lung density that obscure vascular markings, indicate the presence of alveolar edema. Air bronchograms may be observed in severe edema. Because the radiographic signs of interstitial and alveolar edema are determined by gas and blood volumes and their distribution in the lungs in addition to the presence of edema, the recognition and quantification of edema are not precise, and the radiographic appearance of edema is strongly influenced by the lung volume at the time the film is made. The chest roentgenogram score is an integral part of the Lung Injury Score. In this context, considerable interobserver variation has been reported in recognition of alveolar consolidation by clinicians, and the assessment would be better made, whenever possible, by radiologists.[373]

Chest radiography is of very limited value for the diagnosis of pneumonia in mechanically ventilated patients. High false-positive and false-negative ratings for pneumonia result in low diagnostic accuracy.[374]

**Arterial Blood Studies.** Although not specific, the arterial $P_{O_2}$, $P_{CO_2}$, and pH are the most informative laboratory indicators of overall pulmonary function in edema. Arterial blood studies are not sensitive to early edema. Arterial $P_{O_2}$ may actually rise in the earliest stages of increased pressure edema because the increase in vascular pressures distributes blood flow more uniformly to well-ventilated units.[25] Interstitial pulmonary edema does not usually affect oxygen uptake in the lungs beyond modest hypoxemia caused by ventilation-perfusion mismatching. In contrast, alveolar flooding seriously compromises gas exchange. Hypoxemia is due to right-to-left shunting of blood from perfusion of alveoli that cannot be ventilated because they are fluid filled or collapsed. Ventilation-perfusion abnormalities also contribute to the hypoxemia of edema.[179] In dogs, residual blood flow to regions of injured lung was found to correlate better with decreases in oxygenation than with the amount of excess lung water.[375] In two studies of groups of patients with diverse lung injuries, oxygenation also appeared to depend more on the vasoconstrictive ability of the pulmonary circulation (i.e., the ability to reduce perfusion of damaged and edematous areas of the lungs) than on the amount of edema present.[376, 377] However, this finding was not confirmed in another series of patients.[378] Because the technique used in these studies to measure edema (single pass multiple tracer) is highly dependent on perfusion, which affects the surface area available for indicator exchange,[379] edema in poorly perfused areas of the lungs was probably grossly underestimated.

Arterial $P_{CO_2}$ is often low in edema, especially in the early stages, when tachypnea results in alveolar hyperventilation. An elevated $P_{CO_2}$ (more common with severe edema) indicates alveolar hypoventilation, which can be caused by underlying lung disease, increased metabolic production of carbon dioxide (perhaps related to increased work of breathing), increased wasted ventilation (ventilation of poorly perfused alveoli or airways leading to flooded, nonventilatable alveoli), or mechanical impairment caused by weak or tired respiratory muscles struggling to ventilate stiff lungs.[380] Elevated $P_{CO_2}$ does not necessarily indicate a poor prognosis[381] and often resolves with treatment of pulmonary edema.

Acid-base disturbances are common in increased pressure edema but often do not correlate with severity, morbidity, or mortality.[382] When edema is mild, tachypnea results in hyperventilation and consequent respiratory alkalosis (and subsequent compensating metabolic acidosis). When edema is severe or the lungs have been injured, many patients develop metabolic acidosis as a result of tissue hypoxia, increased work of breathing, intrinsic lung lactate production, or all of these.[381, 383–385] Attempts to correct acidosis with parenteral bicarbonate administration are often futile and unnecessary; rather, the underlying cause must be identified and treated appropriately. Respiratory acidosis caused by alveolar hypoventilation is corrected by mechanical ventilation. Metabolic acidosis can often be corrected by alleviating hypoxemia and improving cardiac function; the possibility of underlying disease amenable to surgery (e.g., intestinal ischemia or infarction, perforation of a viscus) or pancreatitis should not be overlooked. Persistent metabolic acidosis on the first day of ARDS is a particularly poor prognostic sign.[386] Refractory acidosis of either type is usually an ominous sign of impending death. Management of life-threatening acid-base disorders was the subject of a comprehensive review.[387]

**Edema Fluid Protein Concentration Measurement.** When florid pulmonary edema is present, measurement of protein concentration in simultaneously collected edema fluid (suctioned through an endotracheal tube or bronchoscope) and plasma provides a rapid, noninvasive method for distinguishing increased pressure edema from increased permeability edema.[199, 388] Because the microvascular barrier is functionally intact in increased pressure edema, plasma proteins remain largely confined to the intravascular space, and edema fluid protein concentration is low relative to plasma protein concentration (the ratio of edema fluid to plasma protein concentration is generally $<0.6$). Because the microvascular barrier is injured and cannot effectively confine plasma proteins to the vascular space in increased permeability edema, edema fluid protein concentration is high relative to plasma protein concentration (ratio of edema fluid to plasma protein concentration is generally $>0.7$). Intermediate values (between 0.6 and 0.7) may indicate that both types of edema are present and suggest the relative contributions of each. Ratios of edema fluid to plasma colloid osmotic pressure give similar information. Measurement of the ratio of edema fluid to plasma protein concentration has been shown to be a simple method for separating the types of pulmonary edema in numerous reported series of patients with pulmonary edema.[90, 199, 229, 389–393] Two studies indicated that an increasing protein concentration in serial measurements of edema fluid in acute lung injuries was a good sign, reflecting an intact epithelial barrier and removal of fluid from the alveoli.[394, 394a] Such measurements would have to be correlated with the patient's clinical condition because an increasing protein concentration in edema fluid over time might also mean that increased permeability edema was complicating what had been increased pressure edema or that the lungs were injured more severely or more extensively as time passed.

Edema fluid can be collected by inserting a standard 14- to 18-gauge catheter through an endotracheal tube and advancing it into a wedged position in the distal air spaces (similar to the procedure for wedging a bronchoscope). Gentle suction is applied as the catheter is slowly withdrawn, and fluid is collected in a small trap. Several attempts may be needed; if no fluid can be suctioned, the clinician should try changing the patient's position. Samples grossly contaminated with airway secretions (which have a very low protein concentration, $<1.0$ g/dL), such as mucus, pus, and debris, should be discarded. Protein concentrations can be measured by the clinical laboratory or estimated quickly at the bedside from the protein scale of a hand-held refractometer. Refractometric readings must be made from the serum-protein scale because the specific-gravity scale (total dissolved solids), calibrated for urine, gives falsely high readings.[395]

Bronchoalveolar lavage is being investigated as a research and diagnostic tool that may also yield useful information about the cellular and biochemical composition of the air space,[388, 396–398] but lavage is not useful as a method to measure alveolar protein concentration, because the instilled saline dilutes alveolar fluid by an uncertain amount.[388] Attempts to quantitate alveolar fluid by measuring the dilution of various markers added to the instilled fluid during lavage lack precision and have not been found to be useful.[399]

**Pulmonary Function Tests.** With the exception of arterial blood analyses, by the time results of conventional tests of pulmonary function are abnormal in patients with pulmonary edema, the diagnosis is usually obvious or the patient is too sick to study. The general sequence of developing abnormalities as edema accumulates was discussed in the sections on pathophysiology of increased pressure edema and increased permeability edema. The earliest abnormality detectable by conventional studies in increased pressure edema is a rise in $D_{LCO}$ caused by an increase in pulmonary capillary blood volume as a result of pulmonary vascular congestion. Closing volume may be greater when interstitial edema is present, but consistent changes in routine pulmonary function tests are generally not found until the alveoli flood and vital capacity begins to diminish. Because pulmonary function tests are neither sensitive nor specific in edema, provide no information for separating the two types of edema, and are difficult to perform in patients who are ill, such tests are not of much use in the diagnosis of pulmonary edema. However, development of techniques to measure pulmonary function successfully in the intensive care unit has made lung mechanics useful to some clinicians in patient management.[400]

**Hemodynamic Measurements.** Pulmonary vascular pressures are sometimes recommended as helpful for differentiating increased pressure edema from increased permeability edema. However, the fundamental difference between the two types of edema is in the integrity of microvascular and alveolar barrier function, not in the vascular pressures in the lungs. Increased pressure edema can occur at normal or low pulmonary vascular pressures (e.g., when osmotic pressure is very low or alveolar surface pressure is very high or when patients have edema caused by salt water near drowning or upper airway obstruction), and it can fail to occur when pulmonary vascular pressures are high (e.g., when patients suffer from chronic congestive heart failure or long-standing mitral stenosis). Increased permeability edema can occur at normal or high pulmonary vascular pressures (e.g., when a patient with an acute lung injury is severely volume overloaded or when the distribution of resistance has shifted to the venous side of the pulmonary circulation, as in sepsis). Measurement of vascular pressures in the lungs is expensive, is invasive, and can be associated with significant morbidity and mortality.[401–404] The problems with measuring and interpreting pulmonary artery occlusion pressures have been reviewed.[403, 405–409] Whether the use of such catheters may be helpful in the management of patients with pulmonary edema is discussed later.

## Measurement of Lung Water

Quantification of the amount of water in the lungs could be of interest both to detect early pulmonary edema and to assess its clinical course and response to treatment. However, no ideal technique is available. Methods in use or under investigation focus on either measurement of lung density or equilibration of tracers with water in the lungs.[1, 363, 364] The advantages and disadvantages of the clinical techniques and uses of lung water measurements have been succinctly summarized[364] and reviewed.[410] Interest in such measurements assumes that accurate knowledge about lung water would be useful in diagnosis and would be beneficial in the treatment of patients with pulmonary edema. Evidence supporting this assumption is meager, and quantification of lung water remains largely a topic of interest for research rather than a clinical tool.

### Lung Density Methods

Because lung density is determined by air and blood as well as extravascular tissue and water contents, densitometric techniques are only semiquantitative, and baseline lung densities vary widely. These techniques are most useful when a series of studies can be compared in order to estimate changes in lung water content. They are of little use in early edema because lung fluid filtration can increase greatly before lung water content actually increases. The most widely used method is the plain chest roentgenogram (discussed earlier): it is readily available, is relatively inexpensive, is noninvasive, and can be repeated frequently at little risk to the patient. Unfortunately, it is insensitive (lung water must increase by ≥30% before being recognized) and nonspecific (other interstitial or alveolar processes produce similar radiographic shadows). More precise density measurements may be made with techniques such as transmission computed tomography,[365, 411, 412] but the problem of separating changes in gas and blood volumes from changes in water content remains. Similar information may be gathered from transthoracic gamma-ray attenuation[413] or Compton scattering.[414] It might be possible to relate changes in sound speed across the lungs to lung water content,[415] but such measurements would also depend on lung volume. A theoretically related technique, transthoracic bioelectric impedance analysis, attempts to relate the resistance to an alternating electrical current passed through the thorax to the amount of water in the lungs.[416] A novel, and conceptually unrelated, technique for the early detection of edema based on alteration of the characteristics of intrinsic lung sounds has been reported[417]; evaluation of its sensitivity and specificity await further research.

Nuclear magnetic resonance imaging[410, 418, 419] and positron emission tomography[410, 420, 421] techniques for measuring lung water are also under investigation. Their theoretical advantages are the noninvasive measurement of density without ionizing radiation (in the case of nuclear magnetic resonance imaging) and lack of effects of ventilation and perfusion abnormalities; their disadvantages are that the hardware for both techniques is expensive and not readily available, and the slow scanning time and cumbersome equipment are not suitable for studying seriously ill patients.

### Tracer Methods

Attempts have been made to quantitate lung water by measuring either the rates of equilibration of a diffusible indicator and an intravascular indicator (multiple-indicator dilution technique) or the uptake of inhaled gases (soluble-gas technique).[1, 364, 410] Both methods have been the subject of considerable investigation, but neither method is in clinical use. These methods suffer from problems of tracer distribution inhomogeneity and the complexity of the equipment needed to make measurements.

**Multiple-Indicator Dilution Techniques.** These are invasive techniques based on measuring differences in transit-time volumes between two indicators, one nondiffusible (restricted to the intravascular space) and one diffusible (able to enter the extravascular space).[422] Suitable tracers are injected into a systemic vein or the right side of the heart, and time-concentration curves are recorded from a systemic artery. Because the diffusible tracer can in theory equilibrate with a much larger volume (extravascular and intravascular volumes) than the nondiffusible tracer (intravascular volume only), the differences in concentrations of the two tracers over time after traveling through the lungs can be used to calculate both blood flow and extravascular mass (mainly water) of the lungs.

Such techniques are limited by several factors: time, which may not allow the diffusible tracer to reach areas of the lungs remote from the microvascular bed; blood flow inhomogeneities, which restrict the tracers to perfused portions of the vascular bed; inhomogeneity of water distribution in the lungs; recirculation of indicator; measurement of mass (e.g., dry lung, blood vessels, heart) in addition to water mass; and a host of technical details concerning the appropriateness of the indicators and the methods of their injection, withdrawal, and measurement, and calculation of concentration over time. The major problems are underestimation of lung water in pulmonary edemas in which uneven distribution of blood flow develops (i.e., in most lung injuries) and insensitivity (a 50% increase in measured lung water may be significant, but edema is obvious by that time).

Two methods have been the subject of considerable research, the thermal dye method[423] and the multiple-isotope method.[424] The thermal dye method has come closest to clinical use, and a refinement of the method (using a fluorescent indicator) allows measurements to be made with an indwelling catheter without blood withdrawal.[425] The major problems are underestimation of lung water, particularly when vascular perfusion inequalities exist in the lungs or large volumes of edema are present, and accuracy of measurement of thermal changes.[426, 427] Prospective evaluations of extravascular lung water measurements by the thermal dye method versus pulmonary artery wedge pressures to guide the hemodynamic management of critically ill patients claimed superiority of the lung-water technique[428, 429]; benefit appears to have accrued as a result of restrained fluid therapy. The multiple-isotope method requires blood withdrawal for tracer measurement and, like the thermal dye method, underestimates water content if there is perfusion inhomogeneity.[430] This latter method appears to provide a better estimation of lung permeability–surface area product than of lung water content.[379]

A new system using heat as the diffusible indicator and sodium and chloride ions as the nondiffusible indicators has been tested in anesthetized sheep.[431] Blood did not have to be withdrawn for measurements to be made. Extravascular lung mass was overestimated in normal lungs and was underestimated in edematous lungs, and small quantities of liquid instilled into the lungs via the airways were not detected. Poor perfusion in edematous areas was a problem, just as with the thermal dye method. Another noninvasive approach, tested in isolated canine lungs, perfused goat lungs, and anesthetized sheep, used heat as the diffusible indicator and air as the nondiffusible indicator.[432] Heat loss was measured during hyperventilation. Temperature difference between the initial and final states was proportional to pulmonary blood flow, and the rate at which the new steady state was achieved was proportional to airway thermal volume, which was found to be close to the total mass of the lungs, including its blood mass. Pulmonary edema and fluid instilled into the airways increased the measured lung mass. The technique was less accurate in severe edema, probably because airways became obstructed, but it might be useful for detection of early edema.

Although indicator-dilution techniques have yet to produce a clinically useful method to measure lung water, considerable ingenuity has been demonstrated in choosing indicators, and lack of progress cannot be attributed to lack of persistence.

**Soluble-Gas Technique.** This technique is based on the fact that when inhaled, a soluble gas dissolves in pulmonary tissue.[433] Measurement of the difference in concentrations of a soluble and an insoluble gas during rebreathing allows the calculation of lung tissue mass; because most of lung tissue is water, measurement of lung tissue mass should reflect lung water content. The technique is quite complex, but measurements have been made in normal subjects and patients with pulmonary edema,[434] and a model has been proposed to improve lung water estimates.[435] There are many technical difficulties in the application of this method,[364] including wide normal variability, selection of suitable gases, measurement of gas solubility coefficients in normal and edematous lung tissue, methods of performance and analysis (e.g., variations in lung volume and extrapolation of disappearance curves to zero time before the soluble gases dissolve in the blood), ventilation-perfusion inhomogeneities in the lungs, and the expensive, temperamental equipment and elaborate computer support necessary to make the measurements and do the calculations.

## Measurement of Barrier Function

Because transvascular fluid flow into the lungs can be abnormal long before lung water content increases, and because the two types of edema can be separated on the basis of differences in barrier function, detection of increased transvascular fluid flow into the lungs and measurement of barrier integrity might be more helpful than measurement of lung water content in edema. The topic has been reviewed.[410] Clinical distinction between increased pressure edema and increased permeability edema is difficult.[436] A simple and practical method exists to evaluate barrier integrity (edema fluid protein concentration measurements, discussed earlier), and many methods are under investigation to detect early edema and changes in barrier function. However, none is in routine clinical use. Two techniques that have been the subject of investigation are measurement of solute movement into the lungs and measurement of solute disappearance from the air spaces.

### Measurement of Solute Movement Into the Lungs

Microvascular barrier function in the lungs can be measured by noninvasive, external radioflux detection.[357, 359, 364, 410, 437–440] Radioisotope-tagged markers are injected intravenously, and either a collimated scintillation detection probe positioned over the chest wall or a gamma camera is used to detect radioactivity in a portion of the lungs or the entire thorax. With the choice of suitable tracers, intravascular volumes from a restricted marker and transvascular accumulation of a diffusible marker relative to the vascular volume under the detector in the regions of interest can be measured. Choice of a labeled protein (e.g., transferrin and albumin) as the diffusible marker allows measurement of its accumulation in the lungs (a result of transvascular protein flux). Measurement of protein flux may allow separation of the types of edema and should permit detection of abnormal lung solute transport before lung water content has increased. Because measurements are often made over a small portion and then extrapolated to whole lung, their relevance depends on the homogeneity of transvascular protein flow into the lungs. Consistent serial measurements with an external probe require placing the probe over the same area of the lung. Limiting features of the technique, as now applied, are the time required to make the measurements (20 to 180 minutes), the need to serially withdraw small amounts of venous blood, the cumulative radiation dose if serial studies are performed, the normal and methodologic variability of measurements, and the rather complex apparatus and data analysis required. The technique was found to be specific and sensitive in dogs.[438] In a small series of patients with established ARDS, the technique was found to be specific but not particularly sensitive[441]; another study compared small groups of patients with the two different types of pulmonary edema.[442] Subsequent studies used the technique to show increased vascular permeability in the re-expanded lungs of a small group of patients,[111] to differentiate sepsis-related lung injury from congestive heart failure and normal controls,[443] and to identify patients at high risk for developing ARDS.[359] Measurements have not been reported from large series of patients with pulmonary edema. It is not known how practical this technique may be in separating increased pressure edema from increased permeability edema. Protein flow into the lungs is increased in both types of edema, and transvascular protein-flux measurements may be most useful if ranges were described and related to driving pressures. This is a promising noninvasive technique that should be tested more widely.

Barrier function in the lungs has also been assessed by measuring the clearance of radioisotopes from blood into suctioned bronchoalveolar secretions.[238, 444] This technique is an elaboration of edema fluid protein concentration measurements (discussed previously). Suitable tracers (e.g., radiolabeled albumin and diethylenetriamine pentaacetic acid [DPTA]) are injected intravenously and their concentrations measured hourly for 4 to 6 hours in venous blood and in bronchial aspirates obtained by inserting long suction catheters through an endotracheal tube deep into the bronchial tree. Clearance of tracers into bronchial aspirate was found to be significantly higher in increased permeability edema than in increased pressure edema; the ratio of small (DPTA) to large (albumin) solute clearance was particularly sensitive for separating the types of edema (relative clearances were close to equal when barrier function was abnormal in increased permeability edema; small solute clearance was much greater than large solute clearance when barrier function was normal in increased pressure edema). The advantage of this technique over simple edema fluid protein concentration measurements was said to be that this technique avoids the protein-rich airway secretions added to edema fluid through the use of injected tracers that gain access to airway fluid only at the alveolar-capillary barrier. This is unlikely; if airway secretions are protein rich, they are also tracer rich. The real advantage is that barrier function can be assessed over a defined period, and the measurements are not a reflection of integrated barrier history. No study has compared this tracer clearance technique to simple edema fluid protein concentration measurements. Disadvantages of the technique include the following: the function of both microvascular and alveolar barriers must be abnormal; the patient must have an endotracheal tube and enough edema fluid to suction; some of the aspirate may be airway secretion and not alveolar edema; inhomogeneity of edema (or airway) fluid distribution might lead to significant sampling errors; and cumulative radiation dose might be a problem if serial measurements were made to follow disease progress. As with other techniques, measurements would be most useful if ranges were described and related to driving pressures. Because considerable edema fluid must be present, this technique is not useful for early detection of altered alveolar-capillary barrier integrity.

### Measurement of Solute Disappearance from the Air Spaces

Another approach to assessing barrier integrity involves measurement of the rate of disappearance of a radiolabeled solute after deposition within the lungs by aerosolization. The technique and experience with it in humans and experimental animals were subjects of a comprehensive review.[445] Development of methods to measure epithelial barrier permeability with tracer molecules introduced into the airways has also been discussed.[446] The basic method is to introduce a stable, chemically inert, electrically neutral, hydrophilic tracer molecule (generally $^{99m}$Tc-DPTA) into the lungs (by aerosolization in humans) and measure its disappearance from the air spaces with an external scintillation detector.[439] A slightly different method, involving the uptake of mannitol from the lungs into venous blood after intratracheal bolus administration, has also been reported.[447] The technique is noninvasive, requires a brief and modest radiation exposure, is relatively simple to perform with equipment found in most hospitals, and appears to be sensitive to changes in barrier permeability.[448] However, aerosolized tracer clearance is not highly specific: clearance is increased in otherwise healthy persons who smoke cigarettes[441, 445, 449] or cocaine[450] and in patients with chronic lung diseases (e.g., pneumoconioses, pulmonary fibroses, granulomatous diseases)[445] as well as in patients with increased pressure edema, increased permeability edema, and acute lung injuries.[451] Clearance was also markedly increased by PEEP[452–454]; this would make measurements difficult to interpret in very sick patients who require aggressive mechanical ventilatory support. Another problem was that clearance remained abnormally rapid despite improvements in chest radiographic appearance and in gas exchange.[455] This technique is safe and simple, but many problems would have to be solved before measurements could be clinically useful.

## Detection of Lung Injury

Because lung injury occurs before measurements of barrier integrity or transvascular fluid flow are abnormal, methods to detect lung injury before the appearance of abnormal liquid and solute transport might be of help. Early detection of lung injury would be especially valuable if therapies were developed on the basis of the mechanisms of lung injuries. Although tests to determine the causes of lung injuries are not available, methods are being investigated that attempt to detect whether lungs have been injured. Promising techniques include measurement of changes in metabolic functions of the lungs and detection of putative markers of lung injury.

### Changes in Metabolic Functions of the Lung

The lungs are involved in the metabolism of a variety of biologically active substances. Because the removal and metabolism of such substances depend on endothelial cell function, alterations in metabolic function in the lungs might be sensitive early tests of endothelial cell injury.[191] Abnormal levels, activities, or uptakes of various substances (e.g., ACE, vasoactive amines, metabolites of arachidonic acid, endothelin-1, drugs) have been detected when the lungs are injured. Unfortunately, the finding of normal or abnormal uptake by the lungs is neither specific nor sensitive for all acute lung injuries; metabolic functions can be influenced by drugs, cardiac output, vascular surface area, and hypoxia or hyperoxia, and serious lung injury can occur without changes in metabolic function. Although alterations in metabolic functions of the lungs are not clinically useful indicators of endothelial cell function at this time, their potential use for early detection of lung injury justifies continuing investigation.

## Markers of Lung Injury

Potential markers of acute lung injury were the subject of two comprehensive reviews.[388, 456] There is considerable interest in finding a simple blood, urine, bronchoalveolar lavage, or other test that could provide insight into the pathogenesis of acute lung injuries, that could identify patients who would go on to develop acute lung injury or patients who were in the earliest stages of acute lung injury, or that could predict the outcome of patients with injured lungs. To be of clinical use, such a marker would have to be practical and inexpensive to measure as well as sensitive and specific for acute lung injury; with the exception of measurements of edema fluid protein concentration relative to plasma protein concentration (discussed earlier), none is available. There may be many reasons for the lack of progress in identifying suitable markers: many (if not most) patients cannot be enrolled into studies of early or predictive markers because they already have injured lungs when they present or injury occurs very soon after the causative insult; ARDS is not a disease, but rather symptoms that may result from multiple different causes; injury to the lungs is often overwhelming, and subtle differences in potential markers may be missed; measurements of potential markers in biologic fluids may not reflect what is happening at the tissue and cellular levels; and there is little or no uniformity among studies in diagnostic criteria and design (e.g., suitable controls, such as patients with increased pressure pulmonary edema and severe lung disease other than acute lung injury are often not studied; measurements of putative markers are often made at a single time, rather than regularly over the course of acute lung injury). The result is that it might never be possible to find a suitable marker or that potentially useful markers already may have been mistakenly regarded as useless.

Products of complement activation were proposed as markers but were later shown to be poorly correlated with lung injury[457–459] (although there is renewed interest in taking another look at C3a[460]). Measurement of circulating endotoxin was not appropriately sensitive or specific for the presence or the risk of developing lung injury.[265] Release or activity of ACE has not been found to be sensitive or specific for acute lung injuries.[461–463] Factor VIII–related antigen appeared to have potential as a plasma marker of impending acute lung injury in septic patients, but early encouraging results could not be generalized to a large group of patients with acute lung injuries, and abnormal levels can be found in many diseases that do not pose risk for acute lung injury.[464] Examples of other possible markers that have been proposed are fibrin- or fibrinogen-related D-antigen,[465] fibronectin,[466] a lung injury–related serine protease,[467] antioxidants (catalase, manganese superoxide dismutase, glutathione),[468–470] and biochemical and physical changes in surfactant.[171, 174, 471–473]

Because PMNs are implicated in the mechanism of many lung injuries, detection of their presence in the lungs, tests of their function, or measurement of their toxic metabolites might be useful. For example, increased hydrogen peroxide has been measured in the breath and urine of patients with acute lung injuries,[474–477] presumably reflecting the presence of oxygen metabolites in their injured lungs. Evidence of oxidant activity was also reported in bronchoalveolar lavage fluid.[478] Other mediators of inflammation might be appropriately considered as well. For example, TNF has been detected in blood[479–481] and bronchoalveolar lavage fluid[481–484] (but an association between TNF and the development of ARDS was not found,[485] and TNF was found to be elevated in patients with severe congestive heart failure[486]); various lipoxygenase products of arachidonic acid metabolism have been detected in pulmonary edema fluid,[487] bronchoalveolar lavage fluid,[488, 489] plasma,[489] and urine[490, 491]; and elastase has been detected in bronchoalveolar lavage fluid.[484, 492–495] It might also be possible to use magnetic resonance imaging to detect abnormal metabolites in the plasma of patients with acute lung injury.[496] The presence of a generalized increase in vascular permeability in the setting of acute lung injury might be detected by increased urinary albumin excretion rate.[497]

In addition to these possible markers, sporadic reports of abnormal substances or abnormal levels of normally occurring substances detected in fluids obtained from small groups of patients with acute lung injury are continually being reported. Usually, there is considerable overlap between levels in patients who have acute lung injuries and those who do not. Because there was no consensus about diagnostic criteria between studies, the results are mainly of interest to show the wide variety of abnormalities that can be detected when the lungs are injured and to suggest the complexity of the underlying pathophysiology. Various abnormalities can be found in increased pressure edema as well as in increased permeability edema: for example, blood TNF can be elevated[486]; platelet-activating factor and PMNs can be elevated in bronchoalveolar lavage fluid[498]; and interleukin-2 receptor and soluble CD8 antigen can be found in blood.[499]

Because acute lung injuries follow a wide variety of insults and range in severity, and because many abnormalities detected in acute lung injury are found in other severe illnesses of diverse etiology that do not involve the lungs, it seems unlikely that any single marker will be found that unequivocally identifies the risk or the presence of acute lung injury. Focus on particular subgroups of patients with common causes of injury and study of much larger groups of better diagnosed patients would be helpful. An approach that has not received much attention is investigation of the sensitivity and specificity of combinations of markers.

## TREATMENT

Treatment of pulmonary edema requires adequate life support followed by specific therapy directed at the factors that led to accumulation of water in the extravascular spaces of the lungs. Rational therapy also requires a correct diagnosis and an understanding of the nature of the underlying disease state and of the strategies that might prove useful in limiting further edema accumulation and favor fluid removal from the lungs.[500]

### Immediate Therapy

Patients with alveolar edema are often severely ill and require immediate treatment for acute respiratory failure. The basic principles of treatment of respiratory failure are discussed in Chapters 91 to 94. Essential requirements for patients with pulmonary edema include preservation of the airway, provision of adequate ventilation, and maintenance of satisfactory oxygenation. Increasingly sophisticated methods for the noninvasive measurement of blood gases have made their continuous monitoring possible, which can be useful in assessing the adequacy of ventilatory support and the effects of therapy. Blood pressure and other forms of circulatory support may also be needed. A large-bore intravenous line should be placed.

If the patient is not hypotensive, morphine sulfate, 5 to 10 mg, should be given intravenously slowly over several minutes (rapid injection can cause pulmonary vasoconstriction via histamine release from the lungs[501]). Morphine is an extremely useful drug in the treatment of pulmonary edema because it is a potent vasodilator, a central nervous system sedative, and a mild inotropic agent. Its vasodilating effects can substantially reduce pulmonary capillary pressure and may improve depressed cardiac output. The work of the heart is lessened by the vasodilating, bradycardic, and sedative effects of this agent. Cautiously administered morphine usually does not cause respiratory failure or aggravate existing carbon dioxide retention associated with acute pulmonary edema, but the patient must be closely watched if he or she is not intubated and receiving assisted ventilation. Hypotension following morphine administration indicates that too much drug was given or the intravascular volume was not as great as suspected. Undesired results of morphine administration can be readily reversed with its antagonist, naloxone, and the patient's condition can then be reassessed.

If medical care is not immediately available, two treatments (often regarded as historical) for increased pressure pulmonary edema can be lifesaving. First, rotating tourniquets can act to reduce blood volume (and thereby pulmonary perfusion pressure) by trapping blood in the extremities, away from the pulmonary circulation. Tourniquets, or blood pressure cuffs inflated to less than systolic pressure, are applied to three of the four extremities and rotated every 15 minutes. The purpose is to decrease venous return, not to stop all blood flow to the extremities. Care must be taken that the tourniquets be rotated and that venous return from any extremity not be obstructed for more than 45 minutes at a time. A study of patients with left ventricular dysfunction following myocardial infarction showed trapping of considerable blood volume in the periphery by tourniquets, but variable and sometimes unfavorable effects on left ventricular function.[502] Second, phlebotomy[503] (100 to 500 mL) can be used to reduce blood volume in acute pulmonary edema when the patient is not in shock and if drugs and supportive care are not available.

When supportive care is available, positive airway pressure, supplied by a tight-fitting face mask[504, 505] or by mechanical ventilation after endotracheal intubation, performs the same function as rotating tourniquets without risking loss of limbs: high pressure in the thorax impedes venous return, trapping blood volume peripherally (which can have the same variable and sometimes unfavorable effects on left ventricular function as tourniquets). A conceptually related maneuver, temporary balloon occlusion of the inferior vena cava for immediate relief of pulmonary edema, has been reported.[506] Positive airway pressure, mechanical ventilation, or both can also help reverse some of the physiologic disturbances that can contribute to the development of pulmonary edema[507]: improved oxygenation can increase myocardial oxygen supply, mechanical ventilation can be of benefit to decrease the work of breathing and thus lower the work of the heart, and left ventricular afterload can be reduced when positive pleural pressure replaces the wide swings in negative pressure that occur with spontaneous ventilation (and might also prevent cyclic reopening and closing of alveoli[508]). However, too much positive pressure can have adverse effects, such as reducing cardiac output; overdistending ventilated alveoli and thereby compressing their blood vessels, thus shifting blood flow to poorly or nonventilated lung; increasing pulmonary vascular resistance by increasing pulmonary venous resistance, which would increase the hydrostatic pressure at the fluid exchange sites in the lungs; and possibly causing mechanical injury to the lungs.

### Major Options

After emergency treatment has been instituted, there are three major therapeutic options: vasodilators, diuretics, and inotropic agents. The goal of therapy with these agents is to lower the hydrostatic pressure at the filtration sites in the pulmonary vascular bed while maintaining adequate systemic delivery of oxygen. The choice of therapy is dictated by the patient's condition.

Perhaps the most controversial and contentious topic in therapy is the role of bedside right-sided heart catheterization. The pulmonary artery flotation catheter is not "therapy," of course, but it has come to be regarded as such by many clinicians. An attempt at a controlled clinical trial of the efficacy of right-sided heart catheterization had to be abandoned because physicians believed that insertion of a pulmonary artery catheter was ethically imperative and would not allow their patients to be randomly assigned.[509] Data supporting such beliefs do not exist. The data that were collected in this abandoned trial showed statistically significant differences in favor of patients not receiving bedside heart catheterization.

Also, a prospective cohort study of critically ill patients showed that flotation heart catheterization was associated with increased 30-, 60-, and 180-day mortality.[404] Subgroup analysis did not reveal any patient group for which right-sided heart catheterization was associated with improved outcome, and patients with acute respiratory failure and multiple organ system failure were at greatest hazard to do worse when a pulmonary artery catheter was placed. This was an observational study, not a randomized clinical trial, and the reasons for lack of benefit from right-sided heart catheterization were not clear: the pulmonary artery catheter might directly worsen outcome, for example, if its risks and deleterious effects outweighed any benefits; benefits might not be realized if interpretations of hemodynamic measurements were incorrect (lack of skill and knowledge is a common problem in the interpretation of such measurements); the pulmonary artery catheter might be a marker for an aggressive style of care that increases mortality; or changes in therapy in response to hemodynamic information from pulmonary artery catheters might increase mortality. The cohort study appeared to rule out the possibility that right-sided heart catheterization was used in sicker patients, thus resulting in higher mortality (the patients with and without pulmonary artery catheters were matched for severity of illness). In addition to increased mortality, bedside heart catheterization was associated, not surprisingly, with increased costs and utilization of resources. As a result of this observational study, the National Heart, Lung, and Blood Institute is sponsoring several trials to assess the clinical usefulness of pulmonary artery catheterization in critically ill patients.

As already noted, measurement of vascular pressures in the lungs is expensive, invasive, and associated with significant morbidity and mortality[401–404]; the problems with measuring and interpreting pulmonary artery occlusion pressures have been reviewed.[403, 405–409] Well-designed, controlled, randomized clinical trials of right-sided heart catheterization in critically ill patients and in patients with acute lung injuries should provide a more rational basis for the use of flotation pulmonary artery catheters in patients with pulmonary edema.

The only relevant vascular pressure in any type of pulmonary edema is that at the fluid exchange sites in the lungs,[151, 510] and this microvascular pressure varies independently from pulmonary artery systolic and diastolic pressures and from pulmonary arterial occlusion pressure ("pulmonary capillary wedge pressure") in many experimental and clinical conditions. The distribution of vascular resistance is usually altered from normal in edema. Venous resistance is often increased. An example is sepsis, in which pulmonary artery occlusion pressure is usually normal or low, but microvascular pressure may be markedly increased. The relevant microvascular pressure in the lungs can be estimated clinically by analysis of pressure transients recorded immediately after pulmonary artery occlusion. The technique uses a ruler to find the point at which the pressure recording after balloon occlusion of the pulmonary artery catheter most obviously deviates from the rapid, immediate fall in pressure to the later, slower decrease down to the wedge pressure. This point corresponds closely to the pulmonary microvascular pressure. There are problems with subjectivity of measurements, artifacts in pressure waveforms, respiratory variations, regional differences measured in heterogeneous conditions (e.g., acute lung injuries), and measurements made in the presence of high PEEP (the pulmonary arterial pressure tracing may reflect alveolar pressure if the catheter tip is not in zone 3 conditions). The same problems, of course, plague measurements of pulmonary arterial occlusion pressures, which provide no relevant information about the hydrostatic pressure at the fluid exchange sites in the lungs.

### Vasodilators

Vasodilators are the most useful pharmacologic agents for treatment of acute increased pressure pulmonary edema. Their effects occur in minutes. Through dilation of veins, capacitance is increased and blood is redistributed peripherally, thereby lowering the driving pressure for fluid filtration in the lungs; through dilation of arteries, systemic vascular resistance (cardiac afterload) falls, cardiac output and stroke volume increase, and the heart works more efficiently.[511] In addition to morphine, three classes of vasodilators may be useful in pulmonary edema: venodilators (e.g., nitrates), arteriolar dilators (e.g., phentolamine, hydralazine), and mixed dilators (e.g., nitroprusside).

Sodium nitroprusside, a direct-acting venous and arteriolar dilator, is the most potent of the widely used agents in acute pulmonary edema. Its advantages are that the effects are immediate, its half-life is short, and cardiac output is maintained by arteriolar dilation and subsequent increased cardiac stroke volume even as central blood volume is lowered (thereby reducing pressure in the pulmonary vascular bed). Its main disadvantage is that invasive hemodynamic monitoring (i.e., an arterial cannula for continuous measurement of systemic blood pressure) is required because the dose must be carefully titrated to avoid profound hypotension. Prolonged infusions can result in cyanide or thiocyanate toxicity; the earliest sign is metabolic acidosis. Arterial oxygenation can deteriorate during therapy with any vasodilator if increased pulmonary blood flow and inhibition of hypoxia-mediated pulmonary vasoconstriction result in relatively increased perfusion of nonventilated, fluid-filled or collapsed lung.[512–515] Therapy with both nitroprusside and nitroglycerin can be complicated by methemoglobinemia, and all nitrates can precipitate increased intracranial or intraocular pressure.

Nitroprusside is started at 10 μg/min and increased by 5 to 10 μg every 3 to 5 minutes until the desired effect is achieved. Arterial pressure should not be allowed to fall below 60 mm Hg diastolic, and peak systolic pressure should be kept higher than 90 mm Hg. Most patients require 50 to 100 μg/min to achieve the desired effects.

Nitroglycerin and other nitrates are also direct-acting vasodilators, but their predominant effect is on the venous capacitance bed.[516] Intravenous nitroglycerin may be particularly useful in patients with increased pressure pulmonary edema associated with acute myocardial infarction or myocardial insufficiency.[511] Nitroglycerin consistently dilates intercoronary collateral vessels, thereby improving blood flow to ischemic or marginally perfused regions of myocardium. Nitroprusside infusion does not consistently have this effect and may actually result in a decrease in collateral blood flow to ischemic regions of the heart. Nitroglycerin may also be useful in patients with borderline hypotension; because its effects (at least at lower infusion rates) are predominantly venodilating, systemic arterial pressure can be preserved while increased venous capacitance leads to lower driving pressures for fluid filtration in the lungs. At higher doses, nitroglycerin also exerts arteriolar dilator effects similar to those of nitroprusside. The major disadvantage of intravenous nitroglycerin is that invasive hemodynamic monitoring is generally required. Ethanol intoxication may also be a complication of high doses of some preparations.[517]

Intravenous nitroglycerin infusion is started at 10 to 15 μg/min and increased 5 to 10 μg/min every 3 to 5 minutes until mean arterial pressure falls (usually by >20 mm Hg), the pulmonary vascular pressure is brought to the desired level (if it is being measured), headache becomes intolerable, or angina (if present) is relieved. Development of tachycardia during nitroglycerin infusion can indicate that cardiac filling pressures and cardiac output have fallen to low levels. Nitroprusside, which preserves cardiac output, might be a more appropriate therapeutic option under this circumstance.

Isosorbide dinitrate can also be given intravenously. In patients with severe pulmonary edema, the combination of high-dose isosorbide dinitrate plus low-dose furosemide was found to be more effective (50% fewer acute myocardial infarctions) than the combination of high-dose furosemide plus low-dose isosorbide dinitrate.[518] The onset of action of intravenous isosorbide dinitrate is rapid (peak vasodilation at 5 minutes), but the short half-life (about half an hour) requires frequent repeat dosing when it is given by bolus injection. Usually, 3 mg is injected intravenously every 5 minutes until oxygen saturation increases, arterial blood pressure falls more than 30%, or systolic pressure is less than 90 mm Hg. The effective cumulative dose is generally around 12 mg.

Other nitrates can also be useful, especially in increased pressure pulmonary edema, if the patient is not so critically ill that urgent intravenous therapy is required. Transdermal nitroglycerin ointment, 0.5 to 2 inches, or oral isosorbide dinitrate, 20 to 100 mg, are effective venodilators with prolonged duration of action (3 to 5 hours). The advantage of ointment is that it can be wiped off if necessary, but both agents have the disadvantage that effects cannot be as precisely controlled as in intravenous therapy. Tolerance to the effects of transdermal nitroglycerin can develop rapidly,[519] but can be restored after a nitrate-free interval (usually overnight).

Other vasodilators may be useful in the treatment of selected cases of acute increased pressure pulmonary edema but have not been widely used. ACE inhibitors,[520] such as captopril and enalapril, act both to reduce pulmonary vascular pressure and to increase cardiac output. The ACE inhibitors have proved to be useful agents in the treatment of more indolent pulmonary edema states.[521] Their use is not recommended, however, in the setting of acute myocardial infarction.[522] A placebo-controlled, randomized, double-blind clinical trial of intravenous enalaprilat (1 mg over 2 hours) in a small number of congestive heart failure patients with acute pulmonary edema showed reduced pulmonary capillary wedge pressure, increased renal blood flow, and slightly improved oxygenation with therapy.[523] Postsynaptic alpha-receptor blocking agents, such as prazosin and trimazosin, should have effects similar to those of ACE inhibitors, but experience in acute pulmonary edema is limited. Diazoxide may be useful in patients with advanced congestive heart failure that is unresponsive to other vasodilators.[524] Phentolamine, a parenteral arteriolar dilator, is expensive and has more serious side effects than nitroprusside and nitroglycerin. Hydralazine and minoxidil are also predominantly arteriolar dilators. Arteriolar dilators are not often used in pulmonary edema, probably because they have little or no beneficial effects on pulmonary pressures.

## Diuretics

Patients with symptoms of pulmonary edema may also benefit from administration of diuretic agents.[525] These drugs may exert a modest immediate effect by increasing venous capacitance and decreasing the relative perfusion of flooded alveoli (acting as vasodilators),[526, 527] but their principal mechanism of action is to increase sodium and water excretion by the kidneys. The resultant diuresis causes a decrease in left ventricular volume and pressure, and thereby a reduction in the pressure at the filtration sites in the lungs. The effects of therapy may be delayed for hours to days. The potent loop diuretic furosemide, 20 to 40 mg by slow intravenous injection, is the most useful agent in pulmonary edema. Furosemide is equally effective when administered by continuous infusion[525, 528]: a loading dose of 80 mg is followed by a continuous infusion at 10 to 20 mg/hr; if there is no response in an hour, the loading dose is given again and the infusion rate is doubled. Equivalent doses of other loop diuretics (bumetanide, torsemide, or ethacrynic acid) should have the same effects. Because these drugs cause excretion of substantial amounts of potassium and chloride in addition to sodium and water, their use can be associated with severe hypokalemic, hypochloremic metabolic alkalosis, and an increased tendency for development of cardiac arrhythmias if potassium balance is not carefully corrected. Oral or parenteral administration of potassium chloride is usually necessary. Potassium-sparing diuretics, such as spironolactone, triamterene, and amiloride, may also be of some benefit, but the delayed onset of their relatively mild diuretic action makes them less useful than the loop diuretics in the treatment of acutely ill patients.

Therapy with loop diuretics is not always successful. If there is no sign of diuresis in the hour after an initial dose, a higher dose may be administered. Usually, the dose is doubled every hour until diuresis begins. It is not a good idea to push the dose of a loop diuretic too high. If the patient fails to respond to 160 to 320 mg of furosemide, further administration of the drug is unlikely to result in diuresis but can have serious side effects.[529] Some patients are resistant to loop diuretics.[530] If the response to loop diuretics is unsatisfactory, one option is to add a small dose of a diuretic that acts on a different portion of the nephron, such as metolazone, 2.5 to 5.0 mg. Metolazone is slowly and erratically absorbed, and multiple doses may have to be given before synergism with furosemide is manifest. Parenteral thiazide can be expected to produce results more quickly. Combination therapy requires caution because it may result in a profound and prolonged diuresis, causing severe hypokalemia and hypovolemic shock.

If the patient is hypotensive or in frank shock, diuretics are usually not of much benefit, because poor renal perfusion limits any effects they might have on the nephron. In this circumstance, improvement in renal blood flow may produce a diuresis. Pressors or inotropic agents (discussed later), especially those that act to increase renal blood flow (such as relatively low doses [2 to 5 μg/kg/min] of dopamine or dobutamine) may be of substantial benefit.

If the patient has severely diseased kidneys, diuresis may not be an option. In this circumstance, continuous arteriovenous hemofiltration with or without countercurrent dialysis[531, 532] or venovenous ultrafiltration[533] should be considered. These techniques represent considerable advances over traditional hemodialysis, which was often impossible in hemodynamically unstable patients (especially those with low cardiac output or hypotension), and peritoneal dialysis, which was both slow and poorly tolerated. Hemofiltration can be instituted, maintained, and managed successfully by intensive care unit nurses and physicians, and it is not complicated by hypotension because the circuits have small volumes, and pressures are low. Considerable fluid (up to 500 mL/hr) can be removed gradually, with the amount being titrated to the patient's cardiovascular status.

Reduction of blood volume by diuresis (or other means) may not be possible or beneficial in all patients. If the patient is hypotensive, responds to intravascular volume reduction with dramatic decreases in cardiac output and delivery of oxygen to tissues, or develops significant tachycardia, another approach to therapy must be considered in addition to, or in combination with, blood volume reduction.

### Inotropic Agents

Patients with pulmonary edema who have poor cardiac output and hypotension may benefit from inotropic agents, which can be useful in managing patients with hypotension that has been caused by cardiac pump failure, mechanical ventilation, or by therapy directed at reducing thoracic blood volume.[511] Inotropic agents increase cardiac output and therefore can lower the driving pressure for fluid filtration in the lungs by improving myocardial contractility. Three classes of positive inotropic agents may be useful in the management of acute pulmonary edema: catecholamines, digitalis, and new nonglycosidic, nonsympathomimetic inotropic-vasodilating agents.

Catecholamines are the most useful agents in the acute situation. Actions of these drugs are related to the magnitude of their effects on alpha- and beta-adrenergic receptors: alpha stimulation results in peripheral vasoconstriction; $beta_1$ stimulation results in cardiac stimulation; and $beta_2$ stimulation results in vasodilation (and bronchodilation). Relatively nonselective agonists, such as norepinephrine, increase cardiac contractility, but their usefulness is somewhat limited by their tendency to raise systemic vascular resistance (which in turn limits the improvement in cardiac output) and to increase myocardial oxygen needs because of higher heart rate and larger afterload. The selective beta-agonist isoproterenol causes large increases in cardiac output and decreases in pulmonary capillary pressure, but its vasodilatory effects often lead to reductions in arterial pressure and increases in heart rate. The myocardium may become increasingly irritable, and myocardial ischemia can be aggravated by reduction of arterial diastolic pressure. The drugs most commonly used to provide short-term, intravenous inotropic support in acute pulmonary edema are dopamine[511, 534] (the immediate precursor in the endogenous synthesis of norepinephrine) and the synthetic catecholamine dobutamine.[511, 535, 536]

At low doses, dopamine increases cardiac contractility, improves cardiac output without causing significant changes in heart rate or myocardial oxygen consumption, reduces systemic vascular resistance, and directly increases renal blood flow by stimulating dopaminergic receptors, thereby increasing urine output and salt and water excretion. It is particularly useful when hypotension complicates pulmonary edema; its vasopressor activity raises systemic blood pressure while cardiac output is maintained or increased. Ventricular filling pressures are often unchanged or even raised by dopamine infusion, however, and the pressure for fluid filtration in the lungs may actually increase. Venoconstriction may aggravate this stronger force for edema accumulation in the lungs by redistributing blood volume toward the thorax.[534] For this reason, a vasodilator (e.g., nitroglycerin and nitroprusside) may also be given in order to reverse some of the undesired vasopressor effects of dopamine. When hypotension is a major concern, a predominant venodilator (e.g., intravenous nitroglycerin, nitroglycerin ointment) can be administered with dopamine to reduce thoracic blood volume while arterial pressure is supported. Dopamine can also be used to counteract hypotension caused by nitroprusside infusions. Because dopamine infusions may have the unwanted effect of raising the hydrostatic pressure for fluid filtration in the lungs, invasive hemodynamic monitoring can be helpful in assessing the effect of therapy. Measurement of pulmonary vascular pressure, in addition to systemic blood pressure, may be helpful when vasodilators are also being infused. At higher doses, dopamine increasingly stimulates alpha receptors and induces release of endogenous norepinephrine from nerve endings. This produces a pressor effect but also causes increases in heart rate, ventricular irritability, and arrhythmias. Increased filling pressures in the heart also aggravate the tendency for edema formation in the lungs.

Intravenous dopamine therapy is started at 2 to 5 μg/kg/min, and the dose is titrated to produce the desired effects. Doses greater than 10 to 15 μg/kg/min are usually associated with prominent alpha effects, and such therapy may be complicated by arteriolar vasoconstriction so intense that digital necrosis may occur.[537] Dopamine must be infused through a large-bore, secure catheter because tissue infiltration results in necrosis. Dopamine can cause the pupils to be fixed and dilated regardless of the patient's neurologic status. In addition to aggravating pulmonary edema by raising pulmonary perfusion pressure, dopamine infusions may cause an increase in shunting in the lungs and a subsequent decrease in arterial $Po_2$. This effect is thought to be caused by reduction of hypoxic vasoconstriction in the lungs, which is caused by an increase in mixed venous $Po_2$ resulting from improved cardiac output.[538–540] This has not been found to be a problem when patients are being ventilated with PEEP, probably because mechanical ventilation acts to reduce shunt by other means.[539, 541, 542] Dopamine might increase alveolar epithelial active transport,[543] and thus the removal of fluid from flooded alveoli, but the clinical relevance of this effect is unknown.

Dobutamine differs from dopamine in that the former does not cause systemic vasoconstriction. It is primarily a positive inotropic agent but also has mild vasodilating ability. Cardiac output increases both because it has a direct inotropic effect and because systemic vascular resistance is decreased. Filling pressures in the heart tend to fall with dobutamine infusions (rather than rise, as with dopamine), a beneficial effect relative to the forces governing fluid filtration in the lungs. Like dopamine, dobutamine might also increase the rate of alveolar fluid clearance,[544] but the clinical relevance of this effect is also unknown. Renal blood flow tends to increase with dobutamine infusions because cardiac output improves (rather than because renal dopaminergic receptors are stimulated, as with dopamine). Dobutamine is particularly useful for the treatment of pulmonary edema due to cardiac decompensation resulting from decreased ventricular contractility. In acute myocardial infarction, this agent is more effective than parenteral digitalis as a positive inotropic agent, and its effects are more controllable and predictable.

Dobutamine infusions are started at 2 to 3 μg/kg/min, and the dose is increased every 10 to 30 minutes until the desired effects are produced. Effects may be delayed several minutes, and the maximal effect of any dose occurs after 10 minutes or more. The usual dose is 5 to 15 μg/kg/min. Problems are common when the dose exceeds 15 μg/kg/min. Arrhythmias may occur. Tachycardia is an undesirable side effect of dobutamine infusion that indicates the dose is too high and stroke volume is not adequate. In this circumstance, myocardial oxygen demands are excessively increased by the rapid heart rate in the presence of positive inotropy, and the supply of oxygen to the heart is decreased because coronary perfusion pressures are reduced and diastolic perfusion time is shortened. Dobutamine therapy is most successful when left ventricular filling pressures are kept at 18 to 20 mm Hg or higher. Dobutamine should be administered cautiously to patients with atrial fibrillation because the drug facilitates atrioventricular nodal conduction and may cause an increase in ventricular rate. Digitalis may be a more appropriate inotropic agent in that circumstance.

Unfortunately, no orally active catecholamine is available for more long-term treatment. Digitalis continues to be prescribed for long-term inotropic therapy, but few data support its use in patients with congestive heart failure who are in sinus rhythm.[521] It is much less useful than dobutamine or dopamine in acute pulmonary edema because its effects are not as great or as predictable. Its use is also complicated by a narrow ratio of therapeutic-to-toxic dose. Rapid injection of digoxin should be avoided because it may cause systemic venoconstriction and thereby worsen pulmonary edema. Because patients with chronic heart failure are frequently treated with digitalis preparations on an outpatient basis, administration of the drug may be hazardous in acute situations, in which the amount of drug present in the body is unknown. The major use of digitalis is in patients with atrial fibrillation and a rapid ventricular response associated with pulmonary edema. Substantial increases in cardiac output and decreases in pulmonary vascular pressures can be achieved by controlling ventricular rate. When the heart rate is extremely slow, cardiac output can also be substantially increased by administering atropine or electrically pacing the heart.

The use of digitalis and non-ACE inhibitor vasodilators in heart failure has been reviewed.[545] New nonglycosidic, nonsympathomimetic, inotropic vasodilators are being studied and introduced, but experience with these agents in pulmonary edema is limited. The bipyridine derivative amrinone[546] and its more potent analogue milrinone[547] are examples. These drugs are believed to act by inhibiting phosphodiesterase activity, thereby raising intracellular cyclic adenosine monophosphate levels. Increases in intracellular calcium are postulated to lead to the positive inotropic effect. Myocardial oxygen consumption is not increased (unlike the situation with dobutamine therapy). In addition, these drugs may have a direct effect on respiratory muscle contraction, leading to improved respiratory muscle function.[546] These drugs are also peripheral and pulmonary vasodilators, lowering systemic vascular resistance (thereby reducing afterload and increasing cardiac output) and pulmonary vascular resistance (thereby decreasing hydrostatic pressure in the lungs). Such effects could be useful in the short-term management of patients with increased pressure pulmonary edema due to heart failure. Intravenous milrinone (loading dose of 50 μg/kg, followed by a continuous infusion at 0.375 to 0.75 μg/kg/min) can be used as an alternative to low-dose dobutamine to temporarily improve cardiac output and renal blood flow.[522] The most serious short-term adverse reactions involve enhanced cardiac automaticity and arrhythmogenesis. The data available indicate that these drugs, at least over the long run, may not improve survival and, in fact, may have a harmful effect.[521, 522]

The lives of a limited number of patients with severe pulmonary edema refractory to immediate drug therapies might be salvaged by temporary mechanical support (i.e., intra-aortic balloon pumps or ventricular assist devices). Extrapulmonary gas exchange[548, 549] or heart transplantation, lung transplantation, or both[550–553] (see Chapter 97) can be appropriately offered to very few patients, but the possibilities can be considered only if all other therapeutic options have been exhausted.

## Therapeutic Strategy

The possible therapeutic options that have been discussed are directed at the immediate salvage of patients with life-threatening pulmonary edema. Therapy must be clearly goal oriented, responsive to the underlying pathophysiology, and frequently reassessed until the patient is stable. Appropriate information about the effects of therapy can be crucial to decisions about how to proceed, but invasive monitoring is useless if it provides only sensory overload to the physician or is collected rather than used. In both types of edema, the central goal of therapy is to reduce the transudation of fluid into the lungs. Because the rate of edema formation increases exponentially with increases in pulmonary vascular pressures,[554] pressure control is crucial for successful therapy.

## Increased Pressure Edema

The acute recognition and management of congestive heart failure has been the subject of comprehensive reviews and recommendations.[511, 522, 555, 556] The goal of therapy is to reduce the hydrostatic pressure causing edema formation in the lungs. Bed rest, adequate oxygenation, and dietary salt restriction are the basic principles of management. The work of the heart must be reduced as much as possible by restricting physical activity and preventing pain and anxiety, which act to increase the work of the heart by stimulating sympathetic discharge. As the heart fails, cardiac performance is reflexly preserved by progressive increases in vascular volumes that act to maximize cardiac stroke volume and work (the Frank-Starling mechanism). This compensatory increase in preload of the left ventricle results in pulmonary venous hypertension and raises the driving pressure for fluid filtration. As heart failure worsens, cardiac output is steadily reduced, pulmonary and systemic venous pressures rise, systemic vascular resistance increases, and edema, both pulmonary and peripheral, becomes the major manifestation of compromised cardiac function. In patients with increased pressure pulmonary edema, reduction of vascular volume and increase in cardiac output cause the driving pressure for edema formation to decrease. Because the normal safety factors protecting the lungs from edema driven by high filtration pressures are intact, the pressure need be lowered only to near normal. At pulmonary capillary wedge pressures less than 20 mm Hg, fluid filtration in the lungs usually should not be sufficient to cause pulmonary edema. Patients with severe cardiac failure may tolerate higher pressures (because baseline barrier permeability is lowered in the lungs[51, 52] and lymphatic removal capability is improved) and may require such pressures to maintain cardiac output. Therapy is directed at reducing the work the heart must perform and at increasing the heart's efficiency for the work it must do. Some patients with severe hydrostatic pulmonary edema require mechanical ventilation with positive pressure ventilation. The resolution of alveolar edema in these patients is not simply a function of lowering lung vascular pressures; other mechanisms that augment alveolar fluid clearance are important.[556a]

Most patients with acute pulmonary edema caused by cardiac failure have systolic dysfunction, but a sizable minority (around 30%) have diastolic dysfunction.[522] Cardiac contraction is normal, but relaxation is impaired. Because the ventricle does not relax normally, end-diastolic pressure is increased, thereby increasing hydrostatic pressure in the blood vessels in the lungs. Acute diastolic dysfunction producing acute pulmonary edema is not an uncommon manifestation of acute myocardial ischemia or uncontrolled hypertension. Other causes include diabetes mellitus, aortic stenosis, infiltrative cardiomyopathies, endocardial fibroelastosis, hypothermia, septic shock, elevated thoracic pressures from mechanical ventilation, and pericardial effusion. Causal or aggravating conditions should be corrected (e.g., revascularization for coronary artery disease, control of systemic hypertension). The goal of therapy in acute diastolic dysfunction is to lower elevated filling pressures (by the cautious use of diuretics and nitrates) without significantly reducing cardiac output. These patients are prone to develop hypotension in response to diuretics and nitrates because adequate cardiac output depends on elevated filling pressures in the heart. Because systolic function is normal, positive inotropic agents do not help and can make things worse by aggravating ischemia.

In the setting of acute increased pressure pulmonary edema, it is especially important that correctable causes of heart failure be identified and treated. Acute myocardial infarction, ongoing myocardial ischemia, arrhythmias, valvular lesions, systemic hypertension, ventricular septal rupture, rheumatic or other inflammatory myocarditis, digitalis intoxication, pulmonary embolism, infection, thyrotoxicosis, or severe anemia may have caused the heart to fail and must be corrected. Cardiac patients presenting with pulmonary edema infrequently complain of chest pain, but most of them have significant coronary artery disease, and pulmonary edema may be the only manifestation of silent myocardial ischemia.[339]

It is also important that the patient not be overtreated. Increased pressure pulmonary edema usually does not continue to accumulate once the patient is positioned upright and given oxygen, a potent diuretic, and anxiety is relieved. Aggressive treatment, especially if the patient is in poor condition, may be more harmful than the pulmonary edema itself.

## Increased Permeability Edema

The strategy for managing patients with acute lung injury and increased permeability pulmonary edema differs from that for patients with increased pressure pulmonary edema because the lungs are directly damaged in the former rather than being affected "bystanders," as in the latter. The urgent problem is not that the driving pressure for edema formation is abnormally high, but that edema will form in great quantities even at low driving pressures. The goals of therapy, which are listed in Table 54.9, are to remove the cause of lung injury, to support life while the lungs are given a chance to heal, to select a ventilator strategy that will not worsen the lung injury, and to reduce as much as possible the driving pressures for fluid movement across the injured barriers into the lungs.

The cause of lung injury often cannot be unequivocally identified. If it is not obvious, the cause should be assumed to be infection, which is the most common treatable underlying cause of acute lung injury. Although the patient is often seriously ill, diagnostic studies must be

**Table 54.9 ACUTE LUNG INJURY: IMPORTANT PRINCIPLES OF MANAGEMENT**

- Minimize edema accumulation
  - Ensure lowest possible pulmonary microvascular pressure
  - Reduce vascular volume
- Find and treat infection
- Supportive therapy
  - Administer oxygen
  - Lung protection ventilation strategy
  - Optimize blood pressure and cardiac output
- Do more good than harm
  - Avoid hypotension
  - Avoid volume overload
  - Avoid oxygen toxicity
  - Avoid infection

performed to identify a possible source of infection, so that appropriate drainage and antimicrobial therapy can be instituted. Plain chest roentgenograms usually are not helpful.[366] Abdominal sonograms and computed tomographic scans can be diagnostically useful. Sepsis from intra-abdominal infection is common and may be especially difficult to identify. Many of these infections require surgical drainage if antimicrobial drug therapy is to be effective. Surgeons are often reluctant to surgically explore a patient who is acutely ill with lung injury and severely compromised pulmonary function, but operation may be the patient's only hope for survival.

Because specific therapy for acute lung injury is not usually available (unless the cause is infection), supportive therapy is all that can be offered. The goal is to keep the patient alive, in the hope that with time, the lungs will repair themselves. Urgent considerations are adequate ventilation and circulation. Patients with acute lung injury may be hemodynamically unstable, and ventilatory support can be complicated by hypotension or frank shock. PEEP, which is required for adequate ventilation, may compound the problem by impeding venous return to the heart and decreasing cardiac function.

Patients with low pulmonary capillary wedge pressures (<6 mm Hg) and systemic hypotension may require fluid resuscitation to support blood pressure and end-organ perfusion. If the patient has active, ongoing blood loss or the hemoglobin concentration is low (<7.0 g/dL), packed red blood cells are effective not only to expand intravascular volume and restore blood pressure but also to increase the oxygen-carrying capacity of the blood. Patients who are not bleeding and who have normal hemoglobin concentrations should be resuscitated with crystalloid solutions. Because the barriers restricting colloid movement from the vascular space into the lungs are not functioning normally when the lungs are injured, osmotic pressure differences favoring fluid movement into the vascular space cannot be established in the lungs; therefore, there is no advantage to fluid resuscitation with expensive colloid solutions.

Patients whose hypotension does not respond to fluid resuscitation or who have normal (6 to 12 mm Hg) or elevated pulmonary capillary wedge pressure may require pressors or positive inotropic agents. If systemic vascular resistance is elevated, dobutamine would be appropriate. Septic shock is a common problem.[557] Because generalized vasodilation resulting in low systemic vascular resistance is the major hemodynamic abnormality in such patients, dopamine, with its vasopressor properties, is the drug of choice to support blood pressure. An alternative approach can be the use of military antishock trousers, which increase peripheral vascular resistance, thereby increasing cardiac afterload, blood pressure, and blood flow to vital organs in the upper body.[558] Increasing cardiac afterload, however, may not be a good idea in certain patients with ischemic myocardium.

Reduction in pulmonary capillary wedge pressure may increase the survival of patients with acute lung injury,[559] and reduction of pulmonary microvascular pressure is the single most important goal of supportive therapy. Pulmonary vascular pressures can be normal, increased, or decreased in patients with acute lung injury. Injured lungs are sensitive to the driving pressure for fluid extravasation because the barriers limiting fluid and protein flow out of the bloodstream are not intact. Greatly elevated pressures are generally incompatible with survival. The goal of therapy is to maintain the lowest possible pulmonary vascular pressures that are consistent with adequate cardiac output and perfusion of vital organs. If cardiac output is adequate, no pulmonary vascular pressure is too low; edema forms readily even at normal pressure in injured lungs. Because small reductions in the driving pressure for fluid accumulation in the lungs can substantially reduce edema, therapy with drugs that lower pulmonary vascular pressures are useful. Nitroprusside may be especially beneficial because cardiac output can increase even as pulmonary vascular pressures fall. If hypotension is a problem, blood pressure can be supported by also infusing dopamine or dobutamine. Some studies have demonstrated that positive fluid balance correlates negatively with successful outcome in patients with acute lung injury.[428, 429, 560, 561] The likely importance of cautious volume administration and reduction of pulmonary microvascular pressure will be tested in clinical trials in the near future.

Acute lung injury is sometimes complicated by associated volume overload or left ventricular failure. In this circumstance, wedge pressure may be modestly elevated (15 to 25 mm Hg), and the therapeutic options available for increased pressure pulmonary edema (vasodilators, diuretics, positive inotropic agents) would appropriately be considered. As just discussed, the goal of therapy is to have the patient as dry as possible.

Therapy must do more good than harm. Aggressive hemodynamic and ventilatory support of critically ill patients can be self-defeating if complications of therapies become more significant problems than the underlying disease itself.[562] Attempts to increase systemic oxygen delivery (e.g., with inotropes, intravascular fluids, and blood transfusions)[563] or to achieve supranormal values for the cardiac index or normal values for mixed venous oxygen saturation[564] do not reduce mortality and may actually be detrimental. Studies fail to document usefulness of goal-oriented hemodynamic therapy in critically ill patients.[408] Further lung injury caused by toxic concentrations of oxygen must be avoided. PEEP should be applied at the lowest level consistent with adequate $P_{O_2}$ (arterial $P_{O_2}$ >60 mm Hg) at nontoxic inspired oxygen concentration ($F_{I_{O_2}}$ <0.6) to avoid adverse effects on cardiac output. Oxygen demand often can be reduced by suppressing fever or sedating and paralyzing the patient[565, 566] (although this can lead to prolonged neuromuscular blockade[567]). Finally, an adequate hemoglobin concentration should be maintained (hemoglobin 7.0 to 9.0 g/dL). A multicenter, randomized, controlled clinical trial of transfusion requirements in critically ill patients with euvolemia after initial treatment showed that a restrictive strategy of red-cell transfusions (in which red cells were transfused if the hemoglobin concentration dropped below 7.0 g/dL and hemoglobin concentrations were maintained at 7.0 to 9.0 g/dL) was at least as effective as and was possibly superior to a liberal transfusion strategy (in which transfusions were given when the hemoglobin concentration fell below 10.0 g/dL and hemoglobin concentrations were maintained at 10.0 to 12.0 g/dL), with the possible exception of patients with active coronary ischemic syndromes (acute myocardial infarction and unstable angina).[568]

Increasing minute ventilation has been shown to increase edema formation,[569] and overexpansion may mechanically injure the lungs.[354, 570–572] In experimental animals, ventilation with high tidal volumes can increase vascular filtration pressures; produce stress fractures of microvascular endothelium, alveolar epithelium, and basement membranes; and cause lung rupture (so-called ventilation-induced lung injury). The injury appears to be due to increased lung excursions at high volumes (so-called volutrauma), not high airway pressure per se, because it can be prevented by limiting thoracic motion (e.g., by placing the chest in a cast). Although the evidence from animal experiments seemed compelling,[573] clinical evidence of such lung injury is lacking, and benefit from altering traditional ventilation practices was not rigorously demonstrated in small studies.[574–576] In mechanically ventilated patients with sepsis-induced ARDS, no significant correlations were found between high ventilatory pressures or volumes and the development of pneumothorax or other lung air leaks, and pneumothorax or other lung air leaks were not associated with a significantly increased mortality rate.[577] Another study found that pulmonary barotrauma in mechanically ventilated patients correlated closely with underlying disease, specifically ARDS, but not with elevated airway pressures.[578] Other studies found that mortality rates were not different in patients with acute lung injuries whether they suffered barotrauma or not,[579] and patients with acute lung injuries who experienced barotrauma but survived had no more functional impairment when they recovered than surviving patients who did not experience barotrauma.[580] Barotrauma appears to be a consequence rather than a cause of the severity of lung injury.

A well-conducted, prospective, randomized clinical trial that compared a "modern approach" (a strategy of reduced airway pressures and tidal volume, including inverse-ratio ventilation and extrapulmonary $CO_2$ removal, when necessary) with conventional ventilation detected no significant outcome difference between them.[581] Two trials of limited ventilation were not in agreement. One trial showed similar incidence of barotrauma, multiple organ dysfunction, organ failure, and mortality when conventional ventilation was compared with pressure- and volume-limited ventilation.[582] The other trial showed reduced barotrauma and improved survival at 28 days (but no significant difference in survival to hospital discharge) for the patients in the limited ventilation group.[583] However, morbidity appeared to be increased in the limited ventilation group when compared with conventional ventilation. Most of the benefit of limited ventilation accrued in the first 3 days of mechanical ventilation and seemed to have been the result of higher PEEP, perhaps preventing the cyclic closing and reopening of alveoli. The mortality was very high (71%) in the conventional ventilation group, well beyond mortality reported from some clinical trials. Possible explanations for the differences between these two trials of limited ventilation were discussed in an accompanying editorial.[584]

New evidence, however, has become available from a large National Heart, Lung, and Blood Institute (NHLBI) clinical trial carried out with 861 patients. In this study, outcomes using traditional (12-mL/kg, "high") tidal volumes were compared with considerably diminished (6-mL/kg, "low") tidal volumes; mortality in the lower tidal volume group (31%) was significantly lower than mortality in the high tidal volume group (39%).[584a] Some details of the study design were posted on ARDSnet (http://hedwig.mgh.harvard.edu/ardsnet), and the NHLBI press release was posted on their web site (http://www.nhlbi.nih.gov). In addition to decreasing mortality in patients with ARDS, the small tidal volume approach was associated with a lower incidence of nonpulmonary organ failure. Interestingly, results from a recent Italian study showed that a low tidal volume strategy in ARDS patients attenuated the inflammatory response in both the lungs and bloodstream, as measured by a reduction in neutrophil and cytokine concentrations in bronchoalveolar lavage and a reduction in cytokines in circulating blood.[584b]

A number of "adjuncts" to conventional mechanical ventilation have been proposed and studied in small numbers of patients,[507, 574, 575] including prone positioning (discussed later), extrapulmonary gas exchange (oxygenation, $CO_2$ removal, or both),[548, 549] liquid ventilation,[585, 586] tracheal gas insufflation, permissive hypercapnea,[587] and high-frequency ventilation.[588] All of these adjuncts are investigational, and their use should be restricted to controlled clinical trials.[150] Repositioning the patient is the simplest and least invasive of these techniques.[589] Turning patients with severe respiratory failure to the prone position can result in improved pulmonary gas exchange,[590–593] probably as a result of increased ventilation of dorsal lung units and more favorable matching of ventilation and perfusion.[594] Turning critically ill, mechanically ventilated patients from the supine to the prone position is not an uncomplicated or easy task, however, and there are risks involved (e.g., extubation, kinked ventilator tubing, disconnection of catheters, hemodynamic instability, pressure sores on the face). Not all patients respond by improving oxygenation.

Even appropriate therapy may be rendered futile if the patient does not receive adequate nutrition[595, 596]; some evidence indicates that enteral feeding is preferable to parenteral nutrition in preserving gastrointestinal tract integrity, thereby preventing translocation of bacteria and endotoxin.[597, 598] However, adequate enteral nutrition can be difficult in patients who are receiving opiates or have slowed gastrointestinal motility for other reasons. Critically ill patients who require mechanical ventilation are at increased risk for clinically significant gastrointestinal bleeding from stress ulcers. Ranitidine is more effective than sucralfate for prophylaxis against gastrointestinal bleeding in patients requiring mechanical ventilation; there was no difference between the two drugs in the incidence of ventilator-associated pneumonia.[599]

Prevention of ventilator-associated pneumonia was the subject of a comprehensive review.[600] Although a relation between gastric colonization with gram-negative bacilli and nosocomial pneumonia in intensive care unit patients has been shown,[601] selective decontamination of the digestive tract does not appear to significantly improve mortality even though respiratory tract infections are prevented.[602–604] Infection must be rigorously avoided and treated if it occurs. Simple precautions, such as meticulous hand washing and removal of unnecessary catheters, should not be overlooked. The most common cause of late death in acute lung injury is infection.[243] If the condition of a patient who has been stabilized begins to deteriorate, pulmonary infection is likely and must be aggressively diagnosed and treated. The situation is unfortunately complicated by the fact that the inflammatory, proliferative phase of acute lung injury can mimic the sepsis syndrome[218, 219] (discussed earlier).

Little attention has been paid to the efficacy and cost-benefit analysis of routine practices in the care of critically ill patients with pulmonary edema. For example, a study of the efficacy of daily, routine chest radiographs in intubated, mechanically ventilated patients uncovered a sharp division of opinion.[605, 606] In addition, until the results of the recent NHLBI clinical trial of low versus high tidal volumes became available, there were no convincing published data indicating that any particular ventilatory support mode is superior for patients with acute lung injuries or ARDS.[607]

The literature from the patients' point of view is sparse: only a few group studies and scattered personal observations about patient experience in intensive care units have been reported.[608–610] No reports of what it is like to have pulmonary edema could be found. A critical care text[611] has sections dealing with nursing perspectives but no section on patient perspective, and both nurses and patients are slighted in this textbook. The limited information available indicates that many patients had significant amnesia for most of their intensive care unit stay and poor insight into their condition. Many survivors experience depression, which tends to diminish over a prolonged recovery time. Some experience posttraumatic stress disorder. Patient experience is an important area that has been neglected by research.

## Specific Therapy

The possibility for pharmacologic treatment of acute lung injury is reviewed regularly.[146–150, 354, 507, 612–614] Therapeutic agents that have a rationale in our incomplete understanding of the pathogenesis of acute lung injuries and that have been studied in patients with acute lung injuries or its frequent precursor, septic disorders, include corticosteroids, ibuprofen, nitric oxide, prostaglandin $E_1$ ($PGE_1$), liposomal prostaglandins $E_1$ and $E_2$, surfactant, antiendotoxin and anti–TNF-α antibodies, platelet activating factor receptor antagonist, interleukin-1 receptor antagonist, ketoconazole, *N*-acetylcysteine, oxothiazolidine carboxylate, and pentoxifylline. None of these agents has shown any benefit on mortality in large-scale, prospective, randomized, controlled clinical trials. There have been sporadic reports indicating that other agents might be useful. The state of clinical trials in ARDS was the subject of conference reports in 1992,[615] in 1998,[354] and again in 2000,[150] which summarized the status of possible therapies and the opportunities and challenges faced in evaluating them. Research on the therapeutic frontier in acute lung injuries is hampered by the lack of generally accepted diagnostic and staging criteria. The establishment of the ARDS clinical trials network by the NHLBI has already fostered the conduct of large, well-designed studies to define the efficacy and appropriate use of therapy for acute lung injury[150, 607]; additional trials on the value of glucocorticoids late in the evolution of ARDS, on the efficacy of reducing lung vascular pressures, and on the utility of high levels of PEEP, prone ventilation, partial liquid ventilation, and surfactant administration are under way or planned.

The question of the wisdom of potential therapy based on interfering with the inflammatory response needs to be addressed. With the current emphasis on the damaging potential of inflammation, it is important to remember that inflammation plays a vital beneficial role in the destruction of invading microorganisms and other foreign cells. If a patient is saved from lung injury only to die of infection, nothing will have been gained. The redundancy and interaction of inflammatory pathways may frustrate any therapeutic blocking potential. Because functions overlap extensively, blocking any one inflammatory mediator (or even multiple mediators) may have little or no effect on the overall inflammatory response. Also, the question of underlying mechanisms for the diverse causes of ARDS has to be addressed in potential therapies. If the mechanisms of lung injury differ among various causes, application of therapy directed at particular mechanisms is not appropriate until clinical diagnoses of underlying mechanisms can be made. The relatively low incidence of severe acute lung injury among patients admitted with high-risk diagnoses[616, 617] complicates the problem. Finally, the timing of therapy might be an important factor. Therapy that is worthless or harmful at one time in the course of the disease may be beneficial at another.[618]

**Corticosteroids.** Of the possible pharmacologic agents for treatment of acute lung injuries, corticosteroids have the longest history and the widest clinical use. Despite a seemingly compelling rationale for use in the setting of acute lung injury or its frequent precursor, septic disorders,[619] four separate, prospective, randomized, double-blind, placebo-controlled trials of high-dose methylprednisolone therapy failed to show any benefit.[234, 235, 620, 621]

Corticosteroid therapy did not prevent the development of acute lung injury, decrease its incidence in the sepsis syndrome, hasten its reversal, lower its mortality rate, or improve respiratory function. Moreover, corticosteroids were associated with a greater 14-day mortality rate in patients who developed acute lung injury and an increased frequency of infections.[234, 620] Corticosteroids also were found not to be of benefit in the sepsis syndrome[622] and may have caused harm. Thus, corticosteroids should not be given to patients with, or at risk for, developing acute lung injuries unless there is some other indication, such as a history of recent steroid therapy or another reason to suspect adrenal insufficiency. One exception may be the fat embolism syndrome. A prospective, randomized, double-blind, placebo-controlled trial of corticosteroid treatment in 64 patients with long-bone fractures showed that high-dose methylprednisolone effectively prevented the development of the fat embolism syndrome,[623] and short-course corticosteroid therapy appears to be appropriate in such patients, particularly in the presence of the characteristic petechial rash. Recommendation for such prophylactic therapy could be stronger were the study confirmed in a larger group of patients.

The generally disappointing results of corticosteroid trials in acute lung injury have not wholly discouraged investigators. Because of the diversity of precipitating causes and the changing character of acute lung injuries as they progress, some investigators believe that corticosteroids might be beneficial in subsets of patients or when given at a particular time (e.g., during the proliferative phase[218]) or for a more sustained period.[624] Results of studies of corticosteroid therapy late in the course of ARDS (so-called rescue therapy) were encouraging,[625–627] and a small, randomized, double-blind, placebo-controlled clinical trial in patients with severe ARDS whose Lung Injury Score had failed to improve by the seventh day of respiratory failure showed improvement in lung injury and other organ dysfunction scores and reduced mortality for the patients treated with prolonged administration of methylprednisolone.[628] A large-scale NHLBI-sponsored trial is now under way.

The decision to employ rescue therapy (with corticosteroids or any other drug or therapeutic maneuver) is based on the assumption that the physician knows the expected outcome with adequate certainty, but such predictions actually are quite uncertain,[607] and the urge to "do something" can hurt patients rather than help. Perhaps the major lesson learned from our experience with corticosteroids as early treatment for acute lung injuries (other than that they are not effective) is that no matter how attractive any agent might be theoretically or how compelling the rationale for use might be based on experimental animal studies, well-designed and executed large-scale clinical trials must be organized and carried out before any promising therapy finds its way into widespread clinical use.

**Surfactant.** The possibility of administering exogenous surfactant in the treatment of acute lung injury has attracted considerable attention.[178, 274, 629–631] The rationale for such therapy is based on abnormalities of surfactant composition and function that have been demonstrated in acute lung injuries (discussed earlier), which have similarities to the infant respiratory distress syndrome (which has been revolutionized by surfactant therapy),[632, 633] and on the approval of an artificial surfactant (colfosceril [Exosurf]) for clinical use. Among the many possible theoretical benefits of surfactant therapy are stabilized alveoli, improved respiratory compliance, decreased work of breathing, improved gas exchange and consequently decreased need to administer toxic concentrations of oxygen, and enhanced phagocytosis and bronchial transport, which combine with surfactant's antibacterial and antiviral activity to reduce the possibility of lung infection. Surfactant might also inhibit the respiratory burst (and the subsequent release of toxic oxygen metabolites) of PMNs[634] and might modulate lung fibroblast and macrophage activity and decrease release of inflammatory mediators.[635]

Results in experimental models have been mixed,[178, 629, 636, 637] but taken as a whole, they appear to indicate that animals were not harmed by surfactant therapy and that improved gas exchange and lung compliance are a reasonable possibility. A preliminary communication indicated that Exosurf could be administered safely to ventilated patients with sepsis-induced ARDS, but no differences were found in any physiologic parameters when compared with control subjects, and a dose-dependent trend in reduction of mortality did not reach statistical significance.[638] The pilot trial was followed by a large-scale, prospective, double-blind, randomized, placebo-controlled clinical trial in patients with sepsis-induced ARDS,[639] which showed no significant effect on 30-day survival, length of stay in the intensive care unit, duration of mechanical ventilation, or physiologic function. A lack of knowledge about normal and artificial surfactant metabolism, turnover, and inactivation in the setting of acute lung injury, as well as about how surfactant can best be delivered (a study in sheep showed that response to exogenous surfactant depended both on the preparation and how it was delivered[640]), appears to be impeding progress in designing effective therapy. One possibility is that surfactant therapy simply may not be sufficient to affect the symptoms and outcome of ARDS: most of the patients who died in the large-scale trial did so from multiple-organ failure, sepsis or septic shock, or cardiac arrest rather than from any respiratory disease that might have been amenable to surfactant therapy. Another possibility is that the dose of surfactant actually delivered to the patients' lungs by the aerosol method employed in the large-scale trial was very small (probably $<5\%$ of the dose administered), and much of the surfactant was likely deposited in less severely injured lung units that were better ventilated.

More encouraging results have been reported in smaller studies of natural surfactants and bolus administration of large doses. A pilot study tested the effects of a natural, bovine surfactant in patients with ARDS.[641] When large volumes (as much as 4 mL/kg every 8 hours) were instilled down patients' endotracheal tubes, a dose-dependent decrease in 28-day mortality was found (19% mortality at the highest dose vs. 44% mortality in control patients). Another bovine surfactant study administering large doses via the bronchoscope in a small number of patients reported only 20% mortality (all nonpulmonary) at 14 days, and shunt was decreased and arterial $Po_2/Fi_{O2}$ was increased by surfactant.[642] This is a novel approach to the treatment of acute lung injury and will be an active area of experimental and clinical research in the years ahead.

**Antioxidants.** Clinically, *N*-acetylcysteine has advanced farther than any other therapeutic strategy on the basis of the hypothetical role of oxidants in the pathogenesis of acute lung injury. *N*-Acetylcysteine is unique among the free-radical scavengers because it is already in widespread clinical use for acetaminophen and paracetamol overdose, conditions for which it has been found to be safe, to have a favorable therapeutic index, and to be effective. It is also novel among anti-inflammatory agents being tested for human therapy because it acts selectively to quench oxygen radicals rather than globally to suppress the function of leukocytes. *N*-Acetylcysteine appears to act both directly, by scavenging oxygen free radicals, and indirectly, by metabolism into glutathione, which is an important endogenous antioxidant.

Experimental animal studies were encouraging, including a report that indicated *N*-acetylcysteine additionally inhibits TNF release (perhaps because glutathione is an endogenous modulator of TNF production).[643] Results from a pilot randomized, double-blind trial in 30 patients with acute lung injury showed that plasma and red blood cell glutathione levels were decreased in the presence of acute lung injury and could be increased by *N*-acetylcysteine administration. Improvements were shown in chest radiograph edema scores, pulmonary vascular resistance, shunt fraction, static compliance, cardiac output, oxygen delivery, and oxygen consumption.[644] Four subsequent small clinical trials in acute lung injury patients examining the effects of *N*-acetylcysteine or oxothiazolidine carboxylate (Procysteine), which also acts to augment glutathione stores, have been reported.[645–648] None of these trials found improved survival, but in one trial, the duration of acute lung injury appeared to be shortened by either drug.[647] Enthusiasm for this type of therapy must be tempered by the possibility that antioxidants could compromise defenses against infection.[649–651] A phase III clinical trial of oxothiazolidine carboxylate was recently stopped for lack of efficacy.[150]

**Pentoxifylline.** Less is known about the therapeutic possibilities in human acute lung injury of pentoxifylline, a phosphodiesterase inhibitor that increases cyclic adenosine monophosphate in PMNs and inhibits their inflammatory function.[652] Interest in this drug stems, at least in part, from its ready availability. It has been in clinical use for many years in the treatment of intermittent claudication, based on its purported ability to increase the flexibility of red blood cells and thereby reduce blood viscosity and increase capillary blood flow. Its link to the pathogenesis of acute lung injury through the role of PMNs and macrophages in the inflammatory process has led to studies in experimental models that have demonstrated prevention or attenuation of various acute lung injuries, apparently by inhibiting PMNs, in various species.[652–657] Of course, not all acute lung injuries involve PMNs in their pathogenesis, and the usual skepticism about the wisdom of interfering with the inflammatory response applies. A related compound, lisofylline, failed to show efficacy in a phase III trial.[150]

**Antiendotoxin and Other Antibodies.** Two different monoclonal antibodies against endotoxin have been investigated as therapy for sepsis, the most common antecedent to acute lung injury and ARDS: HA-1A human (also known as Centoxin or nebacumab)[236] and E5 murine (also known as Xomen).[237, 658] The underlying rationale for therapy with these agents and the two original clinical trials that were reported has been critiqued,[659, 660] an economic assessment of HA-1A monoclonal antibody for gram-negative sepsis has been made,[661] and a detailed analysis of the original trials and the questions raised about them and about the staggering cost and resulting ethical dilemmas[662] was published. The premise on which antiendotoxin antibody therapy is based appears unproved and unclear; entry criteria differed among the trials; there was no overall statistical difference in survival between placebo and monoclonal antibody treatment for all patients in the trials; the subgroups in which the two antibodies possibly were effective were discordant; it is unclear which patients, if any, might benefit from therapy and how they could be identified; and treated patients who did not have gram-negative bacteremia appear to have been harmed. The HA-1A antibody appeared to offer no benefit over adequate antimicrobial therapy.[659]

In patients with sepsis and a documented gram-negative infection who were not in shock, ARDS (as defined previously in a trial of corticosteroids in patients with acute lung injury[621]) occurred in 14% of the patients in the E5 murine trial; 60% (6 of 10) of those treated with the E5 antibody died, compared with 78% (7 of 9) of those treated with placebo.[237] In the second E5 trial, the antibody appeared to offer some protection against development of ARDS in sepsis patients, but this was a secondary end point that had no effect on survival.[658] In the HA-1A trial, acute lung injury (ARDS as defined by the expanded definition of acute lung injury,[345] discussed earlier) occurred in 11% of the patients with documented gram-negative bacteremia; data on the resolution of lung injury were not published, but major complications of sepsis, which included the patients with ARDS, resolved in 62% of the treated patients, compared with 42% of those given placebo.[236] A subsequent publication discussed the results of HA-1A therapy in the 63 septic patients with ARDS from the larger trial: the antibody did not reverse acute respiratory failure or improve long-term survival.[663] Thus, it appears that if monoclonal antibodies against endotoxin might be of some benefit in any patients with acute lung injury caused by sepsis, their promise was not great. Identifying the subset of patients who might benefit is a major problem. The suggestion that patients could be screened for therapy by measuring circulating endotoxin is not credible, because such measurements are neither sensitive nor specific.[265]

In addition to these antiendotoxin antibodies, large-scale clinical trials in patients with sepsis syndrome treated with monoclonal antibodies against TNF-α[664] and interleukin-1[665] have been reported. Neither showed a significant difference in mortality in patients who received placebo as compared with those who received antibody. No differences in the frequency of continuing, improved, or new organ system failures, such as occurs in ARDS, were found in the anti–TNF-α trial. In the interleukin-1 receptor antagonist trial, secondary and retrospective analysis of the results indicated that survival time might have been increased for patients with ARDS (28-day mortality, 44% for placebo and 34% for antibody, the improvement accruing in the sickest patients).

In clinical trials testing the effects of antibodies in sepsis patients, prospective studies focusing on subgroups (identified retrospectively) that might benefit from therapy have had difficulty reproducing expected benefit. Even were some benefit in ARDS found prospectively, it is unclear whether it would justify the high cost of therapy. A commentary summarized the prospective randomized trial results in sepsis,[666] all of which have failed to show efficacy.

Other antibodies might have therapeutic potential in acute lung injuries: for example, monoclonal antibodies directed against the leukocyte adhesion molecules lymphocyte-function–associated antigen-1α and intercellular adhesion molecule-1 administered intratracheally can both prevent and treat acid-aspiration–induced lung injury in rats,[296] and a monoclonal antibody against interleukin-8 prevented reperfusion lung injury in rabbits[667] and also protected against acid-induced lung injury.[335] Although the clinical failures of antibodies to date are discouraging, this will be an area of active research (and high economic stakes) for many years ahead.

**Prostaglandin $E_1$ and Other Vasodilators.** Another potential pharmacologic treatment of acute lung injury was $PGE_1$, a vasodilator with anti-inflammatory properties. However, a 13-center, randomized, double-blind, placebo-controlled clinical trial showed no improvement in survival (mortality rate at 30 days was 60% in the treated group, 48% in the placebo group).[668] Reduction in systemic and pulmonary vascular resistance and evidence of increased oxygen availability and consumption were counterbalanced by such adverse effects as diarrhea, hypotension, fever, and cardiac arrhythmias. The trial was not designed to resolve the role of $PGE_1$ in patients at risk for developing acute lung injury, so the question of any prophylactic benefit was left unanswered. A smaller, independent study from one institution reported in the same year found $PGE_1$ to be an effective vasodilator but did not influence the development of multiple organ failure or affect mortality of patients with acute lung injury.[669] A secondary report from the larger trial emphasized a purported benefit of $PGE_1$ on oxygenation in a subset of patients,[670] even though survival was not improved, but other studies have indicated that the drug causes deterioration of pulmonary gas exchange and aggravation of arterial hypoxemia by increasing perfusion of underventilated or unventilated lung areas.[515, 671] Another secondary report from the trial emphasized purported beneficial effects with $PGE_1$ therapy on hemodynamic performance, hepatic function, and leukocyte availability,[672] but such effects were rather subtle, and their clinical significance was not obvious. Complaints about the methodology of the multicenter trial focused on the need for more aggressive fluid administration,[673] but the evidence is convincing that intravascular volume expansion is not a good idea in patients with acute lung injury (discussed earlier). Also, a recent clinical trial showed that liposomal $PGE_1$ was ineffective.[150]

Inhaled nitric oxide can also improve oxygenation and lower pulmonary vascular pressure in patients with ARDS, but it does not lead to a sustained improvement in oxygenation as compared with conventional therapy,[674] and it has no beneficial effects on mortality.[675, 676] Similar improvements in oxygenation have been reported from limited experience with liposomal $PGE_1$[677] and aerosolized $PGI_2$ (prostacyclin).[678] Use of any of these drugs in acute lung injury cannot be recommended.

**Miscellaneous Agents.** Finally, numerous other pharmacologic agents have been suggested for the specific treatment of acute lung injuries. Most agents are proposed with an anti-inflammatory rationale. Examples include dapsone,[679, 680] mepacrine,[681] phenytoin,[682, 683] and polyethylene-glycol–conjugated superoxide dismutase.[684] Therapy with almitrine, which may be useful to reduce ventilation-perfusion abnormalities in acute lung injury, has also been suggested.[685] Many more experimental models would need to be studied and the pathophysiologic rationale would need to be strengthened before any of these agents could be proposed for clinical trials. Most of these drugs enjoy a long history of clinical use and thus would bypass the enormous start-up costs and clinical uncertainty that attend new technologies.

## OUTCOME

### Resolution of Edema

Much less is known about recovery from pulmonary edema than about its formation. Water (and extravasated proteins and cellular debris) must be removed from the alveoli and the interstitial spaces to restore the lungs to their normal condition. Edema could be cleared from the lungs by five routes: lymphatics, airways, blood vessels, pleural space, and mediastinum. Cellular debris and particulate matter must be removed from the alveoli by macrophages or must be coughed up and expectorated.

The considerable advances in our understanding of the clearance of fluid and solute from the alveoli have been the subject of many reviews.[8, 686–691] Active sodium transport across the alveolar epithelial barrier into the interstitium drives edema fluid removal from the air spaces. The uninjured alveolar epithelium has a remarkable ability to clear fluid from the air spaces rapidly: for example, serial edema fluid protein concentration measurements relative to simultaneous plasma protein concentrations in a salt-water near drowning patient showed that 50% to 60% of excess alveolar fluid in the lungs was removed over the course of just 4 hours.[142] In experimental studies in rabbits, instillation of 4 mg/kg of seawater into the lungs resulted in a 300% increase in alveolar fluid volume in less than 5 minutes from mostly pure water drawn in osmotically from the plasma by the hyperosmolar (881 ± 29 mOsm) instillate, 80% of which was cleared from the alveoli in 6 hours.[692] Equivalent volumes of iso-osmotic (292 ± 6 mOsm) saline instilled into rabbit lungs were cleared at a similar rate. In neither circumstance was there evidence of injury to the alveolar epithelial barrier, which has been found to be more resistant than the endothelial barrier to a wide range of injuries, including ischemia, alveolar and intravenous endotoxin and bacteria, alveolar endotoxin, intravenous oleic acid, acid aspiration, salt water aspiration, hyperoxia, intratracheal bleomycin, septic and hypovolemic shock, and rewarming after severe hypothermia.[8, 687] Even when mild-to-moderate alveolar injury occurs, the capacity to transport salt and water is often preserved; in severe injury, when the barrier is physically disrupted, the capacity to clear edema is lost, of course, and the vascular endothelium becomes the limiting barrier between the vascular and air spaces. Clinically, the ability to resorb some alveolar fluid (as indicated by increase in edema fluid to plasma protein concentration ratio) in the first 12 hours after the development of acute lung injury was a favorable prognostic finding in one study, associated with a mortality of only 20%; in contrast, the inability to resorb alveolar edema fluid early in the course of acute lung injury was associated with a mortality of nearly 80%.[394] Thus, the function of the alveolar epithelial barrier early in the course of acute lung injury may be a useful prognostic index, perhaps because it serves as a marker of the severity and the extent of lung injury.

Lung $Na^+,K^+$-ATPase activity was increased in rats recovering from experimental thiourea-induced increased permeability pulmonary edema.[693] Alveolar fluid clearance can be increased in uninjured, ex vivo human lungs by salmeterol,[694] and experimental studies have shown that alveolar fluid clearance can be increased pharmacologically (e.g., by catecholamines), even in the presence of acute lung injury and alveolar edema,[8, 687] raising the potential of therapy to hasten the resolution of alveolar edema. Whether such a strategy would be clinically useful remains to be determined.

Clearance of protein from flooded alveoli is much slower (1% to 2% per hour) than clearance of fluid (10% to 20% per hour),[686, 691, 695] concentrating the protein left behind.[394] The rising protein concentration in the alveoli as fluid is resorbed does not effect fluid clearance much, because precipitated protein exerts no osmotic pressure and the concentration of soluble macromolecules (a few mmol/L) is too small to counteract the differences in ion concentration resulting from transepithelial transport. Precipitation of protein as water is absorbed is the origin of hyaline membranes, which may serve as a framework for growth of fibrous tissue. Removal of fluid from flooded alveoli may be slowed, especially when vascular permeability is increased, if the fluid clots. Clotting can occur because extravasation of plasma into the air spaces may lead to activation of the clotting system by surfactant.[165, 194]

Fluid cleared from alveolar spaces into the alveolar wall interstitium could leave the lungs by flowing into the lymphatic capillaries or by moving down the prevailing pressure gradient into the loose peribronchovascular connective tissue spaces. Large amounts of fluid in the air spaces may be partially cleared into peribronchovascular cuffs through the hypothesized leaky terminal–airway epithelium,[696, 697] leaving alveolar fluid and solute behind to be cleared more slowly through the more impermeable alveolar epithelium.

Most of the interstitial water in pulmonary edema is in the peribronchovascular loose connective tissue spaces rather than in the alveolar walls. Because the lymphatic capillaries are arranged to drain only the alveolar wall interstitium, this route for edema removal is not significant for most interstitial water. A study in goats showed that lung lymph originated mainly from alveolar wall interstitial fluid; the contribution of the lung lymphatic system to the clearance of interstitial edema in bronchoalveolar cuffs and interlobular septa was small. The maximum possible contribution by lung lymphatics to the clearance of interstitial edema liquid was below 10%, and airway loss of liquid by evaporation was about twice the rate of lymphatic clearance.[698] In a study of in situ perfused sheep lungs with experimental low- and high-protein pulmonary edema, during recovery from pulmonary edema, interstitial liquid was resorbed into the circulation in inverse proportion to its protein concentration, and only a very small fraction of interstitial edema was cleared by the lung lymphatics during recovery from either type of edema.[699] Some fluid from the loose peribronchovascular interstitium may drain directly into the bloodstream by crossing the walls of blood vessels in the lungs: a study of isolated sheep lungs made edematous by raising vascular pressures showed that the primary route of edema clearance was by vascular resorption (60% of filtered water cleared over 3 hours, 42% by resorption into the bloodstream, 18% by lymphatic, pleural, and mediastinal drainage).[700] Edema may also drain into the pleural space. Pleural effusions are more common in increased pressure pulmonary edema (occurring in about 25% to 50% of patients, usually on the right side if the edema is unilateral) but are present in acute lung injuries as well (occurring in about 35% of patients).[701–703] Formation and removal of pleural effusions are discussed in detail in Chapters 73 and 74. As much as 25% to 30% of edema fluid may leave the lungs through the pleural space.[701, 704] A significant portion of the interstitial edema probably follows the prevailing pressure gradient in the lungs to drain into the mediastinum, where it could be picked up by initial lymphatics.

Short-term alveolar protein clearance appears to proceed primarily by paracellular diffusion and is size dependent.[705] Most proteins are cleared intact, not after being degraded into smaller fragments (although a few specific proteins, e.g., vasoactive intestinal peptide and gastrin, are degraded before being cleared). An albumin-binding protein (albondin) is expressed on lung microvascular endothelial cells, and an antibody to this protein reacts with cellular proteins of alveolar epithelial cells, which also appear to have albondin-like binding sites for albumin.[691] A polymeric immunoglobulin receptor has also been described. The significance of these receptors is unclear. The general consensus is that transcytosis (vectoral transport via vesicles) is not a major mechanism for clearing bulk quantities of albumin or other proteins from the alveolar space. Over the long term, cellular mechanisms, principally phagocytosis and catabolism by macrophages (and perhaps PMNs), account for most protein clearance from the alveolar space. All insoluble, precipitated proteins are removed in this way. Macrophages are also ultimately responsible for removing senescent and dead PMNs and other debris. The small ciliated surface area of the distal air spaces seems to indicate that the mucociliary route could account for only a minor fraction of alveolar protein clearance: although proteins might reach the mucociliary escalator along currents in the alveolar fluid layer, even were this to occur, removal would be very slow (half-time for mucociliary clearance of particles from the alveolar space is measured in days). Complete clearance of alveolar protein from pulmonary edema by any route is slow and may take weeks.

Little is known about the mechanisms and signals that regulate endothelial barrier function or how increased endothelial permeability is returned to normal.[706] The mechanisms of resolution of lung inflammation are also poorly understood.[707]

## Increased Pressure Edema

The outcome of increased pressure pulmonary edema is determined by the underlying cause and the skill of the physician's management. Because most increased pressure pulmonary edema is caused by heart disease, outcome is largely determined by the level of the patient's cardiac function. Patients with pulmonary edema that is uncomplicated by acute myocardial infarction can be expected to do well (mortality rate, <10%).[708] In the presence of acute myocardial infarction, the prognosis is much worse: the hospital mortality is 10% to 40% with accompanying acute pulmonary edema, rising to 50% to 100% when further complicated by hypoperfusion.[511, 709, 710] The advent of thrombolytic therapy has not improved the survival of patients with pulmonary edema complicating acute myocardial infarction.[711] Patients who recover from increased pressure pulmonary edema caused by cardiac disease require long-term outpatient management aimed at preventing recurrent episodes.

Some patients develop increased pressure pulmonary edema from noncardiac causes. Most cases are iatrogenic, being caused by massive volume overload or therapeutic misadventures with drugs that can affect cardiac function. This is a common cause of pulmonary edema in pregnant women, as discussed in Chapter 88. These patients can be expected to do well if the cause of the edema can be removed.

## Increased Permeability Edema

The incidence of acute lung injury is unknown. Many authors recite the National Institutes of Health's 1972 speculation that there are about 150,000 new cases each year (an incidence of about 75 cases per 100,000 population per year), but more recent estimates indicate this figure might have been too high.[712] The large numbers of patients enrolled in the NHLBI ARDS clinical trials since 1996, however, suggest that the original NIH estimate may have been the more accurate of the two.[150] Further data on incidence of acute respiratory failure and ARDS will be forthcoming from an ongoing epidemiologic study in Seattle. The outcome of acute lung injury and resultant increased permeability pulmonary edema is determined by the underlying cause, the extent of injury, and the skill with which the patient is managed. Death is considered to be the usual outcome in patients recognized as having ARDS: reported mortality rates range from 20% to 90% and are generally greater than 40% to 50%. Yearly ARDS mortality rates reported from a single institution in the decade between 1983 and 1993 showed a significant decrease over time occurring in patients younger than 60 years and in those with sepsis syndrome as their risk factor for development of ARDS decreased[713] and as the reported mortality in major epidemiologic or therapeutic trials of ARDS in the 20 years between 1975 and 1995 decreased.[356] If mortality is truly decreasing, the reasons why are obscure. The only sound conclusion that can be drawn is that historical controls cannot be used to evaluate the effects of new therapies or the value of current therapies. It is not certain what any mortality rates really mean, because no definition of ARDS has been uniformly accepted and applied, because patient populations vary widely, and because milder forms of acute lung injury and increased permeability pulmonary edema probably have been unrecognized.

Acute lung injury and increased permeability pulmonary edema are often complications that occur late in the natural history of other diseases and their aggressive treatment. The prognosis worsens as the number and the severity of underlying diseases increase.[362, 714, 715] Patients with sepsis have significantly higher mortality than patients with other clinical disorders associated with the development of acute lung injury.[362] Medical patients fare worse than surgical patients.[716] Mortality is much higher in patients with chronic liver disease[362] or histories of chronic alcohol abuse[717]; besides damaging the liver, chronic ethanol ingestion may reduce alveolar type II cell glutathione content and impair surfactant synthesis and secretion.[718] Mortality has been said to increase with age, but the increased mortality of older ARDS patients might be due to age bias that affects decisions to withdraw supportive care, not to the medical futility of life-sustaining therapies for older patients.[719] Respiratory deaths are less common than deaths from the underlying disease, from nonpulmonary organ dysfunction, or from infection.[243, 244, 362, 716] Superimposed pneumonia may be less common than has been supposed in patients with acute lung injuries,[341] and for patients who survive the initial condition precipitating lung injury, the final outcome may be related more to the magnitude and the duration of the host inflammatory response than to the development of nosocomial infection.[219, 245, 720] Patients seem more likely to die with, rather than of, nosocomial infections.[219] Patients with self-limited causes of injury (e.g., venous air emboli,[222] fat emboli,[721] isolated lung contusion and other trauma, massive blood transfusions, postictal pulmonary edema, heroin pulmonary edema) and those with milder degrees of edema have a greater chance of survival and often clear their edema rapidly (Fig. 54.3).

The long-term outlook for patients who survive diffuse lung injury, even if it is severe, is favorable.[722–726] Most recover to have normal chest roentgenograms, no complaints of dyspnea on exertion, normal lung volumes and air flow, and normal resting and exercise arterial blood

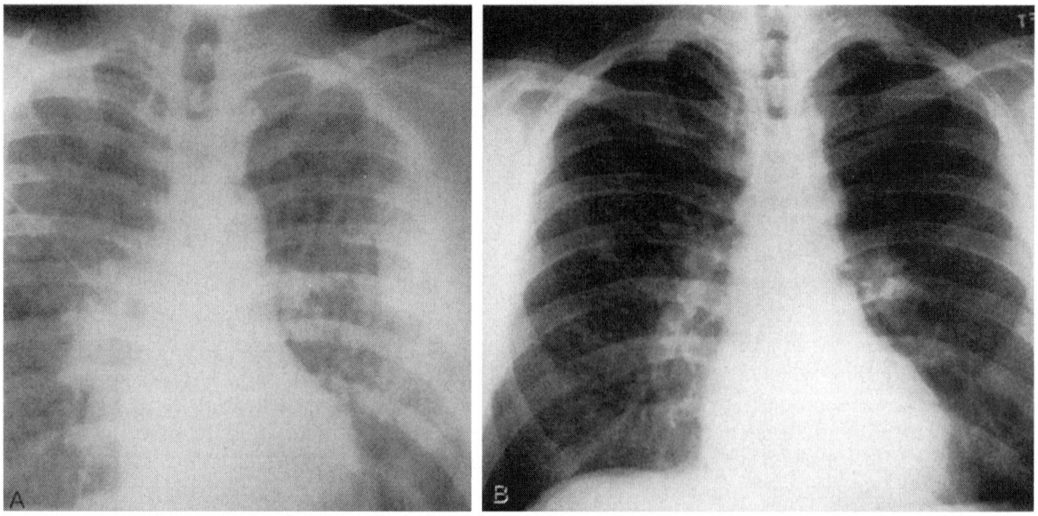


**Figure 54.3** Chest roentgenograms in a patient with heroin-induced increased permeability pulmonary edema. At the time of the initial film *(A)* the heart was not enlarged, the vascular pedicle was normal, and edema was patchy, peripheral, and not gravitationally distributed. Forty-eight hours later, the chest film *(B)* was normal, and the patient had fully recovered. Increased permeability pulmonary edema may resolve rapidly if the initiating agent of lung injury is transient and mild, and the chronic phase of parenchymal lung injury (type II cell hyperplasia, fibrosis, connective tissue deposition, vascular remodeling) does not develop.

gas findings and shunt calculation. Some patients have residual airway hyperreactivity. The most common abnormality is a reduced diffusing capacity, which tends to improve gradually. Not surprisingly, patients with the most days on positive pressure ventilation and those with the lowest static lung compliance during the course of their acute lung injuries are most likely to experience residual pulmonary impairment.[580] Laryngotracheal stenosis, likely a consequence of endotracheal intubation, should be ruled out in patients with persistent exertional dyspnea.[727] Histologic abnormalities may also gradually regress.

Healing often involves some degree of fibrosis.[728] The fibroproliferative reaction to acute lung injury seems to begin much earlier in the course of acute lung injury than has previously been appreciated.[217, 729] Fibrosis can be particularly severe with permanent compromise of respiratory function in patients who require the most aggressive supportive therapy to survive,[730] and patients who develop fibrosis are less likely to survive than those who do not.[731] How much of this problem is due to disease and how much to treatment is not known. It may be possible to modify vigorous fibrotic reactions to lung injury,[638, 732–735] but the consequences of such therapy are unknown. It might also be possible to accelerate reconstitution of alveolar structure in injured lungs: for example, keratinocyte growth factor/fibroblast growth factor-7, which promotes alveolar epithelial hyperplasia in vivo, reduced mortality when given to rats exposed to hyperoxia,[507, 736] and soluble and insoluble fibronectin increased alveolar wound healing in vitro.[737] More information about repair and healing might open new possibilities for therapy.[354, 507, 707, 738]

Although several pharmacologic therapies for ARDS have not been effective in decreasing mortality,[150] the nearly 20% reduction in mortality achieved with a lung protection ventilatory strategy represents a major advance in understanding how to prevent ventilator-induced worsening of lung injury in these patients.[584a]

## SUMMARY

Among the major advances since 1967 has been the acquisition of important new knowledge concerning the physiology of fluid and solute transport in healthy and diseased lungs. Pulmonary edema, or the abnormal accumulation of extravascular fluid, is a pathologic state that occurs when fluid is filtered in the lungs faster than it can be removed. The many causes of pulmonary edema have been grouped into two main pathophysiologic categories: increased pressure edema that results from an increase in the hydrostatic or osmotic forces (or both) that act across the barriers that normally restrict movement of fluid and solutes in the lungs, and increased permeability edema from acute lung injury that results in increased leakiness of those barriers. Although these two basically different types of pulmonary edema share many features, they should be distinguished clinically because they have considerably different treatment requirements and prognoses. This distinction is possible by careful clinical, radiologic, and physiologic evaluation as described in this chapter. Other causes of acute lung injury (e.g., infectious, immunologic, and chemical) are discussed elsewhere in this book.

## References

1. Staub NC: Pulmonary edema. Physiol Rev 54:678–811, 1974.
2. Taylor AE: Capillary fluid filtration: Starling forces and lymph flow. Circ Res 49:557–575, 1981.

3. Staub NC: Pathophysiology of pulmonary edema. *In* Staub NC, Taylor AE (eds): Edema. New York: Raven Press, 1984, pp 719–746.
4. Effros RM: Pulmonary microcirculation and exchange. *In* Renkin EM, Michel CC (eds): Handbook of Physiology. Section 2: The Cardiovascular System. Vol 4: Microcirculation (Part 2). Bethesda, MD: American Physiological Society, 1984, pp 865–915.
5. Taylor AE, Parker JC: Pulmonary interstitial spaces and lymphatics. *In* Fishman AP, Fisher AB (eds): Handbook of Physiology. Section 3: The Respiratory System. Vol 1: Circulation and Nonrespiratory Functions. Bethesda, MD: American Physiological Society, 1985, pp 167–230.
6. Lai-Fook SJ: Mechanical factors in lung liquid distribution. Annu Rev Physiol 55:155–179, 1993.
7. Bhattacharya J: Physiological basis of pulmonary edema. *In* Matthay MA, Ingbar DH (eds): Pulmonary Edema. New York: Marcel Dekker, 1998, pp 1–36.
8. Matthay MA, Folkesson HG, Verkman AS: Salt and water transport across alveolar and distal airway epithelia in the adult lung. Am J Physiol 270:L487–L503, 1996.
9. Matthay MA: Critical role of the alveolar epithelial barrier. *In* Evans TW, Haslett C (eds): ARDS: Acute Respiratory Distress in Adults. London: Chapman & Hall Medical, 1996, pp 345–357.
10. Staub NC: The pathogenesis of pulmonary edema. Prog Cardiovasc Dis 23:53–80, 1980.
11. Cowan GSM, Staub NC, Edmunds LH: Changes in the fluid compartments and dry weights of reimplanted dog lungs. J Appl Physiol 40:962–970, 1976.
12. Cross CE, Shaver JA, Wilson RJ, et al: Mitral stenosis and pulmonary fibrosis: Special reference to pulmonary edema and lung lymphatic function. Arch Intern Med 125:248–254, 1970.
13. Trapnell DH: Radiological appearances of lymphangitis carcinomatosa of the lung. Thorax 19:251–260, 1964.
14. Taylor AE: The lymphatic edema safety factor: The role of edema dependent lymphatic factors (EDLF). Lymphology 23:111–123, 1990.
15. Gropper MA, Wiener-Kronish JP, Hashimoto S: Acute cardiogenic pulmonary edema. Clin Chest Med 15:501–515, 1994.
16. Townsley MI: Hydrostatic pulmonary edema. *In* Matthay MA, Ingbar DH (eds): Pulmonary Edema. New York: Marcel Dekker, 1998, pp 163–202.
17. Erdmann AJ, Vaughan TR, Brigham KL, et al: Effect of increased vascular pressure on lung fluid balance in unanesthetized sheep. Circ Res 37:271–284, 1975.
18. Guyton AC, Lindsey AW: Effect of elevated left atrial pressure and decreased plasma protein concentration on the development of pulmonary edema. Circ Res 7:649–657, 1959.
19. Daluz PL, Shubia H, Weil JV: Pulmonary edema related to changes in colloid osmotic and pulmonary artery pressure in patients after acute myocardial infarction. Circulation 51:350–356, 1975.
20. Allen SJ, Drake RE, Laine GA, et al: Effect of thoracic duct drainage on hydrostatic pulmonary edema and pleural effusion in sheep. J Appl Physiol 71:314–316, 1991.
21. Drake RE, Dhother S, Teague RA, et al: Lymph flow in sheep with rapid cardiac ventricular pacing. Am J Physiol 272:R1595–R1598, 1997.
22. Uhley HN, Leeds SE, Sampson JJ, et al: Role of pulmonary lymphatics in chronic pulmonary edema. Circ Res 11:966–970, 1962.
23. Snapper JR: Lung mechanics in pulmonary edema. Clin Chest Med 6:393–412, 1985.
24. Javaheri S, Bosken CH, Lim SP, et al: Effects of hypohydration on lung function in humans. Am Rev Respir Dis 135:597–599, 1987.
25. Noble WH, Kay JC, Obdrzalek J: Lung mechanics in hypervolemic pulmonary edema. J Appl Physiol 38:681–687, 1975.
26. Lloyd TC: Reflex effects of left heart and pulmonary vascular distension on airways of dogs. J Appl Physiol 49:620–626, 1980.
27. Kikuchi R, Sekizawa K, Sasaki H, et al: Effects of pulmonary congestion on airway reactivity to histamine aerosol in dogs. J Appl Physiol 57:1640–1647, 1984.
28. Lemen R, Jones JG, Graf PD, et al: Closing volume changes in alloxan-induced pulmonary edema in anesthetized dogs. J Appl Physiol 39:235–241, 1975.
29. Klingele TG, Staub NC: Terminal bronchiole diameter changes with volume in isolated, air-filled lobes of cat lung. J Appl Physiol 30:224–227, 1971.
30. Michel RP, Zocchi L, Rossi A, et al: Does interstitial lung edema compress airways and arteries? A morphometric study. J Appl Physiol 62:108–115, 1987.
31. Emery DL, Shown B, Batra G, et al: Changes in collateral ventilation with increased vascular pressure and edema formation. J Appl Physiol 53:70–74, 1982.
32. Ploysongsang Y, Zocchi L, Michel RP, et al: Partitioning of respiratory mechanics in pulmonary interstitial edema in dogs (abstract). Fed Proc 44:1910, 1985.
33. Hughes JMB, Rosenzweig DY: Factors affecting trapped gas volume in perfused dog lungs. J Appl Physiol 29:332–339, 1970.
34. Cook CD, Mead J, Schreiner GL, et al: Pulmonary mechanics during induced pulmonary edema in anesthetized dogs. J Appl Physiol 14:177–186, 1959.
35. Said SI, Longacher JW, Davis RK, et al: Pulmonary gas exchange during induction of pulmonary edema in anesthetized dogs. J Appl Physiol 19:403–407, 1964.
36. Bernard GR, Pou NA, Coggeshall JW, et al: Comparison of the pulmonary dysfunction caused by cardiogenic and noncardiogenic pulmonary edema. Chest 108:798–803, 1995.
37. Bhattacharya J, Nakahara K, Staub NC: Effect of edema on pulmonary blood flow in the isolated perfused dog lung lobe. J Appl Physiol 48:444–449, 1980.
38. Negrini D: Pulmonary microvascular pressure profile during development of hydrostatic edema. Microcirculation 2:173–180, 1995.
39. Muir AL, Hogg JC, Naimark A, et al: Effect of alveolar liquid on distribution of blood flow in dog lungs. J Appl Physiol 39:885–890, 1975.
40. Hughes JMB, Glazier JB, Maloney JE, et al: Effect of extra-alveolar vessels on distribution of blood flow in the dog lung. J Appl Physiol 25:701–712, 1968.
41. Murray JF: Effects of lung inflation on pulmonary arterial pressure in dogs with pulmonary edema. J Appl Physiol 45:442–450, 1978.
42. Julien M, Hakim TS, Vahi R, et al: Effect of hematocrit on vascular pressure profile in dog lungs. J Appl Physiol 58:743–748, 1985.
43. Wang CG, Hakim TS, Michel RP, et al: Segmental pulmonary vascular resistance in progressive hydrostatic and permeability edema. J Appl Physiol 59:242–247, 1985.
44. Muir AL, Hall DL, Despas P, et al: Distribution of blood flow in the lungs in acute pulmonary edema in dogs. J Appl Physiol 33:763–769, 1972.
45. Raj JU, Bland RD, Lai-Fook SJ: Microvascular pressures measured by micropipettes in isolated edematous rabbit lungs. J Appl Physiol 60:539–545, 1986.
46. Hovig T, Nicolaysen A, Nicolaysen G: Ultrastructural studies of the alveolar-capillary barrier in isolated plasma-perfused rabbit lungs: Effects of EDTA and of increased capillary pressure. Acta Physiol Scand 82:417–431, 1971.
47. De Fouw DO, Berendsen PB: Morphological changes in isolated perfused dog lungs after acute hydrostatic edema. Circ Res 43:72–82, 1978.
48. Coalson JJ, Jaques WW, Campbell GS, et al: Ultrastructure of the alveolar-capillary membrane in congenital and acquired heart disease. Arch Pathol 83:377–391, 1967.
49. Hurley JV: Types of pulmonary microvascular injury. Ann NY Acad Sci 384:269–285, 1982.
50. Bachofen H, Bachofen M, Weibel ER: Ultrastructural aspects of pulmonary edema. J Thorac Imaging 3:1–7, 1988.
51. Davies SW, Wilkinson P, Keegan J, et al: Pulmonary microvascular permeability in patients with severe mitral stenosis. Br Heart J 65:89–93, 1991.
52. Davies SW, Bailey J, Keegan J, et al: Reduced pulmonary microvascular permeability in severe chronic left heart failure. Am Heart J 124:137–142, 1992.
53. Townsley MI, Fu Z, Mathieu-Costello O, et al: Pulmonary microvascular permeability: Responses to high vascular pressure after induction of pacing-induced heart failure in dogs. Circ Res 77:317–325, 1995.
54. Felson B: Thoracic calcifications. Chest 56:330–343, 1969.

55. Bachofen H, Schürch S, Michel RP, et al: Experimental hydrostatic pulmonary edema in rabbit lungs: Morphology. Am Rev Respir Dis 147:989–996, 1993.
56. Bachofen H, Schürch S, Weibel ER: Experimental hydrostatic pulmonary edema in rabbit lungs: Barrier lesions. Am Rev Respir Dis 147:997–1004, 1993.
57. Staub NC, Nagano H, Pearce ML: Pulmonary edema in dogs, especially the sequence of fluid accumulation in lungs. J Appl Physiol 22:227–240, 1967.
58. Albertine K: Histopathology of pulmonary edema and the acute respiratory distress syndrome. *In* Matthay MA, Ingbar DH (eds): Pulmonary Edema. New York: Marcel Dekker, 1998, pp 37–83.
59. Crapo JD: New concepts in the formation of pulmonary edema. Am Rev Respir Dis 147:790–792, 1993.
60. Qiao RL, Ying X, Bhattacharya J: Effects of hyperoncotic albumin on endothelial barrier properties of rat lung. Am J Physiol 265:H198–H204, 1993.
61. Wu DXY, Weibel ER, Bachofen H, et al: Lung lesions in experimental hydrostatic pulmonary edema: An electron microscopic and morphometric study. Exp Lung Res 21:711–730, 1995.
62. Abroug F, Ayari M, Nouira S, et al: Assessment of left ventricular function in severe scorpion envenomation: Combined hemodynamic and echo-Doppler study. Intensive Care Med 21:629–635, 1995.
63. Nouira S, Abroug F, Haguiga H, et al: Right ventricular dysfunction following severe scorpion envenomation. Chest 108:682–687, 1995.
64. Chamberlain JJ, Abolnik IZ: Pulmonary edema following a licorice binge. West J Med 167:184–185, 1997.
65. Schraufnagel DE, Patel KR: Sphincters in pulmonary veins: An anatomic study in rats. Am Rev Respir Dis 141:721–726, 1990.
66. Sande MA, Alonso DR, Smith JP, et al: Left atrial tumor presenting with hemoptysis and pulmonary infiltrates. Am Rev Respir Dis 102:258–263, 1970.
67. Charan NB, Turk GM, Hey DH: Effect of increased bronchial venous pressure on lung lymph flow. J Appl Physiol 59:1249–1253, 1985.
68. Lang SA, Maron MB: Hemodynamic basis for cocaine-induced pulmonary edema in dogs. J Appl Physiol 71:1166–1170, 1991.
69. Kato M, Staub NC: Response of small pulmonary arteries to unilobar hypoxia and hypercapnia. Circ Res 19:426–440, 1966.
70. Bland RD, Demling RH, Selinger SL, et al: Effects of alveolar hypoxia on lung fluid and protein transport in unanesthetized sheep. Circ Res 40:269–274, 1977.
71. Landolt CC, Matthay MA, Albertine KH, et al: Overperfusion, hypoxia, and increased pressure cause only hydrostatic pulmonary edema in anesthetized sheep. Circ Res 52:335–341, 1983.
72. van der Werff YD, van der Houwen HK, Heijmans PJM, et al: Postpneumonectomy pulmonary edema: A retrospective analysis of incidence and possible risk factors. Chest 111:1278–1284, 1997.
73. Bärtsch P: High altitude pulmonary edema. Respiration 64:435–443, 1997.
74. Hultgren HN: High-altitude pulmonary edema. *In* Matthay MA, Ingbar DH (eds): Pulmonary Edema. New York: Marcel Dekker, 1998, pp 355–378.
75. Hackett PH, Bertman J, Rodriguez G, et al: Pulmonary edema fluid protein in high-altitude pulmonary edema. JAMA 256:36, 1986.
76. Schoene RB, Swenson ER, Pizzo CJ, et al: The lung at high altitude: Bronchoalveolar lavage in acute mountain sickness and pulmonary edema. J Appl Physiol 64:2605–2613, 1988.
77. Matthay MA, Landolt CC, Staub NC: Differential liquid and protein clearance from the alveoli of anesthetized sheep. J Appl Physiol 53:96–104, 1982.
78. Matthay MA, Berthiaume Y, Staub NC: Long-term clearance of liquid and protein from the lungs of unanesthetized sheep. J Appl Physiol 59:928–934, 1985.
79. West JB, Colice GL, Lee Y-J, et al: Pathogenesis of high-altitude pulmonary oedema: Direct evidence of stress failure of pulmonary capillaries. Eur Respir J 8:523–529, 1995.
80. West JB, Mathieu-Costello O: Vulnerability of pulmonary capillaries in heart disease. Circulation 92:622–631, 1995.
80a. West JBV, Mathiea-Costello O: Structure, strength, failure, and remodeling of the pulmonary blood-gas barrier. Annu Rev Physiol 61:543–572, 1999.
81. Huchon GJ, Hopewell PC, Murray JF: Interactions between permeability and hydrostatic pressure in perfused dogs' lungs. J Appl Physiol 50:905–911, 1981.
82. Jerome EH, Severinghaus JW: High-altitude pulmonary edema. N Engl J Med 334:662–663, 1996.
83. Grissom CK, Zimmerman GA, Whatley RE: Endothelial selectins in acute mountain sickness and high-altitude pulmonary edema. Chest 112:1572–1578, 1997.
84. Hanaoka M, Kubo K, Yamazaki Y, et al: Association of high-altitude pulmonary edema with the major histocompatibility complex. Circulation 97:1124–1128, 1998.
85. Hirai K, Kobayashi T, Kubo K, et al: Effects of denitrogenation on lung fluid balance in awake sheep under 6600m-simulated altitude (abstract). Am Rev Respir Dis 131:A412, 1985.
86. Flick MR, Perel A, Staub NC: Leukocytes are required for increased lung microvascular permeability after microembolization in sheep. Circ Res 48:344–351, 1981.
87. Kleger G-R, Bärtsch P, Vock P, et al: Evidence against an increase in capillary permeability in subjects exposed to high altitude. J Appl Physiol 81:1917–1923, 1996.
88. Kubo K, Hanaoka M, Hayano T, et al: Inflammatory cytokines in BAL fluid and pulmonary hemodynamics in high-altitude pulmonary edema. Respir Physiol 111:301–310, 1998.
89. Maron MB, Pilati CF: Neurogenic pulmonary edema. *In* Matthay MA, Ingbar DH (eds): Pulmonary Edema. New York: Marcel Dekker, 1998, pp 319–354.
90. Smith WS, Matthay MA: Evidence for a hydrostatic mechanism in human neurogenic pulmonary edema. Chest 111:1326–1333, 1997.
91. Maron MB: Analysis of airway fluid protein concentration in neurogenic pulmonary edema. J Appl Physiol 62:470–476, 1987.
92. Simon RP, Bayne LL, Tranbaugh RF, et al: Elevated pulmonary lymph flow and protein content during status epilepticus in sheep. J Appl Physiol 52:91–95, 1982.
93. Jones TA, Townsley MI, Weidner WJ: Effects of intracranial and left atrial hypertension on lung fluid balance in sheep. J Appl Physiol 52:1324–1329, 1982.
94. Simon RP, Bayne LL, Naughton MP: Left atrial pressure elevation recreates the altered lung lymph flow of seizures. J Appl Physiol 53:432–435, 1982.
95. van der Zee H, Neumann PH, Minnear FL, et al: Effects of transient intracranial hypertension on lung fluid and protein exchange. J Appl Physiol 54:178–184, 1983.
96. Peterson BT, Ross JC, Brigham KL: Effect of naloxone on the pulmonary vascular responses to graded levels of intracranial hypertension in anesthetized sheep. Am Rev Respir Dis 128:1024–1029, 1983.
97. Minnear FL, Barie PS, Malik AB: Effects of transient pulmonary hypertension on pulmonary vascular permeability. J Appl Physiol 55:983–989, 1983.
98. Luce JM, Huseby JS, Robertson HT: Increasing intracranial pressure with air causes air embolism, not neurogenic pulmonary edema. J Appl Physiol 50:967–970, 1981.
99. Townsley MI, McClure DE, Weidner WJ: Assessment of pulmonary microvascular permeability in acutely prepared sheep. J Appl Physiol 56:857–861, 1984.
100. Kallet RH, Daniel BM, Gropper M, et al: Acute pulmonary edema following upper airway obstruction: Case reports and brief review. Respir Care 43:476–480, 1998.
101. Vandyke WH, Cure J, Chakko CS, et al: Pulmonary edema after pericardiocentesis for cardiac tamponade. N Engl J Med 309:395–396, 1983.
102. Shenoy MM, Dhar S, Gittin R, et al: Pulmonary edema following pericardiotomy for cardiac tamponade. Chest 86:647–648, 1984.
103. Miller WC, Toon R, Palat H, et al: Experimental pulmonary edema following re-expansion of pneumothorax. Am Rev Respir Dis 108:664–666, 1973.
104. Pavlin J, Cheney FW: Unilateral pulmonary edema in rabbits after reexpansion of collapsed lung. J Appl Physiol 46:31–35, 1979.
105. Trapnell DH, Thurston JGB: Unilateral pulmonary oedema after pleural aspiration. Lancet 1:1367–1369, 1970.
106. Shaw TJ, Caterine JM: Recurrent re-expansion pulmonary edema. Chest 86:784–786, 1984.

107. Libraty DH: Reexpansion pulmonary edema in AIDS. West J Med 156:657–659, 1992.
108. Woodring JH: Focal reexpansion pulmonary edema after drainage of large pleural effusions: Clinical evidence suggesting hypoxic injury to the lung as the cause of edema. South Med J 90:1176–1182, 1997.
109. Marland AM, Glauser FL: Hemodynamic and pulmonary edema protein measurements in a case of reexpansion pulmonary edema. Chest 81:250–251, 1982.
110. Suzuki S, Tanita T, Koike K, et al: Evidence of acute inflammatory response in reexpansion pulmonary edema. Chest 101:275–276, 1992.
111. Wilkinson PD, Keegan J, Davies SW, et al: Changes in pulmonary microvascular permeability accompanying re-expansion oedema: Evidence from dual isotope scintigraphy. Thorax 45:456–459, 1990.
112. Pavlin DJ, Nessly ML, Cheney FW: Increased pulmonary vascular permeability as a cause of re-expansion edema in rabbits. Am Rev Respir Dis 124:422–427, 1981.
113. Jackson RM, Veal CF, Alexander CB, et al: Re-expansion pulmonary edema: A potential role for free radicals in its pathogenesis. Am Rev Respir Dis 137:1165–1171, 1988.
114. Jackson RM, Veal CF, Alexander CB, et al: Neutrophils in reexpansion pulmonary edema. J Appl Physiol 65:228–234, 1988.
115. Jackson RM, Brannen AL, Veal CF, et al: Superoxide dismutase and cytochrome oxidase in collapsed lungs: Possible role in reexpansion edema. J Appl Physiol 65:235–241, 1988.
116. Jackson RM, Veal CF, Beckman JS, et al: Polyethylene glycol-conjugated superoxide dismutase in unilateral lung injury due to re-expansion (re-oxygenation). Am J Med Sci 300:22–28, 1990.
117. Yamazaki S, Ogawa J, Shohzu A, et al: Pulmonary blood flow to rapidly reexpanded lung in spontaneous pneumothorax. Chest 81:118–120, 1982.
118. Heffner JE: Mechanisms underlying ischemia/reperfusion injury of the lung. *In* Matthay MA, Ingbar DH (eds): Pulmonary Edema. New York: Marcel Dekker, 1998, pp 379–412.
119. Allison RC, Kyle J, Adkins WK, et al: Effect of ischemia reperfusion or hypoxia reoxygenation on lung vascular permeability and resistance. J Appl Physiol 69:597–603, 1990.
120. Ward BJ, Pearse DB: Reperfusion pulmonary edema after thrombolytic therapy of massive pulmonary embolism. Am Rev Respir Dis 138:1308–1311, 1988.
121. Modelska K, Pittet J-F: Increased-permeability edema following hemorrhagic and traumatic shock. *In* Matthay MA, Ingbar DH (eds): Pulmonary Edema. New York: Marcel Dekker, 1998, pp 299–318.
122. Albert RK, Lakshminarayan S, Hildebrandt J, et al: Increased surface tension favors pulmonary edema formation in anesthetized dogs' lungs. J Clin Invest 63:1015–1018, 1979.
123. Beck KC, Lai-Fook SJ: Alveolar liquid pressure in excised edematous dog lung with increased static recoil. J Appl Physiol 55:1277–1283, 1983.
124. Dodek PM, Rice TW, Bonsignore MR, et al: Effects of plasmapheresis and of hypoproteinemia on lung liquid conductance in awake sheep. Circ Res 58:269–280, 1986.
125. Parker RE, Wickersham NE, Roselli RJ, et al: Effects of hypoproteinemia on lung microvascular protein sieving and lung lymph flow. J Appl Physiol 60:1293–1299, 1986.
126. Conhaim RL, McGrath AM, Harms BA: Does plasma protein depletion increase lung liquid conductance? Am J Respir Crit Care Med 153:677–683, 1996
127. Dodek P: Does plasma protein depletion increase lung liquid conductance? Am J Respir Crit Care Med 154:1213–1215, 1996.
128. Parker JC, Falgout HJ, Parker RE, et al: The effect of fluid volume loading on exclusion of interstitial albumin and lymph flow in the dog lung. Circ Res 45:440–450, 1979.
129. Parker JC, Falgout HJ, Grimbert FA, et al: The effect of increased vascular pressure on albumin-excluded volume and lymph flow in the dog lung. Circ Res 47:866–875, 1980.
130. Pou NA, Roselli RJ, Parker RE, et al: Effects of air embolism on sheep lung fluid volumes. J Appl Physiol 75:986–993, 1993.
131. Conhaim RL, McGrath AM, Cooler SD, et al: Lung lymph oncotic pressure may not modulate pulmonary vascular filtration in sheep. Am J Respir Crit Care Med 155:971–977, 1997.
132. Bhattacharya J, Groper MA, Staub NC: Interstitial fluid pressure gradient measured by micropuncture in excised dog lung. J Appl Physiol 56:271–277, 1984.
133. Lai-Fook SJ: Mechanics of lung fluid balance. Crit Rev Biomed Eng 13:171–200, 1986.
134. Lai-Fook SJ, Beck KC: Alveolar liquid pressure measured by micropipettes in isolated dog lung. J Appl Physiol 53:737–743, 1982.
135. Nieman GF, Bredenberg CE: High surface tension pulmonary edema induced by detergent aerosol. J Appl Physiol 58:129–136, 1985.
136. Bredenberg CE, Nieman GF, Paskanik AM, et al: Microvascular membrane permeability in high surface tension pulmonary edema. J Appl Physiol 60:253–259, 1986.
137. Bachofen H, Gehr P, Weibel ER: Alterations of mechanical properties and morphology in excised rabbit lungs rinsed with a detergent. J Appl Physiol 47:1002–1010, 1979.
138. Wang C-Z, Barrow RE, Cox CS, et al: Influence of detergent aerosol on lung microvascular permeability. J Appl Physiol 74:1016–1023, 1993.
139. Said SI, Avery ME, Davis RK, et al: Pulmonary surface activity in induced pulmonary edema. J Clin Invest 44:458–464, 1965.
140. Seeger W, Wolf HRD, Stahler G, et al: Alteration of pressure-volume characteristics due to different types of edema induction in isolated rabbit lungs. Respiration 44:273–281, 1983.
141. Goerke J, Clements JA: Alveolar surface tension and lung surfactant. *In* Macklem PT, Mead J (eds): Handbook of Physiology. Section 3: The Respiratory System. Vol 3: Mechanics of Breathing (Part 1). Bethesda, MD: American Physiological Society, 1986, pp 247–261.
142. Cohen DS, Matthay MA, Cogan MG, et al: Pulmonary edema associated with salt water near-drowning: New insights. Am Rev Respir Dis 146:794–796, 1992.
143. Folkesson HG, Effros RM: Aspiration syndromes: Acid, salt water, and fresh water. *In* Matthay MA, Ingbar DH (eds): Pulmonary Edema. New York: Marcel Dekker, 1998, pp 269–297.
144. Ashbaugh DG, Bigelow DB, Petty TL, et al: Acute respiratory distress in adults. Lancet 2:319–323, 1967.
145. Murray JF: Introduction and definition. *In* Evans TW, Haslett C (eds): ARDS: Acute Respiratory Distress in Adults. London: Chapman & Hall Medical, 1996, pp 3–12.
146. Osborne ML, Meyer RJ: Epidemiology. *In* Evans TW, Haslett C (eds): ARDS: Acute Respiratory Distress in Adults. London: Chapman & Hall Medical, 1996, pp 13–23.
147. Kollef MH, Schuster DP: The acute respiratory distress syndrome. N Engl J Med 332:27–37, 1995.
148. Fulkerson WJ, MacIntyre N, Stamler J, et al: Pathogenesis and treatment of the adult respiratory distress syndrome. Arch Intern Med 156:29–38, 1996.
149. Luce JM: Acute lung injury and the acute respiratory distress syndrome. Crit Care Med 26:369–376, 1998.
150. Ware LB, Matthay MA: The acute respiratory distress syndrome. N Engl J Med, in press.
151. Cope DK, Grimbert F, Downey JM, et al: Pulmonary capillary pressure: A review. Crit Care Med 20:1043–1056, 1992.
152. Robbins IM, Newman JH, Brigham KL: Increased-permeability pulmonary edema from sepsis/endotoxin. *In* Matthay MA, Ingbar DH (eds): Pulmonary Edema. New York: Marcel Dekker, 1998, pp 203–245.
153. Gorin AB, Stewart PA: Differential permeability of endothelial and epithelial barriers to albumin flux. J Appl Physiol 47:1315–1324, 1979.
154. Montaner JSG, Tsang J, Evans KG, et al: Alveolar epithelial damage: A critical difference between high pressure and oleic acid-induced low pressure pulmonary edema. J Clin Invest 77:1786–1796, 1986.
155. Pelosi P, Cereda M, Foti G, et al: Alterations of lung and chest wall mechanics in patients with acute lung injury: Effects of positive end-expiratory pressure. Am J Respir Crit Care Med 152:531–537, 1995.
156. Grossman RF, Jones JG, Murray JF: Effects of oleic acid-induced pulmonary edema on lung mechanics. J Appl Physiol 48:1045–1051, 1980.
157. Slutsky AS, Scharf SM, Brown R, et al: The effect of oleic acid-induced pulmonary edema on pulmonary and chest wall mechanics in dogs. Am Rev Respir Dis 121:91–96, 1980.

256. Brogden KA, Cutlip RC, Lehmkuhl HD: Response of sheep after localized deposition of lipopolysaccharide in the lung. Exp Lung Res 7:123–132, 1984.
257. Crocker SH, Eddy DO, Obenauf RN, et al: Bacteremia: Host-specific lung clearance and pulmonary failure. J Trauma 21:215–219, 1981.
258. Guenter CA: Role of leukocytes in the lung after endotoxin administration. Adv Exp Med Biol 23:77–85, 1971.
259. Kinnebrew PS, Parker JC, Falgout HJ, et al: Pulmonary microvascular permeability following *E. coli* endotoxin and hemorrhage. J Appl Physiol 52:403–409, 1982.
260. Chang JC, Lesser M: Quantification of leukocytes in bronchoalveolar lavage samples from rats after intravascular injection of endotoxin. Am Rev Respir Dis 129:72–75, 1984.
261. Heflin AC, Brigham KL: Prevention by granulocyte depletion of increased vascular permeability of sheep lung following endotoxemia. J Clin Invest 68:1253–1260, 1981.
262. Michie HR, Manogue KR, Spriggs DR, et al: Detection of circulating tumor necrosis factor after endotoxin administration. N Engl J Med 318:1481–1486, 1988.
263. Spannhake EW, Colombo JL, Craigo PA, et al: Evidence for modification of pulmonary cyclooxygenase activity by endotoxin in the dog. J Appl Physiol 54:191–198, 1983.
264. Thomas PD, Hampson FW, Hunninghake GW: Bacterial adherence to human endothelial cells. J Appl Physiol 65:1372–1376, 1988.
265. Parsons PE, Worthen GS, Moore EE, et al: The association of circulating endotoxin with the development of the adult respiratory distress syndrome. Am Rev Respir Dis 140:294–301, 1989.
266. LaForce FM, Mullane JF, Boehme RF, et al: The effect of pulmonary edema on antibacterial defenses of the lung. J Lab Clin Med 82:634–648, 1973.
267. Mullane JF, LaForce FM, Huber GL: Variations in lung water and pulmonary host defense mechanisms. Am Surg 39:630–636, 1973.
268. Esrig BC, Fulton RL: Sepsis, resuscitated hemorrhagic shock and shock lung: An experimental correlation. Ann Surg 182:218–227, 1975.
269. Campbell GD, Coalson JJ, Johanson WG: The effect of bacterial superinfection on lung function after diffuse alveolar damage. Am Rev Respir Dis 129:974–978, 1984.
270. Seidenfeld JJ, Mullins RC, Fowler SR, et al: Bacterial infection and acute lung injury in hamsters. Am Rev Respir Dis 134:22–26, 1986.
271. Johanson WG, Higuchi JH, Woods DE, et al: Dissemination of *Pseudomonas aeruginosa* during lung infection in hamsters: Role of oxygen-induced lung injury. Am Rev Respir Dis 132:358–361, 1985.
272. Pison U, Obertacke U, Brand M, et al: Altered pulmonary surfactant in uncomplicated and septicemia-complicated courses of acute respiratory failure. J Trauma 30:19–26, 1990.
273. Coonrod JD, Lester RL, Hsu LC: Characterization of the extracellular bactericidal factors of rat alveolar lining material. J Clin Invest 74:1269–1279, 1984.
274. Morton NS: Exogenous surfactant treatment for the adult respiratory distress syndrome? A historical perspective. Thorax 45:825–830, 1990.
275. Jonsson S, Musher DM, Goree A, et al: Human alveolar lining material and antibacterial defenses. Am Rev Respir Dis 133:136–140, 1986.
276. Shennib H, Chiu RC, Mulder DS, et al: Pulmonary bacterial clearance and alveolar macrophage function in septic shock lung. Am Rev Respir Dis 130:444–449, 1984.
277. Martin TR, Pistorese BP, Hudson LD, et al: The function of lung and blood neutrophils in patients with the adult respiratory distress syndrome: Implications for the pathogenesis of lung infections. Am Rev Respir Dis 144:254–262, 1991.
278. Chollet-Martin S, Jourdain B, Gilbert C, et al: Interactions between neutrophils and cytokines in blood and alveolar spaces during ARDS. Am J Respir Crit Care Med 153:594–601, 1996.
279. Esposito AL: Aspirin impairs antibacterial mechanisms in experimental pneumococcal pneumonia. Am Rev Respir Dis 130:857–862, 1984.
280. Nelson S, Summer WR, Jakab GJ: Aminophylline-induced suppression of pulmonary antibacterial defenses. Am Rev Respir Dis 131:923–927, 1985.
281. Gadek JE, Pacht ER: The interdependence of lung antioxidants and antiprotease defense in ARDS. Chest 110:273S–277S, 1996.
282. Ward PA, Hunninghake GW: Lung inflammation and fibrosis. Am J Respir Crit Care Med 157:S123–S129, 1998.
283. Sibille Y, Reynolds HY: Macrophages and polymorphonuclear neutrophils in lung defense and injury. Am Rev Respir Dis 141:471–501, 1990.
284. Gee MH, Albertine KH: Neutrophil-endothelial cell interactions in the lung. Annu Rev Physiol 55:227–248, 1993.
285. Heffner JE, Repine JE: Pulmonary strategies of antioxidant defense. Am Rev Respir Dis 140:531–554, 1989.
286. Warner AE, Brain JD: The cell biology and pathogenic role of pulmonary intravascular macrophages. Am J Physiol 258:L1–L12, 1990.
287. Hällgren R, Samuelsson T, Venge P, et al: Eosinophil activation in the lung is related to lung damage in adult respiratory distress syndrome. Am Rev Respir Dis 135:639–642, 1987.
288. Allen JN, Davis WB, Pacht ER: Diagnostic significance of increased bronchoalveolar lavage fluid eosinophils. Am Rev Respir Dis 142:642–647, 1990.
289. Rowen JL, Hyde DM, McDonald RJ: Eosinophils cause acute edematous injury in isolated perfused rat lungs. Am Rev Respir Dis 142:215–220, 1990.
290. Hoidal JR: The eosinophil and acute lung injury. Am Rev Respir Dis 142:1245–1246, 1990.
291. MacNee W, Selby C: Neutrophil kinetics in the lungs. Clin Sci 79:97–107, 1990.
292. Hogg JC, Doerschuk CM: Leukocyte traffic in the lung. Annu Rev Physiol 57:97–114, 1995.
293. Mulligan MS, Varani J, Dame MK, et al: Role of endothelial-leukocyte adhesion molecule (ELAM-1) in neutrophil-mediated lung injury in rats. J Clin Invest 88:1396–1406, 1991.
294. Albelda SM: Endothelial and epithelial cell adhesion molecules. Am J Respir Cell Mol Biol 4:195–203, 1991.
295. Harlan JM, Vedder NB, Winn RK, et al: Mechanisms and consequences of leukocyte-endothelial interaction. West J Med 155:365–369, 1991.
296. Nagase T, Ohga E, Sudo E, et al: Intercellular adhesion molecule-1 mediates acid aspiration-induced lung injury. Am J Respir Crit Care Med 154:504–510, 1996.
297. Weiss SJ: Tissue destruction by neutrophils. N Engl J Med 320:365–376, 1989.
298. Cochrane CG: Cellular injury by oxidants. Am J Med 91(Suppl 3C):23S–30S, 1991.
299. Ward PA: Mechanisms of endothelial cell killing by $H_2O_2$ or products of activated neutrophils. Am J Med 91(Suppl 3C):89S–94S, 1991.
300. Deby-Dupont G, Lamy M, Faymonville ME, et al: Proteases and antiproteases in the adult respiratory distress syndrome. *In* Zapol WM, Lemaire F (eds): Adult Respiratory Distress Syndrome. New York: Marcel Dekker, 1991, pp 305–352.
301. Chang S-W, Voelkel NF: Charge-related lung microvascular injury. Am Rev Respir Dis 139:534–545, 1989.
302. Gallin JI: Neutrophil specific granules: A fuse that ignites the inflammatory response. Clin Res 32:320–328, 1984.
303. Kelley J: Cytokines of the lung. Am Rev Respir Dis 141:765–788, 1990.
304. Luster AD: Chemokines: Chemotactic cytokines that mediate inflammation. N Engl J Med 338:436–445, 1998.
305. Glauser FL, Fairman RP: The uncertain role of the neutrophil in increased permeability pulmonary edema. Chest 88:601–607, 1985.
306. Laufe MD, Simon RH, Flint A, et al: Adult respiratory distress syndrome in neutropenic patients. Am J Med 80:1022–1026, 1986.
307. Maunder RJ, Hackman RC, Riff E, et al: Occurrence of the adult respiratory distress syndrome in neutropenic patients. Am Rev Respir Dis 133:313–316, 1986.
308. Nelson S, Belknap SM, Carlson RW, et al: A randomized controlled trial of filgastrim as an adjunct to antibiotics for treatment of hospitalized patients with community-acquired pneumonia. J Infect Dis 178:1075–1080, 1998.
309. Fairman RP, Glauser FL, Falls R: Increases in lung lymph and albumin clearance with ethchlorvynol. J Appl Physiol 50:1151–1155, 1981.

310. Hofman WF, Ehrhart IC: Permeability edema in dog lung depleted of blood components. J Appl Physiol 57:147–153, 1984.
311. Schwartz JS, Spragg RG, Loomis WH, et al: Oleic acid causes high permeability edema in blood-free perfused rabbit lungs (abstract). Clin Res 30:74A, 1982.
312. Martin WJ, Gadek JE, Hunninghake GW, et al: Oxidant injury of lung parenchymal cells. J Clin Invest 68:1277–1288, 1981.
313. Skillrud DM, Martin WJ: Paraquat-induced injury of type II alveolar cells. Am Rev Respir Dis 129:995–999, 1984.
314. Martin WJ: Nitrofurantoin: Evidence for the oxidant injury of lung parenchymal cells. Am Rev Respir Dis 127:482–486, 1983.
315. Schwartz BA, Niewoehner DE, Hoidal JR: Neutrophil depletion does not protect rats from hyperoxic lung injury (abstract). Clin Res 31:746A, 1983.
316. Bowman CM, Butler EN, Repine JE: Hyperoxia damages cultured endothelial cells causing increased neutrophil adherence. Am Rev Respir Dis 128:469–472, 1983.
317. Lindquist P, Saldeen T, Sandler H: Pulmonary damage following pulmonary microembolism in the dog: Effect of various types of treatment. Acta Clin Scand 142:15–19, 1976.
318. Gaynor E: The role of granulocytes in endotoxin-induced vascular injury. Blood 41:797–808, 1973.
319. Pingleton WW, Coalson JJ, Guenter CA: Significance of leukocytes in endotoxin shock (abstract). Clin Res 19:683, 1971.
320. Meyrick B, Berry LC, Christman BW: Response of cultured human pulmonary artery endothelial cells to endotoxin. Am J Physiol 268:L239–L244, 1995.
321. Pingleton WW, Coalson JJ, Guenter CA: Significance of leukocytes in endotoxic shock. Exp Mol Pathol 22:183–194, 1975.
322. Johnson KJ, Ward PA: Acute and progressive lung injury after contact with phorbol myristate acetate. Am J Pathol 107:29–35, 1982.
323. Dyer EL, Snapper JR: Role of circulating granulocytes in sheep lung injury produced by phorbol myristate acetate. J Appl Physiol 60:576–589, 1986.
324. Hamasaki Y, Mojarad M, Saga T, et al: Platelet-activating factor raises airway and vascular pressures and induces edema in lungs perfused with platelet-free solution. Am Rev Respir Dis 129:742–746, 1984.
325. Eiermann GJ, Dickey BF, Thrall RS: Polymorphonuclear leukocyte participation in acute oleic acid-induced lung injury. Am Rev Respir Dis 128:845–850, 1983.
326. Tahamont MV, Malik AB: Granulocytes mediate the increase in pulmonary vascular permeability after thrombin embolism. J Appl Physiol 54:1489–1495, 1983.
327. Heath CA, Lai L, Bizios R, et al: Pulmonary hemodynamic effects of antisheep serum-induced leukopenia. J Leukoc Biol 39:385–397, 1986.
328. Shasby DM, VanBenthuysen KM, Tate RM, et al: Granulocytes mediate acute edematous lung injury in rabbits and isolated rabbit lungs perfused with phorbol myristate acetate: Role of oxygen radicals. Am Rev Respir Dis 125:443–447, 1982.
329. Shasby DM, Fox RB, Harada RN, et al: Reduction of the edema of acute hyperoxic lung injury by granulocyte depletion. J Appl Physiol 52:1237–1244, 1982.
330. Krieger BP, Loomis WH, Czer GT, et al: Mechanisms of interaction between oxygen and granulocytes in hyperoxic lung injury. J Appl Physiol 58:1326–1330, 1985.
331. Laughlin MJ, Wild L, Nickerson PA, et al: Effects of hyperoxia on alveolar permeability of neutropenic rabbits. J Appl Physiol 61:1126–1131, 1986.
332. Turrens JF, Crapo JD, Freeman BA: Protection against oxygen toxicity by intravenous injection of liposome-entrapped catalase and superoxide dismutase. J Clin Invest 73:87–95, 1984.
333. Padmanabhan RV, Gudapaty R, Liener IE, et al: Protection against pulmonary oxygen toxicity in rats by the intratracheal administration of liposome-encapsulated superoxide dismutase or catalase. Am Rev Respir Dis 132:164–167, 1985.
334. Freeman BA, Turrens JF, Mirza Z, et al: Modulation of oxidant lung injury by using liposome-entrapped superoxide dismutase and catalase. Fed Proc 44:2591–2595, 1985.
335. Matthay MA, Rosen GD: Acid aspiration induced lung injury: New insights and therapeutic options. Am J Respir Crit Care Med 154:277–278, 1996.
336. Snashall PD, Chung KF: Airway obstruction and bronchial hyperresponsiveness in left ventricular failure and mitral stenosis. Am Rev Respir Dis 144:945–956, 1991.
337. Hollingsworth HM: Wheezing and stridor. Clin Chest Med 8:231–240, 1987.
338. Hoffman R, Agatston A, Krieger B: Cheyne-Stokes respiration in patients recovering from acute cardiogenic pulmonary edema. Chest 97:410–412, 1990.
339. Graham SP, Vetrovec GW: Comparison of angiographic findings and demographic variables in patients with coronary artery disease presenting with acute pulmonary edema versus those presenting with chest pain. Am J Cardiol 68:1614–1618, 1991.
340. Meduri GU, Wunderink RG, Leeper KV, et al: Management of bacterial pneumonia in ventilated patients: Protected bronchoalveolar lavage as a diagnostic tool. Chest 101:500–508, 1992.
341. Sutherland KR, Steinberg KP, Maunder RJ, et al: Pulmonary infection during the acute respiratory distress syndrome. Am J Respir Crit Care Med 152:550–556, 1995.
342. Warner DO, Warner MA, Divertie MB: Open lung biopsy in patients with diffuse pulmonary infiltrates and acute respiratory failure. Am Rev Respir Dis 137:90–94, 1988.
343. Zaccardelli DS, Pattishall EN: Clinical diagnostic criteria of the adult respiratory distress syndrome in the intensive care unit. Crit Care Med 24:247–251, 1996.
344. Garber BG, Haebert PC, Yelle JD, et al: Adult respiratory distress syndrome: A systemic overview of incidence and risk factors. Crit Care Med 24:687–695, 1996.
345. Murray JF, Matthay MA, Luce JM, et al: An expanded definition of the adult respiratory distress syndrome. Am Rev Respir Dis 138:720–723, 1988. [Erratum, Am Rev Respir Dis 139:1065, 1989].
346. Bernard GR, Artigas A, Brigham KL, et al: The American-European Consensus Conference on ARDS: Definitions, mechanisms, relevant outcomes, and clinical trial coordination. Am J Respir Crit Care Med 149:818–824, 1994.
347. Bone RC: Sepsis, the sepsis syndrome, multi-organ failure: A plea for comparable definitions. Ann Intern Med 114:332–333, 1991.
348. Sands KE, Bates DW, Lanken PN, et al: Epidemiology of sepsis syndrome in 8 academic medical centers. JAMA 278:234–240, 1997.
349. Bone RC, Balk R, Slotman G, et al: Adult respiratory distress syndrome: Sequence and importance of development of multiple organ failure. Chest 101:320–326, 1992.
350. Matuschak GM: Lung-liver interactions in sepsis and multiple organ failure syndrome. Clin Chest Med 17:83–98, 1996.
351. Bihari D, Smithies M, Gimson A, et al: The effects of vasodilation with prostacyclin on oxygen delivery and uptake in critically ill patients. N Engl J Med 317:397–403, 1987.
352. Knaus WA, Draper EA, Wagner DP, et al: APACHE II: A severity of disease classification system. Crit Care Med 13:818–829, 1985.
353. Knaus WA, Wagner DP, Lynn J: Short-term mortality predictions for critically ill hospitalized adults: Science and ethics. Science 254:389–394, 1991.
354. Artigas A, Bernard GR, Carlet J, et al: The American-European Consensus Conference on ARDS, part 2: Ventilatory, pharmacologic, supportive therapy, study design strategies, and issues related to recovery and remodeling. Am J Respir Crit Care Med 157:1332–1347, 1998.
355. Moss M, Goodman PL, Heinig M, et al: Establishing the relative accuracy of three new definitions of the adult respiratory distress syndrome. Crit Care Med 23:1629–1637, 1995.
356. Schuster DP: What is acute lung injury? What is ARDS? Chest 107:1721–1726, 1995.
357. Sinclair DG, Braude S, Haslam PL, et al: Pulmonary endothelial permeability in patients with severe lung injury: Clinical correlates and natural history. Chest 106:535–539, 1994.
358. Groeneveld ABJ, Raijmakers PGHM, Teule GJJ, et al: The $^{67}$gallium pulmonary leak index in assessing the severity and course of the adult respiratory distress syndrome. Crit Care Med 24:1467–1472, 1996.
359. Groeneveld ABJ, Raijmakers PGHM: The $^{67}$gallium-transferrin pulmonary leak index in patients at risk for the acute respiratory distress syndrome. Crit Care Med 26:685–691, 1998.
360. Owens CM, Evans TW, Keogh BF, et al: Computed tomography

in established adult respiratory distress syndrome: Correlation with lung injury score. Chest 106:1815–1821, 1994.
361. Knaus WA, Sun X, Hakim RB, et al: Evaluation of definitions for adult respiratory distress syndrome. Am J Respir Crit Care Med 150:311–317, 1994.
362. Doyle RL, Szaflarski N, Modin GW, et al: Identification of patients with acute lung injury: Predictors of mortality. Am J Respir Crit Care Med 152:1818–1824, 1995.
363. Staub NC: The measurement of lung water content. J Microw Power 18:259–263, 1983.
364. Staub NC: Clinical use of lung water measurements: Report of a workshop. Chest 90:588–594, 1986.
365. Bombino M, Gattinoni L, Pesenti A, et al: The value of portable chest roentgenography in adult respiratory distress syndrome: Comparison with computed tomography. Chest 100:762–769, 1991.
366. Winer-Muram HT, Rubin SA, Miniati M, et al: Guidelines for reading and interpreting chest radiographs in patients receiving mechanical ventilation. Chest 102:565S–570S, 1992.
367. Suh RD, Aberle DR: Radiographic manifestations of pulmonary edema. *In* Matthay MA, Ingbar DH (eds): Pulmonary Edema. New York: Marcel Dekker, 1998, pp 85–119.
368. Coates G, Powles ACP, Morrison SC, et al: The effects of intravenous infusion of saline on lung density, lung volumes, nitrogen washout, computed tomographic scans, and chest radiographs in humans. Am Rev Respir Dis 127:91–96, 1983.
369. Kohen JA, Opsahl JA, Kjellstrand CM: Deceptive patterns of uremic pulmonary edema. Am J Kidney Dis 7:456–460, 1986.
370. Aberle DR, Wiener-Kronish JP, Webb WR, et al: Hydrostatic versus increased permeability pulmonary edema: Diagnosis based on radiographic criteria in critically ill patients. Radiology 168:73–79, 1988.
371. Rocker GM, Rose DH, Manhire AR, et al: The radiographic differentiation of pulmonary oedema. Br J Radiol 62:582–586, 1989.
372. Thomason JWW, Ely EW, Chiles C, et al: Appraising pulmonary edema using supine chest roentgenograms in ventilated patients. Am J Respir Crit Care Med 157:1600–1608, 1998.
373. Beards SC, Jackson A, Hunt L, et al: Interobserver variation in the chest radiograph component of the lung injury score. Anaesthesia 50:928–932, 1995.
374. Winer-Muram HT, Rubin SA, Ellis JV, et al: Pneumonia and ARDS in patients receiving mechanical ventilation: Diagnostic accuracy of chest radiography. Radiology 188:479–485, 1993.
375. Schuster DP, Marklin GF: The effect of regional lung injury or alveolar hypoxia on pulmonary blood flow and lung water measured by positron emission tomography. Am Rev Respir Dis 133:1037–1042, 1986.
376. Brigham KL, Kariman K, Harris TR, et al: Correlation of oxygenation with vascular permeability-surface area but not with lung water in humans with acute respiratory failure and pulmonary edema. J Clin Invest 72:339–349, 1983.
377. Harris TR, Bernard GR, Brigham KL, et al: Lung microvascular transport properties measured by multiple indicator dilution methods in patients with adult respiratory distress syndrome: A comparison between patients reversing respiratory failure and those failing to reverse. Am Rev Respir Dis 141:272–280, 1990.
378. Rinaldo JE, Borovetz HS, Mancini MC, et al: Assessment of lung injury in the adult respiratory distress syndrome using multiple indicator dilution curves. Am Rev Respir Dis 133:1006–1010, 1986.
379. Zelter M, Lipavsky A, Hoeffel JM, et al: Effect of lung injuries on [$^{14}$C]urea permeability-surface area product in dogs. J Appl Physiol 56:1512–1520, 1984.
380. Estenne M, Yernault J-C: The mechanism of $CO_2$ retention in cardiac pulmonary edema. Chest 86:936–938, 1984.
381. Aberman A, Fulop M: The metabolic and respiratory acidosis of acute pulmonary edema. Ann Intern Med 76:173–184, 1972.
382. O'Donovan R, McGowan JA, Lupinacci L, et al: Acid-base disturbances in cardiogenic pulmonary edema. Nephron 57:416–420, 1991.
383. De Backer D, Creteur J, Zhang H, et al: Lactate production by the lungs in acute lung injury. Am J Respir Crit Care Med 156:1099–1104, 1997.
384. Kellum JA, Kramer DJ, Lee K, et al: Release of lactate by the lung in acute lung injury. Chest 111:1301–1305, 1997.
385. Effros RM, Lipchik RJ: Why does lactic acidosis occur in acute lung injury? Chest 111:1157–1158, 1997.
386. Hyers TM: Prediction of survival and mortality in patients with adult respiratory distress syndrome. New Horiz 1:466–70, 1993.
387. Adrogué HJ, Madias NE: Management of life-threatening acid-base disorders. N Engl J Med 338:26–34, 107–111, 1998.
388. Pittet JF, Mackersie RC, Martin TR, et al: Biological markers of acute lung injury: Prognostic and pathogenetic significance. Am J Respir Crit Care Med 155:1187–1205, 1997.
389. Sprung CL, Rackow EC, Fein IA, et al: The spectrum of pulmonary edema: Differentiation of cardiogenic, intermediate, and noncardiogenic forms of pulmonary edema. Am Rev Respir Dis 124:718–722, 1981.
390. Carlson RW, Schaeffer RC, Carpio M, et al: Edema fluid and coagulation changes during fulminant pulmonary edema. Chest 79:43–49, 1981.
391. Katz S, Aberman A, Frand UI, et al: Heroin pulmonary edema: Evidence for increased pulmonary capillary permeability. Am Rev Respir Dis 106:472–474, 1972.
392. Carlson RW, Schaeffer RC, Michaels SG, et al: Pulmonary edema fluid: Spectrum of features in 37 patients. Circulation 60:1161–1169, 1979.
393. Sprung CL, Long WM, Marcial EH, et al: Distribution of proteins in pulmonary edema: The value of fractional concentrations. Am Rev Respir Dis 136:957–963, 1987.
394. Matthay MA, Wiener-Kronish JP: Intact epithelial barrier function is critical for the resolution of alveolar edema in humans. Am Rev Respir Dis 142:1250–1257, 1990.
394a. Ware LB, Golder JA, Finkbeiner WE, et al: Alveolar epithelial fluid transport capacity in reperfusion lung injury after lung transplantation. Am J Respir Crit Care Med 159:980–988, 1999.
395. Light RW: Falsely high refractometric readings for the specific gravity of pleural fluid. Chest 76:300–301, 1979.
396. Fowler AA, Hyers TM, Fisher BJ, et al: The adult respiratory distress syndrome: Cell populations and soluble mediators in the air spaces of patients at high risk. Am Rev Respir Dis 136:1225–1231, 1987.
397. American Thoracic Society: Clinical role of bronchoalveolar lavage in adults with pulmonary disease. Am Rev Respir Dis 142:481–486, 1990.
398. Steinberg KP, Mitchell DR, Maunder RJ, et al: Safety of bronchoalveolar lavage in patients with adult respiratory distress syndrome. Am Rev Respir Dis 148:556–561, 1993.
399. Von Wichert P, Joseph K, Müller B, et al: Bronchoalveolar lavage: Quantitation of intraalveolar fluid? Am Rev Respir Dis 147:148–152, 1993.
400. Marini JJ: Lung mechanics in the adult respiratory distress syndrome: Recent conceptual advances and implications for management. Clin Chest Med 11:673–690, 1990.
401. Connors AF, Castele RJ, Farhat NZ, et al: Complications of right heart catheterization: A prospective autopsy study. Chest 88:567–572, 1985.
402. Altschule MD: A new branch of medicine: Complications of vascular catheters. Chest 89:446, 1986.
403. Matthay MA, Chatterjee K: Bedside catheterization of the pulmonary artery: Risks compared with benefits. Ann Intern Med 109:826–834, 1988.
404. Connors AF, Speroff T, Dawson NV, et al: The effectiveness of right heart catheterization in the initial care of critically ill patients. JAMA 276:889–897, 1996.
405. O'Quinn R, Marini JJ: Pulmonary artery occlusion pressure: Clinical physiology, measurement, and interpretation. Am Rev Respir Dis 128:319–326, 1983.
406. Robin ED: The cult of the Swan-Ganz catheter: Overuse and abuse of pulmonary flow catheters. Ann Intern Med 103:445–449, 1985.
407. Raper R, Sibbald WJ: Misled by the wedge? The Swan-Ganz catheter and left ventricular preload. Chest 89:427–434, 1986.
408. Leibowitz AB: Do pulmonary artery catheters improve patient outcome? No. Crit Care Clin 12:559–568, 1996.
409. Dalen JE, Bone RC: Is it time to pull the pulmonary artery catheter? JAMA 276:916–918, 1996.
410. Schuster DP: Evaluation of pulmonary endothelial barrier function: Quantifying pulmonary edema and lung injury. *In* Matthay MA, Ingbar DH (eds): Pulmonary Edema. New York: Marcel Dekker, 1998, pp 121–161.

411. Stark P, Jasmine J: CT of pulmonary edema. Crit Rev Diagn Imaging 29:245–255, 1989.
412. Forster BB, Müller NL, Mayo JR, et al: High-resolution computed tomography of experimental hydrostatic pulmonary edema. Chest 101:1434–1437, 1992.
413. Simon DS, Murray JF, Staub NC: Measurement of pulmonary edema in intact dogs by transthoracic gamma ray attenuation. J Appl Physiol 47:1228–1233, 1979.
414. Gamsu G, Kaufman L, Swann SJ, et al: Absolute lung density in experimental canine pulmonary edema. Invest Radiol 14:261–269, 1979.
415. Rice DA: Sound speed in pulmonary parenchyma. J Appl Physiol 54:304–308, 1983.
416. Nierman DM, Eisen DI, Fein ED, et al: Transthoracic bioimpedance can measure extravascular lung water in acute lung injury. J Surg Res 65:101–108, 1996.
417. Ploysongsang Y, Michel RP, Rossi A, et al: Early detection of pulmonary congestion and edema in dogs by using lung sounds. J Appl Physiol 66:2061–2070, 1989.
418. Cutillo AG, Goodrich KC, Ganesan K, et al: Lung water measurement by nuclear magnetic resonance: Correlation with morphometry. J Appl Physiol 79:2163–2168, 1995.
419. Caruthers SD, Paschal CB, Pou NA, et al: Regional measurements of pulmonary edema by using magnetic resonance imaging. J Appl Physiol 84:2143–2153, 1998.
420. Schuster DP: Positron emission tomography: Theory and its application to the study of lung disease. Am Rev Respir Dis 139:818–840, 1989.
421. Kaplan JD, Calandrino FS, Schuster DP: A positron emission tomographic comparison of pulmonary vascular permeability during the adult respiratory distress syndrome and pneumonia. Am Rev Respir Dis 143:150–154, 1991.
422. Effros RM: Lung water measurements with the mean transit time approach. J Appl Physiol 59:673–683, 1985.
423. Böck JC, Lewis FR: Clinical relevance of lung water measurement with the thermal-dye dilution technique. J Surg Res 48:254–265, 1990.
424. Chinard FP: Estimation of extravascular lung water by indicator-dilution techniques. Circ Res 37:137–145, 1975.
425. Elings VB, Lewis FR, Briggs J: Indicator dilution using a fluorescent indicator. J Appl Physiol 52:1368–1374, 1982.
426. Allison RC, Carlile PV, Gray BA: Thermodilution measurement of lung water. Clin Chest Med 6:439–467, 1985.
427. Noble WH, Kay JC: Effects of emboli, positive-pressure ventilation, and airway water on lung water measurements. J Appl Physiol 65:156–164, 1988.
428. Eisenberg PR, Hansbrough JR, Anderson D, et al: A prospective study of lung water measurements during patient management in an intensive care unit. Am Rev Respir Dis 136:662–668, 1987.
429. Mitchell JP, Schuller D, Calandrino FS, et al: Improved outcome based on fluid management in critically ill patients requiring pulmonary artery catheterization. Am Rev Respir Dis 145:990–998, 1992.
430. Dawson CA, Bronikowski TA, Linehan JH, et al: Influence of pulmonary vasoconstriction on lung water and perfusion heterogeneity. J Appl Physiol 54:654–660, 1983.
431. Kambara K, Jerome EH, Serikov VB, et al: Reliability of extravascular lung thermal volume measurements by thermal conductivity technique in sheep. J Appl Physiol 73:1449–1456, 1992.
432. Serikov VB, Rumm MS, Kambara K, et al: Application of respiratory heat exchange for the measurement of lung water. J Appl Physiol 72:944–953, 1992.
433. Cander L, Forster RE: Determination of pulmonary parenchymal tissue volume and capillary blood flow in man. J Appl Physiol 14:541–551, 1959.
434. Overland ES, Gupta RN, Huchon GJ, et al: Measurement of pulmonary tissue volume and blood flow in persons with normal and edematous lungs. J Appl Physiol 51:1375–1383, 1981.
435. Burma GM, Saidel GM: Pulmonary blood flow and tissue volume: Model analysis of rebreathing estimation methods. J Appl Physiol 55:205–211, 1983.
436. Sibbald WJ, Cunningham DR, Chin DN: Non-cardiac or cardiac pulmonary edema? A practical approach to clinical differentiation in critically ill patients. Chest 84:452–461, 1983.
437. Gorin AB, Kohler J, DeNardo G: Noninvasive measurement of pulmonary transvascular protein flux in normal man. J Clin Invest 66:869–877, 1980.
438. Dauber IM, Pluss WT, VanGrondelle A, et al: Specificity and sensitivity of noninvasive measurement of pulmonary vascular protein leak. J Appl Physiol 59:564–574, 1985.
439. Staub NC, Hyde RW, Crandall E: Workshop on techniques to evaluate lung alveolar-microvascular injury. Am Rev Respir Dis 141:1071–1077, 1990.
440. Raijmakers PGHM, Groeneveld ABJ, Teule GJJ, et al: Diagnostic value of the gallium-67 pulmonary leak index in pulmonary edema. J Nucl Med 37:1316–1322, 1996.
441. Braude S, Nolop KB, Hughes JMB, et al: Comparison of lung vascular and epithelial permeability indices in the adult respiratory distress syndrome. Am Rev Respir Dis 133:1002–1005, 1986.
442. Mishkin FS, Niden A, Kumar A, et al: Albumin lung/heart ratio change: A simple clinical means of documenting increased pulmonary endothelial permeability to protein. JAMA 257:953–956, 1987.
443. Byrne K, Tatum JL, Henry DA, et al: Increased morbidity with increased pulmonary albumin flux in sepsis-related adult respiratory distress syndrome. Crit Care Med 20:28–34, 1992.
444. Sibbald WJ, Driedger AA, Moffat JD, et al: Pulmonary microvascular clearance of radiotracers in human cardiac and noncardiac pulmonary edema. J Appl Physiol 50:1337–1347, 1981.
445. Effros RM, Mason GR: Measurements of pulmonary epithelial permeability in vivo. Am Rev Respir Dis 127:S59–S65, 1983.
446. Jones JG, Royston D, Minty BD: Changes in alveolar-capillary barrier function in animals and humans. Am Rev Respir Dis 127:S51–S59, 1983.
447. Taylor SM, Downes H, Hirsham CA, et al: Pulmonary uptake of mannitol as an index of changes in lung epithelial permeability. J Appl Physiol 55:614–618, 1983.
448. Coates G, O'Brodovich H, Dolovich M: Lung clearance of $^{99m}$Tc-DPTA in patients with acute lung injury and pulmonary edema. J Thorac Imaging 3:21–27, 1988.
449. Huchon GJ, Russell JA, Barritault LG, et al: Chronic air-flow limitation does not increase respiratory epithelial permeability assessed by aerosolized solute, but smoking does. Am Rev Respir Dis 130:457–460, 1984.
450. Susskind H, Weber DA, Volknow ND, et al: Increased lung permeability following long-term use of free-base cocaine (crack). Chest 100:903–909, 1991.
451. Mason GR, Effros RM, Uszler JM, et al: Small solute clearance from the lungs of patients with cardiogenic and noncardiogenic pulmonary edema. Chest 88:327–334, 1985.
452. Rizk NW, Luce JM, Hoeffel JM, et al: Site of deposition and factors affecting clearance of aerosolized solute from canine lungs. J Appl Physiol 56:723–729, 1984.
453. Marks JD, Luce JM, Lazar NM, et al: Effect of increases in lung volume on clearance of aerosolized solute from human lungs. J Appl Physiol 59:1242–1248, 1985.
454. Barrowcliffe MP, Zanelli GD, Jones JG: Pulmonary clearance of radiotracers after positive end-expiratory pressure or acute lung injury. J Appl Physiol 66:288–294, 1989.
455. Barrowcliffe MP, Jones JG: Pulmonary clearance of 99mTc-DPTA in the diagnosis and evolution of increased permeability pulmonary oedema. Anaesth Intensive Care 17:422–432, 1989.
456. Connelly KG, Repine JE: Markers for predicting the development of acute respiratory distress syndrome. Annu Rev Med 48:429–445, 1997.
457. Weinberg PF, Matthay MA, Webster RO, et al: Biologically active products of complement and acute lung injury in patients with the sepsis syndrome. Am Rev Respir Dis 130:791–796, 1984.
458. Duchateau J, Haas M, Schreyen H, et al: Complement activation in patients at risk of developing the adult respiratory distress syndrome. Am Rev Respir Dis 130:1058–1064, 1984.
459. Parsons PE, Giclas PC: The terminal complement complex (sC5b-9) is not specifically associated with the development of the adult respiratory distress syndrome. Am Rev Respir Dis 141:98–103, 1990.
460. Gama de Abreu M, Kirschfink M, Quintel M, et al: White blood cell counts and plasma C3a have synergistic predictive value in patients at risk for acute respiratory distress syndrome. Crit Care Med 26:1040–1048, 1998.

461. Hollinger MA: Serum angiotensin-converting enzyme: Status report on its diagnostic significance in pulmonary disease. Chest 83:589–590, 1983.
462. Fourrier F, Chopin C, Wallaert B, et al: Angiotensin-converting enzyme in human adult respiratory distress syndrome. Chest 83:593–597, 1983.
463. Krieger B, Schwartz J, Loomis W, et al: Nonspecificity of elevated angiotensin-converting enzyme activity in bronchoalveolar lavage fluid from high permeability lung edema states. Am Rev Respir Dis 129:499–500, 1984.
464. Moss M, Ackerson L, Gillespie MK, et al: von Willebrand factor antigen levels are not predictive for the adult respiratory distress syndrome. Am J Respir Crit Care Med 151:15–20, 1995.
465. Haynes JB, Hyers TM, Giclas PC, et al: Elevated fibrin(ogen) degradation products in the adult respiratory distress syndrome. Am Rev Respir Dis 122:841–847, 1980.
466. Fourrier F, Chopin C, Wallaert B, et al: Compared evolution of plasma fibronectin and angiotensin-converting enzyme levels in septic ARDS. Chest 87:191–195, 1985.
467. Lesser M, Flick MR, Kent B, et al: Proteolytic activity in sheep lung lymph as marker of lung capillary injury. Am Rev Respir Dis 135:643–650, 1987.
468. Pacht ER, Timerman AP, Lykens MG, et al: Deficiency of alveolar glutathione in patients with sepsis and the adult respiratory distress syndrome. Chest 100:1397–1403, 1991.
469. Leff JA, Parsons PE, Day CE, et al: Increased serum catalase activity in septic patients with the adult respiratory distress syndrome. Am Rev Respir Dis 146:985–989, 1992.
470. Leff JA, Parsons PE, Day CE, et al: Serum antioxidants as predictors of adult respiratory distress syndrome in patients with sepsis. Lancet 341:777–780, 1993.
471. Doyle IR, Nicholas TE, Bersten AD: Serum surfactant protein-A levels in patients with acute cardiogenic pulmonary edema and adult respiratory distress syndrome. Am J Respir Crit Care Med 152:307–317, 1995.
472. Shimura S, Masuda T, Takishima T, et al: Surfactant apoprotein-A concentration in airway secretions for the detection of pulmonary oedema. Eur Respir J 9:2525–2530, 1996.
473. Günther A, Siebert C, Schmidt R, et al: Surfactant alterations in severe pneumonia, acute respiratory distress syndrome, and cardiogenic lung edema. Am J Respir Crit Care Med 153:176–184, 1996.
474. Baldwin SR, Simon RH, Grum CM, et al: Oxidant activity in expired breath of patients with adult respiratory distress syndrome. Lancet 1:11–14, 1986.
475. Sznajder JI, Fraiman A, Hall JB, et al: Increased hydrogen peroxide in the expired breath of patients with acute hypoxemic respiratory failure. Chest 96:606–612, 1989.
476. Kietzmann D, Kahl R, Müller M, et al: Hydrogen peroxide in expired breath condensate of patients with acute respiratory failure and with ARDS. Intensive Care Med 19:78–81, 1993.
477. Mathru M, Rooney MW, Dries DJ, et al: Urine hydrogen peroxide during adult respiratory distress syndrome in patients with and without sepsis. Chest 105:232–236, 1994.
478. Cochrane CG, Spragg R, Revak SD: Pathogenesis of the adult respiratory distress syndrome: Evidence of oxidant activity in bronchoalveolar lavage fluid. J Clin Invest 71:754–761, 1983.
479. Marks JD, Marks CB, Luce JM, et al: Plasma tumor necrosis factor in patients with septic shock: Mortality rate, incidence of adult respiratory distress syndrome, and effects of methylprednisolone administration. Am Rev Respir Dis 141:94–97, 1990.
480. Roten R, Markert M, Feihl F, et al: Plasma levels of tumor necrosis factor in the adult respiratory distress syndrome. Am Rev Respir Dis 143:590–592, 1991.
481. Hyers TM, Tricomi SM, Dettenmeier PA, et al: Tumor necrosis factor levels in serum and bronchoalveolar lavage fluid of patients with the adult respiratory distress syndrome. Am Rev Respir Dis 144:268–271, 1991.
482. de Groote MA, Martin MA, Densen P, et al: Plasma tumor necrosis factor levels in patients with presumed sepsis: Results in those treated with antilipid A antibody vs placebo. JAMA 262:249–251, 1989.
483. Millar AB, Foley NM, Singer M, et al: Tumour necrosis factor in bronchoalveolar secretions of patients with adult respiratory distress syndrome. Lancet 2:712–714, 1989.
484. Suter PM, Suter S, Girardin E, et al: High bronchoalveolar levels of tumor necrosis factor and its inhibitors, interleukin-1, interferon, and elastase, in patients with adult respiratory distress syndrome after trauma, shock, or sepsis. Am Rev Respir Dis 145:1016–1022, 1992.
485. Parsons PE, Moore FA, Moore EE, et al: Studies on the role of tumor necrosis factor in adult respiratory distress syndrome. Am Rev Respir Dis 146:694–700, 1992.
486. Levine B, Kalman J, Mayer L, et al: Elevated circulating levels of tumor necrosis factor in severe chronic heart failure. N Engl J Med 323:236–241, 1990.
487. Ratnoff WD, Matthay MA, Wong MYS, et al: Sulfidopeptide-leukotriene peptidases in pulmonary edema fluid from patients with the adult respiratory distress syndrome. J Clin Immunol 8:250–258, 1988.
488. Stephenson AH, Lonigro AJ, Hyers TM, et al: Increased concentrations of leukotrienes in bronchoalveolar lavage fluid of patients with ARDS or at risk for ARDS. Am Rev Respir Dis 138:714–719, 1988.
489. Knöller J, Schönfeld W, König W: Role of leukotrienes in the pathophysiology of ARDS after polytrauma. *In* Sturm JA (ed): Adult Respiratory Distress Syndrome: An Aspect of Multiple Organ Failure. Results of a Prospective Clinical Study. Berlin: Springer-Verlag, 1991, pp 177–192.
490. Fauler J, Tsikas D, Holch M, et al: Enhanced urinary excretion of leukotriene $E_4$ by patients with multiple trauma with or without adult respiratory distress syndrome. Clin Sci 80:497–504, 1991.
491. Bernard GR, Korley V, Chee P, et al: Persistent generation of peptido leukotrienes in patients with the adult respiratory distress syndrome. Am Rev Respir Dis 144:263–267, 1991.
492. Lee CT, Fein AM, Lippmann M, et al: Elastolytic activity in pulmonary lavage fluid from patients with adult respiratory-distress syndrome. N Engl J Med 304:192–196, 1981.
493. McGuire WW, Spragg RG, Cohen AB, et al: Studies on the pathogenesis of the adult respiratory distress syndrome. J Clin Invest 69:543–553, 1982.
494. Idell S, Kucich U, Fein A, et al: Neutrophil elastase-releasing factors in bronchoalveolar lavage from patients with adult respiratory distress syndrome. Am Rev Respir Dis 132:1098–1105, 1985.
495. Wewers MD, Herzyk DJ, Gadek JE: Alveolar fluid neutrophil elastase activity in the adult respiratory distress syndrome is complexed to alpha-2-macroglobulin. J Clin Invest 82:1260–1267, 1988.
496. Kuo C-D, Wu W-G, Wang J-H, et al: Proton nuclear magnetic resonance studies of plasma to determine metabolic status of patients with adult respiratory distress syndrome. Clin Chem 35:667–670, 1989.
497. Pallister I, Gosling P, Alpar K, et al: Prediction of posttraumatic adult respiratory distress syndrome by albumin excretion rate eight hours after admission. J Trauma 42:1056–1061, 1997.
498. Nakos G, Pneumatikos J, Tsangaris I, et al: Proteins and phospholipids in BAL from patients with hydrostatic pulmonary edema. Am J Respir Crit Care Med 155:945–951, 1997.
499. Kurz RW, Stockenhuber F, Gremmel F, et al: Serum concentrations of immune parameters during acute cardiogenic pulmonary edema. Crit Care Med 20:1235–1242, 1992.
500. Staub NC: Pulmonary edema: Physiologic approaches to management. Chest 74:559–564, 1978.
501. Hakim TS, Grunstein MM, Michel RP: Opiate action in the pulmonary circulation. Pulm Pharmacol 5:159–165, 1992.
502. Klein HO, Brodsky E, Ninio R, et al: The effect of venous occlusion with tourniquets on peripheral blood pooling and ventricular function. Chest 103:521–527, 1993.
503. Eiser AR, Lieber JJ, Neff MS: Phlebotomy for pulmonary edema in dialysis patients. Clin Nephrol 47:47–49, 1997.
504. Jasmer RM, Luce JM, Matthay MA: Noninvasive positive pressure ventilation for acute respiratory failure: Underutilized or overrated? Chest 111:1672–1678, 1997.
505. Antonelli M, Conti G, Rocco M, et al: A comparison of noninvasive positive pressure ventilation and conventional mechanical ventilation in patients with acute respiratory failure. N Engl J Med 339:429–435, 1998.
506. Stack RS, Stack RK, Morris KG, et al: Temporary balloon occlu-

sion of the inferior vena cava for immediate reversal of acute pulmonary edema. Am J Cardiol 57:886–887, 1986.
507. Berthiaume Y, Ware LB, Matthay MA: Treatment of acute pulmonary edema and the acute respiratory distress syndrome. *In* Matthay MA, Ingbar DH (eds): Pulmonary Edema. New York: Marcel Dekker, 1998, pp 575–631.
508. Gattinoni L, Pelosi P, Crotti S, et al: Effects of positive end-expiratory pressure on regional distribution of tidal volume and recruitment in adult respiratory distress syndrome. Am J Respir Crit Care Med 151:1807–1814, 1995.
509. Guyatt G, Ontario Intensive Care Study Group: A randomized control trial of right-heart catheterization in critically ill patients. J Intensive Care Med 6:91–95, 1991.
510. Levy MM: Pulmonary capillary pressure: Clinical implications. Crit Care Clin 12:819–839, 1996.
511. Cercek B, Shah PK: Complicated acute myocardial infarction: Heart failure, shock, mechanical complications. Cardiol Clin 9:569–593, 1991.
512. Breen PH, Schumacker PT, Hedenstierna G, et al: How does increased cardiac output increase shunt in pulmonary edema? J Appl Physiol 53:1273–1280, 1982.
513. Sandoval J, Long GR, Skoog C, et al: Independent influence of blood flow rate and mixed venous $Po_2$ on shunt fraction. J Appl Physiol 55:1128–1133, 1983.
514. Breen PH, Schumacker PT, Sandoval J, et al: Increased cardiac output increases shunt: Role of pulmonary edema and perfusion. J Appl Physiol 59:1313–1321, 1985.
515. Radermacher P, Santak B, Becker H, et al: Prostaglandin $E_1$ and nitroglycerin reduce pulmonary capillary pressure but worsen ventilation-perfusion distributions in patients with adult respiratory distress syndrome. Anesthesiology 70:601–606, 1989.
516. Dupuis J: Nitrates in congestive heart failure. Cardiovasc Drugs Ther 8:501–507, 1994.
517. Shook TL, Kirshenbaum JM, Hundley RF, et al: Ethanol intoxication complicating intravenous nitroglycerin therapy. Ann Intern Med 101:498–499, 1984.
518. Cotter G, Metzkor E, Kaluski E, et al: Randomised trial of high-dose isosorbide dinitrate plus low-dose furosemide versus high-dose furosemide plus low-dose isosorbide dinitrate in severe pulmonary oedema. Lancet 351:389–393, 1998.
519. Jordan RA, Seth L, Casebolt P, et al: Rapidly developing tolerance to transdermal nitroglycerin in congestive heart failure. Ann Intern Med 104:295–298, 1986.
520. Brown NJ, Vaughan DE: Angiotensin-converting enzyme inhibitors. Circulation 97:1411–1420, 1998.
521. Furberg CD, Yusuf S: Effect of drug therapy on survival in chronic congestive heart failure. Am J Cardiol 62:41a–45a, 1988.
522. Guidelines for the evaluation and management of heart failure: Report of the American College of Cardiology/American Heart Association Task Force on Practice Guidelines (Committee on Evaluation and Management of Heart Failure). Circulation 92:2764–2784, 1995.
523. Annane D, Bellissant E, Pussard E, et al: Placebo-controlled, randomized, double-blind study of intravenous enalaprilat efficacy and safety in acute cardiogenic pulmonary edema. Circulation 94:1316–1324, 1996.
524. Massie BM, Stern R, Hanlon JT, et al: Beneficial hemodynamic effects of intravenous diazoxide in refractory congestive heart failure. Am Heart J 104:581–586, 1982.
525. Brater DC: Diuretic therapy. N Engl J Med 339:387–395, 1998.
526. Ali J, Wood LDH: Pulmonary vascular effects of furosemide on gas exchange in pulmonary edema. J Appl Physiol 57:160–167, 1984.
527. Dormans TPJ, Pickkers P, Russel FGM, et al: Vascular effects of loop diuretics. Cardiovasc Res 32:988–997, 1996.
528. Schuller D, Lynch JP, Fine D: Protocol-guided diuretic management: Comparison of furosemide by continuous infusion and intermittent bolus. Crit Care Med 25:1969–1975, 1997.
529. Gallagher KL, Jones JK: Furosemide-induced ototoxicity. Ann Intern Med 91:744–745, 1979.
530. Brater DC: Resistance to loop diuretics: Why it happens and what to do about it. Drugs 30:427–443, 1985.
531. Garzia F, Todor R, Scalea T: Continuous arteriovenous hemofiltration countercurrent dialysis (CAVH-D) in acute respiratory failure (ARDS). J Trauma 31:1277–1285, 1991.
532. Reynolds HN, Borg U, Belzberg H, et al: Efficacy of continuous arteriovenous hemofiltration with dialysis in patients with renal failure. Crit Care Med 19:1387–1394, 1991.
533. Susini G, Zucchetti M, Bortone F, et al: Isolated ultrafiltration in cardiogenic pulmonary edema. Crit Care Med 18:14–17, 1990.
534. Molloy WD, Dobson K, Girling L, et al: Effects of dopamine on cardiopulmonary function and left ventricular volumes in patients with acute respiratory failure. Am Rev Respir Dis 130:396–399, 1984.
535. Leier CV, Unverferth DV: Dobutamine. Ann Intern Med 99:490–496, 1983.
536. Duke GJ, Briedis JH, Weaver RA: Renal support in critically ill patients: Low-dose dopamine or low-dose dobutamine? Crit Care Med 22:1919–1925, 1994.
537. Goldbranson FL, Lurie L, Vance RM, et al: Multiple extremity amputations in hypotensive patients treated with dopamine. JAMA 243:1145–1146, 1980.
538. Jardin F, Eveleigh MC, Gurdjian F, et al: Venous admixture in human septic shock: Comparative effects of blood volume expansion, dopamine infusion and isoproterenol infusion on mismatching of ventilation and pulmonary blood flow in peritonitis. Circulation 60:155–159, 1979.
539. Matamis D, Lemaire F, Harf A, et al: Redistribution of pulmonary blood flow induced by positive end-expiratory pressure and dopamine infusion in acute respiratory failure. Am Rev Respir Dis 129:39–44, 1984.
540. Payen DM, Carli PA, Brun-Buisson CJL, et al: Lower body positive pressure vs. dopamine during PEEP in humans. J Appl Physiol 58:77–82, 1985.
541. Malo J, Ali J, Wood LDH: How does positive end-expiratory pressure reduce intrapulmonary shunt in canine pulmonary edema? J Appl Physiol 57:1002–1010, 1984.
542. Dantzker DR, Lynch JP, Weg JG: Depression of cardiac output is a mechanism of shunt reduction in the therapy of acute respiratory failure. Chest 77:636–642, 1980.
543. Barnard ML, Olivera WG, Rutschman DM, et al: Dopamine stimulates sodium transport and liquid clearance in rat lung epithelium. Am J Respir Crit Care Med 156:709–714, 1997.
544. Tibayan FA, Chesnutt AN, Folkesson HG, et al: Dobutamine increases alveolar liquid clearance in ventilated rats by beta-2 receptor stimulation. Am J Respir Crit Care Med 156:438–444, 1997.
545. Chatterjee K: Digitalis and non-ACE inhibitor vasodilators in heart failure. Cardiol Clin 7:99–118, 1989.
546. Takeda S, Takano T, Nakanishi K, et al: Amrinone improves lung compliance in patients receiving mechanical ventilation for cardiogenic pulmonary edema. Acta Anaesth Scand 41:624–628, 1997.
547. Shipley JB, Tolman D, Hastillo A, et al: Milrinone: Basic and clinical pharmacology and acute and chronic management. Am J Med Sci 311:286–291, 1996.
548. Steltzer H, Krafft P, Fridrich P, et al: Severity and outcome of ARDS: The present place of extracorporeal lung assist (ECLA). Int J Artif Organs 18:607–610, 1995.
549. Kolla S, Awad SS, Rich PB, et al: Extracorporeal life support for 100 adult patients with severe respiratory failure. Ann Surg 226:544–556, 1997.
550. Tsang V, Evans TW, Morgan C, et al: Heart-lung transplantation for adult respiratory distress syndrome. Crit Care Med 19:286–287, 1991.
551. Demertzis S, Haverich A, Ziemer G, et al: Successful lung transplantation for posttraumatic adult respiratory distress syndrome after extracorporeal membrane oxygenation support. J Heart Lung Transplant 11:1005–1007, 1992.
552. Egan TM: When is lung transplantation appropriate? J Heart Lung Transplant 11:1008, 1992.
553. Grover FL, Fullerton DA, Zamora MR, et al: The past, present, and future of lung transplantation. Am J Surg 173:523–533, 1997.
554. Ehrhart IC, Hofman WF: Relationship of fluid filtration to lung vascular pressure during edema. J Appl Physiol 70:202–209, 1991.
555. Gheorghiade M, Cody RJ, Francis GS, et al: Current medical therapy for advanced heart failure. Am Heart J 135:S231–S248, 1998.

556. Stevenson LW, Massie BM, Francis GS: Optimizing therapy for complex or refractory heart failure: A management algorithm. Am Heart J 135:S293–S309, 1998.
556a. Verghese GM, Ware LB, Matthay BA, et al: Alveolar epithelial fluid transport and the resolution of clinically severe hydrostatic pulmonary edema. J Appl Physiol 87:1301–1312, 1999.
557. Wheeler AP, Bernard GR: Treating patients with severe sepsis. N Engl J Med 340:207–214, 1999.
558. Kaback KR, Sanders AB, Meislin HW: MAST suit update. JAMA 252:2598–2603, 1984.
559. Humphrey H, Hall J, Sznajder I, et al: Improved survival in ARDS patients associated with a reduction in pulmonary capillary wedge pressure. Chest 97:1176–1180, 1990.
560. Simmons RS, Berdine GG, Seidenfeld JJ, et al: Fluid balance and the adult respiratory distress syndrome. Am Rev Respir Dis 135:924–929, 1987.
561. Schuller D, Mitchell JP, Calandrino FS, et al: Fluid balance during pulmonary edema: Is fluid gain a marker or a cause of poor outcome? Chest 100:1068–1075, 1991.
562. Pingleton SK: Complications of acute respiratory failure. Am Rev Respir Dis 137:1463–1493, 1988.
563. Hayes MA, Timmins AC, Yau EHS, et al: Evaluation of systemic oxygen delivery in the treatment of critically ill patients. N Engl J Med 330:1717–1722, 1994.
564. Gattinoni L, Brazzi L, Pelosi P, et al: A trial of goal-oriented hemodynamic therapy in critically ill patients. N Engl J Med 333:1025–1032, 1995.
565. Manthous CA, Hall JB, Olson D, et al: Effect of cooling on oxygen consumption in febrile critically ill patients. Am J Respir Crit Care Med 151:10–14, 1995.
566. Manthous CA, Hall JB, Kushner R, et al: The effect of mechanical ventilation on oxygen consumption in critically ill patients. Am J Respir Crit Care Med 151:210–214, 1995.
567. Segredo V, Caldwell JE, Matthay MA, et al: Persistent paralysis in critically ill patients after long-term administration of vecuronium. N Engl J Med 327:524–528, 1992.
568. Hébert PC, Wells G, Blajchman MA, et al: A multicenter, randomized, controlled clinical trial of transfusion requirements in critical care. N Engl J Med 340:409–417, 1999.
569. Bshouty Z, Younes M: Effect of breathing pattern and level of ventilation on pulmonary fluid filtration in dog lung. Am Rev Respir Dis 145:372–376, 1992.
570. Dreyfuss D, Saumon G: Ventilator-induced lung injury: Lessons from experimental studies. Am J Respir Crit Care Med 157:294–323, 1998.
571. Slutsky AS, Tremblay LN: Multiple system organ failure: Is mechanical ventilation a contributing factor? Am J Respir Crit Care Med 157:1721–1725, 1998.
572. Sznajder JI, Ridge KM, Saumon G, et al: Lung injury induced by mechanical ventilation. *In* Matthay MA, Ingbar DH (eds): Pulmonary Edema. New York: Marcel Dekker, 1998, pp 413–430.
573. Meade MO, Cook DJ, Kernerman P, et al: How to use articles about harm: The relationship between high tidal volumes, ventilating pressures, and ventilator-induced lung injury. Crit Care Med 25:1915–1922, 1997.
574. Nahum A, Shapiro R: Adjuncts to mechanical ventilation. Clin Chest Med 17:491–511, 1996.
575. Marini JJ: Evolving concepts in the ventilatory management of acute respiratory distress syndrome. Clin Chest Med 17:555–575, 1996.
576. Nelson LD: High-inflation pressure and positive end-expiratory pressure: Injurious to the lung? No. Crit Care Clin 12:603–625, 1996.
577. Weg JG, Anzueto A, Balk RA, et al: The relation of pneumothorax and other air leaks to mortality in the acute respiratory distress syndrome. N Engl J Med 338:341–346, 1998.
578. Gammon RB, Shin MS, Groves RH, et al: Clinical risk factors for pulmonary barotrauma: A multivariate analysis. Am J Respir Crit Care Med 152:1235–1240, 1995.
579. Schnapp LM, Chin DP, Szaflarski N, et al: Frequency and importance of barotrauma in 100 patients with acute lung injury. Crit Care Med 23:272–278, 1995.
580. Suchyta MR, Elliott CG, Jensen RL, et al: Predicting the presence of pulmonary function impairment in adult respiratory distress syndrome survivors. Respiration 60:103–108, 1993.
581. Morris AH, Wallace CJ, Menlove RL, et al: Randomized clinical trial of pressure-controlled inverse ratio ventilation and extracorporeal $CO_2$ removal for adult respiratory distress syndrome. Am J Respir Crit Care Med 149:295–305, 1994 [published erratum appears in Am J Respir Crit Care Med 149:838, 1994].
582. Stewart TE, Meade MO, Cook DJ, et al: Evaluation of a ventilation strategy to prevent barotrauma in patients at high risk for acute respiratory distress syndrome. N Engl J Med 338:355–361, 1998.
583. Amato MBP, Barbas CSV, Medeiros DM, et al: Effect of a protective-ventilation strategy on mortality in the acute respiratory distress syndrome. N Engl J Med 338:347–354, 1998.
584. Hudson LD: Protective ventilation for patients with acute respiratory distress syndrome. N Engl J Med 338:385–387, 1998.
584a. NIH ARDS Network: A trial of traditional versus a lower tidal volume strategy in acute lung injury and the acute respiratory distress syndrome. N Engl J Med, in press.
584b. Ranieri VM, Suter PM, Tortorella C, et al: Effect of mechanical ventilation on inflammatory mediators in patients with acute respiratory distress syndrome. JAMA 282:54–61, 1999.
585. Hirschl RB, Pranikoff T, Wise C, et al: Initial experience with partial liquid ventilation in adult patients with the acute respiratory distress syndrome. JAMA 275:383–389, 1996.
586. Weis CM, Wolfson MR, Shaffer TH: Liquid-assisted ventilation: Physiology and clinical application. Ann Med 29:509–517, 1997.
587. Bidani A, Tzouanakis AE, Cardenas VJ, et al: Permissive hypercapnia in acute respiratory failure. JAMA 272:957–962, 1994.
588. Fort P, Farmer C, Westerman J, et al: High-frequency oscillatory ventilation for adult respiratory distress syndrome: A pilot study. Crit Care Med 25:937–947, 1997.
589. Albert RK: The prone position in acute respiratory distress syndrome: Where we are, and where do we go from here. Crit Care Med 25:1453–1454, 1997.
590. Chatte G, Sab J-M, Dubois J-M, et al: Prone position in mechanically ventilated patients with severe acute respiratory failure. Am J Respir Crit Care Med 155:473–478, 1997.
591. Mure M, Martling C-R, Lindahl SGE: Dramatic effect on oxygenation in patients with severe acute lung insufficiency treated in the prone position. Crit Care Med 25:1539–1544, 1997.
592. Blanch L, Mancebo J, Perez M, et al: Short-term effects of prone position in critically ill patients with acute respiratory distress syndrome. Intensive Care Med 23:1033–1039, 1997.
593. Pelosi P, Tubiolo D, Mascheroni D, et al: Effects of the prone position on respiratory mechanics and gas exchange during acute lung injury. Am J Respir Crit Care Med 157:387–393, 1998.
594. Lamm WJE, Graham MM, Albert RK: Mechanism by which the prone position improves oxygenation in acute lung injury. Am J Respir Crit Care Med 150:184–193, 1994.
595. Rochester DF, Esau SA: Malnutrition and the respiratory system. Chest 85:411–415, 1984.
596. Koretz RL: Breathing and feeding: Can you have one without the other? Chest 85:298–299, 1984.
597. Moore FA, Moore EE, Jones TN, et al: TEN versus TPN following major abdominal trauma: Reduced septic morbidity. J Trauma 29:916–923, 1989.
598. Alexander JW: Nutrition and translocation. J Parent Ent Nutr 14:170s–174s, 1990.
599. Cook D, Guyatt G, Marshall J, et al: A comparison of sucralfate and ranitidine for the prevention of upper gastrointestinal bleeding in patients requiring mechanical ventilation. N Engl J Med 338:791–797, 1998.
600. Kollef MH: The prevention of ventilator-associated pneumonia. N Engl J Med 340:627–634, 1999.
601. Heyland D, Mandell LA: Gastric colonization by gram-negative bacilli and nosocomial pneumonia in the intensive care unit: Evidence for causation. Chest 101:187–193, 1992.
602. Vandenbroucke-Grauls CMJE, Vandenbroucke JP: Effect of selective decontamination of the digestive tract on respiratory tract infections and mortality in the intensive care unit. Lancet 338:859–862, 1991.
603. Cerra FB, Maddaus MA, Dunn DL, et al: Selective gut decontamination reduces nosocomial infections and length of stay but not mortality or organ failure in surgical intensive care unit patients. Arch Surg 127:163–169, 1992.
604. Dematte JE, Sznajder JI: Effects of selective digestive decontami-

nation on lung injury and outcome: The verdict is not yet in. Chest 112:304–306, 1997.
605. Iberti TJ: Daily chest radiographs: The jury is still out (editorial). Crit Care Med 19:597, 1991.
606. Hall JB, White SR, Karrison T: Efficacy of daily routine chest radiographs in intubated, mechanically ventilated patients. Crit Care Med 19:689–693, 1991.
607. Morris AH: Clinical trial issues. *In* Evans TW, Haslett C (eds): ARDS: Acute Respiratory Distress in Adults. London: Chapman & Hall Medical, 1996, pp 451–477.
608. Turner JS, Briggs S, Springhorn HE, et al: Patients' recollection of intensive care unit experience. Crit Care Med 18:966–968, 1990.
609. Weinert CR, Gross CR, Kangas JR, et al: Health-related quality of life after acute lung injury. Am J Respir Crit Care Med 156:1120–1128, 1997.
610. Schelling G, Stoll C, Haller M, et al: Health-related quality of life and posttraumatic stress disorder in survivors of the acute respiratory distress syndrome. Crit Care Med 26:651–659, 1998.
611. Hall JB, Schmidt GA, Wood LDH (eds): Principles of Critical Care. New York: McGraw-Hill, 1992.
612. Metz C, Sibbald WJ: Anti-inflammatory therapy for acute lung injury: A review of animal and clinical studies. Chest 100:1110–1119, 1991.
613. Weinberger SE: Recent advances in pulmonary medicine (second of two parts). N Engl J Med 328:1462–1470, 1993.
614. Griffiths MJD, Evans TW: Prospects for pharmacotherapy. *In* Evans TW, Haslett C (eds): ARDS: Acute Respiratory Distress in Adults. London: Chapman & Hall Medical, 1996, pp 507–523.
615. Petty TL, Bone RC, Gee MH, et al: Contemporary clinical trials in acute respiratory distress syndrome. Chest 101:550–552, 1992.
616. Baumann WR, Jung RC, Koss M, et al: Incidence and mortality of adult respiratory distress syndrome: A prospective analysis from a large metropolitan hospital. Crit Care Med 14:1–4, 1986.
617. Hudson LD, Milberg JA, Anardi D, et al: Clinical risk for development of the acute respiratory distress syndrome. Am J Respir Crit Care Med 151:293–301, 1995.
618. Koizumi M, Frank L, Massaro D: Oxygen toxicity in rats: Varied effect of dexamethasone treatment depending on duration of hyperoxia. Am Rev Respir Dis 131:907–911, 1985.
619. Brigham KL: Corticosteroids in adult respiratory distress syndrome. *In* Zapol WM, Lemaire F (eds): Adult Respiratory Distress Syndrome. New York: Marcel Dekker, 1991, pp 285–304.
620. Weigelt JA, Norcross JF, Borman KR, et al: Early steroid therapy for respiratory failure. Arch Surg 120:536–540, 1985.
621. Bernard GR, Luce JM, Sprung CL, et al: High-dose corticosteroids in patients with the adult respiratory distress syndrome. N Engl J Med 317:1565–1570, 1987.
622. Slotman GJ, Fisher CJ, Bone RC, et al: Detrimental effects of high-dose methylprednisolone sodium succinate on serum concentrations of hepatic and renal function indicators in severe sepsis and septic shock. Crit Care Med 21:191–195, 1993.
623. Schonfeld SA, Ploysongsang Y, DiLisio R, et al: Fat embolism prophylaxis with corticosteroids: A prospective study in high-risk patients. Ann Intern Med 99:438–443, 1983.
624. Hooper RG: ARDS: Inflammation, infections, and corticosteroids. Chest 100:889–890, 1991.
625. Meduri GU, Chinn AJ, Leeper KV, et al: Corticosteroid rescue treatment of progressive fibroproliferation in late ARDS: Patterns of response and predictors of outcome. Chest 105:1516–1527, 1994.
626. Biffl WL, Moore FA, Moore EE, et al: Are corticosteroids salvage therapy for refractory acute respiratory distress syndrome? Am J Surg 170:591–596, 1995.
627. Meduri GU, Headley S, Tolley E, et al: Plasma and BAL cytokine response to corticosteroid rescue treatment in late ARDS. Chest 108:1315–1325, 1995.
628. Meduri GU, Headley AS, Golden E, et al: Effect of prolonged methylprednisolone therapy in unresolving acute respiratory distress syndrome: A randomized controlled trial. JAMA 280:159–165, 1998.
629. Holm BA, Matalon S: Role of pulmonary surfactant in the development and treatment of adult respiratory distress syndrome. Anesth Analg 69:805–818, 1989.
630. Murray JF: Artificial surfactant. Rean Urg 1:49–54, 1992.
631. Lewis JF, Jobe AH: Surfactant and the adult respiratory distress syndrome. Am Rev Respir Dis 147:218–233, 1993.
632. Jobe A, Ikegami M: Surfactant for the treatment of respiratory distress syndrome. Am Rev Respir Dis 136:1256–1275, 1987.
633. Hobar JD, Soll RF, Sutherland JM, et al: A multicenter, randomized, placebo-controlled trial of surfactant therapy for respiratory distress syndrome. N Engl J Med 320:959–965, 1989.
634. Ahuja A, Oh N, Chao W, et al: Inhibition of the human neutrophil respiratory burst by native and synthetic surfactant. Am J Respir Cell Mol Biol 14:496–503, 1996.
635. Thomassen MJ, Antal JM, Barna BP, et al: Surfactant downregulates synthesis of DNA and inflammatory mediators in normal human lung fibroblasts. Am J Physiol 270:L159–L163, 1996.
636. Harris JD, Jackson F, Moxley MA, et al: Effect of exogenous surfactant instillation on experimental acute lung injury. J Appl Physiol 66:1846–1851, 1989.
637. Zelter M, Escudier BJ, Hoeffel JM, et al: Effects of aerosolized artificial surfactant on repeated oleic acid injury in sheep. Am Rev Respir Dis 141:1014–1019, 1990.
638. Weg JG, Balk RA, Tharratt RS, et al: Safety and potential efficacy of an aerosolized surfactant in human sepsis-induced adult respiratory distress syndrome. JAMA 272:1433–1438, 1994.
639. Anzueto A, Baughman RP, Guntupalli KK, et al: Aerosolized surfactant in adults with sepsis-induced acute respiratory distress syndrome. N Engl J Med 334:1417–1421, 1996.
640. Lewis JF, Goffin J, Yue P, et al: Evaluation of exogenous surfactant treatment strategies in an adult model of acute lung injury. J Appl Physiol 80:1156–1164, 1996.
641. Gregory TJ, Steinberg KP, Spragg R, et al: Bovine surfactant therapy for patients with acute respiratory distress syndrome. Am J Respir Crit Care Med 155:1309–1315, 1997.
642. Walmrath D, Günther A, Ghofrani HA, et al: Bronchoscopic surfactant administration in patients with severe adult respiratory distress syndrome and sepsis. Am J Respir Crit Care Med 154:57–62, 1996.
643. Peristeris P, Clark BD, Gatti S, et al: *N*-Acetylcysteine and glutathione as inhibitors of tumor necrosis factor production. Cell Immunol 140:390–399, 1992.
644. Bernard GR: *N*-Acetylcysteine in experimental and clinical acute lung injury. Am J Med 91(Suppl 3C):54S–59S, 1991.
645. Jepsen S, Herlevsen P, Knudsen P, et al: Antioxidant treatment with *N*-acetylcysteine during adult respiratory distress syndrome: A prospective, randomized, placebo-controlled study. Crit Care Med 20:918–923, 1992.
646. Suter PM, Domenighetti G, Schaller M-D, et al: *N*-Acetylcysteine enhances recovery from acute lung injury in man: A randomized, double-blind, placebo-controlled clinical study. Chest 105:190–194, 1994.
647. Bernard GR, Wheeler AP, Arons MM, et al: A trial of antioxidants *N*-acetylcysteine and procysteine in ARDS. Chest 112:164–172, 1997.
648. Domenighetti G, Suter PM, Schaller MD, et al: Treatment with *N*-acetylcysteine during acute respiratory distress syndrome: A randomized, double-blind, placebo-controlled clinical study. J Crit Care 12:177–182, 1997.
649. Johnston RB, Keele BB, Misra HP, et al: The role of superoxide anion generation in phagocytic bactericidal activity: Studies with normal and chronic granulomatous disease leukocytes. J Clin Invest 55:1357–1372, 1975.
650. McDonald RJ, Berger EM, White CW, et al: Effect of superoxide dismutase encapsulated in liposomes or conjugated with polyethylene glycol on neutrophil bactericidal activity in vitro and bacterial clearance in vivo. Am Rev Respir Dis 131:633–637, 1985.
651. Pesanti EL, Nugent KM: Modulation of pulmonary clearance of bacteria by antioxidants. Infect Immun 48:57–61, 1985.
652. Raffin TA: Acute lung injury and pentoxifylline. Crit Care Med 18:1485–1486, 1990.
653. Welsh CH, Lien D, Worthen GS, et al: Pentoxifylline decreased endotoxin-induced pulmonary neutrophil sequestration and extravascular protein accumulation in the dog. Am Rev Respir Dis 138:1106–1114, 1988.
654. Lilly CM, Sandhu JS, Ishizaka A, et al: Pentoxifylline prevents tumor necrosis factor-induced lung injury. Am Rev Respir Dis 139:1361–1368, 1989.

655. Seear MD, Hannam VL, Kaapa P, et al: Effect of pentoxifylline on hemodynamics, alveolar fluid reabsorption, and pulmonary edema in a model of acute lung injury. Am Rev Respir Dis 142:1083–1087, 1990.
656. Hoffmann H, Hatherill JR, Crowley J, et al: Early post-treatment with pentoxifylline or dibutyryl cAMP attenuates *Escherichia coli*–induced acute lung injury in guinea pigs. Am Rev Respir Dis 143:289–293, 1991.
657. McDonald RJ: Pentoxifylline reduces injury to isolated lungs perfused with human neutrophils. Am Rev Respir Dis 144:1347–1350, 1991.
658. Bone RC, Balk RA, Fein AM, et al: A second large controlled clinical study of E5, a monoclonal antibody to endotoxin: Results of a prospective, multicenter, randomized, controlled trial. Crit Care Med 23:994–1006, 1995 [published erratum appears in Crit Care Med 23:1616, 1995].
659. Warren HS, Danner RL, Munford RS: Anti-endotoxin monoclonal antibodies. N Engl J Med 326:1153–1157, 1992.
660. Fang KL: Monoclonal antibodies to endotoxin in the management of sepsis. West J Med 158:393–399, 1993.
661. Schulman KA, Glick HA, Rubin H, et al: Cost-effectiveness of HA-1A antibody for gram-negative sepsis: Economic assessment of a new therapeutic agent. JAMA 266:3466–3471, 1991.
662. Luce JM: Introduction of new technology into critical care practice: A history of HA-1A human monoclonal antibody against endotoxin. Crit Care Med 21:1233–1241, 1993.
663. Bigatello LM, Greene RE, Sprung CL, et al: HA-1A in septic patients with ARDS: Results from the pivotal trial. Intensive Care Med 20:328–334, 1994.
664. Abraham E, Wunderink R, Silverman H, et al: Efficacy and safety of monoclonal antibody to human tumor necrosis factor $\alpha$ in patients with sepsis syndrome: A randomized, controlled, double-blind, multicenter clinical trial. JAMA 273:934–941, 1995.
665. Fisher CJ, Dhainaut J-FA, Opal SM, et al: Recombinant human interleukin-1 receptor antagonist in the treatment of patients with sepsis syndrome: Results from a randomized, double-blind, placebo-controlled trial. JAMA 271:1836–1843, 1994.
666. Bone RC: Why sepsis trials fail. JAMA 276:565–566, 1996.
667. Sekido N, Mukaida N, Harada A, et al: Prevention of lung perfusion injury in rabbits by a monoclonal antibody against interleukin-8. Nature 365:654–657, 1993.
668. Bone RC, Slotman G, Maunder R, et al: Randomized double-blind, multicenter study of prostaglandin $E_1$ in patients with the adult respiratory distress syndrome. Chest 96:114–119, 1989.
669. Russell JA, Ronco JJ, Dodek PM: Physiologic effects and side effects of prostaglandin $E_1$ in the adult respiratory distress syndrome. Chest 97:684–692, 1990.
670. Silverman HJ, Slotman G, Bone RC, et al: Effects of prostaglandin $E_1$ on oxygen delivery and consumption in patients with the adult respiratory distress syndrome: Results from the prostaglandin $E_1$ multicenter trial. Chest 98:405–410, 1990.
671. Mélot C, Lejeune P, Leeman M, et al: Prostaglandin $E_1$ in the adult respiratory distress syndrome: Benefit for pulmonary hypertension and cost for pulmonary gas exchange. Am Rev Respir Dis 139:106–110, 1989.
672. Slotman GJ, Kerstein MD, Bone RC, et al: The effects of prostaglandin $E_1$ on non-pulmonary organ function during clinical acute respiratory failure. J Trauma 32:480–489, 1992.
673. Shoemaker WC: Was a magic bullet aimed in the right direction? Chest 98:257, 1990.
674. Michael JR, Barton RG, Saffle JR, et al: Inhaled nitric oxide versus conventional therapy: Effect on oxygenation in ARDS. Am J Respir Crit Care Med 157:1372–1380, 1998.
675. Dellinger RP, Zimmerman JL, Taylor RW, et al: Effects of inhaled nitric oxide in patients with acute respiratory distress syndrome: Results of a randomized phase II trial. Crit Care Med 26:15–23, 1998.
676. Luhr O, Nathorst-Westfelt U, Lundin S, et al: A retrospective analysis of nitric oxide inhalation in patients with severe acute lung injury in Sweden and Norway 1991–1994. Acta Anaesth Scand 41:1238–1246, 1997.
677. Abraham E, Park YC, Covington P, et al: Liposomal prostaglandin E1 in acute respiratory distress syndrome: A placebo-controlled, randomized, double-blind, multicenter clinical trial. Crit Care Med 24:10–15, 1996.
678. Walmrath D, Schneider T, Schermuly R, et al: Direct comparison of inhaled nitric oxide and aerosolized prostacyclin in acute respiratory distress syndrome. Am J Respir Crit Care Med 153:991–996, 1996.
679. Martin WJ, Kachel DL: Reduction of neutrophil-mediated injury to pulmonary endothelial cells by dapsone. Am Rev Respir Dis 131:544–547, 1985.
680. Theron A, Anderson R: Investigation of the protective effects of the antioxidants ascorbate, cysteine, and dapsone on the phagocytic-mediated oxidative inactivation of human alpha-1-protease inhibitor in vitro. Am Rev Respir Dis 132:1049–1054, 1985.
681. Canham EM, Shoemaker SA, Tate RM, et al: Mepacrine but not methylprednisolone decreases acute edematous lung injury after injection of phorbol myristate acetate in rabbits. Am Rev Respir Dis 127:594–598, 1983.
682. Webster RO, Goldstein IM, Flick MR: Selective inhibition by phenytoin of chemotactic factor-stimulated neutrophil functions. J Lab Clin Med 103:22–33, 1984.
683. Flick MR, Webster RO, Hoeffel JM, et al: Effect of phenytoin on acute lung injuries in unanesthetized sheep. Crit Care Med 21:1563–1571, 1993.
684. Suzuki Y, Tanigaki T, Heimer D, et al: Polyethylene glycol-conjugated superoxide dismutase attenuates septic lung injury in guinea pigs. Am Rev Respir Dis 145:388–393, 1992.
685. Reyes A, Roca J, Rodriguez-Roisin R, et al: Effect of almitrine on ventilation-perfusion distribution in adult respiratory distress syndrome. Am Rev Respir Dis 137:1062–1067, 1988.
686. Folkesson HG, Matthay MA, Weström BR, et al: Alveolar epithelial clearance of protein. J Appl Physiol 80:1431–1445, 1996.
687. Carter EP, Garat C, Sakuma T, et al: Resolution of alveolar edema: In vivo studies. *In* Matthay MA, Ingbar DH (eds): Pulmonary Edema. New York: Marcel Dekker, 1998, pp 431–455.
688. Guo Y, DuVall MD, Matalon S: Biophysical properties of $Na^+$ channels in alveolar epithelial cells. *In* Matthay MA, Ingbar DH (eds): Pulmonary Edema. New York: Marcel Dekker, 1998, pp 457–476.
689. Ingbar DH, Wendt CH, Crandall ED: Na,K-ATPase and the clearance of pulmonary edema fluid. *In* Matthay MA, Ingbar DH (eds): Pulmonary Edema. New York: Marcel Dekker, 1998, pp 477–499.
690. Saumon G: Use of isolated lungs to clarify the mechanisms by which alveolar edema is resolved. *In* Matthay MA, Ingbar DH (eds): Pulmonary Edema. New York: Marcel Dekker, 1998, pp 501–523.
691. Hastings RH, Kim K-J: Alveolar protein clearance. *In* Matthay MA, Ingbar DH (eds): Pulmonary Edema. New York: Marcel Dekker, 1998, pp 549–574.
692. Folkesson HG, Kheradmand F, Matthay MA: The effect of salt water on alveolar epithelial barrier function. Am J Respir Crit Care Med 150:1555–1563, 1994.
693. Zuege D, Suzuki S, Berthiaume Y: Increase of lung sodium-potassium-ATPase activity during recovery from high-permeability pulmonary edema. Am J Physiol 271:L896–L909, 1996.
694. Sakuma T, Folkesson HG, Suzuki S, et al: Beta-adrenergic agonist stimulated alveolar fluid clearance in ex vivo human and rat lungs. Am J Respir Crit Care Med 155:506–512, 1997.
695. Hastings RH, Folkesson HG, Petersen V, et al: Cellular uptake of albumin from lungs of anesthetized rabbits. Am J Physiol 269:L453–L462, 1995.
696. Staub NC: Alveolar flooding and clearance. Am Rev Respir Dis 127:S44–S51, 1983.
697. Conhaim RL: Airway level at which edema liquid enters the air space of isolated dog lungs. J Appl Physiol 67:2234–2242, 1989.
698. Kambara K, Longworth KE, Serikov VB, et al: Effect of interstitial edema on lung lymph flow in goats in the absence of filtration. J Appl Physiol 72:1142–1148, 1992.
699. Fukue M, Serikov VB, Jerome EH: Recovery from increased pressure or increased leakiness edema in perfused sheep lungs. J Appl Physiol 77:184–189, 1994.
700. Pearse DB, Wagner EM, Sylvester JT: Edema clearance in isolated sheep lungs. J Appl Physiol 74:126–132, 1993.
701. Wiener-Kronish JP, Broaddus VC: Interrelationship of pleural and pulmonary interstitial liquid. Annu Rev Physiol 55:209–226, 1993.
702. Wiener-Kronish JP, Matthay MA, Callen PW, et al: Relationship

of pleural effusions to pulmonary hemodynamics in patients with congestive heart failure. Am Rev Respir Dis 132:1253–1256, 1985.
703. Wiener-Kronish JP, Matthay MA: Pleural effusions associated with hydrostatic and increased permeability pulmonary edema. Chest 93:852–858, 1988.
704. Broaddus VC, Wiener-Kronish JP, Staub NC: Clearance of lung edema into the pleural space of volume-loaded anesthetized sheep. J Appl Physiol 68:2623–2630, 1990.
705. Hastings RH, Grady M, Sakuma T, et al: Clearance of different-sized proteins from the alveolar space in humans and rabbits. J Appl Physiol 73:1310–1316, 1992.
706. Lum H, Malik AB: Regulation of vascular endothelial barrier function. Am J Physiol 267:L223–L241, 1994.
707. Haslett C: Mechanisms of resolution of lung inflammation. *In* Evans TW, Haslett C (eds): ARDS: Acute Respiratory Distress in Adults. London: Chapman & Hall Medical, 1996, pp 49–68.
708. Wiener RS, Moses HW, Richeson JF, et al: Hospital and long term survival of patients with acute pulmonary edema associated with coronary artery disease. Am J Cardiol 60:33–35, 1987.
709. Gottlieb S, Moss AJ, McDermott M, et al: Interrelation of left ventricular ejection fraction, pulmonary congestion and outcome in acute myocardial infarction. Am J Cardiol 69:977–984, 1992.
710. Brezins M, Benari B, Papo V, et al: Left ventricular function in patients with acute myocardial infarction, acute pulmonary edema, and mechanical ventilation: Relationship to prognosis. Crit Care Med 21:380–385, 1993.
711. Mueller HS, Cohen LS, Braunwald E, et al: Predictors of early morbidity and mortality after thrombolytic therapy of acute myocardial infarction: Analyses of patient subgroups in the thrombolysis in myocardial infarction (TIMI) trial, phase II. Circulation 85:1254–1264, 1992.
712. Thomsen GE, Morris AH: Incidence of the adult respiratory distress syndrome in the state of Utah. Am J Respir Crit Care Med 152:965–971, 1995.
713. Milberg JA, Davis DR, Steinberg KP, et al: Improved survival of patients with acute respiratory distress syndrome (ARDS): 1983–1993. JAMA 273:306–309, 1995.
714. Gillespie DJ, Marsh HM, Divertie MB, et al: Clinical outcome of respiratory failure in patients requiring prolonged (>24 hours) mechanical ventilation. Chest 90:364–369, 1986.
715. Knaus WA, Wagner DP: Multiple systems organ failure: Epidemiology and prognosis. Crit Care Clin 5:221–232, 1989.
716. Ferring M, Vincent J-L: Is outcome from ARDS related to the severity of respiratory failure? Eur Respir J 10:1297–1300, 1997.
717. Moss M, Bucher B, Moore FA, et al: The role of chronic alcohol abuse in the development of acute respiratory distress syndrome in adults. JAMA 275:50–54, 1996.
718. Holguin F, Moss IM, Brown LAS, et al: Chronic ethanol ingestion impairs alveolar type II cell glutathione homeostasis and function and predisposes to endotoxin-mediated acute edematous lung injury in rats. J Clin Invest 101:761–768, 1998.
719. Suchyta MR, Clemmer TP, Elliott CG, et al: Increased mortality of older patients with acute respiratory distress syndrome. Chest 111:1334–1339, 1997.
720. Meduri GU, Headley S, Kohler G, et al: Persistent elevation of inflammatory cytokines predicts a poor outcome in ARDS: Plasma IL-1β and IL-6 levels are consistent and efficient predictors of outcome over time. Chest 107:1062–1073, 1995.
721. Kraus PA, Lipman J, Lee CCJ, et al: Acute lung injury at Baragwanath ICU: An eight-month audit and call for consensus for other organ failure in the adult respiratory distress syndrome. Chest 103:1832–1836, 1993.
722. Ghio AJ, Elliott CG, Crapo RO, et al: Impairment after adult respiratory distress syndrome: An evaluation based on American Thoracic Society recommendations. Am Rev Respir Dis 139:1158–1162, 1989.
723. Peters JI, Bell RC, Prihoda TJ, et al: Clinical determinants of abnormalities in pulmonary functions in survivors of the adult respiratory distress syndrome. Am Rev Respir Dis 139:1163–1168, 1989.
724. Elliott CG: Pulmonary sequelae in survivors of the adult respiratory distress syndrome. Clin Chest Med 11:789–800, 1990.
725. McHugh LG, Milberg JA, Whitcomb ME, et al: Recovery of function in survivors of the acute respiratory distress syndrome. Am J Respir Crit Care Med 150:90–94, 1994.
726. Hert R, Albert RK: Sequelae of the adult respiratory distress syndrome. Thorax 49:8–13, 1994.
727. Elliott CG, Rasmusson BY, Crapo RO: Upper airway obstruction following adult respiratory distress syndrome: An analysis of 30 survivors. Chest 94:526–530, 1988.
728. Bitterman PB: Pathogenesis of fibrosis in acute lung injury. Am J Med 92:39S–43S, 1992.
729. Pugin J, Verghese G, Widmer M-C, et al: The alveolar space is the site of intense inflammatory and profibrotic reactions in the early phase of acute respiratory distress syndrome. Crit Care Med 27:304–312, 1999.
730. Collins JF, Smith JD, Coalson JJ, et al: Variability in lung collagen amounts after prolonged support of acute respiratory failure. Chest 85:641–646, 1984.
731. Martin C, Papazian L, Payan M-J, et al: Pulmonary fibrosis correlates with outcome in adult respiratory distress syndrome: A study in mechanically ventilated patients. Chest 107:196–200, 1995.
732. Thet LA, Parra SC, Shelburne JD: Repair of oxygen-induced lung injury in adult rats: The role of ornithine decarboxylase and polyamines. Am Rev Respir Dis 129:174–181, 1984.
733. Uitto J, Ryhanen L, Tan EML, et al: Pharmacological inhibition of excessive collagen deposition in fibrotic diseases. Fed Proc 43:2815–2820, 1984.
734. Rennard SI, Bitterman PB, Ozaki T, et al: Colchicine suppresses the release of fibroblast growth factors from alveolar macrophages in vitro: The basis of a possible therapeutic approach to the fibrotic disorders. Am Rev Respir Dis 137:181–185, 1988.
735. Marinelli WA, Henke CA, Harmon KR, et al: Mechanisms of alveolar fibrosis after acute lung injury. Clin Chest Med 11:657–672, 1990.
736. Panos RJ, Bak PM, Simonet WS, et al: Intratracheal instillation of keratinocyte growth factor decreases hyperoxia-induced mortality in rats. J Clin Invest 96:2026–2033, 1995.
737. Garat C, Kheradmand F, Albertine KH, et al: Soluble and insoluble fibronectin increases alveolar epithelial wound healing in vitro. Am J Physiol 271:L844–L853, 1996.
738. Matthay MA: Fibrosing alveolitis in the adult respiratory distress syndrome. Ann Intern Med 122:65–66, 1995.

# 55 Cor Pulmonale

ELLIOT RAPAPORT, M.D.

Introduction
Pulmonary Circulation
Pulmonary Artery Pressure
Pulmonary Artery Wedge Pressure
Pathophysiology of the Pulmonary Circulation
Hypoxic Pulmonary Vasoconstriction
Right Ventricle
Left Ventricle
Neurohormones
Angiotensin II
Natriuretic Peptides
Symptoms and Signs
Chest Radiograph
Electrocardiogram
Echocardiography
Hemodynamics
Differential Diagnosis
Classification of Pulmonary Hypertension
Treatment
Oxygen Therapy
Pulmonary Vasodilators
Angiotensin-Converting Enzyme Inhibition
Nitric Oxide
Endothelin
Prostaglandins
Natural History
Summary

## INTRODUCTION

The term *cor pulmonale,* or pulmonary heart disease, has been used rather loosely over many years to describe three broad groups. They are patients exhibiting pulmonary hypertension resulting in progressive right ventricular hypertrophy, right ventricular dilatation, and eventual cardiac decompensation from (1) disorders that primarily affect ventilatory drive or musculoskeletal respiratory mechanics; (2) pulmonary airway, infiltrative, fibrotic, or vascular diseases; and (3) diseases in which the clinical picture as it affects the lungs and pulmonary circulation is the consequence of a primary cardiovascular disorder. In 1963, an expert committee appointed by the Director General of the World Health Organization recommended a definition based on morbid anatomy. Specifically, the committee defined chronic *cor pulmonale* as "hypertrophy of the right ventricle resulting from diseases affecting the function and/or the structure of the lung, except when these pulmonary alterations are the result of diseases that primarily affect the left side of the heart or congenital heart disease."[1] This definition appears to be an appropriate one for this chapter. Therefore, changes in pulmonary vasculature or pulmonary function related to primary cardiovascular disease are not covered here but are discussed in Chapter 84. Here, the discussion is limited to diseases that primarily affect the air passages, the pulmonary vasculature, or alveolar ventilation.

## PULMONARY CIRCULATION

The major pulmonary arteries normally have less medial thickening than is seen in systemic arteries, reflecting the fact that the pressures in the pulmonary arteries are approximately a fifth to a sixth those normally found in the systemic arteries. In the systemic arteries the ratio of medial thickness to external arterial diameter is 20% to 25%, but in the pulmonary arteries it is closer to 5%.[2] Postmortem casts of the human pulmonary arterial tree show there to be 17 branching orders, from the main pulmonary artery to the alveoli, that follow closely the branching of the bronchial tree.[3, 4] The number of vessels increases by a factor of approximately 3 with each branching order. As these vessels branch, their overall diameter ratio remains relatively constant, ensuring that the resistance to blood flow is minimal.

Muscular branches of the pulmonary artery, vessels with a luminal diameter between 100 and 1000 μm, have circular muscle fibers capable of causing vasoconstriction. These branches also demonstrate muscle hypertrophy in patients with chronic pulmonary hypertension (Fig. 55.1). True pulmonary arterioles, comparable to systemic arterioles, are not seen normally in the pulmonary circulation. Vessels smaller than 100 μm in diameter at the terminal end of the pulmonary arteries are usually referred to as pulmonary arterioles, but they normally have little or no medial smooth muscle. However, with chronic pulmonary hypertension, a single smooth muscle cell layer may extend longitudinally down the vessel. Therefore, pulmonary arterioles lack a true muscular media capable of

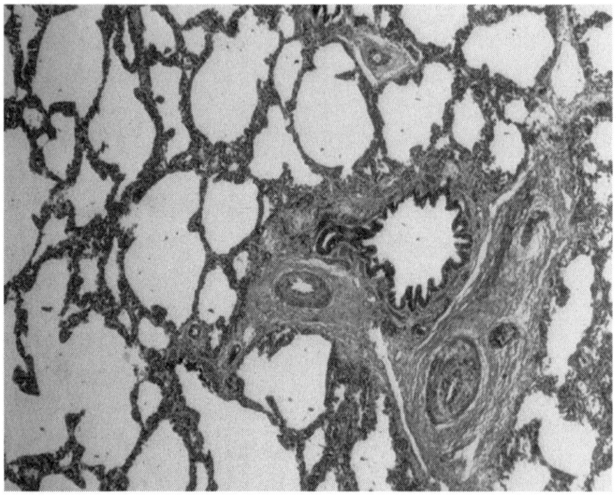

**Figure 55.1** A microscopic section from the lung of a patient who had chronic pulmonary hypertension is shown. The small branches of the pulmonary artery are seen in juxtaposition to a terminal bronchiole. There is intimal thickening and marked medial hypertrophy.

reacting with vigorous vasoconstriction, but they still are capable of distending. The pulmonary vascular resistance is primarily regulated in the very small branches of the pulmonary artery, and these branches are the major site of the muscularization that is seen in patients who develop pulmonary hypertension. These vessels are less distensible to passive increases in pressure, and they can actively vasoconstrict in the presence of hypoxia. The pulmonary capillaries do not have smooth muscle cells within their walls and therefore do not contribute to pulmonary vasoconstriction. They can, however, dilate to some extent as they engorge, as when pulmonary venous pressure rises. Although the pulmonary capillaries, which are literally suspended in air, cannot vasoconstrict, their diameter can decrease in response to increases in intra-alveolar or intrapleural pressure. They may also decrease if there is perivascular inflammation or interstitial transudation of fluid.

## Pulmonary Artery Pressure

Pulmonary artery pressure in the normal resting recumbent adult averages 22/9 mm Hg, with a mean of 15 mm Hg. Pulmonary hypertension in the adult is said to be present when the resting pressure is higher than 30/15 mm Hg or the mean pressure is more than 20 mm Hg. Commonly, pulmonary hypertension observed in cor pulmonale represents the net effect of a variety of different mechanisms. For example, in chronic obstructive pulmonary disease (COPD) resulting from bronchitis and emphysema, the following effects on the pulmonary circulation may be seen: reduction in the cross-sectional area of the pulmonary vasculature, reflecting anatomic loss of pulmonary capillaries as alveoli coalesce; increased pulmonary vascular resistance to pulmonary blood flow due to hypoxic pulmonary vasoconstriction with or without additional vasoconstriction resulting from hypercapnia; medial hypertrophy of muscular pulmonary arteries and muscularization of the arterioles; increased resistance to pulmonary blood flow resulting from polycythemia; increased pulmonary blood flow from systemic arteriolar vasodilation caused by arterial hypoxemia that raises pulmonary artery pressure; and an increase in intra-alveolar pressure with increasing lung inflation that compresses pulmonary capillaries. Pulmonary hypertension may be variable—from mild elevations with exercise returning to normal with rest; to marked elevations in pulmonary artery pressure associated with acute respiratory failure but with restoration to the high-normal or mildly elevated range once ventilatory insufficiency is improved; to fixed severe pulmonary hypertension.

Disturbances in respiratory function ultimately affect the pulmonary circulation predominantly by production of alveolar hypoxia, regardless of whether obstructive or restrictive ventilatory insufficiency (or a combination of the two) is present, whether an abnormality in alveolar-capillary gas exchange is caused by anatomic or functional disturbances, or whether there is a ventilation-perfusion mismatch. In hypoxemia, with or without net hypercapnia, pulmonary artery pressure rises out of proportion to pulmonary capillary pressure, resulting in an increase in the work of the right ventricle and its subsequent hypertrophy.

## Pulmonary Artery Wedge Pressure

The pulmonary artery wedge pressure is normally obtained at cardiac catheterization by occluding a small branch of the pulmonary artery in which the catheter resides, either by inflating a balloon at the end of the catheter or wedging an end-hole catheter into the distal vasculature. This extends the manometric system encompassed by the wall of the catheter, and the static column of fluid within it, to incorporate the walls of the vessel distal to the end of the catheter and the static column of blood within it. The extended manometric system then measures the pressure in the distal capillary-sinusoidal bed of the lung, where blood is still freely flowing (i.e., near the origin of the pulmonary venous system). Because the flow between the pulmonary capillaries and the left atrium normally is a low-resistance network, the pulmonary artery wedge pressure is usually within 1 or 2 mm Hg of left atrial pressure. It is, therefore, possible to estimate the pulmonary vascular resistance by calculating the ratio of the mean pulmonary artery pressure, minus the pulmonary wedge pressure, to the cardiac output.

Although the apexes of the lungs in a person who is sitting or standing are normally in West's zone 2 (see Fig. 50.4 in Chapter 50), if pulmonary artery pressure decreases, zone 1 relationships may develop. Under these conditions, estimates of left atrial pressure from pulmonary artery wedge pressures from these regions are difficult to obtain and may be inaccurate. However, because most measurements of pulmonary artery wedge pressures are made with the patient supine, this is ordinarily not a significant practical problem. Should it be desirable to have measurements of pulmonary vascular resistance or estimations of accurate pulmonary artery wedge pressure while the patient is sitting or standing, the pulmonary artery catheter should be wedged in the inferior portions of the lung: that is, in areas in which the vessel is below the level of the left atrium. Or, alternately, one may reasonably use total pulmonary resistance or the ratio of the mean pulmonary artery pressure to the pulmonary blood flow when studying patients with pulmonary hypertension unrelated to left-sided heart events, in whom pulmonary venous pressures are presumably normal. It should also be noted that the pulmonary artery wedge pressure may not reflect left atrial pressure if a patient is receiving positive-pressure ventilation. If there are wide swings in intrapleural pressure, the wedge pressure should be estimated at end-expiration and not as a mean pressure (Fig. 55.2).

## PATHOPHYSIOLOGY OF THE PULMONARY CIRCULATION

Significant structural changes occur in the pulmonary circulation in patients with COPD. The presence of hypoxemia and chronic ventilatory insufficiency is associated with early evidence of intimal thickening and medial hypertrophy in the smaller branches of the pulmonary arteries.[5] Vascular smooth muscle cells are laid down longitudinally within the intima, and hypertrophy of these cells and smooth muscle cells within the media become prominent. Localized thrombosis in situ can occur, obliterating parts of the pulmonary vascular tree. Coupled with these pathologic changes is pulmonary vasoconstriction arising from the presence of hypoxemia. The structural changes together with the effects of vasoconstriction result in a significant increase in pulmonary vascular resistance. The consequence is pulmonary arterial hypertension, which in itself may further cause structural damage to the smaller branches of the pulmonary circulation and serve as a stimulus for the development of medial hypertrophy and dilation of the larger branches of the pulmonary artery. If these developments are long-standing, prominent atherosclerotic changes may be seen in the main pulmonary artery and its major branches.[6]

Destruction of capillaries that course along alveoli that are being destroyed or coalescing into bullae further diminishes the cross-sectional area of the pulmonary vascular tree. This diminishment in area is likely to occur progressively as hyperinflation worsens. Capillaries may also be destroyed in interstitial fibrosis or parenchymal infiltrative disease.

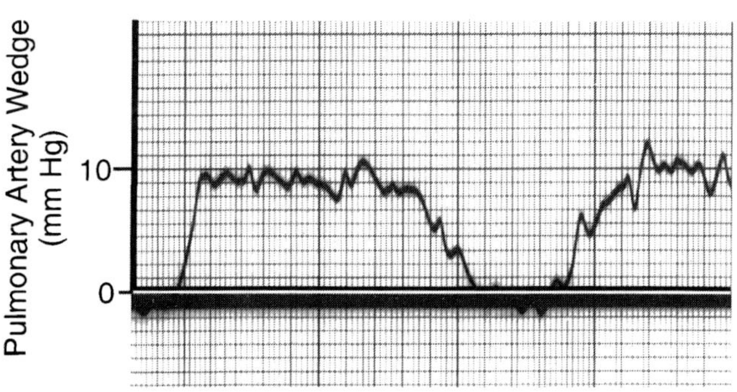


**Figure 55.2** Pulmonary artery wedge pressure in a patient with chronic obstructive lung disease is shown. Note that the wedge pressure is normal. A prominent fall in wedge pressure is observed with the onset of inspiration as intrapleural pressure falls.

Early in the natural history of COPD, the resting pressure in the pulmonary artery is usually normal. It may not be readily apparent that significant capillary destruction is taking place until almost half of the pulmonary vascular tree is destroyed. A large capillary reserve normally exists within the lung. For example, a normal subject exercising may increase cardiac output severalfold with only a small rise in pulmonary perfusing pressure. Similarly, patients with an uncomplicated atrial septal defect can have a pulmonary artery pressure that is still in the normal range despite a pulmonary blood flow that is two to three times normal. Although this undoubtedly means that the cross-sectional area of the pulmonary capillary bed is increased by the distention of partially collapsed capillaries and/or recruitment of capillaries that might be closed were flow less, it should be remembered that pulmonary venous and capillary pressures drop to right atrial levels in patients with atrial septal defect as atrial pressures equilibrate in the presence of the usual large defect. Therefore, the pulmonary arterial minus pulmonary venous pressure gradient is increased despite a normal pulmonary artery pressure.

Finally, this capillary reserve can be demonstrated in the normal person at the time of cardiac catheterization with transient balloon occlusion of the left or right main pulmonary artery. No rise or only a small rise in the resting pulmonary artery pressure results, despite the fact that the entire cardiac output must now go through the pulmonary circulation of one lung.[7, 8] Similarly, patients with pneumonectomy often have only slightly raised resting pulmonary artery pressures after recovery from surgery.

Pulmonary parenchymal disease, particularly idiopathic pulmonary fibrosis, may produce pulmonary hypertension through disturbed gas exchange with the production of pulmonary capillary hypoxemia. This is accomplished through the reduction in pulmonary vascular distensibility by surrounding fibrotic tissue, through mismatching between the distributions of ventilation and perfusion, or directly through destruction or obliteration of a large portion of the pulmonary vascular bed. It is typical for pulmonary hypertension to be produced in patients with chronic pulmonary disease through combinations of anatomic restriction of the pulmonary vascular bed and vasoconstriction due to hypoxia with or without hypercapnia and acidemia.

### Hypoxic Pulmonary Vasoconstriction

Several stimuli may result in precapillary pulmonary vasoconstriction with resultant pulmonary artery hypertension. Of these, the most potent and most important, alveolar hypoxia, may be present under a variety of circumstances. Pulmonary vasoconstriction can occur in perfectly healthy lungs. For example, the pulmonary hypertension observed in persons living at high altitudes is caused by chronic hypoxemia despite the presence of hyperventilation with resultant hypocapnia. Similarly, hypoventilation sufficient to produce alveolar hypoxia and hypercapnia, which may occur in morbidly obese patients, results in pulmonary hypertension secondary to pulmonary vasoconstriction. Other causes of primary hypoventilation, whether it arises centrally or from weakness of the muscles of respiration, may also cause pulmonary hypertension secondary to inadequate alveolar ventilation. Hypercapnia, which is primarily mediated by an increase in hydrogen ion concentration, results in the exacerbation of pulmonary vasoconstriction, augmenting the level expected from a comparable degree of hypoxia alone.

It is of interest to contrast the consequences of hypoxic pulmonary vasoconstriction in healthy residents who are residing at high altitude and in patients with COPD with cor pulmonale who are residing at sea level. In the former case, a combination of alveolar hypoxia, hyperventilation, and hypocapnia is present. In the latter case, hypoxia is often associated with hypoventilation and hypercapnia. Subjects residing at high altitudes have an increased hematocrit and a decreased plasma volume. Their stroke volume and cardiac output tend to be low. In contrast, patients with COPD tend to have normal or increased blood volume, and their cardiac output is generally normal or even increased. Normal subjects, even those residing at very high altitudes, normally do not develop right ventricular failure despite the presence of hypoxia and pulmonary artery hypertension. This suggests that acidemia and hypercapnia are important elements that contribute to impaired right ventricular function in patients with COPD.

Low alveolar $P_{O_2}$ increases pulmonary arterial pressure in a somewhat hyperbolic dose-response curve, with the pressure rising much more rapidly when arterial $P_{O_2}$ values fall below 75 mm Hg. Nevertheless, there is still marked individual variability in the level of pulmonary artery pressure at a given high altitude. In part this may be explained by differences in individual sensitivity to ventilatory drive produced by hypoxia, with some persons hyperventilating more than others. However, some of the variability lies in the difference in pulmonary vasoconstrictive response, which probably reflects an inherited difference in pulmonary vascular reactivity. This latter viewpoint is supported by observations of the high-altitude pulmonary hypertensive disease among cattle known as *brisket disease*.[9] When cattle native to low altitudes are exposed to high altitudes for grazing, pulmonary artery pressure climbs only moderately in some, but in others the pressure climbs steeply. Cattle with either hyporesponsive or hyperresponsive pulmonary vascular reactivity transmit these phenotypes as a genetic trait from parents to offspring.[10]

Just as it has been suggested that genetic traits may play a role in the pulmonary pressor response to the hypoxia of high altitude, one explanation for the observation that some patients with COPD develop pulmonary hypertension, whereas others do not, attributes this variability to inherited differences in the ventilatory sensitivity to hypoxia and carbon dioxide or in pulmonary vascular reactivity, or both.[11]

Most patients who develop resting pulmonary hypertension with COPD are both hypoxemic and hypercarbic; presumably, the hypercarbic patients have a low ventilatory sensitivity to carbon dioxide, because, as noted, hypoxemic residents at high altitudes hyperventilate and are hypocarbic. It is therefore reasoned that some patients who are born with a normal ventilatory sensitivity to carbon dioxide and hypoxia have an increased ventilatory effort in response to obstructive lung disease and therefore maintain relatively normal blood gases. In contrast, a patient who responds with a low ventilatory sensitivity fails to compensate and consequently develops an insufficient ventilatory drive to overcome airway resistance, ultimately causing hypercapnia, hypoxemia, and pulmonary vasoconstriction.

The terms "pink puffers" and "blue bloaters" were applied by clinicians in the past to characterize the differences between two groups that represent extremes in the clinical-physiologic continuum of COPD. As the names imply, the pink puffers were those who were dyspneic from vigorous breathing but maintained their arterial $P_{O_2}$ and $P_{CO_2}$ values in a normal to near-normal range, whereas the blue bloaters were those who became cyanotic and edematous because of hypoventilation with consequent hypoxia and hypercapnia. Originally, it was postulated that these features could be explained by differences in the drive to breathe, excessive in the pink puffers and reduced in the blue bloaters. But that theory was shattered by the results of studies that measured the drive to breathe using the $P_{0.1}$ test (see Chapter 28) in the two groups of patients: compared with healthy subjects, drive to breathe was greatly increased in both pink puffers and blue bloaters, and there was no difference between them.[12] The more severe abnormalities in $P_{O_2}$ and $P_{CO_2}$ that characterize the blue bloaters are now believed to result from differences in the pattern of breathing and, probably, in intrapulmonary gas exchange.[13] It remains true, however, that in general the more abnormal the $P_{O_2}$ and $P_{CO_2}$ values in patients with COPD, the more severe the pulmonary hypertension and polycythemia and the greater the likelihood of cor pulmonale.

## RIGHT VENTRICLE

The normal right ventricle is crescent shaped and has a wall thickness less than 0.6 cm (Fig. 55.3). Its weight is usually less than 65 g in men, less than 50 g in women.[6] Embryologically, the right ventricle develops from two separate components: the bulbus cordis, which becomes the outflow tract, and the sinus venosus, which becomes the inflow tract. These are separated by a muscular ridge, the crista supraventricularis. Normally, the right ventricle contracts almost sequentially from inflow to outflow, thus effectively emptying its volume into the low-impedance pulmonary circulation. In the absence of cardiac disease, the right ventricle plays an almost passive role in maintaining cardiac output in accordance with the venous return and Starling's law of the heart. In fact, in congenital tricuspid atresia, early surgical approaches involved bypass of the right ventricle through anastomosis of the right atrium directly to the pulmonary artery, the so-called Fontan procedure, which resulted in perfusion of the pulmonary circulation from an elevated central venous pressure. However, it should also be noted that a damaged

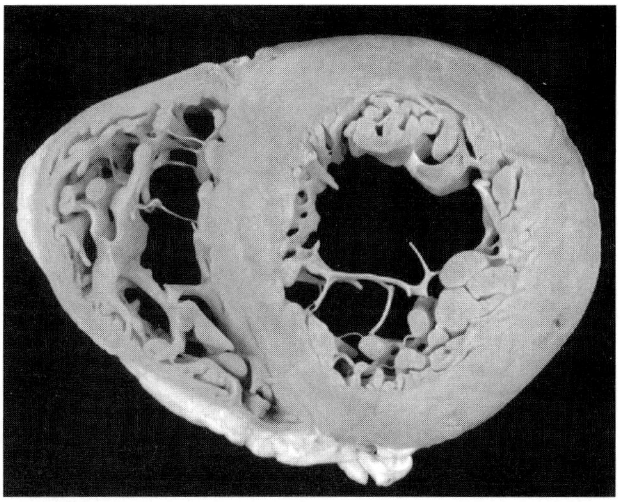

**Figure 55.3** A transverse section through a normal heart illustrates a somewhat crescent-shaped right ventricular cavity, together with the presence of prominent trabeculae carneae. Note that the myocardial thickness of the normal left ventricle is considerably greater than that of the right ventricle.

right ventricle with residual high central venous pressures resulting from an inferior myocardial infarction is associated with a distinctly reduced survival rate.

Because of the shape of the right ventricle, it is difficult to measure the right ventricular volume accurately by radiographic or echocardiographic techniques. In a series of 15 subjects without heart disease, right ventricular end-diastolic volume in the supine position measured by a thermodilution technique, which probably overestimates volumes, averaged 103 ± 24.4 mL/m$^2$.[14] With passive assumption of an upright posture by tilting, right ventricular end-diastolic volume falls due to gravitational pooling of blood within the distensible venous tree. In a separate series of 8 subjects without heart disease, end-diastolic volume fell a mean of 16.3 mL/m$^2$ from a mean baseline of 98.1 ± 23.3 mL/m$^2$. This fall in end-diastolic volume causes less of an end-diastolic fiber stretch and results in a fall in stroke volume with the assumption of an upright position. At the same time, aortic baroreceptor stimulation reflexively increases heart rate by about 12 beats/minute, thus compensating for an average stroke volume fall of approximately 13.3 mL/m$^2$; cardiac output is, therefore, maintained in essentially the same range as in a recumbent patient at rest.[15]

Acute increases in right ventricular afterload result in a significant fall in stroke volume[16]; in contrast, the left ventricle can accommodate an acute increase in afterload with little change in stroke output. Chronic pulmonary hypertension with a corresponding increase in right ventricular work results in a uniform hypertrophy of the right ventricle. As a result, right ventricular weight increases as right ventricular wall myocytes thicken and exhibit enlarged nuclei. Varying degrees of interstitial fibrosis occur. As the ventricle further hypertrophies, it becomes increasingly able to expel the stroke output against high pulmonary arterial resistance and maintain cardiac output. Patients have been observed with primary pulmonary hypertension or with severe mitral stenosis and pulmonary vascular disease in whom the right ventricle maintained a pulmonary artery systolic pressure significantly higher than the systemic pressure.

In patients with COPD, hypoxic vasoconstriction is associated not only with right ventricular hypertrophy but also with right ventricular dilatation. The normal crescent shape of the right ventricle is progressively transformed into a more spherical structure that is better able to generate an increased stroke work (Fig. 55.4).

The increase in right ventricular work associated with hypoxic pulmonary vasoconstriction, with both hypertrophy and dilatation of the right ventricle, produces a significant increase in right ventricular myocardial oxygen consumption. At the same time, an increase in wall thickness tends to decrease right ventricular endocardial coronary perfusion. Furthermore, an increase in end-diastolic pressure occurs as diastolic right ventricular stiffness increases, adding to the compromise of endocardial coronary perfusion. Taken together, these factors result in an imbalance between right ventricular myocardial oxygen demand and supply. Nevertheless, in several studies the end-diastolic pressure-volume relationship, even in the presence of resting pulmonary hypertension, suggested well-preserved right ventricular contractility in patients with COPD. It is only with the additional presence of acidemia or infection that right ventricular failure is precipitated. When chronic hypercapnia with acidosis is pres-

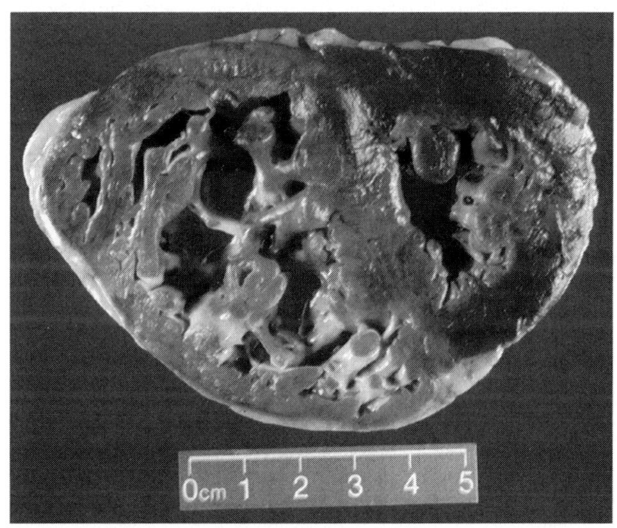


**Figure 55.4** Transverse section of a heart from a patient who had severe pulmonary hypertension showing dilatation of the right ventricular cavity, which has a more spherical shape than the heart shown in Figure 55.3. Marked wall thickness of the right ventricle caused by massive hypertrophy is seen. The trabeculae carneae are also hypertrophied, and endocardial sclerosis is visible on several of them. The left ventricle is relatively normal with protrusion of the posteromedial and anterolateral papillary muscles into the cavity. The bright white patches on the lateral free wall and posterolateral septum are highlight artifacts caused by reflection of the flash during photography.

ent in patients with alveolar hypoventilation, the ability of the right ventricle to increase its work appears to be significantly impaired, and right ventricular end-diastolic pressure increases (i.e., there is a shift to the right in the family of Starling curves). This impairment of myocardial contractility in the presence of hypercapnia probably plays a significant role in producing decompensated pulmonary heart disease in response to acute increases in arterial $Pco_2$ associated with acute decreases in alveolar ventilation or infection. Recordings of right ventricular and pulmonary artery systolic pressures may show pulsus alternans similar to that often seen in left ventricular failure (Fig. 55.5) The development of right ventricular volume overload with ventricular dilatation results in a decreased ejection fraction, because stroke volume tends to be maintained close to the normal range in decompensated pulmonary heart disease.[17] With exercise, patients with COPD significantly raise their right ventricular afterload, with further increases in right ventricular end-diastolic volume and decreases in ejection fraction. It is likely that this deterioration in hemodynamics with exercise is a major factor limiting the ability of such patients to exercise normally.

When congestive heart failure develops and central venous pressure is elevated, the assumption of an upright posture decreases neither right ventricular end-diastolic volume nor stroke volume. Consequently, heart rate does not change. This lack of postural change is attributable to failure of any incremental gravitational pooling of blood in the venous tree because of increased plasma volume, increased tissue pressure from edema with decreasing venous distensibility, and increased venomotor tone.[15]

## LEFT VENTRICLE

Controversy has existed over the years as to whether the left ventricle eventually fails when right ventricular failure results from chronic cor pulmonale. Part of the uncertainty has stemmed from the fact that the early studies of patients with cor pulmonale secondary to COPD included chiefly middle-aged or older men with a history of heavy cigarette smoking, who were likely to have coexisting coronary artery disease. Failure of the left ventricle in some of these patients may have reflected coexisting coronary artery disease rather than the natural history of decompensated pulmonary heart disease. Nevertheless, although left ventricular ejection performance is unimpaired, cardiac catheterization studies have revealed abnormal left ventricular end-diastolic pressure-volume relationships.[18] Echocardiographic studies also showed progressive impairment of left ventricular diastolic function that correlated with the severity of pulmonary hypertension.[18a] It is likely that this results, in large part, from bulging of the interventricular septum from the hypertrophied and dilated right ventricle into the cavity of the left ventricle. As a result, left ventricular diastolic geometry becomes distorted,[19] and filling characteristics may be altered such that a higher filling pressure is required to accomplish the same end-diastolic fiber stretch needed for stroke work, in accordance with Starling's law of the heart. Furthermore, measurements of pulmonary artery wedge pressure as a reflection of left heart filling pressure can be distorted because of the increase in intra-alveolar pressures, as well as the large swings in intrathoracic pressure with resultant large swings in wedge pressure tracings seen in patients with COPD (see Fig. 55.2). This is particularly troublesome when the patient is receiving positive end-expiratory pressure from a respirator. Pulmonary artery wedge pressures should always be estimated at end-expiration rather than attempting to measure the mean wedge pressure.

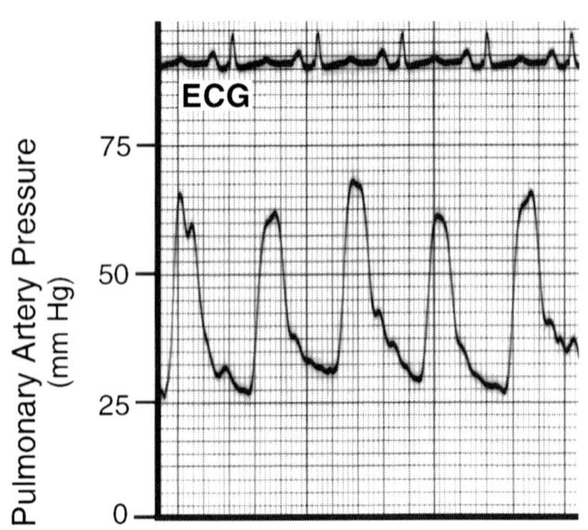


**Figure 55.5** A recording shows the pulmonary artery pressure at the time of cardiac catheterization in a patient with cor pulmonale and heart failure, illustrating pulsus alternans in the pulmonary artery.

## NEUROHORMONES

Plasma catecholamine levels generally rise in patients with decompensated pulmonary heart disease in a manner comparable to that seen in patients with heart failure secondary to primary myocardial disorders. It is clear that increased sympathetic activity is present with decompensation from cor pulmonale, resulting in high levels of circulating catecholamines and stimulation of the renin-angiotensin-aldosterone systems, causing pronounced elevations in plasma levels of these hormones. In the measurements by Anand and associates,[20] vasopressin actually rose to a higher level than was seen in comparable patients in whom failure was not associated with COPD. Because cardiac output is often normal or may even be increased in decompensated pulmonary heart disease, it is likely that the decrease in systemic vascular resistance resulting from both hypercapnia and hypoxia leads to a reflex increase in circulating catecholamines and other neural hormones. Central sympathetic stimulation may also be encouraged by the direct effect of the increased $Pco_2$ on the central nervous system.

## ANGIOTENSIN II

Angiotensin II is a potent vasoconstrictor of the pulmonary vascular bed. The pulmonary vasculature appears to be even more sensitive to the vasoconstrictor effects of angiotensin II than the systemic vascular bed is. This is noteworthy because increased circulating levels of angiotensin II and aldosterone are found in patients with cor pulmonale secondary to COPD who have hypoxia and hypercapnia.[21] It is likely that activation of the renin-angiotensin-aldosterone system, together with hypoxemia, is the underlying major pathophysiologic mechanism responsible for the elevation in pulmonary vascular resistance that is observed in patients with decompensated pulmonary heart disease.

A dose-response relationship of pulmonary vascular resistance to the infusion of angiotensin II has been observed in normal subjects.[22] In patients with pulmonary heart disease, lowering pulmonary vascular resistance and dropping pulmonary artery pressure is an ideal therapeutic goal. Angiotensin II inhibitors might be expected to accomplish this end. They have been demonstrated to improve survival in patients with congestive failure caused by either coronary disease or idiopathic dilated congestive cardiomyopathy. Could such a benefit be expected in patients whose heart failure results from COPD despite the earlier, disappointing experience with vasodilators? Although such vasodilators are capable of reducing pulmonary vascular resistance, they may actually increase hypoxemia. Increased hypoxemia can result from pulmonary vasodilators because perfusion may improve to areas of impaired ventilation, resulting in arterial hypoxemia as a consequence of the ventilation-perfusion mismatch. It is encouraging to note that the angiotensin-converting enzyme (ACE) inhibitor lisinopril has been demonstrated experimentally to attenuate significantly the pulmonary pressor response to hypoxic pulmonary vasoconstriction in healthy human volunteers.[23]

## NATRIURETIC PEPTIDES

The family of natriuretic peptides includes atrial natriuretic peptide (ANP), brain natriuretic peptide (BNP), and c-type natriuretic peptide (CNP). Circulating ANP and BNP levels are elevated many-fold in patients with cor pulmonale, even in the absence of impaired left ventricular function.[24] Presumably, right atrial distention and/or overactivity in response to right ventricular afterload is the stimulus for their release. CNP, which appears to be normal in the usual patient with congestive heart failure, is also elevated, albeit not as extensively as ANP and BNP, in those with cor pulmonale.[25] The elevation of CNP appears to be endothelial in origin, suggesting that its stimulus for release may be either arterial hypoxemia or endothelial damage occurring in cor pulmonale. ANP, BNP, and CNP have approximately equivalent pulmonary vasorelaxant activities. Although atrial natriuretic peptides appear to have little effect on resting vasopulmonary artery tone, they do appear to interact with the vasoactive response of hypoxic pulmonary vasoconstriction. Experimentally, they can attenuate the increased pulmonary hypertension produced by hypoxia.[26]

Patients with cor pulmonale, who demonstrate alveolar hypoxia and elevated circulating angiotensin II levels, have a dose-related decrease in pulmonary artery pressure during an infusion of ANP.[27, 28] The pulmonary pressor response to infused angiotensin II in humans appears to be significantly attenuated by BNP, but not by ANP. A similar effect is noted in response to hypoxic pulmonary pressor changes. It is, therefore, likely that BNP is the predominant natriuretic peptide modulating the response of the pulmonary vasculature to hypoxia and angiotensin II. BNP may play an important role in attenuating the pressor response that is likely to occur in humans because of the actions of alveolar hypoxia and elevated angiotensin II levels. This suggests the possible clinical use of neutral endopeptidase inhibitors that increase circulating levels of endogenous natriuretic peptides by inhibiting their degradation.[29] Such agents might prove useful if added to ACE inhibitors and angiotensin II receptor antagonists in the management of chronic cor pulmonale characterized by alveolar hypoxia and pulmonary hypertension.

## SYMPTOMS AND SIGNS

Small chronic elevations in right ventricular pressure reflecting mild pulmonary hypertension generally produce little in terms of clinical, radiologic, or electrocardiographic findings. When moderate or severe pulmonary hypertension develops, symptoms are often those associated with the underlying pulmonary disease. Most commonly, these are dyspnea on exertion, chronic cough productive of mucoid sputum (particularly in the morning hours), variable degrees of wheezing, and noticeable occasional cyanosis. Clubbing of the fingers, reflecting hypertrophic pulmonary osteoarthropathy, may be present. Moderate or severe pulmonary hypertension by itself (e.g., in patients with primary pulmonary hypertension) may result in only minimal or nonspecific symptoms. Some patients experience dizziness or even exertional syncope, reflecting the inability to increase cardiac output in response to exercise when significant pulmonary vascular disease and pulmonary artery hypertension are present. In addition, these patients frequently display tiredness and easy fatigability.

When resting pulmonary artery pressure is elevated, patients may eventually reach a point at which the right ventricle cannot meet the increased stroke work without a significant increase in right heart filling pressures. The resultant increase in central venous pressure is associated with the developing symptoms of congestive heart failure, such as weight gain, right upper quadrant discomfort, nocturia, peripheral edema, and easy fatigability. On examination, the patient often displays tachypnea, with prominent use of the accessory muscles of respiration, with arms extended holding on to the edges of the mattress, cyanosis, and neck vein distention. In COPD, pulsus paradoxus may be present. The chest may be hyperinflated. There may also be some degree of audible wheezing, particularly if the process of decompensation has been relatively acute and associated with a superimposed respiratory infection. Sinus tachycardia is often present; however, atrial and ventricular arrhythmias are also common.[30] Evidence of fluid retention may include the presence of pleural effusions, some degree of ascites, and dependent edema. The liver is enlarged and tender to palpation, and it may pulsate, reflecting the presence of tricuspid insufficiency. Similarly, the neck veins are distended and may show a large "c-v" wave with rapid y descent, characteristic of tricuspid insufficiency, as well as a prominent "a" wave reflecting the increased force of right atrial contraction.

On examination of the chest, there may be a parasternal systolic lift, reflecting the overactivity of the enlarged right ventricle, and a thud felt over the pulmonary area as the pulmonary valve closes. The heart sounds are often difficult to hear if the patient has underlying COPD. The pulmonic component of the second heart sound (S2) is accentuated and occurs earlier, so that the normal splitting may be abolished and a single loud S2 heard. Normally not heard at the apex, the pulmonic component of S2 may now be clearly heard. A high-pitched systolic ejection click may be heard in the second and third left intercostal spaces next to the sternum. It is often followed by a soft, localized systolic ejection murmur produced by ejection of the stroke volume into a dilated pulmonary artery. An S3 gallop arising from the right side of the heart may be heard in the fourth and fifth interspaces immediately to the left of the sternum. A presystolic S4 gallop may also be heard, reflecting the increased forcible contraction of the right atrium with expulsion of blood into the hypertrophied and dilated right ventricle. Often tricuspid regurgitation is present, and this results in a prominent blowing pansystolic murmur in the same location, which may increase somewhat with inspiration. When prominent pulmonary hypertension is present, a diastolic murmur of pulmonary incompetence may be heard. This murmur, the Graham Steell murmur, is a soft, blowing diastolic murmur usually well localized to the second and third left intercostal spaces next to the sternum.

Acute respiratory failure is characterized by hypoxemia and hypercapnia, or by their worsening if they are chronically present when the patient is stable, and usually requires hospitalization. Dyspnea becomes intense, and the patient is usually bedridden and visibly tachypneic. Coughing is likely to be exacerbated and sputum production increased. Congestive heart failure, if not present earlier, is now clearly evident in most cases. If it was chronically present before the exacerbation of respiratory failure, it will markedly worsen. The patient may exhibit confusion, insomnia, lethargy, and marked fatigue. Fever may be present if the episode has been precipitated or aggravated by an infectious process such as an acute bronchitis.

## Chest Radiograph

The appearance of the chest radiograph depends in large part on the underlying cause for the presence of pulmonary hypertension. Generally, however, the main pulmonary artery segment is enlarged, together with large right and left descending pulmonary arteries. In contrast, there is abrupt tapering of the peripheral vessels, resulting in disproportionately large central pulmonary arteries and attenuated distal vessels. A right descending pulmonary artery with a diameter greater than 16 mm suggests pulmonary hypertension.[31] Enlargement of the right ventricle, which may be observed on echocardiography, is often not appreciated on the chest radiograph. If hyperinflation of the lungs is present, the overall diameter of the cardiac silhouette may not be increased, although the heart may have a globular appearance. Often some encroachment or filling in of the retrosternal space by an enlarged right ventricle may be seen in a lateral view.

Some clinicians have claimed that pleural effusions are not seen in patients presenting with pure cor pulmonale and that their presence indicates that left ventricular dysfunction and failure must also be present. Miserocchi[32] published an extensive analysis of the dynamics of pleural fluid turnover from which he concluded that the early hypothesis by Neergard, based on Starling's hypothesis of fluid exchange, is untenable today in light of current knowledge. Miserocchi's analysis of experimental data leads to the conclusion that pleural fluid filters from the parietal pleural capillaries and adjacent interstitial space into the pleural space, where most of it is drained through parietal pleural lymphatics and not through the visceral pleura or lung lymphatics. This does not negate the fact that increased microvascular filtration through visceral pleura can occur hours after the development of acute pulmonary edema, presumably from an increase in the capillary surface area available for microvascular exchange. As a result, there can be a transient imbalance between capillary fluid exchange and visceral pleural lymphatic drainage, leading to a small transient pleural effusion. (Further discussion about the physiology of pleural liquid formation and removal is presented in Chapter 73.)

This analysis of the dynamics of pleural fluid exchange may seem to be at variance with the usual observation in patients with chronic cor pulmonale and elevated right heart filling pressures. Pleural effusions usually are not seen in these cases despite the fact that the capillary pressures within the parietal pleura presumably are elevated because of the increased systemic venous pressures. Increased fluid transudation into the parietal pleural interstitium and then into the pleural space would be expected. Failure to find pleural effusions under these circumstances probably reflects the capability of the parietal lymphatics to markedly increase their fluid removal capacity, by almost 20-fold, to accommodate the increased flow formation in response to an increase in systemic venous pressure. This would appear to substantiate a prospective study of 37 patients admitted for congestive heart failure in which the presence of pleural effusions correlated with the wedge pressure but not with the right atrial pressure.[33] In a subsequent retrospective study of 18 patients with long-term right atrial and/or pulmonary hypertension but with normal pulmonary artery wedge pressures, no pleural effusions were seen.[34] However, patients have been observed with chronic cor pulmonale and acute exacerbation of cardiac decompensation resulting from a superimposed respiratory infection, who demonstrate small pleural effusions during the acute episode (Fig. 55.6). It is of interest that cattle with brisket disease accumulate transudates in the thoracic cavity as well as in the abdominal cavity and pericardial sac.[35]

In summary, the parietal pleural lymphatic system appears to adjust to chronic marked increases in filtration rates, establishing a steady-state situation that prevents the formation of pleural effusions. However, if there is an acute hemodynamic change, transient filtration can clearly exceed maximum lymphatic drainage, resulting in

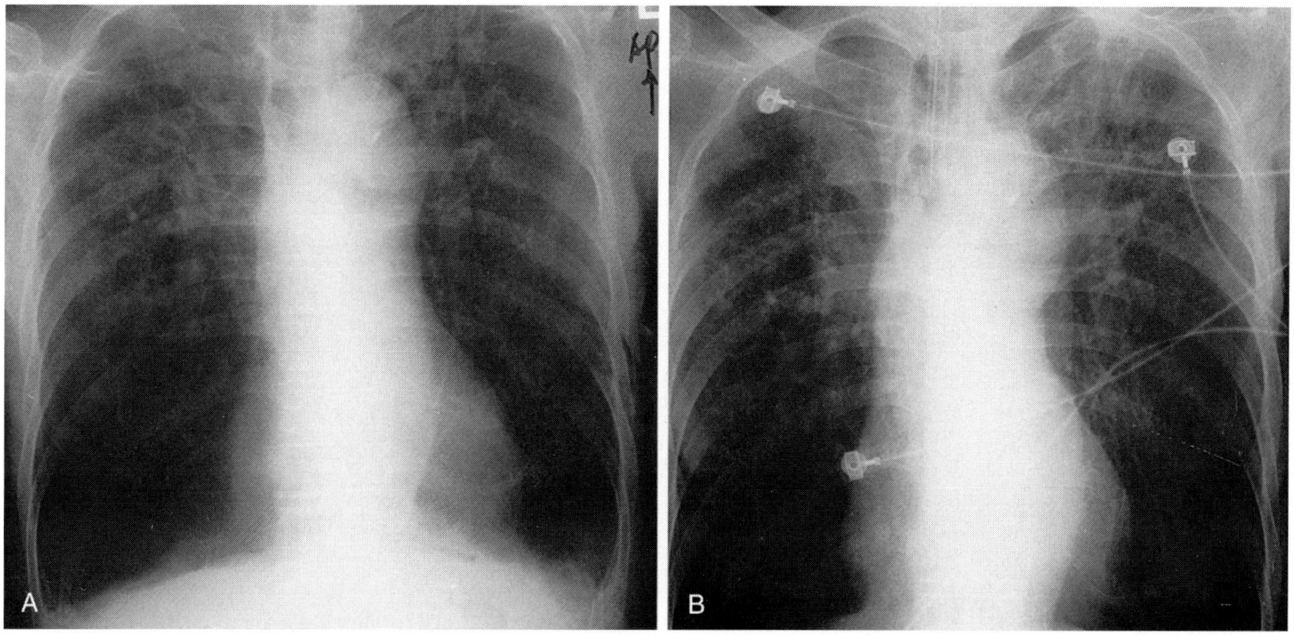


**Figure 55.6** *A,* An upright chest x-ray film of a patient with COPD who had acute cardiac decompensation in association with an upper respiratory infection. Note blunting of both costophrenic angles from the presence of small pleural effusions. *B,* Upright chest x-ray film of the same patient several days later, after restoration of competency, indicating disappearance of the pleural effusions.

a transudate that might take hours to days to clear before a new steady state is established.

## Electrocardiogram

The electrocardiogram can be quite helpful in establishing the presence of chronic cor pulmonale.[36] Characteristically, the P wave has a "p pulmonale" pattern with right-axis deviation resulting in an increase in its amplitude in leads II, III, and aVF to more than 2.5 mm (Fig. 55.7). The P wave may also be tall in the right precordial leads. The QRS vector in the frontal plane often shifts to the right in cor pulmonale, and a low-voltage QRS is common if lung hyperinflation is present. Prominent S waves are seen in leads I, II, and III, probably reflecting hypertrophy of the crista supraventricularis; an incomplete right bundle branch block pattern is also frequently present. When pulmonary artery hypertension is moderate or severe, the more classic findings of right ventricular hypertrophy may dominate the electrocardiogram, which exhibits tall R waves in V1 with an R/S ratio of more than 1, and a prominent S wave in V5 and V6 with an R/S ratio of less than 1. The presence of electrocardiographic evidence of cor pulmonale in patients with COPD is a poor prognostic sign.[36a]

## Echocardiography

Echocardiographic examination can assist the clinician in eliminating various nonpulmonary causes of secondary pulmonary hypertension, such as left ventricular failure from coronary disease or dilated congestive cardiomyopathy, aortic or mitral valve disease, and congenital heart disease with left-to-right shunt. Echocardiographic examination can also be directly useful in the evaluation of a patient with COPD. The actual level of systolic pressure in the pulmonary artery can often be estimated by continuous-wave Doppler echocardiography through analysis of the flow velocity in the presence of tricuspid regurgitation. Additionally, there is usually pulmonic insufficiency detectable by Doppler echocardiography in the presence of pulmonary hypertension; this permits estimation of the pulmonary artery diastolic pressure as well. The size of the right atrium and the right ventricle are readily determined, and the contractile state of the right ventricle can be assessed. If right heart filling pressure is increased, it may be associated with dilatation of the inferior vena cava, which fails to collapse with respiratory maneuvers such as sniffing. Finally, the fact that the left ventricle has a normal contractile state and is of normal size can be verified.

The presence of hyperinflation of the lungs often creates a technical problem that, at times, results in a less than satisfactory examination. Nevertheless, it is useful to try and interrogate cardiac structures with a transthoracic two-dimensional Doppler echocardiographic examination, because a good technician can generally obtain sufficient data to provide useful information for the clinician. There is an 80% to 85% success rate in visualizing cardiac structures adequately by echocardiography in COPD.[37] If sufficient lung hyperinflation prevents an adequate transthoracic examination, one may resort to a transesophageal echocardiogram to clarify the problem. Often patients in this situation are intubated, and a trans-

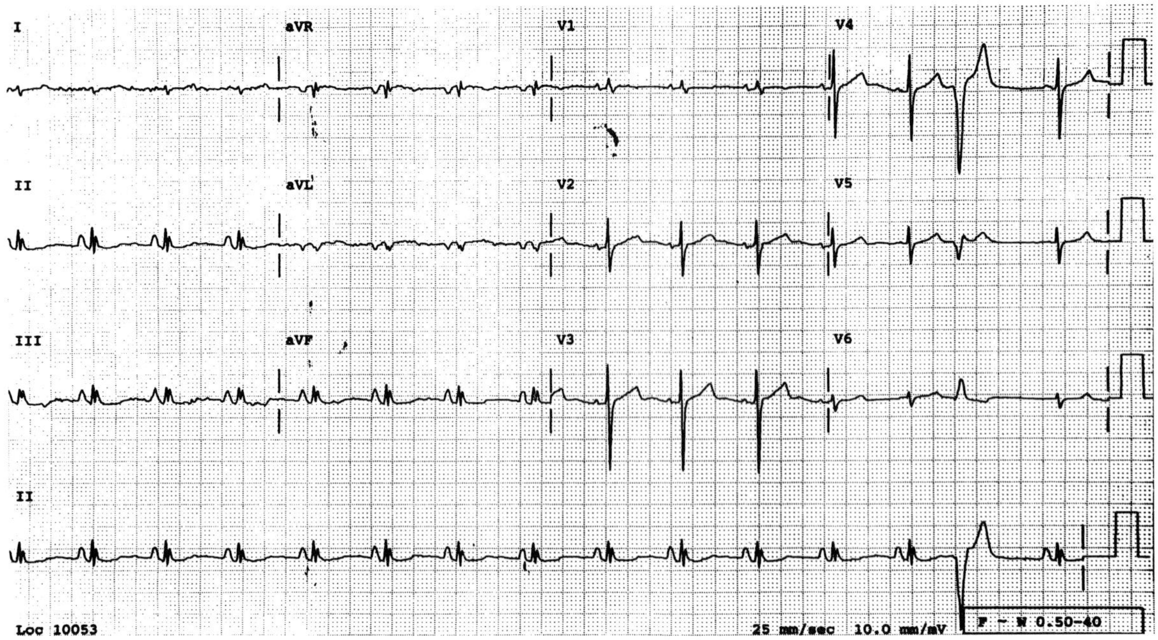


**Figure 55.7** An electrocardiogram in a patient with chronic cor pulmonale reveals prominent ''p pulmonale'' (see text).

esophageal study probe can be slipped into the esophagus with relative ease. A much better delineation of cardiac function and any cardiac pathology can be obtained than is possible with a transthoracic probe.

Figure 55.8 illustrates a Doppler echocardiographic examination in a patient with COPD who presented with severe respiratory distress. The possibility of coexisting coronary disease, which arises frequently in the older male patient, led to the question of whether the patient was in respiratory distress from pulmonary congestion secondary to left ventricular failure or whether the problem reflected pulmonary hypertension and ventilatory in-

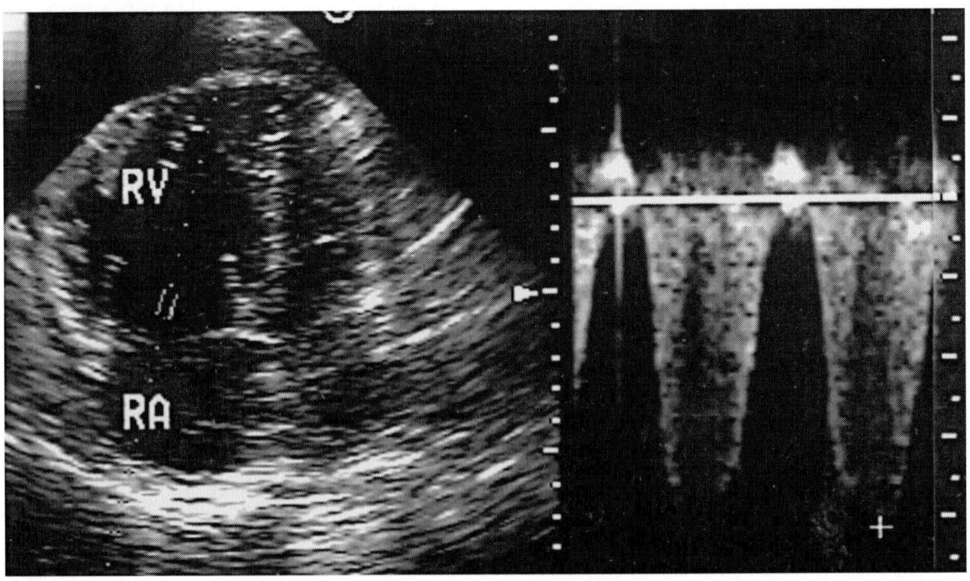


**Figure 55.8** *Left,* Normal left ventricular volume is seen on this echocardiogram of a patient with chronic obstructive pulmonary disease who presented with acute severe respiratory distress. Normal contractility also was observed during recording. The right ventricle is markedly dilated (see text). *Right,* Estimation of the degree of pulmonary hypertension using continuous-wave Doppler measurement of the velocity jet from the tricuspid insufficiency that was present. A 55-mm peak systolic pressure gradient between the right ventricle and right atrium was calculated, indicating moderate-to-severe pulmonary artery hypertension.

sufficiency arising from decompensated pulmonary heart disease. The figure clearly illustrates that the left ventricle was of normal size, and it was seen to have normal contractility during analog recording. On the other hand, the right ventricle was moderately dilated and was observed to have a significantly decreased right ventricular systolic contractile function. Right atrial enlargement was present as well. Although tricuspid insufficiency was not a major clinical problem in this particular patient, there was sufficient tricuspid insufficiency to permit Doppler estimation of the degree of pulmonary hypertension. This is often the case when pulmonary hypertension is present. The right section of Figure 55.8 illustrates a continuous-wave Doppler jet demonstrating that a peak systolic gradient of at least 55 mm Hg was present between the right ventricle and right atrium, indicating moderate-to-severe pulmonary hypertension.

### Hemodynamics

Hemodynamic measurements in patients with decompensated pulmonary heart disease secondary to COPD are subject to error. Use of the direct Fick method to estimate cardiac output at the time of cardiac catheterization is complicated when hypoxemia is present. Hypoxemia may be caused both by shunting across the lungs, from perfusion of unventilated or poorly ventilated alveoli, and by a decrease in oxygen diffusion reflecting alveolar-capillary block from associated fibrosis, parenchymal infiltrative disease, inflammation, and/or edema. Consequently, true pulmonary blood flow, in terms of pulmonary capillary blood flow, is only an approximation when systemic arterial oxygen content is used to calculate the arteriovenous oxygen content across the lungs. Further problems are provided by the fact that there may be difficulty in estimating oxygen consumption if the patient is receiving therapeutic oxygen.

Measurements of pulmonary blood flow by the use of indicator dilution curves such as thermodilution may also be spurious in the presence of pulmonary shunting and in patients with very low outputs. In fact, the clinician should measure the oxygen saturation of pulmonary artery blood from the indwelling pulmonary artery catheter and verify that it is substantially lower than normal before accepting a thermodilution readout that cardiac output is markedly depressed. Within these limitations, however, it would appear that cardiac output in patients with decompensated pulmonary heart disease from hypoxic pulmonary vasoconstriction is generally in the normal range or even increased due to the systemic vasodilation produced by the hypoxemia; this finding contrasts with that in primary pulmonary hypertension, chronic obstructive embolic disease, mitral stenosis with pulmonary vascular disease, or decompensated heart failure caused by primary myocardial disease, in which low-output states are usually present. Hemodynamic studies in COPD patients with and without heart failure consistently show a normal cardiac output.[37, 38]

Measurements performed by Anand and his associates[20] in nine patients with edema due to COPD and in six patients after recovery demonstrated that patients with edema had severe salt and water retention, reduction in renal blood flow and glomerular filtration rate, and a neurohormonal activation comparable to that seen in patients with congestive heart failure due to primary myocardial disease. This was seen despite the fact that mean cardiac output was normal, as was mean pulmonary artery wedge pressure. Therefore, with an increase in arterial $PO_2$ and a fall in $PCO_2$, the patients became free from edema, with a corresponding increase in renal blood plasma flow and normalization of glomerular filtration rate.

Most patients who have chronic cor pulmonale do not need cardiac catheterization to establish a diagnosis. In the absence of a primary pulmonary vascular process, such as repeated pulmonary emboli or primary pulmonary hypertension, the search for effective pulmonary vasodilators is generally considered fruitless. In the case of presumed primary pulmonary hypertension, however, it is customary to take such patients to the cardiac catheterization laboratory or to pass a Swan-Ganz catheter at the bedside to measure pulmonary vascular pressures and to search for responses to acute pulmonary vasodilators such as intravenous prostacyclin, calcium antagonists, acetylcholine, hydralazine, and 100% oxygen. Patients who respond to these agents, particularly prostacyclin, tend to respond to high doses of calcium blockers, and these can be tested for benefit over the next several days, while the patient is on the ward with the Swan-Ganz catheter left in place. Endopeptidase inhibitors have yet to be studied extensively. However, these agents may well prove useful in the future.

## DIFFERENTIAL DIAGNOSIS

There are many causes of pulmonary artery hypertension, as noted in Table 55.1. At times, the underlying cause may be difficult to establish. Specific symptoms and signs of the basic disorder often help to establish the cause of pulmonary hypertension. For example, mitral stenosis noted on physical examination or by echocardiographic examination may represent the underlying cause of pulmonary hypertension. Early in the natural history of mitral stenosis only passive pulmonary hypertension occurs;

**Table 55.1 CLASSIFICATION OF PULMONARY HYPERTENSION**

| |
|---|
| Passive |
| Left ventricular systolic pump failure |
| Decreased left ventricular diastolic compliance, elevated left atrial pressure |
| Mitral stenosis |
| Idiopathic |
| Hyperkinetic |
| Dietary or ingestive pulmonary hypertension |
| Obstructive |
| Obliterative |
| Vasoconstrictive |
| Reflex secondary to chronic pulmonary venous or capillary hypertension |
| Hypoxic |

however, after prolonged elevation of left atrial and pulmonary venous pressure, pulmonary artery pressure rises out of proportion to the raised left atrial pressure from reflex pulmonary vasoconstriction. Radiographic evidence of increased interstitial markings reflecting increased lung vascular volume from high pulmonary blood flow suggests the presence of congenital heart disease with a left-to-right intracardiac shunt. The diagnosis of idiopathic or primary pulmonary hypertension can be made only after other causes of increased obstruction to pulmonary blood flow have been eliminated. Obstructive pulmonary vascular disease caused by appetite suppressants or other toxic substances; pulmonary hypertension associated with occasional cases of decompensated hepatic cirrhosis; silent deep venous thrombotic disease that has resulted in multiple, relatively silent pulmonary emboli with subsequent pulmonary hypertension; and pulmonary vasculitis from systemic lupus erythematosus, scleroderma, or other collagen vascular diseases are but a few examples in which the underlying cause must be sought to explain the basis of the pulmonary hypertension.

The diagnosis of chronic cor pulmonale due to obstructive or restrictive ventilatory insufficiency is usually rapidly established because these patients either have evidence of pulmonary parenchymal disease (e.g., radiographic evidence of pulmonary infiltrative or fibrotic disease, lung hyperinflation, radiologic findings suggesting bronchiectasis) or present with symptoms or physical findings that suggest underlying pulmonary disease (e.g., bronchial wheezing, history of chronic bronchitis with a chronic productive cough). Other patients present with evidence of chest wall deformities that may interfere with respiration (e.g., kyphoscoliosis). Morbid obesity may suggest the presence of the Pickwickian syndrome or primary alveolar hypoventilation. Pulmonary edema on chest radiography, with dilatation of the left side of the heart, should suggest that COPD is not the cause. However, because of increased capillary permeability, the inadequacy of pulmonary lymphatic drainage, and an increase in the pulmonary capillary–to–left atrial pressure gradient, pulmonary edema may be found on occasion in patients with lung disease without overt left ventricular failure.[12] It may also be found in COPD with cor pulmonale in the presence of comorbid conditions affecting the left ventricle.

## CLASSIFICATION OF PULMONARY HYPERTENSION

Table 55.1 presents a simplified classification of pulmonary hypertension. *Passive pulmonary arterial hypertension* results from raised pulmonary venous and capillary pressures that require the pulmonary arterial perfusing pressure to rise correspondingly. In actuality, because of the distensibility of the pulmonary circulation, the mechanical rise in the distending pressure actually causes a diminution in the gradient between mean pulmonary artery and capillary pressure for the same degree of vasomotor tone, despite the overall rise in pulmonary arterial pressure. Passive pulmonary hypertension is most frequently seen when left atrial pressure rises secondary to left ventricular failure or mitral stenosis.

*Hyperkinetic pulmonary hypertension* may arise when there are marked increases in pulmonary blood flow. Normally, the increased cardiac output that is seen in the so-called hyperkinetic states (e.g., severe chronic, normovolemic anemia; generalized Paget's disease; thyrotoxicosis; large arteriovenous fistula) are insufficient to significantly raise the pulmonary artery pressure. However, in congenital heart disease, with very large left-to-right shunts and markedly increased pulmonary blood flow, pulmonary arterial pressure may rise. Therefore, infants and young children with large ventricular septal defects may have systemic pressures in their pulmonary arteries maintained primarily by very large left-to-right shunts and resultant increased pulmonary blood flow.

*Obstructive pulmonary hypertension* refers to a decrease in the cross-sectional area of the pulmonary vascular bed as a result of narrowing or occlusion of distal pulmonary arterioles. This most commonly is caused by repetitive, relatively silent pulmonary emboli arising over time from deep venous thromboses. However, it can also be seen in situations in which vasculitis of the distal pulmonary arterioles produces obstructive pulmonary vascular disease and pulmonary hypertension. Pulmonary hypertension in obstructive pulmonary vascular disease may worsen due to the development of thrombosis in situ in patients with already established pulmonary hypertension and secondary anatomic changes in the smaller branches of the pulmonary circulation. Sickle cell anemia may also be a source of such thromboses. Another cause of obliterative pulmonary vascular disease may be seen in injection drug abusers of drugs such as Ritalin; the talc incorporated in the manufacturing process leads to minute repetitive embolizations. Infective endocarditis on the tricuspid valve with frequent pulmonary emboli can also produce obstructive pulmonary vascular disease.

*Idiopathic or primary pulmonary hypertension,* a relatively infrequent but serious cause of pulmonary hypertension, right ventricular hypertrophy, and eventual congestive heart failure, is discussed in detail in Chapter 52.

*Dietary or ingestive pulmonary hypertension* refers to the ingestion of any of several drugs or substances that have resulted in epidemics of pulmonary hypertension, mimicking primary pulmonary hypertension. One of the most famous of these was the Spanish toxic oil syndrome, which occurred as a result of the ingestion of rapeseed cooking oil that had been adulterated with aniline dye. A large number of children and some adults developed severe pulmonary vascular disease with hypertension as a result.[39, 40] Another example was the occurrence of pulmonary hypertension in Europe caused by ingestion of the appetite suppressant drug aminorex.[41] This chemical produced many cases of pulmonary hypertension in Europe, particularly in Switzerland and Germany, before its toxicity was appreciated and the drug was banned from the market. Ingestion of *Crotalaria* plant seeds has been used to create an animal model of pulmonary hypertension in several species.[42, 43]

*Obliterative pulmonary hypertension* results from a variety of different pulmonary parenchymal processes. It can be seen, for example, in emphysema as bullae coalesce and parts of the capillary bed of the lung are correspondingly obliterated. It may also result from diffuse pulmonary fibrosis and from a variety of parenchymal infiltrative diseases, such as sarcoidosis, advanced tuberculosis, pneumoconiosis, and scleroderma.

*Vasoconstrictive pulmonary hypertension* is the major cause of pulmonary hypertension that is seen in patients with chronic cor pulmonale; it is produced predominantly by alveolar hypoxia. However, patients who develop chronic pulmonary venous and pulmonary capillary hypertension, although they have obligatory passive pulmonary artery hypertension, may develop a reflex pulmonary vasoconstriction that raises pulmonary arterial pressure out of proportion to the passive elevation in pulmonary venous and capillary pressures. This is commonly seen in mitral stenosis: if unrelieved, pulmonary artery pressure climbs out of proportion to the rise in left atrial, pulmonary venous, and pulmonary capillary pressures due to reflex pulmonary vasoconstriction. With opening of the mitral valve by balloon valvotomy or surgery and fall in left atrial pressure toward normal, the process can reverse.

## TREATMENT

Management of patients with decompensated pulmonary heart disease must focus on improvement of the underlying pulmonary disorder if compensation is to be restored. If the clinician simply treats decompensated pulmonary heart disease in the way in which heart failure usually is managed—with diuretics, ACE inhibitors, and digitalis—there will probably be little benefit unless the hypoxia and hypercapnia are also corrected by improved alveolar ventilation and the administration of oxygen. The precipitating event for decompensation in patients with stabilized chronic cor pulmonale from either COPD or infiltrative lung disease is often an associated upper respiratory infection. With increased secretions and infection, this is likely to tip the balance toward further alveolar hypoxemia and hypercapnia, which aggravates pulmonary hypertension and worsens ventricular contractility as a result of acute unbuffered acidemia, resulting in cardiac decompensation.

Improvement in right ventricular performance is best accomplished not only by correcting acidemia but also by reducing the afterload facing the right ventricle (i.e., reducing pulmonary artery pressure). Correction of arterial hypoxemia through the administration of an increased concentration of oxygen in inspired air lowers pulmonary artery pressure in patients with hypoxic pulmonary vasoconstriction. Improvement in alveolar ventilation with intubation and mechanical ventilation helps eliminate the acute hypercapnia and acidemia that depress myocardial contractility. Digoxin therapy improves the contractile strength of the right ventricle and should be instituted if it has not already been started. Digoxin increases pulmonary blood flow and reduces right-sided heart filling pressure. However, it does not lower pulmonary artery pressure.[44] Furthermore, patients with COPD are particularly sensitive to digoxin, and close attention to dosage and electrolyte balance to prevent digitalis toxicity is necessary. Often, an episode of acute cardiac decompensation in a patient who has chronic pulmonary hypertension due to COPD is caused by an underlying pneumonitis or superimposed bronchitis. Patchy areas of atelectasis may also play a role. Empirical antimicrobials, usually a third-generation cephalosporin, should be administered until cultures identify the causative organism and allow more specific treatment to be used. $Beta_2$-agonists such as albuterol are widely accepted as standard management. Not only are they bronchodilators, but they acutely produce a fall in pulmonary artery pressure and a rise in right ventricular ejection fraction with no significant fall in arterial $Po_2$.[45] Anticholinergic drugs such as ipratropium bromide are also useful bronchodilators. Theophylline seems to lessen dyspnea and may be helpful in improving ventilation, but it has considerable toxicity. Finally, corticosteroids appear useful in accelerating recovery from acute respiratory failure in patients with COPD and should be given as early as possible.

If severe polycythemia is present, phlebotomy may be helpful, although clinicians are frequently reluctant to undertake this type of therapy today. In cattle with brisket disease, cardiac output and coronary blood flow increased without a rise in pulmonary artery pressure when phlebotomy was undertaken.[46] Hypoxic patients also show improvement in right ventricular ejection fraction, exercise tolerance, and neuropsychologic function after phlebotomy.[16]

The role of ACE inhibitors in chronic cor pulmonale has not been independently studied in a large randomized, double-blind, clinical trial. However, if a patient presents in severe heart failure associated with chronic pulmonary disease, a trial of ACE inhibitors is warranted, in light of their dramatic benefit in patients with congestive heart failure from other causes.

### Oxygen Therapy

Young adults living at high altitudes have distinctly raised pulmonary arterial pressures that fall to normal if they leave to live at sea level for several years. Such observations, combined with the clinical, pathologic, and physiologic data observed in patients with chronic bronchitis and emphysema, emphasize the importance of hypoxia in the genesis of pulmonary hypertension. It also suggests that continuous domiciliary oxygen therapy might reduce pulmonary arterial hypertension in patients with COPD and thereby improve outcome. Controlled trials evaluating long-term oxygen administration showed improvement in survival, although they failed to demonstrate a clear and consistent reduction in pulmonary hypertension.

Two major randomized trials have been carried out. In the British Medical Research Council evaluation of long-term domiciliary oxygen in chronic hypoxic cor pulmonale, long-term oxygen administration for at least 15 hours/day appeared to prevent further rises in pulmonary arterial pressure, compared with no oxygen administration in control patients.[47] It also lessened mortality. In a National Institutes of Health study in the United States, 12 hours of nocturnal oxygen therapy was compared with continuous therapy. Continuous oxygen therapy proved distinctly more favorable, with a lessened mortality rate at 2 years. Additionally, a decrease was seen in pulmonary vascular resistance, contrasted to a small rise in the group receiving only nocturnal therapy.[48]

Based on the results of these studies, it is clear that

severely hypoxemic patients with COPD should be provided home oxygen therapy, with a goal of continuous therapy but with at least 15 hours/day of oxygen. It must be remembered, however, that the acute administration of high concentrations of oxygen to a patient with hypoxic cor pulmonale can remove an important stimulus to respiration, particularly if the patient is already displaying alveolar hypoventilation as evidenced by hypercapnia. This is important to keep in mind when evaluating a patient's pulmonary hypertensive response to oxygen administration in the catheterization laboratory and when determining the dose for use at home. Patients given domiciliary oxygen need to be observed closely when they are initially being instructed on the use of this therapy to ensure that ventilatory drive is not being substantially impaired and that arterial oxygen saturation actually rises. Further information about the long-term use of oxygen in pulmonary rehabilitation is provided in Chapter 96.

## Pulmonary Vasodilators

Acute evaluation of pulmonary vasodilators has traditionally been done in patients with primary pulmonary hypertension, and less commonly when pulmonary hypertension arises from various causes of secondary obstructive pulmonary hypertension. Ideally, patients are taken to the cardiac catheterization laboratory, where a Swan-Ganz catheter is introduced into the pulmonary circulation and repeat acute trials of various pharmacologic agents are sequentially undertaken while hemodynamic measurements are made. Alternatively, but less desirably, this can be done at the bedside in a monitored bed if skilled nursing care is available. The ideal response when evaluating pulmonary vasodilators is for total oxygen delivery to the systemic circulation to be maintained or increased without a fall in systemic arterial pressure but with a fall in pulmonary artery pressure. Presumably, if this occurs, even with a drop in blood $PO_2$, vasodilators could prove to be useful therapeutic agents when employed chronically. Complete evaluation of such agents usually is not possible with noninvasive techniques. However, if a patient has a significant degree of tricuspid regurgitation, the clinician may be able to evaluate the potential of lowering of the pulmonary arterial pressure through Doppler echocardiographic examination, albeit simultaneous cardiac output measurements would not be available. Many pulmonary vasodilators have been studied over the years. Among the agents that are more commonly evaluated today are oxygen inhalation, ACE inhibitors, calcium antagonists, alpha-adrenergic blockers, beta-adrenergic agonists, hydralazine, inhaled nitric oxide, and prostacyclin. Comparison of the responses to several different drugs may identify a particular agent that can then be used to produce long-term benefit.

It has been far less common to evaluate and subsequently use pulmonary vasodilators as chronic therapy in patients with cor pulmonale due to COPD or diffuse parenchymal disease. Attempts to date have not significantly affected long-term function or survival. One reason is that initial acute pulmonary vasodilating responses to an agent may not persist when the agent is used chronically. For example, in a study of 53 patients with COPD and pulmonary hypertension, the decrease in pulmonary vascular resistance after initial use of the calcium antagonist nifedipine was 23% at rest and 35% during exercise. However, after an average of 13 months of treatment, the decrease in pulmonary vascular resistance was no longer significant.[49]

Another reason for poor long-term benefit may be that pharmacologic reversal of hypoxic pulmonary vasoconstriction with vasodilators may increase pulmonary blood flow to poorly ventilated or nonventilated alveoli, with the net effect that arterial $PO_2$ may fall despite a drop in pulmonary arterial pressure. What is frequently unappreciated is that ventilation-perfusion matching also affects carbon dioxide elimination. Minute ventilation may increase to compensate for the shunting of carbon dioxide and therefore, although arterial $PO_2$ may fall, hypercapnia may not worsen.[50] Another practical problem limiting the use of pulmonary vasodilators is that often they also are systemic vasodilators and may result in significant hypotension. In any case, evaluating individual vasodilating agents with right heart catheterization to test their ability to decrease pulmonary vascular resistance and lower pulmonary arterial pressure is not routinely done today in patients with cor pulmonale due to COPD. Physicians should be on the lookout for the occasional patient with pulmonary hypertension from recurrent pulmonary embolism, because of the considerable benefit from thromboendarterectomy.[50a]

## Angiotensin-Converting Enzyme Inhibition

Studies in the rat exposed to chronic hypoxia in a barochamber and then transferred to an environment of normoxia revealed that enalapril reduced the content and concentration of collagen significantly, suggesting that partial regression of cardiac fibrosis may occur with enalapril, independent of the reduction in pressure load.[51]

In another study of chronically hypoxic rats, the ACE inhibitor quinapril reduced the development of pulmonary hypertension. This was seen both early and after pulmonary hypertension was established. The degree of medial thickness in alveolar duct blood vessels was significantly reduced by quinapril treatment, and stains of vascular smooth muscle cells showed that quinapril appeared to inhibit vascular smooth muscle cell proliferation and/or growth.[52]

Experimental observations in normal volunteers demonstrated that the infusion of saralasin (an angiotensin II receptor blocker) not only produces pulmonary vasodilatation when the renin-angiotensin system has been stimulated but also attenuates pulmonary vasoconstriction in response to acute hypoxia.[53] Studies in patients with chronic cor pulmonale have been inconsistent. When enalapril was added to conventional treatment in 30 patients with chronic cor pulmonale, not only was pulmonary hypertension decreased but renal vascular resistance fell, resulting in increased renal blood flow and an improved glomerular filtration rate.[54] In contrast, the acute effects of captopril were studied in 15 patients with severe COPD who were recovering from right-sided heart failure. Although captopril reduced systemic arterial pressure, it failed to decrease pulmonary vascular resistance in these patients with hypoxic pulmonary hypertension, nor were there any changes in breathing frequency, minute ventilation, or pulmonary gas exchange compared with controls.[55]

Angiotensin II, type I, receptor blockade attenuates the pulmonary vasoconstrictive response of acute hypoxia in normal subjects.[53] This has led to studies of the efficacy of these drugs in patients with COPD with pulmonary hypertension and normal left ventricular systolic function. In an acute study evaluating the response to losartan, an angiotensin II receptor blocker, after at least 1 week of therapy, nine patients with COPD had a significant reduction in both mean pulmonary artery pressure and total pulmonary resistance; this was associated with a significantly lower plasma aldosterone level, compared with patients receiving placebo. Although losartan produced its maximal effects 4 hours after administration, it did not alter oxygen saturation in these patients with hypoxemic cor pulmonale.[56]

The inconsistency in results with ACE inhibition may reflect the small size and short duration of the studies, as well as variations in inclusionary criteria. In the study by Kiely and associates,[56] all patients had documented pulmonary vascular reactivity as assessed by a significant fall in pulmonary artery pressure in response to acute oxygen administration. It is possible that there are other patients in whom failure to demonstrate such vascular reactivity to 100% oxygen would result in a failure to demonstrate benefit from the use of an angiotensin II receptor blocker or ACE inhibitor. At present, there would appear to be no routine role for these agents in COPD. Whether ultimately there may be therapeutic value for their use in patients with cor pulmonale and pulmonary hypertension awaits the results of longer, larger, randomized, double-blind clinical trials.

## Nitric Oxide

Inhaled nitric oxide (NO), or endothelial-derived relaxing factor (EDRF), may affect airway tone through a variety of different mechanisms. It also significantly affects pulmonary vascular tone.[56a] Both pulmonary arterial and venous endothelial cells are capable of producing NO. Using an NO synthase inhibitor in 11 healthy volunteers, Stamler and colleagues[57] demonstrated that NO regulates normoxic pulmonary vascular tone. Furthermore, when volunteers were made hypoxic, inhalation of 40 ppm NO reversed pulmonary vasoconstriction without causing systemic vasodilation.[58]

Endothelial damage with impaired NO production has been proposed as contributing to both acute and chronic pulmonary hypertension.[59] In a study of pulmonary artery rings obtained from 22 patients with COPD undergoing heart-lung transplantation, impaired endothelium-dependent pulmonary artery relaxation (in vitro) was observed and was related to the preoperative levels of hypoxemia and hypercapnia. Additionally, reduced relaxation was significantly correlated to the degree of intimal fibromuscular thickening.[60] The inhalation of NO at 40 ppm reversed pulmonary hypertension caused by breathing a hypoxic gas mixture in awake lambs within 3 minutes.[61]

There is a reduction in the expression of NO synthase in the pulmonary arteries of patients with primary pulmonary hypertension, and the degree of expression is inversely correlated with total pulmonary resistance. Hypoxia markedly lessens NO synthase activity, decreasing NO release, and this deficiency in patients with chronic pulmonary hypertension may contribute to the increase in pulmonary vascular resistance.[62, 63]

In persistent newborn pulmonary hypertension, inhaled NO has proved to be of clinical value.[64, 65] Furthermore, in patients with primary pulmonary hypertension, inhaled NO has been used to predict those patients who might safely and somewhat effectively respond to calcium channel blockers. However, in patients with COPD, intermittent NO inhalations are not commonly used therapeutically, in part because of costs and practical difficulties including toxicity associated with chronic use, but also because of a concern that systemic oxygenation might worsen due to increased local ventilation-perfusion mismatches, as it often does with other vasodilators. However, NO theoretically should vasodilate only those areas it reaches as it is being inhaled, increasing flow only to areas being ventilated and improving ventilation-perfusion match. It would seem reasonable, therefore, to test patients with severe COPD associated with acute respiratory failure (as well as patients with obliterative or primary pulmonary hypertension) for their responsiveness to this potential therapeutic agent as an acute intervention. At present, however, there does not appear to be a clinically meaningful role for its chronic use.

## Endothelin

Endothelins are potent vasoconstrictor peptides synthesized by vascular endothelium. NO inhibits and/or modulates their synthesis. Endothelins play a prominent role in producing vasoconstriction in the coronary circulation. However, pulmonary endothelial cells have not been shown to secrete endothelin in vivo.[66] Therefore, their role, if any, in the genesis of hypoxic pulmonary vasoconstriction has yet to be clarified. In the experimental animal made hypoxic, blockade of NO unmasks a pulmonary vasoconstriction effect of endothelin.[67] Future studies of endothelin antagonists in patients with hypoxic pulmonary vasoconstriction are awaited.

## Prostaglandins

Prostaglandins are synthesized by pulmonary vascular endothelium. Neonatal calves who develop severe pulmonary hypertension when exposed to chronic hypobaric hypoxia have been shown to have a relative deficit in prostaglandin production in their pulmonary arteries. This suggests that prostaglandins may play a role in the development of pulmonary hypertension by the lack of vasodilatory stimuli.[68] Normal subjects exposed acutely to high-altitude hypoxia release both vasoconstrictive and vasoactive eicosanoids, with vasoconstrictors being initially released and vasodilators being released several days later.[69]

Because prostacyclin (epoprostenol) is a powerful pulmonary vasodilator, its therapeutic use in the management of patients with primary pulmonary hypertension has been studied. An early randomized trial in 24 patients with primary pulmonary hypertension revealed that continuous intravenous administration of epoprostenol by portable infusion pump resulted in substantial hemodynamic and symptomatic improvement over 8 weeks.[70] Barst and associates,[71] in a nonblinded study, randomly assigned 81 patients with primary pulmonary hypertension to receive either a continuous intravenous epoprostenol infusion added to conventional therapy or conventional therapy alone. The intravenous dosage given chronically by infusion pump through an implanted catheter was determined by the dosage tolerated in an earlier, short-term, dose-ranging phase of the study. By the end of 12 weeks, epoprostenol resulted in symptomatic and hemodynamic improvement and improved survival.

More recently, a group of 69 patients with primary pulmonary hypertension were similarly given a continuous intravenous infusion of epoprostenol through an implanted catheter using a portable, battery-operated infusion pump, with an initial maximum dose titrated to symptoms or by a drop in systemic blood pressure greater than 10 mm Hg.[72] Patients were monitored up to 3 years, during which time 13 of the patients died, including 3 among 9 patients who underwent single-lung transplantation. However, 18 of the patients were monitored for 330 to 700 days and demonstrated an echocardiographically determined estimated mean fall in the right ventricular minus right atrial systolic pressure gradient from $84.1 \pm 24.1$ to $62.7 \pm 18.2$ mm Hg ($P < .01$). McLaughlin and colleagues[73] evaluated 27 patients with primary pulmonary hypertension who were given epoprostenol over a mean of $16.7 \pm 5.2$ months. By increasing the rate of infusion by an average 2.5 ng/kg/min each month, a 53% decline in pulmonary vascular resistance was achieved at the time of restudy.

All of these studies suggest the desirability of using chronic infusions of epoprostenol in patients with primary pulmonary hypertension. Epoprostenol should be one of the agents routinely evaluated when pulmonary vasodilating agents are being tested acutely in patients with primary pulmonary hypertension.

## NATURAL HISTORY

Chronic bronchitis and emphysema are the cause of chronic cor pulmonale in more than 80% of cases.[74] Therefore, the natural history of cor pulmonale reflects the natural history of COPD. The American Thoracic Society reported that the death rate in 1991 from COPD was 18.6 per 100,000 persons, resulting in its ranking as the fourth leading cause of death. This represented a rise of 32.9% from 1979.[75]

Patients with COPD, whether it is of the bronchitic or emphysematous type, may or may not have pulmonary hypertension at rest. Furthermore, the progression of pulmonary hypertension in COPD is slow.[3] Among patients who are found to have normal pressures at rest, changes in pulmonary hemodynamics are frequently minimal over time. For example, in a group of 61 patients without initial pulmonary arterial hypertension, all of whom had arterial hypoxemia, a second cardiac catheterization on average 93.4 months later revealed an average change in mean pulmonary arterial pressure from $15.5 \pm 2.4$ to $19.6 \pm 7.0$ mm Hg.[76] In a second group of 32 patients, studied earlier by the same researchers,[77] who had pulmonary hypertension on the first catheterization, there was a nonsignificant rise in mean pulmonary arterial pressure, from $27.7 \pm 6.0$ to $31.0 \pm 9.3$ mm Hg, after an average delay of 60 months. Hemodynamic worsening, defined as an increase of 5 mm Hg or more, occurred in approximately one third of patients and was clearly related to worsening of hypoxemia. Mortality in the group with hemodynamic worsening was significantly higher than in those in whom it was not demonstrated. From these observations, it is clear that pulmonary artery hypertension in patients with COPD most closely correlates with the presence of hypoxemia, not necessarily with the extent of emphysema that is present.

There has been relatively little difference in hospital survival rates among patients with acute respiratory failure in modern respiratory intensive care units compared with those managed 10 to 20 years ago, despite the significant advances in respiratory care that have emerged. The hospital survival rates in an international prospective survey of patients who were hypoxemic or hypercarbic while receiving mechanical ventilatory assistance was only 33.3%.[78] Survival rates in this miscellaneous group were higher in patients in whom acute respiratory failure was caused by pneumonia (63%). Nevertheless, the major prognostic factor was the severity of lung injury at entry, with survival as low as 18% for patients with far-advanced lung injury and 67% when acute respiratory failure was associated with less severe lung injury.

A long-term survival experience for COPD in a group initially requiring hospitalization who were in the age range of 50 to 54 years was reported from Finland.[79] Among 2727 new COPD patients, the estimated cumulative survival rate for men with COPD after 10 years was 60.1%, and for women it was 78.0%. However, the primary cause of death among patients initially hospitalized with COPD was ultimately COPD in only 22.1% of cases, with other causes such as coronary artery disease playing a prominent role. Nevertheless, it is clear that the prognosis for COPD patients in their 50s who require hospital treatment is poor.

Prognostic factors in COPD patients receiving long-term oxygen therapy have been analyzed by Oswald-Mammosser and colleagues.[80] Eighty-four patients underwent right-sided heart catheterization before institution of long-term oxygen therapy. These patients had a mean age of 63 years; they had a persistent arterial $P_{O_2}$ of less than 55 mm Hg or an arterial $P_{O_2}$ between 55 and 60 mm Hg and either signs of cor pulmonale or a mean pulmonary artery pressure of 25 mm Hg or greater. When actuarial survival curves were plotted with consideration of a number of variables, it was found that the 5-year survival rate for patients with an initial mean pulmonary artery pressure of 25 mm Hg or less was 62.2%, whereas it was only 36.3% in the 40 remaining patients who had initial pulmonary artery pressures higher than 25 mm Hg. Therefore, it would appear that the level of the pulmonary artery pressure at the time a patient undergoes long-term oxygen therapy is a better prognostic indicator than are such factors as $FEV_1$, the degree of hypoxemia, or the level of hypercapnia.

## SUMMARY

Respiratory disease can result in pulmonary hypertension, which eventually may lead to right ventricular hypertrophy, dilation, and congestive heart failure. Many different mechanisms can contribute to pulmonary hypertension, but most commonly the dominant cause is hypoxic pulmonary vasoconstriction resulting from chronic bronchitis and emphysema. Acute respiratory failure, with the additional burden of further hypoxemia and acidemia, may produce sudden increments in pulmonary artery hypertension as well as impairment in right ventricular contractility leading to acute cardiac decompensation. Effective management requires attention not only to the traditional management of heart failure but also to improvement in the underlying respiratory failure by managing any superimposed infection, improving ventilation, and administering oxygen. Chronic domiciliary oxygen therapy after a patient recovers from acute respiratory failure has been associated with improved survival and some relief of symptoms. Future research needs to address the therapeutic value of the chronic intravenous administration of prostacyclin (epoprostenol) via a portable pump for COPD patients exhibiting moderate to severe pulmonary hypertension in light of its proven benefit in patients with primary pulmonary hypertension.

## References

1. Report of an Expert Committee. Chronic cor pulmonale: Clinical progress. Circulation 27:594, 1963.
2. McGoon MD, Fuster V, Freeman WK, et al: Pulmonary hypertension. *In* Giuliani ER, Gersh BJ, McGoon MD (eds): Mayo Clinic Practice of Cardiology (3rd ed). St Louis: Mosby, 1986, pp. 1815–1836.
3. MacNee W: Pathophysiology of cor pulmonale in chronic obstructive pulmonary disease: Part one. Am J Respir Crit Care Med 150:833–852, 1994.
4. Horsfield K: Morphometry of the small pulmonary arteries in man. Circ Res 42:593–597, 1978.
5. Edwards JE: Pulmonary hypertension of cardiac and pulmonary origins: Pathologic origins. Prog Cardiovasc Dis 9:205–226, 1966.
6. Bove EK, Scott RC: The anatomy of chronic cor pulmonale secondary to intrinsic lung disease. Prog Cardiovasc Dis 9:227–238, 1966.
7. Charms BL, Brofman BL, Elder JC, et al: Unilateral pulmonary artery occlusion in man: II. Studies in patients with chronic pulmonary disease. J Thorac Cardiovasc Surg 35:316–331, 1958.
8. Widimsky J: Pressure, flow and volume changes of the lesser circulation during pulmonary artery occlusion in healthy subjects and patients with pulmonary hypertension. Prog Respir Res 5:224–236, 1970.
9. Hecht HH, Kuida H, Lange RL: Brisket disease: II. Clinical features and hemodynamic observations in altitude-dependent right heart failure in cattle. Am J Med 32:171–183, 1962.
10. Will DH, Horrell JF, Reeves JT, et al: Influence of altitude and age on pulmonary arterial pressure in cattle. Proc Soc Exper Biol Med 150:564–567, 1975.
11. Grover RF: Chronic hypoxic pulmonary hypertension. *In* Fishman AP (ed): The Pulmonary Circulation: Normal and Abnormal. Mechanisms, Management, and the National Registry. Philadelphia: University of Pennsylvania Press, 1990, p. 283.
12. Sorli J, Grassino A, Lorange G, et al: Control of breathing in patients with chronic obstructive lung disease. Clin Sci Mol Med 54;295–304, 1978.
13. Sassoon CSH, Hassell KT, Mahutte CK: Hyperoxic-induced hypercarbia in stable chronic obstructive pulmonary disease. Am Rev Respir Dis 135:907–911, 1987.
14. Rapaport E, Wong M, Ferguson RE, et al: Right ventricular volumes in patients with and without heart failure. Circulation 31:531–541, 1965.
15. Rapaport E, Wong M, Escobar EE, et al: The effect of upright posture on right ventricular volumes in patients with and without heart failure. Am Heart J 71:146–152, 1966.
16. Klinger JR, Hill NS: Right ventricular dysfunction in chronic obstructive pulmonary disease. Chest 99:715–723, 1991.
17. Matthay RA, Berger HJ, Davies RA, et al: Right and left ventricular exercise performance in chronic obstructive pulmonary disease: Radionuclide assessment. Ann Intern Med 93:234–239, 1980.
18. Krayenbuehl HP, Turnia J, Hess O: Left ventricular function in chronic pulmonary hypertension. Am J Cardiol 41:1150–1158, 1978.
18a. Tutar E, Kaya A, Gèulec S, et al: Echocardiographic evaluation of left ventricular diastolic function in chronic cor pulmonale. Am J Cardiol 83:1414–1417, 1999.
19. Schena M, Clini E, Errera D, et al: Echo-Doppler evaluation of left ventricular impairment in chronic cor pulmonale. Chest 109:1446–1451, 1996.
20. Anand IS, Chandrashekhar Y, Ferrari R, et al: Pathogenesis of congestive state in chronic obstructive pulmonary disease. Circulation 86:12–21, 1992.
21. MacNee W: Pathophysiology of cor pulmonale in chronic obstructive pulmonary disease: Part two. Am J Respir Crit Care Med 150:1158–1168, 1994.
22. Lipworth BJ, Dagg KD: Vasoconstrictor effects of angiotensin II on the pulmonary vascular bed. Chest 105:1360–1364, 1994.
23. Cargill RI, Lipworth BJ: Lisinopril attenuates acute hypoxic pulmonary vasoconstriction in humans. Chest: 109:424–429, 1996.
24. Lang CC, Coutie WJ, Struthers AD, et al: Elevated levels of brain natriuretic peptide in acute hypoxaemic chronic obstructive pulmonary disease. Clin Sci 85:529–533, 1992.
25. Cargill RI, Barr CS, Coutie WJ: C-type natriuretic peptide levels in cor pulmonale and in congestive heart failure. Thorax 49:1247–1249, 1994.
26. Zhao L, Hughes JM, Winter RJ: Effects of natriuretic peptides and neutral endopeptidase inhibition in isolated perfused rate lung. Am Rev Respir Dis 146:1198–1201, 1992.
27. Adnot S, Andrivet P, Chabrier PE, et al: Atrial natriuretic factor in chronic obstructive lung disease. J Clin Invest 83:986–993, 1989.
28. Cargill RI, Lipworth BJ: Atrial natriuretic peptide and brain natriuretic peptide in cor pulmonale. Chest 110:1220–1225, 1996.
29. Thompson JS, Morice AH: Neutral endopeptidase inhibitors and the pulmonary circulation. Gen Pharmacol 27:581–585, 1996.
30. Shih H-T, Webb CR, Conway WA: Frequency and significance of cardiac arrhythmias in chronic obstructive lung disease. Chest 94:44–48, 1988.
31. Matthay RA, Schwartz MI, Ellis JH, et al: Pulmonary artery hypertension in chronic obstructive pulmonary disease: Chest radiographic assessment. Invest Radiol 16:95–100, 1981.
32. Miserocchi G: Physiology and pathophysiology of pleural fluid turnover. Eur Respir J 10:219–225, 1997.
33. Wiener-Kronish JP, Matthay MA, Callen PW: Relationship of pleural effusions to pulmonary hemodynamics in patients with congestive heart failure. Am Rev Respir Dis 132:1253–1256, 1985.
34. Wiener-Kronish JP, Goldstein R, Matthay RA, et al: Lack of association of pleural effusion with chronic pulmonary arterial and right atrial hypertension. Chest 92:967–970, 1987.
35. Jensen R, Pierson RE, Braddy PM, et al: Brisket disease in yearling feedlot cattle. J Am Vet Med Assoc 169:515–517, 1976.
36. Phillips RW: The electrocardiogram in cor pulmonale secondary to pulmonary emphysema: A study of 18 cases proved by autopsy. Am Heart J 56:352–371, 1958.
36a. Incalzi RA, Fuso L, De Rosa M, et al: Electrocardiographic signs of chronic cor pulmonale: A negative prognostic finding in chronic obstructive pulmonary disease. Circulation 99:1600–1605, 1999.
37. Murphy ML, Dinh H, Nicholson D: Chronic cor pulmonale. Dis Mon 35:663–718, 1989.

38. Bristow JD, Morris JF, Kloster FE: Hemodynamics of cor pulmonale. Prog Cardiovasc Dis 9:239–258, 1966.
39. Lopez-Sendon J, Gomez Sanchez MAG, Mestre de Juan MJ: Pulmonary hypertension in the toxic oil syndrome. *In* Fishman AP (ed): The Pulmonary Circulation: Normal and Abnormal. Mechanisms, Management, and the National Registry. Philadelphia: University of Pennsylvania Press, 1990, pp. 385–395.
40. Loogen F, Worth H, Schwan G, et al: Long-term follow-up of pulmonary hypertension in patients with and without anorectic drug intake. Cor Vasa 27:111–124, 1985.
41. Gurtner HP: Aminorex pulmonary hypertension. *In* Fishman AP (ed): The Pulmonary Circulation: Normal and Abnormal. Mechanisms, Management, and the National Registry. Philadelphia: University of Pennsylvania Press, 1990, p. 397.
42. McNabb LJ, Baldwin KM: Hemodynamic and metabolic effects of exercise in *Crotalaria*-induced pulmonary hypertension in rats. J Appl Physiol Respir Environ Exercise Physiol 57:1829–1833, 1984.
43. Meyrick BO, Reid LM: *Crotalaria*-induced pulmonary hypertension: Uptake of $^3$H-Thymidine by the cells of the pulmonary circulation and alveolar walls. Am J Pathol 106:84–94, 1982.
44. Ferrer MI, Harvey RM, Cathcart RT, et al: Some effects of digoxin upon the heart and circulation in man: Digoxin in chronic cor pulmonale. Circulation 1:161–186, 1950.
45. MacNee W, Wathen CG, Hannan WJ, et al: Effects of pirbuterol and sodium nitroprusside on pulmonary haemodynamics in hypoxic cor pulmonale. Br Med J 287:1169–1172, 1983.
46. Tsagaris TJ, Sutton RB, Anderson FL: Effect of phlebotomy on coronary blood flow in calves with brisket disease. Proc Soc Exp Biol Med 142:560–563, 1973.
47. Stuart-Harris C, Flenly DC, Bishop JH, et al: Report of the Medical Research Council Working Party: Long-term domiciliary oxygen therapy in chronic cor pulmonale complicating chronic bronchitis and emphysema. Lancet 1:681–686, 1981.
48. Nocturnal Oxygen Therapy Trial Group: Continuous or nocturnal oxygen therapy in hypoxemic chronic obstructive lung disease: A clinical trial. Ann Intern Med 93:391–398, 1980.
49. Gassner A, Sommer G, Fridrich L, et al: Differential therapy with calcium antagonists in pulmonary hypertension secondary to COPD. Chest 98:829–834, 1990.
50. Weinberger SE, Schwartzstein RM, Weiss JW: Hypercapnia. N Engl J Med 321:1223–1231, 1989.
50a. Archibald CJ, Auger WR, Fedullo PF, et al: Long-term outlook after pulmonary thromboendarterectomy. Am J Respir Crit Care Med 160:523–528, 1999.
51. Pelouch V, Kolar F, Ost'adal B, et al: Regression of chronic hypoxia-induced pulmonary hypertension, right ventricular hypertrophy, and fibrosis: Effect of enalapril. Cardiovasc Drugs Ther 11:177–185, 1997.
52. Nong Z, Stassen JM, Moons L, et al: Inhibition of tissue angiotensin-converting enzyme with quinapril reduces hypoxic pulmonary hypertension and pulmonary vascular remodelling. Circulation 94:1941–1947, 1996.
53. Kiely DG, Cargill RI, Lipworth BJ: Angiotensin II receptor blockade and effects on pulmonary hemodynamics and hypoxic pulmonary vasoconstriction in humans. Chest 110:698–703, 1996.
54. Mahajan SK, Sharma VK, Thakral S: Effect of enalapril on renal profile and right ventricular dimensions in chronic cor pulmonale. J Assoc Physicians India 44:323–324, 1996.
55. Zielinski J, Hawrylkiewicz I, Gorecka D, et al: Captopril effects on pulmonary and systemic hemodynamics in chronic cor pulmonale. Chest 90:562–565, 1986.
56. Kiely DG, Cargill RI, Wheeldon NM, et al: Haemodynamic and endocrine effects of type 1 angiotensin II receptor blockade in patients with hypoxaemic cor pulmonale. Cardiovasc Res 33:201–208, 1997.
56a. Hart CM: Nitric oxide in adult lung disease. Chest 115:1407–1417, 1999.
57. Stamler JS, Singel J, Loscaizo J: Biochemistry of nitric oxide and its redox-activated forms. Science 258:1898–1902, 1992.
58. Frostell CG, Blomqvist H, Hedenstierna G, et al: Inhaled nitric oxide selectivity reverses human hypoxic pulmonary vasoconstriction without causing systemic vasodilation. Anesthesiology 78:427–435, 1993.
59. Johns RA: EDRF/Nitric oxide: The endogenous nitrovasodilator and a new cellular messenger. Anesthesiology 75:927–931, 1991.
60. Dinh-Xuan AT, Higenbotham TW, Clelland CA, et al: Impairment of endothelium-dependent pulmonary-artery relaxation in chronic obstructive lung disease. N Engl J Med 324:1539–1547, 1991.
61. Frostell C, Fratacci M-D, Wain J-C: Inhaled nitric oxide: A selective pulmonary vasodilator reversing hypoxic pulmonary vasoconstriction. Circulation 83:2038–2047, 1991.
62. Al-Ali MK, Howarth PH: Nitric oxide and the respiratory system in health and disease. Respir Med 92:702–715, 1998.
63. Dinh-Xuan AT: Endothelial modulation of pulmonary vascular tone. Eur Respir J 5:757–762, 1992.
64. Roberts JD, Polaner DM, Lang P, et al: Inhaled nitric oxide in persistent pulmonary hypertension of the newborn. Lancet 340:818–819, 1992.
65. Kinsella JP, Neish SR, Shaffer E, et al: Low-dose inhalational nitric oxide in persistent pulmonary hypertension of the newborn. Lancet 340:819–820, 1992.
66. Kotlikoff MI, Fishman AP: Endothelin: Mediator of hypoxic vasoconstriction? *In* Fishman AP (ed): The Pulmonary Circulation: Normal and Abnormal. Mechanisms, Management, and the National Registry. Philadelphia: University of Pennsylvania Press, 1990, p. 85.
67. Hubloue I, Leeman M, Pierre S, et al: Interactions between endogenous nitric oxide and endothelins in hypoxic pulmonary vasoconstriction (abstract). Eur Heart J 19:321, 1998.
68. Badesch DB, Orton C, Zapp LM, et al: Decreased arterial wall prostaglandin production in neonatal calves with severe chronic pulmonary hypertension. Am J Respir Cell Mol Biol 1:489–498, 1989.
69. Richalet J-P, Hornych A, Rathat C, et al: Plasma prostaglandins, leukotrienes and thromboxane in acute high altitude hypoxia. Respir Physiol 85:205–215, 1991.
70. Rubin LJ, Mendoza J, Hood M, et al: Treatment of primary pulmonary hypertension with continuous intravenous prostacyclin (epoprostenol). Ann Intern Med 112:485–491, 1990.
71. Barst RJ, Rubin LJ, Long WA, et al: A comparison of continuous intravenous epoprostenol (Prostacylin) with conventional therapy for primary pulmonary hypertension. N Engl J Med 334:296–301, 1996.
72. Shapiro SM, Oudiz RJ, Cao T, et al: Primary pulmonary hypertension: Improved long-term effects and survival with continuous intravenous epoprostenol infusion. J Am Coll Cardiol 30:343–349, 1997.
73. McLaughlin VV, Genthner DE, Panella MM, et al: Reduction in pulmonary vascular resistance with long-term epoprostenol (prostacyclin) therapy in primary pulmonary hypertension. N Engl J Med 338:273–277, 1998.
74. Vance JW: Management of patients with cor pulmonale—acute and chronic. Prog Cardiovasc Dis 9:470–483, 1967.
75. American Thoracic Society: Standards for the diagnosis and care of patients with chronic obstructive pulmonary disease. Am J Respir Crit Care Med 152(Suppl):S77–S120, 1995.
76. Weitzenblum E, Sautegeau A, Ehrhart M, et al: Long-term course of pulmonary arterial pressure in chronic obstructive pulmonary disease. Am Rev Respir Dis 130:993–998, 1984.
77. Weitzenblum E, Loiseau A, Hirth C, et al: Course of pulmonary hemodynamics in patients with chronic obstructive pulmonary disease. Chest 75:656–662, 1979.
78. Vasilyev S, Schaap RN, Mortensen JD: Hospital survival rates of patients with acute respiratory failure in modern respiratory intensive care units. Chest 107:1083–1088, 1995.
79. Keistinen T, Tuuponen T, Kivela S-L: Survival experience of the population needing hospital treatment for asthma or COPD at age 50–54 years. Respir Med 92:568–572, 1998.
80. Oswald-Mammosser M, Weitzenblum E, Quiox E, et al: Prognostic factors in COPD patients receiving long-term oxygen therapy: Importance of pulmonary artery pressure. Chest 107:1193–98, 1995.

SECTION L

# Infiltrative and Interstitial Lung Diseases

# 56 Principles of and Approach to the Patient with Interstitial Lung Disease

MARVIN I. SCHWARZ, M.D. • TALMADGE E. KING, JR., M.D.
REUBEN M. CHERNIACK, M.D.

Introduction
Clinical and Histologic Classification
- Diffuse Alveolar Damage
- Organizing Pneumonia
- Desquamative Interstitial Pneumonia
- Nonspecific Interstitial Pneumonitis
- Usual Interstitial Pneumonia
- Honeycomb Lung
- Lymphocytic Interstitial Pneumonia
- Eosinophilic Pneumonia
- Alveolar Proteinosis
- Diffuse Alveolar Hemorrhage
- Amyloid Deposition
- Granulomatous Pneumonitis

Clinical Features
- Symptoms
- Past History
- Physical Findings
- Radiographic Features
- Functional Assessment
- Laboratory Findings
- Bronchoalveolar Lavage

Tissue Diagnosis
Summary

## INTRODUCTION

The term *interstitial lung disease,* in general, implies inflammatory-fibrotic infiltration of the alveolar walls (septal) resulting in profound effects on the capillary endothelium and the alveolar epithelial lining cells (Fig. 56.1). Under normal conditions, small numbers of interstitial macrophages, fibroblasts, and myofibroblasts reside within the interstitium. Other components of the interstitium include the matrix proteins of the lung, consisting of collagen-related macromolecules and the noncollagenous proteins such as fibronectin and laminin.[1,2] In many of the interstitial lung diseases, interstitial fibrosis appears after injury to the alveolar-capillary basement membranes. It increases the permeability of this structure, enabling the serum contents to enter the alveolar spaces. Fibroblastic proliferation and excessive collagen deposition, the histologic hallmarks of interstitial lung disease, occur either as a direct result of the injury, as a result of an inflammatory cell response that releases proinflammatory and profibrotic cytokines, or as a consequence of the regenerative and reparative processes taking place at the epithelial and endothelial surfaces. Moreover, fibroblastic proliferation and collagen accumulation also occur within airway lumina.[3,4]

*Interstitial lung disease* is a term describing more than 100 entities that injure the distal airways, producing a disease with similar clinical, radiographic, and physiologic features. Many interstitial lung diseases, however, affect not only the alveolar structures but also the lumina and walls of small airways (alveolar ducts, respiratory bronchioles, and terminal bronchioles).[5]

## CLASSIFICATION OF INTERSTITIAL LUNG DISEASE

A clinical classification of the interstitial lung diseases is shown in Figure 56.2 and outlined in detail in Table 56.1.[6,7] Although the diagnosis of interstitial lung disease due to occupational exposure, a medication, or a connective tissue disease may be obvious, the primary and idiopathic interstitial lung diseases are difficult to diagnose on clinical grounds alone. This chapter presents an approach for the evaluation of these patients. An alternative

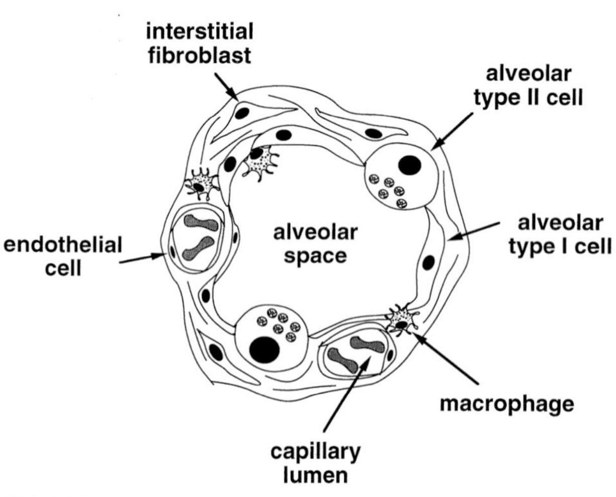


**Figure 56.1** This schematic depiction of the lung parenchyma surrounding an alveolar space shows the major cells that line and lie within the interstitial space.

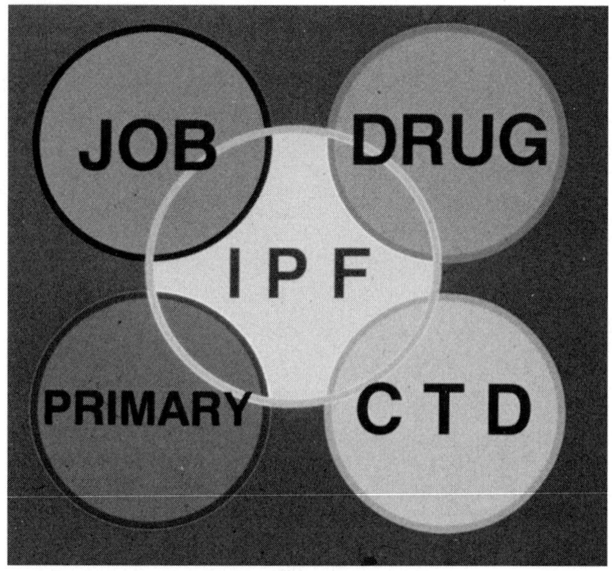


**Figure 56.2** This schematic representation of the major categories of interstitial lung diseases emphasizes the overlap among the various disorders. JOB = occupational diseases; IPF = idiopathic pulmonary fibrosis; DRUG = drug toxicity; CTD = connective tissue disease.

method of classification depends on the resultant histologic pattern. As seen in Figure 56.3, various injuries can produce a variety of histologic patterns, and dissimilar clinical entities depicted in Table 56.1 may result in similar histologies (Table 56.2).

### Diffuse Alveolar Damage

Diffuse alveolar damage develops after an acute injury to the alveolar capillary basement membranes.[8–10] It is most commonly seen in the acute respiratory distress syndrome or in immunosuppressed patients who have received cytotoxic drugs or who have developed diffuse infectious pneumonias.[11,12] After the endothelial-epithelial injury, there is leakage of serum proteins and red blood cells into the alveolar spaces. The alveolar epithelium becomes necrotic and is sloughed, and the interstitium becomes edematous. Hyaline membranes, recognized as eosinophilic debris and consisting of necrotic epithelial cells, protein, and fibrin, form within alveolar spaces (Fig. 56.4). In the reparative or organizing stage of diffuse alveolar damage, there is proliferation and hyperplasia of the alveolar type II epithelial cells, which are capable of differentiating into type I cells. There is also resorption and incorporation of the hyaline membranes and alveolar exudates into the alveolar walls, associated with interstitial intraluminal fibroblast proliferation and collagen deposition. This is known as the *organizing phase* of diffuse alveolar damage. With protracted or repeated parenchymal injury, irreversible fibrosis and honeycomb lung result.[13,14]

### Organizing Pneumonia

Organizing pneumonia is recognized by the appearance in the small airways of intraluminal collections of prolif-

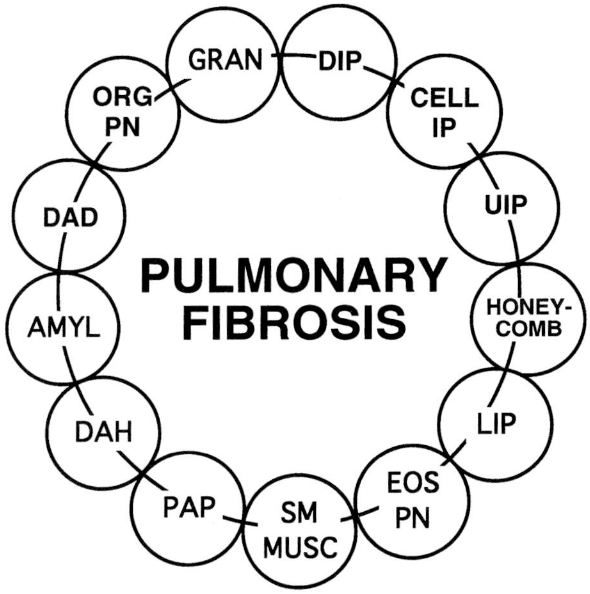


**Figure 56.3** This schematic depiction shows the many different histologic patterns seen in the interstitial lung diseases that are associated with or lead to pulmonary fibrosis. Gran = granulomatous pneumonitis; DIP = desquamative interstitial pneumonia; Cell IP = cellular or nonspecific interstitial pneumonitis; UIP = usual interstitial pneumonitis; LIP = lymphocytic interstitial pneumonitis; Eos Pn = eosinophilic pneumonia; Sm Musc = smooth muscle proliferation; PAP = pulmonary alveolar proteinosis; DAH = diffuse alveolar hemorrhage; Amyl = amyloidosis; DAD = diffuse alveolar damage; Org Pn = organizing pneumonia.

erating fibroblasts that produce mucopolysaccharides and collagen. It is most prominent in the alveolar ducts but extends distally to the alveolar lumina and proximally to membranous bronchioles (Fig. 56.5). This change is accompanied by an interstitial lymphoplasmacytic infiltrate and hyperplasia of the type II epithelial cells. The organizing process, which extends into the membranous bronchioles, produces an intraluminal polypoid bronchiolitis obliterans (Fig. 56.6). If idiopathic, it is called *bronchiolitis obliterans organizing pneumonia* (BOOP), also referred to as *cryptogenic organizing pneumonia*.[15, 16] BOOP should not be confused with the progressive obstructive lung disease known as bronchiolitis obliterans or constrictive bronchiolitis obliterans, which is an irreversible concentric fibrous obliteration of the bronchioles. Organizing pneumonia represents a common reparative response to injury occurring in a variety of interstitial lung diseases (see Table 56.2). If the injury is unresponsive to treatment, progression to irreversible fibrosis and honeycomb lung can result.

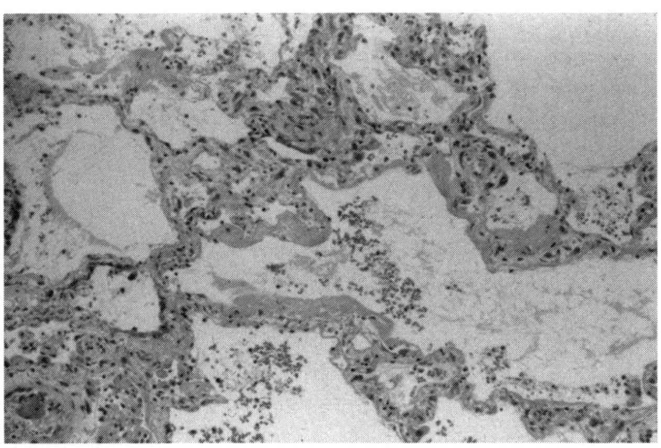

**Figure 56.4.** Photomicrograph shows diffuse alveolar damage. Note the hyaline membranes within alveolar spaces and edema and inflammatory cell infiltration of the alveolar wall. (Original magnification ×10.)

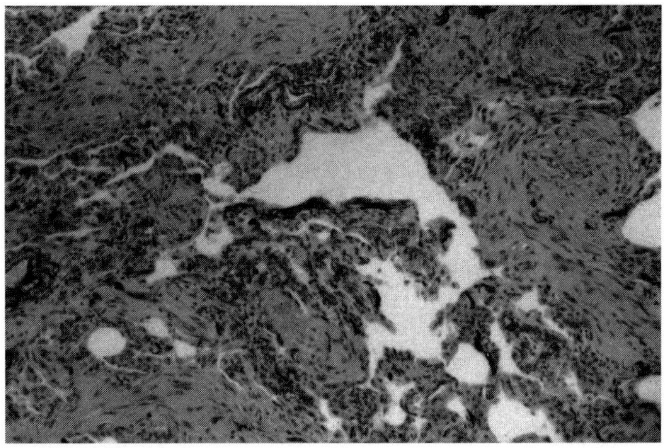

**Figure 56.5** Photomicrograph indicates bronchiolitis obliterans organizing pneumonia. Immature connective tissue and proliferating fibroblasts appearing light blue (pentachrome stain) are present in alveolar ducts and alveolar spaces, and there is an interstitial mononuclear inflammatory cells infiltrate. (Original magnification ×40.)

## Desquamative Interstitial Pneumonia

Desquamative interstitial pneumonia is recognized by dense collections of intraluminal alveolar macrophages

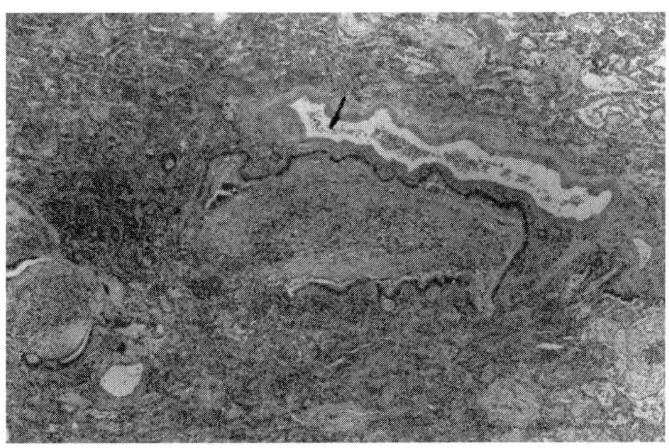

**Figure 56.6** Photomicrograph of bronchiolitis obliterans organizing pneumonia shows a typical inflammatory polyp extending into the lumen of a terminal bronchiole. (Original magnification ×40.)

**Table 56.1 CLINICAL CLASSIFICATION OF THE INTERSTITIAL LUNG DISEASES**

**Connective Tissue Diseases**
Scleroderma
Polymyositis-dermatomyositis
Systemic lupus erythematosus
Rheumatoid arthritis
Mixed connective tissue disease
Ankylosing spondylitis

**Treatment-Related or Drug-Induced Diseases**
Antibiotics (furantoin, sulfasalazine)
Antiarrythmics (amiodarone, tocainide, propranolol)
Anti-inflammatory (gold, penicillamine)
Anticonvulsants (dilantin)
Chemotherapeutic agents (mitomycin C, bleomycin, busulfan, cyclophosphamide, chlorambucil, methotrexate, azathioprine, BCNU (carmustine), procarbazine)
Vitamins (L-tryptophan)
Therapeutic radiation
Oxygen toxicity
Paraquat
Narcotics

**Primary (Unclassified) Diseases**
Sarcoidosis
Eosinophilic granuloma
Amyloidosis
Pulmonary vasculitis
Lipoid pneumonia
Lymphangitic carcinomatosis
Bronchoalveolar carcinoma
Pulmonary lymphoma
Gaucher's disease
Niemann-Pick disease
Hermansky-Pudlak syndrome
Neurofibromatosis
Lymphangioleiomyomatosis
Tuberous sclerosis
Acute respiratory distress syndrome
Acquired immunodeficiency syndrome (AIDS)
Bone marrow transplantation
Postinfectious
Respiratory bronchiolitis
Eosinophilic pneumonia
Alveolar proteinosis
Diffuse alveolar hemorrhage syndromes
Alveolar microlithiasis
Metastatic calcification

**Occupational and Environmental Diseases**
***Inorganic***
Silicosis
Asbestosis
Hard metal pneumoconiosis
Coal worker's pneumoconiosis
Berylliosis
Aluminum oxide fibrosis
Talc pneumoconiosis
Siderosis (arc welder)
Stanosis (tin)
***Organic (Hypersensitivity Pneumonitis)***
Bird breeder's lung
Farmer's lung
(For complete listing see Chapter 67)

**Idiopathic Fibrotic Disorders**
Acute interstitial pneumonitis (Hamman-Rich syndrome)
Idiopathic pulmonary fibrosis
Familial idiopathic pulmonary fibrosis
Desquamative interstitial pneumonitis
Bronchiolitis obliterans organizing pneumonia
Nonspecific interstitial pneumonitis
Lymphocytic interstitial pneumonia (Sjögren's syndrome, connective tissue disease, AIDS, Hashimoto's thyroiditis)
Autoimmune pulmonary fibrosis (inflammatory bowel disease, primary biliary cirrhosis, idiopathic thrombocytopenic purpura, autoimmune hemolytic anemia)

with little interstitial collagen deposition (Fig. 56.7).[17] The original term is misleading in that there is no real desquamation of epithelial cells. There is simply a collection of macrophages in the air spaces. Some believe that idiopathic desquamative interstitial pneumonia is a specific disease entity.[18] There is also evidence to support the notion that desquamative interstitial pneumonia represents an earlier cellular phase of usual interstitial pneumonitis.[19–21] A form of desquamative interstitial pneumonia is known as *giant cell interstitial pneumonitis* because multinucleated giant cells accompany the intraluminal macrophage collections. This condition can be idiopathic, or it can represent a hard metal pneumoconiosis.[22]

## Nonspecific Interstitial Pneumonitis

Nonspecific interstitial pneumonitis refers to either a homogenous infiltration of mononuclear cells that expands the interstitial space or interstitial fibrosis that does not conform to the variegated pattern ascribed to usual interstitial pneumonia. These cells include lymphoplasmacytic cells and interstitial macrophages (Fig. 56.8).[12, 18, 23–25] There is also hyperplasia of type II alveolar lining cells without fibroblastic proliferation or collagen deposition until late in the course. Accumulation of macrophages often accompanies this reaction. The entire spectrum from early inflammation to advanced fibrosis is often seen in lung biopsies of patients with idiopathic pulmonary fibrosis and the interstitial lung diseases associated with connective tissue disease, and there is still disagreement about whether nonspecific interstitial pneumonitis is a distinct entity. It may simply represent a group of interstitial lung diseases that defy classification at this time.

## Usual Interstitial Pneumonia

Usual interstitial pneumonia has been described by some as the transitional phase between a desquamative or nonspecific (cellular) interstitial pneumonia and end-stage honeycomb lung. Others believe that this process appears de novo. Here the number of interstitial inflammatory cells is decreased and the interstitium becomes broadened

**Table 56.2 HISTOLOGIC PATTERNS IN THE INTERSTITIAL LUNG DISEASES AND THEIR DISEASE ASSOCIATIONS**

| Type | Associations |
|---|---|
| Diffuse alveolar damage | Acute respiratory distress syndrome; drugs (cytotoxic agents, heroin, cocaine, paraquat, ethylchlorvynol, aspirin); toxic gas inhalation; radiation therapy; oxygen toxicity; connective tissue disease; infections (legionella, mycoplasma, viral); Hamman-Rich syndrome |
| Organizing pneumonia | Diffuse alveolar damage; diffuse alveolar hemorrhage; drugs (amiodarone, cocaine); infections; connective tissue diseases; hypersensitivity pneumonitis; eosinophilic pneumonia; Wegener's granulomatosis; idiopathic pulmonary fibrosis; bronchiolitis obliterans organizing pneumonia (idiopathic) |
| Desquamative interstitial pneumonia | Idiopathic; connective tissue diseases; respiratory bronchiolitis; eosinophilic granuloma; asbestosis; hard-metal pneumoconiosis (cobalt); Gaucher's disease; Niemann-Pick disease; Hermansky-Pudlak syndrome; drugs (furantoin, amiodarone) |
| Nonspecific interstitial pneumonitis | Idiopathic pulmonary fibrosis; connective tissue diseases; drugs; hypersensitivity pneumonitis; diffuse alveolar damage; infections; acquired immunodeficiency syndrome (AIDS) |
| Usual interstitial pneumonia | Idiopathic pulmonary fibrosis; connective tissue diseases; asbestosis; hypersensitivity pneumonitis; lymphocytic interstitial pneumonia; chronic aspiration pneumonia; chronic radiation pneumonitis; chronic eosinophilic pneumonia; infections; hemosiderosis; Hermansky-Pudlak syndrome; neurofibromatosis; alveolar proteinosis |
| Honeycomb lung | All the entities listed under usual interstitial pneumonia; sarcoidosis; eosinophilic granuloma |
| Lymphocytic interstitial pneumonia | Idiopathic; hypogammaglobulinemia; autoimmune diseases including Hashimoto's thyroiditis, lupus erythematosus, primary biliary cirrhosis, Sjögren's syndrome, myasthenia gravis, and chronic active hepatitis; AIDS; allogeneic bone marrow transplantation |
| Eosinophilic pneumonia | Idiopathic acute and chronic; tropical filarial eosinophilia; parasitic infections; allergic bronchopulmonary aspergillosis; allergic granulomatosis of Churg and Strauss; hypereosinophilic syndrome; AIDS; L-tryptophan |
| Alveolar proteinosis | Pulmonary alveolar proteinosis; acute silicosis; aluminum dust; AIDS; myeloproliferative disorder |
| Diffuse alveolar hemorrhage | |
| With capillaritis | Wegener's granulomatosis, microscopic polyangiitis, systemic lupus erythematosus, polymyositis, scleroderma, rheumatoid arthritis; mixed connective tissue disease, lung transplant, drugs (retinoic acid, propylthiouracil, dilantin); Behçet's disease, cryoglobulinemia, Henoch-Schönlein purpura, pauci-immune glomerulonephritis, immune complex glomerulonephritis) |
| Without capillaritis | Idiopathic pulmonary hemosiderosis; systemic lupus erythematosus; Goodpasture's syndrome, diffuse alveolar damage, pulmonary veno-occlusive disease; mitral stenosis; lymphangioleiomyomatosis |
| Amyloid deposition | Primary amyloidosis; multiple myeloma; lymphocytic interstitial pneumonia |
| Granuloma | Sarcoidosis; hypersensitivity pneumonitis; eosinophilic granuloma; silicosis; intravenous talcosis; berylliosis; lymphocytic interstitial pneumonia; infections |

by proliferating fibroblasts, the laying down of collagen fibers, and, in some instances, smooth muscle proliferation (Fig. 56.9).[26] This process has a predilection for the peripheral (subpleural) and basilar portions of the lung. Alveolar type II cell hyperplasia and intra-alveolar fibrosis are seen. These histologic changes have been referred to clinically as the *midcourse* of interstitial lung disease.[27] "Usual interstitial pneumonia" is the pathologic designation of the clinical disease idiopathic pulmonary fibrosis or cryptogenic fibrosis alveolitis.

## Honeycomb Lung

The term *honeycomb lung* describes a histologic change, often appearing with usual interstitial pneumonitis, that indicates irreversible end-stage disease. Here there is total disruption of the lung architecture by conglomerate fibrosis and the formation of cystic spaces by metaplastic cuboidal epithelium that are devoid of gas exchange function (Fig. 56.10). Mucus that contains acute inflammatory cells collects in the cystic spaces. The metaplastic epithelium has the potential for malignant change (adenocarcinoma or alveolar cell carcinoma). Other findings are proliferation of interstitial smooth muscle cells and pulmonary vascular changes (intimal smooth muscle proliferation and medial hypertrophy), indicating long-standing hypoxic pulmonary vasoconstriction.[28]

## Lymphocytic Interstitial Pneumonia

Lymphocytic interstitial pneumonia is distinguished from the desquamative and nonspecific interstitial pneumonias by the presence of monotonous sheets of lymphocytes infiltrating the interstitium and alveolar lumina.[29] Other features include the interstitial accumulation of macrophages, noncaseating granulomas, perivascular amyloid

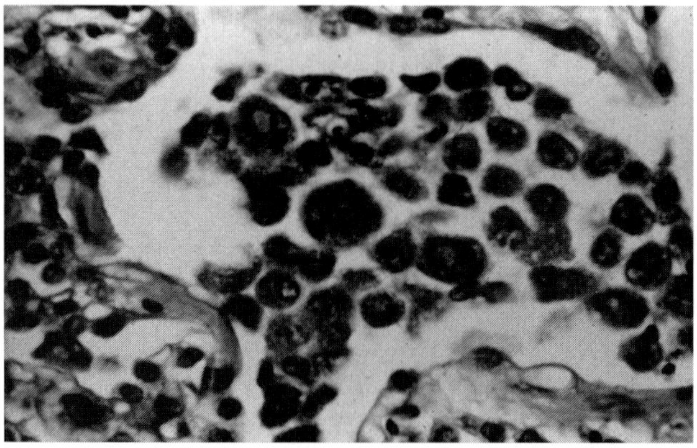

**Figure 56.7** Photomicrograph of desquamative interstitial pneumonia (periodic acid–Schiff stain) shows a characteristic dense collection of macrophages filling the alveolar lumina without alveolar wall collagen. (Original magnification ×100.)

deposits, and germinal lymphoid centers. Conversion to a low-grade pulmonary lymphoma or progression to end-stage honeycomb lung may follow.[30–32]

## Eosinophilic Pneumonia

In eosinophilic pneumonia, there are collections of eosinophils in the interstitium and alveolar spaces. Other prominent features include a lymphoplasmacytic cellular interstitial pneumonia, features of BOOP, and, in chronic cases, usual interstitial pneumonia progressing to honeycomb lung.[33]

## Alveolar Proteinosis

Alveolar proteinosis is characterized by the presence of an amorphous, eosinophilic-staining granular, intra-alveolar exudate.[34] This material is rich in surfactant-associated

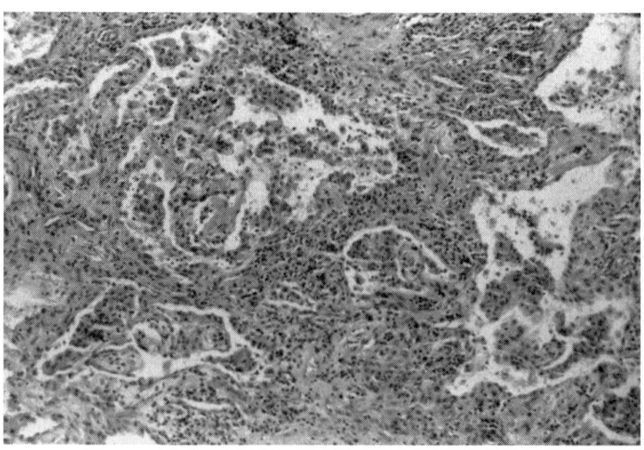

**Figure 56.8** Photomicrograph of nonspecific interstitial pneumonia is shown. Note the lymphoplasmacytic cells expanding the interstitial compartment. Alveolar macrophages are present also. (Original magnification ×10.)

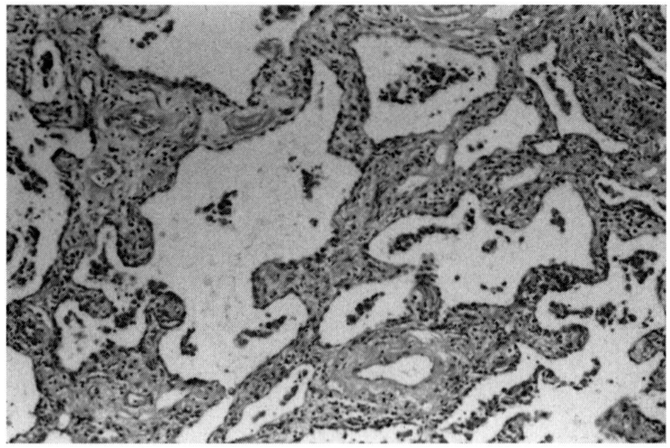

**Figure 56.9** Photomicrograph of usual interstitial pneumonia is shown. Residual lymphoplasmacytic inflammation and collagen deposition broadening alveolar walls. (Original magnification ×10.)

lipids and proteins. Interstitial inflammation is not present, but interstitial fibrosis complicates chronic cases.

## Diffuse Alveolar Hemorrhage

Diffuse alveolar hemorrhage occurs after widespread injury from any of a multitude of causes, often immunologic, to the alveolar capillary membranes.[35] Intra-alveolar red blood cells and hemosiderin-containing macrophages accumulate. In cases of diffuse alveolar hemorrhage associated with pulmonary capillaritis, there is a striking neutrophilic infiltration of the alveolar walls that often results in fibrinoid necrosis.[36] Organization of the hemorrhage occurs, and with repeated episodes progression to interstitial fibrosis may ensue.

## Amyloid Deposition

Amyloid deposition in the lung is seen in primary as opposed to secondary amyloidosis. Light microscopy

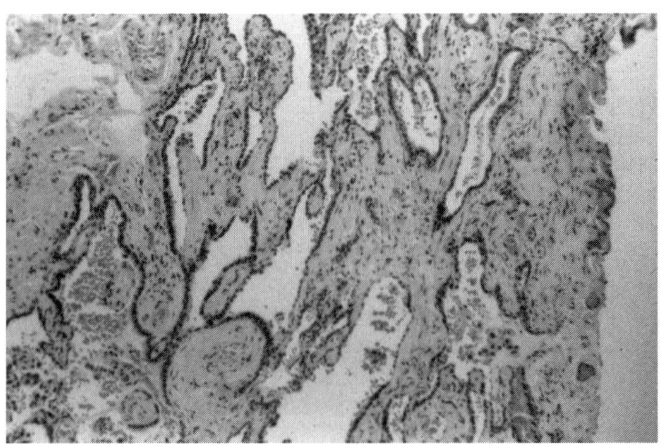

**Figure 56.10** Photomicrograph of honeycomb lung in idiopathic pulmonary fibrosis is shown. There is total disruption of the lung architecture by bands of fibrous tissue forming cystic spaces. The spaces are lined by metaplastic epithelium. (Original magnification ×10.)

demonstrates amorphous material consisting of immunoglobulin light chains infiltrating the alveolar walls and the pulmonary arterioles, arteries, and veins (Fig. 56.11).[37] Electron microscopy indicates that these deposits are most dense within the alveolar capillary basement membranes.[38] Polarized light after Congo red staining reveals the characteristic apple-green birefringence.

## Granulomatous Pneumonitis

The formation of a granuloma represents a local and intense reaction to a foreign antigen. It consists of organized collections of monocytic-macrophagic cells that undergo maturation to form epithelioid cells, the so-called epithelioid granuloma. Within the granuloma there is fusion of the mononuclear phagocytes to form giant cells (Fig. 56.12). At the periphery of the granuloma, collections of lymphocytes are found.[39] Granulomas also contain inclusions such as asteroid bodies, oxalate crystals, cholesterol clefts, and Schaumann's bodies. These features do not distinguish among the various causes of granulomatous lung disease. However, there are features of the granuloma that help in differentiation. Caseous necrosis in most cases indicates granulomatous infection. A bronchocentric distribution of the granuloma is more likely to be found in patients with hypersensitivity pneumonitis and eosinophilic granuloma, whereas in those with berylliosis and sarcoidosis the granulomas follow lymphatic routes.[12] In addition to the granulomatous reaction in this group of diseases, cellular interstitial infiltrates, organizing pneumonia, and usual interstitial pneumonia can be seen.

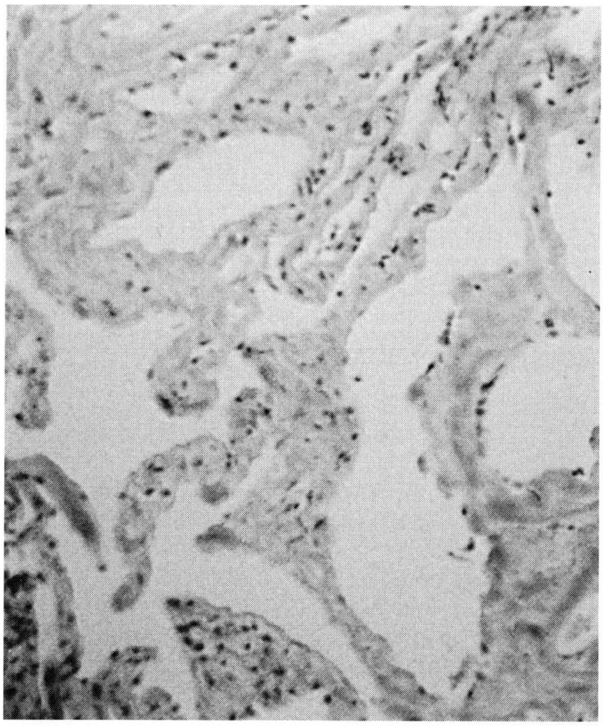

**Figure 56.11** Photomicrograph of amyloid infiltration reveals an amorphous acellular material in the interstitium. (Congo red stain; original magnification ×10.)

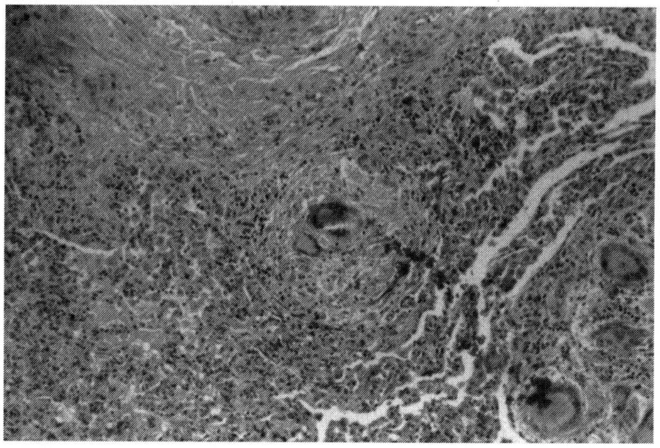

**Figure 56.12** Photomicrograph of sarcoidosis shows granulomas that efface the architecture of the lung. Note the foreign-body giant cells and the inflammatory cells at the periphery of the granulomas. (Original magnification ×10.)

## CLINICAL FEATURES

The hallmarks of an interstitial lung disease are progressive dyspnea and cough, an abnormal chest radiograph, and impaired pulmonary function tests.[7] However, 5% to 10% of symptomatic patients eventually diagnosed as having interstitial lung disease initially have normal chest radiographs.[40, 41] There are also dyspneic patients with or without abnormal chest radiographs in whom routine pulmonary function tests (flows, volumes, and diffusing capacity) are normal.[6] In this situation exercise testing, which measures gas exchange, unmasks abnormalities. Furthermore, high-resolution computed tomographic (HRCT) scans[42–44] and bronchoalveolar lavage[45, 46] can detect abnormalities in the presence of normal radiographs and physiologic tests in patients at high risk for development of interstitial lung disease, such as patients with connective tissue disease, asbestos exposure, or hypersensitivity pneumonitis and patients taking drugs known to injure the lung.

### Symptoms

Progressive dyspnea is usually the most common symptom, but cough can be prominent, particularly in those patients with lymphangitic carcinomatosis in which the bronchial lymphatic channels are infiltrated.[47] Cough is also disturbing in sarcoidosis because the granulomatous reaction may also involve airway walls.[48] Similarly, cough is a prominent symptom in interstitial lung diseases that affect small airways or are bronchocentric in location, such as respiratory bronchiolitis,[49] BOOP,[15] eosinophilic granuloma,[50] and hypersensitivity pneumonitis.[51]

Substernal chest pain, an unusual complaint for most interstitial lung diseases, is frequent in sarcoidosis.[52] Pleuritic-type chest pain may accompany connective tissue and drug-related interstitial lung diseases. The sudden appearance of chest pain due to a pneumothorax can be the presenting manifestation or complicate a preexisting eosinophilic granuloma,[50] lymphangioleiomyomatosis,[53] tuberous sclerosis,[54] or neurofibromatosis.[55] Wheezing, an unusual symptom in interstitial lung disease, has been reported with lymphangitic carcinomatosis,[56] chronic eosinophilic pneumonia,[33] respiratory bronchiolitis,[49] and hypersensitivity pneumonitis due to bird antigens. Hemoptysis is typical for the diffuse alveolar hemorrhage syndromes,[35] lymphangioleiomyomatosis,[53] pulmonary veno-occlusive disease,[57] and long-standing mitral valve disease.[58] However, alveolar hemorrhage may be present without hemoptysis. Hemoptysis occurring in a patient with an established interstitial lung disease raises the possibility of a complicating malignancy.

Symptoms in patients with interstitial lung disease are present for months to years and progress at varying rates. There are several interstitial reactions that are acute (days to several weeks). These are often confused with atypical pneumonias because they cause diffuse radiographic infiltrates and may be associated with fever. Included are acute interstitial pneumonitis (Hamman-Rich syndrome),[59] acute eosinophilic pneumonia,[60] some cases of hypersensitivity pneumonitis,[61] occasionally drug-related interstitial lung diseases, some cases of BOOP,[62] the diffuse alveolar hemorrhage syndromes,[35] and the acute immunologic pneumonias that occur with connective tissue diseases.[63, 64]

## Past History

Interstitial lung disease occurring in a patient with an established connective tissue disease is obvious; there are, however, patients in whom the lung disease precedes the more typical manifestations by months to several years.[64, 65]

**Occupational History.** The occupational history is of obvious importance, and it should be detailed, because a long latency period may exist between exposure and the appearance of clinical disease. The exposure may have been of short duration but high intensity. Hypersensitivity pneumonitis, which can manifest either as recurrent acute or subacute pneumonitis or as an insidious form with slowly progressive dyspnea, must be excluded. There is a growing list of occupational and environmental antigens that can precipitate this granulomatous pneumonitis. Similarly, a drug history is important, and lung disease may appear weeks to years after the drug has been discontinued.[66, 67] Aspiration of gastric contents as a result of gastroesophageal reflux can lead to insidious interstitial infiltrates, as can the nocturnal use of oily nosedrops.[68, 69]

A history of tobacco use is important. More than 90% of patients with eosinophilic granuloma of the lung are smokers at the time of diagnosis; this is also true for respiratory bronchiolitis.[47, 70] Of patients with Goodpasture's syndrome who smoked, 100% had diffuse alveolar hemorrhage, whereas only 20% of a nonsmoking group had pulmonary disease in addition to the renal involvement.[71] Tobacco use also appears to enhance the development of interstitial fibrosis in an asbestos-exposed population. The risk of asbestosis in exposed smokers was 13 times that in a nonsmoking asbestos-exposed cohort.[72, 73] Hypersensitivity pneumonitis, on the other hand, infrequently appears in the active smoker.[74] Also, the incidence of sarcoidosis is higher in nonsmokers.

**Family History.** Family history is occasionally helpful in determining the cause of interstitial lung disease. There is a form of idiopathic pulmonary fibrosis that affects family members in an autosomal-dominant fashion.[75] Familial sarcoidosis is a well-described entity, but its pattern of inheritance is unknown.[76] Other interstitial lung diseases with autosomal-dominant inheritance patterns include tuberous sclerosis[54] and neurofibromatosis.[55] Niemann-Pick disease,[77] Gaucher's disease,[78] and Hermansky-Pudlak syndrome[79] are inherited in an autosomal-recessive fashion.

There are interstitial lung diseases with a sex predilection. Lymphangioleiomyomatosis[53] occurs exclusively in women.[53] In addition, the connective tissue diseases more commonly affect women. Occupational causes are more likely in men. However, transmission of inorganic dust, either from clothes or by living in the vicinity of a manufacturing or mining facility, has resulted in asbestosis and berylliosis in women, children, and men not employed in the industry.[80, 81]

## Physical Findings

The most typical physical finding is bibasilar inspiratory crackles. Crackles are less likely in the granulomatous diseases.[82] Bilateral inspiratory crackles may also be present in a symptomatic patient with a negative chest radiograph. Clubbing of the digits, which in most cases indicates advanced fibrotic disease, is a common finding in patients with the idiopathic or familial forms of pulmonary fibrosis. However, the appearance of digital clubbing in a patient with an established case of interstitial lung disease could indicate an underlying bronchogenic carcinoma. With advanced fibrosis, causing chronic hypoxemia, clinical signs of pulmonary hypertension and cor pulmonale appear. Attention to potential extrapulmonary physical findings supports or suggests a specific diagnosis (Table 56.3).

## Radiographic Features

The chest radiograph remains invaluable for verifying and classifying interstitial lung disease. Although standard chest radiography is not as sensitive for detection as the HRCT scan, it is the logical starting point and the most practical way of identifying and defining disease.

**Plain Roentgenography.** Ziskind and coworkers[83] classified the diffuse lung diseases according to the pattern on chest radiographs. They divided infiltrates into alveolar-filling and primarily interstitial patterns. Alveolar filling is recognized by a homogeneous infiltrate that can be diffuse or patchy and is characterized by confluent nodules with ill-defined outer borders, air bronchograms, and obliteration or silhouetting of normal structures such as the diaphragm, heart, and intrapulmonary blood vessels (Fig. 56.13).[84] Another feature is the acinar rosette or air

**Table 56.3 EXTRAPULMONARY PHYSICAL FINDINGS IN THE INTERSTITIAL LUNG DISEASES**

| FINDING | EXAMPLES |
|---|---|
| Systemic hypertension | Connective tissue disease; neurofibromatosis; some diffuse alveolar hemorrhage syndromes |
| Erythema nodosum | Sarcoidosis; connective tissue disease; Behçet's syndrome |
| Maculopapular rash | Drug-induced; amyloidosis; lipoidosis; connective tissue diseases; Gaucher's disease |
| Heliotrope rash | Dermatomyositis |
| Albinism | Hermansky-Pudlak syndrome |
| Discoid lupus | Idiopathic pulmonary fibrosis; systemic lupus erythematosus |
| Neurofibroma | von Recklinghausen's disease |
| Telangiectasia | Scleroderma |
| Raynaud's phenomenon | Idiopathic pulmonary fibrosis; connective tissue disease |
| Cutaneous vasculitis | Systemic vasculitides; connective tissue disease |
| Subcutaneous nodules | von Recklinghausen's disease; rheumatoid arthritis |
| Calcinosis | Dermatomyositis; scleroderma |
| Uveitis | Sarcoidosis; Behçet's syndrome; ankylosing spondylitis |
| Scleritis | Systemic vasculitis; systemic lupus erythematosus; scleroderma; sarcoidosis |
| Keratoconjunctivitis sicca | Lymphocytic interstitial pneumonia |
| Salivary gland enlargement | Sarcoidosis, lymphocytic interstitial pneumonia |
| Peripheral lymphadenopathy | Sarcoidosis; lymphangitic carcinomatosis; lymphocytic interstitial pneumonia; lymphoma |
| Hepatosplenomegaly | Sarcoidosis; eosinophilic granuloma; connective tissue disease; amyloidosis; lymphocytic interstitial pneumonia |
| Pericarditis | Radiation pneumonitis; connective tissue disease |
| Myositis | Connective tissue disease; drugs (L-tryptophan) |
| Bone involvement | Eosinophilic granuloma; sarcoidosis; Gaucher's disease; lymphangitic carcinomatosis |
| Arthritis | Connective tissue disease; systemic vasculitis; sarcoidosis |
| Diabetes insipidus | Eosinophilic granuloma; sarcoidosis |
| Glomerulonephritis | Systemic vasculitis; connective tissue disease; Goodpasture's syndrome; sarcoidosis |
| Nephrotic syndrome | Amyloidosis; drug-induced (gold, penicillamine); systemic lupus erythematosus |
| Renal mass | Lymphangioleiomyomatosis; tuberous sclerosis |

alveologram, which indicates consolidation of the alveolus and small airways distal to an unobstructed terminal bronchiole (Fig. 56.14). Interstitial lung diseases that are more likely to produce this pattern are listed in Table 56.4. Several (e.g., sarcoidosis, pulmonary lymphoma) have associated hilar adenopathy. In patients with alveolar proteinosis, sparing of the lung parenchyma immediately adjacent to the diaphragm is seen. In chronic eosinophilic pneumonia, the pattern has been referred to as the radiographic negative of pulmonary edema, because the alveolar infiltrates are most prominent in the periphery.[85] A similar alveolar pattern has also been reported to occur in some patients with BOOP (Fig. 56.15).[86]

Radiographic interstitial infiltrates become apparent when the interstitial compartment becomes infiltrated and widened by inflammatory cells, excessive collagen, granulomatous inflammation, or smooth muscle proliferation. In other instances, malignant cells or amyloid deposits expand this compartment. These infiltrates appear as nodules, linear reticular infiltrates, or a combination of linear shadows and nodules (reticulonodular). Miliary nodules accompany infectious granulomas and occasionally noninfectious granulomas (sarcoidosis, eosinophilic granuloma, silicosis, and hypersensitivity pneumonitis) and some malignant diseases (melanoma, hypernephroma, and lymphoma) (Fig. 56.16). Nodules of varying size characterize the granulomatous lung diseases. However, linear infiltrates possibly representing an underlying cellular interstitial infiltrate are also visible.

Linear interstitial changes are seen in most interstitial lung diseases and usually in conjunction with nodular change, the so-called reticulonodular infiltrate (Fig. 56.17). There are, however, several distinctive patterns of linear or reticular interstitial changes (Table 56.5).[84] Short horizontal lines at the lung periphery (Kerley's B lines) representing thickened interlobular septa, are seen after obstruction of the pulmonary lymphatics[87, 88] (Fig. 56.18). The term *radiographic honeycomb lung* refers to a reticular pattern that correlates with the histologic honeycombing.[89] These small cystic structures, which are best seen in the lower and peripheral lung zones, indicate an underlying advanced fibrotic change (Fig. 56.19).

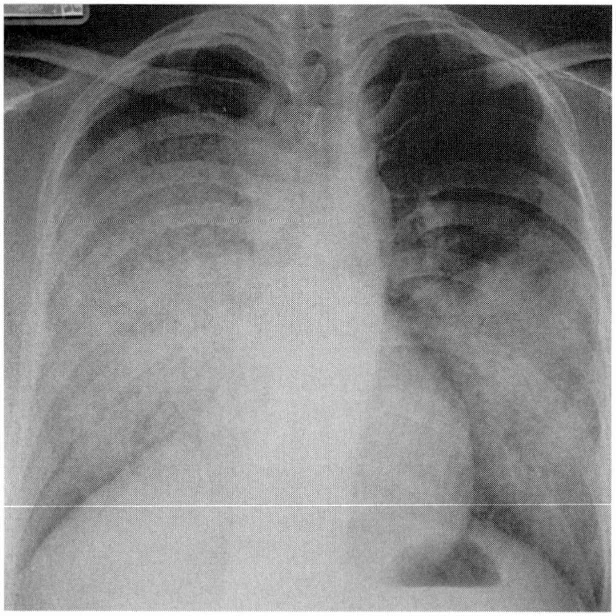

**Figure 56.13** Chest radiograph shows a characteristic pattern of alveolar-filling disease in a patient with diffuse alveolar hemorrhage. Note the homogeneous consolidation with obliteration of the right heart border and the pulmonary vasculature in addition to air bronchograms.

**Table 56.4** INTERSTITIAL LUNG DISEASES PRODUCING AN ALVEOLAR-FILLING PATTERN ON CHEST RADIOGRAPH

| |
|---|
| Alveolar proteinosis (proteinaceous fluid) |
| Alveolar cell carcinoma (malignant cells) |
| Bronchioloalveolar metastases (malignant cells from pancreas, breast) |
| Pulmonary lymphoma (malignant lymphocytes) |
| Lymphocytic interstitial pneumonia (lymphoplasmacytic cells) |
| Alveolar sarcoid (lymphocyte-macrophage alveolitis or confluent granuloma) |
| Desquamative interstitial pneumonia (macrophages) |
| Diffuse alveolar hemorrhage (red blood cells; hemosiderin-filled macrophages) |
| Eosinophilic pneumonia (eosinophils, macrophages; lymphocytes) |
| Alveolar microlithiasis (calcium-phosphate microliths) |
| Bronchiolitis obliterans organizing pneumonia (collagen) |
| Mineral oil aspiration (lipid-filled macrophages) |
| Acute hypersensitivity pneumonia (lymphoplasmacytic cells) |

It is typical for many interstitial lung diseases (e.g., idiopathic pulmonary fibrosis, the connective tissue diseases, asbestosis, cytotoxic drug-induced disorders) to have the greatest concentration of the reticulonodular infiltrates and honeycomb changes in the lower lung zones. In fact, lower lobe volume loss and traction bronchiectasis are typical for the advanced stages of these diseases. There are a group of interstitial diseases (see Table 56.5), often granulomatous, in which the radiographic changes are more prominent in the upper lung zones (Fig. 56.20).

Other radiographic features may point to a diagnosis. For example, diaphragmatic pleural calcification is indicative of asbestos exposure.[90] Pleuritis and pleural effusion may complicate the course of the connective tissue–

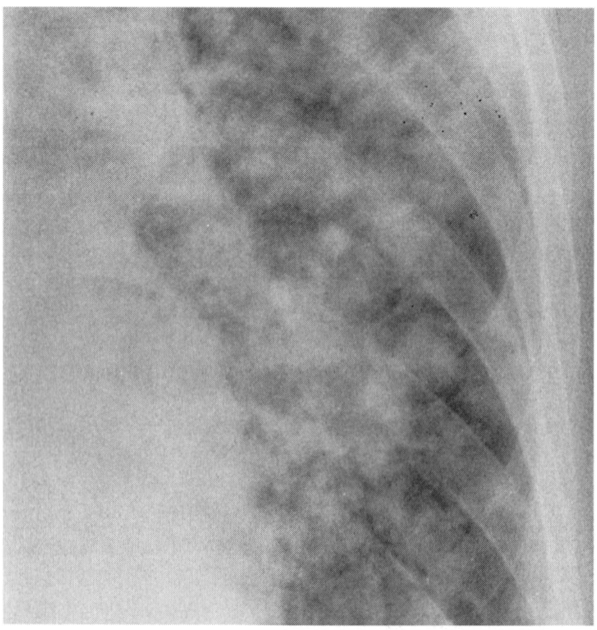

**Figure 56.14** Detailed view of chest radiograph shows alveolar nodules in a patient with alveolar cell carcinoma. Note the ill-defined nodules and distal air alveolograms.

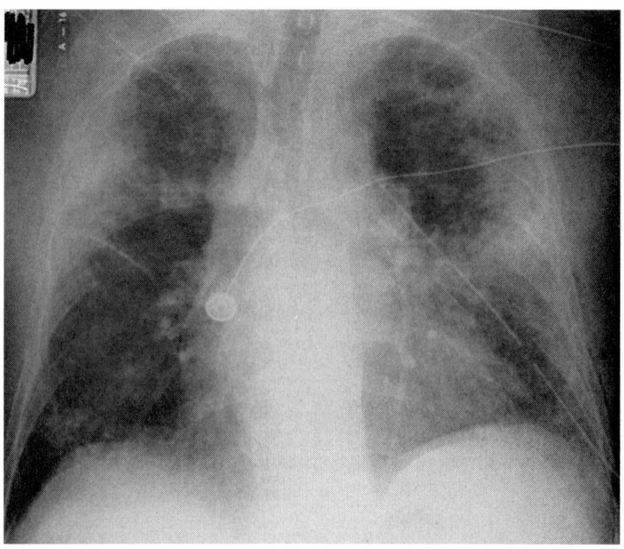

**Figure 56.15** Chest radiograph of a patient with bronchiolitis obliterans organizing pneumonia shows bilateral peripheral alveolar infiltrates. A similar appearance is seen in chronic eosinophilic pneumonia.

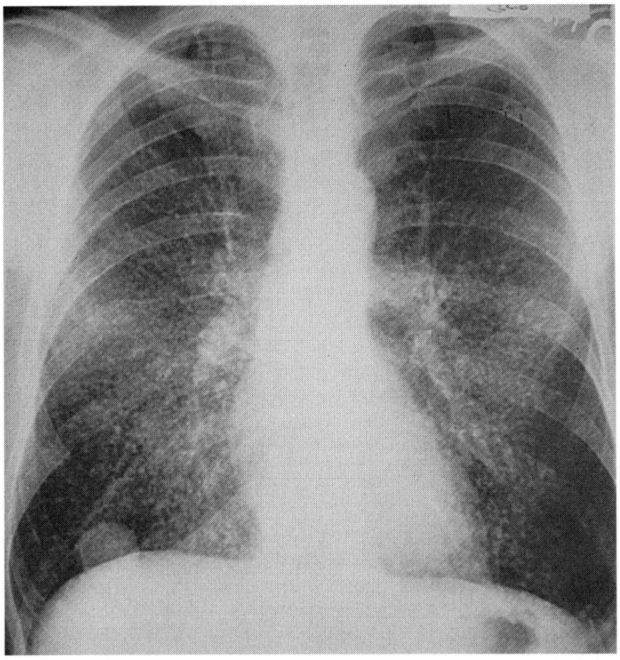

**Figure 56.16** Chest radiograph shows miliary interstitial nodulation in a patient with metastatic malignant melanoma. A large mass is also present in the right lower lobe.

associated interstitial lung diseases. The exception is polymyositis-dermatomyositis.[64] Pneumothorax is often the presenting manifestation of eosinophilic granuloma or lymphangioleiomyomatosis.[88, 91] The majority of interstitial lung diseases result in a gradual reduction of the lung volumes. There are interstitial diseases that are bronchiolocentric, resulting in either maintenance or expansion of the lung volume (see Table 56.5). If an interstitial lung disease is superimposed on emphysema, the lung volumes

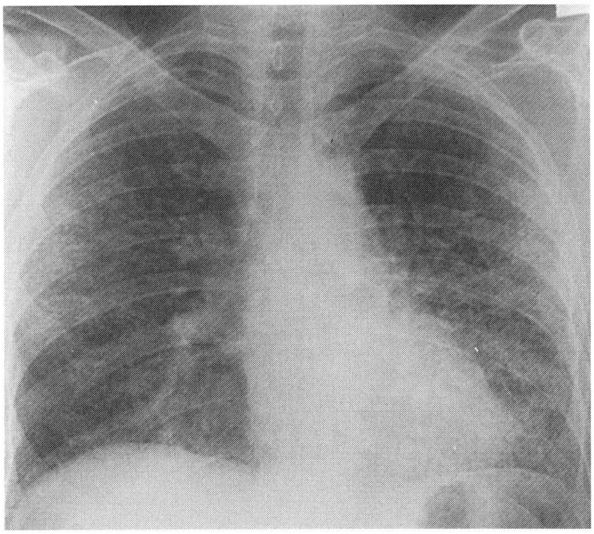

**Figure 56.17** Chest radiograph shows diffuse reticulonodular infiltrates in a patient with idiopathic pulmonary fibrosis.

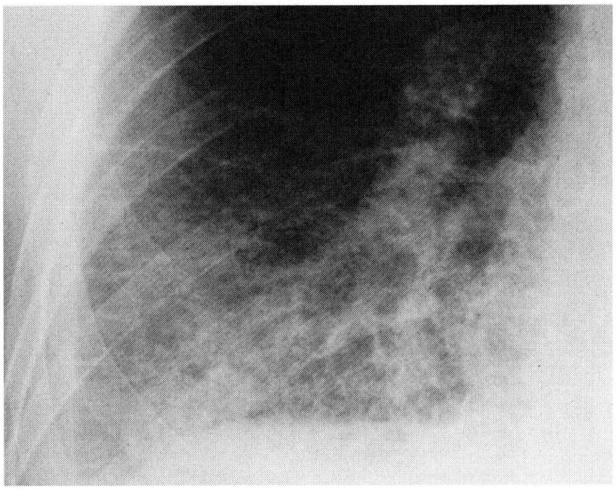

**Figure 56.18** Detailed view of right lung shows Kerley's B lines and pleural effusion in a patient with lymphangitic carcinomatosis.

often are preserved. Prolonged hypoxemia results in radiographic evidence of pulmonary hypertension.

A criticism of the alveolar-interstitial classification is that a mixed pattern is often found. For example, interstitial fibrosis may eventually be superimposed on a disease that was primarily alveolar, such as alveolar proteinosis, diffuse alveolar hemorrhage, eosinophilic pneumonia, or BOOP.[92, 93] Sarcoidosis, a disease characterized by interstitial granuloma, can be alveolar in appearance due to either coalescence of granulomas with compression of adjacent lung or a lymphocytic macrophagic alveolitis.[94] Dense fibrosis from any fibrotic lung disease can compress adjacent lung, producing homogeneous shadows. The appearance of alveolar infiltrates during the course of an interstitial lung disease may represent renewed cellular activity of the primary disease, superimposed infection, or development of alveolar cell carcinoma or adenocarcinoma.[95]

**Computed Tomography.** Conventional chest radiographic assessment for interstitial lung disease may miss up to 10% of cases.[40] Conventional computed tomography (8- to 10-mm slices) offers little more for the detection of radiographic-negative interstitial lung disease.[96, 97] HRCT (2- to 3-mm slices) enables better visualization of fine parenchymal detail and therefore the detection of early air-space filling or interstitial change (Fig. 56.21). In cases of suspected interstitial lung disease with negative conventional radiography, it is important to perform HRCT with prone and supine views. Dependent lung density can mask interstitial change, and vascular engorgement of the dependent portion of lung mimics septal thickening on the supine view.[98–100] Abnormalities that persist on the prone view are indicative of disease.

In patients with abnormal chest radiographs, the diagnostic accuracy increases with HRCT evaluation.[96, 97] In cases of idiopathic pulmonary fibrosis, peripheral reticular opacities, lower-zone subpleural honeycombing, and traction bronchiectasis are seen (Fig. 56.22*A*).[97, 101, 102] The presence of air-space opacification in patients with idio-

**Table 56.5 RADIOGRAPHIC FEATURES OF THE INTERSTITIAL LUNG DISEASES**

| Feature | Diseases |
|---|---|
| Kerley's B lines | Lymphangitic carcinomatosis; lymphangioleiomyomatosis; left atrial hypertension (mitral valve disease, veno-occlusive disease); lymphoma; amyloidosis |
| Radiographic honeycomb lung | Idiopathic pulmonary fibrosis; connective tissue disease; asbestosis; drug induced; lymphocytic interstitial pneumonia: chronic aspiration pneumonia; hemosiderosis; Hermansky-Pudlak syndrome; alveolar proteinosis |
| Upper zone predominant disease | Radiation pneumonitis; neurofibromatosis; chronic sarcoidosis; eosinophilic granuloma; silicosis; chronic hypersensitivity pneumonitis; chronic eosinophilic pneumonia; ankylosing spondylitis; nodular rheumatoid arthritis; berylliosis; drug-induced (amiodarone, gold, BNCU (carmustine)); radiation |
| Lymphadenopathy | Sarcoidosis; lymphoma; lymphangitic carcinomatosis; lymphoid intestitial pneumonia; berylliosis; amyloidosis; Gaucher's disease |
| Pleural disease | Lymphangitic carcinomatosis; connective tissue disease; asbestosis (pleural calcification); lymphangioleiomyomatosis (chylous effusion); drug-induced (furantoin, radiation); sarcoidosis |
| Eggshell calcification of lymph nodes | Silicosis; sarcoidosis; radiation |
| Increased lung volumes | Lymphangioleiomyomatosis; chronic sarcoidosis; chronic eosinophilic granuloma; chronic hypersensitivity pneumonitis; tuberous sclerosis; neurofibromatosis |
| Pneumothorax | Eosinophilic granuloma; lymphangioleiomyomatosis; tuberous sclerosis; neurofibromatosis |

pathic pulmonary fibrosis correlates with active inflammation and is more likely to respond to treatment (Fig. 56.22*B*).[103] In the connective tissue diseases, asbestosis, and some drug-induced interstitial lung disease, the results on HRCT, as on chest radiography, are indistinguishable from those of idiopathic pulmonary fibrosis.[97] In scleroderma, a disease in which the prevalence rate of interstitial lung disease approaches 100% in autopsy series, HRCT detects disease in 45% to 75% of patients when conventional radiography is negative.[42, 104]

In sarcoidosis, in addition to the hilar and mediastinal adenopathy, nodules deposited along bronchovascular bundles and interlobular septa, air-space filling due to the lymphocytic-macrophagic alveolitis, and linear densities secondary to fibrotic scarring can be seen[105–107] (Fig. 56.23). In patients with hypersensitivity pneumonitis, air-

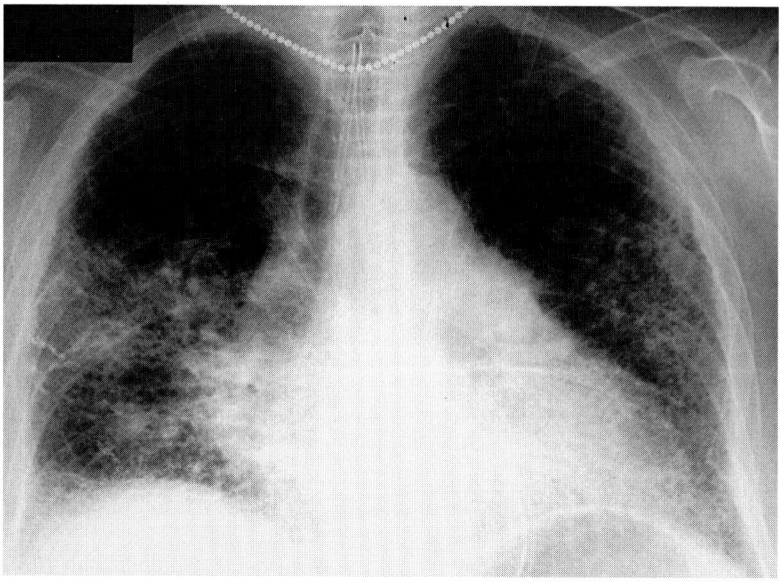

**Figure 56.19** Chest radiograph shows characteristic features of honeycomb lung. A network of 2- to 3-mm cystic spaces is distributed throughout the lung fields. This patient with idiopathic pulmonary fibrosis also had pulmonary hypertension and was receiving oxygen through a transtracheal catheter.

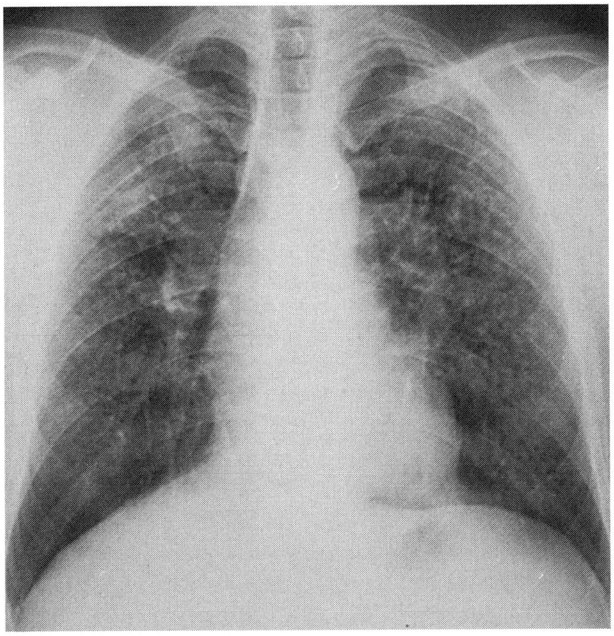

**Figure 56.20** Chest radiograph shows uncomplicated silicosis. Note the nodular interstitial disease with predilection for the middle and upper lung zones.

space–filling centrilobular nodules, and linear opacities without adenopathy are present.[108, 109] The HRCT can be normal in symptomatic patients with biopsy-proved hypersensitivity pneumonitis. In patients with eosinophilic granuloma, the combination of centrilobular nodules and cysts, most prominent in the upper lobes and occasionally accompanied by a pneumothorax, is characteristic[110, 111] (Fig. 56.24). In earlier eosinophilic granuloma, coalescence of the nodules produces an air-space–filling pattern.

In lymphangioleiomyomatosis, the HRCT is typical, revealing rounded, thin-walled cysts throughout[112, 113] (Fig. 56.25). A pneumothorax or pleural effusion (chylous) may accompany this change. Except for the pleural effusion, identical findings are present in tuberous sclerosis.[112] Lymphangitic carcinomatosis produces a beaded-chain appearance of the interlobular septa that correlates with Kerley's B lines detectable by conventional radiography.[114] In asbestos-related disease, noncalcified pleural plaques and early interstitial lung disease are often difficult to detect, and the HRCT is more sensitive then conventional chest radiography.[115, 116]

## Functional Assessment

In interstitial lung disease, there are characteristic alterations of the lungs' mechanical properties[117–119] and impairment of gas exchange at the alveolocapillary interface.[120] Assessment of ventilatory function and the mechanical properties of the lungs, as well as gas exchange, particularly during exercise, are vital components of the initial evaluation of patients with suspected interstitial lung disease. In addition, serial measurements of function enable the physician to determine progression of the disease and the effects of therapeutic intervention.

**Ventilatory Function.** Ventilatory function tests provide an indirect index of alterations to the impedance to respiration offered by the elastic resistance to distention of the lungs and the frictional resistance to air flow in the tracheobronchial tree.[121–123] Clinically, alterations of the mechanical properties of the respiratory system are also reflected in the pattern of breathing that is adopted by the patient. These patients tend to breathe rapidly and

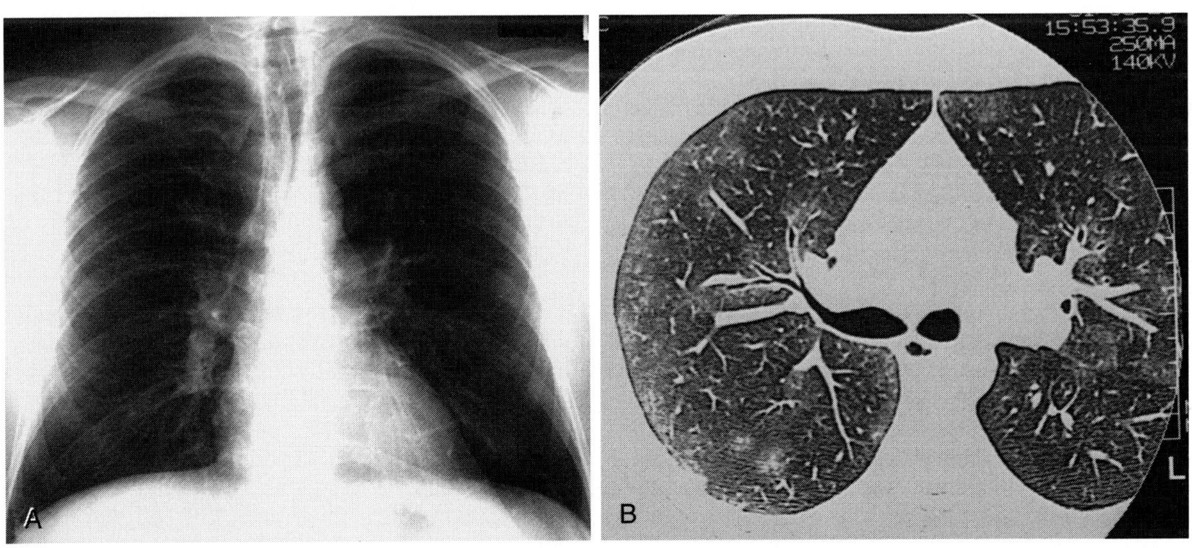


**Figure 56.21** *A,* A normal chest radiograph from a 45-year-old man with established hypersensitivity pneumonitis is shown. At the time, his arterial $P_{O_2}$ while breathing room air was 48 mm Hg. *B,* A high-resolution computed tomographic image of the same patient demonstrates patchy areas of air-space filling.

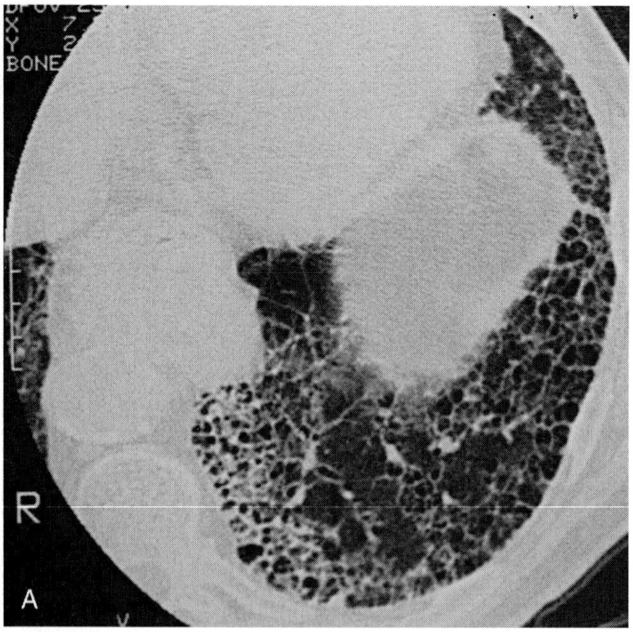


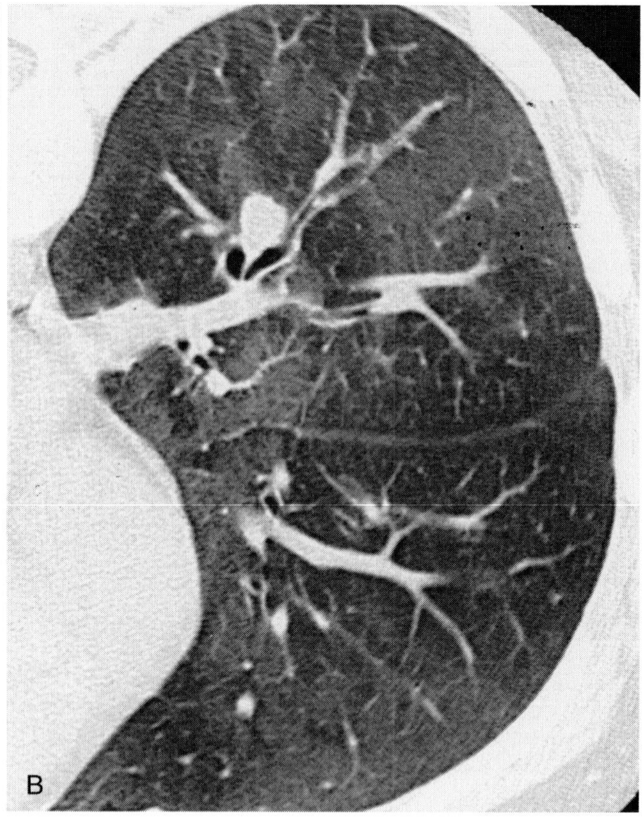


**Figure 56.22** *A,* High-resolution computed tomographic image of advanced idiopathic pulmonary fibrosis shows extensive honeycomb changes. *B,* Cellular and desquamative interstitial pneumonia cause patchy (gray-appearing) air-space disease (ground-glass density).

shallowly, because a larger tidal volume would require an inordinate increase in work of breathing to overcome the greatly increased elastic resistance.[124]

**Elastic Resistance.** Interstitial lung disease is associated with an increase in elastic resistance, and this can be seen in a plot of the static transpulmonary pressure (i.e., at points of no flow) at differing decrements of lung volume from total lung capacity (TLC) to residual volume. In most patients with interstitial lung disease, the plot of the volume-pressure relationship of the lungs is characteristically shifted downward and to the right, with a reduced slope (i.e., compliance is low) and a markedly increased coefficient of elastic recoil (maximum elastic recoil pressure, TLC).[118, 119, 125] On the other hand, as is demonstrated in Figure 56.26, there is significant variation in the position of the volume-pressure curve in patients with idiopathic pulmonary fibrosis and sarcoidosis,[125] and the correlation between alterations of the elastic properties (and lung volume compartments) and the degree of fibrosis present is poor. This is, at least in part, a consequence of the impact of smoking, which appears to differ in the two disorders. In patients with idiopathic pulmonary fibrosis who smoke, the volume-pressure curve is shifted upward and to the left, whereas in smokers with sarcoidosis it is shifted downward and to the right.[125]

Measurements of lung volume reflect changes in position of the volume-pressure curve of the lungs. This is because alterations of the elastic recoil of the lung or chest wall disturb the balance between the elastic forces of the lungs, which act in an expiratory direction, and those of the chest wall, which act in an inspiratory direction. In patients with interstitial lung disease the TLC, functional residual capacity, and residual volume are generally lower than expected (Fig. 56.27). A lower than expected TLC (and vital capacity [VC]) in association with a normal functional residual capacity and a greater than expected residual volume (see Fig. 56.27) generally reflects a mixed restrictive and obstructive disorder. However, because maximum effort is necessary to determine the inspiratory capacity and the expiratory reserve volume, a less than maximal inspiration or expiration, because of either weak respiratory muscles or poor effort, leads to the same findings. Similar qualifications apply to the VC, which is often used as an index of alterations of elastic resistance. In addition, as can be seen in Figure 56.27, a low VC is not specific for restrictive disorders, because it is also lower than expected in patients with air flow limitation (because of an increased residual volume).

**Flow Resistance.** Measurement of lung volume is also important when evaluating air flow resistance. This can be assessed directly from the relationship between the rate of air flow and the resistive component of the transpulmonary pressure.

In clinical practice, various indirect measures of flow resistance can be used: the $FEV_1$; the mean expiratory flow rate between 25% and 75% of the forced vital capacity (FVC), that is, $FEF_{25\text{-}75}$; the maximal expiratory flow rate ($\dot{V}$ max) at a particular proportion (such as 75%, 50%, or 25%) of the FVC (from a flow-volume curve); the $FEV_1$/FVC ratio; or the $FEV_1$/VC ratio. Low flow rates or a low ratio (i.e., less than 70% of predicted)

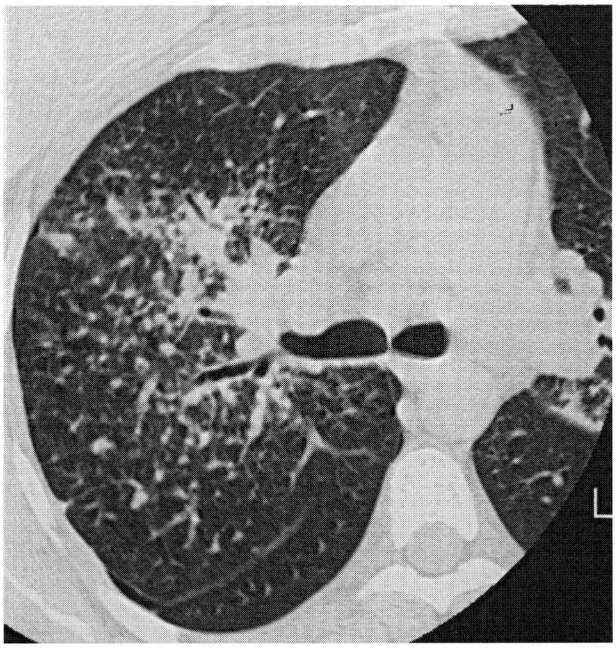


**Figure 56.23** High-resolution computed tomographic image from a patient with sarcoidosis shows hilar lymphadenopathy and nodular disease as well as dense air-space filling.

are believed to indicate expiratory air flow limitation. However, like airway resistance, maximal expiratory flow rates depend on the state of expansion of the airways (i.e., lung volume). The $FEV_1/FVC$ ratio will be overestimated, and the degree of flow limitation underestimated, in the patient who does not exhale fully because of severe dyspnea or muscular weakness, pain, or poor effort.

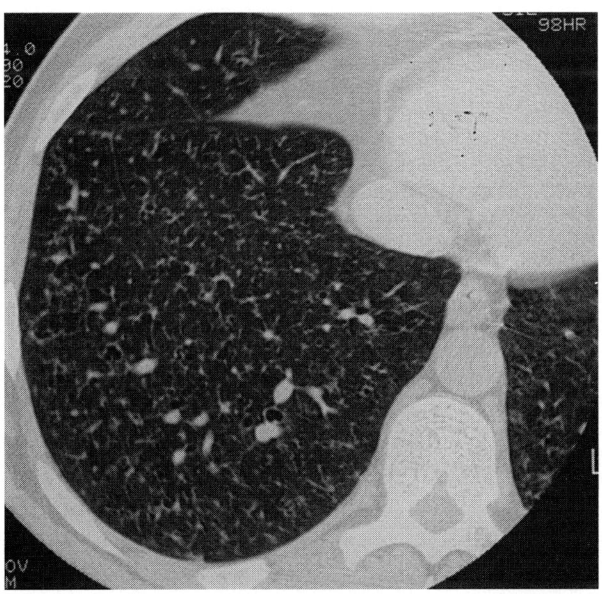


**Figure 56.24** High-resolution computed tomographic image from a patient with eosinophilic granuloma shows diffuse centrilobular nodulation and cyst formation.

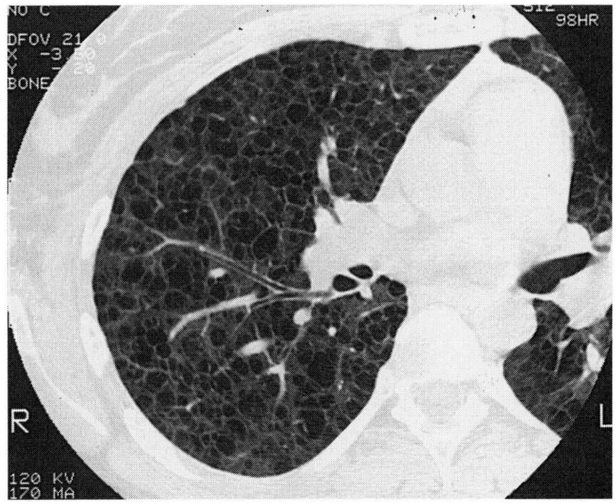


**Figure 56.25** High-resolution computed tomographic image from a patient with lymphangioleiomyomatosis shows characteristic thin-walled cysts throughout the parenchyma.

Air flow resistance is not generally thought to be increased in interstitial lung disease. As is seen in Figure 56.28, $\dot{V}$ max is low in interstitial lung disease, not because of an increase in flow resistance but rather because the flow rates are being achieved at low lung volumes. In fact, in uncomplicated interstitial lung disease, $\dot{V}$ max values are greater than expected at any particular lung volume (isovolume), because the lung elastic recoil pressure, which is the driving pressure for flow in the peripheral airways, is increased.[121] As a corollary, a $\dot{V}$ max lower than expected at a particular lung volume in a patient who is suffering from a restrictive disorder indicates an increase of flow resistance in the more peripheral (upstream) airways. An increase in upstream resistance has been reported in patients with idiopathic pulmonary fibrosis,[126, 127] extrinsic allergic alveolitis, or asbestos exposure.[128]

**Gas Exchange.** Alterations of gas exchange are readily assessed by analysis of the arterial $P_{O_2}$ and $P_{CO_2}$ and calculation of the alveolar-arterial partial pressure gradient for oxygen [$(A-a)P_{O_2}$], both at rest and during exercise.[129]

In patients with interstitial lung disease, arterial blood analysis while at rest usually reveals hypoxemia and an increased $(A-a)P_{O_2}$, along with hypocapnia. In addition, the diffusing capacity for carbon monoxide ($DL_{CO}$) is reduced, primarily because of a reduction in the alveolocapillary surface available for gas exchange. The disturbance of gas exchange generally accompanies abnormalities in ventilatory function,[130] but gas exchange may be normal at rest in a significant number of patients. Similarly, the resting $DL_{CO}$ may be only slightly reduced in patients who demonstrate a mild restrictive disorder or normal gas exchange while at rest, or both.[130]

The $DL_{CO}$ is generally greater than expected in those cases associated with recent pulmonary hemorrhage, because the red blood cells in the pulmonary alveoli take up carbon monoxide readily.[124] Sequential measurements of the $DL_{CO}$ within minutes may aid in the establishment of the diagnosis of alveolar hemorrhage when this disorder is considered in the differential diagnosis.[131] When there is fresh blood in the alveolar spaces, each successive $DL_{CO}$ value will be lower as the hemoglobin in the alveoli becomes saturated with carbon monoxide.

**Exercise.** In most patients, gas exchange is disturbed during exertion, even in those with normal gas exchange at rest. Assessment of gas exchange during exercise provides the best correlation with the severity of disease[132]

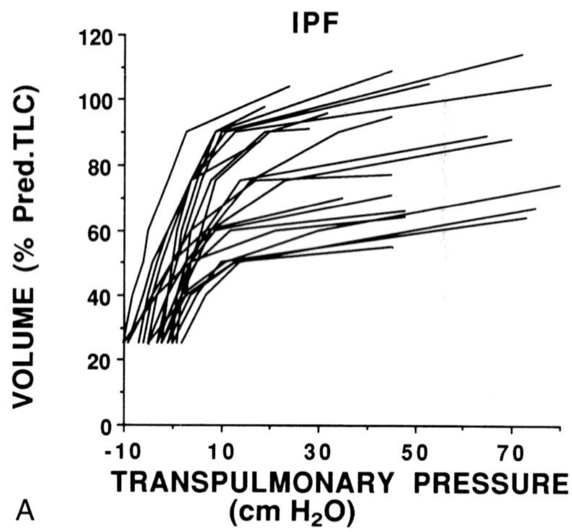


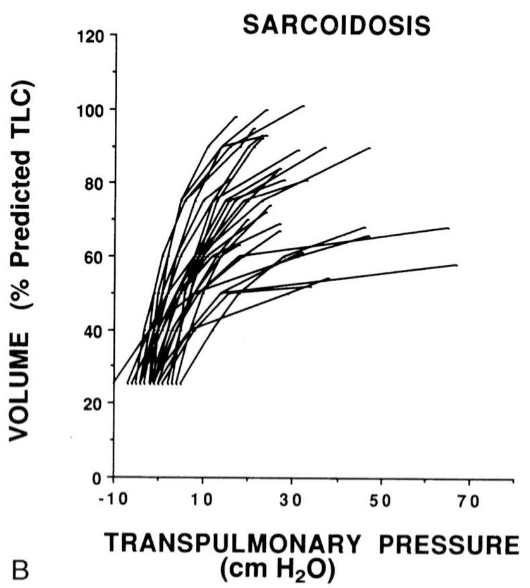


**Figure 56.26** Multiple recordings show volume-pressure characteristics in patients with idiopathic pulmonary fibrosis (IPF) *(A)* and sarcoidosis *(B)*. Note the marked variation of position and shape in both disorders. (Reproduced with permission from Hanley ME, King TE Jr, Schwarz MI, et al: The impact of smoking on mechanical properties of the lungs in idiopathic pulmonary fibrosis and sarcoidosis. Am Rev Respir Dis 144:1102, 1991.)

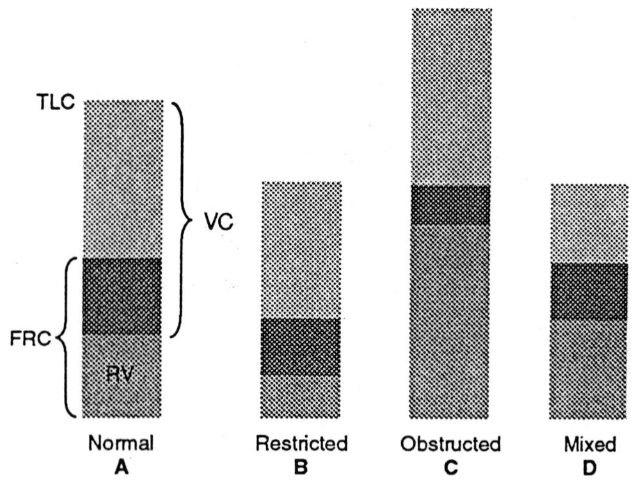


**Figure 56.27** Bar graphs show total lung capacity (TLC) and its subdivisions in healthy persons *(A)* compared with the typical abnormalities found in patients with restrictive disorders *(B)*, obstructive disorders *(C)*, and mixed disorders *(D)*. FRC = functional residual capacity; VC = vital capacity. (Reproduced with permission from Cherniack RM: Pulmonary Function Testing. Philadelphia: WB Saunders, 1992.)

and is probably the most important physiologic determination in patients with interstitial lung disease.

In general, patients with the most severe restrictive disease have the poorest exercise tolerance. As is shown in Figure 56.29, ventilation generally rises excessively during exercise and may approach the ventilatory ceiling. Characteristically, the respiratory frequency rises inordinately with increasing exercise loads because of the increased work that would be required to overcome the elastic resistance of the lungs if the tidal volume were to increase.

The excessive ventilation is frequently preferentially distributed to areas of lung that have normal compliance but diminished perfusion (i.e., high ventilation-perfusion [$\dot{V}/\dot{Q}$] ratio); as a result, unlike the normal response, the calculated dead space ($V_D$) and the ratio of dead space to tidal volume ($V_D/V_T$) rise in association with rapid, shallow breathing. The increase in cardiac output with exercise and the rapid transit of blood through the pulmonary capillaries along with its redistribution in the lungs leads to a greater maldistribution of $\dot{V}/\dot{Q}$ ratios. This results in a rise in $(A-a)P_{O_2}$ and a fall in arterial $P_{O_2}$ (Fig. 56.30). Except for heavy exercise, when the transit through the circulation is exceptionally rapid, it is unlikely that a reduced ability of oxygen to diffuse across a thickened alveolar-capillary membrane plays a significant role in the hypoxemia.

## Laboratory Findings

Table 56.6 summarizes the results of laboratory tests that suggest or support the diagnosis of a specific interstitial lung disease.

## Bronchoalveolar Lavage

Bronchoalveolar lavage (BAL) is a technique employed to sample the distal airways via the instillation of sterile saline through a wedged fiberoptic bronchoscope. After aspiration the contents, which are thought to represent the cellular, immunologic, and biochemical milieu of the alveolar structures, can be analyzed. The use of BAL for the evaluation of interstitial lung disease has been difficult to interpret because of the lack of standardized techniques for both the performance of the procedure and the subsequent analysis of the data. Furthermore, in some of the earlier studies correlative data between lung biopsies and BAL were not obtained. Often the treatment or smoking status of the patient was not considered.[133] A multicenter publication sets forth the methods of performing and analyzing the results of BAL.[134] This study involved a large cohort of normal subjects of varying age and race

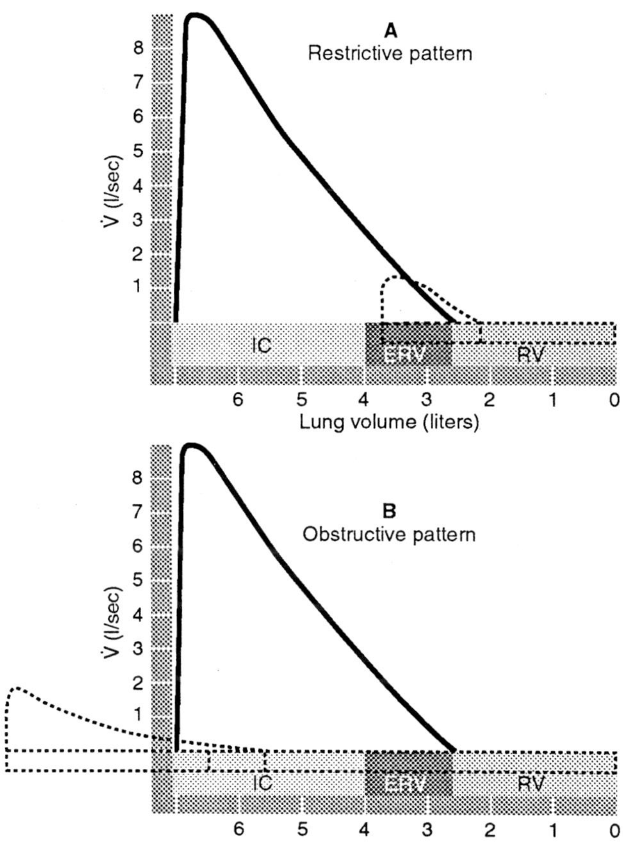


**Figure 56.28** Schematic volume-flow (V̇) curves in a healthy person *(solid line)* are compared with those in patients *(dotted lines)* with a restrictive disorder *(top)* and with an obstructive disorder *(bottom)*. Lung volume is reduced in the restrictive disorder, and maximum expiratory flow rates are low because they are achieved at low lung volumes. Flow rates are higher than expected at low lung volumes because the driving pressure (lung elastic recoil) is increased. (Reproduced with permission from Cherniack RM: Pulmonary Function Testing. Philadelphia: WB Saunders, 1992.)

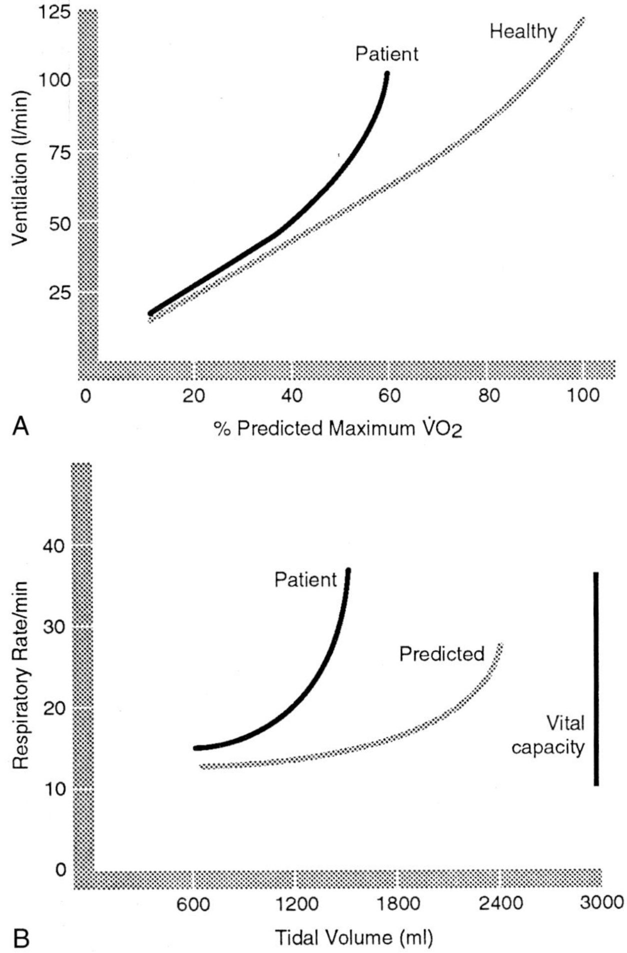


**Figure 56.29** Schematic curves show the ventilatory response *(A)* and respiratory pattern *(B)* during increasing exercise work loads expressed as a percentage of the predicted maximum oxygen uptake ($\dot{V}O_2$) in a healthy person and in a patient with idiopathic pulmonary fibrosis. (Reproduced with permission from Cherniack RM: Pulmonary Function Testing. Philadelphia: WB Saunders, 1992.)

who were compared with patients with documented interstitial lung disease. Smoking affects the BAL results of both normal subjects and patients by amplifying the macrophage and eosinophil populations.[134]

BAL is a useful investigative tool in some interstitial lung diseases.[135, 136] Cytologic analysis of BAL specimens can be diagnostic for lymphangitic carcinomatosis, alveolar cell carcinoma, and pulmonary lymphoma.[137–139] If the eosinophil percentage exceeds 40% (normal, less than 2%), eosinophilic pneumonia is almost always the cause of the diffuse pulmonary infiltration.[33, 60] BAL eosinophilia of a lesser degree may occur with some connective tissue diseases, idiopathic pulmonary fibrosis, or BOOP.[135, 136, 140, 141]

The finding of periodic acid–Schiff–positive lipoproteinaceous bodies in the lavage liquid was originally thought to be diagnostic for pulmonary alveolar proteinosis but has proved to be nonspecific.[142, 143] In cases of the diffuse alveolar hemorrhage syndrome, red blood

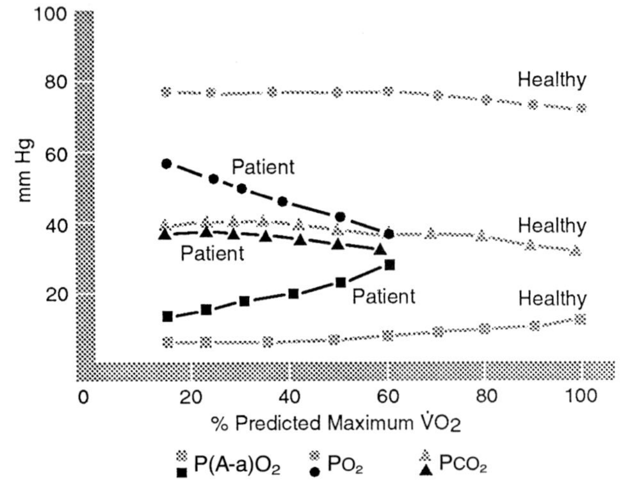


**Figure 56.30** The changes in arterial $Po_2$, alveolar-arterial $Po_2$ difference ($P(A-a)O_2$), and arterial $Pco_2$ during increasing exercise work loads expressed as the percentage of predicted maximum oxygen uptake ($\dot{V}o_2$) in a healthy person and a patient with idiopathic pulmonary fibrosis. (Reproduced with permission from Cherniack RM: Pulmonary Function Testing. Philadelphia: WB Saunders, 1992.)

cells and hemosiderin-laden macrophages dominate the lavage specimen.[35]

There is a group of diseases in which lavage lymphocytosis (more than 35% lymphocytes) predominates. Sarcoidosis and hypersensitivity pneumonitis are most common.[135, 136] Others include lymphocytic interstitial pneumonia, pulmonary lymphoma, berylliosis, and some drug-induced interstitial lung diseases.[144, 145] Smaller but increased percentages of lymphocytes (normal range, 15%) can be seen with these entities in addition to a number of other interstitial lung diseases, including idiopathic pulmonary fibrosis, BOOP, connective tissue diseases, and some pneumoconioses.[145–147] In patients with suspected asbestos-related disease, one or more asbestos bodies per high-powered field of BAL indicates significant exposure, but this does not confirm the diagnosis of asbestosis.[148] Because of the vertical gradient of asbestos bodies recovered in asbestosis, if lavage is used to document previous asbestos exposure, samples should be obtained from a basal segment of one of the lower lobes.[149] A diagnosis of berylliosis is confirmed when lavaged lymphocytes undergo proliferation after exposure to the mineral in vitro.[150]

In the BAL recovered from patients with eosinophilic granuloma, all inflammatory cells are increased even though their percentages remain unchanged. Electron microscopy demonstrates increased numbers of Langerhans' cells. This monocyte, which is thought to be central in the pathogenesis, has a typical pentilaminar body (Birbeck's granule) in the cytoplasm, as revealed by electron microscopy.[50] Langerhans' cells have been described in other fibrotic lung diseases, but not in numbers equivalent to those of eosinophilic granuloma.[151]

Other applications of BAL include disease staging (i.e., cellular infiltrates versus fibrosis on lung biopsies) and the prediction of therapeutic responsiveness. For example, in both the connective tissue diseases and idiopathic pulmonary fibrosis, BAL lymphocytosis is associated with a cellular histology (as opposed to fibrosis) and an improved response to treatment. Furthermore, the overall survival rate in these patients is increased.[152–154] On the other hand, the combination of lavage neutrophilia and eosinophilia without lymphocytosis often portends progressive unresponsive disease.[155, 156] In sarcoidosis, a disease that is characterized by increases in the number of T-helper (CD4+) lymphocytes in the lung, it has been suggested that clinical deterioration may be expected if the BAL lymphocyte exceeds 28%.[157] More recent data indicate that the level of BAL lymphocytes has no value in predicting the clinical outcome in sarcoidosis.[158–160]

The assessment of potential interstitial lung disease in populations at risk is another role for BAL. For example, in patients with scleroderma and rheumatoid arthritis in whom clinical, radiologic, and physiologic evidence of interstitial lung disease is lacking, BAL studies have revealed increases in inflammatory cell populations.[45, 141]

## TISSUE DIAGNOSIS

The final step in the evaluation of a patient with interstitial lung disease is to decide whether tissue is needed for diagnosis. As previously noted, the diagnosis of connective tissue, occupational, or drug-related interstitial lung disease is often obvious after a careful history has been taken. In cases of idiopathic and primary interstitial lung disease (see Table 56.1), the diagnosis may not be as obvious, although clinical, laboratory, and radiologic findings are often suggestive. Furthermore, the diagnosis of idiopathic pulmonary fibrosis, a commonly encountered disorder, in most situations can be established only by lung biopsy. As a matter of practicality, transbronchial biopsy can be performed during the bronchoscopy for BAL. Transbronchial biopsy is relatively safe and is often diagnostic of sarcoidosis, diffuse malignancy, alveolar proteinosis, or eosinophilic pneumonia.[7] Other entities are less frequently confirmed by this procedure. A transbronchial biopsy interpretation, which describes only inflammation, fibrosis, or both, is not evidence for idiopathic pulmonary fibrosis or any other entity listed in Table 56.1. Furthermore, even in clinically confirmed cases of connective tissue or drug-induced interstitial lung disease, several different histologic patterns may evolve (see Table 56.2), and lung biopsy is often undertaken to predict prognosis and therapeutic responsiveness, particularly if BAL and HRCT are inconclusive. If the transbronchial biopsy, clinical, and lavage data are inconclusive and the patient is not at high risk, a video thoracoscopic or open lung biopsy should be performed. Moreover, there is a poor correlation between the results of transbronchial and open lung biopsies unless the transbronchial biopsy yields a specific diagnosis.[161, 162] Therefore, when the transbronchial biopsy is inconclusive and a definitive diagnosis is required, open or thoracoscopic lung biopsy is indicated.[163]

## SUMMARY

The causes of interstitial lung diseases are daunting, but they are linked by many common features: clinical pre-

Table 56.6 LABORATORY FINDINGS IN THE INTERSTITIAL LUNG DISEASES

| FINDING | DISEASES |
|---|---|
| Leukopenia | Sarcoidosis; connective tissue disease; lymphoma; drug-induced |
| Leukocytosis | Systemic vasculitis; hypersensitivity pneumonitis; lymphoma |
| Eosinophilia | Eosinophilic pneumonia; sarcoidosis; systemic vasculitis; drug-induced (sulfa, methotrexate) |
| Thrombocytopenia | Sarcoidosis; idiopathic pulmonary fibrosis; connective tissue disease; drug-induced; Gaucher's disease |
| Hemolytic anemia | Idiopathic pulmonary fibrosis; connective tissue disease; sarcoidosis; lymphoma; drug-induced |
| Normocytic anemia | Diffuse alveolar hemorrhage syndromes; connective tissue disease; lymphangitic carcinomatosis |
| Urinary sediment abnormalities | Connective tissue disease; systemic vasculitis; drug-induced |
| Hypogammaglobulinemia | Lymphocytic interstitial pneumonia |
| Hypergammaglobulinemia | Connective tissue disease; sarcoidosis; systemic vasculitis; idiopathic pulmonary fibrosis; asbestosis; silicosis; lymphocytic interstitial pneumonia; lymphoma |
| Serum autoantibodies | Connective tissue disease; systemic vasculitis; sarcoidosis; idiopathic pulmonary fibrosis; silicosis; asbestosis; lymphocytic interstitial pneumonia |
| Serum immune complexes | Idiopathic pulmonary fibrosis; lymphocytic interstitial pneumonia; systemic vasculitis; connective tissue disease; eosinophilic granuloma |
| Serum angiotensin-converting enzyme | Sarcoidosis; hypersensitivity pneumonitis; silicosis; acute respiratory distress syndrome; Gaucher's disease |
| Antibasement membrane antibody | Goodpasture's syndrome |
| Antineutrophil cytoplasmic antibody | Systemic vasculitis |

sentation, radiographic appearance, physiologic abnormalities, and, in some instances, histologic findings. Nevertheless, a specific diagnosis can be made in many patients from the results of a careful history and certain laboratory tests. Bronchoscopy with bronchoalveolar lavage and, often, transbronchial biopsy are useful in the diagnosis of some causes of interstitial infiltration. Thoracoscopic or open lung biopsy is required for a definitive diagnosis of the remaining cases. Further information about many of the specific members of the interstitial disease family is found in Chapters 57 to 63 in this section. Additional discussion of other causes of interstitial lung disease is found elsewhere in the book: occupational exposure in Chapter 65, environmental inhalants in Chapter 67, and drug toxicity in Chapter 72.

## References


1. Clark JG, Kuhn C, McDonald JA, et al: Lung connective tissue. Int Rev Conn Tissue Res 10:231–249, 1983.
2. Campbell EJ, Senior RM, Welgus HG: Extracellular matrix injury during lung inflammation. Chest 92:161–167, 1987.
3. Burkhardt A: Alveolitis and collapse in the pathogenesis of pulmonary fibrosis. Am Rev Respir Dis 140:513–524, 1989.
4. Fukuda Y, Ishizaki M, Masuda Y, et al: The role of intraalveolar fibrosis in the process of pulmonary structural remodeling in patients with diffuse alveolar damage. Am J Pathol 126:171–182, 1987.
5. Niewoehner DE, Kleinerman J, Rice DB: Pathologic changes in the peripheral airways of young cigarette smokers. N Engl J Med 291:755–758, 1974.
6. Schwarz MI: Idiopathic pulmonary fibrosis. West J Med 149:199–203, 1988.
7. Schwarz MI: Approach to the understanding, diagnosis and management of interstitial lung disease. *In* Schwarz MI, King TE Jr (eds): Interstitial Lung Disease (3rd ed). Hamilton, Ontario: BC Decker, 1998, pp 1–30.
8. Katzenstein A, Bloor C, Liebow AA: Diffuse alveolar damage: The role of oxygen, shock, and related factors. Am J Pathol 85:210–226, 1976.
9. Blennerhassett JB: Shock lung and diffuse alveolar damage: Pathologic and pathogenetic considerations. Pathology 17:239–247, 1985.
10. Olson J, Colby TV, Elliot CG: Hamman Rich syndrome revisited. Mayo Clin Proc 65:1538–1548, 1990.
11. Cooper JAD, White DA, Matthay RA: Drug induced pulmonary disease. Am Rev Respir Dis 133:321–340, 1986.
12. Colby TV, Swenson SJ: Anatomic distribution and histopathologic patterns in interstitial lung disease. *In* Schwarz MI, King TE Jr (eds): Interstitial Lung Disease (3rd ed). Hamilton, Ontario: BC Decker, 1998, pp 31–51.
13. Zapol WM, Trelstad RL, Coffey JW, et al: Pulmonary fibrosis in severe acute respiratory failure. Am Rev Respir Dis 119:547–554, 1979.
14. Churg A, Golden J, Fligiel S, et al: Bronchopulmonary dysplasia in the adult. Am Rev Respir Dis 127:117–120, 1983.

15. Epler GR, Colby TV, McCloud TL, et al: Bronchiolitis obliterans organizing pneumonia. N Engl J Med 312:152–158, 1985.
16. Davison AG, Heard BC, McAllister WAC, et al: Cryptogenic organizing pneumonitis. Q J Med 52:382–394, 1983.
17. Liebow AA, Steer A, Billingsley JG: Desquamative interstitial pneumonia. Am J Med 39:369–404, 1965.
18. Katzenstein ALA, Myers J: Idiopathic pulmonary fibrosis: Clinical relevance of pathologic classification. Am J Respir Crit Care Med 157:1301–1315, 1998.
19. Carrington CB, Gaensler EA, Coutu RE, et al: Natural history and treated course of usual and desquamative interstitial pneumonia. N Engl J Med 298:801–809, 1978.
20. Patchefsky AS, Fraimow W, Hoch WS: Desquamative interstitial pneumonia: Pathologic findings and follow-up in 13 patients. Arch Intern Med 132:222–225, 1973.
21. Tubbs RR, Benjamin SP, Reich NE, et al: Desquamative interstitial pneumonitis: Cellular phase of fibrosing alveolitis. Chest 72:159–165, 1977.
22. Sokolowski JW, Cordray DR, Cantow EF, et al: Giant cell interstitial pneumonitis: Report of a case. Am Rev Respir Dis 105:417–420, 1972.
23. Daniil ZD, Gilchrist FC, Nicholson AG, et al: A histologic pattern of nonspecific interstitial pneumonia is associated with a better prognosis than usual interstitial pneumonia in patients with cryptogenic fibrosing alveolitis. Am J Respir Crit Care Med 160:899–905, 1999.
24. Fujita J, Yamadori I, Suemitsu I, et al: Clinical features of nonspecific interstitial pneumonia. Respir Med 93:113–118, 1999.
25. Kim EY, Lee KS, Chung MP, et al: Nonspecific interstitial pneumonia with fibrosis: serial high-resolution CT findings with functional correlation. AJR Am J Roentgenol 173:949–953, 1999.
26. Colby TV, Churg AC: Patterns of pulmonary fibrosis. Pathol Annu 21:277–310, 1986.
27. Crystal RG, Bitterman PB, Rennard SI, et al: Interstitial lung diseases of unknown cause. N Engl J Med 310:154–166, 1984.
28. Hayes JA, Christensen TG, Gaensler EA: Myointimal plaques in pulmonary vascular sclerosis associated with interstitial lung fibrosis. Lab Invest 41:268–274, 1979.
29. Liebow AA, Carrington CB: Diffuse pulmonary lymphoreticular infiltrations associated with dysproteinemia. Med Clin North Am 57:809–843, 1973.
30. Koss MN, Hochholzer L, Langloss JM, et al: Lymphoid interstitial pneumonia: Clinicopathological and immunopathological findings in 18 cases. Pathology 19:178–185, 1987.
31. Turner RR, Colby TV, Doggett RS: Well differentiated lymphocytic lymphoma: A study of 47 patients with primary manifestation in the lung. Cancer 54:2088–2096, 1984.
32. Strimlan CV, Rosenow EC III, Weiland LH: Lymphocytic interstitial pneumonitis: A review of 13 cases. Ann Intern Med 88:616–621, 1978.
33. Jederlinic PJ, Sicilian L, Gaensler EA: Chronic eosinophilic pneumonia: A report of 19 cases and a review of the literature. Medicine (Baltimore) 67:154–162, 1988.
34. Rosen SH, Castleman B, Liebow AA: Pulmonary alveolar proteinosis. N Engl J Med 258:1123–1142, 1958.
35. Leatherman JW: Immune alveolar hemorrhage. Chest 91:891–897, 1987.
36. Travis WD, Colby TV, Lombard C, et al: A clinicopathologic study of 34 cases of diffuse pulmonary hemorrhage with lung biopsy confirmation. Am J Surg Pathol 14:1112–1125, 1990.
37. Poh SC, Tjia TS, Seah HC: Primary diffuse alveolar septal amyloidosis. Thorax 30:178–185, 1975.
38. Eskon-Wilson K, Friedsen NE, Christensen HE: Primary alveolar septal amyloidosis: A scanning and transmission electron microscopic study. Virchows Arch [A] 371:89–99, 1976.
39. Rosen Y: Sarcoidosis. *In* Dail DH, Hammar SP (eds): Pulmonary Pathology. London: Springer Verlag, 1988, pp. 417–446.
40. Epler GR, McCloud TC, Gaensler EA, et al: Normal chest roentgenograms in chronic diffuse interstitial lung disease. N Engl J Med 298:934–939, 1978.
41. Sahn SA, Schwarz MI: Desquamative interstitial pneumonia with a normal chest radiograph. Br J Dis Chest 68:228–234, 1974.
42. Schurawitzki H, Stiglbauer R, Graninger W, et al.: Interstitial lung disease in progressive systemic sclerosis: High resolution CT versus radiograph. Radiology 176:755–759, 1990.
43. Aberle DR, Gamsu G, Ray CS: High resolution computed CT of benign asbestos related disease: Clinical and radiographic correlation. AJR Am J Roentgenol 151:883–891, 1988.
44. Johkoh T, Muller NL, Cartier Y, et al: Idiopathic interstitial pneumonias: diagnostic accuracy of thin-section CT in 129 patients. Radiology 211:555–560, 1999.
45. Silver RM, Miller KS, Kinsella MD, et al: Evaluation and management of scleroderma lung disease using bronchoalveolar lavage. Am J Med 88:470–476, 1990.
46. Cormier Y, Belanger J, Laviolette M: Persistent bronchoalveolar lavage lymphocytosis in asymptomatic farmers. Am Rev Respir Dis 133:813–847, 1986.
47. Harold JT: Lymphangitis carcinomatosis of the lungs. Q J Med 21:353–360, 1952.
48. Sharma OP, Johnson R: Airway obstruction in sarcoidosis: A study of 123 non-smoking black American patients with sarcoidosis. Chest 94:343–346, 1988.
49. Meyers JL, Veal CF, Myung SS, et al: Respiratory bronchiolitis causing interstitial lung disease: A clinicopathological study of six cases. Am Rev Respir Dis 135:880–884, 1987.
50. Hance AJ, Cadranel J, Soler P, et al.: Pulmonary and extra pulmonary Langerhans cell granulomatosis (histocytosis X). Semin Respir Med 9:349–368, 1988.
51. Coleman A, Colby TV: Histologic diagnosis of extrinsic allergic alveolitis. Am J Surg Pathol 12:514–518, 1988.
52. James DG: Sarcoidosis of the respiratory tract. Semin Respir Med 8:1–111, 1986.
53. Sullivan EJ: Lymphangiomyomatosis: A review. Chest 114:1689–1703, 1998.
54. Dwyer JH, Hickie JB, Garvan J: Pulmonary tuberous sclerosis: Report of three patients and a review of the literature. Q J Med 40:115–125, 1971.
55. Patchefsky AS, Atkinson WG, Hoch HS: Interstitial pulmonary fibrosis and von Recklinghausen's disease: An ultrastructural and immunofluorescent study. Chest 64:459–464, 1973.
56. Sweigert CF, McLaughlin EF, Heath EM: Carcinoma of the pancreas with pulmonary lymphangitic carcinomatosis simulating bronchial asthma: Case report. Ann Intern Med 27:301–303, 1947.
57. Glassroth J, Woodford DW, Carrington CB, et al: Pulmonary veno-occlusive disease in the middle aged. Respiration 47:309–321, 1985.
58. Cortese DA: Pulmonary function in mitral stenosis. Mayo Clin Proc 53:321–326, 1978.
59. Katzenstein A-LA, Myers JL, Mazur MT: Acute interstitial pneumonia: A clinicopathologic, ultrastructural, and kinetic study. Am J Surg Pathol 10:256–267, 1986.
60. Badesch DB, King TE Jr, Schwarz MI: Acute eosinophilic pneumonia: A hypersensitivity phenomenon? Am Rev Respir Dis 139:249–252, 1989.
61. Rose C, King TE Jr: Controversies in hypersensitivity pneumonitis. Am Rev Respir Dis 145:1–2, 1992.
62. Katzenstein A-LA, Myers JL, Prophet WD, et al: Bronchiolitis obliterans and usual interstitial pneumonia: A comparative clinicopathologic study. Am J Surg Pathol 10:373–381, 1986.
63. Matthay RA, Schwarz MI, Petty TL, et al: Pulmonary manifestation of systemic lupus erythematosis: Review of 12 cases of acute lupus pneumonitis. Medicine (Baltimore) 54:397–409, 1975.
64. Schwarz MI, Matthay RA, Sahn SA, et al: Interstitial lung disease in polymyositis and dermatomyositis: Analysis of six cases and review of the literature. Medicine (Baltimore) 55:89–104, 1976.
65. Lomeo RM, Cornella RJ, Shabel S, et al: Progressive systemic sclerosis sine scleroderma presenting as pulmonary interstitial fibrosis. Am J Med 87:525–527, 1989.
66. Elsasser S, Dalquen P, Soler M, et al: Methotrexate induced pneumonitis: Appearance four weeks after discontinuation of therapy. Am Rev Respir Dis 140:1089–1092, 1989.
67. O'Driscoll BR, Haselton PS, Taylor PM, et al: Active lung fibrosis up to 17 years after chemotherapy with carmustine (BCNU) in childhood. N Engl J Med 323:378–382, 1990.
68. Slader A, Zanc AP, Hadnott WH: Aspiration pneumonitis: The sequelae. Chest 59:448–450, 1971.
69. Kennedy JD, Costello P, Balikan JP, et al: Exogenous lipoid pneumonia. AJR Am J Roentgenol 136:1145–1149, 1981.

70. Hance AJ, Basset F, Saumon G, et al: Smoking and interstitial lung disease: The effect of cigarette smoke on the incidence of pulmonary histiocytosis X and sarcoidosis. Ann N Y Acad Sci 465:643–656, 1986.
71. Donaghy M, Rees AJ: Cigarette smoking and lung hemorrhage in glomerulonephritis caused by antibodies to glomerular basement membrane. Lancet 2:390–392, 1983.
72. Blanc PD, Golden JA, Gamsu G, et al: Asbestos exposure cigarette smoking interactions among shipyard workers. JAMA 259:270–273, 1988.
73. Schwartz DA, Galvin JR, Merchant RX, et al: Influence of cigarette smoking on bronchoalveolar lavage cellularity in asbestos-induced lung disease. Am Rev Respir Dis 145:400–405, 1992.
74. Kusaka H, Homma Y, Ogasawara H, et al: Five year followup of *Micropolyspora faeni* antibody in smoking and non-smoking farmers. Am Rev Respir Dis 140:695–699, 1989.
75. Libby DM, Gibofsky A, Fotino M, et al: Immunogenetic and clinical findings in idiopathic pulmonary fibrosis: Association with the B-cell alloantigen HLA-DR2. Am Rev Respir Dis 127:618–622, 1983.
76. Brennan NJ, Crean P, Long JP, et al: High prevalence of familial sarcoidosis in an Irish population. Thorax 39:14–18, 1984.
77. Terry RD, Sperry WM, Brodoff B: Adult lipoidosis resembling Niemann-Pick disease. Am J Pathol 30:263–286, 1954.
78. Schneider EL, Epstein CJ, Kaback MJ, et al: Severe pulmonary involvement in adult Gaucher's disease: Report of three cases and review of the literature. Am J Med 63:475–480, 1977.
79. White DA, Walker Smith GT, Looper JAD, et al: Hermansky-Pudlak syndrome and interstitial lung disease: Report of a case with lavage findings. Am Rev Respir Dis 130:138–141, 1984.
80. Kriebel D, Brain JD, Sprince NL, et al: The pulmonary toxicity of beryllium. Am Rev Respir Dis 137:464–473, 1988.
81. Mossman BT, Gee JBL: Asbestos-related diseases. N Engl J Med 320:1721–1730, 1989.
82. Epler GR, Carrington CB, Gaensler EA: Crackles in the interstitial pulmonary diseases. Chest 73:333–337, 1978.
83. Ziskind MM, Weill H, Buechner HA, et al: Recognition of distinctive radiologic patterns in diffuse pulmonary disease. Arch Intern Med 114:108–112, 1964.
84. Schwarz MI: Radiologic recognition of chronic diffuse lung disease. *In* Schwarz MI, King TE Jr (eds): Interstitial Lung Disease. Philadelphia: BC Decker, 1988, pp. 27–36.
85. Carrington CB, Addington WW, Goff AM, et al: Chronic eosinophilic pneumonia. N Engl J Med 280:787–789, 1969.
86. Bartter T, Irwin RS, Nash G, et al: Idiopathic bronchiolitis obliterans organizing pneumonia with peripheral infiltrates on chest roentgenogram. Arch Intern Med 149:273–279, 1989.
87. Trapnell DH: Radiologic appearances of lymphangitis carcinomatosis of the lung. Thorax 19:251–260, 1964.
88. Corrin B, Liebow AA, Friedman RI: Pulmonary lymphangiomyomatosis: A review. Am J Pathol 79:348–382, 1975.
89. Fulmer JD: An introduction to the interstitial lung diseases. Clin Chest Med 3:457–473, 1982.
90. Becklake MR: Asbestos related diseases of the lung and other organs: Their epidemiology and implications for clinical practice. Am Rev Respir Dis 114:187–227, 1976.
91. Laronique J, Roth C, Battestic JP, et al: Chest radiologic features of pulmonary histiocytosis X: A report based on 50 adult cases. Thorax 37:104–109, 1982.
92. Claque HW, Wallace AC, Morgan WRC: Pulmonary interstitial fibrosis associated with alveolar proteinosis. Thorax 38:865–866, 1983.
93. Bronson SM: Idiopathic pulmonary hemosiderosis in adults: Report of a case and review of the literature. AJR Am J Roentgenol 83:260–271, 1960.
94. Sahn SA, Schwarz MI, Lakshmingarayan S: Sarcoidosis: The significance of an acinar pattern on chest roentgenogram. Chest 65:684–687, 1974.
95. Haddad R, Massaro D: Idiopathic diffuse interstitial fibrosis: A typical epithelial proliferation and lung cases. Am J Med 45:211–219, 1968.
96. Mueller NL, Miller RR: Computed tomography of chronic diffuse lung disease. Am Rev Respir Dis 142:1206–1215, 1990.
97. Mathieson JR, Mayo JR, Staples CA, et al: Chronic diffuse infiltrative lung disease: Comparison of diagnostic accuracy of CT and chest radiography. Radiology 171:111–116, 1989.
98. Aberle DR, Gamsu G, Ray CS: Asbestos-related pleural and parenchymal fibrosis: Detection with high resolution CT. Radiology 166:729–734, 1988.
99. Aberle DR: Current imaging of asbestosis. Curr Opin Radiol 1:9–15, 1989.
100. Lynch D, Gamsu G: Imaging of diffuse parenchymal lung disease. *In* Schwarz MI, King TE Jr (eds): Interstitial Lung Disease (3rd ed). Hamilton, Ontario: BC Decker, 1998, pp 71–102.
101. Mueller NL, Miller RR, Webb WR, et al: Fibrosing alveolitis: CT-pathologic correlation. Radiology 160:585–588, 1986.
102. Westcott JL, Cole SR: Traction bronchiectasis in endstage pulmonary fibrosis. Radiology 161:665–669, 1986.
103. Müller NL, Staples CA, Miller RR, et al: Disease activity in idiopathic pulmonary fibrosis: CT and pathologic correlation. Radiology 165:731–734, 1987.
104. Harrison NK, Glannville AR, Strickland B et al: Pulmonary involvement in systemic sclerosis: The detection of early changes by thin section CT scan, bronchoalveolar lavage and 99mTc-DTPA clearance. Respir Med 83:403–414, 1989.
105. Kuhlman JE, Fishman ER, Hamper VM, et al: The computed radiographic spectrum of thoracic sarcoidosis. Radiographics 9:449–466, 1989.
106. Henry DA, Kiser PE, Scheer CE, et al: Multiple imaging evaluation of sarcoidosis. Radiographics 1:75–95, 1986.
107. Lynch DA, Webb WR, Gamsu G, et al: Computed tomography in sarcoidosis. J Comput Assist Tomogr 13:405–410, 1989.
108. Silvers SF, Müller NL, Miller RR, et al: Hypersensitivity pneumonitis: Evaluation with CT. Radiology 173:441–445, 1989.
109. Hansell D, Moskovic E: High resolution computed tomography in extrinsic allergic alveolitis. Clin Radiol 43:8–12, 1991.
110. Brauner MW, Grenier P, Movelhi MM, et al: Pulmonary histocytosis X: Evaluation with high resolution CT. Radiology 172:255–258, 1989.
111. Moore ADA, Godwin JD, Müller NL, et al: Pulmonary histiocytosis X: Comparison of radiographic and CT findings. Radiology 172:249–254, 1989.
112. Lenoir S, Grenier P, Brauner MW, et al: Pulmonary lymphangiomyomatosis and tuberous sclerosis: Comparison of radiographic and thin section CT findings. Radiology 175:329–334, 1990.
113. Müller NL, Chiles C, Kullnig P: Pulmonary lymphangiomyomatosis: Correlation of CT with radiographic and functional findings. Radiology 175:335–339, 1990.
114. Stein M, Mayo J, Müller NL, et al: Pulmonary lymphangitic spread of carcinoma: Appearance on CT scans. Radiology 162:371–375, 1987.
115. Im J-G, Webb W, Rosen A, et al: Costal pleura: Appearances at high-resolution CT. Radiology 171:125–131, 1989.
116. Aberle DR, Gamsu G, Ray CS, et al: Asbestos related pleural and parenchymal fibrosis: Detection with high resolution CT. Radiology 166:729–734, 1988.
117. Gaensler EA, Carrington CB, Coutu RE, et al: Radiographic-physiologic-pathologic correlations in interstitial pneumonitis. Prog Respir Res 8:233–243, 1975.
118. Gibson GJ, Pride NB: Pulmonary mechanics in fibrosing alveolitis: The effects of lung shrinkage. Am Rev Respir Dis 116:637–647, 1977.
119. Warren CPW, Tse KS, Cherniack RM: Mechanical properties of the lung in extrinsic allergic alveolitis. Thorax 33:315–321, 1978.
120. McCarthy D, Cherniack RM: Regional ventilation-perfusion and hypoxia in cryptogenic fibrosing alveolitis. Am Rev Respir Dis 107:200–208, 1973.
121. Cherniack RM: Pulmonary Function Testing. Philadelphia: WB Saunders, 1992.
122. Cherniack RM: Mechanics of breathing. Semin Respir Med 4:171–179, 1983.
123. Macklem PT: Tests of lung mechanics. N Engl J Med 293:339–342, 1975.
124. Cherniack RM, Cherniack L: Respiration in Health and Disease. Philadelphia: WB Saunders, 1983.
125. Hanley ME, King TE Jr, Schwarz MI, et al: The impact of smoking on mechanical properties of the lungs in idiopathic pulmonary fibrosis and sarcoidosis. Am Rev Respir Dis 144:1102–1106, 1992.
126. Ostrow D, Cherniack RM: A resistance to airflow in patients with diffuse interstitial lung disease. Am Rev Respir Dis 108:205–210, 1973.

127. Fulmer JD, Roberts WC, Von Gal ER, et al: Small airways in idiopathic pulmonary fibrosis: Comparison of morphologic and physiologic observations. J Clin Invest 60:595–610, 1970.
128. Jodoin G, Gibbs GW, Macklem PT, et al: Early effects of asbestos exposure on lung function. Am Rev Respir Dis 104:525–535, 1971.
129. Cherniack RM: Pulmonary ventilation, circulation and gas exchange. Semin Respir Med 4:197–206, 1983.
130. Fulmer JD, Roberts WC, Von Gal ER, et al: Morphologic-physiologic correlates of the severity of fibrosis and degree of cellularity in idiopathic pulmonary fibrosis. J Clin Invest 63:665–676, 1979.
131. Greening AP, Hughes JMB: Serial estimation of carbon monoxide diffusing capacity in intrapulmonary hemorrhage. Clin Sci 60:507–512, 1981.
132. Younes M: Interpretation of clinical exercise testing in respiratory disease. Clin Chest Med 5:189–206, 1984.
133. Watters LC, King TE Jr, Cherniack RM, et al: Bronchoalveolar lavage fluid neutrophils increase after corticosteroid therapy in smokers with idiopathic pulmonary fibrosis. Am Rev Respir Dis 133:104–109, 1988.
134. The BAL Cooperative Steering Committee: Bronchoalveolar lavage constituents in healthy individuals, idiopathic pulmonary fibrosis, and selected comparison groups. Am Rev Respir Dis 141:S169–S202, 1990.
135. Turner-Warwick ME, Haslam PL: Clinical applications of bronchoalveolar lavage: An interim review. Br J Dis Chest 80:105–121, 1966.
136. Reynolds HY: Bronchoalveolar lavage. Am Rev Respir Dis 135:250–263, 1987.
137. Fedullo AV, Ettensohn DB: Bronchoalveolar lavage in lymphangitic spread of adenocarcinoma of the lung. Chest 87:129–131, 1985.
138. Sestini P, Rottoli L, Gotti G, et al: Bronchoalveolar lavage diagnosis of bronchiolo-alveolar carcinomas. Eur J Respir Dis 66:55–58, 1985.
139. Myers JL, Fulmer JD: Bronchoalveolar lavage in the diagnosis of pulmonary lymphoma. Chest 91:642–643, 1987.
140. Konig G, Luderschmid TC, Hammer C, et al: Lung involvement in scleroderma. Chest 85:318–324, 1984.
141. Garcia JGN, Parhami N, Killiam D, et al: Bronchoalveolar lavage fluid evaluation in rheumatoid arthritis. Am Rev Respir Dis 133:450–454, 1986.
142. Martin RJ, Coalson JJ, Rogers RM, et al: Pulmonary alveolar proteinosis: The diagnosis by segmental lavage. Am Rev Respir Dis 121:819–825, 1980.
143. Haslam PL, Hughes DA, Dewar A, et al: Lyoprotein macroaggregates in bronchoalveolar lavage fluid from patients with diffuse interstitial lung disease: Comparison with idiopathic alveolar lipoproteinosis. Thorax 43:140–146, 1988.
144. Helmers RA, Hunninghake GW: Bronchoalveolar lavage in the non-immunocompromised host. Chest 96:1184–1190, 1989.
145. Ettensohn DB, Roberts NJ, Condemi JJ: Bronchoalveolar lavage in gold lung. Chest 85:569–570, 1984.
146. Farber HW, Fairman RP, Glauser FL: Talc granulomatosis: Laboratory findings similar to sarcoidosis. Am Rev Respir Dis 125:258–261, 1982.
147. Epstein PL, Dauber JH, Rossman MD, et al: Bronchoalveolar lavage in a patient with chronic berylliosis: Evidence for hypersensitivity pneumonitis. Ann Intern Med 97:213–216, 1982.
148. Sebastien P, Armstrong B, Minchaux G, et al: Asbestos bodies in bronchoalveolar lavage fluid and in lung parenchyma. Am Rev Respir Dis 137:75–78, 1988.
149. Teschler H, Konietzko N, Schoenfeld B, et al: Distribution of asbestos bodies in the human lung as determined by bronchoalveolar lavage. Am Rev Respir Dis 147:1211–1215, 1993.
150. Newman LS, Kreiss K, King TE Jr, et al: Pathologic and immunologic alterations in early stages of beryllium disease. Am Rev Respir Dis 139:1479–1486, 1989.
151. Kawanami O, Basset F, Ferrans VJ, et al: Pulmonary Langerhans cells in patients with fibrotic lung disorders. Lab Invest 44:227–233, 1981.
152. Rudd RM, Haslam PL, Turner-Warwick M: Cryptogenic fibrosing alveolitis: Relationships of pulmonary physiology and bronchoalveolar lavage to response to treatment and prognosis. Am Rev Respir Dis 124:1–8, 1981.
153. Watters LC, Schwarz MI, Cherniack RM, et al: Idiopathic pulmonary fibrosis: Pretreatment bronchoalveolar lavage cellular constituents and their relationships with lung histopathology and clinical response to therapy. Am Rev Respir Dis 135:696–704, 1987.
154. Karpel JP, Norin AJ: Association of activated cytolytic lung lymphocytes with response to prednisone therapy in patients with idiopathic pulmonary fibrosis. Chest 96:794–798, 1989.
155. Turner-Warwick M, Haslam PL: The value of serial bronchoalveolar lavages in assessing the clinical progress of patients with cryptogenic fibrosing alveolitis. Am Rev Respir Dis 133:26–34, 1987.
156. Peterson MW, Minick M, Hunninghake GW: Prognostic role of eosinophils in pulmonary fibrosis. Chest 92:51–56, 1987.
157. Keogh BA, Hunninghake GW, Line BR, et al: The alveolitis of pulmonary sarcoidosis: Evaluation of natural history and alveolitis dependent changes in lung function. Am Rev Respir Dis 128:256–265, 1983.
158. Israel-Biet D, Venet A, Chrétien J: Persistent high alveolar lymphocytosis as a predictive criterion of chronic pulmonary sarcoidosis. Ann N Y Acad Sci 465:395–406, 1986.
159. Costabel V, Bross BJ, Guzman J, et al: Predictive value of bronchoalveolar T cell subsets for the course of pulmonary sarcoidosis. Ann N Y Acad Sci 465:418–426, 1986.
160. Verstraeten A, Demedts M, Verwilghen J, et al: Predictive value of bronchoalveolar lavage in pulmonary sarcoidosis. Chest 98:560–567, 1990.
161. Gaensler EA, Carrington CB: Open lung biopsy for chronic diffuse infiltrative lung disease: Clinical, roentgenographic, and physiologic correlations in 502 patients. Ann Thorac Surg 30:411–426, 1980.
162. Wall CP, Gaensler EA, Carrington CB, et al: Comparison of transbronchial and open biopsies in chronic infiltrative lung diseases. Am Rev Respir Dis 123:280–285, 1981.
163. Bensard DD, McIntyre RC, Waring BJ: Comparison of video thoracoscope lung biopsy to open lung biopsy in the diagnosis of interstitial lung disease. Chest 103:765–767, 1993.

# 57 Idiopathic Interstitial Pneumonias

Talmadge E. King, Jr., M.D. • Marvin I. Schwarz, M.D.


Introduction
Idiopathic Pulmonary Fibrosis
- Clinical Features
- Blood and Serologic Studies
- Chest Radiography
- Computed Tomography Scan
- Other Imaging Techniques
- Pulmonary Function Tests
- Pulmonary Hemodynamics
- Abnormalities During Sleep
- Histopathology
- Pathogenesis
- Diagnosis
- Staging of Disease Activity
- Management

Familial Idiopathic Pulmonary Fibrosis
Respiratory Bronchiolitis-Associated Interstitial Lung Disease
- Clinical Features
- Pathologic Features
- Clinical Course and Outcome

Acute Interstitial Pneumonia
Cryptogenic Organizing Pneumonia
- Clinical Features
- Pathologic Features
- Clinical Course and Outcome

Lymphocytic Interstitial Pneumonia
- Clinical Features
- Pathologic Features
- Clinical Course and Outcome

Nonspecific Interstitial Pneumonia
- Clinical Features
- Pathologic Features
- Clinical Course and Outcome


## INTRODUCTION

The classification, diagnosis, and management of the idiopathic interstitial pneumonias continue to evolve.[1] Hamman and Rich[2, 3] are credited with the initial description of idiopathic pulmonary fibrosis (IPF): however, their patients contrast sharply with the now classic descriptions of IPF.[4] In fact, their patients experienced a fulminant and rapidly fatal course very unlike that of IPF. As additional clinical and histopathologic studies are reported, it is clearer that most investigators only now identify IPF as cases with the histologic pattern of usual interstitial pneumonia. In addition, it is recognized that distinction of the usual interstitial pneumonia pattern from other histopathologic patterns of the idiopathic interstitial pneumonias identifies patients with differing clinical courses and prognoses.

This chapter describes the major idiopathic interstitial pneumonias (Tables 57.1 and 57.2): IPF (or usual interstitial pneumonia); acute interstitial pneumonia (the proposed synonym for Hamman-Rich syndrome); desquamative interstitial pneumonia; respiratory bronchiolitis-associated interstitial lung disease; bronchiolitis obliterans organizing pneumonia (or cryptogenic organizing pneumonia); lymphocytic interstitial pneumonia; and nonspecific interstitial pneumonia. Lymphocytic interstitial pneumonia is included even though it is a lymphoproliferative disorder often associated with immunodeficiencies.[5] These entities may mimic IPF clinically, physiologically, and radiographically, but are generally associated with a higher response rate to corticosteroid therapy and a better prognosis.[4]

## IDIOPATHIC PULMONARY FIBROSIS

IPF (also called *cryptogenic fibrosing alveolitis*) is a common interstitial lung disease of unknown etiology.[6] It is a well-defined clinical entity that has characteristic clinical, radiographic, physiologic, and pathologic manifestations. The exact prevalence of this condition is unknown but is estimated to be 3 to 5 cases per 100,000 persons, and recent studies show that it might in fact be higher and increasing in several countries.[7–9] The prevalence and incidence of pulmonary fibrosis increase markedly with age.

### Clinical Features

IPF occurs in middle age, usually between 50 and 70 years of age. In fact, it is quite uncommon for a patient

**Table 57.1 CONTRASTING PATHOLOGIC FEATURES OF THE IDIOPATHIC INTERSTITIAL PNEUMONIAS**

| FEATURES | UIP | DIP | RB-ILD | AIP | NSIP | BOOP |
|---|---|---|---|---|---|---|
| Temporal appearance | Variegated | Uniform | Uniform | Uniform | Uniform | Uniform |
| Interstitial inflammation | Scant | Scant | Scant | Scant | Usually prominent | Usually prominent |
| Collagen fibrosis | Yes, patchy | Variable, diffuse | Variable, focal, mild | No | Variable, diffuse | No |
| Fibroblast proliferation | Fibroblast foci prominent | No | No | Diffuse | Occasional, diffuse, or rare fibroblast foci | Diffuse, fibroblastic foci |
| Microscopic honeycomb change | Yes | No | No | No | Rare | No |
| Intra-alveolar macrophage accumulation | Occasional, focal | Yes, diffuse | Peribronchiolar | No | Occasional, patchy | Foamy macrophages common |
| Hyaline membranes | No | No | No | Occasional, focal | No | No |

AIP = acute interstitial pneumonia; BOOP = bronchiolitis obliterans with organizing pneumonia; DIP = desquamative interstitial pneumonia; NSIP = nonspecific interstitial pneumonia; RB-ILD = respiratory bronchiolitis associated with interstitial lung disease; UIP = usual interstitial pneumonia.

Adapted from Katzenstein ALA, Myers JL: Idiopathic pulmonary fibrosis. Clinical relevance of pathologic classification. Am J Respir Crit Care Med 157:1301–1315, 1998; and King TE Jr: Bronchiolitis obliterans. *In* Schwarz MI, King TE Jr (eds): Interstitial Lung Diseases (3rd ed). Hamilton, Ontario: BC Decker 1998, pp 645–684.

to present before the age of 40 years. The typical patient presents with the insidious onset of breathlessness with exertion and a nonproductive cough. Constitutional symptoms are uncommon in IPF alone. Weight loss, fever, fatigue, myalgias, or arthralgia is, however, occasionally present. The onset may be heralded by a flu-like illness, but this is very uncommon, and its presence should suggest another diagnosis. Although patients may present with only a nonproductive cough, all patients experience dyspnea with exertion as the disease progresses. Most patients have these symptoms for months to years before definitive evaluation, usually around 12 to 18 months.

The physical examination is rarely normal. Most patients have bibasilar late inspiratory fine crackles ("Velcro rales") on chest examination. Clubbing of the fingers is seen in 40% to 75% of patients and is a late finding in the disease course. Cardiac examination is usually normal except in the middle or late stages of the disease, when

**Table 57.2 CONTRASTING CLINICAL FEATURES OF THE IDIOPATHIC INTERSTITIAL PNEUMONIAS**

| FEATURES | UIP | DIP | RB-ILD | AIP | NSIP | BOOP |
|---|---|---|---|---|---|---|
| Mean age at onset-years | 60s | 40s | 40s | 50s | 50s | 50s |
| Onset | Insidious | Insidious | Insidious | Acute | Subacute, insidious | Acute or subacute |
| History of cigarette smoking | About two-thirds | Most | Most | Not known | Not known | About half |
| Mortality rate (mean survival) | 68% (5–6 yr) | 27% (12 yr) | 0% | 62% (1–2 mo) | 11% (17 mo) | 10% in 5 years |
| Response to steroids | Poor | Good | Good | Poor | Good | Excellent |
| Complete recovery possible | No | Yes | Yes | Yes | Yes | Yes (up to 70% of patients) |

AIP = acute interstitial pneumonia; BOOP = bronchiolitis obliterans with organizing pneumonia; DIP = desquamative interstitial pneumonia; NSIP = nonspecific interstitial pneumonia; RB-ILD = respiratory bronchiolitis associated with interstitial lung disease; UIP = usual interstitial pneumonia.

Adapted from Katzenstein ALA, Myers JL: Idiopathic pulmonary fibrosis. Clinical relevance of pathologic classification. Am J Respir Crit Care Med 157:1301–1315, 1998; and King TE Jr: Bronchiolitis obliterans. *In* Schwarz MI, King TE Jr (eds): Interstitial Lung Diseases (3rd ed). Hamilton, Ontario: BC Decker, 1998, pp 645–684.

findings of pulmonary hypertension (i.e., augmented $P_2$, right-sided lift, and $S_3$ gallop) and cor pulmonale may become evident. Similarly, cyanosis is a late manifestation indicative of advanced disease. Spontaneous pneumothorax rarely occurs.

## Blood and Serologic Studies

An elevated erythrocyte sedimentation rate, hypergammaglobulinemia, low-titer-positive antinuclear antibodies (21% of patients with only IPF), rheumatoid factor, circulating immune complexes, and cryoimmunoglobulins have been identified in patients. Only circulating immune complexes have been correlated with disease stage or prognosis.[10]

## Chest Radiography

The most common radiographic abnormalities in IPF are a reticular (i.e., net-like) appearance of linear or curvilinear densities. These usually appear as diffuse opacities with a predilection for the lower lung zones (Fig. 57.1). A coarse reticular pattern or multiple cystic or honeycombed areas (i.e., coarse reticular pattern with translucencies measuring 0.5 to 1.0 cm in diameter) are radiographic findings that correlate with advanced disease and poor prognosis (Fig. 57.2). Chest radiographic evidence of reduced lung volumes is usually present unless there is associated obstructive airway disease. Pleural involvement is uncommon in IPF; its presence should suggest another diagnosis, such as collagen vascular disease (especially rheumatoid arthritis or systemic lupus erythematosus), mitral valve disease, congestive heart failure, asbestosis, infection, drug-induced lung disease, or lymphangitic carcinomatosis (see Table 57.5, later).

## Computed Tomography Scan

Increasingly, computed tomography (CT) is being used to evaluate pulmonary parenchymal disease, especially IPF.[11–13] High-resolution CT (HRCT) is useful in the differentiation of IPF from other interstitial lung diseases, the determination of the extent and severity of disease activity, and, most importantly, the detection of disease, especially in patients with normal or minimal change on plain chest radiographs.[13, 14]

HRCT findings in IPF include a marked peripheral and especially subpleural distribution of the interstitial densities. The involvement is patchy, with areas of reticulation intermingled with areas of normal tissue, and this type of involvement is often associated with cystic spaces 2 to 4 mm in diameter (see Fig. 57.2). Correlation of the HRCT findings with the histopathologic manifestations in IPF is incomplete. Early disease appears as either a patchy, predominantly peripheral, air space opacification (i.e., opacified air spaces distinct from reticular densities more than 1 cm in diameter and located away from the fissures), or a hazy increase in lung density (i.e., an increase in CT lung density that does not obscure the underlying lung parenchyma); in addition, the interlobular septa are thickened, and there is prominence of centrilobular core structures. In more advanced disease, there is a predominant reticular pattern in the lower lung zone that consists largely of thickened interlobular septa and intralobular lines, often associated with honeycombing, traction bronchiectasis, and subpleural fibrosis. The HRCT findings of early disease are thought to correlate with alveolar septal inflammation and filling of air spaces by mononuclear cells, although these findings can also be seen in the lungs of patients with features of advanced disease. Those HRCT findings associated with advanced disease presumably represent fibrosis.

Identification of a relationship between pulmonary function testing and HRCT findings remain incomplete. FVC, $D_{L_{CO}}$, and arterial $P_{O_2}$ measured at peak exercise or $O_2$ desaturation during exercise are the physiologic parameters that best correlate with the global extent of disease in HRCT.[15–17] Serial HRCT scanning showed that the changes over time in the total extent of the disease were similar to those changes observed in $D_{L_{CO}}$ and FVC.[17] These data also suggest that FVC, $D_{L_{CO}}$, and gas exchange with exercise are the physiologic variables that best reflect the global extent of disease in IPF and thus may provide significant information for the assessment of the disease's progression, thus potentially limiting the role of serial HRCT scanning in the follow-up of patients with IPF.[17]

HRCT has not replaced lung biopsy in the diagnosis and assessment of most interstitial lung diseases. Connective tissue diseases (particularly scleroderma and rheumatoid arthritis)[18, 19] and asbestosis[20–23] may cause a similar HRCT appearance, except for the presence of parenchymal bands of fibrosis and pleural plaques in patients with asbestosis. Patients with subacute or chronic hypersensitivity pneumonitis can have similar reticular opacity or honeycombing, but often lack the bibasilar predominance seen in IPF.[24] Studies evaluating the ability of HRCT scanning to accurately diagnose IPF have found that HRCT significantly increases the level of diagnostic confidence compared with the chest radiograph. The accuracy of a confident diagnosis of IPF made on HRCT by a trained observer appears to be about 90%.[24–27] Less experienced observers are substantially less accurate than experienced observers.[25]

## Other Imaging Techniques

### Gallium Scanning

Lung scanning with radioactive gallium ($^{67}Ga$) is a noninvasive test for staging the "alveolitis" found in interstitial pulmonary diseases, particularly sarcoidosis. Unfortunately, whether or how the level of $^{67}Ga$ accumulation in the lung correlates with the inflammatory stage of IPF has not been adequately demonstrated. Thus, $^{67}Ga$ lung scanning is not recommended in the routine evaluation of IPF because it is difficult to interpret, it is not specific, and a negative scan does not exclude disease.

### Ventilation-Perfusion Lung Scanning

Ventilation-perfusion lung scanning is not recommended as a routine part of the evaluation. In most parenchymal diseases, ventilation-perfusion scanning reveals an inho-

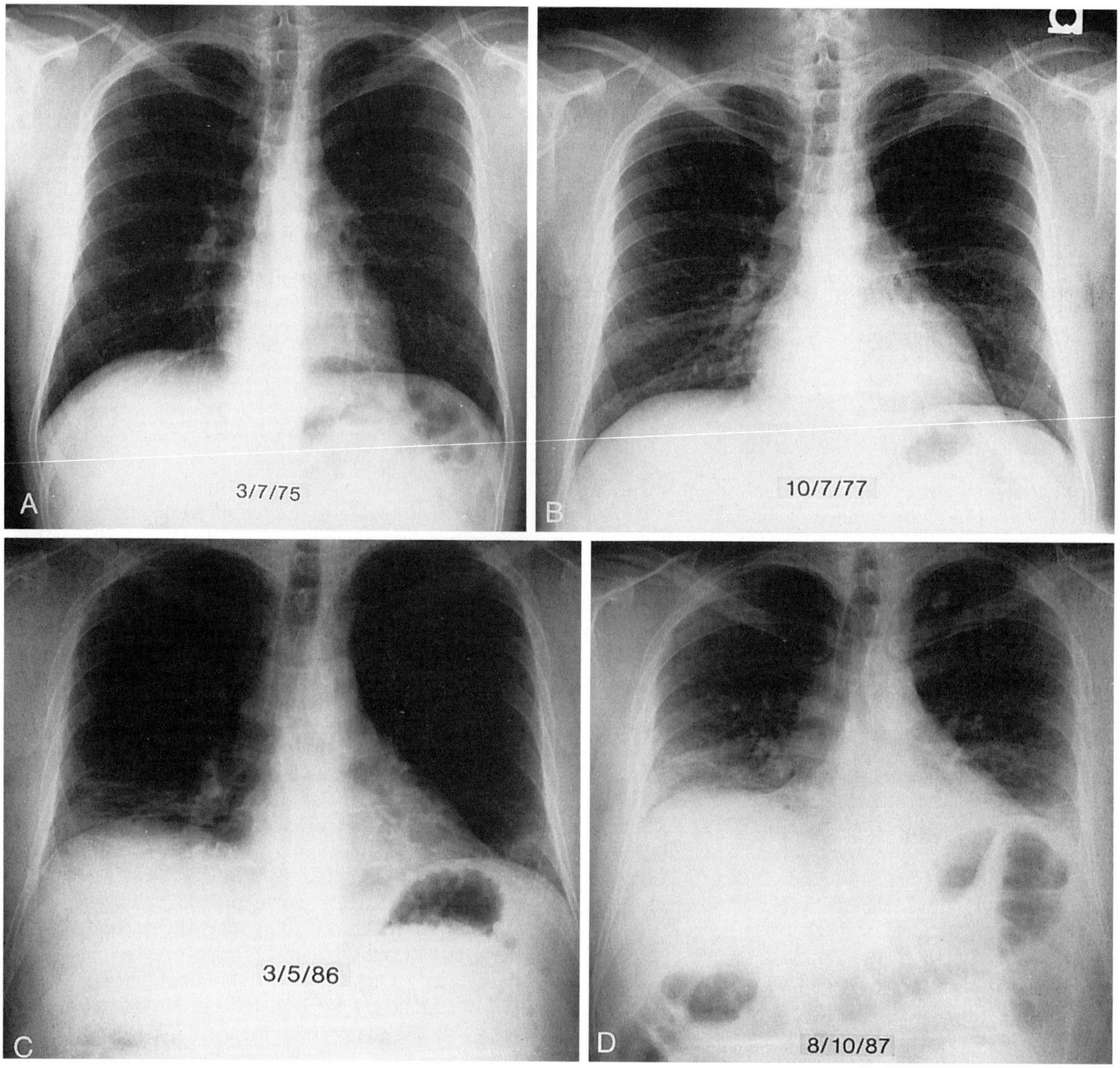


**Figure 57.1** These serial chest radiographs are from a patient with IPF. *A,* The posteroanterior radiograph of the chest was obtained at the time of onset of breathlessness with exercise and mild cough. The chest appears normal. *B,* The follow-up film reveals progressive loss of lung volume and bibasilar, predominantly reticular infiltrates. The patient had stopped regular exercise because of breathlessness with exertion. *C,* Progressive changes are evident, with severe loss of lung volume. Predominantly in the lower lung zone are seen diffuse, bilateral, coarse reticular infiltrates typical of the radiographic appearance of the middle to late stage of pulmonary fibrosis. *D,* Continued disease progression is evident, with honeycombing and pulmonary hypertension. Open lung biopsy revealed usual interstitial pneumonitis with extensive fibrosis and histologic honeycombing. Treatment with corticosteroids and cyclophosphamide (Cytoxan) was started, but the patient experienced a progressive decline in functional status and died 6 months after lung transplantation.

mogeneous reduction of blood flow, ventilation, or both. Two types of perfusion abnormalities occur in IPF: nonsegmental inhomogeneities, which are probably due to a localized loss of the capillary bed, most often in the lower lobes; and increased perfusion of the upper lung zones, resulting from pulmonary hypertension, which induces an upward shift in the gradient of capillary perfusion. Ventilation scans often reveal patchy, nonsegmental areas of decreased ventilation, reflecting regions of airway obstruction or alveolar destruction. Patchy areas of high and

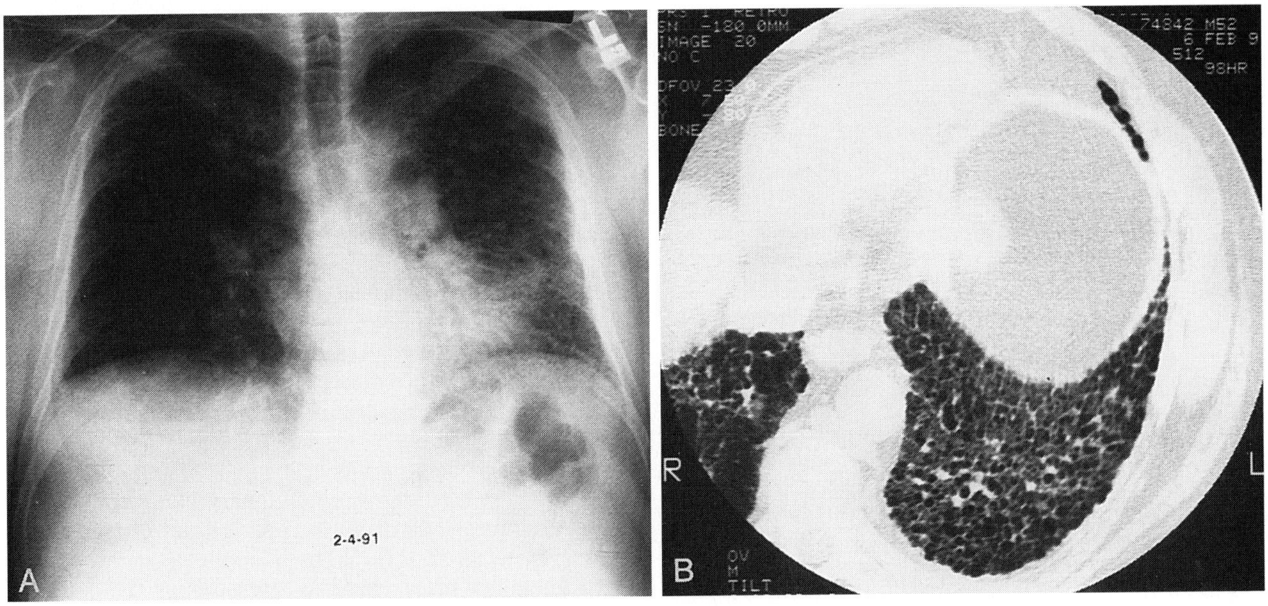


**Figure 57.2** Radiographs show IPF. *A,* Patient with long-standing IPF and diffuse interstitial infiltrates has radiographic evidence of honeycombing. *B,* High-resolution, thin-section CT scan reveals extensive parenchymal involvement with irregular fibrotic changes containing small honeycomb-like air spaces in the left lower lung zones.

low ventilation-perfusion matching usually occur, with a few areas of well-maintained ventilation-perfusion matching. These findings of mismatching of ventilation and blood flow help explain the hypoxemia and high dead space ($V_D$) to tidal volume ($V_T$) ratio found in many of these patients at rest.

## Pulmonary Function Tests

The lung volumes (total lung capacity, functional residual capacity, and residual volume) are reduced. Early in the disease, the lung volumes may be normal, especially in patients with superimposed chronic obstructive pulmonary disease. Lung volumes are higher in smokers with IPF than in those who have never smoked.[28] In general, as the disease progresses, lung compliance decreases and lung volumes fall (Fig. 57.3). A history of smoking alters the pressure-volume relationship, shifting it upward and to the left. Thus, the transpulmonary pressure at any given lung volume in smokers is significantly lower than that in nonsmokers with IPF. As a result, the coefficient of elastic retraction of the lungs is lower in smokers than in nonsmokers with IPF.[28]

Expiratory flow rates, $FEV_1$ and FVC, may be decreased because of the reduction in lung volume, but the $FEV_1$/FVC ratio is maintained. Because of the increased static elastic recoil found in these patients, at any given lung volume, flow rates are often increased (Fig. 57.4).

Patients with IPF are tachypneic, with rapid shallow breaths, probably because of increased work of breathing. This rapid respiratory rate presumably results from altered mechanical reflexes, caused by the increased elastic load, vagal mechanisms, or both, because no defined chemical basis for the hyperventilation has been identified.

The diffusing capacity for carbon monoxide ($DL_{CO}$) is reduced, which may actually precede the loss of lung volume. The decrease in the $DL_{CO}$ results from both a contraction of the pulmonary capillary volume and the presence of ventilation-perfusion abnormalities. The resting arterial blood gases are usually abnormal and reveal hypoxemia and respiratory alkalosis. The major cause of

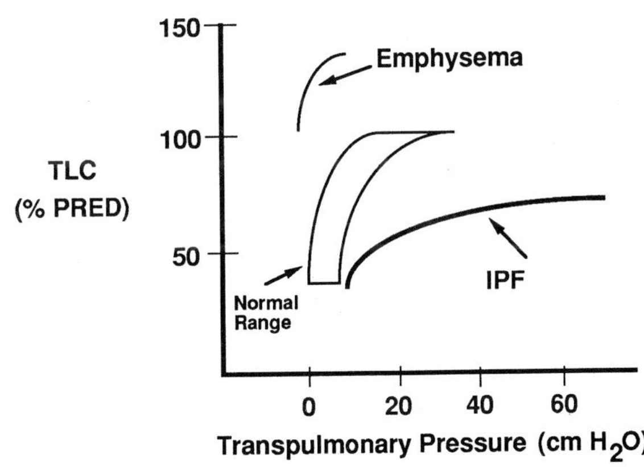


**Figure 57.3** The relationship of the static deflation volume and transthoracic pressure is shown in a patient with IPF. The percentage of predicted total lung capacity (TLC) is plotted against the static transpulmonary pressure for a patient with moderate to severe fibrosis and honeycombing. In general, the compliance, maximum static transpulmonary pressure, and coefficient of retraction (the ratio of maximum transpulmonary pressure to TLC) tend to correlate with the extent of fibrosis observed in open lung biopsy.

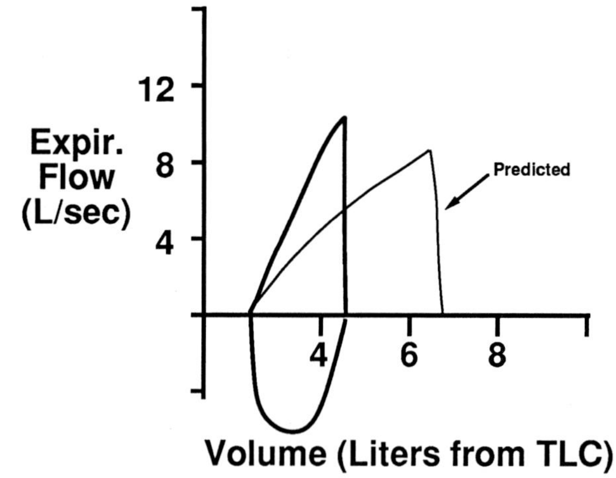


**Figure 57.4** The maximal expiratory flow-volume plot shows results from a patient with IPF. This flow-volume plot of a forced expired vital capacity maneuver and lung volume determination revealed a severe restrictive pattern with increased flow rates at any given lung volume. TLC = total lung capacity.

resting hypoxemia is ventilation-perfusion mismatching, and it is not due to either impaired oxygen diffusion, as was originally suspected, or to anatomic shunts. With exercise, the alveolar-arterial $Po_2$ difference ([A − a]$Po_2$) widens, and the arterial $Po_2$ and oxygen saturation ($So_2$) fall. During maximal exercise, 20% to 30% of the exercise-induced widening of the (A − a)$Po_2$ may be caused by some impairment of oxygen diffusion. Of importance is that the abnormalities identified at rest do not accurately predict the magnitude of the abnormalities that may be seen with exercise (Fig. 57.5). Although these abnormalities can be assessed by oximetry, it has been demonstrated that oxygen saturation determined by this method may not yield as dramatic or significant a change as that obtained by measurement of arterial blood $Po_2$ and $Pco_2$. Exercise testing is more sensitive than assessments at rest in the detection of abnormalities in oxygen transfer. In addition, gas exchange during exercise has been demonstrated to be a sensitive parameter for following the clinical course.

During exercise, patients with IPF have increased minute ventilation primarily because of increased respiratory frequency. This method of increase differs from that in normal subjects, in whom increased ventilation during mild exercise occurs by an increase in the $V_T$ rather than the respiratory rate. Thus, patients with IPF have elevated minute ventilation during exercise that is in part related to the increase in dead space ($V_D$) ventilation. In addition, the ratio of $V_D/V_T$ is increased at rest and is maintained or decreased with exercise. Occasionally, the $V_D/V_T$ ratio increases in interstitial lung disorders that have a prominent pulmonary vascular component, such as scleroderma or pulmonary histiocytosis X.

## Pulmonary Hemodynamics

Pulmonary hypertension rarely occurs at rest but is common during exercise even in the early stages of IPF. When the vital capacity is less than 50% of predicted or the $DL_{CO}$ is less than 45% of predicted, pulmonary hypertension at rest can be expected. In 70% of patients with advanced pulmonary fibrosis, auscultatory findings consistent with pulmonary hypertension are present. The mean pulmonary artery pressure at rest ranges between 23 and 28 mm Hg and rarely exceeds 40 mm Hg. A resting pulmonary artery pressure above 30 mm Hg is associated with a poor prognosis.

The cause of pulmonary hypertension in IPF is multifactorial, with compression and the destruction of pulmonary vessels by the interstitial infiltrative process and vasoconstriction of vessels mediated by hypoxia, acidosis, and autacoids being the most important. The pulmonary artery wedge pressure remains normal in IPF, and cor pulmonale is a late sequela. Oxygen therapy at rest and during exercise improves pulmonary hemodynamics and probably improves exercise capacity and prognosis. Few data exist on the value of vasodilator therapy in the treatment of pulmonary hypertension in the interstitial lung diseases.

## Abnormalities During Sleep

Many patients with IPF, especially those with low daytime arterial $So_2$ or a history of snoring during sleep, develop sleep disturbances that are characterized by reduced rapid eye movement sleep, lighter and more frag-

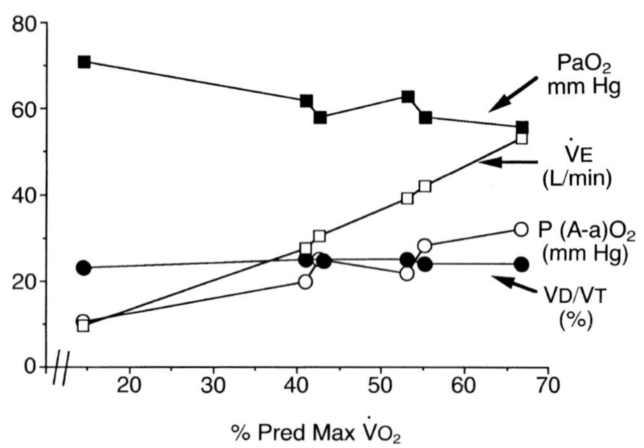


**Figure 57.5.** Exercise testing of IPF is graphed based on results from a patient who complained of dyspnea while running. The chest radiograph was normal, and resting room air arterial blood gas determinations were normal (at elevation 1625 m). The patient performed exercise on a cycle ergometer, and the work rate increased by 10 watts/min to her symptom-limited maximum. Blood was sampled serially from an indwelling arterial catheter. Her resting and exercise electrocardiograms were normal. The patient achieved 65% of predicted maximum workload. The arterial $Po_2$ fell, and the (A − a)$Po_2$ rose. The minute ventilation ($\dot{V}_E$) increased disproportionately with work rate (shown as the percent of predicted maximal $\dot{V}o_2$) and the dead space/tidal volume ratio ($V_D/V_T$) failed to fall. The study was stopped because the patient experienced shortness of breath and leg fatigue.

mented sleep, and hypoxemia during rapid eye movement sleep. Severe hypoxemia occurs in the absence of obstructive sleep apnea or changes in breathing pattern. Tachypnea persists during sleep. Identification and correction of the sleep disturbance may reduce morbidity and improve patient survival.

## Histopathology

The gross appearance of the lungs in IPF reveals a distinctive nodular pleural surface, sometimes with a marked cirrhotic appearance. Microscopic examination demonstrates a spectrum of findings consistent with the pattern of "usual interstitial pneumonia" (UIP) (see Figs. 58.7 to 58.10, later). Important features of UIP include an "alveolitis," characterized by mononuclear cells (predominantly alveolar macrophages and lymphocytes) in the alveolar spaces with relatively intact alveolar walls; derangement of alveolar walls by the presence of edema, fibrinous exudate, mononuclear cell infiltration, and fibroblast proliferation; and connective tissue alterations that occur as the disease advances and cause derangement of parenchymal structures, that is, fibrosis.[5] Cystic spaces lined by metaplastic bronchial epithelium, the so-called honeycombed lung, is an end-stage finding that likely results from damage and scarring of bronchioles as well as holes left behind when alveolar walls disappear.

Katzenstein and Myers[5] emphasize that the earliest change in UIP is the fibroblast focus, characterized by a distinct cluster of fibroblasts and myofibroblasts within the alveolar wall, with little associated interstitial inflammation or intra-alveolar macrophage accumulation. They hypothesize that the fibroblast proliferation occurs in an attempt to repair the damaged alveolus. The process evolves over 1 to 2 weeks and is followed by collagen deposition within a few months. Although an "alveolitis" may be seen in UIP, neither interstitial inflammation nor intra-alveolar macrophage accumulation is a major feature.[5] Because of this latter finding, we no longer adhere to the concept that desquamative interstitial pneumonia or cellular interstitial pneumonitis (now called nonspecific interstitial pneumonia) is the precursor of UIP. We regard desquamative interstitial pneumonia as a separate and distinct entity.

A broad range of extent and severity for most of the histopathologic abnormalities is found in IPF. All patients have evidence of alveolar septal fibrosis.[29] Vasculitis, granulomas, or signs of pneumoconiosis rule out the diagnosis of IPF. Inflammatory airway narrowing, obstructive pneumonitis, and obliterative airway narrowing occur in less than 25% of the patients and are usually of a mild to moderate extent. We have described a quantitative method for the assessment of the histopathologic changes found in IPF[30] and have demonstrated that this correlates with the morphometric findings.[31]

Bronchogenic carcinoma (alveolar cell carcinoma, adenocarcinoma, and oat cell carcinoma) has been identified with increased frequency in advanced IPF. It is postulated that carcinoma arises from the metaplastic bronchiolar epithelium that develops in these patients. Interestingly, a number of the reported cases occurred in patients with familial IPF.

## Pathogenesis

The inciting factors in the development of IPF are unknown. A widely held hypothesis is that this disorder occurs in susceptible individuals after some unknown stimulus. This inciting agent initiates a cascade of events that involves factors controlling inflammatory, immune, and fibrotic processes in the lung. Environmental, viral, immunologic, and genetic factors appear to play important roles.

Cigarette smoking is associated with the development of IPF.[32–34] More patients (72%) than controls (63%) have a history of ever smoking. The odds ratio for ever smoking was 1.6 (95% confidence interval [CI], 1.1 to 2.4) The risk was significantly elevated for former smokers, 1.9 (95% CI, 1.3 to 2.9) and for smokers with 21 to 40 pack-years, 2.3 (95% CI, 1.3 to 3.8).[34] There was no clear exposure-response pattern with cumulative consumption of cigarettes.

Long-term exposure to metal or wood dust has also been shown to be an independent risk factor for IPF. For metal dust, the odds ratio per work-year of exposure was 1.11 (95% CI, 1.06 to 1.16; $P < .001$), and for wood dust the odds ratio per work-year of exposure was 1.12 (95% CI, 1.02 to 1.24; $P < .02$).[33] Steel, brass, and lead were the most common metal dusts.

Infrequently, patients date the onset of their symptoms to a flu-like illness. No convincing cultural, serologic, or morphologic evidence supports prior or persistent viral exposure.[35–43] Increased serum antibodies to Epstein-Barr virus and detectable IgA against viral-capsid antigen are present.[44] The potential role of Epstein-Barr virus or hepatitis C virus in the etiology of IPF is intriguing. Importantly, ultrastructural studies have largely failed to identify viral particles in the lung or in pulmonary secretions. A genetic basis is supported by the findings of familial cases of pulmonary fibrosis.[45]

An important advance in our understanding of interstitial lung disease has been the recognition of the central role of chronic inflammation (alveolitis) in the injury and fibrosis that occurs in the distal airspaces of these patients. Destruction of alveolar units in IPF is mediated by inflammatory and immune processes. The mechanisms by which these inflammatory and immune effector cells injure lung parenchymal cells and induce connective tissue proliferation is conjectural. Clearly, a shift in the types and quantity of inflammatory cells present in the lower respiratory tract occurs in patients with IPF. Considerable heterogeneity does occur, however, with most studies revealing a predominance of neutrophils and macrophages, whereas others suggest that the inflammation is actually the result of other cell types (e.g., lymphocytes or mast cells). Correlative studies of lung parenchymal inflammatory cells and the ultimate course of the disease have suggested that inflammation is a key factor in the prediction of therapeutic responsiveness. Although chronic active inflammation is important, it is the fibrotic and destructive changes that distort the normal lung architecture and result in morbidity. The fibrosis is irreversible and thus plays a central role in the natural history of this disease. Consequently, understanding the mechanisms that modulate both the inflammation and the fibrosis is crucial if clinicians are to develop effective therapeutic regimens.

Activation of macrophages appears to orchestrate the process by the release of neutrophil chemotactic factor and other autokines that are chemotactic for lymphocytes. An increase in the number of fibroblasts also occurs within the alveolar structures, presumably as a result of both the release of a macrophage-derived growth factor and the production of potent chemoattractants for fibroblasts by alveolar macrophages. Data conflict about whether total collagen production is increased per fibroblast or simply reflects the expansion of fibroblast numbers. Similarly, it is not clear whether there is an increased collagen content in the lungs. Yet changes do occur in the type of collagen present such that there is relatively more type I and less type III collagen. Increased type III collagen in patients with active disease has been suggested by the increased levels of type III procollagen peptide (a potential marker of collagen secretion) in the lavage specimens, sera, and tissue of patients with IPF. Finally, the collagen present is altered in location, randomly oriented, thickened, frayed, and twisted, presumably as a result of the destructive effects of proteases such as collagenase.

The quantity and composition of pulmonary surfactant phospholipids recovered by bronchoalveolar lavage are abnormal in IPF.[46, 47] There is a reduced total recovery of surfactant phospholipid, a reduction in the percentage of phosphatidylglycerol, and a slight increase in the percentage of phosphatidylinositol. There is no change in the percentage of saturated phosphatidylcholine. Because phosphatidylglycerol and phosphatidylinositol share a common precursor, CDP-diacylglycerol, their synthesis is related, and the ratio of these two phospholipid species can be used as a marker of surfactant alterations in disease. The protein secretory products of the alveolar type II cell, surfactant proteins A, B, and C are important contributors to the function and metabolism of pulmonary surface active material. McCormack and colleagues[46, 47] have demonstrated that surfactant protein A is reduced in IPF and that decreases in its concentration referenced to total phospholipid (a marker of surfactant to normalize to the surface sampled by lavage and recovery) predicts an adverse clinical outcome. The decrease in surfactant protein A is not disease specific and is found in other interstitial lung diseases.

## Diagnosis

A carefully taken clinical history is the most important step in the diagnosis of IPF because the disorder cannot be diagnosed until known causes of interstitial lung disease have been excluded. Particular emphasis should be placed on possible occupational and environmental exposures. The specific diagnosis cannot rest on the exposure history alone but requires compatible symptoms, physical findings, and radiographic and pulmonary function abnormalities. Additionally, primary interstitial lung diseases occur (e.g., sarcoidosis, eosinophilic granuloma, lymphangitic carcinomatosis, hypersensitivity pneumonitis, respiratory bronchiolitis) that can be differentiated only by their histologic appearance; therefore, a lung biopsy is often required. Connective tissue diseases (see Chapter 58) may be difficult to exclude because the pulmonary manifestations may precede the more typical systemic manifestations by months or years.

The most definitive method of establishing a diagnosis is by surgical lung biopsy.[48] Open or thoracoscopic lung biopsy is indicated because it provides an accurate diagnosis; it excludes neoplastic and infectious processes that occasionally mimic chronic, progressive interstitial disease; it occasionally identifies a more treatable process than originally suspected (e.g., chronic extrinsic allergic alveolitis); and it provides a better assessment of disease activity.[49, 50] Thoracoscopic lung biopsy (see Chapter 27) is the preferred method and is relatively safe with little morbidity and less than 1% mortality. It is performed under general anesthesia; after the procedure, a thoracostomy tube is required for 24 to 48 hours. Recovery is relatively quick, and patients frequently leave the hospital 3 to 5 days after surgery.

We usually do not perform surgical lung biopsy in the elderly (over 70 years of age) or in patients with serious cardiovascular disease, roentgenographic evidence of diffuse honeycombing, severe pulmonary dysfunction, or other major operative risks. In these patients, fiberoptic bronchoscopy with transbronchial biopsy is occasionally performed. In all other patients, however, thoracoscopic lung biopsy is recommended because of the larger quantity of tissue obtained. It is important that the surgeon obtain an adequate sample from several sites. Specifically, the surgeon should avoid obtaining only subpleural tissue (especially if pleuritis is present) and should avoid the dependent segments of the right middle lobe and lingula. This approach decreases the sampling error that often occurs when a single, small piece is obtained by open lung biopsy or the usually small crushed pieces obtained with transbronchial lung biopsy by fiberoptic bronchoscopy. More importantly, it allows the pathologist to better define the extent and severity of the inflammation and fibrosis, factors key to determining prognosis.

## Staging of Disease Activity

### Histopathologic Findings

Examination of lung tissue provides the best estimate of the stage of the disease. Active alveolitis and minimal fibrosis are consistent with early disease. Severe fibrosis and honeycombing with minimal alveolitis are consistent with late stage or end stage disease. If one divides the patients broadly into a cellular (mainly inflammatory) group and a predominantly fibrotic group, one finds similar results. Patients with a more cellular picture tend to be more responsive to corticosteroid treatment and to have a more favorable long-term prognosis than the more fibrotic group (Fig. 57.6). Thus, it is desirable to be able to objectively determine the stage of the disease and the degree of cellularity present.[51, 52]

### Clinical Features

Breathlessness and cough do not identify any particular histopathologic process. Cyanosis and clubbing are more common in fibrotic disease, but their presence does not exclude early inflammatory disease. Patients with a short

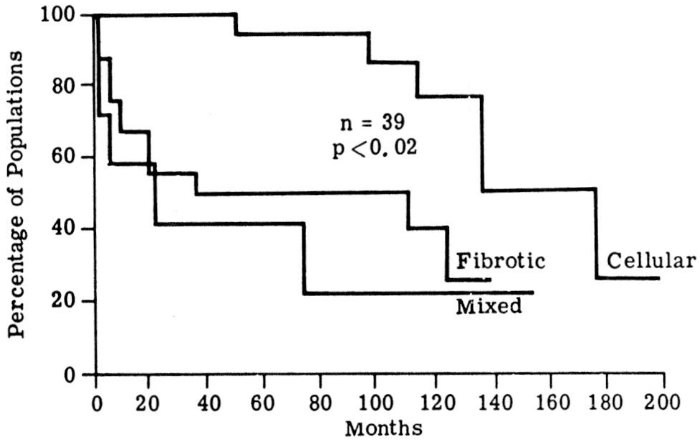


**Figure 57.6** Survival curves are shown for patients with pulmonary fibrosis. The histologic features at the time of diagnosis influenced the prognosis. Patients with more cellular and less fibrotic changes in their lung biopsy samples survive longer. The cases with cellular changes most likely represent nonspecific interstitial pneumonia, whereas the fibrotic or mixed cases represent patients with usual interstitial pneumonia.

duration of symptoms (less than 6 months) before therapy is started tend to achieve the greatest improvement. The type and amount of exertion required to precipitate shortness of breath have been shown to correlate with the roentgenographic profusion of diffuse reticular opacities as well as the reduction in vital capacity. Younger patients tend to have less fibrosis than do older patients, and younger patients and women survive longer than older patients and men.

## Serum Studies

The presence of immunologic markers, including autoantibodies, elevated sedimentation rates, circulating immune complexes and increased serum immunoglobulins, have not been shown to influence the overall natural history of IPF.

## Chest Radiography and CT Scanning

A general pattern of evolution is seen in serial chest radiographs. The early changes include hazy opacities with reduction in lung volumes that progress to a reticular pattern and finally end in coarser, cystic areas of honeycombed lung. A correlation was found between chest radiographic profusion score and the degree of dyspnea at presentation.[52] Patients who have less radiographic abnormalities at presentation survive longer.[53] Unfortunately, the chest radiograph is not a useful monitor of the degree of inflammation present. In fact, only roentgenographic honeycombing correlates with histologic honeycombing. Furthermore, the radiograph may demonstrate no changes even while clinically apparent physiologic deterioration is occurring. Another major problem with using the chest radiograph to follow the disease course or to estimate the stage of disease is that there is considerable interobserver variability in the interpretation.

HRCT scanning in IPF may be useful in staging disease activity. The extent of air space opacification on CT scan correlates with cellularity on the lung biopsy. Patients with IPF who are found to have a higher extent of ground-glass opacities and lower extent of reticular opacities on the initial HRCT are the most likely to respond to corticosteroids.[51]

## Pulmonary Physiologic Tests

Physiologic tests are also neither sensitive nor specific for the presence of inflammation in the lung parenchyma. In fact, in patients with early disease, the routine pulmonary function tests may be normal. Reductions in the vital capacity do correlate with the degree of fibrosis present and show a relationship with the overall histologic derangements. A marked reduction in the vital capacity (less than 50% of predicted) is associated with pulmonary hypertension and a reduced 2 year survival. Reduction of the total lung capacity correlates with neither the histopathologic findings[54] nor the prognosis and survival.[52] The compliance, maximum transpulmonary pressure, and coefficient of elastic retraction of the lung correlate well with the degree of fibrosis but do not exclude the presence of cellularity.[54]

The $DL_{CO}$ has no correlation with the histologic stage of the disease. Patients with normal $DL_{CO}$ values usually do not have significant gas exchange abnormalities, whereas patients with values below 70% of predicted frequently have such changes at rest or with exercise. Survival is longer in patients with a more normal $DL_{CO}$ (more than 45% of predicted value). A marked reduction of the $DL_{CO}$ and resting hypoxemia are associated with pulmonary hypertension and decreased survival. Patients with a predominantly fibrotic process have greater abnormalities of the $(A - a)PO_2$ than those with more cellular changes. Alterations in gas exchange during exercise compared with other indices of lung function correlate best with histopathologic findings. Serial measurements of gas exchange during exercise appear to be the best predictors of responsiveness to treatment. In summary, pulmonary function testing does not correlate with histopathology, especially the degree of alveolitis present, but is nevertheless useful in establishing the presence of impairment in IPF and following its course and response to therapy.

## Bronchoalveolar Lavage

It has been suggested that the bronchoalveolar lavage cellular constituents reflect the state of the pulmonary inflammatory response. Active IPF is characterized by a severalfold increase in the total number of inflammatory cells recovered from the respiratory tract. Unfortunately, many studies have failed to demonstrate a clear distinction between diseases based on the predominant cell type present in the lavage specimens. Moreover, there is no correlation between the percentage of various cell types found in the lavage fluid in patients with IPF and various clinical parameters, serum tests, or pulmonary function studies.[29, 55] On the one hand, in patients with known IPF, bronchoalveolar lavage lymphocytosis is associated with moderate to severe alveolar septal inflammation and with a relative absence of histologic honeycombing. Conversely, bronchoalveolar lavage neutrophilia and eosinophilia tend to occur in patients with more advanced fibrotic disease.

The relationship between bronchoalveolar lavage cellular abnormalities and clinical response to therapy requires additional study. A correlation has, however, been suggested between the percentage of neutrophils or eosinophils in lavage fluid and the prognosis of IPF. That is, increases in these cells are associated with a poor response to corticosteroids. On the other hand, lavage lymphocytosis at the time of presentation predicts a more likely positive response to corticosteroid therapy by both objective and subjective parameters. Importantly, it appears that patients with neutrophilia or eosinophilia or both occasionally respond better to cyclophosphamide therapy. Thus, these data suggest that the initial bronchoalveolar lavage cell counts can help predict response to treatment.

The role and value of serial bronchoalveolar lavage in assessment of the clinical progress of patients with IPF has not been adequately examined. Turner-Warwick and Haslam[56] found that, in patients with definite and sustained clinical improvement, serial lavage cell counts tended to return toward the normal. Interestingly, declines in neutrophil levels in lavage fluid tended to occur in patients who responded to prednisolone, whereas cyclophosphamide response led to a fall in eosinophil counts. Patients who failed to improve had elevated neutrophil and eosinophil counts throughout their course. On the other hand, several of the patients who did not respond appeared to have clinically stable disease and demonstrated persisting neutrophilia, which did not necessarily portend a poor prognosis.

In IPF, changes in the phosphatidylglycerol/phosphatidylinositol ratio are predictive of the cellularity and degree of fibrosis on histopathologic examination of open lung biopsy specimens. In addition, patients with less depression of total phospholipids in lavage fluids improve with corticosteroid therapy, whereas those with more severe decreases in total phospholipids do not. Surfactant protein A is reduced in IPF, and decreases in its concentration referenced to total phospholipid (a marker of surfactant to normalize to the surface sampled by lavage and recovery) predicts an adverse clinical outcome and poorer survival.[46, 47]

In summary, although the data are limited, they appear to support the hypothesis that the initial bronchoalveolar lavage cell counts and phospholipid content can predict the underlying histopathology. Furthermore, monitoring serial lavage cell counts and phospholipid content in individual patients may indicate the clinical course and therefore be useful in establishing the clinical response to treatment and in allowing one to objectively assess the end points in this disease, especially as they relate to reducing the medication used in the treatment.

## Management

Once the diagnosis and the clinical severity are established, most patients require therapy because IPF is a potentially fatal disorder without spontaneous remission. The natural history of IPF has not been appropriately defined: Data obtained from several reports indicate that the median survival after diagnosis, with or without treatment, is less than 5 years. Thus, early diagnosis and treatment are important to prevent the development of irreversible fibrosis. Therapy for IPF, regardless of the agent used, requires 3 to 6 months before its effectiveness can be assessed (Table 57.3). Few adequate randomized, controlled clinical treatment trials of sufficient numbers of patients with IPF have been performed. Consequently, conclusions drawn from the available data need to be confirmed.

### Selecting Patients and Assessing Response to Therapy

Because the clinical course of IPF varies considerably, generalization of the treatment program to be used for an individual patient is often difficult. Neither the patient nor the physician should be lulled into a sense of security by the insidious progression of the disease. Examples abound of slowly progressive, untreated disease that resulted in unresponsive, irreversible fibrosis (see Fig. 57.1) or that developed a rapidly progressive phase.

We believe all patients without contraindications to therapy require treatment at presentation. Those with contraindications, end-stage disease, or without evidence of physiologic impairment, however, may follow a carefully defined and executed program of evaluation at 3- to 6-month intervals to monitor for evidence of deterioration before therapy is started. Equally difficult is the management of elderly patients whose lung biopsy specimens show mainly fibrosis and who have severe pulmonary function abnormalities. In general, these patients receive a brief treatment trial (3 to 6 months) to determine reversibility. Unfortunately, few if any of these patients are likely to have a significant objective response. They also are likely to be at greater risk of experiencing drug-induced side effects. Worse yet, elderly patients have shorter durations of illness before presentation and more rapid downhill courses than do younger patients.[57]

It is often difficult to determine whether treatment is producing the desired effect. In general, the responsive patient reports a decrease in symptoms, demonstrates roentgenographic clearing and physiologic improvement, or shows no further decline in lung function or other parameters of disease activity for prolonged periods. Subjective without objective improvement occurs frequently (up to 70% of treated patients). Objective improvement in physiologic or radiographic abnormalities occurs in 20% to 30% of treated patients. Another problem is that only some parameters may improve. For example, the changes in chest roentgenogram or lung function test results are often divergent. The diffusing capacity may improve considerably, whereas lung volumes may not; the opposite may also occur. Physiologic improvement is defined as a 10% increase in total lung capacity or vital capacity, a 15% increase in single-breath diffusing capacity, and a reduction or normalization of oxygen desaturation during exercise. A composite clinical, roentgenographic, physiologic score (CRP score) has been

**Table 57.3 DRUG TREATMENT IN IDIOPATHIC PULMONARY FIBROSIS**

| Drug | Route | Dose | Duration of Therapy |
|---|---|---|---|
| Glucocorticoids (prednisone) | Oral | Initial, 1–1.5 mg/kg IBW per day<br>At 3 months, 0.5 mg/kg IBW per day<br>At 6 months, 0.25 mg/kg IBW per day<br>At 1 year, taper off* | Optimally, 1 year if tolerated; patients often require ongoing steroid treatment at a low dose (0.25 mg/kg/day) to maintain stability |
| Cyclophosphamide | Oral | 1–2 mg/kg/day (generally do not exceed 150 mg/day; maintain WBC >4000 cells/μL) | At least 3–6 months for adequate trial (usually with low-dose prednisone 0.25 mg/kg/day); if response is improvement, stability, or retardation in rate of deterioration, continue to 1–2 years |
| Azathioprine | Oral | 1–2 mg/kg/day (generally do not exceed 150 mg/day; maintain WBC >4000 cells/μL) | At least 3–6 months for adequate trial (usually with low-dose prednisone 0.25 mg/kg/day); if response is improvement, stability, or retardation in rate of deterioration, continue to 1–2 years |
| Colchicine | Oral | 0.6–1.2 mg bid | At least 3–6 months for adequate trial; if response is improvement, stability, or retardation in rate of deterioration, continue to 1–2 years |

bid = twice a day; IBW = ideal body weight; WBC = white blood count.
*If clinical deterioration occurs, continue dose that maintains stability.

developed that allows a quantification of the clinical course and the impact of therapy in individual patients.[58]

## Corticosteroids

Corticosteroids are the mainstay for the treatment of IPF (see Table 57.3). A favorable clinical response occurs in approximately one third of patients. The rationale for the use of corticosteroids is to suppress the chronic alveolitis. The mechanism by which corticosteroids affect the inflammatory immune effector cells is unknown. Glucocorticoids work by suppressing neutrophil and lymphocyte migration into the lung; decreasing the level of immune complexes; altering alveolar macrophage function by, for example, inhibiting the secretion of proteolytic enzymes or decreasing the amount of chemotactic factors released; and altering the neutrophil adhesion to endothelial surfaces probably mediated by a direct effect on the surface membrane configuration. It is unclear why some patients respond to corticosteroids and others do not. It has been suggested that this may be related to the presence of glucocorticoid surface receptors on the parenchymal cells. This hypothesis is potentially important because the effects of glucocorticoids on target cells are mediated by specific glucocorticoid receptors in the cells.

We initiate therapy with prednisone, 1.0 to 1.5 mg/kg/day, not to exceed a total dose of 100 mg/day; usually a dose of about 60 mg/day is used. This is given as a single oral dose in the morning. Alternate-day therapy is not recommended because no data are available to suggest that it is effective. After approximately 2 to 3 months of daily prednisone therapy, chest roentgenograms and pulmonary physiologic studies are reevaluated. If the patient is responsive, that is, improved or stabilized, prednisone is tapered (by 1 to 2 mg/week) until a maintenance dose of 0.5 mg/kg/day is reached. This dose is continued for an additional 3 to 6 months with the realization that, with clinical and physiologic deterioration, the prednisone dose may have to be raised to previous levels. In general, it is unlikely that corticosteroid therapy can be discontinued, and patients are usually maintained on 0.25 mg/kg/day. In fact, no clear-cut guidelines exist for the length of therapy in IPF. We advocate at least 1 year of therapy with or without another immunosuppressive agent and then a gradual tapering, with regular follow-up (3 to 6 months). Unfortunately, even after this prolonged therapy, one may find that the disease flares up after several months or even years of stability. At this juncture, we generally initiate repeated therapy with the same agents. Many clinicians believe that lifelong treatment is required in the management of IPF that has responded to the initial therapy.

**Table 57.5 COMPLICATIONS OF DISEASE OR THERAPY**

| | |
|---|---|
| **PROGRESSIVE RESPIRATORY FAILURE** | |
| | Mortality, 39% |
| | Findings suggestive of disease progression are multiple and nonspecific |
| **BRONCHOGENIC CARCINOMA** | |
| | Mortality, 10% |
| | Excess risk of 14:1 compared with general population; same histologic distribution as seen in population |
| **CARDIOVASCULAR DISEASE** | |
| | Mortality, 24% |
| | Right ventricular hypertrophy, cor pulmonale due to progressive, long-standing pulmonary hypertension and right-sided heart failure |
| | Left ventricular heart failure usually due to concurrent ischemic heart disease |
| **PULMONARY INFECTION** | |
| | Mortality, 2–4% |
| | Increased incidence; glucocorticoid and cytotoxic therapy may further increase risk |
| **PNEUMOTHORAX** | |
| | Occurs less often than in other interstitial lung disease |
| | May be difficult to manage |
| **PULMONARY EMBOLISM** | |
| | Mortality, 3–7% |
| | Pulmonary angiography frequently required to make diagnosis |

Adapted with permission from Panos RJ, Mortenson RL, Niccoli SA, et al: Clinical deterioration in patients with idiopathic pulmonary fibrosis: Causes and assessment. Am J Med 88:396, 1990.

ing respiratory insufficiency with patients being unable to carry out activities of daily living without extreme distress. Death usually ensues as a result of intractable hypoxemia and respiratory failure.

## FAMILIAL IDIOPATHIC PULMONARY FIBROSIS

The clinical, radiographic, physiologic, and morphologic manifestations of familial IPF are indistinguishable from those of the nonfamilial form. Patients usually present between the ages of 20 and 40 years. The younger the age at the time of presentation, the more aggressive is the disease. There is equal sex distribution (i.e., a ratio of 1.23:1.00 women to men), but women tend to have a more favorable prognosis.[67] An autosomal dominant pattern of inheritance with reduced penetrance has been suggested. Linkage studies have suggested a link between the risk for familial IPF and immunoglobulin gamma (Gm) allotypes. The finding of a significant increase in non-MM protease inhibitor phenotypes, particularly MZ, is additional evidence for a role for chromosome 14 in the increased susceptibility of persons to the development of IPF. There is evidence of a genetic influence in sporadic cases, including conflicting evidence of an increased presence of HLA-B8, HLA-B12, and HLA-B15 and HLA-Dw6 and HLA-DR2 antigens and a decreased incidence of HLA-Dw3. Despite these findings, it remains to be determined if a definite association between an HLA locus and IPF exist.

Bitterman and his coworkers[68] reported the presence of alveolar inflammation in clinically unaffected family members of patients with familial IPF. These family members had increased numbers of neutrophils and activated macrophages that released one or more neutrophil chemoattractants and growth factors for lung fibroblasts and positive gallium-67 lung scans. The significance of these findings is unknown, but the authors speculated that the unaffected family members may be at risk for the development of familial effect.

The role of genetics in the pathogenesis of IPF is further strengthened by the appearance of an IPF-like disease in association with inherited disorders such as neurofibromatosis,[69–71] Hermansky-Pudlak syndrome,[71–75] tuberous sclerosis,[76–80] Gaucher's disease, [81, 82] lymphangiomyomatosis,[83] and the hypocalciuric hypercalcemia syndrome[83](see Chapters 60 and 62).

## RESPIRATORY BRONCHIOLITIS-ASSOCIATED INTERSTITIAL LUNG DISEASE

Respiratory bronchiolitis-associated interstitial lung disease (RB-ILD) and "desquamative" interstitial pneumonia (DIP) are considered together because we believe that they represent different stages of the same process. Also, the term RB-ILD is more anatomically accurate and conveys more important pathogenetic implications that the older term DIP.[5] RB-ILD is a distinct clinical syndrome found in current heavy cigarette smokers.[84–87]

Previously, many investigators considered DIP or RB-ILD to represent an early stage of IPF; however, it is now widely viewed as a distinct clinical and pathologic entity. RB-ILD is uncommon, accounting for less than 10% of the cases of diffuse parenchymal lung disease that we have seen over the last 15 years. Because of the marked differences in clinical course and prognosis, it must be separated from other idiopathic interstitial pneumonias.

## Clinical Features

RB-ILD afflicts primarily cigarette smokers in their fourth or fifth decade of life. There is a male preponderance, with nearly twice as many men as women affected. Patients with the disease commonly present with cough and dyspnea. Coarse, bibasilar end-inspiratory crackles are frequent findings on physical examination. Finger clubbing also occurs in RB-ILD.[5]

The chest radiograph shows less severe changes than in IPF and may be normal in up to 20% of cases. A pattern of fine granular opacities, suggesting an acinar filling process, may be the early finding (see Figs. 56.7 and 56.22*B*). Air bronchograms can be found when this process surrounds the airways. Most often the chest radiograph often reveals diffuse, fine reticular interstitial opacities with normal-appearing lung volumes. Bronchial wall thickening, prominent peribronchovascular interstitium, small regular and irregular opacities, and small peripheral ring shadows are distinctive features of respiratory bronchiolitis. As the disease progresses, linear densities and reticulation occur. The honeycombed pattern is rare.

The CT features of RB-ILD are quite different from those of IPF, showing diffuse bronchial wall thickening, centrilobular nodules, ground-glass opacity, upper lung predominant emphysema, and lower lung predominant air trapping.[88] The ground-glass opacities may be diffuse or patchy, often with a peripheral predominance in the lung.[89] Similar ground-glass opacification, without basal or peripheral predominance, may be found in patients with RB-ILD[90] or hypersensitivity pneumonitis.[24, 91] Even with HRCT, the honeycombed pattern is rarely found.[92, 93]

Pulmonary function testing may be normal but usually shows mild to moderate restriction, normal or slightly reduced diffusing capacity, and mild hypoxemia. A mixed obstructive-restrictive pattern is common, while isolated increases in residual volume may be seen.

## Pathologic Features

The prominent pathologic features (Fig. 57.7) are those of inflammatory processes involving the membranous and respiratory bronchioles, associated with the accumulation of tan-brown pigmented macrophages within respiratory bronchioles as well as neighboring alveolar ducts and alveoli.[85, 87, 94] The bronchiole may be ectatic with mucous stasis, and the walls are mildly thickened. There is frequently evidence of extension of the bronchiolar metaplastic epithelium into the immediately surrounding alveoli. The pulmonary parenchyma away from the airway is usually normal or may demonstrate mild hyperinflation. These findings are sometimes so subtle as to be missed during routine evaluation, and examination of multiple sections may be required to find these abnormalities.[87]

Bedrossian and colleagues[95] coined the term "DIP-like reaction" to identify prominent intra-alveolar macrophage accumulation around space-occupying pulmonary lesions.[5] This DIP-like reaction is usually minimal, however, and does not have the uniform involvement of lung parenchyma as does RB-ILD. This DIP-like pattern can be seen in a number of other processes and is usually easily distinguished from DIP: Eosinophilic granuloma, drug reactions (e.g., amiodarone), chronic alveolar hemorrhage, eosinophilic pneumonia, pneumoconioses (e.g., talcosis, hard metal disease, asbestosis), obstructive pneumonias, and exogenous lipoid pneumonia.

## Clinical Course and Outcome

Because there has not been a longitudinal study of a large group of RB-ILD subjects, the clinical course and prognosis of RB-ILD are unknown. Most studies suggest a favorable response to corticosteroids, with documented improvement in lung function and chest radiographs,[85, 87] and no deaths have been reported.

Patients with the DIP stage of this process also have a good prognosis. Carrington and associates[96] reported a 28% mortality rate after an average survival of 12 years

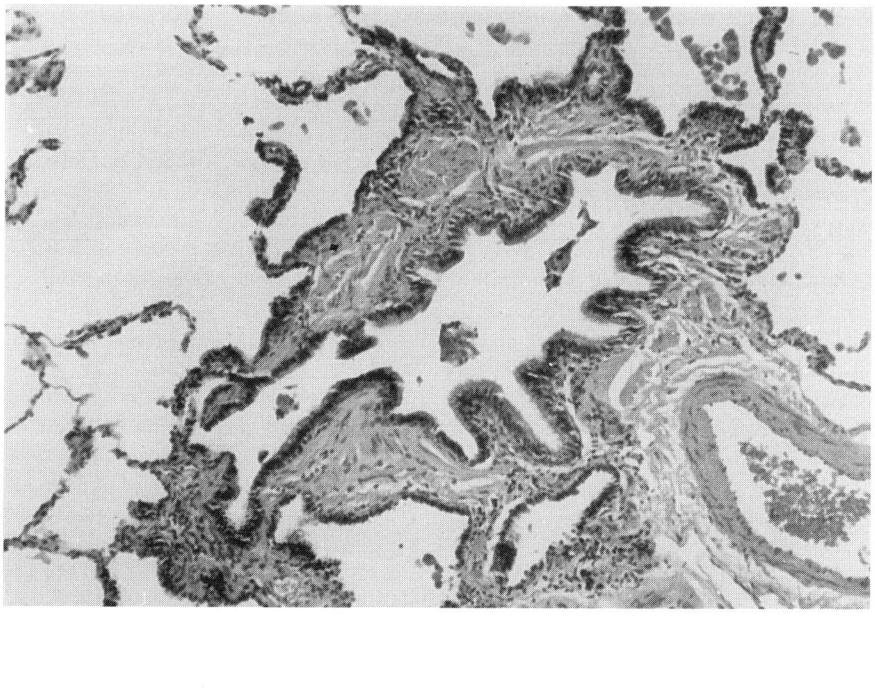

**Figure 57.7** The photomicrograph of respiratory bronchiolitis shows an ectatic small airway, with thickened walls and evidence of extension of the bronchiolar metaplastic epithelium into the immediately surrounding alveoli. Intraluminal macrophages are also present within the peribronchiolar alveolar spaces.

in their series. Other studies have shown similar results, but additional studies of a larger number of subjects are needed.[35, 87, 92, 93] Smoking plays a major role in the pathogenesis, and smoking cessation has been associated with resolution of the symptoms and improvement in the radiographic and physiologic abnormalities. Corticosteroids may be required in refractory or recurrent cases but should not be instituted in the absence of smoking cessation.

## ACUTE INTERSTITIAL PNEUMONIA

Acute interstitial pneumonia (AIP) is a rare fulminant form of lung injury that presents acutely (days to weeks from onset of symptoms), usually in a previously healthy individual.[97] AIP likely represents the subset of cases of idiopathic acute respiratory distress syndrome (ARDS) and is what Hamman and Rich[3] described and termed *acute diffuse interstitial fibrosis.*

Most patients are over the age of 40 years (mean age, 50 years; range, 7 to 83 years). There is no sex predilection. A prodromal illness, lasting usually 7 to 14 days before presentation, is common. The clinical signs and symptoms include fever, cough, and shortness of breath. Routine laboratory studies are nonspecific and generally not helpful.

Diffuse, bilateral, air-space opacification is seen on chest radiograph.[98] CT scans show bilateral, patchy, symmetric areas of ground-glass attenuation. Bilateral areas of air space consolidation may also be present. A predominantly subpleural distribution may be seen. Mild honeycombing, usually involving less than 10% of the lung, may be seen on CT examination. These radiographic findings are similar to those seen in ARDS.

Most patients have moderate to severe hypoxemia and develop respiratory failure. Mechanical ventilation is often required. A surgical lung biopsy is required to confirm the diagnosis of organizing diffuse alveolar damage, the histopathologic counterpart of AIP.[99]

The mortality from AIP is high (more than 60%), with most patients dying within 3 months of presentation. Those who recover, however, usually do not have recurrence of the disease, and most have substantial or complete recovery of lung function. It is not clear that corticosteroid therapy is effective in AIP. The main treatment is supportive care.

## CRYPTOGENIC ORGANIZING PNEUMONIA

Cryptogenic organizing pneumonitis (COP) is a specific clinicopathologic syndrome characterized by a "pneumonia-like" illness, with excessive proliferation of granulation tissue within small airways and alveolar ducts, associated with chronic inflammation in the surrounding alveoli (i.e., bronchiolitis obliterans with organizing pneumonia [BOOP]).[100]

### Clinical Features

The incidence of COP is nearly the same for men (54%) and women (46%). The mean age at presentation is about 58 years (range, 21 to 80 years). Patients with COP are frequently very specific about the time of their disease onset. This is because the disease onset is recent, within usually less than 2 months, and is often dramatic with the development of a flu-like illness, characterized by cough, fever, malaise, fatigue, and weight loss. Inspiratory crackles are frequently present on chest examination. Finger clubbing is rare in patients with COP. Routine laboratory studies are nonspecific. A leukocytosis without increase in eosinophils is seen in approximately half the patients. The initial erythrocyte sedimentation rate is frequently elevated in patients with COP.

The roentgenographic manifestations are distinctive with bilateral, diffuse alveolar opacities in the presence of normal lung volume being characteristic (see Fig. 56.15).[101–103] A peripheral distribution of the infiltrates, very similar to that thought to be "virtually pathognomic" for chronic eosinophilic pneumonia, is commonly seen in COP.[103–105] Irregular linear or nodular interstitial infiltrates are rarely present as the only radiographic manifestation. Honeycombing is rare and is seen only as a late manifestation in the few patients with progressive disease. Other radiographic abnormalities, such as pleural effusion, pleural thickening, hyperinflation, and cavities, are rare. CT scans of the lung reveal patchy air-space consolidation, small nodular opacities, and bronchial wall thickening and dilation, most frequently in the periphery of the lung and often in the lower lung zone.[103, 106–109] Frequently, the CT findings are far more extensive than is expected by review of the plain chest x-ray.

Pulmonary function is usually impaired, with a restrictive defect being most common although an obstructive defect ($FEV_1/FVC$ ratio less than 70%) is found in almost one fifth of subjects with COP, mostly in current or former smokers. Gas exchange abnormalities are extremely common with resting and exercise arterial hypoxemia. The $D_{L_{CO}}$ is reduced (less than 80% of predicted) in three fourths of the patients.

### Pathologic Features

The diagnosis of COP depends on both the clinical setting and the finding of the characteristic pathologic features. Intraluminal fibrotic buds (Masson bodies) seen in respiratory bronchioles, alveolar ducts, and alveoli are the prominent feature (see Figs. 56.5 and 56.6).[64, 86, 110–112] Other pathologic features include foamy cells in the alveolar spaces, prominent type 2 cell hyperplasia, interstitial infiltrates, and fibrinous exudates.

### Clinical Course and Outcome

Corticosteroid therapy results in complete clinical, radiologic, and physiologic recovery in two thirds of patients. One third demonstrate recurrent or persistent disease. In general, clinical improvement is rapid (i.e., within several days or a few weeks). Occasionally recovery was quite dramatic. Relapses can occur when the corticosteroids are withdrawn, usually within 1 to 3 months. Most will improve when retreated with corticosteroids. Spontaneous improvement may occur over 3 to 6 months in some patients.[101, 113] Few of the patients with COP die as a result of this illness, but those prone to develop a rapidly progressive fatal form of BOOP have a clinical course similar to the "Hamman-Rich syndrome."[114] In such patients, the diagnosis is usually delayed or missed.

## LYMPHOCYTIC INTERSTITIAL PNEUMONIA

Lymphocytic interstitial pneumonia (LIP) is an uncommon pathologic process characterized by widespread, monotonous sheets of lymphocytic infiltration in the interstitium of the lung.[115] In addition to being differentiated from IPF, it must be distinguished from lymphocytic infiltrations associated with pseudolymphoma, primary lymphomas, lymphomatoid granulomatosis, benign lymphocytic angiitis and granulomatosis, plasma cell interstitial pneumonia, and angioimmunoblastic lymphadenopathy. LIP is commonly found in association with other immunologic disorders, especially hypogammaglobulinemic or hypergammaglobulinemic conditions and Sjögren's syndrome (Table 57.6).

### Clinical Features

The clinical manifestations of LIP are dominated by those related to the underlying disease, such as Sjögren's syndrome (see Chapter 58). LIP occurs more commonly in women usually in the fourth to sixth decade of life. It is also seen in children, particularly those with hypogammaglobulinemia or the acquired immunodeficiency syndrome (AIDS). Progressive dyspnea and cough are the most common presenting symptoms, while weight loss, pleuritic pain, arthralgias, and fever also occur. Bibasilar rales on chest examination, cyanosis, and finger clubbing are common physical findings. The chest radiograph is nonspecific, with reticular opacities being the most frequent abnormality. As a result of the coalescence of the opacities, a mixed alveolar-interstitial pattern appears as the disease progresses. Cysts, honeycombing, and pulmonary hypertension are also late manifestations.[116] Pleural effusions are infrequent and suggest a complicating lymphoma. A restrictive defect is commonly seen often associated with a reduction in the carbon monoxide diffusing capacity and arterial hypoxemia. A striking T-cell lymphocytosis is seen on bronchoalveolar lavage.

**Table 57.6 DISEASES ASSOCIATED WITH LYMPHOCYTIC INTERSTITIAL PNEUMONITIS**

| |
|---|
| IDIOPATHIC DISEASE WITHOUT DYSPROTEINEMIA |
| DISEASE WITH DYSPROTEINEMIA |
| Hypogammaglobulinemia |
| Monoclonal or polyclonal gammopathy |
| AUTOIMMUNE DISEASES |
| Sjögren's syndrome |
| Chronic active hepatitis |
| Primary biliary cirrhosis |
| Myasthenia gravis |
| Hashimoto's thyroiditis |
| Pernicious anemia |
| Autoimmune hemolytic anemia |
| Systemic lupus erythematosus |
| ALLOGENEIC BONE MARROW TRANSPLANTATION |
| ACQUIRED IMMUNODEFICIENCY SYNDROME |
| MISCELLANEOUS |
| Tuberculosis |
| Celiac sprue |
| Dilantin |

Adapted with permission from Schwartz MI: Lymphocytic infiltrative disorders. *In* Schwarz MI, King TE Jr (eds): Interstitial Lung Diseases. Philadelphia: BC Decker, 1988, p 294.

### Pathologic Features

Open lung biopsy is required for the diagnosis in almost all cases. The lymphocytic infiltration is usually extensive and severe, involving the alveolar septa and peribronchiolar and perivascular interstitium. The lymphocytes are polytypic (both B and T cells may be found), distinguishing them from the monotypic lymphocytic infiltrates characteristic of pulmonary lymphoma. The number of plasma cells and macrophages is also increased in these infiltrates. Other prominent histopathologic features include the accumulation of large interstitial reticuloendothelial cells, mononuclear cells, and giant cells forming noncaseating granulomas; the presence of perivascular and paraseptal amyloid deposition; and well-formed lymphoid germinal centers.

### Clinical Course and Outcome

The clinical course of idiopathic LIP is unknown. When LIP is associated with another disease, the underlying disease largely determines the outcome. Marked improvement or complete resolution followed corticosteroid therapy in many case reports. Progressive pulmonary fibrosis, cor pulmonale, and death can occur despite therapy. Infection is a common complication in these patients, especially those with an associated dysproteinemia. Progression to pulmonary or systemic lymphoma can occur but appears quite rare.

## NONSPECIFIC INTERSTITIAL PNEUMONIA

It is extremely important that the pathologist not use UIP to refer to any nonspecific or nonclassifiable interstitial pneumonia (NSIP). The latter conditions are a heterogeneous group of poorly defined interstitial pneumonias that histologically do not fit with other recognizable clinicopathologic entities.[4, 117, 118] In our experience, some of these cases represent a sampling error as a result of an inadequate lung biopsy. Others have an ill-defined or inadequately evaluated connective tissue disease, drug-induced interstitial lung disease, or chronic hypersensitivity pneumonitis. Patients who are known to be immunocompromised are not included in this group of patients. A number of potential etiologies or associated conditions were identified as connective-tissue diseases (rheumatoid arthritis, systemic lupus erythematosus, polymyositis, scleroderma, and Sjögren's syndrome), hypersensitivity pneumonia, drug-induced lung injury, recent acute lung injury (pneumonia or ARDS), and coronary artery bypass surgery.[5]

## Clinical Features

The presentation is quite similar to that of other forms of idiopathic pneumonias. Most patients have been middle-aged adults, with a subacute onset of symptoms of approximately 8 months before diagnosis.[4, 117–119] There appears to be a slight female predominance (1.4:1). Dyspnea and cough are the most common presenting complaints. Fever and systemic flu-like symptoms are common.[117, 119] The chest radiograph usually shows bilateral reticular opacities. A normal chest radiograph was seen in 7% of cases.[4, 117–119] Bilateral, patchy areas of ground-glass attenuation are characteristic CT findings.[118]

## Pathologic Features

Katzenstein and Myers[5] summarized the main histopathologic features of NSIP. NSIP is characterized by the presence of varying degrees of inflammation and fibrosis within alveolar walls. The changes are temporally uniform, but the process may be patchy with intervening areas of unaffected lung. The process is frequently accentuated in the peribronchiolar interstitium, and the density of the inflammatory infiltrate is considerably greater than that occurring in other idiopathic interstitial pneumonias.[5] Type II cell hyperplasia often accompanies the interstitial inflammation and may be prominent. Except for the uniform nature of the process, some cases with prominent fibrosis characterized by intermingling collagen bundles, lymphocytes, plasma cells, and occasionally fibroblasts may be difficult to distinguish from UIP.[5] Also, fibroblast foci and intraluminal organization characteristic of bronchiolitis obliterans with organizing pneumonia can be found. Patchy intra-alveolar macrophage accumulation occurs in 30% of cases, and the macrophages may be admixed with variable numbers of lymphoid cells.[5] Lymphoid aggregates with germinal centers (so-called lymphoid hyperplasia) were reported in approximately one fourth of NSIP cases.[5] Rarely, poorly formed, nonnecrotizing granulomas accompany the other changes, but they are always focal.

## Clinical Course and Outcome

Patients with NSIP appear to have clinical outcomes different from those of patients with AIP, UIP, DIP, or bronchiolitis obliterans with organizing pneumonia. Importantly, unlike patients with IPF (UIP), most patients with NSIP have a good prognosis, with most showing improvement after treatment with corticosteroids. The prognosis appears to depend on the extent of fibrosis.[5]

## References


1. Schwarz MI, King TE Jr: Interstitial Lung Diseases (3rd ed). Hamilton, Ontario: BC Decker, 1998.
2. Hamman L, Rich AR: Fulminating diffuse interstitial fibrosis of the lungs. Trans Am Clin Climatol Assoc 51:154–163, 1935.
3. Hamman L, Rich AR: Acute diffuse interstitial fibrosis of the lungs. Bull Johns Hopkins Hosp 74:177–212, 1944.
4. Bjoraker JA, Ryu JH, Edwin MK, et al: Prognostic significance of histopathologic subsets in idiopathic pulmonary fibrosis. Am J Respir Crit Care Med 157:199–203, 1998.
5. Katzenstein ALA, Myers JL: Idiopathic pulmonary fibrosis. Clinical relevance of pathologic classification. Am J Respir Crit Care Med 157:1301–1315, 1998.
6. King TE Jr: Idiopathic pulmonary fibrosis. *In* Schwarz MI, King TE Jr (eds): Interstitial Lung Diseases (3rd ed). Hamilton, Ontario: BC. Decker, 1998, 597–644.
7. Coultas DB: Epidemiology of idiopathic pulmonary fibrosis. Semin Respir Med 14:181–196, 1993.
8. Coultas DB, Zumwalt RE, Black WC, et al: The epidemiology of interstitial lung disease. Am J Respir Crit Care Med 150:967–972, 1994.
9. Hubbard R, Johnston IDA, Coultas D, et al: Mortality rates from cryptogenic fibrosing alveolitis is seven countries. Thorax 51:711–716, 1996.
10. Dreisin RB, Schwarz MI, Theofilopoulos AN, et al: Circulating immune complexes in the idiopathic interstitial pneumonias. N Engl J Med 298:353–357, 1978.
11. Wells AU, Hansell DM, Rubens MB, et al: The predictive value of appearances on thin-section computed tomography in fibrosing alveolitis. Am Rev Respir Dis 148:1076–1082, 1993.
12. Wells AU, Rubens MB, du Bois RM, et al: Serial CT in fibrosing alveolitis: Prognostic significance of the initial pattern. AJR Am J Roentgenol 161:1159–1165, 1993.
13. Orens JB, Kazerooni EA, Martinez FJ, et al: The sensitivity of high-resolution CT in detecting idiopathic pulmonary fibrosis proved by open lung biopsy. A prospective study. Chest 108:109–115, 1995.
14. Hiwatari N, Shimura S, Takishima T: Pulmonary emphysema followed by pulmonary fibrosis of undetermined cause. Respiration 60:354–358, 1993.
15. Staples C, Muller N, Vedal S, et al: Usual interstitial pneumonia: Correlation of CT with clinical, functional, and radiographic findings. Radiology 162:377–381, 1987.
16. Wells AU, King AD, Rubens MB, et al: Lone cryptogenic fibrosing alveolitis: A functional-morphologic correlation based on extent of disease on thin-section computed tomography. Am J Respir Crit Care Med 155:1367–1375, 1997.
17. Xaubet A, Agusti C, Luburich P, et al: Pulmonary function tests and CT scan in the management of idiopathic pulmonary fibrosis. Am J Respir Crit Care Med 158:431–436, 1998.
18. Johkoh T, Ikezoe J, Kohno N, et al: High-resolution CT and pulmonary function tests in collagen vascular disease: Comparison with idiopathic pulmonary fibrosis. Eur J Radiol 18:113–121, 1994.
19. Wells AU, Hansell DM, Rubens MB, et al: Fibrosing alveolitis in systemic sclerosis: Indices of lung function in relation to extent of disease on computed tomography. Arthritis Rheum 40:1229–1236, 1997.
20. Aberle DR, Gamsu G, Ray CS, et al: Asbestos-related pleural and parenchymal fibrosis: Detection with high-resolution CT. Radiology 166:729–734, 1988.
21. Aberle DR, Gamsu G, Ray CS: High-resolution CT of benign asbestos-related diseases: Clinical and radiographic correlation. Am J Radiol 151:883–891, 1988.
22. Gamsu G, Aberle DR, Lynch D: Computed tomography in the diagnosis of asbestos-related thoracic disease. J Thorac Imag 4:61–67, 1989.
23. Lynch D, Gamsu G, Aberle D: Conventional and high resolution CT in the diagnosis of asbestos-related diseases. Radiographics 9:523–551, 1989.
24. Lynch DA, Newell JD, Logan PM, et al: Can CT distinguish idiopathic pulmonary fibrosis from hypersensitivity pneumonitis? AJR Am J Roentgenol 165:807–811, 1995.
25. Grenier P, Valeyre D, Cluzel P, et al: Chronic diffuse interstitial lung disease: Diagnostic value of chest radiography and high-resolution CT. Radiology 179:123–132, 1991.
26. Mathieson JR, Mayo JR, Staples CA, et al: Chronic diffuse infiltrative lung disease: Comparison of diagnostic accuracy of CT and chest radiography. Radiology 171:111–116, 1989.
27. Tung KT, Wells AU, Rubens MB, et al: Accuracy of the typical computed tomographic appearances of fibrosing alveolitis. Thorax 48:334–338, 1993.
28. Hanley ME, King TE Jr, Schwarz MI, et al: The impact of smoking on mechanical properties of the lungs in idiopathic pulmonary fibrosis and sarcoidosis. Am Rev Respir Dis 144:1102–1106, 1991.

29. Watters LC, Schwarz MI, Cherniack RM, et al: Idiopathic pulmonary fibrosis: Pretreatment bronchoalveolar lavage cellular constituents and their relationships with lung histopathology and clinical response to therapy. Am Rev Respir Dis 135:696–704, 1987.
30. Cherniack RM, Colby TV, Flint A, et al: Quantitative assessment of lung pathology in idiopathic pulmonary fibrosis. Am Rev Respir Dis 144:892–900, 1991.
31. Hyde DM, King TE Jr, McDermott T, et al: Idiopathic pulmonary fibrosis: The quantitative assessment of lung pathology. Comparison of a semi-quantitative versus a morphometric histopathologic scoring system. Am Rev Respir Dis 146:1042–1047, 1992.
32. Scott J, Johnston I, Britton J: What causes cryptogenic fibrosing alveolitis? A case-control study of environmental exposure to dust. BMJ 301:1015–1017, 1990.
33. Hubbard R, Lewis S, Richards K, et al: Occupational exposure to metal or wood dust and aetiology of cryptogenic fibrosing alveolitis. Lancet 347:284–289, 1996.
34. Baumgartner KB, Samet J, Stidley CA, et al: Cigarette smoking: A risk factor for idiopathic pulmonary fibrosis. Am J Respir Crit Care Med 155:242–248, 1997.
35. Gaensler EA, Goff AM, Prowse CM: Desquamative interstitial pneumonia. N Engl J Med 274:113–128, 1966.
36. Kuisk H, Sanchez JS: Desquamative interstitial pneumonia and idiopathic diffuse pulmonary fibrosis with their advanced final stages as "muscular cirrhosis of the lungs" (diffuse bronchiolectasis with muscular hyperplasia. AJR Am J Roentgenol 107:258–279, 1969.
37. Tubbs RR, Benjamin SP, Osborne DG, et al: Surface and transmission ultrastructural characteristics of desquamative interstitial pneumonitis. Hum Pathol 9:693–703, 1978.
38. Patchefsky AS, Banner M, Freundlich IM: Desquamative interstitial pneumonia significance of intranuclear viral-like inclusion bodies. Ann Intern Med 74:322–327, 1971.
39. Kawanami O, Ferrans VJ, Fulmer JD, et al: Nuclear inclusions in alveolar epithelium of patients with fibrotic lung disorders. Am J Pathol 94:301–312, 1979.
40. Shortland JR, Darke CS, Crane WAJ: Electron microscopy of desquamative interstitial pneumonia. Thorax 24:192–208, 1969.
41. McNary WFJ, Gaensler EA: Intranuclear inclusion bodies in desquamative interstitial pneumonia. Electron microscopic observations. Ann Intern Med 74:404–407, 1971.
42. Kuwano K, Nomoto Y, Kunitake R, et al: Detection of adenovirus E1A DNA in pulmonary fibrosis using nested polymerase chain reaction. Eur Respir J 10:1445–1449, 1997.
43. Egan JJ, Woodcock AA, Stewart JP: Viruses and idiopathic pulmonary fibrosis. Eur Respir J 10:1433–1437, 1997.
44. Vergnon JM, Vincent M, De The G, et al: Cryptogenic fibrosing alveolitis and Epstein-Barr virus: An association? Lancet 2:768–771, 1984.
45. Raghu G, Mageto YN: Genetic predisposition of interstitial lung disease. *In* Schwarz MI, King TE Jr (eds): Interstitial Lung Diseases (3rd ed). Hamilton, Ontario: BC Decker, 1998, pp 119–134.
46. McCormack FX, King TE, Jr, Voelker DR, et al: Idiopathic pulmonary fibrosis: Abnormalities in the bronchoalveolar lavage content of surfactant protein A. Am Rev Respir Dis 144:160–166, 1991.
47. McCormack FX, King TE Jr, Bucher BL, et al: Surfactant protein A predicts survival in idiopathic pulmonary fibrosis. Am J Respir Crit Care Med 152:751–759, 1995.
48. Raghu G: Interstitial lung disease: A diagnostic approach. Are CT scan and lung biopsy indicated in every patient? Am J Respir Crit Care Med 151:909–914, 1995.
49. Bensard DD, McIntyre RC Jr, Waring BJ, et al: Comparison of video thoracoscopic lung biopsy to open lung biopsy in the diagnosis of interstitial lung disease. Chest 103:765–770, 1993.
50. Ferson PF, Landreneau RJ, Dowling RD, et al: Comparison of open versus thorascopic lung biopsy for diffuse infiltrative pulmonary disease. J Thoracic Cardiovasc Surg 106:194–199, 1993.
51. Gay SE, Kazerooni EA, Toews GB, et al: Idiopathic pulmonary fibrosis: Predicting response to therapy and survival. Am J Respir Crit Care Med 157:1063–1072, 1998.
52. Daniil ZD, Gilchrist FC, Nicholson AG, et al: A histologic pattern of nonspecific interstitial pneumonia is associated with a better prognosis than usual interstitial pneumonia in patients with cryptogenic fibrosing alveolitis. Am J Respir Crit Care Med 160:899–905, 1999.
53. Turner-Warwick M, Burrows B, Johnson A: Cryptogenic fibrosing alveolitis: Clinical features and their influence on survival. Thorax 35:171–180, 1980.
54. Fulmer JD, Roberts WC, von Gal ER, et al: Morphologic-physiologic correlates of the severity of fibrosis and degree of cellularity in idiopathic pulmonary fibrosis. J Clin Invest 63:665–676, 1979.
55. Crystal RG, Gadek JE, Ferrans VJ, et al: Interstitial lung disease: Current concepts of pathogenesis, staging, and therapy. Am J Med 70:542–568, 1981.
56. Turner-Warwick M, Haslam PL: The value of serial bronchoalveolar lavages in assessing the clinical progress of patients with cryptogenic fibrosing alveolitis. Am Rev Respir Dis 135:26–34, 1987.
57. Schreiner R, Mortenson RL, Ikle D, et al: Interstitial lung disease in the elderly. *In* Mahler D (ed): Pulmonary Disease in the Elderly (Vol 63). New York: Marcel Dekker 1993, pp 339–385.
58. Watters LC, King TE, Schwarz MI, et al: A clinical, radiographic, and physiologic scoring system for the longitudinal assessment of patients with idiopathic pulmonary fibrosis. Am Rev Respir Dis 133:97–103, 1986.
59. Peters SG, McDougall JC, Douglas WW, et al: Colchicine in the treatment of pulmonary fibrosis. Chest 103:101–104, 1993.
60. Douglas WW, Ryu JH, Swensen SJ, et al: Colchicine versus prednisone in the treatment of idiopathic pulmonary fibrosis. A randomized prospective study. Members of the Lung Study Group. Am J Respir Crit Care Med 158:220–225, 1998.
61. Raghu G, Johnson WC, Lockhart D, et al: Treatment of idiopathic pulmonary fibrosis with a new antifibrotic agent, pirfenidone: Results of a prospective, open-label Phase II study. Am J Respir Crit Care Med 159(4, part 1):1061–1069, 1999.
62. International Guidelines for the Selection of Lung Transplant Candidates. Am J Respir Crit Care Med 158:335–339, 1998.
63. Panos RJ, Mortenson R, Niccoli SA, et al: Clinical deterioration in patients with idiopathic pulmonary fibrosis. Causes and assessment. Am J Med 88:396–404, 1990.
64. Kitaichi M: Pathologic features and the classification of interstitial pneumonia of unknown etiology. Bull Chest Dis Res Inst Kyoto Univ 23:1–18, 1990.
65. Kondoh Y, Taniguchi H, Kawabata Y, et al: Acute exacerbation in idiopathic pulmonary fibrosis. Analysis of clinical and pathologic findings in three cases. Chest 103:1808–1812, 1993.
66. Hiwatari N, Shimura S, Takishima T, et al: Bronchoalveolar lavage as a possible cause of acute exacerbation in idiopathic pulmonary fibrosis patients. Tohoku J Exp Med 174:379–386, 1994.
67. Barzo P: Familial idiopathic fibrosing alveolitis. Eur J Respir Dis 66:350–352, 1985.
68. Bitterman PB, Rennard SI, Keogh BA, et al: Familial idiopathic pulmonary fibrosis. Evidence of lung inflammation in unaffected family members. N Engl J Med 314:1343–1347, 1986.
69. Renzi GD, Lopez-Majano V: Early diagnosis of interstitial fibrosis. Respiration 33:294–302, 1976.
70. Riccardi VM: Von Recklinghausen neurofibromatosis. N Engl J Med. 305:1617–1627, 1981.
71. DePinho RA, Kaplan KL: The Hermansky-Pudlak syndrome. Report of three cases and review of pathophysiology and management considerations. Medicine 64:192–202, 1985.
72. Hermansky F, Pudlak P: Albinism associated with hemorrhagic diatheses and unusual pigmented reticular cells in the bone marrow. Report of two cases of histochemical studies. Blood 14:162–169, 1959.
73. Hoste P, Willems J, Devriendt J, et al: J, Familial diffuse interstitial pulmonary fibrosis associated with oculocutaneous albinism. Report of two cases with a family study. Scand J Respir Dis 60:128–134, 1970.
74. Garay SM, Gardella JE, Fazzini EP, et al: Hermansky-Pudlak syndrome: Pulmonary manifestations of a family study. Am J Med 66:219–232, 1979.
75. Davies BH, Tuddenham EGD: Familial pulmonary fibrosis associated with oculocutaneous albinism and platelet function defect. Q J Med 65:219–232, 1976.
76. Dwyer JM, Hickie JB, Garvan J: Pulmonary tuberous sclerosis.

Report of three patients and a review of the literature. Q J Med 40:115–125, 1971.
77. Berg G, Vejlens G: Maladie kystique du poumon et sclerose tubereuse du cerveau. Acta Paediatr 26:16–30, 1939.
78. Makle SK, Pardee N, Martin CJ: Involvement of the lung in tuberous sclerosis. Chest 58:538–540, 1970.
79. Harris JO, Waltuck BL, Swenson EW: The pathophysiology of the lungs in tuberous sclerosis. A case report and literature review. Am Rev Respir Dis 100:379–387, 1969.
80. Master K, Ting EY, Katz M: Pathophysiology in pulmonary tuberous sclerosis. N Y State J Med 74:2000–2003, 1974.
81. Schneider EL, Epstein CJ, Kaback MJ, et al: Severe pulmonary involvement in adult Gaucher's disease Report of three cases and review of the literature. Am J Med 63:475–480, 1977.
82. Wolson AH: Pulmonary findings in Gaucher's disease. AJR Am J Roentgenol 123:712–715, 1975.
83. Carrington CB, Cergell DW, Gaensler EA, et al: Lymphangioleiomyomatosis. Physiologic-pathologic-radiology correlations. Am Rev Respir Dis 116:977–995, 1977.
84. Wright JL, Lawson LM, Pare PD, et al: Morphology of peripheral airways in current smokers and ex-smokers. Am Rev Respir Dis 127:474–477, 1983.
85. Myers JL, Veal CF, Shin MS, et al: Respiratory bronchiolitis causing interstitial lung disease: A clinicopathologic study of six cases. Am Rev Respir Dis 135:880–884, 1987.
86. Guerry-Force ML, Mueller NL, Wright JL, et al: A comparison of bronchiolitis obliterans with organizing pneumonia, usual interstitial pneumonia, and small airways disease. Am Rev Respir Dis 135:705–712, 1987.
87. Yousem SA, Colby TV, Gaensler EA: Respiratory bronchiolitis-associated interstitial lung disease and its relationship to desquamative interstitial pneumonia. Mayo Clin Proc 64:1373–1380, 1989.
88. Park JS, Brown KK, Hale VA, et al: Respiratory bronchiolitis associated interstitial lung disease: Radiologic features with clinical correlation. Radiology, in press.
89. Hartman TE, Primack SL, Swensen SJ, et al: Desquamative interstitial pneumonia: Thin-section CT findings in 22 patients. Radiology 187:787–790, 1993.
90. Holt RM, Schmidt RA, Godwin D, et al: High resolution CT in respiratory bronchiolitis-associated interstitial lung disease. J Comput Assist Tomogr 17:46–50, 1993.
91. Silver SF, Muller NL, Miller RR, et al: Hypersensitivity pneumonitis: Evaluation with CT. Radiology 173:441–445, 1989.
92. Hartman TE, Primack SL, Kang EY, et al: Disease progression in usual interstitial pneumonia compared with desquamative interstitial pneumonia. Assessment with serial CT. Chest 110:378–382, 1996.
93. Akira M, Yamamoto S, Hara H, et al: Serial computed tomographic evaluation in desquamative interstitial pneumonia. Thorax 52:333–337, 1997.
94. Niewoehner D, Kleinerman J, Rice D: Pathologic changes in the peripheral airways of young cigarette smokers. N Engl J Med 291:755–758, 1974.
95. Bedrossian CW, Kuhn MC III, Luna MA, et al: Desquamative interstitial pneumonia-like reaction accompanying pulmonary lesions. Chest 72:166–169, 1977.
96. Carrington CB, Gaensler EA, Coutu RE, et al: Natural history and treated course of usual and desquamative interstitial pneumonia. N Engl J Med 298:801–809, 1978.
97. Olson J, Colby TV, Elliott CG: Hamman-Rich syndrome revisited. Mayo Clin Proc 65:1538–1548, 1990.
98. Primack SL, Hartman TE, Ikezoe J, et al: Acute interstitial pneumonia: Radiographic and CT findings in nine patients. Radiology 188:817–820, 1993.
99. Askin FB: Acute interstitial pneumonia: Histopathologic patterns of acute lung injury and the Hamman-Rich syndrome revisited [editorial; comment]. Radiology 188:620–621, 1993.
100. Wright L, King TE Jr: Cryptogenic organizing pneumonia (idiopathic bronchiolitis obliterans organizing pneumonia): An update. Clin Pulmonary Med 4:152–158, 1997.
101. Epler GR, Colby TV, McLoud TC, et al: Bronchiolitis obliterans organizing pneumonia. N Engl J Med 312:152–158, 1985.
102. Chandler PW, Shin MS, Friedman SE, et al: Radiographic manifestations of bronchiolitis obliterans with organizing pneumonia versus usual interstitial pneumonia. AJR 147:899–906, 1986.
103. Muller NL, Guerry-Force ML, Staples CA, et al: Differential diagnosis of bronchiolitis obliterans with organizing pneumonia and usual interstitial pneumonia clinical, functional, and radiologic findings. Radiology 162:151–156, 1987.
104. Davison AG, Heard BE, McAllister WAC, et al: Cryptogenic organizing pneumonitis. Q J Med 52:382–394, 1983.
105. Bartter T, Irwin RS, Nash G, et al: Idiopathic bronchiolitis obliterans organizing pneumonia with peripheral infiltrates on chest roentgenogram. Arch Intern Med 149:273–279, 1989.
106. Nishimura K, Itoh H: Is CT useful in differentiating between BOOP and idiopathic UIP? *In* Harasawa M, Fukuchi Y, Morinari H (eds): Interstitial Pneumonia of Unknown Etiology. Tokyo: University of Tokyo Press, 1989, pp 317–324.
107. Muller NL, Staples CA, Miller RR: Bronchiolitis obliterans organizing pneumonia: CT features in 14 patients. AJR Am J Roentgenol 154:983–987, 1990.
108. Muller NL, Miller RR: Computed tomography of chronic diffuse infiltrative lung disease, Part 1. Am Rev Respir Dis 142:1206–1215, 1990.
109. Preidler KW, Szolar DM, Moelleken S, et al: Distribution pattern of computed tomography findings in patients with bronchiolitis obliterans organizing pneumonia. Invest Radiol 31:251–255, 1996.
110. Katzenstein ALA, Myers JL, Prophet DW, et al: Bronchiolitis obliterans and usual interstitial pneumonia. Am J Surg Pathol 10:373–381, 1986.
111. Myers JL, Katzenstein AL: Ultrastructural evidence of alveolar epithelial injury in idiopathic bronchiolitis obliterans-organizing pneumonia. Am J Pathol 132:102–109, 1988.
112. Kuhn C III, Boldt J, King TE Jr, et al: An immunohistochemical study of architectural remodeling and connective tissue synthesis in pulmonary fibrosis. Am Rev Respir Dis 140:1693–1703, 1989.
113. Yamamoto M, Ina Y, Kitaichi M: Bronchiolitis obliterans organizing pneumonia (BOOP): Profile in Japan. *In* Harasawa M, Fukuchi Y, Morinari H (eds): Interstitial Pneumonia of Unknown Etiology. Tokyo: University of Tokyo Press, 1989, pp 61–70.
114. Cohen AJ, King TE Jr, Downey GP: Rapidly progressive bronchiolitis obliterans with organizing pneumonia. Am J Respir Crit Care Med 149:1670–1675, 1994.
115. Koss MN, Hochholzer L, Langloss JM, et al: Lymphoid interstitial pneumonia: Clinicopathological and immunopathologic findings in 18 cases. Pathology 19:178–185, 1987.
116. Ichikawa Y, Kinoshita M, Koga T, et al: Lung cyst formation in lymphocytic interstitial pnuemonia: CT features. J Comput Assist Tomogr 18:745–748, 1994.
117. Katzenstein AL, Fiorelli RF: Nonspecific interstitial pneumonia/fibrosis. Histologic features and clinical significance. Am J Surg Pathol 18:136–147, 1994.
118. Park JS, Lee KS, Kim JS, et al: Nonspecific interstitial pneumonia with fibrosis: Radiographic and CT findings in seven patients. Radiology 195:645–648, 1995.
119. Kim EY, Lee KS, Chung MP, et al: Nonspecific interstitial pneumonia with fibrosis: Serial high-resolution CT findings with functional correlation. AJR Am J Roentgenol 173:949–953, 1999.
120. King TE Jr: Bronchiolitis obliterans. *In* Schwarz MI, King TE Jr (eds): Interstitial Lung Diseases (3rd ed). Hamilton, Ontari: BC Decker, 1998, pp 645–684.
121. Cryer PE, Kissane JM, Clinicopathologic conference: Mixed connective tissue disease. Am J Med 65:833–842, 1978.

# 58 The Lungs and Connective Tissue Diseases

R. M. du Bois, M.D. • A. U. Wells, M.D.

Introduction
Systemic Sclerosis (Scleroderma)
Epidemiology and Risk Factors
Pulmonary Manifestations
Interstitial Pulmonary Fibrosis
Pulmonary Vascular Disease in Systemic Sclerosis
Other Pulmonary Complications
Rheumatoid Arthritis
Epidemiology and Risk Factors
Pulmonary Manifestations
Drug-Induced Lung Disease
Systemic Lupus Erythematosus
Epidemiology and Risk Factors
Pulmonary Manifestations
Sjögren's Syndrome
Epidemiology and Risk Factors
Pulmonary Manifestations
Polymyositis with Dermatomyositis
Epidemiology and Risk Factors
Pulmonary Manifestations
Mixed Connective Tissue Disease
Relapsing Polychondritis
Behçet's Disease
Ankylosing Spondylitis
Marfan's Syndrome

## INTRODUCTION

The lung may be involved in all connective tissue diseases.[1, 2] The involvement may be subclinical, but its true extent may be masked by exercise limitation due to musculoskeletal features of the connective tissue disease. Patterns of lung involvement vary considerably within each connective tissue disease. The differential diagnosis is made even wider after inclusion of the drug-induced pulmonary reactions (Table 58.1) and the opportunistic infections secondary to therapy for the lung disease (Table 58.2), which may present with features indistinguishable from diffuse lung disease.

It is not surprising that the lung is involved frequently in connective tissue disease because these are systemic syndromes, but it is disappointing that little is known about the true incidence and prevalence of lung disease because of the dearth of well-controlled prospective, unselected series. Imprecision of nomenclature also has confused the issue. With this background, the aims of this chapter are to highlight the ways in which the lung may be involved in the most common connective tissue diseases and to indicate, when appropriate, the most usual pattern of lung disease for each connective tissue disease, with an emphasis on approaches to diagnosis and efficient management.

## SYSTEMIC SCLEROSIS (SCLERODERMA)

The preliminary criteria for classification of systemic sclerosis (SSc) require that one major or two or more minor criteria are present (Table 58.3)[3] The skin changes may affect the entire extremity or face, neck, and trunk (thorax and abdomen). Scleroderma is traditionally classified on the basis of skin disease extent: Limited disease can involve the face, but the trunk and limbs proximal to the elbows and knees are spared. Diffuse disease can involve any part of the body.

### Epidemiology and Risk Factors

The incidence of SSc is approximately 2 to $20/10^6$ population/year, with a peak incidence in the fourth to sixth decades. The prevalence is 30 to $120/10^6$, with a 3:1 to 8:1 female preponderance.[4, 5] Mortality rates have been remarkably consistent over the years, varying from 0.9 to 1.5/million for male and 2.1 to 3.8/million for females in the United States. The disease occurs worldwide. Although scleroderma clusters in families with other auto-

**Table 58.1 DRUG TOXICITY: PATTERNS OF LUNG DISEASE THAT HAVE BEEN REPORTED AS ADVERSE EFFECTS OF DRUGS COMMONLY USED TO TREAT CONNECTIVE TISSUE DISEASES**

| Pulmonary Effect | Penicillamine | Methotrexate | Gold | Cyclophosphamide | Sulfasalazine |
|---|---|---|---|---|---|
| Hypersensitivity pneumonitis | | + | + | | |
| Pulmonary infiltrate with eosinophilia | | + | + | | + |
| Interstitial pulmonary fibrosis | | | + | + | |
| Obliterative bronchiolitis | + | | + | | |
| Organizing pneumonia | + | + | + | | + |
| Pleural effusion, thickening | | + | | + | + |
| Alveolar hemorrhage, vasculitis | + | | | | + |

immune disease, there are very few reports of first-degree relatives having SSc. Genetic involvement in the disease has been determined by the identification of chromosomal abnormalities[6] and by studies of the major histocompatibility complex genes.[7] Although many of the early studies were serologic, more recently polymerase chain reaction technology has been employed. With this latter approach, an association between diffuse lung disease and human leukocyte antigens DR3 and DR52a has been recognized.[8]

## Pulmonary Manifestations

More is known about the pulmonary complications of SSc than any other connective tissue disease. Pulmonary involvement has emerged as the major cause of excess morbidity and mortality in SSc. The patterns of lung disease with which systemic sclerosis may present are variable and are shown in Table 58.3.

A variety of agents are known to induce SSc-like pulmonary disease, including D-penicillamine, tryptophan, bleomycin, pentazocine, and (particularly in males) the industrial agents vinyl chloride, benzene, toluene, and trichloroethylene.[9] Silica exposure increases the odds ratio of SSc and silicosis increases the rate even further.[10] The toxic oil syndrome occurred in Madrid in 1981 after ingestion of an adulterated cooking oil that contained rapeseed oil denatured with aniline.[11] This provoked a scleroderma-like syndrome with pulmonary involvement. The association with silicone breast implants is unproved.

## Interstitial Pulmonary Fibrosis

**Pathogenesis.** Of all of the lung problems in the connective tissue diseases, most is known about the pathophysiology of interstitial pulmonary fibrosis SSc. There are several distinct, but related, aspects of pathogenesis.

**Predisposition.** There is good evidence that individuals are predisposed genetically to develop systemic SSc, and there are emerging markers that define risks for diffuse lung disease. Class II major histocompatibility complex associations increase the risk of interstitial pulmonary fibrosis in SSc.[8] The relative risk is increased if the anti–deoxyribonucleic acid (DNA) topoisomerase (Scl70) antibody is present. Recent studies have shown that there is an association between Scl70 and an allele of the major histocompatibility complex DPB1 gene. The importance of genetics to SSc is illustrated in a study of Choctaw Indians residing in southeastern Oklahoma. The prevalence of SSc in full-blooded Choctaws is roughly 1 in 200, which is significantly higher than that found in non–full-blooded Choctaws (1 in 3000) and strikingly higher than the global prevalence of SSc in other Native Americans in Oklahoma (1 in 10,000).[12] The genetic susceptibility probably results in injury and an immune response.[13, 14] It has been shown that there is highly restricted T-cell responses to epitopes of DNA topoisomerase 1 both in healthy individuals and in those with SSc. Thus, the appearance of the autoantibody in individuals with Scl70-responsive T-cell clones is possibly responsible for driving the immune response.[15–17] In the lung, there is an accumulation of "memory-type" CD45 RO lymphocytes and secondary lymphoid follicles with true germinal centers within lung biopsy samples.[18, 19] Furthermore, the T cells present within the lung express cytokines of both the T helper 1 and T helper 2 subsets.[20]

**Inflammation Amplification.** A wide variety of cytokines has been identified in bronchoalveolar lavage fluid that clearly contribute to the cascade of inflammation in the lungs.[21, 22] The most striking of these is interleukin-8 (neutrophil chemoattractant and activator), tumor necrosis factor-α (TNF-α; early cytokine involved in many pathologic processes), macrophage inflammatory protein-1α (MIP-1α) (important in neutrophil chemotaxis), and RANTES (regulated on activation normal T-cell expressed and secreted) (important in T-cell and eosinophil recruitment and activation). It is clear, therefore, that the downstream events of the initiation results in the release of a number of pro-inflammatory cytokines that are responsible for further recruitment and activation of inflammatory cells at disease sites.

**Fibrogenetic Factors.** The hallmark of SSc in both lung and skin is the accumulation of connective tissue matrix cells and proteins.[23–26] Many factors have been studied in this regard, and a wide variety of growth factors have been identified. Perhaps the most striking of these at present is connective tissue growth factor, which appears to depend on transforming growth factor-β (TGF-β) for up regulation and has a potent effect on collagen production as evidenced by collagen gel retraction stud-

**Table 58.2 IMMUNOSUPPRESSIVE THERAPY: COMMON DRUGS USED IN THE TREATMENT OF THE MAJOR PULMONARY COMPLICATIONS OF CONNECTIVE TISSUE DISEASES**

| Drug | Dose | Duration | Comments | Monitoring |
|---|---|---|---|---|
| Azathioprine | 2.5 mg/kg/day<br>Max. 150 mg/day | Continuous | Maximal effect may not be evident for 6–9 months but has better adverse effect profile than cyclophosphamide. May be used long term. Starting dose, 50 mg daily with monitoring full blood count in case of thiopurine methyltransferase deficiency; maintenance dose from 1 month. | Full blood count<br>Liver function tests |
| Cyclophosphamide<br>po<br>iv | <br>2 mg/kg/day to 150 mg/day<br>600 mg/m² monthly for 1–6 months | <br>Variable<br>Variable | Intravenous therapy for rapid induction of remission at 2–4 mg/kg/day for 3–4 days especially for vasculitis. Pulsed iv cyclophosphamide may be given at 1–3 monthly intervals with better adverse effect profile and lower long-term cumulative dose, particularly for nonvasculitic disease. Oral cyclosphamide may be used continuously or substituted at 3 months for azathioprine because of more favorable adverse effect profile in diffuse lung disease. | Full blood count<br>Liver function tests<br>Urinalysis for blood |
| Cyclosporin A | 5 mg/kg/day | Continuous | Bioavailability variable, thus blood monitoring necessary. May be used in combination with prednisolone. | Blood pressure<br>Urea and creatinine<br>Cyclosporin level |
| Methotrexate | 7.5–20 mg/week | Continuous | Little information to support use except as second-line therapy after first-line treatment. Pulmonary toxicity may be limiting. | Full blood counts<br>Liver function tests |
| Prednisolone | 1 mg/kg/day or 20 mg alternate days | Continuous | Prednisolone used alone in high dose for cellular diffuse lung disease and then titrated to control. Used in conjunction with immunosuppressants; for more fibrotic disease, the low dose regimen is used. | Blood pressure<br>Blood glucose<br>Weight |
| Methylprednisolone, iv | 500–1000 mg/day | 3–5 days | Used for aggressive induction of remission particularly for vasculitis or acute pneumonitis, then followed by maintenance therapy of prednisolone or prednisolone plus immunosuppressive agent. | |

iv = intravenous; po = oral.

**Table 58.3 SYSTEMIC SCLEROSIS (SCLERODERMA)**

**Criteria for Diagnosis***
- Major
  - Thickening of the skin of the hands
- Minor
  - Sclerodactyly, i.e., the changes of the major criteria but limited to the fingers
  - Digital pitting scars or loss of substance from the finger pad: depressed areas at tips of fingers or loss of digital pad tissue as a result of ischemia
- Bibasilar pulmonary fibrosis

**Lung Manifestations**
- Interstitial pulmonary fibrosis
- Organizing pneumonia
- Isolated pulmonary vascular disease
- Aspiration pneumonia (secondary to esophageal dysmotility)
- Chest wall restriction

*The major or two or more minor criteria required for diagnosis.

ies.[27–29] TGF-β is found in high amounts in the lungs of patients with SSc[30]; endothelin-1 (ET-1) and coagulation cascade proteins are also present in high amounts in bronchoalveolar lavage fluid.[26, 31] Fibroblasts from patients with lung disease exhibit dysregulated type I collagen biosynthesis and impaired messenger ribonucleic acid (RNA) down regulation. The balance of ET receptors (A and B) is modified in the lung of patients with scleroderma, with there being a consistent decrease in ET-A and an increase in ET-B receptors.[23, 32]

There are a number of events occurring in parallel that result in the development of lung injury and subsequent fibrosis. It is simplistic to target any one of these as being the important factor, but there seems little doubt that the key cytokines in the cascade include TNF-α (because it occurs very early in disease and has been shown in animal models to be a pivotal factor in lung fibrosis)[33–36] and TGF-β (which colocalizes with collagen gene up regulation and has been shown to be important in connective tissue growth factor release).[37] The balance of TH1 to TH2 cytokines is also key because, when the shift is in favor of TH2 cytokines, such as in idiopathic pulmonary fibrosis, the prognosis is worse and is associated with a much higher eosinophil influx into the lung in comparison with patients with SSc, whose TH1/TH2 ratio is balanced and who have less eosinophil influx per unit lung involvement.[20]

**Clinical Features.** The prevalence of lung disease in SSc varies depending on the method used for detection. Dyspnea occurs in roughly 55% of patients (range 21% to 80%).[38] Cough is a less frequently reported symptom, but, when it occurs, it is dry and nonproductive. Hemoptysis may occur in the context of complicating carcinoma or bronchial telangiectasia.[39] Pleuritic chest pain is uncommon. Pneumothorax is even less common. Chest radiographic series identified diffuse lung disease in up to 67% of patients and lung function abnormalities in up to 90%. The lung is involved more commonly in patients with diffuse cutaneous SSc (i.e., involving skin proximal to the elbow), but the extent of skin involvement does not correlate with lung function changes. Patients may often be symptom free. Digital clubbing never occurs because of the poor vasculature of the digits. Fine crackles are heard at the bases and are of a "Velcro" character. Pleural rub is almost never heard. Rarely, scleroderma of the chest wall may cause extrathoracic restriction. Secondary pulmonary hypertension with appropriate clinical features of right ventricular strain, raised jugular venous pressure, and ankle edema may be seen during the terminal stages of the disease.

Lung disease may be the first manifestation of SSc. A history of Raynaud's phenomenon is often helpful. Careful examination of the capillaries in the nail beds reveals the typical feature associated with scleroderma: abnormal loops associated with capillary "fall-out." The presence of autoantibodies, particularly antinuclear antibodies, is helpful in suggesting a connective tissue disease etiology (Table 58.4).

**Imaging.** Chest radiography typically shows a reticulonodular pattern in the bases and periphery in early disease. There is obvious loss of volume with more extensive reticulonodular shadowing in more advanced disease. In this situation, honeycombing may be present (Fig. 58.1*A*).

Computed tomography (CT) has revolutionized the interpretation of the pattern and extent of disease.[40–42] Disease is again localized to the peripheral rim, occurring earliest at the bases and posteriorly. As disease becomes more advanced, it progresses superiorly, centrally, and anteriorly. Esophageal dilation may be apparent, which can be helpful in the diagnosis if the lung disease is the first manifestation of the systemic disease (Fig. 58.1*B* and 1*C*). The pattern may be "ground glass," which reflects a more cellular histopathology or a "reticular" pattern, often with honeycomb features, linear abnormalities, and traction bronchiolectasis.

CT extent correlates extremely well with lung function, particularly gas transfer. Strikingly, the associations with gas exchange show a much greater deficit per unit lung involved on CT scans from individuals with idiopathic pulmonary fibrosis than with SSc.[41] The extent of individual patterns (ground glass vs. reticular) is associated with the type of inflammatory cell found in bronchoalveolar lavage. More extensive reticular (consistent with more fibrosis) disease is associated with high neutrophil numbers, and this influx therefore appears to depend on disease extent regardless of disease type.[43]

Gallium scans provide no added value. Technetium 99m-diethylinetriamine pentacetate clearance has been used in some medical centers to identify early disease and to predict prognosis.[44, 45] A more rapid clearance of this isotope is indicative of a loss of epithelial cell integrity, and rapid clearance indicates uptake from the air space into the circulation. A persistently rapid clearance rate confers an increased risk of subsequent lung function deterioration, and a persistently normal clearance rate predicts lung function stability.

**Lung Function Tests.** The interstitial pulmonary fibrosis of SSc is characterized by a restrictive ventilatory defect of mechanical function, which results in reduced

**Table 58.4** AUTOANTIBODY SPECIFICITY IN CONNECTIVE TISSUE DISEASE

| CTD | Autoantibody | Target | Comments |
|---|---|---|---|
| Systemic sclerosis | Anticentromere | Centromere proteins (CENP A - F) | 20–40% total SSc wide racial variation<br>70–80% limited cutaneous variant with pulmonary hypertension |
| | Scl-70 | DNA topoisomerase 1 | 28–70% total SSc wide racial variation, >30% diffuse cutaneous disease with interstitial lung disease |
| | PM-Scl | — | Scleroderma-myositis overlap syndromes |
| | Antinucleolar | RNA Polymerase 1 | 8–20% SSc suggests poorest 10 year survival, renal crisis |
| | Ku | DNA-binding proteins | Scleroderma-myositis overlap syndromes |
| Rheumatoid arthritis | Rheumatoid factor | IgG | Seropositive disease more frequent with pulmonary disease |
| | ANA | | |
| | Histone | Histone proteins | 5% rheumatoid vasculitis |
| SLE | dsDNA | Double-stranded DNA | 50–75%, strong association with nephritis. |
| | ANA | — | 90–95% |
| | Ro/La | RNA transcription factors | 60%/20% |
| | Histone | Histone proteins | >90% drug-induced lupus, 20–30% primary SLE |
| | Sm | — | 10% Caucasians, and 30% African Americans and Chinese |
| | Lupus anticoagulant | Phospholipid | 20–30% |
| DM/PM | Jo-1 | Histidyl tRNA synthetase | 20–30% inflammatory myopathy but 50–100% when associated with diffuse interstitial lung disease |
| | PL-7 | Threonyl tRNA synthetase | <3% antisynthetase syndrome |
| | PL-12 | Alanyl tRNA synthetase | <3% antisynthetase syndrome |
| | EJ | Glycyl tRNA synthetase | <2% antisynthetase syndrome |
| | OJ | Isoleucyl tRNA synthetase | <2% antisynthetase syndrome<br>Antisynthetase antibodies 25–30% DM/PM (Jo-1 most prevalent) |
| | Mi-2 | Nuclear proteins | <8% DM |
| MCTD | U1-RNP | Small nuclear proteins | Myositis overlap syndromes (10% SSc) |
| | U2-RNP | — | Myositis, SLE, SSc |
| Relapsing polychondritis | Anticartilage | Cartilage | Unknown sensitivity |
| | Anticollagen | Collagen | |
| Sjögrens syndrome | Ro (SS-A) | RNA transcription factors | 40–50% primary Sjögrens syndrome (25–30% SLE) |
| | La (SS-B) | | 50% Sjogrens (10% SLE) |

ANA = antinuclear antibody; CTD = connective tissue disease; DM/PM = dermatomyositis/polymyositis; MCTD = mixed connective tissue diseases; SSc = systemic sclerosis; SLE = systemic lupus erythematosus.

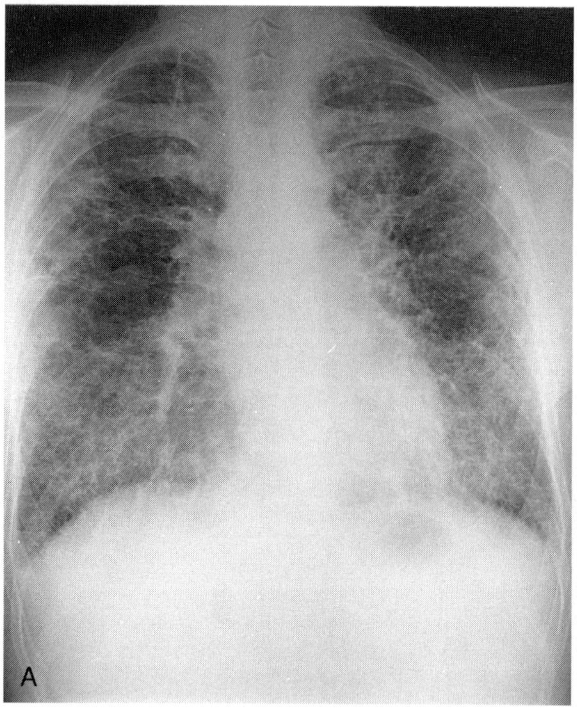


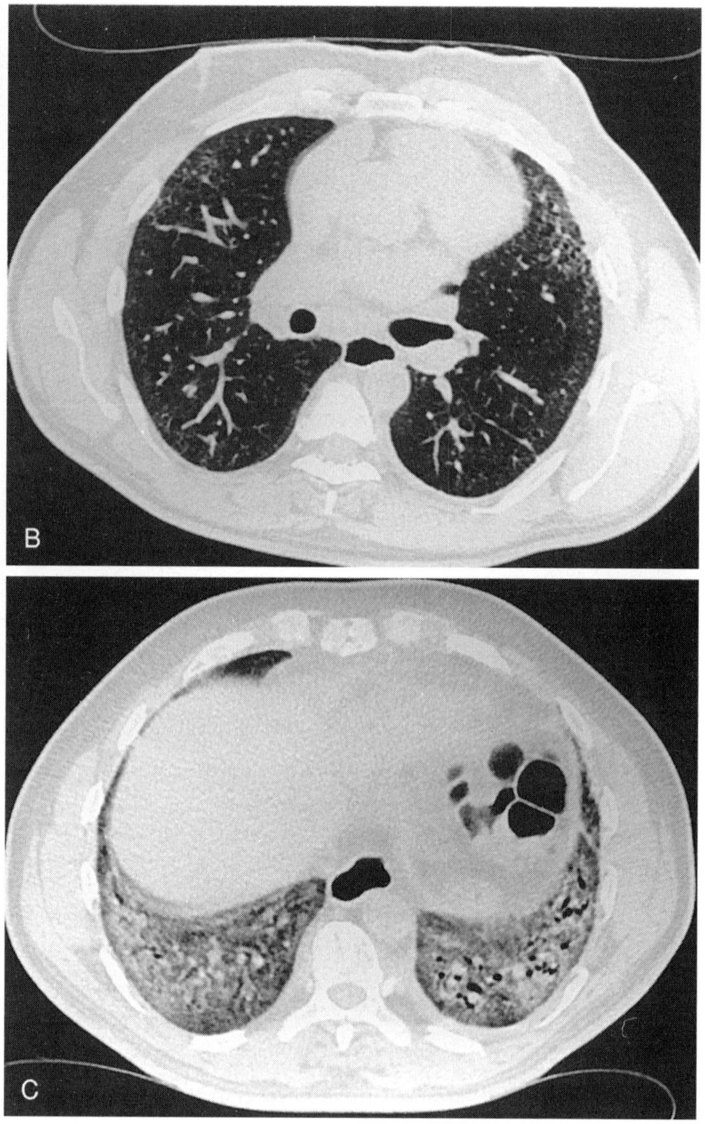


**Figure 58.1** *A,* The chest radiograph was taken from a patient with systemic sclerosis. Note the widespread predominantly peripheral pattern of reticulonodular disease. The heart borders and the diaphragms are obscured. *B,* This CT scan was taken at a level just below the carina in a patient with systemic sclerosis. Note the peripheral reticular pattern that in this case is more prominent anteriorly. In this patient with subtle disease, the dilated esophagus is a clue as to the true cause of the fibrosing lung disease. *C,* This CT scan was taken at the level of the diaphragms in a patient with more extensive interstitial pulmonary fibrosis in the context of systemic sclerosis. Note in particular the very dilated airways, indicating that the apparent ground-glass/consolidation pattern is dense fibrosis. Again, the dilated esophagus indicates that this disease is likely to be part of systemic sclerosis.

pulmonary compliance, vital capacity, and total lung capacity. Residual volume is decreased. Carbon monoxide transfer factor ($DL_{CO}$ is reduced and may be the only abnormality in early disease. Blood gas analysis usually reveals a reduced arterial $PO_2$ with a normal or low arterial $PCO_2$. Hypoxia is usually not marked until very late in the disease process.

There have been a number of studies of rate of change of lung function in SSc.[46–48] These are weakened somewhat by selection criteria, but, on average, it would appear that vital capacity declines three times more rapidly than in normal individuals and that gas transfer declines at twice the rate. In one study 27 of 38 patients lost more than 30 mL of vital capacity per year (the normal rate of decline). A second study showed that vital capacity loss was greater in patients who had evidence of an active alveolitis on bronchoalveolar lavage. Rates of decline are often higher within 2 years of onset of SSc, emphasizing the importance of identifying lung disease early.

Exercise lung function testing increases ventilation-perfusion mismatching and also increases diffusion abnormalities so that hypoxia results with widening of the alveolar-arterial gradient. Minute ventilation increases generally as a consequence of increased ventilation rate rather than tidal volume. Dead space ventilation may increase on exercise, with a rise in the $V_D/V_T$ ratio. For a given degree of lung involvement defined by CT, abnormalities on exercise gas exchange are worse in patients with idiopathic pulmonary fibrosis than in those with interstitial pulmonary fibrosis in association with SSc.

**Bronchoalveolar lavage.** This is a useful tool for identifying alveolitis in systemic sclerosis before the onset of pulmonary symptoms.[45, 49] A neutrophil alveolitis has been described by some authors to predict more progressive disease.[47, 50, 51] It has, however, been shown that an increase in neutrophils reflects an increase in the extent of disease on CT, particularly the reticular pattern, and this increase is, therefore, likely a marker of more extensive disease rather than an independent index of progressive disease.[43]

Bronchoalveolar lavage (BAL) should not be used alone to determine whether treatment should be started. Many patients with apparently normal BAL findings may exhibit progressive disease. Similarly, BAL provides no added value for monitoring disease.

**Biopsy.** If the pattern of disease is at all atypical after review of the less invasive indices, lung biopsy is necessary. No extra information is obtained by a transbronchial biopsy, and surgical biopsy is required in this situation. Examples of circumstances in which biopsy is indicated include an unusual pattern of disease on CT, marked pleural disease, and more than 20% lymphocytes on BAL. Pathologically, the most common pattern is of usual interstitial pneumonia, with thickening of the alveolar walls with inflammatory cells (mononuclear cells, granulocytes, and plasma cells), connective tissue matrix cells, and proteins combined with intra-alveolar inflammation (predominantly by macrophages), type II pneumocyte proliferation, and vascular obliteration. The distribution is subpleural and basal and is maximal in posterior segments, with the macroscopic findings of the lung surface taking on a fine nodular, "cirrhotic" appearance in the early stages and honeycombing with more advanced disease.

Electron microscopy shows evidence of early endothelial and epithelial cell injury, even where there is no abnormality on light microscopy. More recently, some patients have been found to have the pattern of nonspecific interstitial pneumonia. This pattern differs from usual interstitial pneumonia in exhibiting a homogeneous pattern of pathology. One of the hallmark features of usual interstitial pneumonia is the presence of a heterogeneous appearance, with some normal alveoli being seen in the same section as areas of extensive alveolar remodeling. These pathologic differences may reflect different disease subsets with differences in outcome. Autopsy studies have shown some diffuse lung disease in up to 79% of cases and pulmonary vascular disease in 29%.

In some patients who exhibit a more accelerated course of disease, histopathologic examination has shown a diffuse alveolar damage pattern.[52]

**Serologic Investigations.** Although SSc is traditionally defined on the basis of the extent of the skin disease as outlined above, the pattern of autoantibodies appears to be a much stronger determinant of the associated internal organ involvement.[7, 53, 54]

Antinuclear antibodies are found in 90% to 100% of patients with SSc (roughly 30% of normal individuals have antinuclear antibodies at a titer of 1:40), but in 30% the specific antigen is unidentified. Three major autoantibodies include anticentromere, occurring in 57% of patients with limited cutaneous disease; anti-topoisomerase (Scl-70), occurring in 40% of patients with diffuse disease; and PM-Scl, occurring in a small fraction of cases in association with the polymyositis overlap syndrome. It is rare to have both Scl-70 and anticentromere antibodies. Diffuse lung disease is rare in the presence of anticentromere antibodies, and a protective role for this autoantibody has been argued but not substantiated. Interstitial pulmonary fibrosis is strongly associated with the Scl-70 antibody and with diffuse scleroderma. Limited cutaneous disease associates with vascular disease and the anticentromere antibody. Both forms of lung disease may progress to pulmonary hypertension.

**Prognosis.** The prognosis of interstitial pulmonary fibrosis in SSc depends on the extent of disease at presentation. Worse lung function, particularly vital capacity and $DL_{CO}$, indicate a poorer outcome, and similar observations have been made based on extent of disease on CT as the criterion. Several studies have shown an increased decline in lung function in patients with interstitial pulmonary fibrosis compared with normal individuals.[46–48] Although crude mortality rates are 3.9% per year for males and 2.6% per year for females, lung disease remains the most common cause of death in patients with SSc.[55] In one series of causes of death lung disease was the most common, accounting for 21% of all deaths. There is also an increased risk of lung cancer in SSc.[5, 56]

**Treatment.** There are reports of a wide variety of treatments for interstitial pulmonary fibrosis in SSc.[57] Most of these include immunosuppression. None of these studies has, however, been a properly controlled prospective randomized investigation. Despite this, there is a consensus in published reports of an advantage of treatment with cyclophosphamide, together with prednisolone, to improve lung function and prognosis.[58, 59] The treatment regimen used most commonly involves moderately low dosages of prednisolone at 10 mg per day or 20 mg every other day, together with cyclophosphamide at 2 mg/kg/day orally up to a maximum of 150 mg. Close scrutiny with full blood counts, liver function tests, and urine testing for evidence of hemorrhagic cystitis is needed. The question of pneumocystis prophylaxis is not resolved. Some medical centers use cotrimoxazole three times a week if immunosuppressive agents are being given.

End-stage lung disease has been treated with single lung transplantation provided there is no evidence of disease activity in other organs. In terminal disease that is not amenable for transplantation, consideration must be given to regular oxygen therapy, treatment of supervening heart failure, and infection.

## Pulmonary Vascular Disease in Systemic Sclerosis

Unlike the other connective tissue diseases, vascular involvement in SSc is caused by concentric fibrosis of small arterioles replacing the normal intima and media, but the plexiform lesions and fibrinoid necrosis of primary pulmonary hypertension are not seen. Isolated vascular disease occurs mainly in the limited form of SSc. Associated features are those of the CREST syndrome (*c*alcinosis, *R*aynaud's phenomenon, *e*sophageal dysmotility, *s*clerodactyly, *t*elangiectasias) with prominent telangiectasia, esophageal disease, abnormal nailfold capillaries (dilated capillaries and dropout of capillary loops), and a positive anticentromere antibody. Chest radiography, CT scanning, and BAL are all normal. Lung function studies show an isolated fall in $DL_{CO}$. When damage to the pulmonary vascular bed is extensive (gas transfer <50% predicted), the risk of pulmonary hypertension increases.[60] Mortality rates are increased with increasing pulmonary hypertension. Diethylenetriamine penta-acetic acid clearance measurements are usually normal in patients with pure pulmonary vascular disease in scleroderma and help to differentiate vascular disease from early diffuse disease in patients with an isolated fall in $DL_{CO}$.

Doppler echocardiography is a good measure of pulmonary hypertension.[61, 62] It has been shown to correlate with measurements of pulmonary artery pressures made at right heart catheterization but is noninvasive. Qualitative features found on echocardiography may also suggest pulmonary hypertension in the absence of a tricuspid regurgitant jet, precluding measurement of the gradient across the tricuspid valve and thus an estimate of pulmonary artery pressure. These include right ventricular dilation and right ventricular hypertrophy.

Optimal treatment of pulmonary vascular disease in SSc has not been defined. Calcium channel antagonists may be helpful, but often the dosage required to improve pulmonary vasculature causes unacceptable drops in left-sided pressures and peripheral edema. Angiotensin-converting enzyme inhibitors can be helpful. The most promising approach at present is the use of pulses of intravenous prostacyclin.[63] Exact dosage regimens need to be validated, but in acute studies and longer term evaluation (uncontrolled studies), improvements in pulmonary vascular resistance and pulmonary pressures have been shown.

### Other Pulmonary Complications

Aspiration pneumonia is extremely uncommon, particularly considering the prevalence of esophageal dysfunction in systemic sclerosis. Pleural disease is uncommon. Rarely, the extent of skin tightness over the chest wall produces an extrinsic restriction of ventilation. Occasionally, the first manifestation of pulmonary parenchymal disease is organizing pneumonia. This responds well to corticosteroid therapy, as does organizing pneumonia in other contexts.

## RHEUMATOID ARTHRITIS

The American Rheumatism Association revised criteria for the classification of rheumatoid arthritis (RA) require that at least four of the criteria listed in Table 58.5 be satisfied for a minimum of 6 weeks.[64, 65]

### Epidemiology and Risk Factors

The reported incidence of RA ranges from 0.2 to 3.0/1000 person-years (less than 0.5/1000 years in most surveys), with a rising incidence with increasing age into the seventh decade. In adult Caucasians, the prevalence of RA ranges from 0.5% to 2%, with a male to female ratio between 1:2 and 1:4. Depending on disease severity (as judged by disability scales and the need for long-term corticosteroid therapy), the age-matched mortality rate of RA is up to twofold higher than in the general population. The prevalence of RA is similar throughout the world. Evidence in support of a genetic predisposition includes familial and twin clustering and associations between RA and human leukocyte antigen (HLA) DRB1 alleles.[66] Hormonal factors may play a role, judging from the female preponderance of RA and a reduced incidence during pregnancy. Infectious agents and socioeconomic factors have not been shown to be etiologically important.

**Table 58.5 RHEUMATOID ARTHRITIS**

| |
|---|
| **Criteria for Diagnosis*** |
| Morning stiffness (lasting at least 1 hour) |
| Arthritis (soft-tissue swelling or fluid) of three or more joints (PIP, MCP, wrist, elbow, knee, ankle, MTP joints) |
| Arthritis of hand joints (swelling of at least one wrist, MCP, or PIP joint) |
| Symmetric arthritis, i.e., simultaneous arthritis of the same joints on both sides of the body |
| Rheumatoid nodules |
| Serum rheumatoid factor positivity (at a level such that <5% of normal controls are positive) |
| Radiographic hand or wrist changes typical of rheumatoid arthritis |
| **Lung Manifestations** |
| Interstitial pulmonary fibrosis |
| Organizing pneumonia |
| Obliterative bronchiolitis |
| Follicular bronchiolitis |
| Bronchiectasis |
| Vasculitis |
| Nodules |
| Pleural disease |
| Lymphocytic interstitial pneumonia |
| Drug induced |

*At least four criteria for a minimum of 6 weeks.
MCP = metacarpophalangeal; MTP = metatarsophalangeal; PIP = proximal interphalangeal.

### Pulmonary Manifestations

Pleuropulmonary manifestations are multiple and are listed in Table 58.5.

#### Interstitial Pulmonary Fibrosis

The interstitial pulmonary fibrosis of RA has a male predominance (male to female ratio, 3:1), is associated with HLA B8 and HLA Dw3 positivity,[67] and is histologically similar to idiopathic pulmonary fibrosis. Smoking is a risk factor for the development of overt pulmonary fibrosis in RA[68] and has also been associated with subclinical disease.[69] High titers of rheumatoid factor[68] and the presence of rheumatoid nodules[70, 71] are also associated with an increased prevalence of pulmonary fibrosis in RA.

In early disease, a lymphocytic interstitial infiltrate is often the predominant abnormality,[72] and prominent peribronchiolar follicles, containing aggregates of lymphocytes with germinal centers, are often seen.[73] In long-standing disease, fibrosis predominates, often resulting in cystic changes or honeycombing. It is difficult to quantify the prevalence of interstitial pulmonary fibrosis because, in series in which "interstitial fibrosis" is described, histologic appearances are seldom subcategorized. Minor pulmonary fibrosis is common in RA; in one open lung biopsy series performed in volunteers with RA (some without clinical evidence of interstitial lung disease), pulmonary fibrosis was seen in 60% of patients.[74] Reductions in carbon monoxide diffusing capacity are found in 40% of unselected RA patients.[75] Radiologically overt pulmonary fibrosis is, however, found in only 1% to 5% of RA patients (based on three large chest radiographic series).[68, 70, 76]

Severe progressive disease requiring hospitalization may be associated with *cor pulmonale* and respiratory failure and has a poor prognosis with a 5 year survival rate of less than 50%[77]; however, a large subgroup of patients have more indolent disease that progresses little during prolonged follow-up. The most frequent symptom is exertional dyspnea, although this may be masked by a general loss of mobility due to systemic disease. The clinical picture is usually identical to that of idiopathic pulmonary fibrosis with bilateral, predominantly basal crackles and tachypnea, cyanosis, and right heart failure in advanced disease. Finger clubbing, which is occasionally striking, is more prevalent than in other connective tissue diseases.

## Organizing Pneumonia

Organizing pneumonia (bronchiolitis obilterans organizing pneumonia) is characterized by plugs of granulation tissue in the air spaces distal to and including the terminal bronchioles, associated with lymphocytic infiltration within well-preserved bronchiolar walls and the surrounding lung interstitium. The term *bronchiolitis obliterans organizing pneumonia* has caused confusion among clinicians,[78] stimulating the recent use of the term *proliferative bronchiolitis*.[79] Organizing pneumonia has a very different profile from the entity of bronchiolitis obliterans (also found in RA), with a clinical presentation of pneumonia (as opposed to airflow obstruction), multifocal consolidation on chest radiograph and CT, a restrictive functional defect, and a much higher chance of responsiveness to corticosteroids than bronchiolitis obliterans (with a good outcome in 15 of the first 17 reported cases) (Fig. 58.2).[80] Organizing pneumonia is more common in RA than in other connective tissue diseases (with the possible exception of polymyositis). In a series of 40 patients with RA undergoing open lung biopsy, organizing

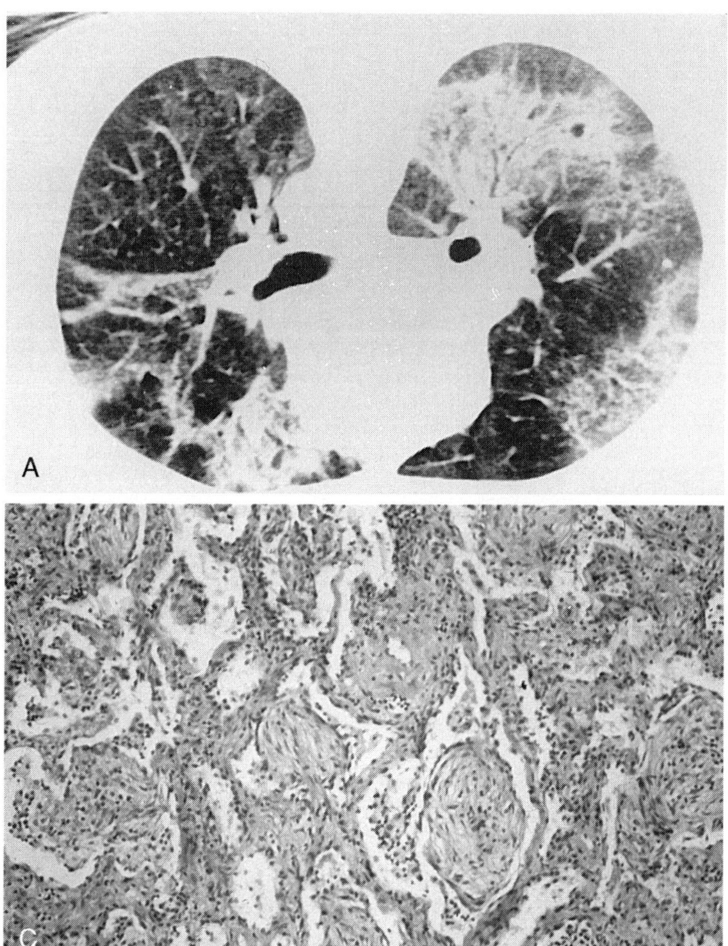


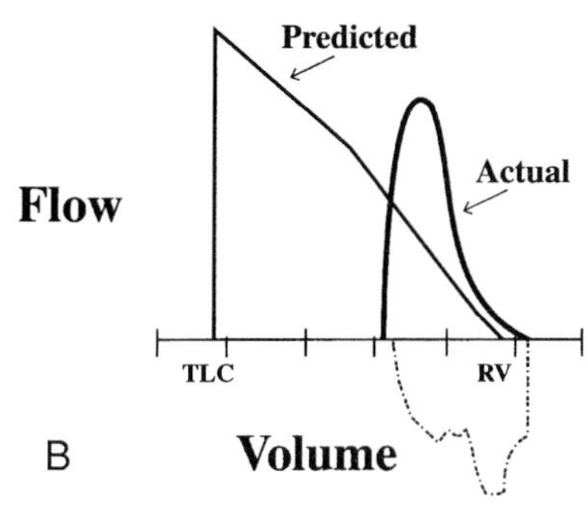


**Figure 58.2** *A,* This CT scan is from a patient with rheumatoid arthritis and organizing pneumonia. Note the pattern of air space consolidation that is bilateral. *B,* A flow volume loop from the same patient as in *A* is shown. The flow volume loop is shifted to the right by comparison with the ideal predicted loop, but the flow rates are relatively well preserved. TLC = total lung capacity; RV = residual volume. *C,* This surgical lung biopsy specimen is from a patient with organizing pneumonia in the context of rheumatoid arthritis. The alveoli and respiratory bronchioles are filled with loosely packed connective tissue.

pneumonia (6 cases) had a similar prevalence to fibrosing alveolitis (5 cases),[81] although organizing pneumonia might have been over-represented due to an acute presentation (and thus a perceived need to reach a definitive histologic diagnosis). The good prognosis generally seen in organizing pneumonia has been emphasized in the medical literature, but a minority of RA patients progress to respiratory failure and death despite treatment.

## Obliterative Bronchiolitis

Obliterative bronchiolitis (OB, synonymous with bronchiolitis obliterans and constrictive bronchiolitis) (Fig. 58.3) is characterized histologically by destruction of the bronchiolar wall by granulation tissue, effacement of the lumen, and eventual replacement of the bronchiole by fibrous tissue. There is circumstantial evidence to suggest that OB may be preceded by an inflammatory exudate; prominent bronchiolar inflammation may be found in patients with the shortest symptomatic course.[82] OB in RA has now been described in numerous case reports and small series. The expression of HLA antigens B40 and DR1 is increased in OB associated with RA (but not in isolated OB).[83] In early descriptions, the hallmark of OB was a rapidly progressive, often fatal course; however, as clinician awareness of the disease was then low, patients with advanced and progressive disease were undoubtedly over-represented. There is great heterogeneity in the

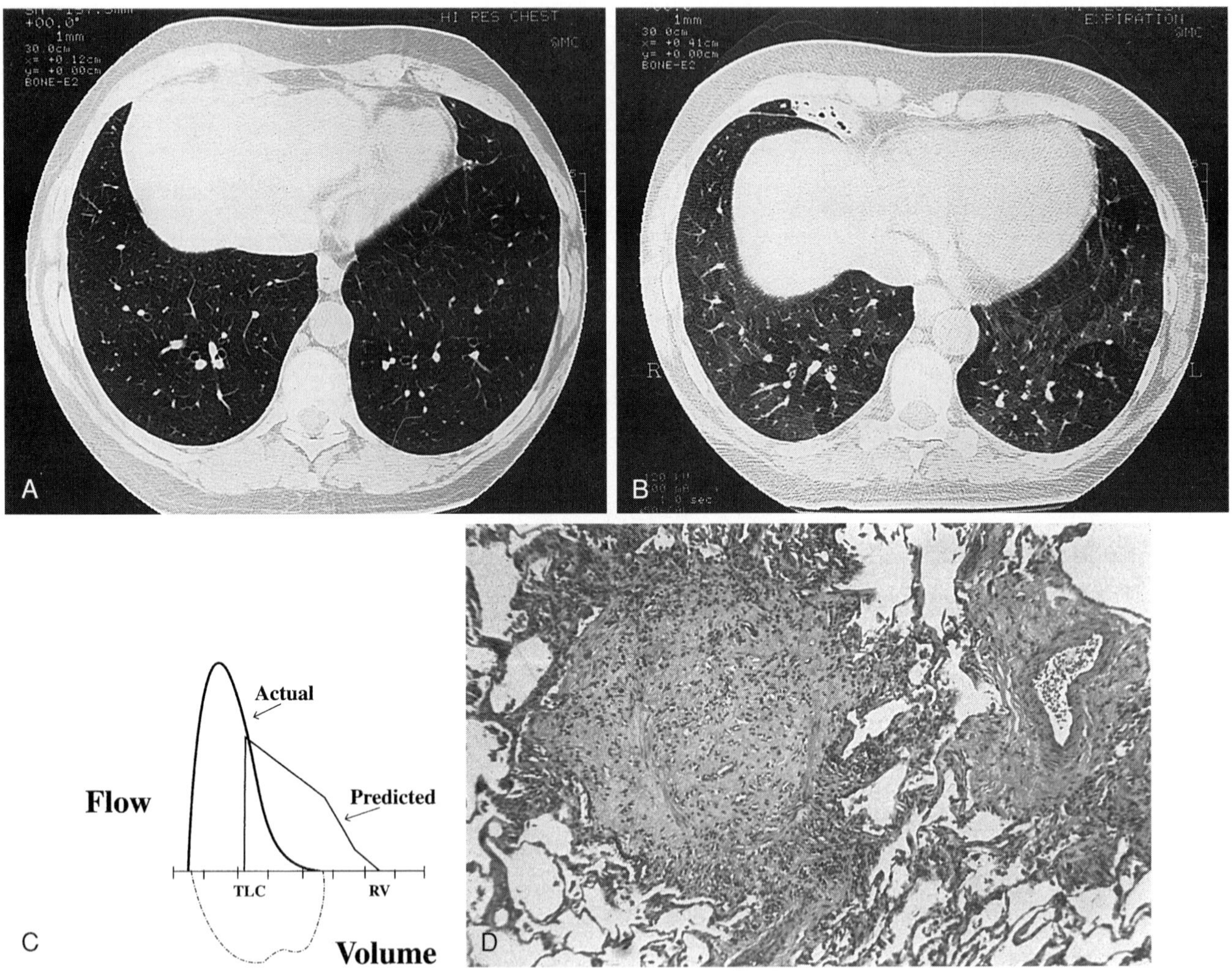


**Figure 58.3** Inspiratory and expiratory CT sections were obtained from a patient with rheumatoid arthritis with obliterative bronchiolitis. *A*, The inspiratory image is essentially normal. *B*, On the expiratory CT scan, there is extensive regional inhomogeneity, the reduced density resulting from regional vasoconstriction or regional gas trapping. *C*, A flow volume curve from the same patient as in *A* and *B* shows marked elevation of total lung capacity (TLC) and residual volume (RV) associated with characteristic concavity of the expiratory limb, indicating airflow obstruction. *D*, This surgical lung biopsy specimen is from a patient with obliterative bronchiolitis. A slit-like residual orifice is visible, but otherwise the whole of this terminal bronchiole is effaced by dense fibrous tissue. Note that the surrounding alveoli are normal.

speed of progression, with some patients having indolent disease[84]; the use of CT in RA patients with suspected pulmonary complications has now identified a subgroup with occult bronchiolitis, often admixed with interstitial lung disease. The prevalence of unsuspected OB in unselected RA patients remains uncertain, with unexplained airflow obstruction identified in a significant minority (including many nonsmokers) in one study[85] but no increase in the prevalence of pulmonary function abnormalities suggestive of isolated small airway disease in two subsequent controlled series.[86, 87]

Two major associations with the development of OB in RA have been reported. It is likely that secondary Sjögren's syndrome is an important predisposing factor, being associated with OB in five of six RA patients in one series[84]; the spectrum of histologic abnormalities in these cases, ranging from peribronchiolar lymphocytic infiltration to small airway destruction, was analogous to changes seen in the parotid gland in Sjögren's syndrome. As the presence or absence of Sjögren's syndrome is not documented in many case reports of OB in RA, the etiologic importance of Sjögren's syndrome remains uncertain.

More contentious is the reported association between OB and the use of penicillamine, first reported in the late 1970s.[88] After a number of case reports and small series, a significantly higher prevalence of OB was identified in RA patients who took penicillamine (3/133) than in other RA patients (0/469) in a large cohort.[82] It is possible that the development of OB and the use of penicillamine are both markers of more aggressive RA and are linked for this reason; however, OB developed less than 1 year after penicillamine was begun in 19 of the first 20 cases,[82] and thus the association is unlikely to be entirely spurious. As OB has been reported in many RA patients not taking penicillamine, it is likely that an underlying predisposition to OB in RA is unmasked by penicillamine (which disrupts collagen linkage and thus interferes with tissue repair).[89] A relationship between OB and gold therapy has been suggested[90] but is not endorsed by recent clinical experience.

## Follicular Bronchiolitis

Follicular bronchiolitis (FB) is characterized by external compression of bronchioles by hyperplastic lymphoid follicles, with variable lymphocytic infiltration of the bronchiolar wall. FB is associated more commonly with RA than with other connective tissue disease[91, 92] and is often found incidentally at lung biopsy in RA patients with interstitial pulmonary fibrosis. No causative mechanism has been identified, and it is unclear whether FB predisposes to the subsequent development of OB. When found in isolation, FB simulates interstitial lung disease, with reticular or reticulonodular abnormalities on chest radiography and a pattern of functional impairment that may be restrictive or obstructive. Clinically significant isolated FB is rare in RA, but its recognition is important because a response to corticosteroid therapy, although not the rule, is much more likely than in OB; in six of the first nine reported cases, disease stabilized or regressed with treatment.[80]

## Bronchiectasis

The prevalence of bronchiectasis is higher in RA than in other connective tissue diseases (Fig. 58.4). A recent literature review identified 289 patients with bronchiectasis associated with RA reported since 1928; however, as respiratory symptoms preceded the systemic manifestations of RA in 90%, it is likely that chance association accounts for a high proportion of early reported cases.[93] Although associated with long-standing RA in one study,[94] bronchiectasis was found on CT in 30% of 50 RA patients with normal chest radiographs on prospective evaluation.[95] Bronchiectasis in RA is not associated with more aggressive systemic disease and is often clinically silent, with little or no sputum production and a less progressive and disabling course than in patients with idiopathic bronchiectasis.

## Pulmonary Vasculitis

It is surprising that pulmonary vasculitis is reported only rarely in RA given the relatively high prevalence of systemic vasculitis in the disease. Pulmonary hypertension resulting from pulmonary vascular disease (as opposed to extensive pulmonary fibrosis) is uncommon, although occasional cases of pulmonary vasculitis have been found at autopsy.[81, 96] Similarly, diffuse alveolar hemorrhage is a rare complication of RA.

## Pulmonary Rheumatoid Nodules

Pulmonary rheumatoid nodules may be single or multiple, are found on chest radiography in less than 1% of RA patients,[71] and are usually associated with rheumatoid nodules elsewhere in the body,[97] although they occasionally precede the development of systemic disease. Nod-

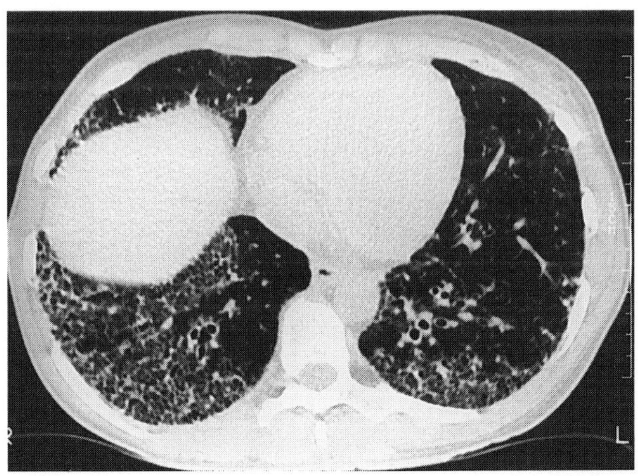


**Figure 58.4** This CT scan was taken at the level of the diaphragm in a patient with rheumatoid arthritis. The typical reticular pattern of fibrosing alveolitis in the context of rheumatoid arthritis can be seen in the right lung. On the left there are similar but less advanced changes. In addition, and notably remote from the fibrotic areas, are airways that are clearly bronchiectatic.

ules are well circumscribed, with central necrotic material contained by palisading epithelioid cells and surrounded by fibrosis and lymphocytic infiltration. Nodule cavitation occasionally causes hemoptysis, and pneumothorax may result from the rupture of subpleural nodules. Diffuse infiltration by small nodules leading to respiratory failure has been reported.[98] Nodules generally, however, present as asymptomatic abnormalities on chest radiography and may vary in size according to underlying rheumatoid activity; thus, when solitary, their growth as judged by chest radiography may simulate malignancy.[99] Caplan's syndrome consists of the association of single or multiple nodules with coal worker's pneumoconiosis,[100] which is often trivial, in keeping with the suggestion that nodule formation results from a hypersensitivity reaction to inhaled coal dust perhaps amplified by immunologic overactivity.

### Pleural Disease

Pleural disease is seen at autopsy in approximately 50% of patients,[71] and 20% give a history of pleuritic chest pain.[101] Pleural effusions are, however, found in less than 5%,[68, 70] usually in males,[97] and are frequently asymptomatic, often being identified on routine chest radiography. In a minority, pleuritic pain and fever are prominent, and the exclusion of empyema (which may be more prevalent in RA[102]) is required. Occasionally, effusions may develop acutely in association with pericarditis or exacerbations of arthritis; more typically, radiographic abnormalities are chronic, often remaining unchanged for years.[103] The fluid is an exudate, with a low glucose level (correlating poorly with serum glucose),[104] a low pH, and, usually, a predominant lymphocytosis (although a neutrophilia is occasionally found). Pleural fluid rheumatoid factor levels tend to mirror serum levels and have little independent diagnostic value.

### Other Pulmonary Complications

Other pulmonary complications of RA are rare. Lymphocytic interstitial pneumonia is an occasional finding at lung biopsy[105] and responds variably to corticosteroid therapy. Apical fibrosis mimicking the lung disease of ankylosing spondylitis has been reported.[106] Extensive apical cavitation in the absence of nodules or other causes of fibrocavitatary disease (including tuberculosis) has been described in a handful of cases and may follow a fulminant course.[107] Lower respiratory tract infection is increased in frequency in RA; bronchopneumonia is a common terminal event, accounting for 15% to 20% of deaths in RA patients.[108, 109]

## Drug-Induced Pulmonary Disease

Drug-induced pulmonary disease is a particular problem in RA because of the widespread use of methotrexate in routine clinical practice, and it has been reported in 3% to 18% of RA patients treated with methotrexate.[110, 111] Methotrexate pneumonitis is potentially life-threatening. It presents with cough, dyspnea, fever, widespread crackles, and pulmonary infiltrates on chest radiography and CT, which may be focal or diffuse.[112] Although the presentation is sometimes explosive, more often the onset is subacute (with symptoms evolving for up to 2 months before diagnosis[112]); 50% of cases are diagnosed within 4 months of initiation of methotrexate therapy. As the clinical and radiographic features are nonspecific, methotrexate-induced lung disease should always be suspected in the treated patient presenting with progressive lung disease. Unfortunately, histologic findings are nonspecific, although prominent lymphocytic infiltration increases the probability of a methotrexate-injured lung.[113] There is conflicting evidence on whether preexisting lung disease predisposes to lung injury caused by methotrexate, but the published evidence does not suggest that functional impairment is an absolute contraindication to its use (although particular caution is warranted when pulmonary reserve is grossly compromised, and patients with previous methotrexate toxicity should not be re-treated).[112, 114] Pulmonary methotrexate toxicity is associated with a mortality rate of 15% to 20%[112]; as the lymphocytic component of disease is wholly or partially reversible, immediate withdrawal of methotrexate and the early institution of steroid therapy are warranted.

Pulmonary toxicity in RA has also been documented with sulfasalazine, gold therapy, and penicillamine (discussed earlier). Pulmonary infiltrates (due to organizing pneumonia) associated with sulfasalazine occur most commonly in the upper lobes; this side effect is rare in RA, with only a handful of cases reported (most cases occurring in ulcerative colitis).[115] Pulmonary disease induced by gold takes the form of alveolar opacities adjacent to bronchovascular bundles, best demonstrated by high-resolution CT, and often associated with fever or skin rash, relatively low rheumatoid factor titers, and a BAL lymphocytosis.[116] In most patients with sulfasalazine or gold toxicity, lung disease largely regresses with withdrawal of the agent and corticosteroid therapy.

## Pulmonary Function Tests

Patterns of functional impairment in RA have been variable in unselected populations, with predominant airflow obstruction a frequent finding in one cohort,[85] but reductions in carbon monoxide diffusing capacity ascribed to occult interstitial fibrosis in at least 40%.[75] Inconsistencies in published data can be ascribed to the confounding effects of smoking and variations in the type and severity of associated pulmonary disease. Airflow obstruction may result from bronchiectasis or OB. Interstitial pulmonary fibrosis, organizing pneumonia, and lymphocytic interstitial pneumonia give rise to restrictive defects. Pleural disease may also be restrictive but is usually distinguished by elevation of KCO.

## Radiologic Features

In chest radiographic series of unselected patients with RA, appearances indicative of interstitial lung disease are found in 1% to 5% of cases.[68, 70, 76] In interstitial pulmonary fibrosis, appearances are indistinguishable from idiopathic pulmonary fibrosis, with symmetric basal interstitial opacification in limited disease and diffuse coarse reticulonodular abnormalities in extensive disease. Rheumatoid nodules are usually radiologically discrete and small, but are often multiple and may reach up to 7 cm in diameter; in Caplan's syndrome, nodules appear in crops, often grow rapidly, and may cavitate. Other chest radiographic findings in RA include focal consolidation (in organizing pneumonia, infectious pneumonia, and lung disease induced by methotrexate), hyperinflation (in OB), and pleural thickening or effusion.

The CT appearances of interstitial pulmonary fibrosis in RA are similar to those in idiopathic pulmonary fibrosis, with the most common abnormality being a reticular pattern (irregular linear opacities with cyst formation or honeycombing, typically subpleural and most extensive posteriorly and at the lung bases, except in extensive disease). Ground-glass attenuation, consisting of a patchy or diffuse increase in lung density, is likely to denote inflammatory histologic appearances, as in idiopathic pulmonary fibrosis. The cardinal CT feature of organizing pneumonia is patchy bilateral air-space consolidation (often with associated ground-glass attenuation), which is often predominantly subpleural,[117] but may have a bronchovascular distribution.[118] Small nodules (up to 1 cm in diameter) are common in organizing pneumonia; small pleural effusions and limited fibrosis (probably resulting from prolonged untreated inflammation) are occasional findings.

In bronchiolitis,[119] bronchiolar structures are occasionally visualized directly on CT as centrilobular micronodular opacities and peripheral branching structures, denoting marked thickening of the bronchiolar wall; this appearance may be most frequent in follicular bronchiolitis. In OB, areas of reduced lung density in a patchy distribution ("mosaic perfusion") are associated with a reduction in the caliber of pulmonary vessels in areas of decreased attenuation, indicative of regional hypoxic vasoconstriction in areas of severe bronchiolitis. Bronchiectasis and bronchial wall thickening on CT are common in constrictive bronchiolitis.

## Treatment of Pulmonary Complications

The treatment of pulmonary disease has usually consisted of corticosteroid therapy, with or without immunosuppressive agents. Due to small numbers, regimens have remained anecdotal. Organizing pneumonia and methotrexate pneumonitis often respond well to treatment. Regression of disease is highly variable in follicular bronchiolitis and lymphocytic interstitial pneumonia and is virtually never seen in OB. Lung function may improve in response to treatment in interstitial pulmonary fibrosis, but more often the goal is to prevent further progression of disease, especially when extensive.

# SYSTEMIC LUPUS ERYTHEMATOSUS

Systemic lupus erythematosus (SLE) is an inflammatory multisystem disorder of unknown etiology with protean clinical and laboratory manifestations and a variable course and prognosis. The 1982 revised American College of Rheumatology criteria for the diagnosis of SLE require that a minimum of four of the criteria listed in Table 58.6 be satisfied (although SLE is sometimes diagnosed with fewer than four criteria).[120]

**Table 58.6 SYSTEMIC LUPUS ERYTHEMATOSIS**

| |
|---|
| **Criteria for Diagnosis*** |
| Malar rash |
| Discoid rash |
| Photosensitivity skin rash |
| Oral or nasopharyngeal ulceration |
| Nonerosive arthritis involving two or more peripheral joints |
| Serositis (pleuritis or pericarditis) |
| Renal disorder (persistent proteinuria or cellular casts) |
| Neurologic disorder (unexplained seizures or psychosis) |
| Hematologic disorder (hemolytic anemia, leukopenia, lymphopenia, or thrombocytopenia) |
| Immunologic disorder (positive LE cell, anti-DNA antibody, anti-Sm antibody, false-positive syphilis serology) |
| Elevated antinuclear antibodies |
| **Lung Manifestations** |
| Diffuse lung disease |
| Extrapulmonary restriction ("shrinking lung syndrome") |
| Diffuse alveolar hemorrhage |
| Pulmonary hypertension |
| Pleural disease |

*Minimum of four criteria required.

## Epidemiology and Risk Factors

SLE occurs throughout the world; the reported prevalence ranges from 12/100,000 to 50/100,000, and the incidence ranges from 1.8/100,000/year to 7.6/100,000/year.[121] There is a 6-fold to 10-fold female excess, and the disease is three times more common in African Americans than in whites. The 5 year survival rate exceeds 90%, but the mortality rate is three times higher than in the general population. Support for a genetic contribution to disease includes a high prevalence in monozygotic twins, familial clustering, and associations between SLE and HLA DR2, DR3, and the C4A null allele.[122] No infectious or other environmental factor has been shown to play a major etiologic role.

## Pulmonary Manifestations

Pleuropulmonary manifestations of SLE are listed in Table 58.6.

### Diffuse Lung Disease

Diffuse lung disease on lung biopsy or at autopsy has been reported in 4%, 33%, and 70% of SLE patients.[123–125] These striking inconsistencies undoubtedly reflect major variations in the histologic diagnostic criteria: In the series with the highest prevalence, trivial interstitial thickening was categorized as "pulmonary fibrosis" but likely represented the minor residuum of infection or inflammatory complications of SLE. Only 3% of SLE patients have clinical evidence of diffuse lung disease at the onset of systemic disease, and a disease resembling interstitial pulmonary fibrosis develops during follow-up in less than 5%.[126] The clinical presentation (dyspnea, cough, predominantly basal crackles, a restrictive lung function defect or isolated reduction in carbon monoxide diffusing capacity, basal infiltrates on chest radiography) is typical of idiopathic pulmonary fibrosis. Features not typical of idiopathic pulmonary fibrosis, however, include variably associated pleuritic pain, a paucity of patients with morphologically extensive or functionally severe lung fibrosis, and the frequent presence of enlarged peribronchiolar lymphoid follicles at lung biopsy (although other histologic findings are indistinguishable from idiopathic pulmonary fibrosis). Partial regression of disease with corticosteroids in 9 of 14 cases in one series[127] suggests that an empirical trial of therapy is usually warranted.

Although seen in less than 2% of SLE patients, acute lupus pneumonitis is often life-threatening, with a mortality rate despite treatment of more than 50% once respiratory failure has supervened.[128] The predominant histologic feature of diffuse alveolar damage is nonspecific, and it has been argued that acute lupus pneumonitis is merely a manifestation of aspiration or bacterial infection.[123] Well-documented striking responses to corticosteroids and immunosuppressive agents after antibiotic failure, however, suggest strongly that the disorder is a true, albeit rare, entity. Acute lupus pneumonitis is not to be confused with organizing pneumonia ("bronchiolitis obliterans organizing pneumonia"), discussed elsewhere in this chapter and reported in only a handful of adult patients with SLE, or lymphocytic interstitial pneumonia, described in a small number of patients with SLE.

## Extrapulmonary Restriction

Extrapulmonary restriction, resulting in exertional dyspnea, a restrictive functional defect, and marked elevation of KCO, is a well-recognized complication of SLE. The "shrinking lung syndrome" was first described in patients with severe restriction and a marked reduction in lung volume on chest radiography, and it is generally ascribed to diaphragmatic weakness (Fig. 58.5).[129, 130] The use of sniff pressures to evaluate diaphragmatic strength may, however, be confounded by concurrent lung restriction or airflow obstruction; in one study, with the use of alternative methods to evaluate diaphragmatic function, the characteristic restrictive defect was attributed to an "unspecified restriction in chest wall expansion."[131] No treatment of proven efficacy currently exists, although a handful of patients have improved in association with corticosteroid or immunosuppressive therapy. The disorder is almost always self-limited, although sometimes it is severe.

## Diffuse Alveolar Hemorrhage

Although seen more frequently in SLE than in other connective tissue disorders, diffuse alveolar hemorrhage is rare in SLE. The typical presentation of acute dyspnea and extensive pulmonary infiltrates on chest radiography may mimic acute lupus pneumonitis, especially in the absence of hemoptysis. Diffuse alveolar hemorrhage is often life-threatening, with a mortality rate similar to that of acute lupus pneumonitis; as the two diseases are both treated empirically with corticosteroid and immunosuppressive therapy, however, the important differential diagnosis is opportunistic infection. Patients with SLE have underlying defects in most arms of the immune system and are at added risk of fulminant infection with the use of corticosteroids or immunosuppressive agents.[132] In this context, a misdiagnosis of acute lupus pneumonitis or diffuse alveolar hemorrhage may lead to a potentially disastrous increase in immunosuppression. Thus, the performance of BAL to exclude opportunistic infection may be crucial in SLE patients with unexplained extensive pulmonary infiltrates.

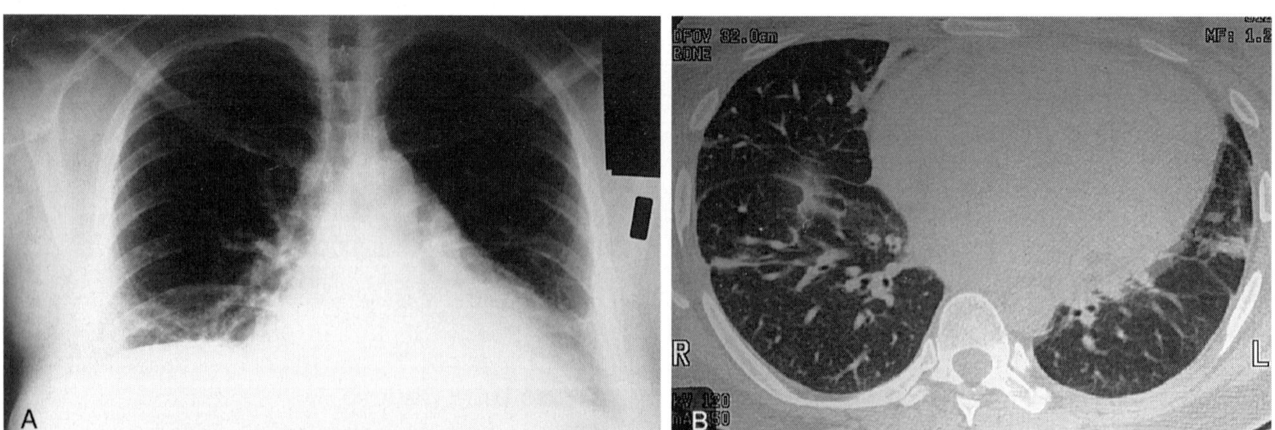


**Figure 58.5** *A,* This chest radiograph from a patient with systemic lupus erythematosis shows marked elevation of both hemidiaphragms, in keeping with "the vanishing lung syndrome." *B,* On a CT scan from the same patient as in *A,* linear abnormalities are seen that denote subsegmental atelectasis resulting from regional hypoventilation (due to diaphragmatic weakness).

### Pulmonary Hypertension

Pulmonary hypertension was once considered rare in SLE, but it is now reported with increasing frequency[133] and has a 2 year survival rate of less than 50% in severe disease. Abnormalities indicative of subclinical pulmonary hypertension are found on echocardiography in 10% of SLE patients, usually in association with Raynaud's phenomenon,[134] and thus it is likely that pulmonary hypertension results from vasoconstriction rather than pulmonary vasculitis (which is seldom identified in SLE); in autopsied patients with pulmonary hypertension, overt vasculitis is rare.

An important alternative mechanism for pulmonary hypertension is thromboembolism, which has a high prevalence in SLE, especially in patients with antiphospholipid antibodies (which cross-react with coagulation factors).[135] In a 1993 study of 842 SLE patients, IgG anticardiolipin antibodies were present more frequently than IgM antibodies (24% vs. 13%), but both were associated with a 30% prevalence of thrombosis (as opposed to 10% in other SLE patients).[136] In view of the multiplicity of mechanisms potentially responsible for pulmonary hypertension, vasodilators, anticoagulation, and corticosteroid or immunosuppressive agents have all been advocated empirically for patients with the pulmonary vascular disease of SLE.

### Pleural Disease

Pleural disease is the most common pulmonary manifestation of SLE. Clinical or radiographic evidence of pleural involvement is seen in 20% of patients at the onset of systemic disease and occurs in at least 50% at some time[137] (with pleural abnormalities at autopsy in 50% to 100%[124, 138]). Pleural disease is often asymptomatic, but pleuritic pain may be recurrent or intractable. The fluid is usually serosanguinous (but occasionally hemorrhagic) and exudative with a neutrophilia in patients with pleurisy but a predominant lymphocytosis in chronic effusions.[137] The nonspecific histologic appearance of fibrinous pleuritis is not diagnostically useful. The identification of lupus erythematosus cells has largely fallen out of favor, as technical difficulties greatly reduce the sensitivity of the test (in confirming that a pleural effusion is due to SLE).[139] The measurement of pleural fluid antinuclear antibody titers may be more diagnostically useful when the etiology of pleural disease is in doubt.[140]

## SJÖGREN'S SYNDROME

Sjögren's syndrome is an autoimmune disorder characterized by lymphocytic infiltration of the lacrimal, salivary, conjunctival, and pharyngeal mucosal glands, with variable involvement of extraglandular tissue. The cardinal clinical features of keratoconjunctivitis sicca (dry eyes) and xerostomia (a dry mouth) may occur in isolation (primary Sjögren's syndrome, typically seen in women older than age 40 years) but are more often associated with connective tissue diseases such as RA, SSc, or SLE (secondary Sjögren's syndrome). Variable diagnostic criteria are used internationally; in one proposed diagnostic algorithm, sicca symptoms are mandatory, with supportive evidence including ocular signs (positive Shirmer's test, Rose Bengal score >3), typical histologic appearances on salivary gland biopsy, antibodies to Ro (SS-A) or LA (SS-B), or reduced salivary flow.[141, 142]

### Epidemiology and Risk Factors

The reported prevalence of primary Sjögren's syndrome ranges from 0.5% to 3.0%. The etiology of the disease is unknown. There is some evidence to suggest a genetic predisposition, including familial clustering and an association with HLA Dw2 and HLA Dw3, but no environmental triggers have been identified.

### Pulmonary Manifestations

Pulmonary involvement is common in Sjögren's syndrome. In early series, primary and secondary Sjögren's syndrome were combined; it is likely that many of the pulmonary abnormalities seen in secondary Sjögren's syndrome were ascribed to the underlying connective tissue disease. Careful evaluation of patients with primary Sjögren's syndrome has shown that cough and dyspnea are common,[143] with objective evidence of pulmonary abnormalities in approximately one fourth of cases.[144] Lung involvement usually consists of lymphocytic infiltration similar to that seen in salivary glands and resulting in tracheobronchial disease or interstitial lung disease, depending on whether involvement is limited to secretory glandular tissue or is more widespread. Population studies of respiratory involvement in Sjögren's syndrome have, however, been hampered by variations in diagnostic criteria, failure to discriminate between primary and secondary Sjögren's syndrome, and failure to control for confounding features such as drug treatment and smoking. Lung manifestations include diffuse lung disease and tracheobronchial disease.

### Diffuse Lung Disease

Although often asymptomatic, diffuse lung disease in Sjögren's syndrome may present with cough, dyspnea, crackles on auscultation, reticular or reticulonodular abnormalities on chest radiography, and a restrictive pattern of functional impairment. Interstitial involvement can be classified as pulmonary fibrosis, lymphocytic interstitial pneumonia, or lymphoma. Pulmonary fibrosis has been reported in up to 10% of patients with primary Sjögren's syndrome[145] and may result from prolonged lymphocytic interstitial infiltration. Although a presentation typical of extensive or progressive interstitial pulmonary fibrosis is rare, and interstitial disease in Sjögren's syndrome is often regarded as clinically insignificant, Gardiner and coworkers[145] found that patients with primary Sjögren's syndrome complaining of dyspnea (approximately 10%) have a high prevalence of histologic abnormalities (fibrosis or lymphocytic infiltration) on transbronchial biopsy.[145]

Lymphocytic interstitial infiltration may take the form of lymphocytic interstitial pneumonia, pseudolymphoma (extensive pulmonary lymphocytic infiltration with the

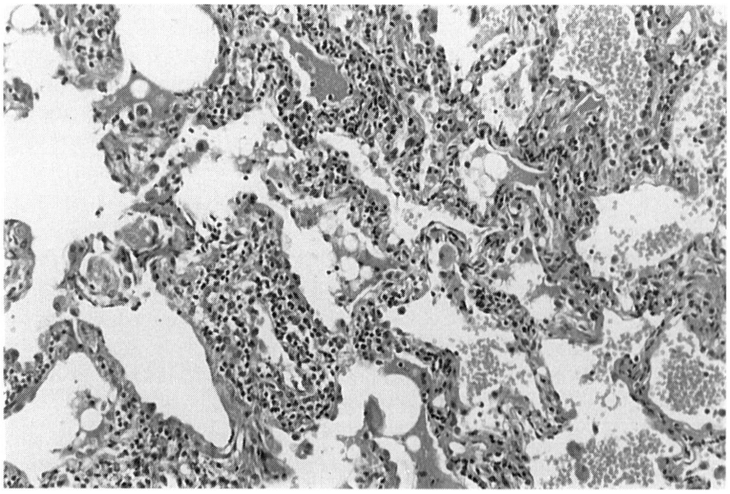

**Figure 58.6** This surgical lung biopsy specimen was taken from a patient with diffuse lung disease in the context of Sjögren's syndrome. Note the dense lymphocytic infiltrate within the interstitium. (Courtesy of Dr. Andrew Nicholson, Royal Brompton Hospital.)

formation of lymphoid follicles), or pulmonary lymphoma. Lymphocytic interstial pneumonia, the most common form of diffuse lung disease in Sjögren's syndrome (Fig. 58.6),[146] is characterized by a diffuse lymphocytic infiltrate, with or without histiocytes and multinucleated giant cells, most prominent around bronchioles. Pseudolymphoma, characterized by pulmonary infiltration, may regress spontaneously and often responds well to corticosteroid therapy; however, some patients progress to pulmonary lymphoma. The prevalence of lymphoma is increased 40-fold to 50-fold in Sjögren's syndrome[147]; pulmonary lymphoma has a highly variable clinical and radiographic presentation, with the spectrum of disease ranging from diffuse interstitial involvement to discrete (often perihilar) masses. It is now believed that all lymphocytic interstitial pneumonia may represent malignant disease of varying nature.

Organizing pneumonia (bronchiolitis obliterans organizing pneumonia) has been reported in Sjögren's syndrome but occurs less frequently than in rheumatoid arthritis or polymyositis. A response to corticosteroid therapy is usual but not invariable.

### Tracheobronchial Disease

Tracheobronchial disease may take the form of loss of mucous secretion in the trachea (xerotrachea), chronic bronchitis, or small airway disease. Xerotrachea occurs in up to 25% of patients with primary Sjögren's syndrome and consists of atrophy of tracheobronchial mucous glands in association with a lymphoplasmocytic infiltrate, manifesting clinically as a relentless dry cough and endobronchial inflammation at bronchoscopy.[148] It is likely that similar histologic abnormalities in bronchi and bronchioles account for an increased prevalence of bronchial hyperresponsiveness, reported in 40% to 60% of patients with primary and secondary Sjögren's syndrome[149, 150]

Subclinical bronchiolitis may be common in Sjögren's syndrome. In the interstitial lung disease of Sjögren's syndrome, lymphocytic infiltration is more prominent around small bronchioles,[151] resulting in a BAL lymphocytosis[152]; thus, it is likely that the occasional cases of isolated lymphocytic bronchiolitis, presenting with a clinical picture of chronic obstructive pulmonary disease, represent a more limited form of lymphocytic infiltration. The evaluation of air flow at low lung volumes in unselected patients with primary and secondary Sjögren's syndrome has demonstrated a high prevalence of small airway dysfunction[143]; aerosol penetration from central airways to the lung periphery is reduced, indicating small airway obstruction.[153] These abnormalities, indicating either obstructive bronchiolitis (OB) or mucous plugging, may contribute to an increased prevalence of bronchopneumonia but do not evolve into severe OB (which is not generally a feature of Sjögren's syndrome, except in occasional cases with associated RA). Follicular bronchiolitis has been reported in a handful of patients with primary Sjögren's syndrome[91] but may occur more frequently in secondary Sjögren's syndrome; in a number of reported cases of follicular bronchiolitis associated with RA, the presence of Sjögren's syndrome is not explicitly excluded. Follicular bronchiolitis and diffuse bronchiolar lymphocytic infiltration may be part of the same spectrum of disease but the relationship between the two disorders is uncertain.

## POLYMYOSITIS WITH DERMATOMYOSITIS

The defining criteria for polymyositis with dermatomyositis are listed in Table 58.7. For polymyositis, a definite diagnosis is made if the first four features are present, a probable diagnosis is made if any three of the first four features are present, and a possible diagnosis is made if any two of the first four features are present. For dermatomyositis, the typical rash must be present, plus any three of the first four for a definite diagnosis, two of the first four for a probable diagnosis, and one of the first four for a possible diagnosis (Bohan and Peter criteria[154]).

The skin problems of dermatomyositis include the presence of scaly cutaneous eruptions affecting extensor surfaces of the finger joints (Gottron's tubercles) or the characteristic edema and violaceous or purplish, heliotrope rash that surrounds the eyelids. Proximal muscle weakness tends to be insidious, progressive, and painless, affecting head, neck, and limb girdles and eventually involving the muscles of the tongue and pharynx and the

**Table 58.7 POLYMYOSITIS WITH DERMATOMYOSITIS**

| |
|---|
| **Criteria for Diagnosis** |
| Symmetric proximal muscle weakness |
| Muscle biopsy material showing myositis |
| Elevation of serum skeletal muscle enzymes |
| Characteristic electromyographic pattern of myositis |
| Typical rash of dermatomyositis |
| **Lung Manifestations** |
| Interstitial pulmonary fibrosis |
| Acute pneumonitis (with diffuse alveolar damage) |
| Organizing pneumonia |
| Aspiration pneumonia |
| Pulmonary vasculitis and alveolar hemorrhage |
| Respiratory muscle weakness |

respiratory muscles. Pulmonary complications occur in approximately 45% of patients and are the most frequent cause of death.

## Epidemiology and Risk Factors

The inflammatory myopathies are relatively rare, affecting 2 to $10/10^6$ population with a female to male predominance of 2.5:1 and with a bimodal age distribution peaking in childhood and in the fourth to fifth decades. Dermatomyositis appears to have a higher expression of HLA B8/DR3, B14, and B40 while polymyositis associates with HLA B8/DR3 and in African-Americans with B7 and DRw6.[155]

There are multiple manifestations of lung disease as listed in Table 58.7. The prevalence of lung disease varies from series to series, and often the respiratory symptoms are masked by muscle fatigue. Nonetheless, pulmonary complications of the disease can be a frequent cause of death. In combined series, the prevalence of diffuse lung disease can be up to 64%.

## Pulmonary Manifestations

### Diffuse Lung Disease

Diffuse lung disease is the most common problem encountered in the context of dermatomyositis with polymyositis. The pattern of diffuse lung disease often mimics that of interstitial pulmonary fibrosis, but an acute, rapidly progressive form of acute pneumonitis can occur. Organizing pneumonia may also be the presenting feature (Fig. 58.7). The histopathologic features associated with these forms of presentation include usual interstitial pneumonia in patients with an interstitial pulmonary fibrosis pattern, diffuse alveolar damage in the acute pneumonitis, and bronchiolitis obliterans together with organizing pneumonia in those patients who have the clinical features of organizing pneumonia.[156–158] More recently, it has been shown that one of the characteristic features of chronic diffuse lung disease in polymyositis with dermatomyositis is a combination of the features of organizing pneumonia and interstitial pulmonary fibrosis on high-resolution CT.[159] One recent report has described an acute presentation of pulmonary capillaritis with alveolar hemorrhage in association with polymyositis.[159, 160]

**Clinical Features.** The clinical features of diffuse lung disease in polymyositis with dermatomyositis depend on the nature of the lung process. Breathlessness on exertion without wheeze is a common presenting symptom, and, if the myopathy is severe, orthopnea may be striking. Hemoptysis may occur if there is capillaritis. Pleural disease is uncommon.

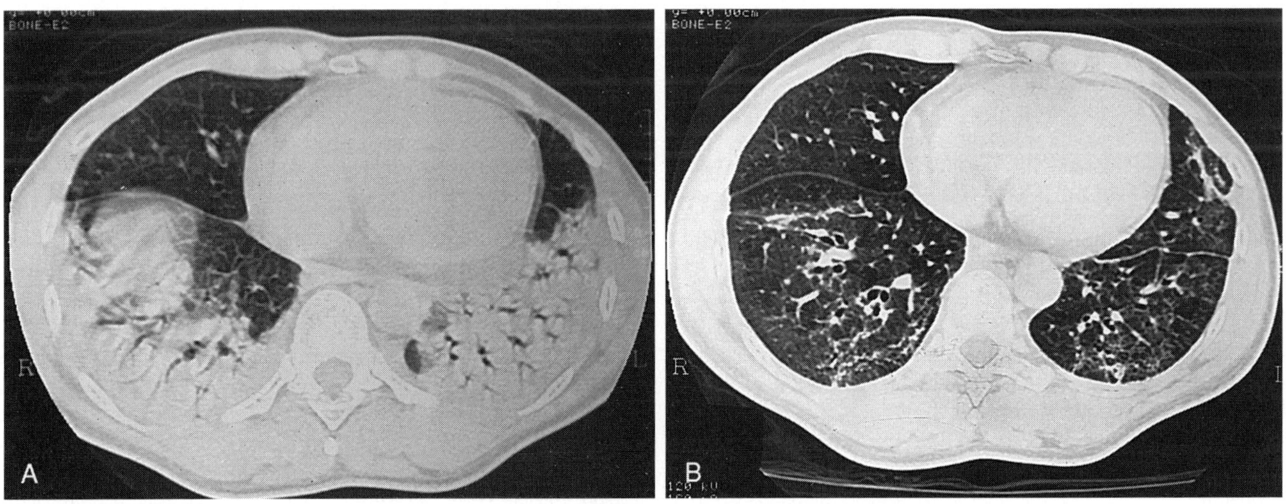


**Figure 58.7** *A,* The CT scan shows dense consolidation that denotes organizing pneumonia in a patient with polymyositis. As shown in this example, the disease tends to be most prominent posteriorly in the lower lobes. *B,* After treatment, the dense consolidation has regressed, but there is extensive residual linear opacification, representing residual fibrosis and resulting in traction bronchiectasis on the right and a restrictive functional defect.

**Imaging.** Chest radiography depends on lung disease. Chronic diffuse lung disease is associated with peripheral reticular nodular opacities, particularly in the bases as for interstitial pulmonary fibrosis. Acute pneumonitis can result in ground-glass opacification on chest radiography and alveolar hemorrhage with areas of consolidation.

CT is much more specific than radiography, highlighting the distributions of the different processes. A combination of consolidation with a peripheral reticular pattern is highly characteristic.

Lung function tests show a restrictive ventilatory defect with reduced gas transfer. In recent hemorrhage or marked myopathy, there may be a disproportionate preservation of a gas transfer index (KCO). It must be remembered, however, that acute hemorrhage can occur in the context of previous chronic disease, and so the KCO may be normal or subnormal but elevated from a level that was previously lower.

Dermatomyositis and polymyositis are well-recognized paraneoplastic phenomena, so it is sometimes difficult to determine which condition presented first.[161] Screening for occult carcinoma is recommended with mammography, abdominal CT, pelvic ultrasonography, and tumor markers.

**Autoantibodies.** Studies of autoantibodies have highlighted the association between the presence of antibodies to aminoacyl tRNA synthetases, inflammatory myopathies, and diffuse lung disease.[162] Jo-1 (antihistidyl tRNA synthetase) is the most common, occurring in 20% to 30% of patients with inflammatory myopathy and in 50% to 100% of cases of inflammatory myopathy and diffuse lung disease in contrast to less than 5% of patients without diffuse lung disease. A variety of novel autoantibodies have been described with affinity for other tRNA synthetase molecules: PL12, PL7, EJ, and OJ. These molecules help define the antisynthetase syndrome: the coexistence of myositis, diffuse lung disease, and arthritis.

In some patients, diffuse lung disease is the presenting feature. Typical CT appearances may suggest the diagnosis. In this situation, typical autoantibodies may be found, confirming a suspicion of dermatomyositis with polymyositis.

### Other Pulmonary Manifestations

Aspiration pneumonia needs to be considered if there is upper airway and pharyngeal muscle weakness. The predilection for posterior segments may suggest this diagnosis.

The treatment of lung disease depends on the histopathologic pattern. Organizing pneumonia responds well to corticosteroids alone. Vasculitis may require a combination of high-dose prednisolone and immunosuppression. More chronic diffuse lung disease may respond to a combination of prednisolone and azathioprine.

## MIXED CONNECTIVE TISSUE DISEASE

Mixed connective tissue disease (MCTD) is defined by the presence of features of SLE, SSc, and polymyositis (Sjögren's syndrome may also be seen) in association with high titers (>1:1600) of autoantibody directed against the extractable nuclear antigen U1-RNP.[163, 164] Criteria that have been suggested for the diagnosis of MCTD include the presence of antibody to the U1 ribonuclear protein together with the clinical features of hand edema, synovitis, Raynaud's phenomenon, acrosclerosis, and myositis. At least three of these clinical features are needed in addition to the autoantibody finding. A fourth clinical feature is required if the initial three are Raynaud's phenomenon, edema, and acrosclerosis. The difference between MCTD and overlap syndrome may be semantic, but the former often presents more acutely and with greater specificity for U1-RNP. MCTD may differentiate into specific rheumatologic diseases. This differentiation may be genetically determined.[165, 166]

The prevalence of the disease is unclear, but it is estimated at 1 in 10,000, with a 9:1 female preponderance.[167] Pleuropulmonary complications occur in 20% to 85% of patients, but diffuse lung disease is the most common lung complication.[168] Survival is better if the diffuse lung disease is associated with U1-RNP positivity than with no U1-RNP. Pulmonary involvement, investigations, and treatment are as for the individual connective tissue diseases.

Other overlap syndromes are reported in which clinical features of more than one connective tissue disease are present in the same patient. Although MCTD tissue disease remains the most clearly definable, other overlap syndromes occur both with and without typical autoantibody association. Of the former, overlapping clinical features found in association with U2-RNP and U3-RNP and the tRNA synthetase-associated diseases (see earlier) can be considered to be part of an overlap syndrome.[167] Antibodies to PM-Scl, KU, and U2-RNP are associated with overlaps of SSc and polymyositis.[164]

Whether these distinctly defined subsets of overlap have implications in terms of prognosis or treatment is uncertain. Treatment depends on the nature of the lung disease and is identical to the approaches used for the other connective tissue diseases.[165]

## RELAPSING POLYCHONDRITIS

The diagnosis of relapsing polychondritis requires the presence of three or more of the following clinical features[170, 171]: bilateral auricular chondritis; nonerosive, seronegative inflammatory polyarthritis; nasal chondritis; ocular inflammation; respiratory tract involvement (either upper or lower respiratory tract); cochlear with or without vestibular abnormality; and positive biopsy specimen. The presence of anticartilage antibodies may be helpful in the diagnosis.

Relapsing polychondritis is rare and is characterized by episodic painful and destructive cartilaginous inflammation. The condition affects men and women equally and has a peak incidence between 40 and 60 years of age. It is considered an autoimmune process, and autoantibodies have been found directed against cartilage and type II collagen. Diagnosis is chiefly clinical but can be confirmed at biopsy of affected cartilage, including tracheal rings.

Relapsing polychondritis is usually multifocal, affecting cartilage of the ear (85% to 94%), nose (54% to 57%) (Fig. 58.8*A*), upper respiratory tract (31% to 48%), and ribs. Additionally, patients frequently suffer ocular inflammation, nonerosive arthropathy (52%), and vestibulocochlear dysfunction.[171, 172] It may occur in association with a wide range of other conditions, especially connective tissue disease and vasculitis. Approximately 30% of patients have a preexisting connective tissue disease.

Respiratory involvement probably accounts for around 10% of deaths in this condition. Pulmonary parenchymal disease is rare, but vasculitis may occur. Destruction and obstruction of the glottis, trachea, and bronchi lead to airway stricture, collapse, and distal infection Fig. 58.8)[173] Lung function testing shows diminution in maximal inspiratory (large, extrathoracic airways) and expiratory (smaller, intrathoracic airways) flow rates, suggesting airway collapse while static recoil pressures are preserved. With dynamic CT scanning showing tracheal ring thickening, collapse on inspiratory maneuvers can help to localize the large airway disease.

Treatment depends on disease severity. Mild cases may be controlled with nonsteroidal anti-inflammatroy drop,

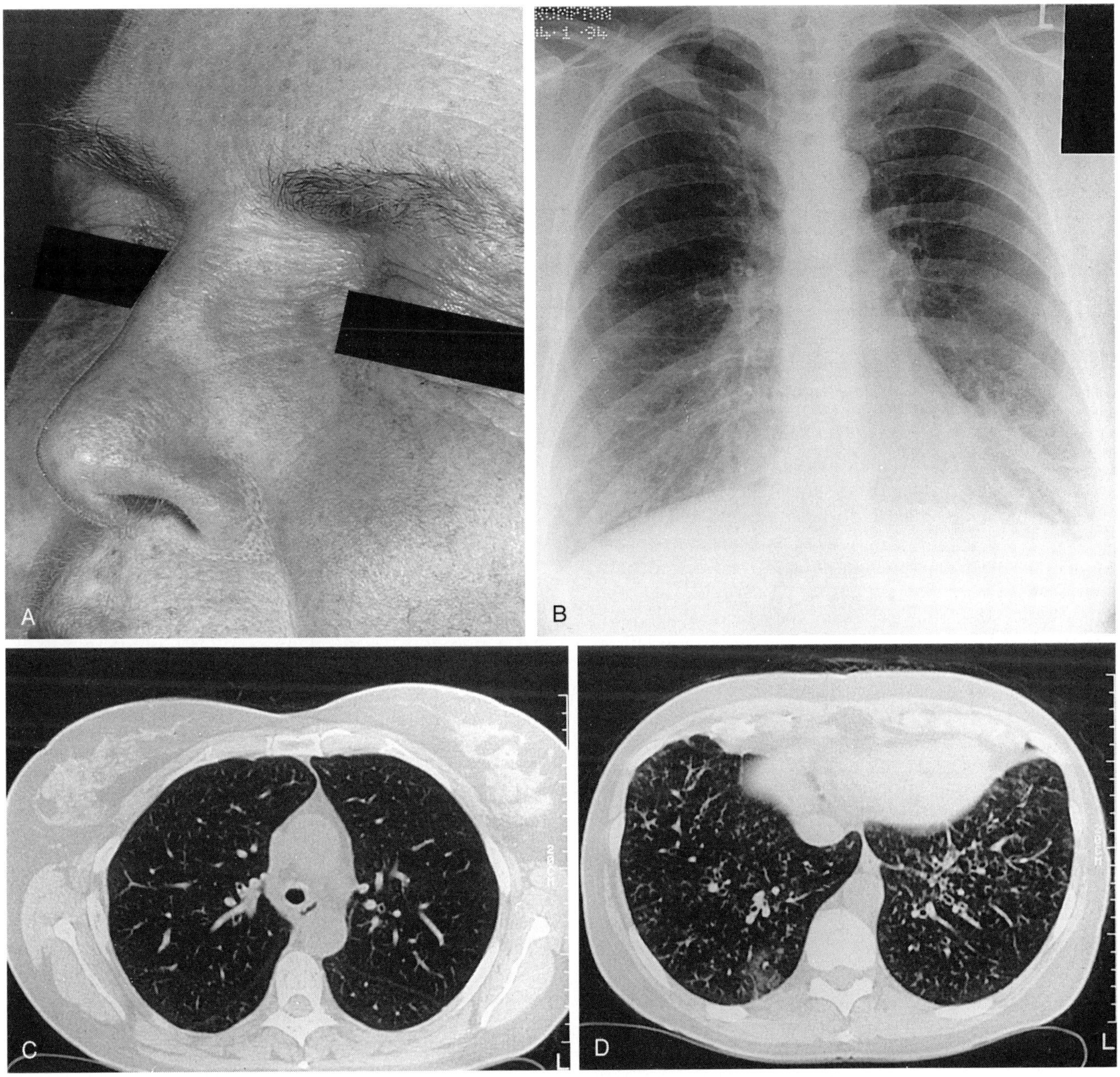

**Figure 58.8** Relapsing polychondritis is shown. *A*, Loss of cartilage in this individual's nose results in a "saddle" deformity. *B*, This chest radiograph of the same individual as in *A* demonstrates tracheal narrowing. *C*, Tracheal narrowing and thickening shown more graphically in the CT scan. *D*, Thickening of the segmental bronchi is seen together with patchy attenuation ("mosaicism"), which indicates small airway involvement.

while troublesome relapses may require short-term high-dose corticosteroid therapy. Steroid-resistant lesions have been treated with immunosuppressive agents such as cyclophosphamide. Tracheostomy and stenting are occasionally indicated, but other surgical treatment is difficult due to the diffuse nature of involvement,[174] In one large review of 159 reported cases, three fourths of the patients required chronic corticosteroid therapy, which, in that series, decreased the frequency, duration, and severity of flare-ups but did not prevent disease progression.[170]

## BEHÇET'S DISEASE

Behçet's disease occurs predominantly in the countries bordering the Mediterranean sea. Prevalence estimates approach 80 to 300/100,000 in Turkey. Males and females are affected equally, and age of onset is usually in the third or fourth decade. There is an association between the HLA B51 allele and more severely affected patients. Herpes simplex type 1 and streptococci have been suggested as causative agents.[175] Diagnosis requires the presence of recurrent aphthous ulceration occurring at least three times in a 12-month period and two of the four minor features listed in Table 58.8.[176]

Mucocutaneous ulceration is the clinical hallmark, with aphthous oral and genital ulceration seen in almost all patients. Other cutaneous features include erythema nodosum, an acneiform rash, and papular lesions of cutaneous vasculitis. Uveitis is the major cause of morbidity, but systemic vasculitis may affect all systems.

Pulmonary involvement is seen in 1% to 7% and tends to affect HLA B51+ younger males (<25 years) more severely. Symptoms include dyspnea, chest pain, and recurrent hemoptysis that can be massive and fatal.[177] Pathology reveals pulmonary arterial aneurysms, arterial and venous thromboses, pulmonary infarcts, and occasionally pleural effusion.[178] Radiography is nonspecific but may demonstrate the features of pulmonary hemorrhage, vascular occlusion, or mass lesions representing arterial aneurysm(s).[179]

Treatment is complex and depends on presentation. Steroids and immunosuppressive agents are used to control vasculitis, and colchicine has been helpful for some patients.[180] Anticoagulants may be required for control of thrombosis, but the risk of hemorrhage is significant. Pulmonary embolization and surgical resection have been reported to be successful, but surgical treatment of aneurysms can result in aneurysms at the anastomosis site.[181]

**Table 58.8 BEHÇET'S SYNDROME**

**Criteria for Diagnosis**

- Major (required)
  - Recurrent aphthous ulceration occurring at least three times in a 12 month period
- Minor (two of four)
  - Recurrent genital ulceration
  - Ocular disease
  - Skin lesions (erythema nodosum, skin ulcers)
  - Positive pathergy test (the development of a papule or pustule 24–48 hours after simple skin trauma such as a skin prick)

## ANKYLOSING SPONDYLITIS

Ankylosing spondylitis (AS) is a seronegative spondyloarthritis developing in 0.05% to 1.5% of the general population and is associated with the major histocompatibility antigen HLA-B27.[182] The cardinal site of disease is the vertebral column, but peripheral joint arthritis is seen in approximately one third of patients, and extra-articular features include aortic regurgitation, uveitis, pulmonary disease, and extrapulmonary restriction.

Fibrotic lung disease on chest radiography, largely or entirely confined to the upper zones, was seen in only 1% to 2% of a series of 2080 patients with AS.[183] On high-resolution CT, however, limited interstitial lung disease, bronchiectasis, or paraseptal emphysema are present in the majority of patients, even when chest radiographic appearances are normal,[184] and a subclinical lymphocytic alveolitis may be evident with BAL.[185] Histologically, lung abnormalities consist of a variable mixture of lymphocytic infiltration, fibrosis, and bullous change.[186] On chest radiography, diffuse reticulonodular infiltrates in the upper zones are usually symmetric and are seldom extensive except in patients with severe spinal disease[187] or a long history of AS.[183, 186] Occasionally apical fibrosis may, however, precede the development of extrapulmonary disease. No proven treatment exists to prevent the development of apical fibrosis; resistance to corticosteroid therapy is the rule.

Cavities may develop within distorted fibrotic apical tissue and are sometimes colonized by mycobacteria or fungi, especially *Aspergillus fumigatus*, which are isolated in up to 60% of AS patients with apical cavitation.[188] Life-threatening hemoptysis is an occasional complication of mycetoma formation within cavities and may be controllable by bronchial artery embolization; the resection of a mycetoma is a treatment of last resort due to the high prevalence of postoperative bronchopleural fistula or empyema. Advanced apical fibrosis is often associated with apical pleural thickening, but pleural disease is seldom seen adjacent to normal lung parenchyma elsewhere in the thorax. There is an increased (up to 10%) prevalence of pneumothorax in AS patients with apical fibrosis,[183] probably due to subpleural bullous degeneration in advancing disease.

Extrapulmonary restriction due to immobilization of the chest wall (costovertebral ankylosis) is an occasional complication of AS, associated with surprisingly little impairment in pulmonary function, perhaps because the diaphragm is able to make a major contribution in the presence of a high resting volume.[189]

## MARFAN'S SYNDROME

Marfan's syndrome (MS) is an autosomal dominant condition of variable penetrance affecting approximately 5/100,000. MS is characterized by abnormalities of fibrous connective tissue (due to mutations on chromosome 15), especially in the skeleton (long limbs, arachnodactyly, pectus excavatum, kyphoscoliosis), eyes (subluxation of the lens), and cardiovascular system (aortic or mitral regurgitation, aortic aneurysm). The reduced life expectancy of MS is largely attributable to cardiac complications; there is no effective treatment to reverse disease or to slow progression.

Respiratory complications can be subdivided into pulmonary and extrapulmonary abnormalities. Localized bulla formation with a predilection for the lung apex[190] is an occasional striking finding in young patients. Generalized emphysema in nonsmoking patients with MS may become evident at any age and is sometimes fatal in childhood.[191]

The high prevalence of pneumothorax in MS of 5% to 10%[192] (over 100-fold higher than in the general population) can be ascribed to the rupture of subpleural bullae; emphysema is present on chest radiography in the majority of MS patients with pneumothoraces,[192, 193] which are often recurrent and bilateral. Underlying apical fibrosis has been reported in a handful of cases. Other less frequent parenchymal manifestations include congenital malformations of the middle lobes (which may be absent or rudimentary) and an increased prevalence of bronchopneumonia.[192]

Isolated pectus excavatum in MS is seldom associated with significant impairment in lung function. However, occasionally kyphoscoliosis is associated with fatal cor pulmonale.[194] It is likely that nocturnal desaturation amplifies hypoxia due to kyphoscoliosis. Increased upper airway collapsibility during sleep was recently shown to be common in MS,[195] accounting for an association between MS and obstructive sleep apnea.

## References


1. Wells AU, Hansell DM, du Bois RM: Interstitial lung disease in the collagen vascular diseases. Semin Respir Med 14:333–343, 1993.
2. Cannon GW, Zimmerman GA, (eds): The Lung in Rheumatic Diseases. New York: Marcel Dekker, 1990.
3. Masi AT, Rodnan GP, Medsger TAJ, et al: Preliminary criteria for the classification of systemic sclerosis (scleroderma). Arthritis Rheum 23:581–590, 1980.
4. Silman AJ, Black CM, Welsh KI: Epidemiology, demographics, genetics. *In* Clements PJ, Furst DE (eds): Systemic Sclerosis. Baltimore: Williams Wilkins, 1996, pp 23–50.
5. Silman AJ: Scleroderma—demographics and survival. J Rheumatol-Suppl 48:58–61, 1997.
6. Artlett CM, Black CM, Briggs DC, et al: Telomere reduction in scleroderma patients: A possible cause for chromosomal instability. Br J Rheumatol 35:732–737, 1996.
7. Fanning GC, Welsh KI, Bunn C, et al: HLA associations in three mutually exclusive autoantibody subgroups in UK systemic sclerosis patients. Br J Rheumatol 37:201–207, 1998.
8. Briggs DC, Vaughan RW, Welsh KI, et al: Immunogenetic prediction of pulmonary fibrosis in systemic sclerosis Lancet 338:661–662, 1991.
9. Silver RM: Scleroderma and pseudoscleroderma: Environmental exposure. *In* Clements PJ, Furst DE (eds): Systemic Sclerosis Baltimore: Williams & Wilkins, 1996, pp 81–98.
10. Rodnan GP, Benedek TG, Medsger TA Jr, et al: The association of progressive systemic sclerosis (scleroderma) with coal miners' pneumoconiosis and other forms of silicosis. Ann Intern Med 66:323–334, 1967.
11. Tabuenca JM: Toxic-allergic syndrome caused by ingestion of rapeseed oil denatured with aniline. Lancet 2:567–568, 1981.
12. Arnett FC, Howard RF, Tan F, et al: Increased prevalence of systemic sclerosis in a Native American tribe in Oklahoma. Association with an Amerindian HLA haplotype. Arthritis Rheum 39:1362–1370, 1996.
13. Yurovsky VV, Wigley FM, Wise RA, et al: Skewing of the CD8+ T-cell repertoire in the lungs of patients with systemic sclerosis. Hum Immunol 48:84–97, 1996.
14. Yurovsky VV, White B: T cell repertoire in systemic sclerosis. Int Rev Immunol 12:97–105, 1995.
15. Kuwana M, Kaburaki J, Mimori T, et al: Autoantigenic epitopes on DNA topoisomerase I. Clinical and immunogenetic associations in systemic sclerosis. Arthritis Rheum 36:1406–1413, 1993.
16. Kuwana M, Medsger TA Jr, Wright TM: Highly restricted TCR-alpha beta usage by autoreactive human T cell clones specific for DNA topoisomerase I: Recognition of an immunodominant epitope. J Immunol 158:485–491, 1997.
17. Kuwana M, Medsger TA Jr, Wright TM: T cell proliferative response induced by DNA topoisomerase I in patients with systemic sclerosis and healthy donors. J Clin Invest 96:586–596, 1995.
18. Wells AU, Lorimer S, Majumdar S, et al: Fibrosing alveolitis in systemic sclerosis: Increase in memory T-cells in lung interstitium. Eur Respir J 8:266–271, 1995.
19. Petrek M, Pantelidis P, Southcott AM, et al: The source and role of RANTES in interstitial lung disease. Eur Respir J 10:1207–1216, 1997.
20. Hamid Q, Majumdar S, Sheppard M, et al: Expression of IL-4, IL-5, INF gamma and IL-2 mRNA in fibrosing alveolitis associated with systemic sclerosis. Am Rev Respir Dis 147:A479, 1993.
21. Majumdar S, Li D, Ansari T, et al: Different cytokine profiles in cryptogenic fibrosing alveolitis and fibrosinig alveolitis associated with systemic sclerosis: a quantitative study of open lung biopsies. Eur Respir J 14:251–257, 1999.
22. Bolster MB, Ludwicka A, Sutherland SE, et al: Cytokine concentrations in bronchoalveolar lavage fluid of patients with systemic sclerosis. Arthritis Rheum 40:743–751, 1997.
23. Shi-Wen X, Denton CP, McWhirter A, et al: Scleroderma lung fibroblasts exhibit elevated and dysregulated type I collagen biosynthesis. Arthritis Rheum 40:1237–1244, 1997.
24. Allen JT, Knight RA, Bloor CA, et al: Enhanced insulin-like growth factor binding protein-related protein 2 (connective tissue growth factor) expression in patients with idiopathic pulmonary fibrosis and pulmonary sarcoidosis. Am J Respir Cell Mol Biol 21:693–700, 1999.
25. Ohba T, McDonald JK, Silver RM, et al: Scleroderma bronchoalveolar lavage fluid contains thrombin, a mediator of human lung fibroblast proliferation via induction of platelet-derived growth factor alpha-receptor. Am J Respir Cell Mol Biol 10:405–412, 1994.
26. Cambrey AD, Harrison NK, Dawes KE, et al: Increased levels of endothelin-1 in bronchoalveolar lavage fluid from patients with systemic sclerosis contribute to fibroblast mitogenic activity in vitro. Am J Respir Cell Mol Biol 11:439–445, 1994.
27. Gauldie J, Jordana M, Cox G: Cytokines and pulmonary fibrosis. Thorax 48:931–935, 1993.
28. Xing Z, Tremblay GM, Sime PJ, et al: Overexpression of granulocyte-macrophage colony-stimulating factor induces pulmonary granulation tissue formation and fibrosis by induction of transforming growth factor-beta 1 and myofibroblast accumulation. Am J Pathol 150:59–66, 1997.
29. Sime PJ, Xing Z, Graham FL, et al: Adenovector-mediated gene transfer of active transforming growth factor-beta 1 induces prolonged severe fibrosis in rat lung. J Clin Invest 100:768–776, 1997.
30. Corrin B, Butcher D, McAnulty BJ, et al: Immunohistochemical localization of transforming growth factor-beta 1 in the lungs of patients with systemic sclerosis, cryptogenic fibrosing alveolitis and other lung disorders. Histopathology 24:145–150, 1994.
31. Gray AJ, Bishop JE, Reeves JT, et al: Partially degraded fibrin(-ogen) stimulates fibroblast proliferation in vitro. Am J Respir Cell Mol Biol 12:684–690, 1995.
32. Abraham DJ, Vancheeswaran R, Dashwood MR, et al: Increased levels of endothelin-1 and differential endothelin type A and B receptor expression in scleroderma-associated fibrotic lung disease. Am J Pathol 151:831–841, 1997.
33. Piguet PF, Collart MA, Grau GE, et al: Requirement of tumour

necrosis factor for development of silica-induced pulmonary fibrosis. Nature 344:245–247, 1990.
34. Piguet PF, Vesin C: Treatment by human recombinant TNF receptor of pulmonary fibrosis induced by bleomycin or silica in mice. Eur Respir J 7:515–518, 1994.
35. Piguet PF, Ribaux C, Karpuz V, et al: Expression and localization of tumor necrosis alpha and its mRNA in idiopathic pulmonary fibrosis. Am J Pathol 143:651–655, 1993.
36. Piguet PF: Is tumor necrosis factor the major effector of pulmonary fibrosis? Eur Cytokine Netw 1:257–258, 1990.
37. Khalil N, O'Connor RN, Unruh HW, et al: Increased production and immunohistochemical localization of transforming growth factor-beta in idiopathic pulmonary fibrosis. Am J Respir Cell Mol Biol 5:155–162, 1991.
38. Alton E, Turner-Warwick M: Lung involvement in scleroderma. *In* Jayson MIV, Black CM (eds): Systemic Sclerosis: Scleroderma. London: John Wiley & Sons, 1988, pp 181–205.
39. Kim JH, Follett JV, Rice JR, et al: Endobronchial telangiectases and hemoptysis in scleroderma. Am J Med 84:173–174, 1988.
40. Wells AU, Hansell DM, Rubens MB, et al: Fibrosing alveolitis in systemic sclerosis: Indices of lung function in relation to extent of disease on computed tomography. Arthritis Rheum 40:1229–1236, 1997.
41. Wells AU, Hansell DM, Rubens MB, et al: Functional impairment in lone cryptogenic fibrosing alveolitis and fibrosing alveolitis associated with systemic sclerosis: A comparison. Am J Respir Crit Care Med 155:1657–1664, 1997.
42. Wells AU, Hansell DM, Rubens MB, et al: Fibrosing alveolitis in systemic sclerosis: Bronchoalveolar lavage findings in relation to computed tomographic appearance. Am J Respir Crit Care Med 150:462–468, 1994.
43. Wells AU, Hansell DM, Haslam PL, et al: Bronchoalveolar lavage cellularity: Lone cryptogenic fibrosing alveolitis compared with the fibrosing alveolitis of systemic sclerosis. Am J Respir Crit Care Med 157:1474–1482, 1998.
44. Wells AU, Hansell DM, Harrison NK, et al: Clearance of inhaled 99m-Tc DTPA predicts the clinical course of fibrosing alveolitis. Eur Respir J 6:797–802, 1993.
45. Harrison NK, Glanville AR, Strickland B, et al: Pulmonary involvement in systemic sclerosis: The detection of early changes by thin section CT scan, bronchoalveolar lavage and 99mTc-DTPA clearance. Respir Med 83:403–414, 1989.
46. Schneider PD, Wise RA, Hochberg MC, et al: Serial pulmonary function in systemic sclerosis. Am J Med 73:385, 1982.
47. Silver RM, Miller KS, Kinsella MB, et al: Evaluation and management of scleroderma lung disease using bronchoalveolar lavage. Am J Med 88:470–476, 1990.
48. Steen VD, Conte C, Owens GR, et al: Severe restrictive lung disease in systemic sclerosis. Arthritis Rheum 37:1283–1289, 1994.
49. Wallaert B: Subclinical alveolitis in immunologic systemic disorders. Lung Suppl 168:974–983, 1990.
50. Witt C, Borges AC, John M, et al: Pulmonary involvement in diffuse cutaneous systemic sclerosis: Broncheoalveolar fluid granulocytosis predicts progression of fibrosing alveolitis. Ann Rheum Dis 58:635–640, 1999.
51. Behr J, Vogelmeier C, Beinert T, et al: Bronchoalveolar lavage for evaluation and management of scleroderma disease of the lung. Am J Respir Crit Care Med 154:400–406, 1996.
52. Muir TE, Tazelaar HD, Colby TV, et al: Organizing diffuse alveolar damage associated with progressive systemic sclerosis. Mayo Clin Proc 72:639–642, 1997.
53. Jacobsen S, Halberg P, Ullman S, et al: A longitudinal study of pulmonary function in Danish patients with systemic sclerosis. Clin Rheumatol 16:384–390, 1997.
54. Spencer-Green G, Alter D, Welch HG: Test performance in systemic sclerosis: Anti-centromere and anti-Scl-70 antibodies. Am J Med 103:242–248, 1997.
55. Bryan C, Howard Y, Brennan P, et al: Survival following the onset of scleroderma: Results from a retrospective inception cohort study of the UK patient population. Br J Rheumatol 35:1122–1126, 1996.
56. Rosenthal AK, McLaughlin JK, Gridley G, et al: Incidence of cancer among patients with systemic sclerosis. Cancer 76:910–914, 1995.
57. Lynch JP 3rd, McCune WJ: Immunosuppressive and cytotoxic pharmacotherapy for pulmonary disorders. Am J Respir Crit Care Med 155:395–420, 1997.
58. Steen VD, Lanz JK Jr, Conte C, et al: Therapy for severe interstitial lung disease in systemic sclerosis. A retrospective study. Arthritis Rheum 37:1290–1296, 1994.
59. Bolster MB, Silver RM: Assessment and management of scleroderma lung disease. Curr Opin Rheumatol 11:508–513, 1999.
60. Black CM, du Bois RM: Organ involvement: Pulmonary. *In* Clements PJ, Furst DE (eds): Systemic Sclerosis. Baltimore: Williams & Wilkins, 299–331, 1996.
61. Cailes JB, Phillips GD, Wells AU, et al: Correlation of echocardiography and right heart catheter in systemic sclerosis. Am J Respir Crit Care Med 149:A43, 1994.
62. Murata I, Kihara H, Shinohara S, et al: Echocardiographic evaluation of pulmonary arterial hypertension in patients with progressive systemic sclerosis and related syndromes. Jpn Circ J 56:983–991, 1992.
63. Menon N, McAlpine L, Peacock AJ, et al: The acute effects of prostacyclin on pulmonary hemodynamics in patients with pulmonary hypertension secondary to systemic sclerosis. Arthritis Rheum 41:466–469, 1998.
64. Arnett FC, Edworthy SM, Bloch DA, et al: The American Rheumatism Association 1987 revised criteria for the classification of rheumatoid arthritis. Arthritis Rheum 31:315–324, 1988.
65. Tanoue LT: Pulmonary manifestations of rheumatoid arthritis. Clin Chest Med 19:667–685, viii, 1998.
66. Nepom GT, Nepom B: Genetics of the major histocompatibility complex in rheumatoid arthritis. *In* Klippel JH, Dieppe PA (eds): Rheumatology. London: Mosby, 7.1–7.12, 1998.
67. Gladman DD, Anhorn KA: HLA and disease manifestations in rheumatoid arthritis—A Canadian experience. J Rheumatol 13:274–276, 1986.
68. Hyland RH, Gordon DA, Broder I, et al: A systematic controlled study of pulmonary abnormalities in rheumatoid arthritis. J Rheumatol 10:395–405, 1983.
69. Gilligan DM, O'Connor CM, Ward K, et al: Bronchoalveolar lavage in patients with mild and severe rheumatoid lung disease. Thorax 45:591–596, 1990.
70. Jurik AG, Davidsen D, Graudal H: Prevalence of pulmonary involvement in rheumatoid arthritis and its relationship to some characteristics of the patients. A radiological and clinical study. Scand J Rheumatol 11:217–224, 1982.
71. Shannon TM, Gale ME: Noncardiac manifestations of rheumatoid arthritis in the thorax. J Thorac Imag 7:19–29, 1992.
72. Scadding JG: The lungs in rheumatoid arthritis. Proc R Soc Med 62:227–238, 1969.
73. DeHoratius RJ, Abruzzo JL, Williams RC Jr: Immunofluorescent and immunologic studies of rheumatoid lung. Arch Intern Med 129:441–446, 1972.
74. Cervantes-Perez C, Toro-Perez AH, Rodriguez-Jurado P: Pulmonary involvement in rheumatoid arthritis. JAMA 243:1715–1719, 1980.
75. Roschmann RA, Rothenberg RJ: Pulmonary fibrosis in rheumatoid arthritis: A review of clinical features and therapy. Semin Arthritis Rheum 16:174–185, 1987.
76. Walker WC, Wright V: Pulmonary lesions and rheumatoid arthritis. Medicine 47:501, 1968.
77. Hakala M: Poor prognosis in patients with rheumatoid arthritis hospitalized for interstitial lung fibrosis. Chest 93:114–118, 1988.
78. du Bois RM, Geddes DM: Obliterative bronchiolitis, cryptogenic organising pneumonitis and bronchiolitis obliterans organizing pneumonia: Three names for two different conditions. Eur Respir J 4:774–775, 1991.
79. Colby TV, Myers JL: Clinical and histologic spectrum of bronchiolitis obliterans organising pneumonia. Semin Respir Med 13:119–133, 1992.
80. Wells AU, du Bois RM: Bronchiolitis in association with connective tissue disorders. Clin Chest Med 14:655–666, 1993.
81. Yousem SA, Colby TV, Carrington CB: Lung biopsy in rheumatoid arthritis. Am Rev Respir Dis 131:770–777, 1985.
82. Wolfe F, Schurle DR, Lin JJ, et al: Upper and lower airway disease in penicillamine treated patients with rheumatoid arthritis. J Rheumatol 10:406–410, 1983.
83. Sweatman MC, Markwick JR, Charles PJ, et al: Histocompatibility antigens in adult obliterative bronchiolitis with or without rheumatoid arthritis. Dis Markers 4:19–26, 1986.

84. Begin R, Masse S, Cantin A, et al: Airway disease in a subset of nonsmoking rheumatoid patients. Characterization of the disease and evidence for an autoimmune pathogenesis. Am J Med 72:743–750, 1982.
85. Geddes DM, Webley M, Emerson PA: Airways obstruction in rheumatoid arthritis. Ann Rheum Dis 38:222–225, 1979.
86. Andonopoulos AP, Constantopoulos SH, Drosos AA, et al: Pulmonary function of nonsmoking patients with rheumatoid arthritis in the presence and absence of secondary Sjögren's syndrome, a controlled study. Respiration 53:251–258, 1988.
87. Sassoon CS, McAlpine SW, Tashkin DP, et al: Small airways function in nonsmokers with rheumatoid arthritis. Arthritis Rheum 27:1218–1226, 1984.
88. Geddes DM, Corrin B, Brewerton DA, et al: Progressive airway obliteration in adults and its association with rheumatoid disease. Q J Med XLVI:427–444, 1977.
89. Nimni ME, Bavetta LA: Collagen defect induced by penicillamine. Science 150:905–907, 1965.
90. Lahdensuo A, Mattila J, Vilppula A: Bronchiolitis in rheumatoid arthritis. Chest 85:705–708, 1984.
91. Fortoul TI, Cano-Valle F, Oliva E, et al: Follicular bronchiolitis in association with connective tissue diseases. Lung 163:305–314, 1985.
92. Yousem SA, Colby TV, Carrington CB: Follicular bronchitis/bronchiolitis. Hum Pathol 16:702–706, 1985.
93. Despaux J, Polio JC, Toussirot E, et al: Rheumatoid arthritis and bronchiectasis. A retrospective study of fourteen cases. Rev Rhum, Eng Ed 63:801–808, 1996.
94. Shadick NA, Fanta CH, Weinblatt ME, et al: Bronchiectasis. A late feature of severe rheumatoid arthritis. Medicine 73:161–170, 1994.
95. Perez T, Remy-Jardin M, Cortet B: Airways involvement in rheumatoid arthritis: Clinical, functional, and HRCT findings. Am J Respir Crit Care Med 157:1658–1665, 1998.
96. Armstrong JG, Steele RH: Localised pulmonary arteritis in rheumatoid disease. Thorax 37:313–314, 1982.
97. Kelly CA: Rheumatoid arthritis: Classical rheumatoid lung disease. Baillieres Clin Rheumatol 7:1–16, 1993.
98. Fellbaum C, Domej W, Popper H: Rheumatoid arthritis with extensive lung lesions. Thorax 44:70–71, 1989.
99. Jolles H, Moseley PL, Peterson MW: Nodular pulmonary opacities in patients with rheumatoid arthritis. A diagnostic dilemma. Chest 96:1022–1025, 1989.
100. Caplan A: Certain unusual radiological appearances in the chest of coal-miners suffering from rheumatoid arthritis. Thorax 8:29, 1953.
101. Walker WC, Wright V: Rheumatoid pleuritis. Ann Rheum Dis 26:467–474, 1967.
102. Jones FL Jr, Blodgett RC Jr: Empyema in rheumatoid pleuropulmonary disease. Ann Intern Med 74:665–671, 1971.
103. Lee PR, Sox HC, North FS, et al: Pleurisy with effusion in rheumatoid arthritis. Arch Intern Med 104:634, 1959.
104. Dodson WH, Hollingsworth JW: Pleural effusion in rheumatoid arthritis. Impaired transport of glucose. N Engl J Med 275:1337–1342, 1966.
105. Yousem SA, Colby TV, Carrington CB: Lung biopsy in rheumatoid arthritis. Am Rev Respir Dis 131:770, 1985.
106. Strohl KP, Feldman NT, Ingram RH Jr: Apical fibrobullous disease with rheumatoid arthritis. Chest 75:739–741, 1979.
107. Yue CC, Park CH, Kushner I: Apical fibrocavitary lesions of the lung in rheumatoid arthritis. Report of two cases and review of the literature. Am J Med 81:741–746, 1986.
108. Mutru O, Koota K, Isomaki H: Causes of death in autopsied RA patients. Scand J Rheumatol 5:239–240, 1976.
109. Koota K, Isomaki H, Mutru O: Death rate and causes of death in RA patients during a period of five years. Scand J Rheumatol 6:241–244, 1977.
110. St Clair EW, Rice JR, Snyderman R: Pneumonitis complicating low-dose methotrexate therapy in rheumatoid arthritis. Arch Intern Med 145:2035–2038, 1985.
111. Alarcon GS, Kremer JM, Macaiuso M, et al: Risk factors for methotrexate-induced lung injury in patients with rheumatoid arthritis. A multicenter, case-control study. Methotrexate-Lung Study Group. Ann Intern Med 127:356–364, 1997.
112. Kremer JM, Alarcon GS, Weinblatt ME, et al: Clinical, laboratory, radiographic, and histopathologic features of methotrexate-associated lung injury in patients with rheumatoid arthritis: A multicenter study with literature review. Arthritis Rheum 40:1829–1837, 1997.
113. Salaffi F, Manganelli P, Carotti M, et al: Methotrexate-induced pneumonitis in patients with rheumatoid arthritis and psoriatic arthritis: Report of five cases and review of the literature. Clin Rheumatol 16:296–304, 1997.
114. Cannon GW: Methotrexate pulmonary toxicity. Rheum Dis Clin North Am 23:917–937, 1997.
115. Camus P, Piard F, Ashcroft T, et al: The lung in inflammatory bowel disease. Medicine 72:151–183, 1993.
116. Tomioka R, King TE Jr: Gold-induced pulmonary disease: Clinical features, outcome, and differentiation from rheumatoid lung disease. Am J Respir Crit Care Med 155:1011–1020, 1997.
117. Alasaly K, Muller N, Ostrow DN, et al: Cryptogenic organizing pneumonia. A report of 25 cases and a review of the literature. Medicine 74:201–211, 1995.
118. Lee KS, Kullnig P, Hartman TE, et al: Cryptogenic organizing pneumonia: CT findings in 43 patients. AJR Am J Roentgenol 162:543–546, 1994.
119. Wells AU: Computed tomographic imaging of bronchiolar disorders. Curr Opin Pulm Med 4:85–92, 1998.
120. Tan EM, Cohen AS, Fries JF, et al: The 1982 revised criteria for the classification of systemic lupus erythematosus. Arthritis Rheum 25:1271–1277, 1982.
121. Gladman DD, Urowitz MB: Systemic lupus erythematosis: Clinical features. *In* Klippel JH, Dieppe PA (eds): Rheumatology. London: Mosby, 1998, pp 1.1–1.17.
122. Reinersten JL, Klippel JH, Johnson AH, et al: Family studies of B lymphocyte alloantigens in systemic lupus erythematosus. J Rheumatol 9:253–262, 1982.
123. Haupt HM, Moore GW, Hutchins GM: The lung in systemic lupus erythematosus. Analysis of the pathologic changes in 120 patients. Am J Med 71:791–798, 1981.
124. Miller LR, Greenberg SD, McLarty JW: Lupus lung. Chest 88:265, 1985.
125. Gross M, Esterly JR, Earle RH: Pulmonary alterations in systemic lupus erythematosus. Am Rev Respir Dis 105:572, 1972.
126. Eisenberg H, Dubois EL, Sherwin RP, et al: Diffuse interstitial lung disease in systemic lupus erythematosus. Ann Intern Med 79:37–45, 1973.
127. Weinrib L, Sharma OP, Quismorio FP Jr: A long-term study of interstitial lung disease in systemic lupus erythematosus. Semin Arthritis Rheum 20:48–56, 1990.
128. Orens JB, Martinez FJ, Lynch JP 3rd: Pleuropulmonary manifestations of systemic lupus erythematosus. Rheum Dis Clin North Am 20:159–193, 1994.
129. Gibson GJ, Edmonds JP, Hughes GRV: Diaphragm function and lung involvement in systemic lupus erythematosus. Am J Med 63:926–932, 1977.
130. Wilcox PG, Stein HB, Clarke SD, et al: Phrenic nerve function in patients with diaphragmatic weakness and systemic lupus erythematosus. Chest 93:352, 1988.
131. Laroche CM, Mulvey DA, Hawkins PN et al: Diaphragm strength in the shrinking lung syndrome of systemic lupus erythematosus. Q J Med 71:429–439, 1989.
132. Nived O, Sturfelt G, Wollheim F: Systemic lupus erythematosus and infection: A controlled and prospective study including an epidemiological group. Q J Med 55:271–287, 1985.
133. Asherson RA, Oakley CM: Pulmonary hypertension and systemic lupus erythematosus [published erratum appears in J Rheumatol 13:840, 1986]. J Rheumatol 13:1–5, 1986.
134. Simonson JS, Schiller NB, Petri M, et al: Pulmonary hypertension in systemic lupus erythematosus. J Rheumatol 16:918–925, 1989.
135. Alarcon-Segovia D, Deleze M, Oria CV et al: Antiphospholipid antibodies and the antiphospholipid syndrome in systemic lupus erythematosus. A prospective analysis of 500 consecutive patients. Medicine 68:353–365, 1989.
136. Cervera R, Khamashta MA, Font J, et al: Systemic lupus erythematosus: Clinical and immunologic patterns of disease expression in a cohort of 1,000 patients. The European Working Party on Systemic Lupus Erythematosus. Medicine 72:113–124, 1993.
137. Good JT Jr, King TE, Antony VB, et al: Lupus pleuritis. Clinical

features and pleural fluid characteristics with special reference to pleural fluid antinuclear antibodies. Chest 84:714–718, 1983.
138. Gross M, Esterly JR, Earle RH: Pulmonary alterations in systemic lupus erythematosus. Am Rev Respir Dis 105:572–577, 1972.
139. Naylor B: Cytological aspects of pleural, peritoneal and pericardial fluids from patients with systemic lupus erythematosus. Cytopathology 3:1–8, 1992.
140. Leechawengwong M, Berger HW, Sukumaran M: Diagnostic significance of antinuclear antibodies in pleural effusion. Mt Sinai J Med 46:137–139, 1979.
141. Vitali C, Bombardieri S, Moutsopoulos HM, et al: Preliminary criteria for the classification of Sjögren's syndrome. Results of a prospective concerted action supported by the European Community. Arthritis Rheum 36:340–347, 1993.
142. Manthrope R, Jacobsson LTH: Sjögren's syndrome. Baillieres Clin Rheumatol 9:483–486, 1995.
143. Papathanasiou MP, Constantopoulos SH, Tsampoulas C, et al: Reappraisal of respiratory abnormalities in primary and secondary Sjögren's syndrome. A controlled study. Chest 90:370, 1986.
144. Gardiner P: Primary Sjögren's syndrome. Baillieres Clin Rheumatol 7:59–77, 1993.
145. Gardiner P, Ward C, Allison A, et al: Pleuropulmonary abnormalities in primary Sjögren's syndrome. J Rheumatol 20:831–837, 1993.
146. Strimlan CV, Rosenow EC, Divertie MB, et al: Pulmonary manifestations of Sjögren's syndrome. Chest 70:354, 1976.
147. Kassan SS, Thomas TL, Moutsopoulos HM, et al: Increased risk of lymphoma in sicca syndrome. Ann Intern Med 89:888–892, 1978.
148. Constantopoulos SH, Drosos AA, Maddison PJ, et al: Xerotrachea and interstitial lung disease in primary Sjögren's syndrome. Respiration 46:310–314, 1984.
149. Gudbjornsson B, Hedenstrom H, Stalenheim G, et al: Bronchial hyperresponsiveness to methacholine in patients with primary Sjögren's syndrome. Ann Rheum Dis 50:36–40, 1991.
150. La Corte R, Bajocchi G, Potena A, et al: Bronchial hyperreactivity in systemic sclerosis patients: Influence of associated Sjögren's syndrome. Ann Rheum Dis 54:636–639, 1995.
151. Liebow AA, Carrington CB: Diffuse pulmonary lymphoreticular infiltrations associated with dysproteinemia. Med Clin North Am 57:809, 1973.
152. Dalavanga YA, Constantopoulos SH, Galanopoulou V, et al: Alveolitis correlates with clinical pulmonary involvement in primary Sjögren's syndrome. Chest 99:1394–1397, 1991.
153. Fairfax AJ, Haslam PL, Pavia D, et al: Pulmonary disorders associated with Sjögren's syndrome. Q J Med 50:279–295, 1981.
154. Bohan A, Peter JB: Polymyositis and dermatomyositis (second of two parts). N Engl J Med 292:403–407, 1975.
155. Medsger TA, Oddis CV: Inflammatory muscle disease. *In* Klippel JH, Dieppe PA (eds): Rheumatology. London: Mosby, 1998, pp 13.1–13.14.
156. Nobutoh T, Kohda M, Doi Y, et al: An autopsy case of dermatomyositis with rapidly progressive diffuse alveolar damage. J Dermatol 25:32–36, 1998.
157. Fata F, Rathore R, Schiff C, et al: Bronchiolitis obliterans organizing pneumonia as the first manifestation of polymyositis. South Med J 90:227–230, 1997.
158. Shinohara T, Hidaka T, Matsuki Y, et al: Rapidly progressive interstitial lung disease associated with dermatomyositis responding to intravenous cyclophosphamide pulse therapy. Intern Med 36:519–523, 1997.
159. Mino M, Noma S, Taguchi Y, et al: Pulmonary involvement in polymyositis and dermatomyositis: Sequential evaluation with CT. AJR Am J Roentgenol 169:83–87, 1997.
160. Schwarz MI, Sutarik JM, Nick JA, et al: Pulmonary capillaritis and diffuse alveolar hemorrhage. A primary manifestation of polymyositis. Am J Respir Crit Care Med 151:2037–2040, 1995.
161. Chow WH, Gridley G, Mellemkjaer L, et al: Cancer risk following polymyositis and dermatomyositis: A nationwide cohort study in Denmark. Cancer Causes Control 6:9–13, 1995.
162. Targoff IN: Humoral immunity in polymyositis/dermatomyositis. J Invest Dermatol 100:116S–123S, 1993.
163. Amigues JM, Cantagrel A, Abbal M, et al: Comparative study of 4 diagnosis criteria sets for mixed connective tissue disease in patients with anti-RNP antibodies. Autoimmunity Group of the Hospitals of Toulouse. J Rheumatol 23:2055–2062, 1996.
164. Maddison PJ: Overlap syndromes and mixed connective tissue disease. Cur Opin Rheumatol 3:995–1000, 1991.
165. Gendi NS, Welsh KI, Van Venrooij WJ, et al: HLA type as a predictor of mixed connective tissue disease differentiation. Ten-year clinical and immunogenetic followup of 46 patients. Arthritis Rheum 38:259–266, 1995.
166. Kallenberg CG: Overlapping syndromes, undifferentiated connective tissue disease, and other fibrosing conditions. Cur Opin Rheumatol 5:809–815, 1993.
167. Venables PJW: Overlap Syndromes. *In* Klippel JH, Dieppe PA (eds): Rheumatology. London: Mosby, 1998, pp 33.1–33.8.
168. Prakash UB: Respiratory complications in mixed connective tissue disease. Clin Chest Med 19:733–746, ix, 1998.
169. Maddison PJ: Overlap syndromes and mixed connective tissue disease. Cur Opin Rheumatol 3:995–1000, 1991.
170. McAdam LP, O'Hanlan MA, Bluestone R, et al: Relapsing polychondritis: Prospective study of 23 patients and a review of the literature. Medicine 55:193–215, 1976.
171. Zeuner M, Straub RH, Rauh G, et al: Relapsing polychondritis: Clinical and immunogenetic analysis of 62 patients. J Rheumatol 24:96–101, 1997.
172. Lee-Chiong TL Jr: Pulmonary manifestations of ankylosing spondylitis and relapsing polychondritis. Clin Chest Med 19:747–757, ix, 1998.
173. Eng J, Sabanathan S: Airway complications in relapsing polychondritis. Ann Thorac Surg 51:686–692, 1991.
174. Shah R, Sabanathan S, Mearns AJ, Featherstone H: Self-expanding tracheobronchial stents in the management of major airway problems. J Cardiovasc Surg 36:343–348, 1995.
175. Yazici H, Yurdakul S, Hamuryudan V: Behçet's syndrome. *In* Klippel JH, Dieppe PA (eds): Rheumatology. London: Mosby, 1998, pp 26.1–26.6.
176. Anonymous: Criteria for diagnosis of Behçet's disease. International Study Group for Behçet's Disease. Lancet 335:1078–1080, 1990.
177. Raz I, Okon E, Chajek-Shaul T: Pulmonary manifestations in Behçet's syndrome. Chest 95:585–589, 1989.
178. Tunaci A, Berkmen YM, Gokmen E: Thoracic involvement in Behçet's disease: Pathologic, clinical, and imaging features. AJR Am J Roentgen 164:51–56, 1995.
179. Ahn JM, Im JG, Ryoo JW, et al: Thoracic manifestations of Behçet's syndrome: Radiographic and CT findings in nine patients. Radiology 194:199–203, 1995.
180. Yazici H, Barnes CG: Practical treatment recommendations for pharmacotherapy of Behçet's syndrome. Drugs 42:796–804, 1991.
181. Tuzun H, Besirli K, Sayin A, et al: Management of aneurysms in Behçet's syndrome: An analysis of 24 patients. Surgery 121:150–156, 1997.
182. Schlosstein L, Terasaki PI, Bluestone R, et al: High association of an HL-A antigen, W27, with ankylosing spondylitis. N Engl J Med 288:704–706, 1973.
183. Rosenow E, Strimlan CV, Muhm JR, et al: Pleuropulmonary manifestations of ankylosing spondylitis. Mayo Clin Proc 52:641–649, 1977.
184. Casserly IP, Fenlon HM, Breatnach E, et al: Lung findings on high-resolution computed tomography in idiopathic ankylosing spondylitis—Correlation with clinical findings, pulmonary function testing and plain radiography. Br J Rheumatol 36:677–682, 1997.
185. Jeandel P, Bonnet D, Chouc PY, et al: Demonstration of subclinical pulmonary alveolitis in spondylarthropathies. [In French.] Rev Rhum Ed Fr 5:301–309, 1994.
186. Wolson AH, Rohwedder JJ: Upper lobe fibrosis in ankylosing spondylitis. AJR Am J Roentgenol Radium Ther Nucl Med 124:466–471, 1975.
187. Chakera TM, Howarth FH, Kendall MJ, et al: The chest radiograph in ankylosing spondylitis. Clin Radiol 26:455–459, 1975.
188. Davies D: Ankylosing spondylitis and lung fibrosis. Q J Med 41:395–417, 1972.
189. Hunninghake GW, Fauci AS: Pulmonary involvement in the collagen vascular diseases. Am Rev Respir Dis 119:471–503, 1979.

190. Turner JA, Stanley NN: Fragile lung in the Marfan syndrome. Thorax 31:771–775, 1976.
191. Dominguez R, Weisgrau RA, Santamaria M: Pulmonary hyperinflation and emphysema in infants with the Marfan syndrome. Pediatr Radiol 17:365–369, 1987.
192. Wood JR, Bellamy D, Child AH, et al: Pulmonary disease in patients with Marfan syndrome. Thorax 39:780–784, 1984.
193. Hall JR, Pyeritz RE, Dudgeon DL, et al: Pneumothorax in the Marfan syndrome: Prevalence and therapy. Ann Thorac Surg 37:500–504, 1984.
194. Wanderman KL, Goldstein MS, Faber J: Letter: Cor pulmonale secondary to severe kyphoscoliosis in Marfan's syndrome. Chest 67:250–251, 1975.
195. Cistulli PA, Sullivan CE: Sleep apnea in Marfan's syndrome. Increased upper airway collapsibility during sleep. Chest 108:631–635, 1995.

# 59 Sarcoidosis

Barry L. Fanburg, M.D. • Otto Villa, M.D., Ph.D.

Introduction
Epidemiology
Genetic Factors
Clinical Presentation
Radiographic Features
Physiologic Alterations
Pathology
Immunologic Features
Diagnosis
Activity of Disease
Course and Prognosis
Therapy
Summary

## INTRODUCTION

Despite an awareness of sarcoidosis since the late 1800s, no etiologic agent for this disease has been identified. Rather, it has been described as a complex of clinical and pathologic abnormalities that blend into an often typical, but sometimes bewildering, pattern of disease. The hallmark of the pathologic process is a granuloma composed of various inflammatory and related cells that may occur in any area of the body. The cellular infiltrate may remit spontaneously or progress to scarring. Combinations of inflammation, scarring, and occasionally associated hypercalcemia may interfere with organ function and lead to life-threatening events. Fortunately, the disease usually remits spontaneously with no significant sequelae.

Some research in animals has suggested the possibility of a transmissible agent in sarcoidosis,[1, 2] but if such an agent exists, it must have extremely low infectivity or a protracted incubation period so that the initial contact goes unrecognized. Some studies using the polymerase chain reaction have found evidence of *Mycobacterium tuberculosis* in tissue from patients with diagnosed sarcoidosis, but the results have been controversial.[3] Because inhalation of beryllium produces a pathologic process quite similar to sarcoidosis, another possible cause of disease is the inhalation of airborne substances, but no supportive evidence of this has been obtained.

The most striking advances in the late 1990s were made in defining the immunologic process in sarcoidosis. The cellular response is primarily one of T lymphocytes, but T-lymphocyte activation and proliferation are dependent on biochemical substances provided by tissue monocytes and alveolar macrophages.[4] Much research is still needed to determine the inciting event, the cell-signaling sequences for histologic alterations, the process by which spontaneous resolution occurs, and the mechanism that causes some cases to progress to extensive scarring.

## EPIDEMIOLOGY

Sarcoidosis occurs worldwide,[5] and the clinical presentation may vary in different localities, but there are more factors in common than there are dissimilarities in the disease throughout the world. Reported prevalence varies widely according to geographic location,[6–8] possibly because surveillance and criteria for diagnosis differ from one country to another. In most countries there is a slight female preponderance, but this finding may be related to sex distribution within the clinic population reported.[8] In the United States, the prevalence of sarcoidosis among blacks has been reported to be 10 to 17 times that of whites in military, Veterans Administration, and large urban clinic populations; however, as with the sex incidence, the racial background of the population studied must be considered when results are interpreted.

## GENETIC FACTORS

The possibility that genetic factors play a role in the disease is supported by the occurrence of sarcoidosis in twins and other family members.[9] However, the penetrance of any such factor must be weak, because the frequency of occurrence in relatives is very low. There seems to be a preponderance of disease in monozygotic over dizygotic twins. Sibling, parent-child, and husband-wife combinations have been reported, but there is no apparent relationship between this clustering of disease and cause.

Despite some associations of human leukocyte antigens (HLA) and sarcoidosis, no definite correlations have been made. A higher frequency of sarcoidosis has been found in black patients with HLA-Bw 15 than in those lacking this antigen.[10] Another study related the presence of

HLA-B8 antigen and spontaneous resolution of disease,[11] and HLA-B8 antigen has also been reported to occur frequently with sarcoid arthritis and erythema nodosum.[12]

## CLINICAL PRESENTATION

Sarcoidosis may affect almost any organ of the body, and the disease may present in an acute, subacute, or chronic form. Onset of disease occurs most commonly between the ages of 20 and 40 years, but sarcoidosis is known to be present in children[13–15] and in geriatric populations.[16] The incidence in childhood may be underestimated because of the infrequency of chest roentgenograms in this age group, and the frequency of onset in the older population is likely overestimated because asymptomatic disease may have been long-standing. In fact, it is difficult to find cases of sarcoidosis with clearly documented onset late in life.

Most typically, sarcoidosis presents in asymptomatic patients who are found to have an abnormal chest roentgenogram that shows hilar and paratracheal adenopathy, evidence of parenchymal disease, or both. Despite the radiographic abnormalities, findings of the physical examination of the chest are usually within normal limits. Generalized symptoms such as fatigue, weight loss, and anorexia occur infrequently. Fever occurs only occasionally.

The symptoms and related organ involvement that lead a patient to the attention of a physician are listed in Table 59.1. Pulmonary symptoms include dyspnea with exertion, cough, and wheezing. Hemoptysis occurs rarely and suggests the presence of a mycetoma. Involvement of the upper airways and posterior pharynx may produce symptoms of upper airway obstruction.[17–19] Vocal cord granulomas produce hoarseness, and granulomas of the nasal mucosa may cause polyps, nasal obstruction, or sinusitis.[20]

Lesions of the skin occur acutely or chronically and are quite varied. Erythema nodosum is a painful nodular panniculitis and vasculitis that is frequently associated with bilateral hilar adenopathy and arthralgias (Löffgren's syndrome) (Fig. 59.1). Other skin lesions are caused by granulomas that present as raised nodules or flat plaques over various areas of the body. Subcutaneous nodules may occur,[21] and severe sarcoid lesions can be confused with those of necrobiosis lipoidica diabeticorum.[22] Among the skin lesions, lupus pernio presents as bluish-purple elevations over the face.

Ophthalmologic manifestations occur in 5% to 10% of patients with sarcoidosis.[23] The lesion most frequently encountered is inflammation of the uveal tract, which may lead to residual synechiae and scarring. Gray "mutton fat" precipitates may be present in the anterior chamber or on the posterior corneal surface. Granulomas also occur on the conjunctiva. The lacrimal gland may be enlarged secondarily to sarcoidosis, and keratoconjunctivitis sicca similar to that found in Sjögren's syndrome may result. Choroiditis and nodular vitreous opacities also occur. Optic neuritis resulting from sarcoidosis has been described. Infiltration of the orbital tissues by granulomas may in rare cases cause exophthalmos.

Arthralgias occurring in sarcoidosis are often associated with erythema nodosum and hilar adenopathy. The arthralgias may be monoarticular or polyarticular and frequently involve the ankles and wrists. Granulomas in skeletal muscle are frequently asymptomatic, but in a small percentage of cases, acute proximal myopathy and marked increase in creatine phosphokinase level occur.[24, 25]

Because almost any region of the nervous system may be affected by sarcoidosis, the neurologic symptoms are quite diverse. It has been estimated that approximately 5% of patients with sarcoidosis have neurologic involvement. The most common presentation is cranial nerve palsy, the facial nerve being involved most frequently. The association of facial nerve palsy with parotitis and uveitis has been referred to as uveoparotid fever (Heerfordt's syndrome). Fluctuating reversible hearing loss and vestibular dysfunction occur in some patients, whereas ischemia secondary to vasculitis results in irreversible damage to the neural tissue in others.[26] Peripheral neurop-

**Table 59.1 CLINICAL FEATURES OF SARCOIDOSIS**

| Organ System Involvement | Symptoms or Presentation |
|---|---|
| Pulmonary | Dyspnea, cough, wheezing, hemoptysis |
| Upper airway | Dyspnea, nasal congestion, polyps, hoarseness |
| Dermatologic | Nodules, papules, plaques |
| Ocular | Photophobia, bearing, pain, loss of vision, lacrimal gland enlargement |
| Rheumatologic | Polyarthropathy, monoarthropathy, myopathy |
| Neurologic | Cranial nerve palsy, headache, hearing loss, paresthesia, seizures, meningitis, encephalopathy, space-occupying lesion |
| Cardiologic | Syncope, dyspnea, conduction disturbance, congestive heart failure, arrhythmias, cardiac tamponade |
| Gastrointestinal | Dysphagia, abdominal pain, jaundice |
| Hematologic | Lymph node enlargement, hypersplenism (thrombocytopenia, leukopenia, anemia) |
| Renal | Kidney failure, calculi |
| Endocrine-metabolic | Diabetes insipidus, hypercalcemia, hypercalciuria, epididymitis |

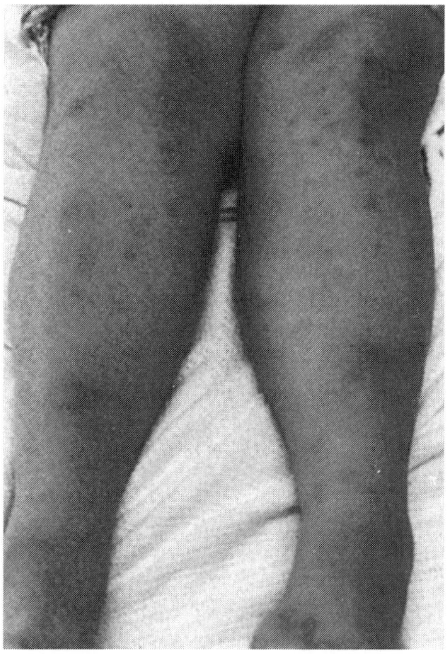

**Figure 59.1** Erythema nodosum occurring widespread over both lower extremities of a patient with arthritis and hilar adenopathy: the classic Löffgren's syndrome.

athy, meningitis, and lesions of the pituitary gland, spinal cord, and cerebellum have also been described, and symptoms and signs of a space-occupying brain lesion occasionally occur.[27] Cerebrospinal fluid findings may be normal or show increased protein, pleocytosis, or hypoglycorrhachia. The cerebrospinal fluid pressure may be elevated.

Although often asymptomatic, cardiac involvement may result in congestive heart failure, heart block, cardiac arrhythmias, angina pectoris, or sudden death.[28] Premature ventricular contractions and ventricular tachycardia are the most frequent arrhythmias. A wide variety of electrocardiographic abnormalities may be present, but it is often difficult to ascribe them exclusively to sarcoidosis. Pericardial effusion occurs infrequently, as does constrictive pericarditis.[29] Cor pulmonale secondary to sarcoidosis-related pulmonary hypertension may be present.

Clinical manifestations of liver disease are infrequent. The most common symptom of hepatic sarcoidosis is prolonged fever, but right upper quadrant pain may occur.[30] Portal fibrosis and obliteration of the hepatic venous bed may produce portal hypertension. Biliary hepatitis and cirrhosis have in rare cases been associated with sarcoidosis.

Dysphagia in patients with sarcoidosis is often secondary to mechanical compression by lymph nodes or infiltration of the esophageal wall by granulomas, but direct involvement of Auerbach's plexus may result in achalasia.[31] Jejunal atrophy and nonnecrotizing granuloma of the stomach, small bowel, and colon in association with malabsorption have been reported.[32] Sarcoidosis involving the appendix mimics acute appendicitis. Acute cholecystitis has been reported, and pancreatitis may present with abdominal pain but without endocrine dysfunction.

Sarcoidosis frequently involves the reticuloendothelial system. Lymph node enlargement is usually minimal and apt to be noted by the physician rather than by the patient. Cervical, supraclavicular, epitrochlear, and inguinal nodes may be enlarged and are usually discrete and movable. On occasion, the nodes are grossly enlarged. Involvement of cervical nodes or parotid glands may prompt the patient to visit a dentist.[33] At times, the liver or spleen is enlarged. Marked splenomegaly occurs with more chronic disease and may have associated thrombocytopenia, leukopenia, or anemia. Pancytopenia may also occur without splenomegaly.[34]

Patients with sarcoidosis may present with kidney failure. Granulomas occur in the kidney, but the usual cause of the kidney failure is related to hypercalcemia and hypercalciuria.[35]

Endocrine and metabolic presentations of sarcoidosis include hypopituitarism, primary polydipsia, inappropriate antidiuretic hormone syndrome, diabetes insipidus, hypercalciuria, and hypercalcemia.[36] Hypercalciuria occurs more frequently than hypercalcemia.[37] Alteration in calcium metabolism has been postulated to be due to increased intestinal absorption of calcium secondary to enhanced sensitivity to vitamin D or to production of active vitamin D metabolites by sarcoid tissue.[38, 39] Serum parathyroid hormone may be reduced, presumably secondary to an elevated serum calcium level.[40] The clinical features of sarcoidosis-associated hypercalcemia and hypercalciuria are not unique, and primary hyperparathyroidism must be considered in the diagnosis. In rare cases, sarcoidosis affects the thyroid, parathyroid, and adrenal glands.

Involvement of the epididymis, testes, and uterus has been reported.[41] Any portion of the genital system may be affected, but asymptomatic testicular enlargement and epididymitis occur most frequently. Uncomplicated sarcoidosis does not appear to influence fertility or pregnancy adversely.[42] The effect of more severe sarcoidosis on pregnancy reflects the extent of physiologic impairment by the disease. The effect of pregnancy on the course of sarcoidosis is uncertain, but some observers believe that there is improvement during pregnancy and exacerbation after delivery.[41]

## RADIOGRAPHIC FEATURES

Certain radiographic findings, although not diagnostic, are highly suggestive of sarcoidosis. The finding of enlarged bilateral and symmetric bronchopulmonary and paratracheal lymph nodes (Fig. 59.2) has been recognized in sarcoidosis since at least 1940.[43–45] There is often an apparent predominance of right hilar and paratracheal lymph nodes, as left-sided nodes are obscured by other structures. The lateral chest roentgenogram may be helpful in identifying the presence of increased radiographic densities in the hilar area (Fig. 59.3). Subtle changes in density may be seen when current and past roentgenograms are compared directly.

The parenchyma of the lung may be normal or may show a variety of abnormalities, including reticulonodular infiltrates and bullous changes. According to the joint statement of the American Thoracic Society, European

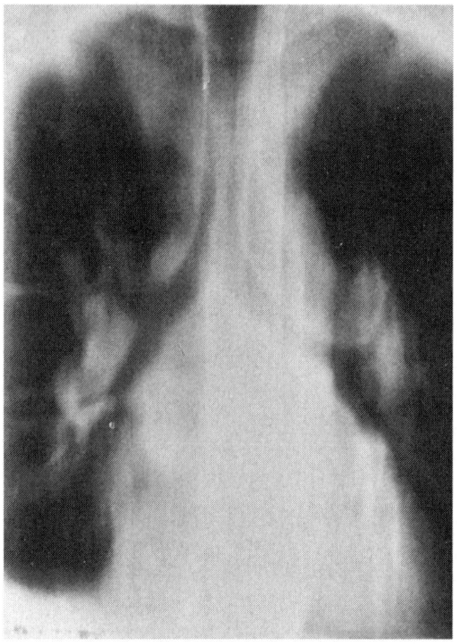

**Figure 59.2** Chest tomogram of a patient with stage 1 sarcoidosis, showing bilateral hilar and right paratracheal adenopathy.

Respiratory Society, and World Association of Sarcoidosis and Other Granulomatous Diseases,[46] there are five roentgenographic stages of intrathoracic sarcoidosis: stage 0 indicates no visible intrathoracic abnormalities; stage I (formerly stage 1) indicates bilateral hilar lymphadenopathy, which may be accompanied by paratracheal adenopathy; stage II (formerly stage 2A) indicates bilateral hilar adenopathy accompanied by parenchymal infiltration; stage III (formerly stage 2B) indicates parenchymal infiltration without hilar adenopathy; and stage IV (formerly stage 3) indicates advanced fibrosis with evidence of honeycombing, hilar retraction, bullae, cysts, and emphysema. It has been estimated that approximately 5% to 10% of patients with sarcoidosis have normal chest radiographs. Intrathoracic lymphadenopathy occurs in approximately 75% to 90% of patients,[47] and patients with lymphadenopathy appear to be equally distributed in the stages of disease classified as Stages I and II. Stage IV radiographic changes, fortunately, occur infrequently. Some general progression of the stages of sarcoidosis is suggested by the fact that parenchymal changes follow those of lymphadenopathy, but it is unusual for enlargement of lymph nodes to occur after parenchymal changes have been noted. Also, it is rare for pulmonary parenchymal or nodal changes to recur after spontaneous radiographic clearing has occurred.

Although lymph node enlargement in sarcoidosis is most frequently observed in the paratracheal region and around large airways, enlarged subcarinal and anterior and posterior mediastinal nodes can now also be recognized with the use of computed tomography.[48, 49] Similarly, lymphadenopathy may be detected by computed tomographic scans in any area of the body. Lymphadenopathy may regress entirely or may remain static for years. Lymph nodes also may enlarge somewhat under observation and be confused with lymphoma.

The most frequent pulmonary parenchymal pattern to occur in sarcoidosis is a reticulonodular one and consists of fine linear densities and small irregular nodules that measure 3 to 5 mm in diameter (Fig. 59.4). The parenchymal pattern may also be a miliary one (Fig. 59.5). At times, the infiltrate consists of large coalescent areas with fluffy margins referred to as an "alveolar pattern," or it may be nodular and confused with tumor. Honeycombing, hilar retraction, volume loss, and bullous changes are associated with scarring of advanced disease (Fig. 59.6).

The typical radiographic manifestations of sarcoidosis

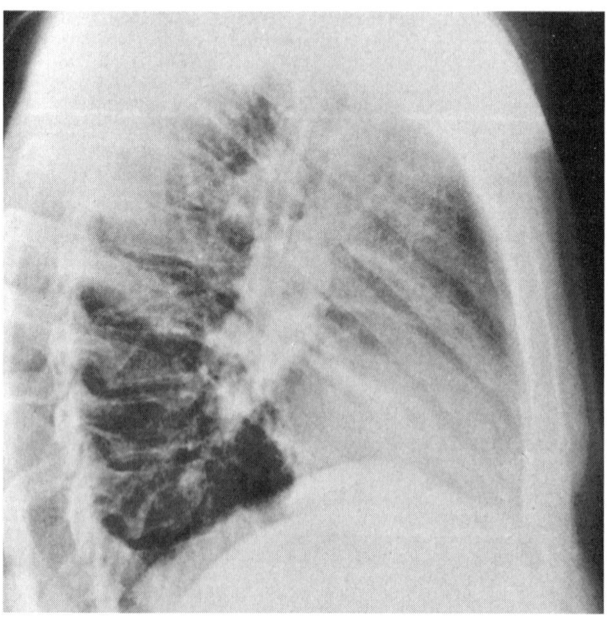

**Figure 59.3** Lateral chest roentgenogram of a patient with stage II sarcoidosis, showing the hilar density of the lymphadenopathy and parenchymal reticulonodular changes.

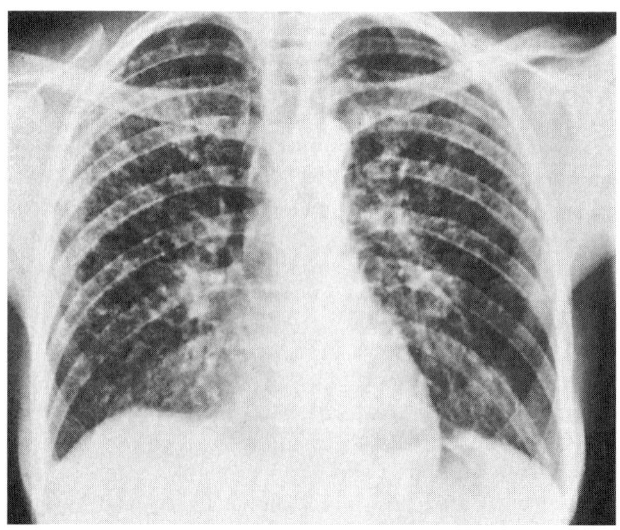

**Figure 59.4** Chest roentgenogram of a patient without adenopathy (stage III disease), showing diffuse reticulonodular changes.

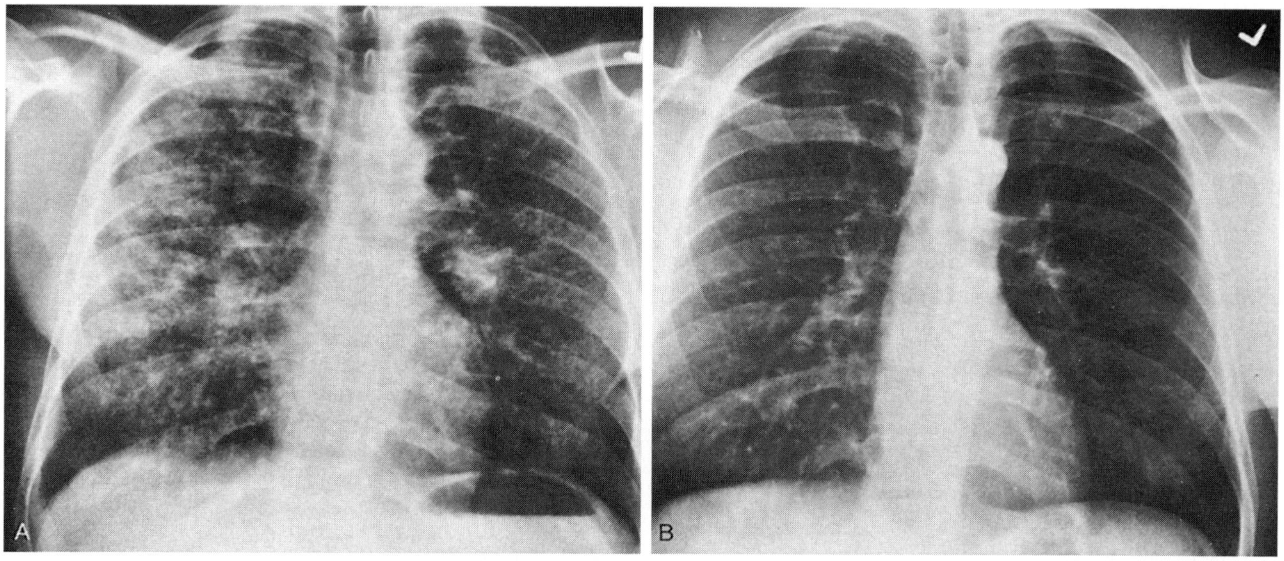


**Figure 59.5** Roentgenograms of the chest of a patient with sarcoidosis, showing *(A)* diffuse granular parenchymal pattern of sarcoidosis with a miliary appearance and, *(B)* 2 years later, complete remission after corticosteroid was discontinued 1 year previously.

are generally recognized. However, there are many unusual manifestations, which have been reviewed by Rockoff and Rohatgi[50] and are noted in Table 59.2.

Although pleural involvement without clinical or radiographic evidence is more common than generally thought,[51] pleural effusions are infrequent.[52] When a pleural effusion is present, it is usually asymptomatic. It may be either unilateral or bilateral and is generally small. However, massive pleural effusion has been reported.[53] The effusion is usually an exudate and is characterized by a predominance of lymphocytes. Other causes of pleural effusion should be excluded (see Chapter 74). Only two cases of sarcoidosis-related chylothorax have been reported.[54, 55]

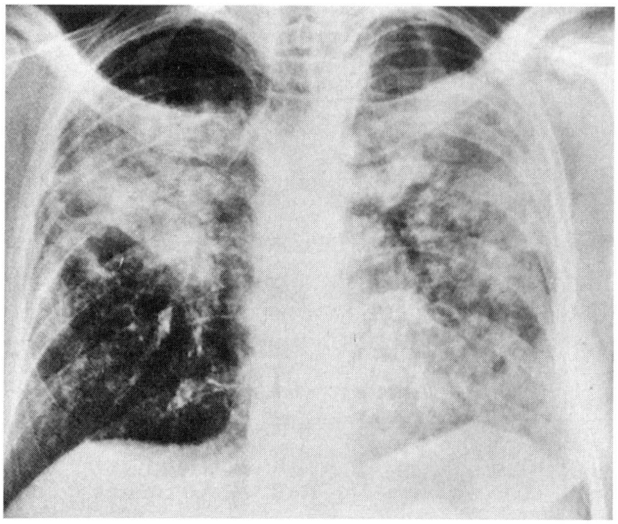

**Figure 59.6** Stage IV sarcoidosis, with conglomerate lesions and hilar retraction.

Most cases of pneumothorax in patients with sarcoidosis occur in association with diffuse fibrocystic disease and are thought to result from a rupture of a subpleural bleb. These pneumothoraces may be recurrent. Pleural thickening may occur in association with sarcoidosis but does not lead to clinical symptoms and may not be noticed by the patient. With apical pleural thickening, consideration should be given to the possibility of underlying aspergillosis and associated mycetoma.[56]

Isolated enlargement of anterior or posterior mediastinal nodes is rare. Calcification of the mediastinal or peribronchial lymph nodes is unusual, but may occur in association with long-standing disease.[57, 58] The configuration of the calcification is not specific and has been described as amorphous, popcorn-like, and eggshell. The cause of the calcification has not been established, but it is known that hypercalcemia is not responsible. Thickening of the tracheal wall may occur in patients with sarcoidosis, and the trachea may also be compressed by enlarged nodes. These abnormalities have been detected only by computed tomographic scanning and are of no clinical significance. Pneumomediastinum is exceedingly rare.

Like mediastinal nodes, hilar nodes may be calcified and retracted upward. Calcification of hilar nodes is more common than that of mediastinal nodes, and eggshell calcification of hilar nodes in patients who have not been exposed to silica or coal dust suggests the diagnosis of sarcoidosis.[59] Unilateral hilar adenopathy occurs in no more than 1% to 3% of patients.[60, 61]

Abnormalities of the airways that occur in sarcoidosis may be detected roentgenographically. Bronchial granulomas or external compression by enlarged nodes may lead to narrowing of the airways. Bronchostenosis may occur in single or multiple locations and causes lobar atelectasis.[62, 63] Although any lobe may be involved, right middle lobe atelectasis is unusual in this setting. Regression of

**Table 59.2 UNUSUAL ROENTGENOGRAPHIC MANIFESTATIONS OF SARCOIDOSIS**

| | |
|---|---|
| **Pleural Lesions** | |
| | Effusion |
| | Chylothorax |
| | Pneumothorax |
| | Pleural thickening |
| **Mediastinum** | |
| | Isolated anterior, middle, or posterior adenopathy |
| | Nodes may be calcified and may show eggshell calcifications |
| | Mediastinal emphysema |
| | Tracheal involvement |
| **Hilum** | |
| | Unilateral hilar adenopathy (1%–3%) and eggshell calcifications |
| **Lung** | |
| | Bronchostenosis or lobar atelectasis, postobstructive bronchiectasis |
| | Cavitation |
| | Mycetoma |
| | Alveolar pattern |
| | "Vanishing lung" |
| | Unilateral alveolar or interstitial pattern |
| | Pulmonary nodule: single or multiple |
| **Cardiovascular Lesions** | |
| | Pulmonary hypertension |
| | Superior vena cava obstruction |
| | Innominate vein obstruction |
| | Pulmonary artery obstruction by granuloma or enlarged lymph node |
| | Cardiomegaly |
| | Pericardial effusion |
| **Bone Lesions, Including Rib, Sternum, Thoracic Vertebra** | |

From Rockoff SD, Rohatgi PK: Unusual manifestations of thoracic sarcoidosis. Am J Radiol 144:513–528, 1985.

the atelectasis may occur spontaneously or after corticosteroid therapy. Bronchiectasis may occur behind the site of obstruction.

Although large bullae or cystic bronchiectasis associated with sarcoidosis may simulate cavitation, true cavities also occur.[64, 65] The walls of the cavities contain granulomas and suggest the presence of ischemic necrosis within conglomerate granulomas or extrusion of ischemic hyaline fibrous tissue. The cavities are either solitary or multiple and may resolve with or without corticosteroid therapy. Mycetomas, usually caused by *Aspergillus* species, sometimes develop and may be associated with hemoptysis, which can be life-threatening.[66, 67] In a 10-year prospective study of 100 patients with histologically proven sarcoidosis, Wollschlager and Khan[68] found 12 patients with serum precipitins to *Aspergillus*, and 10 of these patients had aspergillomas. Two patients died of massive hemoptysis. The patients with aspergillomas represented 50% of those with stage IV cystic parenchymal disease.

Parenchymal nodules may be solitary or multiple, may be quite large and confluent, and may mimic metastatic disease (Fig. 59.7) or pulmonary consolidation.[69] Although roentgenograms usually show bilateral or diffuse disease, unilateral (Fig. 59.8) or lobar infiltrates may occur,[70] and the presence of peripheral infiltrates similar to eosinophilic pneumonia has been reported.[71]

High-resolution computed tomography of the chest has been reported to be helpful in diagnosis and projection of the course of sarcoidosis.[72, 73] It has been proposed that through the use of this technique, pulmonary sarcoidosis can be distinguished from other interstitial infiltrative processes. Patchy nodules or segmental ground-glass opacities have been associated with early and potentially reversible disease, whereas scarring, cystic changes, and distortion of airway structure indicate chronic disease.

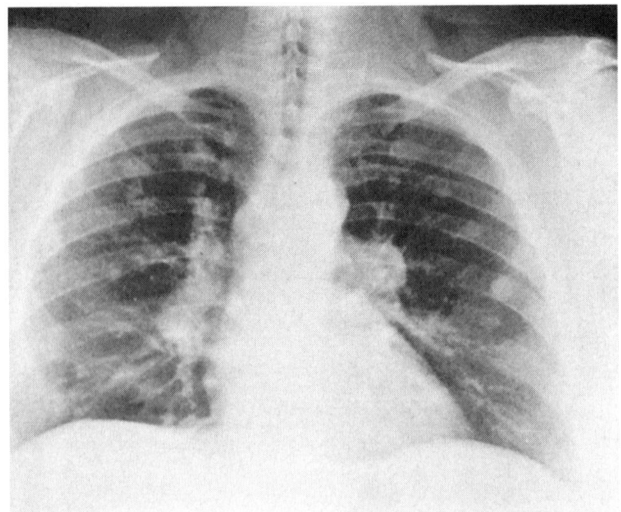

**Figure 59.7** Peripheral parenchymal nodules of sarcoidosis, giving an appearance of metastatic cancer.

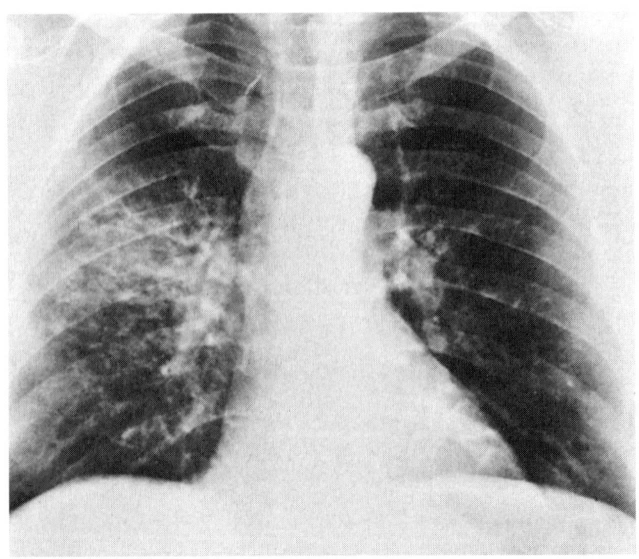

**Figure 59.8** Roentgenogram of chest, showing unusual focal unilateral infiltrate of sarcoidosis.

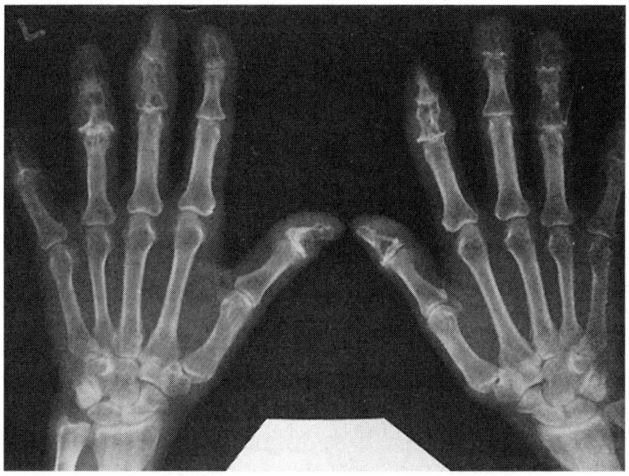

**Figure 59.9** Roentgenogram of the hands of a patient with sarcoidosis, showing typical cystic bone changes and attrition of distal phalanges.

Radiographic changes of the heart or involvement of thoracic blood vessels may be present, and cardiomegaly may be observed. Pulmonary hypertension may be associated with severe fibrocystic disease, but there have been a few case reports of pulmonary hypertension in the absence of severe fibrotic or parenchymal disease. Superior vena cava obstruction occurs in rare instances,[74–76] and there has been one report of innominate vein obstruction.[77] Although sarcoidosis does not usually compress large vessels, narrowing of the pulmonary artery secondary to extrinsic pressure by large intrathoracic nodes of sarcoidosis has been reported.[78]

Involvement of short tubular bones of the hands and feet occurs in approximately 3% of patients with sarcoidosis and is usually associated with skin and visceral disease (Fig. 59.9). Bone lesions may also occur in the ribs, sternum, or thoracic vertebrae[79, 80]; the lesions may be lytic or sclerotic. Asymmetric pseudoclubbing of fingers resulting from bone cysts with associated dactylitis has been described.[81] Radionuclide scanning, with the use of technetium ($^{99m}$Tc)–labeled pyrophosphate or diphosphonate isotope has been reported to be more sensitive than gallium ($^{67}$Ga) citrate scintigraphy or radiographic bone studies in detecting these osseous lesions.[79, 82]

## PHYSIOLOGIC ALTERATIONS

Pulmonary function tests provide an assessment of the extent of pulmonary functional impairment. They correlate poorly with clinical findings because of large pulmonary functional reserve. Similarly, they do not correlate with roentgenographic findings because these abnormalities are produced by three-dimensional changes and do not necessarily represent uniform density of disease. Because physiologic changes may be caused by both fibrosis and granuloma, pulmonary function abnormalities do not reflect activity or reversibility of disease. Nevertheless, they may be useful in helping to decide whether to start treatment and in providing objective data when monitoring patients, either on or off treatment.

The most frequent and earliest abnormalities in pulmonary function in patients with sarcoidosis are reductions in lung volumes (restrictive lung disease) and impairment in diffusing capacity.[83–85] Expiratory flow rates may be reduced, which indicates airway obstruction.[86] Reduction in lung compliance and increased airway resistance may be found with more elaborate testing. On occasion, there are no abnormalities in pulmonary function despite roentgenographically visible infiltrates.[87, 88] Pulmonary functional impairment is closely related to location, extent, and nature (fibrosis or granuloma) of the disease. Functional impairment may improve only minimally with spontaneous resolution of disease, which suggests that the impairment is largely attributable to fibrosis.[84, 89] Also, pulmonary function may gradually deteriorate or may be considerably improved with corticosteroids, which indicates resolution of reversible granulomas.[90]

Reduced diffusing capacity is believed to be caused by a combination of interstitial and pulmonary vascular disease. Usually, there is evidence of coexisting restrictive disease. Significant pulmonary hypertension from sarcoidosis of the lung is usually associated with marked restrictive disease, but there have been a few case reports of pulmonary hypertension without reduction in lung volume, which indicates primary vascular involvement,[91, 92] and spontaneous resolution of pulmonary hypertension in this setting has been reported in one patient.[93]

Arterial hypoxemia occurring at rest suggests more advanced disease.[94] A decrease in arterial oxygen saturation with exercise occurs frequently and is considered to be caused largely by a ventilation-perfusion mismatch. A diffusion defect, if severe, may also contribute to this finding. Arterial $P_{O_2}$ during exercise and total lung capacity have been reported to correlate with right ventricular ejection fraction in patients with restrictive pulmonary disease, whereas left ventricular ejection fraction remains within normal limits. Hypercapnia occurs only in patients with advanced disease. Although arterial $P_{CO_2}$ is usually within the normal range, it may be reduced as a result of hyperventilation.

## PATHOLOGY

Granulomas of sarcoidosis often exist diffusely throughout the body despite a lack of clinical evidence of disease. Histologic features are usually quite typical but not specific. The architecture of the lesion is that of multiple similar granulomas, consisting of whorls of elongated cells (fibroblasts and epithelioid cells) with mononuclear inflammatory cells at their periphery (Fig. 59.10 and Fig. 59.11). Giant cells are located within the granulomas, and multinucleated crystalline or cellular inclusion bodies are frequently found. The individual granulomatous nodules may be distinct as a result of separation by connective tissue or may merge with adjacent nodules. Scarring with fibrosis or hyalinization suggests chronicity, but the time required for development of these changes is uncertain. The presence of central necrosis may cause confusion with tuberculous granulomas, which typically show necrosis. Ultrastructural examinations have not revealed any unique features of the granulomas of sarcoidosis, nor have they been helpful in suggesting the pathogenesis

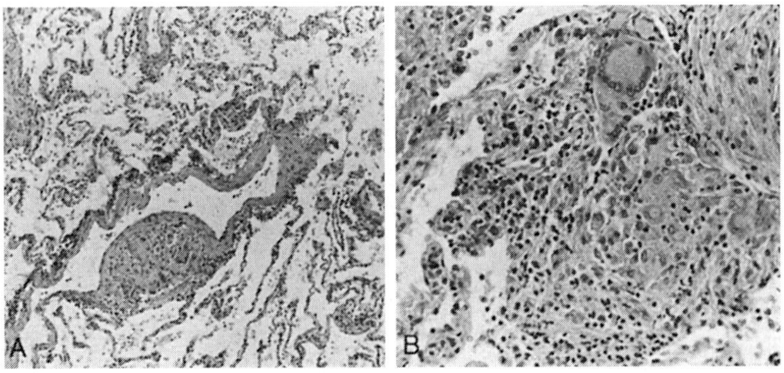


**Figure 59.10** Histologic specimens from an open lung biopsy of a 39-year-old man with pulmonary sarcoidosis, showing *(A)* an interstitial granuloma *(upper left)* and a second granuloma within the wall of a small artery (original magnification × 80) and *(B)* higher power (original magnification × 200) of the interstitial granuloma showing histiocytes, giant cells, fibroblasts, and lymphocytes.

of disease. However, macrophages and lymphocytes of patients with sarcoidosis are larger than normal ones and show distinctive features of their subcellular components.[95]

An association of sarcoidosis with tuberculosis is recorded in the literature,[96–98] but the significance of this observation is uncertain. The distinction between sarcoidosis and tuberculosis is often difficult, and the two diseases are sometimes concurrent. To further complicate the issue, similar granulomas occur in a wide variety of other diseases, such as malignancy or immune deficiencies, fungal disease, berylliosis, and foreign body reactions.[99, 100] These diagnoses should be excluded by clinical assessment, appropriate staining procedures, and examination of tissue by refraction.

## IMMUNOLOGIC FEATURES

Sarcoidosis is characterized by an accumulation of activated T cells that express the cluster of differentiation antigen 4 ($CD4^+$) as well as an accumulation of macrophages and their progeny in the interstitium and alveoli of the lung.[101, 102] Analysis of samples obtained from the lower respiratory tract via bronchoalveolar lavage (BAL) shows an increase in $CD4^+$, with a concomitant decrease in $CD8^+$ T cells, yielding a high $CD4^+/CD8^+$ ratio[102, 103]; $CD8^+$ predominance has also been described.[104, 105] The imbalance in the $CD4^+/CD8^+$ ratio could be due to proliferation of the $CD4^+$ subset, because these cells spontaneously release interleukin (IL)–2,[106, 107] express IL-2 receptor subunits (CD25,[108] CD122, and CD 132[109]), and proliferate in response to exogenous IL-2[108] or IL-15.[109] Further evidence of local cell proliferation is suggested by the fact that BAL lymphocytes express high levels of the activation marker CD45RO, which defines memory cells.[110]

Local proliferation of T cells in an antigen-driven manner is expected to yield increased frequencies of clonotypic T-cell antigen receptor gene products. Indeed, analysis of BAL or biopsies from positive Kveim skin test results demonstrates a bias toward certain polymorphic segments of the T-cell receptor (TCR) $\alpha,\beta$[111–113] and TCR $\gamma,\delta$.[114, 115] Although there may be a dominance in TCR usage in a given patient, considerable variability can be seen among individuals, which could be due to the wide repertoire of human major histocompatibility complex (MHC) molecules of the class II. The issue of T-cell clonality is important, inasmuch as mature $CD4^+$ T cells can be divided into at least two groups of clones: (1) T helper 1 (Th1) cells, which produce interferon gamma (INF-$\gamma$), IL-2, IL-12, and IL-18 and are associated with granulomatous diseases; and (2) T helper 2 (Th2) cells, which produce IL-4, IL-5, IL-6, IL-10, and IL-13; downregulate Th1; and are associated with B-cell class switch and allergic reactions.[116–118] However, it is unclear which phenotype truly predominates in sarcoidosis, inasmuch as some authors have found Th1,[119, 120] some have reported Th2,[121] and others have reported indistinct cytokine profiles.[122, 123]

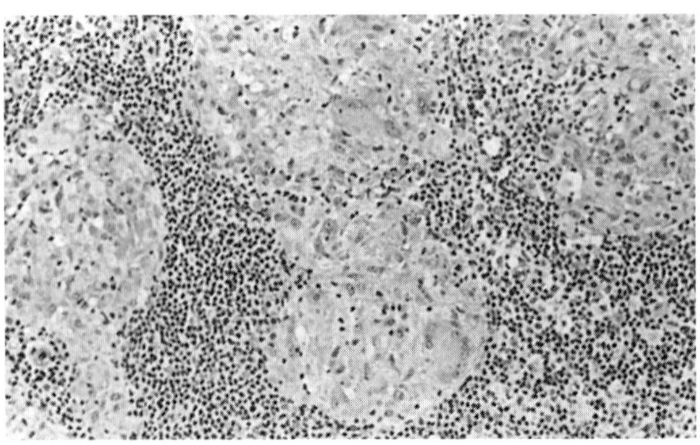

**Figure 59.11** Section of a lymph node of a 34-year-old woman, showing extensive replacement by noncaseating granulomas (original magnification × 200).

T-cell clones arise upon stimulation via the TCR-CD3 complex by a molecule of the MHC plus antigen expressed on the surface of an antigen-presenting cell. There is growing evidence to suggest that alveolar macrophages and their progeny from patients with sarcoidosis, the multinucleated giant cell, are efficient antigen-presenting cells, as opposed to alveolar macrophages from normal individuals that express low levels of accessory molecules and fail to present antigen to HLA-matched T-cell lines.[124] Indeed, alveolar macrophages from sarcoidosis patients express high levels of CD80, CD40, and CD86,[125] which are essential T-cell co-stimulatory molecules, by binding to CD28 or CD152 (previously named CTLA-4) on the T cell. Alveolar macrophages also express CD11/CD18[126] and CD54,[127] which are important in the first recognition that occurs between T cell and antigen-presenting cells. However, the clearest evidence of cooperation between antigen-presenting cells and T cells is that BAL cells of sarcoidosis patients can present antigen to MHC-matched T-cell lines.[128] Alveolar macrophages in sarcoidosis produce not only factors that amplify inflammation, such as tumor necrosis factor (TNF)–α,[129, 130] INF- γ,[131] IL-1,[132] IL-15,[109] and reactive oxygen species,[133] but also chemokines such as induced protein (IP)-10 that stimulate the directional migration of activated T cells.[134] The linkage between alveolar macrophages and multinucleated giant cells is not completely understood; however, in vitro alveolar macrophages transform into multinucleated giant cells when stimulated with macrophage colony-stimulating factor (MCSF) and granulocyte-macrophage (GM)-CSF.[135, 136] Furthermore, multinucleated giant cells may be able to present antigens to T cells, because these cells express the requisite class II–MHC molecules (HLA-DR and HLA-DQ).[137, 138]

Although the cause of sarcoidosis remains unknown, the fact that alveolar macrophages may be acting as antigen-presenting cells and the oligoclonal usage of TCR genes suggest that an antigen could be driving these immune phenomena. Indeed, Boeck postulated in the 19th century that *M. tuberculosis* could be such an antigen.[139] Since then, a number of infectious organisms have been considered, including cell wall–deficient mycobacterium,[140] atypical mycobacterium,[141] *Propionibacterium acnes,*[142] *Tropherema whippelii,*[143, 144] and human herpesvirus type 8.[145] In the 1990s, the diagnosis of sarcoidosis mandated that no microbes grow or can be demonstrated through conventional techniques. One argument against an infectious cause for sarcoidosis is that despite the use of immune-suppressive medication, patients do not die of overwhelming infections by the candidate microbes. On the other hand, a transmissible agent could explain the recurrence of sarcoidosis in lung or liver allografts[126, 146–151] or the appearance of sarcoidosis in a bone marrow recipient from a donor with pulmonary sarcoidosis.[151] Perhaps the clearest evidence in favor of an antigen is that 80% of patients develop a T-cell recall response[152] when injected with the Kveim reagent, which is an extract of granulomatous splenic tissue from patients with sarcoidosis.[153] This test has been validated worldwide, yields less than 1% false positive results, and is available at certain centers around the world.[153] The specific component that elicits oligoclonal accumulation of T cells at sites of Kveim injection is unknown, but it seems to be a complex three-dimensional protein.[154] A number of environmental agents have been proposed to cause sarcoidosis, including clay soil, pine dust, talc, or metals such as beryllium or zirconium; however, the epidemiologic and clinical data do not support these theories.[155]

In addition to T cells and alveolar macrophages, B cells have also been found in association with granulomas,[156] and increased levels of immunoglobulins have been reported in the BAL.[157–159] This antibody response is due to polyclonal B-cell stimulation,[160] which again suggests an antigen-driven process. These antibodies exhibit an array of specificity ranging from viruses[161] to mycobacteria[141] to autoantigens on both $CD4^+$ and $CD8^+$ T cells[162] and even to stress proteins.[163] Whether these antibodies play a role in pathogenesis or merely represent cross reactivity remains to be determined. Sarcoidosis patients also exhibit systemic immunologic alterations, such as the impaired ability to mount a delayed-type hypersensitivity response to cutaneous antigens, including purified protein derivative and mumps.[164] However, some patients may react initially or may convert later, thus requiring further work-up to exclude tuberculosis. On the other hand, most patients react to the intradermal injection of Kveim antigen independently of stage of disease.[153, 165]

## DIAGNOSIS

At times, the clinical presentation is sufficiently typical that the diagnosis can be made without biopsy material. This is the case for the presentation of bilateral symmetric hilar adenopathy in an otherwise asymptomatic person who may or may not have erythema nodosum or uveitis.[166] There is a remote possibility of lymphoma in these patients, but in that case, constitutional symptoms usually develop within a short interval after discovery of the hilar adenopathy. Similarly, sarcoidosis is the likely diagnosis if reticulonodular changes are present on the chest roentgenogram of an asymptomatic 20- to 40-year-old patient with normal findings of a chest examination. Eosinophilic granuloma is an alternative diagnosis.

In addition to lymphoma and eosinophilic granuloma, other diagnoses that are often considered in the differential include tuberculosis, fungal disease, berylliosis, lymphangitic spread of carcinoma, and interstitial fibrosis of various causes. On occasion, sarcoidosis may be confused with asthma when the involvement is primarily of the airways. Depending on the pattern of organ involvement, a large number of other diagnoses are often possible.

It is frequently reassuring to patient and physician to have a tissue diagnosis, and many techniques for obtaining this have been used. The most specific location for obtaining biopsy specimens for diagnosis is the lung. Transbronchial biopsy has become the accepted method for obtaining tissue,[167] and it is positive in approximately 50% to 60% of patients who do not have roentgenographic evidence of parenchymal disease. Among patients with radiographic abnormalities, the positivity rate increases to 85% to 90%.[168] False-positive diagnoses by lung biopsy are exceedingly rare. On the other hand, lymph node and liver biopsies may yield false-positive diagnoses. Skin and conjunctival biopsies have a high specificity for sarcoidosis, but sensitivity is low with grossly normal conjunctivae.[169] Foreign body granulomas can be excluded by examination under polarized light. Biopsy of a variety of other clinically abnormal tissues may provide the diagnosis.

The Kveim reaction has been used for diagnosis, but results vary, depending on the source of antigen. This finding is not surprising, because the antigen is an impure preparation obtained from spleens of various patients with sarcoidosis. Furthermore, the granulomatous response produced by the antigen may be interpreted differently by different investigators. Israel and Goldstein[170] concluded that the Kveim reaction is an immunologic response associated with lymphadenopathy of diverse causes. Because of a 4- to 6-week delay in diagnosis, difficulty in obtaining antigen, and current availability of more specific tests, the Kveim reaction has fallen into disuse.

Elevation of serum angiotensin I–converting enzyme (ACE) in patients with sarcoidosis was first noted by Lieberman.[171] It was hoped that measurement of serum ACE would be a sensitive and specific serum marker, but in a review of extensive subsequent research, Fanburg[172] noted that this enzyme was elevated more than two standard deviations from the normal mean in only 41% to 80% of patients with sarcoidosis. The reason for the wide variation in results is not clear. Furthermore, elevations in serum ACE have been noted in patients with various other diseases, including miliary tuberculosis, histoplasmosis, Gaucher's disease, leprosy, human immunodeficiency virus infection, and hepatitis.[171, 173–175] Measurements of ACE activity in locations other than serum, such as peripheral monocytes[176] or in tears of patients with ocular sarcoidosis, may help in diagnosis, but such specimens are not easy to obtain.[177] Other serum enzymes such as lysozyme and thermolysin-like metallopeptidase have also been reported to be elevated in patients with sarcoidosis,[178, 179] but their usefulness is still not established.

Bronchoalveolar lavage (see Chapter 27) has been used for the diagnosis of sarcoidosis[180] but, again, is not a specific test. The percentage of lymphocytes is elevated.[180] The measurement of ACE levels in BAL fluid has not been particularly helpful in clinical evaluations. Radionuclide scanning with $^{67}$Ga has been used,[181] but $^{67}$Ga is also taken up by the lungs in patients with a large number of other diseases and therefore is not specific for sarcoidosis. Nevertheless, $^{67}$Ga scanning provides some quantitation of the extent of sarcoidosis and may be useful in providing a site for biopsy of granulomatous tissue that would have otherwise gone unrecognized.[182]

Thus, sarcoidosis is still diagnosed by clinical assessment and tissue biopsy. Other findings, such as anergy to delayed hypersensitivity reactions, Kveim positivity, lymphocytosis in BAL fluid, and elevation of serum ACE level, may add support but do not in themselves provide conclusive evidence for the diagnosis.

## ACTIVITY OF DISEASE

Although the concept of "activity" of sarcoidosis is a useful one with regard to prognosis and therapy, it is difficult to define the concept precisely. Activity usually implies potential for deterioration in organ function (i.e., the granulomatous process is still present). "Inactivity" implies clearing of the granulomatous process or progression to fibrosis and hyalinization (conditions incapable of causing further damage). The clinical features of activity or inactivity are vaguely defined. "Active" disease suggests occurrence of clinical changes (i.e., increasing symptoms, progression noted by roentgenographic or pulmonary function evaluation, and clinical evidence of deterioration of function of other organ systems). Thus, if clinical and laboratory findings are the "gold standard" for activity of sarcoidosis, they are very imprecise, and other tests, measured against this standard, suffer from similar imprecision.

There are basically three tests that have been used to assess activity of sarcoidosis: measurement of the percentage of lymphocytes in BAL, $^{67}$Ga scanning, and determination of serum ACE concentration. Another test, the rate of pulmonary clearance of $^{99m}$Tc-diethylenetriamine pentaacetate (DTPA), has been found to correlate better with serum ACE activity than with lavage lymphocytosis and has also been used to monitor activity.[183] Normally, BAL fluid contains mostly alveolar macrophages (approximately 90% of the total cells), few lymphocytes (10%), and small numbers of neutrophils (1% to 2%). In patients with sarcoidosis, there is an increase in the proportion of lymphocytes.[180] Furthermore, there is an increase in T lymphocytes, and with the use of surface markers, it has been established that the increase occurs in $CD4^+$ (helper) lymphocytes.[184] After it was recognized that a lymphocytic alveolitis characterized sarcoidosis, a high-intensity alveolitis was defined as a lymphocyte differential count greater than 28%, and a low-intensity alveolitis was defined as a lymphocyte differential count less than 28%.[180] The lavage cellularity corresponded to cellularity by tissue biopsy. Implicit in the definition of intensity of alveolitis was an assessment of the prognosis of disease. Although some studies have supported this concept,[185] prognostication and assessment of activity as defined on the basis of percentage of lymphocytes in BAL are now less certain.

Similarly, the value of $^{67}$Ga scanning as a noninvasive indicator of outcome is also not clear. Because $^{67}$Ga scanning appears to reflect the lymphocyte differential count of the BAL,[181] it is tempting to consider this examination as an indicator of activity, but the published data are conflicting. A negative $^{67}$Ga scan does suggest inactivity of disease.[186, 187]

The value of serial serum ACE levels as an indicator of activity of sarcoidosis is also uncertain. The rationale for the relationship is that elevated serum ACE in patients with sarcoidosis is produced by granulomatous tissue and that the level of serum ACE reflects the granulomatous "load" of the body. This approach fails to consider the possibility that turnover of serum ACE may also be altered and that despite elevated rates of synthesis and release of ACE, serum levels of this enzyme may remain unchanged in the presence of increased degradation. Nevertheless, it has now been observed in several studies that regardless of the initial level of serum ACE, a decrease in level of the enzyme reflects spontaneous remission of disease or response to corticosteroid therapy.[188–190] A recurrence of elevation in serum ACE may reflect recrudescence of disease.

The rate of clearance from the lungs of $^{99m}$Tc-DTPA (see Chapter 26) is a potentially useful way to monitor activity of pulmonary sarcoidosis. After studies demonstrated that the rate of clearance was increased in nonsmoking patients with sarcoidosis and that the values correlated with serum ACE levels, Dusser and colleagues[183] performed serial studies in 37 patients and showed that accelerated clearance of $^{99m}$Tc-DTPA was useful in predicting subsequent deterioration of pulmonary function and that increased values decreased with corticosteroid therapy. In addition, it has been found that the levels of serum-soluble IL-2 receptor (ssIL-2R) are higher in patients with sarcoidosis whose lung function test results are abnormal than in those whose results are normal[191]; however, the value of ssIL-2R as a predictor of progression remains to be established.

## COURSE AND PROGNOSIS

Although sarcoidosis is usually a self-limited disease, its progression may at times impair activities of patients and can be life-threatening. Special attention should be paid to evaluating pulmonary function and the blood calcium level, because abnormalities in these variables may lead insidiously to functional impairment of vital organs. Other vital organs that may be irreversibly damaged usually manifest their involvement more overtly. For example, the patient with a neurologic or ophthalmologic problem is well aware of having an abnormality.

A decision regarding therapy is often difficult and depends on the risk of vital organ impairment. If the decision is made not to treat, it is necessary for the physician to monitor the patient at regular intervals until it is certain that the disease has remitted or is fully quiescent. Although there is considerable disagreement over what parameters are most important to follow either with or without treatment, it seems reasonable, at least, to observe the patient clinically and to obtain a chest roentgenogram and pulmonary function evaluation every 3 to 6 months for the first 2 years of observation. In patients with intrathoracic sarcoidosis, the combination of parenchymal lesions and functional impairment at the time of initial diagnosis portends an unfavorable prognosis.[191a] Serum ACE levels can be measured with little difficulty and may give some indication of the course of activity of disease. $^{67}$Ga scanning, $^{99m}$Tc-DTPA clearance, and BAL are at present research tools. As further research defines more helpful variables to monitor, those can be substituted for currently used measurements.

## THERAPY

The natural history of sarcoidosis has been reviewed extensively.[192, 193] Thirty to fifty per cent of cases spontaneously remit in a period of up to 3 years. Approximately 30% show progression over the next 5 to 10 years, and 20% to 30% remain relatively stable during this time. There is a negligible mortality rate during the first several years of disease and a low mortality rate thereafter. Because sarcoidosis may become inactive or regress spontaneously and the only effective therapy has significant side effects and is not curative, treatment is frequently withheld. This is certainly an appropriate approach for an asymptomatic patient with no significant interference with organ function.[194] The risk with this approach is that the disease process may insidiously progress to irreversible fibrosis. Therefore, it is necessary to evaluate these patients periodically with the hope that therapy will still be effective if organ functional impairment is detected.

When there is evidence of significant impairment of function of a vital organ (heart, lung, brain, kidney, or eye), therapy should be instituted immediately. Therapy should also be used for persistent hypercalcemia or hypercalciuria and may be required for diffuse cutaneous lesions. A more difficult question regarding the use of therapy arises when there are pulmonary parenchymal infiltrates or when moderate pulmonary functional impairment is present in an asymptomatic person. In these cases, the decision regarding therapy is not clear, although total remission of disease is unlikely. A test that forecasts the likelihood of progression of disease would be useful, but such a test is not available.

Corticosteroids are currently considered the most effective treatment for sarcoidosis.[195, 196] There is no evidence that any other corticosteroid preparation is more effective for sarcoidosis than prednisone,[197] and treatment can usually be started with 30 mg per day or 40 to 60 mg every other day by mouth.[195, 198, 199] On occasion, higher doses are required. When therapy is effective, a clinical or radiologic response is usually obtained in 2 to 4 weeks. If there is no measurable response to steroid therapy in 4 to 6 weeks, it is reasonable to discontinue treatment with the likelihood that the histologic process is primarily fibrosis. Once a response is obtained, the amount of prednisone should be reduced to the lowest effective dose that maintains the response, and an alternate-day schedule should be considered. It is often possible to maintain remission of disease with doses as low as 10 to 15 mg daily or even on alternate days. Administration of corticosteroids by aerosol is not effective in patients with sarcoidosis,[200] but new preparations and delivery devices may provide better results.

The duration of treatment is often uncertain. Usually, treatment is continued for several weeks or months. With recurrence of the features for which it was started, treatment may have to be reinstituted. The natural course of disease seems to be uninfluenced by therapy, and corticosteroid treatment may be required for months or years.

A wide variety of therapies other than corticosteroids have been tried for sarcoidosis with varying degrees of effectiveness (see Lynch and Baughman[201]). These have been used both alone and in combination with steroids and include immunosuppressive agents such as methotrexate and azathioprine, alkylating agents such as cyclophosphamide and chlorambucil, T-cell/cytokine inhibitors such as cyclosporine and pentoxifylline, and antimalarials such as chloroquine and hydrochloroquine. Each of these other therapies has its own side effects, and other therapies will most certainly be tested in the future. Although these agents clearly have been helpful in selected patients,[46, 201a] there are few properly controlled studies on which to base decisions regarding efficacy of these therapies versus conventional corticosteroid therapy. Often when these other therapies are tried, steroids have not been adequately or appropriately utilized. Organ transplantation is currently used to treat end-stage sarcoidosis. When an approach concerning any form of therapy is derived, "minimization of harm for the patient"[202] should be emphasized.

It is possible that less toxic and more effective therapy will become available. Future insights into the pathogenesis of sarcoidosis may allow new approaches for treating a specific causative agent or for utilizing naturally occurring body defense mechanisms that, at times, seem to have a powerful ability to contain the disease.

## SUMMARY

Despite extensive investigation, many questions persist about most aspects of sarcoidosis. Its cause is unknown; its pathogenesis remains mysterious, although $CD4^+$ lymphocytes appear to be involved; and there is no laboratory test or histologic appearance that is pathognomonic. Usually sarcoidosis is a benign, self-limited disease that resolves spontaneously without significant sequelae. Occasionally, however, the disease causes serious functional limitation, which is most often pulmonary and may be life-threatening. Unfortunately, it is impossible by currently available tests to establish in which patients the disease will progress and in which it will subside. Patients with sarcoidosis who require therapy generally respond well to corticosteroids, but the optimum dosage and duration of treatment are still largely empirical.

## References


1. Mitchel DN, Rees RJW: A transmissible agent from sarcoid tissue. Lancet 2:81–84, 1969.
2. Mitchell DN, Rees RJW: An attempt to demonstrate a transmissible agent from sarcoid material. Postgrad Med J 46:510–514, 1970.
3. Fidler HM, Rook GA, Johnson NM, et al: *Mycobacterium tuberculosis* DNA in tissue affected by sarcoidosis. BMJ 306:546–549, 1993.
4. Thomas PD, Hunninghake GW: State of the art. Current concepts of the pathogenesis of sarcoidosis. Am Rev Respir Dis 135:747–760, 1987.
5. James DG, Neville E, Siltzbach LE: A worldwide review of sarcoidosis. Ann N Y Acad Sci 278:321–334, 1976.
6. Levinsky L, Cummiskey J, Romer FK, et al: Sarcoidosis in Europe: A cooperative study. Proceedings of the VIIth International Conference on Sarcoidosis and Other Granulomatous Disorders. Ann N Y Acad Sci 278:335–346, 1976.
7. Hillerdal G, Nou E, Osterman K, et al: Sarcoidosis: Epidemiology and prognosis. A 15-year European study. Am Rev Respir Dis 130:29–32, 1984.
8. Teirstein AS, Lesser, M: Worldwide distribution and epidemiology of sarcoidosis. *In* Fanburg BL (ed): Sarcoidosis and Other Granulomatous Diseases of the Lung (vol 20). New York: Marcel Dekker, 1983, pp 101–134.
9. Selroos O, Sellergren TL, Vuorio M, et al: Sarcoidosis in identical twins. Observations on the course of treated and untreated identical diseases. Am Rev Respir Dis 108:1401–1406, 1973.
10. Al-Arif O, Goldstein RA, Affronti LH, et al: HLA antigen and sarcoidosis in a North American black population. *In* Williams WJ, Davies BH (eds): Eighth Conference on Sarcoidosis. Cardiff, UK: Alpha Omega, 1980, pp 206–212.
11. Smith MJ, Turton CWG, Mitchell DN, et al: Association of HLA B8 with spontaneous resolution in sarcoidosis. Thorax 36:296–298, 1981.
12. James DG: Genetics and familial sarcoidosis. *In* Fanburg BL (ed): Sarcoidosis and Other Granulomatous Diseases of the Lung. New York: Marcel Dekker, 1983, pp 135–146.
13. Kendig EL, Brummer DL: The prognosis of sarcoidosis in children. Chest 70:351–353, 1976.
14. Jasper PL, Denny FW: Sarcoidosis in children with special emphasis on the natural history and treatment. J Pediatr 73:499–512, 1968.
15. Siltzbach LE, Greenberg GM: Childhood sarcoidosis—A study of 18 patients. N Engl J Med 279:1239–1245, 1968.
16. Margolis ML, Israel HL: Sarcoidosis in older patients—Clinical characteristics and course. Geriatrics 38:121–123, 1983.
17. McKelvie P, Gresson C, Pokhrel RP, et al: Sarcoidosis of the upper air passages. Br J Dis Chest 62:200–206, 1968.
18. Paller AS, Surek C, Silva-Walsh I, et al: Cutaneous sarcoidosis associated with sarcoidosis of the upper airway. Arch Dermatol 119:592–596, 1983.
19. Henry DA, Cho SR: Tracheal stenosis in sarcoidosis. South Med J 76:1323–1324, 1983.
20. Selroos O, Niemist M: Sarcoidosis of the nose. Including a report on a patient with large sarcoid polyp of the nasal mucosa. Scand J Respir Dis 58:57–62, 1977.
21. Vainsencher D, Winkelmann RK: Subcutaneous sarcoidosis. Arch Dermatol 120:1028–1031, 1984.
22. Saxe N, Benatar SR, Bok L, et al: Sarcoidosis with leg ulcers and annular facial lesion. Arch Dermatol 120:93–96, 1984.
23. Kataria S, Trevathan GE, Holland JE, et al: Ocular presentation of sarcoidosis in children. Clin Pediatr 22:793–797, 1983.
24. Silverstein A, Siltzbach LE: Muscle involvement in sarcoidosis. Asymptomatic, myositis, and myopathy. Arch Neurol 21:235–241, 1969.
25. Ando DG, Lynch JP III, Fantone JC III: Sarcoid myopathy with elevated creatine phosphokinase. Am Rev Respir Dis 131:298–300, 1985.
26. Babin RW, Liu C, Aschenbrener C: Histopathology of neurosensory deafness in sarcoidosis. Ann Otol Rhinol Laryngol 93:389–393, 1984.
27. Delaney P: Neurologic manifestations in sarcoidosis: Review of the literature with a report of 23 cases. Ann Intern Med 87:336–345, 1977.
28. Roberts WC, McAllister HA Jr, Ferrans VJ: Sarcoidosis of the heart. A clinicopathologic study of 35 necropsy patients (Group I) and review of 78 previously described necropsy patients (Group II). Am J Med 63:86–108, 1977.
29. Garrett J, O'Neill H, Blake S: Constrictive pericarditis associated with sarcoidosis. Am Heart J 107:394, 1984.
30. Israel HL, Margolis ML, Rose LJ: Hepatic granulomatosis and sarcoidosis. Further observations. Dig Dis Sci 29:353–356, 1984.
31. Dufresne CR, Jeyasingham K, Baker RR: Achalasia of the cardia associated with pulmonary sarcoidosis. Surgery 94:32–35, 1983.
32. Sprague R, Harper P, McClain S, et al: Disseminated gastrointestinal sarcoidosis. Case report and review of the literature. Gastroenterology 87:421–425, 1984.
33. Gold RS, Sager E: Oral sarcoidosis: Review of the literature. J Oral Surg 34:237–244, 1976.
34. Knodel AR, Beekman JF: Severe thrombocytopenia and sarcoidosis. JAMA 243:258–259, 1980.
35. Muther RS, McCarron DA, Bennett WM: Renal manifestations of sarcoidosis. Arch Intern Med 141:643–645, 1981.
36. Winnacker JL, Becker KL, Katz S: Endocrine aspects of sarcoidosis. N Engl J Med 278:483–492, 1968.
37. Goldstein RA, Israel HL, Becker KL, et al: The infrequency of hypercalcemia in sarcoidosis. Am J Med 51:21–30, 1971.
38. Bell NH, Gill JR, Bartter FC: On the abnormal calcium absorption in sarcoidosis. Am J Med 36:500–513, 1964.
39. Adams JS, Singer FR, Gacad MA, et al: Isolation and structural identification of 1,25-dihydroxy vitamin $D_3$ produced by cultured alveolar macrophages in sarcoidosis. J Clin Endocrinol Metab 60:960–966, 1985.
40. Cushard WG, Simon AB, Canterbury JM, et al: Parathyroid function in sarcoidosis. N Engl J Med 286:395–398, 1972.
41. Winnacker JL, Becker KL, Katz S: Endocrine aspects of sarcoidosis. N Engl J Med 278:427–434, 1968.
42. Mayock RL, Sullivan RD, Greening RR, et al: Sarcoidosis and pregnancy. JAMA 164:158–163, 1957.
43. Meisels E: The course of Besnier-Boeck's disease of the lungs in serial roentgenograms. Am J Radiol 44:564–567, 1940.
44. Bernstein S, Sussman M: Thoracic manifestations of sarcoidosis. Radiology 44:37–43, 1945.
45. Garland LH: Pulmonary sarcoidosis: The early roentgen findings. Radiology 48:333–354, 1947.
46. American Thoracic Society (ATS), European Respiratory Society (ERS), and World Association of Sarcoidosis and Other Granulomatous Disorders (WASOG): Statement on sarcoidosis. Am J Respir Crit Care Med 160:736–755, 1999.
47. Dunbar RD: Sarcoidosis and its radiologic manifestations. CRC Crit Rev Diagn Imaging 11:185–221, 1978.

48. Bein ME, Putman CE, McLoud TC, et al: A reevaluation of intrathoracic lymphadenopathy in sarcoidosis. Am J Radiol 131:409–415, 1978.
49. Schabel SI, Foote GA, McKee KA: Posterior lymphadenopathy in sarcoidosis. Am J Radiol 129:591–593, 1978.
50. Rockoff SD, Rohatgi PK: Unusual manifestations of thoracic sarcoidosis. Am J Radiol 144:513–528, 1985.
51. Beekman JF, Zimmett SM, Chun BK, et al: Spectrum of pleural involvement in sarcoidosis. Arch Intern Med 136:323–330, 1976.
52. Mayock RL, Bertrand P, Morrison CR, et al: Manifestations of sarcoidosis: Analysis of 145 patients with a review of nine series selected from the literature. Am J Med 35:67–89, 1963.
53. Berte SJ, Pfotenhauer MA: Massive pleural effusion in sarcoidosis. Am Rev Respir Dis 86:261–264, 1962.
54. Aberg H, Bah M, Waters AW: Sarcoidosis complicated by chylothorax. Minn Med 57:1065–1070, 1966.
55. Haegeli A, Keller R: Chylothorax bei sarkoidose. Schweiz Med Wochenschr 111:125–128, 1981.
56. Gorske KJ, Fleming RJ: Mycetoma formation in cavitary pulmonary sarcoidosis. Radiology 95:279–285, 1970.
57. Scadding JG: Further observations on calcification in sarcoidosis. Scand J Respir Dis 49(Suppl):235–242, 1968.
58. Israel HL, Lenchner G, Steiner RM: Late development of mediastinal calcification in sarcoidosis. Am Rev Respir Dis 124:302–305, 1981.
59. Gross BH, Schneider HK, Proto AV: Eggshell calcification of lymph nodes: An update. Am J Radiol 135:1265–1268, 1980.
60. Kirks DR, McCormick VD, Greenspan RH: Pulmonary sarcoidosis: Roentgenographic analysis of 150 patients. Am J Radiol 117:777–786, 1973.
61. Fisher J, Muren O: Sarcoidosis presenting as unilateral hilar mass. South Med J 72:370–371, 1979.
62. Olsson T, Bjornstad-Pettersen HB, Sternberg NL: Bronchostenosis due to sarcoidosis: A cause of atelectasis and airway obstruction simulating pulmonary neoplasm and chronic obstructive pulmonary disease. Chest 75:663–666, 1979.
63. Westcott JL, Noehren TH: Bronchial stenosis in chronic sarcoidosis. Chest 63:893–897, 1973.
64. Rohatgi PK, Schwab LE: Primary acute pulmonary cavitation in sarcoidosis. Am J Radiol 134:1199–1203, 1980.
65. Tellis CJ, Putnam JS: Cavitation in large multinodular pulmonary disease: A rare manifestation of sarcoidosis. Chest 71:792–793, 1977.
66. Fougner AK, Gjone E: Aspergilloma. Nord Med 59:303–305, 1958.
67. Freundlich IM, Libshitz H, Glassman LM, et al: Sarcoidosis: Typical and atypical thoracic manifestations and complications. Clin Radiol 21:376–383, 1970.
68. Wollschlager C, Khan F: Aspergillomas complicating sarcoidosis. A prospective study in 100 patients. Chest 86:585–588, 1984.
69. Onal E, Lopata M, Lourenco RV: Nodular pulmonary sarcoidosis: Clinical, roentgenographic and physiologic course in five patients. Chest 72:296–300, 1977.
70. Demicco WA, Fanburg BL: Sarcoidosis presenting as a lobar or unilateral lung infiltrate. Clin Radiol 33:663–669, 1982.
71. Glazer HS, Levitt RG, Shakelford GD: Peripheral pulmonary infiltrates in sarcoidosis. Chest 86:741–744, 1984.
72. Murdock J, Muller NL: Pulmonary sarcoidosis: Changes on follow-up CT examination. AJR Am J Roentgenol 159:473–477, 1992.
73. Brauner MW, Lenoir S, Granier P, et al: Pulmonary sarcoidosis. CT assessment of reversibility. Radiology 182:345–349, 1992.
74. Brandstetter RD, Hansen DE, Jarowski CI, et al: Superior vena caval syndrome as the initial clinical manifestation of sarcoidosis. Heart Lung 10:101–104, 1981.
75. Morgans WE, Al-Jilahawi AN, Mbatha PB: Superior vena cava obstruction caused by sarcoidosis. Thorax 35:397–398, 1980.
76. Kinney EL, Murthy R, Ascunce G, et al: Sarcoidosis: Rare cause of superior vena cava obstruction. Pa Med 83:31, 1980.
77. Javaheri S, Hales K: Sarcoidosis: Cause of innominate vein obstruction and massive pleural effusion. Lung 157:81–85, 1980.
78. Heitala S, Stinnett RG, Faunce HF: Pulmonary artery narrowing in sarcoidosis. JAMA 237:572–573, 1977.
79. Yaghmai I: Radiographic, angiographic and radionuclide manifestations of osseous sarcoidosis. Radiographics 3:375–396, 1983.
80. Neville E, Carstairs LS, James DG: Bone sarcoidosis. Ann N Y Acad Sci 278:475–487, 1976.
81. Lieberman J, Krauthammer M: Pseudoclubbing in a patient with sarcoidosis of the phalangeal bones. Arch Intern Med 143:1017–1019, 1983.
82. Rohatgi PK: Radioisotope scanning in osseous sarcoidosis. Am J Radiol 134:189–191, 1980.
83. Kanagami H, Katsura T, Shiraishi K, et al: Clinical aspects of sarcoidosis with emphasis on pulmonary function tests. Jpn J Chest Dis 20:853–862, 1961.
84. Sharma OP, Colp C, Williams MH Jr: Pulmonary function studies in patients with bilateral sarcoidosis of hilar lymph nodes. Arch Intern Med 117:436–439, 1966.
85. Young RC Jr, Carr C, Shelton TG, et al: Sarcoidosis: Relationship between changes in lung structure and function. Am Rev Respir Dis 95:224–238, 1967.
86. DeRemee RA, Anderson HA: Sarcoidosis. A correlation of dyspnea with roentgenographic stage and pulmonary function changes. Mayo Clin Proc 49:742–745, 1974.
87. Williams MH Jr: Pulmonary function in Boeck's sarcoid. J Clin Invest 32:909–913, 1953.
88. Romer FK: Sarcoidosis with large nodular lesions simulating pulmonary metastases. An analysis of 125 cases of intrathoracic sarcoidosis. Scand J Respir Dis 58:11–16, 1977.
89. Boushy SF, Kurtzman RS, Martin, ND, et al: The course of pulmonary function in sarcoidosis. Ann Intern Med 62:939–955, 1965.
90. Sharma OP, Colp C, Williams MH Jr: Course of pulmonary sarcoidosis with and without corticosteroid therapy as determined by pulmonary function studies. Am J Med 41:541–551, 1966.
91. Moyer JH, Ackerman AJ: Sarcoidosis: A clinical and roentgenographic study of 28 cases. Am Rev Tuberc 61:299–322, 1959.
92. Smith LJ, Lawrence JB, Katzenstein AA: Vascular sarcoidosis: A rare cause of pulmonary hypertension. Am J Med Sci 285:38–44, 1983.
93. Levine BW, Saldana M, Hutter AM: Pulmonary hypertension in sarcoidosis. Am Rev Respir Dis 103:413–417, 1971.
94. Svanborg N: Studies on the cardiopulmonary function in sarcoidosis. Acta Med Scand 170(Suppl 366):75–117, 1961.
95. Danel C, Dewar A, Corrin B, et al: Ultrastructural changes in bronchoalveolar lavage cells in sarcoidosis and comparison with tissue granuloma. Am J Pathol 112:7–17, 1983.
96. Kent DC, Houk VN, Elliot RC, et al: The definitive evaluation of sarcoidosis. Am Rev Respir Dis 101:721–727, 1970.
97. Greenberg SD, Györkey F, Wegg JG, et al: The ultrastructure of the pulmonary granuloma in sarcoidosis. Am Rev Respir Dis 102:648–652, 1970.
98. Leake ES, Myrvik QN: Osmiophilic structures in granulomatous macrophages and the problem of intracellular mycobacteria. Am Rev Respir Dis 104:132–133, 1971.
99. James DG, Walker AN: All that glitters is not sarcoidosis. *In* Gallopin Y (ed): La Sarcoidose Particulierement dans ses Localisations Extrathoraciques. Rapports du Symposium Européen, September 23–25, 1971. Geneva: Hallwage, 1972, p 113.
100. Brincker H: Sarcoid reactions and sarcoidosis in Hodgkin's disease and other malignant lymphomata. Am Rev Respir Dis 106:600–603, 1972.
101. Rosen Y, Athanassiades TJ, Moon S, et al: Nongranulomatous interstitial pneumonitis in sarcoidosis. Relationship to development of epithelioid granulomas. Chest 74:122–125, 1978.
102. Hunninghake GW, Crystal RG: Pulmonary sarcoidosis: A disorder mediated by excess helper T-lymphocyte activity at sites of disease activity. N Engl J Med 305:429–434, 1981.
103. Schoenfeld N, Schmitt M, Remy N, et al: Activation of bronchoalveolar lavage T lymphocytes and clinical, functional and radiological features in sarcoidosis. Sarcoidosis 12:135–139, 1995.
104. Haneda H, Yamaguchi E, Okazaki N, et al: [A case of pulmonary sarcoidosis with CD8 positive cell dominant alveolitis]. Nippon Kyobu Shikkan Gakkai Zasshi 27:367–372, 1989.
105. Agostini C, Trentin L, Zambello R, et al: CD8 alveolitis in sarcoidosis: Incidence, phenotypic characteristics, and clinical features. Am J Med 95:466–472, 1993.
106. Pinkston P, Bitterman PB, Crystal RG: Spontaneous release of interleukin-2 by lung T lymphocytes in active pulmonary sarcoidosis. N Engl J Med 308:793–800, 1983.

107. Saltini C, Spurzem JR, Lee JJ, et al: Spontaneous release of interleukin 2 by lung T lymphocytes in active pulmonary sarcoidosis is primarily from the Leu3+DR+ T cell subset. J Clin Invest 77:1962–1970, 1986.
108. Konishi K, Moller DR, Saltini C, et al: Spontaneous expression of the interleukin 2 receptor gene and presence of functional interleukin 2 receptors on T lymphocytes in the blood of individuals with active pulmonary sarcoidosis. J Clin Invest 82:775–781, 1988.
109. Agostini C, Trentin L, Facco M, et al: Role of IL-15, IL-2, and their receptors in the development of T cell alveolitis in pulmonary sarcoidosis. J Immunol 157:910–918, 1996.
110. Saltini C, Kirby M, Trapnell BC, et al: Biased accumulation of T lymphocytes with "memory"-type CD45 leukocyte common antigen gene expression on the epithelial surface of the human lung. J Exp Med 171:1123–1140, 1990.
111. Moller DR, Konishi K, Kirby M, et al: Bias toward use of a specific T cell receptor beta-chain variable region in a subgroup of individuals with sarcoidosis. J Clin Invest 82:1183–1191, 1988.
112. Forman JD, Klein JT, Silver RF, et al: Selective activation and accumulation of oligoclonal V beta-specific T cells in active pulmonary sarcoidosis. J Clin Invest 94:1533–1542, 1994.
113. Forrester JM, Wang Y, Ricalton N, et al: TCR expression of activated T cell clones in the lungs of patients with pulmonary sarcoidosis. J Immunol 153:4291–4302, 1994.
114. Balbi B, Moller D, Kirby M, et al: Increased numbers of T lymphocytes with gamma delta-positive antigen receptors in a subgroup of individuals with pulmonary sarcoidosis. J Clin Invest 85:1353–1361, 1990.
115. Gruber R, Pforte A, Beer B, et al: Determination of gamma/delta and other T-lymphocyte subsets in bronchoalveolar lavage fluid and peripheral blood from patients with sarcoidosis and idiopathic fibrosis of the lung. APMIS 104:199–205, 1996.
116. Mosmann TR, Cherwinski H, Bond MW, et al: Two types of murine helper T cell clone: I. Definition according to profiles of lymphokine activities and secreted proteins. J Immunol 136:2348–2357, 1986.
117. Del Prete G: The concept of type-1 and type-2 helper T cells and their cytokines in humans. Int Rev Immunol 16:427–455, 1998.
118. Trinchieri G: Proinflammatory and immunoregulatory functions of interleukin-12. Int Rev Immunol 16:365–396, 1998.
118a. Moller DR: Cells and cytokines involved in the pathogenesis of sarcoidosis. Sarcoidosis Vasc Diffuse Lung Dis 16:24–31, 1999.
119. Moller DR, Forman JD, Liu MC, et al.: Enhanced expression of IL-12 associated with Th1 cytokine profiles in active pulmonary sarcoidosis. J Immunol 156:4952–4960, 1996.
120. Minshall EM, Tsicopoulos A, Yasruel Z, et al: Cytokine mRNA gene expression in active and nonactive pulmonary sarcoidosis. Eur Respir J 10:2034–2039, 1997.
121. Tsuda T, Kita S: Histochemical study of sarcoid granulomatous lesions. Nippon Rinsho 52:1456–1461, 1994.
122. Baumer I, Zissel G, Schlaak M: Th1/Th2 cell distribution in pulmonary sarcoidosis. Am J Respir Cell Mol Biol 16:171–177, 1997.
123. Garlepp MJ, Rose AH, Dench JE, et al: Clonal analysis of lung and blood T cells in patients with sarcoidosis. Thorax 49:577–585, 1994.
124. Chelen CJ, Fang Y, Freeman GJ, et al: Human alveolar macrophages present antigen ineffectively due to defective expression of B7 costimulatory cell surface molecules. J Clin Invest 95:1415–1421, 1995.
125. Nicod LP, Isler P: Alveolar macrophages in sarcoidosis coexpress high levels of CD86 (B7.2), CD40, and CD30L. Am J Respir Cell Mol Biol 17:91–96, 1997.
126. Thomas ED, Ramberg RE, Sale GE, et al: Direct evidence for a bone marrow origin of the alveolar macrophage in man. Science 192:1016–1018, 1976.
127. Striz I, Wang YM, Kalaycioglu O, et al: Expression of alveolar macrophage adhesion molecules in pulmonary sarcoidosis. Chest 102:882–886, 1992.
128. Lem VM, Lipscomb MF, Weissler JC, et al: Bronchoalveolar cells from sarcoid patients demonstrate enhanced antigen presentation. J Immunol 135:1766–1771, 1985.
129. Baughman RP, Strohofer SA, Buchsbaum J, et al: Release of tumor necrosis factor by alveolar macrophages of patients with sarcoidosis. J Lab Clin Med 115:36–42, 1990.
130. Zheng L, Teschler H, Guzman J, et al: Alveolar macrophage TNF-alpha release and BAL cell phenotypes in sarcoidosis. Am J Respir Crit Care Med 152:1061–1066, 1995.
131. Robinson BW, McLemore TL, Crystal RG, et al: Gamma interferon is spontaneously released by alveolar macrophages and lung T lymphocytes in patients with pulmonary sarcoidosis. J Clin Invest 75:1488–1495, 1985.
132. Hunninghake GW: Release of interleukin-1 by alveolar macrophages of patients with active pulmonary sarcoidosis. Am Rev Respir Dis 129:569–572, 1984.
133. Schaberg T, Rau M, Stephan H, et al: Increased number of alveolar macrophages expressing surface molecules of the CD11/CD18 family in sarcoidosis and idiopathic pulmonary fibrosis is related to the production of superoxide anions by these cells. Am Rev Respir Dis 147:1507–1513, 1993.
134. Agostini C, Cassatella M, Zambello R, et al: Involvement of the IP-10 chemokine in sarcoid granulomatous reactions. J Immunol 161:6413–6420, 1998.
135. Lemaire I, Yang H, Lafont V, et al: Differential effects of macrophage- and granulocyte-macrophage colony-stimulating factors on cytokine gene expression during rat alveolar macrophage differentiation into multinucleated giant cells (MGC): Role for IL-6 in type 2 MGC formation. J Immunol 1:5118–5125, 1996.
136. Lemaire I, Yang H, Lauzon W, et al: M-CSF and GM-CSF promote alveolar macrophage differentiation into multinucleated giant cells with distinct phenotypes. J Leukoc Biol 60:509–518, 1996.
137. v Maarsseveen T, Mullink R, Rensen R, et al: HLA-DR antigens in epithelioid cell granulomas of sarcoidosis, using semithin frozen sections. A concept about granuloma formation. Sarcoidosis 2:148–153, 1985.
138. Roncalli M, Servida E: Granulomatous and nongranulomatous lymphadenitis in sarcoidosis. An immunophenotypic study of seven cases. Pathol Res Pract 185:351–357, 1989.
139. Boeck C: Multiple benign sarcoidosis of the skin. J Cutan Dis 17:543, 1899.
140. Almenoff PL, Johnson A, Lesser M, et al: Growth of acid fast L forms from the blood of patients with sarcoidosis. Thorax 51:530–533, 1996.
141. el-Zaatari FA, Naser SA, Markesich DC, et al: Identification of *Mycobacterium avium* complex in sarcoidosis. J Clin Microbiol 34:2240–2245, 1996.
142. Abe C, Iwai K, Mikami R, et al: Frequent isolation of *Propionibacterium acnes* from sarcoidosis lymph nodes. Zentralbl Bakteriol Mikrobiol Hyg [A] 256:541–547, 1984.
143. Diaz Lobato S, Gonzalez Ruiz JM, Granado S, et al: [Sarcoidosis and Whipple's disease: An association or a relationship?]. Rev Clin Esp 190:184–186, 1992.
144. Cho C, Linscheer WG, Hirschkorn, MA, et al: Sarcoidlike granulomas as an early manifestation of Whipple's disease. Gastroenterology 87:941–947, 1984.
145. Di Alberti L, Piattelli A, Artese L, et al: Human herpesvirus 8 variants in sarcoid tissues [see comments]. Lancet 350:1655–1661, 1997.
146. Bjortuft O, Foerster A, Boe J, et al: Single lung transplantation as treatment for end-stage pulmonary sarcoidosis: Recurrence of sarcoidosis in two different lung allografts in one patient. J Heart Lung Transplant 13:24–29, 1994.
147. Fidler HM, Hadziyannis SJ, Dhillon AP, et al: Recurrent hepatic sarcoidosis following liver transplantation. Transplant Proc 29:2509–2510, 1997.
148. Johnson BA, Duncan SR, Ohori NP, et al: Recurrence of sarcoidosis in pulmonary allograft recipients. Am Rev Respir Dis 148:1373–1377, 1993.
149. Martinez FJ, Orens JB, Deeb M, et al: Recurrence of sarcoidosis following bilateral allogeneic lung transplantation. Chest 106:1597–1599, 1994.
150. Padilla ML, Schilero GJ, Teirstein AS: Sarcoidosis and transplantation. Sarcoidosis Vasc Diffuse Lung Dis 14:16–22, 1997.
151. Heyll A, Meckenstock G, Aul C: Possible transmission of sarcoidosis via allogeneic bone marrow transplantation. Bone Marrow Transplant 14:161, 1994.

152. Klein JT, Horn TD, Forman JD, et al: Selection of oligoclonal V beta-specific T cells in the intradermal response to Kveim-Siltzbach reagent in individuals with sarcoidosis. J Immunol 154:1450–1460, 1995.
153. Siltzback LE: The Kveim test in sarcoidosis: A study of 750 patients. JAMA 178:476, 1961.
154. Lyons DJ, Donald S, Mitchell DN, et al: Chemical inactivation of the Kveim reagent. Respiration 59:22–26, 1992.
155. Moller DR: Etiology of sarcoidosis. Clin Chest Med 18:695–706, 1997.
156. Fazel SB, Howie SE, Krajewski AS, et al: B lymphocyte accumulations in human pulmonary sarcoidosis. Thorax 47:964–967, 1992.
157. Bauer W, Gorny MK, Morell A, et al: [Bronchoalveolar immunoglobulins in sarcoidosis]. Schweiz Med Wochenschr 115:103–105, 1985.
158. Oklek K, Ziora D, Niepsuj G, et al: [Cell count and immunoglobulin level in the bronchoalveolar lavage fluid (BALF) in patients with sarcoidosis]. Pneumonol Pol 58:17–25, 1990.
159. Rankin JA, Naegel GP, Schrader CE, et al: Air-space immunoglobulin production and levels in bronchoalveolar lavage fluid of normal subjects and patients with sarcoidosis. Am Rev Respir Dis 127:442–448, 1983.
160. Kurosu K, Yumoto N, Mikata A, et al: Monoclonality of B-cell lineage in primary pulmonary lymphoma demonstrated by immunoglobulin heavy chain gene sequence analysis of histologically non-definitive transbronchial biopsy specimens. J Pathol 178:316–322, 1996.
161. Hillerdal G, Frisk G, Nettelbladt O, et al: High frequency of IgM antibodies to coxsackie B virus in sarcoidosis patients and patients with asbestos-related lesions [see comments]. Sarcoidosis 9:39–42, 1992.
162. Spurzem JR, Saltini C, Crystal RG: Functional significance of anti–T-lymphocyte antibodies in sarcoidosis. Am Rev Respir Dis 137:600–605, 1988.
163. Staton JM, Dench JE, Currie B, et al: Expression and immune recognition of stress proteins in sarcoidosis and other chronic interstitial lung diseases. Immunol Cell Biol 73:23–32, 1995.
164. Quinn EL, Bunch DC, Yagel EM: The mumps skin test and complement fixation test as a diagnostic aid in sarcoidosis. J Invest Dermatol 24:595–598, 1955.
165. Djuric B, Zaumseil I, Eckert H, et al: [Report on the application of various Kveim antigens in diagnostic of sarcoidosis]. Z Erkr Atmungsorgane 149:234–237, 1977.
166. Winterbauer RH, Belic N, Moores KD: A clinical interpretation of bilateral hilar adenopathy. Ann Intern Med 78:65–71, 1973.
167. Koerner SK, Sakowitz AJ, Appelman RI, et al: Transbronchial lung biopsy for the diagnosis of sarcoidosis. N Engl J Med 293:268–270, 1975.
168. Teirstein AS: Fiberoptic bronchoscopy in the diagnosis of sarcoidosis. *In* Fanburg BL (ed): Sarcoidosis and Other Granulomatous Diseases of the Lung. New York: Marcel Dekker, 1983, pp 323–333.
169. James DG: Biopsy of tissues other than the lung in the diagnosis of sarcoidosis. *In* Fanburg BL (ed): Sarcoidosis and Other Granulomatous Diseases of the Lung. New York: Marcel Dekker, 1983, pp 335–345.
170. Israel HL, Goldstein RA: Relation of Kveim-antigen reaction to lymphadenopathy. N Engl J Med 284:345–349, 1971.
171. Lieberman J: Elevation of serum angiotensin-converting enzyme (ACE) level in sarcoidosis. Am J Med 59:365–372, 1975.
172. Fanburg BL: Serum angiotensin-1-converting enzyme in the diagnosis and determination of activity of sarcoidosis. *In* Fanburg BL (ed): Sarcoidosis and Other Granulomatous Diseases of the Lung. New York: Marcel Dekker, 1983, pp 263–272.
173. Silverstein W, Friedland J: Elevated serum and spleen angiotensin converting enzyme and serum lysozyme in Gaucher's disease. Clin Chim Acta 74:21–25, 1977.
174. Ovellete DR, Kelly JW, Anders GT: Serum angiotensin-converting enzyme is elevated in patients with human immunodeficiency virus infection. Arch Int Med 152:321–324, 1992.
175. Fanburg BL, Schoenberger MD, Bachus B, et al: Elevated serum angiotensin 1 converting enzyme in sarcoidosis. Am Rev Respir Dis 114:525–528, 1976.
176. Okabe T, Yamagata K, Fujisawa M, et al: Increased angiotensin converting enzyme in peripheral blood monocytes from patients with sarcoidosis. J Clin Invest 75:911–914, 1985.
177. Sharma OP, Vita JB: Determination of angiotensin-converting enzyme in tears. A noninvasive test for ocular sarcoidosis. Arch Dermatol 101:559–561, 1983.
178. Selroos O, Klockars M: Serum lysozyme in sarcoidosis. Evaluation of its usefulness in determination of disease activity. Scand J Respir Dis 58:110–116, 1977.
179. Almenoff J, Teirstein AS, Thornton JC, et al: Identification of a thermolysin-like metalloendopeptidase in serum: Activity in normal subject and in patients with sarcoidosis. J Lab Clin Med 103:420–431, 1984.
180. Crystal RG, Roberts WC, Hunninghake GW, et al: Pulmonary sarcoidosis: A disease characteristic and perpetuated by activated lung T-lymphocytes. Ann Intern Med 94:73–94, 1981.
181. Line BR, Hunninghake GW, Keogh BA, et al: Gallium-67 scanning to stage the alveolitis of sarcoidosis: Correlation with clinical studies, pulmonary function studies and bronchoalveolar lavage. Am Rev Respir Dis 123:440–446, 1981.
182. Israel HL, Albertine KA, Park CH, et al: Whole-body gallium 67 scans. Role in diagnosis of sarcoidosis. Am Rev Respir Dis 144:1182–1186, 1991.
183. Dusser DJ, Collignon MA, Stanislas-Leguern G, et al: Respiratory clearance of $^{99m}$Tc-DTPA and pulmonary involvement in sarcoidosis. Am Rev Respir Dis 134:493–497, 1986.
184. Hunninghake GW, Crystal RG: Pulmonary sarcoidosis, a disorder mediated by excess helper T-lymphocyte activity at sites of disease activity. N Engl J Med 305:429–434, 1981.
185. Keogh BA, Hunninghake GW, Line BR, et al: The alveolitis of pulmonary sarcoidosis evaluation or natural history and alveolitis-dependent changes in lung function. Am Rev Respir Dis 128:256–265, 1983.
186. Klech H, Kohn H, Kummer F, et al: Assessment of activity of sarcoidosis. Sensitivity and specificity of $^{67}$gallium scintigraphy, serum ACE levels, chest roentgenography and blood lymphocyte subpopulations. Chest 82:732–738, 1982.
187. Gupta RG, Bekerman C, Sicilian L, et al: Gallium 67 citrate scanning and serum angiotensin converting enzyme levels in sarcoidosis. Radiology 144:895–899, 1982.
188. Yotsumoto H: Longitudinal observations of serum angiotensin-converting enzyme activity in sarcoidosis with and without treatment. Chest 82:556–559, 1982.
189. Lieberman J, Schleissner LA, Nosel A, et al: Serum correlations of serum angiotensin-converting enzyme (ACE) in sarcoidosis. A longitudinal study of serum ACE, 67 gallium scans, chest roentgenograms and pulmonary function. Chest 54:522–528, 1983.
190. Ainslie GM, Benatar SR: Serum angiotensin converting enzyme in sarcoidosis: Sensitivity and specificity in diagnosis: Correlations with disease activity, duration, extrathoracic involvement, radiographic type and therapy. Q J Med 55:253–270, 1985.
191. Pforte A, Brunner A, Gais P, et al: Concomitant modulation of serum-soluble interleukin-2 receptor and alveolar macrophage interleukin-2 receptor in sarcoidosis. Am Rev Respir Dis 147:717–722, 1993.
191a. Nagai S, Shigematsu M, Hamada K, et al: Clinical courses and prognoses of pulmonary sarcoidosis. Curr Opin Pulm Med 5:293–298, 1999.
192. Sones M, Israel HL: Course and prognosis of sarcoidosis. Am J Med 29:84–93, 1960.
193. Smallie H, Hoyle C: The natural history of sarcoidosis. QJ Med 53:539–558, 1960.
194. Israel HL, Fouts DW, Beggs RA: A controlled trial of prednisone treatment of sarcoidosis. Am Rev Respir Dis 107:609–614, 1974.
195. Johns CJ, MacGregor MI, Zackery JB, et al: Extended experience in the long-term corticosteroid treatment of pulmonary sarcoidosis. Ann N Y Acad Sci 278:722–731, 1976.
196. Turiaf J, Johns CJ, Teirstein AS, et al: The problem of the treatment of sarcoidosis: Report of the subcommittee on therapy. Ann N Y Acad Sci 278:743–751, 1976.
197. Fanburg BL: Drug therapy reviews. The treatment of sarcoidosis. J Maine Med Assoc 70:37–42, 1979.
198. MacGregor RR, Sheagren JN, Lipsett MB, et al: Alternate-day prednisone therapy. Evaluation of delayed hypersensitivity re-

sponse, control of disease and steroid side effects. N Engl J Med 280:1427–1431, 1969.
199. Harter JG, Reddy WJ, Thorn GW: Studies on intermittent corticosteroid dosage regimen. N Engl J Med 269:591–596, 1963.
200. Williams MH: Pulmonary function in sarcoidosis. *In* Fanburg BL (ed): Sarcoidosis and Other Granulomatous Diseases of the Lung. New York: Marcel Dekker, 1983, pp 77–98.
201. Lynch JP III, Baughman RP: Drug therapy for sarcoidosis: Beyond steroids. J Respir Dis 19:202–215, 1998.
201a. Baughman RP, Lower EE: A clinical approach to the use of methotrexate for sarcoidosis. Thorax 54:742–746, 1999.
202. Hunninghake GW: Goal or treatment for sarcoidosis. Minimize harm for the patient. Am J Respir Crit Care Med 156:1369–1370, 1997.

# 60 Diffuse Alveolar Hemorrhage and Other Rare Infiltrative Disorders

MARVIN I. SCHWARZ, M.D. • REUBEN M. CHERNIACK, M.D.
TALMADGE E. KING, JR., M.D.

Diffuse Alveolar Hemorrhage
- Pathology
- Clinical Presentation
- Physiology
- Laboratory Data

Diffuse Alveolar Hemorrhage with Capillaritis
- Isolated Pulmonary Capillaritis
- Wegener's Granulomatosis
- Microscopic Polyangiitis
- Connective Tissue Disease
- Mixed Cryoglobulinemia
- Behçet's Syndrome
- Henoch-Schönlein Purpura
- Glomerulonephritis and Alveolar Hemorrhage
- Acute Pulmonary Allograft Rejection

Diffuse Alveolar Hemorrhage Without Capillaritis
- Idiopathic Pulmonary Hemosiderosis
- Goodpasture's Syndrome
- Diffuse Alveolar Damage
- Penicillamine
- Trimellitic Anhydride
- Mitral Stenosis
- Coagulation Disorders
- Pulmonary Veno-occlusive Disease
- Pulmonary Capillary Hemangiomatosis
- Lymphangioleiomyomatosis
- Tuberous Sclerosis

Other Rare Infiltrative Disorders
- Neurofibromatosis
- Gaucher's Disease
- Niemann-Pick Disease
- Hermansky-Pudlak Syndrome
- Pulmonary Alveolar Microlithiasis

Summary

## DIFFUSE ALVEOLAR HEMORRHAGE

Hemoptysis usually results from conditions that are focal in either the airways or lung parenchyma. These include bronchitis, bronchiectasis, necrotizing pneumonia, malignancy, pulmonary infarction, and arteriovenous malformations. In these, either the bronchial or the pulmonary circulations are the bleeding sources. The great majority of the alveolar structures are unaffected, although the potential for diffuse aspiration of blood exists. In addition, there are a group of disorders that have adverse effects on the small pulmonary vessels (arterioles, capillaries, and venules), and these vessels are a source of bleeding. In this region the majority of the alveolar capillary surface is affected, producing the syndrome known as diffuse alveolar hemorrhage (DAH). The causes of DAH are divided into those associated with the histologic entity pulmonary capillaritis and those that result from a variety of histologic processes that are not associated with this inflammatory interstitial lesion (Table 60.1). Note that in both the connective tissue diseases and Goodpasture's syndrome, DAH has been described both with and without pulmonary capillaritis.

### Pathology

Pulmonary capillaritis was first described by Spencer in 1957.[1] The term refers to an inflammatory lesion of the alveolar interstitium characterized by neutrophilic infiltration of the alveolar interstitium, with subsequent fibrinoid necrosis. This in turn leads to loss of integrity of the epithelial-endothelial basement membranes and leakage of red blood cells (DAH) and neutrophils into the alveolar spaces (Fig. 60.1 and Fig. 60.2). Many of the neutrophils are fragmented (leukocytoclasis) and appear pyknotic. Nuclear dust accumulates in the lung parenchyma, and small thrombi are often present in capillaries and venules. As for all causes of DAH, intra-alveolar hemosiderin-containing macrophages and collections of

**Table 60.1 CAUSES OF DIFFUSE ALVEOLAR HEMORRHAGE**

| |
|---|
| **With Pulmonary Capillaritis** |
| Wegener's granulomatosis |
| Microscopic polyangiitis |
| Isolated pulmonary capillaritis |
| Connective tissue diseases* |
| Primary antiphospholipid syndrome |
| Mixed cryoglobulinemia |
| Behçet's syndrome |
| Henoch-Schönlein purpura |
| Goodpasture's syndrome* |
| Pauci-immune glomerulonephritis |
| Immune complex–associated glomerulonephritis |
| Drug induced (see text) |
| Acute lung allograft rejection |
| **Without Pulmonary Capillaritis** |
| Idiopathic pulmonary hemosiderosis |
| Systemic lupus erythematosus* |
| Goodpasture's syndrome* |
| Diffuse alveolar damage |
| Penicillamine |
| Trimellitic anhydride |
| Mitral stenosis |
| Coagulation disorders |
| Pulmonary veno-occlusive disease |
| Pulmonary capillary hemangiomatosis |
| Lymphangioleiomyomatosis |
| Tuberous sclerosis |

*In systemic lupus erythematosus and Goodpasture's syndrome, diffuse alveolar hemorrhage has been reported with and without pulmonary capillaritis.

free interstitial hemosiderin appear after the acute hemorrhage. Other histologic features include hyperplasia of the type II alveolar epithelial lining cells, intra-alveolar organization of the DAH (organizing pneumonia), and mononuclear cell infiltration of the alveolar interstitium.[2–4]

In the bland form, the alveolar walls are essentially normal, and the histologic picture is that of DAH. Other histologic processes, such as diffuse alveolar damage, pulmonary veno-occlusive disease, and lymphangioleiomyomatosis, can also be associated with DAH.

## Clinical Presentation

Cough, dyspnea, and hemoptysis are the most prominent symptoms in DAH with or without pulmonary capillaritis. Some patients complain of chest pain. Hemoptysis, however, is not invariably present on presentation and is often delayed even when extensive intra-alveolar bleeding has occurred. In this situation, an unexplained falling hematocrit, acute diffuse pulmonary infiltration that is visible on chest radiograph, and a sequential bloody bronchoalveolar lavage specimen are diagnostic. In general, the symptoms are usually of short duration, being present from days to several weeks before the patient seeks medical attention. Of more importance is that with many of the causes of DAH, the symptoms and signs are recurrent.

Depending on the etiology of DAH, fever and signs and symptoms referring to a systemic vasculitis, such as cutaneous vasculitis, sinusitis, inflammatory ocular disease, arthritis, and glomerulonephritis, often accompany the pulmonary symptoms. The chest radiograph demonstrates diffuse or focal patchy alveolar infiltration, and the computed tomographic (CT) scan confirms the presence of this air space–filling disease (Fig. 60.3 and Fig. 60.4). With recurrent and chronic disease, interstitial infiltrates may appear. Radiographic interstitial infiltrates highlighted by Kerley's B lines become apparent during resolution of the diffuse alveolar bleeding that accompanies mitral stenosis or pulmonary veno-occlusive disease. In patients with DAH in whom extrapulmonary disease is not apparent, an echocardiogram is indicated to rule out mitral valvular disease. An iron-deficiency anemia is the rule, the white blood cell and platelet counts are usually increased, and the erythrocyte sedimentation rate

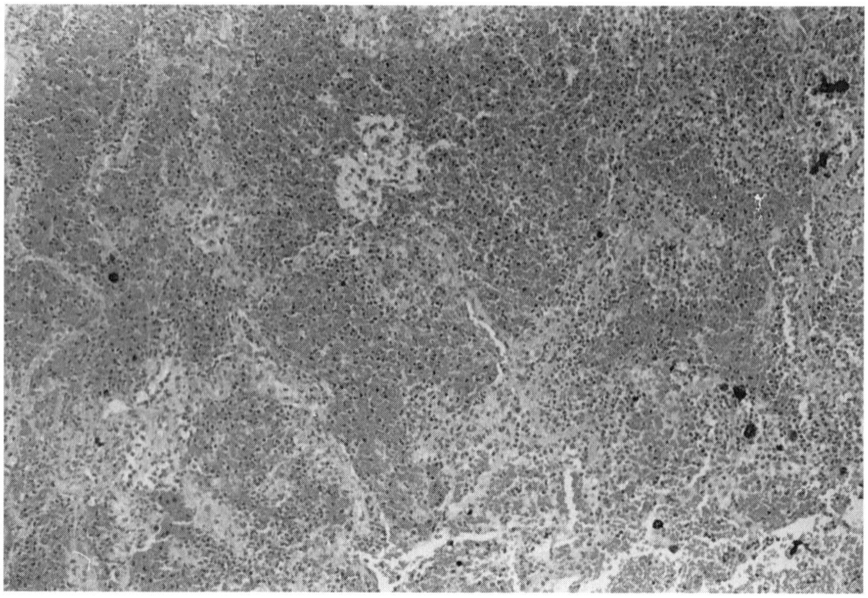

**Figure 60.1** Micrograph showing diffuse alveolar hemorrhage secondary to pulmonary capillaritis. Alveolar spaces are filled with red blood cells as well as nucleated cells. The alveolar interstitium is broadened and infiltrated by neutrophils. Dark-staining hemosiderin collections can be appreciated. (Original magnification × 10.)

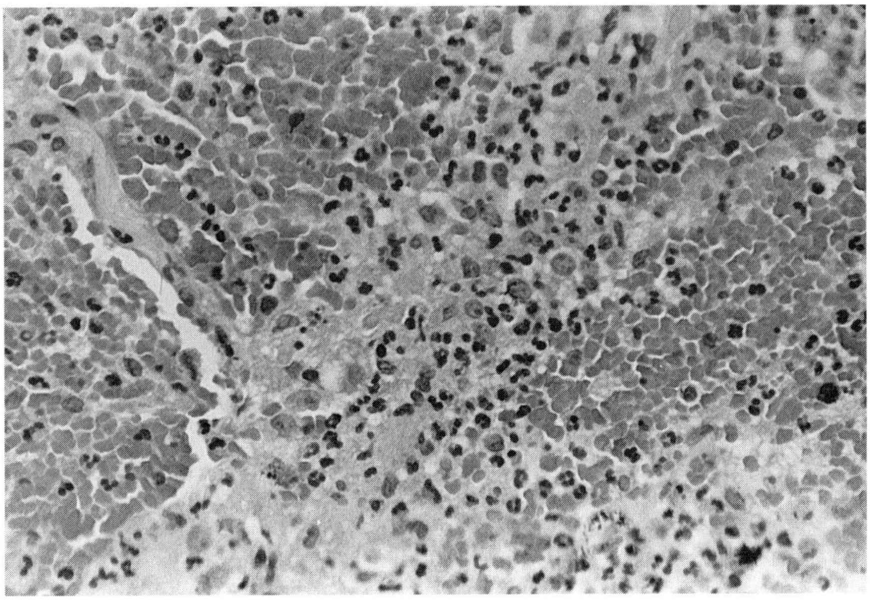

**Figure 60.2** Micrograph showing diffuse alveolar hemorrhage secondary to pulmonary capillaritis. Necrotic edematous alveolar walls are infiltrated by neutrophils that often have pyknotic fragmented nuclei. The alveolar spaces are filled with red blood cells as well as neutrophils. (Original magnification × 40.)

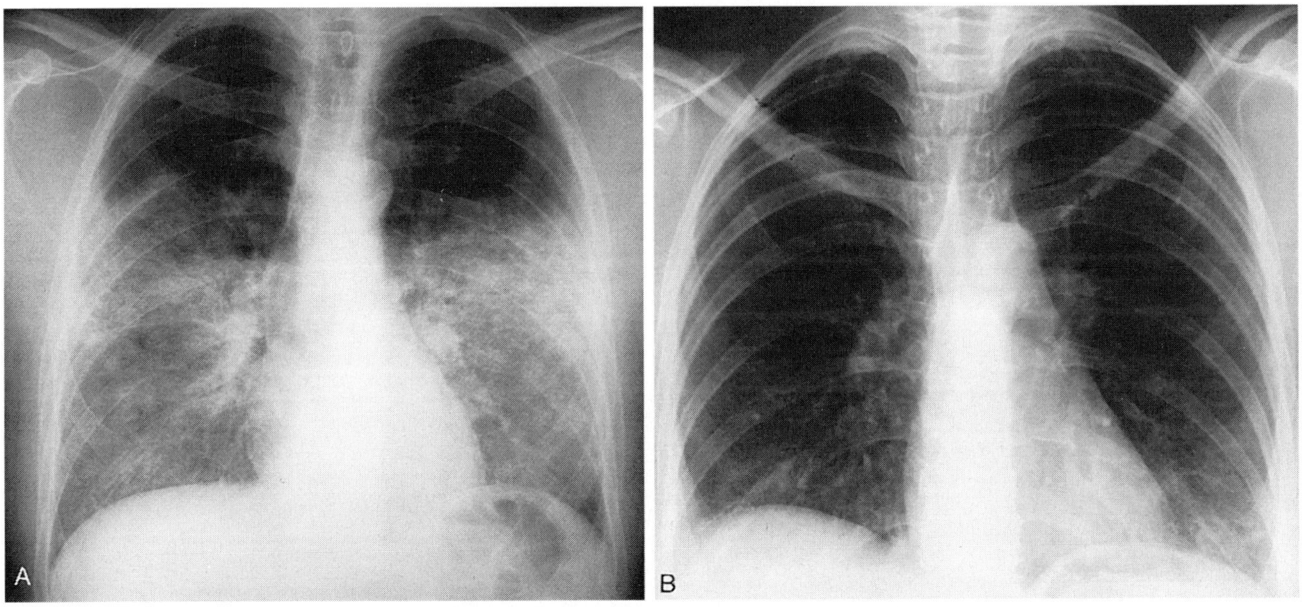


**Figure 60.3** *A,* Chest radiograph showing diffuse alveolar infiltrates after diffuse alveolar hemorrhage secondary to microscopic polyangiitis. Cardiac size is normal. *B,* Chest radiograph showing patchy alveolar infiltrates due to diffuse alveolar hemorrhage in a patient with Wegener's granulomatosis.

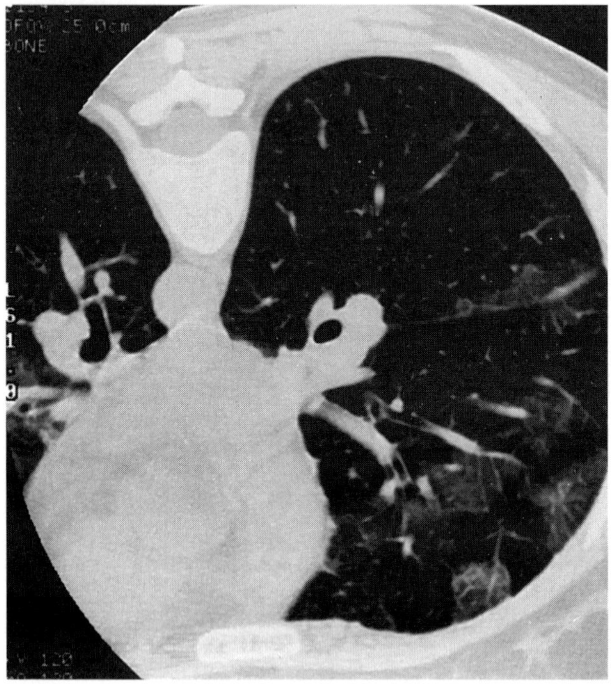

**Figure 60.4** High-resolution computed tomographic scan (prone) of patient in Figure 60.3*B*, confirming the focal nature of the alveolar hemorrhage.

is elevated, particularly in cases of DAH associated with capillaritis. In DAH associated with systemic vasculitis, the connective tissue diseases, and Goodpasture's syndrome, an abnormal urinary sediment and proteinuria, indicating glomerulonephritis, are present. Serum creatinine levels are elevated as well. The renal lesion is a focal segmental necrotizing glomerulitis with crescent formation, and this is a form of rapidly progressive glomerulonephritis (Fig. 60.5).

## Physiology

Varying degrees of hypoxemia result from the ventilation-perfusion abnormalities produced by the alveolar hemorrhage, and patients often require ventilatory support. In less dramatic cases, hemoptysis is intermittent, producing patchy or focal alveolar infiltrates on the chest radiograph with little interference with gas exchange. Serial measurements of the diffusing capacity for carbon monoxide has been suggested as a sensitive indicator for active alveolar bleeding in patients with recurrent DAH.[5] An unexpected increase in the diffusing capacity is the rule in spite of the gas-exchange abnormalities and abnormal chest radiograph. This increase is attributed to the increased binding of carbon monoxide to intra-alveolar hemoglobin. Furthermore, in less obvious cases of diffuse lung disease due to DAH in which there is minimal or no hemoptysis, an unexpected increase in the diffusing capacity leads to the correct initial diagnosis or to the detection of a recurrence in an established case. Bronchoalveolar lavage in a patient with unexplained alveolar infiltration on the chest radiograph and occult DAH reveals a predominance of red blood cells and hemosiderin-containing macrophages.[6]

In several cases of recurrent DAH (especially those that follow Wegener's granulomatosis, microscopic polyangiitis, idiopathic pulmonary hemosiderosis, and mitral stenosis), progression to pulmonary fibrosis and restrictive ventilatory impairment have been documented.[7–9]

## Laboratory Data

Table 60.2 summarizes the differential clinical and laboratory features of the common causes of DAH. The presence of proteinuria and an abnormal urinary sediment (red blood cells and red blood cell casts), which for most causes of DAH belies the underlying focal segmental necrotizing glomerulonephritis, excludes the diagnosis of idiopathic pulmonary hemosiderosis and isolated pulmo-

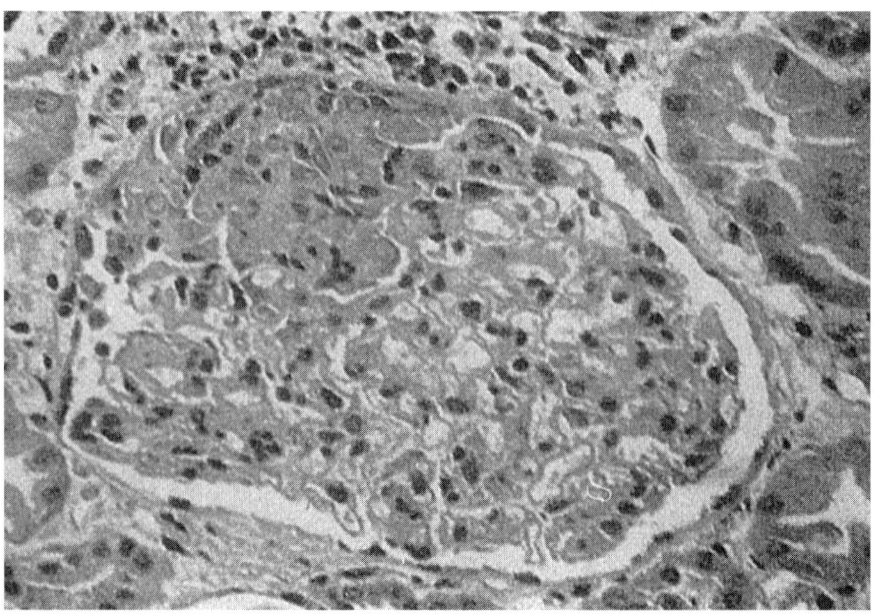

**Figure 60.5** Micrograph of a renal biopsy specimen demonstrating focal segmental necrotizing glomerulonephritis. Note the fibrinoid necrosis at the upper left. (Original magnification × 40.)

**Table 60.2** CLINICAL DIFFERENTIATION OF COMMON DIFFUSE ALVEOLAR HEMORRHAGE SYNDROMES

| Syndrome | Anemia | Renal Disease | Arthritis | Skin Vasculitis | ANA | RF | $C_L$ | ABMA | ANCA | Anti-DNA Antibody | Tissue Antibody Staining |
|---|---|---|---|---|---|---|---|---|---|---|---|
| Wegener's granulomatosis | + | + | + | + | ± | ± | WNL | – | + (c) | – | Granular or – |
| Microscopic polyangiitis | + | + | + | + | ± | ± | WNL | – | + (p) | – | – |
| Systemic lupus erythematosus | + | + | + | ± | + | + | Low | – | – | + | (Granular) immunoglobulin G |
| Goodpasture's syndrome | + | + | – | – | – | – | WNL | + | – | – | (Linear) immunoglobulin |
| Idiopathic hemosiderosis | + | – | – | – | – | – | WNL | – | – | – | – |
| Isolated pulmonary capillaritis | + | – | – | – | – | – | WNL | – | – | – | – |
| Henoch-Schönlein purpura | + | + | + | + | – | – | WNL | – | ± | – | + (Granular) immunoglobulin A |

**Abbreviations:* ABMA = anti-basement membrane antibody; ANA = anti-nuclear antibody; ANCA = antineutrophil cytoplasmic antibody; Anti-DNA = anti-deoxyribonucleic acid antibody; $C_L$ = complement; RF = rheumatoid factor; WNL = within normal limits.

nary capillaritis. If cutaneous lesions are present in the form of either splinter hemorrhages or palpable purpura (leukocytoclastic vasculitis), Goodpasture's syndrome can be ruled out as well. The diagnosis of Goodpasture's syndrome is confirmed by the presence of anti–glomerular basement membrane antibody (anti-GBM Ab) in the serum and the linear deposition of immunoglobulin and complement in basement membranes of the kidney and lung.[10, 11] Active DAH in systemic lupus erythematosus is accompanied by reduced serum complement levels as well as the presence of antinuclear and native anti–deoxyribonucleic acid (anti-DNA) antibodies in the serum. Henoch-Schönlein purpura is characterized by the formation of immunoglobulin A (IgA) immune complexes present in the circulation and also bound to tissue.[12] A positive test result for serum antineutrophil cytoplasmic antibody (ANCA) was first thought to be specific for Wegener's granulomatosis, but it also appears in microscopic polyangiitis.[13] ANCA levels are also elevated in pauci-immune glomerulonephritis, a vasculitis affecting primarily the kidneys and an occasional cause of DAH, and in two systemic vasculitides not usually associated with DAH: Churg-Strauss syndrome and polyarteritis nodosa.[14–17]

Previously, the pathogenesis of DAH, at least for cases associated with pulmonary capillaritis, was thought to be either immune complex mediated (lupus erythematosus, Henoch-Schönlein purpura, and possibly microscopic polyangiitis and Wegener's granulomatosis) or due to an antibody directed against basement membrane (Goodpasture's syndrome). More recently, it has been proposed that not only is ANCA a marker for the presence and activity of the aforementioned systemic vasculitides but also this antibody is pathogenetic, inasmuch as it induces neutrophils and mononuclear phagocytes to undergo both a respiratory burst and degranulation, which could injure the endothelium through the release of proteolytic enzymes and the generation of toxic oxygen products.[15]

Two types of ANCA are measured for clinical use. c-ANCA is specific for the 29-kd component of the cytoplasmic granule of the neutrophil and the monocyte, producing a central granular immunofluorescent staining pattern. This granule has been identified as proteinase 3, which is an elastolytic neutral protease. p-ANCA has specificity for the myeloperoxidase granule of the neutrophil, resulting in a perinuclear or a nuclear staining pattern.[18] The c-ANCA level is more likely to be elevated in the serum of patients with systemic vasculitis if the lungs and sinuses are involved, as in Wegener's granulomatosis, whereas p-ANCA is more likely to appear in the serum in microscopic polyangiitis, pauci-immune glomerulonephritis, and a form of isolated pulmonary capillaritis. There can be crossover.[19, 20]

## DIFFUSE ALVEOLAR HEMORRHAGE WITH CAPILLARITIS

### Isolated Pulmonary Capillaritis

Isolated pulmonary capillaritis is a small vessel vasculitis confined to the lungs and without concomitant systemic involvement.[21] There are two forms: one with serum p-ANCA positivity and the other without positive serology.[22, 23] In one series, the latter type was the most frequent cause of pulmonary capillaritis and DAH.[22] Direct immunofluorescent studies of the lung yielded negative findings in the latter series. Although respiratory failure necessitating ventilatory support was frequent, response to corticosteroids and cyclophosphamide was good, and only one of eight patients did not survive. Recurrences appeared in two subjects. During a 4-year follow-up period, clinical or serologic evidence for a systemic vasculitis or connective tissue disease did not appear.

Isolated forms of pulmonary capillaritis causing DAH must be distinguished from idiopathic pulmonary hemosiderosis, which is not associated with pulmonary capillaritis, lung-limited forms of Goodpasture's syndrome, and mitral stenosis. All patients who present with unexplained DAH should have an echocardiogram and undergo thoracoscopic or open-lung biopsy.

### Wegener's Granulomatosis

DAH secondary to pulmonary capillaritis can either complicate an established case of Wegener's granulomatosis or represent the initial manifestation. Pulmonary capillaritis, therefore, can be the sole histologic finding, or it can occur in combination with the more typical pathologic features of Wegener's granulomatosis. Examination of open-lung biopsy specimens from 87 patients with Wegener's granulomatosis revealed a 31% incidence of capillaritis, but in only 3 was this an isolated finding.[4] In another series, capillaritis was present in 17% of 35 patients, but never as an isolated finding.[24] In a postmortem study of 22 patients, capillaritis was the sole histologic feature in 3 and occurred in conjunction with the more typical granulomatous vasculitis in 7 cases.[25] In cases in which the typical histologic features (granulomatous inflammation, small and medium vessel vasculitis, and parenchymal necrosis) and clinical presentation (sinusitis, cavitary lung lesions) are absent and only DAH with or without a cutaneous leukocytoclastic vasculitis or a focal segmental necrotizing glomerulitis is present, the differentiation from microscopic polyangiitis is difficult. The specific diagnosis then depends on the ANCA pattern. In Wegener's granulomatosis, the characteristic histologic and clinical features may appear months to years after an initial presentation of DAH and capillaritis.[10, 26, 27]

More than 40 cases of Wegener's granulomatosis with DAH and pulmonary capillaritis have been described. The rate of early mortality is 37%, and this mortality is most often due to acute respiratory or renal failure.[4, 10, 23–31] Renal disease in the form of a focal segmental necrotizing glomerulitis, a cutaneous leukocytoclastic vasculitis, and arthritis often accompany the DAH. Treatment with corticosteroids and cyclophosphamide is the recommended therapy and, depending on the severity of the disease, can be initially administered intravenously. Recurrences with tapering of the medications are to be expected. Disease activity is monitored by measurements of sedimentation rates, ANCA levels, and serial diffusing capacity and by microscopic urine examinations.

As previously stated, the differentiation of Wegener's granulomatosis with DAH from microscopic polyangiitis is difficult, because the clinical presentation, histopathologic findings, and serologic findings can be identical.[6, 8, 32] In fact, the response to treatment and the tendency for recurrences are similar. The differentiation can be established only after the development of the more typical upper airway disease and pathologic features in Wegener's granulomatosis.

## Microscopic Polyangiitis

Microscopic polyangiitis is thought to be the small vessel variant of polyarteritis nodosa. It is a frequent cause of pulmonary capillaritis and DAH.[1, 2, 10, 33–38] Microscopic polyangiitis is distinguishable from polyarteritis nodosa by the absence of medium-sized blood vessel involvement, the absence of asthma and systemic hypertension, and the relative sparing of the abdominal viscera. In addition, DAH has not been documented as co-occurring with polyarteritis nodosa.

The most consistent pathologic feature is a focal segmental necrotizing glomerulonephritis, the renal lesion common to all systemic vasculitides. The lungs are involved by capillaritis in 20% to 30% of cases.[35, 38, 39] The lung disease (DAH) tends to be severe and is often life-threatening. Other manifestations include cutaneous vasculitis; musculoskeletal involvement; diarrhea and gastrointestinal bleeding from mucosal vasculitis that is often visible by direct examination; peripheral neuropathy; and, in a few cases, sinusitis.[38] As with other vasculitides, the sedimentation rate is elevated, and nonspecific increases of serum rheumatoid factor and antinuclear antibody are found. Although circulating immune complexes are present in 45% of cases, tissue localization of these complexes is difficult to detect. Anti-DNA antibodies and hypocomplementemia, findings suggestive of systemic lupus erythematosus, are absent. A positive serum p-ANCA finding strongly supports the diagnosis. Antibodies to hepatitis B and C antigen are present in 33% of cases.[40]

Treatment consists of either oral or intravenous corticosteroids combined with cyclophosphamide or azathioprine. Adjuvant treatment with plasmapheresis is recommended by some authors, but its additional efficacy is difficult to determine.[35, 38] Outcome with early initiation of therapy for microscopic polyangiitis is generally good, with a 65% rate of 5-year survival.[37] However, the presence of DAH contributes to a rate of early mortality of 25%.[1, 2, 10, 33–39] There is a tendency for recurrence with tapering of the medications, and both a restrictive lung disease and an obstructive lung disease have been reported in survivors. The transition to pulmonary fibrosis and restrictive ventilatory impairment after recurrent DAH has been described.[8, 15] There have been three cases of severe irreversible airway dysfunction after recurrent episodes of DAH that complicated microscopic polyangiitis.[41] The follow-up period was more than 10 years. It is postulated that the combination of recurrent vascular obliteration from capillaritis and the release of neutral proteases and oxygen radicals from the overwhelming and recurrent burden of neutrophils causes permanent damage to the alveolar septa and results in emphysema.

## Connective Tissue Disease

In the unusual circumstance, DAH and glomerulonephritis occur in patients with rheumatoid arthritis,[42, 43] scleroderma,[44, 45] or mixed connective tissue disease.[46, 47] DAH and pulmonary capillaritis isolated to the lung have also been described in polymyositis, rheumatoid arthritis, and mixed connective tissue disease.[48, 49] In the polymyositis cases, DAH was the presenting manifestation,[48] and in rheumatoid arthritis and mixed connective tissue disease, DAH and capillaritis followed the primary diagnosis (2 to 20 years).[49] The absence of a systemic vasculitis, including glomerulonephritis, was unexpected.

However, among the connective tissue diseases, DAH both with and without pulmonary capillaritis occurs most frequently in systemic lupus erythematosus.[10, 50] This complication is associated with a 50% rate of mortality and is recurrent in survivors.[10, 51–60] Mortality is caused by DAH, a concurrent infection, or another systemic complication of systemic lupus erythematosus, such as renal or central nervous system disease. Histopathologic examination reveals capillaritis in most cases, but in some patients, bland pulmonary hemorrhage and diffuse alveolar damage have been described.[57, 61] Granular deposits of immunoglobulin G (IgG) and complement (C3) are found in the alveolar interstitium and within the walls of intra-alveolar blood vessels (Fig. 60.6).[57–59] However, immune complexes are not uniformly present.[56] Myers and Katzenstein described four patients with systemic lupus erythematosus and massive DAH associated with pulmonary capillaritis; in two of these patients, immune complexes were demonstrated by both light- and electron-microscopic techniques.[60]

It is unusual for DAH to be the initial manifestation of systemic lupus erythematosus,[53] in contrast to acute lupus pneumonitis, in which DAH is often the initial manifestation.[61] In systemic lupus erythematosus, DAH appears

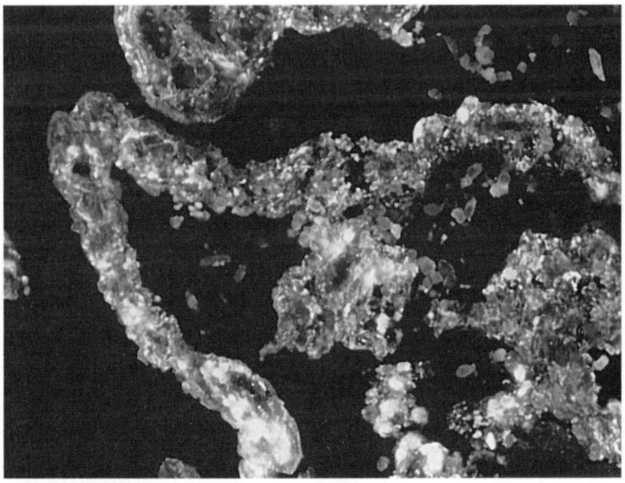

**Figure 60.6** Immunofluorescence study demonstrating granular deposition of immunoglobulin G in the alveolar walls of a patient with systemic lupus erythematosus and diffuse alveolar hemorrhage secondary to pulmonary capillaritis. (Original magnification × 40.)

later in the clinical course.[10, 52] Most patients have active lupus nephritis.[50] The onset of hemoptysis can be quite dramatic, producing severe gas-exchange abnormalities and necessitating assisted ventilation. Reduced complement levels and increased serum titers of antinuclear antibodies confirm the diagnosis.

DAH must be distinguished from other causes of hemoptysis in systemic lupus erythematosus. Acute lupus pneumonitis presents with fever, cough, and dyspnea; in 50% of cases, this is the initial manifestation of systemic lupus erythematosus.[61, 62] In addition to the diffuse alveolar infiltrates on chest radiograph that appear in both conditions, pleural and pericardial effusions are present in acute lupus pneumonitis. Although hemoptysis may accompany acute lupus pneumonitis, significant reductions of the hemoglobin are not to be expected. Histologically, acute lupus pneumonitis is an inflammatory lesion consisting of organizing pneumonia, diffuse alveolar damage, a cellular interstitial pneumonia, and sometimes intra-alveolar hemorrhage. Other diagnostic considerations include infectious pneumonias and pulmonary infarction associated with deep venous thrombosis with or without a circulating anticoagulant.[63–68]

Treatment of DAH caused by systemic lupus erythematosus includes high-dose intravenous therapy with corticosteroids as well as azathioprine or cyclophosphamide. Plasmapheresis has been combined with chemotherapy in some cases, but it probably has little or no utility.[50] Broad-spectrum antibiotic coverage is recommended because of some evidence that infection may trigger the hemorrhage.[50, 62, 66, 67]

## Mixed Cryoglobulinemia

Mixed cryoglobulinemia is a systemic vasculitis that is recognized from the presence of purpura, arthritis, hepatitis, and glomerulonephritis. It is thought to be an immune complex–induced disease, possibly resulting from a hepatitis B or C viral infection. Interstitial lung disease consisting of inflammation and fibrosis of the alveolar walls is the most common pulmonary manifestation.[68, 69] Cutaneous vasculitis appearing as raised purpura is the clinical hallmark of this disease. Histologically, there is a perivascular polymorphonuclear infiltration with tissue extravasation and fragmentation in the dermis. The renal disease is a proliferative glomerulonephritis with positive granular immunofluorescence. There has been only one documented case of DAH with pulmonary capillaritis that complicated mixed cryoglobulinemia.[70]

## Behçet's Syndrome

Behçet's syndrome is a chronic relapsing illness characterized by oral and genital ulceration, iridocyclitis, thrombophlebitis, and a multisystem disease consisting of a cutaneous vasculitis, arthritis, and meningoencephalitis.[71, 72] Immune complexes have been identified in the serum of active cases as well as in lung and other organs.[71–73]

The lung is involved in 5% to 10% of cases. The pulmonary disease is typically a small-vessel vasculitis affecting capillaries, venules, and arterioles. The renal disease is a focal segmental necrotizing vasculitis, as occurs in other systemic vasculitides. Immune complexes composed of IgG and complement have been identified in small pulmonary vessels in several cases.[73] In addition, involvement of larger vessels can lead to aneurysms of the bronchial arteries, which can erode into bronchi, causing massive pulmonary hemorrhage and death.[74–77] Another potential cause for hemoptysis in Behçet's syndrome is pulmonary arterial occlusion with infarction.[73] Efthimiou and associates, in their review of 28 cases of pulmonary involvement in Behçet's syndrome, emphasized several points: pulmonary complaints consisting of cough, hemoptysis, chest pain, and fever were more common in men than in women; pulmonary hemorrhage was the cause of death in 39%; and death usually occurred within 6 years of the first episode of hemoptysis.[75] Other authors have confirmed the seriousness of this complication regardless of its cause.[76–77] Treatment consists of corticosteroids and immunosuppressive therapy.[78]

## Henoch-Schönlein Purpura

Henoch-Schönlein purpura, primarily a disease of children, also occurs in adults.[79, 80] Adults present with the typical palpable purpuric rash (leukocytoclastic vasculitis) and glomerulonephritis.[81] The joints and gastrointestinal tract are commonly involved. Pulmonary involvement is apparently rare. In several large series, pulmonary disease, except for transient chest radiographic infiltrates, was not mentioned.[79–82] There have been two proven cases of DAH with pulmonary capillaritis in patients with Henoch-Schönlein purpura.[83–89] In one, IgA immune complexes were present in the alveolar septa.[84] It is postulated that IgA immune complexes, which are present in the serum and kidneys of these patients, are responsible for the tissue damage that results in the clinical syndrome.[85–87] Corticosteroids are recommended.

## Glomerulonephritis and Alveolar Hemorrhage

Focal segmental necrotizing glomerulonephritis is common to all the systemic vasculitides. There are three types of renal limited vasculitis associated with this lesion and DAH but not necessarily with other manifestations of systemic disease: (1) an immune complex–mediated glomerulonephritis, which is characterized by the granular deposition of immunoglobulin and complement in the glomerulus; (2) a pauci-immune glomerulonephritis, which does not manifest immune complexes but does demonstrate p-ANCA serology; and (3) an anti–glomerular basement membrane antibody disease (Goodpasture's syndrome), which is characterized by the presence of circulating and tissue-bound basement membrane directed against lung and kidney.[19]

Immune complex–related crescentic glomerulonephritis is rarely accompanied by capillaritis and DAH.[3, 88, 89] Although the kidneys demonstrate granular immune deposits, immune complexes were not found in lung tissue.[90, 91]

Pauci-immune crescentic glomerulonephritis lacks any immunoreaction product except for minimal accumulation of fibrin.[13] In this sense, it is histologically and immunologically similar to the glomerulonephritis of microscopic polyangiitis and Wegener's granulomatosis[10, 92] and is considered to represent a form of renal-limited vasculitis.[93, 94] Up to 50% of affected patients develop pulmonary capillaritis and DAH, and a smaller number develop a full-blown systemic vasculitis indistinguishable from microscopic polyangiitis. Another indication that pauci-immune crescentic glomerulonephritis represents a limited form of vasculitis is the presence of serum p-ANCA in these patients.[15] Because clinical manifestations are often limited to the lung and kidney, it can be confused with Goodpasture's syndrome.[10, 85] The two are differentiated by the absence of anti–glomerular basement membrane antibody in the serum and by the negative findings of renal immunofluorescence studies. Treatment with pulse doses of corticosteroids, plus immunosuppressive therapy with either cyclophosphamide or azathioprine, is recommended.

### Acute Pulmonary Allograft Rejection

Pulmonary capillaritis and DAH have been reported after lung transplantation for a variety of underlying diseases.[95] The suspected acute vascular rejection can occur weeks to months after the transplantation. This represents a serious immunologic complication that threatens survival. In addition to standard anti-inflammatory therapy, plasmapheresis may be effective.

## DIFFUSE ALVEOLAR HEMORRHAGE WITHOUT CAPILLARITIS

### Idiopathic Pulmonary Hemosiderosis

Idiopathic pulmonary hemosiderosis (IPH) is a diagnosis of exclusion.[96–98] Efforts to rule out other causes of DAH such as mitral valve disease, systemic vasculitis, or the connective tissue diseases are essential. Clinically, this entity is characterized by recurrent DAH without renal or other systemic disease, and the histologic examination of the lung reveals bland alveolar hemorrhage with hemosiderin accumulation (Fig. 60.7).

The pathologic defect is not understood.[90] Histologic examination of lung tissue reveals hyperplasia of type II alveolar epithelial cells with capillary dilatation and tortuosity.[99, 100] Erythrocytes and hemosiderin-containing macrophages fill alveolar spaces. Hemosiderin collects in the lung interstitium and is thought to be the basis for the collagen proliferation and parenchymal fibrosis that occurs in this disease.[100, 101] The iron content of the lung is increased.[97, 98] Pulmonary immune complexes are absent in the lung, which thus differentiates IPH from a rare presentation of lung-limited Goodpasture's syndrome.[99–101]

Electron-microscopic studies indicate degeneration of type I alveolar epithelial cells with exposure of their basement membranes,[102, 103] breaks in the continuity of the alveolar capillary basement membrane,[104] thickening or reduplication of the membrane,[96] separation of the basement membrane with fibrillar material found in the splits,[100] and focal ruptures of the membrane with collagen deposition.[100] Although nonspecific, these findings indicate a form of diffuse alveolar injury.[101]

Although the pathogenesis remains unclear, evidence suggests an immune disorder. Some cases have occurred in the setting of celiac disease,[105] serum IgA levels are increased in 50% of cases,[106] and there are definite, although few, responses to immunosuppressive therapy.[97, 107]

IPH is predominantly a disease of children; however, adults, usually over 30 years of age, represent 20% of cases.[97, 108] The age range for the onset of disease is 4 months to 62 years. Among adults, men are more often affected, and there are reports of familial cases.[109, 110] IPH is characterized either by recurrent, often life-threatening

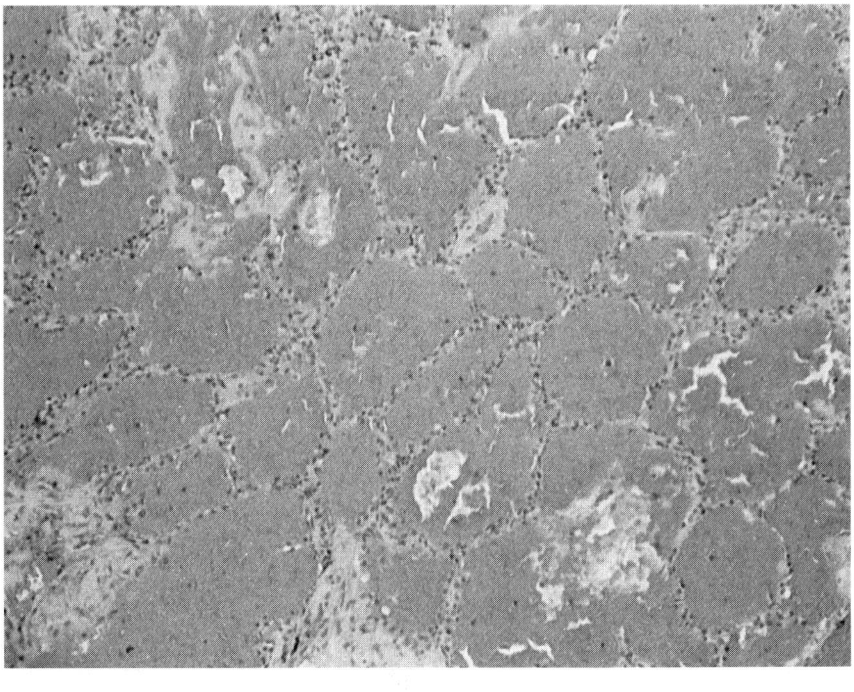

**Figure 60.7** Micrograph showing bland alveolar hemorrhage in a patient with idiopathic pulmonary hemosiderosis. The alveolar walls are of normal thickness, and the apparent increase in cellularity represents type II alveolar cell hyperplasia. (Original magnification × 10.)

hemoptysis or by intermittent blood-streaked sputum. Fever, cough, substernal chest pain, and fatigue secondary to the iron deficiency anemia are also reported. The symptoms do not distinguish IPH from other causes of DAH. As with other DAH etiologies, IPH can present with dyspnea and an abnormal chest radiograph but without an iron deficiency anemia or hemoptysis. Bronchoalveolar lavage reveals a predominance of red blood cells and hemosiderin-containing macrophages, which suggests the diagnosis of DAH.[101] Crackles are heard, and in 20% of pediatric cases, lymphadenopathy and hepatosplenomegaly are found.[111, 112] In chronic recurrent disease, finger clubbing, progressive dyspnea, and progressive pulmonary fibrosis appear.[97, 113]

Pulmonary function testing reveals a restrictive ventilatory defect with an increase in the diffusing capacity for carbon monoxide during periods of active bleeding. With time and superimposition of lung parenchymal fibrosis, the diffusing capacity falls.[112] The chest radiograph reveals bilateral air space filling that is either diffuse or patchy. The alveolar infiltrates tend to resolve slowly over days to weeks, leaving a residual reticulonodular infiltrate that may persist, depending on the chronicity of the disease and the development of interstitial fibrosis. An echocardiogram is needed to rule out mitral valve disease, and a microscopic urinalysis excludes the presence of glomerulonephritis. Measurements of serum antibody, as outlined in Table 60.2, reveal the absence of associated systemic disease. However, in adult cases, lung tissue is needed to exclude the entity of isolated pulmonary capillaritis.[21] It is likely that until the 1990s, cases of isolated pulmonary capillaritis were ascribed to IPH.

Clinical benefit and recovery from the acute hemorrhage after corticosteroid therapy have been reported, but long-term benefit is unlikely.[97, 108, 112, 114] Azathioprine has been successful in several cases.[100, 107] In 75% of cases, the mean length of survival is 3 to 5 years.[97, 108, 115, 116] However, adults have a better prognosis. Approximately 25% of patients are free of disease after the initial episode. Another 25% are free of active disease but have persistent dyspnea and anemia, and another quarter have persistent active disease that leads to fibrosis and severe restrictive lung disease. The remainder have unresponsive disease with repeated massive hemorrhage and an early death from respiratory causes.

## Goodpasture's Syndrome

Whether the case reported by Goodpasture[117] in 1919 describes the syndrome that bears his name is questionable. He described an 18-year-old man who died 6 weeks after an influenza infection and was found to have DAH, pleuritis, glomerulonephritis, splenic infarctions, and vasculitis of the small intestines. In 1965, an antibody to glomerular basement membrane (anti-GBM Ab)—more specifically, type IV collagen—was identified in the kidneys and lungs of some patients with DAH and glomerulonephritis.[118, 119] The diagnosis of Goodpasture's syndrome, also known as anti–basement membrane antibody (ABMA) disease, is reserved for cases of DAH and glomerulonephritis in which this antibody appears in the serum and is found bound to kidney and lung basement membranes in a linear manner.[10, 120] At least 90% of patients with Goodpasture's syndrome have a circulating anti-GBM Ab.[121, 122] The higher the level, the more severe is the renal disease; in general, however, the level of anti-GBM Ab is not considered an accurate index of disease activity.

In 60% to 80% of cases, the lung and renal disease appear simultaneously; in 5% to 10% only the lung is affected; and in the remainder, renal disease exists by itself.[10, 123–125] Men are more commonly affected (60% to 80% of patients are men), and the concentration of cases is greatest between the ages of 20 and 30 years.[118, 126–128] In older populations, however, the sex distribution is equal[129] and the disease tends to be limited to the kidney. Interestingly, DAH is more likely to occur in patients who smoke.[129] The permeability of the lungs is increased in most smokers,[130] and this is thought to be an important factor leading to the DAH in Goodpasture's syndrome. In one study, 100% of smokers with Goodpasture's syndrome developed both DAH and glomerulonephritis, and of the nonsmokers, only 20% developed DAH.[129] Also, resumption of cigarette smoking by patients with Goodpasture's syndrome who are in remission results in recurrent episodes of DAH.[123] In addition, exposure to volatile hydrocarbons is associated with initiation, as well as exacerbations, of DAH.[124, 125, 131–133]

Pulmonary capillaritis is present in some cases of Goodpasture's syndrome, but the usual histologic appearance is bland pulmonary hemorrhage.[133] Alveolar wall necrosis, which is seen with systemic vasculitis, does not occur in Goodpasture's syndrome. The renal histologic findings are a focal segmental necrotizing glomerulonephritis with crescent formation. The major distinction between Goodpasture's syndrome and the other rapidly progressive glomerulonephritides is the presence of an uninterrupted linear deposition of immunoglobulin and complement along the glomerular basement membrane.[134, 135] Identical findings are present on alveolar basement membranes (Fig. 60.8).[136] In 5% to 10% of

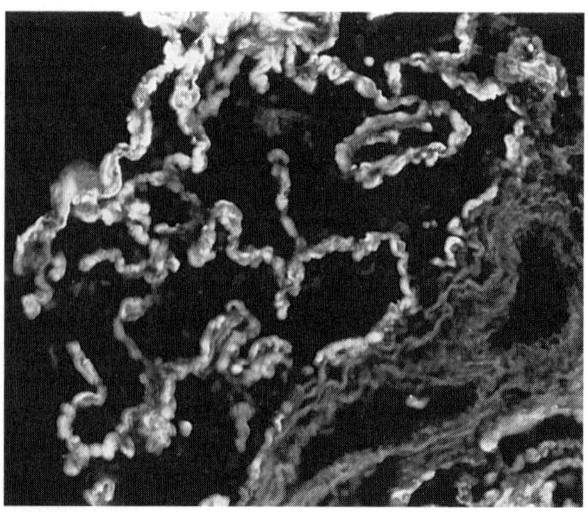

**Figure 60.8** Immunofluorescence study demonstrating linear staining (immunoglobulin G) of alveolar walls in a patient with Goodpasture's syndrome. (Original magnification × 10.)

patients, DAH without renal disease dominates the clinical picture. However, renal biopsy still reveals the typical linear staining.[135, 137, 138]

It is clear that antibody to basement membrane is pathogenetic; however, the stimulus for its production remains unknown.[139] The clinical onset of Goodpasture's syndrome has been temporarily related to infection with influenza A2[140] as well as to other respiratory infections, hydrocarbon exposure, and tobacco use. It is interesting to note that in experimental models, the introduction of anti-GBM Ab produces renal but not pulmonary disease. For deposition of this antibody to occur in the lung in those models, an additional injury that increases alveolar-capillary permeability is required.[124]

The presence of histocompatibility human leukocyte antigen (HLA)–DRw2 and HLA-B7 (90% and 60%, respectively) in patients with Goodpasture's syndrome indicates that susceptible individuals are predisposed to the disease.[141–144] Evidence suggests that patients with Goodpasture's syndrome and HLA-B7 and HLA-DRw2 have unusually severe renal disease and a poor prognosis.[145]

Symptoms most often refer to the respiratory system and consist of hemoptysis, cough, and dyspnea. Fatigue caused by iron deficiency anemia and renal failure may predominate. Microscopic hematuria and proteinuria and increases in the serum creatinine are often present, but gross hematuria and hypertension are unusual. The diffusing capacity is increased during periods of active bleeding and is considered to be a useful monitor of DAH.[146, 147] An increase of 30% above baseline is highly suggestive of an intra-alveolar hemorrhage, and it is possible that this increase may precede pulmonary symptoms or even chest radiographic changes, thereby signaling an exacerbation. It must be remembered that there are patients with Goodpasture's syndrome whose chest radiographs are abnormal but whose urinalyses and renal function test results are normal; these patients show typical linear immunofluorescence in tissue from renal biopsy.[148]

In the few patients without renal disease, DAH responds to corticosteroids either by the oral route or by intravenous pulse dosing.[149, 150] However, glomerulonephritis appears resistant to the anti-inflammatory effects of this monotherapy.[118, 135] Cytotoxic agents have some effect on the rapidly progressive glomerulonephritis but, again, are efficacious mainly for the control of DAH.[121, 126] Bilateral nephrectomy, despite initial encouraging results for the control of DAH, no longer has a role in the management of Goodpasture's syndrome. The combination of plasmapheresis, corticosteroids, and cytotoxic drugs is effective, particularly in patients who do not have oligoanuria and do not require dialysis.[151–158] Plasmapheresis (3 to 6 L daily) is generally continued for 2 weeks. Combinations of cyclophosphamide or azathioprine with corticosteroids lead to a dramatic fall in anti-GBM Ab, which does not necessarily correlate with the rate of improvement in the renal and pulmonary disease.[159] With this combination therapy, even oliguric dialysis-dependent subjects responded to the point at which dialysis could be discontinued.[153, 154, 157] However, anuric patients do not respond to combination therapy, and dialysis and renal transplantation are then necessary.[129]

The survival rate has improved from 80% mortality at 6 months (half dying from DAH and the rest from renal insufficiency) to a more improved disease course.[118, 126] Spontaneous remissions occur in cases without clinical renal disease.[121, 148] Although the 2-year survival rate for all treated patients is approximately 50%, the majority of the deaths occur during the first year.[127] DAH is the usual cause of death, often being precipitated by a concomitant infection.[123, 124] Severe renal failure producing oligoanuria reduces the survival rate to 50% at 6 months. Renal biopsy not only is diagnostic but also has prognostic value. In subjects in whom less than 30% of the glomeruli have undergone crescent formation in conjunction with preserved renal function, there are a significant therapeutic response and prolonged survival. However, when 70% or more of glomeruli have formed crescents along with renal insufficiency, renal failure is progressive and often unresponsive, eventually necessitating dialysis.[153, 159]

## Diffuse Alveolar Damage

Diffuse alveolar damage is the underlying histopathology of the acute respiratory distress syndrome, but it also can have a variety of other etiologies (Table 60.3).[160–162] In severe cases, red blood cells enter the alveolar space after the injury to the alveolar-capillary interface, and this in turn can result in hemoptysis. In addition to the hemorrhagic alveolar fluid, the interstitium of the lung becomes edematous and the type I alveolar epithelial lining cells are sloughed. Even early in this process, chronic inflam-

**Table 60.3 CAUSES OF DIFFUSE ALVEOLAR DAMAGE**

| |
|---|
| **DRUG INDUCED** |
| Cytotoxic agents (bleomycin, BCNU, busulfan, cyclophosphamide) |
| Antibiotics (nitrofurantoin) |
| Analgesics (acetylsalicylic acid) |
| Opiates (heroin, methadone, crack cocaine) |
| Sedatives (ethchlorvynol) |
| Diuretics (hydrochlorothiazide) |
| Insecticides (paraquat) |
| **ACUTE RESPIRATORY DISTRESS SYNDROME** |
| Shock |
| Trauma |
| Oxygen toxicity |
| Aspiration |
| Smoke inhalation |
| Ozone inhalation |
| Nitrogen dioxide inhalation |
| **PNEUMONIA** |
| *Mycoplasma pneumoniae* |
| *Legionella* |
| Viral |
| *Pneumocystis carinii* |
| **RADIATION PNEUMONITIS** |
| **HEAVY METAL FUMES** |
| **CONNECTIVE TISSUE DISEASES** |
| **ACUTE INTERSTITIAL PNEUMONIA (HAMMAN-RICH SYNDROME)** |

mation and fibroblastic proliferation of the alveolar wall are present. Hyaline membranes, which are eosinophilic-appearing debris consisting of necrotic cells, protein, and fibrin, are found adjacent to the alveolar walls. The neutrophilic influx in DAH is not as intense as it is in pulmonary capillaritis. The chronic phases of diffuse alveolar damage are characterized by collagen deposition resembling both a usual interstitial pneumonia and an organizing pneumonia.[163–170] Several drugs (see Chapter 72) may cause diffuse alveolar damage that, if severe, may be accompanied by DAH.

## Penicillamine

Ingestion of penicillamine can result in DAH and an immune complex–mediated glomerulonephritis. Glomerular capillaries display a granular as opposed to a linear immunofluorescent pattern for IgG and the third component of complement.[171, 172] There have been eight reports of this complication in patients receiving treatment for rheumatoid arthritis, Wilson's disease, or primary biliary cirrhosis.[171–176] In general, at least 1 g daily for a minimum of 10 months is necessary, and cases have appeared after 20 years of daily treatment. All patients presented with DAH, and in one case this was the only manifestation. The others had a crescentic glomerulonephritis as well.[175] Systemic involvement other than the lungs or kidneys has not been seen, which prompts some authors to call this a drug-induced Goodpasture's syndrome,[171–173] but the pattern of deposition of immunoglobulin in the kidney clearly differentiates this entity from Goodpasture's syndrome. Three patients recovered after a combination of immunosuppressive therapy and plasmapheresis.[172, 175]

## Trimellitic Anhydride

Trimellitic anhydride is used for the manufacture of paints, epoxy resins, and plastics. A DAH syndrome without renal or other systemic disease reportedly occurs after the inhalation of fumes or the dry powder.[176–178] Antibodies to this compound have been identified in the serum of affected workers. A latent period of 1 to 3 months precedes the development of DAH, and this latent period supports an immunologic basis for this syndrome. With removal from exposure, which most commonly follows the spraying of this product on heated surfaces, the hemorrhage and iron deficiency anemia resolve. Long-term physiologic impairment is not to be expected if further exposure is avoided.

## Mitral Stenosis

Mitral stenosis must be ruled out in any individual who presents with DAH without renal or other systemic manifestations. Mitral stenosis can be relatively silent well into adulthood, and as a result of the pulmonary venous hypertension, intermittent hemoptysis of small to moderate amounts occur. Because mitral stenosis is often misdiagnosed and always recurrent, a hemosiderosis-like picture with organization of the hemorrhage and the appearance of interstitial fibrosis may appear.[179] Massive hemoptysis results from rupture of engorged anastomotic bronchial varicosities as a result of long-standing elevation of the left atrial pressure.[180] Correction of the stenotic valve prevents recurrences.

## Coagulation Disorders

DAH can complicate hemostatic defects, but the physician must always suspect a predisposing underlying parenchymal problem, such as bronchiectasis, malignancy, systemic lupus erythematosus, mitral stenosis, or a condition that injures the alveolar capillary membrane, such as shock or sepsis.[6] Other conditions associated with DAH include disseminated intravascular coagulation,[181] idiopathic thrombocytopenic purpura,[182] and thrombotic thrombocytopenic purpura.[183] In most anticoagulated patients, correction of the defect reverses the DAH.

DAH is common in patients with acute leukemia who have undergone induction chemotherapy and are thrombocytopenic.[184–186] Although the thrombocytopenia is often profound and contributes to the DAH, these patients also have evidence at autopsy of diffuse alveolar damage due to chemotherapy, oxygen toxicity, or infection.

## Pulmonary Veno-occlusive Disease

Pulmonary veno-occlusive disease, a cause of primary pulmonary hypertension that affects all age groups, is most common in children and young adults. The sex distribution is equal.[187–192] As with other forms of pulmonary hypertension, patients with pulmonary veno-occlusive disease present with dyspnea and syncope and with physical findings suggestive of cor pulmonale.[187] Because pulmonary veno-occlusive disease is a postcapillary form of pulmonary hypertension resulting from fibrous obliteration of small veins and venules, hemoptysis, paroxysmal nocturnal dyspnea, and orthopnea occur (Fig. 60.9). Recanalization of the venous lumens suggests the possibility of previous thrombosis. The chest radiograph shows signs of pulmonary hypertension; in some cases, interstitial infiltrates with Kerley's B lines, representing alveolar septal lymphatic edema, are seen (Fig. 60.10).[193] With significant pulmonary venous bleeding, alveolar infiltrates are superimposed. Pulmonary function studies reveal a reduced diffusing capacity for carbon monoxide with preservation of lung volumes, a physiologic picture similar to that found in other causes of primary pulmonary hypertension.

If a pulmonary artery catheter is properly placed, it reveals an elevated pulmonary capillary wedge pressure in addition to pulmonary hypertension. This helps differentiate pulmonary veno-occlusive disease–induced pulmonary hypertension from other causes of primary pulmonary hypertension.[192] In addition, hemoptysis occurring with suspected primary pulmonary hypertension points to a postcapillary lesion. Definitive diagnosis is achieved by lung biopsy, which demonstrates the fibrous intimal obliteration of venules with acute or recanalized thrombi[190, 191] and hemosiderosis.[193]

Although pulmonary veno-occlusive disease occurs as a complication of chemotherapy for malignant disease[194] and of bone marrow transplantation,[195] most cases are idiopathic. The responsible chemotherapeutic agents are

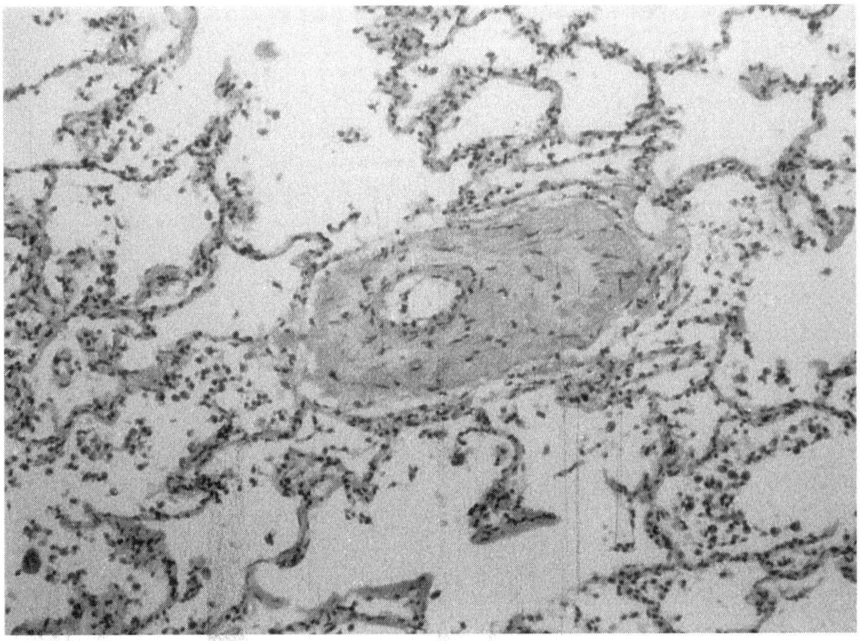

**Figure 60.9** Micrograph showing a pulmonary vein in a patient with pulmonary veno-occlusive disease. Note the proliferation of collagen, resulting in luminal obliteration and partial recanalization. (Original magnification × 10.)

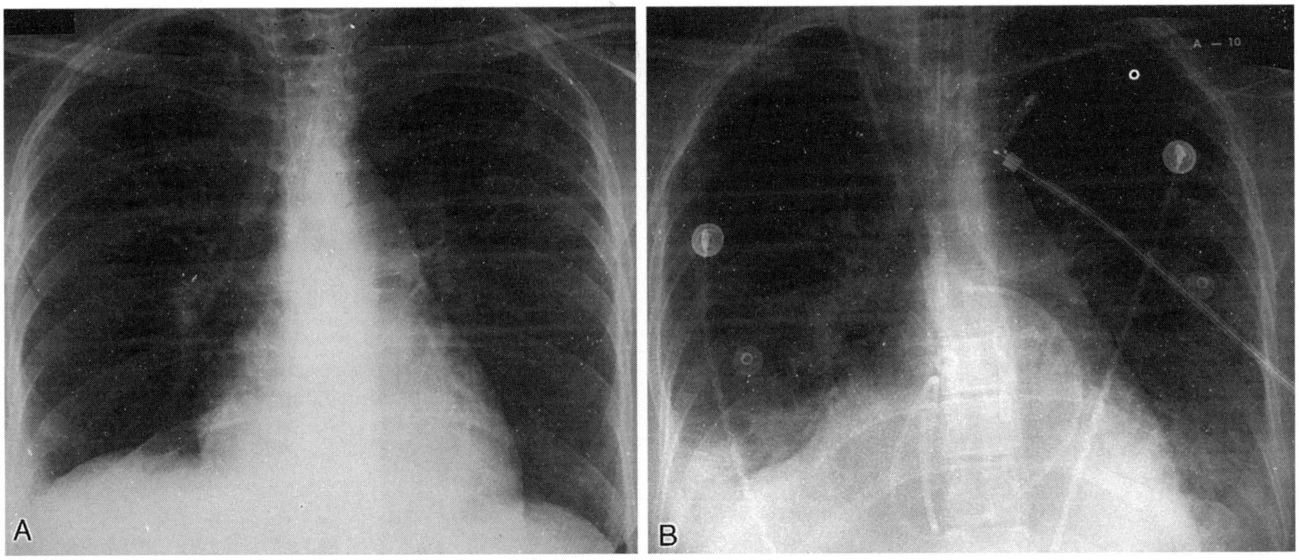


**Figure 60.10** *A,* Chest radiograph of a patient with pulmonary veno-occlusive disease, demonstrating cardiomegaly, enlarged pulmonary arteries, and a prominent right ventricular airflow tract. *B,* Later chest film of the same patient, demonstrating radiographic signs of congestive heart failure. Note the alveolar infiltrates, right-sided pleural effusion, and Kerley's B lines.

bleomycin and carmustine. Some idiopathic cases have autoimmune features such as Raynaud's phenomenon, arthritis, and serum autoantibodies, and cases have been described in patients with systemic lupus erythematosus. Corrin and associates[196] reported electron-dense deposits in one case. Several patients have had clinical responses to azathioprine,[197] and in one patient who developed pulmonary veno-occlusive disease after bone marrow transplantation, there was resolution with corticosteroid treatment.[198] Anticoagulation[199] is temporarily effective in some cases, as is chronic vasodilator therapy.[192, 199, 200] Vasodilator therapy has prolonged survival well beyond the expected 48 months.

## Pulmonary Capillary Hemangiomatosis

Pulmonary capillary hemangiomatosis is a rare cause of pulmonary hypertension associated with DAH. The DAH is severe and recurrent.[201–204] A number of cases occurring in children and young adults have been reported. In one family, three siblings with the disorder were been found.[203] This unique histology is characterized by a proliferation of capillaries, which infiltrate the interstitium and proliferate within walls of pulmonary veins impinging on their lumens, producing a form of pulmonary veno-occlusive disease (Fig. 60.11).[201] Patients present with symptoms of pulmonary hypertension (dyspnea, fatigue, and syncope) as well as hemoptysis. The chest radiograph indicates pulmonary hypertension as well as prominent reticulonodular infiltrates. With active bleeding after rupture of this rich vascular network, alveolar infiltrates appear.

This entity must be distinguished from other causes of primary pulmonary hypertension, particularly pulmonary veno-occlusive disease, which it can mimic. Survival after diagnosis is usually 1 to 5 years, although in one case, treatment with recombinant interferon alpha-2a resulted in marked clinical, physiologic, and radiographic improvement.[205]

## Lymphangioleiomyomatosis

Lymphangioleiomyomatosis (LAM) is an unusual lung disease (see Chapter 62) of premenopausal women. There is proliferation of smooth muscle in the walls of the pulmonary lymphatic vessels, which can lead to obstruction and the formation of chylous pleural effusions. Smooth muscle proliferates within alveolar walls, producing an interstitial lung disease. Involvement of the walls of bronchioles causes progressive airflow limitation and cyst formation (Fig. 60.12). Furthermore, the myoproliferation occludes venules and small veins, resulting in episodes of recurrent but limited alveolar hemorrhage. The abdominal lymphatic channels are sometimes involved, and a benign angiomyolipoma of the kidney may be present.[206–210]

Symptoms first appear in women between the ages of 17 and 47 years. Dyspnea, which eventually occurs in all affected women, is the result of the interstitial process, a chylous pleural effusion, or the obstructive lung disease. Pneumothorax causing acute dyspnea is a frequent complication of this interstitial lung disease and may be the presenting manifestation or a complication in an established case. Pneumothorax results from rupture of the parenchymal cysts and appears in 40% of patients.[206, 208, 209] Intermittent hemoptysis occurs in 40% as a result of the obstruction and rupture of small pulmonary veins. The alveolar bleeding is often focal; extensive DAH is unusual. Pathologic specimens typically demonstrate focal areas of hemorrhage and hemosiderin deposition. Clinically apparent involvement of the abdominal lymphatic channels, a less frequent association, produces a chylous ascites. Other rare clinical manifestations include chyluria, chylopericardium, chyloptyses, and lower-extremity edema.[207–209]

The chest radiographic findings are variable. Early on, the chylous pleural effusion may dominate, or small irregular interstitial opacities representing proliferating interstitial muscle bundles may produce a micronodular or

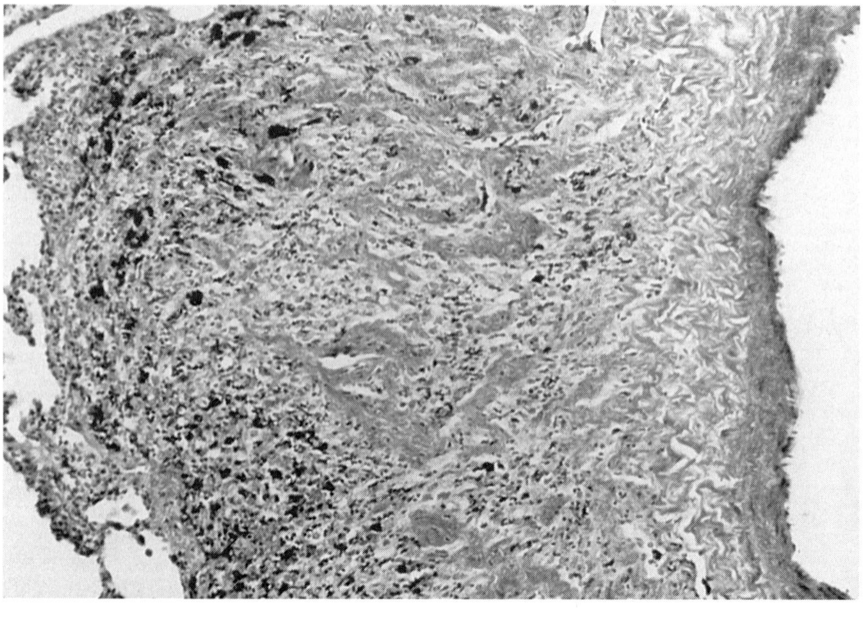

**Figure 60.11** Micrograph showing pulmonary capillary hemangiomatosis. There is capillary proliferation in the wall of this large pulmonary vein. (Original magnification × 100.)

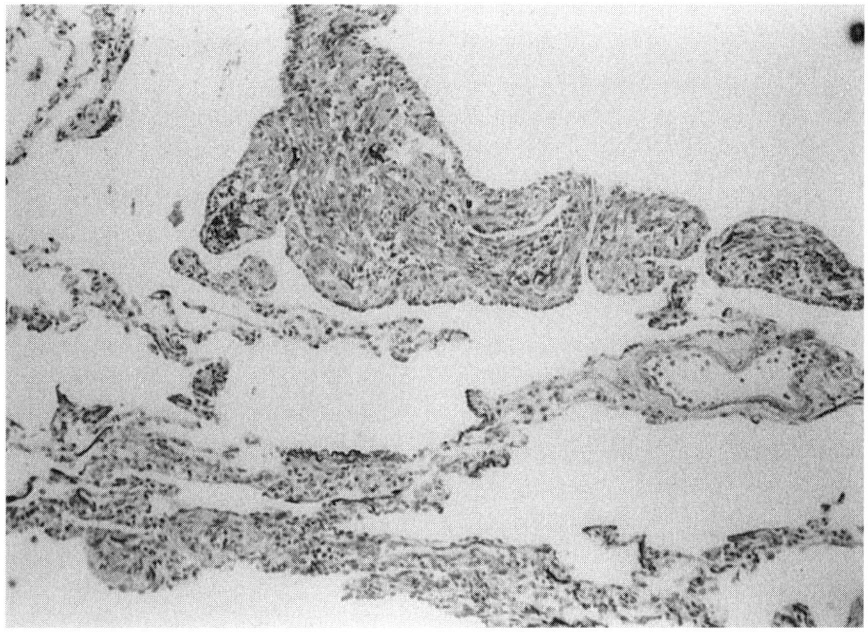

**Figure 60.12** Micrograph showing lymphangioleiomyomatosis. There is smooth muscle proliferating in and broadening the alveolar walls. (Original magnification × 40.)

miliary pattern. Septal lines (Kerley's B lines) due to the lymphatic obstruction appear, producing a coarse reticular pattern. In more advanced disease, the chest radiograph shows hyperinflation, small cystic areas that may be superimposed on a coarse reticular pattern, and sometimes a pneumothorax (Fig. 60.13). The CT scan in the advanced case reveals multiple thin-walled cysts throughout the lung parenchyma (Fig. 60.14).[211]

Although a restrictive ventilatory pattern, due either to the interstitial lung disease or to the pleural effusions, may be seen early on, the most frequent physiologic pattern encountered is the progressive obstructive lung disease with hyperinflation and a reduced diffusing capacity for carbon monoxide. These findings are identical to those found in emphysema,[206, 209, 212–214] but airflow limitation in LAM is probably due to airway narrowing rather than to a loss of elastic recoil.[214]

Because LAM occurs in premenopausal women and because the disease is reported to accelerate both during pregnancy and after estrogen therapy, hormonal influences are thought to be important in its pathogenesis.[215–217] Electron microscopy of the lung in LAM reveals the proliferating smooth muscle cells to be similar to that of the uterine smooth muscle cells.[218] Also, a progestin receptor

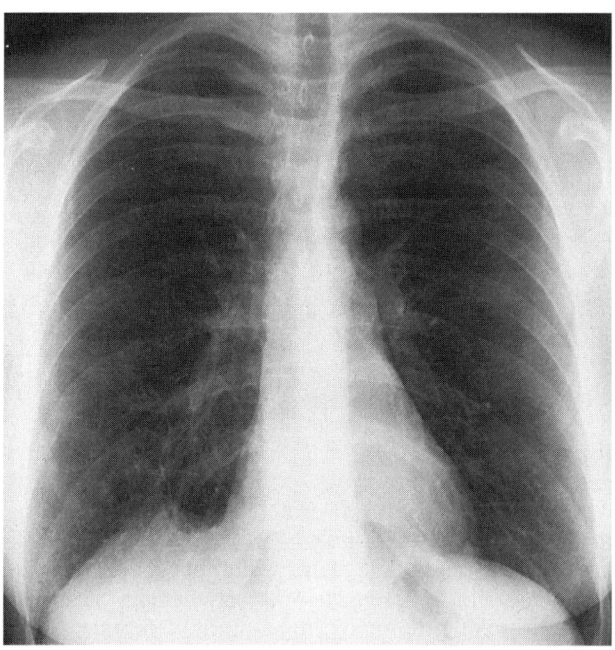

**Figure 60.13** Chest radiograph showing lymphangioleiomyomatosis. Note the hyperinflation and lower-zone interstitial infiltrates.

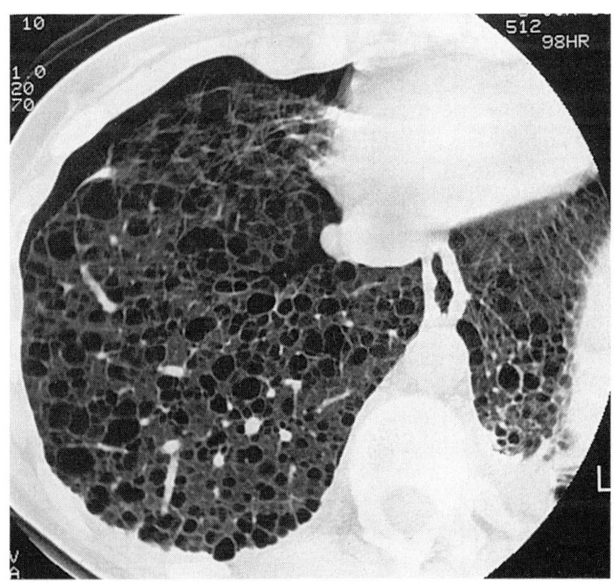


**Figure 60.14** High-resolution CT scan showing lymphangioleiomyomatosis. It demonstrates the network of thin-walled cysts as well as a pneumothorax.

has been identified in the lungs of LAM subjects that is not found in the lungs of unaffected women.[219–221]

Unfortunately, most women die of this disease within 10 years of onset of symptoms, but the course is variable, and lung transplantation offers a promising therapeutic alternative. Most therapies have been directed toward reduction of the circulating estrogen levels, and these include oral and intramuscular medroxyprogesterone, oophorectomy, tamoxifen, or various combinations of the aforementioned treatment.[215, 219, 222–225] Medroxyprogesterone may result in prolonged periods of disease stabilization or even physiologic improvement in some cases, especially when treatment is initiated early (e.g., in the presence of chylous effusions).[207] Single-lung transplantation has also been successful, but recurrences of LAM have been documented.

## Tuberous Sclerosis

Tuberous sclerosis involving the lungs is pathologically identical to LAM and therefore has a similar clinical, radiographic, and physiologic picture. However, in tuberous sclerosis, 20% of patients with pulmonary involvement are male and chylous pleural effusions are rare. In addition, treatment with antiestrogen regimens is not recommended.[226–231]

Tuberous sclerosis is a systemic disease with a clinical triad of mental retardation, epilepsy, and dermal angiofibroma (adenoma sebaceum).[226] Systemic manifestations include calcified cerebral and paraventricular hamartomas, renal angiomyolipomas, cardiac rhabdomyomas, and periungual fibromas. Death occurs in more than 75% of affected individuals by 20 years of age, usually from neurologic complications.[227] Pulmonary disease is rare, appearing in 1% and only in female patients who survive to adulthood. The onset of dyspnea usually occurs during the third decade.[229–232] As in LAM, progressive dyspnea, recurrent spontaneous pneumothoraces, and hemoptysis are to be expected. Hemoptysis is rarely severe enough to result in the syndrome of DAH. There is no recommended treatment.

# OTHER RARE INFILTRATIVE DISORDERS

## Neurofibromatosis

Neurofibromatosis, also known as von Recklinghausen's disease, is an autosomal dominant disease that is recognized by the appearance of cutaneous café-au-lait spots, subcutaneous neurofibromas, and the Lisch nodule in the iris.[232] The thoracic manifestations of neurofibromatosis are listed in Table 60.4. Interstitial lung disease occurs in 25% of affected patients, and dyspnea appears between the third and sixth decades.[233–237] Lower-zone radiographic interstitial infiltrates are the rule, and bullous changes eventually appear in the upper zones. Physiologic testing early in the course of the disease reveals restrictive ventilatory impairment, but with time an obstructive lung disease supervenes, because the fibrotic process in the lung involves not only the interstitium but also the small airways. Scar carcinoma has been reported as a complication of neurofibromatosis.[235]

**Table 60.4 THORACIC MANIFESTATIONS OF NEUROFIBROMATOSIS**

| |
|---|
| **LUNG PARENCHYMAL** |
| Interstitial lung disease |
| Metastatic neural tumor |
| **MEDIASTINAL** |
| Meningocele |
| Vagal nerve neurofibroma |
| **CHEST WALL** |
| Subcutaneous neurofibromas |
| Rib notching (inferior) from intercostal neurofibroma |
| Kyphoscoliosis |
| Apical neurofibroma (Pancoast's syndrome) |

## Gaucher's Disease

The adult form of Gaucher's disease, a hereditary disorder that is most common in Ashkenazi Jews, is relatively benign and is associated with prolonged survival. It presents with hepatosplenomegaly, anemia, thrombocytopenia, long-bone erosions, and an increase in serum acid phosphatase. This is an autosomal recessive disease, the pathologic hallmark being the Gaucher cell. The Gaucher cell is a reticuloendothelial cell containing a foamy cytoplasm due to the accumulation of glucocerebrosides, which results from a deficiency of glucocerebrosidase. This leads to an excessive deposition of glucocerebrosides in the reticuloendothelial system, bone marrow, central nervous system, and occasionally the lung.

The infantile form of this disease is uniformly fatal because of central nervous system involvement. The adult cases are more benign. Pulmonary disease occurs in adult cases.[232–242] The parenchymal disease, which consists of radiographically visible small nodules, appears during the first three decades of life. Pathologic examination reveals masses of alveolar macrophages filled with glucocerebroside infiltrating the interstitium and filling alveolar spaces. There are no acute or chronic inflammatory cells or interstitial fibrosis. In addition to interstitial lung disease, affected patients are susceptible to lung infection. A single case of pulmonary hypertension from diffuse small-vessel obstruction by these cells has been reported.[243] Enzyme replacement (glucocerebrosidase) has some therapeutic promise.

## Niemann-Pick Disease

Because of a genetically determined deficiency of sphingomyelinase, sphingomyelin accumulates in the cells of the reticuloendothelial and central nervous systems.[244] As in Gaucher's disease, there is an infantile form that is rapidly fatal. The adult form, which appears during the second and third decades, is relatively benign, presenting with hepatosplenomegaly, hemostatic defects, platelet dysfunction, and, occasionally, cerebellar ataxia. Interstitial lung disease, which appears as diffuse nodular infiltrates on the chest radiograph, is usually asymptomatic, although a mild restrictive ventilatory defect and reduced diffusing capacity have been reported.[245–247] One case of cor pulmonale in Niemann-Pick disease has been described.[246] As in Gaucher's disease, foamy alveolar macrophages are found on lung biopsy.

## Hermansky-Pudlak Syndrome

Hermansky-Pudlak syndrome is an autosomal recessive disorder found in inhabitants of Puerto Rico and of southern Holland.[248–252] Although the biochemical defect is unknown, there is an accumulation of a chromolipid ceroid related to lipofuscin in the reticuloendothelial system. This results in partial tyrosine-negative oculocutaneous albinism and a qualitative platelet defect. In addition, a granulomatous colitis and progressive pulmonary fibrosis occur. The interstitial lung disease is more likely to occur in women and develops during the second through fourth decades.[249–250] It progresses slowly and is unresponsive to treatment. It results in severe dyspnea because of the increased work of breathing and the gas-exchange abnormalities. Spirometry and measurement of lung volumes reveal a restrictive lung disease. The chest radiograph shows nonspecific reticulonodular infiltrates, which progress to radiographic honeycomb lung and pulmonary hypertension.

The histologic appearance is one of extensive interstitial fibrosis with filling of the alveolar spaces by ceroid-containing macrophages. These macrophages are identified in bronchoalveolar lavage and by subsequent staining with the Fontana-Masson silver reduction technique.[250]

## Pulmonary Alveolar Microlithiasis

Pulmonary alveolar microlithiasis is a rare disease in which concretions collect in alveolar spaces (Fig. 60.15).[253] The concretions are composed of calcium and phosphorus.[254, 255] With time, the alveolar walls become fibrotic, and severe physiologic impairment supervenes.[254] No cause has been identified. A systemic disorder of calcium metabolism has not been identified, nor is there evidence for common exposures or immunologic abnormalities. Most authors believe that the responsible mechanism is an inborn error of calcium metabolism that is confined to the lung and leads to precipitation of the salts.[256, 257] In more than 50% of cases, a familial association, usually in siblings, is found.[254, 258]

Most cases are diagnosed during the third through fifth decades. Among familial cases, women are affected more often than men, but there is an equal distribution among the sporadic cases.[258, 259] Cough and dyspnea are usually reported late in the disease course and are associated with restrictive lung disease and gas exchange impairment.[260] Expectorated microliths are unusual.[254] With the development of interstitial fibrosis, crackles, finger clubbing, and signs of cor pulmonale appear.[254, 261]

The chest radiograph is characteristic and shows a diffuse bilateral calcific infiltrate with predilection for the lower lung zones. This infiltrate is alveolar, producing air bronchograms and radiographic obliteration of the heart borders, pulmonary vessels, and diaphragmatic surfaces (Fig. 60.16).[262] In the later stages, radiographic signs of pulmonary hypertension appear. The chest CT scan confirms the calcified nodules and occasionally demonstrates pleural calcification.[263, 264]

Pulmonary function remains normal or only slightly impaired for a prolonged period after disease detection.[255, 256] With progression and the development of fibrosis, a restrictive ventilatory defect with a reduced diffusing capacity for carbon monoxide and severe gas-exchange abnormalities become obvious, and respiratory failure ensues. Serum calcium and phosphate levels are normal. Erythrocytosis, secondary to hypoxemia, is found in the later stages of the disease.[253]

The chest radiograph is often all that is needed for diagnosis, but technetium ($^{99m}Tc$) bone scintigraphy or transbronchial lung biopsy can provide confirmation.[265, 266]

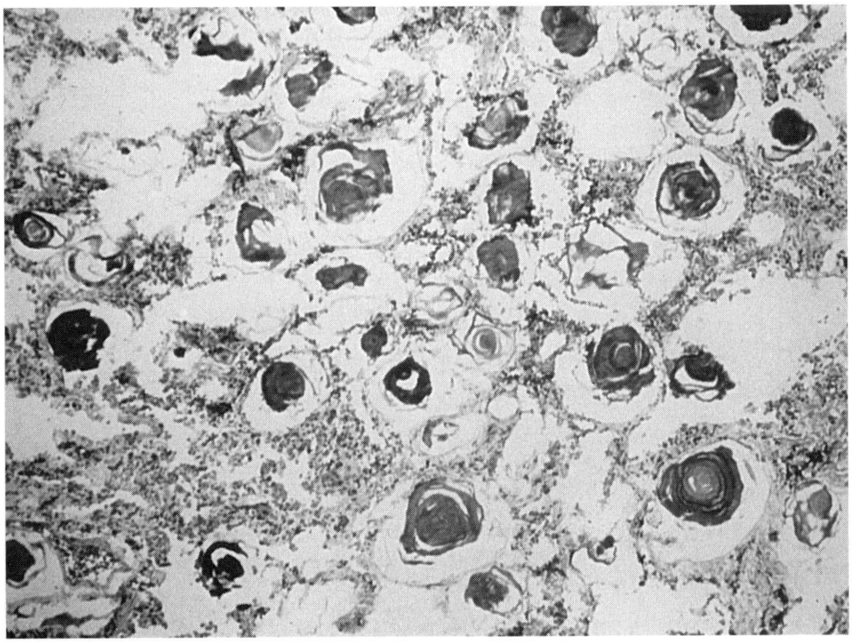

**Figure 60.15** Micrograph showing alveolar microlithiasis. Intra-alveolar calcified microliths are present, and some of the alveolar walls are thickened by inflammation and collagen deposition. (Original magnification × 10.)

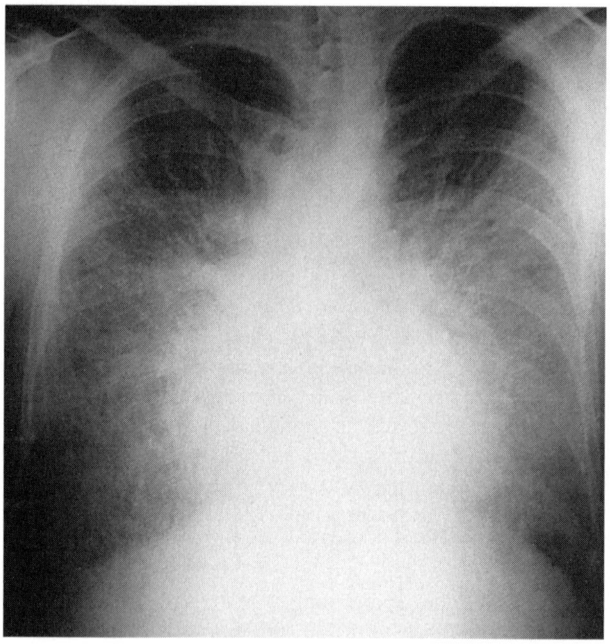

**Figure 60.16** Chest radiograph showing alveolar microlithiasis. There is diffuse alveolar filling, with air bronchograms and obliteration of the heart borders.

Treatment is supportive. Whole-lung lavage, which is effective for pulmonary alveolar proteinosis, has no beneficial effect.[267] Lung transplantation has been successfully performed.

## SUMMARY

DAH is an uncommon but usually striking event that is associated with several different underlying disorders. In this chapter, the causes of DAH are subdivided into those with and without histologic evidence of pulmonary capillaritis. Many of the disorders causing widespread hemorrhage appear to be immunologically mediated, either through injury to the capillary basement membrane by specific autoantibody or through deposition of immune complexes. Most of these syndromes can be diagnosed in the presence of certain accompanying clinical features, laboratory abnormalities, and histologic findings, although overlap occurs. Diagnosis is essential because treatment with corticosteroids, cytotoxic agents, and plasmapheresis, alone or in combinations, is often helpful.

This chapter also provides information about other diffuse interstitial lung diseases that are occasionally complicated by extensive alveolar hemorrhage and other infiltrative disorders. All of these are rare, but most are diagnosable, and treatment is available for a few.

## References


1. Spencer H: Pulmonary lesions in polyarteritis nodosa. Br J Tuberc Dis Chest 51:123–130, 1957.
2. Mark EJ, Ramierez JF: Pulmonary capillaritis and hemorrhage in patients with systemic vasculitis. Arch Pathol Lab Med 109:413–418, 1985.
3. Travis WD, Colby TV, Lombard C, et al: A clinicopathologic study of 34 cases of diffuse pulmonary hemorrhage with lung biopsy confirmation. Am J Surg 14:1112–1125, 1990.
4. Travis WD, Hoffman GS, Leavitt RV, et al: Surgical pathology of the lung in Wegener's granulomatosis: A review of 87 open lung biopsies from 67 patients. Am J Surg Pathol 15:315–333, 1991.
5. Greening AP, Hughes JMB: Serial estimation of carbon monoxide diffusing capacity in intra-pulmonary hemorrhage. Clin Sci 60:507–512, 1981.
6. Drew WL, Finley T. N., Golde DW: Diagnostic lavage and occult pulmonary hemorrhage in thrombocytopenic immunocompromised patients. Am Rev Respir Dis 116:343–361, 1977.
7. Jennette JC, Wilkman AS, Falk RJ: Anti-neutrophil cytoplasmic antibody associated glomerulonephritis and vasculitis. Am J Pathol 135:921–930, 1989.
8. Nada AR, Torres VE, Ryu JH, et al: Pulmonary fibrosis as an unusual clinical manifestation of a pulmonary-renal vasculitis in elderly patients. Mayo Clin Proc 65:847–856, 1990.
9. Bronson SM: Idiopathic pulmonary hemosiderosis in adults: Report of a case and review of the literature. AJR Am J Roentgenol 83:260–271, 1960.
10. Leatherman JW, Davies SF, Hoidal JR: Alveolar hemorrhage syndromes: Diffuse microvascular lung hemorrhage in immune and idiopathic disorders. Medicine 63:343–361, 1984.
11. Beechler CR, Enquist RW, Hunt RR, et al: Immunofluorescence of transbronchial lung biopsies in Goodpasture's syndrome. Am Rev Respir Dis 121:869–872, 1980.
12. Roth DA, Wilz DR, Theil GB: Schönlein-Henoch syndrome in adults. Q J Med 217:145–152, 1985.
13. Davies DJ, Moran JE, Niall JF, et al: Short report. Systemic necrotizing glomerulonephritis with antineutrophil antibody: Possible arbovirus etiology? BMJ 285:606, 1982.
14. Kallenberg CG, Tervaert JW: What is new with anti-neutrophil cytoplasmic antibodies: Diagnostic, pathogenetic and therapeutic implications. Curr Opin Nephrol Hypertens 8:307–315, 1999.
15. Hoffman GS, Kerr GS, Leavitt RY, et al: Wegener granulomatosis: An analysis of 158 patients. Ann Intern Med 116:488–498, 1992.
16. Guillevin L, Durand-Gasselin B, Cevallos R, et al: Microscopic polyangiitis: Clinical and laboratory findings in eighty-five patients. Arthritis Rheum 42:421–430, 1999.
17. Andrasy K, Koderisch J, Waldherr R, et al: Diagnostic significance of anticytoplasmic antibodies in detection of Wegener's granulomatosis and other forms of systemic vasculitis. Nephron 49:257–258, 1988.
18. Falk RJ, Jennette JC: Anti-neutrophil cytoplasmic autoantibodies with specificity for myeloperoxidase in patients with systemic vasculitis and idiopathic necrotizing and crescentic glomerulonephritis. N Engl J Med 318:1651–1657, 1988.
19. Goeken JA: Antineutrophil cytoplasmic antibody—A useful serologic marker for vasculitis. J Clin Immunol 2:161–174, 1991.
20. Walters MDS, Savage COS, Dillon MJ, et al: Antineutrophil cytoplasm antibody in crescentic glomerulonephritis. Arch Dis Child 63:814–817, 1988.
21. Jennings CA, King TE Jr, Tuder RM, et al: Diffuse alveolar hemorrhage with underlying isolated pauciimmune pulmonary capillaritis. Am J Respir Crit Care Med 155:1101–1109, 1997.
22. Bosch X, Font J, Miraquiek E, et al: Antimyeloperoxidase autoantibody-associated necrotizing alveolar capillaritis. Am Rev Respir Dis 146:1326–1329, 1992.
23. Case Records of the Massachusetts General Hospital: Case #12-1986. N Engl J Med 314:834–844, 1986.
24. Mark EG, Matsbaro O, Tan-Liu NS, et al: The pulmonary biopsy in early diagnosis of Wegener's (pathergic) granulomatosis: A study based on 35 open lung biopsies. Hum Pathol 9:1065–1071, 1988.
25. Yoshikawa Y, Watanabe T: Pulmonary lesions in Wegener's granulomatosis: A clinicopathologic study of 22 autopsy cases. Hum Pathol 17:401–410, 1986.
26. Fuller T, Olsen N, Block A, et al: Wegener's granulomatosis: Treatment with heparin in addition to azathioprine and corticosteroids. Nephron 9:225–234, 1972.
27. Hensley MJ, Feldman NT, Lazarus JM, et al: Diffuse pulmonary hemorrhage and rapidly progressive renal failure: An uncommon presentation of Wegener's granulomatosis. Am J Med 60:894–898, 1979.

28. Kjellstrand CM, Simmons RL, Vranga VM, et al: Acute fulminant Wegener's granulomatosis: Therapy with immunosuppression, hemodialysis, and renal transplantation. Arch Intern Med 34:40–43, 1974.
29. Stokes TC, McCann BG, Roes RT, et al: Acute fulminating intrapulmonary hemorrhage in Wegener's granulomatosis. Thorax 37:315–316, 1982.
30. Travis WD, Carpentier HA, Lie ST: Diffuse pulmonary hemorrhage: An uncommon manifestation of Wegener's granulomatosis. Am J Surg Pathol 11:702–708, 1987.
31. Lendud C, DeVuyst RJ, Dupont E, et al: Wegener's granulomatosis presenting as acute respiratory failure with anti-neutrophil cytoplasm antibodies. Chest 96:345–347, 1989.
32. Hall JB, Wadham B, Wood CJ, et al: Vasculitis and glomerulonephritis: A subgroup with an antineutrophil antibody. Aust N Z J Med 14:277–278, 1984.
33. Thomashow BM, Felton CP, Navarrio C: Diffuse intrapulmonary hemorrhage, renal failure, and a systemic vasculitis: A case report and review of the literature. Am J Med 68:299–304, 1980.
34. Imoto EM, Lombard CM, Sachs DPL: Pulmonary capillaritis and hemorrhage: A clue to the diagnosis of systemic necrotizing vasculitis. Chest 96:927–928, 1989.
35. Haworth SJ, Savage COS, Carr D, et al: Pulmonary hemorrhage complicating Wegener's granulomatosis and microscopic polyarteritis. BMJ 290:1775–1778, 1985.
36. Zashin S, Fattor R, Fortin D: Microscopic polyarteritis: A forgotten etiology of hemoptyses and rapidly progressive glomerulonephritis. Ann Rheum Dis 49:53–56, 1990.
37. Doebbeling BN, Bonsib SM, Walher WP: Pulmonary-renal syndrome with "triad" involvement due to small vessel vasculitis. J Rheumatol 17:1087–1090, 1990.
38. Savage COS, Winearls CG, Evans DV, et al: Microscopic polyarteritis: Presentation, pathology, and prognosis. Q J Med 56:467–483, 1985.
39. Leatherman JW: The lung in systemic vasculitis. Semin Respir Infect 3:274–288, 1988.
40. Bocanegra TS, Espinoza LR, Vasey FB, et al: Pulmonary hemorrhage in systemic necrotizing vasculitis associated with hepatitis B. Chest 80:102–103, 1981.
41. Schwarz MI, Mortenson RL, Colby TV, et al: Pulmonary capillaritis. The association with progressive irreversible airflow limitation and hyperinflation. Am Rev Respir Dis 148:507–511, 1993.
42. Ognibene AJ, Dito WR: Rheumatoid disease with unusual pulmonary manifestations. Arch Intern Med 116:567–570, 1966.
43. Smith BS: Idiopathic pulmonary hemosiderosis and rheumatoid arthritis. BMJ 1:1403–1406, 1966.
44. Rallenback J, Prinsloo I, Zwi S: Progressive systemic sclerosis complicated by diffuse pulmonary hemorrhage. Thorax 32:767–770, 1977.
45. Griffin MT, Robb JD, Martin JR: Diffuse alveolar hemorrhage associated with progressive systemic sclerosis. Thorax 45:903–904, 1990.
46. Leatherman JW, Sibley RK, Davies SF: Diffuse intrapulmonary and glomerulonephritis unrelated to antiglomerular basement membrane antibody disease. Am J Med 72:401–406, 1982.
47. Germain M, J., Davidman M: Pulmonary hemorrhage and acute renal failure in a patient with mixed connective tissue disease. Am J Kidney Dis 3:420–424, 1984.
48. Schwarz MI, Sutarik JM, Nick JA, et al: Pulmonary capillaritis and diffuse alveolar hemorrhage: A primary manifestation of polymyositis. Am J Respir Crit Care Med 151:2037–2040, 1995.
49. Schwarz MI, Zamora MR, Hodges TN, et al: Isolated pulmonary capillaritis and diffuse alveolar hemorrhage in rheumatoid arthritis and mixed connective tissue disease. Chest 113:1609–1615, 1998.
50. Zamora MR, Warner ML, Tuder RM, et al: Diffuse alveolar hemorrhage and systemic lupus erythematosus: Clinical presentation, histology, survival and outcome. Medicine 76:192–202, 1997.
51. Leavitt RY, Fauci AS: Pulmonary vasculitis. Am Rev Respir Dis 134:149–166, 1986.
52. Gould DB, Soriano RZ: Acute alveolar hemorrhage in lupus erythematosus. Ann Intern Med 83:836–837, 1975.
53. Eagen JW, Memoli VA, Roberts JL, et al: Pulmonary hemorrhage in systemic lupus erythematosus. Medicine 57:545–560, 1978.
54. Mintz G, Galindo LF, Fernandez-Diez J, et al: Acute massive pulmonary hemorrhage in systemic lupus erythematosus. J Rheumatol 5:39–50, 1978.
55. Marino CT, Pertschuk LP: Pulmonary hemorrhage in systemic lupus erythematosus. Arch Intern Med 141:201–203, 1981.
56. Desnoyers MR, Bernstein S, Cooper AG, et al: Pulmonary hemorrhage in lupus erythematosus without evidence of an immunologic cause. Arch Intern Med 144:1398–1400, 1984.
57. Gertner E: Diffuse alveolar hemorrhage in the antiphospholipid syndrome: Spectrum of disease and treatment. J Rheumatol 26:805–807, 1999.
58. Elliot M, Kuhn C: Idiopathic pulmonary hemosiderosis: Ultrastructural abnormalities in the capillary walls. Am Rev Respir Dis 102:895–904, 1970.
59. Rodriguez-Inturbe B, Garcia R, Rubio L, et al: Immunohistologic findings in the lung in systemic lupus erythematosus. Arch Pathol Lab Med 101:342–344, 1977.
60. Myers JL, Katzenstein AL: Microangiitis in lupus-induced pulmonary hemorrhage. Am J Clin Pathol 85:552–556, 1986.
61. Matthay RA, Schwarz MI, Petty TL, et al: Pulmonary manifestations of systemic lupus erythematosus: A review of 12 cases of acute pneumonitis. Medicine 54:397–409, 1975.
62. Carette S, Macher AM, Nussbaum A, et al: Severe acute pulmonary disease in patients with systemic lupus erythematosus: Ten years of experience at the National Institutes of Health. Semin Arthritis Rheum 14:52–59, 1984.
63. Gladman DD, Urowitz MB: Venous syndromes and pulmonary embolism in systemic lupus erythematosus. Ann Rheum Dis 39:340–343, 1980.
64. Howe HS, Boey ML, Fong KY, et al: Pulmonary hemorrhage, pulmonary infarction, and lupus anticoagulant. Ann Rheum Dis 47:869–872, 1988.
65. Alarcon-Segovia D, Deleze M, Oria CV, et al: Anti-phospholipid antibodies and the anti-phospholipid syndrome in systemic lupus erythematosus: A prospective analysis of 500 consecutive patients. Medicine 68:353–365, 1989.
66. Pines A, Kaplinsky N, Olchovsky D, et al: Pleuropulmonary manifestations of systemic lupus erythematosus: Clinical features of its subgroups. Chest 88:129–135, 1985.
67. Rees AJ, Lockwood CM, Peters DK: Enhanced allergic tissue injury in Goodpasture's syndrome by intercurrent bacterial infection. BMJ 2:723–726, 1977.
68. Bombardieri S, Paoletti P, Ferri C, et al: Lung involvement in essential mixed cryoglobulinemia. Am J Med 66:748–756, 1979.
69. Clinicopathologic Conference: Mixed cryoglobulinemia. Am J Med 61:95, 1976.
70. Ball JA, Young KR Jr: Pulmonary manifestations of Goodpasture's syndrome. Antiglomerular basement membrane disease and related disorders. Clin Chest Med 19:777–791, 1998.
71. O'Duffy JD, Carney JA, Doedhar S: Behçet's disease. Ann Intern Med 75:561–570, 1971.
72. Chajeck T, Fainaru M: Behçet's disease: Report of 41 cases and review of the literature. Medicine 54:179–196, 1975.
73. Gamble CN, Wiesner KG, Shapiro RF, et al: The immune complex pathogenesis of glomerulonephritis and pulmonary vasculitis in Behçet's disease. Am J Med 6:1031–1039, 1979.
74. Cadman EC, Lundberg WB, Mitchell MS: Pulmonary manifestations in Behçet's syndrome. Arch Intern Med 136:944–947, 1976.
75. Efthimiou J, Johnston C, Spiro SG, et al: Pulmonary disease in Behçet's syndrome. Q J Med 227:259–280, 1986.
76. Strickler H, Malinverni R: Multiple large aneurysms of pulmonary arteries in Behçet's disease: Clinical remission and radiologic resolution after corticosteroid therapy. Arch Intern Med 149:925–927, 1989.
77. Raz I, Okon E, Chajek-Shaul T: Pulmonary manifestations in Behçet's syndrome. Chest 95:585–589, 1989.
78. Yazici H, Pazarli H, Barnes CG, et al: A controlled trial of azathioprine in Behçet's syndrome. N Engl J Med 322:281–285, 1990.
79. Cream JJ, Gumpel JM, Peachey RDG: Schönlein-Henoch purpura in the adult. Q J Med 9:219–228, 1978.
80. Bar-On H, Rosenmann E: Schönlein-Henoch syndrome in adults. Isr J Med Sci 8:1702–1715, 1972.
81. Roth DA, Wilz DR, Theil GB: Schönlein-Henoch syndrome in adults. Q J Med 217:145–152, 1985.

82. Counahan R, Cameron JS: Henoch-Schönlein purpura nephritis. Contrib Nephrol 7:143–148, 1977.
83. Weiss VF, Naidu S: Fatal pulmonary hemorrhage in Henoch-Schönlein purpura. Cutis 23:687–688, 1979.
84. Kathuria S, Chejfec G: Fatal pulmonary Henoch-Schönlein purpura. Chest 82:654–656, 1982.
85. Kauffmann RH, Hermann WA, Meyer CJLM, et al: Circulating IgA-immune complexes in Henoch-Schönlein purpura: A longitudinal study of their relationship to disease activity and vascular deposition of IgA. Am J Med 69:859–866, 1980.
86. Baart de la Failk-Ruyper EH, Kater L, Kuijten RH, et al: IgA deposits in cutaneous blood vessel walls and mesangium in Henoch-Schönlein purpura. Lancet 1:892–893, 1973.
87. Levinsky R, Barratt T: IgA immune complexes in Henoch-Schönlein purpura. Lancet 2:1100–1103, 1979.
88. Loughlin GM, Taussig LM, Murphy SA, et al: Immune-complex mediated glomerulonephritis and pulmonary hemorrhage simulating Goodpasture's syndrome. J Pediatr 93:181–184, 1978.
89. Beirne GJ, Kopp WL, Zimmerman SW: Goodpasture's syndrome dissociation from antibodies to glomerular basement membrane. Arch Intern Med 132:261–265, 1973.
90. Clinicopathologic Conference: Proliferative glomerulonephritis and pulmonary hemorrhage. Am J Med 55:199–210, 1973.
91. Lewis EJ, Schur PH, Busch GJ, et al: Immunopathologic features of a patient with glomerulonephritis and pulmonary hemorrhage. Am J Med 54:507–513, 1973.
92. Holdsworth S, Boyce N, Thomson NM, et al: The clinical spectrum of acute glomerulonephritis and lung hemorrhage (Goodpasture's syndrome). Q J Med 216:75–86, 1985.
93. Leatherman JW: Immune alveolar hemorrhage. Chest 91:891–897, 1987.
94. Couser WG: Idiopathic crescentic glomerulonephritis. *In* Massry SG, Glassrock RJ (eds): Textbook of Nephrology. Baltimore: Williams & Wilkins, 1983, pp 6–52.
95. Badesch DB, Zamora MR, Fullerton D, et al: Pulmonary capillaritis: A possible histologic form of acute pulmonary allograft rejection. J Heart Lung Transplant 17:415–422, 1998.
96. Soergel KH, Sommers SC: Idiopathic pulmonary hemosiderosis and related syndromes. Am J Med 32:499–511, 1962.
97. Cohen S: Idiopathic pulmonary hemosiderosis. Am J Med Sci 317:67–74, 1999.
98. Donald RJ, Edwards RL, McEvoy JDS: Alveolar capillary basement membrane lesions in Goodpasture's syndrome and idiopathic pulmonary hemosiderosis. Am J Med 59:642–649, 1975.
99. Case Records of the Massachusetts General Hospital: Case #30-1979. N Engl J Med 301:201–208, 1979.
100. Yeager H, Powell D, Winberg RM, et al: Idiopathic pulmonary hemosiderosis. Ultrastructural studies and response to azathioprine. Arch Intern Med 136:1145–1149, 1976.
101. Katzenstein AL: Idiopathic pulmonary hemosiderosis. *In* Katzenstein AL, Askin FB (eds): Surgical Pathology of Non-neoplastic Lung Disease. Philadelphia: WB Saunders, 1982, p 133.
102. Irwin RS, Cotrell TS, Hsu KC, et al: Idiopathic pulmonary hemosiderosis: An electron microscopic and immunofluorescent study. Chest 65:41–45, 1974.
103. Donlan CJ Jr, Strodes CH, Duffy FD: Idiopathic pulmonary hemosiderosis: Electron-microscopic, immunofluorescent and iron kinetic studies. Chest 68:577–584, 1975.
104. Hyatt RW, Adelstein ER, Halazon JF, et al: Ultrastructure of the lung in idiopathic pulmonary hemosiderosis. Am J Med 52:822–829, 1972.
105. Wright PH, Menzies IS, Pounder RE, et al: Adult idiopathic hemosiderosis and coeliac disease. Q J Med 50:95–102, 1981.
106. Valassir-Adam H, Rouska A, Karpouzac J, et al: Raised IgA in idiopathic pulmonary hemosiderosis. Arch Dis Child 50:320–322, 1976.
107. Byrd RB, Gracey DR: Immunosuppressive treatment of idiopathic pulmonary hemosiderosis. JAMA 226:458–459, 1973.
108. Chryssanthopoulos C, Cassimos C, Panagiotidou C: Prognostic criteria in idiopathic pulmonary hemosiderosis in children. Eur J Pediatr 140:123–125, 1985.
109. Beckerman RC, Taussig LM, Pinnas JL: Familial idiopathic pulmonary hemosiderosis. Am J Dis Child 133:609–611, 1979.
110. Thaell JF, Greipp PR, Stubbs SE, et al: Idiopathic pulmonary hemosiderosis: Two cases in a family. Mayo Clin Proc 53:113–118, 1978.
111. Case Records of the Massachusetts General Hospital: Case #30-1988. N Engl J Med 319:227–237, 1988.
112. Bowley NH, Hughes JBM, Steiner RE: The chest x-ray in pulmonary capillary hemorrhage: Correlation with carbon monoxide uptake. Clin Radiol 30:413–417, 1979.
113. Reppetto G, Lisboa C, Emparanza E, et al: Idiopathic pulmonary hemosiderosis. Clinical, radiological, and respiratory function studies. Pediatrics 40:24–32, 1967.
114. Bailey P, Broden BM: Idiopathic pulmonary hemosiderosis: Report of two cases and review of the literature. Postgrad Med J 55:266–272, 1979.
115. Kjellman B, Elinder G, Garnicz S, et al: Idiopathic pulmonary hemosiderosis in Swedish children. Acta Paediatr Scand 73:584–588, 1984.
116. Albelda SM, Gefter WB, Epstein DM, et al: Diffuse pulmonary hemorrhage: A review and classification. Radiology 154:289–297, 1985.
117. Goodpasture EW: The significance of certain pulmonary lesions in relation to the etiology of influenza. Am J Med Sci 158:863–870, 1919.
118. Duncan DA, Drummond KN, Michael AF, et al: Pulmonary hemorrhage and glomerulonephritis: Report of six cases and study of the renal lesion by the fluorescent antibody technique and electron microscopy. Ann Intern Med 62:920–938, 1965.
119. Hellmark T, Burkhardt H, Wieslander J: Goodpasture disease. Characterization of a single conformational epitope as the target of pathogenic autoantibodies. J Biol Chem 274:25862–25868, 1999.
120. Martinez JS, Kohler PF: Variant "Goodpasture's syndrome"? The need for immunologic criteria in rapidly progressive glomerulonephritis and hemorrhagic pneumonitis. Ann Intern Med 75:67–76, 1971.
121. Wilson CB, Dixon FJ: Antiglomerular basement membrane antibody induced glomerulonephritis. Kidney Int 3:74–89, 1973.
122. Simpson IJ, Doak PB, Williams LC, et al: Plasma exchange in Goodpasture's syndrome. Am J Med Nephrol 2:301–311, 1982.
123. Rees AJ: Pulmonary injury caused by anti-basement membrane antibodies. Semin Respir Dis 5:264–272, 1984.
124. McPhaul JJ, Mullins JD: Glomerulonephritis mediated by antibody to glomerular basement membrane: Immunologic, clinical and histopathological characteristics. J Clin Invest 57:351–361, 1976.
125. Kelly PT, Haponick EF: Goodpasture's syndrome: Molecular and clinical advances. Medicine 73:171–185, 1994.
126. Beirne GJ, Wagnild JP, Zimmerman SW, et al: Idiopathic crescentic glomerulonephritis. Medicine 56:349–381, 1977.
127. Teague CA, Doak PB, Simpson IJ, et al: Goodpasture's syndrome: An analysis of 29 cases. Kidney Int 13:492–504, 1978.
128. Savage COS, Pusey CD, Bowman C, et al: Antiglomerular basement membrane antibody mediated disease in the British Isles 1980–1984. BMJ 292:301–354, 1986.
129. Donaghy M, Rees AJ: Cigarette smoking and lung hemorrhage in glomerulonephritis caused by autoantibodies to glomerular basement membrane. Lancet 1:1390–1392, 1983.
130. Jones JG, Monty BD, Lawler P, et al: Increased alveolar epithelial permeability in cigarette smokers. Lancet 1:66–67, 1980.
131. Beirne GJ, Brennan JT: Glomerulonephritis associated with hydrocarbon solvents mediated by anti-glomerular basement membrane antibody. Arch Environ Health 25:365–369, 1972.
132. Keogh AM, Ibels LS, Allen DH, et al: Exacerbation of Goodpasture's syndrome after inadvertent exposure to hydrocarbon fumes. BMJ 288:188, 1984.
133. Lombard CM, Colby TV, Elliot CG: Surgical pathology of the lung in anti–basement membrane antibody associated with Goodpasture's syndrome. Hum Pathol 20:445–451, 1989.
134. Matthew TH, Hobbs JB, Kalowski S, et al: Normal renal diagnostic findings. Ann Intern Med 82:215–218, 1975.
135. Beirne GJ, Octaviano GN, Kopp WL, et al: Immunohistology of the lung in Goodpasture's syndrome. Ann Intern Med 69:1207–1212, 1968.
136. Abboud RT, Chase WH, Ballon HS, et al: Goodpasture's syndrome: Diagnosis by transbronchial lung biopsy. Ann Intern Med 89:635–638, 1978.
137. Zimmerman CM, Varanasi VR, Hoff B: Goodpasture's syndrome with normal renal function. Am J Med 66:163–171, 1979.

138. Lerner RA, Glassock RJ, Dixon JF: The role of antiglomerular basement membrane antibody in the pathogenesis of human glomerulonephritis. J Exp Med 126:989–1004, 1967.
139. Wilson CB, Smith RC: Goodpasture's syndrome associated with influenza A2 virus infection. Ann Intern Med 76:91–94, 1972.
140. Jennings L, Roholt OA, Pressman D, et al: Experimental anti-alveolar basement membrane antibody–mediated pneumonitis. The role of increased permeability of the alveolar capillary wall induced by oxygen. J Immunol 127:129–134, 1981.
141. Rees AJ, Peters DK, Amos N, et al: The influence of HLA-linked genes on the severity of anti-GBM antibody–mediated nephritis. Kidney Int 26:444–450, 1984.
142. Perl SI, Russell BA, Charlesworth JA, et al: Goodpasture's (anti-GBM) disease and HLA-DRw2. N Engl J Med 305:463–464, 1981.
143. Rees AJ, Peters DK, Compston DAS, et al: Strong association between HLA-DRw2 and antibody-mediated Goodpasture's syndrome. Lancet 1:966–968, 1978.
144. Peters DK, Rees AJ, Lockwood CM, et al: Treatment and prognosis in anti–basement membrane antibody–mediated nephritis. Transplant Proc 14:513–521, 1986.
145. Addelman M, Logan AS, Grossman RF: Monitoring intrapulmonary hemorrhage in Goodpasture's syndrome. Chest 87:119–120, 1985.
146. Ewan PW, Jones HA, Rhodes CG, et al: Detection of intrapulmonary hemorrhage with carbon monoxide uptake. Application in Goodpasture's syndrome. N Engl J Med 295:1391–1396, 1976.
147. Bell DD, Moffatt SL, Singer M, et al: Antibasement membrane antibody disease without clinical evidence of renal disease. Am Rev Respir Dis 142:234–237, 1990.
148. McCormack JR, Kass J, Skewes M: Goodpasture's syndrome. Compr Ther 13:25–32, 1987.
149. Balow JE: Plasmapheresis: Development and application in treatment of renal disorders. Artif Organs 10:324–330, 1986.
150. Stanton MC, Tange JD: Goodpasture's syndrome. Aust Ann Med 7:132–144, 1958.
151. Lockwood CM, Rees AJ, Pearson TA, et al: Immunosuppression and plasma exchange in the treatment of Goodpasture's syndrome. Lancet 1:711–715, 1976.
152. Keller F, Offerman G, Schultz EG, et al: Membrane plasma exchange in Goodpasture's syndrome. Am J Med Sci 287:32–36, 1984.
153. Rosenblatt SG, Knight W, Bannayan GA, et al: Treatment of Goodpasture's syndrome with plasmapheresis. A case report and review of the literature. Am J Med 66:689–696, 1979.
154. Erickson SB, Kurtz SB, Donadio JV, et al: Use of combined plasmapheresis and immunosuppression in the treatment of Goodpasture's syndrome. Mayo Clin Proc 54:714–720, 1979.
155. Shumak KH, Rock GA: Therapeutic plasma exchange. N Engl J Med 310:762–771, 1984.
156. Fort J, Espinel E, Rodriguez JA, et al: Partial recovery of renal function in an oligoanuric patient affected with Goodpasture's syndrome after treatment with steroids, immunosuppressives, and plasmapheresis. Clin Nephrol 22:211–212, 1984.
157. Bygren P, Freiburghaus C, Lindholm T, et al: Goodpasture's syndrome treated with staphylococcal protein A immunoadsorption. Lancet 2:1295–1296, 1985.
158. Johnson JP, Moore J, Austin HA, et al: Therapy of antiglomerular basement membrane antibody disease: Analysis of prognostic significance of clinical, pathologic, and treatment factors. Medicine 64:219–227, 1985.
159. Hind CRK, Lockwood CM, Peters DK, et al: Prognosis after immunosuppression of patients with crescentic nephritis requiring dialysis. Lancet 1:263–265, 1983.
160. Rees AJ, Lockwood CM, Peters DK: Enhanced allergic tissue injury in Goodpasture's syndrome by intercurrent bacterial infection. BMJ 2:723–726, 1977.
161. Katzenstein AL, Bloor C, Liebow AA: Diffuse alveolar damage: The role of oxygen, shock and related factors. Am J Pathol 85:210–226, 1976.
162. Cooper JAD, White DA, Matthay RA: Drug induced pulmonary disease. Am Rev Respir Dis 133:321–340, 1986.
163. Rebello S, Mason JK: Pulmonary histological appearances in fatal paraquat poisoning. Histopathology 2:53–66, 1978.
164. Pratt PC: Pathology of pulmonary oxygen toxicity. Am Rev Respir Dis 110:51–57, 1974.
165. Bils RF: Ultrastructural alterations of alveolar tissue of mice: III. Ozone. Arch Environ Health 20:468–480, 1970.
166. Gross NJ: The pathogenesis of radiation induced lung damage. Lung 159:115–125, 1981.
167. Forrester JM, Steele AW, Waldron JA, et al: Crack lung: An acute pulmonary syndrome with a spectrum of clinical and histopathologic findings. Am Rev Respir Dis 142:462–467, 1990.
168. Murray RJ, Albin RJ, Mergner W, et al: Diffuse alveolar hemorrhage temporally related to cocaine smoking. Chest 93:427–429, 1988.
169. Tomashefski JF Jr: Pulmonary pathology of the adult respiratory distress syndrome. Clin Chest Med 11:593–619, 1990.
170. Gibson T, Burry HC, Ogg C: Goodpasture's syndrome and D-penicillamine. Ann Intern Med 84:100, 1975.
171. Gavaghan TE, McNaught PJ, Ralston M, et al: Penicillamine induced Goodpasture's syndrome: Successful treatment of a fulminant case. Aust N Z Med J 11:261–265, 1981.
172. Sternlieb I, Bennett B, Scheinberg IHD: D-penicillamine induced Goodpasture's syndrome in Wilson's disease. Ann Intern Med 82:673–676, 1975.
173. Hill HFH: Penicillamine in rheumatoid arthritis: Adverse affects. Scand J Rheumatol 28:94–99, 1979.
174. Louie S, Gamble CN, Cross CE: Penicillamine associated pulmonary hemorrhage. J Rheumatol 13:963–966, 1986.
175. Matloff DS, Kaplan MM: D-penicillamine induced Goodpasture's like syndrome in primary biliary cirrhosis: Successful treatment with plasmapheresis and immunosuppressive therapy. Gastroenterology 78:1046–1049, 1980.
176. Zeiss CR, Wolkonsky P, Chacon R, et al: Syndromes in workers opposed to trimellitic anhydride. Ann Intern Med 98:8–12, 1983.
177. Herbert FA, Orford R: Pulmonary hemorrhage and edema due to inhalation of resins containing trimellitic anhydride. Chest 76:546–551, 1979.
178. Ahmad D, Patterson R, Morgan WKC, et al: Pulmonary hemorrhage and hemolytic anemia due to trimellitic anhydride. Lancet 2:328–330, 1979.
179. Cortese DA: Pulmonary function in mitral stenosis. Mayo Clin Proc 53:321–326, 1978.
180. Ramsey HW, de la Torre A, Bartley TD, et al: Intractable hemoptyses in mitral stenosis treated by emergency mitral commissurotomy. Ann Intern Med 67:588–593, 1967.
181. Robboy SJ, Minna JD, Colman RW, et al: Pulmonary hemorrhage syndrome as a manifestation of disseminated intravascular coagulation. Chest 63:718–721, 1973.
182. Buchanan GR, Moore GC: Pulmonary hemosiderosis and immune thrombocytopenia. JAMA 246:861–864, 1981.
183. Martinez AJ, Maltby JD, Hurst DJ: Thrombotic thrombocytopenic purpura seen as pulmonary hemorrhage. Arch Intern Med 143:1818–1820, 1983.
184. Golde DW, Drew WL, Klein HZ, et al: Occult pulmonary hemorrhage in leukemia. BMJ 2:166–168, 1975.
185. Smith LJ, Katzenstein AL: Pathogenesis of massive pulmonary hemorrhage in acute leukemia. Arch Intern Med 142:2149–2152, 1982.
186. Fireman Z, Yust I, Abramov CC: Lethal occult pulmonary hemorrhage in drug-induced thrombocytopenia. Chest 79:358–359, 1981.
187. Wagenvoort CA, Wagenvoort TN, Takahashi T: Pulmonary veno-occlusive disease: Involvement of pulmonary arteries and review of the literature. Hum Pathol 16:1033–1041, 1985.
188. Rosenthal A, Vawter G, Wagenvoort CA: Intrapulmonary veno-occlusive disease. Am J Cardiol 31:78–83, 1973.
189. Case Records of the Massachusetts General Hospital: Case #21-1986. N Engl J Med 314:1435–1445, 1986.
190. Pietra GG, Edwards WD, Kay JM, et al: Histopathology of primary pulmonary hypertension. A qualitative and quantitative study of pulmonary blood vessels from 58 patients in the National Heart, Lung, and Blood Institute, Primary Pulmonary Hypertension Registry. Circulation 80:1198–1206, 1989.
191. Glassroth J, Woodford DW, Carrington CB, et al: Pulmonary veno-occlusive disease in the middle-aged. Respiration 47:309–321, 1985.
192. Palevsky HI, Pietra GG, Fishman AP: Pulmonary veno-occlusive disease and its response to vasodilator agents. Am Rev Respir Dis 142:426–429, 1990.

193. Bjornsson J, Edwards WD: Primary pulmonary hypertension: A histopathologic study of 80 cases. Mayo Clin Proc 60:16–25, 1985.
194. Lombard CM, Churg A, Winokur S: Pulmonary veno-occlusive disease following therapy for malignant neoplasms. Chest 92:871–876, 1987.
195. Troussard X, Bernaudin JF, Cordonnier C, et al: Pulmonary veno-occlusive disease after bone marrow transplantation. Thorax 39:956–957, 1984.
196. Corrin B, Spencer H, Turner-Warwick M, et al: Pulmonary veno-occlusion. An immune complex disease? Virchows Arch 364:81–86, 1974.
197. Sanderson JE, Spiro SG, Henry AT, et al: A case of pulmonary veno-occlusive disease responding to azathioprine. Thorax 32:140–148, 1977.
198. Hackman RC, Madtes DK, Peterson FB, et al: Pulmonary veno-occlusive disease following bone marrow transplantation. Transplantation 47:989–992, 1989.
199. Liu L, Sackler VP: A case of pulmonary veno-occlusive disease. Angiology 23:299–304, 1972.
200. Salzman GA, Rosa UW: Prolonged survival in pulmonary veno-occlusive disease treated with nifedipine. Chest 95:1154–1156, 1989.
201. Faber CN, Yousem SA, Dauber JH, et al: Pulmonary capillary hemangiomatosis: A report of three cases and review of the literature. Am Rev Respir Dis 140:808–813, 1989.
202. Langleben D, Heneghan JM, Batten AP, et al: Familial pulmonary capillary hemangiomatosis resulting in primary pulmonary hypertension. Ann Intern Med 109:106–109, 1988.
203. Vevaina JR, Mark EJ: Thoracic hemangiomatosis masquerading as interstitial lung disease. Chest 93:657–659, 1988.
204. Magee F, Wright JL, Kay JM, et al: Pulmonary capillary hemangiomatosis. Am Rev Respir Dis 132:922–925, 1985.
205. White CW, Sondheimer HM, Crouch EC, et al: Treatment of pulmonary hemangiomatosis with recombinant interferon alpha-2a. N Engl J Med 320:1197–1200, 1989.
206. Taylor JR, Ryu J, Colby TV, et al: Lymphangioleiomyomatosis: Clinical course in 32 patients. N Engl J Med 323:1254–1260, 1990.
207. Urban T, Lazor R, Lacronique J, et al: Pulmonary lymphangioleiomyomatosis. A study of 69 patients. Groupe d'Etudes et de Recherche sur les Maladies "Orphelines" Pulmonaires (GERM"O"P). Medicine 78:321–337, 1999.
208. Johnson S: Rare diseases. 1. Lymphangioleiomyomatosis: Clinical features, management and basic mechanisms. Thorax 54:254–264, 1999.
209. El Allaf DE, Borlee G, Hadjoudj H, et al: Pulmonary lymphangiomyomatosis. Eur J Respir Dis 65:147–152, 1984.
210. Bernstein SM, Newell JD, Adamszy KD, et al: How common are renal angiomyolipomas in patients with lymphangioleiomyomatosis. Am J Respir Crit Care Med 152:2138–2143, 1995.
211. Kirchner J, Stein A, Viel K, et al: Pulmonary lymphangioleiomyomatosis: High-resolution CT findings. Eur Radiol 9:49–54, 1999.
212. Case Records of the Massachusetts General Hospital: Case #24-1988. N Engl J Med 318:1601–1610, 1988.
213. Lie JT, Miller DR, Williams DE: Cystic disease of the lung in tuberous sclerosis: Clinicopathologic correlation including body plethysmographic lung function tests. Mayo Clin Proc 55:547–553, 1980.
214. Burger CD, Hyatt RE, Staats BA: Pulmonary mechanics in lymphangioleiomyomatosis. Am Rev Respir Dis 143:1030–1033, 1991.
215. NHLBI Workshop Summary. Report of workshop on lymphangioleiomyomatosis. National Heart, Lung, and Blood Institute. Am J Respir Crit Care Med 159:679–683, 1999.
216. Yockey CC, Riepe RE, Ryan K: Pulmonary lymphangioleiomyomatosis complicated by pregnancy. Kans Med 87:277–293, 1986.
217. Shen A, Iseman MD, Waldron JE, et al: Exacerbation of pulmonary lymphangioleiomyomatosis by exogenous estrogens. Chest 95:782–785, 1987.
218. Kane PB, Lane BP, Cordice JWV, et al: Ultrastructure of the proliferating cells in pulmonary lymphangioleiomyomatosis. Arch Pathol Lab Med 102:618–622, 1978.
219. McCarty KS, Mossler JA, McLelland R, et al: Pulmonary lymphangioleiomyomatosis responsive to progesterone. N Engl J Med 303:1461–1465, 1980.
220. Berger U, Khaghani A, Pomerance A, et al: Pulmonary lymphangioleiomyomatosis: An immunocytochemical study. Am J Clin Pathol 903:609–614, 1990.
221. Blentani MM, Carvalho CRR, Saldiva PH, et al: Steroid receptors in pulmonary lymphangioleiomyomatosis. Chest 85:96–99, 1984.
222. Adamson D, Heinrichs WL, Raybin DM, et al: A Successful treatment of pulmonary lymphangioleiomyomatosis with oophorectomy and progesterone. Am Rev Respir Dis 132:916–921, 1985.
223. Tomasian A, Greenberg MS, Rummerman H: Tamoxifen for lymphangioleiomyomatosis. N Engl J Med 306:745–746, 1982.
224. Svendsen TL, Viskum K, Hansborg N, et al: Pulmonary lymphangioleiomyomatosis lesion treated with medroxyprogesterone, oophorectomy, and tamoxifen. Br J Dis Chest 78:264–271, 1984.
225. Eliasson AH, Phillips YY, Tenholder MF: Treatment of lymphangioleiomyomatosis. Chest 196:1352–1355, 1989.
226. Marshall D, Saul GB, Sach E: Tuberous sclerosis: A report of 16 cases in two family trees revealing genetic dominance. N Engl J Med 261:1102–1103, 1959.
227. Medley BE, Mcleod AR, Houser OW: Tuberous sclerosis. Semin Roentgenol 11:35–54, 1976.
228. Dwyer JH, Hickie JB, Garvan J: Pulmonary tuberous sclerosis: Report of three patients and a review of the literature. Q J Med 40:115–125, 1971.
229. Capron F, Ameille J, Leclerc P, et al: Pulmonary lymphangioleiomyomatosis and Bourneville's tuberous sclerosis with pulmonary involvement: The same disease? Cancer 52:851–855, 1983.
230. Liberman BA, Chamberlain DW, Goldstein RS: Tuberous sclerosis with pulmonary involvement. Can Med Assoc J 130:287–289, 1984.
231. Maestres CA, Catalan M, Letung E, et al: Tuberous sclerosis and associated pleuropulmonary lesions. Thorac Cardiovasc Surg 31:243–246, 1983.
232. Riccardi VM: von Recklinghausen's neurofibromatosis. N Engl J Med 305:1616–1627, 1981.
233. Massaro D, Katz S: Fibrosing alveolitis: Its occurrence, roentgenographic, and pathologic features in von Recklinghausen's neurofibromatosis. Am Rev Respir Dis 93:934–942, 1966.
234. Webb WR, Goodman PC: Fibrosing alveolitis in patients with neurofibromatosis. Radiology 122:289–293, 1977.
235. Schoerder ID, Elinck W, Renterghenu DV, et al: Desquamative interstitial pneumonia and scar cancer of the lung complicating generalized neurofibromatosis. Eur J Respir Dis 65:623–626, 1984.
236. Patchefsky AS, Atkinson WG, Hoch WS, et al: Interstitial pulmonary fibrosis and von Recklinghausen's disease: An ultrastructural and immunofluorescent study. Chest 64:459–464, 1973.
237. Unger PD, Geller SA, Anderson PJ: Pulmonary lesions in a patient with neurofibromatosis. Arch Pathol Lab Med 108:654–657, 1984.
238. Schneider EL, Epstein CJ, Kaback MJ, et al: Severe pulmonary involvement in Gaucher's disease: Report of three cases and review of the literature. Am J Med 63:475–480, 1977.
239. Wolson AA: Pulmonary findings in Gaucher's disease. AJR Am J Roentgenol 123:712–715, 1975.
240. Fisher MR, Sider L: Diffuse reticulonodular infiltration associated with splenomegaly. Chest 84:609–610, 1983.
241. Terry RD, Sperry WM, Brodoff B: Adult lipoidosis resembling Niemann-Pick disease. Am J Pathol 30:263–286, 1954.
242. Myers B: Gaucher's disease of the lungs. BMJ 2:8–12, 1937.
243. Roberts WC, Fredrickson DS: Gaucher's disease of the lung causing severe pulmonary hypertension with associated acute pericarditis. Circulation 35:783–789, 1967.
244. Lynn R, Terry RD: Lipid histochemistry and electron microscopy in adult Niemann-Pick disease. Am J Med 37:987–991, 1964.
245. Lachman R, Crocker A, Schulman V, et al: Radiologic findings in Niemann-Pick disease. Radiology 108:659–664, 1973.
246. Lever AML, Ryder JB: Cor pulmonale in an adult secondary to Niemann-Pick disease. Thorax 38:873–874, 1983.
247. Long RG, Lake BD, Pettit JE, et al: Adult Niemann-Pick disease. Am J Med 62:627–635, 1977.
248. Hermansky F, Pudlak P: Albinism associated with hemorrhagic diathesis and unusual pigmented cells in the bone marrow: Re-

port of two cases with histochemical study. Blood 14:162–169, 1959.
249. Garay SM, Gardella JE, Fazzini EP, et al: Hermansky-Pudlack syndrome. Pulmonary manifestations of a ceroid storage disorder. Am J Med 66:737–747, 1979.
250. White DA, Walker-Smith GJ, Cooper JAD, et al: Hermansky-Pudlak syndrome and interstitial lung disease: Report of a case with lavage findings. Am Rev Respir Dis 130:138–141, 1984.
251. Schinella RA, Greco MA, Garay SM, et al: Hermansky-Pudlak syndrome: A clinicopathologic study. Hum Pathol 16:366–376, 1985.
252. Depinho RA, Kaplan KL: The Hermansky-Pudlak syndrome: Report of three cases and review of pathophysiology and management considerations. Medicine 64:192–202, 1985.
253. Meyer HH, Gilbert ES, Kent G: A clinical review of pulmonary microlithiasis. JAMA 161:1153–1157, 1956.
254. Prakash UBS, Barham SS, Rosenow EC III, et al: Pulmonary alveolar microlithiasis: A review including ultrastructural and pulmonary function studies. Mayo Clin Proc 58:290–300, 1983.
255. Mitro JM, Moreno A, Coca A, et al: Pulmonary alveolar microlithiasis with an unusual radiographical pattern. Br J Dis Chest 76:91–92, 1982.
256. Caffrey PR, Altmen RS: Pulmonary alveolar microlithiasis occurring in premature twins. Pediatrics 66:758–763, 1965.
257. Yang SP, Lin CC: Pulmonary alveolar microlithiasis: A report of two youngest cases in a family. Dis. Chest 44:163–167, 1963.
258. Josman MC, Dodd GD, Jones WD, et al: The familial occurrence of pulmonary alveolar microlithiasis. AJR Am J Roentgenol 77:947–1012, 1957.
259. Sears MR, Chang AR, Taylor AJ: Pulmonary alveolar microlithiasis. Thorax 26:704–711, 1971.
260. Fuleihan FJD, Abboud RT, Balikan JP, et al: Pulmonary alveolar microlithiasis: Lung function in five cases. Thorax 24:84–90, 1969.
261. Schraufnagel DE, Pate JAP, Wang NS: Micronodular pulmonary pattern: Association with inhaled steroid. AJR Am J Roentgenol 137:57–63, 1981.
262. Balikian JP, Fuleihan JFD, Nucho CN: Pulmonary alveolar microlithiasis: Report of five cases with special reference to roentgen manifestations. AJR Am J Roentgenol 103:509–518, 1968.
263. Pant K, Shah A, Mathur RK, et al: Pulmonary alveolar microlithiasis with pleural calcification and nephrolithiasis. Chest 98:245–246, 1990.
264. Winselberg GG, Boller M, Sachs M, et al: CT evaluation of pulmonary alveolar microlithiasis. J Comput Assist Tomogr 8:1029–1031, 1984.
265. Brown MI, Swee RG, Olson RJ, et al: Pulmonary uptake of Tc-99m diphosphonate in alveolar microlithiasis. AJR Am J Roentgenol 131:703–704, 1978.
266. Cale WF, Petsonk EL, Boyd CB: Transbronchial biopsy of pulmonary alveolar microlithiasis. Arch Intern Med 143:358–359, 1983.
267. Palombini BC, Posto ND, Wallace CU, et al: Bronchopulmonary lavage in alveolar microlithiasis. Chest 80:423–424, 1981.

# 61 Eosinophilic Lung Diseases

EDWARD J. GOETZL, M.D. • JOHN M. LUCE, M.D.

Introduction
Cell Biology and Biochemistry of Eosinophils
- Regulation of Production and Tissue Distribution
- Cellular and Biochemical Characteristics
- Specific Stimuli and Specialized Functions

Eosinophilic Lung Diseases
- History and Classification
- Parasitic Infections
- Drug and Chemical Reactions
- Allergic Bronchopulmonary Aspergillosis
- Chronic Eosinophilic Pneumonia
- Acute Eosinophilic Pneumonia
- Hypereosinophilic Syndrome
- Allergic Granulomatosis and Angiitis

Summary

## INTRODUCTION

Eosinophils are bone marrow–derived granulocytes, which have distinctive cellular properties and functions, and which increase in concentration in the blood and some tissues during diverse types of immunologic reactions, parasitic infections, and many other, apparently unrelated, diseases.[1, 2] Eosinophils are normal constituents of the lungs, and eosinophilia in the blood, airway secretions, and pulmonary tissues is a hallmark of asthma, pulmonary granulomatosis and vasculitis, some interstitial lung disorders, pulmonary parasitic infections, and most of the primary and secondary systemic eosinophilic syndromes.[3] Lung mast cells, T lymphocytes, macrophages, and airway epithelial cells secrete potent soluble factors that attract and activate eosinophils.[3–5] Experimental and clinical studies during the past three decades have expanded our understanding of specific receptors and surface adhesive proteins of eosinophils, defined the properties of their unique cationic protein constituents, revealed the range of lipid and peptide mediators generated by eosinophils, and elucidated their capacity to produce and respond to diverse cytokines. Although there is incomplete knowledge of the mechanisms of many of the protective and deleterious effects of eosinophils in the lungs and other organs, it is clear that they are pathogenetically critical in asthma and many pulmonary inflammatory and fibrosing diseases.

This chapter is divided into two main sections. The first section provides important basic information about the cell biology, biochemistry, regulation, and function of eosinophils. The second section describes the history and classification and the clinical aspects of the most common kinds of eosinophilic lung disease.

## CELL BIOLOGY AND BIOCHEMISTRY OF EOSINOPHILS

The purposes of this section are to discuss recent basic discoveries of the cell biology, biochemistry, and immunology of eosinophils that may contribute to the development and outcome of eosinophilic lung disease and to suggest how this knowledge may lead to new diagnostic tests and treatment modalities.

### Regulation of Production and Tissue Distribution

Most eosinophils in adult mammals are produced in the bone marrow and released into the blood with an emergence time of 60 to 80 hours, enter tissues with site specificity, and disappear from the circulation and tissues with respective half-times of 8 to 12 hours and more than 24 hours.[6] The eosinophil is principally a tissue leukocyte, in contrast to other granulocytes.[7] The number of eosinophils in nonmarrow tissues is nearly equal to that in bone marrow, which exceeds by 200 to 400 times the number in blood. The bone marrow progenitors of eosinophils are distinct from those of other leukocytes and are controlled independently by a separate subset of eosinophilopoietic factors.

A series of cytokines secreted by stimulated T lymphocytes are the predominant eosinophilopoietic factors in animal experimental models and in limited studies of humans. The transfer of immunocompetent T lymphocytes alone reconstitutes depressed eosinophilopoietic responses of rodents with T-lymphocyte–dependent immunodeficiencies caused by genetic defects or irradiation. Normally, the sequential actions of interleukin-3 (IL-3) and granulocyte-macrophage colony-stimulating factor on eosinophil precursors induce initial development and commitment to the eosinophil lineage, after which IL-5 elicits terminal differentiation to mature eosinophils.[8] IL-5 is highly specific for eosinophils, whereas IL-3 and granulocyte-macrophage colony-stimulating factor also stimulate production of other leukocytes. The finding that IL-5 is generated selectively by T lymphocytes of patients with blood eosinophilia after incubation in vitro with IL-2 suggested that an elevated level of IL-5 is the principal stimulus of increased eosinophilopoiesis in the presence of normal levels of IL-3 and granulocyte-macrophage colony-stimulating factor.[9] The dominant role of IL-5 in eosinophilia was confirmed by the demonstration of high eosinophilia in the blood of transgenic mice overexpressing only the IL-5 gene[10] and by the selectively high levels of IL-5 in patients with various reactive eosinophilias and hypereosinophilic syndromes.[11] Furthermore, 16 of 60 patients with the idiopathic hypereosinophilic syndrome were found to have clonal populations of abnormal T cells that produced large amounts of IL-5.[11a]

The entry of blood eosinophils into tissues occurs in at least three steps, including selectin-mediated initial contact with endothelial cells, vascular adherence and transendothelial migration, and attraction to specific tissues. IL-4, IL-1, and tumor necrosis factor all are capable of augmenting eosinophil vascular adherence and transendothelial migration by activating endothelial vascular cell adhesion molecule-1 and thereby facilitating its binding to the very late activation antigen-4 expressed on the surface of eosinophils, but not neutrophils.[12, 13] A wide range of specific chemotactic factors, including some of the immune cytokines, attract marginated and perivascular eosinophils to different tissue sites.

## Cellular and Biochemical Characteristics

Eosinophils are similar to other granulocytes in size and polymorphic shape but have a bilobed nucleus, which lacks a nucleolus, and contain three different types of cytoplasmic granules. The numerous specific or secondary granules are responsible for the tinctorial properties of eosinophils, the primary granules develop earlier in eosinophil maturation and lack the crystalloid cores of specific granules, and a smaller type of granule contains arylsulfatase and other enzymes preferentially.[1, 2] A distinct composite of three classes of cellular constituents distinguishes eosinophils from other leukocytes and endows eosinophils with unique functional capabilities (Table 61.1). The enzymatic constituents include a series of lysosomal hydrolases and a peroxidase, which is structurally different from myeloperoxidase but similarly gener-

**Table 61.1 PRINCIPAL PROTEIN CONSTITUENTS OF HUMAN EOSINOPHILS**

| Constituent | Cellular Location | Structure | Functions |
|---|---|---|---|
| **Enzymes** | | | |
| Peroxidase | Secondary granules | MW = 75,000 | Microbicidal, cytotoxic |
| Lysophospholipase | Plasma membrane | MW = 13,000–17,000 | Degrades lysophospholipids |
| Phospholipase D | Granules | MW = 60,000 | Inactivates PAF |
| Histaminase | Granules | MW = 160,000 | Inactivates histamine |
| **Cationic Proteins** | | | |
| Major basic protein | Core of secondary granules | MW = 9300 | Mast cell activation<br>Helminthotoxicity |
| Eosinophil cationic proteins | Matrix of secondary granules | MW = 21,000–29,000 | Same as MBP; also neurotoxic and alter HF/P |
| Eosinophil-derived neurotoxin | Matrix of secondary granules | MW = 18,000–19,000 | Central neurotoxin |
| **Receptors and Other Surface Proteins** | | | |
| FcγRII | Plasma membrane | CD32 | Eosinophil activation |
| Fcε RII | Plasma membrane | Similar to CD23 | Eosinophil activation |
| Fcα | Plasma membrane | Binds IgAs > IgAm | Unknown |
| CRs | Plasma membrane | Includes C1qR, CR1, CR3 and C5aR | Recognition of ICs and mediators |
| LFA-1 | Plasma membrane | CD11a and CD18 | Cellular adhesiveness |
| VLA-4 | Plasma membrane | CDw49d | Adherence to endothelial cells |
| CD4 | Plasma membrane | 434 aa; 4 Ig-like loops | R for MHC II/HIV/LCF |
| HLA-DR | Plasma membrane | Alpha/beta heterodimer | Antigen presentation |

HF = Hageman's factor; HIV = human immunodeficiency virus; IC = immune complex; IgAm = monomeric IgA; IgAs = secretory IgA; LCF = lymphocyte chemoattractant factor; MBP = major basic protein; MHC = major histocompatibility complex; MW = molecular weight; P = plasminogen; PAF = platelet-activating factor; R = receptor; CR = complement receptor; LFA-1 = type 1 lymphocyte function-associated antigen; VLA = very late activation antigen-4.

**Table 61.2 DISTINCTIVE PULMONARY EFFECTS OF EOSINOPHILS AND EOSINOPHIL CONSTITUENTS AND PRODUCTS**

| MEDIATOR | FUNCTIONS |
|---|---|
| Cationic proteins | |
| Major basic protein | Mast cell activation<br>Transient bronchoconstriction<br>Enhancement of tracheal contractions<br>Nasal epithelial damage<br>Tracheal epithelial damage<br>Inhibition of respiratory airway mucous secretion |
| Eosinophil cationic protein | Tracheal epithelial damage<br>Enhancement of respiratory airway mucous secretion |
| Eosinophil peroxidase | Mast cell activation<br>Nasal epithelial damage<br>Transient bronchoconstriction |
| Cytokines | |
| Il-4, IL-5, Il-8, IL-12, MIF, MCP-1, TGF-α, TGF-β1, TNF-α | Recruit and affect functions of other cells |
| Lipid mediators | |
| Phospholipid platelet-activating factor | Bronchoconstriction<br>Augmentation of respiratory airway contractile sensitivity |
| Leukotriene $C_4$ and leukotriene $D_4$ | Bronchoconstriction<br>Increased vascular permeability<br>Enhancement of respiratory airway mucous secretion |

IL = interleukin; MIF = macrophage inhibition factor; TGF = transforming growth factor; MCP = monocyte chemotactic protein; TNF = tumor necrosis factor.

ates hypohalous acids with microbicidal and cytotoxic effects. Lysophospholipase forms Charcot-Leyden crystals that are the signature of eosinophils in sputum, feces, and some tissues. Histaminase and phospholipase D effectively degrade histamine and the phospholipid platelet-activating factor (PAF), respectively. The abundant major basic protein and eosinophil cationic protein (ECP) of specific granules are broadly cytotoxic.[2, 14] Eosinophil-derived neurotoxin and ECP are members of the same ribonuclease superfamily and have significant structural similarity.[15] ECP is principally a microbial toxin, whereas eosinophil-derived neurotoxin is a potent neurotoxin.

The recognition by eosinophils of fluid-phase molecules and other cells is facilitated by a wide range of surface receptors (see Table 61.1). The interactions of eosinophils with other cells, including lymphocytes, fibroblasts, endothelial cells, and epithelial cells, are mediated by the type 1 lymphocyte function–associated and very late activation antigen-4 adhesive proteins. Other adhesive proteins may become important in viral infections. For example, respiratory syncytial virus infection up-regulates CD11b, but not CD11a or CD11c, on eosinophils and concurrently increases expression of the counterligand intercellular adhesion molecule 1 on respiratory epithelial cells.[16] Eosinophils recognize and respond to immune complexes, and opsonized cells and particles that bind to complement receptors and Fc receptors specific for immunoglobulin G (IgG), IgA, and IgE.[1, 17] Eosinophils in tissues, but not in blood, are exposed to factors that maintain surface expression of CD4 and HLA-DR protein.[1, 2] The expression of HLA-DR protein provides a mechanism for antigen presentation by activated eosinophils to T helper cells. The CD4 on eosinophils not only permits chemotactic responses to lymphocyte chemoattractant factor[18] but also binds to gp120 of human immunodeficiency virus-1.

Eosinophils also generate diverse cytokines and the low-molecular-weight mediators, PAF, leukotriene $C_4$ ($LTC_4$), $LTD_4$, eicosanoids of the 15-lipoxygenase pathway, and some neuropeptides (Table 61.2).[1, 2, 19, 20] The eosinophil-derived quantities and potencies of most such mediators suggest that only $LTC_4$ and its peptidolytic derivatives would contribute significantly to most eosinophilic hypersensitivity and inflammatory reactions. However, some cytokines may emerge as important eosinophil-generated mediators of inflammation and tissue fibrosis.[21]

## Specific Stimuli and Specialized Functions

Many factors from the immune system and other sources stimulate the chemotaxis or directed migration and numerous other functions of eosinophils. In most complex reactions of the lungs, eosinophils accumulate in the airway and parenchymal tissues as a result of the local generation of a mixture of chemotactic factors of different structures. Immune reactions generate diverse eosinophil chemotactic factors, including the lymphocyte chemoattractant factor, the eosinophilotactic chemokines eotaxin MCP-3 and RANTES, IL-2, C5a, the fatty acid $LTB_4$, tetrapeptides of the eosinophil chemotactic factor of anaphylaxis, and the phospholipid PAF.[1–3, 22, 23] Each of these factors is not only capable of stimulating eosinophil chemotaxis but also evokes one or more of a series of other eosinophil responses, including increased adhesiveness, an oxidative burst, degranulation, and greater cytotoxicity. Eotaxin from macrophages and respiratory epithelial cells is responsible for the basal levels of eosinophils in pulmonary and gastrointestinal tissues and is the major stimulus of eosinophil responses to challenges. Delayed apoptosis of eosinophils, principally attributable to IL-5, also contributes directly to pulmonary tissue eosinophilia.[24] The long duration of eosinophil responses may explain their greater capacity to kill multicellular parasites and to induce fibrosis in heart and lung tissues.

The principal beneficial functions of eosinophils are manifested in helminthic parasitic diseases. The eosinophil is especially equipped to adhere to multicellular microorganisms, such as parasites, and to deliver on their surface oxidative metabolites, proteases, and cationic polypeptides, which slowly but effectively achieve a cytotoxic effect. Eosinophils also have two unique effector and regulatory functions. First, eosinophil products, especially cytokines and cationic peptides, evoke specific responses of other cells, as exemplified by noncytotoxic stimulation of mast cells, platelets, and neutrophils, which may contribute to mediation of hypersensitivity and inflammation. Second, eosinophils secrete diverse enzymes, which destroy peptide, lipid, and phospholipid mediators of cellular activities in many types of physiologic and pathologic responses. Thus, eosinophils may contribute to or act to contain and terminate such responses, depending on the cause, location, magnitude, and time course of the reaction. The potential deleterious effects of eosinophils are observed in hypereosinophilic diseases of the skin and fascia, endomyocardial fibrosis, and some pulmonary eosinophilias, which are discussed subsequently.

Eosinophils activated by allergic reactions, parasitic infections, and other diseases with blood and tissue eosinophilia differ morphologically, functionally, and biochemically from those normally found in blood. When activated, eosinophils become less dense, lose granule contents, and show cytoplasmic vacuoles.[25, 26] The heightened activity of such low-density eosinophils is demonstrated by their greater expression of complement and IgG receptors, increased metabolic activity and mediator generation, and more efficient cytotoxicity for helminths, as well as a higher potential for damage to normal cells of mammalian tissues.[1, 2] The process of activation is attributable largely to the action of specific cytokines, which convert normal mature blood eosinophils into low-density–activated eosinophils in vitro. The principal cytokines that evoke eosinophilopoiesis, IL-3, IL-5, and granulocyte-macrophage colony-stimulating factor, as well as gamma interferon, PAF, and some other inflammatory factors, induce all of the characteristics of hypodense activated eosinophils. Activation of eosinophils and an increase in their number are consistent findings in patients with allergic diseases and asthma. Eosinophils also predominate and contribute to late-phase responses in many other hypersensitivity states. The levels of activated eosinophils correlate quantitatively with the activity and severity of these conditions and some other hypereosinophilic diseases.[26]

The specific effects of eosinophils on lung tissues and functions range from transient reversible responses to permanent damage (see Table 62.2). For example, both major basic protein and peroxidase on one end of the spectrum activate pulmonary mast cells and elicit transient bronchoconstriction and on the other end of the spectrum damage or destroy respiratory airway cells.[1, 2] In contrast, the lipid mediator products of eosinophils, PAF and $LTB_4$-$LTC_4$-$LTD_4$, potently alter respiratory vascular tissue, airway smooth muscle, and epithelial and glandular functions without cytotoxic potential. Eosinophil-derived mediators may exert opposing functions in the lung, such as the effects on mucous secretion that include inhibition by major basic protein and enhancement by ECP and $LTC_4$-$LTD_4$.[27] The many pulmonary effects of eosinophils and eosinophil constituents are evident in the ensuing descriptions of eosinophilic lung diseases.

## EOSINOPHILIC LUNG DISEASES

### History and Classification

In 1936, Löffler[28] reported on a series of four Swiss patients with a syndrome of mild and transient fever, malaise, nonproductive cough, wheezing, chest radiographic infiltrates, and peripheral eosinophilia that was subsequently named after him. Weingarten,[29] in 1943, used the term *tropical eosinophilia* to describe patients from India who had a more severe and prolonged course than patients with Löffler's syndrome. In time, Löffler's syndrome and tropical eosinophilia were attributed to infections with *Ascaris* worms and filarial nematodes, respectively; however, patients with more varied clinical presentations and either infection with other parasites or no documented infections were being identified around the world. Such identification prompted Reeder and Goodrich[30] in 1952 to argue that Löffler's syndrome, tropical eosinophilia, and related disorders be subsumed under the more general term *pulmonary infiltrates with eosinophilia* (PIE syndrome).

Also in 1952, Crofton and colleagues[31] proposed that the term *pulmonary eosinophilia* be applied to clinical disorders accompanied by chest radiographic infiltrations and blood eosinophilia. These investigators also proposed a classification of pulmonary eosinophilia, representing a clinical and pathologic continuum from mild to severe. Included in the classification was (1) simple pulmonary eosinophilia (Löffler's syndrome), (2) prolonged pulmonary eosinophilia, (3) pulmonary eosinophilia with asthma, (4) tropical eosinophilia, and (5) polyarteritis nodosa. Crofton and coworkers[31] arbitrarily took a minimum level of 6% of the total white blood cells as indicating peripheral eosinophilia. They assumed that the eosinophilia and the disorder with which it was associated represented hypersensitivity reactions to various identified and unidentified antigens.

In 1969, Liebow and Carrington[32] suggested that the term *eosinophilic pneumonia* replace pulmonary eosinophilia and PIE syndrome. In addition, they used the term to designate not only pulmonary infiltrations associated with eosinophilia, but also "infiltrations of the lung by

**Table 61.3 EOSINOPHILIC LUNG DISEASE**

| |
|---|
| Simple pulmonary eosinophilia (Löffler's syndrome) |
| Chronic eosinophilic pneumonia |
| Acute eosinophilic pneumonia |
| Allergic granulomatosis and angiitis (Churg-Strauss syndrome) |
| Hypereosinophilic syndrome |
| Asthma |
| Allergic bronchopulmonary aspergillosis |
| Bronchocentric granulomatosis |
| Parasitic infections |
| Drug and chemical reactions |

eosinophils that may or may not be accompanied by an excess of these cells in the peripheral blood." These investigators also broadened the classification of Crofton and colleagues[31] to include presumed hypersensitivity reactions attributable to newly identified pathogens, such as *Aspergillus fumigatus,* and emphasized the relative commonness of idiopathic chronic eosinophilic pneumonia, a condition discussed separately by Carrington and associates[33] in the same year.

Other classification systems followed, including that of Allen and Davis,[34] who use the term *eosinophilic lung diseases* to describe the diverse group of pulmonary disorders that have in common an increase in circulating or tissue eosinophils that are of pathogenetic importance. This classification, in the order proposed by Allen and Davis, is outlined in Table 61.3. Because most cases of simple pulmonary eosinophilia are due to parasitic infections or drug or chemical reactions, simple eosinophilia is not considered separately but is dealt with in the other two discussions. Furthermore, parasitic infections and drug reactions are discussed first, followed by allergic bronchopulmonary aspergillosis (ABPA), because their cause is known. Bronchocentric granulomatosis is discussed under ABPA because the conditions appear to be related. Asthma, the most common eosinophilic lung disease (Barnes[35] has called it "chronic eosinophilic bronchitis"), is covered in Chapter 39. This term should not be confused with the different entity *eosinophilic bronchitis*, which, like asthma, includes chronic cough and sputum eosinophilia, but, unlike asthma, does not include airway hyperresponsiveness and expiratory air flow obstruction.[35a]

## Parasitic Infections

An alphabetical listing of some of the parasites that can cause eosinophilic lung diseases is provided in Table 61.4. Of these parasites, *Ancylostoma duodenale, Ascaris* species (particularly *lumbricoides* and *suum), Clonorchis sinensis, Entamoeba histolytica, Necator americanus,* and *Stronglyloides stercoralis* have been reported to cause simple pulmonary eosinophilia or Löffler's syndrome. Tropical pulmonary eosinophilia is caused primarily by the filarial nematodes *Wucheria bancrofti* and *Brugia malayi,* although *A. duodenale, S. stercoralis,* and *Toxocara canis* can produce a similar clinical picture. In this section, only disease caused by *A. lumbricoides* and *W. bancrofti* is commented on. Additional information about parasitic infestations is provided in Chapter 36.

Infection with the roundworm *A. lumbricoides* is present in 25% of the world's population, including Löffler's original four patients, and is the most common cause of pulmonary infiltration and blood eosinophilia in the world.[34] After *Ascaris* eggs are ingested, larvae hatch in the intestine, penetrate the mesenteric lymphatics and venules, migrate to the lungs, mature into adult worms, pass through the alveolar wall, crawl up the airways, are swallowed, and reenter the intestinal tract. The transit of larvae through the lungs has traditionally been thought to invoke the fever, malaise, nonproductive cough, wheezing, dyspnea, occasional chest pain, and rash that characterize Löffler's syndrome. These symptoms, if they occur at all, are accompanied by chest radiographic infiltrates that often are perihilar, a restrictive deficit on pulmonary function testing, and mild blood eosinophilia. Nogami and colleagues[36] suggested that the lung transit of *Ascaris* may not be essential in the pathogenesis of simple pulmonary eosinophilia because when mice sensitized to *Ascaris* are challenged with *Ascaris* extract, eosinophilic infiltrate may develop in the lungs. At any rate, because Löffler's syndrome occurs before the adult worms mature in the lungs, stool examination for *Ascaris* ova is usually negative until the patients' physical and radiographic abnormalities have resolved, which usually takes 2 weeks. *Ascaris* infection is therefore usually diagnosed clinically, although larvae may be present in sputum and bronchoalveolar lavage fluid. Systemic and pulmonary symptoms rarely require treatment, but the intestinal infection should be treated with oral mebendazole, 100 mg twice daily for 3 days.[34]

*W. bancrofti* is a mosquito-borne filarial parasite that preferentially infests lymphatics. There, the adult worms release microfilaria that travel to the lung and elicit a marked inflammatory reaction. Patients infected with *Wucheria* may present with fever, malaise, anorexia, lassitude, nonproductive cough that often is nocturnal, dyspnea, chest pain, and wheezing.[37] Lymphadenopathy and hepatomegaly also may be present. If no treatment is given, symptoms and physical findings may persist for months or may remit spontaneously and then recur months or even years later. Chest radiographs typically reveal a reticulonodular infiltrate; there also may be cavitation and pleural effusions (Fig. 61.1). Pulmonary function tests usually show restrictive changes and, with time,

**Table 61.4 PARASITES CAUSING EOSINOPHILIC LUNG DISEASE**

| | |
|---|---|
| *Ancylostoma* species | *Opisthorchis* species |
| *Ascaris* species | *Paragonimus westermani* |
| *Brugia malayi* | *Schistosoma* species |
| *Clonorchis sinensis* | *Strongyloides stercoralis* |
| *Diroflaria immitis* | *Toxocara* species |
| *Echinococcus* species | *Trichinella spiralis* |
| *Entamoeba histolytica* | *Wucheria bancrofti* |
| *Necator americanus* | |

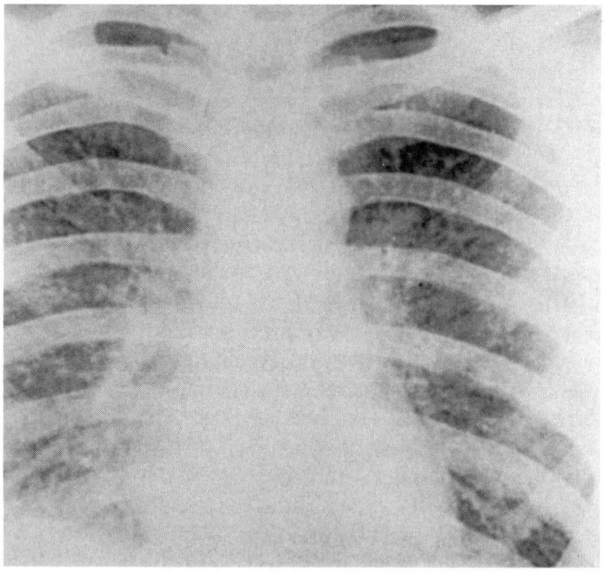

**Figure 61.1** Chest radiograph of 24-year-old Indian student with filarial infection who presented with fever, wheezing, and 70% peripheral blood eosinophils. Chest radiographic infiltrates resolved one week after treatment with diethylcarbamazine. (Courtesy of P. Weller, M.D.)

a reduced diffusion capacity. Blood eosinophils are in the range of 5000 to 60,000 cells/μL, a greater amount than that seen in simple pulmonary eosinophilia, and bronchoalveolar lavage eosinophils may average 50%.[34] High titers of antifilarial antibodies can be detected and are diagnostically useful. Although microfilaria may be demonstrated in the lung, lymph nodes, and liver, tropical eosinophilia usually is diagnosed clinically. Diethylcarbamazine should be given in a dosage of 6 to 12 mg/kg/day for up to 3 weeks. Symptoms should improve within a few days of initiation of therapy, but residual mild symptoms may persist. Clinical relapses after an initial improvement are not uncommon and usually respond to repeated treatment with diethylcarbamazine. Nevertheless, clinical, radiographic, and hematologic abnormalities may last indefinitely in patients who develop chronic interstitial lung disease.

## Drug and Chemical Reactions

Hundreds, if not thousands, of drugs and chemicals have been implicated in causing eosinophilic lung disease through individual case reports. A sample of substances for which a causal relationship with eosinophilic lung disease has been established by means of repeat case reports, rechallenge of affected patients, or both is found in Table 61.5. Other drug-related pulmonary manifestations are described in Chapter 72. Most of the implicated drugs and chemicals have been associated with the development of pulmonary infiltrates, fever (typically low grade), peripheral eosinophilia, and varying degrees of pulmonary symptoms that range from none to severe dyspnea, with or without fever and nonproductive cough. These symptoms may follow initial exposure but often occur only after several doses of a given drug. Typically, reports of these reactions have compared them with Löffler's syndrome.[38–47] In some cases, however, investigators have described more fulminant reactions that resemble those seen with acute eosinophilic pneumonia.[48, 49] Chronic interstitial lung disease also can occur.

Nitrofurantoin is one agent that can cause acute and chronic reactions. Peripheral blood eosinophil counts tend to be higher in the acute variety of nitrofurantoin reactions, which usually occur a few hours to several days after initiation of therapy.[50, 51] Fever, dyspnea, and nonproductive cough are the most common symptoms; wheezing may also be present. The chest radiograph usually shows diffuse interstitial infiltrates, although an alveolar pattern and pleural effusions also have been reported. Despite the peripheral eosinophilia, which is not a universal finding, eosinophils are not generally found in lung tissue or bronchoalveolar lavage fluid. Therefore, diagnosis depends on the suspicion that nitrofurantoin may be responsible and the remission of symptoms, pulmonary infiltrates, and eosinophilia after the drug is withdrawn. Chronic nitrofurantoin reactions generally occur 6 months to years after chronic nitrofurantoin use.[52] This disorder resembles idiopathic pulmonary fibrosis clinically, radiologically, and histologically. A lymphocytic and not eosinophilic alveolitis may be documented by bronchoalveolar lavage. Patients may be given corticosteroids, but their value in this and other reactions to nitrofurantoin is unclear.

The most dramatic recent outbreak of drug and chemical-related eosinophilic lung disease involved the eosinophilia-myalgia syndrome. This syndrome was first reported in 1990 in a series of three patients in New Mexico, all of whom had muscle aches, pain, and tenderness; dyspnea and nonproductive cough; rash; abdominal pain; and mouth ulcers.[53] All three patients had taken L-tryptophan for insomnia and other problems. All had peripheral blood eosinophilia greater than 40%, abnormal

**Table 61.5** DRUGS AND CHEMICALS CAUSING EOSINOPHILIC LUNG DISEASE

| | |
|---|---|
| Aluminum | Methotrexate |
| Ampicillin | Methylphenidate |
| Beclomethasone | Minocycline |
| Bleomycin | Naproxen |
| Carbamazepine | Nickel |
| Captopril | Nitrofurantoin |
| Chlorpromazine | Penicillin |
| Clofibrate | Pencillamine |
| Cocaine | Pentamidine |
| Cobalt | Phenytoin |
| Cromolyn | Pyrimethamine |
| Dapsone | Rapeseed oil |
| Desipramine | Sulfadoxine |
| Diflunisal | Sulfasalazine |
| Fenbufen | Sulindac |
| Granulocyte-macrophage colony-stimulating factor | Tamoxifen |
| | Tetracycline |
| Ibuprofen | Tolazamide |
| Interleukin-2 | L-Tryptophan |

liver function results, and normal creatinine kinase levels. Two patients underwent biopsy, which revealed eosinophilic infiltration of several organs. Although chest radiographs of the three patients were normal, subsequent reports[54, 55] demonstrated radiographic pulmonary infiltration, respiratory muscle weakness, restrictive pulmonary function deficits, and eosinophilic alveolitis. Ultimately, the outbreak of the eosinophilia-myalgia syndrome of 1985 was linked to ingestion of a chemical constituent that was associated with tryptophan-manufacturing conditions at one company.[56] After manufacturing improvements at the company, the syndrome disappeared.

## Allergic Bronchopulmonary Aspergillosis

Allergic bronchopulmonary aspergillosis was first identified in asthmatic patients in England by Hinson and colleagues[57] in 1952 and in the United States by Slavin and associates in 1969.[58] The disorder also occurs in patients with cystic fibrosis[59]; in one report, 2% of 14,210 children with cystic fibrosis had been diagnosed with ABPA.[59a] The diagnostic criteria for ABPA, derived primarily from Rosenberg and colleagues,[60] are shown in Table 61.6. Patients with ABPA also frequently have *A. fumigatus* in their sputum, expectoration of bronchial casts in sputum, central bronchiectasis on chest radiographs or computed tomographic studies, and antibodies to *Aspergillus* in both serum and bronchoalveolar lavage fluid. Allen and Davis[34] consider the IgE level to be the most useful laboratory test in ABPA, noting that the level correlates well with disease activity and that a normal level in a symptomatic patient excludes the diagnosis of ABPA.

Allergic bronchopulmonary fungosis has also been reported with *Aspergillus terreus, Candida albicans, Curvularia lunata, Drechslera hawaiiensis, Stemphylium lanuginosum, Rhizopus, Torolopsis glabrata,* and, most recently, *Fusarium vasinfectum.*[61] Nevertheless, the disorder is most commonly associated with *A. fumigatus,* hence the widespread use of the term ABPA. Because *A. fumigatus* can grow over a wide temperature range, including body temperature, after the spores are inhaled and deposited in secretions in the bronchial tree of susceptible persons, the fungus proliferates and produces hyphae, the branched vegetative form. This provokes an antibody reaction with the production of specific IgE and IgG antibodies, as well as high levels of nonspecific IgE. The markedly elevated amounts of IgE lacking defined antibody activity explain the much higher concentrations of total IgE in asthmatic patients with ABPA in comparison with other asthmatic patients.[62]

**Table 61.6 DIAGNOSTIC CRITERIA FOR ALLERGIC BRONCHOPULMONARY ASPERGILLOSIS**

| |
|---|
| Asthma |
| Blood eosinophilia |
| Chest radiographic infiltrates |
| *Aspergillus* precipitins |
| Positive skin prick test to *Aspergillus* antigens |
| Increased serum immunoglobulin E level |

The immunologic reaction to *A. fumigatus* is probably a combination of type 1 and type 3 hypersensitivity reactions. When *Aspergillus* begins to grow in the bronchial tree, it causes IgE production, either by direct stimulation of B cells capable of producing IgE or indirectly by activation of T cells. The specific IgE and IgG antibodies are believed to combine with some of the *Aspergillus* antigen generated in airway secretions; the resulting immune complexes then cause damage to the bronchial walls and initiate eosinophilic infiltration into the lungs.[63] Mast cells and basophils involved in the type 1 reaction may release eosinophil attractant cytokines resulting in late-phase IgE-dependent eosinophilic reactions. Eosinophils may release mediators, such as ECP, major basic protein, and peroxidase, all of which cause direct tissue damage and two of which may contribute to the development of further bronchoconstriction. Because granulomas, giant cells, and mononuclear cell infiltrates are found in the lungs of patients with ABPA along with an infiltrate of eosinophils, there is a cell-mediated component to the hypersensitivity reaction.[64, 65]

The pulmonary pathologic lesions in patients with ABPA are of two types: (1) marked eosinophilic infiltration of the lung with features of eosinophilic pneumonia and (2) mucous plugging of the airways. The plugs are heavily infiltrated by *Aspergillus* hyphae (Fig. 61.2), but the fungus does not invade the bronchial wall or surrounding lung. The bronchi also contain eosinophils, fibrin, Charcot-Leyden crystals (Fig. 61.3), and Curschmann's spirals. Bronchial occlusion caused by the plugs results in collapse of distal lung. Bronchiectasis occurs in association with these plugs as a consequence of the local immune reaction.[66, 67] The bronchiectasis, which is often proximal and in the upper lobes, represents a major clinical problem in patients with ABPA. In the lung distal to plugs, there may be eosinophilic infiltration with a chronic inflammatory infiltration, including granulomas and multinucleate giant cells.

Although ABPA may occur at any age, it is more common in adults than in children. Males and females are equally affected. Most asthmatic patients are atopic and developed their asthma in childhood, but in some patients, asthma does not develop until years after diagnosis of the ABPA.[62] In some,[68] but not all,[60] series, the episodes of ABPA were more common in autumn and winter when *A. fumigatus* spore counts are at their highest. It is likely that most episodes of pulmonary eosinophilia associated with ABPA are asymptomatic and are undetected. Frequently, the diagnosis is made by routine chest radiographs in asthmatic patients. Sometimes there may be synchronous worsening of their asthma control, and about two thirds of symptomatic patients have a cough that is productive of bronchial casts.[69] In only about 10% of cases,[70] are there systemic features of night sweats, fever, or malaise. Physical signs are usually unhelpful, although fever and wheeze and signs of bronchiectasis and lobar or segmental consolidation or collapse may be present.

The radiologic abnormalities of ABPA were described by Patterson and associates.[70] Segmental, lobar, or pulmo-

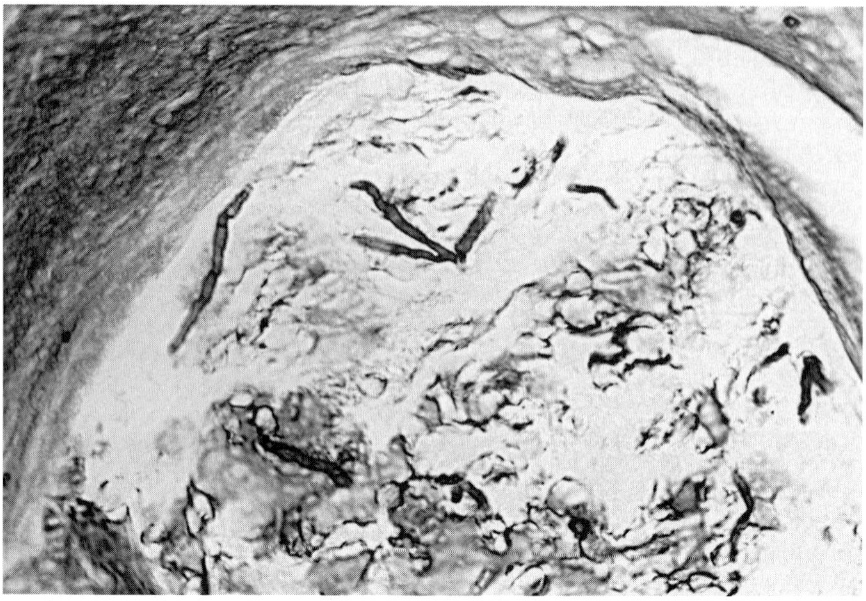

**Figure 61.2** Photomicrograph of a mucous plug in a patient with bronchopulmonary aspergillosis showing *Aspergillus* hyphae. (Grocott's stain; original magnification ×500.)

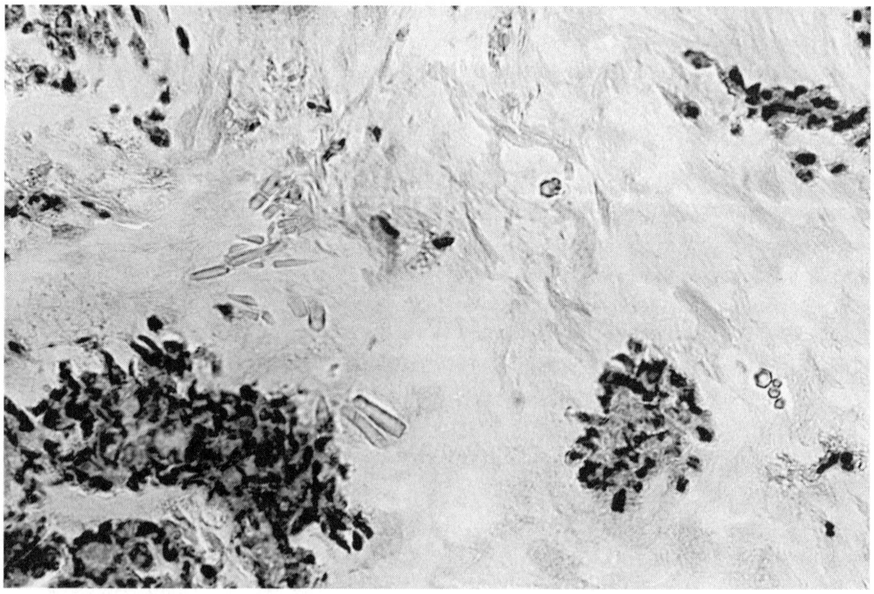

**Figure 61.3** Photomicrograph of a mucous plug in the same patient as in Figure 61.2 with bronchopulmonary aspergillosis showing Charcot-Leyden crystals. (Hematoxylin and eosin stain; original magnification ×500.)

nary collapse is found after mucous plugging of the airways (Fig. 61.4). These usually clear rapidly after steroid therapy or bronchoscopy (Fig. 61.5). However, it is this process that, if untreated, progresses to localized bronchiectasis and scarring, often in the upper lobes (Fig. 61.6 and Fig. 61.7). The radiologic features of bronchiectasis include tramline shadows caused by thickening of the walls of dilated bronchi, ring shadows due to dilated bronchi themselves, and gloved-finger shadows due to trapped distal secretions within dilated bronchi. Most patients with ABPA have radiologic features of bronchiectasis by the time the diagnosis of ABPA is made; the findings on high-resolution computed tomography of bronchiectasis affecting three or more lobes, centrilobular nodules, and mucoid impaction are said to be "highly suggestive" of ABPA.[70a] Pulmonary function testing of patients with ABPA usually reveals air flow obstruction related to underlying asthma and bronchiectasis, with reduction of lung volumes and diffusing capacity during acute episodes.[71]

Bronchocentric granulomatosis was first reported by Liebow[72] in 1973. This disorder is seen in two types of patients: those without an asthmatic history, who do not manifest a blood or pulmonary eosinophilia, and those with asthma, eosinophilia, and *Aspergillus* in their sputum and lung tissue. Katzenstein and coworkers[73] speculated that in the latter group, bronchocentric granulomatosis may represent a form of ABPA or that in vulnerable patients, both disorders may represent hypersensitivity reactions to fungi. Patients with bronchocentric granulomatosis may present with symptoms related to ABPA or underlying asthma. In addition to manifesting the radiologic signs of these disorders, they also may have mass lesions on their chest radiographs.[74] Biopsy of such lesions characteristically reveals a granulomatosis or necrotizing replacement of the bronchi.[34, 73]

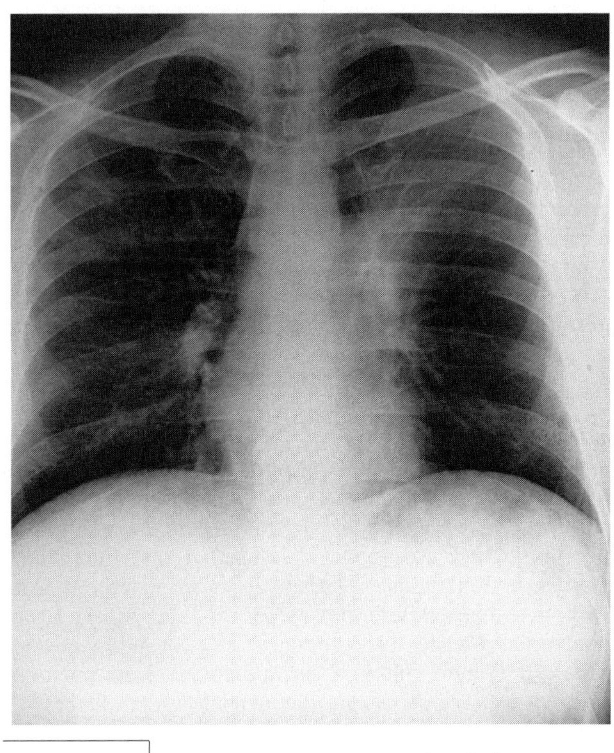

**Figure 61.4** Roentgenogram showing left upper lobe segmental collapse due to mucous plugging in an asthmatic patient with bronchopulmonary aspergillosis.

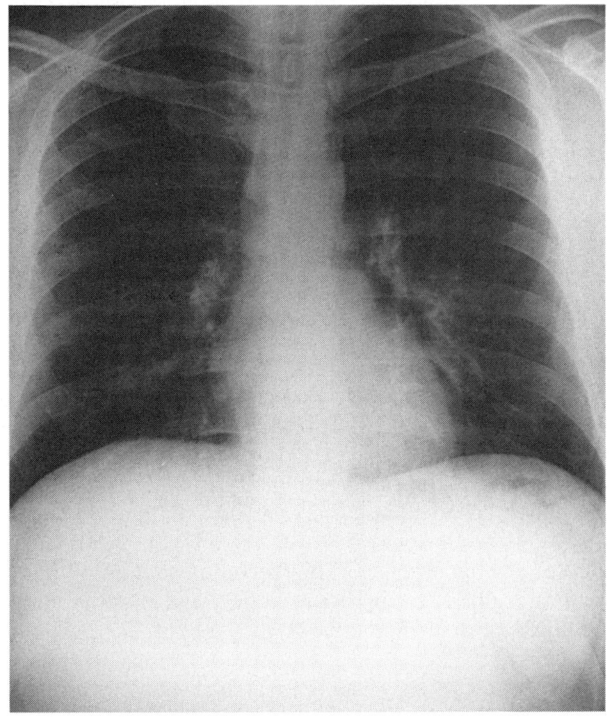

**Figure 61.5** Chest radiograph of same patient as in Figure 61.4 taken 3 weeks later after a course of oral prednisolone, showing re-expansion and clearing of the infiltrate.

Although bronchocentric granulomatosis requires a tissue diagnosis, ABPA is diagnosed by the clinical and laboratory criteria spelled out in Table 61.6. Blood eosinophilia is usually moderate, in the range of 500 to 2000 cells/μL, but occasionally high counts occur. *A. fumigatus* can be found in the sputum of most patients, but this finding is not specific for ABPA. A positive immediate reaction to skin testing with *A. fumigatus* is one of the prerequisites for ABPA, a positive reaction being a wheal of 3 mm or greater maximal diameter within 10 minutes of a skin prick test. Most patients with ABPA have strongly positive immediate reactions, often with negative reactions to other common allergens. Approximately one fifth of patients have delayed type reactions visible 3 to 5 hours after skin prick tests, but nearly all have positive delayed reactions if the *A. fumigatus* extract is injected intradermally. IgG-precipitating antibodies to *A. fumigatus* are found in more than 90% of cases. However, the finding of *Aspergillus* precipitins is not diagnostic of ABPA, because they are also found in about 1% of healthy adults, 14% of adult atopic asthmatic patients, and 20% of patients with farmer's lung.[75] As previously noted, serum IgE is often markedly elevated during acute episodes of ABPA, and serum IgE level has been used to monitor the response to therapy.[70]

The cornerstone of therapy for both ABPA and bronchocentric granulomatosis is oral corticosteroids, which presumably dampen the inflammatory response to fungi and increase the efficacy of killing by the body.[66] An oral steroid such as prednisone should be given emergently when the diagnosis is made and during subsequent exacerbations. The dose used varies widely among centers from 0.5 mg/kg per day in some patients[70] to more than 20 mg/day in others.[76] There is also no definite guide as to the duration of high-dose steroids, with some investigators suggesting 2 weeks at a high dosage before the same dosage is given every second day for 3 months.[70] Others treat at high dose until a clinical response is obtained. Response is normally assessed in terms of radiologic clearing and resolution of blood eosinophilia, but Wang and colleagues,[77] among others, advocate monitoring serum IgE levels as the best index of adequate treatment. Once an adequate initial response has been achieved, it is usual practice in some centers to continue on a low dosage of prednisone (5 to 10 mg/day) in the hope of suppressing recurrences. This recommendation is based on the results of retrospective series, and there is ample evidence that further attacks may occur despite such "suppressive" treatment.[76] On rare occasions, long-term corticosteroid therapy has been associated with dissemination of the aspergillosis.[78] In North America, there is a tendency to stop giving steroids between attacks and to monitor IgE levels as a marker of activity.[70, 77]

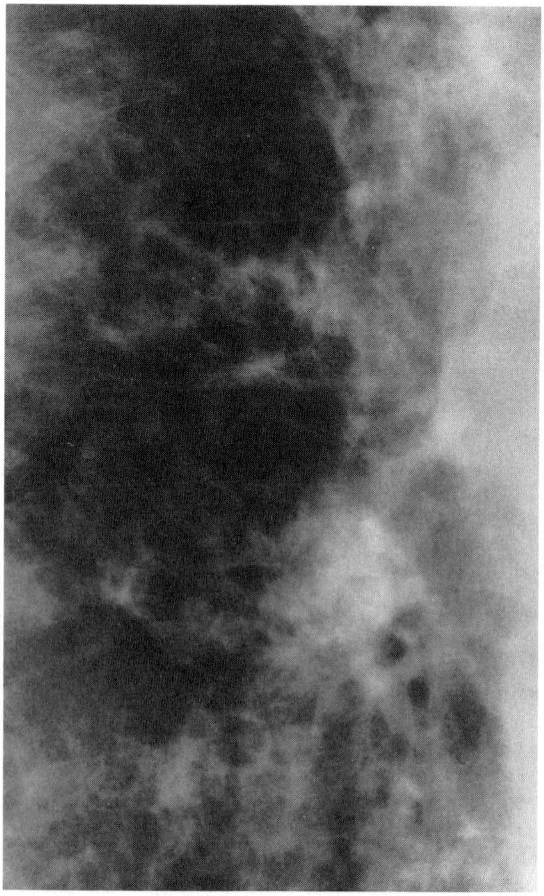

**Figure 61.6** Detail of right perihilar area on chest roentgenogram of a patient with allergic bronchopulmonary aspergillosis and marked proximal bronchiectasis showing extensive ring shadows.

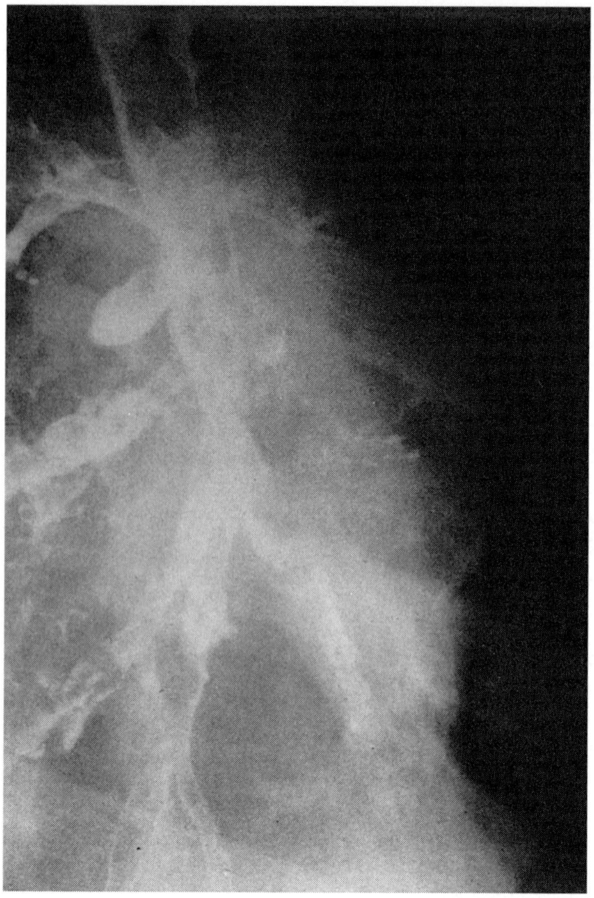

**Figure 61.7** Left-sided bronchogram in patient with proximal bronchiectasis due to allergic bronchopulmonary aspergillosis showing dilated and nontapering bronchi.

The concomitant use of antifungal agents with corticosteroids is gaining favor.[79] Preliminary results from a randomized trial showed that itraconazole, 200 mg twice daily for 16 weeks followed by 200 mg daily for an additional 16 weeks, improved clinical response and was steroid sparing.[79a]

## Chronic Eosinophilic Pneumonia

In 1968, Carrington and associates[33] coined the term *chronic eosinophilic pneumonia* to describe a condition characterized by the coexistence of blood eosinophilia with pulmonary eosinophilic infiltration for which there was no obvious cause. Diagnostic criteria derived from those investigators are presented in Table 61.7. Bronchoalveolar lavage fluid contains 25% or more eosinophils in the acute phase of chronic eosinophilic pneumonia, with normalization occurring after therapy.[34] Eosinophil-active cytokines such as IL-5 and IL-10 also are strikingly elevated in bronchoalveolar lavage fluid from radiographically involved lung segments.[80] Histologic examination reveals an interstitial and alveolar infiltrate with eosinophils, macrophages, and often multinu-

**Table 61.7** DIAGNOSTIC CRITERIA FOR CHRONIC EOSINOPHILIC PNEUMONIA

| |
|---|
| Subacute onset |
| Usually mild hypoxemia |
| Diffuse, usually peripheral radiographic infiltrates |
| Blood and lung eosinophilia |
| Absence of parasitic, fungal, or other lung infection |
| No history of drug reaction |
| Prompt and complete response to corticosteroids |
| Relapse common after corticosteroids are discontinued |

cleate giant cells (Figs. 61.8 and Fig. 61.9). The giant cells frequently contain fragments of eosinophils and small crystals, which are probably precursors of Charcot-Leyden crystals. Occasionally, large Charcot-Leyden crystals also may be found along with features of bronchiolitis obliterans and vasculitis.

Chronic eosinophilic pneumonia occurs most commonly in middle-aged women but can occur at any age in either sex. Cough with mucoid or no sputum, breathlessness, weight loss, fever, and night sweats are the main initial symptoms. Hemoptysis is an occasional feature. Patients may have lymphadenopathy and hepatomegaly. Symptoms may persist for weeks or months if adequate therapy is not given. Asthma coexists in approximately 50% of cases and, when it does, tends to be of recent onset.[81] Although blood eosinophilia is typical, in some cases, this may not occur.[33] There is usually blood neutrophilia and sometimes anemia. The erythrocyte sedimentation rate is raised, often to about 100 mm in the first hour.[82] Serum IgE levels are increased in most patients but may be normal. Eosinophilia may be detected in sputum. Circulating immune complexes may be found during attacks of chronic eosinophilic pneumonia.[82] Increased levels of eosinophilic cationic protein also are commonly found in the serum, although this increase may be found in other eosinophilic lung diseases.[83] The classical radiologic features are of peripheral pulmonary densities, which resemble the photographic negative of pulmonary edema.[84] The shadows may be isolated or widespread and often do not conform to segmental or lobar boundaries (Figs. 61.10 and Fig. 61.11). The densities may spontaneously disappear and reappear in the same or other places on the radiograph. Computed tomographic images confirm the presence of peripheral consolidation and may show hilar adenopathy.[85]

In patients in whom there is diagnostic doubt, open or thoracoscopic lung biopsy may be needed to establish the diagnosis, as was the case in five patients with bronchiolitis obliterans and organizing pneumonia who presented with clinical and radiologic features similar to those of chronic eosinophilic pneumonia.[86] Usually, however, the combination of clinical and radiologic features with blood eosinophilia is sufficient to establish a clinical diagnosis.

Corticosteroids rapidly suppress both the clinical and the radiographic abnormalities.[84] Prednisone therapy, 30 to 60 mg/day, results in radiologic improvement within 3 days and a normal chest roentgenogram within 3 weeks. The corticosteroid dosage can be gradually reduced thereafter, but with caution, because recurrence of the disease is not uncommon.[87] In one series of eight patients, the mean duration of therapy was 5 years, and six patients had been successfully weaned off steroids.[88] Long-term prognosis is good.[87]

## Acute Eosinophilic Pneumonia

Acute eosinophilic pneumonia was first described in 1989 by Allen and colleagues[89] and Badesch and colleagues.[90] The diagnostic criteria for this condition, as suggested by Allen and Davis[34] and by Pope-Harman and associates,[91] are outlined in Table 61.8. Although the cause of acute eosinophilic pneumonia is unknown, it is thought to represent a hypersensitivity reaction to unidentified inhaled antigens.[90] Patients with the condition may be of either gender and of any age, with a range of 13 years[92] to 86 years[93] having been reported. They typically present with symptoms lasting a few hours to a few days, fever that

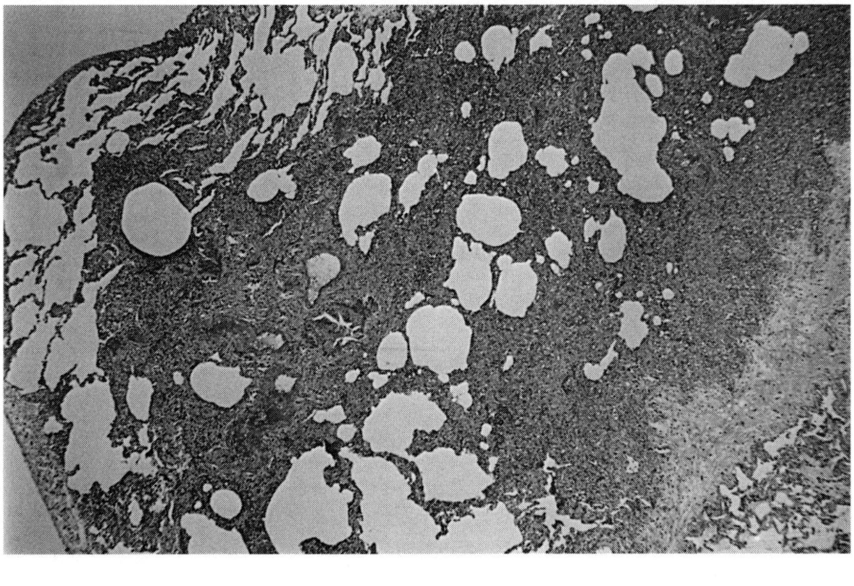

**Figure 61.8** Low-power view of lung tissue obtained from a patient with chronic eosinophilic pneumonia at autopsy showing extensive infiltration with eosinophils and macrophages. (Original magnification ×40.)

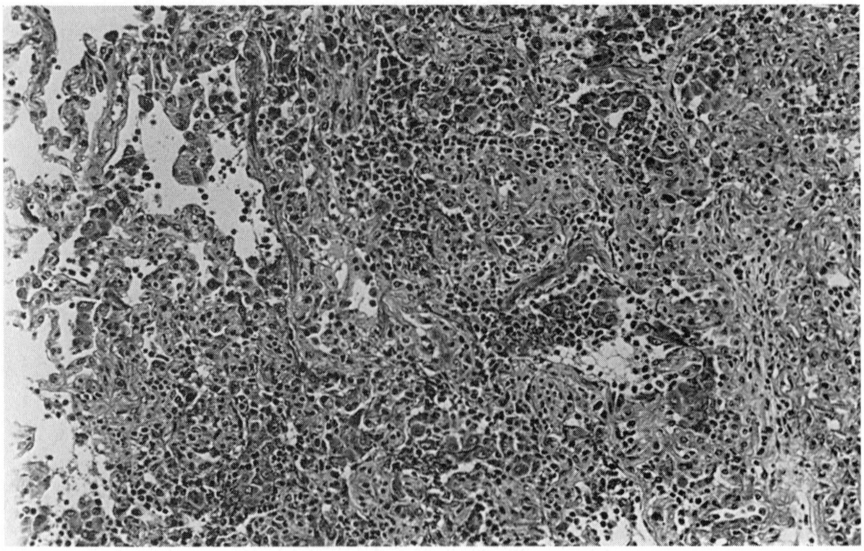

**Figure 61.9** High-power view of the same specimen as in Figure 61.10 demonstrating prominent type II cells, eosinophils, and macrophages in the infiltrate. (Original magnification ×250.)

may be very high, myalgias, and hypoxemia that is so severe that mechanical ventilation may be required.[34] The white blood cell count usually is elevated, but peripheral blood eosinophilia occurs in only one third of patients.[91] For the diagnostic criteria in Table 61.6 to be met, concurrent infection or drug reaction cannot be present.

Chest radiographs in patients with acute eosinophilic pneumonia may progress from minimal infiltrates to diffuse disease.[94] Usually, these infiltrates are not peripheral, in contrast to chronic eosinophilic pneumonia.[95] Computed tomography reveals diffuse parenchymal infiltrates, pleural effusions, and normal lymph nodes. Pulmonary function testing reveals restriction, a low diffusing capacity, and no evidence of obstruction.[34] The bronchoalveolar lavage fluid of patients with acute eosinophilic pneumonia contains large numbers of eosinophils and high concentrations of IL-5 and adhesion molecules, all of which decrease after treatment.[96] As described by Tazelaar and coworkers,[97] lung biopsy specimens contain mononuclear cells, especially eosinophils, in the interstitium and alveoli, accompanied by hyaline membranes and other features of diffuse alveolar damage, the histologic counterpart of the acute respiratory distress syndrome.

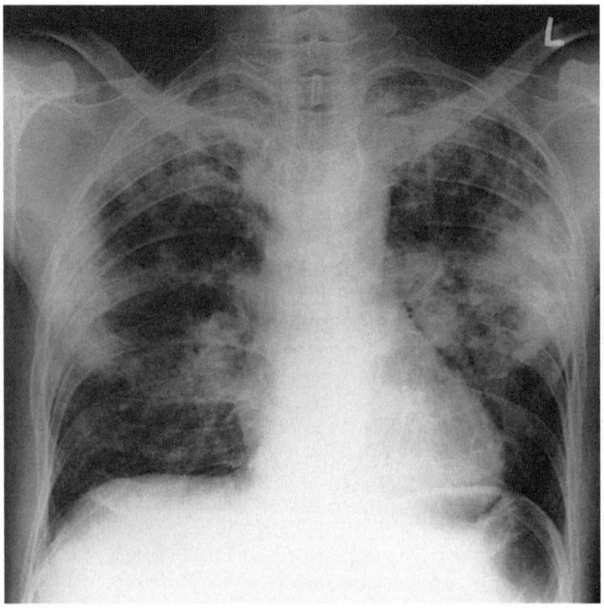

**Figure 61.10** Chest roentgenogram showing extensive peripheral shadowing in a 50-year-old man whose initial symptoms were fever, night sweats, and unproductive cough. Transbronchial biopsy demonstrated chronic eosinophilic pneumonia.

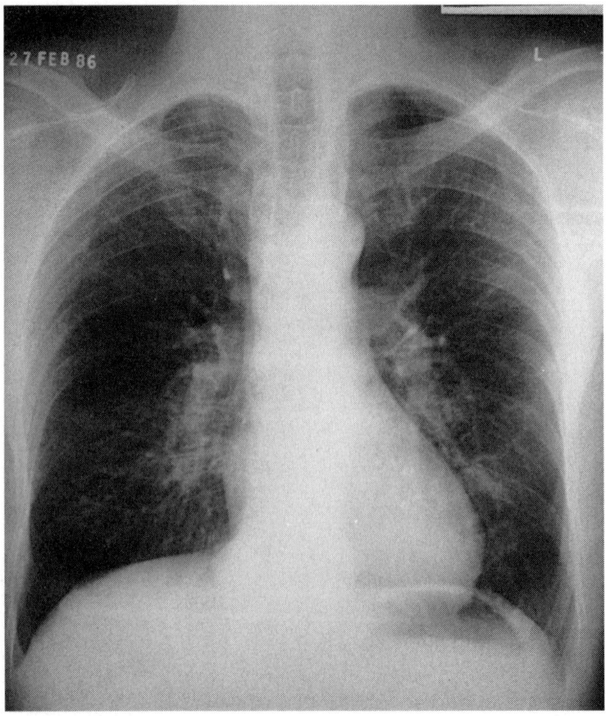


**Figure 61.11** Chest roentgenogram of the same patient as in Figure 61.10, 2 weeks later after a course of oral prednisolone showing marked clearing.

**Table 61.8 DIAGNOSTIC CRITERIA FOR ACUTE EOSINOPHILIC PNEUMONIA**

| |
|---|
| Acute febrile illness |
| Severe hypoxemia |
| Diffuse chest radiographic infiltrates |
| Greater than 25% eosinophils in bronchoalveolar lavage fluid |
| Absence of parasitic, fungal, and other lung infections |
| No history of drug reaction |
| Prompt and complete response to corticosteroids |
| Failure to relapse after corticosteroids are discontinued |

Patients with acute eosinophilic pneumonia usually respond to high doses of corticosteroids, such as 60 to 125 mg of methylprednisolone every 6 hours, within 24 to 48 hours.[34] Because of this, and because the diagnosis of acute eosinophilic pneumonia cannot be made before infections have been ruled out, patients suspected of having acute eosinophilic pneumonia generally should undergo bronchoalveolar lavage or lung biopsy before treatment is begun. After respiratory failure resolves, corticosteroids can be tapered over a 2- to 4-week period. Then, patients should not experience remission unless they have another condition, including chronic eosinophilic pneumonia. Although all patients with acute eosinophilic pneumonia probably should be treated once this diagnosis is made, spontaneous remission of the disease has been reported.[95]

## Hypereosinophilic Syndrome

The hypereosinophilic syndrome was first discussed in detail by Harding and Anderson[98] in 1965; subsequent series were reviewed by Chusid and coworkers[99] in 1975, Fauci and colleagues[100] in 1982, and Spry and coworkers[101] in 1983. The generally accepted diagnostic criteria listed in Table 61.9 were derived from the review of Fauci and associates.[100] They include persistent blood eosinophilia (1500 eosinophils/μL or more) for a prolonged period (or death before eosinophilia can become prolonged), no evidence of another reason for the eosinophilia, and evidence of tissue organ invasion by, and dysfunction because of, eosinophils. The cause of the hypereosinophilic syndrome is unknown, and it is a different clinical entity than the eosinophilic leukemias.[102, 103] Nevertheless, the hypereosinophilic syndrome probably results from T-lymphocyte clonal proliferation in response to unidentified stimuli.[104, 105]

**Table 61.9 DIAGNOSTIC CRITERIA FOR THE HYPEREOSINOPHILIC SYNDROME**

| |
|---|
| Blood eosinophilia for ≥6 months or death before 6 months with appropriate signs and symptoms |
| No evidence of parasites, allergies, or other causes of eosinophilia |
| Signs and symptoms of organ system damage or dysfunction related to eosinophilia |

After reviewing 150 of the first recognized cases, Spry and associates[101] found a 9:1 male dominance among patients with the hypereosinophilic syndrome, with an average onset in the fourth decade. The usual presenting features are fever, anorexia, and weight loss in association with symptoms referable to affected systems. The heart is involved in 60% of cases, with dysrhythmias, cardiac failure, and mitral and tricuspid valve incompetence.[99, 100] Thromboembolic disease is present in two thirds of the patients and hypertension and proteinuria in some. The lungs are involved in about half the patients, many of whom have cough as a prominent feature. Pulmonary consolidation and pleural effusions can occur, and both the infiltrate and the liquid have high eosinophil contents. Winn and colleagues[106] described a patient with ARDS that was attributable to the hypereosinophilic syndrome. Focal neurologic abnormalities may result from thromboembolism or vasculitis, and generalized intellectual deterioration and peripheral neuropathy can also occur. Abdominal pain, polyarthropathy, muscle weakness, and rashes are among the nonspecific presentations. Marked blood eosinophilia is usual, with an average of 20,000 cells/μL, but counts up to 180,000/μL have been recorded. The eosinophils have high levels of eosinophilic cationic protein with increased vacuolization on the peripheral blood smear.[101] There are also greatly increased numbers of the eosinophil series in the bone marrow.

Early studies described a mortality of 77% at 3 years in patients with the hypereosinophilic syndrome. In 1978, however, Parrillo and coworkers[107] reported that of 26 patients with the syndrome, 5 showed no evidence of progressive organ-system dysfunction without treatment, and 6 of 16 treated with corticosteroids had a good response and needed no further therapy. Of eight patients who did not respond to corticosteroids, hydroxyurea produced excellent responses in six and partial responses in two. Overall, the mortality rate among the 26 patients was only 4% at 3 years. Alfa interferon has proved useful in patients who fail to respond to conventional therapy and in patients who are unable to tolerate corticosteroids and those with peptic ulcers.[108, 109] In addition, anticoagulants should be used in patients with thromboembolic disease.

## Allergic Granulomatosis and Angiitis

In 1951, Churg and Strauss[110] described 13 patients with asthma, fever, blood eosinophilia, and clinical evidence of vasculitis involving many organs. Pathologic examination revealed necrotizing eosinophilia and granulomatous vascular changes in addition to extravascular granulomatous lesions. The patients differed from those with polyarteritis nodosa by virtue of their asthma, eosinophilia, and granulomatosis. Churg and Strauss called this disorder *allergic granulomatosis and angiitis*, but it is commonly known as the *Churg-Strauss syndrome*. The diagnostic criteria for this combination are listed in Table 61.10. The presence of these criteria are 85% sensitive and 100% specific for the disease.[111]

Patients with allergic granulomatosis and angiitis usually have asthma and rhinitis or sinusitis for 8 or more years before they develop profound eosinophilia and in-

**Table 61.10** DIAGNOSTIC CRITERIA FOR ALLERGIC GRANULOMATOSIS AND ANGIITIS

| |
|---|
| Asthma |
| Blood eosinophilia > 10% |
| Mononeuropathy or polyneuropathy |
| Chest radiographic infiltrates |
| Paranasal sinus abnormalities |
| Biopsy containing a blood vessel with extravascular eosinophils |

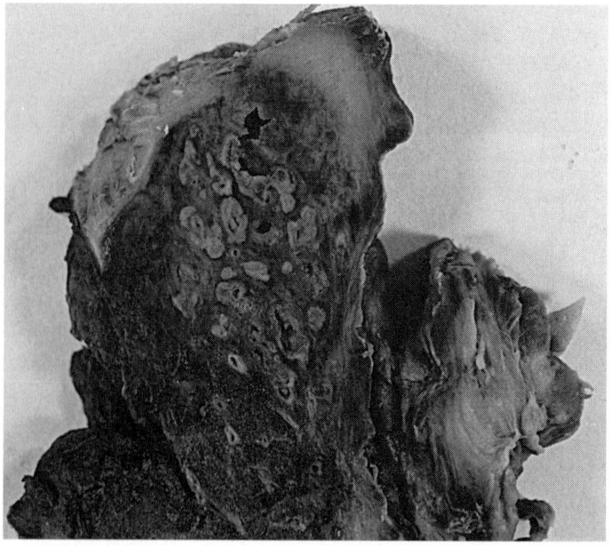

**Figure 61.12** Macroscopic view of resected specimen of lung from a patient with Churg-Strauss syndrome. Note extensive infiltration with granulomatous lesions around the airways.

filtration of organs with eosinophils.[34] Depending on the organ involved, patients may have rashes or nodules, abdominal pain, gastrointestinal bleeding, heart failure, renal insufficiency or failure, single or multiple peripheral nerve deficits, and central nervous system involvement. In a series of 96 patients with Churg-Strauss syndrome, asthma was the most commonly observed manifestation at presentation and mononeuritis multiplex was the second.[111a] Chest radiographs commonly show patchy transient infiltrates or small nodules. Computed tomography reveals nonspecific parenchymal infiltration and nodules.[112] Findings on lung biopsy, which has long been the diagnostic gold standard, include a combination of asthmatic changes with those of eosinophilic pneumonia and also vasculitis and necrotizing granulomas (Figs. 61.12 and 61.13). The eosinophilic vasculitis predominantly affects small and medium-sized arteries and can be found in vessels in other involved organs.

Without treatment, most patients with allergic granulomatosis and angiitis die within months, but the prognosis has improved considerably as a result of early diagnosis and rapid initiation of therapy.[111a, 113] A mean length of survival of 9 years has been reported in patients treated with corticosteroids.[114] Prednisone is customarily given in 40- to 60-mg doses a day for several weeks for treatment of vasculitis; longer courses may be necessary for patients with peripheral or central nervous involvement. Prednisone is continued thereafter at lower doses for up to a year.[34, 115] Patients who do not respond to corticosteroids may benefit from cyclophosphamide[116] or alfa interferon.[117] The presence of renal insufficiency or failure is a poor prognostic sign.[113] Hypertension may be difficult to treat and may persist in patients with Churg-Strauss syndrome.[115]

An interesting association has been made between certain leukotriene receptor antagonists, zafirlukast and montelukast, when used for the treatment of asthma and the development of Churg-Strauss syndrome.[118] The connection between the two events is by no means clear. One theory holds that previously inapparent Churg-Strauss syndrome manifests itself as corticosteroids are withdrawn owing to the steroid-sparing effects of the leuko-

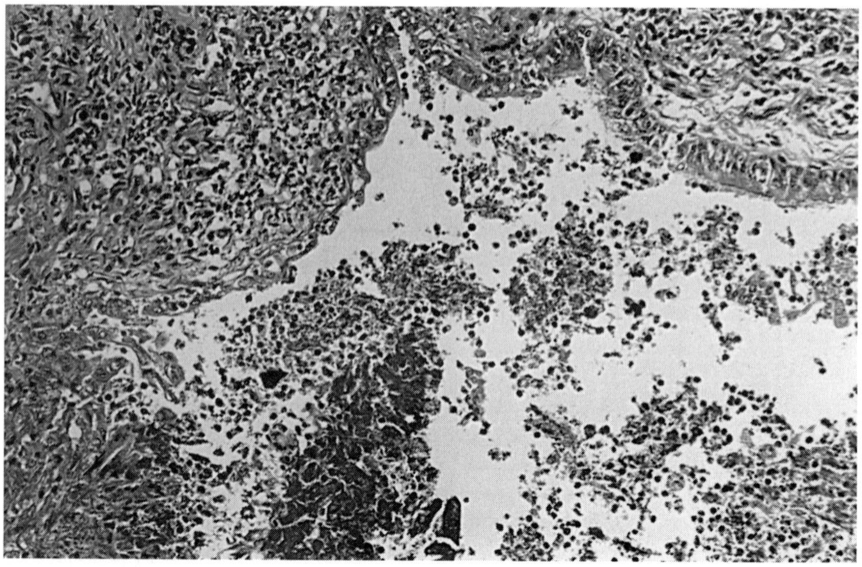

**Figure 61.13** Microscopic view of the same specimen as shown in Figure 61.12 illustrating epithelial destruction and granuloma formation. The dark staining area represents principally eosinophil debris. (Hematoxylin and eosin stain; original magnification ×250.)

triene antagonists[119]; Churg-Strauss syndrome has developed, however, in two patients given zafirlukast who were not receiving corticosteroids.[120] Further experience should define whether this occurrence represents an unmasking of a forme fruste of Churg-Strauss syndrome or a particular type of drug toxicity; meanwhile, however, physicians should know that leukotriene antagonists may possess unique immunologic and eosinophilic properties.

## SUMMARY

The eosinophil is a cell with diverse biologic functions. Eosinophils are major participants in defenses against metazoan parasites, and they may also enhance or inhibit immediate hypersensitivity reactions. Although the pathogenetic mechanisms in the various pulmonary eosinophilic diseases are poorly understood, aberrant hypersensitivity responses appear to play an important role in all of them. Several classifications of eosinophilic lung disease have been suggested, but none is satisfactory. Parasitic infections, drug and chemical reactions, ABPA, chronic eosinophilic pneumonia, acute eosinophilic pneumonia, hypereosinophilic syndrome, and allergic granulomatosis and angiitis all demonstrate tissue eosinophilic infiltration and/or circulating eosinophilia, but they manifest strikingly different clinical, diagnostic, therapeutic, and prognostic features. More information is needed to better characterize these remarkable disorders.

## References


1. Wardlaw AJ, Moqbel R, Kay AB: Eosinophils: Biology and role in disease. Adv Immunol 60:151–266, 1995.
2. Weller PF: Human eosinophils. J Allergy Clin Immunol 100:283–287, 1997.
3. Weller PF, Goetzl EJ: The human eosinophil: Roles in host defense and tissue injury. Am J Pathol 100:793–820, 1980.
4. Henderson WR Jr: Lipid-derived and other chemical mediators of inflammation in the lung. J Allergy Clin Immunol 79:543–553, 1987.
5. Parish WE, Luckhurst E: Eosinophilia VI: Spontaneous synthesis of chemokinetic, chemotactic, and complement receptor-inducing activities for eosinophils by bronchial T-lymphocytes of asthmatic-bronchitic patients. Clin Allergy 12:475–488, 1982.
6. Parwaresch MR, Walle AJ, Arndt D: The peripheral kinetics of human radiolabelled eosinophils. Virchows Arch 21:57–66, 1976.
7. Hudson G: Quantitative study of the eosinophil granulocytes. Semin Hematol 5:166–186, 1968.
8. Clutterbuck EJ, Sanderson CJ: Regulation of human eosinophil precursor production by cytokines: A comparison of recombinant human interleukin-1 (rhIL-1), rhIL-3, rhIL-5, rhIL-6, and rh granulocyte-macrophage colony-stimulating factor. Blood 75:1774–1782, 1990.
9. Enokihara H, Furusawa S, Nakakubo H, et al: T cells from eosinophilic patients produce interleukin-5 with interleukin-2 stimulation. Blood 73:1809–1813, 1989.
10. Dent LA, Strath M, Mellor AL, et al: Eosinophilia in transgenic mice expressing interleukin-5. J Exp Med 172:1425–1431, 1990.
11. Owen WF, Rothenberg ME, Peterson J, et al: Interleukin-5 and phenotypically altered eosinophils in the blood of patients with the idiopathic hypereosinophilic syndrome. J Exp Med 170:343–348, 1989.

11a. Simon H-U, Plötz SG, Dummer R, et al: Abnormal clones of T cells producing interleukin-5 in idiopathic eosinophilia. N Engl J Med 341:1112–1120, 1999.

12. Dobrina A, Mengazzi R, Carlos TM, et al: Mechanisms of eosinophil adherence to cultured vascular endothelial cells: Eosinophils bind to the cytokine-induced endothelial ligand vascular cell adhesion molecule-1 via the late activation antigen-4 integrin receptor. J Clin Invest 88:20–26, 1991.
13. Weller PF, Rand TH, Goelz SE, et al: Human eosinophil adherence to vascular endothelium mediated by binding to vascular cell adhesion molecule 1 and endothelial leukocyte adhesion molecule 1. Proc Natl Acad Sci USA 88:7430–7433, 1991.
14. Ackerman SJ, Gleich GJ, Loegering DA, et al: Comparative toxicity of purified human eosinophil granule cationic proteins for schistosomula of *Schistosoma mansoni*. Am J Trop Med Hyg 34:735–745, 1985.
15. Rosenberg HF, Dyer KD: Eosinophil cationic protein and eosinophil-derived neurotoxin: Evolution of novel function in a primate ribonuclease gene family. J Biol Chem 270:21539–21544, 1995.
16. Olszewska-Pazdrak B, Pazdrak K, Ogra PL, et al: Respiratory syncytial virus-infected pulmonary epithelial cells induce eosinophil degranulation by a CD18-mediated mechanism. J Immunol 160:4889–4895, 1998.
17. Graziano RF, Looney RA, Shen L, et al: Fc gamma R–mediated killing by eosinophils. J Immunol 142:230–235, 1989.
18. Rand TH, Cruikshank WW, Center DM, et al: CD4-mediated stimulation of human eosinophils: Lymphocyte chemoattractant factor and other CD4-binding ligands elicit eosinophil migration. J Exp Med 173:1521–1528, 1991.
19. Turk J, Mass RL, Brash AR, et al: Arachidonic acid 15-lipoxygenase products from human eosinophils. J Biol Chem 257:7056–7067, 1982.
20. Weinstock JV, Blum A, Walder J, et al: Eosinophils from granulomas in murine schistosomiasis mansoni produce substance P. J Immunol 141:961–966, 1988.
21. Rochester CL, Ackerman SJ, Zheng T, et al: Eosinophil-fibroblast interactions: Granule major basic protein interacts with IL-1 and transforming growth factor-beta in the stimulation of lung fibroblast IL-6-type cytokine production. J Immunol 156:4449–4456, 1996.
22. Ponath PD, Qin S, Ringler DJ, et al: Cloning of the human eosinophil chemoattractant, eotaxin. J Clin Invest 97:604–612, 1996.
23. Lilly CM, Nakamura H, Kesselman H, et al: Expression of eotaxin by human lung epithelial cells: Induction by cytokines and inhibition by glucocorticoids. J Clin Invest 99:1767–1773, 1997.
24. Simon H-U, Yousefi S, Schranz C, et al: Direct demonstration of delayed eosinophil apoptosis as a mechanism causing tissue eosinophilia. J Immunol 158:3902–3908, 1997
25. Winqvist I, Olofsson T, Olsson I, et al: Altered density, metabolism and surface receptors of eosinophils in eosinophilia. Immunology 47:531–539, 1982.
26. Frick WE, Sedgwick JB, Busse WW: The appearance of hypodense eosinophils in antigen-dependent late phase asthma. Am Rev Respir Dis 139:1401–1406, 1989.
27. Lundgren JD, Davey RT Jr, Lundgren B: Eosinophil cationic protein stimulates and major basic protein inhibits airway mucus secretion. J Allergy Clin Immunol 87:689–698, 1991.
28. Löffler W: Zur Differential-Diagnose der Lungeninfiltrierungen. II Über flüchtige Succedan-Infiltrate (mir Eosinophilia). Beitr Klin Tuberk 79:368–392, 1932.
29. Weingarten RJ: Tropical eosinophilia. Lancet 1:103–105, 1943.
30. Reeder WH, Goodrich BE: Pulmonary infiltration with eosinophilia (PIE syndrome). Ann Intern Med 36:1217–1240, 1952.
31. Crofton JW, Livingstone JL, Oswald NC, et al: Pulmonary eosinophilia. Thorax 7:1–35, 1952.
32. Liebow AA, Carrington CB: The eosinophilic pneumonias. Medicine (Baltimore) 48:251–285, 1969.
33. Carrington CB, Addington WW, Goff AM, et al: Chronic eosinophilic pneumonia. N Engl J Med 280:787–798, 1969.
34. Allen JN, Davis WB: Eosinophilic lung diseases. Am J Respir Crit Care Med 150:1423–1438, 1994.
35. Barnes PJ: A new approach to the treatment of asthma. N Engl J Med 321:1517–1527, 1989.

35a. Brightling CE, Ward R, Goh K, et al: Eosinophilic bronchitis is an important cause of chronic cough. Am J Respir Crit Care Med 160:406–410, 1999.

36. Nogami M, Suko M, Odudaira H, et al: Experimental pulmonary eosinophilia in mice by *Ascaris suum* extract. Am Rev Respir Dis 141:1289–1295, 1990.
37. Neva FA, Ottersen EA: Current concepts in parasitology: Tropical (filarial) eosinophilia. N Engl J Med 298:1129–1131, 1978.

38. Ho D, Tashkin DP, Bein ME, et al: Pulmonary infiltrates with eosinophilia associated with tetracycline. Chest 76:33–36, 1979.
39. Davies D, Lloyd-Jones JK: Pulmonary eosinophilia caused by penicillamine. Thorax 35:957–958, 1980.
40. Nadir DA, Schillaci RF: Pulmonary infiltrates with eosinophilia due to naproxen. Chest 83:280–282, 1983.
41. Stephen WC, Parks RD, Tempest B: Acute hypersensitivity pneumonitis associated with carbamazepine therapy. Chest 74:463–464, 1978.
42. Nadeem S, Nasir N, Israel RH: Löffler's syndrome secondary to crack cocaine. Chest 105:1599–1600, 1994.
43. Janier M, Guilleuin L, Badellet G: Pulmonary eosinophilia associated with dapsone. Lancet 434:860–861, 1994.
44. Dykhuizen RS, Zaidi AM, Godden DJ, et al: Minocycline and pulmonary eosinophilia. BMJ 310:1520–1521, 1995.
45. Seebach J, Speich R, Fehr J, et al: GM-CSF-induced acute eosinophilic pneumonia. Br J Haematol 90:963–965, 1995.
46. Rich MW, Thomas RA: A case of eosinophilic pneumonia and vasculitis induced by diflunisal. Chest 111:1767–1769, 1997.
47. Schwarz YA, Kivity S, Fischbein A, et al: Eosinophilic lung reaction to aluminium and hard metal. Chest 105:1261–1263, 1994.
48. Mahatma M, Haponik EF, Nelson S, et al: Phenytoin-induced acute respiratory failure with pulmonary eosinophilia. Am J Med 87:93–94, 1989.
49. Salerno SM, Strong JS, Roth BJ, et al: Eosinophilic pneumonia and respiratory failure associated with a trazodone overdose. Am J Respir Crit Care Med 152:2170–2172, 1995.
50. Hailey WJ, Glascock HW, Hewitt WF: Pleuropneumonia reaction to nitrofurantoin. N Engl J Med 281:1087–1090, 1969.
51. Holmberg L, Boman G, Bottiger IE, et al: Reverse reactions to nitrofurantoin: Analysis of 921 reports. Am J Med 69:733–738, 1980.
52. Robinson BWS: Nitrofurantoin-induced interstitial pulmonary fibrosis. Med J Aust 1:72–76, 1983.
53. Hertzman PA, Blevins WL, Mayer J, et al: Association of the eosinophilia-myalgia syndrome with the ingestion of tryptophan. N Engl J Med 322:869–873, 1990.
54. Martin RW, Duffy J, Engel AG, et al: The clinical spectrum of the eosinophilia-myalgia syndrome associated with L-tryptophan ingestion: Clinical features in 20 patients and aspects of pathophysiology. Ann Intern Med 113:124–134, 1990.
55. Tazetaar HD, Myers JL, Drage CW, et al: Pulmonary disease associated with L-tryptophan induced eosinophilic myalgia syndrome: Clinical and pathological features. Chest 97:1032–1036, 1990.
56. Belongia EA, Hedberg CW, Gleich GJ, et al. An investigation of the cause of the eosinophilia-myalgia syndrome associated with tryptophan use. N Engl J Med 323:357–365, 1990.
57. Hinson KFW, Moon AJ, Plummer NS: Broncho-pulmonary aspergillosis: A review and a report of eight new cases. Thorax 7:317–333, 1952.
58. Slavin RG, Stanczyk DJ, Lonigro AJ, et al: Allergic bronchopulmonary aspergillosis: A North American rarity. Am J Med 47:306–313, 1969.
59. Laufer P, Fink JN, Bruno WT, et al: Allergic bronchopulmonary aspergillosis in cystic fibrosis. J Allergy Clin Immunol 73:44–48, 1984.
59a. Geller DE, Kaplowitz H, Light MJ, et al: Allergic bronchopulmonary aspergillosis in cystic fibrosis: Reported prevalence, regional distribution, and patient characteristics. Chest 116:639–646, 1999.
60. Rosenberg M, Patterson R, Mintzer R, et al: Clinical and immunologic criteria for the diagnosis of allergic bronchopulmonary aspergillosis. Ann Intern Med 86:405–414, 1977.
61. Backman KS, Roberts M, Patterson R: Allergic bronchopulmonary mycosis caused by *Fusarium vasinfectum*. Am J Respir Crit Care Med 152:1379–1381, 1995.
62. Patterson R, Fink JN, Pruzansky JJ, et al: Serum immunoglobulin levels in pulmonary allergic aspergillosis and certain other lung diseases with specific reference to immunoglobulin E. Am J Med 54:16–22, 1973.
63. Tomee JFC, Dubois AEJ, Koëter GH, et al: Specific IgG4 responses during chronic and transient antigen exposure in aspergillosis. Am J Respir Crit Care Med 153:1952–1957, 1996.
64. Chauhan B, Santiago L, Kirschmann DA, et al: The association of HLA-DR alleles and T cell activation with allergic bronchopulmonary aspergillosis. J Immunol 159:4072–4076, 1997.
65. Chauhan B, Knutsen AP, Hutcheson PS, et al: T cell subsets, epitope mapping, and HLA-restriction in patients with allergic bronchopulmonary aspergillosis. J Clin Invest 97:2324–2331, 1996.
66. Kauffman HF, Tomee JFC, van der Werf TS, et al: Review of fungus-induced asthmatic reactions. Am J Respir Crit Care Med 151:2109–2116, 1995.
67. Greenberger PA: Immunologic aspects of lung diseases and cystic fibrosis. JAMA 278:1924–1930, 1997.
68. Safirstein BH, D'Souza MF, Simon G, et al: Five year follow-up of allergic bronchopulmonary aspergillosis. Am Rev Respir Dis 108:450–459, 1973.
69. Gilbert R, Patterson R: Pulmonary allergic aspergillosis. Ann Intern Med 72:395–403, 1970.
70. Patterson R, Greenberger PA, Halwig JM, et al: Allergic bronchopulmonary aspergillosis: Natural history and classification of early disease by serologic and roentgenographic studies. Arch Intern Med 146:916–918, 1986.
70a. Ward S, Heyneman L, Lee MJ, et al: Accuracy of CT in the diagnosis of allergic bronchopulmonary aspergillosis. AJR Am J Roentgenol 173:937–942, 1999.
71. Nichols D, Dopico GA, Braun S, et al: Acute and chronic pulmonary function changes in allergic bronchopulmonary aspergillosis. Am J Med 67:631–637, 1979.
72. Liebow AA: Pulmonary angiitis and granulomatosis. Am Rev Respir Dis 108:1–18, 1973.
73. Katzenstein AL, Liebow AA, Friedman PJ: Bronchocentric granulomatosis, mucoid impaction, and hypersensitivity reactions to fungi. Am Rev Respir Dis 111:497–537, 1975.
74. Robinson RG, Wehunt WD, Tsou E, et al: Bronchocentric granulomatosis: Roentgenographic manifestations. Am Rev Respir Dis 125:751–756, 1982.
75. Hoehne JH, Reed CE, Bickie HA: Allergic bronchopulmonary aspergillosis is not rare. Chest 63:177–181, 1973.
76. Capewell S, Chapman BJ, Alexander F, et al: Corticosteroid treatment and prognosis in pulmonary eosinophilia. Thorax 44:925–929, 1989.
77. Wang JLF, Patterson R, Roberts M, et al: The management of allergic bronchopulmonary aspergillosis. Am Rev Respir Dis 120:87–92, 1979.
78. Bodey GP, Glann AS: Central nervous system aspergillosis following steroidal therapy for allergic bronchopulmonary aspergillosis. Chest 103:299–301, 1993.
79. Leon EE, Craig TJ: Antifungals in the treatment of allergic bronchopulmonary aspergillosis. Ann Allergy Asthma Immunol 82:511–516, 1999.
79a. Stevens DA, Lee JY, Jerome D, et al: Randomized double-blind study of itraconazole in allergic bronchopulmonary aspergillosis (abstract). Interscience Conference on Antimicrobial Agents and Chemotherapy, Toronto, Canada, September 1997.
80. Kita H, Sur S, Hunt LW, et al: Cytokine production at the site of disease in chronic eosinophilic pneumonitis. Am J Respir Crit Care Med 153:1437–1441, 1996.
81. Fox B, Seed W: Chronic eosinophilic pneumonia. Thorax 35:570–580, 1980.
82. Demedts M, DeMan F: Circulating immune complexes in chronic eosinophilic pneumonia. Acta Clin Belg 46:75–81, 1991.
83. Shijubo N, Shigehara K, Hirasawa M, et al: Eosinophilic cationic protein in chronic eosinophilic pneumonia and eosinophilic granuloma. Chest 106:1481–1486, 1994.
84. Gaensler EA, Carrington CB: Peripheral opacities in chronic eosinophilic pneumonia: The photographic negative of pulmonary oedema. AJR Am J Roentgenol 128:1–13, 1973.
85. Mayo JR, Mubler NL, Road J, et al: Chronic eosinophilic pneumonia: CT findings in six cases. AJR Am J Roentgenol 153:727–730, 1989.
86. Bartter T, Irwin RS, Nash G, et al: Idiopathic bronchiolitis obliterans organizing pneumonia with peripheral infiltrates on chest roentgenogram. Arch Intern Med 149:273–279, 1989.
87. Naughton M, Fahy J, FitzGerald MX: Chronic eosinophilic pneumonia: A long-term follow-up of 12 patients. Chest 103:162–165, 1993.
88. Pearson DJ, Rosenow EC: Chronic eosinophilic pneumonia (Carrington's): A follow-up study. Mayo Clin Proc 53:73–78, 1978.

89. Allen JN, Pacht ER, Gadek JE, et al: Acute eosinophilic pneumonia as a reversible cause of noninfectious respiratory failure. N Engl J Med 321:569–574, 1989.
90. Badesch DB, King TE, Schwarz MI: Acute eosinophilic pneumonia: A hypersensitivity phenomenon? Am Rev Respir Dis 139:249–252, 1989.
91. Pope-Harman AL, Davis WB, Allen ED, et al: Acute eosinophilic pneumonia: A summary of 15 cases and review of the literature. Medicine (Baltimore) 75:334–342, 1996.
92. Bucheit J, Eid N, Rodgers G, et al: Acute eosinophilic pneumonia with respiratory failure: A new syndrome? Am Rev Respir Dis 145:716–718, 1992.
93. Iwami T, Umemoto S, Ikeda K, et al: A case of acute eosinophilic pneumonia: Evidence for hypersensitivity-like pulmonary reaction. Chest 110:1618–1621, 1996.
94. King MA, Pope-Harman AL, Allen JN, et al: Acute eosinophilic pneumonia: Radiologic and clinical features. Radiology 203:715–719, 1997.
95. Hayakawa H, Sato A, Toyoshima M, et al: A clinical study of idiopathic eosinophilic pneumonia. Chest 105:1462–1466, 1994.
96. Okubo Y, Hossain M, Kai R, et al: Adhesion molecules on eosinophiles in acute eosinophilic pneumonia. Am J Respir Crit Care Med 151:1259–1262, 1995.
97. Tazelaar HD, Linz LJ, Colby TV, et al: Acute eosinophilic pneumonia: Histopathologic findings in nine patients. Am J Respir Crit Care Med 155:296–302, 1997.
98. Hardy WR, Anderson RE: The hypereosinophilic syndromes. Ann Intern Med 68:1003–1010, 1965.
99. Chusid MJ, Dale DC, West BC, et al: The hypereosinophilic syndrome: Analysis of fourteen cases with review of the literature. Medicine (Baltimore) 54:1–27, 1975.
100. Fauci AS, Harley JB, Roberts WC, et al: The idiopathic hypereosinophilic syndrome: Clinical, pathophysiologic, and therapeutic considerations. Ann Intern Med 97:78–92, 1982.
101. Spry CJF, Davies J, Tar PC, et al: Clinical features of 15 patients with the hypereosinophilic syndrome. Q J Med 52:1–22, 1983.
102. Bain BJ: Eosinophilic leukaemias and the idiopathic hypereosinophilic syndrome. Br J Haematology 95:2–9, 1996.
103. Weide R, Rieder H, Mehraein Y, et al: Chronic eosinophilic leukaemia (CEL): A distinct myeloproliferative disease. Br J Haematol 96:117–123, 1997.
104. Logan E, Schandene L, Crusiaux A, et al: Brief report: Clonal proliferation of type 2 helper T cells in a man with the hypereosinophilic syndrome. N Engl J Med 330:535–538, 1994.
105. Malbrain MLNG, Van den Bergh H, Zachée P: Further evidence for the clonal nature of the idiopathic hypereosinophilic syndrome: Complete haematological and cytogenetic remission induced by interferon-alpha in a case with a unique chromosomal abnormality. Br J Haematol 92:176–183, 1996.
106. Winn RE, Kollef MH, Meyer JI: Pulmonary involvement in the hypereosinophilic syndrome. Chest 105:656–660, 1994.
107. Parrillo JE, Fauci AS, Wolff SM: Therapy of the hypereosinophilic syndrome. Ann Intern Med 89:167–172, 1978.
108. Canonica GW, Passalacqua G, Pronzato C, et al: Effective long-term alpha-interferon treatment for hypereosinophilic syndrome. J Allergy Clin Immunol 96:131–133, 1995.
109. Butterfield JH, Gleich GJ: Interferon-alpha treatment of six patients with the idiopathic hypereosinophilic syndrome. Ann Intern Med 121:648–653, 1994.
110. Churg J, Strauss L: Allergic granulomatosis, allergic angiitis, and periarteritis nodosa. Am J Pathol 27:277–301, 1951.
111. Masi AT, Hunder GG, Lie JT, et al: The American College of Rheumatology 1990 criteria for the classification of Churg-Strauss syndrome (allergic granulomatosis and angiitis). Arthritis Rheum 33:1094–1100, 1990.
111a. Guellevin L, Cohen P, Gayrand M, et al: Churg-Strauss syndrome. Clinical study and long-term follow-up of 96 patients. Medicine (Baltimore) 78:26–37, 1999.
112. Worthy SA, Müller NL, Hansell DM, et al: Churg-Strauss syndrome: The spectrum of pulmonary CT findings in 17 patients. AJR Am J Roentgenol 170:297–300, 1998.
113. Guillevin L, Lhote F, Gayraud M, et al: Prognostic factors in polyarteritis nodosa and Churg-Strauss syndrome: A prospective study in 342 patients. Medicine (Baltimore) 75:17–28, 1996.
114. Chumbley LL, Hanson EG, DeRemee RA: Allergen granulomatosis and angiitis (Churg-Strauss syndrome): Report and analysis of 30 cases. Mayo Clin Proc 52:477–484, 1977.
115. Lanham JG, Elkon KB, Puvey CD, et al: Systemic vasculitis with asthma and eosinophilia: A clinical approach to the Churg-Strauss syndrome. Medicine (Baltimore) 63:65–81, 1984.
116. Guillevin L, Lhote F, Cohen P, et al: Corticosteroids plus pulse cyclophosphamide and plasma exchanges versus corticosteroids plus pulse cyclophosphamide alone in the treatment of polyarteritis nodosa and Churg-Strauss syndrome patients with factors predicting poor prognosis: A prospective, randomized trial in sixty-two patients. Arthritis Rheum 38:1638–1645, 1995.
117. Tatsis E, Schnabel A, Gross WL: Interferon-alpha treatment of four patients with the Churg-Strauss syndrome. Ann Intern Med 129:370–374, 1998.
118. Wechsler ME, Garpestad E, Flier SR, et al: Pulmonary infiltrates, eosinophilia, and cardiomyopathy following corticosteroid withdrawal in patients with asthma receiving zafirlukast. JAMA 279:455–457, 1998.
119. Lipworth BJ: Leukotriene-receptor antagonists. Lancet 353:57–62, 1999.
120. Green RL, Vayonis AG: Churg-Strauss syndrome after zafirlukast in two patients not receiving systemic steroid treatment. Lancet 353:725–726, 1999.

# 62 Lymphangioleiomyomatosis

Kenneth G. Kalassian, M.D. • Thomas A. Raffin, M.D.

Introduction
Historical Overview
Pathologic Findings
Lymphangioleiomyomatosis Cell Characteristics
- Genetic Regulation
- Hormone Receptors
- Apoptosis
- Extracellular Milieu

Clinical Characteristics
- Epidemiology
- History, Physical Examination, and Laboratory Findings
- Pulmonary Function Abnormalities
- Radiography and Computed Tomography

Diagnosis
Treatment
- Hormones
- General Considerations
- Chylous Fluid Collections
- Renal Angiomyolipomas
- Lung Transplantation
- Future Directions

Summary

## INTRODUCTION

Lymphangioleiomyomatosis (LAM) is a disease resulting from the proliferation of a unique smooth muscle-like cell type, the LAM cell, involving the small airways, the pulmonary microvasculature, and the intrathoracic and extrathoracic lymphatic structures. Proliferation of LAM cells produces airway obstruction, cystic changes in the lung parenchyma, pulmonary hemorrhage, and chylous fluid collections. Clinical features of the disease at the time of presentation are often nonspecific and, although sophisticated imaging techniques such as high-resolution computed tomography (CT) may reveal findings suggestive of LAM, the chest radiograph may be nondescript. The lack of distinctive characteristics frequently leads to a delay in identification of the disease or to an incorrect diagnosis. The mechanisms of pathogenesis of the disease remain poorly understood. The disease occurs primarily in premenopausal women, and it has long been suspected that hormonal factors play an important role. Despite confirmation of the presence of hormone receptors on the surface of the LAM cell, therapeutic attempts with hormonal manipulation have been disappointing. Most patients have a slow, progressive decline in lung function, culminating in hypoxemic respiratory failure. Lung transplantation still remains the only treatment option for many patients, but recent insights into LAM cell biology have created new possibilities for an effective medical therapy.

## HISTORICAL OVERVIEW

More than 60 years ago, von Stoessel[1] reported the results of an autopsy on a premenopausal woman who died of respiratory failure of unknown etiology. It initially was assumed that the woman died of complications of tuberculosis. The autopsy findings revealed, however, diffuse cystic changes of the lung parenchyma in association with what appeared to be airway smooth muscle proliferation. Dilated intrathoracic lymphatic vessels also were observed. He deemed his findings to be representative of a distinctive pathologic process that he called "muscular cirrhosis" of the lung. In the same year of von Stoessel's report, Burrell and Ross[2] published the case of a patient presenting with a chylous effusion in the setting of findings similar to those of von Stoessel, which Burrell and Ross believed were consistent with the presence of an underlying leiomyosarcoma. The observations of von Stoessel and Burrell and Ross may represent the first published accounts of what currently is known as LAM.

After these initial observations, case reports describing a similar clinicopathologic entity began to appear in the medical literature. Rosendal,[3] in a report that included what may be the first description of the chest radiographic findings in LAM, also was the first to use the term "myomatosis" to describe the abnormal smooth muscle proliferation characteristic of the disease. Roujeau and colleagues[4] submitted a detailed description of the lymphectasia resulting from abnormal smooth muscle proliferation, and Brandt[5] was the first to note that smooth muscle proliferation affected not only the anatomy and the development of airways and lymphatic structures but the pulmonary vasculature as well.

As observational information accumulated, the etiology of the disease process became the focus of speculation. Inglis[6] suggested that the pathogenesis of the disease may be the result of systemic or circulating factors and later hypothesized that the disease was a neoplastic process. Laipply and Sherrick[7] attributed the described clinical and pathologic findings to a purely structural cause, spontaneous rupture of the thoracic duct. It was Cornog and Enterline,[8] in the first published series of patients with LAM, who proposed a theory of LAM pathogenesis concordant with current understanding. Building on the opinion of Henke and Hecht[9] that the pathologic findings of LAM were a result of a "hamartomatous" or a benign proliferative process, and the observation made from their own cases that LAM lacked the fundamental characteristics of a malignancy, Cornog and Enterline[8] presciently suggested that LAM was a non-neoplastic proliferation resulting from a pathologic stimulus under genetic control. They also recognized the similarity between the pathologic characteristics of LAM and tuberous sclerosis complex.

After Cornog and Enterline, numerous additional case reports and small case series of what currently is termed LAM were published, including Wolff's ultrastructural analysis of the LAM cell, Leeds's observation of the relationship between LAM and renal angiomyolipomas, and Bush's report of a therapeutic attempt at hormonal manipulation.[10–12] The first extensive review of LAM was published by Corrin and coworkers[13] and was followed by relatively large case series and literature reviews by Silverstein and associates[14] and Carrington and colleagues.[15] The long-term clinical course of patients with LAM was reported first by Taylor and colleagues,[16] who also exposed the lack of efficacy of hormonal therapy. Burger and coworkers[17] made a detailed analysis of the pulmonary mechanics of patients with LAM. The abnormalities of pulmonary physiology observed in the disease have been detailed by Crausman and colleagues.[18] Kitaichi and coworkers[19] and Urban and coworkers[19a] have reported large clinical series of patients and have provided important information regarding the presentation, clinical course, and prognosis of patients with LAM. These reports, in conjunction with the insights into LAM cell biology afforded by the work of numerous investigators,[20–24] have provided the foundation for future advances in basic and clinical LAM research.

## PATHOLOGIC FINDINGS

Macroscopic examination of the lungs of patients with LAM obtained postmortem reveals a large number of predominantly thin-walled and round cystic structures varying in size from several millimeters to several centimeters in diameter (Fig. 62.1*A*). These cystic structures are distributed diffusely without a predilection for a particular lung zone and without a defined central or peripheral relationship with the pleural surface. Focal areas of hemorrhage within the lung parenchyma may be visualized. Dilated lymphatics form bleb-like lesions on the parietal and visceral pleural surfaces, reflecting underlying lymphatic obstruction. Distention of the larger lymphatic structures, most notably the thoracic duct, is a consequence of such obstruction and results in the development of extensive collateral lymphatic formation, both intrathoracic and extrathoracic, including the lymphatic networks of the retroperitoneum and pelvis. A chylous pericardial effusion, chylous pleural effusions, and chylous ascites may be present. Cyst formation may occur in the extrathoracic lymphatic areas and, when large, may resemble retroperitoneal or pelvic masses. The lymph nodes also undergo morphologic changes. They often are enlarged, pale white or tan in color, and on palpation have been described as spongy and resilient. Gross changes may be apparent in the axillary, cervical, subclavian, mediastinal, para-aortic, and pelvic nodal chains. In addition to lymphatic abnormalities, the other important extrathoracic pathologic feature of LAM is the presence of renal angiomyolipomas, hamartomatous lesions composed of smooth muscle, adipose tissue, and blood vessels.[13, 15]

On light microscopy, the hallmark pathologic finding of LAM is abnormal smooth muscle-like cellular proliferation infiltrating airway, pleural, lymphatic, and vascular structures (see Fig. 62.1*C* and *D*). The pulmonary parenchymal lesions of LAM may be divided into two types: the early, or active, phase lesions and the late lesions.[19] In the early lesions, abnormal accumulations of smooth muscle cells are found in the adventitia of the terminal bronchi with particular prominence at the level of the respiratory bronchioles, in the alveolar walls, and in the pleura. The alveolar-capillary interface is spared during this phase. Involvement of the alveolar walls occurs in association with dilated emphysema-like alveolar spaces. Unlike emphysema, however, there is relatively little frank destruction of alveolar walls. Within the alveoli are found hyperplastic type II pneumocytes and hemosiderin-laden macrophages. In late lesions, the smooth muscle accumulation, in association with increased collagen deposition, forms nodular aggregates. These nodular aggregates have different immunohistochemical properties from the atypical smooth muscle-like proliferation of LAM and, in the case of pulmonary LAM associated with tuberous sclerosis complex, have been designated as a distinct entity termed multifocal micronodular pneumocyte hyperplasia or multifocal alveolar hyperplasia.[25–27] In contrast to early-phase lesions, the markedly dilated alveolar spaces of late-phase lesions contain few hemosiderin-laden macrophages.

Sectioning of grossly dilated lymphatic vessels reveals abnormal smooth muscle proliferation in association with masses of lymphocytes resulting in a marked reduction in luminal diameter. In the larger lymphatics, extensive cord-like collections of atypical smooth muscle-like cells may convey a subdivided, plexiform appearance to these lymph conduits. Atypical smooth muscle-like infiltration often is observed in the subcapsular region of lymph nodes, but the infiltrate may be so extensive as to effectively replace the normal nodal architecture. Similar infiltration is observed in the pulmonary vasculature. Although the integrity of arterial and capillary vessels rarely is compromised, pulmonary veins and venules may be

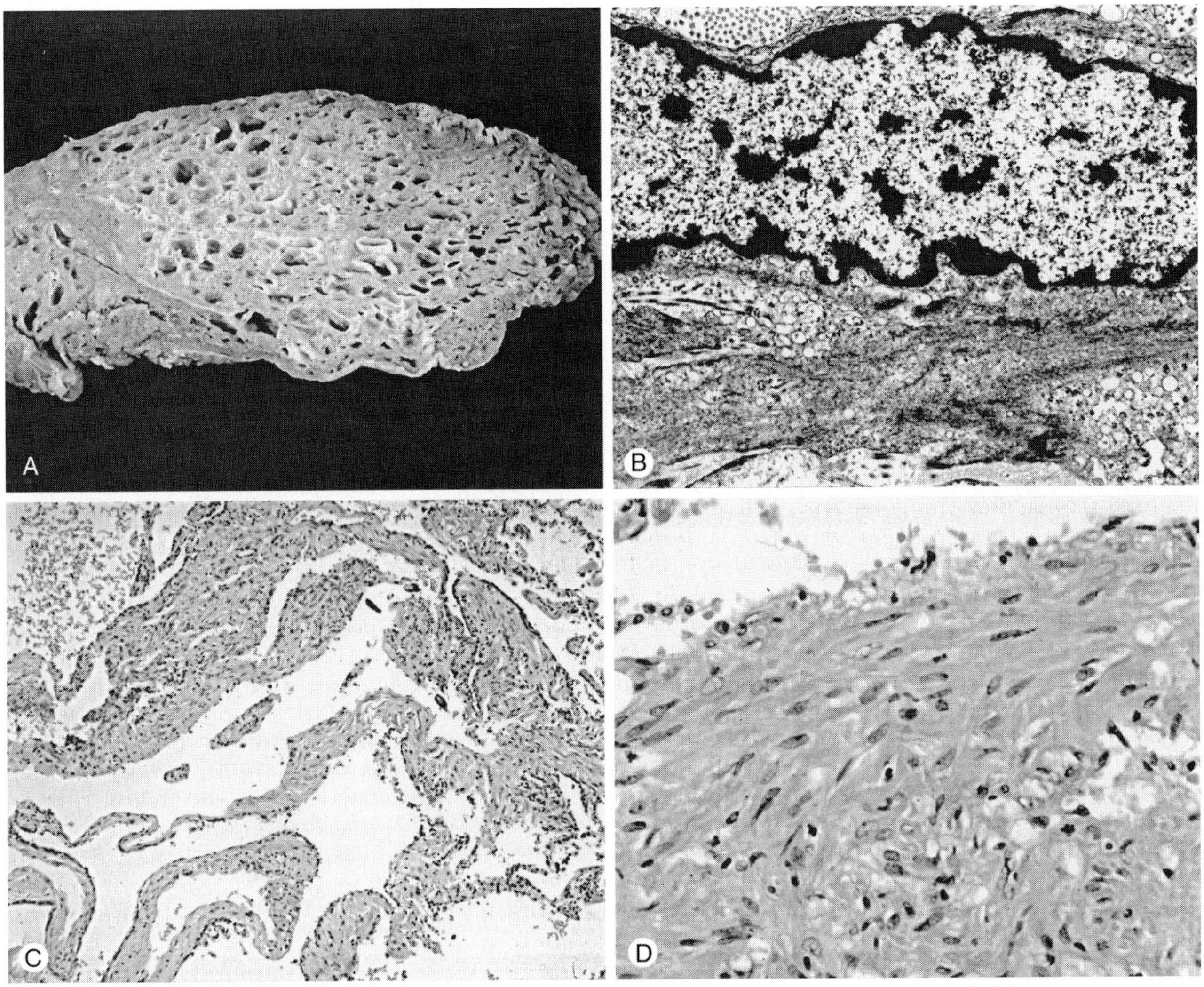


**Figure 62.1** *A,* The classic gross appearance of advanced LAM consisting of numerous small cysts ranging from 0.5 to 1.0 cm. *B,* Transmission electron photomicrograph showing immature smooth muscle cell with irregular nucleus and microfilament bundles with dense bodies in the cytoplasm (× 12,500). *C,* Low-power photomicrograph showing subpleural air-filled cysts containing smooth muscle cells in their walls (hematoxylin and eosin, × 15). *D,* Photomicrograph showing bundles of smooth muscle cells within the interstitium of the cyst walls (hematoxylin and eosin, × 400).

obliterated totally, resulting in widespread veno-occlusion, focal hemorrhage, and hemosiderosis.

## LYMPHANGIOLEIOMYOMATOSIS CELL CHARACTERISTICS

The atypical smooth muscle-like cells found in LAM are cytologically distinctive and phenotypically heterogeneous. Three coexisting cell types have been identified: plump spindle-shaped cells with round or ovoid nuclei and indistinct granular chromatin; small elongated cells with a paucity of cytoplasm and prominent, densely-concentrated chromatin; and large polygonal cells with abundant vacuolated cytoplasm.[23, 28] It has been proposed that this cellular heterogeneity represents various degrees of differentiation of a novel cell type associated with prominent vascular proliferation. The presence of alpha-smooth muscle specific actin in these cells confirms their myoid lineage.[29] Electron microscopy, however, demonstrates (see Fig. 62.1*B*) that LAM cells have features unusual to smooth muscle cells, such as multiply indented nuclei with prominent nucleoli, prominent microfilament bundles with dense bodies, and a well-developed endoplasmic reticulum.[22, 28, 30, 31] Numerous electron-dense membrane-bound granules consisting of fine crystal-like lamellae are evident. Similar cellular features are found in angiomyolipomas of the kidney and liver as well as clear cell tumors of the lung.[32–34]

Along with myoid markers, LAM cells also stain with HMB-45, a monoclonal antibody derived from melanoma hybridomas, which had been considered a specific immunohistochemical marker for melanomas and melanocytic lesions.[35, 36] Given that HMB-45 stains the cytoplasm of LAM cells in an intense granular pattern correlating with the distribution of the electron-dense membrane-bound granules noted on electron microscopy, and that this staining pattern and its ultrastructural correlate are identical among all the HMB-45–reactive cells, suggests that the antigen in LAM and in the cells displaying melanogenesis is the same.

The HMB-45–reactive antigen has been localized to the cytoplasm and in cells of melanocytic lineage is associated with immature melanosomes.[37] Expression cloning of the cDNA of the antigen, with subsequent cDNA sequence analysis and comparison with known sequences in genetic databases, has revealed total homology with *Pmel 17*, a gene important in the regulation of melanin biosynthesis.[38] In conjunction with tyrosinase, which catalyzes the initial steps from L-tyrosine to L-dopa and L-dopa–derived intermediates, the *Pmel 17* gene product controls the distal steps in the eumelanin synthetic pathway.[39]

## Genetic Regulation

The *Pmel 17* cDNA has an 11-nucleotide 5′ untranslated region, a 2007-base pair open-reading frame, and 108-base pair 3′ untranslated region ending in a polyadenosine tail.[40] The amino acid sequence deduced from the open-reading frame encodes a protein of 668 amino acids. The first 23 amino acids of the N-terminus form a signal region characteristic of a membrane-associated protein. Amino acids from position 24-597 constitute the extramembrane domain. Three contiguous repeat motifs of 26 amino acids each are present at positions 315 through 392. Each contains a high number of serine and threonine residues in serine-threonine and threonine-threonine combinations. These repeats are preceded by a histidine-rich region and followed by a region rich in cysteine residues. Five asparagine-related glycosylation sites are dispersed throughout the extracellular domain at positions 81, 106, 11, 321, and 568. The transmembrane region is located near the C-terminal end by charged residues in a configuration consistent with a single helical transmembrane span.

*Gp-100*, a melanocyte lineage-specific antigen, is nearly identical in sequence to *Pmel 17*.[41] The most significant difference is a 21-base pair in-frame deletion on the *gp-100* transcript. Polymerase chain reaction analysis has revealed the presence of a 102-base-pair intron directly next to the 21-base pair insertion in the *Pmel* cDNA. The exon/intron boundaries include consensus 5′ donor and 3′ acceptor splice sequences. The 21-base pair region is located upstream of the 3′ splice sequence and preceded by an alternative 3′ acceptor splice site. This acceptor site lacks a pyrimidine-rich region in the consensus 3′ acceptor site. Such suboptimal RNA processing sites have been implicated in the regulation of alternative RNA processing. This suggests that *Pmel 17* and *gp-100* result from alternative splicing of transcripts from the same gene. Three other nucleotide differences have been observed between *Pmel 17* and *gp-100*. Base pair differences at position 254 and position 577 result in single amino acid substitutions. A nucleotide substitution at position 762 is silent.[42]

The human *Pmel 17/gp-100* gene has been mapped to position 12pter-q21 on chromosome 12. One of the candidate gene loci for tuberous sclerosis complex also has been mapped to chromosome 12.[43] The association of tuberous sclerosis with an increased incidence of LAM has long been recognized. The locus at position 12q22-q24 contains the gene for phenylalanine hydroxylase that is responsible for catalyzing the conversion of phenylalanine to tyrosine. TSC1 and TSC2, the two gene loci formally assigned to tuberous sclerosis, are located at 9q34 and 16p13, respectively.[44] TSC2 at position 16p13 is next to the gene for adult polycystic kidney disease.[45] Loss of heterozygosity at this locus has been demonstrated to be present in renal angiomyolipomas from patients with LAM and tuberous sclerosis.[46] TSC1 contains the gene for dopamine-B-hydroxylase that catalyzes the conversion of L-dopamine to norepinephrine. Thus, putative genes for tuberous sclerosis and LAM are involved in the closely related pathways of catecholamine and melanin synthesis. Further cytogenetic studies may help to define the link between these two clinically associated diseases.

When expression of *Pmel 17/gp-100*, as measured by the degree of HMB-45 staining, is measured in melanocytes, it is found that gene expression is inducible and reversible.[47] Potential growth factors have been identified that may stimulate *Pmel 17* activation; these include insulin-like growth factor-1, epidermal growth factor, adrenal corticosteroids, and pituitary hormones. Under the influence of growth factors, aberrant expression of *Pmel 17/gp-100* could result in the accumulation of eumelanin precursors that are suspected to have mutagenic effects.[48]

## Hormone Receptors

The predilection of LAM for premenopausal women and reports of increased disease activity during pregnancy and with exogenous estrogen administration have stimulated investigation of the role of sex steroids in the abnormal smooth muscle-like proliferation characteristic of the disease.[49–51] Analyses of estrogen and progesterone receptor expression in LAM cells have produced varying results.[52–54] Interpretation is made more difficult by the use of varying techniques, either ligand-binding assays or immunohistochemical methods, of receptor identification. It is unclear whether the variability represents methodologic differences in receptor analysis or true heterogeneity in receptor expression.[55] Recently, more sophisticated techniques of estrogen and progesterone receptor identification have identified estrogen and progesterone receptors on a large proportion of LAM cells and have confirmed the absence of estrogen and progesterone receptors on normal smooth muscle cells.[24]

A detailed model of estrogen receptor function has been created.[56] Estradiol diffuses into the cell nucleus, where it binds to the estrogen receptor in association with heat shock proteins. Hormone binding stimulates dimerization of the estrogen receptors that then bind to the DNA target, the estrogen-response element. The estrogen-response element is a palindromic sequence found near the start sites of transcription of many genes. Activation of these genes may lead to the activation of autocrine and paracrine stimulatory processes. It has been demonstrated that membrane signaling systems, such as those mediated by insulin-like growth factors and epidermal growth factor, have a complex interrelationship with the estrogen receptor in which growth factors may bind to estrogen receptors, activating estrogen receptor-mediated transcription.[57–59] In addition, novel polypeptide mitogens that mediate the effects of sex steroid hormones on smooth muscle growth in uterine leiomyomas have been identified. These findings may have important implications for growth factor regulation of cellular function in LAM.

### Apoptosis

Perturbations in apoptosis, the process of programmed cell death, play an important role in many disorders associated with abnormal cellular proliferation. The protein Bcl-2 and its Bcl-2 family of proteins mediate apoptosis in a variety of hormonally responsive tissues, such as the mammary tissue, the prostate gland, and the endometrium. Members of the Bcl-2 family include both inhibitors and promoters of apoptosis, the expression of which may be under hormonal control. Their action is exerted through the formation of protein dimers with a preponderance of heterodimers of inhibitor and promoter proteins inhibiting the process of programmed cell death and an increased ratio of homodimers of promoter proteins facilitating apoptosis. Bcl-2 also has been shown to suppress apoptosis through inhibition of the apoptotic action of the *myc* oncogene. Bcl-2 and Mcl-1 are among the proteins of the Bcl-2 family that inhibit apoptosis, whereas Bax is one of several that promote cell death. Immunohistochemical analysis suggests that both Bcl-2/Bax and Mcl-1/Bax heterodimers are present in the cytoplasm of LAM cells. The presence of these heterodimers correlates with the presence of estrogen and progesterone receptors, a relationship observed in breast cancer cells. Therefore, the inhibition of apoptosis, possibly regulated by hormonal factors, may contribute to the unchecked cellular proliferation characteristic of LAM.[24]

### Extracellular Milieu

The extracellular matrix of the atypical smooth muscle cell-like infiltration in LAM contains basement membrane components, fibrillar interstitial collagens, and fibronectin.[22] At the periphery of the atypical smooth muscle cell-like infiltrate, intense remodeling activity occurs with degradation of collagen and elastic fibers in early-phase LAM lesions. Fibronectin, the earliest matrix protein found in fibrogenesis, is present in abundance. Resident lung interstitial cells, under the influence of proliferating smooth muscle cells, increase their production of usual matrix proteins. Electron-dense granules containing calcium, iron, and phosphorus are found on epithelial basement membranes, elastic fibers, and collagen fibrils. In late-phase lesions, compaction of collagen into bundles, consistent with the development of fibrosis, is observed. Alpha$_1$-antitrypsin has been identified in proximity to damaged elastic fibers in the extracellular matrix, suggesting that the degradation of extracellular matrix components and parenchymal cyst formation may be related to the same imbalance in the elastase/alpha$_1$-antitrypsin system that may contribute to the pathogenesis of emphysema.[21]

Efforts to identify elastase in the LAM extracellular matrix have been unsuccessful, thereby focusing attention on a different enzyme-inhibitor system, the matrix metalloproteinases, and their tissue inhibitors.[23] Matrix metalloproteinases and their tissue inhibitors regulate the turnover of extracellular matrix components such as collagen, proteoglycans, and elastic fibers. Abnormalities in the matrix metalloproteinase-tissue inhibitor system have been implicated in the pathogenesis of several disease states, including destructive pulmonary and neoplastic processes. The matrix metalloproteinases MMP-2 and MMP-9 have been implicated in the destruction of basement membrane architecture seen with the invasive growth of tumor cells. Both these matrix metalloproteinases as well as MMP-1 have been identified in the extracellular matrix of LAM cells, implicating the matrix metalloproteinase-tissue inhibitor system in the connective tissue destruction and the cyst formation found in LAM.

Infiltration of the airways by LAM cell proliferation and concomitant cystic destruction of the lung parenchyma results in airflow limitation and an obstructive ventilatory defect. The possible mechanism for airflow limitation is either a direct mechanical impediment to airflow secondary to LAM cell infiltration and structured airway narrowing or loss of elastic recoil forces due to extracellular matrix disruption. Formal studies of the pulmonary mechanics of patients with LAM, including measurements of resistance and elastance and the construction of maximal flow-static recoil curves, demonstrate that resistance to airflow is increased markedly and that static compliance also is increased.[17, 18] Calculation of retractile force from the pressure-volume relationship at varying percentages of total lung capacity reveals a relatively modest reduction in elastic recoil forces. Dynamic compliance, in contrast to static compliance, is decreased. The difference in dynamic and static compliance is most likely caused by a wide variance in time constants of individual lung units, resulting in inhomogeneous ventilation. Overall, the reduction in airflow in patients with LAM is much greater in magnitude than the reduction in elastic recoil forces. This suggests that structural airway narrowing secondary to LAM cell infiltration is a more important mechanism in producing airflow obstruction than loss of elastic recoil due to extracellular matrix disruption. However, extracellular matrix disruption, in combination with ventilation-perfusion inequalities, plays an important role in diffusion limitation.

## CLINICAL CHARACTERISTICS

### Epidemiology

The relative rarity of LAM has precluded accurate population-based estimates of the incidence and prevalence of the disease. The small amount of information available relies on census-taking through physician questionnaires, consensus opinions from expert panels, and interstitial lung disease registries. According to approximately 100 Belgian pulmonologists who participated in an interstitial lung disease registry, approximately 1% of all interstitial lung disease diagnosed in that country was attributable to LAM.[60] This percentage, which represents an incidence of approximately 0.8 cases per 1 million of the population, has remained essentially constant since the establishment of the registry in 1990. In comparison, rates of 21 cases per 1 million of population for sarcoidosis, 16 cases per 1 million of population for idiopathic pulmonary fibrosis, 11 cases per 1 million of population for hypersensitivity pneumonitis, and 8 cases per 1 million of population for collagen vascular disease-related interstitial lung disease were found. A questionnaire-based study aimed at defining the relationship between LAM and the use of oral contraception conducted in the United Kingdom identified 23 cases of LAM among a population of 58.5 million, or 0.39 cases per 1 million of the population.[61] An expert panel from a National Institutes of Health-sponsored workshop on LAM conducted in 1995 estimated that there were no more than 3 cases per 1 million of population within the United States.[62] A workshop conducted in 1997 included international participation and provided estimates of prevalence from France, Singapore, and Korea, where 1.8, 0.24, and 0.03 cases per 1 million of the population were observed, respectively.[63]

Most persons afflicted with LAM are premenopausal women. LAM has been reported in a small number of postmenopausal women using exogenous estrogens, the oldest of whom was 72 years of age at the time of diagnosis.[64–66] The mean age at the onset of symptoms in three large series ranged from 32.0 to 38.5 years.[16, 19, 68] A summary of several reported series reported a mean age of onset of 34 years.[68a] The disease has been described in women of black, Asian, and white races. A survey by the LAM Foundation found that more than 90% of patients diagnosed with the disease in the United States are white (LAM Foundation Patient Survey; Sue Byrnes, personal communication, 1996). LAM has been reported in a phenotypic male; however, genotypic confirmation was lacking.[69] A single report of LAM in a nonhuman mammal, a male bottlenose dolphin with a profoundly low testosterone level, also exists.[70]

## History, Physical Examination, and Laboratory Findings

Patients with LAM most commonly present with dyspnea on exertion and nonproductive cough (Table 62.1).[16, 67] The dyspnea on exertion is usually insidious in onset and slowly progressive, as evidenced in the largest patient series by the mean time of 2.8 years between the onset of the patient's symptoms and the first evaluation by a physician.[67] Other symptoms that may be present include dyspnea at rest, chest pain, and hemoptysis. Hemoptysis is usually minor, but a fatal case of hemoptysis has been reported.[71] Marked weight gain and increased abdominal girth may suggest the presence of chylous ascites. Weight gain and increased abdominal girth, in conjunction with lower-extremity edema, may be reported when a patient

**Table 62.1** CLINICAL CHARACTERISTICS OF PATIENTS WITH LAM AT THE TIME OF PRESENTATION AS REPORTED IN TWO LARGE SERIES OF LAM PATIENTS

| CHARACTERISTIC | TAYLOR ET AL[16] (N = 32) (%) | KITAICHI ET AL[19] (N = 46) (%) |
|---|---|---|
| Symptoms | | |
| Dyspnea | | |
| Resting | 0 | 43 |
| Exertional | 47 | 88 |
| Cough | 12 | 41 |
| Chest pain | 12 | 14 |
| Hemoptysis | 9 | 39 |
| Chyloptysis | 0 | 0 |
| Physical findings | | |
| Crackles | NR | 22 |
| Wheezing | 0 | NR |
| Rhonchi | NR | 14 |
| Pleural effusion | 0 | 11 |
| Ascites | 3 | 5 |
| Chest radiography | | |
| Normal | 3 | 10 |
| Reticular or reticulonodular changes | 47 | 85 |
| Cysts or bullae | 12 | 45 |
| Pleural effusion | 0 | 11 |
| Pneumothorax | 53 | 32 |
| Hyperinflation | 0 | 48 |

LAM = Lymphangioleiomyomatosis; NR = not reported.

presents at a relatively late stage in the disease process after cor pulmonale with right heart failure has developed. Lower-extremity edema also may be noted by the patient in the setting of lower-extremity lymphedema. Abdominal pain, flank pain, or hematuria may suggest the presence of an underlying renal angiomyolipoma. If a history of dermatologic or neurologic abnormalities is elicited from the patient, then careful screening should be undertaken to exclude the diagnosis of tuberous sclerosis complex. Chyloptysis and chyluria rarely occur.

Other than with tuberous sclerosis complex, there is no known specific association of LAM with other comorbid diseases. Because worsening of respiratory symptoms and respiratory function has been noted during pregnancy, a reproductive history, with particular attention to the temporal relationship of prior pregnancies to respiratory symptoms, should be obtained. The gynecologic-reproductive history of patients with LAM also may reveal a history of spontaneous abortions and uterine fibroids.[61] A review of the patient's previous and current medication usage should focus on the use of estrogens or estrogen-containing preparations. LAM does not appear to be an inherited disorder; the family history is useful, primarily to exclude alternative diagnoses that may be hereditary in origin. Likewise, there appears to be no known relationship to environmental exposures or personal habits such as smoking, consumption of alcohol, or use of illicit drugs.

The physical examination findings in LAM are nonspecific. Examination of the chest most often reveals mild tachypnea and normal breath sounds, but crackles and rhonchi may be heard in a minority of patients. Hyperresonance to percussion and diminished breath sounds raise suspicion for a pneumothorax. The cardiovascular examination should be directed toward detecting signs of pulmonary hypertension and right-heart dysfunction, such as right ventricular heave, intensified second component of the second heart sound, gallop rhythm, elevated jugular venous pressure, hepatomegaly, and lower-extremity edema.[72] In addition to hepatomegaly, the abdomen should be examined for the presence of ascites as well as a palpable mass in the flanks, such as might be present with a renal angiomyolipoma. A wood-like texture of lower extremity edema, if present, might suggest chronic lymphedema as opposed to cor pulmonal as the etiology. An effort should be made to identify dermatologic lesions characteristic of tuberous sclerosis, such as hypopigmented leaf-shaped spots over the trunk and limbs; adenoma sebaceum over the cheeks, chin, and forehead; and a rough, yellow thickening of the skin over the lumbosacral area, Shagreen's patch. A detailed assessment of the patient's cognitive ability also may be helpful in detecting tuberous sclerosis complex.

Laboratory test results in LAM, like the physical examination findings, are nonspecific. Lymphopenia and electrolyte abnormalities may be observed with repeated or prolonged drainage of chylous pleural effusions, and elevated serum transaminase levels may be found with hepatic congestion secondary to right-heart failure. The complete blood count and serum chemistry values are usually otherwise normal. The urinalysis may reveal red blood cells in the setting of hematuria from a renal angiomyolipoma. Analysis of the pleural fluid or ascites demonstrates the presence of chylomicrons and an elevated triglyceride level consistent with a chylous fluid collection. Although there are anecdotal reports of elevated serum levels of CA-125 in patients with LAM, there is no evidence at present to suggest that its measurement has any clinical utility.[73, 74]

## Pulmonary Function Abnormalities

Obstructive and combined obstructive-restrictive ventilatory defects are observed in patients with LAM.[17, 18] Pulmonary function tests typically show decreased $FEV_1$, $FEV_1$/FVC, and diffusion capacity with normal to increased TLC and increased RV. The degree of airflow limitation is quantified in several series as the ratio of $FEV_1$ to FVC, and the mean value for $FEV_1$/FVC in these series ranges from 37% to 70% of predicted.[13, 15, 17–19, 68] In the largest series of patients, measurements at 1-year intervals over a 5-year period revealed mean values of 64% and 47% of predicted in surviving patients and those who died, respectively.[19] The percentages remained constant from year to year during the 5-year period. The mean TLC in surviving and deceased patients from that same series is 92% and 132% of predicted values. The mean diffusion capacity from the most recent series in which it was reported is 54% of predicted.[68]

Reductions of lung volumes suggesting a concomitant restrictive ventilatory defect are observed in a subset of patients in all series and almost exclusively in patients who have undergone instrumentation of the thoracic cavity for lung biopsy or pleurodesis. Arterial blood gas analysis most often demonstrates hypoxemia with eucapnia or hypocapnia. Hypercapnia is rare. An increased alveolar-arterial oxygen tension difference reflects destruction of the alveolar-capillary interface by the disease process as well as the effects of inhomogeneous ventilation secondary to airway obstruction with resultant ventilation-perfusion inequalities. Cardiopulmonary exercise testing of patients with LAM reveals decreased maximal workload and maximum oxygen consumption. The oxygen pulse at maximal exercise and the anaerobic threshold also are reduced. The maximum minute ventilation is increased significantly for the amount of work performed and, in combination with a low breathing reserve, is consistent with a marked ventilatory limitation to exercise. An increase in the alveolar-arterial oxygen tension difference as well as an abnormally preserved, as opposed to the normally reduced, dead space to tidal volume ratio during exercise suggests that a component of LAM patients' exercise limitation is due to the effect of LAM cell proliferation on the pulmonary vasculature.[18]

## Radiography and Computed Tomography

The spectrum of findings on the chest radiograph of patients with LAM ranges from no discernible abnormality to a honeycomb-like pattern similar to that found in the later stages of several interstitial lung diseases.[15] A diffuse reticular or reticulonodular pattern of increased opacification without predominance for any one lung zone commonly is observed. These opacities have been correlated anatomically to underlying LAM cell proliferation and do not diminish in prominence over time. Additional reticular opacities, described as coarse in appearance and often accompanying septal lines, are attributed to dilatation of lymphatic vessels. These opacities may vary in intensity over time, with changes in the degree of lymphatic engorgement. Small evanescent areas of focal airspace opacification believed to represent areas of hemorrhage may be noted. Cystic changes are observed uncommonly on chest radiograph and, if present, usually are recognized only when the average cyst diameter is greater than 1 cm.[75] They may be indistinguishable from those seen in diseases such as bronchiectasis and emphysema. Coalescence of cystic changes in the later stages of the disease, in combination with increased reticular opacification secondary to LAM cell proliferation, may confer a honeycomb-like appearance to lung zones on the chest radiograph. Although interstitial lung diseases may present with reticular opacification and cystic changes on the chest radiograph similar to that found in LAM, the lung volumes in LAM, in contrast to most interstitial lung diseases, are normal or increased. Serial chest radiographs may demonstrate a subtle increase in lung volumes over time, with elongation of the cardiomediastinal silhouette and flattening of the diaphragmatic contours.[13]

The principal extraparenchymal abnormalities seen on chest radiographs of patients with LAM are pneumothorax and pleural effusion. More than 50% of patients with LAM have radiographic evidence of pneumothorax at the time of presentation, and as many as 80% develop a pneumothorax during the course of the disease.[16, 19] Pneumothorax may be accompanied by extrathoracic evidence of barotrauma, including pneumoperitoneum and pneumoretropharynx.[76, 77] Pleural effusions, almost exclusively chylous in nature, range in extent from blunting of the costophrenic angle to complete opacification of the hemithorax. Both pneumothorax and pleural effusion are usually unilateral, but bilateral presentations have been reported.[78, 79] Enlargement of the cardiac silhouette may occur in the rare case of chylopericardium.

High-resolution computed tomography (HRCT) of the thorax in patients with LAM, even in the earliest stages of the disease, is remarkable for demonstrating numerous thin-walled air-filled cysts diffusely distributed throughout all lung zones.[75, 80–84] The cysts are primarily round but may assume a polygonal or an irregular contour when confluent. The diameter of the cysts varies from 2 to 60 mm, with the thickness of the cyst walls ranging from the lower limits of radiographic resolution to approximately 4 mm. The lung parenchyma between the cysts usually appears normal. The interlobular septa are thickened on rare occasion, but the characteristic polygonal architecture of lymphangitic spread of carcinoma is absent. Focal areas of air space consolidation may be visualized and, as on chest radiograph, probably represent areas of hemorrhage. Other findings that also are seen on chest radiograph include pleural effusions and pneumothoraces. A pericardial effusion may be evident in the setting of chylopericardium. The HRCT findings of LAM may be differentiated from other entities such as emphysema, interstitial fibrosis, and bronchiectasis, even when the ordinary chest film findings are indistinguishable. The one disease that may closely mimic the HRCT abnormalities of LAM is eosinophilic granuloma (Fig. 62.2). Eosinophilic granuloma usually can be distinguished from LAM by the presence of multiple nodular opacities and a predominantly upper lobe, as opposed to a diffuse, distribution of cystic changes. In the more advanced stages of eosinophilic granuloma, however, nodular densities as well as the usual radiographically evident upper-lobe predominance may be absent, resulting in an HRCT appearance not easily differentiated from that of LAM.

If CT imaging is extended through the abdomen and

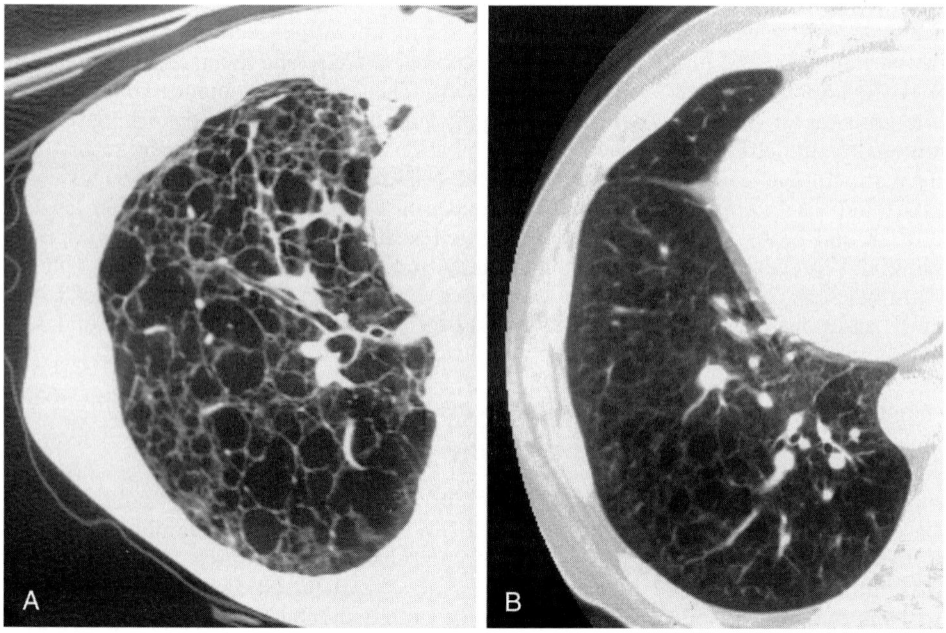


**Figure 62.2** Two high-resolution computed tomograms (HRCTs) of the right side of the chest of patients with two different lung diseases characterized by thin-walled air-filled cysts. *A*, LAM. *B*, Eosinophilic granuloma.

pelvis, renal angiomyolipomas, dilated lymphatic structures, and ascites, if present, are easily recognized. Renal angiomyolipomas appear as heterogeneous renal masses several centimeters in diameter consisting of a mixture of fat and water density areas. They are found in 33% to 57% of patients with LAM and, in contrast to patients with tuberous sclerosis complex, are usually unilateral.[85]

Efforts to correlate chest radiographic findings with pulmonary function abnormalities reveal a low correlation between measured lung function parameters and semiquantitative assessments of radiographic disease extent.[81] HRCT abnormalities do correlate with diffusion capacity values and, to a lesser degree, with the $FEV_1$/FVC ratios. The development of quantitative HRCT employing advanced image processing techniques may result in a better correlation with physiologic measurements of disease severity.[86]

## DIAGNOSIS

The often insidious onset of the disease, in combination with nonspecific clinical and chest radiographic findings, makes initial misdiagnosis of patients with LAM common. The mean interval between the initial symptoms attributable to the disease and its diagnosis was 3.4 years in one series[68] and over 4 years in another.[68a] The initial clinical diagnoses among those patients polled include asthma, spontaneous pneumothorax, emphysema, chronic bronchitis, pulmonary fibrosis, and cancer. Correlation of clinical and radiographic findings may prompt early consideration of LAM in the differential diagnosis by clinicians experienced with the disease, and HRCT results, particularly the presence of a renal angiomyolipoma, may be suggestive of the diagnosis of LAM. In a review of patients undergoing lung transplantation for LAM, nearly 25% of patients were diagnosed by HRCT without a tissue biopsy. The diagnosis of LAM was confirmed in all patients by pathologic examination of the explanted lung.[87] Until the use of HRCT as a sole modality for diagnosis has been formally studied, the implications of a diagnosis of LAM usually mandate tissue confirmation by examination of a biopsy specimen. The diagnosis of LAM has been accomplished by a variety of methods, including open-lung biopsy, thoracoscopic biopsy, transbronchial biopsy, and lymph node biopsy. Case reports of diagnosis by cytologic examination of fine-needle aspirates of lung specimens and of the pleural fluid also exist.[88–90] Open-lung biopsy or thoracoscopic biopsy are traditionally the biopsy methods of choice when LAM is included in the differential diagnosis. The availability of immunohistochemical staining with HMB-45, which in the lung will only stain LAM cells, has improved the usefulness of transbronchial biopsy in the diagnosis of LAM, and transbronchial biopsy is being employed more frequently as a less invasive biopsy technique of first choice.[35] Even when an adequate tissue specimen is obtained, a definitive diagnosis of LAM is not always assured because LAM may mimic other pathologic entities, such as benign metastasizing leiomyoma, mesenchymal cystic hamartoma, pulmonary sarcoma, or native pulmonary muscular proliferation.[91]

## TREATMENT

### Hormones

The predilection of LAM for premenopausal women and the existence of estrogen and progesterone receptors on the surface of LAM cells, unlike normal smooth muscle cells, have led to the assumption that hormonal manipulation may be useful in the treatment of the disease. Ablation of ovarian function by the administration of luteinizing hormone-releasing hormone analogues, radiotherapy, and oophorectomy has resulted in anecdotal reports of clinical benefit.[92–97] The natural history of inexorable clinical deterioration, however, has been altered significantly by these therapies only in rare instances. Antiestrogen therapy with medroxyprogesterone, because of its relatively low morbidity compared with other forms of ablation of ovarian estrogen production, has become the primary form of medical treatment for the disease. Medroxyprogesterone has produced slowing of disease progression and, in a small number of patients, clinical improvement.[66, 98–101] Commonly administered as a monthly or bimonthly intramuscular injection, it also may be given in the oral form as medroxyprogesterone acetate. Interestingly, response to medroxyprogesterone does not correlate with a patient's estrogen or progesterone receptor status but appears to be most efficacious in the patient with a chylous pleural effusion or chylous ascites. It has been suggested that the primary benefit from medroxyprogesterone therapy may be a reduction in chyle production; however, stabilization in the pretreatment rate of decline of airflow measurements on spirometric testing has been observed. An empiric trial of medroxyprogesterone, regardless of whether a chylous fluid collection is present, is warranted in most patents. As an adjunct to treatment with antiestrogen therapy with medroxyprogesterone, administration of exogenous estrogens and of medications with estrogen receptor agonist activity should be discontinued.[49] The hormonal changes of pregnancy have been associated with clinical deterioration, although reports of unchanged disease severity also exist.[50, 51, 102–105] A conservative approach to care of the patient with LAM includes discouragement of pregnancy, and, because pregnancy may occur while the patient is undergoing progesterone therapy, barrier forms of contraception should be used.

A variety of other therapies have been employed in the treatment of LAM. Alkylating chemotherapy agents, such as cyclophosphamide, and interferon-alpha have been abandoned because of their lack of demonstrated benefit and their significant toxicity. Oral corticosteroids have proved to be of no clinical benefit. Treatment with tamoxifen, with its partial estrogen receptor agonist activity, has been associated with both clinical improvement and exacerbation of the disease.[16, 106–110] There are as yet no reports of the use of newer tamoxifen analogues, which lack partial estrogen receptor agonist activity, in the treatment of LAM.

### General Considerations

The principles of care that apply to all patients with chronic lung disease also apply to those with LAM.

Patients with LAM should routinely receive the polyvalent pneumococcal vaccine and annual influenza vaccinations. An appropriate nutritional prescription and a plan to promote cardiorespiratory fitness, through a formal pulmonary rehabilitation program if necessary, should be instituted. If the patient uses tobacco, smoking cessation is essential. As has been learned from the treatment of patients with breast cancer and other life-threatening diseases, participation in patient support groups and frequent contact with the treating physician, with strengthening of the patient-physician bond, results in improvement of quality of life and may result in improved survival. The LAM Foundation, a national patient advocacy and support organization, has proved to be an excellent resource.

The incidence of lower and upper respiratory tract infections in patients with LAM is most likely similar to that of patients with other chronic nonimmunologically mediated respiratory disease. There should be a low threshold for treatment with antibiotics if symptoms suggestive of a bacterial infection are present. Guidelines for the diagnosis and treatment of community-acquired and hospital-acquired bacterial lower respiratory infections in patients with chronic lung disease are also applicable to patients with LAM. Poor dentition, chronic sinusitis, and other abnormalities that predispose patients to lower respiratory tract infections should be addressed aggressively. Acute respiratory failure may be treated with endotracheal intubation and mechanical ventilation, or a trial of noninvasive positive-pressure ventilation, with techniques to minimize dynamic hyperinflation and barotrauma. Pneumothorax is treated in the conventional fashion with tube thoracostomy and, if necessary, chemical or mechanical pleurodesis (see Chapter 75). Pneumothorax has been reported in patients with LAM during air travel, but information to suggest that air travel should be restricted is lacking.[111]

## Chylous Fluid Collections

The effects of a chylous fluid collection may be classified as local, metabolic, or immunologic.[112] The local effects of chylous pleural effusions are similar to other types of pleural fluid collections. Accumulation of chyle in the pleural space may lead to compression of the ipsilateral lung, atelectasis and, in the patient with limited respiratory reserve, acute respiratory failure. When chylous effusions become very large, shift of the mediastinum may occur, with resultant hemodynamic compromise. Chylous ascites may result in an extraparenchymal restrictive ventilatory defect. Repeated drainage of chylous fluid collections results in depletion of proteins, lipids, vitamins, and electrolytes. Hypoalbuminemia, hyponatremia, metabolic acidosis, and hypocalcemia develop, as well as deficiencies of the fat-soluble vitamins A, D, E, and K. Immunologic impairment occurs as a consequence of loss of the depletion of the main cellular element of chyle, T lymphocytes, leading to compromised cell-mediated immunity.[113] The adverse effects of chyle loss relegate the drainage of chylous effusions to those circumstances in which respiratory function is significantly compromised. Losses of proteins, electrolytes, and fat-soluble nutrients should be replaced and may require the use of total parenteral nutrition. To reduce the flow of chyle, lipids are withheld, with the exception of medium-chain triglycerides, which are not transported by the intestinal lacteal system and thus are not a component of chyle.

## Renal Angiomyolipomas

The major complications resulting from the presence of renal angiomyolipomas are retroperitoneal hemorrhage and hypertension resulting from invasion of the renal vein. Renal cell carcinoma also has been reported. Because of the high likelihood of the development of a major complication, it is recommended that symptomatic lesions greater than 4 cm in diameter be treated with embolization, enucleation, or partial nephrectomy.[114] Total nephrectomy rarely is required and is reserved for instances in which other measures have failed. Patients with symptomatic lesions less than 4 cm in diameter should be monitored for prompt resolution of symptoms. If symptoms persist, angiography should be performed and embolization or surgical intervention should be considered. Asymptomatic lesions greater than 4 cm in diameter may be followed with biannual imaging by CT or ultrasound. For asymptomatic lesions less than 4 cm in diameter, imaging on an annual basis is sufficient.

The ideal method of monitoring of patients with LAM and its attendant complications remains to be determined. The insensitivity of routine chest radiography for detecting even marked changes in the lung parenchyma, which are easily observed on HRCT, consigns its role to excluding a supervening process, such as infection, pneumothorax, or chylous effusion, as a cause of acute clinical deterioration. In contrast, HRCT allows detection of even subtle changes in parenchymal abnormalities and is additionally useful in following changes in renal angiomyolipomas. A reasonable approach to monitoring with imaging studies therefore would include an annual HRCT of the thorax and abdomen with an increase in frequency to biannually if asymptomatic renal angiomyolipomas of greater than 4 cm in diameter are detected. Quantitative HRCT, in addition to its potential to assess disease severity, also may find a role as a prognostic tool through its correlation with $FEV_1/FVC$. In addition to a reduction in $FEV_1/FVC$, an increase in TLC has been identified as a poor prognostic factor. Spirometric measurement and measurement of lung volumes therefore constitute important elements in routine periodic evaluation of the patient with LAM. Although change in diffusion capacity has yet to be studied formally as a prognostic factor, it appears to correlate well with disease progression. Its ease of measurement makes it a worthwhile addition to the interval assessment of patients with LAM.

## Lung Transplantation

Despite treatment with antiestrogen therapy and close clinical monitoring, most patients with LAM suffer a slow and inexorable decline in respiratory function, culminating in death from hypoxemic respiratory failure. Kaplan-Meier plots of actuarial survival of patients with LAM in the two most recently reported series reveal a survival at 8.5 years of 78% and 38%, respectively.[16, 19]

The disappointing results of medical therapy have prompted the use of organ transplantation. The first transplantation procedure performed for LAM was a heart-lung transplantation performed in 1983.[115] The first single-lung transplantation occurred in 1988.[116] An extensive retrospective study of lung transplantation for LAM found that nearly 40 transplantation procedures had been performed as of 1995.[87] The mean time from the onset of symptoms to transplantation was 11 years.

Physiologic measurements in this patient population at the time of transplantation included a mean $FEV_1$ of 24% of the predicted value, a mean $FEV_1/FVC$ of 38%, and a mean diffusion capacity of 26% of the predicted value. All but one patient had refractory hypoxemia. Nearly 80% of patients underwent single-lung transplantation, with the remainder undergoing bilateral lung transplantation. Since the first transplantation procedure for LAM, heart-lung transplantation has not been performed again as of the conclusion of the study.[87] Recently, a case of combined lung and kidney transplantation for LAM and large renal angiomyolipoma, causing compromise in renal function in a patient who had undergone prior nephrectomy, has been reported.

The most common intraoperative complication in the retrospective compilation was moderate to severe intrathoracic hemorrhage as a result of pleural adhesions, which occurred in more than 50% of patients. Most patients with pleural adhesions had not undergone instrumentation of the thoracic cavity, which suggests that adhesions and operative hemorrhage were more likely to be related to the underlying disease process rather than prior thoracic surgery. Marked hemodynamic instability, due to dynamic hyperinflation and/or intraoperative pneumothorax, also has been reported.[117, 118] In the case of intraoperative pneumothorax, an unanticipated institution of cardiopulmonary bypass was necessary.

Postoperative morbidity, as in lung transplantation for other diseases, was dominated by rejection and infection (see Chapter 97). At least one acute rejection episode was documented in 82% of patients, and 53% had at least one episode of pneumonia. The microorganisms responsible for infection were similar in type and distribution to those found in other lung transplant populations. The overwhelming majority of infections occurred in the transplanted allograft, with only two infections, both due to *Aspergillus* species, arising from the native lung. Of the patients who suffered acute rejection, 33% went on to develop bronchiolitis obliterans.

Complications that appeared to be related to LAM in particular included native lung pneumothorax in 15% of transplanted patients. In all cases of native lung pneumothorax, no significant respiratory compromise occurred. Recurrent chylous effusions, present in 9% of transplanted patients, were deemed secondary to surgical disruption of mediastinal lymphatic structures during the transplant procedure. Recurrence of LAM in the transplanted lung occurred in one patient in this series, and, as in a subsequently reported case, the transplanted lung was obtained from a male donor.

An improvement in the mean $FEV_1$ to 48% of the predicted value was observed at 6 months after transplantation. The 1- and 2-year survival rates after lung transplantation for LAM were 69% and 58%, respectively, as of 1996. These rates compare favorably with those for lung transplantation overall as well as with disease-specific rates for emphysema and idiopathic pulmonary fibrosis, as reported by the St. Louis International Transplant Registry.

## Future Directions

The rarity of LAM and the lack of a practical animal model or cultured cell line have impeded research into the mechanisms of the disease. Parallels with other disease entities have afforded new insights into LAM cell biology and offer promise for the development of an effective therapy. The HMB-45–associated antigen, *Pmel 17/gp-100*, is being exploited as a target for immunotherapy in the treatment of melanoma. Such immunotherapy techniques may be applicable to the treatment of LAM. The melanin and catecholamine synthetic pathways, the enzymes of which are coded for by putative genes of tuberous sclerosis complex and possibly LAM, likewise may be targeted for therapeutic purposes. If modulation of apoptosis through the Bcl-2 system can be accomplished, LAM cell proliferation may be arrested. As further information regarding LAM cell biology accrues and inroads into the cell biology and treatment of other diseases are made, other concepts for the treatment of LAM will be forthcoming.

The National Institutes of Health, in conjunction with the Cleveland Clinic and six regional centers nationwide, have organized a LAM Registry, which will allow the standardized compilation of clinical data from a relatively large number of patients and the formation of a tissue bank to further basic research.[119] This valuable resource, and the research it will foster, may lead to elucidation of the fundamental mechanisms of pathogenesis of LAM and the creation of an effective medical therapy for a disease that currently is poorly understood.

## SUMMARY

LAM is a rare pulmonary disease that results from the unrestrained proliferation of a smooth muscle-like cell that has unique biologic characteristics. Most patients with LAM are premenopausal women who seek medical attention for worsening dyspnea, the most common complaint, or pneumothorax, chylous fluid collections, or a complication of renal angiomyolipoma. HRCT is helpful in making the diagnosis, but tissue confirmation is usually necessary. Despite the presence of hormonal receptors on the LAM cell, therapeutic manipulation of hormone status has not had much success in halting the inherent tendency for the disease to relentlessly progress. For patients with advanced LAM, lung transplantation offers the only hope at present.

## References

1. von Stoessel E: Uber muskulature cirrhose der Lunge. Beitr Klin Tuberk 90:432–442, 1937.
2. Burrell L, Ross H: A case of chylous effusion due to leiomyosarcoma. Br J Tuberc 31:38–39, 1937.

3. Rosendal T: A case of diffuse myomatosis and cyst formation in the lung. Acta Radiol 23:138–146, 1942.
4. Roujeau J, Delarue J, Depierre R: Lymphangiectasie pulmonaire diffuse, pneumonie chyleuse et chylothorax, apres thrombose puerperale de la veine sous-claviere gauche. J Fr Med Chir Thorac 4:488–503, 1950.
5. Brandt M: Uber angiomyomatose der lungen mit wabenstruktur. Virchows Arch 321:585–598, 1952.
6. Inglis K: The nature and origin of smooth muscle-like neoplastic tissue in the lungs and corresponding lymph nodes in a case of so-called "honeycomb lungs." Arch De Vecchi Anat Patol 31:179–209, 1960.
7. Laipply T, Sherrick J: Intrathoracic angiomyomatous hyperplasia associated with chronic chylothorax. Lab Invest 7:387–400, 1958.
8. Cornog JJ, Enterline H: Lymphangiomyoma, a benign lesion of chyliferous lymphatics synonymous with lymphangiopericytoma. Cancer 19:1909–1930, 1966.
9. Henke D, Hecht A: Chylothorax und ascites chylosus bei neurinomatoser hamartie im bereich des ductus thoracicus. Thoraxchirurgie 6:564–587, 1959.
10. Bush J, McLean R, Sieker H: Diffuse lung disease due to lymphangiomyoma. Am J Med 46:645–654, 1969.
11. Wolff M: Lymphangiomyoma: Clinicopathologic study and ultrastructural confirmation of its histogenesis. Cancer 31:988–1007, 1973.
12. Leeds S, Benioff M, Ortega P: Pulmonary lymphangiomyoma with renal angiomyolipomas. Calif Med 119:74–78, 1973.
13. Corrin B, Liebow AA, Friedman PJ: Pulmonary lymphangiomyomatosis: A review. Am J Pathol 79:348–382, 1975.
14. Silverstein EF, Ellis K, Wolff M, Jaretzki AD: Pulmonary lymphangiomyomatosis. Am J Roentgenol Radium Ther Nucl Med 120:832–850, 1974.
15. Carrington CB, Cugell DW, Gaensler EA, et al: Lymphangioleiomyomatosis: Physiologic-pathologic-radiologic correlations. Am Rev Respir Dis 116:977–995, 1977.
16. Taylor JR, Ryu J, Colby TV, Raffin TA: Lymphangioleiomyomatosis: Clinical course in 32 patients. N Engl J Med 323:1254–1260, 1990.
17. Burger CD, Hyatt RE, Staats BA: Pulmonary mechanics in lymphangioleiomyomatosis. Am Rev Respir Dis 143:1030–1033, 1991.
18. Crausman RS, Jennings CA, Mortenson RL, et al: Lymphangioleiomyomatosis: The pathophysiology of diminished exercise capacity. Am J Respir Crit Care Med 153:1368–1376, 1996.
19. Kitaichi M, Nishimura K, Itoh H, Izumi T: Pulmonary lymphangioleiomyomatosis: A report of 46 patients including a clinicopathologic study of prognostic factors. Am J Respir Crit Care Med 151:527–533, 1995.
19a. Urban T, Lazor R, Lacronique J, et al: Pulmonary lymphangioleiomyomatosis. A study of 69 patients. Medicine (Baltimore) 78:321–337, 1999.
20. Bonetti F, Chiodera P: Lymphangioleiomyomatosis and tuberous sclerosis: Where is the border? Eur Respir J 9:399–401, 1996.
21. Fukuda Y, Kawamoto M, Yamamoto A, et al: Role of elastic fiber degradation in emphysema-like lesions of pulmonary lymphangiomyomatosis. Hum Pathol 21:1252–1261, 1990.
22. Peyrol S, Gindre D, Cordier JF, et al: Characterization of the smooth muscle cell infiltrate and associated connective matrix of lymphangiomyomatosis: Immunohistochemical and ultrastructural study of two cases. J Pathol 168:387–395, 1992.
23. Hayashi T, Fleming MV, Stetler-Stevenson WG, et al: Immunohistochemical study of matrix metalloproteinases (MMPs) and their tissue inhibitors (TIMPs) in pulmonary lymphangioleiomyomatosis (LAM). Hum Pathol 28:1071–1078, 1997.
24. Usuki J, Horiba K, Chu SC, et al: Immunohistochemical analysis of proteins of the Bcl-2 family in pulmonary lymphangioleiomyomatosis: Association of Bcl-2 expression with hormone receptor status. Arch Pathol Lab Med 122:895–902, 1998.
25. Muir TE, Leslie KO, Popper H, et al: Micronodular pneumocyte hyperplasia. Am J Surg Pathol 22:465–472, 1998.
26. Chuah KL, Tan PH: Multifocal micronodular pneumocyte hyperplasia, lymphangiomyomatosis and clear cell micronodules of the lung in a Chinese female patient with tuberous sclerosis. Pathology 30:242–246, 1998.
27. Guinee D, Singh R, Azumi N, et al: Multifocal micronodular pneumocyte hyperplasia: A distinctive pulmonary manifestation of tuberous sclerosis. Mod Pathol 8:902–906, 1995.
28. Bonetti F, Pea M, Martignoni G, et al: Cellular heterogeneity in lymphangiomyomatosis of the lung. Hum Pathol 22:727–728, 1991.
29. Matthews TJ, Hornall D, Sheppard MN: Comparison of the use of antibodies to alpha smooth muscle actin and desmin in pulmonary lymphangioleiomyomatosis. J Clin Pathol 46:479–480, 1993.
30. Basset F, Soler P, Marsac J, Corrin B: Pulmonary lymphangiomyomatosis: three new cases studied with electron microscopy. Cancer 38:2357–2366, 1976.
31. Kane PB, Lane BP, Cordice JW, Greenberg GM: Ultrastructure of the proliferating cells in pulmonary lymphangiomyomatosis. Arch Pathol Lab Med 102:618–622, 1978.
32. Lantuejoul S, Isaac S, Pinel N, et al: Clear cell tumor of the lung: An immunohistochemical and ultrastructural study supporting a pericytic differentiation. Mod Pathol 10:1001–1008, 1997.
33. Gaffey MJ, Mills SE, Zarbo RJ, et al: Clear cell tumor of the lung: Immunohistochemical and ultrastructural evidence of melanogenesis. Am J Surg Pathol 15:644–653, 1991.
34. Bonetti F, Pea M, Martignoni G, et al: Clear cell ("sugar") tumor of the lung is a lesion strictly related to angiomyolipoma—The concept of a family of lesions characterized by the presence of the perivascular epithelioid cells (PEC). Pathology 26:230–236, 1994.
35. Bonetti F, Chiodera PL, Pea M, et al:. Transbronchial biopsy in lymphangiomyomatosis of the lung. HMB45 for diagnosis. Am J Surg Pathol 17:1092–1102, 1993.
36. Hoon V, Thung SN, Kaneko M, Unger PD: HMB-45 reactivity in renal angiomyolipoma and lymphangioleiomyomatosis. Arch Pathol Lab Med 118:732–734, 1994.
37. Esclamado RM, Gown AM, Vogel AM: Unique proteins defined by monoclonal antibodies specific for human melanoma: Some potential clinical applications. Am J Surg 152:376–385, 1986.
38. Wagner SN, Wagner C, Hofler H, et al: Expression cloning of the cDNA encoding a melanoma-associated Ag recognized by mAb HMB-45: Identification as melanocyte-specific Pmel 17 cDNA. Lab Invest 73:229–235, 1995.
39. Kwon BS. Pigmentation genes: The tyrosinase gene family and the pmel 17 gene family. J Invest Dermatol 100:134S–140S, 1993.
40. Kwon BS, Chintamaneni C, Kozak CA, et al: A melanocyte-specific gene, Pmel 17, maps near the silver coat color locus on mouse chromosome 10 and is in a syntenic region on human chromosome 12. Proc Natl Acad Sci USA 88:9228–9232, 1991.
41. Bakker AB, Schreurs MW, Tafazzul G, et al: Identification of a novel peptide derived from the melanocyte-specific gp100 antigen as the dominant epitope recognized by an HLA-A2.1-restricted anti-melanoma CTL line. Int J Cancer 62:97–102, 1995.
42. Kalassian KG, Doyle R, Kao P, et al: Lymphangioleiomyomatosis: New insights. Am J Respir Crit Care Med 155:1183–1186, 1997.
43. Fahsold R, Rott HD, Lorenz P: A third gene locus for tuberous sclerosis is closely linked to the phenylalanine hydroxylase gene locus. Hum Genet 88:85–90, 1991.
44. Sampson JR, Harris PC: The molecular genetics of tuberous sclerosis. Hum Mol Genet 3 Spec No:1477–1480, 1994.
45. Kandt RS, Haines JL, Smith M, et al: Linkage of an important gene locus for tuberous sclerosis to a chromosome 16 marker for polycystic kidney disease. Nat Genet 2:37–41, 1992.
46. Smolarek TA, Wessner LL, McCormack FX, et al: Evidence that lymphangiomyomatosis is caused by TSC2 mutations: Chromosome 16p13 loss of heterozygosity in angiomyolipomas and lymph nodes from women with lymphangiomyomatosis. Am J Hum Genet 62:810–815, 1998.
47. Smoller BR, Hsu A, Krueger J: HMB-45 monoclonal antibody recognizes an inducible and reversible melanocyte cytoplasmic protein. J Cutan Pathol 18:315–322, 1991.
48. Jimbow K, Lee SK, King MG, et al: Melanin pigments and melanosomal proteins as differentiation markers unique to normal and neoplastic melanocytes. J Invest Dermatol 100:259S–268S, 1993.
49. Shen A, Iseman MD, Waldron JA, King TE: Exacerbation of pulmonary lymphangioleiomyomatosis by exogenous estrogens. Chest 91:782–785, 1987.

50. Yockey CC, Riepe RE, Ryan K: Pulmonary lymphangioleiomyomatosis complicated by pregnancy. Kans Med 87:277–278, 293, 1986.
51. Hughes E, Hodder RV: Pulmonary lymphangiomyomatosis complicating pregnancy: A case report. J Reprod Med 32:553–557, 1987.
52. Ohori NP, Yousem SA, Sonmez-Alpan E, Colby TV: Estrogen and progesterone receptors in lymphangioleiomyomatosis, epithelioid hemangioendothelioma, and sclerosing hemangioma of the lung. Am J Clin Pathol 96:529–535, 1991.
53. Berger U, Khaghani A, Pomerance A, et al: Pulmonary lymphangioleiomyomatosis and steroid receptors: An immunocytochemical study. Am J Clin Pathol 93:609–614, 1990.
54. Brentani MM, Carvalho CR, Saldiva PH, et al: Steroid receptors in pulmonary lymphangiomyomatosis. Chest 85:96–99, 1984.
55. Kinoshita M, Yokoyama T, Higuchi E, et al: Hormone receptors in pulmonary lymphangiomyomatosis. Kurume Med J 42:141–144, 1995.
56. Brown M: Estrogen receptor molecular biology. Hematol Oncol Clin North Am 8:101–112, 1994.
57. Korach KS: Insights from the study of animals lacking functional estrogen receptor. Science 266:1524–1527, 1994.
58. Chalbos D, Philips A, Rochefort H: Genomic cross-talk between the estrogen receptor and growth factor regulatory pathways in estrogen target tissues. Semin Cancer Biol 5:361–368, 1994.
59. Ignar-Trowbridge DM, Pimentel M, Teng CT, et al: Cross talk between peptide growth factor and estrogen receptor signaling systems. Environ Health Perspect 103(Suppl 7):35–38, 1995.
60. Roelandt M, Demedts M, Callebaut W, et al: Epidemiology of interstitial lung disease (ILD) in flanders: Registration by pneumologists in 1992–1994. Working group on ILD, VRGT. Vereniging voor Respiratoire Gezondheidszorg en Tuberculosebestrijding. Acta Clin Belg 50:260–268, 1995.
61. Wahedna I, Cooper S, Williams J, et al: Relation of pulmonary lymphangio-leiomyomatosis to use of the oral contraceptive pill and fertility in the UK: A national case control study. Thorax 49:910–914, 1994.
62. National Heart Lung, and Blood Institute. Unpublished Workshop on Lymphangioleiomyomatosis, Bethesda, MD, 1995.
63. Report of workshop on lymphangioleiomyomatosis. Am J Respir Crit Care Med 159:679–683, 1999.
64. Baldi S, Papotti M, Valente ML, et al: Pulmonary lymphangioleiomyomatosis in postmenopausal women: Report of two cases and review of the literature. Eur Respir J 7:1013–1016, 1994.
65. Sinclair W, Wright JL, Churg A: Lymphangioleiomyomatosis presenting in a postmenopausal woman. Thorax 40:475–476, 1985.
66. Zanella A, Toppan P, Nitti D, Lise M: Pulmonary lymphangioleiomyomatosis: A case report in postmenopausal woman treated with pleurodesis and progesterone (medroxyprogesterone acetate). Tumori 82:96–98, 1996.
67. Kitaichi M, Izumi T: Lymphangioleiomyomatosis. Curr Opin Pulm Med 1:417–424, 1995.
68. Chu SC, Horiba K, Usuki J, et al: Comprehensive evaluation of 35 patients with lymphangioleiomyomatosis. Chest 115:1041–1052, 1999.
68a. Johnson S: Lymphangioleiomyomatosis: Clinical features, management and basic mechanisms. Thorax 54:254–264, 1999.
69. Kang HW, Kim CJ, Kang SK, et al: Pulmonary lymphangioleiomyomatosis in a male. J Korean Med Sci 6:83–85, 1991.
70. Rawson AJ, Patton GW, Brooks JS: Lymphangiomyomatosis in the Atlantic bottlenose dolphin (*Tursiops truncatus*). J Wildl Dis 28:323–325, 1992.
71. Fliegel E, Chitkara RK, Azueta V, Steinberg H: Fatal hemoptysis in lymphangiomyomatosis. N Y State J Med 91:66–67, 1991.
72. Kawahara Y, Taniguchi T, Kadou T, et al: Elevated pulmonary arterial pressure in pulmonary lymphangiomyomatosis. Jpn J Med 28:520–522, 1989.
73. Kanbe A, Hajiro K, Adachi Y, et al: Lymphangiomyomatosis associated with chylous ascites and high serum CA- 125 levels: A case report. Jpn J Med 26:237–242, 1987.
74. Zahner J, Strauer BE: CA-125—A tumor marker of lymphangioleiomyomatosis of diagnostic and prognostic importance. Geburtshilfe Frauenheilkd 53:492–494, 1993.
75. Muller NL, Chiles C, Kullnig P: Pulmonary lymphangiomyomatosis: Correlation of CT with radiographic and functional findings. Radiology 175:335–339, 1990.
76. Crausman RS, Mellman D, Bloomfield EC, Jennings CA: Pulmonary barotrauma as the cause of pneumoretropharynx in pulmonary lymphangioleiomyomatosis. Am J Emerg Med 14:297–299, 1996.
77. Tamura K, Satoh Y, Ikoma A, Miyazaki T: Pneumoperitoneum in a patient with lymphangiomyomatosis. Respiration 58:211–213, 1991.
78. Fairfax AJ, McNabb WR, Spiro SG: Chylothorax: A review of 18 cases. Thorax 41:880–885, 1986.
79. Berkman N, Bloom A, Cohen P, et al: Bilateral spontaneous pneumothorax as the presenting feature in lymphangioleiomyomatosis. Respir Med 89:381–383, 1995.
80. Aberle DR, Hansell DM, Brown K, Tashkin DP: Lymphangiomyomatosis: CT, chest radiographic, and functional correlations. Radiology 176:381–387, 1990.
81. Lenoir S, Grenier P, Brauner MW, et al: Pulmonary lymphangiomyomatosis and tuberous sclerosis: comparison of radiographic and thin-section CT findings. Radiology 175:329–334, 1990.
82. Rappaport DC, Weisbrod GL, Herman SJ, Chamberlain DW: Pulmonary lymphangioleiomyomatosis: high-resolution CT findings in four cases. AJR Am J Roentgenol 152:961–964, 1989.
83. Templeton PA, McLoud TC, Muller NL, et al: Pulmonary lymphangioleiomyomatosis: CT and pathologic findings. J Comput Assist Tomogr 13:54–57, 1989.
84. Sherrier RH, Chiles C, Roggli V: Pulmonary lymphangioleiomyomatosis: CT findings [see comments]. AJR Am J Roentgenol 153:937–940, 1989.
85. Blute ML: How common are renal angiomyolipomas in patients with pulmonary lymphangiomyomatosis? Am J Respir Crit Care Med 154:1580–1581, 1996.
86. Crausman RS, Lynch DA, Mortenson RL, et al: Quantitative CT predicts the severity of physiologic dysfunction in patients with lymphangioleiomyomatosis. Chest 109:131–137, 1996.
87. Boehler A, Speich R, Russi EW, Weder W: Lung transplantation for lymphangioleiomyomatosis. N Engl J Med 335:1275–1280, 1996.
88. Itami M, Teshima S, Asakuma Y, et al: Pulmonary lymphangiomyomatosis diagnosed by effusion cytology: A case report. Acta Cytol 41:522–528, 1997.
89. Berner A, Franzen S, Heilo A: Fine needle aspiration cytology as a diagnostic approach to lymphangioleiomyomatosis: A case report. Acta Cytol 41:877–879, 1997.
90. Buhl L, Larsen KE, Bjorn-Hansen L: Lymphangioleiomyomatosis: Is fine needle aspiration cytodiagnosis possible? Acta Cytol 32:559–562, 1988.
91. Wockel W, Meister P, Karg O, Morresi-Hauf A: Native pulmonary muscular proliferation. Pathol Res Pract 193:599–605, 1997.
92. Banner AS, Carrington CB, Emory WB, et al: Efficacy of oophorectomy in lymphangioleiomyomatosis and benign metastasizing leiomyoma. N Engl J Med 305:204–209, 1981.
93. Adamson D, Heinrichs WL, Raybin DM, Raffin TA: Successful treatment of pulmonary lymphangiomyomatosis with oophorectomy and progesterone. Am Rev Respir Dis 132:916–921, 1985.
94. Flandes Aldeyturriaga J, Golpe Gomez A, Perez Rodriguez E: Lymphangioleiomyomatosis: The effectiveness of radiotherapy-induced ovarian function annulment. A case report. Respiration 58:214–218, 1991.
95. Rossi GA, Balbi B, Oddera S, et al: Response to treatment with an analog of the luteinizing-hormone-releasing hormone in a patient with pulmonary lymphangioleiomyomatosis. Am Rev Respir Dis 143:174–176, 1991.
96. Logan RF, Fawcett IW: Oophorectomy for pulmonary lymphangioleiomyomatosis: A case report. Br J Dis Chest 79:98–100, 1985.
97. Winter JA: Oophorectomy in lymphangioleiomyomatosis and benign metastasizing leiomyoma. N Engl J Med 305:1416–1417, 1981.
98. Sawicka EH, Morris AJ: A report of two long-surviving cases of pulmonary lymphangioleiomyomatosis and the response to progesterone therapy. Br J Dis Chest 79:400–406, 1985.
99. McCarty KS Jr, Mossler JA, McLelland R, Sieker HO: Pulmonary lymphangiomyomatosis responsive to progesterone. N Engl J Med 303:1461–1465, 1980.

100. Eliasson AH, Phillips YY, Tenholder MF: Treatment of lymphangioleiomyomatosis: A meta-analysis. Chest 96:1352–1355, 1989.
101. Rajjoub S, Blatt MW, Ritterspach J: Response to treatment with progesterone in a patient with pulmonary lymphangioleiomyomatosis. W V Med J 91:322–323, 1995.
101a. Johnson SR, Tattersfield AE: Decline in lung function in lymphangioleiomyomatosis. Relation to menopause and progesterone treatment. Am J Respir Crit Care Med 160:628–633, 1999.
102. Brunelli A, Catalini G, Fianchini A: Pregnancy exacerbating unsuspected mediastinal lymphangioleiomyomatosis and chylothorax. Int J Gynaecol Obstet 52:289–290, 1996.
103. Murata A, Takeda Y, Usuki J, et al: A case of pulmonary lymphangiomyomatosis induced by pregnancy. Nihon Kyobu Shikkan Gakkai Zasshi 27:1106–1111, 1989.
104. Warren SE, Lee D, Martin V, Messink W: Pulmonary lymphangiomyomatosis causing bilateral pneumothorax during pregnancy. Ann Thorac Surg 55:998–1000, 1993.
105. Yigla M, Bentur L, Ben Izhak O, Rubin AH: Pulmonary lymphangioleiomyomatosis: Prolonged survival despite multiple pregnancies and no hormonal intervention. Respirology 1:213–215, 1996.
106. Anker N, Francis D, Viskum K: Two cases of lymphangioleiomyomatosis treated by hormonal manipulation. Ugeskr Laeger 155:2354–2356, 1993.
107. Hara H, Tono Y, Matsushima T, Manabe T: A case of pulmonary lymphangiomyomatosis with tuberous sclerosis—Treated with tamoxifen. Nihon Kyobu Shikkan Gakkai Zasshi 25:918–923, 1987.
108. Luna CM, Gene R, Jolly EC, et al: Pulmonary lymphangiomyomatosis associated with tuberous sclerosis: Treatment with tamoxifen and tetracycline-pleurodesis. Chest 88:473–475, 1985.
109. Tomasian A, Greenberg MS, Rumerman H: Tamoxifen for lymphangioleiomyomatosis. N Engl J Med 306:745–746, 1982.
110. Clemm C, Jehn U, Wolf-Hornung B, et al: Lymphangiomyomatosis: A report of three cases treated with tamoxifen. Klin Wochenschr 65:391–393, 1987.
111. Sullivan EJ: Lymphangioleiomyomatosis: A review. Chest 114:1689–1703, 1998.
112. Merrigan BA, Winter DC, O'Sullivan GC: Chylothorax. Br J Surg 84:15–20, 1997.
113. Valentine VG, Raffin TA: The management of chylothorax. Chest 102:586–591, 1992.
114. Oesterling JE, Fishman EK, Goldman SM, Marshall FF: The management of renal angiomyolipoma. J Urol 135:1121–1124, 1986.
115. Estenne M, de Francquen P, Wellens F, et al: Combined heart-and-lung transplantation for lymphangioleiomyomatosis. Lancet 1:275, 1984.
116. Sleiman C, Mal H, Jebrak G, et al: Pulmonary lymphangiomyomatosis treated by single lung transplantation. Am Rev Respir Dis 145:964–966, 1992.
117. Popple C, Higgins TL, McCarthy P, et al: Unilateral auto-PEEP in the recipient of a single lung transplant. Chest 103:297–299, 1993.
118. Brusset A, Bonnette P, Hatahet Z, et al: Single lung transplantation for pulmonary lymphangiomyomatosis: Unexpected need for extracorporeal circulation. Chest 107:278–282, 1995.
119. Sullivan EJ, Beck GJ, Cleveland Clinic Foundation, et al: Lymphangioleiomyomatosis registry (letter). Chest 115:301, 1999.

# 63 Pulmonary Alveolar Proteinosis

KARLMAN WASSERMAN, M.D., PH.D.
GREGORY R. MASON, M.D.

Introduction
Pathology
- Histopathology
- Electron Microscopy
- Alveolar Lavage Material

Natural History
Etiology and Pathogenesis
- Genetic Defects
- Defective Alveolar Macrophages
- Surfactant Overproduction or Decreased Clearance
- Unusual Injury Response to Inhaled Agents
- Immunodeficiency State
- Response to Infection

Clinical Presentation
- Physical Signs
- Roentgenographic Findings
- Laboratory Examination
- Respiratory Function

Diagnosis
Treatment
- Whole-Lung Lavage
- Heparin and Acetylcysteine

Prognosis
Summary

## INTRODUCTION

Pulmonary alveolar proteinosis is a disorder in which an amorphous, insoluble, proteinaceous material, rich in phospholipid and surfactant proteins, is deposited in alveoli and bronchioles. This material is unique because it does not appear to stimulate an inflammatory process, and lung fibrosis is minimal. The primary disturbance produced by this disorder is impairment in oxygen transfer to the blood perfusing the involved alveoli. Thus, patients are usually hypoxemic at rest, depending on the degree of involvement of the lungs, and become progressively more hypoxemic with exercise. Death results from the effects of hypoxia, although superinfection by opportunistic organisms may occur.

This disease first was described in 1958 by three eminent pathologists.[1] Because the pathology was sufficiently distinctive and unlikely to have escaped their notice previously, these pathologists believed that the disease might be caused by a new agent in the environment. Four decades after its original description, we are just beginning to gain insight into the cause(s) and mechanism(s) of this disease. There is both light and electron microscopic evidence suggesting that the disease process is linked to pulmonary surfactant.[2] Although pulmonary alveolar proteinosis has occurred in humans in association with silica[3] and aluminum[4] dust exposure, usually there is no exposure history, and the finding of an abnormal accumulation of inorganic dust in the lungs is uncommon.

## PATHOLOGY

Grossly, the lungs of patients with pulmonary alveolar proteinosis are very heavy, containing insoluble yellow material that can exude from cut lung surfaces.[1] The disease affects the lung in patches, taking on an acinar distribution in appearance. Unlike the findings in pulmonary fibrosis, honeycombing is absent and the pleural surfaces appear to be spared.

### Histopathology

There has been little added to our knowledge of the light microscopy histopathology of pulmonary alveolar proteinosis since the original description by Rosen and coworkers.[1] Periodic acid–Schiff (PAS)-positive, amorphous, granular material, rich in lipids, is deposited in the alveolar spaces, rising up into the bronchioles in more severe cases. The alveolar lining cells are often cuboidal and contain PAS-positive cytoplasm (Fig. 63.1). Typically, the alveolar septa do not have significant fibrosis, nor is there evidence of inflammation within the alveolar spaces other than distended foamy macrophages. Granulocytic and lymphocytic cells are very rarely found in the alveolar spaces. The septa may appear normal but often contain an increased number of septal cells. From their histopathologic observations, Rosen and colleagues[1] suggested that the intra-alveolar material originated from

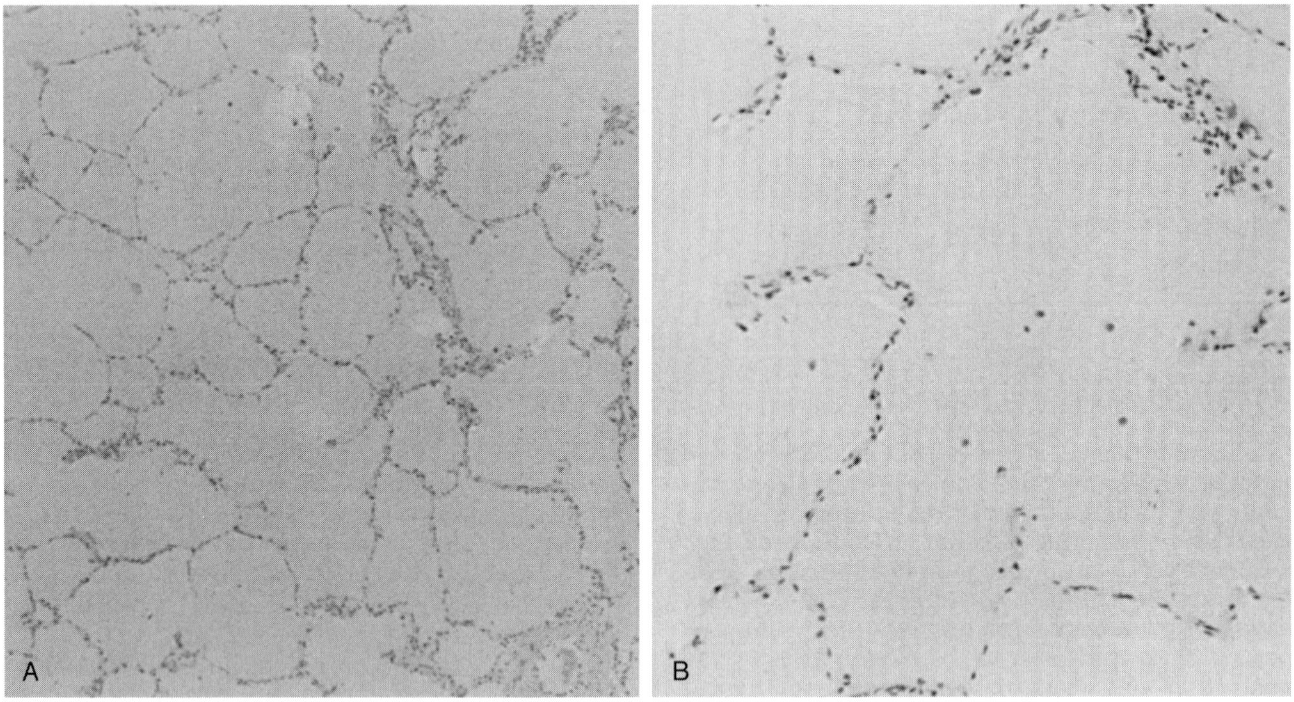


**Figure 63.1** Histopathologic findings in pulmonary alveolar proteinosis. *A,* Alveoli are filled with amorphous PAS-positive staining material without an inflammatory response. (Original magnification × 320.) The septa usually appear normal or have increased numbers of septal cells, as described by Rosen and coworkers.[1] The septal wall is free of fibrosis. *B,* Higher magnification (original ×800). Alveolar macrophages are seen within the amorphous alveolar filling material.

degenerated alveolar cells. Indeed, some lung sections show a marked increase in these alveolar cells, even sheets of them, which appear to be type II pneumocytes. Acicular clefts also are noted frequently in the intra-alveolar material, suggesting that inorganic dust might be present.

The large macrophages commonly found as single cells in the midst of the insoluble alveolar material are interesting because their cytoplasm is PAS positive, like the surrounding material. The macrophages appear to incorporate the alveolar material, to be unable to digest it, and then to become large and relatively immobile. They probably become entrapped in the insoluble, intra-alveolar material and eventually die, becoming "ghost cells." Thus, the macrophage itself might contribute to the lipid-laden, proteinaceous material occupying the alveolar space.

We occasionally observe cases of pulmonary alveolar proteinosis with thickened septa and interstitial fibrosis accompanying the typical alveolar changes of this disease. In some cases, there is a history of recurrent pneumonia and the lung biopsy specimen may have evidence of subacute or chronic inflammation. Indeed, patients with pulmonary alveolar proteinosis may be candidates for repeated lung infections, particularly ones caused by *Nocardia asteroides*. Repeat infections may be responsible for the fibrosis and inflammatory response seen in some patients.

## Electron Microscopy

Electron microscopic findings are striking, revealing many electron-dense, lamellar bodies composed of coiled bilayers of phospholipid that resemble surfactant in the alveolar spaces (Fig. 63.2).[2] These bodies are in the alveolar spaces surrounded by fragments of lamellar bodies and amorphous material (see Fig. 63.2), in alveolar macrophages (Fig. 63.3), and in type II pneumocytes.

## Alveolar Lavage Material

A better description of the alveolar material perhaps can be obtained from analysis of the material removed during lung lavage than from the lung biopsy specimen. The pulmonary alveolar proteinosis material is muddy in texture and has a beige color. It has a relatively high specific gravity and settles to the bottom of a bottle of saline within 20 minutes. It is very insoluble and resists degradation by trypsin, acetylcysteine, and heparin. The soluble component contains serum proteins with elevated concentrations of immunoglobulin G and markedly reduced alpha$_2$-macroglobulin.[5,6] The insoluble component has been shown to contain glycoproteins and phospholipid, primarily dipalmitoylphosphatidylcholine, much of it in the form of myelin structures (see Fig. 63.2) resembling those seen in the lamellar bodies of type II pneumocytes and isolated pulmonary surfactant.[7] Surfactant proteins A and D have been found in large amounts in lavage liquid from patients with pulmonary alveolar proteinosis.[8,9] The material removed from the patient during lavage is almost always sterile when cultured for bacteria, fungi, mycobacteria, and viruses.

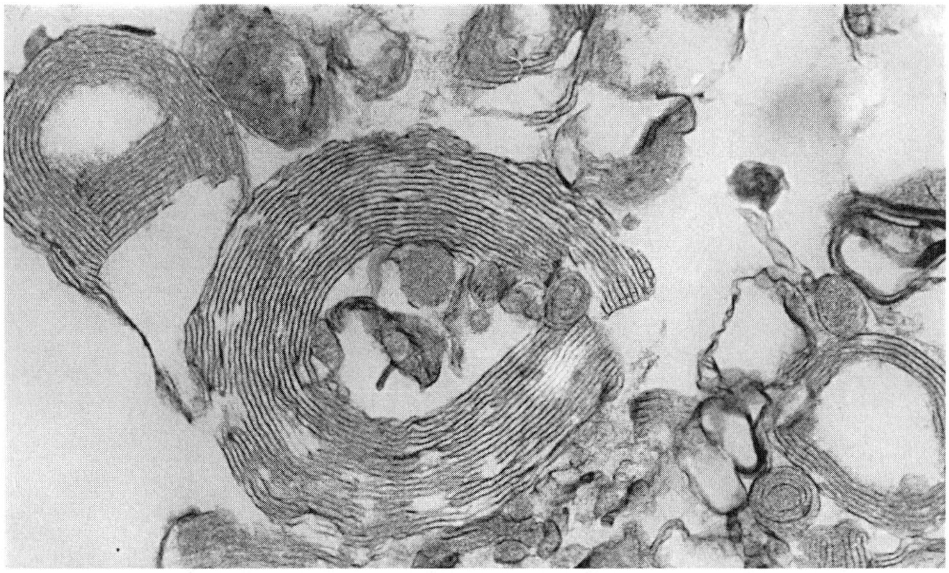

**Figure 63.2** Electron micrograph of alveolar debris. The structure of the material is lamellated, resembling surfactant. (Original magnification ×30,000.)

## NATURAL HISTORY

Without a national registry of this disorder, it is difficult to determine the frequency with which it occurs. However, from the reports in the literature, it is evident that this disease is seen throughout the United States and in virtually all industrialized countries. We estimate that several hundred new cases occur nationwide each year, and several thousand patients with this disease are alive in the United States. Because this disease does not appear to be as rare as once thought and because its etiology is unknown, we believe that a registry for it should be established.

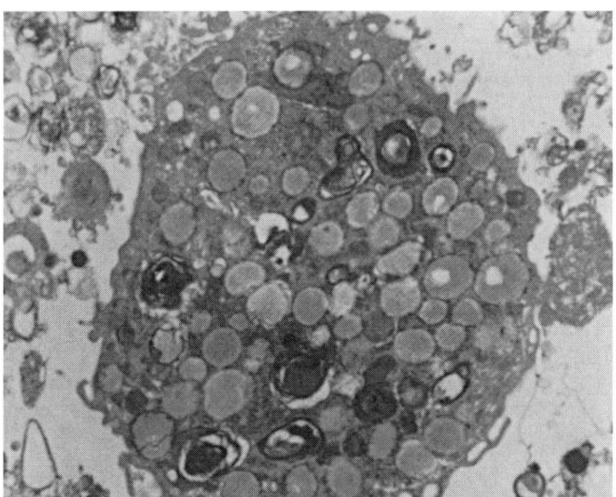

**Figure 63.3** Electron photomicrograph of a pulmonary macrophage from lavage material of a patient with pulmonary alveolar proteinosis. Lamellar material is abundant in the cytoplasm. This same material is found free in the alveolar spaces and lavage effluent of patients with pulmonary alveolar proteinosis. (Original magnification ×9625.)

Larson and Gordinier[10] reviewed 79 cases in the world literature in 1964. They noted that about one third of the patients progressively deteriorated or died, probably from hypoxia or superinfection; another one third appeared to be stable but symptomatic when reported; and the remaining one third appeared to improve, probably spontaneously, because none of the therapeutic modalities in use at the time, such as antibiotics, corticosteroids, potassium iodide, digesting enzymes, and bronchodilators, had been shown to be effective.

When whole-lung lavage was introduced by Ramirez and associates[11] in 1965, the prognosis improved. They observed that one lung could be filled safely with an isotonic saline solution and then be re-aerated. Modifications of this lavage technique were used to treat pulmonary alveolar proteinosis during the next 15 years. Since then, whole-lung lavage has been the method of treatment for the juvenile and adult forms of this disease and usually results in striking improvement clinically, physiologically, and radiologically.

Pulmonary alveolar proteinosis usually is not associated with other diseases, but it has been reported with hematologic malignancies,[10, 12, 13] inorganic dust exposure,[3] and infections in immunocompromised persons.[14] The disease primarily affects young or middle-aged adults, and it occurs in males about twice as often as it does in females; in our series, the ratio was even higher (Table 63.1). It also has occurred in infants,[15, 16] including children of the same family, but not adult siblings, suggesting either a genetic influence or common exposure. These patients do not behave as though they are immunosuppressed. However, because they often are given large doses of corticosteroids, or occasionally have a hematologic malignancy, they may be more susceptible to opportunistic infections than other patients with chronic lung diseases that impair pulmonary clearance mechanisms.

Nocardia pneumonia occurs with relatively high frequency, particularly in immunosuppressed patients.[17] However, it may occur in patients who have not been treated with immunosuppressive drugs and who have no

**Table 63.1 PHYSICAL CHARACTERISTICS AND OCCUPATIONS OF 30 PATIENTS WITH PULMONARY ALVEOLAR PROTEINOSIS**

| Patient | Age (yr) | Sex | Race* | Occupation |
|---|---|---|---|---|
| 1 | 3 | M | W | Child |
| 2 | 4 | M | W | Child |
| 3 | 30 | M | W | White-collar worker |
| 4 | 30 | M | W | Laborer |
| 5 | 30 | M | B | Laborer |
| 6 | 45 | M | W | Sea captain |
| 7 | 40 | M | W | White-collar worker |
| 8 | 17 | F | W | Student |
| 9 | 43 | F | W | Homemaker |
| 10 | 23 | F | W | Beautician |
| 11 | 29 | M | W | Salesman |
| 12 | 31 | M | W | Cement finisher |
| 13 | 22 | M | W | Computer operator |
| 14 | 20 | M | H | Plumber |
| 15 | 34 | M | W | Bakery worker |
| 16 | 44 | M | W | Heavy equipment operator |
| 17 | 35 | M | W | Heavy equipment operator |
| 18 | 30 | M | W | Laborer |
| 19 | 20 | M | H | Student |
| 20 | 37 | M | W | Salesman |
| 21 | 46 | F | W | Machinist |
| 22 | 47 | M | W | Construction worker |
| 23 | 40 | M | W | Maintenance worker |
| 24 | 41 | F | B | Secretary |
| 25 | 57 | F | A | Homemaker |
| 26 | 19 | M | B | Student |
| 27 | 56 | M | H | Construction worker |
| 28 | 27 | M | W | Truck driver |
| 29 | 35 | M | W | Bartender |
| 30 | 43 | F | W | Housekeeper |
| 31 | 9 | F | W | Student |
| 32 | 18 | M | W | Student |
| 33 | 50 | F | W | Housewife |
| 34 | 35 | M | W | Office worker, HIV+ |
| 35 | 50 | M | W | Accountant |

*Code: A = Asian; B = black; H = Hispanic; W = white

clear evidence of immunosuppression or a concomitant disease.

The term "secondary" alveolar proteinosis has been used to describe alveolar proteinosis occurring with malignancies[18] and also has been used to describe the findings in patients with human immunodeficiency virus infection.[19] The term "silicoproteinosis" has been used when histologic features typical of pulmonary alveolar proteinosis occur concurrently with evidence of inorganic dust pulmonary disease.

It has been conjectured that pulmonary alveolar proteinosis might be stimulated by inorganic dusts because it has been found in association with inorganic dust disease.[3, 4] However, pulmonary lavage material and tissue biopsy specimens typically do not contain high concentrations of inorganic dusts. Nevertheless, a disease resembling pulmonary alveolar proteinosis can be produced in animals by exposing them to fine quartz dust.[20]

Table 63.1 lists the occupations and age at diagnosis of 35 patients whom we have evaluated. It would appear that some of the patients had an opportunity to be exposed to a variety of dusts, although others had no history of inorganic dust exposure. Thus, the role of dusts in the naturally occurring form of pulmonary alveolar proteinosis is unclear.

Although usually not preceded by pulmonary alveolar proteinosis, pulmonary fibrosis has been reported in several patients with a classic history of pulmonary alveolar proteinosis.[21, 22] We observed a patient who had a complete remission from pulmonary alveolar proteinosis after whole-lung lavage in 1972 and remained asymptomatic for 10 years. The chest radiograph then changed, and new interstitial markings and honeycombing developed. The progressive loss of pulmonary function evolved to a typical picture of severe restrictive lung disease. The patient became quite symptomatic, with shortness of breath and a cough. Lung lavage produced only scant material, and the fluid was not characteristic of pulmonary alveolar proteinosis. Also, the lavage procedure did not appear to help him. It seemed as though this was a different disease from that which he had experienced 10 years earlier. Of the 35 patients with pulmonary alveolar proteinosis (see

Table 63.1), only this patient developed interstitial pulmonary fibrosis. Hudson and associates[23] reported a virtually identical experience with pulmonary insufficiency secondary to interstitial fibrosis 13 years after open-lung biopsy diagnosis of pulmonary alveolar proteinosis.

## ETIOLOGY AND PATHOGENESIS

A number of hypotheses have been suggested to explain the development of pulmonary alveolar proteinosis. They include genetic defects, defective alveolar macrophages, surfactant overproduction or decreased clearance, an unusual injury response to inhaled agents, immunodeficiency state, and response to infection. Although not used in the original description, "primary" and "secondary" have been applied by some authorities to describe this disorder. The adjective "secondary" is used when coexisting abnormalities, such as infection, hematologic malignancy, or silicosis, are present. Sometimes the term silicoproteinosis has been used when a considerable amount of silica or silicates is found in the air spaces. We believe that the distinction has not been helpful at the state of our current knowledge of the disease, and this classification has not been useful in describing the clinical presentations of the patients that we have seen.

### Genetic Defects

Since 1995, there have been a number of reports on the molecular biology of pulmonary alveolar proteinosis (PAP), particularly in the pediatric age group. At least three different gene defects that result in PAP have been reported: a mutation in the gene responsible for the production of surfactant protein-B (SP-B)[24, 25, 36]; an underexpression of the GM-CSF gene[26, 27]; and the beta-chain of the GM-CSF receptor in peripheral blood monocytes.[28]

Nogee and colleagues[24] reported neonatal PAP in five full-term newborns who died of respiratory failure, three of whom were siblings. Analysis of the pulmonary alveolar material revealed a deficiency in SP-B. This was further studied by de Mello and associates[25] in 10 SP-B–deficient patients in whom a mutation in the SP-B gene was described. It was suggested that the mutation is probably more common than previously appreciated and may account for unexplained neonatal deaths.

PAP also has been shown to result from an underexpression of GM-CSF.[26] In detailed studies in mice with knockout of the gene for GM-CSF, Huffman and coworkers[27] were able to produce the classical picture of PAP, despite structurally normal but abnormally increased amounts of surfactant proteins. Restoring expression of GM-CSF in respiratory epithelium to the transgenic mice corrects the aberrant surfactant homeostasis. The authors conclude that GM-CSF regulates the clearance and the catabolism of the surfactant protein and lipids from alveoli and not the production.

Dirksen and colleagues[28] described eight pediatric patients with PAP, four of whom expressed a defect in the beta-chain GM-CSF receptor of peripheral blood monocytes. These were older pediatric patients than those with SP-B deficiency. None of these patients had a deficiency in SP-B. It was suggested that a defect or deficiency in the beta chain of the GM-CSF receptor causes the alveolar macrophage to be unable to process the surfactant protein normally. These cells, which normally ingest and degrade surfactant, eventually die, causing the accumulation of phospholipid and surfactant protein in the alveoli. This group produced PAP experimentally in knockout mice by deletion of the GM-CSF gene or the common receptor component (beta chain) for GM-CSF, IL-3, and IL-5.[29] Bone marrow transplantation with wild-type bone marrow reversed the established disease in these genetically altered mice.[29] Thus, this mouse model demonstrated the genetic origin of some forms of PAP.

The possibility and likelihood of a defect in the hematopoietic system causing disease in some of the adult forms of PAP is supported by the increased incidence of PAP in hematologic disorders.[12–13, 30] The report of Cordonnier and colleagues[30] provides evidence linking defects in the monocytes (precursor to the alveolar macrophage) to PAP. By analysis of bronchoalveolar lavage (BAL), they showed PAP in 10 (10%) of their patients with myeloid forms of leukemia but none in patients with lymphoid malignancies. The presence of PAP was noted particularly during periods of neutropenia and therefore must be distinguished from active infection. Four of these cases showed the PAP to disappear on repeat BAL, with improvement in the neutrophil count.

Abnormal pulmonary alveolar macrophage function as a possible genetic etiology of pulmonary alveolar proteinosis was hypothesized by Parker and Novotny[31] in their case report of a 41-year-old woman who developed severe PAP. She underwent a double-lung transplantation because of unmanageable symptoms. Three years later, she developed a recurrence of PAP in the transplanted lungs. Because of lack of exposure history, the authors suggested that the disease process did not develop from an inhaled toxin but rather from disturbed function within the patient, most likely an abnormality in the hematopoietic source of the pulmonary alveolar macrophages.

### Defective Alveolar Macrophages

Abnormal macrophage function has been described in patients with pulmonary alveolar proteinosis,[32] and it appears that this is an acquired disturbance caused by ingesting alveolar material by the macrophages.[33] Golde and coworkers[32] suggested that the macrophages become relatively immobile consequent to "overfeeding," causing them to become exceptionally large (>5 to 10 times normal). In culture medium, these macrophages eliminate much of their ingested material and appear to become normally mobile.[34] Peripheral blood monocytes in adults with alveolar proteinosis have normal phagocytic properties.[35]

### Surfactant Overproduction or Decreased Clearance

The chemical similarity between surfactant and pulmonary alveolar proteinosis material first was noted by Larson and Gordinier.[10] They suggested that pulmonary alveolar proteinosis material might result from an overproduction of surfactant or a failure of surfactant removal.

This attractive hypothesis is consistent with electron microscopic findings showing that material in the alveolar spaces and that obtained during whole-lung lavage closely resemble the surfactant-containing lamellar bodies found in and secreted by type II pneumocytes. This suggests that the pulmonary alveolar material possibly originates, at least in part, from these alveolar cells. If there is an excessive rate of secretion or impaired rate of reutilization of surfactant, then this material would accumulate in the alveoli.

### Unusual Injury Response to Inhaled Agents

The case reports of silica[3] and aluminum[4] dust exposure coexisting with pulmonary alveolar proteinosis, and the experimental finding that inhaled fine silica dust in animals can cause a similar disease,[20] lend support to the hypothesis that inhaled dust is responsible for the development of some forms of pulmonary alveolar proteinosis. However, the lack of accumulation of inorganic particles in the alveolar spaces of the lungs in most cases of pulmonary alveolar proteinosis and the lack of epidemiologic support relating occupation to disease occurrence make this hypothesis unsatisfactory for most cases. It is possible that pulmonary alveolar proteinosis has multiple causes and that inhaled dust is but one.

### Immunodeficiency State

The view that pulmonary alveolar proteinosis is an immunologic disorder has limited support. Patients with alveolar proteinosis usually do not have joint, skin, or renal manifestations. They do not have a predilection to infection involving organ systems other than the lungs, nor do they have an abnormal response to infection.

Despite several reports of changes in the lung resembling pulmonary alveolar proteinosis in patients with acquired immunodeficiency syndrome (AIDS), these have been associated with infectious agents. However, we have seen a single human immunodeficiency virus (HIV)-infected patient without AIDS with the typical findings of alveolar proteinosis on lung biopsy. In contrast to *Pneumocystis* pneumonia, proliferation of type II cells was less marked and the granularity of the amorphous material was not coarse. The physiology and clinical response of this patient was similar to that of other noninfected patients with alveolar proteinosis.

### Response to Infection

Because of the histologic similarities between *Pneumocystis carinii* pneumonia and pulmonary alveolar proteinosis, both of which are primarily intra-alveolar processes, Rosen and associates[1] speculated that the disease may be a "burned out" form of pneumocystis. However, despite intensive search, they could not find a single *Pneumocystis* organism in any of their 27 original cases. It is of interest that pulmonary alveolar proteinosis-like ultrastructural abnormalities have been described in bronchoalveolar lavage fluid from patients with various immunosuppressive diseases complicated by *P. carinii* pneumonia.[14] Bacterial infections, particularly *Nocardia asteroides*, have been associated with pulmonary alveolar proteinosis. Other bacterial infections may occur and result from patients' increased susceptibility to infection because of impaired lung clearance mechanisms, immunosuppression from use of corticosteroids for treatment, or an underlying hematologic malignancy. Because lavage fluid cultures are virtually always sterile, it seems unlikely that microorganisms are the stimulus for the pathogenesis of this disorder.

In summary, both the lung biopsy specimen and the BAL material provide us with valuable insights into the pathogenesis of pulmonary alveolar proteinosis. Multiple lung lavage treatments make longitudinal data collection possible and improve our understanding of pathogenesis. The disease appears to originate at the alveolar surface. Type II pneumocytes are involved, either by oversecreting, overreplicating, or failing to reabsorb used surfactant, possibly in response to an inhaled foreign agent. But because the materials in the alveoli are natural products of the body, an inflammatory reaction is not stimulated. Nevertheless, it appears that alveolar proteinosis in the newborn is the result of genetic factors in GM-CSF or its receptor, but a genetic factor in the adult form of the disease is less clear.[36] Because the appearance of the disease is in such a diverse group of patients, pulmonary alveolar proteinosis is likely to be a common manifestation of heterogeneous factors that affect the type II pneumocyte or the alveolar macrophage, or both.

## CLINICAL PRESENTATION

The major symptom of pulmonary alveolar proteinosis is shortness of breath with exercise. Some patients have a mild cough with occasional sputum production described as "white and gummy" or "chunky" in consistency. Chest pain and hemoptysis are extremely unusual, but weight loss, malaise, and fatigue are common. If the patient has fever, either the disease is not pulmonary alveolar proteinosis or the patient has a superinfection.

### Physical Signs

Patients with pulmonary alveolar proteinosis may show few physical signs of disease. The hypoxic patient usually has weight loss and, in severe cases, clubbed fingers, cyanosis, and petechial hemorrhages in the retina. The patient usually breathes comfortably at rest. The chest examination reveals surprisingly little. On deep inspiration, interspace retraction is minimal and chest expansion may be normal, unlike findings in patients with restrictive lung disease secondary to interstitial pulmonary fibrosis. Breath sounds are usually normal. Fine rales at the lung bases may be present, and if so, they are very few. The absence of rales, despite the presence of large amounts of infiltrate on the chest radiograph, can be attributed to the peripheral process of this disorder (i.e., filling of the most peripheral gas spaces). Because gas does not move through the proteinaceous material, there is no operative mechanism for generating rales. If there are prominent rales, a superinfection should be suspected.

## Roentgenographic Findings

The disease process affects both lungs relatively uniformly. The infiltrates generally are more pronounced in the perihilar regions and appear to be less dense peripherally, suggesting the "bat wing" appearance of pulmonary edema, and unlike idiopathic interstitial pulmonary fibrosis. Figure 63.4 demonstrates a characteristic chest roentgenogram and the dramatic clearing in the same patient after whole-lung lavage of both lungs. The pattern of the infiltrate appears to be a combination of acinar filling and increased interstitial markings. Lymphadenopathy and pleural disease are rare.

Computed tomography demonstrates the extent and pattern of regional lung involvement of pulmonary alveolar proteinosis better than the chest roentgenogram. The involved lung may have either dense consolidation or a ground glass appearance. Portions of the healthy lung adjacent to diseased portions provide a mosaic patchy appearance. Thickened lobular septa may give rise to a diffuse "interstitial" pattern. These abnormalities resolve partially or completely after lavage, indicating the absence of true interstitial disease.[37] Although the computed tomographic appearance may be too variable to be diagnostic, it may prove useful in evaluating the evolution of the disease process or the response to therapy.[38] A characteristic appearance should suggest strongly the diagnosis of pulmonary alveolar proteinosis.

## Laboratory Examination

The hematocrit and hemoglobin concentrations are normal or increased. If they are reduced, a complicating illness must be suspected. The white blood cell and differential counts are also normal. The lactate dehydrogenase (LDH) concentration characteristically is increased, but serum glutamic-oxaloacetic transaminase (SGOT) is normal. High levels of pulmonary surfactant protein A have been reported in the sera of patients with pulmonary alveolar proteinosis.[39] Chemical disturbances associated with organ abnormalities other than the lungs are quite unusual.

## Respiratory Function

The diffusing capacity for carbon monoxide ($DL_{CO}$) and $DL_{CO}$ per liter of alveolar volume ($DL_{CO}/VA$) are characteristically reduced.[40] Vital capacity and total lung capacity generally are reduced, although they may be normal. The reduction in these lung volumes is not as striking as the decrease in $DL_{CO}$, possibly reflecting the relative absence of fibrosis. In pulmonary alveolar proteinosis, the reduced $DL_{CO}$ and $DL_{CO}/VA$ probably reflect a relatively pure form of alveolar-capillary block syndrome.

Arterial $PO_2$ and oxygen saturation are reduced (Fig. 63.5). Arterial $PCO_2$ usually is decreased as well (Fig. 63.6), but pH is normal, reflecting a chronic compensated respiratory alkalosis. With exercise, arterial $PO_2$ progressively decreases as work rate is increased incrementally (see Fig. 63.5); before lavage, arterial $PCO_2$ also decreases, but to a lesser degree, and remains essentially unchanged after the lavage (see Fig. 63.6). The minute ventilation required to perform exercise is high because of the low arterial $PCO_2$ set-point maintained by these patients. Performing exercise while breathing 100% oxygen substantially reduces the ventilatory response to exercise (Fig. 63.7), demonstrating a significant hypoxic drive to breathe. After lavage, the ventilatory requirement is re-

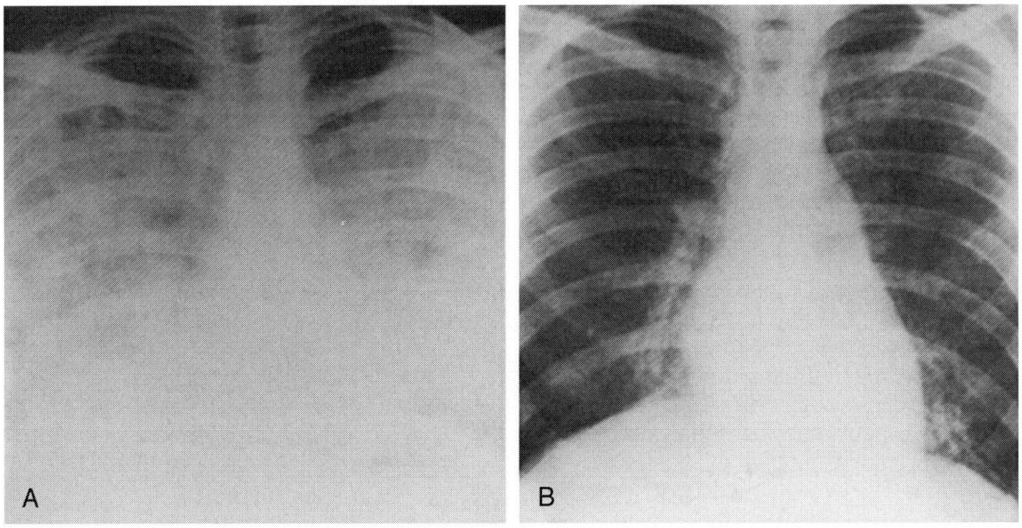


**Figure 63.4** Chest roentgenograms of a 19-year-old patient with severe pulmonary alveolar proteinosis. *A,* At the time of initial diagnosis. *B,* After whole-lung lavage treatment. Although all patients, in our experience, have rapid improvement on the chest roentgenogram after lung lavage, some becoming normal, the improvement is often not quite as striking as that shown.

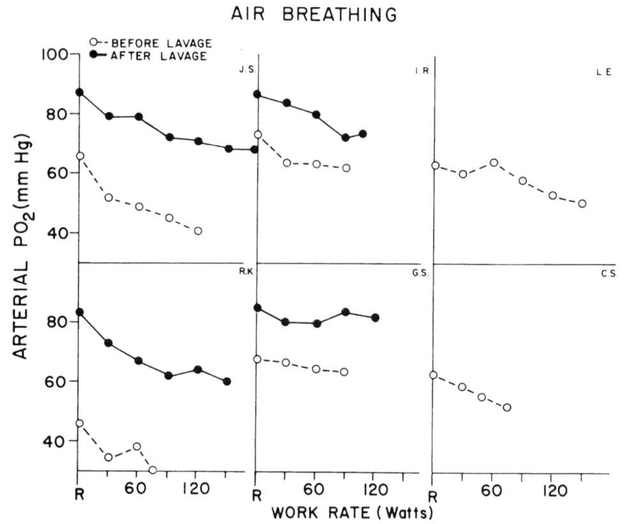


**Figure 63.5** Response of arterial $Po_2$ to exercise in six patients before (and 2 days after) whole-lung lavage treatment. Note the arterial $Po_2$ decreases with increasing work rate before whole-lung lavage and improves after treatment.

duced significantly at the same exercise work rate, and exercise tolerance is improved (see Fig. 63.7).

## DIAGNOSIS

Because the major symptom of shortness of breath and radiologic findings of pulmonary infiltrates are common to many pulmonary disorders, it is worthwhile noting some of the distinctive features of pulmonary alveolar proteinosis. As mentioned previously, these patients generally show no sign of infection or hematologic evidence of chronic or acute disease. The radiologic examination usually cannot distinguish infiltrates of pulmonary alveolar proteinosis from infection.

The diagnosis of pulmonary alveolar proteinosis can be made from BAL or lung biopsy during bronchoscopy, avoiding an open-lung biopsy. BAL of a lung segment produces an effluent which is usually milky in appearance. Under light microscopy, a large amount of amorphous debris with frequent, very large macrophages having prominent cytoplasm that stains deep pink with PAS can be observed. Cells other than macrophages are absent. If there is a neutrophilia or lymphocytosis, an infection or autoimmune response must be considered, but these are rare. Electron microscopy of the lavage fluid sediment shows abundant lamellar bodies and phospholipid organized in coils (see Fig. 63.2). Pulmonary alveolar proteinosis should be considered in the differential diagnosis of an afebrile patient demonstrating perihilar pulmonary infiltrates on the chest roentgenogram with absence of physical signs when the chest is examined. As described previously, the diagnosis is evident from the histopathologic findings on examination of either lung biopsy or BAL fluid by light and electron microscopy.

## TREATMENT

Whole-lung lavage is the only consistently successful treatment for pulmonary alveolar proteinosis and is described in detail. Other forms of treatment that have been used, such as corticosteroids, saturated potassium iodide solution, and aerosolization or instillation of trypsin, acetylcysteine, and heparin into the lungs, have not been shown to be beneficial.

### Whole-Lung Lavage

Ramirez and colleagues[11] took the bold step of using a Carlens tube to separate both lungs, degassing one lung and then flooding it with saline containing heparin and acetylcysteine, while providing gas exchange for the patient with the other lung. The patient was given only local anesthesia and allowed to take deep breaths to mix the acetylcysteine-saline with the material in the alveolar spaces. The solution then was drained, suctioned, and coughed out, resulting in a significant improvement of the patient. With the demonstration that the lung can be flooded and then re-aerated. Wasserman and coworkers[41] modified the technique of Ramirez to perform whole-lung lavage in an anesthetized patient in whom the lung remained degassed for approximately 3 hours while it was lavaged with fresh solutions until the effluent was almost clear. This required 20 L or more of solution for each lung.

Finding that the alveolar proteinosis material was not significantly dissolved by the addition of heparin and acetylcysteine in large amounts in vitro, Wasserman[42] evaluated the efficacy of these substances during whole-lung lavage in two patients with pulmonary alveolar proteinosis. No benefit was found over the use of saline alone when acetylcysteine and heparin were added to the saline. Later, it was found that the yield from whole-lung lavage could be enhanced considerably by chest percussion during the procedure.[41]

A number of techniques have been described for whole-lung lavage, including lavaging each lung on 2

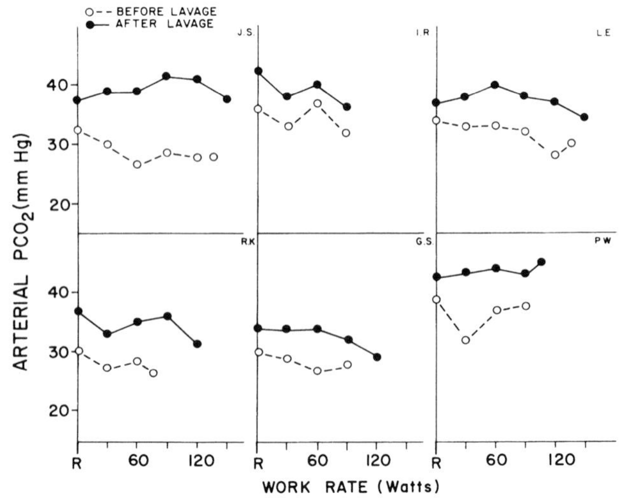


**Figure 63.6** Response of arterial $Pco_2$ to exercise in six patients before (and 2 days after) whole-lung lavage treatment. It should be noted that the patients have a compensated respiratory alkalosis before lavage that quickly disappears after treatment.

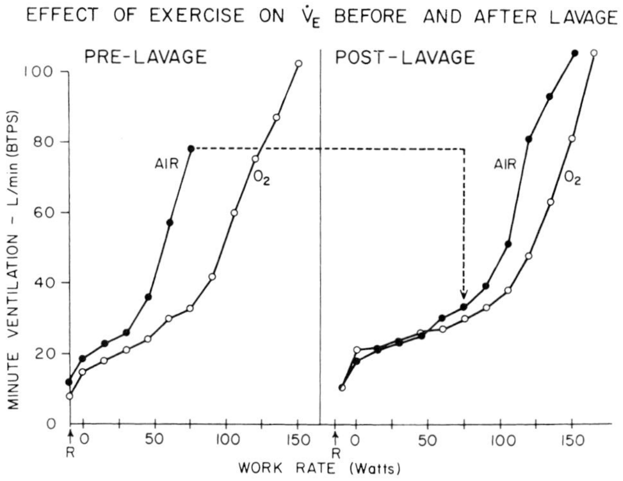


**Figure 63.7** Ventilatory response to incremental exercise before and 2 days after whole-lung lavage while breathing air (and 100% $O_2$ in one patient). The broken line arrow linking the two panels is designed to show the magnitude of the ventilation decrease at 75 W in this patient while breathing air. This treatment obviously provided the patient with a striking relief of his dyspnea.

separate days,[40, 41, 43] one lung at a time on the same day,[44] and, in small children, both lungs while on partial cardiopulmonary bypass.[16, 45] The reader should review these specific reports for the lavage techniques used in special situations. We find the following technique most efficacious for adults.

## Staff

Although the procedure can be accomplished with a smaller team, we find that a team of six people is optimal.

- A physician skilled in the evaluation of the physiologic status of the cardiovascular and respiratory systems is the team leader. This physician oversees the procedure and decides when the tracheal divider is in the correct position, when to start and terminate the lavage, and when the lavaged lung is re-aerated and the patient is ready to leave the operating room for the recovery room. This physician continuously monitors the electrocardiogram, the oxygen saturation by ear oximetry, and breath-to-breath changes in airway pressure and volume. Any unusual change is a reason for stopping the procedure to obtain an understanding of its significance before continuing. This physician is responsible for the overall safety of the patient while the others attend to specific tasks.
- An anesthesiologist anesthetizes the patient, controls the airway gases, and inserts the tracheal divider. He or she also monitors the patient's vital signs, temperature, level of anesthesia, and degree of paralysis.
- Another person is responsible for filling the lung with saline, draining it, and doing this repeatedly during the lavage procedure until there is appropriate clearing of the lavage effluent.
- A scribe is needed to record the airway pressure and the volume of each lung before and after the lavage to compare the compliance of the lavaged to the nonlavaged lung. In addition, this person records the volume of saline instilled and drained from each lung during each individual lavage to ensure that fluid balance is maintained. This provides assurance that saline has not leaked from the lavaged lung into either the pleural space or the contralateral lung. The scribe also records data on arterial oxygen saturation from the ear oximeter and blood gases.
- A respiratory therapist is needed to provide mechanical chest percussion to the side of the chest being lavaged.
- A nurse assistant provides any special supplies or equipment and communicates with outside support personnel (e.g., radiologists).

## Patient Preparation

The procedure is performed in the operating room under general anesthesia with muscle paralysis, and with continuous monitoring of heart rate and rhythm by an electrocardiograph and of arterial oxygen saturation by ear oximetry. The anesthesiologist monitors heart rate, blood pressure, arterial blood gases, level of anesthesia, and degree of motor blockade. The patient is ventilated with oxygen and the anesthetic gas. When the patient is anesthetized, a tracheal divider is passed, allowing separation of the two lungs. A Carlens tube had been used traditionally, but currently a disposable transparent tracheal divider with openings at the same sites (left main stem bronchus and trachea) as in the Carlens tube is used, with its position verified with a pediatric bronchoscope inserted through the tracheal lumen. Because this tracheal divider does not have a hook on it, unlike the Carlens tube, it is easier to pass. But the hook is useful because it facilitates maintenance of the catheter's position during the procedure. The supine position, rather than the decubitus position, is used during the lung lavage procedure to minimize mediastinal and therefore tracheal shifts. In the decubitus position, these shifts are more likely to occur and cause saline to leak into the contralateral lung. Ventilation with 100% oxygen and the anesthetic gas is adjusted so that it adequately regulates arterial $P_{CO_2}$ if only one lung is functioning. This can be tested by clamping the side to be lavaged for several minutes and checking the arterial $P_{CO_2}$.

The dynamic lung compliance is determined for each lung by measuring the inflation volume and pressure of each side while the other side is clamped. If, during the lavage procedure, the compliance of the ventilated side decreases, one should suspect saline spillover from the lavaged side or a herniation of the occluding balloon from the lavage to the ventilated side.

## The Lavage Procedure

An inverted "Y" connector is used to link the lumen of the Carlens tube in the lung to be lavaged with tubing to a saline reservoir and tubing leading to a bottle below the level of the chest that collects the lavage effluent. Before starting the lavage, the tubing system should be filled completely with saline; to obtain the proper siphon effect when draining the lung, care must be taken to avoid trapping air bubbles in the tubing.

Because the lung to be lavaged contains only oxygen, it is degassed within 5 minutes. Unclamping the tubing from the saline reservoir to the lung to be lavaged permits saline to flow into the lung as the oxygen is absorbed. The saline reservoir filling pressure is set at 30 cm $H_2O$. Saline stops flowing into the lung when all the oxygen is absorbed and when the lung has reached approximately its total capacity. The tubing from the saline reservoir then is clamped, and the clamp on the tubing leading to the drainage bottle is released. After drainage of some clear saline from the lung tubing dead space, an opaque beige solution should drain from the lung. The volume of the saline entering the lung should approximate the volume of saline leaving the lung, except for the first inflow, from which about 500 mL is retained in the residual volume. The volume used for each inflow is 1 to 1.5 L in an average adult, and it takes approximately 5 minutes to fill and drain the lung. This information is recorded by the scribe. The respiratory therapist provides percussion to the side of the chest in all lavages after the first. Before the lavage procedure, the chest being lavaged is covered with adhesive flannel to protect the skin from abrasion during percussion. The chest is percussed with a mechanical percussor during the filling and drainage of the lung, except when both the inflow and outflow tubing are clamped, and when the lung is near residual volume. As previously reported by Kao and associates,[43] lung percussion increases the yield of proteinosis material by about fourfold. We do an average of 10 to 15 whole-lung lavages during a single lavage procedure, the total treatment lasting between 1 and 2 hours.

## Lung Re-aeration

We believe that re-aeration of the lavaged lung and restoration of its compliance before sending the patient into the recovery room speed the patient's recovery and minimize chances of infection in the just-lavaged lung. Therefore, once the lavage is terminated, the "Y" tube connected to the tracheal divider is disconnected, and saline and foam are suctioned out of the lavaged lung. The respirator then is attached to both ports of the tracheal divider while ventilating both sides. More foam soon rises up in the channel of the lavaged lung, and suctioning again is needed. When the saline and foam come up more slowly, the unlavaged side is clamped for 5- to 10-breath intervals so that only the just-lavaged lung receives the total ventilation. This provides a deeper inspiration to the just-lavaged side and speeds removal of foam.

After about 15 minutes, we start monitoring the pressure and volume of the two lungs. We continue ventilating only the just-lavaged lung for about 5 breaths after about 10 to 20 breaths of ventilating both lungs. This alternating ventilation is used until the pressure-volume relationship of the lavaged lung is approximately equal, as shown in Figure 63.8. We are then confident that the lavaged lung has regained its surface forces (regenerated surfactant) and will not become atelectatic relative to the unlavaged lung. The lung generally is re-aerated within 1 hour after the lavage is completed, and the patient can be extubated. We attribute our low incidence of postoperative morbidity and the lack of the need for an endotracheal tube to manage the patient after the lavage to the re-aeration procedure.

In the recovery room, the respiratory therapist encourages deep breathing assisted by a positive pressure respirator. The patient is awake but sleepy at this time. In 2 to 3 hours, the patient is awake and stable enough to return to the medical floor. That evening, the patient already notices that it is easier to breathe on the side just lavaged and generally is interested in eating. We allow the patient to have a light meal on the evening of the lavage. For the first 24 hours, we treat the patient with a beta-agonist aerosol and encourage deep breathing and use of an incentive spirometer.

## Other Aspects of Whole-Lung Lavage

Despite having one lung completely filled with isotonic saline for 2 to 3 hours during lung lavage, the changes in serum electrolyte composition are not marked.[41] As one might predict, bicarbonate and potassium are decreased, and chloride is increased. However, these changes are temporary and self-correct within 24 hours.

During the lavage procedure, blood is diverted to the ventilated lung when the lung being lavaged is filled with saline and returns to the lavaged lung when that lung is drained.[41, 46] Monitoring with a reliable ear oximeter or measuring arterial $Po_2$ provides the lavage team with information they might require for making the decision to discontinue the lavage treatment early because of hypoxemia. We have found whole-lung lavage to be safe and effective when the lavage team has a good appreciation of the physiology involved in performing the procedure and re-aerating the lung. In well more than 100 lavage procedures, our morbidity consists of one minor pneumothorax not requiring a chest tube. On this occasion, we deviated from our usual procedure and attempted to reventilate the lung using positive end-expiratory pressure. Although we have had no other complications associated with lung lavage, we have been forced to shorten the lavage procedure on several occasions because of unsatisfactory placement of the Carlens tube. But even on these occasions, the patient experienced considerable improvement in function and symptoms.

After 2 to 3 hours in the recovery room, the patient is sufficiently awake to return to his or her hospital room, breathing supplemental oxygen supplied through nasal prongs. The blood gas measurements by that evening are improved considerably. When patients are questioned about how they feel 6 to 8 hours after the lung lavage, the uniform response is that the lavaged side of the chest feels "much lighter." The use of the weight reference to describe the change in symptomatology is interesting. The amount of solid material removed from each lung is usually at least the weight of the lung itself. Thus, it is easy to understand that there may be a sense of acute

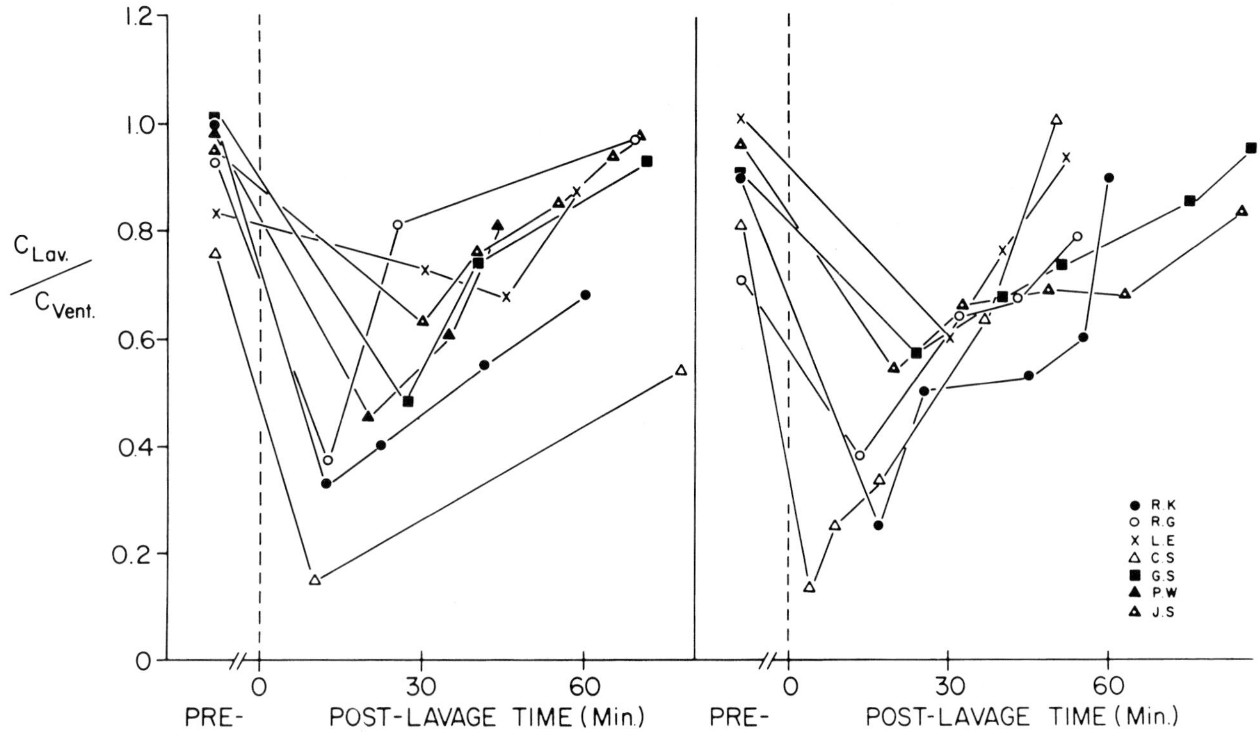


**Figure 63.8** Ratio of dynamic compliance of the just-lavaged lung (and chest wall) ($C_{Lav.}$) to the ventilated lung (and chest wall) ($C_{Vent.}$) at the times indicated after the right lung *(right panel)* and left lung *(left panel)* lavage. The ordinate shows the values before the start of lung lavage (pre), and the abscissa shows the time after discontinuance of the lavage. When the values reach a value of "1," the re-aeration procedure is considered complete, the double-lumen catheter is removed, and the patient is sent to the recovery room.

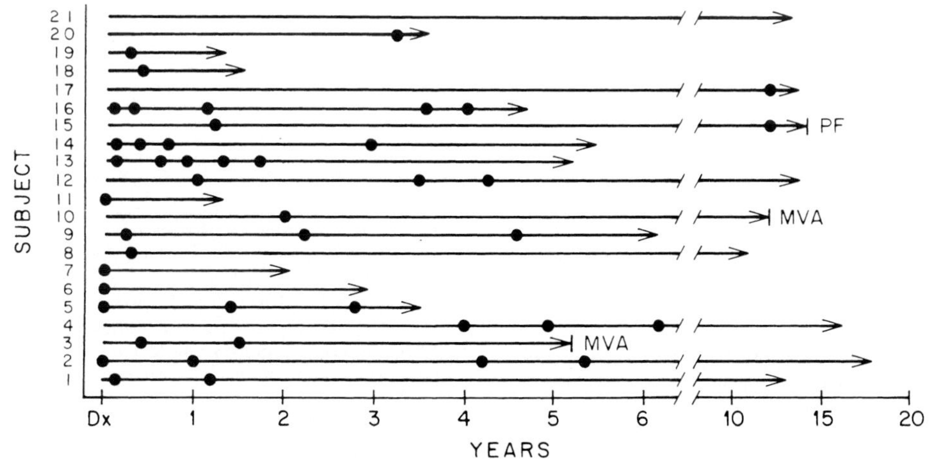


**Figure 63.9** Available follow-up, after diagnosis, on 21 patients with alveolar proteinosis. Two of the three deaths in our patients were due to motor vehicle accidents (MVA) unrelated to their pulmonary alveolar proteinosis. The single patient with pulmonary fibrosis (PF) is the only patient with pulmonary alveolar proteinosis that we have seen develop this disorder. Although only one lavage may be needed for a prolonged remission, some patients may need several lavages at 6- to 12-month intervals before their disease becomes quiescent.

weight change within the chest when breathing after whole-lung lavage.

## PROGNOSIS

Patients with pulmonary alveolar proteinosis treated with whole-lung lavage almost always do well. Some require repeat lung lavage treatments at intervals of 6 to 12 months before the disease process smolders out and becomes quiescent. Figure 63.9 shows the follow-up of 21 patients with pulmonary alveolar proteinosis on whom information was available. All who are living appear to be doing well. Our longest surviving patient with whom one of us has maintained contact (patient 2), is free of symptoms 31 years since her first lavage for an incapacitating illness (resting arterial $P_{O_2} < 40$ mm Hg). Although requiring four lung lavages within the first 5 years after diagnosis, she has not required a repeat lung lavage since 1973. Because there is much that we do not know about this fascinating disease, we believe that these patients should be watched more closely than healthy subjects for detection of complicating illnesses.

## SUMMARY

Pulmonary alveolar proteinosis is a noninflammatory disease of the lungs, primarily involving the alveoli and probably, more specifically, alveolar macrophages and type II pneumocytes. The alveolar spaces are filled with an amorphous, insoluble, proteinaceous lipid material that ultrastructurally contains phospholipid and resembles surfactant. The major symptom is exertional dyspnea caused by impaired diffusion of oxygen from the gas spaces of the lung to the capillary blood. It usually can be treated effectively by whole-lung lavage. The prognosis is good in most patients. Much progress is being made in our understanding of the pathogenesis of this disease. The molecular basis of the disease is being clarified, particularly in neonatal patients. The etiology remains speculative in the adult population probably because of multiple factors that might induce the disease process.

## References


1. Rosen SH, Castleman B, Liebow AA: Pulmonary alveolar proteinosis. N Engl J Med 258:1123–1142, 1958.
2. Hook GER, Gilmore LB, Talley FA: Multi-lamellated structures from the lungs of patients with pulmonary alveolar proteinosis. Lab Invest 50:711–725, 1984.
3. Buechner HA, Ansari A: Acute silicoproteinosis: A new pathologic variant of acute silicosis in sandblasters characterized by histologic features resembling alveolar proteinosis. Dis Chest 55:274–284, 1969.
4. Miller RR, Churg AM, Hutcheon M, Lam S: Case reports: Pulmonary alveolar proteinosis and aluminum dust exposure. Am Rev Respir Dis 130:312–315, 1984.
5. Rupp GH, Wasserman K, Ogawa M, Heiner DC: Bronchopulmonary fluids in pulmonary alveolar proteinosis. J Allergy Clin Immunol 51:227–237, 1973.
6. Bell DY, Hook GER: Pulmonary alveolar proteinosis: Analysis of airway and alveolar proteins. Am Rev Respir Dis 119:979–990, 1979.
7. Hook GER, Bell DY, Gilmore LB, et al: Composition of bronchoalveolar lavage effluents from patients with pulmonary alveolar proteinosis. Lab Invest 39:342–357, 1978.
8. Honda Y, Takahashi H, Shijubo N, et al: Surfactant protein A concentration in bronchoalveolar lavage fluids of patients with pulmonary alveolar proteinosis. Chest 103:496–499, 1993.
9. Crouch E, Persson A, Chang D: Accumulation of surfactant protein D in human pulmonary alveolar proteinosis. Am J Pathol 142:241–248, 1993.
10. Larson RK, Gordinier R: Pulmonary alveolar proteinosis: Report of six cases, review of the literature and formulation of a new theory. Ann Intern Med 62:292–312, 1965.
11. Ramirez J, Kieffer RF Jr, Ball D Jr: Bronchopulmonary lavage in man. Ann Intern Med 63:819–828, 1965.
12. Aymard JP, Gyger M, Lavalee R, et al: A case of pulmonary alveolar proteinosis complicating chronic myelogenous leukemia. Cancer 53:954–956, 1984.
13. Carnovale R, Zornoza J, Goldman AM, Luna M: Pulmonary alveolar proteinosis: Its association with hematologic malignancy and lymphoma. Radiology 122:303–306, 1977.
14. Tran VN, Vojek AM, Bernaudin JF, et al: Pulmonary alveolar proteinosis associated with Pneumocystis carinii: Ultrastructural identification in bronchoalveolar lavage in AIDS and immunocompromised non-AIDS patients. Chest 98:801–805, 1990.
15. Colon AR, Lawrence RD, Mills SD, O'Connell EJ: Childhood pulmonary alveolar proteinosis (PAP). Am J Dis Child 121:481–485, 1971.
16. Sakai Y, Abo W, Yoshimura H, et al: Pulmonary alveolar proteinosis in infants. Eur J Pediatr 158:424–426, 1999.
17. Bedrossian CWM, Luna MA, Conklin RH, Miller WC: Alveolar proteinosis as a consequence of immunosuppression: A hypothesis based on clinical and pathologic observations. Hum Pathol 11(Suppl):527–535, 1980.
18. Green D, Dighe P, Ali NO, Katele GV: Pulmonary alveolar proteinosis complicating chronic myelogenous leukemia. Cancer 46:1763–1766, 1980.
19. Ruben FL, Talamo TS: Secondary alveolar proteinosis in two patients with acquired immune deficiency syndrome. Am J Med 80:1187–1190, 1986.
20. Heppleston AG, Wright NA, Stewart JA: Experimental alveolar lipoproteinosis following the inhalation of silica. J Pathol 101:293–307, 1970.
21. Miller PA, Ravin CE, Walker Smith GJ, Osborne DRS: Pulmonary alveolar proteinosis with interstitial involvement. AJR Am J Roentgenol 137:1060–1071, 1981.
22. Kaplan AI, Sabin S: Case report: Interstitial fibrosis after uncomplicated pulmonary alveolar proteinosis. Postgrad Med 61:263–265, 1977.
23. Hudson AR, Halprin GM, Miller JA, Kilburn KH: Pulmonary interstitial fibrosis following alveolar proteinosis. Chest 65:700–702, 1974.
24. Nogee LM, Garnier G, Dietz HC, et al: A mutation in the surfactant protein B gene responsible for fatal neonatal respiratory disease in multiple kindreds. J Clin Invest 93:1860–1863, 1994.
25. de Mello DE, Nogee LM, Heyman S, et al: Molecular and phenotypic variability in the congenital alveolar proteinosis syndrome associated with inherited surfactant protein B deficiency. J Pediatr 125:43–50, 1994.
26. Hallman M, Meritt TA: Lack of GM-CSF as a cause of pulmonary alveolar proteinosis. J Clin Invest 97:589–590, 1996.
27. Huffman JA, Hull WM, Dranoff G, et al: Pulmonary epithelial cell expression of GM-CSF corrects the alveolar proteinosis in GM-CSF-deficient mice. J Clin Invest 97:649–655, 1996.
28. Dirksen U, Nishinakamura R, Groneck P, et al: Human pulmonary alveolar proteinosis associated with a defect in GM-CSF/IL-3/IL-5 receptor common β chain expression. J Clin Invest 100:2211–2217, 1997.
29. Nishinakamura R, Wiler R, Dirksen U, et al: The pulmonary alveolar proteinosis in granulocyte macrophage colony-stimulating factor/interleukins 3/5 βc receptor-deficient mice is reversed by bone marrow transplantation. J Exp Med 183:2657–2662, 1996.
30. Cordonnier C, Fleury-Feith J, Escudier E, et al: Secondary alveolar proteinosis is a reversible cause of respiratory failure in leukemic patients. Am J Respir Crit Care Med 149:788–794, 1994.
31. Parker LA, Novotny DB: Recurrent alveolar proteinosis following double lung transplantation: Chest 111:1457–1458, 1997.
32. Golde DW, Territo M, Finley TN, Cline MJ: Defective lung macrophages in pulmonary alveolar proteinosis. Ann Intern Med 85:304–309, 1976.

33. Nugent KM, Pesanti EL: Macrophage function in pulmonary alveolar proteinosis. Am Rev Respir Dis 127:780–781, 1983.
34. Spitler L, Keuppers F, Fundenberg HH: Normal macrophages function in pulmonary alveolar proteinosis. Am Rev Respir Dis 102:975–977, 1970.
35. Stratton JA, Sieger L, Wasserman K: The immunoinhibitory activities of the lung lavage materials and sera from patients with pulmonary alveolar proteinosis (PAP). J Clin Lab Immunol 5:81–86, 1981.
36. Kitamura T, Tanaka N, Watanabe J, et al: Idiopathic pulmonary alveolar proteinosis as an autoimmune disease with neutralizing antibody against granulocyte/macrophage colony-stimulating factor. J Exp Med 190:875–880, 1999.
37. Godwin JD, Muller NL, Takasugi JE: Pulmonary alveolar proteinosis: CT findings. Radiology 169:609–613, 1988.
38. Murayama S, Murakami J, Yabuuchi H, et al: "Crazy paving appearance" on high resolution CT in various diseases. J Comput Assist Tomogr 23:749–752, 1999.
39. Kuroki Y, Tsutahara S, Shijubo N, et al: Elevated levels of lung surfactant protein A in sera from patients with idiopathic pulmonary fibrosis and pulmonary alveolar proteinosis. Am Rev Respir Dis 147:723–729, 1993.
40. Selecky PA, Wasserman K, Benfield JR, Lippman M: The clinical and physiological effect of whole-lung lavage in pulmonary alveolar proteinosis: A ten-year experience. Ann Thorac Surg 24:451–461, 1977.
41. Wasserman K, Blank N, Fletcher G: Lung lavage (alveolar washing) in alveolar proteinosis. Am J Med 44:611–617, 1968.
42. Wasserman K: Solutions used for lung lavage in alveolar proteinosis: Respiratory Care Symposium. J Wadsworth Gen Hosp 11:217–221, 1968.
43. Kao D, Wasserman K, Benfield JR, Costley D: Advances in the treatment of pulmonary alveolar proteinosis. Am Rev Respir Dis 111:361–363, 1975.
44. Kariman K, Kylstra JA, Spock A: Pulmonary alveolar proteinosis: Prospective clinical experience in 23 patients for 15 years. Lung 162:223–231, 1984.
45. Freedman AP, Pelias A, Johnston RF, et al: Alveolar proteinosis lung lavage using partial cardiopulmonary bypass. Thorax 36:543–545, 1981.
46. Claypool WD, Rogers RM, Matuschak GM: Update on the clinical diagnosis, management, and pathogenesis of pulmonary alveolar proteinosis (phospholipidosis). Chest 85:550–558, 1984.

SECTION

# M

# Environmental and Occupational Disorders

# 64 General Principles and Diagnostic Approach

PAUL D. BLANC, M.D., M.S.P.H.


Introduction

Importance of Occupational and Environmental Respiratory Disorders

Historical Perspectives

Research Methods

Diagnosis

Prevention

Future Directions

Summary


## INTRODUCTION

Presenting introductory comments on general principles and a diagnostic approach encompassing occupational and environmental respiratory disorders as a *group* is quite a challenge. Other clinical topics in respiratory medicine may be logically discussed according to etiologic agent (such as causes of pulmonary infection), anatomic site (such as vasculature, pleura, or mediastinum), pathologic classification (such as type of malignancy or infiltrative process), or physiologic impairment (such as airway obstruction, respiratory failure). In contrast, occupational and environmental lung disease does not lend itself neatly to any single formulation. In this Section the authors include topics defined by pathology (pneumoconioses, hypersensitivity pneumonitis), by physiology (occupational asthma, obstructive disease), and by etiology (high altitude, diving, drug-induced disease). They also include two other important topics for which the defining rationale is none of these but rather length and degree of exposure: air pollution, which concerns itself with chronic low-level exposures, and acute occupational and environmental respiratory syndromes, which focus on high-level acute inhalational effects.

Although this Section addresses many topics in occupational and environmental lung disease that are likely to be encountered by pulmonary specialists, it is not meant to be all inclusive. There is much that is clearly relevant to occupational and environmental disorders that is not separated out here. In particular, the reader is referred elsewhere in the text to detailed discussions of cigarette smoking (e.g., Chapters 38 and 98). Other specific occupational and environmental topics are included within more general Sections such as those on neoplasms (occupational exposures as well as radiation pneumonitis), infectious diseases (such as tuberculosis risk in health care workers), and infiltrative disorders (including work-related factors in pulmonary hemosiderosis and alveolar proteinosis). Finally, the reader's attention is called to Chapter 30, where the impact of impairment through disability in its social and workplace context is discussed, especially with regard to occupational pulmonary medical practice.

## IMPORTANCE OF OCCUPATIONAL AND ENVIRONMENTAL RESPIRATORY DISORDERS

Given the difficulties in including occupational and environmental respiratory disorders under a single rubric, even in defining the topic by any set of unifying criteria, it is legitimate to ask why an attempt is made to discuss them as an entity at all. The answer is threefold. The first motivation to address occupational and environmental disorders together derives from their importance as disease models. Occupational asthma is a case in point. Exposure to sensitizing agents of both large and small molecular weights in the workplace arguably provides the clearest example we have for the study of the pathophysiology and natural history of human asthma.[1–3] From our experience with these agents, we have gained important information regarding atopy in asthma risk, induction of increased airway responsiveness, progression from specific to nonspecific hyperreactivity, and persistence of increased responsiveness after removal from exposure to its initiator. The pneumoconioses, in particular silicosis[4, 4a] and asbestosis,[4a, 5, 6] serve as another prime example of the usefulness of occupational and environmental lung diseases as model systems from which to gain knowledge about similar pathophysiologic processes when the causative factors are unknown (such as idiopathic pulmonary fibrosis). In both controlled animal exposures and clinical studies in humans, the pneumoconioses have yielded significant insights into mechanisms of lung inflammation, fibroblast proliferation, and collagen deposition. Occupational asthma and the pneumoconioses are two leading but far from isolated examples of the crucial role of the study of occupational and environmental lung disorders in understanding general disease processes.[7] These and other potential models are listed in Table 64.1.

Second, treating occupational and environmental factors as a group serves as a counterbalance to their underemphasis at all levels of medical training, from the undergraduate medical curriculum through postgraduate fellowship.[8] Occupational and environmental medicine is an underfilled specialty relative to service needs. This situation is projected to persist into the foreseeable future, even in the United States, where there is an excess of other medical subspecialists.[9] Because those with lung disease due to environmental or work-related factors are unlikely to be treated initially by occupational or environmental specialists, it is incumbent on pulmonologists generally to be familiar with and to have a high enough index of suspicion to diagnose these disorders.[8, 10]

A third reason to consider these conditions together is their public health and economic importance, underscored by the policy debates encountered frequently in the occupational and environmental arena. For example, the experimental observation that those with underlying increased airway responsiveness bronchoconstrict after inhalation of low levels of sulfur dioxide is more than a scientific finding with interesting implications for the study of mechanisms in asthma.[11, 12] Because a sizable subset of the population may exhibit increased nonspecific airway responsiveness and because sulfur dioxide is a major byproduct of fossil fuel burning, this observation has had a major public health and economic impact through promulgation of air pollution standards. Many other occupational and environmental exposures associated with pulmonary disease, such as to asbestos, radon, coal dust, ozone, and acid aerosols, have also engendered regulatory interventions that are contentiously debated because of their potential public health and economic consequences.

**Table 64.1 OCCUPATIONAL AND ENVIRONMENTAL DISORDERS AS DISEASE MODELS**

| Occupational or Environmental Syndrome | Potential Disease Model |
|---|---|
| Occupational asthma | Asthma |
| Asbestosis, silicosis | Pulmonary fibrosis |
| Irritant inhalant injury | Diffuse alveolar damage (acute respiratory distress syndrome) |
| High-altitude pulmonary edema | Noncardiogenic pulmonary edema |
| Berylliosis | Granulomatous lung disease |
| Spanish toxic oil syndrome | Plexigenic pulmonary arteriopathy |
| Occupational bronchitis | Chronic mucus hypersecretion |
| Paraquat injury | Pulmonary fibrosis |
| Acute silicosis | Pulmonary alveolar proteinosis |
| Chronic cadmium exposure | Emphysema |
| Hard metal disease | Giant cell pneumonia |
| Uranium mining, coke oven work | Lung carcinogenesis |

## HISTORICAL PERSPECTIVES

Concern about the respiratory effects of exposures in the workplace and in the environment is far from a uniquely modern preoccupation. The Egyptian Papyrus Sallier described both the metal worker "grilled at the mouth of the furnace" and the weaver so "doubled up with his knees drawn to his stomach, he cannot breathe."[13] The first treatise devoted solely to occupational health, written in 1473 by Ellenbog, was aptly titled "On the poisonous evil vapors" (Von den gifftigen besen Tempffen und Reuchen).[14] This pamphlet describes inhalational hazards of coal smoke, mercury fume, and acid aerosols among goldsmiths. Although the early history of occupational medicine predominantly reflects concerns with lung diseases among miners and metal workers, Ramazzini, whose classic treatise was first published in 1713, commented on lung disease among a number of additional occupations, including weaving, farming, butchering, and pottery making.[15] With the industrial revolution came a variety of new hazards and new diseases: By 1832, Thackrah[16] was able to document with frightening detail the toll in morbidity and mortality, much of it respiratory, among the working classes.

To emphasize the relationship between occupational illness and exposures in the community, the metaphor of the coal mine canary is often invoked. Just as early toxicity to the canary warns of danger to the miner, so too occupational disease among workers with the highest levels of exposure may presage effects in the community due to lower level airborne contamination beyond the factory gate. Interpretation of past writings on the potential health effects of air pollution is complicated by a conceptual framework that has changed over time from the four humors theory to the germ theory. Moreover, only since the 18th century, with the development of modern analytic methods, has the chemical nature of the atmosphere come to be understood even in general terms. Nonetheless, attention to the potential adverse respiratory effects in the community from airborne toxic materials has a long history, often intertwined with that of occupational health and industrial hygiene.

The modern era in occupational and environmental respiratory health as a unified concern can be dated to the use of poison gas in World War I, predominantly chlorine, phosgene, and mustard gases that acted primarily as respiratory rather than systemic toxins.[17] A body of medical literature after World War I describes potential long-term residual respiratory impairments among survivors of gassing, raising early questions on chemical mechanisms of airway obstruction and chronic bronchitis long before the later epidemiologic recognition of the role of cigarette smoking in these disorders.[17a] World War I also spurred heightened governmental interest in and funding for industrial hygiene. For example, the US Department of Labor supported Hamilton's pioneering studies among munitions workers.[18] From early in the 20th century until the major US regulatory changes were introduced in the 1970s, jurisdiction over study of air pollution was delegated to the Division of Industrial Hygiene in the US Public Health Service, underscoring the interdependence of these two fields.[19]

Because environmental and occupational health were essentially overlapping disciplines, occupational experts were called to investigate three dramatic episodes of air pollution that, more than any others, led to the heightened awareness underpinning our current research and regulatory environment. These occurred in the Meuse Valley, Belgium, from December 1 to 5, 1930; in Donora, Pennsylvania, from October 27 to 31, 1948; and in London, England, from December 5 to 9, 1952.[19, 20] It is worth remembering that the specific identities of the exposures responsible for the morbidity and mortality observed in these incidents were initially not known with certainty, nor had the photochemistry of oxidant smog been delineated at that time.

As a final historical comment on occupational and environmental respiratory disorders, a useful perspective may be gained from the concluding comments made by Schrenk to the Section on Preventive and Industrial Medicine of the American Medical Association in 1949 about his investigations at Donora. As chief scientist of the Environmental Investigation Branch of the Division of Industrial Hygiene, he stated:

> The data available pertain to acute effects or to effects on workers in good health and to exposures of eight hours daily. When dealing with atmospheric contaminants, one must consider continuous exposure over many hours as well as effects on the aged, persons with impaired health, and hypersusceptible and allergic persons. Furthermore, available data are confined almost entirely to the effects of single substances. Little is known of the effects of simultaneous exposure to several toxic substances. The role that extremely fine particles play by absorbing and transporting toxic gases or vapors to the alveoli is almost entirely unexplored. In addition to the direct action of toxic substances, the possible influence of atmospheric pollution on common diseases needs careful and critical analysis.[21]

## RESEARCH METHODS

The research priorities outlined in Schrenk's farsighted comments in large part remain valid today, even if his agenda might be widened to include other concerns as well, such as low-level long-latency carcinogenic effects and, in a time when Bhopal is more familiar than Donora, immediate toxicity from massive overexposure.[22] As the breadth of these topics indicates, the research needs in occupational and environmental respiratory medicine are great.[23, 24] Furthermore, the demands of the field are somewhat specialized relative to pulmonary medicine as a whole. Although investigators of occupational and environmental lung diseases face the same basic scientific challenges as their colleagues who study other respiratory conditions, the nature of research in this area is such that it often relies on disciplines that are less familiar to other pulmonary research investigators. Two disciplines key to occupational and environmental pulmonary research are epidemiology and toxicology.

Pivotal epidemiologic concepts relate to methods of estimating risk. Building from simple descriptive statistics, the epidemiologist estimates risk by examining frequencies among study groups compared with "expected" values. Risk relative to its expectation is one of the primary measures used in occupational and environmental medicine to quantify differences between exposed and unexposed persons. Sometimes relative risk is estimated in terms of an odds ratio; when the effect studied is mortality, the risk estimate can be expressed as a "standardized mortality ratio."[25] An exposure-associated relative risk of 1.4 (e.g., risk of decreased airflow at low lung volumes associated with heavy cigarette smoking after taking into account asbestos exposure)[26] would mean that the rate observed among the exposed was approximately one and a half times greater than that among the nonexposed, or, stated in other terms, a 40% excess of exposure-associated abnormality was observed. A relative risk greater than 2.0 implies that in any single person with both disease and its risk factor, more probably than not the abnormality observed can be attributed to the exposure in question. Relative risk can also be used to evaluate synergistic interactions.[27] In this way, if a relative risk for disease associated with exposure "A" is 5.0 and for exposure "B" is 9.0, while the relative risk for persons with both risk factors compared with neither is 45.0, this risk pattern suggests a multiplicative effect, such as the risk of bronchogenic carcinoma observed with combined radon and cigarette smoking.[28]

Toxicology is no less important to occupational and environmental medicine. Toxicologic concepts of exposure direct much of the methodologic approach to dose response in occupational and environmental research. Examples of exposure-focused research issues in this field include the following: particle size and deposition and the effects of water solubility on the dose delivered to the lung; years employed or years elapsed since first employment and mean or peak ambient air concentrations of substances in parts per million as alternative measures of dose; and the impact of active metabolites and detoxification on the effects of potential toxins.[23, 26, 29] Another concept with important research implications is target organ toxicity. The primary portal of entry to the body for gases, fumes, and dusts is the lungs. Adverse effects due to exposure to these substances may not, however, include respiratory disorders. For example, in the occupational setting, lead poisoning typically occurs through fume inhalation, but the target organs for chronic lead toxicity are the nervous system and the kidneys. Conversely, drug-induced pulmonary disease is a manifestation of lung target organ toxicity, even when exposure occurs through ingestion or parenteral administration.

In both epidemiologic and toxicologic analyses, the study of the effects in populations demands measurement instruments that provide reproducible and comparable data gathered by different observers using large data sets. For these reasons, standardized pulmonary function testing of large groups of subjects has been fundamental to much of occupational and environmental pulmonary research. Although well established methodologically, important challenges in population-based pulmonary function testing remain, including the use of appropriate "normal" expected values, especially among cigarette smokers and nonwhites,[30] assessing possible biases due to exclusion of spirometry "test failures,"[31] and employing self-administered peak-flow meters in field studies.[32, 32a]

Parallel to its reliance on spirometric measurements, occupational and environmental pulmonary research has also used other population-based methods. The survey research method allows assessment by questionnaire of both exposure factors and responses of interest (such as respiratory symptoms) in a standardized and quantifiable manner. Another important research tool is the standardized system developed by the International Labour Organization for scoring chest radiographic abnormalities. This scoring schema is discussed more fully in Chapter 65.

## DIAGNOSIS

For the individual practitioner, identifying an association between an occupational or environmental risk factor and a respiratory disorder is often problem-ridden at best. There are exceptions, as when an exposure is massive and the effect is immediate and unequivocal. Even in these situations, however, the clinician in practice may initially know only that a toxic release occurred, without details of exposure intensity or even the specific identification of the substances involved. At other times, the exposure is identified but is unusual with potential adverse effects that are poorly documented even in specialized toxicologic references.[33]

As an aid to the diagnosis of exposures of the patient at the workplace or to specific drugs, the clinician may attempt a re-exposure by returning the patient to work, by challenge under controlled laboratory conditions, or by reinstitution of therapy. These "individual" clinical trials play a useful role. Caution is warranted, however, because such challenges can present a significant risk to patients even when performed with care at experienced medical centers. Even more infrequent is the opportunity for a diagnostic approach to occupational and environmental disease in which tissue samples or biologic tests provide specific confirmatory data. Examples are birefringent silica in granulomas, beryllium lymphoblast transformation, serum thermophilic precipitants, blood paraquat levels, or fat staining of cells in lipoid pneumonitis.

More commonly, exposure is remote in time and difficult to ascertain directly. The first step in linking an occupational or environmental exposure to the respiratory disorder being evaluated is to entertain such risk factors in the differential diagnosis.[34, 35, 35a] This is not a trivial point. The presentation of occupationally or environmentally caused illness is rarely pathognomonic, either clinically or pathologically. Once the possibility is considered, the clinician must then attempt to elicit the appropriate information when taking the history in a systematic and yet targeted fashion.

Table 64.2 outlines briefly the key features of an occupational history focused on the respiratory system. The primary components include the following: understanding the job process; assessing, albeit indirectly, the degree of exposure; evaluating temporal associations between exposure and disease; delineating protective measures employed; gauging hygienic conditions; and, finally, ruling out certain specific exposures of importance. More detailed formulations for occupational and environmental history taking may serve as a basis for an expanded approach, particularly if a written questionnaire format is appropriate to the clinical context.

## PREVENTION

If one fundamental principle unites all aspects of occupational and environmental respiratory medicine, it is that prevention must be paramount to the practitioner. For virtually none of the disorders discussed in this Section is there any specific efficacious therapeutic intervention, and for many of them even general supportive care may have little impact. In the field of occupational and envi-

**Table 64.2 QUESTIONS TO ASK WHEN TAKING AN OCCUPATIONAL RESPIRATORY HISTORY***

**Job/Process**

- What is your job title? What do you do exactly?
- What do you produce in your workplace?
- Describe the industrial process (equipment) that you work with. If power equipment is used, how is it powered?
- Is the industrial process a closed system or an open system?
- What other processes or work stations are nearby?
- Who does maintenance and how often?

**Exposure Levels**

- Do you see dust or mist in the air?
- Can you see your coworkers or nearby objects clearly?
- Are surfaces dusty or damp? Is the paint or wallpaper peeling, discolored, or damp?
- Is there a strong smell or taste? (Does it then go away?)
- Is there directed ventilation, and where does it come from? Are filters in the air system checked or changed? Is the airflow known?
- Do you blow dust from your nose or cough it up at the end of the day?
- Do you have direct skin contact with the materials you work with?
- Has anyone at your job site ever sampled the air for a specific substance?

**Temporal Aspects**

- Are your symptoms different on the first day of the work week? At the end of the first shift of the week? At the end of the work week? Away from work? On days off? During vacation? Has there been any change in process, product, or your duties?
- Is any kind of mask for respiratory protection available or provided? Do you wear it? When and how often? What kind of mask?
- Disposable paper type? Screw-in cartridge type? (What type of cartridge? How often is the cartridge changed?) Air supplied? (Where is the air intake?)
- Were you ever "fitted" for a mask? Did you undergo pulmonary function testing before getting a mask?

**Epidemiologic Aspects and Hygiene**

- Anyone else symptomatic? If yes, what is their job, location?
- Do you eat in the workplace? Do you smoke in the workplace?
- Are you provided with a uniform? Is it changed and left there? Is there a union? Safety and health committee? How many employees are at your work site?

**Specific Exposures**

- Did you ever work with asbestos? Insulation material? Heat-resistant material? Was it friable? Did you "disturb" it? (Family exposure or neighborhood exposure?)
- Did you ever work with silica? Sand? Mining or quarrying? Ever around sandblasting? (What color was the sand?) Did you do anything to grind or break up rock or dirt?
- Was two-part glue, paint, or coating mixed up just before use? Ever work with urethane?
- Ever work with solvents or degreasers? (Ever become dizzy, nauseated, "high" or have a headache from it?)
- Did you ever perform construction work? Shipyard work? Military service? Crafts, hobbies, or artwork?
- Have you ever performed any dusty work I have not asked about? Any jobs with fumes or gases I have not asked about?

*The standard occupational history delineates all past employment, usually starting with the present and working backward systematically. The occupational history also attempts to include environmental exposures, for example, from hobbies, the neighborhood, or in the home. Realistically, one may not elicit a complete occupational history in many clinical situations. Moreover, in occupational lung disease certain questions are more frequent and of greater potential importance. As a general rule, ask about specific details of the job. Do not be satisfied with a general "occupation" or "trade" such as "machinist," "painter," "electronics worker," or "farmer."

ronmental lung disease, it is critical to promote prevention in its primary, secondary, and tertiary components.[36]

Primary prevention means abrogating the risk factor before illness strikes. In occupational medicine, the preferred prevention strategies are first to substitute less hazardous products wherever possible and second to modify processes to reduce exposures to safe levels. Although the occupational history outlined in Table 64.2 includes several questions related to respiratory protective equipment, this is not the first-line strategy in primary prevention. When respirators are used to protect against inhaling intoxicants, a program for utilizing the apparatus properly is a necessary component. For environmental exposures, prevention policy is also geared to promulgation of standards that protect the population from adverse effects, including the outright banning of certain hazards (e.g., structural asbestos spraying). In drug-related disease, premarket testing and strict indications for use are two clear examples of effective primary preventive strategies. Similarly, assessment of fitness to dive and ascent acclimatization represent primary prevention approaches to disorders caused by underwater and high-altitude environments, respectively.

The pulmonary clinician is more frequently faced with opportunities for secondary than for primary preventive interventions. Medical surveillance is fundamental and is geared to detect adverse exposure effects before they result in impairment leading to significant compromise of the host *and then to take action preventing further deterioration.* Without such action, surveillance deteriorates to a form of documentation of morbidity rather than being a tool for secondary prevention.

In practice, prevention based on surveillance often means prevention of further exposure.[37, 37a] The most straightforward example of this is discontinuation of a drug that has either a cumulative dose-related or a non–

dose-related idiosyncratic adverse pulmonary effect. In the occupational setting, product and process change notwithstanding, secondary prevention is most frequently accomplished through removal of the employee from the work site or, at a minimum, from exposure-related specific job duties. In particular, the diagnosis of occupational asthma mandates aggressive secondary preventive measures because even very low levels of exposure (such as concentrations lower than can be achieved with routine respiratory protection) will induce responses in sensitized persons, and, moreover, continued exposure can be associated with progression to nonspecific increased airway responsiveness that may persist even after removal from the workplace.[38, 39]

Another important aspect of secondary prevention is the identification of others at risk owing to similar exposure. In addition to questioning the index case about others who may also be ill, the treating physician is obligated to report occupational and environmental illnesses through all appropriate mechanisms of surveillance. Under certain circumstances, this may also include direct notification of regulatory authorities. The physician should also view the process of disability evaluation as a meaningful secondary prevention activity, because in many cases recognition of the occupational nature of a chronic disease for the purposes of compensation will trigger investigations into hazardous industries and occupations.

Tertiary prevention subsumes those activities that attempt to slow progression or preclude anticipated complications of previous exposure or of disease that is already established.[36] For occupational and environmental exposures known or suspected to exhibit a synergistic risk for bronchogenic carcinoma, smoking cessation is an important tertiary prevention strategy. Because of the large numbers of former heavily exposed asbestos workers, this has been a population particularly targeted for such prevention activities. Tuberculosis prophylaxis among silicotics represents another form of tertiary prevention.

## FUTURE DIRECTIONS

The chapters that follow in this Section forcefully demonstrate the breadth and depth of the exciting and critically important field of occupational and environmental health. These chapters on the pneumoconioses, hypersensitivity pneumonitis, asthma and obstructive lung disease, acute inhalational syndromes, drug toxicity, diving, and high altitude testify to the rapid development that has occurred in occupational and environmental pulmonary medicine in recent years. An important test for this growing field will come in its response to the current explosion of knowledge in basic cellular and molecular pulmonary biology. The potential role for occupational and environmental disorders to serve as model systems for the study of disease processes highlights the insights that may be gained when clinical and basic science disciplines combine forces to address these questions aggressively.

At the same time, the fundamental charge to the practitioner treating occupational and environmental lung disorders remains the recognition of disease and the reduction of morbidity. As the health advocates of our patients in this field, we are often thrust uncomfortably into roles for which we have been ill-prepared by routine medical training.[40, 41] Moreover, occupational and environmental cases are frequently extremely demanding of time, litigious, and uncertain in the ultimate determination of causality. Partly for these reasons, some clinicians have come to minimize their involvement with such cases or to avoid them altogether. The troubles that plague occupational and environmental pulmonary medicine cannot be separated from their larger social and economic context, and they are unlikely to be solved without the regulatory, tort, and insurance reforms that will undoubtably occur in the future. Modern guidance may be taken by reminding ourselves of Agricola's words on miners' diseases, written almost 500 years ago: "we should always devote more care to maintaining our health, that we may freely perform our bodily functions, than to making profits."[42]

## SUMMARY

Occupational and environmental disorders constitute an important and challenging topic in respiratory medicine. Their diagnosis, treatment, and, most prominently, their prevention have major public health implications. Research methods central to occupational and environmental health, particularly biostatistics and epidemiology, need to become more familiar to pulmonologists. In clinical practice, taking a structured and focused occupational history should be a routine part of patient evaluation. Certain disorders of occupational and environmental respiratory medicine may serve as model systems in which to study general processes of broad concern, such as airway reactivity and interstitial fibrosis.

## References


1. Chan-Yeung M, Malo JL: Occupational asthma. New Engl J Med 333:107–112, 1995.
2. Venables KM, Chan-Yeung M: Occupational asthma. Lancet 349:1465–1469, 1997.
3. Bates DV: Workshop summary: Environmental and occupational asthma. Chest 98:251s–252s, 1990.
4. Silicosis and Silicate Disease Committee: Diseases associated with exposure to silica and nonfibrous silicate minerals. Arch Pathol Lab Med 112:673–720, 1988.
4a. Mossman BT, Churg A: Mechanisms in the pathogenesis of asbestosis and silicosis. Am J Respir Crit Care 157:1666–1680, 1998.
5. Mossman BT, Gee JBL: Medical progress: Asbestos-related diseases. N Engl J Med 320:1721–1730, 1989.
6. Rom WN, Travis WD, Brody AR: State of the art: Cellular and molecular basis of the asbestos-related diseases. Am Rev Respir Dis 143:408–422, 1991.
7. Cullen MR, Cherniack MG, Rosenstock L: Medical progress: Occupational medicine. N Engl J Med 322:594–601, 675–683, 1990.
8. Institute of Medicine: Role of the Primary Care Physician in Occupational and Environmental Medicine. Washington DC, National Academy Press, 1988.
9. Castorina, J, Rosenstock L: Physician shortage in occupational and environmental medicine. Ann Intern Med 113:983–986, 1990.
10. Kilbourne EM, Weiner J: Occupational and environmental medicine: The internist's role. Ann Intern Med 113:974–980, 1990.
11. Nadel JA, Salem H, Tamplin B, et al: Mechanism of bronchoconstriction during inhalation of sulfur dioxide. J Appl Physiol 20:164–167, 1965.
12. Sheppard D, Wong WS, Uehara CF, et al: Lower threshold and

greater bronchomotor responsiveness of asthmatic subjects to sulfur dioxide. Am Rev Respir Dis 122:873–878, 1980.
13. Sigerist HE: Historical background of industrial and occupational diseases. *In* Marti-Ibanez F (ed): Henry E. Sigerist on the History of Medicine. New York: MD Publications, 1960, pp 46–56.
14. Ellenbog U: On the poisonous evil vapors. Lancet 1:230–231, 1932.
15. Ramazzini B: De Morbis Artificum [Diseases of Workers: The Latin Text of 1713 Revised with translation and notes by Wilmer Cave Wright]. Chicago: University of Chicago Press, 1940.
16. Thackrah CT: The Effects of Arts, Trades, and Professions, and of Civic States and Habits of Living on Health and Longevity (2nd ed). London: Longman, Rees, Orme, Brown, Green, and Longman, 1832.
17. Eckert WG: Mass deaths by gas or chemical poisoning. Am J Forensic Med Pathol 12:119–125, 1991.
17a. Blanc PD: The legacy of war gas. Am J Med 106:689–690, 1999.
18. Hamilton A: Exploring the dangerous trades. Boston: Atlantic Brown, 1943.
19. Sellars C: The public health service's office of industrial hygiene and the transformation of industrial medicine. Bull Hist Med 65:42–73, 1991.
20. Logan WPD: Mortality in the London fog incident, 1952. Lancet 1:336–338, 1953.
21. Schrenk HH: Causes, constituents and physical effects of smog involved in specific dramatic episodes. Arch Ind Hyg Occup Med 1:189–194, 1950.
22. Koplan JP, Falk H, Green G: Public health lessons from the Bhopal chemical disaster. JAMA 264:2795–2796, 1990.
23. Brooks SM, Kalica AR: NHLBI workshop summary: Strategies for elucidating the relationship between occupational exposures and chronic air-flow obstruction. Am Rev Respir Dis 135:268–273, 1987.
24. Workshop on Environmental and Occupational Asthma: Research gaps and priorities. Chest 98:246s–248s, 1990.
25. Monson RR: Occupational Epidemiology (2nd ed). Boca Raton, FL: CRC Press, 1990, pp 105–148.
26. Blanc PD, Golden JA, Gamsu G, et al: Asbestos exposure–cigarette smoking interactions among shipyard workers. JAMA 259:370–373, 1988.
27. Kundiev JI, Navakatikyan AO: Study of combined effects. *In* Karvonen M, Mikheev MI (eds): Epidemiology of Occupational Health, WHO Regional Publications Series No. 20. Copenhagen: World Health Organization, 1986, pp 209–230.
28. Axelson O: Occupational and environmental exposures to radon: Cancer risks. Annu Rev Public Health 12:235–255, 1991.
29. National Research Council: Biologic Markers in Pulmonary Toxicology. Washington DC: National Academy Press, 1989.
30. American Thoracic Society: Lung function testing: Selection of reference values and interpretive strategies. Am Rev Respir Dis 144:1202–1218, 1991.
31. Becklake MR: The epidemiology of spirometric test failure. Br J Ind Med 47:73–74, 1990.
32. Quackenboss JJ, Lebowitz M.D, Krzyzanowski M: The normal range of diurnal changes in peak expiratory flow rates. Am Rev Respir Dis 143:323–330, 1991.
32a. Weytjens K, Malo JL, Cartier A, et al: Comparison of peak expiratory flows and $FEV_1$ in assessing immediate asthmatic reactions due to occupational agents. Allergy 54:621–625, 1999.
33. Blanc PD, Golden JA: Unusual occupationally related disorders of the lung: Case reports and a literature review. Occcup Med 7:403–422, 1992.
34. Goldman RH, Peters JM: The occupational and environmental health history. JAMA 246:2831–2836, 1981.
35. The Occupational and Environmental Health Committee: Taking the occupational history. Ann Intern Med 99:641–651, 1983.
35a. Lax MB, Grant WD, Manetti FA, et al: Recognizing occupational disease—Taking an effective occupational history. Am Fam Phys 58:935–944, 1998.
36. Harber P: Pulmonary prevention: Programmatic characterization. Occup Med 6:133–143, 1991.
37. Brooks SM, Discher, DP, Epler GE, et al: Surveillance for respiratory hazards in the occupational setting. Am Rev Respir Dis 126:952–956, 1982.
37a. Fine LJ: Surveillance and occupational health. Int J Occup Environ Health 5:26–29, 1999.
38. Becklake MR: Epidemiology and surveillance. Chest 98:165s–172s, 1990.
39. Cullen MR: Clinical surveillance and management of occupational asthma. Chest 98:196s–201s, 1990.
40. McCally M, Cassel CK: Medical responsibility and global environmental change. Ann Intern Med 113:467–473, 1990.
41. Ducatmam AM: Occupational physicians and occupational medicine. J Occup Med 35:251–259, 1993.
42. Hoover HC, Hoover LH: De Re Metallica. New York: Dover Publications, 1950, p 214.

# 65 Pneumoconioses

MARGARET R. BECKLAKE, M.D. • ROBERT L. COWIE, M.D.

Introduction
- Definitions
- Accumulation of Dust in the Lung and Tissue Reactions
- Exposure-Response Relationships
- Chest Imaging: Roentgenography, Computed Tomography, and Gallium Scintigraphy
- Lung Function Tests
- Clinical Issues and Principles of Management
- Epidemiology and Implications for Clinical Practice

Silicosis
- Definition
- Industries and Occupations Still at Risk
- Pathology
- Pathogenesis
- Epidemiology: Secular Trends and Their Implications for the Clinician
- Clinical Features
- Radiographic and Lung Function Changes
- Diagnosis and Complications
- Management and Control

Coal Workers' Pneumoconiosis
- Definition and Occupations at Risk
- Pathology
- Pathogenesis
- Epidemiology and Natural History
- Clinical Features
- Chest Radiography
- Lung Function
- Diagnosis, Complications, and Management

Asbestos-Related Fibrosis of the Lungs (Asbestosis) and Pleura
- Asbestos Minerals
- Asbestosis (Pulmonary Parenchymal Fibrosis)
- Pleural Plaques
- Pleural Fibrosis and Visceroparietal Reactions
- Benign Asbestos-Related Pleural Effusions
- Management, Prevention, and Health Monitoring

Non-asbestos Mineral Silicates (Fibrous or Not) and Lung Disease

Other Pneumoconioses, Old and New

Beryllium Lung Disease
- Beryllium: Uses, Human Toxicity, and Exposures
- Pathology and Immune Pathogenesis
- Clinical Features
- Diagnosis and Management

Hard Metal Disease

Summary

## INTRODUCTION

### Definitions

*Pneumoconiosis* is a venerable word, coined from the Greek (*pneuma* = air and *konis* = dust) and introduced in the 19th century to describe lung diseases consequent to the inhalation of mineral dusts. Over time, it has been adapted to indicate the nature of the putative dust, for example, silicosis (silica), asbestosis (asbestos), siderosis (iron); or to indicate the occupation at risk, for example, coal workers' pneumoconiosis.[1–5]

In the 1998 edition of its *Encyclopedia of Occupational Health and Safety*,[1] the International Labour Organization (ILO) retains its earlier definition of the term *pneumoconiosis* to describe "the accumulation of dust in the lungs and the tissue reactions to its presence." By "dust" is meant "an aerosol consisting of solid inanimate particles." From the pathologic point of view, tissue reaction may be noncollagenous (when stromal reaction is minimal, consisting of reticulin fibers) or collagenous (when scarring is permanent). Exposure to the same dusts may result in the transition from one form to another, and workplace exposures to mixed dusts with different fibrogenic potential is becoming increasingly common, resulting in pneumoconioses that can range from noncollagenous to collagenous.[1] Not included in the definition of pneumoconiosis are conditions that also develop from inhalation of dust, which causes reactions in the bronchi and lung parenchyma, but in which dust does not accumulate in the lungs in the long term. Examples are asthma, chronic obstructive pulmonary disease (COPD), and farmer's lung.[1–7]

### Accumulation of Dust in the Lung and Tissue Reactions

The deposition of particles in the lungs depends on the particle size, and geometric and aerodynamic properties, and their clearance is determined by the mucociliary escalator and cellular mechanisms, in particular, the macrophage (Chapter 15). Dust accumulation in the lungs is determined by the nature and the amount of dust accumulated and retained in contact with the target cells for a long enough period to evoke a biologic response. Mathematical models predict that for a continuous exposure to 4 μm particles of an inert dust, for instance, equilibrium is predicted to be reached within 293 days, with the lung dust burden after 1 year representing 9% of the total mass that entered the lung.[4] Comparable figures for intermittent exposure (simulating occupational conditions) are 5 years for equilibrium to be reached and 25 years for the lung dust burden to be 1.5% of the total mass that entered the lung.[4] However, retention patterns appear to be dust specific and determine the dose,[1] whereas in addition to dose, tissue responses to inorganic dusts depend on particle size and the biologic activity of the dust, which in turn depends on its surface chemical and physical properties.[1, 2] Thus, some dusts, such as coal, appear relatively inert and may accumulate in considerable amounts with minimal tissue response; others, in particular silica and asbestos, have potent biologic effects in the short and long term. These are illustrated by the now classic studies of Nagelschmidt,[8] shown in Figure 65.1; the footnote elaborates on the relationship of quartz to total dust in the various pneumoconioses illustrated. Parenchymal responses include nodular fibrosis (the classic example is the silicotic islet), diffuse fibrosis (the classic example is asbestosis), and macule formation with focal emphysema (the classic example is the coal dust macule).[1–5] Irregular and mixed fibrotic patterns also have been described as a consequence of mixed exposures involving other mineral dusts or fibers in addition to silica dust exposure.[1] For any given dust exposure, the severity of the tissue reaction appears to be related to the cumulative lung dust burden.[1] In the past decade, exploitation of the techniques for quantitative and qualitative assessment of dust in lungs and in bronchoalveolar lavage (BAL) fluid[9] has not only

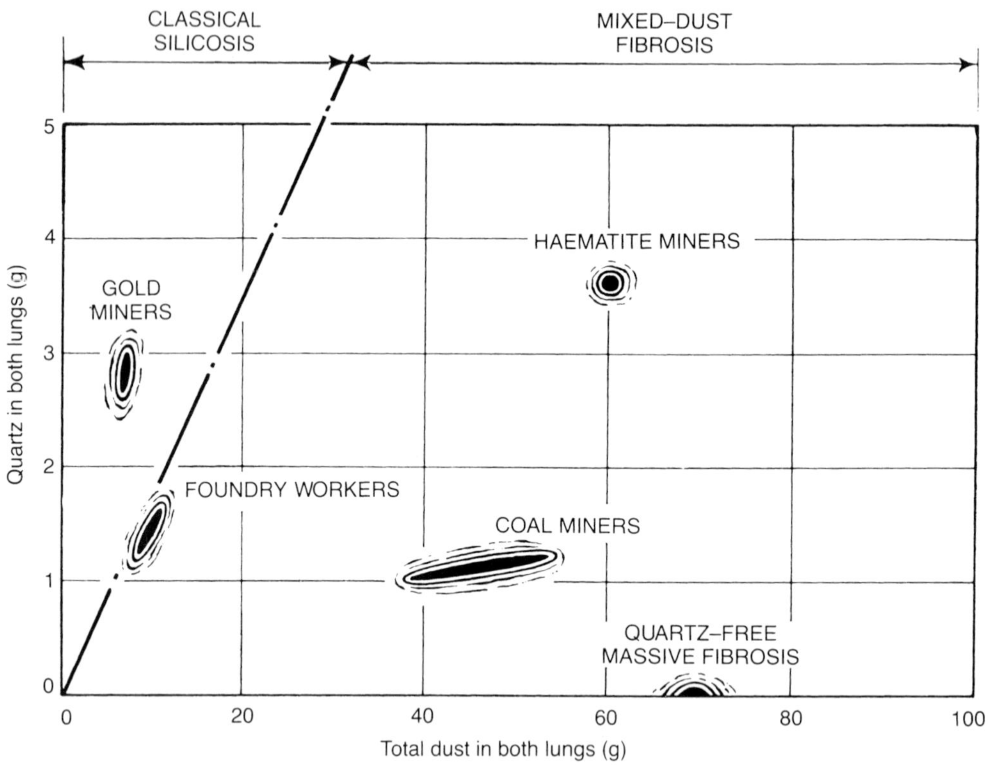


**Figure 65.1** Graph showing the average amounts of total dust and quartz in lungs with advanced forms of different pneumoconioses. The lungs of gold miners with classic silicosis had on average a small total dust load, of which a high proportion was quartz; those of men with coal workers' pneumoconiosis (CWP) had a heavy total dust load with a quartz content half that seen in silicosis; those of foundry workers with mixed dust pneumoconiosis had a small total dust load comparable to that seen in silicosis, with a low quartz content comparable to that seen in CWP. In another mixed dust pneumoconiosis, that of hematite miners, the lungs show a high total dust load, comparable to that seen in CWP, and a high quartz content, comparable to that seen in classic silicosis. Hematite mine dust appears to inhibit, in part, the quartz effect. Massive fibrosis in coal miners may occur in lungs that are quartz free. This figure, frequently reproduced in textbooks, is a tribute to its clear message based on some of the earliest work on lung dust burden, which was carried out by Nagelschmidt. (From Nagelschmidt G: The relation between lung dust and lung pathology in pneumoconiosis. Br J Ind Med 17:247–259, 1960.)

thrown light on exposure-dose relationships but also has clarified the balance between short-term and long-term retention.[10, 10a, 11]

## Exposure-Response Relationships

In population-based studies, the dust burden in the lung, for practical purposes, can be assessed only indirectly. However, exposure can be assessed directly on the basis of job history, on the engineering history of the plant, including the level and efficiency of dust controls, and, where available, from environmental measurements, either personal or static monitors using the strategy of sampling by exposure zone for jobs with similar exposure.[12] Although the exposure history is likely to be no more than an indirect reflection of dose (i.e., lung dust burden),[1] convincing exposure-response relationships for the pulmonary changes of pneumoconiosis can invariably be demonstrated in work force studies.[13, 14] At the public health level, the demonstration of exposure-response relationships is important and is necessary supportive evidence that the abnormality, dysfunction, or disease in question is causally related to the exposure.[13, 14] Figures 65.2 and 65.3 (discussed later) illustrate the relationships of the *prevalence* of silicosis and asbestosis (detected radiologically) to dust levels (based on environmental measurements), derived from data on Ontario hard rock miners[13] and asbestos workers in various industries,[14] respectively.

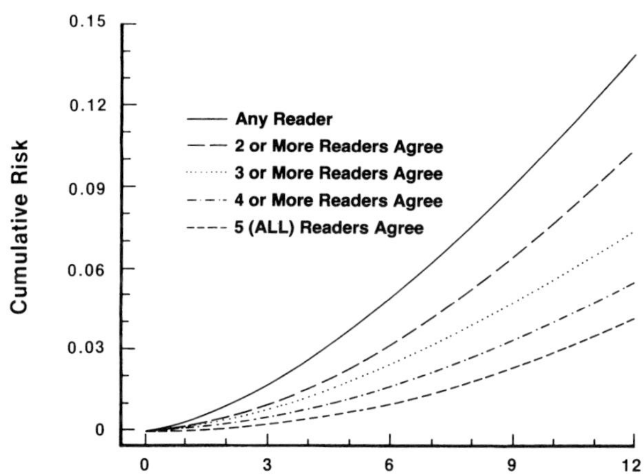


**Figure 65.2** The cumulative risk of developing silicosis in relation to cumulative exposure to respirable silica (mg/m³ × years), lagged by 5 years, among hardrock miners. The cohort consisted of all miners on the Ontario Workmen's Compensation Board's master file of miners who started work between 1941 and 1959 and were followed by chest radiography until their dust exposure ended or until 1982, whichever came first. The figure shows fitted Weibull models for one to five levels of reader consensus. The criterion for silicosis was a chest radiograph reading of small rounded opacities of profusion 1/1 or greater, using the ILO standard reference films, on the miner's most recent film. The films of 32 of 2109 miners were considered by one or more readers to have silicosis and were retained for the purposes of this analysis. (From Muir DCF, Shannon HS, Julian JA, et al: Silica exposure and silicosis among Ontario hardrock miners: III. Analysis and risk estimates. Am J Ind Med 16:29–43, 1989.)

The demonstration of exposure-response relationships also has implications for clinical practice. For instance, a clinical diagnosis of pneumoconiosis is strengthened greatly when there has been exposure to dust levels known to be associated with an increased risk of disease, particularly when environmental standards have been exceeded. Although exposure-response relationships generally describe the events in a work force, there are exceptions at both ends of the spectrum; they include the apparently heavily exposed individuals who remain unaffected and the apparently lightly exposed individuals who are affected. Thus, environmental standards such as threshold limit values are in the nature of hypotheses, or, in the words of the American Conference of Government and Industrial Hygienists (ACGIH) who propose threshold limit values, they are levels that, if respected throughout an individual's working life, are unlikely to be associated with disease. However, dust sampling may be problematic and even in a workplace where average dust concentrations are below the threshold limit value, nearly half the samples exceed this value.[15, 16] Thus, a clinician never should reject outright the diagnosis of a pneumoconiosis (if in his or her judgment this seems the most likely possibility) on the grounds that exposure was too remote, too short, or in a workplace where the threshold limit value was respected. The subject in question may be unusually susceptible, may have had an unusual exposure profile, or may retain more dust than others similarly exposed.

## Chest Imaging: Roentgenography, Computed Tomography, and Gallium Scintigraphy

The use of the ILO standard films for the descriptive interpretation of the radiologic appearance of diffuse parenchymal lung disease is well described in detail elsewhere.[1, 2] The system, originally developed for epidemiologic studies of occupational lung disease, also may assist clinical interpretation. Apart from improving consistency in the reading of parenchymal disease, which is notoriously subject to reader variability,[2] this reading system enables the clinician who uses it to set an individual case in the context of the available epidemiologic information. This may be crucial to the establishment of the work relatedness of disease and is also of value in prognosis. However, the classification was developed for descriptive, not diagnostic purposes, and does not address pattern recognition, a common clinical approach to radiologic diagnosis.

An important feature of the system is that the reader, after noting the quality of the film, is asked to classify "all appearances consistent with those defined and represented in the standard radiographs and guidelines for use of the ILO International Classification of Radiographs of Pneumoconiosis."[1, 2] Small opacities in the parenchyma are classified by shape and size: *p*, *q*, or *r* for rounded opacities (diameter, <1.5 mm, 1.5 to 3 mm, or >3 mm, respectively) and *s*, *t*, or *u* for irregular opacities (of

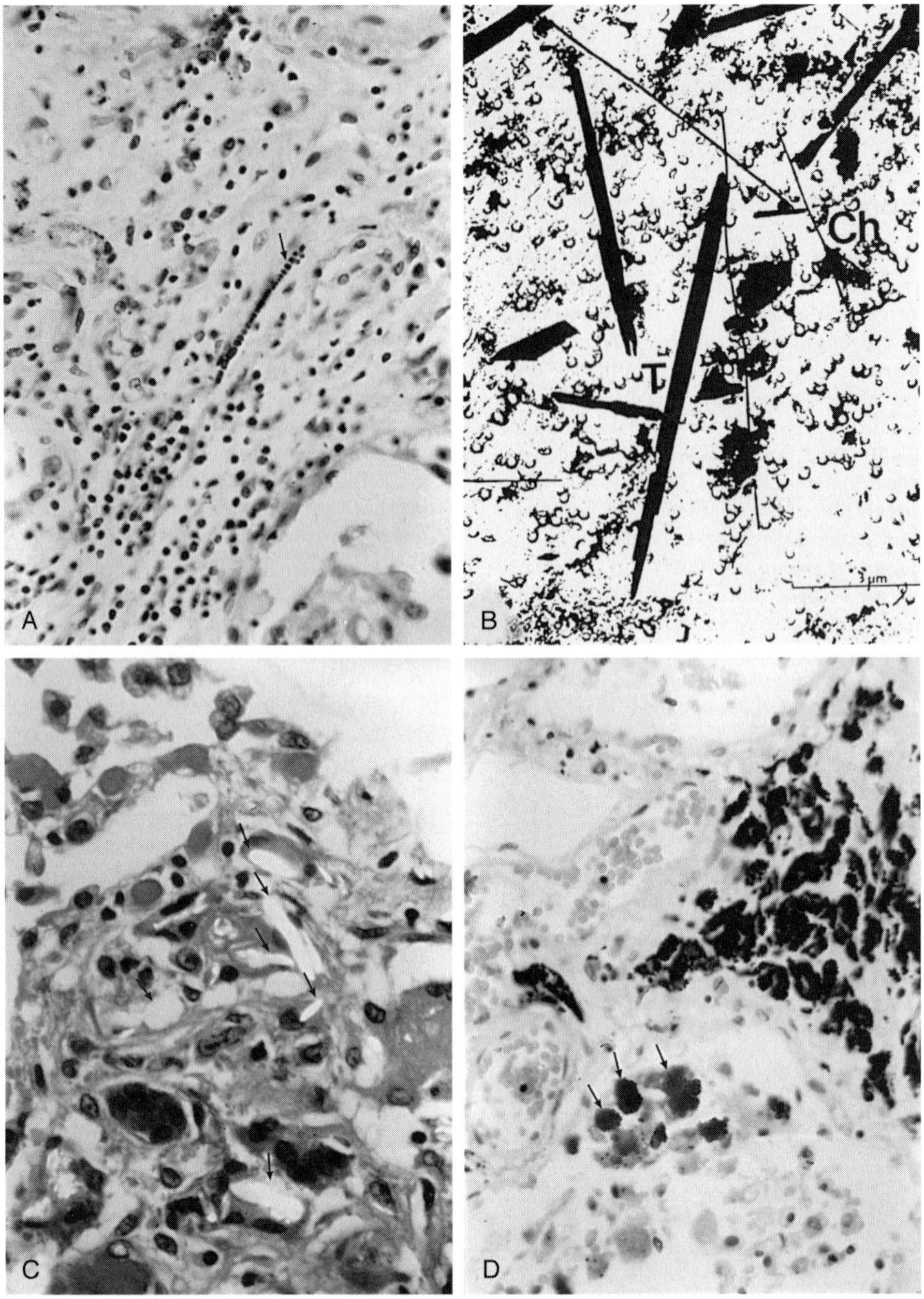


**Figure 65.3** The putative agent in the lung tissue in four cases is demonstrated. *A,* Typical asbestos body *(arrows)* in the lung of a 65-year-old long-term chrysotile asbestos miner with asbestosis, from the Thetford area. (Original magnification $\times$ 250, light microscopy.) *B,* Lung digest from the case of a 67-year-old long-term chrysotile miner with asbestosis from the Thetford area, photographed on a filter of pore diameter 0.2 mm (pores are evident as small punched-out areas in the photograph). The thin fibers labeled Ch were identified as chrysotile using morphologic criteria and energy-dispensive x-ray spectrometry (EDS). The thick fibers labeled T were identified as tremolite by EDS. In this mining area, there is a small amount of tremolite in the mined ore that accumulates preferentially in the lung tissue.[176] Amphiboles such as crocidolite, amosite, or tremolite most frequently form the core of asbestos bodies. For each asbestos body found in lung tissue, the number of uncoated fibers is at least several orders of magnitude greater. (Original magnification $\times$ 10,000, transmission electron microscopy.) *C,* Lung section from a 45-year-old man who died of pulmonary fibrosis due to talc. The talc particles, some examples of which are identified *(arrows),* appear as birefringent *(bright white)* elongated particles. (Original magnification $\times$ 250 by light microscopy using polarizers.) *D,* Lung section from a 65-year-old welder showing amorphous carbon particles *(upper right)* and a cluster of rounded iron-coated particles *(arrows).* Particle clusters like this frequently are seen in the lung sections of welders and of foundry workers who have had exposure to iron dusts and fumes. (Original magnification $\times$ 250, light microscopy.) (Courtesy of Drs. Bruce Case and R. S. Fraser, Department of Pathology, and Dr. Patrick Sébastien, formerly of the School of Occupational Health, McGill University, Montreal.)

width, <1.5 mm, 1.5 to 3 mm, or >3 mm, respectively). Profusion category (or concentration) is next read on a 12-point scale (0/−, 0/0, 0/1 up to 3/2, 3/3, and 3/+) in comparison with the standard radiographs. Large opacities are classified as category A (for one or more such opacities with a diameter of 1 cm but not exceeding a combined diameter of 5 cm), category B (one or more larger than 10 cm in diameter and whose combined area does not exceed one upper zone), and category C (larger than B). Likewise, provision is made to grade pleural thickening for width ($a \leq 5$ mm, $b = > 5$ mm but $< 10$ mm, and $c \geq 10$ mm) and extent (*1* = up to one quarter, *2* = one quarter to one half, and *3* = over one half of the lateral chest wall). The extent of pleural calcification also is graded, and there are provisions for comment on other features. Revised guidelines are in preparation.[1]

In the United States, the National Institute of Occupational Safety and Health (NIOSH) administers the National Coal Workers' Health Surveillance Program, which provides coal miners with the opportunity of a periodic medical examination.[2] The program incorporates quality control in terms of roentgenographic technique and reading procedures using the ILO classification and reader training.[2] This involves training seminars for physicians who may qualify as "A" readers (i.e., attended the seminars) or "B" readers, who passed a comprehensive examination on the basis of 120 roentgenograms read into the ILO classification. Many US clinics and hospitals now also conform to these standards.[2]

Although chest roentgenography remains the cornerstone of surveillance for pneumoconiosis in the workplace, computed tomography (CT) and high-resolution computed tomography (HRCT) have revolutionized clinical case evaluation.[17–19] HRCT is able to characterize lung and pleural lesions, their extent and confluence, with remarkable precision and is considerably more sensitive in detecting disease compared with the conventional chest roentgenogram. For the detection of the early stages of pneumoconiosis, when lesions are relatively few, 1.5-mm or 1-mm rather than 10-mm cuts should be made. HRCT (1-mm cuts) also can provide a quantitative assessment of any emphysema present.[19] The role of gallium scintigraphy in the diagnosis of pneumoconiosis is uncertain.[20] Increased gallium uptake by the lungs is associated with the presence of an active inflammatory reaction and thus may be sensitive although not specific for pneumoconiosis in an active phase.[21]

## Lung Function Tests

Lung function tests are used to assess the degree of impairment caused by pneumoconiosis[22–24]; measurements may be made at rest and during exercise (Chapter 28). Pneumoconiosis may be associated with apparently normal lung function, or with a predominantly obstructive, restrictive, or mixed pattern of dysfunction. In the individual case, interpretation of results in terms of lung function profiles usually is done by the use of reference or predicted values.[23] This is complicated by the need to define the margins of "normality," an elusive concept at the best of times.[23, 24] In addition, published prediction formulas vary considerably primarily because of the differences in the characteristics of the subjects examined to generate the various predicted values.[24] As a result, a 1991 American Thoracic Society statement concluded that no one set of prediction equations is likely to be applicable to all laboratories, in all circumstances, and to all populations.[23] In the individual case, even comparison with pre-employment figures, if these exist (an alternative to using predicted normal values), may not be definitive, given that some technical drift over time is inevitable, although this is probably the most reliable way to detect departures from initial levels in an individual who was previously healthy. In addition, there is good evidence that individuals who undertake dusty occupations on average have higher spirometric lung volumes than the general population, on whom most predicted values are based.[24] Thus, it is not appropriate to minimize the functional significance of pneumoconiosis on the grounds of apparently normal lung function.

## Clinical Issues and Principles of Management

The clinician is faced with two main tasks when evaluating a case of suspected pneumoconiosis.[2–4] First is the meticulous assessment of the nature of the disease process, including its site (airways or pulmonary parenchyma or pleura?), its extent, and whether it has decreased the individual's performance in particular for his or her current job (is there evidence of impairment or disability?).[22] Assessment of impairment is based on symptoms and measurements of pulmonary function at rest and during exercise where indicated (Chapter 28). The clinical and laboratory tools available for this task, discussed in detail elsewhere in this textbook, are the same as those for chronic nonmalignant lung disease, whatever the cause. Assessment of disability is made in the wider context of whether the subject is fit for his or her job, and thus requires expert knowledge of the job content; it usually is made by qualified professionals from the fields of law and economics, as well as in some of the other health sciences.[22]

Second is the need to determine whether there has been environmental or occupational exposure of duration, intensity, and character sufficient to account in full or in part for the patient's present condition. For this task, the key tool is the occupational history, a task for which the clinician's interviewing skills are well suited, even in the absence of personal experience of workplaces or shop floors. This lack can be overcome by using one of the published formats for taking an occupational history.[25, 26] Worth emphasizing is the fact that currently in industrialized countries, and increasingly in industrializing countries, workers are usually able to give the physician a remarkably complete account of their occupation, the materials handled, and the processes involved.[25, 27, 28] Because pneumoconiosis is a reaction to retained dust, it may appear and progress, not only during exposure, but after exposure has ceased,[29] hence the importance of a complete exposure history, including summer jobs as student, military service, and short-term jobs. In addition, in industrialized countries, between 25% and 60% of men and up to 30% of women report exposure to dust or fumes at work,[30] further testimony to the fact that an occupational history is as essential as the smoking history in the practice of respiratory medicine. On occasions, it may be necessary to establish occupational exposure on the basis of analysis of biologic material (sputum, bronchoalveolar lavage, transbronchial or open-lung biopsy specimen) for the putative dust or its breakdown products.[2, 10, 11] This is particularly so in cases in which the exposure is remote and the exposure history incomplete or unreliable. Figure 65.3 presents examples of cases in which the putative dust was demonstrated in the pathologic specimens, and the case record in Figure 65.9 is an example of the use of lung dust burden measurements in establishing attributability.

Tuberculosis was a common complication of the mineral dust pneumoconiosis in the early part of this century, when infection levels were high in parent populations from which work forces were drawn and drug therapy was not yet available.[31] Although now relatively rare in industrialized countries,[31] tuberculosis remains an important issue in industrializing countries and undoubtedly will increase in both in response to the human immunodeficiency virus (HIV) epidemic.[32, 33, 33a]

Pneumoconiosis may appear and progress only after work exposure ceases; for practical purposes, regression does not occur.[34–34] Medical management invariably is limited to symptomatic treatment. Thus, the main issue for the patient, whether to quit the present job, depends on a knowledge of current dust levels in the patient's workplace. This information is not usually available to the treating physician, who nevertheless must ensure that the patient is advised appropriately on this question. Relevant, too, are the patient's age, socioeconomic circumstances, proximity to retirement, and compensation status, all factors to be taken into account in making this difficult and often heartbreaking decision. In the case of silicosis, there is renewed interest in interventions to interrupt the inflammatory pathophysiologic process that leads to chronic silicosis[36]; new as well as previously tried pharmacologic and other approaches are likely to be evaluated in the 21st century (see also under Silicosis; management and control).

The physician also should be aware that each time the diagnosis of pneumoconiosis is substantiated, it carries with it several important legal public health implications. In many jurisdictions, the physician has the legal responsibility for reporting all cases of pneumoconiosis seen.[37] The fact that a case of pneumoconiosis has been diagnosed is a "sentinel health event" and an index of failure of environmental controls in the workplace that may well require intervention by an appropriate authority.[37] There are differences in disease notification practice and in compensation legislation among states and among countries, and physicians should be aware of the appropriate procedure in the location of their practice.[37]

### Epidemiology and Implications for Clinical Practice

Information on the distribution of these diseases within and between work forces and the factors that influence distribution (the essence of epidemiology) provides the scientific base that the physician uses to reach a diagnosis, set prognosis, and plan management. Thus, knowledge of pneumoconiosis rates in the industries located in the local area assists the physician in diagnosis. Likewise, determining prognosis depends on work-force–based information, on knowing which factors influence disease progression favorably and unfavorably, and the likely effect of further exposure even at low levels. The same information dictates management, in particular whether workers should be advised to quit their jobs. Information on the natural history of these diseases is very meager[37] and seldom can be supplied by case studies alone; the physician must supplement this information with information from work-force–based (epidemiologic) studies in which environmental exposure and health events are linked but take into account what has been called the "healthy" worker effect.[38] This refers to the fact that individuals at work tend to enjoy better health than those not at work, the result of health selection in the workplace (men recruited to work in physically demanding jobs have on average better lung function than those in less demanding jobs in the same workplace),[24, 39] as well as health selection out of the workplace (workers who leave employment often do so for reasons of ill health).[2]

In the discussion that follows, the various types of pneumoconioses are considered separately with respect to occupations at risk, pathophysiology, and epidemiology, as well as the clinical issues of diagnosis, prognosis, and management. On all continents and in many countries, there is a substantial proportion of individuals exposed to dust at work and therefore potentially at risk for pneumoconiosis.[30] Lists of occupations and jobs at risk are never exhaustive (Table 65.1) but are meant as a guide for use in general office practice, where it may be more important to raise the suspicion of a diagnosis of pneumoconiosis than to be knowledgeable about the particular exposures a given job title implies. Indeed, the latter often falls into the expertise of the industrial hygienist. For those in occupational health or occupational medicine practice, reference should be made to one of the more specialized texts that describe the occupations at risk in greater detail.[1–5, 40]

## SILICOSIS

### Definition

*Silicosis* is a fibrotic lung disease attributable to the inhalation, retention, and lung reaction to silicon dioxide, or silica, in crystalline form, usually as quartz, and less commonly in other forms such as cristobalite and tridymite.[1] Amorphous or noncrystalline silica, in the form of diatomite and vitreous silica, is relatively nontoxic.[1, 32] Silica in the form of silicates such as asbestos, mica, and talc evokes a different type of pulmonary response[2, 4] and is considered separately.

### Industries and Occupations Still at Risk

Silicosis is an ancient disease and in all likelihood was associated with what might be called the starting point of human progress, when prehistoric humans began to fash-

**Table 65.1** INDUSTRIES AND OCCUPATIONS STILL AT RISK FOR SILICOSIS IN THE 1990s

| Industries, with Examples* | Some Occupations Implicated |
|---|---|
| Mining, tunneling, and excavating | Miner, driller, tunneler, developer, stoper |
| Underground: gold,[1-4, 32] copper,[4] iron,[42] tin,[4] uranium,[52] civil engineering projects[1, 2] | Mobile rig drill operator |
| Surface: coal,[1-4] iron,[42] excavation of foundations[1, 4, 43] | |
| Quarrying | Driller, hammerer, digger |
| Granite,[45, 59] sandstone,[4] slate,[3] sand,[45] chinastone/clay[2, 4] | |
| Stonework | Cutter, dresser, driller, polisher, grinder, mason |
| Granite sheds,[37, 58] monumental masonry[2, 4, 58] | |
| Foundries | Molder, knockout man, fettler, coremaker, caster |
| Ferrous[1-4, 45] and nonferrous metals[2] | |
| Abrasives | Crusher, pulverizer, and mixer; workers in the manufacture of abrasives |
| Production: silica flour,[1, 2] metal polish, and sandpapers,[1, 2] fillers in paint, rubber, and plastics[1, 5] | Operators of high-speed jets |
| Sandblasting: oil rigs,[59, 66] tombstones[36, 58] | |
| Ceramics | Workers at any stage of process if products are dry |
| Manufacture of pottery,[44] stoneware,[4] refractory bricks for ovens and kilns[2, 44] | |
| Others | |
| Glass making,[1-3] boiler scaling,[1, 2] traditional crafts,[2, 53] stone grinders,[4] gemstone workers,[40, 41] dental technicians[2] | |

*Good descriptions of many of these industries can be found in other medical texts.[1-6]

ion flint instruments in the paleolithic period.[32] Hippocrates reported that metal diggers or miners breathed with difficulty; Dutch pathologists in the 1700s noted that the lungs of stone cutters cut like a mass of sand, and the English medical literature of the 19th century contains detailed clinical descriptions of this pneumoconiosis.[4, 32] In the early decades of the 20th century, up until World War II, silicosis remained the major cause of morbidity and mortality in men exposed to silica dust in a variety of occupations, many if not most of which currently remain risk occupations.[1, 32] Table 65.1 provides some common examples but is not exhaustive.[1, 2, 4, 10, 37, 41]

Modern technology, if unaccompanied by modern controls, may result in exposures to finer dust particles than in the traditional industries and jobs. Thus, whenever the earth's crust is broken and silica-containing rock or sand is mined, milled and processed, or used, there are potential risks for the individuals whose occupation(s) involve them in these processes. What often first is reported as a new pneumoconiosis turns out to be silicosis in an industry not previously thought to be at risk[42] or a mixed dust pneumoconiosis in which silica is implicated with other dusts.[43] Furthermore, given the chronic nature of silicosis, including the fact that it may appear, develop, and progress long after the putative exposure has ceased, some of the patients of the 1990s had their exposure in World War II, making it essential that the physician's inquiry into a patient's occupation(s) be assiduous, exhaustive, and complete.

Currently in many countries, including those that have long been industrialized as well as those in the process of industrialization, foundries are the main source of silicosis.[1, 2, 4, 37, 44, 45] In addition, epidemics of acute silicosis continue to occur, even in industrialized countries with developed legislative systems and state environmental surveillance programs. Small industries organized in ignorance of the potential risk and employing people on contract are usually involved. Examples in the early part of the century include the quartz millers in Nevada and tunnelers in West Virginia[46]; more recent examples are tombstone blasters, silica flour millers, the surface or strip miners operating large mobile drill rigs,[37] and gemstone workers.[41, 45]

On a worldwide basis, many individuals are exposed to silica dust at work. For instance, it has been estimated that more than 1 million Americans are so exposed; furthermore, in 30% to 50% of workplaces in different industrial sectors inspected between 1979 and 1992, at least one airborne dust sample contained more than 100 mm/m$^3$ of crystalline silica, the Occupational Safety and Health Administration [OSHA] permissible exposure limit.[44] From these data, the US Department of Labor estimated that 59,000 cases of silicosis could be expected in these 1 million US workers exposed to silica.[48] Numbers at work in mines and quarries and at risk in 14 countries in Europe (excluding Poland and countries of the former USSR) have been estimated at 839,000; in 8 countries in Australasia (excluding China), at 189,000, and in 6 countries in Africa, at 394,000.[30] The prevalence of silicosis in South Africa has been rising,[49] and cases continue to be reported in the United States,[50, 51] Canada,[52] Italy,[53] and Sweden.[54] Thus, clinicians on all continents can expect to see cases of pneumoconiosis in the 21st century.[37]

## Pathology

Three clinicopathologic types of silicosis have been described (Table 65.2): *chronic silicosis*, which typically follows exposure, measured in decades rather than years, to respirable dust usually containing less than 30% quartz; *accelerated silicosis,* which follows shorter, heavier exposure; and *acute silicosis,* which follows intense exposure to fine dust of high silica content for periods measured in months rather than years.[1–3, 5, 48, 55–59]

Figure 65.4*A* to *C* illustrates the pathologic lesions of chronic silicosis. The hallmark of chronic silicosis is the silicotic islet or nodule, one of the few agent-specific lesions in pathology (see Fig. 65.4). The mature lesion is characterized by a cell-free and largely dust-free central area of concentrically arranged, whorled hyalinized collagen fibers, surrounded by an area of concentrically arranged collagen fibers and a more peripheral zone of randomly oriented fibers interspersed with dust-laden macrophages.[56, 60] Less common features include interstitial pulmonary fibrosis and plaque-like lesions involving the visceral pleura often distributed along the anatomic lobulations of the lung.[55, 56] Silicotic nodules develop first in the hilar lymph nodes and may be confined to this area; here they may become encased in calcification and impinge on or erode into airways. The disease process next involves the lung parenchyma, islets often developing in the lymphatic drainage channels of the lung, particularly in the perivascular sheath; there is also a predilection for the upper lobes, at least when the exposure has been in mining.[55] In addition, some of the nodules may take on a granulomatous appearance with giant cells; and there may be a more diffuse type of interstitial reaction with type II cell hyperplasia.[2] In accelerated silicosis, the changes are similar to those seen in the chronic form, the difference being one of degree, severity, amount of lung involved, and incubation time. With continued exposure, the nodules tend to increase in size[56] and, in a minority of cases, may become confluent, leading to the development of *conglomerate silicosis*, also called *progressive massive fibrosis* (PMF). These lesions, which usually involve the upper lobes, tend to obliterate lung structure and may cavitate, which may be an indication of tuberculosis.[56, 60.] Acute silicosis may show all the features of pulmonary alveolar proteinosis (Chapter 63), in addition to an interstitial pneumonitis similar to that seen in the accelerated form of the disease; silica particles and various biomarkers of tissue reaction can be identified in the proteinaceous material from the alveolar spaces as well as in lavage material.[3, 4, 9]

An unusual type of nodule, called the *rheumatoid sili-*

**Table 65.2 CLINICOPATHOLOGIC TYPES OF SILICOSIS**

| Type | Exposure | Pathologic Features | Clinical Features |
|---|---|---|---|
| Chronic | Usually over 20 years,[1, 2, 32] often to dust containing less than 30% quartz | Mainly the classic silicotic islet or nodule; usually involving hilar nodes first, then upper lobes to which it may be limited | Small rounded opacities on roentgenogram[3]; not necessarily associated with increased morbidity or mortality[1, 2]; impairment of pulmonary function may occur,[48, 70] but not invariably[32]; may progress to conglomerate silicosis and be complicated by tuberculosis, particularly in high-prevalence areas[54] |
| Accelerated | 5–15 years,[1, 2] usually to dusts of higher quartz content[55] | Numerous nodules at various stages of development,[56] sometimes with irregular interstitial fibrosis | Irregular upper zone fibrosis with a nodular component; symptomatic with impairment, and often progression to respiratory failure and death; cavitation with infection by atypical mycobacteria not unusual[76] |
| Acute | May be measured in months,[1, 2] usually to very fine dusts of high quartz content[56] | Alveoloproteinosis (air spaces filled with neutrophils, epithelial cells, and proteinaceous materials) with interstitial reactions and early, loosely organized nodules[48, 56] | Resembles acute air space disease on chest roentgenogram; rapid progression to acute respiratory failure; fulminating tuberculosis is a common terminal complication[32, 48, 56] |

*cotic nodule*, may be seen in the lungs of exposed subjects, with or without a background of small rounded opacities on the chest roentgenogram, who during life exhibit rheumatoid arthritis or high levels of circulating rheumatoid factor, or both.[4, 56, 60–63] These nodules are often larger than the usual silicotic lesion and have light gray necrotic centers surrounded by palisades of fibroblasts with a prominent inflammatory reaction. Lung dust in and around the nodules was analyzed in one case report and reflected the exposure.[61] Rheumatoid nodules occur much less frequently in association with silica exposure than with coal dust exposure (see subsequent discussion in this chapter).[62]

Tuberculosis may complicate the disease at any stage, but particularly at risk are cases of acute and accelerated disease.[31, 32, 37, 59] Exposure without silicosis also may predispose individuals to tuberculosis.[64, 65] Although *Mycobacterium tuberculosis* is the usual organism, nontuberculous mycobacteria (NTM) account for a large proportion of the mycobacterial disease not only in acute and accelerated silicosis, but also in chronic silicosis.[37, 66, 66a] The proportion of tuberculosis and of disease caused by NTM in silica-exposed subjects probably reflects the profile of infection in the population from which the particular work force is drawn.[37, 59, 65]

The lungs of exposed individuals, whether or not they show silicosis, also may demonstrate the features of other diseases associated with occupational dust exposure, such as chronic bronchitis and emphysema.[6, 7, 67–69] The pathologic features of these diseases, described in Chapters 18 and 38, are similar whether associated with occupational exposure to dusts and fumes encountered in the workplace or with exposure to cigarette smoke. In contrast to clinical case series,[19] population-based studies[68–69, 70] suggest that emphysema associated with exposure to dusty environments develops independently of silicosis. However, because both are related to cumulative exposure, both often occur in the same individual. Small-airway abnormalities, including fibrosis and pigmentation of respiratory bronchioles, also are seen in association with exposures to a variety of mineral dusts, including those responsible for silicosis.[71]

Extrathoracic manifestations of silicosis include silicotic lesions in the lymph nodes in the neck and abdominal chains and occasionally in organs such as liver, spleen,[2, 4, 37, 55] and bone marrow.[72] There is also an association between exposure to silica and certain connective tissue diseases other than rheumatoid arthritis, such as progressive systemic sclerosis,[2, 4, 37, 73–76] systemic lupus erythematosus,[77] and possibly a nephropathy involving glomerular capillary loops and basement membranes.[2, 4, 37, 56]

More recently, associations between exposure to silica or the presence of silicosis with lung cancer, or both also have been described.[37, 78] The nature of the association is discussed in the section on epidemiology.

## Pathogenesis

The series of reactions that follows the inhalation of quartz particles is complex, involving all cell components of the air-tissue interface as well as systemic changes. (Related matters are discussed in Chapter 19.) An excellent review of this topic summarizes the processes whereby silica produces inflammation and fibrogenesis in the lung.[79] Silica particles of less than 5 μm reach the lower respiratory tract and may enter the alveoli. There is some debate as to whether larger or smaller particles are more fibrogenic but agreement that freshly fractured silica is more toxic to the alveolar macrophages.[80] The surface characteristics of the silica determine their redox potential and ability to react with hydrogen, oxygen, and nitrogen. Coated silica particles have been shown to have a much reduced ability to injure lung: this may explain the relatively nonfibrogenic response to silica in coal and in hematite miners[8] and the observation that the incidence of silicosis is decreased by concomitant exposure to other dusts.[81] The nature of the lung injury also is determined by the intensity of the exposure. Low-intensity exposure generally produces aggregates of fibrosis with relative sparing of the lung architecture, whereas high-intensity exposure causes widespread pulmonary inflammation and collagen deposition.[82] Once silica has been ingested by the alveolar macrophage, oxidants, cytokines, and growth factors are produced. Tumor necrosis factor-alpha (TNF-α) and interleukin 1 (IL-1) are cytokines that play an important role in the initiation of silicosis, and experimental inhibition of these cytokines has been shown to prevent silicosis. Growth factors, including transforming growth factor-beta (TGF-β), are important in fibrogenesis (and also have been implicated in carcinogenesis) in association with silica.[83, 84] Injury to alveolar type I epithelial cells and hyperplasia and hypertrophy of alveolar type II cells occur early in the process. The changes in the alveolar type II cells initially may play a role in repair but with progression are thought to lead to fibrogenesis. Other cells that are implicated in the development of silicosis include neutrophils, T and B lymphocytes, and mast cells. In experimental silicosis, the absence of mast cells is associated with a significant reduction in the severity of the lung lesions.[85] Although the major determinant of silicosis is the level of exposure to silica-containing dust, individual susceptibility to the disease may play a role,[4, 32, 86, 87] a view supported by the observation of variable degrees of silicosis in individuals with apparently similar exposure and by studies on animals.[88] In addition to its clearly powerful fibrogenic potential, epidemiologic studies indicate that silicosis is associated with a significantly increased risk for lung cancer,[37, 78] and the International Agency for Research in Cancer (IARC) classified silica dust as "carcinogenic to humans."[89] (See also the next section.)

## Epidemiology: Secular Trends and Their Implications for the Clinician

In the early decades of this century, silicosis was regarded as a disease that disabled the young and killed them prematurely; it currently is regarded by many as no more than a radiologic abnormality,[2, 4, 32] not associated with impairment or disability and even without effect on longevity[1–3] in many although not all[90–92] populations at risk. These secular trends, supported in general by a decrease in numbers of cases certified and an increase in the average age and length of service at certification in the

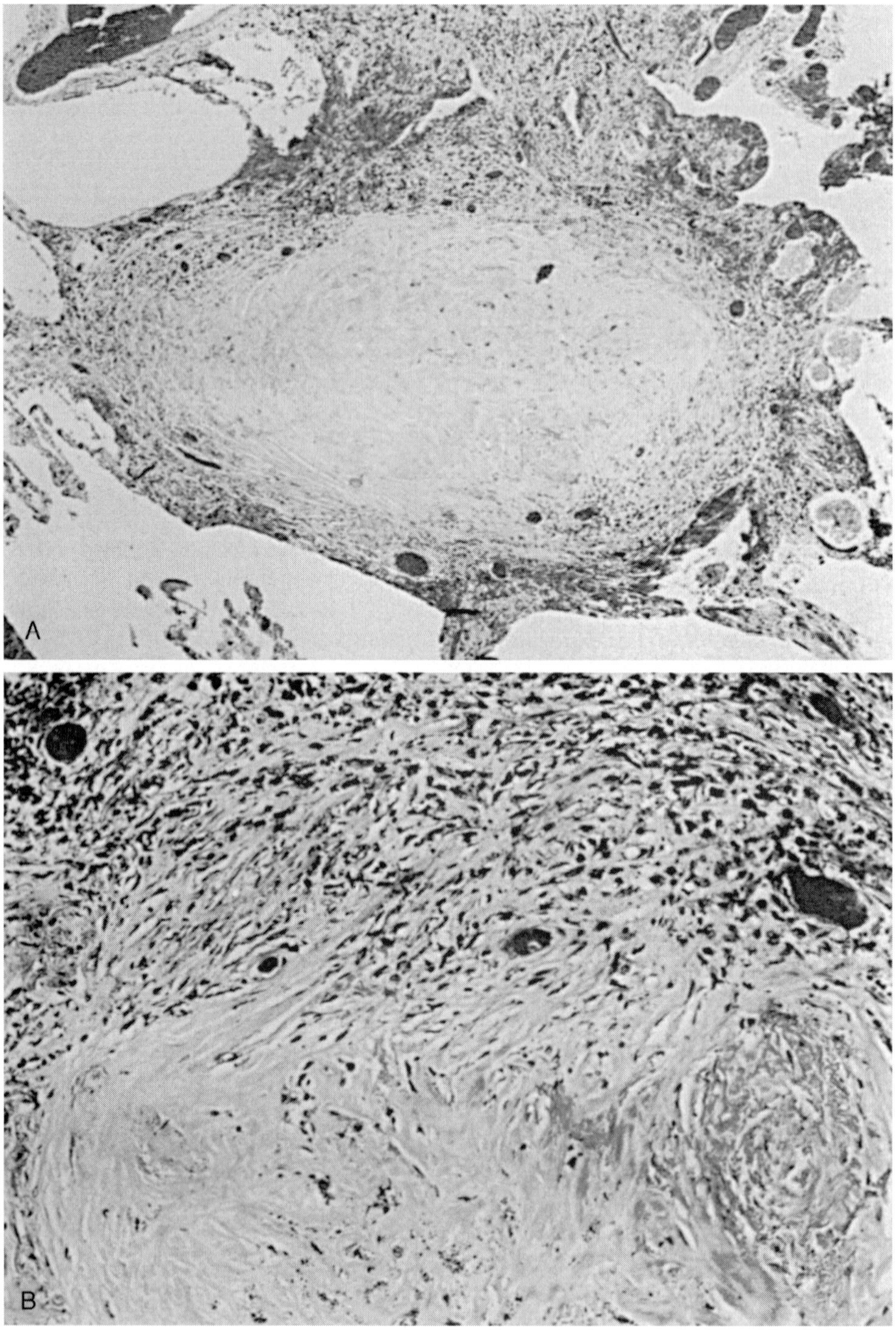


**Figure 65.4** Pathologic lesions of chronic silicosis. *A*, Silicotic nodule characterized by a central zone of a cellular hyalinized collagen with a whorled appearance, and a peripheral zone of macrophages in which abundant foreign material is situated (original magnification × 40, light microscopy). *B*, Silicotic nodule at higher magnification to show these characteristics to better advantage (original magnification × 150, light microscopy).

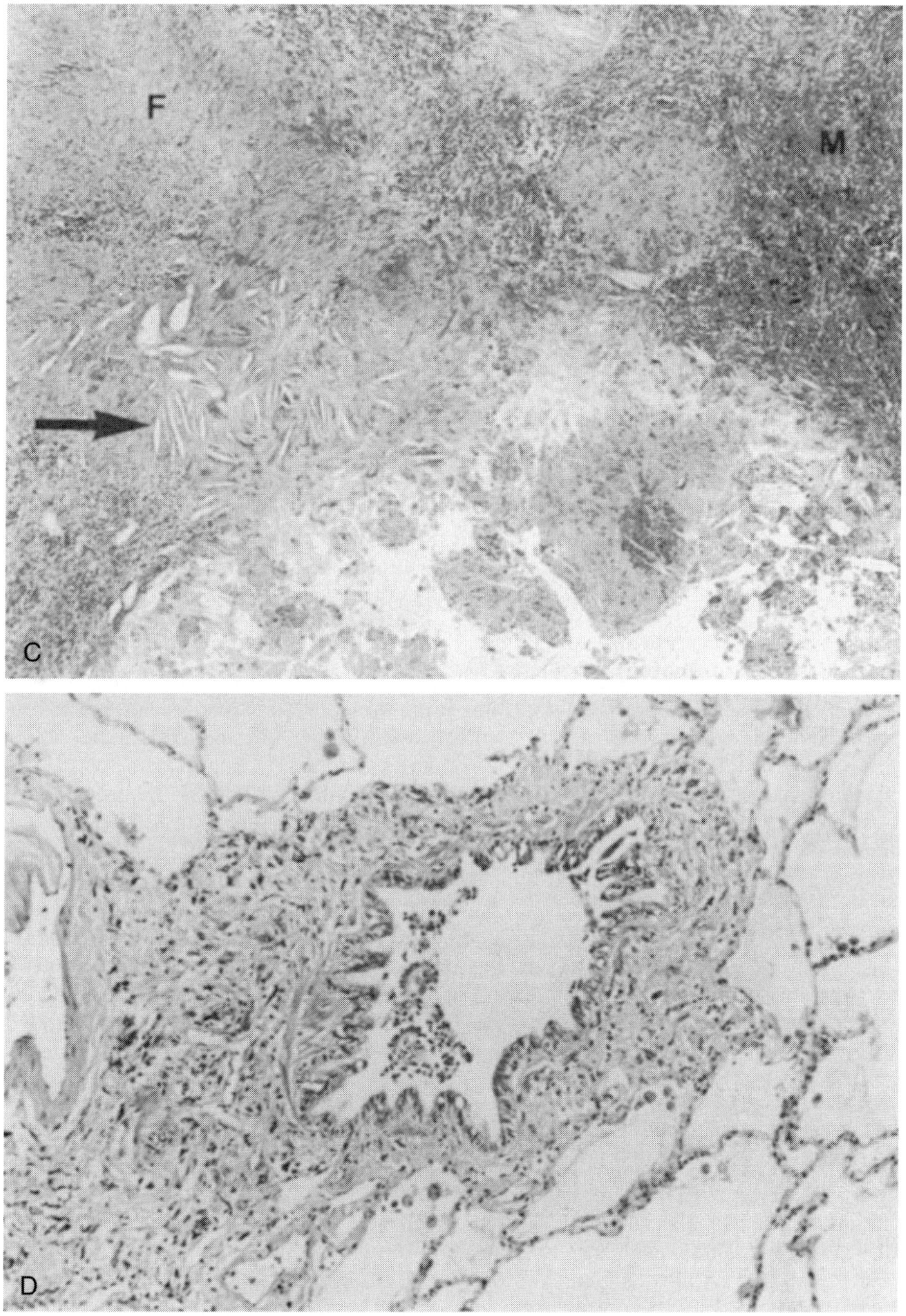


**Figure 65.4** *Continued*
*C,* Progressive massive fibrosis from a case of silicosis showing fibrosis (F), aggregates of pigment laden macrophages (M), and multiple cholesterol clefts *(arrow).* The tissue in the lower half is necrotic and has undergone liquefaction (original magnification × 25, light microscopy). *D,* Mineral dust small airway disease, characterized by peribronchiolar fibrous tissue containing a moderate amount of foreign particulate material; occasional silicotic nodules were present elsewhere in the lung parenchyma (original magnification × 150, light microscopy). (*A* through *C* from Fraser RG, Paré JAP, Fraser RS, Genereux GP: Diagnosis of Diseases of the Chest (3rd ed). Philadelphia: WB Saunders, 1990, pp 2288–2289. *D* courtesy of Dr. R. S. Fraser.)

work forces of many of the industrialized countries,[32] may be the result of a decreasing proportion of acute and subacute cases and an increasing number of chronic cases. Reasons include improved environmental controls, falling rates of tuberculosis, and perhaps the advent of drug therapy for tuberculosis. Notwithstanding these trends, there remains well-warranted concern that this avoidable disease remains a significant cause of morbidity[37, 70, 92] and mortality.[93–96]

The prevalence of silicosis is difficult to estimate, given the large number of industries at risk (see Table 65.1), the irregular nature of employment in many of them, the transient labor force in industrializing as well as in industrialized countries, and the probably frequent appearance of disease after the worker has left the work force.[32, 91] In large controlled industries employing many workers, such as the South African gold mines, and in certain industries that have been subjected to specific studies,[2] rates have fallen but the disease has by no means been eliminated. Nor can the rates from different countries be compared because criteria for calculating both the numerator (i.e., persons with disease) and the denominator (i.e., persons at risk) differ in different jurisdictions.[2, 32] For the clinician in office or hospital practice, therefore, there are few if any countries in the world where silicosis can be relegated to the end of the differential diagnosis list in a patient with nonmalignant respiratory disease and an exposure history. Chest physicians in particular have an obligation to be aware of local industries at risk for silicosis in the area of their practice.[45, 97]

The presence of silicosis in an individual or a work force means that there has been exposure to quartz dust. The risk of developing disease is determined by the lung dust burden, which in turn is related primarily to the intensity, nature, and duration of exposure. Exposure-response relationships have been demonstrated in various industries at risk for silicosis.[2, 32, 98] In calculating an individual's risk for silicosis, duration and intensity of exposure are of primary interest[13, 99] but peak exposure also may be important.[100] The physician should, however, not be inhibited from considering the diagnosis of silicosis when that diagnosis is suggested by clinical and radiologic features, even when exposure appears to have been insignificant or in an occupation not known to be associated with silicosis.

The natural history of silicosis, even in the chronic form, varies greatly. In some series, up to half the cases of simple and conglomerate silicosis progress after exposure has ceased.[91] There also are case examples of conglomerate silicosis that remain radiologically static and clinically silent until death occurs from some other disease; other cases follow a rapidly progressive disabling course. Dust load and residence time in the lung to the point at which disease develops appear to be important determinants of progression.[91] However, population-based studies of the factors influencing progression of disease are limited, despite the fact that this information is crucial to clinical management. An early report of a case-control study based on the Swedish silicosis register indicated that progression of disease was more likely to occur if exposure continued for 2 years or more after the earliest radiologic change was detected than if exposure after detection did not exceed 2 years.[34] Survival in one series also was shown to be reduced in the presence of dyspnea, expectoration, abnormal breath sounds, and a reduced vital capacity.[90] In a 5-year study of South African gold miners, the rate of deterioration of lung function was related to the initial extent of radiologic nodule profusion with annual loss of $FEV_1$ increasing from 57 mL to 128 mL for nodule profusion category 1 to 3, respectively.[92] In that study, nodule profusion increased by one subcategory (e.g., 2/2 to 2/3) during the 5 years, regardless of further exposure to silica.

The association between silicosis and tuberculosis has long been recognized.[1, 2, 4, 37, 101, 102] Rates for active tuberculosis in silicotic subjects range from 5% to 43%, depending on whether radiologic or autopsy criteria are used,[34, 101] an increase varying from 2- to 30-fold more than in nonsilicotic miners. Factors thought to influence the development of tuberculosis in the silicotic subject include the stage and type of disease (acute silicotics appear to be at considerably higher risk),[2, 59] the prevalence of tuberculosis in the population from which the work force was drawn, as well as the age and general health status of the work force.[32, 101, 102] Despite the changing nature of silicosis, the decrease in its incidence, the decreasing rates for tuberculosis in the general population, and improved screening of new recruits into most industries, the association between these two diseases persists.[31, 103] This issue calls for urgent further study particularly because of the worldwide HIV epidemic and the associated increase in prevalence of tuberculosis and in treatment failure.[104, 105] Disease caused by NTM also is recognized increasingly in those with silicosis[37, 59, 66, 66a] and should be recognized to provide appropriate treatment.

The relationship between silica exposure, silicosis, and systemic collagen vascular disease remains to be clarified. Epidemiologic evidence indicates that the presence of rheumatoid arthritis, high levels of circulating rheumatoid factor, or both increases the risk of the exposed individual developing silicosis,[62, 63] that is, the two conditions are associated with each other, the former increasing the risk of developing the latter. By contrast, progressive systemic sclerosis is associated with silica exposure, not with silicosis, that is, the two conditions share a common cause but do not appear to be associated with each other.[73, 74]

Lung cancer is not a rare occurrence in middle-aged miners who smoke, and until the mid-1980s it was thought to occur with equal frequency in those with and without silicosis.[2, 4] However, contrary trends in some work forces led to a re-examination of the question of whether occupational exposures associated with the risk of silicosis (as distinct from the presence of silicosis) increases the lung cancer risk; on balance, the evidence from epidemiologic studies suggests that this is the case.[56, 106–111] As indicated above, when the question was reviewed by the IARC in 1996[110] in light of new data, the agency classified crystalline silica as "carcinogenic to humans." The American Thoracic Society statement on Adverse Effects of Crystalline Silica Exposure was more cautious, concluding that those with silicosis are at increased risk for lung cancer, but that less information is available for workers exposed to silica who do not smoke.[37]

## Clinical Features

The symptoms and signs of chronic silicosis, a disease characterized by focal pulmonary fibrosis, are no different from those of focal pulmonary fibrosis caused by other agents; their evolution and time course are related to type and severity of disease process. The main symptom is breathlessness, first noted under the stress of effort and later at rest as the large working reserve of the lung is diminished.[1–4] In chronic silicosis (see also Table 65.2), and in the absence of other respiratory disease, even this symptom may be absent, and it is not unusual for a patient to present as a symptom-free individual requiring assessment because of an abnormal chest roentgenogram. The appearance of breathlessness also may mark the development of a complication such as progressive massive fibrosis, tuberculosis, or airway disease. Cough, a not infrequent symptom, may be caused by chronic bronchitis, associated with cigarette usage, with the occupational exposure itself (particularly if the dust load is heavy), or with both, or with the presence of reactive airways.[112] This symptom also may signal the development of tuberculosis[2] or lung cancer, and more rarely these days it may be the consequence of hilar node enlargement and impingement on the main airways.[113]

Other airway-related symptoms, such as wheezing and chest tightness, are less common and usually attributable to associated diseases such as bronchitis, emphysema, or COPD. Miners with reactive airways also may be more susceptible to adverse effects from airborne contaminants.[112] Chest pain is not a feature, nor are systemic symptoms such as fever and weight loss, which should be attributed to tuberculosis or HIV (or both), or lung cancer until proven otherwise. In the absence of complications, there may be no physical signs; when complications occur, they may be reflected in the chest examination. Clubbing is not a feature of silicosis.[3]

In accelerated and acute silicosis, the time scale of symptom evolution is in years or months rather than decades (see Table 65.2). In the acute form particularly, breathlessness may become disabling within months, followed by impaired gas exchange and organ failure.

## Radiographic and Lung Function Changes

Uncomplicated silicosis is characterized by the presence of small rounded opacities on the chest roentgenogram, as graded in the ILO classification (as described previously). Rounded opacities on the roentgenogram are produced by the summation of superimposed silicotic nodules, whereas HRCT permits the visualization of individual nodules.[18] Silicotic nodules are usually, although not invariably, symmetrically distributed and tend to occur first in the upper zones, later, although not invariably, involving other zones.[2, 3] Occasionally they are calcified, resembling microlithiasis.[4] Enlargement of the hilar nodes may precede the development of the parenchymal lesions. Eggshell calcification, when present, is strongly suggestive although not pathognomonic of silicosis.[4] Pleural plaques may occur but are not a common feature of silicosis.[56] Complicated silicosis (progressive massive fibrosis) is characterized by the coalescence of small rounded opacities to form larger lesions; they are graded on the ILO scale according to size and extent (categories A to C). CT assessment is superior to the chest roentgenogram in assessing not only the presence and extent of silicotic nodulation, but in particular is able to reveal early conglomeration.[18] With time, the mass lesions tend to contract, usually to the upper lobes, leaving hypertranslucent zones at their margins and often at the lung bases; in this process, small rounded opacities previously evident may disappear, resulting in a picture compatible with tuberculosis on the chest roentgenogram.[2] The rapid development of several large lesions suggests rheumatoid silicosis. For the most part, changing lesions, particularly if cavitated, should be regarded as evidence of mycobacterial disease. Acute silicosis is characterized radiologically by diffuse changes that usually display an air space and interstitial pattern rather than nodularity.[1]

Given the wide variety of clinical and pathologic manifestations of silicosis itself, often affecting vessels and airways as well as parenchyma,[56, 59] and given the coexistence of bronchitis, small airways disease, and emphysema in many cases (whether these are related to the individual's occupational exposure[6, 32, 67, 70] or to cigarette use), it is not surprising that there is no consistent lung function profile associated with silicosis. In chronic silicosis, spirometric tests ($FEV_1$, $FEV_1/FVC$, and maximal midexpiratory flow [$FEF_{25-75}$]) usually reflect airflow limitation.[70, 91, 114] Lung volumes (vital capacity [VC], total lung capacity [TLC]) may be reduced in advanced disease but usually not the functional residual capacity (FRC), and residual volume (RV). Reduction in diffusing capacity is generally apparent in more advanced chronic silicosis.[70, 115, 116] Indeed, the view has been expressed that most of the lung function changes associated with chronic silicosis can be attributed to the associated emphysema.[67, 117] In the accelerated and acute forms, functional changes are more marked and progression is more rapid. In acute silicosis, radiologic progression is accompanied by increasing impairment of function and gas exchange, which leads to organ failure and eventually to death from intractable hypoxemia. This clinical course is more likely to occur when the radiologic picture is predominantly interstitial.[3] Interpretation of pulmonary function tests is discussed in Chapter 28.

## Diagnosis and Complications

In the presence of a history of exposure and the characteristic radiographic changes, the diagnosis of silicosis should present no difficulty.[2, 4] Problems arise when the history of exposure is remote, forgotten, or missed (hence the importance of a careful and comprehensive occupational history) or when the radiologic features are unusual, for example, when the radiologic (including CT) lesions are solitary or few or are confined to fibrotic changes in a single lobe, as in some cases of rapidly developing silicosis.[2] Detection of silica in bronchoalveolar lavage material may raise suspicion. Lung biopsy (transbronchial, transthoracic, or open) may be necessary to clarify the nature of unusual or conglomerate lesions, or both, in which progressive massive fibrosis, lung cancer, and tuberculosis are all possible diagnoses. Biopsy material always should be submitted to microanalysis for dust,[10, 11] including silica, because for the most part the decision to perform a biopsy indicates an element of doubt in the diagnosis. An increase in cells in the bronchial washings,[9] in particular lymphocytes, or an active gallium scan, or both, suggests the presence of an active alveolitis that is likely to progress.

Complications include infection by mycobacteria or fungi, cor pulmonale, spontaneous pneumothorax, broncholithiasis, and tracheobronchial obstruction from polypoid granuloma developing in the neighborhood of eggshell calcification in hilar nodes.[2, 4, 59, 113] Diagnosis of active tuberculosis in the silicotic subject may be more difficult than in the nonsilicotic subject,[2, 31, 101, 102] but in general a good sample of sputum or sputum induced by nebulized hypertonic saline sent for mycobacterial culture provides the diagnosis. The presence of cough, hemoptysis, and systemic symptoms (weight loss, fever) always should raise the suspicion and prompt an active search for organisms or histologic evidence in biologic material from any of the following sources: sputum, bronchoalveolar lavage or lung biopsy material, pleural fluid or biopsy specimens, and urine. The same course of action is indicated if any of the following features develops on the chest roentgenogram: new parenchymal change, especially in the upper zones; coalescence of nodules or rapid growth of a few; cavitation; and pleural or pericardial effusion. In work forces under radiologic surveillance, it is usually the chest roentgenogram, not the other features, that gives the key to the diagnosis.[118]

## Management and Control

Once established, the fibrotic process of chronic silicosis is thought to be irreversible; management of the individual case is thus directed toward preventing progression and the development of complicated disease, which usually is accompanied by impairment and eventual disability. This may include advice on leaving or changing a current job, which should be given in the light of knowledge of the environmental conditions past and present. Such knowledge is often not within the physician's expertise; appropriate counseling should be arranged (see also the discussion on principles of management in the introduction to this chapter).

Interventions to interrupt the inflammatory process that leads to chronic silicosis have been tried in the past several decades and include inhalation of aluminum powder and inhalation or pharmacologic use of polyvinylpynidine-N-oxide (PVNO).[2, 119, 120] There is, however, no evidence that they are of any value in prevention or in the reversal of established disease in humans,[2, 120] and they may even be harmful. More recently, tetrandine, an alkaloid derived from the root of *Stephania tetradandra*, used extensively in traditional Chinese medicine,[36, 120] is considered to hold promise.[36] The use of cytotoxic and anti-inflammatory agents, including steroids, is discussed elsewhere in this volume (Chapter 56) in relation to the treatment of interstitial pulmonary fibrosis; their application to pneumoconiosis in general and silicosis in particular remains to be clarified. Also attracting attention is whole-lung lavage to remove dust, inflammatory cells, and mediator burden.[36] Silica has been removed successfully from the lung (an average of 6.7 mg of quartz per lung lavage in one series)[121]; however, there is as yet no proof that this decreases the progression of the disease.[120, 121]

Management of acute silicosis is described in several case reports.[4, 59, 121] Treatment with bronchoalveolar lavage, steroids, or both, has been used when the disease manifests as alveolar proteinosis.[121, 122] Although alveolar proteinosis occurring in the absence of silica exposure usually resolves spontaneously or responds to bronchoalveolar lavage (Chapter 63), alveolar proteinosis occurring in association with silica exposure may not respond to bronchoalveolar lavage, even though quite large quantities of dust can be removed.[122] Prognosis depends on the extent of parenchymal response to the silica and the vigor of the associated fibrotic lesions; progression to disability, organ failure, and early death is invariable. Treatment should be directed toward control of mycobacterial infection, which is a common complication often involving NTM[2, 4, 59] and other supportive measures. No doubt because of the poor prognosis of accelerated and acute silicosis and the fact that it is often young men with short exposure histories who are affected, patients with this diagnosis were among the early recipients of lung transplants. (For lung transplantation, see Chapter 97.)

Current treatment regimens for tuberculosis that include rifampin have been shown to be effective in the treatment of tuberculosis in subjects with silicosis.[123–125] Treatment compliance and acquired drug resistance remain issues, especially in countries with high prevalence of tuberculosis and of HIV infection in the general population. Tuberculosis, even when treated successfully, is associated with a loss of lung function in those with silicosis,[92] and every attempt should be made to prevent tuberculosis in those with silicosis and a positive tuberculin skin test. To date, attempts at chemoprophylaxis have provided incomplete protection against tuberculosis.[126, 127] When mycobacterial disease is found to be caused by NTM, appropriate therapy should be provided.[128] Tuberculosis and NTM are discussed in Chapter 34.

The most important aspect of the management of silicosis relates to its prevention. To achieve this, a sustained effort must be made to increase awareness of silicosis. It was reported that deaths from silicosis in younger subjects in the United States occurred after exposure in the construction and manufacturing sectors, with none from mining.[96] This suggests a lack of awareness of the hazards of silica outside the traditional occupations associated with silicosis.

# COAL WORKERS' PNEUMOCONIOSIS

## Definition and Occupations at Risk

*Coal workers' pneumoconiosis* (CWP) is a distinct pathologic entity resulting from the deposition of coal dust in the lungs.[1–5, 129] The tissue reactions to deposits of dust

(Fig. 65.5) include the *coal macule*, which when associated with focal emphysema constitutes the *coal nodule*, the characteristic lesion of simple CWP, and complicated CWP, or PMF.[129] Coal miners also may develop silicotic nodules when the coal seams that they mine are in hard rock,[2] for instance, in mines with a high grade of coal such as anthracite,[15] and in specific jobs such as roof bolters and motormen. Coal mining also is associated with chronic (industrial) bronchitis,[2] chronic airflow limitation,[2, 6] and emphysema.[2, 3, 129, 130] For these diseases, distinguishing the contribution of cigarette smoking from that of occupational exposure has proved a difficult task,[2] but the evidence that both bronchitis and emphysema also may be associated causally with coal mining exposure independently of CWP is now broadly based on studies from work forces based in several countries and is sufficiently coherent to have gained wide,[2, 3, 131] although not universal,[132] acceptance.

The term *black lung*, originally a colloquial reference to any lung disorder or disease associated with coal mining, became a legal term in the United States after the introduction of the US 1969 Federal Coal Mine Health and Safety Act, also called the Black Lung Act.[3] This term should be distinguished from the medical, epidemiologic, and pathologic terminology that is used to describe the various disorders and diseases associated with coal mining.[3] In the United Kingdom, recognition of attributability of coal mine dust as a cause of centriacinar emphysema, which can lead to loss of lung function, was contained in a judgment, delivered on January 23, 1998, in the longest and probably the most expensive personal injury court case ever heard in Britain, and the findings have been summarized for medical readers (see also the discussion in the section on epidemiology and natural history).[115, 130, 133, 134]

The main occupation at risk for CWP is coal mining, an industry that in the 1970s, despite modern mechanization, still employed approximately 250,000 people in the United Kingdom, and a comparable number in Western Europe.[30] Estimates of numbers employed in the United States in 1986 were approximately 175,000[135] and decreased to 118,733 in 1992.[15] Coal is also mined in Eastern Europe, India, and China and on the African, Australian, and South American continents.[30] With mechanization, output has increased even though the number of miners has shrunk in most countries[3]; however, dust exposure also may have increased, and former as well as current coal workers are likely to be seen in office medical practice for several decades to come. Other occupations at risk for exposure to coal or carbon dust include coal trimming (which involves loading and stowing coal in stores or ships' holds), the mining and milling of

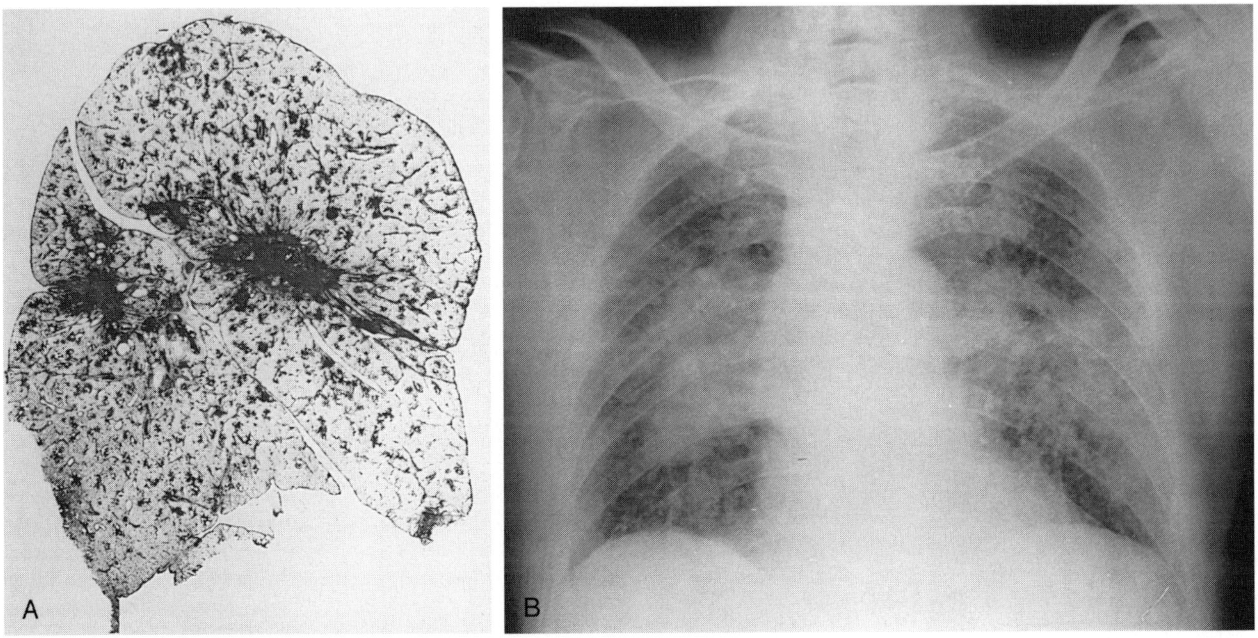


**Figure 65.5** *A,* Whole-lung section of 71-year-old Appalachian coal miner. The miner was a nonsmoker and had worked for 28 years underground, primarily at face work. The midsagittal section of the left lung shows massive lesions in the apical portion of the lower lobe and in the central area of the upper lobe. PMF is seen against a background of simple nodular and macular coal worker's pneumoconiosis. In several areas, there is evidence of coalescence of nodules. There is mild focal emphysema associated with the coal dust macules. *B,* The chest roentgenogram shows features of PMF against a background of nodularity. The mass lesion on the right shows the propensity of PMF to move toward the hilum. The opacities are somewhat atypical for their predominantly lower zone situation. (Case from the NIOSH W. Laqueur collection, courtesy of Drs. V. Vallyathan and F. H. Y. Green.)

graphite in carbon plants and in the manufacture of carbon electrodes, as well as the manufacture and use of carbon black.[2, 4]

## Pathology

The primary lesion in coal workers' pneumoconiosis is the *coal macule*, which can be seen (although not palpated) on macroscopic examination as a small (up to 4 mm) pigmented lesion, distributed evenly initially in the upper lobes, although the lower lobes subsequently may become involved (see Figs. 65.5*A* and *B*).[1–3, 129, 131] On microscopic examination, the coal macule consists of an aggregation of dust, dust-laden macrophages, and fibroblasts accumulated around respiratory bronchioles, often filling contiguous alveoli and extending into the interstitium, with irregular collagen fibrosis (Fig. 65.6*A*).[2, 3, 131, 136] With time, the coal macule may enlarge to become a *coal nodule*, a palpable lesion in which, in addition to dust and many dust-laden macrophages, contains reticulin fibers and irregular collagen fibrosis (see Fig. 65.6*B*).[1, 2, 131] In time, the wall of the respiratory bronchiole weakens and the bronchioles dilate to create an area of *focal emphysema*. This form of centriacinar emphysema in combination with the macule form the characteristic lesion of coal workers' pneumoconiosis.[2, 131] Muscular arteries also may become surrounded by coal dust.[129] Other features include subpleural dust deposits, enlargement of the hilar and mediastinal nodes, and, on occasion, tattooing of the parietal pleural lymphatic channels by coal dust.[4] Classic silicotic lesions are seen in approximately 12% of US coal miners[131] and form when lung dust residue contains 18% or more quartz.[1, 8] Coal nodules have been classified radiologically as micro (up to 7 mm in diameter) and macro (7 to 20 mm in diameter) and usually occur on a background of coal macules.[1] Lesions greater than 1 cm have been accepted as radiologic evidence of PMF, although the College of American Pathologists recommends a minimum diameter of 2 cm.[2, 129] These bulky, often irregular but well-defined, heavily pigmented rubbery black tissue masses usually develop in the posterior segment of the upper lobes or apical segments of the lower lobes.[2] Microscopically, the lesions contain the same elements as the coal nodule and hence are thought by some to develop from the coalescence of perivascularly located coal nodules (see Fig. 65.6*C*). PMF lesions are frequently progressive and massive but not necessarily so.[129] They may impinge on and obliterate airways and vessels and cross interlobar fissures, and cavitation is not uncommon as a consequence of ischemic necrosis or of mycobacterial infection. Vasculitis in the surrounding vessels also may be a feature.[129]

*Rheumatoid pneumoconiosis*, one variant of which is called Caplan's syndrome, is a nodular form of CWP associated with rheumatoid arthritis or a rheumatoid diathesis. It is characterized by necrobiotic nodules that are larger than the coal nodules and have smoother borders. Pigmentation is arranged in concentric laminations and, relative to PMF lesions, contains little dust.[2] These lesions may cavitate or calcify, or do both.[4] The microscopic features are similar to those described for the rheumatoid silicotic lesion (see under the discussion of the pathology

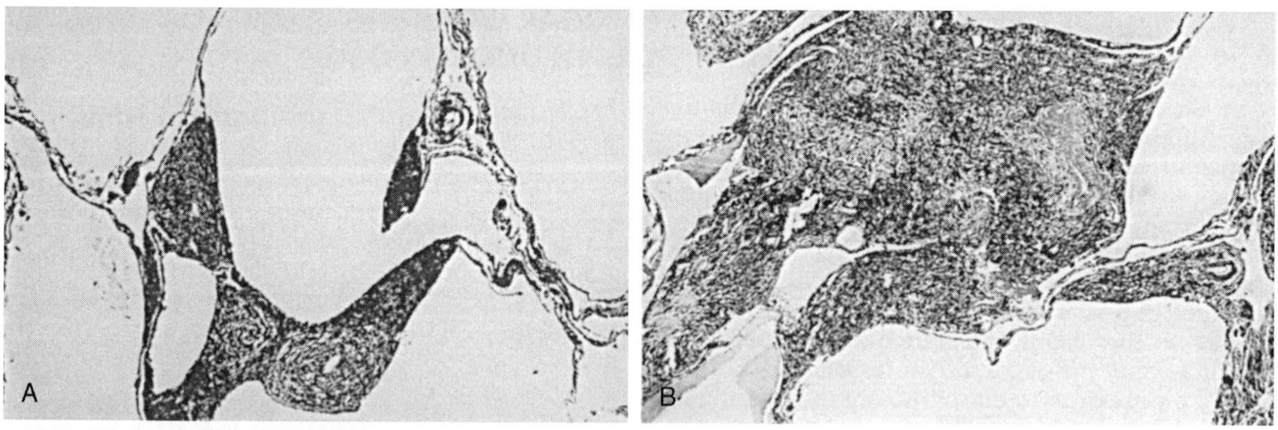


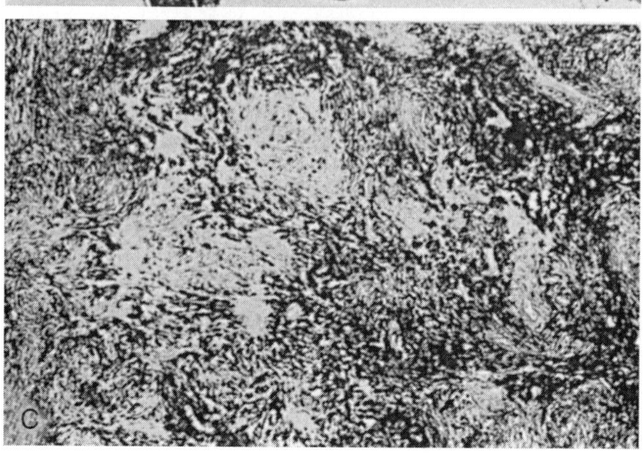


**Figure 65.6** Pathologic lesions of coal workers' pneumoconiosis: examples from South African coal miners. *A,* Dust and dust-laden phagocytes in the wall of a distal airway in which reticulin and collagen fibers were demonstrated. Focal emphysema is associated with the lesion. *B,* Coal macule consisting of dust and dust-laden phagocytes, reticulin, and dense, irregular depositions of collagen. This lesion would be palpable. There also was associated focal emphysema. *C,* Progressive massive fibrosis with coalescence of macules and dense collagen deposition. (Original magnification × 100.) (Courtesy of Dr. B. Goldstein, National Center for Occupational Health, Johannesburg.)

of silicosis). Active areas in the nodules contain dust-laden macrophages, lymphocytes, polymorphonuclear leukocytes, and plasma cells,[5] and when activity ceases, they may collapse or calcify.[5] The surrounding vessels show arteritis or a plasma cell perivascular infiltrate.[129] Rheumatoid pneumoconiosis lesions originally were described in Welsh coal miners and are reported in Belgian coal miners, but are uncommon in North American coal miners.[129]

## Pathogenesis

Coal mine dust contains a variable amount of quartz ranging from negligible to considerable, depending on the nature of ore-bearing rock, the size of the coal seam, the nature of the processes used to mine the seam (including degree of mechanization), and the dust suppression measures used.[4] The effect of coal on the lung also is related to its rank, which is based on its carbon content, with anthracite ranking highest (93%), through bituminous, subbituminous, to the lowest ranked lignite with the least carbon content.[15, 131] In epidemiologic studies, paradoxically, CWP is more common in mines of high-rank coal than in those of low-rank coal. This may relate to the greater relative surface area, higher surface-free radicals, and silica in the high- rather than the low-rank coal.[1, 3, 131, 137]

The coal dust macule and nodule are ascribed to the accumulation of large amounts of relatively inert dust in the lung. As the lung burden of dust increases, alveolar macrophages are activated and reactive oxygen species are released. These in turn trigger the release of cytokines, including interleukins and tumor necrosis factor, which set in motion the processes of inflammation and fibrogenesis that are responsible for the development of pneumoconiosis, and the release of proteases, which contribute to the associated emphysema.[2] The fibrosis, however, is considerably less intense and extensive than that evoked by the more bioactive dusts, such as silica and asbestos.[2, 3, 138] Centriacinar and more generalized forms of emphysema also are associated with coal dust exposure. Indeed one view is that "wherever fibrosis occurs, there is also emphysema"; the lungs of smokers are cited as examples, and the argument made that "there seems to be a common pathway to these two diseases and that coal workers' pneumoconiosis sits halfway between those characterized mainly by fibrosis and those predominantly emphysematous."[115]

Although the exact pathogenetic mechanisms underlying the development of PMF remain in doubt, these lesions are thought to relate to the amount of coal dust accumulated in the lung, the proportion of inhaled silica in the dust and its surface bioactivity, individual immunologic factors, and whether tuberculosis is present.[131, 137] Of these factors, the total dust burden appears to be the most important.[139] In addition, there are striking differences in rates of simple pneumoconiosis and PMF between different coal pits, mining areas, and countries,[135] suggesting that other characteristics of the dust particles, including their shape, size, composition, bioactivity, and durability in lung tissue also make a contribution to the risk of developing PMF.

## Epidemiology and Natural History

Studies in the United States in the 1950s and in the United Kingdom in the 1960s showed that even though the occupation of coal mining was not associated with higher mortality rates than were seen in the general population, mortality rates attributable to respiratory disease, respiratory tuberculosis, and stomach cancer were increased.[2] Nor was it possible to detect an increase in mortality related to simple CWP,[2, 140, 141] although given the "healthy" worker effect, these rates may be underestimates. The post-World War II period saw an improvement in the economic status of coal miners, as well as the recognition of CWP as a distinct disease entity and the introduction of environmental controls and surveillance in the United Kingdom and the United States.[2] At present, the overall life expectancy of coal miners appears to be comparable to that of the general population in many countries, including the United States, the United Kingdom, Germany, and Australia,[2] but not in others including the Netherlands.[140] Furthermore, mortality rates from lung cancer[2, 141] and heart disease[2] appear to be low, the latter perhaps due to competing risks.[2] Studies conducted before the 1980s also established that survival rates for men with PMF were reduced substantially and that this disorder is also associated with increased morbidity, impairment of pulmonary function, and disability.[2]

A comprehensive prospective study of more than 20 pits across the United Kingdom, started in 1959,[115] provided clear evidence of exposure-response relationships for the incidence of CWP, data that have provided the basis for setting environmental standards in the United Kingdom and in the United States.[2, 115] Thus, the main risk factor for CWP was exposure to respirable coal mine dust; risk also increased with coal rank (carbon content) but not with quartz content.[3] Residence time of dust in the lung (reflected in duration at similar exposures) also influenced incidence.[142] There were, however, marked but largely unexplained differences between pits; although explained in part by rank of coal mined, exposure differences that were not reflected in the dust counts used to characterize exposure are also a very reasonable possibility.[142]

The period from the 1950s to the 1980s saw a decline in prevalence rates for CWP in several countries, including the United States, the United Kingdom, and Australia.[1] In the United States, for instance, dust surveillance procedures carried out since 1969 documented a decrease in average dust levels, and rates for simple radiologic CWP (category 1/0 +) fell from between 27% and 40% in 1970 to 1972 to approximately half those levels in 1985 to 1988.[3] However, rates varied considerably between regions (e.g., from 46% in eastern Pennsylvania anthracite miners to <5% in Colorado miners).

Given that PMF is associated with more severe adverse effects on the health and life expectancy of coal miners than simple CWP, an understanding of the factors that enhance attack rates of PMF is of key importance to clinical as well as public health practice. Risk factors include category of CWP, coal rank, and age but not apparently silica content of the dust.[1, 3] For example, in one study in the United Kingdom, the risk of developing

PMF was negligible in active miners with category 2 simple CWP exposed to dust concentrations under 2 mg/m$^3$ but increased to 20% if exposure was 8 mg/m$^3$.[15] In addition, attack rates of PMF also have been shown to be considerably higher in ex-miners compared with current miners, evidence that prevalence studies in current miners underestimate the risk and rates.[137]

Rheumatoid pneumoconiosis (Caplan's syndrome) originally was described as a variant of PMF in coal workers, on the basis of its distinctive radiologic features. Active arthritis or circulating rheumatoid factor were generally found but not always.[1] The association with rheumatoid arthritis has led to the investigation of the immunologic features in coal workers with CWP and PMF, in an attempt to explain the different rates of evolution and progression of these conditions.[143, 144] Rheumatoid factor also has been demonstrated in PMF lesions. At present, most evidence suggests that the presence of rheumatoid arthritis, a rheumatoid diathesis, or both, is a host factor that modifies the response of an individual to coal mine dust exposure. Conversely, dust exposure does not appear to be a risk factor for rheumatoid arthritis.[1]

Although it currently is recognized that silica does not play a primary role in the causation of CWP, coal miners, especially those mining anthracite, may develop the lesions of silicosis. When present, silicosis usually is associated with CWP.[131] Although combined exposure to silica and coal dust may produce less silicosis than would a similar pure exposure to silica, silica exposure is nevertheless thought to contribute to the risk of developing PMF.[15] Interstitial fibrosis recognized by the presence of irregular opacities on the chest roentgenogram also has been reported to occur in association with CWP.[145] Some studies have suggested that interstitial fibrosis occurs more commonly in coal miners than in the general population. These lesions may contain black pigment but are otherwise indistinguishable from usual interstitial fibrosis.[131]

With the generally decreasing rates for CWP in most countries, the focus of interest has shifted to an examination of the relationship of coal mining exposure to chronic bronchitis and emphysema.[1, 2, 146] Earlier studies, cross-sectional in design, were on the whole consistent in demonstrating an association between occupational exposure and tests of airflow limitation[6]; however, the confounding effects of smoking were not uniformly taken into account, and there was reluctance to accept that the association was causal.[147, 148] Part of the reluctance among clinicians to accept that exposure to coal mine dust could cause chronic airflow limitation has no doubt been the practical difficulty in translating this into attributability for compensation purposes in the coal miner who also smokes.[6] However, this was done in a remarkable judgment in a common law action in the United Kingdom in which Mr. Justice Turner concluded that "there was abundant evidence that officials interpreted their duties as requiring the production of coal first and the taking of precautions in respect of health second," that "(1) coal mine dust is a cause of centriacinar emphysema; that (2) said emphysema may, and usually does lead to a loss of $FEV_1$; (3) confirmation that the causes and effects of tobacco smoke are in (1) and (2) above; (4) it is probable . . . there is a common causal pathway to both cigarette and mine dust emphysema which usually gives rise to breathlessness; (5) . . . in a minority of cases [there is] a range of effects from simple impairment, frank disability, and occasionally death; and (6) in the individual smoker, it is not possible to attribute the cause of breathlessness to the one insult or the other."[133]

In the early 1980s, the evidence for causality was strengthened greatly by the publication of two longitudinal studies, one from the United Kingdom[149] and one from the United States,[150] involving approximately 1600 and 1000 men, respectively; both studies showed that mine dust exposure resulted in an $FEV_1$ loss during the follow-up period approximately one third as severe as the effects of smoking, except for the highest exposure levels, for which they were comparable to those of smoking. Subsequent longitudinal and cross-sectional studies have for the most part confirmed the inverse relationship between exposure and $FEV_1$[115, 130, 151, 152] and have shown it to be independent of smoking and of the presence of CWP.[153, 154] The effect may be more marked in younger miners,[153] also may involve gas transfer (reflected in the diffusing capacity), and may be related to exposure during follow-up (as opposed to prior exposure) even at what are considered low levels of exposure.[154] An association between $FEV_1$ decline and mine dust exposure was not demonstrable, however, in a 1990 study in Kentucky miners in whom the exposure variable analyzed was years below ground.[155] By contrast, four other studies based on autopsy material have implicated coal mining exposure in the production of emphysema,[6] which also was shown to be related to the amount of dust accumulated in the lung but not to the presence of CWP.[2, 115, 146] In their comprehensive 1998 review, Coggan and Taylor concluded that (1) the balance of evidence points overwhelmingly to coal mine dust being a cause of impaired lung function; (2) this can be disabling; and (3) the best estimate of the loss of $FEV_1$ in relation to exposure of coal miners, based on the available data, is 0.76 mL/gram hours/m$^3$.[130]

The relationships between hypersecretion of mucus (chronic bronchitis) and chronic airflow limitation (emphysema) on the one hand and the environmental factor of coal mining exposure on the other appear to be similar to those found for cigarette smoking.[146] Both disease processes appear to be related independently to both exposures (coal mining and cigarette smoking) but not necessarily to each other. Whereas the hypersecretion of mucus tends to regress when either environmental exposure ceases, chronic airflow limitation does not. In addition, although exposure-response relationships generally have been shown for chronic airflow limitation with both coal mining and cigarette smoking, not all those exposed to what appear to be comparable levels are affected, pointing to a role for individual susceptibility. The characteristic that makes an individual susceptible may well be the reactivity of his or her airways to an inhaled agent, either cigarettes or pollutants inhaled at work[6] (in Chapters 38 and 64, the natural history of chronic airflow limitation is discussed). In addition, in US coal miners, acute cross-shift changes in ventilatory capacity have been documented,[156] and longitudinal studies have shown that those who exhibit persistent airway hyperresponsiveness to methacholine over a 5-year period also show a greater $FEV_1$ decline compared with those whose airways' hyper-responsiveness reverses over the same time period.[157] This raises the possibility that acute airway reactions to coal mine dust exposure are a determinant of annual $FEV_1$ decline, a widely accepted clinical marker of COPD in population studies[2, 6] and a potentially useful tool in evaluating the impact of environmental controls.[157]

## Clinical Features

Simple coal workers' pneumoconiosis generally is regarded as a disease state without symptoms or physical signs, and diagnosis is based on the chest roentgenogram changes in an individual who has had coal mining exposure.[1–3] There are, however, differences between pits and between geographic areas, and given the findings in a 1990 study in Kentucky suggesting that the FVC may be impaired in simple CWP and account for the symptom of dyspnea,[155] the question needs to be re-examined. The symptoms of cough and sputum reported by most coal miners are likely to be the consequence of dust-induced chronic bronchitis.[2] Most evidence suggests that when it is present, breathlessness on effort is caused by associated chronic airflow limitation or the focal emphysema that is part of the mature coal macule or by the development of PMF.[2] However, even patients with category A PMF (lesions 1 to 5 cm in diameter) may be symptom free. Hemoptysis is not a feature of CWP but occurs not infrequently in chronic bronchitis, whereas coughing of black sputum (melanoptysis) may result from the rupture of a cavitating PMF lesion into an airway but is no longer a common occurrence. Lesions of PMF that impinge on airways may cause abnormal breath sounds.[4] Large or bilateral PMF lesions also may be associated with the signs and symptoms of pulmonary heart disease. The presence of rheumatoid arthritis or subcutaneous rheumatoid nodules raises the possibility of Caplan's syndrome.

## Chest Radiography

The hallmark of simple CWP on the chest roentgenogram is the presence of small rounded opacities in the lung parenchyma.[1, 2, 4] (See the discussion of chest roentgenograms in the introduction to this chapter.) Most commonly observed are type q lesions; types p and r are less common and probably are associated more frequently with focal emphysema. Because the chest roentgenogram has been shown to be insensitive to the presence of macules and micronodules,[158] HRCT may be useful in the early detection of coal nodules. Small rounded opacities usually are seen first in the upper zones and involve the other zones at a later stage; all lung zones are unlikely to be involved unless profusion category 3 is present.[1] Their overall profusion is closely related to the lung dust content at autopsy; the relative contribution of coal dust and other minerals (such as quartz, mica, and kaolin) to the radiographic changes being of the order of 1 to 3.8, corresponding to their radiographic absorption coefficient. Small irregular opacities also occur in a profusion up to 1/0 in association with increasing age and smoking,[159] and in coal workers may relate to coexisting fibrosis and emphysema.[115] Small rounded opacities probably never regress,[142] although the presence of emphysema appears to reduce the reading of profusion on the chest roentgenogram. Progression is difficult to read on roentgenograms taken at intervals of less than 5 years.[2] Some enlargement of hilar nodes is usual, but egg-shell calcification is unusual.[1]

Progressive massive fibrosis is diagnosed radiologically when the parenchymal opacities exceed 1 cm in diameter, a cutoff point that is arbitrary in what is obviously a continuous process, as shown by the pathologic demonstration of PMF without associated radiologic features.[158] Conversely, approximately one third of cases diagnosed as PMF on the roentgenogram have been shown at autopsy to represent other lesions, including tumors, Caplan's nodules, or tuberculosis scars.[158] Progressive massive fibrosis lesions are more common in the upper lobes, situated posteriorly, and are usually well demarcated from the adjacent lung. As PMF becomes more advanced, the lesions are nearly always bilateral. They may take on bizarre shapes; cavitation of such lesions with subsequent closure may occur; dense calcification also may develop.[4] As the lesions shrink to the apex, bullous lesions may be seen in the surrounding lung.[4]

Lesions seen on the chest roentgenogram in Caplan's syndrome are somewhat like those of PMF but display the following features: they are usually multiple and peripherally located and range in diameter from 0.5 to 5.0 cm; they appear within a short time, often weeks; they usually appear on a background of a profusion of small rounded opacities of category 0 or 1, seldom more, in contrast to PMF, in which the background profusion is usually category 1 or 2; the lesions may cavitate, fluid levels may appear, and the cavity may become surrounded by a fine layer of calcification; and in some cases, they disappear, often completely, to be followed at a later date by a fresh crop of lesions.[2] The ILO classification of roentgenograms provides a special notation for lesions thought to be rheumatoid pneumoconiosis. The roentgenographic manifestations of rheumatoid pneumoconiosis usually develop concomitantly with the joint manifestations or after them, but occasionally roentgenographic manifestations may precede joint manifestations by as much as 10 years.[2]

## Lung Function

Most evidence[2, 3] supports the view that simple CWP is a condition with little demonstrable effect on lung function, except in a few susceptible individuals.[130] In part, this may be due to the health selection effect into a dusty job.[6, 39] With profusion category 3 of small rounded opacities and with PMF, deficits of lung function are invariably demonstrable.[152] The lung function deficits in the susceptible individuals with simple CWP include reduction in FVC in the higher categories of profusion; increasing residual volume with increasing profusion category; and occasional abnormalities in indices of gas exchange, for example, dead space to tidal volume ($V_D/V_T$) ratios, in frequency dependence of compliance, in carbon monoxide diffusing capacity ($D_{LCO}$) (particularly in the presence of mixed rounded and irregular opacities), and in decreased elastic recoil.[2] All these abnormalities are usually more frequent and more marked in the presence of PMF, which also is characterized by the development of airflow limitation.[2] Pulmonary hypertension is likely to occur in proportion to the reduction of the vascular bed.[2] In addition, independently of the presence of radiologic CWP, coal miners are at risk for developing exposure-related airflow limitation reflected in reduced $FEV_1$ and $FEV_1$/FVC ratio.[115, 130]

## Diagnosis, Complications, and Management

A history of occupational exposure to coal and a chest roentgenogram are the fundamental elements in the diagnosis of CWP. An HRCT scan of the chest may be used to demonstrate evidence of CWP when the features on the roentgenogram are inconclusive.

Complications include mycobacterial infection, either by *M. tuberculosis* or NTM,[2] although the risk of this complication may be less for coal workers than for those who are at risk for, or have, silicosis.[1] Other complications include Caplan's syndrome, which is associated more commonly with coal mining than with gold mining exposure, and scleroderma, in which the opposite is true.[4] Most evidence suggests that the occupation of coal mining is associated with a decreased risk of lung cancer but an increased risk of stomach cancer.[15, 131, 160]

The principles of management are those summarized in the introduction to this chapter and elaborated in the section on silicosis. Younger subjects with radiologic disease of profusion category 1 or greater should be advised to change their occupation to one in which they are no longer exposed to dust because of their risk of developing PMF. Tuberculin skin testing and chemoprophylaxis for those with CWP that are positive is probably advisable, although no efficacy studies have been published. Surveillance for tuberculosis and its treatment are recommended. The inclusion of rifampin in the initial treatment regimen for tuberculosis in coal workers largely eliminates the less favorable response to treatment caused by the coexistence of CWP and even PMF, and results are almost as favorable as those obtained in cases without these diseases.[161] Management of other dust-related, smoking-related, or dust- and smoking-related diseases, such as chronic bronchitis and emphysema, is less straightforward. Antismoking counseling obviously should given on general principles; although there are no data to show any interaction between smoking and CWP, both coal mining and smoking have the capacity to cause COPD.

# ASBESTOS-RELATED FIBROSIS OF THE LUNGS (ASBESTOSIS) AND PLEURA

## Asbestos Minerals

### History and Uses

Asbestos is an ancient mineral exploited by humans from prehistoric times because of its properties of durability and heat resistance and its fibrous nature, which enabled it to be spun.[1, 3] It was used by the Finns in the fashioning of pottery as early as 2500 B.C.; the Vestal Virgins in Rome used it for the wicks of their oil lamps; and Marco Polo marveled at the fire-resistant cloth made with asbestos by the Chinese he encountered in his Asian travels. Commercial use of asbestos started in the 19th century with open pit mining and grew as mechanization replaced hand cobbing,[1, 2] and growth was exponential between the two world wars. Production peaked at more than 5 million tons per year in 1976 and stabilized at approximately 4 million tons per year in the early 1980s, faltering only in the late 1980s, when the ill health effects of exposure became a matter of increasing public concern.[1] Use in Europe and North America decreased considerably in the 1980s, and the use of substitutes increased proportionately (as of 1999, 25 countries have banned or severely restricted the use of asbestos), while on the African, Asian, and South American continents, asbestos continued to be in demand as a cheap, durable material for use in water reticulation and in housing projects for their rapidly urbanizing populations.

The word *asbestos* (of Greek origin and meaning "*unquenchable*"[3]) is used currently as a collective term for naturally occurring mineral silicates of the serpentine and amphibole group. Despite different origins and physical and chemical properties, these silicates have in common a fibrous habit, that is, they occur naturally in bundles of parallel, radiating, or interlaced fibers that usually can be separated readily.

What is meant by the term *fiber* is of more than pedantic importance, because particle dimensions are determinants, probably important ones, of biologic potency. Thus, to the mineralogist, a fiber is defined as a particle whose length to diameter (called aspect) ratio is equal to or greater than 10:1, whereas the definition used by the Occupational Safety and Health Administration as a basis for standard setting is a particle more than 5 μm in length with an aspect ratio equal to or greater than 3:1. This covers the many needle-like fragments found in the air, where asbestos is being mined, milled, fabricated, or installed commercially.[162, 163]

Table 65.3 lists some of the mineral silicates that have been found in human lung tissue and gives a general (but by no means exhaustive) indication of their commercial uses.[1, 2, 4, 162–165] From the point of view of ill health effects, the most important are the asbestos fibers and the man-made mineral fibers, whose production is increasing commensurate with their growing commercial role as substitutes for asbestos. By contrast, world production of the nonasbestos mineral silicates is approximately 30 million tons per year, almost eightfold greater than that of the asbestos mineral silicates.[163] Note that the presence of fibers in lung tissue does not of itself imply causality in terms of disease, although it often does, as is discussed later. Biologic potency (and disease-producing potential) depends in general on dose delivered to the target organ, fiber dimensions, and durability in the lung tissue. The role of each of these parameters may not be the same for all fibers and all disease entities.[162, 164] Nonfibrous particles greater than 10 μm seldom reach the lung parenchyma, whereas fibers up to 200 μm can be found in the lungs if their diameter is less than 3 μm.[3]

**Table 65.3 MINERAL SILICATES THAT HAVE BEEN FOUND IN HUMAN LUNG TISSUE***

| Mineral: Group and Form | Location of Major Deposits, Commercial or Other | Main Commercial Uses and/or Other Human Exposures |
|---|---|---|
| **Asbestos minerals** | | |
| Serpentine | | |
| Chrysotile† (white asbestos) | Canada (Quebec, British Columbia, Yukon, Newfoundland‡), Russia, China (Szechwan), Brazil, Mediterranean countries (Cyprus, Corsica, Greece, Italy), southern Africa (South Africa, Zimbabwe, Swaziland) | Asbestos cement products (pipes, gutters, tiles, roofing); insulation, fireproofing, reinforced plastics (fan blades, electric switchgear); textiles; friction materials; paper products; filters, spray-on products |
| Amphibole | | |
| Crocidolite (blue asbestos) | South Africa (Northwest Cape‡), western Australia‡ | Used in combination, mostly in cement but also in many of the products listed above |
| Amosite (brown asbestos) | South Africa (northern province, former Transvaal) | |
| Anthophyllite | Finland‡ | Filler in rubber and plastics |
| Tremolite | Contaminates ore in certain asbestos, talc, iron, and vermiculite mines; also found in some agricultural soils | May or may not be removed in processing; has rural domestic uses (e.g., stucco) |
| Cummington-grunerite | Contaminates ore in certain iron mines (often not fibrous) | No commercial use |
| **Nonasbestos mineral silicates** | | |
| Clay minerals (usually fine-grained, powder-like) such as kaolin and montmorillanite (bentonite) | 40 countries, including China, US (Georgia, North Carolina), UK (Cornwall), Czechoslovakia, Germany, Egypt, Japan | Functional filler in paper, plastic, bricks and cement, rubber, paint etc.; fireclays, refractories, ceramics |
| Attapulgite and sepiolite | US (Georgia, Florida), Spain, Australia, South Africa | Oil absorbants; pesticide carriers; pet litter |
| Talcs (usually plate-like but can roll into scrolls) | US (Vermont, Montana, New York, California); Italy, Spain, Norway, China, Japan, Korea, Canada | Ceramics; paper making; cosmetics; pharmaceuticals; animal feed; fertilizer; anticaking; paints; varnishes; plastic reinforcer |
| Micas (usually flaky) | | |
| Muscovite | US (North Carolina, Georgia, and other states); France, Spain, China, India, Italy | Filler in plastics, drill sites, special paints; refractories; semiconductors; insulation; anticorrosion materials; welding rods |
| Vermiculite (expands when heated) | South Africa, US (Montana, Virginia), Australia, Kenya | Absorbant (horticulture); plasters; boards; insulation; fire resistance |
| Wollastonite (occurs as needles or fibers in limestones) | US (California, New York), Japan, former USSR, Finland, Mexico, Australia | Filler/flux in ceramic industry; used in latex and oil-based paint; in welding fluxes; asbestos substitute in hardboard, insulation, and brake linings |
| Zeolite (fibrous), e.g., erionite§ | Turkey (Cappadocia and Anatolia regions): noncommercial deposits | Houses constructed in erionite rock; soil containing fibers mixed with tremolite; sepiolite used in stucco and plaster |
| Other (mainly nonfibrous) | Worldwide (in filling of lava cavities); mined in 16 countries, including several in Europe, in the US, and in Japan | Pollutant and radioactive waste control; also used in catalysts, adsorbants, conditioners |
| **Man-made mineral fibers** | | |
| Glasswool and filament, rock wool, slagwool, ceramic fiber | Production in more than 100 factories around the world | Many uses previously reserved for asbestos: glass filament used in mats, lamination, yarns; glass-rock and slagwool used as insulation in buildings and in car and naval construction; ceramic fiber used in reinforced cloth, discs, brakes, gaskets, board, and paper; high-performance ceramic fiber used in jet engines, spacecraft |

*Abstracted from published information[1-5, 162-165], the list is not exhaustive, and the reader should consult the references for further information. Asbestos minerals invariably exhibit the fibrous habit; nonasbestos mineral silicates also may do so. Most silicate deposits are mineralogically heterogeneous, as are most of the commercial forms of the minerals.[163]

†Accounts for more than 90% of the world's commercial production; other fibers usually are used in combination with chrysotile.

‡Mining no longer in operation.

§One of three epidemics of mesothelioma in Turkish villages implicated erionite; in the other two, tremolite and/or chrysotile were implicated.[165] As of 1999, 25 countries have banned or severely restricted the use of asbestos. Source: The Asbestos Institute, 1200 McGill College Ave, Suite 1640, Montreal, Quebec, Canada H3B4G7.

## Sources of Human Exposure

Given its many uses, the potential sources for human exposure to asbestos are legion even today. Such sources are summarized elsewhere,[1–3, 162–165] and the list given in Table 65.3 should be regarded as a short guide for use in office practice. The discussion that follows deals mainly with exposure to asbestos fibers; the principles, however, apply equally to exposure to other fibers.

In industrialized countries, and increasingly in industrializing countries, human exposure is most likely to be *occupational* and may occur in mining, milling, transporting, manufacturing, and applying or using raw fiber or manufactured products.[164] In World War II, a major source of exposure was in the ship building, repair, or refitting industries; in the post–World War II period, major sources of exposure have been and continue to be in the construction and transport industries.[2] Sources of asbestos-containing materials in post–World War II buildings include boards, panels, surfacing, insulation, tile and floor covering, roofing, and caulking.[3] Exposure also occurs in maintenance operations or demolition of plants and buildings in which asbestos-containing materials have been used.[3, 164] Other sources of human exposure are the removal of asbestos lagging or insulation from ships or buildings and the disposal of industrial waste, such as the dumps of defunct asbestos plants.[2, 164] In most industrialized countries, these sources of exposure have diminished in response to heightened public awareness and control regulations.[2, 162–164]

*Indirect occupational exposure*, also called *bystander exposure*, describes the exposure of those men whose trades require them to work in the vicinity of others who work with asbestos or asbestos-containing materials. Exposure occurred in the ship building, repair, and refitting industries, especially in World War II, and the construction industry, especially in the boom years that followed World War II.[164] This includes insulators and laggers who mix asbestos on site, often in closed spaces, carpenters, plumbers, welders, boiler makers, scrap metal workers, and electricians, all of whom are or were at risk for fiber exposure.[164]

*Domestic exposure* occurred primarily as a consequence of fiber-laden work clothes being laundered at home. The dust they shed settles in the furnishings, carpets, upholstered sofas, and drapes and is resuspended in the air by human activity, in particular house cleaning. Domestic exposure still accounts for a proportion, probably small, of cases of asbestos-related disease, pleural and to a lesser extent parenchymal, and is reported to have accounted for up to 15% of malignant mesothelioma in some series.[162] Given the long incubation period of this tumor (from 20 to 40 years), domestic exposure is likely to be the source of cases presenting well into the 21st century.[1, 3, 164–167]

*Environmental and residential exposure* occurs as a consequence of living in the neighborhood of asbestos mines or mills or plants that use the material and contaminate the environment.[1, 3, 168] This source of exposure was first dramatically brought to medical attention in 1960 in a report of a cluster of 31 cases of malignant mesothelioma among residents as well as crocidolite asbestos miners of the Northwest Cape, South Africa (cases continue to be reported from this area).[1, 2, 166] Environmental exposures from nonindustrial sources also have been documented among residents of rural areas in Eastern Europe, where the soil is contaminated with various fibers.[165] In addition, epidemics of asbestos-related pleural disease, nonmalignant as well as malignant, have occurred among residents of Turkish villages whose homes were constructed in erionite tuff rock or who used erionite and tremolite in stucco and plaster.[2, 164, 165] By contrast, a cohort study comparing the mortality experience of more than 4500 women living in the vicinity of the Quebec chrysotile mines with that of 1.375 million women from 60 reference areas in the province comprising towns of similar size revealed no excess of lung or digestive system cancer; there were, however, seven deaths from mesothelioma.[168]

A major concern since the 1980s has been the potential risk of exposure to occupants of public (including schools), commercial, and residential buildings constructed during the post-World War II period, when many asbestos-containing materials were used in construction.[3, 169] Exposure in buildings is less by an order of magnitude than that encountered in the workplace except for custodians and others responsible for building maintenance (see previous discussion). Public concern in the United States was reflected in directives by the Environmental Protection Agency (EPA) to schools and a health review mandated by the US Congress,[169] which provided estimates of lifetime cancer risk (see Asbestosis, Asbestos Exposure, Lung Cancer, and Mesothelioma).

## The Fate of Inhaled Fibers

Accumulation of fibers in the lung is the outcome of exposure, deposition, clearance, and retention, all processes that depend on fiber dimensions; level, intensity, and profile of exposure are also important.[162, 170, 171] Fiber retention is related to their impaction and accumulation at the bifurcations of small airway junctions and alveolar ducts. Peaks of early and late clearance occur, with preferential clearance of short compared with long fibers, and in the short term of chrysotile compared with amphibole fibers.[172] Retention of fibers is patchy, with greater fiber burden being found in the lung regions with shorter pathways and greater accumulations of longer fibers in lungs that are the site of asbestosis than in lungs in which only airway lesions have developed.[172] Within hours of deposition, these fiber accumulations evoke a macrophagic reaction in the small airways, associated alveoli, and interstitium.[172] Fibers equal to or less than 3 μm are phagocytosed by activated macrophages, then translocated to lymphatic channels, and eventually drained to the pleural space, whereas longer fibers are phagocytosed incompletely, often by more than one macrophage, and become the core of what were called *asbestos bodies* originally because they were seen in association with asbestos exposure.[3] However, although most coated fibers in human lungs have been shown to contain asbestos (usually amphibole) when subject to radiographic diffraction analysis,[5, 11, 14] the term *ferruginous bodies* also has been suggested to underline the fact that other mineral fibers also may undergo coating in human lungs.[172] As yet unexplained are how fibers transmigrate to the parietal pleura to produce pleural plaques.[173]

In the lungs of exposed individuals, the number of uncoated, or bare, fibers (for practical purposes only visible on electron microscopy), exceeds the number of coated fibers (asbestos bodies), visible by light microscopy, by anything from 5- to 10,000-fold.[5, 174] For many years, the coated asbestos fiber *asbestos body* has been considered the hallmark of exposure, past or current, no doubt because of its distinctive structure and because it was readily visible under the light microscope.[2, 172] The presence of more than one coated fiber has been cited (and challenged) as a necessary criterion for the pathologic diagnosis of asbestosis even in a subject with an appropriate exposure history.[174] Asbestos bodies may be found in sputum or in BAL fluid when lung tissue levels are very high. Asbestos bodies in sputum or BAL are found more commonly when dust exposure is recent and with amphibole, rather than chrysotile, exposure.[5, 175, 176]

### Exposure vs. Dose-Response Relationships

Epidemiologic studies consistently have demonstrated exposure-response relationships for asbestos-related parenchymal lung fibrosis (Fig. 65.7).[14, 170] There are differences in the slope of the exposure-response relationships between industrial sectors, probably related to fiber size (mining < various industrial processes), and within industrial processes, probably related to fiber type and between fiber differences in biopersistance (chrysotile < amphiboles such as amosite, crocidolite, and possibly tremolite). For asbestos-related pleural disease also, exposure-response relationships also usually have been demonstrable, although often less clearly so and usually for exposure measurements that reflect residence time of the dust in the lungs rather than cumulative exposure.[171, 173] Direct measurements of lung dust burden have confirmed that urban dwellers carry a substantial fiber burden in their lungs, and that this burden is greater in residents of mining towns.[176] Mineralogic analysis also has shown fibrosis grade to be correlated generally with fiber concentration, both in chrysotile and amosite exposed workers. The toxicity of mineral fibers is thought to be determined by their physical and aerodynamic properties, which determine deposition and retention. The length of fibers is relevant: longer fibers are more toxic than short fibers, but the short fibers may be more important in the pathogenesis of fibrosis than was previously thought.[5] Also relevant in fibrogenesis and probably carcinogenesis is the solubility of the fibers, which determines their survival in lung tissue, and their surface properties and electrical charge, which may affect their toxicity for cell membranes and the formation of free radicals.[2, 3, 79]

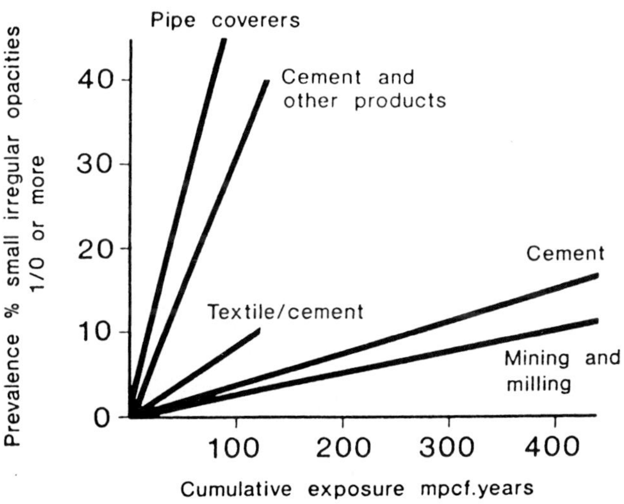


**Figure 65.7** The figure shows the prevalence (%) of small irregular radiographic opacities (1/0 or more) in relation to cumulative exposure in millions of particles per cubic foot × years (mpcf. years) in different work forces exposed to asbestos. Idealized exposure-response relationships are shown for various sectors of the asbestos industry, including mining and milling, cement, and textile production (studies carried out in Quebec), and for cement and other products and pipe covering (studies carried out in the United States). Further details are given elsewhere.[170] (From Becklake MR: Occupational lung disease: Past record and future trend using the asbestos case as an example. Clin Invest Med 6:305–317, 1983.)

## Asbestosis (Pulmonary Parenchymal Fibrosis)

### Pathology and Pathogenesis

Asbestosis tends to be prominent in the lower lobes and in the subpleural areas. When disease is advanced, the lungs are small, streaks of fibrosis outline lobar and interlobar septa, and the visceral pleura invariably is thickened. Honeycombing may be prominent subpleurally and in the lower lobes. Unlike silicosis, the tracheobronchial lymph nodes do not show characteristic changes, and progressive massive fibrosis is unusual.[174] The advanced case of asbestos-related fibrosis is not distinguishable from advanced fibrosis due to any other cause (Fig. 65.8*A* and *B*), except by the presence of asbestos bodies or uncoated asbestos fibers.[5] At the other end of the disease spectrum, the lesions of mild asbestosis may occur only at scattered sites (again, preferentially in the lower lobes and subpleural areas), and they usually consist of foci of peribronchiolar fibrosis,[71] some chronic interstitial inflammation, accumulation of macrophages in the air spaces, and proliferation of type II pneumocytes with foci of fibrosis in the walls, usually of first-order respiratory bronchioles.[174] Second- and third-order bronchioles and alveolar ducts tend to be involved as the disease progresses and the fibrosis spreads to involve the alveolar interstitium (see Fig. 65.8*B*).

In general, the grade of pulmonary fibrosis relates to the fiber burden carried by the lungs.[5] On the basis of animal and human data,[2, 3, 79, 177] the sequence of events leading to asbestosis is thought to commence with an alveolitis that, if the fiber burden is low and cleared, may resolve. If the fiber load is low but retained, a nonprogressive distal airway lesion, mineral dust-induced peripheral airway disease, may develop.[71, 172] If the dust

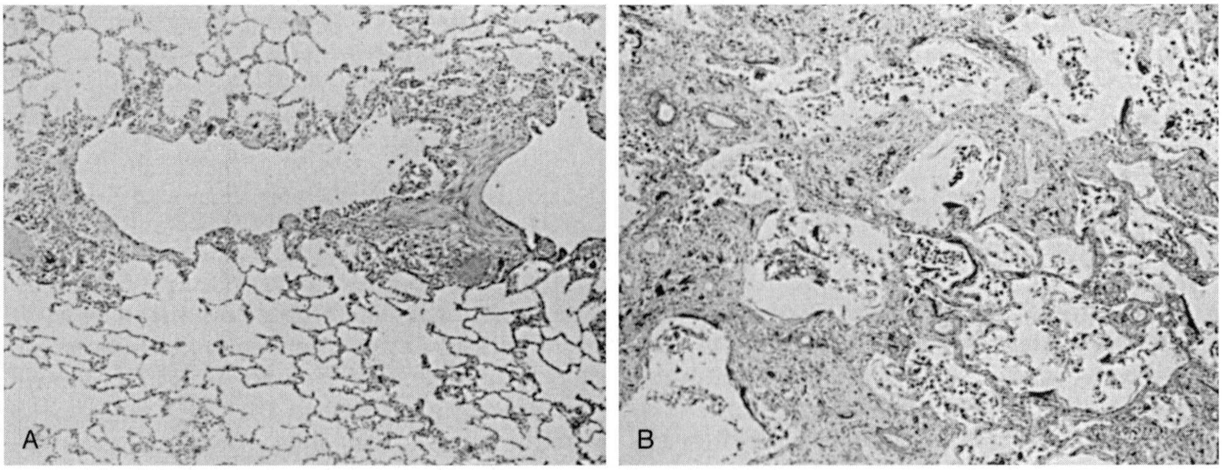


**Figure 65.8** Pathologic features of asbestosis: examples from South African asbestos workers. *A,* Dust-laden phagocytes in the lumen and wall of a terminal bronchiole with commencing fibrosis. Giant cells, fibers, and asbestos bodies also are seen in the lesion. The architecture of the surrounding lung parenchyma is preserved. *B,* Diffuse interstitial fibrosis with destruction of the lung architecture and honeycombing; dust-laden phagocytes, fibers, and asbestos bodies are seen in the air spaces and interstitial tissue. (Original magnification × 100, light microscopy.) (Courtesy of Dr. B. Goldstein, National Center for Occupational Health, Johannesburg.)

load retained is high, and phagocytosis of fibers by alveolar and interstitial macrophages is incomplete, fibronectin is released with other proinflammatory and cytotoxic agents such as free oxygen radicals. These interact with and recruit fibroblasts to the site of the injury, where they proliferate and lay down collagen. If sustained, this leads to irreversible damage, loss of alveolar spaces, and the development of chronic interstitial lung fibrosis—in other words, asbestosis.[172]

## Epidemiology and Natural History

Clinical asbestosis, like clinical silicosis, appears to be becoming less frequent and less severe as exposure levels in workplaces around the world are increasingly meeting currently recommended control levels.[32, 178] Other encouraging evidence includes the static or falling rates of certification of disability for asbestosis (e.g., in the United Kingdom and Canada),[179–181] and the static (in the United States)[135] and decreasing (in the United Kingdom)[179] frequency with which asbestosis is mentioned on the death certificate. When low-level exposure to asbestos has occurred, latency is increased, as seen for instance in indirect occupational (bystander) exposure in both the shipbuilding and ship repair industries and in the transport and building industries.[170] The pattern of exposure also determines the nature of the disease. In occupations in which exposure is intermittent but of high intensity, the ratio of pleural to parenchymal radiologic abnormality may exceed 20 whereas a 2:1 pleural to parenchymal ratio is more usual in occupations in which workers are more consistently exposed.[29, 170, 171] Exposure at a young age is an independent determinant of both attack and progression rates of parenchymal and pleural radiologic abnormality, suggesting that residence time of dust in the lung is important in their pathogenesis.[29, 170, 182] Other determinants of progression are level and duration of exposure, cumulative exposure, fiber type (more frequent if there has been exposure to amphiboles-crocidolite or amosite, or mixtures of amphibole and chrysotile than to chrysotile alone) (see Fig. 65.8), and, in some studies, initial radiologic status.[170, 183] Once established, radiologic asbestosis may remain static or it may progress; rarely has regression been recorded.[29] Radiologic asbestosis also may appear and progress long after exposure ceases; in one study of chrysotile miners and millers in Quebec, "attack" and progression rates of 31% and 9%, respectively, were recorded for pleuroparenchymal disease over an average follow-up period of 17 years since last exposure.[170] Progression in the absence of further exposure relates to cumulative exposure up to the time of quitting and is also considerably more common in individuals with already detectable parenchymal radiologic abnormalities.[170, 182] There is no evidence that human leukocyte antigen (HLA) phenotype influences risk.[4, 170]

Smoking deserves comment because of its role as a universal risk factor for respiratory disease, both malignant and nonmalignant. Thus, the long-term inhalation of cigarette smoke in individuals with no asbestos exposure is associated with bronchiolitis and peribronchiolar fibrosis, and there is some evidence that at least the milder grades of radiologic small irregular opacities (read into the ILO classification) may be caused by smoking.[159] Pathologic studies do not show evidence of an association between asbestosis grade and smoking,[184] although there is evidence to suggest that smoking enhances the retention of fibers in the lungs.[5, 184]

## Clinical Features

Asbestosis has been called a monosymptomatic disease because the earliest, most consistently reported, and most distressing symptom is dyspnea.[164] It occurs first on heavy effort, then at progressively diminishing levels of effort as the disease progresses. Dyspnea often precedes other evidence of disease and therefore may be underrated by the physician because of its subjective nature. However, the consistency of its relationship to exposure levels[170] (and by implication, to early parenchymal asbestosis) in studies of exposed work forces is good reason to take it seriously in any exposed individual. Persistent cough and sputum also are reported commonly, almost as frequently as dyspnea in some series.[173, 185] The cough is, however, usually dry, often occurs with distressing spasms, and has been attributed to the stimulation of lung receptors. A productive cough is usually associated with smoking. Chest tightness or pain, or both, is not uncommon and may be caused by acute asbestos-associated pleural reactions.

Basal crackles, an early and distinctive feature of asbestosis, are fine crisp sounds, often heard first over axillary and basal regions, and then more generally as the disease advances.[1, 4] They are thought to be due to explosive opening of airways to lung regions that close on expiration. Features of note are their persistence (they usually are unaffected by coughing), their timing (at first, at mid to late inspiration, and eventually during most of inspiration), and their high-pitched quality.[186] Other sounds, including coarse crackles and rhonchi, reflect airway disease that may be related to cigarette smoking or to dust in the occupational environment.[6] Clubbing of the fingers and occasionally the toes develops in some subjects. Late manifestations include respiratory and circulatory failure and these, with cancer, are common causes of death.[185]

## Radiographic Features

The posteroanterior chest radiograph remains a key tool in the initial clinical diagnosis of asbestosis, and in the health surveillance of exposed workers. The 1980 ILO classification uses the term "small irregular opacities" to describe the irregular linear shadows that develop in the lung parenchyma and obscure the normal bronchovascular arborization pattern seen in disease-free lungs.[2, 164] The parenchymal opacities usually are seen first in the lower lateral zones between the rib shadows (see the discussion of the chest roentgenogram in the introduction to this chapter). As their profusion increases, the borders of the heart are obscured. Small rounded opacities are unusual when the exposure has been primarily to fibers but are more likely to be seen in workers who also have had silica exposure: for instance, asbestos cement workers.[1–3]

Early fibrotic changes are better visualized by HRCT, particularly for subpleural parenchymal changes that may be obscured by overlying pleural fibrosis on the chest roentgenogram.[17] Visceral pleural involvement, including thickening of the interlobar fissures, is common.[173] Changes in the parietal pleura (discussed subsequently) are also common, and the presence of pleural plaques (particularly if they are bilateral) or of pleural thickening provides useful evidence that the parenchymal disease is asbestos related. Hilar node enlargement is not a feature of asbestosis, and PMF lesions, including rheumatoid pneumoconiosis, are less common than in workers exposed to coal or silica. The radiologic features of well-developed disease seldom present a diagnostic problem; interpretation of the less marked changes is much more subjective and the use of ILO films and of HRCT proportionately more valuable.[17, 187] The CT scan is also useful in characterizing localized pleuropulmonary lesions, including rounded atelectasis, which must be distinguished from lung cancer because it presents as a solid localized lesion (discussed later in this chapter).

## Lung Function

Established asbestosis is often but certainly not always associated with a restrictive lung function profile (Chapter 28).[170] With less advanced radiologic disease, FVC and the diffusing capacity usually are reduced, whereas reduction in flow at low lung volumes (MMEF) is a common finding in keeping with small airway abnormality.[71, 138, 172, 173] In studies of exposed populations, a substantial proportion of subjects (up to half in some series)[29] exhibit a mixed or obstructive function profile, in keeping with the parallel development of airway and parenchymal effects of working in dusty occupations contaminated by mineral dusts.[146] When repeated lung function tests are used to assess evolution of disease, simple volume measurements such as FVC appear to be the most useful.[14, 29, 188]

## Diagnosis and Complications

Criteria for diagnosis depend on the purpose for which a diagnosis is required. Clinical diagnosis depends on establishing the presence, extent, and nature of pulmonary fibrosis (see previous discussion) and whether there has been exposure of a duration and intensity sufficient to put the individual at risk for developing asbestosis.[189] The fewer the features, the less certain the diagnosis; the more trivial the exposure, the less likely that it is causal. When radiologic or lung function changes are marginal, CT or HRCT often reveal the presence of parenchymal abnormality and associated pleural thickening or plaques. In the absence of what appears to be an adequate exposure history, it rarely may be appropriate to perform a biopsy of the lung to establish the nature of the disease and establish the presence and burden of asbestos in the lung (see the previous discussion of fibers in the section on asbestos minerals). BAL also may be useful because the finding of asbestos bodies in BAL is considered to reflect a substantial lung burden on asbestos.[190] However, the presence of asbestos bodies in BAL establishes the exposure, not the disease.[191–193]

Diagnosis of asbestosis for the purpose of legal attributability calls for greater certainty and the use of criteria that vary according to the legal administrative system involved.[2–4] Most published criteria consider histopathology as the best means of establishing the diagnosis.[3, 172] In its absence, the following criteria are proposed: (1) a reliable history of asbestos exposure; (2) an appropriate lag time between exposure and detection; (3) evidence of lung fibrosis on the chest radiograph or HRCT scan; (4) a restrictive pattern of lung function; (5) bilateral fixed inspiratory crackles; and (6) clubbing of the fingers or toes, or both. Of these, history or exposure and evidence (radiographic or HRCT) are considered essential and the others confirmatory.[172]

The individual with asbestosis is at increased risk for cancer of the lung[194, 195] and, by virtue of asbestos exposure, is also at risk for mesothelioma. Working in a dusty occupation (as is the case for most workplaces contaminated by asbestos dust) also puts the worker at risk for developing COPD.[2, 146] Tuberculosis and rheumatoid pneumoconiosis are not common complications of asbestosis.[196]

## Asbestosis, Asbestos Exposure, Lung Cancer, and Mesothelioma

The observation made in the 1930s that lung cancer occurred more frequently in association with asbestosis than with several other types of pneumoconiosis[164] was responsible for first directing attention to the potential of asbestos exposure for carcinogenesis. At first, cancers seen in association with asbestosis were assumed to be scar cancers, analogous to those seen in diffuse interstitial fibrosis from other causes.[195] Consistent with this theory was their location (more common in the lower lobes, where asbestos-related fibrosis tends to be more severe), their often multicentric origin, and possibly their cell type (a preponderance of adenocarcinoma).[4, 174] Subsequently, mortality studies of exposed work forces confirmed the excess lung cancer risk and showed it to be related to the intensity and duration of exposure[5, 14] and to decrease after exposure ceases, thus providing evidence for causality. Autopsy analyses of lung fiber burden in those dying from asbestosis vs. lung cancer were 30 vs. 13 million fibers per gram dry lung.[184]

In 1977, the IARC classified asbestos as a human carcinogen, the target sites being lung, larynx, and pleura.[1, 194] A comment was included in the report to the effect that "as to a relationship between asbestosis and bronchial cancer, there is at present no scientific documentation indicating that these entities are interrelated in any way other than they constitute disease outcomes that may be associated causally with exposure to asbestos as a common environmental factor."[194] In 1982, the IARC classified asbestos as "causally associated with cancer in humans" but did not revisit the issue of asbestosis, asbestos exposure, and lung cancer.[197] Since that date, a considerable body of evidence has accumulated in support of the view that asbestos exposure in the absence of asbestosis is a cause of lung cancer,[198–213] and in 1996, an IARC report on Mechanisms of Fiber Carcinogenesis outlined five possible mechanisms without favoring any one above another.[198] This view is in line with experimental studies (cellular and molecular) suggesting that asbestos may have multiple roles in the pathogenesis of malignancy, a question that touches on the whole issue of the interrelationship of inflammation, fibrogenesis, and carcinogenesis; for instance, profibrotic mediators also may lead to carcinogenicity.[3, 79] Most current opinion supports the conclusions reached in one review[205] that lung cancers can occur in the absence of radiologic asbestosis, although there are dissenting views.[209]

The lung cancer risk is enhanced by cigarette smoking (probably multiplicative rather than additive) but is also demonstrable in nonsmokers.[169, 198] A recent analysis estimated the attributable proportion due to synergy to be as high as one third.[198a] Other factors influencing the risk of lung cancer in exposed work forces include industry (risk greater in the textile vs. the asbestos cement industry), fiber type (risk greater when exposure is to amphibole-crocidolite, amosite or tremolite- or mixed amphibole-chrysotile than when it is only to chrysotile),[195, 209] and fiber dimensions (longer fibers are more carcinogenic than shorter fibers).[172, 195, 199]

The emergence of cancer as an important cause of death in asbestos-exposed individuals can be attributed to workplace controls, introduced in the 1970s and implemented over the latter half of the 20th century, resulting in a decrease in the competing risk from asbestosis, and greater chance of survival into the cancer age group.[164] Lung dust burden studies in workers coming to autopsy with different asbestos-related diseases have confirmed that the dust burden associated with asbestosis is on average several-fold greater than that associated with asbestos-related lung cancer.[5, 213, 213a] For instance, in chrysotile miners in Quebec, the fiber concentrations in those dying of asbestosis vs. those dying of lung cancer vs. nonexposed were 30 vs. 13 vs. 2 million chrysotile fibers per gram dry lung tissue; for those engaged in trades with asbestos exposure in the Pacific Northwest, where amosite was the dominant fiber, the equivalent figures were 10.0 vs. 1.0 vs. 0.7 million fibers per gram of dry lung tissue.[213] In addition, all histologic cell types of lung cancer have been shown to be associated with asbestos exposure, further supporting the direct role of asbestos as a carcinogen. Much,[200, 201] although not all,[195, 203] the evidence from observational studies supports this view,[2, 5] as do the results of several studies specifically designed to test the hypothesis.[202, 204] Several reviews or workshops have reached similar conclusions.[202, 205, 205a]

In addition to its biological importance, the question is also of practical interest in terms of legal attributability, and this varies between jurisdictions. There is obviously a much stronger case for attributing lung cancer in a particular individual to asbestos exposure in the presence of asbestosis and in the absence of a smoking history than in the absence of asbestosis and in the presence of a smoking history. Given the methodologic variation in asbestos fiber and body counting, all available information about exposure should be assembled in such evaluations[207]; in other words, the presence of asbestosis should not be used as the only indicator of important occupational exposure.

Of great concern to the public is the risk of cancer from schooling or working in a building constructed with asbestos-containing materials. The lifetime risk for premature cancer death from exposure at school from age 5 to 18 years has been estimated at 6 per million exposed, and for working in an office building with asbestos-containing material, at 4 per million exposed, compared with a risk of 2000 per million for 20 years employed in a workplace conforming to 0.1 fiber/mL, that is, in compliance with the current permissible exposure limit proposed by the Occupational Safety and Health Administration.[3, 169] However, although malignant mesothelioma has been reported in 16 teachers from different parts of the United States, 12 of whom had no identified exposure outside of school employment,[2] other population studies have failed to show an increase in the incidence of mesothelioma in relation to the use of asbestos in buildings.[169] Residential exposure has, however, been implicated in mesothelioma production.[168]

## Pleural Plaques

### Pathology and Pathogenesis

Pleural plaques are distinctive, smooth, white, raised, irregular lesions usually found on the parietal and rarely on the visceral pleura. They may vary from small to extensive (up to 50 cm$^2$) and are usually nonadherent. Common sites are the lateral and posterior midzones, where they may follow the rib contour and the diaphragm, less often the mediastinum and pericardium, and rarely if ever the apices and costophrenic sulci.[4, 164, 173] On microscopic section, pleural plaques consist of avascular, acellular, laminated collagen fibers arranged parallel to the surface or in whorls, with hyaline changes and occasional fibroblasts. Macroscopic calcification is common, and microscopic calcification extremely common, especially in the parietal lesions.[164] The lesions usually are covered by mesothelium. Fine asbestos fibers are seen on electron microscopy.[173] The lungs of patients from the general population who have plaques have been shown to contain a 50- to 250-fold excess of long, thin, mainly amphibole fibers.[5] In asbestos miners and millers in Quebec, and in those engaged in the Pacific Northwest trades that involve exposure to asbestos, the lung burden is similar to that seen in association with lung cancer (see previous discussion).[213]

Pleural plaques are thought to develop as a result of the release of fibers into the pleural space by mechanisms open to conjecture.[5] Release or escape probably occurs from subpleural accumulations of fibers, usually the short fine ones, which are able to penetrate the deeper lung spaces and are cleared via subpleural lymphatic channels.[5] Within the pleural space, macrophage and cellular interactions may be pivotal to fiber localization and plaque formation, which occur quite rapidly; in the absence of macrophages, the pleural reaction tends to be disorganized and widespread.[210] The parietal location may be due to the fact that for fibers, as for macrophages, the only exit from the pleural space is via stomas that communicate directly with the parietal pleural lymphatic channels, in contrast to pleural fluid, which is absorbed by the visceral pleura after its formation in the parietal pleura. Pleural fibrosis and pleural plaques may have the same pathogenesis.[5]

### Clinical Features

Pleural plaques, in the absence of parenchymal disease, may or may not cause signs and symptoms and often are detected as an incidental finding on a routine chest roentgenogram. Their visualization depends on their thickness and the orientation of the x-ray beam. Only a modest proportion of those seen at autopsy are detected on posteroanterior chest roentgenograms; oblique views increase the yield. CT and HRCT scans can identify plaques at an earlier, less well-developed stage, can differentiate plaques from extra pleural fat pads, and can characterize early fibrotic change[3] in the underlying lung parenchyma (up to 50% in some series).[4] In epidemiologic studies, lung volumes (mainly VC and FVC) are on average modestly but consistently reduced, and the diffusion constant K is increased by the presence of pleural plaques, after associated parenchymal fibrosis has been taken into account.[29, 173, 188]

### Epidemiology

Pleural plaques are currently the most frequent[4, 173] and often the only manifestation of asbestos exposure,[4, 173, 179, 180] and asbestos exposure is the commonest cause of pleural plaques.[3] Bilateral pleural plaques are more likely to be associated with occupational exposure than unilateral plaques, for which other causes should be considered. Age and residence time of dust in the lungs are determinants of these unusual pleural lesions[173]; smoking is a determinant in some[1] but not most studies.[173] Domestic and residential exposures have been implicated in the production of pleural plaques (see the discussion of human exposure in the section on asbestos minerals), with remarkably high rates for pleural calcification (up to 30%) being described in some rural communities in the eastern Mediterranean countries of Corsica, Greece, Cyprus, and Turkey.[164, 165] Of greater concern to the patient and the clinician is the prognostic significance of plaques: in one study, they were associated with alveolitis, as reflected in bronchoalveolar cell counts[210] and by implication with an increased likelihood of developing parenchymal disease. The results of a Swedish cohort mortality study involving 1596 men were interpreted as showing that pleural plaques on the chest radiograph indicated significant exposure to asbestos, as well an increased risk of mesothelioma and possibly also for lung cancer.[211]

## Pleural Fibrosis and Visceroparietal Reactions

### Pathology

Like pleural plaques, pleural fibrosis and visceroparietal pleural reactions may be localized or diffuse, may vary in thickness from a milky discoloration of the lung surface to a thick, white peel encasing much of one or both lungs, commonly may involve the interlobar fissures, and may occur, and be quite severe, in the presence of minimal parenchymal reaction.[173, 174] Occasionally, a localized pleural reaction may fold on itself and the surfaces synthesize, trapping the underlying lung and leading to a well-defined pleuroparenchymal lesion or pseudo tumor, also called *rounded atelectasis*[173] (Fig. 65.9*A* to *C*). Asbestos bodies and fibers usually are found in the visceral pleura, the underlying parenchyma, or both,[173] and the lung dust burden usually reflects the occupational exposure, with total electron microscopic fiber counts considerably less than those seen in asbestosis, but comparable

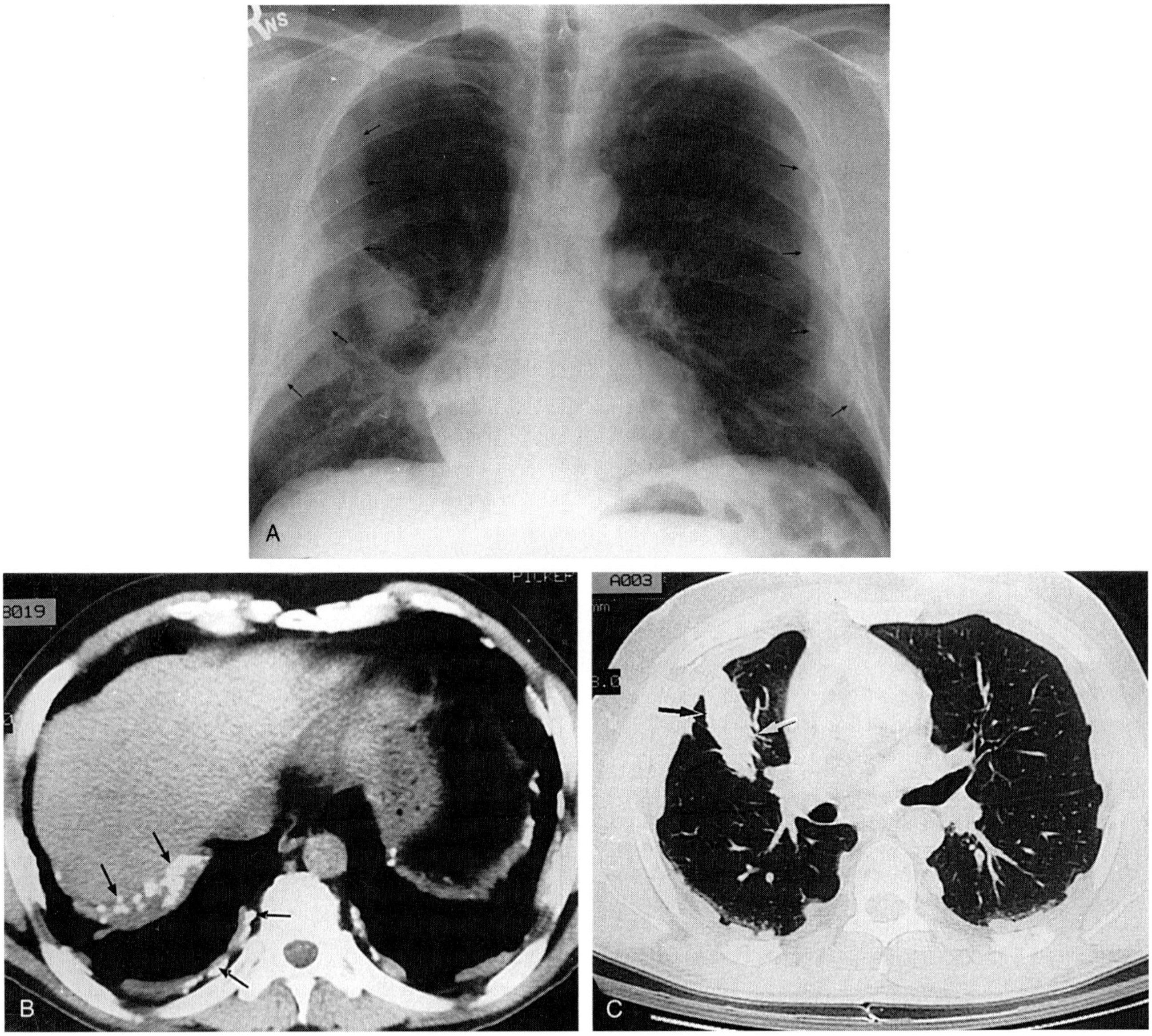


**Figure 65.9** Asbestos-related pulmonary parenchymal and pleural disease (bilateral pleural fibrosis and rounded atalectasis) in a 50-year-old man. The patient had worked as an electrician since the age of 17 years, first in construction for 10 years (with known exposure to asbestos), then briefly on naval ships during World War II, and in a chemical plant (with known exposure to talc) for the past 20 years. His exercise tolerance was excellent and his only complaint was a dry cough. Chest roentgenographic abnormalities had been noted 4 years previously. *A,* The posterior-anterior chest roentgenogram showed bilateral diaphragmatic plaques, extensive bilateral pleural thickening (category c3 using the ILO reference radiographs), and a circumscribed lesion in the right midzone that had increased in size over the past year. *B,* On the CT scan, the pleural plaques *(arrows)* were shown to be much more extensive than appeared from the posterior-anterior chest roentgenogram. *C,* Many plaques *(arrows)* were calcified. In addition, HRCT at multiple levels revealed bands of subpleural fibrosis related to the pleural plaques or thickening, or both. Lung volumes and $D_{L_{CO}}$ were greater than 100% and 98% of predicted values, respectively. Because the circumscribed lesion had enlarged over the past year, it was removed surgically. The lesion, which was nonmalignant and pleural based, consisted of pleural, subpleural, and interstitial fibrosis. Analysis of lung digest revealed the following: 36,000 asbestos bodies/g dry lung tissue, and 7570 fibers/mg dry lung tissue, more than half of which were asbestos fibers and less than 1% were talc. These findings implicated his earlier rather than his more recent occupational exposures as the cause of his pleural disease. (Dr. J. Kosiuk, Department of Radiology, Royal Victoria Hospital, Montreal, carried out the radiographic studies. Dr. A. Dufresne, School of Occupational Health, McGill University, carried out the lung dust analyses.)

to those seen in minimal (or negligible) asbestosis in one series,[212] and to those seen in asbestosis-related lung cancer in other series.[213]

### Epidemiology

Like pleural plaques, pleural fibrosis and visceroparietal reactions may occur in the absence of radiologic parenchymal fibrosis, and they are increasing in frequency.[173] The exposures implicated (see Table 65.3) are often short, heavy, remote, and related to amphiboles. Latency is usually long (>20 years), reflected in the fact that these reactions relate to time since first exposure (a proxy for residence time of dust in the lung) and not to cumulative exposure dose.[29, 171, 173] In one study, the residua of an effusion were almost as commonly responsible for diffuse pleural fibrosis as were confluent plaques.[214] In the United States, radiographic pleural abnormality has been reported in approximately 1% of men without known exposure.[173] Pleural fibrosis also has been reported in association with environmental exposures from mining operations (see previous discussion under sources of human exposure), for example, in Finland and South Africa, and from nonmining (agricultural) operations in Bulgaria, the former Czechoslovakia, Poland, Greece, and Turkey. Epidemiologic studies are also consistent in showing that the presence of pleural fibrosis is associated with reduction in lung function, after any associated parenchymal fibrosis has been taken into account.[29, 173, 188]

### Diagnosis

Diagnosis usually is based initially on the chest roentgenogram.[214] Clinical presentation, like that of pleural plaques, is often as an incidental abnormality detected on a routine chest roentgenogram. After careful inquiry, a remote history of exposure, often quite brief but usually heavy, can be obtained from the subject. Rounded atelectasis also may present as a radiologic abnormality in an asymptomatic subject, usually with a clear history of exposure, past or current. Conversely, some subjects present with breathlessness[173, 214] or chest pain, or both, with or without a history of acute episodes, attributed to benign pleural effusions (see subsequent discussion). Pleural fibrosis restricts the movement of the lungs; in the absence of associated parenchymal disease, clinical signs may be minimal, even though functional impairment is detectable: sometimes, but by no means always, impairment is surprisingly modest in the face of what appears to be quite severe pleural disease.[29, 173, 215] Pleural fibrosis occasionally becomes severe enough to precipitate respiratory and cardiac failure and to require pleurectomy.[173, 216]

The radiologic and CT features of pleural fibrosis were discussed under pleural plaques. Given a history of exposure, obliteration of the costophrenic angle is likely to represent the residua of asbestos pleural effusion[3, 173, 214] and is associated with impairment of lung function (on average a deficit of 0.22 L and 0.40 L for $FEV_1$ and FVC, respectively, in one study).[217] In rounded atelectasis, the CT scan is particularly useful in delineating the relationship of the rounded lesion to other pleural changes including fissures.[17] Nevertheless, the inability to be certain that a mass lesion that is increasing in size in a person exposed to asbestos is not a cancer (even in the presence of a negative needle biopsy result) leads most clinicians to recommend their surgical excision.

## Benign Asbestos-Related Pleural Effusions

Benign asbestos-related pleural effusions may occur in lungs free of other stigmata of asbestos exposure or may mark an increase in the extent or severity of an already present pleural reaction. The term benign does not imply a lack of clinical significance, but that the effusion is not associated with mesothelioma.[173] Benign asbestos-related pleural effusions usually occur within 15 years of the first exposure, even after exposure has ceased.[173] They are more common in men in their 20s and 30s than in older men and may be the most common manifestation of asbestos pleural disease in this age group, more common than plaques or diffuse fibrosis.[3] The episodes are usually transient and may be silent. They also may give rise to chest tightness and, occasionally, pleural pain, fever, and dyspnea.[173] Pleural rubs also have been reported. The effusion is usually small, and the exudate is blood-stained and contains leukocytes.[164] Asbestos bodies rarely are found in the fluid, but they may be seen in the underlying parenchyma on biopsy.[218] The sedimentation rate often is raised.[218]

Diagnosis is by exclusion, and suggested criteria include: (1) an exposure history; (2) the absence of other causes; and (3) absence of tumor in a 3-year follow-up.[172] Because cytologic examination of the pleural fluid is rarely conclusive, a thoracoscopic biopsy invariably is required to exclude other causes; to establish the presence of fibers in the pleural fluid (rarely demonstrable), pleura (sometimes demonstrable), or the underlying lung parenchyma (not infrequently demonstrable); and to rule out malignancy, in particular malignant pleural mesothelioma. The usual pathologic findings in benign asbestos-related pleural effusion are those of chronic fibrous pleurisy with minimal cellularity.

The prognosis of benign asbestos-related pleural effusions is on the whole good; most clear spontaneously, whether it be the first episode or a recurrence.[3] Recurrence may be on the opposite side. Although effusion is a common form of presentation for malignant mesothelioma (Chapter 76), there is no evidence that a benign effusion predisposes to future pleural malignancy. It appears rather to represent a stage in the evolution of asbestos-related pleural fibrosis, and carries the same risk (in one series approximately 10%) of developing parenchymal fibrosis (asbestosis) as chronic pleural fibrosis. These pleural effusions are not considered precursors of mesothelioma.[3]

The pathogenesis is unknown. Both mechanical irritation by fibers permeating the pleura and a direct cytotoxic effect on the surface mesothelial layer have been invoked.[173] Animal models suggest that the exudative pleural reaction to asbestos particles released into the pleural space results in a polymorphonuclear leukocyte response, followed by the release of chemotactic activity from sources other than complement, probably from asbestos-pleural tissue interactions.[219] Asbestos also may directly stimulate pleural mesothelial cells to synthesize interleukin-8, a potent neutrophil chemotactic factor, which may play an important role in mediating asbestos-induced pleural inflammation.[220] To view the mesothelial cell proliferation as a general response to fibrotic lung repair[221] is a less credible hypothesis given the much smaller burden of fibers seen with pleural than with parenchymal reactions to asbestos.[213]

## Management, Prevention, and Health Monitoring

The principles guiding clinical management of all these asbestos-related lung conditions are no different from those guiding this management when there is no history of asbestos exposure. These are discussed in Chapter 57. The specific issues involved in the management of work-related or potentially work-related disease were discussed previously in this chapter. The physician is reminded of the importance of making the appropriate notification of any case of asbestos-related disease. Notification, together with any procedures related to compensation, depends on the local jurisdiction operating in the area of the physician's practice. Another issue that the physician must face is how to advise the individual affected on future employment (assuming it is not out of the question for reasons of disability). Advice should be guided by our knowledge, limited as it is, of the natural history of the disease processes with or without further exposure,[29, 173, 174] of the current exposure levels in the individual's workplace, and of the impact of further exposure on the risks of malignancy, parenchymal or pleural. In particular, it is important to emphasize that, even in the absence of any further exposure whatsoever, progression of all the nonmalignant asbestos-related diseases discussed here may occur on the basis of dust load already in the lungs. Current evidence suggests that once there is definite parenchymal radiologic abnormality, the prudent option is to avoid all further exposure.[138] Furthermore, continued exposure is likely to contribute in maintaining industrial bronchitis, if present, and in increasing the risk of chronic airflow limitation.[6] The possible role of smoking in the initiation and progression of fibrotic parenchymal disease and its established role in multiplying the risk of lung cancer are strong indications for antismoking advice to be given to the individual and for instituting smoking cessation programs in workplaces contaminated by asbestos dust.

No active treatment measures have been shown to influence the course of asbestosis. Corticosteroids and other antiinflammatory and cytotoxic agents advocated for other interstitial lung diseases are less effective in asbestosis possibly because the active agent remains in situ in the lungs. A placebo-controlled trial of beta carotene and retinyl palmate for chemoprevention of lung cancer in a population of 816 asbestos-exposed men with a high rate of smoking showed that raising the serum concentration led to an approximately 100 mL increase of $FEV_1$ and FVC. [222] Patients with end-stage asbestosis also have been the recipients of lung and heart-lung transplants (see the previous discussion on the management of acute silicosis). Lung transplantation is discussed in Chapter 97.

For the nonmalignant asbestos-related pleural disorders, the evidence is now reasonably clear that those with pleural fibrosis (and effusion seems to be a phase in the natural history of pleural fibrosis) are at greater risk for parenchymal fibrosis in the future,[170, 183, 200] with its attendant risks of progression and disablement. It would be wise to avoid any further exposure once pleural fibrosis becomes manifest and probably also (although this is less certain) once a pleural effusion has occurred. The presence of pleural fibrosis or pleural plaques does not increase the individual's risk of malignant pleural mesothelioma any more than the risk associated with the dust load already carried by the lungs. There is, however, a higher risk of developing parenchymal fibrosis (and its attendant health implications) than in the individual with no such stigmata of exposure.[223]

Control and prevention of asbestos-related lung diseases are a public health issue, well discussed elsewhere.[2–4] Success requires control of the work force environment, setting and enforcing of standards, and pre-employment or in-service health examinations for exposed workers as part of a health monitoring program. Implicit in the latter examination, which has the elements of a screening examination, is the hope that early detection might avoid later damaging disease, a hypothesis still to be tested. Nor is the interpretation of small changes between examinations (in physical signs and in radiologic, lung function, and cytologic examinations) an easy task; such examinations still probably are regarded best as biologic monitoring (for the purpose of detecting average trends within a work force) rather than as a method of case identification. Nevertheless, some individuals seek this type of health examination from their personal physician or clinic, and the clinician must make a best judgment on the basis of available information.

There is also some encouraging information for the individual with past exposure. First, only a minority of those exposed are likely to develop radiologic changes, and only a minority of those with radiologic changes develop clinical manifestations and any degree of disablement.[224] Furthermore, the additional chance of developing a carcinoma of the lung in the face of frank asbestosis is likely to be considerably lower than the 10% to 30% quoted on the basis of case data from subjects exposed before the 1960s, when exposure levels were higher and asbestosis was, as far as can be judged, a more severe disease.[185] Quitting cigarette smoking benefits the asbestos-exposed individual even more than the nonexposed individual because of the multiplicative interaction of these two agents.[195, 198, 198a, 225] For the current worker who has never been exposed to more than the present control levels ($\leq$1 fiber/mL for a 50-year working life), ill-health effects are unlikely to be demonstrable by any practicable method of study, according to one expert view.[186] The mesothelioma risk, perhaps more disquieting for those with past occupational exposure, also may be expected to decline with time, but in the UK this may not occur before the second decade of the 21st century.[169, 226, 226a]

## NON-ASBESTOS MINERAL SILICATES (FIBROUS OR NOT) AND LUNG DISEASE

Exposure to some of the non-asbestos mineral silicates listed in Table 65.3 has been associated with lung disease. Silicate dust particles are found in the lungs of most urban dwellers,[14, 56] and in general they appear to have low biologic activity.[163] Disease may develop after long, heavy exposure; in its early stages, it is characterized by accumulation of dust-laden macrophages around respiratory bronchioles, and later by fiber deposits with little mature collagen; the disease appears to progress in relation to lung dust overload.[56, 162, 163, 165] Silicates are used widely for filling materials (kaolin, talc, and chlorite), for insulation (mica, vermiculite), and for absorbents (attapulgite, sepiolite), among other uses.[163] The clay minerals talcs and mica (also called phyllosilicates because of their sheet structure)[163] constitute an important group. World production and use (estimated in 1991 as 5.3 million tons for talc alone) considerably exceeds that of the asbestos minerals, peak annual production of which reached 5 million tons and occurred in the late 1970s. Before a 1989 NATO Workshop, their toxicity as a group for humans had been studied little,[163] although three (talc, attapulgite, and sepiolite) had been evaluated for carcinogenic risk for humans by the IARC.[163] The information in this section is derived from the report of this workshop[163] and other sources.[2–5, 227]

Talc and, more often, mica particles also may form the core of ferruginous bodies. In general, the nonfibrous silicates have pulmonary effects similar to those caused by coal, unless they contain fibrous forms of these minerals or are contaminated by asbestos fibers, in which case their effects are closer to those produced by asbestos. The biological effects of silica (quartz) also are believed to be modulated by the presence of silicates.[56]

Among the clay minerals, the lesions of *kaolin pneumoconiosis* tend to be cellular and dust packed.[163] In its simple form, this pneumoconiosis usually is not associated with clinical or lung function changes, but massive fibrosis, when it occurs, tends to be diffuse and to be accompanied by impairment.[3, 4] In 10 surveys of kaolin-exposed work forces, the radiologic prevalence of simple pneumoconiosis (mostly small round opacities) ranged from less than 1% to 26.3%, whereas complicated pneumoconiosis and pleural change were unusual.[227] In general, prevalence was related to level and duration of dust exposure and probably contamination by other materials, including silica. Adverse effects on lung function were judged to be minor. Although lung cancers have been mentioned in relation to kaolin exposure, no cohort mortality studies had been reported up to 1990.[227]

The lesions of *talc pneumoconiosis* include peribronchial and perivascular interstitial accumulations of dust-filled macrophages, ill-defined nodular lesions in which birefringent talc crystals can be seen,[3] and foreign body granulomas.[4, 163] In general, the disease evolves slowly, and progressive massive fibrosis occurs infrequently; tuberculosis may complicate the condition. Interstitial fibrosis also may occur. A granulomatous arteritis caused by talc embolism is described in drug addicts who use an intravenous route for talc-containing drug tablets. Pleural changes, including plaques, are common; they usually are associated with mining exposures and may be due to contamination of mine dust by fiber (tremolite or anthophyllite).[163] Reactions to talc can be difficult to distinguish from those caused by silica or by asbestos, which often contaminate or even predominate in industrial grade talc.[5] In six surveys of talc-exposed work forces, prevalence of small opacities ranged from less than 1% to 37.2%, the latter in long-time workers and the lower rates in some studies in which exposure was to pure talc.[227, 228] Adverse effects on pulmonary function have been found.[163] In three of seven cohort mortality studies in talc-exposed workers, excess deaths were recorded from nonmalignant respiratory disease, including pneumoconiosis. In addition, an excess of respiratory cancer mortality was found in five of the seven cohorts, but these findings must be interpreted with caution since they were based on only 13 or fewer deaths in each cohort. In four of these, coexposure to other carcinogenic agents (mineral fibers, radon, silica) could have been implicated.[227] Several cases of mesothelioma also were reported, but all in cohorts exposed to fiber-contaminated dusts.[227]

The lesions of *mica pneumoconiosis* comprise dust particles surrounded by reticulin but usually with relatively little cellular reaction, although there are case reports of interstitial fibrosis[229] in which granulomas also have been described.[227] In three surveys of mica-exposed work forces, the prevalence of radiologic pneumoconiosis ranged from 1% to 44%, the latter work force being exposed to quartz-contaminated mica.[227] No mortality studies have been reported, but there has been one case report of a peritoneal mesothelioma in a mica-exposed worker.[227] *Vermiculite*, also a mica, does not appear to be toxic to the lungs of animals. However, in four surveys of vermiculite-exposed mine workers, the prevalence of radiologic pneumoconiosis ranged from less than 1% to 18%, and of pleural changes from 3% to 28%; in a processing plant, rates were higher and were related to cumulative exposure.[163, 227] In one study, lung function was not affected,[230] although health selection may have operated to minimize an exposure effect.[38] Pleural effusions were not infrequent in two of the mica-exposed work forces, in one of which mortality from malignant and nonmalignant respiratory disease was increased in relation to exposure[231]; contamination of the mine ore vermiculite by amphibole was implicated.[227]

The authors of the 1990 epidemiology review[227] concluded that (1) there is little evidence that occupational exposure to pure kaolin, talc, mica, or vermiculite carries any important risk for health; (2) long and heavy exposure to kaolin and mica may result in low-grade radiographic changes, but clinically important pneumoconioses in work forces exposed to these phyllosilicates are likely to be the result of contamination by silica or asbestos fiber; (3) pleural lesions are common in talc-exposed workers but are probably caused by fiber contaminants; and (4) the increased rates of lung cancer or mesothelioma recorded in several exposed work forces are unlikely caused by any of the four phyllosilicates reviewed, but probably result from exposure to fiber or silica contaminants of the ore or milled products.

The production of man-made vitreous fibers (MMVFs)

(including glass fibers and mineral wool, and refractory ceramic fibers as well as man-made mineral fibers such as carbon graphite, Keular-paramid, silicon carbide, and aluminum oxide), has increased markedly since the restriction or banning of asbestos in several countries, including the United States.[1, 3, 232] As with asbestos fibers, determinants of MMVF toxicity are (1) their dimensions (greatest risk with fine, long fibers less than 0.25 in diameter and longer than 8 mm[1]); (2) their biopersistence, which can be altered in the production process according to the end use; and (3) dose to the target organ.[1] MMVFs differ from asbestos fibers in being more soluble, less durable, and less biopersistent along a gradient: glass > rock > ceramic fibers.[232] Fibers are also coarser along a gradient: continuous glass filament > insulation wool > ceramic fibers > special purpose.[232] In addition, human exposure has been to levels 2 to 3 orders of magnitude less than in the early development of the asbestos industry. Human health data, sparse for synthetic mineral fibers, are available for MMVFs and refractory ceramic fibers, and have been the subject of excellent comprehensive review,[232] the prime source for the information presented here. MMVFs and refractory ceramic fibers are produced in more than 100 factories around the world[162] and are useful for more than 3500 applications,[3] some of which are listed in Table 65.3. Most are manufactured by melting the raw material and fiberizing the melt through a nozzle to form a continuous filament or alternating to form fiber wool.[2] Airborne levels in plants manufacturing MMVFs are commonly lower than 1 fiber/mL and lower in most applications except working in attic and loft insulation[232]; airborne fiber diameters are also much greater (over 1 mm) except in the manufacture of ceramic fiber. Within the man-made mineral fiber industry, concentrations are higher in plants making special purpose or ceramic fibers, and in blowing or spraying operations carried out in closed spaces. Despite their intensely irritating effects on skin and mucous membranes, there is no firm evidence that these fibers produce lung fibrosis, pleural lesions, or nonspecific respiratory disease in humans, although exposure to refractory ceramic fibers may enhance the effects of smoking in producing airway disease.[232] However, an increased standardized mortality ratio for lung cancer has been shown in several cohorts exposed to MMVFs, especially in the early technologic phases of rock slag production, during which other carcinogenic agents were also present in many workplaces.[232] There was no evidence of an increased mesothelioma risk for MMVF workers and insufficient epidemiologic data to assess the lung cancer risk in workers exposed to refractory and ceramic fibers. The view that, fiber for fiber, rock/slagwool could be more hazardous than asbestos[162] is not universally accepted.[233] For this reason, continued surveillance of exposed work forces is considered essential, particularly in those end applications such as insulation.[232] An additional handicap to the physician is that unlike asbestos fibers, MMVFs in BAL or biopsy material cannot be used as objective indications of exposure.[232] In the future, in situ confocal laser scanning microscopy may be able to provide detailed information about lung fiber burden in biopsy material.[232a]

## OTHER PNEUMOCONIOSES, OLD AND NEW

The pneumoconioses already discussed account for the majority of cases in most countries of the world. They exemplify a range of pulmonary reactions, from minimal reaction to a large lung particulate dust load (e.g., CWP) to a very specific fibrotic reaction to a comparatively small lung dust particulate load (e.g., silicosis). In the case of mineral fibers, the pulmonary reaction appears to be determined by lung fiber load of a particular size range (the long, fine fiber), as well as by fiber durability.

Several long-recognized, well-catalogued but less common pneumoconioses, which fall into the group in which the dust load is heavy but pulmonary reaction minimal, have not yet been mentioned. They include the pneumoconioses resulting from inhalation of iron in welding fumes or in iron mine or hematite mine dust *(siderosis)*, those that result from the inhalation of barytes by barium miners or workers *(baritosis)*, and those that result from exposure to tin dust *(stannosis)*. Other dusts that fall into this category include bismuth, manganese, Fuller's earth, and titanium. A more comprehensive list can be found elsewhere.[2, 4] At the other end of the scale, what originally have been described as unusual or new forms of pneumoconiosis often turn out to be a form of the oldest pneumoconiosis, silicosis, which escaped recognition because exposure levels to quartz were higher than originally appreciated or the features of the pulmonary response were modified by the presence of other dusts. Examples include Labrador lung (after exposure of iron miners to ore dust containing silica and some anthophyllite fibers)[42, 234] and disease in bentonite workers that also turned out to be silicosis (dust levels were high and contained about 10% quartz).[2, 4] The pneumoconiosis of foundrymen is also an example of a response to mixed dust, in which the proportion of quartz is a key determinant to the character of the response.[4] Careful case reports by observant clinicians continue to identify interstitial lung disease associated with various exposures and thus provide the information to stimulate the epidemiologic studies necessary to place them in proper context. Exposures implicated include those to titanium, vanadium, zirconium, hafnium, and rare earth metals,[3] and polyvinyl chloride polymer.[235] This list is incomplete, and the reader is referred to one of several comprehensive specialized texts[1–4] for descriptions of these other pneumoconioses, old and new.

## BERYLLIUM LUNG DISEASE

### Beryllium: Uses, Human Toxicity, and Exposures

Beryllium is a rare metal that has many applications in modern industry because of its light weight, tensile strength, high melting point (1500°C), excellent alloying properties (beryllium-copper the most widely used),[1] good thermal and electrical conductivity, resistance to corrosion, and ability to reduce the speed of nuclear fission.[3, 4, 236] Major sources are Argentina, Brazil, India, Zimbabwe, South Africa, and the United States.[1] Its toxicity for humans was first recognized in Europe in the 1930s. In the United States, an epidemic of chronic beryllium disease occurred as a result of exposure in the fluorescent light industry during the 1940s, leading to discontinuation of its use in that industry and the institution of engineering controls in other industries handling beryllium.[1] However, the number of cases continued to increase from 300 registered in a US case registry (started in 1952 by Dr Harriet Hardy at the Massachusetts General Hospital to catalogue patient characteristics[1]) to 904 in 1987.[2] Of these 904 cases, 212 had acute disease, 648 chronic, and 44 acute disease that became chronic.[2, 236] The distribution of reported exposures had now changed; only a minority (27.3%) had been exposed in the fluorescent light industry, whereas almost half (48.5%) had been exposed in the manufacture of beryllium metal products (alloys, ceramics, and radiographic and vacuum tubes), and a further 12.1% in the extraction and smelting of beryllium.[2] The number of individuals potentially exposed in the United States in 1987 was estimated between 30,000 and 800,000 in the following industries: aerospace, electronics, ceramics, metal, including refining of scrap metal, nuclear (reactors, weapons) telecommunications, tool and die, and welding.[2, 237] The first case of nonoccupational exposure in 40 years was reported in 1991, in the wife of a worker who handled her husband's work-soiled clothes on only two occasions.[238] Beryllium contamination inside the personal vehicles of workers was subsequently documented.[238a]

The register was archived by the National Institute of Occupational Safety and Health (Cincinnati) in 1978 and has not accepted new cases since then.[2] Nevertheless, it has been estimated that between 200 and 300 individuals have been sensitized since that date (most with disease), according to enhanced work force screening efforts (using the Beryllium Lymphocyte proliferation test and immunologic testing) together with BAL and transbronchial biopsy. With early diagnosis of subclinical disease, the epidemiology of chronic beryllium disease has changed substantially.

## Pathology and Immune Pathogenesis

*Acute beryllium disease* in humans, defined as a disease from which the subject recovers within a year, has been attributed to toxic, dose-related lung injury characterized by acute inflammatory reactions in the upper airways, bronchiolitis, pulmonary edema, and chemical pneumonitis.[1–4] *Chronic beryllium disease* is a multisystem disorder characterized by noncaseating granulomas that occur throughout the body, although their primary manifestation is in the lung.[236] The percentage of those exposed occupationally in the 1980s who became sensitized was probably between 3% and 15%.[240] In a 1997 survey of 646 workers in a beryllium metal alloy and oxide production plant, sensitization was present in 9.4%, and 24 new cases were identified that, together with 5 known cases, resulted in a disease prevalence of 4.6%.[240] On pathologic examination, chronic beryllium disease is characterized by the presence of a lymphocytic (helper/inducer T cells) alveolitis, as well as noncaseating epithelioid granulomas indistinguishable from those of sarcoidosis.[239] There is a variable amount of fibroblastic activity that progresses to interstitial fibrosis as the lesions mature. As in sarcoidosis, granulomatous lesions also are found in other organs, including thoracic and abdominal lymph nodes, spleen, liver, kidneys, and adrenal glands.

Beryllium enters the body by inhalation, and occasionally via the skin, where it acts as a specific antigen (alone or as a hapten through an IL-2 receptor pathway), leading to a proliferation of specific CD4 lymphocytes, release of lymphokines, and granuloma formation.[1] Cell mechanisms are complex.[241, 241a, 241b] Because the agent persists in the lung, its slow release over time explains the appearance and progression of disease,[1] even without further exposure. There is also some evidence for an underlying genetic basis for susceptibility to beryllium disease, linked to a major histocompatibility complex (MHC) class II marker (HLA-DPβ-1 Glu69) carrier status, which adds to the effect of the process (exposure) risk factor.[5, 242] Evidence for delayed hypersensitivity in beryllium disease includes positive reactions to skin testing and in vitro responses of the lymphocytes to stimulation by beryllium, the Beryllium Lymphycyte Proliferation Test (BeLPT).[240] Skin testing, which at one point was thought to activate the pulmonary lesions, largely has been replaced by the BeLPT.[240] Although these reactions are thought to indicate exposure and sensitization, not disease, six of eight sensitized individuals had granulomas on transbronchial biopsy in one series.[243]

Until the early 1990s, the evidence that beryllium was carcinogenic for humans was considered limited and was based mainly on methodologic criticisms of the available mortality studies.[2] Currently, the preponderance of evidence is considered to support the view that beryllium is a human carcinogen, especially in patients with beryllium lung disease,[2] and in 1993 the IARC reclassified beryllium as a class 1 human carcinogen.[244]

## Clinical Features

The clinical features of *acute beryllium disease* include cough, chest pain, blood-tinged sputum, crackles, and patchy air-space disease on the chest radiograph, with resolution within a year. No new case has been reported to the US Beryllium Case Registry since 1987.[2] *Chronic beryllium disease* may follow an acute beryllium pneumonitis, but more usually develops without antecedent events. In the U.K. Beryllium Registry, 59 cases of chronic beryllium disease were recorded to 1993; of these, 5 were acute, 7 had skin lesions only, and 25 of the patients with chronic cases were known to have died.[4]

The clinical features of chronic beryllium disease are similar to those of pulmonary sarcoidosis and include dyspnea, cough, chest pain, weight loss, fatigue, and arthralgias; crackles are not always an early feature.[2, 4] Radiographic changes may precede the development of symptoms. The usual finding is ill-defined nodular or irregular opacities; hilar adenopathy is seen in approximately 40% of cases but is usually mild.[2] In the later stages of the disease, lung volume shrinks, often irregularly, and there is hyperinflation or distortion of adjacent areas and extensive honeycombing. In chronic beryllium disease, pulmonary function usually shows a restrictive defect in advanced disease, but features including obstruction or isolated reduction in carbon monoxide diffusing capacity may occur with mild or moderate disease. Other, nonspecific, laboratory findings include hyperuricemia, hypercalcemia/hypercalcuria, and elevated serum angiotensin-converting enzyme levels. Hypersensitivity to beryllium can be demonstrated by the BeLPT, increasingly used to determine whether exposed individuals have become sensitized.[2]

The clinical course of chronic beryllium disease is variable. Some cases remain stable, some relapse and remit, and some progress inexorably.[2]

### Diagnosis and Management

Criteria for diagnosis, established for entering a case into the US Beryllium Case Registry,[1] were four of the following six features: (1) exposure established on the basis of history, environmental sampling, or other evidence; (2) objective evidence of lower respiratory disease and a clinical course consistent with beryllium disease; (3) radiologic evidence of interstitial fibronodular disease; (4) impairment of lung function (restrictive, obstructive, or diffusion defect); (5) histopathologic changes in lung or lymph nodes (or both) consistent with beryllium disease; and (6) demonstration of the presence of beryllium in biologic material (lung, lymph nodes, or urine).[1] Levels of 0.02 mg beryllium per gram of dried tissue and greater are found in chronic beryllium disease.[4] In the 1980s, improved diagnostic tools in the form of BAL and transbronchial biopsy, together with the BeLPT performed on blood or BAL material, have improved greatly the accuracy of clinical diagnosis, and two additional clinical categories have been suggested: beryllium sensitization (positive blood or BAL BeLPT but negative biopsy) and subclinical beryllium disease (positive BeLPT and biopsy but no clinical or radiologic features of the disease).[239]

Most patients with chronic beryllium disease present in a fashion indistinguishable from pulmonary sarcoidosis, although extrathoracic manifestations of disease (splenomegaly, hilar and mediastinal adenopathy), not unusual in sarcoidosis, are less common in chronic beryllium disease.[4] Evidence of sensitization to beryllium can be obtained in most instances by performing BeLPT on blood or BAL material (the yield from blood is lower than from BAL).[2] BeLPT, however, is only available in a few laboratories, to which specimens may be shipped overnight. During the "epidemic" of beryllium disease during the 1940s and 1950s, chronic beryllium disease was very likely to have been considered in the differential diagnosis of sarcoidosis. Given the potentially long latency time for chronic beryllium disease and despite the generally lower exposures that have occurred since the 1950s and its decreasing frequency, chronic beryllium disease still should remain in the differential diagnosis of sarcoidosis cases seen in the early 21st century. For instance, a cluster of cases associated with exposure in a scrap metal recovery plant came to attention in the 1980s because the index case, aware of the potentially toxic effects of beryllium, referred himself for evaluation for "beryllosis," prompted by the occurrence of several cases of "sarcoidosis" among his coworkers.[237]

The most important step in case management is complete cessation of further exposure to beryllium. Steroid therapy has been recommended in chronic beryllium disease, and long-term steroid therapy is believed to alter the course of the disease favorably, although there are no reports of permanent cure.[2, 4] Greater caution also is required in reducing the dose[4] in chronic beryllium disease than in sarcoidosis because of the risk of serious relapse, attributed to the fact that the causal agent, beryllium, remains permanently in the target tissue as an insoluble protein-bound complex.[4]

Chronic beryllium disease is controlled through the maintenance of the environmental levels in conformity with recommended control levels in all workplaces in which beryllium is used (the Atomic Energy Commission's environmental standards are 2 $\mu g/m^3$ averaged over an 8-hour day, not exceeding a peak of 25 $\mu g/m^3$ for 30 min).[1] The engineering controls that were introduced in the United States in the 1950s have by and large been successful, although, even in the late 1970s there were industries in which the environmental standards were far exceeded,[237] usually in small industries with intermittent use of modern high-technology processes. Peak exposures, usually related to equipment failure or repair, may be more likely to induce sensitization although this also has occurred in plants with median levels below 2 $\mu g/m^3$.[2] Current metrics for measuring the exposure capable of inducing sensitization also may not be appropriate. High-temperature operations are more likely to induce disease than exposure to heavier doses of "cold working" alloys.[237]

Medical surveillance of exposed work forces also plays a role in allowing this versatile mineral to be used safely,[4] both by biologic monitoring for sensitization using blood BeLPT[243] and by case detection. In case detection, a combination of the traditional clinical tools and criteria just referred to is used, as well as bronchoscopy for the harvesting of BAL lymphocytes for the BeLPT and for transbronchial biopsy with tissue analysis. Management of the sensitized individual usually should include advice to avoid further exposure. This advice is based on the likelihood that sensitized individuals usually have granulomas on transbronchial biopsy, even when chest roentgenograms and lung function tests are normal.

## HARD METAL DISEASE

Hard metal disease is a disorder related to modern technology. Hard metal disease, first described in Germany in the 1940s, is now reported from many countries in workers engaged in the manufacture or use of products derived from a sintering process that involves pressurization plus heating to 1500°C a mixture of tungsten carbide powder and 10% cobalt.[1] The resulting sinter consists of a matrix of cobalt into which the metallic tungsten carbide has been incorporated; tantalum, titanium, and aluminum carbides may be layered on the surface and chromium and nickel added.[245] Because of their diamond-like hardness, extreme strength, and heat resistance, "hard metal" products have wide application in industry, as drill tips (from dental to engineering drilling and diamond polishing), cutting and tunneling tools, grinding wheels, molds, jet engines, and ferromagnets. Human exposure occurs both in the manufacturing of hard metal products and in their maintenance and use in the many aforementioned applications. The grinding of sintered pieces generates high dust and cobalt concentrations.

Work-related illness in hard metal workers[245] may be acute (rhinitis and asthma), subacute (fibrosing alveolitis), or chronic (diffuse and progressive interstitial fibrosis). The interstitial fibrosis is characterized by unusual multinucleated giant cells comprising alveolar type II cells and macrophages that can be recovered from BAL. Cognitive behavioral sequelae, including memory deficits, are also associated with hard metal disease in humans.[265] The interstitial lung disease currently is thought to be a hypersensitivity pneumonitis to cobalt, which reacts with metallic carbides to produce active oxygen species.[2, 246] A genetic association with some HLA-DP alleles may also be implicated.[246a] This affords a plausible explanation of why only a small proportion of those exposed develop disease. A 1998 industry-wide cohort study in 10 facilities in France documented an increased mortality from lung cancer associated with simultaneous exposure to cobalt and tungsten carbide.[247] A review of workplace surveys indicates that interstitial disease is quite rare whereas airway disease, including bronchitis and asthma, are both more frequent.[245] Both interstitial and airway disease may of course occur in the same individual. Diagnosis is based on an exposure history, a compatible clinical presentation, and pathologic and mineralogic features on biopsy: tungsten carbide usually can be identified, but not cobalt (because, it is believed, of its solubility).[245] Cobalt exposure can be confirmed by patch test, or in urine or blood samples; lymphocyte (blood or BAL) transformation or leukocyte inhibition factor in response to cobalt also may be useful.[4, 245] Prompt diagnosis and removal from exposure may reverse acute disease, including asthma, and prevent the development of chronic disease.[4] Steroids and cyclophosphamide have been used with success to treat cases of hard metal disease with an acute course.[2] Prevention requires control of exposure; for monitoring work force exposure, urinary cobalt may be useful.

*Silicon-carbide (Carborundum) pneumoconiosis* associated with work exposure in the manufacture of carborundum, which is used for its hardness, is usually a relatively benign condition under current exposure levels.[248] The prevalence of small irregular opacities 1/0 on the chest radiograph was 2.6% in one survey of 1036 workers.[249]

## SUMMARY

This chapter has dealt with the classic pneumoconioses: silicosis, CWP, asbestosis, and asbestos-related pleural disease, as well as with some of the interstitial lung diseases that do not correspond to the ILO definition of pneumoconiosis, in which the agent is not necessarily a dust and does not necessarily remain in the lung (e.g., beryllium and hard metal lung disease). The emphasis has been on providing information pertinent to the office encounter with a patient who is at risk for or may have a pneumoconiosis or other work-related lung disease. From the material presented, it is evident that in the 21st century, the physician should consider the possibility of a workplace exposure as the underlying cause not only for clinical syndromes, suggesting the classical pneumoconioses and interstitial lung disease, but also for clinical syndromes as varied as asthma, alveolitis, hypersensitivity pneumonitis, and acute and chronic airway disease, as well as solid lesions suggesting lung cancer, and lung cancer itself. In other words, all pulmonary disease, nonmalignant and malignant, airway or parenchymal, may be related to workplace exposure(s), and this applies as much to women as it does to men.[6a, 249a]

A striking feature of the material reviewed in this chapter is the variation among workplaces in the slope of exposure-response relationships, indicating striking differences among workplaces in the prevalence of radiologic pneumoconiosis at what appear to be comparable exposure levels (see Fig. 65.2[13] and Fig. 65.7[170]). A plausible explanation, and one for which there is experimental evidence, invokes the interaction between the putative dust(s) and other workplace contaminants, in the form of dusts or fumes; this could account for the different features of a particular pneumoconiosis in different workplaces. Such an explanation also has biological plausibility: the lungs of those exposed must deal with all contaminants of workplace air, and in evaluation of cases the physician should have in mind not only dusts but all potential workplace contaminants, often a very long list, given modern industrial technology.[6, 7]

The current tools for diagnosis are remarkable, the potential for identifying the agent in biologic material is extraordinary, yet the most powerful tool for detection of new work-related diseases or old diseases in workplaces not previously identified as at risk, is simple and clinical, the occupational history. This tool, if used by the physician with sensitivity and imagination and backed by a high index of suspicion and an understanding of scientific principles underlying the practice of chest medicine, still remains the cornerstone of diagnosis for the diseases of occupation just as it was in Ramazzini's day in 18th-century Italy.[250] Lack of knowledge of workplaces or deference to the obviously greater knowledge and expertise of the industrial hygienist or engineer, or both, should not deter the physician from recording a complete occupational history; indeed, few professions are able to offer the interviewing experience that comes with clinical practice.

## References

1. International Labour Office: Encyclopedia of Occupational Health and Safety (4th ed). Geneva: ILO, 1997.
2. Rom WN: Environmental and Occupational Medicine (3rd ed). Philadelphia: Lippincott-Raven, 1998.
3. Harber P, Schenker MB, Balmes JR: Occupational and Environmental Respiratory Disease. St. Louis: Mosby, 1995.
4. Parkes WR: Occupational Lung Disorders (3rd ed). London: Butterworth, 1994.
5. Churg A, Green FHY: Pathology of Occupational Lung Disease (2nd ed). Baltimore: Williams & Wilkins, 1998.
6. Becklake MR: Occupational exposures: Evidence for a causal association with chronic obstructive pulmonary disease. Am Rev Respir Dis 140(Suppl):S85–S89, 1989.

6a. Becklake MR: The work relatedness of airway dysfunction. *In* Proceedings of the 9th International Conference in Epidemiology in Occupational Health, Sept 23–25, 1992, International Commission on Occupational Health, DHHS (NIOSH) Publication no.

94-112. Washington, DC: US Department of Health and Human Services, Public Health Service, Centers for Disease Control and Prevention, National Institute for Occupational Safety and Health, 1994, pp 1–28.
7. Oxman AD, Muir DCF, Shannon HS, et al: Occupational dust exposure and chronic obstructive pulmonary disease. Am Rev Respir Dis 148:38–48, 1993.
7a. US Department of Health and Human Services, Public Health Service, Centers for Disease Control and Prevention, National Institute for Occupational Safety and Health: Atlas of Respiratory Disease Mortality, United States: 1982–1993, DDHS (NIOSH) Publication no. 98-157. Washington, DC: Authors, 1998, pp 23–27.
8. Nagelschmidt G: The relation between lung dust and lung pathology in pneumoconiosis. Br J Ind Med 17:247–259, 1960.
9. American Thoracic Society: Clinical role of bronchoalveolar lavage in adults with pulmonary disease. Am Rev Respir Dis 142:481–486, 1990.
9a. Fireman E, Greif J, Schwarz Y, et al: Assessment of hazardous dust exposure by BAL and induced sputum. Chest 115:1720–1728, 1999.
10. Dufresne A, Begin R, Masse S, et al: Retention of asbestos fibers in lungs of workers with asbestosis, asbestosis and lung cancer, and mesothelioma in Asbestos township. Occup Environ Med 53:801–807, 1996.
10a. Dufresne A, Looserewanich P, Begin R, et al: Tentative explanatory variable of lung dust concentration in gold miners exposed to crystalline silica. J Expos Analysis Epid 8:875–898, 1998.
11. Dufresne A, Perrault G, Yamato H, et al: Clearance of man-made mineral fibers from the lungs of sheep. Occup Environ Med 66:684–690, 1999.
12. Corn M: Strategies of air sampling. *In* McDonald JC (ed): Recent Advances in Occupational Health. Edinburgh: Churchill Livingstone, 1981, pp 199–209.
13. Muir DCF, Julian JA, Shannon HS, et al: Silica exposure and silicosis among Ontario hardrock miners: III. Analysis and risk estimates. Am J Ind Med 16:29–43, 1989.
14. Becklake MR: Asbestos-related diseases of the lung and other organs: Their epidemiology and implications for clinical practice. Am Rev Respir Dis 114:187–227, 1976.
15. National Institute for Occupational Safety and Health [NIOSH]: Occupational Exposure to Respirable Coal Mine Dust. Cincinnati, OH: US Department of Health and Human Services, Public Health Services, Centers for Disease Control and Prevention, NIOSH, 1995, pp 95–106.
16. Gerrity TR, Garrard CG, Geates DB, et al: A mathematical model of particle retention in the airspaces of human lungs. Br J Ind Med 40:121–130, 1983.
17. Gamsu G, Aberle DR, Lynch D: Computed tomography in the diagnosis of asbestos related thoracic disease. J Thorac Imaging 4:61–67, 1989.
18. Bégin R, Ostiguy G, Fillion R, et al: Computed tomography scan in the early detection of silicosis. Am Rev Respir Dis 144:697–705, 1991.
19. Kinsella M, Müller N, Vedal S, et al: Emphysema in silicosis: A comparison of smokers with nonsmokers using pulmonary function testing and computed tomography. Am Rev Respir Dis 141:1497–1500, 1990.
20. Leonard JF, Templeton PA: Pulmonary imaging techniques in the diagnosis of occupational interstitial lung disease. Occup Med 7:241–260, 1992.
21. Harber P, Smitherman J: Asbestosis: Diagnostic dilution. J Occup Med 33:786–793, 1991.
22. American Thoracic Society: Evaluation of impairment and disability. Am Rev Respir Dis 133:1205–1209, 1986.
23. American Thoracic Society: Lung function testing: Selection of reference values and interpretative strategies. Am Rev Respir Dis 144:1202–1218, 1991.
24. Becklake MR, White N: Sources of variation in spirometric measurements. Occup Med 8:241–264, 1993.
25. Abrams HK: The worker as teacher. Am J Ind Med 4:759–768, 1983.
26. The Occupational and Environmental Health Committee of the American Lung Association of San Diego and Imperial Counties: Taking the occupational history. Ann Intern Med 99:641–651, 1983.
27. Fonn S, Groeneveld HT, de Beer M, et al: An environmental and respiratory health survey of workers in a grain mill in the Johannesburg area, South Africa. Am J Ind Med 24:387–400, 1993.
28. Cullen MR, Baloyi RS: Prevalence of pneumoconiosis among coal and heavy metal miners in Zimbabwe. Am J Ind Med 17:677–682, 1990.
29. Becklake MR: Asbestos and other fiber-related diseases of the lungs and pleura: Distribution and determinants in exposed populations. Chest 100:248–254, 1991.
30. Becklake MR: Occupational pollution. Chest 96:372S–378S, 1989.
31. Snider DE: The relationship between tuberculosis and silicosis. Am Rev Respir Dis 118:455–460, 1978.
32. Becklake MR: The mineral dust diseases. Tuberc Lung Dis 73:13–20, 1992.
33. Murray JF: An emerging global programme against tuberculosis: Agenda for research, including the impact of HIV infection. Bull Int Union Tuberc Lung Dis 66:207–209, 1991.
33a. Churchyard GJ, Kleinschmidt I, Corbett EL, et al: Mycobacterial disease in South African gold miners in the era of HIV infection. Int J Tuberc Lung Dis 3:791–798, 1999.
34. Westerholm P: Silicosis: Observations on a case register. Scand J Work Environ Health 6(Suppl 2):1–86, 1980.
35. Westerholm P, Ahlmark A, Maasing R, et al: Silicosis and risk of lung cancer or lung tuberculosis: A cohort study. Environ Res 41:339–350, 1986.
36. Banks DE, Balaan M, Wang M-L: Silicosis in the 1990's revisited. Chest 111:837–838, 1997.
37. American Thoracic Society: Adverse effects of crystalline silica exposure. Am J Respir Crit Care Med 155:761–765, 1997.
38. Eisen EA, Wegman DH, Louis TA, et al: Healthy worker effect in a longitudinal study of one-second forced expiratory volume ($FEV_1$) and chronic exposure to granite dust. Int J Epidemiol 24:1154–1162, 1995.
39. Becklake MR, Lalloo U: The "healthy smoker": A phenomenon of health selection. Respiration 57:137–144, 1990.
40. Castranova V, Vallyathan V, Wallace WE: Silica and Silica-Induced Disease. Boca Raton: CRC Press, 1995.
41. White NW, Chetty R, Bateman ED: Silicosis among gemstone workers in South Africa: Tiger's-eye pneumoconiosis. Am J Ind Med 19:205–213, 1991.
42. Edstrom HW, Rice DMD: "Labrador lung": An unusual mixed dust pneumoconiosis. Can Med Assoc J 126:27–30, 1982.
43. Wagner JC, Pooley FD, Gibbs A, et al: Inhalation of china stone and china clay dusts: Relationship between the mineralogy of dust retained in the lungs and pathological changes. Thorax 41:190–196, 1986.
44. Ehrlich RI, Rees D, Zwi AB: Silicosis in non-mining industry on the Witwatersrand. S Afr Med J 73:704–708, 1988.
45. Valiante DJ, Rosenman KD: Does silicosis still occur? JAMA 262:3003–3007, 1989.
46. Watts WF, Parker DR: Quartz exposure trends in metal and nonmetal mining. Appl Occup Environ Hyg 10:1009–1018, 1995.
47. Rastogi SK, Gupta BN, Chandra H, et al: A study of the prevalence of respiratory morbidity among agate workers. Int Arch Occup Environ Health 63:21–26, 1991.
48. Landrigan P: Silicosis. *In* Rosenstock L (ed): Occupational Pulmonary Disease. Occup Med State Art Rev 2:319–326, 1987.
49. Murray J, Kielkowski D, Reid P: Occupational disease trends in black South African goldminers: An autopsy-based study. Am J Respir Crit Care Med 153:706–710, 1996.
50. National Institute for Occupational Safety and Health [NIOSH]: Alert: Request for Assistance in Preventing Silicosis and Deaths in Rock Drillers, Publication No. 92-107. Cincinnati: NIOSH, 1992.
51. US Department of Health and Human Services, Public Health Service, Centers for Disease Control and Prevention, National Institute for Occupational Safety and Health: Work-Related Lung Disease Surveillance Report, Publication No. 96-134. Cincinnati: DHSS (NIOSH), 1996.
52. Finkelstein MM: Silicosis surveillance in Ontario from 1979 to 1992. Scand J Work Environ Health 21:5507, 1995.
53. Cavariani F, Di Pietro A, Miceli M: The incidence of silicosis among ceramic workers in central Italy. Scand J Work Environ Health 21:58–62, 1995.

54. Gerhardsson L, Ahlmark A: A 50 year survey and follow-up of silicosis in an industrial country: Mineral exposure and pneumoconiosis. *In* Inhaled Particles VI. London: British Occupational Hygiene Society, 1988, pp 697–704.
55. Strachan AS, Simson FW: A preliminary study of silicosis as seen on the Witwatersrand. *In* Silicosis Records of the International Conference Held in Johannesburg, 13 August 1930, Series F, No. 13. Geneva: International Labour Organisation, 1931, pp 223–248.
56. Craighead JE, Kleinerman J: Diseases associated with exposure to silica and nonfibrous silicate minerals. Arch Pathol Lab Med 112:673–720, 1988.
57. Thériault GP, Peters JM, Fine LJ: Pulmonary function in granite shed workers of Vermont. Arch Environ Health 28:18–22, 1974.
58. Costello J, Graham WGB: Vermont granite workers' mortality study. Am J Ind Med 13:483–497, 1988.
59. Ziskind M, Jones R, Weill H: Silicosis. Am Rev Respir Dis 113:463–465, 1976.
60. Gibbs AR, Wagner JC: Diseases due to silica. *In* Churg A, Green FHY (eds): Pathology of Occupational Lung Disease (2nd ed). Baltimore: Williams & Wilkins, 1998, pp 209–233.
61. Anttilla S, Sutinen S, Auako P, et al: Rheumatoid pneumoconiosis in a dolomite worker: A light and electron microscopic and x-ray microanalytic study. Chest 78:195–200, 1984.
62. Sluis-Cremer G, Hessel PA, Hnizdo E, et al: Relationship between silicosis and rheumatoid arthritis. Thorax 41:596–601, 1986.
63. Klockars M, Koskela R-S, Järvinen E, et al: Silica exposure and rheumatoid arthritis: A follow up study of granite workers 1940–81. BMJ 294:997–1000, 1987.
64. Cowie RL, Langton ME, Becklake MR: Pulmonary tuberculosis in South African gold miners. Am Rev Respir Dis 139:1086–1089, 1989.
65. Cowie RL: The epidemiology of tuberculosis in gold miners with silicosis. Am J Respir Crit Care Med 150:1460–1462, 1994.
66. Bailey WC, Brown M, Buechner HA, et al: Silico-mycobacterial disease in sandblasters. Am Rev Respir Dis 110:115–125, 1974.
66a. Corbett EL, Churchyard GJ, Hay M, et al: The impact of HIV infection on *Mycobacterium kansasii* disease in South African gold miners. Am J Respir Crit Care Med 160:10–14, 1999.
67. Cowie RL, Hay M, Thomas RG: Association of silicosis, lung dysfunction and emphysema in gold miners. Thorax 48:746–749, 1993.
68. Becklake MR, Irwig L, Kielkowski D, et al: The predictors of emphysema in South African gold miners. Am Rev Respir Dis 135:1234–1241, 1987.
69. Hnizdo E, Baskind E, Sluis-Cremer GK: Combined effect of silica dust exposure and tobacco smoking on the prevalence of respiratory impairments among gold miners. Scand J Work Environ Health 16:411–422, 1990.
70. Cowie RL, Mabena SK: Silicosis, chronic airflow limitation and chronic bronchitis in South African gold miners. Am Rev Respir Dis 143:80–84, 1991.
71. Wright JL, Cagle P, Churg A, et al: Diseases of the small airways. Am Rev Respir Dis 146:240–262, 1992.
72. Eide J, Glyseth B, Skaug V: Silicotic lesions of the bone marrow: Histopathology and microanalysis. Histopathology 8:693–703, 1984.
73. Sluis-Cremer GK, Hessel PA, Hnizdo E, et al: Silica, silicosis, and progressive systemic sclerosis. Br J Ind Med 42:838–843, 1985.
74. Cowie RL: Silica-dust-exposed mine workers with scleroderma. Chest 92:260–262, 1987.
75. Pelmear PL, Roos JO, Maehle WM: Occupationally-induced scleroderma. J Occup Med 34:20–25, 1992.
76. Rustin MHA, Bull HA, Ziegler V, et al: Silica-associated systemic sclerosis is clinically, serologically and immunologically indistinguishable from idiopathic systemic sclerosis. Br J Dermatol 123:725–734, 1990.
77. Sanchez-Roman J, Wichmann I, Salaberri J, et al: Multiple clinical and biological autoimmune manifestations in 50 workers after occupational exposure to silica. Ann Rheum Dis 52:534–538, 1993.
78. Weill H, McDonald JC: Exposure to crystalline silica and risk of lung cancer: The epidemiologic evidence. Thorax 51:97–102, 1996.
79. Mossman BT, Churg A: Mechanisms in the pathogenesis of asbestosis and silicosis. Am J Respir Crit Care Med 157:1666–1680, 1998.
80. Vallyathan V, Castranova V, Pack D: Freshly fractured quartz inhalation leads to enhanced lung injury and inflammation: Potential role of free radicals. Am J Respir Crit Care Med 152:1003–1009, 1995.
81. Wallace WE, Keane MJ, Harrison JC, et al: Surface properties of silica in mixed dusts. *In* Castranova V, Vallyathan V, Wallace WE (eds): Silica and Silica-Induced Disease. Boca Raton: CRC Press, 1995, pp 107–117.
82. Velan GM, Kumar RK, Cohen DD: Pulmonary inflammation and fibrosis following subacute inhalational exposure to silica: Determinants of progression. Pathology 25:282–290, 1993.
83. Vanhée D, Gosset P, Boitelle A, et al: Cytokines and cytokine network in silicosis and coalworkers pneumoconiosis. Eur Respir J 8:834–842, 1995.
84. Williams AO, Knapton AD, Saffiotti U: Growth factors and gene expression in silica-induced fibrogenesis and carcinogenesis. Appl Occup Environ Hyg 10:1089–1098, 1995.
85. Suzuki N, Horiuchi T, Ohta K: Mast cells are essential for the full development of silica-induced pulmonary inflammation: A study with mast cell-deficient mice. Am J Respir Cell Mol Biol 9:475–483, 1993.
86. Kreiss K, Danilovs JA, Newman LS: Histocompatibility antigens in a population based silicosis series. Br J Ind Med 46:364–369, 1989.
87. Koskinen H, Tilikainen A, Nordman H: Increased prevalence of HLA-Aw19 and of the phenogroup Aw19,B18 in advanced silicosis. Chest 83:848–852, 1983.
88. Ohtsuka Y, Munakata M, Ukita H, et al: Increased susceptibility to silicosis and TNF-alpha production in C57BL/6J mice. Am J Respir Crit Care Med 152:2144–2149, 1995.
89. International Agency for Research in Cancer [IARC]: Silica, Some Silicates, Coal Dust and Para-aramid Fibers. Lyon, France: IARC, 1996.
90. Infante-Rivard C, Armstrong B, Ernst P, et al: Descriptive study of prognostic factors influencing survival of compensated silicotic patients. Am Rev Respir Dis 144:1070–1074, 1991.
91. Ng T-P, Chan S-L, Lam K-P: Radiological progression and lung function in silicosis: A ten year follow up study. BMJ 295:164–168, 1987.
92. Cowie RL: The influence of silicosis on deteriorating lung function in gold miners. Chest 113:340–343, 1998.
93. Steenland K, Brown D: Mortality study of gold miners exposed to silica and nonasbestiform amphibole minerals: An update with 14 more years follow-up. Am J Ind Med 27:217–229, 1995.
94. Goldsmith DF, Beaumont JJ, Morrin LA, et al: Respiratory cancer and other chronic disease mortality among silicotics in California. Am J Ind Med 28:459–467, 1995.
95. Ng TP, Chan SL, Lee J: Predictors of mortality in silicosis. Respir Med 86:115–119, 1992.
96. Anonymous: Silicosis deaths in young adults—United States, 1968–1994. MMWR Morb Mortal Wkly Rep 47:331–335, 1998.
97. Rosenman KD, Reilly MJ, Kalinowski DJ, et al: Silicosis in the 1990's. Chest 111:779–786, 1997.
98. Hughes JM: Radiographic evidence of silicosis in relation to silica exposure. Appl Occup Environ Hyg 10:1064–1069, 1995.
99. Muir DCF, Shannon HS, Julian JA, et al: Silica exposure and silicosis among Ontario hardrock miners: I. Methodology. Am J Ind Med 16:5–11, 1989.
100. Moore E, Martin JR, Edwards EG, et al (eds): Dust Exposure Indices at the Earliest Appearance of Pneumoconiosis: VIIth International Pneumoconiosis Conference, Pittsburgh, 1988. Part I, Publication No. 90-108. US Department of Health and Human Services (NIOSH), Washington, DC: 1990, pp 672–677.
101. Sluis-Cremer GK: Active pulmonary tuberculosis discovered at post-mortem examinations of the lungs of black miners. Br J Dis Chest 74:374–378, 1980.
102. Cowie RL: The five ages of pulmonary tuberculosis and the South African goldminer. S Afr Med J 76:566–567, 1989.
103. Sherson D, Lander F: Morbidity of pulmonary tuberculosis among silicotic and nonsilicotic foundry workers in Denmark. J Occup Med 32:110–113, 1990.
104. Perriens JH, Colebunders RL, Karahungu C, et al: Increased mor-

tality and treatment failure rate amongst human immunodeficiency (HIV) seropositive compared with HIV seronegative patients with pulmonary tuberculosis treated with "standard" chemotherapy in Kinshasa, Zaire. Am Rev Respir Dis 144:750–755, 1991.
105. Guthui W, Nunn P, Juma E, et al: Cohort study of HIV-positive and HIV-negative tuberculosis, Nairobi, Kenya: Comparison of bacteriological results. Tuberc Lung Dis 73:203–209, 1992.
106. Heppleston AG: Silica pneumoconiosis and carcinoma of the lung. Am J Ind Med 7:285–294, 1985.
107. Weill H, McDonald JC: Exposure to crystalline silica and risk of lung cancer: The epidemiologic evidence. Thorax 51:97–102, 1996.
108. Amandus HE, Shy C, Wing S, et al: Silicosis and lung cancer in North Carolina dusty trades workers. Am J Ind Med 20:57–70, 1991.
109. Pairon JC, Brochard P, Jaurand MC, et al: Silica and lung cancer: A controversial issue. Eur Respir J 4:730–744, 1991.
110. International Agency for Research in Cancer [IARC]: Silica, Some Silicates, Coal Dust and Para-aramid Fibrils, Scientific Publication No. 68. Lyon, France: IARC, 1996.
111. Hessel PA, Sluis-Cremer GK, Hnizdo E: Case-control study of silicosis, silica exposure, and lung cancer in white South African gold miners. Am J Ind Med 10:57–62, 1986.
112. Cowie RL: Pulmonary dysfunction in gold miners with reactive airways. Br J Ind Med 46:873–876, 1989.
113. Cahill BC, Harmon KR, Shumway S, et al: Tracheobronchial obstruction due to silicosis. Am Rev Respir Dis 145:719–721, 1992.
114. Bégin R, Ostiguy G, Cantin A, et al: Lung function in silica-exposed workers: A relationship to disease severity assessed by CT scan. Chest 94:539–545, 1988.
115. Seaton A: Coal mining, emphysema, and compensation. Br J Ind Med 47:433–435, 1990.
116. Talini D, Paggiaro PL, Falaschi F, et al: Chest radiography and high resolution tomography in the evaluation of workers exposed to silica dust: Relation to functional findings. Occup Environ Med 52:262–267, 1995.
117. Bergin CJ, Muller NL, Vedal S, et al: CT in silicosis: Correlation with plain films and pulmonary function tests. AJR Am J Roentgenol 146:477–483, 1986.
118. Cowie RL, Escreet BC: The diagnosis of pulmonary tuberculosis. S Afr Med J 57:75–77, 1980.
119. Kennedy MCS: Aluminium powder in the treatment of silicosis of pottery workers and pneumoconiosis of coal-miners. Br J Ind Med 13:85–101, 1956.
120. Banks DE, Cheng YH, Weber SL, et al: Strategies for the treatment of pneumoconiosis. Occup Med 8:205–232, 1993.
121. Desmeules M, Dufresne A, Martel S, et al: Whole lung lavage removes dust and inflammatory cells from the lung in silicosis. Am J Respir Crit Care Med 157:A147, 1998.
122. Mason GR, Abraham JL, Hoffman L, et al: Treatment of mixed-dust pneumoconiosis with whole lung lavage. Am Rev Respir Dis 126:1102–1107, 1982.
123. Escreet BC, Langton ME, Cowie RL: Short-course chemotherapy for silicotuberculosis. S Afr Med J 66:327–330, 1984.
124. Cowie RL: Silicotuberculosis: Long-term outcome after short-course chemotherapy. Tuberc Lung Dis 76:39–42, 1995.
125. Lin TP, Suo J, Lee CN, et al: Short-course chemotherapy of pulmonary tuberculosis in pneumoconiotic patients. Am Rev Respir Dis 136:808–810, 1987.
126. Hong Kong Chest Service/TB Research Centre BMRC: A double-blind placebo-controlled clinical trial of three antituberculosis chemoprophylaxis regimens in patients with silicosis in Hong Kong. Am Rev Respir Dis 145:36–41, 1992.
127. Cowie RL: Short course chemoprophylaxis with rifampicin, isoniazid and pyrazinamide for tuberculosis evaluated in gold miners with silicosis: A double-blind placebo controlled trial. Tuber Lung Dis 77:239–243, 1996.
128. American Thoracic Society: Diagnosis and treatment of disease caused by nontuberculous mycobacteria. Am J Respir Crit Care Med 156:S1–S25, 1997.
129. Kleinerman J, Green F, Harley RA, et al: Pathology standards for coal workers' pneumoconiosis. Arch Pathol Lab Med 103:375–385, 1979.
130. Coggon D, Newman Taylor AN: Coal mining and chronic obstructive pulmonary disease: A review of the evidence. Thorax 53:398–407, 1998.
131. Green FHY, Vallyathan V: Coal workers' pneumoconiosis and pneumoconiosis due to other carbonaceous dusts. *In* Churg A, Green FHY (eds): Pathology of Occupational Lung Disease (2nd ed). Baltimore: Williams & Wilkins, 1998, pp 129–207.
132. Lapp NL, Morgan WKC, Zaldivar G: Airways obstruction, coal mining, and disability. Occup Environ Med 51:234–238, 1994.
133. Rudd R: Coal miners' respiratory disease litigation. Thorax 53:337–340, 1998.
134. Coggon D, Inskip H, Winter P, et al: Contrasting geographical distribution of mortality from pneumoconiosis and chronic bronchitis and emphysema in British coal miners. Occup Environ Med 52:554–555, 1995.
135. US Department of Health and Human Services: Work Related Lung Disease Surveillance Report, Publication No. 91-113. Pittsburgh: National Institute of Occupational Safety and Health, 1991.
136. Churg A, Wright JL, Wiggs B, et al: Small airways disease and mineral dust exposure. Am Rev Respir Dis 131:139–143, 1985.
137. Attfield MD, Seixas NS: Prevalence of pneumoconiosis and its relationship to dust exposure in a cohort of US bituminous coal miners and ex-miners. Am J Ind Med 27:137–151, 1995.
138. Bégin R, Cantin A, Massé S: Recent advances in the pathogenesis and clinical assessment of mineral dust pneumoconioses: Asbestosis, silicosis and coal pneumoconiosis. Eur Respir J 2:988–1001, 1989.
139. Shennan DH, Washington JS, Thomas DJ, et al: Factors predisposing to the development of progressive massive fibrosis in coal miners. Br J Ind Med 38:321–326, 1981.
140. Meijers JMM, Swaen GMH, Slangen JM, et al: Long-term mortality in miners with coal workers' pneumoconiosis in the Netherlands: A pilot study. Am J Ind Med 19:43–50, 1991.
141. Miller BG, Jacobsen M: Dust exposure, pneumoconiosis and mortality of coalminers. J Ind Med 42:723–733, 1985.
142. Hurley JF, Burns J, Copland L, et al: Coalworkers' simple pneumoconiosis and exposure to dust at 10 British coalmines. Br J Ind Med 39:120–127, 1982.
143. Robertson MD, Boyd JE, Collins HPR, et al: Serum immunoglobin levels and humoral immune competence in coalworkers. Am J Ind Med 6:387–393, 1984.
144. Yeh Y-B, Lai Y-R: Influence of rheumatoid factor in coalminers' pneumoconiosis in the Fujian Shaowu colliery, South China. Br J Ind Med 47:143–144, 1990.
145. Cockcroft AE, Wagner JC, Seal EME, et al: Irregular opacities in coalworkers' pneumoconiosis—Correlation with pulmonary function and pathology. Ann Occup Hyg 26:767–787, 1982.
146. Becklake MR: Chronic airflow limitation: Its relationship to work in dusty occupations. Chest 88:608–617, 1985.
147. Humerfelt S, Stensvold I, Kvåale G, et al: Respiratory disorders and lung function among men aged 30–44 years in relation to degree of industrialization in 34 municipalities in Norway (abstract). Eur Respir J 3:168s, 1990.
148. Gevenois PA, De Vuyst P, de Maertelaer V, et al: Comparison of computed density and microscopic morphometry in pulmonary emphysema. Am J Respir Crit Care Med 154:187–192, 1996.
149. Love RG, Miller BG: Longitudinal study of lung function in coal-miners. Thorax 37:193–197, 1982.
150. Attfield MD: Longitudinal decline in $FEV_1$ in United States coal-miners. Thorax 40:132–137, 1985.
151. Seixas NS, Robins TG, Attfield M, et al: Exposure response relationships for coal mine dust and obstructive lung disease following enactment of the Federal Coal Mine Health and Safety Act of 1969. Am J Ind Med 21:715–734, 1992.
152. Attfield M, Hodous TK: Pulmonary function of US coal miners related to dust exposure estimates. Am Rev Respir Dis 145:605–609, 1992.
153. Lewis S, Bennett J, Richards K, et al: A cross sectional study of the independent effect of occupation on lung function in British coal miners. Occup Environ Med 53:125–128, 1996.
154. Carta P, Aru G, Barbieri MT, et al: Dust exposure, respiratory symptoms, and longitudinal decline of lung function in young coal miners. Occup Environ Med 53:312–319, 1996.
155. Cooper K, Johnson TP: Exercise capacity in coalworkers' pneu-

moconiosis: An analysis using causal modelling. Br J Ind Med 47:52–57, 1990.
156. Lapp NL, Hankinson JL, Burgess DB: Changes in ventilatory function in coal miners after a workshift. Arch Environ Health 24:204–208, 1972.
157. Hodgins P, Hennenberger PK, Wang M, et al: Bronchial responsiveness and five-year $FEV_1$ decline: A study in miners and nonminers. Am J Respir Crit Care Med 157:1390–1396, 1996.
158. Vallyathan V, Brower PS, Green FHY, et al: Radiographic and pathologic correlations of coal workers' pneumoconiosis. Am J Respir Crit Care Med 154:741–748, 1996.
159. Blanc PD, Gamsu G: Cigarette smoking and pneumoconiosis: Structuring the debate. Am J Ind Med 16:1–4, 1989.
160. Swaen GM, Meijers JM, Slangen JJ: Risk of gastric cancer in pneumoconiotic coal miners and the effect of respiratory impairment. Occup Environ Med 52:606–610, 1995.
161. Jones FL: Rifampin-containing therapy for pulmonary tuberculosis with coalworkers' pneumoconiosis. Am Rev Respir Dis 125:681–683, 1982.
162. Liddell D, Miller K (eds): Mineral Fibers and Health. Boca Raton: CRC Press, 1991.
163. Bignon J (ed): Health-Related Effects of Phyllosilicates. NATO-ASI Series G: Ecological Sciences Vol G-21. Berlin: Springer-Verlag, 1990, pp 1–448.
164. Selikoff IJ, Lee DHK: Asbestos and Disease. New York: Academic Press, 1978, p. 549.
165. Bignon J, Peto J, Souracci R, et al (eds): Non-occupational Exposure to Mineral Fibers, Scientific Publication No. 90. Lyon, France: International Agency for Research in Cancer, 1989.
166. Zwi AB, Reid G, Landau SP, et al: Mesothelioma in South Africa, 1976–84: Incidence and case characteristics. Int J Epidemiol 18:320–329, 1989.
167. Anderson HA, Lilis R, Dunn SM, et al: Asbestosis among household contracts of asbestos factory workers. Ann N Y Acad Sci 330:387–399, 1980.
168. Camus M, Siemiatycki J, Meek B: Nonoccupational exposure to chrysotile asbestos and the risk of lung cancer. N Engl J Med 338:1565–1571, 1998.
169. Health Effects Institute: Asbestos Research: Asbestos in Public and Commercial Buildings. Cambridge, MA: Health Effects Institute, Asbestos Research, 1991.
170. Becklake MR: Asbestosis. *In* Liddell D, Miller K (eds): Mineral Fibers and Health. Boca Raton: CRC Press, 1991, pp 103–119.
171. Copes R, Thomas D, Becklake MR: Temporal patterns of exposure and nonmalignant pulmonary abnormality in Quebec chrysotile workers. Arch Environ Health 40:80–87, 1985.
171a. Moy EV, Christiani DC: A retired shipyard worker with rapidly progressive pulmonary interstitial fibrosis. Environ Health Persp 107:321–327, 1999.
172. Bégin R, Samet JM, Shaikh RA: Asbestos. *In* Harber P, Schenker MB, Balmes JR (eds): Occupational and Environmental Respiratory Disease. St. Louis: Mosby, 1995, pp 293–329.
173. Ernst P, Zejda J: Pleural and airway disease associated with mineral fibers. *In* Liddell D, Miller K (eds): Mineral Fibers and Health. Boca Raton: CRC Press, 1991, pp 121–134.
174. Craighead JE, Abraham JL, Churg A, et al: The pathology of asbestos-associated diseases of the lungs and pleural cavities: Diagnostic criteria and proposed grading schema. Arch Pathol Lab Med 106:544–596, 1982.
175. Dumortier P, Copl L, de Maertelaer V, et al: Assessment of environmental asbestos exposure in Turkey by bronchoalveolar lavage. Am J Respir Crit Care Med 158:1815–1824, 1998.
176. Case BW, Sébastien P: Environmental and occupational exposures to chrysotile asbestos: A comparative microanalytic study. Arch Environ Health 42:185–191, 1987.
177. Green FH, Harley R, Vallyathan V, et al: Exposure and mineralogical correlates of pulmonary fibrosis in chrysotile asbestos workers. Occup Environ Med 54:549–559, 1997.
178. Bouige D: Dust exposure results in 359 asbestos-using factories from 26 countries. VIIth International Pneumoconiosis Conference, Pittsburgh, 1988, Publication No. 88-108, Part 2. Washington, DC: US Department of Health and Human Services (NIOSH). 1990, pp 1059–1064.
179. Meredith SK, Taylor VM, McDonald JC: Occupational respiratory disease in the United Kingdom 1989: A report to the British Thoracic Society and the Society of Occupational Medicine by the SWORD project group. Br J Ind Med 48:292–298, 1991.
180. Provencher S, De Guire L, Labreche FP: Physician based surveillance system for occupational respiratory diseases: The experience of PROPULSE, Québec, Canada. Occup Environ Med 54:272–276, 1997.
181. Malo J-L: Compensation for occupational asthma in Québec. Chest 98:236S–239S, 1990.
182. Becklake MR, Liddell FDK, Manfreda J, et al: Radiological changes after withdrawal from asbestos exposure. Br J Ind Med 36:23–28, 1979.
183. Cookson W, De Klerk N, Musk AW, et al: The natural history of asbestosis in former crocidolite workers of Wittenoom Gorge. Am Rev Respir Dis 133:994–998, 1986.
184. Becklake MR, Case BW: Fiber burden and asbestos-related lung disease: Determinants of dose-response relationships. Am J Respir Crit Care Med 150:1488–1492, 1994.
185. Huuskonen MS: Clinical features, mortality, and survival of patients with asbestosis. Scand J Work Environ Health 4:265–274, 1978.
186. American Thoracic Society: The diagnosis of non-malignant diseases related to asbestos exposure. Am Rev Respir Dis 134:363–368, 1988.
187. Müller NL, Miller RR: Computed tomography of chronic diffuse infiltrative lung disease. Am Rev Respir Dis 142:1440–1448, 1990.
188. Miller A, Lilis R, Godbold J, et al: Relationship of pulmonary function to radiographic interstitial fibrosis in 2,611 long-term asbestos insulators: An assessment of the international labour office profusion score. Am Rev Respir Dis 145:263–270, 1992.
189. Jones RN: The diagnosis of asbestosis. Am Rev Respir Dis 144:477–478, 1991.
190. De Vuyst P, Dumortier P, Moulin E, et al: Diagnostic value of asbestos bodies in bronchoalveolar lavage fluid. Am Rev Respir Dis 136:1219–1224, 1987.
191. Schwartz DA, Galvin JR, Burmeister LF, et al: The clinical utility and reliability of asbestos bodies in bronchoalveolar fluid. Am Rev Respir Dis 144:684–688, 1991.
192. American Thoracic Society: Clinical role of bronchoalveolar lavage in adults with pulmonary disease. Am Rev Respir Dis 142:481–486, 1990.
193. Sébastien P, Armstrong B, Monchaux G, et al: Asbestos bodies in bronchoalveolar lavage fluid and in lung parenchyma. Am Rev Respir Dis 137:75–78, 1988.
194. International Agency for Research on Cancer [IARC]: Monographs on the Evaluation of Carcinogenic Risk of Chemicals to Man: Asbestos (Vol 14). Lyon, France: IARC, 1977.
195. Hughes JM: Epidemiology of lung cancer in relation to asbestos exposure. *In* Liddell D, Miller K (eds): Mineral Fibers and Health. Boca Raton: CRC Press, 1991, pp 136–145.
196. Segarra-Obiol F, Lopez-Ibãnez P, Nicholas JP: Asbestosis and tuberculosis. Am J Ind Med 4:755–757, 1983.
197. International Agency for Research on Cancer [IARC]: Monographs on the Evaluation of Carcinogenic Risks of Chemicals to Humans (Vols 1–29, Suppl 4). Lyon, France: IARC, 1982.
198. International Agency for Research in Cancer [IARC], Kane AB, Bofetta P, et al (eds): Mechanisms of Fiber Carcinogenesis, Scientific Publication No. 140. Lyon, France: IARC, 1996.
198a. Erren TC, Jacobsen M, Pickarski C: Synergy between asbestos and smoking on lung cancer risks. Epidemiology 10:405–411, 1999.
199. McDonald JC, McDonald AD: Chrysotile, tremolite and carcinogenicity. Ann Occup Hyg 41:699–705, 1997.
200. Liddell FDK, McDonald JC: Radiological findings as predictors of mortality in Quebec asbestos workers. Br J Ind Med 37:257–267, 1980.
201. Hillerdal G, Henderson DW: Asbestos, asbestosis, pleural plaques and lung cancer. Scand J Work Environ Health 23:93–103, 1997.
202. Finkelstein MM: Radiographic asbestosis is not a prerequisite for asbestos-associated lung cancer in Ontario asbestos-cement workers. Am J Ind Med 32:341–348, 1997.
203. De Klerk NH, Musk AW, Eccles JL, et al: Exposure to crocidolite and the incidence of different histological types of lung cancer. Occup Environ Med 53:157–159, 1996.

204. Wilkinson P, Hansell DM, Janssens J, et al: Is lung cancer associated with asbestos exposure when there are no small opacities on the chest radiograph? Lancet 345:1074–1078, 1995.
205. Egilman D, Reinert A: Lung cancer and asbestos exposure: Asbestosis is not necessary. Am J Ind Med 30:398–406, 1996.
205a. Nelson HH, Christiani DC, Wiencke JK, et al: k-*ras* mutation and occupational asbestos exposure in lung adenocarcinoma: Asbestos-related cancer without asbestosis. Cancer Res 15:4570–4573, 1999.
206. Becklake MR: Asbestos-related diseases of the lungs and pleura: Current clinical issues. Am Rev Respir Dis 126:187–194, 1982.
207. Karjalainen A, Nurminen M, Vanhala E, et al: Pulmonary asbestos bodies and asbestos fibers as indicators of exposure. Scand J Work Environ Health 22:34–38, 1996.
208. Churg A: Neoplastic asbestos-induced disease. *In* Churg A, Green FHY (eds): Pathology of Occupational Lung Disease (2nd ed). Baltimore: Williams & Wilkins, 1998, pp 339–391.
209. Hughes JM, Weill H: Asbestosis as a precursor of asbestos related lung cancer: Results of a prospective mortality study. Br J Ind Med 48:229–233, 1991.
210. Constantopoulos SH, Dalavango VA, Sakkalariou K, et al: Lymphocytic alveolitis and pleural calcifications in nonoccupational asbestos exposure. Am Rev Respir Dis 146:1565–1570, 1992.
211. Hillerdal G: Pleural plaques and risk for bronchial carcinoma and mesothelioma: A prospective study. Chest 105:144–150, 1994.
212. Stephens M, Gibbs AR, Pooley FD, et al: Asbestos induced diffuse pleural fibrosis: Pathology and mineralogy. Thorax 42:583–588, 1987.
213. Hnizdo E, Sluis-Cremer GK: Effect of tobacco smoking on the presence of asbestosis at postmortem and on the reading of irregular opacities on roentgenograms in asbestos-exposed workers. Am Rev Respir Dis 138:1207–1212, 1988.
213a. Kayser K, Becker C, Neeburg N, et al: Quantitation of asbestos and asbestos-like fibers in human lung tissue by hot and wet ashing, and the significance of their presence for survival of lung carcinoma and mesothelioma patients. Lung Cancer 24:89–98, 1999.
214. McLoud TC, Woods BO, Carrington CB, et al: Diffuse pleural thickening in an asbestos-exposed population: Prevalence and causes. AJR Am J Roentgenol 144:9–18, 1985.
215. Kilburn KH, Warshaw BA: Pulmonary functional impairment associated with pleural asbestos disease. Chest 98:965–972, 1990.
216. Miller A, Teirstein AS, Selikoff IJ: Ventilatory failure due to asbestos pleurisy. Am J Med 75:911–919, 1983.
217. Bourbeau J, Ernst P, Chrome J, et al: The relationship between respiratory impairment and asbestos-related pleural abnormality in an active work force. Am Rev Respir Dis 142:837–842, 1990.
218. Hillerdal G, Ozesmi M: Benign asbestos pleural effusion: 73 exudates in 60 patients. Eur J Resp Dis 71:113–121, 1987.
219. Shore BL, Daughaday CC, Spilberg I: Benign asbestos pleurisy in the rabbit: A model for the study of pathogenesis. Am Rev Respir Dis 128:481–485, 1983.
220. Boylan AM, Rlauuegg C, Kim KJ, et al: Evidence of a role for mesothelial cell-derived interleukin 8 in the pathogenesis of asbestos-induced pleurisy in rabbits. J Clin Invest 89:1257–1267, 1992.
221. Adamson IVR, Bowden DH: Mesothelial cell proliferation is a general response during fibrotic lung proliferation. Am Rev Respir Dis 147:A910, 1993.
222. Chuwers P, Barnhart S, Blanc P, et al: The protective effect of beta-carotene and retinol on ventilatory function in an asbestos-exposed cohort. Am J Respir Crit Care Med 155:1066–1071, 1997.
223. McMillan GHG, Rossiter CE: Development of radiological and clinical evidence of parenchymal fibrosis in men with non-malignant asbestos-related pleural lesions. Br J Ind Med 39:54–59, 1982.
224. Becklake MR, Thomas D, Liddell FDK, et al: Follow-up respiratory measurements in Quebec chrysotile asbestos miners and millers. Scand J Work Environ Health 1:105–110, 1982.
225. Walker AM: Declining relative risks for lung cancer after cessation of asbestos exposure. J Occup Med 26:422–426, 1984.
226. McDonald JC: Health implications of environmental exposure to asbestos. Environ Hlth Perspect 62:319–328, 1985.
226a. Palo J, Hodgson JT, Matthews FE, et al: Continuing increase in mesothelioma mortality in Britain. Lancet 345:535–539, 1995.
227. Cullinan P, McDonald JC: Respiratory disease from occupational exposure to nonfibrous mineral silicates. *In* Bignon J (ed): The Health-Related Effects of Phyllosilicates. Berlin: Springer-Verlag, 1990, pp 161–178.
228. Wegman DH, Peters JM, Boundy MG, et al: Evaluation of respiratory effects in miners and millers exposed to talc free of asbestos and silica. Br J Ind Med 39:233–238, 1982.
229. Landa SK, Schwartz DA: Mica-associated pulmonary interstitial fibrosis. Am Rev Respir Dis 144:718–721, 1991.
230. Hessel PA, Sluis-Cremer GK: X-ray findings, lung function, and respiratory symptoms in black South African vermiculite workers. Am J Ind Med 15:21–29, 1989.
231. McDonald JC, McDonald AD, Sébastien P, et al: Health of vermiculite miners exposed to trace amounts of fibrous tremolite. Br J Ind Med 45:630–634, 1988.
232. De Vuyst P, Dumortier P, Swaen GM, et al: Respiratory health effects of man-made vitreous (mineral) fibers. Eur Respir J 8:2149–2173, 1995.
232a. Rogers RA, Antonini JM, Brismar H, et al: In situ microscopic analysis of asbestos and synthetic vitreous fibers retained in hamster lungs following inhalation. Environ Health Persp 107:367–375, 1999.
233. Gibbs AR, Wagner JC, Churg A: Diseases due to synthetic fibers. *In* Churg A, Green FHY (eds): Pathology of Occupational Lung Disease (2nd ed). Baltimore: Williams & Wilkins, 1998, pp 393–402.
234. Martin JR, Muir DCF, Moore E, et al: Pneumoconiosis in iron ore surface mining in Labrador. J Occup Med 30:780–784, 1988.
235. White N, Ehrlich RI: Regression of polyvinylchloride polymer pneumoconiosis. Thorax 52:748–749, 1997.
236. Kriebel D, Brain JD, Sprince NL, et al: The pulmonary toxicity of beryllium. Am Rev Respir Dis 137:464–473, 1988.
237. Cullen MR, Kominsky JR, Rossman MD, et al: Chronic beryllium disease in a precious metal refinery: Clinical epidemiologic and immunologic evidence for continuing risk from exposure to low level beryllium fume. Am Rev Respir Dis 135:201–208, 1987.
238. Newman LS, Kreiss K: Nonoccupational beryllium disease masquerading as sarcoidosis: identification by blood lymphocyte proliferative response to beryllium. Am Rev Respir Dis 145:1212–1214, 1992.
238a. Sanderson WT, Henenberger PK, Martyny J, et al: Beryllium contamination inside vehicles of machine shop workers. Appl Occup Environ Hyg 14:223–230, 1999.
239. Newman LS, Kreiss K, King TEJ, et al: Pathologic and immunologic alterations in early stages of beryllium disease: Re-examination of disease definition and natural history. Am Rev Respir Dis 139:1479–1486, 1989.
240. Kreiss K, Mroz MM, Zhen B, et al: Risks of beryllium disease related to work processes at a metal alloy and oxide production plant. Occup Environ Med 54:605–612, 1997.
241. Tinkle SS, Kittle LA, Schumacher BA, et al: Beryllium induces IL-2 and IFN-gamma in berylliosis. J Immunol 158:518–526, 1997.
241a. Comhair SA, Lewis MJ, Bhathena PR, et al: Increased glutathione and glutathione peroxidase in lungs of individuals with chronic beryllium disease. Am J Respir Crit Care Med 159:1824–1829, 1999.
241b. Fontenot AP, Falta MT, Freed BM, et al: Identification of pathogenetic T-cells in patients with beryllium-induced lung disease. J Immunol 163:1019–1025, 1999.
242. Richeldi L, Kreiss K, Mroz MM, et al: Interaction of genetic and exposure factors in the prevalence of berylliosis. Am J Ind Med 32:337–340, 1997.
243. Kreiss K, Mroz MM, Newman LS, et al: Machining risk of beryllium disease and sensitization with median exposures below 2μg/m³. Am J Ind Med 30:16–25, 1996.
244. Meeting of the International Agency for Research on Cancer Working Group on Beryllium, Cadmium, Mercury and Exposures in the Glass Manufacturing Industry. Scand J Work Environ Health 19:360–363, 1993.
245. Balmes JR: Respiratory effects from hard metal dust exposure. *In* Rosenstock L (ed): Occupational Pulmonary Disease. Occup Med State Art Rev, 1987, pp 327–344.

246. Lison D, Lauwerys R, Demedts M, et al: Experimental research into the pathogenesis of cobalt/hard metal lung disease. Eur Respir J 9:1024–1028, 1996.
246a. Potolicchio I, Festucci A, Hausler P, et al. HLA-DP molecules bind cobalt: A possible explanation for the genetic association with hard metal disease. Eur J Immunol 29:2140–2147, 1999.
247. Moulin J-J, Wild P, Romazini S, et al: Lung cancer risk in hard-metal workers. Am J Epidemiol 148:241–248, 1998.
248. Durand P, Bégin R, Samson L, et al: Silicon carbide pneumoconiosis: A radiographic assessment. Am J Ind Med 20:37–47, 1991.
249. Sprince NL, Oliver LC, Eisen EA, et al: Cobalt exposure and lung disease in tungsten carbide production: A cross-sectional study of current workers. Am Rev Respir Dis 138:1220–1226, 1988.
249a. John I, Ahrens W, Bruske-Hohlfeld I, et al: Occupational risk factors for lung cancer in women: Result of a case-control study in Germany. Am J Ind Med 36:90–100, 1999.
250. Ramazzini B, Wright WC (trans): De morbis artificium diatriba Diseases of Workers The Latin Text of 1733 (revised WC Wright, trans). Chicago: University of Chicago Press, 1940, p. 549.

# 66 Occupational Asthma and Byssinosis

JOHN R. BALMES, M.D., M.P.H.

Introduction
Exacerbations of Preexisting Asthma (Work-Aggravated Asthma)
- Irritant Gases
- Allergens
- Other Stimuli

New-Onset Asthma Caused at Work (Occupational Asthma)
- Pathophysiology
- Clinical Features
- Specific Etiologic Agents
- Diagnosis
- Treatment

Byssinosis
- Pathophysiology
- Clinical Features
- Prevention

Summary

## INTRODUCTION

Workplace exposure is an important cause of both new-onset asthma and exacerbations of preexisting disease. Although the term *occupational asthma* usually refers to new-onset asthma caused by exposure at the workplace, exacerbations of preexisting asthma are a potentially more important cause of morbidity at the workplace because there are more workers with *work-aggravated asthma* than work-caused asthma. Both aspects of the relationship between asthma and the workplace are discussed in this chapter.

An accepted operational definition of occupational asthma is variable airflow limitation and airway hyperresponsiveness due to exposure to a specific agent or to conditions in a particular work environment and not to stimuli encountered outside the workplace.[1] This definition includes no reference to the mechanism of asthma induction (Table 66.1) and therefore includes work-related variable airway obstruction caused by antigen-induced hypersensitivity reactions, pharmacologic effects, nonspecific inflammatory processes, and direct airway irritation. Many investigators, however, would restrict occupational asthma to reversible airflow limitation due to sensitization to a substance encountered at work (i.e., *sensitizer-induced asthma*) that involves a latent period and exclude other types of work-related reversible airflow limitation. This restricted definition would exclude, for example, workers who develop persistent symptoms of asthma and nonspecific airway hyperresponsiveness after short-term, high-intensity, inhalational exposure to irritant materials.[2] The argument is that these patients do not have occupational asthma because their disease occurs almost immediately after exposure (with essentially no latent period) and because they are no more sensitive to the offending agent than are other patients with asthma. The term *reactive airway dysfunction syndrome* has been coined to refer to this condition, but *irritant-induced* asthma is used in this chapter. Work-related variable airway obstruction due to organic dusts such as cotton dust (byssinosis) and grain is also not always considered a form of occupational asthma. Different definitions of occupational asthma may be needed for epidemiologic purposes than for medical-

**Table 66.1 POSSIBLE CAUSES OF OCCUPATIONAL ASTHMA**

| MECHANISMS | EXAMPLES |
|---|---|
| **Without "Sensitization"** | |
| Endotoxin effects | Cotton dust |
| Anticholinesterase effect | Organophosphate pesticides |
| Inflammatory response | Ammonia, chlorine |
| Irritant response | Dusts, fumes, vapors, cold |
| **With "Sensitization"** | |
| ***High-Molecular-Weight Compounds*** | |
| IgE mediated (complete allergens) | Animal, plant, bacterial proteins |
| ***Low-Molecular-Weight Compounds*** | |
| IgE mediated (haptens) | Platinum, antibiotics |
| ?Mechanism | Isocyanates, amines, acid anhydrides, plicatic acid |

legal purposes. A more inclusive definition is appropriate for use in a surveillance system in which identification triggers an investigation or intervention. If prevention of work-related asthma disability and loss of productivity is the goal, the definition of occupational asthma should be broadened to include variable airflow limitation and airway hyperresponsiveness caused or aggravated by exposures at the workplace.

## EXACERBATIONS OF PREEXISTING ASTHMA (WORK-AGGRAVATED ASTHMA)

Asthma is a common disease in the general population (affecting approximately 5%).[3] Because many people with asthma have mild disease and can function normally under most circumstances, every common occupation involves a significant number of workers with asthma. Extreme sensitivity of the airways to chemical, physical, and pharmacologic stimuli is a characteristic feature of asthma. Thus, many agents encountered in the workplace that have little or no effect on nonasthmatic workers can cause pronounced symptomatic airflow limitation in workers with asthma.

### Irritant Gases

Although numerous gases that irritate mucous membranes are commonly encountered in industry, little is known about their effects on airway function in people with asthma. Because regulatory standards for exposure at the workplace, unlike air pollution standards, are generally not designed to protect the most susceptible persons, allowable concentrations of irritant gases in the workplace may be orders of magnitude higher than the concentrations needed to cause exacerbations of asthma. An example is sulfur dioxide ($SO_2$) a highly water-soluble gas encountered in significant concentrations in many work sites. On the basis of data showing little effect of $SO_2$ in concentrations under 5 parts per million (ppm) in people with no pulmonary abnormalities, the current US Occupational Safety and Health Administration (OSHA) threshold limit value for $SO_2$ allows exposure to an average concentration of 5 ppm over an 8 hour workshift. Controlled human exposure studies, however, have shown that in persons with mild asthma, pronounced symptomatic airflow limitation can develop after 5 minutes of breathing concentrations of $SO_2$ of 0.5 ppm or less.[4, 5]

The cellular and biochemical mechanisms by which sulfur dioxide causes bronchoconstriction have not been determined. The bronchoconstrictor response does not seem directly related to the irritant properties of the gas because 0.5 ppm is near the sensory detection threshold for sulfur dioxide. In contrast, exposure to a concentration of formaldehyde that causes marked eye and throat irritation does not cause bronchoconstriction in subjects with asthma.[6] Thus, it is not possible to predict the likely bronchoconstrictor response of workers with asthma to a given irritant without directly studying the effects of that material on asthmatic subjects.

### Allergens

Inhalation of specific allergens is a well-recognized cause of exacerbations of asthma. Allergen inhalation not only causes immediate and late-phase airflow limitation but can also cause an increase in nonspecific airway hyperresponsiveness[7] and may thus increase the overall clinical severity of asthma. Specific allergens are an important cause of new-onset asthma caused by occupation and are discussed later, but they are also an important cause of work-associated exacerbations of preexisting asthma. Animal proteins, encountered by laboratory workers, veterinarians, and farmers, are examples of allergens that have been implicated both in exacerbating existing asthma and in causing new-onset asthma.[8]

### Other Stimuli

Many of the other stimuli known to cause bronchoconstriction in patients with asthma may contribute to work-induced exacerbations of asthma. These include environmental tobacco smoke,[9] exercise, particularly in cold or dry environments,[10, 11] and inhalation of high concentrations of respirable dusts.[12] Viral upper respiratory infection, a common cause of exacerbations of asthma in adults, is a well-recognized occupational risk among teachers and childcare workers. Finally, emotional stress is an important component of many jobs that may contribute to exacerbations of asthma.

## NEW-ONSET ASTHMA CAUSED AT WORK (OCCUPATIONAL ASTHMA)

Although exposure at the workplace has been recognized for more than 250 years as a cause of asthma, the incidence and prevalence of work-induced asthma remain unknown, principally because of the lack of an appropriate reporting system in most countries. The proportion of cases of asthma atrributable to occupational exposure has been estimated at 15%.[13–15] Because asthma is a common disease that often presents de novo in adulthood, the association between onset of asthma and exposure to a specific material in the workplace is often missed. By 1994, about 250 specific agents had been found to cause asthma.[16] With the introduction of thousands of new chemicals into workplaces each year, the list of responsible agents is likely to continue to grow. Some commonly encountered sensitizing agents, such as toluene diisocyanate (TDI),[17] flour,[18] and the dust of the western red cedar,[19] cause asthma in 5% or more of exposed workers.

### Pathophysiology

The mechanism by which previously healthy adults develop asthma is poorly understood. Because many who develop asthma in adulthood do not report a family history of asthma or atopic disease, environmental factors are thought to be at least as important as genetic factors in causing adult-onset asthma. In most patients, these presumed "environmental factors" cannot be identified. Patients with work-induced asthma are a notable exception, and work-induced asthma provides a unique opportunity to study the mechanisms underlying the development of adult-onset asthma in general. For further discussion of the pathogenesis of asthma, see Chapter 39.

## Immunologic Mechanisms

Two observations suggest that immunologic mechanisms play an important role in mediating the effects of many, if not most, of the presently recognized causes of occupational asthma. First, affected workers can develop severe airflow limitation after exposure to extremely low concentrations of the responsible agents. For example, concentrations of TDI under 1 part per billion can cause airflow limitation in patients with TDI-induced asthma, whereas a concentration of 20 parts per billion has no effect in asthmatic patients without a history of exposure to TDI.[20] Second, for some agents, like platinum salts[21] and trimellitic anhydride,[22] the presence of specific IgE antibodies and positive skin-prick test responses to the responsible agent correlates with the presence of asthma in exposed workers. For many of the agents known to cause asthma, however, the correlation between evidence of specific IgE antibody and presence of asthma has been either inconsistent (as is the case with TDI)[23] or nonexistent.

Failure to identify specific IgE antibody could be due to difficulty in identifying the appropriate antigen. This problem is particularly likely for low-molecular-weight compounds with a high degree of chemical reactivity, like TDI. Because these compounds are too small to serve as antigens by themselves, the relevant antigen would be expected to be a complex of the chemical and some tissue protein or perhaps an altered tissue protein. It is therefore conceivable that the antigen itself might be different in different workers with asthma caused by the same low-molecular-weight compound. Nonetheless, the failure to identify evidence of specific IgE antibody in most workers with occupational asthma leaves open the possibility that other mechanisms predominate.

## Airway Inflammation

For discussion of the role of inflammation in asthma, see Chapter 39. Airway inflammation and epithelial injury are prominent histologic features in patients who die from severe asthma. Several inflammatory stimuli, including ozone,[24] respiratory viruses,[25, 26] and inhaled antigens,[7] have been shown to induce airway hyperresponsiveness. These agents also produce morphologic evidence of airway injury and inflammatory cell infiltration.[27, 28] Many of the agents known to cause occupational asthma are chemically reactive materials that can also induce airway injury and inflammation. It has therefore been suggested that acute airway inflammation may contribute to the pathogenesis of occupational asthma.

Studies of guinea pigs have shown exposure to TDI to cause inflammatory cell infiltration, airway edema, and an acute increase in airway responsiveness in guinea pigs.[29, 30] The relevance of these findings to clinical TDI-induced asthma is uncertain. On the one hand, the increase in airway responsiveness reported was short-lived, and the concentration of TDI required was many times higher than the current threshold limit for the workplace. On the other hand, epidemiologic studies have shown that workers exposed to frequent spills of TDI are more likely to develop asthma than are workers not exposed to such spills.[31] In the early 1990s, bronchial biopsy specimens from workers with TDI-induced asthma were reported to show inflammation changes similar to those described in asthma of nonoccupational causes.[32]

Agents encountered in the workplace may cause persistent asthma through the induction of inflammation and through the activation of specific immunologic mechanisms. According to this hypothesis, initial injury caused by the direct effects of a workplace chemical could acutely induce airway epithelial injury and at the same time lead to the production of sensitizing antigens consisting of altered tissue proteins with or without conjugation to the inhaled chemical itself. Subsequent exposure to the same chemical may reinduce or potentiate the inflammatory response, both directly and through specific immune mechanisms, leading to the development of more persistent airway hyperresponsiveness. In addition, airway inflammation can increase epithelial and vascular permeability, thus increasing the access of any antigens formed to relevant effector cells. T lymphocytes may be directly involved in mediating the airway inflammatory response to low-molecular-weight sensitizing agents such as TDI.[33] The recent finding of an association between HLA class 2 genes and TDI asthma also suggests that T lymphocytes are important in the pathogenesis of this type of asthma.[34]

That a single episode of severe airway injury can lead to a persistent asthma-like condition is now fairly well accepted. Approximately 50 years ago, four workers were reported to develop new-onset asthma after exposure to high concentrations of sulfur dioxide gas.[35] Since then, anecdotal reports have described patients in whom the onset of asthma was closely related in time to a single high-dose exposure to one or another airborne irritant.[2, 36, 37] Although these reports suggest that a single massive episode of airway injury might cause persistent asthma, convincing evidence that the patients had normal airway hyperresponsiveness before the acute injury occurred is usually lacking. In fact, data collected on persons with inhalational exposure to a respiratory tract irritant who were referred to a poison control center suggest that preexisting wheezing, smoking, or both, are risk factors for persistent asthma after such an episode.[38] A recently reported case series of patients with irritant-induced asthma also suggested that preexisting atopy is an important risk factor.[39] Still controversial is whether irritant-induced asthma can develop after multiple episodes of exposure rather than after a single high-intensity exposure.[40, 41]

## Relationship to Nonspecific Airway Hyperresponsiveness

As discussed previously, increased airway responsiveness to a variety of chemical and physical stimuli is a characteristic feature of asthma.[3] Nonspecific airway hyperresponsiveness is also present in most patients with work-induced asthma and explains the frequent occurrence of symptomatic episodes of airflow limitation from stimuli outside the workplace. One reported series of workers with asthma caused by exposure to the dust of western red cedar found increased airway responsiveness to methacholine in all 55 workers studied.[42] Moreover, when workers were removed from further exposure to red cedar and studied over the next 1 to 9 years, improvement in airway responsiveness paralleled improvement in the clinical severity of the asthma. Those patients who had no improvement in clinical symptoms also had no improvement in airway hyperresponsiveness, whereas in those whose asthma resolved, airway responsiveness returned toward or into the normal range. These findings have been replicated in other studies and suggest that airway responsiveness is an important marker of the clinical course of occupational asthma, as it is for asthma in general.[43]

Of note, however, are the reports of normal airway responsiveness in workers who clearly have work-induced asthma.[44–46] In some of the workers, airway responsiveness has been shown to become abnormal after repeated exposure to the responsible agent (both in the workplace and in the laboratory) and to return to normal again after a period of days to weeks away from such exposure.[47] These observations suggest that nonspecific airway hyperresponsiveness is not a prerequisite for the development of occupational asthma but rather can result from the effects of the responsible agent on previously normal airways.

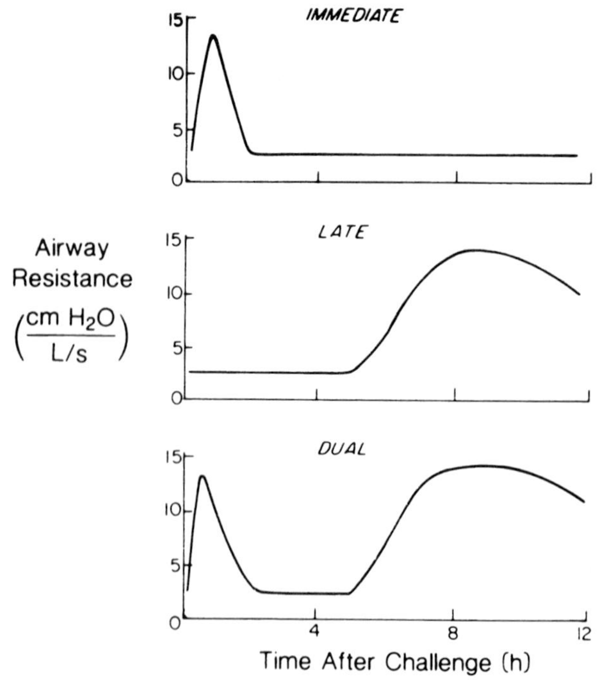


**Figure 66.1** Temporal patterns of increased airway resistance after exposure to agents that cause occupational asthma.

## Clinical Features

A large number of new causes of occupational asthma have been described over the past 20 years, and new chemicals are continually being introduced into the workplace. It is therefore reasonable to assume that many of the agents responsible for occupational asthma have not yet been identified. Furthermore, in many industries workers are exposed to multiple chemicals that can cause asthma, making it difficult to identify the specific chemical responsible for causing asthma in an individual worker. Consequently, the diagnosis of occupational asthma often must be entertained primarily from recognition of the clinical features, particularly the pattern of presentation.

When a worker complains of wheezing and chest tightness occurring primarily at work with improvement during weekends and vacations, most physicians correctly suspect the presence of work-associated asthma. Unfortunately, there are several common variations to this classic presentation that can make the physician's task more difficult. Although asthmatic symptoms often develop immediately after exposure to the responsible agent, immediate symptoms may be minor or even entirely absent, with more pronounced symptoms occurring 4 to 12 hours later. Called the *late asthmatic response,* this pattern (Fig. 66.1) may present with symptoms of asthma occurring primarily in the evenings or on awakening. A dual response (see Fig. 66.1) manifests with symptoms that appear at work, abate, and then recur several hours later. Late and dual responses are more common than simple immediate responses in some forms of work-induced asthma. For example, these patterns occur in up to 80% of workers with asthma caused by dust of the western red cedar.[42] Occasionally, a single exposure to the offending agent can cause repeated asthmatic reactions over several days.[48]

Wheezing is the most widely recognized symptom of asthma, but many workers initially complain primarily of a cough that may or may not be productive.[49] Because coughing is often the earliest symptom of asthma, recognition of this symptom may be important in early diagnosis. As in nonoccupational asthma, rhinitis may precede the onset of work-induced asthma by months or years. Because cough and rhinitis are both common symptoms of other disorders (such as bronchitis and viral upper respiratory infections), their significance is often overlooked. It is important to remember that asthma-induced coughing may be productive of purulent-appearing sputum due to the airway inflammation that is characteristic of the disease. As a result, patients with occupational asthma are often initially misdiagnosed as having recurrent infectious bronchitis. Methacholine or histamine challenge can be useful in supporting the correct diagnosis of asthma in such patients.

Multiple studies suggest that asthma initially caused by workplace exposure can persist for many years after exposure ceases and that the likelihood of persistent asthma increases with an increased duration of symptoms.[43, 50–53] In fact, complete resolution of asthma after exposure ceases may be the exception rather than the rule. Early diagnosis and the removal of affected workers are thus important in preventing long-term morbidity. Serial bronchial biopsies have documented a decrease in subepithelial fibrosis (i.e., airway remodeling) after long-term removal from exposure in TDI-sensitized patients.[54] The early use of inhaled steroid medication may improve the prognosis for resolution of clinical asthma.[55]

Another important and often unrecognized feature of work-induced asthma is that the disease usually does not develop until after relatively long periods from the onset of exposure. In fact, for many agents the incidence of asthma increases with the duration of exposure.[56]

## Specific Etiologic Agents

The large number of agents thus far known to cause occupational asthma through "sensitization" are often divided into two broad categories: low-molecular-weight chemicals and high-molecular-weight (>5 kd) organic materials. It has been assumed that exposure to animals, plants, and their degradation products causes asthma on an antibody-mediated basis because dusts derived from whole plants and animals contain numerous proteins large enough to serve as complete antigens. This assumption is not always correct because these dusts may also contain low-molecular-weight chemicals that can also cause asthma. A partial list of occupational agents known to cause asthma is presented in Table 66.2. The following examples illustrate some important features of occupational asthma due to low-molecular-weight chemicals.

### Western Red Cedar

Inhalation of wood dust is a common cause of asthma among carpenters and sawmill workers. The best-studied causative agent is the dust of the western red cedar *(Thuja plicata),* which has been reported to cause asthma in 5% to 24% of exposed workers.[19, 42, 56, 57] The causative agent in western red cedar appears to be plicatic acid because the inhalation of this chemical causes the same pattern of airflow limitation in affected workers as does inhalation of crude dust. As with a number of other types of work-induced asthma, most affected workers have no history of atopy and skin-test reactivity, and the presence of specific antibodies have not been well correlated with the development of asthma.[57] Long-term follow-up studies have shown that in 50% or more of affected workers symptoms of asthma and nonspecific airway hyperresponsiveness may not improve even after several years away from the offending agent.[51]

### Toluene Diisocyanate

The isocyanates are an important family of chemicals with wide industrial application. In particular, isocyanates are used to make polyurethane plastics, which are almost ubiquitous in modern society. Automobile seat and furniture cushions, automobile dashboards and bumpers, automobile paints, furniture, and floor coatings are just a few examples of the products now commonly made of polyurethane. The isocyanate that previously was most often used to make polyurethane, TDI, has been the focus of extensive research in both laboratory and field studies. Like western red cedar, TDI causes asthma in 5% or more of exposed workers.

In high concentrations, TDI is quite irritating to exposed mucous membranes, and workers with chronic exposure who do not appear to be "sensitized" have been observed to have accelerated annual rates of decline in ventilatory function.[58] In contrast, the concentration range required to cause airflow limitation in some sensitized workers (<0.001 ppm) is orders of magnitude lower. As noted earlier, airway inflammation and nonspecific airway hyperresponsiveness have been induced in guinea pigs after single short-term exposure to TDI at a concentration of 3 ppm, suggesting that immunologic sensitization is not the only etiologic factor.[29, 30] There is also evidence from this guinea pig model[59] and from other in vitro experiments[60] that TDI may trigger bronchoconstriction and nonspecific airway hyperresponsiveness by stimulating capsaicin-sensitive nerves in the airways, leading to the release of potent small peptides (tachykinins).

Like a number of other low-molecular-weight compounds that cause asthma (e.g., phthalic anhydride and trimellitic anhydride), TDI is chemically highly reactive, and its irritant properties are thought to be related to its ability to denature biomolecules. It is possible that such a low-molecular-weight compound, too small to act as a complete antigen, may damage airway cellular proteins and thus secondarily lead to immunologic sensitization to complexes of the chemical with endogenous proteins or to the altered protein itself.[61] TDI is usually only one of many chemicals used in a production process. As such, identification of TDI as the agent responsible for asthma in an individual worker often requires a well-informed worker, a careful history, and thorough exposure assessment of the workplace (including review of material safety data sheets, contacts with the employer and suppliers, and industrial hygiene evaluation).

The widespread use of TDI has led to the recognition of TDI-induced asthma in people who never worked directly with the chemical. One such episode involved a group of office workers exposed to TDI from their office ventilation system, the intake of which was near the exhaust from an adjacent factory.[62] Another report was of police officers accidentally exposed to TDI.[63] Individual cases of TDI-induced asthma have also been identified in people who encountered the material through home use of polyurethane foam[64] or dipping polyurethane-coated wire into solder during electronics assembly home piecework.[65] Because of the health risks associated with TDI, other isocyanate compounds have been used in the manufacture of polyurethane products, such as methylene diphenyl diisocyanate, hexamethylene diisocyanate, and naphthylene diisocyanate. Although it is sometimes alleged that these other isocyanates are less likely to cause occupational asthma than TDI, multiple studies and case reports suggest otherwise.[58, 61]

### Trimellitic Anhydride

Trimellitic anhydride (TMA), another low-molecular-weight compound, is widely used in the manufacture of plastics and as a curing agent in the production of epoxy resin surface coatings and paints. Occupational exposure to this chemical has been reported to cause both immediate and late asthmatic responses.[22] Workers exposed to high concentrations of TMA can also develop a systemic illness characterized by hemoptysis, restrictive lung disease, and anemia.[22, 66] Like TDI, TMA is severely irritating in high concentrations and can cause lacrimation and rhinorrhea in previously unexposed workers.[67] Present

**Table 66.2** SUSPECTED CAUSES OF OCCUPATIONAL ASTHMA

| Material | Industry or Occupation at Risk |
|---|---|
| **Low-Molecular-Weight Chemicals** | |
| ***Isocyanates*** | |
| Toluene diisocyanate | Polyurethane, insulators, laminators, roofers |
| Diphenylmethane diisocyanate | Laminators, polyurethane foam |
| Hexamethylene diisocyanate | Painters, plastics |
| Naphthalene diisocyanate | Chemists, rubber workers |
| ***Anhydrides*** | |
| Trimellitic anhydride | Chemical workers |
| Phthalic anhydride | Paint, plastics |
| Hexahydrophthalic anhydride | Epoxy resins |
| Tetrachlorophthalic anhydride | Epoxy resins |
| ***Metals*** | |
| Chromium | Chrome platers, welders |
| Platinum | Platinum refiners |
| Nickel | Nickel platers, welders |
| Cobalt | Tool grinders, diamond polishers |
| Aluminum? | Aluminum pot-room workers |
| ***Drugs*** | |
| Benzyl penicillin | Pharmaceuticals |
| Ampicillin | Pharmaceuticals |
| Sulfathiazole | Pharmaceuticals |
| Tetracycline | Pharmaceuticals |
| Psyllium | Pharmaceuticals |
| Methyldopa | Pharmaceuticals |
| Salbutamol | Pharmaceuticals |
| Piperazine dihydrochloride | Pharmaceuticals |
| Chloramine T | Pharmaceuticals, laboratory workers |
| Organophosphates | Farm workers, pesticide formulators, fumigators |
| ***Miscellaneous Chemicals*** | |
| Formaldehyde | Laboratory workers, embalmers, insulators, textile workers |
| Glutaraldehyde | Hospital staff (disinfection) |
| Dimethylethanolamine | Paint sprayers |
| Ethylenediamine | Rubber workers, photographic processors |
| Persulfate salts | Chemical workers, beauticians |
| Ethylene oxide | Medical sterilizers |
| Pyrethrin | Fumigators |
| Ammonium thioglycolate | Beauticians |
| Monoethanolamine | Beauticians |
| Hexamethylenamine | Beauticians |
| Polyvinyl chloride vapor | Meat wrappers |
| Aminoethylethanolamine | Aluminum soldering |
| **High-Molecular-Weight Organic Materials** | |
| ***Animals*** | |
| Domestic animals | Farmers, veterinarians, meat processors |
| Birds | Poultry breeders, bird fanciers |
| Bats, mice, guinea pigs | Laboratory workers |
| Sea squirt | Oyster farmers |
| Fish (glue) | Bookbinders, postal workers |
| Silkworms | Silk sericulturers |
| Grain mites, weevils | Grain mill and storage workers, bakers |
| Prawns | Processors |
| Crabs | Processors |
| ***Plants*** | |
| Wheat | Farmers, grain handlers |
| Buckwheat | Bakers |
| Grain dust | Farmers, grain handlers, bakers |
| Rye flour | Bakers |
| Hops | Brewers |
| Tamarind seeds | Millers, spice processors |
| Castor beans | Farmers, castor bean workers |
| Coffee beans | Farmers, coffee bean workers |
| Wool | Textile workers |
| Tobacco dust | Cigarette manufacturers |
| Tea | Food processors |
| Cotton, flax, hemp | Textile workers |
| Latex from natural rubber | Health care workers, food processors |
| ***Vegetable Gums*** | |
| Acacia | Printing |
| Tragacanth | Printing, food processing |
| Karaya | Food processing |
| Arabic | Printing |
| ***Wood Dusts*** | |
| Western red cedar | Woodworkers |
| Cedar of Lebanon | Woodworkers |
| Mahogany | Woodworkers |
| California redwood | Woodworkers |
| Oak | Woodworkers |
| Iroko | Woodworkers |
| Boxwood | Woodworkers |
| Cocabolla | Woodworkers |
| Zebrawood | Woodworkers |
| Mansonia | Woodworkers |
| Mulberry | Woodworkers |
| ***Dyes*** | |
| Anthraquinone | Fabric dyeing |
| Carmine | Cosmetics, dyes |
| Paraphenyl diamine | Fur dyeing |
| Hexafix brilliant yellow | Dye manufacturers |
| Drimaren brilliant blue | Dye manufacturers |
| Cibachrome brilliant scarlet | Dye manufacturers |
| Henna extract | Beauticians |
| ***Fluxes*** | |
| Colophony (soft-core solder) | Solderers, electronics workers |
| ***Enzymes*** | |
| Pancreatic extracts | Pharmaceutical workers |
| *Bacillus subtilis* | Detergent manufacturers |
| Papain | Food processors |
| Trypsin | Plastics and rubber workers |
| Flaviastase | Pharmaceutical workers |
| Bromelain | Food processors |
| Pectinase | Food processors |

evidence suggests that TMA causes asthma by immunologic mechanisms.[22, 67]

A variety of other compounds in the acid anhydride family, including phthalic anhydride, tetrachlorophthalic anhydride (TCPA), hexahydrophthalic anhydride, himic anhydride, and maleic anhydride, have also been shown to cause asthma that is associated with the presence of specific IgE antibodies to protein conjugates.[67] There may be a genetic predisposition to sensitization to TMA, as one study showed an association between sensitization and HLA DR3.[68] Another study of TCPA-exposed workers showed that current smoking status was a significant risk factor for developing both specific IgE antibodies to a TCPA–human serum albumin conjugate and occupational asthma.[69]

## Diagnosis

The most important tool in establishing a diagnosis of work-related asthma is a careful occupational history. The diagnosis of work-related asthma should be considered in every case of adult-onset asthma or aggravation of asthma in adult life. The development of cough, rhinitis, or wheezing (or combinations of these) since the onset of employment, especially if the symptom began after a delay of months to years, should suggests the diagnosis of sensitizer-induced asthma. Work-related conjunctivitis and dermatitis should also prompt consideration of asthma as well. A history of increased symptoms while at work or within several hours after a work shift provides important confirmation. Clear-cut improvement during weekends strongly suggests the diagnosis. Such improvement may not occur if there is chronic airway inflammation as a result of continuous exposure to the sensitizing agent. Improvement with vacations may still occur in this setting. A detailed list of materials encountered in the workplace and in the home workshop may identify a known cause of asthma. A history of atopy is a risk factor for occupational asthma due to high-molecular-weight antigens or haptens that involve IgE-mediated mechanisms, but this is not the case for low-molecular-weight compounds except for acid anhydrides.[70] Smokers may also be at increased risk of asthma due to IgE-inducing agents. Some data suggest that smoking increases the risk of asthma among workers exposed to platinum salts, TCPA, snow crab, ispaghula, and green coffee bean.[70]

Physical examination may reveal wheezing but usually reveals no pulmonary abnormalities if the worker is examined long after the causative workplace exposure. Spirometry carried out before and after a work shift can be diagnostic but will miss most late responses. Measurement of peak expiratory flow with a portable peak flow meter, preferably at regular intervals every day (including weekends) for 2 or more weeks, can be quite helpful in establishing the presence of asthma (suggested by a repeated difference of more than 20% between maximal and minimal values on a given day) and the temporal relationship between airway obstruction and work (Fig. 66.2).[71] The major shortcomings of this measurement are its dependence on patient effort and cooperation and its relative insensitivity to the presence of airflow limitation because of the antecedent deep breath (see Chapter 28).

Occupational asthma, like other forms of asthma, is associated with increased nonspecific airway hyperresponsiveness. Measurement of airway responsiveness by obtaining dose-response curves to inhaled methacholine or histamine often helps confirm the diagnosis.[72] Although these tests do not distinguish work-induced asthma from other forms, the finding of increased airway responsiveness is often sufficient to confirm the diagnosis in workers with a strongly suggestive history. Normal airway responsiveness, however, does not rule out work-related asthma.[44–46] In this circumstance, serial measurement of nonspecific airway responsiveness can be quite useful (see Fig. 66.2). A single exposure to the responsible agent often causes an acute increase in nonspecific airway responsiveness that can persist for days to weeks.[45] Thus, an abrupt increase in airway responsiveness in a worker after either workplace exposure or laboratory exposure to a suspected agent strongly implicates that agent as the cause of the worker's asthma.

When the diagnosis still remains in doubt after these investigations or when an agent not previously known to cause asthma is suspected, specific inhalation challenge testing with the suspected agent may be definitive. In general, the diagnosis of occupational asthma can be firmly established when a 20% or greater decrease in $FEV_1$ occurs after exposure to a subirritant level of the suspected agent. Specific challenge testing is often complicated by a lack of precise information about the agent suspected or the dose required to cause airflow limitation. As a result, except for workers clearly exposed to only one material in the workplace (a rare occurrence), negative results should be interpreted with caution.

Specific challenge testing is a formidable undertaking. Because of the possibility of provoking severe bronchospasm, specific inhalation challenge testing should start with a low level of exposure and should only be performed in a well-equipped clinical facility with adequate resuscitation measures at hand. Because late responses are common and may be severe, hospitalization is recommended for observation and treatment after specific challenges. Finally, proof of the validity of specific challenge testing requires inclusion of appropriate control studies.

In workplaces where exposure occurs to high-molecular-weight antigens (and to certain low-molecular-weight haptens) that cause asthma by IgE-mediated mechanisms, skin testing with the specific antigen(s) in question or detection of specific antibodies in serum, or both, can confirm exposure and sensitization. It should be remembered, however, that positive skin reactions and the presence of specific antibodies can occur in exposed workers without asthma.

## Treatment

The cornerstone of management of occupational asthma is early diagnosis and identification of the responsible material or work process. The primary treatment is then avoidance of further exposure. The approach to treatment of occupational asthma may differ depending on its cause. Workers who continue in jobs with exposure to an agent to which they are sensitized tend to develop increased respiratory symptoms, progressive loss of ventilatory

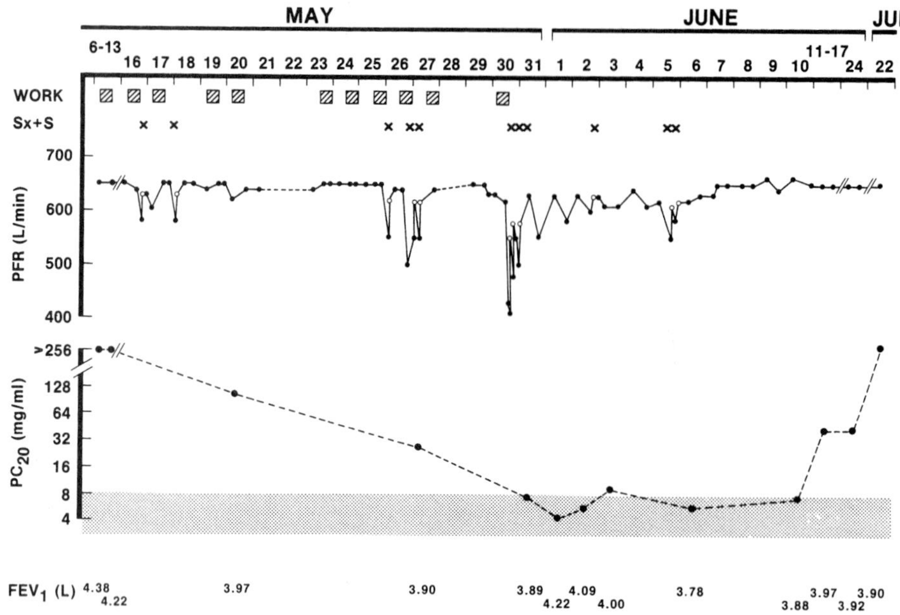


**Figure 66.2** Serial measurements of peak expiratory flow (PFR), $FEV_1$, and airway responsiveness to methacholine before, during, and after periods at work in a worker with toluene diisocyanate–induced asthma. Airway responsiveness is expressed as the concentration of methacholine calculated to cause a 20% fall in $FEV_1$ ($PC_{20}$). Days at work (diagonal lines in boxes) and symptoms (Sx) or the use of inhaled salbutamol (200 μg) (S) are shown at the top. Shaded area at the bottom represents abnormally increased airway responsiveness. Work exposure caused the abrupt onset of symptoms and daily fluctuations in peak expiratory flow. These abnormalities preceded the development of abnormal airway responsiveness. (Courtesy of Dr. FE Hargreave; reproduced with permission from Hargreave FE, Ramsdale EH, Pugsley SO: Occupational asthma without bronchial hyperresponsiveness. Am Rev Respir Dis 130:513–515, 1984.)

function, and increased airway responsiveness.[42, 73] Such deterioration may occur despite suppression of symptoms due to medication, to reduction in intensity of exposure to the sensitizing agent by the use of respiratory protective gear, or to both. Several deaths have been reported among workers with isocyanate asthma who continued to work in jobs with exposure to the agent.[74] On the other hand, personal protective equipment may prevent exacerbations in workers with work-aggravated or irritant-induced asthma.

Because of financial constraints, some patients with occupational asthma cannot leave jobs involving exposure to an agent to which they are sensitized. In such cases, vigorous efforts to reduce exposure to the offending agent are required. Product substitution, enclosure of specific processes, and improved ventilation are preferable to the use of respirators, which are cumbersome and uncomfortable and may leak. If respirators are to be used, however, workers must be medically certified, fit-tested, and properly trained to wear the devices. Careful medical monitoring can help to assess the effectiveness of interventions to reduce exposure.[75] Serial measurement of peak expiratory flow rates can be used to document whether recurrent subclinical airflow limitation is occurring, and serial methacholine challenge can be used to assess whether the level of airway responsiveness is increasing. Patients with deterioration in respiratory symptoms or an accelerated rate of decline in ventilatory function should be strongly encouraged to change jobs. Workers who must leave their jobs because of occupational asthma should be evaluated for degree of disability according to the guidelines published by the American Thoracic Society.[72]

The pharmacologic treatment of occupational asthma is no different than that of nonoccupational asthma. Drug treatment cannot substitute, however, for elimination of exposure in managing occupational asthma.

## BYSSINOSIS

Inhalation of dusts produced by the handling of flax and hemp has been known to cause adverse pulmonary effects for over 250 years. In 1863, acute respiratory symptoms were also described in workers exposed to cotton dust in British textile mills.[76] These symptoms were considered uncommon until the 1950s, when pioneering studies by Schilling and colleagues[77] rekindled interest in the effects of these dusts on the lung.

It is now recognized that inhalation of the dusts of cotton, hemp, flax, and perhaps sisal can produce two distinct patterns of pulmonary response. The best-characterized response is the chest tightness, shortness of breath, or both that occur on the first day of the workweek. Pulmonary function studies have confirmed acute decrements in airway function in affected workers, so the symptoms have been ascribed to bronchoconstriction. Chronic long-term exposure to cotton dust has also been associated with chronic productive cough,[78, 79] an accelerated annual decline in pulmonary function.[78, 80, 81] and respiratory disability.[78] Data from one autopsy series, although based on a small sample, suggest that nonsmoking cotton workers have hypertrophied submucosal glands and goblet cell hyperplasia.[82] Taken together, these observations suggest that long-term exposure to cotton dust can cause a disease resembling chronic bronchitis.

The relationship, if any, between the acute bronchoconstrictor response and this chronic disease remains to be determined. Although one modern study finally confirmed that there is a correlation between the magnitude of acute bronchoconstriction across the workshift and the rate of annual decline in baseline ventilatory function,[83] the use of the term *byssinosis* to describe both responses to vegetable dusts may be misleading.[84, 85]

## Pathophysiology

### Acute Bronchoconstriction

Acute decrements in airway function have been observed during routine workplace exposure to cotton dust in both symptomatic and asymptomatic workers.[86, 87] Qualitatively similar decrements also occur in healthy volunteers exposed to cotton dust in experimental cardrooms.[88, 89] The high prevalence of symptoms and decrements in lung function in workers exposed to crude cotton in cardrooms and the low prevalence of these effects in workers exposed to cleaner-processed cotton suggests that the agent or agents responsible for bronchoconstriction are contained in the cotton bract or trash that contaminates crude cotton rather than in the cotton fibers themselves.[90] Washing or steam-cleaning crude cotton reduces the frequency of bronchoconstrictor responses,[91] suggesting that at least some of the materials responsible are soluble in water. This suggestion was confirmed by the observation that inhalation of an aerosol of water-soluble material extracted from cotton bract causes bronchoconstriction in many normal volunteers.[90, 92] The delayed onset of this response, which is maximal 90 to 120 minutes after exposure, and the tachyphylaxis that occurs with repeated exposure are both features of the bronchoconstrictor response to crude cotton dust.

The nature of the specific component of cotton bract responsible for bronchoconstriction remains controversial. Two separate groups of investigators have shown that the bronchoconstrictor response to cotton dust generated from different batches of cotton in experimental cardrooms correlates closely with the airborne concentration of bacterial endotoxin but not with the concentration of cotton dust.[88, 89] In guinea pigs, inhalation of either endotoxin or cotton dust causes a delayed bronchoconstriction that resembles the pattern of response in humans exposed to cotton dust.[93] Furthermore, the results of at least four studies from Sweden, China, Britain, and Denmark indicate that byssinosis symptoms, baseline $FEV_1$ values, or both among textile mill workers correlate more closely with endotoxin exposure than with dust exposure.[94–97] From these data, some investigators have inferred that endotoxin is the cause of the acute bronconstrictor response to cotton. Another possibility is that bacterial contamination of cotton is a marker for the presence of some other material or materials responsible for causing bronchoconstriction. Inhalation of endotoxin-free aqueous bract extracts has been shown to cause bronchoconstriction in healthy volunteers.[92]

The mechanism by which cotton bract inhalation causes bronchoconstriction also remains undetermined. Extracts of cotton bract stimulate release of histamine from a variety of tissues, including human lung,[98] but the delayed onset of bronchoconstriction and the failure of histamine-receptor antagonists to consistently inhibit bract-induced bronchoconstriction suggest that release of histamine is not the primary mechanism.[99] Pretreatment with cromolyn attenuates the bronchoconstrictor response to extracts of both hemp and cotton dust.[99, 100] This could be interpreted as suggesting that other mast cell–derived mediators might be involved, but the mechanisms of action of cromolyn are poorly understood (see Chapter 11), precluding simple interpretation.

An intriguing hypothesis still largely untested in humans is that the airway obstruction caused by cotton dust inhalation is due to airway inflammation. Cotton dust exposure causes recruitment of polymorphonuclear leukocytes into the airway walls of guinea pigs and hamsters[93, 101] and onto the nasal mucosa of humans.[87] In one guinea pig model, both cotton dust and endotoxin exposures induced increased airway vascular permeability and edema.[93] In a rat model, inhaled endotoxin increased mucous production in nasal and tracheobronchial airway epithelium.[102] Inhalation of cotton bract extract has also been shown to increase polymorphonuclear leukocytes in bronchoalveolar lavage fluid in normal human subjects; the intensity of leukocytosis correlated with the severity of bronchoconstriction.[103] More than one component of cotton bract may contribute to this in vivo recruitment of polymorphonuclear leukocytes, but activation of the fifth component of complement (C5a), one of the most potent chemotactic factors known, appears to play a role. Bacterial endotoxin, although not chemotactic itself, is a potent stimulus to in vivo production not only of C5a but also of interleukin-8, another potent neutrophil chemoattractant. In addition, aqueous preparations of crude cotton dust contain low-molecular-weight substances that are chemotactic for polymorphonuclear leukocytes.[104]

Finally, the chemical components of cotton may cause airway toxicity by additional mechanisms, as through alterations in the function of surfactant or of alveolar macrophages.[105–107]

### Role of Nonspecific Airway Hyperresponsiveness

There is some evidence that acute exposure to cotton dust in naive human subjects induces increased airway responsiveness to methacholine, and it has been suggested that nonspecific airway hyperresponsiveness may be a risk factor for the development of chronic airflow limitation in cotton textile workers.[108] One study of cotton mill workers has shown that workers with byssinosis have increased nonspecific airway hyperresponsiveness compared with nonbyssinotic workers from the same mill and that the cumulative dust exposure was greater among workers with airway hyperresponsiveness.[109] Other studies have reported a significant correlation between responsiveness to inhaled methacholine and responsiveness to cotton bract extract[110] and to cotton dust.[111]

### Chronic Bronchitis and Chronic Airflow Limitation

*Byssinosis* typically refers to the acute bronchoconstrictor response to cotton dust, but there is also considerable epidemiologic evidence of chronic airway responses that may or may not be related to the acute response. Cotton textile workers have a greater prevalence of productive cough than do either community control groups or synthetic textile workers.[80, 81] Although these studies have suggested a relationship between acute chest symptoms and chronic reduction in lung function, none has examined this relationship prospectively. The reported relationship may thus merely reflect an increased prevalence of chest symptoms resulting from reduction in lung function. Weak or absent relationships with cumulative dust exposure, average dust concentration, or length of exposure have been found for bronchitic symptoms and for the annual decline in $FEV_1$.

One study reported significantly greater annual declines in $FEV_1$ in active and retired cotton textile workers than in control subjects in the community, but no dose-response analysis was presented.[78] Most dose response data have come from cross-sectional studies of the acute response. Several reports have provided evidence of a chronic effect of cotton dust on ventilatory function at both high and low dust levels.[83, 112] Longitudinal studies conducted in India, China, and Yugoslavia, where workers were exposed to high concentrations of cotton dust, indicate a clear risk of accelerated loss of lung function.[113–115] Despite the fact that the current US Occupational Safety and Health Administration (OSHA) limits for permissible exposure for US cotton textile mills appear to prevent acute bronchoconstrictor responses, one longitudinal study suggests that a risk for accelerated loss of lung function remains, especially for those workers who also smoke.[112]

## Clinical Features

The diagnosis of byssinosis has traditionally been based on its typical clinical features, especially the history of chest tightness or shortness of breath, or both, that is most prominent on the first day of the workweek in a worker who is exposed to the dust of crude cotton, hemp, flax, or sisal. Workers involved in the initial steps of processing raw cotton, such as opening and carding, have a higher likelihood of developing these symptoms than do workers involved in winding and spinning. Workers exposed solely to finished cotton fabric do not develop this disorder. Documentation of an acute decrement in lung function over a workshift or after exposure to the relevant dust is useful for confirming that the symptoms are due to airway obstruction, but the sensitivity of such a finding has not been evaluated and is likely to be low. Furthermore, it is not clear what degree of decrement in various lung function tests should be considered abnormal. The cotton dust standard adopted by OSHA considers a cross-workshift fall in $FEV_1$ of 5% or 200 mL, whichever is less, to be suggestive of byssinosis. These changes, however, have been shown to be within the expected cross-workshift variation in $FEV_1$ for some workers. Use of this standard thus may be prudent for identifying possible adverse working conditions in cotton-processing plants but can be misleading in identifying significant bronchoconstriction in an individual patient.

As in workers with suspected occupational asthma, chest radiographs and physical examinations usually reveal no abnormalities. For workers who complain of dyspnea, screening pulmonary function tests should include measurement of lung volumes and diffusing capacity in addition to spirometry. Pulmonary function impairment in workers with chronic disease would be expected to resemble that seen in other patients with chronic bronchitis and may involve an increase in residual volume, a decrease in expiratory flow rates, or both. A large reduction in diffusing capacity or in total lung capacity suggests an alternative diagnosis.

## Prevention

Three general approaches to prevention of byssinosis have been proposed. The first is replacement of cotton by synthetic fibers. Although this replacement is occurring to some degree in Europe and the United States, worldwide cotton production continues to increase. A second, more practical approach to prevention is the use of engineering improvements to enclose dusty operations, such as cotton gins and opening, mixing, and carding machines. This approach also requires efficient dust removal from equipment, mill floors, and work surfaces. High-speed carding machines have increased the demand on ventilation systems by increasing the dust output. Nonetheless, the only important impediment to instituting engineering controls is cost. The third major strategy for prevention involves treating cotton plants or raw cotton to eliminate the factor or factors responsible for byssinosis. As noted, washing and steam-cleaning of cotton have been shown to decrease the acute bronchoconstrictor effects of dust inhalation,[91] but those procedures have not been widely instituted. If bacterial endotoxin is proved responsible for these effects, other measures designed to decrease bacterial contamination might prove effective in preventing them.

Medical surveillance of all workers employed in potentially dusty operations also plays an important role in any prevention strategy. Such surveillance provides a method of monitoring the adequacy of dust control and also identifies individual workers who are adversely affected by dust exposure. Surveillance should include an annual respiratory symptom questionnaire and at least annual measurement of spirometry before and after a workshift on the first day of a workweek. The federal OSHA cotton dust standard requires such medical surveillance.

# SUMMARY

Occupational asthma is presently the most common form of occupational lung disease. The prevalence of this disease is likely to remain high for many years, because about 250 industrial agents are known to cause the disease and new chemicals are continuously being introduced into the workplace. The diagnosis is generally established on the basis of a suggestive history of a temporal association between exposure and the onset of symptoms and by objective evidence that these symptoms are related to airflow limitation. Current evidence suggests that early diagnosis, removal from exposure to the responsible agent, and early use of inhaled steroids may play important roles in the prevention of long-term persistence of asthma.

There are two varieties of byssinosis, the disease that results from exposure to the dusts of cotton, hemp, and flax. Acute exposure causes chest tightness from bronchoconstriction. Long-term exposure causes a disease that resembles chronic bronchitis. A relationship between the acute and chronic responses is not fully established. Avoidance of exposure by dust control measures is the best way to prevent the disease. Surveillance of workers is now obligatory in the United States.

## References


1. Bernstein IL, Chan-Yeung M, Malo J-L, et al: Definition and classification of asthma. *In* Bernstein IL, Chan-Yeung M, Malo J-L, et al (eds): Asthma in the Workplace. New York: Marcel Dekker, 1999, pp 1–3.
2. Brooks SM, Weiss MA, Bernstein IL: Reactive airways dysfunction syndrome (RADS). Persistent asthma syndrome after high level irritant exposure. Chest 88: 376–384, 1985.
3. National Asthma Education and Prevention Program Expert Panel Report 2: Guidelines for the diagnosis and management of asthma. Bethesda: U.S. Department of Health and Human Services (NHLBI), publication 97-4051, 1997, p xiii.
4. Horstman DH, Seal E, Folinsbee LJ, et al: The relationship between exposure duration and sulfur dioxide–induced bronchoconstriction in asthmatic subjects. Am Ind Hyg Assoc J 49:38–47, 1988.
5. Balmes JR, Fine JM, Sheppard D: Symptomatic bronchoconstriction after short-term inhalation of sulfur dioxide. Am Rev Respir Dis 136:1117–1121, 1987.
6. Sheppard D, Eschenbacher WL, Epstein J: Lack of bronchomotor response to up to 3 ppm formaldehyde in subjects with asthma. Environ Res 35:133–139, 1984.
7. Cockcroft DW, Ruffin RE, Dolovich J, et al: Allergen-induced increase in non-allergic bronchial reactivity. Clin Allergy 7:503–513, 1977.
8. Cockcroft A, Edwards J, McCarthy P, et al: Allergy in laboratory animal workers. Lancet 1:827–830, 1981.
9. Nadel JA, Comroe JH: Acute effects of inhalation of cigarette smoke on airway conductance. J Appl Physiol 16:713–716, 1961.
10. Deal EC, McFadden ER, Ingram RH, et al: Role of respiratory heat exchange in production of exercise-induced asthma. J Appl Physiol 46:467–475, 1979.
11. Sheppard D, Eschenbacher WL: Airway drying as a stimulus to exercise-induced bronchoconstriction. J Allergy Clin Immunol 73:640–643, 1984.
12. Widdicombe JG, Kent DC, Nadel JA: Mechanism of bronchoconstriction during inhalation of dust. J Appl Physiol 17:613–616, 1962.
13. Blanc P: Occupational asthma in a national disability survey. Chest 92:613–617, 1987.
14. Blanc PD, Cisternas M, Smith S, et al: Occupational asthma in a community-based survey of adult asthma. Chest 109:56–57s, 1996.
15. Blanc PD, Eisner MD, Israel L, et al: The association between occupation and asthma in general medical practice. Chest 115:1259–1264, 1999.
16. Chan-Yeung M, Malo J-L: Etiologic agents in occupational asthma. Eur Respir J 7:346–371, 1994.
17. Butcher BT, Jones RN, O'Neil CE, et al: Longitudinal study of workers employed in the manufacture of toluene-diisocyanate. Am Rev Respir Dis 116:411–421, 1977.
18. Armentia A, Martin-Santos JM, Quintero A, et al: Bakers' asthma: Prevalence and evaluation of immunotherapy with a wheat flour extract. Ann Allergy 65:265–272, 1990.
19. Siracusa A, Kennedy SM, DyBuncio A, et al: Prevalence and predictors of asthma in working groups in British Columbia. Am J Ind Med 28:411–423, 1995.
20. Newman-Taylor AJ: Occupational asthma. Postgrad Med J 64:505–510, 1988.
21. Cromwell O, Pepys J, Parish WE, et al: Specific IgE antibodies to platinum salts in sensitized workers. Clin Allergy 9:109–117, 1979.
22. Grammar LC, Shaughnessy MA, Henderson J, et al: A clinical and immunologic study of workers with trimellitic-anhydride-induced immunologic lung disease after transfer to low exposure jobs. Am Rev Respir Dis 148:54–57, 1993.
23. Karol MH, Tollerud DJ, Campbell TP, et al: Predictive value of airways hyperresponsiveness and circulating IgE for identifying types of responses to toluene diisocyanate challenge. Am J Respir Crit Care Med 149:611–615, 1994.
24. Golden JA, Nadel JA, Boushey HA: Bronchial hyperirritability in healthy subjects after exposure to ozone. Am Rev Respir Dis 118:287–294, 1978.
25. Empey DW, Laitinen LA, Jacobs L, et al: Mechanisms of bronchial hyperreactivity in normal subjects after upper respiratory tract infection. Am Rev Respir Dis 113:131–139, 1976.
26. Little JW, Hall WJ, Douglas RG, et al: Airway hyperreactivity and peripheral airway dysfunction in influenza A infection. Am Rev Respir Dis 118:295–303, 1978.
27. Marsh WR, Irvin CG, Murphy KR, et al: Increases in airway reactivity to histamine and inflammatory cells in bronchoalveolar lavage after the late asthmatic response in an animal model. Am Rev Respir Dis 131:875–879, 1985.
28. Seltzer J, Bigby B, Stulbarg M, et al: Association between airway inflammation and changes in bronchial reactivity induced by ozone in human subjects. J Appl Physiol 60:1321–1326, 1986.
29. Gordon T, Sheppard D, McDonald D, et al: Toluene diisocyanate–induced airway hyperresponsiveness and inflammation of guinea pigs. Am Rev Respir Dis 132:1106–1112, 1985.
30. Sheppard D, Scypinski L, Horn J, et al: Granulocyte mediated airway edema in guinea pigs. J Appl Physiol 60:1213–1220, 1986.
31. Diem JE, Jones RN, Hendrick DJ, et al: Five-year longitudinal study of workers employed in a new toluene diisocyanate manufacturing plant. Am Rev Respir Dis 126:420–428, 1982.
32. Saetta M, Di Stefano A, Mastrelli P, et al: Airway mucosal inflammation in occupational asthma induced by toluene diisocyanate. Am Rev Respir Dis 145:160–168, 1992.
33. Mapp CE, Saetta M, Maesrelli P, et al: Mechanisms and pathology of occupational asthma. Eur Respir J 7:544–554, 1994.
34. Balboni A, Baricordi OR, Fabbri LM, et al: Association between toluene diisocyanate–induced asthma and DQB1 markers: A positive role for aspartic acid at position 57. Eur Respir J 9:207–210, 1996.
35. Romanoff A: Sulfur dioxide poisoning as a cause of asthma. J Allergy 3:166–169, 1938.
36. Alberts WM: Reactive airways dysfunction syndrome. Chest 109:1618–1626, 1996.
37. Kern DG: Outbreak of the reactive airways dysfunction syndrome after a spill of glacial acetic acid. Am Rev Respir Dis 144:1058–1064, 1991.
38. Blanc P, Galbo M, Hiatt P, et al: Morbidity following acute irritant inhalation in a population-based study. JAMA 266:664–669, 1991.
39. Brooks SM, Hammad Y, Richards I, et al: The spectrum of irritant-induced asthma: Sudden and not-so-sudden and the role of allergy. Chest 113:42–49, 1998.
40. Chan-Yeung M, Lam S, Kennedy S, et al: Persistent asthma after repeated exposure to high concentrations of gases in pulp mills. Am J Respir Crit Care Med 149:1676–1680, 1994.
41. Bherer L, Cushman R, Courteau JP, et al: Survey of construction workers repeatedly exposed to chlorine over a three to six month period in a pulp mill: II. Follow-up of affected workers by ques-

tionnaire, spirometry, and assessment of bronchial responsiveness 18 to 24 months after exposure ended. Occup Environ Med 51:225–228, 1994.
42. Chan-Yeung M, Lam S, Koener S: Clinical features and natural history of occupational asthma due to western red cedar *(Thuja plicata)*. Am J Med 72:411–415, 1982.
43. Chan-Yeung M: Evaluation of impairment/disability in patients with occupational asthma. Am Rev Respir Dis 135:950–951, 1987.
44. Smith AB, Brooks SM, Blanchard J: Absence of airway hyperreactivity to methacholine in a worker sensitized to toluene diisocyanate (TDI). J Occup Med 22:227–231, 1980.
45. Hargreave FE, Ramsdale EH, Pugsley SO: Occupational asthma without bronchial hyperresponsiveness. Am Rev Respir Dis 130:513–515, 1984.
46. Mapp C, Dal Vecchio L, Boschetto P, et al: Toluene diisocyanate–induced asthma without airway hyperresponsiveness. Eur J Respir Dis 68:89–95, 1986.
47. Burge PS: Nonspecific bronchial hyperreactivity in workers exposed to toluene diisocyanate, diphenyl methane diisocyanate and colophony. Eur J Respir Dis 123:91–96, 1982.
48. Zammit-Tabona M, Sherkin M, Kijek K, et al: Asthma caused by dimethyl methane diisocyanate in foundry workers. Clinical bronchoprovocation and immunologic studies. Am Rev Respir Dis 128:226–230, 1983.
49. Cullen MR: Clinical surveillance and management of occupational asthma. Chest 98 (Suppl):196S–201S, 1990.
50. Perfetti L, Cartier A, Ghezzo H, et al: Follow-up of occupational asthma after removal from or diminution of exposure to the responsible agent: Relevance of the length of the interval from cessation of exposure. Chest 114:398–403, 1998.
51. Chan-Yeung M, Lam S, Paggiaro PL: A follow-up of 232 patients with occupational asthma due to western red cedar *(Thuja plicata)*. J Allergy Clin Immunol 80:279–284, 1987.
52. Burge PS: Occupational asthma in electronics workers caused by colophony fumes: Follow-up of affected workers. Thorax 37:348–353, 1982.
53. Lozewicz S, Assoufi BK, Hawkins R, et al: Outcome of asthma induced by isocyanates. Br J Dis Chest 81:14–22, 1987.
54. Saetta M, Maestrelli P, Turato G, et al: Airway wall remodeling after cessation of exposure to isocyanates in sensitized asthmatic subjects. Am J Respir Crit Care Med 151:489–494, 1995.
55. Malo J-L, Cartier A, Cote J, et al: Influence of inhaled steroids on recovery from occupational asthma after cessation of exposure: An 18-month double-blind crossover study. Am J Respir Crit Care Med 153:953–960, 1996.
56. Vedal S, Chan-yeung M, Enarson D, et al: Symptoms and pulmonary function in western red cedar workers related to duration of employment and dust exposure. Arch Environ Health 41:179–183, 1986.
57. Chan-Yeung M: Mechanism of occupational asthma due to western red cedar *(Thuja plicata)*. Am J Ind Med 25:13–18, 1994.
58. Musk AW, Peters JM, Wegman DH: Isocyanates and respiratory disease: Current status. Am J Ind Med 13:331–349, 1988.
59. Thompson JE, Scypinski LA, Gordon T, et al: Tachykinins mediate the acute increase in airway responsiveness caused by toluene diisocyanate in guinea pigs. Am Rev Respir Dis 136:43–49, 1987.
60. Mapp CE, Graf PD, Boniotti A, et al: Toluene diisocyanate contracts guinea pig bronchial smooth muscle by activating capsaicin-sensitive sensory nerves. J Pharmacol Exp Ther 256:1082–1085, 1991.
61. Raulf-Heimsoth M, Baur X: Pathomechanisms and pathophysiology of isocyanate-induced diseases: Summary of present knowledge. Am J Ind Med 34:137–143, 1998.
62. Carroll KB, Secombe CJP, Pepys J: Asthma due to nonoccupational exposure to toluene (tolylene) diisocyanate. Clin Allergy 6:99–104, 1976.
63. Luo J-C, Nelsen KG, Fischbein A: Persistent reactive airway dysfunction syndrome after exposure to toluene diisocyanate. Br J Ind Med 47:239–241, 1990.
64. Peters JM, Murphy RLH: Hazards to health: Do-it-yourself polyurethane foam. Am Rev Respir Dis 104:432–433, 1971.
65. Liss GM, Halperin WE, Landrigan PJ: Occupational asthma in a home pieceworker. Arch Environ Health 41:359–360, 1986.
66. Patterson R, Addington W, Banner AS, et al: Anti-hapten antibodies in workers exposed to trimellitic anhydride fumes: A potential immunopathogenetic mechanism for trimellitic anhydride pulmonary disease-anemia syndrome. Am Rev Respir Dis 120:1259–1267, 1979.
67. Venables KM: Low molecular weight chemicals, hypersensitivity, and direct toxicity: The acid anhydrides. Br J Ind Med 46:222–232, 1989.
68. Young RP, Barker RD, Pile KD, et al: The association of HLA-DR3 with specific IgE to inhaled acid anhydrides. Am J Respir Crit Care Med 151:219–221, 1995.
69. Venables KM, Topping MD, Howe W, et al: Interaction of smoking and atopy in producing specific antibody against a hapten protein conjugate. Br Med J 290:201–204, 1985.
70. Venables KM, Chan-Yeung M: Occupational asthma. Lancet 349:1465–1469, 1997.
71. Burge PS, O'Brien IM, Harries MG: Peak flow rate records in the diagnosis of occupational asthma due to colophony. Thorax 34:308–316, 1979.
72. American Thoracic Society: Guidelines for the evaluation of impairment/disability in patients with asthma. Am Rev Respir Dis 147:1056–1061, 1993.
73. Pisati G, Baruffini A, Zedda S: Toluene diisocyanate induced asthma: Outcome according to persistence of cessation of exposure. Br J Ind Med 50:60–64, 1993.
74. Fabbri LM, Danielli D, Crescioli S, et al: Fatal asthma in a subject sensitized to toluene diisocyanate. Am Rev Respir Dis 137:1494–1498, 1988.
75. Balmes JR: Surveillance for occupational asthma. State of the art reviews. Occup Med 6:101–110, 1991.
76. Leach J: Surat cotton, as it bodily affects operatives in cotton mills. Lancet 2:648–649, 1863.
77. Schilling RSF, Hughes JPW, Dingwall-Fordyce I, et al: An epidemiologic study of byssinosis among Lancashire cotton workers. Br J Ind Med 12:217–227, 1955.
78. Beck GJ, Schacter EN, Maunder LR, et al: A prospective study of chronic lung disease in cotton textile workers. Ann Intern Med 97:645–651, 1982.
79. Merchant JA, Kilburn KH, O'Fallon WM, et al: Byssinosis and chronic bronchitis among cotton textile workers. Ann Intern Med 76:423–433, 1972.
80. Berry G, Molyneux MKB, Tombleson JBL: Relationship between dust levels and byssinosis and bronchitis in Lancashire cotton mills. Br J Ind Med 31:18–27, 1974.
81. Bouhuys A, Schoenberg CJ, Beck GJ, et al: Epidemiology of chronic lung disease in a cotton mill community. Lung 154:167–172, 1977.
82. Pratt PC: Comparative prevalence and severity of emphysema and bronchitis at autopsy in cotton mill workers vs. controls. Chest 79 (Suppl):49S–53S, 1981.
83. Glindmeyer HW, Lefant JJ, Jones RN, et al: Cotton dust and across-shift change in $FEV_1$ as predictors of annual change in $FEV_1$. Am J Respir Crit Care Med 149:584–590, 1994.
84. Tockman MS, Baser M: Is cotton dust exposure associated with chronic effects? Am Rev Respir Dis 130:1–3, 1984.
85. Castellan RM: Cotton dust. *In* Harber P, Schenker MB, Balmes JR (eds): Occupational and Environmental Respiratory Disease. St. Louis: Mosby, 1996, pp 401–419.
86. Zuskin E, Valic F, Butkovic D, et al: Lung function in textile workers. Br J Ind Med 32:283–288, 1975.
87. Merchant JA, Halprin GM, Hudson AR, et al: Responses to cotton dust. Arch Environ Health 30:222–229, 1975.
88. Castellan RM, Olenchock SA, Hankinson JL, et al: Acute bronchoconstriction induced by cotton dust: Dose related responses to endotoxin and other dust factors. Ann Intern Med 101:157–163, 1984.
89. Rylander R, Haglind P, Lundholm M: Endotoxin in cotton dust and respiratory function decrement among cotton workers in an experimental cardroom. Am Rev Respir Dis 131:209–213, 1985.
90. Bouhuys A, Lindell SE, Lundin G: Experimental studies on byssinosis. Br Med J 1:324–326, 1960.
91. Merchant JA, Lumsden JC, Kilburn KH, et al: Preprocessing cotton to prevent byssinosis. Br J Ind Med 30:237–247, 1973.
92. Buck MG, Wall JH, Schacter EN: Airway constrictor response to cotton bract extracts in the absence of endotoxin. Br J Ind Med 43:220–226, 1986.

93. Gordon T, Balmes J, Fine J, et al: Airway oedema and obstruction in guinea pigs exposed to inhaled endotoxin. Br J Ind Med 48:629–635, 1991.
94. Haglind P, Lundholm M, Rylander R: Prevalence of byssinosis in Swedish cotton mills. Br J Ind Med 38:138–143, 1981.
95. Kennedy SM, Christiani DC, Eisen EA, et al: Cotton dust and endotoxin exposure relationships in cotton textile workers. Am Rev Respir Dis 135:194–200, 1987.
96. Cinkotai FF, Rigby A, Pickering CAC, et al: Recent trends in the prevalence of byssinotic symptoms in the Lancashire textile industry. Br J Ind Med 45:782–789, 1988.
97. Sigsgaard T, Pederson OF, Juul S, et al: Respiratory disorders and atopy in cotton, wool, and other textile mill workers in Denmark. Am J Ind Med 22:163–184, 1992.
98. Ainsworth SK, Neuman RE, Hanley RA: Histamine release from platelets for assay of byssinogenic substances in cotton mill dust and related materials. Br J Ind Med 36:35–42, 1979.
99. Schachter EN, Brown S, Zuskin E, et al: The effect of mediator modifying drugs in cotton bract–induced bronchospasm. Chest 79(Suppl):73–77, 1981.
100. Zuskin E, Bouhuys A: Protective effect of disodium cromoglycate against airway constriction induced by hemp dust extract. J Allergy Clin Immunol 57:473–479, 1976.
101. Kilburn KH, Lynn WS, Tres LL, et al: Leukocyte recruitment through airway walls by condensed vegetable tannins and quercetin. Lab Invest 28:55–59, 1973.
102. Gordon T, Harkema JR: Effect of inhaled endotoxin on intraepithelial mucosubstances in F344 rat nasal and tracheobronchial airways. Am J Respir Cell Mol Biol 10:177–183, 1994.
103. Cooper JAD, Merrill WW, Buck MG, et al: The relationship between bronchoalveolar neutrophil recruitment and bronchoconstriction induced by a soluble extract of cotton bracts. Am Rev Respir Dis 134:975–982, 1986.
104. Ainsworth SK, Neuman RE: Chemotoxins in cotton mill dust: Possible etiologic agent(s) in byssinosis. Am Rev Respir Dis 124:280–284, 1981.
105. Bates PJ, Ralston NV, Vuk-Pavlovic Z, et al: Calcium influx is required for tannin-mediated arachidonic acid release from alveolar macrophages. Am J Physiol 268:33–40, 1995.
106. DeLucca AJ, Brogden KA, French AD: Agglutination of lung surfactant with glucan. Br J Ind Med 49:755–760, 1992.
107. Kreofsky TJ, Russell JA, Rohrbach MS: Inhibition of alveolar macrophage spreading and phagocytosis by cotton bract tannin. A potential mechanism in the pathogenesis of byssinosis. Am J Pathol 137:263–274, 1990.
108. Rylander R, Schilling RSF, Pickering CAC: Editorial. Effects after acute and chronic exposure to cotton dust: The Manchester criteria. Br J Ind Med 44:577–579, 1987.
109. Fishwick D, Fletcher AM, Pickering CAC, et al: Lung function, bronchial reactivity, atopic status, and dust exposure in Lancashire cotton mill operatives. Am Rev Respir Dis 145:1103–1108, 1992.
110. Schacter EN, Zuskin E, Buck MG: Airway reactivity and cotton bract–induced bronchial obstruction. Chest 87:51–55, 1985.
111. Jacobs RR, Boehlecke B, Van Hage-Hamstein M, et al: Bronchial reactivity, atopy, and airway response to cotton dust. Am Rev Respir Dis 148:19–24, 1993.
112. Glindmeyer HW, Lefante JJ, Jones RN, et al: Exposure-related declines in the lung function of cotton workers: Relationship to current workplace standards. Am Rev Respir Dis 144:675–683, 1991.
113. Kamat SR, Kamat GR, Salpekar VY, Lobo E: Distinguishing byssinosis from chronic obstructive pulmonary disease. Am Rev Respir Dis 124:31–40, 1981.
114. Christiani DC, Wegman DH, Eisen EA, et al: Pulmonary function among cotton textile workers. Chest 105:1713–1721, 1994.
115. Zuskin E, Ivankovic D, Schacter EN, et al: A ten-year follow-up study of cotton textile workers. Am Rev Respir Dis 143:301–305, 1991.

# 67 Hypersensitivity Pneumonitis

CECILE S. ROSE, M.D., M.P.H

Introduction
Etiology
- Microbial Agents
- Animal Proteins
- Chemical Sensitizers

Epidemiology
Occupational and Environmental Exposures
Host Factors
Immunopathogenesis
Histopathology
Clinical Features
- Signs and Symptoms
- Precipitating Antibodies
- Other Laboratory Studies
- Physiology
- Radiology
- Inhalation Challenge
- Bronchoalveolar Lavage
- Lung Biopsy
- Diagnostic Approach

Diagnostic Criteria
Natural History and Prognosis
Treatment
- Antigen Avoidance
- Pharmacologic Therapy

Prevention
Summary

## INTRODUCTION

Hypersensitivity pneumonitis (HP), also known as extrinsic allergic alveolitis, constitutes a spectrum of granulomatous, interstitial, bronchiolar, and alveolar-filling lung diseases resulting from repeated inhalation of and sensitization to a wide variety of organic aerosols and low molecular weight chemical antigens. Previously considered a rare disease, increasing recognition of the ubiquity of environmental antigens, more sensitive diagnostic tools, and better understanding of the limitations of precipitin-based diagnosis have shown that HP is more common than previously thought.

The nature of the inhaled antigen, the circumstances of exposure, and the immunologic reactivity of the host all contribute to the risk for HP. Disease typically is characterized by a lymphocytic alveolitis and granulomatous pneumonitis, with improvement or complete reversibility if antigen exposure ceases. Continued antigen exposure commonly leads to progressive interstitial fibrosis. No single historical or clinical feature is pathognomonic for HP. Rather, diagnosis relies on a strong index of suspicion and a constellation of clinical findings. When the diagnosis is suspected, the clinician must undertake appropriate clinical assessment and environmental intervention to prevent progressive, irreversible lung damage.

## ETIOLOGY

The list of specific agents that cause HP is lengthy, and new exposure circumstances and disease entities continue to be described. The distinctive and often colorful disease names for HP can be organized more simply into three major categories of causal antigens: microbial agents, animal proteins, and low molecular weight chemicals (Table 67.1). Most particulate antigens are of respirable size and deposit in the alveoli; some (such as *Alternaria* spores) are deposited in airways and then solubilized. In addition to triggering a T-lymphocyte alveolitis, intrinsic properties of the antigens capable of causing HP include their nondigestibility by alveolar macrophages and their ability to fix complement and act as adjuvants, thereby enhancing lung immune responses and activating inflammatory cells.[1] There are also an increasing number of pharmacologic agents that have been shown to cause hypersensitivity reactions in the lung,[2] but these are beyond the scope of this chapter and are covered under the subject of drug-induced lung diseases.

### Microbial Agents

Microbial organisms, including bacteria, fungi, and amebae, are the most commonly recognized causes of HP. Microbial contaminants are common in indoor environ-

**Table 67.1 ETIOLOGIC CATEGORIES OF HYPERSENSITIVITY PNEUMONITIS, WITH EXAMPLES**

| |
|---|
| Microbial Agents |
| Bacteria |
| *Examples:* Thermophilic actinomyces, *Bacillus subtilis, Klebsiella, Epicoccum nigrum,* nontuberculous mycobacteria |
| Fungi |
| *Examples: Aspergillus, Penicillium, Cladosporium, Trichosporon, Alternaria, Aureobasidium, Cephalosporium* species |
| Amebae |
| Animal Proteins |
| *Examples:* Avian, fish meal, rat urine, mollusk shell, wheat weevil, silkworm larvae |
| Chemical Sensitizers |
| *Examples:* Isocyanates, acid anhydrides, pyrethrum, Pauli's reagent (sodium diazobenzene sulfate) |

ments and probably cause many more cases of HP than are recognized clinically. Warm, moist environments often provide ideal circumstances for the amplification and proliferation of microbial antigens which, if disseminated and inhaled, can cause sensitizing lung disease.

## Bacteria

Bacteria are unicellular prokaryotic organisms with cell membranes but no organized nuclei or membrane-bound organelles. Most bacteria take the form of rods (bacilli), spheres (cocci), or branched filaments (actinomycetes), and are generally 1 to 5 μm in diameter. Bacteria have adapted to a wide variety of ecologic habitats and segregate under different physical and chemical conditions in indoor and outdoor environments.

Thermophilic actinomycetes, including *Saccharopolyspora rectivirgula* (formerly *Micropolyspora faeni), Thermoactinomyces vulgaris, T. saccharii, T. viridis,* and *T. candidus,* are associated causally with the prototypical example of HP, farmer's lung disease (FLD), first described by Campbell in 1932.[3] These bacteria thrive at 50°C to 55°C temperatures and with moist conditions, secreting enzymes that cause decay of vegetable matter such as hay (FLD), sugar cane (bagassosis), and mushroom compost (mushroom worker's lung).[4–6] They often are found contaminating ventilation and humidification systems (humidifier lung) where temperatures reach 60°C and stagnant water is present.[7]

Indoor bacteria that prefer lower temperatures also can cause HP. An outbreak of *Bacillus subtilis* alveolitis occurred in six family members exposed during renovation to contaminated wood dust from bathroom flooring.[8] The gram-negative bacterium *Klebsiella oxytoca* can cause humidifier lung.[9] Two children developed HP after exposure to an unventilated basement shower contaminated with the bacterium *Epicoccum nigrum.*[10] In addition to gram-negative bacteria themselves, endotoxins contained in their cell walls stimulate the cytokines tumor necrosis factor-alpha (TNF-α) and interleukin-1 (IL-1) and may act as adjuvants, enhancing the inflammatory events leading to alveolitis and granuloma formation.[11]

A spectrum of occupational respiratory diseases including HP occurs with exposure to metalworking fluids. A workshop discussing eight clusters of HP in the automotive industry among metalworking fluid-exposed workers concluded that risk for illness exists where water-based fluids are used and unusual microbial contaminants (probably nontuberculous mycobacteria or fungi) predominate.[12] In one study of 30 affected workers in an automobile engine parts manufacturing plant, 7 workers had HP, with 6 exhibiting serum precipitins to *Acinetobacter lwoffi* .[13]

Recreational as well as occupational exposures to bacterially contaminated water aerosols can cause HP. Nontuberculous mycobacteria contaminating hot tubs cause a granulomatous lung disease with features of HP that may resolve simply with removal from exposure.[14, 15] Bacteria contained in water aerosols were associated with an outbreak of granulomatous pneumonitis termed "lifeguard lung" affecting 33 lifeguards in an indoor swimming pool, with increased levels of airborne endotoxin in comparison with unaffected indoor pools.[16]

## Fungi

Fungi are nonmotile, eukaryotic organisms that have rigid cell walls, lack chlorophyll, and reproduce by means of spores, most of which are designed for airborne transport (disseminators). Fungal spores germinate to produce morphologically diverse forms, including molds and yeasts. Molds are branching hyphal filaments; yeasts are round, oval, or elongated single cells that reproduce mostly by budding and form moist or mucoid colonies. The cell walls of fungi contain polysaccharides (including glucan and chitin) and glycoproteins. Many components of fungi are capable of becoming airborne and acting as antigen sources, including fungal spores, mycelial fragments, metabolites and partially degraded substrates, and fungal toxins.[17]

Fungal spore content in air comes mainly from species adapted to using wind energy for dispersal. The particular species and concentration in air at any given time depend on prevailing winds, temperature, seasonal climatologic factors, circadian patterns of sunlight and darkness, degree of precipitation, availability of substrates, and extent of substrate and atmospheric moisture content. Several U.S. studies have shown that *Cladosporium, Alternaria,* and *Basidiospores* are the most common atmospheric spores.[18] Atmospheric mold counts in Canada found *Alternaria, Cladosporium,* and yeasts to be the most numerous molds, with the peak season between July and October. The indoor pattern of fungal spores reflects both the outdoor spore composition and indoor fungal flora dominated by the *Deuteromycetes,* including *Penicillium, Aspergillus, Rhizopus, Mucor,* and yeasts. Among the interior sites for mold growth are garbage containers, food storage areas, wallpaper, upholstery, areas of increased moisture such as shower curtains, window moldings, window air conditioners, damp basements, and emissions from cool mist vaporizers.[18–25] Saunas, hot tubs, and even tap water also may become contaminated with microorganisms capable of causing hypersensitivity lung disease.[26–28]

Many fungal species have been associated causally with hypersensitivity lung diseases in a wide variety of occupational and environmental circumstances. The respirable conidia of *Aspergillus* species are ubiquitous in nature and commonly found in water, soil, and organic debris. A variety of *Aspergillus* species have been associated with HP in diverse occupational settings, including soy sauce brewers, bird breeders, farmers, and compost, sawmill, mushroom, greenhouse, tobacco, cane mill, grain, and brewery workers,[29–33] and in those exposed to contaminated esparto grass used in the production of ropes, canvas, sandals, mats, baskets, and paper paste.[34, 35] Similarly, a number of *Penicillium* species have been associated with HP, including illness in cork workers (*Penicillium frequentans*), cheese workers (*P. casei, P. roqueforti*), laboratory workers, farmers, and tree cutters.[36–40] *P. citreonigrum* and *Monocillium* species contaminating peat moss were associated with cases of HP among workers in a peat moss processing plant.[41] Fatal HP in three Canadian farmers was traced to *P. brevicompactum* and *P. olivicolor* contaminating agricultural dusts.[42] *Alternaria, Cladosporium, Aureobasidium,* and many other fungal species can cause HP. For example, mixed fungal contaminants in wood dust, bark, and chips have caused HP in sawmill workers, tree cutters, and other wood handlers.[43–46]

Fungal antigens often are implicated in HP cases associated with microbial contamination in homes. Summer-type hypersensitivity pneumonitis, the most prevalent form of HP in Japan, is caused by seasonal mold contamination (mainly *Trichosporon asahii*, formerly *T. cutaneum* serotype II) in the home environment.[47] Domestic fungal exposure associated with decaying wood and damp walls in inner city dwellings is the most common cause of HP in Australia.[29] Multiple fungal species were identified in the homes of individuals with disease, including *Serpula lacrymans, Geotrichum candidum, Penicillium* species, *Alternaria tenuis, Fusarium solani,* and *Aspergillus* species, which suggests that sensitizing microbial exposures may be complex mixtures and disease not always attributable to a single, well-defined antigen. Similarly, *Rhodotorula* species, along with *Aspergillus* and *Candida* species, were implicated in a case of HP from a contaminated home ultrasonic humidifier.[48]

### Amebae

Amebae are small, unicellular eukaryotic organisms that constantly change shape through the formation and retraction of pseudopodia. Free-living amebae can ingest gram-negative bacteria and dissolved organic material, protecting bacteria such as *Legionella* from environmental stresses. Amebae are found in water (especially warm waters such as those used in industrial process fluids, hot springs, swimming pools, and industrial eyewash stations), vegetation, and soil. The amebae *Naegleria gruberi* and *Acanthamoeba castellani* have been implicated in HP from exposure to contaminated humidifiers,[49] but their precise etiologic role awaits further clarification.

## Animal Proteins

Particulates from a variety of animal sources can cause HP when inhaled, with exposure to birds the most clinically important and well recognized. HP from exposure to avian antigens, referred to as bird breeder's or bird fancier's lung, was first described by Plessner in 1960.[50] Avian antigens have been demonstrated in the feathers, droppings, and serum of turkeys, chickens, geese, ducks, parakeets, parrots, budgerigars, pigeons, doves, love birds, canaries, and even native birds and are highly immunogenic.[51, 52] Highest exposures are associated with cleaning out bird lofts, cages, and coops. Bird breeder's lung is the more common form of HP in Great Britain, where approximately 12% of the general population keep budgerigars as pets.[53]

Animal handlers, such as laboratory workers, are at risk for HP from exposure to inhaled animal proteins (including rats and gerbils) in pelts, serum, and excreta.[54, 55] Inhalation of grain infested with the wheat weevil *Sitophilus granarius* can cause a form of HP known as miller's lung.[56] Sericulturists engaged in silk production can develop HP from exposure to larval secretions and cocoon particulates.[57] The dust from mollusk shells cut and polished to make buttons caused HP in production workers.[58] An obsolete form of HP, snuff taker's lung, results from sensitization to the bovine and porcine proteins contained in pituitary snuff used in the past to treat diabetes insipidus.[59]

## Chemical Sensitizers

The chemical-induced forms of HP are probably less common than are microbial and animal protein-induced cases, although some of the inorganic antigens that can cause disease are common in industry.

Isocyanates are used widely for large-scale production of polyurethane polymers in the manufacture of flexible and rigid foams, elastomers, adhesives, and surface coatings. Isocyanates, including toluene diisocyanate, diphenylmethane diisocyanate, and hexamethylene diisocyanate, can cause HP in addition to the more common occupational asthma associated with their exposure.[60–62] More recently, exposure to isocyanate prepolymers (having lower vapor pressures and thus believed to pose a lower risk of sensitization than the diisocyanates) was shown to induce an acute HP-like reaction among workers in automobile parts manufacturing.[63] Specific immunoglobulin G (IgG) antibodies to isocyanates have been detected in the serum and bronchoalveolar lavage (BAL) of affected workers,[64, 65] with a $CD8^+$-predominant T-lymphocyte alveolitis.[66]

Trimellitic anhydride used in plastics, paints, and resins has been associated with an HP-like syndrome often accompanied by anemia.[67] Trimellitic anhydride appears to act as a hapten, combining with endogenous proteins to create new antigenic determinants capable of eliciting IgE or IgG responses.[68] Phthalic anhydride emitted from heated epoxy resin or contained in epoxy paints can cause HP.[69] Rare case reports of HP have been described from exposure to the pesticide pyrethrum; from Pauli's reagent (sodium diazobenzenesulfate) used in chromatography; and from copper sulfate used in Bordeaux mixture to spray vineyards.[70–72]

## EPIDEMIOLOGY

The worldwide prevalence of HP is unknown. Most of the population-based studies of HP focus on the prevalence of illness among agricultural workers. Using a questionnaire survey, Grant and coworkers found the prevalence of FLD in three agricultural areas in Scotland to range from 2.3% to 8.6%.[73] A questionnaire survey of western Wyoming dairy and cattle ranchers elicited a history typical of acute FLD in 3% of those surveyed.[74] A study of Wisconsin farmers described a disease prevalence of 9% to 12% in men exposed to moldy hay.[75] A cross-sectional respiratory morbidity survey of mushroom farm workers found that 20% of the heavily exposed workers reported symptoms consistent with mushroom workers' lung.[32] In Finland, data on clinically confirmed FLD showed a mean annual incidence rate of 44 per 100,000 persons in farming,[76] similar to the rate reported in Sweden of 23 per 100,000. Not surprisingly, HP symptom prevalence rates among agricultural workers are substantially higher than disease prevalence rates based on clinically confirmed cases, which reflects the challenges of HP diagnosis. Similarly, reports of disease outbreaks in microbially contaminated office buildings have described widely varying but usually low attack rates, although in some reports up to 70% of exposed individuals are affected.[77]

The prevalence of HP among bird hobbyists is estimated to range between 0.5% and 21% and probably varies depending on exposure circumstances.[78] A cross-sectional study of nacre-button workers found a 23% prevalence of mollusk-shell HP.[79] Prevalence data for HP associated with exposure to animal proteins is less variable than for the microbially induced hypersensitivity pneumonitides, probably because the measurement of serum precipitins is more reliable in these settings for case confirmation.

Fewer data exist on the prevalence of HP in workers exposed to chemical antigens. Using specific inhalation challenge, Vandenplas and coworkers detected diphenylmethane diisocyanate-induced HP in 8 (4.7%) of 167 workers employed in a wood chipboard manufacturing plant.[80] Interestingly, only one of the eight workers worked continuously near the source of diphenylmethane diisocyanate, indicating that intermittent exposures can lead to illness. Affected subjects were identified through workers' compensation claims, undoubtedly underestimating the actual prevalence of HP in the plant.

Reported disease prevalence and attack rates vary widely and depend on the populations studied, the nature and intensity of antigen exposure, the case definition chosen, and host factors that are poorly understood. However, epidemiologic studies of agricultural workers and bird fanciers suggest that HP may be quite common in some high-risk occupational settings.

## OCCUPATIONAL AND ENVIRONMENTAL EXPOSURES

Although acute symptoms often are attributed to intense, intermittent antigen exposure and chronic forms of HP are thought to result from lower-level, more prolonged exposure, the paucity of environmental exposure data provides little insight into dose-response relationships. Understanding of these relationships is further complicated by the fact that the latency period between exposure to an environmental antigen and onset of HP symptoms may vary from a few weeks to years.

Environmental risk factors, including antigen concentration, duration of exposure before onset of symptoms, frequency and intermittency of exposure, particle size, antigen solubility, use of respiratory protection, and variability in work practices may influence disease prevalence, latency, and severity. FLD is most common in late winter, when stored hay is used to feed cattle, and in regions with heavy rainfall and harsh winter conditions, where feed is likely to become damp and therefore an ideal substrate for microbial proliferation. Summer-type HP in Japan,[81] and more recently described in Korea,[82] is characterized by recurrent seasonal symptoms, familial occurrence of cases, and symptom provocation on occupancy of homes containing *Trichosporon*-contaminated damp and decayed wood and woven straw tatami mats. A longitudinal study of pigeon breeders showed a seasonal variation in specific antibody levels among subjects with pigeon breeder's disease, with a peak in antibody production during late summer when maximum avian exposure was associated with the sporting season.[83] Thus, the most common forms of HP show both seasonal and geographic variation in incidence.

Indirect and apparently trivial antigen exposures can be important in the risk for avian HP. The illness developed in two spouses of pigeon hobbyists, one exposed to her husband's dusty coveralls and the other to a room adjacent to the pigeons.[84] A duvet containing goose feathers was a source of avian antigen-causing HP, and down comforters and pillows can create similar exposure risks.[85] Feathers used for making fishing lures and those contained in decorative wreaths have been associated with cases of HP.[86, 87] These findings suggest that avian antigens are extremely potent inducers of immunologic lung disease, and a careful search for their presence must be included in the history-taking of patients with suspected HP.

## HOST FACTORS

Although many people are exposed to environmental antigens associated with HP, and some develop serum antibodies or BAL lymphocytosis, or both, fewer manifest disease. This suggests that unique host susceptibility or resistance influences individual responses to inhaled antigen. Studies of human leukocyte antigen haplotypes in patients with HP have shown no clear association of disease with a specific histocompatibility locus. No significant association between human leukocyte antigen-A, -B or -C loci antigens and FLD was found in a study of 100 farmers with disease compared with healthy farmers with and without precipitating antibodies.[88] A similar lack of association with human leukocyte antigens is described for bird fancier's disease.[89, 90]

A number of studies have shown that HP occurs more frequently in nonsmokers than in smokers; the mechanisms for this effect are not known.[91, 92] Pigeon fanciers who smoked had a lower incidence of precipitating antibodies to pigeon antigens and lower serum IgG and IgA antibodies to pigeon proteins in enzyme-linked immunosorbent assay in comparison with nonsmoking and ex-smoking pigeon fanciers, which suggests that cigarette smoking depresses both T-independent and T-dependent responses to inhaled antigens.[92] Smokers with FLD had more frequent illness recurrence, were more likely to have insidious than acute symptoms, had lower percent predicted vital capacities, and had poorer 10-year survival in comparison with nonsmokers with FLD.[93] Thus, although HP appears to occur more commonly in nonsmokers, prognosis is poorer in those who smoke, which underlines the importance of smoking cessation or avoidance in those with disease.

HP can occur in infants and children, and diagnosis is often elusive. Avian proteins are the most common antigen associated with HP in the pediatric population. In a study of five children with pigeon breeder's lung, Stiehm and coworkers found that children are more likely to present with the subacute or chronic forms of HP than with acute illness.[94] Microbial antigen exposures are described in case reports of childhood HP. A 5-year-old boy developed a recurrent flu-like illness that progressed to severe respiratory failure over 3 months,[95] confirmed on surgical lung biopsy as HP. Detailed history revealed that the boy's father had arranged a comfortable bed of hay so that the child could rest in the barn during chores; that year, the hay was very moldy and ventilation in the barn was poor. Treatment with corticosteroids and avoidance of the barn resulted in complete clinical resolution. A 10-month-old infant developed wheezing and tachypnea that progressed over 2 months to severe respiratory failure, necessitating mechanical ventilation.[96] Surgical lung biopsy showed histologic findings of HP. Serum precipitins were positive to *Penicillium*. Environmental sampling in the home revealed predominantly *Penicillium* species, the source of which was unclear. Removal from the home and repeated courses of corticosteroids resulted in slow resolution of the child's clinical abnormalities over 14 months. HP should be considered in the differential diagnosis of children with recurrent febrile respiratory illnesses and in those with unexplained interstitial lung disease, and parents should be questioned carefully regarding potential antigen exposures in the home and school.

Pregnancy and delivery appear to trigger symptoms and overt illness in women with pigeon breeder's lung, but the associated hormonal and immunologic changes are not understood.[97]

## IMMUNOPATHOGENESIS

HP is characterized by the presence of activated T lymphocytes in BAL and an interstitial mononuclear cell infiltrate. The pathogenesis of HP involves (1) repeated antigen exposure; (2) immunologic sensitization of the host to the antigen; and (3) immune-mediated damage to the lung (Table 67.2). The immune inflammation resulting in the lymphocytic alveolitis and granulomatous pneumonitis appears to involve a combination of immune complex-mediated, humoral, and, most importantly, cell-mediated or delayed (type IV) immune reactions to inhaled antigen. Despite a rich scientific literature, a full explanation of the complex pathogenesis of HP remains elusive.

Animal models support the importance of cell-mediated immunity in HP. Cultured lymphocytes passively transferred from sensitized animals, including guinea pigs,[98] rats,[99] rabbits,[100] and inbred mice,[101] to unexposed, nonsensitized animals results in disease similar to human HP when the naive animals subsequently are challenged with inhaled or infused intrapulmonary antigens. Similar results occur using passively transferred T lymphocytes that have been activated in vitro with either mitogen or antigen.[102] Interferon-gamma was found to be essential for the expression of HP in studies using "knockout" mice incapable of expressing the gene coding for interferon-gamma, and other experimental studies support the Th1 subset of lymphocytes as important in HP pathogenesis.[101] Enhancement of HP has been shown in mice undergoing repeated intranasal instillation of *S. rectivirgula* and infected concurrently with Sendai virus,[103] suggesting that viral illness may affect host susceptibility to HP.

The cellular and humoral events that characterize HP have been examined using BAL. Within the first 48 hours after exposure of a sensitized host to the antigen, there is an immediate influx of neutrophils,[104] probably stimulated

**Table 67.2 UNIFYING PATHOGENIC CHARACTERISTICS OF HYPERSENSITIVITY PNEUMONITIS**

| |
|---|
| Repeated antigen exposure |
| Immunologic sensitization of host |
| Lung is portal of entry and target organ-mediating response |
| Immune inflammatory pulmonary infiltrate (T lymphocytes) |
| Chronic cellular immune response with ongoing antigen exposure |

by formation of intra-airway immune complexes, activation of the alternative complement pathway, or endotoxin effects of the inhaled antigen.[105–107] Several days later, the local immune response shifts to a T lymphocyte-predominant alveolitis, often with 60% to 70% lymphocytes.[108] Both cellular redistribution from peripheral blood to lung and in situ lymphocyte proliferation contribute to the increased number of lung T cells.[109] Natural killer cells also are increased in BAL from patients with HP in comparison with nonsmokers and with those with sarcoidosis.[110] Mast cell numbers are increased in BAL after antigen exposure, returning to the normal range within 1 to 3 months after removal from exposure.[130] A mild neutrophilia (8% to 10%) may persist.[112] In addition, increased plasma cells have been described in patients with subacute bird breeder's lung.[113]

Examination of BAL lymphocyte subsets in patients with symptomatic HP reveals activated T lymphocytes, often with a predominance of $CD8^+$ cells having suppressor/cytotoxic functions.[114] $CD4^+/CD8^+$ ratios are usually less than 1.[115] However, a number of investigators have shown that these ratios vary widely in patients with HP, with some having normal or increased numbers of $CD4^+$ cells.[116, 117] Reasons for this variability are unclear, but data suggest that the forms of HP (acute vs. chronic) and the timing of last antigen exposure in relation to BAL may affect cellular phenotypes. A $CD4^+$-predominant BAL lymphocytosis has been described in patients with the fibrotic stage of HP.[118] Smoking also affects the cellular phenotypes seen.[119] In a follow-up study of patients with FLD who remained in the agricultural environment but without further exposure to specific antigens at work, Trentin and colleagues described a recovery of $CD4^+$ cells, a decrease in $CD8^+$ cells, and an increase in the $CD4^+/CD8^+$ ratio to the normal range 6 months after initial observation.[120]

Macrophages play a pivotal role in disease pathogenesis by processing and presenting antigen to $CD4^+$ cells in the early phases of the immune response.[121] Early activation of alveolar macrophages by specific antigen/antibody complexes, with release of proinflammatory cytokines such as TNF-α, IL-1, and macrophage-derived lipoxygenase products, sets the stage for the development of HP. Activated T cells of the Th1 phenotype produce IL-2 and interferon-gamma, which can prime macrophages to transcribe and secrete greater amounts of TNF-α and IL-1.[122] Macrophage-derived factors with chemotactic activity for lymphocytes (including IL-1 and IL-8) probably contribute to the influx of $CD8^+$ cells specifically sensitized to antigen in the lungs of affected individuals. These $CD8^+$ (or in some cases, $CD4^+$) T cells may modulate granuloma formation via production of Th1- or Th2-like cytokines.[123] The accumulation of inflammatory and immune effector cells and the release of fibronectin and other matrix proteoglycans by activated alveolar macrophages and myofibroblasts are associated with remodeling of the interstitial matrix and with the lung fibrosis seen in the more chronic form of HP.[124, 125]

In addition to their ability to stimulate a T-cell–mediated response, many of the particulate antigens capable of causing HP are potent immunologic adjuvants.[126] The thermophilic bacterium *S. rectivirgula* capable of causing FLD induces the release of the proinflammatory cytokines IL-1 and TNF-α from human macrophages.[127] Both IL-1 and TNF-α induce fever and inflammation and are important mediators of tissue destruction and remodeling.

## HISTOPATHOLOGY

The histopathology of HP is distinctive, but it is not pathognomonic, and histologic features vary depending on the stage of illness at the time of biopsy.[128] The typical histologic triad of HP includes (1) cellular bronchiolitis (airway-centered inflammation), (2) interstitial mononuclear cell infiltrate, and (3) scattered, small, non-necrotizing granulomas,[129] but an appreciable number of HP cases do not show these classic features.

In the acute and subacute forms of HP, there is a patchy infiltrate of the alveolar walls with mononuclear cells (predominantly lymphocytes and plasma cells) in a bronchiolocentric distribution, usually with accompanying epithelioid granulomas or giant cells (Fig. 67.1). Neutrophils and eosinophils are uncommon, although luminal neutrophils can be seen after acute exposure. Airspace foam cells (foamy macrophages) are a distinctive part of the airway inflammatory process.[130] In a 1982 case series of 60 patients with acute FLD, Reyes and coworkers[131] found interstitial inflammatory infiltrates in 100%, granulomas in 70%, unresolved (organizing) pneumonia in 65%, interstitial fibrosis in 65%, foam cells in 65%, foreign body material (demonstrable by polarized light) in 60%, solitary giant cells in 53%, and bronchiolitis obliterans in 50%. In a study of 475 Japanese patients with summer-type HP, interstitial inflammation was found in 95%, granulomas in 65%, and bronchiolitis obliterans/organizing pneumonia (BOOP) ("Masson bodies") in approximately 30%.

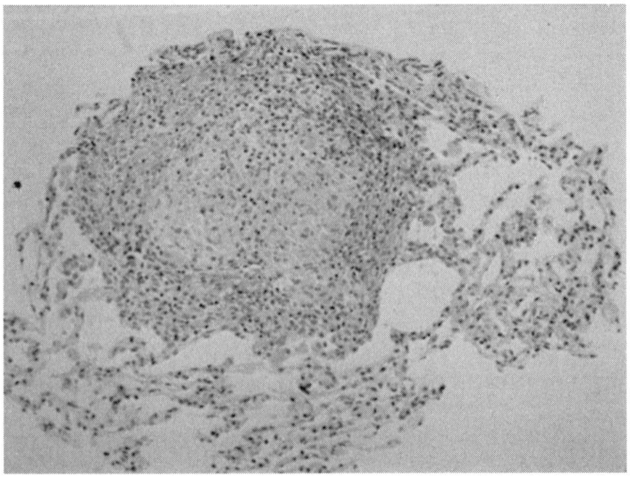

**Figure 67.1** Photomicrograph (original magnification ×40) of a hematoxylin and eosin–stained transbronchial lung biopsy from a patient with hypersensitivity pneumonitis. An interstitial pneumonitis containing epithelioid macrophage aggregates involves a respiratory bronchiole at left. A small, discrete, non-necrotizing interstitial granuloma is present at right.

Interstitial fibrosis with honeycombing is found late in disease, usually accompanying chronic HP, by which time the granulomatous phase may have resolved. The interstitial fibrosis may show airway-centering or may be indistinguishable from a usual interstitial pneumonia pattern. Because the histopathologic findings of HP vary and overlap with other diseases, additional clinical data must be considered in confirming the diagnosis.

## CLINICAL FEATURES

### Signs and Symptoms

Detailed history-taking is the mainstay of HP diagnosis and is essential for planning exposure intervention (Table 67.3). A clinical history suggesting a temporal relationship between symptoms and certain activities is often the first clue to the diagnosis of HP, although such a pattern may not occur in subacute or chronic forms of disease. The work history should include a chronology of current and previous occupations, with a description of specific work processes and exposures. Antigen exposures capable of causing HP can occur in almost any indoor environment under appropriate circumstances, and a simple job title cannot be used to exclude potential risk. For example, a schoolteacher developed chronic HP associated with indoor air quality problems in the school environment; the disease went unrecognized for years.[132]

The environmental history should explore exposure to pets and other domestic animals, particularly birds; hobbies such as gardening and lawn care, which may involve sensitizing chemical exposures like pyrethrins; recreational activities, for example, use of hot tubs and indoor swimming pools from which microbial bioaerosols can be generated; use of humidifiers, cool mist vaporizers, and humidified air conditioners, which can be sources of microbial bioaerosols; moisture indicators such as leaking, flooding, or previous water damage to carpets and furnishings; and visible mold or mildew contamination in occupied spaces. Use of medications (both prescription and nonprescription) should be elicited to assess possible drug-induced lung disease.

The classification of illness into distinct acute, subacute, and chronic forms can be misleading because clinical manifestations frequently overlap. Nevertheless, the varying presentations are associated with variable clinical findings. Acute illness typically begins 4 to 12 hours after exposure, with onset of respiratory and constitutional symptoms of cough, dyspnea, chest tightness, fevers, chills, malaise and myalgias. Symptoms may be accompanied by physical findings of fever, tachypnea, tachycardia, and lung inspiratory crackles. Peripheral blood leukocytosis with neutrophilia and lymphopenia may be present. Eosinophilia is unusual. Acute symptoms of HP are nonspecific and probably frequently are mistaken for infectious respiratory illnesses. Recurrent acute symptom episodes should prompt consideration of hypersensitivity lung disease and a careful historical search for relevant exposures.

The subacute and chronic presentations of illness also require a high degree of clinical suspicion to confirm the diagnosis and initiate appropriate management. Exertional dyspnea and cough are the predominant symptoms, and patients frequently report sputum production, fatigue,

**Table 67.3 COMPONENTS OF AN OCCUPATIONAL AND ENVIRONMENTAL HISTORY FOR PATIENTS WITH SUSPECTED HYPERSENSITIVITY PNEUMONITIS**

| |
|---|
| **Occupational history** |
| Chronology of current and previous occupations |
| Description of job processes and specific work practices |
| List of specific chemicals, dusts, and other aerosol exposures (e.g., grain dust; animal handling; food and plant processing; cooling towers, fountains, and other water sprays; metalworking fluids) |
| Review of material safety data sheets (MSDSs) to identify known chemical sensitizers |
| Reports of industrial hygiene evaluations or environmental testing at the workplace |
| Symptom improvement away from work or symptom worsening with specific workplace exposures |
| Presence of persistent respiratory or constitutional symptoms in exposed coworkers |
| Use of respiratory protection at work |
| **Environmental and residential history** |
| Pets and other domestic animals (especially birds) |
| Hobbies and recreational activities (especially those involving chemicals, feathers or fur, plant materials, and organic dusts) |
| Presence of humidifiers, dehumidifiers, swamp coolers, clothes dryers vented indoors, and other humidity sources |
| Use of hot tubs or saunas |
| Leaking or flooding indoors |
| Water damage to carpets or furnishings |
| Visible fungal growth |
| Feather pillows, comforters, or bedding |
| Similar symptoms in other family members or home occupants |

malaise, anorexia, and weight loss. Physical examination findings may be normal or may reveal basilar crackles. Wheezing occurs in some patients, probably reflecting antigen-mediated inflammatory effects on the airways. Cyanosis and right-sided heart failure may be evident with severe fibrotic disease. Clubbing occurred in approximately half the patients in a case series of pigeon breeder's disease and is associated with a poorer prognostic outcome[133]; however, this is an uncommon finding in other forms of HP.

## Precipitating Antibodies

Although positive precipitating antibodies once were thought to be the hallmark of HP, they are unfortunately neither sensitive nor specific. The finding of specific IgG precipitating antibodies in the serum of a patient with suspected HP indicates exposure sufficient to generate a humoral immunologic response and may be a helpful diagnostic clue. Precipitins appear to have no role in disease pathogenesis but serve as markers of antigen exposure and often are found in individuals without clinically evident disease.[134] Serum precipitins are found in 3% to 30% of asymptomatic farmers and in up to 50% of asymptomatic pigeon breeders.[135, 136] The prevalence of positive tests in asymptomatic individuals fluctuates over time, with subjects testing variably positive or negative at different times, perhaps reflecting variable exposures.[137]

Specific precipitating antibodies frequently are not demonstrable in patients with HP. In one study,[138] 30% to 40% of patients with FLD had no detectable precipitins to commonly tested antigens (*Saccharopolyspora rectivirgula, Aspergillus* species, *and Thermoactinomyces vulgaris*). False-negative results may occur because of poorly standardized antigens, improper quality controls, insensitive techniques, the wrong choice of antigen, or underconcentrated sera.[139] The antibody response in some patients may be too meager to give a precipitin reaction using the traditional Ouchterlony double-immunodiffusion technique. More sensitive assays such as enzyme-linked immunosorbent assay for specific IgG antibodies may lead to confusion because of decreased specificity. Serum precipitins may disappear over variable periods of time after exposure ceases, which adds to the difficulty of antigen-specific diagnosis.[140] In some cases, particularly those associated with complex microbial bioaerosol exposures, disease may not be a reaction to one organism alone but a cumulative reaction to a number of airborne antigens, which may not be reflected in available laboratory antigen panels.

## Other Laboratory Studies

Mild elevations in erythrocyte sedimentation rate, C-reactive protein, and immunoglobulins of IgG, IgM, or IgA isotypes are occasionally evident, reflecting acute or chronic inflammation. Serum angiotensin-converting enzyme concentrations rarely may be increased in patients with recurrent acute symptoms.[141] Antinuclear antibodies and other autoantibodies rarely are detected. Skin tests for both immediate and delayed-type hypersensitivity reactions are unhelpful in diagnosis.

## Physiology

Complete pulmonary function tests (PFTs), including lung volumes, spirometry, and diffusing capacity, should be obtained when feasible in all patients with suspected HP. Lung function abnormalities in acute HP are classically restrictive, with a decrease in FVC, total lung capacity, and diffusion capacity. Hypoxemia is often present, and an exercise-induced decrease in $Po_2$ is an early sign of functional impairment.[142] Four to 6 weeks may be required for complete resolution of these acute abnormalities,[143] PFT results may be normal if performed after resolution of an acute episode but before onset of chronic interstitial fibrosis.

PFT results also may fall within normal limits in subacute forms of HP and may be particularly misleading if no premorbid PFT values are available for comparison. Both restrictive and obstructive defects in pulmonary function occur in subacute and chronic HP, and a combined restrictive and obstructive pattern is common. In 1965, Pepys and Jenkins reported that 10% of 205 patients with FLD showed obstruction alone rather than restriction.[144] Decreased diffusion capacity also is commonly observed. Gas exchange abnormalities, particularly with exercise, may be marked. Nonspecific bronchial hyperreactivity measured by methacholine challenge has been described in 22% to 60% of patients with HP.[145] Thus, HP should be considered in the differential diagnosis of nonsmokers presenting with physiologic findings of emphysema and in patients with airflow limitation and nonspecific bronchial hyperreactivity.

Thus, both rest and exercise PFTs are important components in the diagnostic evaluation of patients with HP, but findings are neither sensitive nor specific. Normal spirometry should not be used to exclude the diagnosis. Once diagnostic confirmation of HP is obtained, serial PFTs should be measured to assess response to therapy and to guide treatment decisions until recovery or stability, or both, of lung function is maintained.

## Radiography

The chest radiograph in acute HP typically reveals a fine micronodular pattern or diffuse ground-glass opacity (Fig. 67.2*A*).[146, 147] Hilar or mediastinal adenopathy rarely is seen on the plain radiograph. The chest film may be normal, particularly in early disease stages, and is a poor screening tool in populations at risk for HP.[148] In one study,[149] 4% of acute cases of FLD had normal films and another 40% to 45% had minimal changes that might easily be overlooked; the extent of radiographic abnormality correlated poorly with the severity of symptoms or functional impairment. Radiographic abnormalities in acute illness regress or resolve over 4 to 6 weeks if further exposure is avoided. In chronic HP, fibrosis may be manifested by linear reticular opacity, volume loss, and honeycombing.

Computed tomographic (CT) scanning is more sensitive than chest radiography in the diagnosis of HP. The most typical CT finding in HP is profuse, diffuse, poorly defined, centrilobular micronodules, probably reflecting a cellular bronchiolitis (see Fig. 67.2*B*).[150–154] Diffuse

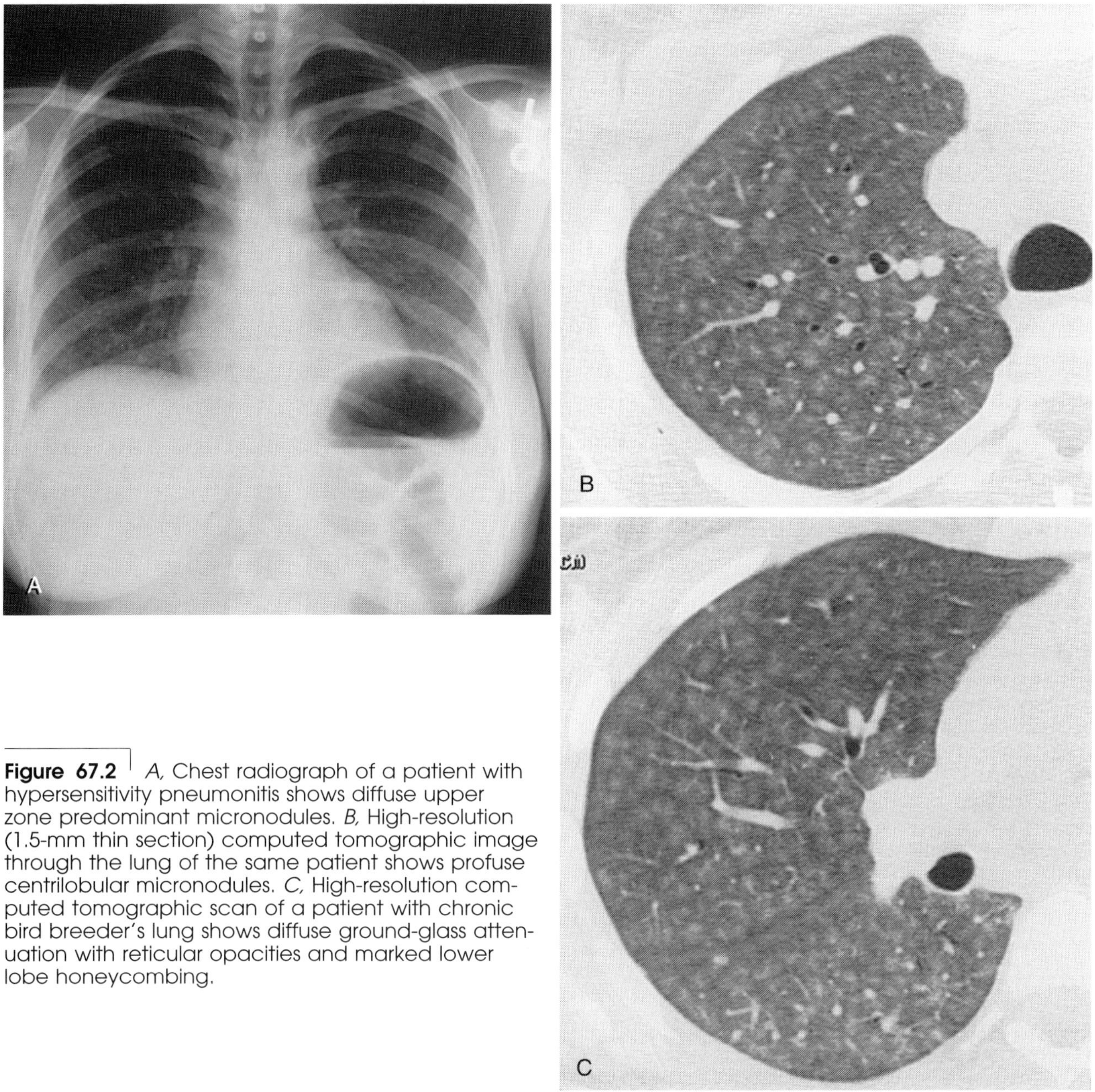


**Figure 67.2** *A,* Chest radiograph of a patient with hypersensitivity pneumonitis shows diffuse upper zone predominant micronodules. *B,* High-resolution (1.5-mm thin section) computed tomographic image through the lung of the same patient shows profuse centrilobular micronodules. *C,* High-resolution computed tomographic scan of a patient with chronic bird breeder's lung shows diffuse ground-glass attenuation with reticular opacities and marked lower lobe honeycombing.

ground-glass attenuation may be the predominant or only CT abnormality in some cases. The CT appearance of HP may be normal if disease is diagnosed early.[150] In chronic HP, findings of lung fibrosis may include reticular opacities, lobar volume loss, or honeycombing (see Fig. 67.2*C*). In one case series, diffuse ground-glass attenuation was observed in most subacute and chronic forms of bird breeder's HP[155]; honeycombing was seen in only 50% of the chronic cases, a number of whom also had concurrent micronodules or ground-glass attenuation, or both. Emphysematous changes have been observed in subacute and chronic HP cases, most of whom were nonsmokers, perhaps related to bronchiolar inflammation and obstruction.[152, 155] Focal areas of hyperlucency (mosaic pattern), perhaps due to bronchiolocentric inflammation with associated air trapping, may be a prominent feature.[156] Mild reactive mediastinal lymphadenopathy is a common CT finding,[157] typically involving only a few nodes with a maximal short axis diameter less than 15 mm.

## Inhalation Challenge

The use of laboratory inhalation challenge in the diagnosis of HP is limited by the lack of standardized antigens and techniques. Inhalation of an aerosolized antigen suspected to be causative is most helpful when acute symptoms and clinical abnormalities are part of the disease presentation and likely to occur within hours after exposure.[158] In experienced laboratories, provocative testing may be useful in discriminating chronic HP induced by avian antigens from other interstitial lung diseases.[159] In some patients with acute symptoms, exposure to the suspect environment with postexposure monitoring of symptoms, temperature, leukocyte count, spirometry, diffusing capacity, and chest radiograph may be preferable to laboratory challenge. Interpretation of results is often difficult, and routine inhalation challenge is not recommended in most patients with suspected HP.[160]

## Bronchoalveolar Lavage

BAL provides a sensitive tool confirming the presence of alveolitis in patients with HP.[161] Typically, a marked lavage lymphocytosis (30% to 70%) without eosinophilia or neutrophilia is found, often but not always with a $CD8^+$ lymphocyte predominance. Total white blood cell numbers are increased, often up to fivefold normal. The absolute number of macrophages is similar to controls, although their percentage in lavage is reduced because of the high number of lymphocytes. Increased numbers of mast cells have been reported in symptomatic patients with HP.[162] Concentrations of IgG, IgM, and IgA antibodies typically are increased in BAL in subjects with HP (although smoking may mitigate this effect), as are total protein and albumin.[163]

The lavage cellular profile may vary considerably depending on the stage of illness and the time interval between BAL and last antigen exposure.[120] The BAL lymphocytosis of HP may persist for years after apparent removal from antigen exposure and despite improvement in other clinical parameters, limiting its utility as a tool to follow the course and progression of disease or to assess adequacy of antigen removal.[164] Individuals exposed to HP antigens but without reported symptoms or other clinical abnormalities may develop a lymphocytic alveolitis,[165, 166] further limiting the diagnostic specificity of BAL. There appears to be little correlation between BAL findings and other clinical abnormalities, including radiographic changes, pulmonary function, and the presence of precipitating antibody.

## Lung Biopsy

Lung biopsy may be indicated in patients without sufficient clinical criteria for definitive diagnosis or to rule out other diseases that necessitate different treatment. Transbronchial biopsies are often sufficient, especially if directed by CT findings, and diagnostic yield increases when 6 to 10 samples are obtained.[167] Interstitial lymphocytic inflammation, granulomas, and bronchiolar inflammation can be seen on transbronchial biopsy; however, appreciation of the airway-centered inflammatory reaction of HP usually requires a surgical lung biopsy. Special stains and cultures are important to distinguish HP from infectious granulomatous conditions, including fungal and mycobacterial diseases. HP differs from sarcoidosis in the finding of inflammatory infiltrates at interstitial sites distant from granulomas, whereas in sarcoidosis such infiltrates generally are found in and around the granulomas.[128, 160] Given the substantial overlap in the histologic appearance of these granulomatous processes, pathology without clinical correlation usually is not sufficient for diagnosis.

**Table 67.4 DIAGNOSTIC APPROACH TO THE PATIENT WITH POSSIBLE HYPERSENSITIVITY PNEUMONITIS (HP)**

| |
|---|
| Obtain detailed occupational and environmental exposure histories, along with regular clinical history |
| Physical examination |
| Pulmonary function, including spirometry, lung volumes, $D_{LCO}$ |
| Chest radiograph, PA and lateral |
| Consider HRCT if chest film is negative or nonspecific |
| Assess exercise ventilatory and gas exchange parameters if exertional dyspnea is prominent |
| Consider serum precipitin analysis; negative results do not rule out HP, but a positive precipitin result helps confirm relevant antigenic exposures |
| Fiberoptic bronchoscopy (FOB) with bronchoalveolar lavage if diagnosis is in doubt; surgical lung biopsy may be indicated if FOB is nondiagnostic |

HRCT = high-resolution computed tomography; PA = posterior-anterior.

## Diagnostic Approach

Because the diagnosis of HP carries such import for prevention of further antigen exposure, we typically perform the following diagnostic studies on all patients with suspected HP (Table 67.4): (1) detailed clinical history; (2) physical examination; (3) chest high-resolution computed tomography (unless the plain film is clearly abnormal); (4) complete PFTs, including lung volumes, pre- and postbronchodilator spirometry, and $D_{LCO}$; and (5) fiberoptic bronchoscopy, usually with BAL and transbronchial biopsies, including special stains and cultures for infectious agents. In patients with exertional dyspnea and normal or minimally abnormal PFTs, exercise physiology is often helpful in defining impairment and important in guiding treatment decisions, including the need for supplemental oxygen. Methacholine challenge does not distinguish asthma from HP and is generally not necessary. Serum precipitins are helpful when positive in confirming the diagnosis in bird breeder's lung and in other circumstances in which the putative antigen has been identified. However, negative precipitins should not be used to exclude the diagnosis.

# DIAGNOSTIC CRITERIA

A number of diagnostic criteria for HP have been proposed. Terho[168] suggested major and minor criteria for FLD, and consider the diagnosis confirmed if the patient fulfills all the major criteria and at least two additional criteria, and if other disease with similar clinical findings have been ruled out. A negative chest film is allowed if the biopsy is positive. The major criteria include: (1) exposure to offending antigens revealed by history, by environmental measurements, or by the presence of antigen-specific IgG antibodies; (2) symptoms compatible with HP appearing several hours after exposure; and (3) abnormal chest radiograph. Additional criteria include:

basilar crepitant rales; decreased diffusion capacity; decreased oxygen tension or saturation at rest or with exercise; abnormal histology compatible with HP; and positive provocation test either by work exposure or controlled inhalation challenge. More recently, Cormier[169] proposed similar diagnostic criteria for HP, including the requirements of appropriate exposure, dyspnea on exertion, inspiratory crackles, and lymphocytic alveolitis (if BAL is done). Proposed supportive criteria include recurrent febrile episodes; infiltrates on chest radiograph; decreased $DL_{CO}$; precipitating antibodies to causative antigens; granulomas on lung biopsy (usually not required); and improvement with contact avoidance. All the proposed diagnostic criteria for HP await validation.

Stringent diagnostic criteria may underestimate milder cases of HP in which the chest radiograph is normal or when symptoms are subtle or insidious. Meta-analysis showed a decline in the sensitivity of the chest radiograph for diagnosis of HP over the years 1950 to 1980.[148] Because a positive exposure history is part of the case definition for disease, absent or inadequate occupational and environmental history-taking probably results in underrecognition of disease. The likelihood that unrecognized HP occurs also is based on several other factors: (1) the signs and symptoms of illness and clinical diagnostic findings are nonspecific and mimic many other diseases, such as asthma, influenza, viral pneumonia, sarcoidosis, and idiopathic pulmonary fibrosis (Table 67.5); (2) early disease may be accompanied by a normal auscultatory lung examination and resting pulmonary function as well as a normal chest radiograph; (3) many of the microbial antigens that cause HP proliferate in common environmental niches, and relevant exposures may be difficult to elicit historically; and (4) precipitating antibodies are often negative and may disappear after exposure ceases, so that a patient with fibrotic lung disease from previous episodes of HP may not be recognized as such.[170]

## NATURAL HISTORY AND PROGNOSIS

The clinical course of HP is variable, but if illness is recognized early, the prognosis for recovery is usually quite good.[171]

In acute HP, symptoms of fever, chills, and cough usually disappear within days after exposure ceases. Malaise, fatigue, and dyspnea may persist for several weeks. There is usually rapid improvement in lung vital capacity and diffusion capacity in the first 2 weeks after an acute attack, but mild abnormalities in pulmonary function often persist for several months. In general, single acute episodes are self-limited. Occasionally, disease may progress despite removal from exposure. Continued symptoms and progressive lung impairment have been reported after recurrent acute attacks and even after a single severe attack.[172, 173]

The subacute or chronic forms of HP, with insidious symptoms and more subtle clinical abnormalities, probably are recognized later in the course of illness and consequently often have a poorer prognosis than acute disease. Symptomatic pigeon breeders monitored for 18 years showed a fourfold average rate of decline in pulmonary function in comparison with the expected rate.[174] Four children and five adults with chronic avian HP were monitored from 6 months to 10 years after treatment with corticosteroids and reduction or elimination of exposure.[175] Only five of the nine were completely asymptomatic, all had persistent positive serum precipitins, several had lung function abnormalities, and one ultimately died of HP after unsuccessful lung transplantation. Fatal diffuse alveolar damage has been described as a compli-

**Table 67.5 DIFFERENTIAL DIAGNOSIS OF HYPERSENSITIVITY PNEUMONITIS***

| | Clinical Presentation | BAL Lymphocytosis | Histopathology |
|---|---|---|---|
| Asthma | ++ | + | − |
| Sarcoidosis | ++ | ++ | + |
| Inhalation fever (e.g., ODTS) | ++ | − | − |
| Viral/mycoplasma pneumonias | ++ | + | − |
| Mycobacterial infections | ++ | ++ | + |
| Fungal infections | + | + | + |
| Other ILD (collagen-vascular, IPF) | + | + | + |
| Chronic beryllium disease | + | ++ | + |
| Lymphoma/leukemia | + | + | + |
| Toxic fume inhalation | + | − | − |

*Designations reflect other illnesses compared with hypersensitivity pneumonitis (acute, subacute, or chronic presentation).

++ = very similar; + = similar; − = dissimilar.

BAL = bronchoalveolar lavage; ILD = interstitial lung disease; IPF = idiopathic pulmonary fibrosis; ODTS = organic duct toxic syndrome.

cation of chronic bird fancier's lung.[176] Overall, long-term mortality rates for patients with chronic HP ranges from 1% to 10%.[177, 178]

Both emphysema (more common in late-stage FLD) and fibrosis (apparently more common as an outcome of bird breeder's lung) are potential sequelae of HP. In a case-control study of 88 farmers with FLD, emphysema was found significantly more often (23%) in those with FLD in comparison with matched control farmers (7%), occurring in 18% of nonsmoking and 44% of smoking FLD patients.[179] Recurrent attacks of FLD were associated in this study with risk for emphysema. In comparison with matched control farmers, those with FLD monitored for 14 years had significant reductions in diffusing capacity and more marked airflow limitation.[180] In another follow-up study of farmers with a history of FLD,[181] obstructive abnormalities from emphysema were the most common findings in those whose disease did not completely resolve; only 50% had no residual disease. In a study of Finnish farmers meeting strict diagnostic criteria for FLD, the risk for asthma necessitating medication was found to increase within the first 3 years after a diagnosis of FLD, with significantly higher asthma prevalence rates in the population with FLD at 5-year follow-up in comparison with the reference population.[182] Patients with HP from avian antigens appear to have a higher risk of developing fibrotic restrictive lung disease in comparison with those with FLD,[183] with a poor 5-year survival similar to that of patients with idiopathic pulmonary fibrosis. Thus, although some patients with HP recover completely, permanent sequelae of the disease include asthma, emphysema, and (sometimes progressive) interstitial fibrosis.

Continued antigen exposure may not lead to clinical deterioration in some cases.[184] Bourke and colleagues found that 18 of 21 individuals with acute pigeon breeder's lung had continued regular exposure to pigeons 10 years after diagnosis, although many used improved ventilation and respiratory protection; only 6 reported continued respiratory symptoms.[185] This phenomenon may be reflected in some animal models of disease, in which repeated antigen inhalation in sensitized animals results in resolution rather than progression of the pulmonary inflammatory response.[186] This modulation of the inflammatory response is not well understood, and there is as yet no role for immunotherapy in disease management.

No functional or biochemical marker exists to predict resolution or progression of disease. The BAL lymphocytosis associated with HP may persist for years after removal from exposure and despite clinical recovery. Age at diagnosis, duration of antigen exposure after onset of symptoms, and total years of exposure before diagnosis seem to have predictive value in the likelihood of recovery from pigeon breeder's lung disease.[187] Pigeon breeders with HP were more likely to improve or recover completely if they had been in contact with birds for less than 2 years. Neither the form of clinical presentation (acute vs. chronic) nor the degree of lung function abnormality at the time of diagnosis was related to recovery in another study of pigeon breeder's disease.[188] Rather, younger age at diagnosis and exposure to antigen for less than 6 months after symptom onset were associated with complete recovery.

## TREATMENT

An accelerated decline in lung function with continued antigen exposure has been demonstrated for most forms of HP. Thus, early diagnosis and avoidance of antigen exposure are the mainstays of treatment, with pharmacologic therapy an important adjunct in some cases.

### Antigen Avoidance

Elimination of a causative antigen from the patient's environment is not only the first step in treatment but also prevents occurrence of hypersensitivity diseases in others exposed. For example, maple bark disease and bagassosis are now quite rare in the United States after changes in the handling of material, which resulted in diminished opportunity for microbial growth. Removal of damaged and colonized areas, disinfection, and elimination of conditions leading to seasonal mold contamination are effective in preventing recurrence of summer-type HP in Japan.[189] An outbreak of HP traced to fungal contamination of an open water-spray ventilation system was controlled by extensive cleaning of the system and corresponding work areas and replacement of the system with a dry (closed-coil) ventilation system.[190] In another large outbreak caused by microbial contamination of a chilled water air-conditioning system, a variety of cleaning and water treatment measures were used to reduce antigen concentration. A solid-phase radioimmunoassay method using antiserum from affected workers was used thereafter to assess levels of airborne antigen and monitor the efficacy of control measures.[191] In cases of home humidifier and hot tub lung, removal of the contaminated sources is usually straightforward.

On-site investigation of the work and home environments by an experienced industrial hygienist may be helpful in cases in which the exposure history is uncertain, particularly when disease is progressive. For fungal contaminants, both area and personal spore sampling and indirect immunofluorescence testing for spore-specific IgG have been used to assess indoor air quality and individual mold sensitization.[192] However, quantitative bioaerosol sampling for indoor microbial antigens is time consuming, expensive, and not readily available to most clinicians, and requires an experienced industrial hygienist and analytical laboratory. Even when properly performed, results are often difficult to interpret.[193] Negative results should not be used to disprove disease or exposure. Settle plates are unreliable in assessing indoor microbial contaminants.

Avoidance of exposure by eliminating the offending antigen from the environment may be difficult in some circumstances. In five homes monitored serially after bird removal, antigen levels measured by inhibition enzyme-linked immunosorbent assay declined gradually despite extensive environmental control measures, with high levels still detectable at 18 months in one home.[194] Avian antigens can be found in homes without birds if wild bird excrement is deposited heavily outside the house and tracked in on shoes. Tannic acid application, used effectively in decreasing indoor cat and mite allergen levels, is not effective in decreasing bird antigen levels in patients with bird breeder's lung.[195]

When elimination of the antigen is not feasible or the etiologic agent is not identified specifically, exposure avoidance usually is accomplished by removing the affected individual from the likely antigen-containing environment. This approach may be simple and adequate for recovery. However, the social consequences and economic disruption to the affected individual may preclude strict abstinence from exposure. A 6-year follow-up study of affected farmers revealed that 50% to 60% remained on the farm[140]; by 15 years, as many as 70% had returned to farming.[178] Especially when antigen exposure avoidance is likely to be inadequate, regular follow-up of pulmonary function, radiography, and symptoms is essential to assess response to treatment, to detect clinical deterioration, and to direct efforts to mitigate ongoing antigen exposure.

## Pharmacologic Therapy

There are anecdotal reports of the beneficial effects of systemic steroids in acute attacks of HP, but controlled clinical trials are lacking. In cases in which pulmonary function abnormalities are minor and spontaneous recovery is likely with removal from exposure, steroids are probably unnecessary. More severe attacks may necessitate treatment with prednisone, typically beginning at 60 mg/day, plus bed rest, supplemental oxygen for hypoxemia, and other appropriate supportive measures. This prednisone dose usually is continued until there is significant symptomatic and functional improvement. Pulmonary function should be monitored within the first 4 weeks after initiation of treatment. If there is objective improvement, a gradual taper to minimum sustaining doses should follow; otherwise, steroids should be tapered and discontinued. Monkare showed that 12 weeks of steroid treatment did not produce better results than 4 weeks of treatment in patients with FLD.[196] Given the paucity of treatment studies and the known side effects of systemic corticosteroids, clinical judgment and careful medical follow-up must guide individual patient management.

The effect of corticosteroids on the long-term course of various forms of HP has received limited attention. In one study, 36 patients, most having suffered only one acute attack of FLD, were assigned randomly to receive prednisolone or placebo for 2 months.[197] The steroid-treated group showed more rapid improvement in physiologic abnormalities (particularly diffusion capacity) at 1-month follow-up, but no differences were found between the treated and untreated groups 5 years later. Interestingly, the group treated with steroids suffered more frequent recurrences of symptomatic FLD during the 5-year follow-up period, although this finding did not reach statistical significance. In a study of pigeon breeders with HP, there were no significant clinical outcome differences between cases who were treated with steroids and those who were not; the mean time for improvement or normalization of pulmonary function after treatment and removal from exposure was 3.4 months.[188]

Inhaled steroids and beta-agonists may be helpful in patients with HP manifested by symptoms of chest tightness and cough and with airflow limitation on pulmonary function.[198] There are as yet no data from controlled clinical trials on the efficacy of inhaled steroids in the treatment of HP.

Cytotoxic agents such as cyclophosphamide, cyclosporine,[199] and azathioprine have been used in patients with refractory progressive HP, but their efficacy is largely unexplored. Lung transplantation may be a last resort in such patients unresponsive to medical therapy.

## Prevention

Recognition of an index case of HP is often a sentinel health event, indicating the need for further investigation and intervention in the implicated environment where others may be at risk and where opportunities for prevention may be identified. For example, indoor microbial contamination often is related to problems with control of moisture. Source, dilution and administrative controls should be used when appropriate to reduce these indoor contaminants. Source control includes preventing leaking and flooding, removing stagnant water sources, eliminating aerosol humidifiers, hot tubs, and vaporizers, and maintaining indoor relative humidity below 70%. If humidifiers are used, frequent cleaning and water changes minimize the risk of microbial growth. Dilution of contaminants can be affected by increasing the amount of outdoor air in a building, and high-efficiency filters can be added to the ventilation system to clean recirculated air.[193] Complete elimination of indoor allergens is probably impossible, and it is often necessary to relocate immunologically sensitized individuals once hypersensitivity lung disease has occurred.

Work practices recommended to reduce the prevalence of FLD include efficient drying of hay and cereals before storage, use of mechanical feeding systems, and better ventilation of farm buildings.[73, 200] In a study of French farmers, the presence of serum precipitins and the risk for FLD was associated with handling of barn-stored cattle fodder.[201] Efforts to diminish disease prevalence were not affected significantly by changing from traditional drying methods to artificial barn fodder drying in this occupational setting.[202] Education of individuals in at-risk occupations in antigen avoidance and early symptom recognition may be helpful.

The efficacy of various types of respirators in preventing antigen sensitization and disease progression once sensitization has occurred is unknown. Helmet-type powered air purifying respirators have been used to prevent episodic exposure in individuals with previous acute episodes of FLD.[203] Respiratory protection has been examined in bird breeders with HP, many of whom are reluctant to abandon their high-risk hobby. Serial measurements of pigeon-specific IgG antibodies were obtained in 22 pigeon fanciers with HP who had ongoing exposure, 13 of whom wore a powered air purifying respirator and 9 who refused respiratory protection.[204] Serum antibody levels declined by 65% over 14 months in those wearing respirators in comparison with no decline in antibody levels in those without respirators; no data were reported on changes in symptoms or pulmonary function in the two groups. Prolonged wearing of respiratory protection is limited by the fact that most respirators are hot and cumbersome. Dust respirators offer substantial, but in some cases incomplete, protection against organic dusts,[205] and are not recommended as preventive measures once sensitization has occurred.

## SUMMARY

Increasing recognition of the ubiquity of environmental antigen exposures and improved diagnostic tools have led to increasing recognition of cases and outbreaks of HP in a wide variety of occupational and nonoccupational settings. HP remains a diagnostic challenge because of the spectrum of clinical findings and the lack of a simple "gold standard" for diagnosis. Rather, the diagnosis depends on a strong clinical index of suspicion, a careful exposure history, and the integration of a constellation of radiographic, physiologic, and histopathologic findings which, by themselves, are nonspecific and mimic a variety of other chest illnesses. HP is both treatable (and even curable if detected early) and preventable (if exposure is recognized and antigen abatement is effective). Unrecognized or untreated, the illness may lead to permanent sequelae including asthma, emphysema, and interstitial fibrosis.[206] Confirmation of the diagnosis often generates broader public health implications regarding the potential risks from ongoing antigen exposure to others sharing the environment. The diagnosis of even one case of HP should prompt a search for additional cases in the shared environment as well as initiation of measures to eliminate further exposure.

## References


1. Salvaggio JE, Millhollon B: Induction and modulation of pulmonary inflammation by organic dusts: Cytokines, immune complexes and "all those things" (editorial). Clin Exp Allergy 22:731–733, 1992.
2. Akoun GM, Cadranel JL, Rosenow EC 3rd, et al: Bronchoalveolar lavage cell data in drug-induced pneumonitis. Allerg Immunol 23:245–252, 1991.
3. Campbell JM: Acute symptoms following work with hay. BMJ 2:1143–1144, 1932.
4. Dickie HA, Rankin J: Farmer's lung: An acute granulomatous interstitial pneumonitis occurring in agricultural workers. JAMA 167:1069–1076, 1958.
5. Pepys J, Jenkins PA, Festenstein GN, et al: Farmer's lung: Thermophilic actinomycetes as a source of "farmer's lung hay" antigen. Lancet 18:182–196, 1963.
6. Buechner H, Prevatt A, Thompson J, et al: Bagassosis: Review with further historical data, studies of pulmonary function, and results of adrenal steroid therapy. Am J Med 25:234–247, 1958.
7. Banaszak EF, Thiede WH, Fink JN: Hypersensitivity pneumonitis due to contamination of an air conditioner. N Engl J Med 283:271–276, 1970.
8. Johnson CL, Bernstein IL, Gallagher JS, et al: Familial hypersensitivity pneumonitis induced by *Bacillus subtilis*. Am Rev Respir Dis 122:339–348, 1980.
9. Kane GC, Marx JJ, Prince DS: Hypersensitivity pneumonitis secondary to *Klebsiella oxytoca:* A new cause of humidifier lung. Chest 104:627–629, 1993.
10. Hogan MB, Patterson R, Pore RS, et al: Basement shower hypersensitivity pneumonitis secondary to *Epicoccum nigrum*. Chest 110:854–856, 1996.
11. Brade H, Brade L, Schade U, et al: Structure, endotoxicity, immunogenicity and antigenicity of bacterial lipopolysaccharides (endotoxins, O-antigens). *In* Levin J (ed): Bacterial Endotoxins: Pathophysiological Effects, Clinical Significance, and Pharmacological Control. New York: Alan R. Liss, 1993, pp 17–45.
12. Kreiss K, Cox-Ganser J: Metalworking fluid-associated hypersensitivity pneumonitis: A workshop summary. Am J Ind Med 32:423–432, 1997.
13. Zacharisen MC, Kadambi AR, Schlueter DP, et al: The spectrum of respiratory disease associated with exposure to metal working fluids. J Occup Environ Med 40:640–647, 1998.
14. Embil J, Warren P, Yakrus M, et al: Pulmonary illness associated with exposure to *Mycobacterium avium* complex in hot tub water: Hypersensitivity pneumonitis or infection? Chest 111:813–816, 1997.
15. Kahana LM, Kay JM, Yakrus MA, et al: *Mycobacterium avium* complex infection in an immunocompetent young adult related to hot tub exposure. Chest 111:242–245, 1997.
16. Rose CS, Martyny J, Newman LN, et al: "Lifeguard lung": Endemic granulomatous pneumonitis in an indoor swimming pool. Am J Public Health 88:1795–1800, 1998.
17. Burge HA: Airborne allergenic fungi: Classification, nomenclature, and distribution. Immunol Allergy Clin North Am 92:307–319, 1989.
18. Fernandez-Caldas E, Fox RW: Environmental control of indoor air pollution. Clin Allergy 76:935–952, 1992.
19. Reynolds SJ, Streifel AJ, McJilton CE: Elevated airborne concentrations of fungi in residential and office environments. Am Ind Hyg Assoc J 51:601–604, 1990.
20. Siersted HC, Gravesen S: Extrinsic allergic alveolitis after exposure to the yeast *Rhodotorula rubra*. Allergy 48:298–299, 1993.
21. Hodges GR, Fink JN, Schlueter DP: Hypersensitivity pneumonitis caused by a contaminated cool-mist vaporizer. Ann Intern Med 80:501–504, 1974.
22. Burke GW, Carrington CB, Strauss R, et al: Allergic alveolitis caused by home humidifiers. JAMA 238:2705–2708, 1977.
23. Robertson AS, Burge PS, Wieland GA, et al: Extrinsic allergic alveolitis caused by a cold water humidifier. Thorax 42:32–37, 1987.
24. Baur X, Richter G, Pethran A, et al: Increased prevalence of IgG-induced sensitization and hypersensitivity pneumonitis (humidifier lung) in nonsmokers exposed to aerosols of a contaminated air conditioner. Respiration 59:211–214, 1992.
25. Fink JN, Banaszak EF, Barboriak JJ, et al: Interstitial lung disease due to contamination of forced air systems. Ann Int Med 84:406–413, 1976.
26. Metzger WJ, Patterson R, Fink J, et al: Sauna-takers disease: Hypersensitivity pneumonitis due to contaminated water in a home sauna. JAMA 236:2209–2211, 1976.
27. Jacobs RL, Thorner RE, Holcomb JR, et al: Hypersensitivity pneumonitis caused by *Cladosporium* in an enclosed hot-tub area. Ann Intern Med 105:204–206, 1986.
28. Muittari A, Kuusisto P, Virtanen P, et al: An epidemic of extrinsic allergic alveolitis caused by tap water. Clin Allergy 10:77–90, 1980.
29. Bryant DH, Rogers P: Allergic alveolitis due to wood-rot fungi. Allergy Proc 12:89–94, 1991.
30. Meeker DP, Gephardt GN, Cordasco EM Jr, et al: Hypersensitivity pneumonitis versus invasive pulmonary aspergillosis: Two cases with unusual pathologic findings and review of the literature. Am Rev Respir Dis 143:431–436, 1991.
31. Tsuchiya Y, Shimokata K, Ohara H, et al: Hypersensitivity pneumonitis in a soy sauce brewer caused by *Aspergillus oryzae*. J Allergy Clin Immunol 91:688–689, 1993.
32. Sanderson W, Kullman G, Sastre J, et al: Outbreak of hypersensitivity pneumonitis among mushroom farm workers. Am J Ind Med 22:859–872, 1992.
33. Yoshida K, Neda A, Yamasaki H, et al: Hypersensitivity pneumonitis resulting from *Aspergillus fumigatus* in a greenhouse. Arch Environ Health 48:260–262, 1993.
34. Moreno-Ancillo A, Padial MA, Lopez-Serrano MC, et al: Hypersensitivity pneumonitis due to inhalation of fungi-contaminated esparto dust in a plaster worker. Allergy Asthma Proc 18:355–357, 1997.
35. Quirce S, Hinojosa M, Blanco R, et al: *Aspergillus fumigatus* is the causative agent of hypersensitivity pneumonitis caused by esparto dust. J Allergy Clin Immunol 102:147–148, 1998.
36. Schlueter D: Cheesewasher's disease: A new occupational hazard? Ann Intern Med 78:606–613, 1973.
37. Avila R, Lacey J: The role of *Penicillium frequentans* in su-

berosis (respiratory disease in workers in the cork industry). Clin Allergy 4:109–117, 1974.
38. Fergusson RJ, Milne LJR, Crompton GK: *Penicillium* allergic alveolitis: Faulty installation of central heating. Thorax 39:294–298, 1984.
39. Van Assendelft AHW, Raitio M, Turkia V: Fuel chip-induced hypersensitivity pneumonitis caused by *Penicillium* species. Chest 87:394–396, 1985.
40. Dykewicz MS, Laufer P, Patterson R, et al: Woodman's disease: Hypersensitivity pneumonitis from cutting live trees. J Allergy Clin Immunol 81:455–460, 1988.
41. Cormier Y, Israel-Assayag E, Bedard G, et al: Hypersensitivity pneumonitis in peat moss processing plant workers. Am J Respir Crit Care Med 158:412–417, 1998.
42. Nakagawa-Yoshida K, Ando M, Etches RI, et al: Fatal cases of farmer's lung in a Canadian family: Probable new antigens, *Penicillium brevicompactum* and *P. olivicolor.* Chest 111:245–248, 1997.
43. Emanuel DA, Wenzel FJ, Lawton BR: Pneumonitis due to *Cryptostroma corticale* (maple-bark disease). N Engl J Med 274:1413–1418, 1996.
44. Sosman AJ, Schlueter DP, Fink JN, et al: Hypersensitivity to wood dust. N Engl J Med 281:977–980, 1969.
45. Belin L: Clinical and immunological data on "wood trimmer's disease" in Sweden. Eur J Respir Dis 107(Suppl):169–176, 1980.
46. Enarson DS, Chan-Yeung M: Characterization of health effects of wood dust exposures. Am J Ind Med 17:33–38, 1990.
47. Ando M, Suga M, Nishiura Y, et al: Summer-type hypersensitivity pneumonitis. Intern Med 34:707–712, 1995.
48. Alvarez-Fernandez JA, Quirce S, Calleja JL, et al: Hypersensitivity pneumonitis due to an ultrasonic humidifier. Allergy 53:210–212, 1998.
49. Edwards JH, Griffiths AJ, Mullins J: Protozoa as sources of antigen in humidifier fever. Nature 264:438–439, 1976.
50. Plessner MM: Une maladie des trieurs de plumes: La fievre du canard. Arch Mal Prof 21:67–69, 1960.
51. Moore VL, Fink JN, Barboriak JJ, et al: Immunologic events in pigeon breeder's disease. J Allergy Clin Immunol 53:319–328, 1974.
52. Kokkarinen J, Tukiainen H, Seppa A, et al: Hypersensitivity pneumonitis due to native birds in a bird ringer. Chest 106:1269–1271, 1994.
53. Boyd G, McSharry C, Banham S, et al: A current view of pigeon fancier's lung. Clin Allergy 12:53–59, 1982.
54. Carrol KB, Pepys J, Longbottom J, et al: Extrinsic allergic alveolitis due to rat serum proteins. Clin Allergy 5:443–456, 1975.
55. Pimental JC: Furrier's lung. Thorax 25:387–398, 1970.
56. Lunn J, Hughes D: Pulmonary hypersensitivity to the grain weevil *(Sitophilus granarius).* Br J Ind Med 24:158–161, 1967.
57. Nakazawa T, Umegae Y: Sericulturist's lung disease: Hypersensitivity pneumonitis related to silk production. Thorax 45:233–234, 1990.
58. Orriols R, Manresa JM, Aliaga JL, et al: Mollusk shell hypersensitivity pneumonitis. Ann Intern Med 113:80–81, 1990.
59. Harper K, Burrell R, Lapp J, et al: Allergic alveolitis due to pituitary snuff. Ann Intern Med 73:581–584, 1970.
60. Vandenplas O, Malo JL, Saetta M, et al: Occupational asthma and extrinsic alveolitis due to isocyanates: Current status and perspectives. Br J Ind Med 50:213–228, 1993.
61. Malo JL, Zeiss CR: Occupational hypersensitivity pneumonitis after exposure to diphyenylmethane diisocyanate. Am Rev Respir Dis 125:113–116, 1982.
62. Yoshizawa Y, Ohtsuka M, Noguchi K, et al: Hypersensitivity pneumonitis induced by toluene diisocyanate: Sequelae of continuous exposure. Ann Intern Med 110:31–34, 1989.
63. Simpson C, Garabrant D, Torrey S, et al: Hypersensitivity pneumonitis–like reaction and occupational asthma associated with 1,3-bis(isocyanatomethyl)cyclohexane pre-polymer. Am J Ind Med 30:48–55, 1996.
64. Selden AI, Belin L, Wass U: Isocyanate exposure and hypersensitivity pneumonitis—Report of a probable case and prevalence of specific immunoglobulin G antibodies among exposed individuals. Scand J Work Environ Health 15:234–237, 1989.
65. Walker CL, Grammer LC, Shaughnessy MA, et al: Diphenylmethane diisocyanate hypersensitivity pneumonitis: A serologic evaluation. J Occup Med 31:315–319, 1989.
66. Bascom R, Kennedy TP, Levitz D, et al: Specific bronchoalveolar lavage IgG antibody in hypersensitivity pneumonitis from diphenylmethane diisocyanate. Am Rev Respir Dis 131:463–465, 1985.
67. Patterson R, Zeiss C, Pruzansky J: Immunology and immunopathology of trimellitic anhydride pulmonary reactions. J Allergy Clin Immunol 70:19–23, 1982.
68. Zeiss CR, Levitz D, Chacon R, et al: Quantitation and new antigenic determinant specificity of antibodies induced by inhalation of trimellitic anhydride in man. Int Arch Allergy Appl Immunol 61:380–388, 1980.
69. Piirila P, Keskinen H, Anttila S, et al: Allergic alveolitis following exposure to epoxy polyester powder paint containing low amounts (< 1%) of acid anhydrides. Eur Respir J 10:948–951, 1997.
70. Carlson JE, Villaveces JW: Hypersensitivity pneumonitis due to pyrethrum. JAMA 237:1718–1719, 1977.
71. Evans W, Seaton A: Hypersensitivity pneumonitis in a technician using Pauli's reagent. Thorax 34:767–770, 1979.
72. Pimental J, Marques S: Vineyard sprayer's lung: A new occupational disease. Thorax 24:678–683, 1969.
73. Grant IW, Blyth W, Wardrop VE, et al: Prevalence of farmer's lung in Scotland: A pilot survey. BMJ 1:530–534, 1972.
74. Madsen D, Klock LE, Wenzel FJ, et al: The prevalence of farmer's lung in an agricultural population. Am Rev Respir Dis 113:171–174, 1976.
75. Marx JJ, Guernsey J, Emanuel DA, et al: Cohort studies of immunologic lung disease among Wisconsin dairy farmers. Am J Ind Med 18:263–268, 1990.
76. Terho EO, Heinonen OP, Lammi S: Incidence of clinically confirmed farmer's lung disease in Finland. Am J Ind Med 10:330, 1986.
77. Hodgson MJ, Morey PR, Simon JS, et al: An outbreak of recurrent acute and chronic hypersensitivity pneumonitis in office workers. Am J Epidemiol 125:631–638, 1987.
78. Christensen LT, Schmidt CD, Robbins L: Pigeon breeder's disease—A prevalence study and review. Clin Allergy 5:417–430, 1975.
79. Orriols R, Aliaga JL, Anto JM, et al: High prevalence of mollusc shell hypersensitivity pneumonitis in nacre factory workers. Eur Respir J 10:780–786, 1997.
80. Vandenplas O, Malo JL, Dugas M, et al: Hypersensitivity pneumonitis-like reaction among workers exposed to diphenylmethane diisocyanate (MDI). Am Rev Respir Dis 147:338–346, 1993.
81. Ando M, Arima K, Yoneda R, et al: Japanese summer-type hypersensitivity pneumonitis. Am Rev Respir Dis 144:765–769, 1991.
82. Yoo CG, Kim YW, Han SK, et al: Summer-type hypersensitivity pneumonitis outside Japan: A case report and the state of the art. Respirology 2:75–77, 1997.
83. McSharry C, Lynch PP, Banham SW, et al: Seasonal variation of antibody levels among pigeon fanciers. Clin Allergy 13:293–299, 1983.
84. Riley DJ, Saldana M: Pigeon breeder's lung: Subacute course and the importance of indirect exposure. Am Rev Respir Dis 107:456–460, 1973.
85. Haitjema T, van Velzen-Blad H, van den Bosch JW: Extrinsic allergic alveolitis caused by goose feathers in a duvet. Thorax 47:990–991, 1992.
86. Kim KT, Dalton JW, Klaustermeyer WB: Subacute hypersensitivity pneumonitis to feathers presenting with weight loss and dyspnea. Ann Allergy 71:19–23, 1993.
87. Meyer FJ, Bauer PC, Costabel U: Feather wreath lung: Chasing a dead bird. Eur Respir J 9:1323–1324, 1996.
88. Flaherty DK, Braun SR, Marx JJ, et al: Serologically detectable HLA-A, -B and -C loci antigens in farmer's lung disease. Am Rev Respir Dis 122:437–446, 1980.
89. Muers MF, Faux JA, Ting A, et al: HLA-A, -B, -C and HLA-DR antigens in extrinsic allergic alveolitis (budgerigar fancier's lung disease). Clin Allergy 12:47–53, 1982.
90. Rodey CF, Fink J, Koethe S, et al: A study of HLA-A, -B, -C and -DR specificities in pigeon breeder's disease. Am Rev Respir Dis 119:755–759, 1979.
91. Warren C: Extrinsic allergic alveolitis: A disease commoner in nonsmokers. Thorax 32:567–573, 1977.
92. Baldwin CI, Todd A, Bourke S, et al: Pigeon fanciers' lung: Ef-

fects of smoking on serum and salivary antibody responses to pigeon antigens. Clin Exp Immunol 113:166–172, 1998.
93. Munakata M, Tanimura K, Ukita H, et al: Smoking promotes insidious and chronic farmer's lung disease, and deteriorates the clinical outcome. Intern Med 34:966–971, 1995.
94. Stiehm ER, Reed CE, Tooley WH: Pigeon breeder's lung in children. Pediatrics 39:904–915, 1967.
95. Bureau MA, Fecteau C, Patriquin H, et al: Farmer's lung in early childhood. Am Rev Respir Dis 119:671–675, 1979.
96. Eisenberg JD, Montanero A, Lee RG: Hypersensitivity pneumonitis in an infant. Pediatr Pulmonol 12:186–190, 1992.
97. Lama MS, Chapela R, Salas J, et al: Hypersensitivity pneumonitis: Cinical approach and an integral concept about its pathogenesis: A Mexican point of view. *In* Lama MS, Barrios R (eds): Interstitial Pulmonary Diseases: Selected Topics. Boca Raton: CRC Press, 1991, pp 171–195.
98. Schuyler M, Cook C, Listrom M, et al: Blast cells transfer experimental hypersensitivity pneumonitis. Am Rev Respir Dis 137:1449–1455, 1988.
99. Richerson HB, Coon JD, Lubaroff D: Adoptive transfer of experimental pneumonitis in the LEW rat. Am J Respir Crit Care Med 151:1205–1210, 1995.
100. Bice DE, Salvaggio JE, Hoffman ED: Passive transfer of experimental hypersensitivity pneumonitis with lymphoid cells in the rabbit. J Allergy Clin Immunol 58:250–262, 1976.
101. Schuyler M, Gott K, Cherne A, et al: Th1 $CD4^+$ cells adoptively transfer experimental hypersensitivity pneumonitis. Cell Immunol 177:169–175, 1997.
102. Schuyler M, Subramanyan S, Hassan MO: Experimental hypersensitivity pneumonitis: Transfer with cultured cells. J Lab Clin Med 109:623–630, 1987.
103. Cormier Y, Samson N, Israel-Assayag E: Viral infection enhances the response to *Saccharopolyspora rectivirgula* in mice prechallenged with this farmer's lung antigen. Lung 174:399–407, 1996.
104. Fournier E, Tonnel AB, Gosset PH, et al: Early neutrophil alveolitis after antigen inhalation in hypersensitivity pneumonitis. Chest 88:563–566, 1985.
105. Yoshizawa Y, Nomura A, Ohdama S, et al: The significance of complement activation in the pathogenesis of hypersensitivity pneumonitis: Sequential changes of complement components and chemotactic activities in bronchoalveolar lavage fluids. Int Arch Allergy Appl Immunol 87:417–423, 1988.
106. Yoshizawa Y, Ohdama S, Tanoue M, et al: Analysis of bronchoalveolar lavage cells and fluids in patients with hypersensitivity pneumonitis: Possible role of chemotactic factors in the pathogenesis of the disease. Int Arch Allergy Appl Immunol 80:376–382, 1986.
107. Rylander R, Haglind P: Airborne endotoxins and humidifier disease. Clin Allergy 14:109–112, 1984.
108. Mornex JF, Cordier G, Pages J, et al: Activated lung lymphocytes in hypersensitivity pneumonitis. J Allergy Clin Immunol 74:719–728, 1984.
109. Semenzato G, Zambello R, Trentin L, et al: Cellular immunity in sarcoidosis and hypersensitivity pneumonitis. Chest 103:139S–143S, 1993.
110. Denis M, Bedard M, Laviolette M, et al: A study of monokine release and natural killer activity in the bronchoalveolar lavage of subjects with farmer's lung. Am Rev Respir Dis 147:934–939, 1993.
111. Bjermer L, Engstrom-Laurent A, Lundgren R, et al: Bronchoalveolar mastocytosis in farmer's lung is related to the disease activity. Arch Intern Med 148:1362–1365, 1988.
112. Haslam P, Dewar A, Butchers P, et al: Mast cells, atypical lymphocytes and neutrophils in bronchoalveolar lavage in extrinsic allergic alveolitis. Am Rev Respir Dis 135:35–47, 1987.
113. Drent M, Wagenaar S, van Velzen-Blad H: Relationship between plasma cell levels and profile of bronchoalveolar lavage fluid in patients wih subacute extrinsic allergic alveolitis. Thorax 48:835–839, 1993.
114. Leatherman JW, Michael AF, Schwartz BA, et al: Lung T cells in hypersensitivity pneumonitis. Ann Intern Med 100:390–392, 1984.
115. Semenzato G, Agostini C, Zambello R, et al: Lung T cells in hypersensitivity pneumonitis: Phenotypic and functional analyses. J Immunol 137:1164–1172, 1986.
116. Cormier Y, Belanger J, Laviolette M: Prognostic significance of bronchoalveolar lymphocytosis in farmer's lung. Am Rev Respir Dis 135:692–695, 1987.
117. Brummond W, Kurup VP, Resnick A, et al: Immunologic response to *Faenia rectivirgula (Micropolyspora faeni)* in a dairy farm family. J Allergy Clin Immunol 82:190–195, 1988.
118. Muryama J, Yoshizawa Y, Ohtsuka M, et al: Lung fibrosis in hypersensitivity pneumonitis. Chest 104:38–43, 1993.
119. Ando M, Konishi K, Yoneda R, et al: Difference in the phenotypes of bronchoalveolar lavage lymphocytes in patients with summer-type hypersensitivity pneumonitis, farmer's lung, ventilation pneumonitis and bird fancier's lung: Report of a nationwide epidemiologic study in Japan. J Allergy Clin Immunol 87:1002–1009, 1991.
120. Trentin L, Marcer G, Chilosi M, et al: Longitudinal study of alveolitis in hypersensitivity pneumonitis patients: An immunological evaluation. J Allergy Clin Immunol 82:577–585, 1988.
121. Stankus RP, Cashner FM, Salvaggio JE: Bronchopulmonary macrophage activation in the pathogenesis of hypersensitivity pneumonitis. J Immunol 120:685–688, 1978.
122. Suga M, Yamasaki H, Nakagawa K, et al: Mechanisms accounting for granulomatous responses in hypersensitivity pneumonitis. Sarcoidosis Vasc Diffuse Lung Dis 14:131–138, 1997.
123. Drent M, Grutters JC, Mulder PG, et al: Is the different T helper cell activity in sarcoidosis and extrinsic allergic alveolitis also reflected by the cellular bronchoalveolar lavage fluid profile? Sarcoidosis Vasc Diffuse Lung Dis 14:31–38, 1997.
124. Teschler H, Thompson AB, Pohl WR, et al: Bronchoalveolar lavage procollagen-III-peptide in recent onset hypersensitivity pneumonitis: Correlation with extracellular matrix components. Eur Respir J 6:709–714, 1993.
125. Bensadoun ES, Burke AK, Hogg JC, et al: Proteoglycans in granulomatous lung diseases. Eur Respir J 10:2731–2737, 1997.
126. Bice DE, Salvaggio JE, Hoffman ED, et al: Adjuvant properties of *Micropolyspora faeni.* J Allergy Clin Immunol 55:267–274, 1976.
127. Denis M, Cormier Y, Tardif J, et al: Hypersensitivity pneumonitis: Whole *Micropolyspora faeni* or antigens thereof stimulate the release of proinflammatory cytokines from macrophages. Am J Respir Cell Biol 5:198–203, 1991.
128. Colby TV, Coleman A: Histological diffferential diagnosis of extrinsic allergic alveolitis. Prog Surg Pathol 10:11–26, 1989.
129. Coleman A, Colby T: Histologic diagnosis of extrinsic allergic alveolitis. Am J Surg Pathol 12:514–518, 1988.
130. Sutinen S, Reijula K, Huhti E, et al: Extrinsic allergic bronchioalveolitis: Serology and biopsy findings. Eur J Respir Dis 64:271–282, 1983.
131. Reyes CN, Wenzel FJ, Lawton BR, et al: The pulmonary pathology of farmer's lung disease. Chest 81:142–146, 1982.
132. Thorn A, Lewne M, Belin L: Allergic alveolitis in a school environment. Scand J Work Environ Health 22:311–314, 1996.
133. Sansores R, Salas J, Chapela R, et al: Clubbing in hypersensitivity pneumonitis: Its prevalence and possible prognostic role. Arch Intern Med 150:1849–1851, 1990.
134. Burrell R, Rylander R: A critical review of the role of precipitins in hypersensitivity pneumonitis. Eur J Respir Dis 62:332–343, 1981.
135. Roberts RC, Wenzel FJ, Emanuel DA: Precipitating antibodies in a midwest dairy farming population toward the antigens associated with farmer's lung disease. J Allergy Clin Immunol 62:518–524, 1976.
136. McSharry C, Banham SW, Lynch PP, et al: Antibody measurement in extrinsic allergic alveolitis. Eur J Respir Dis 65:259–265, 1984.
137. Cormier Y, Belanger J: The fluctuant nature of precipitating antibodies in dairy farmers. Thorax 44:469–473, 1989.
138. Cormier Y, Belanger J, LeBlanc P, et al: Bronchoalveolar lavage in farmers' lung disease: Diagnostic and physiological significance. Br J Ind Med 43:401–405, 1986.
139. Krasnick J, Meuwissen HJ, Nakao MA, et al: Hypersensitivity pneumonitis: Problems in diagnosis. J Allergy Clin Immunol 97:1027–1030, 1996.
140. Barbee RA, Callies Q, Dickie HA, et al: The long-term prognosis in farmer's lung. Am Rev Respir Dis 97:223–231, 1968.
141. Huls G, Lindemann H, Velcovsky HG: Angiotensin converting

enzyme (ACE) in the follow-up control of children and adolescents with allergic alveolitis. Monatsschr Kinderheilkd 137:158–161, 1989.
142. Schwaiblmair M, Beinert T, Vogelmeier C, et al: Cardiopulmonary exercise testing following hay exposure challenge in farmer's lung. Eur Respir J 10:2360–2365, 1997.
143. Cormier Y, Belanger J: Long-term physiologic outcome after acute farmer's lung. Chest 87:796–800, 1985.
144. Pepys J, Jenkins PA: Precipitin (FLH) test in farmer's lung. Thorax 20:21–35, 1965.
145. Freedman PM, Ault B: Bronchial hyperreactivity to methacholine in farmer's lung disease. J Allergy Clin Immunol 67:59–63, 1981.
146. Jaakkola J, Partanen K, Terho EO, et al: Radiographic grading of extrinsic allergic alveolitis: A comparison between a modified ILO classification and a descriptive method. Acta Radiol 32:461–466, 1991.
147. Akira M, Kita N, Higashihara T, et al: Summer-type hypersensitivity pneumonitis: Comparison of high-resolution CT and plain radiographic findings. Am J Roentgenol 158:1223–1228, 1992.
148. Hodgson MJ, Parkinson DK, Karpf M: Chest x-rays in hypersensitivity pneumonitis: A metaanalysis of secular trend. Am J Ind Med 16:45–53, 1989.
149. Monkare S, Ikonen M, Haahtela T: Radiologic findings in farmer's lung: Prognosis and correlation to lung function. Chest 84:460–466, 1985.
150. Lynch DA, Rose CS, Way D, et al: Hypersensitivity pneumonitis: Sensitivity of high-resolution CT in a population-based study. Am J Roentgenol 159:469–472, 1992.
151. Buschman DL, Gamsu G, Waldron JA, et al: Chronic hypersensitivity pneumonitis: Use of CT in diagnosis. Am J Roentgenol 159:957–960, 1992.
152. Adler BD, Padley SP, Muller NL, et al: Chronic hypersensitivity pneumonitis: High-resolution CT and radiographic features in 16 patients. Radiology 185:91–95, 1992.
153. Silver S, Muller N, Miller R, et al: Hypersensitivity pneumonitis: Evaluation with CT. Radiology 173:441–445, 1989.
154. Hansell DM, Moskovic E: High-resolution computed tomography in extrinsic allergic alveolitis. Clin Radiol 43:8–12, 1991.
155. Remy-Jardin M, Remy J, Wallaert B, et al: Subacute and chronic bird breeder hypersensitivity pneumonitis: Sequential evaluation with CT and correlation with lung function tests and bronchoalveolar lavage. Radiology 189:111–118, 1993.
156. Hansell DM, Wells AU, Padley SP, et al: Hypersensitivity pneumonitis: Correlation of individual CT patterns with functional abnormalities. Radiology 199:123–128, 1996.
157. Niimi H, Kang EY, Swong JS, et al: CT of chronic infiltrative lung disease: Prevalence of mediastinal lymphadenopathy. J Comput Assist Tomogr 20:305–308, 1996.
158. Hendrick DJ, Marshall R, Faux JA, et al: Positive "alveolar" responses to antigen inhalation provocation tests: Their validity and recognition. Thorax 35:415–427, 1980.
159. Ramirez-Venegas A, Sansores RH, Perez-Padilla R, et al: Utility of a provocation test for diagnosis of chronic pigeon breeder's disease. Am J Respir Crit Care Med 158:862–869, 1998.
160. Richerson HB, Bernstein IL, Fink JN, et al: Guidelines for the clinical evaluation of hypersensitivity pneumonitis. J Allergy Clin Immunol 839–844, 1989.
161. Drent M, Mulder PGH, Wagenaar SS, et al: Differences in BAL fluid variables in interstitial lung diseases evaluated by discriminant analysis. Eur Respir J 6:803–810, 1993.
162. Laviolette M, Cormier Y, Loiseau A, et al: Bronchoalveolar mast cells in normal farmers and subjects with farmer's lung: Diagnostic, prognostic, and physiologic significance. Am Rev Respir Dis 144:855–860, 1991.
163. Calvanico NJ, Ambegaonkar SP, Schlueter DP, et al: Immunoglobulin levels in bronchoalveolar lavage fluid from pigeon breeders. J Lab Clin Med 96:129–140, 1980.
164. Cormier Y, Belanger J, Laviolette M: Prognostic significance of bronchoalveolar lymphocytosis in farmer's lung. Am Rev Respir Dis 135:692–695, 1987.
165. Cormier Y, Belanger J, Beaudoin J, et al: Abnormal bronchoalveolar lavage in asymptomatic dairy farmers: Study of lymphocytes. Am Rev Respir Dis 130:1046–1049, 1984.
166. Cormier Y, Belanger J, Laviolette M: Persistent bronchoalveolar lymphocytosis in asymptomatic farmers. Am Rev Respir Dis 133:843–847, 1986.
167. Descombes E, Gardiol D, Leuenberger P, et al: Transbronchial lung biopsy: An analysis of 530 cases with reference to the number of samples. Monaldi Arch Chest Dis 52:324–329, 1997.
168. Terho EO: Diagnostic criteria for farmer's lung disease. Am J Ind Med 10:329, 1986.
169. Cormier Y: Hypersensitivity pneumonitis. *In* Rom WN (ed): Environmental and Occupational Medicine. Philadelphia: Lippincott-Raven, 1998, pp 457–466.
170. Rose C, King TE Jr: Controversies in hypersensitivity pneumonitis (editorial). Am Rev Respir Dis 145:1–2, 1992.
171. Monkare S, Haahtela T: Farmer's lung—A 5-year follow-up of eighty-six patients. Clin Allergy 17:143–151, 1987.
172. Chasse M, Blanchette G, Malo JL: Farmer's lung presenting as respiratory failure and homogeneous consolidation. Chest 90:783–784, 1986.
173. Greenberger PA, Pien LC, Patterson R, et al: End-stage lung and ultimately fatal disease in a bird fancier. Am J Med 86:119–122, 1989.
174. Schmidt CD, Jensen RL, Christensen LT, et al: Longitudinal pulmonary function changes in pigeon breeders. Chest 93:359–363, 1988.
175. Grammer LC, Roberts M, Lerner C, et al: Clinical and serologic follow-up of four children and five adults with bird-fancier's lung. J Allergy Clin Immunol 85:655–660, 1990.
176. Tasaka S, Kanazawa M, Kawai C, et al: Fatal diffuse alveolar damage from bird fanciers' lung. Respiration 64:307–309, 1997.
177. Kokkarinen J, Tukiainen H, Terho EO: Mortality due to farmer's lung in Finland. Chest 106:509–512, 1994.
178. Braun SR, doPico GA, Tsiatis A, et al: Farmer's lung disease: Long-term clinical and physiologic outcome. Am Rev Respir Dis 119:185–191, 1979.
179. Erkinjuntti-Pekkanen R, Rytkonen H, Kokkarinen JI, et al: Long-term risk of emphysema in patients with farmer's lung and matched control farmers. Am J Respir Crit Care Med 158:662–665, 1998.
180. Erkinjuntti-Pekkanen R, Kokkarinen JI, Tukiainen HO, et al: Long-term outcome of pulmonary function in farmer's lung: A 14 year follow-up with matched controls. Eur Respir J 10:2046–2050, 1997.
181. Lalancette M, Carrier G, Ferland S, et al: Long term outcome and predictive value of bronchoalveolar lavage fibrosing factors in farmer's lung. Am Rev Respir Dis 148:216–221, 1993.
182. Kokkarinen JI, Tukianinen HO, Terho EO: Asthma in patients with farmer's lung during a five-year follow-up. Scand J Work Environ Health 23:149–151, 1997.
183. Perez Padilla R, Salas J, Chapela R, et al: Mortality in Mexican patients with chronic pigeon breeder's lung compared with those with usual interstitial pneumonia. Am Rev Respir Dis 148:49–53, 1993.
184. Cuthbert OD, Gordon MF: Ten year follow up of farmers with farmer's lung. Br J Indus Med 40:173–176, 1983.
185. Bourke SJ, Banham SW, Carter R, et al: Longitudinal course of extrinsic allergic alveolitis in pigeon breeders. Thorax 44:415–418, 1989.
186. Richerson HB, Richards DW, Swanson PA, et al: Antigen-specific desensitization in a rabbit model of acute hypersensitivity pneumonitis. J Allergy Clin Immunol 68:226–234, 1981.
187. Allen DH, Williams GV, Woolcock AJ: Bird breeder's hypersensitivity pneumonitis: Progress studies of lung function after cessation of exposure to the provoking antigen. Am Rev Respir Dis 114:555–566, 1976.
188. de Gracia J, Morell F, Bofill JM, et al: Time of exposure as a prognostic factor in avian hypersensitivity pneumonitis. Respir Med 83:139–143, 1989.
189. Yoshida K, Ando M, Sakata T, et al: Prevention of summer-type hypersensitivity pneumonitis: Effect of elimination of *Trichosporon cutaneum* from the patients' homes. Arch Environ Health 44:317–322, 1989.
190. Woodard ED, Friedlander B, Lesher RJ, et al: Outbreak of hypersensitivity pneumonitis in an industrial setting. JAMA 259:1965–1969, 1988.
191. Reed CE, Swanson BA, Lopez M, et al: Measurement of IgG antibody and airborne antigen to control an industrial outbreak of hypersensitivity pneumonitis. J Occup Med 25:207–210, 1983.

192. Zwick H, Popp W, Braun O, et al: Personal spore sampling and indirect immunofluroescent test for exploration of hypersensitivity pneumonitis due to mould spores. Allergy 46:277–283, 1991.
193. American Conference of Governmental Industrial Hygienists: Developing an investigation strategy. *In* Macher JM (ed): Bioaerosols Assessment and Control. Cincinnati, OH: American Conference of Government Industrial Hygienists, 1999.
194. Craig TJ: Bird antigen persistence in the home environment after removal of the bird. Ann Allergy 69:510–512, 1992.
195. Craig TJ, Hershey J, Engler RJ, et al: Tannic acid's effect on bird antigen. Ann Allergy Asthma Immunol 75:348–350, 1995.
196. Monkare S: Influence of corticosteroid treatment on the course of farmer's lung. Eur J Respir Dis 64:283–293, 1983.
197. Kokkarinen JI, Tukiainen HO, Terho EO: Effect of corticosteroid treatment on the recovery of pulmonary function in farmer's lung. Am Rev Respir Dis 145:3–5, 1992.
198. Carlsen KH, Leegaard J, Lund OD, et al: Allergic alveolitis in a 12-year-old boy: Treatment with budesonide nebulizing solution. Pediatr Pulmonol 12:257–259, 1992.
199. Losa Garcia JE, Mateos Rodriguez F, Jimenez Lopez A, et al: Effect of cyclosporin A on inflammatory cytokine production by human alveolar macrophages. Respir Med 92:722–728, 1998.
200. Zejda JE, McDuffie HH, Dosman JA: Epidemiology of health and safety risks in agriculture and related industries: Practical applications for rural physicians. West J Med 158:56–63, 1993.
201. Dalphin JC, Toson B, Monnet E, et al: Farmer's lung precipitins in Doubs (a department of France): Prevalence and diagnostic value. Allergy 49:744–750, 1994.
202. Mauny F, Polio JC, Monnet E, et al: Longitudinal study of respiratory health in dairy farmers: Influence of artificical barn fodder drying. Eur Respir J 10:2522–2528, 1997.
203. Nuutinen J, Terho EO, Husman K, et al: Protective value of powered dust respirator helmet for farmers with farmer's lung. Eur J Respir Dis 152:212–220, 1987.
204. Anderson K, Walker A, Boyd G: The long-term effect of a positive pressure respirator on the specific antibody response in pigeon breeders. Clin Exper Allergy 19:45–49, 1988.
205. Hendrick D, Marshall R, Faux J, et al: Protective value of dust respirators in extrinsic allergic alveolitis: Clinical assessment using inhalation provocation tests. Thorax 36:917–921, 1981.
206. Yoshizawa Y, Ohtani Y, Hayakawa H, et al: Chronic hypersensitivity pneumonitis in Japan: A nationwide epidemiologic survey. J Allergy Clin Immunol 103:315–320, 1999.

# 68 Air Pollution

JOHN R. BALMES, M.D. • IRA TAGER, M.D.

Introduction
Pollutants
General Properties, Sources, and Distribution
Defense Against Inhaled Pollutants
Methods of Studying Adverse Effects of Air Pollution
Epidemiologic Studies
Clinical Human Research
Animal Research
Adverse Effects of Specific Pollutants
Sulfur Dioxide and Particulate Matter
Photochemical Oxidants: Ozone and Nitrogen Dioxide
Summary

## INTRODUCTION

Appreciation of a general relationship between disease and breathing air contaminated by the products of human activity is ancient. Steps were taken to regulate the use of coal in England during the reign of Richard II (1377–1399).[1] It later became apparent that the danger was not confined to workers exposed to the highest concentrations of pollutants at sites of production but that those living in the areas immediately surrounding certain industries were also at risk. That whole communities were at risk was most forcefully brought home by a series of episodes: in the Meuse Valley of Belgium in 1930; in Donora, Pennsylvania, in 1948; and in London, England, in 1952.[2] In these episodes, several days of air stagnation resulted in greatly increased concentrations of atmospheric pollutants, especially of sulfur dioxide and particulates, followed by a striking increase in mortality. In the worst of these episodes, in London, the death rate reached a level that had been exceeded in the 20th century only in the influenza pandemic of 1917–1918.[3] Although all age groups shared to some extent in the increase in mortality, most deaths occurred in the very young, the elderly, and persons already suffering from heart or lung disease. The excess mortality was largely due to bronchitis, pneumonia, and other respiratory and cardiac diseases. Individuals seemed also to differ in their sensitivity to the nonlethal consequences of these crises. In Donora, for example, there was one report of exacerbations in 88% of patients with asthma surveyed.[4]

Stimulated by the respiratory health effects of these episodes of extreme ambient air pollution, a large number of investigations have been carried out to define more clearly the impact of ambient air pollution on the respiratory tract and human health. Since 1975, these investigations have identified a variety of respiratory health effects at concentrations that are just above or within the levels set by the US Environmental Protection Agency (USEPA) (Table 68.1).[5]

A comprehensive review of the published research would be encyclopedic, because the effects include not just impairment of human health but also what are collectively termed "welfare" effects, such as reductions in visibility and damage to buildings and structures, to agriculture, and to whole ecosystems. Similarly, the number of pollutants is legion, reflecting the ever-increasing complexity of the production, storage, and destruction of industrial products. Thus this chapter discusses mainly the so-called criteria air pollutants (see Table 68.1), except for lead and carbon monoxide, and reviews what has been learned about the adverse effects of these pollutants on the lungs and airways. Criteria pollutants are those for which the USEPA has determined there is an adequate scientific data base on health effects to justify the regulation of air quality. The regulation of ambient concentration of each specific criteria pollutant is known as the National Ambient Air Quality Standard (NAAQS). The circumscribed nature of this review should be kept in mind, for materials dispersed in the air are not absorbed uniquely through the respiratory tract. Particles settle, for example, on crops and waters destined for ingestion. And even if pollutants are absorbed through the respiratory tract, their adverse effects need not be confined to the lungs and airways, for materials are absorbed through mucosal surfaces into the circulation, and some have been implicated in impairing function of the central nervous system, bone marrow, and other organs.

## POLLUTANTS

The definition of the term *pollutant* is elusive. Some experts consider an air pollutant to be an increase in concentrations of gases or particles to levels above those generally accepted as normal. At some sites, however, gases normally present in the atmosphere, as in caves, may be lethal for humans. Others consider a material to be a pollutant only if it is detectable as an unpleasant or

**Table 68.1 NATIONAL PRIMARY AIR QUALITY STANDARDS IN THE UNITED STATES (CRITERIA POLLUTANTS)**

| Pollutant | Standard | Averaging Period |
|---|---|---|
| Carbon monoxide | 9 ppm (10 mg/m$^3$) | 8 hours |
| | 35 ppm (40 mg/m$^3$) | 1 hour |
| Nitrogen dioxide | 0.053 ppm (100 μg/m$^3$) | 1 year |
| Ozone | 0.12 ppm (235 μg/m$^3$) | 1 hour |
| | 0.08 ppm (157 μg/m$^3$) | 8 hours |
| Particulate <10 μm ($PM_{10}$) | 50 μg/m$^3$ | 1 year |
| | 150 μg/m$^3$ | 24 hours |
| Particulate <2.5 μm ($PM_{2.5}$) | 15 μg/m$^3$ | 1 year |
| | 65 μg/m$^3$ | 24 hours |
| Sulfur dioxide | 0.03 ppm (80 μg/m$^3$) | 1 year |
| | 0.14 ppm (365 μg/m$^3$) | 24 hours |
| Lead | 1.5 μg/m$^3$ | 3 month |

hazardous material. The problem with this definition is apparent, for the definition of a pollutant must now start with the identification of an effect. This is, in fact, the approach that has been taken toward considering products of industrial activity that contaminate the atmosphere, and the definition of what constitutes an "adverse health effect" has been the subject of debate[6] that remains under periodic review. For the purposes of this review, any effect that impairs function or that indicates the initiation of a sequence of events known to result in the impairment of function is considered an "adverse health effect."

Three major types of air pollutants are recognized: the sulfur dioxide and particulate complex, photochemical oxidants, and a miscellaneous category of pollutants arising from industrial and mobile sources (so-called toxic air contaminants). Only the first two of these types of pollution are discussed in this chapter because the primary adverse health effects associated with toxic air contaminants are nonrespiratory cancers and reproductive dysfunction. This conventional method of grouping pollutants is based on the conditions that lead to their production and not necessarily on common biologic effects. For example, atmospheric acids can be generated by by-products of sulfur dioxide (e.g., sulfuric acid) and of oxides of nitrogen (nitric acid). Epidemiologic evidence has implicated atmospheric acidity as a possible contributing factor in the development of adverse respiratory health effects. However, the biologic effects of these acids are quite different from those of the parent compounds from which they are derived. Some of the commonly encountered pollutants associated with adverse pulmonary effects are listed in Table 68.2.

## General Properties, Sources, and Distribution

Sulfur oxides, particulate matter (PM), ozone, and nitrogen dioxide are the most widely encountered pollutants that have been shown to cause adverse pulmonary effects. Sulfur dioxide is produced by the combustion of sulfur contained in fossil fuels such as coal and crude oil, and the major sources of environmental pollution with sulfur dioxide are power plants, oil refineries, smelters, and paper pulp mills. In the United States, sulfur dioxide levels are generally higher in the northeastern and midwestern states, primarily because of the use of high–sulfur-content coal in power plants. Sulfur dioxide itself is a clear, highly water-soluble gas, so it is effectively absorbed by the mucosal surfaces of the upper airways. A very small proportion of inhaled sulfur dioxide reaches the distal regions of the lungs.[7] The sulfur dioxide released into the atmosphere does not, however, remain uniquely in the form of a gas; rather, it undergoes chemical reactions with water, trace metals, and other pollutants to form a variety of particulate aerosols. The nature of particles generated from sulfur-containing fuels varies from place to place, but sulfuric acid and various metallic, acidic, and ammonium sulfates are commonly present. Other nonsulfur products of fossil fuel combustion (soot, fly ash, oxides of iron, zinc, copper, silicates, nitrates) contribute to the type of pollution present in urban areas where coal is burned in many residences and industrial emissions are not well controlled (e.g., London in the 1950s). This mixture of sulfur oxides and small particles may be blown great distances from its site of production, undergoing continuous transformation from gas to particle phase and ultimately becoming "acid rain" capable of profoundly affecting flora and fauna.[8]

In the western United States and many other areas of the world, particulate pollution is not driven by the combustion of sulfur-containing fuels. Atmospheric particulate air pollution arises from a variety of sources, both natural (e.g., sea spray, windblown dust) and synthetic sources (e.g., power plants, motor vehicles).[1, 9, 10] Particulate material that enters the atmosphere can be primary (particles emitted directly) and secondary (particles that form by chemical reactions that involve gas-phase precursors, such as sulfur dioxide and oxides of nitrogen).[4] Particles span a wide range of diameters from 0.003 μm (e.g., from automobiles, power generation) to as large as 1 μm particles produced in the atmosphere. Photochemical processes produce particles in the range of 0.003 to 2 μm in diameter. Windblown dust, pollens, cement dust are generally larger than 2 μm.[11] To date, most studies of the

**Table 68.2 MAJOR POLLUTANTS ASSOCIATED WITH ADVERSE PULMONARY EFFECTS**

| Pollutant | Outdoor Sources | Indoor Sources | Adverse Effects |
|---|---|---|---|
| Sulfur oxides | Power plants, oil refineries, smelters | Kerosene space heaters | Bronchoconstriction |
| Oxides of nitrogen | Motor vehicle exhaust, power plants, oil refineries | Gas stoves and furnaces, kerosene space heaters | Airway injury (respiratory bronchiolitis), impaired lung defenses, enhanced response to allergen |
| Ozone | Motor vehicle exhaust | Aircraft cabins, welding, copiers, ozone generators | Airway injury (respiratory bronchiolitis), decreased lung function, exacerbations of asthma, enhanced response to allergen |
| Particulate matter | Motor vehicle exhaust, power plants | Tobacco and wood smoke | Exacerbations of asthma and chronic obstructive pulmonary disease, increased cardiopulmonary mortality |
| Radon | | Residential basements | Lung cancer |
| Polycyclic hydrocarbons | Diesel exhaust | Tobacco smoke | Lung cancer |

health effects of particles have focused on particle mass. Environmental monitoring before 1987 evaluated particles up to approximately 50 μm in aerodynamic diameter; however, since the 1970s, the focus has been on particle sizes that can be deposited in the human respiratory tract (generally $<$ 10 μm in diameter).[12] Particles classified as "fine" ($<$ 1 μm) can travel for long distances and remain in the atmosphere for days to weeks; coarse particles ($>$ 1 μm) travel for rather short distances and have atmospheric half-lives of minutes to hours.[12] The distribution of the number of particles is inversely rated to particle size.[13] "Fine" mode particles are composed mainly of varying amounts of water and six major components (sulfates, acids, nitrates, elemental carbon, organic carbon, and trace metals), several of which can be further subdivided on the basis of chemical constituents and sources.[12] They are formed from gases by nucleation, condensation, or liquid phase reactions. "Coarse" mode particles are composed primarily of crustal (rock, soil), biologic (pollen, spores), and industrial components; they are formed primarily by mechanical processes that produce small particles from larger particles.

Ozone and nitrogen oxides are primarily products not so much of heavy industrial activity as of the action of sunlight on emissions of internal combustion engines.[14] The most important of these products are unburned hydrocarbons and nitrogen dioxide, an oxidation product of nitrogen oxide, which is in turn a product of the fixation of atmospheric nitrogen with oxygen under conditions of high-temperature combustion. Ultraviolet irradiation of this mixture in the atmosphere results in a complex series of chemical reactions, producing ozone, alkyl nitrates, peroxyacyl nitrates, alcohols, ethers, acids, peroxyacids, and other organic and inorganic compounds that exist in both gas and particulate aerosol phases.[14] This mixture of pollutants typifies the "smog" of areas with large numbers of automobiles and abundant sunlight, such as the Los Angeles basin. Because ozone and nitrogen dioxide are the gases present in highest concentration and because they clearly cause toxic effects in animals and humans excessively exposed to them, they have been the oxidant pollutants most extensively studied. Both gases are relatively insoluble and poorly absorbed by the upper airways. A high proportion of the dose inhaled thus reaches the peripheral portion of the lungs and can cause injury at any site from the upper airways to the alveoli.[15]

Outdoor urban air contains a number of known carcinogens, including polycyclic hydrocarbons, *n*-nitroso compounds, and asbestos. The concentrations of these carcinogens in ambient air, however, are quite low. Epidemiologic studies of exposure to diesel exhaust have provided consistent evidence of an excess risk of lung cancer in workers exposed to diesel exhaust,[16] and diesel exhaust is considered a probable carcinogen in humans by several agencies on the basis of experimental and epidemiologic data.[17] Three large population-based epidemiologic studies also have indicated an increased risk of lung cancer in relation to long-term exposure to ambient concentrations of particulate air pollutants, sulfur dioxide, and ozone.[18–20]

Whereas most attention has been given to pollutants present in outdoor air, it is now apparent that elevated concentrations of airborne contaminants are common inside homes, public buildings, and other indoor microenvironments.[21] Because urban residents typically spend 90% of their time indoors and because some contaminants are present in higher concentrations in indoor air, public health officials have become aware that measurement of outdoor air quality does not adequately characterize the risks of personal exposure.[21] Among the pollutants of indoor air of greatest concern are the by-products of cigarette smoking ("passive smoking" or environmental tobacco smoke), which appear to increase the risk of lower respiratory tract infection and asthma in children and the risk of cardiovascular disease and lung cancer among adults.[22] Nitrogen dioxide, a product of natural gas and kerosene combustion, may be present in indoor air in concentrations many times higher than those in outdoor air.[23] This has been suspected to increase the prevalence of respiratory illnesses in small children in the age range of 5 to 12 years raised in homes with natural gas, rather than electricity, as an energy source for cooking and heating,[24, 25] but not in infants in the first 18 months of life.[26] Sulfur dioxide concentrations can reach levels 20 times higher than the present US primary air quality standard of 0.14 part per million (ppm) in rooms heated by commercially available kerosene-burning space heaters[27]; ozone levels three times or more greater than the permitted level in outdoor air may be encountered in the cabins of high-altitude commercial aircraft[28]; and formaldehyde is released into the air of buildings insulated with urea-formaldehyde foam insulation and in mobile homes in which there is extensive use of plywood.[29]

A pollutant of indoor air that has caused particular concern is radon, a naturally occurring radioactive gas in the decay series of uranium ($^{238}U$) present in building materials made from rocks and soils. Epidemiologic studies of underground miners have provided strong and consistent evidence that radon causes lung cancer, and surveys conducted by the USEPA have documented high levels of radon in some homes in many regions of the United States, especially in the northeastern states.

The lung cancer risk from radon exposure in household air has so far proved difficult to define precisely.[17, 30] There is some suggestion that this risk is consistent with that observed in underground miners.[17] The USEPA has nonetheless estimated that about 15,000 to 20,000 lung cancer deaths annually are attributable to indoor radon.[31] Resolution of the issue may have to await completion of further pooled analyses of existing case-control studies.[17] In the meantime, some experts have suggested that the most cost-efficient way to reduce the incidence of radon-induced lung cancer is through smoking cessation and education of occupants of radon-contaminated homes to take such simple steps as improving the ventilation system, avoiding the use of basements as living areas, and discouraging the display of actinide-containing mineral collections in living areas.

Ironically, the importance of pollution of indoor air became apparent as a result of steps taken to reduce the need for heat production from the combustion of fossil fuels. With more efficient insulation of buildings, the turnover of indoor air is reduced, permitting the accumulation of greater quantities of contaminants.

## DEFENSE AGAINST INHALED POLLUTANTS

Given that the lung is a delicate structure with a large surface area and encounters about 9000 liters of air daily, with each liter containing millions of particles, it is not surprising that an effective system has evolved for removing impurities from the air inhaled and for clearing and destroying particles or microorganisms that gain entry into the respiratory tract. The various mechanisms of defense are interrelated and work in a coordinated manner. A perturbation in any mechanism, whether because of congenital deficiency, disease, or the effect of an inhaled pollutant, may result in the breakdown of the coordinated defense system and in the development of disease. Definition of the mechanisms of defense normally present thus permits the inferential identification of subgroups of the population that may be at particularly high risk for adverse effects from inhaling polluted air.

Air pollutants exist as either gases or suspended particles. As gases, their site of deposition in the respiratory tract is largely a function of their solubility, the duration of exposure, and the airflow pattern of breathing. For highly soluble gases, the nose serves an important defensive function, because the air inhaled transnasally is passed over the large, irregular surface of the turbinates. The promotion of turbulent flow prolongs contact with the mucosal surface, increasing adsorption. Under conditions of quiet breathing, when most air is inspired transnasally, this is an efficient system. For example, the concentration of sulfur dioxide that reaches the glottis is less than 2% of the concentration inspired at the nose.[7] Under other circumstances, the importance of the nose diminishes. The more rapid the inspiratory flow, the smaller the proportion of sulfur dioxide removed.[7] Furthermore, the mouth is substantially less efficient at absorbing gases than is the nose, and the proportion of air inhaled through the mouth increases with the increased ventilatory demands of exercise. Thus the dose of a soluble pollutant delivered to the lower airways is increased by exercise for three reasons: the inspiratory flow is higher, the proportion inhaled through the mouth is increased, and the total quantity inhaled over time is greater (quantity = concentration × volume). The importance of the level of ventilation (in turn a function of the level of exercise) and of the oral-nasal distribution of breathing has perhaps best been shown in studies of the bronchoconstrictor response to sulfur dioxide.[32] Therefore, people with obstructive nasal disease also appear to be at greater risk for adverse respiratory effects of soluble pollutant gases.

For inhaled particles, the duration of retention in the lung, and therefore the likelihood of an adverse effect, is in large part a function of the site of deposition, which is largely determined by the size of the particles themselves.[33] (Deposition and lung clearance are discussed in Chapter 15.) Large particles (diameter $> 10$ μm) are efficiently removed by simple filtration through nasal cilia. Those that are not removed by filtration tend to become deposited by impaction; because of their great inertia, they cannot easily change direction to follow the abrupt changes in the direction of airflow in the nose, pharynx, and tracheobronchial tree; therefore, they impact on the mucosa of the upper respiratory tract and large airways, especially at points of bifurcation. The mechanisms of filtration and impaction are so efficient that few particles more than 10 μm in diameter are deposited in the lower respiratory tract.

The sites of deposition of smaller particles are determined much more by sedimentation and diffusion. Sedimentation, the tendency to fall at a constant rate under the influence of gravity, is influenced by the density and diameter of the particle and by the viscosity of the surrounding gas. Sedimentation probably accounts for the predominant deposition of particles of intermediate size (diameter, 0.5 to 3.0 μm) in the small airways and alveoli. For the smallest particles, diffusion is the mechanism by which deposition occurs. Many of these particles are not deposited at all but remain in suspension in the exhaled air; those that are deposited tend to settle in the terminal bronchioles and alveoli.

To some extent, deposition of particles can be influenced by the pattern of breathing. At the same minute ventilation, small, rapid breaths promote deposition in central airways, whereas slow, deep breaths increase the time for diffusion and sedimentation and favor deposition in the distal airways and alveoli.[34] Because there is intersubject variability in the pattern of breathing adopted to achieve the same increase in ventilation with exercise, it is possible that the sites of deposition, and therefore the effects of particles, differ among people performing similar tasks in the same atmosphere.

For the particles deposited in the tracheobronchial tree, cough and mucociliary clearance are the most important mechanisms of defense. Cough is especially effective in clearing particles deposited in large central airways; it is provoked by stimulation of afferent nerves ("cough receptors"), which are found in greatest density in the mucosa of the larynx and at branch points in the tracheobronchial tree,[35] the sites where particles are most likely to be deposited. (Cough is discussed further in Chapter 21.) The mucociliary system operates over the length of the conducting airways, from the proximal trachea to the terminal bronchioles. The mucus blanket is the product of secretion by goblet and serous cells of the epithelium and by the mucus and serous cells of the submucosal glands (see Chapter 14). The mucus blanket is discontinuous and is propelled mouthward by the cilia of the epithelial cells. The effective removal of particles by the mucociliary system thus requires secretion of glycoproteins by specialized secretory cells, maintenance of liquefaction by the transport of water and solute by airway epithelial cells (discussed in Chapter 14), and coordinated function of airway cilia. Impairment of any of these functions, whether by congenital or acquired diseases affecting mucus or water secretion (e.g., cystic fibrosis, chronic bronchitis) or ciliary function (e.g., dysmotile cilia syndrome), leads to prolongation of the retention time of particles, increasing the likelihood of adverse effects due to the particles themselves or to the materials (e.g., heavy metals) entrained on their surface. Such an impairment of function probably accounts for the finding that exposure to low levels of ozone enhanced pulmonary retention of asbestos fibers in rats.[36]

The clearance of particles deposited beyond the mucociliary blanket, in the distal, gas-exchanging part of the lung, involves primarily the alveolar macrophage. This cell scavenges particles deposited in the alveoli and either digests them or migrates with them to the respiratory bronchiole, where it ascends the mucociliary escalator. A small number of macrophages ingest particles and migrate to peribronchial or perivascular connective tissue. Clearance by this route is slow, and particle-laden macrophages may still be found in lung connective tissue many weeks after exposure.[37]

Although the macrophage usually functions to protect the lungs, it is possible that in some circumstances it contributes to lung injury. It is now hypothesized, for example, that the lung fibrosis caused by silica and asbestos particles is due to the continued attempt by macrophages to ingest and destroy the inhaled fibers. This activity results in the continuous release of connective tissue proteases from the macrophages themselves and in the continuous release of other mediators that secondarily activate lung fibroblasts and attract and activate polymorphonuclear leukocytes.[38]

Appreciation of the macrophage's role as the cell that makes initial contact with inhaled particles and that then communicates with other cells, amplifying the response to challenge, has led to its being regarded as the pivotal cell in lung defense. However, research during the 1990s has led to increased appreciation of the role of airway epithelial cells in mediating lung injury and repair after pollutant exposure.[39]

The function of noncellular mechanisms of lung defense became apparent from observations made on the pathogenesis of emphysema in $alpha_1$-antitrypsin deficiency. These observations led to the theory that the lung's structural proteins require defense against the proteases repeatedly released from inflammatory cells activated to destroy inhaled materials. A deficiency in the containment of proteolytic activity, as from a deficiency in normally circulating antiproteases, results in the destruction of alveolar tissues. This suggests the importance of the discovery that oxidant pollutants cause both a striking increase in polymorphonuclear cells in the lungs and airways[40, 41] and the inactivation of the active site of $alpha_1$-antiprotease.[42] Studies in humans and animals indicate that antioxidant defenses are likely to be important in the expression of air pollutant–induced injury of the respiratory tract.[43–45]

## METHODS OF STUDYING ADVERSE EFFECTS OF AIR POLLUTION

What has been learned about the complex, integrated systems responsible for defending the lungs permits a rational prediction of potential harm from various pollutants and allows inferences about subgroups of the population that might be at greatest risk from harmful effects of different pollutants. However, even sound, scientifically based conjecture is far from an adequate basis for initiating the major industrial and social changes needed to reduce atmospheric pollution. The scientific basis for the actions needed must rest on the demonstration of a high likelihood of harmful effects, as shown by studies of disease in populations exposed to polluted air, acute effects in human subjects after short-term exposure to controlled levels of pollutants in a laboratory, and effects on lung structure and function in animals. Each of these forms of study presents various advantages and disadvantages, and none provides irrefutable proof of harmful effects from a particular pollutant under natural conditions of exposure. Standards are based, therefore, on the coherence of evidence provided by epidemiologic, clinical, and animal research and are set to provide a margin of safety, with the recognition that harmful effects may occur in sensitive subgroups of the population even with exposure to levels below those that have been shown to cause effects in published studies.

### Epidemiologic Studies

Of the three sources of evidence that relate to air pollution health effects, only epidemiologic studies permit the investigation of large numbers of people who are exposed to the ambient air quality conditions that are of interest. The demonstration by such studies of adverse health effects in relation to specific ambient conditions can provide strong support for regulatory intervention. However, by their nature, epidemiologic studies are complex, and to provide valid data, they must overcome certain inherent difficulties.

Many factors other than air pollutants can give rise to acute and chronic respiratory symptoms and functional changes. Modern epidemiologic studies of air pollution health effects do account for the influence of factors such as age, cigarette and other tobacco use, occupational exposures, socioeconomic influences, and underlying medical illnesses. However, it is not possible to be entirely sure that residual effects of such factors have not affected the results of these studies. Since 1990, the use of daily time series studies has increased, inasmuch as these studies provide for control of important confounders that do not change over relatively short periods of time.[46] These studies have led to important advances in the delineation of the potential respiratory health effects of ambient air pollution.

A major difficulty for large-scale epidemiologic studies stems from the fact that many, if not most, ambient environments are complex mixtures of pollutants with potential health effects from a single agent and/or the interaction of several agents. A number of studies have nonetheless been designed to provide the detail necessary to separate out the individual and interactive effects of various pollutants.[47, 48] Such studies, for example, have been able to identify the subcomponent of the particulate component of ambient air pollution that is most strongly associated with the occurrence of chronic respiratory symptoms in children[47] and to distinguish effects of individual pollutants within the complex mixture of ambient pollutants.[49–51]

The assignment of individual exposures and doses also poses a challenge for epidemiologic studies. Factors such as the time spent indoors vs. outdoors and activity patterns are important determinants of exposure and dose. Although still heavily dependent on area-wide monitoring, epidemiologic studies are increasingly capable of providing multiple metrics of exposure (e.g., hourly peaks, hourly averages, 24-hour averages) for a wide variety of pollutants[52] and of evaluating their relationship to the health outcomes of interest. Technologic advances have led to the development of devices that permit personal monitoring of individuals in their breathing zones[53] and offer the prospect of even more refined exposure/dose assignment. Creative epidemiologic designs have led to the study of groups of individuals functioning under well-measured conditions of activity in ambient environments that are dominated by single species of pollutants and that are well characterized in terms of other relevant pollutants,[54–56] temperature, and humidity. Finally, advances in statistical analytic techniques[46, 57] have permitted more realistic modeling of the complex interplay of the components of the environment in relation to health outcomes of interest.

### Clinical Human Research

Experimental studies of human subjects exposed to carefully controlled conditions can demonstrate the occurrence of acute responses to various doses of a single pollutant or pollutant mixture. Such studies can detect the minimal concentrations that induce measurable effects on tests of function and can assess responses in segments of the population predicted to have increased susceptibility to adverse effects under a range of exposure conditions (e.g., rest, vigorous exercise, oral breathing, nasal breathing). These studies are powerful tools for analyzing the effects of a pollutant on an important acute event, such as the precipitation of myocardial ischemia by carbon monoxide in a patient with coronary artery disease[58] or of bronchospasm in a patient with asthma.[59] The limitation of these studies in analyzing the effects of chronic exposure is obvious, and at present the relationship between the effects of low or short-term exposure and the development of disease with long-term exposure is unknown. The finding that a brief exposure to ozone causes acute decrements in lung function does not, for example, necessarily indicate that prolonged or repeated exposure will lead to the development of chronic obstructive lung disease. For even a reasoned guess at the relationship, much more needs to be known about the pathogenesis of chronic obstructive lung disease, about the mechanisms of injury from ozone, and about the mechanisms responsible for tolerance of or adaptation to repeated exposures. With this information, it might be possible to determine whether acute exposure to the pollutant produces an effect known to be a marker indicating the initiation of the pathogenetic sequence responsible for disease.

### Animal Research

Study of animals offers the best opportunity to determine the pathogenetic mechanisms and nature of the changes in lung structure and function that result from chronic exposure to specific pollutants. In addition, animal studies permit assessment of the effects of a range of concentrations, so that a dose-response curve can be constructed: from the dose producing the first measurable change in structure or function to the dose producing a fatal outcome. Studies of animals uniquely offer a means of identifying possible "markers" of events that will lead to disease with chronic exposure, because only in animals is it feasible to relate the changes in measurements of physiologic or biochemical function produced by short-term exposures to the changes in structure and function produced by long-term exposure.

The major limitation of animal studies is that large interspecies variations in the response to pollutants make prediction of human dose-response relationships hazardous. Dogs, for example, can tolerate up to 200 ppm of sulfur dioxide without developing significant bronchoconstriction, whereas guinea pigs appear to be especially sensitive to the bronchomotor effects of the gas,[60] and rodents are relatively insensitive to ozone.[61] Another limitation is that some relatively common human diseases, such as asthma and cystic fibrosis, do not occur in animals, and so the response of people with these diseases cannot be estimated from animal studies.

## ADVERSE EFFECTS OF SPECIFIC POLLUTANTS

### Sulfur Dioxide and Particulate Matter

A large body of accumulated data indicates that many of the health effects that have been attributed to sulfur dioxide in the past may in fact have been due to effects of particulate pollution that includes acid derivatives of sulfur dioxide as well as components that are not related to sulfur dioxide. Nonetheless, these two pollutant categories are discussed together, because many early studies cannot distinguish between their effects.

As mentioned previously, the strongest piece of evidence linking air pollution with adverse health effects is the observation of dramatic increases in mortality during severe episodes of air pollution in the Meuse Valley, Belgium (1930); in Donora, Pennsylvania (1948); and in London, England (1952).[2, 3] During each of these episodes, the concentrations of sulfur dioxide and particulate matter are thought to have been extremely high. For example, during the London episode, it has been estimated that the maximal 24-hour concentration of sulfur dioxide exceeded 1.5 ppm and the concentration of total suspended particulate exceeded 4.4 mg/m$^3$.[62] Both of these values are more than 10-fold higher than the current maximal allowable 24-hour concentrations for these pollutants set by the USEPA (see Table 68.1). Several reanalyses of the London episode have provided evidence that the particulate component and not sulfur dioxide was primarily responsible for the excess deaths that were observed.[63, 64]

Since these episodes, many *epidemiologic studies* have been performed in urban areas around the world to examine the relationship between mortality and fluctuations in the ambient concentrations of sulfur dioxides and particulate matter.[65] Overall, these studies show a consistent pattern of association between increased sulfur oxide and particulate concentrations and mortality.[2, 63–67] Of particular importance is the observation that effects on daily mortality have been observed over ranges of particulate concentrations that are below the current NAAQS.[64, 65, 66, 67–70] Because a high correlation exists between particulate air pollution and components of sulfur pollution ($SO_2$, $H_2SO_4$, $[H^+]$), studies have been undertaken to distinguish the mortality effects of each of these components.[64, 65, 67, 68, 70] The preponderance of evidence suggests that particulate matter (measured either as total suspended particulate [TSP] or particles $< 10\ \mu m$ [$PM_{10}$] or less than $2.5\ \mu m$ [$PM_{2.5}$]) has a greater effect on daily mortality than do various measures of sulfur species.[64, 65, 67, 70–73] Some studies have found $H_2SO_4$ to have the largest effect,[68] and studies from European countries[74] and Canada[75] have identified independent effects for sulfur dioxide. Mortality effects have been observed to occur largely in people 65 years of age or older[69, 76] and in those with underlying cardiopulmonary disease.[76] The mechanisms underlying this excess mortality are not well understood. Increases in plasma viscosity[77] and decreases in heart rate variability (increased risk of fatal arrhythmias)[78] have been suggested as possible mechanisms for the cardiac component. Particle-associated decreases in oxygen saturation[78] and the physical consequences of the deposition of large numbers of particles in the nanometer range as well as the chemical reactivity of the particles have been suggested as contributors to respiratory morbidity and to mortality.[79]

Two cohort studies have provided data to suggest that there are increasing all-cause, cardiopulmonary, and lung cancer mortality rates that are associated with environments that have increasing levels of particle air pollution ($PM_{2.5}$).[19, 20] The only data that related specifically to the respiratory tract were for lung cancer, and these results were not precise enough for a definite conclusion about an effect on lung cancer mortality. No data were provided in these studies on deaths from other respiratory diseases. Some support of these observations is found in a study that reported increases in lung cancer incidence associated with long-term exposure to elevated $PM_{10}$ and in lung cancer incidence among males (not among females).[18] In this same study, sulfur dioxide exposure also was associated with increased incidences of lung cancer in both sexes.

Numerous epidemiologic studies have repeatedly found an association between (1) the presence of acute respiratory symptoms and short-term reductions in pulmonary function and (2) higher concentrations of particulate matter.[80, 81] Results have been less consistent for studies of acid sulfates, although some studies clearly have shown increases in respiratory hospital admissions that are related to sulfur dioxide–derived acid species.[82] The particulate data have been derived from studies that evaluated the effects of different pollutant concentrations on a single population and from studies that compared populations from cities with widely different amounts of ambient pollution.[83] Although early studies did not provide optimal control of variables such as meteorologic factors or smoking,[2, 66] more recent studies have demonstrated increases in respiratory symptoms after careful control of these variables[47, 80, 81, 83] Moreover, the advent of more intensive monitoring networks has permitted investigators to begin to separate potential health effects of particulate matter and sulfur dioxide. In several such studies, acute respiratory health effects have been more closely and consistently associated with the particulate fraction than with gaseous sulfur dioxide.[7, 84, 85]

A number of epidemiologic studies have provided data that acid species derived from sulfur dioxide (e.g., $H_2SO_4$, $NH_4HSO_4$, $[H^+]$) are important contributors to the respiratory health effects associated with particulate pollutions.[47, 86] A detailed panel study of over 200 asthmatics from Denver, Colorado, demonstrated a consistent effect of $[H^+]$ on the occurrence of increased symptoms and worsening asthma.[56] This study controlled for such variables as daily activity, time spent indoors vs. outdoors, and meteorologic factors. Respiratory hospital admissions in 22 acute care hospitals in eastern Canada were found to be associated with increased acid aerosols ($[H^+] > [SO_4^-] >$ fine particles $> PM_{10}$) during summertime haze, and these effects were independent of those related to ambient ozone concentrations.[82]

A large study of the respiratory health effects of acid aerosols in children in 24 North American cities has provided evidence that acids derived from sulfur dioxide have effects on chronic respiratory symptoms and lung function. Levels of sulfate particles were associated with increased prevalence of bronchitis in the previous year, and the sulfate particle effect was identical in magnitude to that for total particle acidity (which includes acids derived from nitrogen dioxide) and greater than that for inhalable particles and total acid.[87] The same study reported small reductions in a variety of lung function measures derived from forced expiratory maneuvers that were related to sulfate particles, but in this analysis the effects related to sulfates were somewhat weaker than those for total particle strong acidity (hydrogen ion concentration).[88] The changes observed were small and seem explainable on the basis of small reductions in forced vital capacity rather than primarily on the basis of measures of flow rates. A 10-year follow-up study of a large population of Seventh Day Adventists in California reported associations between ambient concentrations of suspended sulfates and new cases of adult asthma, which could not be explained by correlations with TSP, sulfur dioxide, or ozone.[89] This is one of a very few studies to provide some evidence of a role for air pollution in the onset of asthma. Moreover, the study provides one of the most comprehensive attempts to estimate personal exposures in a long-term study.

During the Donora, Pennsylvania, air pollution episode in 1948, one study reported respiratory symptoms in 88% of patients with asthma.[4] This observation suggested that patients with asthma are especially sensitive to the adverse effects of sulfur oxide and particulate pollution. Data from the Harvard Six Cities Study has also suggested that asthmatic persons are more likely to have increased respiratory symptoms in relation to particulate matter less than 15 $\mu m$ ($PM_{15}$) than are nonasthmatic persons.[47] Daily hospital emergency room visit rates for asthma in Vancouver, Canada, have also been associated with summer levels of sulfur dioxide and sulfates, but the effects of other pollutants, especially of ozone, could not be completely eliminated.[63] A study of children with wheezing or asthma that employed daily diaries and measures of peak expiratory flow rate (PEFR) for 3 months demonstrated an association of PEFR, respiratory symptoms, and use of asthma medications with levels of $PM_{10}$ (particles $< 10$ $\mu m$)[84]; no wheeze-free children were included in this study. A Canadian study with 18 months of follow-up and a nonasthmatic control group found that children with asthma and exercise-induced decreases in PEFR were more likely than nonasthmatic children to have decreases in PEFR with daily increases in $PM_{10}$.[90] Coughing was increased only in asthmatics. Virtually all daily levels in this study were below the 24-hour $PM_{10}$ NAAQS.[90] Increased use of medications by asthmatic children has been reported to be associated with 5-day mean sulfate levels, and this increased medication use did not alter the reductions in PEFR that were associated with increased sulfates.[91] A study in southern California found that asthma severity and medication use in teenaged asthmatics influenced the response to ambient particulate air pollution.[92] Subjects with more severe asthma were more sensitive to the changes in ambient particle concentrations than were those with less severe asthma, whereas ozone had a greater effect on less symptomatic subjects. Asthmatic children not taking anti-inflammatory medications (inhaled steroids, cromolyn) had the strongest response to particle air pollution.

The acute bronchoconstrictor effects of sulfur dioxide have been well established since the mid-1970s.[93, 94] Inhalation of high concentrations of sulfur dioxide has been repeatedly shown to increase airway resistance in healthy human volunteers.[59, 93, 94] In general, this effect of sulfur dioxide has been observed only after inhalation of concentrations in excess of 5 ppm, well above the concentration found even in the most polluted ambient air. However, multiple studies in humans have shown that subjects with asthma are exquisitely sensitive to the bronchoconstrictor effects of sulfur dioxide.[32, 59, 95] Because sulfur dioxide is highly soluble in water, nearly all of the inspired gas is removed from the upper airways under normal resting conditions. By increasing the delivery of sulfur dioxide to the intrathoracic airways, exercise greatly potentiates sulfur dioxide–induced bronchoconstriction.[32] Concentrations of sulfur dioxide as low as 0.25 ppm can cause symptomatic bronchoconstriction when inhaled during exercise by subjects with asthma.[32, 95, 96] Such concentrations sometimes occur in polluted urban air, especially in the vicinity of point sources such as power plants and smelters. This bronchoconstrictor effect occurs after exposures as brief as 1 minute in duration.[97] Thus, sulfur dioxide–induced bronchoconstriction is not necessarily prevented by the current USEPA standard of

0.14 ppm as a 24-hour maximal average, because this standard does not set limits for maximal concentrations over periods shorter than 24 hours. The 24-hour maximum of 0.14 ppm is far more likely to be exceeded in developing countries than in highly developed countries, because of the use of high sulfur coal and oil in domestic heating, industry, and power plants. Moreover, because the nose is an efficient filter for sulfur dioxide, ambient concentration greatly overestimates the amount of gas that penetrates below the nose. Inhaled submicronic aerosols of sulfuric acid have also been shown to decrease maximal airflow in subjects with asthma.[98, 99] This effect, in contrast to that caused by sulfur dioxide, has been small and not reproducible in laboratories.[100, 101] It is unlikely that the effects of near-ambient concentrations of sulfuric acid on lung function are due to bronchoconstriction, because exposure to concentrations up to two orders of magnitude higher have not led to concentration-dependent effects.[100, 101] Inhaled sulfuric acid aerosol has also been shown to slow the rate of clearance of inhaled particles in normal human subjects.[102] Thus, sulfuric acid in polluted air could prolong the contact time between other inhaled toxins and the respiratory mucosa; however, the clinical significance of this observation is not known.

Another important component of particulate pollution is diesel exhaust particulate. Because of a number of desirable properties of diesel combustion engines (e.g., lower emission of carbon dioxide than gasoline engines), there is intense interest in diesel technology. Diesel exhaust from heavy-duty trucks and diesel-engine cars is a major contributor to particulate air pollution in many parts of the world. Diesel exhaust particles have become the subject of intensive research interest because of reported associations with lung cancer and suggestive data of a role as an "adjuvant" in the production of immunoglobulin E (IgE)–mediated immune responses.

Diesel exhaust is a complex mixture of very small particles (90% $<$ 1 $\mu$g by mass). The particles have hundreds of chemicals adsorbed onto their surfaces, which include known mutagens and carcinogens.[103, 104] A large number of epidemiologic studies have provided estimates of the risk of lung cancer associated with exposure to diesel exhaust in occupational settings.[105] A meta-analysis of 35 studies of occupational exposure to diesel exhaust reported an overall relative risk for lung cancer of 1.33 (95% confidence interval: 1.24 to 1.44) with diesel exhaust exposure. Results were similar for various study designs and in studies that did and did not control for cigarette smoking. Railroad workers and truck drivers were at highest risk.[106] Human epidemiologic data are supported by toxicologic data for rats (but not hamsters and mice) that demonstrate the carcinogenic potential of diesel exhaust, the carbon black component having been identified as an important contributor.[107]

Several studies in mice have shown that repeated intratracheal instillation of diesel exhaust particulate can induce nonspecific airway hyperresponsiveness and enhance the inflammatory response to allergen challenge in previously sensitized animals.[108, 109] There are also data from both from intranasal instillation studies in both mice and humans indicating that diesel exhaust particles can enhance local IgE antibody production.[110–112] As a result of these findings, the potential of diesel exhaust exposures to induce exacerbations of asthma is of increasing research interest.[113]

## Photochemical Oxidants: Ozone and Nitrogen Dioxide

The findings of numerous studies suggesting that air pollution by the sulfur dioxide–particulate complex correlates with mortality and morbidity from lung disease raise the concern that a similar correlation may exist for the photochemical oxidant group of pollutants. This concern is heightened by the broad distribution of photochemical pollution. In 1991, the NAAQS for ozone, 0.12 ppm over 1 hour, was exceeded in 94 of 231 US metropolitan areas, which represent a substantial fraction of the nation's population.[114] The highest levels were recorded in the Los Angeles basin, but the "summer haze" that extends over most of the Northeast of the continent, from northern Florida to southern Ontario, contains high levels of ozone as well as aerosol sulfuric and nitric acids, ammonium sulfate, and nitrates.[115] There have been fewer studies that have shown associations between oxidant pollution and mortality than is the case for particulate pollution. At least one study of the Los Angeles basin, however, did show small but significant associations between daily mortality and three separate environmental factors: temperature, primary motor vehicle–related propellants, and photochemical oxidants.[116]

In terms of morbidity, several epidemiologic studies provided suggestive but far from definitive evidence that photochemical oxidants increase the incidence of chronic obstructive pulmonary disease (COPD).[117–119] An indirect association can be inferred from the findings that lower respiratory tract illness is more common in children raised in homes with natural gas heating and cooking[24, 25] and that lower respiratory tract illness in childhood is more often recalled by patients with COPD than by healthy controls.[120] Direct study of the question has shown that long-term residence in areas with high levels of photochemical oxidants is associated with a greater prevalence of symptoms of respiratory disease, with slight but significant abnormalities in tests of airway function and/or greater rate of decline in ventilatory function.[121–125] Results of a more recent study of college freshmen suggest that lifetime exposure to ozone in southern California can lead to slight but measurable differences in lung function.[126] Whether these abnormalities in pulmonary function tests indicate higher risk for developing the clinical syndromes of chronic obstructive bronchitis and emphysema is not yet known. Because individual susceptibility to developing COPD appears to be so variable, and because cigarette smoking has such a dominant role in causing the disease, considerably more data than are currently available will be needed to implicate or exclude photochemical oxidants definitively as important risk factors for the development of COPD.

Provocative data, however, have been presented from an autopsy study of young people in Los Angeles County who died suddenly without evidence of overt disease. These data suggest the possibility that respiratory bronchiolitis with extension of inflammation into adjacent alveoli in the centriacinar region of the lung may result from residence in a metropolitan area characterized by photochemical oxidant pollution.[127] Another provocative report presented suggestive evidence that chronic exposure to high ambient ozone levels in Mexico City led to nasal mucosal dysplasia.[128] That levels of ozone at or below the old NAAQS for ozone, 0.12 ppm, can cause decrements in lung function in human subjects under "real world" conditions has been shown in multiple studies.[54, 55, 129, 130] The decrements in lung function found in children at summer camps are greater than those found in children exposed to comparable concentrations of ozone in chambers for 1 or 2 hours. Two explanations are possible: the cumulative dose of ozone was greater in the summer camp setting, or the response to ozone was potentiated by other pollutants in the ambient air.[54, 129] In addition to the camp study results, exercising adults have also been shown to have decrements in lung function in response to ambient ozone.[55, 130]

The epidemiologic case for photochemical oxidants as a cause of exacerbation of preexisting respiratory disease is stronger for asthma than for COPD. Several panel studies of asthmatics, in southern California, Houston, and Tucson, have shown that the risk of asthmatic exacerbation was enhanced by an increase in ozone.[131–134] Additional evidence comes from at least four other North American studies that have shown that the number of emergency room visits for asthma exacerbations in Montreal, New Brunswick, Atlanta, and New Jersey was correlated with ozone levels.[135–138] The effect of photochemical oxidants on exacerbations of chronic obstructive pulmonary disease has been less studied. In general, epidemiologic studies have shown that exacerbations of COPD are more strongly associated with levels of sulfur dioxide and particulate mass than with levels of ozone or nitrogen dioxide,[139] and acute exposure studies have not shown patients with COPD to be more responsive to ozone.[140, 141] In fact, smokers tend to be less responsive to ozone than are nonsmokers in terms of acute decrements in lung function.[142] Perhaps the most persuasive evidence that ambient ozone exposure can lead to exacerbations of COPD comes from studies in southern Ontario that found that the number of hospital admissions for all respiratory diseases, including exacerbations of chronic bronchitis and emphysema, correlated with ozone concentrations during summer months.[143, 144] Unfortunately, there is also exposure to other pollutants with "summer haze" in Ontario, so that the effect of ozone cannot be entirely disentangled from that of other pollutants, especially acid sulfate particulate.

Other, less severe consequences have been more firmly linked to atmospheric oxidant levels. Performance in running events decreases in Los Angeles track meets when oxidant concentrations exceed 0.25 ppm, and this has been confirmed in a chamber study of competitive cyclists.[145, 146] Headache, eye irritation, cough, and chest discomfort have all been found more commonly when oxidant levels rise above 0.15 ppm.[147]

Nitrogen dioxide is another of the criteria pollutants named by the USEPA and, in ambient air, is often found in association with ozone or other pollutants. It is less potent as an oxidant, and although the high concentrations found in silos are clearly responsible for the acute and sometimes lethal pulmonary edema of "silo-filler's disease,"[148] the low levels of nitrogen dioxide in outdoor air have not been definitively linked to adverse health effects in epidemiologic studies. The results of several studies, however, have provoked renewed interest in this pollutant.[149, 150] In the late 1970s it became apparent that indoor concentrations often exceeded outdoor concentrations, particularly in homes equipped with gas stoves, and may be extremely high in inner city homes heated by ovens.[23] Because indoor air is relatively free of the other pollutants normally associated with nitrogen dioxide in outdoor air, this discovery enabled epidemiologic study of this potentially important pollutant. Research interest focused on the possibility that exposure to nitrogen dioxide in indoor air might increase the occurrence of respiratory infections,[149] in part because of animal studies showing that nitrogen dioxide exposure reduces the clearance of infecting organisms. Unfortunately, epidemiologic studies of this question have not been definitive.[24–26, 149]

The results of studies of the acute effects of exposure of human volunteers to ozone correspond well, but not perfectly, with the results of epidemiologic studies. At first, these studies focused almost exclusively on symptoms and changes in lung mechanics produced by short (1- to 2-hour) exposure to ozone and nitrogen dioxide. For ozone, the effects most consistently observed are cough, substernal discomfort, decreases in the $FEV_1$ and FVC, a rise in airway resistance, and a fall in lung compliance. These effects were first noted in healthy subjects exposed to 0.30 ppm or more while performing light exercise,[151] but they have also been observed with exposure to concentrations at and below the former NAAQS of 0.12 ppm when the duration of exposure was prolonged to 6 hours and moderate exercise was performed.[152–154] With this longer exposure, the functional decrements became progressively greater after each hour of exposure[152] but returned to baseline by the following day. A wide variability in responsiveness to ozone is found between healthy subjects: $FEV_1$ falls sharply in 20% to 25% of the subjects and not at all in others exposed under identical conditions.[152] The basis for the greater responsiveness of some individuals is unknown, but because responses are highly reproducible within individuals,[155] it appears that there is a subgroup in the healthy population with heightened sensitivity to ozone. With repeated daily exposures to ozone, both the symptoms and the changes in lung mechanics diminish.[156, 157] Without further exposure, this tolerance lasts for 7 to 10 days.

Studies of the effects of nitrogen dioxide on healthy subjects have yielded qualitatively similar results, with the important exception that the concentration needed to produce unequivocal respiratory dysfunction, 2.5 ppm, is well above the levels measured in ambient air during pollution episodes.[158] The effect of concentrations attainable in severe episodes, 0.5 to 1.0 ppm, has been studied in subjects performing moderate exercise; the changes in symptoms and in lung mechanics were modest in comparison with those produced by the levels of ozone likely to be present in the same atmosphere.[158, 159]

In addition to the changes in lung mechanics, increases

in nonspecific airway responsiveness also occur with oxidant exposure. For ozone, it is firmly established that concentrations commonly reached in urban air can increase airway responsiveness, both in healthy subjects and in those with preexisting airway hyperresponsiveness.[153, 154, 160, 161] In some studies, exposure of exercising asthmatic subjects to 0.30 ppm of nitrogen dioxide caused an increase in airway responsiveness, but in others, no such effects were found, even when conducted by the same investigators who had previously found an effect.[162] In view of the results of epidemiologic studies demonstrating an association between increased levels of ozone and increased risk of exacerbations of asthma,[131–138] the possibility that ozone may directly narrow the airways in people with asthma has been examined. Because airway hyperresponsiveness is characteristic of asthma, and because ozone causes increased airway responsiveness in healthy people, it was expected that ozone would cause bronchoconstriction in subjects with asthma. Most studies of asthmatic subjects, however, have shown no increased lung function responses to ozone in comparison to healthy subjects,[163, 164] although at least two studies did show modestly greater changes in expiratory flow rates.[165, 166] This is not really surprising because the acute decrements in lung function in response to ozone are restrictive in nature as a result of neural reflex inhibition of deep inspiration.[167]

The failure of clinical exposure studies to demonstrate a markedly heightened responsiveness of asthmatics to the acute effects of ozone on lung function is not necessarily inconsistent with the epidemiologic findings, for ozone could act by heightening responsiveness to another stimulus. Indeed, prior exposure to ozone has been shown to potentiate the early bronchoconstrictor response of allergic asthmatics to subsequent exposure to antigen.[168, 169] There is also evidence that prior exposure to nitrogen dioxide can enhance both the early and late responses to inhaled antigen in allergic asthmatic subjects.[170, 171] The mechanisms of the effects of ozone on the lungs and airways have been examined by analyzing ozone-induced changes in the cellular and chemical composition of bronchoalveolar lavage (BAL) fluid. In subjects exposed to 0.4 or 0.6 ppm of ozone for 2 hours, the proportion of polymorphonuclear leukocytes in lavage fluid obtained 2 hours later increased strikingly, especially in the subjects in whom airway responsiveness increased most.[172] BAL fluid obtained 18 hours after exposure to 0.4 ppm for 2 hours contains an increased proportion of polymorphonuclear leukocytes and increased concentrations of total protein, albumin, interleukin-6, fibronectin, and several other proteins, which suggests the presence of airway epithelial injury and inflammation.[40] Generically similar changes have been found in BAL fluid obtained 18 hours after 4 hours of exposure to 0.2 ppm or 6.6 hours of exposure of healthy subjects to 0.12 and 0.08 ppm of ozone, as well as in nasal lavage fluid from subjects exposed to 0.5 ppm of ozone.[41, 173, 174] It is thus clear that ozone can initiate inflammatory changes in the airways and is capable of producing tissue damage at "real world" levels.[175] However, the clinical and public health significance of these findings cannot be defined without careful study of basic mechanisms in animals and without correlation with the results of long-term studies of effects in chronically exposed populations. In contrast to their lack of heightened response to the acute effects of ozone on lung function, asthmatic subjects do appear to have enhanced ozone-induced airway inflammation in comparison with healthy subjects.[164, 176]

The inflammatory effect of nitrogen dioxide, like that of ozone, has been studied by examining BAL fluid. Even multihour exposures to a high concentration such as 2.0 ppm over 4 days causes only mild airway inflammation.[177] In view of the hypothesized relationship between nitrogen dioxide exposure and increased risk of respiratory infection, the finding that alveolar macrophages obtained from nitrogen dioxide–exposed subjects are less effective at inactivating influenza virus is particularly interesting.[178]

Because of concerns that nitrogen dioxide enhances susceptibility to infection, attenuated influenza virus was administered intranasally to healthy volunteers exposed to 0, 1, 2, or 3 ppm of nitrogen dioxide for 2 hours on 3 consecutive days.[179] Pulmonary function tests and bronchial reactivity to methacholine were unchanged after nitrogen dioxide exposure, virus infection, or both. The infection rates were high after all exposures but were not significantly higher than in the control group, perhaps because of the relatively small sample size. Numerous studies of the acute effects of ozone and nitrogen dioxide have been undertaken in animals. Death from pulmonary edema results from exposure to high concentrations of both pollutants, as has been reported for humans accidentally exposed to lethal levels. Ozone causes similar types of alterations in lung morphology in all animal species studied.[180] The most affected cells are the ciliated epithelial cells of the airways and type I cells in the gas exchange region. Within the nasal cavity, anterior portions of the respiratory and transitional epithelium are affected.[181] Cilia are lost or damaged; some ciliated cells become necrotic, are lost, and are replaced with nonciliated cells. Mucus-secreting cells are affected as well.

The primary site of injury after brief (<24-hour) exposure to ozone is the centriacinar region of the lung in animals; injury is also evident to a lesser extent in the trachea and proximal bronchi; at equivalent exposures, nonhuman primates appear to be more sensitive than rats.[61] The cellular characteristics of the injury consist of a sloughing of alveolar type I cells, proliferation of alveolar type II cells, and a loss of ciliated cells. Inflammatory cells, mostly macrophages and polymorphonuclear leukocytes, appear in the lumina of the bronchioles and alveolar ducts.[182] With increased duration of exposure, alveolar septa in the centriacinar region thicken as a result of increased matrix, basement membrane, collagen, and fibroblasts and a thickened alveolar epithelium.

In rats and monkeys, ciliated and type I cells become necrotic and are sloughed from the epithelium as early as 2 to 4 hours after exposure to 0.5 ppm.[183] Repair, as shown by increased deoxyribonucleic acid (DNA) synthesis begins by about 18 to 24 hours of exposure, although cell damage continues.[183–185] The lesion is fully developed by 3 days of exposure, after which the rate of repair exceeds the rate of damage. There is an increase in antioxidant activity in the damaged area, presumably because of proliferation of type II cells, which are rich in these enzymes.[186]

With chronic exposure to ozone, the time course of various responses differs.[180, 183] Inflammatory changes peak after a few days of ozone exposure; are still seen, but to a much lesser degree, after months of exposure; and resolve quickly after exposure ceases. Epithelial hyperplasia rapidly increases during the first week of exposure, plateaus as exposure continues, and slowly decreases after exposure ceases. Interstitial fibrosis requires months of exposure to be detectable but may persist after exposure ceases.

Chronic exposures to ozone can lead to distal airway remodeling.[180] So-called bronchiolization of centriacinar alveoli means that bronchial epithelium has replaced type I and II cells typical of alveolar ducts (i.e., increased respiratory bronchioles). Bronchiolization has been observed at exposures as low as 0.25 ppm (8 hours/day for 18 months) in monkeys and can persist for months after exposure ceases.[187] Exposure regimens that have attempted to model ozone "episodes" or "seasons" with intermittent clean-air periods have affected experimental outcomes.[187–189] Although a simple pattern of responses has not emerged from intermittent-exposure studies, it is clear that the basic toxicologic principle of dose (i.e., concentration $\times$ time) is not sufficient to understand the complexity of the ozone dose-response relationship.

Chronic exposures can also lead to thickening of centriacinar alveolar septae, as a result of increased inflammatory cells, fibroblasts, and extracellular matrix, with some evidence of fibrosis (i.e., increased collagen).[188, 190–192] In general, relatively high ozone concentrations ($>$0.5 ppm) administered for long duration (i.e., months) are required to produce evidence of interalveolar fibrosis.[189, 192, 193] However, morphometry and lung function tests in rats exposed to an "urban" pattern involving 9-hour peaks up to only 0.25 ppm ozone (5 days/week for 78 weeks) also yielded evidence of fibrosis.[189, 194] Studies of animals exposed to nitrogen dioxide provide generally similar results, except that morphologic abnormalities are produced by short-term exposure only if the concentrations used are well above those found even in severely polluted outdoor air. Short-term exposures to 5.0 ppm generally produce minimal or no morphologic effects in the rat.[195] Long-term exposures to levels greater than 2.0 ppm nitrogen dioxide are necessary to produce persistent changes in the lungs such as bronchiolitis and collagen deposition.[195, 196]

Multiple studies have shown that nitrogen dioxide enhances susceptibility to bacterial and viral infection, probably mediated at least in part through effects on alveolar macrophages.[195, 197] Infectivity model experiments involving exposure to nitrogen dioxide followed by challenge with viable bacteria or viruses have demonstrated that nitrogen dioxide enhances microbe-induced mortality after short-term exposure to 2.0 ppm or more or after long-term exposure to 0.5 ppm.[195, 198–200] Only cautious extrapolations to human responses can be drawn from these studies of animals. The finding that nitrogen dioxide is less directly toxic than ozone is probably applicable to humans, because it fits with what has been learned from controlled human exposure studies. It is uncertain whether the levels of nitrogen dioxide currently found in outdoor urban air pose a hazard by themselves; however, there are grounds for concern that the high levels of nitrogen dioxide sometimes found in indoor air lead to increased risk of respiratory tract infection. It seems likely that acute exposure to near-ambient concentrations of ozone causes damage in the centriacinar region of the human lung, because this is the site of greatest damage in all the animal species that have been studied. This likelihood may be a cause for concern over the possible interaction of ozone with cigarette smoking in the pathogenesis of COPD, because the changes of chronic bronchitis and emphysema are thought to occur in this region first.

## SUMMARY

The potential of air pollution as a hazard to human health became unmistakable between 1930 and 1952, when a series of air pollution crises caused striking increases in mortality. The properties, sources, and distribution of pollutants have since been defined. Their effects on the lungs and airways have been determined by short-term controlled exposures of human volunteers, by acute and chronic exposures of laboratory animals, and by epidemiologic studies of exposed populations. For major, widespread classes of pollutants, such as the photochemical oxidants, sulfur dioxide, and particulate matter, the effects of high concentrations on healthy subjects have been described, and measures to reduce the production of pollutants at mobile and stationary sources have improved air quality, so that large, acute increases in mortality associated with air pollution crises no longer occur in developed countries. However, epidemiologic data collected since 1990 from multiple urban areas indicate that fluctuations in daily mortality are correlated with current levels of particulate pollution in these countries. Given the increased morbidity from asthma seen in the developed world, concern has also been raised about the potential of both oxidant pollutants and particulate matter (especially diesel exhaust particles) to induce exacerbations of asthma, either through direct effects or enhancement of allergic responses. The interactive effects of pollutants with other inhaled agents, such as antigens, cigarette smoke, and respiratory viruses, are not yet adequately defined.

## References

1. Ayres SM, Evans RG, Buehler ME: Air pollution: a major public health problem. CRC Crit Rev Clin Lab Sci 3:1–40, 1972.
2. Shy CM, Goldsmith JR, Hackney JD, et al: Health Effects of Air Pollution. New York: American Lung Association, 1978.
3. Logan WPD: Mortality in the London fog incident. Lancet 1:336–339, 1953.
4. Schrenk HH, Heiman H, Clayton GD, et al: Air pollution in Donora, Pennsylvania. Epidemiology of the unusual smog episode of October 1948. Washington, DC: US Government Printing Office (Public Health Bulletin), 1949, p. 306.
5. American Thoracic Society: State of the art: Health effects of outdoor air pollution. Am J Respir Crit Care Med 153:3–50, 477–498, 1996.
6. Andrews C, Buist S, Ferris B, et al: Guidelines as to what constitutes an adverse respiratory health effect, with special reference to epidemiologic studies of air pollution. Am Rev Respir Dis 131:666–668, 1985.

7. Frank NR, Yoder RE, Brain JD, et al: $SO_2$ ($^{35}S$-labeled) absorption by the nose and mouth under conditions of varying concentration and flow. Arch Environ Health 18:315–322, 1969.
8. Gorman E, Martin FB, Litzau JT: Acid rain: Ionic correlations in the eastern United States, 1980–1981. Science 225:407–409, 1984.
9. US Environmental Protection Agency: Sources and emissions of atmospheric particles. *In* Air Quality Criteria for Particulate Matter, Vol 1. Washington, DC: National Center for Environmental Assessment Office of Research and Development, US EPA, 1996, pp 5-1 to 5-34.
10. Wark K, Warner CF: Air Pollution: Its Origin and Control. New York: Harper-Collins, 1981, pp 143–151.
11. US Environmental Protection Agency: Physics and chemistry of particulate matter. *In* Air Quality Criteria for Particulate Matter, Vol 1. Washington, DC: National Center for Environmental Assessment Office of Research and Development, US EPA, 1996, pp 3-1 to 3-11.
12. US Environmental Protection Agency: Integrative synthesis of key points: PM exposure, dosimetry, and health effects. *In* Air Quality Criteria for Particulate Matter, Vol 3. Washington, DC: National Center for Environmental Assessment Office of Research and Development, US EPA, 1996, pp 13-1 to 13-28.
13. Peters A, Wichmann HE, Tuch T, et al.: Respiratory health effects are associated with the number of ultrafine particles. Am J Respir Crit Care Med 155:1376–1383, 1997.
14. US Environmental Protection Agency: Tropospheric ozone chemistry. *In* Air Quality Criteria for Ozone and Related Photochemical Oxidants, Vol 1. Washington, DC: National Center for Environmental Assessment Office of Research and Development, US EPA, 1996, pp 3-16 to 3-37.
15. Miller FJ: Similarity between man and laboratory animals in regional pulmonary deposition of ozone. Environ Res 17:84–101, 1978.
16. Cohen AJ, Higgins MWP: Health effects of diesel exhaust: Epidemiology. *In* Diesel Exhaust: A Critical Analysis of Emissions, Exposure, and Health Effects—A Special Report of the Institute's Diesel Working Group (No. 293). Cambridge, MA: Health Effects Institute, 1995, pp 253–288.
17. Samet JM, Cohen AJ: Air Pollution and Lung Cancer. *In* Swift DL, Foster WM (eds): Air Pollutants and the Respiratory Tract. New York: Marcel Dekker, 1999, pp 181–217.
18. Beeson WL, Abbey DE, Knutsen SF: Long-term concentrations of ambient air pollutants and incident lung cancer in California adults: Results from the ASHMOG Study. Environ Health Perspect 106:813–823, 1998.
19. Dockery DW, Pope CA, Xu X, et al: An association between air pollution and mortality in six U.S. cities [see comments]. N Engl J Med 329:1753–1759, 1993.
20. Pope CA, Thun MJ, Namboodiri MM, et al: Particle air pollution as a predictor of mortality in a prospective study of U.S. adults. Am J Respir Crit Care Med 151:669–674, 1995.
21. Lambert WE, Samet JM: Indoor air pollution. *In* Harber P, Schenker M, Balmes J (eds): Occupational and Environmental Respiratory Disease. St. Louis: Mosby–Year Book, 1996 pp 784–807.
22. Hanrahan JP, Weiss ST: Environmental tobacco smoke. *In* Harber P, Schenker M, Balmes J (eds): Occupational and Environmental Respiratory Disease. St. Louis: Mosby–Year Book, 1996, pp 767–783.
23. Spengler JD, Duffy C, Letz R, et al: Nitrogen dioxide inside and outside 137 homes and implications for ambient air quality standards and health effects research. Environ Sci Technol 17:164–168, 1983.
24. Neas LM, Dockery DW, Ware JH, et al: Association of indoor nitrogen dioxide with respiratory symptoms and pulmonary function in children. Am J Epidemiol 134:204–219, 1991.
25. Hasselbad V, Kotchmar JJ, Eddy DM: Synthesis of environmental evidence: Nitrogen dioxide epidemiology studies. J Air Waste Management Assoc 42:662–671, 1992.
26. Samet JM, Lambert WE, Skipper BJ, et al: A study of respiratory illnesses in infants and nitrogen dioxide exposure. Arch Environ Health 47:57–63, 1992.
27. Leaderer BP: Air pollutant emissions from kerosene space heaters. Science 218:1113–1115, 1982.
28. Bennett G: Ozone contamination of high altitude aircraft cabins. Aerospace Med 33:969–973, 1962.
29. Marbury MC, Krieger RA. Formaldehyde. *In* Samet JM, Spengler JD (eds): Indoor Air Pollution. Baltimore: Johns Hopkins University Press, 1991, pp 223–251.
30. Lubin JH, Boice JD: Lung cancer risk from residential radon: Meta-analysis of eight epidemiologic studies. J Natl Cancer Inst 89:49–57, 1997.
31. Puskin JS, Nelson CB: EPA's perspective on risks from residential radon exposure. J Air Pollut Control Assoc 39:915–920, 1989.
32. Bethel RA, Erle DJ, Epstein J, et al: Effect of exercise rate and route of inhalation on sulfur dioxide–induced bronchoconstriction in asthmatic subjects. Am Rev Respir Dis 128:592–596, 1983.
33. Lippman M, Yeates DB, Albert RE: Deposition, retention, and clearance of inhaled particles. Br J Ind Med 37:337–362, 1980.
34. Martin D, Jacobi W: Diffusion of small-sized particles in the bronchial tree. Health Phys 23:23–29, 1972.
35. Fillenz M, Woods RI: Sensory innervation of the airways. *In* Porter R (ed): Ciba Foundation Symposium: Breathing: Herring-Breuer Centenary Symposium. London: Churchill, 1970, pp 101–107.
36. Pinkerton KE, Brody AR, Miller FJ, et al: Exposure to low levels of ozone results in enhanced pulmonary retention of inhaled asbestos fibers. Am Rev Respir Dis 140:1075–1081, 1989.
37. Sorokin SP, Brain JD: Pathways of clearance in mouse lungs exposed to iron oxide aerosols. Anat Rec 181:581–588, 1975.
38. Mossman BT, Churg A: Mechanisms in the pathogenesis of asbestosis and silicosis. Am J Respir Crit Care Med 157:1666–1680, 1998.
39. Devlin RB, McKinnon TL, Noah TL, et al: Cytokine and fibronectin production by human alveolar macrophages and airway epithelial cells exposed to ozone in vitro. Am J Physiol 266:1612–1619, 1994.
40. Koren HS, Devlin RB, Graham DE, et al: Ozone-induced inflammation in the lower airways of human subjects. Am Rev Respir Dis 139:407–415, 1989.
41. Aris RM, Christian D, Hearne PQ, et al: Ozone-induced airway inflammation in human subjects as determined by airway lavage and biopsy. Am Rev Respir Dis 148:1363–1372, 1993.
42. Johnson DA: Ozone inactivation of human $alpha_1$-antiproteinase. Am Rev Respir Dis 121:1031–1038, 1980.
43. Romieu I, Meneses F, Ramirez M, et al: Antioxidant supplementation and respiratory functions among workers exposed to high levels of ozone. Am J Respir Crit Care Med 158:226–232, 1998.
44. Plopper CG, Hatch GE, Wong V, et al: Relationship of inhaled ozone concentration to acute tracheobronchial epithelial injury, site-specific ozone dose, and glutathione depletion in rhesus monkeys. Am J Respir Cell Mol Biol 19:387–399, 1998.
45. Grievink L, Zijlstra AG, Ke X, et al: Double-blind intervention trial on modulation of ozone effects on pulmonary function. Am J Epidemiol 149:306–314, 1999.
46. Schwartz J, Spix C, Touloumi G, et al: Methodologic issues in studies of air pollution and daily counts of deaths or hospital admissions. J Epidemiol Commun Health 50 (Suppl 1):S3–S11, 1996.
47. Dockery DW, Speizer FE, Stram DO, et al: Effects of inhalable particles on respiratory health of children. Am Rev Respir Dis 139:587–594, 1989.
48. Detels R, Tashkin DP, Sayre JW, et al: The UCLA population study of COPD: X. A cohort study of changes in respiratory disease associated with chronic exposure to $SO_x$, $NO_x$, and hydrocarbons. Am J Public Health 81:350–359, 1991.
49. Spix C, Anderson HR, Schwartz J, et al: Short-term effects of air pollution on hospital admissions of respiratory diseases in Europe: A quantitative summary of APHEA study results. Arch Environ Health 53:54–64, 1998.
50. Abbey DE, Burchette RJ, Knutsen SF, et al: Long-term particulate and other air pollutants and lung function in nonsmokers. Am J Respir Crit Care Med 158:289–298, 1998.
51. Burnett RT, Cakmak S, Brook JR, et al: The role of particulate size and chemistry in the association between summertime ambient air pollution and hospitalization for cardiorespiratory diseases. Environ Health Perspect 105:614–620, 1997.
52. Higgins ITT, D'Arcy JB, Gibbons DI, et al: Effect of exposure

to ambient ozone on ventilatory lung function in children. Am Rev Respir Dis 141:1336–1346, 1990.

53. Liu L-JS, Koutrakis P, Olson MP, et al: Evaluation of the Harvard ozone passive sampler on human subjects indoors. Environ Sci Technol 28:915–923, 1994.
54. Spektor DM, Lippmann M, Thurston GD, et al: Effects of ambient ozone on respiratory function in active normal children. Am Rev Respir Dis 137:313–330, 1988.
55. Spektor DM, Lippmann M, Thurston GD, et al: Effects of ambient ozone on respiratory function in healthy adults exercising outdoors. Am Rev Respir Dis 138:821–828, 1988.
56. Ostro BD, Lipsett MJ, Wiener MB, et al: Asthmatic responses to airborne acid aerosols. Am J Public Health 81:694–702, 1991.
57. Zeger SL, Dominici F, Samet JM: Harvesting-resistant estimates of air pollution effects on mortality. Ann Epidemiol 10:171–175, 1999.
58. Aronow WS, Isbell MW: Carbon monoxide effect on exercise-induced angina pectoris. Ann Intern Med 79:392–395, 1973.
59. Sheppard D, Wong SC, Uehara CF, et al: Lower threshold and greater bronchomotor responsiveness of asthmatic subjects to sulfur dioxide. Am Rev Respir Dis 122:873–878, 1980.
60. Amdur MO, Underhill DW: The effect of various aerosols on the response of guinea pigs to sulfur dioxide. Arch Environ Health 16:460–468, 1968.
61. US Environmental Protection Agency: Respiratory tract effects of ozone. *In* Air Quality Criteria for Ozone and Related Photochemical Oxidants, Vol 3. Washington, DC: National Center for Environmental Assessment Office of Research and Development, US EPA, 1996, pp 6-80 to 6-81.
62. Holland WW, Bennett AE, Cameron IR, et al: Health effects of particulate pollution: Reappraising the evidence. Am J Epidemiol 110:527–659, 1979.
63. Thurston GD, Ito K, Lippmann M, et al: Reexamination of London, England, mortality in relation to exposure to acidic aerosols during 1963–1972 winters. Environ Health Perspect 79:73–82, 1989.
64. Schwartz J, Marcus A: Mortality and air pollution in London: A time series analysis. Am J Epidemiol 131:185–194, 1990.
65. Vedal S: Ambient particles and health: Lines that divide. J Air Waste Manage Assoc 47:551–581, 1997.
66. Whittemore AS: Air pollution and respiratory disease. Annu Rev Public Health 2:397–429, 1981.
67. Schwartz, J: Air pollution and daily mortality: A review and meta-analysis. Environ Res 64:36–52, 1994.
68. Ozhaynak H, Thurston DG: Associations between 1980 U.S. mortality rates and alternative measures of airborne particulate concentration. Risk Anal 4:449–461, 1987.
69. Fairley D: The relationship of daily mortality to suspended particulates in Santa Clara County, 1980–1986. Environ Health Perspect 89:159–168, 1990.
70. Dockery DW, Schwartz J, Spengler JD: Air pollution and daily mortality: Associations with particulates and acid aerosols. Environ Res 59:362–373, 1992.
71. Borja-Aburto VH, Loomis DP, Bangdiwals SI, et al: Ozone, suspended particulates and daily mortality in Mexico City. Am J Epidemiol 145:258–268, 1997.
72. Kelsall JE, Samet JM, Zeger SL, et al: Air pollution and mortality in Philadelphia, 1974–1988. Am J Epidemiol 146:750–762, 1997.
73. Schwartz J, Dockery DW, Neas LM: Is daily mortality associated specifically with fine particles? J Air Waste Manage Assoc 46:927–939, 1996.
74. Zmirou D, Schwartz J, Saez M, et al: Time-series analysis of air pollution and cause-specific mortality. Epidemiology 9:495–503, 1998.
75. Brunett RT, Cakmak S, Brook JR: The effect of the urban ambient air pollution mix on daily mortality rates in 11 Canadian cities. Can J Public Health 89:152–156, 1998.
76. Schwartz J: What are people dying of on high air pollution days? Environ Res 64:26–35, 1994.
77. Peters A, Doring A, Wichmann H-E, Koenig W: Increased plasma viscosity during an air pollution episode: A link to mortality. Lancet 349:1582–1587, 1997.
78. Pope CA, Dockery DW, Kanner RE, et al: Oxygen saturation, pulse rate associated with particulate air pollution. Am J Respir Crit Care Med 159:365–372, 1999.
79. Seaton A, MacNee W, Donaldson K, et al: Particulate air pollution and acute health effects. Lancet 345:176–178, 1995.
80. Pope CA, Dockery DW: Epidemiology of particle effects. *In* Holgate ST, Samet JM, Koren HS, Maynard RL (eds): Air Pollution and Health. New York: Academic Press, 1999, pp 673–705.
81. Dockery DW, Pope CA: Acute respiratory effects of particulate air pollution. Annu Rev Public Health 15:107–132, 1994.
82. Thurston GD, Ito K, Hayes CG, et al: Respiratory hospital admissions and summertime haze air pollution in Toronto, Ontario: Consideration of the role of acid aerosols. Environ Res 65:271–290, 1994.
83. Schwartz J: Air pollution and hospital admissions for respiratory disease. Epidemiology 7:20–28, 1995.
84. Pope CA, Dockery DW, Spengler JD, et al: Respiratory health and $PM^{10}$ pollution. Am Rev Respir Dis 144:558–574, 1991.
85. Pope CA: Respiratory hospital admissions associated with $PM^{10}$ pollution in Utah, Salt Lake and Cache Valleys. Arch Environ Health 46:90–97, 1991.
86. Spengler JD, Brauer, M, Koutrakis P: Acid air and health. Environ Sci Technol 24:946–956, 1990.
87. Dockery DW, Cunningham J, Damokosh AI, et al: Health effects of acid aerosols on North American children: Respiratory symptoms. Environ Health Perspect 104:500–505, 1996.
88. Raizenne M, Neas LM, Damokosh AI, et al: Health effects of acid aerosols on North American children: Pulmonary function. Environ Health Perspect 104:506–514, 1996.
89. Abbey DE, Petersen FF, Mills PK, et al: Chronic respiratory disease associated with long term ambient concentrations of sulfates and other air pollutants. J Exp Anal Environ Epidemiol 3:99–115, 1993.
90. Vedal S, Petkau J, White R, et al: Acute effect of ambient inhalable particles in asthmatic and non-asthmatic children. Am J Respir Crit Care Med 157:1034–1043, 1998.
91. Peters A, Dockery DW, Heinrich J, et al: Medication use modifies the health effects of particulate sulfate air pollution in children with asthma. Environ Health Perspect 105:430–435, 1997.
92. Delfino RJ, Zeiger RS, Seltzer JM, et al: Symptoms in pediatric asthmatics and air pollution: differences in effects by symptom severity, anti-inflamatory medication use and particulate averaging time. Environ Health Perspect 106:751–761, 1998.
93. Frank NR, Amdur MO, Worcester J, et al: Effects of acute controlled exposure to $SO_2$ on respiratory mechanics in healthy male adults. J Appl Physiol 17:252–258, 1962.
94. Nadel JA, Salem H, Tamplin, B, et al: Mechanism of bronchoconstriction during inhalation of sulfur dioxide. J Appl Physiol 20:164–167, 1965.
95. Linn WS, Venet TG, Shamoo DA, et al: Respiratory effects of sulfur dioxide in heavily exercising asthmatics: A dose-response study. Am Rev Respir Dis 127:278–283, 1983.
96. Horstman D, Roger LJ, Kehrl H, et al: Airway sensitivity of asthmatics to ozone. Toxicol Ind Health 2:289–298, 1986.
97. Balmes JR, Fine JM, Sheppard D: Symptomatic bronchoconstriction after short-term inhalation of sulfur dioxide. Am Rev Respir Dis 136:1117–1121, 1987.
98. Koenig JQ, Pierson WE, Horike M: The effects of inhaled sulfuric acid on pulmonary function in adolescent asthmatics. Am Rev Respir Dis 128:221–225, 1983.
99. Utell MJ, Morrow PE, Speers DM, et al: Airway responses to sulfate and sulfuric acid aerosols in asthmatics. Am Rev Respir Dis 128:444–450, 1983.
100. Avol EL, Linn WS, Shamoo DA, et al: Respiratory response of young asthmatic volunteers in controlled exposures to sulfuric acid aerosol. Am Rev Respir Dis 142:343–348, 1990.
101. Aris R, Christian D, Sheppard D, et al: Lack of bronchoconstrictor response to sulfuric acid aerosols and fogs. Am Rev Respir Dis 143:744–750, 1991.
102. Leikauf GD, Yeates DB, Wakes KA, et al: Effects of sulfuric acid aerosol on respiratory mechanics and mucociliary particle clearance in healthy nonsmoking adults. Am Ind Hyg Assoc J 42:273–282, 1981.
103. Johnson JH: Automotive emissions. *In* Watson AY, Bates RR, Kennedy D (eds): Air Pollution, The Automobile, and Public

Health. Cambridge, MA: Health Effects Institute, 1988, pp 65–68.
104. Nauss KM: Critical issues in assessing the carcinogenesis of diesel exhaust: A synthesis of current knowledge. *In* Diesel Exhaust: A Critical Analysis of Emissions, Exposure, and Health Effects. Cambridge, MA: Health Effects Institute, 1995, p 14.
105. Cohen AJ, Nikula K: The health effects of diesel exhaust: Laboratory and epidemiologic Studies. *In* Holgate ST, Samet JM, Koren HS, Maynard RL (eds): Air Pollution and Health. New York: Academic Press, 1999, pp 707–475.
106. Bhatia R, Lopipero P, Smith AH: Diesel exhaust exposure and lung cancer. Epidemiology 9:84–91, 1997.
107. Busby WF, Newberne PM: Diesel emissions and other substances associated with animal carcinogenicity. *In* Diesel Exhaust: A Critical Analysis of Emissions, Exposure, and Health Effects. Cambridge, MA: Health Effects Institute, 1995, pp 187–220.
108. Takano H, Yoshikawa T, Ichinose T, et al: Diesel exhaust particles enhance antigen-induced airway inflammation and local cytokine expression in mice. Am J Respir Crit Care Med 156:36–42, 1997.
109. Nel AE, Diaz-Sanchez D, Ng D, et al: Enhancement of allergic inflammation by the interaction between diesel exhaust particles and the immune system. J Allergy Clin Immunol 102:539–557, 1998.
110. Takafuji S, Suzuki S, Koizumi K, et al: Diesel exhaust particulates inoculated by the intranasal route have an adjuvant activity for IgE production in mice. J Allergy Clin Immunol 79:639–645, 1987.
111. Diaz-Sanchez D, Dotson AR, Takenaka H, et al: Diesel exhaust particles induce local IgE production in vivo and alter the pattern of IgE messenger RNA isoforms. J Clin Invest 94:1417–1425, 1994.
112. Takenaka H, Zhang K, Diaz-Sanchez D, et al: Enhanced human IgE production results from exposure to the aromatic hydrocarbons from diesel exhaust: Direct effects on B-cell IgE production. J Allergy Clin Immunol 95:103–115, 1995.
113. Peterson B, Saxon A: Global increases in allergic respiratory disease: The possible role of diesel exhaust particles. Ann Allergy Asthma Immunol 77:263–270, 1996.
114. US Environmental Protection Agency: Environmental concentrations, patterns, and exposure estimates. *In* Air Quality Criteria for Ozone and Related Photochemical Oxidants, Vol 1. Washington, DC: National Center for Environmental Assessment Office of Research and Development, US EPA, 1996, pp 4-15 to 4-19.
115. Bates DV: Ozone: Myth and reality. Environ Res 50:230–237, 1989.
116. Kinney PL, Ozkaynak H: Associations of daily mortality and air pollution in Los Angeles County. Environ Res 54:99–120, 1991.
117. Hodgkin JE, Abbey DE, Euler GL, et al: COPD prevalence in nonsmokers in high and low photochemical air pollution areas. Chest 86:830–838, 1984.
118. Abbey DE, Mills PK, Petersen FF, et al: Long-term ambient concentrations of total suspended particulates and oxidants as related to incidence of chronic disease in California Seventh-Day Adventists. Environ Health Perspect 94:43–50, 1991.
119. Euler GL, Abbey DE, Hodgkin JE, et al: Chronic obstructive pulmonary disease symptom effects of long-term cumulative exposure to ambient levels of total oxidants and nitrogen dioxide in California Seventh-Day Adventist residents. Arch Environ Health, 43:279–285, 1988.
120. Burrows B, Knudson RJ, Lebowitz MD: The relationship of childhood respiratory illness to adult obstructive airway disease. Am Rev Respir Dis 115:751–760, 1977.
121. Detels R, Sayre JW, Coulson AH, et al: The UCLA population studies of chronic obstructive respiratory disease: IV. Respiratory effects of long-term exposure to photochemical oxidants, nitrogen dioxide, and sulfates on current and never-smokers. Am Rev Respir Dis 124:673–680, 1981.
122. Stern B, Jones L, Raizenne M, et al: Respiratory health effects associated with ambient sulfates and ozone in two rural Canadian communities. Environ Res 49:20–39, 1985.
123. Kilburn KH, Warshaw R, Thornton, JC: Pulmonary function impairment and symptoms in women in the Los Angeles Harbor area. Am J Med 79:23–28, 1985.
124. Detels R, Tashkin DP, Sayre JW, et al: The UCLA population studies of chronic obstructive respiratory disease: 9. Lung function changes associated with chronic exposure to photochemical oxidants: A cohort study among newer smokers. Chest 92:594–603, 1987.
125. Schwartz J: Lung function and chronic exposure to air pollution: A cross-sectional analysis of NHANES II. Environ Res 50:309–321, 1989.
126. Kunzli N, Lurmann F, Segal M, et al: Association between lifetime ambient ozone exposure and pulmonary function in college freshman—Results of a pilot study. Environ Res 72:8–23, 1997.
127. Sherwin RP: Air pollution: The pathobiologic issues. J Toxicol Clin Toxicol 29:385–400, 1991.
128. Calderon-Garciduenas L, Osorno-Velasquez A, Bravo-Alvarez H, et al: Histopathologic changes of the nasal mucosa in southwest metropolitan Mexico City inhabitants. Am J Pathol 140: 225–232, 1992.
129. Kinney PL, Thurston GD, Raizenne M: The effects of ambient ozone on lung function in children: A reanalysis of six summer camp studies. Environ Health Perspect 104:170–174, 1996.
130. Korrick SA, Neas LM, Dockery DW, et al: Effects of ozone and other pollutants on the pulmonary function of adult hikers. Environ Health Perspect 106:93–99, 1998.
131. Whittemore AS, Korn EL: Asthma and air pollution in the Los Angeles area. Am J Public Health 70:687–696, 1980.
132. Holguin AH, Buffler PA, Contant CF: The effects of ozone on asthmatics in the Houston area. *In* Lee SD (ed): Evaluation of the Scientific Basis for Ozone/Oxidants Standards. Pittsburgh: Air Pollution Control Association (APCA International Specialty Conference Transactions TR-4), 1982, pp 262–280.
133. Krzyzanowski M, Quackenboss JJ, Lebowitz MD: Relation of peak expiratory flow rates and symptoms to ambient ozone. Arch Environ Health 47:107–115, 1992.
134. Delfino RJ, Coate BD, Zeiger RS, et al: Daily asthma severity in relation to personal ozone exposure and outdoor fungal spores. Am J Respir Crit Care Med 154:633–641, 1996.
135. Steib DM, Burnett RT, Beveridge RC, et al: Association between ozone and asthma emergency department visits in St. John, New Brunswick, Canada. Environ Health Perspect 104:1354–1360.
136. White MC, Etzel RA, Wilcox WD, et al: Exacerbations of childhood asthma and ozone pollution in Atlanta. Environ Res 65:56–68, 1994.
137. Cody RP, Weisel CP, Birnbaum G, et al: The effect of ozone associated with summertime photochemical smog on the frequency of asthma visits to hospital emergency departments. Environ Res 58:184–194, 1992.
138. Delfino RJ, Murphy-Moulton AM, Burnett RT, et al: Effects of air pollution on emergency room visits for respiratory illnesses in Montreal, Quebec. Am J Respir Crit Care Med 155:568–576, 1997.
139. Sunyer J, Anto JM, Murillo C, et al: Effects of urban air pollution on emergency room admissions for chronic obstructive pulmonary disease. Am J Epidemiol 134:277–286, 1991.
140. Linn WS, Shamoo DA, Venet TG, et al: Response to ozone in volunteers with chronic obstructive pulmonary disease. Arch Environ Health 38:278–283, 1983.
141. Gong H, Shamoo DA, Anderson KR, et al: Responses of older men with and without chronic obstructive pulmonary disease to prolonged ozone exposure. Arch Environ Health 52:18–25, 1997.
142. Frampton MW, Morrow PE, Torres A, et al: Ozone responsiveness in smokers and nonsmokers. Am J Respir Crit Care Med 155:116–121, 1997.
143. Bates DV, Sitzo R: Air pollution and hospital admissions in southern Ontario: The acid summer haze effect. Environ Res 43:317–331, 1987.
144. Burnett RT, Dales RE, Raizenne M, et al: Effects of low ambient levels of ozone and sulfates on the frequency of respiratory admissions to Ontario hospitals. Environ Res 65:172–194, 1994.
145. Pierson WE: Impact of air pollutants on athletic performance. Allergy Proc 10:209–214, 1989.
146. Gong H, Bradley PW, Simmons MS, et al: Impaired exercise performance and pulmonary function in elite cyclists during low-level ozone exposure in a hot environment. Am Rev Respir Dis 134:726–733, 1986.

147. Hammer DI, Hasselblad R, Portnoy B, et al: Los Angeles student nurse study: Daily symptom reporting and photochemical oxidants. Arch Environ Health 28:255–260, 1974.
148. Douglas WW, Hepper NG, Colby TV: Silo-filler's disease. Mayo Clin Proc 64:291–304, 1989.
149. Samet JM: Nitrogen dioxide and respiratory infection. Am Rev Respir Dis 139:1073–1074, 1989.
150. Peters JM, Avol E, Gauderman WJ, et al: A study of twelve southern California communities with differing levels and types of air pollution: II. Effects on pulmonary function. Am J Respir Crit Care Med 159:768–775, 1999.
151. Bates DV, Bell GM, Burnham CD, et al: Short-term effects of ozone on the lung. J Appl Physiol 32:176–181, 1977.
152. McDonnell WF, Horstman DH: Pulmonary effects of ozone exposure during exercise: Dose-response characteristics. J Appl Physiol 54:1345–1352, 1983.
153. Horstman DH, Folinsbee LF, Ives PJ, et al: Ozone concentration and pulmonary response relationships for 6.6-hour exposures with five hours of moderate exercise to 0.08, 0.10, and 0.12 ppm. Am Rev Respir Dis 142:1158–1163, 1990.
154. McDonnell WF, Kehrl HR, Abdul-Salaam S, et al: Respiratory response of humans exposed to low levels of ozone for 6.6 hours. Arch Environ Health 46:145–150, 1991.
155. McDonnell WF, Horstmann DH, Abdul-Salaam S, et al: Reproducibility of individual responses to ozone exposure. Am Rev Respir Dis 131:36–40, 1985.
156. Hackney JD, Linn WS, Mohler JG, et al: Adaptation to short-term respiratory effects of ozone in men exposed repeatedly. J Appl Physiol 43:82–85, 1977.
157. Christian DL, Chen LL, Scannell CH, et al: Ozone-induced inflammation is attenuated with multiday exposure. Am J Respir Crit Care Med 158:532–537, 1998.
158. Hackney JD, Triede FC, Linn WS, et al: Experimental studies on human health effects of air pollutants: IV. Short-term physiological and clinical effects of nitrogen dioxide exposure. Arch Environ Health 33:176–181, 1978.
159. Folinsbee LJ, Horvath SM, Bedi JF, et al: Effects of 0.62 ppm $NO_2$ on cardiopulmonary function in young male non-smokers. Environ Res 15:199–205, 1978.
160. Orehek J, Massari JP, Gayrard P, et al: Effect of short-term, low-level nitrogen dioxide exposure on bronchial sensitivity of asthmatic patients. J Clin Invest 57:301–307, 1976.
161. Bauer MA, Utell MJ, Morrow PE, et al: 0.30 ppm nitrogen dioxide potentiates exercise-induced bronchospasm in asthmatics. Am Rev Respir Dis 134:1203–1208, 1986.
162. Samet JM, Utell MJ: The risk of nitrogen dioxide: What have we learned from epidemiological and clinical studies? Toxicol Ind Health 6:247–262, 1990.
163. Balmes JR: The role of ozone exposure in the epidemiology of asthma. Environ Health Perspect 101:219–224, 1993.
164. Scannell C, Chen L, Aris RM, et al: Greater ozone-induced inflammatory responses in subjects with asthma. Am J Respir Crit Care Med 154:24–29, 1996.
165. Kreit JW, Gross KB, Moore TB, et al: Ozone-induced changes in pulmonary function and bronchial responsiveness in asthmatics. J Appl Physiol 66:217–222, 1989.
166. Horstman DH, Ball BA, Brown J, et al: Toxicol Ind Health 11:369–385, 1995.
167. Hazucha MJ, Bates DV, Bromberg PA: Mechanisms of action of ozone on the human lung. J Appl Physiol 67:1535–1541, 1989.
168. Molfino NA, Wright SC, Satz I, et al: Effect of low concentrations of ozone on inhaled allergen responses in asthmatic subjects. Lancet 338:199–203, 1991.
169. Jorres R, Nowak D, Magnussen H: The effect of ozone exposure on allergen responsiveness in subjects with asthma or rhinitis. Am J Respir Crit Care Med 153:56–64, 1996.
170. Tunnicliffe WS, Burge PS, Ayres JG: Effect of domestic concentrations of nitrogen dioxide on airway responses to inhaled allergen in asthmatic patients. Lancet 344:1733–1736, 1994.
171. Strand V, Rak S, Svartengren M, et al: Nitrogen dioxide exposure enhances asthmatic reactions to inhaled allergen in subjects with asthma. Am J Respir Crit Care Med 155:881–887, 1997.
172. Seltzer J, Bigby BG, Stulbarg MS, et al: Ozone-induced change in bronchial reactivity and airway inflammation in human subjects. J Appl Physiol 60:1321–1326, 1986.
173. Devlin RB, McDonnell WF, Mann R, et al: Exposure of humans to ambient levels for 6.6 hours causes cellular and biochemical changes in the lung. Am J Respir Cell Mol Biol 4:72–81, 1991.
174. Graham D, Henderson F, House D: Neutrophil influx measured in nasal lavages of humans exposed to ozone. Arch Environ Health 43:228–233, 1988.
175. Kinney, PL, Nilsen DM, Lippmann M, et al: Biomarkers of lung inflammation in recreational joggers exposed to ozone. Am J Respir Crit Care Med 154:1430–1435, 1996.
176. Basha MA, Gross KB, Gwizdala CJ, et al: Bronchoalveolar lavage neutrophilia in asthmatic and healthy volunteers after controlled exposure to ozone and filtered air. Chest 106:1757–1765, 1994.
177. Blomberg A, Krishna MT, Helleday R, et al: Persistent airway inflammation but accommodated antioxidant and lung function responses after repeated daily exposure to nitrogen dioxide. Am J Respir Crit Care Med 159:536–543 1999.
178. Frampton MW, Smeglin M, Roberts NJ, et al: Nitrogen dioxide exposure in vivo and human alveolar macrophage inactivation of influenza virus in vitro. Environ Res 48:179–192, 1989.
179. Goings SA, Kulle TJ, Bascom R, et al: Effect of nitrogen dioxide exposure on susceptibility to influenza A virus infection in healthy adults. Am Rev Respir Dis 139:1075–1081, 1989.
180. U.S. Environmental Protection Agency. Respiratory tract effects of ozone. *In* Air Quality Criteria for Ozone and Related Photochemical Oxidants, Vol 3. Washington, DC: National Center for Environmental Assessment Office of Research and Development, US EPA, 1996, pp 6-54 to 6-76.
181. Harkema JR, Plopper CG, Hyde DM, et al: Response of the macaque nasal epithelium to ambient levels of ozone: A morphometric study of the transitional and respiratory epithelium. Am J Pathol 128:29–44, 1987.
182. Dungworth DL: Noncarcinogenic responses of the respiratory tract to inhaled toxicants. *In* McClellan RO, Henderson RF (eds): Concepts in Inhalation Toxicology. New York: Hemisphere Publishing, 1989, pp 273–298.
183. Stephens RJ, Sloan MF, Evans MJ, et al: Early response of lung to low levels of ozone. Am J Pathol 74:31–58, 1974.
184. Evans MJ, Johnson LV, Stephens RJ, et al: Cell renewal in the lungs of rats exposed to low levels of ozone. Exp Mol Pathol 24:70–83, 1976.
185. Castleman WL, Dungworth DL, Schwartz LW, et al: Acute respiratory bronchiolitis: An ultrastructural and autoradiographic study of epithelial cell injury and renewal in rhesus monkeys exposed to ozone. Am J Pathol 98:811–840, 1980.
186. Bassett DJP, Bowen-Kelly E, Elbon CL, et al: Rat lung recovery from 3 days of continuous exposure to 0.75 ppm ozone. J Toxicol Environ Health 25:329–347, 1988.
187. Tyler WS, Tyler NK, Last JA, et al: Comparison of daily and seasonal exposures of young monkeys to ozone. Toxicology 50:131–144.
188. Chang L-Y, Huang Y, Stockstill BL, et al: Epithelial injury and interstitial fibrosis in the proximal alveolar regions of rats chronically exposed to a simulated pattern of urban ambient ozone. Toxicol Appl Pharmacol 109:219–234, 1992.
189. Barr BC, Hyde DM, Plopper CG, et al: A comparison of terminal airway remodeling in chronic daily versus episodic ozone exposure. Toxicol Appl Pharmacol 106:384–407, 1990.
190. Barry BE, Mercer RR, Miller FJ, et al: Effect of inhalation of 0.25 ppm ozone on the terminal bronchioles of juvenile and adult rats. Exp Lung Res 14:225–245, 1988.
191. Fujinaka LE, Hyde DM, Plopper CG, et al: Respiratory bronchiolitis following long-term ozone exposure in bonnet monkeys: A morphometric study. Exp Lung Res 8:167–190, 1985.
192. Pickrell JA, Hahn FF, Rebar AH, et al: Changes in collagen metabolism and proteinolysis after repeated inhalation exposure to ozone. Exp Mol Pathol 46:159–167, 1987.
193. Last JA, Greenberg DB: Ozone-induced alterations in collagen metabolism of rat lungs: II. Long-term exposures. Toxicol Appl Pharmacol 55:108–114, 1980.
194. Costa DL, Tepper JS, Stevens MA, et al: Restrictive lung disease in rats exposed chronically to an urban profile of ozone. Am J Respir Crit Care Med 151:1512–1518, 1995.
195. US Environmental Protection Agency: Studies of the effects of

nitrogen compounds on animals. *In* Air Quality Criteria for Oxides of Nitrogen, Vol 3. Washington, DC: National Center for Environmental Assessment Office of Research and Development, US EPA, 1993, pp 13-202 to 13-205.
196. Chang Y-L, Mercer RR, Stockstill BL, et al: Effects of low levels of $NO_2$ on terminal bronchiolar cells and its relative toxicity compared to $O_3$. Toxicol Appl Pharmacol 96:451–464, 1988.
197. Schlesinger RB. Intermittent inhalation of nitrogen dioxide: Effects on rabbit alveolar macrophages. J Toxicol Environ Health 21:127–139, 1987.
198. Ehrlich R, Findlay JC, Fenters JD, et al: Health effects of short-term inhalation of nitrogen dioxide and ozone mixtures. Environ Res 10:217–233, 1977.
199. Ehrlich R, Henry MC: Chronic toxicity of nitrogen dioxide: I. Effect on resistance to bacterial pneumonia. Arch Environ Health 17:860–865, 1968.
200. Rose RM, Fuglestad JM, Skornik WA, et al: The pathophysiology of enhanced susceptibility to murine cytomegalovirus respiratory infection during short-term exposure to nitrogen dioxide. Am Rev Respir Dis 137:912–917, 1988.

# 69 Acute Pulmonary Responses to Toxic Exposures

PAUL D. BLANC, M.D., M.S.P.H.

Introduction
Pathogenesis of Irritant Lung Injury
Other Pathogenic Processes
Acute Management
Chronic Pathologic Sequelae and Residual Effects
Specific Exposures
Chlorine, Chloramine, and Hydrochloric Acid
Oxides of Nitrogen, Ozone, Sulfur Dioxide, and Acid Aerosols
Military and Crowd Control Agents
Cadmium, Mercury, and Other Toxic Metals
Metal Fume Fever, Polymer Fume Fever, and Organic Dust Toxic Syndrome
Hydrocarbon Pneumonitis and Baby Powder Aspiration
Paraquat
Smoke Inhalation
Pharmacologic Syndromes
Other Inhalant Exposures
Summary

## INTRODUCTION

This chapter focuses on the acute effects on the lung after exposure to toxic substances. As used in this chapter, "acute" subsumes short-term exposures (minutes to hours) with the initial onset of pulmonary responses within a similarly rapid time period. As a general rule, the relevant exposures are of high intensity, far in excess of recommended safety limits for the workplace or the environment. Moreover, this chapter does not address brief exposures inducing acute responses mediated by amnestic (e.g., allergic) mechanisms. These responses require prior exposures that already have led to sensitization, such as occupational asthma (Chapter 66) or hypersensitivity pneumonitis (Chapter 67).

For the acute pulmonary responses addressed in this chapter, the lung is the target organ for toxicity. *Target organ* does not equate with *route of exposure*. Although for many acute exposures the route of delivery for toxins is by inhalation, the primary toxic insult is not to the lung (e.g., solvent inhalation that causes central nervous system depression). Inhalation exposures such as these are not addressed here. In contrast, paraquat and hydrocarbon aspiration are examples of ingested toxins with severe acute effects on the lung as the target organ for toxicity and are included.

Acute lung toxicity results from a variety of exposures but is manifest by a fairly narrow repertoire of injury. The pathogenic considerations of acute lung responses, including diffuse alveolar damage, as well as principles of clinical management of the acute toxic pulmonary syndromes are generalizable to a wide variety of exposures. The possible chronic sequelae of acute toxic injury, particularly the potential for altered lung structure or responses, although infrequent, are also largely generic outcomes. Nonetheless, a number of specific occupational and environmental exposures are particularly relevant to respiratory medicine because of their frequency and the severity of their toxicity or because of unusual pathophysiologic mechanisms.

## PATHOGENESIS OF IRRITANT LUNG INJURY

Irritant gases and aerosols represent a group of heterogeneous agents that are capable of causing extensive cell injury throughout the respiratory tract. The primary location of lung injury and the onset of clinical symptoms are partly dependent on the solubility of the gas or aerosol involved. However, overwhelming exposures to any irritant inhalant can cause extensive damage throughout the respiratory tract. Ammonia[1] and sulfur dioxide[2] are examples of substances that are highly soluble in water. Such highly soluble substances cause immediate irritation of the conjunctival mucosa and upper airways. In contrast, oxides of nitrogen,[3] ozone,[4] and phosgene[5] have relatively low water solubility. For this reason, exposure to one of these agents may *not* be characterized by immediate mucous membrane symptoms. This may lead to more prolonged exposures and delays in seeking medical attention. Both more and less soluble irritant exposures can lead to distal lung injury, but in the case of highly soluble materials, a history of severe upper respiratory symptoms should precede the presentation of distal airway and alveolar damage.

In addition to solubility and the amount of gas or aerosol inhaled, other physical properties that may be pertinent to the pathogenesis of acute irritant injury include pH, chemical reactivity, and, in the case of fume or aerosols, particle or droplet physical characteristics. On the cellular level, respiratory tract injury may be mediated through the deposition or formation of an acid, alkali, or free radical. In most cases, the detailed cellular mechanisms of injury from irritant inhalants have not been well delineated or remain controversial. This is true even for relatively common irritants such as chlorine, an agent for which a great deal of human and experiment animal data exist.[6]

Regardless of the cellular mechanisms involved, the most common target of irritant lung damage is airway epithelium. The airway epithelium provides a barrier that protects submucosal structures (nerves, vessels, and smooth muscle) from direct exposure to environmental agents. Many environmental agents cause disruption of the integrity of this protective barrier. Disruption may result in edema, inflammation, smooth muscle contraction, and stimulation of afferent neurons. Compromise of the tight junction interface between epithelial cells may be a common aspect of injury after exposure to a variety of irritant agents.[7] Moreover, damage to the airway epithelium, particularly at tight junctions, may render the respiratory mucosa permeable to further exposure to inhaled substances. These agents then may penetrate the subepithelial mucosal region and interact with effector cells in subepithelial mucosa, leading to smooth muscle contraction or to neurally mediated effects.

Irritants reaching the lower respiratory tract, either because of their inherent physical characteristics or because of exposures that overwhelm the absorptive capacity of the upper airway, can injure alveolar lining cells directly. Alveolar type I epithelial cells, which have a relatively large surface area, appear to be particularly susceptible to chemical injury. The major clinical consequence of injury to the peripheral airways and alveoli is diffuse bronchiolar inflammation with obstruction and alveolar filling (pulmonary edema). Pathophysiologically, irritant injury at this level leads to a nonspecific pattern of diffuse alveolar damage similar to that seen from a variety of different causes (see Chapter 54). The pathologic changes in fatal cases of irritant lung injury include focal and confluent areas of edema with protein-rich fluid in the alveolar spaces, hyaline membrane formation, and denudation of the alveolar epithelium.[8, 9] In addition, mucous membranes of the bronchial and bronchiolar walls may be destroyed or denuded. A component of pulmonary hemorrhage may occur in irritant lung injury but typically is not a major clinical manifestation. Its presence should raise suspicion of other syndromes.[10]

## OTHER PATHOGENIC PROCESSES

Acute irritant injury is the predominant, but not the only, pathophysiologic mechanism underlying acute toxic lung syndromes. Some of the diverse agents causing these syndromes are detailed subsequently in this chapter. After exposure to other toxins, unlike irritant chemical-related injury, it is difficult to delineate a descending, hierarchical pattern from upper airway to lower lung injury. Many of these exposures lead to adult respiratory distress syndrome in their most severe manifestations. This includes heavy metal pneumonitis,[11] hydrocarbon aspiration,[12] and paraquat lung injury.[13] The inhalation fever syndromes mark the principal exception to this general phenomenon.[14] The pathophysiology of these self-limited acute lung syndromes appears to be cytokine mediated, without obvious lung injury.

## ACUTE MANAGEMENT

Diffuse alveolar damage after severe acute toxic lung injury is nonspecific. Therefore, the treatment of acute toxin-related lung injury should be consistent with the basic management of acute respiratory distress syndrome due to other causes (see Chapter 54). If the patient has severe nasopharyngeal edema, a tracheotomy may be needed. The role of corticosteroids in the acute phase of pulmonary edema and diffuse alveolar damage after irritant inhalation and other toxic injuries has not been studied in controlled trials. However, concomitant airway injury with acute bronchospasm often warrants the use of corticosteroids (along with bronchodilators) on the basis of airway obstruction. Prophylactic antibiotic drugs have not been proved efficacious; antibiotics should be reserved for those patients with clinical evidence of infection. In the management of adult respiratory distress syndrome, oxygen toxicity is a particular issue after paraquat exposure because of its specific mechanism of action.[13] Inhalation fever is self-limited, so the principal clinical management issue is to exclude other exposures with less benign outcomes.[14, 15]

## CHRONIC PATHOLOGIC SEQUELAE AND RESIDUAL EFFECTS

Among those surviving symptomatic exposure to acute irritants, persistent structural and functional effects may occur. Long-term follow-up evaluation after recovery from adult respiratory distress syndrome due to heterogeneous causes (predominantly associated with sepsis) suggests that residual deficits in lung volumes, airflow, and gas exchange may persist long after recovery.[16] Follow-up studies of more homogeneous populations evaluated after inhalation injury (with only a minority experiencing severe injury) suggest that airflow obstruction and nonspecific airway hyperresponsiveness are the most common persistent abnormalities after irritant injury. Even so, epidemiologic data suggest that these outcomes only occur in a minority of those exposed.[17–19] The term *reactive airway dysfunction syndrome* (RADS) has been applied to the persistence of airway reactivity after acute exposure to respiratory irritants.[20, 21] The more general term *irritant-induced asthma* also has been used to describe this condition.[22, 23] Insofar as this syndrome represents a form of work-related asthma, it is addressed in Chapter 66.

Other outcomes of inhalation injury are uncommon.

Bronchiolitis obliterans (BO),[24–31] bronchiectasis,[1, 30, 32–35] and bronchiolitis obliterans organizing pneumonia[36] (BOOP) occur but are rare. Irritants have long been known to cause BO.[37] Nitrogen dioxide is the single agent (excluding fire smoke by-products) best documented to do so. Yet even with nitrogen dioxide, BO is an infrequent event; for example, only one case was found in a series of 20 moderate to severe exposures.[24] Pathologically, irritant-induced BO usually is characterized by intrabronchial granulation tissue (to which the term *proliferative BO* is applied), as opposed to constrictive (obliterative) BO.[8, 9]

There are nosologic distinctions between proliferative BO and BOOP; importantly, both tend to be steroid responsive.[38] In addition to syndromes such as BO and BOOP, respiratory complaints after irritant inhalation can be psychogenic manifestations of a somatoform disorder, rather than a pulmonary process.[39, 39a]

## SPECIFIC EXPOSURES

### Chlorine, Chloramine, and Hydrochloric Acid

Among the toxic agents (Table 69.1), chlorine is one of the most common and potent irritant inhalants known.[40, 41] Common forms of exposure include: industrial leaks,[42] environmental releases occurring primarily in transport,[43] water purification,[44] swimming pool-related events,[45] and household-cleaning product misadventures.[46] In the form of a yellow-green acrid gas, industrial and environmental releases typically present clear-cut exposure histories. Because the gas is heavier than air, higher contamination can be expected in low-lying areas (hence its use in trench warfare in World War I).[47] However, other environmental conditions may supervene. Examples include one well-documented case of the gas rising along the heated outside wall of a factory where rooftop workers were exposed.[42] In another case, chlorine initially collected in a basement, but then it was sucked up into the central heating system of a dormitory.[48]

The history of exposure to chlorine may be less straightforward when inhalation occurs after de novo generation of gas from chlorine-containing liquids or powders. The most common *liquid* formulation associated with chlorine gas release is hypochlorite bleach, whereas the active chlorine component of dry *powdered* bleaching cleansers is typically a chlorinated phosphate. In either liquid or powdered bleaches, the liberation of chlorine gas is pH dependent, occurring on contact with acids in

**Table 69.1 SELECTED TOXIC AGENTS CAUSING PULMONARY RESPONSES**

| Agent | Common Exposure Scenarios | References |
|---|---|---|
| Acid aerosols | Plating; microelectronics; other manufacturing | 59, 66–69 |
| Acrolein | Structural or wildland fires; other combustion | 58, 149, 151 |
| Ammonia | Industrial refrigeration leaks; fertilizers | 1, 164, 168 |
| Brevetoxin | Aerosolization of red tide toxin | 161, 162 |
| Bromine | Water treatment; chemical manufacturing | 31, 170, 172 |
| Cadmium fume | Flame cutting soldered or sheet metal materials | 89–91 |
| Chlorine gas | Gas leak; water treatment; bleach + acid mix | 4, 6, 42 |
| Chlorine dioxide | Pulp paper bleaching | 94, 61 |
| Crowd control agents | Military and police training and operations | 83–85 |
| Dimethyl sulfate | Industrial chemical yielding sulfuric acid | 65 |
| Fluoropolymers | Overheating or burning Teflon-type polymers | 71, 104 |
| Hydrocarbons | Aspiration of low viscosity materials | 12, 136 |
| Hydrogen sulfide | Sewers and manure pits; fossil fuel extraction | 176, 178 |
| Mercury vapor | Gold amalgam volatilization | 92–94 |
| Methyl bromide | Pesticide fumigant | 173, 174 |
| Methyl isocyanate | Pesticide manufacturing | 179, 181 |
| Methyl isothiocyanate | Breakdown product of metam sodium fumigant | 182 |
| Mustard gas | Chemical warfare agent | 32, 74 |
| Nickel carbonyl | Nickel processing | 95, 96 |
| Nitrogen dioxide | Silo filling; combustion; welding | 3, 25 |
| Organic dusts/aerosols | Contaminated dust or bioaerosol generation | 15, 117, 119 |
| Organophosphates | Pesticide application; chemical warfare | 78, 79 |
| Ozone | Bleaching; water treatment; plasma welding | 60, 61 |
| Paraquat | Herbicide skin contamination or ingestion | 13, 140, 144 |
| Phosgene | Chlorinated solvent breakdown by-product | 5, 75 |
| Phosphine | Fumigation with aluminum or zinc phosphide | 184, 185 |
| Sulfur dioxide | Refrigeration; cement manufacture; mining | 2, 62, 64 |
| Tributyltin (Bis(tributyltin) oxide) | Paint additive for mold inhibition | 102 |
| Vanadium | Ore processing; fossil fuel by-product | 100 |
| Zinc oxide fume | Welding galvanized steel; brass casting | 106, 125 |

common household products containing muriatic (hydrochloric), phosphoric, or hydrofluoric acid.[46] In contrast, mixing chlorine-containing products with ammonia leads to release of chloramine gas, whose irritant effects are attributed to in situ pulmonary reactions releasing chlorine, hypochlorous acid, and ammonia.[46]

Although de novo release of chlorine or chloramine gas due to product mixing is a major source of exposure in the household, irritant effects after inhalation of hypochlorite aerosols in confined spaces without a history of combining products (not an uncommon scenario when cleaning bathrooms) also can be associated with irritant effects. Similarly, in certain industrial operations, hydrochloric (hydrogen chloride in water) or hypochlorous acid aerosols are also respiratory irritants. Other sources of chlorine exposure occur in specific industrial processes that use a large number of inorganic chlorine derivatives. Worthy of particular mention are chlorine dioxide (used in pulp paper processing),[49] chlorinated silanes (gases used in microelectronics),[50] reactive metal halides (e.g., titanium or antimony chlorides),[11] and thionyl chloride (which breaks down to yield hydrogen chloride and sulfur dioxide).[27, 50a]

For chlorine, chloramine, and hydrochloric acid, the acute respiratory response corresponds to the effective dose delivered to the lungs. All these compounds appear to share final common toxic pathways. As noted in the general discussion of acute toxic inhalations, water solubility is an important determinant of the dose reaching the lower airways. For chlorine and chloramine, lower solubility favors deeper penetration with a more effective delivered dose compared with an equivalent inhalation of acid. However, exposure to any of these compounds is associated with some degree of immediate mucous membrane and upper airway irritation. In fact, the absence of acute irritant effects is not clinically consistent with chlorine gas or related exposures.

Chlorine inhalation may manifest any of the full spectrum of pulmonary irritant effects, from minor mucosal responses to diffuse alveolar damage.[42–48] Persistent airway hyperresponsiveness after irritant exposure has been associated particularly with chlorine gas and chlorine-containing products, although this may reflect the frequency of such exposures, rather than a propensity for chlorine to have this effect.[6, 22, 23, 51, 52]

## Oxides of Nitrogen, Ozone, Sulfur Dioxide, and Acid Aerosols

These inhalants are major air pollutants; the effects of low-level exposure are discussed in detail in Chapter 68. When they are inhaled in high concentrations, these irritants also cause acute lung injury. Because of lower solubility, longer exposure with a greater predilection for lung injury may occur with ozone[4] and, even more commonly, nitrogen dioxide.[54] Nonetheless, with sulfur dioxide and acid aerosols, sufficient intensity of exposure leads to diffuse alveolar damage.

High-intensity exposure to oxides of nitrogen occurs through decomposition of organic matter. Examples include nitrogen dioxide-induced lung injury among farmers (also known as silo filler's disease),[25, 55] use of internal combustion engines in enclosed spaces,[3, 56, 57] thermal degradation of polymers (e.g., in structural fires),[58] explosives or industrial mishaps,[24, 59] and welding by-products, particularly when "gas-shielded" techniques are employed (manual inert gas welding or tungsten inert welding).[60]

High-intensity occupational ozone exposure is unusual, but it can occur with welding conditions associated with oxides of nitrogen.[60] More recently, ozone in water treatment and in pulp paper bleaching also has emerged as a health issue.[61] Important sources of high-level sulfur dioxide exposure include mining and ore refining,[2] Portland cement manufacturing,[62] and industrial releases.[63] Historically, sulfur dioxide also has been important in pulp paper processing[61] and as a refrigerant.[64]

In ambient air pollution, the acid aerosols of primary concern are sulfuric and nitric acids, but they also can be encountered occupationally. Sulfuric acid exposure occurs both through direct use and through the breakdown of a highly toxic industrial chemical, dimethyl sulfate.[65] Nitric acid also has many industrial uses.[59] A number of other inorganic and organic acid vapors and aerosols are also important potential causes of acute lung injury, including chromic,[66] acetic,[67] formic,[68] and hydrofluoric acids.[69]

Hydrofluoric acid (hydrogen fluoride), in addition to nonspecific irritant effects, can induce clinically significant hypocalcemia.[70] Exposures occur in manufacturing of both microelectronics and phosphate fertilizers, in household use of hydrofluoric acid rust removal agents (the mixture of which with hypochlorite bleach can evolve both chlorine and hydrogen fluoride), and in pyrolysis of fluorinated polymers.[71] Hydrogen fluoride is a chronic exposure problem in the aluminum smelting industry. Hydrogen fluoride also is released as a breakdown product of sulfur hexafluoride, an electric-insulating chemical.[72]

## Military and Crowd Control Agents

Unfortunately, these exposures are not of mere historical interest.[47, 73] Of the major World War I chemical weapons, only sulfur mustard (mustard gas) has been used "militarily" since World War II. Classified as a vesicant because of blistering induced by skin contact, mustard gas inhalation causes severe respiratory injury. Survivors exhibit residual tracheobronchitis and bronchiectasis.[32, 74, 74a] Phosgene, another World War I toxic gas, currently is encountered as a thermal breakdown product or ultraviolet photoreactant of chlorinated solvents (e.g., methylene chloride).[5, 75] A common cause of exposure is inadvertent phosgene production from welding metals "degreased" with solvents.[50] Phosgene is the prototypic deeply penetrating inhalant exhibiting a delayed onset of symptoms (12 to 24 hours after exposure). Chloropicrin, another World War I gas, is a low-threshold irritant currently encountered in chemical manufacturing and as a component of fumigants.[76, 77] The modern chemical warfare armamentarium is dominated by systemic toxins developed from organophosphate pesticides.[78, 79] These highly lethal neurotoxins have important respiratory effects, including manifestations of both muscarinic receptor stimulation (bronchorrhea and bronchospasm) and nicotinic receptor depolarization blockade (respiratory muscle paralysis).

Crowd control agents ("tear gases"), as opposed to the war gases, are intended to incapacitate persons via immediate mucous membrane irritation.[80] The agents in greatest use worldwide are chloroacetophenone ("mace"), and orthochlorobenzamalonitrile.[81, 82] In addition to their mucous membrane effects, case reports have implicated these agents in lower respiratory injury with high-intensity exposure (e.g., in enclosed buildings).[83–85] Unlike tear gas, the primary component of "smoke bombs," zinc chloride, is a potent lower respiratory tract irritant.[86] Military and police exposures (including training exercises) have resulted in severe pulmonary edema.[87, 88]

## Cadmium, Mercury, and Other Toxic Metals

Inhalation of certain metal fumes or vapors causes acute pneumonitis.[11] The two metals most important clinically are cadmium and mercury. In both instances, the most important factor in acute pulmonary insult is high-intensity, acute inhalation. With cadmium, exposure typically occurs through welding, brazing (high-temperature soldering), or flame cutting metal under conditions of poor ventilation.[89–91] The usual source of cadmium is the welding rod, brazing solder, or a metal coating, rather than the base metal itself.[60] For mercury, high levels of the relatively volatile metal can be generated effectively from many nonenclosed operations, most notably through heated metal reclamation processes (e.g, home refining of mercury-gold amalgams).[92–94] These short-term, high-level inhalation exposures contrast with other chronic lower-level occupational and environmental exposure toxicities from cadmium or mercury. Other metals, including antimony, manganese, and beryllium, frequently are cited as causes of acute pneumonitis, but there are few reports in the last 50 years providing documentation of such disorders.[11] Nickel carbonyl is an organic metal derivative and potent pulmonary toxin, with exposure primarily limited to nickel refining.[95, 96] Inorganic nickel, although a sensitizer, is not associated with pneumonitis.

Dangerous exposures to cadmium, mercury, and nickel carbonyl occur in part because they are not immediately irritating, analogous to symptoms after phosgene gas inhalation. Patients typically present in respiratory distress 12 to 24 hours after exposure.[89–94] The exposure history often remains occult unless aggressively pursued. Metal pneumonitis from these materials also can include fever as a clinical manifestation of the toxic syndrome. However, the term *metal fume fever* should not be used in this context.[97] The toxic mechanism in heavy metal pneumonitis is presumed to be inhibition of enzymatic and other critical cellular functions. Chelation treatment has not been shown to be effective in heavy metal pneumonitis due to cadmium or mercury. The agent dithiocarb (diethyldithiocarbamate) has been used as a chelating antidote for nickel carbonyl pneumonitis, although this has not been tested in a controlled manner.[98] Disulfiram has been suggested as a potential treatment alternative.[99]

Two other metal compounds are well-documented bronchial irritants in humans, although they are not associated with reports of frank pneumonitis. Vanadium, which is encountered in metal processing and, in lower concentrations, as a fossil fuel by-product, causes acute bronchitis.[100, 101] Tributyltin (bis[tributyltin] oxide), an organotin compound employed as a mildew and mold retardant in paint, is also an airway irritant.[102]

## Metal Fume Fever, Polymer Fume Fever, and Organic Dust Toxic Syndrome

There are a number of febrile flu-like pulmonary syndromes reflecting similar clinical responses to a diverse group of acute inhalational exposures.[14, 103] Their hallmark is chills, fever, malaise, and myalgia with onset 4 to 8 hours after intense inhalation of fumes or dust.[14, 15, 97, 104] Common respiratory complaints include cough or mild dyspnea, but findings of chest radiographic infiltrates or hypoxemia are inconsistent with this disorder. Peripheral leukocytosis usually accompanies the syndrome; bronchoalveolar lavage shows a marked influx of neutrophils.[105–107] These syndromes all are self-limited, resolving clinically within 12 to 48 hours. Signs or symptoms of pneumonitis should suggest alternative, less benign diagnoses, such as cadmium pneumonitis,[90, 91] hypersensitivity pneumonitis (Chapter 67), or inhalation of more toxic temperature-dependent fluoropolymer pyrolysis byproducts (which include hydrogen fluoride and carbonyl fluoride).[71, 108, 109] An outbreak of toxic pneumonitis, which should be distinguished from fume fever, was associated with exposure to fluoropolymer-containing protective sprays for shoes.[110, 111] These exposures did not involve thermal breakdown by-products.

Metal fume fever and organic dust toxic syndrome share a common feature of tachyphylaxis, with a blunted response to daily repeated inhalation (and hence the name "Monday fever") among both brass founders and cotton mill workers.[14, 112, 113] Metal fume fever is associated with zinc oxide inhalation from welding galvanized metal or brass working.[114] There is only limited evidence that other metals (magnesium and copper) cause a similar response,[97, 115] and experimental data from 1997 further discounted magnesium as a potential cause of fume fever.[116] Organic dust toxic syndrome is associated with inhalation of thermophilic bacteria and fungal spores contaminating materials such as wood chips,[117] straw,[118] silage,[119] and textile raw materials.[113] The syndrome includes variously named conditions including pulmonary mycotoxicosis,[120] silo unloader's syndrome,[119] and mill fever.[121] One of the best documented historical outbreaks of organic dust toxic syndrome occurred among individuals who work with stained (contaminated) cotton mattresses.[113] Inhalation of aerosols from contaminated water sources produces a similar syndrome, some of which is attributable to *Legionella* species (Pontiac fever) as well as to other organisms.[14] Polymer fume fever is associated with thermal breakdown products of fluoropolymers (e.g., Teflon and related materials).[104, 122–124] The pathophysiologic mechanisms underlying all these syndromes have not been established, but research since 1993 suggests that pulmonary cytokines may play a key role.[125–132]

## Hydrocarbon Pneumonitis and Baby Powder Aspiration

Hydrocarbon pneumonitis occurs with oral ingestion of hydrocarbons. This is a major public health toxicologic problem in the pediatric age group, accounting for many hospital admissions each year.[41] Common hydrocarbons involved are mineral spirits, mineral seal oil (common in furniture polish), lamp oil, kerosene (paraffin), turpentine (pine oil), gasoline, and lighter fluid.[12, 133–136] Even though these substances have systemic toxic effects such as central nervous system depression, life-threatening complications of ingestion are predominantly the result of concomitant hydrocarbon aspiration and subsequent pulmonary compromise, making the lung the target organ of concern in hydrocarbon ingestion. In contradistinction to aspiration hydrocarbon pneumonitis, the toxicity of hydrocarbon (solvent) inhalation manifests primarily in either central nervous system or cardiac effects. Major pulmonary target organ damage associated with acute hydrocarbon exposure by inhalation is unusual but has been reported.[137]

Hydrocarbon aspiration can occur with initial ingestion or with vomiting. Low viscosity of an ingested hydrocarbon is considered a major factor promoting aspiration (presumably for mechanical reasons), for example, with mineral seal oil.[12, 134] Although theoretical consideration has been given to potential effects on surfactant as being mediators of hydrocarbon aspiration toxicity, the chemical pneumonitis of the syndrome appears to be nonspecific.

Another acute inhalational pediatric syndrome is caused by baby (talcum) powder aspiration.[138, 139] Within hours, the inhaled powder can cause a severe and potentially fatal pneumonitis. The pathophysiology of baby powder pneumonitis may not be specific to talc per se and is distinct from talcosis, a chronic granulomatous lung disease. There is no proposed specific mechanism of the acute syndrome. Pediatricians emphasize prevention through discontinuing the use of such powders in infants, but exposures still occur.

## Paraquat

Paraquat is a widely used herbicide and a potent toxin. Ingestion rather than inhalation is the typical route of exposure associated with human toxicity. Contamination through skin absorption also can occur. The theoretical risk of smoking contaminated materials has never been established clinically. Most paraquat deaths result from suicidal intent.[13, 140, 141] Paraquat ingestion is a relatively uncommon method of suicide in the United States, but its incidence is greater in a number of other countries, perhaps related to patterns of crop utilization and other access factors.[140, 142] Although paraquat ingestion leads to acute gastrointestinal tract necrosis and multiorgan failure, the lung is the target organ for toxicity among those surviving the immediate postingestion period. Diquat, a related dipyridyl herbicide, does not seem to cause acute lung toxicity.[143]

The pulmonary toxicity of paraquat, in contrast to its gastrointestinal effects, does not reflect caustic irritant injury. Rather, paraquat appears to be unique in its ability to induce an accelerated, chemically induced pulmonary fibrosis. After stabilization following acute multiorgan paraquat toxic effects, disease progression is marked by rapidly worsening respiratory distress, hypoxemia, and a restrictive ventilatory defect, with a decrease in severe cases in lung compliance and a decreasing diffusing capacity, ending in death from ventilatory failure within days to weeks.[13, 140] Survivors may demonstrate modest and slow improvement in lung function.[144] Diagnosis of paraquat exposure is usually clear on the basis of the patient's history, but confirmatory blood or urine levels are available through chemical manufacturers. The mechanism of paraquat toxicity is attributed to the generation of superoxide radicals that may be, in part, iron dependent.[145] Consistent with an oxidant mechanism, supplemental oxygen and radiation therapy may worsen the outcome.[140, 146] There are no known antidotes for paraquat poisoning, nor is enhanced elimination (hemoperfusion) efficacious.[13, 140]

## Smoke Inhalation

The generic term *smoke inhalation* includes potential exposure to a wide array of substances because of the complex chemistry of heat decomposition and pyrolysis. Although cytotoxic anoxia from carbon monoxide, cyanide, and oxidants represents a major manifestation of toxic insult from acute smoke inhalation, this *nonpulmonary target organ* effect is not covered here.[58, 147–149] However, there are a number of irritant chemical pyrolysis products that do have significant potential target organ pulmonary toxicity. In contrast to thermal injury to the respiratory tract, which typically is limited to upper airways with laryngeal edema the major potential medical management problem,[150] irritant smoke inhalation injury from fires can severely affect the entire respiratory tract.

In certain cases, irritant chemicals from fires result from liberation of preformed substances, but most commonly, the toxins of concern are formed de novo. These irritants are produced by the thermal degradation of both naturally occurring and synthetic polymers. The predominant by-products of heat breakdown are determined by the nature of the polymers consumed, but the precise mixture of agents released in any specific event may be difficult to predict, varying in particular according to temperature and oxygen availability.[58, 149] As a general rule, the chemical monomer precursor is not a significant polymer breakdown product, although residual monomers can be evolved under certain circumstances. For example, hydrogen chloride rather than vinyl chloride is released when polyvinyl chloride is burned.[58]

Many of the specific chemical irritants that can be released as common thermal breakdown by-products are addressed elsewhere in this chapter. These include the following: hydrochloric acid (hydrogen chloride), hydrofluoric acid (hydrogen fluoride), and other acids; ammonia; phosgene; and oxides of nitrogen. The zinc chloride "smoke" of smoke bombs (in contrast to the heterogeneous character of "natural smoke") also is discussed separately.

Aldehydes merit specific attention, however, because smoke from fires may represent the most common source of high-intensity irritant inhalant injury caused by this group of chemicals. These chemicals include formaldehyde, acetaldehyde, and acrolein. Of these aldehydes, acrolein ($CH_2=CHCHO$), although the most severe irritant, is least familiar to most health-care providers. Acrolein, a highly reactive chemical, is formed as an important pyrolysis product of both synthetic (e.g., acrylic) and natural polymers.[151] The irritant potential of acrolein is reflected in its exposure limit in the workplace in the United States of 0.1 ppm compared with 1 ppm for formaldehyde.[152]

The general considerations concerning irritant exposure discussed previously, including air concentration and water solubility, certainly come into play in smoke inhalation. These are made more complicated by the potential interactive effects of multiple simultaneous exposures, as well as the modifying impact of physical cofactors such as airborne respirable particulates (e.g., soot) that may serve as adsorbent carriers facilitating deep lung penetration. In practice, detailed exposure data delineating the irritant contents of a specific smoke exposure are rarely available. Information that may help to elucidate exposure conditions include identity of the products involved (e.g., specific synthetic polymers, if known), history of inhalation within an enclosed or confined space, evidence of thermal injury, and carboxyhemoglobin and methemoglobin levels as markers of inhalation severity based on other concomitant exposures (carbon monoxide and oxidants).[147–149]

Firefighters (both urban and wildland) and nonoccupationally exposed victims of irritant smoke inhalation have proved important groups in which to study acute inhalational syndromes. Large-scale conflagrations (e.g., urban "wildland" fires) can expose substantial numbers of people to irritant combustion by-products. In particular, such studies have demonstrated acute airflow obstruction and increased nonspecific airway hyperresponsiveness after smoke inhalation.[153–158]

## Pharmacologic Syndromes

Certain natural and synthetic chemical exposures exert acute target organ lung effects that are essentially pharmacologic. These chemicals are site specific for key cellular functions whose impairment is manifest in adverse respiratory effects. As noted previously, the most potent chemical warfare agents act through acetylcholinesterase inhibition, with profound impacts on respiratory function.[78, 79] Similar, albeit less potent, agents have widespread use as agricultural chemicals. Both organophosphate and carbamate pesticides lead to respiratory compromise as a principal toxic effect. For example, in one case series, 40% of 107 poisonings from these pesticides led to respiratory failure, with a high case fatality rate (51%). All the patients without respiratory failure survived.[159]

Inhaled capsaicin, of interest as a research tool to study *substance P*–mediated effects, is associated with cough in occupational settings (e.g., in chili pepper processing).[160] Another naturally occurring toxin with a primary respiratory effect is brevetoxin. This toxin, produced by dinoflagellates, is associated with "red tide" blooms. Environmental inhalation exposure from airborne aerosols of red tide (due to wind and surf action) causes cough, sneeze, and wheeze.[161, 162] The toxin appears to act by stimulating sodium channels in the lung and may behave pharmacologically much as acetylcholine. Respiratory irritation is also a manifestation of *Pfiesteria* dinoflagellate toxin inhalation.[163]

## Other Inhalant Exposures

### Ammonia

Anhydrous ammonia is a gas at room temperature and ambient pressure, although ammonia more commonly is encountered in aqueous form (e.g., in cleaning solutions). In addition to incidents in the chemical industry and in hazardous transportation, commercial refrigeration systems and farming represent important sources of potential exposure to ammonia gas.[1, 164–168] Ammonia has prominent irritant warning properties and is linked with lung injury chiefly in settings of overwhelming exposure or impeded escape. Bronchiectasis has been documented after ammonia exposure.[1] Acute ammonia exposure also has been reported to have residual upper airway effects, including decreased olfactory acuity (hyposmia).[169]

### Bromine and Methyl Bromide

Bromine is an irritant halogen. It usually is handled as a liquid rather than a gas, but it vaporizes readily. Sources of bromine exposure other than environmental releases include chemical synthesis and water purification.[31, 170–172] Methyl bromide is a major industrial fumigant with far greater potential for public exposure. Methyl bromide is also a potent respiratory irritant, but central nervous system effects may account for more important target organ toxicity in typical exposures.[173, 174]

### Ethylene Oxide

Ethylene oxide is a common sterilizing agent used in medical centers.[175] The gas has poor odor-threshold warning properties. Health concerns over nonpulmonary chronic low-level exposure effects have spurred strict exposure controls and detection alarm systems. Nonetheless, ethylene oxide's widespread use provides ample opportunity for nonintentional release. At exposures near its odor threshold, pulmonary injury may occur.[175]

### Hydrogen Sulfide

Hydrogen sulfide is a common by-product of petroleum extraction and refining as well as a potential hazard from the breakdown of organic materials (hence its common name "sewer gas").[176] Hydrogen sulfide is a respiratory irritant, but it is an even more potent cytotoxic asphyxiant, impairing cytochrome oxidase and cellular respiration. Therefore, in cases of severe hydrogen sulfide exposure, rapid cardiovascular collapse and death overshadow any pulmonary organ effects, with irritant symptoms of importance only in lower-intensity exposures.[176–178]

### Methyl Isocyanate and Methyl Isothiocyanate

Methyl isocyanate (MIC) use is restricted to a narrow application in pesticide synthesis. The mass fatalities at

Bhopal, India, make MIC an important toxin for historical reasons. The toxicity of MIC was the result of its severe irritant properties leading to pulmonary edema.[179–181] No cyanide-mediated mechanism was involved. Methyl isothiocyanate, a breakdown product of the soil fumigant metam sodium, is an irritant chemically related to MIC that also has been involved in illness after a less severe mass exposure.[182] Methyl isothiocyanate also has been detected as a low-level contaminant in cigarettes, but its link to potential symptoms is unclear.[183] Urethane exposures do not involve MIC; the isocyanates associated with urethane, such as toluene diisocyanate (TDI), diphenylmethane diisocyanate (MDI), and hexamethylene diisocyanate (HDI), are pulmonary irritants as well as sensitizers (Chapter 66) but do not have toxicity similar to MIC.

### Phosphine

Phosphine is another important commercial fumigant gas with pulmonary and systemic toxicity. Phosphine is generated on site from aluminum or zinc phosphide in agricultural fumigation applications. Phosphine also has industrial applications, particularly in production of microelectronics.[184, 185]

### Miscellaneous Exposures

A number of other occupational and environmental agents result in acute pulmonary syndromes. Examples of such exposures include *diethylaminoethanol* and *cyclohexylamine* (both anticorrosive boiler additives),[186, 187] *amitrole* (a common herbicide component),[188] *sodium azide* (used in a variety of chemical applications but important as a potential inhalant through automobile airbag deployment),[189] *diborane* (an irritant gas used in microelectronics manufacturing),[190, 191] and *hydrogen selenide* (an irritant gas used in several industrial processes).[192, 193] *Acetic anhydride* (used in making epoxy and other resins) also has been associated with acute lung injury.[194] A distinctly different pattern of injury is associated with a related epoxy chemical, *trimellitic anhydride*, which causes a severe pulmonary hemorrhage after subacute exposure.[10] Another outbreak of unusual subacute toxicity occurring after weeks or months of exposure has been linked to *Acramin* textile dyes. Labeled the "Ardystil" syndrome, its principal pulmonary manifestation is rapidly progressive BOOP.[36, 195, 195a]

In addition to these synthetic substances, naturally occurring exposures also are associated with acute and subacute lung responses, although these syndromes are poorly characterized. Epidemiologically, *Stachybotrys atra* mold growth indoors in water-damaged residential structures was associated with a cluster of cases of pulmonary hemorrhage in infants, although a causal link has not been established.[196] Other case reports occasionally have linked other molds or mold by-products with lung injury (as opposed to self-limited organic dust toxic syndrome discussed previously).[197] Lycoperdonosis is a potentially severe, acute pulmonary syndrome following inhalation (usually intentional) of puffball mushroom (*Lycoperdon*) spores.[198] The pathophysiology of the syndrome is not understood, but its high attack rate with heavy exposure suggests a toxic rather than allergic or infective mechanism.

## SUMMARY

Short-term inhalation exposures to toxic substances may have important effects on the lung as the target organ for damage. A number of substances cause acute respiratory tract toxicity, but the repertoire of pulmonary pathologic responses to such injury is limited. Although modified by the solubility and other physical properties of the toxic agent, injury in large part depends on the intensity and duration of exposure. Extensive injury can lead to acute pulmonary edema and diffuse alveolar damage. Specific exposures of importance include chlorine, oxides of nitrogen, sulfur dioxide, acid aerosols, toxic metal fumes, and pyrolysis by-products. Aside from acute irritant or toxic lung insult leading to airway injury and diffuse alveolar damage, other patterns of acute responses include the inhalation fevers (which are self-limited and appear to be cytokine mediated) and certain target-specific effects, such as those elicited by cholinesterase inhibition. In addition, exposure by ingestion of some substances (e.g., hydrocarbons and paraquat) can cause important acute pulmonary target organ toxicity.

## References

1. Leduc D, Gris G, Lheureux P, et al: Acute and long term respiratory damage following inhalation of ammonia. Thorax 47:755–757, 1992.
2. Rabonowitz S, Greyson ND, Weiser W, et al: Case report: Clinical and laboratory features of acute sulfur dioxide inhalation poisoning: Two year follow-up. Am Rev Respir Dis 139:556–558, 1989.
3. Karlson-Stiber C, Hojer J, Sjoholm A, et al: Nitrogen dioxide pneumonitis in ice hockey players. J Int Med 239:451–456, 1996.
4. Menzel DB: Ozone: An overview of its toxicity in man and animals. J Toxicol Environ Health 13:183–204, 1984.
5. Snyder RW, Mishel HS, Christensen GC: Pulmonary toxicity following exposure to methylene chloride and its combustion product, phosgene. Chest 101:860–861, 1992.
6. Das R, Blanc PD: Chlorine gas exposure and the lung. Toxicol Ind Health 9:439–55, 1993.
7. Mathay MA, Folkesson HG, Campagna A, et al: Alveolar epithelial barrier and acute lung injury. New Horizons 1:613–622, 1993.
8. Katzenstein A-LA, Askin FB: Surgical Pathology of Non-neoplastic Lung Disease (2nd ed). Philadelphia: WB Saunders, 1990, pp 9–57.
9. Wright JL, Churg A: Diseases caused by gases and fumes. *In* Churg A, Green FHY (eds): Pathology of Occupational Lung Disease (2nd ed). Baltimore: Williams & Wilkins, 1998, pp 57–76.
10. Blanc PD, Golden JA: Unusual occupationally related disorders of the lung: Case reports and a literature review. Occup Med 7:403–422, 1992.
11. Nemery B: Metal toxicity and the respiratory tract. Eur Respir J 3:202–219, 1990.
12. Truemper E, Reyes De La Rocha S, Atkinson SD: Clinical characteristics, pathophysiology and management of hydrocarbon ingestion: Case report and review of the literature. Pediatr Emerg Care 3:187–193, 1987.
13. Pond SM: Manifestations and management of paraquat poisoning. Med J Aust 152:256–259, 1990.
14. Rose CS, Blanc PD: Inhalation fever. *In* Rom WN (ed): Environmental and Occcupational Medicine (3rd ed). Boston: Little, Brown, 1998, pp 467–480.
15. Von Essen S, Robbins RA, Thompson AB, et al: Organic dust

toxic syndrome: An acute febrile reaction distinct from hypersensitivity pneumonitis. Clin Toxicol 28:389–420, 1990.
16. Suchyta MR, Elliot CG, Jensen RL, et al: Predicting the presence of pulmonary impairment in adult respiratory distress syndrome survivors. Respiration 60:103–106, 1993.
17. Blanc PD, Galbo M, Hiatt P, et al: Morbidity following acute irritant inhalation in a population-based study. JAMA 266:664–669, 1991.
18. Blanc PD, Galbo M, Hiatt P, et al: Symptoms, lung function and airway responsiveness following irritant inhalation. Chest 103:1699–1705, 1993.
19. Blanc PD: Chemical inhalation injury and its sequelae. West J Med 160:2–3, 1994.
20. Brooks SM, Weiss MA, Bernstein IL: Reactive airways dysfunction syndrome (RADS). Chest 88:376–384, 1985.
21. Alberts WM, Do Pico GA: Reactive airways dysfunction syndrome. Chest 109:1618–1626, 1996.
22. Tarlo S, Broder I: Irritant-induced occupational asthma. Chest 96:297–300, 1989.
23. Boulet LP: Increases in airway responsiveness following acute exposure to respiratory irritants: Reactive airway dysfunction syndrome or occupational asthma? Chest 94:476–481, 1988.
24. Yockey CC, Eden BM, Byrd RB: The McConnell missile accident: Clinical spectrum of nitrogen dioxide exposure. JAMA 244:1221–1223, 1980.
25. Zwemer FL, Pratt DS, May JJ: Silo filler's disease in New York State. Am Rev Respir Dis 146:650–653, 1992.
26. Lenci G, Wacker G, Schulz V, et al: Bronciolitis obliteransnach Stickstoffdiozyd ($NO_2$)–Inhalation: Klinisch-roentgenologisch-histologische beobachung [Bronchiolitis obliterans after inhalation of nitrogen dioxide ($NO_2$)—Clinical, radiological, histological observations]. Pneumonologie 44:32–36, 1990.
27. Konichezsky S, Schatter A, Ezri T, et al: Thionyl-chloride-induced lung injury and bronchiolitis obliterans. Chest 104:971–973, 1993.
28. Janigan DT, Kiolp T, Michael R, et al: Bronchiolitis obliterans in a man who used his wood-burning stove to burn synthetic construction materials. Can Med Assoc J 156:1171–1173, 1997.
29. Segev JS, Mason UG, Worthen S, et al: Bronchiolitis obliterans: Report of three cases with detailed physiologic studies. Chest 83:169–174, 1983.
30. Tasaka S, Kanazawa M, Mori M, et al: Long-term course of bronchiectasis and bronchiolitis obliterans as late complication of smoke inhalation. Respiration 62:40–42, 1995.
31. Kraut A, Lilis R: Chemical pneumonitis due to exposure to bromine compounds. Chest 94:208–210, 1988.
32. Emad A, Rezaian GR: The diversity of the effects of sulfur mustard gas inhalation on respiratiry system 10 years after a single, heavy exposure: Analysis of 197 cases. Chest 112:734–738, 1997.
33. Kass I, Zamel N, Dobry CA, et al: Bronchiectasis following ammonia burns of the respiratory tract. Chest 62:282–285, 1972.
34. Breton D, Jouvet P, de Blic J, et al: Toxicite des fumees d'incendie: A propos de deux observations pediatriques [Smoke inhalation injury: Two pediatric cases]. Arch Fr Pediatr 50:43–45, 1993.
35. Mahut B, Delacourt C, de Blic J, et al: Bronchiectasis in a child after acrolein inhalation. Chest 104:1286–1287, 1993.
36. Moya C, Anto JM, Newman Taylor AJ: Outbreak of organizing pneumonia in textile printing sprayers. Lancet 344:498–502, 1994.
37. Wagner JH: Bronchiolitis obliterans following the inhalation of acrid fumes. Am J Med Sci 154:511–522, 1917.
38. Myers JL, Colby TV: Pathologic manifestations of bronchiolitis, constrictive bronchiolitis, cryptogenic organizing pneumonia, and diffuse panbronchiolitis. Clin Chest Med 14:611–622, 1993.
39. Bowler RM, Mergler D, Huel G, et al: Psychological, psychosocial, and psychophysiological sequelae in a community affected by a railroad chemical disaster. J Trauma Stress 7:601–624, 1994.
39a. Shusterman D: Upper and lower airway sequelae of irritant inhalations. Clin Pulm Med 6:18–31, 1999.
40. Blanc PD, Galbo MS, Balmes JR, et al: Occupational factors in work-related inhalations: Inferences for prevention strategy. Am J Ind Med 25:783–791, 1994.
41. Litovitz TL, Smilkstein M, Felberg L, et al: 1996 Annual report of the American Association of Poison Control Centers Toxic Exposure Surveillance System. Am J Emerg Med 15:447–500, 1997.
42. Schwartz DA, Smith DD, Lakshminarayan S: The pulmonary sequelae associated with accidental inhalation of chlorine gas. Chest 97:820–825, 1990.
43. Jones RN, Hughes JM, Glindmeyer H, et al: Lung function after acute chlorine exposure. Am Rev Respir Dis 134:1190–1195, 1986.
44. Fleta J, Calvo C, Zuniga J, et al: Intoxication of 76 children by chlorine gas. Hum Toxicol 5:99–100, 1986.
45. Wood BR, Colombo JL, Benson BE: Chlorine inhalation toxicity from vapors generated by swimming pool chlorinator tablets. Pediatrics 79:427–430, 1987.
46. Centers for Disease Control: Chlorine gas toxicity from mixture of bleach with other cleaning products California. MMWR Morb Mortal Wkly Rep 40:619–621, 627–629, 1991.
47. Eckert WG: Mass deaths by gas or chemical poisoning. Am J Forensic Med Pathol 12:119–125, 1991.
48. Hasan FM, Geshan A, Fuleihan FJD: Resolution of pulmonary dysfunction following acute chlorine exposure. Arch Environ Health 38:76–80, 1983.
49. Salisbury DA, Enarson DA, Chan-Yeung M, et al: First-aid reports of acute chlorine gassing among pulpmill workers as predictors of lung health consequences. Am J Ind Med 20:71–81, 1991.
50. Promisloff RA, Phan A, Lenchner GS, et al: Reactive airway dysfunction syndrome in three police officers following a roadside chemical spill. Chest 98:928–929, 1990.
50a. Dunkel R, Wermke R, Felgenhauer N, et al: Short term thionylchloride exposure causing delayed airway obstruction (abstract). J Toxicol Clin Tox 37:417, 1999.
51. Moore BB, Sherman M: Chronic reactive airway disease following acute chlorine gas exposure in an asymptomatic atopic patient. Chest 100:855–856, 1991.
52. Donnelly SC, FitzGerald MX: Reactive airways dysfunction syndrome (RADS) due to chlorine gas exposure. Irish J Med 159:275–277, 1990.
53. Schonhofer B, Vashaar T, Kohler D: Long-term sequelae following accidental chlorine gas exposure. Respiration 63:155–159, 1996.
54. Ainslie G: Inhalational injuries produced by smoke and nitrogen dioxide. Respir Med 87:169–174, 1993.
55. Douglas WW, Hepper NG, Colby TV: Silo-filler's disease. Mayo Clin Proc 64:291–304, 1989.
56. Hedberg K, Hedberg CW, Iber C, et al: An outbreak of nitrogen dioxide induced respiratory illness among ice hockey players. JAMA 262:3014–3017, 1989.
57. Centers for Disease Control: Nitrogen dioxide and carbon monoxide intoxication in an indoor ice arena—Wisconsin, 1992. MMWR Morb Mortal Wkly Rep 41:383–385, 1992.
58. Prien T, Traber DL: Toxic smoke compounds and inhalation injury—A review. Burns 14:451–460, 1988.
59. Hajela R, Janigan DT, Landrigan PL, et al: Fatal pulmonary edema due to nitric acid inhalation in three pulp-mill workers. Chest 97:487–489, 1990.
60. National Institute for Occupational Safety and Health: Criteria for a Recommended Standard: Welding, Brazing and Thermal Cutting, Publication No. 88-110. Cincinnati: US Department of Health and Human Services, 1988.
61. Toren K, Blanc PD: The history of pulp and paper bleaching with special emphasis on its respiratory health effects. Lancet 349:1316–1318, 1997.
62. Centers for Disease Control: Sulfur dioxide exposure in Portland cement plants. MMWR Morb Mortal Wkly Rep 33:195–196, 1984.
63. Centers for Disease Control: Acute occupational exposure to sulfur dioxide—Missouri. MMWR Morb Mortal Wkly Rep 32:541–542, 1983.
64. Galea M: Fatal sulfur dioxide inhalation. Can Med Assoc J 91:345–347, 1964.
65. Ip M, Wong K-L, Wong K-F, et al: Lung injury in dimethyl sulfate poisoning. J Occup Med 31:141–143, 1989.
66. National Institute for Occupational Safety and Health: Criteria

for a Recommended Standard: Chromic Acid, Publication No. 73-11021. Cincinnati: US Department of Health Education and Welfare, 1973.
67. Kern DG: Outbreak of the reactive airways dysfunction syndrome after a spill of glacial acetic acid. Am Rev Respir Dis 144:1058–1064, 1991.
68. Yelon JA, Simpson RL, Gudjonsson O: Formic acid inhalation injury: A case report. J Burn Care Rehabil 17:241–242, 1996.
69. Wing J, Sanderson LM, Bender JD, et al: Acute health effects in a community after a release of hydrofluoric acid. Arch Environ Health 46:155–160, 1991.
70. Upfal M, Doyle C: Medical management of hydrofluoric acid exposure. J Occup Med 32:726–731, 1990.
71. Zanen AL, Rietveld AP: Inhalation trauma due to overheating in a microwave oven. Thorax 48:300–302, 1993.
72. Kraut A, Lillis R: Pulmonary effects of acute exposure to degradation products of sulphur hexafluoride during electrical cable repair work. Br J Ind Med 47:829–832, 1990.
73. Institute of Medicine, Pechura CM, Rall DP (eds): Veterans at Risk: The Health Effects of Mustard Gas and Lewisite. Washington, DC: National Academy Press, 1993.
74. Freitag L, Firusian N, Stamatis G, et al: The role of bronchoscopy in pulmonary complications due to mustard gas inhalation. Chest 100:1436–1441, 1991.
74a. Blanc PD: The legacy of war gas (editorial). Am J Med 106:689–690, 1999.
75. English JM: A case of probable phosgene poisoning. BMJ 1:38, 1964.
76. TeSlaa G, Kaiser M, Biederman L, et al: Chloropicrin toxicity involving animal and human exposure. Vet Hum Toxicol 28:323–324, 1986.
77. Gonmori K, Muto H, Yamamoto T, et al: A case of homicidal intoxication by chloropicrin. Am J Forensic Med Pathol 8:135–138, 1987.
78. Dunn MA, Sidell FR: Progress in medical defense against nerve agents. JAMA 262:649–652, 1989.
79. Danon YL, Shemer J (eds): Chemical Warfare Medicine: Aspects and Perspectives of the Persian Gulf War. Jerusalem: Gefen Publishing, 1994.
80. Reider MJ: Lacrimators. Clin Toxicol Rev 9:1–4, 1987.
81. Jones GRN: CS and its chemical relatives. Nature 235:257–261, 1972.
82. Beswick FW: Chemical agents used in riot control and warfare. Hum Toxicol 2:247–256, 1983.
83. Spark S, Giammona ST: Toxic effect of tear gas on an infant following prolonged exposure. Am J Dis Child 123:245–246, 1972.
84. Hu H, Fine JM, Epstein P, et al: Tear gas-harassing agent or toxic chemical weapon? JAMA 262:660–663, 1989.
85. Roth VS, Franzblau A: RADS after exposure to a riot-control agent: A case report (letter). J Occup Environ Med 38:863–865, 1996.
86. Brown RFR, Marrs TC, Rice P, et al: The histopathology of rat lung following exposure to zinc oxide/hexachlorethane smoke or instillation of zinc chloride followed by treatment with 70% oxygen. Environ Health Perspect 85:81–87, 1990.
87. Evans EH: Casualties following exposure to zinc chloride smoke. Lancet 2:368–369, 1945.
88. Schenker MR, Speizer FE, Taylor JO: Acute upper respiratory symptoms resulting from exposure to zinc chloride aerosol. Environ Res 25:317–324, 1981.
89. Anthony JS, Zamel N, Aberman A: Abnormalities in pulmonary function after brief exposure to toxic metal fumes. J Can Med Assoc 119:586–588, 1978.
90. Barnhart S, Rosenstock L: Cadmium chemical pneumonitis. Chest 86:789–791, 1984.
91. Fuortes L, Leo A, Ellerbeck PG, et al: Acute respiratory fatality associated with exposure to sheet metal and cadmium fumes. Clin Toxicol 29:279–283, 1991.
92. Levin M, Jacobs J, Polos PG: Acute mercury poisoning and mercurial pneumonitis from gold ore purification. Chest 94:551–556, 1988.
93. Rowens B, Guerrero-Bentacourt D, Gottlieb CA, et al: Respiratory failure and death following acute inhalation of mercury vapor. Chest 99:185–190, 1991.
94. Moromisato DY, Anas N, Goodman G: Mercury inhalation poisoning and acute lung injury in a child: Use of high-frequency oscillatory ventilation. Chest 105:613–615, 1994.
95. Vuopala V, Huhti E, Takkunen J, et al: Nickel carbonyl poisoning: Report of 25 cases. Ann Clin Res 2:214–222, 1970.
96. Zicheng S: Acute nickel carbonyl poisoning: A report of 179 cases. Br J Ind Med 43:422–424, 1986.
97. Blanc P, Boushey HA: The lung in metal fume fever. Semin Respir Med 14:212–225, 1993.
98. Kurta DL, Dean BS, Krenzelok EP: Acute nickel carbonyl poisoning. Am J Emerg Med 11:64–66, 1993.
99. Jenouri GA, Snodgrass W, Shippy A, et al: Severe nickel carbonyl pneumonitis: Survival with disulfiram chelation (abstract). Am J Respir Crit Care Med 157:A146, 1998.
100. Musk AW, Tees JG: Asthma caused by occupational exposure to vanadium compounds. Med J Aust 1:183–184, 1982.
101. Irsigler GB, Visser PJ, Spangenberg PAL: Asthma and chemical bronchitis in vanadium plant workers. Am J Ind Med 35:366–374, 1999.
102. Wax PM, Dockstader L: Tributyltin use in interior paints: A continuing health hazard. Clin Toxicol 33:239–241, 1995.
103. Rask-Andersen A, Pratt DS: Inhalation fever: A proposed unifying term for febrile reactions to inhalation of noxious substances. Br J Ind Med 49:40, 1992.
104. Centers for Disease Control: Polymer-fume fever associated with cigarette smoking and the use of tetrafluoroethylene Mississippi. MMWR Morb Mortal Wkly Rep 36:515–516, 521–522, 1987.
105. Volgelmeier C, Konig G, Bencze K, et al: Pulmonary involvement in zinc fume fever. Chest 92:946–948, 1987.
106. Blanc P, Wong H, Bernstein MS, et al: An experimental model of metal fume fever. Ann Intern Med 114:930–936, 1991.
107. Lecours R, Laviolette M, Cormier Y: Bronchoalveolar lavage in pulmonary mycotoxicosis (organic dust toxic syndrome). Thorax 41:924–926, 1986.
108. Robbins JJ, Ware RL: Pulmonary edema from Teflon fumes. N Engl J Med 271:360–361, 1964.
109. Evans EA: Pulmonary edema after inhalation of fumes from polytetra-fluoroethylene (PTFE). J Occup Med 15:599–601, 1973.
110. Centers for Disease Control: Severe acute respiratory illness linked to use of shoe sprays—Colorado, November 1993. MMWR Morb Mortal Wkly Rep 42:885–887, 1993.
111. Laliberte M, Sanfacon G, Blais R: Acute pulmonary toxicity linked to use of a leather protector. Ann Emerg Med 25:841–844, 1995.
112. Drinker P, Thomson RM, Finn JL: Metal fume fever: II. Resistance acquired by inhalation of zinc oxide on two successive days. J Ind Hyg 9:98–105, 1927.
113. Neal PA, Schneiter R, Camanita BH: Report on acute illness among rural mattress makers using low grade, stained cotton. JAMA 119:1074–1082, 1942.
114. National Institute for Occupational Safety and Health: Occupational Exposure to Zinc (Pub. No. 76-104). Washington, DC: US Department of Health, Education and Welfare, 1976.
115. Drinker P, Thomson RM, Finn JL: Metal fume fever: III. The effects of inhaling magnesium oxide fume. J Ind Hyg 9:187–192, 1927.
116. Kuschner WG, Wong H, D'Alessandro A, et al: Human pulmonary responses to experimental inhalation of high concentration fine and ultrafine magnesium oxide particles. Environ Health Perspect 105:1234–1237, 1997.
117. Centers for Disease Control: Acute respiratory illness following occupational exposure to wood chips—Ohio. MMWR Morb Mortal Wkly Rep 35:483–484, 489–490, 1986.
118. Brinton WT, Vastbinder EE, Greene JW, et al: An outbreak of organic dust toxic syndrome in a college fraternity. JAMA 258:1210–1212, 1987.
119. May JJ, Stallones L, Darrow D, et al: Organic dust toxicity (pulmonary mycotoxicosis) associated with silo unloading. Thorax 41:919–923, 1986.
120. Emanuel DA, Wenzel FJ, Lawton BR: Pulmonary mycotoxicosis. Chest 67:293–297, 1975.
121. Taylor G: Acute systemic effects of inhaled occupational agents. *In* Merchant JA (ed): Occupational Respiratory Diseases. Washington, DC: US Department of Health and Human Services, 1986, pp 607–625.
122. Cavagna G, Finulli M, Vigliani EC: Studio sperimentale sulla pa-

tagenesi della febbre da inaliazaione di fumi di Teflon (politetrafluoroetilene) [Experimental study on the pathogenesis of Teflon fume fever]. Med Lav 52:251–261, 1961.
123. Lewis CE, Kerby GR: An epidemic of polymer fume fever. JAMA 191:375–378, 1965.
124. Wegman D, Peters JM: Polymer fume fever and cigarette smoking. Ann Intern Med 81:55–57, 1974.
125. Blanc PD, Boushey HA, Wong H, et al: Cytokines in metal fume fever. Am Rev Respir Dis 147:134–138, 1993.
126. Kuschner WG, D'Alessandro A, Wintermeyer SF, et al: Pulmonary responses to purified zinc oxide fume. J Invest Med 43:371–378, 1995.
127. Kuschner WG, D'Allesandro A, Wong H, et al: Early pulmonary cytokine responses to zinc oxide fume inhalation. Environ Res 75:7–11, 1997.
128. Wintermeyer SF, Kuschner WG, Wong H, et al: Pulmonary responses following wood chip mulch exposure. J Occup Environ Med 39:308–314, 1997.
129. Wang Z, Malmberg P, Larsson P, et al: Time course of interleukin-6 and tumor necrosis factor-alpha increase in serum following inhalation of swine dust. Am J Respir Crit Care Med 143:147–152, 1996.
130. Cormier Y, Duchaine C, Israel-Assayag E, et al: Effects of repeated swine building exposures on normal naive subjects. Eur Respir J 10:1516–1522, 1997.
131. Deetz DC, Jagielo PJ, Quinn TJ, et al: The kinetics of grain dust-induced inflammation of the lower respiratory tract. Am J Crit Care Med 115:254–259, 1997.
132. Borm PJA, Schins ROF, Derhaag TJJM, et al: Cross-shift changes in blood inflammatory markers occur in the absence of airway obstruction in workers exposed to grain dust. Chest 109:1078–1085, 1996.
133. Beamon RF, Siegel CJ, Landers G, et al: Hydrocarbon ingestion in children: A six year retrospective study. J Am Coll Emerg Physicians 5:771–775, 1976.
134. Klein BL, Simon JE: Hydrocarbon poisonings. Pediatr Clin North Am 33:411–419, 1986.
135. Dice WH, Ward G, Kelly J, et al: Pulmonary toxicity following gastrointestinal ingestion of kerosene. Ann Emerg Med 11:138–142, 1982.
136. Brook MP, McCarron MM, Mueller JA: Pine oil cleaner ingestion. Ann Emerg Med 18:391–395, 1989.
137. Nirenberg DW, Horowitz MB, Harris KM, et al: Mineral spirits inhalation associated with hemolysis, pulmonary edema, and ventricular fibrillation. Arch Intern Med 151:1437–1440, 1991.
138. Gould SR, Bernardo DE: Respiratory distress after talc inhalation. Br J Dis Chest 66:230–233, 1972.
139. Motomatsu K, Adachi H, Uno T: Two infant deaths after inhaling baby powder. Chest 75:448–450, 1979.
140. Bismuth C, Garnier R, Baud FJ, et al: Paraquat poisoning: An overview of the current status. Drug Saf 5:243–251, 1990.
141. Smith JC: Paraquat poisoning by skin absorption: A review. Hum Toxicol 7:15–19, 1988.
142. Im JQ, Lee KS, Han MC, et al: Paraquat poisoning: Findings on chest radiography and CT in 42 patients. AJR Am J Roentgenol 157:697–701, 1991.
143. Smith EA, Oehme FW: A review of selected herbicides and their toxicities. Vet Hum Toxicol 33:596–608, 1991.
144. Lin J-L, Liu L, Leu M-L: Recovery of respiratory function in survivors of paraquat intoxication. Arch Environ Health 50:432–439, 1995.
145. Van Der Wal NAA, Smith LL, Van Oirschot JFLM, et al: Effect of iron chelators on paraquat toxicity in rats and alveolar type II cells. Am Rev Respir Dis 145:180–286, 1992.
146. Saenghirunvattana S, Sermswan A, Piratchvej V, et al: Effect of lung irradiation on mice following paraquat intoxication. Chest 101:833–835, 1992.
147. Summer W, Haponik E: Inhalation of irritant gases. Clin Chest Med 2:273–287, 1981.
148. Schwartz DA: Acute inhalational injury. Occup Med 2:297–318, 1987.
149. Wald PH, Balmes JR: Respiratory effects of short-term, high intensity toxic inhalations: Smoke, gases, and fumes. Intensive Care Med 2:260–278, 1987.
150. Haponik EF, Meyers DA, Munster AM, et al: Acute upper airway injury in burn patients: Serial changes of flow volume curves and nasopharyngoscopy. Am Rev Respir Dis 135:360–366, 1987.
151. Hale CA, Barkin PW, Jung W, et al: Synthetic smoke with acrolein but not HC1 produces pulmonary edema. J Appl Physiol 64:1121–1133, 1988.
152. Occupational Safety and Health Administration: Air Contaminants—Permissible Exposure Limits (Title 29 Code of Federal Regulations Part 1910.1000) (OSHA Pub. No. 3112). Washington, DC: US Department of Labor, 1989.
153. Sheppard D, Distefano S, Morse L, et al: Acute effects of routine firefighting on lung function. Am J Ind Med 9:333–340, 1986.
154. Stenton SC, Kelly CA, Waiters EH, et al: Induction of bronchial hyperresponsiveness following smoke inhalation injury. Br J Dis Chest 82:436–438, 1988.
155. Chia KS, Jeyaratnam J, Chan TB, et al: Airway responsiveness of firefighters after smoke exposure. Br J Ind Med 47:524–527, 1990.
156. Kinsella J, Carter R, Reid WH, et al: Increased airways reactivity after smoke inhalation. Lancet 337:595–597, 1991.
157. Liu D, Tager IB, Balmes JR, et al: The effect of smoke inhalation on lung function and airway responsiveness in wildland fire fighters. Am Rev Respir Dis 146:1469–1473, 1992.
158. Shusterman D, Kaplan JZ, Canabarro C: Immediate health effects of an urban wildfire. West J Med 158:133–138, 1993.
159. Tsao TC-Y, Juang Y-C, Lan R-S, et al: Respiratory failure of acute organophosphate and carbamate poisoning. Chest 98:631–636, 1990.
160. Blanc P, Liu D, Juarez C, et al: Cough in hot pepper workers. Chest 27–32, 1991
161. Asai S, Krzanowski JJ, Anderson WH, et al: Effects of the toxin of red tide, *Ptychodiscus brevis,* on canine tracheal smooth muscle: A possible new asthma-triggering mechanism. J Allergy Clin Immunol 69:418–428, 1982.
162. Krzanowski JJ: Natural products and bronchial asthma. J Fla Med Assoc 1:357–358, 1994.
163. Matuszak DL, Sanders M, Taylor JL, et al: Toxic Pfiesteria and human health. Md Med J 46:515–520, 1997.
164. Walton M: Industrial ammonia gassing. Br J Ind Med 30:78–86, 1973.
165. Sobanya R: Fatal anhydrous ammonia inhalation. Hum Pathol 8:293–299, 1977.
166. Montague TJ, Macneil AR: Mass ammonia inhalation. Chest 77:496–498, 1980.
167. Flury KE, Dines DE, Rodarte JR, et al: Airway obstruction due to inhalation of ammonia. Mayo Clin Proc 64:291–304, 1989.
168. De La Hoz RE, Schlueter DP, Rom WN: Chronic lung disease secondary to ammonia inhalation injury: A report on three cases. Am J Ind Med 29:209–214, 1996.
169. Prudhomme JC, Shusterman DJ, Blanc PD: Acute-onset persistent olfactory deficit resulting from multiple over-exposures to ammonia vapor at work. J Am Board Fam Pract 11:66–69, 1998.
170. Morabia A, Selleger C, Landry JC, et al: Accidental bromine exposure in an urban population: An acute epidemiological assessment. Int J Epidemiol 17:148–152, 1988.
171. Lossos IS, Abolnik I: Pneumomediastinum: A complication of exposure to bromine. Br J Ind Med 47:784, 1990.
172. Burns MJ, Linden CH: Another hot tub hazard: Toxicity secondary to bromine and hydrobromic acid exposure. Chest 111:816–819, 1997.
173. Hertzman J, Cullen MR: Methyl bromide intoxication in four field workers during removal of soil fumigation sheets. Am J Ind Med 17:321–326, 1990.
174. Centers for Disease Control: Unintentional methyl bromide gas release. MMWR Morb Mortal Wkly Rep 38:880–882, 1990.
175. National Institute for Occupational Safety and Heath: Ethylene Oxide, Current Intelligence Bulletin 35 (81-130). Cincinnati: Department of Health and Human Services, 1981.
176. Centers for Disease Control: Occupational fatality following exposure to hydrogen sulphide—Nebraska. MMWR Morb Mortal Wkly Rep 35:533–535, 1986.
177. Jappinen P, Vilkka V, Marttila O, et al: Exposure to hydrogen sulphide and respiratory function. Br J Ind Med 47:824–828, 1990.
178. Parra O, Monso E, Gallego M, et al: Inhalaiton of hydrogen sul-

phide: A case of subacute manifestations and long term sequelae. Br J Ind Med 48:286–287, 1991.
179. Mehta PS, Mehta AS, Mehta SJ, et al: Bhopal tragedy's health effects: A review of methyl isocyanate. JAMA 264:2781–2787, 1990.
180. Dhra VR, Kriebel D: The Bhopal disaster: It's not too late for sound epidemiology (editorial). Arch Environ Health 48:436–438, 1993.
181. Cullinan P, Acquilla S, Ramana Dhara V: Respiratory morbidity 10 years after the Union Carbide gas leak at Bhopal: A cross sectional survey. BMJ 314:338–343, 1997.
182. Cone JE, Wugofski L, Balmes JR, et al: Persistent respiratory health effects after a metam sodium pesticide spill. Chest 106:500–508, 1994.
183. Centers for Disease Control: Recall of Philip Morris cigarettes, May 1995–March 1996. MMWR Morb Mortal Wkly Rep 45:251–254, 1996.
184. Wilson R, Lovejoy FH, Jaeger RJ, et al: Acute phosphine poisoning aboard a grain freighter. JAMA 244:148–150, 1980.
185. Feldstein A, Heumann M, Barnett M: Fumigant intoxication during transport of grain by railroad. J Occup Med 33:64–65, 1991.
186. Centers for Disease Control: Workplace exposures to corrosion-inhibiting chemicals from a steam humidification system—Ohio, 1988. MMWR Morb Mortal Wkly Rep 39:863–865, 1990.
187. Gadon ME, Melius JM, McDonald GJ, et al: New-onset asthma after exposure to the steam system additive 2-diethylaminoethanol. J Occup Med 36:623–626, 1994.
188. Balkisson R, Murray D, Hoffstein V: Alveolar damage due to inhalation of amitrole-containing herbicide. Chest 101:1174–1175, 1992.
189. Gross KB, Haidar AH, Basha MA, et al: Acute pulmonary response of asthmatics to aerosols and gases generated by airbag deployment. Am J Respir Crit Care Med 150:408–414, 1994.
190. Lowe HJ, Freeman G: Boron hydride (Borane) intoxication in man. Arch Ind Health 16:523–533, 1957.
191. Wald PH, Becker CE: Toxic gases used in the micro-electronics industry. Occup Med 1:105–117, 1986.
192. Schecter A, Shanske W, Stenzler A, et al: Acute hydrogen selenide inhalation. Chest 77:554–555, 1980.
193. Banerjee BD, Dwivedi S, Singh S: Acute hydrogen selenide gas poisoning admissions in one of the hospitals in Delhi, India: A case report. Hum Exper Toxicol 16:276–278, 1997.
194. Sinclair JS, McManus DT, Ohara MD, et al: Fatal inhalation injury following an industrial accident involving acetic anhydride. Burns 20:469–470, 1994.
195. Ould Kadi F, Mohammed-Brahim B, Fyad A, et al: Outbreak of pulmonary disease in textile sprayers in Algeria (letter). Lancet 344:962–963, 1994.
195a. Cordero P, Solé A: Bronchiolitis obliterans organizing pneumonia (Ardystil syndrome) and chronic demyelinating disease of the central nervous system. Arch Bronconeumol 31:89–92, 1995.
196. Centers for Disease Control: Update: Pulmonary hemorrhage/hemosiderosis among infants—Cleveland, Ohio, 1993–1996. MMWR Morb Mortal Wkly Rep 46:33–35, 1997.
197. Yoshida K, Masayki A, Araki S: Acute pulmonary edema in a storehouse of moldy oranges: A severe case of the organic dust toxic syndrome. Arch Environ Health 44:382–384, 1989.
198. Centers for Disease Control: Respiratory illness associated with inhalation of mushroom spores—Wisconsin, 1994. MMWR Morb Mortal Wkly Rep 43:525–526, 1994.

# 70 High Altitude

ROBERT B. SCHOENE, M.D. • PETER H. HACKETT, M.D.
THOMAS F. HORNBEIN, M.D.

Introduction
Historical Perspective
Adaptation
- Ventilation: Acute and Chronic Adaptation
- Cardiovascular Adaptation
- Hematologic Adaptation
- Tissue Adaptation
- Central Nervous System Response
- Fluid Homeostasis
- Exercise

Maladaptation
- Problems of Lowlanders on Ascent to High Altitude
- Problems of High-Altitude Residents
- Illnesses Influenced by High Altitude
- Miscellaneous Conditions

Summary

## INTRODUCTION

The survival of a species depends on its ability to adapt to acute and chronic stress. High altitude represents a natural stress where barometric pressure is lower than at sea level and, consequently, a lower $Po_2$ is present. Adaptation to this hypoxia will determine whether a species can thrive and reproduce in such an environment.

Nearly 30 million people live at altitudes greater than 2500 m, primarily in the Rocky Mountains of North America, the Andes Mountains of South America, the Ethiopian Highlands of East Africa, and the Himalaya Mountains of South-Central Asia.[1] Although climatic conditions above 5000 m can be habitable, experience suggests that human populations fail to thrive and reproduce above this altitude. Brief forays above 5000 m are possible, but prolonged survival is not.

Increasing numbers of lowlanders are venturing to high altitudes for recreation and adventure. With modern methods of transportation has come the ability to access remote areas and to ascend to high altitude very rapidly. Consequently, the frequency with which illnesses either caused or exacerbated by high altitude occur is also increasing. And with growing awareness of the risks involved in going to high altitude, persons are seeking advice on traveling to these regions, including often older persons with cardiovascular, pulmonary, or other illnesses and women who are pregnant.

The first purpose of this chapter is to review the compensatory mechanisms that take place in the transport of oxygen from the air to the tissues when barometric pressure is lower—normal adaptation. We discuss both acute and chronic adaptation and explore factors determining the limits of adaptation and performance at high altitude. Our second goal is to review the consequences of maladaptation—the acute and chronic illnesses of high altitude.

## HISTORICAL PERSPECTIVE

For most of its approximately 4.6 billion years, the Earth's atmosphere contained essentially no oxygen. About a half billion years ago photosynthetic activity increased, such that about 100 million years ago the oxygen level became sufficient to permit life of multicellular organisms.[2] Subsequently, the amount of oxygen in the atmosphere up to 110,000 m (69 miles) increased and for some time has remained at about 20.9%.[3] The $Po_2$ in the air we breathe, therefore, is simply $0.2093 \times$ barometric pressure (Table 70.1).

Our awareness of the existence of this life-giving gas and of the consequences of its lack is more recent. In 1590, a Jesuit priest, Father Joseph de Acosta, described both the adaptation and the maladaptation occurring on ascent to Pariacaca, a 4500-m Andean pass in South America.[4] He speculated that it was the "thin air" that was responsible for the sensations of headache, dyspnea, and light-headedness that often occur on acute ascent.

During the 17th century, a phenomenal growth occurred in our understanding of the atmosphere. Air was discovered to have weight. In 1641, Berti and Maignan designed the first water barometer, which they placed against the side of a house. In 1643, Torricelli compressed the device by replacing water with mercury. On September 18, 1648, the French scientist Perier carried a barometer to the summit of Puy-de-Dome (1067 m), where he found the pressure to be 78 mm Hg less than at the base of the mountain.

In 1674, John Mayow set the stage for the discovery of oxygen when he burned a candle in a sealed jar containing mice and found that the mice died when the

**Table 70.1 US STANDARD ATMOSPHERE: ALTITUDE, BAROMETRIC PRESSURE, AND INSPIRED PARTIAL PRESSURE OF OXYGEN***

| ALTITUDE (M) | ALTITUDE (FEET) | BAROMETRIC PRESSURE (MM HG) | INSPIRED $PO_2$ (MM HG) |
|---|---|---|---|
| 0 | 0 | 760.0 | 159.1 |
| 1000 | 3280 | 674.4 | 141.2 |
| 2000 | 6560 | 596.3 | 124.9 |
| 3000 | 9840 | 525.8 | 110.1 |
| 4000 | 13,120 | 462.8 | 96.9 |
| 5000 | 16,400 | 405.0 | 84.8 |
| 6000 | 19,680 | 354.0 | 79.1 |
| 8000 | 26,240 | 267.8 | 56.1 |
| 8848 | 29,028 | 253.0 | 43.1 |

*Values except 8848 m, are taken for mid latitude (45° N). There is greater variation at higher altitudes.

Modified with permission from Altman PL, Dittmer DS (eds): Respiration and Circulation. Bethesda, MD: Federation of American Societies for Experimental Biology, 1971, pp. 12–13.

candle burned out. One hundred years later, Lavoisier in France and Priestley in England were able to generate oxygen, which, they found, constituted about 20% of the atmosphere. Neither man was able to devote a full lifetime to science: Lavoisier was beheaded in the French revolution; Priestley emigrated to America. A French physiologist, Paul Bert, is credited with being the father of high-altitude research. His steel bell chambers allowed simulated ascent by decompression. In 1875, he helped design the experiments for the flight of the hot-air balloon Zenith, in which two of the three scientists ascending to over 8000 m died.[5] The first high-altitude laboratory, the Campana Margherita Hut, erected on Monte Rosa (4580 m), was directed by Angelo Mosso.[6] Field studies were pursued on Pike's Peak[7] and in the Andes,[8] and classic reviews by Schneider,[9] Barcroft,[10] Haldane,[11] and Kellogg[12] give a perspective on the prodigious work that was being done early in the 20th century. West[11a] published an excellent treatise of the history of humans' encounters at high altitude. We will emphasize the past 20 to 30 years of research that have built upon the work of these pioneers.

## ADAPTATION

The $PO_2$ diminishes as the oxygen molecules move from air to blood and then to the tissues that require a constant supply of this vital gas. Ventilation, matching of ventilation with blood flow, diffusion of oxygen from the gas to the blood, circulation, diffusion to and into tissue, and metabolism in the cell are all links in the chain of oxygen transport. A number of compensatory mechanisms improve oxygen delivery when its inspired concentration is reduced.[13]

### Ventilation: Acute and Chronic Adaptation

#### Control of Ventilation

Mechanisms regulating breathing are reviewed in Chapter 8. The ventilatory response to high altitude is the most immediate and noticeable physiologic event to occur on acute ascent. The oxygen and carbon dioxide concentrations in alveolar air are a direct reflection of barometric pressure and alveolar ventilation. Measurement of the partial pressures of alveolar gases by Haldane and Priestley in 1905,[14] Boycott and Haldane in 1908,[15] and, later, Rahn and Otis in 1946[16] clearly demonstrated that as barometric pressure decreases, ventilation increases to minimize the drop in alveolar $PO_2$ (Fig. 70.1). Their studies attempted to predict the pressure of alveolar gases

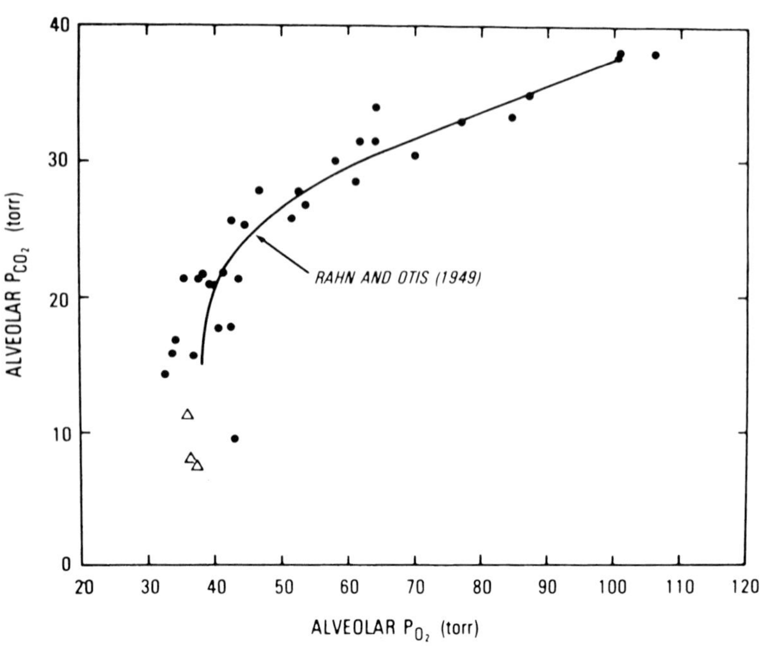


**Figure 70.1** Oxygen–carbon dioxide diagram showing alveolar gas composition in acclimatized subjects at high altitude. At extreme altitudes, marked hyperventilation maintains alveolar $PO_2$ at approximately 35 mm Hg. (From West JB, Hackett PH, Maret KH, et al: Pulmonary gas exchange on the summit of Mt. Everest. J Appl Physiol 55:678–687, 1983. Reprinted with permission.)

at the summit of Mt. Everest (8848 m, barometric pressure about 253 mm Hg), which were measured on the 1981 American Medical Research Expedition to Mt. Everest (see Fig. 70.1). In a single individual, increased breathing resulted in an alveolar $P_{CO_2}$ of 7.5 mm Hg and an alveolar $P_{O_2}$ of 34 mm Hg (inspired $P_{O_2}$ = 43 mm Hg). More recent data collected in a simulated ascent of Mt. Everest in a hypobaric chamber showed slightly higher levels of alveolar $P_{CO_2}$ (11.2 ± 1.7 mm Hg) in six subjects, which also reflects an extraordinary degree of hyperventilation to preserve a viable level of oxygenation.

The ventilatory response to a relatively constant hypoxic stimulus varies over time (Fig. 70.2): the initial increase on ascent, the subsequent course over hours and weeks, and the deacclimatization on descent. In addition, high altitude inhabitants exhibit a different long-term response, which results in lower ventilation at any given altitude than sojourners would demonstrate at smiliar altitudes.

**Acute Response.** With acute hypoxia, ventilation increases immediately, followed 10 to 15 minutes later by

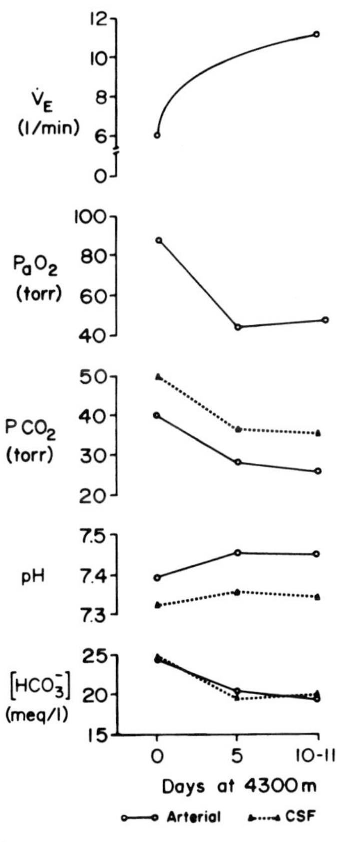


**Figure 70.2** Ventilatory acclimatization during 10- to 11-day sojourn to 4300 m. Ventilation continues to increase as CSF acid-base alterations parallel plasma changes. $\dot{V}_E$ = minute volume of ventilation; $Pa_{O_2}$ = arterial oxygen tension; $P_{CO_2}$ = carbon dioxide tension; $HCO_3^-$ = bicarbonate. (From Forster HV, Dempsey JA, Chosy LW: Incomplete compensation of CSF ($H^+$) in man during acclimatization to high altitude (4300 m). J Appl Physiol 38:1067–1072, 1975. Reprinted with permission.)

a lower level of hyperventilation. As the arterial $P_{O_2}$ decreases from that at sea level to about 60 mm Hg, the increase in ventilation is slight; but as the arterial $P_{O_2}$ drops lower, both carotid chemoreceptor activity and ventilation increase substantially, but with much individual variability in this response. The role of the carotid body in the ventilatory response to hypoxia has been based on extensive direct and indirect evidence. Recording from the whole carotid sinus nerve, Hornbein[17] demonstrated that, like the ventilatory response to hypoxia, neural discharge was related hyperbolically to decreasing $P_{O_2}$ in arterial blood. These results were confirmed on single carotid chemosensor nerve fibers by Biscoe and associates.[18, 19] Surgical ablation of carotid body input results in loss of the ventilatory response to acute hypoxia in ponies,[20] sheep,[21] dogs,[22–24] and calves.[25]

The acute increase in ventilation is inhibited by the resulting respiratory alkalosis and drop in $P_{CO_2}$ at the medullary and peripheral chemosensors.[26, 27] In addition, beginning a few minutes after hypoxic exposure and lasting for perhaps half an hour, a decrease in breathing not explained by hypocapnia is observed; the mechanism causing this transient, hypoxia-induced decrease in breathing, referred to as hypoxia ventilatory decline or "roll off," is the subject of much current investigation. Subsequently, over days, ventilation continues to increase. Although the mechanism is not fully understood, the classic explanation of the progressive increase in ventilation after several days was that renal compensation for the resulting respiratory alkalosis permitted full realization of the hypoxic stimulus to ventilation.[28] However, measurement of blood pH revealed that alkalosis persisted even as ventilation increased. In 1963, Severinghaus and associates[28] examined a possibility suggested by Kellogg[29] that, in spite of persistent peripheral blood alkalinity, the cerebrospinal fluid (CSF) pH affecting the medullary chemosensors might return to normal by virtue of $H^+/HCO_3^-$ regulation across the blood-brain barrier. The sustained hyperventilation on sudden hyperoxia and in the presence of continued alkalinity of blood would be secondary to a relative CSF acidosis.[28, 30]

Although the data presented by Severinghaus and associates[28] indicated restoration of normal CSF pH, subsequent investigators could not confirm these findings. In studies with a larger number of both human and animal subjects, Dempsey, Forster, and their colleagues[31–34] found that not only blood but also lumbar CSF of humans remained alkaline during high-altitude (3100 m) sojourns of up to 3 weeks. Similar findings were documented in cisternal CSF of horses[35] and dogs.[24] During deacclimatization when arterial $P_{CO_2}$, ventilation, and blood and CSF pH have returned toward normal, a sustained hyperventilation persists for days.[35–38]

The inability to account for the ventilatory response at high altitude based on traditional stimuli led some investigators to explore the environment in which the central chemoreceptors exist, namely, the brain interstitial fluid (ISF) and intracellular fluid (ICF). Fencl and coworkers[39] and Pelligrino and associates[40] looked at the ionic and acid-base status of the ISF in goats and the ICF in dogs during hypoxia and reported the occurrence of a more acidic environment in spite of an alkaline CSF. On the other hand, more recent data on anesthetized cats show that brain metabolic acidosis may actually inhibit ventilation and the ventilatory response to hypoxia.[41] Using nuclear magnetic resonance spectroscopy in humans, Goldberg and colleagues[42] looked at brain tissue pH after 7 days at 4300 m in a hypobaric chamber. At the end of the altitude exposure, brain tissue pH was unchanged from before exposure. These results suggest that some mediator(s), other than $H^+$, sustain the hyperventilation during a stay at high altitude.[43–46]

**Subsequent Ventilatory Adaptation.** Over subsequent days to weeks at high altitude, ventilation continues to increase.[16] Data from extreme altitude show that ventilatory change may be ongoing for months or more.[47] A number of factors, such as regulation of brain pH, metabolic rate, and turnover of neurotransmitters, might contribute to this hyperventilation.

One important factor in the progressive hyperventilation may be an increase in the sensitivity over time of the carotid body to hypoxia. This observation has been made in humans[48–50] and in animals.[51–53] This resetting of the hypoxic sensitivity is not understood but may be secondary to a change in neurotransmitters in the carotid body. There also appears to be a role for carbon dioxide sensitivity that is mediated in the brain stem. A number of studies[49, 54, 55] have demonstrated an increase in the ventilatory response to carbon dioxide during and after exposure to high altitude, which suggests that the setpoint for $CO_2$ chemosensitivity changes.

**Ventilation on Descent.** Individuals who have acclimatized to high altitude and who return to low altitude continue to hyperventilate and have increased ventilatory responses to hypoxia and carbon dioxide for several days.[56] Because the subjects are no longer hypoxemic, this continued ventilatory stimulation cannot be attributed to carotid body input. Additionally, it appears that hypocapnia with or without hypoxia is necessary to produce this continued hyperventilation.[32] The persistent hyperventilation on descent could be secondary to a rise in carbon dioxide that results from the loss of hypoxic stimulus to ventilation.[42] This complex interaction of events on descent has not been carefully studied.

**Chronic Ventilatory Adaptation.** With residence at high altitude, ventilation diminishes over that observed in the well-acclimatized sojourner. Resting arterial $P_{CO_2}$, although generally below that at sea level, is higher than that observed in acclimatized lowlanders at high altitude. Most noteworthy is the diminished ventilatory response to an acute hypoxic challenge seen in many high-altitude residents. This diminution of hypoxic chemosensitivity, found in highlanders in the United States,[57] South America,[58–62] and Nepal and Tibet,[63, 64] is an acquired phenomenon associated with prolonged residence. The mechanism for this blunting of hypoxic ventilatory response with chronic hypoxia is not known but occurs in conjunction with hypertrophy of the carotid bodies[65, 66] and may be an adaptive phenomenon in which the disadvantage of the lower arterial $P_{O_2}$ is offset by the lower energy expenditure of the lower ventilation.

More recent evidence suggests that high-altitude natives from the Himalayan Mountains in Tibet and Nepal, populations in which chronic mountain sickness is rare, do not exhibit hypoventilation or blunted hypoxic chemosensitivity to the same extent as South American high-altitude dwellers.[67–69] Huang and coworkers[67] compared three groups of Tibetan highlanders, well-acclimatized sojourners, and sojourners who had developed polycythemia. Highlanders and well-acclimatized sojourners had higher resting minute ventilations, lower arterial $P_{CO_2}$ and higher pH values, higher arterial oxygen saturations, and higher diffusing capacities for carbon monoxide than those with polycythemia. Hackett and colleagues[70] noted similar responses in Sherpas, highland natives living in the Himalaya Mountains, who are descendants of inhabitants of the Tibetan plateau. These results are in contrast to the many studies in South America that have found that high-altitude natives hypoventilate as compared with lowlanders.[57–62, 71–77] Hackett's study, however, included a much larger number of subjects than the earlier studies and therefore may be more representative of this particular high-altitude population. This study[70] also showed that hypoxic chemosensitivity in the Sherpa population, when corrected for their smaller body size, had a normal distribution with a mean and standard deviation comparable to sojourners. These values were similar to those of Tibetan highlanders.[74] These differences between Himalayan and Andean highlanders present an intriguing possibility that these two populations may have adapted differently. The seemingly more successful adaptation of the Tibetans may be a result of their longer exposure to high altitude (perhaps 250,000 vs. 30,000 years).

## Pulmonary Function and Mechanics at Altitude

On ascent, the lung undergoes a number of changes that may alter its function. Vital capacity decreases in the first 24 hours.[75–80] Coates and colleagues[78] also noted an increase in residual volume and in the slope of the alveolar plateau of the single-breath nitrogen test, and Mansell and associates[79] described an increase in residual volume and decrease in lung compliance. These changes are all compatible with an increased interstitial fluid volume, resulting in airway narrowing, gas trapping, and delayed emptying of some lung units. Using transthoracic electrical impedance, Jaeger and associates[80] and Hoon and coworkers[81] reported increased lung water on acute ascent to altitude. In Hoon's study, the increased lung water cleared uneventfully within 24 hours in those subjects who remained asymptomatic but continued to increase in those in whom symptoms of high altitude pulmonary edema developed. These data also suggest that an initial transient increase in intravascular or extravascular lung water may account for the decrease in vital capacity and other mechanical changes. Although hypoxia and hypocapnia may cause airway narrowing, thus increasing airway resistance,[79–82] Gautier and associates[83] found a decrease in resistance at high altitude, presumably secondary to decreased air density.

Chronic exposure causes other changes in the high-altitude dweller. In 1932, Hurtado[84] described "large chests" in the high-altitude natives of Peru, as did Monge and Monge.[85] Hurtado[84] reported larger vital capacities in high-altitude natives (2720 mL/m$^2$ in natives; 2610 mL/m$^2$ in nonnative high-altitude residents, and 2460 mL/m$^2$ in sea-level whites). Similarly, Brody and associates[86] described larger vital capacities in Peruvian highlanders than in lowlanders (5.11 ± 0.64 vs. 3.73 ± 0.32 L). Frisancho and colleagues[87–89] later discovered that the increase in vital capacity was dependent on the age at which the subjects began living at high altitude. Young, growing subjects are more likely to develop larger vital capacities than those who move to high altitude later in life. Young rats[90] and guinea pigs[91] exhibit similar changes. Burri and Weibel[90] made young rats either normoxic, hyperoxic, or hypoxic for 21 days and found significantly greater lung volumes in the hypoxic group. Lechner and Banchero[91] reported that lung hypertrophy was greater the younger the age at which the animal was exposed to hypoxia.

## Gas Exchange

We will discuss alterations of $\dot{V}A/\dot{Q}$ and diffusion that affect gas exchange at high altitude.

**Ventilation and Perfusion.** The ascent of Mt. Everest (8848 m) without supplemental oxygen by Messner and Habeler in 1978 and the subsequent measurements of the barometric pressure and alveolar gas composition on the summit of Mt. Everest by Pizzo[92] have stimulated interest in pulmonary gas exchange during severe hypoxia, but one need not to go such extremes to observe the remarkable adaptations to hypobaric conditions. The initial increase in ventilation during acute exposure is matched by an increase in cardiac output and pulmonary perfusion.[93–95] Additionally, hypoxia causes pulmonary arterial constriction and pulmonary hypertension.[96, 97] At rest at altitude or with regional hypoxia in the lung, this response functions advantageously by improving $\dot{V}A/\dot{Q}$ matching.[95] The increased pulmonary vascular resistance causes redistribution of blood flow such that areas of the lung that are usually poorly perfused at sea level (e.g., nondependent regions) gain perfusion under hypoxic conditions, resulting in greater homogeneity of $\dot{V}A/\dot{Q}$.[98–102] Using radionuclide scanning, Dawson and Grover[103] found that healthy, long-term residents at an altitude of 3100 m had a more uniform $\dot{V}A/\dot{Q}$ distribution than residents at sea level. Gale and coworkers,[95] using the multiple inert gas elimination technique in an altitude chamber, found that $\dot{V}A/\dot{Q}$ matching was optimized at rest up to 4550 m. These studies, using two different techniques, indicate that a normal pulmonary vascular response to hypoxia results in improved gas exchange at rest by optimizing $\dot{V}A/\dot{Q}$ matching. What happens during exercise is discussed later.

**Diffusion.** At high altitude, diffusion of oxygen from alveolus to blood appears to be a major rate-limiting step in oxygen transport. In fact, the higher one goes, the greater the portion of the alveolar-arterial $PO_2$ difference is due to diffusion limitation, especially during exercise. An additional factor at extreme altitudes may be the worsening of the $\dot{V}A/\dot{Q}$ relationship.[104] Oxygen flux is dependent on the pressure gradient for oxygen from the alveolus to capillary blood, gas permeability of the alveolar capillary membrane (DM), capillary blood volume (Vc), and the surface area for gas exchange (discussed in Chapter 28). Several factors serve to limit oxygen transfer. First is the decreasing $PO_2$ as one ascends. Equilibration is time dependent, requiring approximately 0.25 second at sea level. At altitude, even the estimated pulmonary transit time at rest of 0.75 second may not be adequate for end-capillary equilibrium of oxygen to occur, and diffusion limitation is exacerbated during exercise as a consequence of the shortened transit time of blood across the pulmonary capillary and of the fall in mixed venous $PO_2$. Because the low arterial $PO_2$ lies on the steep portion of the oxygen-hemoglobin dissociation curve, a small decrease in $PO_2$ will result in a proportionately greater drop in pulmonary capillary oxygen content than occurs at sea level. All of these factors may result in an increased alveolar-arterial $PO_2$ difference $(A - a)PO_2$ at extreme altitude, which will be accentuated by exercise.

West and Wagner[105] modeled these factors as they pertain to the summit of Mt. Everest, where the barometric pressure was assumed to be about 250 mm Hg. Using assumed reasonable values for hemoglobin concentration, oxygen consumption ($\dot{V}O_2$), diffusion (DM), acid-base status, and capillary transit time, they predicted that at this altitude equilibration of oxygen tension between the alveolus and end-capillary blood is far from complete (Fig. 70.3). Alterations in any single variable, especially DM, could drastically reduce the end-capillary $PO_2$.

With long-term or lifelong residence at high altitude, diffusing capacity of the lung (DL) increases. Whether this increase in DL results from an increased DM and/or Vc is not clear. Attempts to document either an increased alveolar surface area or increased Vc have not been successful. DeGraff and associates[106] thought that the increased diffusing capacity of high-altitude natives was largely due to an increase in Vc, which was one of the advantages of a generalized augmentation of central blood volume at altitude. Vargas and coworkers,[107] studying Andean children, thought that early exposure to high altitude led to improved diffusing capacity in this population. Additionally, either the alveolar-arterial $PO_2$ was found to be lower or the diffusing capacity was found to be higher in high-altitude residents in a number of other studies.[108–114] Dempsey and associates[108] and Schoene and coworkers[115] have obtained data on sojourners and highlanders at rest and during exercise that provide a convincing argument for more efficient oxygen transfer across the lung in long-term dwellers at high altitude. In spite of a modestly lower level of minute ventilation during exercise in high-altitude natives than in sojourners at high altitude, the high-altitude inhabitants exhibited a higher arterial $PO_2$ both at rest and during exercise, suggesting a more efficient oxygen transfer from alveolus to blood.

## Cardiovascular Adaptation

The cardiovascular adaptations to high altitude are numerous and involve changes in cardiac output, the pulmonary and systemic vasculatures, and the microcirculation.

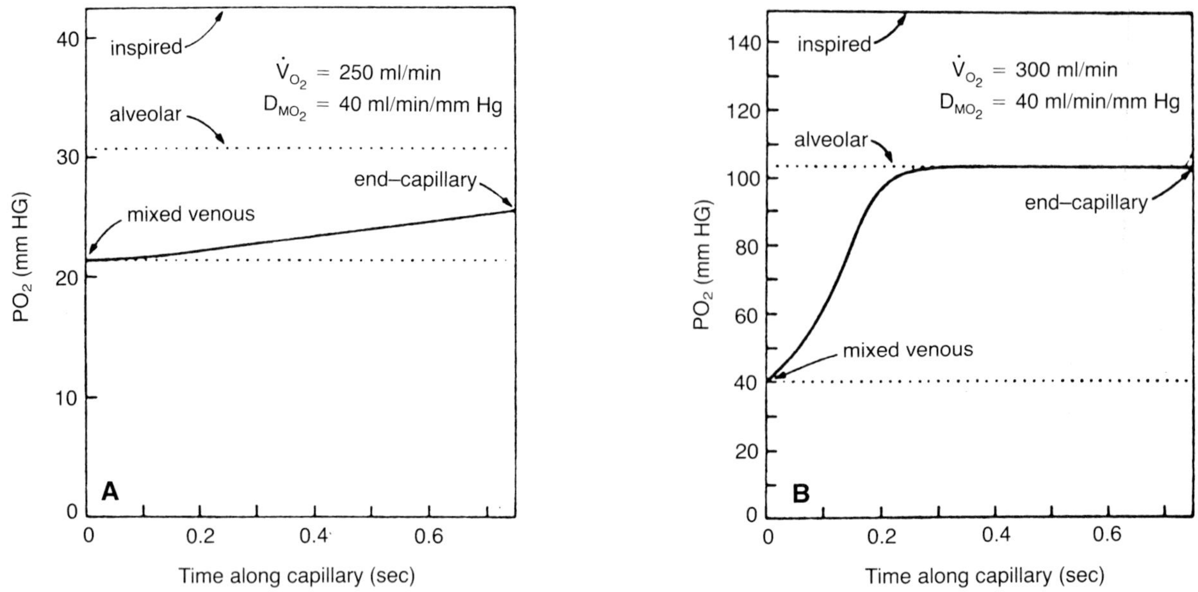


**Figure 70.3** Comparison of the calculated time course of oxygen tension ($Po_2$) in the pulmonary capillary of a climber at rest on the summit of Mt. Everest (barometric pressure = 250 m inspired $Po_2$ = 43 mm Hg) on the left panel to sea-level values (barometric pressure = 760 mm Hg, inspired $Po_2$ = 150 mm Hg) on the right panel. At sea level, there is adequate time for equilibration of alveolar and end-capillary oxygen, whereas at extreme altitude, even at rest, when transit time for the red blood cell is presumably similar to that at sea level, full equilibration is not realized, resulting in end-capillary blood that is not fully saturated. $\dot{V}o_2$ = oxygen consumption; $DMo_2$ = diffusion capacity of the alveolar capillary membrane. (From West JB: Wagner PD: Predicted gas exchange on the summit of Mt. Everest. Respir Physiol 42:1–16, 1980. Reprinted with permission.)

## Cardiac Response

In response to acute hypoxia, an increased cardiac output helps sustain oxygen delivery in spite of the decreased arterial oxygen content.[114, 116–120] The increase in cardiac output is a result of an increased heart rate with little change in stroke volume.[116, 119] The initial increase in cardiac output during hypoxia is mediated by an increase in release of and sensitivity to catecholamines that overrides the augmented parasympathetic tone.[120–124] Over a few days at high altitude, cardiac output decreases, primarily as a result of a decrease in stroke volume, thought to be secondary to a diminished preload from a shrinkage in plasma volume.[125] Heart rate also returns close to its sea-level value. As acclimatization proceeds further, hemoglobin concentration and blood volume increase and oxygen transport is improved by an increase in stroke volume and arterial oxygen content. Steady-state exercise after acclimatization remains constant as blood flow to the muscle decreases and vascular resistance increases.[125a]

Wolfel et al[125b] used beta-adrenergic blockade in subjects acclimatized to 4300 m over 21 days and found that even though oxygen delivery was decreased by a decrease in heart rate that was not compensated for by an increase in stroke volume, total body oxygen consumption was maintained by increased oxygen extraction across the tissue beds, as reflected in mixed venous $Po_2$ values that were as low as documented in studies at simulated 8000 m. This study demonstrates the impressive compensatory mechanisms the body can employ to maintain energy output.

Lowlanders studied over 10 days at 4350 m by Vogel and coworkers[126] showed an increase in systemic blood pressure and greater systemic vascular resistance at rest and exercise after 10 days at high altitude. After prolonged exposure to high altitude, stroke volume, cardiac output, and muscle blood flow are reduced at any given exercise level whereas systemic vascular resistance is increased.[127]

These changes in sojourners at high altitude are not found in healthy people living at high altitude. In fact, a lower systemic blood pressure is generally found in the high-altitude natives in South America, which may be acquired in as little as a year after moving to high altitude.[128] Penaloza and associates[129] speculate that in this population hypoxia has a primary vasodilatory effect on the musculature of the systemic arterial wall.

## Hemodynamic Response

Changes on ascent to high altitude, hypoxic pulmonary vasoconstriction causes pulmonary hypertension, which results in better distribution of blood flow and improved $\dot{V}A/\dot{Q}$ matching.[91–103] However, Wagner and coworkers[104] have shown that $\dot{V}A/\dot{Q}$ heterogeneity develops as one stays for a few days at altitude, presumably secondary to interstitial edema.

On acute exposure to hypoxia, pulmonary artery pressure increases little until the alveolar $Po_2$ drops below 70 mm Hg, then increases markedly (Fig. 70.4). Chronic exposure to high altitude, as documented in the Andes Mountains, results in an even greater increase in pulmonary vascular resistance and pulmonary hypertension, which in some individuals can be severe.[96, 130, 131]

There is both individual and interspecies variation of the hypoxic pulmonary vascular response.[132] For instance, some cattle suffer severe pulmonary hypertension, whereas the Tibetan yak, an animal that has adapted well to high altitude, has no evidence of muscular hypertrophy of the pulmonary arterioles or right ventricular hypertrophy.[133] Months at high altitude (about 3000 m) are required for lowlanders to develop pulmonary hypertension comparable to highlanders'. Once this level of pulmonary hypertension is reached, these lowlanders exhibit a more reactive hypoxic pulmonary vascular response than do the high-altitude natives.[134] As counterpoint, a study by Groves and coworkers[135] reports normal, sea-level values for pulmonary artery pressure in a small sample of native Tibetan highlanders.

Anatomically, pulmonary arterioles are thought to be the site of the constriction that precedes smooth muscle hypertrophy and persistent pulmonary hypertension.[136, 137] Heath and colleagues[138] confirmed these findings in autopsies of humans born and raised at 3800 m, finding distal extension of vascular smooth muscle into pulmonary arterioles as small as 20 μm in diameter. Depending on the severity of changes, particularly intimal fibrosis, the pulmonary hypertension may or may not be reversible, but a return to normal pressures requires months or years at low altitude.[129–131, 139, 140] In contrast, a study of autopsies on high-altitude natives of the Himalaya Mountains of

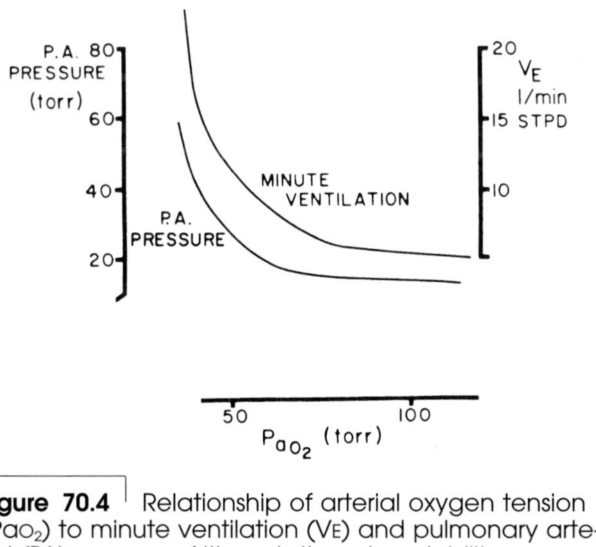


**Figure 70.4** Relationship of arterial oxygen tension ($Pao_2$) to minute ventilation (V̇E) and pulmonary arterial (PA) pressure. Although there is variability among individuals, both the ventilatory and the pulmonary vascular response do not increase until $Pao_2$ falls below 70 mm Hg. (From Reeves JT, Wagner, WW Jr, McMurtry F, et al: Physiological effects of high altitude on the pulmonary circulation. *In* Robertshaw D (ed): International Review of Physiology, Environmental Physiology III. Baltimore: University Park Press, 1979, pp 289–310. Reprinted with permission.)

northern India showed no hypertrophy of pulmonary arteriolar smooth muscle.[141] This finding, along with that of Groves and coworkers,[135] suggests that Himalayan natives who have lived longer at high altitude than have the Andeans have undergone a different pattern of microvascular adaptation in the lung. Thus, there appear to be important ethnic differences in the pulmonary vascular response to sustained hypoxia.

## Hematologic Adaptation

With sustained hypoxia, blood undergoes changes that can improve oxygen transport to tissues. The two basic adaptations are (1) an increased oxygen-carrying capacity from an increase in the number of erythrocytes and (2) an altered affinity of hemoglobin for the oxygen molecule. Recent reviews are available.[142–145] Additionally, there is a decrease in plasma volume over time that is secondary to a water diuresis.

### Erythropoietic Response

Hemoglobin concentration increases within 1 or 2 days of ascent and continues to rise for a number of weeks. The initial rise is due to hemoconcentration resulting from the diuresis that occurs on initial ascent. The continued increase results from increased red blood cell production; this adaptation helps sustain oxygen delivery in the presence of a decreased arterial oxygen saturation.

In 1953, Erslev[146] proposed that a humoral agent, erythropoietin, produced mostly in the kidney[147] and 10% to 15% in the liver,[148] stimulated red blood cell production; hypoxia per se is the primary stimulus for erythropoietin release. Serum erythropoietin levels increase rapidly within 24 to 48 hours of ascent to high altitude, with mean levels being proportional to altitude, and then start to decline within 3 weeks as acclimatization progresses.[148a–151] Both red blood cell volume and total blood volume increase, along with a decrease in plasma volume.[152] The changes increase oxygen content and presumably oxygen delivery at high altitude.[153] The erythropoietic response quickly ceases on descent.[154] A return to sea-level hemoglobin values occurs in approximately 3 weeks.[155]

Marked variability in erythropoiesis exists between individuals, both highlanders and sojourners, and between different highland populations.[56, 145] The difference in erythropoiesis between Andean and Himalayan natives is noteworthy. At 3600 m, the former have hemoglobin levels of 18.2 to 19.0 g/dL[156] versus 14.9 to 17.3 g/dL for the latter.[157]

Whereas the increase in hemoglobin concentration augments arterial oxygen content, a number of changes detrimental to oxygen delivery may also occur. At sea level, a small increase in hemoglobin concentration (1.2 g/dL) improves aerobic performance in trained, elite runners.[158] As hematocrit approaches 60%, viscosity increases and first cardiac output and then oxygen delivery may actually decrease.[159, 160] This decrease in oxygen delivery is thought to be due to an impairment of perfusion of the microcirculation in the exercising muscles as a consequence of increased blood viscosity.

Excessive polycythemia may be deleterious, and phlebotomy may, therefore, be beneficial.[161] In a study on Mt. Everest,[162] four climbers with hematocrits of 60% or greater underwent both psychometric and exercise testing before and after isovolumic hemodilution to produce hematocrits lowered to about 50%. Psychometric test performance improved whereas maximum exercise performance did not change. These results imply that cerebral oxygen delivery may have been improved whereas delivery to exercising muscles was unchanged. The optimal hematocrit remains elusive, but, clearly, high-altitude survival and performance are impaired by an excessive polycythemic response (see Maladaptation later).

## Oxygen-Hemoglobin Affinity

The transport of oxygen by blood is also influenced by the ease with which it is taken up by hemoglobin in the pulmonary capillaries and released from hemoglobin in tissue capillaries. A number of variables affect the process, one of which is the affinity of hemoglobin for oxygen, as defined by the shape and position of the oxygen-hemoglobin dissociation curve. An important feature of the oxygen-hemoglobin relationship is that over a large range of physiologic oxygen partial pressure values (arterial $Po_2$ of 60 to 100 mm Hg), hemoglobin is more than 90% saturated with oxygen. Thus, a change in arterial $Po_2$ within that range has only a modest effect on arterial oxygen content. At arterial $Po_2$ values less than 60 mm Hg, oxygen content of hemoglobin drops precipitously with only small decreases in $Po_2$. At high altitude, certain adaptations of oxygen-hemoglobin affinity occur that may help facilitate oxygen transfer.

The concentration of three substances in blood—hydrogen ion, carbon dioxide, and 2,3-diphosphoglycerate (2,3-DPG)—influence the position of the oxygen-hemoglobin dissociation curve: increases in one or more of these cause a right shift, allowing unloading of oxygen from hemoglobin to the tissues at a higher mean capillary $Po_2$.[163] Although a rightward shift of the oxygen-hemoglobin dissociation curve was initially thought to be advantageous at high altitude,[164–169] not all studies support these results. More precise measurements of the curve[170] have allowed better documentation of human hemoglobin physiology at altitude. Lenfant and coworkers[171–173] and Clench and associates[168] found that humans at altitude in South America have a modestly left-shifted curve. Part of the difficulty in the interpretation of these data resides in the finding of increased 2,3-DPG levels in high-altitude natives. Winslow and colleagues[174] in Peru and Samaja and coworkers[175] in Nepal found increased 2,3-DPG concentrations, which should result in a right shift, but they also found that persistent respiratory alkalosis more than counterbalanced the 2,3-DPG effect, shifting the curve back to normal or slightly to the left.

At very high altitude, a right shift of the oxygen-hemoglobin dissociation curve could be a disadvantage to oxygen transport: the benefit to unloading oxygen from hemoglobin with decreased oxygen affinity at the tissues may be offset by a decrease in loading of oxygen at the lung. A left-shifted curve at extreme altitude would theoretically result in enhanced oxygen loading in the lungs, resulting in a higher arterial oxygen content. Marked respiratory alkalosis and hemoglobin with a high affinity for oxygen both yield a leftward shift of the oxygen-hemoglobin dissociation curve and are two characteristics found in migrating birds, especially bar-headed geese, which can withstand relatively acute exposure to extreme altitude (> 8000 m) while in full flight.[176–179]

Winslow and associates[180] observed the hematologic changes in climbers on Mt. Everest. Two major findings emerged. After 2 months at 6300 m, the polycythemic response (mean hematocrit = 54.4 ± 4.0%) was less than had been anticipated. Although the level of 2,3-DPG increased, the persistent, uncompensated respiratory alkalosis resulted in a much lower $P_{50}$ (Fig. 70.5). As discussed earlier, this leftward shift may convey an important advantage to climbers to extreme altitude.

## Tissue Adaptation

The final stages in the journey of oxygen molecules from ambient air to the mitochondria involve the transfer of oxygen from blood to tissues. Within this critical portion of the oxygen cascade are several steps in the movement of oxygen from within the capillary blood, across the vascular endothelium, through the cytoplasm to the mitochondria, where oxidative phosphorylation occurs. This

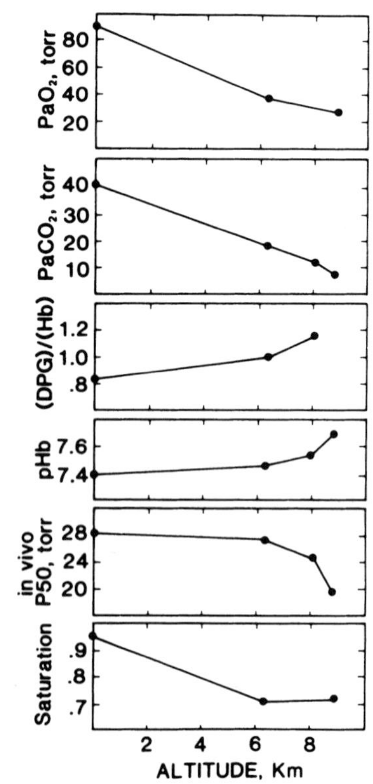


**Figure 70.5** Effectors of oxygen-hemoglobin affinity. The net result at extreme altitude is a protected arterial oxygen saturation. DPG = diphosphoglycerate; for explanation, see text. (From Winslow RM, Samaja M, West JB: Red cell function at extreme altitude on Mount Everest. J Appl Physiol 56:109–116, 1984. Reprinted with permission.)

process depends largely on diffusion and distance. A driving pressure of only 1 to 2 mm Hg is necessary to cause oxygen to diffuse from the cytoplasm to the mitochondria,[181] whereas as much as 10 mm Hg may be needed for sufficient flux from the capillary plasma to the cytoplasm.[182] A $Po_2$ in the capillary blood exists below which the final steps of the oxygen cascade may become impaired.

Certain adaptive changes take place to optimize oxygen transfer from blood to tissue during extreme hypoxia: (1) anatomic changes that minimize the distance for radial diffusion of oxygen from the blood vessel to the mitochondria and (2) biochemical changes that improve the metabolic readiness in the mitochondria. Although human data are scant, some animal studies give some insight into these processes.

### Morphologic Adaptation

A decrease in diffusion distance can be achieved by increasing the concentration of blood vessels in the tissues or increasing the surface area for gas exchange by increasing capillary tortuousity around the muscle cell.[183, 184] Krogh[182] calculated the decreasing maximum distances over which oxygen could diffuse at increasing altitudes to sustain oxidative metabolism. Banchero[185] documented an increase in capillary density and a decrease in the skeletal muscle cell size in dogs after a 3-week exposure to simulated altitude (barometric pressure = 435 mm Hg). Both alterations presumably decrease diffusion distance of oxygen to the mitochondria. But these findings are challenged by recent work.[185a] Decreased diffusion distances were also noted in guinea pigs native to high altitude in Peru,[186] but the technique of cytologic India ink preparation used to define the capillaries did not allow differentiation between formation of new capillaries (angiogenesis) and recruitment of those already present.

Another confounding factor is that during sojourns to altitudes above 5000 m, a decrease in muscle cell size,[187–189] results in a decreased distance for oxygen to diffuse to the mitochondria; it is not clear whether this shrinkage is secondary to decreased physical activity or to a breakdown of muscle protein for fuel induced by severe hypoxia. The functional outcome may be a decrease in muscle strength and aerobic capacity.

The mitochondria are the subcellular structures in which oxidative metabolism takes place. Oxygen consumption depends on mitochondrial numbers and function. The results of morphologic observations vary. Ou and Tenney[190] compared two groups of cattle, one raised at high altitude (4250 m) and the other at sea level, and found mitochondrial density in myocardial cells to be increased by 40% in the high-altitude animals. Using different species and techniques for quantifying mitochondria, other investigators have not noted increases.[191, 192] Human studies both in the field[193] and in the chamber study Operation Everest II[188] described a decrease in mitochondrial volume; at lower altitudes a decrease has not been observed.[185a]

### Biochemical Alterations

Diffusion of oxygen from the blood to the mitochondria of muscle is facilitated by myoglobin, which is an intracellular protein that binds with oxygen at a very low tissue $Po_2$. This molecule may therefore facilitate diffusion of oxygen to muscle mitochondria. Myoglobin concentration correlates quantitatively with the aerobic capacity of the muscle cell and is increased with training.[194] Myoglobin concentration is also elevated in animals native to high altitude[191] and increases in dogs exposed to 435 mm Hg for 3 weeks.[192] The picture was recently complicated by the observation that mice genetically engineered to have no hemoglobin still had normal oxygen consumption at various levels of energy expenditure.[194a]

Investigations of oxidative enzyme alterations during hypoxia have also yielded varied results, depending on the species, the tissue, and the stress.[185a, 195–201] Although the data in animals are inconclusive, the data in humans, particularly at very high altitudes, suggest that the glycolytic capacity, which is responsible for high levels of oxygen consumption, is decreased, whereas fatty acid metabolism, which contributes to endurance exercise, is conserved.

## Central Nervous System Response

The organ most crucially affected by a decrease in oxygenation is the brain. A number of mechanisms exist that optimize oxygen delivery to the brain in spite of profound degrees of hypoxemia, but even these have limits.

### Cerebral Blood Flow

On initial exposure to high altitude the hypoxia-induced increase in cerebral blood flow is in part offset by hypocapnic cerebral vasoconstriction[202–204]; the net result is a modest increase in cerebral blood flow. Severinghaus and colleagues[204] found cerebral blood flow in humans to increase 33% after 12 hours at 3800 m in spite of a fall in arterial $Pco_2$ from 40 to 35 mm Hg. After 4 to 5 days, cerebral blood flow decreased but was still 13% greater than the sea level value. Tibetans, a well-adapted high-altitude population, maintain cerebral blood flow during exercise better than sojourners.[204a]

### Cerebral Function

The flight of the hot-air balloon Zenith in 1875, during which two of the three scientists died after ascending to above 8000 m, is a grim reminder of the potentially catastrophic effect of acute, severe hypoxia. Many other anecdotal accounts of impaired mental function after rapid ascent to high altitude can be cited. As one ascends, motor, sensory, and complex cognitive abilities are progressively impaired. New tasks are learned with difficulty at 3048 m, and simulated altitudes of 6100 m result in a decrement in sensory, perceptual, and motor performance.[205, 206] Even acute, modest decreases in arterial oxygen saturation to 85% impair mental concentration and fine motor coordination; a further decrease to 75% results in poor judgment, irritability, and decreased muscle function.

Lowlanders ascending to 3500 m showed electroencephalographic evidence of cortical depression when compared with natives at that altitude.[207] Forster and colleagues[208] noted that symptoms of anorexia, insomnia, irritability, and depression correlated with the type and rate of change in electroencephalographic activity in seven healthy subjects over a 12-day period at 4300 m.

Several studies have addressed the question of whether the psychometric, behavioral, or cognitive dysfunction persists after return to low altitude. Clark and colleagues[209] did not find residual abnormalities in climbers who had been above 5100 m on Himalayan expeditions. In another pair of studies.[210, 211] subjects who had been at high altitude for 10 months were found to have dysfunction of both motor coordination and speed that resolved over 1 and 2 years, respectively. Individual variation in recovery shortly after descent was found in 30 Polish alpinists on return from 5500 m to sea level.[212] Symptoms compatible with organic brain syndrome were present in half of the climbers, whereas 11 of the 30 had abnormal electroencephalograms on descent. Psychologic tests were mildly to severely abnormal in all of them. Impairment of short-term memory and concentration was documented by Regard et al[212a] in climbers ascending without supplemental oxygen to 8500 m or higher.

From measurements made on climbers before and after an expedition to Mt. Everest and in subjects of Operation Everest II, Hornbein and coworkers[213] found transient deterioration in learning, memory, and expression of verbal material after descent, which returned to baseline 1 year later; however, a symmetric reduction in motor speed, quantified by a finger-tapping test, remained abnormal 1 year later. Of particular interest was that, contrary to expectations, individuals with high hypoxic ventilatory responses (HVRs) and consequently higher arterial oxygen saturations and who performed better physically had more pronounced neuropsychometric dysfunction. One explanation for these findings is that those with a more brisk HVR might have greater hypocapnic cerebral vasoconstriction and, consequently, a lower cerebral oxygen delivery. The bulk of evidence suggests that exposure to very high altitude results not only in acute but also in some residual alterations in neuropsychologic function in certain individuals, as well as possible cortical atrophy after extreme altitude exposure.[213a]

## Respiration and Sleep at High Altitude

Regulation of breathing during sleep is reviewed in Chapter 81. Periodic breathing during sleep at high altitude was described in 1886 by Mosso[214] and is common in sojourners to high altitude. At moderate altitudes, this periodic breathing diminishes over several days as ventilatory acclimatization proceeds.[215] Variability in incidence is thought to be due to differences in individual hypoxic and hypercapnic chemosensitivity.

Several reports review respiration during sleep at high altitude,[216–218] each covering a different aspect of the subject. The consensus is that sleep eliminates most cortical influence on respiration, leaving hypoxemia via carotid chemoreceptors as a more prominent drive. The effect of hypoxically induced changes in $P_{CO_2}$ on hypoxic drive may set up oscillations of ventilation in a poorly damped system (Fig. 70.6).

Lahiri and associates,[219] studying both sojourners and high-altitude natives at 5400 m, observed a direct correlation between hypoxic chemosensitivity and presence of periodic breathing (Fig. 70.7). High-altitude natives, who have lower HVRs, had virtually no periodic breathing. Sojourners' periodic breathing was ablated by administration of oxygen. These findings suggested that those individuals with higher HVRs had greater instability of the peripheral-central oxygen–carbon dioxide interaction, re-

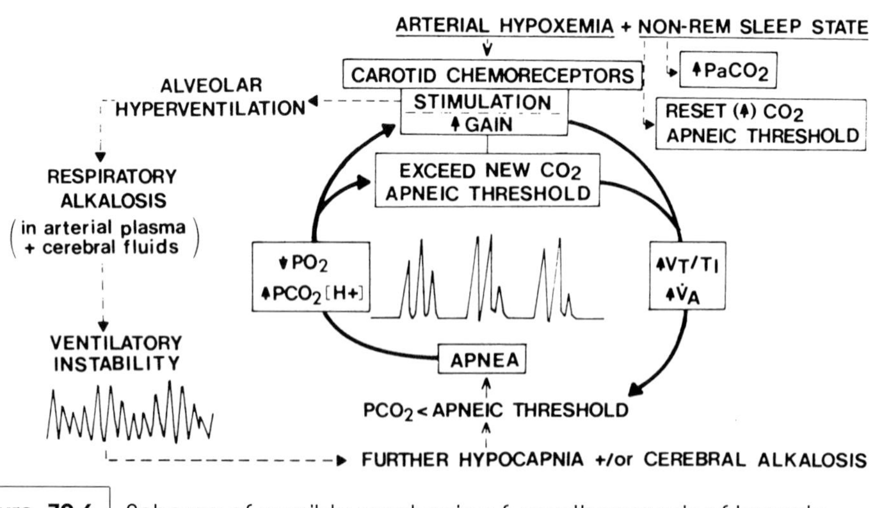


**Figure 70.6** Schema of possible mechanism for pathogenesis of hypoxia-induced periodic breathing during non-REM sleep. Increased peripheral chemoreceptor activity lowers $P_{CO_2}$ and (H+) in arterial plasma and cerebral fluids to near apnea threshold. Subsequent ventilatory oscillations occur with the inherent instability arising from phase delays of the chemical stimuli to the respiratory centers. (From Berssenbrugge A, Dempsey J, Skatrud J: Hypoxic versus hypocapnic effects on periodic breathing during sleep. *In* West JB, Lahiri S (eds): High Altitude and Man. Bethesda, MD: American Physiological Society, 1984, pp 115–128. Reprinted with permission.)

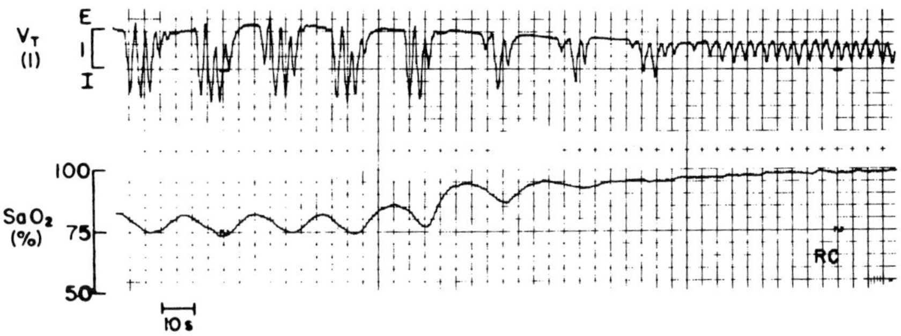


**Figure 70.7** Periodic breathing in lowlander at 5400 m during sleep while breathing ambient air (*left half of tracing*) and oxygen (*right half of tracing*). Upper panel is tidal volume (VT, inspiration downward), and lower panel is arterial oxygen saturation ($Sa_{O_2}$, %). (From Lahiri S, Maret K, Sherpa MG: Dependence of high-altitude sleep apnea on ventilatory sensitivity to hypoxia. Respir Physiol 52:281–301, 1983. Reprinted with permission.)

sulting in more pronounced periodicity. On this same expedition, the climbers who were studied at 6300 m continued to have periodic breathing 6 weeks later, suggesting that the extreme hypoxia at this altitude causes continued instability of the control of ventilation that was not diminished by acclimatization.[220] At moderate altitude, periodic breathing tends to diminish with acclimatization.

Although the mechanism of periodic breathing during sleep at high altitude is not fully understood, it is clear that the most severe hypoxemia experienced by both sojourners and natives occurs during sleep. Marked drops in oxygen saturation during periodic breathing have been noted primarily in sojourners and have been corrected in part by respiratory stimulants such as acetazolamide,[221–223] medroxyprogesterone acetate,[223] and almitrine,[224] each of which may be acting by a different mechanism. The continual wake-sleep cycle may contribute to loss of sleep and inordinate fatigue.

## Fluid Homeostasis

High altitude may induce a dysfunction of osmoregulation, with a difference in fluid homeostasis between healthy persons who ascend to high altitude and those who get altitude illness. The normal response is a diuresis that persists during the stay at high altitude. In the healthy individual, there does not appear to be an alteration in antidiuretic hormone or aldosterone in resting subjects.[225] Exercise over a number of days, on the other hand, activates the renin-angiotensin system.[226] Fluid shifts result in an increase in interstitial and plasma volume and a decrease in intracellular volume.[226] In humans, the overall diuresis may be promoted by a rise in atrial natriuretic peptide. The potential role of fluid balance in the etiology of acute altitude illness is discussed later.

## Exercise

### Maximal Work

Both acute and prolonged exposures to hypoxia result in a decrease in maximal oxygen consumption ($\dot{V}O_{2max}$) and work performance.[95, 227–235] Data from three studies[227, 228, 230] indicate a progressive decline in exercise capacity with increasing altitude, such that $\dot{V}O_{2max}$ decreases about 10% per 1000 meters of altitude gain. At approximately one-half atmosphere, $\dot{V}O_{2max}$ is about half of its sea level value and at one-third atmosphere (as at the summit of Mt. Everest) $VO_{2max}$ is about 23% of that at sea level (Fig. 70.8). A number of factors contribute to this decline in exercise capacity as a function of increasing hypoxia.

### Ventilation

The usual ventilatory response to exercise is further stimulated by hypoxia. This response is proportional to alti-

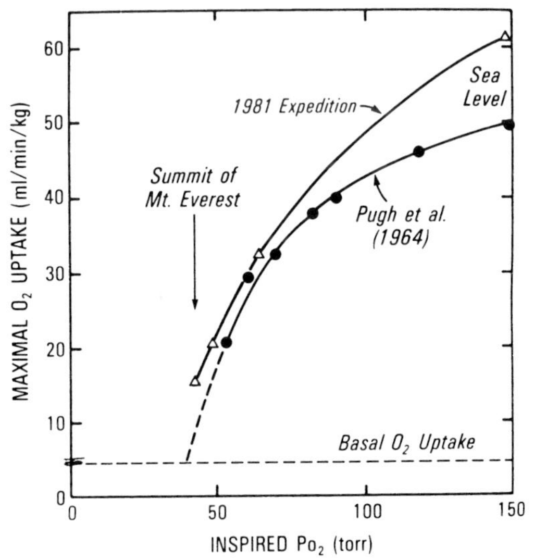


**Figure 70.8** Maximal oxygen uptake ($\dot{V}O_{2max}$) against inspired $P_{O_2}$. There is a predictable decrease in $\dot{V}O_{2max}$ at higher altitudes. The more recent data demonstrate that a small amount of work is possible on the summit of Mt. Everest. (From West JB, Boyer SJ, Graber DJ, et al: Maximal exercise at extreme altitudes on Mount Everest. J Appl Physiol 55:688–702, 1983. Reprinted with permission.)

tude.[228, 236] For instance, the amount of ventilation for a given metabolic rate (the ventilatory equivalent, $\dot{V}E/\dot{V}O_2$) in sojourners to 6300 m is almost four times as great as at sea level (Fig. 70.9).[273] The costs of these extraordinary levels of breathing are both metabolic and subjective. The oxygen cost of exercise hyperpnea at extreme altitude may be as high as 30% to 40% of the overall metabolic rate at high levels of exercise; the aversion to extreme dyspnea may limit both intensity and duration of exercise.

The degree of hyperpnea at moderate levels of exercise is determined both by the magnitude of the hypoxic stimulus and by the individual's hypoxic ventilatory response. In a group of climbers on Mt. Everest, Schoene and associates[236] found that exercise hyperpnea at sea level and at 6300 m correlated with values for HVR obtained at rest at both sea level and after adaptation to 5400 m. These data also demonstrated that those with higher HVRs had less arterial oxygen desaturation during exercise and were able to climb higher. These findings also support an earlier study by Schoene[238] and studies by Oelz and coworkers,[239] Masuyama and colleagues,[240] and Serebrouskaya and Ivashkevich[240a] in which it was observed that most successful climbers to extreme altitude exhibit higher values for HVR at sea level than normal subjects.[238]

On the other hand, chronic or lifelong exposure to high altitude results in a lower ventilatory response to exercise.[115, 241] Dempsey and associates[108] studied sojourners and high-altitude inhabitants in Colorado and found relative hypoventilation (increased $P_{CO_2}$, decreased $\dot{V}E$) during work by the residents. Even so, arterial oxygen saturation was preserved in the high-altitude resident by virtue of a lower $(A - a)P_{O_2}$ that did not increase significantly from rest to exercise. Similar results were described in the Quechua Indians of northern Chile.[115] These findings suggest improved gas exchange in the high-altitude resident, reflected by an increased diffusing capacity at rest and during exercise. This increased diffusing capacity likely results from an increased surface area for gas exchange, diminishing the $(A - a)P_{O_2}$ and enabling a decreased ventilatory work requirement.

## Gas Exchange

In contrast to exercise in most healthy people at sea level, exercise at high altitude results in a decrease in maximal ventilation and heart rate (Fig. 70.10).[228–230] Arterial oxygen saturation decreases acutely[95, 100, 118, 231] (Fig. 70.11) and after prolonged stay at high altitude.[228, 229]

Although $(A - a)P_{O_2}$ increases during hypoxic exercise in sojourners to high altitude,[100, 104, 231] this increase does not appear to occur in high altitude natives.[108, 115] Using the multiple inert gas elimination technique, Torre-Bueno and coworkers[242] noted a substantial role for diffusion limitation as a factor in the widened $(A - a)P_{O_2}$ during exercise at simulated 3030 and 4550 m altitude. Gale and associates[95] also found an increasing contribution of $\dot{V}A/\dot{Q}$ mismatch at these same altitudes and exercise levels, which they believed to be secondary to a nonuniform hypoxic pulmonary vascular response, and which may possibly lead to some interstitial pulmonary edema and thus some $\dot{V}A/\dot{Q}$ heterogeneity and impairment of gas exchange.

These studies, therefore, quantified the contribution of a number of factors to arterial oxygen desaturation during exercise at high altitude. Increasing diffusion limitation is probably secondary to a number of factors, primarily a decreased driving pressure for oxygen from the air to the

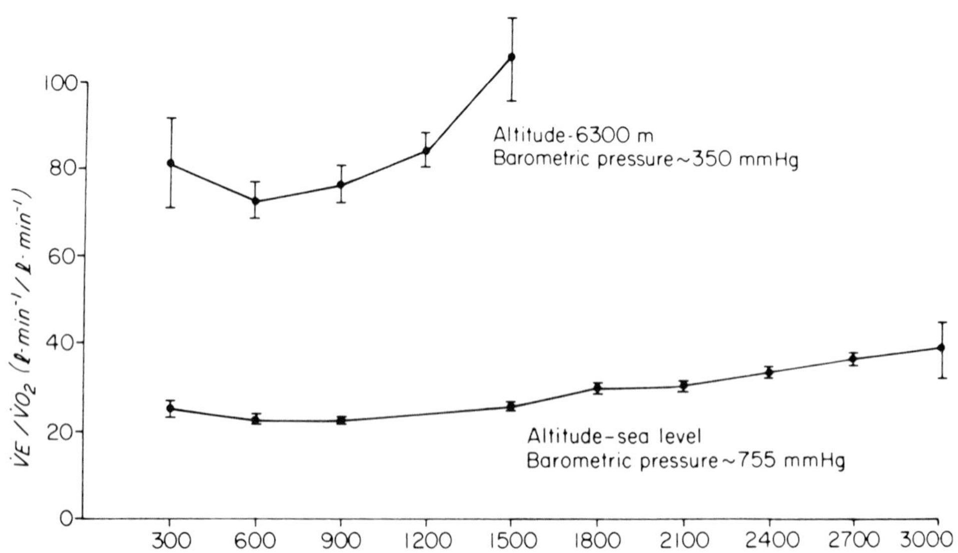


**Figure 70.9** The ventilatory equivalent ($\dot{V}E/\dot{V}O_2$) for given workloads in a group of climbers at sea level *(lower line)* and at 6300 m *(upper line)*. The data demonstrate that the stimulation for ventilation from hypoxia results in a $\dot{V}E/\dot{V}O_2$ that is nearly four times greater than that at sea level. (From Schoene RB: Hypoxic ventilatory response and exercise ventilation at sea level and high altitude. *In* West JB, Lahiri S (eds): High Altitude and Man. Bethesda, MD: American Physiological Society, 1984, pp 19–30. Reprinted with permission.)

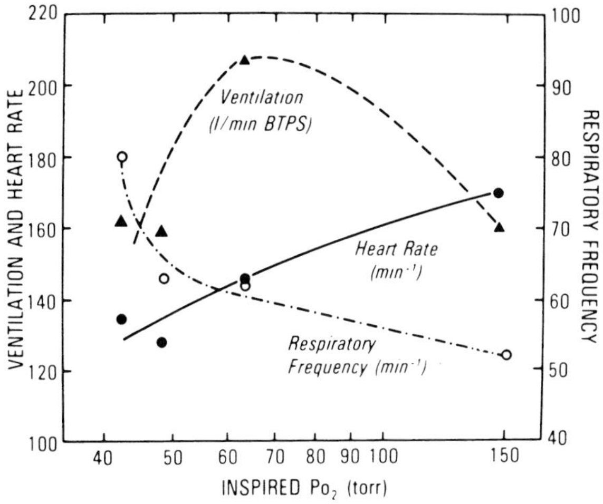


**Figure 70.10** Maximal ventilation ($\dot{V}E_{max}$), respiratory frequency, and heart rate against inspired $Po_2$ at 6300 m. $\dot{V}E_{max}$ is increased because of the stimulation to ventilation from hypoxia as well as a decreased density of the inspired air, whereas at over 8000 m, $\dot{V}E_{max}$ is decreased, probably as a result of a diminished metabolic demand from low work rates. Frequency continues to increase. Maximum heart rate decreases with increasing altitude. (From West JB, Boyer SJ, Graber DJ, et al: Maximal exercise at extreme altitudes on Mount Everest. J Appl Physiol 55:688–702, 1983. Reprinted with permission.)

blood from alveolar hypoxia, coupled with a decreased transit time for blood across the pulmonary capillary from an increased cardiac output with exercise (see Fig. 70.4).

## Cardiovascular Response

With acute exposure to hypoxia, cardiac output and heart rate increase above sea-level values at equivalent submaximal workloads.[119] With prolonged exposure, cardiac output at submaximal workloads is comparable to sea-level values. However, maximum cardiac output is decreased approximately 20% after 2 weeks at 4300 m[243] and 30% after 2 months at 5800 m.[244] Maximal heart rate and stroke volume are decreased with prolonged exposure.[119] The reason for the decrease in maximum heart rate is not understood, but heart rate and cardiac output remain appropriate to the oxygen consumption even up to altitudes of 8000 m. Additionally, during Operation Everest II, echocardiographic studies demonstrated that cardiac contractility was preserved.[245] The decrease in maximum heart rate during exercise is more pronounced in sojourners[227, 228] than it is in high-altitude dwellers,[63, 126, 146] This lower maximum heart rate in sojourners may be secondary to increased vagal tone, but more likely it represents the normal response for a given metabolic demand, which is limited by other factors at high altitude. Maximal cardiac output is decreased at high altitude, probably secondary both to a maximal heart rate that is lower than at sea level and to the decrease in stroke volume.[246]

Pulmonary artery pressures reach high levels during exercise at high altitudes.[247] These pressures did not return to normal when subjects were given oxygen, which suggests some structural changes in the pulmonary vasculature. With the maintenance of a cardiac output appropriate for the level of work rates, the increase in pulmonary vascular resistance in healthy sojourners to high altitude does not seem to limit exercise.

Using data from Operation Everest II, Wagner and colleagues[248] speculated that a diffusion limitation for oxygen from the blood to the muscle might limit its extraction in the peripheral tissues. This hypothesis was tested in an isolated muscle preparation exercised by electrical stimulation by Hogan and associates.[249] Blood flow was held constant, and oxygen delivery was varied at several levels of hypoxia. $\dot{V}o_{2max}$ was related to effluent $Po_2$, oxygen delivery, and calculated capillary $Po_2$, which supports the contention that aerobic function at high altitude may be limited at least in part by limitation of driving pressure or diffusion of oxygen from the blood to the peripheral tissues. The delivery of oxygen from the blood to the mitochondria, however, is a complex interaction of blood flow in the capillary network, the content of oxygen on the hemoglobin, the $P_{50}$ of the blood, and the cell membrane/cytosol/mitochondrial interphase. Hypoxia results in an increase of blood flow, which appears to compensate for the decreased oxygen content,[249a] but Richardson and coworkers[249b] found that blood flow was proportional to work rate in both hypoxic and normoxic conditions.

The importance of the distribution of flow in the capillary network cannot be overlooked. Both athletic training and hypoxic stress result in similar proliferation of capillaries, which would optimize delivery of oxygen.[249c–249f] Hoppeler and colleagues[249g] have begun to unravel the mechanism of the angiogenesis and have noted an increase in messenger ribonucleic acid for vascular endothelial growth factor, a substance that stimulates microvascular growth.

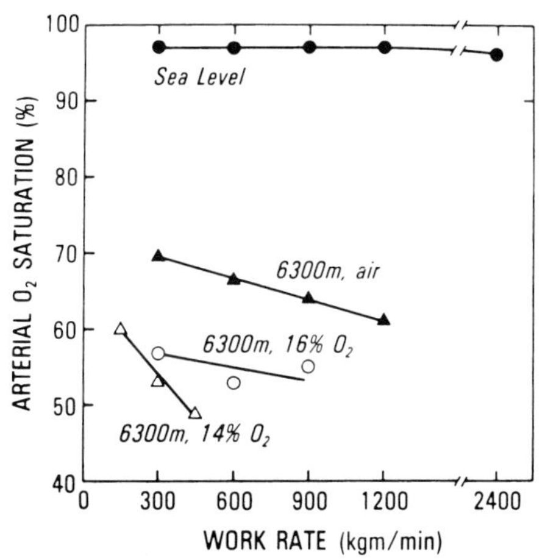


**Figure 70.11** Arterial oxygen saturation (%) does not decrease with exercise at sea level but drops progressively with higher workloads at greater altitudes. There is a diffusion limitation of oxygen transfer across the alveolar-hemoglobin interface. (From West JB, Boyer SJ, Graber DJ, et al: Maximal exercise at extreme altitudes on Mount Everest. J Appl Physiol 55:688–702, 1983. Reprinted with permission.)

The diffusion of oxygen from the blood to the tissue is the final hurdle in the oxygen transport chain. Wagner[249g] has discussed the theoretical reasons why extraction might be limited during hypoxic exercise.[249h–249j] Using mixed venous blood as a reflection of the limits of extraction can be misleading because there are obviously tissue beds that are metabolically much more active during exercise and thus must have a lower oxygen content in the effluent blood than would be reflected in mixed venous blood. Hogan and coworkers[249k] exercised canine gastrocnemius muscle under different levels of hypoxia and found the effluent $Po_2$ to be as low as 11 mm Hg; by keeping flow constant, they found that further extraction was possible. Richardson and colleagues[249l] looked at blood flow during maximal human leg exercise with normoxia and hypoxia and found similar blood flow yet a lower work rate during hypoxic conditions. They concluded that there was diffusion limitation during hypoxia. In an elegant study using nuclear magnetic resonance-spectroscopy during leg extension exercise in humans to determine myoglobin saturation as a reflection of tissue oxygenation, Richardson and coworkers[249b] found that during hypoxia myoglobin saturation was about 50% with a $Po_2$ of about 3 mm Hg. Thus they believed that diffusion of oxygen from the cytosol to the mitochondria encountered less resistance than at the 1 to 5 μm barrier from the red cell sarcolemma.

## Tissue Alterations

The decrease in $\dot{V}o_{2max}$ that remains even after prolonged exposure to high altitude may also be a reflection of factors at the tissue level. Several of the animal studies dealing with morphologic and biochemical changes with hypoxia were discussed earlier; their results pose more questions than they offer answers. Human data are sparse, but Cerretelli and di Prampero[250] studied climbers returning from 2 months at extremely high altitude. After performing muscle biopsies, they found (1) an unchanged ratio of capillaries to muscle fiber; (2) a 10% to 15% decrease in muscle mass, which was secondary to a reduction in fiber diameter; (3) a consequent 20% increase in mitochondria to fiber volume ratio; and (4) a 45% decrease in succinic dehydrogenase activity. Although the radial diffusion distance for oxygen was less, the overall effect was a decrease in oxidative capacity of the muscle after a prolonged sojourn at high altitude. Similar observations were made during Operation Everest II by Green and associates.[251]

Further metabolic changes occur at the muscle cell level that are not understood. On acute exposure to high altitude, blood lactate levels are higher at any given workload than at sea level.[127] This increase in lactate is probably secondary to increased glycogenolysis from the hormonal stresses of tissue hypoxia. Acclimatization, however, results in increased endurance[252–255] and a lower level of muscle and blood lactate than is seen at comparable levels of exercise at sea level.[250, 251] The mechanism of the "lactate paradox" (lower blood lactate concentrations than expected if the tissue during exercise is oxygen supply limited) is not well understood. A number of studies have documented this phenomenon,[255a–255c] and much has been written about it.[255d–255g] It may be a consequence of an inhibition of glycogenolysis during acclimatization, an increased dependence on free fatty acid oxidation for energy, an increased liver and muscle uptake of lactate, or an optimization of the cell-to-cell lactate shuttle.

## Performance and Training at High Altitude.

Maximal oxygen consumption decreases about 3.5% for every 300 m altitude above 1500 m.[254] At moderate altitudes, where many athletic competitions take place, the initial decrease in athletic performance on acute exposure can be partly regained after several weeks of habitation. Pugh[256] studied six world-class international distance runners over a 4-week period in Mexico City (2270 m), the site of the 1968 Olympics. On arrival, the 1- and 3-mile times were 3.6% and 8.5% slower than the times at sea level. After a month's acclimatization, the times were 1.5% and 5.7% slower than the times at sea level. Maximum $\dot{V}o_2$ was reduced 14.4% from sea-level values initially and 9.5% after 1 month. Maximum work at the end of the month actually exceeded sea-level values, which Pugh attributed to increased efficiency. This study and others done at moderate altitudes demonstrate that the initial impairment of performance can be partially overcome by acclimatization. Performance for running events of less than 2 minutes' duration at less than 3000 m altitude is not impaired and may even be slightly improved because of decreased air density. Performances in events of longer duration are predictably diminished and cannot be restored to sea-level capacity with prolonged stay or training at high altitude.

Dill and associates[257] observed a decrement in work performance that was greatest after 2 days at high altitude in spite of a progressive increase in ventilation. These results suggest an initial deterioration of aerobic capacity that improved slowly over several weeks at altitude. High-altitude residents of Leadville, Colorado (3100 m), who had aerobic capacities comparable to those of a control low-altitude group ($\dot{V}o_{2max}$ = 66 to 68 mL/kg min), showed decrements in exercise capacity on reascent from sea level to 3100 m that were similar to those shown by the low-altitude natives.[258] These individuals did not show the relative hypoventilation during exercise that is characteristic of some Himalayan[63] and all Andean[59] high-altitude natives.

Submaximal exercise may be more pertinent to daily life or prolonged athletic events than is rapid and intense exercise to exhaustion. Maher and associates[255] studied eight well-conditioned men after 2 and 12 days' exposure to 4300 m. Exercising at 75% of $\dot{V}o_{2max}$, their endurance time on day 12 was increased significantly as compared with that on day 2, associated with decreased blood lactate concentrations. The authors suggested that endurance improved over time due to improved aerobic capacity as reflected by diminution of anaerobic by-products.

Much controversy existed concerning the benefit of training at high altitude, much of it generated during the 1968 Olympics in Mexico City; subsequently, a number of elite endurance runners have lived and trained at moderate altitude (2000 to 2500 m). The hope was that the beneficial changes bestowed by this exposure would improve performance at low altitude. An early report found enhanced performance after training at altitude.[203] Using a number of different training regimens, Buskirk and associates[254] and Grover and Reeves[259] failed to discern a beneficial effect on performance after return to sea level. The intensity of training at high altitude necessarily was less, provoking the idea that detraining actually took place in sea-level–trained athletes.

Levine and colleagues[260] studied four groups of athletes: (1) those who lived low and trained low (1350 m), (2) those who lived low and trained high (3000 m), (3) those who lived high and trained high, and (4) those who lived high and trained low. Although there were no great differences in the groups, those who lived high and trained low seemed to have gained the benefit of hypoxic conditioning while not losing the intensity of training sessions. This advantage was conveyed presumably by the modestly elevated hemoglobin from the altitude exposure. Of interest was that there was individual variability in the erythropoietic response in that some did and others did not get a rise in hemoglobin and thus no benefit in performance.[260a] This observation is not much different from patients with hypoxic lung disease who have a spectrum of responses with equivalent degrees of hypoxemia that suggests that the stimulus is more subtle and complex than can be discerned from blood partial pressures of oxygen.

A new wrinkle was introduced by Rodriquez and colleagues.[206b] These investigators found that short-term (3 to 5 hours/day for 9 days) exposure to hypobaric hypoxia stimulated erythropoiesis and improved aerobic performance capacity at sea level in healthy subjects.

## MALADAPTATION

Sudden ascent from sea level to the summit of Mt. Everest (8848 m or 29,028 ft) would lead to unconsciousness within minutes and death soon thereafter. Yet mountain climbers ascending over a period of weeks to this altitude can think, perform physical work, and even sleep nearly that high, usually without obvious adverse effects. Rapid ascent to much lower altitudes (2500 to 4000 m), also can lead to problems in some individuals. These acute disorders of high altitude include acute mountain sickness (AMS), high-altitude pulmonary edema (HAPE), and high-altitude cerebral edema (HACE) (Table 70.2). The incidence and severity of illness depend on several factors, including the speed of ascent and amount of altitude gained, the length of stay, and individual susceptibility (Table 70.3).[261] A trip to and from high altitude on the same day is much less stressful than an overnight stay because hypoxia is accentuated during sleep and because of more prolonged exposure. Note the very high incidence of AMS on Mt. Rainier (see Table 70.3) from the rapid rate of ascent (24 hours to 4392 m), yet pulmonary edema or death is rare because the time spent above 3000 m is brief.

### Problems of Lowlanders on Ascent to High Altitude

Susceptibility to altitude illness is highly variable, but for a single individual symptoms are often reproducible given the same rate of ascent and other circumstances. Men and women are equally susceptible to AMS,[261, 261a] but women may be less likely to develop HAPE.[262] Younger adults may be slightly more vulnerable to AMS,[261] but preverbal children recently were found to have the same prevalence as adults.[262a]

In addition to individual differences in susceptibility, factors aggravating hypoxemia, such as alcohol or other respiratory depressants, carbon monoxide poisoning, or respiratory infection, may enhance vulnerability to altitude illness. Although essentially no information exists on how prior or coexisting illnesses might contribute to susceptibility to altitude sickness, one might assume that any condition that causes hypoventilation, hypoxemia, pulmonary hypertension, increased intracranial pressure, or fluid retention could induce or exacerbate altitude illnesses.

#### Acute Mountain Sickness

**Clinical Presentation.** Headache is the most common and prominent symptom of AMS. Typically, the headache occurs within a few hours after ascent to high altitude or

**Table 70.2 DISORDERS ASSOCIATED WITH HIGH ALTITUDE**

| Disorder: In the Unacclimatized | Disorder: In High-Altitude Residents | Problems Potentially Aggravated (Partial List) |
|---|---|---|
| Acute mountain sickness | Chronic mountain sickness | Hypertension |
| Cerebral edema | Reentry pulmonary edema | Arteriosclerotic heart disease |
| Pulmonary edema | Problems of pregnancy | Congestive heart failure |
| Peripheral edema | | Chronic lung disease |
| Retinopathy | | Arteriosclerotic cerebrovascular disease |
| Thromboembolic problems | | Pulmonary hypertension |
| Sleep periodic breathing | | Disorders of pregnancy and childbirth |

**Table 70.3 THE INCIDENCE OF ALTITUDE ILLNESS IN VARIOUS GROUPS**

| Study Group | Sleeping Altitude | Maximum Altitude Reached (m) | Average Rate of Ascent† | AMS (%) | HAPE and/or HACE | Deaths | Reference |
|---|---|---|---|---|---|---|---|
| Colorado skiers | 2400–3000 | 3500 | 1–2 | 15–40 | 0.1–0.01 | ? | 261 |
| Mt. Everest trekkers | 3000–5200 | 5500 | 1–2 (fly in) | 47 | 1.6 | 1:2,500 | 261, 269a |
| | | | 10–13 (walk in) | 23 | .05 | | |
| Mt. McKinley climbers | 3000–5000 | 6195 | 3–7 | 50 | 2–3 | 1:625 | 261 |
| Mt. Rainier climbers | 3000 | 4392 | 1–2 | 67 | 0.1 | 1:10,000 | 77 |
| Indian soldiers | 3000–5000 | 5500 | 1–2 | 1.9 | 2.3–15.5 | ? | 264 |

†Days to sleeping altitude from sea level.
? = data not supplied.
AMS = acute mountain sickness; HACE = high-altitude cerebral edema; HAPE = high-altitude pulmonary edema.

is present on awakening the next morning. Associated symptoms and signs in approximate order of frequency are lassitude, insomnia, anorexia, nausea, dizziness, breathlessness, reduced urination, and vomiting, accompanied by evidence of fluid retention.[263, 264] The early symptoms of AMS are remarkably similar to those of alcohol hangover. Ravenhill,[265] an observant British physician working in a mining camp at 5000 m in the Andes, provided an excellent description of the illness, referred to as *puna,* in 1913:

> It is a curious fact that the symptoms of puna do not usually evince themselves at once. The majority of newcomers have expressed themselves as being quite well on first arrival. As a rule, towards the evening the patient begins to feel rather slack and disinclined for exertion. He goes to bed, but has a restless and troubled night, and wakes next morning with a severe frontal headache. There may be vomiting, frequently there is a sense of oppression in the chest, but there is rarely any respiratory distress or alteration in the normal rate of breathing so long as the patient is at rest. The patient may feel slightly giddy on rising from bed, and any attempt at exertion increases the headache, which is nearly always confined to the frontal region.
>
> On examination the face may be slightly cyanosed; the eyes look dull and heavy, with a tendency to water; the tongue is furred. The pulse is nearly always high, being generally in the neighborhood of 100 [beats per minute] or over; 150 was the highest in my cases. The temperature is normal or slightly under; not often is there any rise of temperature at first, though it may rise towards evening. There is at times reduplication of the pulmonary second sound. The patient feels cold and shivery.
>
> The headache increases towards evening, so also does the pulse rate; all appetite is lost, and the patient wishes to be left alone—to sleep if possible. Generally, during the second night he is able to do so, and as a rule wakes the next morning feeling better; the pulse rate has probably dropped to about 90; the headache is only slight. As the day draws on he probably feels worse again, the symptoms all tending to reappear on any exertion; if however, he keeps to his bed, by the fourth day after arrival he is probably very much better and at the end of the week is quite fit again.

Although Ravenhill mentions tachycardia, Singh and associates[264] found a relative bradycardia (mean heart rate 66 beats per minute) in two thirds of soldiers with AMS. There were no characteristic changes in blood pressure. Localized rales were present in 25% to 35% of the cases.[264] Decreased urine output in spite of adequate hydration is an especially helpful sign if present.[261, 266] Periodic breathing during sleep is normal at altitude, not indicative of AMS, and is therefore not a diagnostic sign. Differential diagnosis includes dehydration, hypothermia, exhaustion, alcohol hangover, carbon monoxide poisoning, and respiratory or cerebral infectious diseases.

Singh described the natural course of the illness in soldiers who were airlifted to between 3300 and 5500 m.[264] Incapacitating illness in 840 soldiers lasted 2 to 5 days. Full recovery, however, took much longer: 38% recovered fully within 3 days, 40% were still ill after 1 week, and 13% had symptoms after 1 month. Three individuals died of pulmonary and cerebral edema. Ski resort tourists sleeping at a more modest altitude of 2700 m exhibited symptoms lasting an average of 15 hours (range: 6 to 94 hours).[267] Most individuals tolerate or treat their own symptoms as the illness resolves over 1 to 3 days while acclimatization occurs, but some persons with AMS seek medical help or are forced to descend. A small percentage of those with AMS (2% to 8%) go on to develop cerebral edema or pulmonary edema, especially if ascent is continued in spite of illness (see Table 70.3). The hallmarks of progression are truncal ataxia and altered mental status, with or without respiratory distress.

**Pathophysiology.** Current concepts of pathophysiology emphasize the cerebral etiology of AMS. Elevated intracranial pressure has been demonstrated in severe illness, and cerebral edema has been noted with various imaging techniques[268–270] and with brain biopsy.[264] The edema observed in these advanced cases of AMS appears to be due to passage of fluid from the intravascular to extravascular space; initially the edema is confined to the white matter.[270] Using magnetic resonance imaging, Hackett and colleagues[270a] found swelling in the white matter and none in the gray matter in patients with HACE, which suggested to them that the extravascular leak was of a vasogenic origin. Whether increased intracranial pressure or brain swelling actually causes the milder symptoms of AMS is, however, not established. One study in subjects with early AMS found no increase in CSF pressure.[271] The classic explanation that the headache and other symptoms of AMS are due to cerebral vasodilation seems unlikely.[272, 273]

The progression of AMS to HACE makes attractive the view that AMS symptoms represent the effect of early cerebral edema with increased intracranial pressure. Although elevated intracranial pressure has been demonstrated in severe illness and cerebral edema has been demonstrated with brain imaging techniques,[268–270] a study in patients with early AMS but nevertheless commonly with significant headache found no increase in CSF pressure.[271] Headache, even severe headache, can be an early symptom of AMS, at a time when edema and significant increases in intracranial pressure are unlikely explanations for its origin. Noting that headaches are generally thought to be due to stimulation of pain fibers in meninges or larger cerebral vessels, the possibility that at least some of the early symptoms of AMS are of a different cause than brain swelling, such as migraine-type of headache, must be considered.[273a]

Interstitial lung edema with impairment of gas exchange,[274] cerebral edema, peripheral edema, and proteinuria all point to a general defect in water homeostasis. Persons susceptible to AMS have elevated aldosterone and antidiuretic hormone levels when compared with controls.[275] In contrast, persons acclimatizing well exhibit diuresis, net water loss, and low antidiuretic hormone values.[275] In addition to this fluid retention, the increased permeability of multiple capillary beds suggests generalized endothelial dysfunction.

Hypoventilation appears to contribute to development of AMS. A brisk increase in ventilation on ascent to altitude is associated with a lower incidence of AMS, and those with AMS tend to have a lower HVR when tested

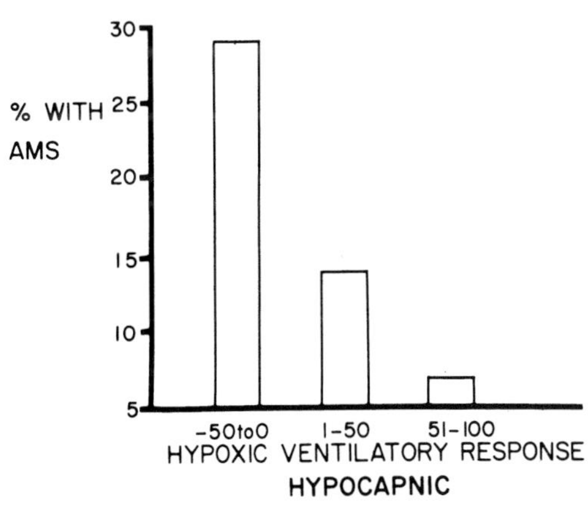


**Figure 70.12** Percentage of subjects who developed acute mountain sickness (AMS), grouped into preascent low, medium, and high hypoxic ventilatory responses. Tests were done without holding carbon dioxide constant. Those with lower hypoxic drives had a higher incidence of illness. (From Hackett PH, Reeves JT, Grover RF, Weil JV: Ventilation in human populations native to high altitude. *In* West JB, Lahiri S (eds): High Altitude and Man. Bethesda, MD: American Physiological Society, 1984, pp 179–191. Reprinted with permission.)

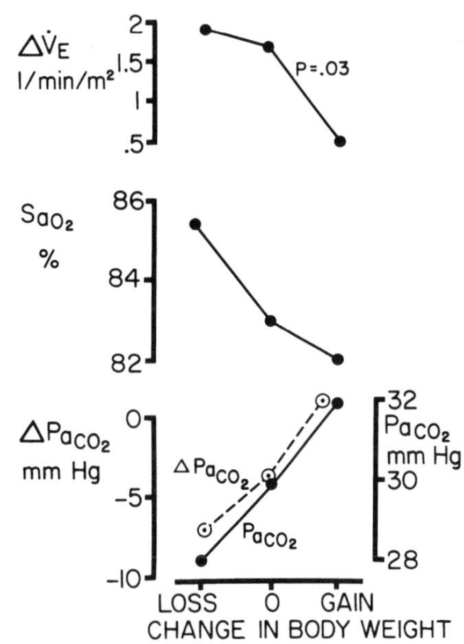


**Figure 70.13** The relationship of $\Delta\dot{V}_E$ (the change in minute ventilation from low to high altitude), $Sa_{O_2}$% (arterial oxygen saturation by ear oximeter), $\Delta Pa_{CO_2}$ (the change in arterial carbon dioxide tension from low to high altitude), and $Pa_{CO_2}$ (arterial carbon dioxide tension) to change in body weight (>2%) on ascent to altitude in trekkers in Nepal. Weight gain was associated with acute mountain sickness. (From Hackett PH, Rennie D, Hofmeister SE, et al: Fluid retention and relative hypoventilation in acute mountain sickness. Respiration 43:321–329, 1982. Reprinted with permission.)

at sea level (Fig. 70.12).[77, 276] Relative hypoventilation enhances hypoxemia, diminishes alkalosis, and has been linked to the fluid retention and weight gain associated with AMS (Fig. 70.13).[277] That acetazolamide, a respiratory stimulant and diuretic, is an effective agent for prevention and treatment reinforces the importance of ventilation, arterial oxygenation, and diuresis (see Fig. 70.13).[77]

**Treatment.** The key to successful treatment is early diagnosis. Persons with mild illness may resolve their symptoms by resting and staying under observation at the same altitude and may respond well to a descent of as little as 300 m, whereas more severe illness requires further descent.[266] Descent should continue until the individual improves and, in severe cases, should not be delayed to wait for a doctor, a rescue team, or a helicopter. At times, field conditions may be such that descent is impractical or impossible or the illness may be mild enough not to warrant the inconvenience of descending.

With the use of a portable hyperbaric chamber, "low altitude" can be brought to the patient. Although chambers have been used for decades in fixed locations, a new lightweight nylon chamber (6 kg) is now being taken on expeditions and treks to high-altitude regions. Pressurization to 2 psi (110 mm Hg) is equivalent to a descent of approximately 1500 m. By means of a foot pump, sufficient gas flow is maintained to keep the carbon dioxide concentration low and the oxygen concentration close to 21%.[278] Supplemental oxygen can also be added to the bag, if it is available and if the patient's condition necessitates it. Studies have documented the chamber to be as effective as administering 26% to 30% oxygen; the critical factor for resolution of illness is the $PO_2$, whether increased by changing the inspired oxygen concentration or the total barometric pressure.[279] These devices are particularly useful when oxygen is not readily available. In ski resorts and other areas with medical facilities, persons suffering from AMS or HAPE prefer oxygen breathing to being treated in a chamber. As with oxygen therapy, relief of symptoms is generally immediate, but treatment is necessary for a number of hours for continued clinical improvement after removal from the chamber. The duration of therapy depends on the severity of illness.[278, 280]

Only a few medications have been evaluated for treatment of AMS. Singh and colleagues[264] found aspirin helpful for headache and promoting sleep, whereas ammonium chloride and potassium chloride were of no value. Ibuprofen and sumatriptin also treat the headache of AMS. Prochlorperazine is useful for treating nausea and vomiting and, unlike some other antiemetics, does not depress ventilation but, rather, may actually increase HVR.[281] Sedative hypnotics, alcohol, opiates, and other ventilatory depressants should be avoided in persons with AMS.

The effectiveness of furosemide in the treatment of AMS remains unclear. Singh and colleagues.[264] reported good results when furosemide was given to 446 soldiers with AMS in doses of 80 mg twice a day for 2 days. Gray and associates,[282] however, reported vascular collapse due to hypovolemia when 40 mg twice a day was given to subjects as prophylaxis for rapid ascent. This report has discouraged its use in North America. No study confirming Singh and coworkers' observation of its value in treatment of AMS has yet been performed. Acetazolamide in doses of 125 to 250 mg every 12 hours has been useful for treatment of AMS and was found effective in a controlled study; the drug improved gas exchange as well as symptoms.[274] Acetazolamide also reduces periodic breathing during sleep, resulting in less arterial hypoxemia.[221] A comparison of acetazolamide and furosemide for treatment would be worthwhile. Dexamethasone, 4 mg every 6 hours, is also effective treatment of AMS, with minimal side effects but with possible rebound when discontinued while still at high altitude.[283–285] Clinicians generally reserve its use for moderate to severe AMS and use acetazolamide for mild illness. Ataxia and altered mental status, which are signs of potential HACE, are considered indications for immediate use of dexamethasone.

Other medications being investigated for treatment of AMS include phenytoin, spironolactone, other diuretics, and other respiratory stimulants. Descent to a lower altitude is still the most reliable treatment.

**Prevention.** A number of measures are effective in preventing or ameliorating AMS. Gradual ascent, with pauses for acclimatization, is the method of choice. The Himalayan Rescue Association recommends an acclimatization day (two nights at the same altitude) for every 600-m gain in sleeping altitude above 3000 m. In one study, a diet high in carbohydrates (>70%) improved oxygenation and reduced symptoms of AMS in soldiers taken to 4200 m.[286] The presumed mechanism of benefit is that carbohydrates increase the respiratory quotient ($\dot{V}CO_2/\dot{V}O_2$), resulting in a higher alveolar $PO_2$.[287] A subsequent study, however, showed no difference in symptom scores or cytokine expression in subjects on a high carbohydrate diet.[287a]

Acetazolamide is a well-established prophylactic agent.[77, 261, 282, 288, 289] Through carbonic anhydrase inhibition, the drug causes a bicarbonate diuresis and a metabolic acidosis, which stimulates ventilation, increasing alveolar $PO_2$ and arterial oxygen saturation, presumably speeding the process of natural acclimatization. The drug is well tolerated, although paresthesias are common. Nausea and drowsiness occasionally occur, and carbonated beverages taste flat, probably secondary to the inhibition of hydration of carbon dioxide on the palette. Acetazolamide has a sulfhydryl group and shares the cautions common to all sulfa drugs. A dosage of 125 mg twice daily for the first 2 to 3 days at altitude, appears to be adequate for most individuals.

Dexamethasone also provides effective prevention when used in a dosage of 4 mg every 6 to 12 hours, starting at least 6 hours before ascent.[290] Studies comparing dexamethasone and acetazolamide have revealed approximately equal effectiveness of the two drugs in preventing AMS.[291–293] Experts generally consider acetazolamide the drug of choice for prophylaxis because of its greater safety and because it enhances acclimatization; dexamethasone does not speed the acclimatization process and may be associated with reappearance of symptoms when discontinued. Dexamethasone should be available, especially in remote areas where rapid treatment of evolving symptoms may keep the victim ambulatory and thus able to ambulate and help him/herself down. The patient is, therefore, much less of a burden to rescuers.

Pharmacologic prophylaxis should probably be reserved for those who are known to be susceptible to AMS or for those who must ascend to altitude quickly (e.g., rescue or military teams) without the benefit of staged ascent. In other circumstances, it is reasonable to delay use of acetazolamide until the symptoms of AMS first develop, at which time acetazolamide can be taken in the usual dosage until symptoms improve.

## High-Altitude Cerebral Edema

High-altitude cerebral edema is defined as the presence of a change in mental status and/or ataxia in a person with AMS, or the presence of both central nervous system abnormalities in a person without AMS who has recently ascended to altitude.

The initial symptoms of HACE are usually those of severe AMS plus neurologic abnormalities. Headache may be incapacitating, nausea and vomiting persistent, and lassitude debilitating. Ataxic gait, usually present and associated with altered mental status, is a reliable diagnostic sign. Among the protean neurologic signs accompanying the illness are papilledema, visual changes, cranial nerve palsies, bladder dysfunction, abnormal reflexes, paresthesias, pareses, aphasia, clonus, hallucinations, seizures, and behavioral changes, terminating in coma and death.[261, 264, 294]

The incidence of HACE is difficult to assess because the boundary of progression from AMS may be hard to define and the symptoms and signs may be similar to those of cerebral hypoxia secondary to *severe* hypoxemia from pulmonary edema. At higher altitudes, HACE may affect 5% to 10% of those experiencing AMS and is more common in those with HAPE.[261, 264] Differential diagnosis includes all other causes of encephalopathy, such as carbon monoxide poisoning, hypertensive crisis, severe cerebral hypoxia secondary to HAPE, cerebral ischemia secondary to thrombosis or hemorrhage, and migrainous encephalopathy. Magnetic resonance imaging reveals a pattern of reversible increased T2-weighted signal in the corpus callosum, especially in the splenum, which may help differentiate HACE from other conditions.[270a]

Pathology reports revealed gross cerebral edema in seven of eight persons who had died of altitude illness; five also had pulmonary edema.[294, 295] Findings included swelling and flattening of the cerebral gyri, compression of the sulci, herniation of cerebellar tonsils and unci, small petechial hemorrhages, and venous and sinus thromboses.

The definitive treatment of HACE is descent. However, recovery is not as rapid as in AMS and HAPE, and a descent in altitude of more than 1000 m may be necessary. Oxygen or hyperbaric therapy may be a lifesaving temporizing measure. In the only study of therapy, severe neurologic symptoms and signs responded to furosemide and betamethasone; the drugs were not studied separately.[264] Dexamethasone is now routinely used in hopes of reducing brain swelling but may be less effective if given after onset of coma. Mannitol and glycerol have been suggested for treatment but are difficult to use safely in the field and have rarely been tried.

## High-Altitude Pulmonary Edema

High altitude pulmonary edema is the most common cause of death from high-altitude illness (see Table 70.3). Although it was probably a problem even when Hannibal's troops crossed the Alps in 217 BC, until recently the condition was misdiagnosed as pneumonia. A physician, "the young, vigorous" Dr. Jacottet, succumbed to HAPE while studying the effect of altitude on Mt. Blanc in 1891. Autopsy revealed a "suffocative catarrh accompanied by acute edema of the lung," the first pathologic description of HAPE. Aleister Crowley, a mountain climber and mystic, may have been the first layman to recognize this entity as edema. On an expedition to K2 in 1902, he described a climber as "suffering from oedema of both lungs and his mind was gone."[296] In 1913, Ravenhill described three individuals with HAPE (two of whom died) and correctly identified high-altitude exposure as the cause, labeling it "cardiac mountain sickness." He attributed the illness to congestive heart failure.[265] Not until reports by Hultgren[296a] and Houston,[297] and subsequent studies by Hultgren and coworkers,[298] was HAPE shown to be a noncardiogenic form of pulmonary edema. Like other noncardiac pulmonary edemas, the exact pathophysiology is still obscure.

**Clinical Presentation.** The following is a typical case history:

> M. E., a 24-year-old man, drove from sea level to a trailhead in the Sierra Nevada and slept at 2440 m. The next day he developed a headache and slight dizziness but was able to keep up with his party as they ascended to 3200 m; his headache was relieved with aspirin, and he slept well. The following afternoon he felt weak and became short of breath when climbing uphill but did fine moving downhill. His headache intensified. He needed assistance making camp and had little appetite. That evening, he noticed raspiness and gurgling in his chest and a dry cough developed. Sleep was difficult, and he became intermittently delirious. The morning of the third day his cough and headache were worse, he was extremely weak, and he became orthopneic. He was assisted down to 2750 m where he improved slightly that night, and the next morning he was evacuated by helicopter to a regional hospital at 1280 m.
>
> M. E. had slept at altitudes greater than 3300 m many times in the past and had had mild AMS on about half of those occasions. He had been running 20 miles a week for the past year and considered himself in excellent condition.
>
> On admission to the emergency department, M. E. was cyanotic; his oral temperature was 38.1°C, blood pressure was 100/78 mm Hg, heart rate was 124 beats per minute, and respiratory frequency was 28 breaths per minute. Rales were present, especially in the right axillary region. Cardiac examination was normal except for an accentuated pulmonic sound. He displayed slight truncal ataxia. Arterial blood gases on room air revealed $P_{O_2}$ of 42 mm Hg, $P_{CO_2}$ of 29 mm Hg, and pH of 7.48. A white blood cell count was 13,200/μL with a left shift. A chest roentgenogram showed extensive, patchy, bilateral pulmonary edema.
>
> He was treated with bed rest and supplemental oxygen and discharged 48 hours later with a nearly normal chest roentgenogram. Arterial blood gases on room air at that time were $P_{O_2}$ of 65 mm Hg, $P_{CO_2}$ of 32 mm Hg, and pH of 7.47. He was advised to ascend more slowly in the future, was taught to recognize the early signs of HAPE, and was given the choice of acetazolamide prophylaxis.

This case illustrates a number of typical aspects of HAPE. Victims are often young, physically fit men who ascend rapidly from sea level and have not had HAPE before in spite of repeated altitude exposures. HAPE occurs within the first 2 to 4 days of ascent to higher altitudes (>2500 m), most commonly on the second night.[266] The earliest indications are decreased exercise performance and slow recovery from exercise. The victim usually notices fatigue, weakness, and dyspnea on exertion, often ascribing these nonspecific symptoms to various other causes. Signs of AMS such as headache, anorexia, and lassitude are frequently present as well. A persistent dry cough develops. Nailbeds become cyanotic. The condition typically worsens at night, and tachycardia and tachypnea develop at rest. Dyspnea at rest and audible congestion in the chest finally signal the presence of a serious pulmonary problem. Orthopnea is common. Pink frothy sputum is a late finding. The severe hypoxemia with or without concomitant cerebral edema may produce mental changes, ataxia, and a decreased level of consciousness. Descents of even 600 m can be lifesaving, but recovery is faster with further descent.

On admission to the hospital, the patient does not generally appear as ill as one would expect based on blood gases and radiographic findings. A temperature of up to 38.5°C is common. Tachycardia is present and correlates with an increased respiratory rate and severity of illness. Rales appear in the right midlung fields first. Concomitant respiratory infection is sometimes present. Radiographs show a patchy, fluffy-type exudate, which may be limited to one area (the right lung field predominating initially) or generalized, depending on the severity of the illness (Fig. 70.14). Pulmonary artery pressure is high, but pulmonary wedge pressure is normal and heart size is not increased.[298]

**Pathologic Findings.** A total of 22 autopsies have been reported in persons dying of HAPE.[264, 295, 299, 300] A proteinaceous exudate with hyaline membranes is characteristic. All had some areas of pneumonitis, with neutrophil accumulation, although none were noted to contain bacteria. Pulmonary veins were not dilated. Most reports mention capillary and arteriolar thrombi and deposits of fibrin, as well as hemorrhage and infarcts. The autopsy findings thus suggest a protein-rich edema and the possibility that clotting abnormalities may play a role in the illness.

Analyses of alveolar fluid in persons with HAPE provide additional insight into the mechanism of HAPE. Schoene and associates[301] obtained brochoalveolar lavage fluids in climbers with AMS and HAPE, as well as in

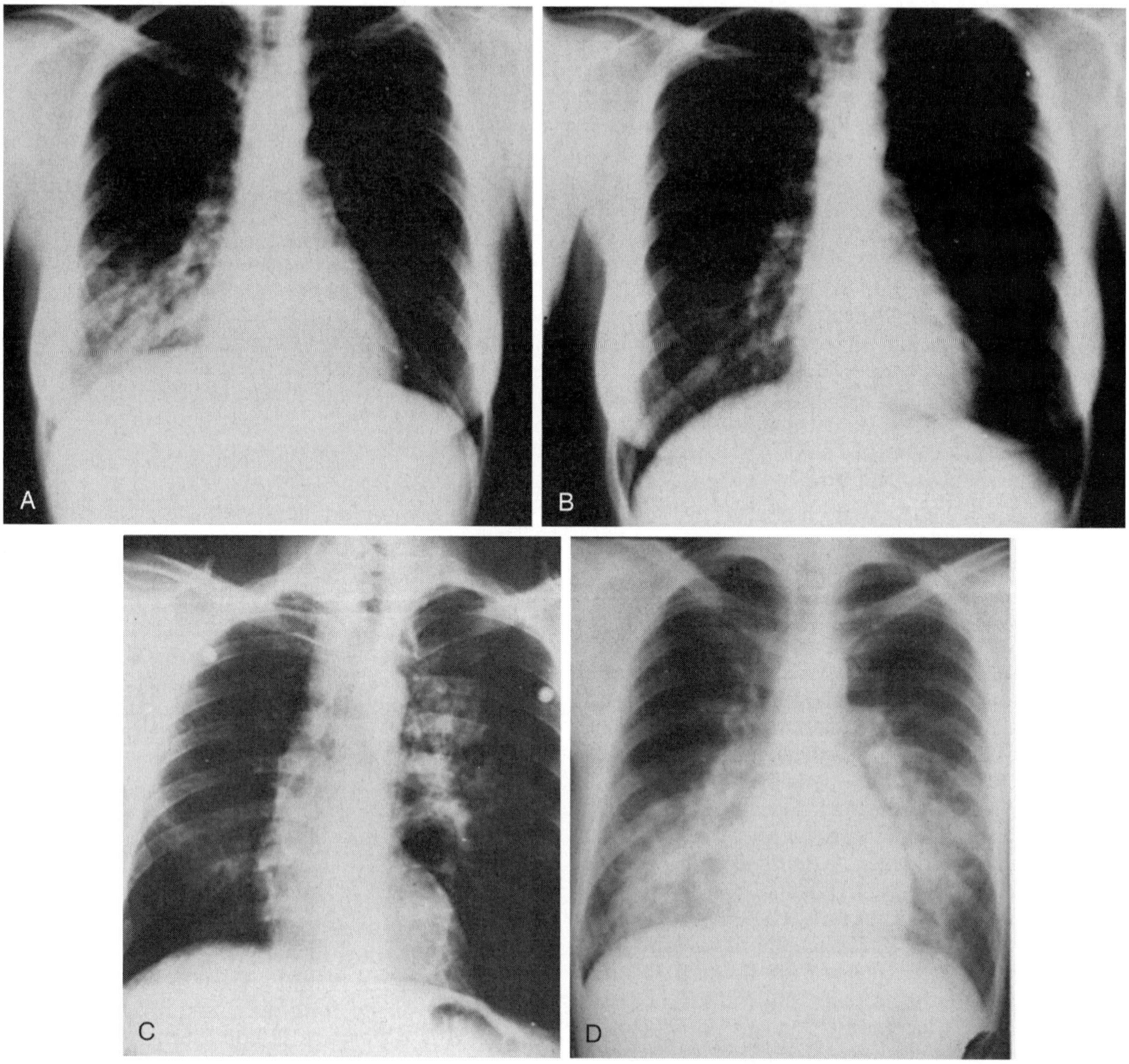


**Figure 70.14** *A,* Typical x-ray film of high-altitude pulmonary edema in a 29-year-old female skier. Note that the edema is unilateral, right-sided, and predominantly in the right middle lobe. *B,* X-ray film of the same patient 1 day later, after descent and oxygen. Note the rapid clearing. *C,* Severe unilateral pulmonary edema in a 21-year-old male with no history of any previous illness. *D,* Severe pulmonary edema of altitude. Note normal heart size.

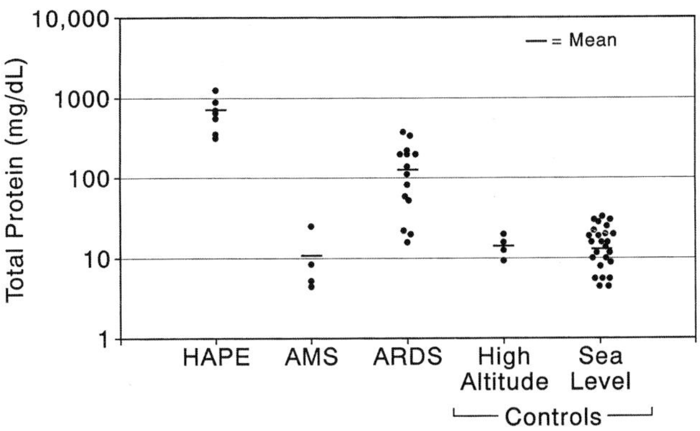


**Figure 70.15** Protein concentration in bronchoalveolar lavage fluid on the vertical axis in high-altitude pulmonary edema (HAPE), acute mountain sickness (AMS), acute respiratory distress syndrome (ARDS), and high-altitude and sea-level controls. (From Schoene RB, Swenson ER, Pizzo CJ, et al: The lung at high altitude: Bronchoalveolar lavage in acute mountain sickness and pulmonary edema. J Appl Physiol 64:2605–2613, 1988. Reprinted with permission.)

healthy subjects. The lavage fluid confirmed that HAPE is a high-protein fluid, higher than in patients with acute respiratory distress syndrome (ARDS), and that the fluid was highly cellular (Fig. 70.15). However, unlike ARDS lavage fluid, which has primarily neutrophils, HAPE fluid contained a higher percentage of alveolar macrophages. Additionally, chemotactic (leukotriene $B_4$) and vasoactive (thromboxane $B_2$) mediators were present in the lavages. The climbers with AMS who had some degree of arterial oxygen desaturation had alveolar fluid that was similar to that of the control subjects. Similar lavage findings emerged from the Japanese Alps in patients with HAPE discovered at moderate altitude in whom cytokines (interleukin [IL]-1, IL-6, IL-8, and tumor necrosis factor-α) were also measured and found to be elevated compared with controls, whereas IL-1α, IL-10, and P-selectin were not.[301a]

**Possible Mechanisms.** Three basic mechanisms for pulmonary edema have been hypothesized: increased microvascular pressure, increased microvascular permeability, or a combination of the two. Because we know HAPE to be due to increased permeability, it is grouped with the pulmonary edemas of noncardiogenic origin: near drowning, narcotic overdose, neurogenic pulmonary edema, and perhaps ARDS (Chapter 54).

In contrast to ARDS, however, rapid clearing of the edema without fibrosis or long-term sequelae is usual in HAPE. This difference is consistent with the presence of architectural lung damage in ARDS as observed at autopsy and by the finding of hydroxyproline in the ARDS lavage fluid and by the absence of these findings in HAPE.[301] Another difference is in the cellular composition of the edema fluid. ARDS lavage fluid contained 97% polymorphonuclear leukocytes, whereas HAPE lavage fluid contained 98% alveolar macrophages. Although the HAPE data are limited, the available evidence suggests that although there are markers of some inflammation in HAPE, it is not the same inflammatory-mediated event as ARDS. It is most likely that high intravascular pressures (see later) initiate a sequence of events that induces a modest post facto inflammatory response that is far less severe than what is seen in ARDS. The roles of high pressure and inflammation and the sequence in which they interact in HAPE are not well delineated.

The search for what triggers the leak continues. In 1967, Hultgren[302] suggested that edema resulted from uneven hypoxic vasoconstriction, resulting in overperfusion of the microvasculature in areas of the lung where arteriolar vasoconstriction failed to protect downstream vessels. Further support for this concept came from Hackett and colleagues,[303] who found a susceptibility to HAPE of persons born without a right pulmonary artery. Staub,[304] in an accompanying editorial, supported the concept of overperfusion of a restricted vascular bed as the cause of the edema. Uneven perfusion is suggested clinically by the typical patchy roentgenographic appearance (see Fig. 70.13) and by nuclear lung scan studies in persons breathing hypoxic gas mixtures,[305] which showed considerable differences in regional perfusion in HAPE-susceptible subjects. Thus, overperfusion of some areas of the pulmonary vasculature in the setting of a generally constricted vascular bed may be a factor involved in the pathogenesis of HAPE. The mechanism of leak in overperfusion edema may be due to high pressure and high flow, subjecting the vascular endothelium to injury from high shear forces. Another postulated mechanism is that of capillary stress failure, in which high pressures transmitted to the capillaries cause them to rupture.[306] The fragility and vulnerability of the pulmonary capillary membrane has been tested as both a primary violator of the capillary barrier as well as an instigator of inflammation.[306a–306c]

Increased pressure may be due to hypoxic pulmonary vasoconstriction, but microemboli are also a possible cause.[295, 300] Indeed, a number of animal studies have failed to produce a permeability edema with overperfusion alone but succeeded when the pulmonary vascular bed was partially embolized. The high intravascular pressures in subjects predisposed to HAPE may also be conveyed to a pulmonary vascular bed that is inherently compromised. Lung diffusion capacity as an indirect marker of capacity for lung perfusion was found to be smaller in HAPE-susceptible individuals.[306d] Furthermore, some patients may have a genetic predisposition to HAPE, as suggested by the finding of HLA alleles (HLA-DR6 and HLA-DQ4) in subjects with pulmonary hypertension and a history of HAPE.[306e]

Markedly elevated pulmonary artery pressure is a consistent finding in HAPE. Persons susceptible to HAPE have an abnormally high pulmonary artery pressure response during hypoxic breathing, as well as on ascent to high altitude,[307, 308] before onset of edema. Increased levels of endothelin-1, a potent pulmonary vasoconstrictor, has been found in HAPE-susceptible subjects, which suggests an inherent characteristic that may help to explain a contributing mechanism to the development of HAPE.[308a] The same group of investigators has postulated that exaggerated postganglionic sympathetic neural discharge, which they have found to occur in susceptible persons, may also contribute to high-altitude pulmonary edema.[308b] In addition, vasodilators, which reduced pulmonary artery pressure 25% to 50% (a reduction similar to that with oxygen), have proven useful for treatment of HAPE,[309, 310] and blocking the pressor response on ascent to altitude with nifedipine also prevented the development of edema in HAPE-susceptible individuals.[311] These findings suggest that the pulmonary hypertension may be causal. On the other hand, similarly high pulmonary arterial pressure has been recorded in persons at altitude without HAPE[308] and in many other conditions as well; thus, pulmonary hypertension is not the sole explanation for HAPE. One hypothesis to explain these facts is that of uneven vasoconstriction; namely, pulmonary hypertension without edema is a uniform constriction with protection of microvessels from high pressures, whereas persons with HAPE have uneven constriction with areas of unprotected downstream vessels. The other possibility is that both pulmonary hypertension and a permeability defect must be present. Certainly, any degree of permeability leak will be worsened when increased arterial pressure is transmitted to the capillaries, as shown by Brigham and coworkers.[312] The use of nitric oxide, a potent pulmonary vasodilator, in patients with HAPE showed improvement in gas exchange, suggesting that $\dot{V}A/\dot{Q}$ heterogeneity is present in HAPE such that improving perfusion to areas that are ventilated and not to areas of shunt improves $\dot{V}A/\dot{Q}$ match and thus overall gas exchange.[312a]

Also, one cannot overlook the potential role of inflammation that may predispose and/or contribute to the microvascular leak. Without sequential data it is not clear whether the inflammatory mediators are present before the evolution of edema or whether their release is stimulated by endothelial damage from exaggerated pulmonary pressures. Subjects with mild to moderate HAPE at a ski resort area in Colorado were found to have high levels of leukotriene $E_4$ in their urine compared with controls, and many had a history of a preceding or intercurrent viral infection.[312b] These findings suggest that there may be some subliminal or even clinically apparent inflammatory process that may make the microvascular endothelium vulnerable to a subsequent increase in pressures.

Another theory of HAPE pathogenesis is that HAPE is a form of neurogenic pulmonary edema. The presence of red blood cells, the spectrum of serum proteins in HAPE lavage fluid, and the absence of architectural damage are all similar to neurogenic pulmonary edema.[313] Also, studies have demonstrated simultaneous cerebral edema in those with HAPE,[270, 314] as well as elevated plasma and urine catecholamines.[275, 315] One component of neurogenic pulmonary edema is thought to be increased microvascular pressure secondary to sympathetically mediated pulmonary venous constriction.[316] Recent work has suggested that alpha-adrenergic blockade may be of value in the treatment of HAPE[317]; the authors speculated that relief of pulmonary venous constriction could play a role because they also found accentuated sympathetic activity in HAPE-susceptible individuals.[308b] Further investigation may help clarify the role of the central and sympathetic nervous systems in HAPE.

As in AMS, but more strongly associated with HAPE, control of ventilation plays a role in the pathophysiology of HAPE.[318] Persons with a low HVR have an increased risk of pulmonary edema, whereas a brisk response may be protective. In addition, dangerous hypoxic depression of ventilation may develop in those who have a low hypoxic drive and who become extremely hypoxic from HAPE.[318] Persons who hypoventilate are more hypoxemic and have greater pulmonary hypertension. More important, however, may be the fact that a low HVR permits hypoxemia, especially during sleep.[319] Supporting this concept is the frequency with which the onset of HAPE occurs during sleep, and indeed sleeping medications may provoke HAPE.[266]

**Treatment.** Proper treatment of HAPE depends on the severity of the illness and the nature of the environment. The sooner the diagnosis is made, the easier the illness can be reversed. In the wilderness, where oxygen and medical expertise may not be available, most persons with HAPE should be evacuated to a lower altitude as soon as possible, keeping in mind the desirability of minimal exertion by the victim. If HAPE is diagnosed early, recovery is rapid with a descent of only 500 to 1000 m, and the victim may be able to reascend cautiously 2 or 3 days later. A portable hyperbaric chamber,[279] or supplemental oxygen, if available, will immediately increase arterial oxygen saturation and reduce pulmonary artery pressure, heart rate, respiratory rate, and symptoms. In situations in which descent is difficult, these treatments can be lifesaving. Rescue groups should make delivery of oxygen to the victim the highest priority if descent may be delayed.

Keeping the patient warm may be important, because cold stress elevates pulmonary artery pressure.[320, 321] The use of an expiratory positive airway pressure mask was shown to improve oxygenation in HAPE and may be useful as a temporizing measure, although its efficacy has not been well evaluated.[322] In high-altitude locations with clinics or hospitals, bed rest alone can be adequate treatment for mild cases, and bed rest with supplemental oxygen generally suffices for moderate and severe illness. Complete resolution of the edema may require 24 to 72 hours of oxygen therapy if treated near the altitude of onset, whereas removing the patient to a lower altitude results in prompter clearing of edema. Curiously, even higher concentrations of oxygen do not seem to be more useful as long as arterial oxygen saturation is maintained above 90%.[279] Apparently, when a threshold $Po_2$ is reached, the pulmonary artery pressure drops and the edema starts to clear, and higher $Po_2$ values do not further accelerate this process. Occasionally, life-threatening HAPE being treated at a medical facility will require descent to a lower altitude as well as a high inspired oxygen concentration if arterial saturation cannot be maintained or if severe encephalopathy develops. Intubation may then be required, as well as therapy directed to the cerebral edema. Pulmonary embolus should also be suspected in patients not responding rapidly to oxygen therapy.

Drugs are not as effective for treatment of HAPE as descent and/or oxygen. Although Singh and colleagues[264] reported good results with furosemide, concerns about hypovolemia and hypotension have constrained its use in North America and by the Himalayan Rescue Association in Nepal. Morphine sulfate, used cautiously and when central nervous system function is intact, can relieve dyspnea, improve oxygenation and comfort, and reduce heart and respiratory rates, much as it does in cardiogenic pulmonary edema.[323] Digitalis, isoproterenol, and corticosteroids have had no demonstrated benefit. Other measures that reduce pulmonary hydrostatic pressure by decreasing venous return may be of value. Vasodilators have recently been shown to lower pulmonary artery pressure and pulmonary vascular resistance, as well as to improve oxygenation.[309] Nifedipine can be given in an initial dose of 10 mg orally, followed by 10-mg doses every 4 hours, or preferably followed by the extended-release preparation, 30 mg, two to three times a day.[309] Experience with hydralazine and phentolamine is limited, and currently nifedipine is the drug therapy of choice. Acetazolamide may be useful, primarily in the early stage of illness. Despite progress in evaluating drug therapy, the best management of this uncommon illness in the back country is early recognition and descent.

**Prevention.** The preventive measures previously described for AMS also apply to HAPE. A fast rate of ascent is an important contributing factor, and graded ascent with adequate time for acclimatization will reduce the risk of HAPE. Menon[323] clearly showed that sedentary men taken abruptly to altitude were just as likely as physically active men to be victims of HAPE. However, once HAPE has developed, exercise, by increasing pulmonary artery pressure and decreasing arterial oxygen saturation, may be detrimental. Because unrecognizable subclinical pulmonary edema might be converted to clinical edema by exercise, avoidance of overexertion, especially when fatigued, may help prevent HAPE. Persons on acetazolamide have occasionally developed HAPE during extremely rapid ascents, but clinical experience suggests that this drug may prevent HAPE in persons with a history of recurrent episodes in the presence of a reasonable rate of ascent. Nifedipine was recently found effective in preventing HAPE in subjects with a past history of the illness[311]; the dose used was 20 mg (slow release) every 8 hours. Because the incidence of HAPE is low, prophylactic nifedipine should be reserved for those known to be susceptible.

## High-Altitude Retinopathy

In 1969, Singh and associates[264] reported blurring of vision and retinal venous engorgement, various degrees of papilledema, and vitreous hemorrhages in soldiers with AMS. At 5350 m on Mt. Logan, Frayser and colleagues[324] noted that the eyegrounds of all those observed showed tortuosity of retinal vessels, vascular engorgement, and optic disc hyperemia; they considered these changes the normal response to hypoxia. They also described retinal hemorrhages in 56% of subjects. Such hemorrhages are now recognized as commonly occurring at altitudes greater than 4500 m (Fig. 70.16). These hemorrhages rarely produce visual changes, although macular hemorrhages have been reported. At lower elevations, retinal

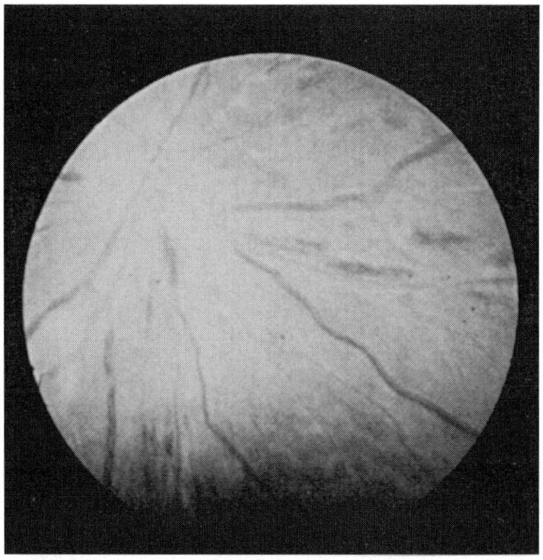

**Figure 70.16** Photograph of the retina of a mountain climber with a visual defect, demonstrating retinal hemorrhages and a cotton-wool exudate.

hemorrhages are associated with AMS.[325] Asymptomatic retinal hemorrhages are self-limited, resolving within 7 to 14 days, and are not considered an indication for descent or other therapy.

The mechanism of high-altitude retinal hemorrhage is not known. Retinal hemorrhages have also been reported in other hypoxic conditions, such as chronic obstructive pulmonary disease (COPD), carbon monoxide poisoning, congenital heart disease, and vaginal birth; hypoxia is certainly the underlying cause at altitude. Hemorrhage can be induced by maximal exercise at high altitude, during which blood pressure is elevated and the arterial oxygen saturation is decreased.[326] The only pathologic specimens reported to date showed hemorrhage from veins and from capillaries but not from arterial vessels.[327] The hemorrhages are similar to those seen on necropsy in the lungs and the brain. Other retinal pathology includes cotton-wool exudates and retinal edema, which can cause blurred vision (see Fig. 70.16).

In persons ascending to high altitude, intermittent blindness may occur without any other symptoms.[328] An intact pupillary reflex suggests that loss of vision may represent a form of cortical blindness.

## Thrombosis: Coagulation and Platelet Changes

The higher than expected incidence of venous thrombosis, pulmonary embolism, and stroke in mountaineers, as well as autopsy findings of widespread thrombi in the brain and lungs, has led to investigations of the clotting mechanism at high altitude. Changes in platelets and in coagulation have been observed in rabbits, mice, rats, calves, and humans on ascent to altitude and have been extensively reviewed.[329]

Hyers and colleagues[330] reported increased fibrinolysis with simulated altitude in both controls and HAPE-susceptible persons, whereas Maher and associates[331] found a fall in factor VIII and a decrease in partial thromboplastin time. Others have not been able to confirm such changes. A remarkable case was reported by O'Bradovich and associates.[332] One of the women in their chamber study developed disseminated intravascular coagulation within 1.5 hours of exposure to hypoxia ($P_B$ = 410 mm Hg). The platelet count had decreased by 100,000/μL,[3] and the partial thromboplastin time had shortened by 10 seconds. She also developed symptoms of AMS, and the study was discontinued.

Coagulation studies on individuals with HAPE are limited. Singh and colleagues[333] reported that HAPE patients had increased fibrinogen levels and prolonged clot lysis times, which they attributed to a breakdown of fibrinolysis. Singh[334] also reported thrombotic, occlusive hypertensive pulmonary vascular disease in soldiers who had recently arrived at altitude. These findings, plus autopsy data, prompted Dickinson and associates[295] to conclude that hypercoagulability of the blood and sequestration of platelets in the pulmonary vascular bed provoke pulmonary thrombosis and may contribute to the pathogenesis of HAPE. Bartsch and associates,[335] on the other hand, with careful longitudinal studies done while subjects were developing HAPE, concluded that platelet and coagulation changes were epiphenomena and not causative.

Taken together, the work done to date does not confirm a causative role for abnormal coagulation in the pathophysiology of altitude illnesses. Peripheral thrombotic events in mountaineers and, therefore, some embolic events may be explained on the basis of dehydration, polycythemia, cold, constrictive clothing, and venous stasis from prolonged periods of weather-imposed inactivity.

### Subacute Mountain Sickness

Recently, two syndromes of pulmonary hypertension and right-sided heart failure have been described in lowlanders who move to high altitude. These may be the human counterpart to brisket disease in cattle, a problem affecting susceptible bovine strains after months of exposure to altitude. Subacute infantile mountain sickness was described in Han Chinese infants who were born at low altitude and then moved to Lhasa, Tibet (3600 m).[336] The adult syndrome was reported by Anand and associates[337] in Indian soldiers posted for over 3 months at altitudes over 5800 m. In both syndromes, congestive heart failure and severe pulmonary hypertension inevitably led to death unless the victim was removed to a lower altitude. Polycythemia is not a feature of the disease in children but was present in the adults. In addition to the pulmonary hypertension, pathogenic features in adults include myocardial dysfunction, fluid and salt retention, and impaired renal function.[338] To date, the syndrome has not been noted in other populations.

## Problems of High-Altitude Residents

### Chronic Mountain Sickness

Chronic mountain sickness occurs in persons born and living at high altitude as well as in lowlanders who move to high altitudes and stay for prolonged periods of time. The entity was first described in Andean dwellers by Monge[339] in 1928 and is often referred to as Monge's disease. Excessive erythrocytosis, that is, a hematocrit above 60% to 70% or more than 2 standard deviations above the average value for healthy residents at a given high altitude, is an essential characteristic of the syndrome; the illness therefore is also referred to as chronic mountain polycythemia, but the term *chronic mountain sickness* is most commonly used. CMS has been reported in North America, China, and the republics of the former Soviet Union, as well as in South America.

The incidence in women before menopause is low but increases appreciably after approximately 45 years of age.[339a] There are geographic and ethnic differences in the prevalence of CMS. It is rarely found in natives of the Tibetan plateau but is frequently encountered in the Andes, in the North American Rockies, and in other mountainous regions where lowlanders have moved.[339, 340] An example is the Han Chinese who have moved to the Tibetan plateau. The reason for this difference is only speculative but is thought possibly to be secondary to more advantageous adaptations that the Tibetans have undergone because of the much greater duration of their existence on the Tibetan plateau (~250,000 years) compared with that of the Andeans (~13,000–15,000 years). Especially important may be the findings that Tibetans have a much lower pulmonary vasoconstrictive response to hypoxia, lower hematocrits, and sea-level birth weights of their children as compared with other high-altitude populations. These fascinating observations invite further unraveling.

**Clinical Presentation.** Symptoms of CMS are similar to those found in persons suffering polycythemia at low altitude: headache, dizziness, lethargy, impaired memory and mentation, and poor sleep. Consistent findings are cyanosis, plethoric appearance, and elevated hematocrit and hemoglobin. The diagnosis can only be established by eliminating all other causes of polycythemia. Indeed, much confusion in the literature regarding incidence and other aspects of CMS may be due to inadequate validation of the diagnosis. Monge, for example, noted a high frequency of bronchial complications in patients with CMS, whereas Kryger and associates[341] found evidence of lung disease in 50% of those with CMS in Leadville, Colorado. Indeed, when viewed as a syndrome, it is possible that many cases represent an interaction between some underlying chronic pathology, such as lung disease, and high altitude. The incidence of cases of pure, or so-called primary, CMS has not been determined.

**Pathophysiology.** Physiologic studies of CMS show a tendency toward excessive hypoxemia in many but not all cases; a blunted HVR; relative hypoventilation; a widened (A − a) $PO_2$; sometimes pulmonary hypertension that can lead to right-sided heart failure; a high-frequency, low-tidal volume breathing pattern with increased dead-space ventilation; an increase in red blood cell mass without an increase in plasma volume; and excessive arterial oxygen desaturation during sleep.[145, 341–344] How all these factors interact in a cause-and-effect role is not clear.

The excessive polycythemia of CMS may be due to greater hypoxemia, but the actual hematocrit values obtained are often higher than expected for the measured arterial oxygen saturation.[343] Thus, an excessive hematopoietic response to a given hypoxic stimulus may be a factor.[344] Hypoventilation appears to be a significant contributor to the greater hypoxemia. Aging, by its effect on hypoventilation and gas exchange, likely explains the increased incidence in the elderly. Although it is tempting to attribute the hypoventilation to loss of the HVR occurring with prolonged residence at high altitude, Kryger and associates[341] demonstrated blunted chemosensitivity in age- and altitude-matched healthy natives similar to that of patients with CMS and concluded that the blunted chemosensitivity played more of a permissive than a causative role. The contribution of ventilation and HVR is reinforced by the very low incidence of CMS in Tibetans, who seem to have a better preserved HVR than Andean natives.[345] Hypoxia itself may ultimately contribute to the ventilatory depression, as evidenced by an increase in ventilation in some natives with CMS when given oxygen to breathe.[341] Severe nocturnal desaturation may also occur (Fig. 70.17).[346] In fact, the Denver investigators thought that the greater hypoxemia during sleep might be adequate to explain the higher hematocrits. These observations also point out that disorders causing mild hypoxemia at sea level, such as sleep apnea or chronic lung disease, can have more serious consequences when superimposed on the hypoxia of high altitude.

**Treatment.** Patients with CMS are treated by reducing red blood cell mass. Improving oxygenation and thereby reducing the hypoxic stimulus for red blood cell production is the most physiologic approach to therapy. Therefore, the definitive treatment for CMS is relocation to a lower altitude. Because a move is not always compatible with the patient's life-style, other treatments are often invoked. Phlebotomy has long been used, not only for CMS but also for any cause of excessive polycythemia. Despite the common clinical practice and prompt subjective improvement, long-term benefits have not been well documented. Low-flow oxygen during sleep is probably effective, especially for those with marked sleep desaturation. Respiratory stimulants, by increasing alveolar $Po_2$, have also been found to be effective in treating CMS. Medroxyprogesterone acetate, given in dosages of 20 to 60 mg/day for 10 weeks, increased tidal volume and minute ventilation, lowered arterial $Pco_2$, and improved oxygenation both awake and asleep.[347] Hematocrit values declined from a mean of 60% to 52%, which is in the normal range for 3100 m. Acetazolamide was also beneficial. The response to respiratory stimulants underscores the contribution of hypoventilation to the pathogenesis of CMS.

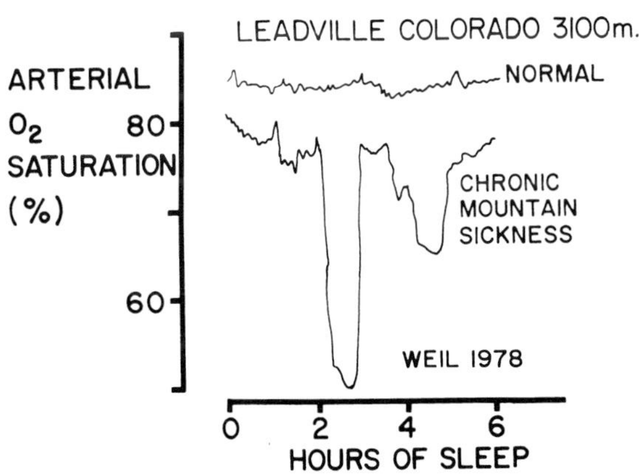


**Figure 70.17** Arterial oxygen saturation (%) by ear oximeter during sleep in a normal resident of Leadville, Colorado, and in a patient with chronic mountain sickness. Severe and prolonged desaturation occurred in the individual with chronic mountain sickness. (From Weil JV, Kryger MH, Scoggin CH: Sleep and breathing at high altitude. *In* Guilleminault C, Dement WC (eds): Sleep Apnea Syndromes. New York: Alan R. Liss, 1978, pp 119–136. Reprinted with permission.)

### Reentry Pulmonary Edema

Some persons living for years at high altitude, who then descend to lower altitudes, develop HAPE on reascent. Authors have suggested that the incidence of HAPE on reascent may be higher than during initial ascent by sojourners,[348, 349] but data on true incidence are lacking. Children and adolescents are more susceptible than adults. Hultgren and Marticorena[348] found in Peruvian natives an incidence of reentry HAPE of 6.4 per 100 exposures in the 1- to 20-year-old age group and 0.4 per 100 exposures in those older than 21. The phenomenon has been most often observed in Peru, where high-altitude residents can return from sea level to high altitude quite rapidly. Cases have also been reported in Leadville, Colorado,[349] but reports are conspicuously absent from Nepal and Tibet, possibly because rapid return to high altitude is not so readily available. Hultgren and Grover[140] have postulated that the increased muscularization of pulmonary arterioles that develops with chronic high-altitude exposure generates an inordinately high pulmonary artery pressure on reascent, causing the edema. Mountaineers have learned that adequate acclimatization to a given altitude will not necessarily protect against HAPE on rapid ascent to a yet higher altitude.

## Illnesses Influenced by High Altitude

Millions of lowlanders of all ages travel to high altitude for work and recreation. Because of increasing ease of travel to these places, this phenomenon has increased a great deal over the past couple of decades. Thus, many low-altitude dwellers with the predictable distribution of diseases compound their maladies with the added stress of hypoxia. Ironically, very few studies have been done to understand what happens to people with various diseases when they visit high-altitude destinations, and even fewer data are available about how to treat them before and after their exposure. The following section, therefore, will cover a number of common medical problems that the practitioner may be asked about, but much of that information will be from flawed clinical studies and anecdotes.

## Hypertension

In sea-level natives who had moved to high altitude, Penaloza and coworkers[129] found a decreased blood pressure in half of 1000 subjects after 2 to 15 years. In contrast, Hu (personal communication) claims that 20% of all lowland Chinese who move to Tibet develop arterial hypertension, and he considers this a form of mountain sickness to be treated by relocating the affected individuals back to low altitude. Also, 25% of 243 Indian soldiers residing for a few months at altitudes of 2500 to 4000 m had blood pressure equal to or greater than 140 mm Hg systolic and/or 100 mm Hg diastolic.[350] Length of time at altitude may explain some of the differences in observations.

Studies of the acute effects of altitude on blood pressure are more consistent. Studies on small numbers of Indian subjects transported to altitude and then controlled for activity as well as diet showed a transient increase in blood pressure: mean 105/66 mm Hg at sea level to 119/77 mm Hg after 3 days, 111/75 mm Hg at 3 weeks, and 102/64 mm Hg on return to sea level.[351] Pugh[352] reported increases in blood pressure in athletes at the Olympic games in Mexico City. Another Indian study showed an increase in 31 of 32 subjects that was maximal at 24 to 48 hours but that persisted for the entire 3 weeks of the study. Mean arterial pressure was 90 mm Hg at sea level, 104 to 105 mm Hg at altitude, and 90 mm Hg on return to sea level.[353] Thus, acute ascent to altitude increases blood pressure slightly.

Little information exists concerning the effect of high altitude on preexisting hypertension. Our clinical impression is that hypertension at altitude is much more common in those with preexisting labile or essential hypertension at sea level, and we recommend that patients on antihypertensive treatment continue their medications while at high altitude. Physicians encountering hypertensive patients living at high altitude may want to consider recommending relocation to a lower altitude if medical management is not successful but a trial descent is.

Hypertension in normally normotensive short-term high-altitude sojourners should be considered transient and need not be treated, because it rarely reaches dangerously high levels and will resolve on descent. Whether hypertensive patients are more susceptible to high-altitude illnesses is unknown.

## Arteriosclerotic Heart Disease

Although high altitude imposes a hypoxic stress on the body, no evidence of myocardial ischemia in individuals without a history of heart disease exists. Numerous electrocardiographic studies in healthy mountain climbers, including studies performed on the summit of Mt. Everest, have failed to show ischemic changes. Of 150 middle-aged males skiing at high altitude, evidence of ischemic changes were seen in 3; only 1, a physician who had suffered an acute myocardial infarction 3 months previously, had symptoms.[354] Grover and coworkers[355] studied three healthy men after 10 days at 3100 m; myocardial oxygen extraction was increased, as coronary blood flow had decreased, but myocardial oxygen tension and consumption remained constant; no such studies have been performed in persons with known heart disease. Grover and coworkers[355] studied 11 patients with known heart disease: 7 had had previous myocardial infarctions, 2 had angina, and 2 had had previous myocardial infarction and had stable exercise-induced angina at the time of the study. Electrocardiograms were obtained during exercise at 1600, 2500, and 3170 m. No patient who had a normal test in Denver had a positive test at altitude, and no patient developed symptoms at altitude who did not have them in Denver.

Morgan and associates,[356] on the other hand, found shorter time to onset of angina in nine men with heart disease on the first day at 3100 m compared with at 1600 m. By the third day, the men were back to their baseline time to onset of angina. Because left ventricular function remained normal, Morgan and coworkers[356] concluded that increased catecholamines and increased left ventricular afterload rather than global ischemia were responsible for the limitations. They recommended that the activity of persons with coronary artery disease be prescribed by heart rate, not by absolute workload, because heart rate at altitude was higher for the same workload.

During a reunion of the US Army 10th Mountain Division group from World War II in Vail, Colorado, 77 men and 20 women (ages 59 to 92 years) were observed.[356a, 356b] Twenty had known coronary artery disease with angina, bypass surgery, or other manifestations, and 38 had abnormal electrocardiograms on arrival. None incurred any further electrocardiographic changes or myocardial events except one individual on the same day after a maximal exercise test who suffered a myocardial infarction. Regardless of this case, the authors concluded that travel to moderate altitude with known, stable heart disease with reasonable activity was safe. Halhuber and colleagues[356c] studied 434 men and women aged 60 to 85 years at altitudes of 1700, 2500, and 3200 m for 4 weeks. The group was chosen because of modest asymptomatic exercise tolerance but also because of known cardiac disease. Except for one myocardial infarction (incidence of 0.2%) there were no other events. These workers also gathered data on 151,000 vacationers to the Alps and found only six deaths, only three of which were cardiac related. The conclusions from these and other studies from even higher altitudes in the Himalaya Mountains[356d, 356e] are that ascent and recreational activity to moderate altitudes is safe.

Little information is available regarding the risk of going to high altitude after surgery for coronary artery disease.[357, 358] Anecdotally, individuals have experienced uneventful treks to high-altitude settings after coronary artery bypass graft surgery. Although these experiences suggest that the additional risk due to coronary artery disease might be low,[357, 358] in fact the magnitude of added risk is not known. A negative stress test would give some reassurance, and a careful plan for acclimatization may help decrease the risk.[358]

## Congestive Heart Failure

One condition that we have observed repeatedly in older persons brought to 2000 m or higher from sea level is decompensation of chronic congestive heart failure. This problem may be difficult to assess because increased breathlessness, especially during exertion, is a normal consequence of exposure to high altitude, and baseline measurements are generally not available. Also, any degree of AMS, with its attendant fluid retention and increased hypoxemia, might aggravate congestive heart failure.

For patients with heart disease who are marginally compensated at sea level and for those with other forms of severe heart disease, supplemental oxygen at high altitude may be an effective means of helping to decrease risks. For example, a person traveling over a high mountain pass or staying only 1 or 2 nights at high altitude can use a liquid oxygen canister or even a compressed gas tank of oxygen to ensure a near-sea-level $Po_2$. Some patients may also need to arrange supplemental oxygen for commercial airline flights because usual cabin pressures are equivalent to 1800 to 2600 m. Further research is necessary to clarify the exact risk of altitude exposure for various subsets of cardiac patients.

## Lung Disease

Surprisingly little is known about the influence of high altitude on lung disease, either as a primary determinant of altitude illness (CMS) or as a cause of exacerbation of lung disease. Moderate high-altitude locations have traditionally been used for recuperation from respiratory diseases such as tuberculosis, both in Europe and in North America, but proof of the efficacy of altitude per se is lacking. Studies of the prevalence of lung disease at altitude are often marred because of the relatively high proportion of miners as well as Third World populations who live in quite smoky houses. A recent report surveying 833 subjects in low- and high-altitude towns in Colorado suggested that lung disease was more common at high altitude.[359] More important, the authors were able to demonstrate a migration of elderly persons from high to low altitude because of heart and lung disease. The migrants' health improved by relocating to lower altitudes. This study suggested an apparently unfavorable interaction of aging, high altitude, and heart and lung disorders. Supporting these results is the report of increased mortality from COPD, also in Colorado high-altitude residents, and the finding that COPD in altitude residents leads to earlier cor pulmonale and higher mortality.[360]

The effects of acute or transient altitude exposure on persons with preexisting lung disease are minimally explored despite the large numbers of such patients at risk. Any person hypoxemic from COPD at sea level will be more hypoxemic at altitude and therefore likely to be more symptomatic. Graham and Houston,[360] however, found that persons with moderate COPD (but without cor pulmonale or carbon dioxide retention) tolerated 2000 m well, complaining only of mild fatigue. Arterial $Po_2$ fell from 66 to 51 mm Hg at rest and from 63 to 46 mm Hg with exercise. Persons with blunted carotid body function from lung disease may not exhibit the normal increase in ventilation on ascent or the usual increased breathlessness associated with more severe hypoxemia. Many patients with chronic airflow obstruction who venture to high altitude report reduced exercise ability at high altitude, and many initiate supplemental oxygen or increase their usual rate of oxygen administration. The effects of altitude on lung disorders is an important area for future research.

Symptomatic pulmonary hypertension, whether primary or secondary, is a contraindication to ascent to high altitude because pulmonary artery pressure will increase further, exacerbating illness and possibly predisposing to HAPE.

Guidelines are available on how to evaluate and treat patients with hypoxemia who are going to travel by air.[360a–360c] The methods to predict air-flight hypoxemia (altitude in cabin approximately 2000 to 2500 m) are tedious and generally not available in most clinical laboratories. It is probably reasonable to prescribe 2 L/min oxygen by nasal prongs for patients with low-altitude oxygen saturations of 88% to 92%, while merely increasing the flow approximately 2 L/min in patients already on oxygen. The one patient who is problematic is the hypoxemic, hypoventilating patient because the addition of oxygen may make him or her hypoventilate even more. Careful titration may be indicated.

## Asthma

Many patients with asthma actually improve on ascent to high altitude, which may seem surprising in that they will encounter more cold, dry air, factors often associated with increased bronchomotor responsiveness. This experience may be secondary to cleaner air with fewer allergens, which has been shown to decrease episodes, especially in children, because they encounter fewer mites and allergens.[360d] In an allergen-free hypobaric chamber, children with exercise-induced bronchospasm were allowed to exercise, and there were no events of exercise-induced bronchospasm.[360e]

We recommend that patients with mild to moderate asthma not be discouraged from going to high altitude. They should be counseled to take their medications with them, and because the margin of safety is less than at low altitude, they should be prepared to use them. However, the experience may be quite surprisingly positive.

## Sleep Apnea

For patients with sleep apnea, the degree of nocturnal desaturation and hypoxemia will be greater at high altitude, which could lead to increased arrhythmias, greater pulmonary hypertension, poorer quality of sleep, and daytime fatigue. Supplemental oxygen, in addition to the patient's standard therapy such as nasal continuous positive airway pressure, may be necessary to maintain adequate oxygenation. On the other hand, sleep apnea might improve on ascent secondary to the hypoxic stimulation of ventilation, but no work has been done in lowlanders with sleep apnea who venture to high altitude.

### Pregnancy

Problems reported in high-altitude natives and especially non-native residents have included reduced fecundity, impaired fertility, slightly increased incidence of congenital malformations, fetal growth retardation, and increased frequency of preeclampsia, neonatal hyperbilirubinemia, and increased infant mortality.[361] The clearest prenatal influence of high altitude is a reduction in infant birth weight of approximately 100 g for each 1000 m increase in elevation. But this lower birth weight appears to be detrimental at high altitude only if the infants are premature or other complications of pregnancy occur.[360] Recent work has suggested that birth weight is related to maternal oxygen transport and that mothers who smoked, were anemic, and had relative hypoventilation also had smaller infants.[362] That the infant mortality rate at 3100 m in Colorado remains twice the rate in Denver is thought to be due largely to increased mortality of preterm infants.[362]

The effects of high altitude on the pregnant sojourner and fetus are not well documented. Studies of experimentally induced acute hypoxia during pregnancy in humans have shown no fetal heart rate change or a slight tachycardia in response to mild hypoxia, whereas severe hypoxia can cause fetal bradycardia.[363] Such severe hypoxemia (inspired oxygen concentrations 8% to 12%) is encountered only at extreme altitudes (>6000 m) or during pulmonary edema at high altitude. Women with complicated pregnancies, however, are more likely to have abnormal fetal heart rate responses to hypoxia. Copher and Huber[364] suggested that an acute hypoxia test may be of value in assessing placental reserve. Anecdotal reports of increased spontaneous abortions at altitude are unconfirmed. The advice given to near-term women to avoid travel by air is based on the desire of the airlines to avoid having passengers go into labor during flights and not on any physiologic data that such flights may be harmful. Until more data become available, it seems prudent to recommend avoiding unnecessary high-altitude exposure for women with complicated pregnancies and no excessively high (>3000 to 4000 m) or prolonged exposures to altitude for lowland women with normal pregnancies.

### Miscellaneous Conditions

The new onset of seizures on ascent to altitude was reported anecdotally (D. Shlim, personal communication); subsequent evaluation revealed epilepsy. Because mild hypoxia has not been shown to induce seizures but hyperventilation is commonly used as a provocative maneuver, it may be that the hyperventilation accompanying altitude exposure can be a trigger in persons with a previously unknown seizure disorder. An increase in seizure activity at altitude in persons on antiepileptic therapy has not, to our knowledge, been reported. Clearly, this is an important area for further inquiry. The consequences of a seizure while in hazardous terrain must also be considered when advising patients with seizure disorders.

Increased difficulty with urination, including complete obstruction, has been noted in individuals with benign prostatic hypertrophy at high altitude. This problem may be due to increased alpha-adrenergic sympathetic tone, perhaps more from cold than from hypoxia. Alpha-adrenergic blockers have been useful for treatment of this condition at sea level and should be beneficial at altitude as well.

A host of other situations in which chronic illness or disability intersect with high altitude pose similar questions of added risk. In almost all instances, our knowledge is limited to anecdotal accounts. The possibility that hypoxia might increase the likelihood or adversity of decompensation is simply unknown, and the individual seeking advice on the risk of going to high altitude should be so informed.

Because high-altitude exposure is commonly associated with remoteness from medical care, even if hypoxia does not exacerbate the incidence or severity of a chronic illness, other risks exist. Among these are the problems involved in evacuating an incapacitated person from a high, remote mountain region to medical assistance. The risk is not only to the victim but also to all those associated with the individual and the task of evacuation, which may involve great risk in itself. Therefore, the risk involved when persons with chronic, nondebilitating diseases travel to high, remote regions is more than an individual one and can affect the health and lives of others as well. This awareness should be considered when decisions are made to embark on such journeys, noting, however, that health risks are often but one of many hazards confronting the traveler and his or her companions.

## SUMMARY

We have reviewed the normal processes that the body undergoes in adapting to the low-oxygen environment of high altitude. These steps optimize the delivery of oxygen from the air to the cell. Additionally, we have discussed the clinical situations in which adaptation is not successful, leading to a spectrum of altitude illnesses, from the milder form, acute mountain sickness, to the more severe manifestations of pulmonary and cerebral edemas. The pathophysiology of acute altitude illnesses is not completely understood, but it is associated with leakage of fluid from the intravascular to the extravascular spaces, primarily in the brain and lungs.

## References


1. Baker PT: The adaptive fitness of high altitude populations. *In* Baker PT (ed): The Biology of High Altitude Peoples. Cambridge, England: Cambridge University Press, 1978, pp. 317–346.
2. Rutten MG: The history of atmospheric oxygen. Space Life Sci 2:5–17, 1970.
3. Frisancho AR: Functional adaptation to high altitude hypoxia. Science 187:313–319, 1975.
4. de Acosta J: Historia Natural y Moral de las Indias, en que le Tratan Las Cosas Notables del Cielo, y Elementos, Metales, Plantas, y Animales Dellas: Y los Ritas, y Ceremonias, Leyes, y Gouierno, y Guerras de los Indios. Seville: Juan de Leon, 1590.
5. Bert P: La Pression Barometrique: Recherches de Physiologie Experimentale. Paris: Masson, 1978.
6. Mosso A: Life of Man in the High Alps (English translation). London: T Fisher Unwin, 1898.
7. Douglas CG, Haldane JS, Henderson Y, et al: Physiologic observations made on Pike's Peak, Colorado, with special reference to

adaptation to low barometric pressures. Philos Trans R Soc Lond Ser B 203:185–318, 1913.
8. Barcroft J, Binger CA, Bock AV, et al: Observations upon the effect of high altitude on the physiological processes of the human body, carried out in the Peruvian Andes, chiefly at Cerro de Pasco. Philos Trans R Soc Lond Ser B 211:351–480, 1923.
9. Schneider EC: Physiological effects of altitude. Physiol Rev 1:631–659, 1921.
10. Barcroft J: The respiratory function of the blood. *In* Lessons from High Altitude. Cambridge, England: Cambridge University Press, 1925.
11. Haldane JS: Acclimatization to high altitude. Physiol Rev 7:363–384, 1927.
11a. West JB: Highlife: A History of High Altitude Physiology and Medicine. Oxford, England: Oxford University Press, 1998.
12. Kellogg RH: Altitude acclimatization: An historical introduction emphasizing the regulation of breathing. Physiologist 11:37–57, 1968.
13. Lenfant C, Sullivan K: Adaptation to high altitude. N Engl J Med 284:1298–1300, 1971.
14. Haldane JS, Priestley JG: The regulation of lung ventilation. J Physiol 32:225–266, 1905.
15. Boycott AE, Haldane JS: The effects of low atmospheric pressure on respiration. J Physiol 37:355–377, 1908.
16. Rahn H, Otis AB: Man's respiratory response during and after acclimatization to high altitude. Am J Physiol 157:445–559, 1946.
17. Hornbein TF: The relationship between stimulus to chemoreceptors and their response. *In* Torrance RW (ed): Arterial Chemoreceptors. Oxford, England, Blackwell Science Publishers, 1968, pp. 65–68.
18. Biscoe TJ, Bradley GW, Purves MJ: The relation between carotid body chemoreceptor discharge, carotid sinus pressure and carotid body venous flow. J Physiol (Lond) 208:99–120, 1970.
19. Biscoe, TJ, Purves MJ, Sampson SR: The frequency of nerve impulses in single carotid body chemoreceptor adherent fibers recorded in vivo with intact circulation. J Physiol (Lond) 208:121–131, 1970.
20. Forster HV, Bisgard GE, Rasmussen B, et al: Ventilatory control in peripheral chemoreceptor denervated ponies during chronic hypoxemia. J Appl Physiol 41:878–885, 1976.
21. Lahiri S, Edelman NH, Cherniack, NS, et al: Role of carotid chemoreflex in respiratory acclimatization to hypoxia in goat and sheep. Respir Physiol 46:367–382, 1981.
22. Bouverot P, Collin R, Favier R, et al: Carotid chemoreceptor function in ventilatory and circulatory $O_2$ convection of exercising dogs at low and high altitude. Respir Physiol 43:147–167, 1981.
23. Bouverot P, Candas V, Libert JP: Role of the arterial chemoreceptors in ventilatory adaptation to hypoxia of awake dogs and rabbits. Respir Physiol 17:209–219, 1973.
24. Bouverot P, Bureau M: Ventilatory acclimatization and CSF acid-base balance in carotid chemodenervated dogs at 3550 m. Pflugers Arch 361:17–23, 1975.
25. Bisgard GE, Vogel JHK: Hypoventilation and pulmonary hypertension in calves after carotid body excision. J Appl Physiol 31:431–437, 1971.
26. Bowes G, Andrey, SM, Kozar LF, et al: Carotid chemoreceptor regulation of expiratory duration. J Appl Physiol 54:1195–1201, 1983.
27. Daristotle L, Berssenbrugge AD, Engwall MJ, et al: The effects of carotid body hypocapnia on ventilation in goats. Respir Physiol 79:123–135, 1990.
28. Severinghaus JW, Mitchell RA, Richardson BW, et al: Respiratory control at high altitude suggesting active transport regulation of CSF pH. J Appl Physiol 18:1155–1166, 1963.
29. Kellogg RH: Effect of altitude on respiratory regulation. Ann NY Acad Sci 109:815–828, 1963.
30. Crawford RD, Severinghaus JW: CSF pH and ventilatory acclimatization to altitude. J Appl Physiol 45:275–283, 1978.
31. Dempsey JA, Forster HV, doPico GA: Ventilatory acclimatization to moderate hypoxemia in man: The role of spinal fluid. J Clin Invest 53:1091–1100, 1974.
32. Dempsey JA, Forster HV, Gledhill N, et al: Effects of moderate hypoxemia and hypocapnia on CSF and ventilation in man. J Appl Physiol 38:665–674, 1975.
33. Dempsey JA, Forster HV, Chosy LW, et al: Regulation of CSF [$HCO_3^-$] during long-term hypoxic hypocapnia in man. J Appl Physiol 44:175–182, 1978.
34. Forster HV, Dempsey JA, Chosy LW: Incomplete compensation of CSF in man during acclimatization to high altitude (4300 m). J Appl Physiol 38:1067–1072, 1975.
35. Orr JA, Bisgard GE, Forster HV, et al: Cerebrospinal fluid alkalosis during high altitude sojourn in unanesthetized ponies. Respir Physiol 25:23–37, 1975.
36. Weiskopf RB, Gabel RA, Fencl V: Alkaline shift in lumbar and intracranial CSF in man after 5 days at high altitude. J Appl Physiol 41:93–97, 1976.
37. Forster HV, Bisgard GE, Dempsey JA, et al: Role of intracranial receptor in physiologic regulation of ventilation in ponies. Chest 73(Suppl):253–255, 1978.
38. Dempsey JA, Forster HV, Bisgard, GE, et al: Role of cerebrospinal fluid in ventilatory deacclimatization from chronic hypoxia. J Clin Invest 64:199–205, 1979.
39. Fencl V, Gabel R, Wolfe D: Composition of cerebral fluids in goats adapted to high altitude. J Appl Physiol 47:508–573, 1979.
40. Pelligrino DA, Musch TI, Dempsey JA: Interregional differences in brain intracellular pH and water compartmentation during acute normoxic and hypoxic hypocapnia in the anesthetized dog. Brain Res 214:387–404, 1981.
41. Neubauer JA, Simone A, Edelman NH: Role of brain lactic acidosis in hypoxic depression of respiration. J Appl Physiol 65:1324–1331, 1988.
42. Goldberg S, Schoene RB, Haynor, D, et al: Brain tissue pH and ventilatory acclimatization to high altitude. J Appl Physiol 72:58–63, 1991.
43. Holtby JG, Berenzanski DJ, Anthonisen NR: Effect of 100% $O_2$ on hypoxic eucapnic ventilation. J Appl Physiol 65:1157–1162, 1988.
44. Olson EB Jr, Dempsey JA: Rat as a model for humanlike ventilatory adaptation to chronic hypoxia. J Appl Physiol 44:763–769, 1978.
45. Robinson KA, Hayner EM: Metabolic effects of exposure to hypoxia plus cold at rest and during exercise in humans. J Appl Physiol 68:720–725, 1990.
46. Morrill CG, Meyer JR, Weil JV: Hypoxic ventilatory depression in dogs. J Appl Physiol 38:143–146, 1975.
47. West JB: Rate of ventilatory acclimatization to extreme altitude. Respir Physiol 74:323–333, 1988.
48. Forster HV, Dempsey JA, Birnbaum MC, et al: Effects of chronic exposure to hypoxia on ventilatory response to $CO_2$ and hypoxia. J Appl Physiol 31:586–592, 1971.
49. Schoene RB, Roach RC, Hackett PH, et al: Operation Everest II: Ventilatory adaptation during gradual decompression to extreme altitude. Med Sci Sports Exerc 22:804–810, 1990.
50. Vizek M, Pickett CK, Weil JV: Increased carotid body hypoxic sensitivity during acclimitization to hypobaric hypoxia. J Appl Physiol 63:2403–2410, 1987.
51. Daristotle L, Engwald MJ, Viu WZ, et al: Ventilatory effects and interactions with change in $Pa_{O_2}$ in awake goats. J Appl Physiol 71:1254–1260, 1991.
52. Bisgard GE, Busch MA, Forster HV: Ventilatory acclimatization to hypoxia is not dependent on cerebral hypocapnic alkalosis. J Appl Physiol 60:1011–1015, 1986.
53. Nielsen AM, Bisgard GE, Vidruk EH: Carotid chemoreceptor activity during acute and sustained hypoxia in goats. J Appl Physiol 65:1796–1802, 1988.
54. Mathew L, Gopinath, PM, Purkayastha SS, et al: Chemoreceptor sensitivity in adaptation to high altitude. Aviat Space Environ Med 54:121–126, 1983.
55. Eger EI II, Kellogg RH, Mines AH, et al: Influence of $CO_2$ on ventilatory acclimatization to altitude. J Appl Physiol 24:607–615, 1968.
56. Winslow RM, Monge C: Hypoxia, Polycythemia, and Chronic Mountain Sickness. Baltimore, Johns Hopkins University Press, 1987.
57. Weil JV, Byrne-Quinn, E, Sodal I, et al: Acquired attenuation of chemoreceptor function in chemically hypoxic man at high altitude. J Clin Invest. 50:186–195, 1971.
58. Sorensen SC, Severinghaus, JW: Irreversible respiratory insensitivity to acute hypoxia in men born at high altitude. J Appl Physiol 25:217–220, 1968.

59. Lahiri S, Kao FF, Velasquez T, et al: Irreversible blunted respiratory sensitivity to hypoxia in high altitude natives. Respir Physiol 6:360–374, 1969.
60. Lahiri S, DeLaney RB, Brody JS, et al: Relative role of environmental and genetic factors in respiratory adaptation to high altitude. Nature 261:133–135, 1976.
61. Chiodi H: Respiratory adaptations to chronic high altitude hypoxia. J Appl Physiol 10:81–87, 1957.
62. Severinghaus JW, Bainton CR, Carcellen A: Respiratory insensitivity to hypoxia in chronically hypoxic man. Respir Physiol 1:308–334, 1966.
63. Lahiri S, Milledge JS, Chattapadhyoy HP, et al: Respiration and heart rate of Sherpa highlanders during exercise. J Appl Physiol 23:545–554, 1967.
64. Milledge JS, Lahiri S: Respiratory control in lowlanders and Sherpa highlanders at altitude. Respir Physiol 2:310–322, 1967.
65. Arias-Stella J: Human carotid body at high altitude (abstract). Am J Pathol 55:82a, 1969.
66. Heath D, Edwards C, Harris P: Postmortem size and structure of the human carotid body: Its relation to pulmonary disease and cardiac hypertrophy. Thorax 25:129–140, 1970.
67. Huang, SY, Ning XH, Zhou, ZN, et al: Ventilatory function in adaptation to high altitude: Studies in Tibet. *In* West JB, Lahiri S (eds): High Altitude and Man. Bethesda, MD: American Physiological Society, 1984, pp. 173–177.
68. Hackett PH, Reeves, JT, Grover RF, et al: Ventilation in human populations native to high altitude. *In* West JB Lahiri S (eds): High Altitude and Man. Bethesda, MD: American Physiological Society, 1984, pp. 179–191.
69. Lahiri S: Respiratory control in Andean and Himalayan high-altitude natives. *In* West JB, Lahiri S (eds): High Altitude and Man. Bethesda, MD: American Physiological Society, 1984, pp. 147–162.
70. Hackett PH, Reeves JT, Reeves CD, et al: Control of breathing in Sherpas at low and high altitude. J Appl Physiol 49:374–379, 1980.
71. Milledge JS, Lahiri S: Respiratory control in lowlanders and Sherpa highlanders at altitude. Respir Physiol 2:310–322, 1967.
72. Cruz J: Mechanisms of breathing in high altitude and sea level subjects. Respir Physiol 17:146–161, 1973.
73. Lahiri S: Alveolar gas pressures in man with lifetime hypoxia. Respir Physiol 4:373–386, 1968.
74. Huang SY, Gu ZZ, Pa CF, et al: Ventilatory control in Tibetan highlanders. *In* Geological and Ecological Studies of Qinghai-Xizang Plateau. New York, Gordon and Breach, 1981, pp. 1363–1369.
75. Tenney SM, Rahn H, Stroud RC, et al: Adaptation to high altitude: Changes in lung volumes during the first seven days at Mt. Evans, Colorado. J Appl Physiol 5:607–613, 1953.
76. Dill DB, Hillyard SD, Miller J: Vital capacity exercise performance, and blood gases at altitude related to age. J Appl Physiol 48:6–9, 1980.
77. Larson EB, Roach RC, Schoene RB, Hornbein TF: Acute mountain sickness and acetazelamide: Clinical efficacy and effect on ventilation. JAMA 248:328–332, 1982.
78. Coates G, Gray G, Mansell A, et al: Changes in lung volume, lung density, and distribution of ventilation during hypobaric decompression. J Appl Physiol 46:752–755, 1979.
79. Mansell A, Poules A, Sutton JR: Changes in pulmonary PV characteristics of human subjects at an altitude of 5366 m. J Appl Physiol 49:79–83, 1980.
80. Jaeger JJ, Sylvester JT, Cymerman A, et al: Evidence for increased intrathoracic fluid volume in man at high altitude. J Appl Physiol 47:670–676, 1979.
81. Hoon RS, Balasubramanio V, Tiwari BC, et al: Changes in transthoracic electrical impedance at high altitude. Br Heart J 39:61–66, 1977.
82. Cruz JC: Mechanics of breathing in high altitude and sea level subjects. Respir Physiol 17:146–161, 1973.
83. Gautier H, Peslin R, Grassine A, et al: Mechanical properties of the lungs during acclimatization to altitude. J Appl Physiol 52:1407–1415, 1982.
84. Hurtado A: Respiratory adaptations in the Indian natives of the Peruvian Andes. Am J Phys Anthropol 17:137–161, 1932.
85. Monge MC, Monge CC: Chronic mountain sickness. *In* High Altitude Diseases: Mechanism and Management. Springfield, IL: Charles C Thomas, 1966, p. 14.
86. Brody JS, Lahiri S Simpsen M et al: Lung elasticity and airway dynamics in Peruvian natives to high altitude. J Appl Physiol 42:245–251, 1977.
87. Frisancho AR: Functional adaptation to high altitude hypoxia. Science 187:313–319, 1975.
88. Frisancho AR, Velasquez T, Sanchez J: Influence of developmental adaptation on lung function at high altitude. Hum Biol 45:583–594, 1973.
89. Frisancho AR, Martinez C, Velasquez T, et al: Influence of developmental adaptation on aerobic capacity at high altitude. J Appl Physiol 34:176–180, 1973.
90. Burri PH, Weibel SR: Environmental oxygen tension and lung growth. Respir Physiol 11:247–264, 1971.
91. Lechner AJ, Banchero N: Lung morphometry in guinea pigs acclimated to hypoxia during growth. Respir Physiol 42:155–169, 1980.
92. West JB, Hackett PH, Maret KH, et al: Pulmonary gas exchange on the summit of Mt. Everest. J Appl Physiol 55:678–687, 1983.
93. Vogel JA, Harris CW: Cardiopulmonary responses of resting man during early exposure to high altitude. J Appl Physiol 22:1124–1128, 1967.
94. Kontos HA, Lavasseur JE, Richardson DW, et al: Comparative circulatory responses to systemic hypoxia in man and in unanesthetized dog. J Appl Physiol 23:281–286, 1967.
95. Gale GE, Torre-Bueno JR, Moon RE, et al: Ventilation-perfusion inequality in normal humans during exercise at sea level and simulated altitude. J Appl Physiol 58:978–988, 1985.
96. Rotta A, Canepa A, Hurtado A, et al: Pulmonary circulation at sea level and at high altitudes. J Appl Physiol 9:328–336, 1956.
97. Fishman AP: Hypoxia and the pulmonary circulation: How and where it acts. Circ Res 38:221–231, 1976.
98. Dawson A: Regional pulmonary blood flow in sitting and supine man during and after acute hypoxia. J Clin Invest 48:301–310, 1969.
99. Dawson A: Regional lung function during early acclimatization to 3100 m altitude. J Appl Physiol 33:218–223, 1972.
100. Sylvester JT, Cymerman A, Gurtner G, et al: Components of alveolar-arterial $O_2$ gradient during rest and exercise at sea level and high altitude. J Appl Physiol 50:1129–1139, 1981.
101. Hansen TN, LeBlanc AL, Gest AL: Hypoxia and angiotensin II infusion redistribution lung blood flow in lambs. J Appl Physiol 58:812–818, 1985.
102. Haab, P, Held DR, Ernst H, et al: Ventilation perfusion relationships during high altitude adaptation. J Appl Physiol 26:77–81, 1969.
103. Dawson A, Grover RF: Regional lung function in natives and long-term residents at 3100 m altitude. J Appl Physiol 36:294–298, 1974.
104. Wagner PD, Sutton JR, Reeves JT, et al: Operation Everest II: Pulmonary gas exchange during simulated ascent of Mt. Everest. J Appl Physiol 63:2348–2359, 1987.
105. West, JB, Wagner PD: Predicted gas exchange on the summit of Mt. Everest. Respir Physiol 42:1–16, 1980.
106. DeGraff AC Jr, Grover RF, Johnson RL Jr, et al: Diffusing capacity of the lung in Caucasians native to 3100 m. J Appl Physiol 29:71–76, 1970.
107. Vargas E, Beard J, Haas J, et al: Pulmonary diffusing capacity in young Andean highland children. Respiration 43:330–335, 1982.
108. Dempsey JA, Reddun WG, Birnbaum ML, et al: Effects of acute through life-long hypoxic exposure in exercise pulmonary gas exchange. Respir Physiol 13:62–89, 1971.
109. Cerny FC, Dempsey JA, Reddan WG: Pulmonary gas exchange in non-native residents of high altitude. J Clin Invest 52:2993–2999, 1973.
110. Hurtado A: Animals in high altitude: Man above 5000 meters—Mountain exploration. *In* Dill DB (ed): Handbook of Physiology. Section 4: Adapation to the Environment. Washington, DC: American Physiological Society, 1964, pp. 843–860.
111. Vincent J, Hellot MF, Vargas E, et al: Pulmonary gas exchange, diffusing capacity in natives and newcomers at high altitude. Respir Physiol 34:219–231, 1978.
112. Guleria JS, Pande JN, Sethi PK, et al: Pulmonary diffusing capacity at high altitude. J Appl Physiol 31:536–543, 1971.

113. Remmers JE, Mithoefer JC: The carbon monoxide diffusing capacity in permanent residents at high altitude. Respir Physiol 6:233–244, 1969.
114. Krueger F, Tenney SM, Mithoeffer JC, et al: Alveolar-arterial oxygen gradient in Andean natives at high altitude. J Appl Physiol 19:13–16, 1964.
115. Schoene RB, Roach RC, Lahiri S, et al: Increased diffusion capacity maintains arterial saturations during exercise in the Quechua Indians of the Chilean Altiplano. Am J Hum Biol 2:663–668, 1990.
116. Klausen K: Cardiac output in man in rest and work during and after acclimatization to 3800 m. J Appl Physiol 21:609–616, 1966.
117. Vogel JA, Harris CW: Cardiopulmonary responses of resting man during early exposure to high altitude. J Appl Physiol 22:1124–1128, 1967.
118. Stenberg J, Ecblom B, Messin R: Hemodynamic response to work at simulated altitude, 4000 m. J Appl Physiol 21:1589–1594, 1966.
119. Vogel JA, Hartley H, Cruz JC, et al: Cardiac output during exercise in sea-level residents at sea level and high altitude. J Appl Physiol 36:169–172, 1974.
120. Manchander SC, Maher JT, Cymerman A: Cardiac performance during graded exercise in acute hypoxia. J Appl Physiol 38:858–862, 1975.
121. Meerson FZ, Pshennikova MG: Effects of adaptation to high altitude hypoxia on the contractile function and adrenoreactivity of the heart. Basic Respir Cardiol 74:142–154, 1979.
122. Rapin JR, Loudert J, Drouet L, et al: Uptake of noradrenaline in high altitude native hearts. Experientia 33:739–740, 1977.
123. Novikova NA, Gorina MS, Kapel Ko, VI: Contractile function of the heart and its reactivity to noradrenaline in the process of the body's adaptation to moderate altitude. Bull Eksp Biol Med 84:5–7, 1977.
124. Cunningham WL, Becker EJ, Krueger F: Catecholamines in plasma and urine at high altitude. J Appl Physiol 20:607–610, 1965.
125. Alexander JK, Grover RF: Mechanism of reduced stroke volume at high altitude. Clin Cardiol 6:301–303, 1983.
125a. Wolfel EE, Groves BM, Brooks GA, et al.: Oxygen transport during steady-state submaximal exercise in chronic hypoxia. J Appl Physiol 70: 1129–1136, 1991.
125b. Wolfel JAP, Wolfel EE, Selland MA, et al: $O_2$ extraction maintains $O_2$ uptake during submaximal exercise with β-adrenergic blockade at 4,300 m. J Appl Physiol 85:1092–1102, 1998.
126. Vogel JA, Hartley H, Cruz JC: Cardiac output during exercise in altitude natives at sea level and high altitude. J Appl Physiol 36:173–176, 1974.
127. Bender PR, Groves BM, McCullough RE, et al: Oxygen transport to exercising leg in chronic hypoxia. J Appl Physiol 65:2592–2597, 1988.
128. Heath D, Williams DR: Systemic circulation. *In* Man at High Altitude: The Pathophysiology of Acclimatization and Adaptation. Edinburgh: Churchill Livingstone, 1977, pp. 161–163.
129. Penaloza D, Arias-Stella J, Sime F, et al: The heart and pulmonary circulation in children at high altitude: Physiological, anatomical and clinical observations. Pediatrics 34:568–582, 1964.
130. Lockhart A, Saiag B: Altitude and the human pulmonary circulation. Clin Sci 60:599–605, 1981.
131. Heath D, Williams DR: Pulmonary hypertension. *In* Man at High Altitude: The Pathophysiology of Acclimatization and Adaptation. Edinburgh: Churchill Livingstone, 1977, pp. 75–88.
132. Reeves JT, Wagner WW Jr, McMurtry F, et al: Physiological effects of high altitude on the pulmonary circulation. *In* Robertshaw D (ed): International Review of Physiology, Environmental Physiology III. Baltimore: University Park Press, 1979, pp. 289–310.
133. Heath D, Williams D, Dickinson J: The pulmonary arteries of the yak. Cardiovasc, Res 18:133–139, 1984.
134. Coudert J: La circulation pulmonaire du natif de la haute altitude à La Paz (3700 m). *In* Anthropologie des Populations Andines, vol. 63. Paris: Inserm, 1976, p. 305.
135. Groves BM, Droma T, Sutton JR, et al: Minimal hypoxic pulmonary hypertension in normal Tibetans at 3658 m. J. App Physiol 74:312–318, 1993.
136. Arias-Stella J, Saldana M: The terminal portion of the pulmonary vascular tree in people native to high altitude. Circulation 28:915–925, 1963.
137. Jaenke RS, Alexander AF: Fine structural alterations of bovine peripheral pulmonary arteries in hypoxia-induced hypertension. Am J Pathol 73:377–390, 1973.
138. Heath D, Smith P, Rios Dalenz J, et al: Small pulmonary arteries in some natives of La Paz, Bolivia. Thorax 36:599–604, 1981.
139. Blount SG, Jr, Vogel JHK: Altitude and the pulmonary circulation. Adv Intern Med 13:11–31, 1967.
140. Hultgren HN, Grover RF: Circulatory adaptation to high altitude. Ann Rev Med 19:119–152, 1968.
141. Gupta ML, Rao KS, Anand IS, et al: Lack of smooth muscle in the small pulmonary arteries of the native Ludakhi: Is the Himalayan highlander adapted? Am Rev Respir Dis 145:1201–1204, 1992.
142. Heath D, Williams DR: The blood. *In* Man at High Altitude: The Pathophysiology of Acclimatization and Adaptation. Edinburgh, Churchill Livingstone, 1977, pp. 39–53.
143. Hlastala MP: Interactions between $O_2$ and $CO_2$: The blood. *In* Sutton JR, Jones NL, Houston CS (eds): Hypoxia: Man at Altitude. New York, Thieme-Stratton, 1982, pp. 17–23.
144. Winslow RM: Red cell function at extreme altitude. *In* West JB, Lahiri S (eds): High Altitude and Man. Bethesda, MD: American Physiological Society, 1984, pp. 59–72.
145. Winslow RM: High altitude polycythemia. *In* West JB, Lahiri S (eds): High Altitude and Man. Bethesda, MD: American Physiological Society, 1984, pp. 163–172.
146. Erslev AJ: Humoral regulation of red cell production. Blood 8:349–357, 1953.
147. Jacobson LO, Goldwasser E, Freed W, et al: Role of kidney in erythropoiesis. Nature (Lond) 179:633, 1957.
148. Erslev A: Erythropoietin coming of age. N Engl J Med 316:101–103, 1987.
148a. Knaupp W, Khilnani S, Sherwood J, et al: Erythropoietin response to acute normobaric hypoxia in humans. J Appl Physiol 73:837–840, 1992.
149. Faura J, Ramos J, Reynafarje C, et al: Effect of altitude on erythropoiesis. Blood 33:668–676, 1969.
150. Abbrecht PH, Littell JK: Plasma erythropoietin in men and mice during acclimatization to different altitudes. J Appl Physiol 32:54–58, 1972.
151. Milledge JS, Coates PM: Serum erythropoietin in humans at high altitude and its relation to plasma renin. J Appl Physiol 59:360–364, 1985.
152. Sanchez C, Merino C, Figallo M: Simultaneous measurements of plasma volume and cell mass in polycythemia of high altitude. J Appl Physiol 28:775–778, 1970.
153. Torrance JC, Lenfant C, Cruz J, et al: Oxygen transport mechanisms in residents at high altitude. Respir Physiol 10:1–12, 1971.
154. Reynafarje C, Ramos J, Faura J, et al: Humoral control of erythropoietic activity in man during and after high altitude exposure. Proc Soc Exp Biol Med 116:649–650, 1964.
155. Milledge JS, Coates PM: Serum erythropoietin in humans at high altitude and its relation to plasma renin. J Appl Physiol 59:360–364, 1985.
156. Arnaud J, Quilici JC, Gutierrez N, et al. Methemoglobin and erythrocyte reducing systems in high-altitude natives. Ann Hum Biol 6:585–592, 1979.
157. Beall CM, Reischman AB: Hemoglobin levels in a Himalayan high altitude population. Am J Phys Anthropol 63:301–306, 1984.
158. Buick FJ, Gledhill N, Froese AB et al: Effect of induced erythrocythemia on aerobic work capacities. J Appl Physiol 48:636–642, 1980.
159. Murray JF, Gold P, Johnson BL Jr: The circulatory effects of hematocrit variations in normovolemic and hypervolemic dogs. J Clin Invest 42:1150–1159, 1963.
160. Fan FC Chen RYZ, Schuessler GB, et al: Effect of hematocrit variations on regional hemodynamics and oxygen transport in the dog. Am J Physiol 238:H545–H552, 1980.
161. Zink RA, Schaffert W, Brendel W, et al: Hemodilution in high altitude climbing (abstract). Anesthesiology 53:93, 1978.
162. Sarnquist FH, Schoene RB, Hackett PH: Exercise tolerance and cerebral function after acute hemodilution of polycythemic mountain climbers. Aviat Space Environ Med 57:313–317, 1986.

163. Finch CA, Lenfant C: Oxygen transport in man. N Engl J Med 296:407–415, 1972.
164. Aste-Salazar H, Hurtado A: The affinity of hemoglobin for oxygen at sea level and high altitude. Am J Physiol 142:733–743, 1944.
165. Moore LG, Brewer GJ: Beneficial effect of rightward hemoglobin-oxygen dissociation curve shift for short-term high altitude adaptations. J Lab Clin Med 98:145–154, 1981.
166. Hoyt RW, Wood SC, Hicks JW, et al: Effects of long distance running at high altitude on the standard oxygen-hemoglobin dissociation curve and red cell 2,3-DPG. Eur J Appl Physiol 51:175–181, 1983.
167. Hurtado A: Animals in high altitude: Resident man. *In* Dill DB, Adolf EF (eds): Handbook of Physiology: Adaptation to the Environment. Washington, DC: American Physiological Society, 1964, pp. 843–860.
168. Clench J, Ferrell RE, Schull WJ: Effect of chronic altitude hypoxia on hematologic and glycolytic parameters. Am J Physiol 242:R447–R451, 1982.
169. Keys A, Hall, FG, Barron ES: The position of the oxygen dissociation curve of human blood. Am J Physiol 115:292–307, 1936.
170. Rossi-Bernardi L, Luzzania M, Samaja M, et al: Continuous determination of the oxygen dissociation curve for whole blood. Clin Chem 21:1747–1753, 1975.
171. Lenfant C, Ways P, Aucutt C, Cruz J: Effect of chronic hypoxic hypoxia on the $O_2$-Hb dissociation curve and respiratory gas transport in man. Respir Physiol 7:7–29, 1969.
172. Lenfant C, Torrance JD, English E, et al: Effect of altitude on oxygen binding by hemoglobin and on organic phosphate levels. J Clin Invest 47:2652–2656, 1968.
173. Lenfant C, Torrance JD, Reynafarje C: Shift of the $O_2$-Hb dissociation curve at altitude: Mechanism and effect. J Appl Physiol 305:625–631, 1971.
174. Winslow RM, Monge CC, Statham NJ, et al: Variability of oxygen affinity of blood: Human subjects native to high altitude. J Appl Physiol 51:1411–1416, 1981.
175. Samaja M, Veicsteinas A, Cerritelli P: Oxygen affinity of blood in altitude Sherpas. J Appl Physiol 47:337–341, 1979.
176. Swan LW: Goose of the Himalaya. Nat Hist 79:68–75, 1970.
177. Petschow D, Wurdinger I, Baumann R, et al: Causes of high blood $O_2$ affinity of animals living at high altitude. J Appl Physiol 42:139–143, 1977.
178. Black CP, Tenney SM: Oxygen transport during progressive hypoxia in high altitude and sea-level waterfowl. Respir Physiol 39:217–239, 1980.
179. Faraci FM, Kilgore DL Jr, Feddle MR: Oxygen delivery to the heart and brain during hypoxia: Peking duck vs. bar-headed goose. Am J Physiol 247:R69–R75, 1984.
180. Winslow RM, Samaja M, West JB: Red cell function at extreme altitude on Mount Everest. J Appl Physiol 56:109–116, 1984.
181. Chance B, Cohen P, Jobsis F, et al: Intracellular oxidation-reduction states in vivo. Science 137:499–508, 1962.
182. Krogh A: Number and distribution of capillaries in muscles with calculations of the oxygen pressure head necessary to supply the tissue. J Physiol (Lond) 52:409–415, 1919.
183. Potter RF, Groom AC: Capillary density and geometry in cardiac and skeletal muscle studied by means of cohesion casts. Microvasc Res 25:68–84, 1983.
184. Mathiew-Costello O: Capillary tortuosity and degree of contraction or extension of skeletal muscle. Microvasc Res 33:98–117, 1987.
185. Banchero N: Capillary density of skeletal muscle in dogs exposed to simulated altitude. Proc Soc Exp Biol Med 148:435–439, 1975.
185a. Green HJ, Sutton JR, Wolfel EE, et al: Altitude acclimatization and energy metabolic adaptations in skeletal muscle during exercise. J Appl Physiol 73:2701–2708, 1992.
186. Valdivia E: Total capillary bed in striated muscle of guinea pigs native to the Peruvian mountains. Am J Physiol 194:585–589, 1958.
187. Bontellier U, Howald H, diPrampero PE, et al: Human muscle adaptation to chronic hypoxia. Prog Clin Biol Res 136:273–281, 1983.
188. MacDougall JD, Green HJ, Sutton JR, et al: Operation Everest II: Structural adaptations in skeletal muscle in response to extreme simulated altitude. Acta Physiol Scand 142:421–427, 1991.
189. Rose MS Houston CS, Fulco CS, et al: Operation Everest II: Nutrition and body composition. J Appl Physiol 65:2545–2551, 1988.
190. Ou LC, Tenney SM: Properties of mitochondria from hearts of cattle acclimatized to high altitude. Respir Physiol 8:151–159, 1970.
191. Tappan DV, Reynafarje B: Tissue pigment manifestations of adaptation to high altitudes. Am J Physiol 190:99–103, 1957.
192. Gimenz M, Sanderson RJ, Reiss OK, et al: Effects of altitude on myoglobin and mitochondrial protein in canine skeletal muscle. Respiration 34:171–176, 1977.
193. Howald J, Pette D, Simoneau JA, et al: Effect of chronic hypoxia on muscle enzyme activities. Int J Sports Med II(Suppl 1):510–514, 1990.
194. Lawrie RA: Effect of enforced exercise on myoglobin concentration in muscle. Nature 171:1069–1071, 1953.
194a. Garry DJ, Ordway GA, Lorrenz JN, et al: Mice without myoglobin. Nature 395:905–908, 1998.
195. Tappan DV, Reynafarje B, Potter VR, et al: Alterations in enzymes and metabolites resulting from adaptation to low oxygen tensions. Am J Physiol 190:93–98, 1957.
196. Nelson BD, Highman B, Altland PD: Oxidative phosphorylation during altitude acclimation in rats. Am J Physiol 213:1414–1418, 1967.
197. Harris P, Castillo Y, Gibson K, et al: Succinic and lactic dehydrogenase activity in myocardial homogenates from animals at high and low altitude. J Mol Cell Cardiol 1:189–193, 1970.
198. Mager M, Blatt WF, Natale PJ, et al: Effect of high altitude on lactic dehydrogenase isozymes of neonatal and adult rats. Am J Physiol 215:5–13, 1968.
199. Pickett CB, Cascarano J, Wilson MA: Acute and chronic hypoxia in rats. J Exp Zool 210:49–58, 1979.
200. Reynafarje B, Green J: Pyridine nucleotide-cytochrome-C reductases in rats exposed to low oxygen tensions. Proc Soc Exp Biol Med 103:224–225, 1960.
201. Hochachka PW, Stanley C, Merkt J, et al: Metabolic meaning of elevated levels of oxidative enzymes in high altitude adapted animals: An interpretive hypothesis. Respir Physiol 52:303–313, 1982.
202. Kety SS, Schmidt CF: The effects of altered arterial tensions of carbon dioxide and oxygen on cerebral blood flow and cerebral oxygen consumption of normal young men. J Clin Invest 27:484–492, 1948.
203. Kogure K, Scheinberg P, Reinmuthon J, et al: Mechanisms of cerebral vasodilation in hypoxia. J Appl Physiol 29:223–229, 1970.
204. Severinghaus JW, Chiodi H, Eger EL II, et al: Cerebral blood flow in man at high altitude: Role of cerebrospinal fluid pH in normalization of flow in chronic hypocapnia. Circ Res 19:274–282, 1966.
204a. Huang SY, Sun S, Droma T, et al: Internal carotid arterial flow velocity during exercise in Tibetan and Han residents of Lhasa (3650 m). J Appl Physiol 73:2638–2642, 1992.
205. Cahoon PL: Simple decision making at high altitude. Ergonomics 14:157–164, 1972.
206. Kobrick JL: Effects of hypoxia on peripheral visual response to dim stimuli. Percept Mot Skills 41:467–474, 1975.
207. Selvamurthy W, Saxena RK, Krishnamurthy N, et al: Changes in EEG pattern during acclimatization to high altitude (3500 meters) in man. Aviat Space Environ Med 49:968–971, 1968.
208. Forster HV, Soto RJ, Dempsey JA, et al: Effect of sojourn at 4300 meters altitude on electroencephalogram and visual evoked response. J Appl Physiol 39:109–113, 1975.
209. Clark CF, Heaton RK, Wiens AN: Neuropsychological functioning after prolonged high altitude exposure in mountaineering. Aviat Space Environ Med 54:202–207, 1983.
210. Sharma VM, Malhotra MS: Ethnic variations in psychological performance under altitude stress. Aviat Space Environ Med 47:248–251, 1976.
211. Sharma, VM, Malhotra MS, Baskoran AS: Variations in psychomotor efficiency during prolonged stay at high altitude. Ergonomics 18:511–516, 1975.
212. Ryn Z: Psychopathology in alpinism. Acta Med Pol 12:453–467, 1976.
212a. Regard M, Oelz O, Brugger P, et al: Persistent cognitive impairment in climbers after repeated exposure to high altitude. Neurology 39:210–213, 1989.

213. Hornbein TF, Townes B, Houston CS: The cost to the central nervous system of climbing to extremely high altitude. N Engl J Med 321:1714–1719, 1989.

213a. Garrido E, Costello A, Ventura JL, et al: Cortical atrophy and other brain magnetic resonance imaging (MRI) changes after extremely high altitude climbs without oxygen. Int J Sports Med 14:232–234, 1993.

214. Mosso A: La respiration periodique et la respiration superflue ou de luxe. Arch Ital Biol 7:48–127, 1886.

215. Sutton JR, Gray GW, Houston CS, et al: Effects of duration at altitude and acetazolamide in ventilation and oxygenation during sleep. Sleep 3:455–464, 1980.

216. Lahiri S, Maret KH, Sherpa MG, et al: Sleep and periodic breathing at high altitude: Sherpa natives versus sojourners. *In* West JB, Lahiri S (eds): High Altitude and Man. Bethesda, MD: American Physiological Society, 1984 pp. 73–90.

217. Berssenbrugge A, Dempsey J, Skatrud J: Hypoxic versus hypocapnic effects on periodic breathing during sleep. *In* West JB, Lahiri, S (eds): High Altitude and Man. Bethesda, MD: American Physiological Society, 1984, pp. 115–128.

218. Badr MS, Skatrud J-B, Simon PM, et al: Effect of hypercapnia on total pulmonary resistance during wakefulness and during NREM sleep. Am Rev Respir Dis 144:406–414, 1991.

219. Lahiri S, Maret K, Sherpa MG: Dependence of high-altitude sleep apnea on ventilatory sensitivity to hypoxia. Respir Physiol 52:281–301, 1983.

220. West JB, Peters RM Jr, Aksnes G, et al: Nocturnal periodic breathing at altitudes of 6300 and 8050 meters. J Appl Physiol 61:280–287, 1987.

221. Sutton JR, Houston CS, Mansele AL, et al: Effect of acetazolamide on hypoxia during sleep at high altitude. N Engl J Med 301:1329–1331, 1979.

222. Swenson ER, Leatham KL, Roach RC, et al: Renal carbonic anhydrase inhibition reduces high altitude periodic breathing. Respir Physiol 86:333–334, 1991.

223. Kryger M, McCullough RE, Collins D, et al: Treatment of chronic mountain polycythemia with respiratory stimulation. Am Rev Respir Dis 117:455–464, 1978.

224. Hackett PH, Roach RC, Harrison G, et al: Respiratory stimulants and sleep periodic breathing at high altitude: Almitrine versus acetazolamide. Am Rev Respir Dis 135:896–898, 1987.

225. Keynes RJ, Smith GW, Slater JDH, et al: Renin and aldosterone at high altitude in man. J Endocrinol 92:131–140, 1982.

226. Williams ES, Ward MP, Milledge JS, et al: Effect of the exercise of seven days hill-walking on fluid homeostasis. Clin Sci 56:305–316, 1979.

227. Pugh LGCE: Cardiac output in muscular exercise at 5800 m (19,000 feet). J Appl Physiol 19:441–447, 1964.

228. West JB, Boyer SJ, Graber DJ, et al: Maximal exercise at extreme altitudes on Mount Everest. J Appl Physiol 55:688–702, 1983.

229. West JB, Lahiri S, Gill MB, et al: Arterial oxygen saturation during exercise at high altitude. J Appl Physiol 17:617–621, 1962.

230. Sutton JR, Reeves JT, Wagner PD, et al: Operation Everest II: Oxygen transport during exercise at extreme simulated altitude. J Appl Physiol 64:1309–1321, 1988.

231. Wagner PD, Gale GE, Moon RE, et al: Pulmonary gas exchange in humans exercising at sea level and simulated altitude. J Appl Physiol 61:280–287, 1986.

232. Dill DB, Myhre LG, Phillips EE Jr, et al: Work capacity in acute exposures to altitude. J Appl Physiol 21:1168–1176, 1966.

233. Stenberg, J, Ekblom B, Messin R: Hemodynamic response to work at simulated altitude. J Appl Physiol 21:1559–1594, 1966.

234. Squires RW, Buskirk ER: Aerobic capacity during acute exposure to simulated altitude 914 to 2286 m. Med Sci Sports Exerc 14:36–40, 1982.

235. Cerretelli P: Limiting factors to oxygen transport on Mount Everest. J Appl Physiol 40:658–667, 1976.

236. Schoene RB, Lahiri S, Hackett, PH, et al: Relationship of hypoxic ventilatory response to exercise performance on Mount Everest. J Appl Physiol 56:1478–1483, 1984.

237. Schoene RB: Hypoxic ventilatory response and exercise ventilation at sea level and high altitude. *In* West JB, Lahiri S (eds): Man at High Altitude. Bethesda, MD: American Physiological Society, 1984, pp. 19–30.

238. Schoene RB: The control of ventilation in climbers to extreme altitude. J Appl Physiol 53:886–890, 1982.

239. Oelz O, Howald H, diPrampero PE, et al: Physiological profile of world-class high-altitude climbers. J Appl Physiol 60:1734–1742, 1986.

240. Masuyama S, Kimura H, Sugita, T, et al: Control of ventilation in extreme-altitude climbers. J Appl Physiol 61:500–506, 1986.

240a. Serebrouskaya TV, Ivashkevich AA: Effect of a 1-year stay at altitude on ventilation, metabolism, and work capacity. J Appl Physiol 73:1749–1755, 1992.

241. Lahiri S, Kao FF, Velasquez T, et al: Respiration of man during exercise at high altitude: Highlanders vs. lowlanders. Respir Physiol 8:361–375, 1970.

242. Torre-Bueno JR, Wagner PD, Saltzman HA, et al: Diffusion limitation in normal humans during exercise at sea level and simulated altitude. J Appl Physiol 58:989–995, 1985.

243. Saltin B, Grover RF, Blomqvist CG, et al: Maximal oxygen uptake and cardiac output after two weeks at 4300 meters. J Appl Physiol 25:400–409, 1968.

244. Pugh LGCE: Cardiac output in muscular exercise at 5800 meters. J Appl Physiol 19:441–447, 1964.

245. Reeves, JT, Groves BM, Sutton JR, et al: Operation Everest II: Preservation of cardiac function at extreme altitude. J Appl Physiol 63:531–539, 1987.

246. Grover RF, Reeves, JT, Grover EB, et al: Muscular exercise in young men native to 3100 m altitude. J Appl Physiol 22:555–564, 1967.

247. Groves BM, Reeves JT, Sutton JR, et al: Operation Everest II: Elevated high altitude pulmonary resistance unresponsive to oxygen. J Appl Physiol 63:521–530, 1987.

248. Roca J, Hogan MC, Story D: Evidence for peripheral tissue diffusion limitation of maximum $O_2$ uptake. J Appl Physiol 67:291–299, 1989.

249. Hogan MC, Roca J, Wagner PD, et al: Limitation of maximal $O_2$ uptake and performance by acute hypoxia in dog muscle in situ. J Appl Physiol 65:815–821, 1988.

249a. Rowell LB, Saltin B, Kiens B, et al: Is peak quadriceps blood flow in humans even higher during exercise with hypoxemia? Am J Physiol 251:H1038–H1044, 1986.

249b. Richardson RS, Noyszewski EA, Kendrick KF, et al: Myoglobin $O_2$ desaturation during exercise: Evidence of a limited $O_2$ transport. J Clin Invest 96:1916–1926, 1995.

249c. Crenshaw AG, Fryden J, Thornell L, et al: Extreme endurance training: Evidence of capillary and mitochondrial compartmentalization in human skeletal muscle. Eur J Appl Physiol 63:173–178, 1991.

249d. Roca J, Agusti AG, Alonso A, et al: Effects of training on muscle $O_2$ transport at $Vo_{2max}$. J Appl Physiol 73:1067–1076, 1992.

249e. Green GA, Danall RA, Bierd TB, et al: Effect of aortic balloon inflation on ventilation and brain stem blood flow in piglets. J Appl Physiol 66:2174–2180, 1989.

249f. Jostarndt-Fogenk, Puntschart A, Hoppeler H, et al: Fiber-type specific expression of fast and slow essential myosin light chain mRNAs in trained human skeletal muscles. Acta Physiol Scand 146:299–308, 1998.

249g. Hoppeler H: Vascular growth in hypoxic skeletal muscle. *In* Roach RC, Wagner PD, Hackett PH (eds): Hypoxia: Into the Next Millennium. New York, Plenum, 1999, pp 277–286.

249h. Wagner PD: Limitations of oxygen transport to the cell. Medicine 21:391–398, 1995.

249i. Wagner PD: Gas exchange and peripheral diffusion limitation. Med Sci Sports Exerc 24:54–58, 1992.

249j. Wagner PD: Determinants of maximal oxygen transport and utilization. Annu Rev Physiol 58:21–50, 1996.

249k. Hogan MC, Bebout DE, Wagner PD, et al: Maximal oxygen uptake of in situ dog muscle during acute hypoxemia with constant profusion. J Appl Physiol 69:570–576, 1990.

249l. Richardson RS, Knight DR, Poole DC, et al: Determinants of maximal exercise $VO_2$ during single leg knee-extensor exercise in humans. Am J Physiol 268:H1453–H1461, 1995.

250. Cerretelli P, di Prampero PE: Aerobic and anaerobic metabolism during exercise at altitude. Med Sport Sci 19:1–19, 1985.

251. Green HJ, Sutton JR, Young P, et al: Operation Everest II: Muscle energetics during maximal exhaustive exercise. J Appl Physiol 66:142–150, 1989.

252. Bigard, AX, Brunet A, Guezennec CY, et al: Skeletal muscle changes after endurance training at high altitude. J Appl Physiol 71:2114–2121, 1991.
253. Horstman D, Weiskopf R, Jackson RE: Work capacity during three-week sojourn at 4300 meters: Effects of relative polycythemia. J Appl Physiol 49:311–318, 1980.
254. Buskirk ER, Kollias J, Akers RF, et al: Maximal performance at altitude and on return from altitude in conditioned runners. J Appl Physiol 23:259–266, 1967.
255. Maher JT, Jones LG, Hartley LH: Effects of high altitude exposure on submaximal endurance capacity of men. J Appl Physiol 37:895–898, 1974.
255a. Edwards HT: Lactic acid in rest and work at high altitude. Am J Physiol 116:367–375, 1936.
255b. West JB: Lactate during exercise at extreme altitude. Fed Proc 45:2953–2957, 1986.
255c. Cerretelli P: Limiting factors to oxygen transport on Mt. Everest. J Appl Physiol 40:658–667, 1976.
255d. Brooks GA, Wolfe E, Groves BM, et al: Muscle accounts for glucous disposal but not blood lactate experience during exercise after acclimatization to 4300 meters. J Appl Physiol 72:2435–2445, 1992.
255e. Brooks GA, Wolfe EE, Butterfield GE, et al: The poor relationship between arterial (lactate) and leg net release during exercise at 4300 meters altitude. Am J Physiol 275:R1192–R1201, 1998.
255f. Reeves JT, Wolfel EE, Green HJ, et al: Oxygen transport during exercise at altitude and the lactate paradox: Lessons from Operation Everest II in Pikes Peak. Exerc Sport Sci Rev 20:275–296, 1992.
255g. Brooks GA, Dubouchaud H, Brown M, et al: Role of mitochondrial lactate dehydrogenates and lactate oxidation in the intercellular lactate shuttle. Proc Natl Acad Sci USA 96:1129–1134, 1999.
256. Pugh LGCE: Athletes at altitude. J Physiol 192:619–646, 1967.
257. Dill DB, Myrhe LG, Phillips EE Jr, et al: Work capacity in acute exposure to altitude. J Appl Physiol 21:1168–1176, 1966.
258. Grover RF, Reeves JT, Grover EB, et al: Muscular exercise in young men native to 3100 meters altitude. J Appl Physiol 22:555–564, 1967.
259. Grover RF, Reeves JT: Exercise performance of athletes at sea level and 3100 meters altitude. Med Thorac 23:129–143, 1966.
260. Levine BD, Stray-Gundersen J: "Living high—training low": Effect of moderate-altitude acclimatization with low-altitude training on performance. J Appl Physiol 83:102–112, 1997.
260a. Chapman RF, Stray-Gunderson J, Levine BD: Individual variation and response to altitude training. J Appl Physiol 85:1448–1456, 1998.
260b. Rodriguez FA, Casas H, Cases M, et al: Intermittent hypobaric hypoxia stimulates erythropoiesis and improves aerobic capacity. Med Sci Sports Exerc 31:264–268, 1999.
261. Hackett PH, Rennie D, Levine HD: The incidence, importance, and prophylaxis of acute mountain sickness. Lancet 2:1149–1154, 1976.
261a. Honignan B, Theis MK, Koziol-McClain J, et al: Acute mountain sickness in a general tourist population at moderate altitudes. Ann Intern Med 118:587–592, 1993.
262. Sophocles AM: High-altitude pulmonary edema in Vail, Colorado, 1975–1982. West J Med 144:569–573, 1986.
262a. Yaron M, Waldman N, Miermeyer S, et al: The diagnosis of acute mountain sickness in pre-verbal children. Arch Pediatr Adolesc Med 152:683–687, 1998.
263. Hackett PH, Rennie D: Acute mountain sickness. Semin Respir Med 5:132–140, 1983.
264. Singh I, Khanna PK, Srivastava MC, et al: Acute mountain sickness. N Engl J Med 280:175–184, 1969.
265. Ravenhill TH: Some experiences of mountain sickness in the Andes. J Trop Med Hyg 16:313–320, 1913.
266. Hackett, PH: Mountain Sickness: Prevention, Recognition and Treatment. New York, American Alpine Club, 1980.
267. Montgomery AB, Mills J, Luce JM: Incidence of acute mountain sickness at intermediate altitude. JAMA 261:732–734, 1989.
268. Levine BD, Yoshimura K, Kobayashi T, et al: Dexamethasone in the treatment of acute mountain sickness. N Engl J Med 321:1707–1713, 1989.
269. Kobayashi T, Koyama S, Kubo K, et al: Clinical features of patients with high altitude pulmonary edema in Japan. Chest 92:814–821, 1987.
269a. Hackett PH, Rennie D: Avoiding mountain sickness. Lancet 2:938, 1978.
270. Hackett PH, Yarnell P, Hill RP: MRI in high altitude cerebral edema: Evidence for vasogenic edema (abstract). *In* Sutton JR, Coates G, Remmers JE (eds): Hypoxia: The Adaptations. Philadelphia, BC Decker, 1990, p. 295.
270a. Hackett PH, Yarnell PR, Hill R, et al: High altitude cerebral edema evaluated with magnetic resonance imaging: Clinical correlation and pathophysiology. JAMA 280:1920–1925, 1998.
271. Hartig GS, Hackett PH: Cerebral spinal fluid pressure and cerebral blood velocity in acute mountain sickness. *In* Sutton JR, Coates G, Houston CS (eds): Hypoxia and Mountain Medicine. Burlington, VT: Queen City Printers, 1992, pp. 260– 265.
272. Jensen JB, Wright AD, Lassen NA, et al: Cerebral blood flow in acute mountain sickness. J Appl Physiol 69:430–433, 1990.
273. Otis SM, Rossman ME, Schneider PA, et al: Relationship of cerebral blood flow regulation to acute mountain sickness. J Ultrasound Med 8:143–148, 1989.
273a. Buzzi MG, Bonamini M, Moskowitz MA: Neurogenic model of migraine. Cephalalgia 15:277–280, 1995.
274. Grissom CK, Roach RC, Sarnquist FH, et al: Acetazolamide in the treatment of acute mountain sickness: Clinical efficacy and effect on gas exchange. Ann Intern Med 116:461–465, 1992.
275. Bartsch P, Maggiorini M, Schobersberger W, et al: Enhanced exercise-induced rise of aldosterone and vasopressin preceding mountain sickness. J Appl Physiol 711:136–143, 1991.
276. Moore LG, Harrison GL, McCullough RE, et al: Low acute hypoxic ventilatory response and hypoxic depression in acute altitude sickness. J Appl Physiol 60:1407–1412, 1986.
277. Hackett PH, Rennie ID, Hofmeister SE, et al: Fluid retention and relative hypoventilation in acute mountain sickness. Respiration 43:321–329, 1982.
278. Taber RL: Protocols for the use of a portable hyperbaric chamber for the treatment of high altitude disorders. J Wilderness Med 1:181–192, 1990.
279. Hackett PH, Roach RC, Goldberg S, et al: A portable, fabric hyperbaric chamber for treatment of high altitude pulmonary edema (abstract). *In* Sutton JR, Coates G, Remmers JE: Hypoxia: The Adaptations. Philadelphia: BC Decker, 1990, p. 291.
280. Kasic JF, Yaron M, Nicholas RA, et al: Treatment of acute mountain sickness: Hyperbaric versus oxygen therapy. Ann Emerg Med 20:1109–1112, 1991.
281. Olson LG, Hensley MJ, Saunders NA: Augmentation of ventilatory response to asphyxia by prochlorperazine in humans. J Appl Physiol 53:637–643, 1982.
282. Gray GW, Bryan AC, Frayser R, et al: Control of acute mountain sickness. Aerospace Med 1:81–84, 1971.
283. Ferrazzini G, Maggiorini M, Kriemler S, et al: Successful treatment of acute mountain sickness with dexamethasone. BMJ 294:1380–1382, 1986.
284. Hackett PH, Roach RC, Wood RA, et al: Dexamethasone for prevention and treatment of acute mountain sickness. Aviat Space Environ Med 59:950–954, 1988.
285. Levine BD, Yoshimura K, Kobayashi T, et al: Dexamethasone in the treatment of acute mountain sickness. N Engl J Med 321:1707–1713, 1989.
286. Hansen JE, Hartley LH, Hogan RP: Arterial oxygen increase by high carbohydrate diet at altitude. J Appl Physiol 33:441–445, 1972.
287. Consolazio CF, Matoush LO, Johnson HL, et al: Effects of a high carbohydrate diet on performance and clinical symptomatology after rapid ascent to high altitude. Fed Proc 28:937–943, 1969.
287a. Swenson ER, MacDonald A, Vathever M, et al: Acute mountain sickness is not altered by a high carbohydrate diet nor associated with elevated circulating cytokines. Aviat Space Environ Med 68:499–503, 1997.
288. Birmingham Medical Research Expeditionary Society Mountain Sickness Study Group: Acetazolamide in control of acute mountain sickness. Lancet 1:180–183, 1981.
289. Greene MK, Kerr AM, McIntosh IB, et al: Acetazolamide in prevention of acute mountain sickness: A double blind controlled cross-over study. BMJ 283:811–813, 1981.

290. Johnson TS, Rock PB, Fulco CS, et al: Prevention of acute mountain sickness by dexamethasone. N Engl J Med 310:683–686, 1984.
291. Ellsworth AJ, Larson EB, Strickland D: A randomized trial of dexamethasone and acetazolamide for acute mountain sickness prophylaxis. Am J Med 83:1024–1030, 1987.
292. Ellsworth AJ, Meyer EF, Larson EB: Acetazolamide and dexamethasone use versus placebo to prevent acute mountain sickness on Mount Rainier. West J Med 154:289–293, 1991.
293. Zell, SC, Goodman PH: Acetazolamide and dexamethasone in the prevention of acute mountain sickness. West J Med 148:541–545, 1988.
294. Houston CS, Dickinson JD: Cerebral form of high altitude illness. Lancet 2:758–761, 1975.
295. Dickinson JD, Heath D, Gosney J, et al: Altitude-related deaths in seven trekkers in the Himalayas. Thorax 38:646–656, 1983.
296. Crowley A, Symonds J, Grant K (eds): The Confessions of Alistair Crowley: An Autobiography. New York, Bantam Books, 1971.
296a. Hultgren H, Spickard W: Medical experiences in Peru. Stanford Med Bull 18:76–95, 1960.
297. Houston CS: Acute pulmonary edema of high altitude. N Engl J Med 263:478–480, 1960.
298. Hultgren HN, Lopez CE, Lundberg E, et al: Physiologic studies of pulmonary edema at high altitude. Circulation 29:393–408, 1964.
299. Nayak NC, Roy S, Narayaran TK: Pathologic features of altitude sickness. Am J Pathol 45:381–391, 1964.
300. Arias-Stella J, Kruger H: Pathology of high altitude pulmonary edema. Arch Pathol 76:4353, 1963.
301. Schoene RB, Swenson ER, Pizzo CJ, et al: The lung at high altitude: Bronchoalveolar lavage in acute mountain sickness and pulmonary edema. J Appl Physiol 64:2605–2613, 1988.
301a. Kubo K, Hanaoka M, Yamaguchi S, et al: Cytokines in bronchoalveolar lavage fluid in patients with high altitude pulmonary oedema at moderate altitude in Japan. Thorax 51:739–742, 1996.
302. Hultgren HN: High altitude pulmonary edema. *In* Hegnauer A (ed): Biomedical Problems of High Terrestrial Altitudes. Springfield, VA, Federal Scientific and Technical Information, 1967, pp. 131–141.
303. Hackett PH, Creagh CE, Grover RF, et al: High altitude pulmonary edema in persons without the right pulmonary artery. N Engl J Med 302:1070–1073, 1980.
304. Staub NC: Overperfusion edema. N Engl J Med 302:1085–1086, 1980.
305. Viswanathan R, Subramanian S, Radha TG: Effect of hypoxia on regional lung perfusion, by scanning. Respiration 37:142–147, 1979.
306. West JBV, Mathiea-Costello O: Structure, strength, failure, and remodeling of the pulmonary blood-gas barrier. Annu Rev Physiol 61:543–572, 1999.
306a. Tsukimoto K, Yoshimura N, Ichioka M, et al: Protein, cell, and leukotriene $B_4$ concentrations of lung edema fluid produced by high capillary pressures in rabbit. J Appl Physiol 76:321–327, 1994.
306b. West JB, Mathieu-Costello O: Strength of the pulmonary blood-gas barrier. Respir Physiol 88:141–148, 1992.
306c. West JB, Tsukimoto K, Mathieu-Costello O, et al: Stress failure in pulmonary capillaries. J Appl Physiol 70:1731–1742, 1991.
306d. Steinacker JM, Tobias P, Mendd E, et al: Lung diffusing capacity and exercise in subjects with previous high-altitude pulmonary oedema. Eur Respir J 11:643–650, 1998.
306e. Hanaoka M, Kubo K, Yamazaki Y, et al: Association of high-altitude pulmonary edema with the major histocompatibility complex. Circulation 97:1124–1128, 1998.
307. Yagi H, Yamada H, Kobayashi T, et al: Doppler assessment of pulmonary hypertension induced by hypoxic breathing in subjects susceptible to high altitude pulmonary edema. Am Rev Respir Dis 142:796–801, 1990.
308. Hultgren HN, Grover RF, Hartley LH: Abnormal circulatory responses to high altitude in subjects with a previous history of high altitude pulmonary edema. Circulation 44:759–770, 1971.
308a. Sartori C, Vollenweider L, Loffler BM, et al: Exaggerated endothelin release in high-altitude pulmonary edema. Circulation 99:2665–2668, 1999.
308b. Duplain H, Vollenweider L, Delabays A, et al: Augmented sympathetic activation during short-term hypoxia and high-altitude exposure in subjects susceptible to high-altitude pulmonary edema. Circulation 99:1713–1718, 1999.
309. Oelz O, Maggiorini M, Ritter M, et al: Nifedipine for high altitude pulmonary edema. Lancet 2:1241–1244, 1989.
310. Hackett PH, Greene ER, Roach RC, et al: Nifedipine and hydralazine for treatment of high altitude pulmonary edema (abstract). *In* Sutton JR, Coates G, Remmers JE (eds): Hypoxia: The Adaptations. Philadelphia, BC Decker, 1990, p. 291.
311. Bartsch P, Maggiorini M, Ritter M, et al: Prevention of high-altitude pulmonary edema by nifedipine. N Engl J Med 325:1284–1289, 1991.
312. Brigham KL, Woolverton WC, Blake LH, Staub NC: Increased sheep lung vascular permeability caused by *Pseudomonas* bacteremia. J Clin Invest 54:792–804, 1974.
312a. Scherrer U, Vollenweider L, Delabays A, et al: Inhaled nitric oxide for high-altitude pulmonary edema. N Engl J Med 334:624–629, 1996.
312b. Kaminsky DA, Jones K, Schoene RB, et al: Urinary leukotriene E4 levels in high-altitude pulmonary edema. A possible role for inflammation. Chest 110:939–945, 1996.
313. Maron MB: Analysis of airway fluid protein concentration in neurogenic pulmonary edema. J Appl Physiol 62:470–476, 1987.
314. Kobayashi T, Koyama S, Kubo K, et al: Clinical features of patients with high altitude pulmonary edema in Japan. Chest 92:814–821, 1987.
315. Koyama S, Kobayashi T, Kubo K, et al: The increased sympathoadrenal activity in patients with high altitude pulmonary edema is centrally mediated. Jpn J Med 27:10–16, 1988.
316. Malik AB: Pulmonary vascular response to increase in intracranial pressure: Role of sympathetic mechanisms. J Appl Physiol 42:335–343, 1977.
317. Hackett PH, Hartig G, Greene D, et al: Sympathetic blockade and high altitude pulmonary edema. FASEB J 6:A1468, 1992.
318. Hackett PH, Roach RC, Schoene RB, et al: Abnormal control of ventilation in high-altitude pulmonary edema. J Appl Physiol 64:1268–1272, 1988.
319. Masuyama B, Kimura H, Kuriyama T, et al: Relationship between disordered breathing during sleep at high altitude and ventilatory chemosensitivities to hypoxia and hypercapnia (abstract). *In* Sutton JR, Houston CS, Coates G (eds): Hypoxia. The Tolerable Limits. Indianapolis, IN: Benchmark Press, 1988, p. 378.
320. Stene J, Gelblum J, McCauley M, et al: Influence of cervical spinal cord transection in ICU patients on pulmonary vascular reflexes to brief cold air (5 degrees C) in the nose (abstract). *In* Sutton JR, Houston CS, Jones NL (eds): Hypoxia, Exercise and Altitude. New York, Alan R. Liss, 1983, pp. 476–477.
321. Chauca D, Bligh J: An additive effect of cold exposure and hypoxia on pulmonary artery pressure in sheep. Res Vet Sci 21:123–124, 1976.
322. Schoene RB, Roach RC, Hackett PH, et al: High altitude pulmonary edema and exercise at 4400 meters on Mount McKinley: Effect of expiratory positive airway pressure. Chest 87:330–333, 1985.
323. Menon ND: High altitude pulmonary edema. N Engl J Med 273:66–72, 1965.
324. Frayser R, Houston CS, Bryan AC, et al: Retinal hemorrhage at high altitude. N Engl J Med 282:1183–1184, 1970.
325. Hackett PH, Rennie ID: Rales, peripheral edema, retinal hemorrhage and acute mountain sickness. Am J Med 67:214–218, 1979.
326. McFadden DM, Houston CS, Sutton JR, et al: High altitude retinopathy. JAMA 245:581–586, 1981.
327. Lubin JR, Rennie ID, Hackett PH, Albert, DM: High altitude retinal hemorrhage: A clinical and pathological case report. Ann Ophthalmol 14:1071–1076, 1982.
328. Hackett PH, Hollingshead KF, Roach R, et al: Cortical blindness in high altitude climbers and trekkers-A report of 6 cases (abstract). *In* Sutton JR, Houston CS, Coates G (eds): Hypoxia and Cold. New York, Praeger Press, 1987, p. 536.
329. Heath D, Williams DR: Man at High Altitude, 2nd ed. Edinburgh, Churchill Livingstone, 1981.
330. Hyers TM, Scoggin CH, Will DH, et al: Accentuated hypoxemia at high altitude in subjects susceptible to high altitude pulmonary edema. J Appl Physiol 46:41–46, 1979.

331. Maher JT, Levine PH, Cymermen A: Human coagulation abnormalities during acute exposure to hypobaric hypoxia. J Appl Physiol 41:702–707, 1976.
332. O'Bradovich H, Andrew M, Gray GW, et al: Hypoxia alters blood coagulation during acute decompression in humans. J Appl Physiol 56:666–670, 1984.
333. Singh I, Chohan IS, Mathew NT: Fibrinolytic activity in high altitude pulmonary edema. Indian J Med Res 57:210–217, 1969.
334. Singh I: Pulmonary Hypertension in New Arrivals at High Altitude. Proceedings of World Health Organization Meeting on Primary Pulmonary Hypertension, October 1973. Geneva, WHO, 1974.
335. Bartsch P, Haeberli A, Franciolli M, et al: PW: Coagulation and fibrinolysis in acute mountain sickness and beginning pulmonary edema. J Appl Physiol 66:2136–2144, 1989.
336. Sui GJ, Liu YH, Cheng XS, et al: Subacute infantile mountain sickness. J Pathol 155:161–170, 1988.
337. Anand IS, Malhotra RM, Chandrashekhar Y, et al: Adult subacute mountain sickness—A syndrome of congestive heart failure in man at very high altitude. Lancet 335:561–565, 1990.
338. Anand IS, Phil D, Chandrashekhar Y: Subacute mountain sickness syndromes: Role of pulmonary hypertension. *In* Sutton JR, Coates G, Houston CS (eds): Hypoxia and Mountain Medicine. Burlington, VT: Queen City Printers, 1992, pp. 241–251.
339. Monge MC: La enfermedad de los Andes: Sindromes eritremicos. Ann Fac Med Univ San Marcos (Lima) 11:1–316, 1928.
339a. Leon-Velarde F, Ramos MA, Hernandez JA, et al: The role of menopause in the development of chronic mountain sickness. Am J Physiol 272(1 Pt 2):R90–R94, 1997.
340. Xie C-F, Pei S-X: Some physiological data on sojourners and native highlanders at three different altitudes in Xizang. *In* Shang LD (ed): Proceedings of Symposium on Tibet Plateau. New York, Gordon and Breach Science Publishers, 1981, pp. 1449–1452.
341. Kryger M, McCullough R, Doekel R, et al: Excessive polycythemia of high altitude: Role of ventilatory drive and lung disease. Am. Rev. Respir. Dis. 118:659–666, 1978.
342. Kryger MH, Grover RF: Chronic mountain sickness. Semin Respir Med 5:164–168, 1983.
343. Monge CC: Natural acclimatization to high altitudes: Clinical conditions in life at high altitudes. Scientific publication No. 140, Washington, DC, Pan American Health Organization, 1996, pp. 46–52.
344. Winslow RM: Relationship between erythropoiesis and ventilation in high altitude natives. *In* Lahiri S, Cherniack NS, Fitzerland RS (eds): Response and Adaptation to Hypoxia. Organ to Organelle. New York, Oxford University Press, 1991, pp. 143–156.
345. Zhuang J, Droma T, Sun S, et al: Hypoxic ventilatory responsiveness in Tibetan compared to Han residents at 3650 m. J Appl Physiol 74:303–311, 1993.
346. Weil JV, Kryger MH, Scoggin CH: Sleep and breathing at high altitude. *In* Guilleminault C, Dement WC (eds): Sleep Apnea Syndromes. New York, Alan R. Liss, 1978, pp. 119–136.
347. Kryger M, McCullough RE, Collins D, et al: Treatment of excessive polycythemia of high altitude with respiratory stimulant drugs. Am Rev Respir Dis 117:455–464, 1978.
348. Hultgren HN, Marticorena EA: High altitude pulmonary edema: Epidemiologic observations in Peru. Chest 74:372–376, 1978.
349. Scoggin CH, Hyers TM, Reeves JT, et al: High altitude pulmonary edema in the children and young adults of Leadville, Colorado. N Engl J Med 297:1269–1273, 1977.
350. Kamat SR, Sitaram S, Raju VRK, et al: A study of some cardiorespiratory parameters in newcomers to high altitude. *In* Malhotra MS (ed.): Human Adaptability to Environments and Physical Fitness. Madras: Defence Institute of Physiology and Allied Sciences, 1966, p. 141.
351. Malhotra MS, Selvamurthy W, Purkayastha, SS, et al: Responses of the autonomic nervous system during acclimatization to high altitude in man. Aviat Space Environ Med 47:1076–1079, 1976.
352. Pugh LGCE: Report of medical research project into effects of altitude in Mexico City. *In* Åstrand PO, Rodahl K (eds): Textbook of Work Physiology. New York, McGraw-Hill, 1977, p. 652.
353. Kamat SR, Banerji BC: Study of cardiopulmonary function on exposure to high altitude: Acute acclimatization to an altitude of 3500 to 4000 meters. Am Rev Respir Dis 106:404–413, 1972.
354. Grover RF, Tucker, CE, McGroarty SR, et al: The coronary stress of skiing at high altitude. Arch Intern Med 150:1205–1208, 1990.
355. Grover RF, Lufschanowski R, Alexander JK: Decreased coronary blood flow in man following ascent to high altitude. Adv Cardiol 5:72–79, 1970.
356. Morgan BJ, Alexander, JK, Nicoli SA, et al: The patient with coronary heart disease at altitude: Observations during acute exposure to 3100 meters. J Wilderness Med 1:147–153, 1990.
356a. Roach RC, Houston CS, Honigman B, et al: How well do older persons tolerate moderate altitude? West J Med 162:32–36, 1995.
356b. Levine BD, Zuckerman JH, deFilippi CR: Effect of high-altitude exposure on the elderly: The Tenth Mountain Division study. Circulation 96:1224–1232, 1997.
356c. Halhaber M, Humpler E, Inama K, et al: Does altitude cause exhaustion of the heart and circulatory system? Med Sport Sci 19:192–202, 1985.
356d. Shlim DR, Gallie J: The causes of death among trekkers in Nepal. Int J Sports Med 13(Suppl 1):S74–S76, 1992.
356e. Dickinson J, Heath D, Gosney J, et al: Altitude-related deaths in seven trekkers in the Himalayas. Thorax 38:646–656, 1983.
357. Rennie ID: Will mountain trekkers have heart attacks? (editorial) JAMA 261:1045–1046, 1989.
358. Hultgren HN: Coronary heart disease and trekking. J Wilderness Med 1:154–162, 1990.
359. Regensteiner JG, Moore LG: Migration of the elderly from high altitudes in Colorado. JAMA 253:3124–3128, 1985.
360. Graham WG, Houston CS: Short-term adaptation to moderate altitude: Patients with chronic obstructive pulmonary disease. JAMA 240:1491–1494, 1978.
360a. Dillard T. Rosenberg A, Berg B, et al: Hypoxemia during altitude exposure. A meta-analysis of chronic obstructive pulmonary disease. Chest 103:422–425, 1993.
360b. Gong H Jr, Tashkin DP, Lee EY, et al: Hypoxia-altitude simulation test. Evaluation of patients with chronic airway obstruction. Am Rev Respir Dis 130:980–986, 1984.
360c. Gong H Jr: Air travel and oxygen therapy in cardiopulmonary patients. Chest 101:1104–1113, 1992.
360d. Simon HU, Grotzer M, Nikolaizik WH, et al: High altitude climate therapy reduces peripheral blood T lymphocyte activation, eosinophilia, and bronchial obstruction in children with housedust mite allergic asthma. Pediatr Pulmonol 17:304–311, 1994.
360e. Matsuda S, Onda T, Iikura Y: Bronchial response of asthmatic patients in an atmosphere-changing chamber: 2. Effects of exercise at high altitude. Int Arch Allergy Immunol 107:402–405, 1995.
361. Moore LG, Regensteiner JG: Adaptation to high altitude. Ann Rev Anthropol 12:285–304, 1983.
362. Moore LG, Rounds SS, Jahnipen D, et al: Infant birth rate is related to maternal arterial oxygenation at high altitude. J Appl Physiol 52:695–699, 1982.
363. Ritchie K: The fetal response to changes in the composition of maternal inspired air in human pregnancy. Semin Perinatol 4:295–299, 1980.
364. Copher DE, Huber CP: Heart rate response of the human fetus to induced maternal hypoxia. Am J Obstet Gynecol 98:320–335, 1967.

# 71 Diving Medicine

ALFRED A. BOVE, M.D., PH.D. • TOM NEUMAN, M.D.


Introduction
- Increased Pressure
- Relation to Altitude
- Water Immersion
- Thermal Exposure
- Energy Needs for Diving

Equipment
- Open Circuit Scuba
- Closed Circuit Scuba
- Surface Supplied Equipment

Nomenclature of the Disorders Related to Diving

Pressure Effects: Boyle's Law
- Relation of Gas Volume to Depth
- Barotrauma
- Pulmonary Barotrauma and Arterial Gas Embolism
- Pathophysiology
- Clinical Manifestations of Arterial Air Embolism
- Middle Ear Barotrauma
- Alternobaric Vertigo
- Inner Ear Barotrauma
- Sinus Barotrauma
- Facial Barotrauma
- Skin Barotrauma
- Tooth Barotrauma
- Gastrointestinal Barotrauma

Dissolved Inert Gas Effects
- Gas Solubility and Henry's Law
- Inert Gas Kinetics
- Gas Supersaturation in Tissues
- Decompression Sickness
- Factors Affecting Risk of Decompression Sickness
- Clinical Manifestations
- Treatment
- Hyperbaric Therapy
- Supplemental Oxygen and Fluids
- Diagnostic Testing
- Emergency Treatment

Inert Gas Narcosis

Medical Qualifications for Diving
- Exercise Requirements
- Sudden Unconsciousness
- Pulmonary Disorders
- Cardiac Disorders

Near Drowning
- Pathophysiology
- Clinical Presentation
- Cardiovascular System
- Pulmonary System
- Neurologic Status
- Treatment
- Prognosis

Summary




## INTRODUCTION

### Increased Pressure

Humans are exposed to increased pressure when submerged underwater and when subjected to elevated pressures in closed pressure vessels. Underwater exposure is experienced by divers who are subject to increasing pressure directly proportional to depth (Table 71.1). Pressure vessels include hyperbaric chambers used for treatment of medical and diving-related diseases, pressurized tunnels and caissons used for underwater construction, and underwater habitats. Divers entering the aquatic environment are also subject to limited mobility and the risk of heat loss. As depth and pressure increase, the diver

**Table 71.1 PRESSURE EQUIVALENTS FOR ALTITUDE AND DEPTH**

| | FEET | ATM | MM HG | PSI |
|---|---|---|---|---|
| Altitude | 12,000 | 0.636 | 483 | 9.3 |
| above | 8000 | 0.742 | 564 | 10.9 |
| sea level | 4000 | 0.863 | 656 | 12.7 |
| —Sea level— | 0 | 1 | 760 | 14.7 |
| | 33 | 2 | 1520 | 29.4 |
| Depth | 66 | 3 | 2280 | 44.1 |
| in | 99 | 4 | 3040 | 58.8 |
| seawater | 132 | 5 | 3800 | 73.5 |

ATM = atmospheres absolute; psi = pounds/square inch.

breathes gas of increased density using breathing equipment that provides oxygen and allows for elimination of carbon dioxide.

## Relation to Altitude

Table 71.1 also shows the effects of altitude on ambient pressure. Excursions to high altitude expose tissues to supersaturation of inert gases and to the risk of free gas formation in blood and tissues (discussed later). Divers with increased inert gas in tissues from diving can develop free gas in tissues when going to altitude after diving even though they follow established protocols for ascent from depth to the surface. Flying after diving is a common occurrence among sport divers who may fly in commercial aircraft (about 8000 ft equivalent altitude) shortly after diving. The excursion above sea level produces inert gas supersaturation, which may cause free gas to form in tissues and blood.

## Water Immersion

Increases in intrathoracic blood volume occur with water immersion.[1] Intrathoracic pressure at end expiration increases from −5 cm $H_2O$ while standing in air to −2 cm $H_2O$ during immersion,[2, 3] while abdominal pressure increases from −6 cm $H_2O$ in air to +12 cm $H_2O$ during immersion.[2, 4] The hydrostatic pressure of the water column prevents blood from pooling in the peripheral veins. The increase in transdiaphragmatic pressure and the absence of venous blood pooling increase venous return during immersion. (In this respect, immersion in water is analogous to a gravity-free state.) The magnitude of the increase in the intrathoracic blood volume during head-out immersion has been estimated to be about 500 mL.[1, 5] The central blood shifts result in an increase in cardiac output[6] and an increase in central venous pressure. The increase in intrathoracic blood volume causes release of natriuretic hormones from the heart and an immersion diuresis.

Although immersion effects are found in all divers, breath-hold divers also exhibit effects from diving while apneic.[7] Breath-hold divers can develop sudden unconsciousness during ascent from long apneic dives.[8, 9] This phenomenon is called *shallow water blackout* and is due to a progressive reduction in arterial $P_{O_2}$ as the breath-hold diver ascends with already reduced arterial $P_{O_2}$ due to metabolic needs.

## Thermal Exposure

Diving exposures can produce temperatures ranging from near the freezing point of seawater (−2.2°C) to the 40°C experienced when divers descend into inactive nuclear reactors for inspection operations. Most diving is done in water with temperature below the skin temperature (30°C), and the diver loses heat throughout the dive. Therefore, hypothermia is a constant hazard in diving and will occur rapidly in the absence of protective garments even in relatively warm water (e.g., 22°C to 23°C). Heat loss is inhibited in divers doing moderate work in water above 30°C, and hyperthermia can develop. A diver must be in 33°C water to be thermoneutral at rest.

As in other forms of hypothermia, initial sensations of cold give way to shivering as a means of heat production. Below 23°C, an unprotected diver will become hypothermic after a short exposure. When body core temperature falls below 35°C, severe shivering is present; muscles of the forearm and hand are stiff, and fine motor function of the hands is impaired.[10] Inability to use the hands may become a safety hazard in cold water diving. Thermal protection for diving generally can be classified as "wet" or "dry." Wet suits are foam neoprene and contain an insulating layer of water situated between the skin and the garment. Dry suits are designed to keep the diver free from water contact. A thin outer garment is an impenetrable barrier. The insulation is derived from undergarments, which utilize trapped air as an insulating medium. The trapped water layer and the nitrogen gas contained in the foam neoprene account for the resistance to heat transfer characteristic of wet suits. Compression of neoprene occurs with increasing depth, however, thereby reducing the effectiveness of the insulation. For example, a wet suit with 9 mm thickness of neoprene at the surface will be compressed to approximately 3 mm at a depth of 3 ATA (66 feet of seawater [fsw]). As a consequence, effective insulation is reduced. The undergarments of a dry suit tend to be compressed less because compressed air is added to the dry suit to maintain a constant suit volume as depth increases. Wearing a wet suit in relatively warm water (25°C) increases the risk of heat injury during physical exertion. Divers wearing no thermal protection in 15°C to 18°C water are able to maintain a normal core temperature during continuous exercise at a $\dot{V}O_2$ of 1.5 to 1.8 L/min. On the other hand, intermittent exercise at an equivalent intensity results in a decrease in core temperature in 25°C water.[11, 12] Likewise, brief periods of exercise at a $\dot{V}O_2$ of 2.4 L/min are insufficient to prevent a decline in rectal temperature in thermally protected divers in 5°C water. Combinations of higher water temperatures, greater or longer exercise intensities, and thermal protection may actually produce an increase in core temperature. Divers face heat loss even in tropical waters, which have temperatures ranging from 29°C to 31°C, and specialized dress for this type of exposure is available.

Diving dress for thermal protection has been developed for different levels of cold exposure. For exposures exceeding 1 to 2 hours with minimal work in 22°C water, a wet suit will provide adequate thermal protection.[13] When water temperature reaches 17°C, a dry suit with an air layer between the diver and the water is required for moderate working exposures; a wet suit can be used for short exposures. When temperature reaches 4°C, a heated wet suit is used to maintain a stable body temperature. When helium is used at depths exceeding 300 ft, some operations also heat the breathing gas to prevent hypothermia from respiratory heat loss. Below 600 ft, breathing gas must be heated.

Cold stress also evokes adaptive thermogenic responses, reflected by changes in $\dot{V}O_2$. The increase in $\dot{V}O_2$ relative to thermoneutral conditions may be immediate upon submersion and persist throughout continuous exercise. A rise in $\dot{V}O_2$ upon exposure to cold water represents an adaptive response that generates additional body heat in order to minimize a change in core temperature. A slower rise in $\dot{V}O_2$ can occur in divers wearing thermal protection. Slow heat loss is often unrecognized until severe hypothermia is present.

Peripheral vasoconstriction occurs in response to the stress of cold water diving. The magnitude of the vasoconstriction is dependent on body core temperature, which, in turn, is affected by the amount of thermal protection and the water temperature. Cold-induced vasoconstriction can persist throughout light to moderate exercise. The same adaptive response can contribute to nonfreezing cold injury when finger or toe temperatures remain below 8°C to 10°C for more than 30 minutes.

### Energy Needs for Diving

A scuba diver swimming underwater at a speed of 1.0 knot (about 100 ft/min) consumes about 25 mL/min/kg of oxygen (Fig. 71.1). This is a high workload and is uncommon in sport scuba diving. Because swimming energy is proportional to the square of velocity,[14] only extremely fit divers tolerate workloads for higher swimming speeds. A diver with a maximum oxygen consumption of 40 mL/min/kg would be able to tolerate swimming at 1.3 knots for a few minutes but would become extremely tachypneic to compensate for lactate production, and fatigue would develop rapidly. Swimming at 60% of maximum oxygen consumption (about 8 mets), a work level that is at or slightly below the anaerobic threshold,[15] can be sustained for long periods of time because lactate does not accumulate in the blood. For a diver with a maximum oxygen consumption of 40 mL/kg/min, sustainable swimming speed, working at 60% to 65% of maximum capacity, would be about 100 ft/min, while the diver with a maximum oxygen consumption of 25 mL/kg/min would be able to sustain a swimming speed of about 70 ft/min. Safety considerations suggest that the sport diver should be able to tolerate a peak work load of about 40 mL/kg/min and a sustained workload of about 24 mL/kg/min (60% of maximum). Scuba divers who maintain this level of physical conditioning can be expected to respond

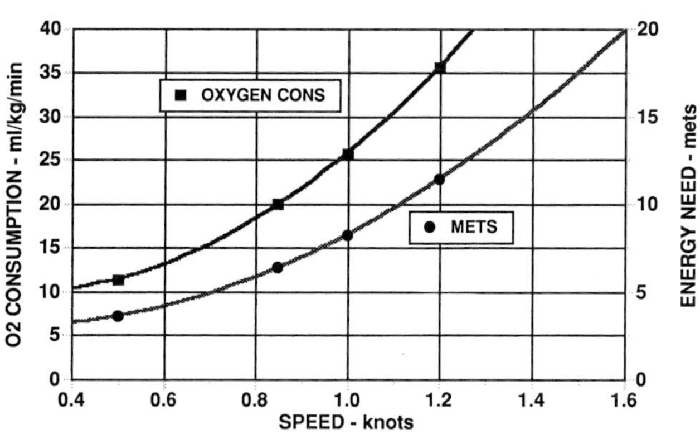


**Figure 71.1** Oxygen consumption and metabolic equivalents (mets) are shown for underwater swimming. Data are from the US Navy Diving Manual (reference 13).

appropriately to most diving workloads. Divers who do not achieve this conditioning level may have difficulty with even minor adverse conditions related to diving. As a result, severe dyspnea may accompany workloads above 65% of maximum aerobic capacity, a physical stress that often leads to panic and increases the risk for drowning.

## EQUIPMENT

### Open Circuit Scuba

The most commonly used breathing support system in diving is the open circuit scuba (self-contained underwater breathing apparatus). This equipment (Fig. 71.2) consists of a pressurized metal cylinder containing compressed air connected to a pressure regulator that lowers pressure first to about 100 psi over ambient pressure and then to ambient pressure in a demand-type regulator with a mouthpiece in the diver's mouth. This device delivers ambient pressure air only when inhalation is initiated and allows flow that matches the minute volume of the diver. The device may not deliver adequate flow at extremes of exercise, but such high flow rates are rarely needed. Their reliability and ease of use have allowed millions of amateur divers to partake in diving as a recreation. Use of open circuit scuba is limited by the amount of compressed air available in the cylinder carried by the diver. A typical scuba cylinder can supply approximately 2100 L of air at the surface (1 ATA). This volume is reduced in direct proportion to ambient pressure. For example, at a depth of 66 fsw (3 ATA) the effective volume of air is decreased to 700 L. With a minute ventilation of 20 L/min, this air supply would last 35 minutes; a 10% increase in minute ventilation will decrease time by about 3 minutes. Open circuit scuba is usually limited to depths above 200 ft because of limited air supply and concern for oxygen toxicity.

### Closed Circuit Scuba

To increase diving exposure time, self-contained equipment has advanced to a form that uses a $CO_2$ absorbent to remove exhaled carbon dioxide and replenishes only the oxygen used per minute. Inert gas is conserved by recycling the exhaled gas through a $CO_2$ absorbent and then adding oxygen before the gas is rebreathed in the closed system (see Fig. 71.2). This equipment has several advantages: little gas is released into the surrounding water, oxygen can be carried in volumes adequate for several hours of exposure, and gas consumption is independent of depth. With a mixture of oxygen and inert gas, some of these units can be used to depths exceeding 300 ft.[16] With 100% oxygen, depth is limited to 25 ft because of oxygen toxicity.

### Surface Supplied Equipment

Commercial diving developed when compressed air pumps were perfected and an appropriate diving helmet was developed. The helmet need only consist of an inverted cylinder closed at the top into which the diver's head is placed. The cylinder usually has several glass side

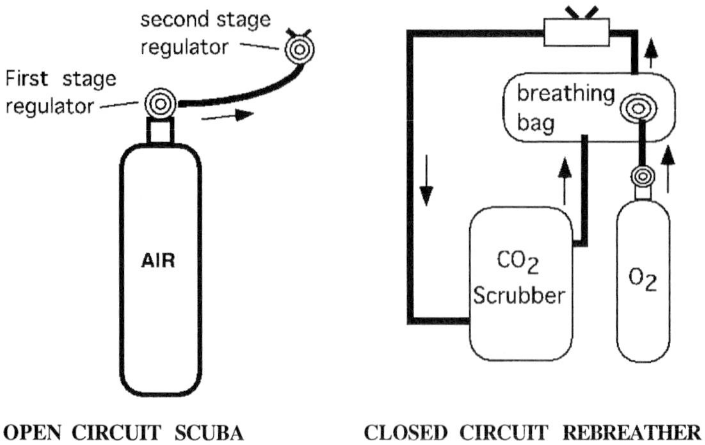


**Figure 71.2** The schematics show two types of self-contained diving systems. The open circuit scuba is the system commonly used for recreational diving. Air is exhaled into the surrounding water. Rebreather systems allow exhaled breathing gas to be recycled through a $CO_2$ scrubber, mixed with additional breathing gas, and returned to the diver through a breathing bag. Breathing gas is replenished via a demand valve. This system can be used with 100% oxygen or oxygen-enriched air mixtures. Other forms of rebreather systems contain separate oxygen and inert gas supplies, and mixing is controlled with a small computer to maintain a constant oxygen partial pressure.

ports for viewing and can be open at the bottom. The diver breathes compressed air pumped from the surface to the helmet, while the excess air flows out through the bottom of the helmet. Commercial divers have used this simple design for nearly two centuries. The modern diving helmet is attached at the collar to a diving dress so that air flows from the helmet into the suit to maintain an air layer for thermal protection. Excess air leaves the closed suit-helmet system via an exhaust valve.

## NOMENCLATURE OF THE DISORDERS RELATED TO DIVING

Golding and coworkers[17] described a scheme for categorizing decompression-related disorders that has become the standard nomenclature for describing pressure-related disorders. They described disorders related to supersaturation of inert gases in tissues with subsequent bubble formation as *decompression sickness.* They described a systemic form of decompression sickness that involves the central nervous system, the lungs, and the circulation ("serious," type II) and a nonsystemic (peripheral) form that involves the skin, bones, and joints ("minor," type I). *Barotrauma* and *arterial gas embolism* were named separately based on different pathophysiologic mechanisms.

Recently several clinical investigators proposed a new method for describing diseases related to decompression. *Decompression illness* is proposed to include disorders previously classified as decompression sickness and arterial gas embolism in a single diagnosis. Francis and Smith[18] provided a list of clinical descriptions that include the location, the symptoms and signs, and the progression of the disorder but not the underlying pathophysiology. They suggest that the two illnesses (decompression sickness and arterial gas embolism) are difficult to separate from one another clinically, and both require the same therapy. Under these circumstances, there is no need to differentiate the pathophysiologic mechanisms of the disease, and symptomatic description is adequate to propose a plan of therapy. In this chapter, we adhere to a pathophysiologic classification of the pressure disorders.

## PRESSURE EFFECTS: BOYLE'S LAW

### Relation of Gas Volume to Depth

Boyle's law states that if the temperature of a fixed mass of gas is kept constant, the relationship between the volume and pressure will vary in such a way that the product of the pressure and volume will remain constant.[19] This relationship is described by the equation $PV = K$, where P is absolute pressure, V is volume, and K is a constant. The temperature and mass are constant. Thus, at a constant temperature and mass, the volume of a gas is inversely proportional to the pressure exerted on that gas. Consequently, when the pressure is doubled, the volume is reduced to one half of the original volume. This relationship is graphically illustrated in Figure 71.3. Two different states of a gas at the same temperature may be denoted by subscripts 1 and 2. With this type of notation, Boyle's law may also be written as

$$P_1V_1 = P_2V_2$$

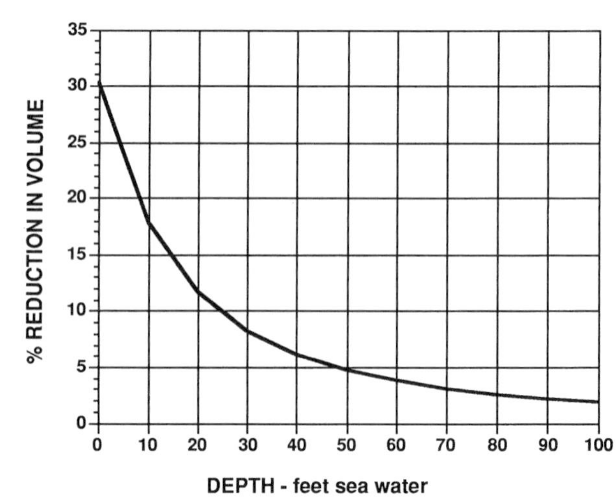


**Figure 71.3** The relation of volume changes to depth underwater is shown. Volume changes are greater per foot of depth change near the surface than in deeper depths.

Because the gas volume is proportional to the absolute pressure, the volume change from 33 to 66 fsw (2 to 3 ATA) is less than the change from the surface to 33 fsw (1 to 2 ATA). Understanding this relationship is important to the diver because it illustrates that changes of depth while in shallow water cause greater volume changes than equivalent changes of depth in deeper water. Rapid volume expansion in shallow water can cause tissue injury.

## Barotrauma

Because of the relation of gas volume to ambient pressure described by Boyle's law, volume in the lungs, middle ear, paranasal sinuses, gut, and so forth all are reduced as pressure increases. Displacement of tissues into the diminishing volume of these spaces causes a phenomenon called *squeeze,* which damages tissues, and may cause dysfunction of the organ involved. Barotrauma can affect a paranasal sinus with a blocked orifice (sinus squeeze), a small residual air pocket left between a tooth filling and the base of the tooth (tooth squeeze), the air space within a diving mask (mask squeeze), or between the skin and a fold in a dry diving suit (suit squeeze). All can produce tissue injury due to displacement of tissues into the diminishing air space. Although lung squeeze is theoretically possible by breath-hold diving to a depth that reduces the lung volume below the residual volume,[5] in practice this has not been observed probably because of the increased intrapulmonary blood volume and compression of the thorax. Squeeze is a common, usually minor consequence of diving. Middle ear barotrauma is the most common diving-related disorder encountered in divers.[20]

## Pulmonary Barotrauma and Arterial Gas Embolism

Injury to the lungs is a potentially lethal complication most often due to poor diving practices. When a diver subjected to increasing pressure breathes from an air supply at depth, the breathing gas is pressurized to the ambient pressure so that pressure gradients from breathing supply to the airways are not altered as the diver descends. Divers in swimming pools at depths greater than 4 ft are susceptible to pulmonary barotrauma. In the 1930s, a number of deaths were observed during submarine escape training in the US Navy. Studies by Behnke,[21] Polak and Adams,[22] and Shilling[23] showed that the mechanism was arterial air embolism caused by pulmonary barotrauma. They reported the features of this injury as separate from the already understood problem of decompression sickness (see later). Subsequently, fatalities were identified in which no evidence of prior pulmonary disease was present but pulmonary barotrauma occurred, resulting in air embolism. In some cases, obstruction of a single bronchus was thought to cause overexpansion of a lung segment.[24] Based on those observations, diving and submarine training was prohibited for subjects with a history of any disease that causes airway obstruction, and asthma was included. Later studies[25–27] provided further insight into mechanisms and prevention of pulmonary barotrauma. Asymptomatic anatomic abnormalities of the lung[22] and asthma[23] were thought to contribute to the risk of barotrauma. Recent data suggest that asthma is not an absolute contraindication (see later).

## Pathophysiology

Under experimental conditions, it has been demonstrated that transpulmonary pressures (i.e., the difference of intratracheal and intrapleural pressures) of 95 to 110 cm $H_2O$ are sufficient to disrupt pulmonary parenchyma and allow gases into the interstitium.[25] Extra-alveolar gas can migrate through the perivascular sheaths of the pulmonary vasculature to cause mediastinal emphysema and pneumothorax.[25] Gas can also dissect into the retroperitoneum and into the subcutaneous tissues of the neck. When intrathoracic pressure drops at the time of the first breath after the pulmonary barotrauma, extra-alveolar gas can pass into ruptured blood vessels, travel to the left side of the heart, and enter the arterial circulation as gaseous emboli.[26, 27] The dissemination of gas bubbles throughout the arterial circulation causes injury to other organ systems and to skeletal muscle, which is evident by a rise in serum creatine kinase level.[28]

Pulmonary barotrauma can occur in divers who would not be considered at risk for lung overpressure. Wilmshurst and coworkers[29] found that occult lung disease and probably smoking increase the risk of pulmonary barotrauma and cerebral air embolism. They also observed cerebral symptoms in individuals with evidence of patent foramen ovale, but considered the mechanism in these individuals to be related to decompression sickness with right to left shunting of bubbles. Tetzlaff and colleagues[30] suggested that prospective pulmonary function testing could be used as a means of separating individuals with a history of asthma who can dive safely from those who might be at risk for pulmonary barotrauma. They identified changes in the flow-volume curve, specifically, reduced midexpiratory flow at 25% of vital capacity in pulmonary barotrauma patients compared with patients who had decompression sickness but not pulmonary barotrauma. $FEV_1$ was similar in both groups. The authors also performed computed tomography (CT) of the chest and found 13 lung abnormalities among the 15 patients with pulmonary barotrauma. Although only four cases in the control group had CT of the chest, none had an abnormal finding. Although these studies are retrospective, both suggest that occult lung disease and asthma may contribute to unexplained cerebral air embolism. Epidemiologic studies, however, have not demonstrated a significant relationship between asthma and an increased risk for pulmonary barotrauma (see later under Medical Qualifications for Diving).

## Clinical Manifestations of Arterial Air Embolism

The most commonly involved organ is the brain where strokelike symptoms are found within minutes after the diver surfaces. Patients may present with varying neurologic and systemic signs and symptoms. The most frequently observed signs are loss of consciousness or stupor and confusion. Also frequently seen are seizures, vertigo, visual disturbances, sensory changes, headache, and circulatory collapse.[31] In a study of pulmonary barotrauma resulting from submarine escape training, Elliott and associates[31] found that most individuals fully recovered if they were promptly recompressed. However, one fourth to one third of victims in this group had recurrence of symptoms during decompression from the initial hyperbaric treatment and required a second recompression treatment. The signs and symptoms of this secondary process are similar to the initial presentation but are more gradual in onset and may include headache, progressive stupor, visual disturbances, and convulsions.

Victims of arterial gas embolism frequently suffer near-drowning episodes when they lose consciousness in the water. Chest radiographs (Fig. 71.4) may show a diffuse lung edema pattern. About 5% of patients immediately develop apnea, unconsciousness, and cardiac arrest. This catastrophic course results from filling of the central vascular bed with air. Many of these individuals are unresponsive to cardiopulmonary resuscitation and advanced life support measures.[32] Harker and coworkers[33] reported the pulmonary findings of 31 patients with cerebral air embolism from diving: 25% demonstrated pneumomediastinum; 10%, subcutaneous emphysema; 6%, pneumocardium; 3%, pneumoperitoneum; and 3%, pneumothorax. Fifty-two percent had pulmonary infiltrates indicating associated near drowning.

Extra-alveolar gas can enter the mediastinum and the subcutaneous spaces of the neck and can enter the pleural space. Mediastinal emphysema is generally associated with mild substernal pain or no symptoms. This pain is described as either a dull ache or tightness and may be exacerbated by inspiration, coughing, or swallowing. The pain may radiate to any portion of the upper torso. Unless massive, this condition is not usually associated with respiratory symptoms. On physical examination, a crunching sound synchronous with cardiac action may be auscultated (Hamman's sign). The chest radiograph confirms the diagnosis. No treatment is usually necessary.

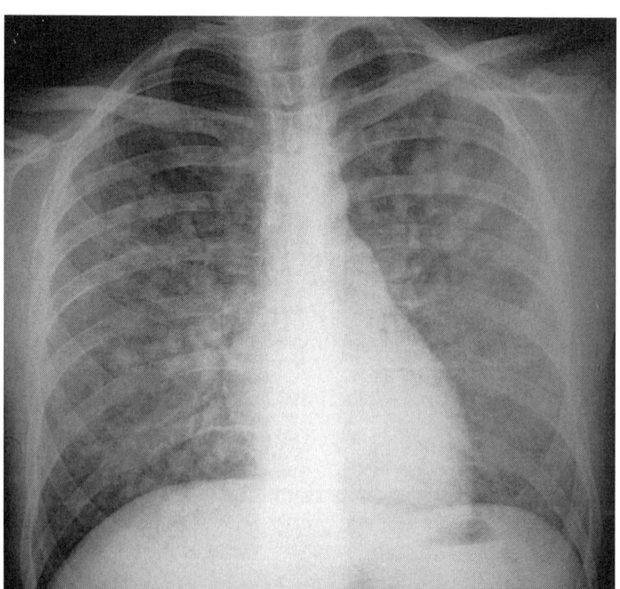

**Figure 71.4** Chest radiograph from a diver shows pulmonary barotrauma and near drowning. The diffuse pulmonary edema pattern is suggestive of water aspiration.

Air dissecting cephalad from the mediastinum causes subcutaneous emphysema in the neck. Swelling and crepitus in the root of the neck and supraclavicular fossa, sore throat, hoarseness, and dysphagia may result. Radiographs may be helpful in detecting subtle cases. When extra-alveolar gas ruptures into the pleural space (either from the mediastinum through the parietal pleura or from the perivascular tissues through the visceral pleura), a pneumothorax results. Laboratory evaluation may show an elevated hematocrit level and elevation of several serum enzyme levels.[28] Treatment for arterial gas embolism requires recompression in a hyperbaric chamber (see later).

## Middle Ear Barotrauma

Middle ear barotrauma ("ear squeeze") occurs when the eustachian tube is blocked or fails to open during descent and the middle ear space cannot equilibrate with the increasing ambient pressure.[34] The tympanic membrane is displaced inward and may ultimately rupture. The middle ear may fill with blood from engorged mucous membranes. Infection and hearing loss are complications. Symptoms occur during descent and include pain in the affected ear that increases with depth. Relief of pain without proper ventilation of the middle ear usually indicates that the tympanic membrane has ruptured. Cold water entering the middle ear when the tympanic membrane ruptures may cause vertigo due to unequal stimulation of the vestibular apparatus. Late complications include acute otitis media, serous otitis media, and chronic tympanic membrane rupture.[20]

Prevention is achieved by ensuring that the eustachian tube is patent and that the ears can be equilibrated at surface pressure before descending. A Valsalva maneuver is commonly used to accomplish this goal. Several grading schemes for middle ear barotrauma have been proposed. The grading by Teed[35] is commonly used for clinical management. Because middle ear barotrauma causes edema and hemorrhage into the middle ear, equalization is usually impossible to achieve until healing is complete. The presence of middle ear barotrauma usually prohibits diving until it is resolved.

## Alternobaric Vertigo

Alternobaric vertigo occurs on ascent when the reduction of middle ear pressure is not uniform in both ears. The pressure imbalance causes differential stimulation of the vestibular apparatus, resulting in vertigo. The phenomenon was first reported by Vorosmarti and Bradley.[36] The sensation of vertigo occurs on ascent, usually within 30 to 40 ft of the surface, and may persist for 1 to 2 hours after diving. Vertigo is self-limiting and usually gradually disappears without therapy. Symptoms are similar to labyrinthitis and can include nausea, vomiting, and generalized malaise. Onset of symptoms underwater may be dangerous due to disorientation, particularly in novice divers.

The disorder must be differentiated from vestibular decompression sickness, which is usually associated with deeper, prolonged diving or saturation diving.[37] Some subjects may be particularly susceptible to alternobaric vertigo if they have had previous injury or infection of the labyrinths. No therapy is required in most cases because the disorder is self-limiting. In susceptible individuals, use of moderate doses of antihistamines or decongestants may prevent symptoms.

### Inner Ear Barotrauma

Inner ear barotrauma occurs on descent in divers who perform a forceful Valsalva maneuver in an attempt to equalize middle ear pressure. If the eustachian tube is blocked, middle ear pressure becomes progressively more negative relative to ambient pressure.[20, 38] When a Valsalva maneuver is performed, intrathoracic pressure, central venous pressure, spinal fluid pressure, and inner ear pressure rise above ambient pressure, thereby increasing the gradient between the inner ear endolymph and the middle ear. If the middle ear pressure is already below ambient pressure, the differential pressure from inner ear to middle ear may become large enough to rupture the round or oval window. When one of these structures ruptures, endolymph flows from the inner ear to the middle ear, and auditory and vestibular dysfunction follows. Symptoms usually follow a forceful Valsalva maneuver while descending with a blocked eustachian tube. They include sudden onset of vertigo, nausea, vomiting, tinnitus, and loss of hearing on the affected side.[39] Severity may vary, and some divers will complain of hearing loss, tinnitus, or vertigo only after diving.

Prevention is by training and attention to eustachian tube function. Treatment varies from conservative therapy to surgical repair of the round or oval window. Vertigo and nausea can be treated with benzodiazepine medications. Tinnitus and reduced hearing may become chronic, particularly if no treatment is provided.

### Sinus Barotrauma

Paranasal sinuses are susceptible to pressure effects similar to the middle ear. When a sinus orifice is blocked, pressure within the sinus becomes negative to ambient pressure, and mucosal blood vessels become engorged and eventually rupture. The resulting mucosal hemorrhage fills the sinus with blood. Symptoms are usually reported as pain over the affected sinus during descent and epistaxis on ascent when the expanding residual air in the sinus discharges the blood in the sinus. Headache following a dive may indicate sphenoid sinus barotrauma. The disorder is self-limiting; treatment is decongestants to re-establish orifice patency and maneuvers to drain the affected sinus. Persistence of blood in the sinus may result in acute bacterial sinusitis, which should be treated with appropriate antibiotics. Prevention is accomplished by avoiding diving with congestion of the nasopharynx and prudent use of decongestants.

### Facial Barotrauma

Facial barotrauma has been called "mask squeeze" by the diving community because it occurs in the distribution of the diving mask. Because diving masks cover the mouth and nose, like other air-containing spaces, they require continuous pressure equilibration by exhaling through the nose into the mask. If pressure within the mask is not equilibrated with ambient pressure, blood vessels in the face and conjunctiva become engorged and eventually rupture.[40] Facial edema, ecchymoses, and conjunctival hemorrhages are noted after diving, usually in novice divers. The disorder is self-limiting; no treatment is needed. Proper training prevents the disorder.

### Skin Barotrauma

An infrequent injury to the skin occurs in divers using air-containing diving suits ("dry suits"). Folds in the suit may become compressed against the skin and allow prolapse of skin into the fold. The result is linear ecchymoses on the trunk or extremities. The injury is self-limiting; no therapy is required.

### Tooth Barotrauma

Barodontalgia occurs on descent when air pockets under fillings or in areas of decay become compressed. Severe toothache results, which is relieved by ascending. Rarely an air pocket under a filling expands on ascent and ejects the filling from the tooth. Treatment is by dental repair. Careful dental work prevents this disorder.[41]

### Gastrointestinal Barotrauma

Air may enter the stomach and intestines during diving due to faulty breathing apparatus or by air swallowing. On ascent, the air will expand and distend the stomach or intestine. Gastric distention can occlude the esophageal gastric junction and prevent eructation. Distention of the stomach may occasionally cause stomach rupture and peritonitis. The diver experiences abdominal pain, which increases during ascent. Treatment may require surgical repair of the ruptured viscus. Divers with previous gastric surgery may be prone to gastric air trapping.[42] The disorder is prevented by attention to equipment maintenance and avoidance of air swallowing.

## DISSOLVED INERT GAS EFFECTS

### Gas Solubility and Henry's Law

Pressure determines the amount of gas that is dissolved in tissues and fluids of the body. A person subjected to increased ambient pressure takes up gases into the tissues of the body according to an exponential kinetic process. At equilibrium, the partial pressure of the gas and the solubility of the gas in the specific tissue (Table 71.2) determine dissolved gas content of tissues. Of the gases involved in diving, oxygen is not a problem with decompression sickness due to its low partial pressure at the cellular level[43]; $CO_2$ does not cause concern for decom-

Table 71.2 CHARACTERISTICS OF INERT GASES*

| GAS | MOLECULAR WEIGHT | LIPID SOLUBILITY† | WATER SOLUBILITY† | NARCOTIC POTENTIAL‡ |
|---|---|---|---|---|
| Helium | 4 | 0.015 | 0.009 | 0.23 |
| Neon | 20 | 0.019 | 0.009 | 0.28 |
| Hydrogen | 2 | 0.036 | 0.018 | 0.55 |
| Nitrogen | 28 | 0.067 | 0.013 | 1.00 |
| Argon | 40 | 0.140 | 0.026 | 2.32 |

*Solubility of the various gases in lipid is related to their narcotic potential. Helium is the least and argon the most narcotic gas in the list. Adapted from Bennett PB: Inert gase narcosis and HPNS. *In* Bove AA (ed): Diving Medicine. Philadelphia: WB Saunders, 1997, pp 117–130.

†Expressed as gas volume/solute volume at 1 bar.

‡Values relative to nitrogen.

pression sickness because of its high solubility and low partial pressure. Inert gases (nitrogen, helium), however, are limiting factors in diving because of their ability to supersaturate quickly and form a gas phase as the diver ascends with increased dissolved gas in the tissues.

## Inert Gas Kinetics

Gases dissolve in tissues, fats, and water according to Henry's law:

$$V = K \cdot P$$

where K, a solubility coefficient, and P, the partial pressure of the gas, determine the quantity (V) of dissolved inert gas. Solubility coefficients for water and lipid are provided in Table 71.2. Although Henry's law determines the amount of gas in the tissue, there is a finite time required for equilibrium to be achieved. Blood flow and gas diffusion affect the rate of gas flow into tissues.

Gases entering tissues approximate a first-order relationship, where rate of gas flow into tissue is proportional to the pressure difference between blood and tissue. Factors that affect the rate of entry include blood flow to the tissue and the rate of diffusion of gases into the tissue.[47] In the body, blood flow is the major factor controlling rate of gas exchange in tissues. The concentration of gas in tissues follows the kinetic equation

$$\frac{dC}{dt} = K \cdot \Delta C$$

where the change in concentration over time (dC/dt) is proportional to a constant (K) times the difference in concentration between blood and tissues ($\Delta C$). Solution of the equation describes an asymptotic curve (Fig. 71.5). In which the tissue gas concentration approaches the maximum concentration for the given pressure after time has elapsed. There is a family of curves for different values of K. These curves represent different tissue compartments, which have different gas exchange characteristics.[44] Similar kinetics control the washout of inert gas from tissues when ambient pressure is reduced (see Fig. 71.5).

The majority of diving is of short duration (i.e., minutes to hours) and shallow exposure (i.e., in depths shallower that 200 ft). Such diving can be performed with self-contained equipment or with breathing gas supplied from the surface through a hose. Such diving exposures allow only a few tissues to reach equilibrium based on Henry's law, while most tissues are not fully saturated. Divers can return to the surface from these short duration dives by following a schedule of ascent based on depth and time.[44] Tables describing decompression protocols are available throughout the world and are usually developed for military or commercial diving needs.[13] Decompression tables have been incorporated into durable wrist-mounted computers, which provide instantaneous information on decompression during diving.

When diving exposure is long enough, all tissues reach equilibrium at the new ambient pressure and are fully saturated with inert gas. An important advance in diving technology resulted from the work of Bond,[45] who conducted habitat experiments with helium-oxygen (heliox) breathing gas. Bond's work demonstrated that divers could spend prolonged periods (weeks) under pressure, with all tissues saturated at the increased pressure, without serious physiologic changes. Working dives conducted with Bond's techniques have been performed at depths over 1000 ft in open sea for periods up to 3 to 4 weeks. Breathing gases for these saturation dives are mixed with extreme care because dives of 1000 ft with normoxic mixtures (0.3 to 0.5 bar oxygen) require that oxygen concentrations be held to tolerances of 0.01% to avoid hypoxia or oxygen toxicity.

## Gas Supersaturation in Tissues

When the diver ascends, pressure is reduced rapidly, inert gases dissolved in tissues cannot equilibrate instantaneously with the lower pressure, and tissues become supersaturated with gas. When the degree of supersaturation becomes excessive, dissolved gas will leave the solution and form bubbles. Boycott and colleagues[46] first demonstrated that a diver could prevent bubble formation by keeping the degree of supersaturation below a certain level. They suggested that a 2:1 ratio of initial to final tissue partial pressure after ascent would prevent bubble formation. Their concept of a critical pressure ratio for

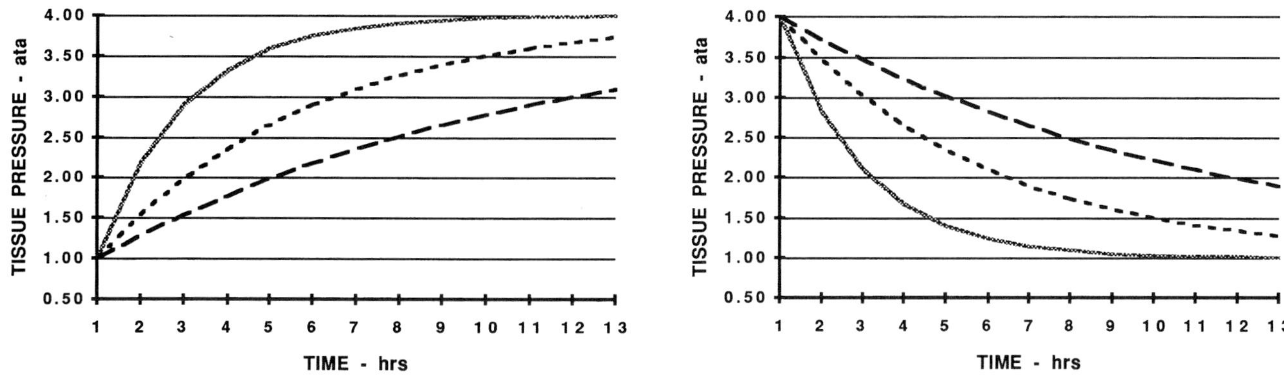


**Figure 71.5** The curves show inert gas uptake *(left)* and washout *(right)* for three theoretical tissue compartments. The gas content of tissues is expressed as a partial pressure.

bubble formation is the basis for decompression tables used to prevent decompression sickness.

Boycott and colleagues[46] assumed that the body could be considered as a set of tissues with different rates of gas diffusion. Although these "tissues" do not represent discrete anatomic structures, they provide a convenient means to understand the kinetics of inert gas exchange. Examples of tissues with rapid gas exchange are blood and lung alveolar cells; those with slow gas exchange are ligaments, tendons, and the vitreous humor of the eye. In most decompression tables, stops during ascent are selected to avoid excess supersaturation in tissues with specific gas exchange rates (Fig. 71.6). Tables have been designed for different inert gases, continuous or staged decompression, saturation exposure, caisson or tunnel exposure, and types of diving such as commercial or recreational. Operations involving exposure to increased partial pressure of inert gas must always consider the decompression procedures as well as the diving procedures. For certain exposures, decompression time far exceeds the exposure time and renders the exposure impractical. For long or deep exposures, the technique of saturation diving is used (see earlier). Decompression procedures are well defined for air and other mixtures of nitrogen and oxygen; helium and oxygen; nitrogen, helium, and oxygen (trimix); hydrogen and oxygen; and a few rare earth gases such as argon and neon used in experimental exposures.

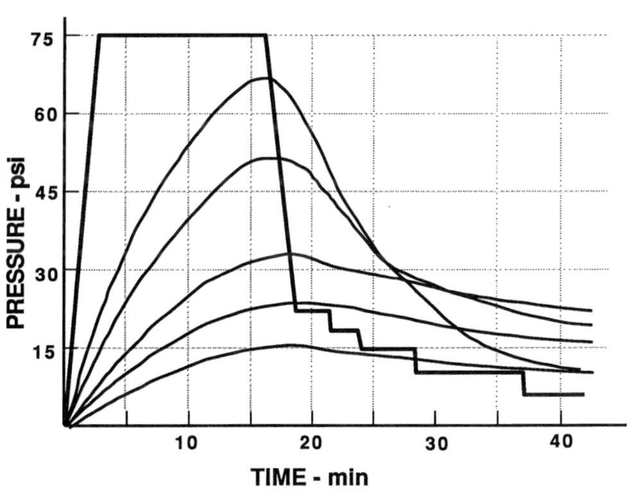


**Figure 71.6** Theoretical nitrogen gas concentrations are expressed in units of pressure for an exposure of 75 psi (5.1 ATA) following the depth-time profile indicated by the heavy line. Curves are shown for five theoretical tissue compartments with different rates of gas exchange. Tissue gas concentration increases during exposure to pressure. When pressure is reduced, gas concentration in tissues begins to fall. Stops during return to baseline allow tissue concentration to fall to a safe level of supersaturation before reducing pressure further.

## Decompression Sickness

Excess supersaturation causes dissolved gases to change phase to the gaseous form, and bubbles form in blood and tissues.[48] Expansion of gases in blood and tissues on ascent results in damage and dysfunction of tissues and organs and venous gas embolism to the lungs. Sudden decompression following a long, deep dive can be fatal, and miscalculation of decompression requirements can cause serious injury to organs and tissues. Decompression sickness (DCS) is the disorder caused by damage to organs and tissues as a result of bubble production and growth.

In the 19th century, Bert[49] described the pathophysiology of DCS. Several investigators in the early 20th century concluded from autopsies on divers and caisson workers that DCS is caused by inert gas bubbles in the blood and tissues.[50, 51] Based on bubble volume and location, they were able to explain the variety and severity of the symptoms. Paralysis resulted from bubbles in the spinal cord, cerebral dysfunction was thought to result from bubbles in the brain, and dyspnea was associated with bubbles in the pulmonary circulation. The causes of musculoskeletal forms of DCS, manifested as joint pain, are less clear. Muscle and joint pain may be due to bubbles in ligaments, fascia, periosteum, or nerve sheaths.

Bubbles also have biochemical effects, which are independent of their mechanical effects. Hallenbeck and colleagues[52] described effects of bubbles in blood and tissues that were not caused by mechanical obstruction. Subsequent studies identified clotting and platelet activation by bubbles,[53] intravascular coagulation, plasma leakage from the intravascular space, hemoconcentration, and hypovolemia[54] as manifestations of bubble surface effects. Hematologic abnormalities are infrequent in mild cases.[55]

Bubbles and tissue injury result in activation of acute inflammation.[56] The inflammatory response alters vascular permeability, causing fluid to leak into the interstitial tissues of the systemic and pulmonary vascular beds.[57, 58] In severe cases, pulmonary edema can occur; hypovolemia with significant plasma loss and hemoconcentration result.

## Factors Affecting Risk of Decompression Sickness

### Silent Bubbles

The use of Doppler ultrasound for intravascular bubble detection has provided insight into the presence of bubbles following diving.[59] Many divers show bubble presence but no manifestations of illness ("silent bubbles"). The concept of a threshold or dose-response effect has been postulated, where a clinical disorder required a certain volume of bubbles; lesser amounts are asymptomatic.[60] The presence of bubbles in asymptomatic divers and aviators, however, is associated with increased risk of developing symptoms of DCS after diving or altitude exposure.[61, 62]

### Patent Foramen Ovale

Moon and coworkers[63] reported 30 patients with a history of DCS who were studied with bubble contrast echocardiography for identification of a patent foramen ovale (PFO). Sixty-one percent of 18 patients with serious DCS had shunting, while a 25% prevalence was seen in normal volunteers. Wilmshurst and associates[64] identified a single patient with paradoxical gas embolism through an atrial septal defect and suggested that the atrial septal defect augmented symptoms of DCS in this patient. Moon and coworkers[65] evaluated 90 divers with previous DCS who were studied using bubble contrast echocardiography and color flow Doppler to detect right to left shunting through a PFO. Fifty-nine of 90 had experienced serious decompression symptoms, while 31 had experienced pain only or mild symptoms. Forty-nine per cent of the serious DCS subjects had evidence of a right to left shunt during either Valsalva maneuver or at rest compared with 19.8% of controls. With musculoskeletal DCS there was no difference in PFO prevalence between the diving subjects and the controls.

Bubble contrast echocardiography appeared to be the most sensitive method for detecting a shunt, whereas color flow Doppler alone appeared to be a poor means of detecting the shunt in a transthoracic echo. Wilmshurst and colleagues[66] found no difference in PFO prevalence when comparing control subjects to divers with onset of neurologic symptoms later than 30 minutes after surfacing or with joint pain. In divers who had neurologic symptoms within 30 minutes of surfacing, the prevalence of shunt was significantly higher than in controls. The prevalence of interatrial shunt was 65% in divers with onset of DCS within 30 minutes of surfacing. The authors point out that cerebral dysfunction is usually thought to be due to cerebral gas embolism. In the presence of a PFO, however, cerebral gas embolism caused by bubbles transiting a PFO may blur the distinction between neurologic DCS and air embolism. Wilmshurst and coworkers[66] found variability in the severity of shunting among different tests and times. They suggest that this variability may occur during diving and would explain the fact that divers with PFO may dive for many years without developing symptoms. De novo formation of bubbles in spinal cord and other tissue remains a well-documented cause of pathogenesis in DCS; however, the presence of a PFO is associated with an increase in the risk of DCS of about twofold.[67]

### Age

Attempts to determine the impact of age on susceptibility to DCS have aroused much debate, but very few persuasive data have resulted. A 10-year study by the US Air Force on flight exposures ranging from 1500 to 30,000 ft show a threefold increase in susceptibility when comparing fliers 18 to 21 years of age with fliers 42 years of age and older.[68] The study suggests a trend toward increased DCS susceptibility in individuals over age 42 because the increased susceptibility for the younger group could be attributed, at least in part, to enhanced risk taking or to a relative lack of experience compared with the older group.

## Clinical Manifestations

Based on the nomenclature proposed by Golding and coworkers,[17] DCS has been divided into a systemic form (type 2) and a nonsystemic, musculoskeletal form (type 1). A more complex symptom-based nomenclature has also been described.[18] Most sport and commercial divers now carry small decompression computers while diving to improve compliance with safe decompression protocols. Divers can, however, suffer DCS even after a "safe profile" is indicated by either diving tables or wrist-mounted computers.

The incidence of DCS varies among different populations (Table 71.3). Sport and military divers have similar rates of type 1 and type 2 DCS. Commercial divers have the highest incidence of DCS.[67] In this population, the incidence of minor DCS is high. In the early 1990s, the incidence of DCS was 1 in 10,000 dives for the sport diver compared with 1 in 100,000 for those who participated in diving for scientific or academic purposes.[69]

There is a spectrum of signs and symptoms in DCS that can mimic a variety of other disorders (Table 71.4). The disease develops after an ascent from depth when a diver does not follow the established procedures for returning to the surface that are designed to prevent effervescence of dissolved inert gas (nitrogen). The formation of free gas in the body has several consequences. Free gas entering the vascular system from the peripheral tis-

Table 71.3 FREQUENCY OF DECOMPRESSION SICKNESS (DCS) IN SPORT, MILITARY, AND COMMERCIAL AIR DIVING POPULATIONS*

| Source | Military | Sport | Commercial | All |
|---|---|---|---|---|
| Total dives† | 648,488 | 2,577,680 | 43,063 | 3,269,231 |
| Total DCS† | 172 | 878 | 152 | 1202 |
| Type II DCS† | 86 | 649 | 9 | 744 |
| Incidence DCS‡ | 2.65 | 3.41 | 35.3 | 3.68 |
| Incidence DCS II‡ | 1.33 | 2.52 | 2.09 | 2.28 |

*DCS incidence is provided in the last two rows. From Bove AA: Risk of decompression sickness with patent foramen ovale. Undersea Hyperbaric Med 25:175–178, 1998.
†Values are numbers of events.
‡Incidence per 10,000 dives. DCS II = DCS type II.

sues will transit the veins and cause varying degrees of pulmonary vascular obstruction. When the free gas volume is large and significant pulmonary obstruction occurs, a classic syndrome (chokes) is described.[71, 72] This syndrome is manifested by chest pain, dyspnea, and cough.[73]

DCS is often associated with free gas in the blood and with mechanical tissue inury from expanding gas. Bubbles and tissue injury result in activation of acute inflammation,[56] damage to vascular endothelium, microvascular occlusion, and focal regions of tissue ischemia. With severe DCS, endothelial damage to blood vessels occurs[73] and focal regions of tissue ischemia are evident. A frequent target organ is the spinal cord in humans.[70, 71] A common manifestation of DCS in divers is evidence of spinal cord dysfunction usually at levels below the diaphragm.[72] Symptoms include paresthesias, muscle weakness, paralysis of the lower extremities, bowel or bladder incontinence, urinary retention, and sexual impotence. In cases of very sudden ascent from deep depth (blowup), usually found in commercial diving exposures, a massive DCS syndrome can occur with both cerebral and spinal neurologic symptoms, unconsciousness, hypovolemic shock, pulmonary edema, and a high mortality rate.[73] A rare but important symptom of systemic (type 2) decompression sickness is sudden acute neurologic hearing loss or vestibular dysfunction. DCS of this type usually occurs from deep, prolonged commercial diving exposures and, if untreated, can result in permanent deafness.[74] Presence of cerebral involvement in DCS has been suggested, but the overlap in cerebral involvement with arterial gas embolism makes unclear the exact etiology of cerebral injury. Presence of a PFO (see earlier) can contribute to cerebral gas embolism in DCS.

The nonsystemic (type 1) form of DCS is manifested by pains in the extremities and joints.[76] Symptoms of local joint pain are often confused with pain from injuries, and the diagnosis of decompression sickness may be missed. In some populations a high incidence of aseptic bone necrosis is found in divers who have experienced DCS of the joints in the distant past or who have experienced deep, prolonged dives in commercial operations[75] and in caisson workers.[76] An erythematous or purpuric skin rash may also be a manifestation of DCS. Leffler and White[77] described their experience with a large diving operation (5000 dives) to salvage a crashed airliner.[77] They treated 19 divers for decompression-related illness, 18 of whom recovered fully.

Table 71.4 FREQUENCY OF DECOMPRESSION SICKNESS (DCS) SYMPTOMS IN 100 CASES*

| Symptom | Percentage of All DCS Symptoms |
|---|---|
| Skin itch | 4 |
| Headache | 11 |
| Fatigue and malaise | 13 |
| Bone and joint pain | 54 |
| Spinal and back pain | 11 |
| Spinal and neurologic pain | 22 |
| Respiratory trouble | 21 |

*Adapted from the Navy Department: US Navy Diving Manual. Vol 1, Rev 3: Air Diving. NAVSEA 0994-LP-001-9110. Washington, DC: US Government Printing Office, 1996.

## Treatment

The clinical manifestations of arterial air embolism and decompression sickness often overlap, and treatment goals for both disorders include recompression and other adjunctive measures. Bubble-induced injury can result in local hemorrhages in the spinal cord, brain, and other organs and direct tissue injury due to distortion as bubbles expand.

The initial treatment of DCS and arterial gas embolism should always be a return to pressure by recompression in a hyperbaric chamber and administration of oxygen at increased ambient pressure (hyperbaric oxygen). Fluid replacement and antiplatelet agents are also a part of the initial treatment. Once stabilized with pressure and oxygen, the patient must be decompressed slowly to permit the inert gas to be carried away from tissues by the circulatory system and then to be exhaled by the lungs. With early treatment, DCS and air embolism generally have an excellent prognosis for recovery, but when delay occurs, permanent injury to the brain or spinal cord may occur.

## Hyperbaric Therapy

Treatment of DCS and arterial gas embolism should be instituted with recompression as soon as possible. A history and physical evaluation, including a neurologic examination and cognitive assessment, should be obtained before treatment when possible. Therapy is provided in a hyperbaric chamber by a trained medical team. Return to depth underwater is not a satisfactory method of recompression for DCS or air embolism. This treatment however, has been used under extreme circumstances with a support team properly equipped and trained in open water treatment of these disorders. Hyperbaric therapy should be postponed for further diagnostic studies only if the findings from such studies could influence the choice of therapy.

The usual practice is to follow the standard protocols for pressure treatment outlined in the US Navy Diving Manual.[13] Treatment for minor or type 1 decompression sickness manifested by symptoms of joint or bone pain is a pressure exposure equivalent to a 60 ft depth in seawater (60 fsw) using intermittent oxygen therapy. Itching and erythema of the skin may also be signs of type 1 DCS but skin findings alone usually do not require recompression therapy.

Two protocols established by the US Navy (USN) have been recommended: USN Treatment Table 5, a 135-minute exposure, and USN Treatment Table 6, a 285-minute exposure with 100% oxygen at 60 fsw with air breaks to avoid pulmonary oxygen toxicity. The designation of these treatment protocols as Treatment Table 5 and Treatment Table 6 is arbitrary and is based on their position in the list of treatment tables published in the US Navy Diving Manual.[13] Treatment Table 5 can be used for treatment of type 1 DCS. Most practitioners, however, use Treatment Table 6 to account for the possibility of accompanying serious signs or symptoms that might be missed on examination. For serious or type 2 DCS, Treatment Table 6 is recommended.

When a diver ascends from extreme depths with significant missed decompression, the medical officer may choose to use recompression tables that pressurize the diver to a "depth of relief," to use alternate gas mixtures (i.e., helium oxygen), or to hold the diver for over 24 hours at a single depth to stabilize the medical status (saturation treatment). Several treatment protocols based on these principles are available.[78] For surface-supplied air and scuba divers, the principal treatment gases are oxygen and air. For treatment depths greater than 60 fsw (18 msw), enriched nitrogen-oxygen (nitrox) or helium-oxygen (heliox) may also be used. Helium-oxygen mixtures are used for treatments deeper than 200 to 220 fsw (60 to 67 msw).

Patients with residual signs or symptoms after the initial hyperbaric treatment may demonstrate incremental improvements with subsequent hyperbaric oxygen treatments. Repeated hyperbaric oxygen treatments can be given although end points for repetitive therapy are not well defined. Treatments can be administered until no further change of symptoms is found or for a fixed number of exposures (e.g., five). Controlled trials to determine efficacy of repetitive treatments, however, are not available, and neurologic injuries may return to normal without further hyperbaric treatment. Treatment of arterial gas embolism follows similar treatment protocols. Recompression to 60 fsw and oxygen therapy are usually successful,[79] but recompression to 165 fsw depth equivalent (5 ATA) is recommended if symptoms persist after recompression to 60 fsw.[13]

## Supplemental Oxygen and Fluids

Early administration of supplemental oxygen on the surface is beneficial for treating both DCS and arterial gas embolism; the optimal inspired concentration of oxygen is 100%. Intravenous fluid administration also is a useful initial treatment. Central nervous system injury may be exacerbated by hyperglycemia, and glucose-containing intravenous solutions should be administered cautiously. Measurement of hematocrit and urine-specific gravity is useful for the quantification of dehydration and plasma leakage from the vascular system.

## Diagnostic Testing

Chest radiography can be used to diagnose pneumothorax, pneumomediastinum associated with pulmonary overpressure accidents, and the pulmonary abnormalities associated with aspiration or capillary leakage associated with "chokes." In most cases, it is not necessary to postpone recompression treatment in order to obtain radiographic studies. If pneumothorax is suspected, a chest radiograph can be helpful in making the decision to insert a chest tube. Neurologic and psychologic testing may be useful in determining response to treatment when brain injury is present. Electronystagmography (ENG) and audiography may be useful in distinguishing inner ear DCS from inner ear barotrauma, for which the treatment is quite different. Inner ear DCS requires recompression, whereas inner ear barotrauma is managed with bedrest, avoidance of straining, and possibly surgical intervention. The circumstances causing the two syndromes are distinct (see earlier) and are helpful in the differential diagnosis; however, in the event the distinction cannot be made, recompression therapy may be of benefit. Central nervous system injury is best diagnosed by magnetic resonance imaging (MRI). Areas of cerebral and spinal cord ischemia or infarction can be identified by MRI and correlate with clinical findings.[80, 81] MRI studies in divers with no history of decompression-related disorders are also found to be abnormal in some studies[82]; however, the significance of MRI findings in these individuals is unclear.

## Emergency Treatment

Because divers may be injured in areas remote from medical care, treatment measures should be instituted during transit to a hyperbaric chamber facility. Emergency treatment before transfer of an injured diver should include 100% oxygen by mask, aspirin by mouth 325 to 975 mg, and Ringer's lactate intravenously. One study of oxygen, aspirin, intravenous fluids, and hydrocortisone intravenously (1 to 2 g) during transit to a hyperbaric chamber found that two thirds of the cases had a favorable outcome.[83] A favorable response to urgent care should not prolong transfer to the closest chamber facility capable of providing recompression therapy.

## INERT GAS NARCOSIS

Inert gas narcosis (nitrogen narcosis) results from breathing air at depths greater than 100 fsw.[84, 85] Symptoms are similar to alcohol inebriation and include loss of fine motor control and high-order mental skills, bizarre and inappropriate behavior, improper response to emotional stress, hostility, and unconsciousness. Symptoms increase with depth from 100 ft, and some individuals may manifest severe symptoms at 130 ft. At 300 to 400 ft, unconsciousness may occur owing to the anesthetic effect of nitrogen at this pressure. In diving deeper than 200 ft, helium replaces nitrogen as the inert gas to prevent narcosis.[86, 87] Fatigue, heavy work, and cold water can augment the narcotic effect of nitrogen. Symptoms disappear immediately on ascending to a shallow depth. Often there is amnesia for the events that occurred below.[84] Nitrogen effects on nervous function are thought to have the same mechanism of action as anesthetic gases. Gas effects on cell membrane function result in reduced cellular activity and, ultimately, general anesthesia. Narcotic potential varies among the inert gases (see Table 71.2).

## MEDICAL QUALIFICATIONS FOR DIVING

The type of diving dictates the medical requirements. Military divers have the most stringent requirements, while recreational divers have the most relaxed requirements. Commercial divers, caisson and tunnel workers, and hyperbaric chamber workers all have unique standards. Because of the stresses of underwater exposure (exercise, cold, increased gas density), divers require a reasonable level of physical fitness and must be free of physical limitations that could compromise safety. In most cases, limitations occur because of conditions that limit physical capacity. Disorders that limit cardiovascular or pulmonary function during exercise, physical deconditioning, metabolic disorders that limit exercise capacity, and certain physical handicaps can compromise diving safety.

### Exercise Requirements

Workloads in diving vary based on the type of diving. A diver swimming underwater at a speed of 1.0 knot consumes about 25 mL/min/kg of oxygen.[88] This is a high workload and is uncommon in recreational diving. A diver with a maximum oxygen consumption of 40 mL/min/kg would be able to tolerate swimming at 1.3 knots for a few minutes. The diver would hyperventilate to compensate for lactate production, and fatigue would develop rapidly. Swimming at 60% of maximum, a work level that is at or slightly below the anaerobic threshold,[15] can be sustained for long periods of time because lactate does not accumulate in the blood. For a diver with a maximum oxygen consumption of 40 mL/kg/min, working at 60% to 65% of maximum capacity, sustainable swimming speed would be about 100 ft/min, whereas the diver with a maximum oxygen consumption of 25 mL/kg/min could sustain a swimming speed of about 70 ft/min. Safety considerations suggest that divers should tolerate a peak workload of about 40 mL/kg/min and a sustained workload of about 24 mL/kg/min to ensure safety under adverse diving conditions. Divers who do not achieve this level of fitness should avoid dives that may require high levels of physical exertion.

### Sudden Unconsciousness

Disorders that cause sudden unconsciousness underwater are considered to be contraindications to diving. Seizure disorders are considered to be a contraindication to diving because increased oxygen partial pressure, hyperventilation, and increased catecholamines during stress all can lower seizure threshold. A diver sustaining an underwater seizure is at risk for drowning and may compromise the safety of others who attempt a rescue. Insulin-dependent diabetes mellitus is considered a contraindication to commercial and military diving due to the risk of hypoglycemia; however, special training for diabetic recreational divers has allowed safe diving for some insulin-dependent sport divers.

### Pulmonary Disorders

Asthma has been a subject of controversy in diving because of possible air trapping and pulmonary overinflation during ascent. An increased risk for pulmonary barotrauma, however, has not been supported by clinical observation. Neuman and coworkers[89] reviewed data on the risk of diving with asthma. They suggested that blanket prohibition is not justified by published data. Criteria for safe diving by patients with a history of asthma include evidence that expiratory air flow at 50% of peak (mid-expiratory flow) is not reduced after exercise by greater than 50%.[90] A more detailed discussion of issues related to asthma and diving has been published.[90] Clinical and operational experience suggests that patients with a history of spontaneous pneumothorax may be at risk for lung collapse and development of a progressively worsening tension pneumothorax during diving. As air in the pleural space expands during ascent, compression of the contralateral lung, heart, and great vessels can cause obstruction of blood flow and shock. Treatment requires immediate decompression of the pleural space through an intercostal needle or chest tube and may be difficult in remote diving sites.

### Cardiac Disorders

Patients with coronary disease may develop manifestations (angina pectoris, myocardial infarction, sudden death) while diving. Mebane and colleagues[91] reported the mortality experience from the Diving Alert Network. Of 33 cases of sudden death while diving, 31 were attributed to coronary disease, one was related to a cerebral vascular accident, and one was related to aortic stenosis. Screening of diving candidates for coronary disease is particularly important in the sport diving community, in which candidates at increased risk for coronary disease due to age and chronic illness may present for training.

Diving candidates with atrial septal defects risk paradoxical embolism of gas bubbles that form in the venous circulation during decompression.[88] The presence of an atrial septal defect is considered to be a contraindication to diving. Ventricular septal defect does not appear to produce a risk for paradoxical embolization of bubbles. In patients with minimal or no symptoms who have either atrial or ventricular septal defects with normal pressures in the central circulation, the shunt will be directed from left to right and no arterial desaturation occurs. Patients with a right to left shunt and arterial hypoxemia will normally have severely limited exercise capacity and should not dive. A detailed treatment of this topic can be found elsewhere.[88]

## NEAR DROWNING

In the approximately 100 to 150 scuba fatalities in the United States each year, drowning is reported as the leading cause of death.[92] In reality, arterial gas embolism may be the precipitating factor or even the cause of death in many of these accidents.[93] Fatigue or panic may also contribute to diving-related drowning by impairing judgment and increasing risk of an improper or inadequate response to adverse changes in the environment. In the United States, drowning of males is approximately five times more common than of females.[94] As with fatal automobile accidents, the single most important factor in drowning incidents involving adults is alcohol. Multiple studies done in widely different geographical areas, such as the United States,[94] New Zealand,[95] Africa,[96] and Australia,[97] reveal that in well over half of the adults who drown, alcohol is a significant contributing factor. With scuba-related drowning or near-drowning incidents, the most common factor is entanglement or the diver running out of air at depth or in a cave.

Although not generally reported in diving fatality statistics, there is strong evidence that intentional hyperventilation before breath-hold diving is associated with both drowning and near-drowning episodes.[8, 9] Hyperventilation reduces the arterial $P_{CO_2}$, so the breath-hold break point is prolonged sufficiently for hypoxemia to occur before the individual is forced to breathe.[98] The hypoxemia in turn causes the individual to lose consciousness, and the submersion incident then occurs.

Hypothermia leading to drowning and near-drowning incidents has been reported frequently; however, in diving fatalities this is an unusual occurrence due to the almost universal use of either wet suits or dry suits by divers for thermal protection. Hypothermia per se is rarely the cause of death for people immersed in water. Hypothermia reduces a person's ability to function until the point of unconsciousness or helplessness is reached. At that time, the victim's head falls into the water, resulting in drowning or near drowning. Maximum breath-hold times of normally clothed individuals drops dramatically in cold water, further compromising their ability to survive in rough water where they may be intermittently submerged. In rare circumstances, however, hypothermia can have a protective effect on the near-drowning victim (see later).

Hypothermia is only one of many conditions that can precipitate drowning by causing unconsciousness. In the case of scuba diving incidents, contamination of the diver's air supply with carbon monoxide produces rapid unconsciousness, and oxygen-induced seizures have been implicated as the cause of death in divers using oxygen-enriched air as a breathing mixture.[99]

### Pathophysiology

Approximately 10% to 15% of near-drowning victims appear not to aspirate fluid during immersion.[100, 101] To account for the lack of aspiration in these individuals, it has been hypothesized that reflex laryngospasm occurs and persists until reflex ventilatory activity ceases. Experimental data to support this hypothesis, however, are lacking. In near-drowning victims who do not aspirate, the period of hypoxemia generally is as long as the immersion incident itself. If ventilation can be re-established before the development of injury secondary to hypoxemia, recovery typically is rapid and uneventful.

When aspiration occurs, the pathophysiologic processes are markedly different, although in the majority of cases the underlying primary process remains hypoxemia due to flooding of the airways with water. Unlike the victim without aspiration, the individual who aspirates remains hypoxemic, even after being removed from the fluid medium and even after ventilation is re-established. As a result, in the latter group the period of hypoxemia is potentially much longer, and secondary damage due to the hypoxemia is more likely to occur. The continuing hypoxemia is most frequently due to direct lung injury from the aspirated fluid, which causes areas of low ventilation/perfusion ($V_A/Q$) ratio to develop.

The mechanisms by which hypoxemia develops have not been completely elucidated. With salt water aspiration, it is believed that hyperosmotic fluid causes transudation of fluid into alveoli, and the aspiration of debris (sand, diatoms, algae, etc.) causes a reactive exudate. As a result, alveoli become filled and are not ventilated, and hypoxemia occurs. In fresh water aspiration, it is believed surfactant is washed out of the lungs, causing areas of focal alveolar collapse, leading to areas of shunt and low $V_A/Q$ ratio, again resulting in hypoxemia. These abnormalities persist until the lung damage resolves or until surfactant can be regenerated.

Victims often swallow large amounts of fluid during the near-drowning episode, so further decreases in ventilatory function may occur as a result of elevation of the diaphragm from gastric distention. Vomiting and aspiration of gastric contents further complicate the near-drowning episode. Hypoxemia and decreased alveolar ventilation produce a number of consequences. Elevations of arterial $P_{CO_2}$ and decreases in pH occur quickly. Metabolic acidosis can be extremely severe because the victim often struggles during the near-drowning episode. Finally, cardiovascular collapse may occur, resulting in cardiac arrest. If hypoxemia and decreased cardiac output persist long enough, anoxic cerebral damage can ensue.[102–104] Although electrolyte disturbances are usually not a significant problem in near drowning, the exception to this situation appears to be submersion victims in the Dead

Sea where electrolyte concentrations are greater than those in usual seawater.[105] Victims of near drowning in that unique environment do have major electrolyte abnormalities, and it is believed that these disturbances are responsible for the fatal arrhythmias that have occurred in that group.[106] The remaining specific consequence of aspiration is pneumonia, which can occur in near-drowning victims. The pathogens and the clinical picture of pneumonia associated with near drowning has recently been reviewed extensively.[107]

Because cardiac arrest is secondary to hypoxemia in near drowning, it presumably takes a significant amount of time to occur. If the water in which the victim is immersed is cold enough during this time, if the surface area to mass ratio of the victim is large enough, and if the victim swallows enough water, core temperature may decrease sufficiently that oxygen demands are markedly decreased. It is unclear, however, whether the above information is adequate to explain the degree of cooling and the amount of cerebral protection that appears to occur in some incidents.

## Clinical Presentation

The clinical presentation of drowning or near-drowning victims is highly variable. The patient who is unconscious and apparently without vital signs at the site of the accident may be hemodynamically stable and neurologically intact in the emergency room, whereas the victim initially hemodynamically stable at the scene might deteriorate significantly before arrival at the hospital.

## Cardiovascular System

Victims of significant near drowning often suffer cardiac arrest, but frequently respond to resuscitative measures. It is not uncommon, however, for a victim to be brought to the emergency room still requiring cardiopulmonary resuscitation. If the patient responds to cardiopulmonary resuscitation with a stable rhythm or if the patient never suffers a cardiac arrest, supraventricular tachycardias are commonly seen. If the patient presents with a viable rhythm, it will most likely be supraventricular tachycardia secondary to hypoxemia and acidosis.[102, 103] Usually the patient is hemodynamically intact (i.e., adequate blood pressure and pulse with a presumably adequate cardiac output).

## Pulmonary System

Patients with water aspiration may present with little or no respiratory complaints or with severe pulmonary edema.[108] This is probably due to direct lung injury and is not usually cardiogenic in origin. Patients who have aspirated any significant quantity of water frequently have a widened alveolar-arterial (A − a) oxygen gradient and anything from mild to severe hypoxemia. Arterial $P_{CO_2}$ can be low or elevated depending on alveolar ventilation (Table 71.5). Chest radiographs can show patchy infiltrates, which are most common in the periphery or in the medial basal regions, or frank pulmonary edema (see Fig. 71.4).[109] The pulmonary edema is a form of the acute respiratory distress syndrome.[109] The clinical course cannot be predicted with certainty by the radiographic picture of lung injury.[110] Victims with clear-cut pulmonary difficulties may show minimal radiographic abnormalities, and those with minimal clinical injury may have severely abnormal radiographic pictures.

**Table 71.5** AVERAGE BLOOD GAS MEASUREMENTS IN HOSPITALIZED NEAR-DROWNING VICTIMS BREATHING ROOM AIR ON ADMISSION*

| | PH | $Pa_{CO_2}$ (MM HG) | $Pa_{O_2}$ (MM HG) | BASE EXCESS (MEQ) |
|---|---|---|---|---|
| Freshwater | 7.26 | 38 | 66 | −9 |
| Seawater | 7.37 | 36 | 56 | −5 |
| All | 7.30 | 37 | 62 | −7 |

Adapted from Modell JH, Davis JH, Giammona ST, et al: Blood gas and electrolyte changes in human near-drowning victims. JAMA 203:337–343, 1968.

## Neurologic Status

The neurologic status of patients can also be quite varied. To compare results among different groups, a classification scheme has been suggested to describe these patients.[111, 112] In this classification system, patients are placed into category A, B, or C based on their initial neurologic status. Category A patients are awake; category B patients are blunted; and category C patients are comatose. Within category C, patients are further classified as C1, C2, or C3, depending on their best motor response. The C1 comatose patient has a decorticate response, the C2 patient has a decerebrate response, and the C3 patient has no motor response at all.

## Treatment

Following cardiac arrest, restoration of normal neurologic function, although unusual, has been described even after prolonged cardiac arrest.[113–116] As cardiac arrest in this setting is invariably due to hypoxemia and acidosis, the first goal must be to establish a reliable airway and to supply as high a fractional inspired oxygen concentration as soon as possible. Until the results of arterial blood gas determinations are available, 100% oxygen should be provided. Aspiration of stomach contents is a constant threat in the comatose patient, so bag-valve-mask oxygenation probably has a limited role in the advanced care of these patients. Endotracheal intubation is the preferred method for establishing an airway. This approach needs to take into account the possibility of a concomitant unstable neck injury and the risk of aspiration. At present there are insufficient data to warrant the routine use of the Heimlich maneuver in near-drowning victims.

Patients with arrest due to near drowning can have a profound metabolic acidosis. The doses of bicarbonate required to reverse such acidosis may be far larger than the doses recommended for patients suffering cardiac arrest from primary heart disease.[117] Generally, in immersion incidents, the cardiac arrest is secondary to hypoxemia and acidosis, whereas, with cardiac arrest secondary to underlying heart disease, acidosis and hypoxemia are secondary to the cardiac arrest itself. As a result, anterial blood gas determinations are necessary to determine more precise bicarbonate dosing. Concurrently, a nasogastric tube should be inserted to decompress the stomach, and body temperature readings should be obtained to rule out hypothermia. In the presence of a significantly lowered body temperature, aggressive rewarming measures should be instituted.

Once an adequate airway has been obtained and spontaneous cardiac activity achieved, adequate oxygen delivery to the tissues needs to be ensured, which requires an adequate arterial $PO_2$. Generally, in the near-drowning victim, hemodynamic stability is relatively easy to achieve; however, occasional patients will have marked decreases in blood pressure and associated decreases in cardiac output. The initial therapy for hypotension of most etiologies is a trial of fluids, but for a near-drowning victim with pulmonary edema, this may not be appropriate. As a result, this group of patients may require invasive hemodynamic monitoring. With knowledge of pulmonary artery wedge pressure and cardiac output, more rational decisions concerning the need for fluids or pressors can then be made.[108] Isolated measurement of the central venous pressure is generally not an accurate method of judging intravascular volume status in the presence of noncardiac pulmonary edema. In addition, changes in central venous pressure, whether up or down, do not necessarily correspond to changes in the pulmonary artery wedge pressure or left ventricular filling pressures. As a result, the use of CVP measurements in the management of the near-drowning victim is extremely limited; direct measurement of pulmonary artery wedge pressure and cardiac output may need to be obtained in addition to the arterial blood gases in patients with hypotension and evidence of pulmonary edema.

Positive endexpiratory pressure has been shown, both experimentally and clinically, to be extremely effective in reversing the abnormal $V_A/Q$ relationships leading to hypoxemia.[118] Usually only modest amounts of pressure are necessary to achieve adequate oxygenation, and the improvement in pulmonary function can be quite dramatic. Positive end-expiratory pressure apparently does not alter the course of the underlying pulmonary injury but rather allows for adequate oxygenation while the lung is recovering. It also allows this recovery to take place at a level of inspired oxygen that is not in itself toxic to the lung.[119] Usually the pulmonary injury resolves over a period of 48 to 72 hours, and ventilatory support in most circumstances is relatively brief, unless infection develops. Consequently, in patients who are able to tolerate it, nasal continuous or bilevel positive airway pressure may be reasonable methods for short-term ventilatory support. The risk of aspiration, however, is not inconsequential with this treatment modality.[117, 120, 121] At present there are insufficient data to warrant the use of inverse ratio ventilation in cases of near drowning.[122] It may be prudent to manage some near-drowning victims with modern high-flow oxygen delivery systems for relatively brief periods before resorting to more invasive methods of providing adequate oxygenation.

The use of antibiotics in the near-drowning victim who aspirates ocean water or swimming pool water is generally necessary only for those individuals who become febrile, develop new pulmonary infiltrates, or develop purulent secretions.[123] Prophylactic antibiotics do not improve mortality or decrease morbidity.[102] Because most pulmonary infections in the near-drowning victim appear to be hospital acquired, prophylactic antibiotics seem to select for more resistant organisms.[124] In addition to clinical experience, experimental evidence also suggests that the use of prophylactic antibiotics is not indicated. If the victim aspirates heavily contaminated water with a known or suspected organism, the use of prophylactic antibiotics may be appropriate. A rare complication of near drowning is the aspiration of sand or gravel.[125] Although bronchoscopy for the routine management of the near-drowning victim is probably not warranted, consideration for this procedure should be made when unexpected difficulties with mechanical ventilation occur.

Adrenocortical steroids to treat the lung injury associated with near drowning are also probably unwarranted. Experimental evidence with this form of aspiration as well as others strongly suggests that steroids do not improve the long-term outcome or short-term morbidity.[126, 127] There is, however, one uncontrolled series of four cases that suggests high-dose steroids may be beneficial to near-drowning victims who present with pulmonary edema.[128] Artificial surfactant has also been used to treat the pulmonary injury associated with near drowning.[129]

Any victim who has more than minimal respiratory symptoms, an abnormal chest radiograph, or abnormal arterial blood gas measurements should be admitted to the hospital, because pulmonary damage may not be clinically manifest for several hours after the incident.[130] Nearly all patients who will demonstrate significant problems of gas exchange, however, will do so by 4 to 8 hours after the incident. In the setting of a diving accident, an unconscious victim may have sustained an air embolism as well. Whenever doubt exists, both conditions should be treated simultaneously.

## Prognosis

The prognosis for the near-drowning victim depends mainly on the duration of immersion, the length of the anoxic period, and the degree of damage secondary to the anoxic episode. Patients who arrive at the hospital neurologically intact have an excellent prognosis and should survive neurologically unimpaired. Additionally, the occurrence of an apparent "cardiac arrest" does not in itself suggest a poor outcome. If the presumed "cardiac arrest" responds to first aid at the scene of the accident, the outcome may be excellent. Cardiac arrest that persists through the period of initial first aid and transport to the hospital is a poor prognostic sign, but the presence of spontaneous respirations on presentation to the emergency department following cardiac arrest in the field is a good prognostic sign.[131] The duration of immersion correlates with the degree of damage secondary to the anoxic episode and therefore with the outcome. No prognostic test has proven a reliable basis for treatment decisions, and predictions concerning outcome cannot be made in the presence of severe hypothermia.

## SUMMARY

Diving and work in compressed air have produced occupational exposure to hazardous environments for over 100 years. In the past 50 years diving has become a recreation participated in by many millions of individuals throughout the world. Besides the medical support for commercial diving and the unique training needed by physicians supporting military diving, any physician may encounter a recreational diver seeking consultation about an illness related to a diving exposure, or medical clearance for diving. Therefore, knowledge of the basic physiology and pathophysiology is important in understanding the patient's illness or evaluation requirements. Occasionally a physician may be confronted with treatment for an acute medical emergency related to diving exposure, such as DCS or near drowning. This chapter provides a basic introduction and a basis for initiating treatment, seeking consultation, or furthering education in this interesting area of environmental medicine.

## Acknowledgment

The authors thank Anne Scheck, Los Angeles, for editorial assistance.

## References

1. Hong SK, Cerretelli P, Cruz JC, et al: Mechanics of respiration during submersion in water. J Appl Physiol 27:537–538, 1969.
2. Agostoni E, Gurtner G, Torri G, et al: Respiratory mechanics during submersion and negative pressure breathing. J Appl Physiol 21:251–258, 1966.
3. Johnson LF, Lin YC, Hong SK: Gastroesophageal dynamics during immersion in water to the neck. J Appl Physiol 38:449–454, 1975.
4. Hong SK, Ting EY, Rahn H: Lung volumes at different depths of submersion. J Appl Physiol 23:18–22, 1967.
5. Craig AB Jr, Ware DE: Effect of immersion in water on vital capacity and residual volume of the lungs. J Appl Physiol 23:423–425, 1967.
6. Arborelius M, Balldin UI, Lidja B, et al: Hemodynamic changes in man during immersion with the head above water. Aerosp Med 43:592–598, 1972.
7. Hong SK, Rahn H, Kang DH, et al: Diving pattern, lung volumes, and alveolar gas in the Korean diving women (Ama). J Appl Physiol 18:457–465, 1963.
8. Craig AB Jr: Underwater swimming and loss of consciousness. JAMA 176:255–258, 1961.
9. Craig AB Jr: Causes of loss of consciousness during underwater swimming. J Appl Physiol 16:583–586, 1961.
10. Mebane GY: Hypothermia. In Bove AA (ed): Diving Medicine. Philadelphia: WB Saunders, 1997, pp 207–216.
11. Pendergast DR, Tedesco M, Nawrocki DM, et al: Energetics of underwater swimming with SCUBA. Med Sci Sports Exerc 28:573–580, 1996.
12. Doubt TJ: Cardiovascular and thermal responses to SCUBA diving. Med Sci Sports Exerc 28:581–586, 1996.
13. Navy Department: US Navy Diving Manual. Vol 1, Rev 3: Air Diving. NAVSEA 0994-LP-001-9110. Washington, DC: US Government Printing Office, 1996.
14. Batchelor FRS: An Introduction to Fluid Dynamics. Cambridge: Cambridge University Press, 1967, pp 255–263.
15. Wasserman K, Whipp BJ, Koyal SN, et al: Anaerobic threshold and respiratory gas exchange during exercise. J Appl Physiol 35:236–247, 1973.
16. Navy Department. US Navy Diving Manual. Vol 2: Mixed Gas Diving. NAVSEA 0994 LP-001-9120. Washington, DC: US Printing Office, 1996, pp 12-1–12-44.
17. Golding FC, Griffiths P, Hempleman HV, et al: Decompression sickness during construction of the Dartford Tunnel. Br J Ind Med 17:167–180, 1960.
18. Francis TJR, Smith DH: Describing Decompression Illness. 42nd UHMS Workshop. Kensington, MD: Undersea and Hyperbaric Medical Society, 1991.
19. Boyle R: New pneumatic experiments about respiration. Philos Trans R Soc Lond 5:2011–2031, 1670.
20. Farmer JC: Ear and sinus problems in diving. *In* Bove AA (ed): Diving Medicine. Philadelphia: WB Saunders, 1997, pp 235–257.
21. Behnke AR: Analysis of accidents occurring in training with the submarine "lung." US Naval Med Bull 30:177–184, 1932.
22. Polak B, Adams H: Traumatic air embolism in submarine escape training. US Naval Med Bull 30:165–177, 1932.
23. Shilling CW: Expiratory force as related to submarine escape training. US Naval Med Bull 31:1–7, 1933.
24. Liebow AA, Stark JE, Vogel J, et al: Intrapulmonary air trapping in submarine escape training casualties. US Armed Forces Med J 10:265–289, 1959.
25. Schaefer KE, Nulty WP, Carey C, et al: Mechanisms in development of interstitial emphysema and air embolism on decompression from depth. J Appl Physiol 13:15–29, 1958.
26. Malhotra MC, Wright CAM: Arterial air embolism during decompression and its prevention. Proc R Soc Med B154:418–427, 1960.
27. Bove AA, Hallenbeck JM, Elliott DH: Circulatory responses to venous air embolism and decompression sickness in dogs. Undersea Biomed Res 1:207–220, 1974.
28. Smith R, Neuman T: Elevation of serum creatine kinase in divers with arterial gas embolism. N Engl J Med 330:19–24, 1994.
29. Wilmshurst P. Davidson C, O'Connell G, et al: Role of cardiorespiratory abnormalities, smoking and dive characteristics in the manifestations of neurological decompression illness. Clin Sci 86(3):297–303, 1994.
30. Tetzlaff K, Reuter M, Leplow B, et al: Risk factors for pulmonary barotrauma in divers. Chest 112:654–659, 1997.
31. Elliott DH, Harrison JAB, Barnard EEP: Clinical and radiographic features of 88 cases of decompression barotrauma. *In* Shilling CW, Beckett MW (eds): Proceedings of the Sixth Symposium on Underwater Physiology. Bethesda: FASEB, 1978, pp 527–535.
32. Neuman TS, Jacoby I, Bove AA: Fatal pulmonary barotrauma due to obstruction of the central circulation with air. J Emerg Med 16:413–417, 1998.
33. Harker CP, Neuman TS, Olson LK, et al: The roentgenographic findings associated with air embolism in sport scuba divers. J Emerg Med 11(4):443–449, 1993.
34. Vail HH: Traumatic conditions of the ear in workers in an atmosphere of compressed air. Arch Otolaryngol 10:113–126, 1929.
35. Teed RW: Factors producing obstruction of the auditory tube in submarine personnel. US Naval Med Bull 44:293–306, 1944.
36. Vorosmarti J, Bradley JJ: Alternobaric vertigo in military divers. Milit Med 135:182–185, 1970.
37. Lundgren C, Tjernstrom O, Ornhagen H: Alternobaric vertigo and hearing disturbances in connection with diving: An epidemiologic study. Undersea Biomed Res 1:251–258, 1974.
38. Freeman P, Edmonds C: Inner ear barotrauma. Arch Otolaryngol 95:556–563, 1972.
39. Pullen FW: Perilymphatic fistula induced by barotrauma. Am J Otol 13:270–272, 1992.
40. Butler FK: Diving and hyperbaric ophthalmology. Surv Ophthalmol 39:347–366, 1995.
41. Kieser J, Holborow D: The prevention and management of oral barotrauma. NZ Dent J 93:114–116, 1997.
42. Hayden JD, Davies JB, Martin IG: Diaphragmatic rupture resulting from gastrointestinal barotrauma in a scuba diver. Br J Sports Med 32:75–76, 1998.

43. Lambertsen CJ: Therapeutic gases: Oxygen, carbon dioxide and helium. In DiPalma JR (ed): Drill's Pharmacology in Medicine (4th ed). New York: McGraw-Hill, 1971, pp 1145–1179.
44. Vann RD: Mechanisms and risk of decompression sickness. *In* Bove AA (ed): Bove and Davis' Diving Medicine. Philadelphia: WB Saunders, 1997, pp 146–158.
45. Bond G: New developments in high pressure living. Arch Environ Health 9:310–314, 1964.
46. Boycott AE, Damant GCC, Haldane J: The prevention of compressed air illness. J Hyg Cambridge 8:342–443, 1908.
47. Kety S: The theory and applications of the exchange of inert gas at the lungs and tissues. Pharmacol Rev 3:1–41, 1951.
48. Harvey EN, Barnes DK, McElroy WD, et al: Bubble formation in animals. I. Physical factors. J Cell Comp Physiol 24:1–22, 1944.
49. Bert P: Barometric Pressure. Researches in Experimental Physiology. Hitchcock MA, Hitchcock FA, trans. Columbus Book Co, 1943. Reprinted by the Undersea Medical Society, Bethesda, MD, 1978.
50. Keays FL Compressed air illness, with a report of 3,692 cases. Dept Med Publ, Cornell Univ Med Coll 2:1–55, 1909.
51. Erdman S: Aeropathy of compressed air illness among tunnel workers. JAMA 49:1665–1670, 1907.
52. Hallenbeck JM, Bove AA, Moquin R, et al: Accelerated coagulation of whole blood and cell free plasma by bubbling in vitro. Aerosp Med 44:712–714, 1973.
53. Philp RB, Inwood MJ, Warren BA: Interaction between gas bubbles and components of the blood: Implications in decompression sickness. Aerosp Med 946–956, 1972.
54. Bove AA, Hallenbeck JM: Changes in blood and plasma volumes in dogs during decompression sickness. Aerosp Med 45:49–55, 1974.
55. Boussuges A, Sainty JM, Juhan-Vague I, et al: Activation of coagulation in decompression illness. Aviat Space Environ Med 69:129–132, 1998.
56. Bove AA: Basis for drug therapy in decompression sickness. Undersea Biomed Res 9:91–112, 1982.
57. Neuman TS, Spragg RG, Howard R, et al: Cardiopulmonary consequences of decompression stress. Am Rev Respir Dis 128:552–559, 1983.
58. Levin LL, Stewart GJ, Lynch PR, et al: Blood and blood vessel wall changes induced by decompression sickness in dogs. J Appl Physiol 50:944–949, 1981.
59. Spencer MP: Decompression limits for compressed air determined by ultrasonically detected blood bubbles. J Appl Physiol 40:227–235, 1976.
60. Butler BD, Robinson R, Fife C, et al: Doppler detection of decompression bubbles with computer assisted digitization of ultrasonic signals. Aviat Space Environ Med 62:997–1004, 1991.
61. Conkin J, Waligora JM, Foster PP, et al: Information about venous gas emboli improves prediction of hypobaric decompression sickness. Aviat Space Environ Med 69:8–16, 1998.
62. Kumar VK, Waligora JM, Billica RD: Utility of Doppler-detectable microbubbles in the diagnosis and treatment of decompression sickness. Aviat Space Environ Med 68:151–158, 1997.
63. Moon RE, Camporesi EM, Kisslo JA: Patent foramen ovale and decompression sickness in divers. Lancet i:513–514, 1989.
64. Wilmshurst PT, Byrne JC, Webb-Peploe MM: Relation between intraatrial shunts and decompression sickness in divers. Lancet 2:1302–1305, 1989.
65. Moon RE, Kisslo JA, Massey EW, et al: Patent foramen ovale (PFO) and decompression illness. Undersea Biomed Res 13(Suppl):15, 1991.
66. Wilmshurst PT, Treacher DF, Crowther A, et al: Effects of a patent foramen ovale on arterial saturation during exercise and on cardiovascular responses to deep breathing, Valsalva manoeuvre, and passive tilt: Relation to history of decompression illness in divers. Br Heart J 71:229–231, 1994.
67. Bove AA: Risk of decompression sickness with patent foramen ovale. Undersea Hyperbaric Med 25:175–178, 1998.
68. Sulaiman ZM, Pilmanis AA, O'Conner RB: Relationship between age and susceptibility to altitude decompression sickness. Aviat Space Environ Med 68:695–698, 1997.
69. Gilliam BC: Dealing with denial: Getting bends out of the closet. Sources. National Association of Underwater Instructors, Tampa, FL, Jan/Feb 41–43, 1992.
70. Hallenbeck JM, Bove AA, Elliott DH: Mechanisms underlying spinal cord damage in decompression sickness. Neurology 25:308–316, 1975.
71. Nix WA, Hopf HC: Central nervous system damage after decompression accidents Deutsch Med Wochenschr 105:302–306, 1980.
72. Neuman TS, Spragg RG, Wagner PD, et al: Cardiopulmonary consequences of decompression sickness. Respir Physiol 41:143–155, 1980.
73. Norman, JN, Childs, CM, Jones, et al: Management of a complex diving accident. Undersea Biomed Res 6:209–216, 1979.
74. Farmer JC, Thomas WG, Youngblood DG, et al: Inner ear decompression sickness. Laryngoscope 86:1315–1326, 1976.
75. Elliott DH: Decompression inadequacy in aseptic bone necrosis. Proc R Soc Med 64:1278–1280, 1971.
76. McCallum RI, Walder DN: Bone lesions in compressed air workers. J Bone Joint Surg 48:207–235, 1966.
77. Leffler CT, White JC: Recompression treatments during the recovery of TWA Flight 800. Undersea Hyperbaric Med 24:301–308, 1997.
78. Moon RE: Treatment of decompression sickness and arterial air embolism. *In* Bove AA (ed): Diving Medicine. Philadelphia: WB Saunders, 1997, pp 184–204.
79. Bove AA, Clark JM, Simon AJ, et al: Successful therapy of cerebral air embolism with hyperbaric oxygen at 2.8 ATA. Undersea Biomed Res 9:76–80, 1982.
80. Reuter M, Tetzlaff K, Hutzelmann A, et al: MR imaging of the central nervous system in diving-related decompression illness. Acta Radiol 38:940–944, 1997.
81. Sparacia G, Banco A, Sparacia B, et al: Magnetic resonance findings in scuba diving-related spinal cord decompression sickness. Magma 5:111–115, 1997.
82. Reul J, Weis J, Jung A, et al: Central nervous system lesions and cervical disc herniations in amateur divers. Lancet 345:1403–1405, 1995.
83. Saumarez RC, Bolt JF, Gregory RJ: Neurologic decompression sickness treated without recompression. Br Med J 1:151–152, 1973.
84. Bennett PB: Inert gas narcosis and HPNS. In Bove AA (ed): Diving Medicine. Philadelphia: WB Saunders, 1997, pp 117–130.
85. Behnke AR, Thompson RM, Motley EP: The psychologic effects from breathing air at 4 atmospheres pressure. Am J Physiol 112:554–558, 1935.
86. End E: The use of new equipment and helium gas in a world record dive. J Ind Hyg Toxicol 20:511–520, 1938.
87. Behnke AR, Willmon TL: USS Squalus: Medical aspects of the rescue and salvage operations and the use of oxygen in deep sea diving. U.S. Navy Med Bull 37:629–640, 1939.
88. Bove AA: Cardiovascular disorders. In Bove AA (eds): Diving Medicine. Philadelphia: WB Saunders, 278–292, 1997.
89. Neuman TS, Bove AA, O'Connor RD, et al: Asthma and Diving. Ann Allergy 73:344–350, 1994.
90. Elliott DE: Are Asthmatics Fit To Dive? Kensington, MD: Undersea and Hyperbaric Medical Society, 1996.
91. Mebane GY, Low N, Dovenbarger J: A review of autopsies on recreational scuba divers: 1989–1992. Undersea Biomed Res 20(Suppl):70, 1993.
92. McAniff JJ: United States underwater fatality statistics, 1970–82, including a preliminary assessment of 1983 fatalities. National Underwater Accident Data Center, University of Rhode Island. Report No. URI-SSR-84-17, 1984.
93. Powers AT, Bass B, Stewart J, et al: A six year review of SCUBA diving fatalities in San Diego County. Undersea Biomed Res 19(Suppl):20, 1992.
94. Dietz PE, Baker SP: Drowning: Epidemiology and prevention. Am J Public Health 64:303–312, 1974.
95. Cairns FJ, Koelmeyer TD, Smeeton WM: Deaths from drowning. NZ Med J 97:65–67, 1984.
96. Davis S, Smith LS: Alcohol and drowning in Cape Town. S Afr Med J 62:931–933, 1999.
97. Plueckhahn VD: The aetiology of 134 deaths due to "drowning" in Geelong during the years 1957–1971. Med J Aust 2:1183–1187, 1972.
98. Lanphier EH, Rahn H: Alveolar gas exchange during breath holding with air. J Appl Physiol 18:478–482, 1963.
99. Divers Alert Network: 1992 Report on Diving Accidents and Fatalities. Duke University Medical Center, Durham, NC: 1994.

100. Modell JH, Davis JH, Giammona ST, et al: Blood gas and electrolyte changes in human near-drowning victims. JAMA 203:337–343, 1968.
101. Cot C: Asphyxia from drowning: Treatment based on experimental findings. Bull Acad Natl Med (Paris) 105:758, 1931.
102. Modell JH, Moya F, Newby EJ, et al: The effects of fluid volume in sea water drowning. Ann Intern Med 67:68–80, 1967.
103. Modell JH, Moya F: Effects of volume of aspirated fluid during chlorinated fresh-water drowning. Anesthesiology 27:662–672, 1966.
104. Giammona ST, Modell JH: Drowning by total immersion: Effects on pulmonary surfactant of distilled water, isotonic saline and sea water. Am J Dis Child 114:612–616, 1967.
105. Alkan ML, Gaszes T, Kotev S, et al: Near drowning in the Dead Sea. Isr J Med Sci 13:290–294, 1977.
106. Yagil Y, Stalnikowicz R, Michaeli J, et al: Near drowning in the Dead Sea: Electrolyte imbalances and therapeutic implications. Arch Intern Med 145:50–53, 1985.
107. Szpilman D: Near-drowning and drowning classification: A proposal to stratify mortality based on the analysis of 1,831 cases. Chest 112:660–665, 1997.
108. Lheureux P, Vincent JL, Brimioulle S: Fulminant pulmonary edema after near drowning: Remarkably high colloid osmotic pressure in tracheal fluid. Intensive Care Med 10:205–207, 1984.
109. Fine NL, Myerson DA, Myerson PJ, et al: Near drowning presenting as the adult respiratory distress syndrome. Chest 65:347–349, 1974.
110. Rosenbaum HT, Thompson WL, Fuller RH: Radiographic pulmonary changes in near drowning. Radiology 83:306–312, 1964.
111. Conn AW, Montes JE, Barker GA, et al: Cerebral salvage in near drowning following neurological classification by triage. Can Anaesth Soc J 27:201–210, 1980.
112. Modell JH, Graves SA, Kuck EJ: Near drowning: Correlation of level of consciousness and survival. Can Anaesth Soc J 27:211–215, 1980.
113. Sekar TS, McDonnell KF, Namsirikul P, et al: Survival after prolonged immersion in cold water without neurologic sequelae. Arch Intern Med 140:775–779, 1980.
114. Siebke H, Breivik H, Rod T, et al: Survival after 40 minutes submersion without cerebral sequelae. Lancet 1:1275–1277, 1975.
115. Wolford JP: Cold water near-drowning response. J Emerg Med Services 3:5–8, 1984.
116. Young RSK, Zaineraitis ED, Dooling EO: Neurologic outcome in cold-water drowning. JAMA 244:1233–1235, 1980.
117. Guidelines for cardiopulmonary resuscitation (CPR) and emergency cardiac care (ECC). JAMA 268:2171–2302, 1992.
118. Van Haeringen JR, Blokzijl EJ, van Dyl W, et al: Treatment of the respiratory distress syndrome following nondirect pulmonary trauma with positive end expiratory pressure with special emphasis on near drowning. Chest 66(Suppl):30S–34S, 1974.
119. Rutledge RR, Flor RJ: The use of mechanical ventilation with positive end expiratory pressure in the treatment of near drowning. Anesthesiology 38:194–196, 1973.
120. Meyer TJ, Hill NS: Noninvasive positive pressure ventilation to treat respiratory failure. Ann Intern Med 120:760–770, 1994.
121. Lapinsky SE, Mount DB, Mackey D, et al: Management of acute respiratory failure due to pulmonary edema with nasal positive pressure support. Chest 105:229–231, 1994.
122. Shanholtz C, Brower R: Should inverse ratio ventilation be used in the adult respiratory distress syndrome: ARRD 149:1354–1358, 1994.
123. Kizer KW: Resuscitation of submersion casualties. Emerg Med Clin North Am 1:643–652, 1983.
124. Hughes JA: Drowning—An overview. J Am Coll Emerg Physicians 6:172, 1977.
125. Dunagan DP, Cox JE, Chang MC, et al: Sand aspiration with near drowning. Radiographic and bronchoscopic findings. Am J Respir Crit Care Med 156:292–295, 1997.
126. Calderwood HW, Modell JH, Ruiz BC: The ineffectiveness of steroid therapy for treatment of fresh-water near drowning. Anesthesiology 43:642–650, 1975.
127. Downs JB, Chapman RL, Modell JH, et al: An evaluation of steroid therapy in aspiration pneumonitis. Anesthesiology 40:129–135, 1974.
128. Sladen A. Zauder HL: Methyl prednisolone therapy for pulmonary edema following near drowning. JAMA 215:1793–1795, 1971.
129. McBrian M, Katumba JJ, Mukhtar AI: Artificial surfactant in the treatment of near drowning. Lancet 342:1485–1486, 1993.
130. Putman CE: Drowning: Another plunge. Am J Roentgenol Radium Ther Nucl Med 125:543–549, 1975.
131. Jacobsen WK, Mason LJ, Briggs BA, et al: Correlation of spontaneous respiration and neurologic damage in near drowning. Crit Care Med 11:487–489, 1983.

# 72 Drug-Induced Pulmonary Disease

ANDREW H. LIMPER, M.D. • EDWARD C. ROSENOW, III, M.D.

Introduction
Mechanisms of Drug-Induced Pulmonary Injury
Chemotherapeutic Agents
- Alkylating Agents
- Antibiotic Agents
- Antimetabolites
- Nitrosoureas
- Other Chemotherapeutic Agents

Immunotherapy
- Interleukin-2
- Tumor Necrosis Factor
- Radiation

Antimicrobial Agents
- Nitrofurantoin: Acute Reaction
- Nitrofurantoin: Chronic Reaction
- Sulfasalazine
- Miscellaneous Antimicrobial Drugs

Illicit Drugs
- Heroin
- Methadone and Propoxyphene
- Methylphenidate
- Cocaine
- Talc Granulomatosis

Cardiovascular Drugs
- Angiotensin-Converting Enzyme Inhibitors
- Amiodarone
- Protamine
- Beta-Adrenergic Antagonists
- Tocainide and Flecainide

Anti-inflammatory Agents
- Aspirin
- Gold
- Methotrexate
- Penicillamine
- Leukotriene Antagonists
- Other Nonsteroidal Anti-inflammatory Drugs
- Corticosteroids

Drug-Induced Systemic Lupus Erythematosus
Inhalants
- Oil
- Oxygen

Transfusion-Related Acute Alveolar Damage
Radiographic Contrast Medium–Induced Leukostasis
Miscellaneous Drugs
- Tocolytic-Induced Pulmonary Edema
- Hydrochlorothiazide
- Methysergide and Bromocriptine
- Dextran
- Appetite Supressants
- Esophageal Variceal Sclerotherapy
- Phenothiazine
- Tricyclic Drug Overdose
- Hydantoin
- Dantrolene

Specific Pulmonary Tissue Responses: Drug-Induced Disease by End-Organ Response
- Bronchospasm
- Pleural Effusion
- Drug-Induced Noncardiogenic Pulmonary Edema and Other Forms of Lung Injury
- Pulmonary Infiltrates and Eosinophilia

Summary

## INTRODUCTION

It is estimated that 2% to 5% of hospitalized patients are admitted because of an adverse drug reaction. An estimated 0.3% of hospital deaths are drug related, resulting in tens of thousands of deaths in the United States per year. Such numbers are notoriously inaccurate[1]; nevertheless, the problems associated with adverse drug reactions, which are for the most part preventable, account for considerable morbidity, mortality, and expense. Table 72.1 lists the classifications of drug reactions. The exact cause of the reaction in any given case, however, is usually unknown.

We also know little about the pharmacokinetic properties of drugs in individual patients. Some metabolites last only a fraction of a second; thus, they do not accumulate and are not measurable. Many drug-related injuries are

**Table 72.1 CLASSIFICATION OF DRUG REACTIONS**

| |
|---|
| Allergic or hypersensitivity reactions |
| Overdosage |
| Intolerance |
| Idiosyncratic reaction |
| Side effects |
| Secondary effects |

not reproducible in animals and therefore cannot be studied in depth. Moreover, if a drug in the therapeutic dose range caused an adverse reaction in most of the patients who received it, the drug would not be usable. Thus, the very success of many drugs, and the fact that only a small percentage of the population reacts adversely to drugs, has also inhibited greater understanding of the reactions. Even though we know the mechanism of injury for some drugs, we do not know why the same injury does not occur in more people. Furthermore, we do not understand why a patient can be rechallenged months and years later with the same drug and not develop the same reaction. What effects do multiple drugs have on production of an adverse reaction? It is uncommon for a hospital patient to be taking a single drug at one time. These deficiencies in our knowledge eventually need to be corrected.

Some minor side effects of drugs are considered an acceptable risk in order to obtain any benefit. Our own study of open lung biopsies in the immunocompromised host disclosed that in 21% of patients with diffuse pulmonary disease, the disease was likely to have been caused by a chemotherapeutic drug. Finally, we know far less than we should because there is no requirement to report adverse drug reactions. We estimate that less than 5% of all adverse drug-induced pulmonary diseases are reported.

There are more than 200 drugs known to affect the lungs adversely; many are listed in Table 72.2. To minimize mortality and significant morbidity, it is incumbent on the clinician to keep in mind at least the more common drugs that may induce pulmonary disease.[2–6]

## MECHANISMS OF DRUG-INDUCED PULMONARY INJURY

Relatively little is known of the mechanisms of drug injury to the lungs. At this time, four mechanisms are recognized: oxidant injury by chronic nitrofurantoin ingestion; direct cytotoxic effects on alveolar capillary endothelial cells by cytotoxic drugs (and these effects may be aggravated by oxidant injuries); deposition of phospholipids within cells, such as produced by amphophilic drugs like amiodarone; and immune system–mediated injury through drug-induced systemic lupus erythematosus.[4, 7–10] Although extensive investigation has been undertaken to look for other forms of immune system–mediated injury, only the systemic lupus erythematosus induced by drugs has been proven.

In addition to their respiratory functions, the lungs are actively involved in the regulation of several important vasoactive endogenous substances, including prostaglandins, angiotensin, serotonin, and bradykinin. Except for angiotensin conversion, however, there has been no proof that inhibition of this metabolic function produces systemic effects; no other specific function of an extrapulmonary organ has been reported to be regulated directly by the lung. Very little is known about the metabolic handling of drugs by the lungs.

Oxidant-mediated injury is thought to play a significant role in several of the drug-induced pulmonary diseases, namely, the chronic reaction to nitrofurantoin and possibly many of the chemotherapeutic drug-induced pulmonary injuries.[7] In vitro, nitrofurantoin is capable of generating toxic oxygen-derived substances such as hydrogen peroxide, hydroxyl radical, superoxide, and singlet oxygen. These oxygen radicals generate singlet electron transfers that disrupt critical cell functions. Nitrofurantoin may produce pulmonary fibrosis by accelerating the generation of oxygen radicals within lung cells, overwhelming the normal antioxidant protective mechanisms. This in turn incites an inflammatory and fibrotic reaction. It may be that some individuals are deficient in the cellular antioxidant glutathione, which normally is protective against oxygen radicals, making them more prone to developing drug-induced lung injury.

It is postulated that chemotherapeutic drug injury represents a direct toxic reaction. Considerable research has been done with bleomycin-induced lung injury. Bleomycin does not have a major effect on the bone marrow or on immunocompetency. The exact mechanism of bleomycin lung injury is unknown. Epithelial cells in the lung and skin, however, contain lower levels of a specific inactivating enzyme against bleomycin than do epithelial cells in other organs. Thus, the drug is allowed to accumulate within the cell and induce DNA fragmentation.[8] Because bleomycin toxicity appears to be related to dosage and age, the toxicity probably is related to the levels of inactivating enzyme in certain individuals. Bleomycin apparently overwhelms this enzyme with a large total dose. It is also likely that there is a relative deficiency of the enzyme in individuals over 70 years of age. Furthermore, some individuals of any age may be relatively deficient in this enzyme and hence especially sensitive to bleomycin lung toxicity.

The first cell to be affected by bleomycin are the type I epithelial cells. Repair of injured type I cells is accomplished by type II cells, which proliferate and differentiate into type I cells to restore the normal air-blood barrier. The vulnerability of the type II cell to bleomycin depends on the state of its cell cycle. If it is in the resting $G_0$ phase, the cell appears resistant to bleomycin injury, whereas if the cell is proliferating or differentiating, atypical exaggerated metaplasia occurs. Consequently, with net loss of type I alveolar epithelial cells, a fibroblastic reparative process is initiated. Bleomycin also stimulates fibroblasts directly to increase collagen synthesis. Type I cells are particularly vulnerable to injury by bleomycin, but in the steady state the type II cell is generally considered to be injury resistant. By dosing bleomycin repeatedly, the likelihood increases that type II cells will be exposed while vulnerable during their proliferative or differentiating periods.

**Table 72.2** CLASSIFICATION OF DRUG-INDUCED AND RELATED PULMONARY DISEASES BY TYPE OF MEDICATION

| | |
|---|---|
| **Chemotherapeutic** | **Cardiovascular** |
| *Cytotoxic* | Amoidarone* |
| Azathioprine | Angiotensin-converting enzyme inhibitors |
| Bleomycin* | Anticoagulants |
| Busulfan | Beta-blockers* |
| Chlorambucil | Dipyridamole |
| Cyclophosphamide | Flecainide |
| Etoposide | Protamine* |
| Interleukin-2 | Tocainide |
| Melphalan | **Inhalant** |
| Mitomycin C* | Aspirated oil |
| Nitrosoamines | Oxygen |
| Procarbazine | **Intravenous** |
| Tumor necrosis factor | Blood* |
| Vinblastine | Ethanolamide maolate (sodium morrhuate)* |
| Zinostatin | Ethiodized oil (lymphangiogram) |
| *Noncytotoxic* | Talc |
| Bleomycin* | **Miscellaneous** |
| Cytosine arabinoside* | Bromocriptine |
| Methotrexate* | Dantrolene |
| Procarbazine* | Hydrocholorothiazide* |
| **Antibiotic** | Methysergide |
| Amphotericin B* | Tocolytic agents* |
| Nitrofurantoin | Tricyclics* |
| Acute* | L-Tryptophan |
| Chronic | Radiation |
| Sulfasalazine | Systemic lupus erythematosus (drug-induced) |
| **Anti-inflammatory** | Complement-mediated leukostasis* |
| Acetylsalicylic acid* | |
| Gold | |
| Methotrexate | |
| Nonsteroidal anti-inflammatory agents | |
| Penicillamine* | |
| **Analgesic** | |
| Heroin* | |
| Methadone* | |
| Naloxone* | |
| Placidyl* | |
| Propoxyphene* | |
| Salicylates* | |

* Typically present as acute or subacute respiratory insufficiency.

It is not known whether bleomycin and other chemotherapeutic drugs stimulate the formation of oxygen radicals as a primary form of injury. It may be that when injury has taken place, the normal antioxidant substances glutathione and superoxide dismutase are damaged or impaired such that breathing supplementary oxygen is sufficient to cause an oxidant injury. Not all of the reactions to chemotherapeutic drugs are as dose and age related as bleomycin. The relationship to aggravation by oxygen also does not appear to be as strong. Thus, the mechanism of toxicity may vary with each drug and each individual.

Amiodarone has brought to light another potential mechanism of drug-induced lung injury. Amiodarone has been demonstrated to produce phospholipidosis in the alveolar macrophage and in type II cells. In individuals who react adversely to this drug, there is a marked accumulation of abnormal alveolar macrophages containing lamellar inclusions with a variety of phospholipids.[7, 7a] It is not known whether this phospholipidosis is a secondary effect or whether phospholipid accumulation primarily incites the interstitial pneumonitis, with accompanying infiltration of polymorphonuclear leukocytes and lymphocytes. There are more than 20 cationic amphophilic drugs known to induce phospholipid storage disorders in cells, particularly in the lungs. It is believed that these drugs induce impairment in phospholipid catabolism. The cells containing these lamellar inclusions are increased in size as well as number. The process is reversible with discontinuation of the drug.

Drug-induced systemic lupus erythematosus (SLE) is another cause of pulmonary disease for which there is moderate understanding of the drug-inducing mechanism.[10] There are two groups of drugs associated with drug-induced SLE. The first group commonly elicits antinuclear antibody formation in a large percentage of the persons taking the drug, but only a small percentage of these develop clinical symptoms of SLE. The second group is made up of numerous drugs that have been reported to induce antinuclear antibodies only rarely, but virtually all those afflicted develop SLE.

In drug-induced SLE, the antibodies are primarily against histones. In contrast, during idiopathic SLE, the antinuclear antibodies are heterogeneous and consist of antibodies to native DNA, histones, and nonhistone ribonuclear proteins, as well as antibodies formed against extranuclear host components such as clotting factors.[10] Exactly how drugs incite antibodies to nuclear protein is not clear because these agents are in themselves nonimmunogenic. A current hypothesis that explains some of these aberrations is that the drug acts as an adjuvant or immunostimulant, producing a disorder in immunity. Autoimmunity then develops from the clonal expansion of cell-reacting lymphocytes, which are ordinarily held in check by a balance of helper and suppressor influences, rather than from an alteration in the cell itself.

## CHEMOTHERAPEUTIC AGENTS

Pulmonary diseases induced by chemotherapeutic agents are a major problem for the pulmonary specialist for two reasons: The diseases can be fatal, and they mimic other pulmonary diseases such as infection because of their related fever and radiographic abnormalities. Chemotherapeutically induced pulmonary disease was first recognized in 1961 in a patient treated with busulfan, but in the last decade it has become a major problem, particularly with bleomycin, methotrexate, and cyclophosphamide. Almost all patients taking these drugs are immunocompromised because of the disease being treated, as well as the effects of the drugs themselves. In addition to the drug-induced effects on the lungs, many of these patients have other pulmonary problems, including susceptibility to a variety of infections and recurrence in the lungs of the disease for which the patient is being treated.

The definitive diagnosis of cytotoxic lung damage depends on a history of drug exposure, histologic evidence of lung damage, and the exclusion of other causes of the lung injury. In many cases it is a diagnosis by exclusion because pathologists are unable to ascribe the observed changes solely to the effects of the drug. Time as well as appropriate histologic studies, however, generally eliminate the possibilities of other conditions producing these effects. Clinicians caring for these patients must be aware of all the drugs that can potentially produce adverse effects on the lungs. Unfortunately, there is no diagnostic blood test or even tissue study that confirms the diagnosis. Overall, less than 10% of the patients taking these various drugs develop pulmonary side effects, and trying to anticipate which patients will be affected has been the goal of most authors in reviewing the numerous reports of these side effects.[2–4, 9, 11–19]

It is obvious that there are many ways that chemotherapeutic drugs can affect the lungs, and even though the end stage of the epithelial cellular atypia seen histologically is similar for many of the drugs, the mechanisms of injury may be quite different. This chapter provides an overview of the various types of presentations seen with each of the drugs listed in Table 72.3 according to their pharmacologic chemotherapeutic action.

The clinical presentations of many drug effects are quite similar, with the exception that some tend to present more acutely and others more chronically. Typically, symptoms of dyspnea, nonproductive cough, and frequently fever begin weeks to years after the drug is first taken. Fever is associated with most chemotherapeutic drug-induced pulmonary disease, but it may not be a consistent fever in that there may be days without obvious fever even though the drug continues to be taken. Chills are usually absent. Weight loss is common. The chest radiograph may be normal for days or weeks before showing typical changes in a diffuse interstitial pattern. Occasionally, there is a diffuse alveolar-interstitial pattern that may be helpful in recognizing an early drug effect, but it is in no way diagnostic (Fig. 72.1). There is no radiographic pattern characteristic of any particular drug-induced pulmonary disease, with the possible exception of hilar lymphadenopathy during methotrexate pneumonitis. Auscultation of the lungs discloses crackles, but this is also nonspecific. Small pleural effusions occur as a consequence of some adverse drug reactions, but not consistently enough to be of diagnostic benefit. Clubbing has not been reported in any of these reactions.

**Table 72.3 PHARMACOLOGIC ACTION OF CHEMOTHERAPEUTIC AGENTS**

| |
|---|
| **Alkylating** |
| Busulfan |
| Cyclophosphamide |
| Chlorambucil |
| Melphalan |
| Vinblastine |
| **Antimetabolite** |
| Methotrexate |
| Mercaptopurine |
| Azathioprine |
| Cytosine arabinoside |
| **Antibiotic** |
| Bleomycin |
| Mitomycin C |
| **Nitrosamines** |
| Bischloroethyl nitrosourea |
| Chloroethyl cyclohexyl nitrosourea (CCNU) |
| Methyl-(CCNU) |
| **Other** |
| Procarbazine |
| Zinostatin |
| Etoposide (VP-16) |
| Tumor necrosis factor |
| Interleukin-2 |

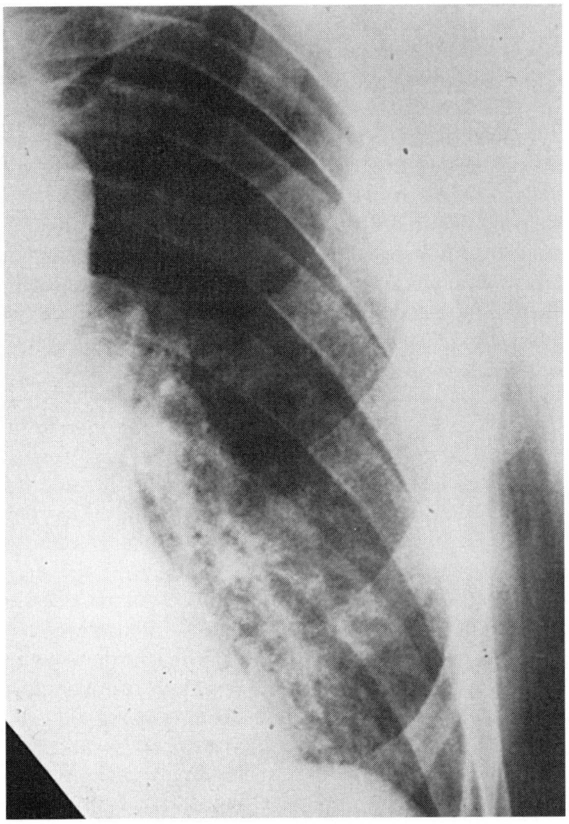

**Figure 72.1** The close-up chest radiograph shows an alveolar and interstitial pattern that is characteristic, but not diagnostic, of cytotoxic lung disease.

The results of pulmonary function studies are abnormal in essentially all patients with chemotherapeutic drug disease when compared with the pretreatment pulmonary function studies. The carbon monoxide diffusing capacity may decrease before volumes are decreased. There is no disproportionate decrease in rates of air flow. The decrease in diffusing capacity may precede the clinical onset of symptoms and radiographic changes by days or weeks. In some prospective studies, diffusing capacity has been used to detect the early onset of pulmonary reaction, at which time the drug or drugs are discontinued to minimize progression into clinical disease. Gallium ($^{67}$Ga) uptake has also been shown to be increased in most of these chemotherapeutic drug reactions, showing that the lungs are affected even before the chest radiograph becomes abnormal.

Bronchoalveolar lavage may be another means of assessing early lung damage from these drugs, but the results are quite variable. What is not known is how often histologic abnormalities occur that do not progress to clinical disease. For example, some studies have shown atypia in the sputum cytology in many patients who have no clinical symptoms.

According to some pathologists, the histologic findings of cytotoxicity in the lungs are characteristic of a chemotherapeutic drug effect by virtue of the marked atypia produced in the type II pneumocyte. Fewer type I cells are present, whereas there are more type II pneumocytes showing what was originally described as "bizarre" changes. The nuclear to cytoplasmic ratio remains normal, however, and there is no increased number of mitotic abnormalities in these cells; therefore, these changes should not be interpreted as malignant. There is a marked inflammatory reaction in the interstitium and a deposition of fibrin and collagen in the septal wall. These can progress to the point of severe fibrosis, resulting in respiratory insufficiency and death.

## Alkylating Agents

**Busulfan.** This drug is useful for the treatment of chronic myeloproliferative disorders. The average interval from the initiation of therapy to the onset of pulmonary symptoms is about 3.5 years, with a range of 8 months to 10 years, but symptoms can occur as early as 6 weeks. The estimated incidence is 6%, with a range of 2.5% to 43%.[20] The onset of dyspnea, cough, and fever is usually more insidious than with other chemotherapeutically induced pulmonary diseases. Symptoms have even been reported to occur months after discontinuation of therapy. The response to discontinuing the drug and to the administration of corticosteroids is quite variable; some patients improve, but in most the disease progresses to death. It is not obvious whether busulfan-related injury is dose dependent. Concomitant radiation therapy may play an adverse role, as it does with some of the other drugs. The chest radiograph, more than in many other drug-induced pulmonary diseases, shows a combination of an alveolar-interstitial process, probably due to a greater degree of desquamation into the alveolar spaces. Alveolar proteinosis has been reported in a number of patients receiving busulfan; it appears to be more refractory to therapeutic lavage than the spontaneous onset type of alveolar proteinosis (Chapter 63).[21–23]

**Cyclophosphamide.** The incidence of cyclophosphamide-induced pneumonitis is grossly underestimated.[24] A retrospective analysis from the Mayo Clinic identified six patients over 20 years in whom cyclophosphamide was the only factor contributing to lung disease.[25] Clinical features of cyclophosphamide-associated pulmonary toxicity include dyspnea, fever, cough, new parenchymal infiltrates, gas exchange abnormalities, and pleural thickening. Two patterns of cyclophosphamide-induced lung toxicity are appreciated: Early onset pneumonitis occurs within the first 1 to 6 months after institution of therapy and generally responds to withdrawal of the drug. In contrast, late onset pneumonitis develops after months to years of cyclophosphamide therapy and is manifested by progressive pulmonary fibrosis and bilateral pleural thickening. Unfortunately, the late onset variety has minimal response to withdrawal of cyclophosphamide and institution of corticosteroid therapy.[25] There does not appear to be a clear relationship between dose and pulmonary disease with cyclophosphamide, nor does there appear to be a clear-cut synergism between cyclophosphamide and other drugs. There has also been a report of a negative rechallenge with cyclophosphamide, that is, the drug was reinstituted without subsequent pulmonary sequelae. This has similarly been reported in methotrexate pneumonitis.

**Chlorambucil.** This drug is used primarily in chronic lymphocytic disorders. The clinical presentation, chest radiographic findings, and histologic findings are similar to those described for other alkylating agent–induced pulmonary reactions. The presentation is generally insidious, occurring 6 months to 1 year or more after therapy is begun.

**Melphalan.** There have been only a few well-documented cases of pulmonary toxicity associated with melphalan, which is used in the treatment of multiple myeloma, although this incidence may be underestimated. The course varies from acute to subacute. There are no particular clues for predicting which patients will develop side effects. There certainly must be a very low incidence of pulmonary side effects, in view of the fact that this is the primary drug used in the treatment of a relatively chronic disease.

## Antibiotic Agents

**Bleomycin.** Bleomycin pulmonary toxicity is the most common chemotherapeutically induced pulmonary disease and the best studied.[26, 26a] Studies based on frequent tests of pulmonary function and chest radiographs disclosed that as many as 20% of treated patients develop clinical pulmonary disease, and 1% die from pulmonary consequences of bleomycin. There is a significant increase in bleomycin-related pulmonary disease in those over 70 years of age and in those who have received a total dose of over 450 U, with a 10% death rate in those having received a total dose greater than 550 U. In these studies, frequent monitoring of the carbon monoxide diffusing capacity predicted subsequent clinical disease. It has been suggested that when there is a progressive fall in the carbon monoxide diffusing capacity, the drug should be withheld.[27]

There is a definite correlation between prior or concomitant thoracic radiotherapy and an increased incidence of severe bleomycin pulmonary toxicity. There is also evidence of a synergistic effect between prior bleomycin exposure and subsequent exposure to a high inspired oxygen concentration, which occurs most commonly during anesthesia and in the postoperative recovery period.[28, 29] It is not known how long after bleomycin exposure that breathing a high inspired oxygen concentration predisposes the patient to bleomycin toxicity, but certainly an interval of fewer than 6 months should be considered highly risky. High inspired oxygen concentrations should be avoided if possible. In addition, there also appears to be synergistic toxicity between bleomycin and cyclophosphamide.

Bleomycin pulmonary toxicity may be reversible if minimal changes have occurred. One study reported that if the patient survives the acute event, the pulmonary findings are reversible.[30] If significant fibrosis is present, however, the process may progress despite the administration of corticosteroids. There is a rare hypersensitivity type of bleomycin toxicity associated with acute onset, fever, and eosinophilia. Discontinuation of the drug and initiation of corticosteroids bring about reversal of the process.

An unusual complication of bleomycin pneumonitis, and unique to this drug, is the presence nodular lesions mimicking metastasis (Fig. 72.2).[31, 32] Histologically, most of these lesions consist of bronchiolitis obliterans with organizing pneumonitis. Computed tomography (CT) of the lung may also be useful to establish an early diagnosis of bleomycin pneumonitis.[33, 34] In one study of 100 patients taking bleomycin, a computed tomographic scan was abnormal in 38%, whereas the chest radiograph was abnormal in only 15%.[33]

**Mitomycin C.** The exact incidence of mitomycin lung disease is unknown, but in one series the incidence was 8%, and in two different series the incidence ranged from 12% to 39%.[35] The clinical presentation, radiographic findings, and histology are similar to those of other adverse alkylating drug reactions reported thus far except that the carbon monoxide diffusing capacity does not decrease before the onset of clinical symptoms.[35] The response to corticosteroids has also been impressive in a number of patients, possibly more so than for other forms of chemotherapy-associated pneumonitis.

In addition to mitocycin-induced pneumonitis, there have now been a number of case reports of a very unusual reaction of a microangiopathic hemolytic anemia associated with renal failure and noncardiogenic pulmonary edema.[36] Most patients developed side effects between 6 and 12 months after starting chemotherapy, with about half of them developing the acute respiratory distress syndrome (Chapter 54). The mortality rate of those with respiratory complications was 95% compared with 50% for patients without lung involvement. Many of these patients had also been given fluorouracil, normally not considered a drug toxic to the lungs. In some patients, the reaction was seemingly precipitated by blood transfu-

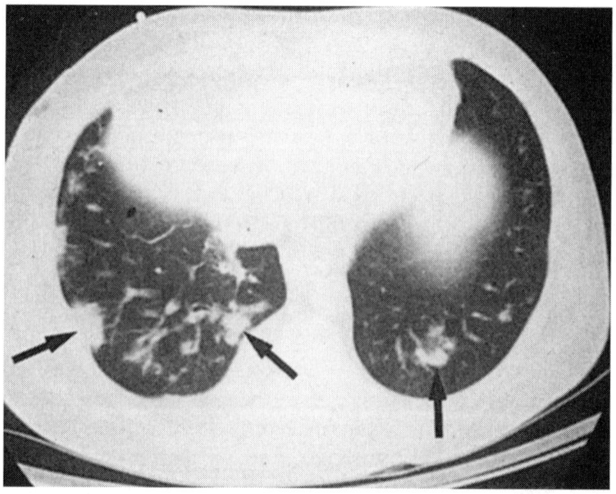

**Figure 72.2** The CT scan of bleomycin pneumonitis shows a nodular pattern. The histologic features of this form of bleomycin-induced lung injury are typical of bronchiolitis obliterans with organizing pneumonitis.

sions. Histologically, microangiopathic changes are seen in the kidneys and lungs: intimal hyperplasia of the arterioles (sometimes associated with complete occlusion of the lumen), along with prominent nuclear atypia of the capillary cells and capillary fibrin thrombi.

## Antimetabolites

**Methotrexate.** This drug is used in many combination programs for neoplasia, as well as for some nonmalignant conditions such as psoriasis and rheumatoid arthritis. Several hundred cases of adverse pulmonary reactions have been reported. Methotrexate pneumonitis is unique and has led to only a few fatalities. The onset of dyspnea, nonproductive cough, and fever may begin a few days to several weeks after initiation of therapy and, in rare cases, a few months or years later.[37] The process is almost always reversible with or without the addition of corticosteroids. Eosinophilia is seen in at least half of the cases, and the disease is believed to be a form of hypersensitivity pneumonitis. (For a discussion of this disease, see Chapter 61). The intriguing feature of this reaction is that the drug may be reinstituted after resolution of methotrexate pneumonitis without subsequent recurrence of symptoms or findings (in essence, a negative rechallenge). In about one third of the patients, weakly formed granulomas occur, also an unusual finding. There is no cellular atypia, such as is seen in other cytotoxic drug reactions.

The chest radiograph shows a more homogeneous infiltrate throughout the lung fields than occurs with the other agents. Hilar adenopathy or pleural effusion occurs in at least 10% to 15% of the patients. Also, in contrast to most of the other adverse chemotherapy reactions, prospective studies of patients taking this drug have not demonstrated a diminished diffusing capacity that might detect subclinical toxicity. The reaction is not dose related. There have been a few reports of fatal reactions occurring either from intrathecal methotrexate or from oral ingestion after previous intrathecal injections.

**Azathioprine.** There are at least six case reports of azathioprine pneumonitis. The incidence must be quite low, considering that this drug is widely used for a number of neoplastic as well as non-neoplastic conditions. Nevertheless, the possibility of azathioprine pneumonitis in any individual treated with this drug should be kept in mind. Azathioprine is metabolized to 6-mercaptopurine; there have been at least four reports of interstitial pneumonitis of the cytotoxic variety in association with this drug.[6] Most of these patients, however, have also received other drugs that potentially could be implicated in the pneumonitis.

**Cytosine Arabinoside.** This cytotoxic drug is used to induce remission of acute leukemia, and it has been associated with fatal noncardiac pulmonary edema (Fig. 72.3). Histologically, there is marked intra-alveolar proteinaceous material without the cellular atypia and mononuclear infiltration described with other cytotoxic drugs. In two large series, 13% to 28% of the patients with side effects developed respiratory distress during the administration of the drug, and nearly one half developed symptoms within a month of discontinuing it.[38, 39] The mechanism underlying this reaction is unknown. It is associated with a high mortality rate.

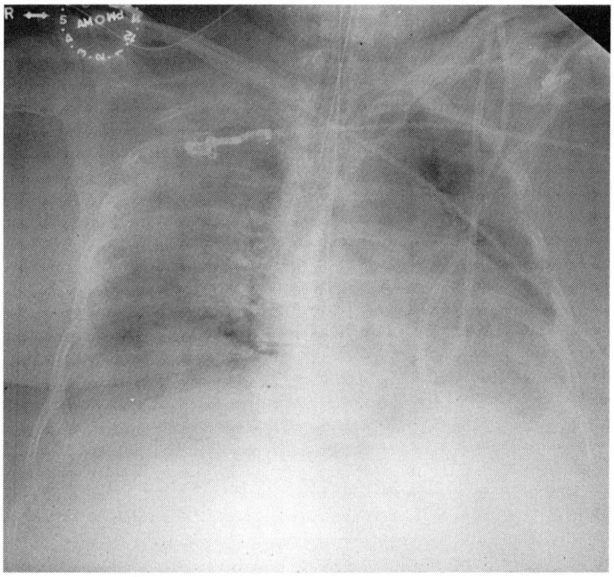

**Figure 72.3** The chest radiograph of a 44-year-old female shows acute noncardiac pulmonary edema that resulted from cytosine arabinoside–induced pulmonary disease. Histologic examination typically demonstrates intense intra-alveolar proteinaceous material forming hyaline membranes, but little other reaction.

## Nitrosoureas

**Bischloroethyl Nitrosourea.** The incidence of pulmonary toxicity associated with the administration of bischloroethyl nitrosourea varies from 1.5% to 20% and appears to be dose related, with up to a 50% risk of lung disease at a total dose of over 1500 mg/m$^2$. There have been reports, however, of pulmonary effects occurring with a much lower dose.[40] The duration of therapy before the onset of pulmonary toxicity has varied from 6 months to 3 years. There may also be a synergistic effect with cyclophosphamide, possibly radiation therapy, and other drugs. The clinical course is similar to that of bleomycin and cyclophosphamide. The outcome is unpredictable and sometimes fatal. There have been a few case reports of pulmonary toxicity with methyl-chloroethyl cyclohexyl nitrosourea and chloroethyl cyclohexyl nitrosourea. Apparently, fever is less commonly associated with this form of pulmonary toxicity than with most of the other chemotherapeutic drugs.

An unusual long-term complication of bischloroethyl nitrosourea toxicity is evidence of upper lobe pulmonary fibrosis many years after the completion of chemotherapy.[41] O'Driscoll and colleagues[41] studied 17 patients for up to 17 years, and 12 of the 17 (71%) developed upper lobe fibrosis. Another complication that is almost exclusively associated with the nitrosoureas is pneumothorax.[42]

### Other Chemotherapeutic Agents

**Procarbazine.** Pulmonary side effects of procarbazine are rather infrequent, with only a few cases of probable procarbazine pneumonitis being reported. This side effects may be cytotoxic. In other patients, toxicity has been related to a rapid onset hypersensitivity reaction associated with eosinophilia that declines after the drug is discontinued.

**Zinostatin.** There are a few reports of zinostatin toxicity occurring after a patient has received the drug for a long time. Unique to this drug is the report of hypertrophy of the pulmonary vasculature that appears to be associated with the cytotoxic effect.

**Etoposide.** This drug (VP-16) is used in combination chemotherapy with cyclophosphamide and methotrexate for small cell carcinoma of the lung. It has not been independently associated with a high incidence of pulmonary cytotoxicity.

**Vinblastine.** This is one of the oldest chemotherapeutic agents and was not associated with pulmonary complications until it was combined with other agents, specifically mitomycin C. This combination has been complicated by asthma, interstitial pneumonitis, and noncardiac pulmonary edema.[43, 44]

## IMMUNOTHERAPY

### Interleukin-2

Interleukin-2 has been used with or without lymphokine-activated killer cells as an experimental drug for treatment of certain malignancies.[45–47] Well over half of the patients in whom interleukin-2 has been used developed one or more pulmonary complications, including acute respiratory distress syndrome, noncardiac pulmonary edema, hyperreactive airway disease, and, on the basis of cardiac toxicity, cardiogenic pulmonary edema.

### Tumor Necrosis Factor

Tumor necrosis factor is a macrophage-produced cytokine that causes necrosis of certain neoplasms and has been used in research protocols.[48, 49] In one study of 27 patients, pulmonary function studies showed a statistically significant decline in carbon monoxide diffusing capacity in all patients studied, beginning about 2 weeks after initiation of therapy. The results of other pulmonary function tests did not change significantly.[49]

### Radiation

The acute effects of radiation can produce histologic changes mimicking cytotoxic lung responses and may occasionally involve areas of lung outside the port of radiation.[49a] The process is generally heralded by fever beginning 3 to 8 weeks after initiation of radiation therapy and may rapidly progress to a fatal outcome despite institution of corticosteroids. The disease may improve spontaneously but usually progresses to chronic radiation effects. Bronchoalveolar lavage predominantly demonstrates lymphocytes not only in the involved lung but also in the contralateral lung.[50] The chronic effects of radiation are well known. They begin 3 to 6 months or later after radiation therapy, and their primary effect is vascular.[51]

## ANTIMICROBIAL AGENTS

### Nitrofurantoin: Acute Reaction

Acute nitrofurantoin pneumonitis may be one of the most common drug-induced pulmonary diseases.[52–56] The Swedish Adverse Drug Reaction Committee reported 921 patients with adverse reactions to this drug: 43% were acute pulmonary reactions, and another 5% were due to chronic interstitial pneumonitis.[52, 53] They estimated that all of these reactions occurred in fewer than 1% of those taking the drug. Seventy-one per cent of all reactions were severe enough to require hospitalization, but only 1% were fatal. The fatalities included 4 of 49 patients with chronic pulmonary fibrosis and 2 of 398 with acute pulmonary reaction.

Acute pulmonary reactions are probably underestimated.[54] Interestingly, of the 921 patients in the Swedish study just mentioned, 172 gave histories of previous use of nitrofurantoin, with over half of these patients having experienced a nonpulmonary adverse reaction before the current exposure! In other series, the incidence was estimated to be anywhere from 1 in 550 to 1 in 5400 individuals.[54] The mechanism of the acute nitrofurantoin reaction is unknown. There are only a few studies on the lung histology in individuals with acute nitrofurantoin pneumonitis, and these have shown a proliferation of fibroblasts and a lymphoplasmocytic infiltrate, occasionally with an intra-alveolar desquamation of cells. Despite peripheral blood eosinophilia, eosinophils are not usually seen in the lung tissue itself.

The typical reaction begins a few hours to several days after initiation of therapy.[3, 54] It appears to be much more common in females, but this is probably because of the increased use of this drug for urinary tract infections in women. Fever is present in most cases, dyspnea is almost always present, and cough is present in about two thirds of cases. Other incidental findings include leukocytosis and eosinophilia in one third and an elevation in sedimentation rate in nearly one half. The chest radiograph shows an alveolar process, an interstitial process, or both. The reaction may be unilateral or asymmetric. It is generally most prominent at the bases. Pleural effusion has been found in one third of patients, most commonly unilaterally. There are no reported laboratory studies of pleural fluid analyses in acute nitrofurantoin reaction. Bronchospasm has been reported in a number of cases, but its incidence is unknown. It may occur in the absence of pulmonary parenchymal or pleural disease.[54]

The onset of the acute symptoms does not appear to be dose related: It has occurred with a single low dose of 25 mg, with the average daily dose being 100 to 150 mg. Pleuritic chest pain occurs in about one third, mimicking acute pulmonary embolism and, in some cases, pneumonitis and myocardial infarction. Rales are heard in most cases. There is no way to diagnose acute nitrofurantoin pneumonitis other than to suspect that the drug is responsible and to stop its administration. Unfortunately, many patients who take the drug do not mention it when asked what drugs they are taking. The patient is frequently admitted to the hospital because of the presence of bilateral pulmonary infiltrates, fever, dyspnea, and hypoxemia. Once all medications are discontinued, the pneumonitis clears spontaneously, and it is assumed that the antimicrobial agents initiated during hospitalization brought about the resolution.

Treatment consists of supportive measures and discontinuation of the medication. It is not known whether corticosteroids accelerate the resolution. There is probably no indication for them. There is also no indication for rechallenge to confirm the diagnosis.

Nitrofurantoin-induced SLE with pleuropulmonary disease and positive antinuclear antibody has also been reported. Little information on this form of lung disease is available at this time.

### Nitrofurantoin: Chronic Reaction

There is no overlap between the acute and chronic pulmonary reactions to nitrofurantoin, probably because the mechanisms are entirely different. Martin[55] showed that lung parenchymal cells incubated with nitrofurantoin exhibit significant cellular injury through production of oxygen radicals (see the earlier discussion of mechanisms of drug-induced pulmonary injury). Chronic reactions occur far less commonly than acute pulmonary reactions. In chronic reactions, fever and eosinophilia are much less common.[52–54, 56, 57] The onset of dyspnea and cough is usually insidious, beginning 6 months to many years after the chronic (either continuous or intermittent) use of nitrofurantoin. These reactions are more common in women.

The chest radiograph shows a diffuse interstitial process.[54, 57, 58] There is no associated bronchospasm or obstructive airway disease. Pulmonary function testing demonstrates a restrictive pattern. Bronchoalveolar lavage usually shows a lymphocytic reaction.[59, 60] Histologic analysis of lung tissue shows inflammatory cells and fibrosis. Clinically, radiologically, and histologically, this condition mimics idiopathic pulmonary fibrosis, with the single exception that these patients have ingested nitrofurantoin chronically.

The literature varies as to the utility of corticosteroids. Our experience is that they are almost always required before significant resolution occurs. Others imply that this infiltrate resolves spontaneously on discontinuation of the medication.[58] Our policy is to observe the patient for 2 to 4 months after discontinuing nitrofurantoin and then to repeat the chest radiograph and pulmonary function studies. If there is no improvement, a trial of corticosteroids is given.

### Sulfasalazine

Sulfasalazine is an antimicrobial drug that has been used for many years for the treatment of inflammatory bowel disease.[61] There appear to be two separate types of reactions: One is a pulmonary infiltrate and eosinophilia and the other a bronchiolitis obliterans with organizing pneumonitis. The onset of symptoms of cough, dyspnea, and, in about half, fever, begins 1 to 8 months after initiation of continuous therapy. The dosage ranges from 1.5 to 4 g/day. The chest radiograph shows a variable pattern of lung infiltrates, ranging from upper lobe alveolar infiltrates to a diffuse interstitial process. Over half of the patients had significant blood eosinophilia, but none had migratory pulmonary infiltrates. Most of the resolution occurs within 1 week to 6 months after the drug is discontinued and, if necessary, corticosteroids are added. Sulfasalazine is metabolized to 5-aminosalicylic acid and sulfapyridine, both of which have been implicated in eosinophilic pneumonitis.

In cases of suspected sulfasalazine-associated pulmonary disorders, it is important to keep in mind that inflammatory bowel disease has been associated with a variety of pulmonary abnormalities independent of sulfasalazine use. Inflammatory bowel disease has been independently linked to airway inflammation, interstitial lung disease including bronchiolitis obliterans with organizing pneumonia, neutrophilic necrotic pulmonary nodules, and serositis.[62] Most of these disorders respond to corticosteroid therapy.

### Miscellaneous Antimicrobial Drugs

There are many scattered reports of unusual reactions to various antimicrobial drugs.[63] Compared with the wide use of these agents, the incidence of reactions is extremely low. Many of these reactions appear to be pulmonary infiltrates with eosinophilia.

The polymyxin and aminoglycoside antibiotics are known to produce respiratory muscle weakness when they reach an excessive level in the blood.[64] Toxic levels in the blood occur in patients to whom these drugs are given by direct instillation into the peritoneal or pleural space, in persons with renal failure, or when the patient receiving them has been given a muscle-relaxing agent at the time of general anesthesia. These effects are reversible with physostigmine.

The combined administration of granulocytes with amphotericin B may predispose some patients to transient deterioration in pulmonary function.[65, 66]

## ILLICIT DRUGS

### Heroin

Although nitrofurantoin appears to be the most commonly reported prescribed drug with adverse pulmonary effects, heroin pulmonary edema may be the most common drug-induced pulmonary disease worldwide. Hospitals in all major cities of the United States receive hundreds of patients with heroin pulmonary edema. Heroin is diacetylmorphine and, because of its increased lipid solubility, it crosses the blood-brain barrier much more readily than morphine.[67–69] There are several postulated mechanisms of heroin-induced noncardiac pulmonary edema. These include a direct toxic effect on the alveolar capillary membrane, leading to an increased permeability and extravasation of fluid into the alveolar spaces; a neurogenic response to central nervous system injury; an allergic or hypersensitivity reaction; and an acute hypoxic effect on the alveolar capillary membrane in association with secondary increased permeability. The hypoxemic theory is the one most commonly touted, but other causes of acute hypoxia, such as barbiturate overdosage with depression of the respiratory center, rarely result in noncardiac pulmonary edema.[67] Immunologic abnormalities have been reported, including depression of total complement, C3 complement component, and immunoglobulins. In other cases, the presence of immune complexes in the alveolar capillary wall has been observed. This is unlikely, however, to be the primary mechanism.

Heroin pulmonary edema can occur with the first intravenous use of the drug. It is believed that the effects of heroin are related to the dose. The exact dose, however, is almost always unknown. Up to 40% of addicts hospitalized for acute drug overdose have acute pulmonary edema with severe hypoxemia and hypercapnia. The noncardiac pulmonary edema is indistinguishable at the outset from other forms of acute respiratory distress syndrome. The pulmonary capillary wedge pressure is usually within normal range. Typically, symptoms of dyspnea and somnolence begin within minutes of the intravenous "push," but reports of delayed onset of hours and even a few days have been published.

The pupils are small. Auscultation of the lungs discloses crackles. The chest radiograph shows changes of noncardiac pulmonary edema. The patient hypoventilates, producing hypoxemia and hypercapnia. Acidosis can be metabolic as well as respiratory.

Up to one half of these patients vomit and aspirate, producing secondary bacterial infection. This should be suspected if the pulmonary infiltrates do not clear within 24 to 48 hours of treatment. Other pulmonary abnormalities include septic emboli from infected thrombophlebitis or tricuspid endocarditis. Treatment consists of assisted ventilation with positive end-expiratory pressure if necessary, oxygen, and intravenous naloxone to reverse the respiratory depression. This is usually sufficient treatment for the noncardiac pulmonary edema, which will reverse with time. Corticosteroids are unnecessary. Because up to half of these patients have aspirated and have bacterial infections, appropriate use of antimicrobial drugs is indicated. Histologic features of acute heroin noncardiac pulmonary edema are nonspecific. In addition to the extensive exudative fluid, variable degrees of atelectasis and alveolar hemorrhage are usually evident.

Bronchiectasis and necrotizing bronchitis in chronic heroin abusers have been reported. These may be more sequelae of recurrent gastric juice aspiration than of the effects of heroin, with or without pulmonary edema. Pulmonary function is abnormal in patients with pulmonary edema, but, even after the radiographic clearance of the edema and the return of lung volume to normal, a reduction in the carbon monoxide diffusing capacity may persist. In chronic abusers of heroin and other illicit drugs, pulmonary function abnormalities are more likely to be related to talc granulomatosis than to sequelae of a single acute injury.

## Methadone and Propoxyphene

Pulmonary sequelae similar to those associated with heroin have been reported with methadone and propoxyphene and likely have similar mechanisms. Treatment is the same as for heroin-induced sequelae. Addicts in drug rehabilitation programs have free access to methadone. They accumulate the drug illegally and dissolve and inject it. Noncardiac pulmonary edema has been reported in cases of both oral and intravenous overdose of both methadone and propoxyphene.

Propoxyphene is a rapidly absorbed drug, and, even after oral ingestion, death can occur within 30 minutes from respiratory depression and arrest and noncardiac pulmonary edema. In some parts of the United States, propoxyphene is a commonly used drug in attempted suicide.

## Methylphenidate

Methylphenidate may have more serious adverse side effects than heroin or cocaine.[70, 71] In one series, all 22 patients had chest pain and wheezing, and most had abnormal pulmonary function tests and hemoptysis.[70] In another series, severe panlobular emphysema was found in seven patients who died as a result of the abnormalities.[71]

## Cocaine

Cocaine use remains a major problem throughout the world, and there are increasing reports of adverse pulmonary effects from both intravenous and inhalation use of the drug. These are over and above the known cardiac effects of cocaine, which produces left ventricular failure with pulmonary congestion and edema. The principal long-term effects of cocaine are infection and aspiration, noncardiac pulmonary edema, particulate embolization, talcosis, diffuse alveolar damage, alveolar hemorrhage, intra-alveolar eosinophilic infiltration, lung mass with or without cavitation, and bronchiolitis obliterans with organizing pneumonia (Table 72.4).[72–74]

## Talc Granulomatosis

Talc (magnesium silicate) is used as a filler in many medications intended for oral use. Addicts who abuse oral medications such as meperidine, methadone, propox-

**Table 72.4 PULMONARY EFFECTS OF COCAINE**

| |
|---|
| Infection and aspiration leading to noncardiac pulmonary edema |
| Particulate embolization |
| Talcosis |
| Diffuse alveolar damage |
| Alveolar hemorrhage |
| Intra-alveolar eosinophilic infiltration |
| Lung mass with or without cavitation |
| Bronchiolitis obliterans with organizing pneumonia |

yphene, methylphenidate, amphetamines, and tripelennamine crush the tablets, mix them with various solutions, and inject them intravenously. This results in the insidious onset of granulomatous interstitial fibrosis, granulomatous pulmonary arterial occlusion, or both.[69, 72, 75–78] This usually does not occur in heroin addicts because heroin is mixed with soluble fillers such as quinine, lactose, or maltose. In large series of consecutive autopsies performed on addicts, depending on the type of addiction, the incidence of talc granulomatosis ranged from 15% to 80%.

Dyspnea is the major symptom, cough occurs in some patients, and, in more advanced stages of pulmonary hypertension, symptoms of exercise-induced syncope, right heart failure, and even sudden death occur. The chest radiograph may be normal in up to half of patients with proven talc granulomatosis. Thus, a normal chest radiograph does not eliminate the possibility of this condition. Pulmonary function studies characteristically show a low diffusing capacity before any other abnormalities are evident because of occlusion of pulmonary blood vessels. This may remain the only abnormality. Chest radiographs of these patients show diffuse micronodular densities varying in size between 1 and 3 mm, which may mimic alveolar microlithiasis.

Histologically, the pulmonary tissue demonstrates granulomatous changes, with multinucleated giant cells, mononuclear inflammatory cells, lymphocytes, and fibrosis.[75, 78] Talc is detected (with polarized light) by the presence of strongly birefringent crystals within the granulomas. Bronchoalveolar lavage shows a lymphocytosis consistent with that reported in other granulomatous diseases. Intracellular and free talc have been identified in the bronchoalveolar lavage. Talc retinopathy occurs in over half of the patients. Talc emboli presenting as small, whitish, glistening foci near the macula within a small vessel are characteristic.

Results of therapy with corticosteroids vary from no response to significant improvement. It is often worth administering steroids for at least a short period of time, if one keeps in mind that these persons are susceptible to infection because of the numerous organisms they have been exposed to in the use of nonsterile intravenous medication.

## CARDIOVASCULAR DRUGS

### Angiotensin-Converting Enzyme Inhibitors

Angiotensin-converting enzyme (ACE) inhibitors are widely used for control of hypertension and in the management of congestive heart failure. Soon after their introduction, these agents were associated with nonproductive cough and, more rarely, with angioneurotic edema.[79, 80] Dry cough occurs in 5% to 20% of patients taking ACE inhibitors, being reported with captopril, enalopril, lisinopril, and virtually all other ACE inhibitors. The mechanisms of ACE inhibitor–induced cough likely involves accumulation of kinins and substance P, which are normally degraded by ACE and related enzymes. The cough generally is reported in the first few weeks of therapy but may not be appreciated for months. ACE cough is usually benign but can be quite annoying, causing half of the patients affected to discontinue these agents. Exacerbation of bronchospasm has been associated with ACE inhibitor use only on very rare occasions. Fortunately, most patients can be switched to other classes of drugs. Rechallenge with a different ACE antagonist is not recommended because the cough will usually recur. Cough generally abates within 4 days of discontinuation of the agent, providing confirmation of the diagnosis. For patients who have no other therapeutic options, baclofen and cromolyn sodium have been employed with some success to suppress ACE-induced cough.

ACE inhibitors cause angioneurotic edema much less frequently, being reported in 0.1% to 0.2% of patients receiving ACE inhibitors. This complication usually occurs within hours to, at most, 1 week after initiation of therapy. This reaction may be mediated by bradykinins but may also involve autoantibodies and complement system components. Treatment involves the use of epinephrine, antihistamines, and corticosteroid administration. The ACE inhibitor must be discontinued and future use by these patients avoided.

### Amiodarone

Amiodarone is an antiarrhythmic agent that has been available in Europe since 1962, but no adverse pulmonary effects were reported until 1980. It has significant benefit for ventricular dysrhythmias in patients who do not respond to most other antiarrhythmic agents. This drug is associated with a number of side effects, which include corneal microdeposits (in nearly 100% of the patients); peripheral neuropathy; liver dysfunction; thyroid dysfunction, including hypothyroidism and hyperthyroidism; and bluish pigmentation of the skin. The most serious side effect, however, is an interstitial pneumonitis, which occurs in up to 6% of patients and may be fatal.[7, 81, 82]

The mechanism of amiodarone toxicity is unknown, but it has peculiar histologic features that may be a clue to the mechanism. The histologic findings generally include foamy alveolar macrophages and type II pneumocytes containing lamellar inclusions. In one half of the patients who take amiodarone and die of nonpulmonary causes, macrophages and type II pneumocytes contain a significant amount of phospholipids.

The incidence of pulmonary toxicity from amiodarone varies widely but probably averages 4% to 6% of those patients taking the drug.[81, 83, 84] The majority of those affected are males, but this may be related to increased use by males. Symptoms consist of insidious dyspnea, nonproductive cough, occasionally a low-grade fever without chills, followed by subtle chest radiographic findings, which initially may be asymmetric or even limited to the upper lobes. If the drug is continued, the process may diffusely involve the lungs with an interstitial or alveolar process (Fig. 72.4). Pleural effusion is uncommon. Pleuritic chest pain occurs in about 10% of patients. Clubbing has not been reported. Crackles may be heard, but it is difficult to be certain whether these are due to pulmonary edema because congestive heart failure is common in these patients. In about 20% of patients

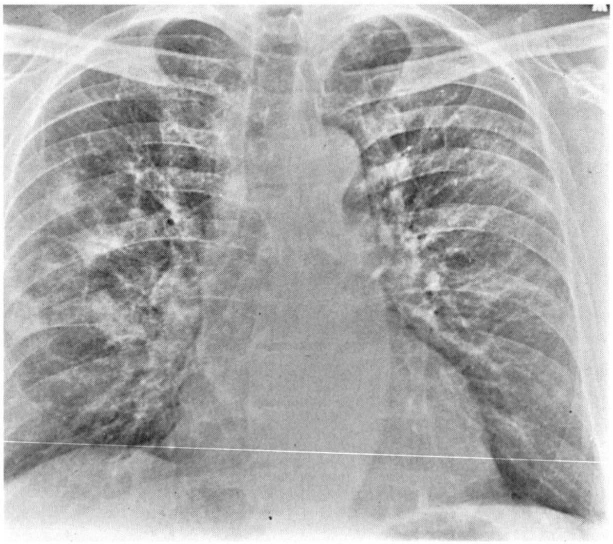

**Figure 72.4** The chest radiograph of a 72-year-old man shows amiodarone-induced lung disease. The pattern is predominantly interstitial and nonuniform.

with amiodarone pneumonitis, the presentation is acute, mimicking pneumonia.

Laboratory studies disclose a normal to mildly elevated leukocyte count, generally no eosinophilia, and an elevated sedimentation rate in the majority, with little or no reactivity to antinuclear antibody. Pulmonary function studies disclose a decrease in total lung capacity and carbon monoxide diffusing capacity as well as hypoxemia. A decrease in the lung volumes and carbon monoxide diffusing capacity, however, can occur as a result of congestive heart failure, and thus a change in these parameters is not diagnostic of impending clinical amiodarone pneumonitis. However, there are several reports of $^{67}$Ga radionuclide lung scanning that demonstrate its benefit in differentiating amiodarone pneumonitis from congestive heart failure.[85, 89] There may be an increased predisposition to amiodarone pneumonitis if either pulmonary function or chest radiographic findings are abnormal before administration of the drug begins.

Most patients who develop amiodarone pneumonitis have been taking the drug for at least 1 month, and some for a few years. Most are receiving at least 400 mg/day. There have been a number of reports, however, of amiodarone pneumonitis occurring with as little as 200 mg/day. There are also reports of patients receiving 200 mg/day for months or even years and not developing amiodarone pneumonitis until the dose is boosted for purposes of better control of the arrhythmia. Generally, the systemic side effects from amiodarone, such as peripheral neuropathy and liver dysfunction, correlate with the serum levels (usually greater than 2.5 mg/L), but this is not necessarily the case with the pulmonary toxicity. Perhaps the greater phospholipid turnover in the lungs explains the greater chance for lung toxicity from amiodarone. The diagnosis of amiodarone pneumonitis is really one of exclusion. Table 72.5 summarizes the approach to the patient who takes amiodarone and has an abnormal chest radiograph.

**Table 72.5 DIAGNOSIS OF AMIODARONE PNEUMONITIS***

| |
|---|
| Bronchoalveolar lavage |
| Presence of phospholipid-filled macrophages† |
| Increased lymphocytes or polymorphonuclear leukocytes |
| Elevated sedimentation rate |
| Positive $^{67}$Ga scan |
| Ga scan |
| Computed tomographic scan showing increased density of infiltrates or lesions |
| Exclusion of other conditions, i.e., congestive heart failure, pulmonary embolism, pneumonia |

*Assumes appropriate clinical setting, i.e., more than 400 mg/day for 2 months.

†The presence of phospholipid-filled macrophages supports the diagnosis but is not diagnostic, whereas their absence excludes the condition.

Normally, amiodarone pneumonitis is thought to be primarily an interstitial or alveolar process (or both), sometimes mimicking eosinophilic pneumonitis with peripheral infiltrates, but there are a number of reports of confluent lesions occurring as a result of amiodarone pneumonitis. Many of these are bronchiolitis obliterans with organizing pneumonitis.[86–88] CT of the lung can further define these processes because amiodarone is an iodinated compound and thus is radiopaque; on a CT scan the amiodarone pneumonitis lesions are denser than the surrounding soft tissue in the chest wall (Fig. 72.5). This latter finding may confirm the diagnosis.[89, 90]

Treatment, consisting of drug withdrawal, leads to a variety of responses. Some patients who were not treated with corticosteroids died of pulmonary fibrosis and respiratory failure. Others died despite being treated with cor-

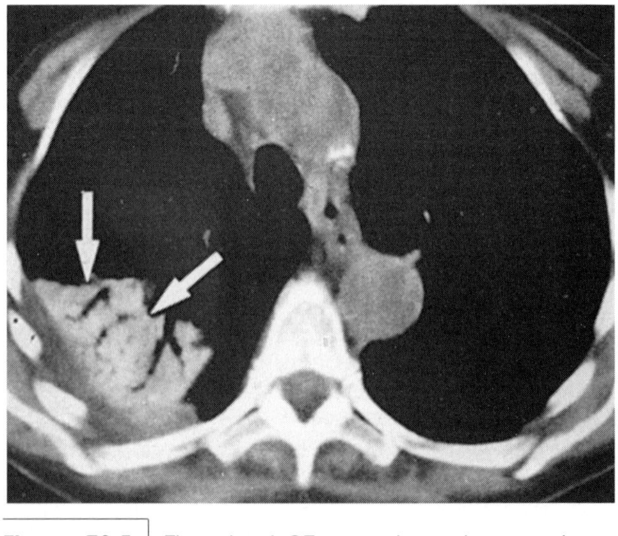

**Figure 72.5** The chest CT scan shows large pulmonary masses from amiodarone pneumonitis. Note that the masses *(arrows)* are appreciably denser than the surrounding soft tissue in the chest wall in this CT scan obtained without contrast.

ticosteroids. The majority respond significantly to the discontinuation of the drug and the addition of corticosteroids, which are usually required for a period of at least 2 and perhaps 6 months or longer. There are many case reports of patients who continued on amiodarone because it was the only drug that controlled their ventricular dysrhythmia and who at the same time were given corticosteroids to suppress their pneumonic reaction.[91]

Initially, it was believed that tissue confirmation by biopsy was necessary to establish a diagnosis, although discontinuation of the drug and addition of corticosteroids may offer a presumptive diagnosis if the process clears. Now, only the absence of foamy cells eliminates the diagnosis. The presence of such foamy macrophages only confirms exposure to the drug; their presence alone does not necessarily indicate amiodarone toxicity. Bronchoalveolar lavage has had mixed results, with some authors reporting a high percentage of lymphocytes or neutrophils and others obtaining normal values.[81] As mentioned, a positive $^{67}Ga$ scan is highly suggestive of an inflammatory pneumonitis rather than congestive heart failure. If the diagnosis has not been established, the clinician must decide whether to proceed with an open lung biopsy to rule out other causes or to consider diminishing the dose or discontinuing the drug, adding corticosteroids, or both. Correlating the response with the change in sedimentation rate may be of some value. A normal wedge pressure rules out left ventricular failure.

There are reports of postoperative acute respiratory distress syndrome in patients treated with amiodarone.[92–95] Several of these patients have died as a result of the acute respiratory distress syndrome, which begins 18 to 72 hours after surgery. In one series, acute respiratory distress syndrome occurred in 50% of the patients who take or have recently taken amiodarone.[95] It has been postulated that the high fraction of inspired oxygen given during the operation and the postoperative period contributed to this complication.

## Protamine

Protamine sulfate is routinely used to reverse the anticoagulant effects of heparin following cardiovascular surgical procedures. Systemic hypotension is not an uncommon sequela of this drug. There have now, however, been a number of cases of noncardiogenic pulmonary edema occurring within minutes to 1 to 2 hours after the administration of the drug.[96, 97] It is frequently associated with an anaphylactic reaction and bronchospasm, an increase in pulmonary artery pressure with normal wedge pressure, and hypotension. In at least half of the patients there is a history of previous use of protamine, either in a similar situation or as protamine zinc insulin. Skin testing can confirm the sensitization.

Death from cardiovascular collapse and noncardiac pulmonary edema may occur as a result of protamine. The anesthesiologist may note significant difficulty ventilating the patient because of severe bronchoconstriction, which occurs in some patients. Therapy is supportive, including reintubation if the patient has been extubated, assisting ventilation with high inspired oxygen concentrations, administering a trial of high-dose corticosteroids, and treating the hypotension with an alpha-adrenergic agonist. For patients whose skin test is positive to protamine or who have a history of reaction to protamine, an alternative method of reversing the effects of heparin is to use intravenous hexadimethrine.[97]

## Beta-Adrenergic Antagonists

The first beta-adrenergic antagonist was synthesized in the late 1950s. Since then, numerous similar agents have been synthesized, and a number are now available for clinical use. They are among the most commonly prescribed drugs. Beta-adrenergic receptors can be divided into excitatory $beta_1$-receptors located in the heart and inhibitory $beta_2$-receptors located in the bronchi. The beta-adrenergic blockers, or beta-blockers, are competitive antagonists. (For a discussion of the adrenergic drugs, see Chapter 11.)

Propranolol was the first beta-adrenergic antagonist introduced. It was quickly recognized that it had adverse effects on individuals with known obstructive lung disease.[98] Studies have also demonstrated increased airway resistance in normal persons and in asymptomatic asthmatic patients who use propranolol.[98] Thus, this agent should be avoided by all patients with known obstructive airway disease, even those who are asymptomatic. The following beta-adrenergic antagonists, presented in decreasing order of bronchoprovocation potential, are available for clinical use in the United States: propranolol, timolol, nadolol, metoprolol, atenolol, pindolol, and labetalol.[99]

There are two features of beta-adrenergic antagonists that predict their potential for bronchoprovocation. The first is their cardioselectivity, and the second is their intrinsic sympathomimetic activity. Generally, cardioselectivity is the more important of the two. If the drug is cardioselective, it has little effect on the inhibitory beta-receptors located in the bronchial walls. Propranolol, timolol, and nadolol have essentially no cardioselectivity.[99] Metoprolol has some cardioselectivity, and atenolol has considerable cardioselectivity, making atenolol the drug of choice for an individual with obstructive airway disease who needs a beta-adrenergic antagonist. The other mechanism important in beta-adrenergic antagonist is intrinsic sympathomimetic activity, with pindolol having strong intrinsic sympathomimetic activity. Labetalol is unique in that it has combined alpha-antagonistic and beta-antagonist effects. It is not cardioselective, nor does it have intrinsic sympathomimetic activity; therefore, it is assumed that it is its alpha-adrenergic antagonist potential that causes it to be bronchoprotective.

Thus, among the seven drugs listed, atenolol and then metoprolol and probably labetalol are the three that can be used with relative safety by persons with obstructive airway disease, if absolutely necessary. These should always, however, be given in conjunction with an aerosolized $beta_2$-adrenergic agent. Calcium channel blockers may be a good alternative to beta-blocking drugs, if indicated, because they also have some bronchodilating capabilities.[100]

Similar findings have been shown to occur in asthmatic patients who use timolol eyedrops for glaucoma. There are many case reports of the adverse effects of topical ocular timolol, including a number of fatal cases of status asthmaticus.[101, 102] Topically applied timolol is absorbed through the conjunctiva and bypasses the liver, resulting in a higher blood concentration than when given orally. A newer ocular beta-adrenergic antagonist, betaxolol, has been shown to be safer in patients with known airway disease. There are scattered reports of beta-blocker-associated interstitial pneumonitis.[103] Propafenone is a new membrane-stabilizing antiarrhythmic agent that is structurally similar to propranolol and has the potential to aggravate bronchospasm.[104]

### Tocainide and Flecainide

Tocainide is used in the treatment of refractory ventricular arrhythmias. There are more than 40 known cases of acute interstitial pneumonitis beginning 3 weeks to several months after initiation of therapy.[105] The response to discontinuation of the drug is good; corticosteroids may be necessary in some cases. Flecainide, another antidysrythmic agent, has been reported to be associated with the acute respiratory distress syndrome[106] and an interstitial lymphocytic pneumonitis.[107]

## ANTI-INFLAMMATORY AGENTS

### Aspirin

Anti-inflammatory agents are among the most commonly used drugs, and many have pulmonary side effects.[108, 109] Aspirin is the most commonly used drug in the world. In the United States, there are over 200 proprietary drugs that contain aspirin. It is estimated that up to 5% of asthmatics are sensitive to aspirin; ingestion may cause fatal aggravation of bronchospasm.[110, 111] The exact cause of aspirin-sensitive asthma is unknown. One theory is that acetylsalicylic acid and similar compounds inhibit cyclooxygenase, and thus prevent the generation of cyclooxygenase products. If bronchodilator prostaglandins (such as prostaglandin $E_2$), are normally released by these subjects, their inhibition could cause bronchospasm.

The aspirin-asthma triad consists of asthma, rhinitis, and nasal polyposis. Almost always there are other associated side effects, such as cutaneous rashes and gastrointestinal symptoms. These adverse reactions are not dose related because they can occur with very small doses. In addition, salicylate-induced noncardiac pulmonary edema can occur when the serum salicylate level is greater than 40 mg/dL. This can occur without an intentional overdosage in patients chronically ingesting salicylates.[112–114] It occurs more commonly in elderly persons who are smokers than in younger nonsmokers. The mechanism is unknown, although it may be a direct effect on the alveolar capillary wall, resulting in an increase in capillary permeability. It may be related to the effect of salicylates on platelets or prostaglandins or occur through a central nervous system effect. It does not occur in every individual with very high serum salicylate levels.

Because of the respiratory center stimulation by salicylates, hyperventilation occurs, resulting in hypocapnea. Despite hyperventilation, the arterial $P_{O_2}$ may be paradoxically low because of the presence of pulmonary edema. In one review of the 177 consecutive patients admitted to an intensive care unit for salicylate intoxication, 47% had respiratory failure.[114] Out of the 177 patients, 94% required mechanical ventilation. Abnormal clotting studies were noted in 38%, and 36% were acidemic. There was a 15% mortality rate. In another report it was found that in 8% of all asthmatic patients who required mechanical ventilation, the intervention was made necessary by ingestion of aspirin or a nonsteroidal anti-inflammatory agent.[111]

Treatment of salicylate-induced noncardiac pulmonary edema depends on the severity of the edema; some patients require intubation and even hemodialysis. Treatment with forced alkaline diuresis is often recommended, but this is dangerous in patients who already have pulmonary edema. (For a discussion of the treatment of pulmonary edema, see Chapter 54.)

Leatherman and Schmitz[115] describe a pseudosepsis syndrome associated with chronic salicylate ingestion. Most patients had fever, leukocytosis, hypotension, and multiple organ failure, including the acute respiratory distress syndrome. This condition is easily missed unless salicylate intoxication is suspected and the blood salicylate level is measured.

### Gold

Gold has been used since ancient times for treating various disorders, rheumatoid arthritis in particular.[108, 109, 116, 117] There are now a number of reports of diffuse interstitial pneumonitis-fibrosis associated with gold use that are thought to be separate from that of rheumatoid lung. Interstitial pneumonitis is more commonly observed in patients taking sodium aurothiomalate than in those taking aurothioglucose, but this may reflect the more common use of the former drug. Symptoms of dyspnea with or without fever begin insidiously several weeks to months after initiation of weekly intramuscular injections of gold. A few reports have demonstrated peripheral blood eosinophilia, but this is uncommon. Pleural effusion is not associated with this reaction.

In diffuse interstitial pneumonitis-fibrosis, the chest radiograph shows a predominantly interstitial process. Bronchoalveolar lavage usually demonstrates a high percentage of lymphocytes.[116] Histologically, the lung demonstrates fibrosis with an interstitial infiltrate of lymphocytes and plasma cells and focal hyperplasia of type II pneumocytes. Electron microscopy demonstrates electron-dense structures within lysosomes of endothelial cells of the alveolar capillaries and interstitial macrophages. Microanalysis with an electron probe shows that these electron-dense structures contain gold, suggesting that a direct toxic effect might be an important mechanism in the pathogenesis of gold-induced pulmonary reactions. There are no control studies, however, of the lungs of patients who are taking gold but do not develop gold pneumonitis.

Other associated complications of gold are often present, such as dermatitis, peripheral neuropathy, and proteinuria. Secondary infections have not been reported as a complication of gold pneumonitis, nor have there been deaths reported from irreversible lung fibrosis. The treatment may be as simple as withdrawing the drug and allowing the process to resolve spontaneously. A number of patients, however, have required corticosteroids for reversal. Gold pneumonitis is not thought to be related to rheumatoid fibrosis in that the parenchymal disease improves spontaneously with discontinuation of the gold or almost always regresses with the use of corticosteroids.

## Methotrexate

Methotrexate is being used increasingly as an anti-inflammatory agent. Pulmonary complications occur in about 5% of patients on low-dose (e.g., 10 mg/week) methotrexate for rheumatoid arthritis.[118, 119] There is no correlation with age or underlying disease. Almost all the complications include fever, crackles, hypoxemia, and dyspnea with cough. There is no eosinophilia. Most patients who undergo open lung biopsies exhibit noncaseating granulomas. All nine patients in one series responded to discontinuing the drug and to taking high doses of prednisone. An interesting possible synergistic relationship is with nitrofurantoin, which was used concomitantly in two of the nine patients. There have been five deaths reported. In addition to inducing lung disease, this agent is immunosuppressive and has been associated with opportunistic infections, including *Pneumocystis carinii* pneumonia.[120]

## Penicillamine

There are three possible pulmonary complications with the use of penicillamine with no apparent overlap: penicillamine-induced SLE, bronchiolitis obliterans, and Goodpasture's syndrome. A fourth entity has been described, namely pneumonitis or alveolitis, but it is likely that this is drug-induced SLE. Some patients with pneumonitis or alveolitis have high titers of antinuclear antibodies. Penicillamine-induced disease appears to be one of the more common causes of drug-induced SLE.[121] This condition should always be considered in patients receiving penicillamine, especially if a pleural effusion is present. A normal concentration of sugar in the effusion fluid eliminates the possibility of a rheumatoid effusion.

Bronchiolitis obliterans is underestimated in its incidence and severity.[122] There have been no studies reported on the pulmonary functions of rheumatoid patients before initiation of penicillamine that compare them with those of patients who subsequently develop bronchiolitis. Perhaps there is a predisposing obstructive lung disease in the rheumatoid patient that is worsened by penicillamine in the form of a bronchiolitis obliterans. Corticosteroids have little benefit in treating this condition, which usually presents in an advanced state. Bronchiolitis is discussed in Chapter 43.

There have been several case reports of penicillamine-induced Goodpasture's syndrome (Chapter 60) with diffuse alveolar hemorrhage.[123] If recognized early enough, appropriate therapy with hemodialysis, plasmapheresis, and immunosuppression may prevent a fatal outcome.

## Leukotriene Antagonists

Recent reports have associated zafirlukast and related leukotriene antagonists with manifestations of Churg-Strauss syndrome.[124, 125] These potent agents have been employed to treat asthma. As zafirlukast is added to an asthmatic treatment regimen, corticosteroids are frequently tapered. A number of patients have been described who exhibit pulmonary infiltrates, cardiomyopathy, and eosinophilia while receiving zafirlukast. It is currently unknown whether these medications actually trigger these reactions or whether they unmask a preexistent infiltrative eosinophilic disorder as the corticosteroids are withdrawn. In either event, the pulmonary reaction responds to discontinuation of zafirlukast and reinstitution of corticosteroids.

## Other Nonsteroidal Anti-inflammatory Drugs

Most of the nonsteroidal anti-inflammatory agents can produce the same side effects as aspirin, including aggravation of asthma, noncardiac pulmonary edema, drug-induced SLE, and pulmonary infiltrates with eosinophilia. Naproxen may be more commonly associated with an infiltrate and eosinophilia than are the other agents.[126] A few agents can cause hypervolemia and, in turn, pulmonary edema through the mechanism of increased sodium retention through the kidneys.

## Corticosteroids

Corticosteroids given in immunosuppressive doses are well known for predisposing patients to the development of opportunistic infections (Chapter 83). A most unusual adverse effect of corticosteroids is the production of mediastinal lipomatosis, that is, the deposition of mediastinal fat, which produces a widening of the mediastinum that mimics lymphadenopathy or other neoplasms (Fig. 72.6). Clinically, these patients have a "cushinglike" appearance, with round facies and a buffalo hump. The same kind of fat that deposits in the buffalo hump occurs in the mediastinum. The chest radiograph does not show the lumpiness usually expected with adenopathy. CT can usually make this diagnosis by establishing radiographic fat density throughout the mediastinal mass (see Fig. 72.6).[127] Mediastinal lipomatosis does not necessitate tapering corticosteroids because the fat does not compromise vital structures.

# DRUG-INDUCED SYSTEMIC LUPUS ERYTHEMATOSUS

There are over 40 drugs that have been reported to induce the SLE syndrome, but only 5 regularly induce antinuclear antibodies in patients taking them: hydralazine, procainamide, isoniazid, hydantoins, and penicillamine.[10, 128, 129] Only a small percentage of the patients taking these drugs develop the clinical syndrome which involves the pleuropulmonary system in over half the cases (see the earlier discussion on mechanisms of drug-induced injury). It is thought that patients who develop antinuclear antibodies to these drugs are "slow acetylators." Symptoms almost always begin insidiously after the patient has been taking the drug for many months or even years. Systemic signs and symptoms of polyarthralgia, myalgia, fever,

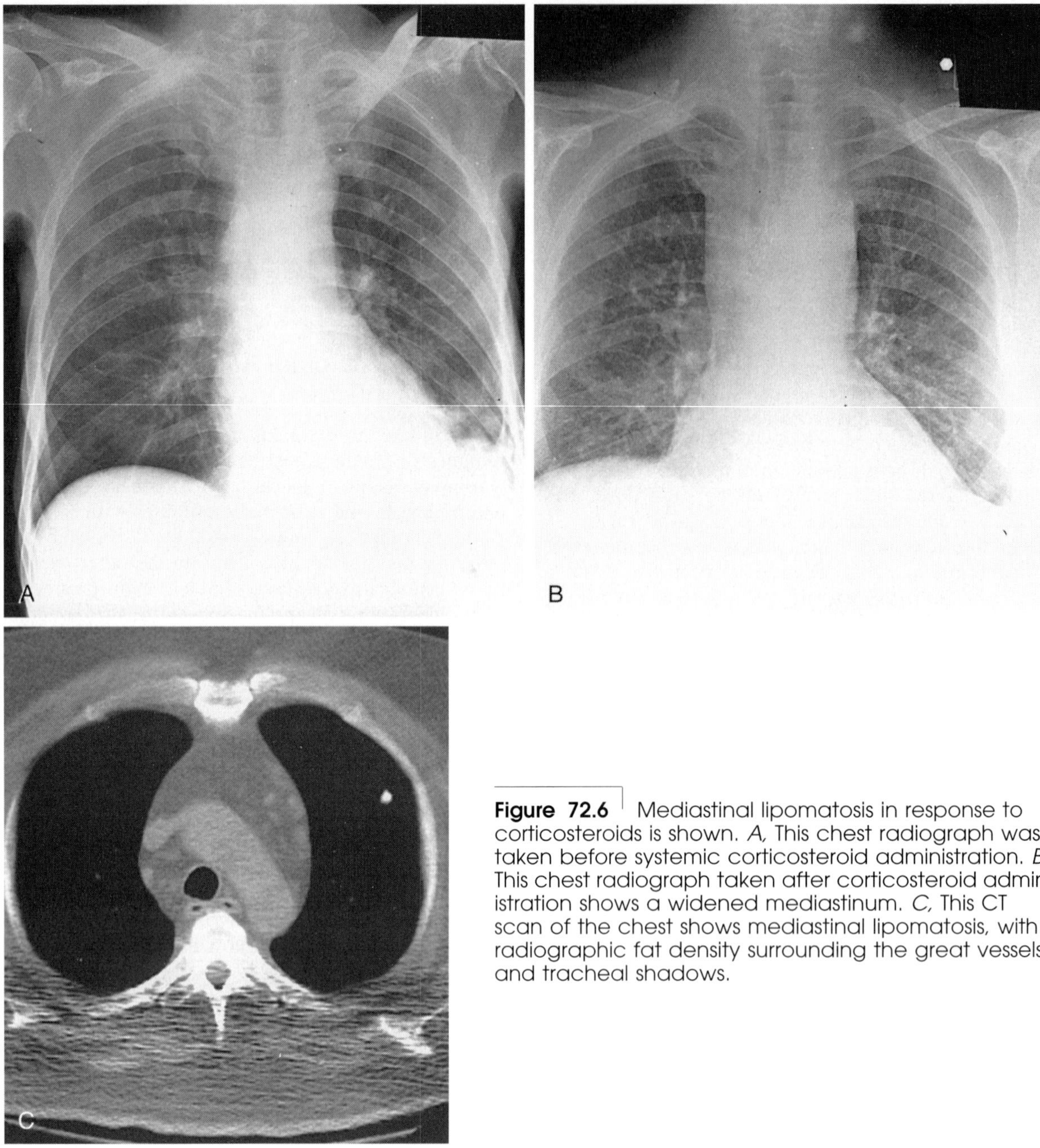

**Figure 72.6** Mediastinal lipomatosis in response to corticosteroids is shown. *A,* This chest radiograph was taken before systemic corticosteroid administration. *B,* This chest radiograph taken after corticosteroid administration shows a widened mediastinum. *C,* This CT scan of the chest shows mediastinal lipomatosis, with radiographic fat density surrounding the great vessels and tracheal shadows.

pleurisy, and cutaneous lesions are common. Renal disease is very uncommon, however, possibly because complement is not as often involved in the drug-induced form of SLE as in the spontaneous type.

The antinuclear antibody assay is positive in all patients with drug-induced SLE. The test for anti-native (anti-double-stranded) DNA, however, is negative. The complement level may or may not be abnormal. The Coombs' test is positive in about one third of patients. An elevated erythrocyte sedimentation rate and hypergammaglobulinemia are common nonspecific findings.

The chest radiographic findings of the drug-induced form of the disease are indistinguishable from spontaneous onset SLE and include pleural effusions in one third of patients, basilar infiltrates, pneumonitis with atelectasis, and apparent cardiomegaly from pericardial effusion. Pleural fluid glucose level is normal or at least correlates with the blood glucose level.

The symptoms usually resolve after the drug is discontinued. Occasionally, however, it is necessary to add corticosteroids for more rapid resolution of disabling symptoms. If the offending drug cannot be discontinued for clinical reasons, the lowest dose should be used, along with the addition of corticosteroids.

## INHALANTS

### Oil

Aspirated oil can produce a variety of pulmonary diseases, ranging from an asymptomatic solitary nodule to diffuse disease with severe respiratory insufficiency.[130, 131] Most commonly, however, the diseases present in an asymptomatic individual with an incidental finding of an abnormality on the chest radiograph that often mimics a more serious process such as bronchogenic carcinoma. Because patients rarely consider oily nose drops, oily eye lubricants, or mineral oil as a medication, they rarely volunteer that they are taking oil-containing medications.

There are three types of oil: mineral oils, neutral oils, and animal fats. Mineral oils are the most commonly aspirated oils. Oily droplets are taken up by macrophages that eventually disintegrate and release the oil, which in turn inhibits ciliary activity.[130] Thus, the oil is not expectorated and the cycle is repeated again. Eventually, a fibrotic or granulomatous reaction occurs. Neutral or vegetable oils (e.g., olive or castor oil) do not elicit a local reaction and are removed by expectoration. Animal fats (e.g., milk, butter) are rapidly hydrolyzed, with the liberated fatty acids producing tissue necrosis followed by fibrosis. Milk and butter are not commonly aspirated, probably because they do not suppress the cough reflex like mineral oils do.

The diagnosis can be established with the demonstration of oil in the lung tissue. CT has been used to diagnose lipoid-induced infiltrates.[131] Treatment involves the discontinuation of the oil-containing medication. Once this occurs, progression is unlikely.

## Oxygen

Exposure to high concentrations of oxygen may contribute to or aggravate the acute respiratory distress syndrome.[132–138] There are two theories as to the mechanisms of oxygen-induced pulmonary disease. The first is that a high fraction of inspired oxygen induces formation and release of free oxidant radicals. These short-lived molecules damage DNA, destroy lipid membranes, and inactivate intracellular enzymes.[132] The other theory is that hyperoxia produces a direct injury to endothelial cells and type I epithelial cells, resulting in an alveolar-capillary leak.[133]

Lavage fluid shows an increase in albumin and transferrin as well as alveolar macrophage release of fibronectin and alveolar macrophage-derived growth factor.[133] Bronchoalveolar lavage does not show a change in the type or number of inflammatory cells in the first 24 to 48 hours, but after this there is an influx of polymorphonuclear leukocytes. Eventually, hyperoxia increases the number of fibroblasts in the alveolar walls, resulting in fibrosis.[133, 136]

Results of studies in volunteers show that breathing 100% oxygen for 6 to 48 hours produces variable effects, but in some a tracheobronchitis occurs, with symptoms of substernal burning, chest tightness, and nonproductive cough.[137] It also produces a reduction in vital capacity and carbon monoxide diffusing capacity.[134] The development of tolerance to hyperoxia appears to be related to the ability of the individual to increase the production of antioxidants, a mechanism that may be determined genetically.[132]

The sequelae of oxygen toxicity are separable into two phases, the acute, or exudative, phase and the subacute proliferative phase; however, there is considerable overlap between the two phases, with the proliferative phase beginning after the fourth to seventh day. The exudative phase begins within 48 to 72 hours, depending on the fraction of inspired oxygen, and is associated with perivascular, interstitial, and alveolar edema with atelectasis, as well as alveolar hemorrhage. This phase appears to be reversible.

The proliferative phase is characterized by progressive resorption of exudates and hyperplasia of type II cells. This is followed by the deposition of collagen and elastin in the interstitium and hyaline membrane deposition. This is usually an irreversible phase. Clinically, hypoxemia and diminished compliance progress, requiring a greater fraction of inspired oxygen and assisted ventilation, further aggravating the problem. The chest radiograph shows an alveolar-interstitial pattern in an irregular distribution, with evidence of moderate loss of volume from patchy atelectasis.

There is no clinical way of diagnosing oxygen toxicity. A lung biopsy specimen may show changes consistent with oxygen toxicity, but its primary value is to exclude other causes. Keeping the arterial $Po_2$ less than 80 mm Hg or the inspired fraction of oxygen below 0.40 to 0.50 minimizes the chance of oxygen toxicity developing.

## TRANSFUSION-RELATED ACUTE ALVEOLAR DAMAGE

Acute alveolar damage as a result of transfusion reaction is probably one of the more rarely recognized adverse drug reactions, if one considers transfused blood or its products a form of drug. The damage is usually the result of donor antibodies against leukocyte antigens or donor leukocyte-specific immune cells reacting against the recipient's leukocytes.[139] In about 5% of the cases, the recipient's antileukocyte antibodies react against the donor's leukocytes. The acute alveolar damage reaction is not a hemolytic transfusion reaction or an anaphylactic reaction.

The clinical presentation is that of onset of dyspnea, cough, fever, and hypotension within a few hours of receiving a transfusion. An urticarial rash occurs in about half of these patients. The onset of symptoms can occur in response to as little as 50 mL of transfused blood or blood products. The pulmonary artery wedge pressure is always normal. Any blood product containing plasma and plasma proteins can produce this form of reaction.

The source of the antibodies is almost always blood taken from multiparous women who have had three or more pregnancies. Approximately 7% of all multiparous women carry human leukocyte antigen antibodies in their blood.[139] It is recommended that donor blood of all multiparous women be screened for these antibodies and, if found, only the frozen or washed erythrocytes used.

The treatment of leukoagglutinin-mediated noncardiac pulmonary edema is supportive, including assisted ventilation if necessary and supplemental oxygen. It is unknown whether a short course of high-dose corticosteroids is of benefit, but it is certainly worth considering. The course of the noncardiac pulmonary edema is usually limited to 72 hours or less.

## RADIOGRAPHIC CONTRAST MEDIUM–INDUCED LEUKOSTASIS

The symptoms and signs produced by complement-induced granulocyte aggregation associated with radiographic contrast media are frequently attributed to an allergic reaction that may cause noncardiac pulmonary edema.[140–142] Anaphylaxis as a cause can be eliminated by the absence of urticaria or other rash and by the absence of significant laryngeal edema or bronchospasm. Histologic examination of the lungs demonstrates aggregates of granulocytes obstructing microscopic pulmonary arterioles and capillaries. These can be overlooked if not carefully sought or if the autopsy or examination of lung tissue is not done within a few hours of the reaction.

Clinically, the onset of symptoms of dyspnea and hypoxemia begins within a few minutes to an hour of the injection of the radiographic contrast medium. There is not necessarily a history of an allergic reaction to iodine. Treatment is supportive and includes a trial of high-dose corticosteroids, although this may be ineffective.

The activation of complement and, in turn, the generation of C5a stimulates granulocytes to aggregate and to adhere to endothelium, releasing proteases and toxic oxygen compounds. These, in turn, produce endothelial damage and capillary leakage. One study found high postmortem plasma histamine levels, which were thought to represent mast cell activation.[142]

## MISCELLANEOUS DRUGS

### Tocolytic-Induced Pulmonary Edema

Tocolytics are agents that have been widely used in the treatment of premature labor by inhibiting uterine contractions. The most commonly used drugs are terbutaline, albuterol, ritodrine, and other beta-mimetic drugs. There are many reports of these agents inducing pulmonary edema in otherwise healthy women.[143] The incidence varies from 0.5% to 5% of those receiving these drugs. Predisposing factors include the use of corticosteroids, twin gestation, fluid overload (particularly with saline), and anemia. The beta-mimetic drugs typically stimulate beta$_2$-adrenergic receptors, increasing the maternal pulse rate and the cardiac output and producing a peripheral vasodilation. Hemodilution occurs and can be detected by a drop in the hemoglobin, hematocrit, and albumin levels. The blood pressure may drop as a result of the peripheral vasodilation and may be a sign that too much tocolytic has been given.

A typical clinical scenario is as follows. Despite the tocolytic agent, labor continues, the tocolytic agent is stopped, and corticosteroids are added to accelerate fetal lung maturation. With the discontinuation of the tocolytic, the vasodilated vessels return to normal tone with a reduction of the intravascular volume. During delivery, further autotransfusion due to uterine contractions occurs, with the resultant development of pulmonary edema, usually in the postpartum period.

There are conflicting reports of the wedge pressure ranging from normal to elevated. In one study, those with an elevated wedge pressure had normal left ventricular function studies by echocardiography. At this point, it is uncertain whether the pulmonary edema is truly cardiac or noncardiac in origin.

The treatment is oxygen and diuresis. In certain cases, consideration has been given to resuming the tocolytic agent merely to reproduce the peripheral vasodilation and to allow the resumption of the intravascular volume that was present before the tocolytic agent was withdrawn. Corticosteroids aggravate the situation by their mineralocorticoid effect, which promotes fluid retention. The differential diagnosis includes aspiration of gastric contents, left heart failure, amniotic fluid embolism, and overtransfusion. Further discussion about tocolytic-induced pulmonary edema is provided in Chapter 88.

### Hydrochlorothiazide

There are over 30 reported cases of acute onset of diffuse pulmonary infiltrates associated with the ingestion of hydrochlorothiazide.[144, 145] It may begin with the first dose or days later; 90% of cases occur in women who take the drug intermittently rather than daily, presumably for fluid retention. Symptoms consist of fairly rapid onset of dyspnea that clears within 48 to 72 hours of discontinuation of the drug. A low-grade fever may be present. There is no eosinophilia and no positive antinuclear antibodies. The chest radiograph shows a diffuse bilateral alveolar-interstitial infiltrate. In the few cases studied, the pulmonary capillary wedge pressure was normal.

### Methysergide and Bromocriptine

Methysergide, bromocriptine, and cabergoline are structurally similar and produce similar pleuropulmonary reactions.[146–148] Methysergide is now rarely used to treat vascular headaches because there are better alternative drugs, whereas bromocriptine and cabergoline are used for the treatment of Parkinson's disease. The pleuropulmonary disease produced by both of these agents has an insidious onset. The predominant feature is pleural thickening and effusion, which is reversible by discontinuing the medication. Effusions, are rarely large, not commonly associated with pleuritic pain, and may show lymphocytosis.[146]

### Dextran

Hyskon is a low-molecular-weight dextran that is capable of producing noncardiac pulmonary edema.[149] It is used principally in hysteroscopic (endoscopic uterine) surgery, most often for improving fertility, during which the endometrial cavity is distended with approximately 500 mL of low-molecular-weight dextran. An average of 500 mL of dextran expands a circulating volume by more than 800 mL if it gets into the general circulation. The incidence of noncardiac pulmonary edema increases significantly if the following events occur: more than 500 mL is used, surfaces are excessively irritated, and the procedure lasts more than 45 minutes. In addition to the noncardiac pulmonary edema, coagulopathy can also occur.

### Appetite Suppressants

In the 1960, excess cases of pulmonary hypertension were associated with the potent anorexogen aminorex fumarate.

More recently, pulmonary hypertension has been associated with dexfenfluramine, fenfluramine, and phentermine.[150] In addition, valvular heart disease has also been associated with these agents.[151] A careful drug history must be taken for patients presenting with dyspnea, cardiovascular symptoms, or heart murmurs to exclude this possibility. Drug-associated pulmonary hypertension may be progressive and fatal despite discontinuation of the agents.[150]

## Esophageal Variceal Sclerotherapy

Recent reports testified to the potential complications of esophageal variceal sclerotherapy with sodium morrhuate, sodium tetradecyl sulfate, or ethanolamine oleate.[152, 153] Typically, about 1 mL of one of these substances is injected into or around the varices, and up to 15 to 20 injections are made during a single procedure. The chest radiograph taken shortly after the procedure was abnormal in 85% of the cases studied at the Mayo Clinic, but this was rarely of clinical significance.[151] Pleural effusion occurred in about 25% of patients, mediastinal widening in 33%, atelectasis in 12%, and pulmonary infiltrates in 9%. Fever, chest pain, and difficulty in swallowing were common after the procedure but rarely amounted to a serious problem.

In the literature, pleural effusion occurred in anywhere from 0% to 50% of the patients; most of these patients were asymptomatic.[152] Effusions were more common when a large volume of fluid was injected and the volume per site was increased, but not always when the number of sites was increased. Serious complications such as mediastinitis or frank esophageal rupture are rare, but should be suspected if the fever persists for more than 24 hours, if pleural effusion is large, or if there is persistent chest pain. Acute respiratory distress syndrome can occur but happens in less than 1% of the patients in whom the procedure is carried out.

## Phenothiazine

Overdosage with phenothiazine can produce noncardiac pulmonary edema. This is possibly caused by a neurogenic mechanism.[154]

## Tricyclic Drug Overdose

Tricyclic drug overdose is one of the more common causes of drug emergencies seen in the emergency room setting. About one third of the pulmonary complications that these patients develop are either noncardiac pulmonary edema or aspiration. If hypotension results, cardiac pulmonary edema can occur.[155–157] Nearly 80% of the patients have an initially widened alveolar-arterial $Po_2$ difference. Mechanical ventilation may be required in up to three fourths of patients. The higher the drug level, the more likely the patient is to develop pulmonary complications. Nearly one half of the patients have an abnormal chest radiograph, and in about 10% acute respiratory distress syndrome develops.

## Hydantoin

There has been much confusion in the literature as to whether hydantoin produces parenchymal pulmonary disease and mediastinal adenopathy. Reports in the affirmative have been followed by a more detailed patient study refuting the possibility of pulmonary parenchymal disease.[158, 159] The only two hydantoin-induced pulmonary diseases are drug-induced SLE and a few rare cases of hypersensitivity pneumonitis that show a predominance of lymphocytes found in the bronchoalveolar lavage fluid or biopsied tissue. The facts that hydantoin is one of the more commonly used drugs over extremely long periods of time and that it has not shown an obvious relationship to the induction of significant pulmonary disease make it unlikely that there is a true relationship of any consequence.

## Dantrolene

Dantrolene is a long-acting skeletal muscle relaxant used to treat patients with spastic neurologic disorders.[160] There have been several case reports of chronic pleural effusion or pericarditis, or both, associated with this drug. Peripheral blood eosinophilia was seen in some patients taking dantrolene.

# SPECIFIC PULMONARY TISSUE RESPONSES: DRUG-INDUCED DISEASE BY END-ORGAN RESPONSE

## Bronchospasm

Table 72.6 lists the drugs known to be associated with bronchospasm. Most have already been discussed. Dipyridamole, a drug used as a coronary vasodilator in thallium testing, is associated with severe bronchospasm in less than 1% of patients.[161, 162] These patients almost always have asthma or emphysema. A reaction can be prevented or treated with aminophylline. Nebulized pen-

**Table 72.6 DRUGS OR AGENTS ASSOCIATED WITH THE INDUCTION OF BRONCHOSPASM**

| |
|---|
| Acetylsalicylic acid |
| Beta-blockers |
| Cocaine |
| Contrast agents |
| Dipyridamole |
| Hydrocortisone |
| Interleukin-2 |
| Nebulized drugs |
| Pentamidine |
| Beclomethasone |
| Propellants |
| Nitrofurantoin (acute) |
| Nonsteroidal anti-inflammatory agents |
| Propafenone |
| Protamine |
| Vinblastine/mitomycin |

**Table 72.7 DRUGS OR AGENTS ASSOCIATED WITH THE INDUCTION OF PLEURAL EFFUSION**

| |
|---|
| Amiodarone |
| Bromocriptine |
| Chemotherapeutic agents |
| Dantrolene |
| Sclerosing agents for esophageal varices |
| Interleukin-2 |
| L-Tryptophan |
| Methysergide |
| Nitrofurantoin (acute) |
| Systemic lupus erythematosus (drug-induced) |
| Tocolytics |

tamidine, used in the prevention or treatment of *P. carinii* pulmonary infection, produced a significant drop in the $FEV_1$ in 26% to 34% of patients.[163, 164] The preventive or therapeutic benefits from nebulized salbutamol or ipratropium vary, depending on the study. Even drugs used for the treatment of asthma have been implicated in worsening of asthma, such as beclomethasone and isoproterenol.

## Pleural Effusion

Table 72.7 lists the drugs known to be associated with pleural effusion[165–167]; most of these were discussed earlier. It is rare that a drug-induced pleural effusion is large or massive. Pleural effusion may also be associated with drug-induced SLE.

**Table 72.8 DRUGS, DISORDERS, AND SUBSTANCES ASSOCIATED WITH THE INDUCTION OF ACUTE-ONSET* PULMONARY INSUFFICIENCY**

| |
|---|
| Amphotericin B |
| Acetylsalicylic acid |
| Bleomycin/$O_2$ |
| Bleomycin† |
| Blood or blood products |
| Complement-mediated leukostasis |
| Epinephrine |
| Ethchlorvynol |
| Fat emulsion |
| Fibrinolysis |
| Heroin |
| Hydrochlorothiazide |
| Hyskon (dextran-70) |
| Interleukin-2 |
| Intrathecal methotrexate |
| Methotrexate† |
| Mitomycin |
| Nitrofurantoin |
| Procarbazine† |
| Protamine |
| Tricyclic antidepressants |
| Tumor necrosis factor |

*Less than 48 hours.
†Hypersensitivity with eosinophilia.

**Table 72.9 DRUGS AND DRUG-INDUCED DISORDERS ASSOCIATED WITH THE INDUCTION OF SUBACUTE RESPIRATORY FAILURE**

| |
|---|
| Amiodarone |
| Chemotherapeutic agents |
| L-Tryptophan |
| Nitrofurantoin (chronic) |
| Systemic lupus erythematosus (drug-induced) |

## Drug-Induced Noncardiogenic Pulmonary Edema and Other Forms of Lung Injury

Drugs known to be associated with the induction of acute respiratory failure, including noncardiogenic pulmonary edema, are listed in Table 72.8; most have been discussed earlier.[168, 169] Table 72.9 enumerates the medications that can induce respiratory failure on a subacute chronic basis. Finally, Table 72.10 lists drugs known to be capable of inducing bronchiolitis obliterans with organizing pneumonitis (Chapter 43). This pathologic entity also occurs after viral infections, with connective tissue disorders, and after organ or bone marrow transplantation. It is therefore important to keep in mind that medications can also cause this.

## Pulmonary Infiltrates and Eosinophilia

Drugs known to be associated with peripheral blood or bronchoalveolar lavage fluid eosinophilia are listed in Table 72.11. A differential blood count should be performed in any patient with peripheral lung infiltrates.

There are over 30 drugs known to be associated with the pulmonary infiltrates and eosinophilia syndrome

**Table 72.10 DRUGS OR TREATMENT ASSOCIATED WITH THE INDUCTION OF BRONCHIOLITIS OBLITERANS WITH ORGANIZING PNEUMONITIS**

| |
|---|
| Gold |
| Penicillamine |
| Sulfasalazine |
| Bleomycin |
| Radiation |
| Amiodarone |
| Methotrexate |
| Mitomycin C |
| Cyclophosphamide |
| Cocaine |

| Table 72.11 | DRUGS ASSOCIATED WITH THE INDUCTION OF RADIOGRAPHIC PULMONARY INFILTRATIONS AND EOSINOPHILIA* |
|---|---|
| | Beclomethasone (inhaled) |
| | Capoten |
| | Carbamazepine |
| | Chlorpropamide |
| | Clofibrate |
| | Desipramine |
| | Imipramine |
| | Methotrexate |
| | Methylphenidate |
| | Minocycline |
| | Naproxyn |
| | Nitrofurantoin |
| | Para-aminosalicylic acid |
| | Penicillin |
| | Sulfonamides |
| | Tetracycline |
| | Tolazamide |

*Either peripheral blood eosinophilia or greater than 10% eosinophils in bronchoalveolar lavage or both.

(Chapter 61). Some of the more common ones include nitrofurantoin, methotrexate, salicylates, the sulfonamides, penicillins, and naproxen. A patient with an unexplained pulmonary process should always have a differential blood count. The findings of bronchoalveolar lavage in these patients may be suggestive, but unfortunately not diagnostic. As in other drug-induced lung disease, bronchoalveolar lavage may be helpful in excluding other causes, including infection.

## SUMMARY

Clinicians must maintain a high index of suspicion that an unexplained pulmonary disease may be caused by a medication. Most drug-induced pulmonary reactions are reversible if the drug is stopped in time. If necessary, additional measures such as judicious use of corticosteroids may be useful. There are almost no diagnostic studies available that will confirm the presence of a drug-induced lung disease. Rechallenging the patient with the suspected drug is dangerous and generally not indicated. If there is a question of whether a medication can be the cause of a particular pulmonary abnormality, one option is to call the medical director of the drug manufacturer listed in the *Physicians' Desk Reference.* In addition, a timely website containing pertinent information on drug-induced lung disease can be accessed at www.pneumotox.com.

## References


1. Classen DC, Pestotnik SL, Evans RS, et al: Computerized surveillance of adverse drug events in hospital patients. JAMA 266:2847–2851, 1991.
2. Akoun GM, White JP: Treatment-induced respiratory disorders. *In* Dukes MNG (ed): Drug-Induced Disorders. Vol 3. Amsterdam: Elsevier, 1989, pp 1–377.
3. Rosenow EC III, Martin WJ II: Drug-induced interstitial lung disease. *In* Schwarz MI, King TE Jr (eds): Interstitial Lung Disease. Toronto: BC Decker, 1988, pp 123–137.
4. Myers JL: Pathology of drug-induced lung disease. *In* Katzenstein AL, Askin F (eds): Surgical Pathology of Non-neoplastic Lung Disease (2nd ed). Philadelphia: WB Saunders, 1990, pp 97–127.
5. Rosenow EC III, Myers JL, Swensen SJ, et al: Drug-induced pulmonary disease. An update. Chest 102:239–250, 1992.
6. Cooper JAD Jr, White DA, et al: Drug-induced pulmonary disease: Part 1: Cytotoxic drugs. Part 2: Noncytotoxic drugs. Am Rev Respir Dis 133:321–340, 488–505, 1986.
7. Martin WJ II, Rosenow EC III: Amiodarone pulmonary toxicity. Recognition and pathogenesis (Part 2). Chest 93:1242–1248, 1988.

7a. Carol JW, Leeder RG, Racz WJ, et al: Effects of vitamin E supplementation on pulmonary morphology and collagen deposition in amiodarone treated hamsters. Toxicology 133:75–84, 1999.

8. Adamson IY: Drug-induced pulmonary fibrosis. Environ Health Perspect 55:25–36, 1984.
9. Ernst P, Sorenson PG: Cytotoxic lung damage. Int Soc Exp Hematol 12:8–11, 1984.
10. Schoen RT, Trentham DE: Drug-induced lupus: An adjuvant disease. Am J Med 71:5–8, 1981.
11. Rosenow EC III: Chemotherapeutic drug-induced pulmonary disease. Semin Respir Med 2:89–96, 1980.
12. Collis CH: Lung damage from cytotoxic drugs. Cancer Chemother Pharmacol 4:17–27, 1980.
13. Snyder LS, Hertz MI: Cytotoxic drug-induced lung injury. Semin Respir Infect 3:217–228, 1988.
14. Scheulen ME: Reduction of pulmonary toxicity. Cancer Treat Rev 14:241–243, 1987.
15. Lehne G, Lote K: Pulmonary toxicity of cytotoxic and immunosuppressive agents. Acta Oncol 29:113–124, 1990.
16. Twohig KJ, Matthay RA: Pulmonary effects of cytotoxic agents other than bleomycin. Clin Chest Med 11:31–54, 1990.
17. Brooks BJ Jr, Seifter EJ, Walsh TE, et al: Pulmonary toxicity with combined modality therapy for limited stage small cell lung cancer. J Clin Oncol 4:200–209, 1986.
18. Ginsberg SJ, Comis RL: The pulmonary toxicity of antineoplastic agents. Semin Oncol 9:34–51, 1982.
19. Klein DS, Wilds PR: Pulmonary toxicity of antineoplastic agents: Anaesthetic and postoperative implications. Ann Anesth Soc J 30:399–405, 1983.
20. Massin F, Fur A, Reybet-Degat O, et al: Busulfan-induced pneumopathy. Rev Mal Respir 4:3–10, 1987.
21. Bedrossian CWM, Luna MA, Conklin RH, et al: Alveolar proteinosis as a consequence of immunosuppression. Hum Pathol 11:527–535, 1980.
22. Aymard JP, Gyger M, Lavallee R, et al: A case of pulmonary alveolar proteinosis complicating chronic myelogenous leukemia. Cancer 53:954–956, 1984.
23. Watanabe K, Sueishi K, Tanaka K, et al: Pulmonary alveolar proteinosis and disseminated atypical mycobacteriosis in a patient with busulfan lung. Acta Pathol Jpn 40:63–66, 1990.
24. Morgan M, Dodds A, Atkinson K, et al: The toxicity of busulphan and cyclophosphamide as the preparative regimen for bone marrow transplantation. Br J Haematol 77:529–534, 1991.
25. Malik SW, Myers JL, DeRemee RA, et al: Lung toxicity with cyclophosphamide use: Two distinct patterns. Am J Respir Crit Care Med 154:1851–1856, 1996.
26. Jules-Elysee K, White DA: Bleomycin-induced pulmonary toxicity. Clin Chest Med 11:1–20, 1990.

26a. Real E, Roca MJ, Vinuales A, et al: Life-threatening lung toxicity induced by low doses of bleomycin in a patient with Hodgkin's disease. Haematologica 84:667–668, 1999.

27. Wolkowicz J, Sturgeon MB, Rawji M, et al: Bleomycin-induced pulmonary function abnormalities. Chest 101:97–101, 1992.
28. Ingrassia TS III, Ryu JH, Trastek VF, et al: Oxygen-exacerbated bleomycin pulmonary toxicity. Mayo Clin Proc 66:173–178, 1991.
29. Goldiner PL, Carlon GC, Cvitkovic E, et al: Factors influencing postoperative morbidity and mortality in patients treated with bleomycin. BMJ 1:1664–1667, 1978.
30. Van Barneveld RWC, Sleijfer DT, VanDerMark TW, et al: Natu-

ral course of bleomycin-induced pneumonitis. A follow-up study. Am Rev Respir Dis 135:48–51, 1987.
31. Santrach PJ, Askin FB, Wells RJ, et al: Nodular form of bleomycin-related pulmonary injury in patients with osteogenic sarcoma. Cancer 64:806–811, 1989.
32. Cohen MB, Austin JH, Smith-Vaniz A, et al: Nodular bleomycin toxicity. Am J Clin Pathol 92:101–104, 1989.
33. Bellamy EA, Husband JE, Blaquiere RM, et al: Bleomycin-related lung damage: CT evidence. Radiology 156:155–158, 1985.
34. Mills P, Husband J: Computed tomography of pulmonary bleomycin toxicity. Semin Ultrasound CT MR 11:417–422, 1990.
35. Verweij J, van Zanten T, Souren T, et al: Prospective study on the dose relationship of mitomycin C–induced interstitial pneumonitis. Cancer 60:756–761, 1987.
36. Sheldon R, Slaughter D: A syndrome of microangiopathic hemolytic anemia, renal impairment, and pulmonary edema in chemotherapy-treated patients with adenocarcinoma. Cancer 58:1428–1436, 1986.
37. Hasan FM, Mark EJ: A 28-year-old man with increasing dyspnea, dry cough, and fever after chemotherapy for lymphoma. N Engl J Med 323:737–747, 1990.
38. Andersson BS, Luna MA, Yee C, et al: Fatal pulmonary failure complicating high-dose cytosine arabinoside therapy in acute leukemia. Cancer 65:1079–1084, 1990.
39. Jehn J, Göldel N, Rienmuller R, et al: Noncardiogenic pulmonary edema complicating intermediate and high-dose Ara C treatment for relapsed acute leukemia. Med Oncol Tumor Pharmacother 5:41–47, 1988.
40. Smith AC: The pulmonary toxicity of nitrosoureas. Pharmacol Ther 41:443–460, 1989.
41. O'Driscoll BR, Hasleton PS, Taylor PM, et al: Active lung fibrosis up to 17 years after chemotherapy with carmustine (BCNU) in childhood. N Engl J Med 323:378–382, 1990.
42. Durant JR, Norgard MJ, Murad TM, et al: Pulmonary toxicity associated with bischloroethyl nitrosourea (BCNU). Ann Intern Med 90:191–194, 1979.
43. Rao SX, Ramaswamy G, Levin M, et al: Fatal acute respiratory failure after vinblastine-mitomycin therapy in lung carcinoma. Arch Intern Med 145:1905–1907, 1985.
44. Hoelzer KL, Harrison BR, Luedke SW, et al: Vinblastine-associated pulmonary toxicity in patients receiving combination therapy with mitomycin and cisplatin. Drug Intell Clin Pharm 20:287–289, 1986.
45. Lazarus DS, Kurnick JT, Kradin RL: Alterations in pulmonary function in cancer patients receiving adoptive immunotherapy with tumor-infiltrating lymphocytes and interleukin-2. Am Rev Respir Dis 141:193–198, 1990.
46. Saxon RR, Klein JS, Bar MH, et al: Pathogenesis of pulmonary edema during interleukin-2 therapy: Correlation of chest radiographic and clinical findings in 54 patients. AJR 156:281–285, 1991.
47. Conant EF, Fox KR, Miller WT: Pulmonary edema as a complication of interleukin-2 therapy. AJR 152:749–752, 1989.
48. Hocking DC, Phillips PG, Ferro TJ, et al: Mechanisms of pulmonary edema induced by tumor necrosis factor-alpha. Circ Res 67:68–77, 1990.
49. Kuei JH, Tashkin DP, Figlin RA: Pulmonary toxicity of recombinant human tumor necrosis factor. Chest 96:334–338, 1989.
49a. Prakash UBS: Radiation-induced injury in the non-irradiated lung. Eur Respir J 13:715–717, 1999.
50. Roberts CM, Foulcher E, Zaunders JJ, et al: Radiation pneumonitis: A possible lymphocyte-mediated hypersensitivity reaction. Ann Intern Med 118:696–700, 1993.
51. Boyars MC: Clinical management of radiation-induced lung disease. J Respir Dis 11:167–183, 1990.
52. Holmberg L, Boman G, Bottiger IE, et al: Adverse reactions to nitrofurantoin. Analysis of 921 reports. Am J Med 69:733–738, 1980.
53. Holmberg L, Boman G: Pulmonary reactions to nitrofurantoin: 447 cases reported to the Swedish Adverse Drug Reaction Committee 1966–1976. Eur J Respir Dis 62:180–189, 1981.
54. Prakash UBS: Pulmonary reaction to nitrofurantoin. Semin Respir Dis 2:71–75, 1980.
55. Martin WJ II: Nitrofurantoin: Evidence for the oxidant injury of lung parenchymal cells. Am Rev Respir Dis 127:482–486, 1983.
56. Pearsall HR, Ewalt J, Tsoi MS, et al: Nitrofurantoin lung sensitivity: Report of a case with prolonged nitrofurantoin sensitivity and interaction of nitrofurantoin-stimulated lymphocytes with alveolar cells. J Lab Clin Invest 83:728–737, 1974.
57. Jayasundera NS, Johnson RD, Nicholson DP: Chronic pulmonary reaction to nitrofurantoin. JAMA 243:769, 1980.
58. Robinson BWS: Nitrofurantoin-induced interstitial pulmonary fibrosis. Med J Aust 1:72–76, 1983.
59. Brutinel WM, Martin WJ II: Chronic nitrofurantoin reaction associated with T-lymphocyte alveolitis. Chest 89:150–152, 1986.
60. Akoun GM, Cadranel JL, Rosenow EC III, et al: Bronchoalveolar lavage cell data in drug-induced pneumonitis. Allergy Immunol 23:245–252, 1991.
61. Boyd O, Gibbs AR, Smith AP: Fibrosing alveolitis due to sulphasalazine in a patient with rheumatoid arthritis. Br J Rheumatol 29:222–224, 1990.
62. Camus P, Piard F, Ashcroft T, Gal AA, et al: The lung in inflammatory bowel disease. Medicine 72:151–183, 1993.
63. Kohno S, Yamaguchi K, Yasuoka A, et al: Clinical evaluation of 12 cases of antimicrobial drug-induced pneumonitis. Jpn J Med 29:248–254, 1990.
64. Warner WA, Sanders E: Neuromuscular blockade associated with gentamicin therapy. JAMA 215:1153–1154, 1971.
65. Dutcher JP, Kendall J, Norris D, et al: Granulocyte transfusion therapy and amphotericin B. Am J Hematol 31:102–108, 1989.
66. Levine SJ, Walsh TJ, Martinez A, et al: Cardiopulmonary toxicity after liposomal amphotericin B infusion. Ann Intern Med 114:664–666, 1991.
67. Brashear RE: Effects of heroin, morphine, methadone, and propoxyphene on the lung. Semin Respir Med 2:59–69, 1980.
68. Heffner JE, Harley RA, Schabel SI: Pulmonary reactions from illicit substance abuse. Clin Chest Med 11:151–162, 1990.
69. O'Donnell AE, Pappas LS: Pulmonary complications of intravenous drug abuse. Chest 94:251–253, 1988.
70. Parran TV Jr, Jasinski DR: Intravenous methylphenidate abuse. Arch Intern Med 151:781–783, 1991.
71. Schmidt RA, Glenny RW, Godwin JD, et al: Panlobular emphysema in young intravenous ritalin abusers. Am Rev Respir Dis 143:649–656, 1991.
72. McCarroll KA, Roszler MH: Lung disorders due to drug abuse. J Thorac Imaging 6:30–35, 1991.
73. Forrester JM, Steele AW, Waldron JA, et al: Crack lung: An acute pulmonary syndrome with a spectrum of clinical and histopathologic findings. Am Rev Respir Dis 142:462–467, 1990.
74. Kline JN, Hirasuna JD: Pulmonary edema after free-base cocaine smoking—Not due to an adulterant. Chest 97:1009–1010, 1990.
75. Crouch E, Churg A: Progressive massive fibrosis of the lung secondary to intravenous injection of talc. A pathologic and mineralogic analysis. Am J Clin Pathol 80:520–526, 1983.
76. Radow SK, Nachamkin I, Morrow C, et al: Foreign body granulomatosis. Clinical and immunologic findings. Am Rev Respir Dis 127:575–580, 1983.
77. Waller BF, Brownlee WJ, Roberts WC: Self-induced pulmonary granulomatosis. A consequence of intravenous injection of drugs intended for oral use. Chest 78:90–94, 1980.
78. Pare JP, Cote G, Fraser RS: Long-term follow-up of drug abusers with intravenous talcosis. Am Rev Respir Dis 139:233–241, 1989.
79. Israili ZH, Hall WD: Cough and angioneutrotic edema associated with angiotensin-converting enzyme inhibitor therapy. A review of the literature and pathophysiology. Ann Intern Med 117:234–242, 1992.
80. Alderman CP: Adverse effects of the angiotensin converting enzyme inhibitors. Ann Pharmacother 30:55–61, 1996.
81. Martin WJ II, Rosenow EC III: Amiodarone pulmonary toxicity (Part 1). Chest 93:1067–1075, 1988.
82. Kennedy JI Jr: Clinical aspects of amiodarone pulmonary toxicity. Clin Chest Med 11:119–129, 1990.
83. Dean PJ, Groshart KD, Porterfield JG, et al: Amiodarone-associated pulmonary toxicity. A clinical and pathologic study of eleven cases. Am J Clin Pathol 87:7–13, 1987.
84. Dusman RE, Stanton MS, Miles WM, et al: Clinical features of amiodarone-induced pulmonary toxicity. Circulation 82:51–59, 1990.
85. Xaubet A, Roca J, Rodriguez-Roisin R, et al: Bronchoalveolar la-

vage cellular analysis and gallium lung scan in the assessment of patients with amiodarone-induced pneumonitis. Respiration 52:272–280, 1987.
86. Arnon R, Raz I, Chajek-Shaul T, et al: Amiodarone pulmonary toxicity presenting as a solitary lung mass. Chest 93:425–427, 1988.
87. Camus P, Lombard JN, Perrichon M, et al: Bronchiolitis obliterans organizing pneumonia in patients taking acebutolol or amiodarone. Thorax 44:711–715, 1989.
88. Piccione W Jr, Faber LP, Rosenberg MS: Amiodarone-induced pulmonary mass. Ann Thorac Surg 47:918–919, 1989.
89. Ren H, Kuhlman JE, Hruban RH, et al: CT-pathology correlation of amiodarone lung. J Comput Assist Tomogr 14:760–765, 1990.
90. Kuhlman JE, Teigen C, Ren H, et al: Amiodarone pulmonary toxicity: CT findings in symptomatic patients. Radiology 177:121–125, 1990.
91. Zaher C, Hamer A, Peter T, et al: Low-dose steroid therapy for prophylaxis of amiodarone-induced pulmonary infiltrates [letter to the editor]. N Engl J Med 308:779, 1983.
92. Kay GN, Epstein AE, Kirklin JK, et al: Fatal postoperative amiodarone pulmonary toxicity. Am J Cardiol 62:490–493, 1988.
93. Nalos PC, Kass RM, Gang ES, et al: Life-threatening postoperative pulmonary complications in patients with previous amiodarone pulmonary toxicity undergoing cardiothoracic operations. J Thorac Cardiovasc Surg 93:904–912, 1987.
94. Tuzcu EM, Maloney JD, Sangani BH, et al: Cardiopulmonary effects of chronic amiodarone therapy in the early postoperative course of cardiac surgery patients. Cleve Clin J Med 54:491–495, 1987.
95. Greenspon AJ, Kidwell GA, Hurley W, et al: Amiodarone-induced postoperative adult respiratory distress syndrome. Circulation 84:III-407–415, 1991.
96. Just-Viera JO, Fischer CR, Gago O, et al: Acute reaction to protamine. Its importance to surgeons. Am Surg 50:52–60, 1984.
97. Doolan L, McKenzie I, Krafchek J, et al: Protamine sulphate hypersensitivity. Anaesth Intensive Care 9:147–149, 1981.
98. Chester EH, Schwartz HJ, Fleming GM: Adverse effect of propranolol on airway function in nonasthmatic chronic obstructive lung disease. Chest 79:540–544, 1981.
99. Reynolds RJ, Burford JG, George RB: Using beta-blockers safely in asthma and COPD patients. J Respir Dis 3:95–113, 1982.
100. Middleton E: Airway smooth muscle, asthma and calcium ions. J Allergy Clin Immunol 73:643–650, 1984.
101. Weinreb RN, van Buskirk EM, Cherniack R, et al: Long-term betaxolol therapy in glaucoma patients with pulmonary disease. Am J Ophthalmol 106:162–167, 1988.
102. Everitt DE, Avorn J: Systemic effects of medications used to treat glaucoma. Ann Intern Med 112:120–125, 1990.
103. Gauthier-Rahman S, Akoun GM, Milleron BJ, et al: Leukocyte migration inhibition in propranolol-induced pneumonitis. Chest 97:238–241, 1990.
104. Shen EN: Propafenone: A promising new antiarrhythmic agent. Chest 98:434–441, 1990.
105. Feinberg L, Travis WD, Ferrans V, et al: Pulmonary fibrosis associated with tocainide. Am Rev Respir Dis 141:505–508, 1990.
106. Hanston P, Evrard P, Mahieu P, et al: Flecainide-associated interstitial pneumonitis. Lancet 337:371–372, 1991.
107. Akoun GM, Cadranel JL, Israel-Biet D, et al: Flecainide-associated pneumonitis. Lancet 337:49, 1991.
108. Zitnik RJ, Cooper JA Jr: Pulmonary disease due to antirheumatic agents. Clin Chest Med 11:139–150, 1990.
109. Cannon GW: Pulmonary complications of antirheumatic drug therapy. Semin Arthritis Rheum 19:353–364, 1990.
110. Ameisen JC, Capron A: Aspirin-sensitive asthma. Clin Exp Allergy 20:127–129, 1990.
111. Picado C, Castillo JA, Montserrat JM, et al: Aspirin-intolerance as a precipitating factor of life-threatening attacks of asthma requiring mechanical ventilation. Eur Respir J 2:127–129, 1989.
112. Heffner JE, Sahn SA: Salicylate-induced pulmonary edema: Clinical features and prognosis. Ann Intern Med 95:405–409, 1981.
113. McGuigan MA: A two-year review of salicylate deaths in Ontario. Arch Intern Med 147:510–512, 1987.
114. Thisted B, Krantz T, Strom J, et al: Acute salicylate self-poisoning in 177 consecutive patients treated in ICU. Acta Anaesthesiol Scand 31:312–316, 1987.
115. Leatherman JW, Schmitz PG: Fever, hyperdynamic shock, and multiple-system organ failure. A pseudo-sepsis syndrome associated with chronic salicylate intoxication. Chest 100:1391–1396, 1991.
116. Ettensohn DB, Roberts NJ Jr, Condemi JJ: Bronchoalveolar lavage in gold lung. Chest 85:569–570, 1984.
117. Evans RB, Ettensohn DB, Fawaz-Estrup F, et al: Gold lung: Recent developments in pathogenesis, diagnosis, and therapy. Semin Arthritis Rheum 16:196–205, 1987.
118. Carson CW, Cannon GW, Egger MJ, et al: Pulmonary disease during the treatment of rheumatoid arthritis with low dose pulse methotrexate. Semin Arthritis Rheum 16:186–195, 1987.
119. Gispen JG, Alarcon GS, Johnson JJ, et al: Toxicity of methotrexate in rheumatoid arthritis. J Rheumatol 14:73–79, 1987.
120. Duerksen DR, Blondel-Hill E, Bailey RJ: *Pneumocystis carinii* pneumonia complicating methotrexate treatment of primary sclerosing cholangitis. Am J Gastroenterol 90:1886–1887, 1995.
121. Chalmers A, Thompson D, Stein HB, et al: Systemic lupus erythematosus during penicillamine therapy for rheumatoid arthritis. Ann Intern Med 97:659–663, 1982.
122. Murphy KC, Atkins CJ, Offer RC, et al: Obliterative bronchiolitis in two rheumatoid arthritis patients treated with penicillamine. Arthritis Rheum 24:557–560, 1981.
123. Peces R, Riera JR, Arboleya LR, et al: Goodpasture's syndrome in a patient receiving penicillamine and carbimazole. Nephron 45:316–320, 1987.
124. Wechsler ME, Garpestad E, Flier SR, et al: Pulmonary infiltrates, eosinophilia, and cardiomyopathy following corticosteroid withdrawal in patients with asthma receiving zafirlukast. JAMA 279:455–457, 1998.
125. Knoell DL, Lucas J, Allen JN: Churg-Strauss syndrome associated with Zafirlukast. Chest 114:332–334, 1998.
126. Londino AV Jr, Wolf GL, Calabro JJ, et al: Naproxen and pneumonitis [letter to the editor]. JAMA 252:1853, 1984.
127. Bien ME, Mancuso AA, Mink JH, et al: Computed tomography in the evaluation of mediastinal lipomatosis. J Comput Assist Tomogr 2:379–383, 1978.
128. Totoritis MC, Rubin RL: Drug-induced lupus. Postgrad Med 78:149–161, 1985.
129. Hess EV, Mongey AB: Drug-related lupus. Bull Rheum Dis 40:1–8, 1991.
130. Lipinski JK, Weisbrod GL, Sanders DE: Exogenous lipoid pneumonitis. J Can Assoc Radiol 31:92–98, 1980.
131. Prakash UB, Rosenow EC III: Pulmonary complications from ophthalmic preparations. Mayo Clin Proc 65:521–529, 1990.
132. Frank L, Massaro FL: Oxygen toxicity. Am J Med 69:117–126, 1980.
133. Davis WB, Rennard SI, Bitterman PB, et al: Pulmonary oxygen toxicity: Early reversible changes in human alveolar structures induced by hyperoxia. N Engl J Med 309:878–883, 1983.
134. Jackson RM: Pulmonary oxygen toxicity. Chest 88:900–905, 1985.
135. Bowman CM, Butler EN, Repine JE: Hyperoxia damages cultured endothelial cells causing increased neutrophil adherence. Am Rev Respir Dis 128:469–472, 1983.
136. Fox RB, Hoidal JR, Brown DM, et al: Pulmonary inflammation caused by oxygen toxicity: Involvement of chemotactic factors and polymorphonuclear leukocytes. Am Rev Respir Dis 123:521–523, 1981.
137. Sackner MA, Landa J, Hirsch J, et al: Pulmonary effects of oxygen breathing. A 6-hour study in normal men. Ann Intern Med 82:40–43, 1975.
138. Coalson JJ, King RJ, Winter VT, et al: Oxygen and pneumonia-induced lung injury. J Appl Physiol 67:346–356, 1989.
139. Popovsky MA, Abel MD, Moore SB: Transfusion-related acute lung injury associated with passive transfer of antileukocyte antibodies. Am Rev Respir Med 128:185–189, 1983.
140. Schneiderman H, Hammerschmidt DE, McCall AR, et al: Fatal complement-induced leukostasis after diatrizoate injection. Principles of clinicopathologic diagnosis. JAMA 250:2340–2342, 1983.
141. Boden WE: Anaphylactoid pulmonary edema (shock lung) and hypotension after radiologic contrast media injection. Chest 81:759–761, 1982.
142. Vandenplas O, Hantson P, Dive A, et al: Fulminant pulmonary edema following intravenous administration of radiocontrast media. Acta Clin Belg 45:334–339, 1990.

143. Pisani RJ, Rosenow EC III: Pulmonary edema associated with tocolytic therapy. Ann Intern Med 110:714–718, 1989.
144. Kavaru MS, Ahmad M, Amirthalingam KN: Hydrochlorothiazide-induced acute pulmonary edema. Cleve Clin J Med 57:181–184, 1990.
145. Biron P, Dessureault J, Napke E: Acute allergic interstitial pneumonitis induced by hydrochlorothiazide. Can Med Assoc J 145:28–34, 1991.
146. Kinnunen E, Viljanen A: Pleuropulmonary involvement during bromocriptine treatment. Chest 94:1034–1036, 1988.
147. Ling LL, Ahlskog JE, Munger TM, et al: Constrictive pericarditis and pleuropulmonary disease associated with cabergoline therapy for Parkinson's disease. Mayo Clin Proc 74:371–375, 1999.
148. Rosenow EC III: Miscellaneous DIPD. Semin Roentgenol 2:76–88, 1980.
149. McLucas B: Hyskon complications in hysteroscopic surgery. Obstet Gynecol Surv 46:196–200, 1991.
150. Mark EJ, Patalas ED, Chang HT, et al: Fatal pulmonary hypertension associated with the short-term use of fenfluramine and phenteramine. N Engl J Med 337:602–606, 1997.
151. Connolly HM, Crary JL, McGoon MD, et al: Valvular heart disease associated with fenfluramine-phenteramine. N Engl J Med 337:581–588, 1997.
152. Zeller FA, Cannon CR, Prakash UBS: Thoracic manifestations after esophageal variceal sclerotherapy. Mayo Clin Proc 66:727–732, 1991.
153. Edling JE, Bacon BR: Pleuropulmonary complications of endoscopic variceal sclerotherapy. Chest 99:1252–1257, 1991.
154. Li C, Gefter WB: Acute pulmonary edema induced by overdosage of phenothiazines. Chest 101:102–104, 1992.
155. Roy TM, Ossorio MA, Cipolla LM, et al: Pulmonary complications after tricyclic antidepressant overdose. Chest 96:852–856, 1989.
156. Varnell RM, Godwin JD, Richardson ML, et al: Adult respiratory distress syndrome from overdose of tricyclic antidepressants. Radiology 170:667–670, 1989.
157. Shannon M, Lovejoy FH Jr: Pulmonary consequences of severe tricyclic antidepressant ingestion. J Toxicol Clin Toxicol 25:443–461, 1987.
158. Michael JR, Rudin ML: Acute pulmonary disease caused by phenytoin. Ann Intern Med 95:452–454, 1981.
159. Chamberlain DW, Hyland RH, Ross DJ: Diphenylhydantoin-induced lymphocytic interstitial pneumonia. Chest 90:458–460, 1986.
160. Miller DH, Haas LF: Pneumonitis, pleural effusion and pericarditis following treatment with dantrolene. J Neurol Neurosurg Psychiatry 47:553–554, 1984.
161. Houben JJG: The role of dipyridamole in bronchospasm. Chest 98:253–254, 1990.
162. Ranhosky A, Kempthorne-Rawson J: The safety of intravenous dipyridamole thallium myocardial perfusion imaging. Circulation 81:1205–1209, 1990.
163. Quieffin J, Hunter J, Schechter MT, et al: Aerosol pentamidine-induced bronchoconstriction. Predictive factors and preventive therapy. Chest 100:624–627, 1991.
164. Katzman M, Meade W, Iglar K, et al: High incidence of bronchospasm with regular administration of aerosolized pentamidine. Chest 101:79–81, 1992.
165. Sahn SA: The pleura. Am Rev Respir Dis 138:184–234, 1988.
166. Miller WT Jr: Drug-related pleural and mediastinal disorders. J Thorac Imaging 6:36–51, 1991.
167. Byrd RP, Morris CJ, Roy TM: Drug-induced pleural effusions. J Ky Med Assoc 89:71–73, 1991.
168. Reed CR, Glauser FL: Drug-induced noncardiogenic pulmonary edema. Chest 100:1120–1124, 1991.
169. Rosenow EC III, Pisani RJ: Acute drug-induced lung injury. *In* Carlson RW, Geheb MA (eds): Principles and Practice of Medical Intensive Care. Philadelphia: WB Saunders, 1993, pp 896–902.

SECTION N

# Disorders of the Pleura

# 73 General Principles and Diagnostic Approach

V. COURTNEY BROADDUS, M.D. • RICHARD W. LIGHT, M.D.

Introduction
Function of the Pleural Space
Embryology and Anatomy
- Blood Supply
- Lymphatics
- Nerve Supply

Physiology of the Pleural Space
- Normal Pleural Liquid and Protein Turnover
- Pleural Pressure

Pathophysiology of the Pleural Space
- Pleural Effusions
- Effects of Pleural Effusions on Lung Function

Approach to Patients with Pleural Effusion
- Differential Diagnosis of Pleural Effusion
- Separation of Exudates from Transudates
- Differentiating Exudative Pleural Effusions
- Other Diagnostic Tests for Pleural Fluid
- Useful Radiographic Tests in Patients with Suspected Pleural Disease
- Invasive Tests in Patients with Undiagnosed Exudative Pleural Effusions

Summary

## INTRODUCTION

The pleura consists of two membranes, the visceral pleura covering the lung and the parietal pleura covering the chest wall and diaphragm. These two pleural membranes meet at the hilar root of the lung. In the sheep, an animal with a pleural anatomy similar to that of humans, the surface area of the visceral pleura of one lung, including that invaginating into the lung fissures, is similar to that of the parietal pleura of one hemithorax, approximately 1000 $cm^2$.[1] The normal pleural space is approximately 18 to 20 μm in width, although it widens at its most dependent areas.[1] Although this idea was at one time controversial, it is now clear that pleural membranes do not touch each other and that the pleural space is a real, not a potential, space[1] (Fig. 73.1).

## FUNCTION OF THE PLEURAL SPACE

It is likely that the primary function of the pleural membranes is to allow extensive movement of the lung relative to the chest wall. If the lung adhered directly to the chest wall, its expansion and deflation would be more limited. Encased in its slippery coat, the lung, although still coupled mechanically to the chest wall, is able to expand across a breadth of several intercostal spaces. Nonetheless, in clinical and experimental studies, pleural symphy-

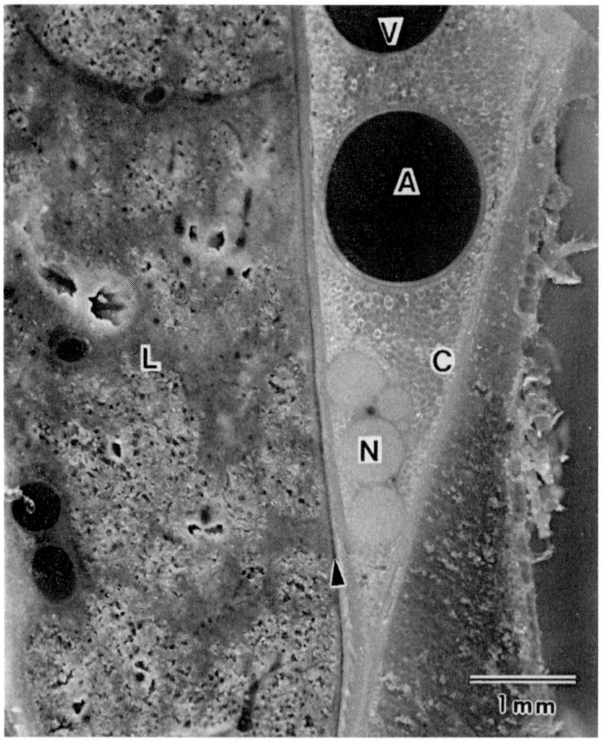


**Figure 73.1** The pleural space is depicted in a frozen sheep thorax by reflected-light microscopy. The pleural space is seen as a continuous dark band *(arrowhead)* between the lung (L) and the chest wall (C). Because the section was removed from beneath a rib, the intercostal vein (V), artery (A), and nerve (N) are seen. (From Albertine KH, Wiener-Kronish JP, Bastacky J, et al: No evidence for mesothelial cell contact across the costal pleural space of sheep. J Appl Physiol 70:123–134, 1991.)

sis has not been associated with large abnormalities in lung function.[2] The most common findings have been a decrease in volume of the affected lung[3] and, in one study, of the opposite lung as well.[4] If pleural thickening accompanies pleural symphysis, abnormalities of lung function may result more from fibrothorax than from obliteration of the pleural space alone.[2]

The visceral pleura may also provide mechanical support for the lung: contributing to the shape of the lung,[5] providing a limit to expansion,[6] and contributing to the work of deflation.[7] Because the submesothelial connective tissue is continuous with the connective tissue of the lung parenchyma, the visceral pleura may help to distribute the forces produced by negative inflation pressures evenly over the lung. In this way, overdistention of alveoli at the pleural surface may be avoided, lessening the chance of rupture and pneumothorax.

One function of the pleural space is to provide a route by which edema can escape the lung.[8–10] As has been shown in several experimental studies of either hydrostatic or increased permeability lung edema,[9–11] the pleural space can function as an additional safety factor protecting against the development of alveolar edema. The formation of transudative effusions in patients with congestive heart failure apparently reflects the movement of edema from the lung to a space where its effects on lung function are relatively small.[12]

## EMBRYOLOGY AND ANATOMY

The pleural, pericardial, and peritoneal spaces begin to form from the mesoderm by the third week of gestational age.[13] Interestingly, the pleural space enlarges independent of lung growth. By 9 weeks, the pleural cavity has become separated from both the pericardial and the peritoneal spaces. Various cysts, diverticula, and defects can result from incomplete partitioning of the three mesodermal spaces. At this time, the lung buds invaginate into the visceral pleura and henceforth retain a pleural covering.

The pleural membranes are smooth glistening coverings for the constantly moving lung. Overlying each pleural membrane is a single cell layer of mesothelial cells. These cells can vary in shape from flat to cuboidal or columnar, perhaps according to the degree of stretching of the underlying submesothelial tissue. These cells, the most numerous of the pleural space, may have a variety of functions that are important to pleural biology. Mesothelial cells can secrete the macromolecular components of the extracellular matrix and organize them into mature matrix,[14] phagocytose particles,[15, 16] produce fibrinolytic and procoagulant factors,[17–19] and secrete neutrophil and monocyte chemotactic factors[20, 21] that may be important for inflammatory cell recruitment into the pleural spaces.[22] On their surface are microvilli, which are irregularly distributed over the pleural surfaces. In general, microvilli are more dense over the visceral than over the parietal pleura and in caudal regions than in cranial regions.[23] Although microvilli presumably exist to increase surface area for metabolic functions, the function of these prominent structures is unknown. Mesothelial cells produce hyaluronan but not mucin, express keratin microfilaments, and stain negatively with epithelial-specific antibodies (Ber-EP4, B72.3, Leu.M1, and CEA), all features that are important for histochemical and immunohistochemical identification of the cells in pleural effusions.[24]

The cells lie on a thin basement membrane overlying a varying region of connective tissue that contains mostly collagen and elastin. Although the parietal pleural connective tissue layer is of a consistent thickness, the visceral connective tissue layer varies greatly. In a single individual, the visceral pleura varies from a thinner layer at the cranial region to a thicker layer at the caudal region.[25] The visceral pleura varies among species from a thin pleura with little connective tissue and no bronchial blood supply in smaller animals to the thick pleura with its own bronchial blood supply found in larger animals, including humans.[26] Analysis of the constituents of the visceral pleura has shown that there is more collagen relative to elastin than is found in the lung parenchyma, a finding consistent with a mechanical role for the pleura.[27] This connective tissue layer contains blood vessels and lymphatics and joins with the connective tissue of the lung.

### Blood Supply

The parietal pleura is supplied by intercostal arteries[28] (Fig. 73.2*A*). The visceral pleura in humans, like that in

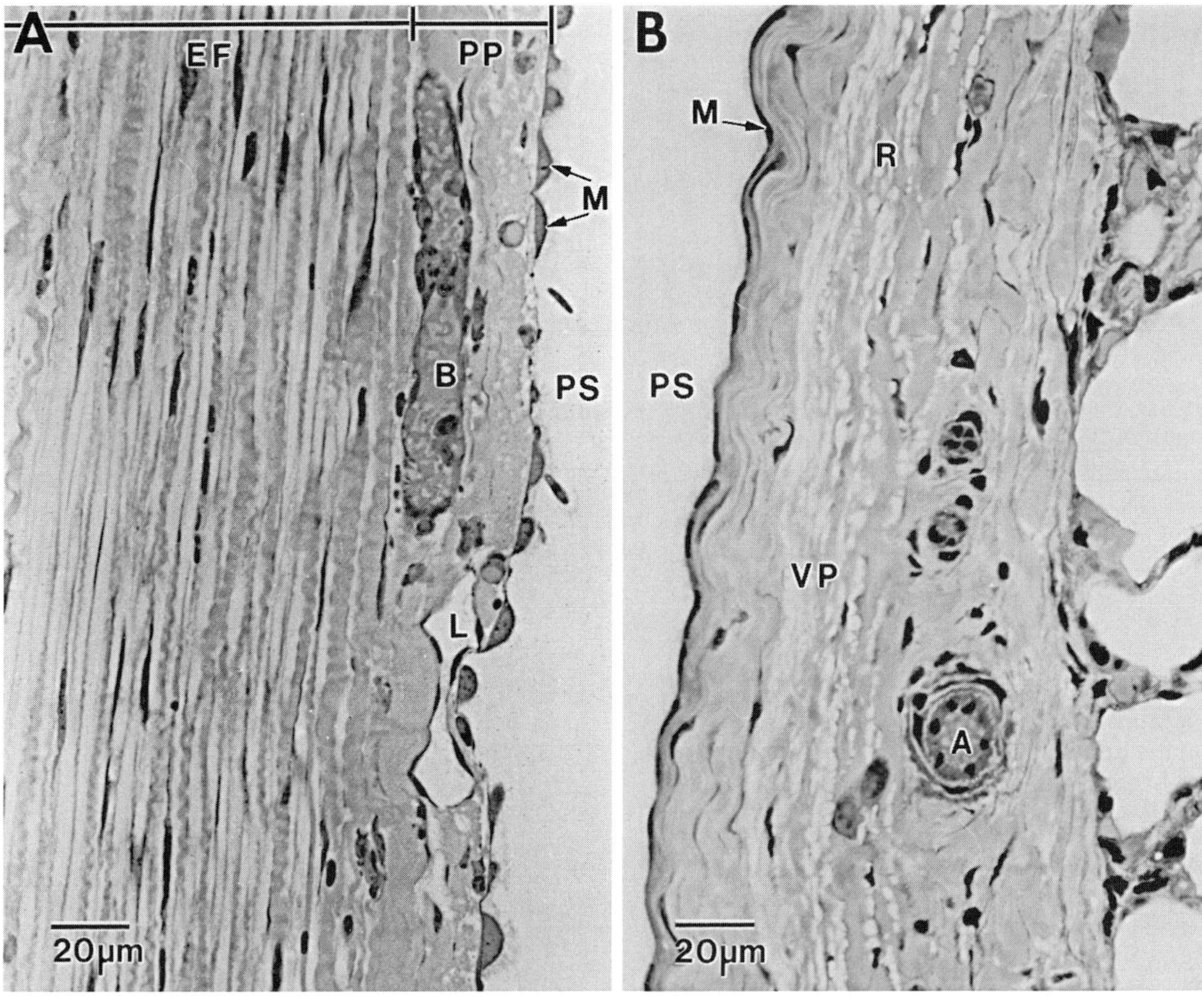


**Figure 73.2** Light micrograph showing the parietal and visceral pleurae of the sheep, an animal with a similar pleural anatomy to that of humans. Both membranes are covered by a single layer of mesothelial cells (M). *A,* The parietal pleura (PP) is the layer of loose connective tissue between the pleural space (PS) and the dense connective tissue of the endothoracic fascia (EF). Within the loose connective tissue are blood microvessels (B) from the intercostal arteries and lymphatic lacunae (L) which open into the pleural space via stomata. *B,* The visceral pleural (VP) lies between the pleural space (PS) and the alveoli. The blood supply to the visceral pleura is via the bronchial arteries (A), which drain into pulmonary veins. The pleura contains dense bands of elastin and collagen. (From Staub NC, Wiener-Kronish JP, Albertine KH: Transport through the pleura: Physiology of normal liquid and solute exchange in the pleural space. *In* Chrétien J, Bignon J, Hirsch A (eds): The Pleura in Health and Disease. New York: Marcel Dekker, 1985, pp 174–175.)

sheep, is exclusively supplied by the bronchial circulation, which drains into pulmonary veins[25] (see Fig. 73.2*B*). The drainage route via pulmonary veins may have contributed to earlier confusion about whether the visceral pleural blood supply was from a systemic (bronchial) or a pulmonary circulation. Both pleurae in humans, therefore, have a systemic circulation, although the visceral pleural bronchial circulation may have a slightly lower perfusion pressure than the parietal pleural intercostal circulation because of its drainage into a lower-pressure pulmonary venous system.

## Lymphatics

After injecting carbon particles into the pleural space as a visible marker of lymphatic drainage pathways, one finds that the black carbon has been taken up into lymphatics on the parietal side, but not on the visceral side (Fig. 73.3). The visceral pleura has extensive lymphatics, but they do not connect to the pleural space.[25] Demonstrated in rabbits, sheep, and now in humans, the parietal pleural lymphatics connect to the pleural space via stomas, holes 8 to 10 μm in diameter that are formed by

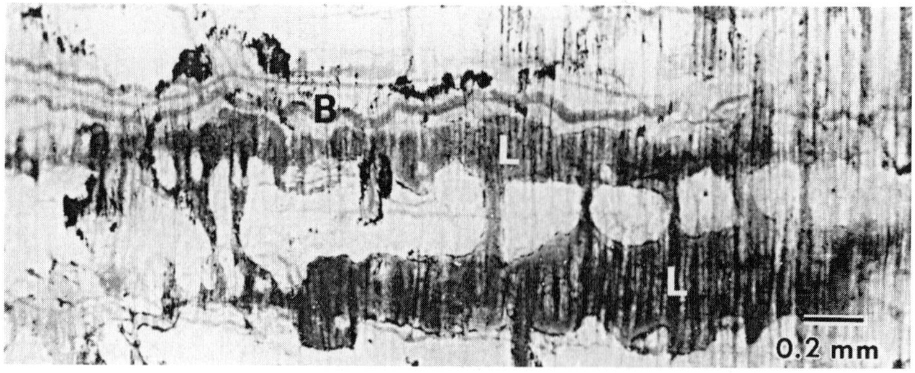


**Figure 73.3** Macroscopic photograph of lymphatic lacunae in the parietal pleura over an intercostal space. Colloidal carbon was instilled into the pleural space to label the draining lymphatics. When one looks down upon the pleura, the lymphatic lacunae (L) appear as broad cisterns. B = blood vessel. (Original magnification ×39.) (Reprinted by permission of Wiley-Liss, a division of Wiley and Sons, Inc., copyright owner. © From Albertine KH, Wiener-Kronish JP, Staub NC: The structure of the parietal pleura and its relationship to pleural liquid dynamics in sheep. Anat Rec 208:406, 1984.)

discontinuities in the mesothelial layer where mesothelium joins to the underlying lymphatic endothelium.[29, 30] The stomas can accommodate particles as large as erythrocytes. In various experimental studies, these lymphatic channels have been shown to be the major route of exit of liquid from the pleural space.[31] From the stomas, liquid drains to lacunae, spider-like submesothelial collecting lymphatics, which then drain to infracostal lymphatics, to parasternal and periaortic nodes, to the thoracic duct, and into the systemic venous system.

Lymphoid cells have been described lying within aggregates along the mediastinum underneath morphologically different mesothelial cells, forming raised structures called *Kampmeier's foci.*[32] These foci may have an immune function.[33]

### Nerve Supply

Only the parietal pleura contains sensory nerve fibers, supplied by the intercostal and the phrenic nerves. The costal and peripheral diaphragmatic regions are innervated by the intercostal nerves, and pain from these regions is referred to the adjacent chest wall. The central diaphragmatic region is innervated by the phrenic nerve, and pain from this region is referred to the ipsilateral shoulder. The visceral pleura does not contain sensory nerve fibers; therefore, pain, whether from inflammation, tumor, or catheters advanced far out in the lung during bronchoscopy, indicates involvement of the adjacent parietal pleura.

## PHYSIOLOGY OF THE PLEURAL SPACE

### Normal Pleural Liquid and Protein Turnover

There have been conflicting theories concerning the entry and exit of pleural liquid, including theories that pleural liquid was secreted by pleural mesothelial cells and that pleural liquid entered from the parietal (high-pressure) pleura and was absorbed on the visceral (low-pressure) pleura. Since the 1980s, a consensus has developed that pleural liquid arises from the systemic pleural vessels in both pleurae, flows across the leaky pleural membranes into the pleural space, and exits the pleural space via the parietal pleural lymphatics[34] (Fig. 73.4). In this way, the pleural space is analogous to any interstitial space of the body. There are several lines of evidence for this newer explanation.

1. Intrapleural pressure is lower than the interstitial pressure of either of the pleural tissues.[35] This pressure difference constitutes a gradient for liquid movement into, but not out of, the pleural space.
2. The pleural membranes are leaky to liquid and protein. Whether tested in vitro[36, 36a] or in situ,[37] the pleura offers little resistance to protein movement.
3. Mesothelial cells have not been shown to generate an electric potential difference, as would be expected if there were active transport across them.[38] Although pleural liquid has been reported to be alkaline with a higher bicarbonate than plasma,[39] there is no evidence for mesothelial participation in generating a bicarbonate gradient. If, indeed, the mesothelial layer is leaky, it is difficult to explain how mesothelial cells could maintain such a gradient.
4. The entry of pleural liquid is slow and is compatible with known interstitial flow rates. By noninvasive studies of the equilibration of radiolabeled albumin, the entry rate of pleural liquid is approximately 0.01 mL/kg per hour in a sheep, or about 0.5 mL hourly in a grown man.[40] The half-time of pleural liquid turnover in sheep and rabbits is 6 to 8 hours.[40, 41]
5. The protein concentration of normal pleural liquid is low in sheep[40] and probably in humans, which implies sieving of the protein across a high-

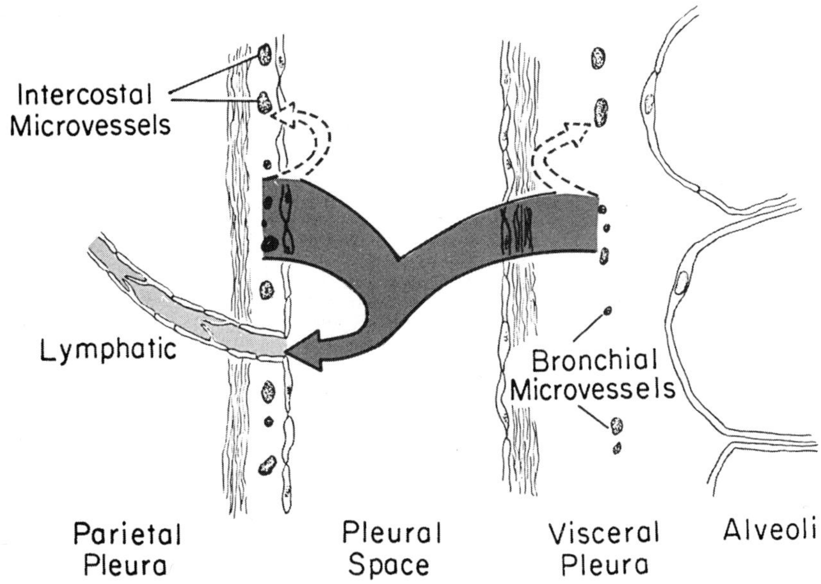


**Figure 73.4** Schema showing normal pleural liquid turnover. The initial microvascular filtrate in the parietal and visceral pleura is partly reabsorbed *(dashed arrows)*. The remaining low-protein interstitial liquid flows across the leaky pleural mesothelial layers into the pleural space. The pleural liquid exits the pleural space via the parietal pleural lymphatic stomata. (From Staub NC, Wiener-Kronish JP, Albertine KH: Transport through the pleura: Physiology of normal liquid and solute exchange in the pleural space. *In* Chrétien J, Bignon J, Hirsch A (eds): The Pleura in Health and Disease. New York: Marcel Dekker, 1985, p 182.)

pressure gradient. The protein concentration of sheep pleural liquid (10 g/L) and the pleural-to-plasma protein concentration ratio (0.15) are similar to those of filtrates from high-pressure systemic vessels. By comparison, a filtrate from low-pressure pulmonary vessels has a higher protein concentration (45 g/L) and ratio (lymph-to-plasma protein concentration ratio, 0.69).[42]

6. Most liquid exits the pleural space by bulk flow, not by diffusion. This is evident because the protein concentration of pleural effusions does not change as the effusion is absorbed, as is expected with bulk flow. If liquid were absorbed by diffusion, then proteins would diffuse at a slower rate, and the protein concentration would progressively increase. In addition, erythrocytes instilled into the pleural space are absorbed intact[43, 44] and in almost the same proportion as the liquid and protein.[31] This indicates that the major route of exit is via holes large enough to accommodate sheep erythrocytes (6- to 8-μm diameter). The only possible exit is via the parietal pleural stomas (10- to 12-μm diameter) and the pleural lymphatics. Of note, these lymphatics have a large capacity for absorption. When artificial effusions were instilled into the pleural space of awake sheep, the exit rate (0.28 mL/kg per hour) was nearly 30 times the baseline exit rate (0.01 mL/kg per hour).[31]

## Pleural Pressure

A controversy has existed over whether there are two pleural pressures, or one.[45] Two pressures had been proposed to explain a discrepancy between two ways of measuring pleural pressure. One pressure, a liquid pressure measured using catheters, varied at 1 cm $H_2O$/cm lung height, as would a static column of liquid. The other pressure, a surface pressure measured using surface balloons and suction cups, varied by less than 1 cm $H_2O$/cm height and was equal and opposite to pulmonary recoil pressure. It appears now that the controversy arose because of the difficulty of measuring pleural pressure with catheters. The catheters were large relative to the narrow pleural space, distorted the space, and created a static column of liquid. With the use of relatively noninvasive micropipets, it is clear that pleural pressure is the same in the liquid as on the pleural surface and varies by approximately 0.5 cm $H_2O$/cm height.[45] The existence of this vertical pressure gradient implies that pleural liquid does not form a static column but slowly flows from the top to the bottom of the space.

The actual pleural pressure in humans is approximately $-5$ cm $H_2O$ at midchest at functional residual capacity and $-30$ cm $H_2O$ at total lung capacity.[46] If the lung were less compliant at these volumes, these pressures would be more negative. In one study of patients undergoing thoracentesis, those with more negative pleural pressures had a smaller improvement in lung volume than those with less negative pressures, presumably reflecting the presence of underlying diseased, noncompliant lung.[47]

Although the pleural space pressure is negative, gases do not accumulate there. The sum of all partial pressures of gases in capillary blood is approximately 700 mm Hg, or 60 mm Hg below atmospheric pressure ($P_{H_2O}$ = 47, $P_{CO_2}$ = 46, $P_{N_2}$ = 570, and $P_{O_2}$ = 40 mm Hg). The subatmospheric pressure of dissolved gases in capillary blood helps to maintain the pleural space free of gas and facilitates absorption of any gas that does enter the pleural space. Of note, to increase the gradient to augment absorption of gas, one can lower the partial pressure of nitrogen in the blood by having a patient breathe increased concentrations of inspired oxygen. The oxygen displaces alveolar nitrogen, thereby lowering the partial pressure of nitrogen in capillary blood; because of the limited absorption of oxygen that results from the plateau of the oxygen-hemoglobin dissociation curve, however, the increase in inspired oxygen does not add greatly to the partial pressure of oxygen in capillary blood.

## PATHOPHYSIOLOGY OF THE PLEURAL SPACE

### Pleural Effusions

For pleural liquid to accumulate, either the entry rate of liquid must increase to a sustained rate more than 30 times normal (to exceed the reserve lymphatic removal capacity), the exit rate of liquid must decrease, or both rates must change. In the clinical setting, it is most likely that excess pleural liquid accumulates as a result of changes in both entry and exit rates. Although clinicians are more aware of the problem of an increased entry rate of liquid, many of the causes of pleural effusions probably also decrease the exit rate of pleural liquid by interfering with pleural lymphatic drainage. The lymphatic exit rate may be decreased by obstruction of the parietal pleural stomas, inhibition of lymphatic contractility, infiltration of draining parasternal lymph nodes, or elevation of the systemic venous pressure into which the lymph drains. Decreases in lymphatic clearance have been confirmed in patients with tuberculous and malignant effusions[48] and in those with the yellow-nail syndrome, a disease of lymphatic function.[49]

To determine the origin of effusions, a classic and useful distinction is that between transudates and exudates.[50] Transudates (protein ratio [pleural:plasma] $\leq 0.50$ and lactate dehydrogenase ratio [pleural:plasma] $\leq 0.60$) form by leakage of liquid across an intact barrier as a result of increases in hydrostatic pressures or decreases in osmotic pressures across that barrier. Transudates generally indicate that the pleural membranes are not themselves abnormal. Exudates (protein ratio $> 0.50$ or lactate dehydrogenase [LDH] ratio $> 0.60$) form from leakage of liquid and protein across an altered barrier with increased permeability.

The circulatory barrier across which the liquid and protein leak is not always obvious. Most transudates are caused by congestive heart failure and originate from the capillary circulation of the lungs. The pleural effusions form from leakage of edema from the pulmonary interstitium across the leaky visceral pleura into the pleural space.[8, 9, 12, 51] Other transudates, those associated with the nephrotic syndrome or atelectasis, may form because of altered pressures (osmotic or hydrostatic) across the pleural capillaries. Some transudates may develop because of an isolated decrease in exit rate, as may happen with the superior vena cava syndrome. Finally, hepatic hydrothorax and effusions from peritoneal dialysis develop when liquid flows from the peritoneal space into the lower pressure pleural space across macroscopic holes in the diaphragm.

Exudates arise from injured capillary beds in the lung, the pleura, or adjacent tissues. Most exudates, such as those associated with pneumonia or pulmonary embolism, probably form after lung inflammation and injury when a high-protein lung edema leaks into the pleural space. Another large category of exudates arises from pleural injury due to inflammation, infection, or malignancy. Exudates can form when exudative liquid in the mediastinum (esophageal rupture or chylothorax), retroperitoneum (pancreatic pseudocyst), or peritoneum (ascites from spontaneous bacterial peritonitis or Meigs' syndrome) finds its way into the lower-pressure pleural space.

For either transudates or exudates, lymphatic obstruction may contribute to the accumulation of the effusion.[8] Nonetheless, because lymphatic clearance does not alter the pleural fluid protein concentration, the protein concentration gives information about the formation of the fluid, not about its removal.

### Effects of Pleural Effusions on Lung Function

In the presence of a space-occupying liquid in the pleural space, the lung recoils inward and the chest wall recoils outward. If the lung and chest wall have normal compliances, the decrease in lung volume accounts for approximately a third of the volume of the pleural effusion, and the increase in chest wall position accounts for the remaining two thirds. As a result, lung volumes are reduced by less than the pleural effusion volume. If the lung is otherwise normal, there is no evidence that an effusion causes significant hypoxemia, perhaps because ventilation and perfusion are reduced similarly. In fact, in one study, hypoxemia was noted only after liquid was removed by thoracentesis,[52] when perfusion presumably was restored whereas ventilation remained impaired.

Common symptoms of patients with effusions are pleuritic chest pain, cough, and dyspnea. It appears that the three symptoms have different causes. Pleuritic chest pain derives from inflammation of the parietal pleura, the site of pleural pain receptors. Occasionally, this symptom is accompanied by an audible or palpable pleural friction rub, reflecting the movement of abnormal pleural tissues. Cough may be due to distortion of the lung, in the same way that cough follows lung collapse from a pneumothorax. Dyspnea is most likely caused by the mechanical inefficiency of the respiratory muscles that are stretched by the outward displacement of the chest wall and the downward displacement of the diaphragm. After the removal of large pleural effusions, dyspnea is generally relieved promptly, although the reduction in pleural liquid volume is associated with only small increases in lung volume and little improvement, or an actual decrease, in oxygenation. In one study, nine patients underwent removal of more than 1800 mL of pleural liquid, and despite increases in vital capacity of only 300 mL, all patients experienced immediate relief of dyspnea.[53] Although the vital capacity changed little, patients could generate a more negative pleural pressure at the same lung volume after thoracentesis than before. This ability to generate a more negative pleural pressure was evidence of an improved efficiency of the respiratory muscles after the return of the chest wall to a more normal position after thoracentesis. This improved efficiency of breathing may explain the relief of dyspnea after removal of pleural liquid.

## APPROACH TO PATIENTS WITH PLEURAL EFFUSION

The possibility of a pleural effusion should be considered whenever a patient with an abnormal chest radiograph is evaluated. Increased densities on the chest radiograph are frequently attributed to parenchymal infiltrates when they actually represent pleural fluid. Free pleural fluid gravitates to the most dependent part of the thoracic cavity, which is the posterior costophrenic sulcus when the patient is upright. Therefore, if the posterior costophrenic angle is blunted or if the posterior part of the diaphragm is not visible on the lateral chest radiograph, bilateral decubitus chest radiographs should be obtained to ascertain whether free pleural fluid is present. If the distance between the inside of the thoracic cavity and the outside of the lung is less than 10 mm, the pleural effusion is not likely to be clinically significant and, in any case, would be difficult to sample by thoracentesis. If the distance is greater than 10 mm, an effort should be made to determine the cause of the pleural effusion.

## Differential Diagnosis of Pleural Effusion

Many different diseases may have an accompanying pleural effusion (Table 73.1). The vigor with which a diagnosis is pursued should depend on the likelihood that the person has that particular disease. Table 73.2 shows rough estimates of the annual incidence of the most common causes of pleural effusions. Congestive heart failure, pulmonary embolism, and cirrhosis are responsible for almost all transudative pleural effusions. Pneumonia, malignant pleural disease, pulmonary embolism, and gastrointestinal disease account for at least 90% of all exudative pleural effusions.

## Separation of Exudates from Transudates

A diagnostic thoracentesis should be performed on nearly every patient with free pleural fluid that measures more than 10 mm on the decubitus radiograph. If the patient has obvious congestive heart failure, consideration can be given to postponing the thoracentesis until the heart failure is treated. However, if the patient is febrile or has pleuritic chest pain or if the effusions are not of comparable size on both sides, a thoracentesis should be performed without delay.

The first question that should be answered with the diagnostic thoracentesis is whether the patient has a transudative or an exudative pleural effusion. The identification of transudates or exudates is made by analysis of the levels of protein and LDH in the pleural fluid and the serum. Exudative pleural effusions meet at least one of the following criteria, whereas transudative pleural effusions meet none[50]: (1) pleural fluid protein/serum protein greater than 0.50, (2) pleural fluid LDH/serum LDH greater than 0.60, and (3) pleural fluid LDH greater than two thirds of the upper normal limit for serum. If none of these criteria is met, the patient has a transudative pleural effusion, and the pleural surfaces can be ignored

**Table 73.1** DIFFERENTIAL DIAGNOSES OF PLEURAL EFFUSIONS

| | |
|---|---|
| TRANSUDATIVE PLEURAL EFFUSIONS | Collagen vascular diseases |
| Congestive heart failure | Rheumatoid pleuritis |
| Pericardial disease | Systemic lupus erythematosus |
| Cirrhosis | Drug-induced lupus |
| Nephrotic syndrome | Immunoblastic lymphadenopathy |
| Peritoneal dialysis | Sjögren's syndrome |
| Myxedema | Churg-Strauss syndrome |
| Fontan procedure | Wegener's granulomatosis |
| Pulmonary emboli | Postpericardiectomy or postmyocardial infarction syndrome |
| Sarcoidosis | Coronary artery bypass surgery |
| EXUDATIVE PLEURAL EFFUSIONS | Asbestos exposure |
| Neoplastic diseases | Sarcoidosis |
| Metastatic disease | Uremia |
| Mesothelioma | Meigs' syndrome |
| Infectious diseases | Yellow nail syndrome |
| Pyogenic bacterial infections | Drug-induced pleural disease |
| Tuberculosis | Nitrofurantoin |
| Actinomycosis and nocardiosis | Dantrolene |
| Fungal infections | Methysergide |
| Viral infections | Bromocriptine |
| Parasitic infections | Procarbazine |
| Pulmonary embolism | Amiodarone |
| Gastrointestinal disease | Trapped lung |
| Esophageal perforation | Radiation therapy |
| Pancreatic disease | Electric burns |
| Intra-abdominal abscesses | Urinary tract obstruction |
| Diaphragmatic hernia | Iatrogenic injury |
| Postabdominal surgery | Hemothorax |
| Postendoscopic variceal sclerotherapy | Chylothorax |

effusion. Pleural fluid white blood cell counts above 10,000/μL are most common with empyemas and parapneumonic effusions, but are also seen with pancreatitis, pulmonary embolism, and collagen vascular diseases, and occasionally, with malignancy and tuberculosis.[57]

The differential white cell count on the pleural fluid is much more useful than the absolute cell count itself. When the pleural fluid differential cell count is performed, the cells should be partitioned into the following categories: polymorphonuclear leukocytes, eosinophils, small lymphocytes, mesothelial cells, and other mononuclear cells. Pleural effusions due to an acute disease process, such as pneumonia, pulmonary embolization, pancreatitis, intra-abdominal abscess, and early tuberculosis, contain predominantly polymorphonuclear leukocytes. Pleural effusions due to a chronic disease process contain predominantly mononuclear cells.

Pleural fluid eosinophilia (≥10% eosinophils by differential count) is more common in benign inflammatory conditions but does not eliminate the possibility of malignant or tuberculous disease. Although retrospective studies have found that eosinophilia is associated with benign disease,[73] a prospective study in a population with a high prevalence of malignancy has found that eosinophilic effusions were as likely to be malignant as were noneosinophilic effusions.[74] Patients with pleural tuberculosis can sometimes have pleural fluid eosinophilia.[75] Most patients with pleural fluid eosinophilia have either air or blood in their pleural space.[76] On occasions when no pleural fluid eosinophils are found in the initial thoracentesis liquid but many eosinophils are seen in a subsequent specimen, the most likely explanation is a small pneumothorax caused by the initial thoracentesis.[73]

Blood in the pleural space is associated with pleural fluid eosinophilia. With traumatic hemothorax, pleural fluid eosinophilia does not occur until the second week.[76] The cause appears to be the production of interleukin-5 by $CD4^+$ T cells within the pleural space.[77] At times, the pleural fluid eosinophilia associated with a hemothorax can lead to eosinophilia in the peripheral blood.[78] The bloody pleural effusion complicating pulmonary embolism frequently contains many eosinophils.[57, 76]

If the cause of the eosinophilia is not evident, several unusual diagnoses should be considered. Benign asbestos pleural effusions are frequently eosinophilic. In one series, 15 of 29 patients (52%) with benign asbestos pleural effusions had pleural fluid eosinophilia.[73] Patients with pleural effusions secondary to drug reactions (nitrofurantoin or dantrolene) typically have pleural fluid eosinophilia.[60] The pleural fluid of patients with pleural paragonimiasis is typically eosinophilic with low glucose level, low pH, and high LDH level.[79] The Churg-Strauss syndrome is the only other disease that produces this constellation of pleural fluid findings.[80]

No cause is ever determined for approximately 20% of exudative pleural effusions. Interestingly, pleural fluid eosinophilia is found in approximately 40% of these effusions.[73] Therefore, if pleural fluid eosinophilia is found at the time of the initial thoracentesis and no obvious diagnosis is obtained after routine studies looking for the diagnoses just discussed, the subsequent workup should be relatively nonaggressive, after the presence of pulmonary embolism is excluded.

Mesothelial cells are the cells that line the pleural cavities. It is unusual to find mesothelial cells in effusions caused by tuberculosis; in one series of 65 patients with tuberculous pleuritis, only one patient had more than one mesothelial cell/1000 cells.[76] However, the absence of mesothelial cells is also common with other conditions in which the pleura becomes coated with fibrin, such as a complicated parapneumonic effusion.

The demonstration that more than 50% of the white blood cells in an exudative pleural effusion are small lymphocytes indicates that the patient probably has a malignant or a tuberculous pleural effusion. Ninety of 96 (94%) exudative pleural effusions in two series[57, 81] with more than 50% small lymphocytes were due to tuberculosis or malignant disease. Because these two diseases can be diagnosed with needle biopsy of the pleura, the presence of pleural fluid lymphocytosis should alert the physician to consider needle biopsy of the pleura for diagnosis. In general, separation of pleural lymphocytes into T and B lymphocytes has not been useful diagnostically, because the pleural fluid contains a higher percentage of T lymphocytes (~70%), a lower percentage of B lymphocytes (~10%), and a higher percentage of null cells (~20%) than the corresponding peripheral blood.[82, 83] Such partitioning can be useful diagnostically, however, when a diagnosis of chronic lymphocytic leukemia or lymphoma is suspected.[84] With these diseases, all the pleural lymphocytes are of the same type.

**Pleural Fluid Cytology.** A pleural fluid specimen from every patient with an undiagnosed exudative pleural effusion should be sent for cytopathologic studies. The first pleural fluid cytologic study is positive for malignant cells in up to 60% of the effusions caused by pleural malignancy.[57] If three separate specimens are submitted, up to 90% with pleural malignancy have positive cytopathology. The percentage of cases in which cytologic study of the pleural fluid establishes the diagnosis of a malignant pleural effusion ranges from 40% to 87%.[57, 85, 86] The frequency of positive pleural fluid cytologic tests is dependent on the tumor type. For example, less than 25% of patients with Hodgkin's disease have positive cytologic findings,[87] whereas most patients with adenocarcinomas have positive cytologic findings.[86] The percentage of positive diagnoses is higher if both cell blocks and smears are prepared and examined. Each additional sample may increase diagnostic yield in part by providing a higher percentage of fresher cells as older degenerated cells are largely removed by the earlier thoracenteses. The percentage of positive diagnoses is obviously dependent on the skill of the cytologist.

Positive pleural cytologic change has been shown to occur even without a pleural effusion; preresectional lavage of the pleural space during thoracotomy can demonstrate malignant cells in up to 14% of patients with stage I lung cancer.[87a] This otherwise inapparent involvement of the pleural space may explain the poor survival rate of patients after resection for early-stage lung cancer.

**Other Diagnostic Tests for Malignancy.** Cytologic studies may be nondiagnostic either because of a problem of specificity (for instance, the malignant cells cannot be differentiated from reactive mesothelial cells and "atypical" benign cells) or because of a problem of sensitivity (for instance, the malignant cells are rare). Several assays are being evaluated for their ability to increase the specificity of cytology for diagnosis of malignancy. Fluorescent in situ hybridization with chromosome-specific probes can confirm hyperdiploidity of specific chromosomes, thereby confirming that abnormal cells are indeed malignant.[88] Chromosomal analysis is, at times, still useful for the diagnosis of pleural leukemia or lymphoma.[89] Flow cytometry for DNA content can also show increased DNA content and abnormal cell cycle but is cumbersome and requires a high number of cells. Argylophilic nucleolar organizing regions, areas of nuclear DNA coding for ribosomal RNA, are found in greater numbers and in larger size in malignant cells than in benign reactive cells, although the degree of overlap limits the diagnostic value.[90] In addition, many assays have been tested in an attempt to increase sensitivity for the diagnosis of malignancy. Many of these tests, such as the detection of tumor markers in pleural liquid, are limited by their lack of specificity for malignant effusions. Future directions, such as detection by a polymerase chain reaction (PCR)-based assay of tumor-specific activities, such as those of telomerase, may hold promise.[91, 91a]

**Immunohistochemical and Other Studies for Diagnosing Malignancy.** Numerous papers have been published during the past few years on the diagnostic utility of monoclonal antibodies in the diagnosis of pleural malignancy.[92, 93] Adenocarcinoma is currently separated from mesothelioma or reactive mesothelial cells by the use of a panel of monoclonal antibodies directed against epithelial antigens. Adenocarcinoma can be expected to stain with B72.3, Leu-M1, anticarcinoembryonic antigen, and the newer Ber-EP4, whereas mesothelioma or reactive mesothelial cells usually stain with none.[24, 94]

**Culture and Bacteriologic Stains.** Pleural fluid from patients with undiagnosed exudative pleural effusions should be cultured for bacteria (both aerobically and anaerobically), mycobacteria, and fungi. Gram's stain should also be obtained. In the case of a probable complicated parapneumonic effusion with an initial negative Gram's stain, the sediment of the pleural fluid should be stained because the bacteria are precipitated in the sediment along with the white blood cells and the debris.

One potentially useful adjunct to culture is countercurrent immunoelectrophoresis, which can identify some bacterial antigens in pleural fluid of parapneumonic effusions. This may be especially useful in children, whose common pathogens, *Staphylococcus aureus, Streptococcus pneumoniae,* and *Haemophilus influenzae,* have antigens available for identification by countercurrent immunoelectrophoresis.[95] The antigens for anaerobic bacteria, the more common pathogen in adults, are not available.

## Other Diagnostic Tests for Pleural Fluid

**Pleural Fluid pH and $P_{CO_2}$.** The pleural fluid pH can be reduced to less than 7.20 by 10 different conditions: (1) complicated parapneumonic effusion, (2) esophageal rupture, (3) rheumatoid pleuritis, (4) tuberculous pleuritis, (5) malignant pleural disease, (6) hemothorax, (7) systemic acidosis, (8) paragonimiasis, (9) lupus pleuritis, and (10) urinothorax.[60] With exudative pleural effusions, the decreased pleural fluid pH appears to result from lactic acid and carbon dioxide accumulation in the pleural fluid.[96] With transudative pleural effusions, the pleural fluid has a slightly higher pH than the blood.[97]

The pleural fluid pH is most useful in determining whether chest tubes should be inserted in patients with parapneumonic effusions.[61] A fall in the pleural fluid pH appears to be a sensitive indicator that the patient has a highly inflammatory parapneumonic pleural effusion that will require drainage.

The routine measurement of pleural fluid pH is recommended only in patients with parapneumonic effusions. In general, pleural fluids with a low pH also have a low glucose level and a high LDH level.[96] In many institutions, pleural fluid glucose is used as an alternative to the pH measurement. When the pleural fluid pH is used as a diagnostic test, it must be measured with the same care as arterial pH. The fluid should be collected anaerobically in a heparinized syringe and placed on ice. If the sample is left open to air, a spuriously high pH value can be obtained because of the rapid loss of carbon dioxide. The pH must be measured with a blood gas machine; a pH meter or an indicator paper is not sufficiently accurate.[98]

**Tests for Collagen Vascular Diseases.** About 5% of patients with rheumatoid arthritis[99] and 50% of patients with systemic lupus erythematosus[100] have a pleural effusion sometime during the course of their disease. At times, the effusions may be the first manifestation of the disease; therefore, these diagnostic possibilities should be considered in patients with undiagnosed exudative pleural effusion.

Measurement of the ANA titer is the best screening test for lupus pleuritis, although it is now evident that a positive pleural fluid ANA result is not specific for the diagnosis. Although all patients with lupus pleuritis have a positive pleural liquid ANA ($>$ 1:40), a positive ANA finding has been found between 11% and 27% of all other effusions.[101, 102] In one prospective study, the titer of ANA, the ratio of pleural:plasma ANA, or the pattern of staining did not increase the specificity for systemic lupus erythematosus.[102] In fact, a positive pleural fluid ANA finding in patients without systemic lupus erythematosus may be associated with malignancy.[102]

When a rheumatoid pleural effusion is suspected, the clinical picture usually establishes the diagnosis. If any question exists, the level of rheumatoid factor in the pleural fluid should be measured. Only patients with rheumatoid pleuritis have a pleural fluid rheumatoid factor titer equal to or greater than 1:320 and equal to or greater than the serum titer.[103]

**Adenosine Deaminase.** Adenosine deaminase (ADA), a product of activated lymphocytes, catalyzes the conversion of adenosine to inosine and is important for normal immune function. The pleural fluid ADA levels are elevated in almost all patients with tuberculous pleuritis, but not with other conditions.[104] An occasional patient with empyema, lymphoma, or leukemia may have elevated pleural fluid ADA levels; clinically, however, these entities should be relatively easy to differentiate from tuberculosis. The specificity of ADA for the diagnosis of tuberculosis is increased if a high value is combined with pleural fluid lymphocytosis (lymphocyte/neutrophil ratio $> 0.75$).[105] Assays for ADA are not readily available in the United States.

**Interferon Gamma.** Interferon gamma, a T-cell lymphokine, plays a critical role in the effective clinical response to *Mycobacterium tuberculosis.* Pleural liquid interferon gamma is elevated almost exclusively in tuberculous effusions[106] and may be more specific for tuberculosis than ADA.[107] It also retains its diagnostic utility for tuberculosis in human immunodeficiency virus–positive patients, whereas the ADA may not.[107]

**Polymerase Chain Reaction Amplification for *Mycobacterium tuberculosis.*** A 123-base pair DNA sequence IS6110 is specific to *M. tuberculosis* and is amplified by PCR to provide evidence for the presence of *M. tuberculosis.* The potential of the test is great for providing a rapid, highly sensitive and specific diagnosis of mycobacterial infection. In practice, although PCR techniques should be able to detect a single target genome, PCR amplification of clinical samples has been limited by a low sensitivity, often little better than culture itself.[108] The decreased sensitivity may be due to degradation of the target DNA by sample processing or by inhibitors of amplification in clinical fluids. Before wide application of PCR assays, considerations must include its cost and its potential to identify antibiotic resistance of the organism.

**Other Enzymes and Proteins.** Over the past several years, many articles have been written on the utility of measuring various enzymes and proteins in the pleural space, including hyaluronic acid, lysozyme or its components, mucoproteins, mucopolysaccharides, $\beta_2$-microglobulin, alpha-fetoprotein, aldolase, glutamic oxaloacetic transaminase, glutamic pyruvic transaminase, and alkaline and acid phosphatase. None has proved to be of value in the differential diagnosis or management of patients with pleural effusions.[60]

## Useful Radiographic Tests in Patients with Suspected Pleural Disease

The possibility of a pleural effusion should be considered whenever a patient with an abnormal chest radiograph is evaluated. Two main factors influence the distribution of free fluid in the pleural space. First, the fluid collects in the most dependent part of the thoracic cavity because the lung is less dense than the pleural fluid. Second, because of their elastic recoil, the lobes of the lung maintain their traditional shape at all stages of collapse.

When the patient is upright, the fluid first accumulates between the inferior surface of the lower lobe and the diaphragm. If less than 75 mL of fluid is present, it may occupy only this position without overflowing into the costophrenic sinuses. When more fluid accumulates, it spills over into the posterior costophrenic angle and obliterates the posterior part of the diaphragm on the lateral projection. The possibility of a pleural effusion should be suspected whenever the posterior part of one or both hemidiaphragms is obscured. The presence of a clinically significant amount of free pleural fluid can be excluded if both posterior costophrenic angles are clear.

When there are larger amounts of pleural fluid, the lateral costophrenic angle on the posteroanterior radiograph becomes blunted. Collins and associates[109] demonstrated that at least 175 mL of pleural fluid had to be injected into the pleural space of cadavers before the lateral costophrenic angle was blunted. In some of their cases, more than 500 mL of pleural fluid could be present without blunting the lateral costophrenic angle. As more fluid accumulates, the entire outline of the hemidiaphragm on the affected side is lost, and the fluid extends upward around the anterior, lateral, and posterior thoracic walls, producing opacification of the lung base and the typical meniscus shape of the fluid.

The changes just discussed are suggestive rather than diagnostic of the presence of pleural fluid. Lateral decubitus radiographs should be obtained in most instances when free pleural fluid is suspected. If the entire hemithorax is opacified, decubitus radiographs are of no use because there is no air-containing lung in the hemithorax. The basis for the use of the lateral decubitus view is that free fluid gravitates to the most dependent part of the pleural space. When a patient is placed in the lateral recumbent position, the free pleural fluid on the dependent side accumulates between the chest wall and the lung (Fig. 73.5). As little as 5 mL of pleural fluid can be demonstrated with properly exposed decubitus radiographs.[110] The amount of pleural fluid can be semiquantitated by measuring the distance between the inner border of the chest wall and the outer border of the lung (Fig. 73.5). As already stated, when this distance is less than 10 mm, the amount of pleural fluid is small, and a diagnostic thoracentesis is usually not attempted.

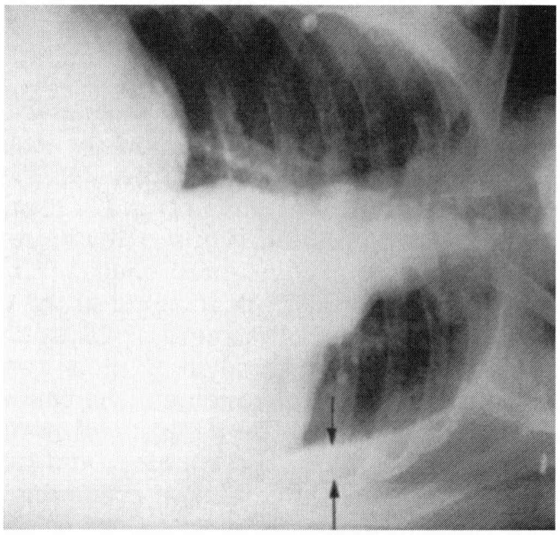

**Figure 73.5** Left lateral decubitus chest radiograph demonstrating the presence of free pleural fluid. The amount of pleural fluid can be semiquantified by measuring the distance between the two arrows.

It is frequently useful to obtain bilateral decubitus radiographs when free pleural fluid is suspected. When the radiograph is obtained with the suspect side superior, the fluid gravitates toward the mediastinum. This facilitates the evaluation of the underlying lung for infiltrates or atelectasis. In addition, if the lateral costophrenic angle is blunted on the posteroanterior view and is clear on the decubitus view with the suspect side superior, the blunting can be attributed to pleural fluid.

Pleural fluid may become encapsulated by adhesions anywhere between the parietal and the visceral pleurae or in the interlobar fissures. Such loculation occurs most frequently in association with conditions that cause intense pleural inflammation, such as complicated parapneumonic effusion, hemothorax, and tuberculous pleuritis. When the loculation is situated between the lung and the chest wall, there is a characteristic radiographic picture. The loculation is D-shaped, with the base of the D against the chest wall and the smooth convexity protruding inward toward the lung (Fig. 73.6). The absence of air bronchograms helps differentiate a loculated pleural effusion from a parenchymal infiltrate. A definite diagnosis of loculated pleural effusion is best established by ultrasonography. The demonstration of one locule should serve as an indication to search for additional locules because multiple locules are common.

**Ultrasonography.** One way to document and locate loculated pleural fluid is with ultrasonography. In the presence of pleural fluid, the proximal echoes from the skin, intercostal muscles, and parietal pleura are separated from the distal echoes arising from the visceral pleura and the lung by a central echo-free space. The advantages of ultrasonography over computed tomography (CT) are the ease and speed with which the examination can be performed, the lack of ionizing radiation, the relatively low cost, and the ability to provide continuous guidance for thoracentesis or pleural biopsy.[111, 111a]

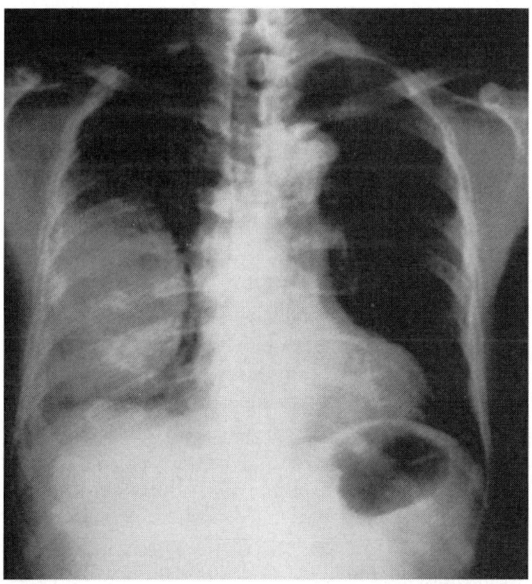

**Figure 73.6** Posteroanterior chest radiograph demonstrating a D-shaped density with the base of the D against the right lateral chest wall. No free pleural fluid was demonstrated with the lateral decubitus radiograph in this patient. (From Light RW: Pleural Diseases (3rd ed). Philadelphia: Lea & Febiger, 1995, p 26.)

However, it should be emphasized that ultrasonic examination of the pleura is not without difficulties. In one study, pleural abnormalities in 42 of 59 patients were characterized as echo-free, but fluid could be obtained from only 31 of these 42 patients. The radiographic abnormalities contained echoes in the other 17 patients, and despite the presence of internal echoes or septations, the thoracentesis was successful in all 17 patients.[112]

The appropriate site for a thoracentesis can be identified by use of ultrasonography, although its routine use is probably not cost effective. If a patient has a moderate or large effusion, ultrasonography is indicated only if no fluid is obtained after two or three attempts.[113] When ultrasonography is used to identify the site for thoracentesis, it is important to perform the thoracentesis during the ultrasonic examination. If the skin is marked and the patient is returned to his or her room, thoracentesis is frequently unsuccessful because the relationship between the skin and the pleural fluid may have changed. In addition, when the thoracentesis is performed at the time of the ultrasonic examination, the ultrasonographer receives immediate feedback concerning the accuracy of the procedure. This immediate feedback is valuable in improving the skill of the ultrasonographer.

**Computed Tomography.** CT is currently the best way to visualize the pleural space.[114] Frequently, the presence of pleural fluid makes it difficult to evaluate the status of the underlying pulmonary parenchyma with routine chest radiography. CT of the chest has its greatest utility in demonstrating parenchymal abnormalities in patients with extensive pleural disease. At times, it is difficult to distinguish parenchymal abnormalities from pleural abnormalities with CT; in such instances, the bolus injection of intravenous contrast medium is indicated because the unaerated perfused lung parenchyma enhances, whereas the pleural abnormality does not.[111a, 115]

Chest CT is useful in distinguishing a parenchymal lung abscess located near the chest wall from an empyema with an air-fluid level. The most distinctive features are the margins of the abnormality. With empyema, the cavity walls are of uniform thickness both internally and externally, and the adjacent lung is usually compressed. With lung abscess, the walls of the cavity are not of uniform thickness, and the adjacent lung is not compressed. In addition, most empyemas have a lenticular shape and demonstrate the "split pleura" sign (see Fig. 74.2).[116]

The diagnosis of pleural mesothelioma (Chapter 76) is usually strongly suggested by a chest CT that demonstrates a thickened pleura with an irregular, often nodular, internal margin. These changes are most pronounced at the base of the lung. In addition, the major fissure is usually markedly thickened because of a combination of fibrosis, tumor, and associated fluid.[24, 117]

**Magnetic Resonance Imaging.** This imaging technique has generated considerable interest as a safe and sensitive method for imaging human pathologic conditions (see Chapter 25). Pleural effusions generally have long T1 and T2 values. The intensity of pleural effusions is therefore low to extremely low on T1-weighted images.[118] However, at the present time, magnetic resonance imaging of the chest is less satisfactory than ultrasonography or CT in identifying the presence of pleural fluid. It is possible that with improved magnetic resonance technology, the characteristics of pleural fluid can be determined noninvasively. At the present time, respiratory and cardiac motion are the major limitations in evaluating specific intensity patterns of fluid collections of various compositions.[119]

**Other Studies.** Pulmonary embolism (see Chapter 51) is one of the leading causes of pleural effusion. Because the pleural effusion with pulmonary embolization can be either a transudate or an exudate, the diagnosis of pulmonary embolization should be considered in every patient with a pleural effusion.

The standard approach has incorporated lung ventilation-perfusion scanning. However, the interpretation of the perfusion lung scan is difficult in patients with pleural fluid.[120] Areas of the hemithorax occupied by the pleural fluid are poorly perfused. With a large effusion, perfusion to the entire ipsilateral lung may be attenuated owing to reflex vasoconstriction. In addition, if perfusion scans are obtained with the patient recumbent, the fluid can gravitate into the fissure to produce large perfusion defects. If the ventilation lung scan is subsequently performed with the patient erect, areas of gross mismatching of the ventilation and perfusion may be seen; these are due merely to the shift of the pleural fluid as the position of the patient changes. Therefore, the difficulties inherent in interpretation of lung scanning are exacerbated in the presence of pleural effusions. As an alternative to lung scanning, it is reasonable to select spiral CT angiography as an initial study in these patients. Spiral CT angiography is highly sensitive and specific for pulmonary emboli in the proximal, segmental pulmonary arteries.[121] In contrast to lung scanning, spiral CT can establish alternate diagnoses as well.[122] Where spiral CT is not available, lung scanning can be used, perhaps after efforts to improve accuracy by withdrawing as much pleural liquid as possible. The indications for duplex ultrasonography, pulmonary angiography, and other diagnostic modalities are considered in Chapter 51.

## Invasive Tests in Patients with Undiagnosed Exudative Pleural Effusions

In the patient with an undiagnosed exudative pleural effusion, several invasive tests might be considered, including needle biopsy of the pleura, bronchoscopy, thoracoscopy, and open biopsy of the pleura. No diagnosis is ever established for approximately 20% of all exudative pleural effusions, and many resolve spontaneously, leaving no residua.[123] In patients with undiagnosed exudative pleural effusions, three factors should influence the vigor with which one pursues the diagnosis with invasive tests:

1. The symptoms and the clinical course of the patient; if the symptoms of the patient are minimal or if the symptoms are improving with time, a less aggressive approach is indicated.
2. The trend of the pleural fluid LDH level with time; if the pleural fluid LDH increases with serial thoracenteses, a more aggressive approach is indicated.
3. The attitude of the patient; if the patient is anxious to know the cause of the pleural effusion, an aggressive approach should be taken.

**Needle Biopsy of the Pleura.** Small specimens of the parietal pleura can be obtained with needle biopsy. The needles most commonly used for this procedure are the Cope needle and the Abrams needle.[60, 124] Because needle biopsy of the pleura is useful mainly to establish the diagnosis of malignant or tuberculous pleural effusions, this procedure should be considered when one of these diagnoses is suspected.

The results of needle biopsy of the pleura are positive in 40% to 60% of patients with malignant pleural disease.[123, 125] Overall, the yield from pleural fluid cytology tends to be higher. In one series of 281 patients with malignant pleural effusions, the pleural biopsy result was positive in 43%, whereas the pleural fluid cytologic result was positive in 58%. In only 7% was the pleural biopsy result positive and the pleural fluid cytologic result negative.[123] However, in a second series of 189 patients with malignant pleural effusions, the pleural biopsy result was positive in 60%, whereas the cytologic result was positive in 52%. Both pleural fluid cytologic and biopsy results were positive in 33%, only the biopsy result was positive in 27%, and only the cytologic result was positive in 19%.[125] A prudent approach to the patient with a suspected malignant pleural effusion is to obtain a pleural biopsy specimen only if the cytologic sample obtained at the time of the initial diagnostic thoracentesis is nondiagnostic.

Needle biopsy of the pleura has its greatest utility in diagnosing tuberculous pleuritis. The initial biopsy is positive for granulomas in 50% to 80% of patients.[126] The demonstration of granulomas on the pleural biopsy is virtually diagnostic of tuberculous pleuritis; caseous necrosis or acid-fast bacilli need not be demonstrated, although on rare occasions fungal diseases, sarcoidosis, or rheumatoid pleuritis can produce granulomatous pleuritis. When tuberculous pleuritis is suspected, a portion of the pleural biopsy specimen should be cultured for mycobacteria. In one series of 21 patients with tuberculous pleuritis, cultures of the biopsy specimens were positive for *M. tuberculosis* in 16 (76%), and 5 of those with positive cultures did not reveal granulomas on microscopic examination.[127] In this series, either the microscopic examination or the biopsy culture was positive in 20 of the 21 patients (95%).[127] If the initial biopsy is nondiagnostic and the patient has tuberculous pleuritis, a second biopsy is diagnostic 10% to 40% of the time.[126, 128]

In addition to helping establish the diagnosis, cultures of needle biopsy specimens from patients with tuberculous pleurisy can be used for drug susceptibility testing. Often, the presentation of a patient with a recent positive protein derivative conversion and an exudative pleural effusion with lymphocytosis is classic and is unlikely to be due to any diagnosis other than tuberculous pleurisy. The diagnosis can be further supported by measurements, where available, of pleural fluid ADA or interferon gamma. In those cases, treatment for tuberculosis can be offered with confidence without needle biopsy confirmation. However, when the patient may have been exposed to drug-resistant organisms, needle biopsy increases the likelihood of obtaining organisms for culture and is recommended.

The two major complications of needle biopsy of the pleura are pneumothorax and bleeding. Pneumothoraces large enough to require a chest tube occur in only about 1% of pleural biopsies.[123, 129] It is likely that many pneumothoraces develop because of leakage of air through the biopsy needle and do not necessarily indicate puncture of the lung. A hemothorax can result if an intercostal artery or a vein inadvertently undergoes biopsy. In one series, a fatal hemothorax occurred in 2 of 227 biopsy procedures.[129] The pleural biopsy needle can also be mistakenly inserted into the liver, spleen, or kidney, which can lead to hemorrhage in these organs. However, bleeding complications are rare.

If no diagnosis is obtained after routine laboratory tests that included cytology and one-needle biopsy of the pleura, what can be said concerning the patient? Poe and coworkers[129] followed up 143 such patients for 12 to 72 months, during which time 29 patients were diagnosed with malignant pleural disease and one patient with tuberculous pleuritis. In all 29 cases in which malignancy was eventually diagnosed, the diagnosis of malignant neoplasm was suggested by clinical criteria, such as weight loss, constitutional symptoms, and history of previous cancer. These authors concluded that most patients with undiagnosed exudative pleural effusions in whom the clinical picture does not suggest malignancy are best managed by observation. In those with symptoms suggestive of malignancy, thoracoscopy is probably the procedure of choice.

**Bronchoscopy.** Another procedure that should be considered in the patient with an undiagnosed pleural effusion is bronchoscopy (see Chapter 27). If the patient has an associated parenchymal lesion or hemoptysis, fiberoptic bronchoscopy will provide a diagnosis in nearly 75%.[130] If the patient has neither a parenchymal abnormality nor hemoptysis, a diagnosis for the pleural effusion is established less than 10% of the time.[131] At the present time, CT scan of the chest should be performed in all patients with undiagnosed exudative pleural effusions. Bronchoscopy should then be performed only if CT demonstrates parenchymal abnormalities or if the patient has hemoptysis. At the time of bronchoscopy, special attention is paid to those portions of the lung in which the parenchymal abnormalities were demonstrated.

**Thoracoscopy.** Thoracoscopy may be useful diagnostically in patients in whom the origin of a pleural effusion remains unclear after routine fluid analysis and needle biopsy of the pleura. In many cases, especially for the evaluation of malignancy, thoracoscopy may supplant needle biopsy because of a greater diagnostic yield and the added ability to provide pleural sclerosis. Thoracoscopy can be performed by pulmonologists using local anesthesia and conscious sedation for direct visualization of the pleural surfaces, tissue sampling, and pleurodesis; thoracoscopy performed by thoracic surgeons, generally referred to as video-assisted thoracoscopic surgery, utilizes general anesthesia and single-lung ventilation by double-lumen intubation and allows greater access to the pleura and lung for surgical procedures.[132] After a pneumothorax is induced on the side of the pleural effusion, the thoracoscope is introduced through the chest wall into the pleural space. The only absolute contraindication for the use of thoracoscopy is the lack of an adequate pleural space for placing and manuevering the thoracoscope; relative contraindications include hypoxemia not caused by the pleural effusion and likely to limit the ability to collapse one lung for the procedure. In the past few years, there has been a dramatic improvement in the equipment and in the expertise of operators so that in some institutions, thoracoscopy is now the procedure of choice for the diagnosis and management of diseases of the pleura.[133]

Two separate studies, each with 102 patients, reported diagnostic yields of 93%[134] and 80%,[135] respectively. However, when the studies are examined in detail, one finds that the only diagnosis that is definitely established with thoracoscopy is malignancy. In the two series the diagnosis was established in 99 of 117 patients (85%) with malignancy, including 51 of 56 (91%) of those with mesothelioma.[134, 135]

Which patients with undiagnosed pleural effusions should undergo thoracoscopy? A diagnosis can be established in more than 80% of patients with malignancy, including those with mesothelioma. Moreover, talc can be insufflated at the time of the procedure, and this practice controls the effusion in the most patients. Nonetheless, the procedure has minor risks; a need for postprocedure chest tube or tubes and a procedure cost should be considered. Thoracoscopy is therefore recommended, assuming that the technical expertize and facilities are available, for the patient with an undiagnosed pleural effusion after diagnostic thoracentesis and needle biopsy of the pleura in whom the diagnosis of malignancy is strongly suspected and in whom one wishes to establish this diagnosis.

**Open Biopsy of the Pleura.** Thoracotomy with direct biopsy of the pleura provides the best visualization of the pleura and the best biopsy specimens. Nowadays, the less invasive thoracoscopy can replace thoracotomy in most instances. The main indication for open pleural biopsy is progressive undiagnosed pleural disease that cannot be approached by, or has failed to be diagnosed by, thoracoscopy. In the past, for example, the diagnosis of malignant mesothelioma was usually made with open biopsy of the pleura, but now the diagnosis can be established with thoracoscopy in most cases.

Open pleural biopsy does not always provide a diagnosis in patients with pleural effusions. Douglass and associates[136] reported that thoracotomy failed to provide a specific diagnosis for 7 of 21 patients with undiagnosed pleural effusion. Over the 11-year period from 1962 to 1972, 51 patients with pleural effusion at the Mayo Clinic had no diagnosis after an open pleural biopsy.[137] In 31 of these patients (61%), there was no recurrence of the pleural effusion, and no cause ever became apparent. However, 13 of the patients were eventually proven to have malignancy; 6 had lymphoma and 4 had malignant mesothelioma. Thus, observation of patients with undiagnosed pleural effusions is often warranted unless there is compelling reason to pursue the diagnosis of malignancy.

## SUMMARY

Disorders of the pleura are common medical problems that often bring patients to their physicians or complicate the course of patients already under medical care. In this chapter, the anatomy and physiology of the pleural membranes and pleural space have been reviewed. In addition, the initial diagnostic approach to the patient with pleural disease, especially pleural effusion, was discussed. The subsequent three chapters provide specific clinical details about pleural effusion (see Chapter 74); pneumothorax, chylothorax, hemothorax, and fibrothorax (see Chapter 75); and tumors of the pleura (see Chapter 76).

## References

1. Albertine KH, Wiener-Kronish JP, Bastacky J, et al: No evidence for mesothelial cell contact across the costal pleural space of sheep. J Appl Physiol 70:123–134, 1991.
2. Gaensler EA: Parietal pleurectomy for recurrent spontaneous pneumothorax. Surg Gynecol Obstet 102:293–308, 1956.
3. Deschamps C, Rodarte JR: Effects of unilateral pleural symphysis on respiratory system mechanics and gas exchange in anesthetized dogs. Am Rev Respir Dis 137:1385–1389, 1988.
4. Davidson FF, Glazier JB: Unilateral pleuritis and regional lung function. Ann Intern Med 77:37–42, 1972.
5. Stamenovic D: Mechanical properties of pleural membrane. J Appl Physiol 57:1189–1194, 1984.
6. Humphrey JD: A possible role of the pleura in lung mechanics. J Biomech 20:773–777, 1987.
7. Hajji MA, Wilson TA, Lai-Fook SJ: Improved measurements of shear modulus and pleural membrane tension of the lung. J Appl Physiol 47:175–181, 1979.
8. Broaddus VC, Light RW: What is the origin of transudates and exudates? Chest 102:658–659, 1992.
9. Broaddus VC, Wiener-Kronish JP, Staub NC: Clearance of lung edema into the pleural space of volume-loaded, anesthetized sheep. J Appl Physiol 68:2623–2630, 1990.
10. Wiener-Kronish JP, Matthay MA, Callen PW, et al: Relationship of pleural effusions to pulmonary hemodynamics in patients with heart failure. Am Rev Respir Dis 132:1253–1256, 1985.
11. Miller KS, Harley RA, Sahn SA: Pleural effusions associated with ethchlorvynol lung injury result from visceral pleural leak. Am Rev Respir Dis 140:764–770, 1989.
12. Wiener-Kronish JP, Broaddus VC: Interrelationship of pleural and pulmonary interstitial liquid. Annu Rev Physiol 55:209–226, 1993.
13. Gray SW, Skandalakis JE. Development of the pleura. *In* Chretien J, Bignon J, Hirsch A, (ed): The Pleura in Health and Disease. Vol 30. New York: Marcel Dekker, 1985, pp 3–19.
14. Rennard SI, Jaurand M-C, Bignon J, et al: Role of pleural mesothelial cells in the production of the submesothelial connective tissue matrix of lung. Am Rev Respir Dis 130:267–274, 1984.
15. Jaurand M-C, Kaplan H, Thiollet J, et al: Phagocytosis of chrysotile fibers by pleural mesothelial cells in culture. Am J Pathol 94:529–538, 1979.
16. Boylan AM, Sanan DA, Sheppard D, et al: Vitronectin enhances internalization of crocidolite asbestos by rabbit pleural mesothelial cells via the integrin $\alpha v\beta 5$. J Clin Invest 96:1987–2001, 1995.
17. Idell S, Zwieb C, Kuman A, et al: Pathways of fibrin turnover of human pleural mesothelial cells in vitro. Am J Respir Cell Mol Biol 7:414–426, 1992.
18. Sitter T, Toet K, Fricke H, et al: Modulation of procoagulant and fibrinolytic system components of mesothelial cells by inflammatory mediators. Am J Physiol 172:R1256–R1263, 1996.
19. Kumar A, Koenig KB, Johnson AR, et al: Expression and assembly of procoagulant complexes by human pleural mesothelial cells. Thromb Haemost 71:587–592, 1994.
20. Goodman RB, Wood RG, Martin TR, et al: Cytokine-stimulated human mesothelial cells produce chemotactic activity for neutrophils including NAP-1/IL-8. J Immunol 148:457–465, 1992.
21. Antony VB, Hott JW, Kunkel SL, et al: Pleural mesothelial cell expression of C-C (monocyte chemotactic peptide) and C-X-C (interleukin-8) chemokines. Am J Respir Cell Mol Biol 12:581–588, 1995.
22. Boylan AM, Hébert CA, Sadick M, et al: Interleukin-8 is a major component of pleural liquid chemotactic activity in a rabbit model of endotoxin pleurisy. Am J Physiol 267:L137–L144, 1994.
23. Wang NS: The regional difference of pleural mesothelial cells in rabbits. Am Rev Respir Dis 110:623–633, 1974.
24. Nishimura SL, Broaddus VC: Asbestos-induced pleural disease. Clin Chest Med 19:311–329, 1998.
25. Albertine KH, Wiener-Kronish JP, Roos PJ, et al: Structure, blood supply, and lymphatic vessels of the sheep's visceral pleura. Am J Anat 165:277–294, 1982.
26. McLaughlin RF, Tyler WS, Canada RO: Subgross pulmonary anatomy of the rabbit, rat, and guinea pig, with additional notes on the human lung. Am Rev Respir Dis 94:380–387, 1966.
27. Oldmixon EH, Hoppin FGJ: Comparison of amounts of collagen and elastin in pleura and parenchyma of dog lung. J Appl Physiol 56:1383–1388, 1956.
28. Albertine KH, Wiener-Kronish JP, Staub NC: The structure of the parietal pleura and its relationship to pleural liquid dynamics in sheep. Anat Rec 208:401–409, 1984.
29. Wang N-S: The preformed stomas connecting the pleural cavity and the lymphatics in the parietal pleura. Am Rev Respir Dis 111:12–20, 1975.
30. Li J: Ultrastructural study on the pleural stomata in human. Funct Develop Morphol 3:277–280, 1993.
31. Broaddus VC, Wiener-Kronish JP, Berthiaume Y, et al: Removal of pleural liquid and protein by lymphatics in awake sheep. J Appl Physiol 64:384–390, 1988.
32. Wang N-S: Anatomy of the pleura. *In* Antony VB (ed): Diseases of the Pleura. Philadelphia: WB Saunders, 1998, pp 229–240.
33. Pereira ADD, Aguas AP, Oliveira MJ, et al: Experimental modulation of the reactivity of pleural milky spots (Kampmeier's foci) by Freund's adjuvants, betamethasone and mycobacterial infection. J Anat 185:471–479, 1994.
34. Staub NC, Wiener-Kronish JP, Albertine KH: Transport through the pleura: Physiology of normal liquid and solute exchange in the pleural space. *In* Chrétien J, Bignon J, Hirsch A, (eds): The Pleura in Health and Disease. Vol 30. New York: Marcel Dekker, 1985, pp 169–193.
35. Bhattacharya J, Gropper MA, Staub NC: Interstitial fluid pressure gradient measured by micropuncture in excised dog lung. J Appl Physiol 56:271–277, 1984.
36. Kim KJ, Critz AM, Crandall ED: Transport of water and solutes across sheep visceral pleura. Am Rev Respir Dis 120:883–892, 1979.
36a. Parameswaran S, Brown LV, Ibbott GS, et al: Hydraulic conductivity, albumin reflection and diffusion coefficients of pig mediastinal pleura. Microvasc Res 58:114–127, 1999.
37. Negrini D, Townsley MI, Taylor AE: Hydraulic conductivity of the canine parietal pleura in vivo. J Appl Physiol 69:438–442, 1990.
38. Payne DK, Kinasewitz GT, Gonzalez E: Comparative permeability of canine visceral and parietal pleura. J Appl Physiol 65:2558–2564, 1988.
39. Rolf LL, Travis DM: Pleural fluid-plasma bicarbonate gradients in oxygen-toxic and normal rats. Am J Physiol 224:857–861, 1973.
40. Wiener-Kronish JP, Albertine KH, Licko V, et al: Protein egress and entry rates in pleural fluid and plasma in sheep. J Appl Physiol 56:459–463, 1984.

41. Broaddus VC, Araya M: Liquid and protein dynamics using a new, minimally invasive pleural catheter in rabbits. J Appl Physiol 72:851–857, 1992.
42. Erdmann AJ, Vaughan TR, Brigham KL, et al: Effect of increased vascular pressure on lung fluid balance in unanesthetized sheep. Circ Res 37:271–284, 1975.
43. Wilson JL, Herrod CM, Searle GL, et al: The absorption of blood from the pleural space. Surgery 48:766–774, 1960.
44. Courtice FC, Morris B: The effect of diaphragmatic movement on the absorption of protein and of red cells from the pleural cavity. Aust J Exp Biol 31:227–238, 1953.
45. Lai-Fook SJ, Rodarte JR: Pleural pressure distribution and its relationship to lung volume and interstitial pressure. J Appl Physiol 70:967–978, 1991.
46. Murray JF: The Normal Lung. Philadelphia: WB Saunders, 1986, pp 377.
47. Light RW, Stansbury DW, Brown SE: The relationship between pleural pressures and changes in pulmonary function after therapeutic thoracentesis. Am Rev Respir Dis 133:658–661, 1986.
48. Leckie WJH, Tothill P: Albumin turnover in pleural effusions. Clin Sci 29:339–352, 1965.
49. Runyon BA, Forker EL, Sopko JA: Pleural-fluid kinetics in a patient with primary lymphedema, pleural effusions, and yellow nails. Am Rev Respir Dis 119:821–825, 1979.
50. Light RW, MacGregor MI, Luchsinger PC, et al: Pleural effusions: The diagnostic separation of transudates and exudates. Ann Intern Med 77:507–513, 1972.
51. Allen S, Gabel J, Drake R: Left atrial hypertension causes pleural effusion formation in unanesthetized sheep. Am J Physiol 257:H690–H692, 1989.
52. Brandstetter RD, Cohen RP: Hypoxemia after thoracentesis: A predictable and treatable condition. JAMA 242:1060–1061, 1979.
53. Estenne M, Yernault J-C, de Troyer A: Mechanism of relief of dyspnea after thoracocentesis in patients with large pleural effusions. Am J Med 74:813–819, 1983.
54. Assi Z, Caruso JL, Herndon J, et al: Cytologically proved malignant pleural effusions: Distribution of transudates and exudates. Chest 113:1302–1304, 1998.
55. Burgess LJ, Maritz FJ, Taljaard JJF: Comparative analysis of the biochemical parameters used to distinguish between pleural transudates and exudates. Chest 107:1604–1609, 1995.
56. Peterman TA, Speicher CE: Evaluating pleural effusions: A two-stage approach. JAMA 252:1051–1053, 1984.
57. Light RW, Erozan YS, Ball WC: Cells in pleural fluid: Their value in differential diagnosis. Arch Intern Med 132:854–860, 1973.
58. Staats BA, Ellefson RD, Budahn LL, et al: The lipoprotein profile of chylous and nonchylous pleural effusions. Mayo Clin Proc 55:700–704, 1980.
59. Light RW, Ball WC: Lactate dehydrogenase isoenzymes in pleural effusions. Am Rev Respir Dis 108:660–664, 1973.
60. Light RW: Pleural Diseases (3rd ed). Baltimore: Williams & Wilkins, 1995.
61. Light RW, Girard WM, Jenkinson SG, et al: Parapneumonic effusions. Am J Med 69:507–512, 1980.
62. Lillington GA, Carr DT, Mayne JG: Rheumatoid pleurisy with effusion. Arch Intern Med 128:764–768, 1971.
63. Good JTJ, King TE, Antony VB, et al: Lupus pleuritis: Clinical features and pleural fluid characteristics with special reference to pleural fluid antinuclear antibodies. Chest 84:714–718, 1983.
64. Sahn SA, Good JTJ: Pleural fluid pH in malignant effusions: Diagnostic, prognostic, and therapeutic implications. Ann Intern Med 108:345–349, 1988.
65. Reeder LB, DeFilippi VJ, Ferguson MK: Current results of therapy for esophageal perforation. Am J Surg 169:615–617, 1995.
66. Abbott OA, Mansour KA, Logan WD, et al: Atraumatic so-called "spontaneous" rupture of the esophagus. J Thorac Cardiovasc Surg 59:67–83, 1970.
67. Sherr HP, Light RW, Merson MH, et al: Origin of pleural fluid amylase in esophageal rupture. Ann Intern Med 76:985–986, 1972.
68. Maulitz RM, Good JTJ, Kaplan RL, et al: The pleuropulmonary consequences of esophageal rupture: An experimental model. Am Rev Respir Dis 120:363–367, 1979.
69. Lankisch PG, Droge M, Becher R: Pleural effusions: A new negative prognostic parameter for acute pancreatitis. Am J Gastroenterol 89:1849–1851, 1994.
70. Rockey DC, Cello JP: Pancreaticopleural fistula: Report of 7 patients and review of the literature. Medicine (Baltimore) 69:332–344, 1990.
71. Light RW, Ball WC: Glucose and amylase in pleural effusions. JAMA 225:257–260, 1973.
72. Kramer MR, Ceperao RJ, Pitchenik AE: High amylase in neoplasm-related pleural effusion. Ann Intern Med 110:567–569, 1989.
73. Adelman M, Albelda SM, Gottlieb J, et al: Diagnostic utility of pleural fluid eosinophilia. Am J Med 77:915–920, 1984.
74. Rubins JB, Rubins HB: Etiology and prognostic significance of eosinophilic pleural effusion: A prospective study. Chest 110:1271–1274, 1996.
75. Bassiri AG, Morris W, Kirsch CM: Eosinophilic tuberculous pleural effusion. West J Med 166:277–279, 1997.
76. Spriggs AI, Boddington MM: The Cytology of Effusions. New York: Grune & Stratton, 1968, pp 5–11.
77. Schandene L, Namias B, Crusiaux A, et al: IL-5 in post-traumatic eosinophilic pleural effusion. Clin Exp Immunol 93:115–119, 1993.
78. Maltais F, Laberge F, Cormier Y: Blood hypereosinophilia in the course of posttraumatic pleural effusion. Chest 98:348–351, 1990.
79. Johnson RJ, Johnson JR: Paragonimiasis in Indochinese refugees. Am Rev Respir Dis 128:534–538, 1983.
80. Erzurum SE, Underwood GA, Hamilos DL, et al: Pleural effusion in Churg-Strauss syndrome. Chest 95:1357–1359, 1989.
81. Yam LT: Diagnostic significance of lymphocytes in pleural effusions. Ann Intern Med 66:972–982, 1967.
82. Pettersson T, Klockars M, Hellstrom P-E, et al: T and B lymphocytes in pleural effusions. Chest 73:49–51, 1978.
83. Lucivero G, Pierucci G, Bonomo L: Lymphocytes subsets in peripheral blood and pleural fluid. Eur Respir J 1:337–340, 1988.
84. Domagala W, Emerson EE, Kos LG: T and B lymphocytes enumeration in the diagnosis of lymphocyte-rich pleural fluids. Acta Cytol 25:471–477, 1981.
85. Jarvi OH, Kunnas RJ, Laitio MT, et al: The accuracy and significance of cytologic cancer diagnosis of pleural effusions. Acta Cytol 16:152–157, 1972.
86. Dekker A, Bupp PA: Cytology of serous effusions: An investigation into the usefulness of cell blocks versus smears. Am J Clin Pathol 70:855–860, 1978.
87. Melamed MR: The cytological presentation of malignant lymphomas and related diseases in effusions. Cancer 16:413–431, 1963.
87a. Dresler CM, Fratelli C, Babb J: Prognostic value of positive pleural lavage in patients with lung cancer resection. Ann Thorac Surg 67:1435–1439, 1999.
88. Florentine BD, Sanchez B, Raza A, et al: Detection of hyperdiploid malignant cells in body cavity effusions by fluorescent in situ hybridization on ThinPrep slides. Cancer 81:299–308, 1997.
89. Dewald G, Dines DE, Weiland LH, et al: Usefulness of chromosome examination in the diagnosis of malignant pleural effusions. N Engl J Med 295:1494–1500, 1976.
90. Bethwaite PB, Delahunt B, Holloway LJ, et al: Comparison of silver-staining nucleolar organizer region (AgNOR) counts and proliferating cell nuclear antigen (PCNA) expression in reactive mesothelial hyperplasia and malignant mesothelioma. Pathology 27:1–4, 1995.
91. Yang C-T, Lee M-H, Lan R-S, et al: Telomerase activity in pleural effusions: Diagnostic significance. J Clin Oncol 16:567–573, 1998.
91a. Mu XC, Brian TP, Lowry CV, et al: Telomerase activity in benign and malignant cytologic fluids. Cancer 87:93–99, 1999.
92. Wick MR, Loy T, Mills SE, et al: Malignant epithelioid pleural mesothelioma versus peripheral pulmonary adenocarcinoma: A histochemical, ultrastructural, and immunohistologic study of 103 cases. Hum Pathol 21:759–766, 1990.
93. Wirth PR, Legier J, Wright GLJ: Immunohistochemical evaluation of seven monoclonal antibodies for differentiation of pleural mesothelioma from lung adenocarcinoma. Cancer 67:655–662, 1991.
94. Bailey ME, Brown RW, Mody DR, et al: Ber-EP4 for differentiating adenocarcinoma from reactive and neoplastic mesothelial

cells in serous effusions: Comparison with CEA, B72.3, and Leu-M1. Acta Cytol 40:1212–1216, 1996.
95. Coonrod JD, Wilson HD: Etiologic diagnosis of intrapleural empyema by counterimmunoelectrophoresis. Am Rev Respir Dis 113:637–641, 1976.
96. Potts DE, Willcox MA, Good JTJ, et al: The acidosis of low-glucose pleural effusions. Am Rev Respir Dis 117:665–671, 1978.
97. Light RW, MacGregor MI, Ball WCJ, et al: Diagnostic significance of pleural fluid pH and PCO2. Chest 64:591–596, 1973.
98. Cheng D-S, Rodriguez RM, Rogers J, et al: Comparison of pleural fluid pH values obtained using blood gas machine, pH meter and pH indicator strip. Chest 114:1368–1172, 1998.
99. Walker WC, Wright V: Rheumatoid pleuritis. Ann Rheum Dis 26:467–474, 1967.
100. Winslow WA, Ploss LN, Loitman B: Pleuritis in systemic lupus erythematosus: Its importance as an early manifestation in diagnosis. Ann Intern Med 49:70–88, 1958.
101. Khare V, Baethge B, Lang S, et al: Antinuclear antibodies in pleural fluid. Chest 106:866–871, 1994.
102. Wang DY, Yang PC, Yu WL, et al: Antinuclear antibodies in pleural and pericardial fluid: A prospective study, in press.
103. Halla JT, Schrohenloher RE, Volanakis JE: Immune complexes and other laboratory features of pleural effusions. Ann Intern Med 92:748–752, 1980.
104. Banales JL, Pineda PR, Fitzgerald JM, et al: Adenosine deaminase in the diagnosis of tuberculous pleural effusions: A report of 218 patients and review of the literature. Chest 99:355–357, 1991.
105. Burgess LJ, Maritz FJ, Le Roux I, et al: Combined use of pleural adenosine deaminase with lymphocyte/neutrophil ratio: Increased specificity for the diagnosis of tuberculous pleuritis. Chest 109:414–419, 1996.
106. Ribera E, Ocana I, Martinez-Vazquez JM, et al: High level of interferon gamma in tuberculous pleural effusion. Chest 93:308–311, 1988.
107. Villena V, López-Encuentra A, Echave-Sustaeta J, et al: Interferon-gamma in 388 immunocompromised and immunocompetent patients for diagnosing pleural tuberculosis. Eur Respir J 9:2635–2639, 1996.
108. Forbes BA: Critical assessment of gene amplification approaches on the diagnosis of tuberculosis. Immunol Invest 26:105–116, 1997.
109. Collins JD, Burwell D, Furmanski S, et al: Minimal detectable pleural effusions. Radiology 105:51–53, 1972.
110. Moskowitz H, Platt RT, Schachar R, et al: Roentgen visualization of minute pleural effusion. Radiology 109:33–35, 1973.
111. vanSonnenberg E, Wittich GR, Goodacre BW, et al: Percutaneous drainage of thoracic collections. J Thorac Imaging 13:74–82, 1998.
111a. Levin DL, Klein JS: Imaging techniques for pleural space infections. Semin Respir Infect 14:31–38, 1999.
112. Laing FC, Filly RA: Problems in the application of ultrasonography for the evaluation of pleural opacities. Radiology 126:211–214, 1978.
113. Kohan JM, Poe RH, Israel RH, et al: Value of chest ultrasonography versus decubitus roentgenography for thoracentesis. Am Rev Respir Dis 133:1124–1126, 1986.
114. McLoud TC: CT and MR in pleural disease. Clin Chest Med 19:261–276, 1998.
115. Henschke CI, Yankelevitz DF, Davis SD: Pleural diseases: Multimodality imaging and clinical management. Curr Prob Diagn Radiol 20:155–181, 1991.
116. Stark DD, Federle MP, Goodman PC, et al: Differentiating lung abscess and empyema: radiography and computed tomography. AJR Am J Roentgenol 141:163–167, 1983.
117. Kreel L: Computed tomography in mesothelioma. Semin Oncol 8:302–312, 1981.
118. Gamsu G, Sostman D: Magnetic resonance imaging of the thorax. Am Rev Respir Dis 139:254–274, 1989.
119. Bittner RC, Felix R: Magnetic resonance (MR) imaging of the chest: State-of-the-art. Eur Respir J 1392–1404, 1998.
120. Goddard P, Henson J, Davies ER: Pleural effusion causing unmatched ventilation defects in ventilation and perfusion scanning. Clin Radiol 37:285–286, 1986.
121. Remy-Jardin M, Remy J, Deschildre F, et al: Diagnosis of pulmonary embolism with spiral CT: Comparison with pulmonary angiography and scintigraphy. Radiology 200:699–706, 1996.
122. Garg K, Welsh CH, Geyerabend AJ, et al: Pulmonary embolism: Diagnosis with spiral CT and ventilation-perfusion scanning—Correlation with pulmonary angiographic results or clinical outcome. Radiology 208:201–208, 1998.
123. Prakash UBS, Relman HM: Comparison of needle biopsy with cytologic analysis for the evaluation of pleural effusion: Analysis of 414 cases. Mayo Clin Proc 60:158–164, 1985.
124. Kirsch CM, Kroe M, Jensen WA, et al: A modified Abrams needle biopsy technique. Chest 108:982–986, 1995.
125. Bueno CE, Clemente G, Castro BC, et al: Cytologic and bacteriologic analysis of fluid and pleural biopsy specimens with Cope's needle. Arch Intern Med 150:1190–1194, 1990.
126. Scerbo J, Keltz H, Stone DJ: A prospective study of closed pleural biopsies. JAMA 218:377–380, 1971.
127. Levine H, Metzger W, Lacera D, et al: Diagnosis of tuberculous pleurisy by culture of pleural biopsy specimens. Arch Intern Med 126:269–271, 1970.
128. Von Hoff DD, LiVolsi V: Diagnostic reliability of needle biopsy of the parietal pleura. Am J Clin Pathol 64:200–203, 1975.
129. Poe RH, Israel RH, Utell MJ, et al: Sensitivity, specificity, and predictive values of closed pleural biopsy. Arch Intern Med 144:325–328, 1984.
130. Chang SC, Perng RP: The role of fiberoptic bronchoscopy in evaluating the causes of pleural effusions. Arch Intern Med 149:855–857, 1989.
131. Feinsilver SH, Barrows AA, Braman SS: Fiberoptic bronchoscopy and pleural effusion of unknown origin. Chest 90:516–519, 1986.
132. Hartman DL, Antony VB: Thoracoscopy: The pulmonologist's role. Semin Respir Crit Care Med 16:354–360, 1995.
133. Loddenkemper R: Thoracoscopy: State-of-the-art. Eur Respir J 11:213–221, 1998.
134. Menzies R, Charbonneau M: Thoracoscopy for the diagnosis of pleural disease. Ann Intern Med 114:271–276, 1991.
135. Hucker J, Bhatnagar ND, al-Jailaihawi AN, et al: Thoracoscopy in the diagnosis and management of recurrent pleural effusions. Ann Thorac Surg 52:1145–1147, 1991.
136. Douglas BE, Carr DT, Bernatz PE: Diagnostic thoracotomy in the study of "idiopathic" pleural effusion. Am Rev Tuberc 74:954–957, 1956.
137. Ryan CJ, Rodgers RF, Unni KK, et al: The outcome of patients with pleural effusion of indeterminate cause at thoracotomy. Mayo Clin Proc 56:145–149, 1981.

# 74 Pleural Effusion

Richard W. Light, M.D. • V. Courtney Broaddus, M.D.

Introduction
Transudative Pleural Effusions
- Congestive Heart Failure
- Pericardial Disease
- Hepatic Hydrothorax
- Nephrotic Syndrome
- Peritoneal Dialysis
- Myxedema
- Fontan's Procedure
- Other Causes of Transudative Pleural Effusions

Exudative Pleural Effusions
- Parapneumonic Effusions and Empyema
- Tuberculous Pleuritis
- Actinomycosis
- Nocardiosis
- Fungal Diseases of the Pleura
- Viral Infections
- Parasitic Diseases
- Pulmonary Embolism
- Abdominal Diseases
- Miscellaneous Diseases

Summary

## INTRODUCTION

Pleural effusion is the most common manifestation of disorders of the pleura. The differential diagnosis and the approximate annual incidence of pleural effusion were presented in the preceding chapter (see Tables 73.1 and 73.2). As emphasized, the diagnostic workup of patients with a clinically significant pleural effusion nearly always begins with a thoracentesis. Then, on the basis of whether the fluid is a transudate or an exudate, diagnostic insight is provided, and further evaluation can proceed as indicated. Exudative pleural effusions meet at least one of the following criteria, whereas transudative effusions meet none: pleural fluid protein-serum protein ratio of more than 0.5, pleural fluid lactate dehydrogenase (LDH)–serum LDH ratio of more than 0.6, and pleural fluid LDH more than two thirds of the upper normal limit for serum.[1]

## TRANSUDATIVE PLEURAL EFFUSIONS

Transudative pleural effusions, as defined by the criteria in the preceding paragraph, frequently accompany many common clinical disorders. It is noteworthy that the primary abnormality in most cases of transudative pleural effusions originates in organs other than the pleura or lungs, especially the heart, liver, and kidneys. This association emphasizes the fact that although patients may visit their physicians for respiratory complaints, these symptoms may be caused by extrapulmonary disorders. Further discussion of the pulmonary manifestations of primary diseases in extrapulmonary organ systems is found in Chapters 82 to 90.

### Congestive Heart Failure

Congestive heart failure is the most common cause of pleural effusion.[2] The incidence of pleural effusion in patients with congestive heart failure is high. In one series of 114 patients with left ventricular failure, 58% of the patients had a pleural effusion.[3] In an autopsy series of 402 patients with congestive heart failure at the Mayo Clinic, 290 of the patients (72%) had pleural effusions with volumes greater than 250 mL.[4]

**Pathophysiology.** It appears that the pleural fluid that accumulates with congestive heart failure is related to the clearance of pulmonary interstitial fluid across a leaky mesothelium into the pleural space.[5] In studies in which sheep lungs were isolated in situ, volume loading led to an increase in transudation across the lung into the pleural space. The pleural fluid contained the same protein concentration as that in the lung lymph and the interstitial edema liquid in the lung. The volume of pleural fluid constituted about 25% of all edema formed in the lung.[6] In other experiments in sheep with high-pressure pulmonary edema, pleural fluid accumulated only after pulmonary edema had developed.[7] In the clinical situation, patients with congestive heart failure are much more likely to have a pleural effusion if there is radiologically apparent pulmonary edema.[8] In addition, the presence of pleural effusions on ultrasound correlates more closely with the pulmonary venous pressure than with either systemic venous pressure or pulmonary artery pressure.[8]

**Clinical Manifestations.** Patients with pleural effusion resulting from congestive heart failure usually have symptoms and signs of heart failure, such as dyspnea on exertion, orthopnea, nocturia, peripheral edema, distended

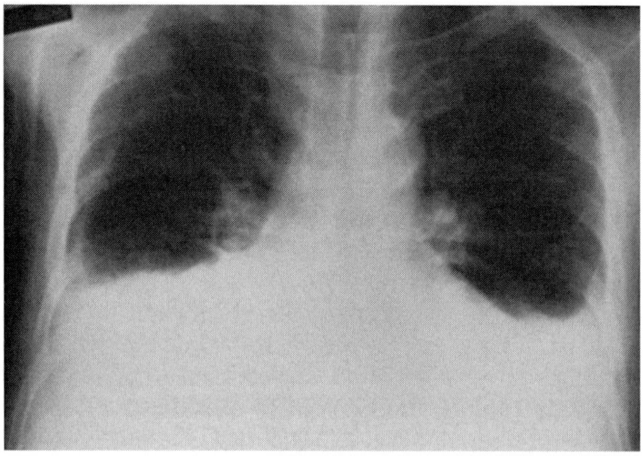

**Figure 74.1** Posteroanterior chest roentgenogram from a patient with congestive heart failure demonstrating bilateral pleural effusions and cardiomegaly.

neck veins, crackles, and a cardiac gallop. The chest radiograph almost always reveals cardiomegaly in addition to the pleural effusion.

The pleural effusions that occur with congestive heart failure tend to be bilateral (Fig. 74.1). In an autopsy study of 250 patients with congestive heart failure and pleural effusion, 88% of the patients had bilateral pleural effusions. In addition, the mean volume of pleural fluid in the right pleural space (1084 mL) was only slightly greater than the mean volume of fluid in the left pleural space (913 mL).[4] Moreover, of the 35 patients who did have unilateral pleural effusions, 46% had either pulmonary embolism or pneumonia.[4] Peterman and Brothers[9] reviewed the records of 55 consecutive patients with the diagnosis of congestive heart failure and a transudative effusion on thoracentesis and reported that the effusions were equal bilaterally in 19 patients, predominantly right sided in 18, and predominantly left sided in 17. Weiss and Spodick[10] reported that 73% of 51 patients with congestive heart failure had bilateral effusions, 19% had unilateral right-sided effusions, and 9% had unilateral left-sided effusions.

Although congestive heart failure is by far the most common cause of bilateral pleural effusions, an alternate explanation should be sought if there is no cardiomegaly. In one series of 78 patients with bilateral effusions but a normal-sized heart, only 4% of the effusions were caused by congestive heart failure.[11]

**Diagnosis and Management.** The diagnosis is usually suggested by the clinical picture of congestive heart failure. The initial decision that should be made is whether or not a diagnostic thoracentesis should be performed. In a patient with congestive heart failure and a pleural effusion, a diagnostic thoracentesis should be performed if the pleural effusion is unilateral, if bilateral effusions are not comparable in size, if the patient is febrile, if the patient has pleuritic chest pain, or if the patient does not have cardiomegaly. If none of these conditions is met, one can treat the congestive heart failure and perform a diagnostic thoracentesis only if the effusion does not resolve. The biochemical characteristics of the pleural fluid change little over a few days despite vigorous diuresis.[12]

The pleural fluid from a patient with congestive heart failure is usually a transudate, as defined previously.[1] If congestive heart failure is suspected, the most cost-effective approach to diagnosis is to order only protein and LDH levels initially. Other tests are ordered only if the fluid turns out to be an exudate.[13] However, the pleural fluid of approximately 20% of patients with congestive heart failure meets exudative criteria.[14] If a patient has congestive heart failure clinically but the pleural fluid meets exudative criteria, the difference in the concentrations of albumin between the pleural fluid and the serum should be measured. If this difference is more than 1.2 g/dL, then the pleural effusion is probably due only to the heart failure.[14] If the pleural fluid is transudative, one should not exclude the diagnosis of pulmonary embolism because patients with this disorder may have a transudative pleural effusion.[15]

Patients with congestive heart failure and pleural effusion should be treated with afterload reduction, diuretics, and inotropes, as needed. When the heart failure is successfully managed, the pleural effusion usually resolves. If the patient is markedly dyspneic when first evaluated, a therapeutic thoracentesis to relieve the dyspnea should be considered. Rarely, despite intensive therapy of the congestive heart failure, a patient has persistent large effusions. If such patients are dyspneic and if their dyspnea is relieved by a therapeutic thoracentesis, consideration can be given to controlling the effusions with a pleurodesis using a sclerosing agent, such as doxycycline or talc slurry[16]; further details about pleurodesis are provided in Chapter 76.

## Pericardial Disease

There is a high incidence of pleural effusion in patients with pericardial disease. In one series of 35 patients with constrictive pericarditis, 60% of the patients had radiologically demonstrable pleural effusions.[17] Weiss and Spodick[18] reviewed 124 patients with pericardial disease and found that 35 (28%) had a pleural effusion. In this series the pleural effusions tended to be left sided. Of the 35 patients, 21 had only a left-sided pleural effusion, whereas only 2 had a right-sided pleural effusion; the remaining 12 effusions were bilateral. However, in another series of 21 patients with constrictive pericarditis and pleural effusion, the pleural effusion was right sided only in 9 (43%) and was bilateral in the remaining 12 (57%).[17]

The mechanism responsible for the pleural effusion associated with pericardial disease is not clear. The obvious explanation is that the pulmonary and systemic capillary pressures are elevated secondary to the pericardial disease, resulting in a transudative pleural effusion, and this probably is the mechanism in patients with constrictive pericarditis. This does not appear to be the complete explanation in patients with inflammatory pericardial disease, however, because the pleural effusion in these patients tends to be left sided; if the effusion were due to elevated pressures, one would expect it to be bilateral.

The characteristics of the pleural fluid in patients with inflammatory pericardial disease have not been well delineated. It is probable that the pericardial inflammation itself is related to the development of the left pleural effusion, possibly by extension of the inflammation to the adjacent pleura.[18]

## Hepatic Hydrothorax

Patients with cirrhosis of the liver may develop a pleural effusion. The incidence of pleural effusion is much higher if ascitic fluid also is present. In one series of 330 patients with cirrhosis and ascites, 18 (6%) had a pleural effusion.[19] In a second series, 6% of 200 patients with cirrhosis had a pleural effusion, but none of the 54 patients without ascites had demonstrable pleural fluid, even though the serum albumin level was below 25 g/L in 11 of the patients.[20] However, there is no obvious ascitic fluid in some patients with hepatic hydrothorax, presumably because the ascitic fluid moves almost entirely to the pleural space because of prevailing pressure gradients.[21]

**Pathophysiology.** The predominant mechanism leading to a pleural effusion in a patient with cirrhosis and ascites appears to be the movement of the ascitic fluid from the peritoneal cavity through defects in the diaphragm into the pleural space.[22] The decreased plasma oncotic pressure is only a secondary factor.

The diaphragmatic defects have been demonstrated in many ways. Lieberman and coworkers[19] introduced 500 to 1000 mL of air into the peritoneal cavity of five patients with cirrhosis, ascites, and pleural effusions and found that a pneumothorax developed in all patients within 48 hours. In addition, they were able to demonstrate air bubbles coming through an otherwise undetectable diaphragmatic defect at thoracoscopy in one of their patients. In two of their patients, diaphragmatic defects were demonstrated at postmortem examination.[19] Mouroux and coworkers[23] performed thoracoscopy on eight patients and were able to identify diaphragmatic defects in six. There are no lymphatic connections between the peritoneal and the pleural spaces. Thus, the connections between the spaces are either preexisting developmental defects or are defects caused by trauma or stretching.

**Clinical Manifestations.** The clinical situation in patients with pleural effusions from cirrhosis and ascites is usually dominated by the cirrhosis and ascites. At times, however, the presence of a large pleural effusion may produce severe dyspnea. The pleural effusion associated with cirrhosis and ascites is frequently large and can occupy the entire hemithorax. The large effusions occur because the diaphragmatic defect permits fluid to flow from the peritoneal cavity into the pleural cavity until the pleural pressure approaches the peritoneal pressure. The pleural pressures in patients with pleural effusions secondary to ascites are higher than those in patients with other transudative pleural effusions.[24] The pleural effusions are usually right sided (67%) but occasionally are left sided (16%) or bilateral (16%).[19, 20]

**Diagnosis and Treatment.** It is usually easy to establish the diagnosis of hepatic hydrothorax from the clinical picture. Both a paracentesis and a thoracentesis should be performed to confirm that the ascites and the pleural fluid are both transudates. The protein level in the pleural fluid is usually higher than that in the ascitic fluid but is still below 30 g/L.[19] If the polymorphonuclear cell count is greater than 500 cells/μL, the diagnosis of spontaneous bacterial pleuritis in conjunction with spontaneous bacterial peritonitis should be considered.[25]

The initial management of the pleural effusion associated with cirrhosis and ascites should be directed toward treatment of the ascites. The patient should be given a low-salt diet and treated with diuretics. If diet and diuretics do not control the effusion, the best approach is probably implantation of a transjugular intrahepatic portal systemic shunt. Transjugular intrahepatic portal systemic shunt is usually effective in the management of hepatic hydrothorax, but randomized studies have not been reported,[26] and the procedure is not universally successful. In the largest series, 5 of 24 patients (21%) developed worsening liver function and died within 45 days.[26] The best treatment for these patients is probably liver transplantation.

If neither transjugular intrahepatic portal systemic shunt nor liver transplantation is feasible, the best alternative treatment is probably videothoracoscopy with closure of the diaphragmatic defects and talc insufflation. Mouroux and associates[23] performed this procedure in eight patients. Diaphragmatic defects were found and closed in six patients, and none of these patients had a recurrent pleural effusion. No defects were found in the remaining two patients, but after talc insufflation, the effusions occupied only the lower one third of the hemithorax. An alternative treatment is tube thoracostomy, with care being taken to avoid rapid fluid shifts, followed by the injection of a sclerosing agent, such as doxycycline or talc. Another alternative treatment is the insertion of a peritoneojugular shunt; this may be ineffective because the pleural pressure is lower than the central venous pressure.

### Spontaneous Bacterial Pleuritis

Spontaneous bacterial pleuritis is, by definition, infection of a preexisting hepatic hydrothorax in which a parapneumonic infection has been excluded. Originally termed *spontaneous bacterial empyema,* we prefer the term *pleuritis* to emphasize its similarity to spontaneous bacterial peritonitis, and to indicate that its treatment does not require tube thoracostomy. In one series in Spain, 16 of 120 patients (13%) admitted with a diagnosis of hepatic hydrothorax had a spontaneous bacterial pleuritis.[25] The diagnosis is made if the pleural fluid culture is positive and the pleural fluid neutrophil count is greater than 250 cells/μL and a pneumonic process has been excluded. If the pleural fluid neutrophil count is greater than 500 cells/μL and the pleural fluid cultures are negative, culture-negative spontaneous bacterial pleuritis is diagnosed.[25] In the series from Spain, 10 of 24 episodes (43%) of spontaneous bacterial empyema were not associated with bacterial peritonitis.[25] Appropriate treatment of spontaneous bacterial pleuritis requires systemic antibiotics, but tube thoracostomy does not appear to be necessary.[25] It remains to be seen whether spontaneous bacterial pleuritis is a common occurrence in the United States.

## Nephrotic Syndrome

There is a high incidence of pleural effusion in patients with the nephrotic syndrome. In one study of 52 patients, 21% had pleural effusions.[27] The mechanism responsible for the transudative pleural effusion associated with the nephrotic syndrome is probably the combination of decreased plasma oncotic pressure and increased hydrostatic pressure. The increased hydrostatic pressure is due to salt retention, which produces hypervolemia.[28] The pleural effusions in patients with a nephrotic syndrome are usually bilateral and are frequently infrapulmonary in location.[27]

A diagnostic thoracentesis should be performed in all patients with the nephrotic syndrome and a pleural effusion to prove that the pleural fluid is a transudate. Nonetheless, the possibility of pulmonary embolism should always be considered in patients with the nephrotic syndrome and a pleural effusion. In one series of 36 patients with the nephrotic syndrome, 22% had pulmonary emboli.[29] Because the pleural fluid secondary to pulmonary embolism can be either a transudate or an exudate, a scintigraphic lung scan or a spiral computed tomographic (CT) scan should be obtained in all patients with the nephrotic syndrome and pleural effusion.

The treatment of the pleural effusion associated with the nephrotic syndrome should be aimed at increasing the level of protein in the serum by decreasing the protein loss in urine. A pleurodesis with a sclerosing agent should be considered in selected patients who are symptomatic from the pleural effusion.[30]

## Peritoneal Dialysis

Peritoneal dialysis is occasionally complicated by the development of an acute hydrothorax. In a review of 3195 patients receiving continuous ambulatory peritoneal dialysis in Japan, 1.6% developed a pleural effusion as a result of the movement of the dialysate from the peritoneal cavity into the pleural cavity.[31] The effusion developed within 30 days of initiation of the dialysis in 50% of the patients, but 18% had been receiving dialysis for more than a year before the effusion developed.[31]

The pleural fluid in these patients is characterized by a glucose level intermediate between that of the dialysate and the serum, a protein level below 10 g/L, and a low LDH level. Although the communication closes spontaneously in some patients, a surgical approach is usually required if continuous ambulatory peritoneal dialysis is to be continued. The treatment of choice is probably thoracoscopy with closure of the diaphragmatic defects, followed by pleurodesis.[32] Alternative treatments are pleurodesis alone or thoracotomy with repair of the diaphragmatic defects.

## Myxedema

A pleural effusion sometimes occurs as a complication of myxedema.[33] Most patients with myxedema and pleural effusion have a concomitant pericardial effusion. In one series of 25 patients with pericardial effusions secondary to myxedema, 13 of the patients (52%) had concomitant pleural effusion.[34] When the pleural effusion occurs simultaneously with a pericardial effusion, the pleural fluid is usually a transudate.[35] The isolated pleural effusion seen in conjunction with myxedema can be either a transudate or an exudate.[33] Thyroid replacement is the obvious treatment for pleural effusions associated with myxedema.

## Fontan's Procedure

With Fontan's procedure, an anastomosis is created between the superior vena cava, the right atrium, or the inferior vena cava and the pulmonary artery to bypass the right ventricle, usually because of tricuspid atresia or a univentricular heart. Pleural effusion occurs in many patients after surgery and contributes significantly to postoperative morbidity. Pleural effusions are more likely to occur in patients who have significant aortopulmonary collateral vessels before surgery[36]; thus, Spicer and colleagues recommended that these vessels be embolized during preoperative angiography.[36] The treatment of choice for these effusions is usually insertion of a pleuroperitoneal shunt.[37] Alternative treatments are creation of a late fenestration to create a right-to-left shunt[38] or chemical pleurodesis.

## Other Causes of Transudative Pleural Effusions

Pulmonary embolism and sarcoidosis have been reported to be associated with transudative pleural effusions. However, because exudative pleural effusions are more common with both of these conditions, they are discussed later in this chapter. Formation of transudative effusions in these diseases is likely a result of extrapleural effects, including increased systemic venous pressure, decreased pleural pressure, or obstruction of lymphatic drainage. Pleural amyloidosis is associated with transudative effusions, but because, these patients almost always have cardiac amyloid, the effusions are probably due to heart failure.[28]

# EXUDATIVE PLEURAL EFFUSIONS

Exudative pleural effusions, defined according to the criteria in the introductory paragraph, are common clinical problems. These effusions may develop as a result of inflammation, injury, or malignancy, which can involve the pleural surfaces, the adjacent lung, or more distant tissues, such as mediastinal and abdominal organs. Further discussion of effusions secondary to pleural tumors is presented in Chapter 76, and special types of effusions (chylothorax and hemothorax) are discussed in Chapter 75.

## Parapneumonic Effusions and Empyema

A parapneumonic effusion is any pleural effusion associated with bacterial pneumonia, lung abscess, or bronchiectasis. Parapneumonic effusions are probably the most common exudative pleural effusion in the United States. The annual incidence of bacterial pneumonia in the United States is estimated to be 4 million.[39] Approximately 40% of patients with bacterial pneumonia have an accompanying pleural effusion.[40] The morbidity and mortality in patients with pneumonia and pleural effusion are higher than in patients with pneumonia alone. In one study of patients with community-acquired pneumonia, the relative risk of mortality was 7.0 times higher for patients with bilateral pleural effusions and 3.4 times higher for patients with unilateral pleural effusions of moderate or greater size than that in other patients with community-acquired pneumonia.[41] At least some of the increase in morbidity and mortality may be due to improper management of the pleural effusion.

When one is managing a patient with a parapneumonic effusion, the main decision to make is whether or not chest tubes should be inserted. The term *complicated parapneumonic effusion* is used to refer to those effusions that require tube thoracostomy for their resolution. An empyema is, by definition, pus in the pleural space, and this entity is also discussed in Chapter 33. Approximately 60% of empyemas are complicated parapneumonic effusions, whereas 20% occur after thoracic surgical procedures, and the remaining 20% occur as complications of various conditions, such as thoracic trauma, esophageal perforation, thoracentesis, and subdiaphragmatic infection.[42]

**Pathophysiology.** The evolution of a parapneumonic pleural effusion can be divided into three stages, which are not sharply defined but rather represent a continuous spectrum.[43] In the first stage, the exudative stage, a focus of parenchymal infection leads to increased pulmonary interstitial fluid, some of which traverses the visceral pleura and causes the accumulation of a small sterile pleural effusion. The pleural fluid in this stage is an exudate with primarily polymorphonuclear leukocytes, a normal glucose level, and a normal pH. With institution of appropriate antibiotic therapy during this stage, both the pneumonic process and the pleural effusion resolve.

The next stage is the fibropurulent stage, characterized by infection of the previously sterile pleural fluid with the offending bacteria. In this stage, more pleural fluid accumulates and contains many polymorphonuclear leukocytes, bacteria, and cellular debris. In addition, fibrin is deposited as continuous sheets that cover both the visceral and the parietal pleura in the involved area. As this stage progresses, there is a tendency for the fibrin membranes to partition the involved pleural space into multiple locules. This loculation prevents extension of the empyema but makes complete drainage of the pleural space with chest tubes increasingly difficult. The pleural fluid pH and glucose level decrease, and the LDH level increases progressively as this stage evolves.

In the last stage, the organization stage, fibroblasts grow into the exudate from both the visceral and the parietal pleural surfaces to produce an inelastic membrane. This membrane, sometimes called a *pleural peel,* can encase the lung and hinder the re-expansion of the underlying lung when the pleural fluid is evacuated. If the underlying lung cannot re-expand, consideration should be given to decortication, because it is virtually impossible to eradicate the infection if the space persists after the fluid is evacuated. However, if the infection is already controlled, the peel frequently resolves spontaneously over the ensuing 3 to 6 months.

**Bacteriology.** Before the antibiotic era, *Streptococcus pneumoniae* or hemolytic streptococci were responsible for most empyemas.[44] Then, between 1955 and 1965, *Staphylococcus aureus* was the bacterium most commonly isolated from pleural fluid.[44] In the 1970s anaerobic organisms were most commonly isolated,[45] but this study used meticulous methods to isolate these organisms. It appears, however, that aerobic organisms are now responsible for most empyema.[42]

In a patient with a bacterial pneumonia, the incidence of associated pleural effusion and the frequency with which the pleural fluid becomes infected depend on the infecting organism.[42] For example, approximately 35% of patients with anaerobic pneumonia have a culture-positive pleural effusion,[45] whereas fewer than 5% of patients with pneumococcal pneumonia have culture-positive pleural effusions.[40]

**Clinical Manifestations**

***Aerobic Bacterial Infections.*** Patients with aerobic bacterial pneumonia and pleural effusion initially have an acute febrile illness consisting of chest pain, sputum production, and leukocytosis. The incidence of pleuritic chest pain and the degree of leukocytosis are comparable whether or not there is an accompanying pleural effusion.[40]

***Anaerobic Bacterial Infections.*** Patients with anaerobic bacterial infections involving the pleural space usually present with a subacute illness. In one series, the duration of symptoms before presentation averaged 10 days, with 70% of the patients having symptoms for more than 7 days.[46] Most patients with anaerobic pleuropulmonary infections have significant weight loss (mean: 13.2 kg in one series),[46] as well as leukocytosis and mild anemia.[46] In addition, most patients have risk factors for aspiration of an anaerobic inoculum; these risk factors include alcoholism, an episode of unconsciousness, and infected gums.

Because of the nonspecificity of the symptoms associated with empyema, the diagnosis may not be considered, and accordingly, it is delayed. In one series of 119 patients from England in the late 1980s, empyema was considered the most likely diagnosis by the admitting doctor in only 35 patients (29%).[47] In this same series, the diagnosis was delayed for more than 1 week in 28 patients and for more than 1 month after admission in 5 patients.[47] In this series, the most common symptom was malaise (73%), and only 56% of the patients were febrile.

**Diagnosis.** The possibility of a parapneumonic effusion should be considered whenever a patient with a bacterial pneumonia is initially evaluated. The presence of a significant amount of pleural fluid is usually suggested by the appearance of the lateral chest radiograph.

When the patient is upright, the lowest part of the hemithorax is the posterior costophrenic angle; hence, free pleural fluid first collects there. If either of the posterior costophrenic angles is blunted or if the diaphragm is not visible throughout its length, bilateral decubitus chest radiographs should be obtained. The view with the involved side superior provides useful information because when the free pleural fluid is next to the mediastinum, one can assess how much of the increased radiodensity is due to the fluid and how much is due to the parenchymal infiltrate.

With the involved side dependent, the amount of free pleural fluid can be semiquantitated by measuring the distance between the inside of the chest wall and the outside of the lung. If this distance is less than 10 mm, the effusion is not clinically significant, and thoracentesis is not indicated.[40] If the thickness of the fluid exceeds 10 mm, then a thoracentesis should be performed immediately. Only by examining the pleural fluid can one distinguish a complicated from an uncomplicated parapneumonic effusion. The pleural fluid should be examined grossly for color, turbidity, and odor. Aliquots are sent for determination of the pleural fluid glucose, LDH, amylase, and protein levels; pH; a differential and total leukocyte count; Gram's stain; and aerobic and anaerobic bacterial cultures. If one is to obtain accurate values for the pleural fluid pH, the fluid must be maintained anaerobically until it is analyzed, and the analysis must be made with a blood gas machine—values obtained with a pH meter or pH indicator strip paper are not accurate because of the escape of carbon dioxide and the fact that pH meters measure the pH at 25°C rather than 37°C.[48] In most instances, the pleural fluid should also be submitted for mycobacterial and fungal smears and cultures.

Not all patients with an acute illness, parenchymal infiltrates, and pleural effusion have an acute bacterial pneumonia. This clinical picture may also be seen with pulmonary embolization, acute pancreatitis, tuberculosis, Dressler's syndrome, and other diseases. The diagnostic workup of each patient should be individualized based on the clinical situation.

Patients with empyema may have mediastinal lymphadenopathy secondary to the empyema. Haramati and associates[49] obtained chest CT scans in 27 patients with nontuberculous empyema. They reported that 13 of the patients (48%) had at least one lymph node greater than 1 cm in its short axis. The lymphadenopathy was unilateral and ipsilateral in seven patients, bilateral in five, and unilateral and contralateral in one.[49] Four patients had follow-up radiographs, and the lymphadenopathy had decreased or resolved in all.[49]

**Treatment.** When a patient with pneumonia and a pleural effusion is initially evaluated, an appropriate antibiotic must be selected, and the decision whether to initiate invasive therapy for the pleural effusion must be made. Bacterial cultures of the sputum, blood, and pleural fluid should be obtained before antibiotic therapy is instituted. Antibiotic therapy for bacterial pneumonia is discussed in Chapter 33.

***Prognostic Factors.*** Findings that suggest that a more aggressive approach will be necessary for a parapneumonic effusion are listed in Table 74.1. The more purulent the pleural fluid, the lower the glucose level, and the lower the pH, the more likely the patient is to require increasingly invasive procedures for complete drainage.

**Table 74.1 FACTORS SUGGESTING THAT A MORE INVASIVE APPROACH WILL BE NECESSARY FOR THE RESOLUTION OF A PARAPNEUMONIC EFFUSION***

1. Thick pus is present in the pleural space.
2. Pleural fluid Gram's stain is positive.
3. Pleural fluid glucose level is < 60 mg/dL.
4. Pleural fluid pH is < 7.20.
5. Pleural fluid culture is positive.
6. Pleural fluid lactate dehydrogenase level is > 3 × upper normal limit for serum.
7. Pleural fluid is loculated.

*Listed in order of decreasing seriousness.

***Overall Treatment Plan.*** The treatment options for patients with parapneumonic effusions and empyema, in order of increasing invasiveness, are diagnostic thoracentesis, therapeutic thoracentesis, tube thoracostomy, tube thoracostomy with thrombolytics, thoracoscopy, and thoracotomy with decortication. If the patient has any of the poor prognostic factors, it is likely that one of these treatments will be necessary. It is important to not continue any one treatment that is not working for more than a day or so.[50, 50a]

The effectiveness of a given treatment is evaluated by the clinical status of the patient together with the amount and the characteristics of the pleural fluid. If the patient appears to be responding, if the amount of pleural fluid is not large, and if the characteristics of the fluid are improving, the treatment should be considered successful. More invasive procedures are not indicated for pleural thickening alone. Chest CT scans are very useful in evaluating the adequacy of drainage of the pleural space.

Patients with effusions that measure more than 10 mm in thickness on the decubitus radiograph, or which are loculated, should have a thoracentesis within hours of admission. If poor prognostic factors are present, one should attempt to remove all the fluid with a therapeutic thoracentesis or tube thoracostomy on the day of admission. If these maneuvers are unsuccessful, thrombolytics or thoracoscopy should be tried within 48 hours. If the drainage is still unsuccessful, surgical consultation concerning decortication should be obtained.

***Diagnostic Versus Therapeutic Thoracentesis.*** To determine whether the patient has any of the prognostic factors listed in Table 74.1, a thoracentesis must be performed. Should a therapeutic or a diagnostic thoracentesis initially be performed? Because the risks of a diagnostic thoracentesis and a therapeutic thoracentesis are comparable, a therapeutic thoracentesis should be performed initially in patients with parapneumonic effusions. If the pleural fluid never recurs, one need not worry about the pleural fluid. If the pleural fluid recurs after a therapeutic thoracentesis, poor prognostic findings in the pleural fluid indicate the need for more drainage—either an additional therapeutic thoracentesis or a tube thoracostomy. The absence of poor prognostic findings in a patient who is improving clinically indicates that additional drainage is not necessary. No more than three therapeutic thoracenteses are recommended.

If the pleural fluid cannot be completely removed because it is loculated, tube thoracostomy should be performed if any of the other poor prognostic factors listed in Table 74.1 are present.

***Therapeutic Thoracentesis.*** Although therapeutic thoracentesis is not commonly used in the treatment of parapneumonic effusions, a few studies suggest that it may have a role. Sasse and coworkers[51] reported that therapeutic thoracentesis was at least as good as chest tube placement in the treatment of early pleural infections in a rabbit model of empyema. In a human study, Storm and associates[52] reported that 48 of 51 patients (94%) with empyema (purulent pleural fluid or positive microbiologic studies on the pleural fluid) were managed successfully with daily thoracentesis. There have been no controlled studies comparing therapeutic thoracentesis with small-tube thoracostomy in the treatment of patients with complicated parapneumonic effusions. Obviously, therapeutic thoracentesis will not be adequate if the pleural fluid is loculated or if the fibrinous coating over the visceral pleura prevents the underlying lung from expanding.

***Chest Tubes.*** Once it is decided that tube thoracostomy is necessary, there should be no delay in its performance, because a complicated parapneumonic effusion can progress from free-flowing pleural fluid to loculated pleural fluid within hours. In one series of 47 anaerobic empyemas, five patients died, and all deaths were attributed to a delay in obtaining adequate pleural drainage.[46] In a subsequent series, a delay in instituting chest tube drainage resulted in a mortality increase from 3.4% to 16%.[53] The chest tube should be positioned in the most dependent part of the effusion.

In the past, it was recommended that relatively large (26 to 36F) chest tubes be used in the treatment of parapneumonic effusions because of the belief that smaller tubes would become obstructed by the thick fluid. However, it appears that many patients can be managed with much smaller tubes. When two series are combined, 41 of 53 patients (77%) were managed successfully with smaller chest tubes (8.3 to 16F).[54, 55] These results are as good as those reported in some series in which larger tubes were utilized.[53, 56] The small chest tubes in the aforementioned two series were inserted percutaneously by interventional radiologists. It is likely that the excellent results are related to accurate image-guided placement of the catheter. If the pleural fluid is frank pus, it is still preferable to insert a large chest tube.[50] The chest tube should be left in place until the volume of the pleural drainage per 24 hours is less than 50 mL and until the draining fluid becomes clear yellow.

Successful closed-tube drainage of a complicated parapneumonic effusion is associated with improvement in the clinical and radiologic status of the patient within 24 to 48 hours. If there is no significant improvement after this period, either the pleural drainage is unsatisfactory or the patient is receiving the wrong antibiotic. In such situations, the culture results should be reviewed and the adequacy of the pleural drainage should be assessed by chest radiographs, CT scans, or ultrasonic examination. If the pleural space is found to be inadequately drained, another chest tube should be inserted, a fibrinolytic agent should be injected intrapleurally, or a more extensive surgical procedure should be performed. Inadequate drainage can be caused by poor positioning of the tube, obstruction of the chest tube, loculated pleural fluid, or inadequate expansion of the underlying lung caused by coating of the visceral pleura.

***Intrapleural Thrombolytic Agents.*** These agents have been recommended in the treatment of loculated parapneumonic effusions because they possibly facilitate drainage as a result of their fibrinolytic action. In the past several years, there have been several uncontrolled studies that purported to show the utility of streptokinase[57–60] or urokinase[57, 59, 61] in the treatment of multiloculated pleural infections. The usual dose of streptokinase is 250,000 U, in 30 to 60 mL of normal saline given intrapleurally via the chest tube. The usual dose of urokinase is 100,000 U diluted in the same manner. The chest tube is clamped for 1 to 2 hours after instillation. The administration of these agents intrapleurally has no effect on the systemic bleeding parameters and can be repeated daily for up to 14 days.

There have been three controlled studies on the use of thrombolytics for loculated parapneumonic effusions.[62–64] In one study, streptokinase, 250,000 U daily (the number of days determined by the clinical response), was compared with no thrombolytic agent in the management of 52 patients with loculated parapneumonic effusion. This study was not randomized or blinded in that the patients received no thrombolytics for the first half of the study and streptokinase for the latter half of the study. In this study, there was no significant difference in the need for more invasive surgery or the mortality rate between the two groups.[62] In the second study, 24 patients were randomly assigned to receive streptokinase, 250,000 IU daily, or control saline flushes for up to 3 days. The streptokinase group had a significantly greater reduction in the size of the pleural fluid collection and greater improvement in the chest radiograph.[63] In the third study, 31 patients were randomly assigned to receive either intrapleural urokinase or normal saline for 3 days. The group that received urokinase had significantly greater improvement in the chest radiographs and a significantly reduced need for surgery.[64]

At the present time, a trial of intrapleural thrombolytic therapy can be considered for patients with complicated parapneumonic effusions who have inadequate drainage after 24 hours of treatment with tube thoracostomy. Alternatively, one can proceed directly to thoracoscopy. A successful response to the thrombolytic therapy is indicated by an improvement in the chest radiograph, not just increased drainage from the chest tube. If improvement is not noted after the first one or two doses, considerations should be given to more invasive procedures, such as thoracoscopy and thoracotomy. Fibrinolytic agents are less likely to be effective if the process has been ongoing for more than 7 days or if the pleural fluid is very purulent. It appears that streptokinase and urokinase are probably equally effective.

***Thoracoscopy.*** Thoracoscopy, which includes breakdown of adhesions and complete drainage of the pleural space, is the procedure of choice when tube thoracostomy (with or without thrombolytics) fails. One study has demonstrated that proceeding directly to thoracoscopy was more cost effective than using an intermediate step with thrombolytics.[65] Before thoracoscopy, a chest CT should be obtained[66] to provide anatomic information about the size and the extent of the empyema cavity. The finding of a thickened visceral pleural peel without septations suggests that the empyema may be chronic and probably will not be amenable to thoracoscopic débridement alone.[66] Most patients who undergo thoracoscopy need no additional therapy. In one series of 44 patients who presented for the surgical treatment of complicated parapneumonic effusion, 30 patients (68%) needed no further procedure, and 14 patients required open thoracotomy with decortication.[67] Thoracoscopy can be effective in patients who have had prolonged symptoms for more than 30 days.[67] An alternative to thoracoscopy is a mini-thoracotomy to permit the manual breakdown of adhesions and the placement of one or more chest tubes.

***Decortication.*** This procedure should be considered in patients who require additional drainage after tube thoracostomy or thoracoscopy.[68] With this procedure, a full thoracotomy is performed to remove all fibrous tissue and pus from the pleural space. Decortication eliminates the pleural sepsis and allows the underlying lung to expand. Decortication is major thoracic surgery and should not be performed on patients who are markedly debilitated. It should not be performed just to remove thickened pleura, because such thickening usually resolves spontaneously over several months. After 6 months, however, if the pleural thickening persists and the pulmonary function is sufficiently reduced to limit the patient's activities, decortication should be considered.

***Open Drainage (Eloesser's flap).*** With this relatively minor surgical procedure, which can be performed under local anesthesia, a U-shaped incision is made to provide a skin flap overlying the lower part of the empyema collection; the exposed rib segments and underlying parietal pleura are excised to open the empyema cavity; then, the skin flap is sutured inside the cavity to create a semipermanent opening into which one or more large-bore short tubes are inserted. The open-drainage procedure allows more complete drainage and frees the patient from attachment to chest-tube bottles. After the procedure, the cavity should be irrigated daily with a mild antiseptic solution, and the drainage from the tubes can be collected in a colostomy bag placed over the tubes. Open drainage is preferred to decortication only in those patients who are thought to be too ill to tolerate the more extensive procedure. Patients treated by open drainage can expect to have an open chest wound for a prolonged period. In one series of 33 patients treated by an open-drainage procedure, the median time for healing the drainage site was 142 days.[46]

## Bronchopleural Fistula Complicating Empyema

When an empyema is complicated by the presence of a bronchopleural fistula, adequate pleural drainage is crucial. The pleural fluid that is not drained exteriorly with chest tubes is likely to drain interiorly throughout the tracheobronchial tree, producing a severe diffuse pneumonia. A bronchopleural fistula should be suspected whenever the chest radiograph reveals an air-fluid level or when the patient expectorates copious quantities of sputum while lying on one side (as the empyema drains into the bronchial tree) and not while lying on the other side.

At times, it is difficult to determine whether an air-fluid level is in the lung or in the pleural space. It is important to make this differentiation because a lung abscess should be treated with antibiotics alone, whereas it is imperative to drain the pleural space if a bronchopleural fistula exists. Chest CT is quite valuable in making this differentiation. On CT, a lung abscess is characterized by thick and irregular cavity walls, no compression of the adjacent lung, and no separation of the thickened visceral pleura from the parietal pleura. An empyema cavity has walls that, at least in part, are distinctly thin, uniform, and smooth on both the luminal margin and the exterior surface; the adjacent lung can be compressed; and the thickened visceral pleura is separated from the parietal pleura, the "split pleura" sign.[69] A frame from the CT series of a patient with bronchopleural fistula complicating a loculated empyema is shown in Figure 74.2. However, CT is not infallible in distinguishing empyemas from lung abscesses by use of these criteria. However, the differentiation can usually be made after intravenous injection of contrast material. The demonstration of vessels within a lesion unequivocally identifies the lesion as parenchymal. Moreover, pulmonary parenchyma is enhanced after a bolus administration of contrast materials, whereas most pleural lesions show minimal or no enhancement.[70]

## Postpneumonectomy Empyema

The incidence of empyema after pneumonectomy varies from 2% to 16%.[71, 72] This diagnosis should be suspected in any patient who undergoes pneumonectomy and becomes febrile, starts expectorating large amounts of sputum, has purulent drainage from the thoracotomy wound, or has a mediastinum that is midline or shifted to the contralateral side. The diagnosis is established with a diagnostic thoracentesis that reveals organisms on Gram's stain or culture.

A postpneumonectomy empyema is an extremely serious complication because it is impossible to eliminate the space containing the infection and, consequently, it is difficult to sterilize the pleural space. Approximately 80% of patients with postpneumonectomy empyema have a bronchopleural or an esophagopleural fistula.[72] Therefore,

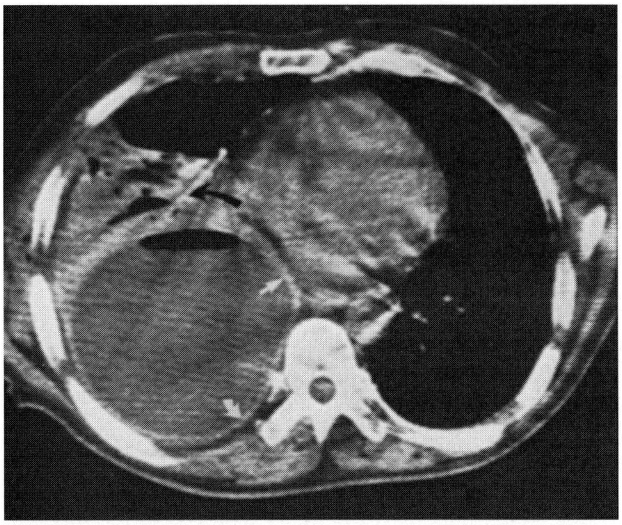

**Figure 74.2** A computed tomographic scan from a patient with empyema and bronchopleural fistula. Large empyema is round and forms acute angles with chest wall. Compressed lung and distorted bronchi *(curved black arrow)* are draped over empyema. "Split pleura" sign is formed by thickened visceral pleura *(straight white arrow)* that is separated from parietal pleura *(curved white arrow).* Note air-fluid level within empyema cavity. (From Stark DD, Federle MP, Goodman PC, et al: Differentiating lung abscess and empyema: Radiography and computed tomography. AJR Am J Roentgenol 141:163–167, 1983. © 1983, American Roentgen Ray Society.)

all patients with this complication should undergo a chest CT scan and a bronchoscopy.

The treatment of a postpneumonectomy empyema involves two different aspects, draining the infected pleural fluid and closing the bronchopleural fistula. The pleural fluid is best drained by tube thoracostomy if the empyema occurs in the first few days after pneumonectomy. Subsequently, most patients require open drainage. If the patient does not have a bronchopleural fistula, operative irrigation and filling of the residual space with an antibiotic-containing solution may be curative.[72]

If a bronchopleural fistula is present, it must be treated. Attempts can be made to close the fistula with fibrin sealant and decalcified spongy calf bone administered bronchoscopically,[73] but a thoracotomy and surgical closing of the fistula by use of an intrathoracic muscle transposition[71] or a pedicled omental flap are usually required.[72]

## Tuberculous Pleuritis

In many parts of the world, the most common cause of an exudative pleural effusion is tuberculosis. However, in the United States, the annual incidence of tuberculous pleural effusion is only about 1000 patients. Approximately 1 in every 30 cases of tuberculosis is tuberculous pleuritis, and this ratio has remained constant even after the advent of the acquired immunodeficiency syndrome (AIDS).[74] In some countries, however, the percentage of patients with tuberculosis who have a pleural effusion exceeds 30%.[75]

A pleural effusion as a manifestation of tuberculosis has been likened to a primary chancre as a manifestation of syphilis. Both are self-limited and of little immediate concern, but both may lead to serious disease many years later. Most instances of pleural effusion secondary to tuberculosis resolve spontaneously; however, if patients are not treated with antituberculous therapy, they have about a 50% likelihood of developing active tuberculosis in the subsequent 5 years.[76, 77]

**Pathogenesis.** A tuberculous pleural effusion can either be a sequela to a primary infection acquired 3 to 6 months previously or represent reactivation tuberculosis.[78] As discussed in Chapter 34, two different pathogenetic mechanisms can lead to tuberculous pleural effusions. By far, the more common is the entry of only a few *Mycobacterium tuberculosis* into the pleural space; in the presence of specific cell-mediated immunity, tubercle bacilli provoke an intense hypersensitivity reaction and outpouring of fluid.[79] Chest radiographs may or may not reveal associated parenchymal involvement. In the second variety, a subpleural caseous focus or cavity ruptures into the pleural space and causes what is sometimes called a *tuberculous empyema* because the fluid contains many bacilli. Chest radiographs nearly always show parenchymal abnormalities.

As just mentioned, delayed hypersensitivity appears to play a large role in the pathogenesis of tuberculous pleuritis. In animal models, the intrapleural injection of tuberculous protein in sensitized animals results in the rapid appearance of an exudative pleural effusion.[79] When the animals are given antilymphocyte serum, the development of the effusion is suppressed. It is probable that delayed hypersensitivity also plays a large role in the development of tuberculous pleural effusions in humans. The mycobacterial burden in the pleural space is low because the pleural fluid cultures from only about 35% of patients with tuberculous pleuritis are positive.[80] T lymphocytes specifically sensitized to tuberculous protein are present in the pleural fluid.[79]

Although delayed hypersensitivity to tuberculous protein is believed to be primarily responsible for tuberculous pleuritis, approximately one third of patients with tuberculous pleuritis have a negative tuberculin skin test result when first evaluated.[80] This anergy to purified protein derivative appears to be due to an antigen-specific extrapleural immunosuppression. Occasionally, the immunosuppression may result from a relative depletion of the circulating purified protein derivative–reactive lymphocytes as they sequester in the pleural space. More commonly, immunosuppression is thought to be due to suppressor cells, either adherent monocytes or Fc-bearing lymphocytes, that are found in the blood but not in the pleural space.[79]

**Clinical Manifestations.** Tuberculous pleuritis occurs as an acute illness in about two thirds of cases and as a chronic illness in the remaining one third. The acute illness is marked by cough and chest pain in about 75% of patients and often mimics a bacterial pneumonia with

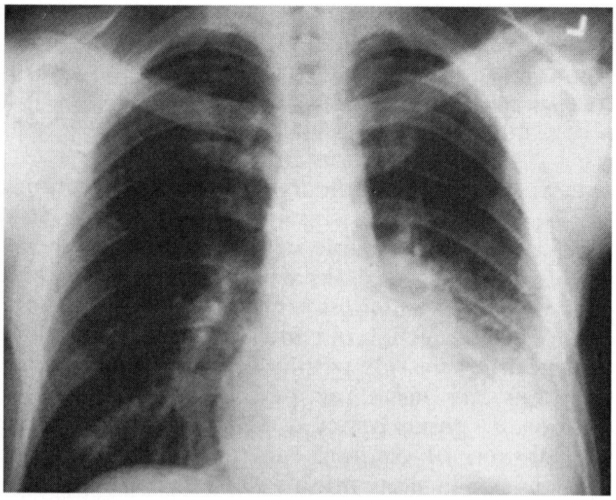

**Figure 74.3** Posteroanterior chest roentgenogram from a patient with tuberculous pleuritis and left-sided pleural effusion.

parapneumonic effusion. The chronic form is characterized by low-grade fever, weakness, and weight loss.[81]

Pleural effusions secondary to tuberculous pleuritis are almost always unilateral (Fig. 74.3) and are usually small to moderate in size, although they may occupy the entire hemithorax.[82] About 50% of patients have smooth pleural thickening of greater than 1 cm on CT scan.[82] About one third of patients have coexisting parenchymal disease. In such patients, the pleural effusion is almost always on the side of the parenchymal infiltrate and invariably indicates active parenchymal disease.[81] It is likely that even in cases with no radiographic evidence of parenchymal involvement, the effusion is associated with a subpleural focus of infection.

***Pleural Fluid.*** The pleural fluid from patients with tuberculous pleuritis is an exudate that usually contains predominantly small lymphocytes. If symptoms have been present only a few days, neutrophils may be predominant. The pleural fluid glucose level is usually similar to that of serum, but at times, it is reduced. A pleural fluid protein level above 5.0 g/dL is suggestive of tuberculous pleuritis.

**Diagnosis.** The possibility of tuberculous pleuritis should be considered in every patient with an undiagnosed exudative pleural effusion, even though only a small percentage of such effusions are due to tuberculosis in the United States.[2] For the past 40 years, the most common way to establish the diagnosis of tuberculous pleuritis has been through needle biopsy of the pleura. However, in recent years, three tests that can be performed on pleural fluid have been developed that may be useful in establishing or excluding the diagnosis of tuberculous pleuritis[82a]: (1) the level of adenosine deaminase (ADA) in the pleural fluid, (2) the level of interferon gamma in the pleural fluid, and (3) the polymerase chain reaction (PCR) for mycobacterial DNA. One disadvantage of these tests is that they do not provide bacteria for antibiotic sensitivity testing.

Adenosine deaminase is predominantly a T-lymphocyte enzyme that catalyzes the conversion of adenosine to inosine. When a cutoff of 47 U/L is used, the pleural fluid ADA level appears to be a very sensitive test for the diagnosis of tuberculous pleuritis. When the results of two studies with a total of 397 patients with tuberculosis were combined, the pleural fluid ADA was above 47 U/L in 383 (96.5%).[80, 83] Pleural fluid ADA levels are frequently not elevated in human immunodeficiency virus–positive patients with tuberculous pleuritis.[83] An elevated pleural fluid ADA level is also seen with empyema and with rheumatoid pleuritis, but these conditions should be relatively easy to distinguish from tuberculous pleuritis clinically. The specificity of the pleural fluid ADA level for tuberculosis can be increased it if is combined with a pleural fluid lymphocyte/neutrophil ratio of $> 0.75$.[83] The ADA can be used to exclude the diagnosis of tuberculosis. In one study, none of 19 patients with a positive tuberculin skin test result, an ADA below 45 IU/L, and an exudative pleural effusion followed up without treatment for a mean of 62 months developed tuberculosis.[84]

Interferon gamma is a lymphokine produced by T lymphocytes in response to antigen stimulation. In one study, 72 of 73 patients (99%) with tuberculous pleuritis had pleural fluid interferon gamma levels above 3.7 U/mL.[85] The specificity of an elevated interferon gamma level is greater than that of an elevated ADA level.[85] Importantly, pleural fluid interferon gamma levels are elevated in patients with tuberculosis who are human immunodeficiency virus positive.[85] The primary advantage of ADA over interferon gamma is the lower cost of ADA. However, it is difficult to find commercial laboratories that measure ADA in the United States.

A PCR test for tuberculous DNA on pleural fluid may be useful in the diagnosis of tuberculous pleuritis. In one study, the sensitivity and specificity of PCR were similar to those of ADA,[86] but in another study, the sensitivity was only 42%.[85] It is likely that the results with PCR will improve as its technology is refined.

All patients with an undiagnosed exudative pleural effusion should undergo mycobacterial cultures of their pleural fluid and should have one of the aforementioned three tests performed on their pleural fluid. If the culture of the fluid is positive, treatment for tuberculosis should be initiated. If one of the other tests is positive for tuberculosis, the patient should also be treated for tuberculosis unless the patient has a disease that is known to be associated with a positive result or if there is no pleural fluid lymphocytosis. In areas with a high likelihood of resistant tuberculosis, one may also want to obtain pleural tissue for cultures via needle biopsy of the pleura or thoracoscopy. If the patient does not respond to therapy, then further investigations are warranted. Needle biopsy of the pleura can be performed in questionable cases, but unless the likelihood of tuberculosis is high, the invasive diagnostic test of choice is usually thoracoscopy (see Chapter 73).

**Treatment.** Patients with tuberculous pleuritis should be treated with antituberculous medications in the same treatment regimens that are administered to patients with pulmonary tuberculosis; these are fully discussed in Chapter 34. With treatment, patients generally become afebrile within about 2 weeks, and the pleural effusion resolves within 6 weeks. On occasion, the pleural effusion worsens after antituberculous therapy is initiated. In this situation, the possibility of a wrong diagnosis must be considered, but paradoxical worsening can occur with the correct diagnosis and appropriate antituberculous medications.[87] Mild degrees of pleural fibrosis are present a year after therapy is begun in about 50% of patients. The presence of fibrosis is not related to the initial pleural fluid findings and is of limited clinical significance.[88]

The role of systemic corticosteroids in the treatment of tuberculous pleuritis remains controversial. There were no benefits with the use of systemic corticosteroids in two controlled studies in which therapeutic thoracentesis was also performed,[89, 90] but the duration of fever and the time required for fluid resorption were decreased in a third study in which no therapeutic thoracentesis was performed.[91] Therapeutic thoracentesis is indicated if the patient has a moderate-sized or larger pleural effusion producing symptoms. Use of corticosteroids may be necessary for those who are markedly symptomatic, but only after the institution of appropriate antituberculosis therapy.

## Actinomycosis

More than 50% of patients with thoracic actinomycosis have pleural involvement.[92] In one series of 15 patients, 6 had pleural effusion, and an additional 6 had marked pleural thickening.[92] The characteristic chest radiographic finding is a localized lung lesion extending to the chest wall with pleural thickening or effusion. The pleural fluid with actinomycosis may be either frank pus with predominantly polymorphonuclear leukocytes or serous fluid with predominantly lymphocytes.

The diagnosis of actinomycosis should be considered when a chronic infiltrative pulmonary lesion extends to adjacent lobes through intralobar fissures. The presence of chest wall abscesses or draining sinus tracts suggests the diagnosis, as do bone changes consisting of periosteal proliferation or bone destruction. The definitive diagnosis is established with the demonstration of *Actinomyces israelii* by anaerobic cultures. Patients with pleural actinomycosis should be treated with high doses of penicillin or another suitable antimicrobial (Chapter 33) for prolonged periods. The management of the pleural effusion is similar to that for patients with any other bacterial pneumonia.

## Nocardiosis

Pleural effusions develop in approximately 50% of patients with pulmonary nocardiosis.[93] Patients with pleural effusion secondary to nocardiosis almost always have an associated parenchymal infiltrate. The pleural fluid can range from serous fluid to frank pus, and pleural fluid cultures may or may not be positive. Because most patients who develop nocardiosis are immunosuppressed,[93] this diagnosis should be considered in the immunosuppressed patient with a parenchymal infiltrate and a pleural effusion. The diagnosis is established with aerobic cultures, which should be observed for at least 2 weeks, because *Nocardia asteroides* is a slow-growing organism. Patients with pleural nocardiosis should be treated with sulfonamides or suitable alternative antimicrobials (Chapter 33), and the pleural effusion should be managed as any pleural effusion complicating a pneumonia.

## Fungal Diseases of the Pleura

Fungal infections of the lungs are discussed in Chapter 35. This section considers the pleural complications of aspergillosis, blastomycosis, coccidioidomycosis, cryptococcosis, and histoplasmosis.

### Aspergillosis

The pleural space occasionally becomes infected with *Aspergillus,* usually *Aspergillus fumigatus.*[94] Pleural aspergillosis usually occurs in one of two settings. Most commonly, it occurs in patients who were treated in the past with artificial pneumothorax therapy for tuberculosis. Pleural aspergillosis may also complicate lobectomy or pneumonectomy, in which situation a bronchopleural fistula is almost always present.[95]

The diagnosis of pleural aspergillosis should be suspected in any patient with a history of artificial pneumothorax therapy for tuberculosis who has signs and symptoms of a chronic infection, such as weight loss, malaise, low-grade fever, and chronic cough. The chest radiograph reveals increasing degrees of pleural thickening and usually an air-fluid level in the pleural space, indicating the presence of a bronchopleural fistula.[94] In some patients, fungus balls may be evident in either the lungs or the pleural space. The diagnosis is confirmed by the demonstration of *Aspergillus* on fungal cultures of the pleural fluid. Patients with pleural aspergillosis almost always have positive precipitin blood test results for antibodies against *Aspergillus.*

The optimal treatment for pleural aspergillosis is surgical removal of the involved pleura and resection of the involved lobe or the entire ipsilateral lung, if necessary.[94] Lung resection is usually necessary because the infection tends to invade and destroy the underlying lung. Surgery should be performed as early as possible to avoid progressive destruction of the lung. Itraconazole or amphotericin B should be administered systemically before and after the surgery to prevent postoperative pleural infection with *Aspergillus.*[96] Some patients with pleural aspergillosis are too debilitated to undergo a major surgical procedure. Such patients should undergo open-window thoracostomy with daily insertion of gauze impregnated with amphotericin B.[97]

The clinical picture of postoperative *Aspergillus* pleural infections is similar to that of other postpneumonectomy infections. Once the diagnosis is established, a chest tube should be inserted, and the pleural space should be irrigated daily with 25 mg of amphotericin B or 75,000 U of nystatin.[98] Over an extended period, most patients are cured with this treatment.

### Blastomycosis

Infection with *Blastomyces dermatitidis* produces a pleural effusion in about 10% of patients, and an additional

40% or more have pleural thickening.[99] Patients with pleural blastomycosis have signs and symptoms similar to those of tuberculous pleuritis. The pleural fluid is usually an exudate with predominantly small lymphocytes, although polymorphonuclear leukocytes may predominate.[100] Because pleural biopsy may reveal noncaseating granulomas, one should consider the diagnosis of blastomycosis in patients with a clinical picture compatible with tuberculous pleuritis and granulomas on pleural biopsy. The diagnosis is established by demonstrating the organism in secretions, pleural fluid, or histologic sections. Patients with pleural blastomycosis should be treated with itraconazole or amphotericin B, as described in Chapter 35.

### Coccidioidomycosis

Two types of pleural disease occur in association with coccidioidomycosis. The first is associated with a primary benign infection and may or may not have concomitant parenchymal involvement. The second occurs when a coccidioidal cavity ruptures to produce a hydropneumothorax.

**Primary Coccidioidomycosis.** The incidence of pleural effusion with symptomatic primary coccidioidomycosis is about 7%.[101] Most patients are febrile and have pleuritic chest pain, and nearly 50% have either erythema nodosum or erythema multiforme.[101] The pleural effusion is almost always unilateral, often occupying more than 50% of the hemithorax.[101] There is a coexisting parenchymal infiltrate in about 50%. The pleural fluid is an exudate containing predominantly small lymphocytes and has a glucose level above 60 mg/dL (3.33 mmol/L).[101] Pleural fluid cultures are positive for *Coccidioides immitis* in about 20%, whereas cultures of pleural biopsy specimens are almost always positive.

Most patients with primary coccidioidomycosis and pleural effusion require no systemic antifungal therapy. Only patients with a negative skin test result or other evidence of dissemination should be treated. The complement fixation titers are usually high in patients with coccidioidal pleural effusion, and a high titer alone should not be used as an indication for treatment.

**Rupture of Coccidioidal Cavity.** Hydropneumothoraces develop in 1% to 5% of patients with chronic cavitary coccidioidomycosis. The rupture of the cavity into the pleural space is usually heralded by the development of an acute illness with systemic signs of toxicity. These patients should undergo tube thoracostomy immediately to drain the air and fluid from the pleural space. Most patients require a thoracotomy with a partial or total lobectomy, and most require some degree of decortication. The administration of antifungal drugs does not appear to be required.[102]

### Cryptococcosis

Pleural involvement with cryptococcosis appears to result from extension of a primary subpleural cryptococcal nodule into the pleural space. About 50% of patients with pleural cryptococcosis have disseminated disease, and most have an accompanying parenchymal abnormality.[103] Most patients who have a cryptococcal pleural effusion are immunosuppressed, and many of the patients have AIDS.[104, 105] The pleural fluid is an exudate, usually with a predominance of small lymphocytes.

Not all patients with pleural cryptococcosis require treatment with systemic antifungal therapy.[106] Treatment should be initiated in patients with cryptococcal antigen in their blood or cerebrospinal fluid; in immunosuppressed patients, including those with AIDS; and in those with enlarging effusions, especially if pleural cell counts and LDH concentrations are increasing.[104]

### Histoplasmosis

Pleural effusion is rare with histoplasmosis. In one review of 259 patients with pulmonary histoplasmosis, only one had a pleural effusion.[107] Patients with pleural effusions secondary to histoplasmosis usually have a subacute illness characterized by low-grade fever and pleuritic chest pain. The chest radiograph usually reveals an infiltrate or a subpleural nodule in addition to the pleural effusion.[108] The pleural fluid is an exudate in which lymphocytes predominate, and the pleural biopsy usually reveals noncaseating granulomas. No systemic treatment is usually necessary for a pleural effusion secondary to histoplasmosis because the effusion normally resolves spontaneously over several weeks. Systemic therapy should be administered if the effusion persists over 3 to 4 weeks or if the patient is immunosuppressed (see Chapter 35).

## Viral Infections

Viral infections probably account for a sizable percentage of undiagnosed exudative pleural effusions. However, the diagnosis is rarely established because it usually depends on the isolation of the virus or the demonstration of a significant increase in antibody titers to the virus. These studies are not routinely obtained on patients with undiagnosed pleural effusions.

### Primary Atypical Pneumonia

The incidence of pleural effusions with so-called primary atypical pneumonia (usually caused by *Mycoplasma* or viruses) is as high as 20%.[109] The effusions associated with atypical pneumonia are usually small, are exudative, and contain predominantly neutrophils. Thoracentesis should be performed in such patients to exclude a complicated parapneumonic effusion.

### Other Viruses

Viral infection is probably responsible for a much higher percentage of pleural effusion without parenchymal infiltrates than is generally recognized. In one epidemic, 559 soldiers in Turkey had an acute febrile illness characterized by pleuritic chest pain and a mononuclear cell–predominant pleural effusion without parenchymal infiltrates. No pathogens were demonstrated, and it was assumed that this self-limited disease was due to a virus, although serologic studies were not performed.[110]

A pleural effusion can occur with infectious hepatitis. In one prospective study of 156 hepatitis patients, 70% had at least a small pleural effusion.[111] In this situation the pleural fluid is an exudate with predominantly mononuclear cells.[112] One must be careful in handling pleural fluid when infectious hepatitis is suspected because the infectious hepatitis B antigen has been demonstrated in pleural fluid.

Almost all patients with the hantavirus pulmonary syndrome (see Chapter 32) have a pleural effusion. Initially, the fluid is a transudate, probably resulting from cardiac dysfunction, but subsequently, the fluid becomes exudative.[113] Almost all patients with severe cases of dengue hemorrhagic fever also have pleural effusions, which are either right sided or bilateral.[114] Pleural effusions have also been reported to result from infection with infectious mononucleosis, respiratory syncytial virus, influenza viruses, measles after the administration of inactivated virus vaccine, cytomegalovirus, herpes simplex virus, and Lassa fever virus.

### Acquired Immunodeficiency Syndrome

As discussed in Chapter 82, pleural effusions occur in patients with AIDS but are less common than are parenchymal infiltrates. The distribution of the diseases responsible for pleural effusions in patients with AIDS varies widely from series to series.[115] In series from industrialized countries that included predominantly intravenous drug users, the most common cause is parapneumonic effusions; in contrast, in series with predominantly homosexuals, the most common cause is Kaposi's sarcoma. In series from Africa, tuberculosis is the most common cause.[115] Other causes of pleural effusions in patients with AIDS include body-cavity lymphoma (see Chapter 76), *Pneumocystis carinii,* opportunistic infections, renal failure, and congestive heart failure.[115]

Patients with AIDS and parapneumonic effusions should be managed as would any patient with a parapneumonic effusion, but the incidence of complicated parapneumonic effusion is higher in patients with AIDS.[116] The incidence of pleural effusion with pulmonary Kaposi's sarcoma is approximately 50%.[115] Most patients with a pleural effusion due to Kaposi's sarcoma have bilateral parenchymal infiltrates. The diagnosis of pleural involvement is difficult and often depends on the demonstration of pulmonary Kaposi's sarcoma, either by bronchoscopic examination or by high-resolution CT or chest radiographic findings. The pleural fluid is an exudate that is usually serosanguineous or hemorrhagic. Pleural fluid cytologic examinations are invariably negative with pleural Kaposi's sarcoma; pleural biopsy results are also usually negative because the parietal pleura is not involved.[115]

Patients with AIDS with an exudative pleural effusion should have a diagnostic thoracentesis which includes bacterial, mycobacterial, and fungal cultures and possibly a test for either interferon gamma or PCR for tuberculosis. If this does not establish a diagnosis, consideration should be given to performing thoracoscopy, at which time a pleurodesis may be considered in symptomatic patients.

## Parasitic Diseases

Parasitic infections of the lungs are discussed in Chapter 36. Those that may involve the pleura, amebiasis, echinococcosis, and paragonimiasis, are also considered in this section.

### Amebiasis

Pleural effusions arise by two different mechanisms in conjunction with amebic liver abscess. First, an amebic liver abscess may irritate the diaphragm and produce a sympathetic pleural effusion in a manner analogous to that of pyogenic liver abscess. Second, a pleural effusion develops when the amebic liver abscess ruptures into the pleural space through the diaphragm.[117]

The sympathetic effusion in amebic liver abscess is more common than rupture of an abscess through the diaphragm.[117] Patients with sympathetic effusions frequently have pleuritic chest pain referred to the tip of the scapula or the shoulder. The chest radiograph reveals a small to moderate-sized pleural effusion and often elevation of the hemidiaphragm with platelike atelectasis.[118] The pleural fluid has not been well characterized. The diagnosis can be established by positive gel diffusion and indirect hemagglutination tests, the results of which are positive in more than 98% of patients with extraintestinal invasive amebiasis.[119] Patients with amebic abscess and a sympathetic pleural effusion should be treated with antiamebic drugs, as described in Chapter 36.

The transdiaphragmatic rupture of an amebic liver abscess is usually heralded by an abrupt exacerbation of pain in the right upper quadrant and may be accompanied by a tearing sensation.[118] Shortly thereafter, progressive respiratory distress, sepsis, and occasionally shock develop. The pleural effusion is frequently massive, with opacification of the entire hemithorax and shift of the mediastinum to the contralateral side.[118] The diagnosis of amebic abscess with transdiaphragmatic rupture is suggested by the discovery of "anchovy paste"– or "chocolate sauce"–like pleural fluid on diagnostic thoracentesis.

Patients with transdiaphragmatic rupture should undergo tube thoracostomy. Large-bore tubes should be used because the pleural fluid can be quite thick.[118] The patients should also be treated with the same drugs recommended for patients with sympathetic effusions. Most patients are cured with the drugs plus pleural drainage.[120] Because bacterial infection of the pleural space complicates the process in about one third of patients,[119] bacterial cultures of the pleural fluid should be obtained routinely. If bacterial infection is present, appropriate antibiotic therapy should be initiated.

### Echinococcosis

Pleural involvement with hydatid disease can occur in one of three situations: a hepatic hydatid cyst, or, on rare occasions, a splenic cyst may rupture through the diaphragm into the pleural space; a pulmonary hydatid cyst may rupture into the pleural space; or the pleura maybe be primarily involved by the slowly enlarging cyst.[121] Less than 5% of hepatic or pulmonary hydatid cysts rupture into the pleural space.

When a hydatid cyst ruptures into the pleural space, the patient develops acute symptoms, with sudden tearing chest pain, dyspnea, and shock from the antigenic challenge to the body.[122] The cyst frequently also ruptures into the tracheobronchial tree, producing a bronchopleural fistula with a hydropneumothorax that may become secondarily infected.

The diagnosis of pleural echinococcosis is established by the demonstration of echinococcal scolices with hooklets in the pleural fluid or the pleural biopsy specimen. Eosinophils are frequently present in the pleural fluid unless it is secondarily infected.[123] Patients with pleural echinococcosis should be immediately subjected to thoracotomy to remove the parasite, to excise the original cyst, and to close the bronchopleural fistula.[122]

### Paragonimiasis

Pleural disease is common with paragonimiasis. In one series of 71 patients, 43 (61%) had pleural disease, including 20 with unilateral pleural effusions, 6 with bilateral pleural effusions, 6 each with unilateral and bilateral hydropneumothorax, and 5 with pleural thickening.[124] In a review of 25 Indochinese refugees with paragonimiasis, 48% had pleural effusions, which were massive in 6 patients and the sole manifestation in 5.[125] Paragonimiasis can occur in natives of the United States who have never left the country.[126]

Patients with pleural paragonimiasis present with a chronic illness. There is also a parenchymal infiltrate in approximately 50% of patients. The pleural fluid in patients with pleural paragonimiasis is characteristic. It is an exudate with a glucose level of less than 10 mg/dL (0.56 mmol/L), an LDH level of more than three times the upper limit of normal for serum, a pH below 7.10, and a differential revealing a high percentage of eosinophils.[125] In addition, cholesterol crystals are frequently present.[125] Pleural paragonimiasis is one of only two conditions in which the pleural fluid is characterized by a low pH, a low glucose level, and many eosinophils; the other is the Churg-Strauss syndrome.[127] Usually, there are no ova in the pleural fluid.

The diagnosis of pleural paragonimiasis is strongly suggested by the unique pleural fluid findings of low glucose level, low pH, and pleural fluid eosinophilia. The diagnosis is established definitively by demonstrating the typical operculated eggs in sputum, stool, or pleural fluid. A complement fixation titer above 1:8 for *Paragonimus westermani* is strongly suggestive of the diagnosis.[125]

The treatment of choice for paragonimiasis is praziquantel, 25 mg/kg body weight three times a day for 3 days.[128] If the pleural disease has been present for such a prolonged period that the pleural surfaces are abnormally thickened, penetration of antiparasitic agents into the pleural space is insufficient to eradicate the infection, and thoracotomy with decortication may be necessary.[129]

### *Pneumocystis carinii*

Pleural effusions are rare in patients with *P. carinii* pneumonia, but they have been reported. The pleural effusion appears to be an extension of the pulmonary process, and concurrent pneumothoraces are common.[130] The pleural fluid is an exudate with a relatively low protein level but an LDH level above the upper normal limit for serum.[130] At times, organisms can be visualized in the pleural fluid.

## Pulmonary Embolism

The diagnosis most commonly overlooked in the differential diagnosis of a patient with an undiagnosed pleural effusion is pulmonary embolism. It has been estimated that at least 250,000 persons are hospitalized annually in the United States with venous thromboembolism.[131] Because between 30% and 50% of patients with pulmonary emboli have an associated pleural effusion,[132] approximately 100,000 pleural effusions secondary to pulmonary emboli should occur annually. Therefore, one should expect to see more cases of pleural effusion secondary to pulmonary embolization than to bronchogenic carcinoma. Nevertheless, in most large series, pulmonary embolization accounts for fewer than 5% of pleural effusions. This discrepancy probably occurs because the diagnosis is frequently not considered in patients with undiagnosed pleural effusions. The diagnosis and treatment of pulmonary embolism are discussed in Chapter 51.

**Pathophysiology.** The mechanism by which pulmonary embolization produces pleural effusions is unknown. The pleural fluid in association with a pulmonary embolus can be either transudative or exudative.[15] Transudative effusions, which account for the minority of the effusions, may result from increased central venous pressure or decreased intrapleural pressure. Exudative effusions indicate an increase in the permeability of the capillaries either in the lung or in the pleura as a result of ischemia or inflammation. Soluble factors, such as vascular endothelial growth factor, may play a role in at least some patients because the pleural fluid vascular endothelial growth factor level was very high in one patient with pulmonary embolism.[133]

**Clinical Manifestations.** Patients with pulmonary embolism can be divided into three categories, depending on their presenting symptoms: (1) pleuritic pain or hemoptysis, (2) isolated dyspnea, and (3) circulatory collapse. In the PIOPED study, 56% of the patients with pleuritic pain or hemoptysis had pleural effusion, 26% of those with isolated dyspnea had pleural effusion, but none of the patients with circulatory collapse had pleural effusion.[134]

Approximately 50% of patients with paraembolic effusions have parenchymal infiltrates.[134a] The infiltrates are usually in the lower lobes, are pleura based, and are convex toward the hilum. Paraembolic effusions are usually small; in one series, 48 of 56 patients (86%) had only blunting of the costophrenic angle, and no patient had an effusion that occupied more than one third of a hemithorax.[132] Patients with parenchymal infiltrates tend to have larger effusions.[134a] The pleural effusions are usually unilateral, but in one series, chest CT demonstrated bilateral pleural fluid in 6 of 13 patients with pulmonary embolization.[135]

Pleural fluid analysis is of limited value in establishing the diagnosis of paraembolic effusion because there is nothing characteristic about the fluid. The pleural fluid is an exudate in 75% and a transudate in 25%.[15] The pleural fluid red blood cell count exceeds 100,000/μL in fewer than 20% and is below 10,000/μL in at least 30%. The pleural fluid white blood cell count can vary from under 100 to over 50,000/μL. The differential white blood cell count may reveal predominantly polymorphonuclear leukocytes or lymphocytes.

**Diagnosis.** The possibility of pulmonary embolization should be considered in every patient with a pleural effusion, even if the patient has obvious congestive heart failure. In an autopsy series of 290 patients with congestive heart failure and pleural effusion, 60 (21%) had pulmonary emboli.[4] When a paraembolic effusion is suspected, the initial diagnostic study is usually a perfusion lung scan or a spiral CT. Lung scans must be interpreted with even more than the usual amount of caution in patients with pleural effusions. A large effusion may severely compress portions of the underlying lung and cause shifts of perfusion to other regions of the ipsilateral lung or to the contralateral lung.[136] Small mobile effusions of any cause may gravitate to different regions of the pleural space, depending largely on the position of the patient at the time of the examination. Fluid may enter a major fissure when the patient lies supine for a perfusion scan, causing a perfusion defect. Then, when the patient stands erect for a chest radiograph, no comparable defect is seen on the radiograph. Similarly, mismatched ventilation and perfusion defects may be produced by pleural fluid of any cause when the scans are obtained with the patient in different positions.[137] For these reasons, a therapeutic thoracentesis should be performed before obtaining the lung scan if a moderate or large effusion is present.[137] If the perfusion scan is abnormal, a ventilation lung scan should then be obtained. Because of these difficulties in the interpretation of lung scanning, spiral CT with bolus contrast is probably the preferable test, where it is available.[137a] If doubt exists concerning the diagnosis after these tests, a pulmonary arteriogram should be performed.

**Treatment.** The treatment of the patient with a paraembolic effusion is the same as for any patient with pulmonary emboli (see Chapter 51). The presence of bloody pleural fluid is not a contraindication to the administration of heparin or, if indicated, thrombolytic therapy. Bynum and Wilson[134a] treated three patients who had pleural fluid red blood cell counts above 100,000/mm$^3$ with intravenous heparin and observed no increase in the size of the effusion.

Paraembolic effusions usually reach their maximum size within the first 3 days.[15] If the effusion increases in size after this time, the patient probably has recurrent emboli or another complication. Bynum and Wilson[134a] reported two patients in whom an enlarging ipsilateral effusion developed; one had recurrent pulmonary emboli, whereas the other had a pleural infection. Of two additional patients in whom contralateral pleural effusions developed, both had recurrent emboli. A diagnostic thoracentesis is therefore indicated in patients in whom the effusion enlarges after therapy is instituted. If bloody pleural fluid is discovered, a pleural fluid hematocrit value should be obtained. If the pleural fluid hematocrit value is greater than 50% of the peripheral hematocrit, a hemothorax is present that cannot be attributed to pulmonary embolism. If this is the case, anticoagulation should be discontinued, and tube thoracostomy should be performed.[138]

With treatment, paraembolic effusions gradually resolve. The resolution is much more rapid in patients without parenchymal infiltrates; in most of these patients, complete resolution occurs within 7 days. In contrast, resolution is rarely complete within 7 days in those with parenchymal infiltrates.

## Abdominal Diseases

As discussed in Chapter 85, many abdominal diseases can cause pulmonary signs and symptoms. This section describes the most important of these disorders that cause pleural effusion. The development of pleural effusions in patients with chronic liver disease and ascites and in those with infectious hepatitis has already been considered.

### Esophageal Perforation

The diagnosis of esophageal rupture should always be considered in the differential diagnosis of exudative pleural effusions because if this condition is not rapidly treated, the mortality approaches 100%. Approximately 60% of patients with esophageal perforation have a pleural effusion, whereas about 25% have a pneumothorax.[139] The pleural effusion is usually left sided (Fig. 74.4), but it may be right sided or bilateral.

Esophageal perforation most commonly occurs as a complication of esophagoscopy and is more likely to occur when there is an attempt to remove a foreign body or to dilate an esophageal stricture.[140] Overall, the

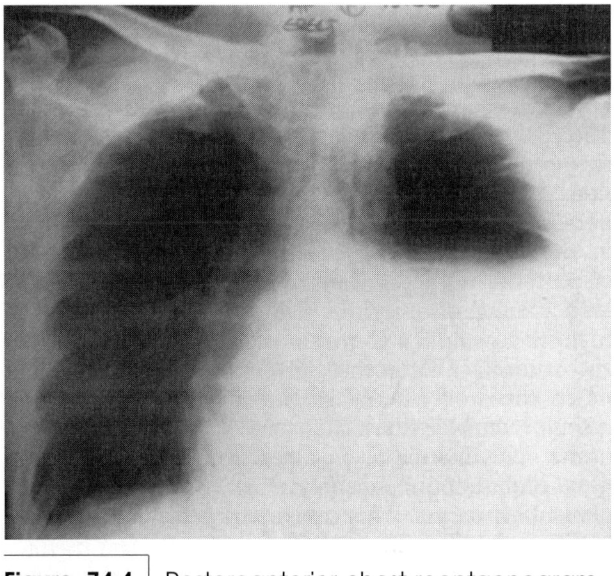

**Figure 74.4** Posteroanterior chest roentgenogram from a patient with a perforated esophagus demonstrating a left hydropneumothorax, air in the mediastinum, and subcutaneous emphysema.

incidence of esophageal perforation with esophagoscopic examination is 0.15% to 0.70%.[139]

The insertion of a Blakemore-Sengstaken tube for esophageal varices is sometimes complicated by esophageal rupture. Frequently, the diagnosis is missed in these patients because of the severity of their illness and the multiple coexisting problems.[139] Esophageal perforation may also result from foreign bodies, esophageal carcinoma, gastric intubation, chest trauma, chest surgery, or vomiting (Boerhaave's syndrome).

**Clinical Manifestations.** The symptoms associated with esophageal perforation result from the acute mediastinitis produced by contamination of the mediastinum by the oropharyngeal contents. Most of the morbidity from esophageal perforation is caused by infection of the mediastinum and the pleural space by the oropharyngeal bacterial flora.[141]

A patient with an esophageal perforation is usually acutely ill. With a spontaneous rupture, there is frequently a sensation of tearing or bursting in the lower part of the chest or the epigastrium. The chest pain is characteristically excruciating and is often unrelieved by opiates.[142] Dyspnea is frequently a prominent symptom. More than 50% of patients have small amounts of hematemesis.[143] The presence of subcutaneous emphysema in the suprasternal notch is suggestive of the diagnosis. However, less than 10% of patients have subcutaneous emphysema within the first 4 hours of rupture.[143] When the esophagus is perforated during esophagoscopy, the endoscopist generally does not realize it; however, the patients usually develop persistent chest or epigastric pain within a few hours after completion of the procedure.

**Diagnosis.** The diagnosis of esophageal rupture should be considered in all acutely ill patients with an exudative pleural effusion because the mortality increases considerably when treatment is delayed for more than 24 hours. The best screening test for esophageal rupture appears to be the level of amylase in the pleural fluid.[143] In the experimental model, the pleural fluid amylase level is elevated within 2 hours of rupture.[141] Only one patient has been reported in the literature who had a perforated esophagus without an elevated pleural fluid amylase level. This patient was unable to produce saliva because of Sjögren's syndrome with keratoconjunctivitis sicca.[144] The pleural fluid amylase level is elevated owing to saliva, with its high amylase content, entering the pleural space.[145]

The pleural fluid pH is usually decreased below 7.00 in patients with pleural effusion secondary to esophageal perforation.[146] The mechanism for the low pleural fluid pH appears to be the intense inflammatory response resulting from the mediastinitis and not the regurgitation of gastric juice into the pleural space.[146] The demonstration of either squamous epithelial cells or food particles in the pleural fluid is highly suggestive of the diagnosis.[147]

The diagnosis is established when esophageal perforation is confirmed by contrast studies of the esophagus. Hexabrix (ioxaglate meglumine and ioxaglate sodium) is the contrast agent of choice because it does not elicit much of an inflammatory reaction or bronchospasm.[148]

**Treatment.** The treatment of mediastinitis from esophageal perforation and other causes is discussed in detail in Chapter 78. Prompt surgical exploration of the mediastinum with primary repair of the esophageal tear and drainage of the pleural space and the mediastinum should be carried out.[149] Parenteral antibiotics should be given to treat the mediastinitis and pleural infection. If exploration of the mediastinum is delayed for more than 48 hours after rupture, primary repair is usually not possible because of the damaged tissue. Such patients are probably best managed with T-tube intubation of the esophageal defect.[149]

## Pancreatic Disease

Three different types of nonmalignant pancreatic disease can have an accompanying pleural effusion: acute pancreatitis, chronic pancreatitis with pseudocyst, and pancreatic ascites.

**Acute Pancreatitis.** In a study of 133 patients with their first attack of acute pancreatitis, 66% of the patients had a pleural effusion.[150] The effusion was bilateral in 51 (77%), unilateral left sided in 10 (15%), and unilateral right sided in 5 (8%). On the side with the largest effusion, the thickness of the fluid was less than 10 mm in 32 (48%), 10 to 20 mm in 18 (27%), and more than 20 mm in 16 (24%). Patients with acute pancreatitis who develop a pleural effusion tend to have more severe disease and a higher likelihood of subsequently developing a pseudocyst than do those without effusions.[150] The exudative pleural effusion accompanying acute pancreatitis results from the diaphragmatic inflammation and transdiaphragmatic transfer of the exudative fluid arising from acute pancreatic inflammation.

The clinical picture is usually dominated by abdominal symptoms, including pain, nausea, and vomiting. However, at times, respiratory symptoms consisting of pleuritic chest pain and dyspnea may dominate the clinical picture. For this reason, pleural fluid amylase level should be measured in all acutely ill patients with exudative pleural effusions. In addition to the small to moderate-sized pleural effusion, the chest radiograph may reveal an elevated diaphragm and basilar infiltrates.[151] Demonstration of an elevated pleural fluid amylase level is highly suggestive of the diagnosis, but the diagnosis of esophageal rupture must be excluded. The pleural fluid is an exudate with predominantly polymorphonuclear leukocytes and a normal glucose level.

Patients with pancreatitis and a pleural effusion should be treated for their pancreatitis in the usual manner (see Chapter 85). If the pleural effusion does not resolve within 2 weeks of the initiation of treatment, the possibility of a pancreatic abscess or a pancreatic pseudocyst must be considered.

**Chronic Pancreatic Pleural Effusion.** Patients with chronic pancreatic disease sometimes have a large chronic pleural effusion. Most of these patients have a pancreatic pseudocyst. When the pancreatic ductal system is disrupted, a pseudocyst may form in the pancreas. A sinus tract may extend from the pseudocyst through the aortic or esophageal hiatus into the mediastinum. Once the sinus tract reaches the mediastinum, the process may be contained to form a mediastinal pseudocyst or it may rupture into one or both pleural spaces (Fig. 74.5), resulting in a large chronic pleural effusion.[152]

The clinical picture of patients with chronic pancreatic disease and pleural effusion is usually dominated by chest symptoms, such as dyspnea, cough, and chest pain. Most patients do not have abdominal symptoms because the pancreaticopleural fistula decompresses the pseudocyst. The pleural effusion is usually massive and recurs rapidly after thoracentesis.[152] The effusion is usually left sided but may be right sided or bilateral.

The key to the diagnosis is a markedly elevated pleural fluid amylase level. Patients with chronic pancreatic pleural disease must be differentiated from those with malignant pleural effusion, who also may have an elevated pleural fluid amylase level. The amylase level is usually much higher with the pseudocyst. In rare cases in which the differentiation is not obvious, it can be made by measuring amylase isoenzymes because the amylase with malignancy is the salivary type.[153] The serum level of amylase is often mildly elevated in patients with chronic pancreatitis. Both ultrasound and CT are useful in establishing the diagnosis of pancreatic pseudocyst. Endoscopic retrograde cholangiopancreatography usually documents the fistulous tract or other pancreatic pathology.

Patients with chronic pancreatic pleural effusions should be given a trial of conservative therapy for 2 to 3 weeks that consists of nasogastric suction, no oral intake, suppression of pancreatic secretion with atropine, and repeated therapeutic thoracenteses.[152] The administration of a continuous infusion of somatostatin may decrease the secretions through the fistula and facilitate closure.[154] Conservative treatment is successful within 4 weeks in about 40% of patients. If conservative treatment fails, a laparotomy should be performed. The anatomy of the pancreatic ductal system should be assessed before surgery with endoscopic retrograde cholangiopancreatography or at the time of operation with operative pancreatograph. If a sinus tract is found, it should be ligated or excised. The pancreas should be partially resected, drained with a Roux-en-Y loop, or both, depending on the pancreatographic findings.[152] An alternative approach is to attempt percutaneous abdominal pseudocyst drainage by use of CT guidance.[155] Decortication of the pleura may be necessary for some patients in order to remove the thick pleural peel created by the intense inflammation caused by the presence of pancreatic enzymes.

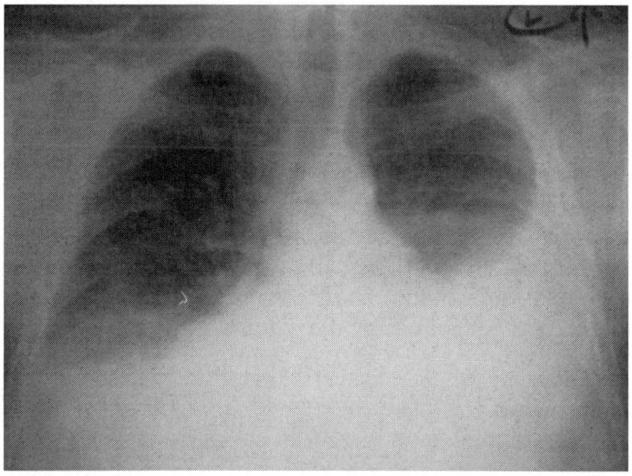

**Figure 74.5** Chest roentgenogram of a 35-year-old man with chronic pancreatitis showing bilateral, amylase-rich pleural effusions. Computed tomography showed pseudocyst with extension in the mediastinum.

**Pancreatic Ascites.** Some patients with pancreatic disease develop ascites characterized by high amylase and protein levels. If such patients should happen to have or develop a defect in their diaphragm, they develop a large pleural effusion as a result of the flow of fluid from the peritoneal cavity to the pleural cavity. The treatment for pancreatic ascites is the same as for pancreatic pleural effusion, except serial paracenteses rather than serial thoracenteses are performed.[156]

## Intra-Abdominal Abscesses

Pleural effusions frequently occur with intra-abdominal abscesses. The possibility of an intra-abdominal abscess should be considered strongly in any patient with an undiagnosed exudative pleural effusion containing predominantly polymorphonuclear leukocytes, particularly when there are no pulmonary parenchymal infiltrates. The mechanism responsible for the development of the exudative pleural effusion is probably diaphragmatic irritation.

Subphrenic abscess is the intra-abdominal abscess most commonly associated with a pleural effusion; pleural effusions occur in approximately 80% of patients with subphrenic abscess.[157] The approximate incidence of effusions with other intra-abdominal abscesses is 40% in pancreatic abscesses,[158] 30% in splenic abscess,[159] 20% in intrahepatic abscesses.[160] With pancreatic abscess, the pleural fluid has a high amylase level.

**Clinical Manifestations.** Subphrenic abscess most commonly develops as a postoperative complication 1 to 3 weeks after intra-abdominal surgery.[157] Splenectomy and gastrectomy are particularly likely to be complicated by left subphrenic abscess. There is no antecedent abdominal surgery in approximately 10% of patients with subphrenic abscess.[157] The abscess may result from perforation of the stomach, duodenum, appendix, colon, or a diverticulum, or from diverticulitis, cholecystitis, pancreatitis, or trauma. The diagnosis is not established before death in more than 50% of patients with subphrenic abscess without antecedent surgery. Most patients have fever, leukocytosis, and abdominal pain, but frequently, there are no localizing signs or symptoms. Most patients with pyogenic intrahepatic abscesses have fever and anorexia. Abdominal pain is common, but frequently, it is not localized to the right upper quadrant. On physical examination, an enlarged, tender liver can be demonstrated. Laboratory tests reveal leukocytosis, anemia, elevated alkaline phosphatase levels, and hyperbilirubinemia.[160]

Pancreatic abscess usually follows an episode of acute pancreatitis. This diagnosis should be suspected if the patient does not respond to the initial therapy or if fever, abdominal pain, and leukocytosis develop within 3 weeks of the episode of acute pancreatitis.[158] Splenic abscess is uncommon and usually occurs in patients with systemic infection. Bacterial endocarditis is the most common underlying infection.[159]

The pleural fluid that accumulates in patients with intra-abdominal abscesses is an exudate with predominantly polymorphonuclear leukocytes. The pleural fluid white blood cell count may exceed 50,000/μL but the pleural fluid pH and glucose concentration usually remain above 7.20 and 60 mg/dL (3.33 mmol/L), respectively. Only rarely does the pleural fluid become infected.

**Diagnosis and Treatment.** The diagnosis of intra-abdominal abscess is best established with an abdominal CT scan,[161] which should be obtained in every patient with an undiagnosed exudative pleural effusion characterized by predominantly polymorphonuclear leukocytes if there are no parenchymal infiltrates. The appropriate treatment for a patient with an intra-abdominal abscess and a pleural effusion is drainage of the abscess combined with parenteral antibiotics.[162]

## Diaphragmatic Hernia

Hernias through the diaphragm are important in two ways in the differential diagnosis of patients with suspected pleural disease. First, they may mimic a pleural effusion, and second, a pleural effusion is usually present with a strangulated diaphragmatic hernia. The possibility of a diaphragmatic hernia should be considered whenever an apparent pleural effusion has an atypical shape or location. If air is present in the herniated intestine, the diagnosis is easily established. If no air is present, an upper gastrointestinal series and a small bowel follow-through, a barium enema, or both, may be required to establish the diagnosis.

Most patients with a strangulated diaphragmatic hernia have a pleural effusion. Usually, diaphragmatic hernias are traumatic in origin, but the strangulation may not occur for months to years after the original injury, which usually is an automobile accident.[163] More than 90% of strangulated diaphragmatic hernias are on the left side, perhaps because the liver protects the right hemidiaphragm. Strangulation usually occurs suddenly and progresses rapidly, and the patient presents with signs of intestinal obstruction. Left shoulder pain is typically present owing to diaphragmatic irritation. The diagnosis is suggested by the presence of air-fluid levels in the strangulated viscera within the left pleural space. The pleural fluid is a serosanguineous exudate with predominantly polymorphonuclear leukocytes. The proper treatment is immediate surgery to prevent gangrene of the strangulated viscera.[163]

## Abdominal Surgery

Approximately 50% of patients undergoing abdominal surgery develop a pleural effusion in the first few days after surgery.[164, 165] The incidence of postoperative pleural effusion is greater in patients undergoing upper abdominal surgery, in patients with postoperative atelectasis, and in those patients with free abdominal fluid at surgery.[164, 165] The accumulation of pleural fluid within the first 72 hours after abdominal surgery is probably related to either diaphragmatic irritation or transdiaphragmatic movement of intra-abdominal fluid. A postoperative patient with a significant amount of pleural fluid, particularly when associated with fever, should have a diagnostic thoracentesis to rule out pleural infection as a cause of the effusion. In addition, the possibility of pulmonary embolization should be considered. If the effusion develops more than 72 hours after surgery, it is probably not related to the surgical procedure itself, and alternative explanations must be sought, such as pulmonary embolization, intra-abdominal abscess, and hypervolemia.

## Endoscopic Variceal Sclerotherapy

Endoscopic variceal sclerotherapy has become one of the principal forms of therapy for patients who bleed from ruptured esophageal varices. Small pleural effusions complicate the procedure up to 50% of the time.[166, 167] The pleural effusion is thought to result from the extravasation of the sclerosant into the esophageal mucosa, which results in an intense inflammatory reaction in the mediastinum and pleura. The effusions can be right sided, left sided, or bilateral, and the fluid is exudative. If the effusion persists for more than 24 to 48 hours and is accompanied by fever, or if the effusion occupies more than 25% of the hemithorax, a thoracentesis should be performed to rule out an infection, a chylothorax, or an esophagopleural fistula.[166] The latter diagnosis is suggested by a high pleural fluid amylase level.

## Liver Transplantation

Almost all patients who undergo an orthotopic liver transplantation develop a pleural effusion after surgery. In one study, 40 of 42 patients (95%) developed a right-sided pleural effusion within 72 hours of transplantation.[168] The effusions are bilateral in about one third of patients, but the amount of fluid is almost always greater on the right side.[169] The effusions are large enough to require therapeutic thoracentesis or tube thoracostomy in a sizeable percentage of patients. The natural history of these effusions is that they increase in size over the first 3 postoperative days and then gradually resolve over several weeks to several months.[169] The pathogenesis of these effusions is probably related to injury or irritation of the right hemidiaphragm caused by the extensive right upper quadrant dissection. These pleural effusions can be largely prevented if a fibrin sealant is sprayed on the undersurface of the diaphragm around the insertion of the liver ligaments at the time of the transplantation.[170]

## Bilious Pleural Effusion

Bilious pleural effusions are due to a fistula from the biliary tree to the pleural space.[171] The fistula may be secondary to trauma, suppurative complications of biliary tract infections, or surgery, particularly when biliary obstruction is present. The diagnosis should be suspected in any patient with an obstructed biliary tract. The pleural fluid usually appears bilious, but at times, the diagnosis may depend on the demonstration that the ratio of pleural fluid to serum bilirubin is greater than 1.0. Appropriate treatment consists of re-establishment of biliary drainage. The incidence of empyema with bilious pleural effusion is approximately 50%. Most patients who have a bilious pleural effusion require decortication and diaphragmatic repair.[171]

## Miscellaneous Diseases

### Rheumatoid Pleuritis

The pleura is occasionally involved in the course of rheumatoid arthritis. Approximately 5% of patients with rheumatoid arthritis have a pleural effusion, and approximately 20% experience pleuritic chest pain.[172, 173] Rheumatoid pleurisy has a striking male predominance, despite the higher prevalence of rheumatoid disease in women; more than 10% of men, but less than 2% of women, with rheumatoid disease have a pleural effusion.[172, 173] Additional information about rheumatoid pleuritis and other pulmonary manifestations of rheumatoid arthritis is found in Chapter 58.

The pathogenesis of the pleuritis or the pleural effusion associated with rheumatoid arthritis is not definitely known but probably involves cellular immune reactions. Evidence for this immune mechanism include elevated pleural fluid levels of soluble interleukin-2 receptor, T lymphocytes, and adenosine deaminase.[174] Autopsy examination usually reveals only thickened pleura, with nonspecific chronic inflammation. The thickened visceral pleural surfaces are frequently studded with small nodules with the histologic features of rheumatoid nodules.

**Clinical Manifestations.** Rheumatoid pleural effusions classically occur in the older male patient with rheumatoid arthritis and subcutaneous nodules. Almost all patients with rheumatoid pleural effusions are older than 35 years; moreover, approximately 80% are men and approximately 80% have subcutaneous nodules. The pleural effusion usually develops only after the arthritis has been present for several years.[173]

Patients with rheumatoid pleuritis may be symptomatic with pleuritic chest pain or fever,[173, 175] and some patients experience dyspnea secondary to the presence of pleural fluid. In most patients, the chest radiograph reveals a small or moderate-sized pleural effusion. In approximately 25% of patients, the effusion is bilateral.[173] With time, the effusion may alternate from one side to the other or may come and go on the same side. Other intrathoracic manifestations of rheumatoid disease are present in up to one third of patients.[173]

**Diagnosis.** The diagnosis is suggested by the clinical picture of rheumatoid arthritis and the presence of a pleural effusion. The pleural fluid with rheumatoid pleuritis is distinctive, characterized by a glucose level less than 30 mg/dL (1.67 mmol/L), a high LDH level (>700 IU/L), a low pH (<7.20), and a high rheumatoid factor titer (>1:320).[175] Occasionally, the pleural fluid glucose is not reduced when the patient is first seen, but serial pleural fluid glucose determinations reveal progressively lower pleural fluid glucose levels. Another interesting characteristic of rheumatoid pleural effusions is their tendency to contain cholesterol crystals or high levels of cholesterol.[176]

With the characteristic pleural fluid findings, the primary alternative diagnosis to exclude is complicated parapneumonic effusion. The incidence of complicated parapneumonic effusion is high in patients with rheumatoid pleuritis,[177] so this differentiation is important. It is particularly important to examine the Gram stain of the pleural fluid and to culture the fluid both aerobically and anaerobically.

**Prognosis and Treatment.** The natural history of rheumatoid pleuritis varies. Most patients experience a spontaneous resolution within 3 months, but the effusion is persistent in an occasional patient, and massive pleural thickening sometimes develops.[171] There are no studies that demonstrate that anti-inflammatory therapy has any influence on the course of rheumatoid pleuritis. The results after intrapleural corticosteroids have been mixed.[178] Decortication should be considered in patients with thickened pleura, who are symptomatic with dyspnea. This procedure is particularly difficult in patients with rheumatoid pleuritis because it is not easy to develop a plane of dissection between the lung and the fibrous peel.[179]

### Lupus Pleuritis

Patients with either systemic or drug-induced lupus erythematosus may develop a pleural effusion. Approximately 40% of patients with systemic lupus erythematosus or drug-induced lupus have a pleural effusion during the course of their disease.[180]

**Clinical Manifestations.** Most patients with lupus pleuritis have arthritis or arthralgias before the development of a pleural effusion. However, in one series of 21 patients, the pleuritis preceded any other symptom in 6 of the patients (29%).[178] Almost all patients with lupus pleuritis have pleuritic chest pain, and the majority are also febrile.[175] Lupus pleuritis frequently develops in association with an exacerbation of the underlying disease. The pleural effusions secondary to lupus are usually small and are bilateral in about 50% of patients.[180]

Many medications have been incriminated for producing drug-induced lupus erythematosus (see Chapter 72). Hydralazine, procainamide, isoniazid, phenytoin, and chlorpromazine are the ones most commonly associated with drug-induced lupus.[181] The presenting signs, symptoms, and radiographic abnormalities are similar, whether the pleuritis is due to spontaneous or to drug-induced lupus. The symptoms associated with drug-induced lupus characteristically abate within days of discontinuing the offending drug.

**Diagnosis.** The possibility of lupus pleuritis should be considered in any patient with an exudative pleural effusion of unknown cause. The pleural fluid can contain a predominance of either polymorphonuclear or mononuclear cells, depending on the timing of the thoracentesis in relation to the development of the symptoms.[182] Although it was believed in the past that elevated antinuclear antibody titers in the pleural fluid were diagnostic of lupus pleuritis, it appears that such elevated titers are neither specific nor sensitive for diagnosing lupus pleuritis.[183, 184] Likewise, because the presence of lupus erythematosus cells in pleural fluid is not specific for lupus pleuritis, this test should not be ordered.[185] The diagnosis is based primarily on the clinical picture and the serologic findings for lupus.

**Treatment.** In contrast to rheumatoid pleuritis, the pleuritis with systemic lupus responds to corticosteroid administration. It is recommended that patients with lupus pleuritis be treated with oral prednisone, 80 mg every other day, with rapid tapering once the symptoms are controlled. At times, the effusion is large, is symptomatic, and does not respond to corticosteroid therapy. In such a situation, consideration should be given to chemical pleurodesis.[186] Of course, if the patient has drug-induced lupus, the offending drug should be withdrawn.[181]

### Postcardiac Injury Syndrome

This syndrome, which is also known as the postpericardiectomy or the postmyocardial infarction (Dressler's) syndrome, is characterized by combinations of pericarditis, pleuritis, and pneumonitis that develop after injury to the myocardium or pericardium. The postcardiac injury syndrome has occurred after myocardial infarction, cardiac surgery, blunt chest trauma, percutaneous left ventricle puncture, and implantation of a pacemaker.[187] The incidence of the postcardiac injury syndrome is approximately 1% after myocardial infarction and is somewhat higher after cardiac surgery.[187] The exact pathogenesis of this syndrome is unknown, but it appears to have an immunologic basis. Engle and colleagues[188] reported that there was a close relationship between the development of the syndrome and the presence of antiheart antibodies, but it is unclear whether the antiheart antibodies precipitate or result from the syndrome.

**Clinical Manifestations.** The syndrome typically develops about 3 weeks after the injury, but it can occur any time between 3 days and 1 year later. The two cardinal symptoms are fever and chest pain. The chest pain often precedes the onset of fever and can vary from an agonizing crush to a dull ache. At times, it may have a pleuritic component. Most patients have a pericardial friction rub, and echocardiography can demonstrate pleural fluid in more than 50% of the patients.[189] Pulmonary infiltrates are present in about 50% of patients, and laboratory evaluation reveals leukocytosis with an elevated erythrocyte sedimentation rate.[189–191]

A pleural effusion occurs in about two thirds of patients with the postcardiac injury syndrome.[191] The pleural effusions are bilateral and small in most patients.[189, 191] The pleural fluid is an exudate that is frequently serosanguineous or bloody.[189] The pleural fluid glucose level exceeds 60 mg/dL (3.33 mmol/L), and the pH is usually above 7.40.[189] The pleural fluid differential may reveal either predominantly polymorphonuclear leukocytes or mononuclear cells, depending on the acuteness of the process.[189]

**Diagnosis.** The diagnosis of the postcardiac injury syndrome should be considered in any patient who develops a pleural effusion after injury to the heart. The diagnosis of the syndrome is established by the clinical picture and by the ruling out of congestive heart failure, pulmonary embolism, and pneumonia. A spiral CT scan or a perfusion lung scan should be obtained to exclude the diagnosis of pulmonary embolization. An advantage of spiral CT is that it can also document pericardial and parenchymal involvement or an alternative diagnosis.

**Treatment.** The postcardiac injury syndrome usually responds to treatment with anti-inflammatory agents, such as aspirin and indomethacin. Corticosteroids may be necessary in more severe cases. It is important to consider the diagnosis in patients who have undergone coronary artery bypass procedures because the pericarditis may cause graft occlusion. Such patients should be treated with prednisone, 30 mg per day for a week, with tapering doses thereafter.[190]

### Coronary Artery Bypass Surgery

The prevalence of pleural effusion in the few days after coronary artery bypass graft (CABG) surgery exceeds 40%.[192, 193] The effusions are usually small and are predominantly left sided.[192, 193] Most of the effusions gradually disappear in the weeks after CABG. The pathogenesis of these small effusions is unknown, but it is probably related to the trauma of the surgery.[189]

In contrast to the small, almost universally occurring effusions in the immediate postoperative period, a few patients develop larger symptomatic pleural effusions after CABG. In one series, 29 of 320 patients had effusion that occupied more than 25% of the chest 28 days after surgery.[194] Most of these larger effusions cannot be explained by congestive heart failure, pleural infection, pulmonary embolism, the postcardiac injury syndrome, or chylothorax, all of which can cause pleural effusions after CABG.

The larger effusions that occur after CABG can be divided into those that are bloody and those that are serous. The bloody effusions are probably secondary to bleeding into the pleural space. They reach their maximal size within 30 days of surgery, are frequently associated with pleural fluid and/or peripheral eosinophilia, have a high pleural fluid LDH level, and respond to one or two therapeutic thoracenteses. In contrast, the cause of the serous pleural effusions is unknown. They tend to reach their maximal size more than 30 days after surgery, have more than 50% small lymphocytes, and have a relatively low pleural fluid LDH level.[195] They are more difficult to manage. If the effusions recur after one or two therapeutic thoracenteses in conjunction with anti-inflammatory agents, consideration should be given to tube thoracostomy with pleural sclerosis.

## Lung Transplantation

With lung transplantation, the lymphatics that normally drain the lung are severed. Accordingly, the fluid that normally leaves the lung via these lymphatics drains through the pleural space. The presence of chest tubes in the first few days after lung transplantation prevents the accumulation of pleural fluid. However, patients who develop complications after lung transplantation are likely to develop pleural effusions. In one study, pleural effusions occurred with 14 (74%) of 19 episodes of acute rejection, 7 (88%) of 8 instances of chronic rejection, 6 (55%) of 11 episodes of infection, and 3 (75%) of 4 instances of lymphoproliferative disease.[196] (More details about lung transplantation are provided in Chapter 97.)

## Bone Marrow Transplantation

In one review, 7 (0.4%) of 1905 patients who had received a bone marrow transplant developed at least two significant effusions for which there was no clear-cut explanation involving the pleural, peritoneal, or pericardial cavities. This complication was seen only in children and only in recipients of allogeneic transplants. The effusions are large, require chest tubes, and are transudates. It appears that the effusions are due to either acute or chronic graft-versus-host disease.[197]

## Asbestos Exposure

An otherwise unexplained pleural effusion may occur after exposure to asbestos, which may have been brief or intermittent, and in the immediate or distant past. Epler and coworkers[198] reviewed the medical histories of 1135 asbestos workers whom they had followed up for several years and found that 35 (3%) of the workers had pleural effusions for which there was no other ready explanation. The heavier the asbestos exposure, the more likely the patient is to develop a pleural effusion. The pleural effusion sometimes develops within 5 years, but in one large series, the mean latency was 30 years.[198]

The pathogenesis of the pleural effusion occurring after asbestos exposure is unknown.[199] Asbestos fibers, both long and short, may move from the lung to the pleural space and lodge in the parietal pleura, where they appear to be concentrated in specific locations that correlate with the lymphatic drainage. Here, their presence leads to a continuous low-grade inflammation.[199] This chronic inflammation can either decrease the lymphatic clearance of the pleural space or increase the permeability of the capillaries in the parietal pleura, either of which could lead to the development of an exudative pleural effusion. An immune mechanism has been invoked to explain the fluctuations in the degree of pleuritis with time.[200]

**Clinical Manifestations.** Patients with pleural effusion secondary to asbestos exposure have surprisingly few symptoms. In the series of Epler and coworkers,[198] 66% had no symptoms. The chest roentgenogram usually reveals a small to moderate-sized effusion, which is bilateral in about 10%. The pleural fluid is an exudate, and the pleural fluid differential can reveal either predominantly polymorphonuclear leukocytes or mononuclear cells.[201] Interestingly, pleural fluid eosinophilia was present in 15 (52%) of the 29 patients with asbestos pleural effusions for whom pleural fluid differentials were reported.[202]

**Diagnosis.** The diagnosis of benign asbestos effusion is one of exclusion. It requires the following criteria: history of direct or indirect exposure to asbestos; exclusion of other causes, notably infection, pulmonary embolism, and malignancy; and follow-up of at least 2 years to verify that the effusion is benign.[200]

**Prognosis.** The natural history of the patient with an asbestos pleural effusion is one of chronicity with frequent recurrences and sometimes the development of extensive fibrosis of the parietal pleura.[198, 201] On average, the pleural effusion persists for 3 months but eventually clears and leaves no residual pleural disease. Massive pleural fibrosis develops in about 20% of patients, and ipsilateral blunting of the costophrenic angle occurs in another 20%.[198, 201] Rounded atelectasis also develops in about 10% of patients.[201] There is no known treatment for asbestos pleural effusion. Further information about asbestos-induced lung disease is provided in Chapter 65.

## Other Collagen Vascular Diseases

The Churg-Strauss syndrome is characterized by hypereosinophilia and systemic vasculitis in patients with asthma and allergic rhinitis (see Chapter 61).[203] Pleural effusions occur in approximately 30% of patients with this syndrome. The associated pleural fluid is distinctive in that it has a very high LDH level, a low glucose level, a low pH, and a high percentage of eosinophils.[203] The other disease with comparable findings is paragonimiasis.[125] This syndrome responds well to corticosteroids.

Pleural effusions occasionally occur in the course of Wegener's granulomatosis, Sjögren's syndrome, and angioimmunoblastic lymphadenopathy, which are described in detail elsewhere (see Chapters 47, 52, and 58). The pleural disease that occurs with these diseases constitutes a relatively minor portion of the clinical picture. The pleural fluid findings with each of the disorders have not been adequately described.

## Sarcoidosis

A pleural effusion occasionally occurs in patients with sarcoidosis (see Chapter 59). The incidence of pleural effusion with sarcoidosis is probably between 1% and 2%,[204, 205] although it has been reported to be as high as 7%.[206] Patients with sarcoid pleural effusion usually have extensive parenchymal sarcoidosis and, frequently, extrathoracic sarcoidosis.[204, 206] The symptoms of pleural involvement with sarcoidosis vary; many patients have no symptoms, although an equal number have pleuritic chest pain or dyspnea.[204]

The pleural effusions with sarcoidosis are usually small and are bilateral in approximately one third of cases. The pleural fluid is almost always an exudate, and its differential is characterized by predominantly small lymphocytes.[207]

The diagnosis of sarcoidosis depends initially on histologic demonstration of noncaseating granulomas in biopsy specimens from conventional sites. In the patient with known sarcoidosis, one can attribute the presence of the pleural effusion to sarcoid only when other causes of exudative lymphocyte-predominant pleural effusions, such as tuberculosis, are excluded. The pleural biopsy with sarcoid pleural effusion may reveal noncaseating granulomas. The pleural effusion secondary to sarcoidosis may resolve spontaneously, or corticosteroid therapy may be required for its resolution.[207]

## Uremia

Uremia may be complicated by a fibrinous pleuritis and pleural effusion.[208, 209] The pathogenesis of the pleural effusion associated with uremia is unclear. It is probably somewhat analogous to that for uremic pericarditis because more than half of the patients with uremic pleuritis also have uremic pericarditis. The incidence of pleural effusions with uremia is approximately 3%.[209] A close relationship does not appear to exist between the degree of uremia and the occurrence of a pleural effusion.

The pleural effusion seen with uremia frequently occupies more than 50% of the hemithorax and is bilateral in about 20% of patients.[209] More than 50% of patients are symptomatic from the pleural disease, with fever (50%), chest pain (30%), cough (35%), and dyspnea (20%) being the most common symptoms. The pleural fluid is an exudate that is frequently serosanguineous or bloody. The glucose level is within normal limits, and the differential white blood cell count reveals predominantly lymphocytes.[209] Pleural biopsy specimens invariably reveal chronic fibrinous pleuritis.

The diagnosis of uremic pleuritis is one of exclusion in the patient with chronic renal failure. After beginning dialysis, the effusion gradually disappears within 4 to 6 weeks in about 75% of patients. In the remaining patients, the effusion persists, progresses, or recurs. An occasional patient develops marked pleural thickening that may require decortication.[210]

## Urinary Tract Obstruction

Obstruction of the urinary tract resulting in a retroperitoneal urine collection (urinoma) can lead to a pleural effusion.[211] The mechanism by which the pleural fluid accumulates is unknown, but it is thought that this retroperitoneal fluid drains into the pleural space. The collection of fluid actually represents urine, and the pleural fluid smells like urine. The diagnosis can be established with simultaneous measurement of the creatinine levels in the pleural fluid and serum. Only patients with urinary tract obstruction have higher pleural fluid creatinine levels.[211] When the urinary tract obstruction is relieved, the pleural effusion rapidly disappears.[211]

## Meigs' Syndrome

Meigs and Cass[212] originally described a syndrome characterized by ascites and pleural effusion in association with solid benign ovarian tumors. Subsequently, it has become apparent that a similar syndrome can occur with benign cystic ovarian tumors, with benign tumors of the uterus (fibromyomas), and with low-grade ovarian malignant tumors without evidence of metastases.[187] The ascites appears to result from the secretion of large amounts of fluid by the tumors.[187] It is thought that the pleural effusion results from the ascitic fluid passing through defects in the diaphragm into the pleural space.[213]

Patients with Meigs' syndrome usually have a chronic illness characterized by weight loss, pleural effusion, ascites, and a pelvic mass. It is important to realize that not all patients with this constellation of symptoms have a disseminated malignancy. Approximately 70% of the effusions are right sided, and 20% are bilateral. The pleural fluid is usually an exudate with a relatively low white blood cell count ($<1000/\mu L$) and occasionally is bloody.

The diagnosis of Meigs' syndrome should be considered in all women who have a pelvic mass, ascites, and a pleural effusion. If the cytology of the pleural fluid is negative in such patients, a diagnostic laparoscopy or an exploratory laparotomy should be performed to determine whether there are peritoneal metastases. The diagnosis is confirmed when the ascites and the pleural fluid resolve after the primary neoplasm is removed and do not recur. The pleural fluid disappears from the chest within the first 2 weeks after surgery.

## Endometriosis

An occasional patient with severe endometriosis presents with massive ascites. In one review, 10 of 27 patients (37%) also had a pleural effusion.[214] The effusions are usually right sided but may be bilateral. The pleural fluid is a bloody or a chocolatey exudate. The serum carcinoembryonic antigen level may be elevated, suggesting ovarian carcinoma. Hormonal therapy, including gonadotropin-releasing hormone agonists, may be attempted, but frequently it is ineffective, and many patients require total abdominal hysterectomy plus bilateral salpingo-oophorectomy.[214]

## Ovarian Hyperstimulation Syndrome

This syndrome is a serious complication of ovulation induction. The dramatic clinical picture is characterized by massive ovarian enlargement and multiple cysts, hemoconcentration, and third-space accumulation of fluid.[214a] The full-blown syndrome may be complicated by renal failure, hypovolemic shock, thromboembolic episodes, acute respiratory distress syndrome, and death. Although the pathophysiology of this syndrome is incompletely understood, it is likely that the increased capillary permeability is due to the secretion of powerful vasoactive substances by the ovaries, which are stimulated by the exogenous human chorionic gonadotropin.[215]

Patients with the syndrome present within 2 to 3 weeks of receiving the human chorionic gonadotropin. Patients typically present with abdominal pain and distention, nonproductive cough, and dyspnea caused by ascites, pleural effusion, or both. The pleural effusion is usually bilateral, and the pleural fluid is an exudate with predominantly neutrophils and a relatively low LDH level.[216] The treatment of severe cases requires restoration of intravascular volume, correction of electrolyte abnormalities, and venous thromboembolism prophylaxis.[216]

## Extramedullary Hematopoiesis

Patients with severe chronic anemia may develop pleural effusions as a result of extramedullary hematopoiesis of the pleura.[217] Thoracentesis reveals a bloody pleural fluid with granulocytic, erythroid progenitors and megakaryocytes.[217] Management of the effusions is difficult, but pleurodesis with talc has been successful.[217]

## Yellow-Nail Syndrome

This syndrome consists of the triad of deformed yellow nails, lymphedema, and pleural effusions. The three entities may become manifest at widely disparate times and therefore are not all concurrently present in every patient.[217] One patient developed lymphedema in childhood, chronic nail changes at age 78 years, and a pleural effusion in her ninth decade.[217] The basic abnormality responsible for this syndrome appears to be hypoplasia of the lymphatic vessels.[217, 218]

Typically, the nails are pale yellow to greenish in color and are excessively curved from side to side. They are also thickened and may show transverse ridging or onycholysis (separation of nail from bed). The pleural effusions are bilateral in about 50% and can be massive. Once a pleural effusion has developed with this syndrome, it tends to persist and to recur rapidly after thoracentesis.[217] The pleural fluid is usually a clear exudate with predominantly lymphocytes.[217]

The diagnosis is usually established by the presence of the triad of pleural effusion, lymphedema, and yellow nails. The diagnosis may be difficult to establish if the pleural effusion is the first manifestation of the syndrome. There is no specific treatment for the syndrome, but if the effusion is large and is producing symptoms, the effusion can be treated with pleurodesis, parietal pleurectomy, or a pleuroperitoneal shunt.[187]

## Drug Reactions Producing Pleural Effusions

Lupus-like syndromes occur in conjunction with the administration of many different medications and have been discussed earlier in this chapter and in Chapter 72. Although there are case reports of pleural disease following the administration of many drugs,[219, 219a] the following drugs definitely induce pleural disease.

**Nitrofurantoin.** Pleuropulmonary reactions occasionally result from the administration of nitrofurantoin. Such reactions can have an acute or a chronic presentation.[220] The acute presentation occurs within 1 month of initiation of therapy and is manifested by dyspnea, nonproductive cough, and fever. About 20% of patients have an infiltrate and an effusion, and about 3% have only an effusion. Most patients have both peripheral eosinophilia ($>350/\mu L$) and lymphopenia ($<1000/\mu L$).[221] Pleural fluid analysis revealed 17% eosinophils in the one patient for whom pleural fluid analysis was reported.[221]

The chronic syndrome occurs when the patient has been taking nitrofurantoin for 2 months to 5 years and is much less common than the acute syndrome. Pleural effusion occurs in less than 10% of patients, and no patient with the chronic syndrome has had a pleural effusion without an infiltratc.[220]

The diagnosis of nitrofurantoin pleuropulmonary reaction should be suspected in all patients with a pleural effusion who are taking nitrofurantoin. If the drug is discontinued, the patient usually improves clinically within 1 to 4 days, and the chest radiograph becomes normal within a week with the acute syndrome, whereas the time course is much longer for the chronic syndrome.[220]

**Dantrolene.** Dantrolene sodium is a long-acting skeletal muscle relaxant with a chemical structure similar to that of nitrofurantoin. Its administration can lead to the development of pleural or pericardial disease.[222] The pleural effusion is unilateral and develops 2 months to 12 years after the initial administration of dantrolene. Patients may be febrile and may have pleuritic chest pain. The pleural fluid is an eosinophilic exudate with a normal glucose level.[222] When dantrolene is discontinued, the patient improves symptomatically within days, but it may take several months for the pleural effusion to resolve completely.

**Methysergide.** The administration of methysergide can lead to a pleuropulmonary disease similar to that seen with nitrofurantoin.[223] Symptoms consisting of chest pain, dyspnea, and fever develop 1 month to 3 years after methysergide therapy is initiated. The chest radiograph commonly shows bilateral loculated pleural effusions and pleural thickening.[223, 224] When methysergide is discontinued, the symptoms of the patients improve. However, in one series of 13 patients, severe pleural fibrosis persisted in the 2 patients who had continued to take the drug for the longest period (18 and 36 months) after the onset of the pleurisy.[223]

**Bromocriptine.** The long-term administration of bromocriptine mesylate, a dopamine receptor agonist, which is sometimes used in the treatment of Parkinson's disease or prolactin-secreting pituitary adenomas, can lead to pleuropulmonary changes.[225] As of 1988, a total of 23 patients had been reported. All the patients were men, and the drug had been taken for 6 months to 4 years before symptoms developed. Two per cent to 5% of patients receiving long-term bromocriptine therapy develop pleuropulmonary disease. The incidence of pleural disease is higher if the patient has previous exposure to asbestos.[226] The chest radiograph reveals unilateral or bilateral pleural thickening or effusion in most patients. Analysis of the pleural fluid reveals an exudate with predominantly lymphocytes and frequently eosinophilia.[225] The natural history of pleuropulmonary disease during bromocriptine therapy is unclear. The disease progresses only in some of the patients who continue taking the drug.[225]

**Procarbazine.** There have been two detailed case reports in which pleuropulmonary reactions consisting of chills, cough, dyspnea, and bilateral pulmonary infiltrates with pleural effusion occurred after treatment with procarbazine.[227, 228] In both cases, symptoms developed within hours after procarbazine therapy; in both instances, rechallenge with procarbazine again produced the infiltrates and pleural effusions. With discontinuation of the drug, the symptoms and radiographic changes resolved within several days.

**Amiodarone.** Amiodarone is an antiarrhythmic that may produce severe pulmonary toxicity (see Chapter 72). Pleural effusions occur as a manifestation of amiodarone toxicity, but they are uncommon. Most cases have concomitant parenchymal involvement,[229] but cases have been reported in which there is none.[230] The pleural fluid is an exudate and may have predominantly lymphocytes, macrophages, or polymorphonuclear leukocytes.[229, 230]

## Trapped Lung

As a result of inflammation, a fibrous peel may form over the visceral pleura. This peel can prevent the underlying lung from expanding fully, thereby "trapping" the underlying lung. The resulting negative pleural pressure leads to the development of a chronic pleural effusion.[24, 187]

A patient with a chronic pleural effusion secondary to trapped lung may experience shortness of breath or may be asymptomatic. Symptoms of acute pleural inflammation, such as pleuritic chest pain and fever, are distinctly uncommon, but the patient often gives a history of such events in the past. One characteristic of the pleural effusion secondary to trapped lung is that the amount of fluid is remarkably constant from one study to another. With trapped lung, the pleural fluid is a borderline exudate; the ratio of pleural fluid to serum protein is about 0.5, and the ratio of pleural fluid LDH to serum LDH is about 0.6.[187]

The diagnosis of pleural effusion secondary to trapped lung should be suspected in any patient with a stable, chronic pleural effusion, particularly if the patient has a history of pneumonia, pneumothorax, hemothorax, or thoracic operation. The thickened visceral pleura can be demonstrated if 200 to 400 mL of air is injected into the pleural space at the time of a thoracentesis. Alternatively, the thickened pleura can be demonstrated by CT of the chest. Measurement of the pleural pressure as fluid is withdrawn during therapeutic thoracentesis is useful diagnostically. With trapped lung compared with normal lung, the pleural pressure is low initially and decreases more rapidly as fluid is removed.[24]

The definitive therapy for trapped lung is thoracotomy with decortication. However, this major surgery is indicated only in patients who are symptomatic from the disease. If the patient is asymptomatic or minimally symptomatic, the patient can be observed if the clinical picture, pleural fluid findings, and pleural pressure measurements are all compatible with the diagnosis.[24]

## Therapeutic Radiation Exposure

Radiotherapy to the chest can cause the development of a pleural effusion. Bachman and Macken[231] followed up 200 patients treated with 4000 to 6000 rads to the hemithorax for breast carcinoma and reported that 11 patients (6%) developed a pleural effusion. The pleural effusion developed in all patients within 6 months of the completion of the radiotherapy, and every patient had concomitant radiation pneumonitis. The pleural effusion tends to be small and to resolve gradually over many months.[231] The pleural fluid is an exudate with many mesothelial cells.[232] It is important to recognize that this entity exists, and that the development of a pleural effusion in a patient after radiotherapy does not necessarily indicate that the patient has a recurrence of the malignancy. Radiation-induced injury to the lung is discussed further in Chapter 46.

## Iatrogenic Pleural Effusions

The iatrogenic pleural effusions that are secondary to various pharmacologic agents, radiotherapy, endoscopic esophageal sclerotherapy, coronary artery bypass surgery, abdominal surgery, and fluid overload are discussed earlier in this chapter. However, pleural effusions can result from misplacement of a percutaneously inserted catheter or a nasogastric catheter, both of which are discussed here.

Both internal jugular and subclavian vein catheterization can be complicated by the development of a pleural effusion. The pleural fluid may have the characteristics of the intravenous fluid, or it may be bloody from laceration of the blood vessels.[233] The diagnosis of a misplaced central venous catheter should be considered in all patients with such lines who rapidly develop pleural effusions, and the patients should be evaluated by diagnostic thoracentesis. Small pleural effusions may also develop after translumbar aortographic examination and after percutaneous transhepatic coronary vein occlusion. The effusions in these circumstances are usually small and resolve spontaneously.

In the past several years, the development of soft, flexible, small-bore polyurethane feeding tubes has made nasogastric and nasoenteric feeding more practical and comfortable for patients. However, misplacement of these tubes can lead to serious pleural complications. Pneumothorax is the most common complication,[234] but infusion of the enteral formula into the pleural space, or the development of an empyema, or both, also occur relatively frequently.[234] These small flexible tubes are inserted with a stylet in place that enables easier advancement of the device. However, with the stylet in place, the tubing becomes stiff enough that it can perforate structures relatively easily. The risk is much greater if the patient has an endotracheal tube in place or is obtunded.[234] To prevent these complications, these tubes should be inserted only by experienced persons, and the tube should be immediately removed if the patient starts coughing. The tube should not be advanced if resistance is felt, and before feeding is initiated, the position of the tip of the tube must be confirmed radiographically.[235] If enteral solutions enter the pleural space, tube thoracostomy should be performed to remove the solution. In addition, the patient should be carefully observed for the development of an empyema.[234]

## SUMMARY

Pleural effusion is a common clinical finding that occurs in patients with underlying disease of the neighboring lung or of the pleura itself. Pleural effusion is also a common manifestation of extrapulmonary disorders, particularly thromboembolism and diseases of the heart (congestive heart failure) or abdominal organs; unilateral or bilateral effusion is found in certain connective tissue diseases, especially rheumatoid arthritis and lupus erythematosus, and may complicate the administration of many different drugs. The evaluation of a patient with clinically significant pleural effusion of unknown cause begins with a diagnostic thoracentesis and measurement of the protein and LDH levels to differentiate a transudate from an exudate. This distinction helps guide subsequent workup, if necessary, with the goal of defining the underlying disorder that led to the accumulation of the fluid. Treatment varies considerably and depends on the specific cause. Cure is possible in many instances, and symptomatic relief can be provided for nearly all patients with pleural effusion.

## References


1. Light RW, MacGregor MI, Luchsinger PC, et al: Pleural effusions: The diagnostic separation of transudates and exudates. Ann Intern Med 77:505–513, 1972.
2. Light RW: Approach to the patient. *In* Pleural Diseases (3rd ed). Baltimore: Williams & Wilkins, 1995, pp 75–82.
3. Logue RB, Rogers JV Jr, Gay BB Jr: Subtle roentgenographic signs of left heart failure. Am Heart J 65:464–473, 1963.
4. Race GA, Scheifley CH, Edwards JE: Hydrothorax in congestive heart failure. Am J Med 22:83–89, 1957.
5. Broaddus VC, Light RW: What is the origin of pleural transudates and exudates? Chest 102:658–659, 1992.
6. Broaddus VC, Wiener-Kronish JP, Staub NC: Clearance of lung edema into the pleural space of volume-loaded anesthetized sheep. J Appl Physiol 68:2623–2630, 1990.
7. Allen SJ, Gabel JC, Drake RE: Left atrial hypertension causes pleural effusion formation in unanesthetized sheep. Am J Physiol 257:H690–H692, 1989.
8. Wiener-Kronish JP, Matthay MA, Callen PW, et al: Relationship of pleural effusions to pulmonary hemodynamics in patients with congestive heart failure. Am Rev Respir Dis 132:1253–1256, 1985.
9. Peterman TA, Brothers SK: Pleural effusions in congestive heart failure and in pericardial disease (letter). N Engl J Med 309:313, 1984.
10. Weiss JM, Spodick, DH: Brief reports: Laterality of pleural effusions in chronic congestive heart failure. Am J Cardiol 53:951, 1984.
11. Rabin CB, Blackman NS: Bilateral pleural effusions: Its significance in association with a heart of normal size. J Mt Sinai Hosp NY 24:45–63, 1957.
12. Shinto RW, Light RW: The effects of diuresis upon the characteristics of pleural fluid in patients with congestive heart failure. Am J Med 88:230–233, 1990.
13. Peterman TA, Speicher CE: Evaluating pleural effusions: A two-stage laboratory approach. JAMA 252:1051–1053, 1984.
14. Burgess LJ, Maritz FJ, Taljaard JJ: Comparative analysis of the biochemical parameters used to distinguish between pleural transudates and exudates. Chest 107:1604–1609, 1995.
15. Bynum LJ, Wilson JE III: Characteristics of pleural effusions associated with pulmonary embolism. Arch Intern Med 136:159–162, 1976.
16. Spicer AJ, Fisher JA: Recurring pleural effusion in congestive heart failure treated by pleurodesis. J Irish Med Assoc 62:177–178, 1969.
17. Plum GE, Bruwer AJ, Clagett OT: Chronic constrictive pericarditis: Roentgenologic findings in 35 surgically proved cases. Mayo Clin Proc 32:555–566, 1957.
18. Weiss JM, Spodick DH: Association of left pleural effusion with pericardial disease. N Engl J Med 308:696–697, 1983.
19. Lieberman FL, Hidemura R, Peters RL, et al: Pathogenesis and treatment of hydrothorax complicating cirrhosis with ascites. Ann Intern Med 64:341–351, 1966.
20. Johnston RF, Loo RV: Hepatic hydrothorax: Studies to determine the source of the fluid and report of thirteen cases. Ann Intern Med 61:385–401, 1964.
21. Hahn MH, Hahn PY, Gadallah SF, et al: Hepatic hydrothorax: Possible etiology of recurring pleural effusion. Am Fam Physician 56:523–527, 1997.
22. Kirschner PA: Porous diaphragm syndromes. Chest Surg Clin North Am 8:449–472, 1998.
23. Mouroux J, Perrin C, Venissac N, et al: Management of pleural effusion of cirrhotic origin. Chest 109:1093–1096, 1996.
24. Light RW, Jenkinson SG, Minh V, et al: Observations on pleural pressures as fluid is withdrawn during thoracentesis. Am Rev Respir Dis 121:799–804, 1980.
25. Xiol X, Castellvi JM, Guardiola J, et al: Spontaneous bacterial empyema in cirrhotic patients: A prospective study. Hepatology 23:719–723, 1996.
26. Gordon FD, Anastopoulos HT, Crenshaw W, et al: The successful treatment of symptomatic, refractory hepatic hydrothorax with transjugular intrahepatic portosystemic shunt. Hepatology 25:1366–1369, 1997.
27. Cavina G, Vichi G: Radiological aspects of pleural effusions in medical nephropathy in children. Ann Radiol Diagn 31:163–202, 1958.
28. Kinasewitz GT: Transudative effusions. Eur Respir J 10:714–718, 1997.
29. Llach F, Arieff AI, Massry SG: Renal vein thrombosis and nephrotic syndrome: A prospective study of 36 adult patients. Ann Intern Med 83:8–14, 1975.
30. Jenkins PG, Shelp WD: Recurrent pleural transudate in the nephrotic syndrome: A new approach to treatment. JAMA 230:587–588, 1974.
31. Nomoto Y, Suga T, Nakajima K, et al: Acute hydrothorax in continuous ambulatory peritoneal dialysis: A collaborative study of 161 centers. Am J Nephrol 9:363–367, 1989.
32. Di Bisceglie M, Paladini P, Voltolini L, et al: Videothoracoscopic obliteration of pleuroperitoneal fistula in continuous peritoneal dialysis. Ann Thorac Surg 62:1509–1510, 1996.
33. Gottehrer A, Roa J, Stanford GG, et al: Hypothyroidism and pleural effusions. Chest 98:1130–1132, 1990.
34. Marks PA, Roof BS: Pericardial effusion associated with myxedema. Ann Intern Med 39:230–240, 1953.
35. Smolar EN, Rubin JE, Avramides A, et al: Cardiac tamponade in primary myxedema and review of the literature. Am J Med Sci 272:345–352, 1976.
36. Spicer RL, Uzark KC, Moore JW, et al: Aortopulmonary collateral vessels and prolonged pleural effusions after modified Fontan procedures. Am Heart J 131:1164–1168, 1996.
37. Sade RM, Wiles HB: Pleuroperitoneal shunt for persistent pleural drainage after Fontan procedure. J Thorac Cardiovasc Surg 100:621–623, 1990.
38. Rychik J, Rome JJ, Jacobs ML: Late surgical fenestration for complications after the Fontan operation. Circulation 96:33–36, 1997.
39. Neiderman MS, Bass JB, Campbell GD, et al: Guidelines for the initial management of adults with community-acquired pneumonia: Diagnosis, assessment of severity, and initial antimicrobial therapy. Am Rev Respir Dis 148:1418–1426, 1993.
40. Light RW, Girard WM, Jenkinson SG, et al: Parapneumonic effusions. Am J Med 69:507–511, 1980.
41. Hasley PB, Albaum MN, Li Y-H, et al: Do pulmonary radiographic findings at presentation predict mortality in patients with community-acquired pneumonia? Arch Intern Med 156:2206–2212, 1996.
42. Light RW: Parapneumonic effusions and infections of the pleural space. *In* Pleural Diseases (3rd ed). Baltimore: Williams & Wilkins, 1995, pp 129–153.
43. Andrews NC, Parker EF, Shaw RR, et al: Management of nontuberculous empyema. Am Rev Respir Dis 85:935–936, 1962.

44. Finland M, Barnes MW: Changing ecology of acute bacterial empyema: Occurrence and mortality at Boston City Hospital during 12 selected years from 1935 to 1972. J Infect Dis 137:274–291, 1978.
45. Bartlett JG, Gorbach SL, Thadepalli H, et al: Bacteriology of empyema. Lancet 1:338–340, 1974.
46. Bartlett JG, Finegold SM: Anaerobic infections of the lung and pleural space. Am Rev Respir Dis 110:56–77, 1974.
47. Ferguson AD, Prescott RJ, Selkon JB, et al: The clinical course and management of thoracic empyema. QJM 89:285–289, 1996.
48. Cheng D-S, Rodriguez RM, Rogers J, et al: Comparison of pleural fluid pH values obtained using blood gas machine, pH meter and pH indicator strip. Chest 114:1368–1372, 1998.
49. Haramati LB, Alterman DD, White CS, et al: Intrathoracic lymphadenopathy in patients with empyema. J Comput Assist Tomogr 21:608–611, 1997.
50. Light RW, Rodriguez RM: Management of parapneumonic effusions. Clin Chest Med 19:373–382, 1998.
50a. Lim TK, Chin NK: Empirical treatment with fibrinolysis and early surgery reduces the duration of hospitalization in pleural sepsis. Eur Respir J 13:514–518, 1999.
51. Sasse SA, Nguyen TK, Kwok RY, et al: Utility of daily therapeutic thoracentesis for the treatment of empyema, in press.
52. Storm HKR, Krasnik M, Bang K, et al: Treatment of pleural empyema secondary to pneumonia: Thoracocentesis regimen versus tube drainage. Thorax 47:821–824, 1992.
53. Ashbaugh DG: Empyema thoracis: Factors influencing morbidity and mortality. Chest 99:1162–1165, 1991.
54. Silverman SG, Mueller PR, Saini S, et al: Thoracic empyema: Management with image-guided catheter drainage. Radiology 169:5–9, 1988.
55. Kerr A, Vasudevan VP, Powell S, et al: Percutaneous catheter drainage for acute empyema: Improved cure rate using CAT scan, fluoroscopy, and pigtail drainage catheters. NY State J Med 91:4–7, 1991.
56. Ali I, Unruh H: Management of empyema thoracis. Ann Thorac Surg 50:355–359, 1990.
57. Bouros D, Schiza S, Patsourakis G, et al: Intrapleural streptokinase versus urokinase in the treatment of complicated parapneumonic effusions: A prospective, double-blind study. Am J Respir Crit Care Med 155:291–295, 1997.
58. Laisaar T, Puttsepp E, Laisaar V: Early administration of intrapleural streptokinase in the treatment of multiloculated pleural effusions and pleural empyemas. Thorac Cardiovasc Surg 44:252–256, 1996.
59. Temes RT, Follis F, Kessler RM, et al: Intrapleural fibrinolytics in management of empyema thoracis. Chest 110:102–106, 1996.
60. Roupie E, Bouabdallah K, Delclaux C, et al: Intrapleural administration of streptokinase in complicated purulent pleural effusion: A CT-guided strategy. Intensive Care Med 22:1351–1353, 1996.
61. Moulton JS, Moore PT, Mencini RA: Treatment of loculated pleural effusions with transcatheter intracavitary urokinase. AJR Am J Roentgenol 153:941–945, 1989.
62. Chin NK, Lim TK: Controlled trial of intrapleural streptokinase in the treatment of pleural empyema and complicated parapneumonic effusions. Chest 111:275–279, 1997.
63. Davies RJO, Traill ZC, Gleeson FV: Randomised controlled trial of intrapleural streptokinase in community acquired pleural infection. Thorax 52:416–421, 1997.
64. Bouros D, Schiza S, Tzanakis N, et al: Intrapleural urokinase vs normal saline in the treatment of complicated parapneumonic effusions and empyema: A randomized, double-blind study. Am J Respir Crit Care Med 159:37–42, 1999.
65. Wait MA, Sharma S, Hohn J, Dal Nogare A: A randomized trial of empyema therapy. Chest 111:1548–1551, 1997.
66. Silen ML, Naunheim KS: Thoracoscopic approach to the management of empyema thoracis: Indications and results. Chest Surg Clin North Am 6:491–499, 1996.
67. Lawrence DR, Ohri SK, Moxon RE, et al: Thoracoscopic debridement of empyema thoracis. Ann Thorac Surg 64:1448–1450, 1997.
68. Thurer RJ: Decortication in thoracic empyema: Indications and surgical technique. Chest Surg Clin North Am 6:461–490, 1996.
69. Stark DD, Federle MP, Goodman PC, et al: Differentiating lung abscess and empyema: Radiography and computed tomography. AJR Am J Roentgenol 141:163–167, 1983.
70. Bressler EL, Francis IR, Glazer GM, et al: Bolus contrast medium enhancement for distinguishing pleural from parenchymal lung disease: CT features. J Comput Assist Tomogr 11:435–440, 1987.
71. Deschamps C, Pairolero PC, Allen MS, et al: Management of postpneumonectomy empyema and bronchopleural fistula. Chest Surg Clin North Am 6:519–527, 1996.
72. Wain JC: Management of late postpneumonectomy empyema and bronchopleural fistula. Chest Surg Clin North Am 6:529–541, 1996.
73. Hollaus PH, Lax F, el-Nashef BB, et al: Natural history of bronchopleural fistula after pneumonectomy: A review of 96 cases. Ann Thorac Surg 63:1391–1396, 1997.
74. Mehta JB, Dutt A, Harvill L, et al: Epidemiology of extrapulmonary tuberculosis. Chest 99:1134–1138, 1991.
75. Mlika-Cabanne N, Brauner M, Mugusi F, et al: Radiographic abnormalities in tuberculosis and risk of coexisting human immunodeficiency virus infection. Am J Respir Crit Care Med 152:786–793, 1995.
76. Roper WH, Waring JJ: Primary serofibrinous pleural effusion in military personnel. Am Rev Respir Dis 71:616–634, 1955.
77. Patiala J: Initial tuberculous pleuritis in the Finnish Armed Forces in 1939–1945 with special reference to eventual postpleuritic tuberculosis. Acta Tuberc Scand 36(Suppl):1–57, 1954.
78. Moudgil H, Sridhar G, Leitch AG: Reactivation disease: The commonest form of tuberculous pleural effusion in Edinburgh, 1980–1991. Respir Med 88:301–304, 1994.
79. Ellner JJ, Barnes PF, Wallis RS, et al: The immunology of tuberculous pleurisy. Semin Respir Infect 3:335–342, 1988.
80. Valdés L, Alvarez D, San Jose E, et al: Tuberculous pleurisy: A study of 254 cases. Arch Intern Med 158:2017–2021, 1998.
81. Berger HW, Mejia E: Tuberculous pleurisy. Chest 63:88–92, 1973.
82. Yilmaz MU, Kumcuoglu Z, Utkaner G, et al: Computed tomography findings of tuberculous pleurisy. Int J Tuberc Lung Dis 2:164–167, 1998.
82a. Light RW: Useful tests on the pleural fluid in the management of patients with pleural effusions. Curr Opin Pul Med 5:245–249, 1999.
83. Burgess LJ, Maritz FJ, Le Roux I, et al: Combined use of pleural adenosine deaminase with lymphocyte/neutrophil ratio: Increased specificity for the diagnosis of tuberculous pleuritis. Chest 109:414–419, 1996.
84. Ferrer JS, Munoz XG, Orriols RM, et al: Evolution of idiopathic pleural effusion: A prospective, long-term follow-up study. Chest 109:1508–1513, 1996.
85. Villena V, Lopez-Encuentra A, Echave-Sustaeta J, et al: Interferon-gamma in 388 immunocompromised and immunocompetent patients for diagnosing pleural tuberculosis. Eur Respir J 9:2635–2639, 1996.
86. Querol JM, Minguez J, Garcia-Sanchez E, et al: Rapid diagnosis of pleural tuberculosis by polymerase chain reaction. Am J Respir Crit Care Med 152:1977–1981, 1995.
87. Al-Majed SA: Study of paradoxical response to chemotherapy in tuberculous pleural effusion. Respir Med 90:211–214, 1996.
88. Barbas CS, Cukier A, de Varvalho CR, et al: The relationship between pleural fluid findings and the development of pleural thickening in patients with pleural tuberculosis. Chest 100:1264–1267, 1991.
89. Wyser C, Walzl G, Smedema JP, et al: Corticosteroids in the treatment of tuberculous pleurisy: A double-blind, placebo-controlled, randomized study. Chest 110:333–338, 1996.
90. Galarza I, Canete C, Granados A, et al: Randomised trial of corticosteroids in the treatment of tuberculous pleurisy. Thorax 50:1305–1307, 1995.
91. Lee CH, Wang WJ, Lan RS, et al: Corticosteroids in the treatment of tuberculous pleurisy: A double-blind, placebo-controlled, randomized study. Chest 94:1256–1259, 1988.
92. Flynn MW, Felson B: The roentgen manifestations of thoracic actinomycosis. AJR Am J Roentgenol 110:707–716, 1970.
93. Feigin DS: Nocardiosis of the lung: Chest radiographic findings in 21 cases. Radiology 159:9–14, 1986.
94. Hillerdal G: Pulmonary aspergillus infection invading the pleura. Thorax 36:745–751, 1981.
95. Wex P, Utta E, Drozdz W: Surgical treatment of pulmonary and

pleuropulmonary *Aspergillus* disease. Thorac Cardiovasc Surg 41:64–70, 1993.
96. Klein NC, Cunha BA: New antifungal drugs for pulmonary mycoses. Chest 110:525–532, 1996.
97. Shirakusa T, Ueda H, Saito T, et al: Surgical treatment of pulmonary aspergilloma and *Aspergillus* empyema. Ann Thorac Surg 48:779–782, 1989.
98. Colp CR, Cook WA: Successful treatment of pleural aspergillosis and bronchopleural fistula. Chest 68:96–98, 1975.
99. Kinasewitz GT, Penn RL, George RB: The spectrum and significance of pleural disease in blastomycosis. Chest 86:580–584, 1985.
100. Failla PJ, Cerise FP, Karam GH, et al: Blastomycosis: Pulmonary and pleural manifestations. South Med J 88:405–410, 1995.
101. Lonky SA, Catanzaro A, Moser KM, et al: Acute coccidioidal pleural effusion. Am Rev Respir Dis 114:681–688, 1976.
102. Cunningham RT, Einstein H: Coccidioidal pulmonary cavities with rupture. J Thorac Cardiovasc Surg 84:172–177, 1982.
103. Young EJ, Hirsh DD, Fainstein V, et al: Pleural effusions due to *Cryptococcus neoformans:* A review of the literature and report of two cases with cryptococcal antigen determinations. Am Rev Respir Dis 121:743–747, 1980.
104. Wasser L, Talavera W: Pulmonary cryptococcosis in AIDS. Chest 92:692–695, 1987.
105. Conces DJ Jr, Vix VA, Tarver RD: Pleural cryptococcosis. J Thorac Imaging 5:84–86, 1990.
106. Duperval R, Hermans PE, Brewer NS, et al: Cryptococcosis, with emphasis on the significance of isolation of *Cryptococcus neoformans* from the respiratory tract. Chest 72:13–19, 1977.
107. Connell JV Jr, Mumh JR: Radiographic manifestations of pulmonary histoplasmosis: A 10-yr review. Radiology 121:281–285, 1976.
108. Weissbluth M: Pleural effusion in histoplasmosis. J Pediatr 88:894–895, 1976.
109. Fine NL, Smith LR, Sheedy PF: Frequency of pleural effusions in mycoplasma and viral pneumonias. N Engl J Med 283:790–793, 1970.
110. Alptekin F: An epidemic of pleurisy with effusion in Bitlis, Turkey: Study of 559 cases. US Armed Forces Med J 9:1–11, 1958.
111. Sposito M, Petroni VA, Valeri L: Importanza diagnostica dei piccoli versamenti pleurici nella virus epatite. Epatologia 12:228–231, 1966.
112. Gross PA, Gerding DN: Pleural effusion associated with viral hepatitis. Gastroenterology 60:898–902, 1971.
113. Bustamante EA, Levy H, Simpson SQ: Pleural fluid characteristics in hantavirus pulmonary syndrome. Chest 112:1133–1136, 1997.
114. Setiawan MW, Samsi TK, Wulur H, et al: Dengue haemorrhagic fever: Ultrasound as an aid to predict the severity of the disease. Pediatr Radiol 16:28:1–4, 1998.
115. Light RW, Hamm H: Pleural disease and the acquired immune deficiency syndrome. Eur Respir J 10:2638–2643, 1997.
116. Suay V, Cordero PJ, Martinez E, et al: Parapneumonic effusions secondary to community-acquired bacterial pneumonia in human immunodeficiency virus-infected patients. Eur Respir J 8:1934–1939, 1995.
117. Reed SI: Amebiasis: An update. Clin Infect Dis 15:385–393, 1992.
118. Ibarra-Perez C: Thoracic complications of amebic abscess of the liver. Chest 79:672–676, 1981.
119. Cameron EWJ: The treatment of pleuropulmonary amebiasis with metronidazole. Chest 73:647–650, 1978.
120. Baijal SS, Agarwal DK, Roy S, et al: Complex ruptured amebic liver abscesses: The role of percutaneous catheter drainage. Eur J Radiol 20:65–67, 1995.
121. Aguilar X, Fernandez-Muixi J, Magarolasm R, et al: An unusual presentation of secondary pleural hydatidosis. Eur Respir J 11:243–245, 1998.
122. Xanthakis DS, Katsaras E, Efthimiadis M, et al: Hydatid cyst of the liver with intrathoracic rupture. Thorax 36:497–501, 1981.
123. Barzilai A, Pollack S, Kaftori JK, et al: Splenic echinococcal cyst burrowing into left pleural space. Chest 72:543–545, 1977.
124. Im JG, Whang HY, Kim WS, et al: Pleuropulmonary paragonimiasis: Radiologic findings in 71 patients. AJR Am J Roentgenol 159:39–43, 1992.
125. Johnson RJ, Johnson JR: Paragonimiasis in Indochinese refugees. Am Rev Respir Dis 128:534–538, 1983.
126. Pachucki CT, Levandowski RA, Brown VA, et al: American paragonimiasis treated with praziquantel. N Engl J Med 311:582–583, 1984.
127. Erzurum SE, Underwood GA, Hamilos DL, et al: Pleural effusion in Churg-Strauss syndrome. Chest 95:1357–1359, 1989.
128. Sharma OP: The man who loved drunken crabs: A case of pulmonary paragonimiasis. Chest 95:670–672, 1989.
129. Dietrick RB, Sade RM, Pak JS: Results of decortication in chronic empyema with special reference to paragonimiasis. J Thorac Cardiovasc Surg 82:58–62, 1981.
130. Horowitz ML, Schiff M, Samuels J, et al: *Pneumocystis carinii* pleural effusion: Pathogenesis and pleural fluid analysis. Am Rev Respir Dis 148:232–234, 1993.
131. Goldhaber SZ: Pulmonary embolism. N Engl J Med 339:93–104, 1998.
132. Stein PD, Henry JW: Clinical characteristics of patients with acute pulmonary embolism stratified according to their presenting syndromes. Chest 112:974–979, 1997.
133. Cheng DS, Rodriguez RM, Perkett EA, et al: Vascular endothelial growth factor (VEGF) in pleural fluid. Am J Respir Dis Crit Care Med 115:760–765, 1999.
134. PIOPED Investigators: Value of the ventilation/perfusion scan in acute pulmonary embolism. Results of the prospective investigation of pulmonary embolism diagnosis (PIOPED). JAMA 263:2753–2759, 1990.
134a. Bynum LJ, Wilson JE III: Radiographic features of pleural effusions in pulmonary embolism. Am Rev Respir Dis 117:829–834, 1978.
135. Coche EE, Muller NL, Kim KI, et al: Acute pulmonary embolism: Ancillary findings at spiral CT. Radiology 207:753–758, 1998.
136. Baum S, Vincent NR, Lyons KP, et al: Atlas of Nuclear Medicine Imaging. New York: Appleton-Century-Crofts, 1981.
137. Light RW: Pleural effusion due to pulmonary embolism. *In* Pleural Diseases (3rd ed). Baltimore: Williams & Wilkins, 1995, pp 187–191.
137a. Shah AA, Davis SD, Gamsu G, et al: Parenchymal and pleural findings in patients with and patients without acute pulmonary embolism detected at spiral CT. Radiology 211:147–153, 1999.
138. Rostand RA, Feldman RL, Block ER: Massive hemothorax complicating heparin anticoagulation for pulmonary embolus. South Med J 70:1128–1130, 1977.
139. Michel L, Grillo HC, Malt RA: Operative and nonoperative management of esophageal perforations. Ann Surg 194:57–63, 1981.
140. Bufkin BL, Miller JI Jr, Mansour KA: Esophageal perforation: Emphasis on management. Ann Thorac Surg 61:1447–1451, 1996.
141. Maulitz RM, Good JT Jr, Kaplan RL, et al: The pleuropulmonary consequences of esophageal rupture: An experimental model. Am Rev Respir Dis 120:363–367, 1979.
142. Tesler MA, Eisenberg MM: Spontaneous esophageal rupture. Int Abstr Surg 117:1–9, 1963.
143. Abbott OA, Mansour KA, Logan WD, et al: Atraumatic so-called "spontaneous" rupture of the esophagus. J Thorac Cardiovasc Surg 59:67–83, 1970.
144. Rudin JS, Ellrodt AG, Phillips EH: Low pleural fluid amylase associated with spontaneous rupture of the esophagus. Arch Intern Med 143:1034–1035, 1983.
145. Sherr HP, Light RW, Merson MH, et al: Origin of pleural fluid amylase in esophageal rupture. Ann Intern Med 76:985–986, 1972.
146. Good JT, Antony VB, Reller LB, et al: The pathogenesis of the low pleural fluid pH in esophageal rupture. Am Rev Respir Dis 127:702–704, 1983.
147. Eriksen KR: Oesophagopleural fistula diagnosed by microscopic examination of pleural fluid. Acta Chir Scand 128:771–777, 1964.
148. Ginai AZ: Experimental evaluation of various available contrast agents for use in the gastrointestinal tract in case of suspected leakage: Effects on pleura. Br J Radiol 59:887–894, 1986.
149. Bufkin BL, Miller JI Jr, Mansour KA: Esophageal perforation: Emphasis on management. Ann Thorac Surg 61:1447–1451, 1996.

150. Lankisch PG, Groge M, Becher R: Pleural effusions: A new negative prognostic parameter for acute pancreatitis. Am J Gastroenterol 89:1849–1851, 1994.
151. Roseman DM, Kowlessar OD, Sleisenger MH: Pulmonary manifestations of pancreatitis. N Engl J Med 263:294–296, 1960.
152. Rockey DC, Cello JP: Pancreaticopleural fistula: Report of 7 patients and review of the literature. Medicine 69:332–344, 1990.
153. Kramer MR, Saidana MJ, Cepero RJ, et al: High amylase levels in neoplasm-related pleural effusion. Ann Intern Med 110:567–569, 1989.
154. Pederzoli P, Bassi C, Falconi M, et al: Conservative treatment of external pancreatic fistulas with parenteral nutrition alone or in combination with continuous intravenous infusion of somatostatin, glucagon or calcitonin. Surg Gynecol Obstet 163:428–432, 1986.
155. Lang EK, Paolini RM, Pottmeyer A: The efficacy of palliative and definitive percutaneous versus surgical drainage of pancreatic abscesses and pseudocysts: A prospective study of 85 patients. South Med J 84:55–64, 1991.
156. Lipsett PA, Cameron JL: Internal pancreatic fistula. Am J Surg 163:216–220, 1992.
157. van der Sluis RF: Subphrenic abscess. Surg Gynecol Obstet 158:427–430, 1984.
158. Miller TA, Lindenauer SM, Frey CF, et al: Pancreatic abscess. Arch Surg 108:545–551, 1974.
159. Johnson JF, Raff MJ, Barnwell PA, et al: Splenic abscess complicating infectious endocarditis. Arch Intern Med 143:906–912, 1983.
160. Rubin RH, Swartz MN, Malt R: Hepatic abscess: Changes in clinical, bacteriologic and therapeutic aspects. Am J Med 57:601–610, 1974.
161. Haaga JR, Weinstein AJ: CT-guided percutaneous aspiration and drainage of abscesses. AJR Am J Roentgenol 135:1187–1194, 1980.
162. Voros D, Gouliamos A, Kotoulas G, et al: Percutaneous drainage of intra-abdominal abscesses using large lumen tubes under computed tomographic control. Eur J Surg 162:895–898, 1996.
163. Aronchick JM, Epstein DM, Gefter WB, et al: Chronic traumatic diaphragmatic hernia: The significance of pleural effusion. Radiology 168:675–678, 1988.
164. Light RW, George RB: Incidence and significance of pleural effusion after abdominal surgery. Chest 69:621–626, 1976.
165. Nielsen PH, Jepsen SB, Olsen AD: Postoperative pleural effusion following upper abdominal surgery. Chest 96:1133–1135, 1989.
166. Edling JE, Bacon BR: Pleuropulmonary complications of endoscopic variceal sclerotherapy. Chest 99:1252–1257, 1991.
167. Parikh SS, Amarapurkar DN, Dhawan PS, et al: Development of pleural effusion after sclerotherapy with absolute alcohol. Gastrointest Endosc 39:404–405, 1993.
168. Spizarny DL, Gross BH, McLoud T: Enlarging pleural effusion after liver transplantation. J Thorac Imaging 8:85–87, 1993.
169. Afessa B, Gay PC, Plevak DJ, et al: Pulmonary complications of orthotopic liver transplantation. Mayo Clin Proc 68:427–434, 1993.
170. Uetsuji S, Komada Y, Kwon AH, et al: Prevention of pleural effusion after hepatectomy using fibrin sealant. Int Surg 79:135–137, 1994.
171. Delco F, Domenighetti G, Kauzlaric D, et al: Spontaneous biliothorax (thoracobilia) following cholecystopleural fistula presenting as an acute respiratory insufficiency: Successful removal of gallstones from the pleural space. Chest 106:961–963, 1994.
172. Horler AR, Thompson M: The pleural and pulmonary complications of rheumatoid arthritis. Ann Intern Med 51:1179–1203, 1959.
173. Walker WC, Wright V: Rheumatoid pleuritis. Ann Rheum Dis 26:467–474, 1967.
174. Pettersson T, Soderblom T, Nyberg P, et al: Pleural fluid soluble interleukin 2 receptor in rheumatoid arthritis and systemic lupus erythematosus. J Rheumatol 21:1820–1824, 1994.
175. Halla JT, Schrohenloher RE, Volanakis JE: Immune complexes and other laboratory features of pleural effusions. Ann Intern Med 92:748–752, 1980.
176. Ferguson GC: Cholesterol pleural effusion in rheumatoid lung disease. Thorax 21:577–582, 1966.
177. Jones FL, Blodgett RC: Empyema in rheumatoid pleuropulmonary disease. Ann Intern Med 74:665–671, 1971.
178. Chapman PT, O'Donnell JL, Moller PW: Rheumatoid pleural effusion: Response to intrapleural corticosteroid. Rheumatology 19:478–480, 1992.
179. Yarbrough JW, Sealy WC, Miller JA: Thoracic surgical problems associated with rheumatoid arthritis. J Thorac Cardiovasc Surg 68:347–354, 1975.
180. Winslow WA, Ploss LN, Loitman B: Pleuritis in systemic lupus erythematosus: Its importance as an early manifestation in diagnosis. Ann Intern Med 49:70–88, 1958.
181. Light RW: Pleural effusion due to drug reaction. *In* Pleural Diseases (3rd ed). Baltimore: Williams & Wilkins, 1995, pp 219–223.
182. Good JT Jr, King TE, Antony VB, et al: Lupus pleuritis: Clinical features and pleural fluid characteristics with special reference to pleural fluid antinuclear antibodies. Chest 84:714–718, 1983.
183. Khare V, Baethge B, Lang S, et al: Antinuclear antibodies in pleural fluid. Chest 106:866–871, 1994.
184. Wang DY, Yang PC, Yu WL, et al: Antinuclear antibodies in pleural and pericardial fluid. Chest, in press.
185. Chao TY, Huang SH, Chu CC: Lupus erythematosus cells in pleural effusions: Diagnostic of systemic lupus erythematosus? Acta Cytol 41:1231–1233, 1997.
186. Vargas FS, Milanez JR, Filomeno LT, et al: Intrapleural talc for the prevention of recurrence in benign or undiagnosed pleural effusion. Chest 106:1771–1775, 1994.
187. Light RW: Pleural effusion due to miscellaneous diseases. *In* Pleural Diseases (3rd ed). Baltimore: Williams & Wilkins, 1995, pp 224–241.
188. Engle MA, Zabriskie JB, Senterfit LB, et al: Post pericardiotomy syndrome: A new look at an old condition. Mod Concep Cardiovasc Dis 44:59–64, 1975.
189. Stelzner TJ, King TE Jr, Antony VB, et al: The pleuropulmonary manifestations of postcardiac injury syndrome. Chest 84:383–388, 1983.
190. Urschel HC Jr, Razzuk MA, Gardner M: Coronary artery bypass occlusion secondary to postcardiotomy syndrome. Ann Thorac Surg 22:528–531, 1976.
191. Dressler W: The post-myocardial infarction syndrome. Arch Intern Med 103:28–42, 1959.
192. Peng MJ, Vargas FS, Cukier A, et al: Postoperative pleural changes after coronary revascularization: Comparison between saphenous vein and internal mammary artery grafting. Chest 101:327–330, 1992.
193. Hurlburt D, Myers ML, Lefcoe M, et al: Pleuropulmonary morbidity: Internal thoracic artery versus saphenous vein graft. Ann Thorac Surg 50:959–964, 1990.
194. Rodriguez RM, Moyers JP, Rogers JT, et al: Incidence of pleural effusions 30 days post coronary artery bypass surgery. Chest 114:387S, 1998.
195. Light RW, Rogers JT, Cheng D-S, et al: Large pleural effusions occurring after coronary artery bypass grafting. Ann Intern Med 130:891–896, 1999.
196. Medina LS, Siegel MJ, Bejarano PA, et al: Pediatric lung transplantation: Radiographic-histologic correlation. Radiology 187:807–810, 1993.
197. Seber A, Khan SP, Kersey JH: Unexplained effusions: Association with allogeneic bone marrow transplantation and acute or chronic graft-versus-host disease. Bone Marrow Transplant 17:207–211, 1996.
198. Epler GR, McLoud TC, Gaensler EA: Prevalence and incidence of benign asbestos pleural effusion in a working population. JAMA 247:617–622, 1982.
199. Nishimura SL, Broaddus VC: Asbestos-induced pleural disease. Clin Chest Med 19:311–329, 1998.
200. Hillerdal G: Nonmalignant pleural disease related to asbestos exposure. Clin Chest Med 6:141–152, 1985.
201. Hillerdal G, Ozesmi M: Benign asbestos pleural effusion: 73 exudates in 60 patients. Eur J Respir Dis 71:113–121, 1987.
202. Adelman M, Albelda SM, Gottlieb J, et al: Diagnostic utility of pleural fluid eosinophilia. Am J Med 77:915–920, 1984.
203. Lanham JG, Elkon KB, Pusey CD, et al: Systemic vasculitis with asthma and eosinophilia: A clinical approach to the Churg-Strauss syndrome. Medicine 63:65–81, 1984.
204. Chusid EL, Siltzbach LE: Sarcoidosis of the pleura. Ann Intern Med 81:190–194, 1974.

205. Beekman JF, Zimmet SM, Chun BK, et al: Spectrum of pleural involvement in sarcoidosis. Arch Intern Med 136:323–330, 1976.
206. Wilen SB, Rabinowitz JG, Ulreich S, et al: Pleural involvement in sarcoidosis. Am J Med 57:200–209, 1974.
207. Nicholls AJ, Friend JAR, Legge JS: Sarcoid pleural effusion: Three cases and review of the literature. Thorax 35:277–281, 1980.
208. Nidus BD, Matalon R, Cantacuzino D, et al: Uremic pleuritis: A clinicopathological entity. N Engl J Med 281:255–256, 1969.
209. Berger HW, Rammohan G, Neff MS, et al: Uremic pleural effusion: A study in 14 patients on chronic dialysis. Ann Intern Med 82:362–364, 1975.
210. Rodelas R, Rakowski TA, Argy WP, et al: Fibrosing uremic pleuritis during hemodialysis. JAMA 243:2424–2425, 1980.
211. Baron RL, Stark DD, McClennan BL, et al: Intrathoracic extension of retroperitoneal urine collections. AJR Am J Roentgenol 137:37–41, 1981.
212. Meigs JV, Cass JW: Fibroma of the ovary with ascites and hydrothorax. Am J Obstet Gynecol 33:249–267, 1937.
213. Kirschner PA: Porous diaphragm syndromes. Chest Surg Clin North Am 8:449–472, 1998.
214. Muneyyirci-Delale O, Neil G, Serur E, et al: Endometriosis with massive ascites. Gynecol Oncol 69:42–46, 1998.
214a. Abramov Y, Eichalal U, Schenker JG: Pulmonary manifestations of severe ovarian hyperstimulation syndrome: a multicenter study. Fertil Steril 71:645–651, 1999.
215. Elchalal U, Schenker JG: The pathophysiology of ovarian hyperstimulation syndrome: Views and ideas. Hum Reprod 12:1129–1137, 1997.
216. Mukherjee D, Lange P, Sferry C, et al: Dyspnea, cough, and chest pain in a 35-year-old pregnant woman. Chest 107:1460–1462, 1995.
217. Beer DJ, Pereira W Jr, Snider GL: Pleural effusion associated with primary lymphedema: A perspective on the yellow nail syndrome. Am Rev Respir Dis 117:595–599, 1978.
218. Lewis M, Kallenbach JA, Zaltzman M, et al: Pleurectomy in the management of massive pleural effusion associated with primary lymphoedema: Demonstration of abnormal pleural lymphatics. Thorax 38:637–639, 1983.
219. Antony VB: Drug-induced pleural disease. Clin Chest Med 19:331–340, 1998.
219a. Morelock SY, Sahn SA: Drugs and the pleura. Chest 116:212–221, 1999.
220. Holmberg L, Boman G: Pulmonary reactions to nitrofurantoin: 447 cases reported to the Swedish adverse drug reaction committee, 1966–1976. Eur J Respir Dis 62:180–189, 1981.
221. Geller M, Flaherty DK, Dickie HA, et al: Lymphopenia in acute nitrofurantoin pleuropulmonary reactions. J Allergy Clin Immunol 59:445–448, 1977.
222. Petusevsky ML, Faling LJ, Rocklin RE, et al: Pleuropericardial reaction to treatment with dantrolene. JAMA 242:2772–2774, 1979.
223. Kok-Jensen A, Lindeneg O: Pleurisy and fibrosis of the pleura during methysergide treatment of hemicrania. Scand J Respir Dis 51:218–222, 1970.
224. Graham JR: Cardiac and pulmonary fibrosis during methysergide therapy for headache. Am J Med Sci 254:1–12, 1967.
225. McElvaney NG, Wilcox PG, Churg A, et al: Pleuropulmonary disease during bromocriptine treatment of Parkinson's disease. Arch Intern Med 148:2231–2236, 1988.
226. Hillerdal G, Lee J, Blomkvist A, et al: Pleural disease during treatment with bromocriptine in patients previously exposed to asbestos. Eur Respir J 10:2711–2715, 1997.
227. Jones SE, Moore M, Blank N, et al: Hypersensitivity to procarbazine (Matulane) manifested by fever and pleuropulmonary reaction. Cancer 29:498–500, 1972.
228. Ecker MD, Jay B, Keohane MF: Procarbazine lung. AJR Am J Roentgenol 131:527–528, 1978.
229. Gonzalez-Rothi RJ, Hannan SE, Hood I, et al: Amiodarone pulmonary toxicity presenting as bilateral exudative pleural effusions. Chest 92:179–182, 1987.
230. Stein B, Zaatari GS, Pine JR: Amiodarone pulmonary toxicity: Clinical, cytologic and ultrastructural findings. Acta Cytol 31:357–361, 1987.
231. Bachman AL, Macken K: Pleural effusions following supervoltage radiation for breast carcinoma. Radiology 72:699–709, 1959.
232. Fentanes de Torres E, Guevara E: Pleuritis by radiation: Report of two cases. Acta Cytol 25:427–429, 1981.
233. Duntley P, Seiver J, Forwess ML, et al: Vascular erosin by central venous catheter. Clinical features and outcomes. Chest 101:1633–1638, 1992.
234. Roubenoff R, Ravich WJ: Pneumothorax due to nasogastric feeding tubes: Report of four cases, review of the literature, and recommendations for prevention. Arch Intern Med 149:184–188, 1989.
235. Miller KS, Tomlinson JR, Sahn SA: Pleuropulmonary complications of enteral tube feedings. Chest 88:231–233, 1985.

# 75 Pneumothorax, Chylothorax, Hemothorax, and Fibrothorax

RICHARD W. LIGHT, M.D. • V. COURTNEY BROADDUS, M.D.


Introduction
Pathophysiology of Pneumothorax
Primary Spontaneous Pneumothorax
- Incidence
- Etiologic Factors
- Clinical Manifestations
- Diagnosis
- Recurrence Rates
- Treatment

Secondary Spontaneous Pneumothorax
- Incidence
- Etiologic Factors
- Clinical Manifestations
- Diagnosis
- Recurrence Rates
- Treatment
- Pneumothorax Secondary to *P. carinii* in Patients with AIDS
- Pneumothorax Secondary to Tuberculosis

Iatrogenic Pneumothorax
- Diagnosis
- Treatment

Traumatic (Noniatrogenic) Pneumothorax
- Mechanism
- Diagnosis and Treatment

Neonatal Pneumothorax
- Pathogenesis
- Clinical Manifestations
- Treatment

Catamenial Pneumothorax
- Pathogenesis
- Diagnosis and Treatment

Tension Pneumothorax
- Pathophysiology
- Clinical Manifestations
- Diagnosis and Treatment

Re-expansion Pulmonary Edema
- Pathophysiology
- Clinical Manifestations
- Prevention

Chylothorax
- Pathophysiology
- Etiology
- Clinical Manifestations
- Diagnosis
- Treatment
- Pulmonary Lymphangiomyomatosis

Chyliform Pleural Effusions and Pseudochylothorax
- Pathogenesis
- Clinical Manifestations
- Diagnosis
- Treatment

Hemothorax
- Traumatic Hemothorax
- Iatrogenic Hemothorax
- Nontraumatic Hemothorax
- Hemothorax Complicating Anticoagulant Therapy

Fibrothorax
- Diagnosis
- Treatment

Summary


## Introduction

By definition, a pneumothorax is present when there is air in the pleural space. Pneumothoraces are classified as *spontaneous pneumothoraces,* which occur without preceding trauma or other obvious cause, and *traumatic pneumothoraces,* which occur as a result of direct or indirect trauma to the chest, sometimes as a result of a diagnostic or therapeutic maneuver (*iatrogenic pneumothorax*). Spontaneous pneumothoraces are subclassified as *primary* or *secondary spontaneous pneumothoraces.* A primary spontaneous pneumothorax occurs in an otherwise healthy person without underlying lung disease. A secondary spontaneous pneumothorax is a complication of an underlying lung disease, most commonly chronic obstructive pulmonary disease.

Most pleural effusions prove to be either an exudate or a transudate according to the criteria provided in Chapter 73. Occasionally, the liquid contents turn out to be chyle, chylous fluid, or blood. This chapter also describes the pathogenesis and clinical manifestations of chylothorax, chyliform pleural effusions and pseudochylothorax, and hemothorax. In addition, the sequelae of chronic organizing pleural disease of any origin—fibrothorax—is also considered.

## PATHOPHYSIOLOGY OF PNEUMOTHORAX

In normal people, the pressure in the pleural space is negative with respect to the alveolar pressure during the entire respiratory cycle. The pressure gradient between the alveoli and the pleural space, the transpulmonary pressure, is the result of the inherent elastic recoil of the lung. During spontaneous breathing, the pleural pressure is also negative with respect to the atmospheric pressure. The functional residual capacity, or resting end-expiratory volume of the lung, is the volume at which the inherent outward pull of the chest wall is equal to, but opposite in direction to, the inward pull (recoil) of the lung.[1]

When a communication develops between an alveolus or other intrapulmonary air space and the pleural space, air will flow from the alveolus into the pleural space until there is no longer a pressure difference or until the communication is sealed. Similarly, when a communication develops through the chest wall between the atmosphere and the pleural space, air will enter the pleural space until the pressure gradient is eliminated or the communication is closed. The influence of a pneumothorax on the volume of the hemithorax and the lung is illustrated in Figure 75.1. When sufficient air enters the pleural space to increase the pleural pressure from −5 to −2.5 cm $H_2O$, the transpulmonary or recoil pressure decreases from 5 to 2.5 cm $H_2O$. The amount of air necessary to effect this change in the pleural pressure is equal to 33% of the patient's vital capacity. The largest

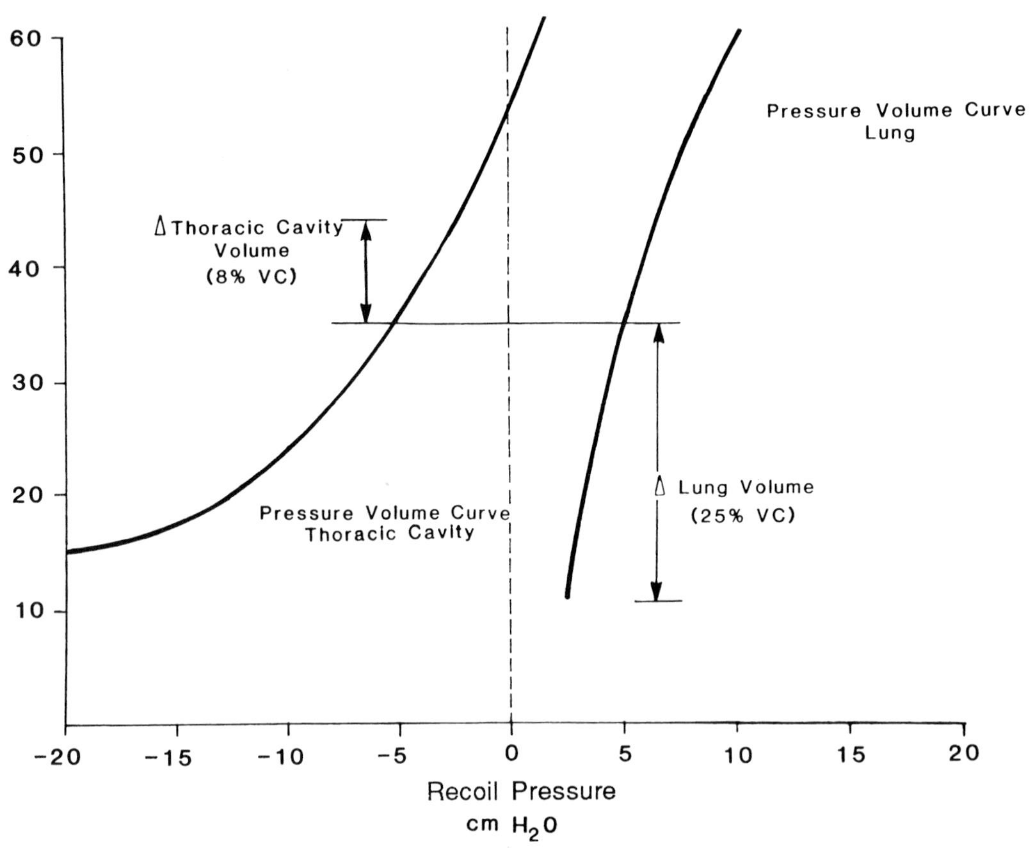


**Figure 75.1** Influence of a pneumothorax on the volumes of the lung and hemithorax. Note that the volume of a hemithorax becomes larger as the volume of the lung becomes smaller because of the changes in recoil pressure. The changes in volumes of the thoracic cavity and lung are unequal because of differences in the slopes of their respective pressure-volume curves. VC = vital capacity. (Reproduced with permission from Light RW: Pleural Diseases (3rd ed). Baltimore: Williams & Wilkins, 1995, p 244.)

portion of this pleural air displaces air from the lung as the functional residual capacity decreases from 35% to 10% of the original vital capacity. The increase in pleural pressure also changes the recoil pressure acting across the chest wall, which allows the thoracic cavity to expand along its pressure-volume curve. The increase in the pleural pressure also causes a shift of the mediastinum to the contralateral side, an enlarged hemithorax, and a depressed hemidiaphragm. These findings do not necessarily indicate that a tension pneumothorax is present.[1]

The main physiologic consequences of a pneumothorax are a decrease in the vital capacity (as illustrated in Fig. 75.1) and a decrease in the arterial $Po_2$. In patients with primary spontaneous pneumothorax, the decrease in the vital capacity is usually well tolerated. If the lung function of the patient is abnormal before the development of the pneumothorax, however, the decrease in vital capacity may lead to respiratory insufficiency with alveolar hypoventilation and respiratory acidosis.

Most patients with a pneumothorax have a reduced arterial $Po_2$ and an increase in the alveolar-arterial oxygen tension difference. In a series of 12 patients with spontaneous penumothorax, the arterial $Po_2$ was below 80 mm Hg in 9 (75%) and was below 55 mm Hg in 2 patients, both of whom had secondary spontaneous pneumothorax.[2]

The reduction in arterial $Po_2$ appears to be caused by areas with low ventilation-perfusion ratios, anatomic shunts, and, occasionally, alveolar hypoventilation. Norris and coworkers[2] reported that the average right-to-left shunt in their 12 patients with spontaneous pneumothorax was over 10% while the patients were breathing 100% oxygen. Larger pneumothoraces were associated with greater shunts. When the pneumothorax occupied less than 25% of the hemithorax, the shunt was not increased.[2]

After air is evacuated from the pleural space, the arterial $Po_2$ usually improves, but the improvement may take several hours. Norris and colleagues[2] evacuated the pleural air from three patients with a pneumothorax and an initial anatomic shunt above 20%; within 90 minutes, the shunt had decreased below 10%, but it still remained above 5% in all patients. The delay in improvement may be related to the duration of the pneumothorax.

## PRIMARY SPONTANEOUS PNEUMOTHORAX

### Incidence

Each year, approximately 9000 persons in the United States develop a primary spontaneous pneumothorax. This estimate is based on a study of the residents of Olmsted County, Minnesota, between 1959 and 1978.[3] During this period, when the population of the county averaged 60,000, 77 cases of primary pneumothorax were reported. The age-adjusted incidence was 7.4/100,000/year for men and 1.2/100,000/year for women. When these figures are extrapolated to the entire US population, the annual estimate of 9000 persons is obtained.

### Etiologic Factors

Primary spontaneous pneumothorax is believed to result from rupture of a subpleural emphysematous bleb, which is usually located in the apex of the lung.[4] Blebs can be found in more than 75% of patients undergoing thoracoscopy for treatment of primary spontaneous pneumothorax.[4] The pathogenesis of these subpleural blebs is unclear. Such blebs have been attributed to congenital abnormalities, inflammation of the bronchioles, and disturbances of the collateral ventilation.[4] There is a strong association between smoking and the development of a primary spontaneous pneumothorax. When four separate series of patients with primary spontaneous pneumothorax are combined, 461 of 505 patients (91%) with primary spontaneous pneumothorax were smokers or ex-smokers.[1] The occurrence of a spontaneous pneumothorax is related to the level of cigarette smoking. In men the relative risk of a pneumothorax is 7 times higher in light smokers (1 to 12 cigarettes/day), 21 times higher in moderate smokers (13 to 22 cigarettes/day), and 102 times higher in heavy smokers (>22 cigarettes/day) than in nonsmokers.[5] It is probable that smoking-induced disease of small airways contributes to the development of the subpleural blebs.

Patients with primary spontaneous pneumothorax tend to be taller and thinner than control persons. In one study of military recruits with primary spontaneous pneumothorax, persons with a pneumothorax were on the average 2 inches taller and 25 pounds lighter than the typical military recruit.[6] An increased length of the chest may contribute to the formation of the subpleural blebs. Because pleural pressure falls about 0.20 cm $H_2O$ per cm vertical height, pleural pressure will be more negative at the apex of the lung in taller than shorter people; accordingly, the alveoli at their lung apex are subjected to a greater mean distending pressure. Over an extended period, this could lead to the formation of subpleural blebs in those tall people who are genetically predisposed to bleb formation.

A tendency for the development of a primary spontaneous pneumothorax can be inherited. Some cases are due to an autosomal dominant gene with incomplete penetrance, the penetrance being lower in women (21%) than in men (50%). There also appears to be an inheritance due to an X-linked recessive gene.[7]

### Clinical Manifestations

Primary spontaneous pneumothorax usually develops while the patient is at rest, and only rarely do the initial symptoms occur during heavy exercise.[8] Surprisingly, many patients with spontaneous pneumothorax do not seek medical attention immediately after the development of symptoms. In one series, 18% of patients waited more than 1 week after development of symptoms before obtaining medical help.[9]

Chest pain and dyspnea are the two main symptoms associated with the development of primary spontaneous pneumothorax. In one series of 39 patients with primary spontaneous pneumothorax, every patient had chest pain or dyspnea, and both symptoms were present in 25 of 39 patients (64%).[10] The chest pain usually has an acute onset and is localized to the side of the pneumothorax. A rare complication of spontaneous pneumothorax is Horner's syndrome, which is thought to result from traction on the sympathetic ganglion produced by a shift of the mediastinum.[11]

On physical examination, the vital signs are usually normal, with the exception of a moderate tachycardia. A tension pneumothorax should be suspected if the pulse rate exceeds 140 beats/min or if hypotension, cyanosis, or electromechanical dissociation is present. On examination of the chest, the side with pneumothorax is larger than the contralateral side and moves less during the respiratory cycle. Tactile fremitus is absent, the percussion note is hyperresonant, and the breath sounds are absent or reduced on the affected side. The lower edge of the liver may be shifted inferiorly with a right-sided pneumothorax. With a large pneumothorax, the trachea may be shifted toward the contralateral side.

The presence of a pneumothorax may elicit electrocardiographic changes. With left pneumothorax, all of the following changes have been noted: rightward shift of the frontal QRS axis, diminution of precordial R voltage, decrease in QRS amplitude, and precordial T-wave inversion. With right pneumothorax, the following changes have been noted: diminution of precordial QRS voltage, right axis deviation, and a prominent R wave in lead $V_2$ with associated loss of S-wave voltage, mimicking posterior myocardial infarction.[12] All these changes are thought to be due to mechanical effects and should not be mistaken for cardiac ischemia or infarction.

## Diagnosis

The diagnosis is usually suggested by the clinical history and the physical examination. The diagnosis is established by demonstrating a pleural line on the chest radiograph (Fig. 75.2). In doubtful cases, lateral decubitus films may facilitate the diagnosis. Expiratory films are no more sensitive than inspiratory films in detecting pneumothoraces and are not recommended.[4] A small pleural effusion is associated with a primary spontaneous pneumothorax in approximately 15% of cases and is manifested radiographically as an air-fluid level.[9, 10]

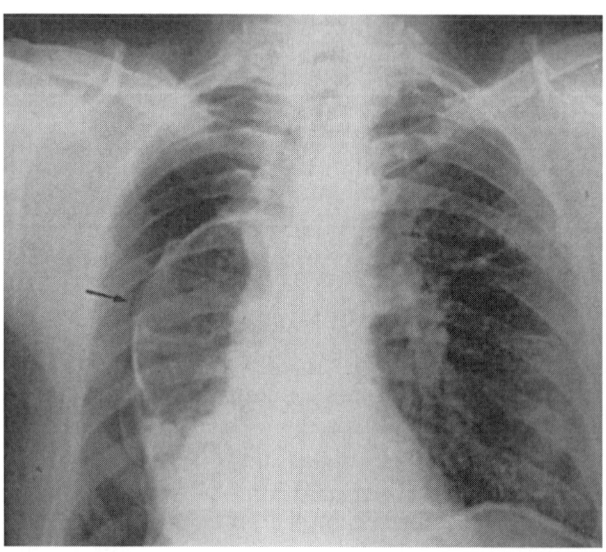

**Figure 75.2** Posteroanterior radiograph demonstrating a pneumothorax on the right side. Note the obvious pleural line (*arrow*) that separates the lung from the air in the pleural space. (Reproduced with permission from Light RW: Pleural Diseases (1st ed). Philadelphia: Lea & Febiger, 1983, p 29.)

The amount of lung collapse should be semiquantitated when one is managing a patient with a pneumothorax. Because the volumes of the lung and the hemithorax are roughly proportional to the cube of their diameters, one can estimate the degree of collapse (PNX %) by measuring average diameters of the lung and the hemithorax, cubing these diameters, and using the following equation:

$$\text{PNX \%} = 100[1 - \text{lung}^3/\text{hemithorax}^3] \quad (1)$$

## Recurrence Rates

Following a primary spontaneous pneumothorax, a patient is at risk of recurrence particularly in the months immediately after the first episode. Sadikot and associates[13] followed up 153 patients with primary spontaneous pneumothorax for a mean of 54 months and reported that 39% had a recurrent ipsilateral pneumothorax, most within the first year. Once a patient has a primary spontaneous pneumothorax there is also an increased risk of having a pneumothorax on the contralateral side. In the report of Sadikot and coworkers,[13] 15% of their 153 patients developed a pneumothorax on the contralateral side as well.

There have been several attempts to predict who will develop recurrent pneumothorax. Patients who are tall and those who continue to smoke are more likely to have a recurrence.[13] Yet, there is no relationship between the number of blebs or the size of the blebs on computed tomography (CT)[14] or the appearance of the lung at thoracotomy[15] and the risk of recurrence. Once a patient has had one recurrence, the risk of another recurrence increases to more than 50%.[16]

## Treatment

There are two goals to managing a patient with a primary spontaneous pneumothorax: to rid the pleural space of its air and to decrease the likelihood of a recurrence. There are several different approaches to the treatment of patients with primary spontaneous pneumothorax. These include observation, supplemental oxygen, simple aspiration of the pneumothorax, simple tube thoracostomy, tube thoracostomy with instillation of a sclerosing agent, thoracoscopy with oversewing of the blebs and pleurodesis, and open thoracotomy. When the appropriate treatment for any given patient is selected, it should be remembered that primary spontaneous pneumothorax is mainly a nuisance and rarely life-threatening to the patient.

**Observation.** Once the communication between the alveoli and the pleural space is eliminated, the air in the pleural space will be gradually reabsorbed. The rate of spontaneous reabsorption is slow. Kircher and Swartzel[17] estimated that 1.25% of the volume of the hemithorax is absorbed each 24 hours. Therefore, if a patient has a 20%

pneumothorax, it will take 16 days for pleural air to be absorbed spontaneously. For this reason, it is recommended that only patients with pneumothoraces occupying less than 15% of the hemithorax be considered for this type of treatment. If the patient is hospitalized, supplemental oxygen should be administered to increase the rate of pleural air absorption.

**Supplemental Oxygen.** In pneumothorax, gases move in and out of the pleural space from the capillaries in the visceral and parietal pleura. The movement of each gas depends on the gradient between its partial pressure in the capillaries and in the pleural space, the blood flow per unit surface area available for gas exchange, and the solubility of each gas in the surrounding tissues. Normally, the sum of all the partial pressures in the capillary blood with a patient breathing room air is about 706 mm Hg ($P_{H_2O} = 47$, $P_{CO_2} = 46$, $P_{N_2} = 573$, and $P_{O_2} = 40$ mm Hg). If it is assumed that the pleural pressure is approximately 0 when there is a pneumothorax, then the net gradient for gas absorption is only 54 mm Hg ($760 - 706$). If the patient is placed on 100% oxygen, however, the sum of all the partial pressures in the capillary blood will probably fall below 200 mm Hg (the $P_{N_2}$ will approach 0, whereas the $P_{O_2}$ will remain under 100 mm Hg). Accordingly, the net gradient for gas absorption will exceed 550 mm Hg or be 10 times greater than it was with the patient breathing room air.[1]

Indeed, the administration of supplemental oxygen accelerates the rate of pleural air absorption in clinical and experimental situations. Chernick and Avery[18] demonstrated that the administration of humidified 100% oxygen to rabbits with experimentally induced pneumothoraces increased the rate of absorption by about sixfold. Subsequent studies in patients with spontaneous pneumothorax have demonstrated that pleural air is absorbed about four times faster when the patients are given high concentrations of supplemental oxygen to breathe.[19] It is recommended that hospitalized patients with any type of pneumothorax who are not subjected to aspiration or tube thoracostomy be treated with supplemental oxygen at high concentrations.

**Simple Aspiration.** The initial treatment for patients with primary spontaneous pneumothoraces greater than 15% of the volume of the hemithorax should probably be simple aspiration.[20, 21] This procedure is successful in approximately 65% of patients with spontaneous pneumothorax. The advantages of this procedure are that, if successful, hospitalization is not required and the small tube is less painful than a large tube. The recurrence rates appear to be similar after simple aspiration and after tube thoracostomy.[20, 21]

With this procedure a relatively small needle (~16 gauge) with an internal polyethylene catheter is inserted into the second anterior intercostal space at the midclavicular line after local anesthesia. An alternative site is selected if the pneumothorax is loculated or if adhesions are present. After the needle is inserted, it is extracted, leaving the catheter tip in the pleural space. A three-way stopcock and a 60-mL syringe are attached to the catheter. Air is manually withdrawn until no more can be aspirated. The catheter is then occluded for several hours. If the chest radiograph confirms that there has been no recurrence, the catheter is removed and the patient is discharged. Alternatively, the patient can be observed in the hospital overnight or can be discharged with a Heimlich valve attached to the catheter. If the total volume of air aspirated exceeds 4 L and no resistance has been felt, it is assumed that there has been no expansion, and alternative procedures are initiated.

It is recommended that most patients with their first primary spontaneous pneumothorax be managed initially with simple aspiration on an outpatient basis. For patients who reside more than 15 minutes from the hospital, consideration can be given to observing them overnight in the hospital. Patients should return in 24 to 72 hours for a follow-up chest radiograph. If aspiration is unsuccessful, then either thoracoscopy or tube thoracostomy should be undertaken. Because a patient with a first primary spontaneous pneumothorax has less than a 50% likelihood of developing a recurrent ipsilateral spontaneous pneumothorax and because a pneumothorax is primarily a nuisance rather than life-threatening, there is little reason to go to great lengths to prevent a recurrence. Simple aspiration is not recommended for patients with secondary spontaneous pneumothoraces or for recurrent primary spontaneous pneumothoraces.

**Tube Thoracostomy.** For the past several decades, most patients with primary spontaneous pneumothorax have been managed initially with tube thoracostomy. This procedure is recommended if simple aspiration proves ineffective and thoracoscopy is not readily available; it rapidly results in the re-expansion of the underlying lung and does not require prolonged hospitalization. In one series of 81 patients treated with tube thoracostomy, the average duration of hospitalization was only 4 days, with a range of 3 to 6 days. Only three patients (4%) had persistent air leaks after several days of chest tube drainage.[9] Indeed, it has been demonstrated that patients with primary spontaneous pneumothorax can be managed as outpatients with Heimlich valves.[22]

When a spontaneous pneumothorax is managed with tube thoracostomy, relatively small tubes (12 to 16 Fr) appear to be as effective as larger tubes.[22] Because the risk of re-expansion pulmonary edema is greater when the lung is re-expanded rapidly, it is probably better to use water seal and to avoid suction for the first 24 hours of tube thoracostomy.[23]

After the lung has re-expanded and the air leak has ceased for 24 hours, the chest tube can be removed. There is probably no reason to clamp the tube before its removal. If the lung remains unexpanded or if there is a persistent air leak 72 hours after tube thoracostomy, consideration should be given to performing thoracoscopy or thoracotomy. There is no evidence that the intrapleural injection of a sclerosing agent facilitates closure of a bronchopleural fistula.[24]

**Tube Thoracostomy with Instillation of a Sclerosing Agent.** Because many patients with an initial primary spontaneous pneumothorax will have a recurrence, efforts have been made to diminish the recurrence rates by injecting sclerosing agents into the pleural space at the time of initial episode. The two agents most commonly used are doxycycline and talc slurry. The administration of one of these agents will reduce the recurrence rates from approximately 40% to 25% (Fig. 75.3).[24, 25] However, because thoracoscopy with stapling of blebs and pleural abrasion reduces the recurrence rate to less than 5%,[26] the thoracoscopic procedure is preferred if it is readily available. Because the administration of talc intrapleurally may be associated with the development of the acute respiratory distress syndrome,[27, 27a] a tetracycline derivative (e.g., doxycycline 500 mg) is probably the agent of choice. Bleomycin is not recommended for pneumothoraces because animal studies have demonstrated that it does not produce a pleurodesis when the pleura is normal.[28, 29]

The procedure for the intrapleural instillation of doxycycline is outlined in Chapter 76 in the discussion of malignant pleural effusions. Because the injection of a tetracycline derivative can be very painful, particularly in a patient with a pneumothorax and a relatively normal pleura, heavy sedation should be given before sclerosis.

**Thoracoscopy.** As video-thoracoscopy becomes more widely available, patients with spontaneous pneumothorax are increasingly being managed with thoracoscopy. It is the procedure of choice if aspiration fails or if the patient has a recurrent pneumothorax. During video-thoracoscopy, attempts are made to eliminate the blebs responsible for the pneumothorax and to create a pleurodesis. The primary means by which the blebs have been treated is with endo-stapling. The disadvantage of endo-stapling is that it is expensive. When this is a concern, the apical blebs and bullae can be managed by thoracoscopic suturing.[30] Pleurodesis is probably best induced by pleural abrasion.[31]

Primary spontaneous pneumothorax is managed well with video-thoracoscopy. When three series with a total of 384 patients are combined, only 14 (3.6%) of the patients had a recurrence with a follow-up period of more than 1 year.[31–33] The median duration of hospitalization for patients treated with thoracoscopy is about 3 days. The most common complication of video-thoracoscopy for the treatment of primary spontaneous pneumothorax is a persistent air leak, which occurs in less than 5%.[32] Video-thoracoscopy is preferred to thoracotomy because the hospitalization times are shorter and there is less morbidity.[34]

**Open Thoracotomy.** When video-thoracoscopy is not available, open thoracotomy with oversewing of the blebs and pleural abrasion is a reasonable alternative. It should be considered when an air leak persists or the lung remains unexpanded after 3 days of chest tube drainage, or if a patient has had more than one recurrent primary spontaneous pneumothorax.

Thoracotomy is effective in preventing recurrences.[35, 36] In one large series of 362 patients undergoing parietal pleurectomy, there were only two documented ipsilateral recurrences with an average follow-up period of 4.5 years in 310 patients.[35] There was a single death attributable to the operative procedure, and the average postoperative period of hospitalization was only 6 days.[35] Various methods have been used for scarification of the pleural surfaces, ranging from visceral and parietal pleurectomy to abrasion of the pleura with dry sponges. Because all appear to be equally effective, pleural abrasion with dry

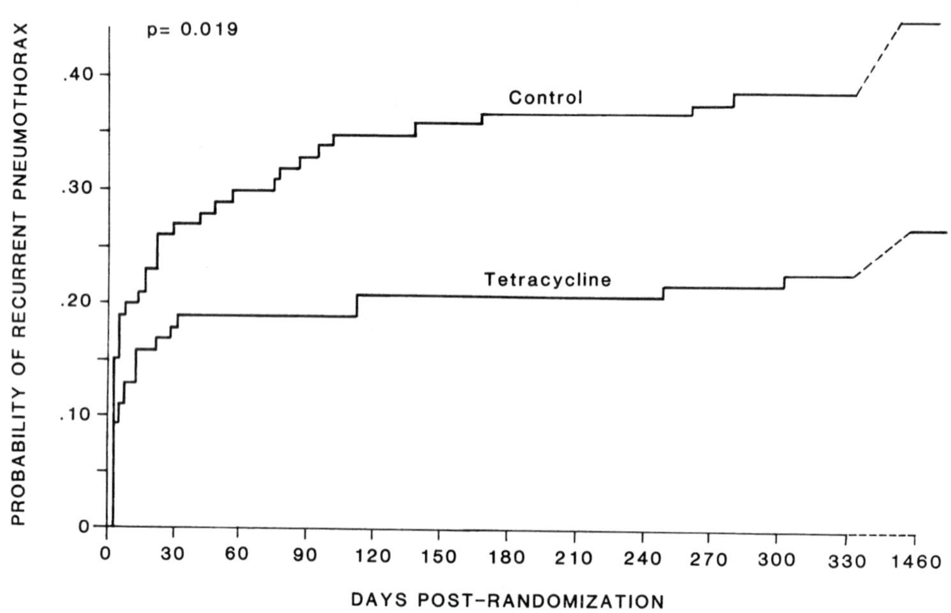


**Figure 75.3** Probability of recurrent pneumothorax after assignment to the tetracycline or the control group in the Veterans Administration cooperative study on spontaneous pneumothorax. (Reproduced with permission from Light RW, O'Hara VS, Moritz TE, et al: Intrapleural tetracycline for the prevention of recurrent spontaneous pneumothorax. JAMA 264:2224–2230, 1990.)

gauze is recommended because it is less traumatic than pleurectomy and does not affect a subsequent thoracotomy.[37]

In summary, most patients with their first primary spontaneous pneumothorax should be managed initially with simple aspiration of the pleural air with a plastic catheter. If this is ineffective, thoracoscopy should be performed promptly, with endo-stapling of blebs and pleural abrasion to create a pleurodesis. Patients with recurrent primary spontaneous pneumothorax should undergo thoracoscopy. When thoracoscopy is unavailable, patients who fail aspiration should be managed with tube thoracostomy with an attempt at pleurodesis with either doxycycline or talc. If, after 3 days of thoracostomy drainage, there is a persistent air leak or the lungs have not re-expanded, thoracotomy should be considered.

## SECONDARY SPONTANEOUS PNEUMOTHORAX

A secondary spontaneous pneumothorax is more serious than a primary spontaneous pneumothorax because it further decreases the pulmonary function of a patient whose reserve is already diminished. In addition, the presence of the underlying lung disease makes management of the pneumothorax more difficult.

### Incidence

The incidence of secondary spontaneous pneumothorax is similar to that of primary spontaneous pneumothorax. It has been estimated that there are about 8000 new cases of secondary spontaneous pneumothorax in the United States each year. Secondary spontaneous pneumothoraces are three times more common in men than in women.[3]

### Etiologic Factors

Chronic obstructive pulmonary disease (COPD) is the most common underlying disease in patients with secondary spontaneous pneumothorax, although almost any lung disease can lead to secondary spontaneous pneumothorax. In one series of 45 patients with secondary spontaneous pneumothorax, 30 patients had COPD, 6 had tuberculosis, 4 had sarcoidosis, and 5 had miscellaneous diseases.[38] Among patients with COPD, the incidence of secondary spontaneous pneumothorax increases with progressive severity of the COPD. In the Veterans Administration cooperative study[24] on pneumothorax, 27% of the 229 participants had an $FEV_1$/FVC ratio below 0.40. In the last few years, one of the diseases most commonly associated with secondary spontaneous pneumothorax has become acquired immunodeficiency syndrome (AIDS)–associated *Pneumocystis carinii* infection.[39–41] There is also a high incidence of spontaneous pneumothorax in patients with cystic fibrosis. In a series of 144 patients older than 10 years with cystic fibrosis, 12.5% had experienced a secondary spontaneous pneumothorax.[42]

### Clinical Manifestations

In general, the clinical symptoms associated with secondary spontaneous pneumothorax are more severe than are those associated with primary spontaneous pneumothorax. In the series of 57 patients with COPD and pneumothorax reported by Dines and coworkers,[43] all patients complained of shortness of breath, 74% had chest pain on the side of the pneumothorax, 9% were cyanotic, and 7% were hypotensive. Although earlier studies reported a mortality rate that exceeded 10% with pneumothorax secondary to COPD,[43–45] in the large Veterans Administration cooperative study the mortality rate from pneumothorax was only 1%.[24]

### Diagnosis

The possibility of a pneumothorax should be considered in every patient with COPD who suddenly has increasing shortness of breath, particularly if there is associated chest pain. The physical examination of a patient with a secondary spontaneous pneumothorax is less helpful in establishing the diagnosis than it is in a patient with a primary spontaneous pneumothorax. The patients with underlying disease may already have hyperexpanded lungs, decreased tactile fremitus, a hyperresonant percussion note, and distant breath sounds over both lung fields. Accordingly, when a pneumothorax develops, side-to-side differences in the physical examination may not be apparent.

The diagnosis of secondary spontaneous pneumothorax is established by the demonstration of a pleural line on the chest radiograph. It is sometimes difficult to see this line in radiographs of patients with COPD because the hyperlucent emphysematous lung shows little difference in radiodensity with the pneumothorax. Frequently, the presence of the pneumothorax is overlooked on the initial chest radiograph, particularly when the film is overexposed. In patients with lung disease, the radiographic appearance of the pneumothorax can be altered by the underlying abnormalities. Areas of normal lung collapse more evenly and completely than do diseased areas with large bullae or severe emphysema, which have a decreased elastic recoil and may trap gas.

It is important to distinguish a spontaneous pneumothorax from a large, thin-walled, air-containing bulla in patients with COPD. The apparent pleural line with a large bulla is usually concave toward the lateral chest wall, whereas the pleural line with a pneumothorax is usually oriented convexly toward the lateral chest wall. At times CT examination of the chest is necessary to make this differentiation.[46]

### Recurrence Rates

It appears that the recurrence rates for secondary spontaneous pneumothoraces are somewhat higher than are those for primary spontaneous pneumothoraces if the patients are not treated with sclerosing agents or thoracotomy. In two series of patients with both primary and secondary spontaneous pneumothoraces, the recurrence rates were somewhat higher in the patients with secondary spontaneous pneumothorax (~45%) than they were in patients with primary spontaneous pneumothorax (~30%) over a 3 to 5 year observation period.[24, 47]

## Treatment

Urgent evaluation is indicated for any patient suspected of having a secondary spontaneous pneumothorax. Patients with secondary spontaneous pneumothoraces occasionally die before a chest tube can be inserted. Such deaths were reported in 3 of 57 patients (5%) with pneumothorax secondary to COPD[43] and in 3 of 15 patients (20%) with cystic fibrosis.[48] The high immediate mortality rate emphasizes that an important secondary treatment goal for these patients is reducing the likelihood of a recurrence.

The initial treatment for nearly every patient with a secondary spontaneous pneumothorax should be tube thoracostomy. Simple aspiration should not be performed because it frequently is ineffective and, in addition, does not decrease the likelihood of a recurrence. The evacuation of even a small pneumothorax can lead to a rapid improvement in symptoms. If respiratory failure occurs, necessitating mechanical ventilation, a chest tube should be placed immediately because the pneumothorax is likely to enlarge during mechanical ventilation.

It is more difficult to expand the lung and air leaks persist longer in patients with secondary spontaneous than in patients with primary spontaneous pneumothorax who are treated with tube thoracostomy. In secondary spontaneous pneumothorax caused by COPD, the median time for lung expansion is 5 days compared with 1 day for primary spontaneous pneumothorax,[43] and more patients require prolonged chest tube drainage.[49] In one series, 35% of patients with cystic fibrosis required multiple chest tubes[48]; similarly, in another series, 29% of patients with COPD required more than one chest tube.[44] After 7 days of tube thoracostomy drainage, the lung remains unexpanded or the air leak persists in about 20% of patients with secondary spontaneous pneumothorax.[43, 48]

A case can be made for subjecting most patients with secondary spontaneous pneumothorax to thoracoscopy soon after admission.[26] Thoracoscopy should certainly be performed in patients with a persistent air leak or an unexpanded lung after 72 hours of tube thoracostomy. If the lung expands and the air leak ceases within the first 48 hours, an attempt should be made to prevent a recurrence. Because recurrence rates after chemical pleurodesis are about 20% whereas those after thoracoscopy are less than 5%, the better approach is clearly thoracoscopy. If one is planning thoracoscopy, however, there is no reason to delay. If thoracoscopy is not available, it is recommended that either doxycycline (500 mg) or talc slurry (5 g) be instilled into the pleural space in an attempt to prevent a recurrent pneumothorax. If thoracoscopy is unavailable and there is a persistent air leak or an unexpanded lung after 5 days, consideration should be given to thoracotomy. In patients with either COPD or cystic fibrosis, the mortality rate from thoracotomy is about 10%.[42, 43]

One consideration for patients with secondary spontaneous pneumothorax is the effect that a pleural sclerosing agent might have on a future lung transplant. In the past, if attempts at pleurodesis had been made on the side of the proposed transplant, patients were excluded from lung transplantation due to the risk of excess bleeding. In 1998, however, a consensus conference statement on lung transplantation in cystic fibrosis stated that pleurodesis is not a contraindication to lung transplantation.[50]

## Pneumothorax Secondary to *P. carinii* in Patients with AIDS

Patients with AIDS and *P. carinii* infection have a relatively high incidence of spontaneous pneumothorax. Approximately 5% of patients with AIDS who receive prophylactic pentamidine will have a spontaneous pneumothorax.[51] Most patients with AIDS who have a spontaneous pneumothorax have a history of *P. carinii* infection, many are taking prophylactic pentamidine, and most have a recurrence of their *P. carinii* infection.[40, 41] Pentamidine is much less used now than previously but pneumothorax remains a serious problem in AIDS patients with *P. carinii* pneumonia.[51a] The explanation for the high incidence of spontaneous pneumothorax in these patients appears to be the presence of multiple subpleural lung cavities, which are associated with subpleural necrosis.[52] Once one of these patients has a pneumothorax, he or she is likely to have another one on the opposite side. This occurred in 13 of 20 patients (65%) in one series.[40] It should be noted that iatrogenic pneumothoraces, particularly those related to mechanical ventilation or pulmonary procedures, are also common in patients with AIDS.[39]

Due to the necrotic lung surrounding the ruptured cavity, the spontaneous pneumothorax associated with AIDS and *P. carinii* infection is notoriously difficult to treat. In one report of 20 patients, the median duration of tube thoracostomy was 20 days; 11 patients had sclerotherapy, whereas 5 patients had thoracotomy.[40]

It is recommended that patients with AIDS and a spontaneous pneumothorax be treated with tube thoracostomy. If the air leak persists for more than a few days, there are two options: a Heimlich valve or video-thoracoscopy. The intrapleural injection of a sclerosing agent has not been shown to be effective in expediting closure of the leak. In general the Heimlich valve is preferred because the patient can be managed as an outpatient. In one recent series, 8 of 25 patients were successfully managed as outpatients with a Heimlich valve.[52] If the patient cannot be managed with a Heimlich valve, video-thoracoscopy can be performed. Wait[53] has reported that 30 of 32 patients (94%) with AIDS and spontaneous pneumothorax were managed successfully with talc insufflation without endo-stapling. If operative intervention is planned, it has been recommended that this be carried out early to avoid the prolonged air leak, hospitalization, and morbidity that nearly always occur.[54]

## Pneumothorax Secondary to Tuberculosis

Between 1% and 3% of patients hospitalized for pulmonary tuberculosis will have a pneumothorax.[55] All such patients should be treated with tube thoracostomy. In one series of 28 patients, 11 were treated by observation or repeated pleural aspiration and 7 (64%) died.[55] In contrast, only 1 of 17 patients (6%) treated with tube thoracostomy died. In this series, the median duration of the tube thoracostomy was 50 days. Obviously, antituberculous chemotherapy should be given concomitantly with the tube thoracostomy. Open thoracotomy should not be considered until the patient has received antituberculous therapy for at least 6 weeks.

## IATROGENIC PNEUMOTHORAX

Iatrogenic pneumothoraces are probably more common than primary and secondary spontaneous pneumothoraces combined. Between 1950 and 1974, there were 102 instances of iatrogenic pneumothorax in Olmsted County, Minnesota, compared with 77 cases of primary and 64 cases of secondary spontaneous pneumothorax.[3] The relative incidence of iatrogenic pneumothorax has probably increased over the past few decades because of the increased use of invasive procedures such as transbronchial biopsy, percutaneous lung aspiration, ventilation with high levels of positive end-expiratory pressure, and central vein catheterization, all of which are associated with a high incidence of pneumothorax. Indeed, in the period between November 1, 1983, and January 1, 1989, at the Veterans Administration Hospital in Long Beach, California, there were 108 instances of iatrogenic pneumothorax compared with 90 instances of spontaneous pneumothorax. The causes of the 108 cases of iatrogenic pneumothorax at that facility were as follows: transthoracic needle aspiration in 35, thoracentesis in 31, insertion of subclavicular intravenous line in 23, positive-pressure ventilation in 6, transbronchial biopsy in 3, and miscellaneous in 10.[56]

Currently, the leading cause of iatrogenic pneumothorax is transthoracic needle aspiration. The incidence of iatrogenic pneumothorax with this procedure is about 20%, and 10% of these patients require tube thoracostomy.[57, 58] This procedure is more likely to result in a pneumothorax if the patient has COPD or if the lesion is deep within the lung.[58]

One of the more common causes of iatrogenic pneumothorax is mechanical ventilation. In one early series of 553 patients undergoing mechanical ventilation, 4% developed a pneumothorax.[59] The frequency of the pneumothorax was increased if the patient had aspiration pneumonia (37%), was treated with positive end-expiratory pressure (15%), had intubation of the right main-stem bronchus (13%), or had COPD (8%).[59] In a more recent study, the incidence of pneumothorax in 725 patients with the acute respiratory distress syndrome was 6.9%.[60]

Other common causes of iatrogenic pneumothorax (with approximate incidences) are thoracentesis (5%),[61] pleural biopsy (8%),[62] and transbronchial lung biopsy (6%).[63] Iatrogenic pneumothorax also frequently complicates cardiopulmonary resuscitation. Other procedures associated with the development of an iatrogenic pneumothorax include subclavian or internal jugular vein catheterization, tracheostomy, intercostal nerve block, mediastinoscopy, liver biopsy, and the insertion of small nasogastric tubes.[1]

### Diagnosis

The diagnosis of iatrogenic pneumothorax should be suspected in any patient treated by mechanical ventilation whose clinical condition suddenly deteriorates. A sensitive indicator of the development of a pneumothorax in such patients is increased peak and plateau pressures if the patient is on a volume-cycled ventilator or a decreased tidal volume if the patient is on a pressure-cycled ventilator. The diagnosis should also be suspected in any patient who becomes more dyspneic after a medical or surgical procedure that is known to be associated with the development of a pneumothorax. It should be emphasized that the pneumothorax may not be evident immediately after thoracic procedures, and symptoms may not develop for 24 hours or longer.[64, 65] The diagnosis is readily confirmed by a chest radiograph. In patients with extensive pulmonary infiltrates, there may be little evidence of lung collapse, but the air in the pleural space may instead be indicated by the "deep sulcus sign" (Fig. 75.4).

### Treatment

The treatment of iatrogenic pneumothorax differs from that of spontaneous pneumothorax in that one does not have to worry about preventing a recurrent pneumothorax. The symptoms can vary from none to severe respiratory distress when an iatrogenic pneumothorax develops after a procedure. If the patient has at most minimal symptoms and the pneumothorax occupies less than 15% of the volume of the hemithorax, the patient can be observed. The administration of supplemental oxygen increases the rate at which the pneumothorax is absorbed for the reasons described in the previous section. If the patient has more than minimal symptoms or if the pneumothorax occupies more than 15% of the hemithorax, the procedure of choice is simple aspiration with a plastic catheter,[66] as described for primary spontaneous pneumothorax. If simple aspiration does not control the pneumothorax, then tube thoracostomy should be performed. Small-bore chest tubes (gauge 7 to 9 Fr) with Heimlich valves are quite effective in this situation.[67, 68]

The management of patients with an iatrogenic pneumothorax secondary to positive-pressure mechanical ventilation should include tube thoracostomy to prevent the evolution of a tension pneumothorax. Tension pneumothorax develops because the positive pressure during inspiration forces more air into the pleural space than exits during expiration. If the patient continues to receive mechanical ventilation, the chest tube should be left in place for at least 48 hours after the air leak stops. At times, a bronchopleural fistula is so large that a high percentage of the total inspired volume exits through the chest tube. This volume still provides effective ventilation, however, because the air that egresses from the chest tube often contains levels of carbon dioxide similar to exhaled gas.[69, 70] Although the use of high-frequency ventilators has been recommended in this situation,[71] two studies in adults[72, 73] have demonstrated that high-frequency ventilation does not improve gas exchange or decrease the flow through the fistula.

## TRAUMATIC (NONIATROGENIC) PNEUMOTHORAX

The incidence of pneumothorax after blunt trauma depends on the severity of the trauma. The incidence of pneumothorax has exceeded 35% in some series.[74]

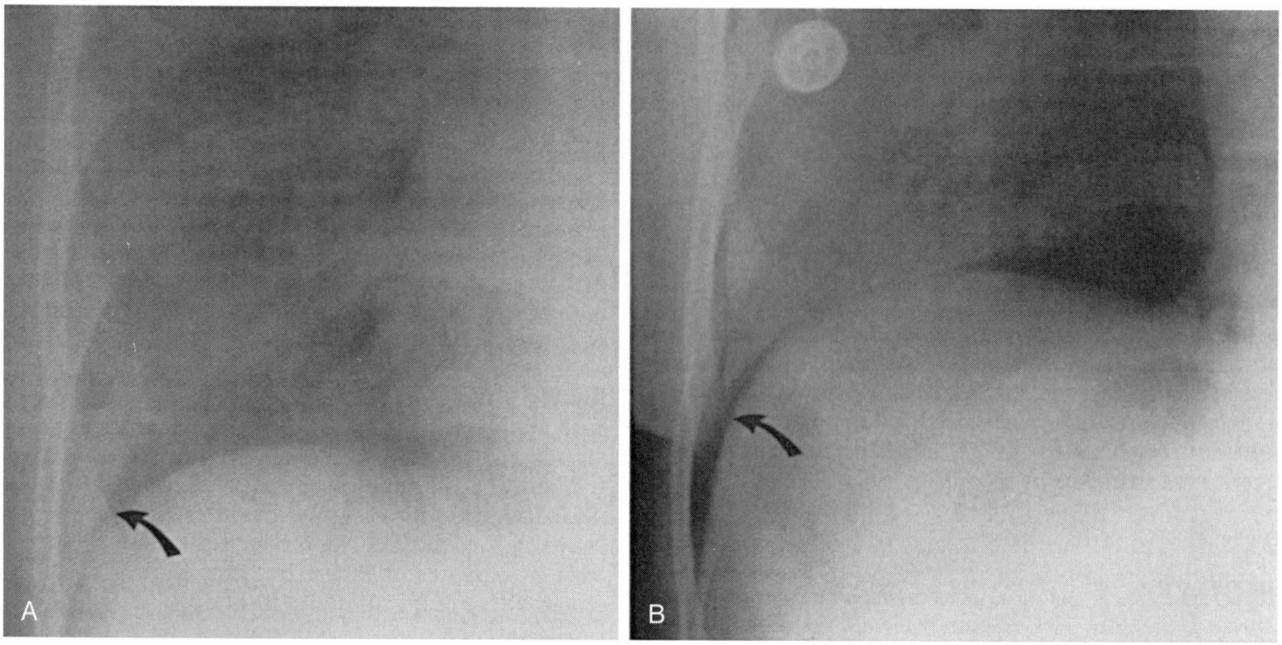

**Figure 75.4** Detailed views of right costophrenic angle from successive chest roentgenograms before *(A)* and after *(B)* the development of a pneumothorax. Both illustrations show diffuse infiltrations in the right lower lung field. Note change in costophrenic angle *(curved arrows)* caused by air in the pleural space between the diaphragm and the chest wall: the "deep sulcus sign."

## Mechanism

A traumatic pneumothorax can result from either penetrating or nonpenetrating chest trauma. With penetrating chest trauma, the mechanism of the pneumothorax is easily understood because the wound allows air to enter the pleural space directly through the chest wall or through the visceral pleura from the tracheobronchial tree.

With nonpenetrating trauma, a pneumothorax may develop if the visceral pleura is lacerated secondary to a rib fracture or dislocation. In the majority of patients with pneumothorax secondary to nonpenetrating trauma, however, there are no associated rib fractures. In this instance, it is thought that the sudden chest compression abruptly increases the alveolar pressure, which may cause alveolar rupture. Once the alveolus is ruptured, air enters the interstitial space and dissects toward either the visceral pleura or the mediastinum. A pneumothorax develops when either the visceral or the mediastinal pleura ruptures, allowing air to enter the pleural space.

## Diagnosis and Treatment

The diagnosis of pneumothorax is made by the chest radiograph or the chest CT. A pneumothorax that is apparent on the chest CT, but not on the chest radiograph, is called an *occult* pneumothorax.[75, 75a] About 40% of traumatic pneumothoraces are occult.[75]

Most traumatic pneumothoraces should be treated with tube thoracostomy. If the patient has an occult pneumothorax or if the distance between the lung and chest wall does not exceed 1.5 cm, however, tube thoracostomy is probably not indicated unless the patient is receiving mechanical ventilation. In one series, 333 patients with pneumothoraces less than 1.5 cm were initially managed without chest tubes, and only 33 (10%) subsequently required tube thoracostomy.[76] The lung usually expands, and the air leak ceases within 24 hours of thoracostomy in traumatic pneumothorax.[76] If the leak persists for more than a few days, consideration should be given to performing thoracoscopy. Carrillo and associates[77] performed thoracoscopy in 11 such patients and were able to identify and repair the site of the air leak in 10 of the 11 patients. In the eleventh patient, a chemical pleurodesis was performed. There were no further air leaks in any of the patients, and all chest tubes were removed within 24 hours.[77]

Two uncommon diagnoses, both of which are indications for immediate thoracotomy, should be considered for any patient with a traumatic pneumothorax. Fracture of the trachea or a major bronchus can lead to a pneumothorax. This usually occurs in the presence of an anterior or lateral fracture of one or more of the first three ribs. Most patients will have at least some hemoptysis.[78] In patients with a traumatic pneumothorax, the presence of a large pneumothorax with continued leakage of air into the pleural space after tube thoracostomy, a fracture of one or more of the first three ribs, or hemoptysis should serve as an indication for fiberoptic bronchoscopy to assess the possibility of a bronchial tear.[78] Primary surgical repair of the tear usually results in full restoration of function of the distal lung.[78]

The second diagnosis that should be considered is traumatic rupture of the esophagus; a hydropneumothorax almost always accompanies this condition. A reliable screening test for esophageal rupture is measurement of the pleural fluid amylase concentration.[79] If this level is elevated, contrast radiographic studies of the esophagus should be performed. It is important to establish the diagnosis of esophageal rupture expeditiously because the mortality approaches 100% if surgical treatment is not carried out promptly.

## NEONATAL PNEUMOTHORAX

A spontaneous pneumothorax is present shortly after birth in 1% to 2% of all infants, and the pneumothorax is symptomatic in approximately half of these.[18, 80] The incidence of spontaneous neonatal pneumothorax is twice as high in male as in female infants. Affected infants are usually full term or post term.[18] Usually, the infant has had a history of fetal distress requiring resuscitation or a difficult delivery with evidence of aspiration of meconium, blood, or mucus.[18]

There is a high incidence of pneumothorax in infants with neonatal respiratory distress syndrome. In one series of 295 newborn infants with the syndrome, 19% had a pneumothorax.[81] Pneumothorax developed in 29% of those requiring intermittent positive-pressure ventilation with positive end-expiratory pressure, 11% of those requiring continuous positive airway pressure, and in only 4% of those not requiring respiratory assistance.[81]

### Pathogenesis

The development of a spontaneous neonatal pneumothorax is related to the mechanical problems of expanding the lung for the first time. During the first few breaths of life, the transpulmonary pressures average 40 cm $H_2O$, with occasional pressures as high as 100 cm $H_2O$.[82] At birth, the alveoli usually open in rapid sequence, but, if bronchial obstruction is present from the aspiration of blood, meconium, or mucus, high transpulmonary pressures may lead to rupture of the lung. A transpulmonary pressure of 60 cm $H_2O$ ruptures an adult lung,[18] whereas a transpulmonary pressure of 45 cm $H_2O$ ruptures a neonatal rabbit lung.[83]

### Clinical Manifestations

With neonatal spontaneous pneumothorax, the signs vary from none to severe acute respiratory distress, depending on the size of the pneumothorax. With a small pneumothorax, there may be mild apneic spells with some irritability or restlessness. With a large pneumothorax, there may be severe respiratory distress with marked tachypnea, grunting, retractions, and cyanosis.[18] In newborn babies, the detection of pneumothorax by physical examination is often difficult. Because breath sounds are widely transmitted in the small neonatal thorax, diminished breath sounds on the affected side may be difficult to appreciate. The most reliable sign is a shift of the apical heart impulse away from the side of the pneumothorax.[18] The diagnosis of neonatal spontaneous pneumothorax is confirmed by a high-quality chest radiograph.

The development of a pneumothorax in a patient with neonatal respiratory distress syndrome is usually heralded by a change in the vital signs. In one series of 49 patients, cardiac arrest marked the development of the pneumothorax in 12 patients (24%); most of the other patients had a decrease in the blood pressure, pulse, or respiratory rate.[81] In another series, however, the earliest signs were an increase in the blood pressure, heart rate, or pulse pressure.[84]

### Treatment

An infant with a spontaneous pneumothorax who is asymptomatic or mildly symptomatic can be treated by close observation because the pneumothorax will resolve in the majority of infants over a few days. It is necessary to observe the patient closely because of the possibility that the pneumothorax will enlarge or that a tension pneumothorax will develop.[18] Supplemental oxygen can hasten the resolution of the pneumothorax, but it should be administered with care because of the dangers of retrolental fibroplasia.[18] Tube thoracostomy should be performed on any neonate who is more than mildly symptomatic. The air leak almost always stops within 24 hours.[18] Tube thoracostomy should be performed in virtually all infants with the neonatal respiratory distress syndrome and pneumothorax because the pneumothorax further compromises the ventilatory status of the patient and tends to increase in size.

## CATAMENIAL PNEUMOTHORAX

A catamenial pneumothorax is a pneumothorax that occurs in conjunction with menstruation (Fig. 75.5). This is an uncommon entity; only 80 cases had been reported by 1996.[85] With catamenial pneumothorax, respiratory symptoms usually develop within 24 to 48 hours of the

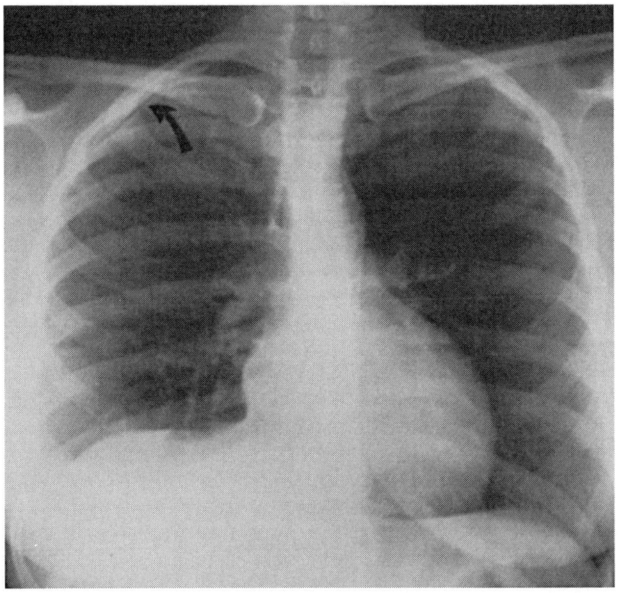

**Figure 75.5** Posteroanterior chest roentgenogram from a 32-year-old woman showing a small right-sided pneumothorax *(arrow)*. This was the fourth episode with onset during menses. (Courtesy of Dr. Louis S. Lehman, San Francisco.)

onset of the menstrual flow.[85] The initial pneumothorax usually does not occur until the woman is at least 30 years of age. Most pneumothoraces are right sided, but left-sided and even bilateral pneumothoraces have been reported.[85] Catamenial pneumothoraces tend to be recurrent unless there is a definite therapeutic intervention. On the average, patients have about five pneumothoraces before the diagnosis is recognized.

### Pathogenesis

The pathogenesis of catamenial pneumothorax is not definitely established. When the syndrome was initially described by Maurer and colleagues,[86] it was hypothesized that air gained access to the peritoneal cavity during menstruation and then entered the pleural cavity through a diaphragmatic defect. In a subsequent review of 18 patients who had undergone thoracotomy, however, diaphragmatic defects were demonstrable in only three, whereas six had pleural or diaphragmatic endometriosis.[87] These reviewers concluded that the most plausible explanation was leakage of air from the lung owing to subpleural endometrial implants.[87] In a review of the reported cases of catamenial pneumothorax, 8 of 61 patients (13%) had pleural endometriosis, 16 (26%) had diaphragmatic defects, and 14 (23%) had blebs or cysts. No abnormalities were found in 15 (25%).[85] Because most of these patients do have pelvic endometriosis,[85] it seems likely that endometriosis (either pelvic or thoracic) is responsible for the syndrome in most patients.

### Diagnosis and Treatment

Any woman over the age of 25 years who has a spontaneous pneumothorax within the first 48 hours of her menstrual period should be suspected of having a catamenial pneumothorax. The treatment of catamenial pneumothorax is aimed at treating endometriosis, known or suspected, by suppressing the ectopic endometrium. This can be attempted by suppression of ovulation with oral contraceptives or suppression of gonadotropins with danazol or gonadotropin-releasing hormone to produce a medical oophorectomy.[85] These measures, however, are effective in less than 50% of patients.[85] Alternative treatments include thoracoscopy with stapling of blebs, closure of diaphragmatic defects and parietal abrasion or pleurectomy,[88] or chemical pleurodesis.[85]

## TENSION PNEUMOTHORAX

A tension pneumothorax is said to be present when the intrapleural pressure exceeds the atmospheric pressure throughout expiration and often during inspiration as well. Most patients who develop a tension pneumothorax are receiving positive pressure to their airways, either during mechanical ventilation or during resuscitation.[88a] For a tension pneumothorax to develop in a spontaneously breathing person, some type of one-way valve mechanism must be present. During inspiration, when the pleural pressure is most negative, air moves from the lung into the pleural space while the opening is patent. Then, during expiration, the communication between the lung and the pleural space may become partially or totally occluded, and air accumulates in the pleural space under positive pressure.

### Pathophysiology

The development of a tension pneumothorax is usually heralded by a sudden deterioration in the cardiopulmonary status of the patient. The explanation for this sudden deterioration is probably related to the combination of a decreased cardiac output due to impaired venous return and profound hypoxia due to ventilation perfusion mismatches. Carvalho and associates[89] induced tension pneumothorax with a mean pleural pressure of +25 cm $H_2O$ in 10 adult mechanically ventilated sheep. They found that the mean cardiac output decreased from 3.5 L/min to 1.1 L/min. In their preparation, the arterial $Po_2$ fell from a baseline value of 159 to 59 mm Hg. Barton and associates[89a] induced tension pneumothoraces in pigs and found that, at a pleural pressure of +10 cm $H_2O$, there was profound hypoxemia (arterial $So_2$ fell from 97% to 55%) and a moderate decrease in the cardiac output (2.8 to 1.8 L/min). In patients on mechanical ventilation who develop tension pneumothorax, there is a large drop in the cardiac output.[90]

### Clinical Manifestations

Patients most commonly have a tension pneumothorax while they are receiving positive-pressure mechanical ventilation or during cardiopulmonary resuscitation.[91] Tension pneumothorax has also been reported to occur as a complication of hyperbaric oxygen therapy.[92] Occasionally, a tension pneumothorax will evolve during the course of a spontaneous pneumothorax. Cases have been reported in which the tension pneumothorax developed due to improper connection of one-way flutter valves with small-caliber chest tubes.[93]

The clinical picture associated with the development of a tension pneumothorax is striking. The patient appears distressed with rapid labored respirations, cyanosis, marked tachycardia, and profuse diaphoresis. The physical findings are those of a very large pneumothorax. Arterial blood gases reveal marked hypoxemia and sometimes respiratory acidosis.

Tension pneumothorax should be suspected in patients receiving mechanical ventilation who suddenly deteriorate clinically. In this situation, the peak pressures on the ventilator usually increase markedly if the patient is on volume-type ventilation, whereas the tidal volumes decrease markedly if the patient is on pressure-support ventilation. Tension pneumothorax should also be suspected in any patient undergoing cardiopulmonary resuscitation in whom ventilation is difficult. In one series of 3500 autopsies, an unsuspected tension pneumothorax was found in 12 cadavers; 10 of these had been receiving mechanical ventilation, and 9 had undergone cardiopulmonary resuscitation.[91] Tension pneumothorax should also be suspected in any patient who deteriorates suddenly who already has a pneumothorax or who has undergone a procedure known to cause a pneumothorax.

## Diagnosis and Treatment

A tension pneumothorax is a medical emergency. One should not waste time trying to establish the diagnosis of tension pneumothorax radiologically because the clinical situation and the physical findings are usually sufficient to strongly suggest the diagnosis. When the diagnosis is suspected, the patient should immediately be given a high concentration of supplemental oxygen to alleviate the hypoxia. A large-bore needle should be immediately inserted into the pleural space through the second anterior intercostal space. This is best done with a catheter needle. After the catheter needle is inserted into the chest, the needle is removed. Then a large syringe containing a few milliliters of sterile saline is attached to the catheter. The plunger is then pulled out of the syringe. If air bubbles through the saline after the plunger is withdrawn, the diagnosis of tension pneumothorax is established. If the fluid enters the pleural space from the syringe, the patient does not have a tension pneumothorax and the catheter should be removed.

If the procedure just described confirms the diagnosis of a tension pneumothorax, the catheter should be left in place and in communication with the atmosphere until air ceases to exit through the syringe. Additional air can be withdrawn from the pleural space with the syringe and the three-way stopcock. The patient should be prepared for immediate tube thoracostomy.

# RE-EXPANSION PULMONARY EDEMA

Unilateral pulmonary edema may develop in certain patients whose lung has been rapidly reinflated after a varied period of collapse secondary to a pneumothorax or a pleural effusion.[94] This entity, called *re-expansion pulmonary edema*, is further discussed in Chapter 54. Patients with re-expansion pulmonary edema have various degrees of hypoxia and hypotension. On occasion, the pulmonary edema becomes bilateral, and the patient requires intubation and mechanical ventilation. On rare occasions, the syndrome is fatal[95]; the seriousness of the syndrome is emphasized by the fact that it has been fatal in otherwise healthy, young persons.[96, 97] Although the incidence of re-expansion pulmonary edema is not known, it is probably relatively low because there were no instances of re-expansion pulmonary edema in the Veterans Administration cooperative study of more than 200 patients with spontaneous pneumothorax.[24] In a retrospective study of 320 episodes of pneumothorax, re-expansion pulmonary edema occurred in 3 patients (1.0%).[98] In 1988, Mahfood and associates[99] reviewed the literature on re-expansion pulmonary edema and were able to find only 53 cases; however, the syndrome was fatal in 11 (21%).

## Pathophysiology

Re-expansion pulmonary edema appears to be due to increased permeability of the pulmonary vasculature. In both experimental animals[100] and humans,[101] the edema fluid has a high protein content, suggesting that it is leakiness of the capillaries rather than increased hydrostatic pressure that is responsible for the edema formation. It has been hypothesized that the mechanical stresses applied to the lung during re-expansion damage the capillaries and lead to pulmonary edema.[100] Reperfusion injury due to oxygen-free radicals is another possibility. Three separate studies[102–104] demonstrated that the administration of oxygen-scavenging compounds such as dimethylthiourea, catalase, or superoxide dismutase all partially inhibit the neutrophilic infiltration associated with the development of re-expansion pulmonary edema, but do not impressively decrease the amount of edema in the experimental situation.

In experimental animals, re-expansion pulmonary edema occurs only if the lung has been collapsed for several days and only if negative pressure is applied to the pleural space. In humans, most cases of re-expansion pulmonary edema develop when the pneumothorax or pleural effusion has been present for at least 3 days[99] and when negative pressure has been applied to the pleural space.[96, 105]

## Clinical Manifestations

Patients with re-expansion pulmonary edema typically have pernicious coughing or chest tightness during or immediately after tube thoracostomy or thoracentesis. The symptoms usually progress for 12 to 24 hours, and serial chest radiographs reveal progressive ipsilateral pulmonary edema, which may progress to involve the contralateral lung. If the patient does not die within the first 48 hours, recovery is usually complete. Treatment is primarily supportive, with the administration of supplemental oxygen and diuretics, and intubation and mechanical ventilation when necessary. One report suggested that the syndrome could be aborted if the patient is treated with continuous positive airway pressure within the first hour of the development of the syndrome.[106] Obviously, chest tubes should be placed to water-seal drainage if the syndrome develops.

## Prevention

Because re-expansion pulmonary edema can be fatal, it is important to prevent it when possible. The possibility of its development should be considered in any patient with a large pneumothorax or pleural effusion who is going to be subjected to tube thoracostomy or thoracentesis. When tube thoracostomy is performed for spontaneous pneumothorax, the tubes should initially be connected to an underwater-seal drainage apparatus rather than to negative pleural pressure. If underwater-seal drainage does not cause re-expansion of the underlying lung within 24 to 48 hours, then negative pressure can be applied to the pleural space.[1]

When a thoracentesis is performed, the amount of pleural fluid withdrawn should be limited to 1000 mL unless pleural pressures are monitored. At times during therapeutic thoracentesis, the pleural pressure falls rapidly, reaching levels of $-50$ cm $H_2O$ or even lower in some patients.[107] Sometimes the patient has no immediate symptoms attributable to this low pleural pressure, and the operator cannot perceive the highly negative pleural pressure. It is hypothesized that the large negative pleural pressures and the resulting mechanical stresses on the lung may lead to re-expansion pulmonary edema. Light and colleagues[107] showed that as long as the pleural pressure does not fall below $-20$ cm $H_2O$, thoracentesis can be continued safely without the development of re-expansion pulmonary edema. Indeed, with pressure monitoring, it is possible to remove more than 5000 mL pleural fluid from some patients. It is therefore recommended that the amount of pleural fluid withdrawn should be limited to 1000 mL unless pleural pressures are monitored. With monitoring, thoracentesis can be continued until the pleural pressure falls below $-20$ cm $H_2O$.[107]

## CHYLOTHORAX

Pleural fluid is occasionally found to be milky or at least turbid. When this cloudiness persists after centrifugation, it is almost always due to a high lipid content in the pleural fluid. Two different situations bring about the accumulation of high levels of lipid in pleural liquid. In one, chyle enters the pleural space as a result of disruption of the thoracic duct, producing a chylothorax or a chylous pleural effusion. In the second, large amounts of cholesterol or lecithin-globulin complexes accumulate in a long-standing pleural effusion to produce a pseudochylothorax or a chyliform pleural effusion.[108] It is important to differentiate these two conditions because their prognosis and management are completely different.

### Pathophysiology

A chylothorax forms when the thoracic duct becomes disrupted. Ligation of the thoracic duct does not, by itself, produce a chylothorax in experimental animals, presumably because of the many collateral vessels and lymphaticovenous anastomoses.

Dietary fats in the form of long-chain triglycerides are conveyed to the blood via the thoracic duct in the form of chylomicrons. After the chylomicrons are formed, they enter the intestinal lacteal vessels and are then transported to the cisterna chyli. The thoracic duct leaves the cisterna chyli and passes through the aortic hiatus of the diaphragm on the anterior surface of the vertebral body between the aorta and the azygos vein into the posterior mediastinum. The thoracic duct then ascends extrapleurally in the posterior mediastinum along the right side of the anterior surface of the vertebral column. Between the level of the fourth and sixth thoracic vertebrae, the duct crosses to the left side of the vertebral column and continues cephalad to enter the superior mediastinum between the aortic arch and the subclavian artery and the left side of the esophagus. Once the thoracic duct passes the thoracic inlet, it arches above the clavicle and passes anterior to the subclavian artery, vertebral artery, and thyrocervical trunk to terminate in the region of the left jugular and subclavian veins. Although this course is the typical one, there are wide anatomic variations in all portions of the duct.

Chyle, the drainage from the thoracic duct, is a milky, opalescent fluid that usually separates into three layers on standing: a creamy uppermost layer containing chylomicrons, a milky intermediate layer, and a dependent layer containing cellular elements. Chyle is bacteriostatic and resists becoming infected even if it stands at room temperature for several weeks. In addition, chyle is not irritating and usually does not evoke thickening of the pleural membrane.

The thoracic duct normally conveys between 1500 and 2500 mL of chyle daily.[109] The flow varies considerably, depending on the diet of the person. The ingestion of fat can increase the flow of lymph in the thoracic duct by a factor of 2 to 10 for several hours. The ingestion of protein or carbohydrate has little effect on the flow, but the ingestion of liquid does increase the flow. The electrolyte composition of chyle is similar to that of serum, and the protein content is usually above 3 g/dL (30 g/L).[108] The primary cellular component of chyle is the T lymphocyte.[108] Prolonged loss of chyle results in severe nutritional depletion, water and electrolyte loss, hypolipemia, and lymphopenia of T cells with resulting immunosuppression.[110–112]

### Etiology

The factors responsible for chylothorax in five separate series totaling 143 patients are shown in Table 75.1. More than 50% of chylothoraces are caused by tumors, and of those due to tumors, lymphoma is found in approximately 75%. In recent years, chylothorax has been reported in several patients with AIDS and Kaposi's sarcoma.[113–115]

Trauma, most often due to a cardiovascular or thoracic surgical procedure, is the second leading cause of chylothorax. The incidence of chylothorax after cardiovascular operations is about 0.5%. Surgical procedures that involve mobilization of the left subclavian artery are particularly likely to be complicated by chylothorax.[116] Chylothorax complicates about 4% of esophageal resections and is particularly common with transhiatal resections.[117] Chylothorax has also been reported as a complication of esophagoscopy, stellate ganglion blockade, thoracic sympathectomy, high translumbar aortography, cervical node dissection, pneumonectomy, and spinal surgery.[108]

Nonsurgical trauma can also lead to chylothorax. The

**Table 75.1 CAUSES OF CHYLOTHORAX FROM FIVE SEPARATE SERIES***

| Cause | N | % |
|---|---|---|
| **Tumor** | 76 | 54 |
| Lymphoma | 57 | |
| Other | 19 | |
| **Trauma** | 36 | 25 |
| Surgical | 31 | |
| Other | 5 | |
| **Idiopathic** | 22 | 15 |
| Congenital | 8 | |
| Other | 14 | |
| **Miscellaneous** | 9 | 6 |

*Adapted with permission from Light RW: Pleural Diseases (3rd ed). Baltimore: Williams & Wilkins, 1995, p 285.

thoracic duct may be disrupted with penetrating injuries involving the neck or thorax. Nonpenetrating trauma in which the spine is hyperextended or a vertebra is fractured can lead to chylothorax, particularly if the injury occurs shortly after the ingestion of a fatty meal. Less impressive traumas such as weight lifting, straining, severe bouts of coughing or vomiting, childbirth, and vigorous stretching while yawning have been reported to cause chylothorax. Chylothoraces secondary to closed trauma are usually on the right side, with the site of rupture being in the region of the ninth or tenth thoracic vertebra.

Chylothorax is the most common type of neonatal pleural effusion.[118, 119] These chylothoraces may be due to rupture of the thoracic duct from trauma during delivery or to developmental abnormalities of the thoracic duct.[119] Before milk feeding, the pleural fluid is clear in appearance; once the infant begins milk feeding, the pleural fluid takes on the milky appearance of chyle.

Chylothoraces can also arise from chylous ascites that moves across the diaphragm into the pleural space. Causes of chylous ascites include many of the causes of chylothorax. In addition, cirrhosis may be a cause of chylous ascites and associated chylothorax. Romero and coworkers[120] described five cirrhotic patients in whom chylothorax was associated with chylous ascites; when a radioisotope was injected into the peritoneal cavity of these patients, it rapidly appeared in the pleural cavity. Interestingly, these chylothoraces were transudative, suggesting that the chyle was diluted in low protein cirrhotic ascites fluid.

There are many other causes of chylothorax, but, even when all are grouped together, they account for only a small percentage of all chylothoraces. Pulmonary lymphangiomyomatosis is the most common other cause of chylothorax and is discussed later in this chapter. Other disease entities associated with chylothorax are abnormalities of the lymphatic vessels, such as intestinal lymphangiectasis or reticular hyperplasia, superior vena caval or subclavian vein thrombosis, filariasis, lymph node enlargement, mediastinal tuberculosis, lymphangitis of the thoracic duct, aneurysms of the thoracic aorta that erode the duct, tuberous sclerosis, amyloidosis,[107] and Gorham's syndrome (disappearing bone disease).[121]

If no cause can be found for the chylothorax, it is labeled *idiopathic*. Before attaching this label, however, lymphoma should be excluded. In one series the diagnosis of lymphoma was not established in four patients until at least 6 months after they presented with a chylothorax.[122] In the adult, most cases of idiopathic chylothorax are probably related to minor trauma such as coughing, stretching, or hiccuping after the ingestion of fatty meals.

## Clinical Manifestations

The symptoms, physical findings, and roentgenographic features of chylothorax are the same as those encountered in patients with comparably sized pleural effusions of any cause. Pleuritic chest pain and fever are rare because chyle is not irritating to the pleural surface. With nontraumatic chylothorax, the onset of symptoms is usually gradual, with the patient complaining of fatigue, dyspnea on exertion, and chest heaviness and discomfort on the affected side.

With traumatic chylothorax, there is usually a latent period of 2 to 10 days between the trauma and the development of the pleural effusion.[123] During this latent period, chyle accumulates in the posterior mediastinum to form a chyloma, which may be visible on the chest radiograph as a posterior mediastinal mass.[108] The mass disappears when the mediastinal pleura ruptures and the chylothorax is formed. Hypotension, cyanosis, and extreme dyspnea may develop when the chyloma ruptures into the pleural space.[108]

Neonatal chylothorax may present with respiratory distress in the first few days of life. Fifty per cent of the infants have symptoms within the first 24 hours, whereas 75% have symptoms by the end of the first week.[115] Most neonatal chylothoraces are either right sided or bilateral; only rarely are they left sided.[119] There is a high frequency of neonatal chylothoraces in infants with hydramnios.[119] With neonatal chylothorax, the appearance of the pleural fluid is serous until milk feedings have begun.[119]

The main threat to life with chylothorax is inanition from malnutrition if the chyle is drained externally. The daily loss of 1500 to 2500 mL of fluid containing substantial amounts of protein, fats, electrolytes, and lymphocytes will rapidly make any patient malnourished and immunocompromised.

## Diagnosis

It is usually easy to establish the diagnosis of chylothorax because chyle has a distinctive white odorless milky appearance. Chylous pleural fluid must be differentiated from empyema fluid and chyliform pleural fluid. In empyema, the milky appearance is caused by suspended white blood cells and debris which will sediment upon centrifugation leaving a clear supernatant. In chyliform pleural effusion from a pseudochylothorax, the milky appearance is also caused by high lipid levels and the supernatant will remain cloudy after centrifugation, as does chyle. The lipids in chyliform effusion are cholesterol or lecithin-globulin complexes rather than chylomicrons.

Usually it is relatively easy to differentiate chylous from chyliform pleural fluid by the clinical picture. In contrast to a chylous effusion, a chyliform pleural effusion usually has been long-standing (5 years or more). The patient with a pseudochylothorax has markedly thickened pleura on CT scan, whereas the pleura with chylothorax is normal. Examination of the pleural liquid can easily demonstrate the cholesterol crystals that are present in some patients with pseudochylothorax.[108]

It should be emphasized that the pleural fluid with chylothorax does not always look like typical chyle. In a series of 24 patients reported by Romero and associates,[120] 14 were milky, 5 were bloody, 3 were turbid yellow, and 2 were clear yellow. The possibility of a chylothorax should be considered whenever a turbid, serosanguineous, or bloody pleural fluid is obtained during a diagnostic thoracentesis. Such fluids should be centrifuged. If turbidity persists in the supernatant, the possibility of a chylothorax should be explored.

When doubt exists as to whether a patient has a chylo-

effusion have pleural surfaces that are markedly thickened and sometimes calcified, and most have had a pleural effusion for at least 5 years. Most of the cholesterol in chyliform pleural effusions is associated with high-density lipoproteins in contrast to the cholesterol in acute exudates, which is mostly bound to low-density lipoproteins.[136] It has been hypothesized that the cholesterol that enters the pleural space with acute pleural inflammation becomes trapped in the pleural space and undergoes a change in lipoprotein-binding characteristics. Then the thickened pleura results in a very slow transfer of cholesterol out of the pleural space.[136] Serum cholesterol levels and systemic cholesterol metabolism appear to be normal in patients with pseudochylothorax.

The three most common situations in which a chyliform pleural effusion occurs are after tuberculous pleurisy, after therapeutic pneumothorax, or in chronic rheumatoid pleurisy.[109, 135a] Pseudochylothorax is particularly likely to develop in patients who have been treated with artificial pneumothorax for pulmonary tuberculosis and who have a chronic pleural effusion secondary to the atelectatic lung.[137] Pleural paragonimiasis may also be associated with chyliform pleural effusion,[138] as can any disease state that is associated with thickened pleura and chronic pleural effusion.

### Clinical Manifestations

Pseudochylothorax occurs in patients with long-standing pleural effusions.[109] The mean duration of the effusion is 5 years before it turns chyliform, but an occasional pleural effusion has become chyliform within 1 year of onset. Many patients with chyliform pleural effusions are asymptomatic or at least no more symptomatic than when they initially developed the pleural effusion. When symptoms do occur, they are usually related to the underlying disease process or to the impairment of pulmonary function produced by the effusion and the thickened and sometimes calcified pleura.

### Diagnosis

The diagnosis of chyliform pleural effusion is usually not difficult. The pleural effusion is long-standing, and the pleura is thickened or calcified. In such patients, the two other diagnostic possibilities are empyema and chylothorax. The pleural surfaces are usually normal, however, if the patient has a chylothorax. If the patient has an empyema, centrifugation of the pleural fluid will produce a clear supernatant. If the supernatant remains turbid, the sediment should be examined for cholesterol crystals because their presence is diagnostic of pseudochylothorax. The cholesterol crystals give a distinct satin-like sheen to the pleural fluid. Microscopically, these crystals have a typical rhomboid appearance.[108] Not all patients with chyliform pleural effusion have cholesterol crystals in their pleural fluid; however, most have an elevated pleural fluid cholesterol level (>250 mg/dL or 6.45 mmol/L).[108]

### Treatment

The possibility of tuberculosis should always be considered when a patient is found to have a chyliform pleural effusion. If the patient has a history of tuberculosis and has never been treated with antituberculous therapy, isoniazid and rifampin should be given for 9 months. If the patient has only a positive purified protein derivative skin test, he or she should also be treated with antituberculous medications as discussed in Chapter 34.

When the patient's exercise capacity is limited by shortness of breath, a therapeutic thoracentesis should be performed. Hillerdal[137] reported that the removal of several hundred milliliters of pleural fluid from patients with pseudochylothorax resulted in a markedly improved exercise tolerance. Decortication should be considered if the patient is symptomatic and the underlying lung is believed to be functional.[139]

## HEMOTHORAX

Hemothorax is the presence of blood in the pleural space. The term *hemothorax* is reserved for those cases in which the hematocrit of the pleural fluid is at least 50% that of the peripheral blood.[140] When bloody pleural fluid is obtained with a diagnostic thoracentesis, the hematocrit should always be measured. Frequently, even though the pleural fluid appears to be pure blood, the hematocrit of the fluid will be less than 5%.

### Traumatic Hemothorax

Blood may enter the pleural space from injury to the chest wall, diaphragm, lung, blood vessels, or mediastinum. On entering the pleural space, the blood coagulates rapidly, but, presumably as a result of the physical agitation produced by movement of the heart and lungs, the clot may be defibrinated. Loculation occurs early in the course of hemothorax.

**Diagnosis.** The diagnosis of traumatic hemothorax should be suspected in any patient with penetrating or nonpenetrating trauma of the chest (Fig. 75.7). It should be emphasized that the hemothorax may not be apparent on the initial chest radiograph. In one series of 130 patients with hemothorax secondary to nonpenetrating trauma, the hemothorax was not appreciated on the initial chest radiograph in 24% of the patients.[141] Although the hemothorax was missed in some of the patients because the initial radiograph was obtained with the patient supine, other patients had no evidence of a hemothorax on the upright radiograph.[141] The CT scan is more sensitive than the chest radiograph in detecting hemothoraces. In a study of 103 patients, published in 1997, Trupka and coworkers[142] demonstrated that thoracic CT detected a hemothorax in 21 patients (20%) in whom the routine chest radiograph showed no pleural fluid. When patients experience severe thoracic trauma, a CT scan of the chest is indicated not only for its ability to identify hemothorax but also for its capability to identify pneumothorax, lung contusion, and bone fractures.[142] The diagnosis is established by demonstration of a pleural fluid hematocrit greater than 50% of that of the peripheral blood.

**Treatment.** A patient with a traumatic hemothorax should undergo immediate tube thoracostomy for the fol-

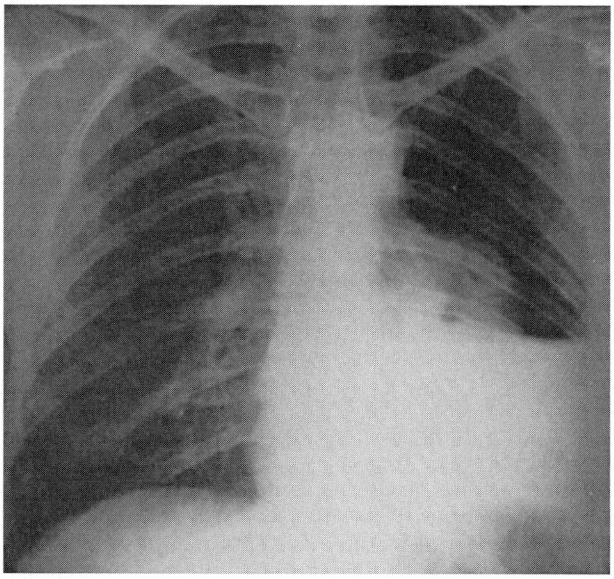

**Figure 75.7** This posteroanterior chest radiograph is from a patient who suffered multiple injuries in an automobile accident. The patient has a hemopneumothorax. With the prompt institution of tube thoracostomy, the air and blood were evacuated from the pleural space, and the chest radiograph was normal 1 week later.

lowing reasons: It permits nearly complete evacuation of the blood from the pleural space. It can stop the bleeding if the bleeding is from pleural lacerations by bringing the two pleural surfaces in apposition. It enables quantitation of the degree of continued bleeding. It may decrease the incidence of subsequent empyema.[143] The blood drained from the pleural space may be autotransfused.[144] The rapid evacuation of the blood from the pleural space is believed to decrease the incidence of subsequent fibrothorax.[145]

It is recommended that the chest tube be inserted relatively high (fourth or fifth intercostal space) in the midaxillary line because the ipsilateral hemidiaphragm may be elevated secondary to the trauma.[143] Large-bore chest tubes should be used because the blood frequently clots. Chest tubes should be removed as soon as they stop draining or cease to function because they can serve as conduits for pleural infection. Although attempts can be made to clear the chest tubes via saline flushes or thrombolytic agents in the tube, the injection of fibrinolytics into the pleural space should be avoided.

Approximately 20% of patients with hemothorax require thoracotomy. Immediate thoracotomy is indicated for suspected cardiac tamponade, vascular injury, pleural contamination, debridement of devitalized tissue, sucking chest wounds, or major bronchial air leaks.[146] Continued pleural hemorrhage is another indication for prompt thoracotomy. Before thoracotomy is performed for this reason, it is important to ascertain that the bleeding is not from a misplaced central venous catheter. This diagnosis is readily established by examining the appearance of the pleural drainage when the character of the infusion fluid is changed.[147] There are no precise criteria for the amount of pleural bleeding that should serve as an indication for thoracotomy, and each case must be individualized; however, if the bleeding is more than 200 mL/hr and shows no signs of slowing, thoracotomy should be seriously considered. At some medical centers, hemodynamically stable patients with persistent bleeding are subjected to thoracoscopy rather than thoracotomy.[148]

**Complications.** The four main pleural complications of traumatic hemothorax are the retention of clotted blood in the pleural space, pleural infection, pleural effusion, and fibrothorax. Most patients with small to moderate amounts of clotted blood remaining in their pleural space have no residual pleural abnormalities even if no intervention is undertaken.[146] If more than 30% of the hemithorax is occupied by clotted blood, the hemithorax should be evacuated; decisions regarding thoracoscopic evacuation should not be made from the plain chest radiograph alone and require CT studies.[148a] It appears that removal is most easily done with thoracoscopy.[149] The clotted blood should be evacuated within 7 days because after this time it begins to become organized and is much more difficult to remove.[149] In a prospective, randomized trial, video-assisted thoracoscopy was more effective than thoracostomy tube drainage for removing retained hemothoraces. In this study, both the length of hospital stay (7 vs. 3.6 days) and the duration of tube drainage (4.5 vs. 2.5 days) were shorter in the group receiving video-assisted thoracoscopy.[150]

Empyema occurs in 1% to 4% of patients with traumatic hemothorax.[143, 146] Empyema is more frequent in patients who are admitted in shock, have gross contamination of their pleural space, have associated abdominal injuries, or undergo prolonged pleural drainage.[145, 146] The administration of prophylactic antibiotics (e.g., cefazolin 500 mg every 6 hours until tube removal) results in a significant decrease in the incidence of pleural infection.[151] The treatment of empyema complicating hemothorax is similar to that of any bacterial infection of the pleural space (see Chapters 33 and 74). Because many patients with traumatic hemothorax and empyema are young and physically fit, thoracoscopy with the breakdown of adhesions or thoracotomy with decortication should be considered if tube thoracotomy does not rapidly resolve the pleural infection.

In more than 10% of patients with traumatic hemothorax, a pleural effusion will develop after the chest tubes are removed.[146] Most such pleural effusions resolve spontaneously, leaving no residual pleural abnormalities. It is important to perform a diagnostic thoracentesis in such patients, however, to verify that no pleural infection is present.

Fibrothorax develops in less than 1% of patients with hemothorax. Fibrothorax appears to develop more frequently when a hemopneumothorax is present or when a hemothorax becomes infected. The definitive treatment for fibrothorax is decortication. Decortication for fibrothorax should be delayed for several months after the injury, however, to allow time for spontaneous resolution of the pleural thickening, which is often considerable.

### Iatrogenic Hemothorax

Whenever a hemothorax is discovered, the possibility of an iatrogenic origin should be considered. The most common cause of iatrogenic hemothorax is thoracic surgery, while the second most common cause is perforation of a central vein or artery by a percutaneously inserted catheter[152] or leaking from the aorta after translumbar aortographic study. Iatrogenic hemothorax can also follow thoracentesis, pleural biopsy, percutaneous lung aspiration or biopsy, transbronchial biopsy, and endoscopic esophageal variceal therapy.[153] Patients with iatrogenic hemothorax should be managed, as are patients with traumatic hemothoraces, with chest tubes and thoracoscopy or thoracotomy as needed.

### Nontraumatic Hemothorax

Nontraumatic hemothoraces are distinctly uncommon. The most common cause is metastatic pleural disease,[154] whereas the second most common cause is a complication of anticoagulation therapy for pulmonary embolization.[155] A spontaneous hemothorax may result from rupture of an abnormal intrathoracic blood vessel such as an aortic aneurysm,[156] a pulmonary artery aneurysm, a patent ductus arteriosus, or a coarctation of the aorta.[140] Other causes of spontaneous hemothorax include a complication of a bleeding disorder such as hemophilia or thrombocytopenia, a complication of spontaneous pneumothorax, rupture of a splenic artery aneurysm through the diaphragm, bronchopulmonary sequestration, thoracic endometriosis,[157] chickenpox pneumonia,[158] and intrathoracic extramedullary hematopoiesis.[159] The cause of the hemothorax in some patients remains unknown despite exploratory thoracotomy.[160]

Chest tubes should be inserted into patients with spontaneous hemothorax to remove the blood from the pleural space and to quantitate the degree of continued bleeding. An attempt should be made to determine the cause of the hemothorax. If brisk (>100 mL/hr) bleeding persists, emergency thoracotomy should be performed.

### Hemothorax Complicating Anticoagulant Therapy

By 1977, 11 cases of hemothorax complicating anticoagulant therapy had been reported.[155] Of the 11 patients reported, 5 were receiving only heparin, 4 were receiving heparin and warfarin, and 2 were receiving only warfarin. The hemothorax usually becomes apparent 4 to 7 days after anticoagulation therapy is initiated, but it may occur only after several months. When the hemothorax develops, the coagulation studies are usually within the acceptable therapeutic range. Patients with spontaneous hemothorax complicating anticoagulant therapy should discontinue the anticoagulants and should have chest tubes inserted in an attempt to remove all the blood from the pleural space.[155]

## FIBROTHORAX

A dense layer of fibrous tissue may be deposited over the pleural surface when there is intense inflammation of the pleural space. A fibrothorax most commonly develops as a complication of an empyema or a hemothorax. Fibrothorax has also developed as a complication of tuberculo-

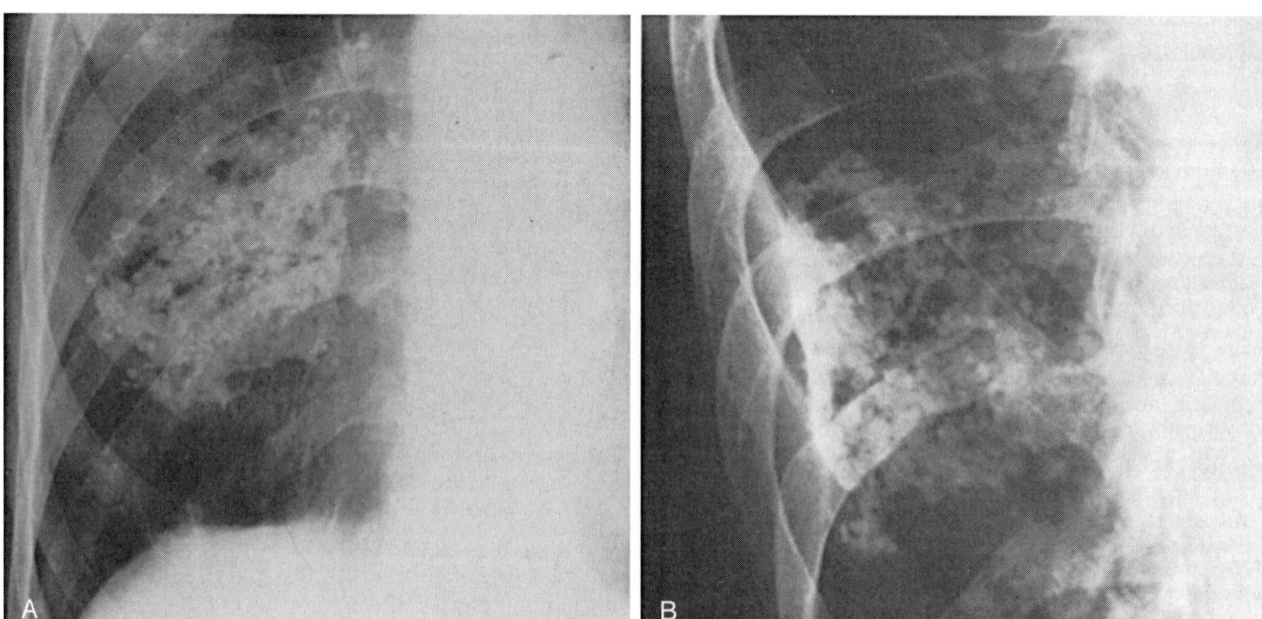


**Figure 75.8** Detailed views from posteroanterior (*A*) and oblique (*B*) chest roentgenograms of a 62-year-old man showing localized fibrothorax with calcified plaque on the right. The patient had had right-sided empyema 32 years before. (Reproduced with permission from Hinshaw HC, Murray JF: Diseases of the Chest. Philadelphia: WB Saunders, 1980, p 912.)

sis, pancreatitis, collagen vascular disease, uremia, and paragonimiasis. In all of these instances, the fibrothorax occurs on the side of the previous inflammatory pleural disease through the deposition of fibrous tissue on the visceral pleural surface. Asbestos exposure may also lead to fibrothorax.[161] In this instance, the deposition of fibrous tissue involves both the parietal and visceral surfaces, obliterating the pleural space. Pleural fibrosis appears to be particularly common in patients who have developed recurrent benign asbestos effusions.[161]

## Diagnosis

The diagnosis of fibrothorax is usually easily made from the roentgenographic findings plus a history of an old injury or infection consistent with a chronic hemothorax or empyema. Radiologically, a peel of uniform thickness surrounds the lung. Calcification occurs frequently on the inner aspect of the peel (Fig. 75.8) and provides an indicator by which the thickness of the peel may be accurately measured.

Routine pulmonary function testing reveals mild-to-severe restrictive ventilatory dysfunction. The blood flow is reduced more than is the ventilation on the side of the fibrothorax. In one study of 127 patients, the mean oxygen uptake on the affected side was 19% of the total, whereas the mean ventilation was 33% of the total.[162] Pulmonary function may be severely compromised in patients with extensive fibrothorax. As a result of the marked pleural thickening, the hemithorax becomes contracted, and its mobility is reduced.[162] As the fibrothorax progresses, the intercostal spaces may narrow, the size of the involved hemithorax may diminish, and the mediastinum may be displaced ipsilaterally. In patients with bilateral fibrothorax resulting from asbestos exposure, respiratory failure with carbon dioxide retention may develop.[163]

## Treatment

Decortication is the only treatment available for fibrothorax. In decortication, the fibrous peel is removed from the pleural surface. The degree of improvement after decortication varies; the most important factor is the condition of the underlying lung.[162, 164] The vital capacity may improve more than 50% after decortication if the underlying lung is normal, but the vital capacity may even decrease after decortication in patients with extensive parenchymal disease. The duration of the fibrothorax does not seem important in predicting the outcome. In one case report, there was a marked subjective improvement after decortication in a patient who had a fibrothorax for 44 years.[164]

It should be emphasized that patients with a recent hemothorax, empyema, or tuberculous pleuritis frequently show marked spontaneous improvement in their symptoms and the degree of pleural thickening in the 3 to 6 months after the acute episode. Therefore, decortication should be considered only if the pleural thickening has been present for several months and if the lifestyle of the patient is compromised by exertional dyspnea. If previous chest radiographs demonstrated extensive parenchymal disease or if CT scans of the chest revealed significant parenchymal disease, decortication may not be advisable. The results of decortication in patients with bilateral fibrothorax secondary to asbestos exposure have been disappointing; this is probably because of the presence of concomitant parenchymal disease.[165] Finally, decortication is a major surgical procedure and should not be performed on patients debilitated by other diseases.

## SUMMARY

Pneumothorax is increasing in frequency mainly because of the large number of diagnostic or therapeutic maneuvers that enable air to enter the pleural space. Spontaneous pneumothorax in otherwise healthy persons and traumatic (noniatrogenic) pneumothorax continue to be common and sometimes serious clinical problems. Tension pneumothorax is often life-threatening and requires immediate relief. A less common, but also serious complication is re-expansion pulmonary edema. These and other aspects of pneumothorax are described in detail in this chapter.

Chylothorax is not a common disorder, but it is important to recognize when it occurs. Most cases are caused by tumor, especially lymphoma, with trauma accounting for most of the remainder. Chylothorax can usually be differentiated from pseudochylothorax by differences in the clinical picture. With chylothorax, symptoms are acute and the pleural surfaces are normal, whereas with pseudochylothorax symptoms are chronic and the pleural surfaces are thickened. Bloody pleural fluid with a hematocrit more than 50% of that in peripheral blood is called a *hemothorax,* which is usually caused by trauma, either accidental or iatrogenic. A few cases are spontaneous in origin or are related to anticoagulant therapy. Fibrothorax most commonly develops as a complication of empyema or hemothorax, which organizes into a thick fibrous layer on one or both pleural surfaces.

## References

1. Light RW: Pneumothorax. *In* Pleural Diseases (3rd ed). Baltimore: Williams & Wilkins, 1995, pp 242–277.
2. Norris RM, Jones JG, Bishop JM: Respiratory gas exchange in patients with spontaneous pneumothorax. Thorax 23:427–433, 1968.
3. Melton LJ, Hepper NG, Offord KP: Incidence of spontaneous pneumothorax in Olmsted County, Minnesota: 1950 to 1974. Am Rev Respir Dis 120:1379–1382, 1979.
4. Schramel FM, Postmus PE, Vanderschueren RG: Current aspects of spontaneous pneumothorax. Eur Respir J 10:1372–1379, 1997.
5. Bense L, Eklung G, Wiman LG: Smoking and the increased risk of contracting spontaneous pneumothorax. Chest 92:1009–1012, 1987.
6. Withers JN, Fishback ME, Kiehl PV, et al: Spontaneous pneumothorax. Am J Surg 108:772–776, 1964.
7. Abolnik IZ, Lossos IS, Zlotogora J, et al: On the inheritance of primary spontaneous pneumothorax. Am J Med Genet 40:155–158, 1991.
8. Bense L, Wiman LG, Hedenstierna G: Onset of symptoms in spontaneous pneumothorax: Correlations to physical activity. Eur J Respir Dis 71:181–186, 1987.
9. Seremetis MG: The management of spontaneous pneumothorax. Chest 57:65–68, 1970.
10. Vail WJ, Alway AE, England NJ: Spontaneous pneumothorax. Chest 38:512–515, 1960.
11. Aston SJ, Rosove M: Horner's syndrome occurring with spontaneous pneumothorax. N Engl J Med 287:1098, 1972.

12. Alikhan M, Biddison JH: Electrocardiographic changes with right-sided pneumothorax. South Med J 91:677–680, 1998.
13. Sadikot RT, Greene T, Meadows K, et al: Recurrence of primary spontaneous pneumothorax. Thorax 52:805–809, 1997.
14. Mitlehner W, Friedrich M, Dissmann W: Value of computer tomography in the detection of bullae and blebs in patients with primary spontaneous pneumothorax. Respiration 59:221–227, 1992.
15. Janssen JP, Schramel FM, Sutedja TG, et al: Videothoracoscopic appearance of first and recurrent pneumothorax. Chest 108:330–334, 1995.
16. Gobbel WG Jr, Rhea WG Jr, Nelson IA, et al: Spontaneous pneumothorax. J Thorac Cardiovasc Surg 46:331–345, 1963.
17. Kircher LT Jr, Swartzel RL: Spontaneous pneumothorax and its treatment. JAMA 155:24–29, 1954.
18. Chernick V, Avery ME: Spontaneous alveolar rupture at birth. Pediatrics 32:816–824, 1963.
19. Northfield TC: Oxygen therapy for spontaneous pneumothorax. BMJ 4:86–88, 1971.
20. Harvey J, Prescott RJ: Simple aspiration versus intercostal tube drainage for spontaneous pneumothorax in patients with normal lungs. British Thoracic Society Research Committee. BMJ 309:1338–1339, 1994.
21. Andrivet P, Djedaini K, Teboul J-L, et al: Spontaneous pneumothorax. Comparison of thoracic drainage vs immediate or delayed needle aspiration. Chest 108:335–340, 1995.
22. Ponn RB, Silverman HJ, Federico JA: Outpatient chest tube management. Ann Thorac Surg 64:1437–1440, 1997.
23. Shaw TJ, Caterine JM: Recurrent re-expansion pulmonary edema. Chest 86:784–786, 1984.
24. Light RW, O'Hara VS, Moritz TE, et al: Intrapleural tetracycline for the prevention of recurrent spontaneous pneumothorax. JAMA 264:2224–2230, 1990.
25. Almind M, Lange P, Viskum K: Spontaneous pneumothorax: Comparison of simple drainage, talc pleurodesis, and tetracycline pleurodesis. Thorax 44:627–630, 1989.
26. Light RW: Diseases of the pleura. The management of pneumothorax. Curr Opin Pulm Med 3:303–304, 1997.
27. Milanez Campos JR, Werebe EC, Vargas FS, et al: Respiratory failure due to insufflated talc. Lancet 349:251–252, 1997.
27a. Rehse DH, Aye RW, Florence MG: Respiratory failure following talc pleurodesis. Am J Surg 177:437–440, 1999.
28. Sahn SA, Good JT: The effect of common sclerosing agents on the rabbit pleural space. Am Rev Respir Dis 124:65–67, 1981.
29. Vargas FS, Wang N-S, Lee HM, et al: Effectiveness of bleomycin in comparison to tetracycline as pleural sclerosing agent in rabbits. Chest 104:1582–1584, 1993.
30. Yim AP: Video-assisted thoracoscopic suturing of apical bullae. An alternative to staple resection in the management of primary spontaneous pneumothorax. Surg Endosc 9:1013–1016, 1995.
31. Bertrand PC, Regnard JF, Spaggiari L, et al: Immediate and long-term results after surgical treatment of primary spontaneous pneumothorax by VATS. Ann Thorac Surg 61:1641–1645, 1996.
32. Yim AP, Liu HP: Video assisted thoracoscopic management of primary spontaneous pneumothorax. Surg Laparosc Endosc 7:236–240, 1997.
33. Naunheim KS, Mack MJ, Hazelrigg SR, et al: Safety and efficacy of video-assisted thoracic surgical techniques for the treatment of spontaneous pneumothorax. J Thorac Cardiovasc Surg 109:1198–1203, 1995.
34. Crisci R, Coloni GF: Video-assisted thoracoscopic surgery versus thoracotomy for recurrent spontaneous pneumothorax. A comparison of results and costs. Eur J Cardiothorac Surg 10:556–560, 1996.
35. Deslauriers J, Beaulieu M, Despres J-P, et al: Transaxillary pleurectomy for treatment of spontaneous pneumothorax. Ann Thorac Surg 30:569–574, 1980.
36. Nkere UU, Griffin SC, Fountain SW: Pleural abrasion: A new method of pleurodesis. Thorax 46:596–598, 1991.
37. O'Hara VS: Spontaneous pneumothorax. Milit Med 143:32–35, 1978.
38. O'Rourke JP, Yee ES: Civilian spontaneous pneumothorax. Treatment options and long-term results. Chest 96:1302–1306, 1989.
39. Byrnes TA, Brevig JK, Yeoh CB: Pneumothorax in patients with acquired immunodeficiency syndrome. J Thorac Cardiovasc Surg 98:546–550, 1990.
40. Sepkowitz KA, Telzak EE, Gold JW, et al: Pneumothorax in AIDS. Ann Intern Med 114:455–459, 1991.
41. Newsome GS, Ward DJ, Pierce PF: Spontaneous pneumothorax in patients with acquired immunodeficiency syndrome treated with prophylactic aerosolized pentamidine. Arch Intern Med 150:2167–2168, 1990.
42. Luck SR, Raffensperger JG, Sullivan HJ, Gibson LE: Management of pneumothorax in children with chronic pulmonary disease. J Thorac Cardiovasc Surg 74:834–839, 1977.
43. Dines DE, Clagett OT, Payne WS: Spontaneous pneumothorax in emphysema. Mayo Clin Proc 45:481–487, 1970.
44. Shields TW, Oilschlager GA: Spontaneous pneumothorax in patients 40 years of age and older. Ann Thorac Surg 2:377–383, 1966.
45. George RB, Herbert SJ, Shames JM, et al: Pneumothorax complicating pulmonary emphysema. JAMA 234:389–393, 1975.
46. Bourgouin P, Cousineau G, Lemire P, Herber G: Computed tomography used to exclude pneumothorax in bullous lung disease. J Can Assoc Radiol 36:341–342, 1985.
47. Lippert HL, Lund O, Blegvad S, et al: Independent risk factors for cumulative recurrence rate after first spontaneous pneumothorax. Eur Respir J 4:324–331, 1991.
48. Boat TF, Di Sant'Agnese PA, Warwick WJ, et al: Pneumothorax in cystic fibrosis. JAMA 209:1498–1504, 1969.
49. Videm V, Pillgram-Larsen J, Ellingsen O, et al: Spontaneous pneumothorax in chronic obstructive pulmonary disease: Complications, treatment and recurrences. Eur J Respir Dis 71:365–371, 1987.
50. Yankaskas MR, Mallory GB Jr, and the Consensus Committee: Lung transplantation in cystic fibrosis. Chest 113:217–226, 1998.
51. Leoung GS, Feigal DW Jr, Montgomery AB, et al: Aerosolized pentamidine for prophylaxis against *Pneumocystis carinii* pneumonia. N Engl J Med 323:769–775, 1990.
51a. Boiselle PM, Crans CA Jr, Kaplan MA: The changing face of *Pneumocystis carinii* pneumonia in AIDS patients. AJR Am J Roentgenol 172:1301–1309, 1999.
52. Light RW, Hamm H: Pleural disease and the acquired immune deficiency syndrome. Eur Respir J 10:2638–2643, 1997.
53. Wait MA: AIDS-related pneumothorax. Ann Thorac Surg 64:290–291, 1997.
54. Horowitz MD, Oliva H: Pneumothorax in AIDS patients: Operative management. Am Surg 59:200–204, 1993.
55. Wilder RJ, Beacham EG, Ravitch MM: Spontaneous pneumothorax complicating cavitary tuberculosis. J Thorac Cardiovasc Surg 43:561–573, 1962.
56. Despars JA, Sassoon CSH, Light RW: Significance of iatrogenic pneumothoraces. Chest 105:1147–1150, 1994.
57. Li H, Boiselle PM, Shepard JO, et al: Diagnostic accuracy and safety of CT-guided percutaneous needle aspiration biopsy of the lung: Comparison of small and large pulmonary nodules. AJR Am J Roentgenol 167:105–109, 1996.
58. Vitulo P, Dore R, Cerveri I, et al: The role of functional respiratory tests in predicting pneumothorax during lung needle biopsy. Chest 109:612–615, 1995.
59. DeLatorre FJ, Tomasa A, Klamburg J, et al: Incidence of pneumothorax and pneumomediastinum in patients with aspiration pneumonia requiring ventilatory support. Chest 72:141–144, 1977.
60. Weg JG, Anzueto A, Balk RA, et al: The relation of pneumothorax and other air leaks to mortality in the acute respiratory distress syndrome. N Engl J Med 338:341–346, 1998.
61. Doyle JJ, Hnatiuk OW, Torrington KG, et al: Necessity of routine chest roentgenography after thoracentesis. Ann Intern Med 124:816–820, 1996.
62. Poe RH, Israel RH, Utell MJ, et al: Sensitivity, specificity, and predictive values of closed pleural biopsy. Arch Intern Med 144:325–328, 1984.
63. Herf SM, Suratt PM, Arora NS: Deaths and complications associated with transbronchial lung biopsy. Am Rev Respir Dis 115:708–711, 1977.
64. Levy H, Kallenbach JM, Feldman C, et al: Delayed pneumothorax after transbronchial lung biopsy. Thorax 41:647–648, 1986.
65. Plaus WJ: Delayed pneumothorax after subclavian vein catheterization. J Parenter Enteral Nutr 14:414–415, 1990.
66. Hamilton AAD, Archer GJ: Treatment of pneumothorax by simple aspiration. Thorax 38:934–936, 1983.

67. Conces DJ Jr, Tarver RD, Gray WC, et al: Treatment of pneumothoraces utilizing small caliber chest tubes. Chest 94:55–57, 1988.
68. Laub M, Milman N, Muller D, et al: Role of small calibre chest tube drainage for iatrogenic pneumothorax. Thorax 45:748–749, 1990.
69. Bishop MJ, Benson MS, Pierson DJ: Carbon dioxide excretion via bronchopleural fistulas in adult respiratory distress syndrome. Chest 91:400–402, 1987.
70. Powner DJ, Cline CD, Rodman GH: Effect of chest-tube suction on gas flow through a bronchopleural fistula. Crit Care Med 13:99–101, 1985.
71. Carlson GC, Kahn RC, Howland WS, et al: Clinical experience with high frequency jet ventilation. Crit Care Med 9:1–6, 1981.
72. Bishop MJ, Benson MS, Sato P, et al: Comparison of high frequency jet ventilation with conventional mechanical ventilation for bronchopleural fistula. Anesth Analg 66:833–838, 1987.
73. Albelda SM, Hansen-Flaschen JH, Taylor E, et al: Evaluation of high-frequency jet ventilation in patients with bronchopleural fistulas by quantitation of the airleak. Anesthesiology 63:551–554, 1985.
74. Trupka A, Waydhas C, Hallfeldt KK, et al: Value of thoracic computed tomography in the first assessment of severely injured patients with blunt chest trauma: Results of a prospective study. J Trauma 43:405–411, 1997.
75. Bridges KG, Welch G, Silver M, et al: CT detection of occult pneumothorax in multiple trauma patients. J Emerg Med 11:179–186, 1993.
75a. Wolfman NT, Myers WS, Glauser SJ, et al: Validity of CT classification on management of occult pneumothorax: A prospective study. AJR Am J Roentgenol 171:1317–1320, 1998.
76. Knottenbelt JD, van der Spuy JW: Traumatic pneumothorax: A scheme for rapid patient turnover. Br J Accident Surg 21:77–80, 1990.
77. Carrillo EH, Schmacht DC, Gable DR, et al: Thoracoscopy in the management of posttraumatic persistent pneumothorax. J Am Coll Surg 186:636–639, 1998.
78. Guest JL, Anderson JN: Major airway injury in closed chest trauma. Chest 72:63–66, 1977.
79. Sherr HP, Light RW, Merson MH, et al: Origin of pleural fluid amylase in esophageal rupture. Ann Intern Med 76:985–986, 1972.
80. Steele RW, Metz JR, Bass JW, et al: Pneumothorax and pneumomediastinum in the newborn. Radiology 98:629–632, 1971.
81. Ogata ES, Gregory GA, Kitterman JA, et al: Pneumothorax in the respiratory distress syndrome: Incidence and effect on vital signs, blood gases, and pH. Pediatrics 58:177–183, 1976.
82. Karlberg P, Cherry RB, Escardo F, et al: Respiratory studies on newborns. II. Pulmonary ventilation and mechanics of breathing in the first minutes of life including the onset of respiration. Acta Pediatr 51:121–136, 1962.
83. Adler SM, Wyszogrodski I: Pneumothorax as a function of gestational age: Clinical and experimental studies. J Pediatr 87:771–775, 1975.
84. Goldberg RN: Sustained arterial blood pressure elevation associated with pneumothoraces: Early detection via continuous monitoring. Pediatrics 68:775–777, 1981.
85. Joseph J, Sahn SA: Thoracic endometriosis syndrome: New observations from an analysis of 110 cases. Am J Med 100:164–170, 1996.
86. Maurer ER, Schaal JA, Mendez FL: Chronic recurrent spontaneous pneumothorax due to endometriosis of the diaphragm. JAMA 168:2013–2014, 1958.
87. Lillington GA, Mitchell SP, Wood GA: Catamenial pneumothorax. JAMA 219:1328–1332, 1972.
88. Van Schil PE, Vercauteren SR, Vermeire PA, et al: Catamenial pneumothorax caused by thoracic endometriosis. Ann Thorac Surg 62:585–586, 1996.
88a. Barton ED. Tension pneumothorax. Curr Opin Pulm Med 5:269–274, 1999.
88b. Strange C: Pleural complications in the intensive care unit. Clin Crit Care Med 20:317–327, 1999.
89. Carvalho P, Hilderbrandt J, Charan NB: Changes in bronchial and pulmonary arterial blood flow with progressive tension pneumothorax. J Appl Physiol 81:1664–1669, 1996.
89a. Barton ED, Rhee P, Hutton KC, et al: The pathophysiology of tension pneumothorax in ventilated swine. J Emerg Med 15:147–153, 1997.
90. Beards SC, Lipman J: Decreased cardiac index as an indicator of tension pneumothorax in the ventilated patient. Anesthesiology 49:137–141, 1994.
91. Ludwig J, Kienzle GD: Pneumothorax in a large autopsy population. Am J Clin Pathol 70:24–26, 1978.
92. Murphy DG, Sloan EP, Hart RG, et al: Tension pneumothorax associated with hyperbaric oxygen therapy. Am J Emerg Med 9:176–179, 1991.
93. Mainini SE, Johnson FE: Tension pneumothorax complicating small-caliber chest tube insertion. Chest 97:759–760, 1990.
94. Pavlin DJ, Nessly ML, Cheney FW: Increased pulmonary vascular permeability as a cause of re-expansion edema in rabbits. Am Rev Respir Dis 124:422–427, 1981.
95. Olcott EW: Fatal reexpansion pulmonary edema following pleural catheter placement. J Vasc Intervent Radiol 5:176–178, 1994.
96. Trapnell DH, Thurston JGB: Unilateral pulmonary edema after pleural aspiration. Lancet 1:1367–1369, 1970.
97. Peatfield RC, Edwards RR, Johnson NM: Two unexpected deaths from pneumothorax. Lancet 1:356–358, 1979.
98. Rozenman J, Yellin A, Simansky DA, et al: Re-expansion pulmonary oedema following spontaneous pneumothorax. Respir Med 90:235–238, 1996.
99. Mahfood S, Hix WR, Aaron BL, et al: Reexpansion pulmonary edema. Ann Thorac Surg 45:340–345, 1988.
100. Pavlin J, Cheney FW Jr: Unilateral pulmonary edema in rabbits after re-expansion of collapsed lung. J Appl Physiol Respir Environ Exerc Physiol 46:31–35, 1979.
101. Sprung CL, Loewenherz JW, Baier H, et al: Evidence for increased permeability in re-expansion pulmonary edema. Am J Med 71:497–500, 1981.
102. Jackson RM, Veal CF, Beckman JS, et al: Polyethylene glycol–conjugated superoxide dismutase in unilateral lung injury due to re-expansion (re-oxygenation). Am J Med Sci 300:22–28, 1990.
103. Jackson RM, Veal CF, Alexander CB, et al: Re-expansion pulmonary edema. A potential role for free radicals in its pathogenesis. Am Rev Respir Dis 137:1165–1171, 1988.
104. Doerschuk CM, Allard MF, Oyarzun MJ: Evaluation of reexpansion pulmonary edema following unilateral pneumothorax in rabbits and the effect of superoxide dismutase. Exp Lung Res 16:355–367, 1990.
105. Henderson AF, Banham SW, Moran F: Re-expansion pulmonary oedema: A potentially serious complication of delayed diagnosis of pneumothorax. BMJ 291:593–594, 1985.
106. Smolle-Juettner FM, Prause G, Ratzenhofer B, et al: The importance of early detection and therapy of reexpansion pulmonary edema. Thorac Cardiovasc Surg 39:162–166, 1991.
107. Light RW, Jenkinson SG, Minh V, et al: Observations on pleural pressures as fluid is withdrawn during thoracentesis. Am Rev Respir Dis 121:799–804, 1980.
108. Light RW: Chylothorax and pseudochylothorax. *In* Pleural Diseases (3rd ed). Baltimore: Williams & Wilkins, 1995, pp 284–298.
109. Hillerdal G: Chylothorax and pseudochylothorax. Eur Respir J 10:1157–1162, 1997.
110. Machleder HI, Paulus H: Clinical and immunological alterations observed in patients undergoing long-term thoracic duct drainage. Surgery 84:157–165, 1978.
111. Breaux JR, Marks C: Chylothorax causing reversible T-cell depletion. J Trauma 28:705–707, 1988.
112. McKenna MJ, Chu JW, Kahkonen DM: Disturbances in lipid metabolism associated with chylothorax and its management. Henry Ford Hosp Med J 39:49–51, 1991.
113. Judson MA, Postic B: Chylothorax in a patient with AIDS and Kaposi's sarcoma. South Med J 83:322–324, 1990.
114. Pennington DW, Warnock ML, Stulbarg MS: Chylothorax and respiratory failure in Kaposi's sarcoma. West J Med 152:421–422, 1990.
115. Bogner JR, Gross M, Zietz C, et al: Chylothorax as fatal complication in fulminating Kaposi's sarcoma in a patient with AIDS. Klin Wochenschr 69:134, 1991.
116. Strausser JL, Flye MW: Management of nontraumatic chylothorax. Ann Thorac Surg 31:520–526, 1981.

117. Dougenis D, Walker WS, Cameron EW, et al: Management of chylothorax complicating extensive esophageal resection. Surg Gynecol Obstet 174:501–506, 1992.
118. Chernick V, Reed MH: Pneumothorax and chylothorax in the neonatal period. J Pediatr 76:624–632, 1970.
119. Van Aerde J, Campbell AN, Smyth JA, et al: Spontaneous chylothorax in newborns. Am J Dis Child 138:961–964, 1984.
120. Romero S, Martin C, Hernandez L, et al: Chylothorax in cirrhosis of the liver: Analysis of its frequency and clinical characteristics. Chest 114:154–159, 1998.
121. Tie MLH, Poland GA, Rosenow EC III: Chylothorax in Gorham's syndrome. A common complication of a rare disease. Chest 105:208–213, 1994.
122. Roy PH, Carr DT, Payne WS: The problem of chylothorax. Mayo Clin Proc 42:457–467, 1967.
123. Miller JI Jr: Diagnosis and management of chylothorax. Chest Surg Clin North Am 6:139–148, 1996.
124. Staats BA, Ellefson RD, Budahn LL, et al: The lipoprotein profile of chylous and nonchylous pleural effusions. Mayo Clin Proc 55:700–704, 1980.
125. Browse NL, Allen DR, Wilson NM: Management of chylothorax. Br J Surg 84:1711–1716, 1997.
126. Little AG, Kadowaki MH, Ferguson MK, et al: Pleuro-peritoneal shunting. Alternative therapy for pleural effusions. Ann Surg 208:443–450, 1988.
127. Murphy MC, Newman BM, Rodgers BM: Pleuroperitoneal shunts in the management of persistent chylothorax. Ann Thorac Surg 48:195–200, 1989.
128. Rheuban KS, Kron IL, Carpenter MA, et al: Pleuroperitoneal shunts for refractory chylothorax after operation for congenital heart disease. Ann Thorac Surg 53:85–87, 1992.
129. Cerfolio RJ, Allen MS, Deschamps C, et al: Postoperative chylothorax. J Thorac Cardiovasc Surg 112:1361–1365, 1996.
130. Vargas FS, Milanez JR, Filomeno LT, et al: Intrapleural talc for the prevention of recurrence in benign or undiagnosed pleural effusion. Chest 106:1771–1775, 1994.
131. Janssen JP, Joosten HJ, Postmus PE: Thoracoscopic treatment of postoperative chylothorax after coronary bypass surgery. Thorax 49:1273, 1994.
132. Robinson CLN: The management of chylothorax. Ann Thorac Surg 39:90–95, 1985.
132a. Mares DC, Mathur PN: Medical thoracoscopic talc pleurodesis for chylothorax due to lymphoma: A case series. Chest 114:731–735, 1998.
133. Perry RE, Hodgman J, Cass AB: Pleural effusion in the neonatal period. J Pediatr 62:838–843, 1963.
133a. Engum SA, Rescorla FJ, West KW, et al: The use of pleuroperitoneal shunts in the management of persistent chylothorax in infants. J Pediatr Surg 34:286–290, 1999.
134. Taylor JR, Ryu J, Colby TV, et al: Lymphangioleiomyomatosis: Clinical course in 32 patients. N Engl J Med 323:1254–1260, 1990.
135. Kalassian KG, Doyle R, Kao P, et al: Lymphangioleiomyomatosis: New insights. Am J Respir Crit Care Med 155:1183–1186, 1997.
135a. Garcia-Zamalloa A, Ruiz-Irastorza G, Aguayo FJ, et al: Pseudochylothorax. Report of 2 cases and review of the literature. Medicine 78:200–207, 1999.
136. Hamm H, Pfalzer B, Fabel H: Lipoprotein analysis in a chyliform pleural effusion. Implications for pathogenesis and diagnosis. Respiration 58:294–300, 1991.
137. Hillerdal G: Chyliform (cholesterol) pleural effusion—Eleven new cases. Chest 86:426–428, 1985.
138. Johnson JR, Falk A, Iber C, et al: Paragonimiasis in the United States. A report of nine cases in Hmong immigrants. Chest 82:168–171, 1982.
139. Goldman A, Burford TH: Cholesterol pleural effusion: A report of three cases with a cure by decortication. Dis Chest 18:586–594, 1950.
140. Light RW: Hemothorax. *In* Pleural Diseases (3rd ed). Baltimore: Williams & Wilkins, 1995, pp 278–283.
141. Drummond DS, Craig RH: Traumatic hemothorax: Complications and management. Am Surg 33:403–408, 1967.
142. Trupka A, Waydhas C, Hallfeldt KK, et al: Value of thoracic computed tomography in the first assessment of severely injured patients with blunt chest trauma: Results of a prospective study. J Trauma 43:405–411, 1997.
143. Beall AC Jr, Crawford HW, DeBakey ME: Considerations in the management of acute traumatic hemothorax. J Thorac Cardiovasc Surg 52:351–360, 1966.
144. Barriot P, Riou B, Viars P: Prehospital autotransfusion in life-threatening hemothorax. Chest 93:522–526, 1988.
145. Griffith GL, Todd EP, McMillin RD, et al: Acute traumatic hemothorax. Ann Thorac Surg 26:204–207, 1978.
146. Wilson JM, Boren CH, Peterson SR, et al: Traumatic hemothorax: Is decortication necessary? J Thorac Cardiovasc Surg 77:489–495, 1979.
147. Mattox KL, Fisher RG: Persistent hemothorax secondary to malposition of a subclavian venous catheter. J Trauma 17:387–388, 1977.
148. Liu DW, Liu HP, Lin PJ, et al: Video-assisted thoracic surgery in treatment of chest trauma. J Trauma 42:670–674, 1997.
148a. Velmahos GC, Murray JA, Asensio JA, et al: Predicting the need for thoracoscopic evacuation of residual traumatic hemothorax: Chest radiograph is insufficient. J Trauma 46:65–70, 1999.
149. Carrillo EH, Richardson JD: Thoracoscopy in the management of hemothorax and retained blood after trauma. Curr Opin Pulm Med 4:243–246, 1998.
150. Meyer DM, Jessen ME, Wait MA, et al: Early evacuation of traumatic retained hemothoraces using thoracoscopy: A prospective, randomized trial. Ann Thorac Surg 64:1396–1400, 1997.
151. Brunner RG, Vinsant GO, Alexander RH, et al: The role of antibiotic therapy in the prevention of empyema in patients with an isolated chest injury (ISS 9-10): A prospective study. J Trauma 30:1148–1153, 1990.
152. Krauss D, Schmidt GA: Cardiac tamponade and contralateral hemothorax after subclavian vein catheterization. Chest 99:517–518, 1991.
153. Hussain A, Raja AJ: Occurrence of hemothorax (unilateral) after sclerotherapy [letter]. Am J Gastroenterol 86:1553–1554, 1991.
154. Berliner K: Hemorrhagic pleural effusion: An analysis of 120 cases. Ann Intern Med 14:2266–2284, 1941.
155. Rostand RA, Feldman RL, Block ER: Massive hemothorax complicating heparin anticoagulation for pulmonary embolus. South Med J 70:1128–1130, 1977.
156. Huddy SP, Joyce WP, Pepper JR: Leaking thoraco-abdominal aortic aneurysm presenting with a massive left haemothorax: A clinical trap. Postgrad Med J 66:292–293, 1990.
157. Joseph J, Sahn SA: Thoracic endometriosis syndrome: New observations from an analysis of 110 cases. Am J Med 100:164–170, 1996.
158. Rodriguez E, Martinez MJ, Javaloyas M, et al: Haemothorax in the course of chickenpox. Thorax 41:491, 1986.
159. Smith PR, Manjoney DL, Teitcher JB, et al: Massive hemothorax due to intrathoracic extramedullary hematopoiesis in a patient with thalassemia intermedia. Chest 94:603–608, 1988.
160. Yung CM, Bessen SC, Hingorani V, et al: Idiopathic hemothorax. Chest 103:638–639, 1993.
161. Epler GR, McCloud CT, Gaensler EA: Prevalence and incidence of benign pleural effusion: Diagnosis and cause. JAMA 267:617–622, 1982.
162. Gaensler EA: Lung displacement: Abdominal enlargement, pleural space disorder, deformities of the thoracic cage. *In* Fenn WD, Rahn H (eds): Handbook of Physiology. Section 3: Respiration. Vol 2. Washington, DC: American Physiological Society, 1965, pp 1623–1661.
163. Miller A, Teristein A, Selikoff RJ: Ventilatory failure due to asbestos pleurisy. Am J Med 75:911–913, 1983.
164. Hughes RL, Jensik RJ, Faber LP, et al: Evaluation of unilateral decortication: A patient successfully treated 44 years after onset of tuberculosis. Ann Thorac Surg 19:704–715, 1975.
165. Hillerdal G: Non-malignant asbestos pleural disease. Thorax 36:669–675, 1981.

# 76 Tumors of the Pleura

RICHARD W. LIGHT, M.D. • V. COURTNEY BROADDUS, M.D.

Introduction
Malignant Mesothelioma
- Etiologic Factors
- Incidence
- Pathologic Features
- Clinical Manifestations
- Diagnosis
- Treatment

Benign Fibrous Mesothelioma
- Pathology
- Clinical Manifestations
- Diagnosis and Treatment

Primary Effusion Lymphoma
Pyothorax-Associated Lymphoma
Metastatic Pleural Disease
- Etiology
- Pathogenesis
- Clinical Manifestations
- Diagnosis
- Treatment
- Prognosis

Summary

## INTRODUCTION

The main primary tumors that involve the pleura are malignant mesothelioma, benign fibrous mesothelioma, primary effusion lymphoma, and pyothorax-associated lymphoma. These four tumors are all relatively uncommon. Much more commonly, the tumors that involve the pleura are metastatic. The four primary tumors and the metastatic tumors that involve the pleura are reviewed in this chapter.

## MALIGNANT MESOTHELIOMA

Malignant mesotheliomas are thought to arise from the mesothelial cells lining the pleural cavities. Malignant mesothelioma, with its dismal prognosis, should be differentiated from benign mesothelioma, which is also discussed in this chapter; it has an excellent prognosis. About 20% of mesotheliomas arise in the peritoneal cavity, but only pleural mesotheliomas are discussed here.

### Etiologic Factors

Without doubt, asbestos exposure is responsible for most cases of malignant mesothelioma. The role of asbestos in the etiology of mesothelioma was first convincingly documented by Wagner and colleagues[1] in 1960 with the observation that 45 of 47 South African patients with this rare malignancy had a history of contact with asbestos. In laboratory animals, mesotheliomas can be induced by the intrapleural instillation of asbestos.[2] In one study of 300 autopsies of asbestos workers, 3% had mesothelioma.[3] Overall, asbestos contact can be documented in approximately two thirds of all patients with malignant mesothelioma.[4] Because asbestos is found in a variety of industrial products, including insulation, roofing and ceiling tiles, brake linings, and numerous small appliances, however, many persons are unaware of their exposure to this substance. Further discussion about asbestos-induced pleural and pulmonary disorders is provided in Chapter 65.

All types of asbestos fibers with the exception of anthophyllite have been implicated in the pathogenesis of mesothelioma. The risk is not, however, the same for each fiber. The greatest risk is associated with crocidolite and amosite exposure and the least with chrysotile and tremolite exposure.[5, 6] Chrysotile accounts for about 90% of the commercial asbestos, but probably is related to the development of mesothelioma only when the level of exposure is high.[6] The latent period between the first exposure to asbestos and the emergence of the tumor is usually 30 to 45 years.[7] The incidence of mesothelioma observed in various groups of exposed persons is proportional to the duration and the severity of the exposure.

Not all mesotheliomas can be attributed to asbestos exposure. An unusually high incidence of mesothelioma has been observed in the Cappadocian region of Turkey, where approximately 1% of the population dies each year from malignant mesothelioma.[8] Because the atmosphere in this location contains increased amounts of erionite, a mineral of the silicate zeolite family, the increased incidence of mesothelioma has been attributed to the inhalation of this substance.[8]

Mesotheliomas have also been reported after radiation exposure, but a recent population study suggested that this relationship[9] was not strong. Chronic pleural disease may also lead to mesothelioma; in one series, 3 of 35 patients with malignant mesothelioma had a history of calcific pleural tuberculosis but not of exposure to asbestos.[10]

## Incidence

Malignant mesothelioma is still a relatively rare tumor, but its incidence has increased over the past few decades. In the United States, the incidence of mesothelioma in men is expected to peak at an annual rate of 2300 cases before the year 2000 and then drop toward 500 cases over the next 50 years. The incidence of mesothelioma in women has remained constant at about 500 cases per year.[11] These trends mirror the US trend in raw asbestos utilization.[11]

## Pathologic Features

In the earliest stages, malignant mesotheliomas appear grossly as multiple minute, round, gray, flat macules or tiny gray nodules.[12] With further development of the tumor, the pleural surface becomes progressively thicker and nodular in appearance, as the growing tumor extends in all directions to form a continuous layer encasing the lung and leading to contraction of the involved hemithorax. In advanced stages, the diaphragm, liver, pericardium, heart, contralateral pleura, and other mediastinal structures may be involved. Hematogenously disseminated metastases are present in about 50% of patients at autopsy, but these are usually clinically silent.[12]

Microscopically, malignant mesotheliomas are characterized by marked variation within a single tumor or among different tumors with a similar gross appearance.[11] Histologically, malignant mesotheliomas are classified as epithelial, sarcomatous, or mixed tumors.[12] In the epithelial form, the neoplastic cells show various epithelial arrangements such as papillary, tubular, tubulopapillary, cordlike, or sheetlike. The sarcomatous form resembles a spindle cell sarcoma in that the cells are spindle shaped with a parallel arrangement and have ovoid or elongated nuclei with well-developed nucleoli. The mixed form contains features of both the epithelial and the sarcomatous forms.[12]

The frequency of the three main histologic types varies from series to series. In a review of 819 cases from the literature, 50% of the mesotheliomas were epithelial, 34% were mixed, and 16% were sarcomatous.[13] The more biopsy specimens examined from a given tumor, the more likely the tumor is to be classified as mixed.

## Clinical Manifestations

The mean age of patients with malignant mesothelioma is about 60 years, with the majority between 50 and 70 years.[14] The most common presenting symptom is chest pain.[14] The chest pain is usually nonpleuritic and is frequently referred to the upper abdomen or shoulder because of diaphragmatic involvement. Dyspnea is present in about 40% of patients at presentation.[14] Other common symptoms are fever, chills, sweats, weakness, and malaise. At the time of presentation, more than 50% of patients have a large pleural effusion. Those presenting with large pleural effusions tend to have prominent dyspnea, whereas those presenting without large effusions are more likely to have chest pain, weight loss, and fever, along with evidence of tumor on examination.[15] Occasionally, the patient presents with either intermittent hypoglycemia or hypertrophic pulmonary osteoarthropathy,[16] but these conditions are much more common with benign than with malignant mesothelioma.

The clinical findings depend partly on whether the mesothelioma is epithelial or sarcomatous. Epithelial and mixed mesotheliomas often are associated with a large pleural effusion, while sarcomatous tumors usually are associated with a small or no pleural effusion. Patients with the epithelial type are more likely to have supraclavicular or axillary lymph node involvement and extension to the pericardium, contralateral pleura, and peritoneum. Distant metastases and bone metastases are more common with the sarcomatous tumors.[17]

**Radiographic Findings.** The chest radiograph reveals a pleural effusion in about 75% of patients.[18] The effusion is frequently large, occupying more than 50% of the hemithorax (Fig. 76.1). Pleural plaques are evident in the opposite hemithorax in about one third of patients. As the disease progresses, the tumor encases the ipsilateral lung, shifting the mediastinum toward the side of the tumor and contracting the involved hemithorax. In the late stages of the disease, the chest radiograph may show mediastinal widening, enlargement of the cardiac shadow owing to infiltration of the pericardium, soft-tissue masses, or destruction of the ribs.

Chest computed tomography (CT) scans are extremely useful in the evaluation of patients suspected of having malignant mesothelioma[18, 19] because the CT can demon-

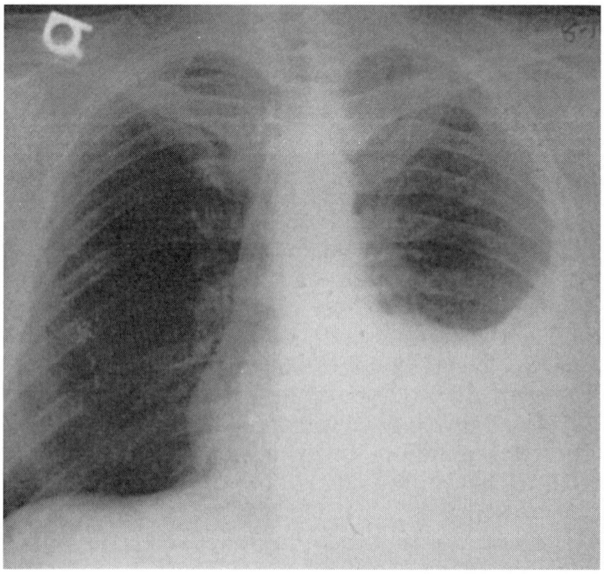

**Figure 76.1** Posteroanterior chest radiograph from a patient with a malignant mesothelioma demonstrating a left pleural effusion and thickening of the pleura over the upper left lung. (Reproduced with permission from Light RW: Pleural Diseases (3rd ed). Philadelphia: Lea & Febiger, 1995, p 120.)

strate the pleural disease, which would otherwise be obscured by pleural fluid on standard chest radiographs. The CT scan reveals that the pleura is thickened, with an irregular, often nodular internal margin that serves to distinguish this tumor from other types of pleural thickening. The major fissure is usually markedly thickened because of a combination of fibrosis, tumor, and associated fluid. In addition, it may appear nodular because of cancerous infiltration.[19] Often the CT scan will reveal intrapulmonary nodules that are not apparent on the standard chest radiograph.[19]

**Pleural Fluid.** The pleural fluid associated with mesothelioma is an exudate that is serosanguineous in about half the patients.[20] If the tumor is large, the pleural fluid glucose level and the pH may be reduced.[20] Patients with a low pleural fluid glucose or pH level have shorter survival times.[20] The pleural fluid is generally cellular, containing a mixture of normal mesothelial cells, malignant mesothelial cells, and various numbers of lymphocytes and polymorphonuclear leukocytes.[21] Cytologic examination of the pleural fluid is diagnostic of mesothelioma in about 25% of cases.[22] Although it was thought that mesotheliomas tended to have high levels of pleural fluid hyaluronic acid, it appears that measurement of the hyaluronic acid levels in the pleural fluid is not useful diagnostically.[23]

## Diagnosis

The diagnosis of malignant mesothelioma should be considered for any patient with an exudative pleural effusion, particularly if the patient has a history of asbestos exposure. The chest CT scan will usually be suggestive of the diagnosis. Although cytologic smears, needle biopsies, and sections from cell blocks of pleural fluid can establish the diagnosis of malignancy, they usually cannot distinguish between a metastatic adenocarcinoma and a mesothelioma.[24]

If the patient has skin deposits, these should be biopsied in an attempt to establish the diagnosis. In general, the diagnosis of malignant mesothelioma is best made with thoracoscopy.[22] If thoracoscopy is unavailable, open thoracotomy is usually required to make the diagnosis. With either procedure, generous specimens from several different areas should be obtained because the microscopic features can vary within a single tumor, even though the mass looks the same on gross examination. When pleural biopsy, tube thoracostomy, or thoracoscopy is performed in patients with mesothelioma, there is a high incidence (20%) of seeding of the operative tract with malignant mesothelioma. This seeding can be prevented if three daily sessions of radiotherapy at a dosage of 7 Gy/day are delivered 10 to 15 days after the procedure.[22, 25]

During the past decades, three techniques have been developed that establish the diagnosis of mesothelioma with greater certainty. These three techniques are immunocytochemistry, electron microscopy, and histochemical staining. To obtain these special studies, biopsy specimens should be immediately fixed in neutral buffered formalin, and a small piece should be fixed in glutaraldehyde for electron microscopy.[26]

Immunohistochemical studies with a panel of monoclonal antibodies are now most often used to differentiate metastatic adenocarcinomas from mesotheliomas. Many different antibodies have been developed,[24] but the four that appear to be the most useful are carcinoembryonic antigen, B72.3, Leu M1, and, most recently, Ber (EP4). If two or three of these tests are positive, the patient in all probability has adenocarcinoma. If none of the tests is positive, the patient in all probability has mesothelioma. It should be noted that these tests are also negative with benign mesothelial cells.[27]

Histochemical studies are used to identify adenocarcinomas by the presence of mucin-containing vacuoles and to identify mesotheliomas by their hyaluronan-containing vacuoles. These findings are not, however, absolute in distinguishing the two entities. In practice, histochemical studies are used in combination with the newer immunohistochemical approaches for the diagnosis of mesothelioma.[24]

Electron microscopy can also distinguish mesotheliomas from metastatic adenocarcinomas, but it is more time consuming and expensive than histochemical or immunohistochemical studies. The ultrastructural features of mesothelioma, especially the better-differentiated epithelial forms, are so characteristic as to be virtually diagnostic.[28] These characteristics include the absence of microvillus core rootlets, glycocalyceal bodies, and secretory granules; the presence of intracellular desmosomes, junctional complexes, and intracytoplasmic lumina; and characteristic microvilli. The appearance of the microvilli is the most important diagnostically: In mesothelioma, microvilli are numerous and are characteristically long and thin, whereas in adenocarcinoma they are typically much less frequent and are usually short and stubby.[28, 29]

In view of the dismal results with the different therapeutic modalities for malignant mesothelioma, the need to establish a definitive diagnosis might be questioned. The alternative diagnosis is usually metastatic adenocarcinoma, also for which no definitive therapy exists. At times, however, especially when the malignancy is extensive, the most prudent course is to treat the patient symptomatically without ever establishing the diagnosis. Making a diagnosis is essential if the patient contemplates litigation or entering a clinical trial for the treatment of mesothelioma. As treatment outcomes and options improve for mesothelioma, accurate histologic determination and staging will become more crucial.

## Treatment

The primary hope for a cure with malignant mesothelioma is surgery in conjunction with chemotherapy and radiotherapy. In the earliest stages of the disease, complete remissions have been reported with intrapleural interferon-gamma.[30]

**Staging.** Several staging systems have been proposed, but none is ideal.[31] One of the more practical staging systems is the four-stage system proposed by Sugarbaker and coworkers:[31] Stage I consists of resectable tumors without lymph node involvement; stage II consists of resectable tumors with positive lymph nodes; stage III includes unresectable tumors due to local extension of the tumor into the mediastinal structures or across the diaphragm; and stage IV consists of tumors with hematogenous dissemination. Survival is related to the stage of the disease. The median survival times with treatment were 22 months for those with stage I disease, 17 months for stage II disease, and 11 months for stage III disease.[31] Factors associated with a poor prognosis are a low performance status, chest pain, nonepithelial histology, and an age greater than 75 years.[4]

**Surgical Treatment.** The primary hope for cure for patients with malignant mesothelioma is multimodality therapy consisting of an extrapleural pneumonectomy followed by combination chemotherapy and radiotherapy. Sugarbaker and associates[32] performed this type of surgery on 120 patients between 1980 and 1995 who were stage I or II. All patients also received postoperative chemotherapy consisting of cyclophosphamide, adriamycin, and cisplatin and radiotherapy to the ipsilateral empty hemithorax. Patients were excluded if their left-ventricular ejection fraction was less than 45%, if the arterial $Po_2$ level was less than 65 mm Hg, or if their predicted postoperative $FEV_1$ was less than 1 L. The surgical resection included en bloc removal of the lung, parietal pleura, ipsilateral pericardium, and ipsilateral diaphragm.

Extrapleural pneumonectomy requires extensive surgery, which has a postoperative mortality rate of 5% and substantial postoperative morbidity. The overall median survival was 21 months, with 2 and 5 year survival rates of 45% and 22%, respectively. The survival rates were highest in patients with epithelial types, whose 2 and 5 year survival rates were 65% and 27%, respectively. The status of the lymph nodes was also important prognostically. The 2 and 5 year survival rates in the 39 patients with epithelial-type tumors and negative nodes were 74% and 39%, respectively.[32] Interestingly, gross residual tumor, microscopically positive margins, and tumor involving either the pericardium or diaphragm did not significantly affect survival. If a patient is not a candidate for extrapleural pneumonectomy, pleurectomy/decortication in conjunction with chemotherapy can be tried.[33]. It remains to be demonstrated, however, whether this therapy prolongs median survival.

**Chemotherapy.** The role of chemotherapy in the treatment of malignant mesothelioma appears to be limited. Doxorubicin and mitomycin appear to be the most active single agents against mesothelioma,[34] but response rates are usually less than 20%.[34] The response rates to multiple drug regimens containing doxorubicin or mitomycin are slightly higher than with the single drugs, but the response rates are still less than 30%.[34] Because there is no evidence that chemotherapy prolongs overall survival, it is recommended only if it is part of a clinical trial.

**Radiotherapy.** The results with external radiotherapy as the sole treatment for malignant mesothelioma have been disappointing, and at the present time it is not recommended.[35] There may be a place for internal radiation therapy in the management of malignant mesothelioma.[36] Over the past several years, patients with malignant mesothelioma at the Memorial Sloan–Kettering Cancer Center have undergone pleurectomy with the implantation of permanent radioactive iodine ($^{125}I$) sources in residual tumor. Postoperatively, the patients receive external radiation therapy with or without chemotherapy. The median survival rate of the 33 patients treated since 1977 exceeds 21 months.[36]

**Immunotherapy.** One series has shown a good response to intrapleural interferon-gamma.[30] In this series, 89 patients were treated with intrapleural interferon-gamma on an outpatient basis, and there were 8 complete responses and 9 partial responses. Most of the responses were obtained in patients with early stage disease.

**Palliative Therapy.** The two chief symptoms of patients with mesothelioma are dyspnea and chest pain. Most patients with a malignant mesothelioma have a large pleural effusion, which accumulates rapidly after aspiration.[15] In certain patients, this contributes to the dyspnea, and, if a therapeutic thoracentesis alleviates the dyspnea, chemical pleurodesis or the insertion of a pleuroperitoneal shunt pump should be considered.[15] Pleurectomy should also be considered for those patients with large pleural effusions that cannot be controlled with chemical pleurodesis. If those procedures fail, or if the dyspnea is not relieved with a thoracentesis, as is frequently the case, the dyspnea should be managed symptomatically with opiates, supplemental oxygen, or both.

Chest pain is probably the most difficult symptom to manage in patients with malignant mesothelioma. It is frequently severe and unremitting in the terminal stages of the disease. Radiotherapy appears to be of no benefit in the management of the pain.[15] Sufficient analgesics, including opiates when necessary, should be given to alleviate suffering.

## BENIGN FIBROUS MESOTHELIOMA

Benign fibrous mesotheliomas are localized pleural tumors that appear to arise from the multipotential subserosal cells and usually express mesenchymal differentiation.[37] They appear to be unrelated to previous asbestos exposure.[16] They are uncommon tumors, with fewer than 1100 cases reported. Patients with this benign tumor have an excellent prognosis.

### Pathology

Benign fibrous mesotheliomas appear as firm, encapsulated, and lobulated masses with a characteristic whorled appearance.[16] On occasion, these tumors invade the lung and chest wall locally.[38] Benign mesotheliomas arise from the visceral pleura in about 70% of patients and from the parietal pleura in the remaining 30%. Microscopically, these tumors are characterized by uniform, elongated spindle cells and varied amounts of collagen and reticulum fibers in bundles of many sizes.[16]

## Clinical Manifestations

Approximately half of the patients with benign fibrous mesotheliomas are asymptomatic, with the chest mass discovered on a routine chest radiograph.[16] Symptoms, when present, include cough, chest pain, and dyspnea, each of which occurs in about 40% of symptomatic patients. Fever without evidence of infection occurs in about 25% of patients with symptoms.

Two paraneoplastic syndromes occur frequently in patients with benign fibrous mesotheliomas, namely, hypertrophic pulmonary osteoarthropathy and hypoglycemia. Hypertrophic pulmonary osteoarthropathy occurs in approximately 20% of patients with benign mesotheliomas. Most patients with this syndrome have tumors greater than 7 cm in diameter.[16] When the tumor is removed, the symptoms of hypertrophic pulmonary osteoarthropathy are usually relieved immediately. It is important to realize that pulmonary hypertrophic osteoarthropathy in conjunction with a large chest mass may not indicate inoperable bronchogenic carcinoma.

Symptomatic hypoglycemia occurs in about 4% of patients with benign fibrous mesothelioma.[39] The mechanism responsible for the hypoglycemia appears to be the production of high levels of insulin-like growth factor II by the tumor.[40] The increased production of this insulin-like substance leads to an increased metabolism of glucose by peripheral tissues and perhaps by the tumor. Surgical removal of the tumor cures the hypoglycemia. For further discussion of hypertrophic pulmonary osteoarthropathy, hypoglycemia, and other paraneoplastic syndromes, the reader is referred to Chapters 23 and 46.

Benign fibrous mesotheliomas appear radiologically as solitary, sharply defined, discrete masses located at the periphery of the lung (Fig. 76.2) or adjacent to a fissure.[41] Frequently the mass is loculated. There is an associated pleural effusion in about 10%, but the presence of the pleural effusion does not adversely affect the prognosis.[41] Occasionally, the mass may be so large that it occupies the entire hemithorax and shifts the heart and mediastinum toward the contralateral side. The CT scan is suggestive of the diagnosis because the tumor is large, noninvasive, sometimes heterogeneous, and enhanced after the administration of intravenous contrast material. Contrast enhancement is usually intense, as a result of the rich vasculature of the tumor.[41] Magnetic resonance imaging (MRI) may suggest the diagnosis because benign fibrous mesotheliomas have low signal intensity (as do all masses with a high collagen content) on all MR-sequence images, whereas malignant mesotheliomas and other malignant diseases have high signal intensity on the T2-weighted images.[41]

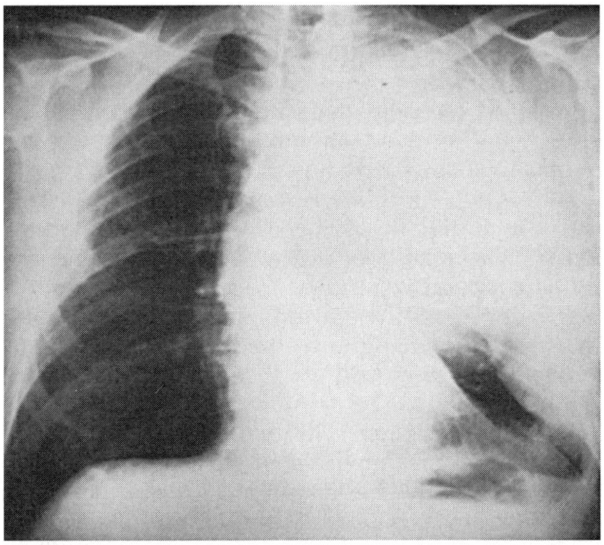

**Figure 76.2** Posteroanterior roentgenogram from a 64-year-old man who had mesothelioma-associated hypoglycemia. Note the large left-sided pleural-based mass and small pleural effusion.

## Diagnosis and Treatment

The diagnosis is usually made at thoracotomy, and the treatment of choice is surgical removal. Most patients are cured with surgical resection, but the disease recurs in approximately 10%. Recurrences have been reported more than 10 years after the initial resection. Patients who have undergone surgical resection for benign fibrous mesothelioma should have annual chest radiographs to detect recurrences at a time when they may still be operable.

# PRIMARY EFFUSION LYMPHOMA

Primary effusion lymphoma is an uncommon type of lymphoma that grows in body cavities and presents as a malignant lymphomatous effusion without an identifiable contiguous tumor mass.[42] These tumors usually occur in homosexual men with acquired immunodeficiency syndrome and contain the Kaposi's sarcoma–associated human herpes virus-8 (KSHV or HHV8), but they may occur in human immunodeficiency virus–negative organ transplant recipients.[43] Most cases are also characterized by the presence of the Epstein-Barr virus.[42]. The primary effusion lymphoma has a distinctive morphology, bridging large cell immunoblastic lymphoma and anaplastic large cell lymphoma. The pleural fluid is a lymphocytic exudate characterized by a very high lactate dehydrogenase level. The diagnosis can usually be established with pleural fluid cytology. The optimal treatment for these lymphomas remains to be established,[44] but the median survival is only 4 to 6 months.

# PYOTHORAX-ASSOCIATED LYMPHOMA

Pyothorax-associated lymphoma is a new entity, and only about 60 cases have been reported, mostly from Japan.[45] Pyothorax-associated lymphoma occurs almost exclusively in patients who, several decades earlier, received artificial pneumothorax for the treatment of long-standing pulmonary tuberculosis. Thus, because of the lack of active pyothorax, the name should actually be *pneumothorax-associated* lymphoma. Most of these lymphomas are of B-cell lineage. The Epstein-Barr virus genome has been detected in all of the tumors tested.[45]

The male to female ratio of patients with this disease

is 5.2:1. Common presenting symptoms are chest pain, productive cough, fever, and dyspnea. Some patients present with a tumor of the chest wall. CT scans reveal pleural masses without effusions in the majority of patients.[46]

## METASTATIC PLEURAL DISEASE

Malignant pleural effusions secondary to metastatic disease are second only to infections as a cause of exudative pleural effusion. It is estimated that 200,000 malignant pleural effusions occur annually in the United States.[47]

### Etiology

The three tumors that cause approximately 75% of all malignant pleural effusions are lung carcinoma (30%), breast carcinoma (25%), and lymphomas (20%). Metastatic ovarian carcinoma is responsible for about 6%, and sarcomas, particularly melanoma, account for about 3%. No other single tumor accounts for more than 1% of malignant pleural effusions. The primary tumor is never identified in about 6% of patients with malignant pleural effusion.[48]

### Pathogenesis

A malignant tumor can lead to the development of a pleural effusion by several different mechanisms (Table 76.1). The presence of pleural metastases may increase the permeability of the pleural surfaces so that more fluid and protein enter the pleural space. The increased fluid formation may be due to the elaboration of vascular endothelial growth factor from the metastatic tumors.[49] Decreased clearance of fluid may contribute to the formation of pleural fluid, but it certainly is not the primary mechanism. If decreased clearance of fluid were responsible, one would expect patients to have a transudative pleural effusion, and the total amount of fluid accumulating each day should be less than 15 mL.[50] This certainly is not the case for many patients with malignant effusions.

**Table 76.1 TEN MECHANISMS BY WHICH MALIGNANT DISEASE MAY LEAD TO PLEURAL EFFUSION**

1. Pleural metastases with increased permeability
2. Pleural metastases with obstruction of pleural lymphatic vessels
3. Mediastinal lymph node involvement with decreased pleural lymphatic drainage
4. Bronchial obstruction (decreased pleural pressures)
5. Postobstructive pneumonitis
6. Thoracic duct interruption (chylothorax)
7. Pericardial involvement
8. Hypoproteinemia
9. Pulmonary embolism
10. Postradiation therapy

Modified with permission from Light RW: Pleural Diseases (3rd ed). Philadelphia: Lea & Febiger, 1995, p 99.

If a lobar or main-stem bronchus becomes obstructed by a tumor, the lung distal to the obstruction becomes atelectatic. Accordingly, the remaining lung has to overexpand or the ipsilateral hemithorax has to contract, both of which lead to a more negative pleural pressure, which can cause a pleural effusion. A parapneumonic effusion can result if postobstructive pneumonia develops distal to a partially occluded bronchus.

A chylothorax may accumulate if the thoracic duct is obstructed; the majority of chylothoraces that are not traumatic in origin are secondary to neoplastic involvement of the thoracic duct, particularly by lymphomas (see Chapter 75). If the hydrostatic pressures in the systemic and pulmonary circulation become elevated because of pericardial involvement by the tumor, a transudative pleural effusion may result. Patients with malignancy may also have a pleural effusion secondary to hypoproteinemia, pulmonary embolism, or radiation therapy.

In patients with bronchogenic carcinoma, pleural metastases are thought to arise from tumor emboli seeding via the pulmonary artery to the ipsilateral pleura.[51, 52] In one autopsy study,[52] the pleural metastases were exclusively ipsilateral in 17 of 24 cases of bronchogenic carcinoma. The parietal pleura rarely is involved without visceral pleural involvement,[51, 52] suggesting that metastases extend directly from the visceral to the parietal pleura. It is thought that contralateral pleural metastases usually indicate hepatic involvement with tumor and tertiary spread from the hepatic metastases to the contralateral pleura.[51]

In patients with nonbronchogenic carcinoma, pleural metastases are usually due to tertiary spread from secondary hepatic tumors. In Meyer's series[51] of 23 patients with malignant pleural disease from nonbronchogenic carcinoma, 19 (83%) had hepatic metastases. Moreover, 11 of these 19 patients had only visceral pleural metastases.[51]

Only about 50% of patients with pleural metastases will have a pleural effusion.[51, 52] The presence of a pleural effusion is more closely related to neoplastic invasion of the mediastinal lymph nodes than to the extent of pleural involvement by nodular metastases.[51]

### Clinical Manifestations

The most common symptom reported by patients with malignant pleural effusion is dyspnea, occurring in more than 50% of people with metastatic pleural disease.[53] Only about 25% of patients with malignant pleural effusion have chest pain, which is usually dull and aching rather than pleuritic. Many patients have symptoms attributable to the tumor itself, such as weight loss, malaise, and anorexia. Approximately 20% of patients are asymptomatic when the pleural effusion is first discovered.[53]

Malignant pleural effusions vary in size from a few milliliters that cause minimal blunting of the costophrenic angle to several liters that completely opacify the hemithorax and shift the mediastinum to the contralateral side. If a hemithorax is opacified and the mediastinum is not shifted toward the contralateral side, it is likely that the patient has bronchogenic carcinoma with obstruction of a main-stem bronchus, a fixed mediastinum owing to tumor involvement, or a malignant mesothelioma. If the mediastinum is shifted toward the side of the effusion, the pleural pressure on the side of the effusion is more negative than on the contralateral side. The inability of this negative pressure to reinflate the lung strongly suggests that the lung cannot reinflate, and pleurodesis via tube thoracostomy is unlikely to be successful.

The chest radiograph of a patient with a pleural effusion secondary to bronchogenic carcinoma usually reveals a parenchymal lesion (Fig. 76.3), although at times a therapeutic thoracentesis must be performed before the pulmonary abnormality is evident. During the course of their disease, at least half the patients with disseminated lung cancer will develop a pleural effusion. Although pleural effusions can be caused by all types of lung carcinoma, malignant effusions are most frequently due to adenocarcinoma.[53] With lung carcinoma, the pleural effusion is usually on the same side as the primary tumor but at times can be bilateral. The pleural effusion is often present at the time of diagnosis or shortly thereafter.[54]

Approximately 50% of patients with disseminated breast carcinoma will develop a pleural effusion during the course of their disease.[55] The pleural effusion is on the same side as the original breast tumor in 60%, on the contralateral side in 25%, and bilateral in 15%.[55] The mean interval between the development of the primary tumor and the appearance of the pleural effusion is more than 2 years and can be as long as 20 years.[54] Less than 10% of patients have radiographically evident pulmonary metastases.[56]

Approximately 16% of patients with non-Hodgkin's lymphoma or Hodgkin's disease have pleural effusion during the course of their disease. In most of these patients, the effusion is present at the time of the initial diagnosis.[57] Pleural effusion is usually not an isolated finding but is associated with disease elsewhere. With Hodgkin's disease, 90% of the effusions have associated mediastinal lymphadenopathy. With non-Hodgkin's lymphoma, 20% to 70% have evidence of mediastinal disease, and 90% have evidence of disease elsewhere. About 20% of the effusions are chylothoraces in patients with non-Hodgkin's lymphoma, but only 3% are chylothoraces with Hodgkin's disease.[57]

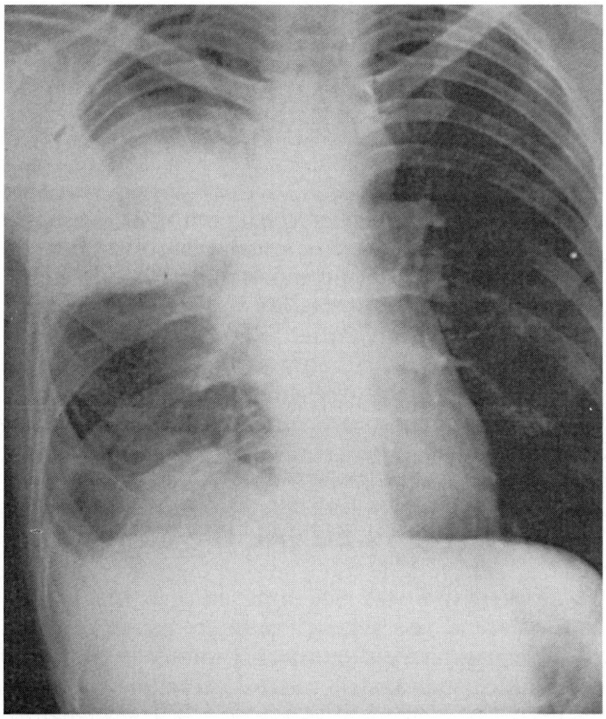

**Figure 76.3** Posteroanterior chest radiograph demonstrating a right pleural effusion and a large chest mass. The parenchymal lesion is not this dramatic in all patients with pleural effusion secondary to bronchogenic carcinoma.

The pleural fluid from a malignant pleural effusion is an exudate.[58] Most pleural effusions that meet exudative criteria by the quantity of lactic dehydrogenase in the fluid but not by the protein or lactic dehydrogenase ratio are malignant.[58] Although malignant pleural disease is probably the most common cause of a grossly bloody pleural fluid, nearly 50% of malignant pleural effusions do not appear to be bloody and have pleural fluid red blood cell counts under 10,000/μL.[59] The differential cell count can reveal a predominance of small lymphocytes, other mononuclear cells, or neutrophils.[59] Although it has been stated in the past that pleural fluid eosinophilia is uncommon with malignant pleural effusions,[60] a recent article questions this conclusion.[61] In this study of 460 pleural effusions, 20% of eosinophilic effusions were malignant and 20% of noneosinophilic effusions were malignant.[61]

The pleural fluid glucose level is reduced to below 60 mg/dL (3.33 mmol/L) in approximately 20% of malignant pleural effusions.[62, 63] Malignant pleural effusions with a low glucose level also tend to have a low pH. Patients with these findings usually have a large tumor burden in their pleural space; accordingly, their prognosis is poor, with a median survival rate of only about 1 to 2 months.[62, 63] The pleural fluid amylase level is elevated in approximately 10% of patients with malignant pleural effusion, and usually the primary tumor in such patients is not in the pancreas.[64] Pancreatic disease can be differentiated from malignant disease with a high pleural fluid amylase level because the amylase with malignant disease is of the salivary type.[64]

## Diagnosis

The diagnosis of a malignant pleural effusion is established by demonstration of malignant cells in the pleural fluid or in the pleura itself. In most instances, the diagnosis is established by cytologic examination of the pleural fluid or biopsy of the pleura via thoracoscopy.

**Pleural Fluid Cytology.** Pleural fluid cytology is positive in 60% to 90% of patients with pleural malignancy.[65, 66] The incidence of positive cytology depends on the stage of the tumor, the type of the tumor, and the skill of the cytologist. Cytologic findings are frequently negative if the tumor involvement of the pleura is minimal. The results are usually positive if the patient has an adenocarcinoma, but they are nondiagnostic in more than 80% of patients with squamous cell carcinoma, lymphoma, or mesothelioma. The cytologic findings will also be negative if the effusion is not related to malignant involvement of the pleura but rather is secondary to another factor, such as congestive heart failure, pulmonary emboli, pneumonia, lymphatic blockade, or hypoproteinemia.

With cytologic examination, the neoplasm can generally be classified into a histologic type such as adenocarcinoma, but the primary site of the tumor cannot usually be inferred from the cytologic findings.[67] If the cytologic report suggests adenocarcinoma, the diagnosis of mesothelioma should be considered because, on cytologic examination, the epithelial form of mesothelioma is frequently misinterpreted as adenocarcinoma.

**Pleural Biopsy.** Over the past few decades, the diagnosis of pleural malignancy has frequently been established with needle biopsy of the pleura. With improvements in cytologic examination of pleural fluid and with the increasing availability of thoracoscopy, however, needle biopsy is not generally recommended when pleural malignancy is suspected.[66] In one series from the Mayo Clinic, only 20 of 118 patients (17%) with pleural malignancy and nondiagnostic cytology had a positive needle biopsy test of the pleura.[68]

**Thoracoscopy.** The diagnosis of malignancy can be established by thoracoscopy in more than 90% of patients with malignant pleural disease.[69, 70] An important advantage of establishing the diagnosis of malignancy with thoracoscopy is that the effusion can be controlled via pleurodesis with the same procedure.[66] The best means by which to achieve pleurodesis in this situation is with the insufflation of 2 to 5 g of talc.[71]

**Other Diagnostic Tests.** There have been numerous papers published in the past several years advocating measurement of various tumor markers in the pleural fluid to establish the diagnosis of malignant pleural effusions. Markers recommended to be measured include carcinoembryonic antigen; carbohydrate antigens 19-9, 15-3, 72-4, and 125; tissue polypeptide antigen; alpha-fetoprotein; $alpha_1$-acid glycoprotein; and $beta_2$-microglobulin.[72] In general, the mean levels of all these tumor markers are higher in malignant than in benign effusions. There are, however, false-positive results with all of these tumor markers.[73] Because the consequences of making a wrong diagnosis of pleural malignancy are profound, the use of tumor markers in the diagnosis of pleural malignancy is not recommended.[66]

As discussed earlier in this chapter, immunohistochemical staining with monoclonal antibodies directed toward various antigens is useful in differentiating malignant mesothelioma from metastatic adenocarcinoma. The DNA content of malignant cells tends to be abnormal, and quantitation of nuclear DNA via flow cytometry has been advocated for the diagnosis of pleural malignancy. When flow cytometric analysis is compared with cytologic diagnosis, however, the flow cytometric analysis is both less sensitive and less specific and is therefore not recommended.[74] Flow cytometry can be used to establish the cell lineage of lymphocytes (T or B cells) and the clonality of a population of lymphocytes and is therefore useful in the diagnosis of pleural lymphoma.[75]

**Positive Cytology with Unknown Primary.** The source of the primary tumor in 75% of patients with malignant pleural effusion is the lung, the breast, or a lymphoma, with the majority of the remaining primary tumors originating in the abdomen. Patients with malignant pleural effusions and an unknown primary tumor should therefore undergo CT scanning of the chest and abdomen, mammography, and pelvic examination. If, after these tests, there is still no clue as to the origin of the tumor, no further diagnostic tests are indicated. Patients with a malignant pleural effusion have a limited life expectancy (mean, 3 months), and it serves no purpose to keep them in the hospital for a prolonged period in an attempt to establish the source of the primary tumor. The primary tumor is never identified in 6% of all patients with malignant pleural effusion.

## Treatment

The initial step in the management of a patient with a malignant pleural effusion is to attempt to identify the site of the primary tumor. The main reason for this is to decide whether to administer systemic chemotherapy.[76] The presence of a malignant pleural effusion indicates disseminated tumor; therefore, the only hope for cure is systemic chemotherapy, which will control the pleural effusion in approximately 40% of patients with metastatic breast carcinomas[56] and in 35% of patients with small cell lung carcinoma.[77]

**Chemical Pleurodesis.** Chemical pleurodesis should be considered for patients with malignant pleural effusions who are not candidates for systemic chemotherapy or who have failed systemic chemotherapy. The objective is to eradicate the pleural space and thus prevent the accumulation of pleural fluid, not to diminish the tumor burden. Therefore, only patients who are symptomatic from their pleural effusion should be considered candidates for chemical pleurodesis and then only if their symptoms have been shown to be relieved by a therapeutic thoracentesis. If the patient is asymptomatic, it does not make sense to put the patient through the trauma of a pleurodesis just to make the chest radiograph look better. Similarly, if the patient is moribund from disseminated tumor, he or she should not be made uncomfortable with chest tubes for the last few days of life.

Before a pleurodesis is attempted, the position of the mediastinum should be evaluated. If the mediastinum is shifted toward the side of the effusion, pleurodesis is contraindicated.[47] A shift of the mediastinum toward the side of the effusion indicates that the underlying lung is unable to expand normally and that the pleural pressure is more negative on the side of the effusion. Therefore, if a chest tube is inserted, it is unlikely that the visceral and parietal pleura can be brought into apposition for a successful pleurodesis.[47]

The goal of a chemical pleurodesis is to obliterate the pleural space so that there is no room for the pleural fluid to reaccumulate.[47] This is accomplished by injecting an agent into the pleural space that will create an intense inflammatory response, resulting in fusion of the visceral and parietal pleurae and obliteration of the intervening space. Therefore, it is important to evacuate the pleural fluid with a chest tube before the procedure is attempted and to maintain the apposition of the pleural surfaces after the sclerosing agent is injected. The visceral and parietal pleurae will not fuse if they are not touching each other after the sclerosing agent is injected. Pleurodesis is more effective when chest tubes are inserted than when the fluid is merely aspirated.[78] It should be noted that if a small chest tube is placed intrapleurally, spontaneous pleurodesis will occur in approximately 50% of patients at a median time of 3 to 4 weeks after chest tube insertion.[79]

***Choice of Sclerosing Agent.*** Although many substances have been used during the past 50 years as sclerosing agents, the three agents used most commonly at the present time are the tetracycline derivatives, talc slurry, or bleomycin. In a review article, Walker-Renard and coworkers[80] reported that, of these three agents, talc was most effective, the tetracycline derivatives were next, and bleomycin was last. The excellent results (~90%) reported with talc were, however, influenced by the fact that many of the patients patients had received insufflated talc at the time of thoracoscopy. If patients are found to have a trapped lung or loculated fluid at thoracoscopy, talc is usually not administered. Accordingly, this selection bias probably contributed to the better results for talc.

Talc, tetracycline, and bleomycin all have their proponents but none is ideal.[80a] We prefer doxycycline 500 mg because it is efficacious,[81, 82] widely available, and inexpensive. The primary disadvantage of talc is that its intrapleural administration has been associated with the development of the acute respiratory distress syndrome and death.[82, 83] At autopsy, talc particles are found distributed throughout the body.[83] It has been speculated that this syndrome is more likely to result from the use of talc with a small median particle size.[84] The primary disadvantage of bleomycin is that it is much more expensive (about $1000) than the other agents. It is likely that within the next few years a more specific pleural sclerosant such as a cytokine cocktail will be developed.[85]

***Technique.*** Once it is determined that a patient is a candidate for a chemical pleurodesis, tube thoracostomy should be performed. Because the patient has a limited life expectancy (median, ~90 days), this therapy ideally should be done on an outpatient basis. The feasibility of outpatient therapy has been demonstrated by Patz and coworkers,[86] who drained the effusions via gravity drainage into a collection bottle, and by Putnam and coworkers,[87] who drained the effusions by connecting the indwelling catheter to suction bottles on an as-needed basis.[87] If outpatient therapy is selected, the sclerosant can be injected through the indwelling catheter after the volume of the drainage is less than 100 mL/day and a chest radiograph demonstrates that the lung is fully expanded. If inpatient therapy is undertaken, the sclerosant can be injected as soon as the lung is fully expanded with no loss of effectiveness.[81] If successful re-expansion of the lung cannot be accomplished with tube thoracostomy, sclerosing agents should not be injected into the pleural space. Their injection can only lead to more thickening of the visceral pleura and consequent further compromise of the underlying lung.

Because pleurodesis with a tetracycline derivative at times is quite painful, it is recommended that treated patients be given medications such as lorazepam or midazolam to produce conscious sedation. After the sclerosing agent is injected into the pleural space through the chest tube, 50 mL of saline is subsequently injected through the tube to clear the agent.[88] Afterward, the chest tube is clamped for about 2 hours. Although we recommended in the past that the patient be moved into different positions after the intrapleural injection, we no longer do these maneuvers. In both animals and humans, the dispersal of radioisotopes injected intrapleurally is similar whether or not rotation is performed.[88] Nonetheless, for a particulate such as talc, rotation may assist its distribution in the pleural space. The optimal duration for suction postinjection is not known, but there is no evidence success rates are increased if suction is prolonged beyond 48 hours.

Pleurodesis effectively controls the pleural effusions in 70% to 90% of properly selected patients.[80, 88] Most failures occur when sclerosis is attempted in patients in whom the mediastinum is shifted toward the side of the effusion or in whom the underlying lung does not reexpand after tube thoracostomy. Pleurodesis more commonly fails when the pleural fluid glucose level is below 60 mg/dL (3.33 mmol/L) or the pleural fluid pH is less than 7.30.[62, 63] Because the procedure will be effective in some patients with low glucose or pH, however, sclerosis should still be attempted in such individuals if the indications outlined above are met.

**Alternative Therapies.** Alternative therapies to chemical pleurodesis include insertion of a chronic indwelling catheter, insertion of a pleuroperitoneal shunt, symptomatic therapy with opiates and oxygen (discussed earlier for malignant mesothelioma), serial therapeutic thoracentesis, and pleurectomy.

***Chronic Indwelling Catheter.*** Patients with recurring malignant pleural effusions can be managed as outpatients with a chronic indwelling catheter. With one commercially available system, the indwelling catheter has a special adaptor on its distal end through which the patient drains the effusion as needed. Although sclerosis occurs spontaneously in about 50% of such patients, consideration should be given to instilling sclerosants through the access catheter if high (>1000 mL/week) levels of drainage persist after 2 weeks, because these patients are unlikely to achieve a spontaneous pleurodesis.[79]

***Pleuroperitoneal Shunt.*** This device consists of two catheters connected with a valved pump chamber that is tunneled under the skin so that one catheter is in the pleural space and the other in the peritoneal space. The shunt can be inserted during an outpatient procedure. The pleural effusion is then controlled by the patient's manual compression of the pump chamber to move the pleural fluid from the pleural space to the peritoneal cavity. The two primary problems with the shunt are the need for frequent pumping each day and the tendency for the shunt to become occluded. The pleuroperitoneal shunt is probably the treatment of choice for the patient with a trapped lung in whom the accumulation of fluid causes dyspnea.[47]

***Thoracentesis.*** Serial therapeutic thoracenteses are usually not warranted for patients with malignant pleural effusion. After a therapeutic thoracentesis, a malignant pleural effusion will usually reaccumulate rapidly, frequently within 1 to 3 days. Serial therapeutic thoracenteses should only be performed in moribund patients for whom the procedures offer symptomatic relief.

***Pleurectomy.*** Pleurectomy may be used to control a malignant pleural effusion in two different situations. First, if a patient undergoes a diagnostic thoracotomy for an undiagnosed pleural effusion and malignant disease is present, a parietal pleurectomy can be performed to induce a pleurodesis.[90] Second, pleurectomy should be considered for the symptomatic patient with a persistent pleural effusion and trapping of the ipsilateral lung. Pleurectomy, which includes decortication of the trapped lung in conjunction with parietal pleurectomy, controls the malignant pleural effusions in more than 90% of cases, but it is a substantial surgical procedure with a mortality rate of about 10%.[89] Parietal pleurectomy in conjunction with decortication is recommended only for those patients who are in good overall condition, whose primary tumor is either under control or progressing slowly, and who are symptomatic from the effusion. Patients who meet these criteria are rarely seen.

## Prognosis

Patients with malignant pleural effusions have a poor prognosis. In one series of 96 patients, the mean survival rate after diagnosis was only 3.1 months, with a 54% mortality rate within 1 month and an 84% mortality at 6 months.[53] The mean survival for the 30 patients with lung cancer was only 2.2 months, whereas the mean survival of 13 patients with breast cancer was 7.3 months.[53] In more recent series,[62, 63] the survival rate of patients with low pleural fluid glucose or pH level is very short (1 to 2 months), but for patients with pleural fluid glucose levels above 60 mg/dL (3.33 mmol/L) and a pH above 7.30, survival averages 6 months.

## SUMMARY

Malignant mesothelioma is an uncommon tumor, but it appears to be increasing in incidence. Because of its frequent association with previous exposure to asbestos, the diagnosis of malignant mesothelioma raises important worker's compensation issues that the attending physician must consider (Chapter 65). Benign fibrous mesothelioma is even rarer than malignant mesothelioma, but it is curable by surgical resection and is sometimes attended by striking paraneoplastic manifestations (clubbing of the digits or hypoglycemia). Two rare lymphomas, primary effusion lymphoma and pyothorax-associated lymphoma, arise in the pleural space and appear to be due to viral infections. Pleural effusions due to metastatic disease are a common clinical problem that are usually caused by spread from bronchogenic carcinoma, cancer of the breast, or lymphoma. Metastatic malignancy may lead to pleural effusion by several mechanisms, but in most instances the pleura is directly involved. Most patients with malignant pleural effusion should be subjected to a pleurodesis procedure designed to obliterate the pleural space.

## References


1. Wagner JC, Sleggs EA, Marchand P: Diffuse pleural mesothelioma and asbestos exposure in the North Western Cape Province. Br J Ind Med 17:260–271, 1960.
2. Wagner JC, Berry G, Timbrell V: Mesothelioma in rats after inoculation with asbestos and other materials. Br J Cancer 28:173–185, 1973.
3. Selikoff IJ, Churg J, Hammond, EC: Relation between exposure to asbestos and mesothelioma. N Engl J Med 272:560–565, 1965.
4. Herndon JE, Green MR, Chahinian AP, et al: Factors predictive of survival among 337 patients with mesothelioma treated between 1984 and 1994 by the Cancer and Leukemia Group B. Chest 113:723–731, 1998.
5. Churg A: Chrysotile, tremolite, and malignant mesothelioma in man. Chest 93:621–628, 1988.
6. Churg A: Asbestos-related disease in the workplace and the environment: Controversial issues. Monogr Pathol 36:52–77, 1993.
7. Pisani RJ, Colby TV, Williams DE: Malignant mesothelioma of the pleura. Mayo Clin Proc 63:1234–1244, 1988.
8. Baris I, Simonato L, Artvinli, M, et al: Epidemiological and environmental evidence of the health effects of exposure to erionite fibres: A four-year study in the Cappadocian region of Turkey. Int J Cancer 39:10–17, 1987.
9. Cavazza A, Travis LB, Travis WD, et al: Post-irradiation malignant mesothelioma. Cancer 77:1379–1385, 1996.
10. Roviaro GC, Sartori F, Calabro F, et al: The association of pleural mesothelioma and tuberculosis. Am Rev Respir Dis 126:569–571, 1982.
11. Price B: Analysis of current trends in United States mesothelioma incidence. Am J Epidemiol 145:211–218, 1997.
12. Corson JM: Pathology of diffuse malignant pleural mesothelioma. Semin Thorac Cardiovasc Surg 9:347–355, 1997.
13. Hillerdal G: Malignant mesothelioma 1982: Review of 4710 published cases. Br J Dis Chest 77:321–343, 1983.
14. Light RW: Malignant and benign mesotheliomas. *In* Pleural Diseases (3rd ed): Baltimore: Williams & Wilkins, 1995, pp 117–128.
15. Law MR, Hodson ME, Turner-Warwick M: Malignant mesothelioma of the pleura: Clinical aspects and symptomatic treatment. Eur J Respir Dis 65:162–168,1984.
16. Robinson LA, Reilly RB: Localized pleural mesothelioma. The clinical spectrum. Chest 106:1611–1615, 1994.
17. Law MR, Hodson ME, Heard BE: Malignant mesothelioma of the pleura: Relation between histological type and clinical behaviour. Thorax 37:810–815, 1982.
18. Kawashima A, Libshitz HI: Malignant pleural mesothelioma: CT manifestations in 50 cases. AJR 155:965–969, 1990.
19. Kreel L: Computed tomography in mesothelioma. Semin Oncol 8:302–312, 1981.
20. Gottehrer A, Taryle, DA, Reed CE, et al: Pleural fluid analysis in malignant mesothelioma. Chest 100:1003–1006, 1991.
21. Klempman S: The exfoliative cytology of diffuse pleural mesothelioma. Cancer 15:691–704, 1962.
22. Boutin C, Rey F: Thoracoscopy in pleural malignant mesothelioma: A prospective study of 188 consecutive patients. Part 1: Diagnosis. Cancer 72:389–393, 1993.
23. Hillerdal G, Lindqvist U, Engstrom-Laurent A: Hyaluronan in pleural effusions and in serum. Cancer 67:2410–2414, 1991.
24. Dejmek A: Methods to improve the diagnostic accuracy of malignant mesothelioma. Respir Med 90:191–199, 1996.
25. Boutin C, Rancoise R, Viallat J-R: Prevention of malignant seeding after invasive diagnostic procedures in patients with pleural mesothelioma. Chest 108:754–758, 1995.
26. Antman KH, Corson JM: Benign and malignant mesothelioma. *In* Light RW (ed): Clinics in Chest Medicine, Symposium on Pleural Diseases. Philadelphia: WB Saunders, 1985, pp 141–152.

27. Brown RW, Clark GM, Tandon AK, et al: Multiple-marker immunohistochemical phenotypes distinguishing malignant pleural mesothelioma from pulmonary adenocarcinoma. Hum Pathol 24:347–354, 1993.
28. Coleman M, Henderson DW, Mukherjee TM: The ultrastructural pathology of malignant pleural mesothelioma. Pathol Ann. 24:303–353, 1989.
29. Warhol MJ, Hunter NJ, Corson JM: An ultrastructural comparison of mesotheliomas and adenocarcinomas of the ovary and endometrium. Int J Gynecol Pathol 1:125–134, 1982.
30. Boutin C, Nussbaum E, Monnet I, et al: Intrapleural treatment with recombinant gamma-interferon in early stage malignant pleural mesothelioma. Cancer 74:2460–2467, 1994.
31. Sugarbaker DJ, Norberto JJ, Swanson SJ: Surgical staging and work-up of patients with diffuse malignant pleural mesothelioma. Semin Thorac Cardiovasc Surg 9:356–360, 1997.
32. Sugarbaker DJ, Garcia JP, Richards WG, et al: Extrapleural pneumonectomy in the multimodality therapy of malignant mesothelioma. Results in 120 consecutive patients. Ann Surg 224:288–296, 1996.
33. Rusch VW: Pleurectomy/decortication in the setting of multimodality treatment for diffuse malignant pleural mesothelioma. Semin Thorac Cardiovasc Surg 9:367–372, 1997.
34. Taub RN, Antman KH: Chemotherapy for malignant mesothelioma. Semin Thorac Cardiovasc Surg 9:361–366, 1997.
35. Linden CJ, Mercke C, Albrechtsson U, et al: Effect of hemithorax irradiation alone or combined with doxorubicin and cyclophosphamide in 47 pleural mesotheliomas: A nonrandomized phase II study. Eur Respir J 9:2565–2572, 1996.
36. Martini N, McCormack PM, Bains MS, et al: Pleural mesothelioma. Ann Thorac Surg 43:113–120, 1987.
37. Steinetz C, Clarke R, Jacobs GH, et al: Localized fibrous tumors of the pleura: Correlation of histopathological, immunohistochemical and ultrastructural features. Pathol Res Pract 186:344–357, 1990.
38. Ellis K, Wolff M: Mesotheliomas and secondary tumors of the pleura. Semin Roentgenol 12:303–311, 1977.
39. Briselli M, Mark EJ, Dickersin GR: Solitary fibrous tumors of the pleura: Eight new cases and review of 360 cases in the literature. Cancer 47:2678–2689, 1981.
40. Axelrod L, Ron D: Insulin-like growth factor II and the riddle of tumor-induced hypoglycemia. N Engl J Med 319:1477–1478, 1988.
41. Ferretti GR, Chiles C, Cox JE, et al: Localized benign fibrous tumors of the pleura: MR appearance. J Comput Assist Tomogr 21:115–120, 1997.
42. Nador RG, Cesarman E, Chadburn A, et al: Primary effusion lymphoma: A distinct clinicopathologic entity associated with the Kaposi's sarcoma–associated herpes virus. Blood 88:645–656, 1996.
43. Jones D, Ballestas ME, Kaye KM, et al: Primary-effusion lymphomas and Kaposi's sarcoma in a cardiac-transplant recipient. N Engl J Med 339:444–449, 1998.
44. Light RW, Hamm H: Pleural disease and the acquired immune deficiency syndrome. Eur Respir J 10:2638–2643, 1997.
45. Taniere P, Manai A, Charpentier R, et al: Pyothorax-associated lymphoma: Relationship with Epstein-Barr virus, human herpes virus-8 and body cavity–based high grade lymphomas. Eur Respir J 11:779–783, 1998.
46. Kanno H, Ohsawak M, Iuchi K, et al: Appearance of a different clone of Epstein-Barr virus genome in recurrent tumor of pyothorax-associated lymphoma (PAL) and a mini-review of PAL. Leukemia 12:1288–1294, 1998.
47. Light RW: Malignant pleural effusions. *In* Pleural Diseases (3rd ed): Baltimore: Williams & Wilkins, 1995, pp 94–116.
48. Spriggs AI, Boddington MM: The Cytology of Effusions (2nd ed): New York: Grune & Stratton, 1968.
49. Cheng C-S, Rodriguez RM, Perkett EA, et al: Vascular endothelial growth factor in pleural fluid. Chest 115:760–765, 1999.
50. Light RW, Hamm H: Malignant pleural effusion: Would the real cause please stand up? Eur Respir J 10:1701–170, 1997.
51. Meyer PC: Metastatic carcinoma of the pleura. Thorax 21:437–443, 1966.
52. Rodriguez-Panadero F, Borderas Naranjo F, Lopez Mejias J: Pleural metastatic tumours and effusions. Frequency and pathogenic mechanisms in a post-mortem series. Eur Respir J 2:366–369, 1989.
53. Chernow B, Sahn SA: Carcinomatous involvement of the pleura. Am J Med 63:695–702, 1977.
54. van de Molengraft FJ, Vooijs GP: The interval between the diagnosis of malignancy and the development of effusions, with reference to the role of cytologic diagnosis. Acta Cytol 32:183–187, 1988.
55. Goldsmith HS, Bailey HD, Callahan EL, et al: Pulmonary lymphangitic metastases from breast carcinoma. Arch Surg 94:483–488, 1967.
56. Fentiman IS, Millis R, Sexton S, et al: Pleural effusions in breast cancer: A review of 105 cases. Cancer 47:2087–2092, 1981.
57. Berkman N, Breuer R, Kramer MR, et al: Pulmonary involvement in lymphoma. Leuk Lymph 20:229–237, 1996.
58. Light RW, MacGregor MI, Luchsinger PC, et al: Pleural effusions: The diagnostic separation of transudates and exudates. Ann Intern Med 77:507–513, 1972.
59. Light RW, Erozan YS, Ball WC: Cells in pleural fluid: Their value in differential diagnosis. Arch Intern Med 132:854–860, 1973.
60. Adelman M, Albelda SM, Gottlieb J, et al: Diagnostic utility of pleural fluid eosinophilia. Am J Med 77:915–920, 1984.
61. Rubins JB, Rubins HB: Etiology and prognostic significance of eosinophilic pleural effusions. A prospective study. Chest 110:1271–1274, 1996.
62. Rodriguez-Panadero F, Lopez-Mejias L: Survival time of patients with pleural metastatic carcinoma predicted by glucose and pH studies. Chest 95:320–324, 1989.
63. Sahn SA, Good JT Jr: Pleural fluid pH in malignant effusions. Ann Intern Med 108:345–349, 1988.
64. Kramer MR, Saidana MJ, Cepero RJ, et al: High amylase levels in neoplasm-related pleural effusion. Ann Intern Med 110:567–569, 1989.
65. Sahn SA: Pleural diseases related to metastatic malignancies. Eur Respir J 10:1907–1913, 1997.
66. Light RW: Closed needle biopsy of the pleura is a valuable diagnostic procedure. Con: closed needle biopsy. J Bronchol 5:332–336, 1998.
67. Naylor B, Schmidt RW: The case for exfoliative cytology of serous effusions. Lancet 1:711–712, 1964.
68. Prakash UBS, Reiman HM: Comparison of needle biopsy with cytologic analysis for the evaluation of pleural effusions: Analysis of 414 cases. Mayo Clin Proc 60:158–164, 1985.
69. Menzies R, Charbonneau M: Thoracoscopy for the diagnosis of pleural disease. Ann Intern Med 114:271–276, 1991.
70. Hucker J, Bhatnagar NK, Al-Jilaihawi AN, et al: Thoracoscopy in the diagnosis and management of recurrent pleural effusions. Ann Thorac Surg 52:1145–1147, 1991.
71. Milanez RC, Vargas FS, Filomeno LB, et al: Intrapleural talc for the treatment of malignant pleural effusions secondary to breast cancer. Cancer 75:2688–2692, 1995.
72. Villena V, Lopez-Encuentra A, Echave-Sustaeta J, et al: Diagnostic value of CA 72-4, carcinoembryonic antigen, CA 15-3, and CA 19-9 assay in pleural fluid. Cancer 78:736–740, 1996.
73. Garcia-Pachon E, Padilla-Navas I, Dosda D, et al: Elevated level of carcinoembryonic antigen in nonmalignant pleural effusions. Chest 111:643–647, 1997.
74. Rodriguez de Castro F, Molero T, Acosta O, et al: Value of DNA analysis in addition to cytological testing in the diagnosis of malignant pleural effusions. Thorax 49:692–694, 1994.
75. Moriarty AT, Wiersema L, Snyder W, et al: Immunophenotyping of cytologic specimens by flow cytometry. Diagn Cytopathol 9:252–258, 1993.
76. Grossi F, Pennucci MC, Tixi L, et al: Management of malignant pleural effusions. Drugs 55:47–58, 1998.
77. Livingston RB, McCracken JD, Trauth CJ, et al: Isolated pleural effusions in small cell lung carcinoma: Favorable prognosis. Chest 81:208–211, 1982.
78. Leahy BC, Honeybourne D, Brear SG, et al: Treatment of malignant pleural effusions with intrapleural *Corynebacterium parvum* or tetracycline. Eur J Respir Dis 66:50–54, 1985.
79. Rodriguez RM, Putnam JB, Glassfor D, et al: Predicting spontaneous pleurodesis in patients with malignant pleural effusion treated with an indwelling catheter. Am J Respir Crit Care Med 157:A65, 1998.

80. Walker-Renard PB, Vaughan LM, Sahn SA: Chemical pleurodesis for malignant pleural effusions. Ann Intern Med 120:56–64, 1994.
80a. Mitchem RE, Herndon BL, Fiorella RM, et al: Pleurodesis by autologous blood, doxycycline, and talc in a rabbit model. Ann Thorac Surg 67:917–921, 1999.
81. Villanueva AG, Gray AW Jr, Shahian DM et al: Efficacy of short term versus long term tube thoracostomy drainage before tetracycline pleurodesis in the treatment of malignant pleural effusions. Thorax 49:23–25, 1994.
82. Patz EF Jr, McAdams HP, Erasmus JJ et al: Sclerotherapy for malignant pleural effusions: A prospective randomized trial of bleomycin vs doxycycline with small-bore catheter drainage. Chest 113:1305–1311, 1998.
83. Milanez Campos JR, Werebe EC, Vargas FS, et al: Respiratory failure due to insufflated talc. Lancet 349:251–252, 1997.
83a. Rehse DH, Aye RW, Florence MG: Respiratory failure following talc pleurodesis. Am J Surg 177:437–440, 1999.
84. Ferrer J, Villarino MA, Tura JM et al: Comparison of size and composition of nine different talcs. Its relevance for pleurodesis. Am J Respir Crit Care Med 157:A66, 1998.
85. Lane K, Cheng D-W, Rogers J, et al: An innovative method by which pleurodesis can be produced in rabbits. Chest 114:364S, 1998.
86. Patz, EF Jr McAdams HP, Goodman PC, et al: Ambulatory sclerotherapy for malignant pleural effusions. Radiology 199:133–135, 1996.
87. Putnam JB, Light RW, Rodriguez RM, et al: A randomized comparison of indwelling pleural catheter and doxycycline pleurodesis in the management of malignant pleural effusions. Cancer 86:1992–1999.
88. Light RW, Vargas FS: Pleural sclerosis for the treatment of pneumothorax and pleural effusion. Lung 175:213–223, 1997.
89. Martini N, Bains MS, Beattie EJ, Jr: Indications for pleurectomy in malignant effusion. Cancer 35:734–738, 1975.

# Disorders of the Mediastinum

SECTION O

# 77 General Principles and Diagnostic Approach

DAVID R. PARK, M.D. • DAVID J. PIERSON, M.D.

Introduction
Normal Mediastinum
Clinical Settings and Presentations of Mediastinal Disease
- Asymptomatic Mass
- Effects of Compression or Invasion of Adjacent Tissues
- Systemic Symptoms and Syndromes
- Pneumomediastinum and Mediastinitis
- Investigation of the Mediastinum in Patients with Malignancy

Techniques for Visualizing the Mediastinum and its Contents
- Conventional Radiographic Techniques
- Computed Tomography
- Magnetic Resonance Imaging
- Ultrasonography
- Radionuclide Imaging

Techniques for Obtaining Mediastinal Tissue
- Needle Aspiration and Biopsy
- Mediastinoscopy, Anterior Mediastinotomy, and Thoracoscopy

General Approach to Diagnostic Investigation
- Evaluation of a Mediastinal Mass
- Mediastinal Evaluation to Stage Bronchogenic Carcinoma

Summary

## INTRODUCTION

The mediastinum is the region in the chest between the pleural cavities; it contains the heart and other thoracic viscera except for the lungs. It is bounded laterally by the parietal pleurae, anteriorly by the sternum, posteriorly by the vertebral column and paravertebral gutters, superiorly by the thoracic inlet, and inferiorly by the diaphragm. Interest in the mediastinum as a separate body region stems from the diversity and vital importance of the structures it contains and from the multiplicity of disease processes by which it can be affected. The nonspecific nature of the clinical manifestations of most of these disorders and the mediastinum's inaccessibility for diagnostic examination result in considerable challenge to the clinician evaluating mediastinal disease.

After the contents of the mediastinum and the clinical manifestations produced by disease in this region are described, this chapter focuses on the techniques available for diagnostic investigation. These techniques include imaging the mediastinal contents and obtaining tissue for cytologic or histologic examination. A general approach to the clinical evaluation of mediastinal disease is then presented that considers the risks and potential benefits of the available techniques in light of their overall impact on clinical management.

## NORMAL MEDIASTINUM

The anatomy of the mediastinum can be described in several ways, depending on whether it is being considered from the point of view of the radiologist[1–3] or of the operating surgeon.[4–6] Most clinicians simply divide the mediastinum into anterior, middle, and posterior compartments, as seen on the lateral chest roentgenogram (Fig. 77.1).[7] The anterior compartment consists of everything lying forward of and superior to the heart shadow; its boundaries are the sternum, the first rib, and an imaginary curved line following the anterior heart border and brachiocephalic vessels from the diaphragm to the thoracic inlet. Within the anterior compartment lie the thymus gland and lymphatic tissue (Table 77.1).

**Table 77.1 NORMAL MEDIASTINAL CONTENTS**

| |
|---|
| Anterior compartment |
| Thymus gland |
| Substernal extensions of thyroid and parathyroid glands |
| Lymphatic vessels and lymph nodes |
| Areolar connective tissue |
| Middle compartment |
| Heart |
| Pericardium |
| Aortic arch and great vessels |
| Innominate veins and superior vena cava |
| Trachea and main bronchi |
| Hila |
| Lymph nodes |
| Phrenic and upper vagus nerves |
| Areolar connective tissue |
| Posterior compartment |
| Esophagus |
| Descending aorta |
| Azygos and hemiazygos veins |
| Thoracic duct |
| Lymph nodes |
| Vagus nerves (lower portions) |
| Sympathetic chains |
| Areolar connective tissue |

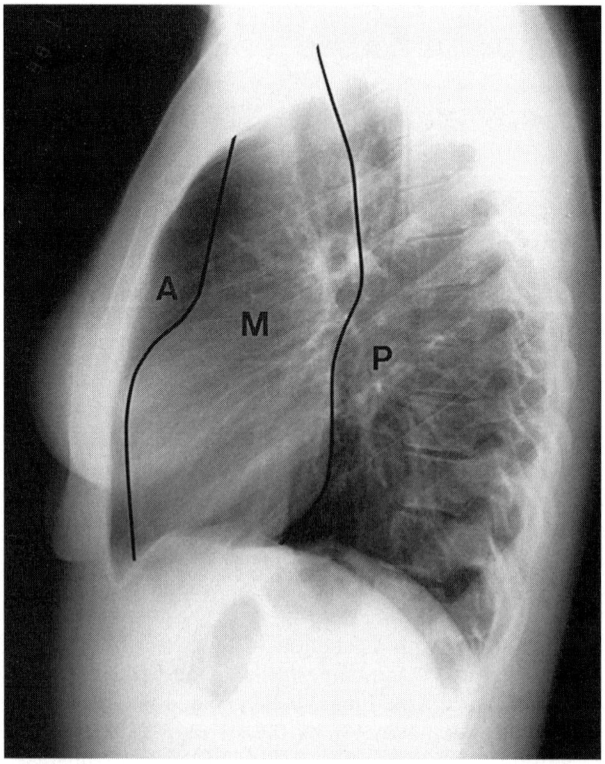


**Figure 77.1** By convention, the mediastinum is divided into anterior (A), middle (M), and posterior (P) compartments, according to its appearance on the lateral chest roentgenogram. Although other, more complex subdivisions exist, this one is most helpful to the clinician.

Dorsal to the anterior mediastinum is the middle compartment, extending from the lower edge of the sternum along the diaphragm and then cephalad along the posterior heart border and posterior wall of the trachea. It contains the heart, pericardium, and trachea, plus the aortic arch and its major branches, pulmonary arteries, innominate veins, pulmonary hila, and several groups of lymph nodes. In addition, the phrenic and upper vagus nerves course through the middle mediastinal compartment.

The posterior mediastinum occupies the space between the back of the heart and trachea and the front of the posterior ribs and paravertebral gutters on each side. It extends from the diaphragm cephalad to the first rib. In it are the esophagus, descending aorta, azygos and hemiazygos veins, paravertebral lymph nodes, and thoracic duct. The lower portions of the vagus nerve and sympathetic chains are also within the posterior mediastinum.

The three-compartment model just described is consistent with embryonic development of the region and also with the characteristic distribution of individual disorders encountered clinically. Other classifications exist, however. Some authors include the most superior portion of the anterior mediastinum as a separate, fourth compartment. Heitzman[1] subdivides the mediastinum into seven distinct regions: thoracic inlet, anterior mediastinum, supra-aortic area, infra-aortic area, supra-azygos area, infra-azygos area, and hila. This classification has been praised for enabling radiologists to localize lesions more accurately and for permitting more precise differential diagnosis,[8] but it seems unnecessarily complicated for the clinician. A similar categorization, based on surgical landmarks, is used for the mapping of lymph node locations during mediastinal staging of bronchogenic carcinoma.[9]

Separation of mediastinal structures into anterior, middle, and posterior compartments follows logically from the appearance of the chest on conventional roentgenography and, because evaluation of a mediastinal abnormality nearly always starts with a conventional chest roentgenogram, these compartments will likely remain the fundamental anatomic units of the mediastinum. The anatomic relationships of the mediastinal viscera and tissue planes, however, are best appreciated on axial images such as those produced by computed tomography scans and as shown schematically in Figure 77.2.[10] The anatomy of tissue planes in the mediastinum and their continuity with spaces in the neck and abdomen are discussed further in Chapters 78 and 79.

## CLINICAL SETTINGS AND PRESENTATIONS OF MEDIASTINAL DISEASE

### Asymptomatic Mass

The incidental discovery of a mediastinal mass that has produced no symptoms is the most common setting in which the clinician encounters primary mediastinal disease, and most asymptomatic masses are benign.[6, 11] Table 77.2 lists the disorders that present as a mediastinal mass and the compartments in which they characteristically occur. Each is discussed in more detail in Chapter 79.

**Table 77.2 DISORDERS PRESENTING AS A MASS IN THE MEDIASTINUM**

- Anterior mediastinum
  - Thymic neoplasms
  - Germ cell tumors
    - Teratoma
    - Seminoma
    - Nonseminomatous germ cell tumors
      - Embryonal cell carcinoma
      - Choriocarcinoma
  - Lymphoma
    - Hodgkin's disease
    - Non-Hodgkin's lymphoma
  - Thyroid neoplasms
  - Parathyroid neoplasms
  - Mesenchymal tumors
    - Lipoma
    - Fibroma
    - Lymphangioma
    - Hemangioma
    - Mesothelioma
    - Others
  - Diaphragmatic hernia (Morgagni)
  - Primary carcinoma
  - Angiofollicular lymphoid hyperplasia (Castleman's disease)
- Middle mediastinum
  - Lymphadenopathy
    - Reactive and granulomatous inflammation
    - Metastasis
  - Lymphoma
  - Developmental cysts
    - Pericardial cyst
    - Foregut duplication cysts
      - Bronchogenic cyst
      - Enteric cyst
    - Others
  - Vascular enlargements
  - Diaphragmatic hernia (hiatal)
- Posterior mediastinum
  - Neurogenic tumors
    - Arising from peripheral nerves
    - Arising from sympathetic ganglia
    - Arising from paraganglionic tissue
  - Meningocele
  - Esophageal lesions
    - Carcinoma
    - Diverticula
  - Diaphragmatic hernia (Bochdalek)
  - Miscellaneous

### Effects of Compression or Invasion of Adjacent Tissues

Masses or inflammation in the mediastinum can produce a wide variety of symptoms. Chest pain, from traction on mediastinal tissues, tissue invasion, or bone erosion, is common. Cough also occurs frequently because of extrinsic compression of the trachea or main-stem bronchi or erosion into the airway itself. Either of these processes predisposes to postobstructive pneumonia. Hemoptysis also may be part of the clinical presentation. Invasion or irritation of the pleural surface may produce a pleural effusion and can cause pain and dyspnea. Compression or direct invasion of the esophagus may lead to dysphagia, which can be the presenting symptom of a mediastinal mass in the posterior compartment. In granulomatous mediastinitis and mediastinal fibrosis, esophageal involvement is second in frequency only to superior vena caval obstruction in terms of clinical effects.[12]

The superior vena cava is especially vulnerable to extrinsic compression and obstruction because it is thin walled, its intravascular pressure is low, and it is relatively confined by lymph nodes and other more rigid structures. A distinct *superior vena cava syndrome* results from increased venous pressure in the upper thorax, head, and neck[6, 13, 14] and is characterized by dilation of collateral veins in the upper portion of the thorax and neck; edema and plethora of the face, neck, and upper torso; suffusion and edema of the conjunctiva; and cerebral symptoms, such as headache, disturbance of consciousness, and visual distortion.[13, 14] Tinnitus and epistaxis also may occur, and all symptoms are exacerbated in the supine position. Tuberculous mediastinitis and syphilitic aneurysms were once the most common causes of superior vena cava obstruction. In more recent series, bronchogenic carcinoma is by far the most common etiology,[6, 14] and fewer than 20% of cases are due to nonmalignant disease such as thrombosis or mediastinal fibrosis.[15]

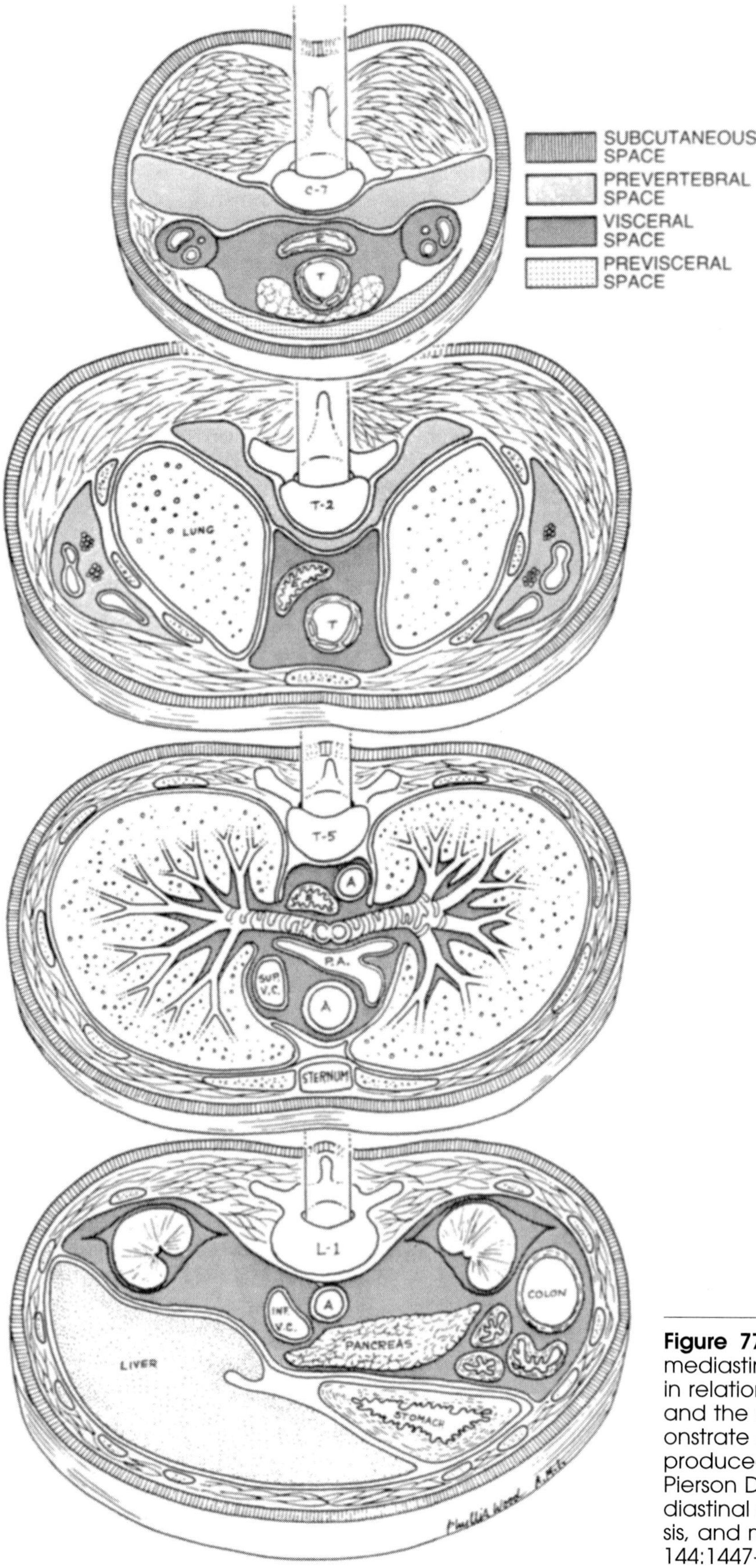


**Figure 77.2** Soft-tissue compartments of the mediastinum (levels of T-2 and T-5) are shown in relation to those of the neck (level of C-7) and the upper abdomen (level of L-1) to demonstrate continuity of the visceral space. (Reproduced with permission from Maunder RJ, Pierson DJ, Hudson LD: Subcutaneous and mediastinal emphysema: Pathophysiology, diagnosis, and management. Arch Intern Med 144:1447–1453, 1984.)

Mediastinal masses can produce a variety of symptoms by invading or compressing nerves. These include hoarseness from recurrent laryngeal nerve involvement, Horner's syndrome from involvement of sympathetic ganglia, dyspnea from diaphragmatic paralysis, and clinical manifestations of spinal cord or nerve root compression.

### Systemic Symptoms and Syndromes

Fever, anorexia, weight loss, and other systemic symptoms are nonspecific features of malignancy and granulomatous inflammation that occur frequently in patients with mediastinal disease. In addition, primary mediastinal tumors are associated with a wide array of distinctive systemic syndromes, including Cushing's syndrome, hypertension, gynecomastia, hypoglycemia, and hypercalcemia.[6, 11] Thymoma is notorious for its association with myasthenia gravis; less commonly, pure red cell aplasia, hypogammaglobulinemia, and myocarditis occur with this neoplasm.

### Pneumomediastinum and Mediastinitis

Air in the mediastinum (pneumomediastinum) is a common complication of mechanical ventilation and may also be encountered in spontaneously breathing patients under a wide variety of circumstances. Pain is the most common symptom[10, 16–18] and presumably results from stretching of mediastinal tissues. It is characteristically substernal and aggravated by breathing and changes in position. Other manifestations of air in the mediastinum include dyspnea, dysphagia, dysphonia with the characteristic "hot potato" voice, and subcutaneous crepitation. Acute inflammation within the confined space of the mediastinum causes a dramatic clinical picture dominated by substernal chest pain, chills, high fever, and prostration. Pneumomediastinum and mediastinitis are discussed further in Chapter 78.

### Investigation of the Mediastinum in Patients with Malignancy

The most common clinical circumstance under which the clinician's attention is focused on the mediastinum is in the staging of patients with lung cancer. Bronchogenic carcinoma is the most common malignancy in the United States, with 170,000 new cases and nearly 160,000 deaths per year.[19] Crucial to the management of patients with non–small cell carcinoma, affecting both initial therapy and ultimate survival, is whether and to what extent the mediastinum is involved.[20, 21] Considerable controversy surrounds the question of whether ipsilateral lymph node metastasis should preclude surgical resection for cure.[22, 23] Although metastatic involvement of the mediastinum has been considered a contraindication for surgery, recent reports cite improved survival with resection in ipsilateral metastatic disease,[24–27] and increasing attention is being focused on combined surgical and chemotherapeutic treatment approaches.[28, 29] With any of these philosophies, careful preoperative evaluation of the mediastinum is crucial to the decision-making process.[30–32] (See Chapter 46 for further discussion of bronchogenic carcinoma.)

Nonthoracic malignancies also may metastasize to the mediastinum. This is particularly common with tumors originating in the head and neck, the genitourinary tract, the breasts, and the skin (malignant melanoma).[2]

## TECHNIQUES FOR VISUALIZING THE MEDIASTINUM AND ITS CONTENTS

The diagnostic approach to disorders of the mediastinum may be divided into two phases; noninvasive imaging techniques and invasive procedures for obtaining tissue samples. The former category includes conventional radiographic studies, computed tomography (CT), magnetic resonance imaging (MRI), transthoracic and endoscopic ultrasonography, and various radionuclide studies. Characteristic mediastinal imaging findings that suggest specific diagnoses are listed in Table 77.3.

### Conventional Radiographic Techniques

Standard posteroanterior and lateral chest roentgenograms are the means through which most mediastinal abnormalities are first detected. A stable appearance, in comparison with older films, can obviate the need for further investigation. If old roentgenograms are not available, however, or if the abnormality has appeared or enlarged since the last film, further evaluation is usually required. Special conventional roentgenographic views, fluoroscopy, and tomography may provide additional information about a mass, but these have largely been replaced by CT and MRI.[33]

In the appropriate clinical settings, contrast studies remain important diagnostic tools in mediastinal disease. Barium esophagrams can demonstrate extrinsic compression, tumor invasion,[11] or fistula formation; and angiography may be helpful in discerning solid or cystic from vascular structures, can identify the vascular supply of tumors, and can sample blood for hormonal localization of certain tumors. Myelography may help to delineate intraspinal extension of posterior mediastinal tumors and to differentiate neurogenic neoplasms from meningoceles, but it has largely been supplanted by CT and MRI.

Air contrast studies are seldom used intentionally in the United States today. These studies include diagnostic pneumothorax, to show whether a mass is adherent to the mediastinum or chest wall[34, 35], diagnostic pneumoperitoneum, which can demonstrate diaphragmatic herniation through the foramens of Morgagni (anterior) or Bochdalek (posterior); and diagnostic pneumomediastinum, to distinguish between thymic hyperplasia and thymoma.[11]

### Computed Tomography

Evaluation of mediastinal disease has changed dramatically since the advent of CT imaging. The transaxial plane of CT is well suited for assessment of mediastinal structures, most of which are oriented perpendicularly to this plane. Certain patterns and densities on CT images are virtually pathognomonic. These include high-density calcified tissue and contrast-enhanced blood vessels; and fat, whose characteristic low density enables it to be identified with certainty (Fig. 77.3).[36–38] Normal anatomic variations and fluid-filled cysts can be distinguished con-

**Table 77.3 SOME CHARACTERISTIC ROENTGENOGRAPHIC FINDINGS IN MEDIASTINAL DISEASE**

| FEATURE | LIKELY ETIOLOGY |
|---|---|
| Huge mass on initial presentation | Neurogenic tumor<br>Meningocele<br>Mesenchymal tumor |
| Teardrop-shaped mass within interlobar fissure | Pericardial or bronchogenic cyst |
| Fat density on CT scan | Mediastinal lipomatosis or lipoma |
| Calcification in mass | In rim of mass<br>Cystic thymoma or thyroid adenoma<br>Aneurysm<br>Silicosis (``eggshell'' calcification)<br>In center of mass<br>Thyroid adenoma<br>Teratoma |
| Teeth or bone | Teratoma |
| Phleboliths | Hemangioma |
| Air-fluid level in mass | Esophageal disease<br>Diaphragmatic hernia<br>Developmental cyst<br>Cystic teratoma<br>Abscess |
| Mass with associated parenchymal infiltrate | Granulomatous infection<br>Metastatic bronchogenic carcinoma<br>Lymphoma with direct extension into lung<br>Esophageal abnormality with aspiration |
| Pneumonitis | Bronchial compression by primary mediastinal mass |
| Mass wtih associated pleural effusion | Metastatic malignancy with pleural involvement<br>Granulomatous inflammation of lymph nodes |
| Superior vena cava obstruction | Recent onset<br>Bronchogenic carcinoma<br>Lymphoma<br>Catheter-associated thrombosis<br>Long-standing<br>Mediastinal fibrosis |
| Erosion or destruction of bone | Arterial aneurysm<br>Tumors of peripheral nerves or sympathetic ganglia<br>Meningocele |
| Spine or rib deformity | Enteric cyst |

fidently from other processes, and the site of origin of mediastinal masses can be better identified.[2, 36] Characteristic CT findings in a variety of mediastinal disorders have now been described, including thymoma[39] and other thymic disorders,[40] pericardial cysts,[41] thyroid goiters,[41a] abnormalities at the right cardiophrenic angle,[42] and a variety of benign conditions.[43]

Despite its numerous advantages for mediastinal imaging, CT also has several limitations. Although vertically oriented structures (e.g., those in the paratracheal area), are well seen on cross-sectional CT images, horizontally oriented structures and boundaries are much more difficult to evaluate.[22] Abnormalities in the aortopulmonary window area and the subcarinal region are examples. Certain distinctions cannot be made reliably by CT, such as between the proximity of a mass and its invasion of central structures, between tumor invasion of the lung parenchyma and associated atelectasis or consolidation,[22] and between benign and malignant causes of mediastinal lymph node enlargement.

Lymph nodes are readily identifiable on CT scan and can be categorized as normal in size and shape, enlarged, coalescent, or grossly replaced by tumor mass.[2] For practical purposes, most authors consider mediastinal lymph nodes more than 1.0 cm in diameter as abnormal. In recent studies of mediastinal lung cancer staging confirmed by surgical exploration, however, the sensitivity of the 1.0 cm cut-off value for detecting cancerous nodes by CT has ranged from 27% to 90%.[44–61] The specificity of the 1.0 cm cut-off value in these studies ranged from 43% to 93%, with most well under 90%. Mediastinal lymph nodes more than 2.0 cm in diameter are virtually always abnormal,[62, 63] and most nodes more than 2.0 cm in diameter in patients with lung cancer contain metastatic disease.[63] Even in series of patients with proven bronchogenic carcinoma, however, benign findings were present in 10% of lymph nodes more than 2.0 cm in diameter or with evidence of central necrosis[44] and in 37% of lymph nodes 2 to 4 cm in diameter.[46] Thus, normal-appearing nodes often contain metastatic cancer, and even markedly enlarged nodes with an abnormal appearance may not.

Despite these limitations, CT has become the imaging

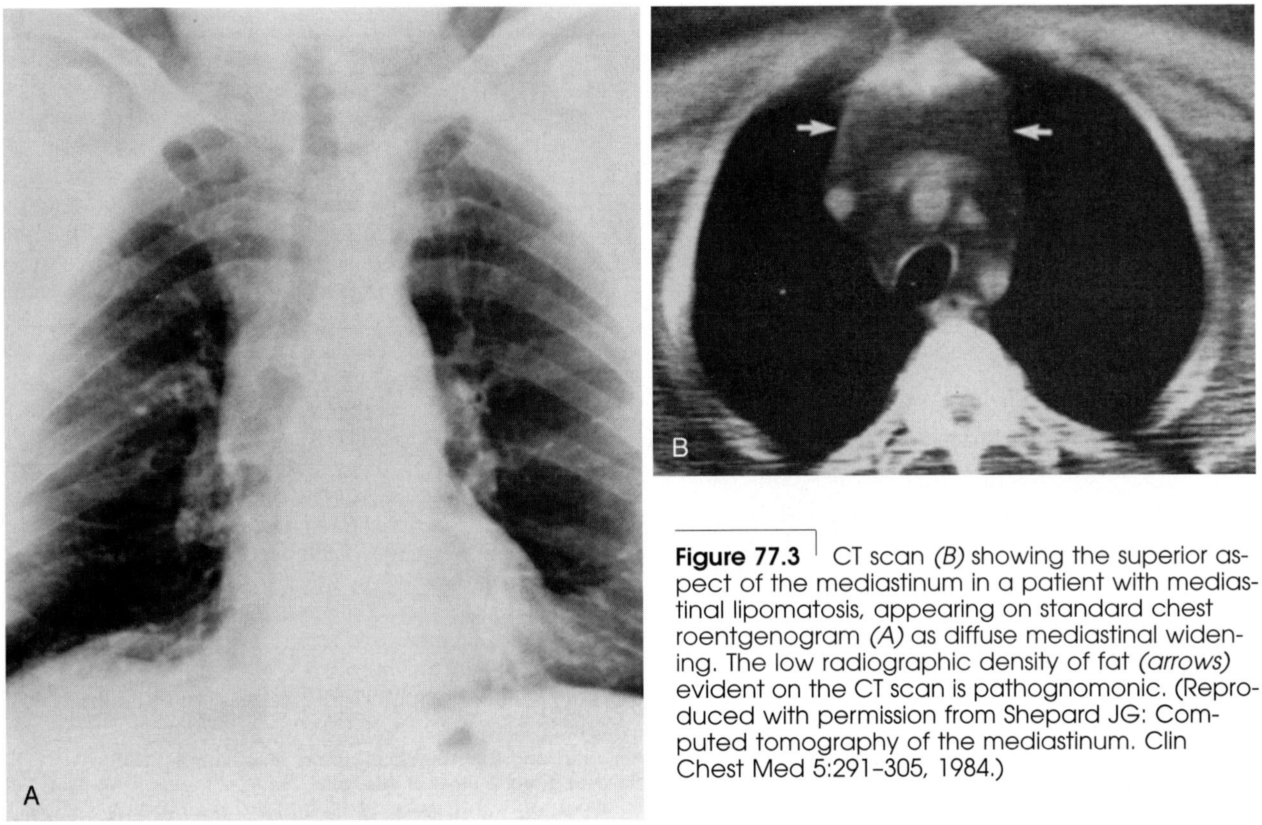


**Figure 77.3** CT scan *(B)* showing the superior aspect of the mediastinum in a patient with mediastinal lipomatosis, appearing on standard chest roentgenogram *(A)* as diffuse mediastinal widening. The low radiographic density of fat *(arrows)* evident on the CT scan is pathognomonic. (Reproduced with permission from Shepard JG: Computed tomography of the mediastinum. Clin Chest Med 5:291–305, 1984.)

procedure of choice for the evaluation of the mediastinum in patients with lung cancer.[64–68] In the majority of patients with bronchogenic cancer presumed to be resectable on clinical grounds, CT neither proves unresectability nor confidently excludes the possibility of mediastinal lymph node metastases. It can be helpful, however, either by confirming a clinical suspicion of extensive mediastinal involvement or visceral organ invasion, which precludes consideration of curative resection, or by precisely defining mediastinal anatomy and guiding invasive staging procedures.

## Magnetic Resonance Imaging

MRI assesses tissues by measuring radiofrequency-induced nuclear resonance emissions instead of the attenuation of transmitted ionizing radiation as used by conventional roentgenography and CT (see additional discussion in Chapter 25). This facilitates the construction of MR images not only in axial cross section (Fig. 77.4) but also in coronal and sagittal planes better suited to evaluating vertically oriented structures and tissue boundaries (Figs. 77.5 and 77.6).[22, 69] MR images of blood vessels are readily identifiable without the need for contrast enhancement (see Fig. 77.6),[22, 70] and metallic objects that cause artifacts on CT scans do not interfere with MRI.[33]

There are at present few known hazards to MRI, although cardiac pacemaker function may be altered and some metallic devices may be subjected to magnetic forces.[71] Several other disadvantages exist. Data acquisition time is long, and respiratory motion blurs spatial resolution and image sharpness in the chest. The long acquisition times and confined nature of the apparatus contribute to the sense of claustrophobia experienced by some patients, although newer open-sided scanners may help to alleviate this problem.

MRI is being increasingly used to evaluate the mediastinum in both general applications in chest disease[2, 69, 72, 73] and more specific circumstances such as bronchogenic carcinoma,[22, 66, 67, 74–77] lymphoma,[78] and various benign conditions.[69, 79] Whether current MRI techniques are superior to CT for staging the mediastinum for resectability in lung cancer remains unclear. A large multicenter study comparing the two techniques found similar accuracies for the detection of mediastinal node involvement, although MRI was superior for detecting direct mediastinal tumor invasion.[45] Based on this experience and on numerous smaller studies, most authorities now recommend CT for routine staging purposes and MRI for defining anatomy in special circumstances such as before surgical resection of superior sulcus tumors or those invading the mediastinum, chest wall, or diaphragm.[65–67, 77] If MRI is used, gadolinium enhancement can improve its sensitivity for detecting abnormal nodes.[74, 80]

Like CT, MRI has limitations. Both distinguish poorly between hilar masses and adjacent collapsed or consolidated lung.[22] Both can accurately demonstrate vertebral invasion, but neither detects rib invasion ideally.[81] Both can also show displacement or compression of the esophagus or trachea by tumor, but often they are unable to indicate whether there is also invasion of these structures.[22] Most importantly, neither technique reliably dis-

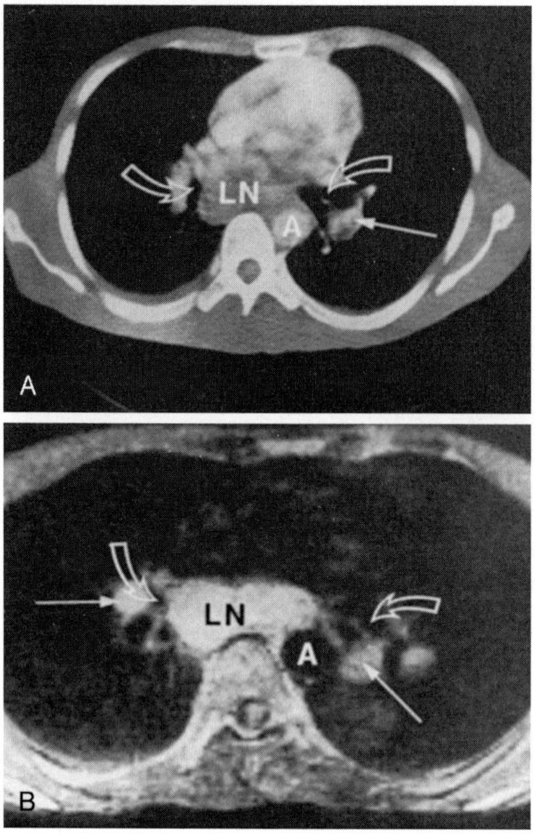


**Figure 77.4** Comparison between CT *(A)* and MRI *(B)* showing mediastinal and hilar lymph nodes in a patient with metastatic adenocarcinoma. Both scans are at the level of the subcarinal space and show enlarged subcarinal lymph nodes (LN). The CT scan is contrast enhanced. *Open curved arrows* indicate bronchi; *straight arrows* indicate hilar lymph nodes. The better contrast between the heart and descending aorta (A) and the subcarinal node in the MRI makes the latter more apparent. That the hilar lymph nodes are bilaterally enlarged is also better recognized with MRI than with CT. (Reproduced with permission from Dooms GC, Hricak H: Radiologic imaging modalities, including magnetic resonance, for evaluating lymph nodes. West J Med 144:49–57, 1986.)

tinguishes between benign and malignant causes of lymph node enlargement.

## Ultrasonography

Ultrasonography may be useful in confirming the cystic nature of mediastinal masses. Successful diagnosis of pericardial[82] and other[83] developmental cysts has been accomplished with this technique, although it cannot readily distinguish between benign and malignant cystic lesions. Both transthoracic and endoscopic ultrasound probes may be useful in the evaluation of mediastinal disease.[84–86]

## Radionuclide Imaging

Radionuclide imaging studies rely on the localization of markers based on specific metabolic or immunologic properties of the target tissue. Compared with CT or MRI, the spatial resolution of radionuclide scans is relatively poor, but the overall accuracy may be greatly improved over that of anatomic or morphologic images if a sufficiently specific probe is available. An additional appeal is the potential ability to diagnose and stage a malignancy and to identify distant metastases with a single scan of the entire body. Unfortunately, this ideal has not yet been fully realized.

Planar imaging with gallium ($^{67}Ga$) has been used in preoperative mediastinal assessment of patients with bronchogenic carcinoma, but early enthusiasm was eventually replaced by disenchantment with this technique.[33, 87, 88] In their comparison of $^{67}Ga$ scans with standard chest roentgenograms and CT, Dooms and Hricak[33] determined that the radionuclide test was the least sensitive, specific, and accurate. $^{67}Ga$ scans produced too many false-positive results because of nonspecific uptake by benign inflammatory nodes, and they missed small neoplastic nodes.[33] In general, results with planar imaging of thallium ($^{201}Tl$) tracer have been similarly disappointing. (Various radionuclide techniques and their results are discussed further in Chapter 26.)

Radionuclide imaging techniques are occasionally helpful in the evaluation of the mediastinum under other circumstances. For instance, $^{67}Ga$ scans have been used in the evaluation of patients with sarcoidosis. Characteristic "lambda" and "panda" signs result from uptake in the lacrimal and salivary glands and the mediastinal lymph nodes.[89] The lack of specificity, however, has relegated the use of $^{67}Ga$ scans to selected cases with high pretest probability or to detect subclinical extrathoracic sites of involvement.[90] Radioiodine scanning may detect ectopic thyroid tissue, a positive result of which is pathognomonic for that condition.[11] Various radionuclide studies that may be used to characterize primary mediastinal tumors and cysts are discussed further in Chapter 79.

Immunolocalization is another theoretically appealing means of specifically targeting a probe to tumor tissues. Experience with technetium-labeled antibodies, however, has been disappointing due to a high rate of false-positive signals in the mediastinum.[91, 92]

Single photon emission computed tomography (SPECT) permits imaging of standard gamma-emitting probes in a cross-sectional fashion similar to conventional CT. This results in improved sensitivity, resolution, and anatomic information relative to planar images. The accuracy of $^{201}Tl$-SPECT for determining mediastinal node involvement by lung cancer compares favorably with that of CT but is not sensitive or specific enough to supplant surgical staging.[93, 94]

Positron emission tomography (PET) is perhaps the most promising imaging technique available for use in the evaluation of lung cancer.[90, 95] PET technology relies on high-energy photon-emitting probes such as $^{18}F$-fluorodeoxyglucose, which are metabolically trapped within tumor cells. The result is a high signal-to-background

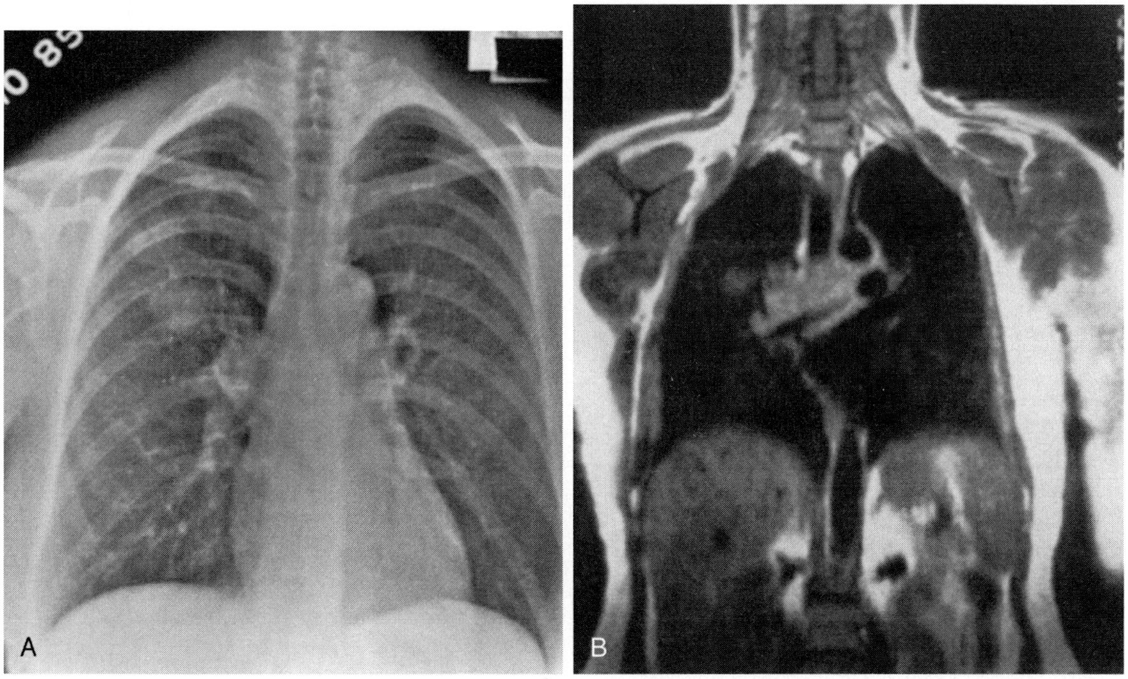


**Figure 77.5** Chest roentgenogram *(A)* and coronal MRI *(B)* of a patient with adenocarcinoma of the right upper lung field, showing metastases to the right hilum and mediastinum. (Reproduced with permission from Martini N, Heelan R, Westcott J, et al: Comparative merits of conventional, computed tomographic, and magnetic resonance imaging in assessing mediastinal involvement in surgically confirmed lung carcinoma. J Thorac Cardiovasc Surg 90:639–648, 1985.)

ratio, excellent spatial resolution, and a highly accurate test (Fig. 77.7). Preliminary studies of $^{18}$F-fluoro-deoxyglucose and PET for the mediastinal staging of lung cancer showed the promise of this technique but did not use objective signal quantification and routine CT anatomic correlation to optimize the results.[49, 50, 52, 54, 96, 97] When both of these refinements have been incorporated in prospective studies, PET has detected mediastinal metastases with sensitivities and specificities ranging from 93% to 100% and 98% to 100%, respectively.[55, 56, 58] Unfortunately, PET technology is costly and not universally available, and efforts to use modified SPECT equipment have failed to match the performance of dedicated PET scanners.[98] The role of PET in mediastinal staging remains to be determined. With further technical refinements and larger confirmatory studies, PET may obviate the need for invasive preoperative staging.[99]

## TECHNIQUES FOR OBTAINING MEDIASTINAL TISSUE

Most patients with a mediastinal mass or adenopathy eventually require an invasive diagnostic approach. Primary mediastinal tumors usually require biopsy to determine the cause. Because many primary mediastinal masses should be removed regardless of their cause, however, consideration should be given to surgical resection as the initial invasive approach in the appropriate settings.[99a] Mediastinal tissue sampling is central to the man-

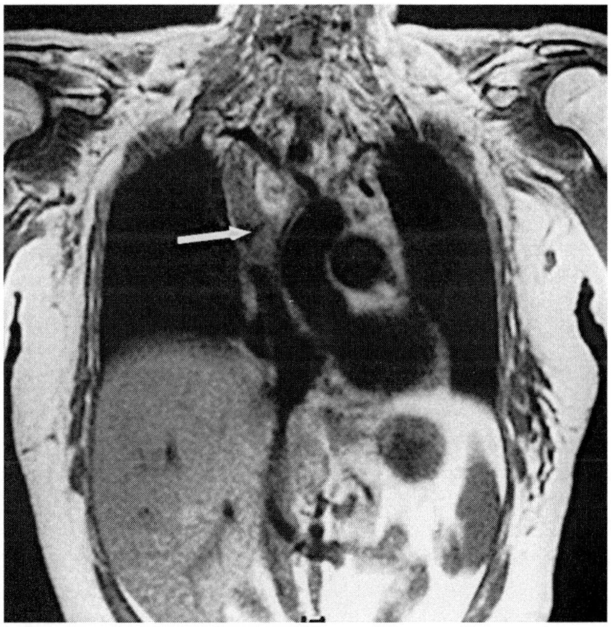

**Figure 77.6** Coronal MRI obtained from a 52-year-old woman with multiple myeloma, experiencing symptoms of superior vena cava obstruction following placement of an indwelling central venous catheter in preparation for bone marrow transplantation. Black ''flow void'' is present within the heart and great vessels, and the superior vena cava is completely obstructed by thrombus *(arrow)*.

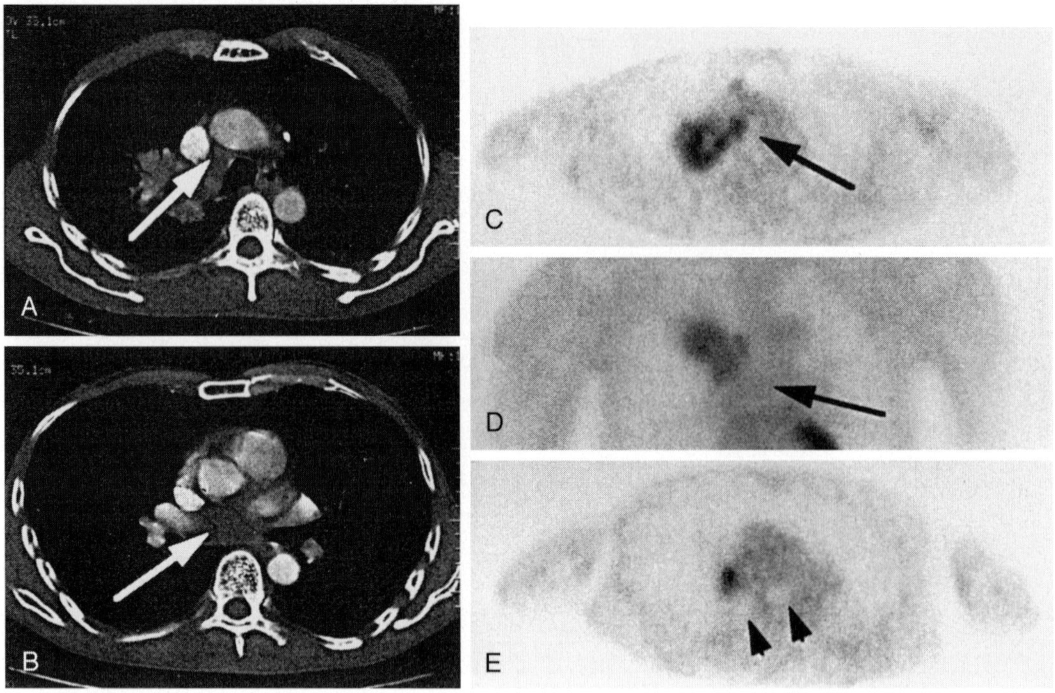


**Figure 77.7** CT and PET scans obtained from a patient with right upper lobe squamous cell carcinoma. The primary tumor and right paratracheal adenopathy *(A)* and subcarinal adenopathy *(B)* are evident on the standard CT images *(white arrows)*. PET images reveal probe uptake in the primary tumor and right paratracheal nodes on axial *(black arrow) (C)* and coronal *(D)* views, but not in the subcarinal node on coronal *(black arrow) (D)* and axial *(E)* views. The *arrowheads* in *E* point to the main bronchi. At mediastinoscopy, the right paratracheal nodes were found to be malignant, and the subcarinal nodes were enlarged but benign. (Reproduced with permission from Vansteenkiste JF, Stroobants SG, De Leyn PR, et al: Mediastinal lymph node staging with FDG-PET scan in patients with potentially operable non-small cell lung cancer: A prospective analysis of 50 cases. Leuven Lung Cancer Group. Chest 112:1480–1486, 1997.)

agement of bronchogenic carcinoma because noninvasive assessment of the mediastinum usually cannot definitively confirm or exclude the presence of metastases and because findings of mediastinal metastases may drastically alter the surgical and therapeutic options.

## Needle Aspiration and Biopsy

Transbronchial needle aspiration (TBNA) via the fiberoptic bronchoscope is an appealing technique because it can yield definitive proof of the presence of malignancy in the mediastinum through the use of a procedure that is less hazardous and costly than mediastinoscopy (see additional discussion in Chapter 27).[100] In the setting of bronchogenic carcinoma, TBNA focuses on the subcarinal lymph nodes and on right paratracheal nodes, both of which are common metastatic sites that can produce false-negative results when sampled by mediastinoscopy.[101, 102] The procedure was initially carried out via the rigid bronchoscope and then adapted for use through the flexible fiberoptic bronchoscope.[103, 104] Subsequently, larger needles were developed that can yield tissue fragments suitable for histologic evaluation.[105–107] Despite the proximity of major vessels and lung parenchyma to the areas routinely biopsied, TBNA appears to be a safe procedure; only two significant complications (pneumothorax and hemomediastinum) have been reported in more than 1500 reported procedures.

Experience with TBNA for assessing mediastinal lymph node metastases in bronchogenic carcinoma has been reported mostly in terms of the "yield" of positive results, without definitive surgical confirmation of both positive and negative TBNA results.[108–112] A careful prospective study found that only 15% of patients with the established diagnosis of lung cancer had a positive result from TBNA, but in 69% of these the TBNA specimen was the only preoperative evidence for mediastinal metastases.[109] The true sensitivity and specificity of TBNA appears to range from 14% to 50% and 96% to 100%, respectively.[113, 114] Thus, negative results require definitive operative confirmation, but the risk of false-positive TBNA results appears to be quite low. Of four false-positive results reported in the literature, two were thought to have resulted from aspiration of the primary tumor adjacent to a major airway, and two were attributed to tumor cells picked up from tracheobronchial secretions.[113, 115, 116] Nevertheless, it is sensibly recommended that TBNA be performed before bronchial exploration or biopsy of any endobronchial lesions.[108, 109]

To achieve comparable results in clinical practice,

training and experience with TBNA are necessary,[117, 118] along with appropriate selection of patients. The yield is improved in patients with visible endobronchial lesions or with widening or erythema of the carina.[108, 109, 119] Mediastinal adenopathy on plain roentgenograms and subcarinal adenopathy on CT also are associated with improved yield,[120] and real-time CT guidance of the biopsy needle placement can improve the sensitivity of the procedure.[121]

Finally, TBNA may have utility in other clinical situations such as in the diagnosis of a variety of primary mediastinal masses and cysts, metastases from extrathoracic malignancies, miscellaneous benign conditions,[100, 111] and the evaluation of mediastinal adenopathy associated with human immunodeficiency virus infection.[122]

Percutaneous needle aspiration and biopsy of mediastinal masses, used sporadically for several decades, has experienced renewed utilization with CT guidance (Fig. 77.8).[123–127] When performed by experienced clinicians, this procedure can be done with acceptable morbidity and yields results comparable with those from percutaneous biopsy of pulmonary lesions. As with TBNA, serious bleeding is seldom encountered,[123, 126, 127] and accurate diagnosis of a wide variety of lesions has been reported.[124, 125, 128–129a] Accuracy undoubtedly varies with the skill and persistence of the operator and is enhanced when immediate cytopathologic examination determines whether an adequate sample has been obtained.[127]

Endoscopic ultrasonography-guided needle aspiration and biopsy is a relatively new technique that relies on the availability of endoscopic ultrasound probes to guide the placement of biopsy needles, which are passed through the working channel of a gastroscope. The proximity of the esophagus to areas of the mediastinum relatively inaccessible to mediastinoscopy, such as the subcarinal lymph nodes, make this approach particularly appealing. Preliminary studies suggest that it is highly accurate and well tolerated.[85, 86, 130] In selected cases, endoscopic ultrasonography-guided biopsy can confirm the presence of mediastinal metastases and obviate the need for surgical-staging procedures.[131]

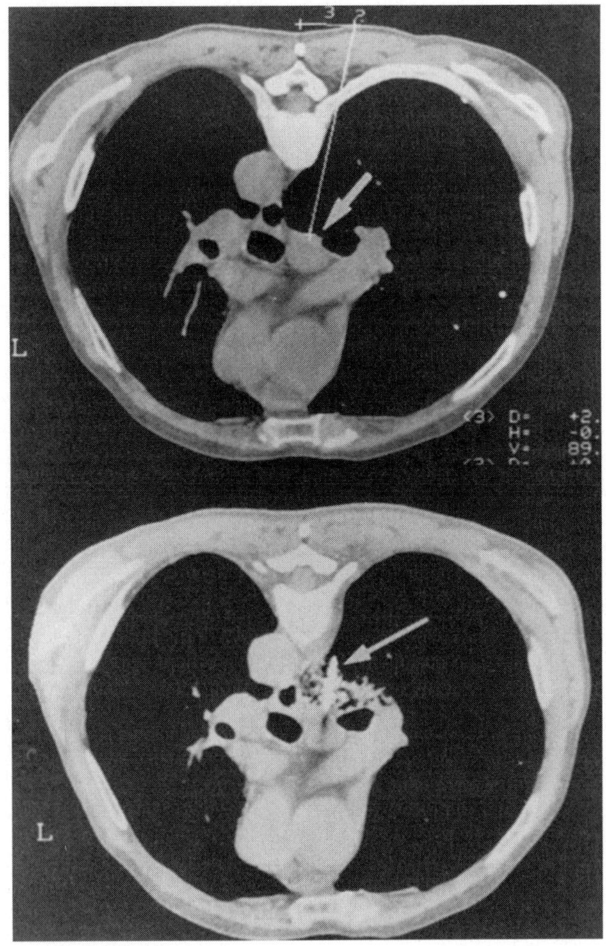


**Figure 77.8** CT-guided needle aspiration of a mediastinal mass is illustrated. The upper image shows the planned course of the biopsy needle, entering the left paraspinal area to reach a subcarinal lymph node *(top arrow)*. The lower image shows the tip of the needle extending into the mass *(bottom arrow)*. (Reproduced with permission from Akamatsu H, Terashima M, Koike T, et al: Staging of primary lung cancer by computed tomography-guided percutaneous needle cytology of mediastinal lymph nodes. Ann Thorac Surg 62:352–355, 1996.)

## Mediastinoscopy, Anterior Mediastinotomy, and Thoracoscopy

Suprasternal mediastinoscopy is a procedure that allows direct inspection and biopsy of lymph nodes or other masses in the superior portion of the anterior mediastinum.[6, 132] In its present form, it was introduced by Carlens[133] in 1959. Although more invasive than any of the techniques discussed previously in this chapter, mediastinoscopy can provide large specimens for histologic examination, including entire lymph nodes, rather than the cellular aspirates or small tissue fragments produced by needle biopsy techniques.

Mediastinal anatomy from the mediastinoscopist's perspective is different from that based on the lateral chest roentgenogram as described earlier: Structures are considered according to whether they lie anterior, posterior, or immediately to the right or left of the trachea.[8, 9] Not all of the mediastinal lymph nodes can be reached by the mediastinoscope. Those readily accessible include the right paratracheal nodes to the level of the tracheal bifurcation and the left paratracheal nodes as far as the aortic arch.[2, 132] Most subcarinal nodes and nodes in aortic and para-aortic locations cannot be reached via the cervical approach, but are accessible with anterior mediastinoscopy or mediastinotomy through an incision in the left second intercostal space.[2, 132] Mediastinoscopy and anterior mediastinotomy usually require general anesthesia, but may be performed as outpatient procedures when subsequent thoracotomy is not planned immediately.[134]

Mediastinoscopy has utility in evaluating mediastinal adenopathy or mass lesions in a variety of settings, including the evaluation of complications of human immunodeficiency virus infection.[135] Its most frequent application, however, is in the staging of bronchogenic carcinoma.[136] Surgeons debate whether to perform this procedure at the time of thoracotomy or to schedule thoracotomy at a later time, after final pathologic results are available. The former approach has the disadvantages of extending anesthesia time and relying on preliminary histologic examination in the determination of resectability, whereas the latter approach requires two separate episodes of anesthesia and postoperative recuperation. Recent evidence suggests that either frozen section or imprint cytology methods can provide rapid and accurate results, thereby facilitating immediate decisions about the feasibility of curative resection.[137, 138]

Precise indications for mediastinoscopy in lung cancer are controversial. To do the procedure automatically in all patients with this diagnosis would seem excessive, but neither CT nor MRI reliably excludes metastatic lymph node involvement, which sometimes occurs at only a microscopic level. The presence of enlarged nodes is also an important indication for mediastinoscopy so that patients with resectable tumors are not incorrectly assumed to have inoperable metastatic spread.[139] In an attempt to reduce the incidence of unnecessary mediastinoscopy, some authors would omit mediastinoscopy if all nodes were less than 1.0 or 1.5 cm diameter by CT scan[2, 24, 32] or if the primary tumor were small or located in either of the lower lobes.[48, 140] Despite these guidelines, the decision of whom to subject to mediastinoscopy or anterior mediastinotomy for lung cancer staging remains a variable one that depends on local resources, personal experience, and the patient's wishes as well as on published clinical data.

In addition to limitations in the nodal groups it can reliably sample,[101, 102] imperfect overall sensitivity,[48, 114, 141] and the necessity for general anesthesia, mediastinoscopy has numerous potential complications. Serious complications (death, major bleeding, and permanent damage to the recurrent laryngeal nerve) occurred in 1.2% of 600 procedures in one series.[142] Other complications included pneumothorax, lesser degrees of hemorrhage, transient recurrent nerve paralysis, and elevation of one hemidiaphragm in about 1% each. Injury to the trachea, esophageal perforation, thoracic duct laceration, air embolism, and mediastinitis have also been reported as complications of mediastinoscopy. The presence of superior vena cava obstruction has been considered a relative contraindication until recently.[142a] Morbidity and mortality from anterior mediastinotomy in 62 patients were 16.1% and 1.6%, respectively.[143]

Thoracoscopy, usually considered a tool for the evaluation of pleural and lung abnormalities, also can be helpful in the management of mediastinal diseases. After dissection through the parietal mediastinal pleura, mediastinal lymph nodes can be sampled to aid in the staging of malignancies such as esophageal carcinoma[144] and for the diagnosis and resection of primary mediastinal tumors and cysts.[145–152]

## GENERAL APPROACH TO DIAGNOSTIC INVESTIGATION

### Evaluation of a Mediastinal Mass

Mass lesions in the mediastinum require a tissue diagnosis unless optimal management can be definitively decided on the basis of clinical information and noninvasive test results alone. Only a few masses fall into this category. These include mediastinal thyroid tissue, which can be identified by radioactive iodine scans; certain granulomatous lesions that are densely calcified and have remained unchanged on serial roentgenograms; and mediastinal lipomatosis with typical CT findings. Lymphoma or other malignancy diagnosed by biopsy of tissues outside the thorax does not require separate demonstration that it is also the cause of a mediastinal mass. Confirmed active pulmonary tuberculosis or sarcoidosis usually warrants a trial of therapy and a period of observation before invasive approaches are used to evaluate coexistent mediastinal abnormalities. For most mediastinal masses, however, thorough diagnostic evaluation must lead to examination of tissue obtained from the lesion.

In fact, most primary mediastinal masses must be surgically removed whether they are benign or malignant. Resection of benign neoplasms is advisable because they may subsequently enlarge, compress mediastinal structures, cause bleeding, rupture, become infected, or, with varying degrees of likelihood, undergo malignant degeneration (discussed further in Chapter 79). Because of this, the preoperative workup should aim to assess the patient's general health and suitability for curative operation and should provide laboratory and radiographic clues to a specific diagnosis, plus the mass's size, location, density, homogeneity, and gross involvement of surrounding tissues. Imaging by CT or MR will more completely depict the lesion than standard chest roentgenograms and will also help guide the surgeon. The need for specialized studies such as a thyroid scan will be dictated by the clinical setting and when a specific diagnosis is suspected. Otherwise, if the patient is a candidate for potentially curative surgical resection, this should be the next step in most cases.

### Mediastinal Evaluation to Stage Bronchogenic Carcinoma

The extent to which a bronchogenic carcinoma has spread anatomically is the primary determinant of prognosis in this disease.[20, 21] Thus, in patients who appear to be candidates for surgical resection, staging consists of a deliberate search for metastases in the mediastinal lymph nodes.[30–32, 153] Ideally, determination of the presence or absence of nodal metastases should be done without subjecting patients to invasive procedures, especially if nodal metastasis that alters the therapeutic approach has already occurred. Unfortunately, the clinician's ability to achieve such an ideal is hampered by the failure of noninvasive techniques to indicate for certain that a given node contains malignant cells. The clinician is thus faced with a series of judgments that can be guided but not dictated by the reported experiences of others. To refuse surgery for a patient with curable disease (Fig. 77.9) is a greater loss than to perform mediastinoscopy or even thoracotomy on another who is unresectable. It thus seems logical to progress through the staging process from diagnosis to imaging of the mediastinum, to examination of nodal tissue, to surgical exploration, stopping the sequence on

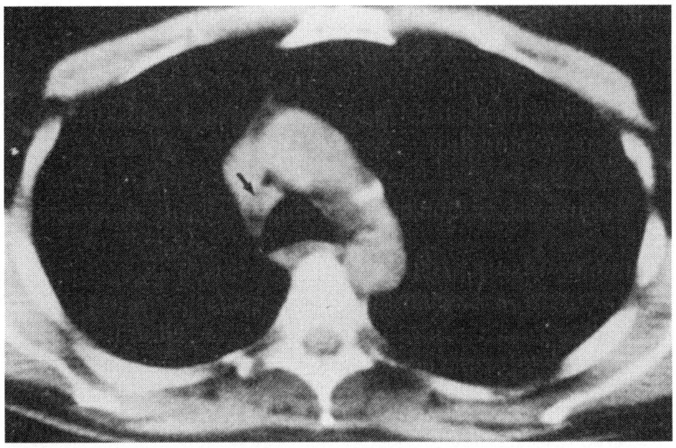

**Figure 77.9** Computed tomogram of a patient with lung cancer showing a false-positive lymph node. The pretracheal node *(arrow)* was 1.5 cm in greatest diameter, but proved to be anthracotic without a trace of tumor. (Reproduced with permission from Heitzman ER: The role of computed tomography in the diagnosis and management of lung cancer. Chest 89:237S–241S, 1986.)

the confident discovery of metastatic disease but otherwise proceeding to resection.

Which imaging procedure or procedures to employ, how to obtain diagnostic tissue, and what constitutes the confident identification of metastases that contraindicate surgery are decisions that must be made but in the absence of absolute answers. Most clinicians would currently favor delineating the extent of the primary tumor and the location and size of mediastinal lymph nodes with CT, followed by mediastinoscopy or mediastinotomy in the majority of patients both to confirm metastases in those with enlarged nodes and to look with more sensitivity at those normal in size. The local availability of CT or MRI, access to special expertise and imaging techniques, and clinical experience with TBNA, mediastinoscopy, or other procedures will all influence the individual clinician's approach.

Finally, the general condition and wishes of the patient with lung cancer must enter into the clinical staging process. Evidence that curative resection is not an option for many patients can be detected through a systematic extrathoracic assessment[32] either because the patient has obvious signs of distant metastases or because severe chronic pulmonary, cardiac, or other systemic disease renders aggressive, curative therapy unfeasible.

## SUMMARY

The mediastinum contains numerous vital structures that may be involved by a variety of diseases. This chapter reviews the compartments of the mediastinum and their contents, the clinical manifestations of common diseases that affect the organs and structures within the region, and the available imaging and invasive techniques that are helpful in evaluating patients with mediastinal disorders. Emphasis is placed on the evaluation of the mediastinum in the staging of bronchogenic carcinoma. The remaining chapters in this section describe the principal disorders that affect the mediastinum: pneumomediastinum and mediastinitis (Chapter 78) and tumors and cysts of the mediastinum (Chapter 79).

## References

1. Heitzman ER: The Mediastinum: Radiologic Correlations with Anatomy and Pathology (2nd ed). New York: Springer-Verlag, 1988.
2. Naidich DP, Zerhouni EA, Siegelman SS: Computed Tomography and Magnetic Resonance of the Thorax (2nd ed). New York: Raven Press, 1991.
3. Proto AV: The chest radiograph: Anatomic considerations. Clin Chest Med 5:213–246, 1984.
4. Foster ED, Munro DD, Dobell ARC: Mediastinoscopy: A review of anatomical relationships and complications. Ann Thorac Surg 13:273–286, 1972.
5. Mast WR, Jafek BW: Mediastinal anatomy for the mediastinoscopist. Arch Otolaryngol 101:596–599, 1975.
6. Beszniak I, Szende B, Lapis K: Mediastinal Tumors and Pseudotumors. Basel: S Karger, 1984.
7. Fraser R, Pare J, Fraser R, et al: The normal chest. *In* Fraser R, Pare J, Fraser R, et al (eds): Synopsis of Diseases of the Chest (2nd ed). Philadelphia: WB Saunders, 1994, pp 1–116.
8. Marchevsky AM, Kaneko M: Surgical Pathology of the Mediastinum. New York: Raven Press, 1984, pp 1–3.
9. Clinical staging of primary lung cancer. American Thoracic Society node mapping scheme. Am Rev Respir Dis 127:659–669, 1983.
10. Maunder RJ, Pierson DJ, Hudson LD: Subcutaneous and mediastinal emphysema: Pathophysiology, diagnosis, and management. Arch Intern Med 144:1447–1453, 1984.
11. Silverman NA, Sabiston DCJ: Mediastinal masses. Surg Clin North Am 60:757–777, 1980.
12. Schowengerdt CG, Suyemoto R, Main FB: Granulomatous and fibrous mediastinitis: A review and analysis of 180 cases. J Thorac Cardiovasc Surg 57:365–379, 1969.
13. Urschel HC, Paulson DL: Superior vena caval obstruction. Dis Chest 49:155–164, 1966.
14. Lokich JJ, Goodman R: Superior vena cava syndrome: Clinical management. JAMA 231:58–61, 1975.
15. Yellin A, Rosen A, Reichert N, et al: Superior vena cava syndrome: The myth—The facts. Am Rev Respir Dis 141:1114–1118, 1990.
16. Munsell WP: Pneumomediastinum. JAMA 202:689–693, 1967.
17. Yellin A, Gapany-Gapanavicius M, Lieberman Y: Spontaneous pneumomediastinum: Is it a rare cause of chest pain? Thorax 38:383–385, 1983.
18. Holmes KD, McGuirt WF: Spontaneous pneumomediastinum: Evaluation and treatment. J Fam Pract 31:422, 425–426, 1990.
19. Fry WA, Menck HR, Winchester DP: The National Cancer Data Base report on lung cancer. Cancer 77:1947–1955, 1996.
20. Mountain CF: Revisions in the International System for Staging Lung Cancer. Chest 111:1710–1717, 1997.
21. Naruke T, Tsuchiya R, Kondo H, et al: Implications of staging in lung cancer. Chest 112:242S–248S, 1997.
22. Martini N, Heelan R, Westcott J, et al: Comparative merits of conventional, computed tomographic, and magnetic resonance imaging in assessing mediastinal involvement in surgically confirmed lung carcinoma. J Thorac Cardiovasc Surg 90:639–648, 1985.
23. Pearson F: Lung cancer: The past twenty-five years. Chest 89:200S–205S, 1986.
24. Daly BD, Mueller JD, Faling LJ, et al: N2 lung cancer: Outcome in patients with false-negative computed tomographic scans of the chest. J Thorac Cardiovasc Surg 105:904–910, 1993.
25. Miller DL, McManus KG, Allen MS, et al: Results of surgical resection in patients with N2 non–small cell lung cancer. Ann Thorac Surg 57:1095–1100, 1994.
26. Goldstraw P, Mannam GC, Kaplan DK, Michail P: Surgical management of non–small-cell lung cancer with ipsilateral mediastinal node metastasis (N2 disease). J Thorac Cardiovasc Surg 107:19–27, 1994.
27. Ginsberg RJ: Resection of non–small cell lung cancer: How much and by what route. Chest 112:203S–205S, 1997.

28. Rusch VW: Adjuvant and neoadjuvant therapy for stages I through III non–small cell lung cancer. Ann Thorac Surg 58:899–900, 1994.
29. Einhorn LH: Neoadjuvant and adjuvant trials in non–small cell lung cancer. Ann Thorac Surg 65:208–211, 1998.
30. Pretreatment evaluation of non–small-cell lung cancer. The American Thoracic Society and The European Respiratory Society. Am J Respir Crit Care Med 156:320–332, 1997.
31. Miller JD, Gorenstein LA, Patterson GA: Staging: The key to rational management of lung cancer. Ann Thorac Surg 53:170–178, 1992.
32. Spiro SG, Goldstraw P: The staging of lung cancer. Thorax 39:401–407, 1984.
33. Dooms GC, Hricak H: Radiologic imaging modalities, including magnetic resonance, for evaluating lymph nodes. West J Med 144:49–57, 1986.
34. Watanabe A, Shimokata K, Saka H, et al: Chest CT combined with artificial pneumothorax: Value in determining origin and extent of tumor. Am J Roentgenol 156:707–710, 1991.
35. Yokoi K, Mori K, Miyazawa N, et al: Tumor invasion of the chest wall and mediastinum in lung cancer: Evaluation with pneumothorax CT. Radiology 181:147–152, 1991.
36. Brown K, Aberle D, Batra P, et al: Current use of imaging in the evaluation of primary mediastinal masses. Chest 98:466–473, 1990.
37. Mendez GJ, Isikoff MB, Isikoff SK, et al: Fatty tumors of the thorax demonstrated by CT. Am J Roentgenol 133:207–212, 1979.
38. Shepard JO: Computed tomography of the mediastinum. Clin Chest Med 5:291–305, 1984.
39. Brown LR, Muhm JR, Gray JE: Radiographic detection of thymoma. Am J Roentgenol 134:1181–1188, 1980.
40. Baron RL, Lee JKT, Sagel SS, et al: Computed tomography of the abnormal thymus. Radiology 142:127–134, 1982.
41. Pugatch RD, Braver JH, Robbins AH, et al: CT diagnosis of pericardial cysts. Am J Roentgenol 131:515–516, 1978.
41a. Buckley JA, Stark P: Intrathoracic mediastinal thyroid goiter: Imaging manifestations. AJR Am J Roentgenol 173:471–475, 1999.
42. Modic MT, Janicki PC: Computed tomography of mass lesions of the right cardiophrenic angle. J Comput Assist Tomogr 4:521–526, 1980.
43. Pugatch RD, Faling LJ, Robins AH, et al: CT diagnosis of benign mediastinal abnormalities. Am J Roentgenol 134:685–694, 1980.
44. Ratto GB, Frola C, Cantoni S, et al: Improving clinical efficacy of computed tomographic scan in the preoperative assessment of patients with non–small cell lung cancer. J Thorac Cardiovasc Surg 99:416–425, 1990.
45. Webb WR, Gatsonis C, Zerhouni EA, et al: CT and MR imaging in staging non–small cell bronchogenic carcinoma: Report of the Radiologic Diagnostic Oncology Group. Radiology 178:705–713, 1991.
46. McLoud TC, Bourgouin PM, Greenberg RW, et al: Bronchogenic carcinoma: Analysis of staging in the mediastinum with CT by correlative lymph node mapping and sampling. Radiology 182:319–323, 1992.
47. Seely JM, Mayo JR, Miller RR, et al: T1 lung cancer: Prevalence of mediastinal nodal metastases and diagnostic accuracy of CT. Radiology 186:129–132, 1993.
48. Dillemans B, Deneffe G, Verschakelen J, et al: Value of computed tomography and mediastinoscopy in preoperative evaluation of mediastinal nodes in non–small cell lung cancer. A study of 569 patients. Eur J Cardiothorac Surg 8:37–42, 1994.
49. Wahl RL, Quint LE, Greenough RL, et al: Staging of mediastinal non–small cell lung cancer with FDG PET, CT, and fusion images: Preliminary prospective evaluation. Radiology 191:371–377, 1994.
50. Scott WJ, Schwabe JL, Gupta NC, et al: Positron emission tomography of lung tumors and mediastinal lymph nodes using [$^{18}$F]fluorodeoxyglucose. The Members of the PET-Lung Tumor Study Group. Ann Thorac Surg 58:698–703, 1994.
51. Bollen EC, Goei R, van't Hof Grootenboer BE, et al: Interobserver variability and accuracy of computed tomographic assessment of nodal status in lung cancer. Ann Thorac Surg 58:158–162, 1994.
52. Valk PE, Pounds TR, Hopkins DM, et al: Staging non–small cell lung cancer by whole-body positron emission tomographic imaging. Ann Thorac Surg 60:1573–1581, 1995.
53. Chin R Jr, Ward R, Keyes JW, et al: Mediastinal staging of non–small-cell lung cancer with positron emission tomography. Am J Respir Crit Care Med 152:2090–2096, 1995.
54. Patz EF Jr, Lowe VJ, Goodman PC, et al: Thoracic nodal staging with PET imaging with 18FDG in patients with bronchogenic carcinoma. Chest 108:1617–1621, 1995.
55. Scott WJ, Gobar LS, Terry JD, et al: Mediastinal lymph node staging of non–small-cell lung cancer: A prospective comparison of computed tomography and positron emission tomography. J Thorac Cardiovasc Surg 111:642–648, 1996.
56. Sazon DA, Santiago SM, Soo Hoo GW, et al: Fluorodeoxyglucose-positron emission tomography in the detection and staging of lung cancer. Am J Respir Crit Care Med 153:417–421, 1996.
57. Arita T, Matsumoto T, Kuramitsu T, et al: Is it possible to differentiate malignant mediastinal nodes from benign nodes by size? Reevaluation by CT, transesophageal echocardiography, and nodal specimen. Chest 110:1004–1008, 1996.
58. Vansteenkiste JF, Stroobants SG, De Leyn PR, et al: Mediastinal lymph node staging with FDG-PET scan in patients with potentially operable non–small cell lung cancer: A prospective analysis of 50 cases. Leuven Lung Cancer Group. Chest 112:1480–1486, 1997.
59. Gdeedo A, Van Schil P, Corthouts B, et al: Prospective evaluation of computed tomography and mediastinoscopy in mediastinal lymph node staging. Eur Respir J 10:1547–1551, 1997.
60. Gdeedo A, Van Schil P, Corthouts B, et al: Comparison of imaging TNM [(i)TNM] and pathological TNM [pTNM] in staging of bronchogenic carcinoma. Eur J Cardiothorac Surg 12:224–227, 1997.
61. Dales RE, Stark RM, Raman S: Computed tomography to stage lung cancer. Approaching a controversy using meta-analysis. Am Rev Respir Dis 141:1096–1101, 1990.
62. Schnyder PA, Gamsu G: CT of the pretracheal retrocaval space. Am J Roentgenol 136:303–308, 1981.
63. Baron RL, Levitt RG, Sagel SS, et al: Computed tomography in the preoperative evaluation of bronchogenic carcinoma. Radiology 145:727–732, 1982.
64. Colice GL: Chest CT for known or suspected lung cancer. Chest 106:1538–1550, 1994.
65. Pugatch RD: Radiologic evaluation in chest malignancies. A review of imaging modalities. Chest 107:294S–297S, 1995.
66. Quint LE, Francis IR, Wahl RL, et al: Preoperative staging of non–small-cell carcinoma of the lung: Imaging methods. AJR Am J Roentgenol 164:1349–1359, 1995.
67. Bonomo L, Ciccotosto C, Guidotti A, et al: Lung cancer staging: The role of computed tomography and magnetic resonance imaging. Eur J Radiol 23:35–45, 1996.
68. Shaffer K: Radiologic evaluation in lung cancer: Diagnosis and staging. Chest 112:235S–238S, 1997.
69. Gamsu G, Sostman D: Magnetic resonance imaging of the thorax. Am Rev Respir Dis 139:254–274, 1989.
70. Hansen ME, Spritzer CE, Sostman HD: Assessing the patency of mediastinal and thoracic inlet veins: Value of MR imaging. AJR Am J Roentgenol 155:1177–1182, 1990.
71. Dujovny M, Alp MS, Dujovny N, et al: Aneurysm clips: Magnetic quantification and magnetic resonance imaging safety. Technical note. J Neurosurg 87:788–794, 1997.
72. Weinreb JC, Naidich DP: Thoracic magnetic resonance imaging. Clin Chest Med 12:33–54, 1991.
73. Link KM, Samuels LJ, Reed JC, et al: Magnetic resonance imaging of the mediastinum and its contents. J Thorac Imaging 8:34–53, 1993.
74. Kono M, Adachi S, Kusumoto M, et al: Clinical utility of Gd-DTPA-enhanced magnetic resonance imaging in lung cancer. J Thorac Imaging 8:18–26, 1993.
75. Templeton PA, Caskey CI, Zerhouni EA: Current uses of CT and MR imaging in the staging of lung cancer. Radiol Clin North Am 28:631–646, 1990.
76. Cohen AM, Creviston S, LiPuma JP, et al: NMR evaluation of hilar and mediastinal lymphadenopathy. Radiology 148:739–742, 1983.
77. Grover FL: The role of CT and MRI in staging of the mediastinum. Chest 106:391S–396S, 1994.

78. Bonomo L, Ciccotosto C, Guidotti A, et al: Staging of thoracic lymphoma by radiological imaging. Eur Radiol 7:1179–1189, 1997.
79. Gamsu G, Stark DD, Webb WR, et al: Magnetic resonance imaging of benign mediastinal masses. Radiology 151:709–713, 1984.
80. Crisci R, Di Cesare E, Lupattelli L, et al: MR study of N2 disease in lung cancer: Contrast-enhanced method using gadolinium-DTPA. Eur J Cardiothorac Surg 11:214–217, 1997.
81. Pennes DR, Glazer GM, Wimbish KJ, et al: Chest wall invasion by lung cancer. Limitations of CT evaluation. AJR Am J Roentgenol 144:507–511, 1985.
82. Hynes JK, Tajik AJ, Osborn MJ, et al: Two-dimensional echocardiographic diagnosis of pericardial cyst. Mayo Clin Proc 58:60–63, 1983.
83. Koch PC, Kronzon I, Winer HE, et al: Displacement of the heart by a giant mediastinal cyst. Am J Cardiol 40:445–448, 1977.
84. Wernecke K, Diederich S: Sonographic features of mediastinal tumors. AJR Am J Roentgenol 163:1357–1364, 1994.
85. Wiersema MJ, Kochman ML, Cramer HM, et al: Preoperative staging of non–small cell lung cancer: Transesophageal US-guided fine-needle aspiration biopsy of mediastinal lymph nodes. Radiology 190:239–242, 1994.
86. Pedersen BH, Vilmann P, Folke K, et al: Endoscopic ultrasonography and real-time guided fine-needle aspiration biopsy of solid lesions of the mediastinum suspected of malignancy. Chest 110:539–544, 1996.
87. McKenna RJ, Haynie TP, Libshitz HI, et al: Critical evaluation of 67-gallium scan for surgical patients with lung cancer. Chest 87:428–431, 1985.
88. Friedman PJ, Feigin DS, Liston SE, et al: Sensitivity of chest radiography, computed tomography, and gallium scanning to metastasis in lung carcinoma. Cancer 54:1300–1306, 1984.
89. Sulavik SB, Spencer RP, Weed DA, et al: Recognition of distinctive patterns of gallium-67 distribution in sarcoidosis. J Nucl Med 31:1909–1914, 1990.
90. Man'a J: Nuclear imaging. 67Gallium, 201thallium, 18F-labeled fluoro-2-deoxy-D-glucose positron emission tomography. Clin Chest Med 18:799–811, 1997.
91. Vansant JP, Johnson DH, O'Donnell DM, et al: Staging lung carcinoma with a Tc-99m labeled monoclonal antibody. Clin Nucl Med 17:431–438, 1992.
92. Rusch V, Macapinlac H, Heelan R, et al: NR-LU-10 monoclonal antibody scanning. A helpful new adjunct to computed tomography in evaluating non–small-cell lung cancer. J Thorac Cardiovasc Surg 106:200–204, 1993.
93. Matsuno S, Tanabe M, Kawasaki Y, et al: Effectiveness of planar image and single photon emission tomography of thallium-201 compared with gallium-67 in patients with primary lung cancer. Eur J Nucl Med 19:86–95, 1992.
94. Yokoi K, Okuyama A, Mori K, et al: Mediastinal lymph node metastasis from lung cancer: Evaluation with Tl-201 SPECT—Comparison with CT. Radiology 192:813–817, 1994.
95. Lowe VJ, Naunheim KS: Positron emission tomography in lung cancer. Ann Thorac Surg 65:1821–1829, 1998.
96. Sasaki M, Ichiya Y, Kuwabara Y, et al: The usefulness of FDG positron emission tomography for the detection of mediastinal lymph node metastases in patients with non–small cell lung cancer: A comparative study with x-ray computed tomography. Eur J Nucl Med 23:741–747, 1996.
97. Guhlmann A, Storck M, Kotzerke J, et al: Lymph node staging in non–small cell lung cancer: Evaluation by [18F]FDG positron emission tomography (PET). Thorax 52:438–441, 1997.
98. Shreve PD, Steventon RS, Deters EC, et al: Oncologic diagnosis with 2-[fluorine-18]fluoro-2-deoxy-D-glucose imaging: Dual-head coincidence gamma camera versus positron emission tomographic scanner. Radiology 207:431–437, 1998.
99. Gambhir SS, Hoh CK, Phelps ME, et al: Decision tree sensitivity analysis for cost-effectiveness of FDG-PET in the staging and management of non–small-cell lung carcinoma. J Nucl Med 37:1428–1436, 1996.
99a. Esposito G: Diagnosis of mediastinal masses and principles of surgical tactics and technique for the treatment. Semin Pediatr Surg 8:54–60, 1999.
100. Shure D: Transbronchial needle aspiration—current status. Mayo Clin Proc 64:251–254, 1989.
101. Hashim SW, Baue AW, Geha AS: The role of mediastinoscopy and mediastinotomy in lung cancer. Clin Chest Med 3:353–359, 1982.
102. Carlens E, Larsson S: Mediastinoscopy in lung cancer. Semin Respir Med 3:176–183, 1982.
103. Oho K, Kato H, Ogawa I, et al: A new needle for transfiberoptic bronchoscopic use. Chest 76:492, 1979.
104. Wang KP, Terry PB: Transbronchial needle aspiration in the diagnosis and staging of bronchogenic carcinoma. Am Rev Respir Dis 127:344–347, 1983.
105. Wang KP: Flexible transbronchial needle aspiration biopsy for histologic specimens. Chest 88:860–863, 1985.
106. Mehta AC, Kavuru MS, Meeker DP, et al: Transbronchial needle aspiration for histology specimens. Chest 96:1228–1232, 1989.
107. Schenk DA, Strollo PJ, Pickard JS, et al: Utility of the Wang 18-gauge transbronchial histology needle in the staging of bronchogenic carcinoma. Chest 96:272–274, 1989.
108. Wang KP, Brower R, Haponik EF, et al: Flexible transbronchial needle aspiration for staging of bronchogenic carcinoma. Chest 84:571–576, 1983.
109. Shure D, Fedullo PF: The role of transcarinal needle aspiration in the staging of bronchogenic carcinoma. Chest 86:693–696, 1984.
110. Harrow EM, Oldenburg FA Jr, Lingenfelter MS, et al: Transbronchial needle aspiration in clinical practice. A five-year experience. Chest 96:1268–1272, 1989.
111. Gay PC, Brutinel WM: Transbronchial needle aspiration in the practice of bronchoscopy. Mayo Clin Proc 64:158–162, 1989.
112. Utz JP, Patel AM, Edell ES: The role of transcarinal needle aspiration in the staging of bronchogenic carcinoma. Chest 104:1012–1016, 1993.
113. Schenk DA, Bower JH, Bryan CL, et al: Transbronchial needle aspiration staging of bronchogenic carcinoma. Am Rev Respir Dis 134:146–148, 1986.
114. Ratto GB, Mereu C, Motta G: The prognostic significance of preoperative assessment of mediastinal lymph nodes in patients with lung cancer. Chest 93:807–813, 1988.
115. Cropp AJ, DiMarco AF, Lankerani M: False-positive transbronchial needle aspiration in bronchogenic carcinoma. Chest 85:696–697, 1984.
116. Carlin BW, Harrell JH, Fedullo PF: False-positive transcarinal needle aspirate in the evaluation of bronchogenic carcinoma. Am Rev Respir Dis 140:1800–1802, 1989.
117. Haponik EF, Cappellari JO, Chin R, et al: Education and experience improve transbronchial needle aspiration performance. Am J Respir Crit Care Med 151:1998–2002, 1995.
118. Rodriguez de Castro F, Diaz Lopez F, Serda GJ, et al: Relevance of training in transbronchial fine-needle aspiration technique. Chest 111:103–105, 1997.
119. Shields GW, Coggeshall JW, Witt WS, et al: Transbronchoscopic needle aspiration in the diagnosis and staging of lung cancer. South Med J 79:694–695, 1986.
120. Harrow E, Halber M, Hardy S, et al: Bronchoscopic and roentgenographic correlates of a positive transbronchial needle aspiration in the staging of lung cancer. Chest 100:1592–1596, 1991.
121. Rong F, Cui B: CT scan directed transbronchial needle aspiration biopsy for mediastinal nodes. Chest 114:36–39, 1998.
122. Harkin TJ, Ciotoli C, Addrizzo-Harris DJ, et al: Transbronchial needle aspiration (TBNA) in patients infected with HIV. Am J Respir Crit Care Med 157:1913–1918, 1998.
123. Westcott JL: Needle aspiration biopsy of pulmonary, hilar, and mediastinal masses. Clin Chest Med 5:365–377, 1984.
124. Moinuddin SM, Lee LH, Montgomery JH: Mediastinal needle biopsy. AJR Am J Roentgenol 143:531–532, 1984.
125. Weisbrod GL, Lyons DJ, Tao LC, et al: Percutaneous fine-needle aspiration biopsy of mediastinal lesions. AJR Am J Roentgenol 143:525–529, 1984.
126. Akamatsu H, Terashima M, Koike T, et al: Staging of primary lung cancer by computed tomography–guided percutaneous needle cytology of mediastinal lymph nodes. Ann Thorac Surg 62:352–355, 1996.
127. Belfiore G, Camera L, Moggio G, et al: Middle mediastinum lesions: Preliminary experience with CT-guided fine-needle aspiration biopsy with a suprasternal approach. Radiology 202:870–873, 1997.

128. Westcott JL: Transthoracic biopsy and drainage procedures. *In* Freundlich I, Bragg D (eds): A Radiologic Approach to Diseases of the Chest. Baltimore: Williams & Wilkins, 1992, pp 374–386.
129. Rosenberger A, Adler OB: Mediastinal biopsy. *In* Dondelinger R, Rossi P, Kurdziel J, et al (eds): Interventional Radiology. New York: Thieme, 1990, pp 18–26.
129a. Zinzani PL, Corneli G, Cancellieri A, et al: Core needle biopsy is effective in the initial diagnosis of mediastinal lymphoma. Haematologica 84:600–603, 1999.
130. Silvestri GA, Hoffman BJ, Bhutani MS, et al: Endoscopic ultrasound with fine-needle aspiration in the diagnosis and staging of lung cancer. Ann Thorac Surg 61:1441–1445, 1996.
131. Gress FG, Savides TJ, Sandler A, et al: Endoscopic ultrasonography, fine-needle aspiration biopsy guided by endoscopic ultrasonography, and computed tomography in the preoperative staging of non-small-cell lung cancer: A comparison study. Ann Intern Med 127:604–612, 1997.
132. Goldstraw P: Mediastinal exploration by mediastinoscopy and mediastinotomy. Br J Dis Chest 82:111–120, 1988.
133. Carlens E: Mediastinoscopy: A method for inspection and tissue biopsy in the superior mediastinum. Dis Chest 36:343–352, 1959.
134. Vallieres E, Pag'e A, Verdant A: Ambulatory mediastinoscopy and anterior mediastinotomy. Ann Thorac Surg 52:1122–1126, 1991.
135. Mouroux J, Riquet M, Padovani B, et al: Surgical management of thoracic manifestations in human immunodeficiency virus-positive patients: Indications and results. Br J Surg 82:39–43, 1995.
136. Ginsberg RJ: Evaluation of the mediastinum by invasive techniques. Surg Clin North Am 67:1025–1035, 1987.
137. de Montpr'eville VT, Dulmet EM, Nashashibi N: Frozen section diagnosis and surgical biopsy of lymph nodes, tumors and pseudotumors of the mediastinum. Eur J Cardiothorac Surg 13:190–195, 1998.
138. Clarke MR, Landreneau RJ, Borochovitz D: Intraoperative imprint cytology for evaluation of mediastinal lymphadenopathy. Ann Thorac Surg 57:1206–1210, 1994.
139. Pearson EG: Evaluation of tomography and mediastinoscopy for the detection of mediastinal lymph nodes metastases. Ann Thorac Surg 37:441–442, 1984.
140. Mentzer SJ, Swanson SJ, DeCamp MM, et al: Mediastinoscopy, thoracoscopy, and video-assisted thoracic surgery in the diagnosis and staging of lung cancer. Chest 112:239S–241S, 1997.
141. Funatsu T, Matsubara Y, Ikeda S, et al: Preoperative mediastinoscopic assessment of N factors and the need for mediastinal lymph node dissection in T1 lung cancer. J Thorac Cardiovasc Surg 108:321–328, 1994.
142. Kliems G, Savic B: Complications of mediastinoscopy. Endoscopy 1:9–12, 1979.
142a. Mineo TC, Ambrogi V, Nofroni I, et al: Mediastinoscopy in superior vena cava obstruction: Analysis of 80 consecutive patients. Ann Thorac Surg 68:223–226, 1999.
143. Best LA, Munichor M, Ben-Shakhar M, et al: The contribution of anterior mediastinotomy in the diseases of the mediastinum and lung. Ann Thorac Surg 43:78–81, 1987.
144. Krasna MJ: Advances in staging of esophageal carcinoma. Chest 113:107S–111S, 1998.
145. Prinz RA, Lonchyna V, Carnaille B, et al: Thoracoscopic excision of enlarged mediastinal parathyroid glands. Surgery 116:999–1004, 1994.
146. Smythe WR, Bavaria JE, Hall RA, et al: Thoracoscopic removal of mediastinal parathyroid adenoma. Ann Thorac Surg 59:236–238, 1995.
147. Knight R, Ratzer ER, Fenoglio ME, et al: Thoracoscopic excision of mediastinal parathyroid adenomas: A report of two cases and review of the literature. J Am Coll Surg 185:481–485, 1997.
148. Hazelrigg SR, Landreneau RJ, Mack MJ, et al: Thoracoscopic resection of mediastinal cysts. Ann Thorac Surg 56:659–660, 1993.
149. Naunheim KS, Andrus CH: Thoracoscopic drainage and resection of giant mediastinal cyst. Ann Thorac Surg 55:156–158, 1993.
150. Naunheim KS: Video thoracoscopy for masses of the posterior mediastinum. Ann Thorac Surg 56:657–658, 1993.
151. Sugarbaker DJ: Thoracoscopy in the management of anterior mediastinal masses. Ann Thorac Surg 56:653–656, 1993.
152. Roviaro G, Rebuffat C, Varoli F, et al: Videothoracoscopic excision of mediastinal masses: Indications and technique. Ann Thorac Surg 58:1679–1683, 1994.
153. Kerr KM, Lamb D, Wathen CG, et al: Pathological assessment of mediastinal lymph nodes in lung cancer: Implications for non-invasive mediastinal staging. Thorax 47:337–341, 1992.

# 78 Pneumomediastinum and Mediastinitis

DAVID R. PARK, M.D. • DAVID J. PIERSON, M.D.

Introduction
General Anatomic Considerations
Pneumomediastinum
- Pathophysiology
- Clinical Settings and Syndromes
- Clinical Manifestations and Diagnosis
- Approach to Management
- Sequelae

Mediastinitis
- Acute Mediastinitis
- Chronic "Granulomatous" Mediastinitis and Mediastinal Fibrosis

Summary

## INTRODUCTION

Pneumomediastinum (air in the mediastinum) and mediastinitis (infection or inflammation in the mediastinum) are disorders that predominantly involve the potential spaces and interstitial and lymphatic tissues of the mediastinum rather than the visceral organs. Although both may occur together, for example, after esophageal rupture, the term *pneumomediastinum* usually refers to the presence of aberrant air in the mediastinum without accompanying infection or inflammatory disorder. *Mediastinitis* is the appropriate term when infection or inflammation is the primary disease process regardless of the variable presence of air. These conditions are each seen in a variety of unique clinical circumstances. Both, however, tend to result from breaches in the integrity of mediastinal structures or from the continuity of mediastinal tissue planes with sites of pathologic involvement elsewhere in the body. Thus anatomic considerations are similar for the two processes and are considered together at the beginning of this chapter. The pathophysiology, clinical settings, management approaches, and impact on patient well-being of pneumomediastinum and mediastinitis are quite different and are discussed separately.

## GENERAL ANATOMIC CONSIDERATIONS

The mediastinum is traversed by air-filled structures (trachea and esophagus), which also may contain colonizing microorganisms. In addition, mediastinal lymph nodes drain the airways and lung parenchyma where inhaled organisms, antigens, and dusts are encountered. Consequently, entry of air or inflammatory and infectious materials into the mediastinum is readily accomplished by breaches in the integrity of these mediastinal structures or when materials deposited in the airways or distal lung enter the lymphatic system.

How air reaches the mediastinum from ruptured alveoli or from outside the chest, and its physiologic and clinical effects once it is there, can be understood by referring to the soft-tissue compartments of the neck, thorax, and abdomen, as illustrated in Figure 77–2. The same anatomic relationships that permit air to dissect freely throughout the mediastinum also predispose to the spread of infection and other inflammatory processes.[1–3] The visceral space surrounding the trachea, esophagus, and great vessels of the neck continues into the chest to envelop the mediastinal structures and passes through the diaphragm with the esophagus to communicate with the retroperitoneal space. A continuum thus connects the viscera-containing portions of the neck, chest, and retroperitoneal space.[1] A similar continuum exists between the endothoracic fascia of the outer chest wall and the abdominal transversalis fascia.[4] Furthermore, within the mediastinum, the vessels and airways of the pulmonary hilum are surrounded by an interstitial space, which extends distally into the lung and eventually merges with the space surrounded by bronchovascular sheaths (see Fig. 77–2).[2]

Thus, it is possible for air that originates within any of the structures mentioned, or inflammation originating at any site in the mediastinum, to dissect around or spread to involve any of these structures. Although air in the mediastinum does not usually cause serious clinical consequences unless it is under tension, the proximity of the mediastinal tissue planes to many vital organs makes the mediastinum uniquely vulnerable to inflammatory injury. Consequently, mediastinal inflammation can give rise to widely varying manifestations that are related more to the functions of the affected structures than to symptoms or signs of the inflammation itself. In the remainder of this chapter, pneumomediastinum and related forms of extra-alveolar air and then the various forms of mediastinitis are discussed.

## PNEUMOMEDIASTINUM

Pneumomediastinum consists of air or other gas in the mediastinum. Also known as mediastinal emphysema, it is one of several forms of extra-alveolar air or air outside the confines of the respiratory and gastrointestinal tracts; the others are pulmonary interstitial emphysema, pneumopericardium, subcutaneous emphysema, pneumoperitoneum, and pneumoretroperitoneum. Pneumothorax, the most common life-threatening form of extra-alveolar air, is discussed in Chapter 75 and mentioned only briefly here.

Extra-alveolar air in the form of pneumomediastinum and subcutaneous emphysema occurs in a wide variety of clinical settings, the earliest of which to be recognized was during childbirth. In her "Observations" of 1617 (as cited by Gordon[5]), Louise Bourgeois, midwife to the queen of France, wrote, "I saw that she tried to stop crying out, and I implored her not to stop, for fear that her throat might swell." According to Faust,[6] the first formal medical documentation of pneumomediastinum and subcutaneous emphysema following Valsalva's maneuver during labor was by Simmons in 1784, and this association was reported in more than 130 patients by 1927.[5] Within two decades thereafter, Hamman[7,8] had thoroughly established the clinical features of spontaneous pneumomediastinum, and Macklin and Macklin[9] had elegantly elucidated its pathophysiology. Although little has been added to the pioneering descriptions of these investigators, pneumomediastinum and other forms of extra-alveolar air are encountered today in an increased variety of clinical circumstances. These include mechanical ventilation and other aspects of critical care, decompression in diving and other settings, chest trauma, asthma, and numerous other situations in addition to childbirth.[1,10]

### Pathophysiology

The pathophysiology of pneumomediastinum depends on the clinical circumstances in which it is encountered. Pneumomediastinum most commonly results from microscopic alveolar rupture but can also result from air escaping from the upper respiratory tract, intrathoracic airways, or gastrointestinal tract. Gas can be generated by bacteria causing infection of the visceral space, and outside air can reach the mediastinum after trauma or surgery. These potential sources for mediastinal emphysema are summarized in Table 78.1 and discussed in the following sections.

#### Air Originating in the Upper Respiratory Tract

Mediastinal air dissecting downward from the head and neck can originate in several ways. Retropharyngeal ab-

**Table 78.1 POSSIBLE SOURCES OF AIR IN THE MEDIASTINUM**

| |
|---|
| Upper respiratory tract |
| Head and neck infection (odontogenic, salivary glands, cervical adenitis, tonsillitis, peritonsillar abscess, osteomyelitis of facial bones) |
| Fractures (involving paranasal sinuses, orbit, mandibles, other facial bones) |
| Other mucosal disruption (trauma, surgery, attempted endotracheal intubation) |
| Dental procedures (extractions, air-turbine drilling) |
| Intrathoracic airways |
| Blunt or penetrating chest trauma |
| Foreign body |
| Iatrogenic (bronchoscopy, bronchial brushing, transbronchial biopsy, needle aspiration) |
| Neoplasm |
| Lung parenchyma |
| Direct disruption of alveoli (penetrating trauma, surgery, transbronchial biopsy, needle aspiration) |
| "Spontaneous" alveolar rupture (shearing force between alveolus and adjacent bronchovascular sheath)* |
| Gastrointestinal tract |
| Esophageal perforation |
| Via pneumoperitoneum or pneumoretroperitoneum (gastric or intestinal perforation, diverticulitis, pneumatosis cystoides intestinalis, endoscopy, biopsy, infection) |
| Infection with gas-producing organisms |
| Acute bacterial mediastinitis |
| Head and neck infections |
| Air from outside the body |
| Penetrating trauma to neck or chest |
| Surgical procedures (tracheotomy, mediastinoscopy, sternotomy) |
| Via subcutaneous emphysema in association with chest tube insertion |
| Artificial pneumothorax |
| Artificial pneumoperitoneum |

*See Table 78.2 for clinical settings.

scess is a long-established cause of gas in the neck,[11] but other infections, including dental abscess, cervical adenitis, salivary gland infection, tonsillitis, and osteomyelitis of the facial bones can also produce this finding.[1, 3, 12, 13] Odontogenic infections are said to be the most common of these.[14]

Dental extractions or drilling, especially in the lower molar teeth[12, 15] and especially if an air-turbine drill is used,[16–18] can be followed by pneumomediastinum.[19] Although drilling has been considered necessary for this to occur, pneumomediastinum can be massive and associated with complications after simple dental extraction in the absence of drilling.[20] Passage of air into the soft tissues from the socket of an extracted tooth can be increased dramatically if positive pressure is applied at the mouth—as illustrated by the case of a soldier whose neck swelled on resumption of his duties as a bugler immediately after a tooth extraction.[21]

Injury to the paranasal sinuses, orbit, mandible, and other facial bones adjacent to the upper airways can provide access of air to the fascial planes of the neck,[22, 23] especially after nose blowing.[12] Surgical procedures involving the upper respiratory tract may produce air in the neck via breaches in either the oropharyngeal mucosa,[24] or in the trachea and skin.[25] Pneumomediastinum and subcutaneous emphysema are common after tracheotomy.[26] These findings were noted in 43% of the cases in one pediatric series[27] and in 13% in a prospective series in adults.[28]

Pneumomediastinum can also occur after attempts at endotracheal intubation or after overinflation of the endotracheal tube cuff when the hypopharyngeal mucosa or membranous trachea is injured.[29, 30] Tracheal injury and esophageal rupture leading to pneumomediastinum can happen also when air is forced into the open mouth.[31–33]

## Air Originating in the Intrathoracic Airways

Blunt thoracic trauma, particularly deceleration injury as sustained in motor vehicle accidents, may lacerate or fracture the trachea or main bronchi and allow air to enter the mediastinum.[34] Although this may occur in the proximal trachea,[35] most such injuries are within 3 cm of the carina, probably owing to the relative fixation of the airway at the carina and the development of a shearing force when the more mobile parts are displaced by the sudden impact.[34, 36, 37]

Other potential sources of mediastinal air from the major intrathoracic airways include perforation by an aspirated foreign body and erosion by bronchogenic or esophageal neoplasm.[38] Although bronchoscopy is much less frequently associated with visceral perforation than is esophagoscopy, increasing use of endobronchial therapies for bronchial obstruction and bronchoscopic biopsy techniques render this source for mediastinal air increasingly likely.

## Air Originating in the Lung Parenchyma

Most instances of pneumomediastinum are the result of alveolar disruption. This may occur after direct injury to the lung parenchyma, which allows air to escape from torn alveoli and terminal bronchioles after penetrating thoracic trauma, or from cut surfaces during surgery. The lung may be nicked in the course of tracheotomy[25] or central venous access procedures, and this mechanism may also be the source of extra-alveolar air after percutaneous or transbronchial lung biopsy. Most cases, however, probably follow "spontaneous" alveolar rupture.

**Mechanism of Alveolar Rupture.** Disruption of alveolar walls and entry of air into the bronchovascular sheath can result when a sudden increase in alveolar pressure, or a fall in perivascular interstitial pressure, establishes a gradient of sufficient magnitude to disrupt the alveolar walls at their bases and introduce air into the pulmonary interstitium (Fig. 78.1). This mechanism is readily understood in the case of extra-alveolar air after deceleration injury,[39, 40] and is the likely genesis in most other clinical settings as well.[1, 9] Although it has been speculated that a sufficient increase in intrapulmonic pressure was capable of producing alveolar rupture,[41] animal experiments have demonstrated that an increase in alveolar volume, due to increased transpulmonary pressure, is a more important determinant of disruption of the alveolar walls.[42] This finding may explain the rarity of alveolar rupture after coughing and sneezing, acts that buttress the chest and abdominal walls to counter the transient high intrapulmonic pressures.[43]

High alveolar volumes undoubtedly contribute to alveolar rupture after sudden decompression.[43, 44] The mechanism of alveolar rupture presumably relates to overdistention due to the expansion of gas trapped in the lungs during ascent. Accordingly, alveolar rupture is especially

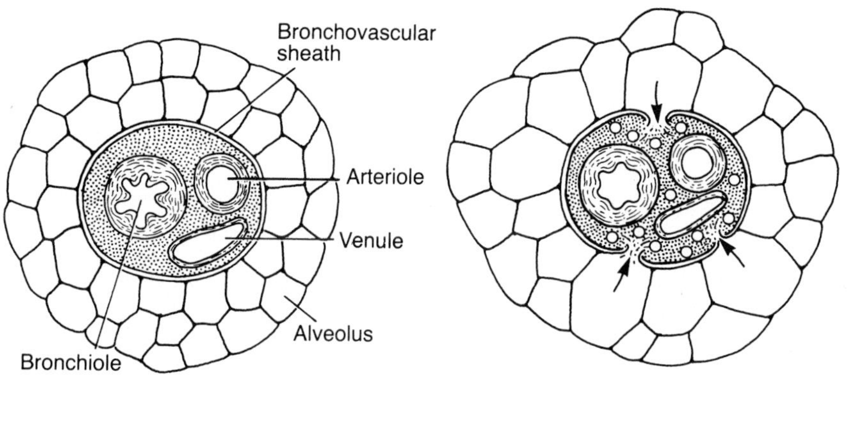


**Figure 78.1** Schematic diagram showing the mechanism of alveolar rupture into the bronchovascular sheath resulting from a momentary pressure gradient between them. (Reproduced with permission from Maunder RJ, Pierson DJ, Hudson LD: Subcutaneous and mediastinal emphysema: Pathophysiology, diagnosis, and management. Arch Intern Med 144:1447–1453, 1984.)

prevalent after sudden ascent from shallow depths, as the proportional volume expansion of intrathoracic gas is greater: Ascent from 99 to 66 feet beneath the surface increases gas volume by 33%, whereas rising from 33 feet to the surface doubles it.[45–47]

Pneumomediastinum and other forms of ventilator-related barotrauma are almost always associated with parenchymal abnormality in the affected lung,[43, 48–50] and this is also the case in most instances occurring during spontaneous ventilation.[1, 9] In both circumstances, alveolar rupture occurs by the same mechanism: a transient but increased pressure gradient between the alveolus and the interstitial space within the bronchovascular sheath. Periacinar and paraseptal blebs are often found at autopsy in the lungs of otherwise healthy persons,[51] and the blebs could predispose such individuals to alveolar rupture through this sequence.[52]

**Spread of Air After Alveolar Rupture.** Entry of air within the confines of the bronchovascular sheath, as depicted schematically in Figure 78.1, produces pulmonary interstitial emphysema. This is the initial consequence of alveolar rupture (Fig. 78.2) and may be the only overt manifestation of extra-alveolar air, especially in neonates with infantile respiratory distress syndrome.[53–55] According to Munsell,[56] Laennec called this condition *interlobular emphysema*. The clinical description of pulmonary interstitial emphysema, which is rarely observed in adults,[43] is attributed to Hamman.[57]

Because the mean pressure in the mediastinum, like that in the pleural space, is always somewhat negative with respect to the pressure in the alveoli and adjacent parenchyma, the pressure difference causes air to move centripetally, facilitated by the pumping action of breathing.[36, 58] This is illustrated in Figure 78.2 and was convincingly described in the 1944 paper by Macklin and

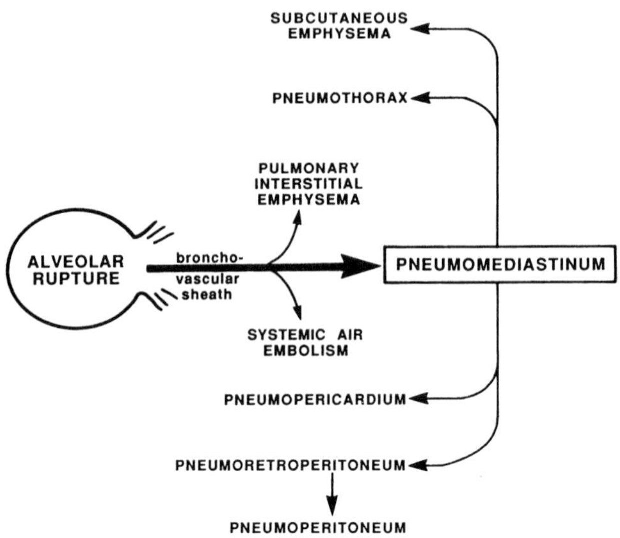


**Figure 78.2** The pathogenesis of the different forms of extra-alveolar air resulting from alveolar rupture is shown.

Macklin,[9] who first confirmed the sequence in experimental animals:

> [T]he first step . . . was air passing through numerous minute ruptures in the strained bases of the alveoli of the overinflated region into the underlying vascular sheaths. The air bubbles, at the very first minute, moved along the vascular sheaths, coalescing and gaining in size. This streaming of air through the pulmonic interstitium reminded one of the flow of a river that ever increases in size by addition of new tributaries as it proceeds on its course. Reaching the root of the lung, the train of air bubbles passed into and distended the mediastinum. With continued insufflation an actual overflow into the retroperitoneum, anterior mediastinum and subcutaneous tissues of the root of the neck and axillae occurred. In extreme cases the mediastinal wall ruptured, producing a pneumothorax.

These classic observations have since been confirmed in other studies,[59] but little has been added conceptually. In animal experiments, lower sustained inflation-hold pressures are required to produce pulmonary interstitial emphysema than to create a pneumomediastinum or pneumothorax,[53] and radiographic evidence of pneumomediastinum often precedes pneumothorax in mechanically ventilated patients with acute respiratory distress syndrome (ARDS).[60]

Extra-alveolar air may enter pulmonary blood vessels as well as the interstitium, with resultant *arterial air embolism*.[44, 45] This complication is particularly common in the setting of decompression illness,[45, 61] yet is relatively rare as a complication of mechanical ventilation, despite a high incidence of alveolar rupture and other forms of aberrant air.[62, 63]

Why is air embolism recognized commonly in decompression illness and rarely during mechanical ventilation, despite the occurrence of alveolar rupture in both circumstances? Perhaps the explanation relates to the volume of air entering the circulation at a given moment; to varying degrees of injury to the pulmonary venules and veins, where aberrant air would enter the systemic circulation; to the difficulty in recognizing subtle forms of air embolism in critically ill patients; or to the upright posture of ascending divers, favoring clinically overt cerebral embolization of any air entering the systemic circulation. Also, bubbles may form directly within systemic circulation during decompression, leading to arterial air embolism in the absence of pulmonary barotrauma.

Although commonly believed to require septal defects or pulmonary arteriovenous shunts, systemic air embolism without the overt presence of such defects can follow introduction of air into the venous system.[64, 65]

Pneumothorax after alveolar rupture occurs most commonly through the sequence depicted in Figure 78.2. Once in the mediastinum, air follows the path of least resistance and may rupture through the delicate mediastinal fascia and overlying pleura into the pleural space. The observation that pneumomediastinum preceded pneumothorax in most mechanically ventilated patients in one series lends substantial support to this model.[60] Another mechanism for pneumothorax after alveolar rupture has been proposed by Newton and Adams,[66] in which air dissects toward the periphery of the lung rather than toward the mediastinum and ruptures via subpleural blebs through the visceral surface of the lung. Which of these most often accounts for "spontaneous" pneumothorax is uncertain.

Extra-alveolar air originating from disrupted alveoli may appear below the diaphragm in the form of either *pneumoperitoneum* or *pneumoretroperitoneum*.[67–69] To reach the retroperitoneal space, and thence into the peritoneal cavity, air from the mediastinum usually extends via the loosely packed paraesophageal areolar tissue to pass through and beneath the diaphragm. An alternative route directly through the diaphragm has also been suggested.[70] In a review of 28 cases of pneumoperitoneum occurring during mechanical ventilation, Hillman[10] noted subcutaneous emphysema in 19, pneumothorax in 18, and pneumomediastinum in only 13. Pneumoperitoneum has also occurred without evidence of pneumomediastinum after emergency ascent during scuba diving.[71]

### Air Originating in the Gastrointestinal Tract

Mediastinal air can be of gastrointestinal origin, either from above or from below the diaphragm, although this is less common than the spread of mediastinal air into the abdomen. In *Boerhaave's syndrome*,[72] rupture of the esophagus allows air and other material to enter the mediastinum. In this circumstance, pneumomediastinum is usually accompanied by acute mediastinitis, as described later in this chapter. Pneumomediastinum can also be a consequence of esophageal perforation during upper gastrointestinal endoscopy[73] or after the ingestion of a caustic substance such as paraquat.[74]

Air or other gas originating in the retroperitoneal space also can spread to the mediastinum,[1, 4] although this is rare. Possible causes of pneumomediastinum from this sequence include perforation of a duodenal ulcer, ulcerative colitis, sigmoid diverticulitis, pneumatosis cystoides intestinalis, "rectal barotrauma,"[75] and procedures such as sigmoidoscopy, colonoscopy, and barium enema.[76]

### Air Originating from External and Miscellaneous Sources

Pneumomediastinum can arise from air entering the body from external sources, particularly if positive pressure is applied to the subcutaneous planes. Air can enter the cervical soft tissues during tracheotomy[25–29] or the chest wall during arthroscopic shoulder surgery[77, 78] and subsequently reach the mediastinum. Pneumothorax can be the source of mediastinal air by an unusual mechanism when treated with tube thoracostomy,[79, 80] as first described by Sauerbruch.[81] Once a connection is established from pleural space to skin by means of a chest tube, air can enter the subcutaneous tissues, dissect to the neck, and penetrate into the mediastinum from above. Air introduced into the pleural space under tension, as in the era of therapeutic pneumothorax for treatment for tuberculosis, could conceivably enter the mediastinum directly across the parietal pleura.[82]

Pneumomediastinum has also been observed after the deliberate insufflation of air into the peritoneal cavity during both the treatment of tuberculosis[83] and the course of modern era laparoscopy.[84, 85] Presumably, air introduced into the peritoneal cavity by any mechanism could migrate, by the reverse of the sequence shown in Figure 78.2, to the mediastinum. This would include air entering the peritoneal cavity via the female genital tract during pelvic examination,[86] douche,[87] postpartum exercise,[88] or blowing into the vagina,[89, 90] especially during pregnancy.[91, 92]

Gas can form in the mediastinum during acute bacterial mediastinitis caused by gas-producing organisms. More commonly, pneumomediastinum associated with mediastinitis is due to communication with the gastrointestinal tract (as in Boerhaave's syndrome), respiratory tract (as in necrotizing pneumonia or head and neck soft-tissue infection), or outside air (as in traumatic or poststernotomy mediastinitis). These conditions are described in more detail in the second part of this chapter.

## Clinical Settings and Syndromes

Pneumomediastinum after alveolar rupture is encountered clinically in two general setting: *spontaneous* mediastinal emphysema and *barotrauma* (or pneumomediastinum occurring during positive-pressure ventilation or associated with other externally applied distending pressure). Two dramatic clinical syndromes deserve separate discussion: pneumopericardium, in which the mediastinal air is confined to the pericardium, sometimes with profound physiologic effects, and systemic air embolism, in which morbid microvascular complications are common.

### Pneumomediastinum During Spontaneous Breathing

Alveolar rupture can sometimes be induced by voluntarily manipulating the breathing pattern such that lung volume is increased or sudden pressure changes occur. A typical example is pneumomediastinum reported after marijuana smoking.[93] Vigorous straining against a closed glottis, after inhaling to total lung capacity, is the assumed mechanism. The same complication has occurred after inhaling free-base cocaine,[94–96] during which users sometimes add additional external airway pressure by having an accomplice blow vigorously into their mouths through a cardboard tube.[97] Pneumomediastinum has also been reported in two college fraternity brothers after the recreational inhalation of nitrous oxide from disposable canisters.[98]

Mediastinal and subcutaneous emphysema occurred in a medical student after pulmonary function testing,[52] and these findings have also been observed in other healthy young individuals after dancing,[99] strenuous shouting, yelling, and singing during the course of basic training for the US Marines.[100] Other circumstances in which healthy persons have developed pneumomediastinum include playing the trumpet,[101] inflating a balloon,[101, 102] and mountain climbing.[103] In mountaineers, alveolar rupture may be related to "voluntary pressure breathing," a practice originally proposed for fliers during World War II that consists of slow, deep inhalations followed by forced exhalation through tightly pursed lips. This maneuver has been advocated by some climbers as a means of getting more oxygen into the blood, but it could well lead to alveolar rupture. The cases reported by Vosk and Houston[103] were members of the same climbing party, and both had practiced "voluntary pressure breathing" during ascent.

Much more common than the voluntary maneuvers just discussed is the inadvertent manipulation of the breathing pattern in the course of straining or exertion. As mentioned earlier, the first recorded pneumomediastinum occurred during childbirth,[5] and this complication of labor has been cited many times.[6, 56, 104–107] It has also been noted after vomiting in association with bulimia,[108] hyperemesis gravidarum,[109] diabetic ketoacidosis,[110–112] and other settings. Prolonged straining during convulsive seizures can be followed by mediastinal emphysema,[113] as can athletic competition,[114, 115] and violent coughing.[116] It is reasonable to expect that any activity producing large momentary swings in intrathoracic pressure could result in alveolar rupture and pneumomediastinum; other authors have listed sneezing, hiccuping, and straining at stool among such predispositions.[1, 9, 56]

Localized airway obstruction, resulting in regional overdistention of lung tissue, can lead to burst alveoli and all the reported forms of extra-alveolar air. This is easiest to visualize in the case of an obstructing foreign body,[117] blood clot,[118] or tumor,[119] but it may also explain the observation of extra-alveolar air in obstructive and parenchymal lung diseases. Pneumomediastinum is well described as a complication of acute asthma, both in children[120–124] and in adults.[125–130] Although chest roentgenograms are not routinely obtained during attacks of asthma, pneumomediastinum is not infrequent, having been noted in 5.4% of 479 roentgenograms of children admitted with asthma attacks.[123]

Parenchymal lung diseases associated with pneumomediastinum include atelectasis,[9] bronchiolitis,[131, 132] pneumonia,[122, 133] influenza,[9, 56] measles,[134] and large hematogenous metastases from primary soft-tissue malignancies.[135]

As mentioned earlier, alveolar rupture is a relatively common complication of sudden decompression.[44, 45, 136] Extra-alveolar air may be the presenting symptom of dysbarism after scuba diving[71, 137] or decompression in a hyperbaric chamber,[138] and it could also follow sudden atmospheric pressure changes during air travel.

Although a history of a potential predisposing event or disease process is elicited in most patients with "spontaneous" pneumomediastinum or other forms of extra-alveolar air, cases without such associations do occur and are known as *Hamman's syndrome*. Hamman's original patient was a 51-year-old physician in whom no predisposing factor could be identified.[57] Hamman[7] later reported several additional cases of truly "idiopathic" pneumomediastinum.

## Pneumomediastinum Associated with External Positive Pressure

Externally applied positive intrathoracic pressure is another general category of clinical settings associated with extra-alveolar air (Table 78.2). Most familiar within this category is "barotrauma" during mechanical ventilation[139]; however, this term is in part a misnomer because alveolar overinflation, rather than high airway pressures per se, probably plays a major role.[43]

Whether abetted by positive-pressure ventilation or occurring as a result of severe lung dysfunction, extra-alveolar air is common in mechanically ventilated patients.[48, 49, 62, 140] As previously discussed, alveolar rupture during positive-pressure ventilation is thought to occur as a result of overdistention in an area of lung with abnormal airways or parenchyma.[48, 49] Delivered tidal volumes in excess of 15 mL/kg, particularly when combined with high levels of positive end-expiratory pressure (PEEP), predispose to barotrauma, although the disease processes traditionally managed in this fashion are themselves associated with alveolar rupture.[43] In fact, Gammon and associates[60] found that the acute respiratory distress syndrome was the lung disease most commonly associated with barotrauma, and was the only independently associated risk factor for barotrauma among all ventilated patients.[50] The authors attribute previously reported univariate associations between airway pressures and barotrauma to the fact that airway pressures serve as a marker of the severity of lung injury (or dysfunction) rather than a direct risk factor for pulmonary barotrauma.[50] Further supporting this hypothesis is evidence from a recent study that found that the generally modest airway pressures and delivered volumes used were no different among those patients with acute respiratory distress syndrome who developed and did not develop barotrauma.[141] In fact, it is likely that both the severity of underlying lung injury or airway obstruction and particular styles of ventilator management that result in higher pressures and overdistention are responsible.[142]

Several distinct modes of mechanical ventilation have been introduced with the main purpose of decreasing the incidence of barotrauma. These include pressure-limited modes of mechanical ventilation (e.g., inspiratory-pressure support; pressure-control ventilation; airway-pressure release ventilation), and high-frequency ventilation.[142] The hope that barotrauma would be lessened by these modes is based on rational theory,[143] but no controlled clinical trials comparing the incidence of barotrauma with pressure-limited vs. volume-limited ventilation have been reported.[139] In infants, high-frequency jet ventilation appears to reduce the incidence of pulmonary interstitial emphysema but not actual air leak.[144] No differences in pulmonary barotrauma were observed in other studies of high-frequency ventilation for pediatric[145, 146] and adult patients.[147]

An alternative approach is the use of conventional volume-limited ventilatory modes with parameters selected to avoid overdistention (and also the repetitive opening and collapse of lung units). Such "protective" ventilatory strategies, designed to reduce microscopic ventilator-induced lung injury, might also reduce the incidence of barotrauma. Two randomized trials have compared this approach with more traditional ventilatory parameters, but the results thus far regarding overt barotrauma are contradictory and thus inconclusive.[148, 149]

**Table 78.2 ALVEOLAR RUPTURE: REPORTED CLINICAL SETTINGS**

| |
|---|
| Deliberate alteration in breathing pattern |
| Marijuana smoking, cocaine inhalation |
| Pulmonary function testing |
| Mountain climbing |
| Wind instrument playing |
| Yelling, shouting, singing |
| Straining and other involuntary alterations in breathing pattern |
| Childbirth |
| Vomiting |
| Seizures, status epilepticus |
| Violent coughing, sneezing, hiccuping |
| Heavy lifting, athletic competition |
| Straining at stool |
| Intrinsic lung disease |
| Asthma |
| Atelectasis |
| Bronchiolitis |
| Pneumonia |
| Influenza |
| Measles |
| Tuberculosis |
| Silicosis |
| Foreign body |
| Tumor |
| Decompression, gas expansion |
| Scuba diving |
| Air travel |
| Positive intrathoracic pressure of external origin |
| Mechanical ventilation |
| Continuous positive airway pressure |
| Manual ventilation during resuscitation, anesthesia, or transport |
| Equipment malfunction or misconnection in anesthesia or oxygen therapy |
| Heimlich maneuver |
| Deceleration injury |
| Idiopathic (Hamman's syndrome) |

Theoretic analysis[150] and studies on experimental animals[151] suggest that a gradual inhalation, followed by a pause at peak inflation, produces optimum intrapulmonary gas distribution and oxygenation. However, in clinical practice this is of dubious value and may be hazardous. Long inspiratory times may so reduce the time available for lung emptying that air trapping and intrinsic PEEP ensue, especially when airflow obstruction or high minute ventilation needs are present.[152, 153] This "dynamic air trapping" results in overinflation and can produce alveolar rupture and overt barotrauma. Clinical observations suggest that in the setting of severe asthma, any attempt to increase total minute volume (regardless of the specific ventilatory pattern) is associated with increased intrinsic PEEP and barotrauma.[154]

Noninvasive forms of positive-pressure ventilation are less often associated with barotrauma than is conventional mechanical ventilation. This is probably because of the lower airway pressures used, and the less severe lung diseases being treated. Although intermittent positive-pressure breathing has been associated with fatal pneumothorax when used in the management of severe asthma,[128] it does not carry the same risk of alveolar rupture associated with other forms of mechanical ventilation,[155] Similarly, continuous positive airway pressure (CPAP) applied by mask was associated with pneumomediastinum in only 1 of 331 applications of this therapy cited in one review.[156]

Barotrauma is especially likely when inappropriate excessive manual ventilation or insufflation of air or oxygen under high pressure are performed. Barotrauma is a well-documented complication of manual ventilation during cardiopulmonary resuscitation,[157, 158] not only from lung puncture during attempted line placement but also from excessive lung distention. Improperly connected oxygen tubing for in-hospital transport of intubated patients, such that exhalation is prevented, has resulted in life-threatening barotrauma,[159] as have similar errors after anesthesia and surgery.[160] A variety of other anesthesia-related causes of alveolar rupture can occur,[66] most of which are attributable to inadvertent overinflation or mechanical obstruction to exhalation.

Deceleration injury commonly results in extra-alveolar air, even when there is no open chest wound or displaced rib fracture.[39] Although motor vehicle accidents are currently the most common setting for such injuries, they can also follow blows to the chest or falls into water

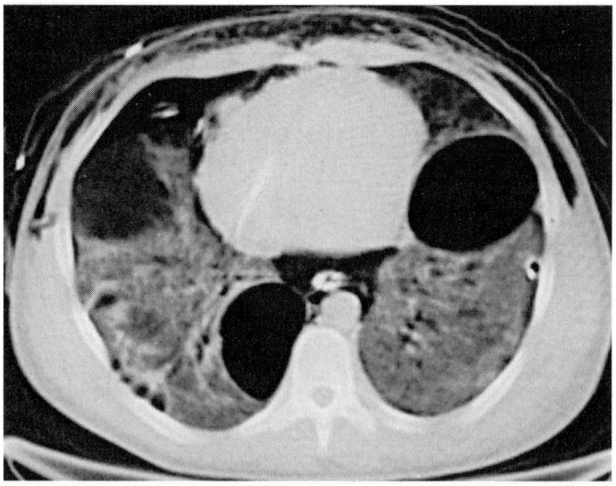

**Figure 78.5** Computed tomogram showing the pneumomediastinum associated with subcutaneous emphysema in a patient undergoing mechanical ventilation for severe acute respiratory distress syndrome. Mediastinal air can be seen in both the middle and posterior mediastinal compartments.

of alveolar rupture during positive-pressure ventilation are important clinical danger signals, as half or more will go on to pneumothorax.[60, 192]

Finally, as many as half of all radiographically detectable instances of pneumomediastinum may be undetected if only a posteroanterior exposure is made.[114] Careful examination of routine films may yield adequate information in many cases,[185] but computed tomography (CT) is probably more accurate than plain roentgenography for detecting aberrant air in all its forms and should be considered when important management decisions rest on a given distinction.

## Approach to Management

### Natural History of Pneumomediastinum

In most cases of pneumomediastinum, the air tends to spread throughout the mediastinum and to vent out of the thorax into the subcutaneous tissue planes.[1, 193] Subcutaneous emphysema can become massive and prove distressing to both patient and physician, but it is seldom dangerous in itself. Surgical relief of subcutaneous air collections is unnecessary, and they will resolve spontaneously once the primary air leak has sealed. Depending on the circumstances, other forms of aberrant air may require intervention, virtually always for the relief of mechanical physiologic compromise.

### Management of Spontaneous Pneumomediastinum

Most cases of spontaneous pneumomediastinum can be linked to one or more predisposing factors such as bronchospasm, infection, or foreign body, and treatment or removal of these is followed by gradual resolution of the aberrant air. Pain and other symptoms should be alleviated, but specific therapy for pneumomediastinum is rarely needed. Some authors have recommended breathing supplemental oxygen in high concentration to hasten reabsorption,[56, 105, 127] but only modest supplementation would probably work as well if it substantially increased arterial oxygen tension, and even this would seem unnecessary in most cases. Treatment in a hyperbaric chamber has been carried out in cases related to submarine training,[194] but pneumomediastinum is not one of the currently accepted indications for hyperbaric therapy.[46, 47]

Although pneumomediastinum rarely becomes physiologically significant, in rare instances it can produce life-threatening cardiovascular collapse.[5, 9, 195] Two recorded deaths have been attributed to this phenomenon.[5] Puncture or incision of the skin and subcutaneous tissues to allow the air to escape is often mentioned but seldom actually needed. An early, well-documented incident was, however, described by Laennec more than 150 years ago, as related by Munsell.[56] The great French clinician was called to see a small boy who had been run over by a dung cart: Laennec described how his 4-year-old patient was placed in a tent; with a candle for light, Laennec inserted sticks into the boy's neck, supraclavicular areas, and anterior portion of the chest. A subsequent, rapid, large outpouring of air extinguished the candle, and the boy, previously in extremis, recovered. Modern medicine can add little more to this emergency decompression regimen except for the substitution of sterile needles for sticks.

Other equally convincing if less eloquently described instances of life-threatening pneumomediastinum and its immediate surgical relief have been recorded.[195] Although surgical treatment of massive or symptomatic subcutaneous emphysema has been advocated,[196] a careful examination of the literature reveals very few instances in which this has actually been carried out. Techniques that have been used include aspiration of the mediastinum with needles,[8, 105, 197] cervical mediastinotomy,[116, 127, 193, 195, 198, 199] infraclavicular incisions,[200] and splitting or completely excising the sternum.[104] Tracheotomy has also been advocated by some,[104, 201] although others believe this is contraindicated.[127] Most experienced clinicians reserve invasive therapy for cases of increasing airway impingement or for cardiovascular compromise such as shock or acute superior vena cava syndrome. In these instances, which must be exceedingly rare, a small suprasternal incision into the mediastinal fascia seems to be the most prudent approach.

### Management of Pneumomediastinum During Positive-Pressure Ventilation

The appearance of mediastinal or subcutaneous air in a patient receiving positive-pressure ventilation is always a cause for concern. Although not usually physiologically significant without associated tension pneumothorax, pneumomediastinum may progress rapidly to the latter.[60] Pneumothorax in a mechanically ventilated patient requires prompt tube thoracostomy, and some clinicians favor "prophylactic" chest tube placement when extra-alveolar air first appears. This practice is probably not justified because of the hazards and complications of chest tube drainage in such patients, but a tube thoracostomy tray should be kept at the bedside for prompt use if the clinical picture of tension pneumothorax should appear.

Discontinuation of positive-pressure ventilation, if feasible, would seem advantageous for patients with ventilator-related extra-alveolar air in any form. Short of this, several adjustments should theoretically diminish the tendency of air to enter the mediastinum, although no clinical studies support these recommendations. Delivered tidal volume should be kept no larger than 10 to 12 mL/kg. Positive end-expiratory pressure should be reduced or discontinued if possible, and mean intrathoracic pressure should be minimized through adjustment of inspiratory flow and timing. Patient-triggered pressure-limited ventilation (e.g., inspiratory pressure support) or low-rate intermittent mandatory ventilation would probably be preferable to mandatory volume-limited ventilation if clinically feasible.[143] Monitoring of total effective thoracic compliance, especially during therapy with PEEP, may help to minimize the likelihood of additional alveolar rupture.[43, 202]

Occult PEEP, or "intrinsic PEEP," can augment air leakage, and steps to minimize this complication should be taken when it occurs[153]; these would include reducing minute ventilation and minimizing inspiratory time by increasing peak inspiratory flow rate and using ventilatory circuitry of low compressible volume. Finally, bronchospasm and other potentially reversible contributors to air trapping during mechanical ventilation should be treated vigorously.

Tracheobronchial disruption causing extra-alveolar air requires prompt diagnosis and surgical repair.[34, 36, 203] This condition should be considered in a patient with blunt thoracic trauma in the presence of extensive soft-tissue emphysema, airway bleeding, or nonresolving pneumothorax,[1, 39, 203, 204] especially if on chest roentgenography the collapsed lung tissue appears to have fallen away from the hilum.[205] When these findings are present, emergent bronchoscopy should be carried out to establish the diagnosis.[1, 39, 203, 206]

Pneumopericardium in the neonate during mechanical ventilation is considered a medical emergency that should be treated with prompt evacuation.[207] Most authors recommend drainage with a pericardial tube.[207, 208] Although much less common, tension pneumopericardium in the adult may be adequately relieved by pericardiocentesis, followed by close observation.[163]

### Sequelae

Pneumomediastinum subsides uneventfully in most instances once the precipitating event or process has resolved. Recurrence of spontaneous mediastinal emphysema is most unusual, although it has been described in both children[123] and adults.[103, 175]

Air in the pleural space can induce localized eosinophilic inflammation called *reactive eosinophilic pleuritis*.[209] A presumed mediastinal analogue to this phenomenon has also been described.[210] Diagnostic pneumomediastinum was performed 1 week before thymectomy in 63 patients with myasthenia gravis, and the thymuses of 29 of them contained "histioeosinophilic" granulomas.[210] This interesting observation suggests that pneumomediastinum in other clinical settings could be followed by similar changes, although whether they persist or could have clinical significance is unknown.

## MEDIASTINITIS

The term *mediastinitis* encompasses a number of loosely related processes that involve inflammation of mediastinal structures and its sequelae. Most forms of mediastinitis are infectious in etiology, and variations in their clinical presentation depend more on the chronicity of the underlying process than on the specific microbial cause. Thus, it seems logical to classify this family of disorders according to "acute" and "chronic" forms rather than into more specific etiologic categories. For largely anatomic reasons, acute mediastinitis is a distinct, usually catastrophic disorder. The chronic forms of mediastinal inflammation comprise a spectrum of disease, defined usually by radiographic or histologic features, that ranges from active granulomatous inflammation to "burned-out" mediastinal fibrosis. In the remainder of this chapter, acute mediastinitis is discussed, and then the various forms of chronic mediastinitis are dealt with as parts of a continuum rather than as separate disease processes.

### Acute Mediastinitis

Acute mediastinitis was once a rare and dramatic condition of a fulminating and usually fatal course seen after rupture of the esophagus from forceful vomiting or in conjunction with penetrating trauma. Beginning in the 1950s and 1960s, however, with the proliferation of endoscopic procedures, and since the 1970s with the rise of cardiac surgery via median sternotomy, acute mediastinitis has become somewhat more common and certainly more varied in its clinical presentation. Because of this new clinical variation, which may include relatively indolent infections, the term *suppurative mediastinitis* has been proposed as more accurate than *acute*. In either case, a distinction is drawn between these disorders and chronic *granulomatous* mediastinitis.

#### Clinical Classification

Involvement of different mediastinal regions tends to have typical causes: Infection in the superior mediastinum is most often the result of direct extension from neck infection; anterior mediastinal infection usually occurs after surgery or penetrating wounds to the anterior thorax; and posterior mediastinal abscesses are characteristic for tuberculous or pyogenic spinal infections.[211] Because the clinical picture of acute mediastinitis is influenced most strongly by the route and circumstances of infection, however, classification according to these factors seems most reasonable. This discussion follows the classification

**Table 78.3 ACUTE MEDIASTINITIS: ETIOLOGIES AND CLINICAL SETTINGS**

| |
|---|
| Perforation of a thoracic viscus |
| Esophagus |
| ''Spontaneous'' forceful vomiting (Boerhaave's syndrome), pneumatic trauma |
| Direct penetrating trauma |
| Impacted foreign body |
| Instrumentation: esophagoscopy, sclerotherapy, esophageal obturator airway |
| Erosion of carcinoma, necrotizing infection |
| Trachea or main bronchi |
| Direct penetrating trauma |
| Instrumentation: bronchoscopy, intubation |
| Foreign body |
| Erosion of carcinoma |
| Laser therapy |
| Direct extension of infection from elsewhere |
| Intrathoracic: lung; pleura, pericardium, lymph node, paraspinous abscess |
| Extrathoracic |
| From above: retropharyngeal space, odontogenic |
| From below: pancreatitis |
| ''Primary'' mediastinal infection: inhalation anthrax |
| Mediastinitis following sternotomy for cardiothoracic surgery |

according to the mechanism of mediastinal entry given in Table 78.3.

## Clinical Features

The classic clinical description of acute mediastinitis, as is seen after spontaneous esophageal rupture, is as follows: Onset is sudden and dramatic, with chills, high fever, and prostration. Patients are restless and irritable, with a sense of impending doom. Tachycardia, tachypnea, and signs of systemic toxicity are prominent. Most patients complain of severe substernal chest pain, worsened by breathing or coughing, and unrelieved by opiates. The pain may be referred into the neck and ear if the process involves the superiormost part of the mediastinum, whereas posterior or inferior mediastinal involvement may cause radicular pain radiating around the chest and pain between the scapulae. Examination may reveal supraclavicular fullness and tenderness over the sternum or sternoclavicular joints and crepitus, and other signs of mediastinal and subcutaneous emphysema may be prominent. Hamman's sign (a crunching sound synchronous with cardiac systole, heard over the anterior thorax) is characteristic but not always present. Later, tracheal deviation, cervical venous distention, and other signs of compression of mediastinal structures may appear.

The manifestations of localized mediastinal abscess are often related to mass effect. Symptoms and signs may include hoarseness (from impingement on a recurrent laryngeal nerve), diaphragmatic weakness or paralysis (from phrenic nerve involvement), Horner's syndrome (resulting from dysfunction of a stellate ganglion), and tachycardia secondary to vagus nerve involvement.[212]

The clinical picture just described, which is typical for esophageal rupture in Boerhaave's syndrome, varies in other settings today.[213] Acute mediastinitis is now less often "spontaneous" and more frequently iatrogenic; its manifestations are also modified by current pre-endoscopic preparations, surgical practice, and widespread use of antibiotics. The following discussion characterizes the clinical picture and management of acute mediastinitis in each of the four general settings listed in Table 78.3.

### Mediastinitis Resulting from Visceral Perforation

*Boerhaave's syndrome* refers to esophageal rupture associated with forceful vomiting, classically after overeating or excessive drinking. It is the most familiar example of acute mediastinitis[214–217] although no longer the most common. In addition to the clinical manifestations described above, hematemesis may be present before the actual rupture and tends to diminish or stop after rupture occurs.[218] Unilateral or bilateral hydropneumothorax is common and quickly progresses to empyema (Fig. 78.6). Spontaneous esophageal rupture can be difficult to diagnose, especially in the patient with altered sensorium who may delay seeking medical attention and who may not be able to relate a clear history. Adding to the clinician's confusion is the fact that lower esophageal rupture may be mistaken for an abdominal catastrophe.[218]

The mechanism of esophageal rupture, as elucidated by Rogers and associates,[204] involves hydrostatic forces that overcome the tensile strength of the normal esophageal wall. A momentary rise in intragastric pressure, as in vomiting, trauma, seizure, or other straining, accompanied by relaxation of the lower esophageal sphincter, permits gastric contents to enter and distend the lower esophagus. If the upper sphincter does not open so that regurgitation of esophageal contents can occur, hydrostatic pressure within the esophagus may rise to the point that its wall gives way at its weakest point. Rupture usually occurs in the lower left posterolateral wall, where the muscle bundles in the longitudinal layer of the esophagus separate, which allows a bubble of mucosa to protrude through into the mediastinum and burst. This mech-

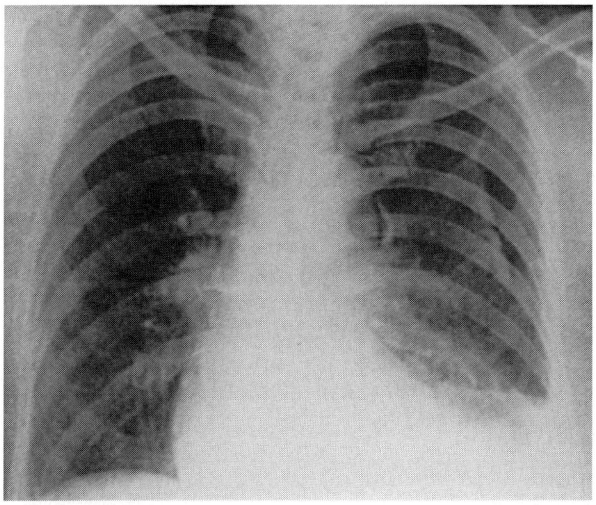

**Figure 78.6** This chest roentgenogram from a 64-year-old woman was taken 16 hours after traumatic perforation of the esophagus. The classic features of pneumomediastinum and left-sided hydropneumothorax are evident.

anism may be similar to that in pneumatic esophageal rupture, a bizarre occurrence related to biting and puncturing an automobile tire inner tube or closing the mouth around the leaking valve of an automobile tire.[32, 33, 219]

Penetrating chest injuries may result in acute mediastinitis, especially if the wound is grossly contaminated or causes visceral injury, or if there has been a delay in reaching medical attention. In such instances the diagnosis of acute mediastinitis may not be apparent if the patient has other serious injuries.

In the present era, the most common cause of acute mediastinitis is esophageal perforation during diagnostic or therapeutic endoscopic procedures.[211, 214, 220] In a review of 30 years of experience with esophageal perforation before the widespread use of flexible fiberoptic endoscopy, 77% of cases were due to endoscopy.[221] Actual passage of the instrument may be less traumatic today, but perforation of the diseased esophagus is still a recognized complication.

In a review by Wesdorp and associates[222] of 54 esophageal perforations related to endoscopy or instrumentation, 35 instances occurred during intubation with plastic prostheses in patients with malignancy. Of 19 perforations in patients with nonmalignant disease, 6 occurred during fiberoptic endoscopy and 13 during dilation procedures. The diagnosis was made within 2 hours in 94% of these patients. Fourteen of the 19 patients with benign disease were treated conservatively, and 5 were treated with surgery; there were no deaths among these patients, probably reflecting the influence of an empty gut lumen, prompt recognition of the complication, and immediate treatment.

Endoscopic injection sclerotherapy is associated with mediastinal complications in a significant number of patients who have the procedure, particularly with repeated treatments.[220, 223] Frank perforation, associated with necrosis of the esophageal wall and usually occurring 2 to 14 days after the procedure, has been reported in approximately 6% of patients.[223, 224] More common is pleural effusion, presumably associated with subclinical chemical mediastinitis without actual perforation, which has been noted in up to 14% of patients.[220, 225] In most instances, this complication is benign and self-limited, responding to conservative therapy in this generally ill patient population.[225]

Other reported causes of traumatic esophageal perforation include the esophageal obturator airway[215] and swallowed foreign bodies, particularly if the swallowed object is chosen with self-inflicted injury as the intent. One series describes six inmates who swallowed hypodermic needles fashioned in the shape of "stars" to win temporary reprieves from prison.[226] Unfortunately, all required surgical management, and one patient experienced a lengthy and complicated hospital course. Similarly, ingestion of caustic solutions such as lye or paraquat can lead to esophageal perforation.[74]

The diagnosis of esophageal perforation depends on an appropriate degree of clinical suspicion. On the chest roentgenogram, the hallmarks are diffuse mediastinal widening and the presence of air in the mediastinum and elsewhere in soft tissues. Mediastinal air-fluid levels may be seen, and pneumothorax or hydropneumothorax may be present. CT can delineate these abnormalities more clearly, but may not be necessary if the picture is characteristic and the patient gravely ill. Passage of ingested contrast material into the periesophageal space or pleura is diagnostic when observed.[227, 228] The diagnosis is usually established at operation, however, although percutaneous mediastinal aspiration with a subxyphoid approach is advocated by some as a means of earlier diagnosis.[229]

Successful management of frank esophageal perforation requires early surgical repair, drainage of the mediastinum and often the pleural space, and administration of appropriate antibiotics.[212, 214, 215, 230, 231] Percutaneous catheter aspiration of mediastinal abscesses, under CT guidance, has been used when the infection is localized and the clinical setting is less urgent.[232]

Complications of acute mediastinitis after esophageal rupture may include localized abscess formation, extensive pleural empyema, and persistent esophagocutaneous fistulas.[214] A prolonged stormy course is usual, and reexploration may be necessary to ensure adequate drainage. Prolonged parenteral hyperalimentation is often required.

Mortality reported due to acute mediastinitis after esophageal disruption has ranged from 10% to 20%[221, 233] to as high as 40% to 50%[218, 233]; these variations are attributable to differences in patient selection and management approaches. Timing of surgical drainage has been of prime importance in determining the clinical outcome; in one series of 39 cases, mostly after esophagoscopy, survival was 70% when surgery was performed within 24 hours of injury and 20% when done after 24 hours.[233] More recent series, reporting consistently aggressive surgical management, cite 89% to 90% survival rate after spontaneous esophageal rupture[234, 235] even when surgery was delayed beyond 24 hours after onset of symptoms.[234]

Other potential iatrogenic causes of mediastinitis include bronchoscopy and migration of indwelling central venous catheters. Bronchoscopy is a much less frequently reported cause of mediastinitis than esophagoscopy; however, increasing use of the Nd-YAG laser and mechanical endobronchial procedures, often performed in the setting of malignancy with chronic airway colonization or postobstructive pneumonia, adds to the likelihood of potential mediastinal complications. Intravascular catheters may be another source of acute mediastinitis when the catheter tip erodes through the vessel wall into the mediastinum. Mediastinal inflammation may result from chemical rather than infectious causes if the liquid being infused is hyperosmotic,[236] vessicant, or vasoactive (Fig. 78.7).

## Direct Extension of Infection from Other Sites

Direct extension of infection into the mediastinum from elsewhere has become rare in the antibiotic era.[237] Earlier in the 20th century, however, it was more frequent, and a series of 100 patients with suppurative mediastinitis reported in 1938 included 21 patients in whom it was secondary to oropharyngeal infection.[11] Infection originating in periodontal tissues, in the tonsillar region, or after pharyngeal perforation may extend via the prevertebral, visceral, or pretracheal spaces or in the carotid sheaths,[3, 214, 238] although the usual route is via the retropharyngeal space to the posterior mediastinum.[14, 239] Mediastinal infection occurring in this fashion, which has been given the name *descending necrotizing mediastinitis*, is perhaps the most clinically devastating form of the disorder.[14, 240]

Odontogenic infection is consistently the most common source of descending necrotizing mediastinitis.[14, 237] Most cases are mixed infections with both aerobic and anaerobic organisms on culture,[14, 241] and purulent pleural and pericardial involvement is common.[14, 237]

In addition to the clinical signs described previously for acute mediastinitis after esophageal perforation, patients with this form of the disease may have widening of the retropharyngeal space, with or without associated air-fluid levels, anterior displacement of the tracheal air column, and loss of the normal cervical spine lordosis on lateral films of the neck.[14] CT scans of the neck can be definitive in otherwise equivocal cases. Despite aggressive surgical drainage, usually by the cervical route, overall mortality remains 23% to 42%.[14, 237] Although thoracoscopic[242] and percutaneous drainage approaches have been described, aggressive open drainage and irrigation remain the standard approach. Extensive mediastinal exposure is usually necessary in patients with involvement below the tracheal bifurcation or with progressive disease.[237] Such a policy of aggressive surgical drainage via a thoracic approach in 12 patients with descending necrotizing mediastinitis reduced mortality to 16.5%.[242a]

Direct extension of infection from elsewhere in the chest is a rare cause of acute mediastinitis, but can occur with eroding neoplasms. Extension from anterior chest wall and neck infections have been described in injection drug users,[237, 243] and acute purulent mediastinitis has also been reported after closed-chest cardiopulmonary resuscitation,[244] although the pathogenesis in such a case is unclear. A less acute form, one that can occur as a

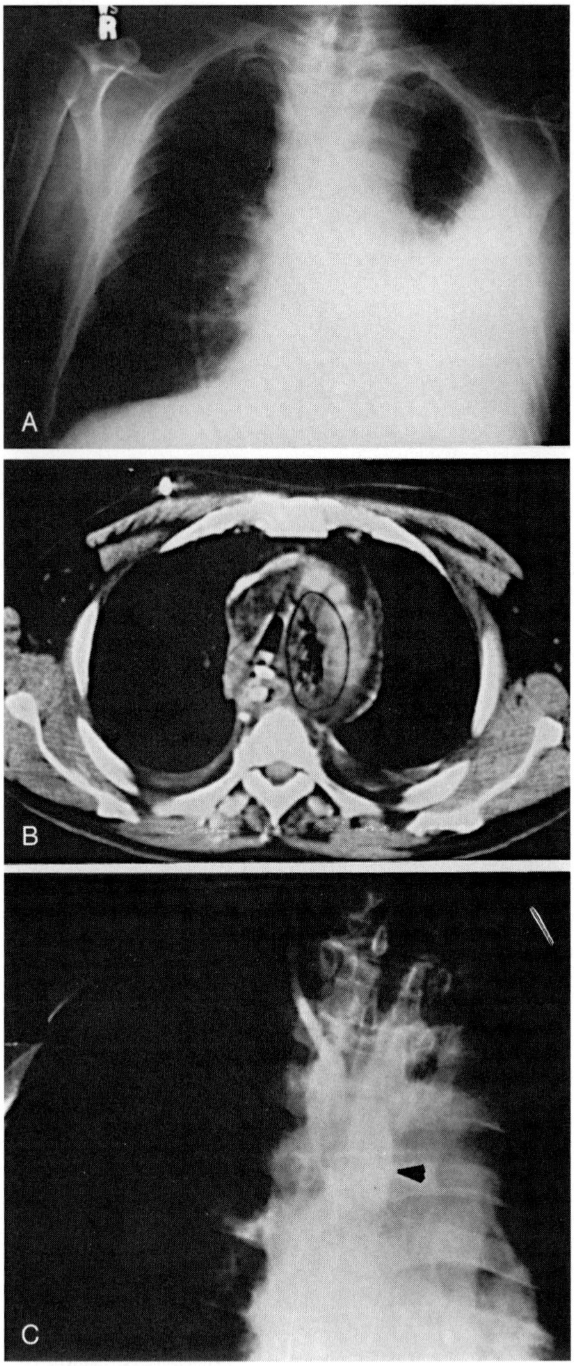


**Figure 78.7** These films are from of a 74-year-old man with mediastinitis due to erosion of an indwelling central venous catheter tip into the mediastinum. *A*, The chest roentgenogram shows mediastinal widening, radiolucency in the left upper mediastinum, left pleural effusion, and medial deviation of the catheter tip. *B*, The chest CT shows a gas-containing mediastinal abscess between the trachea and contrast-enhanced great vessels (an indelible elliptical line was drawn around the area on the original film). *C*, Although blood could be aspirated from the catheter, contrast material injected through the catheter passed directly into the mediastinum *(arrowhead)*.

complication of vertebral or costal tuberculous infection,[14] also is rare today in developed countries.

Pancreatitis has been reported to extend into the mediastinum, presenting as acute mediastinal widening with the clinical picture of mediastinitis.[245] Spread in such a circumstance would presumably be via the aortic and esophageal hiatuses and could also explain the reported occurrence of pancreatic pseudocysts in the mediastinum.[211]

## "Primary Mediastinitis": Inhalation Anthrax

Anthrax, caused by infection with *Bacillus anthracis*, is primarily a disease of cattle, sheep, and goats and is most prevalent in the Middle East. Human infection usually results from handling hides or hair from infected animals. Ninety per cent of cases are the cutaneous form of the disease, which is contracted by direct inoculation. A less common form is inhalation anthrax, or *woolsorter's disease*, which is contracted by inhaling *B. anthracis* spores. Their deposition in the distal air spaces is followed by ingestion by alveolar macrophages and transport to the mediastinal lymph nodes. A hemorrhagic mediastinitis rapidly evolves, followed by bacteremia, overwhelming sepsis, and usually death.[246]

Clinically, patients first experience a flulike illness for 2 or 3 days, followed by rapid development of the picture of acute mediastinitis, with severe respiratory distress, chest pain, and prostration.[247] Chest roentgenograms show mediastinal widening, and the diagnosis is established by demonstration of the gram-positive, boxcar-shaped bacilli in tissue specimens. A direct fluorescent antibody test is available for confirmation. High-dose intravenous penicillin G is the treatment of choice,[246] although penicillin-resistant strains have been reported.[248] Because of the virulence of the organism in this setting, inhalation anthrax is a devastating disease even with appropriate treatment: 12 of 13 well-documented cases in the United States had fatal outcomes.[249] The disease is fortunately rare, with one report documenting only two confirmed cases in this country in 25 years.[250] Nevertheless, anthrax remains a very real concern because of its devastating clinical effects and its ominous potential as an agent of biologic warfare.[251]

## Mediastinitis After Cardiac Surgery

Whereas some other forms of acute mediastinitis have been decreasing in frequency, bacterial mediastinitis after median sternotomy for coronary artery bypass, valve replacement, or correction of congenital heart disease has become an increasingly important entity,[212, 252–254] and several cases of acute bacterial mediastinitis have occurred after heart and heart-lung transplantation.[255–257] Along with its occurrence as a complication of endoscopy, this form illustrates the predominately iatrogenic character of acute mediastinitis in the present era.

The incidence of mediastinal infection after cardiac surgery has been variously reported at 0.4% to 5.0%, but figures of 0.7% to 1.4%[254, 258] are probably representative; in a comprehensive review, Sarr and colleagues[252] reported an incidence of 1.3% (151 cases of mediastinitis in 11,967 procedures). Poststernotomy mediastinitis has become a substantial clinical problem not because of a high case incidence, but because cardiac surgery via median sternotomy has become such a widely used procedure.

Factors that appear to predispose to development of mediastinitis after cardiac surgery include the presence of serious disease in other organ systems,[253, 254, 258] a history of previous sternotomy,[252, 254, 258, 259] the duration of the surgical procedure[252, 260, 261] and of perfusion time,[254, 259, 261] as well as when multiple valve replacement accompanies coronary artery bypass.[252, 258] Whether the operation is coronary artery surgery, valve replacement, or correction of congenital heart defects does not, however, otherwise affect the likelihood of this complication.[252] A low cardiac output state in the early postoperative period[252, 258, 259] and the amount of postoperative bleeding are other important risk factors[252]; 53% of cases in one series had lost more than 1250 mL of blood postoperatively.[259] The incidence of postoperative mediastinitis is further increased if reoperation is required to control bleeding[253, 254, 259] or if the patient requires more than 48 hours of mechanical ventilation postoperatively.[254] Preoperative use of beta-adrenergic drugs was associated with mediastinitis in one study and was attributed to their being a marker for obstructive lung diseases and the increased stress placed on sternal wounds in the presence of airflow obstruction and cough[261]; a more recent study also identified chronic obstructive pulmonary disease as predisposing to postoperative mediastinitis.[261a] Preoperative cardiac dysfunction, high New York Heart Association functional class, and obesity were predictive of postoperative mediastinitis in some studies[260, 261] but not in another.[258] Age and gender do not appear to influence the incidence[258]; postoperative mediastinitis has been reported in children[262] as well as in adults.

The bacteriology of postoperative mediastinitis varies and parallels that of early prosthetic valve endocarditis.[253] *Staphylococcus epidermidis* and *Staphylococcus aureus* have been the most frequent organisms in several series.[252, 253, 259] As many as 40% of cases have mixed infections,[252] with gram-positive and gram-negative organisms reported with nearly equal frequencies. Anaerobes are rare,[252] and *Candida* species[252, 263] and atypical mycobacteria *(Mycobacterium chelonei* and *Mycobacterium fortuitum)*[212] are infrequent, but have been reported. Infection with the last two groups tends to be more indolent and to involve the sternum or costochondral tissues.

Most cases appear to result from direct contamination of the mediastinum at the time of operation,[253] and the epidemiology of cases within an institution suggests that sound general infection control and careful asepsis in the operating room remain the most effective means of prevention.[252] Although definitive proof of their efficacy is still lacking, prophylactic antibiotics are widely used in the perioperative management of cardiac surgery patients. This practice has influenced the bacteriology and clinical manifestations of poststernotomy mediastinitis: Infecting organisms are usually resistant to whichever antimicrobial drugs have been given prophylactically.[253]

Mediastinitis may occur as early as 3 days or as late as 6 months after surgery,[253] although most cases occur within 2 weeks.[252] Presentation within the first postoperative week is more often associated with gram-negative infection and also more likely to be accompanied by bacteremia, while presentation after the second week increases the likelihood that *Staphylococcus* is the infecting agent.[253]

Acute mediastinitis occurring after cardiac surgery tends to be less devastating than that seen in the settings described previously, perhaps because it remains relatively localized longer and tends to be recognized earlier. Only 4 of the 21 patients in the series of Bor and coworkers[253] developed the classic signs of mediastinitis. Typically, the clinical course consists of fever and systemic signs on the first day, followed by bacteremia on the second, and then local signs of wound infection on the third day.[253] Drainage from the sternotomy incision and other localizing findings are present in most patients.[252, 253]

The diagnosis is usually made at the time of reexploration of the sternotomy wound and, thus, rests on high clinical suspicion in the appropriate setting. Distinguishing between superficial and deep wound infections may be difficult, especially if the clinical signs of infection are modest. A variety of diagnostic tests have been used in reported series, including gallium scanning, ultrasonography, and CT. CT is particularly helpful in identifying and discerning soft-tissue swelling, fluid collections, and sternal erosion or dehiscence.[264] The first two findings are, however, common in the early postoperative period, and their significance is much clearer when they persist or develop after 14 days.[264, 265] Some authors use subxyphoid[229] or trans-sternotomy[259] needle aspiration in suspected cases, although, as with the other tests mentioned, the potential exists for delayed diagnosis in a condition that can progress rapidly. Patients with fever, positive blood cultures, and wound abnormalities in the poststernotomy period should probably be explored.[253]

As in other settings, therapy for poststernotomy mediastinitis consists of early surgical exploration, debridement and drainage, and prolonged administration of systemic antibiotics.[252, 266] There has been disagreement in the past as to whether the incision should be left open or closed around drains for irrigation. Most authors now advocate early closure, even though re-exploration may be necessary. This approach avoids respiratory and cardiovascular compromise from the open chest wound, and, although mortality rates are the same, patients managed with their wounds left open stay substantially longer in the hospital.[252, 258, 267, 268] Catheter drainage alone may be effective for carefully selected cases.[269]

Reported mortality from mediastinitis after cardiac surgery varies considerably,[252, 260] partly because of varying incidence of coexisting disease, different treatment regimens, use of prophylactic antibiotics, and when the patients were seen—in one series extending back to the 1950s.[258] Currently, most patients should survive, with mortality rates of 20% to 40%.[253, 267] Hospitalization of survivors is usually prolonged by this complication[270]; the mean duration in one large series was 46 days for patients with mediastinitis compared with 23 days for noninfected subjects.[253]

Spread of infection to contiguous prosthetic material or valves is a devastating complication that usually portends a fatal outcome.[253] Infection may occasionally spread to adjacent pericardium, lung, or chest wall. Sternal osteomyelitis or costochondritis, once seen in as many as one third of cases,[271] has become a less common complication with earlier aggressive management.

The possibility of progressive mediastinal fibrosis and other disabling long-term sequelae in survivors has recently been addressed in a series of patients evaluated at a mean of 50 months after surgery.[272] Five of the 11 patients had pleural thickening on the chest roentgenogram, but there were no significant clinical or physiologic sequelae.

## Chronic "Granulomatous" Mediastinitis and Mediastinal Fibrosis

Mediastinal disease in adults that is chronic in nature and not the result of malignancy may be considered in the broad categories of granulomatous mediastinitis and mediastinal fibrosis. These conditions are not so much separate disease processes, however, as they are two ends of a spectrum of chronic inflammation and fibrosis. This pathophysiologic continuum is not evident in most of the literature, which mainly reports groups of cases at one or another end of the spectrum, collected according to differing criteria. Among the larger series, some have been based on pathologic material, selected according to the presence of granulomas[273] or fibrosis[274, 275]; others have reported only cases of proven etiology,[276, 277] with mediastinal widening or mass on the chest roentgenogram,[278] or who presented with superior vena cava obstruction.[279–281] Attempts to garner large numbers of cases from the literature[282, 283] have necessarily been hampered by this lack of uniformity in selection, which is not always evident. Furthermore, because nearly all published series are retrospective, the clinical descriptions of chronic mediastinitis are imperfect, to say the least.

Disorders falling along the continuum from active granulomatous mediastinitis to pure mediastinal fibrosis have been designated by the following terms, among others: mediastinal adenitis, mediastinal granulomatosis, sclerosing mediastinitis, mediastinal collagenosis, and fibrosing mediastinitis. Conceptually, all these processes may be thought of as variations of a common process that differ in the nature of the host response and in the point in their natural history at which they are examined (Fig. 78.8).[283a]

### Pathophysiology and Etiologies

The pathogenesis of granulomatous mediastinitis and mediastinal fibrosis, and of their varying manifestations, is most easily understood using histoplasmosis or tuberculosis as an example. Infection begins as a primary focus in the lung, after which regional lymph nodes draining the focus become involved, and then mediastinal adenitis ensues. This is accompanied by some degree of periadenitis and, eventually, a cluster of caseating lymph nodes, which breaks down into an irregular mass and which

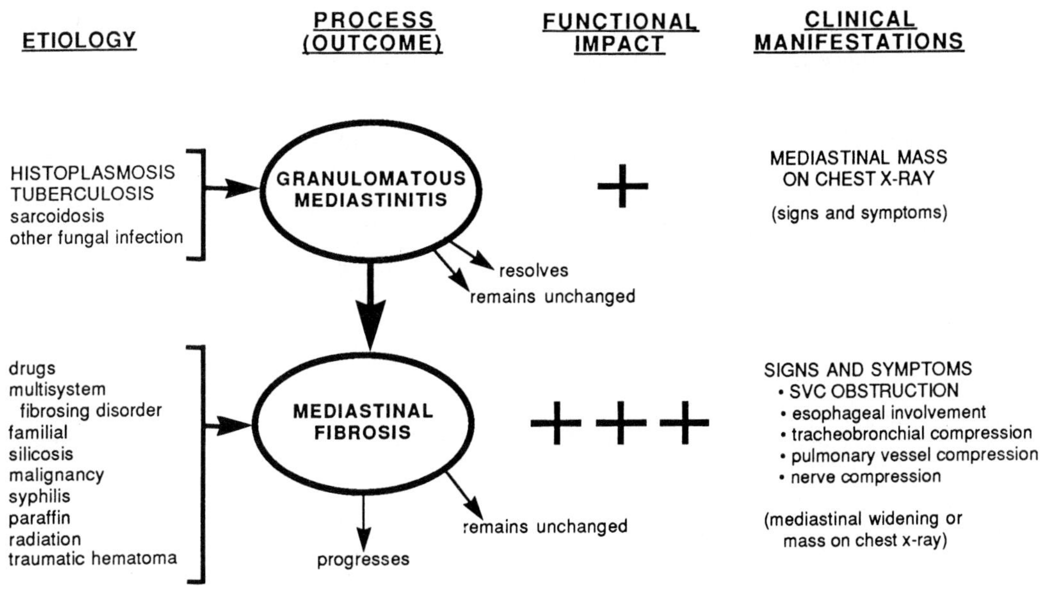


**Figure 78.8** The pathophysiologic relationships between granulomatous mediastinitis and mediastinal fibrosis are outlined. The predominant etiologies and clinical manifestations for each process are shown in capital letters. SVC = superior vena cava.

heals by fibrous encapsulation. In some cases, dense calcification may occur within this mass (Fig. 78.9). In most instances, the mediastinal mass is 4 to 6 cm in diameter, although it may be as large as 10 cm.[212] The thickness of the fibrotic capsule is the main determinant of the clinical picture[276]: In perhaps 75% of cases, it is 2 to 5 mm in thickness and has little clinical impact, whereas in 25% the capsule reaches 6 to 9 mm and invades or engulfs adjacent tissues.[212] This benign localized process produces physiologically important effects because of the compact nature of the mediastinum and the importance and vulnerability of the structures it contains.

Symptoms and physiologic effects of this process are determined based on which lymph nodes are involved.[215] Most commonly, they are in the right perihilar region, perhaps accounting in part for the high prevalence of the superior vena cava syndrome observed in this condition. Later, if the process progresses to generalized fibrosis, the entire upper portion of the mediastinum may be involved.

Why inflammation and fibrosis progress in some patients and not in others has been the subject of considerable debate. Goodwin and associates[276] postulated that prolonged gradual seepage of some soluble antigen or other substance from the involved lymph nodes, at least in patients with histoplasmosis, causes fibrosis. This theory is supported by the finding of stronger histoplasmin skin test reactivity in patients with mediastinal fibrosis than in others with chronic histoplasmosis[276] and by the observation that coccidioidomycosis, which also produces an exuberant granulomatous mediastinal lymphadenitis, is virtually never associated with mediastinal fibrosis.[215] Other authors reject this theory in favor of an abnormality in collagen organization that, provoked by various stimuli, leads to mediastinal fibrosis.[274] Whether either of these concepts or some other mechanism is responsible, it is evident that the nature and vigor of the host's response is vitally important.

The occurrence of mediastinal and retroperitoneal fibrosis in the same patients,[227, 275, 284] and of idiopathic isolated mediastinal fibrosis in others,[285] has led some investigators to postulate an autoimmune mechanism.[286] The finding of mediastinal and retroperitoneal fibrosis, along with other forms of fibrosis in members of the same family, has led to the term *familial multifocal fibrosclerosis*.[287] Fibrosing processes elsewhere in the body that could be related, in at least some cases, to mediastinal fibrosis, include retroperitoneal fibrosis, Riedel's thyroiditis, sclerosing cholangitis, orbital pseudotumor, sclerosing cervicitis, ligneous perityphlitis of the cecum, and keloids.[274, 287] Others have pointed out dissimilarities between mediastinal and retroperitoneal fibrosis and disagree with this unitary concept.[276]

Most cases of granulomatous mediastinitis are caused by histoplasmosis (especially in North America) or tuberculosis,[212, 227, 273, 274, 276, 282] although, as the disease progresses from active caseous inflammation to largely acellular fibrosis, it becomes more and more difficult to establish the cause with certainty. In 180 cases reviewed by Schowengerdt and colleagues,[282] a definite diagnosis could be established in 33 of 103 examples of "granulomatous mediastinitis" but in only 3 of 77 cases categorized as "mediastinal fibrosis." Histoplasmosis and tuberculosis together accounted for 83% of the confirmed diagnoses.[282] Geographic and ethnic factors affect the frequencies of these infections: Histoplasmosis is most often diagnosed in North America, whereas tuberculosis may produce mediastinal involvement more frequently in persons of Asian than of Northern European descent.[277]

Other reported infectious causes of mediastinal fibrosis include actinomycosis,[288] syphilis,[288, 289] nematode infec-

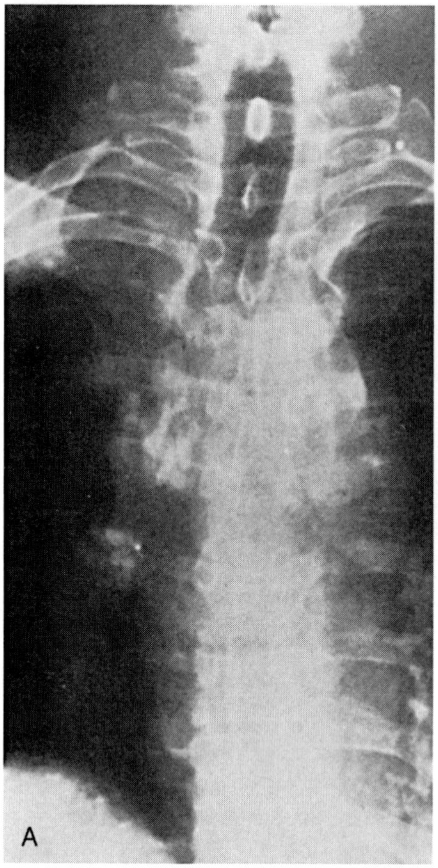


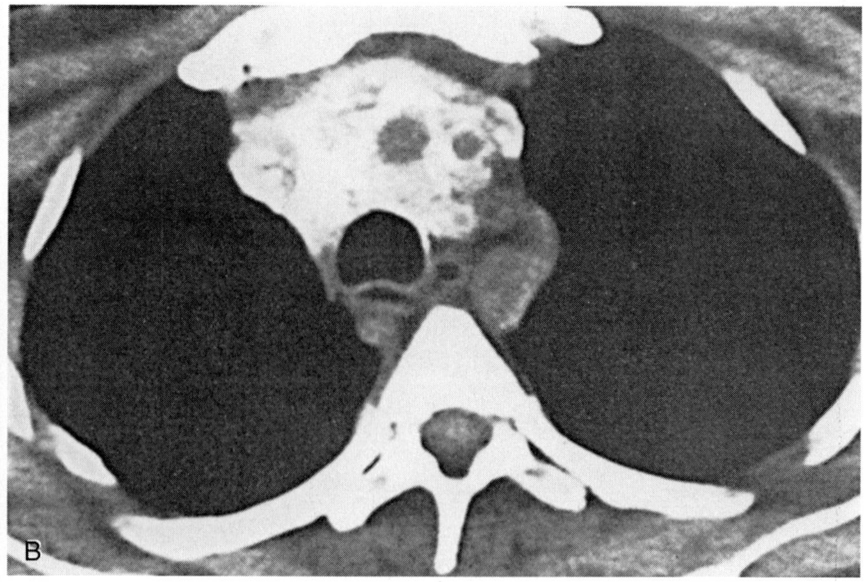


**Figure 78.9** Two films showing mediastinal widening due to chronic granulomatous mediastinitis from histoplasmosis: *A,* A frontal radiograph and *B,* a CT section. Dense calcification is present within the mass. (Reproduced with permission from Naidich DP, Zerhouni EA, Siegelman SS: Computed Tomography and Magnetic Resonance of the Thorax (2nd ed). New York: Raven Press, 1991, p 75.)

tion with *Wuchereria bancrofti,*[290] and "pyogenic" causes,[289] although it appears that the last of these (acute mediastinitis) seldom results in chronic sequelae.[272]

Granulomatous infection is the usual cause of mediastinal fibrosis as diagrammed in Figure 78.8. The same histologic and clinical picture can, however, be the ultimate result of other disease processes. Fibrosis associated with use of methysergide (Sansert), a drug used in the control of severe vascular headache, is perhaps the best known of these. Graham and associates[291] reported 27 patients treated with methysergide in whom retroperitoneal fibrosis developed; three of these patients also had pulmonary and mediastinal involvement. Perhaps because the offending agent can be completely removed from the body, the symptoms and signs of methysergide-induced fibrosis regress or remit completely in most patients when the drug is stopped.[291] Hydralazine was mentioned in one review article as another drug that can cause mediastinal fibrosis,[274] although documentation was not given.

In addition to accounting for 11% of the cases of granulomatous mediastinitis of known cause in the review by Schowengerdt and colleagues,[282] sarcoidosis has been reported as a cause of superior vena caval obstruction owing to mediastinal fibrosis.[292] Other reported noninfectious causes of mediastinal fibrosis include silicosis,[293] paraffin (as a late complication of plombage for tuberculosis), and traumatic mediastinal hematoma.[212, 275] Nodular sclerosing Hodgkin's disease also may masquerade as mediastinal fibrosis,[294] which emphasizes the importance of careful review of adequately representative biopsy samples when evaluating a mediastinal mass. Although there is a report of superior vena caval obstruction thought to be caused by mediastinal irradiation,[295] radiotherapy as a cause of mediastinal fibrosis must be distinctly unusual in view of its widespread use and the absence of other documentation of this complication.[296]

## Clinical Manifestations

On the continuum from active granulomatous mediastinitis to burned-out mediastinal fibrosis, the former tends to be asymptomatic and to be discovered incidentally by chest roentgenography, and the latter tends to cause clinical manifestations. In the largest collection of cases to date, 74% of the patients with granulomatous mediastinitis were asymptomatic, whereas all but 17% with fibrosis presented with symptoms or signs.[282] In 52 patients with mediastinal fibrosis and evidence of histoplasmosis reviewed by Loyd and coworkers,[283] initial symptoms included cough in 41%, dyspnea in 32%, hemoptysis in 31%, and chest pain in 23%. Clinical manifestations develop either because the fibrotic process invades or compresses mediastinal structures or because a calcified mass erodes into adjacent structures. In approximate order of frequency, these manifestations can be grouped into those related to involvement of the superior vena cava,[297] the esophagus, the trachea or main bronchi, the major pulmonary vessels, and mediastinal nerves. In some cases, findings are present in more than one of these categories.

**Superior Vena Cava Obstruction.** This is the most common complication of granulomatous mediastinitis and mediastinal fibrosis. Most patients with this finding have malignancy: Depending on the case selection criteria used, benign causes comprise about 3% to 6% of large published series[279, 298] of which most are due to granulomatous mediastinitis or mediastinal fibrosis.[227] Superior vena caval obstruction can occur at any stage of granulomatous or fibrotic involvement[212, 273, 276, 282]; this complication was present in 77% of symptomatic patients designated as having granulomatous mediastinitis and in 52% of those with symptoms in the setting of mediastinal fibrosis in Schowengerdt's series.[282]

The typical presentation is with all or part of the *superior vena cava syndrome* (described in Chapter 77).[297] Because obstruction develops gradually, collateral channels tend to divert much of the venous flow (Fig. 78.10). Therefore, symptoms may be less prominent than might be expected and may improve with time.[215, 227, 273] Even chronic superior vena caval obstruction can, however, cause serious complications such as hemorrhage from esophageal varices,[298a] recurrent upper extremity thrombophlebitis, and postphlebitic syndrome.[215]

Less commonly, the inferior vena cava can be involved,[282] as can the azygos vein.[212] Thoracic duct obstruction is rare[282] but can produce chylothorax[215] and its associated clinical manifestations (see Chapter 75).

**Esophageal Involvement.** Esophageal involvement is second in frequency only to obstruction of the superior vena cava as a cause of symptoms in patients with granulomatous mediastinitis or mediastinal fibrosis,[282] and it can consist of extrinsic compression, traction diverticulae, disturbances of esophageal motility, or bleeding.[212] Symptoms of dysphagia, chest pain, and eructation are experienced by perhaps one third of patients who have any complaints from their disease.[273, 282]

**Airway Involvement.** Clinical manifestations due to involvement of the trachea or major bronchi are common but are less often encountered than superior vena caval and esophageal complications. Airway complications were present in 7 of 29 patients in one report,[274] and they constituted the most common indication for surgical intervention in another.[299] Any of the main airways may be compromised, but involvement of the right middle lobe is reported as most frequent and is often accompanied by features of the *right middle lobe syndrome*.[212] Bronchoesophageal fistula is rare but has been observed,[277, 282] and it may be heralded by simultaneous hemoptysis and hematemesis.[300] Symptomatic mediastinal adenitis can occur, especially in children, with a characteristic "brassy" cough resulting from tracheal or bronchial compression[212]; this syndrome is self-limited and lasts for several weeks to a few months.

**Pulmonary Vascular Involvement.** Mediastinal fibrosis can involve major vessels on either side of the heart.[274, 276, 282] When this occurs, prognosis is not as benign as in the other clinical presentations already discussed.[215] Progressive obstruction of one or both main pulmonary arteries can result in pulmonary hypertension, cor pulmonale, and refractory right-sided heart failure (Fig. 78.11).[215, 301] Patients with pulmonary hyperten-

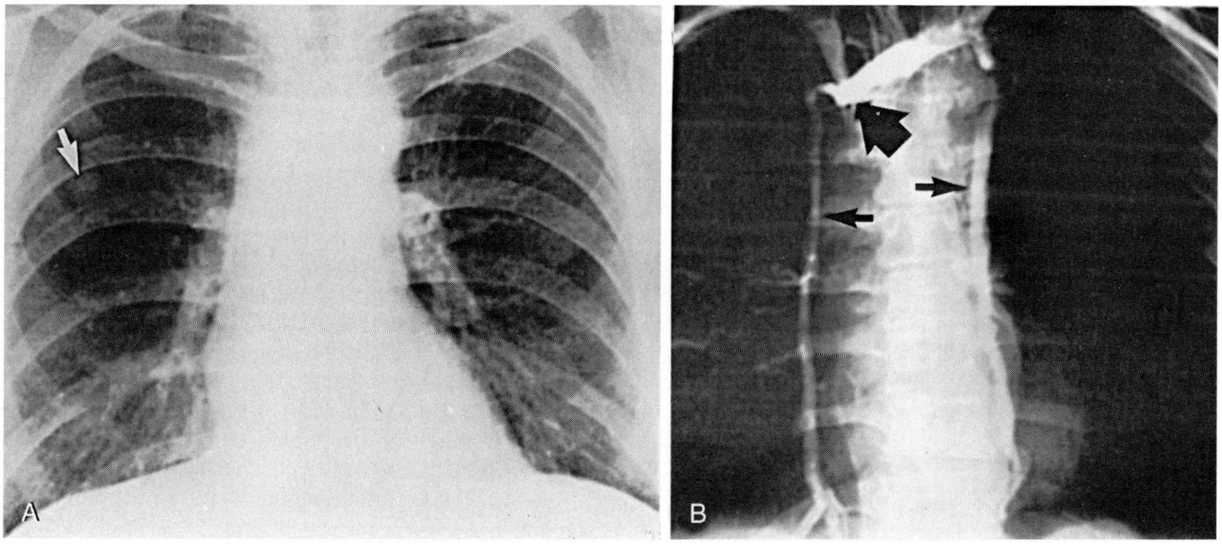


**Figure 78.10** Mediastinal fibrosis (in this instance, from histoplasmosis) with superior vena cava obstruction with extensive collateral circulation. *A*, The standard frontal radiograph shows smooth widening of the superior mediastinum with a peripheral granuloma in the right lung *(arrow)*. *B*, Another film taken just after rapid injection of contrast material into an antecubital vein shows complete obstruction of the superior vena cava *(thick arrow)*, with filling of the internal mammary veins bilaterally *(thin arrows)*. (Reproduced with permission from Fraser RG, Paré JAP, Paré PD, et al: Diagnosis of Diseases of the Chest (3rd ed, Vol II). Philadelphia: WB Saunders, 1990, p 955.)

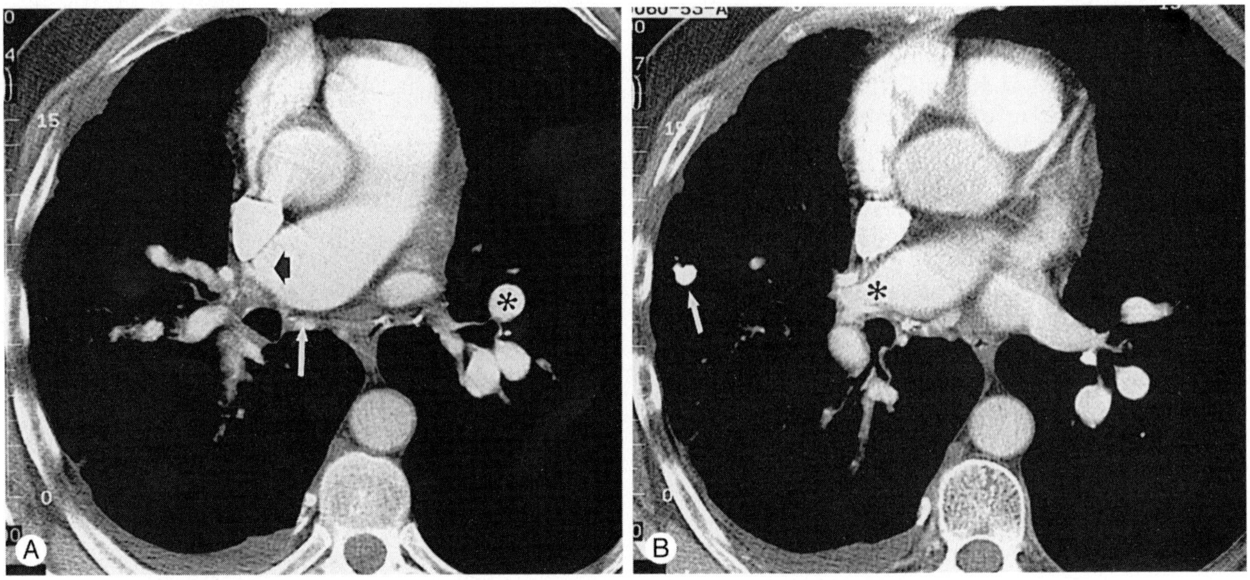


**Figure 78.11** Computed tomographic scans from a 45-year-old man with pulmonary hypertension caused by fibrosing mediastinitis due to histoplasmosis. *A,* At the level of the main pulmonary artery, findings include calcification within the middle mediastinum *(white arrow),* pleural thickening and calcification, smooth tapering stenosis of the right pulmonary artery (black arrow), and post-stenotic dilatation of the left lower lobe pulmonary artery branches *(asterisk).* Stenosis of the left pulmonary artery was also present but not clearly demonstrated on a single image. *B,* At a lower level, a calcified pulmonary granuloma *(white arrow)* and stenosis of the superior pulmonary veins *(asterisk)* are evident.

sion from fibrosing mediastinitis may have clinical and radiographic features in common with chronic thrombotic obstruction of major pulmonary arteries.[302] Stenosis of proximal pulmonary veins can cause a clinical picture similar to severe valvular mitral stenosis, with pulmonary venous hypertension and recurrent episodes of hemoptysis.[215] Pulmonary venous hypertension can be unilateral when the veins from only one lung are involved, and thus may result in unilateral pulmonary fibrosis.[212]

**Mediastinal Nerve Involvement.** Additional manifestations may result from the involvement of mediastinal nerves. Entrapment or compression of one of the recurrent laryngeal nerves can produce hoarseness.[274, 282] Other possible manifestations include diaphragmatic paralysis owing to involvement of one or both phrenic nerves, Horner's syndrome from impingement on autonomic ganglions or nerves, and persistent tachycardia from damage to the vagus nerve.

## Diagnosis and Management

In most instances, surgical exploration is necessary to distinguish between benign and malignant causes for the superior vena caval syndrome, localized mediastinal mass, or other manifestation that brings the patient to the physician's attention. When less invasive procedures are nondiagnostic in patients with the superior vena cava syndrome, mediastinoscopy is said to be "simple, low risk, and effective."[302a] In occasional cases, radiographs from previous years documenting an unchanged appearance, or dense calcification within the mass, will allow a confident diagnosis without operation.

Chest roentgenograms are abnormal in most patients. Granulomatous mediastinitis more often presents as a localized mass, usually in the right paratracheal area, and the later fibrotic state more frequently produces generalized widening of the superior portion of the mediastinum, but these characteristics vary.[227, 273, 274] Mass lesions tend to be smooth and lobulated,[227] and contrast studies in cases of superior vena caval obstruction typically show the affected area to be smooth and tapered[274] in contrast to the more ragged appearances usually seen with cancer. Positron emission tomography was recently reported as positive in one patient with sclerosing mediastinitis and thus cannot be relied on to differentiate benign and malignant causes of mediastinal compression.[302b] In some cases, the mediastinum is normal in appearance on standard chest films, and venography or CT is necessary to demonstrate the anatomic basis of a clinically evident obstruction.[227]

The role of specific medical therapy for granulomatous mediastinitis or mediastinal fibrosis is unclear.[299] Some evidence suggests that selected cases with active inflammation associated with histoplasmosis may benefit from antifungal therapy,[303, 304] but specific indications, if any, for antifungal therapy remain unknown. A similarly conservative approach should be taken to tuberculosis-related mediastinal complications unless sputum or tissue samples are positive for mycobacteria or convincing clinical evidence of active tuberculosis is present.

The clinical manifestations of this disease appear to be

the result of host factors as much as the infection itself. Accordingly, therapy directed at the host inflammatory response has also been attempted. Anecdotal reports of treatment of mediastinal and retroperitoneal fibrosis with corticosteroids have reached opposite conclusions.[305, 306] It appears that diffuse forms of fibrosis may be more likely to respond.[307] As in the case of antimicrobial therapy, the appropriate role for anti-inflammatory therapy for granulomatous mediastinitis and mediastinal fibrosis is presently unknown.

At the time of exploration for diagnosis, some surgeons advise removal of as much of the inflammatory or fibrous mass as possible to reduce its bulk and perhaps diminish its later impact on adjacent tissues.[273, 308] Despite the difficulties presented by fibrotic and granulomatous encasement, bronchoplastic procedures may be quite successful in these patients.[299] Surgery to bypass an obstructed vena cava is technically difficult and not always effective,[273] although this may still be considered if bleeding esophageal varices or recurrent upper-extremity phlebitis is present.[215] Endovascular stent placement is another option.[309] Obstruction of major pulmonary vessels is a poor prognostic sign. Therapeutic options are limited, but angiographic dilation and stent placement may be successful in selected cases (Fig. 78.12).

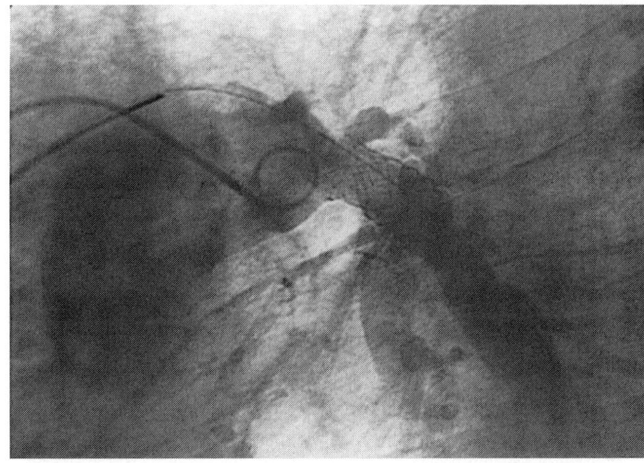

**Figure 78.12** Digital subtraction angiogram (from same patient as in Fig. 78.11) showing the left pulmonary artery immediately after insertion of an expandable wire mesh stent that eliminated the pressure gradient between the main pulmonary artery and left lobar pulmonary arteries. The stent and guidewire lie across the area of previous stenosis, and a pigtail catheter is in the prestenotic pulmonary artery.

## SUMMARY

Pneumomediastinum, the presence of air or other gas in the mediastinum, is not a common clinical disorder, even though it may occur in a wide variety of different circumstances. The gas that causes pneumomediastinum usually originates from the lungs but may arise from the upper respiratory tract or the gastrointestinal tract (especially the esophagus). Less often, pneumomediastinum follows penetrating injuries or complicates infection by gas-forming bacilli. Substernal chest pain signals the onset of mediastinal emphysema, and the diagnosis is usually established by detecting the presence of gas radiographically. Treatment depends primarily on successful management of the underlying disease process, although rarely direct intervention is indicated to decompress air in the mediastinum or pericardium.

Acute mediastinitis is usually a sudden and severe disease that is now most commonly caused by perforation of the esophagus during endoscopic procedures. "Spontaneous" rupture of the esophagus during attacks of vomiting remains an important cause of acute mediastinitis, and infectious complications after surgical procedures that incorporate sternotomy incisions are being encountered with increasing frequency. All forms of acute mediastinitis are life-threatening and require prompt diagnosis, surgical drainage, and antimicrobial treatment.

Chronic mediastinitis is less common than the acute variety and generally is related to granulomatous involvement of the mediastinum and its fibrotic sequelae. Complications include superior vena caval syndrome, esophageal disorders, bronchial obstruction, and pulmonary vessel obstruction. Management is aimed at relief of these mechanical complications. The role of anti-inflammatory and antimicrobial therapy is presently unclear.

## References


1. Maunder RJ, Pierson DJ, Hudson LD: Subcutaneous and mediastinal emphysema: Pathophysiology, diagnosis, and management. Arch Intern Med 144:1447–1453, 1984.
2. Marchand P: The anatomy and applied anatomy of the mediastinal fascia. Thorax 6:359–368, 1951.
3. Moncada R, Warpeha R, Pickleman J, et al: Mediastinitis from odontogenic and deep cervical infection: Anatomic pathways of propagation. Chest 73:497–500, 1978.
4. Meyers MA: Radiological features of the spread and localization of extraperitoneal gas and their relationship to its source. Diagn Radiol 111:17–26, 1974.
5. Gordon CA: Respiratory emphysema in labor: With two new cases and a review of 130 cases in the literature. Am J Obstet Gynecol 14:633–646, 1927.
6. Faust RC: Subcutaneous emphysema during labor. Northwest Med 39:24–26, 1940.
7. Hamman L: Spontaneous mediastinal emphysema. Bull Johns Hopkins Hosp 64:1–21, 1939.
8. Hamman L: Mediastinal emphysema. JAMA 128:1–6, 1945.
9. Macklin MT, Macklin CC: Malignant interstitial emphysema of the lungs and mediastinum as an important occult complication in many respiratory diseases and other conditions: An interpretation of the clinical literature in the light of laboratory experiment. Medicine 23:281–352, 1944.
10. Hillman KM: Pneumoperitoneum—A review. Crit Care Med 10:476–481, 1982.
11. Pearse HEJ: Mediastinitis following cervical suppuration. Ann Surg 108:588–604, 1938.
12. Thawley SE: Air in the neck. Laryngoscope 9:1445–1453, 1974.
13. Schweitzer V: Osteolytic sinusitis and pneumomediastinum: Deceptive otolaryngologic complications of cocaine abuse. Laryngoscope 96:206–210, 1986.
14. Estrera AS, Landay MJ, Grisham JM, et al: Descending necrotizing mediastinitis. Surg Gynecol Obstet 157:545–552, 1983.
15. Romph RF: Subcutaneous and mediastinal emphysema. Ann Emerg Med 1:35–37, 1972.
16. Hunt RB, Sahler OD: Mediastinal emphysema produced by air turbine dental drills. JAMA 205:101–102, 1968.
17. Meyerhoff WL, Nelson R, Fry WA: Mediastinal emphysema after oral surgery. Oral Surg 31:477–479, 1973.
18. Nahlieli O, Neder A: Iatrogenic pneumomediastinum after end-

odontic therapy. Oral Surg Oral Med Oral Pathol 71:618–619, 1991.
19. Shackelford D, Casani JA: Diffuse subcutaneous emphysema, pneumomediastinum, and pneumothorax after dental extraction. Ann Emerg Med 22:248–250, 1993.
20. Sandler CM, Libshitz HI, Marks G: Pneumoperitoneum, pneumomediastinum, and pneumopericardium following dental extraction. Radiology 115:539–540, 1975.
21. Turnbull A: A remarkable coincidence in dental surgery. BMJ 1:1131, 1900.
22. Flood TR: Mediastinal emphysema complicating a zygomatic fracture: A case report and review of the literature. Br J Oral Maxillofac Surg 26:141–148, 1988.
23. Henry CH, Hills EC: Traumatic emphysema of the head, neck, and mediastinum associated with maxillofacial trauma: Case report and review. J Oral Maxillofac Surg 47:876–882, 1989.
24. Gudlaugsson O, Geirsson AJ, Benediktsd'ottir K: Pneumoparotitis: A new diagnostic technique and a case report. Ann Otol Rhinol Laryngol 107:356–358, 1998.
25. Padovan IF, Dawson CA, Henschel EO, et al: Pathogenesis of mediastinal emphysema and pneumothorax following tracheotomy. Chest 66:553–556, 1974.
26. Stauffer JL, Silvestri RC: Complications of endotracheal intubation, tracheostomy, and artificial airways. Respir Care 27:417–434, 1982.
27. Rabuzzi DD, Reed GF: Intrathoracic complications following tracheotomy in children. Trans Am Laryngol Rhinol Otol Soc 74:71–79, 1971.
28. Stauffer JL, Olson DE, Petty TL: Complications and consequences of endotracheal intubation and tracheotomy: A prospective study of 150 critically ill patients. Am J Med 70:65–76, 1981.
29. Hirsch M, Abramowitz HB, Shapira S, et al: Hypopharyngeal injury as a result of attempted endotracheal intubation. Radiology 128:37–39, 1978.
30. Marty An'e CH, Picard E, Jonquet O, et al: Membranous tracheal rupture after endotracheal intubation. Ann Thorac Surg 60:1367–1371, 1995.
31. Frascone RJ, Cicero JJ, Sturm JT: Pneumopericardium occurring during a high-speed motorcycle ride. J Trauma 23:163–164, 1983.
32. Buntain WL, Lynn HB: Traumatic pneumatic disruption of the esophagus. J Thorac Cardiovasc Surg 63:553–560, 1972.
33. Curci MR, Dibbins AW, Grimes CK: Compressed air injury to the esophagus: Case report. J Trauma 29:1713–1715, 1989.
34. Wiot JF: Tracheobronchial trauma. Semin Roentgenol 18:15–22, 1983.
35. Chitre VV, Prinsley PR, Hashmi SM: Pneumopericardium: An unusual manifestation of blunt tracheal trauma. J Laryngol Otol 111:387–388, 1997.
36. Bertelson S, Howitz P: Injuries of the trachea and bronchi. Thorax 27:188–194, 1972.
37. Kirsch MM, Sloane H: Blunt Chest Trauma: General Principles of Management. Boston: Little, Brown, 1977.
38. Sridhar KS, Hussein AM, Patten JE: Spontaneous pneumomediastinum in esophageal carcinoma. Am J Clin Oncol 13:527–531, 1990.
39. Robertson HT, Lakshminarayan S, Hudson LD: Lung injury following a 50-metre fall into water. Thorax 33:175–180, 1978.
40. Alveolar rupture [editorial]. Lancet 2(8081):137–138, 1978.
41. Joannides M, Tsoulsos GD: The etiology of interstitial and mediastinal emphysema. Arch Surg 21:333–339, 1930.
42. Schaefer KE, McNulty WPJ, Carey C, et al: Mechanisms in development of interstitial emphysema and air embolism on decompression from depth. J Appl Physiol 13:15–29, 1958.
43. Pierson DJ: Alveolar rupture during mechanical ventilation: Role of PEEP, peak airway pressure, and distending volume. Respir Care 33:472–483, 1988.
44. Peirce ECI: Cerebral gas embolism (arterial) with special reference to iatrogenic accidents. Hyperbaric Oxygen Rev 1:161–184, 1980.
45. Strauss RH: Diving medicine. Am Rev Respir Dis 119:1001–1023, 1979.
46. Melamed Y, Shupak A, Bitterman H: Medical problems associated with underwater diving. N Engl J Med 326:30–35, 1992.
47. Grim PS, Gottlieb LJ, Boddie A, et al: Hyperbaric oxygen therapy. JAMA 263:2216–2220, 1990.
48. Kumar A, Pontoppidan H, Falk KI: Pulmonary barotrauma during mechanical ventilation. Crit Care Med 1:181–186, 1973.
49. Rohlfing BM, Webb WR, Schlobohm RM: Ventilator-related extra-alveolar air in adults. Radiology 121:25–31, 1976.
50. Gammon RB, Shin MS, Groves RH Jr, et al: Clinical risk factors for pulmonary barotrauma: A multivariate analysis. Am J Respir Crit Care Med 152:1235–1240, 1995.
51. Reid L: The Pathology of Emphysema (Vol 29). London: Lloyd-Luke, 1967.
52. Varkey B, Kory RC: Mediastinal and subcutaneous emphysema following pulmonary function tests. Am Rev Respir Dis 108:1393–1396, 1973.
53. Crosfield JL, Boger D, Clatworthy HW: Hemodynamic and manometric observations in experimental air-block syndrome. J Pediatr Surg 6:339–344, 1971.
54. Madansky DL, Lawson EE, Chernick V, et al: Pneumothorax and other forms of pulmonary air leak in newborns. Am Rev Respir Dis 120:729–737, 1979.
55. Taylor J, Dibbins A, Sobel DB: Neonatal pneumomediastinum: Indications for, and complications of, treatment. Crit Care Med 21:296–298, 1993.
56. Munsell WP: Pneumomediastinum. JAMA 202:689–693, 1967.
57. Hamman L: Spontaneous interstitial emphysema of the lungs. Trans Assoc Am Physicians 52:311–319, 1937.
58. Macklin CC: Transport of air along sheaths of blood vessels from alveoli to mediastinum: Clinical implications. Arch Intern Med 64:913–926, 1939.
59. Donahoe PK, Stewart DR, Osmond JDI, et al: Pneumoperitoneum secondary to pulmonary air leak. J Pediatr 81:797–800, 1972.
60. Gammon RB, Shin MS, Buchalter SE: Pulmonary barotrauma in mechanical ventilation. Patterns and risk factors. Chest 102:568–572, 1992.
61. Ingvar DH, Adolfson J, Lindemark C: Cerebral air embolism during training of submarine personnel in free escape: An encephalographic study. Aerosp Med 44:628–635, 1973.
62. Zwillich CW, Pierson DJ, Creagh CE, et al: Complications of assisted ventilation: A prospective study of 354 consecutive episodes. Am J Med 57:161–174, 1974.
63. Marini JJ, Culver BH: Systemic gas embolism complicating mechanical ventilation of adult respiratory distress syndrome. Ann Intern Med 110:699–707, 1989.
64. Spencer MP, Oyama Y: Pulmonary capacity for dissipation of venous gas emboli. Aerosp Med 42:822–827, 1971.
65. Baskin SE, Wozniak R: Hyperbaric oxygenation in the treatment of hemodialysis associated air embolism. N Engl J Med 293:184–185, 1975.
66. Newton NI, Adams AP: Excessive airway pressure during anesthesia: Hazards, effects, and prevention. Anaesthesia. 33:689–699, 1978.
67. Turner W, Fry WJ: Pneumoperitoneum complicating mechanical ventilation therapy. Arch Surg 112:723–726, 1977.
68. Powner DJ, Snyder JV, Morris CW, et al: Retroperitoneal air dissection associated with mechanical ventilation. Chest 69:739–742, 1976.
69. Gutkin Z, Iellin A, Meged S, et al: Spontaneous pneumoperitoneum without peritonitis. Int Surg 77:219–223, 1992.
70. Brown DR, Keenan WJ: Pneumoperitoneum without gastrointestinal perforation in a neonate. J Pediatr 85:377–379, 1974.
71. Rose DM, Jarczyk PA: Spontaneous pneumoperitoneum after scuba diving. JAMA 239:223, 1978.
72. Jaworski A, Fischer R, Lippmann M: Boerhaave's syndrome. Arch Intern Med 148:223–224, 1988.
73. Minocha A, Richards R: Pneumomediastinum as a complication of upper gastrointestinal endoscopy. J Emerg Med 9:325–329, 1991.
74. Chen KW, Wu MH, Huang JJ, et al: Bilateral spontaneous pneumothoraces, pneumopericardium, pneumomediastinum, and subcutaneous emphysema: A rare presentation of paraquat intoxication. Ann Emerg Med 23:1132–1134, 1994.
75. Mirzayan R, Cepkinian V, Asensio JA: Subcutaneous emphysema, pneumomediastinum, pneumothorax, pneumopericardium, and pneumoperitoneum from rectal barotrauma. J Trauma 41:1073–1075, 1996.

76. Bakker J, van Kersen F, Bellaar-Spruyt J: Pneumopericardium and pneumomediastinum after polypectomy. Endoscopy 23:46–47, 1991.
77. Lee HC, Dewan N, Crosby L: Subcutaneous emphysema, pneumomediastinum, and potentially life-threatening tension pneumothorax: Pulmonary complications from arthroscopic shoulder decompression. Chest 101:1265–1267, 1992.
78. Lau KY: Pneumomediastinum caused by subcutaneous emphysema in the shoulder. A rare complication of arthroscopy. Chest 103:1606–1607, 1993.
79. Liebig S, Siemoneit KD: Mediastinalemphysem und Begleitpneumothorax: Entstehung und Behandlung. Prax Pneumol 28:1133–1138, 1974.
80. Siemoneit KD: Retroperitoneal air dissection and mechanical ventilation. Chest 71:431–432, 1977.
81. Sauerbruch F: Die Bedeutung des Mediastinalemphysems in der Pathologie des Spannungspneumothorax. Beitr Klin Chir 60:450–478, 1908.
82. Banyai A: Direct and indirect pneumoperitoneum incidental to artificial pneumothorax. Am J Med Sci 186:513–518, 1933.
83. Simmonds F: Air embolism and pneumomediastinum in artificial pneumoperitoneum. Lancet 1:530–533, 1946.
84. Glauser FL, Bartlett RH: Pneumoperitoneum in association with pneumothorax. Chest 66:536–540, 1974.
85. Chui PT, Gin T, Chung SC: Subcutaneous emphysema, pneumomediastinum and pneumothorax complicating laparoscopic vagotomy. Report of two cases. Anaesthesia 48:978–981, 1993.
86. Cass LJ, Dow EC, Brooks JR: Pneumoperitoneum following pelvic examination. Am J Gastroenterol 45:209–211, 1966.
87. Walker MA: Pneumoperitoneum following a douche. J Kans Med Soc 43:55, 1942.
88. Lozman H, Newman AJ: Spontaneous pneumoperitoneum occurring during postpartum exercises in the knee-chest position. Am J Obstet Gynecol 72:903–905, 1956.
89. Ashai S, Lipton D, Colon A, et al: Pneumoperitoneum secondary to cunnilingus. N Engl J Med 295:117, 1976.
90. Varon J, Laufer MD, Sternback GL: Recurrent pneumoperitoneum following vaginal insufflation. Am J Emerg Med 9:447–448, 1991.
91. Aronson ME, Nelson PK: Fatal air embolism in pregnancy resulting from an unusual sex act. Obstet Gynecol 30:127–130, 1967.
92. Fyke FEI, Kazmier FJ, Harms RW: Venous air embolism: Life-threatening complication of orogenital sex during pregnancy. Am J Med 78:333–336, 1985.
93. Miller WE, Spiekerman RE, Hepper NG: Pneumomediastinum resulting from performing Valsalva maneuvers during marijuana smoking. Chest 62:233–234, 1972.
94. Shesser R, Davis C, Edelstein S: Pneumomediastinum and pneumothorax after inhaling alkaloidal cocaine. Ann Emerg Med 10:213–215, 1981.
95. Seaman ME: Barotrauma related to inhalational drug abuse. J Emerg Med 8:141–149, 1990.
96. Sullivan TP, Pierson DJ: Pneumomediastinum after freebase cocaine use. Am J Roentgenol 168:84, 1997.
97. Adrouny A, Magnusson P: Pneumopericardium from cocaine inhalation. N Engl J Med 313:48–49, 1985.
98. LiPuma JP, Wellman J, Stern H: Nitrous oxide abuse: A new cause for pneumomediastinum. Radiology 145:602, 1982.
99. Jabourian Z, McKenna EL, Feldman M: Spontaneous pneumomediastinum and subcutaneous emphysema. J Otolaryngol 17:50–53, 1988.
100. McMahon DJ: Spontaneous pneumomediastinum. Am J Surg 131:550–551, 1976.
101. Lorge HJ: The etiology of idiopathic pneumothorax. Am J Med Sci 199:635–641, 1940.
102. Mumford AD, Ashkan K, Elborn S: Clinically significant pulmonary barotrauma after inflation of party balloons. BMJ 313:1619, 1996.
103. Vosk A, Houston CS: Mediastinal emphysema in mountain climbers: Report of two cases and review. Heart Lung 6:799–805, 1977.
104. Zukerman H, Sadovsky E, Frankel M, et al: Subcutaneous and mediastinal emphysema during labor. Gynaecologia 153:12–18, 1962.
105. Brandfass RT, Martinez DM: Mediastinal and subcutaneous emphysema in labor. South Med J 69:1554–1555, 1976.
106. Karson EM, Saltzman D, Davis MR: Pneumomediastinum in pregnancy: Two case reports and a review of the literature, pathophysiology, and management. Obstet Gynecol 64:39S–43S, 1984.
107. Seidl JJ, Brotzman GL: Pneumomediastinum and subcutaneous emphysema following vaginal delivery. Case report and review of the literature. J Fam Pract 39:178–180, 1994.
108. Mitchell JE, Seim HC, Colon E, et al: Medical complications and medical management of bulimia. Ann Intern Med 107:71–77, 1987.
109. Schwartz M, Rossoff L: Pneumomediastinum and bilateral pneumothoraces in a patient with hyperemesis gravidarum. Chest 106:1904–1906, 1994.
110. Beigelman PM, Miller LV, Martin HE: Mediastinal and subcutaneous emphysema in diabetic coma with vomiting. JAMA 208:2315–2318, 1969.
111. Girard DE, Carlson V, Natelson EA, et al: Pneumomediastinum in diabetic ketoacidosis: Comments on mechanism, incidence, and management. Chest 60:455–459, 1971.
112. Watson JP, Barnett AH: Pneumomediastinum in diabetic ketoacidosis. Diabetic Med 6:173–174, 1989.
113. Kistner RW: Acute mediastinal emphysema complicating eclampsia. N Engl J Med 244:873–875, 1951.
114. Millard CE: Pneumomediastinum. Chest 56:297–300, 1969.
115. Morgan EJ, Henderson DA: Pneumomediastinum as a complication of athletic competition. Thorax 36:155–156, 1981.
116. Kobak AJ, Abrams RH: Pregnancy complicated by massive subcutaneous emphysema of mediastinal origin (Hamman's syndrome). Am J Obstet Gynecol 57:789–792, 1949.
117. Gay BB: Radiologic evaluation of the nontraumatized child with respiratory distress. Radiol Clin North Am 16:91–112, 1978.
118. Popovich J, Babcock R: Intraluminal blood cast causing obstructive emphysema and recurrent pneumothorax. Crit Care Med 10:482–483, 1982.
119. Janetos GP, Ochsner SF: Bilateral pneumothorax in metastatic osteogenic sarcoma. Am Rev Respir Dis 88:73–76, 1963.
120. McGovern JP, Singleton EB, Ozkaragoz K, et al: Pneumomediastinum and subcutaneous emphysema complicating bronchial asthma in children: A report of four cases. Ann Allergy 19:1139–1145, 1961.
121. Jorgensen JR, Falliers CJ, Bukantz SC. Pneumothorax and mediastinal and subcutaneous emphysema in children with bronchial asthma. Pediatrics 31:824–832, 1963.
122. Ozonoff MB: Pneumomediastinum associated with asthma and pneumonia in children. Am J Roentgenol 95:112–117, 1965.
123. Eggleston PA, Ward BH, Pierson WE, et al: Radiographic abnormalities in acute asthma in children. Pediatrics 54:442–449, 1974.
124. Pellinen TJ, Karjalainen JE: Spontaneous pneumomediastinum. Acta Med Scand 211:139–140, 1982.
125. Cooley JC, Gillespie JB: Mediastinal emphysema: Pathogenesis and management. Chest 49:104–108, 1966.
126. Kirsch MM, Orvald TO: Mediastinal and subcutaneous emphysema complicating acute bronchial asthma. Chest 57:580–581, 1970.
127. Steffey WR, Cohn AM: Spontaneous subcutaneous emphysema of the head, neck, and mediastinum. Arch Otolaryngol 100:32–35, 1974.
128. Karetsky MS: Asthma mortality: An analysis of one year's experience, review of the literature, and assessment of current modes of therapy. Medicine 54:471–484, 1975.
129. Dattwyler RJ, Goldman MA, Bloch KJ: Pneumomediastinum as a complication of asthma in teenage and young adult patients. J Allergy Clin Immunol 63:412–416, 1979.
130. Zegel HG, Miller WT: Subcutaneous emphysema in a young man. JAMA 241:1273–1274, 1979.
131. Wohl MEB, Chernick V: Bronchiolitis. Am Rev Respir Dis 118:759–781, 1978.
132. Gapany-Gapanavicius M, Yellin A, Almog S, et al: Pneumomediastinum: A complication of chlorine exposure from mixing household cleaning agents. JAMA 248:349–350, 1982.
133. Greenberg LF, Benham Kahn S: *Klebsiella* pneumonia with pneumothorax, pneumomediastinum, and pneumoperitoneum. Dis Chest 43:546–550, 1963.

134. Odita JC, Akamaguna AI: Mediastinal and subcutaneous emphysema associated with childhood measles. Eur J Pediatr 142:33–36, 1984.
135. Sharma S, Rajani M, Aggarwal S, et al: Spontaneous pneumothorax and pneumothorax in metastatic lung disease. Indian J Chest Dis Allied Sci 30:125–132, 1988.
136. Elliott DH, Harrison JAB, Barnard EEP: Clinical and radiological features of 88 cases of decompression barotrauma. *In* Shilling CW, Beckett MW (eds): Underwater Physiology VI. Bethesda: Federation of American Societies of Experimental Biology, 1978, pp 1011–1013.
137. Boettger ML: Scuba diving emergencies: Pulmonary overpressure accidents and decompression sickness. Ann Emerg Med 12:563–567, 1983.
138. Unsworth IP: Pulmonary barotrauma in a hyperbaric chamber. Anaesthesia 28:675–678, 1973.
139. Pierson DJ: Barotrauma and bronchopleural fistula. *In* Tobin MJ (ed): Principles and Practice of Mechanical Ventilation. New York: McGraw-Hill, 1994, pp 813–836.
140. Peterson GW, Baier H: Incidence of pulmonary barotrauma in a medical ICU. Crit Care Med 11:67–69, 1983.
141. Weg JG, Anzueto A, Balk RA, et al: The relation of pneumothorax and other air leaks to mortality in the acute respiratory distress syndrome. N Engl J Med 338:341–346, 1998.
142. Kacmarek RM: Methods of providing mechanical ventilatory support. *In* Pierson D, Kacmarek R (eds): Foundations of Respiratory Care. New York: Churchill Livingstone, 1992, pp 953–972.
143. Kacmarek RM: Management of the patient-ventilator system. *In* Pierson D, Kacmarek R (eds): Foundations of Respiratory Care. New York: Churchill Livingstone, 1992, pp 973–998.
144. Keszler M, Donn SM, Bucciarelli RL, et al: Multicenter controlled trial comparing high-frequency jet ventilation and conventional mechanical ventilation in newborn infants with pulmonary interstitial emphysema. J Pediatr 119:85–93, 1991.
145. Arnold JH, Hanson JH, Toro Figuero LO, et al: Prospective, randomized comparison of high-frequency oscillatory ventilation and conventional mechanical ventilation in pediatric respiratory failure. Crit Care Med 22:1530–1539, 1994.
146. Gerstmann DR, Minton SD, Stoddard RA, et al: The Provo multicenter early high-frequency oscillatory ventilation trial: Improved pulmonary and clinical outcome in respiratory distress syndrome. Pediatrics 98:1044–1057, 1996.
147. Hurst JM, Branson RD, Davis K Jr, et al: Comparison of conventional mechanical ventilation and high-frequency ventilation. A prospective, randomized trial in patients with respiratory failure. Ann Surg 211:486–491, 1990.
148. Amato MB, Barbas CS, Medeiros DM, et al: Effect of a protective-ventilation strategy on mortality in the acute respiratory distress syndrome. N Engl J Med 338:347–354, 1998.
149. Stewart TE, Meade MO, Cook DJ, et al: Evaluation of a ventilation strategy to prevent barotrauma in patients at high risk for acute respiratory distress syndrome. Pressure- and Volume-Limited Ventilation Strategy Group. N Engl J Med 338:355–361, 1998.
150. Jansson L, Johson B: A theoretical study on flow patterns of ventilators. Scand J Respir Dis 53:237–246, 1972.
151. Modell HI, Cheney FW: Effects of inspiratory flow pattern on gas exchange in normal and abnormal lungs. J Appl Physiol Respir Environ Exerc Physiol 46:1103–1107, 1979.
152. Pepe PE, Marini JJ: Ocult positive and end-expiratory pressure in mechanically ventilated patients with airflow obstruction. Am Rev Respir Dis 114:166–169, 1982.
153. Benson MS, Pierson DJ: Auto-PEEP during mechanical ventilation of adults. Respir Care 33:557–565, 1988.
154. Williams TJ, Tuxen DV, Scheinkestel CD, et al: Risk factors for morbidity in mechanically ventilated patients with acute severe asthma. Am Rev Respir Dis 146:607–615, 1992.
155. Shapiro BA, Peterson J, Cane RD: Complications of mechanical aids to intermittent lung inflation. Respir Care 27:467–470, 1982.
156. Branson RD, Hurst JM, DeHaven CBJ: Mask CPAP: State of the art. Respir Care 30:846–857, 1985.
157. McClure JN, Skardasos GM, Brown JM: Cardiac arrest in the operating area. Am Surg 38:241–242, 1972.
158. Atcheson SG, Peterson GV, Fred HL: Ill effects of cardiac resuscitation: Report of two unusual cases. Chest 67:615–616, 1975.
159. Vestal BK, Vestal RE: Iatrogenic pneumothorax: An unusual cause. JAMA 235:1879–1880, 1976.
160. Chiles DG, Mannheimer WN, Miller FE: Pneumothorax, pneumomediastinum, and massive subcutaneous emphysema after general anesthetic: Report of a case. J Oral Surg 28:845–847, 1970.
161. Agia G, Hurst E. Pneumomediastinum following the Heimlich maneuver. Ann Emerg Med 8:473–475, 1979.
162. Hurd TE, Novak R, Gallagher TJ: Tension pneumopericardium: A complication of mechanical ventilation. Crit Care Med 12:200–201, 1984.
163. Cummings RG, Wesly RLR, Adams DH, et al: Pneumopericardium resulting in cardiac tamponade. Ann Thorac Surg 37:511–517, 1984.
164. McEachern RC, Patel RG: Pneumopericardium associated with face-mask continuous positive airway pressure. Chest 112:1441–1443, 1997.
165. Crosfield JL, Clatworthy HW, Frye TR: Surgical therapy in neonatal air-block syndrome. J Thorac Cardiovasc Surg 60:392–401, 1970.
166. Weiss LD, Van Meter KW: Cerebral air embolism in asthmatic scuba divers in a swimming pool. Chest 107:1653–1654, 1995.
167. Bowen F, Chandra R, Avery G: Pulmonary interstitial emphysema with gas embolization in hyaline membrane disease. Am J Dis Child 126:117–118, 1973.
168. Banagle R: Massive intracranial air embolism: A complication of mechanical ventilation. Am J Dis Child 134:799–800, 1980.
169. Graham JM, Beall ACJ, Mattox KL, et al: Systemic air embolism following penetrating trauma to the lung. Chest 72:449–454, 1977.
170. Thomas AN, Stephens BG: Air embolism: A cause of morbidity and death after penetrating chest trauma. J Trauma 14:633–637, 1974.
171. Donato AT, Arciniegas E, Lam CR: Fatal air embolism during thoracotomy for gunshot injury to the lung. J Thorac Cardiovasc Surg 69:296–298, 1975.
172. Pao BS, Hayden SR: Cerebral gas embolism resulting from inhalation of pressurized helium. Ann Emerg Med 28:363–366, 1996.
173. O'Quin RJ, Lakshminarayan S: Venous air embolism. Arch Intern Med 142:2173–2176, 1982.
174. Zaugg M, Kaplan V, Widmer U, et al: Fatal air embolism in an airplane passenger with a giant intrapulmonary bronchogenic cyst. Am J Respir Crit Care Med 157:1686–1689, 1998.
175. Yellin A, Gapany-Gapanavicius M, Lieberman Y: Spontaneous pneumomediastinum: Is it a rare cause of chest pain? Thorax 38:383–385, 1983.
176. Versteegh FG, Broeders IA: Spontaneous pneumomediastinum in children. Eur J Pediatr 150:304–307, 1991.
177. Holmes KD, McGuirt WF: Spontaneous pneumomediastinum: Evaluation and treatment. J Fam Pract 31:422, 425–426, 1990.
178. Smith BA, Ferguson DB: Disposition of spontaneous pneumomediastinum. Am J Emerg Med 9:256–259, 1991.
179. Karns JR, Daue EOJ: Mediastinotomy in spontaneous mediastinal emphysema. JAMA 136:622–623, 1948.
180. Shuster MJ: Pneumomediastinum as a cause of dysphagia and pseudodysphagia. Ann Emerg Med 10:648–651, 1981.
181. Draper AJ: Spontaneous mediastinal emphysema and pneumothorax. Am J Med 5:59–68, 1948.
182. Aisner M, Franco JE: Mediastinal emphysema. N Engl J Med 241:818–825, 1949.
183. Littman D: Electrocardiographic phenomena associated with spontaneous pneumothorax and mediastinal emphysema. Am J Med Sci 212:682–690, 1946.
184. Levin B: The continuous diaphragm sign. Radiology 24:337–338, 1973.
185. Bejvan SM, Godwin JD: Pneumomediastinum: Old signs and new signs. Am J Roentgenol 166:1041–1048, 1996.
186. Whitley MA, Pierson DJ: Does this patient have a pneumomediastinum? Respir Care 31:1151–1153, 1986.
187. Lane EJ, Proto AV, Phillips TW: Mach bands and density perception. Radiology 121:9–17, 1976.
188. Friedman AC, Lautin EM, Rothenberg L: Mach bands and pneumomediastinum. J Can Assoc Radiol 32:232–235, 1981.
189. Campbell RE: Interstitial pulmonary emphysema: A complication of hyaline membrane disease. Am J Roentgenol 110:449–456, 1970.

190. Fletcher BD, Outerbridge EW, Dunbar JS: Pulmonary interstitial emphysema in the newborn. J Can Assoc Radiol 21:273–279, 1970.
191. Westcott JC, Cole SR: Interstitial pulmonary emphysema in children and adults: Roentgenographic features. Radiology 111:367–378, 1974.
192. Zimmerman JE, Dunbar BS, Klingenmaier CH: Management of subcutaneous emphysema, pneumomediastinum, and pneumothorax during respirator therapy. Crit Care Med 3:69–73, 1975.
193. Van Stiegmann G, Brantigan CO, Hopeman AR: Tension pneumomediastinum. Arch Surg 112:1212–1215, 1977.
194. Norman J, Rizzolo P: Subcutaneous, mediastinal, and probable subpericardial emphysema treated with recompression. N Engl J Med 261:269–272, 1959.
195. Beg MH, Reyazuddin N, Ansari MM: Traumatic tension pneumomediastinum mimicking cardiac tamponade. Thorax 43:576–577, 1988.
196. Hill GJ II: Outpatient Surgery (2nd ed). Philadelphia: WB Saunders, 1980, p 262.
197. Jewett TC, Adler RH, Taheri SA: Tension pneumomediastinum in the newborn. J Thorac Cardiovasc Surg 43:540–547, 1962.
198. Webb WR, Johnston JH, Geisler JW: Pneumomediastinum: Physiologic observations. J Thorac Cardiovasc Surg 35:309–315, 1958.
199. Rydell JR: Emergency cervical mediastinotomy for massive mediastinal emphysema. Arch Surg 70:647–653, 1955.
200. Herlan DB, Landreneau RJ, Ferson PF: Massive spontaneous subcutaneous emphysema: Acute management with infraclavicular "blow holes." Chest 102:503–505, 1992.
201. Pecora DV, Yegian D, Hochwald A: Tracheotomy in the treatment of severe mediastinal emphysema. JAMA 166:354–356, 1958.
202. Craig KC, Pierson DJ, Carrico CJ: The clinical use of positive end-expiratory pressure in the adult respiratory distress syndrome. Respir Care 30:184–201, 1985.
203. Kirsch MM, Orringer MB, Behrendt DM, et al: Management of tracheobronchial disruption secondary to nonpenetrating trauma. Ann Thorac Surg 22:93–101, 1976.
204. Rogers LF, Puig AW, Dooley BN, et al: Diagnostic considerations in mediastinal emphysema: A pathophysiologic-roentgenologic approach to Boerhaave's syndrome and spontaneous pneumomediastinum. Am J Roentgenol 115:495–511, 1972.
205. Oh KS, Fleischner FG, Wyman SM: Characteristic pulmonary finding in traumatic complete transection of a main-stem bronchus. Radiology 92:371–372, 1969.
206. Grover FL, Ellestad C, Arom KV, et al: Diagnosis and management of major tracheobronchial injuries. Ann Thorac Surg 28:384–391, 1979.
207. Emery RW, Landes RG, Lindsay WG, et al: Surgical treatment of pneumopericardium in the neonate. World J Surg 2:631–637, 1978.
208. Cohen DJ, Baumgart S, Stephenson LW: Pneumopericardium in neonates: Is it PEEP or is it PIP? Ann Thorac Surg 35:179–183, 1983.
209. Askin FB, McCann BG, Kuhn C: Reactive eosinophilic pleuritis: A lesion to be distinguished from pulmonary eosinophilic granuloma. Arch Pathol Lab Med 101:187–19l, 1977.
210. Halicek F, Rosai J: Histioeosinophilic granulomas in the thymuses of 29 myasthenic patients: A complication of pneumomediastinum. Hum Pathol 15:1137–1144, 1984.
211. Forrest JV, Shackelford GD, Bramson RT, et al. Acute mediastinal widening. Am J Roentgenol Radiol Ther Nucl Med 117:881–885, 1973.
212. Goodwin RAJ: Disorders of the mediastinum. *In* Fishman AP (ed): Pulmonary Diseases and Disorders. New York: McGraw-Hill, 1980, pp 1479–1486.
213. Henderson JAM, Peloquin AJM: Boerhaave revisited: Spontaneous esophageal perforation as a diagnostic masquerader. Am J Med 86:559–567, 1989.
214. Kent EM, Magovern GJ: The mediastinum. *In* Blades B (ed): Surgical Diseases of the Chest (3rd ed). St. Louis: CV Mosby, 1974, pp 202–204.
215. Rohwedder JJ: Neoplastic disease and mediastinal disorders. *In* Guenter CA, Welch MH (eds): Pulmonary Medicine (2nd ed). Philadelphia: JB Lippincott, 1982, pp 880–883.
216. Bjerke HS: Boerhaave's syndrome and barogenic injuries of the esophagus. Chest Surg Clin North Am. 4:819–825, 1994.
217. Brauer RB, Liebermann Meffert D, Stein HJ, et al: Boerhaave's syndrome: Analysis of the literature and report of 18 new cases. Dis Esophagus 10:64–68, 1997.
218. Marston EL, Valk HL: Spontaneous perforation of the esophagus: Review of the literature and report of a case. Ann Intern Med 51:590–607, 1959.
219. Bar-Maor J, Hayari L: Pneumatic perforation of the esophagus in children. J Pediatr Surg 27:1532–1533, 1992.
220. Edling JE, Bacon BR: Pleuropulmonary complications of endoscopic variceal sclerotherapy. Chest 99:1252–1257, 1991.
221. Berry BE, Ochsner JL: Perforation of the esophagus: A 30-year review. J Thorac Cardiovasc Surg 65:1–7, 1973.
222. Wesdorp ICE, Bartelsman JFWM, Huibregtse K, et al: Treatment of instrumental esophageal perforation. Gut: 25:398–404, 1984.
223. Schuman BM, Beckman JW, Tedesco FJ, et al: Complications of endoscopic injection sclerotherapy: A review. Am J Gastroenterol 82:823–830, 1987.
224. Perino LE, Gholson CF, Goff JS Esophageal perforation after fiberoptic variceal sclerotherapy. J Clin Gastroenterol 9:286–289, 1987.
225. Baydur A, Korula J: Cardiorespiratory effects of endoscopic esophageal variceal sclerotherapy. Am J Med 89:477–482, 1990.
226. Vassilev BN, Kazandziev PK, Losanoff JE, et al: Esophageal "stars": a sinister foreign body ingestion. South Med J 90:211–214, 1997.
227. Fraser R, Pare J, Pare P, et al: Diagnosis of Diseases of the Chest (3rd ed, Vol IV). Philadelphia: WB Saunders, 1991.
228. Gollub MJ, Bains MS. Barium sulfate: A new (old) contrast agent for diagnosis of postoperative esophageal leaks. Radiology 202:360–362, 1997.
229. Sarr MG, Watkins LJ, Stewart JR: Mediastinal tap as a useful method for the early diagnosis of mediastinal infection. Surg Gynecol Obstet 159:79–81, 1984.
230. Loop FD, Groves LK: Esophageal perforations. Ann Thorac Surg 10:571–587, 1971.
231. Krizek TJ, Lease JG: Surgical management of suppurative mediastinitis. *In* Sabiston DJ (ed): Textbook of Surgery (14th ed.) Philadelphia: WB Saunders, 1991, pp 1796–1800.
232. Gobien RP, Stanley JH, Gobien BS, et al: Percutaneous catheter aspiration and drainage of suspected mediastinal abscess. Radiology 151:69–71, 1984.
233. Craddock DR, Logan A, Mayell M: Traumatic rupture of the esophagus and stomach. Thorax 23:657–662, 1968.
234. Ohri SK, Liakakos TA, Pathi V, et al: Primary repair of iatrogenic thoracic esophageal perforation and Boerhaave's syndrome. Ann Thorac Surg. 55:603–606, 1993.
235. Sakamoto Y, Tanaka N, Furuya T, et al: Surgical management of late esophageal perforation. Thorac Cardiovasc Surg 45:269–272, 1997.
236. Keung YK, Gendreau J, Barber A, et al: Acute mediastinitis secondary to leakage of parenteral nutrition from a migrated central venous catheter in a patient undergoing autologous bone marrow transplant. Bone Marrow Transplant 17:871–872, 1996.
237. Kiernan PD, Hernandez A, Byrne WD, et al: Descending cervical mediastinitis. Ann Thorac Surg 65:1483–1488, 1998.
238. Garatea-Crelgo J, Gay-Escoda C: Mediastinitis from odontogenic infection: Report of three cases and review of the literature. Int J Oral Maxillofac Surg 20:65–68, 1991.
239. Cogan MIC: Necrotizing mediastinitis secondary to descending cervical cellulitis. Oral Surg 36:307–320, 1973.
240. Wheatley MJ, Stirling MC, Kirsh MM, et al: Descending necrotizing mediastinitis: Transcervical drainage is not enough. Ann Thorac Surg 49:780–784, 1990.
241. Brook I, Frazier EH: Microbiology of acute purulent pericarditis. A 12-year experience in a military hospital. Arch Intern Med 156:1857–1860, 1996.
242. Roberts JR, Smythe WR, Weber RW, et al: Thoracoscopic management of descending necrotizing mediastinitis. Chest 112:850–854, 1997.
242a. Marty-Anâe CH, Berthet JP, Alric P, et al: Management of descending necrotizing mediastinitis: An aggressive treatment for an aggressive disease. Ann Thorac Surg 68:212–217, 1999.
243. Dreyfuss D, Djedaini K, Bidault Lapomme C, et al: Nontrau-

matic acute anterior mediastinitis in two HIV-positive heroin addicts. Chest 101:583–585, 1992.
244. Mensah GA, Gold JP, Schreiber T, et al: Acute purulent mediastinitis and sternal osteomyelitis after closed-chest cardiopulmonary resuscitation: A case report and review of the literature. Ann Thorac Surg 46:353–355, 1988.
245. Poppel MH: Some migratory aspects of inflammatory collections of pancreatic origin. Radiology 72:323–329, 1959.
246. LaForce FM. Anthrax. Clin Infect Dis. 19:1009–1013, 1994.
247. Plotkin SA, Brachman PS, Utel M, et al: An epidemic of inhalation anthrax, the first in the 20th century. Am J Med. 29:992–1001, 1960.
248. Lalitha MK, Thomas MK: Penicillin resistance in *Bacillus anthracis*. Lancet 349:1522, 1997.
249. LaForce FM: *Bacillus anthracis* (anthrax). *In* Mandell GL, Douglas RGJ, Bennett JE (eds): Principles and Practice of Infectious Diseases (3rd ed). New York: John Wiley, 1990, pp 1593–1595.
250. Brachman PS: Inhalation anthrax. Ann NY Acad Sci 353:83–93, 1980.
251. Pile JC, Malone JD, Eitzen EM, et al: Anthrax as a potential biological warfare agent. Arch Intern Med 158:429–434, 1998.
252. Sarr MG, Gott VL, Townsend TR: Mediastinal infection after cardiac surgery. Ann Thorac Surg 38:415–423, 1984.
253. Bor DH, Rose RM, Modlin JF, et al: Mediastinitis after cardiovascular surgery. Rev Infect Dis 5:885–897, 1983.
254. Newman LS, Szczukowski LC, Bain RP, et al: Suppurative mediastinitis after open heart surgery. Chest 94:546–553, 1988.
255. Karwande S, Renlund D, Olsen S, et al: Mediastinitis in heart transplantation. Ann Thorac Surg 54:1039–1045, 1992.
256. Baldwin R, Radovancevic B, Sweeney M, et al: Bacterial mediastinitis after heart transplantation. J Heart Lung Transplant 11:545–549, 1992.
257. Bassiri AG, Girgis RE, Theodore J: *Actinomyces odontolyticus* thoracopulmonary infections. Two cases in lung and heart-lung transplant recipients and a review of the literature. Chest 109:1109–1111, 1996.
258. Rutledge R, Applebaum RE, Kim BJ: Mediastinal infection after open heart surgery. Surgery 97:88–92, 1985.
259. Culliford AT, Cunningham JJ, Zeff RH, et al: Sternal and costochondral infections following open-heart surgery: A review of 2594 cases. J Thorac Cardiovasc Surg 72:714–725, 1976.
260. Milano CA, Kesler K, Archibald N, et al: Mediastinitis after coronary artery bypass graft surgery. Risk factors and long-term survival. Circulation 92:2245–2251, 1995.
261. Bitkover CY, Gardlund B: Mediastinitis after cardiovascular operations: A case–control study of risk factors. Ann Thorac Surg 65:36–40, 1998.
261a. Baskett RJ, MacDougall CE, Ross DB: Is mediastinitis a preventable complication: A 10-year review. Ann Thorac Surg 67:462–465, 1999.
262. Barois A, Grosbuis S, Simon N, et al: Treatment of mediastinitis in children after cardiac surgery: A study of 20 cases. Intensive Care Med 4:35–39, 1978.
263. Glower DD, Douglas JMJ, Gaynor JW, et al: Candida mediastinitis after a cardiac operation. Ann Thorac Surg 49:157–163, 1990.
264. Misawa Y, Fuse K, Hasegawa T: Infectious mediastinitis after cardiac operations: Computed tomographic findings. Ann Thorac Surg 65:622–624, 1998.
265. Jolles H, Henry DA, Roberson JP, et al: Mediastinitis following median sternotomy: CT findings. Radiology 201:463–466, 1996.
266. Craver JM, Rand RP, Bostwick JI, et al: Management of postcardiotomy mediastinitis. *In* Waldhausen J, Orringer M (eds): Complications in Thoracic Surgery. St Louis: Mosby–Year Book, 1991, pp 125–131.
267. El Oakley RM, Wright JE: Postoperative mediastinitis: Classification and management. Ann Thorac Surg 61:1030–1036, 1996.
268. El Gamel A, Yonan NA, Hassan R, et al: Treatment of mediastinitis: Early modified Robicsek closure and pectoralis major advancement flaps. Ann Thorac Surg 65:41–46, 1998.
269. Calvat S, Trouillet JL, Nataf P, et al: Closed drainage using Redon catheters for local treatment of poststernotomy mediastinitis. Ann Thorac Surg 61:195–201, 1996.
270. Lazar HL, Fitzgerald C, Gross S, et al: Determinants of length of stay after coronary artery bypass graft surgery. Circulation 92:II-20–II-24, 1995.
271. Englemam RM, Williams CD, Gouge TH, et al: Mediastinitis following open-heart surgery: Review of two years experience. Arch Surg 107:772–778, 1973.
272. Grigas D, Bor DH, Kosinski E, et al: Cardiopulmonary function following postcardiac surgical mediastinitis. Chest 85:729–732, 1984.
273. Strimlan CV, Dines DE, Payne WS: Mediastinal granuloma. Mayo Clin Proc 50:702–705, 1975.
274. Feigin DS, Eggleston JC, Siegelman SS: The multiple roentgen manifestations of sclerosing mediastinitis. Johns Hopkins Med J 144:1–8, 1979.
275. Light AM: Idiopathic fibrosis of the mediastinum: A discussion of three cases and review of the literature. J Clin Pathol 31:78–88, 1978.
276. Goodwin RA, Nickell JA, DesPrez RM: Mediastinal fibrosis complicating healed primary histoplasmosis and tuberculosis. Medicine 51:227–246, 1972.
277. Bloomberg TJ, Dow CJ: Contemporary mediastinal tuberculosis. Thorax 35:392–396, 1980.
278. Rabinowitz JG, Prater W, Silver J, et al: Mediastinal histoplasmosis. Mt Sinai J Med 47:356–363, 1980.
279. Lokich JJ, Goodman R: Superior vena cava syndrome: Clinical management. JAMA 231:58–61, 1975.
280. Schechter MM: The superior vena cava syndrome. Am J Med Sci 227:46–56, 1954.
281. Mahajan V, Strimlan V, van Ordstrand HS, et al: Benign superior vena cava syndrome. Chest 68:32–35, 1975.
282. Schowengerdt CG, Suyemoto R, Main FB: Granulomatous and fibrous mediastinitis: A review and analysis of 180 cases. J Thorac Cardiovasc Surg 57:365–379, 1969.
283. Loyd JE, Tillman BF, Atkinson JB, et al: Mediastinal fibrosis complicating histoplasmosis. Medicine 67:295–310, 1988.
283a. Flieder DB, Suster S, Moran CA: Idiopathic fibroinflammatory (fibrosing/sclerosing) lesions of the mediastinum: A study of 30 cases with emphasis on morphologic heterogeneity. Mod Pathol 12:257–264, 1999.
284. Cameron DD, Ing ST, Boyle M, et al: Idiopathic mediastinal and retroperitoneal fibrosis. Can Med Assoc J 85:227–232, 1961.
285. Cunningham T, Farrell J, Veale D, et al Anterior mediastinal fibrosis with superior vena caval obstruction complicating the synovitis-acne-pustulosis-hyperostosis-osteomyelitis syndrome. Br J Rheumatol 32:408–410, 1993.
286. Kalweit G, Huwer H, Straub U, et al: Mediastinal compression syndromes due to idiopathic fibrosing mediastinitis–report of three cases and review of the literature. Thorac Cardiovasc Surg 44:105–109, 1996.
287. Comings DE, Skubi K-B, Eyes JV, et al: Familial multifocal fibrosclerosis. Ann Intern Med 66:884–892, 1967.
288. McIntire FT, Sykes EMJ: Obstruction of the superior vena cava: A review of the literature and report of two personal cases. Ann Intern Med 30:925–960, 1949.
289. Ochsner A, Dixon JL: Superior vena cava thrombosis: Review of the literature and report of cases of traumatic and infectious origin. J Thorac Surg 5:641–672, 1936.
290. Gilbert HM, Hartman BJ: Short report: a case of fibrosing mediastinitis caused by *Wuchereria bancrofti*. Am J Trop Med Hyg 54:596–599, 1996.
291. Graham JR, Suby HI, LeCompte PR, et al: Fibrotic disorders associated with methysergide therapy for headache. N Engl J Med 274:359–368, 1966.
292. Gordonson J, Trachtenberg S, Sargent EN Superior vena cava obstruction due to sarcoidosis. Chest 63:292–293, 1973.
293. Ray RL, Truscott DE: Silicosis as a cause of superior vena cava obstruction. Br J Dis Chest 57:210–212, 1963.
294. Flannery MT, Espino M, Altus P, et al: Hodgkin's disease masquerading as sclerosing mediastinitis. South Med J 87:921–923, 1994.
295. Smith AR, Richards V: Superior vena cava obstruction. Am J Surg 96:353–359, 1958.
296. Gross NJ: Pulmonary effects of radiation therapy. Ann Intern Med. 86:81–92, 1977.
297. Yellin A, Rosen A, Reichert N, et al: Superior vena cava syndrome: The myth—The facts. Am Rev Respir Dis 141:1114–1118, 1990.
298. Wychulis AR, Payne WS, Clagett OT, et al: Surgical treatment

of mediastinal tumors: A 40-year experience. J Thorac Cardiovasc Surg 62:379–391, 1971.

298a. Basaranoglu M, Ozdemir S, Celik AF, et al: A case of fibrosing mediastinitis with obstruction of superior vena cava and downhill esophageal varices: A rare cause of upper gastrointestinal hemorrhage. J Clin Gastroenterol 28:268–270, 1999.

299. Mathisen DJ, Grillo HC: Clinical manifestation of mediastinal fibrosis and histoplasmosis. Ann Thorac Surg: 54:1053–1057, 1992.

300. Kefri M, Dyke S, Copeland S, et al: Hemoptysis and hematemesis due to a broncholith: Granulomatous mediastinitis. South Med J 89:243–245, 1996.

301. Espinosa RE, Edwards WD, Rosenow EC, et al: Idiopathic pulmonary hilar fibrosis: An unusual cause of pulmonary hypertension. Mayo Clin Proc 68:778–782, 1993.

302. Berry DF, Buccigrossi D, Peabody J, et al: Pulmonary vascular occlusion and fibrosing mediastinitis. Chest 89:296–301, 1986.

302a. Mineo TC, Ambrogi V, Nofroni I, et al: Mediastinoscopy in superior vena cava obstruction: Analysis of 80 consecutive patients. Ann Thorac Surg 68:223–226, 1999.

302b. Imran MB, Kubota K, Yoshioka S, et al: Sclerosing mediastinitis: Findings on fluorine-18 fluorodeoxyglucose positron emission tomography. Clin Nucl Med 24:305–308, 1999.

303. Urschel HC Jr, Razzuk MA, Netto GJ, et al: Sclerosing mediastinitis: Improved management with histoplasmosis titer and ketoconazole. Ann Thorac Surg 50:215–21, 1990.

304. Maholtz MS, Dauber JH, Yousem SA: Case report: Fluconazole therapy in histoplasma mediastinal granuloma. Am J Med Sci 307:274–277, 1994.

305. Field C, Arnold W, Gloster ES, et al: Steroid therapy as treatment for idiopathic fibrosis of the retroperitoneum and mediastinum. Pediatrics 78:936–938, 1986.

306. Gran JT: Chronic idiopathic mediastinal fibrosis presenting with malaise, pleuritis and thoracic back pain. Br J Rheumatol 32:757–759, 1993.

307. Sherrick AD, Brown LR, Harms GF, et al: The radiographic findings of fibrosing mediastinitis. Chest 106:484–489, 1994.

308. Dunn EJ, Ulicny KS Jr, Wright CB, et al: Surgical implications of sclerosing mediastinitis. A report of six cases and review of the literature. Chest 97:338–346, 1990.

309. Dodds GA, Harrison JK, O'Laughlin MP, et al: Relief of superior vena cava syndrome due to fibrosing mediastinitis using the Palmaz stent. Chest 106:315–318, 1994

# 79 Tumors and Cysts of the Mediastinum

DAVID R. PARK, M.D. • DAVID J. PIERSON, M.D.

Introduction
General Considerations
Classification and Incidence of Mediastinal Masses
Clinical Presentation
Diagnostic Considerations
Lesions Occurring Typically in the Anterior Mediastinum
Thymic Neoplasms
Germ Cell Tumors
Lymphoma
Thyroid
Parathyroid
Mesenchymal Tumors
Lesions Occurring Typically in the Middle Mediastinum
Lymphadenopathy
Developmental Cysts
Vascular Masses and Enlargements
Diaphragmatic Hernia
Lesions Occurring Typically in the Posterior Mediastinum: Neurogenic Tumors
Miscellaneous Mediastinal Masses
Primary Carcinoma and Sarcoma
Other Tumors
Summary

## INTRODUCTION

This chapter discusses lesions that present as a mass in the mediastinum, whether discovered incidentally or identified during evaluation of thoracic or systemic symptoms. Although they meet this definition, mediastinal metastases or tumors invading the mediastinum from other intrathoracic sites are customarily omitted from consideration. Likewise, primary lesions of the trachea, heart, or esophagus, even though they lie within the mediastinum, are not included here. Several of the masses covered in this chapter, such as thyroid and fat, are not tumors or even disease processes per se but are instead aberrantly located or overabundant normal tissues. Justification for their inclusion comes from their similar presentation to that of mediastinal tumors and from the fact that in most instances they require the same evaluation as any other mediastinal mass. The clinical problem is a "mediastinal mass," and this chapter focuses on the main disease processes that cause this presentation. Diseases that are unique to the mediastinum, such as thymic neoplasms and developmental cysts, are discussed in some detail. Other conditions that commonly arise elsewhere in the body, such as lymphoma, are considered mainly in terms of the features of their presentation in the mediastinum.

Mediastinal tumors and cysts have been the subject of numerous reviews, including notable contributions from before 1960[1–3] and during the 1960s,[4, 5] the 1970s,[6–8] the 1980s,[9–11] and 1990s.[12–15] For more extensive discussions of the subject, the reader is referred especially to the works of Silverman and Sabiston,[9] LeRoux and associates,[10] Beszniak and coworkers,[11] Shields,[12] and Strollo and colleagues.[14–15a] Mediastinal tumors in children have also been the subject of several reviews.[16–20]

## GENERAL CONSIDERATIONS

### Classification and Incidence of Mediastinal Masses

The most practical classification of mediastinal masses from a clinical standpoint is by location, grouping together lesions that are characteristically found in the anterior, middle, and posterior mediastinal compartments. This simple scheme is outlined in Table 77.2 and is followed in this chapter, recognizing that such a classification ignores embryologic or histologic similarities between some lesions,[11, 21] and the fact that mediastinal masses often present in mediastinal compartments other than their most typical location.

Primary mediastinal masses are not uncommon, although their real incidence is difficult to ascertain reliably. An overall incidence of 1 case per 100,000 population per year may be a reasonable estimation.[4] The tumors and cysts that account for this incidence individually occur much less frequently. Table 79.1 lists the estimated relative frequencies of the most common mediastinal tumors and cysts, based on the collection by Silverman and

Table 79.1 RELATIVE FREQUENCIES OF MEDIASTINAL MASSES IN ADULTS AND CHILDREN

| LESION | ADULTS (%) | CHILDREN (%) |
|---|---|---|
| Thymoma | 19 | — |
| Developmental cysts | 21 | 18 |
| Bronchogenic | 7 | 8 |
| Pericardial | 7 | <1 |
| Enteric | 3 | 8 |
| Other cysts | 4 | 2 |
| Neurogenic tumors | 21 | 40 |
| Lymphoma | 13 | 18 |
| Germ cell tumors | 11 | 11 |
| Endocrine (thyroid, parathyroid, carcinoid) | 6 | — |
| Mesenchymal tumors | 7 | 9 |
| Primary carcinoma | — | — |
| Other malignancies | 3 | 4 |

Data from N.A. Silverman and D.C. Sabiston and are based on their review of reported mediastinal masses in 1950 adults and 437 children. Curr Probl Cancer 2:1–55, 1977.

Sabiston[9] of nearly 2400 cases from the literature. More recent series suggest a similar pattern,[22–24] although Cohen and associates[24] have observed a rising incidence of mediastinal masses in general and an increasing proportion of lymphoma and malignant neurogenic tumors over the course of their 45 year survey. The precise frequencies of individual disorders vary among series probably because of differences in referral sources and patient populations, but neurogenic tumors, thymomas, and developmental cysts account for around 60% of all mediastinal masses. Lymphomas and germ cell tumors such as teratoma and seminoma account for about one fourth, and a large number of other lesions, both benign and malignant, constitute the remaining 15%.

There are some differences in the incidences of mediastinal masses in adults and children: Thymoma and thyroid masses rarely occur in infants and children, whereas neurogenic tumors are less common in adults. The likelihood of malignancy is higher in infants and children than in adults: In the latter group, about one fourth of all mediastinal mass lesions are malignant, whereas the percentage in children is 40% to 45%.[9] In addition, the presence of human immunodeficiency virus (HIV) infection substantially alters the spectrum of mediastinal disease; granulomatous inflammation due to mycobacterial and other infections, lymphoma, and other opportunistic processes are common, and multiple diseases may be present simultaneously,[25, 26] including bronchogenic carcinoma.[27] Finally, surgical case series are likely to underrepresent causes of mediastinal masses that do not routinely lead to surgical intervention, such as goiter and vascular abnormalities.

## Clinical Presentation

At least half of all mediastinal masses are asymptomatic and detected by chest roentgenography performed for unrelated reasons. Of lesions that are asymptomatic, about 80% are benign, whereas more than half are malignant if they have produced symptoms.[6, 7, 9, 10, 22, 24, 28]

Symptoms in patients with mediastinal mass lesions are usually due to compression by mass effect or to invasion of adjacent intrathoracic structures. Most frequent are complaints of cough, dyspnea, dysphagia, chest pain, and symptoms related to superior vena caval obstruction.[9, 10] Other symptoms arising in the chest are hoarseness, stridor, and those of Horner's syndrome, phrenic nerve involvement and spinal cord compression. Rarely, anterior mediastinal tumors can cause pericarditis or pericardial tamponade,[29] and masses in the middle mediastinum can produce right ventricular outflow obstruction and cor pulmonale.[29, 30]

Mediastinal tumors as a group are frequently associated with systemic syndromes (Table 79.2).[9, 10] Some typically have endocrine function: thyrotoxicosis in those with intrathoracic goiter; Cushing's syndrome associated with thymomas and carcinoid tumors; gynecomastia in patients with human chorionic gonadotropin–secreting germ cell tumors; hypertension, typical in patients with pheochromocytoma but also reported in patients with ganglioneuroma; hypercalcemia, observed in patients with parathyroid adenoma and lymphoma; and diarrhea, often present in children with neuroblastoma and ganglioneuroma. Hypoglycemia in patients with certain mesotheliomas, teratomas, fibrosarcomas, and neurosarcomas is also believed to be the result of tumor products with endocrine activity.

Thymomas are associated with numerous systemic syndromes, most of which appear to be autoimmune in origin.[9, 10, 31] The most familiar of these is myasthenia gravis; others include pure red blood cell aplasia, myocarditis, and hypogammaglobulinemia. Patients with thymoma also have an increased incidence of collagen vascular disease, Whipple's disease, and malignancy elsewhere in the body.

Other mediastinal tumors associated with systemic syndromes or diseases include carcinoid and parathyroid adenoma (multiple endocrine neoplasia), neurofibromas (neurofibromatosis), and lymphomas (fever of unknown origin and alcohol-induced pain). Osteoarthropathy is a known feature of mesothelioma, neurofibroma, and neurilemoma. Finally, neuroblastoma is often associated with opsomyoclonus, thought to be caused by an autoantibody against cerebellar tissues.[32]

## Diagnostic Considerations

The initial diagnostic evaluation of a patient with a mediastinal mass should include these associated clinical syndromes and the anatomic location of the mass (Table 77.2) as clues to the diagnosis. In most cases, however, symptoms are absent or nonspecific as are the effects of the mass on adjacent normal structures. Furthermore, although each of these lesions occurs characteristically in one or another mediastinal compartment, the location is not invariable, and essentially any of them may be encountered in any region of the mediastinum. The basic focus of the diagnostic evaluation of a mediastinal mass is an orderly preparation for obtaining a tissue diagnosis.

Conventional chest roentgenograms are the first diagnostic test for all cases, and certain mediastinal mass lesions have characteristic appearances.[10] For example, teratomas are usually anterior and may contain areas of calcium (sometimes teeth or bone), fat, and soft tissue. Neural tumors are usually far posterior, with sharply delineated margins. Pericardial cysts usually lie against the pericardium, on the diaphragm, or against the anterior chest wall. Foregut duplications of the type commonly called *bronchogenic cysts* tend to lie against the trachea, carina, or main bronchus. Other such associations exist (see Table 77.3).

Computed tomographic (CT) scans can provide clues to the thyroid origin of a mass and can be helpful in identifying lipomatous, vascular, and cystic causes. A recent report described 100% specificity for the CT appearance of teratomas, thymolipomas, and omental fat herniation, but the overall accuracy for predicting the cause of all mediastinal masses was only 48%.[33] With the possible exception of teeth in a teratoma, few clinical or radiographic features are pathognomonic.

Routine laboratory testing can indirectly suggest the endocrine function of a mass, and specific tests for certain tumor products may be helpful. For instance, elevated thyroid hormone levels suggest goiter. Identification of functioning mediastinal thyroid tissue on radionuclide scanning is one of the few circumstances that may preclude tissue examination. Elevated human chorionic gonadotropin or alpha-fetoprotein levels can suggest the presence of a malignant germ cell tumor, and antiacetylcholine receptor antibodies can identify even asymptomatic patients with myasthenia gravis due to thymoma. These distinctions may be important because, as in the case of lymphoma, a biopsy result confirming a malignant germ cell tumor may prompt combined radiation and chemotherapy rather than radical surgical resection. Awareness of the possibility of thymoma and myasthenia gravis can help the surgeon and anesthesiologist to avoid or recognize perioperative complications of neuromuscular weakness.

In general, even lesions discovered to be benign must be removed.[9–11] Benign tumors may continue to enlarge, thus compromising vital structures; they may rupture into adjacent tissues or cavities, hemorrhage, or become infected. Bizarre complications of benign lesions, such as one case of fatal air embolism resulting from the rupture of an air-containing bronchogenic cyst during ascent in

**Table 79.2 SYSTEMIC SYNDROMES ASSOCIATED WITH MEDIASTINAL MASSES**

| Syndrome | Associated Conditions |
|---|---|
| Endocrine effects | |
| Hypothyroidism or hyperthyroidism | Mediastinal goiter |
| Hypercalcemia | Parathyroid adenoma, lymphoma |
| Hypertension | Pheochromocytoma, ganglioneuroma, chemodectoma |
| Cushing's syndrome | Carcinoid, thymoma |
| Hypoglycemia | Mesenchymal tumor |
| Gynecomastia | Germ cell tumor |
| Diarrhea | Ganglioneuroma, neuroblastoma |
| Autoimmune effects | |
| Opsomyoclonus | Neuroblastoma |
| Myasthenia gravis | Thymoma |
| Red cell aplasia | Thymoma |
| Myocarditis | Thymoma |
| Hypogammaglobulinemia | Thymoma |
| Congenital syndromes | |
| Neurofibromatosis | Neurofibroma |
| Multiple endocrine neoplasia | Parathyroid adenoma, pheochromocytoma |
| Unknown causes | |
| Alcohol-induced pain | Hodgkin's disease |
| Fever and night sweats | Lymphoma |

Nonseminomatous mediastinal germ cell tumors have been classified variously[10] but may be grouped into *embryonal cell carcinoma* and *choriocarcinoma*.[9, 79] These highly malignant aggressive tumors often secrete human chorionic gonadotropin, alpha-fetoprotein, or carcinoembryonic antigen, which can also produce clinical manifestations, such as gynecomastia, in 50% of patients.[10] Associations have been noted with Klinefelter's syndrome[92, 93] and with hematologic malignancy.[94, 95] Like seminoma, these tumors occur mainly in men in the third and fourth decades and are usually symptomatic. Although most patients present with disseminated disease and the prognosis has been less favorable than for seminoma,[10] cisplatin-based treatment regimens have markedly improved the outcome, with over 50% of patients achieving long-term survival.[84, 95]

A nonseminomatous malignancy usually grouped with embryonal cell carcinoma or endodermal sinus or yolk sac tumor has recently been treated with high-dose combination chemotherapy with encouraging results.[96, 97] Even disseminated and refractory malignant germ cell tumors may respond to aggressive chemotherapy[98] and salvage regimens involving bone marrow transplantation.[99, 100]

## Lymphoma

Lymphoma is a common cause of a mediastinal mass in both adults and children and represents between 10% and 20% of cases in most series.[9–11, 22, 24] *Hodgkin's disease* has a bimodal age distribution, occurring in adolescents and young adults and in those older than 50 years, whereas *non-Hodgkin's lymphomas* occur most commonly in older adults. Although 50% to 60% of patients with Hodgkin's disease have mediastinal lymph node involvement at the time of diagnosis[101] and non-Hodgkin's lymphomas involve the mediastinum in only 20% of cases,[102] Hodgkin's disease accounts for only one third of all cases of mediastinal lymphoma, the majority being non-Hodgkin's lymphomas.[9] Approximately 5% of patients with either type of lymphoma have disease confined to the mediastinum.[101, 103] Lymphoma is especially common as a thoracic complication in HIV-infected patients.[104–106] HIV-associated lymphomas are usually immunoblastic,[104] although Hodgkin's disease also is more common in patients with HIV infection than in the general population.[105, 107]

Incidental discovery of a mass on a chest roentgenogram is a common presentation of lymphoma, although many patients have systemic symptoms or more localized complaints such as cough and chest pain. Tracheal compromise and superior vena caval obstruction are common, as are pericardial and pleural involvement,[103, 108] and Hodgkin's disease often involves the hilar nodes and lung parenchyma as well.[108] Resection is usually not a necessary part of therapy, but anterior thoracotomy or mediastinoscopy is usually required to confirm the diagnosis if adenopathy is not accessible outside the mediastinum. The prognosis of Hodgkin's and other lymphomas has improved strikingly in the last two decades as more effective and less toxic combinations of radiotherapy and chemotherapy have evolved,[109, 110] and effective salvage regimens including bone marrow transplantation have been developed to treat relapsed disease.[110, 111] More detailed discussions of Hodgkin's disease and non-Hodgkin's lymphomas in pediatric and adult populations are available in several excellent reviews.[112–117]

## Thyroid

Ectopic thyroid glands account for fewer than 10% of mediastinal masses in surgical series but are probably more common in clinical practice. Thyroid tissue within the mediastinum is of two distinct origins. Most commonly, a *cervical goiter* extends substernally into the anterior mediastinum. Primary *intrathoracic goiter*, presumably originating from a rest of heterotopic thyroid tissue, is rarer. Most such goiters are in the anterior mediastinum, but they may occur in the middle or posterior mediastinum as well.[9, 10] Intrathoracic goiter occurs predominantly in women of middle age or older; it is usually asymptomatic, although hoarseness, cough, or swelling of the face and arms may occur. Intrathoracic thyroid tissue is easily recognized by radioactive iodine scanning[118] and may be suspected on the basis of high radiodensity on CT scans, particularly after iodinated contrast injection.[119, 120] Mediastinal goiter need not be resected unless there are symptoms of airway, vessel, nerve, or esophageal compression.

## Parathyroid

Mediastinal parathyroid tissue is said to account for as many as 10% of cases of hyperparathyroidism,[121] and the mediastinum is the most common site for ectopic *parathyroid adenomas* in surgically resistant hyperparathyroidism.[122, 123] Half of ectopic parathyroid adenomas lie in the anterior mediastinum, usually near the thymus.[124] Parathyroid cysts may enlarge sufficiently to appear as a mass on the chest roentgenogram and to produce symptoms[125–128]; in one review, 39 (42%) of 93 patients with parathyroid cysts had functioning hyperthyroidism.[128a] Otherwise, location of aberrant functioning parathyroid tissue can be a difficult clinical problem that may be aided preoperatively by CT, ultrasonography, or MRI.[124, 129–131] Selective angiography and venous sampling for parathormone levels have largely been supplanted by radionuclide scans unless therapeutic embolization is anticipated.[130]

$^{99m}$Technetium sestamibi scanning is highly accurate in the detection of aberrant parathyroid tissue,[131, 132] and its routine use has been proposed as cost effective because it may lessen the chance of protracted or failed cervical explorations in cases of primary hyperparathyroidism.[133] Another study, however, found no differences in meaningful perioperative variables or outcomes of patients who did and did not undergo preoperative localization studies.[134] Localization studies may be better justified for patients who have failed a prior attempt at resection in whom an aberrantly located adenoma would be more likely.[131, 135, 136] Parathyroid adenomas are cured by complete removal, and thoracoscopic resection is increasingly advocated.[137–139]

*Parathyroid carcinoma* is often functional, resulting in varying degrees of hyperparathyroidism, but is also locally invasive and may metastasize.[140] Cure is possible with aggressive surgical management.[141]

## Mesenchymal Tumors

Mesenchymal tumors are unusual mediastinal masses such as lipomas, fibromas, mesotheliomas, lymphangiomas, and several other rare tumors (see Table 77.2).[9] They arise from connective tissue, fat, smooth muscle, striated muscle, blood vessels, or lymphatic channels and can occur in any region of the mediastinum. Histologically and clinically, they are not substantially different from their counterparts elsewhere in the body. Unless the lesion is very large, the presence of symptoms usually means that the lesion is malignant.[9, 38]

*Lipoma* is the most common mesenchymal tumor of the mediastinum and is most often anterior. It may be encapsulated or unencapsulated, but in either case it is smooth and rounded with sharply defined margins. The characteristic low density of lipomas on CT images (Fig. 79.3) permits a confident diagnosis unless there is associated inhomogeneity, invasion of surrounding tissues, or poor demarcation of the mass's perimeter, in which case malignancy (liposarcoma or lipoblastoma) or teratoma must be ruled out.[38, 142]

Considerably more common than lipoma is *mediastinal lipomatosis*, or generalized overabundance of histologically normal unencapsulated fat.[143–147] The presence of some fat in the anterior mediastinum is normal, usually in and around the thymus. Accumulation of excess fat is associated with generalized obesity or Cushing's syndrome, with the use of exogenous corticosteroids and other drugs,[148] and in some cases without explanation.[147] Mediastinal lipomatosis appears on the conventional radiograph as a smooth widening or bulging of normal mediastinal contours, and its low homogeneous CT density confirms the diagnosis.[38] Compression or displacement of other mediastinal structures does not occur.[143–145]

Multiple symmetric lipomatosis is a rare disorder distinct from those just described that can cause tracheal compression.[149] This disorder, however, generally does not affect the anterior mediastinum, cardiophrenic angles, or paraspinal areas.

Sarcomas involving the mediastinum are rare. Nerve sheath sarcoma, spindle cell sarcoma, leiomyosarcoma, and liposarcoma are the four most common types.[150] Prior radiation therapy appears to be a predisposing factor in some cases.[151, 152]

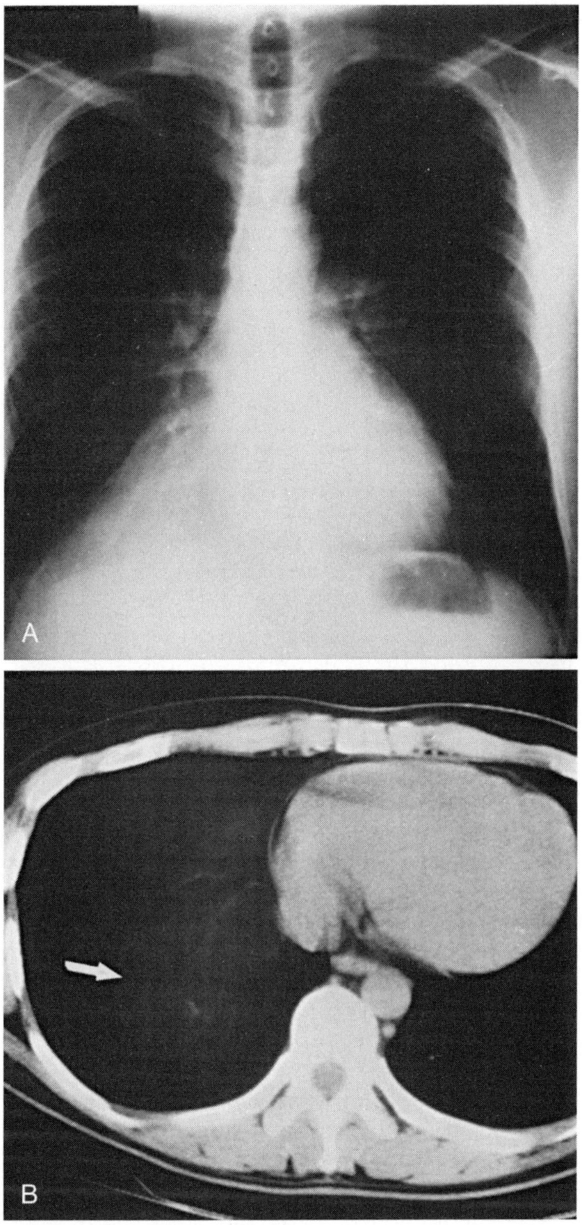


**Figure 79.3.** *A,* The chest roentgenogram from a 31-year-old man shows an abnormality at the right cardiophrenic angle noted as an incidental finding. *B,* The CT scan demonstrates a well-circumscribed homogeneous fat-density mass characteristic of mediastinal lipoma extending into the right hemithorax *(arrow).*

# LESIONS OCCURRING TYPICALLY IN THE MIDDLE MEDIASTINUM

## Lymphadenopathy

Enlargement of lymph nodes represents one of the most common causes of mediastinal abnormality on chest roentgenograms. Numerous anatomic classifications exist for the mediastinal lymph nodes, a comprehensive example of which is the 11 region scheme of the American Thoracic Society.[153] Figure 79.4 presents a simplified grouping of the main mediastinal nodes that corresponds to findings on conventional radiography and CT scans.[154] Nodes in the subcarinal, paratracheal, and hilar areas tend to be larger than those elsewhere,[38, 155, 156] but most authors consider 1.0 cm to be the upper limit of normal size.

Mediastinal lymph node enlargement is most often due to three general categories of disease process: lymphoma,[157, 158] metastatic cancer (discussed in Chapter 77),[154] and granulomatous inflammation (discussed in Chapter 78). Numerous less common causes are described, including Castleman's disease or *angiofollicular lymphoid hyperplasia*. Mediastinal adenopathy is common in HIV-infected patients and is usually infection

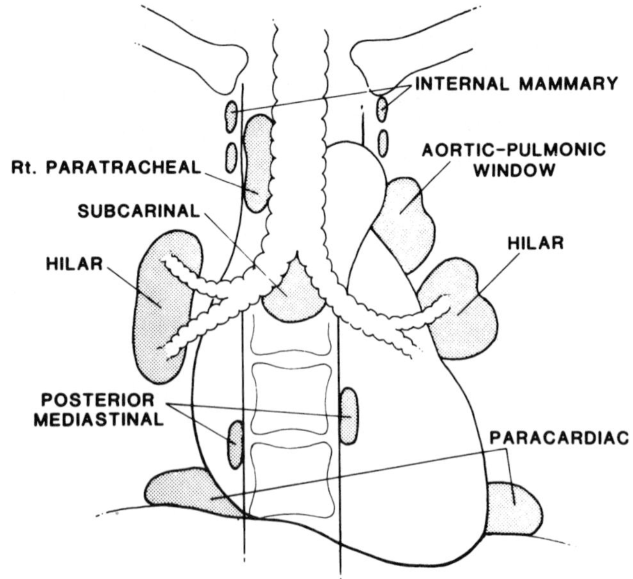


**Figure 79.4.** Simplified diagram depicting typical locations of mediastinal lymph nodes. (Reproduced with permission from McLoud TC, Meyer JE: Mediastinal metastases. Radiol Clin North Am 20:453–468, 1982.)

related, although lymphoma, Kaposi's sarcoma, and other processes may be responsible.[26] Although lymph node enlargement can be detected accurately by CT and MRI, imaging studies cannot reliably distinguish between and among benign and malignant causes of node enlargement. The results serve primarily to guide invasive testing.

## Developmental Cysts

Developmental cysts of various sorts constitute 10% to 20% of all mediastinal masses in both adults and children.[9, 35, 36, 159] Although some are histologically unclassifiable, most can be identified as pericardial, bronchogenic, or enteric on the basis of their lining tissues.[9, 160] Bronchogenic and enteric cysts are often referred to as *foregut duplication cysts* because of their origin from aberrant portions of the ventral and dorsal foregut, respectively.

*Pericardial cysts* account for about one third of cystic masses in adults but are much less common in children (see Table 79.1). They typically lie against the pericardium, diaphragm, or anterior chest wall in the right cardiophrenic angle. Rarely, pericardial cysts may communicate with the pericardium. Although typically harmless, pericardial cysts may enlarge to cause right ventricular outflow obstruction[161] or rupture and hemorrhage to cause pericardial tamponade[162] or sudden cardiac death.[163]

*Bronchogenic cysts* are typically found near the large airways, often just posterior to the carina, although they may be attached to the esophagus or even inside the pericardium.[9] The cyst wall often contains cartilage and respiratory epithelium. Most are discovered incidentally and cause no symptoms; however, they may communicate with the tracheobronchial tree and become infected[37]; some enlarge to cause airway obstruction (especially in infants),[164] pulmonary artery compression,[165] hemodynamic collapse,[166] and even fatal myocardial infarction.[166a] Rupture, with disastrous consequences,[34] and spillage of cyst contents into the airway during anesthesia have been reported.[167]

*Enteric* (or enterogenous) *cysts* are similar in location and appearance to bronchogenic cysts but have digestive tract epithelium. They are relatively uncommon in adults but are the most common cysts found in infants and children, in whom they may be associated with spinal extension and malformations of the vertebral column (called *neurenteric* cysts). Enteric cysts can occasionally be multiple and associated with duplications of other portions of the gastrointestinal tract.

Developmental cysts can usually be identified by CT or ultrasonography, and the diagnosis may be confirmed by aspiration cytology. MRI is valuable in cases of suspected spinal extension. In the appropriate clinical setting, benign cysts need not be resected unless they cause symptoms.[168] Most authorities, however, favor resection because of diagnostic uncertainties and the potential for development of complications.[35–37, 169] Alternatives to thoracotomy include therapeutic aspiration[170, 171] and thoracoscopic or mediastinoscopic excision.[172–174] Resection is usually curative, although cases of recurrence are described.[175, 176]

## Vascular Masses and Enlargements

Although not technically masses, a variety of vascular lesions must be considered in the differential diagnosis of mediastinal enlargement seen on the chest roentgenogram.[10, 177, 178] These include poststenotic aortic dilation, aneurysms or tortuosity of the aorta and great vessels, aortic coarctation, innominate vein and superior vena caval aneurysms, persistent left vena cava, azygos and hemiazygos vein enlargement, anomalous pulmonary venous return, pulmonary venous varix, and cardiophrenic angle varices associated with portal hypertension.[179] Idiopathic dilation of the pulmonary trunk and pulmonary arterial hypertension of any cause may appear as a mediastinal mass, and traumatic aortic transection and more subtle injuries may result in mediastinal hematoma.

Angiography has been the traditional means of diagnosing mediastinal masses of vascular origin, but CT imaging with intravenous contrast injection permits more convenient detection in most cases today.[180, 181] MRI shows great promise in enabling definitive diagnosis without radiation or contrast exposure.[182–184] Both CT and MRI can, however, be misleading if the vascular lumen is obscured.[185]

## Diaphragmatic Hernia

The protrusion of omental fat or other abdominal contents through the diaphragm may occur via several potential routes, and mediastinal mass lesions in any compartment can be the result.[38] A *Morgagni's hernia* produces an anterior cardiophrenic angle mass, usually on the right side. *Bochdalek's hernia*, in the posterior mediastinum, generally appears on the left side, presumably because the liver prevents herniation on the right. Herniation of fat around the esophagus is believed to precede hiatal hernia formation, and either may appear as a mediastinal mass. In the latter instance, an air-fluid level is intermittently seen on horizontal beam films. Fine linear densities are often demonstrable in diaphragmatic fat herniations on CT imaging; thought to represent omental vessels within the hernia, they may help differentiate the former from a lipoma.[38, 186] Although diaphragmatic herniations are usually incidental radiographic findings, traumatic diaphragmatic hernias may protrude into the mediastinum and result in cardiac compromise.[187, 188]

## LESIONS OCCURRING TYPICALLY IN THE POSTERIOR MEDIASTINUM: NEUROGENIC TUMORS

Neoplasms arising from neural tissues constitute the largest single group of mediastinal masses,[9, 10, 189–191] accounting for about 20% of adult cases and twice that number in children (see Table 79.1). They are classified (Table 79.3) according to their specific tissue of origin: peripheral nerves, sympathetic ganglia, and paraganglionic (chemoreceptor) tissue.[190] As a group, neurogenic tumors usually appear radiographically as a unilateral paravertebral mass.[9] Most are benign and asymptomatic in adults, but in children more than half are malignant and symptomatic.[191] Clinical manifestations include chest pain from nerve or bone erosion, dyspnea secondary to tracheal compression, and neurologic deficits resulting from spinal cord compression by intraspinal tumor extension. In addition, many neurogenic tumors are hormonally active.

Tumors arising from peripheral nerves include neurofibromas, neurilemomas or schwannomas, and neurosarcomas.[142, 142a] *Neurofibromas* contain both nerve sheath cells and nerve elements and are the most common tumor of this group. They are incompletely encapsulated and may grow quite large, producing symptoms by nerve compression or space occupation. Mediastinal neurofibroma may be one manifestation of von Recklinghausen's disease (neurofibromatosis), and, as with these tumors elsewhere, malignant degeneration into neurosarcoma eventually occurs in 10% to 15% of patients.[10] Although patients with von Recklinghausen's neurofibromatosis develop mediastinal neurofibromas, meningocele is said to be a more likely cause of a posterior mediastinal mass in such persons.[9]

*Neurilemoma*, or schwannoma, is another common neurogenic tumor that arises from the neural sheath. Most often seen in the third to fifth decades of life, neurilemoma usually causes no symptoms and appears as a well-circumscribed, homogeneous density on chest roentgenogram and CT (Figs. 79.5*A* and 79.5*B*).[9, 10, 142] It is always completely encapsulated and does not invade surrounding tissues, although neurilemomas may extend into intervertebral foramina (Fig. 79.5*C*). They occasionally calcify, and cyst formation may occur, with subsequent mucoid degeneration or hemorrhage. Treatment of both neurilemoma and solitary neurofibroma is resection.

**Table 79.3 NEUROGENIC TUMORS OF THE MEDIASTINUM**

| |
|---|
| Neoplasms arising from peripheral nerves |
| Neurofibroma |
| Neurilemoma (schwannoma) |
| Neurosarcoma |
| Neoplasms arising from sympathetic ganglia |
| Ganglioneuroma |
| Ganglioneuroblastoma |
| Neuroblastoma |
| Sympathicoblastoma |
| Neoplasms arising from paraganglionic tissue |
| Pheochromocytoma |
| Paraganglioma (chemodectoma) |

Malignant tumors of nerve sheath origin are also known as malignant neurofibroma, malignant schwannoma, or neurogenic fibrosarcoma. These tumors behave aggressively, with both local invasion and distant metastasis. Half occur in patients with neurofibromatosis.[15, 192] Treatment requires wide excision and usually adjuvant radiation.[15]

Tumors arising from nerve cells in sympathetic ganglia display a spectrum of neoplastic behavior ranging from *ganglioneuroma*, a benign tumor occurring mainly in children, to the malignant tumors ganglioneuroblastoma and neuroblastoma. Ganglioneuromas cause symptoms merely by mass effect and are usually cured by surgical excision. Ganglioneuroblastomas have intermediate behavior and can invade locally but are less likely to metastasize.[10] *Neuroblastoma* rapidly displaces and invades adjacent structures and may be widely metastatic at the time of presentation.[193, 194] Neuroblastoma accounts for 13% to 23% of childhood mediastinal masses and is the second or third most common cause after the lymphomas.[195, 196] One series of older patients found that 13% of primary tumors were found in the mediastinum,[197] and some authors report that neuroblastoma arising in the mediastinum has a somewhat more favorable prognosis than the same malignancy elsewhere in the body.[198–200] These tumors often elaborate endocrine peptides and catecholamines and are associated with diarrhea, fever, anorexia, and weight loss.[9] The propensity to produce catecholamines is used to advantage by imaging tumor uptake of the catecholamine precursor $^{123}$I-MIGB for purposes of diagnosis and identification of distant tumor metastases.[201] Treatment of neuroblastoma involves surgical resection of stage I disease and combination chemotherapy and radiation for advanced stages.[202] Radical excision of mediastinal neuroblastoma appears to offer no advantages over standard therapy.[199]

Neoplasms arising from paraganglionic or chemoreceptor tissue include *pheochromocytomas*, which are rare in the mediastinum and indistinguishable clinically or histologically from their counterparts in the abdomen, and *paragangliomas* (chemodectomas).[73, 203, 204] Paragangliomas may secrete catecholamines just as do pheochromocytomas. They appear benign under the microscope and

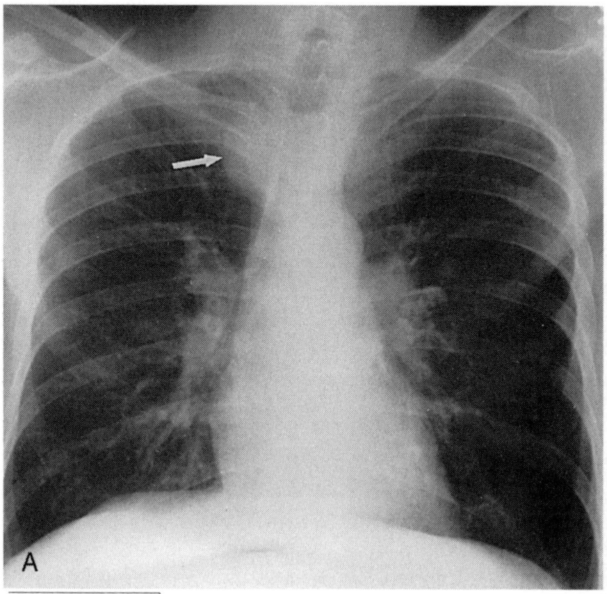


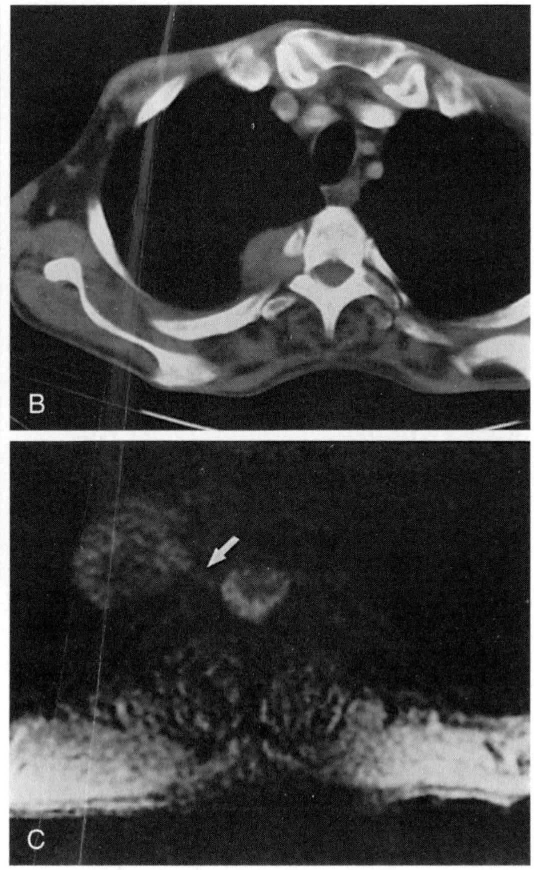


**Figure 79.5.** Series of imaging studies of a 64-year-old asymptomatic man with a surgically proved neurilemoma. *A,* The posteroanterior chest roentgenogram shows an incidental finding of a discrete mass behind the right clavicular head *(arrow).* *B,* The CT scan shows a homogeneous, well-circumscribed appearance and posterior location adjacent to the vertebral column. *C,* The MRI shows extension of the tumor into the neural foramen *(arrow).*

seldom metastasize, but spread locally in an aggressive fashion and thus have high morbidity and mortality rates.[9, 204]

## MISCELLANEOUS MEDIASTINAL MASSES

### Primary Carcinoma and Sarcoma

Numerous rare causes of mass lesions in the mediastinum have been described.[10, 205] These include malignancies known as primary carcinoma and sarcoma of the mediastinum.[9, 206] Primary carcinoma usually occurs in the anterior or middle mediastinum and is believed to be distinct from bronchogenic carcinoma and from other primary mediastinal neoplasms. It occurs primarily in adults, usually in men, and has an aggressive, rapidly fatal course with little response to therapy. Primary mediastinal sarcoma is a rare lesion of children that otherwise clinically resembles primary carcinoma. Poorly differentiated carcinoma of the mediastinum ("Adkins tumor"[207]) is a rare neoplasm whose histology does not permit identification of a likely tissue or site of origin.[206]

### Other Tumors

Miscellaneous benign causes of a mediastinal mass have been described. *Pancreatic pseudocysts* may extend into the mediastinum, usually through the aortic or esophageal hiatus.[10, 205, 208] They have been reported in all three mediastinal compartments. *Hydatid cysts* also occur in the mediastinum, but this is said to be one of the least frequent sites for this type of lesion.[10, 205] The posterior mediastinum is occasionally the site of a thoracic duct cyst.[9] Also, *extramedullary hematopoiesis* in patients with chronic hemolytic anemia may appear as a mediastinal mass, often in a posterior location. *Meningoceles*, outgrowths of spinal meninges that protrude along the course of a spinal nerve, produce posterior mediastinal masses. Finally, it must be remembered that masses found within any of the mediastinal compartments may be lesions more commonly found in another mediastinal compartment or may occasionally have extended from another area in the mediastinum (Fig. 79.6).

## SUMMARY

Mediastinal tumors and cysts are conveniently characterized by location within the mediastinum: anterior, middle, or posterior. At least half the patients with mediastinal tumors are asymptomatic, and the lesions are detected as an incidental finding on a chest roentgenogram obtained for other purposes. Asymptomatic lesions tend to be benign; symptoms are usually caused by compression or invasion of neighboring structures. Occasionally, mediastinal tumors are associated with paraneoplastic manifestations, which are typically endocrine in origin. The workup involves special imaging, usually CT, but definitive diagnosis requires examination of tissue. Most mediastinal masses are treated by surgical resection, and rapidly evolving experience with radiation and combination chemotherapy is improving the outlook for many patients with advanced malignant mediastinal tumors.

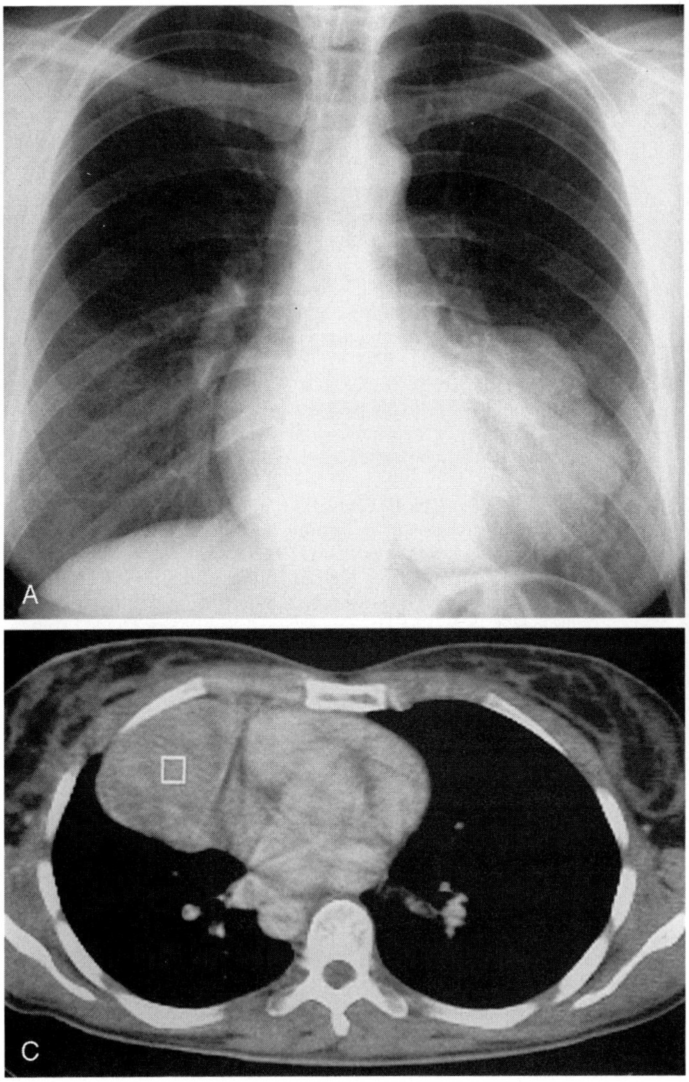


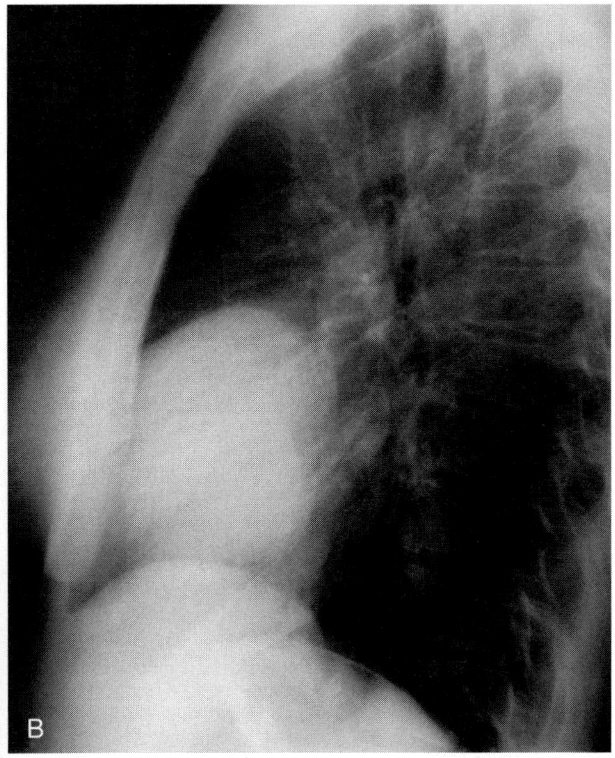


**Figure 79.6.** Typical findings on chest roentgenograms (*A*, posteroanterior; *B*, lateral view) and thoracic CT (*C*) of a mass presenting in the middle mediastinum. At surgery, this mass proved to be a benign thymoma, originating in the anterior mediastinum and extending by a slender stalk into the middle radiographic compartment. (Reproduced courtesy of Dr. Robert Stevens, Wenatchee, WA.)

## References

1. Bradford ML, Mahon HW, Grow JB: Mediastinal cysts and tumors. Surg Gynecol Obstet 85:467–491, 1947.
2. Sabiston DC, Scott HW: Primary neoplasms and cysts of the mediastinum. Ann Surg 136:777–797, 1952.
3. Lyons HA, Calvy GL, Sammons BP: The diagnosis and classification of mediastinal masses: A study of 782 cases. Ann Intern Med 51:897–932, 1959.
4. LeRoux BT: Cysts and tumors of the mediastinum. Surg Gynecol Obstet 115:695–703, 1962.
5. Boyd DP, Midell AI: Mediastinal cysts and tumors. Surg Clin North Am 48:493–505, 1968.
6. Benjamin SP, McCormack LJ, Effler DB, et al: Primary tumors of the mediastinum. Chest 62:297–303, 1972.
7. Rubush JL, Gardner IR, Boyd WC, et al: Mediastinal tumors: A review of 186 cases. J Thorac Cardiovasc Surg 65:216–222, 1973.
8. Silverman NA, Sabiston DC: Primary tumors and cysts of the mediastinum. Curr Probl Cancer 2:1–55, 1977.
9. Silverman NA, Sabiston DCJ: Mediastinal masses. Surg Clin North Am 60:757–777, 1980.
10. LeRoux BT, Kallichurum S, Shama DM: Mediastinal cysts and tumors. Curr Probl Surg 21:1–76, 1984.
11. Beszniak I, Szende B, Lapis K: Mediastinal Tumors and Pseudotumors. Basel: S. Karger, 1984.
12. Shields T: Primary mediastinal tumors and cysts and their diagnostic investigation. *In* Shields T (ed): Mediastinal Surgery. Philadelphia: Lea & Febiger, 1991, pp 111–117.
13. Hoffman OA, Gillespie DJ, Aughenbaugh GL, et al: Primary mediastinal neoplasms (other than thymoma). Mayo Clin Proc 68:880–891, 1993.
14. Strollo DC, Rosado de Christenson ML, Jett JR: Primary mediastinal tumors. Part I: Tumors of the anterior mediastinum. Chest 112:511–522, 1997.
15. Strollo DC, Rosado de Christenson ML, Jett JR: Primary mediastinal tumors: Part II. Tumors of the middle and posterior mediastinum. Chest 112:1344–1357, 1997.

15a. Temes R, Chavez T, Mapel D, et al: Primary mediastinal malignancies: Findings in 219 patients. West J Med 170:161–166, 1999.

16. Haller JAJ, Mazur DO, Morgan WWJ: Diagnosis and management of mediastinal masses in children. J Thorac Cardiovasc Surg 28:385–393, 1969.
17. Grosfield JL, Weinberger M, Kilman JW, et al: Primary mediastinal neoplasms in infants and children. Ann Thorac Surg 12:179–190, 1971.
18. Whittaker LDJ, Lynn HB: Mediastinal tumors and cysts in the pediatric patient. Surg Clin North Am 53:893–904, 1973.
19. Pokorny WJ, Sherman JO: Mediastinal masses in infants and children. J Thorac Cardiovasc Surg 68:869–875, 1974.
20. Filler RM, Simpson JS, Ein SH: Mediastinal masses in infants and children. Pediatr Clin North Am 26:677–690, 1979.
21. Schlumberger HG: Tumors of the Mediastinum: Atlas of Tumor

Pathology (Section V, Fasc 18). Washington, DC: Armed Forces Institute of Pathology, 1951.
22. Davis RD Jr, Oldham HN Jr, Sabiston DC Jr: Primary cysts and neoplasms of the mediastinum: Recent changes in clinical presentation, methods of diagnosis, management, and results. Ann Thorac Surg 44:229–237, 1987.
23. Blegvad S, Lippert H, Simper LB, et al: Mediastinal tumours. A report of 129 cases. Scand J Thorac Cardiovasc Surg 24:39–42, 1990.
24. Cohen AJ, Thompson L, Edwards FH, et al: Primary cysts and tumors of the mediastinum. Ann Thorac Surg 51:378–384, 1991.
25. Mouroux J, Riquet M, Padovani B, et al: Surgical management of thoracic manifestations in human immunodeficiency virus–positive patients: Indications and results. Br J Surg 82:39–43, 1995.
26. Haramati LB, Choi Y, Widrow CA, et al: Isolated lymphadenopathy on chest radiographs of HIV-infected patients. Clin Radiol 51:345–349, 1996.
27. Fishman JE, Schwartz DS, Sais GJ, et al: Bronchogenic carcinoma in HIV-positive patients: Findings on chest radiographs and CT scans. AJR Am J Roentgenol 164:57–61, 1995.
28. Wychulis AR, Payne WS, Clagett OT, et al: Surgical treatment of mediastinal tumors: A 40-year experience. J Thorac Cardiovasc Surg 62:379–391, 1971.
29. Oldham HJN, Sabiston DCJ: Primary tumors and cysts of the mediastinum: Lesions presenting as cardiovascular abnormalities. Arch Surg 96:71–75, 1968.
30. Marshall ME, Trump DL: Acquired extrinsic pulmonic stenosis caused by mediastinal tumors. Cancer 49:1496–1499, 1982.
31. Shields TW: Thymic tumors. *In* Shields T (ed): Mediastinal Surgery. Philadelphia: Lea & Febiger, 1991, pp 153–173.
32. Connolly AM, Pestronk A, Mehta S, et al: Serum autoantibodies in childhood opsoclonus-myoclonus syndrome: An analysis of antigenic targets in neural tissues. J Pediatr 130:878–884, 1997.
33. Ahn JM, Lee KS, Goo JM, et al: Predicting the histotogy of anterior mediastinal masses: Comparison of chest radiography and CT. J Thorac Imaging 11:265–271, 1996.
34. Zaugg M, Kaplan V, Widmer U, et al: Fatal air embolism in an airplane passenger with a giant intrapulmonary bronchogenic cyst. Am J Respir Crit Care Med 157:1686–1689, 1998.
35. St. Georges R, Deslauriers J, Duranceau A, et al: Clinical spectrum of bronchogenic cysts of the mediastinum and lung in the adult. Ann Thorac Surg 52:6–13, 1991.
36. Patel SR, Meeker DP, Biscotti CV, et al: Presentation and management of bronchogenic cysts in the adult. Chest 106:79–85, 1994.
37. Ribet ME, Copin MC, Gosselin B: Bronchogenic cysts of the mediastinum. J Thorac Cardiovasc Surg 109:1003–1010, 1995.
38. Naidich DP, Zerhouni EA, Siegelman SS: Computed Tomography and Magnetic Resonance of the Thorax (2nd ed). New York: Raven Press, 1991.
39. Rosenow ECI, Hurley BT: Disorders of the thymus: A review. Arch Intern Med 144:763–770, 1984.
40. Appelqvist P, Kostiainen S, Franssila K, et al: Treatment and prognosis of thymoma: A review of 25 cases. J Surg Oncol 20:265–268, 1982.
41. LeGolvan DP, Abell MR: Thymomas. Cancer 39:2142–2157, 1977.
42. Verstandig AG, Epstein DM, Miller WT Jr, et al: Thymoma—report of 71 cases and a review. Crit Rev Diagn Imaging 33:201–230, 1992.
43. Cooper JD: Current therapy for thymoma. Chest 103:334S–336S, 1993.
44. Debono DJ, Loehrer PJ: Thymic neoplasms. Curr Opin Oncol 8:112–119, 1996.
45. Kohman LJ: Controversies in the management of malignant thymoma. Chest 112:296S–300S, 1997.
45a. Strollo DC, Rosado-de-Christenson ML: Tumors of the thymus. J Thorac Imaging 14:152–171, 1999.
46. Tao L-C: Guides to Clinical Aspiration Biopsy: Lung, Pleura, and Mediastinum. New York: Igaku-Shoin, 1988, pp. 273–328.
47. Morgenthaler TI, Brown LR, Colby TV, et al: Thymoma. Mayo Clin Proc 68:1110–1123, 1993.
48. Lennon VA, Lambert EH: Myasthenia gravis induced by monoclonal antibodies to acetylcholine receptors. Nature 285:238–240, 1980.
49. Beekman R, Kuks JB, Oosterhuis HJ: Myasthenia gravis: Diagnosis and follow-up of 100 consecutive patients. J Neurol 244:112–118, 1997.
50. Rosado de Christenson ML, Galobardes J, et al: Thymoma: Radiologic-pathologic correlation. Radiographics 12:151–168, 1992.
51. Janssen RS, Kaye AD, Lisak RP, et al: Radiologic evaluation of the mediastinum in myasthenia gravis. Neurology 33:534–539, 1983.
52. Baron RL, Lee JKT, Sagel SS, et al: Computed tomography of the normal thymus. Radiology 142:121–125, 1982.
53. Baron RL, Lee JKT, Sagel SS, et al: Computed tomography of the abnormal thymus. Radiology 142:127–134, 1982.
54. Heiberg E, Wolverson MK, Sundaram M, et al: Normal thymus: CT characteristics in subjects under age 20. AJR Am J Roentgenol 138:491–494, 1982.
55. Kiyosue H, Miyake H, Komatsu E, et al: MRI of cervical masses of thymic origin. J Comput Assist Tomogr 18:206–208, 1994.
56. Sakai F, Sone S, Kiyono K, et al: MR imaging of thymoma: Radiologic-pathologic correlation. AJR Am J Roentgenol 158:751–756, 1992.
57. Lastoria S, Vergara E, Palmieri G, et al: In vivo detection of malignant thymic masses by indium-111-DTPA-D-Phe1-octreotide scintigraphy. J Nucl Med 39:634–639, 1998.
58. Liu RS, Yeh SH, Huang MH, et al: Use of fluorine-18 fluorodeoxyglucose positron emission tomography in the detection of thymoma: A preliminary report. Eur J Nucl Med 22:1402–1407, 1995.
59. Lewis JE, Wick MR, Scheithauer BW, et al: Thymoma. A clinicopathologic review. Cancer 60:2727–2743, 1987.
60. Blumberg D, Port JL, Weksler B, et al: Thymoma: A multivariate analysis of factors predicting survival. Ann Thorac Surg 60:908–913, 1995.
61. Bernatz PE, Khonsari S, Harrison EGJ, et al: Thymoma: Factors influencing prognosis. Surg Clin North Am 53:885–892, 1973.
62. Sugarbaker DJ. Thoracoscopy in the management of anterior mediastinal masses. Ann Thorac Surg 56:653–656, 1993.
63. Curran WJ Jr, Kornstein MJ, Brooks JJ, et al: Invasive thymoma: The role of mediastinal irradiation following complete or incomplete surgical resection. J Clin Oncol 6:1722–1727, 1988.
64. Loehrer PJ Sr, Kim K, Aisner SC, et al: Cisplatin plus doxorubicin plus cyclophosphamide in metastatic or recurrent thymoma: Final results of an intergroup trial. The Eastern Cooperative Oncology Group, Southwest Oncology Group, and Southeastern Cancer Study Group. J Clin Oncol 12:1164–1168, 1994.
65. Loehrer PJ Sr, Chen M, Kim K, et al: Cisplatin, doxorubicin, and cyclophosphamide plus thoracic radiation therapy for limited-stage unresectable thymoma: An intergroup trial. J Clin Oncol 15:3093–3099, 1997.
66. Busch C, Machens A, Pichlmeier U, et al: Long-term outcome and quality of life after thymectomy for myasthenia gravis. Ann Surg 224:225–232, 1996.
67. Cosi V, Romani A, Lombardi M, et al: Prognosis of myasthenia gravis: A retrospective study of 380 patients. J Neurol 244:548–555, 1997.
68. Welch KJ, Tapper D, Vawter GP: Surgical treatment of thymic cysts and neoplasms in children. J Pediatr Surg 14:691–697, 1979.
69. Mok CK, Ho FCS, Nandi P, et al: Lipothymoma. Med J Austr 1:272–274, 1980.
70. Rosado de Christenson ML, Pugatch RD, Moran CA, et al: Thymolipoma: Analysis of 27 cases. Radiology 193:121–126, 1994.
71. Hsu CP, Chen CY, Chen CL, et al: Thymic carcinoma. Ten years' experience in twenty patients. J Thorac Cardiovasc Surg 107:615–620, 1994.
72. Weide LG, Ulbright TM, Loehrer PJ Sr, et al: Thymic carcinoma. A distinct clinical entity responsive to chemotherapy. Cancer 71:1219–1223, 1993.
73. Wick MR, Rosai J: Neuroendocrine neoplasms of the mediastinum. Semin Diagn Pathol 8:35–51, 1991.
74. Economopoulos GC, Lewis JW Jr, Lee MW, et al: Carcinoid tumors of the thymus. Ann Thorac Surg 50:58–61, 1990.
75. Salyer WR, Salyer DC, Eggleston JC: Carcinoid tumors of the thymus. Cancer 37:958–973, 1976.
76. Wick MR, Carney JA, Bernatz PE, et al: Primary mediastinal carcinoid tumors. Am J Surg Pathol 6:195–205, 1982.

77. Edington H, Salwitz J, Longo DL, et al: Thymic hyperplasia masquerading as recurrent Hodgkin's disease: Case report and review of the literature. J Surg Oncol 33:120–123, 1986.
78. Burns DE, Schiffman FJ: Beguiled by the gallium. Thymic rebound in an adult after chemotherapy for Hodgkin's disease. Chest 104:1916–1919, 1993.
79. Knapp RH, Hurt RD, Payne WS, et al: Malignant germ cell tumors of the mediastinum. J Thorac Cardiovasc Surg 89:82–89, 1985.
80. Trastek VF, Pairolero PC: Benign germ cell tumors of the mediastinum. *In* Shields T (ed): Mediastinal Surgery. Philadelphia: Lea & Febiger, 1991, pp 205–210.
81. Dehner LP: Germ cell tumors of the mediastinum. Semin Diagn Pathol 7:266–284, 1990.
81a. Weidner N: Germ-cell tumors of the mediastinum. Semin Diagn Pathol 16:42–50, 1999.
82. Gonzalez-Crussi F: Extragonadal Teratomas. Atlas of Tumor Pathology (Fasc 18). Washington, DC: Armed Forces Institute of Pathology, 1982.
83. Nichols CR, Fox EP: Extragonadal and pediatric germ cell tumors. Hematol Oncol Clin North Am 5:1189–1209, 1991.
84. Nichols CR: Mediastinal germ cell tumors. Semin Thorac Cardiovasc Surg 4:45–50, 1992.
85. Lewis BD, Hurt RD, Payne WS, et al: Benign teratomas of the mediastinum. J Thorac Cardiovasc Surg 86:727–731, 1983.
86. Parker D, Holford CP, Begent RHJ, et al: Effective treatment for malignant mediastinal teratoma. Thorax 38:897–902, 1983.
87. Dulmet EM, Macchiarini P, Suc B, et al: Germ cell tumors of the mediastinum. A 30-year experience. Cancer 72:1894–1901, 1993.
88. Hurt RD, Bruckman JE, Farrow GM, et al: Primary anterior mediastinal seminoma. Cancer 49:1658–1663, 1982.
89. Hainsworth JD, Greco FA: Clinical features of malignant germ cell tumors and primary seminomas of the mediastinum. *In* Shields T (ed): Mediastinal Surgery. Philadelphia: Lea & Febiger, 1991, pp 211–218.
90. Bukowski RM, Wolf M, Kulander BG, et al: Alternating combination chemotherapy in patients with extragonadal germ cell tumors. A Southwest Oncology Group study. Cancer 71:2631–2638, 1993.
91. Bukowski RM: Management of advanced and extragonadal germ-cell tumors. Urol Clin North Am 20:153–160, 1993.
92. Dexeus FH, Logothetis CJ, Chong C, et al: Genetic abnormalities in men with germ cell tumors. J Urol 140:80–84, 1988.
93. Nichols CR, Heerema NA, Palmer C, et al: Klinefelter's syndrome associated with mediastinal germ cell neoplasms. J Clin Oncol 5:1290–1294, 1987.
94. Nichols CR, Hoffman R, Einhorn LH, et al: Hematologic malignancies associated with primary mediastinal germ-cell tumors. Ann Intern Med 102:603–609, 1985.
95. Nichols CR, Roth BJ, Heerema N, et al: Hematologic neoplasia associated with primary mediastinal germ-cell tumors. N Engl J Med 322:1425–1429, 1990.
96. Rusch VW, Logothetis C, Samuels M: Endodermal sinus tumor of the mediastinum: Report of apparent cure in two patients with extensive disease. Chest 86:745–747, 1984.
97. Vogelzang NJ, Anderson RW, Kennedy BJ: Successful treatment of mediastinal germ cell/endodermal sinus tumors. Chest 88:64–69, 1985.
98. Nichols CR, Catalano PJ, Crawford ED, et al: Randomized comparison of cisplatin and etoposide and either bleomycin or ifosfamide in treatment of advanced disseminated germ cell tumors: An Eastern Cooperative Oncology Group, Southwest Oncology Group, and Cancer and Leukemia Group B Study. J Clin Oncol 16:1287–1293, 1998.
99. Nichols CR, Andersen J, Lazarus HM, et al: High-dose carboplatin and etoposide with autologous bone marrow transplantation in refractory germ cell cancer: An Eastern Cooperative Oncology Group protocol. J Clin Oncol 10:558–563, 1992.
100. Nichols CR, Saxman S: Primary salvage treatment of recurrent germ cell tumors: Experience at Indiana University. Semin Oncol 25:210–214, 1998.
101. Vaeth JM, Moskowitz SA, Green JP: Mediastinal Hodgkin's disease. AJR Am J Roentgenol 126:123–126, 1976.
102. Jones SE, Fuks Z, Bull M, et al: Non-Hodgkin's lymphomas. IV. Clinicopathologic correlation in 405 cases. Cancer 31:806–823, 1973.
103. Levitt LJ, Aisenberg AC, Harris NL, et al: Primary non-Hodgkin's lymphoma of the mediastinum. Cancer 50:2486–2492, 1982.
104. Wang CY, Snow JL, Su WP: Lymphoma associated with human immunodeficiency virus infection. Mayo Clin Proc 70:665–672, 1995.
105. Straus DJ: Human immunodeficiency virus–associated lymphomas. Med Clin North Am 81:495–510, 1997.
106. Klencke B, Kaplan L: Advances and future challenges in non-Hodgkin's lymphoma. Curr Opin Oncol 10:422–427, 1998.
107. L'Evy R, Colonna P, Tourani JM, et al: Human immunodeficiency virus associated Hodgkin's disease: Report of 45 cases from the French Registry of HIV-Associated Tumors. Leuk Lymphoma 16:451–456, 1995.
108. Strickler JG, Kurtin PJ: Mediastinal lymphoma. Semin Diagn Pathol 8:2–13, 1991.
109. Davis TA, Horning SJ: Advances in the management of Hodgkin's and non-Hodgkin's lymphoma. Curr Opin Hematol 5:259–263, 1998.
110. Aisenberg A: Problems in Hodgkin's disease management. Blood 93:761–779, 1999.
111. Salzman DE, Briggs AD, Vaughan WP: Bone marrow transplantation for non-Hodgkin's lymphoma: A review. Am J Med Sci 313:228–235, 1997.
112. Jacobs P: Hodgkin's disease and the malignant lymphomas. Dis Mon 39:213–297, 1993.
113. DeVita VT Jr, Hubbard SM: Hodgkin's disease. N Engl J Med 328:560–565, 1993.
114. Armitage JO: Treatment of non-Hodgkin's lymphoma. N Engl J Med 328:1023–1030, 1993.
115. Sandlund JT, Downing JR, Crist WM: Non-Hodgkin's lymphoma in childhood. N Engl J Med 334:1238–1248, 1996.
116. Hudson MM, Donaldson SS: Hodgkin's disease. Pediatr Clin North Am 44:891–906, 1997.
117. Shad A, Magrath I: Non-Hodgkin's lymphoma. Pediatr Clin North Am 44:863–890, 1997.
118. Park HM, Tarver RD, Siddiqui AR, et al: Efficacy of thyroid scintigraphy in the diagnosis of intrathoracic goiter. AJR Am J Roentgenol 148:527–529, 1987.
119. Glazer GM, Axel L, Moss AA: CT diagnosis of mediastinal thyroid. AJR Am J Roentgenol 138:495–498, 1982.
120. Bashist B, Ellis K, Gold RP: Computed tomography of intrathoracic goiters. Am J Roentgenol 140:455–460, 1983.
121. Yousem DM, Scheff AM: Thyroid and parathyroid gland pathology. Role of imaging. Otolaryngol Clin North Am 28:621–649, 1995.
122. Jaskowiak N, Norton JA, Alexander HR, et al: A prospective trial evaluating a standard approach to reoperation for missed parathyroid adenoma. Ann Surg 224:308–320, 1996.
123. Shen W, Duren M, Morita E, et al: Reoperation for persistent or recurrent primary hyperparathyroidism. Arch Surg 131:861–867, 1996.
124. Stark DD, Gooding GA, Moss AA, et al: Parathyroid imaging: Comparison of high-resolution CT and high-resolution sonography. AJR Am J Roentgenol 141:633–638, 1983.
125. Rangnekar N, Bailer WJ, Ghani A, et al: Parathyroid cysts. Report of four cases and review of the literature. Int Surg 81:412–414, 1996.
126. Gurbuz AT, Peetz ME: Giant mediastinal parathyroid cyst: An unusual cause of hypercalcemic crisis—Case report and review of the literature. Surgery 120:795–800, 1996.
127. Hauet EJ, Paul MA, Salu MK: Compression of the trachea by a mediastinal parathyroid cyst. Ann Thorac Surg 64:851–852, 1997.
128. Landau O, Chamberlain DW, Kennedy RS, et al: Mediastinal parathyroid cysts. Ann Thorac Surg 63:951–953, 1997.
128a. Shields TW, Immermann SC: Mediastinal parathyroid cysts revisited. Ann Thorac Surg 67:581–590, 1999.
129. Hopkins CR, Reading CC: Thyroid and parathyroid imaging. Semin Ultrasound CT MR 16:279–295, 1995.
130. Moinuddin M, Whynott C: Ectopic parathyroid adenomas: Multi-imaging modalities and its management. Clin Nucl Med 21:27–32, 1996.

131. Fayet P, Hoeffel C, Fulla Y, et al: Technetium-99m sestamibi scintigraphy, magnetic resonance imaging and venous blood sampling in persistent and recurrent hyperparathyroidism. Br J Radiol 70:459–464, 1997.
132. Caixas A, Berna L, Hernandez A, et al: Efficacy of preoperative diagnostic imaging localization of technetium 99m-sestamibi scintigraphy in hyperparathyroidism. Surgery 121:535–541, 1997.
133. Sofferman RA, Nathan MH: The ectopic parathyroid adenoma: A cost justification for routine preoperative localization with technetium Tc 99m sestamibi scan. Arch Otolaryngol Head Neck Surg 124:649–654, 1998.
134. Roe SM, Brown PW, Pate LM, et al: Initial cervical exploration for parathyroidectomy is not benefited by preoperative localization studies. Am Surg 64:503–507, 1998.
135. Blanco I, Carril JM, Banzo I, et al: Double-phase Tc-99m sestamibi scintigraphy in the preoperative location of lesions causing hyperparathyroidism. Clin Nucl Med 23:291–297, 1998.
136. Sarfati E, Billotey C, Halimi B, et al: Early localization and reoperation for persistent primary hyperparathyroidism. Br J Surg 84:98–100, 1997.
137. Prinz RA, Lonchyna V, Carnaille B, et al: Thoracoscopic excision of enlarged mediastinal parathyroid glands. Surgery 116:999–1004, 1994.
138. Smythe WR, Bavaria JE, Hall RA, et al: Thoracoscopic removal of mediastinal parathyroid adenoma. Ann Thorac Surg 59:236–238, 1995.
139. Knight R, Ratzer ER, Fenoglio ME, et al: Thoracoscopic excision of mediastinal parathyroid adenomas: A report of two cases and review of the literature. J Am Coll Surg 185:481–485, 1997.
140. Cordeiro AC, Montenegro FL, Kulcsar MA, et al: Parathyroid carcinoma. Am J Surg 175:52–55, 1998.
141. V'Azquez Quintana E: Parathyroid carcinoma: Diagnosis and management. Am Surg 63:954–957, 1997.
142. Swanson PE: Soft tissue neoplasms of the mediastinum. Semin Diagn Pathol 8:14–34, 1991.
142a. Marchevsky AM: Mediastinal tumors of peripheral nerve origin. Semin Diagn Pathol 16:65–78, 1999.
143. Koerner HF, Sun DIC: Mediastinal lipomatosis secondary to steroid therapy. Am J Roentgenol Radiol Ther Nucl Med 98:461–464, 1966.
144. Price JF, Rigler LG: Widening of the mediastinum resulting from fat accumulation. Radiology 96:497–500, 1970.
145. Lee WJ, Fattal G: Mediastinal lipomatosis in simple obesity. Chest 70:308–309, 1976.
146. Bein NE, Manusco AA, Mink JH, et al: Computed tomography in the evaluation of mediastinal lipomatosis. J Comput Assist Tomogr 2:379–383, 1978.
147. Homer JM, Wechsler RJ, Carter BL: Mediastinal lipomatosis. Radiology 128:657–661, 1978.
148. Miller WTJ: Drug-related pleural and mediastinal disorders. J Thorac Imaging 6:36–51, 1991.
149. Enzi G, Biondetti PR, Fiore D, et al: Computed tomography of deep fat masses in multiple symmetrical lipomatosis. Radiology 144:122–124, 1982.
150. Burt M, Ihde JK, Hajdu SI, et al: Primary sarcomas of the mediastinum: Results of therapy. J Thorac Cardiovasc Surg 115:671–680, 1998.
151. Killion MJ, Brodovsky HS, Schwarting R: Pericardial angiosarcoma after mediastinal irradiation for seminoma. A case report and a review of the literature. Cancer 78:912–917, 1996.
152. Ducatman BS, Scheithauer BW: Postirradiation neurofibrosarcoma. Cancer 51:1028–1033, 1983.
153. Clinical staging of primary lung cancer American Thoracic Society node mapping scheme. Am Rev Respir Dis 127:659–669, 1983.
154. McLoud TC, Meyer JE: Mediastinal metastases. Radiol Clin North Am 20:453–468, 1982.
155. Genereux GP, Howie JL: Normal mediastinal lymph node size and number: CT and anatomic study. AJR Am J Roentgenol 142:1095–1100, 1984.
156. Glazer GM, Gross BH, Quint LE, et al: Normal mediastinal lymph nodes: Number and size according to American Thoracic Society mapping. AJR Am J Roentgenol 144:261–265, 1985.
157. Filly R, Blank M, Castellino RA: Radiographic distribution of intrathoracic disease in previously untreated patients with Hodgkin's disease and non-Hodgkin's lymphoma. Radiology 120:277–281, 1976.
158. Burgener FA, Hamlin D: Intrathoracic histiocytic lymphoma. AJR Am J Roentgenol 136:499–504, 1981.
159. Cioffi U, Bonavina L, De Simone M, et al: Presentation and surgical management of bronchogenic and esophageal duplication cysts in adults. Chest 113:1492–1496, 1998.
160. Salyer DC, Salyer WR, Eggleston JC: Benign developmental cysts of the mediastinum. Arch Pathol Lab Med 101:136–139, 1977.
161. Ng AF, Olak J: Pericardial cyst causing right ventricular outflow tract obstruction. Ann Thorac Surg 63:1147–1148, 1997.
162. Borges AC, Gellert K, Dietel M, et al: Acute right-sided heart failure due to hemorrhage into a pericardial cyst. Ann Thorac Surg 63:845–847, 1997.
163. Fredman CS, Parsons SR, Aquino TI, et al: Sudden death after a stress test in a patient with a large pericardial cyst. Am Heart J 127:946–950, 1994.
164. Lippmann M, Solit R, Goldberg SK, et al: Mediastinal bronchogenic cyst. A cause of upper airway obstruction. Chest 102:1901–1903, 1992.
165. Worsnop CJ, Teichtahl H, Clarke CP: Bronchogenic cyst: A cause of pulmonary artery obstruction and breathlessness. Ann Thorac Surg 55:1254–1255, 1993.
166. Fratellone PM, Coplan N, Friedman M, et al: Hemodynamic compromise secondary to a mediastinal bronchogenic cyst. Chest 106:610–612, 1994.
166a. Kennebeck GA, Wong AK, Berry WR, et al: Mediastinal bronchogenic cyst manifesting as a catastrophic myocardial infarction. Ann Thorac Surg 67:1789–1791, 1999.
167. Politis GD, Baumann R, Hubbard AM: Spillage of cystic pulmonary masses into the airway during anesthesia. Anesthesiology 87:693–696, 1997.
168. Bolton JW, Shahian DM: Asymptomatic bronchogenic cysts: What is the best management? Ann Thorac Surg 53:1134–1137, 1992.
169. Kirwan WO, Walbaum PR, McCormack RJ: Cystic intrathoracic derivatives of the foregut and their complications. Thorax 28:424–428, 1973.
170. Schwartz AR, Fishman EK, Wang KP: Diagnosis and treatment of a bronchogenic cyst using transbronchial needle aspiration. Thorax 41:326–327, 1986.
171. Tobert DG, Midthun DE: Bronchogenic cyst. J Bronch 3:295–299, 1996.
172. Hazelrigg SR, Landreneau RJ, Mack MJ, et al: Thoracoscopic resection of mediastinal cysts. Ann Thorac Surg 56:659–660, 1993.
173. Urschel JD, Horan TA: Mediastinoscopic treatment of mediastinal cysts. Ann Thorac Surg 58:1698–1700, 1994.
174. Smythe WR, Bavaria JE, Kaiser LR: Mediastinoscopic subtotal removal of mediastinal cysts. Chest 114:614–617, 1998.
175. Read CA, Moront M, Carangelo R, et al: Recurrent bronchogenic cyst. An argument for complete surgical excision. Arch Surg 126:1306–1308, 1991.
176. Gharagozloo F, Dausmann MJ, McReynolds SD, et al: Recurrent bronchogenic pseudocyst 24 years after incomplete excision. Report of a case. Chest 108:880–883, 1995.
177. Kelley MJ, Mannes EJ, Ravin CE: Mediastinal masses of vascular origin: A review. J Thorac Cardiovasc Surg 76:559–572, 1978.
178. Backer CL: Vascular masses of the mediastinum. *In* Shields T (ed): Mediastinal Surgery. Philadelphia: Lea & Febiger, 1991, pp 138–149.
179. Wachsberg RH, Yaghmai V, Javors BR, et al: Cardiophrenic varices in portal hypertension: Evaluation with CT. Radiology 195:553–556, 1995.
180. Marotta R, Franchetto AA: The CT appearance of aortic transection. AJR Am J Roentgenol 166:647–651, 1996.
181. Gavant ML, Menke PG, Fabian T, et al: Blunt traumatic aortic rupture: Detection with helical CT of the chest. Radiology 197:125–133, 1995.
182. Berlin SC: Magnetic resonance imaging of the cardiovascular system and airway. Pediatr Clin North Am 44:659–679, 1997.
183. Burkill GJ, Burn PR, Padley SP: Aneurysm of the left brachiocephalic vein: An unusual cause of mediastinal widening. Br J Radiol 70:837–839, 1997.

184. Soler R, Rodriguez E, Requejo I, et al: Magnetic resonance imaging of congenital abnormalities of the thoracic aorta. Eur Radiol 8:540–546, 1998.
185. Podbielski FJ, Sam ADN, Halldorsson AO, et al: Giant azygos vein varix. Ann Thorac Surg 63:1167–1169, 1997.
186. Rohlfing BM, Korobkin N, Hall AD: Computed tomography of intrathoracic omental herniation and other mediastinal fatty masses. J Comput Assist Tomogr 1:181–183, 1977.
187. D'Cruz IA, Sugathan P: Compression of right atrium by traumatic diaphragmatic hernia. Am Heart J 133:380–383, 1997.
188. Colliver C, Oller DW, Rose G, Brewer D: Traumatic intrapericardial diaphragmatic hernia diagnosed by echocardiography. J Trauma 42:115–117, 1997.
189. Gale AW, Jelihovsky T, Grant AF, et al: Neurogenic tumors of the mediastinum. Ann Thorac Surg 17:434–443, 1974.
190. Reed JC, Hallet KK, Feigin DS: Neural tumors of the thorax: Subject review from the AFIP. Radiology 126:9–17, 1978.
191. Saenz NC, Schnitzer JJ, Eraklis AE, et al: Posterior mediastinal masses. J Pediatr Surg 28:172–176, 1993.
192. Matsui I, Tanimura M, Kobayashi N, et al: Neurofibromatosis type 1 and childhood cancer. Cancer 72:2746–2754, 1993.
193. Shields TW, Reynolds M: Neurogenic tumors of the thorax. Surg Clin North Am 68:645–648, 1988.
194. Matthay KK: Neuroblastoma: A clinical challenge and biologic puzzle. CA Cancer J Clin 45:179–192, 1995.
195. Simpson I, Campbell PE: Mediastinal masses in childhood: A review from a paediatric pathologist's point of view. Prog Pediatr Surg 27:92–126, 1991.
196. Grosfeld JL, Skinner MA, Rescorla FJ, et al: Mediastinal tumors in children: Experience with 196 cases. Ann Surg Oncol 1:121–127, 1994.
197. Franks LM, Bollen A, Seeger RC, et al: Neuroblastoma in adults and adolescents: An indolent course with poor survival. Cancer 79:2028–2035, 1997.
198. Filler RM, Traggis DG, Jaffe N: Favorable outlook for children with mediastinal neuroblastoma. J Pediatr Surg 7:136–143, 1972.
199. Adams GA, Shochat SJ, Smith EI, et al: Thoracic neuroblastoma: A Pediatric Oncology Group study. J Pediatr Surg 28:372–377, 1993.
200. Morris JA, Shochat SJ, Smith EI, et al: Biological variables in thoracic neuroblastoma: A Pediatric Oncology Group study. J Pediatr Surg 30:296–302, 1995.
201. Rufini V, Fisher GA, Shulkin BL, et al: Iodine-123-MIBG imaging of neuroblastoma: Utility of SPECT and delayed imaging. J Nucl Med 37:1464–1468, 1996.
202. Katzenstein HM, Cohn SL: Advances in the diagnosis and treatment of neuroblastoma. Curr Opin Oncol 10:43–51, 1998.
203. Shapiro B, Orringer MB, Gross MD: Mediastinal paragangliomas and pheochromocytomas. *In* Shields T (ed): Mediastinal Surgery. Philadelphia: Lea & Febiger, 1991, pp 254–271.
204. Marchevsky AM, Kaneko M: Surgical Pathology of the Mediastinum. New York: Raven Press, 1984, pp 1–3.
205. Pantoja E, Kattan KR, Thomas HA: Some uncommon lower mediastinal densities. Radiol Clin North Am 22:633–646, 1984.
206. Hainsworth JD, Greco FA: Poorly differentiated carcinoma of the mediastinum. *In* Shields T (ed): Mediastinal Surgery. Philadelphia: Lea & Febiger, 1991, pp 225–227.
207. Adkins RBJ, Maples MD, Hainsworth JD: Primary malignant mediastinal tumors. Ann Thorac Surg 38:648–653, 1984.
208. Jaffe BM, Ferguson TB, Holtz S: Mediastinal pancreatic pseudocysts. Am J Surg 124:600–606, 1972.

SECTION P

# Disorders in the Control of Breathing

# 80 Hypoventilation and Hyperventilation Syndromes

ELIOT A. PHILLIPSON, M.D. • ARTHUR S. SLUTSKY, M.D.


Introduction
Hypoventilation Syndromes
- General Principles and Diagnostic Approach
- Primary Alveolar Hypoventilation
- Summary

Hyperventilation Syndromes
- Introduction
- Pathogenesis
- Physiologic and Clinical Features
- Diagnosis
- Management
- Summary


## INTRODUCTION

As outlined in Chapter 8, breathing is regulated by two anatomically distinct but functionally integrated elements referred to as the metabolic (or automatic) and the behavioral (or voluntary) respiratory control systems. The metabolic system, whose integrating neurons and motor neurons are located in the medulla and pons, is concerned primarily with acid-base balance and blood gas homeostasis. Appropriate to this function, it receives afferent input from peripheral and central chemoreceptors that are sensitive to pH, $P_{CO_2}$, and $P_{O_2}$ and from bronchopulmonary mechanoreceptors that are sensitive to the degree of lung stretch and rate of airflow. In contrast, the behavioral control system, whose neural elements originate in supramedullary and cortical structures,[1] utilizes the ventilatory apparatus for functions whose primary purpose is not gas exchange, the most notable examples being speaking and singing.

Disorders in the control of breathing can arise because of disturbances in either of these two control systems. In broad terms, defects in the behavioral system result in dysphasia, dyspraxia, or alveolar *hyper*ventilation syndromes but do not produce clinically important *hypo*ventilation syndromes.[2, 3] Rather, hypoventilation disorders arise because of either defects in the metabolic control system or defects in the respiratory neuromuscular apparatus, chest wall, lungs, or airways. Such disorders can be acute or chronic. Acute hypoventilation disturbances, which represent life-threatening emergencies, are considered in Chapters 91 to 94. This chapter deals with disturbances in respiratory control that result in chronic hypoventilation or chronic hyperventilation syndromes.

## HYPOVENTILATION SYNDROMES

### General Principles and Diagnostic Approach

#### Pathogenesis

Alveolar hypoventilation exists when arterial $P_{CO_2}$ increases above the normal range of 37 to 43 mm Hg. In clinically important hypoventilation syndromes, arterial $P_{CO_2}$ is 45 mm Hg or higher and typically ranges from 50 to 70 mm Hg.[4–7] Numerous disease entities can result in chronic alveolar hypoventilation (Table 80.1), but in all cases the underlying mechanism involves a defect in either the sensors or the integrating neurons of the metabolic respiratory control system or in the effector organs of breathing (i.e., the neuromuscular system or the ventilatory apparatus) (Table 80.2).

Defects in the metabolic control system result in hypoventilation because abnormalities in blood gases and cerebral acid-base status are not sensed or, if sensed, do not produce an appropriate change in motor output of the brain-stem respiratory neurons. Patients with such defects fail to breathe normally in response to metabolic respiratory stimuli, but because the behavioral control system, respiratory motor pathways, and ventilatory apparatus are intact, they are capable of voluntarily driving respiration. As a result, patients with defects in the metabolic control system typically demonstrate normal ventilatory mechanics, but they have impaired responses to metabolic respiratory stimuli and often hypoventilate severely during sleep, when ventilation is critically dependent on the metabolic control system.[4, 8–13] As a result of chronic hypoventilation, such patients have a primary respiratory acidosis leading to a secondary increase in extracellular bicarbonate concentration.[14, 15] In contrast, patients with a primary metabolic alkalosis may develop secondary hypoventilation as a compensatory response. This type of hypoventilation represents not a defect in respiratory control but rather an appropriate response of the metabolic control system to a disturbance in acid-base status. It can be said that patients with metabolic alkalosis "shouldn't" breathe, in contrast to those with control defects, who "won't" breathe, and those with mechanical defects, who "can't" breathe. However, the degree of hypoventilation that develops in response to metabolic alkalosis depends on several factors, including associated electrolyte disturbances and the sensitivity of the metabolic control system to the accompanying hypoxia.[16, 17] Thus, patients with weak hypoxic responsiveness tend to hypoventilate more than do patients with a brisk hypoxic responsiveness that continues to drive ventilation despite the alkalosis.

Chronic hypoventilation resulting from defects in effector elements of the respiratory system (see Table 80.2) represents disturbances of ventilatory motor and mechanical function and do not in themselves mean that the

**Table 80.2 MECHANISMS UNDERLYING CHRONIC ALVEOLAR HYPOVENTILATION**

| Mechanism Involved | Site or Type of Defect | Major Distinguishing Features |
|---|---|---|
| Sensors | Metabolic alkalosis | Alkaline pH |
| | Peripheral chemoreceptors | Impaired response to hypoxia |
| | Central chemoreceptors | Impaired response to hypercapnia |
| Controller | Brain-stem respiratory neurons or networks | Impaired chemoresponses<br>Sleep-induced hypoventilation<br>Normal ventilatory mechanics |
| Effectors | Neuromuscular apparatus | Reduced maximal respiratory pressures |
| | Ventilatory apparatus | Impaired ventilatory mechanics |

**Table 80.1 CLASSIFICATION OF DISORDERS ASSOCIATED WITH CHRONIC ALVEOLAR HYPOVENTILATION**

DISORDERS OF CHEMOSENSITIVITY
- Carotid body dysfunction, trauma[79]
- Prolonged hypoxia[80, 81]
- Metabolic alkalosis[16]

DISORDERS OF BRAIN-STEM–INTEGRATING AND RHYTHM-GENERATING NETWORKS AND BRAIN-STEM MOTOR NEURONS
- Bulbar poliomyelitis, encephalitis[40, 49–51]
- Infarction[41]
- Neoplasms[82]
- Sarcoidosis[52]
- Demyelinating disorders[53]
- Chronic drug administration[83]
- Primary alveolar hypoventilation syndrome[9, 84]

DISORDERS OF SPINAL CORD, PERIPHERAL NERVES, AND RESPIRATORY MUSCLES
- Poliomyelitis[6, 22]
- Motor neuron disease[23, 55, 56]
- Peripheral neuropathy[85]
- Myasthenia gravis[6, 24]
- Muscular dystrophy[6, 24, 61, 62]
- Chronic myopathy[6, 24, 25, 61, 62]

DISORDERS OF CHEST WALL STRUCTURE
- Obesity-hypoventilation syndrome[5]
- Kyphoscoliosis[86]
- Fibrothorax[86]
- Post-thoracoplasty[86]
- Ankylosing spondylitis[86]

DISORDERS OF LUNGS AND AIRWAYS
- Chronic obstructive pulmonary disease (Chapter 38)
- Cystic fibrosis (Chapter 40)
- Laryngeal and tracheal stenosis[87, 88]
- Obstructive sleep apnea syndrome[31, 33]

metabolic control system is defective. Because the same effector elements also serve the behavioral control system, such patients are usually unable to breathe normally even when consciously attempting to do so. Hence, such defects are characterized either by reductions in the maximum respiratory pressures that can be generated voluntarily or by impairment of lung volumes and flow rates.[7] In the presence of such neural or mechanical defects, coexisting disturbances in respiratory control are often difficult to identify, because the neuromuscular or mechanical defect may preclude normal responses to chemical respiratory stimuli even when the control system is intact.

## Physiologic and Clinical Consequences

Regardless of the underlying cause, the fundamental disturbance in all hypoventilation syndromes is a global reduction in the level of alveolar ventilation, resulting in an increase in alveolar $P_{CO_2}$ and therefore in arterial $P_{CO_2}$. Because of the inverse relationship between alveolar $P_{CO_2}$ and $P_{O_2}$ defined by the alveolar air equation, the rise in alveolar $P_{CO_2}$ produces an obligatory decrease in alveolar $P_{O_2}$, resulting in hypoxemia (Fig. 80.1). These disturbances are typically magnified during sleep because of further reductions in alveolar ventilation secondary to a reduction in overall respiratory drive (Chapter 81).

The primary disturbances produced by alveolar hypoventilation lead to a series of secondary physiologic responses that in turn produce the clinical features of chronic hypoventilation (see Fig. 80.1). These features consist predominantly of hematologic, cardiovascular, and neurologic manifestations. There is considerable debate as to whether the cardiovascular and neurologic features of hypoventilation result from the chronic hypercapnia or from the chronic hypoxemia, but it appears likely that both disturbances play a role. For example, alleviation of hypoxemia alone by the administration of supplemental oxygen reverses the polycythemia and may attenuate the severity of pulmonary hypertension, but supplemental oxygen can also aggravate the degree of hypercapnia and the severity of neurologic complaints.[7, 11, 18, 19]

## Laboratory Assessment

The investigation of the patient with chronic alveolar hypoventilation involves the use of a series of laboratory tests that examine one or more components of the respiratory system (Fig. 80.2). Analysis of the pattern of test results usually enables localization of the site of the underlying defect to the metabolic control system, the respiratory neuromuscular system, or the ventilatory apparatus.

**Defects in Metabolic Control.** The patient with a defect in the chemoreceptors or brain-stem integrating neurons and motor neurons that constitute the metabolic

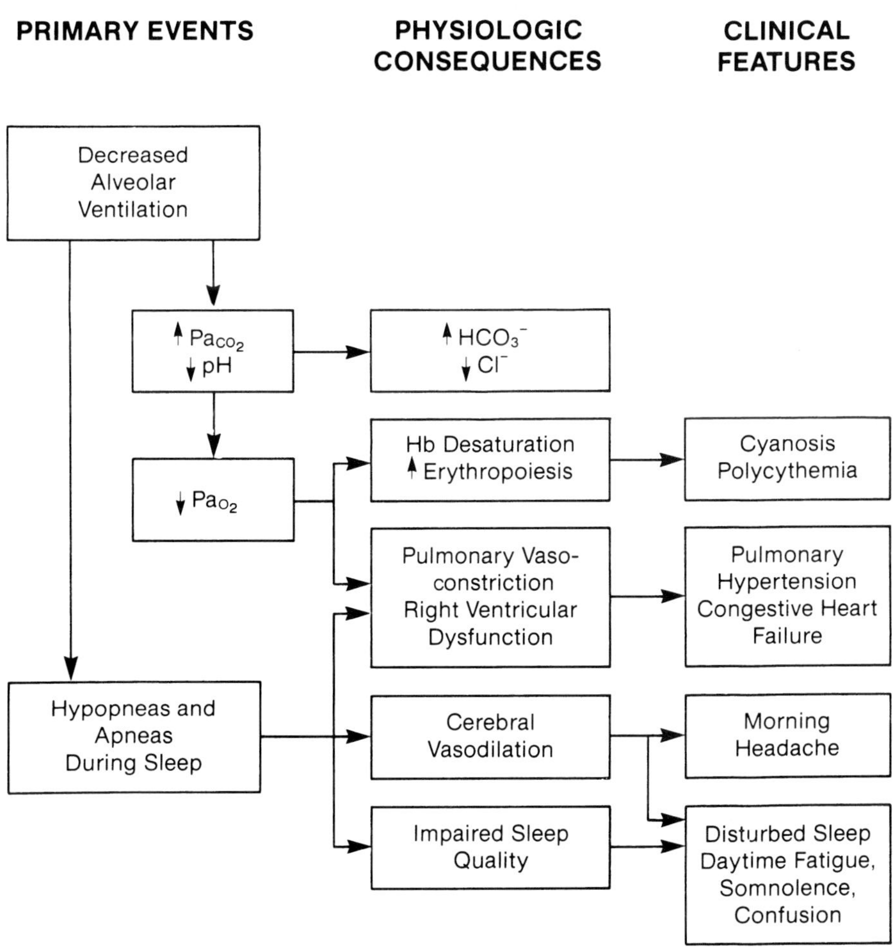


**Figure 80.1** Schema showing the primary events, physiologic responses, and clinical features resulting from alveolar hypoventilation. $Pa_{CO_2}$ = arterial $P_{CO_2}$; $Pa_{O_2}$ = arterial $P_{O_2}$.

with frequent episodes of central hypopnea or outright apnea followed by arousal or awakening. These sleep-related events presumably account for the clinical complaints of disturbed sleep and morning headache; they contribute to daytime fatigue, lethargy, and somnolence; and they play a role in the development of polycythemia and pulmonary hypertension. Support for this concept is derived from the fact that the daytime symptoms of primary alveolar hypoventilation, as well as the polycythemia and pulmonary hypertension, can be alleviated by improving nocturnal ventilation alone.[8, 11, 12]

## Differential Diagnosis

Primary alveolar hypoventilation, in which there is no other identifiable neurologic disease, must be distinguished from central alveolar hypoventilation secondary to underlying neurologic disease (see Table 80.1), although the clinical and laboratory features of the two disorders are often very similar. This distinction requires a careful neurologic history and examination for evidence of other brain-stem or autonomic disturbances. The classic example of chronic alveolar hypoventilation secondary to brain-stem disease is that which follows bulbar poliomyelitis or encephalitis.[40, 49–51] The disorder has also been reported in association with brain-stem vascular insufficiency, infections, neoplasms, sarcoidosis, multiple sclerosis, and autonomic insufficiency syndromes.[3, 41, 52, 53] These secondary causes of central alveolar hypoventilation are usually signified by the other features of the underlying disease process and by the fact that the patient may not be able to increase the level of ventilation voluntarily. A form of subacute central alveolar hypoventilation that follows cervical cordotomy for pain and that follows other forms of spinal surgery has also been described.[54]

Primary alveolar hypoventilation can be confused with chronic disorders of the respiratory neuromuscular system (Chapter 89) that are often unrecognized clinically (see Table 80.1). Increasingly common in this group of disorders is the post-polio syndrome, a form of chronic respiratory insufficiency that typically develops 20 to 30 years after recovery from poliomyelitis.[22] In addition to the history of polio many years earlier, such patients demonstrate weakness of the respiratory muscles (see Fig. 80.2), and many have developed kyphoscoliosis. Motor neuron disease, an idiopathic degeneration of motor neurons from anterior horn cells to cortex, can manifest as chronic respiratory failure, particularly when the phrenic motor neurons are involved.[23, 55, 56] The disease typically occurs in men aged 50 to 70 years and is distinguished from primary alveolar hypoventilation by the presence of muscle weakness and atrophy, often with fasciculation and spasticity. Laboratory investigation reveals a pattern of test results typical of respiratory neuromuscular disease (see Fig. 80.2). Furthermore, the abnormalities are progressive, as is the clinical course of the disease; death, from respiratory complications, usually occurs 2 to 5 years after onset of the disease.

Unilateral diaphragmatic paralysis can result from phrenic nerve trauma, inflammation, or neoplastic infiltration, but in most cases the cause is unknown.[57–60] Patients with unilateral diaphragmatic paralysis are often asymptomatic and do not usually hypoventilate. Bilateral diaphragm weakness or paralysis can result from phrenic neuropathy or from intrinsic diaphragmatic disease, including muscular dystrophies, polymyositis, and acid-maltase deficiency.[6, 24, 25, 61–63] Bilateral diaphragmatic disease may lead to severe chronic alveolar hypoventilation. Distinguishing features include the presence of orthopnea, paradoxical movement of the abdomen in the supine posture, deterioration in lung volumes and in arterial blood gas values in the supine posture, rapid deterioration in ventilation during a maximum voluntary ventilation maneuver, and reduction of the maximum inspiratory pressures that can be generated against an occluded airway. Transdiaphragmatic pressures, calculated from simultaneous measurement of esophageal and gastric pressures, are reduced or absent, and the EMG response of the diaphragm, recorded by an esophageal electrode, reveals a reduction in diaphragm discharge in response to transcutaneous phrenic nerve stimulation in the neck.[6, 63–65]

## Management

Patients with primary alveolar hypoventilation must be cautioned against the use of sedative medications, which may readily induce acute respiratory failure. Respiratory stimulants may be useful in some patients. Several pharmacologic agents, including methylxanthines and analeptics, have been used to treat patients with primary alveolar hypoventilation (Table 80.3), with variable but generally disappointing results. Long-term administration of progesterone has been beneficial in some patients, particularly those with mechanical ventilatory defects and an element of reduced respiratory drive, such as the obesity-hypoventilation syndrome and hypercapnic obstructive lung disease.[66–68] Acetazolamide is effective in increasing respiratory drive in patients with primary metabolic alkalosis superimposed on chronic carbon dioxide retention[69] but is not indicated in pure respiratory acidosis. A few patients with primary alveolar hypoventilation have responded favorably to long-term nocturnal oxygen administration, which suggests that cerebral hypoxia during sleep was aggravating the hypoventilation disorder.[12, 19] In the majority of patients, however, supplemental oxygen aggravates the degree of nocturnal hypoventilation and further increases arterial carbon dioxide levels by removing hypoxic ventilatory drive.

In most patients with primary alveolar hypoventilation or neuromuscular disease, mechanical ventilatory assistance is required for effective management (see Table

**Table 80.3 MANAGEMENT OF PRIMARY ALVEOLAR HYPOVENTILATION**

| | |
|---|---|
| Pharmacologic techniques | Respiratory stimulants (progesterone, acetazolamide) |
| | Supplemental oxygen |
| Mechanical techniques | Rocking bed |
| | Negative-pressure ventilator |
| | Positive-pressure ventilator |
| | Phrenic nerve stimulation |

80.3). Some patients respond favorably to a rocking bed,[7, 18] but most require negative-pressure ventilation in a tank or cuirass,[6, 32, 55, 56, 70, 71] positive-pressure ventilation through a tracheostomy or nose mask,[7, 70, 72–76] or diaphragmatic pacing by electrophrenic stimulation.[8, 77, 78] In most patients, the administration of such treatment only during sleep produces dramatic clinical improvement, with alleviation of daytime symptoms, reversal of polycythemia and pulmonary hypertension, and lowering of daytime arterial $P_{CO_2}$ values.

## Summary

Alveolar hypoventilation can result from numerous disease entities but is ultimately attributable to defects in the metabolic respiratory control system, the respiratory neuromuscular system, or the ventilatory apparatus. Detailed clinical and laboratory investigations can generally distinguish among these underlying mechanisms and locate the site of the defect. In most patients, alveolar hypoventilation is secondary to obstructive airway disease, mechanical chest wall disturbances, neurologic disease affecting the brain stem or spinal cord, or respiratory muscle weakness. In a small percentage of cases, no underlying cause can be found, and such patients are said to have primary alveolar hypoventilation, which is considered to represent failure of the metabolic respiratory control system. Patients with primary alveolar hypoventilation are able to hyperventilate voluntarily, but during sleep, hypoventilation becomes more severe and central apneas are common. Management of patients with primary alveolar hypoventilation, as well as those with respiratory neuromuscular disorders, usually involves mechanical ventilatory assistance. Administration of such treatment only during sleep often produces dramatic clinical improvement and alleviates daytime symptoms.

# HYPERVENTILATION SYNDROMES

## Introduction

*Hyperventilation* refers to an increase in the rate of alveolar ventilation that is excessive for the rate of metabolic carbon dioxide production, resulting in a decrease in arterial $P_{CO_2}$ to below the normal range of 37 to 43 mm Hg. Hyperventilation should be distinguished from *tachypnea*, an increase in respiratory frequency, and from *hyperpnea*, an increase in minute volume of ventilation. Neither of these conditions derives from nor implies a change in arterial $P_{CO_2}$. Hyperventilation is often associated with dyspnea, but not all patients with hyperventilation complain of shortness of breath; conversely, patients with dyspnea need not be hyperventilating.

## Pathogenesis

Alveolar hyperventilation arises from excessive ventilatory drive that is mediated through either the behavioral or metabolic control systems (Fig. 80.3). Many pathophysiologic conditions and diseases can result in an increase in respiratory drive (Table 80.4). In some cases, the mechanism involved is well understood (e.g., hypoxemic activation of the peripheral chemoreceptors); in other cases, several potential mechanisms have been postulated but as yet have not been clearly established (e.g., hyperventilation associated with hepatic failure). Therefore, hyperventilation syndromes are best considered through the use of a clinical rather than mechanistic approach (see Table 80.4).

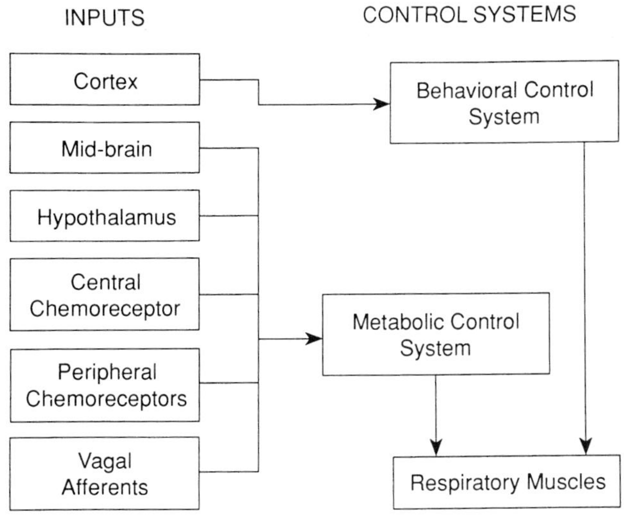


**Figure 80.3** Schematic diagram showing the mechanisms involved in alveolar hyperventilation.

## Hypoxemia

In most clinical settings, hypoxemia is a potent ventilatory stimulus and results in hyperventilation by virtue of its action on the peripheral chemoreceptors (i.e., the carotid bodies; see Chapter 8). The response of minute volume of ventilation (or alveolar ventilation) to decreases in arterial $P_{O_2}$ is not linear: it is substantially greater when arterial $P_{O_2}$ falls below 60 mm Hg.[89] In contrast, although the oxygen content per se of arterial blood is not the primary hypoxic stimulus of the carotid bodies, the ventilatory response to hypoxemia is relatively linear with regard to decreases in arterial oxygen saturation.[89, 90] However, the magnitude of response is attenuated by reduced levels of arterial $P_{CO_2}$ and increased levels of arterial pH.[91] The hyperventilation associated with hypoxia can be dramatic, particularly in persons with normal ventilatory mechanics. For example, at the summit of Mount Everest, where arterial $P_{O_2}$ was estimated to be 27 mm Hg, alveolar $P_{CO_2}$ was reduced to 7.5 mm Hg.[92, 93] Clinically, however, impaired mechanical properties of the chest wall or lungs often attenuate the degree of alveolar hyperventilation induced by hypoxia. Conversely, in many pulmonary disorders that produce hypoxemia, the associated hypocapnia may not be due to the hypoxia and persists even when the hypoxia is alleviated with supplemental oxygen.[94]

The degree of alveolar hyperventilation induced by hypoxia is highly variable; the variation is determined, at least in part, by genetic factors.[95] In addition, there also appears to be a temporal influence that may, in part,

**Table 80.4 HYPERVENTILATION SYNDROMES**

| |
|---|
| **Hypoxemia** |
| High altitude |
| Pulmonary disease |
| Cardiac shunts |
| **Pulmonary Disorders** |
| Pneumonia |
| Interstitial pneumonitis, fibrosis, and edema |
| Pulmonary embolic or vascular disease |
| Bronchial asthma |
| Pneumothorax |
| Chest wall disorders |
| **Cardiovascular Disorders** |
| Congestive heart failure |
| Hypotension |
| **Metabolic Disorders** |
| Acidosis (diabetic, renal, lactic) |
| Hepatic failure |
| **Neurologic and Psychogenic Disorders** |
| Psychogenic or anxiety hyperventilation |
| Central nervous system infection, tumors |
| **Drug-Induced** |
| Salicylates |
| Methylxanthine derivatives |
| Beta-adrenergic agonists |
| Progesterone |
| **Miscellaneous** |
| Fever, sepsis |
| Pain |
| Pregnancy |

From Phillipson EA: Disorders of ventilation. *In* Fauci AS, Braunwald E, Isselbacher KJ, et al (eds): Harrison's Principles of Internal Medicine (14th ed). New York: McGraw-Hill, 1998, pp 1476–1480.

reflect the effects of hypoxia on cerebral blood flow, metabolism, and release of excitatory and inhibitory neuromodulators, all of which secondarily affect breathing.[96–98] Typically, the ventilatory response to acute hypoxia is initially brisk but then decreases after several minutes,[99, 100] only to increase again after 12 to 24 hours as the longer term process of respiratory acclimatization comes into play (see Chapters 8 and 70). However sustained hypoxemia of many years' duration, as occurs in long-time residents at high altitudes and in patients with cyanotic congenital heart disease, is associated with considerable attenuation of hypoxic ventilatory drive.[101–103]

## Pulmonary Disorders

One of the most common causes of hyperventilation in patients with pulmonary disease is stimulation of bronchopulmonary receptors that reflexly increase ventilatory drive and, directly or indirectly, contribute to the sensation of dyspnea (see Chapter 20). These receptors, which are sensitive to a variety of mechanical and chemical stimuli, send impulses to the central nervous system through the afferent vagus nerves, resulting in cough, bronchoconstriction, and hyperventilation.[104] Direct evidence implicating these receptors in the alveolar hyperventilation of lung disease is derived largely from animal studies,[105, 106] but there are also supportive studies in a few patients who have undergone vagal blockade.[107] Indirect support for this notion is derived from the fact that administration of supplemental oxygen to patients with hypoxemic interstitial or pulmonary vascular disease does not necessarily abolish the hyperventilation.[94, 108–110]

Stimulation of chest-wall receptors may contribute to the hyperventilation that accompanies asthma, pulmonary fibrosis, and restrictive chest wall disorders.[105, 111] The mechanisms involved have not been clearly established but are thought to include stimulation of respiratory muscle spindles and other chest-wall receptors. The same mechanisms may also play a role in the pathogenesis of dyspnea in these disorders.[110–112]

## Cardiovascular Disorders

Patients with congestive heart failure and states of low cardiac output typically hyperventilate at rest, during exercise, and even during sleep.[113–117] The mechanisms involved probably include stimulation of pulmonary vascular and interstitial receptors as a result of pulmonary congestion.[104, 118] In addition, low cardiac output states and hypotension stimulate breathing through the arterial baroreceptors[119] and may also stimulate breathing secondary to "stagnant hypoxia" of the carotid body chemoreceptor cells, which normally have a high rate of blood flow in proportion to metabolism.[91]

## Metabolic Disorders

Alveolar hyperventilation is a well-described compensatory response to metabolic acidosis. Although respiratory compensation is generally effective, physiologic compensation for metabolic acidosis is not complete. For example, in a severe metabolic acidosis that reduces serum bicarbonate levels to 8 mEq/L, the uncompensated arterial pH would be 6.92; with hyperventilation to 20 mm Hg (a typical response), pH increases to 7.22. The degree of compensation varies among patients, depending on differences in chemosensitivity and ventilatory mechanics, but in general a decrease in $[HCO_3^-]$ of 1 mEq/L results in a compensatory decrease in arterial $P_{CO_2}$ of about 1 mm Hg.[120, 121] The specific mechanisms involved in the hyperventilation of metabolic acidosis are controversial, but they probably include stimulation of both the peripheral and central chemoreceptors.[92, 122–128] Metabolic acidosis also increases the sensitivity of the peripheral chemoreceptors to hypoxia.[91]

Hyperventilation is a common feature in patients with severe liver disease.[129, 130] Several possible mechanisms have been proposed, including increased blood levels of progesterone, ammonia, and vasoactive intestinal peptide and increased brain levels of ammonia and glutamine, all of which may stimulate respiration.[98, 129, 130] In addition, patients with severe hepatocellular dysfunction or portal hypertension may develop small pulmonary arteriovenous anastomoses ("spider nevi" of the lungs) or portal-pulmonary venous shunts, resulting in hypoxemia and hyperventilation due to stimulation of the peripheral chemoreceptors.

### Neurologic and Psychogenic Disorders

Psychogenic hyperventilation[131–133] is thought to arise from anxiety or stress, both of which act on the behavioral respiratory control system (see Fig. 80.3). In support of this mechanism is the fact that this type of hyperventilation typically abates during sleep, when the behavioral control system is quiescent and breathing is driven by the metabolic system.[48, 133] Apart from psychogenic causes, central neurogenic hyperventilation is relatively rare.[3] Indeed, in most patients with intracranial disturbances who are hyperventilating, the immediate cause is either pulmonary edema or hypoxemia.[134, 135] In rare cases, however, disorders of the midbrain and hypothalamus induce hyperventilation.[3] In addition, patients with head trauma or intracranial hemorrhage may hyperventilate as a secondary reaction to red blood cell glycolysis and acidosis in the cerebrospinal fluid, and patients with brain-stem infiltration by tumor may hyperventilate as a result of lactic acidosis produced by the malignant cells.[134, 136–138] In other rare cases, severe cerebrovascular insufficiency is associated with hyperventilation, possibly by interference with the inhibitory influence normally exerted by cortical structures on the brain-stem respiratory neurons.[139, 140]

### Drug-Induced Hyperventilation

Several drugs cause hyperventilation[141] by stimulating the peripheral or central chemoreceptors or by direct action on the brain-stem respiratory neurons (see Table 80.4). The acid-base disturbance resulting from salicylate overdose is biphasic, consisting of an initial primary respiratory alkalosis followed by a metabolic acidosis that induces secondary hyperventilation.[142, 143]

### Miscellaneous Causes

Fever and sepsis, even in the absence of hypotension, are commonly associated with hyperventilation, over and above any associated increase in metabolic rate.[144–146] The mechanisms involved are not clear, but they could include either carotid body or hypothalamic stimulation by increased temperature. Pain is also frequently accompanied by hyperventilation.[147] The mechanisms involved may include adrenergic stimulation of the peripheral and central chemoreceptors.[91, 148, 149] In addition, painful stimuli may act through the behavioral control system. From a practical clinical standpoint, there is often concern that a painful arterial puncture required for blood gas assessment could result in a spuriously low arterial $P_{CO_2}$ and inappropriate diagnosis of hyperventilation. However, there is little difference in arterial $P_{CO_2}$ between samples obtained with and without the use of local anesthetic.[150] Chronic hyperventilation is a normal feature of pregnancy and of the luteal phase of the menstrual cycle[151] and may result from the effects of progesterone (and perhaps other hormones) acting directly on the brain-stem respiratory neurons.[152, 153]

## Physiologic and Clinical Features

### Respiratory

Because hyperventilation involves an increase in respiratory drive, respiratory muscle effort, and minute volume of ventilation, the most frequent symptom associated with hyperventilation is dyspnea. However, there is considerable discrepancy between the degree of hyperventilation, as assessed by arterial $P_{CO_2}$, and the degree of dyspnea.

From a physiologic standpoint, hyperventilation is clearly beneficial in patients who are hypoxemic because the alveolar hypocapnia is associated with an increase in alveolar $P_{O_2}$ and with a varied increase in arterial $P_{O_2}$ (dependent on pulmonary ventilation-perfusion inhomogeneities). The relationship among these variables is governed by the alveolar air equation (see Chapter 4). This physiologic consequence of hyperventilation is clinically important in patients with hypoxemic pulmonary disease and in healthy persons at high altitude. Indeed, the successful ascent of Mount Everest without the use of supplemental oxygen was critically dependent on the increase in alveolar and arterial $P_{O_2}$ generated by profound alveolar hyperventilation.[92, 93]

Conversely, alveolar hyperventilation can also have detrimental respiratory effects, including a decrease in or loss of respiratory drive immediately after cessation of the hyperventilation, secondary to the low arterial and cerebral $P_{CO_2}$. Under these conditions, hypoxemia can develop quickly without an associated return of respiratory drive or a sensation of dyspnea, because of the persisting hypocapnia that reverses at a considerably slower rate. This sequence of events has been implicated in the deaths of healthy underwater divers who, in advance of diving, voluntarily hyperventilate to decrease alveolar $P_{CO_2}$ and increase alveolar oxygen stores, and thereby prolong underwater breath-holding time. A less dramatic but more common clinical problem resulting from hyperventilation during wakefulness is periodic breathing during sleep, with or without associated central sleep apnea. This sequence of events gives rise to the most common type of central sleep apnea syndrome (see Chapter 81).

### Blood

Respiratory alkalosis produces a leftward shift in the oxygen-hemoglobin dissociation curve (the Bohr effect), which increases loading of oxygen onto hemoglobin in the lungs but decreases release of oxygen at the tissue level. This change can be beneficial or detrimental, depending on the specific conditions. In general, the detrimental effects of impaired oxygen release at the tissues outweigh the beneficial effects of increased oxygen loading in the lungs, because even under conditions of moderate hypoxemia, hemoglobin is well saturated with oxygen without a leftward shift of the dissociation curve (e.g., at an arterial $P_{O_2}$ of 60 mm Hg, hemoglobin is 90% saturated). However, under conditions of severe hypoxia, as at very high altitudes or in utero, the loading of oxygen onto hemoglobin becomes critical to survival, and therefore a respiratory alkalosis and the resulting leftward shift of the dissociation curve can be beneficial.

Respiratory alkalosis also results in several electrolyte shifts that are clinically important, including hypokalemia, hypophosphatemia, and decreased ionizable calcium.[154–157] These shifts contribute to many of the clinical features of hyperventilation, including dizziness, peripheral paresthesias, carpopedal spasm, tetany, and muscle weakness.

### Cardiovascular and Cerebrovascular

The most important clinical consequences of alveolar hyperventilation are those related to vasoconstriction, that is secondary to alkalemia.[158–162] Severe alkalemia can induce cardiac arrhythmias (possibly related to electrolyte disturbances) and cardiac ischemia, which probably results from both the acute coronary vasoconstriction and the increased oxygen affinity of hemoglobin.[160, 162] Alkalemia also induces intense cerebrovascular constriction that can result in dizziness, visual impairment, syncope, and seizures.[96, 132, 163] Acutely, every 1–mm Hg decrease in arterial $P_{CO_2}$ reduces cerebral blood flow by 2%,[164] resulting in cerebral hypoxia, as assessed by metabolic, electroencephalographic, and corneoretinal indices and by direct measurements of cerebral $P_{O_2}$.[165–169] In patients with sickle-cell disease, the degree of cerebral hypoxia may be sufficient to induce red blood cell sickling and cerebral infarction.[170] In general, the severity of cerebral vasoconstriction induced by hyperventilation decreases within hours, as the degree of cerebral alkalosis is attenuated.[132, 171]

## Diagnosis

Although hyperventilation may be suspected clinically in the presence of tachypnea or noticeable hyperpnea, the diagnosis can be confirmed only by analysis of arterial blood gases and pH. The key measurements are the arterial $P_{CO_2}$, a decrease which indicates the presence of hyperventilation, and the pH, which determines whether the disorder is classified as a primary respiratory alkalosis (increased pH) or a primary metabolic acidosis (decreased pH).[120, 121] However, in mixed acid-base disorders, arterial pH may not be alkalemic despite primary alveolar hyperventilation. Measurement of arterial $P_{O_2}$ and calculation of the alveolar-arterial $P_{O_2}$ difference $(A - a)P_{O_2}$ is also helpful, because a widened $(A - a)P_{O_2}$ suggests a pulmonary disorder as the underlying cause of the hyperventilation. The finding of a decreased serum bicarbonate concentration establishes the chronic nature of the disorder and points to an organic cause, as opposed to psychogenic hyperventilation. In patients with suspected psychogenic hyperventilation, measurements of minute volume of ventilation and of arterial or transcutaneous $P_{CO_2}$ during sleep can be useful because the hyperventilation does not usually persist during sleep.

Once the presence of alveolar hyperventilation has been established, the underlying cause can generally be identified on the basis of history, physical examination, and knowledge of coexisting medical disorders (see Table 80.4). Two disorders may not be readily apparent clinically and frequently give rise to "unexplained hyperventilation": pulmonary vascular disease (particularly chronic or recurrent thromboembolism) and psychogenic or anxiety hyperventilation.[132] However, the two disorders can usually be identified and distinguished on the basis of clinical and laboratory features. Hyperventilation secondary to pulmonary vascular disease is invariably accompanied by exertional dyspnea and often by exertional presyncope and clinical signs of pulmonary arterial hypertension. In addition, such patients usually have a widened $(A - a)P_{O_2}$, often have a reduced pulmonary diffusing capacity for carbon monoxide, and usually maintain their hyperventilation during exercise. In contrast, patients with psychogenic hyperventilation typically complain of the need to sigh frequently and of dyspnea at rest and not necessarily during exercise.[133, 172] Symptoms of acute hyperventilation, including paresthesias, carpopedal spasm, and tetany, are frequent, and anxiety is often prominent.[172] Half the patients present with cardiovascular symptoms, including palpitation, tachycardia, and chest pain, and about 25% present with neurologic complaints, including lightheadedness, headache, or memory impairment.[132, 172] In contrast to pulmonary vascular disease, in psychogenic hyperventilation the $(A - a)\ P_{O_2}$ and pulmonary function tests yield normal results, and during mild-to-moderate exercise, the hyperventilation tends to disappear. However, during exercise, heart rate and cardiac output may be high in relation to metabolic rate.

## Management

Alveolar hyperventilation can usually be managed by appropriate treatment of the underlying cause (see Table 80.4). However, in the few patients in whom alkalemia is thought to be inducing acute cerebral vasoconstriction, cardiac arrhythmias or ischemia, or paresthesias and tetany, inhalation of a low concentration of carbon dioxide can provide relief.

The long-term management of patients with disabling psychogenic hyperventilation can be problematic. Careful explanation of the basis of the symptoms is helpful and reassures the patient that no serious cardiac or cerebral disorder is present. Such reassurance is often sufficient to allay the patient's anxiety. If not, more intense psychotherapy or medications that relieve anxiety may be required.[135, 173, 174] Some patients have responded well to beta-adrenergic antagonists or to an exercise program.[149, 175]

## Summary

Hyperventilation can result from several diseases that produce an increase in respiratory drive, including disorders associated with hypoxemia, pulmonary vascular and interstitial disease, congestive heart failure, metabolic acidosis, intracranial disorders, anxiety, and drugs. Patients who are hyperventilating may complain of dyspnea, but there is often a considerable discrepancy between the degree of hyperventilation, as assessed by arterial $P_{CO_2}$, and the degree of dyspnea. Hyperventilation may produce important secondary effects on respiratory drive, on the unloading of oxygen from hemoglobin at the tissue level, and on cardiac and cerebral function. The underlying cause of hyperventilation can often be identified by the associated clinical features and measurements of arterial blood gases, pH, bicarbonate, and the alveolar-arterial $Po_2$ difference. The two disorders that most frequently give rise to "unexplained hyperventilation" are pulmonary vascular disease and anxiety, or psychogenic hyperventilation. Treatment of hyperventilation is generally directed at the underlying disorder.

## References


1. Murphy K, Corfield DR, Guz A, et al: Cerebral areas associated with motor control of speech in humans. J Appl Physiol 83:1438–1447, 1997.
2. Plum F: Neurological integration of behavioural and metabolic control of breathing. *In* Porter R (ed): Breathing: Hering-Breuer Centenary Symposium. London: Churchill, 1970, pp 159–181.
3. Plum F, Leigh RJ: Abnormalities of central mechanisms. *In* Hornbein TF (ed): Regulation of Breathing (Part 2). Vol 17: Lung Biology in Health and Disease. New York: Marcel Dekker, 1981, pp 989–1067.
4. Mellins RB, Balfour HH Jr, Turino GM, et al: Failure of automatic control of ventilation (Ondine's curse). Medicine 49:487–504, 1970.
5. Rochester DF, Enson Y: Current concepts in the pathogenesis of the obesity-hypoventilation syndrome. Am J Med 57:402–420, 1974.
6. Newsom Davis J, Goldman M, Loh L, et al: Diaphragm function and alveolar hypoventilation. Q J Med 45:87–100, 1976.
7. Goldstein RS: Hypoventilation: Neuromuscular and chest wall disorders. Clin Chest Med 13:507–521, 1992.
8. Hyland RH, Jones NL, Powles ACP, et al: Primary alveolar hypoventilation treated with nocturnal electrophrenic respiration. Am Rev Respir Dis 117:165–172, 1978.
9. Rodman T, Close HP: The primary hypoventilation syndrome. Am J Med 26:808–817, 1959.
10. Rhoads GG, Brody JS: Idiopathic alveolar hypoventilation: Clinical spectrum. Ann Intern Med 71:271–278, 1969.
11. Hyland RH, Hutcheon MA, Perl A, et al: Upper airway occlusion induced by diaphragm pacing for primary alveolar hypoventilation: Implications for the pathogenesis of obstructive sleep apnea. Am Rev Respir Dis 124:180–185, 1981.
12. McNicholas WT, Carter JL, Rutherford R, et al: Beneficial effect of oxygen in primary alveolar hypoventilation with central sleep apnea. Am Rev Respir Dis 125:773–775, 1982.
13. Gozal D, Marcus CL, Shoseyof D, et al: Peripheral chemoreceptor function in children with the congenital hypoventilation syndrome. J Appl Physiol 74:379–387, 1993.
14. Schwartz WB, Brackett NC Jr, Cohen JJ: The response of extracellular hydrogen ion concentration to graded degrees of chronic hypercapnia: The physiologic limits of the defense of pH. J Clin Invest 44:291–301, 1965.
15. Goldring RM, Turino GM, Heinemann HO: Respiratory-renal adjustments in chronic hypercapnia in man. Am J Med 51:772–784, 1971.
16. Goldring RM, Cannon PJ, Heinemann HO, et al: Respiratory adjustment to chronic metabolic alkalosis in man. J Clin Invest 47:188–202, 1968.
17. Heinemann HO, Goldring RM: Bicarbonate and the regulation of ventilation. Am J Med 57:361–370, 1974.
18. Barlow PB, Bartlett D Jr, Hauri P, et al: Idiopathic hypoventilation syndrome: Importance of preventing nocturnal hypoxemia and hypercapnia. Am Rev Respir Dis 121:141–145, 1980.
19. Bubis MJ, Anthonisen NR: Primary alveolar hypoventilation treated by nocturnal administration of $O_2$. Am Rev Respir Dis 118:947–953, 1978.
20. Farmer WC, Glenn WWL, Gee JBL: Alveolar hypoventilation syndrome: Studies of ventilatory control in patients selected for diaphragm pacing. Am J Med 64:39–49, 1978.
21. Bradley TD, Phillipson EA: Central sleep apnea. Clin Chest Med 13:493–505, 1992.
22. Lane DJ, Hazleman B, Nicholas PJR: Late onset respiratory failure in patients with previous poliomyelitis. Q J Med 43:551–568, 1974.
23. Gupta RG: Respiratory dysfunction in motor neuron disease. *In* Weiner WJ (ed): Respiratory Dysfunction in Neurologic Disease. Mount Kisco, NY: Futura, 1980, pp 71–81.
24. Gibson GJ, Pride NB, Newsom Davis J, et al: Pulmonary mechanics in patients with respiratory muscle weakness. Am Rev Respir Dis 115:389–395, 1977.
25. Rosenow EC III, Engel AG: Acid maltase deficiency in adults presenting as respiratory failure. Am J Med 64:485–491, 1978.
26. Black LF, Hyatt RE: Maximal respiratory pressures: Normal values, and relationship to age and sex. Am Rev Respir Dis 99:696–701, 1969.
27. Whitelaw WA, Derenne JP, Milic-Emili J: Occlusion pressure as a measure of respiratory center output in conscious man. Respir Physiol 23:181–199, 1975.
28. Altose MD, McCauley WC, Kelsen SG, et al: Effects of hypercapnia and inspiratory flow-resistive loading on respiratory activity in chronic airways obstruction. J Clin Invest 59:500–507, 1977.
29. Gelb AF, Klein E, Schiffman P, et al: Ventilatory response and drive in acute and chronic obstructive pulmonary disease. Am Rev Respir Dis 116:9–16, 1977.
30. Lourenco RV, Miranda JM: Drive and performance of the ventilatory apparatus in chronic obstructive lung disease. N Engl J Med 279:53–59, 1968.
31. Park SS: Respiratory control in chronic obstructive pulmonary diseases. Clin Chest Med 1:73–84, 1980.
32. Riley DJ, Santiago TV, Daniele RP, et al: Blunted respiratory drive in congenital myopathy. Am J Med 63:459–466, 1977.
33. Bradley TD, Rutherford R, Lue F, et al: Role of diffuse airway obstruction in the hypercapnia of obstructive sleep apnea. Am Rev Respir Dis 134:920–924, 1986.
34. Lopata M, Onal E: Mass loading, sleep apnea, and the pathogenesis of obesity hypoventilation. Am Rev Respir Dis 126:640–645, 1982.
35. Rapoport DM, Garay SM, Epstein H, et al: Hypercapnia in the obstructive sleep apnea syndrome: A reevaluation of the "Pickwickian syndrome." Chest 89:627–635, 1986.
36. Mountain R, Zwillich C, Weil J: Hypoventilation in obstructive lung disease: The role of familial factors. N Engl J Med 298:521–525, 1978.
37. Schiffman PL, Westlake RE, Santiago TV, et al: Ventilatory control in parents of victims of sudden-infant-death syndrome. N Engl J Med 302:486–491, 1980.
38. Tankersley CG, Fitzgerald RS, Levitt RC, et al: Genetic control of differential baseline breathing pattern. J Appl Physiol 82:874–881, 1997.
39. O'Donnell CP, Schaub CD, Haines AS, et al: Leptin prevents respiratory depression in obesity. Am J Respir Crit Care Med 159:1477–1484, 1999.
40. Plum F, Swanson AG: Abnormalities in central regulation of respiration in acute and chronic convalescent poliomyelitis. Arch Neurol Psychiatr 80:267–285, 1958.
41. Devereaux MW, Keane JR, Davis RL: Automatic respiratory failure associated with infarction of the medulla. Arch Neurol 29:46–52, 1973.
42. Baker AB, Matzke HA, Brown JR: Poliomyelitis: III. Bulbar poliomyelitis: A study of medullary function. Arch Neurol Psychiatr 63:257–281, 1950.
43. Levin BE, Margolis G: Acute failure of automatic respirations secondary to a unilateral brainstem infarct. Ann Neurol 1:583–586, 1977.
44. Bannister R, Gibson W, Michaels L, et al: Laryngeal abductor paralysis in multiple system atrophy. Brain 104:351–368, 1981.
45. Cole S, Lindenberg LB, Galioto FM Jr, et al: Ultrastructural abnormalities of the carotid body in sudden infant death syndrome. Pediatrics 63:13–17, 1979.
46. Bowes G, Andrey S, Kozar L, et al: Effect of chronic carotid body denervation on respiratory drive and stability in sleeping dogs. Am Rev Respir Dis 129(Suppl):A244, 1984.
47. Moore GC, Zwillich CW, Battaglia JD, et al: Respiratory failure associated with familial depression of ventilatory response to hypoxia and hypercapnia. N Engl J Med 295:861–865, 1976.
48. Phillipson EA, Bowes G: Control of breathing during sleep. *In* Cherniack NS, Widdicombe JG (eds): Handbook of Physiology. Section 3: The Respiratory System (Part II). Vol 2: Control of

Breathing. Bethesda, MD: American Physiological Society, 1986, pp 649–689.

48a. Shea SA: Life without ventilatory chemosensitivity. Respir Physiol 110:199–210, 1997.

49. Garlind T, Linderholm H: Hypoventilation syndrome in a case of chronic epidemic encephalitis. Acta Med Scand 162:333–349, 1958.

50. Cohn JE, Kuida H: Primary alveolar hypoventilation associated with western equine encephalitis. Ann Intern Med 56:633–644, 1962.

51. Solliday NH, Gaensler EA, Schwaber JR, et al: Impaired central chemoreceptor function and chronic hypoventilation many years following poliomyelitis. Respiration 31:177–192, 1974.

52. Daum JJ, Canter HG, Katz S: Central nervous system sarcoidosis with alveolar hypoventilation. Am J Med 38:893–898, 1965.

53. Bloor JW, Johnson RJ, Canales L, et al: Reversible paralysis of automatic respiration in multiple sclerosis. Arch Neurol 34:686–689, 1977.

54. Krieger AJ, Rosomoff HL: Sleep-induced apnea: I. A respiratory and autonomic dysfunction syndrome following bilateral percutaneous cervical cordotomy. J Neurosurg 39:168–180, 1974.

55. Sivak ED, Streib EW: Management of hypoventilation in motor neuron disease presenting with respiratory insufficiency. Ann Neurol 7:188–191, 1980.

56. Thorpy MJ, Schmidt-Nowara WW, Pollak CP, et al: Sleep-induced nonobstructive hypoventilation associated with diaphragmatic paralysis. Ann Neurol 12:308–311, 1982.

57. Arborelius M Jr, Lilja B, Senyk J: Regional and total lung function studies in patients with hemidiaphragmatic paralysis. Respiration 32:253–264, 1975.

58. Ridyard JB, Stewart RM: Regional lung function in unilateral diaphragmatic paralysis. Thorax 31:438–442, 1976.

59. Easton PA, Fleetham JA, De La Rocha A, et al: Respiratory function after paralysis of the right hemidiaphragm. Am Rev Respir Dis 127:125–128, 1983.

60. Riley EA: Idiopathic diaphragmatic paralysis. Am J Med 32:404–416, 1962.

61. Inkley SR, Oldenburg FC, Vignos PJ Jr: Pulmonary function in Duchenne muscular dystrophy related to stage of disease. Am J Med 56:297–306, 1974.

62. Coccagna G, Mantovani M, Parchi C, et al: Alveolar hypoventilation and hypersomnia in myotonic dystrophy. J Neurol Neurosurg Psychiatr 38:977–984, 1975.

63. Derenne JP, Macklem PT, Roussos C: The respiratory muscles: Mechanics, control, and pathophysiology, Part III. Am Rev Respir Dis 118:581–601, 1978.

64. Newsom Davis J: Phrenic nerve conduction in man. J Neurol Neurosurg Psychiatr 30:420–426, 1967.

65. Loh L, Goldman M, Newsom Davis J: The assessment of diaphragm function. Medicine 56:165–169, 1977.

66. Lyons HA, Hwang CT: Therapeutic use of progesterone in alveolar hypoventilation associated with obesity. Am J Med 44:881–888, 1968.

67. Sutton FD Jr, Zwillich CW, Creagh CE, et al: Progesterone for outpatient treatment of Pickwickian syndrome. Ann Intern Med 83:476–479, 1975.

68. Skatrud JB, Dempsey JA, Bhansali P, et al: Determinants of chronic carbon dioxide retention and its correction in humans. J Clin Invest 65:813–821, 1980.

69. Bear R, Goldstein M, Phillipson E, et al: Effect of metabolic alkalosis on respiratory function in patients with chronic obstructive lung disease. Can Med Assoc J 117:900–903, 1977.

70. Garay SM, Turino GM, Goldring RM: Sustained reversal of chronic hypercapnia in patients with alveolar hypoventilation syndromes. Long term maintenance with noninvasive nocturnal mechanical ventilation. Am J Med 70:269–274, 1981.

71. Goldstein RS, Molotiu N, Skrastins R, et al: Reversal of sleep-induced hypoventilation and chronic respiratory failure by nocturnal negative pressure ventilation in patients with restrictive ventilatory impairment. Am Rev Respir Dis 135:1049–1055, 1987.

72. Hoeppner VH, Cockcroft DW, Dosman JA, et al: Nighttime ventilation improves respiratory failure in secondary kyphoscoliosis. Am Rev Respir Dis 129:240–243, 1984.

73. Ellis ER, Bye PTP, Bruderer JW, et al: Treatment of respiratory failure during sleep in patients with neuromuscular disease: Positive pressure ventilation through a nose mask. Am Rev Respir Dis 135:148–152, 1987.

74. Kerby GR, Mayer LS, Pingleton SK: Nocturnal positive pressure ventilation via nasal mask. Am Rev Respir Dis 135:738–740, 1987.

75. Bach JR, Alber AS: Management of chronic alveolar hypoventilation by nasal ventilation. Chest 97:52–57, 1990.

76. Goldstein RS, De Rosie JA, Avendano MA, et al: Influence of non-invasive positive pressure ventilation on inspiratory muscles. Chest 99:408–415, 1991.

77. Glenn WWL, Holcomb WG, Gee JB, et al: Central hypoventilation: Long term ventilatory assistance by radiofrequency electrophrenic respiration. Ann Surg 172:755–773, 1970.

78. Langou RA, Cohen LS, Sheps D, et al: Ondine's curse: Hemodynamic response to diaphragm pacing (electrophrenic respiration). Am Heart J 95:295–300, 1978.

79. Wade JG, Larson CP Jr, Hickey RF, et al: Effect of carotid endarterectomy on carotid chemoreceptor and baroreceptor function in man. N Engl J Med 282:823–829, 1970.

80. Severinghaus JW, Bainton CR, Carcelen A: Respiratory insensitivity to hypoxia in chronically hypoxic man. Respir Physiol 1:308–334, 1966.

81. Weil JV, Byrne-Quinn E, Sodal IE, et al: Acquired attenuation of chemoreceptor function in chronically hypoxic man at high altitude. J Clin Invest 50:186–195, 1971.

82. Hughes JMB: Central respiratory failure reversed by treatment. Brain 90:675–680, 1967.

83. Marks CE Jr, Goldring RM: Chronic hypercapnia during methadone maintenance. Am Rev Respir Dis 108:1088–1093, 1973.

84. Fishman AP, Turino GM, Bergofsky EH: The syndrome of alveolar hypoventilation. Am J Med 23:333–339, 1957.

85. Goldstein RL, Hyde RW, Lapham LW, et al: Peripheral neuropathy presenting with respiratory insufficiency as the primary complaint. Am J Med 56:443–449, 1974.

86. Bergofsky EH: Respiratory failure in disorders of the thoracic cage. Am Rev Respir Dis 119:643–669, 1979.

87. Shim C, Corro P, Park SS, et al: Pulmonary function studies in patients with upper airway obstruction. Am Rev Respir Dis 106:233–238, 1972.

88. Proctor DF: The upper airways: II. The larynx and trachea. Am Rev Respir Dis 115:315–342, 1977.

89. Weil JV, Byrne-Quinn E, Sodal ID, et al: Hypoxic ventilatory drive in normal man. J Clin Invest 49:1061–1072, 1970.

90. Rebuck AS, Campbell EJM: A clinical method for assessing the ventilatory response to hypoxia. Am Rev Respir Dis 109:345–350, 1974.

91. Fitzgerald RS, Lahiri S: Reflex responses to chemoreceptor stimulation. *In* Cherniack NS, Widdicombe JG (eds): Handbook of Physiology. Section 3: The Respiratory System (Part II). Vol 2: Control of Breathing. Bethesda, MD: American Physiological Society, 1986, pp 313–362.

92. West JB: Human physiology at extreme altitudes on Mount Everest. Science 223:784–788, 1984.

93. West JB, Hackett PH, Maret KH, et al: Pulmonary gas exchange on the summit of Mount Everest. J Appl Physiol 55:678–687, 1983.

94. Anthonisen NR, Cherniack RM: Ventilatory control in lung disease. *In* Hornbein TF (ed): Regulation of Breathing (Part II). New York: Marcel Dekker, 1981, pp 965–987.

95. Kawakami Y, Yamamoto H, Yoshikawa T, et al: Chemical and behavioral control of breathing in adult twins. Am Rev Respir Dis 129:703–707, 1984.

96. Kety SS, Schmidt CF: The effects of active and passive hyperventilation on cerebral blood flow, cerebral oxygen consumption, cardiac output, and blood pressure in normal young men. J Clin Invest 25:107–119, 1946.

97. Lee LY, Milhorn HT: Central ventilatory response to $O_2$ and $CO_2$ at three levels of carotid chemoreceptor stimulation. Respir Physiol 25:319–333, 1975.

98. Neubauer JA, Melton JE, Edelman NH: Modulation of respiration during hypoxia. J Appl Physiol 68:441–451, 1990.

99. Easton PA, Slykerman LJ, Anthonisen NR: Ventilatory response to sustained hypoxia in normal adults. J Appl Physiol 61:906–911, 1986.

100. Easton PA, Slykerman LJ, Anthonisen NR: Recovery of the venti-

latory response to hypoxia in normal adults. J Appl Physiol 64:521–528, 1988.
101. Severinghaus JW: Hypoxic respiratory drive and its loss during chronic hypoxia. Clin Physiol 2:57–59, 1972.
102. Edelman NH, Lahiri S, Broudo L, et al: The blunted ventilatory response to hypoxia in cyanotic congenital heart disease. N Engl J Med 282:405–411, 1970.
103. Weil JV: Ventilatory control at high altitude. *In* Cherniack NS, Widdicombe JG (eds): Handbook of Physiology. Section 3: The Respiratory System (Part II). Vol 2: Control of Breathing. Bethesda, MD: American Physiological Society, 1986, pp 703–728.
104. Coleridge HM, Coleridge JCG: Reflexes evoked from tracheobronchial tree and lungs. *In* Cherniack NS, Widdicombe JG (eds): Handbook of Physiology. Section 3: The Respiratory System (Part II). Vol 2: Control of Breathing. Bethesda, MD: American Physiological Society, 1986, pp 395–429.
105. Phillipson E, Murphy E, Kozar LF, et al: Role of vagal stimuli in exercise ventilation in dogs with experimental pneumonitis. J Appl Physiol 39:76–85, 1975.
106. Cotton DJ, Bleecker ER, Fisher SP, et al: Rapid shallow breathing after *Ascaris suum* antigen inhalation: Role of vagus nerves. J Appl Physiol 42:101–106, 1977.
107. Guz A, Noble MI, Eisele JH, et al: Experimental results of vagal blockade in cardiopulmonary disease. *In* Porter R (ed): Breathing: Hering-Breuer Centenary Symposium. London: J. A. Churchill, 1970, pp 315–329.
108. Lourenco RV, Turino GM, Davidson LAG, et al: The regulation of ventilation in diffuse pulmonary fibrosis. Am J Med 38:199–216, 1965.
109. Jones NL, Rebuck AS: Tidal volume during exercise in patients with diffuse fibrosing alveolitis. Bull Eur Physiopathol Respir 15:321–328, 1979.
110. DiMarco AF, Kelsen SG, Cherniack NS, et al: Occlusion pressure and breathing pattern in patients with interstitial lung disease. Am Rev Respir Dis 127:425–430, 1983.
111. von Euler C: On the role of proprioceptors in perception and execution of motor acts with special reference to breathing. *In* Pengelly LD, Rebuck AS, Campbell EJM (eds): Loaded Breathing. Edinburgh: Churchill-Livingstone, 1974, pp 139–149.
112. Killian KJ, Campbell EJ: Dyspnea and exercise. Annu Rev Physiol 45:465–479, 1983.
113. Takasaki Y, Orr D, Popkin J, et al: Effect of nasal continuous positive airway pressure on sleep apnea in congestive heart failure. Am Rev Respir Dis 140:1578–1584, 1989.
114. Dowdell WT, Javaheri S, McGinnis W: Cheyne-Stokes respiration presenting as sleep apnea syndrome. Am Rev Respir Dis 141:871–879, 1990.
115. Bradley TD: Right and left ventricular functional impairment and sleep apnea. Clin Chest Med 13:459–479, 1992.
116. Naughton M, Benard D, Tam A, et al: Role of hyperventilation in the pathogenesis of central sleep apneas in patients with congestive heart failure. Am Rev Respir Dis 148:330–338, 1993.
117. Lorenzi-Filho G, Rankin F, Bies I, et al: Effects of inhaled carbon dioxide and oxygen on Cheyne-Stokes respiration in patients with heart failure. Am J Respir Crit Care Med 159:1490–1498, 1999.
118. Tkacova R, Hall MJ, Liu PP, et al: Left ventricular volume in patients with heart failure and Cheyne-Stokes respiration during sleep. Am J Respir Crit Care Med 156:1549–1555, 1997.
119. De Burgh Daly M: Interactions between respiration and circulation. *In* Cherniack NS, Widdicombe JG (eds): Handbook of Physiology. Section 3: The Respiratory System (Part II). Vol 2: Control of Breathing. Bethesda, MD: American Physiological Society, 1986, pp 529–594.
120. Arbus GS, Hebert LA, Levesque RR, et al: Characterization and clinical application of the "significance band" for acute respiratory alkalosis. N Engl J Med 280:117–123, 1969.
121. Gennari FJ, Goldstein MB, Schwartz WB: The nature of the renal adaptation to chronic hypocapnia. J Clin Invest 51:1722–1730, 1972.
122. Mitchell RA: The regulation of respiration in metabolic acidosis and alkalosis. *In* Brooks CM, Rao FF, Lloyd BB (eds): Cerebrospinal Fluid and Regulation of Ventilation. Oxford, UK: Blackwell, 1965, pp 109–131.
123. Pappenheimer JR, Fencl V, Hersey SR, et al: Role of cerebral fluids in control of respiration as studied in unanesthetized goats. Am J Physiol 208:436–450, 1965.
124. Hamilton RW, Epstein PE, Henderson LW, et al: Control of breathing in uremia: Ventilatory response to $CO_2$ after hemodialysis. J Appl Physiol 41:216–222, 1976.
125. Berger AJ, Mitchell RA, Severinghaus JW: Regulation of respiration. N Engl J Med 297:194–201, 1977.
126. Kaehny WD, Jackson JT: Respiratory response to HCL acidosis in dogs after carotid body denervation. J Appl Physiol 46:1138–1142, 1979.
127. Forster HV, Dempsey JA: Ventilatory adaptations. *In* Hornbein TF (ed): Regulation of Breathing. New York: Marcel Dekker, 1981, pp 845–904.
128. Teppema LJ, Barts PW JA, Folgering HT, et al: Effects of respiratory and (isocapnic) metabolic arterial acid base disturbances on medullary extracellular fluid pH and ventilation in cats. Respir Physiol 53:379–395, 1983.
129. Stanley NN, Salisbury BG, McHenry LC Jr, et al: Effect of liver failure on the response of ventilation and cerebral circulation to carbon dioxide in man and in the goat. Clin Sci Mol Med 49:157–169, 1975.
130. Karetzky MS, Mithoefer JC: The cause of hyperventilation and arterial hypoxia in patients with cirrhosis of the liver. Am J Med Sci 254:797–804, 1967.
131. Lum LC: The syndrome of habitual chronic hyperventilation. *In* Hill O (ed): Modern Trends in Psychosomatic Medicine. London: Butterworths, 1976, pp 196–230.
132. Margarian GJ: Hyperventilation syndromes: Infrequently recognized common expressions of anxiety and stress. Medicine 61:219–236, 1982.
133. Brashear RE: Hyperventilation syndrome. Lung 161:257–273, 1983.
134. Plum F, Posner JB: The Diagnosis of Stupor and Coma. Philadelphia: FA Davis, 1966.
135. Plum F, Swanson AG: Central neurogenic hyperventilation in man. Arch Neurol Psychiatr 81:535–544, 1959.
136. Froman C, Crampton-Smith A: Hyperventilation associated with low pH of cerebrospinal fluid after intracranial hemorrhage. Lancet 1:780–782, 1966.
137. North JB, Jennett S: Abnormal breathing patterns associated with acute brain damage. Arch Neurol 31:338–344, 1974.
138. Leigh RF, Shaw DA: Rapid respiration in unconscious patients. Arch Neurol 33:356–361, 1976.
139. Fink BR, Katz R, Reinhold H, et al: Suprapontine mechanisms in regulation of respiration. Am J Physiol 202:217–220, 1962.
140. Tenney SM, Ou LC: Ventilatory response of decorticate and decerebrate cats to hypoxia and $CO_2$. Respir Physiol 29:81–92, 1976.
141. Hickey RF, Severinghaus JW: Regulation of breathing: Drug effects. *In* Hornbein TF (ed): Regulation of Breathing (Part II). New York: Marcel Dekker, 1981, pp 1251–1312.
142. Tenney SM, Miller RM: Respiratory and circulatory actions of salicylate. Am J Med 19:498–508, 1955.
143. Millhorn DE, Eldridge FL, Waldrop TG: Effects of salicylate and 2,4–dinitrophenol on respiration and metabolism. J Appl Physiol 53:925–929, 1982.
144. Cunningham DJC, Oriordan JLH: The effect of a rise in temperature on the respiratory response to carbon dioxide. Q J Exp Physiol 42:329–345, 1957.
145. Simmons DH, Nicoloff J, Guze LB: Hyperventilation and respiratory alkalosis as signs of gram-negative bacteremia. JAMA 174:2196–2199, 1960.
146. Gaudio R Jr, Abramson N: Heat-induced hyperventilation. J Appl Physiol 25:742–746, 1968.
147. Aronson PR: Hyperventilation from organic disease. Ann Intern Med 50:554–559, 1959.
148. Joels N, White H: The contribution of the arterial chemoreceptors to the stimulation of respiration by adrenaline and noradrenaline in the cat. J Physiol (Lond) 197:1–23, 1968.
149. Heistad DD, Wheeler RC, Mark AL, et al: Effects of adrenergic stimulation on ventilation in man. J Clin Invest 51:1469–1475, 1972.
150. Morgan EJ, Baidwan B, Petty TL, et al: The effects of unanesthetized arterial puncture on $P_{CO_2}$ and pH. Am Rev Respir Dis 120:795–798, 1979.

151. Lyons HA: Respiratory effects of gonadal hormones. *In* Salhanick HA, Kipnis DM, Van de Wiele RL (eds): Metabolic Effects of Gonadal Hormones and Contraceptive Steroids. New York: Plenum, 1969, pp 394–402.
152. Skatrud JB, Dempsey JA, Kaiser DG: Ventilatory response to medroxyprogesterone acetate in normal subjects: Time course and mechanism. J Appl Physiol 44:939–944, 1978.
153. Bayliss DA, Millhorn DE: Central neural mechanisms of progesterone action: Application to the respiratory system. J Appl Physiol 73:393–404, 1992.
154. Brown EB: Physiological effects of hyperventilation. Physiol Rev 33:445–471, 1953.
155. Mostellar ME, Tuttle EP Jr: Effects of alkalosis on plasma concentration and urinary excretion of inorganic phosphate in man. J Clin Invest 43:138–149, 1964.
156. Fitzgerald F: Clinical hypophosphatemia. Annu Rev Med 29:177–189, 1978.
157. Brautbar N, Leibovici H, Finlander P, et al: Mechanism of hypophosphatemia during acute hyperventilation (abstract). Clin Res 28:387A, 1980.
158. Richardson DW, Kontos HA, Raper AJ, et al: Systemic circulatory responses to hypocapnia in man. Am J Physiol 223:1308–1312, 1972.
159. Neill WA, Hattenhauer M: Impairment of myocardial $O_2$ supply due to hyperventilation. Circulation 52:854–858, 1975.
160. Yasue H, Nagao M, Omote S, et al: Coronary arterial spasm and Prinzmetal's variant form of angina induced by hyperventilation and Tris-buffer infusion. Circulation 58:56–62, 1978.
161. Neill WA, Pantley GA, Nakornchai V: Respiratory alkalemia during exercise reduces angina threshold. Chest 80:149–153, 1981.
162. Yasue H, Omote S, Takizawa A, et al: Alkalosis-induced coronary vasoconstriction: Effects of calcium, diltiazem, nitroglycerin and propranolol. Am Heart J 102:206–210, 1981.
163. Hauge A, Thoresen M, Walloe L: Changes in cerebral blood flow during hyperventilation and $CO_2$ breathing measured transcutaneously in humans by a bidirectional, pulsed, ultrasound Doppler blood velocity meter. Acta Physiol Scand 110:167–173, 1980.
164. Raichle ME, Posner JB, Plum F: Cerebral blood flow during and after hyperventilation. Arch Neurol 23:394–403, 1970.
165. Reivich MP, Cohen PJ, Greenbaum L: Alterations in the electroencephalogram of awake man produced by hyperventilation effects of 100% oxygen at 3 atmospheres pressure. Neurology 16:304, 1966.
166. Kogure K, Busto R, Matsumoto A, et al: Effect of hyperventilation on dynamics of cerebral energy metabolism. Am J Physiol 228:1862–1867, 1975.
167. Rebuck AS, Davis C, Longmire D, et al: Arterial oxygenation and carbon dioxide tensions in the production of hypoxic electroencephalographic changes in man. Clin Sci Molec Med 50:301–306, 1976.
168. Siesjo BK, Johannsson H, Ljunggren B, et al: Brain dysfunction in cerebral hypoxia and ischemia. *In* Plum F (ed): Brain Dysfunction and Metabolic Disorders. New York: Raven Press, 1977, pp 75–112.
169. Kennealy JA, McLennan JE, Loudon RG, et al: Hyperventilation-induced cerebral hypoxia. Am Rev Respir Dis 122:407–412, 1980.
170. Arnow PM, Panwalker A, Garvin JS, et al: Aspirin, hyperventilation, and cerebellar infarction in sickle–cell disease. Arch Intern Med 138:148–149, 1978.
171. Severinghaus JW: The role of cerebrospinal fluid pH in normalization of cerebral blood flow in chronic hypocapnia. Acta Neurol Scand 14(Suppl):116–120, 1965.
172. Lewis BI: Hyperventilation syndrome. A clinical and physiological evaluation. Calif Med 21:259–271, 1959.
173. Rosenbaum JF: Current concepts in psychiatry. The drug treatment of anxiety. N Engl J Med 306:401–404, 1982.
174. Van Doorn P, Folgering H, Colla P: Control of end-tidal $P_{CO_2}$ in the hyperventilation syndrome: Effects of biofeedback and breathing instructions compared. Bull Eur Physiopathol Respir 18:829–836, 1982.
175. Folgering H, Rutlen H, Roumen Y: Beta-blockade in the hyperventilation syndrome. A retrospective assessment of symptoms and complaints. Respiration 44:19–25, 1983.

# 81 Sleep Disorders

T. DOUGLAS BRADLEY, M.D. • ELIOT A. PHILLIPSON, M.D.

Introduction
- Impact of Sleep on Breathing
- Impact of Sleep on Cardiovascular Function
- Arousal Responses
- Physiologic and Clinical Consequences
- Laboratory Assessment

Obstructive Sleep Apnea
- Pathogenesis
- Clinical Features
- Cardiovascular Complications
- Diagnosis
- Management

Periodic Breathing and Central Sleep Apnea
- Pathogenesis
- Clinical Features
- Diagnosis
- Management

## INTRODUCTION

Since 1990, respiratory disturbances during sleep have come to be recognized as extremely common disorders with important clinical consequences. In addition to affecting the quality of sleep, there is a growing realization that respiratory-related sleep disturbances can interact closely with, and even contribute to, several common cardiovascular disorders. Thus, a new chapter has been opened in the rapidly evolving field of sleep medicine, which has now firmly entered the mainstream of clinical practice.

### Impact of Sleep on Breathing

Sleep is not a homogeneous phenomenon but rather consists of two distinct states, referred to as non-rapid eye movement (non-REM) or quiet sleep and rapid eye movement (REM) or active sleep.[1–5] The two states are distinguished by a combination of behavioral and electrographic criteria. Non-REM sleep consists of four stages that are thought to represent progressively deeper sleep, with the deepest stages (3 and 4) being referred to as slow-wave sleep. REM sleep, during which dreaming occurs, is characterized by intense cerebral metabolic activity and central nervous system excitation, despite which incoming sensory information and outgoing motor activity are actively inhibited. In the normal adult, non-REM sleep and REM sleep alternate cyclically, with periods of REM sleep lasting 10 to 20 minutes and occurring every 90 to 120 minutes.

Non-REM sleep and REM sleep have several important physiologic influences on breathing, particularly on respiratory drive, stability, and ventilatory mechanics.[6] Overall respiratory drive is decreased during non-REM sleep, owing to loss of the stimulatory effect of wakefulness on breathing and to a reduction in chemosensitivity. As a result, during stages 1 and 2 of non-REM sleep, as the central nervous system state fluctuates between awake and asleep, there is a fluctuation in respiratory drive that predisposes to periodic breathing. Once slow-wave sleep is fully established, nonchemical respiratory inputs are minimized, and breathing is regulated by the metabolic respiratory control system. Under these conditions, overall respiratory drive is usually stable but less than during wakefulness. As a result, minute volume of ventilation is reduced by 1 to 2 L/min compared with wakefulness, arterial $P_{CO_2}$ is increased by 2 to 8 mm Hg, and arterial $P_{O_2}$ is decreased by 5 to 10 mm Hg.

During REM sleep, respiratory drive is often irregular, ventilatory responses to chemical and mechanical respiratory stimuli may be transiently reduced or abolished, and short periods of central apnea lasting 10 to 20 seconds are relatively common. In addition, intercostal and accessory muscle activity is reduced coincident with the generalized inhibition of skeletal muscle tone characteristic of this state. As a result, thoracoabdominal coupling may be diminished, resulting in further decreases in ventilation, and functional residual capacity may be reduced. The influences of non-REM and REM sleep on respiratory drive and muscle activity are exerted on the muscles of the upper airway in addition to those of the chest wall.[7] Therefore, upper airway resistance is increased during non-REM sleep compared with wakefulness, and increased even more during REM sleep.

The physiologic impact of sleep on breathing is of little consequence in healthy persons. In patients with disturbances of respiratory structure or function, however, the imposition of these sleep-related changes on the underlying disturbance may have important clinical consequences. For example, in patients with defects in metabolic respiratory drive, such as occur in the primary alveolar hypoventilation syndrome, withdrawal of the stimulatory effect of wakefulness on breathing may result in marked hypoventilation or apnea. In patients with diaphragmatic weakness or paralysis, inhibition of intercostal and accessory respiratory muscle activity during REM sleep may result in profound hypoventilation. In persons with a structurally small oropharyngeal cavity, reduced activation of the upper airway muscles during non-REM sleep and further inhibition in REM sleep may predispose to upper airway collapse.

## Impact of Sleep on Cardiovascular Function

The shift of central nervous system state from wakefulness to non-REM sleep is normally accompanied by progressive reductions in metabolic rate, sympathetic nervous system activity, heart rate, stroke volume, cardiac output, and systemic blood pressure, and by a progressive increase in vagal tone.[8–11] An important consequence of these physiologic changes is a reduction in myocardial workload. Compared to wakefulness, non-REM sleep is a time of relative autonomic and circulatory stability. This stability is disrupted from time to time by brief microarousals from sleep that provoke sudden transient increases in sympathetic nervous activity, heart rate, and blood pressure.[11, 12]

The effects of REM sleep on cardiovascular activity are more complex than those of non-REM sleep. In animals, renal sympathetic nerve activity decreases during REM sleep, but in humans sympathetic outflow to skeletal muscle vasculature increases and blood pressure rises to levels comparable to those of wakefulness.[9, 11] Whether these differences are species-related or are caused by nonuniform activation of various branches of the sympathetic nervous system remains to be determined. Despite these changes, since adults spend approximately 80% to 85% of their total sleep time in non-REM sleep, the overall effect of sleep is to rest the cardiovascular system. Disruptions of sleep, as occur in such disorders as sleep apnea, interfere with this state of cardiovascular quiescence and, in so doing, stress the heart and circulation.

## Arousal Responses

The ability to awaken from sleep or to arouse to a lighter stage of sleep is an important element of several sleep-related respiratory disturbances. The arousal response, which requires reticular and cortical activation, results in a number of physiologic responses that are of potential benefit.[13] These include immediate increases in respiratory drive and level of ventilation, which serve to correct any preceding hypoventilation; activation of the upper airway dilator and abductor muscles, which serves to terminate obstructive apneas; activation of the cough reflex, which serves to protect the lower airways and lungs from aspiration; and initiation of behavioral responses that may protect life, such as escape from a smoke-filled room. However, the role of the arousal response in the pathogenesis of respiratory disturbances related to sleep is complex. For example, arousal in response to an episode of apnea terminates the respiratory event and limits the degree of asphyxic exposure, but arousal also interferes with the continuity of sleep and over time may expose the individual to the complications of sleep fragmentation or deprivation. Similarly, arousal from sleep may result in transient surges in blood pressure that represent an added burden on the cardiovascular system. Therefore, although the arousal response may be of immediate protective value, it can be maladaptive in the long term and may contribute to the pathophysiology of sleep-related respiratory disturbances.

## Physiologic and Clinical Consequences

Disorders of ventilation during sleep can result in several physiologic and clinical disturbances (Table 81.1). In broad terms, these complications are thought to arise either because of interference with the quality, quantity, or structure of sleep or because of recurrent nocturnal hypoxemia or asphyxia. The disturbances in sleep structure result in neuropsychiatric and behavioral manifestations rather than respiratory complaints, whereas the complications of nocturnal hypoxemia or asphyxia are predominantly cardiovascular and respiratory in nature.

## Laboratory Assessment

Because the clinical consequences of sleep-related respiratory disturbances are thought to arise either from disruptions in sleep quality and architecture or from derangements in blood gases, the laboratory assessment of such disorders is designed to focus on sleep structure and respiratory function. The simplest type of laboratory investigation is the continuous monitoring of arterial oxygen saturation using an ear or finger oximeter. The response time of such instruments is sufficiently rapid to detect transient falls in saturation, such as might occur

**Table 81.1 CONSEQUENCES OF RESPIRATORY DISTURBANCES DURING SLEEP**

| Physiologic Disturbance | Clinical Consequences |
|---|---|
| Fragmentation of sleep by frequent arousals; loss of slow-wave sleep | Recurrent awakenings<br>Restless sleep<br>Unrefreshing sleep<br>Morning headache<br>Daytime sleepiness<br>Cognitive impairment<br>Personality changes |
| Recurrent nocturnal hypoxemia or asphyxia; increased cardiac afterload | Nocturnal cardiac arrhythmias<br>Paroxysmal nocturnal dyspnea<br>Nocturnal angina<br>Pulmonary hypertension<br>Systemic hypertension<br>Left-ventricular dysfunction<br>Chronic respiratory failure |

during an apnea episode lasting 10 to 20 seconds. The pattern of saturation recorded during overnight oximetry can be highly characteristic of specific respiratory disturbances (Fig. 81.1),[14] but the diagnostic accuracy of oximetry as a screening test for any specific disease is relatively low. The addition of transcutaneous $P_{CO_2}$ monitoring to an overnight screening test provides information regarding changes in the mean level of arterial $P_{CO_2}$ over a period of several minutes but cannot detect fluctuations in arterial $P_{CO_2}$ on a breath-by-breath basis or during the course of a single apnea episode. Nevertheless, such information can be helpful in assessing overall trends in alveolar ventilation during sleep (see Fig. 81.1). Overnight Holter monitoring of heart rate and rhythm can also be a useful screening procedure,[15] but abnormalities of cardiac rhythm are neither sufficiently sensitive nor specific enough to stand alone as a screening test for any particular respiratory disturbance during sleep.

Full overnight sleep studies, referred to as polysomnography, involve the recording of several electrographic variables, including the electroencephalogram, electrooculogram, and submental electromyogram (EMG), which allow sleep to be staged and quantitated and brief arousals or awakenings from sleep to be identified.[5] The tibialis EMG is also usually recorded to determine the presence of periodic leg movements during sleep (nocturnal myoclonus).[16] Standard respiratory measurements include arterial oxygen saturation by ear or finger oximetry, often transcutaneous $P_{CO_2}$, and recordings of breathing movements that permit the identification of apneas or hypopneas and their classification as obstructive or nonobstructive (Fig. 81.2).[17] The latter distinction can usually be made with appropriate surface transducers such as the respiratory inductive plethysmograph.[18] In some cases more sensitive techniques may be required, such as measurement of intrapleural pressure swings (with an esophageal catheter) or diaphragm EMG response.[19, 20]

## OBSTRUCTIVE SLEEP APNEA

The clinical importance of sleep apnea arises from the fact that it is one of the leading causes of excessive daytime sleepiness[21, 22] and may contribute to the development of several cardiorespiratory disturbances, including pulmonary hypertension, right-sided heart failure, systemic hypertension, left-ventricular dysfunction, chronic respiratory failure, nocturnal cardiac arrhythmias, and possibly sudden death during sleep.[23–28] During the past decade it has come to be recognized as a common disorder, affecting at least 2% of middle-aged women and 4% of middle-aged men.[29] Prevalence rates in the elderly appear to be even higher.[30]

Sleep apnea is defined as cessation of airflow at the nose and mouth during sleep.[23] In obstructive sleep apnea, airflow ceases because of complete occlusion of the upper airway at the oropharyngeal level, despite continued activation of the inspiratory muscles.[31, 32] In contrast, in central sleep apnea, airflow ceases because drive to all the respiratory muscles is transiently abolished. Isolated central apneas may occur in healthy subjects, particularly during REM sleep.[6] Obstructive apneas are generally considered to be pathologic. In patients with clinically important obstructive sleep apnea, there are usually at least 15 obstructive apnea and hypopnea episodes per hour of sleep. However, evidence has emerged that a high upper airway resistance during sleep (manifested by snoring) that is accompanied by recurrent arousals from sleep, even in the absence of outright apneas and hypopneas, can also result in a clinically important "sleep apnea" syndrome.[33, 34] Therefore, the absence of apneas and hypopneas in a symptomatic patient does not unequivocally exclude a sleep-related respiratory disorder.

### Pathogenesis

The definitive event in obstructive sleep apnea is posterior movement of the tongue and palate into apposition with the posterior pharyngeal wall, resulting in occlusion of the nasopharynx and oropharynx.[31, 32] The resulting airway obstruction initiates a primary sequence of events (Fig. 81.3) that may repeat itself hundreds of times each night. With the onset of sleep the upper airway occludes, resulting in cessation of airflow despite continuing respira-

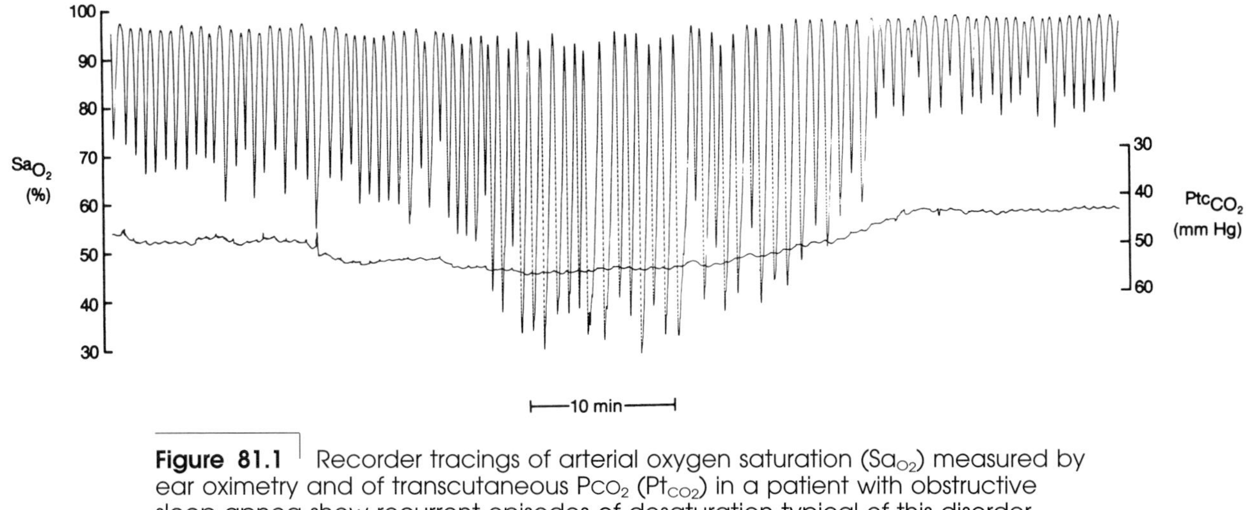


**Figure 81.1** Recorder tracings of arterial oxygen saturation ($Sa_{O_2}$) measured by ear oximetry and of transcutaneous $P_{CO_2}$ ($Pt_{CO_2}$) in a patient with obstructive sleep apnea show recurrent episodes of desaturation typical of this disorder. (From Stradling JR, Phillipson EA: Breathing disorders during sleep. QJM 58:3–18, 1986.)

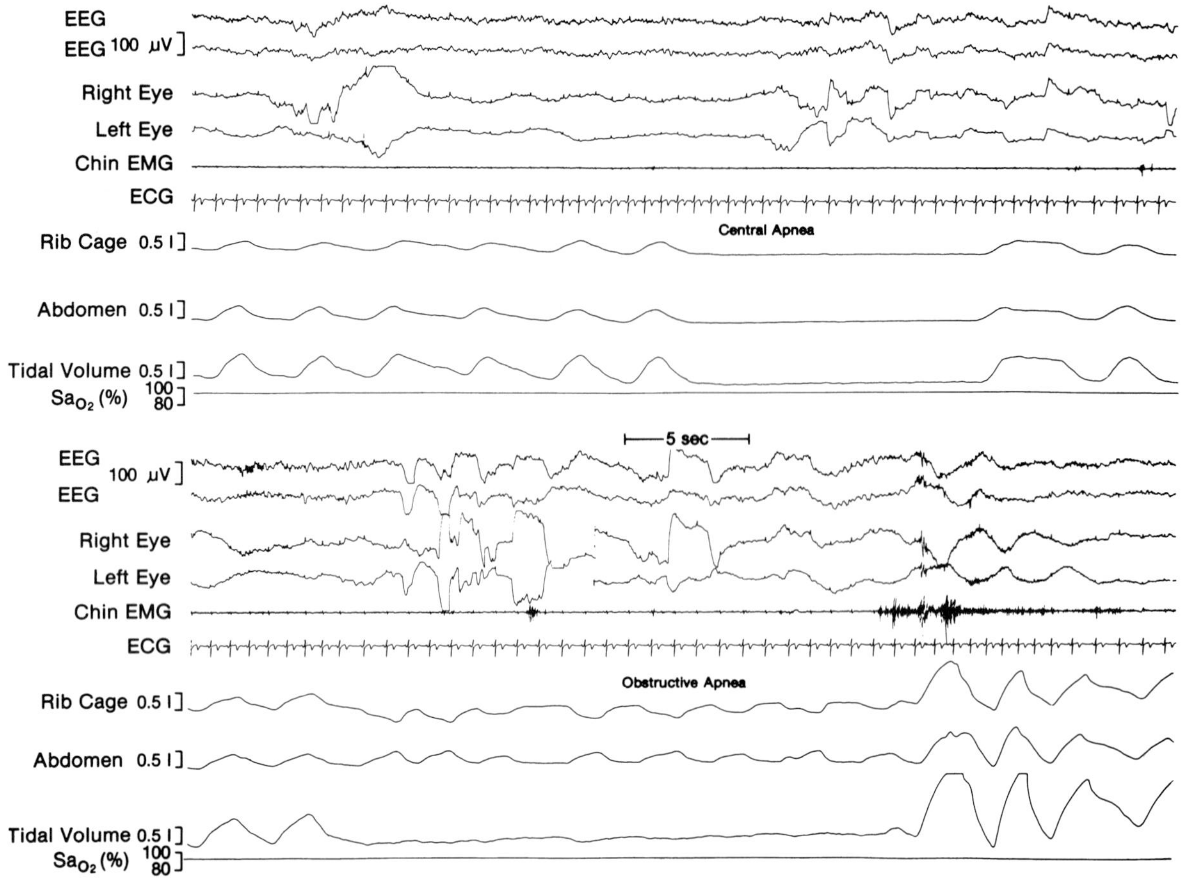


**Figure 81.2** Recorder tracings during polysomnographic study show distinction between central and obstructive apneas, using a respiratory inductive plethysmograph. Upper and lower panels form a continuous record in rapid eye movement (REM) sleep. Channels from the top down show the following: electroencephalogram (EEG), right and left eye movements, submental electromyogram (EMG), electrocardiogram (ECG), movements of rib cage and abdomen, tidal volume, and arterial oxygen saturation ($Sa_{O_2}$). Note that during central apnea the absence of tidal volume excursion was accompanied by absence of rib cage and abdominal movements; during obstructive apnea, paradoxical rib cage and abdominal movements were present. (From Phillipson EA, Bowes G: Sleep disorders. *In* Fishman AP (ed): Update of Pulmonary Diseases and Disorders. New York: McGraw-Hill, 1982, pp 256–273.)

tory efforts. As a result of apnea, progressive asphyxia develops, until there is a brief arousal from sleep, restoration of upper airway patency, and resumption of airflow. With the relief of asphyxia, the patient quickly returns to sleep, only to have the sequence of events repeated over and over again.[35]

Several underlying mechanisms contribute to the onset and termination of upper airway occlusion during sleep. In general terms, upper airway collapse occurs when the subatmospheric pharyngeal pressure generated during inspiration exceeds by some critical amount the stabilizing forces generated by the dilator and abductor muscles of the upper airway.[7, 36–38] Both structural and functional factors contribute to the development of a critical airway-collapsing pressure.[39] A minority of patients have obvious anatomic narrowing of the upper airway, as a result of micrognathia and retrognathia, adenotonsillar hypertrophy, macroglossia, or acromegaly.[40–42] However, in the majority of patients who are free of such disorders, the structural defect is subtle but can be demonstrated during wakefulness by a variety of imaging techniques, including computed tomographic (CT) scanning of the upper airway, acoustic reflection measurements of the pharyngeal area, cephalometric roentgenography, magnetic resonance imaging, and videoendoscopy.[7, 31, 43–48] Obesity frequently contributes to the upper airway narrowing.[43, 48–51] In addition to a reduction in oropharyngeal size, the compliance of the upper airway may be increased, resulting in a tendency for the airway to be floppy and to collapse when subjected to a negative pressure.[37, 38, 52–54]

Because the apneas occur only during sleep, it is obvious that the state of the central nervous system plays an important role in pathogenesis of the disorder. During wakefulness, upper airway muscle activity is greater than normal in patients with obstructive sleep apnea, presumably to compensate for airway narrowing and a high

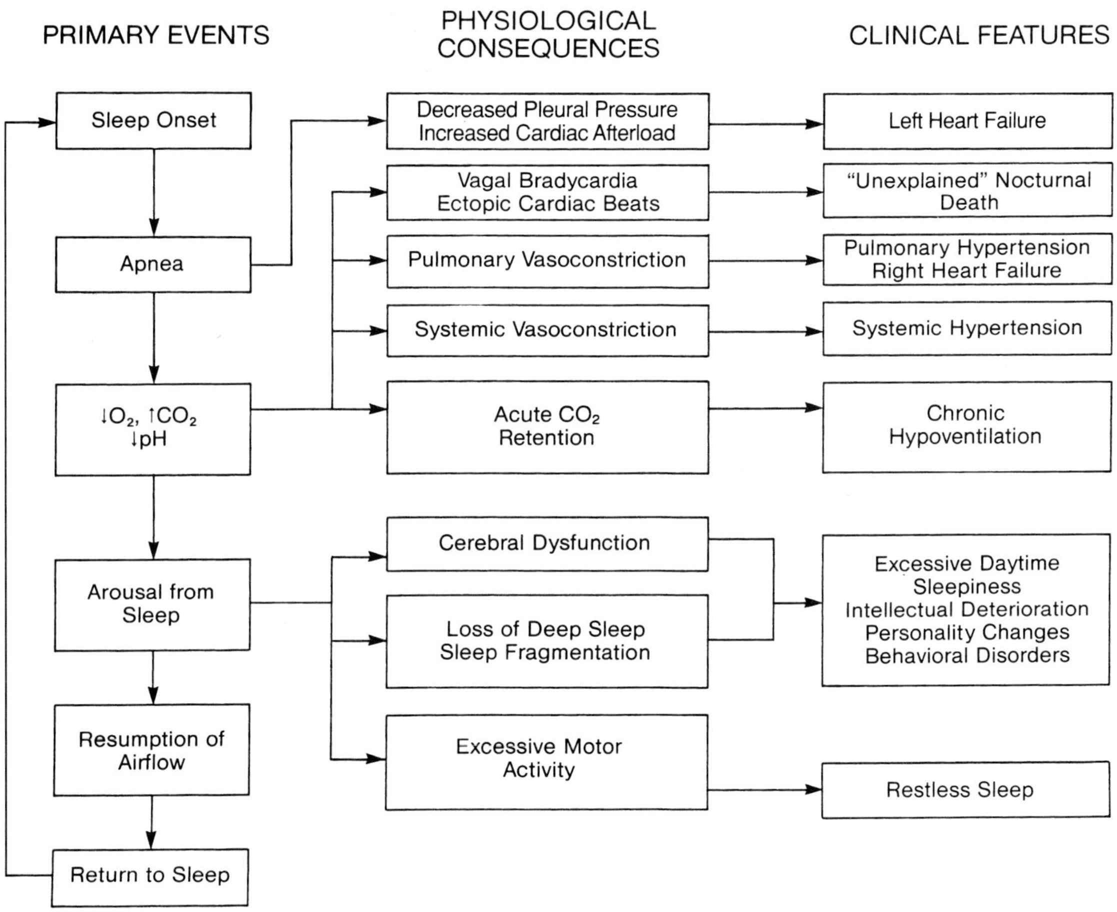


**Figure 81.3** Schema shows the primary sequence of events, physiologic responses, and clinical features of obstructive sleep apnea. (Modified from Phillipson EA: Sleep apnea. Med Clin North Am 23:2314–2323, 1982.)

airway resistance.[55, 56] The normal decrease in upper airway muscle activity that occurs at onset of sleep[7, 57, 58] may be sufficient to allow the development of a critical airway-collapsing pressure during inspiration in susceptible individuals.[7] In addition, the fluctuation of central nervous system state that normally occurs at the onset of sleep results in a transient instability in respiratory drive (characterized by periodic breathing) that is also exerted on the muscles of the upper airway.[59, 60] As a result, the transient reductions in upper airway muscle activity may be excessive in relation to the reductions in diaphragmatic activity.[61–64] Under these conditions, the negative airway pressure generated during inspiration can become sufficient to collapse the pharynx. Therefore, sleep can be considered to exert a permissive influence on upper airway function that predisposes to upper airway collapse in persons who are susceptible because of a small airway lumen.

Physiologic reductions in upper airway muscle activity are particularly marked during REM sleep, which probably accounts for the tendency for obstructive sleep apnea to first develop in this stage of sleep.[6, 52] Alcohol and other sedatives that selectively depress upper airway muscle activity may also promote upper airway collapse in susceptible individuals.[65–68] In many of these patients, varying degrees of nasal obstruction are also present. The resulting high upstream resistance predisposes to upper airway collapse by increasing the degree of subatmospheric pressure generated in the pharynx during inspiration, because the strength of diaphragmatic contraction is increased to overcome airflow resistance in the nose.

Termination of obstructive apnea depends on a brief arousal to a lighter stage of sleep, which is accompanied by activation of the upper airway dilator and abductor muscles and restoration of airway patency.[7, 23, 36, 69] In some cases there may be an outright awakening from sleep. The specific factors involved in the arousal response probably involve chemical stimuli related to asphyxia and mechanical stimuli related to breathing against an occluded airway.[13, 70, 71] Carotid body defects markedly prolong obstructive apneas in experimental animals[72] and are thought to play a similar role in hypercapnic patients with this condition.[73] Arousal can also be delayed by factors that interfere with reticular activation, such as REM sleep, which probably accounts for the fact that apneas are typically longer and associated with more severe degrees of asphyxia in this stage of sleep.[13, 73] Alcohol, sedative medications, and chronic sleep deprivation also impair central nervous system arousability and prolong obstructive apneas.[65, 67, 74, 75]

## Clinical Features

The primary sequence of nocturnal events that characterizes obstructive sleep apnea elicits a series of secondary physiologic responses, which in turn give rise to the clinical features and complications of the syndrome (see Fig. 81.3). In broad terms, the clinical manifestations segregate into two groups: one group is predominantly neuropsychiatric and behavioral and is thought to arise ultimately from the recurrent arousals that terminate each apnea, although recurrent cerebral hypoxia may also play a role;[76] the second group, predominantly cardiorespiratory, is related largely but not exclusively to the recurrent episodes of nocturnal asphyxia.[77]

The most common manifestations of obstructive sleep apnea are neuropsychiatric and behavioral, with excessive daytime sleepiness being the most common complaint.[23–25] Initially, daytime sleepiness develops under passive conditions such as watching television and reading, but as the disorder progresses, sleepiness encroaches progressively into all daily activities and can become severely disabling and dangerous. Tests of driving ability reveal significant impairment in patients with obstructive sleep apnea, and rates of motor vehicle accidents among these patients are considerably increased compared with those among control subjects.[78–82] Frequently associated with excessive daytime sleepiness are signs of intellectual impairment, memory loss, poor judgment, and personality changes.[83–86] Although these manifestations of obstructive sleep apnea are probably related to nocturnal sleep fragmentation and loss of the deeper stages of sleep, patients with apparently similar nocturnal disturbances may demonstrate widely varying degrees of daytime impairment. Furthermore, the patient is frequently unaware of excessive daytime sleepiness or intellectual deterioration; therefore, questioning of family members is an important aspect of history taking.

The most common nocturnal symptom is loud snoring, indicative of upper airway narrowing. Typically, snoring has been present for many years before other symptoms develop, at which time the snoring takes on a temporal character, being interrupted periodically by episodes of silence corresponding to the occlusive events. The termination of each apnea episode is usually heralded by a very loud snoring gasp, accompanied by body movement and flailing of the limbs. The patient may be unaware of these events but often complains of a disturbed or restless sleep, as does the bed partner. Occasionally, the patient awakens fully and may complain of choking, air hunger, or insomnia. Most patients complain of an unrefreshing sleep, mental fogginess and disorientation, and, occasionally, a headache on arising in the morning.[23–25]

## Cardiovascular Complications

Systemic blood pressure may rise transiently during obstructive apneas or at apnea termination as a result of sympathetic activation and reflex vasoconstriction secondary to asphyxia, arousal from sleep, and changes in intrathoracic pressure[87–91] (Fig. 81.4). However, blood pressure usually falls towards baseline on resumption of breathing. Nevertheless, unlike healthy subjects, patients with obstructive sleep apnea fail to lower their overall blood pressure during sleep.[87, 92] Furthermore, more than 50%

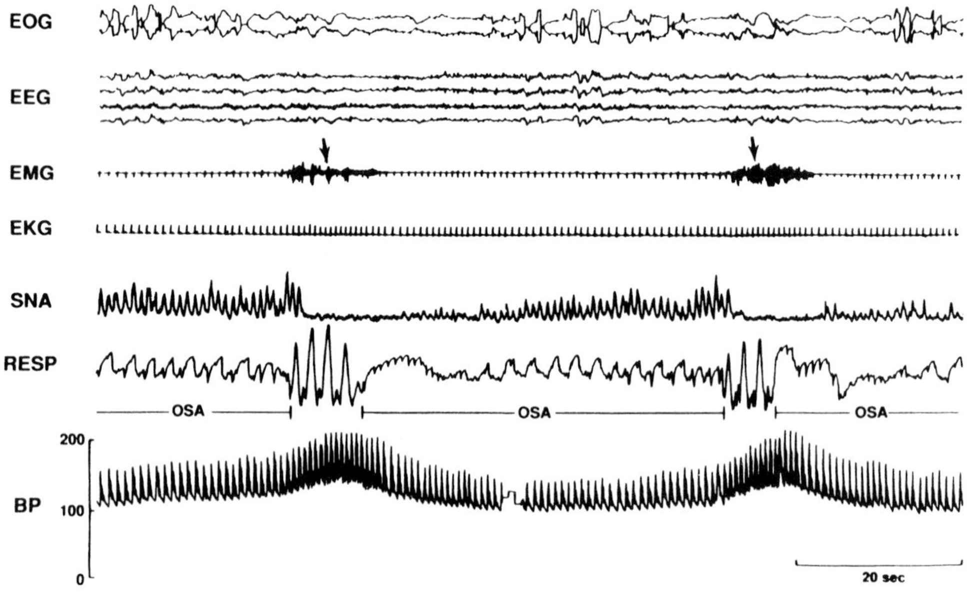


**Figure 81.4** Recordings of sympathetic activity (from the peroneal nerve) and of arterial blood pressure in a patient with obstructive sleep apnea (OSA) are shown. Muscle sympathetic nerve activity (SNA) is suppressed at the beginning of the apnea but increases as arterial $O_2$ saturation (not shown) decreases, reaching a peak at termination of the apnea, after which it is abruptly inhibited by lung inflation. Surges in blood pressure (BP) peak shortly after peak muscle SNA and arousal from sleep *(arrows)*. (From Somers VK, Dyken ME, Clary MP, et al: Sympathetic neural mechanisms in obstructive sleep apnea. J Clin Invest 96:1897–1904, 1995.)

of patients with obstructive sleep apnea have systemic hypertension,[23–25, 93] possibly related to chronically excessive sympathetic nervous system activity and elevated plasma norepinephrine concentrations.[89, 91, 94–96] Some, but not all, epidemiologic studies identify an association between obstructive sleep apnea and systemic hypertension,[97–101] and studies in an animal model of the disorder directly demonstrate that obstructive sleep apnea can lead to sustained increases in waking blood pressure.[102]

In addition to systemic hypertension, there is mounting clinical and experimental evidence that obstructive sleep apnea may adversely affect left-ventricular function both acutely and chronically. Acutely, the exaggerated negative intrathoracic pressure generated during obstructive apneas reduces stroke volume and cardiac output by increasing left-ventricular afterload and reducing left-ventricular preload.[103, 104] Negative intrathoracic pressure, which can reach as much as $-90$ cm $H_2O$ ($-65$ mm Hg),[28] increases left-ventricular transmural pressure, an important determinant of left-ventricular afterload,[103, 105, 106] and reduces left-ventricular preload through its effect on ventricular interactions.[107–110] These adverse effects of exaggerated negative intrathoracic pressure on stroke volume are more pronounced in patients with underlying left-ventricular dysfunction than in healthy subjects,[105, 111] probably because the diseased myocardium is less capable of compensating for the increased afterload.[112] The acute hemodynamic disturbances induced by obstructive apneas could play a role in the development of nocturnal angina and pulmonary edema that have been reported in patients with obstructive sleep apnea.[113–116]

Intermittent hypoxia during obstructive apneas can also adversely affect left-ventricular performance through its effects on preload, afterload, and contractility. Elevations in pulmonary artery pressure due to apnea-related hypoxia impede right-ventricular emptying and reduce the rate of relaxation of both ventricles.[117] These effects, along with those related to negative intrathoracic pressure, can compromise left-ventricular filling.[108, 109, 118, 119] Hypoxia can also contribute to acute elevations in systemic blood pressure through stimulation of the sympathetic nervous system.[120] As a result of these elevations in left-ventricular afterload and in sympathetic cardiac stimulation, the oxygen demands of the myocardium are likely to be increased, which could precipitate myocardial ischemia, nocturnal angina, and cardiac arrhythmias in patients with underlying coronary artery disease.[91, 113, 115, 116, 121–124] Given these associations, there has developed the notion that obstructive sleep apnea can result in sudden death during sleep,[115, 125] but rigorous data in support of this notion are lacking.

Emerging data also point to an association between obstructive sleep apnea and chronic left-ventricular dysfunction, although it has not been established that obstructive sleep apnea can result in overt left-ventricular failure in the absence of chronic hypertension, coronary artery disease, or underlying myocardial dysfunction.[126, 127] Nevertheless, alleviation of obstructive sleep apnea in some patients with congestive heart failure has produced a remarkable improvement in left-ventricular ejection fraction and a decrease in exertional dyspnea.[28] Furthermore, studies in a canine model of obstructive sleep apnea have demonstrated a decrease in left-ventricular ejection fraction after 1 to 3 months of exposure to recurrent upper airway occlusion during sleep.[106] Muscle sympathetic nerve activity and plasma norepinephrine concentrations are chronically increased in patients with obstructive sleep apnea.[89, 91, 95, 96] It is known that survival of patients with congestive heart failure is inversely proportional to cardiac sympathetic nerve activity and plasma norepinephrine concentration,[128, 129] providing a possible explanation for the deleterious effects of obstructive sleep apnea in patients with congestive heart failure.

Ten per cent to 15% of patients with obstructive sleep apnea develop sustained pulmonary hypertension leading to right-sided heart failure.[23, 25, 130] Acute pulmonary vasoconstriction has been well documented during obstructive apneas, but pulmonary arterial pressure during wakefulness is typically normal.[15, 87, 88] The development of sustained pulmonary hypertension appears to require the presence of daytime hypoxemia and hypercapnia in addition to severe nocturnal desaturation.[130–132] The daytime blood gas disturbances can generally be attributed to the combined effects of obesity, diffuse airway obstruction, and reduced respiratory drive. In contrast, there is little evidence that severe nocturnal hypoxemia alone is associated with the development of right-sided heart failure. Ten per cent to 15% of patients with obstructive sleep apnea also develop chronic hypercapnia.[133] When they also have right-sided heart failure, obesity, and daytime sleepiness, such patients can be said to have the *Pickwickian* or obesity-hypoventilation syndrome. The development of chronic carbon dioxide retention appears to require the presence of obesity, mild-to-moderate diffuse airway obstruction, and reductions in ventilatory chemosensitivity and respiratory drive.[133–135] The weakness in respiratory drive can be attributed to genetic influences, the effects of chronic hypoxia, or the effects of chronic sleep fragmentation.[136–138] Together, these disturbances attenuate the normal hyperpnea that typically develops between nocturnal obstructive events, thereby preventing correction of the blood gas disturbances that develop during the apnea episodes.[134]

## Diagnosis

The typical patient with obstructive sleep apnea is a middle-aged or elderly man or woman, mildly to moderately overweight and hypertensive, who presents with a history of snoring, restless sleep, nocturnal choking or dyspnea, and excessive daytime sleepiness.[23–25] The disease is less common in premenopausal women, children, young men, and nonobese individuals. Because the symptoms of obstructive sleep apnea may resemble those of congestive heart failure, sleep apnea is frequently overlooked in patients with underlying cardiac disease, an important oversight that should be avoided, given the increased rate of mortality that sleep apnea confers on such patients.[139, 140] In the patient with a typical clinical picture and a high pretest probability of obstructive sleep apnea, the diagnosis can often be confirmed by overnight screening tests (see Laboratory Assessment), particularly the finding of recurrent episodes of arterial oxygen desaturation (see Fig. 81.1). In contrast, negative screening test results do not exclude the diagnosis.[141, 142] Therefore, the definitive diagnosis often requires a detailed polysomnographic study (see Laboratory Assessment) to demonstrate recurrent episodes of airflow cessation accompanied by continuing respiratory effort (see Fig. 81.2). More simplified studies that measure only cardiorespiratory variables (and delete electrographic measurements) appear to be effective in confirming a diagnosis of obstructive sleep apnea.[143] Such studies are typically performed in the patient's home, unattended by a technician, and are therefore less expensive than laboratory-based polysomnography. However, cardiorespiratory measurements alone may underestimate the severity of sleep apnea and are unable to detect nonrespiratory sleep disorders.

A common clinical dilemma in the investigation of possible obstructive sleep apnea is the patient with a history of mild snoring who is otherwise completely asymptomatic and in good health and in whom no apnea episodes have been witnessed by the bed partner. Although some of these patients may well have a mild degree of sleep apnea, it has not been clearly established that snoring per se or even mild sleep apnea is associated with long-term health complications.[144] Hence, there is no firm indication for sleep studies in such patients, because management, which consists of counseling regarding the need for reduction of weight and of alcohol consumption (where appropriate), cessation of smoking, and avoidance of sleeping in the supine posture,[145, 146] is unlikely to be changed by the demonstration of a few obstructive events during sleep.

## Management

The indications for treatment of patients with obstructive sleep apnea have not been firmly established, but useful guidelines have been developed.[147] There is general agreement that patients with neuropsychiatric or cardiorespiratory complications of the disorder warrant treatment. In contrast, there is uncertainty regarding the approach to treatment in patients who snore but are completely asymptomatic, most of whom will be found to have an increased upper airway resistance during sleep but fewer than 10 apneas and hypopneas and arousals per hour of sleep. This uncertainty relates to the fact that the natural history of untreated snoring or very mild obstructive sleep apnea has not been defined. However, even in the absence of such definitive knowledge, because snoring can be highly disruptive to the sleep of the bed partner, at minimum asymptomatic snorers should receive preventive counseling that is designed to alleviate snoring and to delay its progression to outright sleep apnea. This counseling includes measures that are similar to those prescribed for patients with mild-to-moderate symptoms, including weight reduction (where appropriate), avoidance of alcohol and sedatives, and avoidance of sleeping in the supine posture (to the extent possible).[145, 146]

More invasive approaches to asymptomatic snoring include oral appliances that are designed to keep the tongue forward or to advance the entire mandible. The efficacy of such devices in abolishing snoring has been reported to be 55% to 100%.[148–150] Nasal continuous positive airway pressure (nasal CPAP, to be described later) is highly effective in relieving snoring but is generally not well accepted by asymptomatic snorers.[151] Apart from the conservative measures already noted, currently the most popular invasive treatment for simple snoring is pharyngeal surgery, including both traditional uvulopalatopharyngoplasty[152] and laser-assisted uvulopalatoplasty.[153] Relief of snoring has been reported in up to 80% of patients.

Several different treatments are currently prescribed for patients with symptomatic obstructive sleep apnea, including intraoral appliances, surgery, and nasal CPAP during sleep. Intraoral appliances are designed to keep the mandible and tongue forward and thereby increase the size of the upper airway lumen. Several devices have been demonstrated to be of benefit in selected cases.[148–150, 154] Surgical approaches include uvulopalatopharyngoplasty, which is designed to increase the size of the oropharyngeal lumen by removing redundant soft tissue.[152] The rate of overall long-term cure is less than 50%,[155] but higher rates of success can be achieved by more discriminating selection of appropriate patients.[155–157] Other surgical approaches, including mandibular advancement, hyoid osteotomy, and similar procedures, have a more limited application but higher rates of success in selected patients.[155]

At present, the most effective and widespread treatment for obstructive sleep apnea is nasal CPAP,[147] which provides a pneumatic splint to the airway and prevents development of a critical subatmospheric collapsing pressure.[158] Nasal CPAP is highly effective in the sleep laboratory and is well tolerated by most patients (60% to 85%), even over a period of years.[159, 160] In some centers, nasal CPAP treatment is initiated during the diagnostic study night once the diagnosis has been established,[161] but proper patient training and education on a subsequent day are critically important to ensure long-term compliance. Patients who are unable to tolerate conventional nasal CPAP despite an adequate trial may respond well to second- and third-generation devices that provide more flexible algorithms in titrating the airway pressure.[147, 162]

The only treatment for obstructive sleep apnea that has been tested specifically in patients with cardiac disease is nasal CPAP. In patients with ischemic heart disease and nocturnal angina who are receiving appropriate pharmacologic therapy for angina, treatment of obstructive sleep apnea with CPAP can markedly reduce the frequency of nocturnal cardiac ischemic events.[116] Similarly, in patients with obstructive sleep apnea and congestive heart failure, CPAP has immediate beneficial effects, including improvements in nocturnal oxygenation, reductions in the frequency of arousals, consolidation of sleep, and augmentation of cardiac output.[28] In addition, long-term treatment with nocturnal nasal CPAP results in marked improvements in left-ventricular ejection fraction during the daytime.[28] Because the beneficial effects of unloading the heart at night lead to improvements in left-ventricular function and cardiac functional status that are sustained throughout the day, CPAP should be considered the treatment of choice for obstructive sleep apnea in patients with ischemic heart disease or congestive heart failure.

In patients with severe obstructive sleep apnea in whom all other treatment approaches are ineffective or not tolerated, tracheostomy is indicated and provides immediate relief by bypassing the site of oropharyngeal obstruction during sleep.[163, 164] In such cases, the tracheostomy needs to be opened only at night and can be plugged during waking hours. However, tracheostomy is now performed very rarely in most centers, having been replaced by other treatment modalities, notably nasal CPAP during sleep.

## PERIODIC BREATHING AND CENTRAL SLEEP APNEA

*Central sleep apnea* is defined as a cessation of breathing during sleep that results from transient abolition of drive to the respiratory muscles. *Periodic breathing* refers to a regular waxing and waning of ventilation as a result of fluctuations in central respiratory drive. In some persons, the waning phase of periodic breathing may include a short period of outright apnea that is typically central in type (Cheyne-Stokes respiration). In such cases, central sleep apnea can be considered a manifestation and exaggeration of periodic breathing. Because this form of central sleep apnea is the type most frequently encountered in clinical practice and shares common underlying mechanisms with periodic breathing,[61, 165] these two sleep-related breathing disturbances are best considered together.

### Pathogenesis

Central sleep apnea is not a single disease entity but rather includes several disorders in which the definitive event is the withdrawal of effective central drive to the respiratory muscles.[165, 166] The resulting decrease in ventilation initiates a primary sequence of events similar to those that occur in the obstructive sleep apnea syndrome (see Fig. 81.3). On the basis of theoretical, experimental, and clinical considerations, two distinct underlying mechanisms have been invoked to account for cessation of central respiratory output during sleep. First are outright defects in the respiratory control system or in the respiratory neuromuscular apparatus. Such defects generally result in a chronic alveolar hypoventilation syndrome, manifested by some degree of daytime hypercapnia (see Chapter 80). However, the full impact of such defects usually becomes apparent only during sleep, when the stimulatory influence of behavioral, cortical, and reticular inputs to the brain-stem respiratory neurons (referred to as the waking neural drive to breathing[167]) is minimized and breathing becomes critically dependent on the defective metabolic respiratory control system.[6, 168]

In contrast to central sleep apnea that results from underlying defects in the respiratory controller or neuromuscular systems are central apneic disorders that arise from transient fluctuations or instabilities in an otherwise intact respiratory control system. These instabilities, manifested by periodic breathing (Cheyne-Stokes respiration), typically occur only during drowsiness and light sleep, and because there is no defect in respiratory control or drive, arterial $P_{CO_2}$ levels during steady-state wakefulness or slow-wave sleep are normal or even low.[165, 166] Several theoretical and experimental models have been developed to account for such transient fluctuations in central respiratory drive.[168–173] Common to all these models is a $P_{CO_2}$ level during sleep that falls transiently below the critical threshold value required for maintenance of respiratory rhythm.

Such transient discrepancies in $P_{CO_2}$ levels arise in a number of conditions, the most common of which is the transition from wakefulness to sleep. Because of the waking neural drive to breathing, ventilation is higher and $P_{CO_2}$ levels are lower during wakefulness than during established sleep.[6] Withdrawal of this drive at the transition from wakefulness to sleep results in a $P_{CO_2}$ level that (although appropriate for wakefulness) is below the steady-state value appropriate for sleep (Fig. 81.5). If this $P_{CO_2}$ level of wakefulness is below the threshold value for rhythm generation during sleep, an outright apnea will ensue at onset of sleep until $P_{CO_2}$ rises to the critical threshold value. If sleep becomes firmly established at this point, regular breathing follows without further apneas or hypopneas, as typically occurs in children and adolescents.[174, 175] In adults and in the elderly, however, the transition from waking to sleep is characterized by repeated fluctuations in central nervous system state between "awake" and "asleep." With each momentary arousal from sleep toward wakefulness, the $P_{CO_2}$ levels that were present during sleep represent a hypercapnic

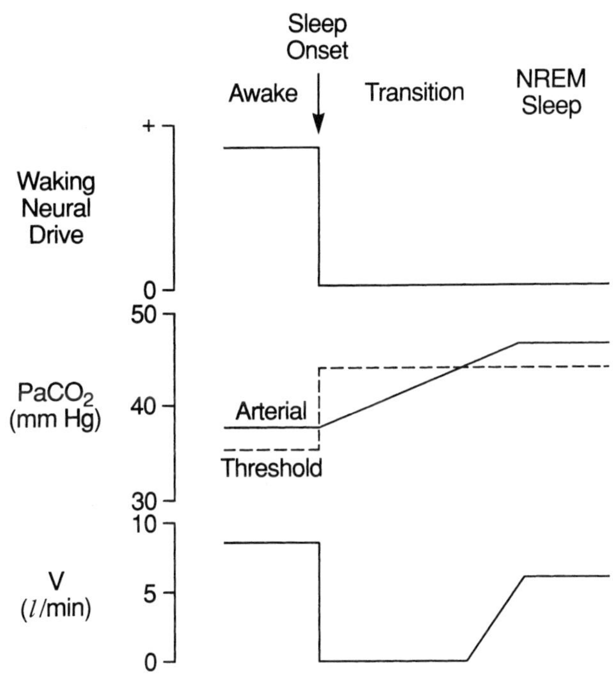


**Figure 81.5** Schematic diagram shows a proposed mechanism underlying central sleep apnea at sleep onset. With the loss of the waking neural drive to breathing at sleep onset, there is an increase in the arterial threshold $P_{CO_2}$ required to maintain respiratory rhythm. As a result, the arterial $P_{CO_2}$ ($Pa_{CO_2}$) that was present during wakefulness may be below the threshold $P_{CO_2}$ for rhythm generation in sleep; hence, ventilation (V) falls to zero and apnea ensues until arterial $P_{CO_2}$ rises above the threshold level for rhythm generation in sleep, whereupon rhythmic breathing resumes. NREM = non-REM. (From Bradley TD, Phillipson EA: Central sleep apnea. Clin Chest Med 13:493–505, 1992.)

stimulus during wakefulness, and ventilation therefore increases in accordance with the awake response to carbon dioxide, resulting in the hyperpneic phase of periodic breathing. The changes in ventilation from the sleeping to the waking phase are a mirror image of those that occur in the waking-to-sleeping phase. This cycle of hypopnea (or apnea) alternating with hyperpnea (Cheyne-Stokes respiration) is repeated until sleep becomes established.

In this scheme, the magnitude of fluctuation in ventilation with changes in central nervous system state depends on the difference between the awake and sleeping values of $P_{CO_2}$ and the steepness of the ventilatory response to carbon dioxide during wakefulness. Any factor that magnifies these variables enhances the tendency to periodic breathing and central sleep apnea. For example, at high altitude, the alveolar hyperventilation that results from hypoxia drives arterial and cerebral $P_{CO_2}$ levels well below the critical threshold value required for maintenance of respiratory rhythm during sleep.[176, 177] Hypoxia may also increase the steepness of the ventilatory response to carbon dioxide. As a result, periodic breathing, characterized by brief central apneas alternating with vigorous hyperpneas, is typical among sojourners at high altitude.[178] Similarly, any cardiac or pulmonary disorder that results in hypoxia and alveolar hyperventilation during wakefulness is likely to be associated with periodic breathing and central apnea during light sleep.

### Central Sleep Apnea in Patients with Left-Ventricular Heart Disease

Periodic breathing and central sleep apnea are frequently observed in patients with congestive heart failure.[179] In contrast to obstructive sleep apnea, central sleep apnea appears to result from, rather than to cause, congestive heart failure. Nevertheless, central sleep apnea can have secondary pathologic consequences for patients with heart failure.

The key factor in the pathogenesis of central sleep apnea in congestive heart failure is similar to that described previously and involves oscillations in arterial $P_{CO_2}$ below and above the threshold for apnea.[180, 181] Reductions in arterial $P_{CO_2}$ below the threshold transiently shut off the central respiratory drive and trigger central apnea, the length of which is proportional to the preceding degree of hyperventilation and the magnitude of reduction of arterial $P_{CO_2}$ below the apnea threshold.[172, 182] For the same degree of left-ventricular systolic dysfunction, patients with central sleep apnea hyperventilate more and have a lower arterial $P_{CO_2}$ both awake and asleep than do patients without central sleep apnea.[180, 183] The higher ventilation and lower arterial $P_{CO_2}$ are associated with higher left-ventricular end-diastolic volume and filling pressures but not necessarily with hypoxia.[184] The chronic hyperventilation is probably caused, therefore, mainly by stimulation of pulmonary vagal receptors by pulmonary congestion.[185] As a result of the chronic hyperventilation, the arterial $P_{CO_2}$ levels in patients with central sleep apnea are very close to the apneic threshold. Under these conditions, abrupt increases in ventilation, frequently triggered by arousals from sleep, drive arterial $P_{CO_2}$ below the threshold, precipitating central apneas.[180, 182] The critical role of reductions in arterial $P_{CO_2}$ in precipitating central apneas is demonstrated by the observation that raising the $P_{CO_2}$ by just 1 to 3 mm Hg (e.g., by inhalation of a carbon dioxide–enriched gas mixture) abolishes central sleep apnea in patients with and without congestive heart failure[181, 186] (Fig. 81.6).

As in patients with obstructive sleep apnea, sleep fragmentation due to arousals at the termination of apneas is probably an important cause of excessive daytime sleepiness and fatigue in patients with congestive heart failure and central sleep apnea.[187, 188] Hypoxia and arousals from sleep are also associated with stimulation of the sympathetic nervous system.[11, 89, 91, 189] Nocturnal and daytime norepinephrine concentrations are markedly higher in congestive heart failure patients with central sleep apnea than in those without sleep apnea and are directly proportional to the frequency of arousals from sleep and the degree of apnea-related hypoxia, but not to left-ventricular ejection fraction.[190] Therefore, it appears that central sleep apnea can trigger sympathetic activation in patients with congestive heart failure and thereby exert a secondary deleterious effect on the underlying disorder.

## Clinical Features

In some persons, recurrent central apneas during sleep are not associated with any clinical manifestations or physiologic disturbances and are therefore of little clinical importance.[191] In others, the primary sequence of nocturnal events that characterize central apnea may give rise to a series of clinical features and complications that are similar to those resulting from obstructive sleep apnea (see Fig. 81.3). Because several different mechanisms can produce central apnea, the associated clinical manifestations are variable.

In patients whose central apnea is a manifestation of an underlying defect in respiratory control or in neuromuscular function, the clinical picture is usually dominated by recurrent episodes of respiratory failure and features of a chronic alveolar hypoventilation syndrome, including carbon dioxide retention, hypoxemia, pulmonary hypertension, right-sided heart failure, and polycythemia.[165, 166] Restless sleep, morning headache, chronic fatigue, and daytime sleepiness are also common in these patients, presumably as a consequence of nocturnal aggravation of hypoxemia and hypercapnia and disruption of normal sleep patterns. In contrast, patients whose central apnea is caused by transient fluctuations in respiratory drive during sleep do not have daytime hypercapnia and do not develop the cardiopulmonary complications of sleep apnea.[165, 166] Rather, they typically present with features of disturbed sleep, including recurrent nocturnal awakenings, morning fatigue, and daytime sleepiness.[165, 166, 192, 193] Because many of these patients also have a history of nasal obstruction and snoring, they are often initially thought to have obstructive sleep apnea. Patients with this type of central sleep apnea may present without any other associated clinical disorder (idiopathic central sleep apnea), but in many the central sleep apnea is secondary to the presence of congestive heart failure.[165, 194] Some of the fatigue that characterizes the heart failure

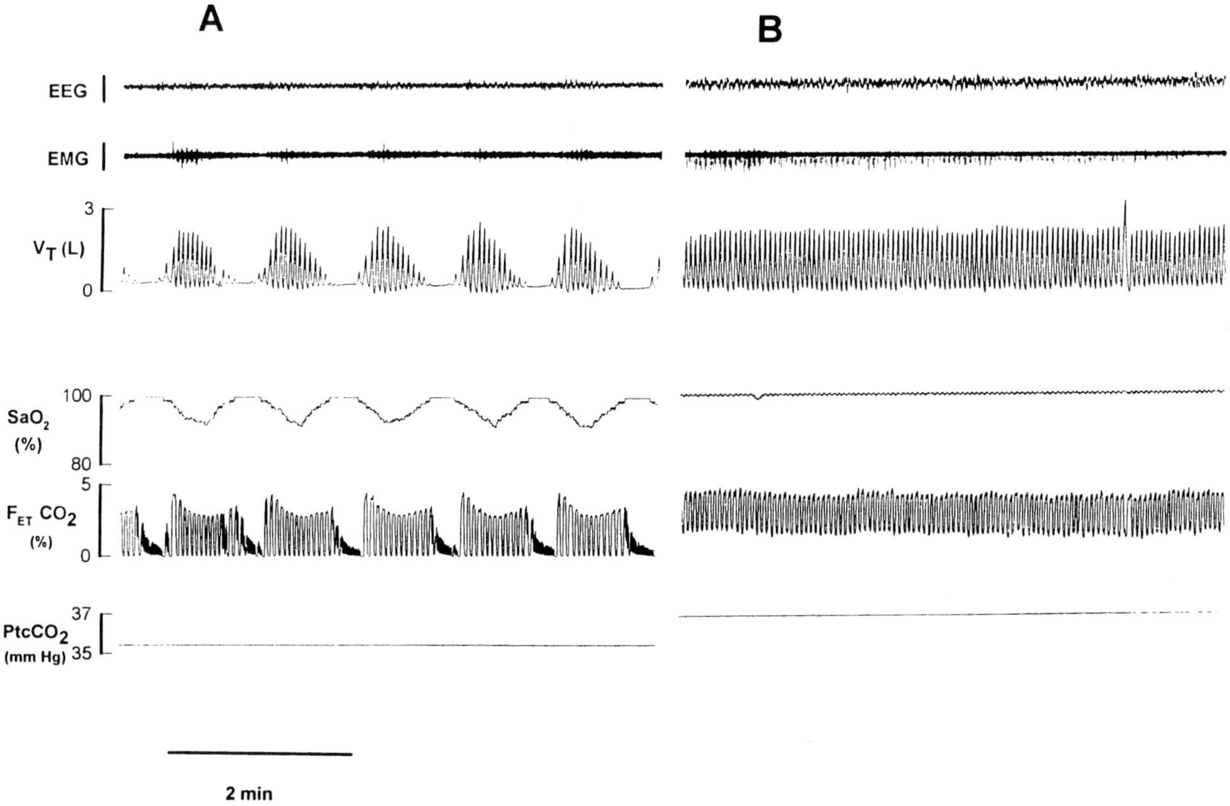


**Figure 81.6** Polysomnographic recordings are shown from a patient during stage 2 sleep while breathing air (A) and 1% carbon dioxide in air (B). Note abolition of central apneas on the tidal volume ($V_T$) trace and of recurrent decreases in arterial oxygen saturation ($Sa{O_2}$) during carbon dioxide inhalation, in association with an increase in transcutaneous $P{CO_2}$. ($Ptc{CO_2}$) of 1.6 mm Hg. EEG-electroencephalogram; EMG-submental electromyogram; $F_{ET}{CO_2}$, end-tidal carbon dioxide concentration. (From Lorenzi-Filho G, Rankin F, Bies I, et al: Effects of inhaled carbon dioxide and oxygen on Cheyne-Stokes respiration in patients with heart failure. Am J Respir Crit Care Med 159:1490–1498, 1999.)

syndrome may be a result of sleep apnea rather than heart failure per se. Patients with heart failure and central sleep apnea may also complain of insomnia and paroxysmal nocturnal dyspnea.[179, 187, 195–197]

The increased nocturnal and daytime sympathetic nervous activity associated with central sleep apnea in patients with congestive heart failure can aggravate myocardial dysfunction and contribute to disease progression.[124, 190] For example, congestive heart failure patients with central sleep apnea have a higher rate of ventricular tachycardia than do patients without sleep apnea, and the timing of ventricular ectopic beats is linked to the central sleep apnea ventilatory cycle and its associated dips in arterial $O_2$ saturation.[198, 199] The underlying cause of this relationship is unknown, but it could be a result of the apnea-related hypoxia, greater sympathetic nervous activity, recurrent surges in systemic blood pressure, or larger left-ventricular volume in patients with central sleep apnea.[124, 184, 190, 200] Because one third of patients with congestive heart failure die suddenly, presumably as a result of cardiac arrhythmias,[201] these relationships deserve further investigation. One or more of these factors may contribute to the increased mortality reported in congestive heart failure patients who have sleep apnea, compared with those who do not.[202]

## Diagnosis

The definitive diagnosis of a central sleep apnea disorder requires a polysomnographic study to demonstrate recurrent episodes of apnea accompanied by an absence of ventilatory effort. The latter criterion can best be confirmed by recording of pleural pressure swings with an esophageal catheter[19] (Fig. 81.7). In most patients, however, the cessation of respiratory drive can be reliably inferred from the coincident absence of ribcage and abdominal movements and of electromyographic activity of the diaphragm (recorded with surface electrodes).

In addition to confirming the presence of central sleep apnea, the polysomnographic findings usually provide an indication of whether the disorder is secondary to defects or to instabilities in the respiratory control system. In patients with defective metabolic respiratory control or neuromuscular disorders, there is a gradual reduction in ventilation to the point of apnea as the waking neural drive to breathing is withdrawn. The hypopneas and ap-

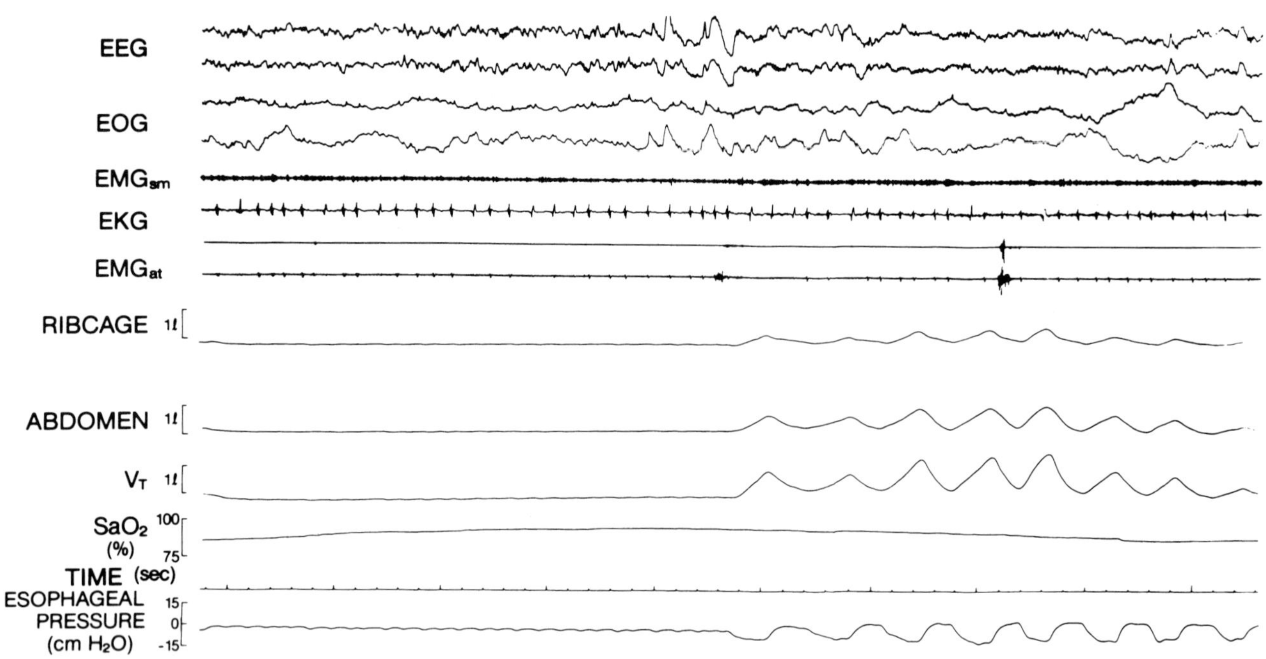


**Figure 81.7** Polysomnographic recording of a central sleep apnea in a patient with congestive heart failure is shown. Note the absence of rib cage and abdominal motion and of esophageal pressure excursions when there is no tidal volume ($V_T$) excursion, indicating an absence of central respiratory drive. (From Takasaki Y, Orr D, Popkin J, et al: Effect of nasal continuous positive airway pressure on sleep apnea in congestive heart failure. Am Rev Respir Dis 140:1578–1584, 1989.)

neas are generally distributed across all stages of sleep but are more prolonged in REM sleep.[166] Furthermore, the reductions in ventilation are usually accompanied by marked decreases in arterial $O_2$ saturation and by increases (often of 10 to 20 mm Hg) in $P_{CO_2}$ that can be measured continuously with a transcutaneous sensor. In contrast to these findings, in patients whose central sleep apnea is secondary to transient instabilities in respiratory drive, the apneas and hypopneas are typically associated with the transition from wakefulness to sleep and alternate with recurrent episodes of hyperpnea associated with arousals from sleep. Once sleep is established, breathing usually becomes regular, so that during slow-wave and REM sleep apneas and hypopneas are distinctly unusual. In most patients with this type of central sleep apnea, the apneic events are associated with only mild degrees of arterial oxygen desaturation and usually a small decrease in $P_{CO_2}$ (Fig. 81.8). The *decrease* in $P_{CO_2}$ related to state transitions plays a critical role in *generating* central apneas during sleep (see Pathogenesis), whereas in patients with defective respiratory control or muscle function, the *increase* in $P_{CO_2}$ that occurs during sleep is the *result* of the central apneas.

## Management

The management of central sleep apnea syndrome depends on the presence or absence of an underlying defect in respiratory drive or neuromuscular function. In patients with such defects, the management is usually the same as for a chronic alveolar hypoventilation syndrome (see Chapter 80). It is important that the patient be cautioned against the use of sedative medications that can aggravate the central sleep apnea and induce acute respiratory failure. Patients are occasionally improved by respiratory stimulant drugs, particularly medroxyprogesterone.[203] Supplemental nocturnal oxygen is of benefit in attenuating nocturnal hypoxemia but may result in more severe hypoventilation and prolongation of apnea episodes.[204–206] In a few patients, oxygen increases ventilation and abolishes apneas, presumably by relieving hypoxic cerebral depression.[207] Despite such measures, the majority of patients with severe nocturnal hypoventilation and central apnea require some type of ventilatory assistance. For those with central alveolar hypoventilation syndromes, electrophrenic pacing of the diaphragm during sleep can be extremely effective.[208, 209] When phrenic stimulation is not available or is inappropriate (as in neuromuscular disorders), mechanical ventilation is usually required, by means of either a positive-pressure ventilator applied through a tracheostomy or nose mask or a negative-pressure ventilator applied to the chest wall.[210–212] The administration of such treatment only during sleep often produces dramatic clinical improvement, with alleviation of daytime symptoms, lowering of daytime arterial $P_{CO_2}$, and reversal of cardiovascular complications.[213, 214]

The management of nonhypercapnic central sleep apnea disorders has not been clearly defined. As would be expected from knowledge of the underlying mechanisms (see Pathogenesis), patients who are hypoxemic generally respond well to supplemental oxygen,[215] and others have benefited, at least in the short term, from acidification

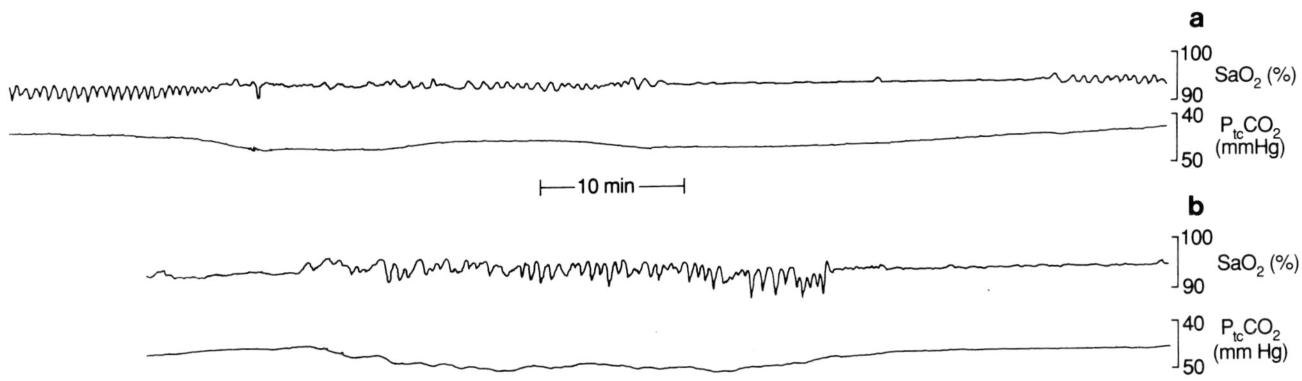


**Figure 81.8** Compressed records of nocturnal arterial oxygen saturation ($Sa_{O_2}$ and transcutaneous $P_{CO_2}$ ($Ptc_{CO_2}$) in a patient *(a)* with idiopathic central sleep apnea, and in a patient *(b)* with obstructive sleep apnea. Record reads from right to left. Note that in patient *a* the segments containing recurrent apneas (indicated by oscillations in $Sa_{O_2}$) are preceded by a small decrease in $Ptc_{CO_2}$. In contrast, in patient *b* the segment containing recurrent apneas is accompanied by a small increase in $Ptc_{CO_2}$. (From Bradley TD, Phillipson EA: Central sleep apnea. Clin Chest Med 13:493–505, 1992.)

with acetazolamide.[193] More recently, this condition has been effectively managed with nasal CPAP, as for obstructive sleep apnea.[216, 217] The mechanisms whereby nasal CPAP abolishes idiopathic central sleep apnea are not entirely clear but may involve an increase in $P_{CO_2}$ above the apneic threshold as a result of the increase in expiratory mechanical load. Nasal CPAP is particularly effective in patients with central sleep apnea associated with congestive heart failure and results in improvements in daytime exercise tolerance and cardiac function, as well as sleep quality.[187, 188, 218] Randomized clinical trials of 1 to 3 months' duration have shown that nasal CPAP has a beneficial effect on several surrogate markers of mortality in patients with congestive heart failure, including increases in left-ventricular ejection fraction, reductions in functional mitral regurgitation, and decreases in atrial natriuretic peptide and norepinephrine concentrations.[187, 188, 190, 219, 220] These findings suggest the potential for nasal CPAP to improve survival in patients with congestive heart failure and central sleep apnea.

## References


1. Aserinsky E, Kleitman N: Regularly occurring periods of eye motility, and concomitant phenomena, during sleep. Science 118:273–274, 1953.
2. Dement WC, Kleitman N: Cyclic variations in EEG during sleep and their relation to eye movements, body motility, and dreaming. Electroencephalogr Clin Neurophysiol 9:673–690, 1957.
3. Jouvet M: Neurophysiology of the sleep states. Physiol Rev 47:117–177, 1967.
4. Parmeggiani PL, Morrison A, Drucker-Colin R, et al: Brain mechanisms of sleep: An overview of methodological issues. *In* McGinty DJ, Drucker-Colin R, Morrison A, et al (eds): Brain Mechanisms of Sleep. New York: Raven Press, 1985, pp 1–33.
5. Rechtschaffen A, Kales A: A Manual of Standardized Terminology: Techniques and Scoring System for Sleep Stages of Human Subjects, Publication No. 204. Washington, DC: National Institutes of Health, 1968.
6. Phillipson EA, Bowes G: Control of breathing during sleep. *In* Cherniack NS, Widdicombe JG (eds): Handbook of Physiology. Section 3: The Respiratory System. Vol 2: Control of Breathing. Bethesda: American Physiological Society, 1986, pp 649–689.
7. Horner RL: Motor control of the pharyngeal musculature and implications for the pathogenesis of obstructive sleep apnea. Sleep 19:827–853, 1996.
8. White DP, Weil JV, Zwillich CW: Metabolic rate and breathing during sleep. J Appl Physiol 59:384–391, 1985.
9. Somers VK, Dyken ME, Mark AL, et al: Sympathetic-nerve activity during sleep in normal subjects. N Engl J Med 328:303–307, 1993.
10. Shepard JW Jr: Gas exchange and hemodynamics during sleep. Med Clin North Am 69:1243–1264, 1985.
11. Hornyak M, Cejnar M, Elam M, et al: Sympathetic muscle nerve activity during sleep in man. Brain 114:1281–1295, 1991.
12. Davies RJ, Belt PJ, Roberts SJ, et al: Arterial blood pressure responses to graded transient arousal from sleep in normal humans. J Appl Physiol 74:1123–1130, 1993.
13. Bowes G, Phillipson EA: Arousal responses to respiratory stimuli during sleep. *In* Saunders NA, Sullivan CE (eds): Lung Biology in Health and Disease. Vol 21: Sleep and Breathing. New York: Marcel Dekker, 1984, pp 137–161.
14. Stradling JR, Phillipson EA: Breathing disorders during sleep. Q J Med 58:3–18, 1986.
15. Motta J, Guilleminault C, Schroeder JS, et al: Tracheostomy and hemodynamic changes in sleep-induced apnea. Ann Intern Med 89:454–458, 1978.
16. Coleman RM: Periodic movements in sleep (nocturnal myoclonus) and restless legs syndrome. *In* Guilleminault C (ed): Sleep and Waking Disorders: Indications and Techniques. Menlo Park, CA: Addison-Wesley, 1982, pp 265–295.
17. Phillipson EA, Bowes G: Sleep disorders. *In* Fishman AP (ed): Update of Pulmonary Diseases and Disorders. New York: McGraw-Hill, 1982, pp 256–273.
18. Stradling JR, Chadwick GA, Quirk C, et al: Respiratory inductance plethysmography: Calibration techniques, their validation and the effects of posture. Bull Eur Physiopathol Respir 21:317–324, 1985.
19. Staats BA, Bonekat HW, Harris CD, et al: Chest wall motion in sleep apnea. Am Rev Respir Dis 130:59–63, 1984.
20. Onal E, Lopata M, Ginzburg AS, et al: Diaphragmatic EMG and transdiaphragmatic pressure measurements with a single catheter. Am Rev Respir Dis 124:563–565, 1981.
21. Coleman RM, Roffwarg HP, Kennedy SJ, et al: Sleep-wake disorders based on polysomnographic diagnosis. JAMA 247:997–1003, 1982.
22. National Commission on Sleep Disorders Research: Wake up America: A National Sleep Alert. Washington, DC: Government Printing Office, 1993.
23. Guilleminault C, Tilkian A, Dement WC: The sleep apnea syndromes. Annu Rev Med 27:465–484, 1976.

24. Lugaresi E, Coccagna G, Mantovani M: Hypersomnia with Periodic Apneas. New York: Spectrum, 1978.
25. Strohl KP, Saunders NA, Sullivan CE: Sleep apnea syndromes. *In* Saunders NA, Sullivan CE (eds): Lung Biology in Health and Disease. Vol 21: Sleep and Breathing. New York: Marcel Dekker, 1984, pp 365–402.
26. Kosvenuo M, Kaprio J, Partinen M, et al: Snoring as a risk factor for hypertension and angina pectoris. Lancet 1:393–396, 1985.
27. Kosvenuo M, Kaprio J, Telakivi T, et al: Snoring as a risk factor for ischemic heart disease and stroke in men. BMJ 294:16–19, 1987.
28. Malone S, Liu PP, Holloway R, et al: Obstructive sleep apnoea in patients with dilated cardiomyopathy: Effects of continuous positive airway pressure. Lancet 338:1480–1484, 1991.
29. Young T, Palta M, Dempsey J, et al: The occurrence of sleep-disordered breathing among middle-aged adults. N Engl J Med 328:1230–1235, 1993.
30. Ancoli-Israel S, Kripke DF, Klauber MR, et al: Sleep disordered breathing in community-dwelling elderly. Sleep 14:486–495, 1991.
31. Suratt PM, Dee P, Atkinson RL, et al: Fluoroscopic and computed tomographic features of the pharyngeal airway in obstructive sleep apnea. Am Rev Respir Dis 127:487–492, 1983.
32. Hudgel DW: Variable site of airway narrowing among obstructive sleep apnea patients. J Appl Physiol 61:1403–1409, 1986.
33. Guilleminault C, Stoohs R, Clerk A, et al: Cause of excessive daytime sleepiness: The upper airway resistance syndrome. Chest 104:781–787, 1993.
34. Guilleminault C, Beck J, Carillo O: EEG arousal and upper airway resistance syndrome. Electroencephalogr Clin Neurophysiol 103:501, 1999.
35. Bradley TD, Phillipson EA: Pathogenesis and pathophysiology of the obstructive sleep apnea syndrome. Med Clin North Am 69:1169–1185, 1985.
36. Remmers JE, de Groot WJ, Sauerland EK, et al: Pathogenesis of upper airway occlusion during sleep. J Appl Physiol 44:931–938, 1978.
37. Smith PL, Wise RA, Gold AR, et al: Upper airway pressure-flow relationships in obstructive sleep apnea. J Appl Physiol 64:789–795, 1988.
38. Schwartz AR, Smith PL, Wise RA, et al: Effect of positive nasal pressure on upper airway pressure-flow relationships. J Appl Physiol 66:1626–1634, 1989.
39. Hudgel DW: The role of upper airway anatomy and physiology in obstructive sleep apnea. Clin Chest Med 13:383–398, 1992.
40. Bear SE, Priest JH: Sleep apnea syndrome: Correction with surgical advancement of the mandible. J Oral Maxillofac Surg 35:543–549, 1980.
41. Mezon BJ, West P, Maclean JP, et al: Sleep apnea in acromegaly. Am J Med 69:615–618, 1980.
42. Orr WC, Martin RJ: Obstructive sleep apnea associated with tonsillar hypertrophy in adults. Arch Intern Med 141:990–992, 1981.
43. Haponik EF, Smith PL, Bohlman ME, et al: Computerized tomography in obstructive sleep apnea. Am Rev Respir Dis 127:221–226, 1983.
44. Riley R, Guilleminault C, Herran J, et al: Cephalometric analyses and flow-volume loops in obstructive sleep apnea patients. Sleep 6:303–311, 1983.
45. Rivlin J, Hoffstein V, Kalbfleisch J, et al: Upper airway morphology in patients with idiopathic obstructive sleep apnea. Am Rev Respir Dis 129:355–360, 1984.
46. Lowe AA, Gionhaker N, Takeuchi K, et al: Three dimensional CT reconstructions of tongue and airway in adult subjects with obstructive sleep apnea. Am J Orthod Dentofacial Orthop 90:364–374, 1986.
47. Larsson S-G, Gislason T, Lindholm CE: Computed tomography of the oropharynx in obstructive sleep apnea. Acta Radiol 29:401–405, 1988.
48. Horner RL, Mohiaddin RH, Lowell DG, et al: Sites and sizes of fat deposits around the pharynx in obese patients with obstructive sleep apnoea and weight matched controls. Eur Respir J 2:613–622, 1989.
49. Fleetham JA: Upper airway imaging in relation to obstructive sleep apnea. Clin Chest Med 13:399–416, 1992.
50. Smith PL, Gold AR, Meyers DA, et al: Weight loss in mildly to moderately obese patients with obstructive sleep apnea. Ann Intern Med 103:850–855, 1985.
51. Davies RJO, Stradling JR: The relationship between neck circumference, radiographic pharyngeal anatomy, and the obstructive sleep apnea syndrome. Eur Respir J 3:509–514, 1990.
52. Issa FG, Sullivan CE: Upper airway closing pressures in obstructive sleep apnea. J Appl Physiol 57:520–527, 1984.
53. Brown IG, Bradley TD, Phillipson EA, et al: Pharyngeal compliance in snoring subjects with and without obstructive sleep apnea. Am Rev Respir Dis 132:211–215, 1985.
54. Bradley TD, Brown IG, Grossman RF, et al: Pharyngeal size in snorers, non-snorers, and patients with obstructive sleep apnea. N Engl J Med 315:1327–1331, 1986.
55. Mezzanotte WS, Tangel DJ, White DP: Waking genioglossal electromyogram in sleep apnea patients versus normal controls (a neuromuscular compensatory mechanism). J Clin Invest 89:1571–1579, 1992.
56. Hendricks JC, Petrof BL, Panckeri K, et al: Compensatory hyperactivity of an upper airway dilator in bulldogs. Am Rev Respir Dis 148:185–194, 1993.
57. Sauerland EK, Harper RM: The human tongue during sleep: Electromyographic activity of the genioglossus muscle. Exp Neurol 51:160–170, 1976.
58. Wheatley JR, Mezzanote WS, Tangel DJ, et al: Influence of sleep on genioglossus muscle activation by negative pressure in normal men. Am Rev Respir Dis 148:597–605, 1993.
59. Onal E, Lopata M, O'Connor T: Pathogenesis of apneas in hypersomnia-sleep apnea syndrome. Am Rev Respir Dis 125:167–174, 1982.
60. Onal E, Lopata M: Periodic breathing and the pathogenesis of occlusive sleep apneas. Am Rev Respir Dis 126:676–680, 1982.
61. Cherniack NS: Sleep apnea and its causes. J Clin Invest 73:150–156, 1984.
62. Hudgel DW, Chapman KR, Faulks C, et al: Changes in inspiratory muscle electrical activity and upper airway resistance during periodic breathing induced by hypoxia during sleep. Am Rev Respir Dis 135:899–906, 1987.
63. Parisi RA, Neubauer JA, Frank MM, et al: Correlation between genioglossal and diaphragmatic responses to hypercapnia during sleep. Am Rev Respir Dis 135:378–382, 1987.
64. Hudgel DW, Harasick T: Fluctuations in timing of upper airway and chest wall inspiratory muscle activity in obstructive sleep apnea. J Appl Physiol 69:443–450, 1990.
65. Taasan VC, Block AJ, Boysen PG, et al: Alcohol increases sleep apnea and oxygen desaturation in asymptomatic men. Am J Med 71:240–245, 1981.
66. Dolly FR, Block AJ: Effect of flurazepam on sleep-disordered breathing and nocturnal oxygen desaturation in asymptomatic subjects. Am J Med 73:239–243, 1982.
67. Issa FG, Sullivan CE: Alcohol, snoring and sleep apnea. J Neurol Neurosurg Psychiatr 45:353–359, 1982.
68. Krol RC, Knuth SL, Bartlett D Jr: Selective reduction of genioglossal muscle activity by alcohol in normal human subjects. Am Rev Respir Dis 129:247–250, 1984.
69. Martin RJ, Pennock BE, Orr WC, et al: Respiratory mechanics and timing during sleep in occlusive sleep apnea. J Appl Physiol 48:432–437, 1980.
70. Vincken W, Guilleminault C, Silvestri L, et al: Inspiratory muscle activity as a trigger causing the airways to open in obstructive sleep apnea. Am Rev Respir Dis 135:372–377, 1987.
71. Yasuma F, Kozar LF, Kimoff RJ, et al: Interaction of chemical and mechanical respiratory stimuli in the arousal response to hypoxia in sleeping dogs. Am Rev Respir Dis 143:1274–1277, 1991.
72. Bowes G, Townsend ER, Bromley SM, et al: Role of the carotid body and of afferent vagal stimuli in the arousal response to airway occlusion in sleeping dogs. Am Rev Respir Dis 123:644–647, 1981.
73. Sullivan CE, Issa FG, Berthon-Jones M, et al: Pathophysiology of sleep apnea. *In* Saunders NA, Sullivan CE (eds): Lung Biology in Health and Disease. Vol 21: Sleep and Breathing. New York: Marcel Dekker, 1984, pp 299–363.
74. Bowes G, Woolf GM, Sullivan CE, et al: Effect of sleep fragmentation on ventilatory and arousal responses of sleeping dogs to respiratory stimuli. Am Rev Respir Dis 122:899–908, 1980.

75. Guilleminault C, Rosekind M: The arousal threshold: Sleep deprivation, sleep fragmentation, and obstructive sleep apnea syndrome. Bull Eur Physiopathol Respir 17:341–349, 1981.
76. Martin SE, Engleman HM, Deary IJ, et al: The effect of sleep fragmentation on daytime function. Am J Respir Crit Care Med 153:1328–1332, 1996.
77. Phillipson EA: Sleep apnea. Med Clin North Am 23:2314–2323, 1982.
78. George CF, Nickerson PW, Hanly PJ, et al: Sleep apnoea patients have more automobile accidents. Lancet 2:447, 1987.
79. Findley L, Unverzagt M, Suratt P: Automobile accidents in patients with obstructive sleep apnea. Am Rev Respir Dis 138:337–340, 1988.
80. Findley L, Fabrizio M, Thommi G, et al: Severity of sleep apnea and automobile crashes. N Engl J Med 320:868–869, 1989.
81. Barbe F, Pericas J, Munoz A, et al: Automobile accidents in patients with sleep apnea syndrome. Am J Respir Crit Care Med 158:18–22, 1998.
82. Teran-Santos J, Jiminez-Gomez A, Cordero-Guevara J: The association between sleep apnea and the risk of traffic accidents. N Engl J Med 340:847–851, 1999.
83. Findley L, Barth JT, Powers DC, et al: Cognitive impairment in patients with obstructive sleep apnea and associated hypoxemia. Chest 90:686–690, 1986.
84. Telakivi T, Kajaste S, Partinen M, et al: Cognitive function in middle-aged snorers and controls: Role of excessive daytime somnolence and sleep related hypoxic events. Sleep 11:454–462, 1988.
85. Bedard MA, Montplaisir J, Richer F, et al: Obstructive sleep apnea syndrome: Pathogenesis of neuropsychological deficits. Clin Exp Neuropsychol 13:950–964, 1991.
86. Naegele B, Thouvard V, Pepin JL, et al: Deficits of cognitive executive functions in patients with sleep apnea syndrome. Sleep 18:43–52, 1995.
87. Coccagna G, Mantovani M, Brignani F, et al: Continuous recording of the pulmonary and systemic arterial pressure during sleep in syndromes of hypersomnia with periodic breathing. Bull Eur Physiopathol Respir 8:1159–1172, 1972.
88. Tilkian AG, Guilleminault C, Schroeder JS, et al: Hemodynamics in sleep-induced apnea. Ann Intern Med 85:714–719, 1976.
89. Hedner J, Ejnell H, Sellgren J, et al: Is high and fluctuating muscle nerve sympathetic activity in the sleep apnoea syndrome of pathogenetic importance for the development of hypertension? J Hypertens 6(Suppl 4):S529–S531, 1988.
90. Morgan BJ, Denahan T, Ebert TJ: Neurocirculatory consequences of negative intrathoracic pressure vs. asphyxia during voluntary apnea. J Appl Physiol 74:2969–2975, 1993.
91. Somers VK, Dyken ME, Clary MP, et al: Sympathetic neural mechanisms in obstructive sleep apnea. J Clin Invest 96:1897–1904, 1995.
92. Mateika JH, Mateika S, Slutsky AS, et al: The effect of snoring on mean arterial blood pressure during non-REM sleep. Am Rev Respir Dis 145:141–146, 1992.
93. Millman RP, Redline S, Carlisle CC, et al: Daytime hypertension in obstructive sleep apnea: Prevalence and contributing risk factors. Chest 99:861–866, 1991.
94. Fletcher EC, Miller J, Schaaf JW, et al: Urinary catecholamines before and after tracheostomy in patients with obstructive sleep apnea and hypertension. Sleep 10:35–44, 1987.
95. Carlson JT, Hedner J, Elam M, et al: Augmented resting sympathetic nerve activity in awake patients with obstructive sleep apnea. Chest 103:1763–1768, 1993.
96. Narkiewicz K, van de Borne PJ, Cooley RL, et al: Sympathetic activity in obese subjects with and without obstructive sleep apnea. Circulation 98:772–776, 1998.
97. Silverberg DS, Oksenberg A: Essential hypertension and abnormal upper airway resistance during sleep. Sleep 20:794–806, 1997.
98. Hoffstein V, Rubinstein I, Mateika S, et al: Determinants of blood pressure in snorers. 2:992–994, 1988.
99. Warley ARH, Mitchell JH, Stradling JR: Prevalence of nocturnal hypoxaemia amongst men with mild to moderate hypertension. QJM 256:637–644, 1988.
100. Stradling JR, Crosby JH: Relation between systemic hypertension and sleep hypoxaemia or snoring: Analysis in 748 men drawn from general practice. BMJ 300:75–78, 1990.
101. Young T, Peppaard P, Palta M, et al: Population-based study of sleep-disordered breathing as a risk factor for hypertension. Arch Intern Med 157:1746–1752, 1997.
102. Brooks D, Horner RL, Kozar LF, et al: Obstructive sleep apnea as a cause of systemic hypertension: Evidence from a canine model. J Clin Invest 99:106–109, 1997.
103. Buda AJ, Pinsky MR, Ingels NBJ, et al: Effect of intrathoracic pressure on left ventricular performance. N Engl J Med 301:453–459, 1979.
104. Bradley TD, Holloway RM, McLaughlin PR, et al: Cardiac output response to continuous positive airway pressure in congestive heart failure. Am Rev Respir Dis 145:377–382, 1992.
105. Scharf SM, Bianco JA, Tow DE, et al: The effects of large negative intrathoracic pressure on left ventricular function in patients with coronary artery disease. Circulation 63:871–875, 1981.
106. Parker JD, Brooks D, Kozar LF, et al: Acute and chronic effects of airway obstruction on canine left ventricular performance. Am J Respir Crit Care Med 160:1888–1896, 1999.
107. Buda AJ, Schroeder JS, Guilleminault C: Abnormalities of pulmonary artery wedge pressures in sleep-induced apnea. Int J Cardiol 1:67–74, 1981.
108. Scharf SM, Graver LM, Balaban K: Cardiovascular effects of periodic occlusions of the upper airways in dogs. Am Rev Respir Dis 146:321–329, 1992.
109. Peters J, Fraser C, Stuart RS, et al: Negative intrathoracic pressure decreases independently left ventricular filling and emptying. Am J Physiol 257:H120–H131, 1989.
110. Virolainen J, Ventila M, Turto H, et al: Effect of negative intrathoracic pressure on left ventricular pressure dynamics and relaxation. J Appl Physiol 79:455–460, 1995.
111. Hall MJ, Ando SI, Floras JS, et al: Magnitude and time course of hemodynamic responses to Mueller maneuvers in patients with congestive heart failure. J Appl Physiol 85:1476–1484, 1998.
112. Ross JJ: Afterload mismatch and preload reserve: A conceptual framework for the analysis of ventricular function. Prog Cardiovasc Dis 18:254–264, 1976.
113. Hanly P, Sasson Z, Zuberi N, et al: ST-segment depression during sleep in obstructive sleep apnea. Am J Cardiol 71:1341-1345, 1993.
114. Chaudhary BA, Ferguson DS, Speir WA: Pulmonary edema as a presenting feature of sleep apnea syndrome. Chest 82:122–124, 1982.
115. Chan HS, Chiu HF, Tse LK, et al: Obstructive sleep apnea presenting with nocturnal angina, heart failure, and near-miss sudden death. Chest 99:1023–1025, 1991.
116. Franklin KA, Nilsson JB, Sahlin C: Sleep apnoea and nocturnal angina. Lancet 345:1085–1087, 1995.
117. Cargill RI, Kiely DG, Lipworth BJ: Adverse effects of hypoxaemia on diastolic filling in humans. Clin Sci 89:165–169, 1995.
118. Tolle FA, Judy WV, Yu PL, et al: Reduced stroke volume related to pleural pressure in obstructive sleep apnea. J Appl Physiol 55:1718–1724, 1983.
119. Stoohs R, Guilleminault C: Cardiovascular changes associated with obstructive sleep apnea syndrome. J Appl Physiol 72:583–589, 1992.
120. Somers VK, Mark AL, Zavala DC, et al: Contrasting effects of hypoxia and hypercapnia on ventilation and sympathetic activity in humans. J Appl Physiol 67:2101–2106, 1989.
121. Galatius-Jensen S, Hansen J, Rasmussen V, et al: Nocturnal hypoxaemia after myocardial infarction: Association with nocturnal myocardial ischaemia and arrhythmias. Br Heart J 72:23–30, 1994.
122. Miller WP: Cardiac arrhythmias and conduction disturbances in the sleep apnea syndrome. Am J Med 73:317–321, 1982.
123. Shepard JW Jr, Garrison MW, Guther DA, et al: Relationship of ventricular ectopy to nocturnal $O_2$ desaturation in patients with obstructive sleep apnea. Chest 88:325–340, 1985.
124. Daly PA, Sole MJ: Myocardial catecholamines and the pathophysiology of heart failure. Circulation 82:I35–I43, 1990.
125. Seppala T, Partinen M, Penttila A, et al: Sudden death and sleeping history among Finnish men. J Intern Med 229:23–28, 1991.
126. Hender J, Ejnell H, Caidahl K: Left ventricular hypertrophy independent of hypertension in patients with obstructive sleep apnea. J Hypertens 8:941–946, 1990.
127. Hanly P, Sasson Z, Zuberi N, et al: Ventricular function in snor-

ers and patients with obstructive sleep apnea. Chest 102:100–105, 1992.
128. Kaye DM, Lambert GM, Lefkovits J, et al: Neurochemical evidence of cardiac sympathetic activation and increased central nervous system norepinephrine turnover in severe congestive heart failure. J Am Coll Cardiol 23:570–578, 1994.
129. Cohn JN, Levine TB, Olivary MT, et al: Plasma norepinephrine as a guide to prognosis in patients with congestive heart failure. N Engl J Med 311:819–823, 1984.
130. Bradley TD, Rutherford R, Grossman RF, et al: Role of daytime hypoxemia in the pathogenesis of right heart failure in the obstructive sleep apnea syndrome. Am Rev Respir Dis 131:835–839, 1985.
131. Weitzenblum E, Krieger J, Apprill M, et al: Daytime pulmonary hypertension in patients with obstructive sleep apnea syndrome. Am Rev Respir Dis 138:345–349, 1988.
132. Whyte KF, Douglas NJ: Peripheral edema in sleep apnea/hypopnea syndrome. Sleep 14:354–356, 1991.
133. Bradley TD, Rutherford R, Lue F, et al: Role of diffuse airway obstruction in the hypercapnia of obstructive sleep apnea. Am Rev Respir Dis 134:920–924, 1986.
134. Garay SM, Rapoport D, Sorkin B, et al: Regulation of ventilation in the obstructive sleep apnea syndrome. Am Rev Respir Dis 124:451–457, 1981.
135. Lopata M, Onal E: Mass loading, sleep apnea, and the pathogenesis of obesity hypoventilation. Am Rev Respir Dis 126:640–645, 1982.
136. Weil JV, Byrne-Quinn E, Sodal IE, et al: Acquired attenuation of chemoreceptor function in chronically hypoxic men at high altitude. J Clin Invest 50:186–195, 1971.
137. Mountain R, Zwillich C, Weil J: Hypoventilation in obstructive lung disease: The role of familial factors. N Engl J Med 298:521–525, 1978.
138. White DP, Douglas NJ, Pickett CK, et al: Sleep deprivation and the control of ventilation. Am Rev Respir Dis 128:984–986, 1983.
139. Lavie P, Herer P, Peled R, et al: Mortality in sleep apnea patients: A multivariate analysis of risk factors. Sleep 18:149–157, 1995.
140. Ancoli-Israel S, Kripke DF, Klauber MR, et al: Morbidity, mortality and sleep disordered breathing in community dwelling elderly. Sleep 19:277–282, 1996.
141. Gyulay S, Olson LG, Hensley MR, et al: A comparison of clinical assessment and home oximetry in the diagnosis of obstructive sleep apnea. Am Rev Respir Dis 147:50–53, 1993.
142. Series F, Marc I, Cormier Y, et al: Utility of nocturnal home oximetry for case finding in patients with suspected sleep apnea syndrome. Ann Intern Med 119:449–453, 1993.
143. Whittle AT, Finch SP, Mortimore IL, et al: Use of home sleep studies for diagnosis of the sleep apnoea/hypopnoea syndrome. Thorax 52:1068–1073, 1997.
144. Hoffstein V: Is snoring dangerous to your health? Sleep 19:506–516, 1996.
145. Bloom JW, Kaltenborn WT, Quan SF: Risk factors in the general population for snoring: Importance of cigarette smoking and obesity. Chest 93:678–683, 1988.
146. Braver HM, Block AJ, Perri MG: Treatment for snoring: Combined weight loss, sleeping on the side, and nasal spray. Chest 107:1283–1288, 1995.
147. American Thoracic Society: Indications and standards for use of nasal continuous positive airway pressure (CPAP) in sleep apnea syndromes. Am J Respir Crit Care Med 150:1738–1745, 1994.
148. O'Sullivan RA, Hillman DR, Mateljan, et al: Mandibular advancement splint: An appliance to treat snoring and obstructive sleep apnea. Am J Respir Crit Care Med 151:194–198, 1995.
149. Ferguson KA, Ono T, Lowe A, et al: A randomized cross-over trial of an oral appliance vs. nasal continuous positive airway pressure in the treatment of mild-moderate obstructive sleep apnea. Chest 109:1269–1275, 1996.
150. Stradling JR, Negus TW, Smith D, et al: Mandibular advancement devices for the control of snoring. Eur Respir J 11:447–450, 1998.
151. Engleman HE, Kingshott RN, Wraith PK, et al: Randomized placebo-controlled crossover trial of continuous positive airway pressure for mild sleep apnea/hypopnea syndrome. Am J Respir Crit Care Med 159:461–467, 1999.
152. Fujita S, Conway W, Zorick F, et al: Surgical correction of anatomic abnormalities in obstructive sleep apnea syndrome: Uvulopalatopharyngoplasty. Otolaryngol Head Neck Surg 89:923–934, 1981.
153. Kamami YV: Laser $CO_2$ for snoring: Preliminary results. Acta Otorhinolaryngol Bclg 44:451–456, 1990.
154. Schmidt-Nowara WW, Meade TE, Hays MB: Treatment of snoring and obstructive sleep apnea with a dental orthosis. Chest 99:1378–1385, 1991.
155. Sher AE, Schechtman KB, Piccirillo JF: The efficacy of surgical modifications of the upper airway in adults with obstructive sleep apnea syndrome. Sleep 19:156–177, 1996.
156. Ryan CF, Lowe AA, Li D, et al: Three dimensional upper airway computed tomography in obstructive sleep apnea: A prospective study in patients treated by uvulopalatopharyngoplasty. Am Rev Respir Dis 144:428–432, 1991.
157. Launois SH, Feroah TR, Campbell WN, et al: Site of pharyngeal narrowing predicts outcome of surgery for obstructive sleep apnea. Am Rev Respir Dis 147:182–189, 1993.
158. Sullivan CE, Issa FG, Berthon-Jones M, et al: Reversal of obstructive sleep apnea by continuous positive airway pressure applied through the nares. Lancet 1:862–865, 1981.
159. Sullivan CE, Issa FG, Berthon-Jones M, et al: Home treatment of obstructive sleep apnea with continuous positive airway pressure applied through a nose-mask. Bull Eur Physiopathol Respir 20:49–54, 1984.
160. Hoffstein V, Viner S, Mateika S, et al: Treatment of obstructive sleep apnea with nasal continuous positive airway pressure: Patient compliance, perception of benefits, and side effects. Am Rev Respir Dis 145:841–845, 1992.
160a. McArdle N, Devereux G, Heidarnejad H, et al: Long-term use of CPAP therapy for sleep apnea/hypopnea syndrome. Am J Respir Crit Care Med 159:1108–1114, 1999.
160b. Pepin JL, Kreiger J, Rodenstein D, et al: Effective complicance during the first 3 months of continuous positive airway pressure. Am J Respir Crit Care Med 160:1124–1129, 1999.
161. Iber C, O'Brien C, Schluter J, et al: Single night studies in obstructive sleep apnea. Sleep 14:383–385, 1991.
162. Sanders MH, Kern N: Obstructive sleep apnea treated by independently adjusted inspiratory and expiratory positive airway pressures via nasal mask. Chest 98:317–324, 1990.
163. Weitzman ED, Kahn E, Pollack CP: Quantitative analysis of sleep and sleep apnea before and after tracheostomy in patients with the hypersomnia-sleep apnea syndrome. Sleep 3:407–423, 1980.
164. Guilleminault C, Simmons FB, Motta J, et al: Obstructive sleep apnea syndrome and tracheostomy: Long-term followup experience. Arch Intern Med 141:985–988, 1981.
165. Bradley TD, Phillipson EA: Central sleep apnea. Clin Chest Med 13:493–505, 1992.
166. Bradley TD, McNicholas WT, Rutherford R, et al: Clinical and physiologic heterogeneity of the central sleep apnea syndrome. Am Rev Respir Dis 134:217–221, 1986.
167. Orem J: The nature of the wakefulness stimulus to breathing. *In* Issa FG, Suratt PM, Remmers JE (eds): Progress in Clinical and Biological Research. Vol 345: Sleep and Respiration. New York: Wiley-Liss, 1990, pp 23–31.
168. Phillipson EA: Control of breathing during sleep. Am Rev Respir Dis 118:909–939, 1978.
169. Longobardo G, Gothe B, Goldman MD, et al: Sleep apnea considered as a control system instability. Respir Physiol 50:311–333, 1982.
170. Khoo MCK, Kronauer RE, Strohl KP, et al: Factors inducing periodic breathing in humans: A general model. J Appl Physiol 53:644–659, 1982.
171. Skatrud JB, Dempsey JA: Interaction of sleep state and chemical stimuli in sustaining rhythmic ventilation. J Appl Physiol 55:813–822, 1983.
172. Datta AK, Shea SA, Horner RL, et al: The influence of induced hypocapnia and sleep on the endogenous respiratory rhythm in humans. J Physiol (Lond) 440:17–33, 1991.
173. Khoo MCK, Gottschalk A, Pack AI: Sleep-induced periodic breathing and apnea: A theoretical study. J Appl Physiol 70:2014–2024, 1991.
174. Carskadon MA, Harvey K, Dement WC, et al: Respiration during sleep in children. West J Med 128:477–481, 1978.

175. Tabachnik E, Muller NL, Bryan AC, et al: Changes in ventilation and chest wall mechanics during sleep in normal adolescents. J Appl Physiol 51:557–564, 1981.
175a. Dunai J, Kleiman J, Trinder J: Ventilatory instability during sleep onset in individuals with high peripheral chemoreceptor chemosensitivity. J Appl Physiol 87:661–672, 1999.
176. Berssenbrugge A, Dempsey J, Iber C, et al: Mechanisms of hypoxia-induced periodic breathing during sleep in humans. J Physiol (Lond) 343:507–524, 1983.
177. Lahiri S, Maret K, Sherpa MG: Dependence of high altitude sleep apnea on ventilatory sensitivity to hypoxia. Respir Physiol 52:281–301, 1983.
178. Weil JV: Sleep at high altitude. Clin Chest Med 6:615–621, 1985.
179. Javaheri S, Parker TJ, Liming JD, et al: Sleep apnea in 81 ambulatory male patients with stable heart failure. Circulation 97:2154–2159, 1998.
179a. Sin DD, Fitzgerald F, Parker JD, et al: Risk factors for central and obstructive sleep apnea in 450 men and women with congestive heart failure. Am J Respir Crit Care Med 160:1101–1106, 1999.
180. Naughton M, Benard D, Tam A, et al: Role of hyperventilation in the pathogenesis of central sleep apneas in patients with congestive heart failure. Am Rev Respir Dis 148:330–338, 1993.
181. Lorenzi-Filho G, Rankin F, Bies I, et al: Effects of inhaled carbon dioxide and oxygen on Cheyne-Stokes respiration in patients with heart failure. Am J Respir Crit Care Med 159:1490–1498, 1999.
182. Xie A, Wong B, Phillipson EA, et al: Interaction of hyperventilation and arousal in the pathogenesis of idiopathic central sleep apnea. Am J Respir Crit Care Med 150:489–495, 1994.
182a. Javaheri S: A mechanism of central sleep apnea in patients with heart failure. N Engl J Med 341:949–954, 1999.
183. Hanly P, Zuberi N, Gray R: Pathogenesis of Cheyne-Stokes respiration in patients with congestive heart failure: Relationship to arterial $P_{CO_2}$. Chest 104:1079–1084, 1993.
184. Tkacova R, Hall MJ, Liu PP, et al: Left ventricular volume in patients with heart failure and Cheyne-Stokes respiration during sleep. Am J Respir Crit Care Med 156:1549–1555, 1997.
185. Churchill ED, Cope O: The rapid shallow breathing resulting from pulmonary congestion and edema. J Exp Med 49:531–537, 1929.
186. Xie A, Rankin F, Rutherford R, et al: Effects of inhaled $CO_2$ and added dead space on idiopathic central sleep apnea. J Appl Physiol 82:918–926, 1997.
187. Takasaki Y, Orr D, Popkin J, et al: Effect of nasal continuous positive airway pressure on sleep apnea in congestive heart failure. Am Rev Respir Dis 140:1578–1584, 1989.
188. Naughton MT, Liu PP, Bernard DC, et al: Treatment of congestive heart failure and Cheyne-Stokes respiration during sleep by continuous positive airway pressure. Am J Respir Crit Care Med 151:92–97, 1995.
189. van de Borne P, Oren R, Abouassaly C, et al: Effect of Cheyne-Stokes respiration on muscle sympathetic nerve activity in severe congestive heart failure secondary to ischemic or idiopathic dilated cardiomyopathy. Am J Cardiol 81:432–436, 1998.
190. Naughton MT, Benard DC, Liu PP, et al: Effects of nasal CPAP on sympathetic activity in patients with heart failure and central sleep apnea. Am J Respir Crit Care Med 152:473–479, 1995.
191. Shore ET, Millman RP, Silage DA, et al: Ventilatory and arousal patterns during sleep in normal young and elderly subjects. J Appl Physiol 59:1607–1615, 1985.
192. Guilleminault C, Eldridge FL, Dement WC: Insomnia with sleep apnea: A new syndrome. Science 181:856–858, 1973.
193. White DP, Zwillich CW, Pickett CK, et al: Central sleep apnea: Improvement with acetazolamide therapy. Arch Intern Med 142:1816–1819, 1982.
194. Bradley TD: Right and left ventricular functional impairment and sleep apnea. Clin Chest Med 13:459–479, 1992.
195. Harrison TR, King CE, Calhoun JA, et al: Cheyne-Stokes respiration as the cause of paroxysmal dyspnea at the onset of sleep. Arch Intern Med 53:891–910, 1934.
196. Hanly PJ, Millar TW, Steljes DG, et al: Respiration and abnormal sleep in patients with congestive heart failure. Chest 96:480–488, 1989.
197. Dowdell WT, Javaheri S, McGinnis W: Cheyne-Stokes respiration presenting as sleep apnea syndrome: Clinical and polysomnographic features. Am Rev Respir Dis 141:871–879, 1990.
198. Findley LJ, Blackburn MR, Goldberger AL, et al: Apneas and oscillation of cardiac ectopy in Cheyne-Stokes breathing during sleep. Am Rev Respir Dis 130:937–939, 1984.
199. Javaheri S, Corbett WS: Association of low $PaCO_2$ with central sleep apnea and ventricular arrhythmias in ambulatory patients with stable heart failure. Ann Intern Med 128:204–207, 1998.
200. Francis CS: Development of arrhythmias in the patient with congestive heart failure: Pathophysiology, prevalence and prognosis. Am J Cardiol 57:3B–7B, 1986.
201. Goldman S, Johnson G, Cohn JN, et al: Mechanism of death in heart failure: The vasodilator-heart failure trials. Circulation 87:VI-24–VI-31, 1993.
202. Hanly PJ, Zuberi-Khokhar NS: Increased mortality associated with Cheyne-Stokes respiration in patients with congestive heart failure. Am J Respir Crit Care Med 153:272–276, 1996.
203. Sutton FD Jr, Zwillich CW, Creagh CE, et al: Progesterone for outpatient treatment of Pickwickian syndrome. Ann Intern Med 83:476–479, 1975.
204. Bubis MJ, Anthonisen NR: Primary alveolar hypoventilation treated by nocturnal administration of $O_2$. Am Rev Respir Dis 118:947–953, 1978.
205. Motta J, Guilleminault C: Effects of oxygen administration in sleep-induced apneas. *In* Guilleminault C, Dement WC (eds): Sleep Apnea Syndromes. New York: Alan R. Liss, 1978, pp 137–144.
206. Barlow PB, Bartlett D Jr, Hauri P, et al: Idiopathic hypoventilation syndrome: Importance of preventing nocturnal hypoxemia and hypercapnia. Am Rev Respir Dis 121:141–145, 1980.
207. McNicholas WT, Carter JL, Rutherford R, et al: Beneficial effect of oxygen in primary alveolar hypoventilation with central sleep apnea. Am Rev Respir Dis 125:773–775, 1982.
208. Farmer WC, Glenn WWL, Gee JBL: Alveolar hypoventilation syndrome: Studies of ventilatory control in patients selected for diaphragm pacing. Am J Med 64:39–49, 1978.
209. Hyland RH, Jones NL, Powles ACP, et al: Primary alveolar hypoventilation treated with nocturnal electrophrenic respiration. Am Rev Respir Dis 117:165–172, 1978.
210. Garay SM, Turino GM, Goldring RM: Sustained reversal of chronic hypercapnia in patients with alveolar hypoventilation syndromes. Am J Med 70:269–274, 1981.
211. Goldstein RS, Molotiu N, Skrastins R, et al: Reversal of sleep-induced hypoventilation and chronic respiratory failure by nocturnal negative pressure ventilation in patients with restrictive ventilatory impairment. Am Rev Respir Dis 135:1049–1055, 1987.
212. Ellis ER, Bye PTP, Bruderer JW, et al: Treatment of respiratory failure during sleep in patients with neuromuscular disease: Positive pressure ventilation through a nose mask. Am Rev Respir Dis 135:148–152, 1987.
213. Bach JR, Alber AS: Management of chronic alveolar hypoventilation by nasal ventilation. Chest 97:52–57, 1990.
214. Goldstein RS, Avendano MA, DeRosie JA, et al: Influence of non-invasive positive pressure ventilation on inspiratory muscles. Chest 99:408–415, 1991.
215. Martin RJ, Sanders MH, Gray BA, et al: Acute and long-term ventilatory effects of hypoxia in the adult sleep apnea syndrome. Am Rev Respir Dis 125:175–180, 1982.
216. Issa FG, Sullivan CE: Reversal of central sleep apnea using nasal CPAP. Chest 90:165–171, 1986.
217. Hoffstein V, Slutsky AS: Central sleep apnea reversed by continuous positive airway pressure. Am Rev Respir Dis 135:1210–1212, 1987.
218. Bradley TD, Holloway R, McLaughlin P, et al: Cardiac output response to continuous positive airway pressure in congestive heart failure. Am Rev Respir Dis 145:377–382, 1992.
219. Tkacova R, Liu PP, Naughton MT, et al: Effect of continuous positive airway pressure on mitral regurgitant fraction and atrial natriuretic peptide in patients with heart failure. J Am Coll Cardiol 30:739–745, 1997.
220. Naughton MT, Bradley TD: Sleep apnea in congestive heart failure. Clin Chest Med 19:99–113, 1998.

# Respiratory Manifestations of Extrapulmonary Disorders

SECTION Q

# 82 Pulmonary Complications of Human Immunodeficiency Virus Infection

LAURENCE HUANG, M.D. • JOHN D. STANSELL, M.D.


Introduction
Epidemiology
Immunologic Abnormalities
Diagnostic Approach
- Evaluation of Human Immunodeficiency Virus Infection
- Evaluation of Human Immunodeficiency Virus–Associated Pulmonary Disease

Infectious Complications
- Bacteria
- Mycobacteria
- Fungi
- Viruses
- Parasites

Noninfectious Disorders
- Malignancies
- Interstitial Pneumonitides
- Other Disorders

Summary


## INTRODUCTION

In 1981, the first remarkable cases of the acquired immunodeficiency syndrome (AIDS) were reported.[1, 2] A few years later, scientists at the Pasteur Institute and National Institutes of Health discovered the first of the causative viruses, human immunodeficiency virus type-1 (HIV-1), and developed an accurate test to detect its presence in humans.[3, 4] Since then, a second virus (HIV-2) has been discovered, and our understanding of HIV disease and its myriad infectious and noninfectious complications has increased enormously. Furthermore, antiretroviral drugs that can suppress HIV viral replication below the limit of quantitation and therapies that can treat and prevent HIV-associated complications have become available. These medications have resulted in a decline in the incidence of new AIDS cases and in the number of AIDS-associated deaths in those countries where they are available. Unfortunately, access to these medications is far from universal, and a cure for HIV or an HIV vaccine of proven effectiveness remains in the future. Therefore, efforts to prevent the spread of new HIV infection and to identify and treat those persons who are already HIV-infected continue to be worldwide priorities.

The lungs are one of the chief target organs of HIV disease and, accordingly, a major source of morbidity and mortality. The spectrum of pulmonary manifestations is broad, and many infectious and noninfectious complications have been recognized (Table 82.1).[5–7] These complications include diseases that are AIDS defining or, if not AIDS defining, then HIV associated, as well as disorders whose association with HIV is inconclusive or coincidental. This chapter provides a brief review of the epidemiology of HIV infection and its immunologic abnormalities. Then, a diagnostic approach to the evaluation of HIV infection and HIV-associated pulmonary disease is detailed, followed by a discussion of the major HIV-associated pulmonary diseases, with emphasis on clinical features, diagnosis, treatment, and prevention.

**Table 82.1 SPECTRUM OF PULMONARY COMPLICATIONS**

| |
|---|
| **Infections** |
| ***Bacteria**** |
| *Streptococcus pneumoniae* |
| *Haemophilus* species |
| *Pseudomonas aeruginosa* |
| Other bacteria |
| ***Mycobacteria*** |
| *Mycobacterium tuberculosis*† |
| *Mycobacterium avium* complex‡ |
| *Mycobacterium kansasii*‡ |
| Other mycobacteria‡ |
| ***Fungi*** |
| *Pneumocystis carinii*§ |
| *Cryptococcus neoformans*‡ |
| *Histoplasma capsulatum*‡ |
| *Coccidioides immitis*‡ |
| *Aspergillus* species |
| *Blastomyces dermatitidis* |
| *Penicillium marneffei* |
| ***Viruses*** |
| Cytomegalovirus§ |
| Other viruses |
| ***Parasites*** |
| *Toxoplasma gondii*‖ |
| Other parasites |
| **Malignancies** |
| Kaposi's sarcoma§ |
| Non-Hodgkin's lymphoma§ |
| Bronchogenic carcinoma |
| **Interstitial pneumonitides** |
| Lymphocytic interstitial pneumonitis¶ |
| Nonspecific interstitial pneumonitis |
| **Other** |
| Chronic obstructive pulmonary disease |
| Pulmonary hypertension |
| Alveolar proteinosis |
| Diffuse alveolar damage |
| Bronchiolitis obliterans organizing pneumonia |
| Sarcoidosis |

*AIDS-defining diagnosis in adults and adolescents (>13 years) if recurrent (≥2 episodes in 12 months). Not applicable as AIDS-defining diagnosis in children.
†AIDS-defining diagnosis in adults and adolescents. AIDS-defining diagnosis in children if extrapulmonary or disseminated.
‡AIDS-defining diagnosis if extrapulmonary or disseminated.
§AIDS-defining diagnosis.
‖AIDS-defining diagnosis if central nervous system is involved.
¶AIDS-defining diagnosis in children. Not applicable as AIDS-defining diagnosis in adults or adolescents.
Modified with permission from Murray JF, Mills J: Pulmonary infectious complications of human immunodeficiency virus infection. Am Rev Respir Dis 141:1356–1372, 1582–1598, 1990.

## EPIDEMIOLOGY

The AIDS epidemic has had a major impact in the United States. From the dawn of the epidemic through June 1999, the Centers for Disease Control and Prevention (CDC) report that 711,344 cases of and 420,201 deaths from AIDS have occurred in the United States and its territories.[8] The annual incidence of AIDS-defining opportunistic illnesses increased each year until 1996, when it decreased for the first time, declining 6.5%.[8, 9] In 1996, the number of AIDS deaths also decreased for the first time, declining by a staggering 25%.[9] Since the decline in AIDS deaths has exceeded the decline in new AIDS cases, more people are living with AIDS in the United States than ever before. The national incidence and prevalence of HIV infection can only be estimated because confidential reporting of HIV infection is conducted in only 25 states. Nevertheless, as of December 1997, the CDC estimated that there were at least 40,000 new HIV infections per year and 650,000 to 900,000 people living with HIV in the United States.[10]

Male homosexuality and injection drug use are the main risk factors for acquiring HIV infection in the United States and account for more than 80% of the cumulative AIDS cases in adults and adolescents.[8] A much lower percentage of cases are attributable to heterosexual contact or to transfusion of contaminated blood, blood components, or tissue. Intrauterine or perinatal transmission from mother to fetus or child is responsible for most of the pediatric cases. The demographics of AIDS in the United States have changed. Women comprise an increasing percentage of adult AIDS cases (currently 22% of adult cases), as do African-Americans and Hispanics (currently 65% of adult cases).[10] The percentage of cases resulting from male homosexuality is declining relative to those from injection drug use and heterosexual contact. In addition, the epidemic has shifted from its initial predominance in large urban cities along the East and West coasts to increasingly include smaller cities and towns throughout the United States, the South, and the Midwest.

Although the US statistics and estimates, among the most accurate available, paint an improving picture, the global picture is worsening at a staggering rate. As of June 1998, the Joint United Nations Programme on HIV/AIDS estimated that there were 33.4 million people living with HIV/AIDS throughout the world and that 13.9 million people died from AIDS since the epidemic began. In 1997, it was estimated that 5.8 million people became infected with HIV, nearly 16,000 new infections a day, and that 2.3 million people died from AIDS.[11] If these current trends continue, the Global AIDS Policy Coalition projects that 60 to 70 million adults will have been infected with HIV by the end of the year 2000.

In contrast to the situation in the United States, heterosexual contact is the predominant mode of HIV transmission worldwide.[11] Women comprise 43% of the adult AIDS cases worldwide, resulting in increasing numbers of children being orphaned by AIDS. Sadly, it is estimated that one in every three children orphaned by this disease is under the age of 5 years, and an estimated 8.2 million children have been orphaned by AIDS since the epidemic began.

More than 95% of all the HIV-infected people in the world live in developing countries.[11] Most of these people are unaware that they are infected with HIV, a fact that promotes the continued spread of the disease. Sub-Saharan Africa is the hardest-hit region, with an estimated 20.8 million people living with HIV/AIDS, but substantial increases are occurring in Asia and Latin America and are expected in Eastern Europe. Accompanying the regional differences in AIDS prevalence are differences in the prevalences of HIV-associated pulmonary diseases. For example, *Pneumocystis carinii* pneumonia (PCP), the most common AIDS-defining opportunistic infection and one of the most common HIV-associated pulmonary infections in the United States, is rare in sub-Saharan Africa. Conversely, tuberculosis, the sovereign HIV-associated infection in Africa, has a considerably smaller impact in the United States. *Penicillium marneffei,* the third most common HIV-associated opportunistic infection in northern Thailand, is practically unheard of outside of Southeast Asia.

## IMMUNOLOGIC ABNORMALITIES

After infection with HIV and without effective antiretroviral therapy, HIV-infected persons experience a gradual but inexorable loss of host immunity that has been characterized as a syndrome of immune dysregulation, dysfunction, and deficiency, involving many components of the immune system.[12] Prominent among these are a depletion of $CD4^+$ T lymphocytes, suppression of host responses to T-cell–dependent antigens, and abnormal activation of B cells.

The most important clinical consequence of HIV infection is the resulting progressive loss of $CD4^+$ lymphocytes. The mechanism of destruction of $CD4^+$ cells is complex and incompletely understood, with both direct and indirect HIV-mediated effects postulated. Single-cell killing, syncytia formation and cell killing, virally mediated suppression of immune cell function, and modulation of the virus-host cell interaction are among the potential mechanisms.[13]

HIV infection suppresses the host response to T-cell–dependent antigens.[14, 15] After encountering a pathogen, T cells normally undergo clonal expansion, which amplifies their response. In HIV-infected patients, however, this proliferation is attenuated in response to both mitogens and viruses to which patients have serologic evidence of prior exposure.

HIV infection results in abnormal activation of B cells. B-cell activation was initially believed to be "polyclonal" in nature because the response included antibodies reactive to many different antigens.[16] Evidence indicates that HIV infection induces both virus-specific and polyclonal B-cell activation. Moreover, these two responses appear to be regulated independently of each other. The HIV-specific responses decrease as the severity of the HIV-induced disease worsens, whereas the polyclonal responses increase; only the polyclonal responses correlate with the number of $CD4^+$ cells and the ratio of $CD4^+$ to $CD8^+$ cells.[17]

## DIAGNOSTIC APPROACH

When a patient seeks medical attention for new respiratory complaints, the differential diagnosis may include HIV infection and one of its complications. In these cases, the physician faces two problems: first, to determine whether the patient is infected with HIV and, second, to elucidate the nature of the respiratory complaints that prompted the visit. Each of these two responsibilities is briefly considered.

### Evaluation of Human Immunodeficiency Virus Infection

The diagnosis of HIV infection itself is made by detection of specific antibodies to the virus with a screening enzyme-linked immunosorbent assay (ELISA) test followed by a confirmatory test such as the Western blot. After acute HIV infection, however, there is a delay of several weeks until the development of detectable antibodies. In these patients, measurement of the plasma HIV ribonucleic acid (RNA, viral load) may indicate acute HIV infection that should be confirmed by repeated HIV antibody testing. Confirmation is necessary because the plasma HIV RNA may be falsely positive at low titers; thus, this test should never be used to establish the diagnosis of HIV infection.

Several laboratory tests have been used to document the stage of HIV disease and to predict the development of AIDS. Currently, the most widely used tests are the determination of the absolute number or percentage of circulating $CD4^+$ lymphocytes and the measurement of plasma HIV RNA. The $CD4^+$ lymphocyte count has proved to be especially useful in the evaluation of HIV-associated complications (including pulmonary disease), as it predicts the development of these diseases.[18] The plasma HIV RNA level has proved to be useful in guiding the management of HIV infection. In addition, evidence suggests that the plasma HIV RNA level is a predictor for the development of AIDS and death due to infection independent of the $CD4^+$ lymphocyte count.[19–21]

### Evaluation of Human Immunodeficiency Virus–Associated Pulmonary Disease

The evaluation of an HIV-infected patient with pulmonary disease is aimed at making a specific diagnosis. In general, definitive diagnosis is preferred to empirical therapy for a number of reasons. Although each of the HIV-associated pulmonary diseases has characteristic clinical and radiographic features, these features overlap. Occasionally, the features are atypical, or more than one pulmonary disease is present. Without appropriate therapy, HIV-infected patients with pneumonia can progress rapidly to respiratory failure and death. Therapies used to treat HIV-associated pulmonary diseases have important toxicities and interactions with other medications that a patient may be receiving. Thus, empirical therapy without an attempted diagnostic evaluation is seldom justified.

The evaluation should begin with the history and physical examination. Laboratory testing should be performed and a chest radiograph obtained from patients with suspected pulmonary disease. Frequently, the results of this evaluation suggest a specific differential diagnosis and management plan. Occasionally, additional studies, including pulmonary function testing, chest computed tomography (CT), high-resolution computed tomography (HRCT), and $^{67}$gallium scanning, are needed to narrow the differential diagnosis and to refine the management plan.

Once the differential diagnosis is established, empirical therapy for the suspected diagnosis should be initiated while the results of diagnostic studies are awaited. The diagnostic studies chosen depend on a number of factors, including the specific diagnosis being considered, the sensitivity and specificity of the diagnostic tests, and the availability (including cost) of the tests. In most cases, sputum and blood cultures should be performed. Depending on the suspected diagnosis, bronchoscopy should be performed if sputum results are nondiagnostic. The decision to perform bronchoalveolar lavage (BAL) with or without transbronchial biopsies (TBBX) depends on the suspected diagnosis and the sensitivities of these procedures for that diagnosis. Thoracentesis (and possibly pleural biopsy) should be considered for patients with pleural effusion. At institutions with expertise, CT-guided transthoracic needle aspiration or surgical procedures such as thoracoscopy or mediastinoscopy can be used. Occasionally, open-lung biopsy is required. The choice of specific diagnostic tests relies on an accurate differential diagnosis derived from a number of factors.

## Prevalence of Pulmonary Diseases

The prevalence of each of the HIV-associated pulmonary diseases depends on a number of factors, especially the clinical setting where the patient is seen and the patient's CD4$^+$ lymphocyte count.

**Clinical Setting.** The clinical setting where the patient is seen influences the prevalence of pulmonary diseases observed. The Pulmonary Complications of HIV Infection Study (PCHIS) was a prospective, observational cohort study that followed more than 1150 HIV-infected subjects for approximately 5 years at six sites across the United States.[22] The investigators found that ambulatory HIV-infected subjects presenting to a clinic with respiratory complaints had upper respiratory tract infections (URIs) and acute bronchitis more often than pneumonia due to bacteria, mycobacteria, *P. carinii,* fungi, viruses, and parasites *combined.*[23] Wallace and colleagues[23] of the PCHIS reported an annual incidence of URI ranging from 35 to 52 episodes per 100 person-years, totaling 1810 episodes during the study period. This exceeded the annual incidence and total number of episodes of bacterial pneumonia (3.9 to 7.3 cases per 100 person-years, 232 total cases), PCP (2.8 to 9.5 cases per 100 person-years, 220 total cases), and pneumonias due to other opportunistic infections (69 total cases) *combined.* Patients with URI or acute bronchitis are, however, usually treated as outpatients, whereas patients with opportunistic pneumonia often require hospitalization. Over the course of the AIDS epidemic, the frequencies of specific pulmonary diseases among HIV-infected patients have changed. Early in the epidemic, PCP accounted for the vast majority of pneumonias seen.[24, 25] More recently, bacterial pneumonia has become the leading pneumonia observed. At San Francisco General Hospital, bacterial pneumonia is currently the most common pulmonary disease seen in hospitalized HIV-infected patients, followed by PCP, tuberculosis, pulmonary Kaposi's sarcoma, and cryptococcal pneumonia (L. Huang, unpublished data). In published series of critically ill HIV-infected patients, PCP remains the most common pulmonary disease seen.[26, 27]

**CD4$^+$ Lymphocyte Count.** The CD4$^+$ lymphocyte count is an excellent indicator of an HIV-infected patient's risk of developing a specific opportunistic infection or neoplasm and is therefore an essential element of the evaluation of pulmonary disease. Many of the HIV-associated pulmonary diseases usually present at or below a characteristic CD4$^+$ lymphocyte count and seldom occur above that count.[18] The exceptions are diseases that can present in persons with or without HIV infection, such as bacterial pneumonia, tuberculosis, and non-Hodgkin's lymphoma. In HIV-infected persons, these diseases can present at any CD4$^+$ lymphocyte count, although their incidence increases and their characteristic presentation changes as the CD4$^+$ count declines.

At CD4$^+$ lymphocyte counts less than 200 cells/μL, bacterial pneumonia is often accompanied by bacteremia, and *Mycobacterium tuberculosis* disease is often extrapulmonary or disseminated. Moreover, below this CD4$^+$ count, *P. carinii* and *Cryptococcus neoformans* pneumonia become important considerations, whereas neither typically occurs in a patient with a count significantly higher than 200 cells/μL. At CD4$^+$ lymphocyte counts below 100 cells/μL, *Pseudomonas aeruginosa, Staphylococcus aureus,* and *Toxoplasma gondii* pneumonias and pulmonary Kaposi's sarcoma become increasingly frequent. Finally, at CD4$^+$ lymphocyte counts less than 50 cells/μL, diseases caused by endemic *(Histoplasma capsulatum, Coccidioides immitis)* and nonendemic (*Aspergillus* species, usually *A. fumigatus*) fungi, certain viruses (cytomegalovirus), and nontuberculous mycobacteria (*Mycobacterium avium* complex) become important considerations. At this degree of immunosuppression, many of these diseases present with extrapulmonary or disseminated manifestations that may dominate the clinical presentation.

Antiretroviral combinations can reverse the previously inexorable decline in a patient's CD4$^+$ lymphocyte count. In many cases, patients experience a dramatic increase in their CD4$^+$ count, an increase that has been sustained for months or even years. This result has produced a number of unanswered questions concerning whether a patient's risk for specific opportunistic infection is lessened by the increase in CD4+ lymphocyte count and, if so, can specific prophylaxis be discontinued. As clinical experience accumulates, many experts increasingly suspect that the risk of opportunistic infections is better reflected by the current CD4+ lymphocyte count. Several large, prospective observational studies suggest that *P. carinii* prophylaxis can be safely discontinued in patients whose CD4+ lymphocyte counts increase above 200 cells/μL.[27a–27c] Prospective, randomized studies to confirm this observation are, however, still in progress. Nevertheless, the 1999 USPHS/IDSA Guidelines for the Prevention of Opportunistic Infections in Persons Infected with Human Immunodeficiency Virus state that "although optimal criteria for discontinuing PCP prophylaxis are still being assessed, providers may wish to discontinue (primary) prophylaxis when patients have sustained a CD4+ T-lymphocyte count >200 cells/μL for at least 3–6 months."[28] Because the published studies mainly included patients who were receiving primary *P. carinii* prophylaxis, the USPHS/IDSA Guidelines state that "although patients receiving secondary prophylaxis (prior episode of PCP) might also be at low risk for PCP when their CD4+ T-lymphocyte counts increase to >200 cells/μL, inadequate numbers of patients have been evaluated to warrant a recommendation to discontinue prophylaxis in such patients."[28] Similar to PCP, observational studies in small numbers of patients suggest that primary prophylaxis for *T. gondii* and *M. avium* complex can also be discontinued in selected individuals.[28] Definitive answers to these questions await the prospective, randomized studies in progress. In either case, the CD4+ lymphocyte count cannot replace the history and physical examination, laboratory tests, and chest radiograph in the diagnostic evaluation.

## History and Physical Examination

Many aspects of the history and physical examination can provide important diagnostic clues to the cause of HIV-associated pulmonary disease.

**Symptoms.** In general, respiratory symptoms are nonspecific; all of the HIV-associated pulmonary diseases can present with cough, dyspnea, and, less commonly, pleuritic chest pain. A productive cough with purulent sputum, however, suggests a bacterial process, whereas a nonproductive cough and dyspnea are more characteristic of PCP. The duration of symptoms can also be useful in distinguishing bacterial pneumonia (usually 3 to 5 days of symptoms) from PCP (usually 2 to 4 weeks of symptoms).

Constitutional symptoms such as fever, night sweats, and weight loss, while nonspecific, often suggest the presence of a systemic or disseminated infection or represent "B" symptoms of non-Hodgkin's lymphoma.

Extrapulmonary symptoms may suggest a disease that has both pulmonary and extrapulmonary manifestations. For example, cryptococcal disease causing both pneumonia and meningitis should be strongly considered in an HIV-infected patient whose CD4+ lymphocyte count is below 200 cells/μL and who presents with cough, dyspnea, and headache.

**Past Medical History.** Many aspects of the past medical history can provide important diagnostic clues to the cause of HIV-associated pulmonary disease.

**HIV Risk Category and Habits.** Men who have sex with men (MSM) have a significantly higher incidence of Kaposi's sarcoma than do patients without this risk factor, and approximately 95% of HIV-associated Kaposi's sarcoma occurs in MSM.[29] Injection drug users have a higher incidence of bacterial pneumonia and tuberculosis than do persons without a history of injection drug use.[30–33] In addition, injection and other illicit drug use can cause important non–HIV-associated pulmonary illnesses such as aspiration pneumonia secondary to altered sensorium, endocarditis-related septic pulmonary emboli, pulmonary vascular disease, and drug-induced pulmonary edema.[34]

As in the general population, HIV-infected patients who are cigarette smokers are at an increased risk for a variety of pulmonary illnesses. Cigarette smokers have a higher incidence of both bacterial bronchitis and bronchopneumonia than do nonsmokers or former smokers, especially if their CD4+ lymphocyte count is below 200 cells/μL.[30] Although it is currently debated whether HIV infection itself is associated with an increased risk of bronchogenic carcinoma, cigarette smokers are more likely than nonsmokers to develop this disease.[29] In addition, patients with a long history of cigarette smoking may present with manifestations of chronic obstructive pulmonary disease as the cause of their respiratory symptoms.[35]

**Residence and Travel.** A history of residence in or travel to a geographic region that is endemic for fungi such as *H. capsulatum, C. immitis, Blastomyces dermatitidis* or *P. marneffei* is a strong determinant of the risk of disease.[36] Patients without such a history are unlikely to develop these diseases. Tuberculosis is more common in certain geographic areas and in certain populations.[37] Patients who were born in or have traveled to a country with a high prevalence of *M. tuberculosis* and patients who are homeless, unstably housed, or previously incarcerated are at high risk of *M. tuberculosis* infection.[33]

**Prior Pulmonary Diseases and Prophylaxis Use.** As is discussed later in the chapter, many of the HIV-associated opportunistic infections recur, especially in the absence of secondary prophylaxis or suppressive therapy. Thus, knowledge of a patient's prior pulmonary history may suggest the etiology of the current illness. Patients who fail to receive or to adhere to recommended prophylaxis have an increased risk for HIV-associated opportunistic infections such as PCP.

**Signs.** As with symptoms, vital signs are nonspecific. Patients with pneumonia may be febrile, tachycardic, and tachypneic. Evidence of systemic hypotension suggests a fulminant disease process (e.g., bacterial septicemia and disseminated histoplasmosis) and is cause for concern. Pulse oximetry often reveals a decrease in the oxygen saturation and provides an estimate of disease severity.

Physical examination of the chest may provide important diagnostic clues. Focal lung findings are detected more often in patients with bacterial pneumonia than in those with PCP, most of whom have a normal examination. Occasionally, chest findings are the result of nonpulmonary disease. For example, rales in association with an S3 cardiac gallop and elevated jugular venous pressure suggest a cardiac etiology.

The remainder of the physical examination is often suggestive of a specific pulmonary disease. Headache or altered mental status suggests *C. neoformans,* whereas a focal neurologic examination usually implicates *T. gondii.* Concurrent visual and respiratory complaints may indicate cytomegalovirus. New cutaneous lesions may be a manifestation of disseminated fungal, bacterial, or mycobacterial disease, and mucocutaneous Kaposi's sarcoma lesions are seen in most patients with pulmonary Kaposi's sarcoma. The absence of mucocutaneous Kaposi's sarcoma lesions does not, however, preclude the presence of pulmonary disease. Hepatosplenomegaly or peripheral lymphadenopathy may be signs of disseminated mycobacterial or fungal disease or non-Hodgkin's lymphoma.

## Laboratory Tests

Laboratory tests may provide important diagnostic clues. HIV-infected patients often, however, have a host of laboratory abnormalities that are nonspecific or are due to conditions unrelated to the pulmonary disease. Laboratory tests that may be useful include the white blood cell count (WBC) and differential and serum lactate dehydrogenase (LDH) and arterial blood gas (ABG) measurements. The last two tests are better as prognostic markers and as baseline values for subsequent measurements than as diagnostic tests. Serial measurements are useful whenever a patient fails to exhibit a clinical response or deteriorates despite appropriate therapy.

**White Blood Cell Count.** When a $CD4^+$ lymphocyte count is unavailable, the WBC and differential (percentage of lymphocytes) can be used to estimate the stage of HIV disease and the risk of specific diseases. The WBC is frequently elevated (or, if normal, elevated relative to the patient's baseline value) in patients with bacterial pneumonia. These patients often have an associated "left shift." Neutropenia is a risk factor for bacterial and certain fungal infections such as *Aspergillus.* Pancytopenia may suggest the presence of mycobacterial or fungal disease or non-Hodgkin's lymphoma involving the bone marrow. With other pulmonary diseases, the WBC more often reflects the stage of the HIV disease or the use of bone marrow suppressive medications than the presence of a specific disease.

**Serum Lactate Dehydrogenase.** The serum LDH level is often elevated in patients with PCP.[35] It is also elevated in many other pulmonary and nonpulmonary conditions, however, limiting its diagnostic use. In patients with PCP, the degree of LDH elevation correlates with prognosis and response to therapy. Those patients with an initial LDH level that is markedly elevated have a worse prognosis than do patients whose LDH is normal or mildly elevated. With successful therapy, the LDH level declines; an increasing LDH level in a patient who is receiving PCP treatment is often a sign of therapeutic failure.

**Arterial Blood Gas.** Values of ABG analysis are frequently abnormal for patients with pulmonary disease. Although nonspecific, the ABG results can be an important factor in the decision whether to hospitalize a patient and are used to determine whether adjunctive corticosteroids are indicated for patients with PCP.

## Chest Radiograph

In the absence of respiratory symptoms, chest radiographic screening for pulmonary disease is rarely useful.[38] Patients who have new-onset symptoms or signs suggestive of pulmonary disease should have a posteroanterior and lateral chest radiograph. The most common chest radiographic features of each of the pulmonary diseases are discussed separately. In general, the distribution (unilateral or bilateral, focal, multifocal, diffuse, specific lung zone[s]) and pattern (interstitial/reticular, granular, alveolar/consolidation, nodular) of any parenchymal abnormalities and the presence or absence of associated findings such as nodules, masses, cysts, cavities, pleural effusions, or intrathoracic adenopathy provide important diagnostic clues and help to direct subsequent evaluation. No constellation of radiographic abnormalities is, however, specific for a particular pulmonary disease; the patterns seen only suggest a differential diagnosis.

## Pulmonary Function Tests

Many of the indications for pulmonary function testing are the same for HIV-infected persons as for any person and are discussed in Chapter 28. In HIV-infected patients, pulmonary function testing, specifically measurement of the diffusing capacity for carbon monoxide ($DL_{CO}$), can be useful in the evaluation of suspected PCP.[39] The $DL_{CO}$ is a sensitive but nonspecific test for PCP in patients with clinically suspected PCP who have a normal or unchanged chest radiograph. Patients whose $DL_{CO}$ is greater than 75% of predicted are unlikely to have PCP; for these patients, neither diagnostic procedures to detect *P. carinii* nor empirical PCP therapy is indicated, and clinical observation or evaluation for another pulmonary process is recommended. Patients whose $DL_{CO}$ is 75% or below of predicted require a diagnostic procedure for *P. carinii,* usually sputum induction or bronchoscopy.

Although the $DL_{CO}$ value has clinical utility in the evaluation of suspected PCP, it should only be obtained when there is a reasonable suspicion for this disease, and it has no role as a screening test to detect early PCP in asymptomatic persons. In an evaluation of 64 HIV-infected patients who had a decline of 20% or more in their $DL_{CO}$ value from a baseline value—in the absence of new respiratory symptoms or new chest radiographic findings—none of the patients had PCP (or another opportunistic infection) diagnosed on sputum induction, bronchoscopy, or clinical follow-up.[40]

## Chest Computed Tomography

Many of the indications for chest CT or HRCT scans are the same for HIV-infected patients as for any patient and are discussed in Chapter 25. Clearly, a chest CT is more sensitive than a chest radiograph for detecting the presence and describing the characteristics and extent of pulmonary disease. Chest CT is also useful in directing invasive diagnostic procedures. In HIV-infected patients, usually the clinical and chest radiographic presentations are sufficient to suggest a specific diagnosis. Occasionally, however, the presentation is confusing. In these cases, chest CT or HRCT scans can be extremely useful because each of the HIV-associated pulmonary diseases has a characteristic CT/HRCT appearance that often allows radiologists to provide a confident diagnosis.[41, 42]

In the experience of Naidich and McGuinness,[41] CT can be especially useful in the identification of occult pulmonary disease, the characterization of diffuse parenchymal disease such as PCP or pulmonary Kaposi's sarcoma, and the identification and characterization of mediastinal lymphadenopathy. In our experience at San Francisco General Hospital, CT can also be useful in the evaluation of multiple pulmonary nodules.[43] Finally, a normal CT scan makes pulmonary opportunistic infection or neoplasm unlikely.[42]

## Radionuclide Imaging

As described in Chapter 26, three radionuclides have been used to study the lungs in HIV-infected persons: gallium citrate ($^{67}$Ga-citrate), technetium diethylenetriamine pentaacetate ($^{99m}$Tc-DTPA), and thallium ($^{201}$Tl). Similar to pulmonary function testing, $^{67}$Ga-citrate was used extensively during the early years of the AIDS epidemic as a guide to further diagnostic studies. Specifically, both of these tests were recommended in cases of clinically suspected pulmonary disease, most often PCP, where the chest radiograph was normal. Currently, a chest CT scan is probably preferred over a $^{67}$gallium scan in most instances because it has a higher sensitivity and specificity than $^{67}$gallium.[44] The clearance of $^{99m}$Tc-DTPA, after it has been inhaled as an aerosol and deposited in the lungs, has been shown to be greatly accelerated in patients with PCP.[45] Occasionally, $^{201}$Tl scintigraphy is useful for patients with pulmonary Kaposi's sarcoma.[46]

## Sputum

Studies of sputum, either expectorated or induced, can establish the diagnosis of many of the HIV-associated pulmonary diseases. Most patients with pyogenic pneumonia complain of a cough productive of purulent sputum. In these cases, an expectorated sputum specimen can be useful in focusing the diagnostic evaluation and selecting the initial antimicrobial therapy.

Most patients with PCP complain of a nonproductive cough. In these cases, examination of induced sputum, obtained by inhalation of a hypertonic saline aerosol generated by an ultrasonic handheld nebulizer, is a sensitive technique for diagnosing PCP and decreases the need for invasive diagnostic procedures.[47] The sensitivity of induced sputum examination for *P. carinii* varies by institution; at San Francisco General Hospital, the sensitivity has remained consistent throughout the AIDS epidemic in the range of 74% to 83%.[47, 48] This range of sensitivities, however, implies that a significant percentage of patients (17% to 26%) will have a false-negative induced sputum examination for *P. carinii* and that further diagnostic studies are indicated in these cases.

Sputum examination and culture are the foundations for the diagnosis of tuberculosis.[33, 49] Several studies report that the sensitivity of sputum acid-fast bacilli (AFB) smear and culture in HIV-infected patients is similar to the sensitivity in the overall population.[50–53] Other studies, however, report a lower sensitivity of sputum smear or culture in HIV-infected patients.[54, 55] Most patients with tuberculosis can produce expectorated specimens suitable for examination and culture; in those patients who are unable to provide an adequate expectorated specimen, induced sputum can be used.

Although the experience and published literature about the value of sputum studies in other infections are limited compared with those for PCP and tuberculosis, sputum examination and culture can establish the diagnosis of a number of HIV-associated pulmonary infections, including those due to nontuberculous mycobacteria (e.g., *Mycobacterium kansasii*), fungi (e.g., *C. neoformans, H. capsulatum, C. immitis, P. marneffei* but not *Aspergillus*), and parasites (e.g., *T. gondii*) but not cytomegalovirus.

## Bronchoscopy

Fiberoptic bronchoscopy is a cornerstone in the evaluation of HIV-associated pulmonary disease. In general, bronchoscopy should be considered for any known or suspected HIV-infected patient with pulmonary disease whose severity warrants a prompt and accurate diagnosis, for patients with suspected pulmonary Kaposi's sarcoma, for patients with suspected non-Hodgkin's lymphoma (if other diagnostic procedures are thought to be more hazardous or less likely to provide the diagnosis), for patients whose diagnosis remains unknown despite less invasive diagnostic studies (e.g., sputum), and for patients whose empirical therapy is failing.

The decision to perform BAL with or without TBBX depends on the suspected diagnosis and on the sensitivities of these procedures for that diagnosis. At the beginning of the AIDS epidemic, both BAL and TBBX were usually performed during the initial bronchoscopy. Studies demonstrated that the yield from these two procedures was complementary in identifying pathogens: The sensitivity of BAL was 86% and that of TBBX 87%; when the two procedures were combined, the sensitivity was 98% for all pathogens and 100% for *P. carinii*.[56] Currently, at San Francisco General Hospital, in cases where PCP is the suspected pathogen, we perform only BAL during the initial bronchoscopy.[48, 57] Our experience is that the sensitivity of BAL fluid examination for *P. carinii* is 97% or higher and, therefore, a negative BAL fluid examination for *P. carinii* rules out the diagnosis of PCP in all but the rarest of cases. To estimate the sensitivity of BAL for PCP, Huang and colleagues[48] reviewed the medical records of 100 randomly selected HIV-infected patients who had both a negative induced sputum test and a negative BAL fluid examination for *P. carinii* and had no other diagnosis established. The authors found that two patients were diagnosed with PCP in the 60 days after their negative BAL, one 46 days and the other 51 days after the negative bronchoscopy. Furthermore, TBBX rarely provided the sole diagnosis of PCP. In this series of 992 cases of PCP over a 4-year period, TBBX was the sole diagnostic procedure in only two cases (0.2%).

In contrast to PCP, TBBX improves the sensitivity of bronchoscopy for diagnosing a number of other important pathogens, including tuberculosis and endemic fungal pneumonias. Furthermore, tissue confirmation from TBBX or another biopsy specimen is mandatory to establish the diagnosis of invasive aspergillosis, cytomegalovirus pneumonia, and pulmonary non-Hodgkin's lymphoma. Therefore, when the clinical and radiographic features suggest one of these pulmonary diseases, it seems prudent to perform both BAL and TBBX during the initial bronchoscopy.

### Other Procedures

Several other procedures have been used in the diagnostic evaluation of patients with HIV-associated pulmonary disease. Diagnostic thoracentesis should be considered for any HIV-infected patient with pleural effusion in whom other studies are nondiagnostic or in whom there is a concern about empyema. Although the addition of pleural biopsy increases the sensitivity of this procedure for tuberculosis, pleural fluid culture alone is often sufficient to establish the diagnosis of bacterial and fungal infections, and pleural fluid cytology can establish the diagnosis of non-Hodgkin's lymphoma. Transthoracic needle aspiration of the lungs can be used to diagnose focal mass lesions and mediastinal adenopathy.[58–60] Video-assisted thoracoscopy has made a number of important contributions. As a result, open-lung biopsy is only occasionally indicated in the evaluation of HIV-associated pulmonary disease. However, when used, open-lung biopsy can establish a diagnosis in most cases.[61–63]

## INFECTIOUS COMPLICATIONS

The hallmark of advancing HIV disease is progressive immunosuppression and, ultimately, the development of one or more complications, most of which are infectious. The lungs are the principal target of the many infections that lead to a diagnosis of AIDS and are often involved in earlier stages of HIV disease as well. In this section, the major pulmonary infectious complications of HIV disease are reviewed according to the category of infectious microorganism that causes them (see Table 82.1).

### Bacteria

Early in the AIDS epidemic, bacterial pneumonia accounted for only a small proportion of pulmonary diseases seen. In 1984, the National Heart, Lung, and Blood Institute conducted a workshop on AIDS-associated pulmonary complications, the purpose of which was to report on the shared experiences of six institutions that had considerable experience with AIDS.[24] Although PCP, either alone or with coexisting infection, accounted for 373 of the 441 (85%) serious pulmonary diseases reported, pyogenic bacterial pneumonia was seen in only 11 (2.5%) cases. Another study of 130 AIDS patients found that bacterial pneumonia was seen in 4 of 61 (7%) patients who developed pulmonary disease over a 4-year period.[64] Subsequently, bacterial pneumonia became recognized as a frequent complication of HIV infection and one that often preceded other opportunistic infections. Multiple retrospective studies cited an increased risk of bacterial infection among HIV-seropositive persons. These studies found a 5- to 80-fold higher risk of bacterial pneumonia in HIV-seropositive than HIV-seronegative people. The recognition that the incidence of bacterial pneumonia is increased in HIV-infected persons and is frequently recurrent led to the inclusion of recurrent bacterial pneumonia (defined as two or more episodes within 12 months) as an AIDS-defining illness in the 1993 CDC Expanded Surveillance Case Definition for AIDS.[65]

Hirschtick and colleagues[30] of the PCHIS confirmed the increased incidence of bacterial pneumonia in HIV-infected persons and provided important new insights into the relationship between bacterial pneumonia and HIV infection. In this study, there were 5.5 episodes of bacterial pneumonia per 100 person-years in the HIV-infected cohort compared with 0.9 episodes per 100 person-years in the HIV-seronegative control cohort ($P < 0.001$). Bacterial pneumonia was more common in HIV-infected patients than in the HIV-seronegative controls, even in the subset of HIV-infected patients with $CD4^+$ lymphocyte counts above 500 cells/μL ($P = 0.004$). Furthermore, the rate of bacterial pneumonia increased as the $CD4^+$ lymphocyte count declined. The authors also found that the incidence of bacterial pneumonia was greater in injection drug users (11.1 episodes per 100 person-years) than in either MSM (4.1 episodes per 100 person-years, $P < 0.001$) or female partners (3.8 episodes per 100 person-years, $P < 0.003$). Cigarette smoking was also associated with an increased incidence of bacterial pneumonia, especially in HIV-infected subjects with a $CD4^+$ lymphocyte count below 200 cells/μL. Osmond and colleagues[31a] of the PCHIS found that patients who developed bacterial or *P. carinii* pneumonia had a significantly shorter median duration of survival compared with $CD4^+$ count–matched control subjects without one of these pneumonias.

Overall, *Streptococcus pneumoniae* and *Haemophilus* species are the two most frequently identified bacteria causing community-acquired pneumonia in HIV-infected persons. More recently, *P. aeruginosa* has emerged as a major community-acquired bacterial pathogen among HIV-infected persons. Other bacteria are occasionally identified as causes of pneumonia in HIV-infected persons, including *Legionella* species, *Rhodococcus equi,* and *Nocardia* species.

#### *Streptococcus pneumoniae* and *Haemophilus* Species

Similar to published series of community-acquired bacterial pneumonia in other populations, *S. pneumoniae* and *Haemophilus* species are the most frequently identified pathogens in HIV-infected persons.[30, 66, 67] Burack and colleagues[66] found that *S. pneumoniae* and *Haemophilus influenzae* were the two most common bacteria seen in their series of 216 cases. Streptococci, usually *S. pneumoniae,* were responsible for 81 cases (37.5%) of bacterial pneumonia, and *Haemophilus* species accounted for an additional 46 cases (21%). Mundy and coworkers[67] also reported that *S. pneumoniae* and *H. influenzae* were the most common bacteria seen in their series of 180 hospitalized HIV-infected patients with pneumonia. Finally, Hirschtick and coworkers[30] of the PCHIS noted that these two bacteria comprised 54% of the bacteria identified in their study of 237 cases of bacterial pneumonia.

**Clinical Features.** In HIV-infected persons, the clinical and radiographic features of bacterial pneumonia are similar to those in immunocompetent persons with a few important exceptions, which are detailed.

***$CD4^+$ Lymphocyte Count.*** Bacterial pneumonia can occur throughout the course of HIV infection and at any $CD4^+$ lymphocyte count. As the $CD4^+$ count declines, however, the incidence of bacterial pneumonia and the rate of bacteremia increase. Hirschtick and coworkers[30] of the PCHIS found that the rate of bacterial pneumonia increased from 2.3 episodes per 100 person-years in HIV-infected subjects with a $CD4^+$ count above 500 cells/μL to 10.8 episodes per 100 person-years in subjects with a $CD4^+$ count below 200 cells/μL. The rate of pneumococcal bacteremia in HIV-infected patients has been estimated to be almost 100 times greater than that in age-matched non–HIV-infected persons.[68] Bacterial pneumonia characteristically presents with fever (in 90% to 100%), cough (in 90% to 100%) that is often productive (60% to 100%), dyspnea (in 45% to 75%), and pleuritic chest pain (in 50% to 70%).[31] The onset of symptoms is usually acute (3 to 5 days). Physical examination of the chest frequently reveals signs of focal lung consolidation or pleural effusion. The WBC count is typically elevated or, if normal, is elevated relative to the patient's baseline value, and there is often an accompanying "left shift."

***Chest Radiograph.*** The chest radiograph characteristically reveals focal consolidation that tends to involve segments or lobes; a single focus is usually seen, but multifocal disease appears more common than in non–HIV-infected persons.[68a] Studies suggest that this "classic" presentation may be seen more frequently in pneumonias due to *S. pneumoniae* and, to a lesser extent, *Haemophilus* species than in those due to community-acquired *P. aeruginosa.* Several of the published series on HIV-associated bacterial pneumonia presented radiographic findings without regard to specific bacteria. One such study reported that 40% of 55 HIV-infected patients with bacterial pneumonia presented with focal, segmental or lobar, alveolar infiltrates, while 38% had diffuse reticulonodular infiltrates, 16% had focal reticulonodular infiltrates, and 5% had nodular or cavitary infiltrates on chest radiograph.[69] A more recent study found that 54% of 99 HIV-infected patients with bacterial pneumonia had a lobar infiltrate, 17% had an interstitial infiltrate, 10% had a nodular infiltrate, and only 1% had a cavitary infiltrate on their radiograph.[70] In this study, multivariate analysis demonstrated that the presence of a lobar infiltrate on chest radiograph was an independent predictor of bacterial pneumonia (odds ratio [OR] = 5.8, 95% confidence interval = 2.1–16.1, $P < 0.001$). It is important to point out, however, that these studies considered all bacterial pathogens together. Numerous reports as well as clinical experience demonstrate that the frequency of certain radiographic findings depends on the specific causative bacteria.

*S. pneumoniae* and *H. influenzae* pneumonia usually present with focal consolidation on chest radiograph, although *H. influenzae* may also present with bilateral interstitial or mixed interstitial-alveolar infiltrates similar to PCP. A review of all English-language published articles and abstracts from 1981 to 1990 about *S. pneumoniae* disease in HIV-infected persons found that three fourths of bacterial pneumonias due to *S. pneumoniae* presented with segmental, lobar, or multilobar consolidation on chest radiograph.[71] Garcia-Leoni and coworkers[72] reported a focal alveolar pattern in 67% and a diffuse alveolar pattern in 10% of the radiographs from 21 HIV-infected patients with *S. pneumoniae* pneumonia. Schlamm and Yancovitz[73] found similar proportions in 34 HIV-infected patients with *H. influenzae* pneumonia where focal or diffuse lobar infiltrates were noted in 74% of the radiographs. Another series of 12 HIV-infected patients with *H. influenzae* pneumonia, however, discovered that the presentation was clinically and radiographically indistinguishable from that of PCP.[74] Patients complained of nonproductive cough and dyspnea with a median symptom duration of 4 weeks. All presented with bilateral interstitial or bilateral mixed interstitial-alveolar infiltrates similar to those in PCP.

**Diagnosis.** The diagnostic approach to bacterial pneumonia is the same for HIV-infected as for non–HIV-infected persons; most patients should have sputum Gram's stain and culture.[75] Blood cultures are specific and should be obtained. Studies have documented a significantly higher rate of bacteremia, especially pneumococcal, among HIV-infected persons.[72, 76–80] In HIV-infected patients, 25% to 80% of those with pneumococcal pneumonia presented with bacteremia, and 5% to 25% of those with *H. influenzae* pneumonia presented with bacteremia. Given these findings, blood cultures should be performed in most, if not all, cases. Finally, thoracentesis should be considered for patients with pleural effusion, especially if the effusion is large or if there is concern about possible empyema. At institutions where drug-resistant bacteria are frequent, attempts to culture the causative bacteria to enable drug susceptibility testing are especially important.

**Treatment.** The principles of the treatment of patients with community-acquired pneumonia are the same for HIV-infected as for non–HIV-infected persons.[75] The choice of antimicrobial agent should be based on a number of factors, such as the results of a sputum Gram's stain, the presence of comorbid conditions (e.g., chronic obstructive pulmonary disease, alcohol use), the clinical and radiographic presentation, and the severity of the pneumonia. Initial empirical therapy should include coverage against frequently identified organisms (e.g., *S. pneumoniae* and *Haemophilus* species). Prevailing drug-resistance patterns must be considered when the antibiotic is selected. For patients with CD4+ lymphocyte counts less than 100 cells/μL, especially if associated with recent hospitalization, neutropenia, and broad-spectrum antimicrobial use, consideration should be given for including coverage against *P. aeruginosa.* The duration of therapy is similar for HIV-infected and non–HIV-infected persons, and the response rates appear to be comparable.

**Prevention.** Despite successful treatment, 25% to 50% of patients with HIV-associated bacterial pneumonia will have a recurrence, sometimes with the same strain of bacteria that caused the original infection. The USPHS/IDSA[28] recommends that pneumococcal vaccine be given to all patients with HIV infection, but the effectiveness of this policy is uncertain, and failures have been reported. The vaccine should be administered as early in the course of HIV disease as possible (e.g., CD4+ lymphocyte count ≥200 cells/μL) to increase the probability of development of a protective antibody response. Although the question of whether (and when) to readminister pneumococcal vaccine in HIV-infected persons remains unanswered, revaccination 5 years after the initial vaccination, or sooner if the initial vaccination was given when the patient's CD4+ lymphocyte count was below 200 cells/μL and his or her current CD4+ count is above 200 cells/μL on antiretroviral therapy, has been suggested.[28] Patients who are cigarette smokers or who use injection drugs should be encouraged to quit. Patients who are receiving trimethoprim-sulfamethoxazole for *P. carinii* or *T. gondii* prophylaxis or clarithromycin or azithromycin for disseminated *M. avium* complex prophylaxis will receive added benefit in that these antimicrobial agents also offer protection against many bacterial infections. Because neutropenia is a strong risk factor for bacterial pneumonia, the use of granulocyte colony-stimulating factor in HIV-infected patients with an absolute neutrophil count below 500 cells/μL has been suggested.[28]

### *Pseudomonas aeruginosa*

During the second decade of the AIDS epidemic, *P. aeruginosa* has been increasingly described as a cause of community-acquired bacterial pneumonia in HIV-infected persons. In contrast to non–HIV-infected persons, the classic risk factors for *P. aeruginosa* infection are often absent in HIV-infected patients, and the disease is often recurrent.

*P. aeruginosa* infection produces a wide spectrum of disease in HIV-infected persons. The two most common presentations are pneumonia and bacteremia.[81–91] Unlike pneumonia due to *S. pneumoniae* and *Haemophilus* species, however, pneumonia due to *P. aeruginosa* usually occurs at more profound degrees of immunosuppression, and the chest radiograph often reveals cavitary infiltrates.

**CD4+ Lymphocyte Count.** Most cases of *P. aeruginosa* pneumonia occur in patients with a CD4+ lymphocyte count less than 100 cells/μL, usually less than 50 cells/μL. In one series of 16 HIV-infected patients with *P. aeruginosa* bronchopulmonary infection, the mean CD4+ count was 25 cells/μL, and only one patient had a CD4+ count above 50 cells/μL (56 cells/μL).[84] Another series of 15 HIV-infected patients with community-acquired *P. aeruginosa* pneumonia reported a mean CD4+ count of 27 cells/μL and noted that 80% had a CD4+ count less than 50 cells/μL.[88] The usual symptoms include fever and cough that is productive, with dyspnea and pleuritic chest pain seen less frequently.[88]

**Chest Radiograph.** Although the chest radiograph may resemble that seen in pneumococcal or *Haemophilus* pneumonias with focal consolidation, a significant proportion of radiographs demonstrate cavitary infiltrates. Schuster and Norris[88] reported that half of the 16 HIV-infected patients with *Pseudomonas* pneumonia had cavitary infiltrates on their admission chest radiograph, and another three (19%) patients had cavities on subsequent radiographs. Less striking results were noted in a study of 58 HIV-infected patients with *P. aeruginosa* infection in which 24% of the 25 patients who had pneumonia had cavitary infiltrates on chest radiograph.[89]

### Other Bacteria

*Legionella* species were originally thought to be an important cause of community-acquired bacterial pneumonia in HIV-infected patients. In the National Heart, Lung, and Blood Institute workshop, *Legionella* species either alone or with coexisting PCP accounted for 19 of the 441 (4.3%) serious pulmonary diseases seen.[24] In an update a few years later, it was noted that *Legionella* pneumonia was seldom seen.[25] There have been only a few series of *Legionella* pneumonia in HIV-infected patients.[92, 93] One series reported eight cases of *Legionella pneumophila* pneumonia occurring in seven HIV-infected patients (1.7% of the patients with Walter Reed stage 5 or 6 in their cohort).[93] The median CD4+ lymphocyte count was 83 cells/μL (range 38 to 155 cells/μL). Five of the cases were nosocomial. Fever (8/8), cough (8/8), and dyspnea (4/8) were the most common symptoms. The chest radiograph revealed lobar infiltrates in six cases and diffuse infiltrates in two. However, six of the eight patients had a concurrent pulmonary opportunistic infection; four had concomitant PCP and two had *R. equi,* which limits interpretation of the radiographic findings. The diagnosis of *L. pneumophila* was established by direct fluorescent antibody in five cases, antibody seroconversion in two, and the combination in one case. All of the patients responded to standard *Legionella* therapy or high doses of trimethoprim-sulfamethoxazole. Although *L. pneumophila* is the most common species identified, other *Legionella* species have also been reported.[94, 95]

There have been a number of reports of *R. equi* (formerly *Corynebacterium equi*) pulmonary disease occurring in HIV-infected persons.[96–101] Most cases present when the CD4+ lymphocyte count is less than 200 cells/μL and usually below 100 cells/μL. In one series of 12 HIV-infected patients with *R. equi* infection, the mean CD4+ count was 48 cells/μL (range 2 to 164 cells/μL) and only one patient had a CD4+ count above 100 cells/μL.[100] Fever (12/12), cough (6/12), and weight loss (4/12) were the most common symptoms. The chest radiograph often reveals cavitary lesions that may mimic tuberculosis or nocardiosis, or focal consolidation that may mimic bacterial pneumonia. Donisi and colleagues[100] reported cavitary lesions in 5 of 12 (42%) radiographs and lobar consolidation in four (33%). Sputum testing or bronchoscopy can establish the diagnosis of *R. equi* pneumonia.[100, 101] Blood cultures are often positive. The optimum treatment regimen and duration have yet to be defined. Combination antibiotic therapy is used, and active agents include rifampin, erythromycin, vancomycin, ciprofloxacin, and imipenam. Treatment is often longer than 2 months. Relapses are common, so long-term maintenance therapy is probably indicated. HIV-infected patients should avoid exposure to aerosolized soil containing farm animal manure.

There have been a handful of reports of *Nocardia* species infection in HIV-infected patients.[102–105] *N. asteroides* is the most common species identified, and the lung is the most commonly affected site. Most cases present when the CD4$^+$ lymphocyte count is below 200 cells/μL. In one series of 30 HIV-infected patients with nocardiosis, the mean CD4$^+$ count was 109 cells/μL (median = 92 cells/μL, range 12 to 266 cells/μL).[105] The presenting symptoms often mimicked tuberculosis. Fever (30/30), a productive cough (22/30), and weight loss (21/30) were most common.[105] The chest radiograph usually reveals cavitary lesions or lobar or multilobar infiltrates, especially in the upper lung zones. In one series of 21 HIV-infected patients, cavitary lesions were seen in 62%, lobar or multilobar consolidation in 52%, reticulonodular infiltrates in 33%, solitary masses in 24%, and pleural effusions in 33% of radiographs. Upper lobe involvement was seen in 71%.[106] Uttamchandani and coworkers[105] reported alveolar infiltrates in 64%, reticulonodular infiltrates in 9%, and mixed reticulonodular-alveolar infiltrates in 27% of radiographs. Upper lobe involvement was seen in 64%, associated cavitation was noted in 18%, pleural effusions in 14%, and adenopathy in 9% of radiographs. Sputum or bronchoscopy can establish the diagnosis of pulmonary nocardiosis. A modified acid-fast stain may provide an early presumptive diagnosis in the proper clinical setting. Trimethoprim-sulfamethoxazole is the treatment of choice.

## Mycobacteria

Early in the AIDS epidemic, mycobacteria were recognized as major sources of HIV-associated morbidity and mortality. Initially, HIV-infected patients were noted to develop disseminated *M. avium* complex. Subsequently, the relationship between HIV and *M. tuberculosis* became clearer, and, more recently, *M. kansasii* has increased in incidence.

### *Mycobacterium tuberculosis*

Tuberculosis is the major opportunistic infection complicating the HIV epidemic worldwide.[107–108a] Although other pathogens may predominate in individual areas, no other pathogen poses as great a global threat to those immunocompromised by HIV infection as *M. tuberculosis.* Moreover, unlike most of the HIV-associated opportunistic infections, *M. tuberculosis* is transmissible from person to person; it is also curable and preventable.[109, 110]

The AIDS epidemic has contributed to a veritable explosion of tuberculosis in sub-Saharan Africa and other developing regions. Developed countries, including the United States, however, have also been affected.[111] Before 1984, the incidence of tuberculosis in the United States declined by 5% to 6% per year. As late as 1987, the possibility of completely eliminating tuberculosis as a major health threat in the United States was contemplated. Epidemiologic evidence suggests that the AIDS epidemic contributed substantially to the increased numbers of tuberculosis cases seen in the United States in the middle to late 1980s and early 1990s.[112, 113] Defining the precise frequency of coexisting HIV and tuberculosis in the United States, however, is limited by incomplete HIV reporting for persons with tuberculosis. Estimates of the magnitude of dual infection, derived by linking AIDS and tuberculosis registries, reveal that 14% of the people diagnosed with tuberculosis in 1993 to 1994 (and 27% of persons aged 25 to 44 years) also appeared on the AIDS registry.[111]

There is now no doubt that HIV infection significantly increases the likelihood that latent *M. tuberculosis* infection will progress to active tuberculous disease. Studies have reported an annual rate of tuberculosis among untreated, tuberculin skin test–positive, HIV-infected persons in the United States of 1.7 to 7.9 cases per 100 person-years.[32, 37, 114] These rates were 4 to 26 times higher than the rates among comparable tuberculin skin test–negative HIV-infected persons, and they are 170 to 790 times higher than the rate among the US population overall (0.01%).[111] Instead of a 5% lifetime risk of "reactivation" disease, the HIV-infected person with latent, untreated *M. tuberculosis* infection risks almost certain active tuberculosis as immune competence wanes.[32] The risk of "reactivation" disease among HIV-infected persons has been estimated at 7% to 10% *per year.*

In addition, the emergence of multidrug-resistant tuberculosis as a public health threat poses a particularly grim prospect for the HIV-infected person.[115] The risk of drug-resistant tuberculosis is greater among HIV-infected patients than among others.[111, 116] In a multivariate analysis, HIV infection was found to be an independent risk factor for at least isoniazid resistance, for both isoniazid and rifampin resistance, and for rifampin monoresistance.[117] Studies with restriction fragment length polymorphism analysis have shown that multidrug-resistant tuberculosis can occur as a result of both failure to adhere to tuberculous therapy and exogenous reinfection from a multidrug-resistant source.[118] This latter sequence is probably an expression of the increased risk of developing active new-onset tuberculosis among HIV-infected patients in these instances after exposure to a patient with multidrug-resistant organisms. Transmission of multidrug-resistant tuberculosis to health care workers and prison guards has been documented; several of these workers, many of whom were HIV seropositive, have developed multidrug-resistant tuberculosis and some have died.[119, 120]

**Clinical Features.** The initial studies of HIV and *M. tuberculosis* dual infection demonstrated the impact of

HIV infection on the natural progression of tuberculosis. More recently, it has also become increasingly apparent that the host immune response to *M. tuberculosis* enhances HIV replication and may accelerate the natural progression of HIV disease.[121–121b] Nakata and colleagues[121] performed BAL in 11 HIV-infected patients with tuberculosis and 10 patients without pulmonary disease and found that the HIV viral load was significantly higher in BAL fluid from the affected lung than from the unaffected lung and the lungs of the control patients without pulmonary disease. In addition, the BAL HIV viral load was higher than the plasma viral load, possibly indicating local production of HIV. Even more compelling direct evidence was provided by Goletti and colleagues,[121a] who showed that the onset of tuberculosis in HIV-infected patients caused an increase in plasma viremia associated with a 5- to 160-fold increase in viral replication and that this, in turn, was correlated with the level of cellular activation.

***$CD4^+$ Lymphocyte Count.*** Tuberculosis can occur throughout the course of HIV infection and at any $CD4^+$ lymphocyte count. Theuer and colleagues[50] reported a median $CD4^+$ count of 326 cells/μL (range 23 to 742 cells/μL) among 11 HIV-infected persons with tuberculosis. Jones and associates[122] found a median $CD4^+$ count of 97 cells/μL among 85 consecutive HIV-infected patients with tuberculosis; 63 patients had a $CD4^+$ count equal to or less than 200 cells/μL, and 22 had a count above 200 cells/μL. The clinical expression of tuberculosis in HIV-infected persons is largely dependent on the degree of host immunosuppression (Table 82.2).[49] HIV-infected persons with relatively early HIV disease typically present with a picture suggestive of reactivation tuberculosis.[123] In these patients, tuberculosis classically presents with fevers, cough that is usually productive, night sweats, malaise, and weight loss. Disease is usually limited to the lung, and signs of extrapulmonary disease are typically absent. In contrast, HIV-infected persons with more advanced HIV disease typically present with a picture reminiscent of primary pulmonary tuberculosis or disseminated tuberculosis.[123] In these patients, symptoms and signs of extrapulmonary disease are often present. In a series of 97 HIV-infected patients with tuberculosis, Jones and coworkers[122] reported that extrapulmonary tuberculosis was seen in 30 of 43 (70%) patients with a $CD4^+$ count of 100 cells/μL or less, 10 of 20 (50%) patients with a count between 101 and 200 cells/μL, 7 of 16 (44%) patients with a count between 201 and 300 cells/μL, and only 5 of 18 (28%) patients with a $CD4^+$ count above 300 cells/μL. Virtually any extrapulmonary site may be involved; common sites include lymph nodes (usually cervical, supraclavicular, and axillary), bone marrow, genitourinary tract, central nervous system, and liver.[124] Although nonspecific, laboratory tests such as the complete blood cell count (CBC) and liver transaminases, when abnormal, are often indicative of tuberculous involvement.[124]

***Chest Radiograph.*** The prevalences of specific chest radiograph features of tuberculosis also depend on the degree of host immunosuppression.[51, 122, 125–127] Disease occurring early in the course of HIV infection mirrors that encountered in immunocompetent persons: upper lung zone infiltrates, often with cavitation on chest radiograph. Tuberculosis occurring later in the course of HIV infection, however, often presents with middle and lower lung zone infiltrates (Fig. 82.1), with diffuse infiltrates, including a miliary pattern, or with a normal radiograph. Greenberg and associates[51] noted a normal radiograph in 19 of 133 (14%) HIV-infected patients with tuberculosis. As the $CD4^+$ lymphocyte count declines, cavitation becomes less common, while intrathoracic adenopathy (Fig. 82.2) becomes more common on chest radiograph. Jones and colleagues[122] reported that adenopathy was seen on the radiographs of 20 of the 58 (34%) HIV-infected patients with a $CD4^+$ count of 200 cells/μL or less compared with 4 of the 29 (14%) patients with a $CD4^+$ count above 200 cells/μL ($P = .04$). Abouya and coworkers[125] found significant differences in the proportion of chest radiographs that showed cavitary infiltrates and those with intrathoracic adenopathy as the $CD4^+$ count declined: In 111 patients coinfected with HIV and *M. tuberculosis,* the proportion of radiographs with cavitary infiltrates decreased from 63% to 44% to 29% as the $CD4^+$ cell count declined from 400 cells/μL and above to 200 to 399 cells/μL and then to below 200 cells/μL ($P < 0.05$); in contrast, the proportion of radiographs with noncavitary infiltrates (33%, 44%, and 58%, respectively) and with intrathoracic adenopathy (0%, 14%, and 20%, respectively) increased as the $CD4^+$ count declined (both $P < 0.05$).

Slow recognition of late "atypical" HIV-associated tuberculosis delays institution of specific chemotherapy and

**Table 82.2** MANIFESTATIONS OF TUBERCULOSIS IN "EARLY" AND "LATE" HIV INFECTION

| Feature | Early | Late |
|---|---|---|
| Skin test | Positive | Negative |
| Distribution | Upper lung zones | Lower and middle lung zones |
| Cavitation | Common | Uncommon |
| Adenopathy | Uncommon | Common |
| Extrapulmonary | 10%–15% | More than 50% |

Adapted from Murray JF: Cursed duet: HIV infection and tuberculosis. Respiration 57:210–220, 1990, with permission from S. Karger AG, Basel, Switzerland.

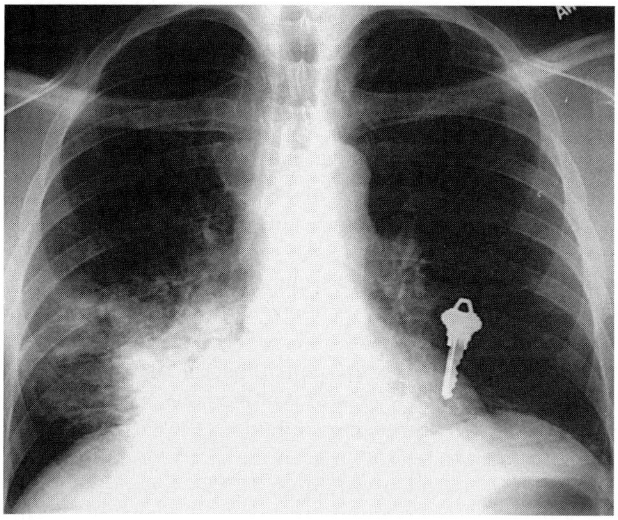

**Figure 82.1** Posteroanterior chest radiograph of HIV-seropositive patient showing focal right lung consolidation with air bronchograms. Culture of sputum revealed *M. tuberculosis* that was monorifampin resistant. Knowledge of the patient's CD4$^+$ lymphocyte count (<50 cells/μL) and understanding that tuberculosis can present with middle to lower lung zone consolidation during "late" HIV infection were instrumental in making the diagnosis of tuberculosis. The key was in the patient's pocket. (Reproduced with permission from L. Huang.)

increases the likelihood of transmission. A high index of suspicion should always be maintained when evaluating HIV-infected populations at high risk for tuberculosis, as the clinical and radiographic presentations vary. The key to the diagnosis is knowledge of the person's CD4$^+$ lymphocyte count and understanding the role that host immunosuppression has in the presentation.

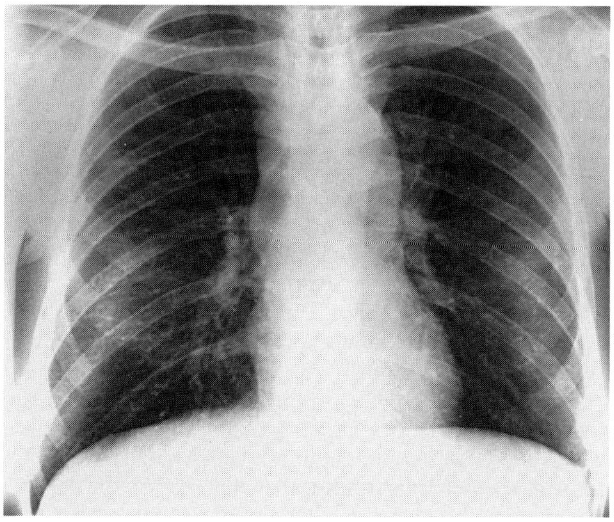

**Figure 82.2** Posteroanterior chest radiograph of HIV-seropositive patient showing mediastinal adenopathy. Culture of biopsy material revealed *M. tuberculosis.* (Reproduced with permission from Murray JF, Mills J: Pulmonary complications of HIV infection. Am Rev Respir Dis 141:1356–1372, 1582–1598, 1990.)

**Diagnosis.** The diagnostic approach to tuberculosis is the same for HIV-infected as for non–HIV-infected persons. Sputum AFB smears are the initial diagnostic tests. As described previously, several studies report that the sensitivity of sputum AFB smear and culture in HIV-infected patients is similar to the sensitivity in the overall population. The detection of AFB on smear, regardless of the source, is an indication for empirical antituberculosis treatment but cannot be considered diagnostic of tuberculosis. Several nontuberculous mycobacteria may present in HIV-infected persons and may be the cause of a smear-positive specimen. Molecular techniques, including the Roche Amplicor polymerase chain reaction and the Gen-Probe Amplified *Mycobacterium tuberculosis* Direct Test, are approved for use in the identification of *M. tuberculosis* in AFB smear-positive specimens. These tests are more sensitive than either acid-fast staining or auramine-rhodamine fluorescence for detecting *M. tuberculosis.* Sputum AFB smears are negative in a significant percentage (about 50%) of cases of tuberculosis. Even three negative AFB smears cannot exclude the diagnosis of tuberculosis. Therefore, patients with clinically suspected tuberculosis should remain on antituberculosis therapy while awaiting the results of culture and/or further diagnostic testing.

The "gold standard" diagnostic test for tuberculosis remains isolation and identification of *M. tuberculosis* by culture. Virtually any specimen can be examined for AFB and cultured for mycobacteria, including sputum, BAL fluid, TBBX specimen, Wang needle aspirate, pleural fluid or biopsy specimen, fine-needle aspirate of lymph node or other lesion, bone marrow aspirate or biopsy specimen, urine, cerebrospinal fluid, and biopsy specimen of other suspicious sites (e.g., liver). Blood cultures are specific and should be obtained, especially from persons with a CD4$^+$ lymphocyte count below 200 cells/μL. The results of drug susceptibility studies are useful in tailoring definitive treatment and essential in cases of drug resistance.

**Treatment.** Because tuberculosis is transmissible, detection of AFB on smear or in culture, regardless of the source, is an indication for empirical antituberculosis treatment while final identification is awaited.[111] The joint CDC and American Thoracic Society guidelines recommend a 6-month treatment regimen for HIV-infected patients with drug-susceptible tuberculosis.[128] HIV-infected patients who experience a delayed clinical and bacteriologic response should, however, be considered candidates for an extension of the duration of therapy. An expert panel recently agreed that a 6-month regimen can be used where patients are usually treated with directly observed therapy and where response to antituberculosis therapy can be monitored.[111] Clearly, HIV-infected patients with drug-resistant tuberculosis require a longer duration of therapy, and expert consultation should be sought in these cases.

HIV-infected persons with suspected tuberculosis should be started on four antituberculous drugs: isoniazid, rifampin, pyrazinamide, and ethambutol.[111] If a strong clinical suspicion exists for *M. avium* complex, multidrug therapy that is active against both tuberculosis and *M. avium* complex can be initiated simultaneously (e.g., adding a macrolide, either clarithromycin or azithromycin, to the above four-drug regimen). All cultures positive for *M. tuberculosis* should be submitted for susceptibility testing. Monoresistance to rifampin is more common in HIV-infected patients than in immunocompetent patients, but the reason for the excess is unclear.[128a] When results of susceptibility testing are available, drug therapy can be tailored. As in the treatment of all patients with tuberculosis, compliance is essential to a successful result. The response to therapy and the time to convert sputum cultures from positive to negative appear to be similar in HIV-infected and non–HIV-infected patients.[111] A retrospective analysis of HIV-infected patients with drug-susceptible tuberculosis found that conventional antituberculosis regimens and duration were appropriate.[129] Patients compliant with medications showed the expected rate of sputum culture conversion (median 10 weeks until negative), radiographic improvement (within 3 months), and low rates of relapse (5%).

HIV-infected patients with tuberculosis are more likely to experience toxicity from antituberculosis drugs than are non–HIV-infected persons. Among the conventionally used drugs, rifampin is most likely to cause adverse reactions,[129] whereas in Africa there is an increased incidence of side effects from thiacetazone, a drug widely used in resource-poor countries because of its low cost.[130, 131] HIV-infected patients with tuberculosis who begin dual therapy for *M. tuberculosis* and HIV infection may develop paradoxical reactions, a temporary exacerbation of clinical and radiographic features, that appear to be related to decreases in plasma HIV RNA and increases in the $CD4^+$ lymphocyte count.[132] The diagnosis of paradoxical reaction is one of exclusion. Patients with paradoxical reactions rarely require change or discontinuation of antituberculous or antiretroviral therapies, and symptomatic therapy is recommended.[111]

HIV-infected patients who are receiving or who are initiating antiretroviral therapy at the time that tuberculosis is diagnosed pose a special problem for the treatment of tuberculosis.[128a] Current guidelines for the treatment of HIV infection recommend the use of combinations of antiretroviral therapies.[133] The recommended combinations include dual nucleoside reverse transcriptase inhibitors (NRTI) combined with either a protease inhibitor (PI) or a non-nucleoside reverse transcriptase inhibitor (NNRTI). Once begun, it is crucial that antiretroviral therapy be continued without interruption for optimum, durable results.[133]

Both PIs and NNRTIs have significant interactions with the rifamycins, principally related to the induction or inhibition (or both) of the hepatic cytochrome P-450 (CYP450) enzyme system.[111] In general, induction of the CYP450 results in decreased drug levels, whereas inhibition results in increased levels. Decreased drug levels are associated with the development of resistance in both HIV and *M. tuberculosis,* whereas increased levels are correlated with toxicity. Of the rifamycins, rifampin is the most potent CYP450 inducer, followed by rifapentine and then rifabutin. The concomitant use of rifampin with a PI results in a 35% to 92% reduction in the area under the concentration-time curve (AUC) of the PI, and its use with an NNRTI results in a 13% to 96% reduction in the AUC of the NNRTI.

Reductions in either drug's AUC is associated with the development of resistance of HIV to that drug. Furthermore, resistance to a single drug often conveys cross-resistance to other drugs in the same class. Therefore, the use of rifampin to treat tuberculosis is contraindicated for an HIV-infected patient receiving or initiating PI therapy, NNRTI therapy, or both.[111] Current recommendations are that HIV-infected patients with tuberculosis who are on PI or NNRTI therapy should continue their antiretroviral therapy and should receive rifabutin, at a decreased daily dose (from 300 to 150 mg) if on a PI or the NNRTI delavirdine, instead of rifampin.[111] The reduction in the daily dose of rifabutin is required because all of the currently available PIs are inhibitors of CYP450 and the concomitant use of a PI and rifabutin will result in a 173% to 293% increase in the AUC of rifabutin.

Compared with the data on the interaction among the PIs and rifabutin, those for NNRTIs and rifabutin are limited. However, nevirapine is a CYP450 inducer, delavirdine is an inhibitor, and efavirenz is both an inducer and an inhibitor. HIV-infected patients with tuberculosis who are to begin concurrent therapy for HIV and *M. tuberculosis* should receive the optimum antiretroviral therapy (usually a combination of dual NRTIs plus either a PI or an NNRTI) and an antituberculosis regimen containing rifabutin. Alternatively, a streptomycin-containing antituberculosis regimen, instead of rifabutin, has been suggested for these patients. Only those HIV-infected patients who decline antiretroviral therapy or who are taking a non-PI, non-NNRTI–containing antiretroviral regimen should receive an antituberculosis regimen containing rifampin. Fortunately, the NRTIs are not metabolized by CYP450, and the other first-line antituberculosis medications are not CYP450 inducers, and thus no dose adjustments or changes are required.

**Prevention.** The tuberculin skin test remains the best screening tool to document *M. tuberculosis* exposure. HIV-infected persons with $CD4^+$ lymphocyte counts above 400 cells/μL are likely to have a positive response to purified protein derivative (PPD) skin testing in the presence of *M. tuberculosis* infection. The magnitude of the delayed hypersensitivity response is, however, likely to be less than that seen in HIV-seronegative persons. Accordingly, 5 mm induration (rather than the conventional 10 mm) is currently recommended as the cut point for prophylaxis in HIV-infected persons. Despite this modification, there is a higher incidence of false-negative tests as the $CD4^+$ count declines. Markowitz and coworkers[37] of the PCHIS found the sensitivity of delayed hypersensitivity/anergy testing to fall off after the $CD4^+$ lymphocyte count declined below 400 cells/μL. At present, routine anergy testing is not generally recommended for HIV-infected patients.[134, 135]

HIV-infected persons with a positive response to PPD or a history of a positive response to PPD who have not received prior prophylaxis should receive isoniazid for 9 months.[111] This is a change from previous recommendations, which called for 12 months of prophylaxis. An alternative is a short-course, multidrug regimen of rifampin plus pyrazinamide for 2 months.[111] At present, the routine use of preventive therapy in anergic or PPD-negative, HIV-infected persons is not generally recommended.[111] Some authorities, however, recommend primary preventive therapy for anergic or PPD-negative, HIV-infected residents of institutions who pose an ongoing significant risk for exposure to *M. tuberculosis* (e.g., prisons, jails, homeless shelters).[111] In addition, HIV-infected persons, including HIV-infected health care workers, who have experienced a significant tuberculosis exposure (sufficient to cause PPD conversions in immunocompetent persons), should be offered appropriate prophylaxis. Several studies document that the risk of reactivation tuberculosis is virtually eliminated if an HIV-infected person who has been infected with a drug-susceptible organism takes adequate prophylaxis.[111] HIV-seropositive persons who have converted their PPD after exposure to multidrug-resistant tuberculosis or anergic HIV-seropositive persons who have experienced a significant contact with multidrug-resistant tuberculosis should be offered prophylaxis based on the susceptibilities of the multidrug-resistant tuberculosis to which they were exposed. Paramount in the management of such patients is the active involvement of an expert in the treatment of multidrug-resistant tuberculosis.

Although concern has been raised about the safety and efficacy of vaccination with bacille Calmette-Guérin (BCG), data suggest that the incidence of local complications (ulceration and lymphadenitis) did not differ among HIV-infected babies who received BCG compared with non–HIV-infected infants.[136] Moreover, the World Health Organization (WHO) and International Union Against Tuberculosis and Lung Diseases (IUATLD) continue to recommend using BCG in developing countries where there is a high prevalence of HIV infection but state that the vaccine should not be given to symptomatic HIV-infected children or adults.

### *Mycobacterium avium* Complex

*M. avium* complex (MAC) consists of several related *Mycobacterium* species, including *M. avium* and *M. intracellulare.* Until 1980, only 24 cases of disseminated MAC had been reported.[137] With the AIDS epidemic, the number of cases rose dramatically. More recently, however, our experience at San Francisco General Hospital and that at many other institutions is that the incidence of disseminated MAC has declined since 1996.[138]

The pathogenesis of disseminated MAC is not completely understood, but it is believed to result from primary acquisition of the microorganism, which is ubiquitous in the environment, rather than reactivation of latent infection, as occurs with most HIV-associated diseases.[139] These mycobacteria probably enter the body chiefly through the gastrointestinal tract and occasionally through the lungs.[140–142] Nearly all cases of disseminated MAC are caused by *M. avium* serotypes, which suggests that there are important differences in exposure to or virulence of these particular strains.[143–145]

**Clinical Features.** Although the lungs are an important potential portal of entry for MAC into the bloodstream, MAC pulmonary disease is rare.[146–148] The most common clinical presentation of disseminated MAC disease is a febrile, wasting syndrome consisting of fever, night sweats, fatigue, anorexia, and weight loss; other manifestations include abdominal pain and chronic diarrhea, hepatosplenomegaly, lymphadenopathy, progressive anemia, and, rarely, extrabiliary obstructive jaundice.[33, 149–151]

***CD4$^+$ Lymphocyte Count.*** More than 95% of cases of disseminated MAC occur in patients whose CD4$^+$ count is 50 cells/μL or less.[152] Patients with disseminated MAC characteristically have nonspecific symptoms, signs, and laboratory abnormalities. Constitutional features dominate the clinical presentation, and respiratory symptoms are usually absent. Physical examination usually reveals evidence of weight loss. Hepatosplenomegaly and lymphadenopathy may also be seen. Laboratory abnormalities include anemia, often severe, and an elevated alkaline phosphatase level. The chest radiograph is typically normal, even when the organism is cultured from respiratory tract secretions.[141] Focal pneumonia has been reported but is extremely rare.[146–148] More frequently seen but still uncommon are endobronchial lesions without pneumonia.[153, 154] These endobronchial lesions appear to be submucosal "pearls" that on biopsy are teeming with acid-fast organisms.

**Diagnosis.** MAC can be cultured from numerous sites, but the most productive sources are blood, bone marrow, liver, or lymph nodes. Blood cultures for MAC are a sensitive method for establishing the diagnosis of disseminated disease.[33] The sensitivity of blood cultures for disseminated MAC has ranged from 86% to 98% of cases in which disseminated disease was confirmed by autopsy. The diagnosis of disseminated MAC can also be established by cultures from any normally sterile body site. Often, MAC is cultured from respiratory specimens such as sputum or BAL fluid, but this finding cannot be considered indicative of either pulmonary or disseminated disease.[141] The pathological findings of MAC infection are characteristic but not definitive. AFBs are remarkably abundant and are often packed within foamy macrophages or histiocytes; granulomas are usually absent or poorly formed.

**Treatment.** Although there are a number of efficacious treatment regimens, the optimal one for treating disseminated MAC is still debated.[155] The key to any regimen is the inclusion of a macrolide, either clarithromycin (500 mg twice daily) or azithromycin (500 to 600 mg daily). One of these should be combined with ethambutol (15 mg/kg/day). Some experts favor the addition of rifabutin (300 to 600 mg daily) to this combination.[155a] As with tuberculosis, the dose of rifabutin must be decreased with concurrent administration of a PI. In the past, disseminated MAC treatment was considered lifelong. In the setting of combination antiretroviral therapy with increases in the CD4$^+$ lymphocyte count to above 100 cells/μL, however, clinicians have discontinued therapy without relapse.[156]

**Prevention.** There are a number of different MAC prophylaxis regimens available. Choices include clarithromycin (500 mg twice daily), azithromycin (1200 mg weekly), rifabutin (300 mg daily), or the combination of azithromycin plus rifabutin; one of the first two regimens is the preferred prophylaxis.[28] The USPHS/IDSA guidelines recommend that MAC prophylaxis be administered to HIV-infected patients with a $CD4^+$ lymphocyte count less than 50 cells/μL and no clinical evidence of disseminated MAC.

### *Mycobacterium kansasii*

Before the AIDS epidemic, infection and disease due to *M. kansasii* were uncommon. In 1980, the incidence of *M. kansasii* infection was estimated to be 0.52 cases per 100,000 persons.[157] Subsequent estimates have documented a dramatic increase in the incidence, which has been related to HIV infection. *M. kansasii* has a particular geographic distribution predominantly in the southern and central United States.[155] We have, however, seen an increase in the number of cases in San Francisco, a nonendemic area. Bloch and associates[158] found a cumulative incidence of *M. kansasii* infection of 2.4 cases per 100,000 HIV-infected adults, a rate that is almost five times higher than the national rate. Although *M. kansasii* pulmonary disease can be clinically indistinguishable from tuberculosis, no person-to-person transmission has been documented, and infection is thought to occur from environmental sources.[155, 158]

**Clinical Features.** *M. kansasii* is the second most common cause of nontuberculous pulmonary disease in the United States.[155] During the second decade of the AIDS epidemic, *M. kansasii* infection has been increasingly described in HIV-infected patients.[158–167b] As mentioned, some of these cases have occurred outside of the endemic area.

***$CD4^+$ Lymphocyte Count.*** Similar to tuberculosis, *M. kansasii* pneumonia can occur at any $CD4^+$ lymphocyte count. Most HIV-infected patients with *M. kansasii*, however, have evidence of severe immunosuppression.[33] Witzig and colleagues[165] found a mean $CD4^+$ count of 62 cells/μL (median $CD4^+$ count was 24 cells/μL) among 49 HIV-infected patients with *M. kansasii* disease, and only four (8%) patients had a $CD4^+$ count above 200 cells/μL. In the study by Bloch and colleagues[158] that included 187 HIV-infected patients, the median $CD4^+$ lymphocyte count was 20 cells/μL (range 0 to 541 cells/μL), and 94% had an AIDS diagnosis. *M. kansasii* disease usually manifests itself with pulmonary involvement; accompanying disseminated disease or only extrapulmonary involvement is seen at the lowest $CD4^+$ lymphocyte counts. Witzig and colleagues[165] found that 32 of 49 (65%) HIV-infected patients with *M. kansasii* had isolated pulmonary disease (mean $CD4^+$ count 75 cells/μL), whereas the remainder had documented disseminated disease (mean $CD4^+$ count 28 cells/μL). The characteristic symptoms of *M. kansasii* include fever, cough that is often productive, dyspnea, and constitutional symptoms such as weight loss, fatigue, and night sweats. Chest pain and hemoptysis are seen in a minority of cases. Physical examination of the chest may be normal, or findings such as crackles and wheezes can be appreciated. Peripheral lymphadenopathy, hepatosplenomegaly, and new cutaneous lesions are extrapulmonary signs of disease.

***Chest Radiograph.*** The chest radiographic findings of *M. kansasii* are varied. The most common radiographic findings include alveolar infiltrates, diffuse infiltrates, and cavities; masses, intrathoracic adenopathy, and pleural effusions have also been reported. In a series of 49 HIV-infected patients with *M. kansasii,* alveolar infiltrates were noted in 55%, interstitial infiltrates in 22%, cavitation in 22%, and mass lesions in 8%.[165] In 8%, the radiograph was normal, and these patients had disseminated disease. The radiographic findings were unilateral in 49% and bilateral in 43%, and the distribution was apical in 35%, mid-lung in 18%, and lower lung in 12%.[165]

**Diagnosis.** The diagnosis of *M. kansasii* rests on its isolation and identification by culture. Pulmonary disease can be diagnosed by all of the techniques used for the diagnosis of tuberculosis. Unlike tuberculosis, however, where identification of *M. tuberculosis* is diagnostic of disease, the identification of *M. kansasii* can occasionally represent colonization rather than disease. To assist clinicians, the American Thoracic Society outlined criteria for the diagnosis of nontuberculous mycobacterial pulmonary disease.[155] These criteria apply to both HIV-infected and non–HIV-infected persons and presume that the patient is symptomatic and has chest radiograph or HRCT evidence of parenchymal disease. The criteria for diagnosis are (1) if three sputum/bronchial wash results are available from the previous 12 months: three positive cultures or two positive cultures and one positive AFB smear; (2) if only one bronchial wash is available: positive culture with a strongly positive AFB smear or heavy growth on solid media (≥2+ for each); (3) if sputum/bronchial wash results are nondiagnostic or another concurrent disease cannot be excluded: transbronchial or lung biopsy specimen revealing *M. kansasii* or biopsy specimen demonstrating mycobacterial histopathologic features and at least one sputum or bronchial wash that is positive (even 1+).

**Treatment.** The American Thoracic Society recommends that a regimen consisting of isoniazid (300 mg daily), rifampin (600 mg daily), and ethambutol (25 mg/kg daily for the first 2 months, then 15 mg/kg daily) be used for treatment of *M. kansasii* pulmonary disease.[155] Patients who are taking PI (or NNRTI) therapy for HIV infection should receive rifabutin or clarithromycin in place of rifampin. Pyrazinamide is unacceptable as an alternative drug because all *M. kansasii* isolates are resistant. Patients should receive treatment for 18 months or a minimum of 12 months after their cultures are converted to negative.

### Other Mycobacteria

Virtually all nontuberculous mycobacterial infections complicating HIV disease are caused by MAC and, increasingly, *M. kansasii.* Other mycobacteria, however, including *M. xenopi, M. fortuitum, M. chelonei, M. malmoense, M. gordonae,* and *M. terrae,* have been occasionally identified.[168] The reason or reasons for this striking disparity are unknown. Increased frequency of exposure or the presence of specific defects in host defenses might account for the predominance of MAC and to a lesser extent *M. kansasii* in AIDS patients. The American Thoracic Society recently summarized the diagnosis and treatment of nontuberculous mycobacterial disease.[155] Readers are referred to this summary as well as to Chapter 34 for details.

## Fungi

Early in the AIDS epidemic, fungi were recognized as major sources of morbidity and mortality. Despite the overall decline in HIV-associated opportunistic infections in the United States, fungi remain frequent causes of HIV-associated disease. Indeed, nearly one fourth of all US AIDS-defining diagnoses in adults and adolescents are due to fungi.[8] Several fungi can cause pulmonary disease in HIV-infected persons. *P. carinii,* previously classified as a protozoan but currently considered a fungus, remains the most common AIDS-defining opportunistic infection in the United States and is a common cause of HIV-associated pneumonia. *C. neoformans,* the most common cause of meningitis in HIV-infected persons, often presents with an associated pneumonia. The endemic fungi *H. capsulatum, C. immitis, P. marneffei,* and to a lesser extent *B. dermatitidis* are among the chief causes of HIV-associated disease seen in their particular geographic regions, and all have important pulmonary presentations. Finally, invasive aspergillosis is often a devastating pulmonary disease seen in HIV-infected persons with severe immunosuppression. Further information is provided in Chapter 35.

### *Pneumocystis carinii*

*P. carinii* pneumonia (PCP) remains the most common AIDS-defining opportunistic infection in the United States, among both children and adults/adolescents.[8] Its overall incidence is, however, declining.[169] Early in the AIDS epidemic, PCP accounted for nearly two thirds of AIDS-defining diagnoses, and an additional 15% to 20% of patients developed PCP at some time during their HIV disease.[170] Currently, however, two factors, the use of combination antiretroviral therapy and *P. carinii* prophylaxis, have combined to dramatically reduce the overall number of cases. At San Francisco General Hospital, we diagnosed between 200 and 290 cases of PCP annually from 1990 to 1994. In 1995 and 1996, the number of cases was below 200; and since 1997, the number has been below 100 (L. Huang, unpublished data). Coincident with this decline was the increasing use of dual nucleoside reverse transcriptase inhibitors and subsequently the introduction of PIs into clinical practice.

**History and Epidemiology.** Identified early in the twentieth century by Chagas, *P. carinii* was first recognized as a human pathogen in the 1950s.[171] Despite over 40 years' experience and an explosion of PCP cases since 1981, we still have very little understanding of this omnipresent organism. In fact, it was only in 1988 that initial homology studies indicated that *P. carinii* was a fungus rather than a protozoan, as previously classified.[172–174] One major obstacle that has impeded further advances has been the inability to reliably culture *P. carinii* f. sp. *hominis* in vitro, forcing researchers to rely on animal models for growth and testing. Although mammals are the only known hosts of *P. carinii* and a number of mammals are susceptible to infection, *P. carinii* has been demonstrated to be species specific.[175–178] Although *P. carinii* can be easily transmitted between mammals of the same species, studies that have attempted to transmit *P. carinii* from one species to another have been unsuccessful. Thus, the animal models used for research may or may not reproduce an accurate human condition.

The ecologic niche for *P. carinii* and its mode of transmission are unknown. The inability to maintain *P. carinii* in culture suggests that *P. carinii* itself may be unable to grow outside of its mammalian host. Given its species specificity, it is doubtful that other mammals are the reservoir for *P. carinii* f. sp. *hominis.* This host-species specificity also implies coevolution of host and *P. carinii* that, in turn, implies long-term carriage in its human host. It has been shown that infection with *P. carinii* is almost ubiquitous. Up to 85% to 100% of the US population have specific antibodies directed against *P. carinii* by the age of 3 years.[179–181] Clearly, most of these individuals never develop PCP. In the setting of severe immunosuppression, such as occurs in HIV infection, however, PCP can affect significant proportions of people. These studies and others suggest that reactivation of latent infection is the cause of most *P. carinii* disease among immunocompromised hosts. Reports of newly acquired infection after de novo exposure to persons with PCP have, however, been documented; these outbreaks occurred among immunocompromised persons in pediatric wards, cancer clinics or wards, transplant units, and other confined spaces and suggest possible person-to-person transmission of *P. carinii* and rapid development of disease.[180, 182–185] In addition, the development of PCP in HIV-infected infants would favor the possibility of recent infection.

Transmission of *P. carinii* probably occurs via inhalation of a *Pneumocystis*-containing aerosol. Hughes[186] and Hughes and colleagues[187] demonstrated that immunocompromised axenic rats maintained in germ-free isolators did not develop PCP despite 3 months of immunosuppression with dexamethasone. In a selective manner, these rats were then exposed to potential sources of *P. carinii,* including air, food, and water. Rats who were exposed to filtered (sterile) air and to regular (unsterile) food and water did not develop PCP. Rats exposed to room (unsterile) air but maintained on sterile food and water did, however, develop PCP, implying that *P. carinii* is acquired as an airborne disease from de novo infection in the setting of immunocompromise. The duration of exposure necessary for transmission may be short. Soulez and coworkers[188] housed *P. carinii*-free SCID mice near corticosteroid-treated non-SCID mice and found that a 1-day exposure was sufficient for transmission of *P. carinii* to the SCID mice.

*P. carinii* infection is overwhelmingly a pulmonary disease. After inhalation, *P. carinii* establishes residence in the alveolus. There, it attaches itself to alveolar type I cells. Although *P. carinii* is closely interdigitated with the type I cell, no fusion of the cellular membranes occurs. Attachment may facilitate access to nutrients directly from the alveolar-capillary bed, however, and appears to be necessary for replication. Over time, the alveolar type I cells become damaged, and the alveoli become increasingly filled with a foamy, eosinophilic exudate. Eventually, impairment of gas exchange occurs, and patients present with hypoxemia.

**Clinical Features.** Setting aside the open question of whether person-to-person transmission of *P. carinii* is an important problem, the risk factors for the development of PCP among HIV-infected persons are clear. These risk factors for adults include a $CD4^+$ lymphocyte count less than 200 cells/μL (see below for infants and children), a history of PCP, and 2 or more weeks of unexplained fever or the presence of oropharyngeal candidiasis.[189, 190]

***$CD4^+$ Lymphocyte Count.*** Approximately 95% of cases of PCP occur in HIV-infected adult patients whose $CD4^+$ lymphocyte count is below 200 cells/μL.[190] The Multicenter AIDS Cohort Study found a markedly increased risk for PCP among HIV-infected subjects with a $CD4^+$ lymphocyte count of 200 cells/μL or less at study entry.[189] These subjects had a nearly fivefold greater risk of developing PCP than did subjects who had a $CD4^+$ lymphocyte count higher than 200 cells/μL at study entry (OR = 4.9, 95% CI = 3.1–8.0, $P < 0.001$). This study also demonstrated that the presence of fever for 2 weeks or more and the development of thrush were independent predictors for PCP. Stansell and coworkers[190] found that the incidence of PCP increased as the $CD4^+$ lymphocyte count declined. Subjects with a $CD4^+$ count between 101 and 200 cells/μL had an incidence of 5.95 cases of PCP per 100 person-years, whereas those with a $CD4^+$ count of 100 cells/μL or less had 11.13 cases per 100 person-years.

Concerning infants and children, a significant percentage of cases of PCP in HIV-infected infants 6 months of age or younger occur when the $CD4^+$ lymphocyte count is above 1500 cells/μL.[191] Furthermore, in these infants, the $CD4^+$ lymphocyte count can decline rapidly (700–1200 cells/μL) in the 3 months preceding PCP.[191] Accordingly, the guidelines for *P. carinii* prophylaxis differ for infants, children, and adults/adolescents (see subsequent section on Prevention).[28]

HIV-infected adults, unlike other immunocompromised persons, usually have a prolonged prodromal illness associated with PCP. Kovacs and colleagues[192] found nearly 1 month of symptoms before presentation in most HIV-infected patients with PCP. In this study, the median duration of symptoms in 40 HIV-infected patients was 28 days, which was significantly longer than the median duration of 5 days seen in the 37 patients with other immunosuppressive diseases ($P < 0.0002$). Kales and colleagues[193] reported a median duration of symptoms of 3 weeks in 143 HIV-infected patients with PCP and found that 72 patients (50%) had a duration of symptoms of 2 weeks or longer. This duration of symptoms can be used to distinguish *P. carinii* from pyogenic pneumonia, which typically presents with 3 to 5 days of symptoms.

Classically, PCP presents with fever, a nonproductive cough, and dyspnea on exertion. In one series of 145 HIV-infected patients with PCP, fever was noted in 86%, cough in 91%, and dyspnea in 95% of patients.[193] High fevers, rigors, purulent sputum, and pleuritic chest pain are uncommon and can be used to distinguish *P. carinii* from pyogenic pneumonia. In a multivariate analysis, Selwyn and colleagues[70] found that the presence of purulent sputum (OR = 2.46, 95% CI = 1.1–5.4, $P = 0.03$) or pleuritic chest pain (OR = 2.99, 95% CI = 1.4–6.6, $P = 0.01$) was an independent predictor of bacterial pneumonia rather than of PCP or tuberculosis.

Physical examination of the chest may be normal. In the series reported by Kales and coworkers,[193] 78 patients (54%) with PCP had a normal lung examination. When abnormal, the most frequent findings on lung auscultation are inspiratory crackles; the presence of crackles has been reported to be associated with a greater disease severity and an increased mortality.[193]

Numerous studies have shown that the serum LDH level is increased in patients with PCP. An elevated serum LDH level does not, however, establish the diagnosis of PCP, nor does a normal serum value rule out the diagnosis.

***Chest Radiograph.*** Classically, PCP presents with bilateral, symmetric reticular or granular opacities (Fig. 82.3).[194] These opacities typically begin in the perihilar region and extend outward as the disease severity increases. Occasionally, the opacities will be unilateral or asymmetric. Our experience has taught us that the pattern seen (reticular, granular) is more important in suggesting the diagnosis of PCP than the distribution (bilateral versus unilateral, symmetric versus asymmetric, diffuse versus focal). Thin-walled cysts or pneumatoceles are seen in 10% to 20% of cases (see Fig. 82.3).[195–196a] Pneumatoceles may be present at the time of diagnosis or may develop during PCP therapy. Pneumatoceles may be single or multiple in number, small or large in size, and predispose patients to pneumothorax, which is another radiographic presentation of PCP. Usually, pneumatoceles resolve but occasionally persist despite successful therapy.

Virtually every possible radiographic finding, including focal, lobar, or segmental consolidation, nodules with or without cavitation, and a miliary pattern, can be seen occasionally.[196] Apical or upper lung zone disease that mimics tuberculosis is associated with aerosolized pentamidine prophylaxis, although this presentation can be seen as well in patients taking oral prophylaxis or no preventive therapy (Fig. 82.4). Intrathoracic adenopathy and pleural effusions are rarely due to PCP. These radiographic findings should prompt a search for an alternate or at least a coexisting process such as bacterial pneumonia, tuberculosis, fungal pneumonia, or pulmonary Kaposi's sarcoma.

PCP may present with a normal chest radiograph. Published studies report the incidence of a normal radiograph to range from 0% to 39%.[194, 196, 197] In our experience, PCP presents with a normal chest radiograph in less than 5% of cases.

**Diagnosis.** At San Francisco General Hospital, patients with a clinical presentation suggestive of PCP and a compatible chest radiograph undergo sputum induction (SI).[35, 198] If SI examination is negative for *P. carinii* and other organisms, patients then undergo bronchoscopy with bronchoalveolar lavage (BAL). In our experience, a negative BAL rules out the diagnosis of PCP in all but the rarest of cases. (This may not be true in other institutions that have not had extensive experience with this method.)

Patients with a suggestive clinical presentation but a normal or unchanged radiograph undergo either pulmonary function testing or chest HRCT to determine who warrants diagnostic testing (e.g., SI). On pulmonary function testing, patients with PCP often display a restrictive ventilatory defect with decreased lung volumes and increased air flow. A more sensitive indicator of PCP, however, is a decrease in the $DL_{CO}$, which is caused by alveolar-capillary block.[199] The $DL_{CO}$ is a sensitive indicator of PCP.[200, 201] Huang and coworkers[39] of the PCHIS demonstrated that a decreased $DL_{CO}$ (defined as ≤75% of the predicted value, corrected for hemoglobin) detected 90% of the cases of PCP in patients whose chest radiograph was normal or unchanged. Moreover, the combination of a normal or unchanged radiograph and a $DL_{CO}$ of more than 75% of predicted virtually rules out the possibility of PCP. Thus, these patients should probably be clinically observed without further evaluation or treatment for *P. carinii,* or they should be evaluated and treated for another process. One drawback to the $DL_{CO}$ is its lack of specificity. The same study that reported a $DL_{CO}$ sensitivity of 90% also found a specificity of 53%.[39] Therefore, a decreased $DL_{CO}$ is not diagnostic of PCP, and patients with clinically suspected PCP who have a decreased $DL_{CO}$ undergo SI in our institution.

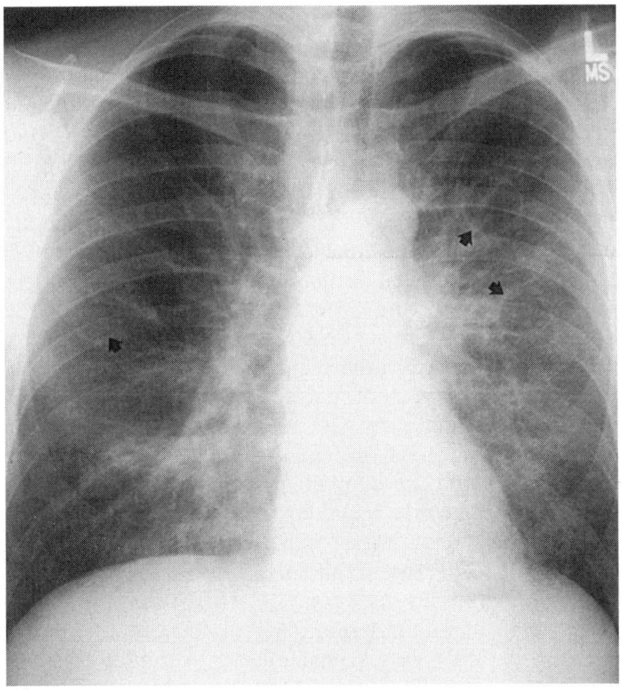

**Figure 82.3** Posteroanterior chest radiograph of HIV-seropositive patient with *P. carinii* pneumonia showing bilateral, predominantly perihilar, granular opacities and three pneumatoceles *(arrows).* (Reproduced with permission from L. Huang.)

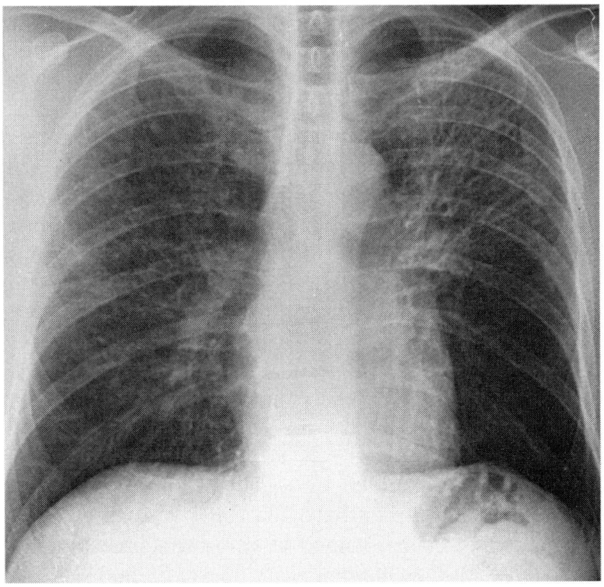

**Figure 82.4** Posteroanterior chest radiograph of HIV-seropositive patient who had been receiving aerosolized pentamidine showing reticular infiltration, predominantly of the upper lung zones, secondary to relapsed PCP. (Reproduced with permission from Murray JF, Mills J: Pulmonary complications of HIV infection. Am Rev Respir Dis 141:1356–1372, 1582–1598, 1990.)

An alternate test to the $DL_{CO}$ is chest HRCT. PCP has a characteristic appearance on HRCT: patchy areas of ground-glass opacity through which vessels are seen and a background of interlobular septal thickening.[41, 42, 202–204] We found that HRCT was a sensitive test for persons with clinically suspected PCP who had a normal, unchanged, or equivocal chest radiograph.[205] In this study of 51 HIV-infected patients with clinically suspected PCP but a normal, unchanged, or equivocal chest radiograph, all patients with PCP diagnosed by either SI or BAL had an HRCT with ground-glass opacities (sensitivity was 100%). In addition, none of the patients whose HRCT was without ground-glass opacities was found to have PCP on SI, BAL, and clinical follow-up. Thus, an HRCT without these lesions rules out the diagnosis of PCP, and these patients should probably be clinically observed without further evaluation or treatment for *P. carinii,* or they should be evaluated and treated for another process. Although HRCT has a better specificity than does $DL_{CO}$ (89% versus 53%), patients with suspected PCP and an HRCT with typical ground-glass densities still must undergo SI in our institution.

$^{67}$Gallium citrate scanning is a highly sensitive but nonspecific test for *P. carinii,* and a negative $^{67}$gallium scan makes the diagnosis of PCP unlikely. Hence, some institutions may choose to use $^{67}$gallium scans, in place of pulmonary function tests or HRCT, for patients with suspected PCP but whose chest radiograph is normal or unchanged. $^{67}$Gallium scans, however, suffer from a relatively high cost, an inherent time delay in obtaining the imaging, and the baseline mild to moderate (1+ to 2+) $^{67}$gallium uptake in the lungs of HIV-infected persons without active pulmonary infection. In our opinion, these factors, combined with the availability and sensitivity of both pulmonary function testing and HRCT scanning, render the nuclear imaging test rarely necessary for the diagnosis of PCP.

The diagnosis of PCP rests on the microscopic visualization of the characteristic *P. carinii* cysts and/or trophic forms on stained respiratory specimens. *P. carinii* can be detected in expectorated[206] or induced sputum; in pulmonary secretions obtained by nasotracheal suction, BAL, or percutaneous aspiration of the lung parenchyma; and in pulmonary tissue obtained by transbronchial, thoracoscopic, or open-lung biopsy.[5, 6] Of these, SI and BAL are the most widely used. The standard method for detection of *P. carinii* has been with cyst wall stains such as toluidine blue-O and methenamine silver or with Giemsa and Diff-Quik, which stain the intracystic sporozoites and the trophic forms.[207] Recently, monoclonal antibodies to *P. carinii* f. sp. *hominis,* which react with both cysts and trophic forms, have been used.[207] Polymerase chain reaction (PCR)-based techniques have also been employed and have been reported to be more sensitive but also less specific than either of the other methods.[207]

A number of studies have examined the impact of prophylaxis against *P. carinii* on the sensitivity of induced sputum and BAL examination for detecting the organisms.[208–215] Some authors reported a lower yield of diagnostic studies for *P. carinii* among patients who were receiving aerosolized pentamidine compared with those having no prophylaxis, whereas others found no difference between the two groups. In patients undergoing bronchoscopy, the yield for *P. carinii* may be improved by performing upper lobe lavage or multiple lobe lavage with or without a more sensitive staining technique (e.g., monoclonal antibodies).[213–215] Our practice is to perform BAL in the most affected lobe visualized on chest radiograph. For patients with diffuse radiographic disease, we usually perform a single lavage in the right middle lobe. For patients with, for example, an upper lung zone predominance on radiograph, however, we often lavage both an upper lobe and the right middle lobe. Despite the widespread use of trimethoprim-sulfamethoxazole and dapsone for *P. carinii* prophylaxis, no studies have evaluated whether the yield of diagnostic studies is changed. Our clinical experience suggests that while the severity of chest radiograph abnormalities may be milder in patients receiving prophylaxis than in those receiving no prophylaxis, the yields from SI and BAL remain the same.

**Treatment.** The standard duration of PCP therapy is 21 days. The choice of specific treatment depends in part on the severity of disease (Table 82.3).

Trimethoprim-sulfamethoxazole (TMP-SMX) remains the treatment of choice for patients with mild, moderate, and severe PCP and is the regimen against which all others are measured. TMP and SMX act in concert to inhibit different steps in folate metabolism. TMP inhibits dihydrofolate reductase, preventing the synthesis of tetrahydrofolate from dihydrofolate, and SMX inhibits dihydropteroate synthase, preventing the conversion of *para*-aminobenzoate to dihydrofolate. TMP-SMX possesses many benefits, including availability in both an intravenous and an oral form, availability as a single drug combination, excellent oral bioavailability, and activity against many community-acquired bacteria that may cause concomitant pyogenic infection. The usual dose of TMP is 15 (range 15–20) mg/kg/day and that of SMX is 75 (range 75–100) mg/kg/day, divided into three or four daily doses. Dosing may be intravenous (recommended for patients with moderate or severe PCP) or oral. In general, we avoid a TMP dose exceeding 320 mg every 8 hours, instead increasing the frequency to every 6 hours. Unfortunately, adverse effects from TMP-SMX are frequent and include rash, fever, gastrointestinal complaints (nausea, vomiting), elevated liver transaminases, hyperkalemia, and bone marrow suppression, especially anemia and neutropenia. Often these effects develop during the second week of therapy. In a significant proportion of HIV-infected patients, the side effects are treatment limiting. Rare adverse reactions include Stevens-Johnson syndrome, toxic epidermal necrolysis, and a clinical syndrome resembling septic shock with hypotension, fever, pulmonary infiltrates, and renal and hepatic dysfunction.

***Trimethoprim-Sulfamethoxazole Versus Pentamidine.*** Three prospective, randomized studies compared TMP-SMX with pentamidine, an aromatic deamidine; two found no significant difference between the two regimens, whereas the third favored TMP-SMX.

Wharton and colleagues[216] studied 40 patients with their first episode of PCP in a prospective, randomized trial of TMP-SMX (20 mg/kg/day of TMP component) versus pentamidine (4 mg/kg/day). Subjects in both groups had similarly decreased arterial oxygenation. Of 20 patients randomized to TMP-SMX, 25% died during the treatment period and 50% required a switch in therapy owing to adverse drug reaction. In comparison, of the 20 patients who received pentamidine as initial therapy, 5% died ($P = 0.09$) and 55% required a switch owing to adverse reaction ($P = 0.9$). The authors found no significant differences in the two treatment arms in the rates of clinical improvement, pulmonary function test results, or $^{67}$gallium uptake by the lungs at the completion of therapy among survivors and concluded that TMP-SMX and pentamidine are equivalent in terms of efficacy and frequency of adverse reactions.

Sattler and associates[217] reported on 69 patients with PCP in a prospective, randomized, noncrossover trial of TMP-SMX (15–20 mg/kg/day of TMP component, dose adjusted to maintain serum TMP concentration between 5 and 8 μg/mL) versus pentamidine (4 mg/kg/day, dose reduced for rise in serum creatinine). One third of the patients in both groups had an arterial $Po_2$ below 60 mm Hg on entry. Of the 36 patients randomized to TMP-SMX, 14% died during the treatment period compared with 39% of the 33 patients randomized to pentamidine ($P = 0.03$). In addition, the authors found that patients

**Table 82.3** TREATMENT REGIMENS FOR *PNEUMOCYSTIS CARINII* PNEUMONIA*

| TREATMENT REGIMEN | DOSES AND FREQUENCY | TOXICITIES |
|---|---|---|
| **Mild PCP** ($PaO_2$ >70 mm Hg *and* alveolar − arterial $PO_2$ difference <35 mm Hg)† | | |
| Trimethoprim (TMP)-sulfamethoxazole | 15 mg/kg (TMP component) daily (q 6–8 hours) | Fever, dermatologic, gastrointestinal, hematologic |
| TMP plus dapsone | 15 mg/kg daily (q 6–8 hours)<br>100 mg once daily | Dermatologic, gastrointestinal, hematologic |
| Clindamycin plus primaquine | 1800 mg daily (q 6–8 hours)<br>30 mg (base) once daily | Dermatologic, gastrointestinal, hematologic |
| Atovaquone | 750 mg thrice daily | Dermatologic, gastrointestinal |
| **Moderate to Severe PCP** ($PaO_2$ ≤70 mm Hg *or* alveolar − arterial $PO_2$ difference ≥35 mm Hg)‡ | | |
| TMP-sulfamethoxazole | 15 mg/kg (TMP component) daily (q 6–8 hours) | Fever, dermatologic, gastrointestinal, hematologic |
| Pentamidine | 3–4 mg/kg once daily | Renal, pancreatic |
| Clindamycin plus primaquine | 1800–2400 mg (q 6–8 hours)<br>30 mg (base) (orally (po)) once daily | Dermatologic, gastrointestinal, hematologic |
| Trimetrexate plus leucovorin§ ± dapsone | 45 mg/$m^2$ once daily<br>+ 20 mg/$m^2$ q 6 hours<br>± 100 mg (po) once daily | Hematologic, dermatologic, fever |

*Recommended duration of therapy is 21 days.
†Oral route is preferred for patients with mild PCP who are treated as outpatients.
‡Intravenous route is preferred (at least until clinical improvement) for patients with moderate to severe PCP. Adjunctive corticosteroids (prednisone 40 mg, po, twice daily for 5 days; then 40 mg, po, once daily for 5 days; then 20 mg, po, once daily for 11 days; or potency equivalent solumedrol intravenously) should also be administered.
§Leucovorin (folinic acid) must be given concomitantly and for 2–3 days after trimetrexate is stopped.

treated with TMP-SMX appeared to respond more rapidly to therapy than did those who received pentamidine with a more rapid improvement in alveolar-arterial $PO_2$. Patients treated with TMP-SMX had higher rates of rash (44%) and anemia (39%), whereas those treated with pentamidine had higher rates of nephrotoxicity (64%), hypotension (27%), and hypoglycemia (21%). On the basis of these results, the authors concluded that TMP-SMX was superior to pentamidine in terms of increased survival and a more rapid improvement in oxygenation.

Klein and coworkers,[218] in the largest series comparing these two regimens, studied 160 patients with PCP in a prospective, randomized trial of TMP-SMX (20 mg/kg/day of TMP component) versus pentamidine (4 mg/kg/day). The mean alveolar-arterial $PO_2$ was similar in both groups. Of 92 patients randomized to TMP-SMX, mortality was 33% during the treatment period. In addition, 42% required a switch in therapy because of treatment failure, and 34% required a switch because of adverse drug reaction. These proportions were similar in the 68 patients randomized to pentamidine where mortality was 26% ($P$ = 0.4), 40% required a switch because of treatment failure ($P$ = 0.7), and 25% required a switch because of adverse drug reaction ($P$ = 0.2). In this large trial, the authors concluded that TMP-SMX and pentamidine are equivalent in terms of efficacy and frequency of treatment-limiting side effects.

These three studies used a dose of TMP-SMX (20 mg/kg/day of TMP component) that is higher than the dose that we currently use (15 mg/kg/day). In addition, the studies were conducted before the recommendations for adjunctive corticosteroid for moderate to severe PCP were implemented, perhaps explaining the frequency of treatment-limiting adverse effects seen with TMP-SMX and the high mortality rate.

***Trimethoprim-Sulfamethoxazole Versus Aerosolized Pentamidine.*** Given the tolerability of aerosolized pentamidine for *P. carinii* prophylaxis, its use for PCP treatment was studied. Montgomery and colleagues[219] studied 303 patients with confirmed (n = 287) or presumed (n = 16) PCP in a prospective, randomized trial of TMP-SMX (15 mg/kg/day of TMP component) versus aerosolized pentamidine (600 mg daily via Respirgard II nebulizer). All subjects had mild or moderate PCP as defined by a resting room air alveolar-arterial $PO_2$ of 55 mm Hg or less. Of the patients randomized to TMP-SMX, 17 died, compared with 12 patients who received aerosolized pentamidine ($P$ = 0.28). Ninety-four patients randomized to aerosolized pentamidine, however, required a switch in therapy due to treatment failure compared with 22 patients who received TMP-SMX ($P$ = 0.002). In addition, the authors found that the arterial $PO_2$ improved more rapidly among patients randomized to TMP-SMX. Although aerosolized pentamidine was better tolerated than TMP-SMX, the authors concluded that TMP-SMX has fewer therapeutic failures, more rapid improvement in oxygenation, and a lower rate of relapse.

***Trimethoprim-Sulfamethoxazole Versus Dapsone or Trimethoprim Plus Dapsone.*** Given the frequency of treatment-limiting adverse effects with both TMP-SMX and intravenous pentamidine, regimens were sought that were better tolerated. Dapsone, a dihydropteroate synthase inhibitor, used as a single agent was found to be a suboptimal treatment. One study by Mills and colleagues[220] found that 7 of 18 (39%) patients treated with dapsone (100 mg/day) required a switch to an alternate therapy because of clinical failure. Safrin and coworkers[221] found similar results using a higher dapsone dose (200 mg/day). In this study, all seven (100%) patients with PCP and an arterial $Po_2$ greater than 60 mm Hg required a switch to an alternate regimen because of clinical failure, including two patients who progressed to respiratory failure necessitating intubation, both of whom eventually died.

In contrast, the addition of TMP to dapsone is an effective regimen. Leoung and colleagues[222] found that trimethoprim (20 mg/kg/day) plus dapsone (100 mg/day) was an effective combination and that all 15 patients treated with this regimen survived, although two patients developed severe rash that required a switch to TMP-SMX. Medina and associates[223] studied 60 patients with their first episode of PCP in a prospective, randomized trial of TMP-SMX (20 mg/kg/day of TMP component) versus TMP (20 mg/kg/day) plus dapsone (100 mg/day). All subjects had mild to moderate PCP defined as an arterial $Po_2$ greater than 60 mm Hg. Of the 30 patients assigned to TMP-SMX, one died, three required a switch to intravenous pentamidine because of treatment failure, and 17 required a switch because of adverse drug reaction. TMP plus dapsone was similar in efficacy, with none of the 30 patients dying and two requiring a switch because of treatment failure. This combination was better tolerated, however, with significantly fewer patients (9) requiring a switch because of adverse reactions ($P$ = 0.025). The authors concluded that TMP plus dapsone was equal in efficacy to TMP-SMX but was associated with fewer treatment-limiting side effects.

***Trimethoprim-Sulfamethoxazole Versus Clindamycin Plus Primaquine.*** The combination of clindamycin, a lincosamide, plus primaquine, a dihydrofolate reductase inhibitor, is an effective regimen. Noskin and associates[224] used clindamycin (usually 900 mg every 8 hours) plus primaquine (30 mg/day) successfully as salvage therapy in patients with PCP. In this study, 26 patients who experienced 28 episodes of PCP were treated with this combination; all had been unresponsive to or intolerant of other regimens. The authors found that therapy was successful in 24 episodes (86%), including four patients who had respiratory failure and were mechanically ventilated. Black and colleagues[225] of the AIDS Clinical Trials Group (ACTG) studied 60 patients with PCP in a prospective, noncomparative study of clindamycin (intravenous 900 mg every 8 hours, followed by 450 mg every 6 hours in 22 patients and 600 mg every 8 hours in 38 other patients) plus primaquine (30 mg base/day). Subjects had mild to moderate PCP as defined by an alveolar-arterial $Po_2$ less than 40 mm Hg. The authors reported that 92% of patients responded and that 77% were able to complete a full course of therapy, and they concluded that clindamycin plus primaquine is an effective regimen.

Toma and colleagues[226] studied 65 patients with their first episode of PCP in a prospective, randomized trial of TMP-SMX (240 mg of TMP component every 6 hours for patients weighing less than 60 kg; 320 mg every 6 hours for patients weighing more than 60 kg) versus clindamycin (450 or 600 mg every 6 hours depending on whether the patient weighed less than or more than 60 kg, respectively) plus primaquine (15 mg base/day). Of the 22 patients with confirmed PCP randomized to TMP-SMX, 1 patient (5%) died within the 2-month follow-up compared with 2 of the 27 patients (7%) who received clindamycin plus primaquine ($P$ = 1.0). Two of the patients (9%) treated with TMP-SMX required a switch because of therapeutic failure, and four patients (18%) required a switch because of drug intolerance. This was similar to patients given clindamycin plus primaquine where three patients (11%) switched because of failure and six patients (22%) switched because of intolerance ($P$ = 1.0 for both comparisons).

***Trimethoprim-Sulfamethoxazole Versus Trimethoprim Plus Dapsone Versus Clindamycin Plus Primaquine.*** Safrin and coworkers[227] of the ACTG compared these three regimens for the treatment of mild to moderate PCP. They studied 181 patients with PCP in a prospective, randomized trial of TMP-SMX (patients weighing 36–50 kg: one and a half double-strength [DS] tablets three times daily; 51–80 kg: two DS tablets three times daily; >80 kg: two and a half DS tablets three times daily) versus trimethoprim (patients weighing 36–50 kg: 200 mg three times daily; 51–80 kg: 300 mg three times daily; >80 kg: 400 mg three times daily) plus dapsone (100 mg daily) versus clindamycin (600 mg three times daily) plus primaquine (30 mg base/day). The study was limited to patients whose room air alveolar-arterial $Po_2$ was 45 mm Hg or less; those whose alveolar-arterial $Po_2$ was 35 to 45 mm Hg received adjunctive corticosteroids. Ninety percent of the subjects had no history of PCP. Of the 64 patients randomized to TMP-SMX, 4 (6%) died during the 81-day study period compared with 2 of the 59 patients (3%) randomized to trimethoprim plus dapsone and 2 of the 58 patients (3%) randomized to clindamycin plus primaquine ($P > 0.2$). In addition, the proportion of subjects who were able to complete the entire 21-day treatment course on their initial regimen was similar ($P > 0.2$). Finally, the authors found no significant differences among the three regimens in terms of the proportions of patients who required a switch in therapy owing to either therapeutic failure ($P > 0.2$) or treatment-limiting toxicity ($P > 0.2$). Although the number of patients enrolled was insufficient to conclusively demonstrate the equality of these regimens, the authors recommend that clinicians consider the differences in the expected toxicities associated with each regimen when selecting which regimen to use.

***Trimethoprim-Sulfamethoxazole Versus Atovaquone.*** Atovaquone, a 1,4-hydroxynaphthoquinone, was shown by Hughes and coworkers[228] to be at least as effective as TMP-SMX in the treatment and prevention of murine PCP. This led Hughes and colleagues[228a] to study 322 patients with PCP in a prospective, randomized

trial of TMP-SMX (two DS tablets three times daily) versus atovaquone (750 mg tablets three times daily). The study was limited to patients with mild to moderate PCP whose room air arterial $Po_2$ level was 60 mm Hg or higher and whose alveolar-arterial $Po_2$ was 45 mm Hg or less; those whose alveolar-arterial $Po_2$ was 35 to 45 mm Hg received adjunctive corticosteroids. Of the 146 evaluable patients randomized to TMP-SMX, lack of therapeutic efficacy was seen in 10 (7%) compared with 28 of the 138 evaluable patients (20%) who received atovaquone ($P = 0.002$). This clinical benefit of TMP-SMX was, however, offset by a significantly higher rate of treatment-limiting toxicity, which occurred in 33 (20%) TMP-SMX–treated patients compared with 11 (7%) atovaquone-treated ones ($P = 0.001$). The authors found that diarrhea at entry was associated with lower plasma atovaquone concentrations and that the plasma concentration was strongly associated with clinical outcome. In this study, 46 of 70 patients (66%) with a plasma steady-state concentration of less than 15 μg/mL responded to atovaquone; in the 43 patients with a concentration of 15 μg/mL or greater, 42 (98%) responded. The poor bioavailability of the atovaquone tablets led to a reformulation of atovaquone as a suspension. Although comparative studies of the suspension have not been performed, the standard dosing is 750 mg three times daily.

***Trimethoprim-Sulfamethoxazole Versus Trimetrexate.*** Trimetrexate is a potent dihydrofolate reductase inhibitor and has been shown to bind to *P. carinii* dihydrofolate reductase up to 1500-fold more avidly than does trimethoprim.[229] Leucovorin (5-formyltetrahydrofolate) must be coadministered to protect the host against the cytotoxic effects of trimetrexate (leucovorin cannot enter *P. carinii*). In the initial study of trimetrexate, Allegra and colleagues[230] studied 49 patients with PCP. Trimetrexate was used as salvage therapy for 16 patients in whom TMP-SMX and pentamidine either had failed or could not be tolerated as initial therapy in 16 patients with a history of sulfonamide intolerance and as initial therapy with sulfadiazine in 17 patients. The authors found a mortality rate of 12% to 31% in the three groups.

In a subsequent comparative study, Sattler and coworkers[231] of the ACTG studied 215 patients with PCP in a prospective, randomized trial of TMP-SMX (20 mg/kg/day of TMP component) versus trimetrexate (45 $mg/m^2$ daily, with leucovorin 20 $mg/m^2$ every 6 hours). The study enrolled patients with moderate to severe PCP as defined by an alveolar-arterial $Po_2$ greater than 30 mm Hg. This study was terminated by the Data and Safety Monitoring Board based on a survival advantage for patients randomized to TMP-SMX (log rank test, $P = .028$). By the end of the 21-day treatment period, 21 of the 103 patients (20%) randomized to TMP-SMX had required a switch in therapy owing to therapeutic failure compared with 38 of the 100 patients (38%) who received trimetrexate ($P = 0.008$). The authors concluded that trimetrexate was an inferior regimen compared with TMP-SMX but speculated that the combination of trimetrexate plus a dihydropteroate synthase inhibitor such as dapsone might have better efficacy than trimetrexate alone.

***Intravenous Versus Aerosolized Pentamidine.*** A few studies have compared two non–TMP-SMX regimens to each other. Soo Hoo and colleagues[232] studied 21 patients with PCP in a prospective, randomized trial of intravenous (4 mg/kg/day) versus inhaled (8 mg/kg/day via Respirgard II nebulizer) pentamidine. All 10 patients randomized to intravenous pentamidine responded to therapy compared with 55% of the 11 patients who received inhaled treatment ($P = 0.02$). Two of the five patients in whom inhaled pentamidine failed eventually died. A subgroup analysis of the inhaled pentamidine group revealed that nonresponders had a greater severity of illness than responders as shown by a lower mean arterial $Po_2$ and a higher alveolar-arterial $Po_2$, suggesting that aerosolized pentamidine may be an option for patients with mild PCP.

Conte and associates[233] reported on 38 patients with PCP in a prospective, randomized trial of intravenous (3 mg/kg/day) versus inhaled (600 mg/day via Respirgard II nebulizer) pentamidine. Of the 17 patients randomized to inhaled pentamidine, 2 (12%) experienced failure during initial therapy (1 died), 6 (35%) had recrudescence of symptoms within 28 days (mean 15 days after cessation of therapy), and 4 (24%) had relapse of PCP within 3 months after cessation of therapy. In comparison, 4 of the 21 (19%) patients who received intravenous pentamidine failed during initial therapy (none died), and none had either recrudescence of symptoms within 28 days ($P = 0.02$) or relapse of PCP within 3 months after cessation of therapy ($P = 0.03$). There was no significant difference in the rates of significant toxicity. The authors concluded that intravenous pentamidine (3 mg/kg/day) is superior to inhaled pentamidine.

***Intravenous Pentamidine Versus Atovaquone.*** Dohn and coworkers[234] of the Atovaquone Study Group evaluated 109 patients with PCP in a prospective, randomized trial of intravenous pentamidine (3 to 4 mg/kg/day) versus atovaquone (750 mg tablets three times daily). Patients had mild to moderate PCP as defined by an arterial $Po_2$ level of 60 mm Hg or greater and an alveolar-arterial $Po_2$ level of 45 mm Hg or less. Patients with an arterial $Po_2$ level between 60 and 70 mm Hg or an alveolar-arterial $Po_2$ level between 35 and 45 mm Hg received adjunctive corticosteroids. Of the 53 patients randomized to pentamidine, 4 (8%) died within 4 weeks after therapy and 9 (17%) died within 8 weeks compared with 7 (12.5%) deaths within 4 weeks and 9 (16%) deaths within 8 weeks among the 56 patients who received atovaquone ($P > 0.5$ for both). There were no significant differences between the two regimens in terms of therapeutic failure, but the atovaquone-treated group had significantly fewer treatment-limiting adverse effects (4%) than the pentamidine-treated group (36%) ($P < 0.001$). The authors concluded that intravenous pentamidine and oral atovaquone have similar rates for successful treatment but that atovaquone has significantly fewer treatment-limiting adverse effects.

***Corticosteroid Therapy.*** Despite the availability of effective treatment regimens, the mortality from PCP remains appreciable. Most of these deaths result from progressive lung disease culminating in intractable hypoxemic respiratory failure. By 1990, three published clinical trials and two preliminary studies supported the use of adjunctive corticosteroids to mitigate the characteristic deterioration in oxygenation seen several days into treatment.[235–237]

Montaner and colleagues[235] conducted a prospective, randomized, double-blind, placebo-controlled trial in 38 patients with a first episode of PCP. Patients had either an oxygen saturation of 85% to 90% at rest or a 5% drop in oxygen saturation during exercise. Prednisone (or placebo) was begun within 48 hours of specific PCP treatment. The study was terminated prematurely when an interim analysis revealed that an early deterioration in oxygen saturation occurred in 8 of 19 placebo-treated patients (42%) compared with 1 of 18 steroid-treated patients (6%) ($P = 0.02$). Patients treated with corticosteroids had an improvement in their median oxygen saturation on day 3 (from 90% to 94%) compared with those who received placebo in whom a worsening in oxygen saturation (from 90% to 87%) was noted ($P = 0.0003$).

Gagnon and associates[236] performed a prospective, randomized, double-blind, placebo-controlled trial in 23 patients with severe PCP as defined by a respiratory rate of more than 30 breaths/minute, a room air alveolar-arterial $P_{O_2}$ level greater than 30 mm Hg, and an arterial $P_{O_2}$ level less than 75 mm Hg on an $F_{I_{O_2}}$ of 0.35 (face mask) but greater than 60 mm Hg on an $F_{I_{O_2}}$ of 1.0. Intravenous methylprednisolone (or placebo) was begun within 72 hours of specific PCP treatment. Similar to Montaner and coworkers' study, this study was terminated prematurely when it was found that 9 of 11 placebo-treated patients (82%) died compared with 3 of 12 steroid-treated ones (25%) ($P < 0.008$). Fewer patients treated with corticosteroids experienced a 20 mm Hg or more decrease in their arterial $P_{O_2}$ at day 7 than those who received placebo ($P < 0.03$).

Bozzette and coworkers[237] of the California Collaborative Treatment Group conducted a prospective, randomized trial in 251 patients with confirmed ($n = 225$) or presumed ($n = 26$) mild, moderate, or severe PCP. Patients were randomized to standard therapy or standard therapy plus corticosteroids. Oral prednisone or intravenous methylprednisolone was begun within 36 hours of specific PCP treatment. Patients randomized to the standard therapy plus corticosteroid group compared with the standard therapy alone group had a lower cumulative risk of respiratory failure at 31 days (0.14 versus 0.30, $P = 0.004$) and of death (0.11 versus 0.23, $P = 0.009$). The patients with moderate or severe PCP had the most benefit from corticosteroids, whereas clinical benefit was not demonstrated for those with mild PCP.

Based on these studies, the National Institutes of Health–University of California Expert Panel for Corticosteroids as Adjunctive Therapy for Pneumocystis Pneumonia[238] concluded that adjunctive corticosteroid therapy "can clearly reduce the likelihood of death, respiratory failure, or deterioration of oxygenation in patients with moderate-to-severe pneumocystis pneumonia." The panel recommended that adjunctive corticosteroids be given to adults or adolescents with documented or suspected PCP if they have an arterial $P_{O_2}$ level less than 70 mm Hg or an alveolar-arterial $P_{O_2}$ difference greater than 35 mm Hg. Adjunctive corticosteroids, either oral prednisone or intravenous methylprednisolone, should be started when specific antipneumocystis treatment is begun.

Early in the AIDS epidemic, it was realized that acute respiratory failure secondary to PCP, if severe enough to warrant mechanical ventilation, had a mortality rate of 86% or greater.[24, 238] Subsequent reports from individual hospitals confirmed this gloomy prognosis; 39 of 45 patients who were intubated and ventilated for PCP at San Francisco General Hospital from 1981 to 1985 died, a mortality rate of 87%.[239] Accordingly, many institutions, including our own, actively discouraged aggressive treatment of PCP-associated acute respiratory failure. The outcome is no longer as dismal as it used to be. The reasons for the reduced mortality are not entirely clear, but early treatment with corticosteroids, recognition of the need for strict fluid management, and progress along the "learning curve" undoubtedly contribute.

**Prevention.** Patients with a history of PCP are at high risk for recurrence. As discussed, adult and adolescent patients with a $CD4^+$ lymphocyte count less than 200 cells/μL or with unexplained fevers or oropharyngeal candidiasis are also at high risk for PCP. Adult or adolescent patients meeting any of these criteria should be offered *P. carinii* prophylaxis.[28] These guidelines also recommend that infants from birth to 1 year of age who are known or suspected to be HIV infected, HIV-infected children aged 1 to 5 years with a $CD4^+$ lymphocyte count below 500 cells/μL (or $CD4^+$ percentage <15%), and HIV-infected children aged 6 to 12 years with a $CD4^+$ lymphocyte count lower than 200 cells/μL all receive *P. carinii* prophylaxis.[28]

TMP-SMX, dapsone, atovaquone suspension, and aerosolized pentamidine are the standard options for *P. carinii* prophylaxis (Table 82.4). TMP-SMX is the first-line prophylaxis choice, both primary and secondary, against *P. carinii.* For those patients intolerant of TMP-SMX, dapsone and atovaquone are both oral drugs that can be used. Many authorities would add pyrimethamine to these drugs for patients with a history of PCP and/or a $CD4^+$ lymphocyte count less than 100 cells/μL. For patients who are *T. gondii* IgG antibody positive, pyrimethamine must be added. Aerosolized pentamidine remains an effective and well-tolerated prophylaxis option. Caution must, however, be exercised when using this drug for secondary prophylaxis or for a patient with a $CD4^+$ lymphocyte count below 100 cells/μL.

Multiple studies have convincingly documented the benefit of prophylaxis over placebo in preventing PCP and extending life. Many studies have compared these regimens with placebo and with each other using different dosages and dosing intervals for primary and secondary prophylaxis. What emerges from these studies is that all of these regimens have specific advantages and disadvantages. Nevertheless, no regimen has been shown to be superior to TMP-SMX for prevention of PCP. Two large studies, one of primary prophylaxis and one of secondary, best illustrate this point.

Bozzette and coworkers[240] of the ACTG conducted a

**Table 82.4 PREVENTION OF *PNEUMOCYSTIS CARINII* PNEUMONIA**

| PREVENTION REGIMENS | ALTERNATIVE DOSING | COMMENTS |
|---|---|---|
| Trimethoprim-sulfamethoxazole 1 double strength (DS) tablet daily | 1 DS tablet thrice weekly; 1 single-strength tablet daily | Also effective prophylaxis against *Toxoplasma gondii* and many bacterial pathogens |
| Dapsone 100 mg daily | | Combine with pyrimethamine and leucovorin in persons who are *T. gondii* IgG antibody positive. Consider combining with pyrimethamine and leucovorin when used for secondary prophylaxis |
| Atovaquone suspension 1500 mg daily, divided into 1–2 doses | | Improved bioavailability compared with tablets |
| Aerosolized pentamidine 300 mg every 4 weeks via RespirGard II nebulizer | | May be associated with increased risk of extrapulmonary disease |

prospective open-label, randomized trial that compared the effectiveness of the three (at the time) approved *P. carinii* prophylaxis regimens for preventing a first episode of PCP in HIV-infected persons with a $CD4^+$ lymphocyte count less than 200 cells/μL. The study compared TMP-SMX (one DS tablet twice daily), dapsone (50 mg twice daily), and aerosolized pentamidine (300 mg every 4 weeks). Persons experiencing adverse effects underwent dose reduction (TMP-SMX and dapsone) first and then were switched to an alternative therapy in a predefined manner if intolerance persisted. During the study, there were 137 cases of PCP in the 842 patients (16%) studied for a median of 39 months. The estimated 36-month risk of PCP for TMP-SMX, dapsone, and aerosolized pentamidine ($P$ = NS) was 18%, 17%, and 21%, respectively. For patients with a $CD4^+$ lymphocyte count lower than 100 cells/μL at study entry, however, the risk was 19%, 22%, and 33%, respectively, for TMP-SMX, dapsone, and aerosolized pentamidine ($P = .04$). Furthermore, an "as-treated" (instead of "intent-to-treat") analysis revealed that only 4 of the 34 (12%) patients in the TMP-SMX arm who developed PCP did so while actually receiving the drug. In contrast, 21 of the 34 (62%) patients in the dapsone arm and 37 of the 38 (97%) patients in the aerosolized pentamidine arm who developed PCP did so "on therapy." Thus, TMP-SMX appeared to be superior for *P. carinii* prophylaxis. Unfortunately, only 21% of the TMP-SMX group and 25% of the dapsone group completed the study on their originally assigned drug compared with 88% of the aerosolized pentamidine group. Twenty-eight percent of the TMP-SMX group and 33% of the dapsone group required dose reduction only during the course of the study. This study clearly demonstrated the advantage of systemic therapy, particularly TMP-SMX, over inhalation therapy in preventing PCP. Other studies found similar benefits to those with TMP-SMX prophylaxis strategies at either attenuated doses or different dosing intervals compared with dapsone (with or without pyrimethamine) or aerosolized pentamidine. The bottom line is that TMP-SMX at any dose from 80 mg TMP (single-strength tablet) per day to 160 mg TMP (one double-strength tablet) three times weekly or per day is the first-line choice for primary *P. carinii* prophylaxis. Alternatives include other systemic therapies, usually dapsone with or without pyrimethamine, but also clindamycin plus primaquine, clindamycin plus pyrimethamine, and combinations with the extended-spectrum macrolides, clarithromycin and azithromycin. One study comparing azithromycin with rifabutin for MAC prophylaxis in patients who were virtually all on *P. carinii* prophylaxis found that azithromycin provided additional protection against PCP beyond that from standard *P. carinii* prophylaxis, especially in those patients who had never had an episode of PCP previously.[240a] More recently, atovaquone has been added to the list of available prophylaxis regimens.[241, 241a] El-Sadr and coworkers[241] of the Community Program for Clinical Research on AIDS (CPCRA) and the ACTG conducted a prospective open-label, randomized trial that compared atovaquone (1500 mg suspension daily) with dapsone (100 mg daily) for patients intolerant to TMP-SMX. These regimens were used for both primary and secondary *P. carinii* prophylaxis. During the study, there were 257 cases of PCP in the 1057 patients (24%). Of the 536 patients randomized to atovaquone, PCP developed in 122 (15.7 cases per 100 person-years) compared with 135 of the 521 patients who received dapsone (18.4 cases per 100 person-years) ($P = 0.2$). Aerosolized pentamidine should be considered for possible use by the less-immunocompromised patient but clearly lacks the efficacy of systemic therapy for persons with a $CD4^+$ lymphocyte count below 100 cells/μL.

Similar findings document the superiority of TMP-

SMX for secondary *P. carinii* prophylaxis (maintenance therapy) of AIDS patients after an initial episode of PCP. Hardy and coworkers[242] of the ACTG conducted a prospective randomized study that compared TMP-SMX (one DS tablet daily) or aerosolized pentamidine (300 mg every 4 weeks) for secondary *P. carinii* prophylaxis. All patients received zidovudine (AZT), and the median follow-up was 17.4 months. There were 14 (9%) PCP recurrences among 154 patients assigned to TMP-SMX compared with 36 (23%) recurrences among the 156 patients randomized to aerosolized pentamidine ($P < 0.001$). By an "intent-to-treat" analysis, the risk of recurrence (adjusted for initial CD4$^+$ count) was 3.25 times higher in the aerosolized pentamidine-treated group than in the TMP-SMX–treated group ($P < 0.001$). In fact, only four of the subjects who received TMP-SMX for more than 3 weeks and tolerated the drug actually developed recurrent disease. In contrast, all of the PCP recurrences in the aerosolized pentamidine-treated group occurred while the patients were taking the drug. Furthermore, the time to a first bacterial infection was significantly longer for the patients assigned to TMP-SMX ($P = 0.02$). As expected, aerosolized pentamidine was the better tolerated of the two regimens. Only 4% of the pentamidine group required crossover compared with 27% of the TMP-SMX group. These data establish the primacy of TMP-SMX for secondary *P. carinii* prophylaxis in AIDS patients. Certainly, the first choice to prevent recurrent PCP, as with primary *P. carinii* prophylaxis, should always be systemic antibiotics. Aerosolized pentamidine should be considered only for those patients intolerant of all systemic options.

## *Cryptococcus neoformans*

Cryptococcosis is a disease caused by the budding encapsulated yeast *C. neoformans.* It is the only encapsulated fungus that infects humans, and India ink or mucicarmine staining can identify its polysaccharide capsule.[36] *C. neoformans* infection occurs after inhalation of a yeast-containing aerosol. The yeast is global in distribution and is most commonly isolated from bird excrement, decaying fruit, and soil. Unlike with *H. capsulatum* and *C. immitis,* however, no clear-cut exposure–disease association exists. In addition, no human-to-human or animal-to-human transmission has been documented.[243]

Early in the AIDS epidemic, approximately 5% to 8% of HIV-infected patients developed cryptococcal disease. Cryptococcosis occurred in 7% of the first 2087 AIDS patients seen at San Francisco General Hospital.[244] Our experience and that of many other institutions, however, is that the incidence of cryptococcosis has dramatically declined since 1996.[138]

**Clinical Features.** Although the portal of entry is the lung, cryptococcal pulmonary infection is often asymptomatic or minimally symptomatic, and the most commonly encountered manifestation of cryptococcal disease is meningitis.[244–258a] In a large series of 106 HIV-infected patients with cryptococcal disease, 89 patients (84%) had meningitis, and only four patients (4%) had isolated pneumonia.[244]

***CD4$^+$ Lymphocyte Count.*** Most cases of cryptococcosis occur in patients with a CD4$^+$ lymphocyte count less than 200 cells/$\mu$L, usually below 100 cells/$\mu$L. One review of 76 patients with cryptococcal disease found a mean CD4$^+$ count of 46 cells/$\mu$L with a range of 2 cells/$\mu$L to 220 cells/$\mu$L in the 65 patients with meningitis.[258] The clinical presentation of cryptococcal disease is often subtle and nonspecific. The most common symptoms are fever, malaise, and headaches. Chuck and Sande[244] reported fever in 65%, malaise in 76%, and headache in 73% of the 89 patients with meningitis. Classic symptoms of meningitis such as nausea or vomiting (42%), altered mental status (28%), stiff neck (22%), and photophobia (18%) were present in only a minority.

Pulmonary cryptococcosis is often clinically silent. Most cases of pulmonary cryptococcal infection are discovered serendipitously on routine chest radiograph rather than as a result of specific symptoms or signs. Chuck and Sande[244] reported respiratory complaints (either cough or dyspnea) in 31% of their 89 patients with cryptococcal meningitis. When present, the most frequent respiratory complaints are cough and dyspnea. Numerous studies have focused on HIV-infected patients with cryptococcal pneumonia.[248–257] In these series, cough and dyspnea were the most common respiratory symptoms, but pleuritic chest pain and productive cough were also reported, perhaps distinguishing pulmonary cryptococcosis from PCP. Batungwanayo and associates[254] noted cough in 94%, dyspnea in 46%, and pleuritic pain in 30% of 37 HIV-infected patients with cryptococcal pneumonia.

Similar to the symptoms, the signs of cryptococcal infection are often nonspecific. Chuck and Sande[244] reported that 56% of 89 patients with meningitis were febrile on examination, 27% had nuchal rigidity, and less than 20% had altered mentation or focal neurologic deficits. Papilledema is rare in patients with normal sensorium. In patients with pneumonia, tachypnea and fine rales may be encountered.[253] Occasionally, cutaneous lesions mimicking molluscum contagiosum[259] or Kaposi's sarcoma[260] may be seen.

***Chest Radiograph.*** Cryptococcal pneumonia most commonly presents with diffuse bilateral interstitial infiltrates.[261] In a series of 37 HIV-infected patients with cryptococcal pneumonia, diffuse interstitial or interstitial-alveolar infiltrates were seen in 76%.[254] Meyohas and colleagues[255] reported the radiographic findings of cryptococcal pneumonia in 17 patients and reviewed the findings in another seven studies that included a total of 75 cases; interstitial infiltrates were seen in 60 of the 92 radiographs (65%). In addition to bilateral interstitial infiltrates, a unilateral interstitial infiltrate, focal consolidation (13%), nodular opacities (11%), cavitation (11%) (Fig. 82.5), pleural effusion (14%), and hilar adenopathy (27%) were all noted in their review. Case reports also document the occurrence of a miliary pattern,[262] solitary pulmonary nodules,[263] isolated pleural effusion,[249] and pneumothorax[264] due to *Cryptococcus.* Finally, cryptococcal pneumonia may also present with a normal radiograph. In the review by Meyohas and associates,[255] a normal chest radiograph was seen in 11% of the 92 cases.

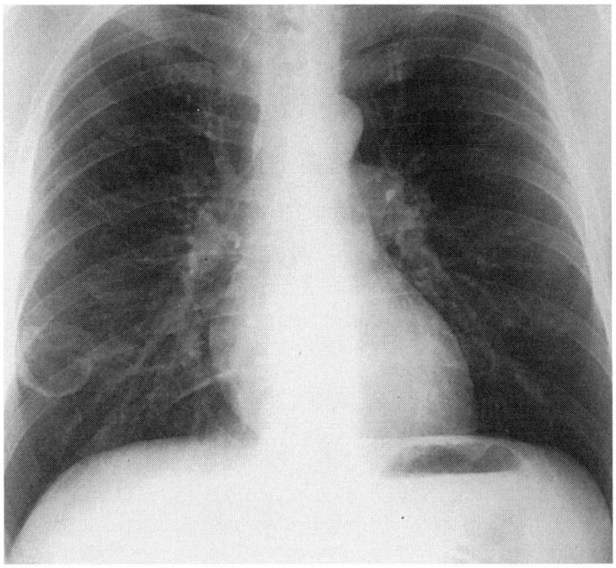

**Figure 82.5** Posteroanterior chest radiograph of HIV-seropositive patient showing a solitary cavitary lesion in the right lower lung field. Culture of bronchoalveolar lavage fluid revealed *C. neoformans*. (Reproduced with permission from Stansell JD: Fungal disease in HIV-infected persons: Cryptococcosis, histoplasmosis, and coccidioidomycosis. J Thorac Imaging 6:28–35, 1991.)

**Diagnosis.** The diagnosis of cryptococcal infection begins with the cryptococcal antigen (CRAG) test. The test can be performed on serum, cerebrospinal fluid, urine, BAL fluid,[265] or pleural fluid. The serum CRAG is sensitive and specific for cryptococcemia. A negative serum CRAG virtually rules out the diagnosis of cryptococcal meningitis but can be seen in cases of isolated pulmonary cryptococcosis. A positive serum CRAG should prompt an evaluation for disseminated disease, especially meningitis, but can be seen in the presence of rheumatoid factor or infection with *Trichosporon beigelii.* Blood fungal cultures are specific and should be obtained as part of the diagnostic evaluation. New cutaneous lesions may be signs of dissemination, and their sudden appearance should prompt consideration for biopsy.

The diagnosis of pulmonary cryptococcosis is usually established by culture of sputum or BAL fluid and occasionally from pleural fluid. Biopsy specimens from transbronchial biopsy and pleural biopsy can also be diagnostic.[248–251, 253–257, 266] Batungwanayo and coworkers[254] found that BAL diagnosed 27 of 33 cases (sensitivity was 82%) of cryptococcal pneumonia compared with transbronchial biopsy, which diagnosed 10 of 21 cases (sensitivity was 48%). In some cases cultures are negative, but BAL or pleural fluid CRAG can establish the diagnosis.[255] Alternatively, because the treatment is identical, the diagnosis of pneumonia may be inferred in the presence of disseminated cryptococcal disease (e.g., meningitis) and a compatible clinical and radiographic presentation. Caution must, however, be exercised with this approach because other opportunistic infections such as PCP may be present concurrently and can demonstrate identical radiographic findings.

**Treatment.** In contrast to cryptococcal meningitis, no treatment guidelines exist for HIV-infected patients presenting with isolated cryptococcal pneumonia or with concurrent cryptococcal pneumonia and meningitis. Some authorities would treat isolated cryptococcal pneumonia that is mild in severity with fluconazole alone (400 mg daily). Patients with clinically significant cryptococcal pneumonia should, however, be considered at high risk for early deterioration and should be offered the best available therapy (Table 82.5). Amphotericin B plus 5-fluorocytosine is the treatment of choice for HIV-infected patients with cryptococcal meningitis. In patients with isolated moderate to severe pneumonia or those with concurrent meningitis, this regimen should be used. Treatment should be continued until the patient is clinically improved, at which point the patient can be switched to fluconazole to complete a 10- to 12-week course. The patient should then be maintained on fluconazole for life. Twice to thrice weekly amphotericin B is another alternative.

**Prevention.** Fluconazole is effective primary prophylaxis against cryptococcosis.[267] Long-term fluconazole administration, however, raises a number of concerns, including the development of drug-resistant fungi. This, combined with clinical studies that failed to show a survival benefit resulting from a reduction in cryptococcal disease,[268] lessens the utility of fluconazole as primary prophylaxis. In fact, the 1999 USPHS/IDSA guidelines do not recommend fluconazole for primary *C. neoformans* prophylaxis.[28]

### *Histoplasma capsulatum*

Histoplasmosis is a disease caused by the dimorphic, soil-dwelling fungus *H. capsulatum.* The fungus is found on all continents except Antarctica, but it is most endemic to North America and the Caribbean basin.[243] The heaviest concentration is found in the Mississippi, Ohio, and St. Lawrence River valleys. In these areas, the fungus exists in microfoci related to the enrichment of the soil with bird or bat excrement. In soil, the fungus exists in a mycelial form with characteristic tuberculate macroconidia.[36] The hyphae also have microconidia that are easily aerosolized when disturbed. Inhalation of these microconidia leads to primary pulmonary infection that is usually clinically silent.

Once deposited in the distal airways and alveoli, *H. capsulatum* transforms into its yeast (or parasitic) form, and an area of pneumonitis develops. During this period before cell-mediated immunity develops, the organism spreads to regional lymph nodes and to the reticuloendothelial organs. Two to 3 weeks after exposure, about 40% of immunocompetent individuals develop a flu-like syndrome with fever, chills, myalgias, a nonproductive cough, and chest pain. Ninety-nine per cent of these cases spontaneously resolve with the development of specific cell-mediated immunity. In contrast, progressive disseminated histoplasmosis develops in HIV-infected persons lacking cell-mediated immunity. Although most cases of HIV-associated histoplasmosis appear to result from de novo exposure, reactivation disease does occur. These

**Table 82.5 TREATMENT OF FUNGAL DISEASE**

| Fungus | Moderate to Severe Disease | Mild Disease | Maintenance/ Suppression |
|---|---|---|---|
| *Cryptococcus neoformans* | Amphotericin B (0.7–0.8 mg/kg daily) plus 5-fluorocytosine (100 mg/kg/day, four divided doses) until clinical improvement (minimum 2 weeks), followed by fluconazole (400 mg daily) for total 10–12 weeks | Fluconazole (800–1200 mg daily) plus 5-fluorocytosine (100 mg/kg/day, four divided doses) for 4 weeks, followed by fluconazole (400 mg daily) for total 10–12 weeks | Fluconazole (200 mg daily). Amphotericin B (0.7–0.8 mg/kg twice to thrice weekly) |
| *Histoplasma capsulatum* | Amphotericin B (0.8–1.0 mg/kg/day) until clinical improvement (total induction dose 1.0–1.5 g) | Itraconazole (300 mg twice daily × 3 days, then 200 mg twice daily) | Itraconazole (200 mg twice daily).* Amphotericin B (0.8–1.0 mg/kg twice to thrice weekly) |
| *Coccidioides immitis* | Amphotericin B (1.0–1.2 mg/kg/day) until clinical improvement (total induction dose 1.0–2.5 g) | Fluconazole (400–1200 mg daily) | Fluconazole (400 mg daily). Amphotericin B (1.0–1.2 mg/kg twice to thrice weekly) |
| *Aspergillus* species (usually *A. fumigatus*) | Amphotericin B (0.8–1.0 mg/kg/day) until clinical improvement | Itraconazole (300 mg twice daily × 3 days, then 200 mg twice daily) | Itraconazole (200 mg twice daily).* Amphotericin B (0.8–1.0 mg/kg twice to thrice weekly) |
| *Blastomyces dermatitidis* | Amphotericin B (0.8–1.0 mg/kg/day) until clinical improvement | Itraconazole (300 mg twice daily × 3 days, then 200 mg twice daily) | Itraconazole (200 mg twice daily)* |
| *Penicillium marneffei* | Amphotericin B (0.6 mg/kg/day for 2 weeks), followed by itraconazole (200 mg twice daily) for additional 10 weeks | Itraconazole (300 mg twice daily × 3 days, then 200 mg twice daily) | Itraconazole (200 mg daily) |

*Dose modification may be necessary to maintain adequate itraconazole serum levels above 2 mg/L.

cases account for the histoplasmosis seen in nonendemic areas such as San Francisco or New York.[269]

**Clinical Features.** Although the portal of entry is the lung, disseminated histoplasmosis most often presents as a febrile wasting illness in HIV-infected persons.[270–277] In a large series of 72 HIV-infected patients with disseminated histoplasmosis, 69 patients (96%) presented with fever and weight loss.[274]

***CD4⁺ Lymphocyte Count.*** Most cases of disseminated histoplasmosis occur in patients with a $CD4^+$ lymphocyte count less than 100 cells/μL and often below 50 cells/μL. The clinical presentation of histoplasmosis is frequently subtle and nonspecific. The most common symptoms are fever and weight loss. Occasionally, the presentation is dramatic with a sepsis-like syndrome associated with hypotension, respiratory failure, liver and renal failure, and coagulopathy. Wheat and colleagues[274] reported a sepsis-like syndrome in 12.5% of 72 patients with disseminated histoplasmosis and noted its presence in 10% of 51 other cases reviewed.

The most frequent respiratory complaints are cough and dyspnea. These symptoms are usually found in patients with chest radiograph abnormalities and are often absent in patients with normal radiographs. A review of 51 cases of HIV-associated progressive disseminated histoplasmosis found that 16% presented with respiratory complaints. Subsequent series of 72 cases and 64 cases found that 53% and 38%, respectively, had respiratory complaints at presentation.[274, 275]

Similar to symptoms, the signs of histoplasmosis are

often nonspecific and most often reveal fever and wasting. Examination of the chest may reveal crackles. Hepatomegaly (26% to 29%), splenomegaly (12% to 35%), lymphadenopathy (17% to 37%), central nervous system findings (14% to 18%), and cutaneous lesions (1% to 18%) may also be seen.[274] As described, a sepsis-like syndrome is present in 10% to 12.5% of cases and portends a poor outcome.[274]

***Chest Radiograph.*** Disseminated histoplasmosis will present with a normal chest radiograph in a significant proportion of cases.[261, 274, 275, 278] Wheat and coworkers[274] reported normal radiographs in 43% of their 72 HIV-infected patients and in 36% of the patients in the literature reviewed. In a series of 50 HIV-infected patients with disseminated histoplasmosis, Conces and colleagues[278] found that 54% had a normal radiograph. The most common radiographic findings are diffuse, often coarse reticular or reticulonodular (Fig. 82.6), occasionally alveolar infiltrates.[261] Wheat and associates[274] found diffuse infiltrates in 44% of their 72 patients, whereas Conces and colleagues[278] found diffuse nodular opacities or diffuse linear opacities in 13 of 50 patients (26% overall but 57% of the patients with an abnormal radiograph). Focal opacities are less common but are found in 7% to 11% of cases.[274] Hilar and mediastinal adenopathy and calcified granulomata are found in less than 5% of patients, attesting to the low incidence of reactivation disease.[274]

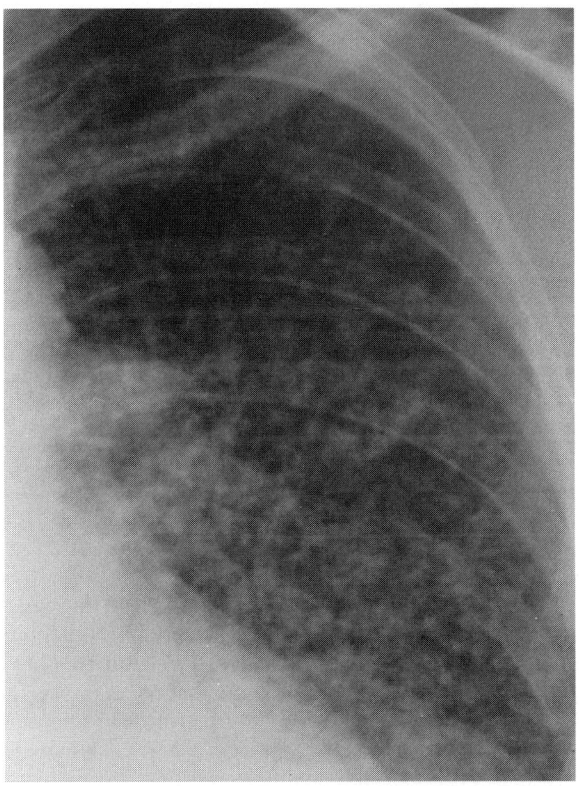

**Figure 82.6** Posteroanterior chest radiograph close-up of the left mid-lung of HIV-seropositive patient showing a medium to coarse reticulonodular pattern characteristic of disseminated fungal disease. (Reprinted with permission from Stansell JD: Fungal disease in HIV-infected persons: Cryptococcosis, histoplasmosis, and coccidioidomycosis. J Thorac Imaging 6:28–35, 1991.)

**Diagnosis.** The diagnosis of histoplasma infection begins with the histoplasma polysaccharide antigen (HPA) test. The test can be performed on urine, serum, cerebrospinal fluid, or BAL fluid. Although the urine HPA is sensitive in disseminated histoplasmosis, it is often negative in isolated pulmonary disease. With successful therapy HPA values fall, and during relapses HPA values rise (usually by ≥2 HPA units), which are useful features for assessing response to therapy and for evaluating possible relapse.[279] A false-positive HPA can occur in patients with other disseminated fungal diseases (blastomycosis, paracoccidioidomycosis, and penicilliosis).[36] Definitive diagnosis requires isolation and identification of the fungus by culture. Blood fungal cultures are specific and should be obtained as part of the diagnostic evaluation. Wheat and coworkers[274] reported that fungal blood cultures were positive in 65 of their 72 cases (90%). Occasionally, the peripheral blood smear reveals intracellular yeast. Other potential diagnostic sources include bone marrow, lymph node, and skin.

The diagnosis of pulmonary histoplasmosis can be established by direct examination and culture of sputum, BAL fluid,[280] or transbronchial biopsy.

**Treatment.** Amphotericin B is the treatment of choice for HIV-infected patients with moderate to severe disease, whereas itraconazole is an alternative for patients with mild disease (Table 82.5). Treatment with amphotericin B should be continued to a cumulative induction dose of 1.0 to 1.5 g. Patients who have responded can be switched to itraconazole. The patient should then be maintained on lifelong suppressive therapy with itraconazole, which is superior to fluconazole.[281] Twice to thrice weekly amphotericin B is another alternative.

**Prevention.** In those areas endemic for *H. capsulatum,* patients should avoid activities that will potentially increase their exposure, such as cleaning chicken coops, disturbing native soil beneath bird-roosting sites, and exploring caves. Primary prophylaxis for persons living in or traveling to an endemic area is not generally recommended.[28]

### *Coccidioides immitis*

Coccidioidomycosis is a disease caused by the dimorphic, soil-dwelling fungus *C. immitis. C. immitis* causes an uncommon, but devastating, disseminated disease that is often fatal in HIV-infected persons. The fungus is endemic to the semiarid regions of North America, notably the southwestern United States and northern Mexico.[243, 281a] It is also found in South America, especially central Argentina. In soil, the fungus exists in a mycelial form with characteristic arthrospores.[36] These arthrospores are easily aerosolized when disrupted. After inhalation and deposition in the distal airways and alveoli, the arthrospores transform into spherules that may develop several hundred endospores. Rupture of the spherules allows widespread dissemination of the endospores, which then form additional spherules, replicating the cycle. Although most cases of HIV-associated coccidioidomycosis appear to result from de novo exposure, reactivation disease does occur.

**Clinical Features.** Although the portal of entry is the lung, coccidioidomycosis often presents with disseminated disease and meningitis.[282–287]

***CD4⁺ Lymphocyte Count.*** Most cases of disseminated coccidioidomycosis occur in patients with a $CD4^+$ lymphocyte count below 100 cells/μL and often less than 50 cells/μL. One review of 91 patients with coccidioidal disease found a mean $CD4^+$ count of 55 cells/μL among patients with diffuse pulmonary disease.[287] The clinical presentation is often nonspecific. Fever, chills, night sweats, and weight loss are common. Singh and colleagues[287] reported fever and chills in 68%, weight loss in 50%, and night sweats in 36% of the 91 patients with coccidioidomycosis. The most frequent respiratory complaint in these patients was cough, which was noted in 64%; dyspnea was less common, only 10%.

Similar to symptoms, the signs of coccidioidomycosis are often nonspecific. Fever and wasting are often present. Examination of the chest may reveal crackles. Lymphadenopathy (24%) and splenomegaly (<10%) may also be seen.[287]

***Chest Radiograph.*** Coccidioidal pneumonia most commonly presents with diffuse reticulonodular infiltrates.[261] In a series of 91 HIV-infected patients with coccidioidomycosis, diffuse reticulonodular infiltrates were seen in 65%.[287] Focal opacities were less common but occurred in 14% of cases and consisted of focal infiltrates, single or multiple nodules, and cavities.[287] Pleural effusion and hilar adenopathy were also reported. Coccidioidomycosis also presents with a normal chest radiograph.

**Diagnosis.** Unlike cryptococcosis and histoplasmosis, there is no specific antigen test available for diagnosing coccidioidomycosis. Thus, definitive diagnosis requires isolation and identification of the fungus by culture or identification of pathognomonic giant spherules in cytologic or histologic preparations. Although skin testing with coccidioidin or spherulin has little diagnostic value, serologic tests can be extremely useful in the evaluation of suspected coccidioidomycosis. Several studies have found an 80% to 90% sensitivity of complement fixation and tube precipitin tests.[283, 284, 287] False-negative titers most often occurred in the most severely immunocompromised patients with diffuse pulmonary disease. In those with positive tests, the titer appeared to reflect the disease activity and was useful for monitoring response to therapy.[284]

Direct examination and culture of sputum, BAL fluid, or transbronchial biopsy can establish the diagnosis of pulmonary coccidioidomycosis. Singh and coworkers[287] found that sputum culture (13 of 19, 68%) and cytology (8 of 11, 73%) were often diagnostic. BAL fluid culture diagnosed 29 of 42 cases (69%), and BAL fluid cytology diagnosed 32 of 48 cases (67%); in addition, transbronchial biopsy culture diagnosed 8 of 10 cases (80%), and biopsy histology diagnosed all 14 cases (100%).

**Treatment.** Amphotericin B is the treatment of choice for HIV-infected patients with disseminated coccidioidomycosis (see Table 82.5). Treatment with amphotericin B should be continued to a cumulative induction dose of 1.0 to 2.5 g.[288] Patients who have responded can be switched to fluconazole. The patient should then be maintained on lifelong suppressive therapy with fluconazole. Twice to thrice weekly amphotericin B is another alternative. The prognosis for pulmonary disease is related to its severity. Fish and associates[283] found that the 31 patients with diffuse pulmonary disease had a significantly higher mortality rate than the 20 with focal disease in one series. Singh and colleagues[287] reported similar results.

**Prevention.** In those areas endemic for *C. immitis,* patients should avoid activities that will potentially increase their exposure, such as visits to construction projects or sites where the soil is disturbed. Primary prophylaxis for persons living in or traveling to an endemic area is generally not recommended.[28]

### *Aspergillus* species

*Aspergillus* species are found worldwide, and exposure is universal. Disease, however, is infrequent unless phagocyte number or function is reduced. Although invasive aspergillosis is a well-documented complication of various immunosuppressive disorders, particularly in patients with hematologic malignancy or organ transplantation, it is an uncommon problem in patients with HIV disease. In 13 patients reported by Denning and coworkers,[289] pulmonary aspergillosis followed the diagnosis of AIDS by a median of 25 months; in these patients, risk factors for the development of aspergillosis besides HIV-induced immunosuppression included use of corticosteroids, neutropenia, marijuana, and broad-spectrum antimicrobial drugs.

**Clinical Features.** The entire spectrum of *Aspergillus*-related lung disease has been observed in HIV-infected persons, from colonization of the respiratory tract[290] or a pre-existing cavity[291, 292] to tracheobronchitis or obstructing bronchial aspergillosis,[293] to invasive aspergillosis.[289, 290, 294–299] We have also seen a case of allergic bronchopulmonary aspergillosis in an HIV-infected asthmatic patient, a case of an *Aspergillus* empyema, and an *Aspergillus* lung mass. We concentrate here on the most severe manifestation of *Aspergillus* pulmonary disease, invasive aspergillosis. Although most patients with invasive aspergillosis have a $CD4^+$ lymphocyte count lower than 50 cells/μL, the classic risk factors for the disease relate more to phagocyte number and function (as determined by neutropenia and use of corticosteroids or broad-spectrum antibiotics) than to absolute $CD4^+$ counts. Patients with aspergillosis present with fever, cough, dyspnea, and occasionally pleuritic chest pain. The chest radiographic abnormalities are variable and include unilateral or bilateral infiltrates, cavitary lesions, nodular and pleural-based densities, and pleural effusions.[300]

**Diagnosis.** The definitive diagnosis of aspergillosis requires both demonstration of tissue invasion and isolation of the organism by culture. Neither sputum nor BAL is sufficient. Microscopy alone cannot distinguish *Aspergillus* species from *Fusarium* or *Pseudallescheria* species. The results of transbronchial biopsy are usually negative, but specimens from sputum, BAL, or percutaneous aspirates are often positive on culture. The absence of histologic proof of tissue invasion is always somewhat disquieting, especially in attempting to distinguish invasive disease from possible colonization of damaged airways. Repeated isolation of the fungus in large numbers with a compatible clinical setting makes the diagnosis more tenable.

**Treatment.** Compared with the fungi previously discussed, there is relatively little experience treating HIV-infected patients with aspergillosis.[289, 290, 297, 299, 301, 302] Usually, amphotericin B or intraconazole has been administered with variable results (see Table 82.5). We have also used liposomal amphotericin B for a few patients with similar outcomes. Even with the prompt institution of therapy, the prognosis is poor, undoubtedly in large part because aspergillosis, when it occurs, is nearly always a late complication of advanced HIV disease.

**Prevention.** Given the ubiquitous nature of *Aspergillus* species, it is impossible to prevent exposure to the organism. Patients with advanced HIV disease should, however, avoid activities that will potentially increase their exposure, including being near decaying vegetation (e.g., composting) and soil.

### *Blastomyces dermatitidis*

Blastomycosis is a disease caused by the endemic, dimorphic fungus *B. dermatitidis.* Blastomycosis is coendemic with histoplasmosis throughout much of the central United States. It is much less common than histoplasmosis, however, and reports of HIV-associated blastomycosis are uncommon.[36, 303]

**Clinical Features.** The largest case series reported 15 cases of HIV-associated blastomycosis.[303] All but one had a $CD4^+$ lymphocyte count less than 200 cells/μL. The authors noted two distinct patterns of disease. Although 12 of 15 patients (80%) had evidence of pulmonary involvement, one group of patients had disease clinically limited to the respiratory system. The other group had disseminated blastomycosis, commonly involving multiple organ systems, including the lungs. Eleven of 15 (73%) had abnormal chest radiographs, with diffuse interstitial or miliary disease (55%) being the most common radiographic finding.

**Treatment.** Amphotericin B is the treatment of choice for HIV-infected patients with severe disease (see Table 82.5).[303] Treatment with amphotericin B should be continued to a cumulative induction dose of 1 g. Patients who have improved can then be switched to itraconazole maintenance therapy for life, whereas those without improvement should continue taking amphotericin B. With prompt institution of therapy, most patients with disease limited to the lungs responded well; in contrast, patients with disseminated disease did poorly (40% mortality in 30 days).[303]

### *Penicillium marneffei*

Penicilliosis is a disease caused by *P. marneffei,* a dimorphic, soil-dwelling fungus. With expansion of the HIV epidemic into southeastern Asia has come a dramatic increase in cases of penicilliosis.[304–311] *P. marneffei* is endemic in southeastern Asian countries,[309] and, in Northern Thailand, it is the third most common opportunistic infection (after tuberculosis and cryptococcosis) in HIV-infected patients with AIDS, accounting for 15% to 20% of all AIDS-related illnesses. Disease is related to soil exposure, especially during the rainy season (May to October), but not to consumption of bamboo rats, the only known nonhuman hosts of *P. marneffei.*[312, 313] Infection is probably acquired via inhalation.

**Clinical Features.** The clinical presentation is often mistaken for tuberculosis, cryptococcosis, or histoplasmosis. The most common symptoms include fever, weight loss, cough, and generalized papular skin lesions, usually with central umbilication. Anemia is a prominent laboratory finding. In one series of 92 patients with *P. marneffei,* fever was present in 92%, weight loss in 76%, and skin lesions in 71%.[306]

**Diagnosis.** *P. marneffei* is most commonly a disseminated disease in HIV-infected patients, and the diagnosis is usually made by blood fungal cultures. Other sites of diagnosis include the skin, bone marrow, and respiratory specimens. In contrast to other *Penicillium* species that cause disease in humans, *P. marneffei* converts to a yeast form in its host, and yeast-laden macrophages can often be seen in peripheral blood, bone marrow aspirates, and touch preparations from tissue biopsies.

**Treatment.** Amphotericin B, followed by itraconazole, is the standard treatment for *P. marneffei* infection (see Tabel 82.5).[314] The duration of amphotericin B treatment is 2 weeks, followed by an additional 10 weeks of itraconazole. This regimen is reported to have a greater than 97% response rate for disseminated *P. marneffei* infection.[314] Without secondary prophylaxis, however, most patients will suffer a relapse within 6 to 12 months.

**Prevention.** The result of a recent prospective double-blind, placebo-controlled trial determined that itraconazole (200 mg daily) is an effective secondary prophylaxis against *P. marneffei.*[315] In this study, none of the 36 patients randomized to itraconazole had a relapse of *P. marneffei* within 1 year compared with 20 of the 35 patients (57%) assigned to placebo. Given the strong association with soil exposure, especially during the rainy season, HIV-infected patients living in or traveling to endemic areas should avoid activities that will potentially increase their exposure. Although formal recommendations are lacking, similar to the other endemic fungi, primary prophylaxis for persons living in or traveling to an endemic area is probably not indicated.

### *Candida* species

Despite the high frequency of mucocutaneous candidiasis in HIV-infected patients, pulmonary candidiasis is distinctly uncommon and is rarely diagnosed during life.[316] Because of the small number of documented cases of pulmonary candidiasis, neither the clinical features nor the treatment is well established. It is clear, however, that tissue invasion must be demonstrated by biopsy for a convincing diagnosis; the mere identification of the fungus in respiratory secretions by culture alone is insufficient.

## Viruses

Many viruses are known to cause pulmonary disease in immunosuppressed persons, including members of the herpesvirus family (cytomegalovirus [CMV], herpes simplex virus, varicella-zoster virus, and Epstein-Barr virus), influenza virus, parainfluenza virus, respiratory syncytial virus, measles virus, adenovirus, and rhinovirus.[317] All of these viruses have been identified in HIV-infected patients; however, only CMV is regarded as an important agent of pulmonary disease. Although clearly the source of significant pathologic conditions in the retina, gastrointestinal tract, and nervous system, the role of CMV in producing pulmonary disease in HIV-infected persons is open to question.[318] Many consider this ubiquitous virus a "passenger" rather than a pathogen in most instances. However, there are also instances where documented pulmonary disease results from CMV.[319–321]

### Cytomegalovirus

CMV is a beta-herpesvirus. The risk of exposure to CMV increases with age, and evidence of CMV infection is extremely common in healthy persons. The results of serologic studies indicate that more than 50% to 70% of all adults and virtually 100% of male homosexuals are infected with the virus.[322] CMV is excreted in saliva, respiratory secretions, urine, and semen. In HIV-infected patients, CMV disease is believed to result chiefly from reactivation of latent infection. Disease has, however, been documented from de novo infection in recipients of solid organs, bone marrow, and blood, which raises the possibility that new infection or superinfection from exogenous sources may also occur in HIV-infected persons.

**Clinical Features.** Retinitis and gastrointestinal disease are the most common forms of HIV-associated CMV disease.[323] CMV is a frequent isolate from the BAL fluid of patients with advanced immunosuppression who undergo evaluation for opportunistic infections, notably *P. carinii.* Because CMV may be shed in respiratory secretions, its mere presence in BAL fluid cannot be construed as diagnostic of CMV pulmonary disease. When dual pulmonary infection is discovered, treatment directed against the coexisting disease and not against CMV usually results in clinical resolution.[324, 325] There are, however, clearly instances when CMV causes pulmonary disease, and the challenge clinicians face is to recognize when these occur.

***$CD4^+$ Lymphocyte Count.*** Most cases of CMV disease occur in patients with a $CD4^+$ lymphocyte count less than 50 cells/μL. In one study of 18 patients with biopsy-proven CMV pneumonia, the median $CD4^+$ count was 4 cells/μL.[321]

The most common symptoms of CMV pneumonia are cough, dyspnea, and fever. In the study by Salomon and colleagues,[321] these were seen in 94%, 94%, and 89%, respectively, of the 18 patients reported. Respiratory symptoms were present for up to 2 weeks in 50% and up to 4 weeks in 94%. Physical examination of the chest may be normal or may reveal crackles or evidence of pleural effusion. The serum LDH has been reported to be elevated in CMV pneumonia.[321]

***Chest Radiograph.*** The chest radiograph findings of CMV pneumonia vary and include reticular or ground-glass opacities, alveolar infiltrates, and nodules or nodular opacities.[321] Pleural effusions may be seen as well.

**Diagnosis.** When suspected CMV pulmonary disease occurs in conjunction with other end-organ disease (e.g., retinitis), CMV therapy must be initiated. Treatment of one end-organ CMV disease in fact treats all, although the length of therapy can differ by organ system. The therapeutic dilemma is much greater when only the lungs appear to be afflicted. Patients suspected of having CMV pneumonitis should undergo careful retinal examination, even if there are no ocular complaints. CMV is usually a disseminated disease and commonly involves multiple organ systems in a single host. The only precise criterion for diagnosis of CMV pulmonary disease is the demonstration of widespread specific cytopathic changes in the lungs. Neither culture of BAL fluid[326, 327] nor cytopathic inclusions on transbronchial biopsy specimens are sufficient to make the diagnosis of CMV pneumonitis.

**Treatment.** Ganciclovir (dihydropropylguanosine), foscarnet (trisodium phosphonoformate, Foscavir), and cidofovir are the principal treatment options for CMV disease. With these drugs, an initial course of induction therapy is used. Unlike retinal and gastrointestinal disease, however, the length of induction therapy for CMV pneumonia is undetermined. Certainly, induction therapy should be continued until clinical improvement occurs as with gastrointestinal disease. Ganciclovir is administered intravenously at 5 mg/kg twice a day for induction therapy followed by 5 mg/kg once a day for maintenance therapy. The usefulness of maintenance therapy in preventing relapse of CMV pneumonitis is unclear. The principal toxicity of ganciclovir is myelosuppression (neutropenia in 20% to 40% and thrombocytopenia in 5%). Patients receiving ganciclovir must have their complete blood counts monitored closely. For patients who develop significant neutropenia, the addition of granulocyte colony-stimulating factor may permit continuation of ganciclovir. Those with persistent neutropenia despite granulocyte colony-stimulating factor should be switched to an alternate therapy such as foscarnet.

Foscarnet must also be administered intravenously at 90 mg/kg twice a day for induction therapy and 90 to 120 mg/kg once a day for maintenance therapy. Because it can bind with calcium and lower ionized calcium levels, foscarnet is usually administered by infusion pump over at least 1 hour. Too rapid an infusion may cause seizures and death. The principal toxicity of foscarnet is nephrotoxicity and electrolyte disturbance. Patients receiving foscarnet must have their renal function and electrolytes monitored closely.

Cidofovir is another alternative. One benefit of cidofovir is that it does not require phosphorylation by virus-induced enzyme and is therefore active against most ganciclovir-resistant viruses that have resistance mutations in the phosphorylating gene. Cidofovir has an extremely long half-life. The principal toxicity of cidofovir is nephrotoxicity that can be diminished by aggressive prehydration and concurrent probenecid therapy. Patients receiving cidofovir must have their renal function monitored closely.

**Prevention.** Oral ganciclovir is licensed for the prevention of CMV disease in HIV-infected patients. This regimen is, however, associated with a high pill burden, high cost, and significant toxicities. In addition, the specter of the development of ganciclovir resistance has combined to limit the general use of this prophylaxis regimen.[28] HIV-infected patients who are CMV IgG negative should be given CMV-negative blood in the event that a transfusion is necessary.

### Other Viruses

Symptomatic pulmonary viral infection other than CMV is uncommon.[328] Herpes simplex virus, while frequently cultured from BAL fluid, is usually a contaminant from upper airway carriage. Lower respiratory tract involvement is rare in HIV-infected persons (0.2% to 4% of autopsy cases) and appears to be more frequent in other immunosuppressed hosts. Herpes simplex virus pulmonary disease causes a focal pneumonia or a diffuse interstitial pneumonitis.[329] The focal pneumonias appear to result from contiguous spread of herpes simplex virus to lung parenchyma and are often associated with necrotizing tracheobronchitis, whereas the diffuse interstitial pneumonias appear to be a manifestation of hematogenous herpes simplex virus dissemination.

Varicella-zoster virus is a rare cause of pneumonia in HIV-infected adult patients.[330] Epstein-Barr virus DNA has been identified in lung biopsy specimens of infants and children with lymphocytic interstitial pneumonitis, but the precise role of the virus in this disease is uncertain.[331] Influenza has been isolated from HIV-infected patients.[332] In this small series,[332] neither the clinical presentation of influenza nor the rate of secondary complications appeared to be different from that in healthy persons. Nevertheless, it is generally recommended that all HIV-infected persons be vaccinated annually.[28] A randomized, double-blind, placebo-controlled study of 102 HIV-infected persons found that influenza vaccine resulted in significant decreases in laboratory-confirmed influenza and respiratory symptoms and no substantial changes in $CD4^+$ lymphocyte count or HIV RNA.[332a] However, some HIV-infected patients, those with $CD4^+$ lymphocyte counts below 100 cells/μL and/or HIV RNA levels above 100,000 copies/mL, are unable to mount a protective antibody response.[332b] HIV itself is present in the lungs of HIV-infected patients during all stages of disease.[333–335] Its pathogenic role in HIV-associated pulmonary disease is, however, presently unclear.

## Parasites

Several unicellular and multicellular parasites cause pulmonary disease in HIV-infected hosts. Of these, *T. gondii* is the most frequent.

### *Toxoplasma gondii*

*T. gondii* is an intracellular protozoan. Toxoplasmosis is a zoonosis with domestic cats as its definitive host but an infectious reservoir that encompasses all animals. Transmission to humans occurs when raw or undercooked meat that contains *T. gondii* is eaten. Domestic cat feces in litter boxes are an additional source of potential infection. Vertical transmission can occur from mother to fetus. In HIV-infected patients, the overwhelming majority of cases of toxoplasmosis result from reactivation of chronic, latent infection. Thus, the keys to preventing toxoplasmosis are prevention of exposure for those not yet infected and prophylaxis for those already seropositive. The seroprevalence of *Toxoplasma* antibodies varies. In the United States, the seroprevalence is 10% to 50%, whereas in Western Europe, the seroprevalence may be as high as 90%.

**Clinical Features.** *T. gondii* encephalitis is a well-recognized complication of advanced HIV disease and is an AIDS-defining condition. Although toxoplasmosis is the most common cause of focal brain abscesses in patients with AIDS, pulmonary involvement is uncommon. Pulmonary disease may occur in patients with central nervous system or disseminated disease or with isolated pulmonary involvement.[336–339]

***$CD4^+$ Lymphocyte Count.*** Toxoplasmosis presents at the lower range of $CD4^+$ lymphocyte counts. In a large study of 64 patients with pulmonary toxoplasmosis conducted in France, the mean (± SD) $CD4^+$ count was 40 (± 75) cells/μL.[339] Pulmonary toxoplasmosis characteristically presents with cough, usually nonproductive, dyspnea, and fever. Physical examination of the chest may be normal or may reveal crackles. Focal neurologic findings are common. Hepatosplenomegaly can be seen.

***Chest Radiograph.*** The chest radiograph usually reveals bilateral infiltrates, either fine reticulonodular infiltrates indistinguishable from PCP or a coarser nodular pattern similar to that seen with tuberculosis or fungal pneumonias.[340] Pleural effusions can be seen, and a variety of other radiographic findings have also been described.[338]

**Diagnosis.** The diagnosis of pulmonary toxoplasmosis is usually established by bronchoscopy with BAL. In one review, BAL was diagnostic in 16 of 17 immunocompromised patients with pulmonary disease.[338]

**Treatment.** The treatment for pulmonary toxoplasmosis is identical to that for central nervous system toxoplasmosis. Traditionally, treatment is with either pyrimethamine and sulfadiazine or pyrimethamine and clindamycin. Leucovorin (folinic acid) should be co-administered. A recent pilot study of 77 patients with central nervous system toxoplasmosis compared TMP-SMX with pyrimethamine and sulfadiazine and found no significant difference in efficacy.[341] In addition, atovaquone has been used with reasonable success as salvage therapy for patients failing or intolerant to the standard treatment options.[342]

**Prevention.** Approximately 30% to 40% of HIV-infected patients who are *Toxoplasma* antibody positive will develop toxoplasmosis if they are not treated prophylactically. Accordingly, these persons should receive primary prophylaxis once their $CD4^+$ lymphocyte count falls below 100 cells/μL.[28] As a practical matter, this is often accomplished when the $CD4^+$ count reaches 200 cells/μL or less because the prophylaxis of choice (TMP-SMX) is also the prophylaxis of choice for *P. carinii.* For patients intolerant of TMP-SMX, dapsone plus pyrimethamine (and leucovorin) can be used. Because relapses are common, patients who recover from toxoplasmosis should receive secondary prophylaxis with either pyrimethamine, sulfadiazine, and leucovorin or pyrimethamine, clindamycin, and leucovorin.[28] Atovaquone (with or without pyrimethamine) is another option.

HIV-infected patients who have cats should either have someone else change the litter box or, if unable to find someone, clean the litter box daily and wash their hands thoroughly afterward.[28] In addition, cats should be kept indoors, should not be allowed to hunt, and should not be fed raw or undercooked meat. Patients themselves should similarly avoid eating raw or undercooked meat.

### Other Parasites

Several cases of both pulmonary cryptosporidiosis and pulmonary microsporidiosis in HIV-infected patients with concurrent intestinal disease have been reported.[343–353] In these cases, aspiration from the gastrointestinal tract appears to be the most probable route of pulmonary infection. Occasionally, patients have presented with disseminated disease, raising the possibility of hematogenous spread. The most common respiratory symptoms are cough, dyspnea, and pleuritic chest pain. One review of the literature found that these symptoms were present in 77%, 58%, and 33%, respectively, of patients with cryptosporidial pulmonary disease.[353] The diagnosis of pulmonary disease can be made by either sputum study or bronchoscopy.

The hyperinfection syndrome with *Strongyloides stercoralis* has been reported in HIV-infected patients.[354–363a] *Strongyloides* hyperinfection does not, however, appear to be an important HIV-associated complication, even in countries where the parasite is endemic.[364] We have encountered several cases of pulmonary strongyloidiasis as part of disseminated disease. All patients were from regions with a high incidence of helminthic infection. Fever with concurrent gastrointestinal and respiratory symptoms was typical. The diagnosis was made by sputum or BAL fluid study. The patients were treated successfully with either albendazole or ivermectin; however, relapses were common, and retreatment was often necessary.

## NONINFECTIOUS DISORDERS

The initial evaluation of respiratory complications usually focuses on the diagnosis of HIV-associated opportunistic infections because of their frequency, the need for prompt therapy, and, in the case of tuberculosis, the concern for transmission to other persons, both HIV infected and non-HIV infected. HIV-infected patients are, however, also susceptible to a number of noninfectious complications, which have been reviewed elsewhere.[7, 29]

### Malignancies

Two quite different HIV-associated malignancies, Kaposi's sarcoma and non-Hodgkin's lymphoma, may involve the lungs: parenchyma, airways, pleura, or hilar or mediastinal lymph nodes. Intrathoracic disease from either neoplasm is usually a manifestation of disease already recognized elsewhere, but occasionally both Kaposi's sarcoma and non-Hodgkin's lymphoma may present with isolated pulmonary disease.

#### Kaposi's Sarcoma

The most common HIV-associated malignancy is Kaposi's sarcoma. One of the truly striking features of the AIDS epidemic in the early 1980s was the explosion of cases of this previously rare disease. Although the incidence of Kaposi's sarcoma has decreased dramatically since then, significant advances have been made in our understanding of its pathogenesis, including its association with a novel human herpesvirus, HHV-8.

The incidence of HIV-associated Kaposi's sarcoma has always been higher in male homosexuals than in other HIV risk groups. Approximately 90% to 95% of cases occur in male homosexuals. It has been estimated that there is a 20,000- to 73,000-fold increased incidence of Kaposi's sarcoma in HIV-infected homosexual men than in the overall population.[365] These observations suggested the presence of a possible sexually transmitted cofactor. In 1994, Chang and colleagues[366] identified DNA fragments present in HIV-associated Kaposi's sarcoma specimens but absent in most non-Kaposi's specimens. The nucleotide sequence of these fragments demonstrated homology to two known gamma-(lymphotropic) herpesviruses, suggesting that the fragments derived from a novel herpesvirus, subsequently named human herpesvirus-8 (HHV-8) or Kaposi's sarcoma-associated herpesvirus

(KSHV).[367] Subsequently, HHV-8 has also been found in specimens from non–HIV-infected persons with classic, endemic (African), and transplant-associated Kaposi's sarcoma. These and other findings argue for a central role of HHV-8 in the pathogenesis of Kaposi's sarcoma and provide new avenues for possible treatment of this disease.

**Clinical Features.** Pulmonary Kaposi's sarcoma is detected clinically in approximately one third of patients with known Kaposi's sarcoma, with the proportion detected at autopsy approaching 50% to 75%.[7, 29]

***CD4⁺ Lymphocyte Count.*** Pulmonary Kaposi's sarcoma presents at the lower range of $CD4^+$ lymphocyte counts. In one study of 168 patients with pulmonary Kaposi's sarcoma, the median $CD4^+$ count was 19 cells/μL; 68% had a $CD4^+$ lymphocyte count below 50 cells/μL, and only 4% had a $CD4^+$ count higher than 200 cells/μL.[368] Most but not all patients with clinically diagnosed pulmonary Kaposi's sarcoma have concomitant mucocutaneous disease. Huang and colleagues[368] found that 85% of 168 consecutive patients diagnosed with pulmonary Kaposi's sarcoma by bronchoscopy had evidence of mucocutaneous involvement at the time of bronchoscopy. The 15% without mucocutaneous involvement had pulmonary disease that ranged from isolated tracheal lesions to diffuse endobronchial involvement that was ultimately fatal. A significant proportion of patients with pulmonary Kaposi's sarcoma also have concurrent opportunistic infection.[7] For example, Huang and colleagues[368] found that 45 of the 168 patients (27%) with pulmonary Kaposi's sarcoma had accompanying opportunistic infection, most frequently PCP. These observations underscore the need to evaluate each patient with Kaposi's sarcoma who presents with respiratory symptoms not only for pulmonary Kaposi's sarcoma but also for opportunistic infection. Patients with pulmonary Kaposi's sarcoma who develop opportunistic infection may also experience a rapid progression of their Kaposi's sarcoma.

Pulmonary Kaposi's sarcoma characteristically presents with nonproductive cough, dyspnea, and fever. Chest pain and hemoptysis are less frequently noted and, in our experience, presage a precipitous clinical decline. Symptoms will usually be present for weeks but may also progress rapidly in a manner indistinguishable from opportunistic infection. Physical examination of the chest is often normal, but crackles, generalized or localized wheezes, and signs of pleural effusion can be observed.

***Chest Radiograph.*** Pulmonary Kaposi's sarcoma characteristically presents with bilateral opacities in a central or perihilar distribution (Fig. 82.7). Typical findings include linear densities, nodules or nodular opacities of varying size, pleural effusions, and intrathoracic adenopathy. Gruden and colleagues[369] reviewed the chest radiographic presentation of 76 consecutive patients with pulmonary Kaposi's sarcoma diagnosed by bronchoscopy whose BAL was negative for infectious organisms. In this study, 95% of the radiographs had peribronchial cuffing and "tram track" opacities, with or without more extensive perihilar coalescent opacities. Small nodules or nodular opacities were seen in 78%, Kerley's B lines in 71%, and pleural effusions in 53% of the radiographs. Of note, no chest radiograph had either Kerley's B lines or pleural effusions without concurrent parenchymal findings. Sixteen per cent of the radiographs had hilar or mediastinal lymph node enlargement. Although this constellation of radiographic findings strongly suggests the diagnosis of pulmonary Kaposi's sarcoma in an HIV-infected male homosexual, no radiograph is diagnostic for Kaposi's sarcoma. Therefore, patients with suspected pulmonary Kaposi's sarcoma should have their diagnosis confirmed.

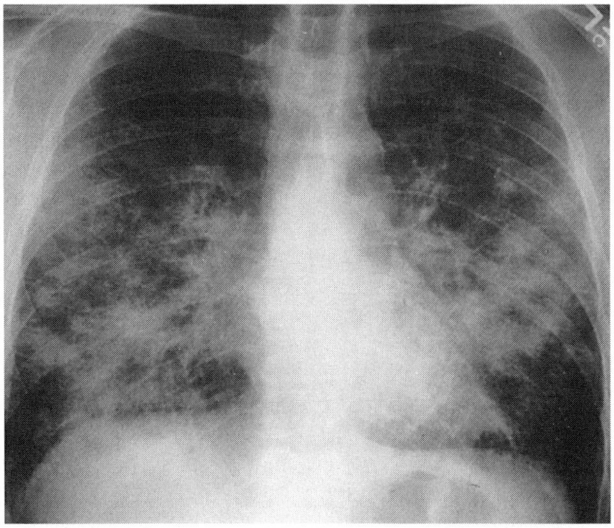

**Figure 82.7** Posteroanterior chest radiograph of HIV-seropositive patient with pulmonary Kaposi's sarcoma diagnosed by bronchoscopy showing the characteristic bilateral, perihilar distribution of abnormalities consisting of nodules and nodular opacities. (Reproduced with permission from L. Huang.)

**Diagnosis.** The diagnosis of pulmonary Kaposi's sarcoma is usually established by bronchoscopy. The finding of characteristic endobronchial, red or violaceous, flat or slightly raised lesions is sufficient to diagnose pulmonary disease (Fig. 82.8). The presence of these lesions does not, however, preclude a concurrent infection, nor does their absence in the observable airway preclude more distal disease or parenchymal, pleural, or nodal involvement. Although endobronchial or transbronchial biopsy of the airway or parenchymal abnormalities, respectively, is usually unnecessary, we have occasionally established the diagnosis by transbronchial biopsy in patients in whom there was a strong clinical suspicion for pulmonary Kaposi's sarcoma but who had no endobronchial lesions detected. Patients with cutaneous Kaposi's sarcoma who develop new respiratory complaints should undergo evaluation according to the algorithm (sputum induction, followed by bronchoscopy) previously described. Patients in whom there is a strong clinical suspicion for pulmonary Kaposi's sarcoma should, however, undergo an initial bronchoscopy.

Patients with pleural effusion may be considered candi-

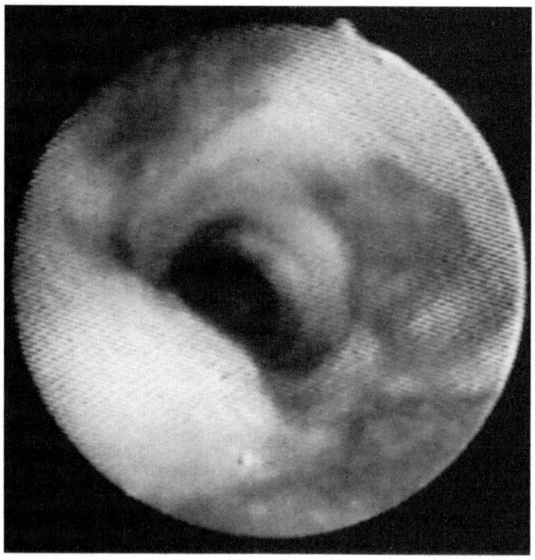

**Figure 82.8** Characteristic Kaposi's sarcoma lesions in trachea of HIV-seropositive patient seen via bronchoscopy. (Reproduced with permission from L. Huang.)

dates for thoracentesis, primarily to exclude the presence of a pyogenic, mycobacterial, or fungal infection, but also to provide symptomatic relief if the effusion is large. Although most Kaposi's sarcoma effusions are exudative, effusions may be transudate or exudate, serous, serosanguineous, or even frankly bloody.[7, 29] We have even seen chylous effusions due to lymphatic obstruction from Kaposi's sarcoma.

Kaposi's sarcoma is $^{67}$gallium scan negative. In contrast, opportunistic infections and non-Hodgkin's lymphoma are $^{67}$gallium avid. Among HIV-associated pulmonary disease, this unique feature of Kaposi's sarcoma has created a niche for the use of $^{67}$gallium scans. In the absence of either a bronchoscopic or tissue diagnosis of pulmonary Kaposi's sarcoma, its presence may be inferred by the finding of significant chest radiographic abnormalities and a negative $^{67}$gallium scan.

**Treatment.** Treatment of pulmonary Kaposi's sarcoma has seen tremendous advancement. Earlier in the AIDS epidemic, treatment was controversial. Many patients found to have pulmonary Kaposi's sarcoma also had a concurrent opportunistic infection. In many of these patients, treatment of the infection resulted in resolution of the respiratory symptoms. Given the significant toxicities of Kaposi's chemotherapy regimens, oncologists often reserved treatment for pulmonary Kaposi's sarcoma to those moderately to severely symptomatic patients without concurrent opportunistic infection.

With advances in treatment for Kaposi's sarcoma and for HIV infection itself, several possibilities currently exist for treating pulmonary disease. One option is to use liposomal anthracycline (doxorubicin or daunorubicin) therapy. These regimens have surpassed the combination of doxorubicin, bleomycin, and vincristine (ABV) as first-line therapy. Paclitaxel (Taxol) has been used as second-line therapy for those with refractory disease. Another option is to aggressively treat the HIV disease with combination antiretroviral therapy. We have seen a number of cases in which this approach has resulted in dramatic improvement and/or resolution of pulmonary symptoms and chest radiographic abnormalities. For selected patients, a stepwise approach of aggressive antiretroviral therapy, followed by chemotherapy against Kaposi's sarcoma if the patient fails to respond to antiretroviral therapy, may be reasonable.

## Non-Hodgkin's Lymphoma

There are some interesting similarities and differences between Kaposi's sarcoma and non-Hodgkin's lymphoma. Both have been documented as complications of other immunosuppressive disorders. In HIV-infected patients, both predominate in male homosexuals, and both can be extremely aggressive in their clinical behavior. In contrast, intrathoracic involvement is more common in Kaposi's sarcoma than in non-Hodgkin's lymphoma, and the incidence of HIV-associated Kaposi's sarcoma is decreasing, whereas that of HIV-associated non-Hodgkin's lymphoma appears to be increasing. One hypothesized explanation for this observation is that the use of antiretroviral therapy and opportunistic infection prophylaxis, by improving the overall survival for HIV-infected patients, may thereby also provide an opportunity for these patients to develop previously less common diseases.[370]

Almost all HIV-associated non-Hodgkin's lymphomas are of B-cell origin. Most are intermediate-grade or high-grade lymphomas, the majority classified as either large cell (60%) or small, noncleaved (Burkitt's) (25% to 30%). The etiology of non-Hodgkin's lymphoma is unknown. Although Epstein-Barr virus has been implicated in the pathogenesis of the primary central nervous system lymphomas and is often present in the body cavity lymphomas, it is found in only a minority of HIV-associated non-Hodgkin's lymphomas.

**Clinical Features.** Most patients with non-Hodgkin's lymphoma present with widely disseminated disease and extranodal involvement. Frequent extranodal sites include the liver, spleen, bone marrow, meninges, gastrointestinal tract, and pericardium. Intrathoracic involvement is seen in a smaller proportion. The reported incidence of intrathoracic disease varies from 0% to 31% of patients at the time of clinical diagnosis and is usually higher at the time of autopsy.[7, 29] Occasionally, the lung is the only site involved.

***$CD4^+$ Lymphocyte Count.*** Non-Hodgkin's lymphoma can present at a wide range of $CD4^+$ lymphocyte counts. The median $CD4^+$ T lymphocyte cell count is approximately 100 cells/μL, and 75% of patients have a $CD4^+$ lymphocyte cell count above 50 cells/μL. In one study of 38 patients with non-Hodgkin's lymphoma, the mean (± SD) $CD4^+$ count was 67 (± 65) cells/μL.[371]

When the lungs are involved, the most common symptoms are cough and dyspnea, with pleuritic chest pain and hemoptysis occurring in a minority. Eisner and colleagues[371] found that these symptoms were present in 71%, 63%, 26%, and 11%, respectively, of the 38 patients reported. Systemic symptoms such as fever, sweats, and weight loss are common. Physical examination of the chest may reveal a variety of findings, including crackles, rhonchi, wheezes, dullness to percussion, decreased breath sounds, and egophony.

***Chest Radiograph.*** The most common chest radiograph parenchymal findings include multiple nodular opacities or masses, lobar infiltrates, and diffuse interstitial infiltrates.[371, 372] Occasionally, a solitary pulmonary nodule (Fig. 82.9) or mass is seen. More rarely, cases of endobronchial lesions have been reported.[373, 374] Pleural effusions are the most common radiographic abnormality, occurring in 40% to 70% of cases.[371, 375] Hilar and mediastinal adenopathy can be found in up to 60% of patients. It must be noted, however, that isolated intrathoracic adenopathy without identifiable extrathoracic nodal involvement is a rare presentation for HIV-associated non-Hodgkin's lymphomas.[376] Among HIV-associated pulmonary complications, the appearance of well-defined single or multiple parenchymal nodules is unique to pulmonary non-Hodgkin's lymphoma. These nodules can vary in size (usually >1 cm) and grow rapidly. The distinct margin of the nodules distinguishes them from the poorly defined margins of pulmonary Kaposi's sarcoma, whereas their size distinguishes them from infectious etiologies. Chest CT scan can be useful in determining the diagnostic procedure.

**Diagnosis.** The diagnosis of non-Hodgkin's lymphoma requires demonstration of malignant lymphocytes on cytology or biopsy specimens. Most often the diagnosis is made by needle aspiration or biopsy of an extrathoracic site. Persons who present with isolated intrathoracic involvement should undergo bronchoscopy with Wang needle biopsy, if abnormal nodes are within reach through the bronchoscope, and with transbronchial biopsies.[371] For lesions outside the sampling distance of the bronchoscope, fluoroscopic or CT-guided fine-needle aspiration should be considered. Other options include mediastinoscopy and open-lung biopsy. In all cases, the presence of a pathologist in the procedure room to immediately evaluate the adequacy of samples seems to improve the best diagnostic yield. For patients with pleural effusions, pleural fluid cytology, biopsy, or both are often diagnostic.[371, 375, 377]

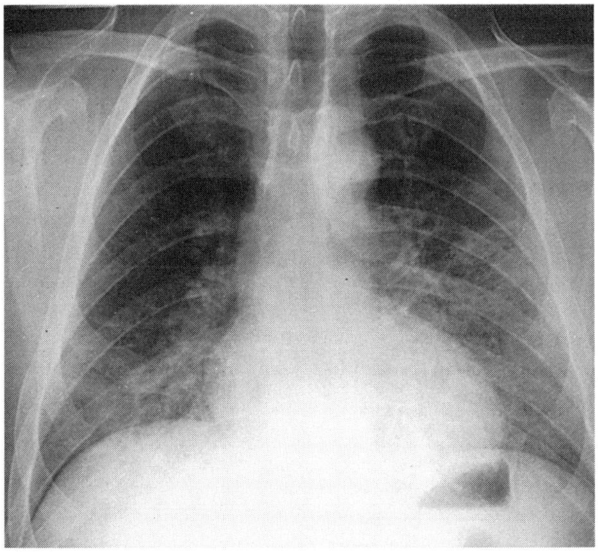

**Figure 82.9** Posteroanterior chest radiograph of HIV-seropositive patient showing focal consolidation in the right mid-lung zone. The wires and clips are from previous coronary artery bypass surgery. Final diagnosis at autopsy was non-Hodgkin's lymphoma. (Reproduced with permission from Murray JF, Mills J: Pulmonary complications of HIV infection. Am Rev Respir Dis 141:1356–1372, 1582–1598, 1990.)

**Treatment.** Standard chemotherapy is usually mBACOD or CHOP, often with adjunctive colony-stimulating factors (granulocyte or granulocyte-macrophage).[378] Treatment of non-Hodgkin's lymphoma is frequently complicated by the development of opportunistic infections and by the presence of decreased bone marrow reserve, which results in a decreased chemotherapy dose intensity. A complete response is seen in 33% to 62%, but relapse occurs in approximately one fourth of the initial responders, usually within the first 6 months. The reported median survival is 4 to 8 months, with approximately half the patients dying from their lymphoma and half dying of opportunistic infection. Because of the frequency of death from opportunistic infection, specifically, PCP, *P. carinii* prophylaxis is warranted in all cases, regardless of $CD4^+$ T lymphocyte cell count. Because these studies were conducted before the widespread use of combinations of antiretroviral therapies, it remains to be seen whether the declines observed for PCP will result in changes to this protocol.

## Bronchogenic Carcinoma

There is significant debate about whether other malignancies that involve the lung, namely, Hodgkin's disease[379] and especially bronchogenic carcinoma,[380–387] are also associated with HIV disease.

**Epidemiology.** In contrast to Kaposi's sarcoma and non-Hodgkin's lymphoma, there is no increase in bronchogenic carcinoma in persons with non–HIV-associated immunosuppressive disorders. Nevertheless, there are a number of reports that suggest that bronchogenic carcinoma is increased in frequency, occurs at a younger age, and has a more aggressive course in HIV-infected patients. One study that cross-matched the HIV/AIDS and cancer registries in Texas found a 6.5-fold increased incidence of bronchogenic carcinoma in HIV/AIDS patients compared with the overall US population.[387] The PCHIS found an observed rate of bronchogenic carcinoma of approximately 180 cases per 100,000 person-years in its HIV-infected cohort.[388] Other studies, however, found no significant increase.[365, 384]

**Clinical Features.** Most HIV-infected patients who develop bronchogenic carcinoma are cigarette smokers. Although all pathologic types are seen, adenocarcinoma has been the most frequent type reported, similar to that seen in non–HIV-infected patients younger than 40 years of age who develop bronchogenic carcinoma. Bronchogenic carcinoma can develop at a wide range of $CD4^+$ lymphocyte counts. In the PCHIS study, the range of $CD4^+$ counts among the patients who developed lung cancer was 127 to 1026 cells/μL.[388] The characteristic presentation of bronchogenic carcinoma is familiar and includes respiratory symptoms such as cough, occasionally with hemoptysis, dyspnea, and chest pain. Constitutional symptoms such as fatigue and weight loss may also be present. The chest radiographic presentation appears to include parenchymal nodules or masses, pleural effusion, and central parenchymal or hilar masses and mediastinal adenopathy.[389–392] Chest CT scans provide additional important details.

**Diagnosis and Treatment.** The diagnosis and treatment of bronchogenic carcinoma in an HIV-infected patient is similar to that in a non–HIV-infected individual. HIV infection should be considered an important concurrent underlying medical problem, much the same as one would consider underlying cardiopulmonary disease. Surgical resection should be considered for any patient whose staging and medical condition support such an approach.[393] The prognosis, however, is poor. The median survival in the reported cases has ranged from 1 to 6 months.

## Interstitial Pneumonitides

Although opportunistic infection and neoplasia dominate the clinical spectrum of HIV-associated pulmonary disease, a small number of patients present with signs and symptoms attributable to one of the interstitial pneumonitides, lymphocytic interstitial pneumonitis (LIP) or nonspecific interstitial pneumonitis (NIP).

### Lymphocytic Interstitial Pneumonitis

Although described by Carrington and Liebow[394] over 30 years ago, it remains speculative whether LIP is a pathogenically distinct entity or whether it is a disorder of multiple causes that all produce a similar pathologic reaction. The facts that LIP occurs with increased frequency in HIV-infected persons (albeit rarely in adults) and is diagnostic of AIDS when it occurs in an HIV-infected child younger than 13 years of age favor the diverse-origin theory. Histologic abnormalities of LIP consist of diffuse infiltration of the alveolar septa and peribronchiolar and perivascular interstitium by lymphocytes. Plasma cells and macrophages can also be seen.[395] An apparently related disorder, pulmonary lymphoid hyperplasia, has similar features, but the aggregates of lymphoid cells, with or without germinal centers, are more conspicuous and are located in peribronchovascular regions.[396]

**Clinical Features.** The most striking feature of HIV-associated LIP is the effect of age on its incidence. Earlier in the AIDS epidemic, one third to one half of AIDS-defining diagnoses in children were due to LIP. More recently, LIP accounted for 17% of these AIDS-defining diagnoses.[8] In contrast, LIP is rare in adults. We have encountered only a handful of biopsy-proven LIP adult cases in our experience with several thousand AIDS patients at San Francisco General Hospital, and there are scattered case reports throughout the literature.[7, 395, 397–400]

The symptoms of LIP include slowly progressive dyspnea, nonproductive cough, and fever. Lung examination may be normal or may reveal inspiratory crackles. These clinical features are indistinguishable from opportunistic infection (e.g., PCP). In children, additional physical examination findings include clubbing, salivary gland enlargement, hepatosplenomegaly, and lymphadenopathy.

The chest radiograph presentation of LIP is nonspecific and characteristically shows bilateral reticulonodular "interstitial" infiltrates with a lower lung zone predominance (Fig. 82.10).[401] Areas of alveolar opacity believed to result from bronchial compression caused by more severe lymphocytic infiltration have been reported.[402] Hilar or mediastinal adenopathy is occasionally seen. Pulmonary function tests often reveal a restrictive ventilatory defect and a decreased diffusing capacity. Chest CT scans may reveal small (2 to 4 mm) nodules often in a peribronchovascular distribution or diffuse areas of ground-glass opacity.[403, 404] Gallium scintigraphy may detect diffuse pulmonary uptake, indistinguishable from PCP, although all patterns have been described.[402]

**Diagnosis.** The diagnosis of LIP requires histologic confirmation by biopsy.[405, 406]

**Treatment.** There are so few cases of LIP among HIV-infected adults that neither definitive therapy nor benefit of therapy has been determined. The clinical course of LIP in adults ranges from mild disease with spontaneous resolution to progressive disease and respiratory failure.

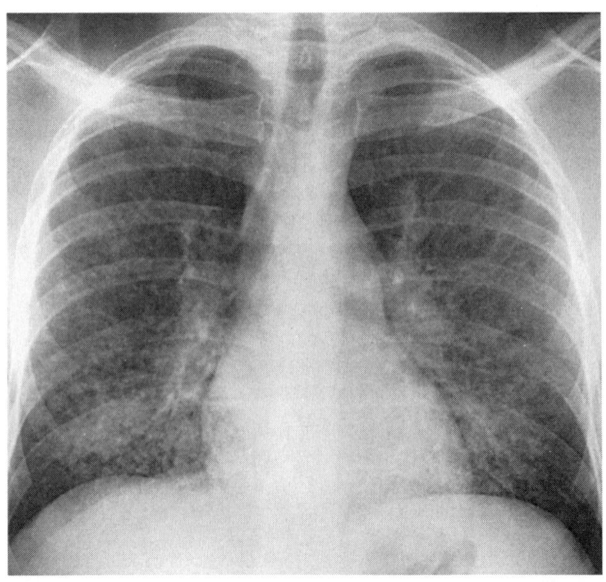

**Figure 82.10** Posteroanterior chest radiograph of HIV-seropositive patient showing diffuse reticulonodular infiltration. Biopsy specimen revealed lymphocytic interstitial pneumonitis.

In the face of progressive illness, however, a trial of corticosteroids seems well justified.

### Nonspecific Interstitial Pneumonitis

NIP is a pulmonary disorder characterized histologically by infiltration of mononuclear cells, predominantly lymphocytes and plasma cells, into the peribronchiolar and perivascular interstitium. In contrast to LIP, the alveolar septa are less frequently involved.[395] NIP has been reported with various frequencies in HIV-infected patients. Because it is a histologic diagnosis, its incidence depends on the frequency with which biopsy is performed during the diagnostic evaluation.

**Clinical Features.** The symptoms of NIP include dyspnea, nonproductive cough, and fever.[407–410] Lung examination may be normal. These clinical features are indistinguishable from those of PCP. However, NIP may present at $CD4^+$ lymphocyte counts above 200 cells/μL, whereas PCP rarely (≤5%) does.[409, 410] In one large series of 67 HIV-infected patients with NIP, the mean $CD4^+$ count in the patients with NIP was 492 cells/μL compared with 57 cells/μL for the matched control subjects with PCP.[410]

The chest radiographic presentation of NIP is nonspecific and usually indistinguishable from that of PCP. As with PCP, NIP can present with a normal radiograph. One study of patients with NIP found that 16 of 36 (44%) had a normal radiograph.[411] The most common radiographic abnormality seen was a diffuse interstitial pattern. Other abnormalities include pleural effusions, alveolar infiltrates, and nodules.[402, 411] Pulmonary function tests often reveal a mildly decreased diffusing capacity.[408]

**Diagnosis.** The diagnosis of NIP requires histologic confirmation and the exclusion of other etiologies.[412]

**Treatment.** The natural history of HIV-associated NIP is poorly understood, but it usually resolves or stabilizes without therapy.[409, 410] Observation is all that is required, with the proviso that, if the patient becomes severely ill, repeat bronchoscopy and biopsy are indicated to look for a different, usually infectious, disorder.

## Other Disorders

### Obstructive Lung Disease

Obstructive lung disease occurs frequently in HIV-infected patients, and a variety of pulmonary function test abnormalities can be seen. The PCHIS performed serial pulmonary function tests in their more than 1100 HIV-infected subjects and demonstrated that advanced HIV infection, characterized by a $CD4^+$ lymphocyte count less than 200 cells/μL or HIV-associated symptoms, race, cigarette smoking, and injection drug use are all associated with reductions in diffusing capacity.[413] A PCHIS multivariate analysis found that both PCP and bacterial pneumonia were independently associated with an accelerated decline in the forced expiratory volume in one second ($FEV_1$) (Stansell, unpublished data). Other investigators have found that significant proportions of HIV-infected subjects have evidence of airflow obstruction.[414] In this one study, 33 of 99 persons with AIDS had decreased forced expiratory flow rates; 20 of the 33 (61%) experienced a significant response to inhaled bronchodilators.

HIV-infected patients may have asthma that precedes their HIV infection.[35] In one clinic-based study, a history of asthma was reported in 21% and current asthma in 17% of 136 patients attending a primary care clinic for HIV infection.[415] On questioning, 61% of the current asthmatic patients reported subjective worsening of their asthma after becoming HIV infected. Whether this worsening was secondary to an increase in upper respiratory tract illnesses or acute bronchitis resulting from HIV infection or whether HIV itself played a role is unclear.

Obstructive airway disease, chronic bronchitis, and bronchiectasis are all well-recognized sequelae of opportunistic infection.[416–418] However, Diaz and coworkers[419] reported four patients without antecedent pneumonia or opportunistic infection who presented with progressive dyspnea. Chest radiographs showed no infiltrations, and pulmonary function tests revealed increased functional residual capacity and residual volumes and decreased diffusing capacity suggestive of emphysema. Only minimal airflow obstruction, however, was noted. Chest HRCT scans revealed emphysema-like bullous changes even though known causes of emphysema were absent in these patients. Whether these cases represent a chance association or whether HIV itself played a role is unclear. More recently, Diaz and colleagues[419a] examined HIV-infected persons with unexplained decreases in diffusing capacity by chest HRCT and by separation of the diffusing capacity into its Dm and Vc components. The authors found HRCT evidence of early emphysema that correlated well with values of both diffusing capacity and its Vc subdivision.

### Pulmonary Hypertension

Numerous reports of primary pulmonary hypertension (PPH) in HIV-infected patients are scattered in the literature.[420–437] The largest single series compared 20 HIV-infected patients with PPH to 93 non–HIV-infected patients with PPH.[431] At PPH diagnosis, the HIV-infected patients were significantly younger and the proportion with New York Heart Association functional class III or IV was significantly lower (50% versus 75%, $P < 0.01$). Pulmonary hypertension was thought to be the cause of death in 8 of the 10 HIV-infected patients who died within 1 year after the diagnosis of pulmonary hypertension. Pathologic findings resembled plexogenic pulmonary arteriopathy. The role, if any, that HIV plays in pulmonary hypertension has yet to be defined. We have seen a number of cases of HIV-infected patients with pulmonary hypertension. In these patients, multiple potential factors, including injection drug use, cigarette use, history of underlying cardiac or pulmonary disease, and prior pulmonary opportunistic infections, have complicated the clinical picture.

### Pulmonary Alveolar Proteinosis

Two cases of "secondary pulmonary alveolar proteinosis" have been reported.[438] Both patients had HIV-associated opportunistic infections. When they failed to improve, histologic examination revealed extensive intra-alveolar deposits of a lipoproteinaceous material that stained strongly with periodic acid–Schiff. The authors speculate that the alveolar proteinosis was secondary to infection, as has been reported in non–HIV-infected persons. Another report demonstrated that both light and ultrastructural examinations of BAL fluid from 9 of 26 patients with PCP showed lipoproteinaceous material highly suggestive of that described in pulmonary alveolar proteinosis.[439] In comparison, none of the BAL fluid samples from 11 patients without PCP had these findings.

### Diffuse Alveolar Damage and Interstitial Fibrosis

Diffuse alveolar damage is a nonspecific pattern of response resulting from acute injury to the alveolar epithelium and endothelium; in contrast, interstitial fibrosis may result from chronic injury. Given the potential severity of HIV-associated opportunistic infections (e.g., PCP) and their tendency to recur, pathologic findings of diffuse alveolar damage and interstitial fibrosis can be expected.[405, 440, 441]

### Bronchiolitis Obliterans with Organizing Pneumonia

Bronchiolitis obliterans with organizing pneumonia has been reported in a handful of HIV-infected patients.[442–445] The clinical and radiographic presentation, diagnosis, and clinical course with corticosteroid therapy were similar to those of bronchiolitis obliterans with organizing pneumonia in non–HIV-infected persons.

### Sarcoidosis

Sarcoidosis is one of the last disorders that one might expect to find among the pulmonary complications of HIV infection. In many respects, the coexistence of these two diseases is seemingly incompatible: Sarcoidosis is characterized by granuloma formation, which HIV infection inhibits; moreover, sarcoid-induced alveolitis consists predominantly of $CD4^+$ lymphocytes, whereas HIV-associated lymphocytic alveolitis consists chiefly of $CD8^+$ lymphocytes.[446] Nevertheless, several cases of sarcoidosis in HIV-infected patients have been reported.[447–450] In these cases, clinical improvement was noted with corticosteroid therapy.

As more HIV-infected persons are treated with potent combinations of antiretroviral therapies with resultant improvement in immune function, it is quite possible that more cases of pulmonary disease will occur in which the invigorated immune system plays an important pathogenetic role. Already, two cases of a sarcoid-like pulmonary disorder have been reported in persons treated with antiretroviral therapy in whom BAL analysis revealed an intense $CD4^+$ alveolitis and histopathology demonstrated noncaseating granulomas.[450a] In addition, we have seen a striking case of acute hypersensitivity pneumonitis (to avian antigen) in a patient who only developed symptoms after she experienced a dramatic increase in her $CD4^+$ lymphocyte count as a result of potent antiretroviral therapy.[450b] In this case, removal of the birds resulted in resolution of her symptoms and radiographic abnormalities.

## SUMMARY

The lungs are one of the chief target organs of HIV disease. This chapter reviews the current epidemiology of HIV/AIDS both in the United States and worldwide, contrasting the two. An overview of the immunologic abnormalities seen in HIV disease as well as an approach to the evaluation of HIV infection and HIV-associated pulmonary disease is provided. Finally, the chapter discusses the major infectious and noninfectious pulmonary complications of HIV infection, with an emphasis on their clinical features, diagnosis, treatment, and prevention.

## References

1. Gottlieb MS, Schroff R, Schanker HM, et al: *Pneumocystis carinii* pneumonia and mucosal candidiasis in previously healthy homosexual men: Evidence of a new acquired cellular immunodeficiency. N Engl J Med 305:1425–1431, 1981.
2. Masur H, Michelis MA, Greene JB, et al: An outbreak of community-acquired *Pneumocystis carinii* pneumonia: Initial manifestation of cellular immune dysfunction. N Engl J Med 305:1431–1438, 1981.
3. Barre-Sinoussi F, Chermann JC, Rey F, et al: Isolation of a T-lymphotropic retrovirus from a patient at risk for acquired immune deficiency syndrome (AIDS). Science 220:868–871, 1983.
4. Popovic M, Sarngadharan MG, Read E, Gallo RC: Detection, isolation, and continuous production of cytopathic retroviruses (HTLV-III) from patients with AIDS and pre-AIDS. Science 224:497–500, 1984.
5. Murray JF, Mills J: Pulmonary infectious complications of human immunodeficiency virus infection. Part I. Am Rev Respir Dis 141:1356–1372, 1990.
6. Murray JF, Mills J: Pulmonary infectious complications of human immunodeficiency virus infection. Part II. Am Rev Respir Dis 141:1582–1598, 1990.
7. White DA, Matthay RA: Noninfectious pulmonary complications of infection with the human immunodeficiency virus. Am Rev Respir Dis 140:1763–1787, 1989.
8. Centers for Disease Control and Prevention: HIV/AIDS Surveillance Report. 11:1–42, 1999.
9. Centers for Disease Control and Prevention: HIV/AIDS Surveillance Report. 8:1–39, 1996.
10. Centers for Disease Control and Prevention: Trends in the HIV and AIDS Epidemic. 10:1–14, 1998.
11. UNAIDS and WHO: Report on the Global HIV/AIDS Epidemic. Geneva: WHO, December 1997, pp 1–26.
12. Edelman AS, Zolla-Pazner S: AIDS: A syndrome of immune dysregulation, dysfunction, and deficiency. FASEB J 3:22–30, 1989.
13. Staprans SI, Feinberg MB: Natural history and immunopathogenesis of HIV-1 disease. *In* Sande MA, Volberding PA (eds): The Medical Management of AIDS (5th ed). Philadelphia: WB Saunders, 1997, pp 29–55.
14. Beck JM, Shellito J: Effects of human immunodeficiency virus on pulmonary host defenses. Semin Respir Infect 4:75–84, 1989.
15. Agostini C, Semenzato G: Immunologic effects of HIV in the lung. Clin Chest Med 17:633–645, 1996.
16. Lane HC, Masur H, Edgar LC, et al: Abnormalities of B-cell activation and immunoregulation in patients with the acquired immunodeficiency syndrome. N Engl J Med 309:453–458, 1983.
17. Shirai A, Cosentino M, Leitman-Klinman SF, et al: Human im-

munodeficiency virus infection induces both polyclonal and virus-specific B cell activation. J Clin Invest 89:561–566, 1992.
18. Hanson DL, Chu SY, Farizo KM, et al: Distribution of CD4+ T lymphocytes at diagnosis of acquired immunodeficiency syndrome-defining and other human immunodeficiency virus–related illnesses. The Adult and Adolescent Spectrum of HIV Disease Project Group. Arch Intern Med 155:1537–1542, 1995.
19. O'Brien WA, Hartigan PM, Martin D, et al: Changes in plasma HIV-1 RNA and CD4+ lymphocyte counts and the risk of progression to AIDS. Veterans Affairs Cooperative Study Group on AIDS. N Engl J Med 334:426–431, 1996.
20. Mellors JW, Munoz A, Giorgi JV, et al: Plasma viral load and CD4+ lymphocytes as prognostic markers of HIV-1 infection. Ann Intern Med 126:946–954, 1997.
21. Vlahov D, Graham N, Hoover D, et al: Prognostic indicators for AIDS and infectious disease death in HIV-infected injection drug users: Plasma viral load and CD4+ cell count. JAMA 279:35–40, 1998.
22. The Pulmonary Complications of HIV Infection Study Group: Design of a prospective study of the pulmonary complications of human immunodeficiency virus infection. J Clin Epidemiol 46:497–507, 1993.
23. Wallace JM, Hansen NI, Lavange L, et al: Respiratory disease trends in the Pulmonary Complications of HIV Infection Study cohort. Pulmonary Complications of HIV Infection Study Group. Am J Respir Crit Care Med 155:72–80, 1997.
24. Murray JF, Felton CP, Garay SM, et al: Pulmonary complications of the acquired immunodeficiency syndrome. Report of a National Heart, Lung, and Blood Institute workshop. N Engl J Med 310:1682–1688, 1984.
25. Murray JF, Garay SM, Hopewell PC, et al: NHLBI workshop summary. Pulmonary complications of the acquired immunodeficiency syndrome: An update. Report of the second National Heart, Lung and Blood Institute workshop. Am Rev Respir Dis 135:504–509, 1987.
26. Wachter RM, Luce JM, Hopewell PC: Critical care of patients with AIDS. JAMA 267:541–547, 1992.
27. Rosen MJ, Clayton K, Schneider RF, et al: Intensive care of patients with HIV infection: Utilization, critical illnesses, and outcomes. Pulmonary Complications of HIV Infection Study Group. Am J Respir Crit Care Med 155:67–71, 1997.
27a. Schneider MM, Borleffs JC, Stolk RP, et al: Discontinuation of prophylaxis for *Pneumocystis carinii* pneumonia in HIV-1-infected patients treated with highly active antiretroviral therapy. Lancet 353:201–203, 1999.
27b. Weverling GJ, Mocroft A, Ledergerber B, et al: Discontinuation of *Pneumocystis carinii* pneumonia prophylaxis after start of highly active antiretroviral therapy in HIV-1 infection. EruoSIDA Study Group. Lancet 353:1293–1298, 1999.
27c. Furrer H, Egger M, Opravil M, et al: Discontinuation of primary prophylaxis against *Pneumocystis carinii* pneumonia in HIV-1-infected adults treated with combination antiretroviral therapy. Swiss HIV Cohort Study. N Engl J Med 340:1301–1306, 1999.
28. USPHS/IDSA: 1999 USPHS/IDSA guidelines for the prevention of opportunistic infections in persons infected with human immunodeficiency virus. U.S. Public Health Service (USPHS) and Infectious Diseases Society of America (IDSA). MMWR Morb Mortal Wkly Rep 48:1–59, 61–66, 1999.
29. White DA: Pulmonary complications of HIV-associated malignancies. Clin Chest Med 17:755–761, 1996.
30. Hirschtick RE, Glassroth J, Jordan MC, et al: Bacterial pneumonia in persons infected with the human immunodeficiency virus. Pulmonary Complications of HIV Infection Study Group. N Engl J Med 333:845–851, 1995.
31. Noskin GA, Glassroth J: Bacterial pneumonia associated with HIV-1 infection. Clin Chest Med 17:713–723, 1996.
32. Selwyn PA, Hartel D, Lewis VA, et al: A prospective study of the risk of tuberculosis among intravenous drug users with human immunodeficiency virus infection. N Engl J Med 320:545–550, 1989.
33. Chin DP, Hopewell PC: Mycobacterial complications of HIV infection. Clin Chest Med 17:697–711, 1996.
34. O'Donnell AE, Selig J, Aravamuthan M, et al: Pulmonary complications associated with illicit drug use. An update. Chest 108:460–463, 1995.
35. Huang L, Stansell JD: AIDS and the lung. Med Clin North Am 80:775–801, 1996.
36. Davies SF, Sarosi GA: Fungal pulmonary complications. Clin Chest Med 17:725–744, 1996.
37. Markowitz N, Hansen NI, Hopewell PC, et al: Incidence of tuberculosis in the United States among HIV-infected persons. The Pulmonary Complications of HIV Infection Study Group. Ann Intern Med 126:123–132, 1997.
38. Schneider RF, Hansen NI, Rosen MJ, et al: Lack of usefulness of radiographic screening for pulmonary disease in asymptomatic HIV-infected adults. Pulmonary Complications of HIV Infection Study Group. Arch Intern Med 156:191–195, 1996.
39. Huang L, Stansell JD, Osmond D, et al: Performance of an algorithm to detect *Pneumocystis carinii* pneumonia in HIV-infected patients. Pulmonary complications of HIV infection study group. Chest 115:1025–1032, 1999.
39a. Osmond DH, Chin DP, Glassroth J, et al: Impact of bacterial pneumonia and *Pneumocystis carinii* pneumonia on human immunodeficiency virus disease progression. Clin Infect Dis 29:536–543, 1999.
40. Kvale PA, Rosen MJ, Hopewell PC, et al: A decline in the pulmonary diffusing capacity does not indicate opportunistic lung disease in asymptomatic persons infected with the human immunodeficiency virus. Pulmonary Complications of HIV Infection Study Group. Am Rev Respir Dis 148:390–395, 1993.
41. Naidich DP, McGuinness G: Pulmonary manifestations of AIDS. CT and radiographic correlations. Radiol Clin North Am 29:999–1017, 1991.
42. Hartman TE, Primack SL, Muller NL, Staples CA: Diagnosis of thoracic complications of AIDS: Accuracy of CT. AJR Am J Roentgenol 162:547–553, 1994.
43. Edinburgh KJ, Jasmer RM, Huang L, et al: Multiple pulmonary nodules in AIDS: Utility of CT in distinguishing among potential etiologies. Radiology (in press).
44. Kirshenbaum KJ, Burke R, Fanapour F, et al: Pulmonary high-resolution computed tomography versus gallium scintigraphy: Diagnostic utility in the diagnosis of patients with AIDS who have chest symptoms and normal or equivocal chest radiographs. J Thorac Imaging 13:52–57, 1998.
45. Mason GR, Duane GB, Mena I, et al: Accelerated solute clearance in *Pneumocystis carinii* pneumonia. Am Rev Respir Dis 135:864–868, 1987.
46. Lee VW, Rosen MP, Baum A, et al: AIDS-related Kaposi sarcoma: Findings on thallium-201 scintigraphy. AJR Am J Roentgenol 151:1233–1235, 1988.
47. Ng VL, Gartner I, Weymouth LA, et al: The use of mucolysed induced sputum for the identification of pulmonary pathogens associated with human immunodeficiency virus infection. Arch Pathol Lab Med 113:488–493, 1989.
48. Huang L, Hecht FM, Stansell JD, et al: Suspected *Pneumocystis carinii* pneumonia with a negative induced sputum examination. Is early bronchoscopy useful? Am J Respir Crit Care Med 151:1866–1871, 1995.
49. Hopewell PC: Impact of human immunodeficiency virus infection on the epidemiology, clinical features, management, and control of tuberculosis. Clin Infect Dis 15:540–547, 1992.
50. Theuer CP, Hopewell PC, Elias D, et al: Human immunodeficiency virus infection in tuberculosis patients. J Infect Dis 162:8–12, 1990.
51. Greenberg SD, Frager D, Suster B, et al: Active pulmonary tuberculosis in patients with AIDS: Spectrum of radiographic findings (including a normal appearance). Radiology 193:115–119, 1994.
52. Smith RL, Yew K, Berkowitz KA, Aranda CP: Factors affecting the yield of acid-fast sputum smears in patients with HIV and tuberculosis. Chest 106:684–686, 1994.
53. Finch D, Beaty CD: The utility of a single sputum specimen in the diagnosis of tuberculosis. Comparison between HIV-infected and non–HIV-infected patients. Chest 111:1174–1179, 1997.
54. Pitchenik AE, Burr J, Suarez M, et al: Human T-cell lymphotropic virus-III (HTLV-III) seropositivity and related disease among 71 consecutive patients in whom tuberculosis was diagnosed. A prospective study. Am Rev Respir Dis 135:875–879, 1987.
55. Klein NC, Duncanson FP, Lenox TH 3d, et al: Use of mycobacterial smears in the diagnosis of pulmonary tuberculosis in AIDS/ARC patients. Chest 95:1190–1192, 1989.

56. Broaddus C, Dake MD, Stulbarg MS, et al: Bronchoalveolar lavage and transbronchial biopsy for the diagnosis of pulmonary infections in the acquired immunodeficiency syndrome. Ann Intern Med 102:747–752, 1985.
57. Golden JA, Hollander H, Stulbarg MS, et al: Bronchoalveolar lavage as the exclusive diagnostic modality for *Pneumocystis carinii* pneumonia. A prospective study among patients with acquired immunodeficiency syndrome. Chest 90:18–22, 1986.
58. Scott WW Jr, Kuhlman JE: Focal pulmonary lesions in patients with AIDS: Percutaneous transthoracic needle biopsy. Radiology 180:419–421, 1991.
59. Gruden JF, Klein JS, Webb WR: Percutaneous transthoracic needle biopsy in AIDS: Analysis in 32 patients. Radiology 189:567–571, 1993.
60. Falguera M, Nogues A, Ruiz-Gonzalez A, et al: Transthoracic needle aspiration in the study of pulmonary infections in patients with HIV. Chest 106:697–702, 1994.
61. Pass HI, Potter D, Shelhammer J, et al: Indications for and diagnostic efficacy of open-lung biopsy in the patient with acquired immunodeficiency syndrome (AIDS). Ann Thorac Surg 41:307–312, 1986.
62. Fitzgerald W, Bevelaqua FA, Garay SM, Aranda CP: The role of open lung biopsy in patients with the acquired immunodeficiency syndrome. Chest 91:659–661, 1987.
63. LoCicero J 3rd: Does every patient with enigmatic lung disease deserve a lung biopsy? The continuing dilemma. Chest 106:706–708, 1994.
64. Stover DE, White DA, Romano PA, et al: Spectrum of pulmonary diseases associated with the acquired immune deficiency syndrome. Am J Med 78:429–437, 1985.
65. Centers for Disease Control and Prevention: From the Centers for Disease Control and Prevention. 1993 revised classification system for HIV infection and expanded surveillance case definition for AIDS among adolescents and adults. JAMA 269:729–730, 1993.
66. Burack JH, Hahn JA, Saint-Maurice D, et al: Microbiology of community-acquired bacterial pneumonia in persons with and at risk for human immunodeficiency virus type 1 infection. Implications for rational empiric antibiotic therapy. Arch Intern Med 154:2589–2596, 1994.
67. Mundy LM, Auwaerter PG, Oldach D, et al: Community-acquired pneumonia: Impact of immune status. Am J Respir Crit Care Med 152:1309–1315, 1995.
68. Daley CL: Bacterial pneumonia in HIV-infected patients. Semin Respir Infect 8:104–115, 1993.
68a. Feldman C, Glatthaar M, Morar R, et al: Bacteremic pneumococcal pneumonia in HIV-seropositive and HIV-seronegative adults. Chest 116:107–114, 1999.
69. Magnenat JL, Nicod LP, Auckenthaler R, et al: Mode of presentation and diagnosis of bacterial pneumonia in human immunodeficiency virus–infected patients. Am Rev Respir Dis 144:917–922, 1991.
70. Selwyn PA, Pumerantz AS, Durante A, et al: Clinical predictors of *Pneumocystis carinii* pneumonia, bacterial pneumonia and tuberculosis in HIV-infected patients. Aids 12:885–893, 1998.
71. Janoff EN, Breiman RF, Daley CL, et al: Pneumococcal disease during HIV infection. Epidemiologic, clinical, and immunologic perspectives. Ann Intern Med 117:314–324, 1992.
72. Garcia-Leoni ME, Moreno S, Rodeno P, et al: Pneumococcal pneumonia in adult hospitalized patients infected with the human immunodeficiency virus. Arch Intern Med 152:1808–1812, 1992.
73. Schlamm HT, Yancovitz SR: *Haemophilus influenzae* pneumonia in young adults with AIDS, ARC, or risk of AIDS. Am J Med 86:11–14, 1989.
74. Moreno S, Martinez R, Barros C, et al: Latent *Haemophilus influenzae* pneumonia in patients infected with HIV. Aids 5:967–970, 1991.
75. Bartlett JG, Breiman RF, Mandell LA, et al: Community-acquired pneumonia in adults: Guidelines for management. The Infectious Diseases Society of America. Clin Infect Dis 26:811–838, 1998.
76. Simberkoff MS, El Sadr W, Schiffman G, et al: *Streptococcus pneumoniae* infections and bacteremia in patients with acquired immune deficiency syndrome, with report of a pneumococcal vaccine failure. Am Rev Respir Dis 130:1174–1176, 1984.
77. Polsky B, Gold JW, Whimbey E, et al: Bacterial pneumonia in patients with the acquired immunodeficiency syndrome. Ann Intern Med 104:38–41, 1986.
78. Whimbey E, Gold JW, Polsky B, et al: Bacteremia and fungemia in patients with the acquired immunodeficiency syndrome. Ann Intern Med 104:511–514, 1986.
79. Witt DJ, Craven DE, McCabe WR: Bacterial infections in adult patients with the acquired immune deficiency syndrome (AIDS) and AIDS-related complex. Am J Med 82:900–906, 1987.
80. Krumholz HM, Sande MA, Lo B: Community-acquired bacteremia in patients with acquired immunodeficiency syndrome: Clinical presentation, bacteriology, and outcome. Am J Med 86:776–779, 1989.
81. Nelson MR, Shanson DC, Barter GJ, et al: *Pseudomonas* septicaemia associated with HIV. Aids 5:761–763, 1991.
82. Kielhofner M, Atmar RL, Hamill RJ, et al: Life-threatening *Pseudomonas aeruginosa* infections in patients with human immunodeficiency virus infection. Clin Infect Dis 14:403–411, 1992.
83. Franzetti F, Cernuschi M, Esposito R, et al: *Pseudomonas* infections in patients with AIDS and AIDS-related complex. J Intern Med 231:437–443, 1992.
84. Baron AD, Hollander H: *Pseudomonas aeruginosa* bronchopulmonary infection in late human immunodeficiency virus disease. Am Rev Respir Dis 148:992–996, 1993.
85. Mendelson MH, Gurtman A, Szabo S, et al: *Pseudomonas aeruginosa* bacteremia in patients with AIDS. Clin Infect Dis 18:886–895, 1994.
86. Fichtenbaum CJ, Woeltje KF, Powderly WG: Serious *Pseudomonas aeruginosa* infections in patients infected with human immunodeficiency virus: A case-control study. Clin Infect Dis 19:417–422, 1994.
87. Shepp DH, Tang IT, Ramundo MB, et al: Serious *Pseudomonas aeruginosa* infection in AIDS. J Acquir Immune Defic Syndr 7:823–831, 1994.
88. Schuster MG, Norris AH: Community-acquired *Pseudomonas aeruginosa* pneumonia in patients with HIV infection. Aids 8:1437–1441, 1994.
89. Dropulic LK, Leslie JM, Eldred LJ, et al: Clinical manifestations and risk factors of *Pseudomonas aeruginosa* infection in patients with AIDS. J Infect Dis 171:930–937, 1995; erratum J Infect Dis 172:327, 1995.
90. Doyle RL, Doherty JJ, Zimmerman LH: Recovery of *Pseudomonas aeruginosa* in respiratory specimens from HIV positive patients being evaluated for *Pneumocystis carinii* pneumonia. Thorax 50:548–550, 1995.
91. Ali NJ, Kessel D, Miller RF: Bronchopulmonary infection with *Pseudomonas aeruginosa* in patients infected with human immunodeficiency virus. Genitourin Med 71:73–77, 1995.
92. Bangsborg JM, Jensen BN, Friis-Moller A, et al: Legionellosis in patients with HIV infection. Infection 18:342–346, 1990.
93. Blatt SP, Dolan MJ, Hendrix CW, et al: Legionnaires' disease in human immunodeficiency virus–infected patients: Eight cases and review. Clin Infect Dis 18:227–232, 1994.
94. Johnson KM, Huseby JS: Lung abscess caused by *Legionella micdadei*. Chest 111:252–253, 1997.
95. Harris A, Lally M, Albrecht M: *Legionella bozemanii* pneumonia in three patients with AIDS. Clin Infect Dis 27:97–99, 1998.
96. Takasugi JE, Godwin JD: Lung abscess caused by *Rhodococcus equi*. J Thorac Imaging 6:72–74, 1991.
97. Cury JD, Harrington PT, Hosein IK: Successful medical therapy of *Rhodococcus equi* pneumonia in a patient with HIV infection. Chest 102:1619–1621, 1992.
98. Shapiro JM, Romney BM, Weiden MD, et al: *Rhodococcus equi* endobronchial mass with lung abscess in a patient with AIDS. Thorax 47:62–63, 1992.
99. Magnani G, Elia GF, McNeil MM, et al: *Rhodococcus equi* cavitary pneumonia in HIV-infected patients: An unsuspected opportunistic pathogen. J Acquir Immune Defic Syndr 5:1059–1064, 1992.
100. Donisi A, Suardi MG, Casari S, et al: *Rhodococcus equi* infection in HIV-infected patients. Aids 10:359–362, 1996.
101. Arlotti M, Zoboli G, Moscatelli GL, et al: *Rhodococcus equi* infection in HIV-positive subjects: A retrospective analysis of 24 cases. Scand J Infect Dis 28:463–467, 1996.
102. Rodriguez JL, Barrio JL, Pitchenik AE: Pulmonary nocardiosis

in the acquired immunodeficiency syndrome. Diagnosis with bronchoalveolar lavage and treatment with non-sulphur containing drugs. Chest 90:912–914, 1986.
103. Kim J, Minamoto GY, Grieco MH: Nocardial infection as a complication of AIDS: Report of six cases and review. Rev Infect Dis 13:624–629, 1991.
104. Javaly K, Horowitz HW, Wormser GP: Nocardiosis in patients with human immunodeficiency virus infection. Report of 2 cases and review of the literature. Medicine (Baltimore) 71:128–138, 1992.
105. Uttamchandani RB, Daikos GL, Reyes RR, et al: Nocardiosis in 30 patients with advanced human immunodeficiency virus infection: Clinical features and outcome. Clin Infect Dis 18:348–353, 1994.
106. Kramer MR, Uttamchandani RB: The radiographic appearance of pulmonary nocardiosis associated with AIDS. Chest 98:382–385, 1990.
107. Murray JF: The white plague: Down and out, or up and coming? J. Burns Amberson lecture. Am Rev Respir Dis 140:1788–1795, 1989.
108. Murray JF: Tuberculosis and HIV infection: Global perspectives. Respirology 2:209–213, 1997.
108a. Dye C, Sheele S, Dolin P, et al: Consensus statement. Global burden of tuberculosis: estimated incidence, prevalence, and mortality by country. WHO Global Surveillance and Monitoring Project. JAMA 282:677–686, 1999.
109. Murray JF: Cursed duet: HIV infection and tuberculosis. Respiration 57:210–220, 1990.
110. Murray JF: Tuberculosis and HIV infection. A global perspective, Respiration 65:335–342, 1998.
111. Centers for Disease Control and Prevention: Prevention and treatment of tuberculosis among patients infected with human immunodeficiency virus: Principles of therapy and revised recommendations. MMWR 47:1–58, 1998.
112. Daley CL, Small PM, Schecter GF, et al: An outbreak of tuberculosis with accelerated progression among persons infected with the human immunodeficiency virus. An analysis using restriction-fragment-length polymorphisms. N Engl J Med 326:231–235, 1992.
113. Small PM, Hopewell PC, Singh SP, et al: The epidemiology of tuberculosis in San Francisco. A population-based study using conventional and molecular methods. N Engl J Med 330:1703–1709, 1994.
114. Daley CL, Hahn JA, Moss AR, et al: Incidence of tuberculosis in injection drug users in San Francisco: Impact of anergy. Am J Respir Crit Care Med 157:19–22, 1998.
115. Bradford WZ, Daley CL: Multiple drug-resistant tuberculosis. Infect Dis Clin North Am 12:157–172, 1998.
116. Bradford WZ, Martin JN, Reingold AL, et al: The changing epidemiology of acquired drug-resistant tuberculosis in San Francisco, USA. Lancet 348:928–931, 1996.
117. Moore M, Onorato IM, McCray E, et al: Trends in drug-resistant tuberculosis in the United States, 1993–1996. JAMA 278:833–837, 1997.
118. Small PM, Shafer RW, Hopewell PC, et al: Exogenous reinfection with multidrug-resistant *Mycobacterium tuberculosis* in patients with advanced HIV infection. N Engl J Med 328:1137–1144, 1993.
119. Dooley SW, Jarvis WR, Martone WJ, et al: Multidrug-resistant tuberculosis. Ann Intern Med 117:257–259, 1992.
120. Pearson ML, Jereb JA, Frieden TR, et al: Nosocomial transmission of multidrug-resistant *Mycobacterium tuberculosis.* A risk to patients and health care workers. Ann Intern Med 117:191–196, 1992.
121. Nakata K, Rom WN, Honda Y, et al: *Mycobacterium tuberculosis* enhances human immunodeficiency virus-1 replication in the lung. Am J Respir Crit Care Med 155:996–1003, 1997.
121a. Goletti D, Weissman D, Jackson RW, et al: Effect of *Mycobacterium tuberculosis* on HIV replication. Role of immune activation. J Immunol 157:1271–1278, 1996.
121b. Del Amo J, Malin AS, Pozniak A, et al: Does tuberculosis accelerate the progression of HIV disease? Evidence from basic science and epidemiology. AIDS 13:1151–1158, 1999.
122. Jones BE, Young SM, Antoniskis D, et al: Relationship of the manifestations of tuberculosis to CD4 cell counts in patients with human immunodeficiency virus infection. Am Rev Respir Dis 148:1292–1297, 1993.
123. Telzak EE: Tuberculosis and human immunodeficiency virus infection. Med Clin North Am 81:345–360, 1997.
124. Shafer RW, Kim DS, Weiss JP, et al: Extrapulmonary tuberculosis in patients with human immunodeficiency virus infection. Medicine (Baltimore) 70:384–397, 1991.
125. Abouya L, Coulibaly IM, Coulibaly D, et al: Radiologic manifestations of pulmonary tuberculosis in HIV-1 and HIV-2–infected patients in Abidjan, Cote d'Ivoire. Tuberc Lung Dis 76:436–440, 1995.
126. Post FA, Wood R, Pillay GP: Pulmonary tuberculosis in HIV infection: Radiographic appearance is related to $CD4^+$ T-lymphocyte count. Tuberc Lung Dis 76:518–521, 1995.
127. Perlman DC, el-Sadr WM, Nelson ET, et al: Variation of chest radiographic patterns in pulmonary tuberculosis by degree of human immunodeficiency virus–related immunosuppression. The Terry Beirn Community Programs for Clinical Research on AIDS (CPCRA). The AIDS Clinical Trials Group (ACTG). Clin Infect Dis 25:242–246, 1997.
128. Bass JB Jr, Farer LS, Hopewell PC, et al: Treatment of tuberculosis and tuberculosis infection in adults and children. American Thoracic Society and The Centers for Disease Control and Prevention. Am J Respir Crit Care Med 149:1359–1374, 1994.
128a. Havlir DV, Barnes PF: Tuberculosis in patients with human immunodeficiency virus infection. N Engl J Med 340:367–373, 1999.
129. Small PM, Schecter GF, Goodman PC, et al: Treatment of tuberculosis in patients with advanced human immunodeficiency virus infection. N Engl J Med 324:289–294, 1991.
130. Colebunders RL, Ryder RW, Nzilambi N, et al: HIV infection in patients with tuberculosis in Kinshasa, Zaire. Am Rev Respir Dis 139:1082–1085, 1989.
131. Eriki PP, Okwera A, Aisu T, et al: The influence of human immunodeficiency virus infection on tuberculosis in Kampala, Uganda. Am Rev Respir Dis 143:185–187, 1991.
132. Narita M, Ashkin D, Hollender ES, et al: Paradoxical worsening of tuberculosis following antiretroviral therapy in patients with AIDS. Am J Respir Crit Care Med 158:157–161, 1998.
133. Department of Health and Human Services and the Henry J. Kaiser Family Foundation: Guidelines for the use of antiretroviral agents in HIV-infected adults and adolescents. Ann Intern Med 128:1079–1100, 1998.
134. Chin DP, Osmond D, Page-Shafer K, et al: Reliability of anergy skin testing in persons with HIV infection. The Pulmonary Complications of HIV Infection Study Group. Am J Respir Crit Care Med 153:1982–1984, 1996.
135. Centers for Disease Control and Prevention: Anergy skin testing and preventive therapy for HIV-infected persons; revised recommendations. MMWR 46:1–10, 1997.
136. Lallemant-Le Coeur S, Lallemant M, Cheynier D, et al: Bacillus Calmette-Guerin immunization in infants born to HIV-1–seropositive mothers. Aids 5:195–199, 1991.
137. Horsburgh CR Jr, Mason UGD, Farhi DC, et al: Disseminated infection with *Mycobacterium avium-intracellulare.* A report of 13 cases and a review of the literature. Medicine (Baltimore) 64:36–48, 1985.
138. Holtzer CD, Jacobson MA, Hadley WK, et al: Decline in the rate of specific opportunistic infections at San Francisco General Hospital: 1994–1997. AIDS 12:1931–1933, 1998.
139. Horsburgh CR Jr, Selik RM: The epidemiology of disseminated nontuberculous mycobacterial infection in the acquired immunodeficiency syndrome (AIDS). Am Rev Respir Dis 139:4–7, 1989.
140. Damsker B, Bottone EJ: *Mycobacterium avium–Mycobacterium intracellulare* from the intestinal tracts of patients with the acquired immunodeficiency syndrome: Concepts regarding acquisition and pathogenesis. J Infect Dis 151:179–181, 1985.
141. Horsburgh CR Jr, Metchock BG, McGowan JE Jr, et al: Clinical implications of recovery of *Mycobacterium avium* complex from the stool or respiratory tract of HIV-infected individuals. Aids 6:512–514, 1992.
142. Chin DP, Hopewell PC, Yajko DM, et al: *Mycobacterium avium* complex in the respiratory or gastrointestinal tract and the risk of *M. avium* complex bacteremia in patients with human immunodeficiency virus infection. J Infect Dis 169:289–295, 1994.

143. Crawford JT, Bates JH: Analysis of plasmids in *Mycobacterium avium-intracellulare* isolates from persons with acquired immunodeficiency syndrome. Am Rev Respir Dis 134:659–661, 1986.
144. Hampson SJ, Portaels F, Thompson J, et al: DNA probes demonstrate a single highly conserved strain of *Mycobacterium avium* infecting AIDS patients. Lancet 1:65–68, 1989.
145. Yakrus MA, Good RC: Geographic distribution, frequency, and specimen source of *Mycobacterium avium* complex serotypes isolated from patients with acquired immunodeficiency syndrome. J Clin Microbiol 28:926–929, 1990.
146. Rigsby MO, Curtis AM: Pulmonary disease from nontuberculous mycobacteria in patients with human immunodeficiency virus. Chest 106:913–919, 1994.
147. Kalayjian RC, Toossi Z, Tomashefski JF Jr, et al: Pulmonary disease due to infection by *Mycobacterium avium* complex in patients with AIDS. Clin Infect Dis 20:1186–1194, 1995.
148. Hocqueloux L, Lesprit P, Herrmann JL, et al: Pulmonary *Mycobacterium avium* complex disease without dissemination in HIV-infected patients. Chest 113:542–548, 1998.
149. Horsburgh CR Jr: *Mycobacterium avium* complex infection in the acquired immunodeficiency syndrome. N Engl J Med 324:1332–1338, 1991.
150. Jacobson MA, Hopewell PC, Yajko DM, et al: Natural history of disseminated *Mycobacterium avium* complex infection in AIDS. J Infect Dis 164:994–998, 1991.
151. Chaisson RE, Moore RD, Richman DD, et al: Incidence and natural history of *Mycobacterium avium* complex infections in patients with advanced human immunodeficiency virus disease treated with zidovudine. The Zidovudine Epidemiology Study Group. Am Rev Respir Dis 146:285–289, 1992.
152. Chin DP, Reingold AL, Horsburgh CR Jr, et al: Predicting *Mycobacterium avium* complex bacteremia in patients infected with human immunodeficiency virus: A prospectively validated model. Clin Infect Dis 19:668–674, 1994.
153. Packer SJ, Cesario T, Williams JH Jr: *Mycobacterium avium* complex infection presenting as endobronchial lesions in immunosuppressed patients. Ann Intern Med 109:389–393, 1988.
154. Mehle ME, Adamo JP, Mehta AC, et al: Endobronchial *Mycobacterium avium-intracellulare* infection in a patient with AIDS. Chest 96:199–201, 1989.
155. Wallace RJ, Glassroth J, Griffith DE, et al: Diagnosis and treatment of disease caused by nontuberculous mycobacteria. Am J Respir Crit Care Med 156:S1–S25, 1997.
155a. Gordin FM, Sullam PM, Shafran SD, et al: A randomized, placebo-controlled study of rifabutin added to a regimen of clarithromycin and ethambutol for treatment of disseminated infection with *Mycobacterium avium* complex. Clin Infect Dis 28:1080–1085, 1999.
156. Aberg JA, Yajko DM, Jacobson MA: Eradication of AIDS-related disseminated *Mycobacterium avium* complex infection after 12 months of antimycobacterial therapy combined with highly active antiretroviral therapy. J Infect Dis 178:1446–1449, 1998.
157. Good RC, Snider DE Jr: Isolation of nontuberculous mycobacteria in the United States, 1980. J Infect Dis 146:829–833, 1982.
158. Bloch KC, Zwerling L, Pletcher MJ, et al: Incidence and clinical implications of isolation of *Mycobacterium kansasii:* Results of a 5-year, population-based study. Ann Intern Med 129:698–704, 1998.
159. Levine B, Chaisson RE: *Mycobacterium kansasii:* A cause of treatable pulmonary disease associated with advanced human immunodeficiency virus (HIV) infection. Ann Intern Med 114:861–868, 1991.
160. Carpenter JL, Parks JM: *Mycobacterium kansasii* infections in patients positive for human immunodeficiency virus. Rev Infect Dis 13:789–796, 1991.
161. Valainis GT, Cardona LM, Greer DL: The spectrum of *Mycobacterium kansasii* disease associated with HIV-1 infected patients. J Acquir Immune Defic Syndr 4:516–520, 1991.
162. Connolly MG Jr, Baughman RP, Dohn MN: *Mycobacterium kansasii* presenting as an endobronchial lesion. Am Rev Respir Dis 148:1405–1407, 1993.
163. Bamberger DM, Driks MR, Gupta MR, et al: *Mycobacterium kansasii* among patients infected with human immunodeficiency virus in Kansas City. Kansas City AIDS Research Consortium. Clin Infect Dis 18:395–400, 1994.
164. Quieffin J, Poubeau P, Laaban JP, et al: *Mycobacterium kansasii* infection presenting as an endobronchial tumor in a patient with the acquired immune deficiency syndrome. Tuberc Lung Dis 75:313–315, 1994.
165. Witzig RS, Fazal BA, Mera RM, et al: Clinical manifestations and implications of coinfection with *Mycobacterium kansasii* and human immunodeficiency virus type 1. Clin Infect Dis 21:77–85, 1995.
166. Campo RE, Campo CE: *Mycobacterium kansasii* disease in patients infected with human immunodeficiency virus. Clin Infect Dis 24:1233–1238, 1997.
167. Fishman JE, Schwartz DS, Sais GJ: *Mycobacterium kansasii* pulmonary infection in patients with AIDS: Spectrum of chest radiographic findings. Radiology 204:171–175, 1997.
167a. Lortholary O, Deniel F, Boudon P, et al: *Mycobacterium kansasii* infection in a Paris suburb: Comparison of disease presentation and outcome according to human immunodeficiency virus status. Groupe d'Etude des Mycobacteries de la Seine-Saint-Denis. Int J Tuberc Lung Dis 3:68–73, 1999.
167b. Corbett EL, Churchyard GJ, Hay M, et al: The impact of HIV infection on *Mycobacterium kansasii* disease in South African gold miners. Am J Respir Crit Care Med 160:10–14, 1999.
168. El-Solh AA, Nopper J, Abdul-Khoudoud MR, et al: Clinical and radiographic manifestations of uncommon pulmonary nontuberculous mycobacterial disease in AIDS patients. Chest 114:138–145, 1998.
169. Palella FJ Jr, Delaney KM, Moorman AC, et al: Declining morbidity and mortality among patients with advanced human immunodeficiency virus infection. HIV Outpatient Study Investigators. N Engl J Med 338:853–860, 1998.
170. Guidelines for prophylaxis against *Pneumocystis carinii* pneumonia for persons infected with human immunodeficiency virus. MMWR Morbid Mortal Weekly Rep 38(Suppl)5:1–9, 1989.
171. Gajdusek D: *Pneumocystis carinii*—Etiologic agent of interstitial plasma cell pneumonia of premature and young infants. Pediatrics 19:543–565, 1957.
172. Edman J, Kovacs J, Masur H: Ribosomal RNA sequence shows *Pneumocystis carinii* to be a member of the fungi. Nature 334:519–522, 1988.
173. Stringer SL, Stringer JR, Blase MA, et al: *Pneumocystis carinii:* Sequence from ribosomal RNA implies a close relationship with fungi. Exp Parasitol 68:450–461, 1989.
174. Stringer SL, Hudson K, Blase MA, et al: Sequence from ribosomal RNA of *Pneumocystis carinii* compared to those of four fungi suggests an ascomycetous affinity. J Protozool 36:14S–16S, 1989.
175. Gigliotti F: Antigenic variation of a major surface glycoprotein of *Pneumocystis carinii.* J Protozool 38:4S–5S, 1991.
176. Gigliotti F: Host species-specific antigenic variation of a mannosylated surface glycoprotein of *Pneumocystis carinii.* J Infect Dis 165:329–336, 1992.
177. Gigliotti F, Haidaris PJ, Haidaris CG, et al: Further evidence of host species-specific variation in antigens of *Pneumocystis carinii* using the polymerase chain reaction. J Infect Dis 168:191–194, 1993.
178. Gigliotti F, Harmsen AG, Haidaris CG, et al: *Pneumocystis carinii* is not universally transmissible between mammalian species. Infect Immun 61:2886–2890, 1993.
179. Meuwissen JH, Tauber I, Leeuwenberg AD, et al: Parasitologic and serologic observations of infection with *Pneumocystis* in humans. J Infect Dis 136:43–49, 1977.
180. Pifer LL, Hughes WT, Stagno S, et al: *Pneumocystis carinii* infection: Evidence for high prevalence in normal and immunosuppressed children. Pediatrics 61:35–41, 1978.
181. Peglow SL, Smulian AG, Linke MJ, et al: Serologic responses to *Pneumocystis carinii* antigens in health and disease. J Infect Dis 161:296–306, 1990.
182. Singer C, Armstrong D, Rosen PP, et al: *Pneumocystis carinii* pneumonia: A cluster of eleven cases. Ann Intern Med 82:772–777, 1975.
183. Ruebush TKD, Weinstein RA, Baehner RL, et al: An outbreak of pneumocystis pneumonia in children with acute lymphocytic leukemia. Am J Dis Child 132:143–148, 1978.
184. Chave JP, David S, Wauters JP, et al: Transmission of *Pneumocystis carinii* from AIDS patients to other immunosuppressed pa-

tients: A cluster of *Pneumocystis carinii* pneumonia in renal transplant recipients. AIDS 5:927–932, 1991.
185. Cheung YF, Chan CF, Lee CW, et al: An outbreak of *Pneumocystis carinii* pneumonia in children with malignancy. J Paediatr Child Health 30:173–175, 1994.
186. Hughes WT: Natural mode of acquisition for de novo infection with *Pneumocystis carinii.* J Infect Dis 145:842–848, 1982.
187. Hughes WT, Bartley DL, Smith BM: A natural source of infection due to *Pneumocystis carinii.* J Infect Dis 147:595, 1983.
188. Soulez B, Palluault F, Cesborn JY, et al: Introduction of *Pneumocystis carinii* in a colony of SCID mice. J Protozool 38:123S–125S, 1991.
189. Phair J, Munoz A, Detels R, et al: The risk of *Pneumocystis carinii* pneumonia among men infected with human immunodeficiency virus type 1. Multicenter AIDS Cohort Study Group. N Engl J Med 322:161–165, 1990.
190. Stansell JD, Osmond DH, Charlebois E, et al: Predictors of *Pneumocystis carinii* pneumonia in HIV-infected persons. Pulmonary Complications of HIV Infection Study Group. Am J Respir Crit Care Med 155:60–66, 1997.
191. Simonds RJ, Lindegren ML, Thomas P, et al: Prophylaxis against *Pneumocystis carinii* pneumonia among children with perinatally acquired human immunodeficiency virus infection in the United States. *Pneumocystis carinii* Pneumonia Prophylaxis Evaluation Working Group. N Engl J Med 332:786–790, 1995.
192. Kovacs JA, Hiemenz JW, Macher AM, et al: *Pneumocystis carinii* pneumonia: A comparison between patients with the acquired immunodeficiency syndrome and patients with other immunodeficiencies. Ann Intern Med 100:663–671, 1984.
193. Kales CP, Murren JR, Torres RA, et al: Early predictors of in-hospital mortality for *Pneumocystis carinii* pneumonia in the acquired immunodeficiency syndrome. Arch Intern Med 147:1413–1417, 1987.
194. DeLorenzo LJ, Huang CT, Maguire GP, et al: Roentgenographic patterns of *Pneumocystis carinii* pneumonia in 104 patients with AIDS. Chest 91:323–327, 1987.
195. Sandhu JS, Goodman PC: Pulmonary cysts associated with *Pneumocystis carinii* pneumonia in patients with AIDS. Radiology 173:33–35, 1989.
196. Kennedy CA, Goetz MB: Atypical roentgenographic manifestations of *Pneumocystis carinii* pneumonia. Arch Intern Med 152:1390–1398, 1992.
196a. Boiselle PM, Crans CA, Kaplan MA: The changing face of *Pneumocystis carinii* pneumonia in AIDS patients. AJR Am J Roentgenol 172:1301–1309, 1999.
197. Opravil M, Marincek B, Fuchs WA, et al: Shortcomings of chest radiography in detecting *Pneumocystis carinii* pneumonia. J Acquir Immune Defic Syndr 7:39–45, 1994.
198. Huang L, Hopewell PC: Bronchoscopy versus sputum induction as the initial procedure for the diagnosis of *Pneumocystis carinii* pneumonia in patients infected with HIV. J Bronchol 5:163–168, 1998.
199. Sankary RM, Turner J, Lipavsky A, et al: Alveolar-capillary block in patients with AIDS and *Pneumocystis carinii* pneumonia. Am Rev Respir Dis 137:443–449, 1988.
200. Coleman DL, Dodek PM, Golden JA, et al: Correlation between serial pulmonary function tests and fiberoptic bronchoscopy in patients with *Pneumocystis carinii* pneumonia and the acquired immune deficiency syndrome. Am Rev Respir Dis 129:491–493, 1984.
201. Hopewell PC, Luce JM: Pulmonary involvement in the acquired immunodeficiency syndrome. Chest 87:104–112, 1985.
202. Bergin CJ, Wirth RL, Berry GJ, et al: *Pneumocystis carinii* pneumonia: CT and HRCT observations. J Comput Assist Tomogr 14:756–759, 1990.
203. Moskovic E, Miller R, Pearson M: High resolution computed tomography of *Pneumocystis carinii* pneumonia in AIDS. Clin Radiol 42:239–243, 1990.
204. Rotondo A, Guidi G, Catalano O, et al: High resolution computed tomography (HRCT) of pulmonary infections in AIDS patients. Rays 19:208–215, 1994.
205. Gruden JF, Huang L, Turner J, et al: High-resolution CT in the evaluation of clinically suspected *Pneumocystis carinii* pneumonia in AIDS patients with normal, equivocal, or nonspecific radiographic findings. AJR Am J Roentgenol 169:967–975, 1997.
206. Metersky ML, Aslenzadeh J, Stelmach P: A comparison of induced and expectorated sputum for the diagnosis of *Pneumocystis carinii* pneumonia. Chest 113:1555–1559, 1998.
207. Shelhamer JH, Gill VJ, Quinn TC, et al: The laboratory evaluation of opportunistic pulmonary infections. Ann Intern Med 124:585–599, 1996.
208. Levine SJ, Masur H, Gill VJ, et al: Effect of aerosolized pentamidine prophylaxis on the diagnosis of *Pneumocystis carinii* pneumonia by induced sputum examination in patients infected with the human immunodeficiency virus. Am Rev Respir Dis 144:760–764, 1991.
209. Metersky ML, Catanzaro A: Diagnostic approach to *Pneumocystis carinii* pneumonia in the setting of prophylactic aerosolized pentamidine. Chest 100:1345–1349, 1991.
210. Fahy JV, Chin DP, Schnapp LM, et al: Effect of aerosolized pentamidine prophylaxis on the clinical severity and diagnosis of *Pneumocystis carinii* pneumonia. Am Rev Respir Dis 146:844–848, 1992.
211. Ng VL, Geaghan SM, Leoung G, et al: Lack of effect of prophylactic aerosolized pentamidine on the detection of *Pneumocystis carinii* in induced sputum or bronchoalveolar lavage specimens. Arch Pathol Lab Med 117:493–496, 1993.
212. Jules-Elysee KM, Stover DE, Zaman MB, et al: Aerosolized pentamidine: Effect on diagnosis and presentation of *Pneumocystis carinii* pneumonia. Ann Intern Med 112:750–757, 1990.
213. Levine SJ, Kennedy D, Shelhamer JH, et al: Diagnosis of *Pneumocystis carinii* pneumonia by multiple lobe, site-directed bronchoalveolar lavage with immunofluorescent monoclonal antibody staining in human immunodeficiency virus–infected patients receiving aerosolized pentamidine chemoprophylaxis. Am Rev Respir Dis 146:838–843, 1992.
214. Baughman RP, Dohn MN, Shipley R, et al: Increased *Pneumocystis carinii* recovery from the upper lobes in *Pneumocystis carinii* pneumonia. The effect of aerosol pentamidine prophylaxis. Chest 103:426–432, 1993.
215. Read CA, Cerrone F, Busseniers AE, et al: Differential lobe lavage for diagnosis of acute *Pneumocystis carinii* pneumonia in patients receiving prophylactic aerosolized pentamidine therapy. Chest 103:1520–1523, 1993.
216. Wharton JM, Coleman DL, Wofsy CB, et al: Trimethoprim-sulfamethoxazole or pentamidine for *Pneumocystis carinii* pneumonia in the acquired immunodeficiency syndrome. A prospective randomized trial. Ann Intern Med 105:37–44, 1986.
217. Sattler FR, Cowan R, Nielsen DM, et al: Trimethoprim-sulfamethoxazole compared with pentamidine for treatment of *Pneumocystis carinii* pneumonia in the acquired immunodeficiency syndrome. A prospective, noncrossover study. Ann Intern Med 109:280–287, 1988.
218. Klein NC, Duncanson FP, Lenox TH, et al: Trimethoprim-sulfamethoxazole versus pentamidine for *Pneumocystis carinii* pneumonia in AIDS patients: Results of a large prospective randomized treatment trial. Aids 6:301–305, 1992.
219. Montgomery AB, Feigal DW Jr, Sattler F, et al: Pentamidine aerosol versus trimethoprim-sulfamethoxazole for *Pneumocystis carinii* in acquired immune deficiency syndrome. Am J Respir Crit Care Med 151:1068–1074, 1995.
220. Mills J, Leoung G, Medina I, et al: Dapsone treatment of *Pneumocystis carinii* pneumonia in the acquired immunodeficiency syndrome. Antimicrob Agents Chemother 32:1057–1060, 1988.
221. Safrin S, Sattler FR, Lee BL, et al: Dapsone as a single agent is suboptimal therapy for *Pneumocystis carinii* pneumonia. J Acquir Immune Defic Syndr 4:244–249, 1991.
222. Leoung GS, Mills J, Hopewell PC, et al: Dapsone-trimethoprim for *Pneumocystis carinii* pneumonia in the acquired immunodeficiency syndrome. Ann Intern Med 105:45–48, 1986.
223. Medina I, Mills J, Leoung G, et al: Oral therapy for *Pneumocystis carinii* pneumonia in the acquired immunodeficiency syndrome. A controlled trial of trimethoprim-sulfamethoxazole versus trimethoprim-dapsone. N Engl J Med 323:776–782, 1990.
224. Noskin GA, Murphy RL, Black JR, et al: Salvage therapy with clindamycin/primaquine for *Pneumocystis carinii* pneumonia. Clin Infect Dis 14:183–188, 1992.
225. Black JR, Feinberg J, Murphy RL, et al: Clindamycin and primaquine therapy for mild-to-moderate episodes of *Pneumocystis carinii* pneumonia in patients with AIDS: AIDS Clinical Trials Group 044. Clin Infect Dis 18:905–913, 1994.

226. Toma E, Fournier S, Dumont M, et al: Clindamycin/primaquine versus trimethoprim-sulfamethoxazole as primary therapy for *Pneumocystis carinii* pneumonia in AIDS: A randomized, double-blind pilot trial. Clin Infect Dis 17:178–184, 1993.
227. Safrin S, Finkelstein DM, Feinberg J, et al: Comparison of three regimens for treatment of mild to moderate *Pneumocystis carinii* pneumonia in patients with AIDS. A double-blind, randomized, trial of oral trimethoprim-sulfamethoxazole, dapsone-trimethoprim, and clindamycin-primaquine. ACTG 108 Study Group. Ann Intern Med 124:792–802, 1996.
228. Hughes WT, Gray VL, Gutteridge WE, et al: Efficacy of a hydroxynaphthoquinone, 566C80, in experimental *Pneumocystis carinii* pneumonitis. Antimicrob Agents Chemother 34:225–228, 1990.
228a. Hughes W, Leoung G, Kramer F, et al: Comparison of atovaquone (566C80) with trimethoprim-sulfamethoxazole to treat *Pneumocystis carinii* pneumonia in patients with AIDS. N Engl J Med 328:1521–1527, 1993.
229. Allegra CJ, Kovacs JA, Drake JC, et al: Activity of antifolates against *Pneumocystis carinii* dihydrofolate reductase and identification of a potent new agent. J Exp Med 165:926–931, 1987.
230. Allegra CJ, Chabner BA, Tuazon CU, et al: Trimetrexate for the treatment of *Pneumocystis carinii* pneumonia in patients with the acquired immunodeficiency syndrome. N Engl J Med 317:978–985, 1987.
231. Sattler FR, Frame P, Davis R, et al: Trimetrexate with leucovorin versus trimethoprim-sulfamethoxazole for moderate to severe episodes of *Pneumocystis carinii* pneumonia in patients with AIDS: A prospective, controlled multicenter investigation of the AIDS Clinical Trials Group Protocol 029/031. J Infect Dis 170:165–172, 1994.
232. Soo Hoo GW, Mohsenifar Z, Meyer RD: Inhaled or intravenous pentamidine therapy for *Pneumocystis carinii* pneumonia in AIDS. A randomized trial. Ann Intern Med 113:195–202, 1990; erratum, Ann Intern Med 1;113:561, 1990.
233. Conte JE Jr, Chernoff D, Feigal DW Jr, et al: Intravenous or inhaled pentamidine for treating *Pneumocystis carinii* pneumonia in AIDS. A randomized trial. Ann Intern Med 113:203–209, 1990.
234. Dohn MN, Weinberg WG, Torres RA, et al: Oral atovaquone compared with intravenous pentamidine for *Pneumocystis carinii* pneumonia in patients with AIDS. Atovaquone Study Group. Ann Intern Med 121:174–180, 1994.
235. Montaner JS, Lawson LM, Levitt N, et al: Corticosteroids prevent early deterioration in patients with moderately severe *Pneumocystis carinii* pneumonia and the acquired immunodeficiency syndrome (AIDS). Ann Intern Med 113:14–20, 1990.
236. Gagnon S, Boota AM, Fischl MA, et al: Corticosteroids as adjunctive therapy for severe *Pneumocystis carinii* pneumonia in the acquired immunodeficiency syndrome. A double-blind, placebo-controlled trial. N Engl J Med 323:1444–1450, 1990.
237. Bozzette SA, Sattler FR, Chiu J, et al: A controlled trial of early adjunctive treatment with corticosteroids for *Pneumocystis carinii* pneumonia in the acquired immunodeficiency syndrome. California Collaborative Treatment Group. N Engl J Med 323:1451–1457, 1990.
238. The National Institutes of Health–University of California Expert Panel for Corticosteroids as Adjunctive Therapy for Pneumocystis Pneumonia. Consensus statement on the use of corticosteroids as adjunctive therapy for *Pneumocystis* pneumonia in the acquired immunodeficiency syndrome. N Engl J Med 323:1500–1504, 1990.
239. Wachter RM, Luce JM, Turner J, et al: Intensive care of patients with the acquired immunodeficiency syndrome. Outcome and changing patterns of utilization. Am Rev Respir Dis 134:891–896, 1986.
240. Bozzette SA, Finkelstein DM, Spector SA, et al: A randomized trial of three antipneumocystis agents in patients with advanced human immunodeficiency virus infection. NIAID AIDS Clinical Trials Group. N Engl J Med 332:693–699, 1995.
240a. Dunne MW, Bozzette S, McCutchan JA, et al: Efficacy of azithromycin in prevention of *Pneumocystis carinii* pneumonia: A randomised trial. California Collaborative Treatment Group. Lancet 354:891–895, 1999.
241. el-Sadr WM, Murphy RL, McCabe Yurik T, et al: Atovaquone compared with dapsone for the prevention of *Pneumocystis carinii* pneumonia in patients with HIV infection who cannot tolerate trimethoprim, sulfonamides, or both. N Engl J Med 339:1889–1895, 1998.
241a. Chan C, Montaner J, Lefebvre EA, et al: Atovaquone suspension compared with aerosolized pentamidine for prevention of *Pneumocystis carinii* pneumonia in human immunodeficiency virus-infected subjects intolerant of trimethoprim or sulfonamides. J Infect Dis 180:369–376, 1999.
242. Hardy WD, Feinberg J, Finkelstein DM, et al: A controlled trial of trimethoprim-sulfamethoxazole or aerosolized pentamidine for secondary prophylaxis of *Pneumocystis carinii* pneumonia in patients with the acquired immunodeficiency syndrome. AIDS Clinical Trials Group Protocol 021. N Engl J Med 327:1842–1848, 1992.
243. Stansell JD: Pulmonary fungal infections in HIV-infected persons. Semin Respir Infect 8:116–123, 1993.
244. Chuck SL, Sande MA: Infections with *Cryptococcus neoformans* in the acquired immunodeficiency syndrome. N Engl J Med 321:794–799, 1989.
245. Kovacs JA, Kovacs AA, Polis M, et al: Cryptococcosis in the acquired immunodeficiency syndrome. Ann Intern Med 103:533–538, 1985.
246. Zuger A, Louie E, Holzman RS, et al: Cryptococcal disease in patients with the acquired immunodeficiency syndrome. Diagnostic features and outcome of treatment. Ann Intern Med 104:234–240, 1986.
247. Eng RH, Bishburg E, Smith SM, et al: Cryptococcal infections in patients with acquired immune deficiency syndrome. Am J Med 81:19–23, 1986.
248. Wasser L, Talavera W: Pulmonary cryptococcosis in AIDS. Chest 92:692–695, 1987.
249. Newman TG, Soni A, Acaron S, et al: Pleural cryptococcosis in the acquired immune deficiency syndrome. Chest 91:459–461, 1987.
250. Chechani V, Kamholz SL: Pulmonary manifestations of disseminated cryptococcosis in patients with AIDS. Chest 98:1060–1066, 1990.
251. Clark RA, Greer DL, Valainis GT, et al: *Cryptococcus neoformans* pulmonary infection in HIV-1–infected patients. J Acquir Immune Defic Syndr 3:480–484, 1990.
252. Clark RA, Greer D, Atkinson W, et al: Spectrum of *Cryptococcus neoformans* infection in 68 patients infected with human immunodeficiency virus. Rev Infect Dis 12:768–777, 1990.
253. Cameron ML, Bartlett JA, Gallis HA, et al: Manifestations of pulmonary cryptococcosis in patients with acquired immunodeficiency syndrome. Rev Infect Dis 13:64–67, 1991.
254. Batungwanayo J, Taelman H, Bogaerts J, et al: Pulmonary cryptococcosis associated with HIV-1 infection in Rwanda: A retrospective study of 37 cases. Aids 8:1271–1276, 1994.
255. Meyohas MC, Roux P, Bollens D, et al: Pulmonary cryptococcosis: Localized and disseminated infections in 27 patients with AIDS. Clin Infect Dis 21:628–633, 1995.
256. Driver JA, Saunders CA, Heinze-Lacey B, et al: Cryptococcal pneumonia in AIDS: Is cryptococcal meningitis preceded by clinically recognizable pneumonia? J Acquir Immune Defic Syndr Hum Retrovirol 9:168–171, 1995.
257. Friedman EP, Miller RF, Severn A, et al: Cryptococcal pneumonia in patients with the acquired immunodeficiency syndrome. Clin Radiol 50:756–760, 1995; erratum, Clin Radiol 51(1):80, 1996.
258. Darras-Joly C, Chevret S, Wolff M, et al: *Cryptococcus neoformans* infection in France: Epidemiologic features of and early prognostic parameters for 76 patients who were infected with human immunodeficiency virus. Clin Infect Dis 23:369–376, 1996.
258a. Hajjeh RA, Conn LA, Stephans DS, et al: Cryptococcosis: Population-based multistate active surveillance and risk factors in human immunodeficiency virus-infected persons. Cryptococcal Active Surveillance Group. J Infect Dis 179:449–454, 1999.
259. Picon L, Vaillant L, Duong T, et al: Cutaneous cryptococcosis resembling molluscum contagiosum: A first manifestation of AIDS. Acta Derm Venereol 69:365–367, 1989.
260. Jones C, Orengo I, Rosen T, et al: Cutaneous cryptococcosis simulating Kaposi's sarcoma in the acquired immunodeficiency syndrome. Cutis 45:163–167, 1990.
261. Stansell JD: Fungal disease in HIV-infected persons: Cryptococ-

cosis, histoplasmosis, and coccidioidomycosis. J Thorac Imaging 6:28–35, 1991.
262. Douketis JD, Kesten S: Miliary pulmonary cryptococcosis in a patient with the acquired immunodeficiency syndrome. Thorax 48:402–403, 1993.
263. Miller KD, Mican JA, Davey RT: Asymptomatic solitary pulmonary nodules due to *Cryptococcus neoformans* in patients infected with human immunodeficiency virus. Clin Infect Dis 23:810–812, 1996.
264. Torre D, Martegani R, Speranza F, et al: Pulmonary cryptococcosis presenting as pneumothorax in a patient with AIDS. Clin Infect Dis 21:1524–1525, 1995.
265. Baughman RP, Rhodes JC, Dohn MN, et al: Detection of cryptococcal antigen in bronchoalveolar lavage fluid: A prospective study of diagnostic utility. Am Rev Respir Dis 145:1226–1229, 1992.
266. Malabonga VM, Basti J, Kamholz SL: Utility of bronchoscopic sampling techniques for cryptococcal disease in AIDS. Chest 99:370–372, 1991.
267. Singh N, Barnish MJ, Berman S, et al: Low-dose fluconazole as primary prophylaxis for cryptococcal infection in AIDS patients with CD4 cell counts of < or = 100/mm$^3$: Demonstration of efficacy in a positive, multicenter trial. Clin Infect Dis 23:1282–1286, 1996.
268. Powderly WG, Finkelstein D, Feinberg J, et al: A randomized trial comparing fluconazole with clotrimazole troches for the prevention of fungal infections in patients with advanced human immunodeficiency virus infection. NIAID AIDS Clinical Trials Group. N Engl J Med 332:700–705, 1995.
269. Huang CT, McGarry T, Cooper S, et al: Disseminated histoplasmosis in the acquired immunodeficiency syndrome. Report of five cases from a nonendemic area. Arch Intern Med 147:1181–1184, 1987.
270. Bonner JR, Alexander WJ, Dismukes WE, et al: Disseminated histoplasmosis in patients with the acquired immune deficiency syndrome. Arch Intern Med 144:2178–2181, 1984.
271. Taylor MN, Baddour LM, Alexander JR: Disseminated histoplasmosis associated with the acquired immune deficiency syndrome. Am J Med 77:579–580, 1984.
272. Wheat LJ, Slama TG, Zeckel ML: Histoplasmosis in the acquired immune deficiency syndrome. Am J Med 78:203–210, 1985.
273. Johnson PC, Khardori N, Najjar AF, et al: Progressive disseminated histoplasmosis in patients with acquired immunodeficiency syndrome. Am J Med 85:152–158, 1988.
274. Wheat LJ, Connolly-Stringfield PA, Baker RL, et al: Disseminated histoplasmosis in the acquired immune deficiency syndrome: Clinical findings, diagnosis and treatment, and review of the literature. Medicine (Baltimore) 69:361–374, 1990.
275. Sarosi GA, Johnson PC: Disseminated histoplasmosis in patients infected with human immunodeficiency virus. Clin Infect Dis 14:S60–S67, 1992.
276. Bradsher RW: Histoplasmosis and blastomycosis. Clin Infect Dis 22:S102–S111, 1996.
277. McKinsey DS, Spiegel RA, Hutwagner L, et al: Prospective study of histoplasmosis in patients infected with human immunodeficiency virus: Incidence, risk factors, and pathophysiology. Clin Infect Dis 24:1195–1203, 1997.
278. Conces DJ Jr, Stockberger SM, Tarver RD, et al: Disseminated histoplasmosis in AIDS: Findings on chest radiographs. AJR Am J Roentgenol 160:15–19, 1993.
279. Wheat LJ, Connolly-Stringfield P, Kohler RB, et al: *Histoplasma capsulatum* polysaccharide antigen detection in diagnosis and management of disseminated histoplasmosis in patients with acquired immunodeficiency syndrome. Am J Med 87:396–400, 1989.
280. Wheat LJ, Connolly-Stringfield P, Williams B, et al: Diagnosis of histoplasmosis in patients with the acquired immunodeficiency syndrome by detection of *Histoplasma capsulatum* polysaccharide antigen in bronchoalveolar lavage fluid. Am Rev Respir Dis 145:1421–1424, 1992.
281. Wheat J, MaWhinney S, Hafner R, et al: Treatment of histoplasmosis with fluconazole in patients with acquired immunodeficiency syndrome. National Institute of Allergy and Infectious Diseases Acquired Immunodeficiency Syndrome Clinical Trials Group and Mycoses Study Group. Am J Med 103:223–232, 1997.
281a. Galgiani JN: Coccidioidomycosis: A regional disease of national importance. Rethinking approaches for control. Ann Intern Med 130:293–300, 1999.
282. Bronnimann DA, Adam RD, Galgiani JN, et al: Coccidioidomycosis in the acquired immunodeficiency syndrome. Ann Intern Med 106:372–379, 1987.
283. Fish DG, Ampel NM, Galgiani JN, et al: Coccidioidomycosis during human immunodeficiency virus infection. A review of 77 patients. Medicine (Baltimore) 69:384–391, 1990.
284. Galgiani JN, Ampel NM: Coccidioidomycosis in human immunodeficiency virus-infected patients. J Infect Dis 162:1165–1169, 1990.
285. Ampel NM, Dols CL, Galgiani JN: Coccidioidomycosis during human immunodeficiency virus infection: Results of a prospective study in a coccidioidal endemic area. Am J Med 94:235–240, 1993.
286. Jones JL, Fleming PL, Ciesielski CA, et al: Coccidioidomycosis among persons with AIDS in the United States. J Infect Dis 171:961–966, 1995.
287. Singh VR, Smith DK, Lawerence J, et al: Coccidioidomycosis in patients infected with human immunodeficiency virus: Review of 91 cases at a single institution. Clin Infect Dis 23:563–568, 1996.
288. Stevens DA: Coccidioidomycosis. N Engl J Med 332:1077–1082, 1995.
289. Denning DW, Follansbee SE, Scolaro M, et al: Pulmonary aspergillosis in the acquired immunodeficiency syndrome. N Engl J Med 324:654–662, 1991.
290. Pursell KJ, Telzak EE, Armstrong D: *Aspergillus* species colonization and invasive disease in patients with AIDS. Clin Infect Dis 14:141–148, 1992.
291. Hohler T, Schnutgen M, Mayet WJ, et al: Pulmonary aspergilloma in a patient with AIDS. Thorax 50:312–313.
292. Addrizzo-Harris DJ, Harkin TJ, McGuinness G, et al: Pulmonary aspergilloma and AIDS. A comparison of HIV-infected and HIV-negative individuals. Chest 111:612–618, 1997.
293. Kemper CA, Hostetler JS, Follansbee SE, et al: Ulcerative and plaque-like tracheobronchitis due to infection with *Aspergillus* in patients with AIDS. Clin Infect Dis 17:344–352, 1993.
294. Klapholz A, Salomon N, Perlman DC, et al: Aspergillosis in the acquired immunodeficiency syndrome. Chest 100:1614–1618, 1991.
295. Decker CF, Parenti DM: Invasive aspergillosis in patients with HIV infection: Report of two patients and a review of the literature. J Acquir Immune Defic Syndr 4:603–606, 1991.
296. Minamoto GY, Barlam TF, Vander Els NJ: Invasive aspergillosis in patients with AIDS. Clin Infect Dis 14:66–74, 1992.
297. Lortholary O, Meyohas MC, Dupont B, et al: Invasive aspergillosis in patients with acquired immunodeficiency syndrome: Report of 33 cases. French Cooperative Study Group on Aspergillosis in AIDS. Am J Med 95:177–187, 1993.
298. Miller WT Jr, Sais GJ, Frank I, et al: Pulmonary aspergillosis in patients with AIDS. Clinical and radiographic correlations. Chest 105:37–44, 1994.
299. Mylonakis E, Barlam TF, Flanigan T, et al: Pulmonary aspergillosis and invasive disease in AIDS: Review of 342 cases. Chest 114:251–262, 1998.
300. Staples CA, Kang EY, Wright JL, et al: Invasive pulmonary aspergillosis in AIDS: Radiographic, CT, and pathologic findings. Radiology 196:409–414, 1995.
301. Denning DW, Lee JY, Hostetler JS, et al: NIAID Mycoses Study Group Multicenter Trial of Oral Itraconazole Therapy for Invasive Aspergillosis. Am J Med 97:135–144, 1994; erratum, Am J Med 97:497, 1994.
302. Khoo SH, Denning DW: Invasive aspergillosis in patients with AIDS. Clin Infect Dis 19:S41–S48, 1994.
303. Pappas PG, Pottage JC, Powderly WG, et al: Blastomycosis in patients with the acquired immunodeficiency syndrome. Ann Intern Med 116:847–853, 1992.
304. Supparatpinyo K, Chiewchanvit S, Hirunsri P, et al: *Penicillium marneffei* infection in patients infected with human immunodeficiency virus. Clin Infect Dis 14:871–874, 1992.
305. Hilmarsdottir I, Meynard JL, Rogeaux O, et al: Disseminated

*Penicillium marneffei* infection associated with human immunodeficiency virus: A report of two cases and a review of 35 published cases. J Acquir Immune Defic Syndr 6:466–471, 1993.
306. Supparatpinyo K, Khamwan C, Baosoung V, et al: Disseminated *Penicillium marneffei* infection in southeast Asia. Lancet 344:110–113, 1994.
307. Heath TC, Patel A, Fisher D, et al: Disseminated *Penicillium marneffei:* Presenting illness of advanced HIV infection; a clinicopathological review, illustrated by a case report. Pathology 27:101–105, 1995.
308. Remadi S, Lotfi C, Finci V, et al: *Penicillium marneffei* infection in patients infected with the human immunodeficiency virus. A report of two cases. Acta Cytol 39:798–802, 1995.
309. Duong TA: Infection due to *Penicillium marneffei,* an emerging pathogen: Review of 155 reported cases. Clin Infect Dis 23:125–130, 1996.
310. Cooper CR Jr, McGinnis MR: Pathology of *Penicillium marneffei.* An emerging acquired immunodeficiency syndrome–related pathogen. Arch Pathol Lab Med 121:798–804, 1997.
311. Hung CC, Hsueh PR, Chen MY, et al: Invasive infection caused by *Penicillium marneffei:* An emerging pathogen in Taiwan. Clin Infect Dis 26:202–203, 1998.
312. Chariyalertsak S, Sirisanthana T, Supparatpinyo K, et al: Seasonal variation of disseminated *Penicillium marneffei* infections in northern Thailand: A clue to the reservoir? J Infect Dis 173:1490–1493, 1996.
313. Chariyalertsak S, Sirisanthana T, Supparatpinyo K, et al: Case-control study of risk factors for *Penicillium marneffei* infection in human immunodeficiency virus–infected patients in northern Thailand. Clin Infect Dis 24:1080–1086, 1997.
314. Sirisanthana T, Supparatpinyo K, Perriens J, et al: Amphotericin B and itraconazole for treatment of disseminated *Penicillium marneffei* infection in human immunodeficiency virus–infected patients. Clin Infect Dis 26:1107–1110, 1998.
315. Supparatpinyo K, Perriens J, Nelson KE, et al: A controlled trial of itraconazole to prevent relapse of *Penicillium marneffei* infection in patients infected with the human immunodeficiency virus. N Engl J Med 339:1739–1743, 1998.
316. Welch K, Finkbeiner W, Alpers CE, et al: Autopsy findings in the acquired immune deficiency syndrome. JAMA 252:1152–1159, 1984.
317. Wallace JM: Viruses and other miscellaneous organisms. Clin Chest Med 17:745–754, 1996.
318. Millar AB, Patou G, Miller RF, et al: Cytomegalovirus in the lungs of patients with AIDS. Respiratory pathogen or passenger? Am Rev Respir Dis 141:1474–1477, 1990.
319. Rodriguez-Barradas MC, Stool E, Musher DM, et al: Diagnosing and treating cytomegalovirus pneumonia in patients with AIDS. Clin Infect Dis 23:76–81, 1996.
320. Waxman AB, Goldie SJ, Brett-Smith H, Matthay RA: Cytomegalovirus as a primary pulmonary pathogen in AIDS. Chest 111:128–134, 1997.
321. Salomon N, Gomez T, Perlman DC, et al: Clinical features and outcomes of HIV-related cytomegalovirus pneumonia. Aids 11:319–324, 1997.
322. Mintz L, Drew WL, Miner RC, et al: Cytomegalovirus infections in homosexual men. An epidemiological study. Ann Intern Med 99:326–329, 1983.
323. Jacobson MA, Mills J: Serious cytomegalovirus disease in the acquired immunodeficiency syndrome (AIDS). Clinical findings, diagnosis, and treatment. Ann Intern Med 108:585–594, 1988.
324. Miles PR, Baughman RP, Linnemann CC Jr: Cytomegalovirus in the bronchoalveolar lavage fluid of patients with AIDS. Chest 97:1072–1076, 1990.
325. Jacobson MA, Mills J, Rush J, et al: Morbidity and mortality of patients with AIDS and first-episode *Pneumocystis carinii* pneumonia unaffected by concomitant pulmonary cytomegalovirus infection. Am Rev Respir Dis 144:6–9, 1991.
326. Mann M, Shelhamer JH, Masur H, et al: Lack of clinical utility of bronchoalveolar lavage cultures for cytomegalovirus in HIV infection. Am J Respir Crit Care Med 155:1723–1728, 1997.
327. Uberti-Foppa C, Lillo F, Terreni MR, et al: Cytomegalovirus pneumonia in AIDS patients: Value of cytomegalovirus culture from BAL fluid and correlation with lung disease. Chest 113:919–923, 1998.
328. Connolly MG Jr, Baughman RP, Dohn MN, et al: Recovery of viruses other than cytomegalovirus from bronchoalveolar lavage fluid. Chest 105:1775–1781, 1994.
329. Ramsey PG, Fife KH, Hackman RC, et al: Herpes simplex virus pneumonia: Clinical, virologic, and pathologic features in 20 patients. Ann Intern Med 97:813–820, 1982.
330. Fraisse P, Faller M, Rey D, et al: Recurrent varicella pneumonia complicating an endogenous reactivation of chickenpox in an HIV-infected adult patient. Eur Respir J 11:776–778, 1998.
331. Andiman WA, Eastman R, Martin K, et al: Opportunistic lymphoproliferations associated with Epstein-Barr viral DNA in infants and children with AIDS. Lancet 2:1390–1393, 1985.
332. Safrin S, Rush JD, Mills J: Influenza in patients with human immunodeficiency virus infection. Chest 98:33–37, 1990.
332a. Tasker SA, Treanor JJ, Paxton WB, et al: Efficacy of influenza vaccination in HIV-infected persons. A randomized, double-blind, placebo-controlled trial. Ann Intern Med 131:430–433, 1999.
332b. Fuller JD, Craven DE, Steger KA, et al: Influenza vaccination of human immunodeficiency virus (HIV)-infected adults: Impact on plasma levels of HIV type 1 RNA and determinants of antibody response. Clin Infect Dis 28:541–547, 1999.
333. Chayt KJ, Harper ME, Marselle LM, et al: Detection of HTLV-III RNA in lungs of patients with AIDS and pulmonary involvement. JAMA 256:2356–2359, 1986; erratum appears in JAMA 16;257:317, 1987.
334. Linnemann CC Jr, Baughman RP, Frame PT, et al: Recovery of human immunodeficiency virus and detection of p24 antigen in bronchoalveolar lavage fluid from adult patients with AIDS. Chest 96:64–67, 1989.
335. Clarke JR, Krishnan V, Bennett J, et al: Detection of HIV-1 in human lung macrophages using the polymerase chain reaction. AIDS 4:1133–1136, 1990.
336. Oksenhendler E, Cadranel J, Sarfati C, et al: *Toxoplasma gondii* pneumonia in patients with the acquired immunodeficiency syndrome. Am J Med 88:18N–21N, 1990.
337. Schnapp LM, Geaghan SM, Campagna A, et al: *Toxoplasma gondii* pneumonitis in patients infected with the human immunodeficiency virus. Arch Intern Med 152:1073–1077, 1992.
338. Pomeroy C, Filice GA: Pulmonary toxoplasmosis: A review. Clin Infect Dis 14:863–870, 1992.
339. Rabaud C, May T, Lucet JC, et al: Pulmonary toxoplasmosis in patients infected with human immunodeficiency virus: A French National Survey. Clin Infect Dis 23:1249–1254, 1996.
340. Goodman PC, Schnapp LM: Pulmonary toxoplasmosis in AIDS. Radiology 184:791–793, 1992.
341. Torre D, Casari S, Speranza F, et al: Randomized trial of trimethoprim-sulfamethoxazole versus pyrimethamine-sulfadiazine for therapy of toxoplasmic encephalitis in patients with AIDS. Italian Collaborative Study Group. Antimicrob Agents Chemother 42:1346–1349, 1998.
342. Torres RA, Weinberg W, Stansell J, et al: Atovaquone for salvage treatment and suppression of toxoplasmic encephalitis in patients with AIDS. Atovaquone/Toxoplasmic Encephalitis Study Group. Clin Infect Dis 24:422–429, 1997.
343. Forgacs P, Tarshis A, Ma P, et al: Intestinal and bronchial cryptosporidiosis in an immunodeficient homosexual man. Ann Intern Med 99:793–794, 1983.
344. Ma P, Villanueva TG, Kaufman D, et al: Respiratory cryptosporidiosis in the acquired immune deficiency syndrome. Use of modified cold Kinyoun and Hemacolor stains for rapid diagnoses. JAMA 252:1298–1301, 1984.
345. Brady EM, Margolis ML, Korzeniowski OM: Pulmonary cryptosporidiosis in acquired immune deficiency syndrome. JAMA 252:89–90, 1984.
346. Weber R, Kuster H, Keller R, et al: Pulmonary and intestinal microsporidiosis in a patient with the acquired immunodeficiency syndrome. Am Rev Respir Dis 146:1603–1605, 1992.
347. Schwartz DA, Visvesvara GS, Leitch GJ, et al: Pathology of symptomatic microsporidial *(Encephalitozoon hellem)* bronchiolitis in the acquired immunodeficiency syndrome: a new respiratory pathogen diagnosed from lung biopsy, bronchoalveolar lavage, sputum, and tissue culture. Hum Pathol 24:937–943, 1993.
348. Weber R, Kuster H, Visvesvara GS, et al: Disseminated microsporidiosis due to *Encephalitozoon hellem:* Pulmonary coloni-

zation, microhematuria, and mild conjunctivitis in a patient with AIDS. Clin Infect Dis 17:415–419, 1993.
349. Remadi S, Dumais J, Wafa K, et al: Pulmonary microsporidiosis in a patient with the acquired immunodeficiency syndrome. A case report. Acta Cytol 39:1112–1116, 1995.
350. Gunnarsson G, Hurlbut D, DeGirolami PC, et al: Multiorgan microsporidiosis: Report of five cases and review. Clin Infect Dis 21:37–44, 1995.
351. Dore GJ, Marriott DJ, Hing MC, et al: Disseminated microsporidiosis due to *Septata intestinalis* in nine patients infected with the human immunodeficiency virus: Response to therapy with albendazole. Clin Infect Dis 21:70–76, 1995.
352. Meynard JL, Meyohas MC, Binet D, et al: Pulmonary cryptosporidiosis in the acquired immunodeficiency syndrome. Infection 24:328–331, 1996.
353. Clavel A, Arnal AC, Sanchez EC, et al: Respiratory cryptosporidiosis: Case series and review of the literature. Infection 24:341–346, 1996.
354. Maayan S, Wormser GP, Widerhorn J, et al: *Strongyloides stercoralis* hyperinfection in a patient with the acquired immune deficiency syndrome. Am J Med 83:945–948, 1987.
355. Schainberg L, Scheinberg MA: Recovery of *Strongyloides stercoralis* by bronchoalveolar lavage in a patient with acquired immunodeficiency syndrome. Am J Med 87:486, 1989.
356. Kramer MR, Gregg PA, Goldstein M, et al: Disseminated strongyloidiasis in AIDS and non-AIDS immunocompromised hosts: Diagnosis by sputum and bronchoalveolar lavage. South Med J 83:1226–1229, 1990.
357. Harcourt-Webster JN, Scaravilli F, Darwish AH: *Strongyloides stercoralis* hyperinfection in an HIV positive patient. J Clin Pathol 44:346–348, 1991.
358. Gompels MM, Todd J, Peters BS, et al: Disseminated strongyloidiasis in AIDS: Uncommon but important. AIDS 5:329–332, 1991.
359. Makris AN, Sher S, Bertoli C, et al: Pulmonary strongyloidiasis: An unusual opportunistic pneumonia in a patient with AIDS. AJR Am J Roentgenol 161:545–547, 1993.
360. Torres JR, Isturiz R, Murillo J, et al: Efficacy of ivermectin in the treatment of strongyloidiasis complicating AIDS. Clin Infect Dis 17:900–902, 1993.
361. Lessnau KD, Can S, Talavera W: Disseminated *Strongyloides stercoralis* in human immunodeficiency virus–infected patients. Treatment failure and a review of the literature. Chest 104:119–122, 1993.
362. Celedon JC, Mathur-Wagh U, Fox J, et al: Systemic strongyloidiasis in patients infected with the human immunodeficiency virus. A report of 3 cases and review of the literature. Medicine (Baltimore) 73:256–263, 1994.
363. Nomura J, Rekrut K: *Strongyloides stercoralis* hyperinfection syndrome in a patient with AIDS: Diagnosis by fluorescent microscopy. Clin Infect Dis 22:736, 1996.
363a. Ferreira MS, Nishioka S, Borges AS, et al: Strongyloidiasis and infection due to human immunodeficiency virus: 25 cases at a Brazilian teaching hospital, including seven cases of hyperinfection syndrome. Clin Infect Dis 28:154–155, 1999.
364. Lucas SB: Missing infections in AIDS. Trans R Soc Trop Med Hyg 84(Suppl 1):34–38, 1990.
365. Biggar RJ, Burnett W, Mikl J, et al: Cancer among New York men at risk of acquired immunodeficiency syndrome. Int J Cancer 43:979–985, 1989.
366. Chang Y, Cesarman E, Pessin MS, et al: Identification of herpesvirus-like DNA sequences in AIDS-associated Kaposi's sarcoma. Science 266:1865–1869, 1994.
367. Moore PS, Chang Y: Detection of herpesvirus-like DNA sequences in Kaposi's sarcoma in patients with and without HIV infection. N Engl J Med 332:1181–1185, 1995.
368. Huang L, Schnapp LM, Gruden JF, et al: Presentation of AIDS-related pulmonary Kaposi's sarcoma diagnosed by bronchoscopy. Am J Respir Crit Care Med 153:1385–1390, 1996.
369. Gruden JF, Huang L, Webb WR, et al: AIDS-related Kaposi sarcoma of the lung: Radiographic findings and staging system with bronchoscopic correlation. Radiology 195:545–552, 1995.
370. Pluda JM, Yarchoan R, Jaffe ES, et al: Development of non-Hodgkin lymphoma in a cohort of patients with severe human immunodeficiency virus (HIV) infection on long-term antiretroviral therapy. Ann Intern Med 113:276–282, 1990.
371. Eisner MD, Kaplan LD, Herndier B, et al: The pulmonary manifestations of AIDS-related non-Hodgkin's lymphoma. Chest 110:729–736, 1996.
372. Goodman PC: Non-Hodgkin's lymphoma in the acquired immunodeficiency syndrome. J Thorac Imaging 6:49–52, 1991.
373. Judson MA, Sahn SA: Endobronchial lesions in HIV-infected individuals. Chest 105:1314–1323, 1994.
374. Keys TC, Judson MA, Reed CE, et al: Endobronchial HIV associated lymphoma. Thorax 49:525–526, 1994.
375. Sider L, Horton ES: Pleural effusion as a presentation of AIDS-related lymphoma. Invest Radiol 24:150–153, 1989.
376. Kaplan LD, Abrams DI, Feigal E, et al: AIDS-associated non-Hodgkin's lymphoma in San Francisco. JAMA 261:719–724, 1989.
377. Knowles DM, Chamulak GA, Subar M, et al: Lymphoid neoplasia associated with the acquired immunodeficiency syndrome (AIDS). The New York University Medical Center experience with 105 patients (1981–1986). Ann Intern Med 108:744–753, 1988.
378. Kaplan LD, Straus DJ, Testa MA, et al: Low-dose compared with standard-dose m-BACOD chemotherapy for non-Hodgkin's lymphoma associated with human immunodeficiency virus infection. National Institute of Allergy and Infectious Diseases AIDS Clinical Trials Group. N Engl J Med 336:1641–1648, 1997.
379. Fajac I, Cadranel JL, Mariette X, et al: Pulmonary Hodgkin's disease in HIV-infected patient. Diagnosis by bronchoalveolar lavage. Chest 102:1913–1914, 1992.
380. Remick SC: Lung cancer. An HIV-related neoplasm or a coincidental finding? Chest 102:1643–1644, 1992.
381. Fraire AE, Awe RJ: Lung cancer in association with human immunodeficiency virus infection. Cancer 70:432–436, 1992.
382. Sridhar KS, Flores MR, Raub WA Jr, et al: Lung cancer in patients with human immunodeficiency virus infection compared with historic control subjects. Chest 102:1704–1708, 1992.
383. Karp J, Profeta G, Marantz PR, et al: Lung cancer in patients with immunodeficiency syndrome. Chest 103:410–413, 1993.
384. Chan TK, Aranda CP, Rom WN: Bronchogenic carcinoma in young patients at risk for acquired immunodeficiency syndrome. Chest 103:862–864, 1993.
385. Tenholder MF, Jackson HD: Bronchogenic carcinoma in patients seropositive for human immunodeficiency virus. Chest 104:1049–1053, 1993.
386. Aaron SD, Warner E, Edelson JD: Bronchogenic carcinoma in patients seropositive for human immunodeficiency virus. Chest 106:640–642, 1994.
387. Parker MS, Leveno DM, Campbell TJ, et al: AIDS-related bronchogenic carcinoma: Fact or fiction? Chest 113:154–161, 1998.
388. Johnson CC, Wilcosky T, Kvale P, et al: Cancer incidence among an HIV-infected cohort. Pulmonary Complications of HIV Infection Study Group. Am J Epidemiol 146:470–475, 1997.
389. Braun MA, Killam DA, Remick SC, et al: Lung cancer in patients seropositive for human immunodeficiency virus. Radiology 175:341–343, 1990.
390. White CS, Haramati LB, Elder KH, et al: Carcinoma of the lung in HIV-positive patients: Findings on chest radiographs and CT scans. AJR Am J Roentgenol 164:593–597, 1995.
391. Fishman JE, Schwartz DS, Sais GJ, et al: Bronchogenic carcinoma in HIV-positive patients: Findings on chest radiographs and CT scans. AJR Am J Roentgenol 164:57–61, 1995.
392. Gruden JF, Webb WR, Yao DC, et al: Bronchogenic carcinoma in 13 patients infected with the human immunodeficiency virus (HIV): Clinical and radiographic findings. J Thorac Imaging 10:99–105, 1995.
393. Thurer RJ, Jacobs JP, Holland FW 2nd, et al: Surgical treatment of lung cancer in patients with human immunodeficiency virus. Ann Thorac Surg 60:599–602, 1995.
394. Carrington C, Liebow A: Lymphocytic interstitial pneumonia. Am J Pathol 48:36, 1966.
395. Schneider RF: Lymphocytic interstitial pneumonitis and nonspecific interstitial pneumonitis. Clin Chest Med 17:763–766, 1996.
396. Joshi VV, Oleske JM, Minnefor AB, et al: Pathology of suspected acquired immune deficiency syndrome in children: A study of eight cases. Pediatr Pathol 2:71–87, 1984.
397. Grieco MH, Chinoy-Acharya P: Lymphocytic interstitial pneumonia associated with the acquired immune deficiency syndrome. Am Rev Respir Dis 131:952–955, 1985.

398. Solal-Celigny P, Couderc LJ, Herman D, et al: Lymphoid interstitial pneumonitis in acquired immunodeficiency syndrome-related complex. Am Rev Respir Dis 131:956–960, 1985.
399. Morris JC, Rosen MJ, Marchevsky A, et al: Lymphocytic interstitial pneumonia in patients at risk for the acquired immune deficiency syndrome. Chest 91:63–67, 1987.
400. Itescu S, Brancato LJ, Buxbaum J, et al: A diffuse infiltrative CD8 lymphocytosis syndrome in human immunodeficiency virus (HIV) infection: A host immune response associated with HLA-DR5. Ann Intern Med 112:3–10, 1990.
401. Oldham SA, Castillo M, Jacobson FL, et al: HIV-associated lymphocytic interstitial pneumonia: Radiologic manifestations and pathologic correlation. Radiology 170:83–87, 1989.
402. Conces DJ Jr, Tarver RD: Noninfectious and nonmalignant pulmonary disease in AIDS. J Thorac Imaging 6:53–59, 1991.
403. Carignan S, Staples CA, Muller NL: Intrathoracic lymphoproliferative disorders in the immunocompromised patient: CT findings. Radiology 197:53–58, 1995.
404. McGuinness G, Scholes JV, Jagirdar JS, et al: Unusual lymphoproliferative disorders in nine adults with HIV or AIDS: CT and pathologic findings. Radiology 197:59–65, 1995.
405. Travis WD, Pittaluga S, Lipschik GY, et al: Atypical pathologic manifestations of *Pneumocystis carinii* pneumonia in the acquired immune deficiency syndrome. Review of 123 lung biopsies from 76 patients with emphasis on cysts, vascular invasion, vasculitis, and granulomas. Am J Surg Pathol 14:615–625, 1990.
406. Saldana MJ, Mones JM: Pulmonary pathology in AIDS: Atypical *Pneumocystis carinii* infection and lymphoid interstitial pneumonia. Thorax 49:S46–S55, 1994.
407. Suffredini AF, Ognibene FP, Lack EE, et al: Nonspecific interstitial pneumonitis: a common cause of pulmonary disease in the acquired immunodeficiency syndrome. Ann Intern Med 107:7–13, 1987.
408. Ognibene FP, Masur H, Rogers P, et al: Nonspecific interstitial pneumonitis without evidence of *Pneumocystis carinii* in asymptomatic patients infected with human immunodeficiency virus (HIV). Ann Intern Med 109:874–879, 1988.
409. Griffiths MH, Miller RF, Semple SJ: Interstitial pneumonitis in patients infected with the human immunodeficiency virus. Thorax 50:1141–1146, 1995.
410. Sattler F, Nichols L, Hirano L, et al: Nonspecific interstitial pneumonitis mimicking *Pneumocystis carinii* pneumonia. Am J Respir Crit Care Med 156:912–917, 1997.
411. Simmons JT, Suffredini AF, Lack EE, et al: Nonspecific interstitial pneumonitis in patients with AIDS: Radiologic features. AJR Am J Roentgenol 149:265–268, 1987.
412. Travis WD, Fox CH, Devaney KO, et al: Lymphoid pneumonitis in 50 adult patients infected with the human immunodeficiency virus: Lymphocytic interstitial pneumonitis versus nonspecific interstitial pneumonitis. Hum Pathol 23:529–541, 1992.
413. Rosen MJ, Lou Y, Kvale PA, et al: Pulmonary function tests in HIV-infected patients without AIDS. Pulmonary Complications of HIV Infection Study Group. Am J Respir Crit Care Med 152:738–745, 1995.
414. O'Donnell CR, Bader MB, Zibrak JD, et al: Abnormal airway function in individuals with the acquired immunodeficiency syndrome. Chest 94:945–948, 1988.
415. Lin RY, Lazarus TS: Asthma and related atopic disorders in outpatients attending an urban HIV clinic. Ann Allergy Asthma Immunol 74:510–515, 1995.
416. Verghese A, al-Samman M, Nabhan D, et al: Bacterial bronchitis and bronchiectasis in human immunodeficiency virus infection. Arch Intern Med 154:2086–2091, 1994.
417. McGuinness G, Gruden JF, Bhalla M, et al: AIDS-related airway disease. AJR Am J Roentgenol 168:67–77, 1997.
418. Bard M, Couderc LJ, Saimot AG, et al: Accelerated obstructive pulmonary disease in HIV infected patients with bronchiectasis. Eur Respir J 11:771–775, 1998.
419. Diaz PT, Clanton TL, Pacht ER: Emphysema-like pulmonary disease associated with human immunodeficiency virus infection. Ann Intern Med 116:124–128, 1992.
419a. Diaz PT, King MA, Pacht ER, et al: The pathophysiology of pulmonary diffusion impairment in human immunodeficiency virus infection. Am J Respir Crit Care Med 160:272–277, 1999.
420. Goldsmith GH Jr, Baily RG, Brettler DB, et al: Primary pulmonary hypertension in patients with classic hemophilia. Ann Intern Med 108:797–799, 1988.
421. Himelman RB, Dohrmann M, Goodman P, et al: Severe pulmonary hypertension and cor pulmonale in the acquired immunodeficiency syndrome. Am J Cardiol 64:1396–1399, 1989.
422. Coplan NL, Shimony RY, Ioachim HL, et al: Primary pulmonary hypertension associated with human immunodeficiency viral infection. Am J Med 89:96–99, 1990.
423. Legoux B, Piette AM, Bouchet PF, et al: Pulmonary hypertension and HIV infection. Am J Med 89:122, 1990.
424. Speich R, Jenni R, Opravil M, et al: Primary pulmonary hypertension in HIV infection. Chest 100:1268–1271, 1991.
425. Rhodes J, Schiller MS, Montoya CH, et al: Severe pulmonary hypertension without significant pulmonary parenchymal disease in a pediatric patient with acquired immunodeficiency syndrome. Clin Pediatr (Phila) 31:629–631, 1992.
426. Jacques C, Richmond G, Tierney L, et al: Primary pulmonary hypertension and human immunodeficiency virus infection in a non-hemophiliac man. Hum Pathol 23:191–194, 1992.
427. Mette SA, Palevsky HI, Pietra GG, et al: Primary pulmonary hypertension in association with human immunodeficiency virus infection. A possible viral etiology for some forms of hypertensive pulmonary arteriopathy. Am Rev Respir Dis 145:1196–1200, 1992.
428. Polos PG, Wolfe D, Harley RA, et al: Pulmonary hypertension and human immunodeficiency virus infection. Two reports and a review of the literature. Chest 101:474–478, 1992.
429. Diaz PT, Clanton TL: Marked pulmonary function abnormalities in a case of HIV-associated pulmonary hypertension. Chest 104:313–315, 1993.
430. Mani S, Smith GJ: HIV and pulmonary hypertension: A review. South Med J 87:357–362, 1994.
431. Petitpretz P, Brenot F, Azarian R, et al: Pulmonary hypertension in patients with human immunodeficiency virus infection. Comparison with primary pulmonary hypertension. Circulation 89:2722–2727, 1994.
432. de Chadarevian JP, Lischner HW, Karmazin N, et al: Pulmonary hypertension and HIV infection: New observations and review of the syndrome. Mod Pathol 7:685–689, 1994.
433. Weiss JR, Pietra GG, Scharf SM: Primary pulmonary hypertension and the human immunodeficiency virus. Report of two cases and a review of the literature. Arch Intern Med 155:2350–2354, 1995.
434. Morse JH, Barst RJ, Itescu S, et al: Primary pulmonary hypertension in HIV infection: An outcome determined by particular HLA class II alleles. Am J Respir Crit Care Med 153:1299–1301, 1996.
435. Cool CD, Kennedy D, Voelkel NF, et al: Pathogenesis and evolution of plexiform lesions in pulmonary hypertension associated with scleroderma and human immunodeficiency virus infection. Hum Pathol 28:434–442, 1997.
436. Mesa RA, Edell ES, Dunn WF, et al: Human immunodeficiency virus infection and pulmonary hypertension: Two new cases and a review of 86 reported cases. Mayo Clin Proc 73:37–45, 1998.
437. Humbert M, Monti G, Fartouckh M, et al: Platelet-derived growth factor expression in primary pulmonary hypertension: Comparison of HIV seropositive and HIV seronegative patients. Eur Respir J 11:554–559, 1998.
438. Ruben FL, Talamo TS: Secondary pulmonary alveolar proteinosis occurring in two patients with acquired immune deficiency syndrome. Am J Med 80:1187–1190, 1986.
439. Tran Van Nhieu J, Vojtek AM, Bernaudin JF, et al: Pulmonary alveolar proteinosis associated with *Pneumocystis carinii*. Ultrastructural identification in bronchoalveolar lavage in AIDS and immunocompromised non-AIDS patients. Chest 98:801–805, 1990.
440. Askin FB, Katzenstein AL: Pneumocystis infection masquerading as diffuse alveolar damage: A potential source of diagnostic error. Chest 79:420–422, 1981.
441. Ramaswamy G, Jagadha V, Tchertkoff V: Diffuse alveolar damage and interstitial fibrosis in acquired immunodeficiency syndrome patients without concurrent pulmonary infection. Arch Pathol Lab Med 109:408–412, 1985.
442. Allen JN, Wewers MD: HIV-associated bronchiolitis obliterans organizing pneumonia. Chest 96:197–198, 1989.

443. Leo YS, Pitchon HE, Messler G, et al: Bronchiolitis obliterans organizing pneumonia in a patient with AIDS. Clin Infect Dis 18:921–924, 1994.
444. Sanito NJ, Morley TF, Condoluci DV: Bronchiolitis obliterans organizing pneumonia in an AIDS patient. Eur Respir J 8:1021–1024, 1995.
445. Zahraa J, Herold B, Abrahams C, et al: Bronchiolitis obliterans organizing pneumonia in a child with acquired immunodeficiency syndrome. Pediatr Infect Dis J 15:448–451, 1996.
446. Semenzato G: Immunology of interstitial lung diseases: Cellular events taking place in the lung of sarcoidosis, hypersensitivity pneumonitis and HIV infection. Eur Respir J 4:94–102, 1991.
447. Coots LE, Lazarus AA: Sarcoidosis diagnosed in a patient with known HIV infection. Chest 96:201–202, 1989.
448. Lowery WS, Whitlock WL, Dietrich RA, et al: Sarcoidosis complicated by HIV infection: Three case reports and a review of the literature. Am Rev Respir Dis 142:887–889, 1990.
449. Amin DN, Sperber K, Brown LK, et al: Positive Kveim test in patients with coexisting sarcoidosis and human immunodeficiency virus infection. Chest 101:1454–1456, 1992.
450. Newman TG, Minkowitz S, Hanna A, et al: Coexistent sarcoidosis and HIV infection. A comparison of bronchoalveolar and peripheral blood lymphocytes. Chest 102:1899–1901, 1992.
450a. Naccache JM, Antoine M, Wislex M, et al: Sarcoid-like pulmonary disorder in human immunodeficiency virus-infected patients receiving antiretroviral therapy. Am J Respir Crit Care Med 159:2009–2013, 1999.
450b. Morris AM, Nishimura S, Huang L: Hypersensitivity pneumonitis in an HIV-infected woman. Thorax, in press.

# 83 Pulmonary Complications of Organ Transplantation and Primary Immunodeficiencies

STEVEN R. DUNCAN, M.D. • THOMAS A. RAFFIN, M.D.

Introduction
Overview of Immune Defenses
- Immune Responses to Extracellular Bacteria
- Immune Responses to Intracellular Bacteria
- Immune Responses to Viruses

Allogeneic Organ Transplantation
- General Aspects
- Early Infectious Complications
- Complications 1 to 6 Months After Transplantation
- Late Complications

Primary Immunodeficiencies
Disorders of Immunoglobulin Production
- X-Linked Agammaglobulinemia
- Common Variable Immunodeficiency
- Selective Immunoglobulin Defects
- Hypogammaglobulinemia with Hyperimmunoglobulin M
- Rare Miscellaneous Immunoglobulin Deficiencies

Complement Deficiencies
Abnormalities of Phagocytes
- Inadequate Numbers of Granulocytes
- Chronic Granulomatous Disease
- Chédiak-Higashi Syndrome
- Leukocyte Adhesion Defects
- Job's Syndrome

Defects of Cellular Immunity
- DiGeorge's Syndrome
- Purine Nucleoside Phosphorylase Deficiency
- Severe Combined Immunodeficiency Disorders
- Ataxia-Telangiectasia
- Wiskott-Aldrich Syndrome

Summary

## INTRODUCTION

Preservation of normal respiratory tract function depends on complex homeostatic mechanisms that neutralize and eliminate an extremely diverse range of potential pathogens. Although physical barriers and other mechanical properties (e.g., airway angulation and secretions, ciliary clearance) subserve important protective functions (see Chapter 15), the critical role of immunologic defenses is attested by the frequency of respiratory tract infections in persons with deficient immune responses. The most dramatic and prevalent examples of pulmonary complications due to immune dysfunction are seen among patients with advanced human immunodeficiency virus (HIV) infection, discussed fully in Chapter 82. In a growing number of cases, the underlying failure of immune mechanisms is an adverse complication of modern medical interventions, including the use of global immunosuppressive agents that are necessary to prevent allograft rejection. Finally, a small number of persons have inherent genetic abnormalities that result in defects in one or more components of the immune system.

The management of pulmonary problems associated with immunodeficiencies is a challenging task for clinicians. Diagnostic accuracy is necessary for successful treatment of these complications, because mistreatment results in a high probability for rapid and fatal progression. Noninvasive clinical assessments are confounded by the broad range of potential pathogens, particularly among patients with defects of cellular immunity. Moreover, diverse infections in these patients often have overlapping or atypical presentations, and they cannot reliably be discriminated by noninvasive methods or distinguished from noninfectious pulmonary complications.[1] The potential diversity of possible pathogens, each requiring specific and potentially toxic antimicrobial therapy, confounds or precludes all-encompassing empirical treatments. Consequently, management of immunodeficient patients with pulmonary problems often requires definitive diagnosis by invasive specimen acquisition, through fine-needle aspiration, thoracoscopy, open thoracotomy, or fiberoptic bronchoscopy.[1a]

Despite the limitations of noninvasive assessments, the ability to deduce the most likely cause of pulmonary dysfunction in an immunodeficient patient is of immeasurable value in the design of diagnostic approaches and treatment options. In general, the most probable infectious agents can often be reasonably estimated by knowledge of the specific underlying immune defect and, among transplant recipients in particular, by understanding of the temporally defined range of pathogens.

The first section of this chapter briefly reviews selected aspects of immune defenses with important clinical relevance for the management of pulmonary complications in immunodeficient patients. The following section is an overview of infectious and noninfectious complications of transplantation procedures other than bone marrow or lung allografts (which are described in Chapter 86 and Chapter 97, respectively). The final section of this chapter discusses primary deficiencies of immunity, emphasizing disorders that are notable for the prominence of their pulmonary complications and the prototypic examples in which the defect is especially illustrative of immune functions. Although patients with primary immunodeficiencies are seldom seen outside referral centers and are most often encountered initially in pediatric practices, the study of these disorders has not only resulted in more effective treatments and increased survival of these patients but has also yielded valuable insights into cellular and molecular mechanisms of the immune system.

## OVERVIEW OF IMMUNE DEFENSES

Although a detailed and definitive description of the field of immunology is beyond the scope and purpose of this discussion (see Chapter 17), a rudimentary understanding of defense mechanisms against pathogenic microbes facilitates clinical management of immunodeficient patients. For purposes of illustration and discussion, the various components of the immune system are presented as isolated entities. As should be readily apparent, however, immune elements are notable for their high degree of complex synergies and intricate regulatory interactions. Consequently, defects in one arm of the immune system may result in multiple dysfunctions that disable a broad range of defense mechanisms.

Responses to foreign substances, including components of microbial pathogens in respiratory or other tissues, can be initiated by either innate (natural) or specific (cognate or acquired) mechanisms. *Innate defenses* do not require previous exposures, are not enhanced by multiple exposures to the same agent, and, for the most part, do not discriminate among diverse foreign substances. Examples of innate defenses include phagocytosis of foreign particles (including microbes) by macrophages, dendritic cells, and granulocytes; complement activation by binding on the surface of infectious organisms (alternative pathway); and nonspecific lysis of virally infected cells by natural killer (NK) cells.

In contrast, *specific immune mechanisms* are stimulated by exposure to a particular molecular component of a foreign substance (an antigen), and the responses are augmented by repeated exposures to that distinct antigen (immunization). Specific immunity is mediated by lymphocytes. Each lymphocyte bears a unique surface receptor, either an immunoglobulin (on B cells) or an antigen receptor (on T cells), that has a limited range of specificities against microbial or other antigens. This receptor specificity is determined by random combinatorial rearrangements of genes encoding variable (V), diversity (D), and joining (J) segments of the receptors during lymphocyte maturation.[2] Although any particular lymphocyte has limited antigen specificity, the large number of these cells, each with a randomly constructed receptor, ensures that each individual has a repertoire that covers an enormous potential range of antigens. Under appropriate conditions, stimulation of these surface receptors by specific antigen binding and cross-linking results in activation and clonal proliferation of the lymphocyte. These clonal expansions produce a large number of effector cells with activity against the particular antigen, as well as a subpopulation of relatively quiescent "memory cells" that are available to respond promptly to subsequent challenge with the same antigen. For purposes of description, the specific immune system is typically further subdivided into *humoral defense,* consisting of antibody elaboration by B lymphocytes, and *cell-mediated immunity,* which is generally used to denote responses of T lymphocytes.

### Immune Responses to Extracellular Bacteria

A broad range of bacteria capable of reproduction outside host cells are important pathogens of the respiratory tract; these include the pyogenic gram-positive cocci *Streptococcus* and *Staphylococcus,* gram-negative bacilli (Enterobacteriaceae, *Haemophilus, Proteus,* and *Pseudomonas*), and various anaerobic bacteria (*Bacteroides, Fusobacterium,* and anaerobic streptococci).

Microbial engulfment and killing by cytotoxic products of phagocytes (e.g., lysosomal enzymes, reactive oxygen and nitrogen species) are first lines of defense against extracellular bacteria[3] (Fig. 83.1). In addition to these direct effector responses, phagocytic cells elaborate a variety of cytokines, such as interferon-alpha (IFN-$\alpha$), tumor necrosis factor-alpha (TNF-$\alpha$), interleukin (IL)-1, IL-6, and IL-8, that both recruit and activate other in-

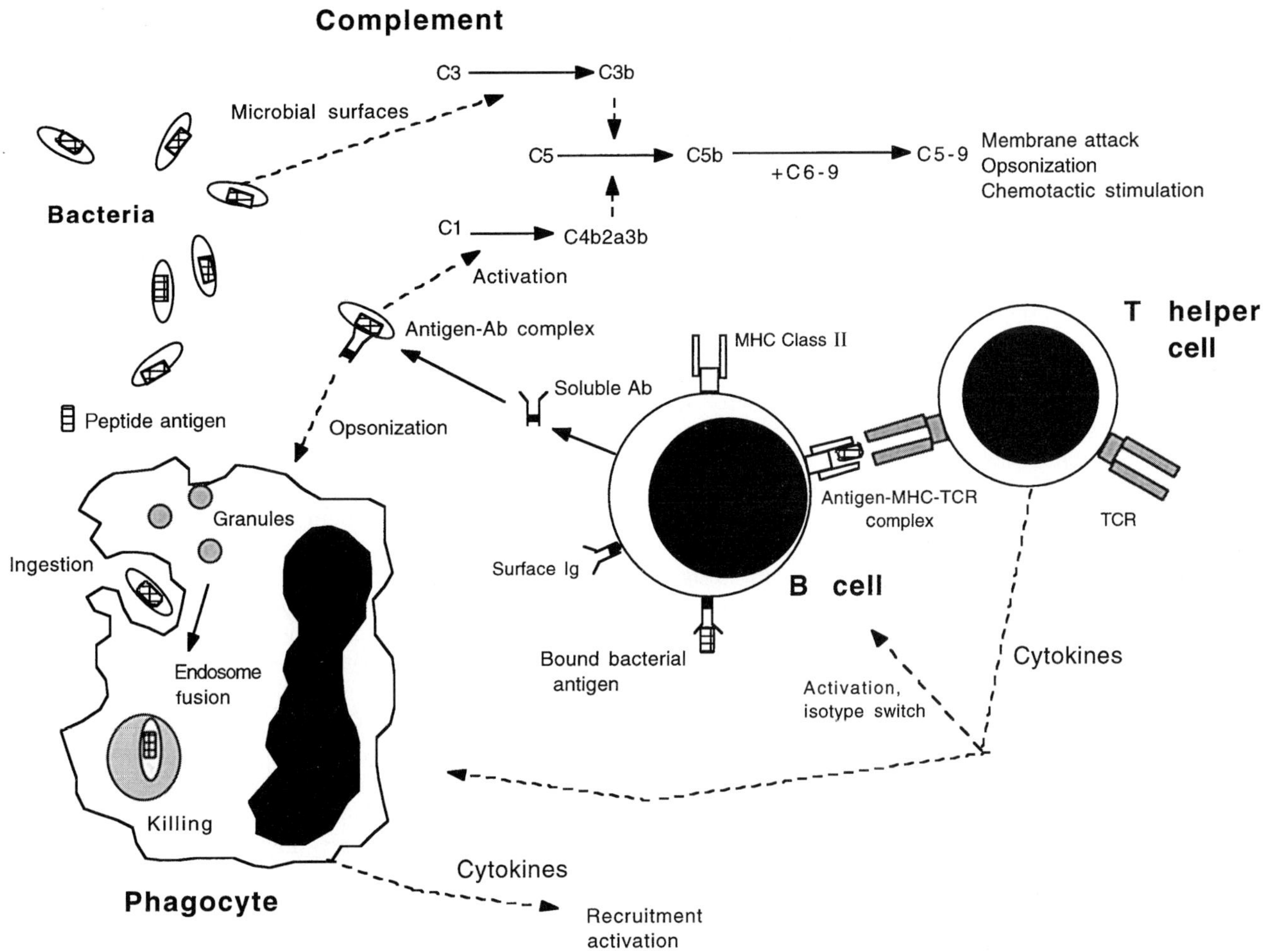


**Figure 83.1** Immune responses to extracellular bacteria. Microbes undergo lysis and opsonization and attract immune effector cells (chemotaxis) through direct activation of complement by surface components. Phagocytes ingest and kill bacteria by enzymatic digestion, iron and metabolite depletion, and generation of oxygen and nitrogen reactive reductive products. Phagocytosis is facilitated by opsonization with antibodies produced by B cells. Other defensive functions of antibodies include neutralization and complement activation. Antibody production is enhanced by cognate interactions between B and T helper cells (usually $CD4^+$ cells), and by cytokine elaboration by the latter. Various cytokines produced by T cells and phagocytes are proinflammatory, with activating and chemotactic functions. Dotted lines denote positive feedback mechanisms. Ab = antibody; MHC = major histocompatibility complex; Ig = immunoglobulin; TCR = T-cell antigen receptor.

flammatory cells and mediate systemic effects of infection (e.g., fever, cachexia, sepsis).[4] Another potent innate defense against these organisms is activation of complement by bacterial cell wall components, notably peptidoglycans of gram-positive cocci and gram-negative bacillary lipopolysaccharides, which results in formation of opsonizing (phagocytosis-enhancing), lytic, and chemotactic end products.[5]

The most important component of specific immune defense against extracellular bacteria is the elaboration of antibodies. Bacterial cell wall polysaccharides and lipids, as well as microbial nucleic acids, are capable of polyclonal binding to and cross-linking of surface-bound immunoglobulins on a large number of B cells.[6] Despite the absence of specific T-cell help, these activated B lymphocytes undergo a series of ordered growth and differentiation steps leading to proliferation of daughter progeny that now secrete the unique immunoglobulins (antibody) determined by the gene rearrangements of the stimulated cells. The end result is a strong and often effective production of pentameric immunoglobulin M (IgM) antibodies with avidity against the microbial antigens.

These antibodies, in turn, help neutralize cell adhesive functions of bacteria by binding and steric hindrance of specific microbial receptors; they also activate complement by the classic pathway, with resultant bactericidal effects described previously. In at least some cases, B cells activated by polyclonal stimulation are capable of undergoing isotype switching by cytokines elaborated by other immune effectors, resulting in production of antibodies with additional opsonification and microbicidal effects. The daughter progeny of B lymphocytes stimulated with polyclonal (T cell–independent) activators do not, however, develop into memory cells capable of effecting rapid and augmented secondary immune responses with antigen reexposure.

T helper cells (usually $CD4^+$) are capable of enhancing the effectiveness of humoral responses by facilitating antibody production of B lymphocytes (see Fig. 83.1). T cells, unlike B lymphocytes, are stimulated only by peptides. After ingestion and partial catabolism, microbial peptides are externally presented by the major histocompatibility (MHC) molecules (usually MHC class II) of antigen-presenting cells. Activated mononuclear phagocytes and B cells are capable of presenting antigens to T cells, although dendritic cells are even more effective at antigen presentation.[7] T cells bearing antigen receptors with avidity to the specific peptide-MHC complex become stimulated to undergo proliferation, again resulting in large pools of effector and memory lymphocytes. Activated T helper cells are potent stimulators of B cells by direct physical contacts (cognate interactions) and by elaboration of T helper type 2 (Th2) cytokines (IL-4, IL-5, IL-6, and TNF).[8] Both cognate T cell–B cell interactions and, to a lesser extent, Th2 cytokines, promote increased antibody production by B cells, development of memory B cells, and isotype switching of antibody from IgM to dimeric IgG (and in some cases IgA and IgE). Even though antigenic specificities of the IgM and IgG antibodies are unchanged by the isotype switch, the latter immunoglobulin is a more effective antimicrobial that, in addition to activating complement, is capable of opsonizing bacteria and triggering target cell lysis by NK cells (known as antibody-dependent cell-mediated cytotoxicity [ADCC]).

## Immune Responses to Intracellular Bacteria

A number of microbes that survive and proliferate in eukaryotic host cells are important pathogens of the respiratory tract, including diverse bacteria (e.g., *Mycobacterium, Mycoplasma, Legionella, Chlamydia*) and several fungi (e.g., *Coccidioides, Histoplasma*). The hallmark of these pathogens is their ability to resist intracellular killing after engulfment by phagocytes. Moreover, in many cases the development of antibody responses does little to alter the course of these infections and does not confer protection against reinfection. The difficulty with which the intracellular organisms are eliminated accounts for their frequent chronic and recrudescent manifestations.

Cell-mediated immune responses are the primary defense against intracellular pathogens (Fig. 83.2). T cells with specificity against microbial peptides become activated after engagements with the peptide-MHC complex presented by antigen-presenting cells, as described previously. $CD4^+$ T cells recognize soluble microbial peptides that are presented by MHC class II molecules, whereas $CD8^+$ T cells recognize intracellular microbial peptides in the context of MHC class I. Although both T-cell subsets are important in these responses, the respective roles of the subtypes are not certain. Subsequently, T cells elaborate the Th1 cytokines IL-2, IFN-γ, TNF, and leukotriene.[8] The net result is comparable to a delayed-type hypersensitivity reaction (e.g., positive tuberculin test), with accumulations of successive waves of neutrophils, T cells, and monocytes and localized edema resulting from loss of capillary integrity and fibrin deposition.[9] Under the influence of extracellular matrix proteins and proinflammatory cytokines, and in particular IFN-γ, local monocytes and macrophages undergo a complex series of transcriptionally regulated changes that result in their activation. Activated macrophages have greatly augmented microbicidal capabilities[3] and are ultimately the effector cell in defense against intracellular pathogens. Despite often intense reactions, however, in many cases the pathogens are not completely eradicated, owing to microbial resistance or limited host responses. Chronic stimulation, activation, and effector responses result in granulomas, which are composed of foci of activated macrophages, or more injurious lesions such as granulomatous inflammation with attendant necrosis and fibrosis.

## Immune Responses to Viruses

As was the case with intracellular bacteria, the innate immune system plays little if any significant role in responses to viral infections. The first important line of defense against respiratory tract viruses are specifically avid neutralizing antibodies in secretions (IgA) that bind to and hinder viral adherence receptors. Early infections can be countered by specific antiviral IgG molecules that act to neutralize and opsonize virions, and the effectiveness of these responses is the basis for therapeutic immunizations.

Effective eradication of established, intracellular viral infections depends on cellular immune mechanisms (Fig. 83.3). Responses similar to those of delayed-type hypersensitivity reaction, as described in the preceding section, occur with activation of T cells bearing antigen receptors against viral-peptide-MHC complexes. Nonetheless, the most important cellular immune response against virus-infected cells is mounted by cytolytic T lymphocytes. Cytolytic T cells, which are primarily $CD8^+$, are activated by direct contact with specific, endogenously synthesized viral peptides presented by MHC class I molecules of infected cells. Although $CD4^+$ T cells are only rarely cytolytic per se, they too subserve important roles in viral defenses by cytokine elaborations that facilitate activation and differentiation of cytolytic precursors. Cytolytic T cells kill by exocytosis of granules containing a membrane pore–forming enzyme and by induction of apoptosis through engagements of Fas on target cells.[10] This killing, although fratricidal and often a significant cause of the tissue injury that occurs with infection, acts to disrupt viral maturation and replication.

# ALLOGENEIC ORGAN TRANSPLANTATION

## General Aspects

Modern immunosuppressive regimens for allogeneic transplant recipients were developed to counter rejection

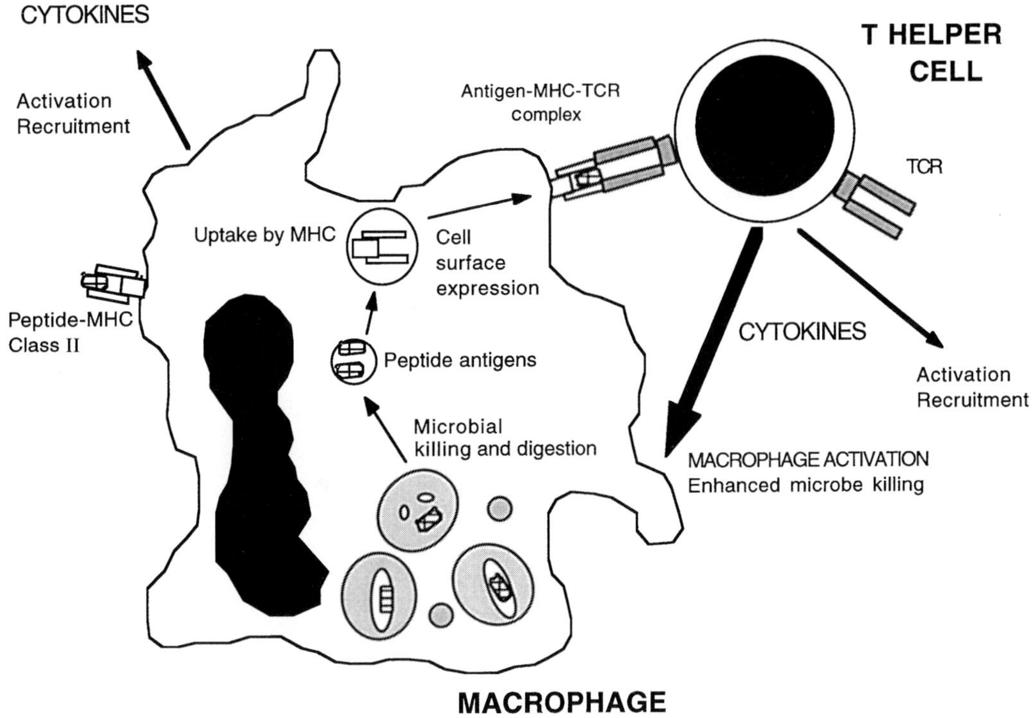


**Figure 83.2** Immune defenses to intracellular bacteria. Macrophages engulf and digest microbes, particularly after opsonization by antibodies and complement (see Fig. 83.1). Bacterial peptide antigens from digests are incorporated into major histocompatibility complex (MHC) class II molecules undergoing assembly. The interactions of peptide-MHC complexes with specific T-cell receptors (TCR) on T helper cells results in elaboration of activating cytokines, particularly interferon-gamma (IFN-$\gamma$), which greatly augment the microbicidal functions of macrophages. Other cytokines released by these cells have diverse proinflammatory effects.

responses directed against foreign MHC molecules by cellular immune mechanisms.[11] Because the precursor frequency of potentially alloreactive T cells is so high,[12] these responses are far stronger than those against most other foreign antigens, particularly antigens of microbial origin. Accordingly, allograft viability can be sustained only at the expense of complicated and intense treatments that severely impair cellular immunity.[13] As outlined in preceding sections, cell-mediated responses play central roles in defenses against virtually all classes of microbial pathogens and are the sole effective counters to intracellular bacterial and viral infections. Allograft recipients are among the most severely immunocompromised patients encountered in clinical practice; depending on the intensity of their rejection therapies, they are at risk for almost the entire range of respiratory tract pathogens. In early series, before the advent of more effective preventive and diagnostic techniques, pulmonary infections occurred in almost half of allograft recipients and accounted for or contributed to 50% to 80% of the mortality in these populations. As many as half of these deaths were caused by opportunistic pathogens.[14–19]

Not only are pulmonary infections more varied and more virulent in transplant recipients, but the host response is so atypical that the usual clinical features are often nonspecific or otherwise confounded by coexistent pulmonary abnormalities. As a notable example, radiographic characteristics of pneumonitis, so often central in the diagnosis of other pulmonary disorders, are almost typically nondiscriminatory among transplant recipients.[20–24] In some other immunosuppressed populations, notably those with isolated deficiencies of granulocytes (e.g., acute nonlymphocytic leukemia), infections are limited almost exclusively to a comparatively small spectrum of pathogens, and initial reliance on empirical therapy may be justified.[20, 25] In contrast, because patients with severe defects of cellular immunity (including transplant recipients) are at risk for serious infections with varied or often multiple organisms having nonspecific features,[26, 27] most experienced clinicians maintain a very low threshold for early use of definitive, albeit invasive, diagnostic modalities.

Perhaps the most useful tool for the initial assessment of pulmonary complications in these patients is awareness of the posttransplantation intervals during which each of the distinct problems tends to be most prevalent (Fig. 83.4). This timetable is remarkably similar, at least in general details, among the many different solid organ transplantation procedures.[28] Although reference to these outlines should not supplant appropriate diagnostic procedures, clinicians armed with an appreciation for the relative likelihood of the potential problems can more wisely

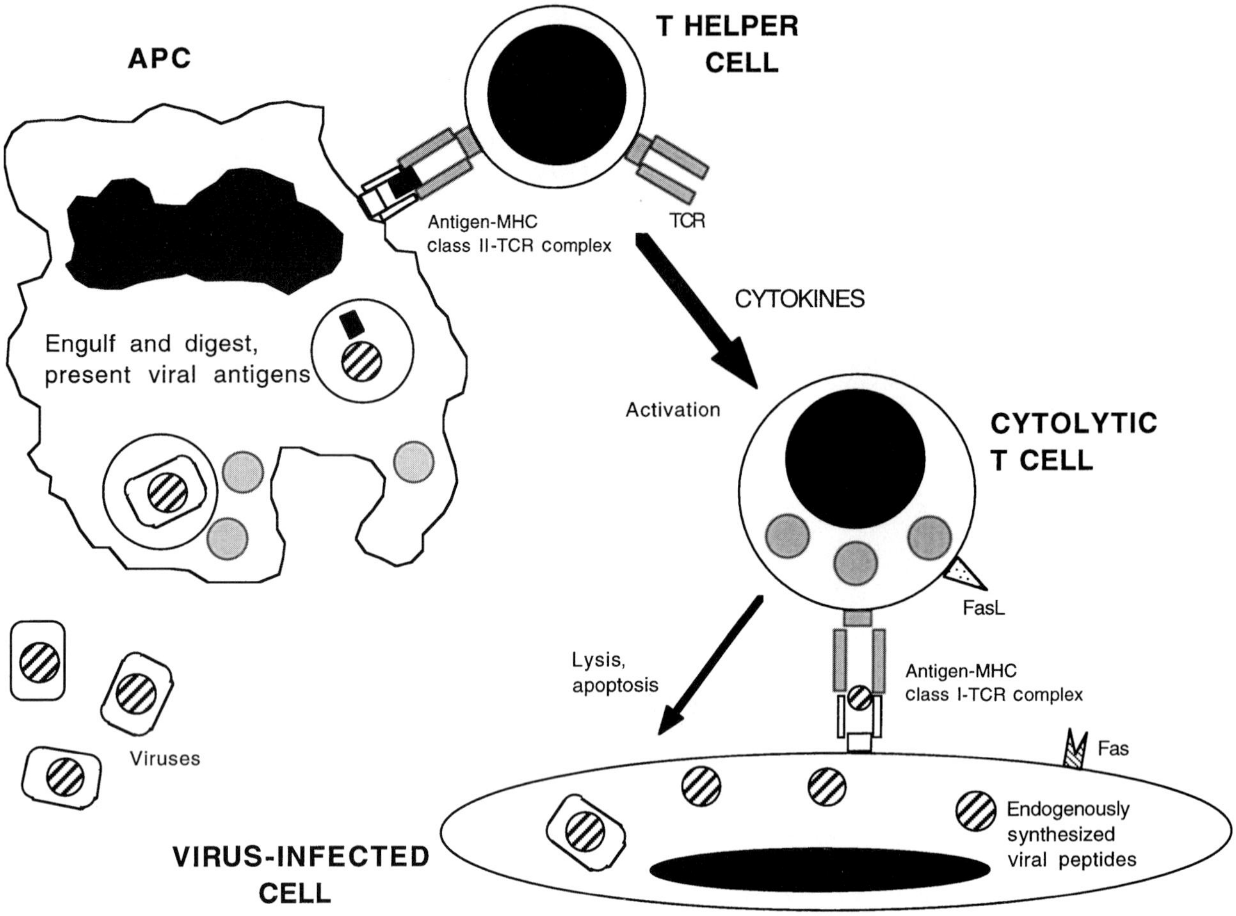


**Figure 83.3** Defenses against viral infection. The main effectors are cytolytic T cells (primarily $CD8^+$) that induce cell lysis and programmed cell death (apoptosis) after specific T-cell receptor (TCR) engagements with newly synthesized viral peptides, presented in the context of the target-cell major histocompatibility complex (MHC) class I molecules. Activation of cytolytic T cells is greatly enhanced by cytokines produced by T helper cells. The latter are stimulated by viral peptides presented by antigen-presenting cells (APC), which include mononuclear phagocytes, B cells, and (particularly) dendritic cells.

tailor diagnostic efforts and implement appropriate empirical therapy while awaiting test results. Furthermore, realistic appraisal of these probabilities is an invaluable aid in assessing the need for subsequent stratagems when results of the initial invasive evaluations are nonspecific.

## Early Infectious Complications

Bacteria are overwhelmingly the most frequent cause of pulmonary infections among virtually all populations of allograft recipients during the first month after transplantation. Organisms typical for nosocomial infections (Enterobacteriaceae, *Pseudomonas aeruginosa,* and lesser numbers of *Staphylococcus aureus*) are predominant.[16, 19, 20, 23, 28–34] In general, the early bacterial pneumonias in transplant recipients manifest acutely, tend to be rapidly progressive, and are usually (but not invariably) accompanied by fairly typical radiographic findings. Various investigators have identified a number of risk factors for bacterial infections, including recipient age older than 40 years, high prednisone doses, leukopenia, and, perhaps most important, other antecedent or concomitant pulmonary problems, such as prolonged intubation.[14, 16, 28, 35] Because of improvements in preventive practices, including antibacterial prophylaxis regimens, the overall frequency of bacterial pneumonias has been somewhat reduced among solid organ recipients.

For the most part, the relative risk of bacterial pneumonias after transplantation is a function of the inherent risk of the surgical procedure for development of postoperative pulmonary complications. Rates of early pneumonias tend to be particularly low among renal allograft recipients and may affect fewer than 10% of these patients.[15, 16, 31, 36] The relatively lesser incidence of early bacterial pneumonias after renal transplantation is largely a consequence of the lower number of postoperative pulmonary complications associated with the low abdominal incision used for these patients. Another factor that may partially account for the lower overall infection rate among renal transplant patients, in comparison with liver and heart

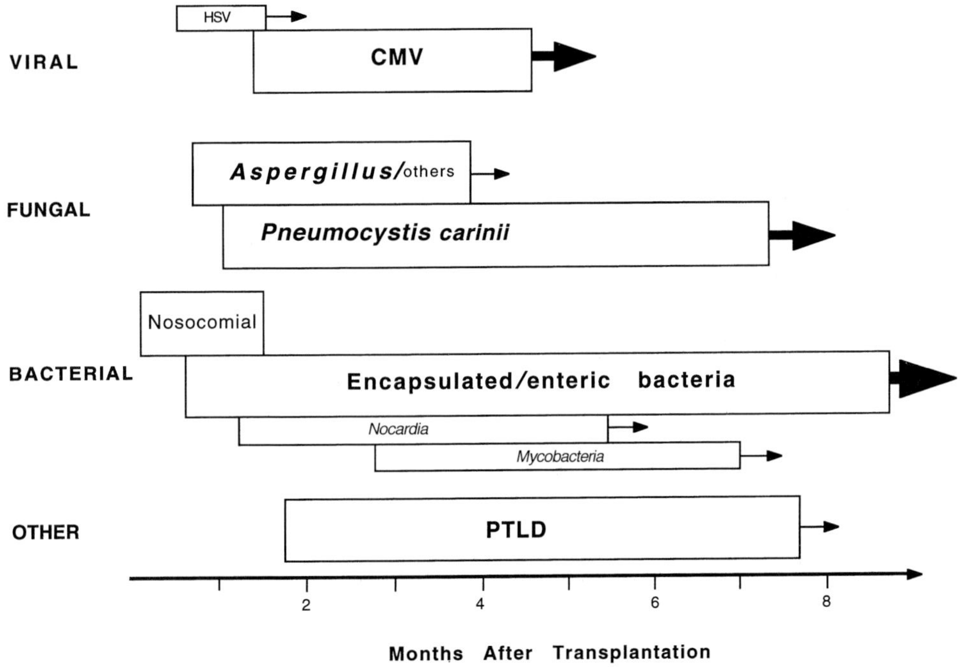


**Figure 83.4** Common time course of pulmonary infections after allogeneic organ transplantation. Note that prophylaxis may delay the usual onset of these infections. HSV = herpes simplex virus; CMV = cytomegalovirus; PTLD = posttransplant lymphoproliferative disease.

allograft recipients, is the ability to survive allograft failure through reinstitution of dialysis. Accordingly, the intensity of immunosuppression regimens tends to be lower in renal transplantation patients and, if absolutely indicated by the presence of other complications, the allograft can be sacrificed by further reductions of these medications.

In contrast, bacterial pneumonias complicate the early course of approximately twice this proportion of liver allograft recipients.[28–30, 32–34, 37–41] Liver transplantation involves extensive surgery in the upper abdomen and is associated with much higher incidences of postoperative pulmonary complications, wound infections, and bacteremia.[33, 39] Selective bowel decontamination has been reported to decrease the overall incidence of bacterial pneumonias after liver transplantation, if at the cost of increasing the relative proportion of infections caused by gram-positive cocci.[37, 40] Another notable and potentially confounding pulmonary complication in these patients in the early posttransplantation period is persistent hypoxemia caused by vascular abnormalities of the hepatopulmonary syndrome.[41, 42]

Heart transplant recipients are even more predisposed to postoperative pneumonias because of risks associated with the thoracic surgical procedure, such as pulmonary atelectasis and retained secretions due to painful, ineffectual cough and shallow respirations, as well as left hemidiaphragmatic and other inspiratory muscle paresis.[17–23, 43–46] A small proportion of these patients also develop postoperative incisional infections or mediastinitis, often with dire results.[47]

*Aspergillus* infection occasionally occurs during the first month after transplantation,[48–51] as do geographically endemic fungal infections, as a result of reactivation or transmission with the donor organ.[52, 53] Sporadic cases of legionellosis, often caused by contaminated hospital water systems, also occur during the first and subsequent weeks.[54, 55]

Isolation of herpes simplex viruses is fairly common during the first few weeks after transplantation, and prophylaxis (or treatment) with either acyclovir or ganciclovir is highly effective.[56] Most often, isolation of this virus from bronchoalveolar lavage or other respiratory tract specimens represents asymptomatic shedding or upper airway mucocutaneous infection, and identification of the virus in patients with acute pulmonary problems should not necessarily lead to complacency that the definitive diagnosis has been established.

## Infectious Complications 1 to 6 Months After Transplantation

Opportunistic pathogens assume increasing importance among transplant recipients with continued cellular immunosuppression during the second and later months after the procedure. This period represents the greatest overall risk for opportunistic infections caused by *Aspergillus,* locally endemic fungi, *Nocardia,* and viruses,[14–24, 26–32, 34–45, 48–52, 55, 57] as well as rare cases of parasitic disease.[58–59]

### Fungal Infections

Fungal pneumonias are especially dreaded complications that tend to have insidious initial presentations, frequently metastasize to other organs, and are associated with high rates of mortality despite even the most aggressive medical therapy.[48–52, 57] Susceptibility to *Aspergillus* and other opportunistic infections has been clearly correlated with the intensity of immunosuppression and treatment for rejection.[28, 60] Chest radiographs of transplant recipients with fungal pneumonias most typically reveal peripheral focal or multifocal infiltrates. Upper-lobe predominance is common with *Aspergillus,* although by no means universal, whereas nocardial infiltrates most frequently involve the lower lung fields. *Aspergillus* lesions tend to cavitate, reflecting the predilection of this organism for angiocentric invasion, thrombosis, and necrosis. Again, however, unusual infiltrates are frequently associated with fungal infections,[27, 57] and other opportunists, including cytomegalovirus (CMV), *Legionella,* and *Pneumocystis,* may also be found in the same lesions.

Unlike most of the other microbial pathogens of immunosuppressed patients, the predominant interstitial and perivascular location of *Aspergillus* often renders recovery by bronchoalveolar lavage or transbronchial biopsies problematic. Accordingly, false-negative rates of these techniques may be as great as 25% to 50% and 85% to 90%, respectively.[61] Conversely, the presence of *Aspergillus* in bronchoalveolar lavage specimens may denote merely airway colonization, although more than one half of transplant recipients with these findings develop invasive disease.[28] Overall, fine-needle transthoracic aspiration appears to be more sensitive than bronchoscopy for diagnosis of aspergillosis, particularly when lesions are small and peripheral.[62]

### *Pneumocystis carinii*

The implementation of prophylaxis with trimethoprim-sulfamethoxazole or other effective agents[63] has resulted in the near-elimination of disease caused by *P. carinii* and has reduced the number of infections caused by susceptible bacteria (including *Nocardia*) and parasites.[64–66] Once a cause of immeasurable morbidity and high mortality rates in early series, these infections are now largely of historical interest among treated recipients. Nonetheless, occasional cases of *P. carinii* occur among patients with medication intolerance or poor compliance. Yield of *P. carinii* organisms from bronchoalveolar lavage fluid in cardiac and probably other transplant recipients may be somewhat lower than the near-perfect yields reported in HIV patients (at least those not receiving prophylaxis).[67] This relatively reduced yield is probably attributable to lesser absolute pathogen burdens and a tendency for *P. carinii* to be localized primarily to the pulmonary interstitium during early infections.[68] Use of transbronchial biopsies in conjunction with bronchoalveolar lavage is likely to increase the sensitivity for bronchoscopic diagnosis of *P. carinii* in these patients.[67]

### Cytomegalovirus

CMV is the single most frequent, serious, and complex pathogen of virtually every allogeneic transplantation population.[16, 20, 24, 26, 28, 31, 43, 65, 69] CMV is a double-stranded herpesvirus. Thousands of genetically different strains are found worldwide in humans, who are the only known reservoir for this pathogen. Asymptomatic infections or mild mononucleosis syndromes are the rule among immunocompetent hosts; the full spectrum of CMV–induced diseases is discussed in Chapter 32. Infection is acquired throughout life via exchanges of virtually any bodily secretion or excretion, and approximately 50% of adult transplantation candidates have serologic evidence of prior infection. Once infection is acquired, lifelong latency is established, after which the virus usually remains dormant, primarily among leukocytes.

Immunosuppression of the intensity necessary for allogeneic transplantation leads to disappearance of cell-mediated responses in the recipient (although anti-CMV antibodies persist), and the virus is able to proliferate. Although the exact nature of the trigger for CMV replication in these patients is unknown, a role for TNF-α has been implicated by associations between circulating levels of the cytokine and disease onset[70] and by findings showing that the cytokine has stimulatory effects on the CMV immediate-early enhancer-promoter.[71] The putative role of this proinflammatory cytokine in CMV reactivation correlates with clinical observations that viral infections are often temporally associated with systemic infections and inflammation, including episodes of allograft rejection.

The epidemiology of CMV disease is remarkably similar among all allograft recipients: infection occurs in about 75% of patients who are at risk (i.e., antecedent viral infection among either recipient or donor or transfusion with CMV-positive blood products); pulmonary involvement is evident in approximately one third of these infections; and, in the absence of antiviral prophylaxis, initial onset is usually between 1 and 4 months after transplantation. Furthermore, predisposing factors for CMV infections are remarkably similar among recipients of different organs[72–76] (Table 83.1).

The spectrum of CMV manifestations among transplant recipients is protean, ranging from asymptomatic viral shedding to various symptomatic mononucleosis-like syndromes to overt pneumonitis with nonspecific dyspnea, hypoxemia, and diffuse interstitial infiltrates that progress in severity over a few hours or days. In general, primary CMV infections of previously uninfected compromised recipients are associated with a much worse prognosis than are reactivations of a latent virus. In addition, many cases of CMV infection in seropositive recipients of solid organs are caused by superinfection with strains derived from the donor or from administered blood products. Superinfecting strains may exhibit antigenic as well as genomic variances from those of the latent virus, and these infections tend to have a worse prognosis than do simple secondary (reactivation) infections.

**Table 83.1 RISK FACTORS FOR CYTOMEGALOVIRUS (CMV) INFECTION IN ALLOGENEIC TRANSPLANT RECIPIENTS**

| |
|---|
| Prior CMV infections in either donor or recipient |
| Transfusion with CMV-positive blood products |
| Intensified immunosuppression |
| Allograft rejection |
| Increased age of recipient |
| Multiple donor-recipient major histocompatibility complex mismatches |
| Decreased or absent CMV-specific cellular cytotoxic responses |

The natural history of early CMV pulmonary infection has not been particularly well described among recipients of solid organ transplants. In the absence of typical histologic or cytopathic findings, mere recovery of virus by shell vial or conventional cultures of bronchoalveolar lavage specimens, or by detection of antigenemia, does not unequivocally establish the diagnosis of ongoing pneumonitis or exclude the possibility of other ongoing processes. Whereas CMV identification by bronchoalveolar lavage in even asymptomatic patients portends pneumonitis among allogeneic bone marrow recipients,[77] isolation of virus from the lungs of recipients of solid organ transplants does not necessarily presage the eventual development of cytopathic disease.[69, 72–74, 78]

In addition to direct cytopathic tissue injuries, CMV infections in transplant recipients are associated with deleterious (and often delayed) secondary effects, notably exacerbations of allograft rejection.[24, 73, 78–81] CMV has been demonstrated to have myriad effects on transcriptional regulation of infected cells, including up-regulated expression of major histocompatibility complex molecules in allografts (increasing their immunogenicity) and increased expression of cell adhesion molecules and inflammatory cytokines, all of which augment cytotoxic activities of recipient $CD8^+$ lymphocytes.[81–84] Peptide products of the viral genome also have sequence and antigenic homologies with MHC class II DR beta chains and with alpha chains of MHC class I molecules and therefore may trigger rejection responses by viral mimicry.[85, 86] In addition, research findings suggest that CMV has superantigenic activity, whereby extremely large numbers of T cells are promiscuously activated independently of their antigen specificities.[87] According to general hypotheses of superantigenic immunopathogenesis,[88] many of the nonspecifically stimulated T cells have intrinsic alloantigen avidities,[12] and these highly activated effectors are capable of producing heightened rejection responses.

CMV infections also heighten propensities for superinfections with *Aspergillus, P. carinii,* and diverse bacterial and viral pathogens.[73–75, 78, 89–93] Mechanisms by which CMV decreases host defenses against other pathogens, thereby promoting concomitant superinfections, are likely to include depression of lymphocyte counts and reversal of normal CD4:CD8 ratios, associated production of immune complexes with anti-idiotypic activities, and suppression of lymphocyte and NK responses to activating cytokines.[94–97] Observations also suggest that CMV has evolved mechanisms to evade intrinsic defense responses, including inhibition of early antigen peptide presentation by MHC of the infected cells, which limits killing of these organisms by cytotoxic T cells.[98]

Intravenous ganciclovir for 2 to 4 weeks is generally the treatment of choice for established pneumonias or other cytopathic CMV infections. Resistant strains can be treated with foscarnet or with multidrug combinations.[99] The role of concomitant immunoglobulin therapy in established infections among solid organ transplant recipients has not been clearly established, although combined therapy is demonstrably more efficacious among bone marrow recipients with viral pneumonia.[100–102] Optimal dosing of immunosuppression is another difficult issue in the management of CMV infections in transplant recipients for which clear guidelines have not been established. On the one hand, reductions of immunosuppression can be postulated to enable some recovery of antiviral cellular immune function, but this consideration must be balanced by the propensity for increased allograft rejection associated with these infections.

The optimal management of viral shedding, in the absence of overt cytopathic disease, is also highly controversial.[69] Effective antiviral therapy is expensive, cumbersome, and associated with toxicities. In most centers the finding of asymptomatic shedding is treated with expectant waiting or with more frequent surveillance. However, many of the adverse indirect CMV effects can apparently occur with simple viral shedding and, possibly, in the absence of virion replication per se.[73, 78–80, 96, 102] Furthermore, although therapies that act by inhibition of viral DNA synthesis (e.g., ganciclovir) may lead to clinical resolution of acute CMV infections, they do not necessarily ameliorate the increased risk and severity of rejection or superinfections after CMV infection.

Clearly, primary prevention of CMV infections in transplant recipients is highly desirable, and a number of agents have been tested for prophylactic efficiency. Trials with intravenous immunoglobulin in solid-organ allograft recipients showed disparate results; the greatest prophylactic benefit was seen with high-titer anti-CMV globulin.[103] Most studies showed that acyclovir had minimal therapeutic effect for established CMV infections, but the efficacy of the agent as primary prophylaxis was suggested by a large trial in renal transplant recipients.[104] Other investigations, however, were unable to demonstrate significant protective effects of acyclovir prophylaxis, particularly in comparison with the more efficacious ganciclovir.[105–110] In general, the most favorable results with ganciclovir prophylaxis were seen when the drug was administered in protracted courses during the period of greatest risk for CMV infections. In addition to prevention of primary CMV infections, there are some indications that ganciclovir prophylaxis diminishes the incidence of allograft rejection and other opportunistic infections, including Epstein-Barr virus (EBV). The efficacy of oral ganciclovir has not been established, although concerns have been raised that the low serum levels attained with this treatment promote the development of drug-resistant CMV.[28]

## Epstein-Barr Virus

A number of other viruses are significant pathogens of transplant recipients during the intermediate period. Reactivation or initial infection with EBV occurs in the majority of patients during the first few weeks after transplantation.[111] Like CMV, EBV is a herpesvirus with a ubiquitous distribution and high prevalence among adults. EBV specifically binds to the type 2 complement receptors of B lymphocytes, with subsequent intracellular entry mediated by endocytosis. Infections of transplant recipients may manifest with severe clinical syndromes resembling mononucleosis, although most cases are probably asymptomatic. The true importance of EBV infection in transplant recipients, however, is the causal role it plays in the development of posttransplantation lymphoproliferative disorder (PTLD).

PTLD is overwhelmingly the most frequent transplant-associated malignancy, occurring in 2% to 10% of solid organ recipients,[112–116] and it may have an even greater prevalence among pediatric transplant recipients.[117] The median time of onset in most series is between 2 and 4 months after transplantation, although cases have been reported as early as 6 weeks. PTLDs are high-grade lymphomas, generally of B-cell origin, that may manifest with either focal or multifocal involvement and often grow insidiously. The malignancy is associated with serologic evidence of primary or reactivated EBV infection, and viral genomes can be identified in the majority of tumors.[118, 119] Peripheral blood smears reveal nonspecific atypical lymphocytes. Most cases among renal and liver transplant recipients involve primarily abdominal viscera and retroperitoneal areas; tumors are found only occasionally in the pulmonary parenchyma. The proportion of lymphoma episodes involving the lungs or mediastinum is considerably greater, however, among heart transplant recipients.

B-cell lymphoproliferative disorders are recognized sequelae of severe deficiencies of cellular-mediated immunity of various causes (e.g., congenital, medication-induced, HIV-induced). The development of these tumors has been compellingly linked to disordered T-cell regulation of proliferation among EBV-infected B lymphocytes.[1] T-cell depletion or inactivation by drugs (notably cyclosporine) readily enables transformation of B lymphocytes with EBV in vitro. The risk for development of these malignancies is closely correlated with the intensity of immunosuppressive treatments[120] and is further markedly increased by concomitant or prior CMV infection.[118, 121] Even though many of these tumors undergo at least partial remission with decreases of immunosuppression, the ultimate mortality rate among affected patients in most series, particularly those with monoclonal or oligoclonal PTLD, tends to be greater than 80%. Treatment by conventional lymphoma management stratagems has been successful in only a small proportion of cases.[113–115, 122, 123]

### Other Viruses

Varicella zoster virus is a pathogen in approximately 10% of transplant recipients during the second and later months after their procedure.[124] Infections with this agent are manifested primarily by cutaneous lesions and dermatomal pain syndromes, although sporadic dissemination with pulmonary involvement has also been reported. A small number of pneumonias caused by adenoviruses have been documented among transplant recipients.[125] In addition to the potential seriousness of these infections, the virus is notable for possible transmission by the allograft. A number of lower respiratory tract infections in adult and pediatric transplant recipients are attributable to respiratory syncytial virus.[126–128] These infections are unique in that they may manifest with acute airflow obstruction and are amenable to treatment with relatively nontoxic specific antiviral therapies. Scattered cases of herpesvirus-6 interstitial pneumonias have also been reported.[129] The epidemiology and drug sensitivity of this virus appear be similar to those of CMV. Transmission of HIV with the transplanted organ (see Chapter 82) is also possible, although scrupulous adherence to detailed donor evaluations, including viral screening, should render this infection a rare complication of transplantation.

## Late Complications

The incidence of infections usually begins to diminish 6 months to 1 year after transplantation. Nonetheless, the relative risk for pulmonary infections among these patients remains several times greater than in normal populations.[130] Accordingly, prompt attention to initial signs or symptoms of respiratory tract abnormalities in these patients is always warranted. Sporadic pneumonias caused by opportunistic microbes, particularly CMV and *P. carinii*, may occur 1 year or longer after transplantation, particularly among those with chronic allograft rejection.[23, 24, 73, 130] *Cryptococcus* is a notable late pathogen of transplant recipients, although pulmonary involvement in these cases tends to be overshadowed by central nervous system manifestations.[131] In general, bacterial pathogens predominate as causes of pneumonias among allograft recipients during this period. Community-acquired pneumonias that occur after hospital discharge among renal allograft patients, and probably in other transplant populations as well, tend to manifest with clinical features and causes similar to those observed in immunologically competent patients.[16]

A special predilection for mycobacterial infections has been noted among allograft recipients. Although these infections can occur at any time, peak prevalences are generally at least several months after transplantation.[132–135] Mycobacterial disease in this population is also notable for the frequency of infections with atypical species (as many as one third of cases), the propensity for unusual clinical and radiographic presentations, and the large proportion of cases with extrapulmonary involvement.

These infections usually respond to conventional chemotherapies, although longer than usual courses of treatment may be necessary to effect cure.[134–136] Initial recommendations called for use of prophylactic isoniazid therapy in virtually all tuberculin-positive transplant recipients (particularly those with renal allografts); more recently, however, a more conservative approach based on close surveillance in low-risk, reliable patients has been advocated.[28]

The possibility of neoplasm should be considered in the differential diagnosis of slowly growing pulmonary infiltrates in long-term survivors.[137] In addition to increased frequencies of carcinomas and other neoplasms that are prevalent among normal populations, Kaposi's sarcoma (associated with human herpesvirus-8) occurs in a markedly disproportionate number of transplant recipients and, in rare cases, manifests with significant lung involvement.[138]

# PRIMARY IMMUNODEFICIENCIES

Although primary immune defects are usually apparent in infancy or early childhood (Table 83.2), certain disor-

Table 83.2 PROTOTYPICAL PRIMARY IMMUNODEFICIENCIES

| SYNDROME | ABNORMALITY | PULMONARY PATHOGENS |
|---|---|---|
| ***Antibody Deficiencies*** | | |
| X-linked agammaglobulinemia | B-cell maturation block | Encapsulated bacteria, *Pneumocystis carinii*, mycoplasma, viruses |
| Common variable immunodeficiency (CVI) | Various B-cell maturation defects | Encapsulated bacteria, various others, depending on abnormality of immunoglobulin (Ig) |
| IgA and IgG subclass deficiencies | Similar to CVI | Encapsulated bacteria |
| Hypogammaglobulin-hyper-IgM | Isotype switch block | Encapsulated bacteria, *P. carinii* |
| ***Complement Defects*** | Multiple abnormalities described | Encapsulated bacteria, Enterobacteriaceae |
| ***Abnormal Phagocytosis*** | | |
| Chronic granulomatous disease | Defects of microbicidal $O_2^-$ and $H_2O_2$ generation | Staphylococci, Enterobacteriaceae, fungi, mycobacteria, occasional *P. carinii*, cytomegalovirus, *Nocardia* |
| Chédiak-Higashi syndrome | Defects of cytoplasmic granule processing | Encapsulated bacteria |
| Leukocyte adhesion defects | Failures of leukocyte recruitment to inflammatory sites | Encapsulated bacteria, fungi |
| Job's syndrome | Abnormal phagocyte chemotaxis, hyper-IgE | Staphylococci, other bacteria |
| ***Cellular Immune Defects*** | | |
| DiGeorge's syndrome | Impaired T cell responses, secondary defects of Ig | Viruses, *P. carinii*, fungi, bacteria |
| Severe combined immunodeficiency | Multiple defects of cytokine, antigen receptor, or presentation signals, critical enzymes | Most opportunistic pathogens, bacteria, fungi |
| Ataxia-telangiectasia | DNA strand-break repair | Encapsulated bacteria |

ders may have delayed onset or partial expression and otherwise elude diagnosis until adolescence or even adulthood; this is particularly true for common variable immunodeficiency (CVI) syndromes and immunoglobulin subclass deficiencies. The last few years have seen remarkable progress in understanding of the molecular defects that underline these diseases, as well as new approaches to treatment, including gene therapies.[139, 140]

Depending on the nature of the immune deficiency, affected patients characteristically present with fungal or recurrent bacterial infections of the gastrointestinal or respiratory tract (especially the sinuses), or of the skin, or with unusual, severe, and repetitive viral infections (as distinct from the common mild viral upper respiratory tract infections that occur in normal persons). The most important step in evaluation of suspected cases is a thorough medical and family history. Ultimate documentation of the underlying abnormality often requires complex laboratory techniques, the details of which are beyond the scope of this chapter.[141] Nonetheless, use of a few relatively simple tests (Table 83.3) is almost always sufficient either to exclude these problems with a high degree of confidence or to draw attention to areas that may require additional detailed studies.

## DISORDERS OF IMMUNOGLOBULIN PRODUCTION

Deficiencies of immunoglobulin production can result from defects in any of the complex steps necessary for the elaboration of these proteins, from initial stages of B-lymphocyte activation to final secretion of the antibody. Deficiencies of immunoglobulin result in impairment of functions subserved by these effectors, notably microbial agglutination, opsonization, and complement activation.[142] Patients affected with antibody deficiencies are particularly prone to recurrent or refractory infections of the sinopulmonary tract and skin with extracellular encapsulated bacteria. Many of these disorders are also associated with extraordinarily increased risks of autoimmune abnormalities and hematologic malignancies.

In general, regular replacement of missing immunoglobulins through intravenous administration of gamma globulin has been shown to be beneficial for prevention and treatment of infections in these patients.[143] Antibiotics are obviously indicated at the first signs of infection. Chronic or recurrent courses of prophylactic antimicrobial agents have the potential to exert selective pressures for resistant organisms, however, and use of these agents can be supported only in certain specific circumstances. Regular chest physiotherapy, including postural drainage, is routinely employed for immunoglobulin-deficient patients with chronic suppurative airway disease. As in patients with cystic fibrosis (see Chapter 40), promotion of clearance of respiratory tract secretions by physical means is useful for symptomatic improvement and may possibly decrease the frequency of pulmonary parenchymal infections.

**Table 83.3 SCREENING TESTS FOR IMMUNE SYSTEM ABNORMALITIES**

| Suspected Defect | Test | Comments |
|---|---|---|
| Immunoglobulins (Ig) | Quantitative IgG, IgM, IgA | Normal results exclude hypogammaglobulinemias |
| | Quantitative IgG subclasses | Normal results exclude subclass defects |
| | Antibody titers: diphtheria, tetanus toxoid, after immunization | Normal results indicated by specific antibodies |
| | Antibody titers before and after immunization with *Haemophilus influenzae* and *Streptococcus pneumoniae* | Normal increase shows ability to mount response to polysaccharide antigens |
| | Antibody titers to allogenic blood types | Normal result (after age 6 mo) shows ability to mount specific antibody responses |
| Phagocytes | Absolute neutrophil count | Normal result excludes neutropenia and most severe chemotactic defects |
| | Nitroblue tetrazolium reduction | Normal result excludes chronic granulomatous disease |
| Complement | 50% hemolyzing dose of complement ($CH_{50}$) | Normal result excludes most deficiencies; if abnormal, consider assays for individual components |
| Cellular immunity | Lymphocyte counts and subsets, delayed hypersensitivity to intradermal *Candida* antigen | Normal results exclude primary T-cell defects |
| | Platelet count | Normal result excludes Wiskott-Aldrich syndrome |

## X-Linked Agammaglobulinemia

X-linked agammaglobulinemia, also known as Bruton's agammaglobulinemia, is a disorder of B lymphocyte maturation that was initially described in 1952 and, as such, was the first recognized inborn error of immunity.[144] The inheritance of this condition was shown, in classic investigations of a small number of pedigree analyses, to be sex-linked recessive. This relatively common disease (estimated to be present in 1 of every 50,000 live births) has served as the prototype for defects of B-cell development and was useful in proving the origin of antibodies in B lymphocytes. X-linked agammaglobulinemia has been found to be the result of diverse mutations of a complex gene encoding a cytoplasmic tyrosine kinase (Bruton tyrosine kinase, or BTK) involved in signal transduction.[145] BTK is expressed in all hematopoietic lineages but appears to be down-regulated in T cells and in fully differentiated B lymphocytes (plasma cells). Functional defects of BTK result in a block in the normal maturation of B-cell precursors into functional immunoglobulin-producing lymphocytes.[146]

This disease is manifested by low (albeit detectable) levels of immunoglobulins and deficient antibody responses to immunizations. Clinical findings include hypoplasia of lymph node germinal centers, absence of tissue plasma cells, and severe reduction in the number of fully differentiated B cells.[145–149] In contrast to the B-lymphocyte abnormalities that characterize this disorder, T-cell numbers and functions do not appear to be adversely affected.

Disease manifestations may be present shortly after birth, but more typically they are delayed until at least 4 to 6 months of age, when levels of passively transferred maternal immunoglobulins decrease. Affected infants develop refractory or recurrent sinopulmonary infections, meningitis, otitis media, and eczema with pyogenic encapsulated bacteria and *P. aeruginosa.* Immunoglobulin deficiencies appear to predispose for infections with mycoplasma, and several cases of disease due to *Ureaplasma urealyticum* have been described in patients with Bruton's syndrome.[150, 151] Pulmonary infection with *P. carinii* has also been sporadically reported.[152] Most viral and fungal infections do not present unusual problems, but the presence of nonspecific granulomatous interstitial pneumonitis may cause diagnostic confusion.[152a] Patients with X-linked agammaglobulinemia have an apparent predilection for enterovirus infections that have resulted in devastating central nervous system and gastrointestinal tract disease.[150, 153] Vaccination of these patients with attenuated live virus vaccines has led to the development of serious infections.[154] Rheumatoid arthritis and other autoimmune diseases develop in as many as 20% of surviving patients, and lymphoma eventually occurs in approximately 5%.

Many of these patients live well into the second decade of life. Chronic bronchiectasis, hypoxemia, pulmonary fibrosis, and cor pulmonale are frequent sequelae of the recurrent respiratory infections. Regular replacement of immunoglobulin by intravenous infusions decreases the incidence and severity of bacterial and viral infections in these patients.[155]

Varying penetrance (or heterogeneity of the syndrome) is suggested by findings that relatives of index cases may present with less extreme deficiencies of antibody responses or have onset of disease late in life.[156] Furthermore, a clinically indistinguishable syndrome with apparent autosomal recessive inheritance affects a small number of women.[157]

## Common Variable Immunodeficiency

The CVI syndromes are relatively frequently encountered and represent various types of B-cell activation or differentiation defects.[158] In contrast to Bruton's agammaglobulinemia, clinical manifestations of CVI most often develop during late childhood or early adult life, although disease can occur at earlier ages.[159, 160] The spectrum of bacterial infections in the two immunodeficiency disorders is similar, although persistent enterovirus infections are less frequent in CVI. Furthermore, inheritance of CVI appears to be autosomal recessive, and both sexes are equally affected. An association with Epstein-Barr virus infections has also been described.[161] The underlying defect has been postulated to be mutations in a susceptibility gene of the MHC class III region of chromosome 6, a locus that has also been implicated in isolated IgA deficiency.[162–164]

Serum levels of IgG are low or virtually absent in affected patients, whereas IgA and IgM are variably depressed. In many cases, B cells appear able to proliferate but fail to differentiate normally. Patients with CVI often have normal total numbers of B cells, hyperplastic lymphoid follicles, and preserved responses to mitogens. Fully differentiated B lymphocytes are not present, however, either in lymphoid tissues or in peripheral blood.[165]

In addition to frequent sinopulmonary infections and recurrent otitis media with encapsulated bacteria, these patients are prone to sprue-like malabsorption that is often attributable to *Giardia* infestation. A number of patients have developed unusual pulmonary abnormalities characterized by parenchymal lymphocytic infiltrations or sarcoid-like granulomas.[166] Chronic bronchiectasis and other debilitating airway diseases occur in as many as 40%, although early diagnosis and scrupulous medical management appear to prevent many of these sequelae. The overall frequency of cancer in these patients is approximately 10 times greater than in normal persons, and women with CVI have a very high relative risk for lymphomas.[167] Various autoimmune disorders are also common complications of CVI.[168] CVI (or a clinically indistinguishable syndrome) occurs in as many as 10% of patients with malignant thymomas.[169]

Maintenance gamma globulin replacement, as described previously, decreases the frequency and severity of infections in patients with CVI. However, immunoglobulin administration to IgA-deficient CVI patients is associated with the possibility of anaphylactic reactions mediated by IgE antibodies with isotypic activity against IgA.[170] Accordingly, preparations that contain low levels of IgA should be used in patients who are at risk.

## Selective Immunoglobulin Defects

Isolated deficiency of IgA is the most frequent inborn defect of humoral immunity, occurring in as many as 1 in 700 persons and accounting for more than 1% of pediatric patients with recurrent infections.[150] The frequency of disease is greatest among Caucasians and is slightly more prevalent in males. Most often, this disorder is autosomal dominant with incomplete penetrance, although pedigrees with recessive inheritance have also been described. CVI occurs with increased frequency among relatives of these patients and, in a few cases, the more severe deficiency has eventually developed in patients who initially presented with isolated IgA defects. Seemingly de novo cases have been attributed to intrauterine infections caused by rubella, CMV, or exposure to various drugs (e.g., phenytoin, gold, D-penicillamine, sulfasalazine).[171]

The clinical features of IgA deficiency are highly varied, and most of those affected are probably asymptomatic.[172–174] Serious systemic infections are unusual in these patients. A minority have intermittent respiratory tract infections or diarrhea, the latter often the result of *Giardia lamblia* infection. Recurrent or chronic respiratory tract infections that result in bronchiectasis occur in a distinctly small proportion of IgA-deficient persons.[172] As with other primary disorders of immunoglobulin production, however, the risk of autoimmune diseases appears to be significantly increased in people with IgA deficiency. The absence of IgA also appears to be linked with increased frequencies of allergies and asthma, an association that has prompted speculation that the antibody is a defense against ingress of allergens across mucocutaneous surfaces.

Typically, peripheral blood counts of patients with IgA deficiency show normal numbers of mature B lymphocytes and normal numbers and proportions of $CD4^+$ and $CD8^+$ cells. Serum IgA levels are usually less than 50 μg/mL, whereas IgG and IgM concentrations are often elevated. Circulating B cells may express surface IgA with normal alpha heavy chains, but they are unable to secrete antibody or differentiate into plasma cells.[174] Accordingly, the defect is assumed to be a differentiation block affecting IgA-committed B cells, with the genetic defect localized to the same area involved in CVI.[162–164]

A number of cases of selective IgG subclass deficiencies have also been described, with or without concomitant defects of IgA production.[175–181] Persons with low or absent $IgG_2$ and $IgG_4$ appear to be particularly predisposed to recurrent or severe pneumonias and middle ear infections, whether IgA is deficient or not. Isolated $IgG_4$ deficits have also been described, and patients with these deficits appear to have increased risks for eventual development of chronic airway disease. A few cases of isolated $IgG_3$ deficiencies have been reported, and these patients may also be at considerable risk for development of recurrent pneumonias. Because total serum IgG levels are often normal in patients with selective subclass deficiencies, the diagnosis of these disorders in suspected cases requires quantitative IgG subclass determinations.

The presence of low levels of isolated immunoglobulin subclasses, however, is by no means an invariable predictor of disease. Manifestations of IgG subclass defects appear to be varied. Isolated $IgG_1$ defects are occasionally detected by routine serum electrophoresis ($IgG_1$ constitutes the largest proportion of Ig), and many patients with very low levels of $IgG_2$ are asymptomatic. Accordingly, indications for immunoglobulin replacement should be based on clinical findings of recurrent infections, rather than isolated laboratory abnormalities. Immunoglobulin administration has reportedly been beneficial for IgA-deficient patients with recurrent infections, even though very little of the antibody can subsequently be demonstrated in secretions.[182]

### Hypogammaglobulinemia with Hyperimmunoglobulin M

Like Bruton's syndrome, hypogammaglobulinemia with increased IgM is caused by a defect in the normal ontogeny of B lymphocytes. Unlike X-linked agammaglobulinemia, however, the block that characterizes the hyperimmunoglobulin M disorder occurs at a much later stage of lymphocyte development.[183–185] Both X-linked and autosomal-recessive syndromes have been described, as well as rare cases in which the condition was acquired later in life. The developmental block has been shown in X-linked cases to be the result of defects in the CD40 ligand (CD40L) gene.[186] CD40L is a $CD4^+$ T-cell receptor that is involved in contact-mediated stimulation of B cells to undergo isotype switching.

Accordingly, patients with the hyperimmunoglobulin M syndrome have absent or markedly reduced IgA and IgG. Antibody protection for the alimentary and respiratory tracts is normally provided by IgA and IgG isotypes, because IgM is too large to readily diffuse into the secretions that blanket luminal surfaces. Consequently, patients with the hypogammaglobulinemia–hyperimmunoglobulin M syndrome are especially prone to respiratory and gastrointestinal infections. Pyogenic organisms predominate, as in other immunoglobulin deficiencies. Affected patients are also predisposed to *P. carinii* pneumonia. Persistent enteroviral infection, a recognized complication of X-linked agammaglobulinemia, has also been described in patients with the hyperimmunoglobulin M syndrome.[186a] Treatment of the syndrome centers on routine gamma globulin replacement, as described earlier. As in other immunoglobulin deficiencies, patients with the hyperimmunoglobulin M syndrome have extraordinarily high rates of lymphoproliferative and autoimmune disorders.

### Rare Miscellaneous Immunoglobulin Deficiencies

Selective IgM deficiency, an unusual autosomal-dominant disorder that appears to be caused by abnormal T-cell function, results in increased susceptibility to meningitis and sepsis with gram-negative bacteria.[187] Deficient antibody responses to polysaccharide antigens, despite the presence of normal serum concentrations of immunoglobulins, have been found in rare patients with recurrent encapsulated bacterial infections.[188]

## COMPLEMENT DEFICIENCIES

Primary deficiencies of complement components are rare causes of immune system dysfunction.[189] C2 deficiency, the most frequent of these abnormalities, is linked with a marked propensity to development of systemic lupus erythematosus (SLE) and other vasculitides but has not been described in most series as a significant risk for recurrent infections. Deficiencies of C1q, C1r, C1s, or C4 have also been associated with SLE, and these defects may impair defenses against bacteria.[190]

C3 and C5 hydrolysis products mediate important host defenses against extracellular microbes, including opsonification (C3b, C5b) and phagocyte chemotaxis and adherence (C3a, C5a). C3 deficiency results in a predisposition for infections with encapsulated bacteria and Enterobacteriaceae that is even more severe than that of agammaglobulinemic patients.[189, 191, 192] Functionally inactive C5 has been reported in a small number of infants with severe skin, gastrointestinal tract, and other infections caused by Enterobacteriaceae and fungi.[193] More commonly, deficiencies of C3 and C5 are secondary sequelae of systemic diseases, particularly SLE, nephrotic syndrome, and hepatic failure. Patients with congenital deficiencies of terminal complement components (i.e., C6 to C8) are uniquely prone to recurrent and disseminated infections with *Neisseria* species and, to a lesser extent, *S. pneumoniae*.[194]

Primary deficiencies of either C3 or C5 can be ameliorated with infusions of fresh-frozen plasma, although the lability of the latter factor requires replacement with plasma that has been stored for less than 24 hours.

## ABNORMALITIES OF PHAGOCYTES

Phagocytosis by polymorphonuclear leukocytes and macrophages is a critical component of respiratory defense against extracellular bacteria. The efficiency of phagocytosis depends on a complex series of antibody, complement, and other mediator functions that lead to microbial opsonization and to phagocyte activation, recruitment, and adherence. The infectious complications of antibody or complement deficiencies result in part from failures to facilitate phagocytosis. Consequently, the spectrum of microbial pathogens in primary phagocyte abnormalities overlaps considerably with those of the humoral and complement deficiencies. The most frequently encountered primary deficiencies of phagocytes that manifest with life-threatening bacterial or fungal respiratory infections are the result of absolute reductions in number of granulocytes. In turn, these defects are most commonly consequences of leukemias or of treatments with myeloid suppressive drugs, as detailed in Chapter 86. The following discussion focuses on the relatively rare innate disorders of phagocyte production or abnormal function.

## Inadequate Numbers of Granulocytes

Inherited or de novo *chronic neutropenia,* characterized by absolute polymorphonuclear lymphocyte counts as low as 50 to 200 cells/μL, has been described in a small number of cases.[195] In marked distinction to patients with comparable degrees of granulocytopenia attributable to acute leukemias or chemotherapy, serious infections among all but the most severely affected persons with chronic primary neutropenia are infrequent. Similarly, patients with *cyclic neutropenia,* a distinct syndrome of intermittent reductions in granulocyte counts with a 21-day periodicity, may be prone to development of fevers, oral ulcers, and cervical adenopathy during neutrophil nadirs, but visceral infections are uncommon.[196]

In part, the low incidence of severe respiratory infections among patients with these primary disorders of neutrophil numbers may be attributed to the presence of compensatory monocytosis. Moreover, aside from the reductions in number, phagocyte functions of patients with chronic or cyclic neutropenia generally appear to be preserved, and defensive epithelial barriers of the skin, respiratory system, and gastrointestinal tract are normal. In contrast, intrinsic functional defects have been demonstrated among the remaining neutrophils of patients with leukemia and those treated with chemotherapy, and these patients often develop subacute mucositis that promotes aspiration and disrupts normal epithelial integrity.

Close surveillance for infectious complications and early treatment with antibiotics are important management stratagems that suffice for the majority of patients with chronic or cyclic neutropenia. Isolated cases have responded to treatment with corticosteroids, androgens, or splenectomy, although these therapies should be reserved for the most severely affected patients.

## Chronic Granulomatous Disease

Chronic granulomatous disease (CGD) is a rare syndrome (1 in 1,000,000 births) caused by metabolic defects that selectively impair the intracellular killing mechanisms of phagocytes.[197–199] Neutrophils and monocytes of affected persons are able to normally ingest opsonized microbes and particulates, but they cannot produce the superoxide anion ($O_2^-$), hydrogen peroxide, or other reductive products of oxygen that are necessary for killing of certain microbial species.[199a] In addition to direct microbicidal properties, these highly reactive oxidants are substrates for myeloperoxidase-catalyzed halogenation reactions with proteins and nucleic acids of ingested pathogens. The X-linked recessive variant, accounting for two thirds of CGD cases, has been shown to be caused by various mutations resulting in deletions or deficiencies of the 91-kd subunit of neutrophil cytochrome *b*. The abnormality of autosomal-recessive forms has been localized to a smaller cytosolic protein component of the reduced nicotinamide adenine dinucleotide phosphate (NADPH)–oxidase system encoded by the q25 region of chromosome 1.

In most cases, the immunodeficiency of CGD is evident during infancy or early childhood, but onset has been reported as late as age 16 years. Affected persons present with severe recurrent lymphadenitis and infections of the oropharynx, skin, gastrointestinal tract, and respiratory system.[198] Numerous aggregates of granulomas may form in a variety of organs, a presumed response of activated macrophages to microbial persistence and chronic antigenic stimulation. Because surgical incisions and wounds often heal poorly, open diagnostic procedures in these patients should be avoided.

Pathogens associated with CGD tend either to be catalase positive, and thus are able to neutralize the minute amount of hydrogen peroxide produced as a by-product of microbial metabolism, or are not able to intrinsically synthesize hydrogen peroxide. The most frequent bacterial causes of disease in CGD patients include S. *aureus,* various Enterobacteriaceae, and *Staphylococcus epidermidis.*[198–200] Occasional pneumonias may be caused by *P. aeruginosa, M. tuberculosis,* or atypical mycobacteria. Fungal infections are also prevalent.[201] *Aspergillus* pneumonia is an especially common manifestation of CGD that is lethal in approximately 50% of cases. Much less commonly, pneumonias among CGD patients are caused by CMV, *Nocardia,* or *P. carinii.* Bacterial species that endogenously synthesize reactive oxygen species (e.g., *Streptococcus* species, *H. influenzae)* are killed normally by CGD phagocytes.

Prophylaxis with trimethoprim-sulfamethoxazole has been shown to decrease the frequency of bacterial infections in affected patients by twofold to threefold.[200, 202] Trials of human recombinant IFN-γ in CGD patients have been prompted by discoveries that this cytokine product of T cells stimulates macrophage oxidative burst activity by increasing transcription of cytochrome *b*. Treatment with this agent has been shown to result in decreased frequency and severity of infections associated with CGD.[203] Bone marrow and stem cell transplantations can result in reconstitution of normal phagocytes in patients with suitable potential donors.[204] Because cellular immune defenses are intact in CGD, however, immunosuppressive agents must be administered to prevent graft-versus-host disease (GVHD). Therefore, patients undergoing this procedure exchange the immunodeficiency of CGD for the quite different risks of infectious and other complications associated with allogeneic marrow transplantation (see Chapter 86). Trials have been conducted with novel gene therapies to correct the underlying molecular defects through the use of autologous hematopoietic cells, with some encouraging initial results.[205–206a]

## Chédiak-Higashi Syndrome

Chédiak-Higashi syndrome (CHS) is a rare autosomal-recessive defect of phagocytic activity that is characterized by abnormal fusion of cytoplasmic granules. Among affected patients, the azurophilic lysosomes of neutrophils, as well as cytoplasmic granules of monocytes and lymphocytes, appear to have fused into giant organelles.[207–209] The defect of CHS also results in cytoplasmic defects among diverse granule-containing cells; albinism among affected patients, for instance, is caused by abnormal fusion of melanocyte pigment organelles.

The most prominent clinical features of CHS are recurrent skin and respiratory tract infections with *S. aureus* and other encapsulated bacteria. Phagocytes of affected patients have impaired microbicidal activity due to deficiencies of lysosomal enzymes, including neutral proteases and myeloperoxidase. In addition, neutrophil counts of these patients tend to be reduced, probably because of accelerated turnover. Chemotactic defects and impaired NK-cell activity have also been described. An accelerated phase characterized by lymphohistiocytic infiltration of viscera has been reported to respond to vincristine and prednisone. An analogous syndrome in mutant beige mice has been successfully reversed by allogeneic bone marrow transplantation, raising the possibility that this therapy may have applicability in humans affected with CHS.

### Leukocyte Adhesion Defects

Leukocyte adhesion defects represent a rare autosomal-recessive abnormality of P2 integrins, essential glycoprotein constituents of the CD11/CD18 receptor complex that mediates leukocyte adhesion.[210–212] In general, defects are localized to the 95-kd P chain (CD18) of the complex that, when noncovalently associated with a subunit, forms the CD11 family of adhesion receptors on almost all bone marrow–derived cells. Both complete and partial forms of the deficiency have been identified.

Affected patients present with recurrent bacterial and fungal infections of skin and upper and lower airways, peritonitis, and perirectal abscesses. These defects do not result in increased frequencies of viral infections or malignancies, presumably because of the existence of alternative adherence mechanisms among T lymphocytes and NK cells.

### Job's Syndrome

The defining abnormality of Job's syndrome, also known as hyperimmunoglobulin E syndrome, has most often been attributed to deficiencies of polymorphonuclear leukocyte and monocyte chemotaxis.[213–216] In some cases at least, the chemotactic abnormality appears to be caused by the presence of plasma inhibitors or other immune system defects that could, in fact, be the sequelae of abnormal lymphocyte regulation. Persons with this unusual syndrome typically present with impaired primary and secondary antibody responses (especially to *S. aureus)* and blunted in vitro cellular immune responses. However, lymphocyte numbers and phenotype ratios are usually normal. Serum concentrations of polyclonal IgE (and usually IgD) are markedly elevated, and eosinophilia is common. Affected patients present in infancy with severe skin and respiratory tract infections. Furunculosis, often with cold abscess formation, is an invariable feature, and pneumonias are common. The pulmonary injuries from repeated lung infections become increasingly problematic among the patients who survive into adulthood. Patients with this syndrome tend to have severe allergic responses to a variety of antigens.[217] Heredity of the syndrome appears to be autosomal dominant with incomplete penetrance.

## DEFECTS OF CELLULAR IMMUNITY

Because virtually all effector limbs of the immune system are coordinately regulated by T cells, the defects described in this section are also characterized by concomitant abnormalities of humoral or phagocyte defense mechanisms. Like allogeneic transplant recipients, patients with these defects are therefore predisposed to infections by a broad range of microbial organisms. Similarly, the generally most serious and complex infections in patients with primary cellular immune defects are those that are caused by opportunistic pathogens, including *P. carinii, Legionella* species, mycobacteria, *Nocardia, Listeria,* and various viruses, particularly members of the herpes family.

### DiGeorge's Syndrome

DiGeorge's syndrome is a constellation of abnormalities caused by embryonal dysmorphogenesis of the third and fourth pharyngeal pouches.[218–220] The failure of neural crest cells to migrate normally into or otherwise interact with these structures during embryogenesis leads to congenital hypoplasia of the thymic and parathyroid glands. Clinical manifestations include craniofacial deformities, great vessel anomalies, and congenital cardiac defects. Most of the early deaths of patients with this syndrome result from cardiovascular abnormalities or neonatal hypocalcemic tetany. The genetic defect of this disorder is a chromosomal deletion that results in monosomy 22q11. Most cases represent spontaneous mutations, although a small number of patients with autosomal-dominant inheritance have been described. Resemblances of the clinical features of DiGeorge's syndrome to those of fetal alcohol syndrome and vitamin A deficiency have also been noted.

Affected infants who do not die from their congenital abnormalities present with an immunodeficiency that is limited to defects of cell-mediated defenses. T-cell numbers are typically reduced, but phenotype proportions tend to be preserved. In vitro and in vivo functions of T cells are depressed to varying degrees, and severe cases may be phenotypically indistinguishable from cases of severe combined immunodeficiency (SCID). These profoundly affected persons lack T-cell responses to mitogens and mixed lymphocyte reactions and have anergy in skin tests of delayed hypersensitivity. In contrast, B-lymphocyte counts are usually normal, and antibody production is impaired in proportion to the degree that T-cell activation is deficient. In most cases, immunoglobulin concentrations are normal, although some patients have low levels of IgA or elevations of serum IgE. Affected patients are prone to severe viral pneumonias, especially with herpes group viruses and measles. Pneumonias caused by fungi, gram-negative bacilli and, to a much lesser degree, *P. carinii* also occur in these patients.

Bone marrow transplantation has been shown to correct the deficiency.[221] Implants of allogenic thymus have also been able to reconstitute T-lymphocyte function.[222]

### Purine Nucleoside Phosphorylase Deficiency

Another immunodeficiency syndrome that primarily involves cellular immune functions is caused by a deficiency of purine nucleoside phosphorylase (PNP).[223, 224] Absence of the enzyme results in accumulations of purine metabolites that have preferentially toxic effects on cellular division of T lymphocytes. Thymuses of these patients are hypoplastic, but the other craniofacial and cardiovascular defects of DiGeorge's syndrome are absent. PNP deficiency is most often characterized by marked lymphopenia and susceptibilities for disseminated viral infections (especially with *Varicella*), *P. carinii* pneumonias, mucocutaneous candidiasis, and chronic diarrhea. Furthermore, more than half of those affected also have some manifestations of neurologic disorders. Although numbers of T cells are severely reduced and cellular immune functions are absent, the overall immunoglobulin levels are usually normal. More than one third of patients with PNP deficiency develop autoimmune diseases.

Pharmacologic attempts at enzyme replacement in PNP-deficient patients have been futile, and persons affected with this disorder do not survive their second decade. Bone marrow transplantation may be curative.[225, 226] In the future, treatment of this disorder, like those of other immunodeficiencies with isolated defects, will probably center on replacement of the abnormal gene.

## Severe Combined Immune Deficiency Disorders

SCID is a syndrome of heterogeneous lymphocyte stem-cell defects that deleteriously affect both T- and B-cell functions. Common features of these disorders include deficient antibody responses to immunization, low serum immunoglobulin levels, and virtual absence of in vitro or in vivo measures of cellular immunity.[227, 228] Severe lymphopenia of both B and T cells is typical in these patients, although some have near-normal absolute counts due to increased numbers of immature lymphocytes.

Infants with SCID present with a triad of mucocutaneous candidiasis, intractable diarrhea, and *P. carinii* pneumonia. Most cases become evident shortly after birth, but onset in a few patients is delayed for 6 to 9 months. Another sentinel feature of this disease is the development of a morbilliform rash within a few days after birth; this is probably a manifestation of GVHD from passively transferred maternal lymphocytes.[165] Transfusions of blood containing viable MHC-mismatched lymphocytes have in some cases led to fatal GVHD in infants with this disorder.

SCID is associated with high frequencies of infections with a wide range of microbes. Viral pathogens, particularly various herpesviruses, adenoviruses, measles, and influenza, are common causes of pneumonias and other diseases. Disseminated *Legionella* is also a reported complication of SCID.[229] Administration of attenuated live virus vaccines or bacille Calmette-Guérin is likely to result in fatal infection. Growth retardation in SCID is correlated with the development of recurrent infections. Death usually occurs within 2 years after birth, unless the patient is isolated in a pathogen-free environment or undergoes bone marrow transplantation.

Several genetic anomalies resulting in the SCID syndrome have been delineated. About half of the cases in the United States are caused by X-linked recessive variants, in which the single most common abnormalities are various mutations in IL2RG, the gamma chain of the IL-2 receptor, which is found in multiple cytokine receptors, including IL-2, IL-4, IL-7, IL-9, and IL-15.[230] Somewhat less frequently, mutations with virtually identical immunodeficiency phenotypes have been identified, such as Janus kinase 3 (JAK3), a downstream transducer of cytokine activation pathways.[231] Even more sporadic mutations of diverse, critical cell-signaling mechanisms have been reported,[232–234] and undoubtedly others capable of severe immune impairments remain to be discovered. About half of the autosomal-dominant cases are attributable to deficiency of adenosine deaminase, an enzyme that catalyzes the irreversible deamination of adenosine and deoxyadenosine.[235, 235a] Although distributed widely, the enzyme appears to be especially active in lymphocytes; toxic effects of accumulations of adenosine metabolite (deoxyadenosine triphosphate) are primarily evident in the developing lymphocytes (and occasionally in chondrocytes).

SCID patients with immunoglobulin deficiencies are logical candidates for gamma globulin replacement. Blood products used in these patients should be irradiated to eliminate the risk of GVHD. Enzyme replacement by infusion of normal red blood cells or repeated administrations of polyethylene glycol–bonded adenosine deaminase have ameliorated B- and T-cell defects of SCID patients with adenosine deaminase deficiency.[235] SCID variants with characterized genetic abnormalities may also be treatable in the near future by transfection with normal human genes. Pending future advances in these therapies, however, allogeneic bone marrow or stem cell transplantations remain the definitive therapy.[236]

## Ataxia-Telangiectasia

This autosomal-recessive syndrome of AT is manifested by profound deficiencies of cellular immunity, variously impaired humoral responses, and a constellation of progressive cerebellar ataxia, telangiectasias, and high incidences of malignancies.[237–239] T-cell responses to mitogens, alloantigens, and skin-test antigens are invariably depressed. In vitro production of all antibody isotypes is also reduced, but these abnormalities can largely be reversed by cocultivation of patient B lymphocytes with normal T cells. The specific defect has been identified in the AT-mutated protein kinase. This kinase has critical functions in multiple mechanisms involved in DNA strand breaks, including T-cell antigen receptor VDJ recombinations.[240] One or more impairments of DNA-repair mechanisms in AT have long been suggested, based on observations of the high rate of associated malignancies and the exquisite radiosensitivities of cells cultured from affected persons.

Despite the often profound deficiencies of cellular immunity, most of these patients are not affected adversely by live-virus vaccination and do not develop GVHD after transfusion of MHC-mismatched blood products; nor does there appear to be an increased risk for *P. carinii* infections. Toddlers with AT do have increased incidences of bacterial and viral sinopulmonary infections, and many eventually develop chronic bronchiectasis. The frequency of serious respiratory tract infections among these patients may be related to the concomitant presence of IgG subclass deficiencies.[241] Ataxia is usually detected during the second year of life, whereas telangiectasias usually have a somewhat later onset. The relative risk for malignancies (especially non-Hodgkin's lymphomas) is increased 100-fold among patients with the syndrome, and unaffected family members may also be at significant risk for the development of neoplasms.[239, 242, 243]

## Wiskott-Aldrich Syndrome

The Wiskott-Aldrich syndrome (WAS) is a rare X-linked recessive disorder (4 infants per 1,000,000 male births) that is typified by not only frequent opportunistic infections but development of thrombocytopenia, eczema, and an increased risk of hematologic malignancies.[244, 245] Despite the myriad other serious complications of this disorder, infection accounts for the majority of deaths among affected persons. Encapsulated pyogenic bacteria and, less commonly, herpesviruses and *P. carinii* are the most frequent pathogens of these patients.

The abnormal phenotype of this syndrome results from various mutations of the *WAS* gene, localized on the short arm of the X chromosome.[246] WAS protein is differentially expressed in hematopoietic cells, where it is a cytoskeletal regulator, important in the polarization of T cells during interactions with B lymphocytes. WAS characteristically results in severely impaired production of antibodies to polysaccharide antigens, varied reductions of T-cell numbers, and impaired mitogen responses that tend to worsen with age. Most of those affected have abnormalities of serum immunoglobulin levels: low levels of IgM and IgG are typical, whereas concentrations of IgA and IgE tend to be increased. Bone marrow transplantation can successfully reverse the various hematologic and immune defects associated with this disorder.[247]

## SUMMARY

Disorders associated with immunodeficiency diseases are becoming increasingly common in clinical medicine, chiefly because of the prevalence of HIV infection (discussed fully in Chapter 82) and immunosuppression resulting from disease or treatment of disease. Compared with these secondary causes of immunodepression, primary causes, usually genetically determined immunologic disorders, are considerably less frequent. The special complications of bone marrow transplantation are discussed in Chapter 86, and those of lung transplantation in Chapter 97. The most frequent and serious complications of immunodeficiency disorders are infectious in origin, and the most likely pathogens can often be predicted from the type and time course of the underlying immunologic abnormality.

## References


1. Crawford SW: Noninfectious lung disease in the immunocompromised host. Respiration 66:385–395, 1999.

1a. Stover DE, Zaman MB, Hajdu SI, et al: Bronchoalveolar lavage in the diagnosis of diffuse pulmonary infiltrates in the immunosuppressed host. Ann Intern Med 101:1–7, 1984.

2. Rodewald HR, Fehling HJ: Molecular and cellular events in early thymocyte development. Adv Immunol 69:1–112, 1998.

3. Aliprantis AO, Diez-Rouz G, Mulder LC, et al: Do macrophages kill through apoptosis? Immunol Today 12:573–576, 1996.

4. Ali H, Haribabu B, Richardson RM, et al: Mechanisms of inflammation and leukocyte activation. Med Clin North Am 81:1–28, 1997.

5. Haeney MR: The role of the complement cascade in sepsis. J Antimicrob Chemother 41:41–46, 1998.

6. Krieg AM, Yi AK, Matson S, et al: CpG motifs in bacterial DNA trigger direct B-cell activation. Nature 374:546–549, 1995.

7. Banchereau J, Steinman RM: Dendritic cells and the control of immunity. Nature 392:245–252, 1998.

8. Mosmann TR, Li L, Hengartner H, et al: Differentiation and function of T cell subsets. Ciba Found Symp 204:148–154, 1997.

9. Tsuyuguchi I: Regulation of the human immune response in tuberculosis. Infect Agents Dis 5:82–97, 1996.

10. Shresta S, Pham CT, Thomas DA, et al: How do cytotoxic lymphocytes kill their targets? Curr Opin Immunol 10:581–587, 1998.

11. Duncan SR, Valentine V, Pekny KW, et al: T-cell clonal proliferations in lung transplant recipients with obliterative bronchiolitis. J Clin Invest 97:2642–2650, 1996.

12. Krensky AM, Weiss A, Crabtree G, et al: T-lymphocyte-antigen interactions in transplant recipients. N Engl J Med 322:510–517, 1990.

13. Turka LA: What's new in transplant immunology: Problems and prospects. Ann Intern Med 128:946–948, 1998.

14. Simmons RL, Uranga VM, LaPlante ES, et al: Pulmonary complications in transplant recipients. Arch Surg 105:260–268, 1972.

15. Munda R, Alexander JW, First MR, et al: Pulmonary infections in renal transplant recipients. Ann Surg 187:126–133, 1978.

16. Ramsey PG, Rubin RH, Tokoff-Rubin N, et al: The renal transplant patient with fever and pulmonary infiltrates: Etiology, clinical manifestations and management. Medicine (Baltimore) 59:206–222, 1980.

17. Remington JS, Gaines JD, Griepp RB, et al: Further experience with infection after cardiac transplantation. Transplant Proc 4:699–705, 1972.

18. Pennock JL, Oyer PE, Reitz BA, et al: Cardiac transplantation in perspective for the future. J Thorac Cardiovasc Surg 83:168–177, 1982.

19. Cooper DKC, Lanza RP, Oliver S, et al: Infectious complications after heart transplantation. Thorax 38:822–828, 1983.

20. Ettinger NA, Trulock EP: Pulmonary considerations of organ transplantation: Part 1. Am Rev Respir Dis 143:1386–1405, 1991.

21. Schulman LL: Cytomegalovirus pneumonitis and lobar consolidation. Chest 91:558–561, 1978.

22. Austin JHM, Schulman LL, Mistrobattista JD: Pulmonary infection after cardiac transplantation: Clinical and radiologic correlations. Radiology 172:259–265, 1989.

23. Cook DJ, Chan J, Dunn CJ, et al: Late occurring pneumonia in heart transplant recipients (abstract). Am Rev Respir Dis 141:A604, 1990.

24. Duncan SR, Cook DJ: Survival of ganciclovir-treated heart transplant recipients with cytomegalovirus pneumonitis. Transplantation 52:910–913, 1991.

25. O'Hanley R, Easaw J, Rugo H, et al: Infectious disease management of adult leukemic patients undergoing chemotherapy: 1982 to 1986 experience at Stanford University Hospital. Am J Med 87:605–613, 1989.

26. Rubin RH, Green R: Clinical approach to the compromised host with fever and pulmonary infiltrates. *In* Rubin RH, Young LS (eds): Clinical Approach to Infection in the Compromised Host (3rd ed). New York: Plenum, 121–162, 1994.

27. Paterson DL, Singh N, Gayowksi T, et al: Pulmonary nodules in liver transplant recipients. Medicine (Baltimore) 77:50–58, 1998.

28. Fishman JA, Rubin RH: Infection in organ-transplant recipients. N Engl J Med 338:1741–1751, 1998.

29. Hesse UJ, Fryd DS, Chatterjee SN, et al: Pulmonary infections: The Minnesota randomized prospective trial of cyclosporine vs azathioprine-antilymphocyte globulin for immunosuppression in renal allograft recipients. Arch Surg 121:1056–1060, 1986.

30. Kusne S, Dummer JS, Singh N, et al: Infections after liver transplantation: An analysis of 101 consecutive cases. Medicine (Baltimore) 67:132–143, 1988.

31. Rubin RH: Infectious disease complications of renal transplantation. Kidney Int 44:221–236, 1993.
32. Hadley S, Samore MH, Lewis WD, et al: Major infectious complications after orthotopic liver transplantation and comparision of outcomes in patients receiving cyclosporine or FK506 as primary immunosuppression. Transplantation 59:851–859, 1995.
33. Mazariegos GV, Molmenti EP, Kramer DJ: Early complications after orthotopic liver transplantation. Surg Clin North Am 79:109–129, 1999.
34. Torbensons M, Wang J, Nichols L, et al: Causes of deaths in autopsied liver transplant patients. Mod Pathol 11:37–46, 1998.
35. Anderson RJ, Schafer LA, Olin DB, et al: Infectious risk factors in the immunosuppressed host. Am J Med 54:453–460, 1973.
36. Marmol A, Hernandez VC, Alfonso J, et al: Infectious disease complication post renal transplant in 220 patients. Transplantation Proc 28:3304, 1996.
37. Pay CV, Hermans PE, Washington JA, et al: Incidence, distribution, and outcome of episodes of infection in 100 orthotopic liver transplantations. Mayo Clin Proc 64:555–564, 1989.
38. Thompson AB, Rickard KA, Shaw BW, et al: Pulmonary complications and disease severity in adult liver transplant recipients. Transplant Proc 20:646S–649S, 1988.
39. Ekberg H, Tranberg KG, Anderson R, et al: Major liver resection: Perioperative course and management. Surgery 100:1–7, 1986.
40. Colonna JD, Winston DJ, Brill JE, et al: Infectious complications in liver transplantation. Arch Surg 123:360–364, 1988.
41. O'Brien JD, Ettinger NA: Pulmonary complications of liver transplantation. Clin Chest Med 17:99–114, 1996.
42. Krowka MJ, Porayko MK, Plevak DJ, et al: Hepatopulmonary syndrome with progressive hypoxemia as an indication for liver transplantation. Mayo Clin Proc 72:44–53, 1997.
43. Dummer JS: Infectious complications of transplantation. *In* Thompson, ME (ed): Cardiac Transplantation. Philadelphia: FA Davis, 1990, pp 163–178.
44. Brooks RG, Remington JS: Transplant-related infections. *In* Bennett, JV, Brachman PS (eds): Hospital Infections (2nd ed). Boston: Little, Brown, 1986, pp 581–618.
45. Hofflin JM, Potasman I, Baldwin JC, et al: Infectious complications in heart transplant recipients receiving cyclosporine and corticosteroids. Ann Intern Med 106:209–216, 1987.
46. Tisi GM: Preoperative evaluation of pulmonary function: Validity, indications, and benefits. Am Rev Respir Dis 119:293–310, 1979.
47. Trento A, Dummer JS, Hardesty RL, et al: Mediastinitis following heart transplantation: Incidence, treatment, and results. Heart Transplant 3:336–340, 1984.
48. Collins LA, Samore MH, Roberts MS, et al: Risk factors for invasive fungal infections complicating orthotopic liver transplantation. J Infect Dis 170:644–652, 1994.
49. Hadley S, Karchmer AW: Fungal infections in solid organ transplant recipients. Infect Dis Clin North Am 9:1045–1054, 1995.
50. Warnock DW: Fungal complications of transplantation: Diagnosis, treatment, and prevention. J Antimicrob Chemother 36(Suppl B):73–80, 1995.
51. Zeluff BJ: Fungal pneumonia in transplant recipients. Semin Respir Infect 5:80–87, 1990.
52. Hall KA, Copeland JG, Zukoski CF, et al: Markers of coccidioido-myxosis before cardiac or renal transplantation and the risk of recurrent infection. Transplantation 55:1422–1426, 1993.
53. Ooi BS, Chen BTM, Lim CH, et al: Survival of a patient transplanted with a kidney infected with *Cryptococcus neoformans*. Transplantation 11:428–429, 1971.
54. Gump DW, Frank RO, Winn WC, et al: Legionnaires' disease in patients with associated serious disease. Ann Intern Med 90:538–542, 1979.
55. Redd SC, Schuster DM, Quan J, et al: Legionellosis in cardiac transplant recipients: Results of a nationwide survey. J Infect Dis 158:651–656, 1988.
56. Ramsey PG, Fife KH, Hackman RC, et al: Herpes simplex virus pneumonia. Ann Intern Med 97:813–820, 1982.
57. Wheat LJ, Smith EJ, Sathapatayavongs B, et al: Histoplasmosis in renal allograft recipients: Two large urban outbreaks. Arch Intern Med 143:703–707, 1983.
58. Morgan JS, Schaffner W, Stone WJ: Opportunistic strongyloidiasis in renal transplant recipients. Transplantation 42:518–524, 1986.
59. Luft BJ, Naot Y, Araujo FG, et al: Primary and reactivated *Toxoplasma* infection in patients with cardiac transplants. Ann Intern Med 99:27–31, 1983.
60. Bach MC, Adler JL, Breman J, et al: Influence of rejection therapy on fungal and nocardial infections in renal transplant recipients. Lancet 1:180–184, 1973.
61. Saito H, Anaissie EJ, Morice RC, et al: Bronchoalveolar lavage in the diagnosis of pulmonary infiltrates in patients with acute leukemia. Chest 94:745–749, 1988.
62. Castellino RA, Blank N: Etiologic diagnosis of focal pulmonary infection in immunocompromised patients by fluoroscopically guided percutaneous needle aspiration. Radiology 132:563–567, 1979.
63. St. Georgiev V: *Pneumocystis carinii. In* Infectious Diseases in Immunocompromised Hosts. New York: CRC Press, 1997, pp 1149–1166.
64. Munoz P, Munoz RM, Palomo J, et al: *Pneumocystis carinii* infection in heart transplant recipients: Efficacy of a weekend prophylaxis schedule. Medicine (Baltimore) 76:415–422, 1997.
65. Rubin RH, Tolkoff-Rubin NE: Antimicrobial strategies in the care of organ transplant recipients. Antimicrob Agents Chemother 37:619–624, 1993.
66. Sullivan KM, Deeg HJ, Sanders JE, et al: Late complications after marrow transplantation. Semin Hematol 21:53–63, 1984.
67. Dunn C, Chan J, Rizk N, et al: Diagnosis of pneumonia in heart transplant recipients using fiberoptic bronchoscopy (abstract). Chest 94:S395, 1988.
68. Limper AH, Offord KP, Smith TF, et al: *Pneumocystis carinii* pneumonia: Differences in lung parasite number and inflammation in patients with and without AIDS. Am Rev Respir Dis 140:1204–1209, 1989.
69. Avery RK: Prevention and treatment of cytomegalovirus infection and disease in heart transplant recipients. Curr Opin Cardiol 13:122–129, 1998.
70. Humbert M, Roux-Lombard P, Cerrina J, et al: Soluble TNF receptors in lung allograft recipients displaying cytomegalovirus pneumonitis. Am J Respir Crit Care Med 149:1681–1686, 1994.
71. Fietze E, Prosch S, Reinke P, et al: Cytomegalovirus infection in transplant recipients: The role of tumor necrosis factor. Transplantation 58:675–670, 1994.
72. Dummer JS, White LT, Ho M, et al: Morbidity of cytomegalovirus infection in recipients of heart or heartlung transplants who received cyclosporine. J Infect Dis 152:1182–1191, 1985.
73. Duncan SR, Paradis IL, Yousem SA, et al: Sequelae of cytomegalovirus pulmonary infections in lung allograft recipients. Am Rev Respir Dis 146:1213–1215, 1992.
74. Rubin RH, Cosimi AB, Tolkoff-Rubin NE, et al: Infectious disease syndromes attributable to cytomegalovirus and their significance among renal transplantation recipients. Transplantation 24:458–464, 1977.
75. Peterson PK, Balfour HH, Marker SC, et al: Cytomegalovirus disease in renal allograft recipients: A prospective study of the clinical features, risk factors, and impact on renal transplantation. Medicine (Baltimore) 59:283–300, 1980.
76. Chou S: Acquisition of donor strains of cytomegalovirus by renal transplant recipients. N Engl J Med 314:1418–1423, 1986.
77. Schmidt GM, Horak DA, Niland JC, et al: A randomized, controlled trial of prophylactic ganciclovir for cytomegalovirus pulmonary infection in recipients of allogeneic bone marrow transplants. N Engl J Med 324:1005–1011, 1991.
78. Simmons RL, Matas AJ, Rattazzi LC, et al: Clinical characteristics of the lethal cytomegalovirus infection following renal transplantation. Surgery 82:537–546, 1977.
79. Grattan MT, Moreno-Cabral CE, Starnes VA, et al: Cytomegalovirus infection is associated with cardiac allograft rejection and atherosclerosis. JAMA 261:3561–3566, 1989.
80. Pouteil-Noble C, Ecochand R, Landrivon G, et al: Cytomegalovirus infection: An etiological factor for rejection? Transplantation 55:851–857, 1993.
81. von Willebrand E, Pettersson E, Ahonen J, et al: CMV infection, class II antigen expression, and human kidney allograft rejection. Transplantation 42:364–367, 1986.
82. van Es A, Baldwin WM, Oijans PJ, et al: Expression of HLA-

DR on T lymphocytes following renal transplantation, and association with graft-rejection episodes and cytomegalovirus infection. Transplantation 37:65–69, 1984.
83. Lebrancho Y, al Najjar A, Kapahi P, et al: The association of increased soluble VCAM-1 levels with CMV disease in human kidney allograft recipients. Transplant Proc 27:960, 1995.
84. Humbert M, Delattre RM, Fattal S, et al: In situ production of interleukin-6 within human lung allografts displaying rejection or cytomegalovirus pneumonia. Transplantation 56:623–627, 1993.
85. Fujinami RS, Nelson JA, Walker L, et al: Sequence homology and immunologic cross-reactivity of human cytomegalovirus with HLA-DR b chain: A means for graft rejection and immunosuppression. J Virol 62:100–105, 1988.
86. Beck S, Barrell BJ: Human cytomegalovirus encodes a glycoprotein homologous to MHC class I antigens. Nature 331:269–272, 1988.
87. Huber BT, Hsu PN, Sutkowski N: Virus-encoded superantigens. Microbiol Rev 60:473–482, 1996.
88. Scherer MT, Ignatowicz L, Winslow GM, et al: Superantigens: Bacterial and viral proteins that manipulate the immune system. Ann Rev Cell Biol 9:101–128, 1993.
89. Ho M: Cytomegalovirus infection and indirect sequelae in the immunocompromised transplant patient. Transplant Proc 23:2–7, 1991.
90. Falagas ME, Snydman DR, Griffith J, et al: Exposure to cytomegalovirus from the donated organ is a risk factor for bacteremia in orthotopic liver transplant recipients. Clin Infect Dis 23:468–474, 1996.
91. Hornef MW, Bein G, Fricke L, et al: Coincidence of Epstein-Barr virus reactivation, cytomegalovirus infection, and rejection episodes in renal transplant recipients. Transplantation 60:474–480, 1994.
92. van den Berg AP, Klompmaker IJ, Haagsma EB, et al: Evidence for an increased rate of bacterial infections in liver transplant patients with cytomegalovirus infection. Clin Transplant 10:224–231, 1996.
93. Patel R, Portela D, Badley AD, et al: Risk factors of invasive *Candida* and non-*Candida* fungal infection after liver transplantation. Transplantation 62:926–934, 1996.
94. Carney WP, Rubin RH, Hoffman RA, et al: Analysis of T lymphocyte subsets in cytomegalovirus mononucleosis. J Immunol 126:2114–2116, 1981.
95. Baldwin WM, Claas FHJ, Van Gemert GW, et al: Studies on lymphocytotoxins and rheumatoid factors in renal transplant recipients with cytomegalovirus disease. Transplant Proc 17:616–617, 1985.
96. Schrier RD, Rice GPA, Oldstone MBA: Suppression of natural killer cell activity and T cell proliferation by fresh isolates of cytomegalovirus. J Infect Dis 153:1084–1091, 1986.
97. van den Berg AP, Meyaard L, Otto SA, et al: Cytomegalovirus infection associated with a decreased proliferative capacity and increased rate of apoptosis in peripheral blood lymphocytes. Transplant Proc 27:936–938, 1995.
98. Gilbert MJ, Riddell SR, Plachter B, et al: Cytomegalovirus selectively blocks antigen processing and presentation of its immediate-early gene product. Nature 383:720–722, 1996.
99. Manion DJ, Vivhagool A, Chou T-C, et al: Susceptibility of human cytomegalovirus to two-drug combinations in vitro. Antiviral Ther 1:237–245, 1996.
100. Reed EC, Bowden RA, Dandliker PS, et al: Treatment of cytomegalovirus pneumonia with ganciclovir and intravenous cytomegalovirus immunoglobulin in patients with bone marrow transplants. Ann Intern Med 109:783–788, 1988.
101. Emanuel D, Cunningham I, Jules-Elysee K, et al: Cytomegalovirus pneumonia after bone marrow transplantation successfully treated with the combination of ganciclovir and high dose intravenous immune globulin. Ann Intern Med 109:777–782, 1988.
102. Grundy JE, Shanley JD, Griffiths PD: Is cytomegalovirus interstitial pneumonitis in transplant recipients an immunopathological condition? Lancet 11:996–999, 1987.
103. Snydman DR, Werner BG, Heinze-Lacey B, et al: Use of cytomegalovirus immune globulin to prevent cytomegalovirus disease in renal transplant recipients. N Engl J Med 317:1049–1054, 1987.
104. Balfour HH, Chace BA, Stapleton JT, et al: Randomized, placebo controlled trial of oral acyclovir for the prevention of cytomegalovirus disease in recipients of renal allografts. N Engl J Med 320:1381–1387, 1989.
105. Duncan SR, Paradis LJ, Dauber JD, et al: Ganciclovir prophylaxis for cytomegalovirus infections in pulmonary allograft recipients. Am Rev Respir Dis 146:1419–1425, 1992.
106. Wong T, Toupance O, Chanard J: Acyclovir to prevent cytomegalovirus infection after renal transplantation. Ann Intern Med 115:68, 1991.
107. Paya CV, Marin E, Keating M, et al: Solid organ transplantation: Result and implications of acyclovir use in liver transplants. J Med Virol 1:123–127, 1993.
108. Martin M, Manez R, Linden P, et al: A prospective randomized trial comparing sequential ganciclovir-high dose acyclovir to high dose acyclovir for prevention of cytomegalovirus disease in adult liver transplantation. Transplantation 58:779–786, 1994.
109. Singh N, Yu VL, Mieles L, et al: High-dose acyclovir compared with short-course preemptive ganciclovir therapy to prevent cytomegalovirus disease in liver transplant recipients: A randomized trial. Ann Intern Med 120:375–381, 1994.
110. Merigan TC, Renlund DG, Keay S, et al: A controlled trial of ganciclovir to prevent cytomegalovirus disease after heart transplantation. N Engl J Med 326:1182–1186, 1992.
111. Strauch B, Andrews L, Miller G, et al: Oropharyngeal excretion of Epstein-Barr virus by renal transplant recipients and other patients treated with immunosuppressant drugs. Lancet 1:234–237, 1974.
112. Penn I: Lymphomas complicating organ transplantation. Transplant Proc 15:2790–2797, 1983.
113. Starzl TE, Porter KA, Iwatsuki S, et al: Reversibility of lymphomas and lymphoproliferative lesions developing under cyclosporine-steroid therapy. Lancet 1:583–587, 1984.
114. Cleary ML, Warnke R, Sklar J: Monoclonality of lymphoproliferative lesions in cardiac-transplant recipients. N Engl J Med 310:477–482, 1984.
115. Nalesnik MA, Jaffe R, Starzl TE: The pathology of posttransplant lymphoproliferative disorders occurring in the setting of cyclosporine A-prednisone immunosuppression. Am J Pathol 133:173–192, 1988.
116. Ying AJ, Myerowitz PD, Marsh WL: Posttransplant lymphoproliferative disorder in cardiac transplant allografts. Ann Thoracic Surg 64:1822–1824, 1997.
117. Boyle GL, Michaels MG, Webber SA, et al: Posttransplant lymphoproliferative disorder in pediatric thoracic organ recipients. J Pediatr 131:309–313, 1997.
118. Ho M, Miller GR, Atchison RW, et al: Epstein-Barr virus infections and DNA hybridization studies in posttransplantation lymphoma and lymphoproliferative lesions: The role of primary infection. J Infect Dis 152:876–886, 1985.
119. Hanto DW, Frizzera G, Gajl-Peczalska KJ, et al: Epstein-Barr virus, immunodeficiency, and B cell lymphoproliferation. Transplantation 39:461–472, 1985.
120. Swinnen LI, Costanzo-Nordin MR, Fisher SG, et al: Increased incidence of lymphoproliferative disorder after immunosuppression with the monoclonal antibody OKT3 in cardiac transplant recipients. N Engl J Med 323:1723–1728, 1990.
121. Basgoz N, Preiksaitis J: Post-transplant lymphoproliferative disorder. Infect Dis Clin North Am 9:901–923, 1995.
122. Randhawa PS, Yousem SA, Paradis IL, et al: The clinical spectrum, pathology, and clonal analysis of Epstein-Barr virus-associated lymphoproliferative disorders in heart-lung transplant recipients. Am J Clin Pathol 92:177–185, 1989.
123. Swinnen LJ: Treatment of organ transplant-related lymphoma. Hematol Oncol Clin North Am 11:963–973, 1997.
124. Fischer A, Blanche S, Le Bidois J, et al: Anti-B-cell monoclonal antibodies in the treatment of severe B-cell lymphoproliferative syndrome following bone marrow and organ transplantation. N Engl J Med 324:1451–1456, 1991.
125. Hierholzer JC: Adenoviruses in the immunocompromised host. Clin Microbiol Rev 5:262–274, 1992.
126. Pohl C, Green M, Wald ER, et al: Respiratory syncytial virus in pediatric liver transplant recipients. J Infect Dis 165:166–170, 1992.
127. Englund JA, Sullivan CJ, Jordan MC, et al: Respiratory syncytial virus infection in immunocompromised adults. Ann Intern Med 109:203–207, 1988.

128. Krinzman S, Basgoz N, Kradin R, et al: Respiratory syncytial virus-associated infections in adult recipients of solid organ transplants. J Heart Lung Transplant 17:202–210, 1998.
129. Ljungman P: Herpes virus infections in immunocompromised patients: Problems and therapeutic interventions. Ann Med 25:329–336, 1993.
130. Duncan SR, Raffin TA: Pulmonary complications of immunodeficiencies. *In* Murray JF (ed): Pulmonary Complications of Systemic Disease. New York: Marcel Dekker, 1992, pp 63–148.
131. Hooper DC, Pruitt AA, Rubin RH: Central nervous system infections in the chronically immunosuppressed. Medicine (Baltimore). 61:166–188, 1982.
132. Riska H, Gronhagen-Riska C, Ahonen J: Tuberculosis and renal allograft transplantation. Transplant Proc 19:4096–4097, 1987.
133. Coutts II, Jegarajah S, Stark JE: Tuberculosis in renal transplant recipients. Br J Dis Chest 73:141–148, 1979.
134. Aguada JM, Herrero JA, Gavalda J, et al: Clinical presentation and outcome of tuberculosis in kidney, liver, and heart transplant recipients in Spain. Transplantation 63:1278–1286, 1997.
135. Lichtenstein LH, MacGregor RR: Mycobacterial infections in renal transplant recipients: Report of five cases and review of the literature. Rev Infect Dis 5:216–226, 1983.
136. Dautzenberg B, Grosset J, Fechner J, et al: The management of thirty immunocompromised patients with tuberculosis. Am Rev Respir Dis 129:494–495, 1984.
137. Penn I: Risk of cancer in the transplant patient. *In* Flye M (ed): Principles of Organ Transplantation. Philadelphia: WB Saunders, 1989, pp 634–643.
138. Chanez P, Mourad G, Aubas P, et al: Kaposi's sarcoma of the bronchial tree in a renal transplant recipient. Respiration 53:259–261, 1988.
139. Smart BA, Ochs HD: The molecular basis and treatment of primary immunodeficiency disorders. Curr Opin Pediatr 9:570–576, 1997.
140. Candotti F, Blaese RM: Gene therapy of primary immunodeficiencies. Springer Semin Immunopathol 19:493–508, 1998.
141. Holland SM, Gallin JI: Evaluation of the patient with recurrent bacterial infections. Annu Rev Med 49:185–199, 1998.
142. Burton DR: Structure and function of antibodies. *In* Calabi F, Neuberger MS (eds): Molecular Genetics of Immunoglobulins. Amsterdam: Elsevier Science, 1987.
143. Buckley RH, Schiff RL: The use of intravenous immune globulin in immunodeficiency diseases. N Engl J Med 325:110–117, 1991.
144. Bruton OC: Agammaglobulinemia. Pediatrics 9:722–728, 1952.
145. Ochs HD, Smith CI: X-linked agammaglobulinemia: A clinical and molecular analysis. Medicine (Baltimore) 75:287–299, 1996.
146. Conley M: B cells in patients with X-linked agammaglobulinemia. J Immunol 134:3070–3074, 1985.
147. Campana D, Farrant J, Inamdar N, et al: Phenotypic features and proliferative activity of B cell progenitors in X-linked agammaglobulinemia. J Immunol 145:1675–1680, 1990.
148. Pearl ER, Vogler LB, Okos AJ, et al: B lymphocyte precursors in human bone marrow: An analysis of normal individuals and patients with antibody-deficient states. J Immunol 120:1169–1175, 1978.
149. Lederman HM, Winkelstein JA: X-linked agammaglobulinemia: An analysis of 96 patients. Medicine (Baltimore) 64:145–156, 1985.
150. Rosen FS, Cooper MD, Wedgwood RJP: The primary immunodeficiencies: I. N Engl J Med 311:235–242, 1994.
151. Roffman C, Pandu Rao C, Lederman H, et al: Increased susceptibility to *Mycoplasma* infection in patients with hypogammaglobulinemia. Am J Med 80:590–594, 1986.
152. Saulsbury FT, Bernstein MT, Winkelstein JA: *Pneumocystis carinii* pneumonia as the presenting infection in congenital hypogammaglobulinemia. J Pediatr 95:559–561, 1979.
152a. Walsh G, Flower CD, Nassu S, et al: Granulomatous interstitial pneumonitis in association with primary hypogammaglobulinemia: Computed tomography appearances. J Thorac Imaging 14:207–209, 1999.
153. Wilfert CM, Buckley RH, Mohanakumar T, et al: Persistent and fatal central nervous system echovirus infections in patients with agammaglobulinemia. N Engl J Med 296:1485–1489, 1977.
154. Wright PF, Hatch MH, Kasselbert AJ, et al: Vaccine-associated poliomyelitis in a child with sex-linked agammaglobulinemia. J Pediatr 91:408–412, 1977.
155. Cunningham-Rundles C, Siegal F, Smithwick E, et al: Efficacy of intravenous immunoglobulin in primary humoral immunodeficiency disease. Ann Intern Med 101:435–439, 1984.
156. Buckley RH, Sidbury JB: Hereditary alterations in the immune response: Coexistence of "agammaglobulinemia," acquired hypogammaglobulinemia and selective immunoglobulin deficiency in a sibship. Pediatr Res 2:72–84, 1968.
157. Hoffman T, Winchester R, Schulkind M, et al: Hypogammaglobulinemia with normal T cell function in female siblings. Clin Immunol Immunopathol 7:364–371, 1977.
158. Spickett GP, Farrant J, North ME, et al: Common variable immunodeficiency: How many diseases? Immunol Today 18:325–328, 1997.
159. Cunningham-Rundles C: Clinical and immunological analysis of 103 patients with common variable immunodeficiency. J Clin Immunol 9:22–33, 1989.
160. Sneller MC (moderator): New insights into common variable immunodeficiency. Ann Intern Med 118:720–730, 1993.
161. Provisor AJ, Lacuone JJ, Chilcote RR, et al: Acquired agammaglobulinemia after a life-threatening illness with clinical and laboratory features of infectious mononucleosis in three related male children. N Engl J Med 293:62–65, 1975.
162. Conley ME, Cooper MD: Genetic basis of abnormal B cell development. Curr Opin Immunol 10:399–406, 1988.
163. Howe HS, So AKL, Farrant J, et al: Common variable immunodeficiency is associated with polymorphic markers in the human major histocompatability complex. Clin Exp Immunol 84:387–390, 1991.
164. Schaffer FM, Nonteiro RC, Volanakis JE, et al: IgA deficiency. Immunodefic Rev 3:15–44, 1991.
165. Rosen FS, Cooper MD, Wedgwood RJP: The primary immunodeficiencies: II. N Engl J Med 311:300–309, 1984.
166. Fasano MB, Sullivan KE, Sarpong SB, et al: Sarcoidosis and common variable immunodeficiency. Medicine (Baltimore) 75:251–261, 1996.
167. Cunningham-Rundles C, Siegal FP, Cunningham-Rundles S, et al: Incidence of cancer in 98 patients with common varied immunodeficiency. J Clin Immunol 7:294–299, 1987.
168. Itescu S: Adult immunodeficiency and rheumatic disease. Rheum Dis Clin North Am 22:53–73, 1996.
169. Rosenow EC, Hurley BT: Disorders of the thymus: A review. Arch Intern Med 144:763–770, 1994.
170. Burks AW, Sampson HA, Buckley RH: Anaphylactic reactions after gamma globulin administration in patients with hypogammaglobulinemia: Detection of IgE antibodies to IgA. N Engl J Med 314:560–564, 1986.
171. Seager J, Jamison DL, Wilson J, et al: IgA deficiency, epilepsy, and phenytoin treatment. Lancet 2:632–635, 1975.
172. Ammann AJ, Hong R: Selective IgA deficiency: Presentation of 30 cases and a review of the literature. Medicine (Baltimore) 50:223–236, 1971.
173. Conley ME, Cooper MD: Immature IgA B cells in IgA deficient patients. N Engl J Med 305:495–497, 1981.
174. Strober W, Krakauer R, Klaeveman HL, et al: Secretory component deficiency: A disorder of the IgA immune system. N Engl J Med 294:351–356, 1976.
175. Umetsu D, Ambosino D, Quinti L, et al: Recurrent sinopulmonary infection and impaired antibody response to bacterial capsular polysaccharide antigen in children with selective IgG subclass deficiency. N Engl J Med 313:1247–1251, 1985.
176. Shackelford PJ, Polmar S, Mayus J, et al: Spectrum of $IgG_2$ subclass deficiency in children with recurrent infections: Prospective study. J Pediatr 108:647–653, 1986.
177. Preud'Homme JL, Hanson LA: IgG subclass deficiency. Immunodefic Rev 2:129–149, 1990.
178. Oxelius VA, Laurell AB, Lindquist B, et al: IgA subclasses in selective IgA deficiency: Importance of $IgG_2$-IgA deficiency. N Engl J Med 304:1476–1477, 1981.
179. Heiner DC: Significance of immunoglobulin G subclasses. Am J Med 76(Suppl 3A):1–6, 1984.
180. Reynolds HY: Immunoglobulin G and its function in the human respiratory tract. Mayo Clin Proc 63:161–174, 1988.
181. Shakleford PJ, Granoff DM, Madassery JV, et al: Clinical and im-

munologic characteristics of healthy children with subnormal serum concentrations of $IgG_2$. Pediatr Res 27:16–21, 1990.
182. South MA, Cooper MD, Wollheim FA, et al: The IgA system: II. The clinical significance of IgA deficiency: Studies in patients with agammaglobulinemia and ataxiatelangiectasia. Am J Med 44:168–178, 1978.
183. Notarangelo LD, Duse M, Ugazio AG: Immunodeficiency with hyper-IgM. Immunodefic Rev 3:101–121, 1992.
184. Fuleihan RL: The X-linked hyperimmunoglobulin M syndrome. Semin Hematol 35:321–331, 1998.
185. Levy J, Espanol-Boren T, Thomas C, et al: Clinical spectrum of X-linked hyper-IgM syndrome. J Pediatr 131:47–54, 1997.
186. Allen RC, Armitage RC, Conley ME, et al: CD40 ligand gene defects responsible for x-linked hyper-IgM syndrome. Science 259:990–993, 1993.
186a. Cunningham CK, Bonville CA, Ochs HD, et al: Enteroviral meningoencephalitis as a complication of X-linked hyper IgM syndrome. J Pediatr 134:584–588, 1999.
187. Faulk WP, Kiyasu WS, Cooper MD, et al: Deficiency of IgM. Pediatrics 47:399–404, 1971.
188. Ambrosino DM, Siber GR, Chilmonczyk BA, et al: An immunodeficiency characterized by impaired antibody responses to polysaccharides. N Engl J Med 316:790–793, 1987.
189. Ross SC, Densen P: Complement deficiency states and infection: Epidemiology, pathogenesis, and consequences of neisserial and other infections in an immune deficiency. Medicine (Baltimore) 63:243–273, 1984.
190. Reid KB: Deficiency of the first component of human complement. Immunodefic Rev 1:247–260, 1988.
191. Hauptmann G, Tappeiner G, Schifferli JA: Inherited deficiency of the fourth component of human complement. Immunodefic Rev 1:3–22, 1988.
192. Ballow M, Shira JE, Harden L, et al: Complete absence of the third component of complement in man. J Clin Invest 56:703–710, 1975.
193. Miller ME, Nilsson UR: A familial deficiency of the phagocytosis-enhancing activity of serum related to a dysfunction of the fifth component of complement (C5). N Engl J Med 282:354–358, 1970.
194. Wurzner R, Orren A, Lachmann PJ: Inherited deficiencies of the terminal components of human complement. Immunodefic Rev 3:123–147, 1992.
195. Dale DC, DuPont G IV, Wewerka JR, et al: Chronic neutropenia. Medicine (Baltimore) 58:128–144, 1979.
196. Price TH, Dale DC: The selective neutropenias. Clin Hematol 7:501–521, 1978.
197. Smith RM, Curnutte JT: Molecular basis of chronic granulomatous disease. Blood 77:673–686, 1991.
198. Babior BM, Woodman RC: Chronic granulomatous disease. Semin Hematol 27:247–259, 1990.
199. Malech HL, Nauseef WM: Primary inherited defects in neutrophil function: Etiology and treatment. Semin Hematol 34:279–290, 1997.
199a. Klebanoff SJ: Myeloperoxidase. Proc Assoc Am Physician 111:383–389, 1999.
200. Mouy R, Fisher A, Vilmer E, et al: Incidence, severity and prevention of infections in chronic granulomatous disease. J Pediatr 114:550–560, 1989.
201. Cohen MS, Isturiz RE, Malech HL, et al: Fungal infection in chronic granulomatous disease. Am J Med 71:59–66, 1981.
202. Margolis DM, Melnick DA, Alling SW, et al: Trimethoprim-sulfamethoxazole in the management of chronic granulomatous disease. J Infect Dis 162:723–726, 1990.
203. Ezekowitz A, Phil D, Dinauer M, et al: Partial correction of the phagocyte defect in patients with X-linked chronic granulomatous disease by subcutaneous interferon gamma. N Engl J Med 319:146–150, 1988.
204. Lenarsky C, Parkman R: Bone marrow transplantaion for the treatment of immune deficiency states. Bone Marrow Transplant 6:361–369, 1990.
205. Becker S, Wasser S, Hauses M, et al: Correction of respiratory burst activity in X-linked chronic granulomatous cells to therapeutically relevant levels after gene transfer into bone marrow $CD34^+$ cells. Hum Gene Ther 9:1561–1570, 1998.
206. Li LL, Dinauer M: Reconstitution of NADPH oxidase activity in human X-linked chronic granulomatous disease myeloid cells after stable gene transfer using a recombinant adeno-associated virus 2 vector. Blood Cells Mol Dis 24:522–538, 1998.
206a. Malech HL: Progress in gene therapy for chronic granulomatous disease. J Infect Dis 179(suppl 2):S318–S325, 1999.
207. Root RK, Rosenthal AS, Balestra DJ: Abnormal bactericidal, metabolic, and lysosomal functions of Chédiak-Higashi syndrome leukocytes. J Clin Invest 51:649–665, 1972.
208. Vassalli JD, Franelli-Piperno A, Griscelli C, et al: Specific protease deficiency in polymorphonuclear leukocytes of Chédiak-Higashi syndrome and beige mice. J Exp Med 147:1285–1290, 1978.
209. Gallin JL, Wright DG, Malech HL, et al: Disorders of phagocyte chemotaxis. Ann Intern Med 92:520–538, 1980.
210. Anderson DC, Springer TA: Leukocyte adhesion deficiency: An inherited defect in the Mac-1, LFA-1, and p150, 95 glycoproteins. Annu Rev Med 38:175–194, 1987.
211. Fischer A, Lisowska-Grospierre B, Anderson DC, et al: Leukocyte adhesion deficiency: Molecular basis and functional consequences. Immunodefic Rev 1:39–54, 1988.
212. Lipnick RN, Iliopoulos A, Salata K, et al: Leukocyte adhesion deficiency: Report of a case and review of the literature. Clin Exp Rheum 14:95–98, 1996.
213. Van Scoy RE, Hill HR, Ritts RE, et al: Familial neutrophil chemotaxis defect, recurrent bacterial infections, mucocutaneous candidiasis and hyperimmunoglobulin E. Ann Intern Med 82:766–771, 1975.
214. Donabedian H, Gallin JL: The hyperimmunoglobulin E recurrent-infection (Job's) syndrome. Medicine (Baltimore) 62:195–208, 1983.
215. Leung DY, Ambrosino DM, Arbeit RD, et al: Impaired antibody responses in the hyperimmunoglobulinemia E syndrome. J Allergy Clin Immunol 81:1082–1087, 1988.
216. Del Prete G, Tiri A, Maggi E, et al: Defective in vitro production of gamma-interferon and tumor necrosis factor-alpha by circulating T cells from patients with the hyperimmunoglobulin E syndrome. J Clin Invest 84:1830–1835, 1989.
217. Jacobs JC, Norman ME: A familial defect of neutrophil chemotaxis with asthma, eczema, and recurrent skin infections. Pediatr Res 11:732–736, 1977.
218. Hong R: The DiGeorge anomaly (CATCH 22, DiGeorge/velocardiofacial syndrome). Semin Hematol 35:282–290, 1998.
219. Lischner HW: DiGeorge syndrome(s). J Pediatr 81:183–192, 1972.
220. Fibison WJ, Budarf M, McDermid H, et al: Molecular studies of DiGeorge syndrome. Am J Hum Genet 46:888–895, 1990.
221. Borzy MS, Ridgway D, Nowa FJ, et al: Successful bone marrow transplantation with split lymphoid chimerism in DiGeorge syndrome. J Clin Immunol 9:386–392, 1989.
222. Maret ML, Kostyu DD, McLaughlin TM, et al: Successful formation of a chimeric human thymus allograft following transplantation of a cultured postnatal human thymus. J Immunol 158:998–1005, 1997.
223. Markert ML: Purine nucleoside phosphorylase deficiency. Immunodefic Rev 3:45–81, 1991.
224. Hirschhorn R: Inherited enzyme deficiencies and immunodeficiency: Adenosine deaminase (ADA) and purine nucleoside phosphorylase (PNP) deficiencies. Clin Immunol Immunopathol 40:157–165, 1986.
225. Broome CB, Graham ML, Saulsbury FT, et al: Correction of purine nucleoside phosphorylase deficiency by transplantation of allogeneic bone marrow from a sibling. J Pediatr 128:373–376, 1996.
226. Carpenter PA, Ziegler JB, Vowels MR: Late diagnosis and correction of purine nucleoside phosphorylase deficiency with allogeneic bone marrow transplantation. Bone Marrow Transplant 17:121–124, 1996.
227. Buckley RH: Immunodeficiency. J Allergy Clin Immunol 72:627–641, 1983.
228. Buckley RH, Schiff RI, Schiff SE, et al: Human severe combined immunodeficiency: Genetic, phenotypic, and functional diversity in one hundred eight infants. J Pediatr 130:378–387, 1997.
229. Cutz E, Throner PS, Rao CP, et al: Disseminated *Legionella pneumophila* infection in an infant with severe combined immunodeficiency. J Pediatr 100:760–762, 1982.

230. Puck JM, Basile G, Schwarz K, et al: IL2RGbase: A database of dc-chain defects causing human X-SCID. Immunol Today 11:507–511, 1996.
231. Johnston JA, Bacon CM, Riedy MC, et al: Signalling by IL-2 and related cytokines: JAKs, STATs, and relationship to immunodeficiency. J Leuk Biol 60:441–452, 1996.
232. Elder ME: ZAP-70 and defects of T-cell receptor signalling. Semin Hematol 35:310–320, 1998.
233. Steimle V, Reith W, Mach B: Major histocompatibility complex class II deficiency: A disease of gene regulation. Adv Immunol 61:327–340, 1996.
234. Puel A, Ziegler SF, Buckley RH, et al: Defective IL7R expression in T(−)B(+)NK(+) severe combined immunodeficiency. Nat Genet 20:394–397, 1998.
235. Resta R, Thompson LF: SCID: The role of adenosine deaminase deficiency. Immunol Today 18:371–374, 1997.
235a. Hershfield MS: Adenosine deaminase deficiency: Clinical expression, molecular basis, and therapy. Semin Hematol 35:291–298, 1998.
236. Buckley RH, Schiff SE, Schiff RI, et al: Hematopoietic stem-cell transplantation for the treatment of severe combined immunodeficiency. N Engl J Med 340:508–516, 1999.
237. Gatti RA, Boder E, Vinters HV, et al: Ataxia-telangiectasia: An interdisciplinary approach to pathogenesis. Medicine (Baltimore) 70:99–117, 1991.
238. Crawford TO: Ataxia telangiectasia. Semin Pediatr Neurol 5:287–294, 1998.
239. Yuille MA, Coignet LJ: The gene in familial and sporadic cancer. Recent Results Cancer Res 154:156–173, 1998.
240. Rotman G, Shiloh Y: ATM: From gene to function. Hum Mol Genet 7:1555–1563, 1998.
241. Oxelius VA, Berkel AI, Hanson LA: $IgG_2$ deficiency in ataxia-telangiectasia. N Engl J Med 306:515–517, 1982.
242. Kersey JH, Shapiro RS, Filipovich AH: Relationship of immunodeficiency to lymphoid malignancy. Pediatr Infect Dis J 7(Suppl):S10–S12, 1988.
243. Swift M, Sholman L, Perry M, et al: Malignant neoplasms in the families of patients with ataxia-telangiectasia. Cancer Res 36:209–215, 1976.
244. Perry GS, Spector BD, Schuman LM, et al: The Wiskott-Aldrich syndrome in the United States and Canada (1892–1979). J Pediatr 97:72–80, 1980.
245. Sullivan KE, Mullen CA, Blasse RM, et al: The Wiskott-Aldrich syndrome. J Pediatr 125:876–885, 1994.
246. Schwarz K, Nonoyama S, Peitsch MC, et al: WASPbase: A database of WAS- and XLT-causing mutations. Immunol Today 17:496–502, 1996.
247. Rimm IJ, Rappeport JM: Bone marrow transplantation for the Wiskott-Aldrich syndrome: Long-term follow-up. Transplantation 50:617–620, 1990.

# 84 Pulmonary Complications of Heart Disease

J. Michael B. Hughes, D.M., F.R.C.P.

Introduction
Causes and Consequences of Raised Pulmonary Venous Pressure
- Interstitial and Alveolar Edema
- Histopathology of Chronic Pulmonary Venous Hypertension
- Hemodynamics
- Lung Volumes
- Diffusing Capacity (Transfer Factor)
- Pulmonary Function After Lowering Pulmonary Venous Pressure
- Lung Compliance
- Airway Resistance
- Respiratory Muscle Function
- Regional Lung Function
- Pulmonary Gas Exchange
- Exercise Responses
- Sleep

Mechanisms of Dyspnea
- Acute Pulmonary Edema
- Orthopnea
- Exercise Dyspnea

Summary

## INTRODUCTION

The main way in which the heart influences the lungs is through the level of pulmonary venous pressure. Acute elevation of pulmonary venous pressure caused by mitral stenosis or inadequate left ventricular contraction leads to pulmonary edema once a mean pulmonary capillary pressure of 25 to 30 mm Hg has been exceeded. More common, nowadays, is the mild-to-moderate pulmonary venous hypertension of chronic treated heart failure, accompanied by profound dyspnea on exertion, a limited exercise capacity, and structural damage to the lungs. This chapter focuses on the pulmonary dysfunction associated with acute and chronic left-sided heart failure and discusses possible mechanisms for the breathlessness and exercise limitation that are the patients' main complaints.

Other causes of pulmonary hypertension are described in Chapter 52; for a discussion of the effects of intracardiac shunts on lung function, the reader is advised to consult the review by Broaddus.[1]

## CAUSES AND CONSEQUENCES OF RAISED PULMONARY VENOUS PRESSURE

### Interstitial and Alveolar Edema

The causes of increased venous pressure are listed in Table 84.1. The effects on the lungs are common to all, but they vary according to the severity of the pressure elevation and the chronicity of the condition. Further information about the pathogenesis of pulmonary edema is provided in Chapter 54.

As pulmonary venous pressure rises, so do pulmonary capillary and arterial pressures. Distention and recruitment of alveolar septal capillaries[2] and recruitment of arteriolar domains occur.[3] An increasing proportion of the lung (in the gravity axis) is in West's zone 3,[4] in which pulmonary venous pressure exceeds alveolar pressure. (See Chapter 4 for more information about the effect of gravity on the lungs.) In accordance with Starling's principle, microvascular filtration and lymph flow increase when capillary pressure rises.[5] Before reaching the lymphatics, the filtrate accumulates in the interstitial spaces of the lung, first in the alveolar septa (where space is limited) and then in the loose peribronchial and perivascular tissue[6] and pleural space.[7] The latter two act as a sump or safety valve to prevent an excessive rise in interstitial pressure, which would flood the alveoli with edema fluid and impair gas exchange. In an experimental study of hydrostatic edema,[7] only one third of the microvascular filtrate was removed by the lymphatic vessels, the remainder being accommodated in the lungs (43%) and in the pleural space (23%). Pulmonary edema fluid is eventually cleared in the systemic venous system via the lymphatics; the elevation of systemic venous pressure in patients with congestive heart failure (CHF) slows lymph flow[8] even

**Table 84.1 COMMON CAUSES OF A RAISED PULMONARY VENOUS PRESSURE**

| Site | Cause: Acute | Cause: Chronic |
|---|---|---|
| Left ventricle | Myocardial infarction<br>Paroxysmal tachycardia<br>Myocarditis<br>Pericardial tamponade | Congestive heart failure<br>Cardiomyopathy (restrictive/ obstructive)<br>Pericardial constriction |
| Mitral valve | Endocarditis<br>Ruptured papillary muscles or chordae tendineae | Mitral stenosis<br>Mitral regurgitation |
| Left atrium | Myxoma<br>Ball-valve thrombus | Myxoma |
| Pulmonary veins | | Veno-occlusive disease<br>Mediastinitis/ fibrosis |

though lymphatic vessels have valves and contract actively, producing intralymphatic pressures up to 30 mm Hg. Pleural transudates are a reflection of pulmonary edema, correlating better with increases in wedge pressure[9] than with rises in systemic venous pressure.[10]

## Histopathology of Chronic Pulmonary Venous Hypertension

**Alveolar Damage.** The earliest histologic changes arising from increases in pulmonary venous and capillary pressures occur in the alveolar-capillary wall,[11] which becomes edematous, particularly in the thicker, collagen-containing parts of the septum. The thinnest part of the alveolar barrier, consisting of the fused basement membranes of the epithelial and endothelial cells, is unaffected, leaving gas exchange unimpaired. The interstitial edema becomes organized and "hyaline" with the formation of a mucopolysaccharide ground substance. There is swelling of endothelial cells and proliferation of connective tissue (reticulin and elastin) in the interstitium and of epithelial type II cells, the last being a stereotyped response to injury.

The initial response to an elevation of capillary pressure is edema with a low protein content and distention of perivascular lymphatics. In experimental models (isolated perfused rabbit lungs), capillary hypertension leads to alveolar damage with endothelial and epithelial cell rupture (breaks or fractures), seen on transmission[12] and scanning[13] electron microscopy. The distribution of edema fluid and its protein content is very inhomogeneous.[14, 15] Clearly, vascular barotrauma induced by elevated left atrial pressures can increase capillary permeability,[16] with leak of protein and erythrocytes into the interstitial and alveolar spaces. The extravascular red blood cells disintegrate, and their hemosiderin is ingested by tissue macrophages (see Fig. 18.11 in Chapter 18). Progressive fibrosis with collagen formation leads to obliteration of pulmonary capillaries.

The increased intraluminal pressure also leads to hypertrophy and fibrous change in the pulmonary arteries and veins. The main changes are medial hypertrophy of the muscular pulmonary arteries with intimal fibrosis and peripheral extension of the muscle coat into the smaller branches of the pulmonary arterial tree. The pulmonary veins show similar changes.[17] The basic pathophysiologic mechanism in acute heart failure is the same as in mitral stenosis, but progression to alveolar hyalinization and fibrosis and medial hypertrophy of vessels has not yet occurred, and a greater degree of functional reversibility can be expected.

**Vascular Remodeling.** The remodeling that occurs in pulmonary hypertension has been studied in detail in experimental models.[18, 19] In vessel segments exposed to 50 mm Hg of mechanical stress, collagen messenger ribonucleic acid (mRNA) expression and synthesis are increased, provided the endothelium is present.[18] Pulmonary smooth muscle cells in culture, from hypertensive animals exposed to chronic hypoxia, produce mRNA for elastin and elastogenic factors that stimulate elastin production.[19] Further information is available in a 1997 review.[20] The extracellular matrix production and cell hypertrophy can regress after reduction of the elevated pulmonary artery pressure; this is associated with recruitment of collagenase-producing mast cells into the outer walls of the pulmonary arteries.[21] Clinically, regression of pulmonary hypertension after reduction of pulmonary venous pressure by mitral valve surgery or cardiac transplantation is substantial but incomplete (Table 84.2).

**Blood-Gas Barrier.** In chronic pulmonary venous hypertension, marked thickening of the basement membranes of the capillary endothelial cells and alveolar epithelial cells occurs. West and Mathieu-Costello[22] reviewed the subject of *stress failure* of the pulmonary capillaries. The integrity of the blood-gas barrier on its thin (0.2 to 0.3 μm in width) gas-exchanging side depends on the lamina densa, the central core of the fused basement membranes of the alveolar epithelial and capillary endothelial cells. The lamina densa comprises a thin (50 nm) layer of type IV collagen. The thickness (and strength) of this layer of collagen varies according to the vascular stress imposed upon it. In the systemic circulation, there is a progression in capillary basement membrane thickness from the thigh to the calf, in keeping with the higher hydrostatic pressures in the lower leg,[23] and a similar thickening in pulmonary capillaries develops in patients with long-standing pulmonary venous hypertension,[11] as already mentioned. Changes in gene expression for extracellular matrix proteins ($\alpha_1$ III and $\alpha_2$ IV procollagen, fibronectin, fibroblast growth factor, and transforming growth factor-beta) occur in response to the increase in capillary wall stress.[24] In addition to conditions associated with high pulmonary venous pressures, pulmonary capillary stress failure with breakdown of the alveolar-capillary membranes occurs consistently in galloping thor-

**Table 84.2** PULMONARY HEMODYNAMICS BEFORE (PRE) AND AFTER (POST) REDUCTION OF PULMONARY VENOUS PRESSURE BY SURGERY (MITRAL VALVULOPLASTY OR CARDIAC TRANSPLANTATION) AND BY INFUSION OF PROSTAGLANDIN $E_1$ ($PGE_1$)

| | Mitral Stenosis (Percutaneous Valvuloplasty, 14 Patients) | | Congestive Heart Failure (Cardiac Transplantation, 11 Patients) | | |
|---|---|---|---|---|---|
| Parameter | Pre | Post (7 mo) | Pre | Post (1 mo) | Post + $PGE_1$ |
| Pulmonary artery pressure (mm Hg) | 51 | 35 | 43 | 23 | 19 |
| Pulmonary wedge pressure (mm Hg) | 26 | 19 | 29 | 11 | 10 |
| Pulmonary artery minus wedge pressure (mm Hg) | 25 | 16 | 14 | 12 | 9 |
| Cardiac output (L/min) | 3.7 | 4.3 | 3.4 | 4.9 | 5.7 |
| Pulmonary vascular resistance (PVR) (mm Hg per L/min) | 7.9 | 3.5 | 4.3 | 2.4 | 1.7 |
| PVR (post/pre %) | — | 44 | — | 56 | 4 |

Data on mitral stenosis from Levine MJ, Weinstein JS, Diver DJ, et al: Progressive improvement in pulmonary vascular resistance after percutaneous mitral valvuloplasty. Circulation 79:1061–1067, 1989. Data on congestive heart failure from Naeije R, Lipski A, Abramowicz M, et al: Nature of pulmonary hypertension in congestive heart failure: Effects of cardiac transplantation. Am J Respir Crit Care Med 149:881–887, 1994.

oughbred racehorses, in intense exercise by elite human athletes, in neurogenic and high-altitude pulmonary edema, and in overinflation of the lung.[22]

## Hemodynamics

**Pressures at Rest and with Exercise.** Table 84.3 contrasts the pulmonary hemodynamic response at rest and with exercise in patients with severe chronic CHF and in young healthy subjects.[25] Half the patients with CHF had idiopathic cardiomyopathy, and only two had valvular lesions; all had cardiomegaly. Nevertheless, the pressure changes in mitral stenosis[17] were the same as in CHF. The obvious points in Table 84.3, in terms of ratios of CHF to normal (columns 3 and 6), are the low ratios (less than 0.35) with maximum exercise for oxygen uptake and

**Table 84.3** PULMONARY HEMODYNAMICS AT REST AND ON MAXIMAL EXERCISE

| | Rest (Mean Values) | | | Exercise* (Mean Values) | | |
|---|---|---|---|---|---|---|
| Parameter | CHF (n = 28) | Normal (n = 29) | CHF/Normal | CHF (n = 28) | Normal (n = 6) | CHF/Normal |
| Oxygen uptake (mL/min per kg) | 4 | 5.3†‡ | — | 12 | 57 | 0.21 |
| Pulmonary artery pressure (mm Hg) | 30 | 14 | 2.15 | 53 | 35 | 1.52 |
| Pulmonary wedge pressure (mm Hg) | 20 | 5 | 4.0 | 38 | 24 | 1.58 |
| Cardiac index (L/min per m²) | 2.5 | 3.55† | 0.7 | 4.54 | 14† | 0.33 |
| Pulmonary vascular resistance (mm Hg L⁻¹ min) | 7§ | 1.5 | 4.65 | 7§ | 0.5 | 14 |
| Pulmonary artery − wedge pressure (mm Hg per L/min) | 10 | 9 | 1.11 | 15 | 11 | 1.38 |

CHF = congestive heart failure.
*Sitting posture: cycle ergometer.
†Assuming body weight of 70 kg and body surface area of 1.83 m².
‡Not really basal.
§New York Heart Association Class II (n = 6), III (n = 19), and IV (n = 3).
Data on CHF from Franciosa JA, Leddy CL, Wilen M, et al: Relation between hemodynamic and ventilatory responses in determining exercise capacity in severe congestive heart failure. Am J Cardiol 53:127, 1984. Data on normal subjects from Reeves JT, Grover RF, Dempsey JA: Pulmonary circulation during exercise. *In* Weir EK, Reeves JT (eds): Lung Biology in Health and Disease Series. Vol. 38. Pulmonary Vascular Physiology and Pathophysiology. New York: Marcel Dekker, 1988, pp. 110–111.

**Table 84.4 POSTURAL EFFECTS ON PULMONARY MECHANICS IN NORMAL SUBJECTS AND IN PATIENTS WITH CONGESTIVE HEART FAILURE (CHF)**

| Pulmonary Variable | Patients with CHF (n = 10) | | Normal Subjects (n = 10) | |
|---|---|---|---|---|
| | Sitting | Supine | Sitting | Supine |
| Visual analog score of breathlessness | 2.2 | 3.9* | 0 | 0 |
| Vital capacity (L) | 2.6 | 2.4* | 4.5 | 4.4 |
| Functional residual capacity (L) | 3.3 | 3.1 | 3.7 | 3.05† |
| $FEV_1$ (% predicted) | 76 | 66† | 103 | 97† |
| $MEF_{50\%}$ VC ($L\ s^{-1}$) | 2.2 | 1.6† | 3.0 | 2.8 |
| Total respiratory resistance (Rrs) (forced oscillation at 6 Hz, cm $H_2O\ L\ s^{-1}$) | 3.4 | 6.1‡ | 2.6 | 3.4† |
| Specific total respiratory resistance (SRrs) (Rrs × midtidal lung volume) | 12.1 | 21‡ | 10.2 | 11.8 |
| ΔSRrs (before ipratropium minus after ipratropium) | 0.9 | 2.2 | 0.7 | 0.7 |

Data from Yap JCH, Moore D, Cleland JGF, et al: Mechanisms of the supine increase in airflow resistance in chronic left ventricular failure (abstract). Am Rev Respir Dis 143:A345, 1991.
*$P < .05$ (sitting versus supine).
†$P < .01$ (sitting versus supine).
‡$P < .001$ (sitting versus supine).

nary Function after Lowering of Pulmonary Venous Pressure) and the engorged pulmonary vessels and extra interstitial fluid probably add another 100 mL at least,[46] making thoracic volume some 600 mL greater than in normal subjects during resting tidal breathing. In the supine posture, because the gas volume in heart failure (at FRC) does not fall as it does in normal subjects, the total thoracic volume may be 800 to 1000 mL greater. Unless there are compensatory increases in the compliances of the lung and chest wall, which is unlikely, the elastic work of breathing must increase and additional work must be done by the inspiratory muscles to maintain the thoracic volume at levels well above the relaxation volume of the system. In fact, the work of breathing, compared with that in normal subjects, is increased 2.5 times in the sitting position and threefold in the supine posture.[47]

## Diffusing Capacity (Transfer Factor)

The extensive literature on the carbon monoxide diffusing capacity ($DL_{CO}$) or its European equivalent transfer factor ($TL_{CO}$) in the early 1960s, mostly dealing with mitral stenosis, was reviewed by Yu[48] and by Harris and Heath.[17] In several studies $DL_{CO}$ (the overall alveolar-capillary conductance) was partitioned (using the Roughton-Forster approach) into membrane diffusive conductance (DM) and the reactive conductance, which is proportional to pulmonary capillary volume (Vc). Table 84.5 summarizes the results from two series.[49, 50] Worsening NYHA functional class is accompanied by a progressive fall in $DL_{CO}$, which is related to a fall in DM rather than to any change in Vc. The reciprocal (1/DM) is the diffusive resistance due to the alveolar capillary membranes. The proportion of the total resistance residing in the membranes rises from 50% in healthy controls to 60% in patients in NYHA grade II functional class and then to 80% in those in NYHA grade III.[50] Lung volumes (e.g., vital capacity, see Table 84.5) are smaller, but the volume-corrected membrane diffusing capacity (DM/VA) also falls in patients with CHF compared with normal controls, to 50% in NYHA grade III.[50] There was a 13% reduction ($p < .005$) in DM in patients with asymptomatic heart failure (NYHA I) after acute saline infusion (10 mL/kg), accompanied by a 9% fall in $FEV_1$; no changes were seen in control subjects.[51] The patients remained asymptomatic, and there was a return to baseline function when the tests were repeated 24 hours later.[51] This implies that acute reductions of DM may be an index of alveolar septal edema. The long-term and irreversible reduction of DM is probably a reflection of stress failure (discussed earlier) of the alveolar-capillary interface induced by pulmonary capillary hypertension[22]—not so much the mean level of capillary pressure, but the peak levels reached on exertion.[28]

Structure-function correlations (lingula biopsy at the time of mitral valvotomy) have shown a good correlation between reduction of $DL_{CO}$ and extent of pulmonary vascular changes, especially intimal fibrosis and luminal narrowing,[52] but not a good correlation with alveolar fibrosis.[53] In patients with NYHA class IV, destruction of the pulmonary vascular bed contributes to the large rise in PVR (see Table 84.5).

The $DL_{CO}$ is more severely affected than are lung volumes.[39] In the study of Rhodes and coworkers,[39] the mean value was 74% of predicted, in contrast to 87% of predicted for vital capacity. The alveolar efficiency for carbon monoxide uptake (KCO or $DL_{CO}$/VA) was somewhat less abnormal, with a mean of 93% of predicted. Because $DL_{CO} = KCO \times VA$, a low VA must have been contributing to the reduction of $DL_{CO}$ through a loss of functioning alveolar tissue. Nevertheless, in a situation of pure loss of units (after lobectomy or pneumonectomy), there is always a compensatory increase in the KCO. Therefore, the reduction in KCO in patients with mitral stenosis, although modest, suggests a significant degree of alveolar destruction or disorganization.

**Table 84.5** PULMONARY HEMODYNAMICS AND CARBON MONOXIDE DIFFUSING CAPACITY ($DL_{CO}$) AND ITS SUBDIVISIONS (MEMBRANE DIFFUSING CAPACITY AND CAPILLARY VOLUME) IN PATIENTS WITH CONGESTIVE HEART FAILURE, BY NEW YORK HEART ASSOCIATION GRADE

| | Gazioglu and Yu | | | Puri et al | | |
|---|---|---|---|---|---|---|
| Parameter | II | III | IV | II | III | Normal |
| No. patients | 11 | 40 | 11 | 40 | 10 | 14 |
| Mean pulmonary artery pressure (mm Hg) | 27 | 31 | 48 | 30 | — | 13 |
| Left atrial pressure (mm Hg) | 16 | 20 | 25 | 21 | — | 8 |
| Pulmonary vascular resistance (mm Hg per L/min) | 2.9 | 3.4 | 10 | 2.9 | — | 1.2 |
| Vital capacity (% predicted) | — | — | — | 82 | 76 | — |
| $DL_{CO}$ (% predicted) | 79 | 74 | 47 | 80 | 72 | — |
| $DL_{CO}$ per unit volume (DL/VA or KCO, % predicted) | — | — | — | 95 | 85 | — |
| Membrane diffusing capacity (% predicted) | 100 | 71 | 61 | 65 | 35 | — |
| Capillary volume (% predicted) | 89 | 91 | 50 | 90 | 124 | — |

Data from Gazioglu K, Yu PN: Pulmonary blood volume and pulmonary capillary blood volume in vascular heart disease. Circulation 35:701, 1967; and Puri SP, Baker BL, Dutka DP et al. Reduced alveolar-capillary membrane diffusing capacity in chronic heart failure. Circulation 91; 2769–2774, 1995.

## Pulmonary Function After Lowering of Pulmonary Venous Pressure

Thoracotomy and sternotomy themselves lead to a temporary (6-week) decrease in vital capacity.[54] Ten weeks after mitral valve surgery, there are, overall, no significant changes in lung volumes or diffusing capacity. There is a small improvement in function over the next 3 months.[55] A fall in residual volume has been observed.[41] Irreversible structural changes (hyalinization of interstitial edema, collagen deposition, and fibrosis) are the reason why pulmonary function fails to improve.

On the other hand, lung volumes do improve after cardiac transplantation. Hosenpud[56] reported an average increase of 0.36 L in $FEV_1$ and 0.55 L in forced vital capacity (FVC) in 17 patients studied 15 $\pm$ 10 months after transplantation. The change in FVC correlated with the decrease in cardiac volume ($r = 0.83$). Table 84.6 summarizes the lung function changes at 1 year after transplantation for two series.[57, 58] Bussieres and colleagues[58] made serial measurements and noted that it was 3 months before $FEV_1$ improved (note the effect of sternotomy[54]) and that there was a further increase at 1 year. Table 84.6 shows significant increases in lung volumes ($FEV_1$, FVC, and total lung capacity), related to cardiac volume changes, but not in the $DL_{CO}$; residual volume (not shown) did not change.

## Lung Compliance

**Effect of Acute Vascular Distention.** The effects of an acute elevation of pulmonary venous pressure on lung compliance were investigated in normal subjects by rapid infusion of 2 L of saline, which is sufficient to raise pulmonary artery diastolic pressure (referred to the lung base) from 23 to 30 mm Hg.[59] There was no fall in lung compliance, nor did the subjects report chest discomfort or dyspnea. This contrasts with the findings of Pepine and Wiener,[33] who induced (by pacing) tachycardia and anginal symptoms in 16 patients with proved ischemic heart disease. Lung compliance did not fall with tachycardia alone, but only when anginal symptoms supervened and left-ventricular end-diastolic pressure rose (Table

**Table 84.6** CHANGES IN PULMONARY FUNCTION IN PATIENTS WITH CONGESTIVE HEART FAILURE BEFORE (PRE) AND 12 MONTHS AFTER (POST) HEART TRANSPLANTATION

| | Bussieres et al | | Niset et al | |
|---|---|---|---|---|
| Parameter | Pre | Post | Pre | Post |
| $FEV_1$ (L) | 2.8 | 3.7 | 2.4 | 2.9 |
| $FEV_1$ (% predicted) | 80 | 105 | 69 | 83 |
| Vital capacity (% predicted) | 85 | 112 | 75 | 94 |
| $FEV_1$/FVC ratio | 0.77 | 0.75 | 0.75 | 0.72 |
| TLC (L) | 5.4 | 6.5 | 5.2 | 6.4 |
| TLC (% predicted) | 80 | 97 | 79 | 98 |
| $DL_{CO}$ (% predicted) | 61 | 68 | 64 | 67 |
| KCO (DL/VA) (% predicted) | 57 | 56 | 65 | 58 |

Data from Bussieres LM, Pflugfelder PW, Ahmad D, et al: Evolution of resting lung function in the first year after cardiac transplantation. Eur Respir J 8:959–962, 1995; and Niset G, Ninane V, Antoine M, et al: Respiratory dysfunction in congestive heart failure: Correction after heart transplantation. Eur Respir J 6:1197–1201, 1993.

84.7). The effect on lung compliance was reversed after sublingual administration of nitroglycerin. During the anginal episode, there was a fall in specific airway conductance (see Table 84.7), which was less impressive than the fall in compliance, and a minimal increase in resting lung volume. Pepine and Wiener[33] could not reproduce the fall in compliance in normal control subjects by inducing chest pain through electric stimulation. The rapidly reversible fall in lung compliance during angina must be linked with vascular distention rather than interstitial or alveolar edema; to date, their findings have not been reproduced. A similar instantaneous fall in compliance (also about 30%) occurs on changing from sitting to supine position.[47]

In excised lungs of rabbits and cats, acute vascular distention (without the induction of pulmonary edema) causes a subtle change in the pressure-volume curve, shifting it to the right above FRC and to the left below FRC.[60] The right shift at high lung volumes can be explained by air displacement due to vascular distention, whereas the left shift at low lung volumes (increase in volume for the same lung recoil pressure and reduction in compliance, $\Delta V/\Delta P$) is thought to be caused by the von Basch effect (the erectile nature of engorged capillaries, which was described in 1887). These effects have been reproduced in normal subjects with elevations of central venous pressure[61] and in patients with pulmonary plethora (atrial septal defect) or with mitral valve disease (Fig. 84.2). Notice that the shift to the right is more pronounced in mitral valve disease than in atrial septal defect (where it is similar to the effects of vascular distention in animal lungs).

**Chronic Changes.** The reduction in static compliance in mitral stenosis correlates with the reduction in vital capacity and total lung capacity.[62] This may reflect the alveolar destruction and fibrosis produced by chronic elevation of pulmonary venous pressure. In contrast to pulmonary fibrotic disease, maximum lung recoil pressure is not increased (see Fig. 84.2). This is related to respiratory muscle weakness (see later discussion). In eight patients with acute pulmonary edema (on a background of CHF), lung compliance was severely reduced, averaging 0.037 L cm $H_2O^{-1}$ (normal, greater than 0.2), rising to 0.09 after recovery.[63]

## Airway Resistance

**Mitral Stenosis.** Although wheezing is a common feature and there is an increase in residual volume, there are only minor increases in airflow resistance in patients with chronic elevation of pulmonary venous pressure. In nonsmokers[39] the mean $FEV_1/FVC$ and total lung capacity values were within normal limits. On a maximum expiratory flow-volume curve, flows at all lung volumes were reduced by about 30%,[40] and airway resistance was increased twofold (equivalent to an average reduction of 13% in bronchial diameter). Frequency dependence of lung compliance was found in only 4 of 14 patients with mitral valve disease.[40] This test is regarded as a sensitive index of peripheral airflow obstruction. There was, in addition, no evidence of delayed nitrogen washout during 100% oxygen breathing.[38]

**Acute Heart Failure.** In cases of acute left-ventricular dysfunction (after myocardial infarction) reviewed by Hales and Kazemi,[42] airflow obstruction shown by a reduced $FEV_1/FVC$ ratio was a frequent finding. Light and George[44] reported a ratio of 0.66 in 15 nonsmokers with acute congestive failure, which improved to 0.71 after treatment and recovery. The ratio was the same in a similar number of smokers who also had heart failure, but they showed no improvement after recovery. Sharp and coworkers[63] studied seven patients with severe pulmonary edema and again after recovery; inspiratory resistance by the von Neergaard and Wirz method averaged 9.1 cm $H_2O$ $L^{-1}$ sec (330% of predicted), falling slightly to 8.7 after treatment. This rise in resistance is probably caused by a fall in FRC (geometric narrowing) and an increase in vagal tone (bronchoconstriction).[64] Peribronchial cuffs of edema fluid do not contribute to the airway narrowing.[65]

**Chronic Heart Failure.** Using an esophageal balloon technique, Cherniack and associates[47] found that airway resistance (seated) was 2.5 times higher in patients with CHF than in normal subjects. In a more recent study,[45] total respiratory resistance (seated) was only slightly higher (1.3 times) and maximal mid-expiratory flow ($MEF_{50\%}$) only slightly lower (0.8 times). The $FEV_1/FVC$ ratio in these patients was normal. Interesting changes

**Table 84.7** EFFECT OF CARDIAC PACING, BEFORE AND DURING ANGINA PECTORIS, ON MEAN HEART RATE, LEFT-VENTRICULAR END-DIASTOLIC PRESSURE, SPECIFIC AIRWAY CONDUCTANCE, AND LUNG COMPLIANCE

| Observation Period | No. Patients | Heart Rate (beats/min) | Left-Ventricular End-Diastolic Pressure (mm Hg) | Specific Airway Conductance (L $sec^{-1}$ cm $H_2O$) | Lung Compliance (L cm $H_2O^{-1}$) |
|---|---|---|---|---|---|
| Control | 24 | 72 | 12.4 | 0.307 | 0.184 |
| Pacing | 16 | 125 | 10.3 | 0.49 | 0.172 |
| Pacing + angina | 6 | 132 | 17.5 | 0.195 | 0.13 |
| Postpacing (no angina) | 6 | 70 | 10.7 | 0.35 | 0.176 |
| Normal subjects | 10 | — | — | 0.303 | — |

Data from Pepine CJ, Wiener J: Relationships of anginal symptoms to lung myocardial ischemia. Circulation 46:863–869, 1972.

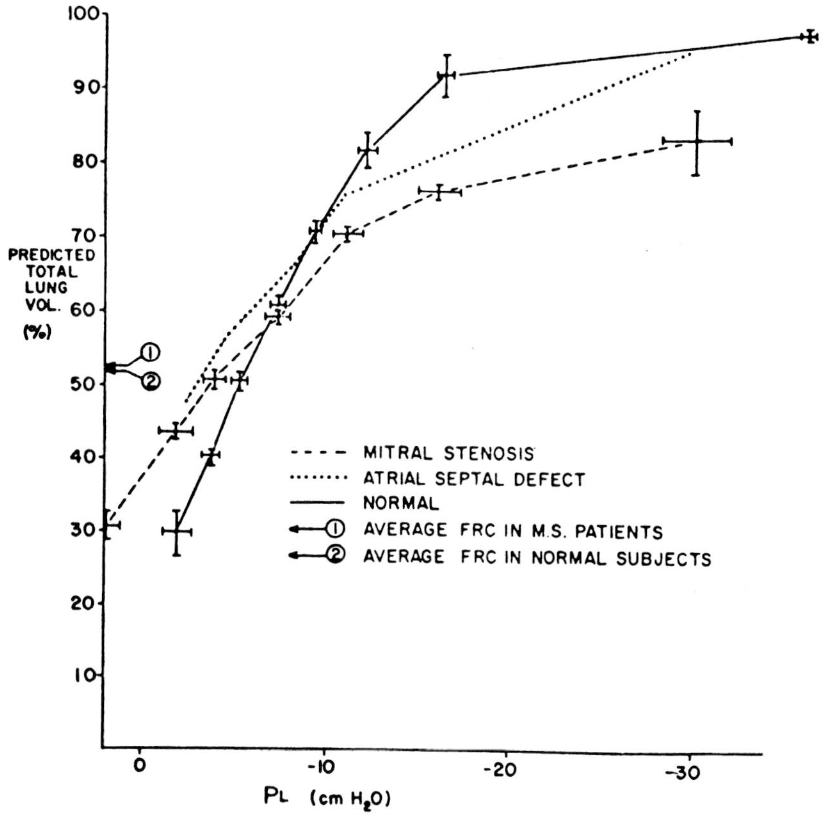


**Figure 84.2** Static pressure (PL)–volume curves (expiration) for normal subjects (n = 9) and for patients with mitral stenosis (n = 23) or atrial septal defect (n = 3). FRC = functional residual capacity; VOL = volume. (From Wood TE, McCleod P, Anthonisen NR, et al: Mechanics of breathing in mitral stenosis. Am Rev Respir Dis 104:52–60, 1971.)

occurred in the supine posture[45] (see Table 84.4). First, there was evidence of orthopnea (increase in breathlessness score); second, there was a fall in $FEV_1$ (although FVC fell equally) and in $MEF_{50\%}$; and third, there was a significant rise in total respiratory resistance, just as in normal subjects. The rise in resistance in the supine posture in normal subjects was accounted for by the fall in FRC, because specific resistance (Rrs times midtidal lung volume) did not rise, whereas it did in the heart failure patients.

**Pathogenesis.** The rise in airway resistance in patients with mitral stenosis and heart failure, which is more marked in the recumbent posture, is not severe. The increase in resistance in the supine posture (see Table 84.4) awaits a good explanation. It is not related to a change in lung volume, nor to vagally-induced bronchoconstriction, because there was no effect after inhaled ipratropium. Generalized mucosal swelling or airway wall edema with narrowing rather than closure of the bronchial lumen could lead to an increase in airway resistance without the regional inhomogeneity of ventilation that is characteristic of asthma and chronic obstructive pulmonary disease (but is absent in heart disease).

**Bronchial Hyperreactivity.** This issue has been reviewed by Snashall and Chung.[66] The studies of Cabanes and coworkers[67] and Rolla and associates[68, 69] showed increased methacholine hyperresponsiveness in patients with CHF[68] and mitral stenosis,[69] in smokers and nonsmokers alike. Cabanes and coworkers[67] inhibited the methacholine-induced bronchoconstriction almost completely by pretreatment with an alpha-adrenergic vasoconstrictor, methoxamine. Inhalation of a beta-agonist reversed 50% of the fall in $FEV_1$ induced by methacholine. They suggested that methacholine caused bronchial vasodilation and mucosal edema, which were prevented by prior treatment with methoxamine.[67] The hypothesis is a provocative one. There have been reports (reviewed by Snashall and Chung[66]) that failed to find bronchial hyperresponsiveness in patients with heart failure; the incidence overall is about 30%, and the predisposing factors are still under investigation.

Conversely, the antimuscarinic drug, ipratropium, when inhaled, causes more bronchodilatation ($\Delta FEV_1$, 11%) in acute cardiac decompensation than after intensive treatment ($\Delta FEV_1$, 4%), implying that airway edema increases cholinergic tone.[68]

## Respiratory Muscle Function

**Mitral Valve Disease.** These patients have a reduced elastic lung recoil pressure at maximum inflation (PL[el]-max), which is similar to that in patients with neuromuscular disease. This decrease in PL(el)max is proportional to the reduction in pressure generated by the inspiratory muscles (PImax) over the whole range of the lung volume.[70]

**Heart Failure.** In patients with CHF there is abundant evidence of structural, biochemical, and functional abnormalities in skeletal muscle, including the respiratory muscles, in particular atrophy of the type I (slow-twitch) fibers (see reviews by Stassijns and colleagues[71] and Piepoli and associates[72]). Recovery of muscle phosphocreatine, studied with nuclear magnetic resonance spectroscopy,[73] is delayed after exercise, and the rate of utilization during exercise is increased; this is compatible with a metabolic defect.

Respiratory muscle endurance is reduced based on a reduction in the maximal sustainable ventilatory capacity on exercise.[74] As heart failure becomes more severe, static respiratory muscle strength, at first unimpaired, becomes progressively less, as shown in Table 84.8, in which the vital capacity is used as a surrogate marker of the severity of CHF.[75–79] In this table, PEmax reflects the strength of the truncal muscles involved in a Valsalva maneuver; PImax tests the inspiratory muscles, predominantly the diaphragm. Table 84.8 shows that there is a global myopathy in heart failure, which is progressive as the patients' condition deteriorates. Twelve months after heart-lung transplantation (for Eisenmenger's syndrome or primary pulmonary hypertension), muscle pressures had improved but remained abnormal (see Table 84.8); the persistence of muscle weakness may reflect, in part, the effects of immunosuppressive drugs including corticosteroids.

The assessment of the severity of muscle weakness depends upon which test of muscle function is used. In a study of 20 patients with CHF, the majority being in NYHA grade 3, Hughes and colleagues[69a] found respiratory muscle strength varied from 72% of control values for PLmax to 90% of control values for esophageal pressure measured during a maximal sniff. PEmax was 80% of control values, and VC was 91% of predicted. There was no correlation between VC and any test of respiratory muscle strength, including transdiaphragmatic pressure (both maximum voluntary and twitch-induced). A just significant correlation was found between VC and maximum quadriceps twitch tension (Polkey MI, personal communication).

The precise reason for the muscle weakness in heart failure is not clear. Ischemia from a low cardiac output and high skeletal muscle vascular resistance is not thought to be the cause. Deconditioning may be a factor, although this is unlikely in the case of the respiratory muscles. Piepoli and coworkers[72] suggested that left-ventricular dysfunction and inactivity activate catabolic factors (tumor necrosis factor production, insulin resistance) and reduce anabolic ones, leading to a myopathic state that is only partially reversed by training programs.

## Regional Lung Function

### Distribution of Blood Flow

***Mitral Stenosis.*** A reversal of the normal blood flow gradient in the erect position, with apical flow equaling or exceeding basal flow, was clearly described in the 1960s in several studies using different radioisotopic techniques.[80] This flow pattern is relatively fixed; although oxygen breathing,[81] vasodilator (acetylcholine) infusion,[82] and raising lung volume[82] increase the proportion of flow to the lower zones, the effect is relatively small. In physiologic terms (Fig. 84.3), there is an increase in the extent of zone 4 in mitral stenosis,[83] with the point of maximum blood flow at total lung capacity and FRC being shifted 6 cm up the lung toward rib 2, compared with normal subjects. At FRC, the level of maximum flow in terms of distance below rib 2 correlates strongly with the level of left atrial pressure (range, 14 to 29 mm Hg) ($r = 0.9$). Friedman and Braunwald[84] found a correlation between lower-zone flow reduction and left atrial pressure. The mechanism of the increased lower-zone vascular resistance is related to the luminal narrowing of pulmonary arteries and veins, which is more severe histologically in the lower lobes. In a positron emission tomographic study, there was an increase in extravascular density (compatible with edema) and a reduction in pulmonary blood volume in the dorsal regions in patients with chronic heart failure.[85]

***Acute Pulmonary Edema.*** In patients with postmyocardial infarction (without clinical heart failure), there is

**Table 84.8** MEASUREMENT OF SKELETAL MUSCLE STRENGTH IN RELATION TO VITAL CAPACITY IN PATIENTS WITH CONGESTIVE HEART FAILURE

| Parameter | McParland et al | Mancini et al | Ambrosino et al | Hammond et al | Ambrosino et al | |
|---|---|---|---|---|---|---|
| | | | | | Pre-HLT | Post-HLT |
| No. patients | 15 | 10 | 45 | 16 | 11 | 11 |
| Vital capacity (% predicted) | 93 | 86 | 80 | 60 | 60 | 77 |
| Hand grip (% controls) | 100 | | | 74 | | |
| Max expiratory pressure (PEmax) (% controls) | 100 | 80 | 78 | 49 | 40 | 50 |
| Max inspiratory pressure PImax) (% controls) | 81 | 76 | 76 | 40 | 50 | 88 |

Pre-HLT = before heart-lung transplantation; Post-HLT = 12 months after heart-lung transplantation.
Data from McParland C, Resch EF, Krishnan B, et al: Inspiratory muscle weakness in chronic heart failure: Role of nutrition and electrolyte status and systemic myopathy. Am J Respir Crit Care Med 151:1101–1107, 1995; Mancini D, Henson D, LaManca J, et al: Respiratory muscle function and dyspnea in patients with chronic congestive heart failure. Circulation 86:909–918, 1992; Ambrosino N, Opasich C, Crotti P, et al: Breathing pattern, ventilatory drive and respiratory muscle strength in chronic heart failure. Eur Respir J 7:17–22, 1994; Hammond MD, Bauer KA, Sharp JT, et al: Respiratory muscle strength in congestive heart failure. Chest 98:1091–1094, 1990; and Ambrosino N, Bruschi C, Callegari G, et al: Time course of exercise capacity, skeletal and respiratory muscle performance after heart-lung transplantation. Eur Respir J 9:1508–1514, 1996.

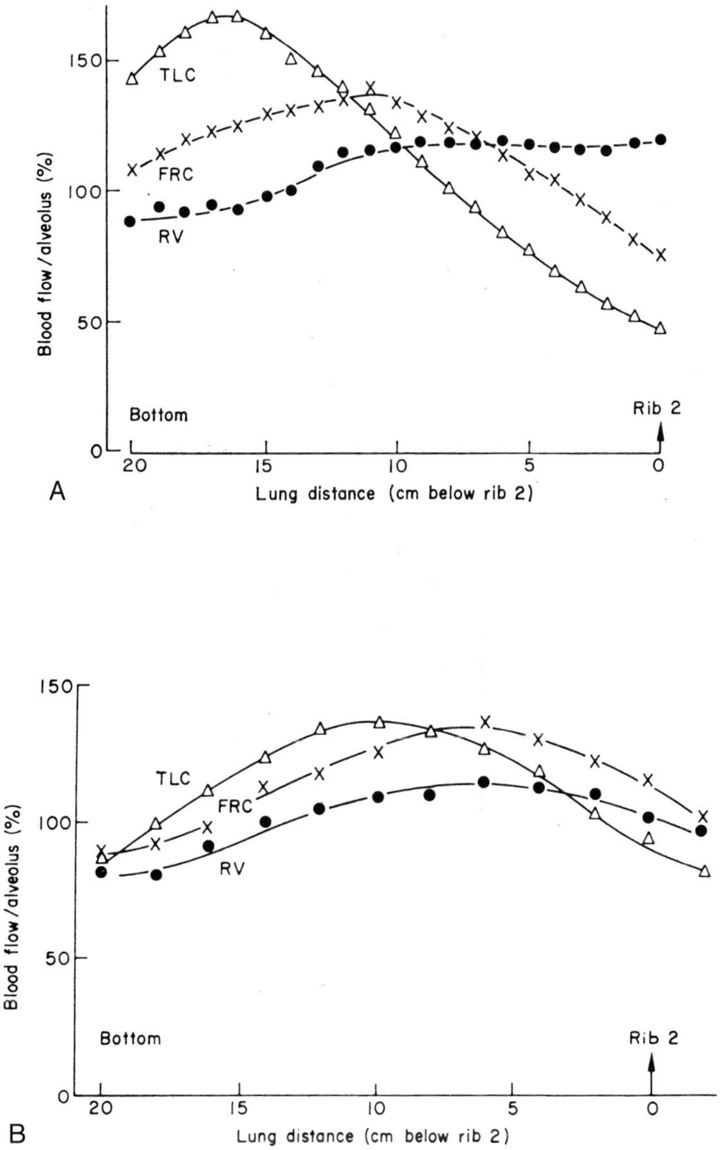


**Figure 84.3** Regional blood flow plotted against lung distance at three lung volumes from maximum (TLC) to minimum (RV) in erect posture. *A,* Mean values in nine normal subjects. Note the shift of the point of maximum blood flow at functional residual capacity (FRC) toward the base at TLC. (Modified from Hughes JMB, Glazier JB, Maloney JE, et al: Effect of lung volume on the distribution of pulmonary blood flow in man. Respir Physiol 4:58, 1968.) *B,* Mean values for eight patients with raised pulmonary venous pressure. Point of maximum flow at FRC and TLC has shifted 6 cm up the lung toward rib 2, compared with normal subjects. (Modified from Hughes JMB, Glazier JB, Rosenzweig DY, et al: Factors determining the distribution of pulmonary blood flow in patients with raised pulmonary venous pressure. Clin Sci 37:847–858, 1973.)

relative hypoperfusion of the lung bases,[86] which is less severe than in patients with mitral stenosis. The distribution is not fixed and returns to normal 2 to 3 weeks later. Understandably, there are no clinical studies of blood flow distribution in patients with acute pulmonary edema. In a study of five patients with a history of recent left-ventricular failure, Wollmer and colleagues,[87] using positron emission tomography, found a large increase in extravascular density (compatible with edema) in the dorsal regions in supine subjects, but normal values for regional vascular volume (except for a reduction in one patient who had gross alveolar edema). This suggests that pulmonary blood flow is not redistributed in patients with acute pulmonary edema.

### Distribution of Ventilation

In patients with chronic heart failure, nitrogen washout tends to be normal, which is consistent with the normal $FEV_1/FVC$ ratio and the mild increase in airway resistance. In one study, nitrogen washout was prolonged in 11 of 18 postmyocardial infarction patients,[88] but the smoking status of the group was not given. Regional ventilation, studied with radioactive gases, is normal in patients with mitral stenosis[82] and postmyocardial infarction.[86]

### Effect of Cardiomegaly

Most patients with CHF have cardiomegaly, and it is not uncommon to find a reduction in regional ventilation (in the sitting position). In a series of 180 patients, there was a significant relationship between heart size and reduced left lower lobe ventilation[89] (assessed with krypton-81m gas). Wiener and associates[90] used single photon emission computed tomography (SPECT) to assess ventilation distribution in patients with CHF and cardiomegaly in recumbent postures. In all seven patients, but not in control subjects, there was a reduction in left lower lobe ventilation in the supine posture, which was reversed by turning the patient prone (Fig. 84.4). No effect was seen in the upper zones.

**Table 84.10 VENTILATORY AND CIRCULATORY INDICES, ARTERIAL OXYGEN SATURATION, AND VISUAL ANALOGUE SCORE OF BREATHLESSNESS (VAS)*†**

| INDEX | AIR (MEAN ± SD) | 50% OXYGEN (MEAN ± SD) |
|---|---|---|
| Minute ventilation (L $min^{-1}$) | 36 ± 8.6 | 28 ± 5.9* |
| Cardiac output (L $min^{-1}$) | 7.3 ± 2.3 | 6.5 ± 1.9* |
| Heart rate (beats/min) | 112 ± 21 | 107 ± 21* |
| $O_2$ delivery (L $min^{-1}$) | 1.4 ± 0.4 | 1.4 ± 0.4 |
| Arterial $O_2$ saturation (%) | 94.6 ± 1.9 | 97.5 ± 1.3* |
| VAS | 13.9 ± 13.1 | 11.5 ± 3.5* |

*In 12 patients with congestive heart failure during steady-state exercise at 45 w breathing air or 50% oxygen ($P < .05$).
†$P < .05$
Modified from Moore DP, Weston AR, Hughes JMB, et al: Effects of increased inspired oxygen concentrations on exercise performance in chronic heart failure. Lancet 339:850, 1992, with permission.

(548 to 632 seconds) by oxygen breathing.[92] Under these circumstances, oxygen delivery might have been enhanced by hyperoxia, but it was not possible to measure it.

**Effect of Alpha-Agonists.** A similar increase in exercise duration (from 526 to 578 seconds) occurred after inhalation of 10 mg of methoxamine, an alpha-agonist.[103] Methoxamine inhibits methacholine-induced bronchoconstriction in patients with CHF[67] (described earlier). Cabanes and coworkers[103] proposed that methoxamine selectively vasoconstricts the bronchial mucosal vessels, preventing exercise-induced bronchial wall edema: a mechanism of great interest, if substantiated.

**Causes of Exercise Hyperventilation.** There are many suggestions and theories but no consensus concerning the mechanisms.[104] Wasserman and associates[105] proposed a "metabolic" analysis on the basis of the alveolar air equation for carbon dioxide:

$$\dot{V}E = \dot{V}CO_2 \times 863/[PaCO_2 \times (1 - VD/VT)]$$

where $\dot{V}E$ and $\dot{V}CO_2$ are minute ventilation and metabolic carbon dioxide production (in liters or milliliters per minute), respectively; 863 is the correction factor from BTPS conditions (body temperature, ambient pressure, saturated with water) to STPD conditions (standard temperature and pressure, dry); and VD/VT is the physiologic dead space as a fraction of the tidal volume. In Wasserman's study,[105] a subset of 20 subjects with moderate heart failure (peak $\dot{V}O_2$ less than 12 mL $min^{-1}$ $kg^{-1}$) had mean peak $\dot{V}O_2$ of 0.77 L $min^{-1}$; $\dot{V}CO_2$, 1.093 L $min^{-1}$; $\dot{V}E$, 51.8 L $min^{-1}$; VD/VT, 0.48; and arterial $PCO_2$ ($PaCO_2$), 35 mm Hg. At the same $\dot{V}O_2$, the values for control subjects were $\dot{V}CO_2$, 0.743; $\dot{V}E$, 22.5; VD/VT, 0.25; and arterial $PCO_2$, 38. The increase in minute ventilation in the CHF group compared with normal subjects (51.8 versus 22.5 L $min^{-1}$) can be apportioned roughly as follows: $\Delta\dot{V}CO_2$, 55%; $\Delta$VD/VT, 36%; and $\Delta PaCO_2$, 9%. Putting Wasserman's arguments very simply, the high minute ventilation in patients with heart failure is a response to (1) excess carbon dioxide production due to the buffering of lactic acid with bicarbonate and carbon dioxide; (2) a high physiologic dead space (wasted ventilation in terms of gas exchange); and (3) a metabolic acidosis which through chemoreceptors lowers arterial $PCO_2$ and restores blood pH to normal (pH was maintained within 0.02 units of resting values).

This analysis explains the *how* of the exercise hyperventilation in heart failure but not the *why*. It requires tight coupling between the dynamics of lactate production by exercising muscles and excess carbon dioxide production, and between arterial $PCO_2$ and arterial pH, which in the unsteady state of fast ramp exercise tests may not be warranted. It also leaves unanswered the question of the cause of the high physiologic dead space. If, for example, there were a neural stimulus to the respiratory center on exercise (either from the periphery or central), this would in itself increase ventilation and secondarily lower arterial $PCO_2$ and increase VD/VT.[101]

Others[72] believe that chemorceptor ("metabolic") feedback is not the sole reason for the hyperventilation observed with exercise in patients with heart failure. Piepoli and colleagues[72] focused on the abnormalities in skeletal muscle in heart failure (see "Respiratory Muscle Function" section) and the "ergoreflex" arising from unmyelinated and small myelinated afferents in muscle, which are sensitive to metabolic changes related to work (ergoreceptors). This reflex can be augmented by occluding an exercising limb immediately on cessation of exercise; this fixes the metabolic state of the muscle and prolongs the activation of the ergoreflex. This reflex promotes the sympathetic vasoconstrictor drive and stimulates ventilation. Compared with control subjects, patients with heart failure maintained their exercise (hand gripping) ventilation throughout the 3-minute period of postexercise limb occlusion, whereas only 63% was maintained by normal subjects. Training the forearm for 6 weeks damped down the ergoreflex.

What other stimuli could contribute to the hyperventilation seen with exercise in patients with CHF? There must be some hypoxic drive, because ventilation at 45 W was 22% less when 50% oxygen was inspired (see Table 84.10), although it was still increased in comparison with control values.[102] Mixed venous $PO_2$ and pH are lower in CHF patients at the same workload than in normal subjects, but metabolic receptors on the right side of the heart or in the pulmonary arteries have never been found. The $\dot{V}E/\dot{V}CO_2$ ratio returns toward normal after cardiac transplantation[98] (see Table 84.9), and the anaerobic threshold is set at a higher $\dot{V}O_2$ level, although still far from normal.[98] Further analysis of changes in physiologic dead space and the ergoreflex before and after cardiac transplantation would be of interest and might increase understanding of the mechanisms of exercise hyperventilation in heart failure.

## Sleep

Periodic breathing (apnea and/or hypopnea, alternating with hyperpnea) is frequently observed in patients with chronic heart failure. It is usually severe and associated with a higher pulmonary wedge pressure than that in other patients with CHF.[105a] Another characteristic pattern of altered breathing is Cheyne-Stokes respiration (CSR), in which tidal volume gradually increases and then decreases, with each cycle interrupted by a period of apnea. CSR occurs during sleep and is a form of central sleep apnea (CSA). Both periodic breathing and CSR occur in healthy subjects, especially men and the elderly, at high altitude. The situation is analogous to the "hunting" seen in servocontrolled systems. Normally the midbrain and cortex smooth out such oscillations. The patient with CSR and central sleep apnea in chronic heart failure has a poor prognosis.[105b] Treatment with nasal continuous positive pressure (CPAP), oxygen, or theophylline may be helpful.[105c]

Another form of sleep-related apnea–hypopnea is the obstructive sleep apnea (OSA) syndrome, which occurs most often in obese men. Progressive collapse of the pharyngeal aperture, when complete, causes apnea (defined as cessation of airflow > 10 seconds). Asynchronous chest and abdominal wall movements are seen during the apneic periods in OSA but are absent in CSA. Apneas are terminated by an arousal reflex, which may be explosive in OSA when the pharynx suddenly opens. At the end of apnea, severe arterial hypoxemia may occur. In OSA and CSA, frequent arousal leads to sleep fragmentation with daytime sleepiness and poor concentration. Systemic blood pressure rises during arousal. There is also sympathetic nervous system activation with increased nocturnal urinary norepinephrine excretion.[105d] OSA may be a risk factor in ischemic heart disease and probably worsens the patient's prognosis of CHF.

In one study using polysomnography of 81 patients with stable CHF, Javaheri and colleagues[105e] found an incidence of CSA of 40% and of OSA of 11%, which is considerably greater than expected in this age group (2% to 4%). Patients with CSA and OSA were more likely to have atrial fibrillations, ventricular arrhythmias, and lower left-ventricular ejection fractions. Their lowest nocturnal arterial oxygen saturation values were 76% ± 12% (SD) compared with 89% ± 4% in those without apneas. There was no difference in daytime oxygenation. The OSA patients were also more likely to be overweight and to snore than the CSA patients. There was no difference in the severity of oxygen desaturation and frequency of arousal. Treatment of OSA in the standard way with nasal CPAP improves left ventricular function.[105d] A full discussion of the pathophysiology and treatment of sleep disorders is provided in Chapter 81.

# MECHANISMS OF DYSPNEA

## Acute Pulmonary Edema

In patients with acute heart failure, breathlessness at rest is associated with an acute elevation of pulmonary venous pressure sufficient to cause interstitial and alveolar edema. The mechanism of the dyspnea, although clearly linked to these changes, is far from clear. (Additional discussion of the mechanisms and clinical features of dyspnea is provided in Chapter 20.) Experimentally, an acute rise in pulmonary vascular pressures increases neural activity in unmyelinated C fibers (arising according to Paintal[106] from juxtapulmonary capillary or J receptors), but a relationship with reflex tachypnea has not been established. Wead and associates[107] concluded (from their own observations and a review of previous data) that intrapulmonary vascular congestion failed to stimulate C fibers or other nerve endings (e.g., irritant, stretch) sufficiently to change central inspiratory activity, nor was there experimental evidence in support of left atrial or pulmonary venous distention as a source. Of course, these experiments are carried out in anesthetized and often partially isolated animal preparations. Snashall and Chung, in their review,[66] marshaled the evidence in favor of intrapulmonary interstitial pressure receptors, but their role in pulmonary edema remains in doubt.

In humans, the induction of an attack of angina pectoris by atrial pacing (Pepine and Wiener[33]), which increased left atrial pressure and decreased lung compliance, caused "chest tightness, substernal discomfort, pressure or constriction," but not dyspnea. Measurements of ventilation and ventilatory pattern were not made. It may be wrong to seek a single cause for the dramatic "air hunger" of patients with acute left-ventricular failure, because factors such as arterial hypoxemia, low cardiac output, and tissue acidosis may combine with the rise of pulmonary interstitial pressure to produce the response. Another possibility is that the reflex tachypnea of acute pulmonary edema arises from expansion of the chest cage. In patients with acute left-ventricular failure, the thorax might have to accommodate 500 mL or more of extra blood and new edema fluid. Unless FRC falls by a similar amount, the chest cage must expand. This increases the elastic work of breathing in a situation in which oxygen delivery to the respiratory muscles may already be compromised, and might contribute to the dyspnea and discomfort of the patient. A similar mechanism may contribute to the sensation of orthopnea (see next section).

## Orthopnea

Dyspnea, relieved in part by sitting upright, is a common symptom in patients with acute or chronic heart failure. Christie and Meakins,[108] who were the first to show, using intrapleural catheters, a decreased lung compliance in CHF, believed that pulmonary vascular congestion stimulated the Hering-Breuer reflex. Sitting up diminished the congestion and relieved the dyspnea. In fact, the fall in pulmonary blood volume in stable patients with CHF on sitting at 45 degrees is quite small (less than 100 mL).[46] There is, on the other hand, an increase in airway resistance (see Table 84.4) and work of breathing[47] in patients with CHF in the supine posture that may be contributing to the symptom of orthopnea. The increase in the visual analogue score of perceived breathlessness when patients changed from the sitting to the supine position was somewhat less after inhalation of the antimuscarinic drug, ipratropium, although the effect on respiratory resistance was only moderate.

In addition, there is a degree of hyperinflation, because FRC does not fall, as it does in normal subjects, when the patient changes to a supine posture (see Table 84.4). Thoracic volume (gas + tissue + edema + intrapulmonary and intracardiac blood volume) during tidal breathing in the supine posture is 750 to 1000 mL greater in these patients than in healthy subjects. The higher the midtidal lung volume, the greater the elastic work of breathing.[47] Afferent signals from the inspiratory muscles, which are working at a shorter length and therefore at a mechanical disadvantage, may contribute to the sensation of orthopnea.

## Exercise Dyspnea

Analysis of the sensation of dyspnea on exercise is complex. Dyspnea may relate to *ventilatory demand*, in terms of excessive ventilation compared with what is expected; the origin of this demand may lie in abnormalities of exercising muscle (structure or blood flow) and excess lactate production. On the other hand, exertional dyspnea may relate to *ventilatory difficulty* in terms of an increase in the elastic or resistive work of breathing; this difficulty may have a peripheral component if there is respiratory muscle weakness and/or fatigue. Perceived dyspnea in heart failure correlates with respiratory muscle weakness ($P_{Imax}$ and $P_{Emax}$), with the work of breathing (tension time index of the diaphragm) and with $FEV_1$.[76]

After cardiac transplantation, the demand for ventilation at a given $\dot{V}O_2$ declines[98] (note the fall in $\dot{V}E/\dot{V}CO_2$ in Table 84.9), and perceived dyspnea falls. The reduced sensation of dyspnea is not accompanied by any fall in the work of breathing,[109] suggesting that the lungs remain stiff and noncompliant. The residual dyspnea in posttransplantation patients may relate to impaired lung mechanics and to skeletal muscle atrophy and deconditioning (see Table 84.8).

## SUMMARY

In patients with heart disease, acute rises of pulmonary venous pressure increase the pulmonary blood volume, reduce lung compliance, and increase (moderately) airway resistance. Microvascular filtration and lymph flow increase. If the pressure increase is sufficient to exceed the rate of clearance of filtrate, alveolar edema ensues. Lung volumes decrease, and gas exchange is compromised (arterial $P_{O_2}$ and $DL_{CO}$ are reduced). Acutely (e.g., after acute myocardial infarction), these changes are reversible. Chronic elevation of pulmonary venous pressure, from whatever cause, leads to alveolar and vascular damage with loss of lung volume, a reduction in the diffusing capacity, and pulmonary hypertension. Gas exchange is well preserved in the absence of alveolar edema. The rise in airway resistance is not as severe in patients with heart disease as in patients with chronic obstructive pulmonary disease, but a proportion of the former also have bronchial hyperreactivity. Respiratory and skeletal muscle function is impaired.

The origin of the symptoms of dyspnea and orthopnea in patients with CHF is not yet understood. An intrapulmonary stimulus seems unlikely, and reflexes arising from overexpansion of the chest wall must be considered. Exercise capacity is limited, primarily because of a low cardiac output, high muscle vascular resistance, and atrophy and deconditioning of the exercising muscles. Accordingly, arterial $P_{O_2}$ is usually within the normal range, but mixed venous $P_{O_2}$ and pH are lower and lactate is higher than in healthy persons. Oxygen breathing improves exercise capacity and duration. The cause of the hyperventilation with exercise is largely peripheral, arising from excess lactate production and an augmented ergoreceptor reflex in exercising muscle. The symptom of dyspnea on exercise is related to increases in the work of breathing and to fatigue of the respiratory muscles.

Reduction of pulmonary venous pressure (e.g., by surgical correction of mitral stenosis), reduces pulmonary hypertension by 50% but does not improve pulmonary function. Cardiac transplantation is accompanied by improvements in PVR, lung volumes (but not diffusing capacity), respiratory muscle function, and exercise capacity and a reduction in exercise hyperventilation and in the sensation of dyspnea; nevertheless, most indices remain at about two thirds of normal values, those most improved being the PVR and lung volumes.

## References

1. Broaddus VC: Cardiac diseases. *In* Murray JF (ed): Pulmonary Complications of Systemic Disease. New York: Marcel Dekker, 1992, pp 149–190.
2. Glazier JB, Hughes JMB, Maloney JE, et al: Measurements of capillary dimensions and blood volume in rapidly frozen lungs. J Appl Physiol 26:65–76, 1969.
3. Warrell DA, Evans JW, Clarke RO, et al: Pattern of filling in the pulmonary capillary bed. J Appl Physiol 32:346–356, 1972.
4. West JB, Dollery CT, Naimark A: Distribution of blood flow in isolated lung: Relation to vascular and alveolar pressures. J Appl Physiol 19:713–724, 1964.
5. Erdmann J, Vaughan T, Brigham K, et al: Effect of increased vascular pressure or lung fluid balance in unanesthetized sheep. Circ Res 37:271–284, 1975.
6. Staub NC, Nagano H, Pearce ML: Pulmonary edema in dogs, especially the sequence of fluid accumulation in lungs. J Appl Physiol 22:227–240, 1967.
7. Broaddus VC, Wiener-Kronish JP, Staub NC: Clearance of lung edema into the pleural space of volume-loaded anesthetized sheep. J Appl Physiol 68:2623–2630, 1990.
8. Drake RE, Giesler M, Laine G, et al: Effect of outflow pressure on lung lymph flow in unanesthetized sheep. J Appl Physiol 58:70–76, 1985.
9. Wiener-Kronish JP, Matthay MA, Callen PW, et al: Relationship of pleural effusions to pulmonary hemodynamics in patients with congestive heart failure. Am Rev Respir Dis 132:1253–1256, 1985.
10. Wiener-Kronish JP, Goldstein R, Matthay MA, et al: Lack of association of pleural effusion with chronic pulmonary arterial and right atrial hypertension. Chest 92:967–970, 1987.
11. Haworth SG, Hall SM, Patel M: Peripheral pulmonary vascular and airway abnormalities in adolescents with rheumatic mitral stenosis. Int J Cardiol 18:405–416, 1988.
12. Tsukimoto K, Mathieu-Costello O, Prediletto R, et al: Ultrastructural appearances of pulmonary capillaries at high transmural pressures. J Appl Physiol 71:573–582, 1991.
13. Costello ML, Mathieu-Costello O, West JB: Stress failure of alveolar epithelial cells studied by scanning electron microscopy. Am Rev Respir Dis 145:1446–1455, 1992.
14. Bachofen H, Schürch S, Michel RP, et al: Experimental hydrostatic pulmonary edema in rabbit lungs: Morphology. Am Rev Respir Dis 147:989–996, 1993.

15. Bachofen H, Schürch S, Weibel ER: Experimental hydrostatic pulmonary edema in rabbit lungs: Barrier lesions. Am Rev Respir Dis 147:997–1004, 1993.
16. Crapo JD: New concepts in the formation of pulmonary edema (editorial). Am Rev Respir Dis 147:790–792, 1993.
17. Harris P, Heath D: The Human Pulmonary Circulation (3rd ed). New York: Churchill Livingstone, 1986.
18. Tozzi CA, Poiani GJ, Harangozo AM, et al: Pressure-induced connective tissue synthesis in pulmonary artery segments is dependent on intact endothelium. J Clin Invest 84:1005–1012, 1989.
19. Mecham RP, Whitehouse LA, Wrenn DS, et al: Smooth muscle-mediated connective tissue remodeling in pulmonary hypertension. Science 237:423–426, 1987.
20. Stenmark KR, Mecham RP: Cellular and molecular mechanisms of pulmonary vascular remodeling. Annu Rev Physiol 59: 89–144, 1997.
21. Tozzi CA, Thakker-Varia S, Yu SY, et al: Mast cell collagenase correlates with regression of pulmonary vascular remodeling in the rat. Am J Respir Cell Mol Biol 18:497–510, 1998.
22. West JB, Mathieu-Costello O: Structure, strength failure, and remodeling of the pulmonary blood-gas barrier. Annu Rev Physiol 61:543–572, 1999.
23. Williamson JR, Vogler NJ, Kilo C: Regional variations in the width of the basement membrane of muscle capillaries in man and the giraffe. Am J Pathol 63:359–370, 1971.
24. Berg JT, Fu Z, Breen EC, et al: High lung inflation increases mRNA levels of ECM components and growth factors in lung parenchyma. J Appl Physiol 83:120–128, 1997.
25. Reeves JT, Grover RF, Dempsey JA: Pulmonary circulation during exercise. *In* Weir EK, Reeves JT (eds): Lung Biology in Health and Disease. Vol 3: Pulmonary Vascular Physiology and Pathophysiology. New York: Marcel Dekker, 1988, pp 107–133.
26. Franciosa JA, Ziesche RN, Wilen M: Functional capacity of patients with chronic left ventricular failure: Relationship of bicycle exercise performance to clinical hemodynamic characterization. Am J Med 67:460–466, 1979.
27. Maseri A, Caldini P, Howard P, et al: Determinants of pulmonary vascular volume: Recruitment versus distensibility. Circ Res 31:218–228, 1972.
28. Harf A, Pratt T, Hughes JMB: Regional distribution of $\dot{V}A/\dot{Q}$ in man at rest and with exercise measured with krypton-81m. J Appl Physiol 44:115–123, 1978.
29. Granath A, Jonsson B, Strandell T: Circulation in healthy old men, studied by right heart catheterization at rest and during exercise in supine and sitting position. Acta Med Scand 176:425–446, 1964.
30. Hultgren H, Lopez C, Lundberg E, et al: Physiologic studies of pulmonary edema at high altitude. Circulation 29:393–408, 1964.
31. Jebavy P, Widimsky J, Stanek V: Distribution of inspired gas and pulmonary diffusing capacity at rest and during graded exercise in patients with mitral stenosis. Respiration 28:216–235, 1971.
32. Taylor AE, Barnard JW, Barman SC, et al: Fluid balance. *In* Crystal RG, West JB, et al (eds): The Lung. Vol 1: Scientific Foundations. New York: Raven Press, 1991, pp 1147–1161.
32a. Townsley MI, Fu Z, Mathieu-Costello O, et al: Pulmonary microvascular permeability: responses to high vascular pressure after induction of pacing-induced heart failure in dogs. Circ Res 77:317–325, 1995.
33. Pepine CJ, Wiener J: Relationships of anginal symptoms to lung myocardial ischemia. Circulation 46:863–869, 1972.
33a. Agostoni PG, Marenzi GC, Pepi M, et al: Isolated ultrafiltration in moderate congestive heart failure. J Am Coll Cardiol 21:424–431, 1993.
34. Gibbs JSR, Keegan J, Wright C, et al: Pulmonary artery pressure changes during exercise and daily activities in chronic heart failure. J Am Coll Cardiol 15:52–61, 1990.
35. Levine MJ, Weinstein JS, Diver DJ, et al: Progressive improvement in pulmonary vascular resistance after percutaneous mitral valvuloplasty. Circulation 79:1061–1067, 1989.
36. Naeije R, Lipski A, Abramowicz M, et al: Nature of pulmonary hypertension in congestive heart failure: Effects of cardiac transplantation. Am J Respir Crit Care Med 149:881–887, 1994.
37. Folz BD, Hessel EA, Ivey TD: The early course of pulmonary hypertension in patients undergoing mitral valve replacement with cardioplegic arrest. J Thorac Cardiovasc Surg 88:238–247, 1984.
38. Frank NR, Cugell DW, Gaensler EA, et al: Ventilatory studies in mitral stenosis. Am J Med 15:60–76, 1953.
39. Rhodes KM, Evemy K, Nariman S, et al: Relation between severity of mitral valve disease and routine lung function tests in nonsmokers. Thorax 37:751–755, 1982.
40. Wood TE, McCleod P, Anthonisen NR, et al: Mechanics of breathing in mitral stenosis. Am Rev Respir Dis 104:52–60, 1971.
41. Richards DGB, Whitfield AGW, Arnott WM, et al: The lung volume in low output cardiac syndromes. Br Heart J 13:381–386, 1951.
42. Hales CA, Kazemi H: Pulmonary function after uncomplicated myocardial infarction. Chest 72:350–358, 1977.
43. Morris MJ, Smith MM, Clarke BG: Lung mechanics after cardiac valve replacement. Thorax 35:453–460, 1980.
44. Light RW, George RB: Serial pulmonary function in patients with acute heart failure. Arch Intern Med 143:429–433, 1983.
45. Yap JCH, Moore D, Cleland JGF, et al: Mechanisms of the supine increase in airflow resistance in chronic left ventricular failure (abstract). Am Rev Respir Dis 143:A345, 1991.
46. Hannan WJ, Vojacek J, Connell HM, et al: Radionuclide determined pulmonary blood volume in ischaemic heart disease. Thorax 36:922–927, 1981.
47. Cherniack RM, Cuddy TE, Armstrong JB: Significance of pulmonary elastic and viscous resistance in orthopnea. Circulation 15:859–864, 1957.
48. Yu PN: Pulmonary Blood Volume in Health and Disease. Philadelphia: Lea & Febiger, 1969, pp 224–246.
49. Gazioglu K, Yu PN: Pulmonary blood volume and pulmonary capillary blood volume in vascular heart disease. Circulation 35:701–709, 1967.
50. Puri SP, Baker BL, Dutka DP, et al: Reduced alveolar-capillary membrane diffusing capacity in chronic heart failure. Circulation 91:2769–2774, 1995.
51. Puri S, Dutka DP, Baker BL, et al: Acute saline infusion reduces alveolar-capillary membrane conductance and increases airflow obstruction in patients with left ventricular dysfunction. Circulation 99:1190–1196, 1999.
52. Aber CP, Campbell JA: Significance of changes in the pulmonary diffusing capacity in mitral stenosis. Thorax 20:135–145, 1965.
53. Jordan SC, Hicken P, Watson DA, et al: Pathology of the lungs in mitral stenosis in relation to respiratory function and pulmonary haemodynamics. Br Heart J 28:101–107, 1966.
54. Estenne M, Yernault J-C, De Smet J-M, et al: Phrenic and diaphragm function after coronary artery bypass grafting. Thorax 40:293–299, 1985.
55. Mustafa KY, Nour MM, Shuhaiber H, et al: Pulmonary function before and sequentially after valve replacement surgery with correlation to preoperative haemodynamic data. Am Rev Respir Dis 130:400–406, 1984.
56. Hosenpud JD: Abnormal pulmonary function specifically related to congestive heart failure: Comparison of patients before and after cardiac transplantation. Am J Med 88:493–496, 1990.
57. Niset G, Ninane V, Antoine M, et al: Respiratory dysfunction in congestive heart failure: Correction after heart transplantation. Eur Respir J 6:1197–1201, 1993.
58. Bussieres LM, Pflugfelder PW, Ahmad D, et al: Evolution of resting lung function in the first year after cardiac transplantation. Eur Respir J 8:959–962, 1995.
59. Muir AL, Flenley DC, Kirby BJ, et al: Cardiorespiratory effects of rapid saline infusion in normal man. J Appl Physiol 38:786–793, 1975.
60. Frank NR: Influence of acute pulmonary vascular congestion on recoiling force of excised cat's lung. J Appl Physiol 14:905–908, 1959.
61. Bondurant S, Mead J, Cook CD: A re-evaluation of effects of acute central congestion on pulmonary compliance in normal subjects. J Appl Physiol 15:875–877, 1960.
62. Frank NR, Lyons HA, Siebens AA, et al: Pulmonary compliance in patients with cardiac disease. Am J Med 22:516–523, 1957.
63. Sharp JT, Griffith GT, Bunnell IL, et al: Ventilatory mechanics in pulmonary edema in man. J Clin Invest 37:111–117, 1958.
64. Chung KF, Keyes SJ, Morgan BM, et al: Mechanisms of airway

narrowing in acute pulmonary edema in dogs: Influence of the vagus and lung volume. Clin Sci 65:289–296, 1983.
65. Michel RP, Zocchi L, Rossi A, et al: Does interstitial lung edema compress airways and arteries? A morphometric study. J Appl Physiol 62:108–115, 1987.
66. Snashall PD, Chung KF: Airway obstruction and bronchial hyperresponsiveness in left ventricular failure and mitral stenosis. Am Rev Respir Dis 144:945–955, 1991.
67. Cabanes LR, Weber SN, Matran R, et al: Bronchial hyperresponsiveness to methacholine in patients with impaired left ventricular function. N Engl J Med 320:1317–1322, 1989.
68. Rolla G, Bucca C, Brussino L, et al: Bronchodilating effect of ipratropium bromide in heart failure. Eur Respir J 6:1492–1495, 1993.
69. Rolla G, Bucca C, Caria E, et al: Bronchial responsiveness in patients with mitral valve disease. Eur Respir J 3:127–131, 1990.
69a. Hughes PD, Polkey MI, Hams ML, et al: Diaphragm strength in chronic heart failure. Am J Respir Crit Care Med 160:529–534, 1999.
70. De Troyer A, Estenne M, Yernault JC: Disturbance of respiratory muscle function in patients with mitral valve disease. Am J Med 69:867–873, 1980.
71. Stassijns G, Lysens R, Decramer M: Peripheral and respiratory muscles in chronic heart failure. Eur Respir J 9:2161–2167, 1996.
72. Piepoli M, Clark AL, Volterrani M, et al: Contribution of muscle afferents to the hemodynamic, autonomic and ventilatory responses to exercise in patients with chronic heart failure. Circulation 93:940–952, 1996.
73. Mancini DM, Walter G, Reichnek N, et al: Contribution of skeletal muscle atrophy to exercise intolerance and altered muscle metabolism in heart failure. Circulation 85:1364–1373, 1992.
74. Mancini DM, Henson D, LaManca J, et al: Evidence of reduced muscle endurance in patients with heart failure. J Am Coll Cardiol 24:972–981, 1994.
75. McParland C, Resch EF, Krishnan B, et al: Inspiratory muscle weakness in chronic heart failure: Role of nutrition and electrolyte status and systemic myopathy. Am J Respir Crit Care Med 151:1101–1107, 1995.
76. Mancini D, Henson D, LaManca J, et al: Respiratory muscle function and dyspnea in patients with chronic congestive heart failure. Circulation 86:909–918, 1992.
77. Ambrosino N, Opasich C, Crotti P, et al: Breathing pattern, ventilatory drive and respiratory muscle strength in chronic heart failure. Eur Respir J 7:17–22, 1994.
78. Hammond MD, Bauer KA, Sharp JT, et al: Respiratory muscle strength in congestive heart failure. Chest 98:1091–1094, 1990.
79. Ambrosino N, Bruschi C, Callegari G, et al: Time course of exercise capacity, skeletal and respiratory muscle performance after heart-lung transplantation. Eur Respir J 9:1508–1514, 1996.
80. Hughes JMB, Glazier JB, Rosenzweig DY, et al: Factors determining the distribution of pulmonary blood flow in patients with raised pulmonary venous pressure. Clin Sci 37:847–858, 1969.
81. Dawson A, Kaneko K, McGregor M: Regional lung function in patients with mitral stenosis studied with xenon133 during air and oxygen breathing. J Clin Invest 44:999–1008, 1965.
82. Glazier JB, Dollery CT, Hughes JMB: The effects of acetylcholine on regional pulmonary blood flow in patients with mitral stenosis. Circulation 38:136–146, 1968.
83. Hughes JMB, Glazier JB, Maloney JE, et al: Effect of lung volume on the distribution of pulmonary blood flow in man. Respir Physiol 4:58–72, 1968.
84. Friedman WF, Braunwald E: Alterations in regional pulmonary blood flow in mitral valve disease studied by radioscope scanning. Circulation 34:363–376, 1966.
85. Wollmer P, Rhodes CG, Allan RM, et al: Regional extravascular lung density and fractional pulmonary blood volume in patients with chronic pulmonary venous hypertension. Clin Physiol 3:241–256, 1983.
86. Kazemi H, Parsons EF, Valenca LM, et al: Distribution of pulmonary blood flow after myocardial ischemia and infarction. Circulation 41:1025–1030, 1976.
87. Wollmer P, Rhodes CG, Deanfield J, et al: Regional extravascular density of the lung in patients with acute pulmonary edema. J Appl Physiol 63:1890–1895, 1987.
88. Pain MCF, Stannard M, Sloman G: Disturbances of pulmonary function after acute myocardial infarction. Br Med J 2:591–594, 1967.
89. Alexander MSM, Arnot RN, Lavender JP: Left lower lobe ventilation and its relation to cardiomegaly and posture. Br Med J 229:94, 1989.
90. Wiener C, Henderson B, McKenna WJ, et al: Left lower lobe ventilation is reduced in patients with cardiomegaly in the supine but not the prone position. Am Rev Respir Dis 141:150–155, 1990.
91. Fillmore SJ, Shapiro M, Killip T: Arterial oxygen tension in acute myocardial infarction: Serial analysis of clinical state and blood gas changes. Am Heart J 79:620–629, 1976.
92. Franciosa JA, Leddy CL, Wilen M, et al: Relation between hemodynamic and ventilatory responses in determining exercise capacity in severe congestive heart failure. Am J Cardiol 53:127–134, 1985.
93. Scheinman MM, Evans GT: Right to left shunt in patients with acute myocardial infarction. Am J Cardiol 29:757–766, 1972.
94. Rubin SA, Brown HA, Swan HJC: Arterial oxygenation and arterial oxygen transport in chronic myocardial failure at rest, during exercise and after hydrallazine treatment. Circulation 66:143–148, 1982.
95. Fink LI, Wilson JR, Ferraro N: Exercise ventilation and pulmonary artery wedge pressure in chronic stable congestive heart failure. Am J Cardiol 57:249–253, 1986.
96. Sullivan MJ, Higginbotham MB, Cobb FR: Increased exercise ventilation in patients with chronic heart failure: Intact ventilatory control despite hemodynamic and pulmonary abnormalities. Circulation 77:552–559, 1988.
97. Al-Rawas OA, Carter R, Richens D, et al: Ventilatory and gas exchange abnormalities on exercise in chronic heart failure. Eur Respir J 8:2022–2028, 1995.
98. Marzo KP, Wilson JR, Mancini DM: Effects of cardiac transplantation on ventilatory response to exercise. Am J Cardiol 69:547–553, 1992.
99. Mandak JS, Aaronson KD, Mancini DM: Serial assessment of exercise capacity after heart transplantation. J Heart Lung Transplant 14:468–478, 1995.
100. D'Arsigny C, Webb KA, Raj S, et al: Ventilatory constraints contribute to exercise limitation and dyspnea in stable congestive heart failure (abstract). Am J Respir Crit Care Med 159:A418, 1999.
101. West JB: Ventilation-perfusion inequality and overall gas exchange in computer models of the lung. Respir Physiol 7:88–110, 1969.
102. Moore DP, Weston AR, Hughes JMB, et al: Effects of increased inspired oxygen concentrations on exercise performance in chronic heart failure. Lancet 339:850–853, 1992.
103. Cabanes L, Costes F, Weber S, et al: Improvement in exercise performance by inhalation of methoxamine in patients with impaired left ventricular function. N Engl J Med 326:1661–1665, 1992.
104. Clark A, Coats A: The mechanisms underlying the increased ventilatory response to exercise in chronic stable heart failure. Eur Heart J 13:1698–1708, 1992.
105. Wasserman K, Zhang YY, Gitt A, et al: Lung function and exercise gas exchange in chronic heart failure. Circulation 96:2221–2227, 1997.
105a. Solin P, Bergin P, Richardson M, et al: Influence of pulmonary capillary wedge pressure on central apnea in heart failure. Circulation 99:1574–1579, 1999.
105b. Lanfranchi PA, Braghivoli A, Bosimini E, et al: Prognostic value of nocturnal Cheyne-Stokes respiration in chronic heart failure. Circulation 99:1435–1440, 1999.
105c. Wilcox I, McNamara SG, Wessendorf T, et al: Prognosis and sleep disordered breathing in heart failure. Thorax 53(suppl 3):533–536, 1998.
105d. Naughton MT, Bradley TD: Sleep apnea in congestive heart failure. Clin Chest Med 19:99–113, 1998.
105e. Javaheri S, Parker TJ, Liming JD: Sleep apnea in 81 ambulatory patients with stable heart failure. Circulation 97:2145–2159, 1998.

106. Paintal AS: Mechanism of stimulation of type J pulmonary receptors. J Physiol 203:511–532, 1969.
107. Wead WB, Cassidy SS, Coast JR, et al: Reflex cardiorespiratory responses to pulmonary vascular congestion. J Appl Physiol 62:870–879, 1987.
108. Christie RV, Meakins JC: The intrapleural pressure in congestive heart failure and its clinical significance. J Clin Invest 13:323–345, 1934.
109. Mancini DM, LaManca J, Donchez L, et al: The sensation of dyspnea during exercise is not determined by the work of breathing in patients with heart failure. J Am Coll Cardiol 28:391–395, 1996.

# 85 Pulmonary Complications of Abdominal Disease

ROBERT RODRIGUEZ-ROISIN, M.D. • JOAN ALBERT BARBERÀ, M.D.

Introduction
Gastroesophageal and Gastrointestinal Disorders
- Gastroesophageal Reflux
- Inflammatory Bowel Disease

Hepatic Diseases
- Pleural Effusion
- Pulmonary Functional Disturbances
- Hepatopulmonary Syndrome
- Portopulmonary Hypertension
- Primary Biliary Cirrhosis
- Chronic Active Hepatitis
- Sclerosing Cholangitis
- Alpha$_1$-Antitrypsin Deficiency

Pancreatitis
- Respiratory Failure
- Pleural Effusion

Chronic Renal Failure
- Pulmonary Edema
- Pleural Disease
- Pulmonary Calcification
- Sleep Apnea
- Hemodialysis-Induced Hypoxemia

Summary

## INTRODUCTION

This chapter is devoted to the pulmonary complications of abdominal disease and begins with a discussion of the most relevant esophageal and bowel disorders. Then the lung-liver syndromes and the specific liver disorders associated with particular pulmonary complications are reviewed. Finally, the respiratory consequences of diseases of the pancreas and kidney are described. The objective in each section is the same: to update the most relevant clinical, pathophysiologic, pathogenetic, and therapeutic aspects of the principal abdominal disease states and thereby assist the clinician in diagnosing and managing these sometimes complex and challenging pulmonary complications.

## GASTROESOPHAGEAL AND GASTROINTESTINAL DISORDERS

### Gastroesophageal Reflux

Gastroesophageal reflux is defined as the retrograde movement of gastric contents into the esophagus. The prevalence of gastroesophageal reflux is common, with more than one third of the population having intermittent complaints of this disorder.[1] Gastroesophageal reflux has long been associated with respiratory symptoms and diseases. These range from overt aspiration pneumonia to more chronic insidious respiratory disorders in which the relationship with gastroesophageal reflux is often difficult to establish. The latter subset includes some forms of bronchitis, bronchiectasis, pulmonary fibrosis, asthma, and chronic cough. The association of gastroesophageal reflux with asthma and chronic cough has been clearly documented, and the possible coexistence of gastroesophageal reflux must be considered especially in patients with refractory cough or wheezing.[2–4]

The prevalence of gastroesophageal reflux in patients with asthma is greater than in the general population, with reported values that range from 33% to 90%, depending on the technique used to define gastroesophageal reflux. Using esophageal manometry and 24 hours ambulatory esophageal pH monitoring, Sontag and colleagues[5] observed that 82% of asthmatics had abnormal amounts of acid reflux. Furthermore, the use of 24-hour ambulatory esophageal pH monitoring revealed that gastroesophageal reflux may be the cause of chronic cough in up to 40% of patients with the symptom.[6, 7] It is also important to note that patients with asthma or chronic cough can have significant reflux without referring the classic reflux symptoms. Irwin and associates[8] reported that gastroesophageal reflux was clinically silent in 24% of patients with difficult-to-control asthma.

## Pathogenesis

The pathogenesis of respiratory abnormalities associated with gastroesophageal reflux can be divided into three basic mechanisms. First, gross aspiration–linked pulmonary syndromes are usually the result of free esophageal reflux with large-volume retrograde flow. Frequently, there is reduced basal lower-esophageal tone and impaired esophageal motility and clearance.[9] These patients may have recurrent pneumonia, bronchiectasis, or pulmonary infiltrates. The endoscopic examination usually reveals severe anatomic changes, such as grade 3 or 4 esophagitis or Barrett's epithelialization of the mucosa.

A second pathogenic mechanism is related to the microaspiration of gastric contents from the proximal (upper) esophagus. This results from small-volume aspirate that produce an exudative mucosal reaction in the larynx and in the tracheobronchial tree. Respiratory symptoms are less apparent and range from hoarseness or chronic cough to difficult-to-control asthma. Jack and coworkers,[10] using simultaneous tracheal and esophageal pH measurements in asthmatics with gastroesophageal reflux, showed that episodes of reflux that were followed by a fall in intratracheal pH resulted in a marked fall in peak expiratory flow rate (PEFR), which was several times greater than that observed when reflux was not followed by tracheal aspiration (Fig. 85.1). This indicates that microaspiration into the bronchial tree not only occurs but induces an important increase in airway resistance. Nevertheless, reflux episodes that do not reach the upper sphincter, and hence are without aspiration, may also induce changes in airway resistance.

The third pathogenic mechanism is produced by gastroesophageal reflux activation of a vagal reflex between the distal (lower) esophagus and the tracheobronchial tree. This reflex mechanism has been described both in patients with bronchial asthma and in those with persistent cough. It was first suggested by Mansfield and Stein,[11] who demonstrated in patients with asthma that the infusion of chlorhidric acid into the esophagus induced an increase in airflow resistance that was rapidly reversed by antacids. These changes occurred even with maximal bronchodilator therapy. In a later study in a canine model, a similar increase in airflow resistance that disappeared after bilat-

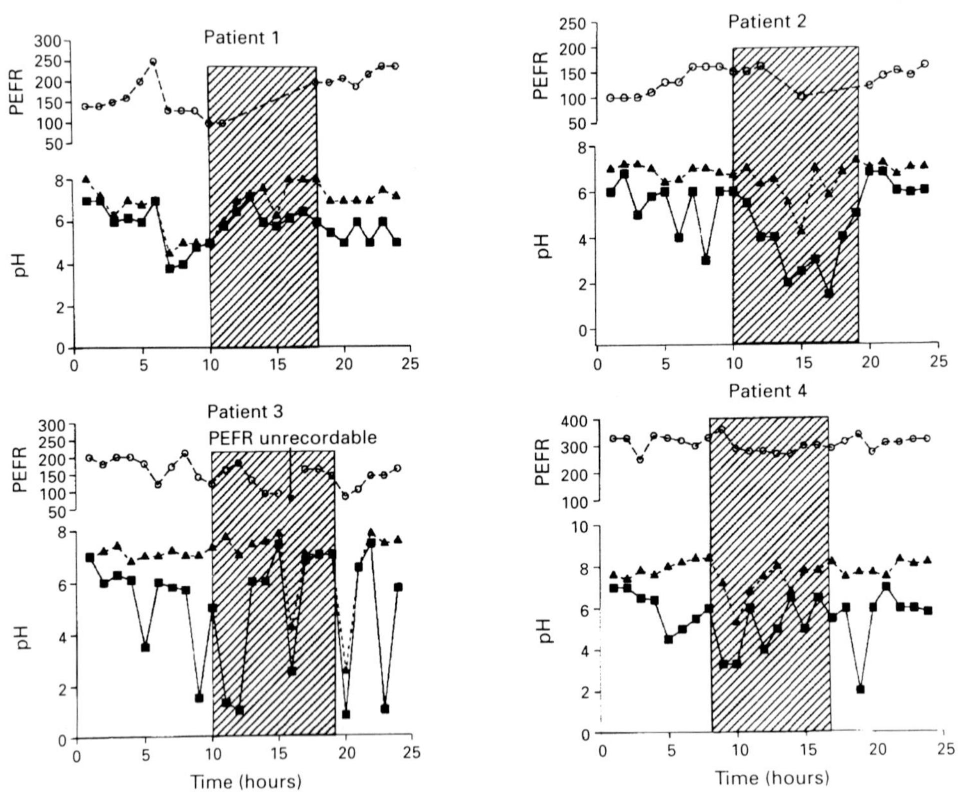


**Figure 85.1** The graphs show simultaneous esophageal (solid squares) and tracheal (solid triangles) pH measurements in four patients with both gastroesophageal reflux and asthma, along with recordings of peak expiratory flow rate (PEFR), over a 24-hour period. There were 37 significant falls in esophageal pH suggestive of gastroesophageal reflux. Five of these episodes were followed by a fall in tracheal pH and were associated with a significant decrease in PEFR (mean change, $-84 \pm 16$ L/min), whereas during the remaining 32 episodes of gastroesophageal reflux without tracheal aspiration the mean change in PEFR was minimal ($-8 \pm 4$ L/min). (From Jack CI, Calverley PMA, Donnelly RJ, et al: Simultaneous tracheal and oesophageal pH measurements in asthmatic patients with gastro-oesophageal reflux. Thorax 50:201–204, 1995.)

eral interruption of the vagal nerves was reported,[12] indicating that it was a vagally mediated mechanism. Supporting the role of a vagal reflex in gastroesophageal reflux–induced bronchoconstriction are the results of Wright and colleagues,[13] who showed that the decrement in $FEV_1$ induced by acid infusion into the esophagus was abolished by pretreatment with intramuscular atropine.

However, not all asthmatic patients show significant changes in airflow resistance after esophageal acid infusion.[14] Mansfield and Stein[11] noted that the increase in airway resistance elicited by esophageal acid infusion was present only in those asthmatics with evidence of esophagitis (positive Bernstein test), suggesting that prior esophageal mucosal injury is necessary to elicit acid-induced changes in airway resistance. Studies using dual-electrode esophageal pH testing seem to confirm this observation. In a study by Schan and coworkers,[15] PEFR decreased after esophageal acid infusion in control subjects, asthmatics with gastroesophageal reflux, asthmatics without gastroesophageal reflux, and subjects with gastroesophageal reflux alone; however, esophageal acid clearance improved PEFR in all groups except the asthmatics with gastroesophageal reflux, who had a further decrease in PEFR. These effects did not depend on acid exposure of the upper esophagus, a prerequisite for microaspiration, and were partially reversed by vagolytic doses of intravenous atropine, implying the importance of a vagally mediated reflex.[3] The stimulation of acid-sensitive esophageal receptors may also enhance bronchial hyperreactivity, as shown by Hervé and colleagues,[16] who demonstrated a reduction in the dose of methacholine required to induce a fall in $FEV_1$ of 20% after esophageal acid infusion. Similarly, the vagus nerve may also play a role in the bronchoconstriction induced by microaspiration. In a cat model, Tuchman and coworkers[17] showed that the increase in lung resistance induced by intratracheal infusion of acid, which was several times greater than that induced by intraesophageal infusion, was abolished after bilateral vagotomy. The logical conclusions from these observations are that gastroesophageal reflux may induce bronchial changes via a vagally mediated reflex originating in the lower esophagus and that these effects are further amplified if reflux reaches the upper esophagus and microaspiration occurs.

The relationship between gastroesophageal reflux and respiratory disorders is further complicated by the fact that physiologic alterations associated with asthma or cough, or with bronchodilator therapy, may themselves promote gastroesophageal reflux. Episodes of bronchospasm and cough are accompanied by an increase in the negative pressure within the thorax, and hence in the esophagus, that may promote reflux. In addition, hyperinflation and air trapping may lead to flattening of the diaphragm, allowing the lower esophageal sphincter to be drawn up into the thorax and impairing the antireflux barrier. Bronchodilator therapy may also promote gastroesophageal reflux. Theophylline increases gastric acid secretion and decreases lower esophageal sphincter tone. Indeed, asthmatics with gastroesophageal reflux who receive theophylline show an increase in esophageal acid exposure and reflux symptoms.[18] Specific beta-adrenergic agents relax smooth muscle tone throughout the body, entailing the potential to promote gastroesophageal reflux. A decrease in lower esophageal sphincter pressure has been shown with beta-adrenergic drugs administered orally or intravenously,[19] but not when these agents were given by inhalation.[20]

## Diagnosis

The possibility of associated gastroesophageal reflux should be suspected in patients with refractory chronic cough or difficult-to-treat asthma. Patients should be questioned about symptoms of gastroesophageal reflux, which include heartburn, regurgitation, or dysphagia. Some patients may complain of atypical chest pain, sore throat, or hoarseness. It is also important to record whether asthma or cough worsens with recumbency, after meals, or during alcohol ingestion. If the clinical history is consistent with gastroesophageal reflux, no further diagnostic workup is necessary and a trial of antireflux therapy should be started.

Gastroesophageal reflux is clinically silent in a significant number of patients. In these cases, different methods have been used to document its presence. Barium swallow techniques and esophageal manometry have low sensitivity for detection of gastroesophageal reflux. Endoscopy is indicated for those patients in whom empirical therapy is unsuccessful and those in whom complicated gastroesophageal reflux (e.g., esophagitis, Barrett's esophagus) is suspected.[3] Scintigraphic monitoring documents pulmonary aspiration of gastric contents; however, as discussed earlier, it has limited value in evaluating patients with respiratory symptoms, which may be provoked by other factors. Ambulatory esophageal pH monitoring is the most sensitive and specific test for gastroesophageal reflux.[3] However, demonstration of reflux by pH monitoring shows an association but not always a cause-and-effect relationship.[2, 21] It has been proposed that if respiratory symptoms and acid reflux episodes occur together more than 75% of the time, then the probability of a causal association is high.[22]

## Treatment

Therapy for gastrointestinal reflux should be instituted by recommending several changes in lifestyle, such as raising the head of the bed, avoiding meals before bedtime, eating low-fat foods, and eliminating caffeine and alcohol. Pharmacologic strategies for treating gastroesophageal reflux include antacids, which can be used for symptomatic relief; histamine-receptor blockers (cimetidine, ranitidine, famotidine), which partially block gastric acid secretion; proton pump inhibitors (omeprazole, lansoprazole), which directly inhibit gastric acid secretion; and prokinetic agents (cisapride), which improve esophageal contractility, increase lower esophageal sphincter pressure, and increase gastric emptying. Surgical interventions include the Nissen-Toupet-Belsey fundoplication and the Hill gastropexy. Larrain and colleagues[23] evaluated the long-term effects of surgery and cimetidine, compared with placebo; after 5 years, only the patients treated with surgery were free of symptoms, whereas those treated with cimetidine or placebo had persistent clinical abnormalities. Laparoscopic antireflux surgery has been developed and was shown to be effective in a series of 195 patients, all of whom had failed to respond to omeprazole.[23a]

A recommended approach for treating patients with respiratory complications of gastroesophageal reflux would be to start with empirical therapy that includes both conservative antireflux measures and acid-suppressive therapy. Administration of high doses of proton pump inhibitors (e.g., omeprazole, 20 mg twice a day) for 3 months is recommended, because some patients treated with lower doses or with histamine-receptor blockers may not show adequate acid suppression.[3, 24, 24a] If the patient's condition improves, then long-term therapy should be considered. Maintenance therapy can include a histamine-receptor blocker or a proton pump inhibitor at the lowest dose necessary to control symptoms, a level that must be determined individually. A prokinetic agent can be added. In patients not responding to the initial trial and in those who report only partial improvement of their symptoms, ambulatory pH testing under acid-suppressive therapy is indicated. If symptoms persist and there is no evidence of esophageal reflux, the test is considered negative and respiratory symptoms are unlikely to be caused by gastroesophageal reflux. If the test confirms the persistence of reflux, then surgery should be considered.[20, 25] Furthermore, the surgical option should be discussed with all patients who require a proton pump inhibitor to control gastroesophageal reflux, especially young patients, because there are still unanswered questions about the long-term safety of these drugs.[3, 21]

## Inflammatory Bowel Disease

Inflammatory bowel disease has been associated with a variety of extraintestinal manifestations, although pulmonary complications are considered to be infrequent. In an analysis of 1400 patients with inflammatory bowel disease by Rogers and colleagues,[26] only 6 patients (0.4%) had unexplained concurrent pulmonary disease. Nevertheless, the prevalence of pulmonary involvement in patients with inflammatory bowel disease may be higher than indicated by Rogers, because pulmonary function abnormalities have been reported in a significant number of patients in the absence of respiratory symptoms.[27–30]

Most of the reported patients with pulmonary complications associated with inflammatory bowel disease had ulcerative colitis (88%),[31] and the remainder had Crohn's disease. Respiratory involvement can occur at any age and seems to be more prevalent in women than in men. Frequently, respiratory complications are associated with other extraintestinal manifestations, such as arthritis, skin changes, or pericarditis. In most cases, respiratory symptoms develop after the diagnosis of inflammatory bowel disease has been made, frequently several years afterward. Nonetheless, in some cases respiratory symptoms antedate or are concomitant with those of the bowel disease.[31]

Various patterns of respiratory impairment in inflammatory bowel disease have been described (Table 85.1).[31] The one most frequently observed is airway disease (51% of cases). Unexplained purulent bronchitis, with or without bronchiectasis, in patients with inflammatory bowel disease was first reported by Kraft and associates[32] in 1976. Subsequent studies confirmed this association.[31, 33, 34] Unexplained productive cough is the predominant symptom; in some instances, it developed dramatically after proctocolectomy.[31] Involvement of the airways can occur at various levels of the tracheobronchial tree and can take the form of tracheal stenosis, chronic bronchitis, bronchiectasis, or bronchiolitis (see Table 85.1). Endoscopic examination shows marked erythema, swelling of the mucosa, and deformation of the airway lumen. Biopsy specimens have revealed mucosal ulceration, thickening of the basement membrane, and marked infiltration by neutrophils and plasma cells.[31, 34] Some authors have found histologic similarities between the inflammatory infiltrate of the airways and that of the colon, suggesting that the bronchial disease may result from a common abnormality in immune regulation that affects both the bowel and the bronchial tree, organs with a common embryologic origin.[31–34] Pulmonary function testing in patients with airway involvement usually reveals an obstructive ventilatory defect.[34] One study demonstrates small airways dysfunction (obstruction) in patients with ulcerative colitis who had normal spirometric measurements, suggesting that subclinical abnormalities in the airways may be more prevalent than suspected in these patients.[30] In some cases, the inflammatory process in the subglottic area can take the form of pseudotumoral lesions, with the potential of producing life-threatening acute upper airway obstruction requiring aggressive airway management.[31, 35]

Interstitial lung disease associated with inflammatory bowel disease has been less frequently observed (28% of cases).[31] Yet, such an association has occasionally been reported with other interstitial disorders, such as bronchi-

**Table 85.1 PATTERNS OF RESPIRATORY INVOLVEMENT IN INFLAMMATORY BOWEL DISEASE**

| Disease Type | No. Cases | % |
|---|---|---|
| Airway disease | | |
| Subglottic stenosis | 6 | 5.7 |
| Chronic bronchitis | 18 | 17.0 |
| Chronic bronchial suppuration | 7 | 6.6 |
| Bronchiectasis | 20 | 18.9 |
| Chronic bronchiolitis | 3 | 2.8 |
| Interstitial lung disease | | |
| BOOP | 11 | 10.4 |
| ILD-pulmonary sarcoidosis | 16 | 15.1 |
| Pulmonary infiltrates and eosinophilia | 3 | 2.8 |
| Necrobiotic nodules | 5 | 4.7 |
| Pleural disease | | |
| Pleural effusion | 4 | 3.8 |
| Pleuropericarditis | 13 | 12.3 |
| TOTAL | 106 | 100.1 |

BOOP = bronchiolitis obliterans with organizing pneumonia; ILD = interstitial lung disease.

From Camus P, Piard F, Ashcroft T, et al: The lung in inflammatory bowel disease. Medicine (Baltimore) 72:151–183, 1993.

olitis obliterans with organizing pneumonia (BOOP),[31, 36] sarcoidosis,[37, 38] and desquamative interstitial pneumonitis,[39] and in the form of the syndrome of pulmonary infiltrates and eosinophilia.[31] Because drugs used to treat ulcerative colitis and Crohn's disease (e.g., sulfasalazine, 5-aminosalicylic acid) may also induce interstitial pulmonary disease (e.g., BOOP, syndrome of pulmonary infiltrates, and eosinophilia)[31] it can be difficult to establish whether the pulmonary involvement is a result of the treatment or of the disease itself. Nonetheless, interstitial lung disorders have been reported in untreated patients, indicating that such an association may occur without exposure to drugs. A reduction in carbon monoxide diffusing capacity ($DL_{CO}$) during the active phases of the disease has been reported,[30, 39, 39a] which also suggests that subclinical pulmonary parenchymal involvement may be more prevalent than previously suspected. Furthermore, bronchoalveolar lavage examination in patients with Crohn's disease revealed the presence of a lymphocytic alveolitis, chiefly owing to an increase of CD4-positive T lymphocytes, in patients who did not have clinical evidence of pulmonary involvement.[40, 41]

Necrobiotic nodules, corresponding histologically to aggregates of neutrophils with areas of necrosis, have been reported in a few patients.[31] Serositis affecting the pleura or the pericardium, or both, has been reported in a small number of cases, especially during the periods of increased disease activity.[31]

Glucocorticosteroids given by inhalation or by mouth usually result in a rapid control of symptoms,[31, 33, 34] especially in those patients who do not have severe structural impairment (e.g., bronchiectasis). In some cases of severe respiratory compromise associated with inflammatory bowel disease, lung transplantation has been performed.[31]

## HEPATIC DISEASES

### Pleural Effusion

Between 5% and 10% of patients with cirrhosis of the liver develop pleural effusion, in the absence of a coexisting cardiopulmonary disease. This effusion, traditionally referred to as *hepatic hydrothorax*, is a transudate (as defined in Chapter 74) unless the pleural fluid is complicated by an infection. Although pleural effusions, which are most commonly located in the right hemithorax but which may also be left-sided or bilateral, are strongly associated with pronounced ascites, there is a small percentage of patients in whom ascites is almost undetectable.[42] The effusion is usually mild to moderate in size and asymptomatic, but in some cases it can be massive and provoke shortness of breath.[43] The mechanism is basically related to the presence of communications (usually small diaphragmatic defects) and to the normal pressure gradient between the abdominal and pleural cavities that facilitates the movement of the liquid into the chest. The presence of pleural fluid disturbs lung mechanics, resulting in decreased lung volumes and pulmonary compliance and positive pleural pressures. Accordingly, pulmonary gas exchange becomes abnormal and causes moderate hypoxemia and increased alveolar-arterial $PO_2$ difference ($[A - a]PO_2$), caused by both slight right-to-left intrapulmonary shunt and mild ventilation-perfusion imbalance; most of these abnormalities do not easily reverse after thoracentesis.[44]

The clinical management of pleural effusion in the context of liver disease is often rather difficult. Repeated thoracenteses may have transitory effects only, and thoracic drainage may result in substantial protein loss. The use of transjugular intrahepatic portosystemic shunting to decrease portal hypertension, which in turn could reduce the size of the hydrothorax, seems to be more promising, at least at short-term.[45]

### Pulmonary Function Disturbances

The most common abnormal lung function test result in patients with end-stage hepatic disease is a decreased $DL_{CO}$; likewise, both obstructive and restrictive ventilatory defects have been observed.[46] The coexistence of massive ascites can decrease lung compliance, increase pleural pressure, and reduce diaphragmatic motility. Altogether these pathophysiologic alterations restrict ventilatory capacity and reduce the efficiency of gas exchange, causing increased $(A - a)PO_2$ values with or without associated hypoxemia.[47]

### Hepatopulmonary Syndrome

Mild-to-moderate arterial hypoxemia is relatively common in the setting of chronic liver diseases. Yet, severe hypoxemia (arterial $PO_2$ less than 60 mm Hg) is less frequent in the absence of intrinsic cardiopulmonary disease; a 9% to 29% prevalence was detected in a population of more than 1100 patients with end-stage liver disease.[48–50] Accordingly, the presence of severe hypoxemia in a patient with chronic hepatic disease alone should strongly suggest the hepatopulmonary syndrome (HPS). Because patients with advanced liver disorders characteristically hyperventilate and are hypocapnic, measurement of the $(A - a)PO_2$ becomes the most sensitive way to detect gas exchange disturbances in HPS. Using this technique, the prevalence of gas exchange defects in patients with advanced liver disease increases markedly, up to 69%.[48–50]

HPS is defined as a syndrome characterized by a clinical triad: advanced chronic liver disease; gas exchange abnormalities, which lead ultimately to severe arterial hypoxemia; and widespread intrapulmonary vascular dilatations, in the absence of intrinsic cardiopulmonary disease.[51, 52] Although HPS is more prevalent in patients with all categories of hepatic cirrhosis, it also occurs in those with other common chronic liver diseases, such as chronic active hepatitis. In rare cases, HPS has been documented in other unusual liver disorders (noncirrhotic portal hypertension, $alpha_1$-antitrypsin deficiency, and Wilson's disease).[53] Nevertheless, the term HPS does not encompass all pleuropulmonary disorders that may subsist with many categories of liver disorders. At present, there is a special clinical interest in HPS because of its high prevalence (an estimated 20%) among patients with end-stage hepatic disease, its life-threatening nature, the lack of beneficial

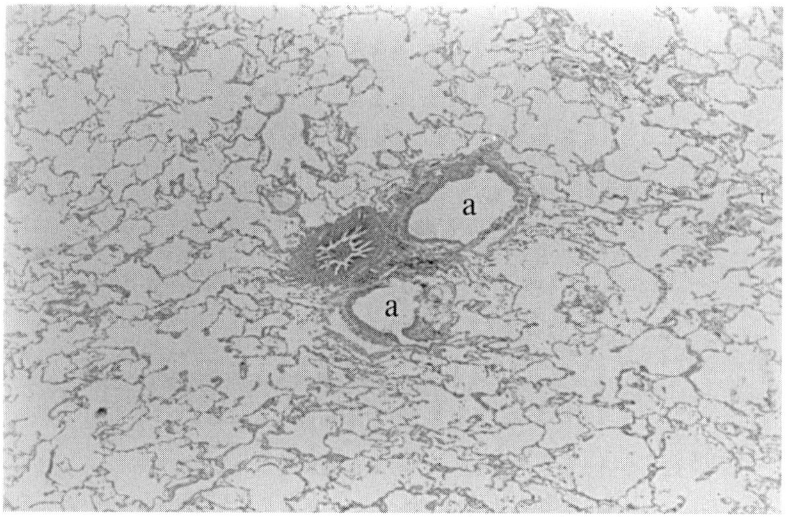


**Figure 85.2** A photomicrograph of a lung biopsy from a patient with hepatopulmonary syndrome is shown. Note the central presence of dilated pulmonary arteries (a) with a neighboring normal terminal bronchiole surrounded by an otherwise structurally intact pulmonary architecture. (Original magnification × 100.) (With permission from Rodriguez-Roisin R, Roca J: Hepatopulmonary syndrome: The paradigm of liver-induced hypoxaemia. Ballière's Clin Gastroenterol 11:387–406, 1997.)

medical therapy, and its unique improvement or full resolution after liver transplantation.[50]

The most conspicuous pathologic finding is a pronounced vasodilation of all peripheral branches of the pulmonary vasculature, at both the precapillary and capillary levels of the lung (15 to 150 μm in diameter), near the gas exchange area.[54] Pleural spider nevi may also be evident, but clear pulmonary arteriovenous communications are seldom visible. More importantly, this widespread pulmonary vasodilation is immersed in an otherwise intact pulmonary structure (Fig. 85.2).

## Pathogenesis

Pathogenically, it can be hypothesized that chronic liver disease associated with portal hypertension and perhaps with portosystemic shunting may cause hepatic failure, thereby inducing widespread vasodilation and a hyperkinetic status that results ultimately in HPS. Yet, the precise mechanism underlying HPS remains uncertain despite numerous investigations. Whether the mechanism of hemodynamic disturbances is related to failure of metabolism, to insufficiency of production of one or more circulating vasoactive substances by the injured liver, or to altered metabolism of some of the vasodilator molecules produced by endothelial cells[55] remains concealed. Circulating humoral vasodilating substances such as glucagon and prostacyclin have been investigated and may contribute to the development of vascular abnormalities in patients with chronic hepatitis, including a blunted hypoxic pulmonary vasoconstrictor response. However, clear evidence of their involvement in HPS is not available.[56, 57]

Nitric oxide (NO), a ubiquitous biologic agent considered to be a fine-tuner of vascular tone, has been presumed to be a pivotal signaling molecule of potential importance in the pathobiology of HPS.[58, 59] Persistent induction of NO synthase (NOS) could account for the hyperkinetic circulatory hallmarks of HPS.[59] Both the constitutive isoform of NOS (cNOS), expressed in endothelial cells (eNOS or type III NOS),[60] and the inducible NOS (iNOS or type II NOS), expressed in target tissues after exposure to proinflammatory cytokines such as human bronchial epithelial cells,[61] have been implicated in animal experimental settings in the pathogenesis of HPS. In keeping with this contention, increased levels of exhaled NO have been observed in patients with advanced unstable hepatic cirrhosis, and also in those with HPS.[62, 63] Moreover, there have been significant decrements in exhaled NO on recovery from the liver disease[64] or after interventions such as administration of methylene blue[65] or performance of lung transplantation.[66] More recently it was shown in patients with liver cirrhosis that there are close correlations between exhaled NO concentration and Child-Pugh score, alkaline phosphatase, bilirubin, aspartate and alanine aminotransferase, and albumin, suggesting that activation of pulmonary NO formation may be triggered by stimulating factors normally inactivated by the liver.[64]

Clinically, most of the patients with HPS are cyanotic, show conspicuous finger clubbing, may complain of shortness of breath and platypnea (increased dyspnea in the upright position relieved by recumbency), and have a hyperkinetic circulation. The majority of the patients exhibit the typical clinical and functional stigmata of advanced liver failure, including those of portal hypertension; in a few cases, severe pulmonary abnormalities may antedate those of hepatic dysfunction.[50, 51] The presence of abundant cutaneous spider angiomata has been postulated as a clinical marker of the severity of both systemic and pulmonary circulatory and gas exchange abnormalities observed in HPS.[67] The more severe the hepatic failure, the greater the severity of HPS, as suggested by a prospective study in cirrhotic patients in which the hypoxemic subpopulation exhibited more severe liver failure as well as higher Child-Pugh scores and hepatic venous pressure gradients.[68] Unlike hereditary hemorrhagic telangiectasia (see Chapter 53), hemoptysis and paradoxic emboli are extremely uncommon clinical manifestations of HPS. A single case of brain abscess has been reported.[68a] When the syndrome coexists with either a chronic obstructive or a restrictive respiratory disorder, the prevailing clinical and functional pulmonary features are those of HPS.[68b]

## Diagnosis

The diagnostic criteria for HPS are as follows[51]: presence of chronic liver disease, ideally without unrelated cardiac or pleuropulmonary disease; normal or near-normal results (basal medium-sized nodular or reticulonodular opacities) on chest roentgenogram; gas exchange abnormalities, more specifically an increased $(A - a)P_{O_2}$ (more than 15 mm Hg), with or without concomitant arterial hypoxemia (arterial $P_{O_2}$ less than 80 mm Hg); and a positive contrast-enhanced echocardiogram (CE-ECO) or an abnormal intravenous radiolabeled perfusion lung scan (i.e., presence of radioactivity in extrapulmonary sites such as liver, spleen, kidneys, and brain) or both. Other additional features that can be useful for further establishing the diagnosis of HPS include decreased $D_{L_{CO}}$, dyspnea with or without platypnea and orthodeoxia (worsened arterial hypoxemia while standing), and a hyperkinetic circulatory status (high cardiac output and low systemic arterial pressures) with normal or low pulmonary artery pressures (PPA).

Two-dimensional CE-ECO appears to be the most sensitive and accurate noninvasive diagnostic procedure to identify right-to-left shunts of blood by finding microbubbles of air (or indocyanine green) in the left heart cavities within three to six beats of their visualization in the right-sided chambers[50, 51] (Fig. 85.3). Normally, echogenicity in the left chambers is not detected because the intravenously injected microbubbles (60 to 90 μm in diameter) are trapped in the pulmonary capillaries. Although CE-ECO cannot distinguish among the different forms of pulmonary vascular deformities (i.e., precapillary, capillary, and pleural dilatations versus direct arteriovenous anastomoses), it can clearly differentiate them from intracardiac communications, such as a patent foramen ovale. Alternatively, the demonstration of radionuclide technetium 99m–macroaggregated albumin ($^{99m}$Tc-MAA) activity over extrapulmonary organs, again after intravenous injection, strongly suggests the presence of right-to-left intrapulmonary shunting, because under normal conditions the albumin macroaggregates (20 to 60 μm in diameter) are trapped in the pulmonary capillary bed. From a pulmonary function viewpoint, the spectrum of gas exchange abnormalities is wide and includes severe hypoxemia at rest (conventionally measured while breathing room air in the upright position), low arterial $P_{CO_2}$, increased $(A - a)P_{O_2}$,[49] and a decreased $D_{L_{CO}}$. In general, expiratory flow rates and lung volumes are within normal limits.

To date the exact prevalence of HPS remains unknown. Using CE-ECO as the gold-standard tool to identify intrapulmonary vascular dilatations, the prevalence of a positive CE-ECO test in patients with chronic liver disease is approximately 20%.[49, 69] However, the relevance of a positive CE-ECO result in patients without coexisting gas exchange disturbances, some of whom may have a normal $(A - a)P_{O_2}$, remains unsettled. These patients are considered to have a *forme fruste* of HPS.[69, 70]

Systemic hypotension, a normal or low PPA with normal or low pulmonary vascular resistance (PVR) (less than 1.5 mm Hg/L per minute),[50] an inordinately high cardiac output, and a reduced pulmonary vascular reactivity are the four hemodynamic hallmarks of HPS. When the constellation of hypoxemia, normal or low PPA, and finger clubbing are observed in a patient with advanced liver disease, the diagnosis of HPS is strongly suggested.

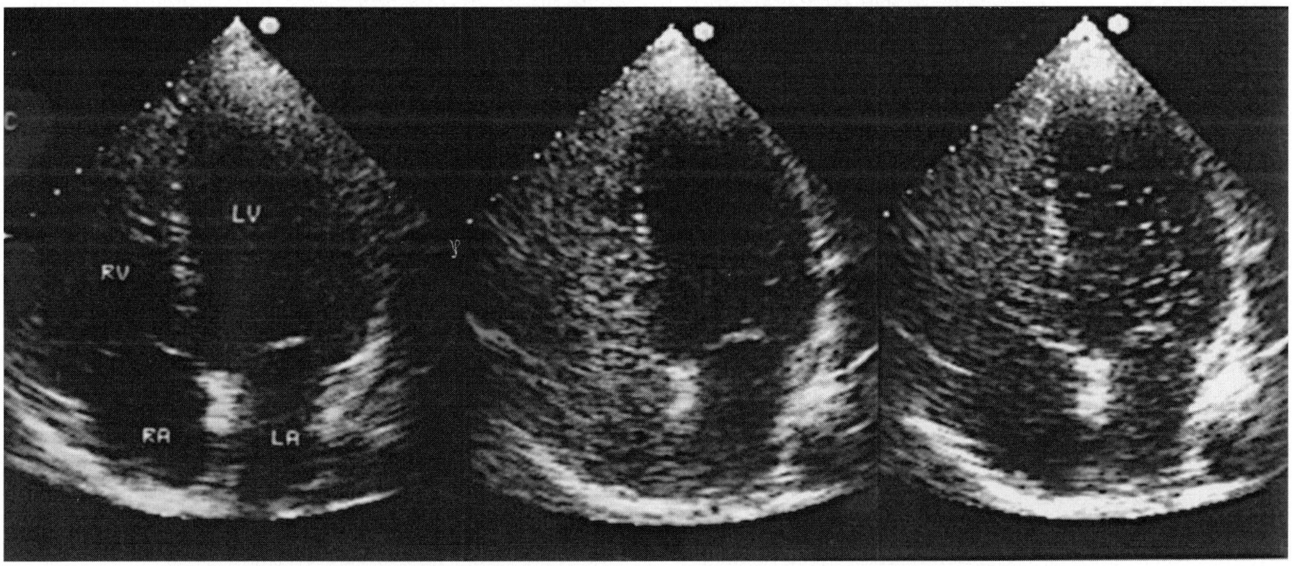


**Figure 85.3** Contrast-enhanced echocardiograms in a patient with hepatopulmonary syndrome are shown. *Left,* Normal four-chamber view (RA = right atrium; RV = right ventricle; LV = left ventricle; LA = left atrium). *Center,* Both RA and RV are occupied by microbubbles. *Right,* delayed opacification of RV and LV. The demonstration of microbubbles in the left cardiac chambers is highly suggestive of the presence of intrapulmonary vascular dilatations or, alternatively, of anatomic arteriovenous malformations. (Courtesy of Dr. C. Paré, Hospital Clinic, Barcelona.)

Although data describing the natural history of HPS are scant, it appears that HPS worsens progressively and has an adverse outcome, with an estimated significant mortality rate (4 out of 7 patients) within a 4-year period after initial diagnosis.[71]

## Gas Exchange Abnormalities

The multiple inert gas elimination technique has been used extensively to investigate the contribution of ventilation-perfusion ($\dot{V}A/\dot{Q}$) mismatching to pulmonary gas exchange abnormalities in patients with HPS and also in a wide spectrum of patients with liver cirrhosis and varying degrees of abnormal hypoxemia.[67, 72–76] When HPS is mild to moderate, the predominant mechanism of hypoxemia is $\dot{V}A/\dot{Q}$ inequality, essentially due to the presence of areas in which ventilation is preserved but perfusion is profoundly increased (i.e., low $\dot{V}A/\dot{Q}$ ratios). In contrast, when HPS is severe, increased intrapulmonary shunt ($\dot{V}A/\dot{Q}$ ratio $= 0$) is the primary abnormality, and alveolar-capillary diffusion limitation to oxygen can coexist. The response of arterial $PO_2$ to 100% oxygen breathing may be helpful to the clinician to estimate the principal intrapulmonary mechanism of hypoxemia in HPS. If arterial $PO_2$ remains basically unaltered during hyperoxic breathing, the major mechanism of abnormal arterial oxygenation should be a marked right-to-left intrapulmonary shunt, most likely due to the presence of arteriovenous malformations. If the arterial $PO_2$ increases but to less than 500 mm Hg, intrapulmonary shunting cannot be excluded. Conversely, a substantial increase of arterial $PO_2$ (greater than 600 mm Hg) rules out the existence of intrapulmonary shunt and indicates that $\dot{V}A/\dot{Q}$ heterogeneity is the main factor causing low arterial oxygenation.

Equally important, the inert gas studies have confirmed the presence of reduced pulmonary vasopressor tone, as previously shown,[67, 77, 78] and have also established that some pulmonary vasoconstriction remains, a condition consistent with altered pulmonary vascular tone favoring the development of alveolar units with low $\dot{V}A/\dot{Q}$ ratios. If the site of hypoxic pulmonary vasoconstriction is supposed to be in small arteries, possibly those smaller than 500 μm in diameter, then the vascular derangement observed in HPS necessarily impairs the ability of these pulmonary vessels to contract in response to vasoconstricting agents. Collectively, as the severity of the liver dysfunction advances, the greater the systemic and pulmonary vasodilation, the lower the hypoxic pulmonary vascular response, and the greater the degree of $\dot{V}A/\dot{Q}$ inequalities, including increased intrapulmonary shunt.[67, 72–76]

A "diffusion-perfusion defect" has also been postulated to explain a diffusion gradient for oxygen in dilated pulmonary capillaries.[79, 80] The contention is that vasodilation induces $\dot{V}A/\dot{Q}$ mismatching, namely areas of alveolar units with low $\dot{V}A/\dot{Q}$ ratios, and also causes inadequate diffusion of oxygen to the center of the enlarged capillary; this, in turn, would lead to alveolar-capillary disequilibrium for oxygen. Moreover, the coexistence of a hyperkinetic status and the resulting shorter transit time of red blood cells would exaggerate further this diffusion-induced gas exchange abnormality. Nowadays, this "diffusion-perfusion defect" can be viewed as a variant of $\dot{V}A/\dot{Q}$ imbalance, possibly with an additional degree of oxygen diffusion limitation, rather than a diffusion impairment for oxygen per se.[50]

## Treatment

Therapeutically, a vast armamentarium of pharmacologic agents has been tested in patients with HPS, with disappointing results overall. These agents include bismesilate almitrine, cyclophosphamide, garlic preparation, indomethacin, long-term oxygen therapy, methylene blue, propranolol, prostaglandin, and somatostatin.[50, 51] In principle, all these approaches held promise because of their efficacy in enhancing pulmonary vasoconstriction (e.g., bismesilate almitrine) or ablating vasodilation (e.g., propranolol). More aggressive palliative procedures, such as embolization of pulmonary fistulas, portal decompression after transjugular intrahepatic portosystemic shunting, or plasma exchange, have not been successful or have at most shown modest effects that warrant further studies.[81] By contrast, liver transplantation has proved to be a much more encouraging alternative approach for HPS.[82–85] In theory, replacement of the damaged organ should prevent all HPS-induced systemic and pulmonary effects, hence resolving or ameliorating gas exchange abnormalities. Although a full comprehensive experience with liver transplantation in the setting of HPS is still unclear, it is currently estimated that approximately two thirds of both pediatric and adult patients with HPS show significant clinical and functional respiratory improvement after this radical surgical procedure.[86] Youth, a good arterial $PO_2$ response to 100% oxygen breathing, and the severity of presurgical hypoxemia are all factors that seem to predict a favorable response to liver transplantation.[85] Collectively, these elements may indicate a more reactive pulmonary vasculature, less profound intrapulmonary shunt, and more $\dot{V}A/\dot{Q}$ inequality as the principal determinants of gas exchange abnormalities.

# Portopulmonary Hypertension

Pulmonary hypertension (PH) associated with portal hypertension or portopulmonary hypertension (PHPH) is, along with HPS, the other mysterious pulmonary vascular disorder that appears to be associated with chronic hepatic disease. Because both the diagnosis and the outcome of PHPH, particularly in relation to the therapeutic benefits of liver transplantation, appear to be substantially different from those of HPS, it is important to highlight the distinctions between the two disorders.[87] Currently, PH is defined as a mean PPA exceeding 25 mm Hg at rest or 30 mm Hg during exercise, in the presence of a normal pulmonary capillary wedge pressure.[88, 89]

It is diagnostically important, however, to note that as many as 20% of patients with advanced liver disease exhibit increased PPA.[86] Moreover, the interplay among PPA, PVR, and cardiac output in hepatic patients is especially complex. Increases in the pressures within the pulmonary circulation can be caused by three mechanisms: first, by "high-flow status," induced passively by a hyperkinetic circulation in which the increased PPA is predominantly attributable to a remarkably high cardiac output and despite the fact that PVR is low,[90] hemodynamic characteristics that are compatible with the diagnosis of HPS. A second mechanism, which is found in almost half of the candidates for liver transplantation and is manifested during exercise[76] or in the setting of rapid volume shifts,[91] is associated with an increased pulmonary capillary wedge pressure, possibly reflecting impaired left–ventricular contractility. The third scenario represents true PHPH, a condition that leads to histologic features identical to those of plexogenic pulmonary arteriopathy (see Chapter 52), including medial hypertrophy, concentric intimal fibrosis, and plexiform lesions of the small arteries, with or without secondary thrombotic changes.[92] According to Castro and coworkers,[86] PHPH should be suspected in patients with chronic liver disease who have an increased $P_{PA}$ (more than 25 mm Hg), an increased PVR (more than 1.5 mm Hg/L per minute or 120 dynes·sec/cm$^5$), and a normal pulmonary capillary wedge pressure.[89]

In the classic retrospective postmortem studies, the prevalence of PH in patients with liver cirrhosis or portal hypertension (or both) ranged between 0.25% and 0.73%[92]; by contrast, PH was detected in only 0.13% of a noncirrhotic population. These data lend further support to the likelihood of a causal association between the two conditions. Subsequently, two prospective studies identified a higher incidence of PH, about 2%, in patients with chronic liver disease,[93, 94] and more recently, two other groups of investigators observed a considerably higher figure, approximately 4%.[86, 95] Furthermore, PHPH has been classified as a category of secondary PH in the consensus statement of the American College of Chest Physicians (ACCP).[96] In a case-control study conducted by the International Primary Hypertension Study Group to investigate the incidence of primary PH, the condition was found in 7.3% of patients with cirrhosis, 3.1% of those with human immunodeficiency virus infection, 2.1% of those with a family history of primary PH, and none of the controls.[97]

From a histopathologic viewpoint, the vascular lesions are indistinguishable from those identified in primary PH, namely isolated medial hypertrophy, plexogenic pulmonary arteriopathy, and thrombotic pulmonary arteriopathy.[98] According to Hervé and colleagues,[89] vasoconstriction, remodeling of the walls of muscular pulmonary arteries, and in situ microthrombosis combine to cause an increase in vascular resistance in PHPH. It is postulated that the portosystemic shunting of vasoactive agents such as thromboxanes, serotonin, bradykinin, and neuropeptide Y, which are normally metabolized by the healthy liver into the pulmonary circulation, may result in arterial vasoconstriction.[91] As in primary PH, an attractive alternative pathogenic hypothesis that cannot be ruled out is pulmonary endothelial dysfunction, more specifically decreased production of the endogenous vasodilator, NO.[91]

The most common symptom is shortness of breath on exertion; chest pain, syncope, and hemoptysis also occur.[94, 99] Radiographically, both enlarged cardiac silhouette and pulmonary artery prominence are noted in approximately two thirds of patients with hemodynamic confirmation of PHPH.[99]

Overall, maximal airflow rates and lung volumes are within or near normal limits, whereas $DL_{CO}$, arterial $P_{O_2}$, and $(A - a)P_{O_2}$ are reduced, although not to the strikingly low levels observed in HPS.[86, 100] Compared with patients with primary PH, mean $P_{PA}$ is lower in patients with PHPH, and cardiac index and mixed venous oxygen saturation are significantly higher.[89] The CE-ECO does not show echogenicity in the left-sided cavities unless there is an abnormal communication at atrial level.[100] Although data are scant, it is suggested that the pulmonary component of PHPH is progressive, with a two- to threefold increase in $P_{PA}$ during a period of 1 to 2 years.[94] Although it is generally assumed that patients with PHPH have a shorter survival time, they actually lived longer than those with other categories of primary PH.[86]

Patients with a clinical suspicion of PHPH, like all patients with primary PH, should have a pharmacologic vasodilator test to assess the degree of reversibility of the pulmonary vasculature in response to common drugs such as nifedipine, NO, and prostacyclin. A 20% reduction in both $P_{PA}$ and PVR is considered to be a criterion of vascular responsiveness. In the series reported by Hervé and colleagues[89] already alluded to, none of the patients with PHPH showed a positive vasodilator response.

Oral vasodilator agents deserve a therapeutic trial in those patients whose vasodilator response has been positive. In addition, continuous infusion of the more powerful vasodilator, epoprostenol (prostacyclin), has been shown to be beneficial in some patients with PHPH.[89, 91, 100a] As in patients with HPS, liver transplantation has been tried but with conflicting results; pediatric patients seem to show a better response than adults.[87] Unlike HPS, however, PHPH is not a current indication for liver transplantation, because these patients are considered to bc at extremely high risk with this elective surgical procedure.[86, 89] There is one case report of a successful outcome after orthoptic liver transplantation in an adult with PHPH associated with a strikingly hyperdynamic circulatory state.[100b]

## Primary Biliary Cirrhosis

Primary biliary cirrhosis (PBC), considered to be an autoimmune disease, is characterized by a chronic, cholestatic, granulomatous and destructive process that involves the intrahepatic bile ducts.[101] When severe, these processes result in cholestasis, cirrhosis, and liver failure. The autoimmunologic basis is reflected in the presence of several immunologic alterations, such as depressed T-suppressor cell function, hypergammaglobulinemia, and the presence of antimitochondrial antibodies. Connective tissue diseases such as the Sicca complex, Sjögren's syndrome, and scleroderma are frequently associated with PBC.[101, 102] Several respiratory diseases have been associated with PBC: interstitial lung disorders, such as lymphocytic interstitial pneumonitis and fibrosing alveolitis; subclinical intrapulmonary granulomas that mimic sarcoidosis[103]; increased numbers of $CD4^+$ lymphocytes in the bronchoalveolar lavage fluid; and obstructive airway disease, such as bronchiectasis.[45] Occasionally, the pulmonary manifestations precede the liver involvement.[104] In addition, thoracic wall deformities secondary to osteopenic vertebral complications induced by abnormal vitamin D metabo-

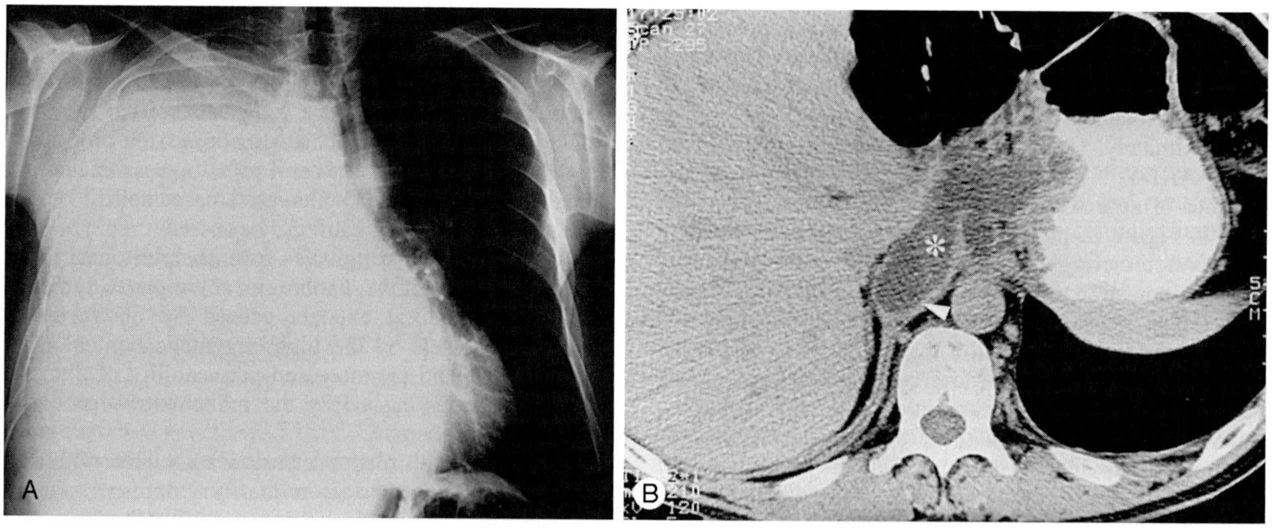

**Figure 85.4** This massive pleural effusion is associated with a pancreatic pseudocyst. *A*, Chest radiograph demonstrates a massive pleural effusion that occupies the right hemithorax. *B*, Computed tomography scan of the upper abdomen, performed after pleural drainage, shows the cephalad extension of the pseudocyst *(asterisk)* through the right crural insertion *(arrow)* and the esophageal hiatus. (Courtesy of Dr. S. Navarro, Hospital Clinic, Barcelona.)

tomographic scanning of the chest and abdomen usually reveal the presence of a pseudocyst and occasionally may even show the pancreaticopleural fistula[137] (see Fig. 85.4). Endoscopic retrograde cholangiopancreatography (ERCP) provides additional information on ductal structures and may demonstrate passage of contrast material from the pancreatic duct or a pseudocyst into the peritoneal cavity, although visualization of the fistula may be difficult.[135, 137] ERCP and computed tomographic scanning together provide complementary information, which is useful, especially if the patient has to undergo surgical intervention.

Patients with chronic pancreatic pleural effusions should be treated initially with nasogastric tube placement, no oral intake, parenteral nutrition, and repeated therapeutic thoracenteses. Inhibition of pancreatic secretion with octreotide has been shown to be useful in promoting the closure of pancreaticopleural fistula in some cases.[138] Nonetheless, if after 2 to 3 weeks of medical therapy the pleural fluid continues to accumulate and the patient remains symptomatic, surgery should be considered.

## CHRONIC RENAL FAILURE

Chronic renal diseases are associated with a variety of respiratory manifestations. Pulmonary edema, pleural disease, pulmonary calcification, and sleep apnea syndrome have been documented in patients with chronic renal failure. Furthermore, treatment with hemodialysis also produces transient changes in pulmonary gas exchange. These disorders are discussed in this section. Systemic necrotizing vasculitis and diseases associated with autoantibodies, which usually affect both the lung and the kidney, are considered in Chapters 58 and 60.

### Pulmonary Edema

Pulmonary edema is common in patients with acute or chronic renal failure. A variety of conditions may favor edema formation: fluid overload, left-ventricular failure, hypoalbuminemia, and increased pulmonary microvascular permeability. The relative importance of increased microvascular permeability versus left-ventricular failure in the pathogenesis of pulmonary edema in renal failure has been largely a subject of controversy. Autopsy findings showing the presence of protein-rich edema fluid, hyaline membranes, and alveolar hemorrhage[139, 140] all pointed to an increased vascular permeability to proteins as the likely mechanism of pulmonary edema formation. The demonstration of an increased protein content in edema fluid sampled directly by endotracheal aspiration reinforced this hypothesis.[141] Furthermore, pulmonary edema has been reported in the absence of volume overload and in the presence of normal intracardiac and pulmonary wedge pressures. However, studies using a double-isotope technique failed to show a significant accumulation of a radiolabeled plasma protein (transferrin) in patients with renal failure and pulmonary edema.[142] The rate of protein accumulation in patients with renal failure was similar to that in patients with cardiogenic pulmonary edema and in normal volunteers, and significantly lower than in patients with ARDS; these observations suggest that pulmonary edema associated with renal failure was probably not related to increased pulmonary vascular permeability to proteins.[142]

Conceivably, heart failure plays an important role in the development of pulmonary edema associated with renal failure. Cardiac disorders are common in end-stage renal disease, and a variety of factors, including hypertension, diabetes mellitus, anemia, surgical arteriovenous fistulas, and ischemic heart disease, may affect adversely cardiac function.[143, 144] Left-ventricular dysfunction may be reversible after dialysis or renal transplantation, which suggests that patients with chronic renal failure may have a specific "uremic cardiomyopathy."[143, 145, 146]

Subclinical lung congestion in patients with chronic renal failure may produce a reduction in lung volumes and in maximal expiratory flow rates that usually reverses after hemodialysis.[147–149] In contrast to the findings in patients with left-ventricular dysfunction,[150] subclinical pulmonary edema in renal failure is not associated with bronchial hyperresponsiveness; no changes in bronchial reactivity have been documented in these patients before and after hemodialysis.[151]

From a clinical standpoint, most instances of pulmonary edema associated with renal failure should be considered to involve elevation of intravascular volume and abnormal left-ventricular function. Accordingly, its treatment should essentially consist of removal of the excess of body fluid with dialysis.

## Pleural Disease

Approximately 20% to 40% of patients who die from chronic renal failure have fibrinous pleuritis detected at autopsy.[139, 152] This fibrinous pleuritis can be manifested as pleuritic chest pain with pleural rubs,[153] pleural effusion,[154] or fibrothorax.[155, 156]

Pleural effusions are present in 3% of patients with chronic renal failure.[154] No relationship exists between the development of pleural effusion and the degree of uremia, the adequacy and duration of dialysis, or the interdialysis interval.[153, 154] Patients may be asymptomatic, or they may present with fever, chest pain, cough, or dyspnea. The effusions usually are unilateral and in some cases may be large, occupying more than 50% of the hemithorax. The pleural fluid is an exudate with either a serosanguineous or a frankly hemorrhagic appearance.[157] The leukocyte count reveals predominance of lymphocytes, and the biopsy specimens usually demonstrate chronic fibrinous pleuritis.[133] The pathogenesis of pleural disease associated with renal failure is not known, but it is probably related to the effect of retained metabolic toxins.

The effusion usually disappears gradually after several weeks of dialysis. In about 25% of patients, it may persist, progress, or recur. If fibrothorax develops and produces a restrictive ventilatory impairment, surgical decortication should be considered.[155, 156]

## Pulmonary Calcification

Metastatic calcification is a complication of chronic renal failure that may affect many visceral and extravisceral organs.[158] Pulmonary involvement is common, but it is usually undetectable by chest radiography and asymptomatic.[159] At times, the chest radiograph may show infiltrates composed of nodular opacities less than 2 mm in diameter that can be diffuse or localized. The infiltrates are relatively stable, in contrast to infectious processes. Pulmonary function tests may reveal a restrictive ventilatory defect or reduction in $D_{LCO}$.

The pathogenesis of pulmonary calcification in patients with chronic renal failure is not known. It has been suggested that it is produced by a process of calciphylaxis, a mechanism by which soft tissues respond to a variety of chemical sensitizers with calcium deposition.[160] The patient's age, the type of underlying renal disease, and the duration of dialysis do not appear to be important in the development of this complication.[159]

The diagnosis of pulmonary calcification can be made by technetium 99m–diphosphonate scanning.[160] Treatment is generally unsatisfactory. Reduction of vitamin D or calcium intake has occasionally been successful.[160, 161] Renal transplantation has been suggested as a therapeutic alternative.[158]

## Sleep Apnea

Disturbed sleep has classically been recognized in patients with end-stage renal disease treated with hemodialysis. Other causes of sleep apnea are described in Chapter 81. Obstructive sleep apnea syndrome and periodic limb movements during sleep appear to be prevalent in patients with chronic renal failure. Using polysomnography, Kimmel and Miller[162] found that sleep apnea was present in 16 (73%) of 22 patients with chronic renal failure whose history was suggestive of sleep apnea; these patients accounted for an overall prevalence of 7.2% of the entire hemodialysis population. Sleep disturbances consist of apneas and hypopneas, both central and obstructive types.[163] The prevalence of sleep apnea among patients with chronic renal failure is similar before and after the initiation of hemodialysis treatment.[162]

Various mechanisms have been proposed to explain the high prevalence of sleep apnea in patients with chronic renal failure: narrowing of the upper airway by submucosal edema[164]; the effect of uremic toxins on the central nervous system[164]; an insufficient stimulus to breathe owing to the decreased arterial $P_{CO_2}$ in patients with chronic metabolic acidosis[165]; or an abnormal ventilatory responsiveness due to a resetting of the threshold level of hydrogen ion concentration necessary for respiratory stimulation secondary to chronic acidosis.[166] Both hemodialysis[164] and renal transplantation[167] have been shown to improve sleep apnea. Nasal continuous positive airway pressure has also shown to be effective in improving daytime symptoms in some patients.[168]

## Hemodialysis-Induced Hypoxemia

During hemodialysis, the majority of patients develop a reduction in arterial $P_{O_2}$. The arterial $P_{O_2}$ falls within a few minutes of initiation of dialysis by 10 to 15 mm Hg, reaches a nadir after 30 to 60 minutes, and persists for the duration of the procedure.[169–171] The severity of hypoxemia varies according to the type of dialysis membrane and the chemical nature of the dialysate buffer.[172] Several mechanisms have been proposed to explain the decrease in arterial $P_{O_2}$: (1) a shift in the oxyhemoglobin dissociation curve caused by the increase in pH during the procedure; (2) depression of central respiratory output due to alkalosis; (3) oxygen diffusion impairment; (4) $\dot{V}_A/\dot{Q}$ mismatching due to stasis of leukocytes in small pulmonary vessels; and (5) hypoventilation due to carbon dioxide excretion via the dialysate. Among these, the most relevant appear to be the two latter mechanisms.

Exposure of blood to dialysis membranes activates the alternative complement pathway, and within minutes C3a and C5a are generated. Complement activation may induce intrapulmonary sequestration of leukocytes and a fall in circulating leukocytes. Based on the temporal association between onset of hypoxemia and the transient leukopenia, it has been postulated that the decrease in arterial $Po_2$ results from $\dot{V}A/\dot{Q}$ mismatching due to leukostasis in small pulmonary vessels.[173] Supporting this suggestion is the observation that bioincompatible membranes (cuprophan) produce more hypoxemia than do biocompatible membranes (polyacrylonitrile, cellulose).[172] However, studies performed specifically to measure $\dot{V}A/\dot{Q}$ distributions during hemodialysis using the multiple inert gas elimination technique have ruled out $\dot{V}A/\dot{Q}$ mismatching as the mechanism of hypoxemia.[174–176] On the contrary, Romaldini and colleagues[175] showed a tendency for $\dot{V}A/\dot{Q}$ balance to improve during the dialysis procedure, which was most likely explained by the dialysis-induced decrease in extravascular lung water.[175] Furthermore, the fact that hypoxemia is also seen during dialysis with membranes that do not cause leukopenia,[177] and the fact that use of bicarbonate buffer or bubbling of carbon dioxide through the dialysate prevents the hypoxemia despite of the development of leukopenia, suggest that factors other than pulmonary leukocyte aggregation account for hemodialysis-associated hypoxemia.

The most accepted explanation for the decrease in arterial $Po_2$ during hemodialysis is the decrease in both alveolar ventilation and the respiratory exchange ratio that is associated with the removal of carbon dioxide in the dialysate. During hemodialysis, carbon dioxide is normally excreted into the dialysis fluid and the amount of carbon dioxide output through the lung is reduced. The result of this nonrespiratory removal of carbon dioxide is a decrease in both the minute ventilation and the respiratory exchange ratio (the ratio between carbon dioxide production and oxygen consumption).[171, 178] According to the alveolar air equation, the implication of a decrease in this ratio is a decrease in the alveolar $Po_2$; other factors being equal, this results in a decreased arterial $Po_2$.[168, 171] The $(A - a)Po_2$ value during hemodialysis actually remains stable despite a significant fall in arterial $Po_2$.[168, 175] The amount of carbon dioxide "unloading" into the dialysate buffer depends on its composition; it is substantial with acetate buffer but appears to be minimal with bicarbonate buffer.[179] In addition, acetate buffer may further reduce respiratory carbon dioxide elimination due to carbon dioxide consumption during acetate metabolism.[180] An additional consequence of the nonrespiratory carbon dioxide "unloading" is to destabilize resting ventilation, because the reduced overall ventilation is frequently accompanied by an irregular breathing pattern, with the development of periodicity and sometimes apneas.[181, 182]

The decrease in arterial $Po_2$ during hemodialysis is unlikely to be important in patients with normal cardiopulmonary function, but it may be clinically relevant in those with preexisting lung disease.[183, 184] Accordingly, the composition of the dialysis membrane and the chemical nature of the dialysate buffer should be considered when dialyzing patients who have cardiopulmonary disease. In these patients, cellulose or polyacrylonitrile filters and a bicarbonate bath are preferred. In addition, supplemental oxygen may be necessary during hemodialysis in some patients.

## SUMMARY

The principal disorders highlighted in this review are the respiratory consequences of gastroesophageal reflux, the pulmonary vascular disease states associated with portal hypertension, and the pleural and lung parenchymal complications of acute pancreatitis. In addition, other pulmonary problems related to specific liver, gastrointestinal, and renal diseases are discussed. Over the last few years, the knowledge and understanding of some of these syndromes, particularly the hepatopulmonary syndrome and pulmonary hypertension associated with portal hypertension, has improved substantially and has offered promising therapeutic approaches.

## References

1. Nebel OT, Fornes MF, Castell DO: Symptomatic gastroesophageal reflux: Incidence and precipitating factors. Am J Dig Dis 21:953–956, 1976.
2. Sontag SJ: Gastroesophageal reflux and asthma. Am J Med 103:84S–90S, 1997.
3. Harding SM, Richter JE: The role of gastroesophageal reflux in chronic cough and asthma. Chest 111:1389–1402, 1997.
4. Hamilos DL: Gastroesophageal reflux and sinusitis in asthma. Clin Chest Med 16:683–697, 1995.
5. Sontag SJ, Schnell TG, Miller TQ, et al: Prevalence of oesophagitis in asthmatics. Gut 33:872–876, 1992.
6. Irwin RS, Curley FJ, French CL: Chronic cough: The spectrum and frequency of causes, key components of the diagnostic evaluation, and outcome of specific therapy. Am Rev Respir Dis 141:640–647, 1990.
7. Mello CJ, Irwin RS, Curley FJ: Predictive values of the character, timing, and complications of chronic cough in diagnosing its cause. Arch Intern Med 156:997–1003, 1996.
8. Irwin RS, Curley FJ, French CL: Difficult-to-control asthma: Contributing factors and outcome of a systematic management protocol. Chest 103:1662–1669, 1993.
9. DeMeester TR, Bonavina L, Iascone C, et al: Chronic respiratory symptoms and occult gastroesophageal reflux: A prospective clinical study and results of surgical therapy. Ann Surg 211:337–345, 1990.
10. Jack CI, Calverley PMA, Donnelly RJ, et al: Simultaneous tracheal and oesophageal pH measurements in asthmatic patients with gastro-oesophageal reflux. Thorax 50:201–204, 1995.
11. Mansfield LE, Stein MR: Gastroesophageal reflux and asthma: A possible reflex mechanism. Ann Allergy 41:224–226, 1978.
12. Mansfield LE, Hameister HH, Spaulding HS, et al: The role of the vagus nerve in airway narrowing caused by intraesophageal hydrochloric acid provocation and esophageal distention. Ann Allergy 47:431–434, 1981.
13. Wright RA, Miller SA, Corsello BF: Acid-induced esophagobronchial-cardiac reflexes in humans. Gastroenterology 99:71–73, 1990.
14. Tan WC, Martin RJ, Pandey R, et al: Effects of spontaneous and simulated gastroesophageal reflux on sleeping asthmatics. Am Rev Respir Dis 141:1394–1399, 1990.
15. Schan CA, Harding SM, Haile JM, et al: Gastroesophageal reflux-induced bronchoconstriction: An intraesophageal acid infusion study using state-of-the-art technology. Chest 106:731–737, 1994.
16. Hervé P, Denjean A, Jian R, et al: Intraesophageal perfusion of acid increases the bronchomotor response to methacholine and to isocapnic hyperventilation in asthmatic subjects. Am Rev Respir Dis 134:986–989, 1986.

17. Tuchman DN, Boyle JT, Pack AI, et al: Comparison of airway responses following tracheal or esophageal acidification in the cat. Gastroenterology 87:872–881, 1984.
18. Ekstrom T, Tibbling L: Influence of theophylline on gastro-oesophageal reflux and asthma. Eur J Clin Pharmacol 35:353–356, 1988.
19. DiMarino AJ, Cohen S: Effect of an oral beta-2 adrenergic agonist on lower esophageal sphincter pressure in normals and in patients with achalasia. Dig Dis Sci 27:1063–1066, 1982.
20. Schindlbeck NE, Heinrich C, Huber RM, et al: Effects of albuterol (salbutamol) on esophageal motility and gastroesophageal reflux in healthy volunteers. JAMA 260:3156–3158, 1988.
21. Pope CE: Acid-reflux disorders. N Engl J Med 331:656–660, 1994.
22. Wiener GJ, Richter JE, Cooper JB, et al: The symptom index: A clinically important parameter of ambulatory 24-hour esophageal pH monitoring. Am J Gastroenterol 83:358–361, 1988.
23. Larrain A, Carrasco E, Galleguillos F, et al: Medical and surgical treatment of nonallergic asthma associated with gastroesophageal reflux. Chest 99:1330–1335, 1991.
23a. Allan CJ, Anvari M: Gastro-oesophageal reflux–related cough and its response to laparoscopic fundoplication. Thorax 53:963–968, 1998.
24. Simpson WG: Gastroesophageal reflux disease and asthma: Diagnosis and management. Arch Intern Med 155:798–803, 1995.
24a. Ing AJ, Ngu MC: Cough and gastro-oesophageal reflux. Lancet 353:944–946, 1999.
25. Ayres JG, Miles JF: Oesophageal reflux and asthma. Eur Respir J 9:1073–1078, 1996.
26. Rogers BHG, Clark L, Kirsher JP: The epidemiologic and demographic characteristics of inflammatory bowel disease: An analysis of a computerized file of 1400 patients. J Chronic Dis 24:743–773, 1971.
27. Eade OE, Smith CL, Alexander JR: Pulmonary function in patients with inflammatory bowel disease. Am J Gastroenterol 73:154–156, 1980.
28. Heatley RV, Thomas V, Prokipchuk EJ, et al: Pulmonary function abnormalities in patients with inflammatory bowel disease. Q J Med 51:241–250, 1982.
29. Munck A, Murciano D, Pariente R, et al: Latent pulmonary function abnormalities in children with Crohn's disease. Eur Respir J 8:377–380, 1995.
30. Tzanakis N, Samiou M, Bouros D, et al: Small airways function in patients with inflammatory bowel disease. Am J Respir Crit Care Med 157:382–386, 1998.
31. Camus P, Piard F, Ashcroft T, et al: The lung in inflammatory bowel disease. Medicine (Baltimore) 72:151–183, 1993.
32. Kraft SC, Earle RH, Roesler M, et al: Unexplained bronchopulmonary disease with inflammatory bowel disease. Arch Intern Med 136:454–459, 1976.
33. Butland RJ, Cole P, Citron KM, et al: Chronic bronchial suppuration and inflammatory bowel disease. Q J Med 50:63–75, 1981.
34. Higenbottam T, Cochrane GM, Clark TJH, et al: Bronchial disease in ulcerative colitis. Thorax 35:581–585, 1980.
35. Rickli H, Fretz M, Hoffman A, et al: Severe inflammatory upper airway stenosis in ulcerative colitis. Eur Respir J 7:1899–1902, 1994.
36. Swinburn CR, Jackson GJ, Cobden I, et al: Bronchiolitis obliterans with organising pneumonia in a patient with ulcerative colitis. Thorax 43:735–736, 1988.
37. Barr GD, Shale DJ, Jewell DP: Ulcerative colitis and sarcoidosis. Postgrad Med J 62:341–345, 1986.
38. Fries W, Grassi SA, Leone L, et al: Association between inflammatory bowel disease and sarcoidosis: Report of two cases and review of the literature. Scand J Gastroenterol 30:1221–1223, 1995.
39. Teague WG, Sutphen JL, Fechner RE: Desquamative interstitial pneumonitis complicating inflammatory bowel disease of childhood. J Pediatr Gastroenterol Nutr 4:663–667, 1985.
39a. Kuzela L, Vavrecka A, Prikazska M, et al: Pulmonary complications in patients with inflammatory bowel disorders. Hepatogastroenterology 46:1714–1719, 1999.
40. Smiejan JM, Cosnes J, Chollet-Martin S, et al: Sarcoid-like lymphocytosis of the lower respiratory tract in patients with active Crohn's disease. Ann Intern Med 104:17–21, 1986.
41. Wallaert B, Colombel JF, Tonnel AB, et al: Evidence of lymphocyte alveolitis in Crohn's disease. Chest 87:363–367, 1985.
42. Lieberman F, Hidemura R, Peters RL, et al: Pathogenesis and treatment of hydrothorax complicating cirrhosis with ascites. Arch Intern Med 64:341–351, 1966.
43. Alberts WM, Salem AJ, Solomon DA, et al: Hepatic hydrothorax: Cause and management. Arch Intern Med 151:2383–2388, 1991.
44. Agustí AGN, Cardús J, Roca J, et al: Ventilation-perfusion mismatch in patients with pleural effusion: Effects of thoracentesis. Am J Respir Crit Care Med 156:1205–1209, 1997.
45. Krowka MJ: Recent pulmonary observations in alpha$_1$-antitrypsin deficiency, primary biliary cirrhosis, chronic hepatitis C, and other hepatic problems. Clin Chest Med 17:67–82, 1996.
46. Hourani M, Bellamy PE, Tashkin DP, et al: Pulmonary dysfunction in advanced liver disease: Frequent occurrence of an abnormal diffusing capacity. Am J Med 90:693–700, 1991.
47. Agustí AGN, Roca J, Bosch J, et al: The lung in patients with cirrhosis. J Hepatol 10:251–257, 1990.
48. Krowka MJ, Dickson ER, Wiesner RH, et al: A prospective study of pulmonary function and gas exchange following liver transplantation. Chest 102:1161–1166, 1992.
49. Martinez-Pallí G, Barberà JA, Visa J, et al: Hepatopulmonary syndrome: Prevalence and clinical markers (abstract). Eur Respir J 9:179s, 1996.
50. Rodriguez-Roisin R, Roca J: Hepatopulmonary syndrome: The paradigm of liver-induced hypoxaemia. Ballière's Clin Gastroenterol 11:387–406, 1997.
51. Rodriguez-Roisin R, Agustí AGN, Roca J: The hepatopulmonary syndrome: New name, old complexities. Thorax 47:897–902, 1992.
52. Rodriguez-Roisin R: Síndrome hepatopulmonar: Un nuevo concepto. ¿Un tratamiento nuevo? Med Clin (Barc) 105:269–274, 1995.
53. Krowka MJ, Cortese DA: Hepatopulmonary syndrome. Chest 98:1053–1054, 1990.
54. Berthelot P, Walker JG, Sherlock S, et al: Arterial changes in the lungs in cirrhosis of the liver-lung spider nevi. N Engl J Med 274:291–298, 1966.
55. Vanhoutte PM: The endothelium-moderator of vascular smooth muscle tone. N Engl J Med 319:512–513, 1998.
56. Groszmann RJ: Vasodilatation and hyperdynamic circulatory state in chronic liver disease. *In* Bosch J, Groszmann RJ (eds): Portal Hypertension: Pathophysiology and Treatment. Oxford, UK: Blackwell Scientific, 1994, pp 17–26.
57. Sikuler E, Groszmann RJ: Hemodynamic studies in long and short term portal hypertensive rats: The relation to systemic glucagon levels. Hepatology 6:414–418, 1986.
58. Moncada S, Higgs A: The L-arginine-nitric oxide pathway. N Engl J Med 329:2002–2012, 1993.
59. Vallance P, Moncada S: Hyperdynamic circulation in cirrhosis: A role for nitric oxide? Lancet 337:776–778, 1991.
60. Sogni P, Moreau R, Gadano A, et al: The role of nitric oxide in the hyperdynamic circulatory syndrome associated with portal hypertension. J Hepatol 23:218–224, 1995.
61. Fallon MB, Abrams GA, Ifou Z, et al: The role of endothelial nitric oxide synthase in the pathogenesis of a rat model of hepatopulmonary syndrome. Gastroenterol 113:606–614, 1997.
62. Matsumoto A, Ogura K, Hirata Y, et al: Increased nitric oxide in the exhaled air of patients with decompensated liver cirrhosis. Ann Intern Med 123:110–113, 1995.
63. Sogni P, Garnier P, Adano A, et al: Endogenous pulmonary nitric oxide production measured from exhaled air is increased in patients with hepatic cirrhosis. J Hepatol 23:471–473, 1995.
64. Söderman C, Leone A, Furst V, et al: Endogenous nitric oxide in exhaled air from patients with liver cirrhosis. Scand J Gastroenterol 32:591–597, 1997.
65. Cremona G, Higenbottam T, Mayoral V, et al: Elevated exhaled nitric oxide in patients with hepatopulmonary syndrome. Eur Respir J 8:1883–1885, 1995.
66. Rolla G, Bucca C, Brussino L: Methylene blue in the hepatopulmonary syndrome (letter). N Engl J Med 331:1098, 1994.
67. Rodriguez-Roisin R, Roca J, Agustí AGN, et al: Gas exchange and pulmonary vascular reactivity in patients with liver cirrhosis. Am Rev Respir Dis 135:1085–1092, 1987.

171. Patterson RW, Nissenson AR, Miller J, et al: Hypoxemia and pulmonary gas exchange during hemodialysis. J Appl Physiol 50:259–264, 1981.
172. De Backer WA, Verpooten GA, Borgongjon DJ, et al: Hypoxemia during hemodialysis: Effects of different membranes and dialysate compositions. Kidney Int 23:738–743, 1983.
173. Craddock PR, Fehr J, Brigham KL, et al: Complement and leukocyte-mediated pulmonary dysfunction in hemodialysis. N Engl J Med 296:769–774, 1977.
174. Ralph DD, Ott SM, Sherrard DJ, et al: Inert gas analysis of ventilation-perfusion matching during hemodialysis. J Clin Invest 73:1385–1391, 1984.
175. Romaldini H, Rodriguez-Roisin R, Lopez FA, et al: The mechanisms of arterial hypoxemia during hemodialysis. Am Rev Respir Dis 129:780–784, 1984.
176. Rodriguez-Roisin R, Wagner PD: Clinical relevance of ventilation-perfusion inequality determined by inert gas elimination. Eur Respir J 3:469–482, 1990.
177. Dumler F, Levin NW: Leukopenia and hypoxemia: Unrelated effects of hemodialysis. Arch Intern Med 139:1103–1106, 1979.
178. Dolan MJ, Whipp BJ, Davidson WD, et al: Hypopnea associated with acetate hemodialysis: Carbon dioxide-flow-dependent ventilation. N Engl J Med 305:72–75, 1981.
179. Cardoso M, Vinay P, Vinet B, et al: Hypoxemia during hemodialysis: A critical review of the facts. Am J Kidney Dis 11:281–297, 1988.
180. Oh MS, Uribarri J, Del Monte ML, et al: A mechanism of hypoxemia during hemodialysis: Consumption of $CO_2$ in metabolism of acetate. Am J Nephrol 5:366–371, 1985.
181. De Backer WA, Heyrman RM, Wittesaele WM, et al: Ventilation and breathing patterns during hemodialysis-induced carbon dioxide unloading. Am Rev Respir Dis 136:406–410, 1987.
182. Heyrman RM, De Backer WA, Van Waeleghem JP, et al: Effect of oxygen administration on the breathing pattern during hemodialysis in man. Eur Respir J 2:972–976, 1989.
183. Peces-Serrano R, Fernandez-Vega F, Alvarez-Grande A: Hypoxemia during hemodialysis in patients with impairment in pulmonary function. Nephron 42:14–18, 1986.
184. Pitcher WD, Diamond SM, Henrich WL: Pulmonary gas exchange during dialysis in patients with obstructive lung disease. Chest 96:1136–1141, 1989.

# 86 Pulmonary Complications of Hematologic Disease

JOHN V. WEIL, M.D. • STEPHEN CRAWFORD, M.D.
PHILIP BROMBERG, M.D.

Introduction
Red Blood Cell Disorders
- Erythrocytosis
- Sickle Cell Disease
- Sickle Cell Trait
- Other Hemoglobin Disorders

Leukocyte Disorders
- Leukemia
- Transfusion-Related Lung Injury
- Other Disorders

Lymphomas
Malignant Plasma Cell Dyscrasias
- General Features
- Multiple Myeloma
- Waldenström's Macroglobulinemia

Coagulopathies
- Hereditary Clotting Factor Deficiencies
- Platelet Disorders
- Disseminated Intravascular Coagulation

Amyloidosis of the Respiratory Tract
- Systemic Amyloidosis
- Localized Amyloidosis

Bone Marrow and Stem Cell Transplantation
- General Features
- Temporal Sequence
- Common Clinical Presentations
- Noninfectious Causes
- Infectious Causes

Summary

## INTRODUCTION

Because of the central position of the lungs in the circulation, this organ is constantly exposed to normal and abnormal circulating elements in the bloodstream; these interactions may lead to pulmonary disease that is often serious, albeit not particularly common. For example, the abnormal red blood cells in patients with sickle cell disease and white blood cells in patients with various types of leukemia may be unable to complete their obligatory circuit through the pulmonary vasculature; the resulting microvascular occlusion causes diffuse lung injury. Severe anemia affects oxygen transport and exercise capacity; erythrocytosis, the opposite condition, is a common compensatory response to chronic hypoxia, and polycythemia vera is a known risk factor for venous thrombosis and pulmonary embolism. Lymphomas may involve the lung parenchyma as well as the mediastinal nodes, and the chemotherapy or radiotherapy that these patients undergo is commonly associated with severe or even fatal pulmonary complications, both infectious and noninfectious. Coagulopathies of various types can cause respiratory tract hemorrhage and pose a significant hazard for invasive diagnostic procedures. Immunoglobulin-producing plasma cell dyscrasias such as myeloma are associated with frequent pulmonary infections, extensive rib involvement, and other phenomena such as alveolar septal amyloidosis derived from perivascular deposition of specific polypeptide fragments of proteolytically cleaved immunoglobulin light chain. Localized airways and parenchymal and nodal amyloidosis, although uncommon, pose unusual problems and potential risks when they occur. Finally, a wide range of both infectious and noninfectious lung diseases frequently complicate hematopoietic stem cell transplantation, including bone marrow transplantation.

The wide-ranging variety of pulmonary complications associated with the major hematologic diseases are reviewed in this chapter. Further information about the lymphomas and lymphoproliferative diseases is available in Chapter 47. Additional information about solid organ transplantation and immunodeficiency disorders is presented in Chapter 83, and lung transplantation is considered separately in Chapter 97.

## RED BLOOD CELL DISORDERS

### Erythrocytosis

Erythrocytosis, or an excess number of circulating red blood cells, is defined by the presence of a red blood cell mass greater than 36 mL/kg in men or 32 mL/kg in women. The degree of resulting elevation in hematocrit and hemoglobin depends on the plasma volume, but hematocrit values higher than 54% in men or 51% in women are considered abnormal. Erythrocytosis is usually classified as either primary or secondary, depending on its cause. It is important to distinguish the two because primary erythrocytosis, chiefly *polycythemia vera,* represents a clonal proliferation of bone marrow lineages that leads to increases in leukocytes and platelets in addition to erythrocytes; this disorder has a different prognosis and requires special treatment. Most cases of secondary erythrocytosis are related to excess secretion of the glycoprotein hormone erythropoietin, an essential growth factor for the red blood cell lineage. Erythropoietin is produced principally in the kidneys, where its synthesis and secretion is regulated by the degree of renal tissue oxygenation, which is probably sensed by a reversible oxygen-binding heme protein. The lower the renal oxygen tension, the greater is the secretion of erythropoietin. Erythropoietin targets erythroid precursors (but not white blood cell precursors or megakaryocytes) in the bone marrow.[1] Erythropoietin-dependent erythrocytosis occurs in chronically hypoxemic normal persons residing at high altitude, in patients with chronic hypoxemic lung or cyanotic heart disease, in patients with conditions including tobacco smoking that cause increased carboxyhemoglobin, and in patients with genetically altered hemoglobins with high oxygen affinity.[2, 3] Secondary erythrocytosis is also seen in patients with erythropoietin-secreting tumors of the liver, kidney, adrenal gland, and cerebellum. In these patients, the erythropoietin production is physiologically inappropriate.

Regardless of the cause, when the hematocrit value exceeds 55%, whole blood viscosity begins to increase in a progressively increasing fashion; this causes an increase in pulmonary vascular resistance and decreases in cardiac output and cerebral blood flow[4, 5] and may lead to vascular thrombosis. Patients with polycythemia vera are especially prone to the latter complication because of their associated thrombocytosis. Erythrocytosis has been shown to impair the vasodilator response to acetylcholine but not to nitric oxide in patients with chronic hypoxic lung disease, which suggests that high hematocrit levels inhibit endothelium-dependent vasodilation, possibly through inactivation of endothelial-derived nitric oxide.[6] Supplemental oxygen is the mainstay of long-term treatment of erythrocytosis in patients with chronic hypoxemia, especially those with chronic obstructive pulmonary disease and sleep disorders[7]; theophylline may also be beneficial.[8] Phlebotomy is well tolerated and is used, when necessary, to reduce the hematocrit to the range of 50% to 55%. Patients with smoking-induced secondary polycythemia respond to smoking cessation, which stops the carboxyhemoglobin-producing activity. Phlebotomy has also been used for patients with polycythemia vera, although they are best treated with chemotherapeutic agents such as hydroxyurea or, especially, anagrelide to reduce the high risk of thrombocytosis-induced thrombosis.

### Sickle Cell Disease

The evolution of knowledge concerning the genetic and molecular basis of sickle cell anemia has been reviewed by Feldman and Tauber.[9] As early as 1910, sickle-shaped red blood cells were seen in the circulation, and by the 1920s the clinical syndrome of sickle cell anemia had been linked to these cells and was known to have increased prevalence in the black population. The chance observation of preferential sickling at the bottom of a test tube of blood led to the linkage between sickling and deoxygenation, and the absence of sickling in red blood cell ghosts indicated the role of hemoglobin. By the next decade, an appreciation of the newly recognized laboratory and clinical features had produced the view that the clinical disorder reflected vascular clogging by sickled cells. Despite the earlier understanding that sickling probably indicated an abnormal feature of hemoglobin, it was only later, in 1949, that Pauling noted the altered electrophoretic mobility of sickle hemoglobin. This led to the recognition that the cause of sickle cell disease was a specific, heritable abnormality in the chemical and physical nature of the hemoglobin molecule. Subsequently, Ingram, in 1956, identified the discrete amino acid substitution that is now recognized as the root cause of the disease. Although this discovery inaugurated an enormous growth in studies concerning the molecular basis of the disease, the knowledge gained in the ensuing 40 years has had little impact on clinical management of the disorder until recently.[10]

#### Pathophysiology

The term *sickle cell disease* is generally used to describe patients with clinical manifestations of the sickle hemoglobinopathy: most commonly, patients with homozygosity for the sickle gene (Hb-SS), but also those with hemoglobin SC and Sβ-thalassemia genotypes.

The sickle abnormality is caused by an alteration of one nucleotide that substitutes valine for glutamic acid at a single site in the hemoglobin beta chain. Heterozygosity produces the relatively benign *sickle trait,* which has been linked to improved survival in children with falciparum malaria. This beneficial effect is thought to have produced the selective pressure responsible for the high worldwide incidence of this most prevalent of genetic disorders and the repeated propagation of the same mutational event in several discrete geographic loci in Africa, Asia, and the Mediterranean.

The critical amino acid substitution reduces hemoglobin solubility, especially in the deoxy state. Homozygosity for hemoglobin S produces a disorder characterized by circulating red blood cells with abnormal shape, stiffness, and membrane characteristics, which leads to accelerated red blood cell destruction (hemolysis) and attendant anemia. These abnormalities also produce the vaso-occlusive features of the disorder, which account for most of the considerable morbidity. Early observation of delayed onset of vascular complications of the disorder after birth led to the discovery that this delay was linked to the persistence of hemoglobin F, which exerts a protective action, possibly as a result of its high oxygen affinity-induced inhibition of polymerization of sickle hemoglobin. This has provided a rationale for several current therapeutic strategies aimed at increasing hemoglobin F levels so as to reduce sickling and its complications.

## General Features

Vaso-occlusion, a central feature of sickle cell disease, was originally attributed to vascular plugging by rigid, misshapen sickle red blood cells. However, subsequent findings suggest important additional contributions from abnormalities in the red blood cell membrane, altered ion transport and red blood cell volume, and enhanced endothelial adherence of sickle red blood cells.[11, 12] Vaso-occlusion is most common in beds with low or sluggish flow and low levels of oxygenation, such as spleen, bone, and certain regions of the lungs. Events in the spleen are of particular importance because of the common piecemeal or abrupt splenic infarction that occurs early in life and leads to functional asplenia; this condition probably contributes to the marked increase in susceptibility to pneumococcal sepsis, a dominant cause of morbidity and mortality in children with sickle cell disease.

Other common vaso-occlusive features include bone infarcts, stroke, renal medullary destruction, and leg ulcers. Ischemic events in bone manifest as vaso-occlusive pain crises, a major source of morbidity and mortality. They are thought to be related to a combination of sluggish flow in marrow sinuses and possibly to increased metabolic demands arising from marrow activity stimulated by anemia. Although most vaso-occlusive events have been ascribed to microvascular occlusion, stroke has been linked to obstruction of large cerebral vessels, which suggests a possible role of endothelial injury with subsequent thrombosis in vascular occlusion.

A striking feature of sickle cell disease is the impressive variation in clinical severity of the disorder among patients who have a single, well-defined genetic abnormality. Some patients have few clinical episodes and near-normal survival, whereas others experience frequent vaso-occlusive episodes, organ dysfunction, and early death. Reasons for this interpatient variation are uncertain but may relate to socioeconomic factors, differences in levels of hemoglobin F, influence of other genetic loci such as beta-s globin haplotype, or interpatient differences in adherence of red blood cells to endothelium.[13, 14]

## Pulmonary Manifestations

Pulmonary manifestations are experienced by most patients with sickle cell disease and are leading causes of morbidity and mortality. Pulmonary syndromes fall primarily into two categories: acute chest syndrome and chronic lung disease.[14a]

**Acute Chest Syndrome.** This syndrome is broadly defined as the onset of new chest symptoms such as cough or chest pain, with a new infiltrate on chest radiograph and often with fever and leukocytosis.[15–18a] The acute chest syndrome is the leading cause of death in sickle cell disease and is second only to vaso-occlusive episodes as the most frequent cause of hospitalization. The disorder occurs in persons with hemoglobin SS, SC, or Sβ-thalassemia genotypes.

The syndrome is most common in young children and in persons with low levels of hemoglobin F, higher hemoglobin levels, or higher steady-state white blood cell or platelet counts. It is also more common in those with a history of episodes of acute chest syndrome. Vaso-occlusive episodes precede the onset of acute chest syndrome 5% to 10% of the time in children and 50% of the time in adults.[19] Specific causes of the syndrome are debated and vary among patient populations (children versus adults), but it is thought to represent mainly episodes of infection, infarction, lung injury, or atelectasis.

***Infection.*** In the 1970s, pneumonia was believed to account for almost 80% of episodes of acute chest syndrome[20]; by the mid-1980s this estimate had decreased to 36%,[21] and by 1997 infection was implicated in only 13%,[22] perhaps as a result of enhanced vigilance for, and prophylaxis against, infections. Currently, an infectious cause seems to be most frequent among children, in whom episodes often begin with fever and cough, most commonly in winter months. The syndrome is less often preceded by painful episodes in children than in adults. The syndrome also seems milder in children, with a mortality rate one quarter of that in adults. Predisposing factors are thought to include increased incidence of infections due to functional asplenia and preexisting lung disease. However, the exact role of infection in most cases remains uncertain because clinical, laboratory, and radiographic findings are collectively insufficient to provide definitive evidence for or against an infectious cause.[23]

In the past, pneumonia due to *Streptococcus pneumoniae* was considered a dominant cause of acute chest syndrome in children, but this complication has greatly decreased in Western countries, presumably because of the use of prophylactic antibiotics and immunization. Current estimates implicate pneumonia in fewer than 20% of cases of acute chest syndrome, with *S. pneumoniae* the most frequent cause and with *Mycoplasma pneumoniae* and *Chlamydia pneumoniae* also often implicated.[23, 24] However, the absence of available definitive tests for infectious causes presents a problem for timely detection and treatment of instances of the syndrome caused by virulent, antibiotic-susceptible organisms.

Although pneumonia is most common in children, it is implicated in only a minority of instances of the acute chest syndrome and is uncommonly caused by detectable bacterial pathogens. However, this situation may change as antibiotic-resistant strains become more prevalent. Among children, early treatment with parenteral broad-spectrum antibiotics is the usual practice. In adults, the relative rarity of antibiotic-susceptible pneumonia, the lack of definitive clinical indicators, and the importance of restricting the use of antibiotics greatly complicate decision-making concerning the appropriate use of antibiotics for treatment of the acute chest syndrome.

***Infarction.*** Because of the nature of the sickling abnormality with its potential for vascular stasis and thrombosis, pulmonary embolism and infarction have been suspected contributors to pulmonary events in sickle cell disease. Although some postmortem observations found pulmonary thromboemboli in a majority of cases,[25] most other series found mainly bone marrow emboli, with only a few occlusive thrombi or pulmonary infarcts.[26] There are no published series of the prevalence of scintigraphic indicators of thromboembolic events and, because the hyperosmolality of contrast agents promotes sickling, angiography is considered to be contraindicated. Therefore, there is little clear evidence in support of a role for thromboembolism in pulmonary complications of sickle cell disease and no evidence to support the use of anticoagulant prophylaxis.

***Lung Injury.*** Several features of the acute chest syndrome suggest that pulmonary vascular injury plays an important causative role, particularly in adults. In many cases the disorder resembles the acute respiratory distress syndrome by virtue of its multilobar distribution, occasional progression to diffuse pulmonary edema, and multiorgan failure.[27, 28] An inflammatory mechanism is suggested by the increased occurrence of the syndrome in patients with elevated leukocyte counts during stable intervals[17] and by the apparent beneficial effects of glucocorticoids.[29] However, unlike usual acute respiratory distress, the acute chest syndrome is often rapidly reversible, as is seen after transfusion-related lung injury (discussed later).

As mentioned, painful crises precede almost half of the episodes of acute chest syndrome in adults, often occurring 2 to 3 days before the development of pulmonary involvement. This suggests that a factor of peripheral origin may mediate the lung injury. Because painful episodes in sickle cell disease are often attributed to bone infarction, a role for bone marrow or fat embolism has been suspected. Further, many associated features of the fat embolism syndrome, including fever, anemia, respiratory distress, multisystem organ dysfunction, and encephalopathy,[30] resemble those of the acute chest syndrome.[31] Findings at autopsy commonly include histologic evidence of pulmonary marrow emboli,[26, 32] and bronchoalveolar lavage (BAL) contains fat-laden macrophages suggestive of fat embolism in 44% of children[31] and 60% of adults[33] with acute chest syndrome. In patients with the acute chest syndrome, findings suggestive of fat embolism are associated with more frequent antecedent bone pain, neurologic symptoms, chest pain, greater declines in hematocrit and platelet count, and longer hospitalizations.[31]

If bone infarction with fat embolism is related to the development of acute chest syndrome, fatty acids would seem to be likely mediators of this linkage, because they are well known to readily induce experimental lung injury and edema.[34] Circulating fatty acids may be increased in patients with both the acute chest syndrome and multisystem organ failure, compared with levels in normal subjects or in patients with clinically stable sickle cell disease.[35] Generation of fatty acids from fats is largely dependent on lipases, and findings suggest that serum concentrations of phospholipase $A_2$, which may contribute to generation of fatty acids as well as to arachidonate-derived inflammatory mediators, are markedly increased in patients with the acute chest syndrome and are correlated with the clinical severity of the episode.[36] These elevations may precede the development of clinical manifestations of the syndrome and therefore may have predictive value for risk stratification and preemptive treatment.

***Atelectasis-Edema.*** Other potential causes of infiltrates and hypoxemia in the acute chest syndrome include atelectasis and pulmonary edema. Scintigraphic evidence suggests that rib infarction may be common in the acute chest syndrome,[37] and attendant splinting of the thorax together with the ventilatory suppressant action of narcotic analgesics may promote the development of atelectasis. Pulmonary edema may also occur as a consequence of the blood volume expansion produced by vigorous intravenous hydration, a frequent feature of management of vaso-occlusive episodes. Although there may be a cardiogenic contribution to pulmonary edema in the acute chest syndrome, left-ventricular function seems generally well preserved in sickle cell disease.[38–40]

***Physical Examination and Laboratory Results.*** Findings include fever, which is more common in infants (64%) than in adults (15%). Chest examination reveals dullness to percussion, crackles, rhonchi, or wheezing in two thirds of cases and is normal in the remainder.[19] Hematologic measurements show moderate declines in hemoglobin concentration from steady state values and leukocytosis. Arterial blood gases measured while the patient is breathing room air show hypoxemia (average $Po_2$, 71 mm Hg) with mild hypocapnia (average $Pco_2$, 35 mm Hg).[19]

Chest radiography commonly reveals infiltrates, most often in a single upper or middle lobe in children but more often lower-lobar or multilobar in adults, and are frequently associated with pleural effusion.[19, 22, 41] Two chronologic patterns of chest radiography are reported: prompt resolution within 24 hours is seen in older patients (median age, 14 years) with no evidence of pneumonia, and persistent changes that last several days to weeks are found in younger patients (median age, 2 years) with a diagnosis of pneumonia.[22] There are no published series reporting results of ventilation-perfusion scans.

***Treatment.*** The changing views concerning optimum treatment of the acute chest syndrome have been reviewed elsewhere.[10, 42, 43] Although there has been little systematic study of the utility of specific measures, the usual approaches include use of antibiotics, supplemental oxygen, hydration, analgesics, and transfusion.

Antibiotics are often used in children, in whom pneumonia is more common than in adults, but there are to date no definitive findings or tests to predict their value in specific cases. In adults, the question of whether to use antibiotics is becoming increasingly difficult because of the importance of reducing their unnecessary use to limit the emergence of resistant bacterial strains. Supplemental oxygen is used to correct hypoxemia and to reduce sickling, but with little clear demonstration of utility.

Hydration may be used to maintain euvolemia, both to induce dilutional reduction of the circulating concentration of sickle red blood cells and perhaps to decrease the intraerthyrocytic concentration of hemoglobin, a determinant of sickling. As mentioned, the potential risk of hydration is that the attendant expansion of blood volume might raise pulmonary microvascular pressure and contribute to edema formation in a setting of pulmonary vascular injury. There are no systematic studies of the value of hydration, but the favorable experience with transfusion (discussed later) suggests that volume expansion may not be a major problem.

Analgesics are commonly used to relieve the pain of sickle crises and to reduce chest splinting and atelectasis. However, there is concern that their ventilatory depressant action may contribute to increased atelectasis and hypoxemia.[23]

Transfusion is generally viewed as the single most effective element in the treatment of the acute chest syndrome.[44] Transfusion commonly results in impressive improvement in hypoxemia within a few hours to days, a change not seen in nontransfused patients.[45] However, there seems to be little effect on other features of the syndrome, such as duration of fever, tachypnea, or hospital stay. Current findings suggest that simple transfusion is as effective and carries fewer complications than exchange transfusion, but the issue remains moot.[45] The mechanism of benefit is unclear but is generally ascribed to dilution of the circulating concentration of sickle red blood cells.

Other, less well documented treatments have been reported. Administration of glucocorticoids has been shown to reduce severity of sickle crises[46] and the acute chest syndrome[29] but may lead to recurrence after discontinuation of treatment. As in other acute respiratory distress syndromes, inhaled nitric oxide has been used with apparent success,[47] as has extracorporeal membrane oxygenation,[48] but experience with these modalities is extremely limited and neither should be considered routine.

***Prevention.*** In addition to influenza and pneumococcal immunizations and administration of prophylactic antibiotics, chronic preventive regimens include transfusion and administration of hydroxyurea; the latter is intended to raise levels of hemoglobin F but perhaps also to act through other mechanisms, such as reduction of the leukocyte count. These measures produce as much as a 50% reduction in recurrence of the acute chest syndrome.[49, 50] The increased risk for development of this syndrome in the perioperative period prompted a study to evaluate the utility of more aggressive preoperative transfusion, which was found to provide no advantage over that achieved with usual chronic transfusion regimens.[51]

**Chronic Lung Disease.** Because this syndrome is generally found in older patients, it is assuming growing importance as survival to adulthood in sickle cell disease increases. Clinical features of chronic lung disease were reviewed by Powars and associates,[40] who noted an average age at diagnosis of 25 years and who found that survival after diagnosis averaged 7 years. However, the authors of a multicenter study questioned the contribution of chronic lung disease to mortality in adults with sickle cell disease.[52]

***Clinical Features.*** The earliest features are abnormalities in pulmonary function, which commonly precede chronic pulmonary symptoms. These include a restrictive ventilatory pattern with decreased vital and total lung capacities. Hypoxemia, generally mild to moderate, is common and is attributable mainly to ventilation-perfusion imbalance with contributions from right-to-left shunting and impaired diffusion, from both decreased membrane and capillary volume components.[40, 53] Chest radiography shows interstitial lung disease with predominantly patchy, basal distribution and vascular attenuation; this is especially evident on high-resolution thin-section computed tomography.[41, 53]

Although many patients with chronic lung disease are asymptomatic, some develop dyspnea during exertion or even at rest. In such instances, pulmonary hypertension is often evident. Early studies using cardiac catheterization found pulmonary hypertension to be a rare but strong predictor of mortality, the median survival time after diagnosis being 30 months.[54] Subsequent studies with echocardiography, however, showed an age-related increase in incidence ranging from mild (57%) to severe pulmonary hypertension (5%) in young adults (average age, 26 years).[38] Severe pulmonary hypertension was found in 20% of older patients (average age, 38 years) with a mortality rate of 42% over the next 2 years, fivefold greater than in patients with no evidence of pulmonary hypertension.[55] Echocardiography during increased cardiac output with exercise or stimulation by dobutamine might allow detection of mild pulmonary hypertension and measurement of rates of progression. This could be used to identify patients with early pulmonary vascular changes and to evaluate potential therapeutic regimens. However, there are no reports that have considered such an approach.

Views concerning the pathophysiologic mechanisms that are responsible for chronic lung dysfunction in sickle cell disease were originally based on autopsy findings, which showed alveolar wall necrosis and fibrosis associated with intravascular sickled red blood cells.[26] These observations led to the belief that chronic lung disease reflected the cumulative effects of microvascular occlusion and consequent local ischemia. However, more recent studies noted that the disorder most commonly develops in patients with a history of frequent prior episodes of acute chest syndrome and that temporal clusters of the syndrome often precede its development.[40, 53, 56] These results suggest that the disorder may reflect the cumulative effects of repeated episodes of acute lung injury.

***Treatment-Prevention.*** There are no systematic studies of measures that might reverse existing manifestations or prevent the development of chronic lung disease in patients with sickle cell disease. On the basis of the view that sickling or episodes of acute chest syndrome (or

## Systemic Amyloidosis

Lung involvement in both the myeloma-associated and idiopathic varieties is usually of the diffuse alveolar septal type that leads to progressive diffuse parenchymal infiltrates, restrictive disease, and impairment of gas exchange.[123–127] Concomitant cardiac amyloidosis is almost invariably present and generally dominates the clinical picture or interacts with the effects of the diffuse pulmonary process.[135] In the largest series reported to date, 55 patients seen at the Mayo Clinic from 1980–1993 were retrospectively identified as having biopsy- or autopsy-proven amyloidosis involving the lung.[121] Thirty-five had "primary" systemic amyloidosis (5 in association with multiple myeloma). This designation implies immunoglobulin light chain (AL-type) amyloidosis, and 30 of the 35 had a monoclonal light chain in serum or urine, or both. Twenty of the 35 had interstitial pulmonary infiltrates of whom 4 had coexisting pleural effusions; 10 had effusions (bilateral in 8) without infiltrates; 1 had pleural thickening; 4 had unremarkable chest radiographs. The presence and severity of accompanying cardiac amyloidosis were not specified. The appearance of this process on high-resolution computed tomography of the chest has been described and the detection of small areas of calcification noted.[128] This tendency toward calcification can be detected with $^{99m}$Tc-labeled bone-seeking agents, but the finding is not specific for alveolar septal amyloidosis and its sensitivity is unknown.[129] Pulmonary hypertension with diffuse pulmonary vascular infiltration has been described.[130]

Massive infiltration of the tongue can cause obstructive sleep apnea, which has been treated with nasal continuous positive airway pressure.[131] Amyloid infiltration of the diaphragm may result in respiratory failure.[132–134] Myocardial amyloidosis can cause restrictive myocardiopathy, conduction abnormalities, and congestive heart failure with transudative pleural effusion.[135]

Rectal mucosal or abdominal subcutaneous fat biopsies are safe and relatively sensitive for systemic amyloid light chain (AL-type) amyloidosis. Although successful transbronchial biopsy has been described,[121] the procedure seems to carry an increased risk of bleeding in the presence of alveolar septal and pulmonary vascular amyloidosis and should therefore be undertaken only after careful consideration. Spontaneous hemoptysis with medial dissection of medium-size pulmonary arteries involved by amyloid has been described,[136] and fatal hemorrhage and air embolism immediately after transbronchial biopsy of a patient with diffuse parenchymal amyloidosis has occurred.[137]

In the past, with rare exceptions, the downhill course of diffuse interstitial pulmonary amyloidosis has been inexorable. Median survival in the Mayo Clinic series was 16 months.[121] Colchicine treatment of amyloidosis of the AA type associated with familial Mediterranean fever has proven to be efficacious,[121a] but this is not the case for AL amyloidosis.[121b, 121c] Reduction of the production of the amyloidogenic light chains by clonal plasma cells is a logical approach. Indeed, melphalan and glucocorticoid administration, inspired by the precedent of myeloma therapy, can be efficacious if M protein production is inhibited.[121b, 121c] More radical treatment with high-dose intravenous melphalan followed by autologous blood stem cell rescue shows substantial promise, although diffuse pulmonary infiltration was not specifically studied.[121d] A different approach involves administration of an iodinated anthracycline,[121e] which binds to amyloid and may block fresh deposition of amyloidogenic polypeptides.[121f]

## Localized Amyloidosis

Two types of localized pulmonary amyloidosis have been described: tracheobronchial and parenchymal. In the Mayo Clinic series described previously, 4 patients had tracheobronchial involvement, whereas 7 had nodular parenchymal amyloid.[121]

### Tracheobronchial

Localized tracheobronchial amyloidosis is uncommon. The lesions may be single or multiple and consist of submucosal plaques or tumor-like masses; the latter variety may impinge on the airway lumen and causes chronic wheezing, dyspnea, cough (these features leading to confusion with asthma), hemoptysis, atelectasis, and chronic infection. Multiple areas of ridging and stenosis covered by pale mucosa are found endoscopically. Over time, the involved areas may develop calcification and even ossification, thus resembling a condition known as *tracheobronchopathia osteoplastica*.[138] Endobronchial biopsy and appropriate histologic examination of the tissue establishes the diagnosis. Treatment by repeated transbronchoscopic piecemeal removal of the occluding plaques may provoke severe hemoptysis. Laser ablation appears to provide a safer and more effective alternative.[121]

### Parenchymal

Pulmonary amyloidosis localized to the lung parenchyma is usually asymptomatic (although spontaneous hemoptysis can occur) and usually manifests as one or more nodules that are easily visible on chest radiographs; diffuse parenchymal infiltration is rare. Resected nodules have shown a surrounding mononuclear infiltrate with a polyclonal surface immunoglobulin pattern in several cases.[139] Nodules may grow slowly and cavitate or become calcified. Two groups of authors have reported multiple amyloid nodules in the lungs of intravenous drug abusers infected with HIV.[140, 141] Resection is generally unnecessary, although this decision must be individualized. Single nodules are usually removed to rule out carcinoma. Diagnosis by percutaneous needle biopsy has been described,[142] but the danger of bleeding must be considered.

A pulmonary arteriovenous fistula developing spontaneously within a large amyloid nodule has been reported.[143] More diffuse lung disease, with multiple thin-walled cysts up to 5 cm in diameter, irregular noncavitating nodules, and lymphoplasmacytic infiltrates, associated with amyloidosis has been described in several patients with Sjögren's syndrome.[144–145a] Massive mediastinal calcified amyloidosis, developing in relation to nodes previously involved by an extramedullary plasmacytoma, caused fatal major airways obstruction in one case.[146] Amyloid unrelated to lymphoma or plasmacytoma occasionally causes hilar and mediastinal adenopathy that may be massive and undergo calcification,[147] resembling in this respect certain cases of sarcoidosis and silicosis.

Finally, amyloid pleural involvement with effusion has been reported,[148, 149] although it rarely appears to be the sole source of clinical problems and usually occurs in the context of more widespread intrathoracic involvement. Cardiac amyloidosis with congestive heart failure is the probable cause of most amyloid-related pleural effusions.

## BONE MARROW AND STEM CELL TRANSPLANTATION

Significant advances have been made in the technique of hematopoietic stem cell transplantation, and the indications for the procedure continue to broaden. Sources of donor stem cells that can serve as a marrow graft have expanded from autologous (same patient), syngeneic (identical twin), and allogeneic (sibling) bone marrow to include a pool of unrelated marrow donors, fetal cord blood, and growth factor–stimulated peripheral blood. The procedures are often referred to as hematopoietic stem cell transplantation (HSCT), stem cell transplantation (SCT), or blood and marrow transplantation (BMT), rather than bone marrow transplantation, in view of the widening sources of these precursors.

### General Features

BMT is used in the treatment of two categories of disease. First, it serves as replacement for dysfunctional hematopoietic or lymphoreticular precursors and congenital enzyme deficiencies. Typical of these diseases are aplastic anemia, thalassemia, and congenital immune deficiency syndromes for which BMT may be considered standard treatment. The second category is malignant diseases, in which BMT is a "salvage" therapy to restore marrow function after lethal, marrow-ablating doses of radiochemotherapy used to eradicate malignant cells.

Antigenic determinants that mediate tissue-graft rejection responses are primarily the HLAs encoded by genes of the major histocompatibility complex. Efforts are made to match the donor marrow as closely as possible to the recipient for these antigens, to avoid graft rejection and graft-vs.-host disease (GVHD).

The procedure entails conditioning of the recipient with marrow-ablative doses of chemotherapy (and, often, radiotherapy) and intravenous infusion of the donor cells. Donor cells may be processed by stem-cell enrichment techniques and may be cryopreserved before administration. Refinements in the technique of BMT include eradication of malignant cells before transplantation with biologic-response modifiers (e.g., interleukins), targeted monoclonal antibodies, or treatment of autologous marrow after harvest to destroy malignant cells and acceleration of engraftment of the transplanted marrow with growth factors (e.g., granulocyte-macrophage colony-stimulating factor) or positive selection of hematopoietic stem cells from the marrow or peripheral blood.

### Temporal Sequence

Host defense abnormalities related to BMT are predictable in extent and duration. After BMT, specific complications tend to occur within specific time periods that are defined by the pattern of reconstitution of the host defenses to infection.[150]

Intensive radiochemotherapy conditioning regimens abolish recipient marrow, but some host alveolar and tissue macrophages persist for an interim period before being replaced by donor cells during the succeeding weeks to months. Host immunoglobulins may circulate for up to 3 months after conditioning. Reconstitution of host defenses after BMT recapitulates the immune system development of a newborn. Recovery of circulating granulocytes usually occurs within the first 2 to 3 weeks after marrow infusion. Recovery of lymphocyte function follows; normal numbers are seen within 1 month after BMT, but antibody production is often delayed until 3 months after BMT. Levels of IgM and IgG are usually normal at 1 year, but IgA concentrations remain low for a longer period. Production of T-dependent antigens, response to vaccination, and cell-mediated skin reactivity to antigens may be delayed for months to years. Patients with chronic GVHD have persistent defects in cell-mediated immunity and poor antigen-specific responses. As a result, they are at continued risk for opportunistic infection as well as dissemination of encapsulated bacteria.

Specific pulmonary complications may be grouped according to their time of presentation relative to the day of transplantation (Table 86.3). "Early" events occur within the first 100 days after transplantation and "late" events beyond day 100. The classification in part reflects the fact that chronic GVHD occurs beyond day 100 after allogeneic transplantation. The early period can be further subdivided into the stage of profound neutropenia, which exists for a variable period after transplantation, and that of acute GVHD, which begins 2 to 3 weeks after allogeneic transplantation and extends approximately to day

**Table 86.3** TEMPORAL SEQUENCE OF THE USUAL PULMONARY COMPLICATIONS OF BONE MARROW TRANSPLANTATION

| Temporal Sequence | Approximate Incidence (%) |
|---|---|
| **Early Complications (<100 Days)** | |
| Pulmonary edema syndromes | 0–50 |
| Infectious pneumonia | 20–30 |
| Bacterial | 2–30 |
| Fungal | 4–13 |
| Viral | 4–10 |
| Protozoan | <5 |
| Idiopathic pneumonia | 7–12 |
| Oral mucositis | 50–70 |
| Pulmonary veno-occlusive disease | Rare |
| **Late Complications (>100 Days)** | |
| Bronchopneumonia | 20–30 |
| Idiopathic pneumonia | 10–20 |
| Viral pneumonia | 0–10 |
| Airflow obstruction (obliterative bronchiolitis) | 2–11* |

*Obstructive airflow among marrow recipients with chronic graft-vs.-host disease.

100. Although this division is clinically useful, overlap occurs in the timing of specific complications.

The occurrence of GVHD is the most important characteristic that separates patients receiving allograft from those receiving syngeneic or autologous marrow or stem cells. Syngeneic and autograft recipients share early risk factors, such as neutropenia, with patients receiving allogeneic transplants and are at risk for early pulmonary complications, such as bacterial or fungal pneumonia and noninfectious treatment-related pulmonary injury. Allogeneic marrow recipients with GVHD have continued abnormalities in immune function that increase the risk of opportunistic infections by mechanisms that are incompletely understood but that include suppressive agents to treat the condition. Among patients with chronic GVHD, infection and pneumonia due to encapsulated organisms (e.g., *S. pneumoniae*, *Haemophilus influenzae*) and *Staphylococcus aureus* appear to be related to deficiencies in specific antibody production or perhaps to continued defects in macrophage function.

## Common Clinical Presentations

The incidence of pulmonary disease is higher among specific transplant recipients, such as those receiving allogeneic compared with syngeneic or autologous transplants, those receiving total body irradiation or high-dose chemotherapy, those with malignancy (especially lymphoma) rather than aplastic anemia, and those of older age. The incidence of pulmonary complications associated with peripheral stem cell transplantation appears comparable to that of marrow transplantation when the intensity of radiochemotherapy and GVHD are considered. A shorter duration of neutropenia associated with peripheral stem cell transplantation may decrease fungal infections. Diffuse noninfectious pulmonary injury, putatively caused by intensive cytoreductive chemotherapy and irradiation, is the most common cause of pneumonia.

A significant proportion of recipients develop pulmonary dysfunction months to years after successful transplantation. Airflow obstructive defects occur in at least 10% of allogeneic marrow recipients with chronic GVHD.[151] The obstruction, often caused by obliterative bronchiolitis, may progress to profound respiratory insufficiency and death. Additionally, up to 20% of recipients develop restrictive lung disease months to years after transplantation.

Signs and symptoms of pulmonary disorders related to BMT are often nonspecific. Tachypnea is common, as are fever, cough, and crackles. However, any or all of these may be absent at the time of presentation of pulmonary complications. Routine chest radiographs are obtained frequently in the first weeks during neutropenia and often provide the first indication of pulmonary involvement. The strategy for evaluating pulmonary abnormalities is based on the timing after marrow infusion and the pattern of radiographic abnormalities.

### Pulmonary Function Tests

Pulmonary function abnormalities after BMT include declines in lung volumes, gas diffusion, and airflow, which tend to be more pronounced among patients who survive pneumonia after transplantation. The reductions are not significantly different between patients receiving autologous versus allogeneic transplants when acute GVHD is accounted for.[152] The decline in lung volume may be at least partially reversible within 2 years after transplantation, whereas the low diffusing capacity reportedly persists for several years. Development of airflow obstruction has been seen in approximately 10% of allogeneic marrow recipients in the presence of chronic GVHD and most often is related to obliterative bronchiolitis.

The results of pulmonary function tests are correlated with mortality. Badier and colleagues[153] noted that both relapses of malignancy and overall mortality correlated with falls in lung volumes and diffusion 1 year after BMT. Poor pulmonary function test results at 3 months after transplantation were shown to be associated with nonrelapse mortality.[115] At 3 months after transplantation, a restrictive lung defect or a significant decline (15%) in total lung capacity from baseline is associated with a twofold increased risk of nonrelapse mortality. In contrast, neither airflow obstruction nor impairment in diffusing capacity is associated with an increased risk. Abnormalities of total lung capacity at 3 months after transplantation are associated with death with respiratory failure, but not with an increased risk of chronic GVHD. On the basis of these results, it is reasonable to routinely evaluate lung function at 3 months and every 12 months after BMT.

### Respiratory Failure

Regardless of cause, respiratory failure is a serious complication of transplantation. In most centers, only about 3% of adult marrow recipients receiving mechanical ventilation survive to 6 months after transplantation, and the same poor prognosis is reported for pediatric marrow transplant recipients.[154–156] The prognosis may be better after autologous than after allogeneic transplantation.[156a] Age older than 40 years and respiratory failure within 90 days after transplantation have been noted as indicators of poor outcome in some studies. In addition, nonsurvivors of respiratory failure utilize the vast majority of blood products administered in the intensive care unit.

Data suggest that severe lung injury combined with hemodynamic instability or hepatic-renal insufficiency is a sensitive and highly specific predictor of death in mechanically ventilated marrow transplant recipients.[157] Using these factors, an accurate prediction of death can be made within 4 days after initiation of mechanical ventilation in 90% of nonsurvivors. These scenarios are probably more common among older patients and those in the early period after transplantation. Patients and families should be counseled regarding the expected outcomes of such situations, and life support measures should be withdrawn when there is virtually no likelihood of survival, such as with severe respiratory failure in the presence of multiorgan failure.

### Diffuse Infiltrates

Although they are common after BMT, diffuse infiltrates most often are nonspecific findings. Infectious causes for diffuse infiltrates have been documented in fewer than 20% of marrow recipients undergoing open lung biopsy within 30 days after marrow transplantation.[158] Within this early time period, pulmonary edema syndromes predominate. The edema may be associated with cardiac decompensation or intravascular volume excess, or with ARDS and pulmonary capillary leak due to treatment-related toxicities or sepsis syndrome. Infections causing diffuse infiltrates within the first weeks after transplantation include community respiratory viruses, such as respiratory syncytial virus (RSV), but cytomegalovirus (CMV) infection is uncommon. Alveolar hemorrhage may contribute to the radiographic infiltrates in the presence of thromocytopenia regardless of the cause of the lung injury.

Between 30 days and 180 days after BMT, idiopathic pneumonia is the most common cause for diffuse radiographic abnormalities.[159] CMV was common in the past but now is unusual in patients receiving appropriate prophylaxis.

### Focal Lesions

Focal parenchymal infiltrates are frequently caused by infection regardless of the time of presentation after transplantation and are related to local fungal infection in 80% of marrow transplant recipients receiving broad-spectrum antibiotics. Other causes include *Legionella* species, *Nocardia,* relapse of lymphoma in patients undergoing transplantation for that condition, bronchiolitis obliterans with organizing pneumonia (BOOP), and, in rare cases, infarction due to thromboembolic disease.

### Mucositis and Aspiration

Desquamation of the oral-pharyngeal mucosa is a frequent complication after intensive chemotherapy. Often referred to as *mucositis,* it develops within the first week after radiotherapy and reaches its greatest severity after 10 to 14 days. Impaired mucociliary clearance is also common.[160, 161]

Recurrent aspiration of oral-pharyngeal contents is frequent among transplant recipients with oral mucositis because of sedation, poor cough reflex, and dysphagia. These patients may present with basilar infiltrates or consolidation. The history is usually suggestive of recurrent aspiration. Typically, cough is induced by attempts at swallowing or there are nocturnal paroxysms of cough in the setting of severe mucositis. The appropriate approach to such patients is conservative: moderation of the administration of sedatives, encouragement of pulmonary toilet, and avoidance of mucosal bleeding through adequate platelet support. Most patients receive broad-spectrum antibiotics. In rare cases, tracheal intubation is required to avoid massive aspiration in a profoundly obtunded patient or acute airway obstruction in the presence of severe upper airway bleeding.

### Pleural Effusions

Radiographically detectable pleural effusions are common in the first weeks after marrow transplantation, are often bilateral, and are rarely related to an identifiable infectious source. They may be associated with fluid retention of any cause and especially with ascites secondary to hepatic veno-occlusive disease.[162] Characteristics include weight gain within the first weeks after transplantation and elevation of the serum bilirubin, which usually precede the development of effusions. Pleural effusions in the presence of weight gain can be approached conservatively without diagnostic thoracentesis. Cautious diuresis often produces satisfactory results. Small effusions are common and may be linked to treatment-related pleuropericarditis or thromboembolic events, but a specific cause is rarely determined. A large unilateral or rapidly accumulating effusion in the presence of fever or ipsilateral chest pain may represent hemorrhage or infection and should be evaluated promptly by thoracentesis.

## Noninfectious Causes

The many noninfectious causes of lung injury after BMT, as in other severely immunocompromised hosts, involve a spectrum of syndromes, including idiopathic pneumonia, alveolar hemorrhage, pulmonary edema, obliterative bronchiolitis, and BOOP.[162a] Idiopathic pneumonia is characterized as a syndrome of hypoxemia and radiographic nonlobar infiltrates in the absence of congestive heart failure and without evidence of an infectious origin. Most noninfectious causes of lung injury are attributed to treatment-related toxicities. Alkylating chemotherapy agents and ionizing radiation are likely contributors, but ARDS secondary to sepsis syndrome also may occur.

### Idiopathic Pneumonia Syndrome

Idiopathic lung injury after BMT has been recognized as a syndrome (idiopathic pneumonia syndrome [IPS]) in recognition of the probability of multiple causes and the varied clinical presentation.[163–165] The diagnosis of IPS is defined by a BAL that fails to reveal infection, in the presence of nonlobar radiographic infiltrates and physiologic changes consistent with pneumonia.

Causes of the diffuse idiopathic pneumonia are probably multiple and include treatment-related toxicities due to radiation or chemotherapeutic agents, or both. However, sepsis-related lung injury may account for a proportion of cases of diffuse idiopathic pneumonia with histology consistent with ARDS. Although GVHD is associated with an increased incidence of idiopathic lung injury, it is unclear whether this is a cell-mediated immune response to the lung or related to an increased incidence of sepsis in these immunosuppressed patients. Also, administration of large volumes of blood products during the transplantation procedure may lead to pulmonary vascular injury through leukoagglutination reactions or other mechanisms described earlier in this chapter. Other unusual causes for noninfectious diffuse pneumonia after marrow transplantation include leukemic infiltration due to relapse of primary malignancy, seeding of malignant cells retained in reinfused autologous marrow, and fat embolization due to marrow infusion.

The clinical presentation of IPS is nonspecific, usually with fever, nonproductive cough, and tachypnea. Hypoxemia with hyperventilation is common. The onset is most often rapid, occurring over a few days, but may occasionally be insidious and similar to that of idiopathic pulmonary fibrosis. Onset is usually within the first 3 weeks after transplantation but may occur up to months later. The chest radiograph shows diffuse intra-alveolar or interstitial infiltrates, or both. The presentation is not sufficiently distinct to be readily differentiated from that of pulmonary edema syndromes or diffuse infectious pneumonia. Marked tachypnea in the absence of radiographic infiltrates should raise the suspicion of obstructive airway disease or pulmonary veno-occlusive disease rather than idiopathic pneumonia.

The incidence within 3 months of transplantation of IPS as presently defined is 7%.[166] There is no significant difference in incidence between allogeneic and autologous marrow recipients. Seventy percent of cases progress rapidly to respiratory failure. The mortality rate of idiopathic lung injury after BMT remains greater than 70%, and two thirds of all deaths are associated with progressive respiratory failure.[167] In one quarter of cases the pneumonia resolves. Infection (especially fungal) is present at autopsy in more than one quarter of cases.

The histologic spectrum of IPS ranges from a primarily interstitial reaction with diffuse or focal widening of the alveolar septa and interstitial spaces by mononuclear inflammatory cells and edema to diffuse alveolar damage with alveolar epithelial necrosis, intra-alveolar hyaline membranes, edema, hemorrhage, and type 2 cell hyperplasia.[168, 169] The predominantly interstitial presentation has been referred to as *idiopathic interstitial pneumonia,* whereas the pathology in diffuse alveolar damage is identical to that seen in ARDS.

BOOP has been reported in three children 2 to 3 months after they had HLA-mismatched or unrelated donor marrow transplants.[170] The onset was associated with fever, cough, and patchy radiographic infiltrates. The syndrome resolved over 1 to 2 months in two of the children after treatment with corticosteroids. Confirmation of the diagnosis requires lung biopsy.

Diagnosis of idiopathic lung injury rests largely on the results of BAL. Lung biopsy (transbronchial, thoracoscopic, or open) appears to add little to the diagnostic sensitivity of BAL for infection in the presence of diffuse parenchymal infiltrates. At present, histopathology does not help to direct therapy in idiopathic lung injury after hematopoietic stem cell transplantation. Lung biopsy should be considered for patients with patchy or multifocal infiltrates because of the higher incidence of infection and concern for false-negative results from BAL.

There are no randomized studies of treatment of idiopathic lung injury after BMT. High-dose corticosteroids (1 to 16 mg/kg/day of methylprednisolone) are commonly used, and anecdotal reports suggest successful outcomes. However, not all retrospective analyses have supported a beneficial effect. Corticosteroid administration has been reported to be effective in diffuse lung injury related to BCNU-containing treatment protocols.

## Pulmonary Hemorrhage

Robbins and coworkers[171] described a specific form of idiopathic pneumonia, known as diffuse alveolar hemorrhage (DAH). The syndrome consisted of progressive dyspnea, hypoxemia, cough, and a progressively bloodier return from BAL in autologous marrow recipients, usually within 2 weeks after transplantation. It was associated with age older than 40 years, high fever, transplantation for a solid tumor, severe mucositis, white blood cell recovery, and renal insufficiency. Thrombocytopenia was common, and patients with DAH received more platelet transfusions than did patients without DAH. The Memorial Sloan-Kettering Cancer Center reported an 8% incidence of noninfectious DAH in 77 consecutive lymphoma patients treated with high-dose therapy and autologous marrow transplantation.[172] There was an association between DAH and prior booster doses of thoracic irradiation, but not between DAH and renal failure.

It is unclear whether this hemorrhagic pneumonia represents a unique syndrome or is a manifestation of severe lung injury (i.e., IPS) in the presence of a bleeding diathesis. Supporting the latter view, studies of quantification of hemosiderin-containing alveolar macrophages obtained by BAL in immunosuppressed patients, as well as an autopsy study, found no relationship between alveolar bleeding and the specific diagnosis or outcome, but hemorrhage was associated with thrombocytopenia and bleeding diatheses.[173, 174] There is little that distinguishes patients with alveolar hemorrhage associated with idiopathic pneumonia clinically from other marrow recipients with IPS.

High-dose corticosteroid administration is commonly used to treat alveolar hemorrhage after BMT. Chao and associates[175] reported on four patients with DAH who had undergone autologous marrow transplantation for leukemia and who recovered after receiving methylprednisolone in initial doses of 1 g/day. In a retrospective study, Metcalf and associates[176] found that the mortality of DAH declined from 92% to 67% with administration of methylprednisolone at a dosage of at least 30 mg/day. The effectiveness of this treatment remains unproved. Supportive care is indicated, including correction of coagulation disorders, platelet support, supplemental oxygen, and careful fluid management.

## Airflow Obstruction and Obliterative Bronchiolitis

Obliterative bronchiolitis was identified histopathologically in 2% of allogeneic marrow transplant recipients and in 6% of patients with chronic GVHD, whereas pulmonary function tests detected an obstructive airflow defect (i.e., $FEV_1$/FVC less than 70%) in 14% of patients 1 year after transplantation.[177, 178] Among recipients of allogeneic grafts who develop chronic GVHD, at least 11% have a significant decline in airflow ($FEV_1$/FVC decrease of more than 15%), compared with pretransplantation values.[179] The incidence of airflow obstruction may be higher in children after transplantation, possibly because of their smaller airway diameters.

Onset of progressive airflow obstruction beyond 100 days after BMT is strongly related to the development of chronic GVHD after allogeneic marrow grafting.[180] There is a higher incidence of decreased levels of IgG among patients with obliterative bronchiolitis than among other marrow recipients. This hypogammaglobulinemia may be a manifestation of the immunologic lesion responsible for the airway disease, or it may be related merely to the presence of chronic GVHD.

The cause of obliterative bronchiolitis after BMT is unknown. Possible causes include those recognized in otherwise normal hosts, including recurrent aspiration; viral infection with influenza, adenovirus, or measles; and bacterial or mycoplasmal infection. None of these factors has been found consistently in affected marrow recipients. However, the strong association between chronic GVHD and the development of airflow obstruction suggests an immunologic mechanism that includes bronchial epithelial injury. The lung epithelium may be the target of immune-mediated injury in chronic GVHD through the expression of Ia antigen and subsequent activation of donor cytotoxic T cells.

The usual clinical manifestation of new-onset airflow obstruction is the insidious onset of tachypnea, dyspnea on exertion, and dry, nonproductive cough. Chest auscultation may be normal or may reveal scattered expiratory wheezing and occasionally diffuse inspiratory crackles. Arterial blood gas analysis reveals moderate hypoxemia and, in the later stages, hypercapnia. Chest radiographs are commonly interpreted as normal, but high-resolution chest computed tomography often reveals parenchymal hypoattenuation and segmental bronchial dilatation. When the presentation is beyond 150 days after marrow grafting, evidence of chronic GVHD is usually present. The major differential diagnosis of the gradual onset of nonspecific respiratory symptoms in the presence of a normal chest radiograph includes pulmonary veno-occlusive disease and pulmonary embolism. Obliterative bronchiolitis is characterized by reduction in expiratory airflow on spirometry and increases in residual lung volumes not found in these other two diseases.

Prospective evaluation of pulmonary function test results after BMT identifies marrow recipients with variable courses of disease progression. Patients with onset of airflow obstruction within the first 150 days after BMT tend to have a rapid decline in pulmonary function and a fatal outcome. These patients might not survive long enough to develop manifestations of chronic GVHD, but they usually display acute GVHD after marrow grafting. It is possible that infection plays a role in the development of airflow obstruction in some of these patients. Marrow recipients with onset of airflow obstruction beyond 150 days after transplantation tend to have a more gradual decline in lung function. Airflow may stabilize in 50% of these patients. Because up to 50% of reported cases include a respiratory infection noted at the time of diagnosis of airflow obstruction, evaluation including BAL may be warranted before treatment is initiated.

There are no prospective trials of treatment for new-onset airflow obstruction. At present, the accepted approach is to aggressively control the chronic GVHD that most often accompanies the airflow obstruction with immunomodulating agents. This usually entails increased immunosuppression with corticosteroids, often with the addition of cyclosporine and azathioprine in severe or progressive cases. Reversal of the airflow obstruction is reported in only 8% of cases; the usual goal of management is stabilization of the obstruction. For this reason, prompt recognition and treatment for this progressive process is critical. Supportive measures include prophylaxis against *P. carinii* pneumonia and *S. pneumoniae* infection, inhaled bronchodilators, supplemental immunoglobulin administration to maintain normal serum levels, and prompt treatment of intercurrent infections.

### Pulmonary Veno-occlusive Disease

Pulmonary veno-occlusive disease is a rare complication that occurs after chemotherapeutic regimens and, very uncommonly, after marrow grafting.[181] The primary histologic lesion, obstruction of the pulmonary veins and venules by loose intimal fibrous proliferation, may be difficult to detect with hematoxylin and eosin stain alone, and specific stains for elastic tissues (e.g., Verhoeff–van Gieson stain) are often required to demonstrate the fibrotic reaction in the veins.

The typical presentation of pulmonary veno-occlusive disease is that of insidious dyspnea on exertion and resting tachypnea within 3 to 4 months after transplantation. Significant hypoxemia may occur along with hyperventilation. Auscultation of the lungs is often normal, although scattered inspiratory crackles may be heard. On cardiac examination, there is evidence of pulmonary hypertension. The chest radiograph is often unrevealing. Noninvasive examinations, echocardiography, perfusion-ventilation nucleotide scans, and electrocardiography are nondiagnostic. Pulmonary function testing may be consistent with mild restrictive defect, but airflow obstruction, suggesting obliterative bronchiolitis, is absent. BAL has failed to demonstrate pathogens or inflammatory cells. Right-sided heart catheterization with pulmonary angiography, the diagnostic procedure of choice, reveals increased pulmonary artery pressure with normal pulmonary artery wedge pressures and excludes the presence of thrombi as a cause for the pulmonary hypertension.

In most patients presenting after treatment for malignancy, the disease has followed an insidious course with progressive hypoxemia and dyspnea on exertion due to pulmonary hypertension. The reported high mortality rate may, in part, be related to the late recognition of the disease at autopsy. Two of three patients diagnosed after BMT recovered from their pulmonary symptoms with high-dose corticosteroid therapy (methylprednisolone, 2.0 mg/kg/day).[182]

## Infectious Causes

Patients undergoing BMT are extremely vulnerable to infections, both during the conditioning treatment, when immunosuppression is deliberately induced, and after receiving the transplant, when immunosuppression is maintained. Moreover, because these patients are hospitalized, they are exposed to a variety of nosocomial pathogens, and they have indwelling vascular cannulas and bladder catheters, which disrupt normal protective barriers.

### Viruses

**Cytomegalovirus.** The incidence of CMV pneumonia has declined significantly since the late 1980s. The incidence now appears to be approximately 4% for both allogeneic and autologous transplantation. The decline is attributable to effective prophylaxis and preemptive treatment. It is presumed that most, if not all, CMV infections occurring in seropositive patients are a result of reactivation of latent infection.

The clinical presentation of CMV pneumonia is not distinct from that of other causes of diffuse pneumonia. The patient may have nonproductive cough, dyspnea, hypoxemia, or fever with a median onset of 60 days after BMT. Onset within the first 2 weeks is unusual. The period of risk for CMV pneumonia generally ends by the fourth or fifth month after transplantation, although later cases occur among patients with chronic GVHD or after autologous transplantation. Chest roentgenograms usually show bilateral infiltrates and, in the later stages, diffuse consolidation. Unilateral, focal, and even nodular infiltrates have been described in the early stages.

The hallmark of CMV pneumonia is the Cowdry type A intracytoplasmic inclusion bodies within the areas of inflammation. The presence of these eosinophilic bodies appears to be related to the duration of infection and may be absent early in the process. Immunohistologic probes may detect CMV-specific DNA and antigen in cases of histologically occult CMV pneumonia. The pneumonia may be primarily a mononuclear interstitial disease, or it may be associated with diffuse alveolar epithelial desquamation with hyaline membrane formation. Both diffuse parenchymal and multifocal patterns have been described.

Currently, survival rates of 30% to 70% can be expected with treatment that incorporates the combination of ganciclovir and intravenous immunoglobulins.[183–185] Ganciclovir is started at a dose of 5.0 mg/kg every 12 hours, with appropriate adjustments for renal function, and is administered for 14 days; this treatment is referred to as *induction.* If the patient has improved by the end of that time, the dosage is reduced to 5.0 mg/kg, given once daily for 30 days or longer; this is the "maintenance" phase. Induction is continued beyond 14 days if the patient has not responded, defined as improved oxygenation and decreased respiratory rate. Maintenance may be given for longer than 30 days, depending on individual patient characteristics. Although the improved survival rates are encouraging, it remains possible that this change is in part attributable to treatment earlier in the disease course. Survival of patients with respiratory failure at the time of initial treatment remains uncommon.

Efforts to prevent CMV pneumonia have been directed primarily at preventing CMV infection and preemptively treating patients who are at highest risk for pneumonia. CMV pneumonia can be eliminated by the use of screened seronegative blood products for allograft recipients who are seronegative before transplantation and who have seronegative marrow donors.[186] This preventive approach is less successful for seronegative patients with seropositive marrow donors, because the marrow itself serves as a source of infection. High-dose acyclovir delays reactivation of latent virus and reduces the probability of CMV pneumonia by approximately 50% in seropositive allogeneic transplant recipients, but not in those receiving autologous transplants.

CMV pneumonia can be prevented with the prophylactic administration of ganciclovir to all seropositive recipients; however, this treatment failed to improve overall survival because of increased sepsis related to the ganciclovir-induced neutropenia. An additional theoretical concern with this approach is a delay in the reestablishment of CMV-specific cytotoxic T lymphocytes and, consequently, an increased risk of CMV pneumonia at a later time. The majority of seropositive patients who are at highest risk for development of CMV pneumonia can be prospectively identified by routine cultures of body fluids. Patients with positive blood, throat, urine, or BAL cultures have a significantly increased probability of developing CMV pneumonia. Treatment of patients at the time of viral excretion significantly decreases the incidence of CMV pneumonia and improves survival, but 30% of marrow recipients develop CMV pneumonia without recognized excretion and are missed by this approach.[187–189] Detection of CMV antigens in blood leukocytes (using peroxidase-labeled monoclonal antibodies) and detection of CMV DNA in plasma or blood leukocytes (using polymerase chain reaction) are sensitive and specific techniques to identify patients at highest risk for CMV pneumonia. The negative predictive value of such testing approaches 100%. Preemptive treatment with ganciclovir on the basis of surveillance polymerase chain reaction or antigenemia studies decreases the incidence of CMV pneumonia.

**Other Viruses.** Adenovirus infection occurs in 5% of patients within the first 3 months after transplantation and is attributable in almost all cases to reactivation of latent virus. Approximately 20% of marrow transplant recipients with adenovirus infection develop pneumonia.[190] Most patients with adenovirus pneumonia have a progressive course leading to death over days to weeks, usually with multisystem disease. In others the diagnosis is recognized only at postmortem examination. There is no proven treatment for adenovirus infection, although interferon remains a theoretical possibility and intravenous ribavirin has been tried.

Pneumonia due to herpes simplex virus (HSV) or varicella-zoster virus (VZV) is uncommon. HSV pneumonia is usually caused by contiguous spread of virus to the trachea or by aspiration from the oropharynx, although it may in rare cases be a manifestation of generalized infection with viremia.[191] VZV pneumonia occurs among patients with disseminated infection and viremia. Both situations have become exceedingly uncommon since the advent of acyclovir treatment and, in the case of HSV, acyclovir prophylaxis.

Human herpesvirus 6 (HHV-6), the cause of childhood roseola (exanthem subitum), has been detected in the lungs of some patients with idiopathic pneumonia.[192] It is unclear whether this virus is a cause of pneumonia or merely latently reactivated, because virtually all adults are seropositive for the virus.

Pneumonia due to ordinary community respiratory viruses, including parainfluenza types 1 and 3, influenza A and B, and RSV, occur sporadically in these patients, as in other immunocompromised patients and in normal persons. With the exception of parainfluenza type 1, these infections are more common during the winter months, and nosocomial transmission from infected healthcare workers has been documented. Several epidemics of respiratory viral infections have been reported among transplant recipients concurrent with infection in the community.[193, 194] Most patients developed upper respiratory infections with fever, coryza, and cough. Approximately one half of these progressed to lower respiratory tract disease with radiographic infiltrates and hypoxemia. The mortality rate approached 80% despite treatment with aerosolized ribavirin. Although parainfluenza infections are seemingly less common, both upper and lower respiratory tract involvement may occur, and mortality is high in the latter form, particularly if respiratory failure occurs.[195]

Mortality rates for patients with RSV pneumonia are 50% to 80%, but survival may be better among patients in whom onset occurs later after transplantation. Patients with parainfluenza have a lower mortality rate unless respiratory failure occurs.[195] Finally, the course of disease in patients with VZV or, presumably, HSV pneumonia should be similar to that seen in other circumstances, and these patients should respond to acyclovir treatment over several days to 1 week with ultimate survival expected.

With the exception of acyclovir treatment for HSV or VZV infection, proven effective therapy for viral pneumonias is not available. Intravenous acyclovir should be given at the dose of 500 mg/m$^2$ every 8 hours with appropriate adjustment for renal function. Treatment should be continued for a minimum of 7 days. Longer courses may be necessary if new lesions continue to form in patients with VZV infection and depending on the clinical response of the patient. Both ribavirin and leukocyte interferon have been used to treat adenovirus infection, with unclear results.

Aerosolized ribavirin has been given to treat parainfluenza and RSV pneumonia. Patients with RSV pneumonia who survived tended to develop disease after marrow engraftment and were treated before the onset of respiratory failure. Combined therapy with aerosolized ribavirin and intravenous immunoglobulin (IVIG, 500 mg every other day) led to survival in eight of nine patients who were treated before the onset of respiratory failure.[196] Prompt screening of nasal-throat specimens by rapid culture and viral detection method (e.g., fluorescence antibody stain, enzyme-linked immunosorbent assay) in patients with upper respiratory tract symptoms is critical to identify infected patients. Those with signs or symptoms of lower respiratory tract disease should be aggressively evaluated with BAL and treated before the development of significant hypoxemia. Handwashing and segregation of infected patients and staff are important measures to stem the spread of infection.

## Fungi

Fungal infections have emerged as a major clinical problem after BMT and may be present in as many as 30% of all fatal cases. *Aspergillus* infection is documented in 4% to 13% of marrow recipients, but *Mucormycosis, Fusarium, Rhizopus,* and *Scedosporium* are also seen.[197] Disseminated yeast infection, especially with *Candida albicans* or *Candida tropicalis,* is reported in more than 20% of patients receiving therapy for hematologic malignancies, and approximately 50% of patients with invasive *Candida* infection have pulmonary involvement.[198] In contrast to the limited pulmonary involvement in yeast infections, most patients infected with filamentous fungi have lung involvement. Many of these diagnoses are made at autopsy, because the premortem diagnosis may be difficult to establish.

Major risk factors for invasive fungal infections are the level and duration of neutropenia, the patient's age, the presence of GVHD, the total number of other infections, and the use of corticosteroids after marrow grafting. The frequency of *Aspergillus* infection is similar between recipients of allogeneic and autologous transplants, but it occurs after engraftment in the former group and during periods of neutropenia before engraftment in the latter.[199] Autologous recipients have fewer *Candida*, but not *Aspergillus,* infections compared with allograft recipients.

The mortality rate for pulmonary infection with filamentous fungi among marrow transplant recipients is estimated at 94%. Early diagnosis and treatment may improve survival rates. Favorable outcome with pulmonary filamentous fungal infection has occurred after treatment with amphotericin at 1 mg/kg/day to a total dose of 2 g or more. The optimal therapy and dosing for invasive aspergillosis has not been established but probably includes amphotericin. Some centers administer the drug at doses up to 1.5 mg/kg/day and add 5-fluorouracil to the course of therapy. Recovery from myelosuppression appears to be critical to recovery from these infections. Although most successful treatment of these pulmonary fungal infections after BMT has also included surgical resection, the precise role of surgery is not clear. Recovery by marrow recipients without complete surgical resection has been noted. Adjunctive therapy with granulocyte transfusions or granulocyte colony-stimulating factor, or both, CSF remains investigational.

Treatment for invasive *Candida* infection also is largely empirical. Amphotericin in doses of at least 0.5 mg/kg/day until clinical response occurs is commonly employed.

## Bacteria

Pathologic specimens rarely confirm bacterial bronchopneumonia after BMT. However, this may represent a selection bias of patients undergoing biopsy, because bacterial pneumonia has been reported in as many as 28% of autopsies of marrow recipients in some centers.[199a] The distribution of bacteria responsible for pulmonary infections during the neutropenic period is unknown. Aerobic gram-negative organisms are frequently detected in episodes of bacterial pulmonary infection. Half of the bacteremic cases after BMT are caused by gram-positive organisms, especially coagulase-negative *Staphylococcus*, and the remainder are caused primarily by aerobic gram-negative enterobacteria.

The manifestations of bacterial pneumonia in patients who have undergone BMT are similar to those in other neutropenic hosts. Fevers occur frequently after transplantation, as do pulmonary infiltrates. Bacterial pneumonia after BMT may appear as patchy or confluent bilateral alveolar consolidation that progresses rapidly. During the early posttransplantation period, the difficulty lies more in the similarities in presentation of bacterial and nonbacterial pulmonary diseases (e.g., oral aspiration). Sputum production is rare among the profoundly neutropenic patients, and diagnosis relies on the clinical response to empirical therapy, blood cultures, or invasive diagnostic procedures such as bronchoscopy or lung biopsy.

Although infection by *Legionella* species among marrow recipients has been an uncommon finding, its clinical manifestations are similar to those seen in other patient groups. Focal infiltrates and spiking fevers unresponsive to broad-spectrum antibiotics are often reported. *Legionella micdadei* pulmonary infection has been reported, manifesting as focal radiographic lesions, occasionally with few systemic symptoms.[200] This clinical appearance should also prompt consideration of invasive pulmonary fungal disease or pulmonary infarct due to embolus.

## Other Infections

**Pneumocystis.** *P. carinii* pneumonia occurred in as many as 10% of marrow transplant recipients before the introduction of trimethoprim-sulfamethoxazole prophylaxis, although the rate varied by region and institution.[201] Routine prophylaxis has markedly reduced the occurrence of this pneumonia. Currently the predominant, if not the exclusive, occurrence of *P. carinii* is among patients who fail to receive prophylaxis after transplantation because of poor engraftment or documented allergy to trimethoprim-sulfamethoxazole.

The median onset of *P. carinii* pneumonia is 60 days after transplantation. The clinical signs and symptoms are not distinct from those of other causes of diffuse pneumonia in immunocompromised patients. Treatment of *P. carinii* pneumonia after marrow transplantation is similar to treatment in other patients. Best results have been achieved with intravenous trimethoprim-sulfamethoxazole at 15 to 20 mg/kg/day of the trimethoprim component, given as divided doses every 6 to 8 hours for a period of 14 to 21 days. Oral administration may be used later in the treatment course, but the initial therapy should be given intravenously. Intravenous pentamidine at recommended doses is the major alternative agent for patients with documented, severe allergy to trimethoprim-sulfamethoxazole.

**Toxoplasmosis.** Most BMT patients with *Toxoplasma gondii* infection have had only central nervous system disease diagnosed and treated during life. However, other patients have had more generalized disease diagnosed at autopsy involving the myocardium, lungs, and brain. Chest radiographs in these patients showed diffuse, patchy involvement. These patients also had concomitant bacterial or viral infection, and the contribution of *Toxoplasma* to either the signs or symptoms of pulmonary disease is uncertain. Most infections have been fatal. Diagnosis and treatment are similar to those in HIV-infected patients (see Chapter 82).

**Mycobacterial Infections.** Both typical and atypical mycobacterial infections have been reported in a small number of patients. Although infection with *Mycobacterium avium* complex has been reported in transplantation patients in Texas, this organism has otherwise been uncommon. Clinical signs and symptoms have been similar to those in other immunocompromised patients (see Chapter 34).

## SUMMARY

This chapter describes the various pulmonary complications associated with major hematologic diseases. An attempt is made to provide sufficient background information about the underlying disease to set the stage for an understanding of the features of greatest interest and importance to the pulmonologist. Red blood cell disorders (erythrocytosis and anemia) are discussed with emphasis on the complex pulmonary manifestations of sickle cell disease. The discussion of white blood cell disorders focuses on the pulmonary effects of the interaction of granulocytes with the lungs and on malignant diseases of lymphocytes, including leukemia, lymphoma, and myeloma. Coagulopathies are discussed with special reference to invasive procedures. Then, the contrasting manifestations of systemic and localized pulmonary amyloidosis are discussed. Finally, the complexities and uncertainties of the rapidly evolving world of bone marrow transplantation are presented from the standpoint of the protean pulmonary complications of this fascinating biologic process that has now become a mainstay of clinical practice.

## References


1. Jelkmann W: Erythropoietin: Structure, control of production, and function. Physiol Rev 72:449–489, 1992.
2. Balcerzak SP, Bromberg PA: Secondary polycythemia. Semin Hematol 12:353–382, 1975.
3. DiMarco AT: Carbon monoxide poisoning presenting as polycythemia (letter). N Engl J Med 319:874, 1988.
4. Thomas DJ, Marshall J, Russell RW, et al: Effect of haematocrit on cerebral blood-flow in man. Lancet 2:941–943, 1977.
5. Rosenthal A, Nathan DG, Marty AT, et al: Acute hemodynamic effects of red cell volume reduction in polycythemia of cyanotic congenital heart disease. Circulation 42:297–308, 1970.
6. Defouilloy C, Teiger E, Sediame S, et al: Polycythemia impairs vasodilator response to acetylcholine in patients with chronic hypoxemic lung disease. Am J Respir Crit Care Med 157:1452–1460, 1998.
7. Douglas NJ: Sleep in patients with chronic obstructive pulmonary disease. Clin Chest Med 19:115–125, 1998.
8. Oren R, Beeri M, Hubert A, et al: Effect of theophylline on erythrocytosis in chronic obstructive pulmonary disease. Arch Intern Med 157:1474–1478, 1997.
9. Feldman SD, Tauber AI: Sickle cell anemia: Reexamining the first "molecular disease." Bull Hist Med 71:623–650, 1997.
10. Steinberg MH: Management of sickle cell disease. N Engl J Med 340:1021–1030, 1999.
11. Hebbel RP: Beyond hemoglobin polymerization: The red blood cell membrane and sickle disease pathophysiology (review). Blood 77:214–237, 1991.
12. Hebbel RP: Perspectives series: Cell adhesion in vascular biology. Adhesive interactions of sickle erythrocytes with endothelium. J Clin Invest 99:2561–2564, 1997.
13. Powars D, Chan LS, Schroeder WA: The variable expression of sickle cell disease is genetically determined. Semin Hematol 27:360–376, 1990.
14. Nagel RL: Sickle cell anemia is a multigene disease: Sickle painful crises, a case in point. Am J Hematol 42:96–101, 1993.
14a. Knight J, Murphy TM, Browning I: The lung in sickle cell disease. Pediatr Pulmonol 28:205–216, 1999.
15. Charache S, Scott JC, Charache P: "Acute chest syndrome" in adults with sickle cell anemia: Microbiology, treatment, and prevention. Arch Intern Med 139:67–69, 1979.
16. Golden C, Styles L, Vichinsky E: Acute chest syndrome and sickle cell disease. Curr Opin Hematol 5:89–92, 1998.
17. Castro O, Brambilla DJ, Thorington B, et al: The acute chest syndrome in sickle cell disease: Incidence and risk factors. The Cooperative Study of Sickle Cell Disease. Blood 84:643–649, 1994.
18. Vichinsky E, Styles L: Pulmonary complications. Hematol Oncol Clin North Am 10:1275–1287, 1996.
18a. Quinn CT, Buchanan GR: The acute chest syndrome of sickle cell disease. J Pediatr 134:416–422, 1999.
19. Vichinsky EP, Styles LA, Colangelo LH, et al: Acute chest syndrome in sickle cell disease: Clinical presentation and course. Cooperative Study of Sickle Cell Disease. Blood. 89:1787–1792, 1997.
20. Barrett-Connor E: Acute pulmonary disease and sickle cell anemia. Am Rev Respir Dis 104:159–165, 1971.
21. Poncz M, Kane E, Gill FM: Acute chest syndrome in sickle cell disease: Etiology and clinical correlates. J Pediatr 107:861–866, 1985.
22. Martin L, Buonomo C: Acute chest syndrome of sickle cell disease: Radiographic and clinical analysis of 70 cases. Pediatr Radiol 27:637–641, 1997.
23. Dreyer ZE: Chest infections and syndromes in sickle cell disease of childhood. Semin Respir Infect 11:163–172, 1996.

24. Kirkpatrick MB, Haynes J Jr, Bass JB Jr: Results of bronchoscopically obtained lower airway cultures from adult sickle cell disease patients with the acute chest syndrome. Am J Med 90:206–210, 1991.
25. Oppenheimer EH, Esterly JR: Pulmonary changes in sickle cell disease. Am Rev Respir Dis 103:858–859, 1971.
26. Haupt HM, Moore GW, Bauer TW, et al: The lung in sickle cell disease. Chest 81:332–337, 1982.
27. Hassell KL, Eckman JR, Lane PA: Acute multiorgan failure syndrome: A potentially catastrophic complication of severe sickle cell pain episodes. Am J Med 96:155–162, 1994.
28. Haynes J Jr, Allison RC. Pulmonary edema: Complication in the management of sickle cell pain crisis. Am J Med 80:833–840, 1986.
29. Bernini JC, Rogers ZR, Sandler ES, et al: Beneficial effect of intravenous dexamethasone in children with mild to moderately severe acute chest syndrome complicating sickle cell disease. Blood 92:3082–3089, 1998.
30. Levy D: The fat embolism syndrome: A review. Clin Orthop (261):281–286, 1990.
31. Vichinsky E, Williams R, Das M, et al: Pulmonary fat embolism: A distinct cause of severe acute chest syndrome in sickle cell anemia. Blood 83:3107–3112, 1994.
32. Shelley WM, Curtis EM: Bone marrow and fat embolism in sickle cell anemia and sickle cell-homoglobin C disease. Bull Johns Hopkins Hosp 103:8–26, 1958.
33. Godeau B, Schaeffer A, Bachir D, et al: Bronchoalveolar lavage in adult sickle cell patients with acute chest syndrome: Value for diagnostic assessment of fat embolism. Am J Respir Crit Care Med 153:1691–1696, 1996.
34. Schuster DP: ARDS: Clinical lessons from the oleic acid model of acute lung injury. Am J Respir Crit Care Med. 149:245–260, 1994.
35. Kuypers FA, Styles LA, Schalkwijk CG, et al: Decreased serum levels of phospholipase $A_2$ and free fatty acid in sickle cell disease associated with acute chest syndrome (ACS). New Trends in Therapy for Hemoglobinopathies, 1994.
36. Styles LA, Schalkwijk CG, Aarsman AJ, et al: Phospholipase A2 levels in acute chest syndrome of sickle cell disease. Blood 87:2573–2578, 1996.
37. Rucknagel DL, Kalinyak KA, Gelfand MJ: Rib infarcts and acute chest syndrome in sickle cell diseases. Lancet 337:831–833, 1991.
38. Simmons BE, Santhanam V, Castaner A, et al: Sickle cell heart disease: Two-dimensional echo and Doppler ultrasonographic findings in the hearts of adult patients with sickle cell anemia. Arch Intern Med 148:1526–1528, 1988.
39. Santoli F, Zerah F, Vasile N, et al: Pulmonary function in sickle cell disease with or without acute chest syndrome. Eur Respir J 12:1124–1129, 1998.
40. Powars D, Weidman JA, Odom-Maryon T, et al: Sickle cell chronic lung disease: Prior morbidity and the risk of pulmonary failure. Medicine (Baltimore) 67:66–76, 1988.
41. Leong CS, Stark P: Thoracic manifestations of sickle cell disease. J Thorac Imaging 13:128–134, 1998.
42. Charache S: Treatment of sickling disorders. Curr Opin Hematol 3:139–144, 1996.
43. Bunn HF: Pathogenesis and treatment of sickle cell disease. N Engl J Med 337:762–769, 1997.
44. Davies SC, Roberts-Harewood M: 1997. Blood transfusion in sickle cell disease. Blood Rev 11:57–71, 1997.
45. Emre U, Miller ST, Gutierez M, et al: Effect of transfusion in acute chest syndrome of sickle cell disease. J Pediatr 127:901–904, 1995.
46. Griffin TC, McIntire D, Buchanan GR: High-dose intravenous methylprednisolone therapy for pain in children and adolescents with sickle cell disease. N Engl J Med 330:733–737, 1994.
47. Atz AM, Wessel DL: Inhaled nitric oxide in sickle cell disease with acute chest syndrome. Anesthesiology 87:988–990, 1997.
48. Pelidis MA, Kato GJ, Resar LM, et al: Successful treatment of life-threatening acute chest syndrome of sickle cell disease with venovenous extracorporeal membrane oxygenation. J Pediatr Hematol Oncol 19:459–461, 1997.
49. Styles LA, Vichinsky E: Effects of a long-term transfusion regimen on sickle cell-related illnesses. J Pediatr 125:909–911, 1994.
50. Charache S, Terrin ML, Moore RD, et al: Effect of hydroxyurea on the frequency of painful crises in sickle cell anemia. Investigators of the Multicenter Study of Hydroxyurea in Sickle Cell Anemia. N Engl J Med 332:1317–1322, 1995.
51. Vichinsky EP, Haberkern CM, Neumayr L, et al: A comparison of conservative and aggressive transfusion regimens in the perioperative management of sickle cell disease. The Preoperative Transfusion in Sickle Cell Disease Study Group. N Engl J Med 333:206–213, 1995.
52. Platt OS, Brambilla DJ, Rosse WF, et al: Mortality in sickle cell disease: Life expectancy and risk factors for early death. N Engl J Med 330:1639–1644, 1994.
53. Aquino SL, Gamsu G, Fahy JV, et al: Chronic pulmonary disorders in sickle cell disease: Findings at thin-section CT. Radiology 193:807–811, 1994.
54. Collins FS, Orringer EP: Pulmonary hypertension and cor pulmonale in the sickle hemoglobinopathies. Am J Med 73:814–821, 1982.
55. Sutton LL, Castro O, Cross DJ, et al: Pulmonary hypertension in sickle cell disease. Am J Cardiol 74:626–628, 1994.
56. Bowen EF, Crowston JG, De Ceulaer K, et al: Peak expiratory flow rate and the acute chest syndrome in homozygous sickle cell disease. Arch Dis Child 66:330–332, 1991.
57. Maddern BR, Reed HT, Ohene-Frempong K, et al: Obstructive sleep apnea syndrome in sickle cell disease. Ann Otol Rhinol Laryngol 98:174–178, 1989.
58. Samuels MP, Stebbens VA, Davies SC, et al: Sleep related upper airway obstruction and hypoxaemia in sickle cell disease. Arch Dis Child 67:925–929, 1992.
59. Brooks LJ, Koziol SM, Chiarucci KM, et al: Does sleep-disordered breathing contribute to the clinical severity of sickle cell anemia? J Pediatr Hematol Oncol 18:135–139, 1996.
60. Leong MA, Dampier C, Varlotta L, et al: Airway hyperreactivity in children with sickle cell disease. J Pediatr 131:278–283, 1997.
61. Sears DA: The morbidity of sickle cell trail: A review of the literature. Am J Med 64:1021–1036, 1978.
62. Heller P, Best RR, Nelson RB, et al: Clinical implications of sickle-cell trait and glucose-6-phosphate dehydrogenase deficiency in hospitalized black male patients. N Engl J Med 300:1001–1005, 1979.
63. Murray MJ, Evans P: Sudden exertional death in a soldier with sickle cell trait. Milit Med 161:303–305, 1996.
64. Benz EJ: Hemoglobin variants associated with hemolytic anemia, altered oxygen affinity, and methemoglobinemia. *In* Hoffman R, Benz EJ Jr, Shatil SJ, et al (eds). Hematology: Basic Principles and Practice (2nd ed). New York: Churchill Livingstone, 1995, pp 652–655.
65. Haab PE, Durand-Arczynska WY: Carbon monoxide effects on oxygen transport. *In* Crystal RG, West JB (eds). The Lung: Scientific Foundations. New York: Raven Press, 1991, pp 1267–1275.
66. Griffin JP: Methaemoglobinaemia. Adverse Drug React Toxicol Rev 16:45–63, 1997.
67. Repine JE: Scientific perspective on adult respiratory distress syndrome. Lancet 339:466–469, 1992.
68. Hughes WT, Armstrong D., Bodey GP, et al: 1997 Guidelines for the use of antimicrobial agents in neutropenic patients with unexplained fever. Infectious Diseases Society of America. Clin Infect Dis 25:551–573, 1997.
69. McKee LC Jr, Collins RD: Intravascular leukocyte thrombi and aggregates as a cause of morbidity and mortality in leukemia. Medicine (Baltimore) 53:463–478, 1974.
70. Wardman AG, Milligan DW, Child JA, et al: Pulmonary infiltrates and adult acute leukaemia: Empirical treatment and survival related to the extent of pulmonary radiological disease. Thorax 39:568–571, 1984.
71. Kelly KM, Lange B: Oncologic emergencies. Pediatr Clin North Am 44:809–830, 1997.
72. Goodnough LT, Brecher ME, Kanter MH, et al: Transfusion medicine: Blood transfusion. N Engl J Med 340:438–447, 1999.
73. Silliman CC, Voelkel NF, Allard JD, et al: Plasma and lipids from stored packed red blood cells cause acute lung injury in an animal model. J Clin Invest 101:1458–1467, 1998.
74. Leach M, Vora AJ, Jones DA, et al: Transfusion-related acute lung injury (TRALI) following autologous stem cell transplant for relapsed acute myeloid leukaemia: A case report and review of the literature. Transfus Med 8:333–337, 1998.
75. Popovsky MA, Moore SB: Diagnostic and pathogenetic considerations in transfusion-related acute lung injury. Transfusion 25:573–577, 1985.

marrow transplantation before and after the introduction of prophylactic ganciclovir therapy in 1989. Bone Marrow Transplant 21:691–695, 1998.
160. Schubert MM, Williams BE, Lloid ME, et al: Clinical assessment scale for the rating of oral mucosal changes associated with bone marrow transplantation: Development of an oral mucositis index. Cancer 69:2469–2477, 1992.
161. Sisson JH, Reed EC, Robbins RA, et al: Impairment of nasal mucociliary clearance during bone marrow transplantation. University of Nebraska Medical Center Bone Marrow Transplantation Pulmonary Study Group. Bone Marrow Transplant 13:631–633, 1994.
162. McDonald GB, Shulman HM, Wolford JL, et al: Liver disease after human marrow transplantation. Semin Liver Dis 7:210–229, 1987.
162a. Crawford SW: Noninfectious lung disease in the immunocompromised host. Respiration 66:385–395, 1999.
163. Wingard JR, Sostrin MB, Vriesendorp HM, et al: Interstitial pneumonitis following autologous bone marrow transplantation. Transplantation 46:61–65, 1988.
164. Wingard JR, Mellits ED, Sostrin MB, et al: Interstitial pneumonitis after allogeneic bone marrow transplantation: Nine-year experience at a single institution. Medicine (Baltimore) 67:175–186, 1988.
165. Clark JG, Hansen JA, Hertz MI, et al: Idiopathic pneumonia syndrome following bone marrow transplantation. NHLBI Workshop. Am Rev Respir Dis 147:1601–1606, 1992.
166. Kantrow SP, Hackman RC, Boeckh M, et al: Idiopathic pneumonia syndrome: Changing spectrum of lung injury after marrow transplantation. Transplantation. 63:1079–1086, 1997.
167. Crawford SW, Hackman RC: Clinical course of idiopathic pneumonia after bone marrow transplantation. Am Rev Respir Dis 147:1393–1400, 1993.
168. Hackman RC: Lower respiratory tract. *In* Sale GE, Shulman HM (eds): The Pathology of Bone Marrow Transplantation. New York: Masson, 1984, pp 156–170.
169. Sloane JP, Depledge MH, Powles RL, et al: Histopathology of the lung after bone marrow transplantation. J Clin Pathol 36:546–554, 1983.
170. Mathew P, Bozeman P, Krance RA, et al: Bronchiolitis obliterans organizing pneumonia (BOOP) in children after allogeneic bone marrow transplantation. Bone Marrow Transplant 13:221–223, 1994.
171. Robbins RA, Linder JL, Stahl MR, et al: Diffuse alveolar hemorrhage in autologous bone marrow transplant recipients. Am J Med 87:511–518, 1989.
172. Jules-Elysee K, Stover DE, Yahalom J, et al: Pulmonary complications in lymphoma patients treated with high-dose therapy autologous bone marrow transplantation. Am Rev Respir Dis 146:485–491, 1992.
173. Agusti C, Ramirez J, Picado C, et al: Diffuse alveolar hemorrhage in allogeneic bone marrow transplantation: A postmortem study. Am J Respir Crit Care Med 151:1006–1010, 1995.
174. De Lassence A, Fleury-Feith J, Escudier E, et al: Alveolar hemorrhage: Diagnostic criteria and results in 194 immunocompromised hosts. Am J Respir Crit Care Med 151:157–163, 1995.
175. Chao NJ, Duncan SR, Long GD, et al: Corticosteroid therapy for diffuse alveolar hemorrhage in autologous bone marrow transplant recipients. Ann Intern Med 114:145–146, 1991.
176. Metcalf JP, Rennard SI, Reed EC, et al: Corticosteroids as adjunctive therapy for diffuse alveolar hemorrhage associated with bone marrow transplantation. University of Nebraska Medical Center Bone Marrow Transplant Group. Am J Med 96:327–334, 1994.
177. Holland HK, Wingard JR, Beschorner WE, et al: Bronchiolitis obliterans in bone marrow transplantation and its relationship to chronic graft-v-host disease and low serum IgG. Blood 72:621–627, 1988.
178. Springmeyer SC, Flournoy N, Sullivan KM, et al: Pulmonary function changes in long-term survivors of allogeneic marrow transplantation. Recent Advances in Bone Marrow Transplantation. New York: Alan R Liss, 1983, pp 343–353.
179. Clark JG, Schwartz DA, Flournoy N, et al: Risk factors for airflow obstruction in recipients of bone marrow transplants. Ann Intern Med 107:648–656, 1987.
180. Chan CK, Hyland RH, Hutcheon MA, et al: Small-airways disease in recipients of allogeneic bone marrow transplants: An analysis of 11 cases and a review of the literature. Medicine (Baltimore) 66:327–340, 1987.
181. Troussard X, Bernaudin JR, Cordonnier C, et al: Pulmonary veno-occlusive disease after bone marrow transplantation. Thorax 39:956–957, 1984.
182. Hackman RC, Madtes DK, Petersen FB, et al: Pulmonary venoocclusive disease following bone marrow transplantation. Transplantation 47:989–992, 1989.
183. Emanuel D, Cunningham I, Jules-Elysee K, et al: Cytomegalovirus pneumonia after bone marrow transplantation successfully treated with the combination of ganciclovir and high-dose intravenous immune globulin. Ann Intern Med 109:777–782, 1988.
184. Reed EC, Bowden RA, Dandliker PS, et al: Treatment of cytomegalovirus pneumonia with ganciclovir and intravenous cytomegalovirus immunoglobulin in patients with bone marrow transplants. Ann Intern Med 109:783–788, 1988.
185. Schmidt GM, Kovacs A, Zaia JA, et al: Ganciclovir/immunoglobulin combination therapy for the treatment of human cytomegalovirus-associated interstitial pneumonia in bone marrow allograft recipients. Transplantation 46:905–907, 1988.
186. Bowden RA, Sayers M, Flournoy N, et al: Cytomegalovirus immune globulin and seronegative blood products to prevent primary cytomegalovirus infection after marrow transplantation. N Engl J Med 314:1006–1010, 1986.
187. Goodrich JM, Mori M, Gleaves CA, et al: Early treatment with ganciclovir to prevent cytomegalovirus disease after allogeneic bone marrow transplantation. N Engl J Med 325:1601–1607, 1991.
188. Goodrich JM, Bowden RA, Fisher L, et al: Ganciclovir prophylaxis to prevent cytomegalovirus disease after allogeneic marrow transplant. Ann Intern Med 118:173–178, 1993.
189. Schmidt GM, Horak DA, Niland JC, et al: A randomized, controlled trial of prophylactic ganciclovir for cytomegalovirus pulmonary infection in recipients of allogeneic bone marrow transplants. The City of Hope-Stanford-Syntex CMV Study Group. N Engl J Med 324:1005–1011, 1991.
190. Shields AF, Hackman RC, Fife KH, et al: Adenovirus infections in patients undergoing bone-marrow transplantation. N Engl J Med 312:529–533, 1985.
191. Ramsey PG, Fife KH, Hackman RC, et al: Herpes simplex virus pneumonia: Clinical, virologic, and pathologic features in 20 patients. Ann Intern Med 97:813–820, 1982.
192. Cone RW, Hackman RC, Huang ML, et al: Human herpesvirus 6 in lung tissue from patients with pneumonitis after bone marrow transplantation. N Engl J Med 329:156–161, 1993.
193. Harrington RD, Hooton TM, Hackman RC, et al: An outbreak of respiratory syncytial virus in a bone marrow transplant center. J Infect Dis 165:987–993, 1992.
194. Hertz MI, Englund JA, Snover D, et al: Respiratory syncytial virus-induced acute lung injury in adult patients with bone marrow transplants: A clinical approach and review of the literature. Medicine (Baltimore) 68:269–281, 1989.
195. Wendt CH, Weisdorf DJ, Jordan MC, et al: Parainfluenza virus respiratory infection after bone marrow transplantation. N Engl J Med 326:921–926, 1992.
196. Whimbey E, Champlin RE, Englund JA, et al: Combination therapy with aerosolized ribavirin and intravenous immunoglobulin for respiratory syncytial virus disease in adult bone marrow transplant recipients. Bone Marrow Transplant 16:393–399, 1995.
197. Wingard JR, Beals SU, Santos GW, et al: *Aspergillus* infections in bone marrow transplant recipients. Bone Marrow Transplant 2:175–181, 1987.
198. Goodrich JM, Reed EC, Mori M, et al: Clinical features and analysis of risk factors for invasive candidal infection after marrow transplantation. J Infect Dis 164:731–740, 1991.
199. Wald A, Leisenring W, van Burik JA, et al: Epidemiology of *Aspergillus* infections in a large cohort of patients undergoing bone marrow transplantation. J Infect Dis 175:1459–1466, 1997.
199a. Cordonnier C, Bernardin J-F, Fleury J, et al: Diagnostic yield of bronchoalveolar lavage in pneumonitis occurring after allogeneic bone marrow transplantation. Am Rev Respir Dis 132:1118–1123, 1985.
200. Schwebke JR, Hackman R, Bowden R: *Legionella micdadei* in bone marrow transplant recipients. Rev Infect Dis 12:824–828, 1990.
201. Dummer JS: *Pneumocystis carinii* infections in transplant recipients. Semin Respir Infect 5:50–57, 1990.

# 87

# Pulmonary Complications of Endocrine Diseases

LESLIE ZIMMERMAN, M.D.

Introduction
Diabetes Mellitus
Thyroid Disorders
  Hyperthyroidism
  Hypothyroidism
Parathyroid Diseases
Adrenal Diseases
Acromegaly
Summary

## INTRODUCTION

Common endocrine disorders can affect the respiratory system in a variety of ways, from an increased risk of specific infections in diabetic patients to upper airway compression in patients with goiter. Many studies of pulmonary physiology have been done on patients with endocrine disorders, some of which have revealed clinically significant abnormalities. For example, complications of sleep-disordered breathing are found in several endocrine diseases.[1] In other studies, however, physiologic abnormalities do not translate into clinical dysfunction, but they help add to our understanding of lung parenchyma growth and development, response to extrathoracic influences, and perhaps even aging. This chapter reviews the effects of various endocrine abnormalities on the pulmonary system.

## DIABETES MELLITUS

Diabetes mellitus is the most common of all endocrine disorders and affects 120 million people worldwide. Because of their chronic metabolic derangements, many diabetic patients develop cardiovascular and end-organ dysfunction. The effects of diabetes on the respiratory system are numerous (Table 87.1), but data are mixed concerning the effect of diabetes on pulmonary function. Some studies have revealed lower than predicted vital capacity,[2] total lung capacity,[2,2a] diffusion capacity for carbon monoxide,[2] carbon monoxide transfer factor,[3,4] maximal oxygen uptake,[2] and inspiratory muscle strength.[5] These mild functional abnormalities have been ascribed to premature aging of the lungs in a fashion similar to the microangiopathic changes that occur in other affected organs in diabetic persons.[6] The results of other studies, however, showed no significant impairment in total lung capacity,[3,4,7–9] diffusion capacity for carbon monoxide,[7,8] vital capacity,[3,4,7–9] pulmonary distensibility,[7] or maximal inspiratory pressure.[10] At most, the reported degree of pulmonary dysfunction is slight in diabetic persons, not uniform, and may only reflect a small sample size or the variable inclusion of smokers in studied populations. Overall, diabetes mellitus does not appear to cause clinically significant pulmonary impairment, and routine pulmonary function testing in patients with diabetes is not warranted.

**Table 87.1 PULMONARY COMPLICATIONS OF DIABETES MELLITUS**

| |
|---|
| Pulmonary function abnormalities (typically minor) |
| ↓ Vital capacity |
| ↓ Total lung capacity |
| ↓ Diffusion capacity for carbon monoxide |
| ↓ Carbon monoxide transfer factor |
| ↓ Maximal oxygen uptake |
| ↓ Inspiratory muscle strength |
| Left-ventricular dysfunction |
| Pleural effusions |
| Obstructive sleep apnea |
| Infections |
| Poorer outcome with |
| Community-acquired pneumonia |
| *Legionella* pneumonia |
| Increased risk of |
| Aspiration pneumonia |
| Mucormycosis infection |
| Tuberculosis |

There does appear to be an increased frequency of heart failure in diabetic persons not explained by coronary artery disease or hypertension. Left-ventricular systolic and diastolic dysfunction with exercise appears to be more common in insulin-dependent diabetics than in nondiabetic persons.[11, 12] In addition, when compared with patients with similar degrees of left-ventricular dysfunction, pleural effusions are more common in diabetic patients.[13] Cases of noncardiogenic pulmonary edema (acute respiratory distress syndrome) have been reported as a complication of diabetic ketoacidosis.[14, 15] Because obesity aggravates both noninsulin-dependent diabetes and obstructive sleep apnea, the incidence and prevalence of obstructive sleep apnea may be higher in people with diabetes.[16, 17]

In previous decades, newborn babies of diabetic mothers were at increased risk for neonatal respiratory distress syndrome. Now, with better metabolic control and more accurate estimations of gestational age, most pregnant diabetic mothers deliver at or near term, which may account for the current low rate of respiratory distress syndrome in this population.[18, 19]

Bacterial pneumonia may or may not be more frequent in diabetic persons. In a study[20] of over 4000 elderly inhabitants in one township, diabetes mellitus was not an independent risk factor for community-acquired pneumonia. Moreover, in a separate study,[21] diabetes was not an independent risk factor for nosocomial pneumonia. Nonetheless, diabetes may be a risk factor for poorer outcome in those persons that develop pneumonia. In a meta-analysis,[22] diabetes was found to be a risk factor for higher mortality in community-acquired pneumonia. Given the high prevalence of and mortality from pneumococcal pneumonia, the demonstrated efficacy of the pneumococcal vaccine and the increasing prevalence of penicillin resistance in pneumococcal strains, the policy of continuing to target people with diabetes for pneumococcal vaccine seems prudent. Diabetes appears to be a risk factor for the high mortality from *Legionella* pneumonia, which requires admission to the intensive care unit.[23] Diabetic patients may also be predisposed to aspiration pneumonia because of pharyngeal dysfunction and diabetic gastroparesis.[24]

People with diabetes are particularly predisposed to mucormycosis, a group of infections caused by fungi in the *Mucor* or *Rhizopus* genera. These ubiquitous, saprophytic fungi are found in soil and decaying food. Infection typically occurs during or after an episode of diabetic ketoacidosis, perhaps because the fungus grows best in an acidic, hyperglycemic environment. Five infectious manifestations of this organism have been described: rhinocerebral, pulmonary, disseminated, cutaneous, and gastrointestinal.[25] Rhinocerebral infection is the most common form, especially in diabetics. Presentation includes sudden periorbital or paranasal swelling and pain, bloody nasal discharge, and black necrotic nasal mucosa. Characteristic findings on computed tomography (CT) are helpful in suggesting the diagnosis.[25a] Treatment requires control of the diabetes, antifungal therapy, and often aggressive surgical debridement. Mortality remains high, especially in those with intracranial involvement. Pulmonary infection mimics invasive aspergillosis and occurs mostly in neutropenic patients, although diabetes mellitus appears to be a risk factor as well. Inhaled mold spores penetrate bronchiole walls, invade arterioles, and cause thrombosis and ischemia. Patients develop nonspecific cough, fever, pleuritic chest pain, and, occasionally hemoptysis. Chest radiographic patterns are nondiagnostic. Treatment requires antifungal therapy (see Chapter 35) and, if localized, surgical resection. Bronchial stenosis is a potential sequela.

Diabetes mellitus is also an independent risk factor for tuberculosis.[26, 27] The radiographic location of tuberculosis in diabetes, which was originally believed to differ, appears to be similar to that in nondiabetic patients.[28]

## THYROID DISORDERS

### Hyperthyroidism

Many patients with hyperthyroidism complain of rest and exertional dyspnea. Hyperthyroid patients may have decreased vital capacity,[29, 30] decreased respiratory muscle strength,[29–32] and an elevated resting minute ventilation[32, 33] (perhaps due to increased central ventilatory drive) that becomes excessive with exercise.[32] Anaerobic thresholds are typically lower than those of age-matched controls.[32, 33] With treatment, vital capacity and respiratory muscle strength improve,[29–31] although some patients have persistent dyspnea.[31, 32] Hyperthyroidism may also lead to cardiomyopathy and congestive heart failure, thereby contributing to dyspnea and exercise limitation.[34] Although the report of a case series of five patients suggested an association between hyperthyroidism and worsening of asthma control,[35] bronchial hyperreactivity in response to methacholine challenge does not appear to be common in most patients with hyperthyroidism.[32] Patients with coincident asthma and thyrotoxicosis may, however, have worsening of asthma control if beta-blocker agents are used to control hyperthyroid manifestations.

### Hypothyroidism

Hypothyroidism has been associated with dyspnea on exertion, respiratory muscle weakness, alveolar hypoventilation, respiratory failure, central and obstructive sleep apnea, and pleural effusions. Lung volumes are generally normal or mildly decreased in mixed populations of obese and nonobese hypothyroid patients.[36–38] Lung volumes typically, though not uniformly, improve with thyroid replacement. In one case series,[38] a subset of hypothyroid, nonobese patients had normal lung volumes and arterial blood gases; however, the diffusion capacities for carbon monoxide were significantly reduced at baseline and improved to near normal after therapy. In the same series,[38] moderate pulmonary restriction was found in the hypothyroid, obese patients, which normalized with weight loss. Both obese and nonobese hypothyroid patients may develop diaphragmatic muscle weakness that can range from mild impairment, which limits exercise tolerance, to severe dysfunction, with marked resting dyspnea and chronic hypercarbia.[36] Although lung function is not seriously impaired in the majority of patients with hypothyroidism, hypoventilation and even respiratory failure have

**Table 87.2** ETIOLOGIES OF PLEURAL EFFUSIONS IN HYPOTHYROID PATIENTS (n = 28)

| Etiology | No. |
|---|---|
| Nonhypothyroid-associated pleural effusions | 22 |
| Pneumonia | 7 |
| Congestive heart failure | 7 |
| Malignancy | 4 |
| Atelectasis | 2 |
| Pancreatitis | 1 |
| Cirrhosis with ascites | 1 |
| Hypothyroid pleural effusion | 5 |
| Hypothyroid-associated effusion due to pericardial involvement | 1 |

Modified with permission from Gottehrer A, Roa J, Stanford GG, et al: Hypothyroidism and pleural effusions. Chest 98:1130–1132, 1990.

been reported.[39] The most consistent finding in both obese and nonobese hypothyroid patients is that some have a markedly blunted ventilatory response to hypoxia,[38, 40, 41] which improves significantly and often within weeks of initiation of thyroid replacement. This improvement is not associated with changes in spirometric function or maximal voluntary ventilation, thus suggesting a central nervous system cause for the abnormal ventilatory response. Hypercapneic ventilatory response is also blunted in some, but not all, patients with hypothyroidism.[40, 41]

Although up to 25% of patients with hypothyroidism have been found to have radiographic evidence of a pleural effusion, most patients also have underlying congestive heart failure (Table 87.2).[42] A small percentage of hypothyroid patients do not have another disease process that would explain the effusion. In these patients, the hypothyroid-related effusions tend to be small, less than one third of the chest cavity, unilateral or bilateral, serous or serosanginous, and transudates or exudates, although generally noninflammatory.[42] Hypothyroid-related effusions typically resolve with treatment of the hypothyroidism.[42]

Hypothyroidism can predispose patients to sleep apnea,[43–45] possibly from narrowing of the upper airway from mucopolysaccharide and protein deposition in the tongue and oropharynx[46] or from abnormalities in ventilatory control.[40] In a case series,[45] only 3.1% of patients with proven obstructive sleep apnea were found to have hypothyroidism; however, 25% of newly diagnosed hypothyroid patients were found to have obstructive sleep apnea (see Chapter 81 for full discussion of sleep apnea). In this group of patients, the ventilatory responses to hypoxia and hypercapnea were blunted in the hypothyroid/obstructive sleep apnea patients. Age and body weight were the best predictors of associated obstructive sleep apnea. All these patients with obstructive sleep apnea and hypothyroidism had significant improvement in their sleep respiratory disturbance index and their awake ventilatory response to hypoxia and hypercapnea with thyroid replacement; another series,[44] however, found less than full improvement with therapy. Grunstein and Sullivan[44] found that, although the mean apnea duration and mean minimum oxygen saturation improved, only two of eight hypothyroid/obstructive sleep apnea patients had enough improvement after thyroid replacement to no longer need to be treated with continuous positive airway pressure. Central sleep apnea also occurs in hypothyroid patients. In a case report[43] of a patient with central sleep apnea and hypothyroidism, a blunted ventilatory response to hypoxia was seen, which improved with thyroid replacement.

Thyroid hormones play an important role in the growth and development of the lung and in the maturation of the lungs' surfactant system.[47, 48] Although previous studies[49, 50] suggested that thyroid hormone levels are decreased in premature infants who develop respiratory distress syndrome, this may be due to decreased thyroxine binding to proteins, similar to the "euthyroid sick" syndrome seen in other acute illnesses.[51] The addition of maternal antenatal thyrotropin-releasing hormone, which increases fetal thyroid hormone levels, to corticosteroids did not decrease the frequency or severity of respiratory distress syndrome in premature babies in a large multicenter trial.[52]

Although most patients with goiter are asymptomatic, goiter can cause airway compression with symptoms of dyspnea, stridor, wheezing, hoarseness, and cough (Fig. 87.1).[53, 54] The degree of airway narrowing can be assessed by recording a flow-volume loop. Surgical resection relieves compressive symptoms[53] in patients with large compressive goiter. Radioactive iodine[55] is an alternative therapeutic approach for elderly patients who are poor surgical candidates.

Iodinated glycerol is a mucolytic agent sometimes used in the management of chronic obstructive pulmonary disease. Use of this medication has been associated with iodine-induced hyperthyroidism,[56, 57] hypothyroidism,[57] and goiter.[58]

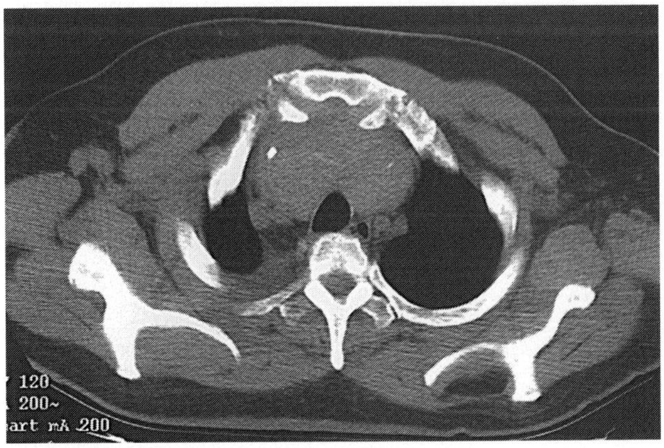


**Figure 87.1** A substernal goiter was found in a 69-year-old man who presented with nonproductive cough and mild dyspnea on exertion. The chest radiograph revealed a superior mediastinal mass. A CT scan revealed a large substernal goiter, confirmed to be thyroid by nuclear medicine scan. (Courtesy of Marcia McCowin, MD.)

## PARATHYROID DISEASES

Hyperparathyroidism, typically secondary hyperparathyroidism in patients with end-stage renal disease, may cause diffuse metastatic calcification in the lungs. Metastatic calcification is the deposition of calcium salts in previously normal tissue. This is in contrast to dystrophic calcification in which there is calcification of diseased or abnormal tissue. Despite phosphate diet restriction, administration of phosphate binders, and hemodialysis, renal failure patients are at risk for metastatic calcification, especially if the calcium-phosphorus double product increases above 70 $mg^2/dL^2$. Pulmonary metastatic calcific nodules occur predominantly in the alveolar septa and are associated with varying degrees of fibrosis and septal thickening. Calcification may also occur in pulmonary arterial and bronchial walls. This phenomenon appears to be quite common; up to 60% of chronic dialysis patients have autopsy evidence of pulmonary metastatic calcification.[59] Most patients are asymptomatic and have normal chest radiographs and pulmonary function; the presence of pulmonary calcification is detected only by autopsy. Patients with heavy deposition of calcific nodules may, however, complain of dyspnea and nonproductive cough. Pulmonary function tests in patients with extensive metastatic calcification may show ventilatory restriction with hypoxemia and low diffusion capacity for carbon monoxide.[59, 60] Radiographically, those patients with more extensive calcification typically have numerous nodules about 3 to 10 mm in size,[61] which are usually better visualized on computed tomography (CT) scans than on plain chest films (Fig. 87.2). In addition to the nodular densities, patchy consolidation and ground-glass attenuation may be seen that may mimic pneumonia or pulmonary edema. The calcific nature of the nodules is often not apparent on plain radiographic or even CT images, perhaps due the small size of the calcium deposits. Radionuclide bone scans, however, usually reveal intense uptake in the lungs and other affected organs (Fig. 87.3).[62, 63] Metastatic calcification has a predilection for the apical portions of the lungs, the stomach, and the kidneys. Because calcium salts tend to precipitate in areas of changing pH, the relatively alkaline areas of lung apices may account for this predilection.[60] Other common sites of deposition include soft tissues and the skin. Parathyroidectomy or treatment with new vitamin D analogs[64] can decrease the calcium-phosphorus double product, reverse bone scan abnormalities and organ deposition, and presumably improve pulmonary function. Metastatic calcification can also rarely occur in primary hyperparathyroidism.[65, 66]

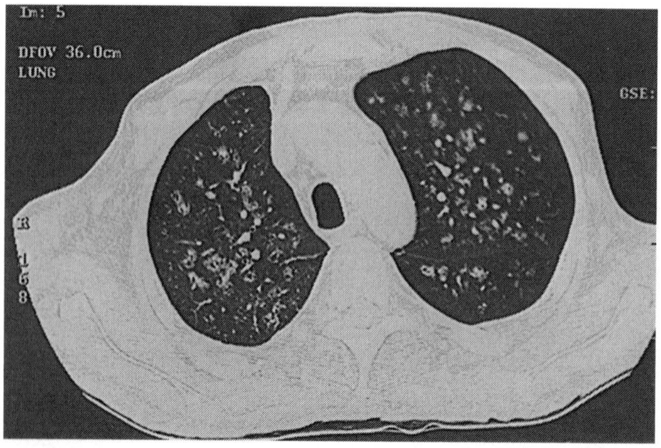


**Figure 87.2** Metastatic calcification occurred in the lungs because of chronic renal failure. A 59-year-old man with end-stage renal disease for 5 years complained of chronic progressive shortness of breath. The serum calcium level was 9.9 mg/dL (normal range, 8.5 to 10.5 mg/dL) and the parathyroid hormone level was 271 pg/mL (normal for the laboratory, 11 to 54 pg/mL). High-resolution CT scan revealed numerous nodular ground-glass densities in a peribronchial pattern, most prominently in the upper lobes. (Courtesy of Marcia McCowin, MD.)

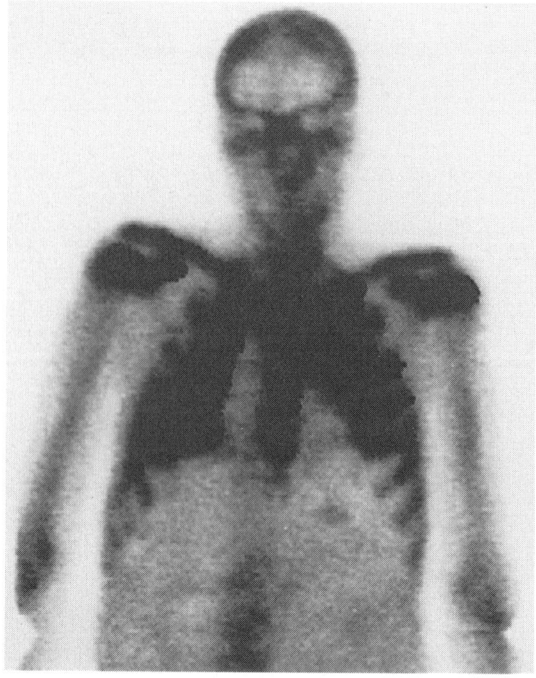

**Figure 87.3** Metastatic calcification in the lungs was caused by chronic renal failure. This is the same patient as in Figure 87.2. Whole-body bone imaging revealed diffuse soft-tissue avidity in both lungs.

Rarely, enlarged mediastinal parathyroid cysts may cause tracheal compression with stridor and/or vocal cord impingement and hoarseness. Surgical excision is the treatment of choice.[67]

## ADRENAL DISEASES

Hypercortisolism from endogenous Cushing's syndrome is a risk factor for mucocutaneous fungal infections and opportunistic pulmonary infections. Endogenous Cushing's syndrome may be due to ectopic adrenocorticotropic hormone production from small cell lung cancer, bronchial carcinoid, thymic carcinoid, islet cell carcinoma of the pancreas, adrenal neoplasia, and pituitary Cushing's disease. Cortisol levels tend to be much higher with ectopic adrenocorticotropic hormone production and adrenal neoplasia than in pituitary Cushing's disease and so pose a much greater hazard for infections. The most common pulmonary infections associated with endogenous Cushing's syndrome are caused by *Cryptococcus, Aspergillus, Nocardia, Pneumocystis*, and *Mycobacterium tuberculosis*.[68–71] *Pneumocystis carinii* pneumonia tends to occur in patients with the highest morning cortisol levels.[71] Correction of hypercortisolism is an important adjunct to antimicrobial therapy.

Adrenal insufficiency via the hypothalamic-pituitary axis may be seen in stressed, very-low-birth-weight infants and make them more susceptible to bronchopulmonary dysplasia.[72, 73] In industrialized countries, 70% to 80% of cases of Addison's disease are "idiopathic" in origin; in contrast, in resource-poor countries, tuberculosis remains by far the most common cause.[73a] Nonmalignant causes of Addison's disease, including tuberculosis and histoplasmosis, are said to have "characteristic" CT abnormalities.[73b]

## ACROMEGALY

Acromegaly, a disorder of excess growth hormone secretion from a pituitary adenoma, is characterized by additional bone growth, soft-tissue hypertrophy, and coarsening of facial features. Macroglossia, oropharyngeal airway narrowing, and vocal cord restriction and fixation may also occur. Total lung capacity and vital capacity are typically increased in patients with acromegaly compared with controls.[74–77] In one study,[76] the elevation of the total lung capacity correlated with the duration of acromegaly. Possible causes for the increased lung volumes in these patients include overdistention of alveoli, hypertrophy or enlargement of individual alveoli, or an increase in the number of alveoli.[74, 77] Diffusion capacity for carbon monoxide may be within normal limits[74, 77] or elevated.[75] Clinical respiratory manifestations of acromegaly include sleep apnea, extrathoracic airway obstruction, and vocal cord dysfunction.

Patients with acromegaly have an increased prevalence of heavy snoring, central sleep apnea, and obstructive sleep apnea.[78, 79] In one study, patients with acromegaly and central sleep apnea were found to have higher growth hormone levels than patients with acromegaly and obstructive sleep apnea.[78] Patients with acromegaly and central sleep apnea also had higher hypercarbic ventilatory response than patients with acromegaly and obstructive sleep apnea or normal controls.[80] These central sleep apnea patients typically had intermittent apneas with normal arterial $P_{CO_2}$ levels rather than hypoventilation and increased $P_{CO_2}$ values. Obstructive sleep apnea is more common than central apnea in acromegaly. Patients with acromegaly may be predisposed to obstructive apneas because of a narrowed upper airway from osseous enlargement, swelling and hyperplasia of tissues in the oropharynx, and macroglossia. A recent study documented anatomic abnormalities, especially at the base of the tongue, in all five patients with acromegaly who had sleep-disordered breathing.[80a] Some patients' obstructive sleep apnea improves with treatment of acromegaly with pituitary ablation[81] or with octreotide.[81a]

Evidence of a variable extrathoracic airway obstruction on flow-volume loops in seen in 30% to 50% of patients with acromegaly.[76, 82] Intubation may be more difficult in patients with acromegaly because of vocal cord fixation, prolapse of an enlarged tongue, and soft-tissue thickening of the oropharynx.[83]

## SUMMARY

Hypothyroidism and diabetes mellitus are very common medical conditions that can also affect the respiratory system. Manifestations include respiratory muscle weakness in hypothyroidism to fulminate life-threatening infection with mucormycosis in poorly controlled diabetes. Other less common endocrine disorders also have specific, common, and fascinating effects on the lung. This chapter has reviewed the effects of these various endocrine disorders on the respiratory system.

## References

1. Rosenow R, McCarthy V, Caruso AC: Sleep apnea in endocrine diseases. J Sleep Res 7:3–11, 1998.
2. Niranjan V, McBrayer DG, Ramirez LC, et al: Glycemic control and cardiopulmonary function in patients with insulin-dependent diabetes mellitus. Am J Med 103:504–513, 1997.
2a. Schnapf BM, Banks RA, Silverstein JH, et al: Pulmonary function in insulin-dependent diabetes mellitus with limited joint mobility. Am Rev Respir Dis 130:930–932, 1984.
3. Weir DC, Jennings PE, Hendy MS, et al: Transfer factor for carbon monoxide in patients with diabetes with and without microangiopathy. Thorax 43:725–726, 1988.
4. Sandler M, Bunn AE, Stewart RI: Pulmonary function in young diabetic patients. Chest 90:670–675, 1986.
5. Wanke T, Formanek D, Auinger M, et al: Inspiratory muscle performance and pulmonary function changes in insulin-dependent diabetes mellitus. Am Rev Respir Dis 143:97–100, 1991.
6. Sandler M: Is the lung a "target organ" in diabetes mellitus? Arch Intern Med 150:1385–1388, 1990.
7. Maccioni FJ, Colebatch HJH: Lung volume and distensibility in insulin-dependent diabetes mellitus. Am Rev Respir Dis 143:1253–1256, 1991.
8. Fuso L, Cotroneo P, Basso S, et al: Postural variations of pulmonary diffusing capacity in insulin-dependent diabetes mellitus. Chest 110:1009–1013, 1996.
9. Sandler M, Bunn AE, Stewart RI: Cross-section study of pulmonary function in patients with insulin-dependent diabetes mellitus. Am Rev Respir Dis 135:223–229, 1987.
10. Enright PL, Kronmal RA, Manolio TA, et al: Respiratory muscle strength in the elderly. Am J Respir Crit Care Med 149:430–438, 1994.
11. Mustonen JN, Uusitupa MIJ, Tahvanainen K, et al: Impaired left ventricular systolic function during exercise in middle-aged insulin-dependent and noninsulin-dependent diabetic subjects without clinically evident cardiovascular disease. Am J Cardiol 62:1273–1279, 1988.
12. Jermendy G, Khoor S, Koltai MZ, et al: Left ventricular diastolic dysfunction in type 1 (insulin dependent) diabetic patients during exercise. Cardiology 77:9–16, 1990.
13. Chertow BS, Kadzielawa R, Burger AJ: Benign pleural effusions in long standing diabetes. Chest 99:1108–1111, 1991.
14. Russel J, Follansbee S, Matthay MA: Adult respiratory distress syndrome complicating diabetic ketoacidosis. West J Med 135:148–150, 1981.
15. Powner D, Synder JV, Grenwich A: Altered pulmonary capillary permeability recovering from diabetic ketoacidosis. Chest 68:253–256, 1975.
16. Katsumata K, Okada T, Miyao M, et al: High incidence of sleep apnea syndrome in a male diabetic population. Diabetes Res Clin Pract 13:45–51, 1991.
17. Brooks B, Cistulli PA, Borkman M, et al: Obstructive sleep apnea in obese noninsulin-dependent diabetic patients: Effects of continuous positive airway pressure treatment on insulin responsiveness. J Clin Endocrinol Metab 79:1681–1685, 1994.

# 88 The Lungs in Obstetric and Gynecologic Disease

NORMAN W. RIZK, M.D.

Introduction
Physiologic Alterations During Normal Pregnancy
- Alterations in Respiratory Physiology
- Alterations in Cardiovascular Physiology

Obstetric Disorders and the Lung
- Obstructive Airway Disease
- Infectious Diseases
- Pulmonary Edema and Pulmonary Vascular Disease
- Acute Lung Injury in Pregnancy

Gynecologic Disorders and the Lung
- Catamenial Pneumothorax
- Endometriosis
- Lymphangioleiomyomatosis
- Trophoblastic Embolization

Summary

## INTRODUCTION

Both respiratory physiology and the respiratory tract's susceptibility to disease are uniquely altered in gynecologic and obstetric conditions, including normal pregnancy. This chapter summarizes normal physiologic alterations during pregnancy and then considers pathologic diseases and disorders that arise during pregnancy. Airway disorders, infectious diseases, pulmonary vascular and embolic disorders, and acute lung injury are considered in turn. Finally, pleural and parenchymal diseases that arise as a consequence of gynecologic conditions are addressed.

## PHYSIOLOGIC ALTERATIONS DURING NORMAL PREGNANCY

Profound alterations of respiratory function and cardiovascular physiology accompany pregnancy; these conditions contribute to many of the disorders of the lung during pregnancy. The adaptive changes during the gravid period are designed to support maternal and fetal well-being during the special stresses of fetal growth and parturition, but they exacerbate some disorders and confuse interpretation of laboratory and imaging studies used to assess many other common conditions.

### Alterations in Respiratory Physiology

Upper airway, particularly nasal, mucosal edema is a common finding in normal pregnancy. About 30% of gravid women complain of rhinitis symptoms,[1] conventionally attributed to the effects of estrogen on mucosal congestion. Animal studies appear to support this attribution.[1, 2] The symptoms begin in the first trimester and persist throughout gestation. Many patients thought to have rhinitis of pregnancy may actually have other or coincident causes of rhinitis.[1] An important implication of nasal mucosal edema in pregnancy is that it predisposes to nosebleeds from nasal intubations, so that an oral approach is favored at the time of delivery.

Chest wall configuration is also altered, partially due to a 50% increase in the average costal angle,[3] and partially due to an increase in the circumference of the lower chest wall. Diaphragmatic position is elevated 4 to 5 cm, but excursion does not diminish.[3] Muscle strength, as measured by maximum transdiaphragmatic pressure, does not appear to be diminished from its usual mean value of about 95 cm $H_2O$,[4] allowing reserve for both the augmented minute ventilation of pregnancy and the stresses of delivery.

Important changes occur in lung function and lung volumes. Because the loss of lung volume resulting from elevation of the diaphragm is only partially offset by the smaller increase in chest wall diameter, functional residual capacity (FRC) is usually diminished by about 18%, or 300 to 500 mL.[5] The FRC diminution is partitioned almost equally between the expiratory reserve volume and the residual volume.[3, 5] The loss of FRC at term is made worse by recumbency, when diaphragm elevation is greatest because of the higher intra-abdominal pressure. Increased pulmonary blood volume in pregnancy may also serve to lower the FRC.[6] This reduction in FRC is associated clinically with increased uptake and eliminastudy has documented this association, and the NAEP Working Group thinks that independent confirmation is required before concluding that epinephrine is teratogenic.[15] Acceptable beta$_2$-agonists in pregnancy include metaproterenol, albuterol, pirbuterol, bitolterol, and terbutaline.

Theophylline has a long history of use during pregnancy and is considered safe, but the therapeutic range in plasma should be adjusted to 8 to 12 μg/mL because of diminished protein binding during pregnancy. Theophylline passes freely to the fetus, and newborns occasionally show signs of theophylline toxicity, particularly when maternal blood levels are high. Theophylline is also transmitted into breast milk, with a serum-to-milk ratio of about 0.73,[25] but in general, less than 1% of the maternal dose is transferred to the infant.

Although animal studies have shown an increased incidence of cleft palate with use of corticosteroids, no human data support this association. Systemic corticosteroids have been reported to cause intrauterine growth retardation but of a relatively modest degree.[26] Halogenated corticosteroids do not cross the placenta easily, and so fetal and neonatal adrenal suppression is not a major concern with these compounds.[15] Among the inhaled steroids, beclomethasone is preferred because of its long history of use in pregnancy and the absence of any demonstrated toxicity to the fetus.

Labor and delivery are especially hazardous for asthmatic patients, partly because of the drugs commonly administered. Narcotics other than fentanyl release histamine, which may worsen bronchospasm. Lumbar epidural analgesia is generally preferred, but if general anesthesia is to be used, pretreatment with atropine and glycopyrrolate assists bronchodilation; ketamine is the preferred anesthetic, although halogenated anesthetics at low concentrations may provide bronchodilatation as well.[15] Preterm labor may be treated with nifedipine or magnesium sulfate safely.[16] Oxytocin is the optimal labor induction agent and is useful for postpartum hemorrhage, but 15-methyl prostaglandin $F_2$–alpha, methylergonovine, and ergonovine may cause bronchospasm and should be avoided if possible.

### Cystic Fibrosis

Cystic fibrosis (CF), occurring in about 1 in 1500 whites and 1 in 17,000 blacks, is a common genetic disease. With improved therapy, median survival has now improved to 30 years of age,[27] and the Cystic Fibrosis Foundation found that 4% of female CF patients between the ages of 17 and 37 were pregnant in 1990.[27a] This occurs despite the frequent infertility of women due to delayed sexual development and the common occurrence of azoospermia in men. Pregnancy in CF patients, as might be anticipated, has been associated with adverse fetal and maternal outcomes.[28] In a review of 215 pregnancies reported between 1960 and 1991, Kent and Farquharson[29] showed that although more than 80% progressed to at least 20 weeks, one fourth of these delivered preterm, and the perinatal death rate was 14%. In this study, there were three maternal deaths, and by 2 years after delivery, 14% of mothers had died.[29] More recent studies suggest that risk stratifies according to severity of illness.[28, 30] In one study of 38 pregnancies, 34 were completed, but there were two preterm deliveries, one neonatal death from sepsis, and one neonate with restricted growth.[30] In this group of less ill patients, only one mother died within 2 years of delivery. Prepregnancy counseling, particularly for women with more severe disease, is essential in limiting excessive maternal and fetal risk. In this regard, it has been suggested that an $FEV_1$ below 60% of predicted is a poor prognostic factor for both mother and infant.[28]

## Infectious Diseases

### Bacterial Pneumonia

Pneumonia is a leading cause of maternal and fetal morbidity and mortality.[31–35] Maternal mortality from pneumonia in nonimmunocompromised hosts ranged from 0% to 4% in series published since 1980.[31–33] The reported incidence varies widely, from 1 per 367 to 1 per 2388 deliveries[31–34]; one report indicated that pneumonia may be increasing in incidence, with human immunodeficiency virus (HIV) and chronic disease the major risk factors.[34]

Pregnancy increases the risk for major complications of pneumonia. In the series by Madinger and colleagues[33] of 25 patients culled from 25,000 deliveries, 40% suffered major complications, including five intubations, two empyemas, one pneumothorax, and one pericardial tamponade. Similarly, in the series by Briggs and associates[36] of 34 patients, 7 required mechanical ventilation, and 2 died. Gestation is also threatened; preterm labor occurs in 4% to 44%.[31–34] The small-for-gestational-age rate is as high as 12%,[31] and intrauterine and neonatal death rates have ranged from 2.6% to 12%.[32, 33] In all series, underlying chronic illness in the mother has been a powerful predictor of adverse outcome in both fetus and mother.

Pneumonia in pregnancy is most commonly bacterial in origin; the microbiologic spectrum mirrors community-acquired pneumonia, with *Streptococcus pneumoniae* and *Haemophilus influenzae* the most common organisms.[31–33] Other common organisms include *Mycoplasma pneumoniae* and *Chlamydia pneumoniae*. As in other community-acquired pneumonias, the causative agent is identified in only about half the cases.

### Viral Pneumonia

Viral pneumonia remains a serious concern in pregnancy. In the influenza pandemic of 1918 to 1919, the maternal rate of mortality from pneumonia was as high as 50%. In the more recent epidemic of 1957 to 1958, pregnant women accounted for 10% of fatalities, and about half of women of childbearing age who died were pregnant.[37] Since the epidemic of 1957 to 1958, the maternal mortality rate from influenza A and B has been low, and the Centers for Disease Control and Prevention (CDC) do not currently recommend the killed virus vaccine for influenza in otherwise healthy women during pregnancy. Although influenza virus does cross the placenta, current opinion holds that it is not likely to be teratogenic to the fetus, despite isolated reports that link influenza with neural tube and other malformations. Amantadine (FDA category C) has been used in pregnancy successfully, both as treatment and as prophylaxis. The chief risk of influenza in the modern era probably resides in its dreaded complication of superimposed staphylococcal or gram-negative bacillary pneumonia.

Varicella pneumonia, caused by a virus of the DNA herpesvirus group, has also been linked to particularly adverse outcomes during pregnancy. In one review, Haake and coworkers[38] reported a 35% mortality rate in pregnant subjects, compared with 10% in other adults. Treatment with acyclovir appear to reduce mortality in gravid patients.[39] Use of varicella-zoster immunoglobulin, which can attenuate or prevent infection when administered within 72 hours of exposure to susceptible people, is not recommended by the CDC for routine use in pregnant women, although some authors contest the wisdom of this approach. The currently licensed attenuated live virus against varicella is contraindicated in pregnancy.

Rubeola viral infection, often complicated by viral and then superimposed bacterial pneumonia, has also been associated with adverse outcomes, including preterm labor, spontaneous abortion, and perinatal mortality.[40] Fetal malformation does not appear to be a risk of the disease. Nonimmune, exposed pregnant patients can receive passive immunoprophylaxis with immunoglobulin within 6 days of exposure; the live viral vaccine is contraindicated during pregnancy.

Hantavirus, which usually presents as a hemorrhagic fever and renal syndrome, can be accompanied by pneumonitis and adult respiratory distress syndrome. It has been reported in pregnancy,[41] but whether it is more severe in pregnancy has not been established.

### Fungal Pneumonias

Fungal pneumonias are uncommon in pregnancy. Although there is no evidence that blastomycosis and histoplasmosis are more severe during pregnancy, it does appear that coccidiomycosis is more likely to disseminate in pregnancy.[42] In the Southwest United States, about 1 in 5000 pregnancies is complicated by this deep mycosis.[43] Dissemination is most likely in the third trimester and has been related both to subtle impairment of cell-mediated immunity and to a stimulatory effect of progesterone and 17-beta-estradiols on fungal proliferation.[44] Amphotericin (FDA category B) is the accepted therapy for disseminated coccidiomycosis.

### Tuberculosis

Tuberculosis does not appear to be more common or severe in pregnancy. Isoniazid, rifampin, and ethambutol have acceptable safety profiles in pregnancy are part of the standard treatment regimens advised by the CDC and American Thoracic Society (ATS) for pregnant women.[45] There is less collective experience with pyrazinamide, and the CDC-ATS statement discourages its use. Worldwide data are accumulating, however, and pyrazinamide appears to be emerging as a drug that can be considered for treating multidrug-resistant tuberculosis. Streptomycin, by contrast, is clearly associated with congenital deafness and is contraindicated during pregnancy.

## Pulmonary Edema and Pulmonary Vascular Disease

Gravid women are at special risk for pulmonary edema for a variety of reasons, including the hypervolemia and high cardiac output of pregnancy, diminished colloid oncotic pressure, occasional need for tocolytic drugs that affect the vascular bed, and unique vascular and endothelial disorders of pregnancy.

### Hydrostatic (Cardiogenic) Pulmonary Edema

The cardiovascular adaptations to pregnancy have already been summarized. Their effects on underlying cardiac disorders are predictable.[46] Stenotic lesions are particularly poorly tolerated.[47] Of these, mitral stenosis is the most common symptomatic valvular disease in pregnancy and frequently presents with pulmonary edema, not only during gestation but also immediately postpartum, because of the large shifts in intravascular volume associated with delivery. The gradient across a stenotic mitral valve is augmented by the increases in blood volume, cardiac output, and heart rate that occur during gestation and the puerperium. In aortic stenosis, the increase in cardiac output required for pregnancy worsens the gradient across the valve. As a compensatory mechanism, end-diastolic volume increases, but the low SVR in aortic stenosis impairs diastolic coronary artery filling and can precipitate ischemic syndromes. The reduction in SVR of pregnancy mitigates the consequences of mitral and aortic regurgitation and of the left-to-right intracardiac shunts of endocardial cushion defects, but worsens the consequences of Eisenmenger's syndrome and uncorrected tetralogy of Fallot. Depending on the cardiac disorder, perturbations of pregnancy can alter fractional shunts, induce hypoxemia, and precipitate pulmonary edema.

A special problem of pregnancy is peripartum cardiomyopathy, a disorder that occurs in 1 of 1500 to 4000 deliveries, may present with congestive heart failure, and is associated with a special propensity for pulmonary and systemic embolization during the last month of pregnancy and for up to 6 months thereafter.[48] An inflammatory subset of this disorder that responds to immunosuppressive therapy can be identified by endomyocardial biopsy.[49]

### Tocolysis-Associated Pulmonary Edema

The systemic administration of $beta_2$-sympathomimetic agents to retard premature labor has been associated with a 0% to 4.4% incidence of pulmonary edema.[50] The etiology of this disorder is controversial.[51] One speculation is that it is due to myocardial dysfunction from prolonged sympathetic stimulation, but descriptions of cases in which hemodynamic measurements were made report normal pulmonary capillary wedge pressures. The idea that increased vascular permeability may contribute to the syndrome is given weight by its association with maternal infection.[52] Some authors have speculated that the disorder requires a coexisting condition, such as volume overload, sepsis, or preeclampsia.[53] It usually presents after at least 24 hours of beta-adrenergic therapy

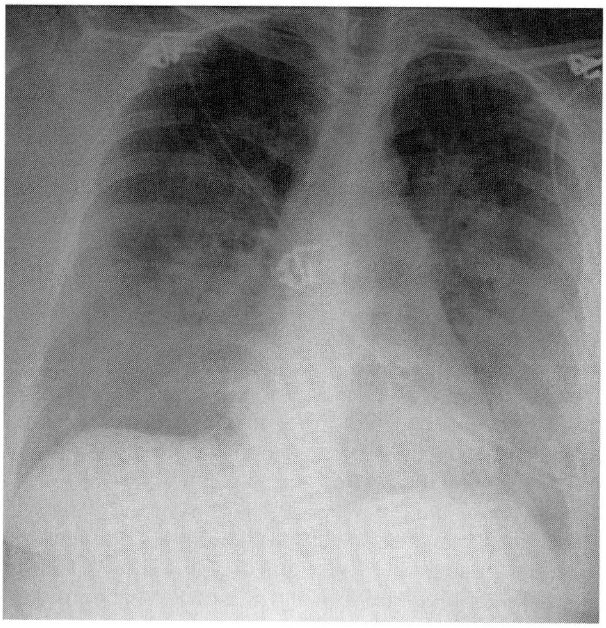

**Figure 88.3** Tocolysis-associated pulmonary edema in a 38-year-old woman in premature labor.

with relatively acute onset of dyspnea and pulmonary edema seen on chest radiograph (Fig. 88.3). Simple discontinuation of beta-adrenergic therapy often results in rapid improvement; whether diuretics need to be given is unresolved, but furosemide is usually administered.

## Pulmonary Edema Associated with Preeclampsia

About 2.9% of patients with preeclampsia or eclampsia develop pulmonary edema.[54] The spectrum of hemodynamic findings associated with pregnancy-induced hypertension and preeclampsia is wide, but in general, left ventricular preload is normal or low, afterload is high, and cardiac output is normal or low (Fig. 88.4). Systolic and diastolic function may also be impaired.[55] The pulmonary edema commonly first occurs in the postpartum period,[54, 55] reflecting fluid administration at delivery. Low colloid oncotic pressure and abnormal vascular permeability likely contribute as well. Hemodynamic monitoring of these patients is probably warranted if oliguria complicates the picture.

## Pulmonary Embolism

Pulmonary embolism is a leading cause of maternal mortality,[56] accounting for 11% of 1453 pregnancy-related deaths in the United States between 1987 and 1990.[57] Even though the risk for pulmonary embolism in pregnant women is about five times as great as in age-matched and sex-matched nongravid controls,[58] it is still relatively rare. A Danish population-based study of 63,000 deliveries found a cumulative incidence of 0.85 in 1000 deliveries from 1984 to 1994.[59] In this study, the incidence of detected pulmonary embolism increased to 1.23 in 1000 deliveries after the introduction of ultrasound, demonstrating that its reported incidence may depend on the adequacy of diagnostic procedures employed. Other studies have reported rates of 0.5 to 1.3 per 1000.[60]

The risk for thrombosis is increased in pregnancy, partly because of the increase in the coagulation factors, particularly $V_c$, $VIII_c$, $X_c$, and von Willebrand factor Ag, and partly because of a marked fall in protein S.[60a] Venous stasis, an important contributor to thrombosis, occurs because of uterine compression of the inferior vena cava and the left iliac vein. Local trauma to pelvic veins at the time of delivery probably accounts for the peak incidence of thromboembolism in the postpartum period, especially after cesarean section. Specific risk factors for thromboembolism include previous thromboembolism during pregnancy or while taking oral contraceptives, prolonged bed rest, a complicated or cesarean delivery, and inherited coagulation defects. These include deficiencies of factor S, factor C, and antithrombin III or the presence of antiphospholipid antibodies, factor V Leiden, and prothrombin 20210A.[60, 60a] The first two risk factors probably warrant prophylactic subcutaneous heparin administration throughout pregnancy.

Diagnosis of deep vein thrombosis during pregnancy and the puerperium is exceptionally difficult because of the peripheral edema associated with pregnancy and the asymmetric compression of the left-sided common iliac vein by the gravid uterus. The initial diagnostic test should be real-time B-mode venous ultrasonography; if the clinical suspicion for venous thrombus is high, impedance plethysmography should also be done to detect isolated iliac vein thrombosis. Compression ultrasonography appears to be the more accurate of the two tests,[61] but use of both in a sequential fashion may improve diagnostic yield. The gold standard for detection of lower extremity thrombosis remains venography, but in pregnancy, thrombosis is typically confined to the iliac veins and may be hard to visualize, even by this technique. When venous thrombosis of the lower extremity is documented, it is usually left-sided, as it was in 58 of 60 cases reported by Ginsberg and colleagues.[62]

The diagnosis of pulmonary embolism in pregnant women is relatively straightforward. Both ventilation-perfusion scanning and pulmonary angiography can be performed during pregnancy in a modified fashion. Estimated fetal radiation exposure for a standard technetium-labeled macroaggregated albumin perfusion scan is about 0.018 cGy,[63] and this can be reduced further by simply halving the dose, without greatly impairing resolution. There is no need for the ventilation portion of the study if perfusion is normal. Similarly, pulmonary angiography, when performed by the brachial route, exposes the fetus to only about 0.050 cGy.[64] Computed tomographic angiography, a newer technique, is also emerging as an acceptable imaging modality but is unreliable for detecting emboli in subsegmental arteries and arteries that course horizontally in the lingula and right middle lobe. Its use in pregnancy has not yet been well studied. Magnetic resonance imaging with gadolinium contrast also has promise because it can image pelvic and lower extremity veins as well as the pulmonary arteries and has no contrast-associated toxicity. Its widespread use requires availability of ultrafast scanners and more experience in its accuracy.

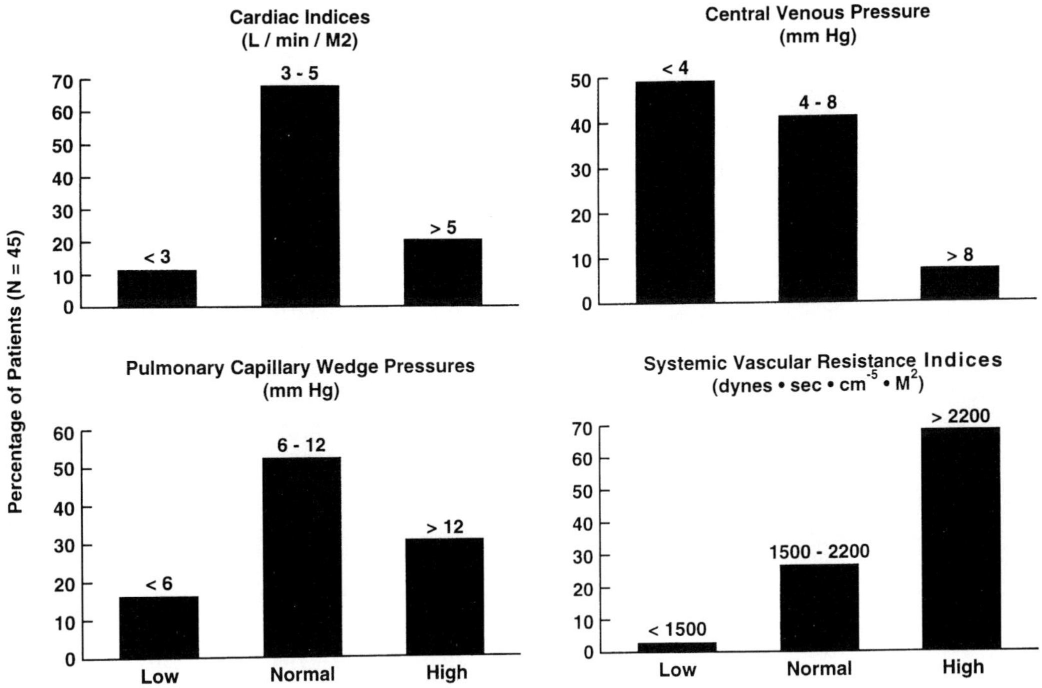


**Figure 88.4** Spectrum of hemodynamic profiles seen in 45 women with severe pregnancy-induced hypertension, one of the disorders sometimes complicated by pulmonary edema. Pulmonary edema in pregnancy-induced hypertension usually does not reflect simple volume overload. (From Clark SC, Cotton DB, Lee W, et al: Hemodynamic profile of severe pregnancy-induced hypertension. Am J Obstet Gynecol 158:523, 1988.)

Embolism in pregnancy is treated with heparin because warfarin crosses the placenta and causes nasal, ophthalmologic, and central nervous system abnormalities. Standard therapy of thromboembolism antepartum encompasses continuous intravenous heparin for 5 to 7 days, followed by subcutaneous adjusted-dose heparin every 12 hours until 24 hours before elective induced delivery. If labor begins unexpectedly, reversal of the heparin effect with protamine is advisable. A major concern about use of longer-term heparin during pregnancy is its tendency to induce osteopenia in as many as 15% of patients.[65] Whether low-molecular-weight heparin fractions are superior is not yet clear, although they appear to be safe and are known not to cross the placenta.[66] Postpartum, warfarin can be given safely during lactation.

## Amniotic Fluid Embolism

Small amounts of amniotic fluid may enter the circulation during uncomplicated pregnancy, but in 1 of 20,000 to 80,000 deliveries, the catastrophic syndrome of amniotic fluid embolism, first described by Steiner and Lushbaugh,[67] occurs. The onset is usually during labor and delivery or immediately after uterine manipulations, when severe dyspnea, hypoxemia, and then seizures and cardiovascular collapse or arrest occur. If the patient survives the initial insult, disseminated intravascular coagulation and acute respiratory distress syndrome usually supervene.[68] Risk factors include older maternal age, high parity, cesarean section, low uterine segment laceration, and meconium staining of amniotic fluid.[53] Abruptio placentae is present in 50% of cases, and fetal demise occurs in 40%.[68] The maternal mortality rate has been as high as 86%[69] but has appeared more recently to be as low as 26%[69a]; overall, amniotic fluid embolism may account for 10% of all maternal deaths.

In a US registry of cases, 78% of the patients with amniotic fluid embolism had ruptured membranes, and several had just undergone intrauterine procedures,[70] clearly implicating traumatic opening of uterine vessels in the pathogenesis. The exact quantity or constituent of the amniotic fluid required to initiate the syndrome is unknown. Pathologically, fetal squamous cells are found in the maternal pulmonary circulation at autopsy (Fig. 88.5), but even in symptom-free patients, fetal cells may be recovered from pulmonary artery catheters placed for other reasons.[71] Hemodynamically, the process is often biphasic, with pulmonary hypertension initially, followed by left ventricular failure.[72] These changes may be caused by leukotrienes and arachidonic acid metabolites, particularly prostaglandin $F_2$, which appears in amniotic fluid during labor. An immunologic basis for some of the changes seems likely because women with male fetuses are more likely to acquire the disorder.[73] Clark and associates[70] have seized on the similarities to anaphylaxis and suggested the disorder be renamed *anaphylactoid syndrome of pregnancy.*

Radiographically, the patients usually develop pulmonary edema, then acute lung injury. Treatment consists of supportive care for the associated disseminated intravas-

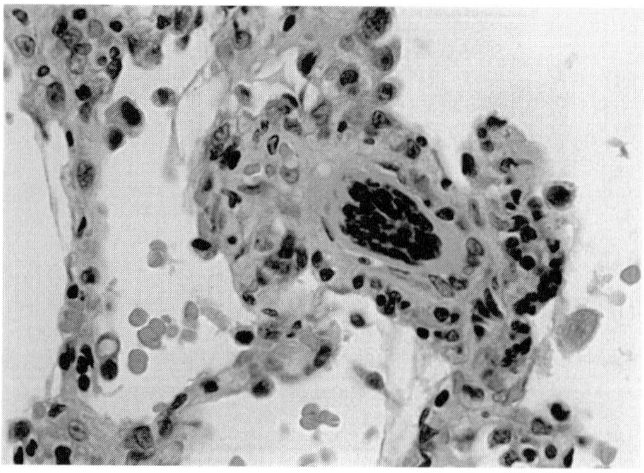

**Figure 88.5** Small pulmonary vessel filled and distended by fetal squamous cells from a fatal case of amniotic fluid embolism in a 39-year-old woman who succumbed within 4 hours of delivery. (Keratin stain; original magnification × 400.) (Courtesy of Dr. Gerald Berry, Department of Pathology, Stanford University, Stanford, CA.)

cular coagulation and left ventricular and respiratory failure. If the fetus survives the initial insult and is intrauterine, it should be promptly delivered. In cases of maternal demise, emergency postmortem or periresuscitative cesarean section is warranted, as in other instances of cardiopulmonary resuscitation in pregnancy.[74]

### Air Embolism

Occasionally, venous air embolism occurs during pregnancy, presumably through the subplacental venous sinuses.[75] This disorder has been clearly documented during labor and delivery, during abortions, in patients with placenta previa, and in those engaging in orogenital sex during pregnancy.

## Acute Lung Injury in Pregnancy

### Aspiration Pneumonitis

Since Mendelson's[76] original report of 66 cases of gastric aspiration in 44,016 deliveries between 1932 and 1945 (an incidence of 0.15%), aspiration has continued to be a major cause of maternal morbidity and mortality. Increased intra-abdominal pressure due to the gravid uterus, the inhibitory effect of progesterone on the tone of the esophageal sphincter, and the assumption of the supine position for delivery all contribute. Eating during labor increases the volume of emesis.[79a] Aspiration of gastric contents with a pH of 2.5 or lower is known to cause chemical pneumonitis and permeability edema. Both in Mendelson's original report and today, about two thirds of cases of aspiration occur in the delivery suite. Emergency intubation of the obstetric airway is particularly difficult,[77] and failed intubation in the delivery suite occurs at a rate eight times that in the general surgical population.[78] To reduce the risk for aspiration and to minimize the chance of acid aspiration at intubation, oral administration of histamine-2 blockers or 0.3 mol/L sodium citrate administered before intubation, in conjunction with a formal airway assessment, is desirable. Identified risk factors in intubation include a high Mallampati class, a short neck, protruding maxillary incisors, and a receding mandible.[79]

### Acute Respiratory Distress Syndrome

Acute respiratory distress syndrome occurs relatively frequently in pregnancy; in one obstetric intensive care unit, it was the leading cause of maternal death during a 6-year period.[80] The three most common nonobstetric causes are pneumonia, sepsis, and aspiration. Common obstetric causes include chorioamnionitis, amniotic fluid embolism, and trophoblastic embolism.[81] Ventilator management is unaltered in pregnancy; prognosis also appears to be the same, with an anticipated 40% to 75% survival rate.[81, 81a]

# GYNECOLOGIC DISORDERS AND THE LUNGS

## Catamenial Pneumothorax

Lillington and colleagues[82] introduced in 1972 the term *catamenial pneumothorax* to describe the already reported phenomenon of spontaneous pneumothorax occurring within 24 to 72 hours after onset of menses. More than 100 cases have been reported. It appears to account for about 2.8% to 5.6% of spontaneous pneumothoraces in women,[83, 84] most often affecting women in the third or fourth decade of life. About 30% to 60% of cases are attributable to thoracic endometriosis, as judged by inspection at thoracotomy,[85] but other cases are more obscure in etiology, so that a number of theories have been advanced. First, during menstruation, the absence of the normal cervical mucus plug permits an open connection between ambient air and the abdominal cavity through the uterus and fallopian tubes. Air can move transdiaphragmatically through right-sided diaphragmatic fenestrations into the pleural space, as it sometimes does during abdominal laparoscopy. This may account for the condition's 90% to 95% right-sided predominance.[86] A second proposal is that high levels of prostaglandin $F_{2\alpha}$ during menstruation causes bronchospasm with attendant air trapping and pneumothorax, but wheezing is not a common symptom of this disorder. A third theory is that pleural blebs or bullae are more susceptible to rupture during menstruation because of hormonal changes,[85, 86] but visceral pleural leaks are rarely found at surgery.

For cases of endometriosis-associated pneumothorax, a trial of gonadotropin-releasing hormones is warranted if the phenomenon is repetitive but not life-threatening. Oral contraceptives, other progestational agents, and tubal ligation have also been used with some success. For cases not clearly associated with systemic endometriosis, thoracoscopy serves to define the etiology and can be used to achieve pleurodesis.

## Endometriosis

Endometriosis probably affects about 10% of women, shows no clear ethnic differences in prevalence, and is most commonly diagnosed at 25 to 29 years of age.[87] Although pelvic pain, dysmenorrhea, and infertility are its predominant manifestations, atypical locations, including diaphragmatic, pleural, and endobronchial sites, have been documented. As described previously, endometriosis can result in recurrent catamenial pneumothorax, but it also has been associated with right-sided pleural pain, pleuritic effusions, and hemothorax. Inspection at thoracotomy or thoracoscopy typically reveals blue-brown nodules on the pleural surface, sometimes in a "gunshot" distribution.[88] The absence of known pelvic endometriosis is not helpful in excluding the diagnosis because only 20% to 70% of cases have associated pelvic disease.[89] Rarely, the implants are found in lung parenchyma, accounting for catamenial hemoptysis. Most pleural and diaphragmatic disease is thought to arise from transdiaphragmatic spread from retrograde menses,[87] even when abdominal disease is not evident. Massive ascites is sometimes related, although only 27 cases have been reported.[90] Pneumothoraces may be attributed to cyclical sloughing of implants on key surfaces, like the visceral pleura,[85] or to air trapping from airway involvement or compression.[82] Pulmonary parenchymal disease may be embolic in origin, as it is presumed to be in the central nervous system. The diagnosis can be established only by biopsy showing the characteristic ectopic endometrial glands in involved sites. Medical therapy consists of progestational agents or gonadotropin-releasing hormones; surgical approaches include excision or local laser ablation.

### Lymphangioleiomyomatosis

Lymphangioleiomyomatosis (LAM) is a rare disorder, with only about 300 reported cases, that afflicts premenopausal women almost exclusively.[91, 92] It is fundamentally a disorder of smooth muscle proliferation that results in functional obstruction of vessels, lymphatics, and airways. (See Chapter 62 for a complete discussion of LAM.) Involvement of pulmonary vascular structures is responsible for the hemoptysis, whereas lymphatic obstruction accounts for the chylous effusions. Mediastinal and retroperitoneal lymphatic proliferation may be a feature of the disease as well. LAM is also associated with renal angiomyolipomas, another hamartomatous disorder. Conventional therapy has included oophorectomy or progestational agents, mainly medroxyprogesterone acetate. Lung transplantation has been performed in more than 60 patients with this disorder, but it has clearly recurred in some of them. Current research centers on growth factors and genetic factors that have been implicated in the disease's causation.[92]

### Trophoblastic Embolization

Trophoblastic embolism is a rare complication of hydatidiform mole. In one series, only 2.6% of 189 patients with hydatidiform mole had an embolic event, so that most episodes of respiratory distress in patients with molar gestations are not caused by embolic events but rather by pulmonary edema, anemia, or another complicating event.[93] Embolization, when it does occur, is most common at the time of evacuation of the mole. Chorionic neoplasms that arise during gestation are suggested by a large discrepancy between gestational date and uterine size and should be evaluated by transvaginal ultrasonography.[93a] Moles can also arise outside of gestation from the gonads of either sex.

## SUMMARY

Obstetric and gynecologic disorders alter the structure, hormonal milieu, and physiologic function of the lung in ways that determine and condition a variety of pulmonary diseases. Some disorders are unique to pregnancy, such as pulmonary edema associated with tocolytic therapy or amniotic fluid embolism. Other conditions, such as mitral stenosis, pulmonary embolism, or coccidiomycosis, are clearly exacerbated by gestation. Still others, such as obstructive airway disease and acute lung injury, are neither more frequent nor more severe in pregnancy but require expert care to optimize maternal and fetal outcome.

Disorders associated with gynecologic function and disease are rare but distinctive. The causation of many of them, like catamenial pneumothorax, thoracic endometriosis, and LAM, remains obscure but is linked to gonadal function. Because of their recurrent and sometimes malign natural history, they require a definitive diagnosis, which is facilitated by awareness of their distinctive features.

## References


1. Mabry RL: Rhinitis of pregnancy. South Med J 79:965–971, 1986.
2. Schatz M, Zieger RS: Diagnosis and management of rhinitis during pregnancy. Allergy Proc 9:545–554, 1988.
3. Weinberger SE, Weiss ST, Cohen WR, et al: Pregnancy and the lung: State of the art. Am Rev Respir Dis 121:559–581, 1980.
4. Contreras G, Gutierrez M, Berioza T, et al: Ventilatory drive and respiratory function in pregnancy. Am Rev Respir Dis 144:837–841, 1991.
5. Cugell DW, Frank NR, Gaensler EA: Pulmonary function in pregnancy. I. Serial observations in normal women. Am Rev Tuberc 67:568–597, 1953.
6. Gilroy RJ, Mangura BT, Lavietes MH: Ribcage and abdominal volume displacements during breathing in pregnancy. Am Rev Respir Dis 137:668–672, 1988.
7. Skatrud JB, Bempsey JA, Kaiser DG: Ventilatory response to medroxyprogesterone acetate in normal subjects: Time course and mechanism. J Appl Physiol 44:939, 1978.
8. Lucius H, Gahlenbeck HO, Kleine O, et al: Respiratory functions, buffer system, and electrolyte concentrations of blood during human pregnancy. Respir Physiol 9:311–317, 1970.
9. Pritchard JA, Baldwin RM, Dickey JC, et al: Blood volume changes in pregnancy and the puerperium. Am J Obstet Gynecol 84:1271–1281, 1962.
10. Silver HM, Seebeck M, Carlson R: Comparison of total blood volume in normal, preeclamptic and nonproteinuric gestational hypertensive pregnancy by simultaneous measurement of red blood cell and plasma volumes. Am J Obstet Gynecol 179:87–93, 1998.
11. Crapo RO: Normal cardiopulmonary physiology during pregnancy. Clin Obstet Gynecol 39:3–16, 1996.
12. Clark SL, Cotton DB, Lee W, et al: Central hemodynamic assessment of normal near term pregnancy. Am J Obstet Gynecol 161:1439–1442, 1989.
13. Hunter S, Robson SC: Adaptation of the maternal heart in pregnancy. Br Heart J 68:540–543, 1992.
14. Rizk N, Kalassian K, Gilligan T, et al: Obstetric complications in pulmonary and critical care medicine. Chest 110:791–809, 1996.

# 89 The Lungs and Neuromuscular Diseases

Thomas K. Aldrich, M.D. • Dudley F. Rochester, M.D.

Introduction
The Respiratory Muscles
- Upper Airway Muscles
- Ventilatory Muscles

Respiratory Dysfunction in Neuromuscular Disease
- Pulmonary Function
- Altered Ventilatory Drive
- Sleep-Related Breathing Disorders
- Aspiration and Cough
- Upper Airway Obstruction
- Kyphoscoliosis
- Pulmonary Embolism

Evaluation of Respiratory Function in Neuromuscular Disease
- Physical Examination
- Arterial Blood Gas Composition
- Pulmonary Function Tests
- Tests of Respiratory Muscle Strength
- Tests of Ventilatory Drive
- Sleep Studies

Diaphragmatic Paralysis
- Etiology
- Clinical Features
- Diagnosis
- Differential Diagnosis
- Treatment
- Postoperative Diaphragmatic Dysfunction

Spinal Cord Injury
- General Aspects
- High Cervical Spinal Cord Injury
- Middle and Lower Cervical Spinal Cord Injury
- Thoracic Spinal Cord Injury

Other Focal Respiratory Muscle Paralyses
- Hemiplegia
- Poliomyelitis

Diffuse Neuromuscular Disease
- Diseases of Acute Onset
- Diseases of Gradual Onset

Treatment of Ventilatory Failure
- Treatment of Underlying Disease
- Supportive Therapy

Syndromes of Inappropriate Respiratory Muscle Contraction
- Hiccups
- Respiratory Myoclonus
- Respiratory Dyskinesias
- Convulsive Disorders

Summary

## INTRODUCTION

Neuromuscular diseases have a major impact on the lungs and respiratory system. The principal respiratory manifestations of neuromuscular disease are pneumonia and respiratory failure.[1, 2] Few generalized neuromuscular diseases spare the respiratory muscles, and neuromuscular disease is a leading cause of ventilatory failure.

Neuromuscular diseases are associated with restrictive defects in ventilatory function, coming about because weakened respiratory muscles are unable to generate either the negative intrathoracic pressure necessary for full inspiration or the positive pressure needed for full expiration. Furthermore, patients with neuromuscular weakness tend to breathe with a rapid, shallow pattern that compromises their ventilatory function by increasing the ratio of dead space to tidal volume. Rapid, shallow breathing also predisposes to basilar atelectasis and perhaps more generalized microatelectasis. Finally, both children and adults with neuromuscular disease have abnormally low chest wall compliance, possibly because of chronically impaired chest wall mobility.[3]

Neuromuscular diseases can affect the respiratory muscles at multiple sites in the neuromuscular apparatus, from the spinal cord to the peripheral nerves, the neuromuscular junctions, and the muscles themselves. Table 89.1 lists the most commonly encountered neuromuscular diseases that affect respiration; several reviews provide

**Table 89.1 NEUROMUSCULAR DISEASES THAT INVOLVE THE RESPIRATORY MUSCLES, CLASSIFIED ACCORDING TO SITE OF NEUROLOGIC OR MUSCULAR INVOLVEMENT**

| SITE | DISEASE |
|---|---|
| Spinal cord | Trauma |
| | Space-occupying lesions |
| | Tumor |
| | Syringomyelia |
| | Anterior horn cell diseases |
| | Poliomyelitis |
| | Amyotrophic lateral sclerosis |
| | Blockade of inhibiting neurons |
| | Tetanus |
| | Strychnine poisoning |
| Motor nerves | Trauma |
| | Peripheral neuropathy |
| | Infectious |
| | Diabetes mellitus |
| | Chronic alcoholism |
| | Idiopathic |
| Neuromuscular junction | Myasthenia gravis |
| | Botulism |
| | Organophosphate poisoning |
| | Antibiotic toxicity |
| Muscle | Progressive dystrophies |
| | Myotonia |
| | Myopathy |
| | Inflammatory |
| | With collagen vascular disease |
| | Congenital |
| | Nutritional |
| | Metabolic |
| | Other |

more exhaustive coverage.[4–8] This chapter reviews the diseases that weaken or paralyze the respiratory muscles and their principal respiratory complications. Neurologic diseases that primarily affect the control of breathing are discussed in Chapters 80 and 81.

## THE RESPIRATORY MUSCLES

### Upper Airway Muscles

The muscles of respiration include not only the muscles in the neck, rib cage, and abdomen that perform the mechanical pumping function but also the muscles that maintain patency of the upper airway to allow airflow to proceed unimpeded.[9] During quiet breathing, this task is accomplished primarily by the vocal cord abductor muscles. At higher levels of ventilatory effort, elevators of the palate, dilators of the pharynx, retractors of the tongue, and even the masseters and the dilators of the nose become active. All help to maintain upper airway caliber and to prevent undue obstruction. The upper airway muscles derive their innervation from cranial nerves V, VII, IX, X, XI, and XII.

### Ventilatory Muscles

#### Inspiratory Muscles

The muscles of the ventilatory pump can be divided into inspiratory and expiratory muscles.[10–12] The principal inspiratory muscles are the diaphragm, the parasternal intercostal muscles, and the scalene muscles in the neck (Table 89.2). The sternomastoids and the lateral external intercostals also contribute to the inspiratory effort. Even the trapezius and serratus superior may assist the inspiratory effort under some circumstances.[12] The diaphragm is innervated by the phrenic nerves, which derive from cervical roots 3 to 5 in humans. The high level of innervation of this primary inspiratory muscle accounts for the survival of many victims of cervical spine injuries; if the diaphragm received its innervation from spinal roots closer to its anatomic position, virtually no inspiratory muscle activity would be left in a person who suffered a cervical spine transection.

#### Expiratory Muscles

The principal expiratory muscles are those of the anterolateral wall of the abdomen. The external and internal oblique muscles and the transversus abdominis are most important in terms of ventilation, whereas the rectus abdominis serves more to restrain the abdominal contents. The lateral internal intercostal muscles and the transversus thoracis (triangularis sterni) may also assist the expiratory effort.

#### Muscle Recruitment

Normally, during quiet supine breathing, the diaphragm alone is responsible for most of the inspiratory effort, whereas the expiratory phase is virtually entirely passive, with the necessary energy for expiratory airflow contributed by inward elastic recoil of the lungs and chest wall. Immediately on sitting or standing upright, the scalene and parasternal intercostal muscles come into play to

**Table 89.2 INNERVATION OF THE RESPIRATORY MUSCLES**

| MUSCLE GROUP | SPINAL CORD LEVEL | NERVE(S) |
|---|---|---|
| **Inspiratory muscles** | | |
| Diaphragm | C-3 to C-5 | Phrenic |
| Parasternal intercostals | T-1 to T-7 | Intercostal |
| Lateral external intercostals | T-1 to T-12 | Intercostal |
| Scalenes | C-4 to C-8 | |
| Sternocleidomastoid | XI, C-1, C-2 | |
| **Expiratory muscles** | | |
| Lateral internal intercostals | T-1 to T-12 | Intercostal |
| Rectus abdominis | T-7 to L-1 | Lumbar |
| External and internal obliques | T-7 to L-1 | Lumbar |
| Transversus abdominis | T-7 to L-1 | Lumbar |

enhance the generation of inspiratory vacuum, and low-level abdominal muscle activity begins to assist expiratory airflow. As higher levels of ventilatory effort become necessary, either because of a higher minute volume requirement or because of the need to overcome airway obstruction or a stiff respiratory system, additional muscle groups are recruited.

At high levels of ventilatory effort, abdominal muscle contraction at the end of expiration actually assists the subsequent inspiration. With abdominal muscle contraction, the diaphragm is pushed higher into the chest and lengthened, improving its position on its length-tension curve and providing a mechanical advantage. Moreover, at the very onset of inspiration, sudden relaxation of the abdominal muscles allows for inspiratory airflow by means of gravity and recoil pressure.

## RESPIRATORY DYSFUNCTION IN NEUROMUSCULAR DISEASE

### Pulmonary Function

Paralysis or paresis of some or all of the inspiratory muscles results in a reduced ability to generate intrathoracic vacuum. When severe, inspiratory muscle weakness causes ventilatory failure even in the absence of lung or chest wall dysfunction. When combined with lung or chest wall diseases, even relatively minor inspiratory muscle weakness can result in ventilatory failure.[13] Because elastic recoil of the respiratory system provides a driving pressure for expiratory airflow, weakness of the expiratory muscles causes less severe impairments of pulmonary mechanical and ventilatory function.

Stiffness (reduced compliance) of the lungs or chest wall is another common complication of neuromuscular disease.[3, 14, 15] The reduction in pulmonary compliance appears to be closely linked to the reduction in lung volumes that is characteristic of neuromuscular disease.[14] The cause may be microatelectasis, reduced surface tension, alterations in the elastic fibers of the pulmonary interstitium, or a combination of one or more of these factors, each of which may result from habitually low lung volumes.[14] Evidently, lung compliance falls only with relatively long-standing disease; the fact that lung compliance is virtually normal in curarized normal subjects[15] indicates that brief periods of respiratory muscle weakness are not sufficient to stiffen the lungs.

### Altered Ventilatory Drive

#### Increased Ventilatory Drive

In most cases of neuromuscular disease, even those complicated by ventilatory failure, respiratory drive is normal or somewhat increased[17–19]; the same phenomenon is observed in curarized normal subjects.[20] However, because of respiratory muscle weakness and abnormal chest wall mechanics, the ventilatory response to the increased drive is often inadequate.[21]

#### Decreased Ventilatory Drive

Patients with quadriplegia have reduced ventilatory drive, manifested as blunted ventilation and airway occlusion pressure responses to hypercapnia.[22] Ventilatory drive may be decreased in a few patients with congenital myopathy[23, 24] or myotonic dystrophy.[25] The cause may be abnormalities of carotid body or medullary chemoreceptor function. These patients usually have only mild to moderate respiratory muscle weakness, and their voluntary ventilatory capacity and ventilatory response to exercise are often well preserved. Hypercapnia may be present during wakefulness and sleep or only during sleep.

### Sleep-Related Breathing Disorders

Sleep disorders are common in neuromuscular diseases; 42% of an unselected neuromuscular disease clinic population[26] and 27.5% of a representative sample of patients with chronic quadriplegia[27] had respiratory disturbance indices greater than 15 per hour. High rates of primarily central apneas and hypopneas have been demonstrated in a wide variety of neuromuscular illnesses, including diaphragmatic paralysis,[28] postpolio syndrome,[29] amyotrophic lateral sclerosis,[30] and myotonic dystrophy.[31] Primarily obstructive apneas are common in quadriplegic patients[27] and in children with many types of neuromuscular disease.[32] Duchenne's muscular dystrophy is characterized by high rates of both obstructive and central apneas.[33, 34]

Hypopnea and oxygen desaturation are most apt to occur during rapid-eye-movement (REM) sleep, when the neck and rib cage muscles are inhibited.[35] The major consequences of sleep-disordered breathing in adults with neuromuscular disease are hypoxemia and the resulting impairments in right ventricular and cognitive function.[36] Bicarbonate retention, sometimes with associated worsening of daytime hypercapnia, may also result. Probably because obstructive sleep apnea and the consequent frequent arousals from sleep are not common in neuromuscular disease, hypersomnolence is often not present to alert the clinician to the presence of a sleep disturbance.[26]

Sleep disordered breathing is discussed in detail in Chapter 81.

### Aspiration and Cough

Many patients with neuromuscular diseases are susceptible to recurrent aspiration, especially in conditions with prominent bulbar involvement such as amyotrophic lateral sclerosis, myasthenia gravis, and multiple sclerosis. The consequence can be acute upper airway obstruction, acute pneumonia, or more chronic syndromes of lipoid pneumonia, basilar fibrosis, or bronchiectasis.

The importance of the expiratory muscles in the generation of an effective cough means that expiratory muscle weakness or paralysis seriously impairs clearance of secretions and compromises the defense against pulmonary infection. Effective coughing requires, first, an intact sensory limb of the cough reflex,[36a] and, second, functioning inspiratory, laryngeal, and expiratory muscles. To cough, one takes an initial deep inspiration, followed by adduction of the vocal cords. Subsequently, vigorous contraction of the abdominal muscles creates a strongly positive intrathoracic pressure.[37] The vocal cords are then abruptly opened narrowly, leading to explosive decompression of the thorax through a small orifice, with generation of rapid linear velocity of expiratory airflow.[38] Thus, weakness of any of the respiratory muscles, including the laryngeal muscles, inspiratory muscles, and especially expiratory muscles, compromises the ability to cough effectively.[39, 40] The physiology of cough and cough-related abnormalities is described further in Chapter 21.

## Upper Airway Obstruction

Patients with neuromuscular disease are at risk for upper airway obstruction from aspirated food or foreign bodies. In addition, patients with weakness of bulbar muscles are susceptible to a functional type of upper airway obstruction caused by inadequate abduction of upper airway structures during the inspiratory phase of respiration.[41, 42]

## Kyphoscoliosis

Because of critical and unbalanced weakness of postural muscles of the spine, kyphoscoliosis is a common complication of certain neuromuscular diseases, particularly poliomyelitis and Duchenne's muscular dystrophy. When severe, kyphoscoliosis results in major increases in the oxygen cost of breathing; the combination of respiratory muscle weakness and kyphoscoliosis results in particular susceptibility to ventilatory failure.

## Pulmonary Embolism

Pulmonary embolism is a constant threat to any immobilized patient, including patients with neuromuscular disease. Patients with spinal cord injury and resulting paralysis appear to be at particularly high risk; Myllynen and associates[43] found evidence for deep vein thrombosis by iodine ($^{125}I$)–labeled fibrinogen scanning in 23 consecutive patients with spinal cord injury, and pulmonary embolism occurred in 9%. Prophylactic use of anticoagulation is highly effective and, although associated with significant risk of hemorrhagic complications, reduces overall mortality rates.[44]

# EVALUATION OF RESPIRATORY FUNCTION IN NEUROMUSCULAR DISEASE

## Physical Examination

The level of consciousness and the pattern of breathing may provide clues to the risk for aspiration or to the presence or absence of impending or overt hypoxemia or acidosis. Dyspnea and tachypnea at rest are signs of severe ventilatory dysfunction. The lung examination may reveal evidence of complicating atelectasis or pneumonia, or it may demonstrate differential expansion of the lungs, as in unilateral diaphragmatic paralysis. The accessible respiratory muscles, sternomastoids, scalenes, intercostals, and abdominals may be palpated directly to assess their level of activity and the presence or absence of atrophy. Inspiratory motion of the abdomen, best assessed in the supine position, often provides information regarding the adequacy of diaphragmatic contraction. Paradoxical, inward movement of the abdomen with inspiration indicates weak diaphragmatic contraction because of paresis or fatigue.[45, 46]

## Arterial Blood Gas Composition

Pulse oximetry is widely used to detect hypoxemia and is of value when there is nocturnal hypopnea or apnea. However, oximetric measurement of arterial oxyhemoglobin saturation (arterial $So_2$) is an inadequate test of awake ventilatory function because it cannot discriminate between hypoventilation and other causes of hypoxemia. Any patient with neuromuscular disease who is suspected of having impending or overt ventilatory failure should have an arterial blood gas analysis with measurement of pH and partial pressures of carbon dioxide (arterial $Pco_2$) and oxygen (arterial $Po_2$).

## Imaging Techniques

The chest radiograph provides essential information regarding the presence or absence of complicating pneumonia, atelectasis, kyphoscoliosis, or other conditions. Occasionally, specific neuromuscular problems, such as unilateral phrenic nerve palsy, are suggested by the finding of an elevated hemidiaphragm. Because apparent or real elevation of a hemidiaphragm may also result from a number of unilateral pulmonary or pleural abnormalities, such as lobar atelectasis, diaphragmatic herniation, or subpulmonic pleural effusion, it is often useful to test the functional status of the phrenic nerve and diaphragm, by using fluoroscopic or, preferably, ultrasonic[47, 48] monitoring of diaphragmatic motion. During a sniff, which represents a brief but powerful contraction of the diaphragm, the healthy hemidiaphragm descends sharply while the resulting intrathoracic negative pressure causes the paralyzed side to rise.

## Pulmonary Function Tests

Testing of pulmonary function is described in detail in Chapter 28. The characteristic finding in most neuromuscular diseases is of a restrictive pattern with well-preserved forced expiratory flow rates[49] because lung recoil is often increased and the airways are usually patent. On spirometry, the ratio of forced expiratory volume in 1 second to forced vital capacity ($FEV_1/FVC$) is usually normal or even higher than normal. The FVC is reduced owing to weakness of inspiratory or expiratory muscles, coupled with decreased compliance of both lung and chest wall. A decrease of 25% or more in FVC shifting from upright to supine is a sign of diaphragmatic weakness.[50]

Maximum voluntary ventilation (MVV) is usually reduced as much as or more than the vital capacity (VC). Patients with bulbar involvement and weakness of muscles responsible for patency of the upper airways may show flattening of the inspiratory limb of the flow–volume loop suggestive of variable extrathoracic upper airway obstruction. This pattern is seen only when inspiratory muscle function is reasonably good, and similar patterns may be seen in patients with inspiratory muscle weakness and in those who make a poor effort.[41] Fallat and coworkers[51] have pointed out that reductions in FVC and MVV by as much as 50% are frequently missed by routine clinical evaluation; therefore, all patients with neuromuscular disease should undergo pulmonary and respiratory muscle function evaluation by objective tests.

Measurement of lung volumes shows that total lung capacity (TLC) is often reduced, mainly from inspiratory muscle weakness. Residual volume (RV) is increased, not because of airway obstruction, but because weak expiratory muscles cannot overcome the outward recoil of the chest wall below functional residual capacity (FRC).[13] Indeed, elevation of RV in the absence of airway obstruction is a sensitive test for weakness of the expiratory muscles.[52] The diffusing capacity for carbon monoxide ($DL_{CO}$) may be normal or low, but it is normal when corrected for the lung volume at which it is measured ($DL_{CO}$/VA).

The motion of the chest and abdomen can also be analyzed by using magnetometry or respiratory inductance plethysmography. These techniques not only can detect paradoxical inspiratory inward movement of the abdomen due to diaphragmatic weakness[53] but also can show asynchronous breathing patterns that result from recruitment of neck inspiratory and abdominal expiratory muscles.[54] These patterns are characteristic of increased ventilatory drive necessitated either by increased work of breathing or severe muscle weakness.

## Tests of Respiratory Muscle Strength

In neuromuscular diseases, the respiratory muscles are almost always affected, and their weakness may be more prominent than is weakness of limb muscles. Because pulmonary function abnormalities occur only when respiratory muscle weakness is severe, it is desirable to test respiratory muscle strength directly. The simplest method is to measure the maximal inspiratory and expiratory pressures (PImax and PEmax) that can be produced by voluntary efforts against a closed airway. The inspiratory effort for PImax should be made after exhaling down to a low lung volume, whereas the expiratory effort for PEmax should be made after inhaling as fully as possible.[55] To avoid spuriously strong PImax results due to suction by pharyngeal muscles, a small leak is provided in the apparatus. For PEmax, a large-bore mouthpiece with lips pursed inside is recommended; if the patient uses a regular mouthpiece, the cheeks should be held rigid with the hands.[56]

The results of both PImax and PEmax are strongly influenced by lung volume because respiratory system elastic recoil provides additional positive pressure below and negative pressure above FRC, because translation of intramuscular tension to pressure is affected by lung volume, and because muscle tension–generating ability (strength) is markedly influenced by muscle fiber length, which, in turn, depends on lung volume.[57] Thus, when PImax or PEmax is measured, lung volume must be controlled.[55]

Unfortunately, the results of maximal respiratory pressure tests are highly dependent on technique and patient effort.[55] They are even more influenced by poor effort than are the results of spirometry, and reproducibility of maximal pressures does not verify that maximal efforts have been made.[58] Nevertheless, PImax and PEmax provide "lower-limit" estimates of inspiratory and expiratory muscle strength, which are usually adequate for clinical decision making.

One way to get around the problem of patient effort is to record the pressures inside the chest (Pes) by using an esophageal balloon catheter. Inspiratory muscle strength can be assessed from the Pes recorded when the subject sniffs sharply,[59] and expiratory pressure can be assessed by recording Pes during a cough.[60] A second balloon catheter can be advanced into the stomach to measure gastric pressure (Pga). The pressure across the diaphragm, transdiaphragmatic pressure (Pdi), can then be recorded as the difference between Pga and Pes, and the strength of diaphragmatic contraction can be assayed as the change in Pdi during an inspiratory effort. Voluntary maximal change in Pdi, generated by maximal inspiratory efforts against a closed airway, is normally greater than 100 cm $H_2O$, at RV or FRC. To determine whether the patient may be using a pattern of breathing that predisposes to fatigue, it is useful to measure Pes and Pdi during a tidal breath. When Pes or Pdi during a tidal breath is more than 40% of PImax, inspiratory muscle fatigue is likely to ensue.

To avoid the discomfort of esophageal and gastric balloon catheter placement, it may be possible to use substitute sites. For example, the pressure recorded by means of a catheter in the urinary bladder is a reasonable estimate of Pga, provided the catheter is clamped and the bladder is partially full.[61] Central venous pressure may not be as good an indicator of Pes because the pressure amplitude is damped.[62]

A more objective test, at least specifically for diaphragm strength, is to measure Pes and Pdi (or less optimally, occluded mouth pressure) in response to electrical[63, 64] or magnetic[65, 66] stimulation of the phrenic nerves. In normal subjects, twitch Pdi measurements average about 25 to 35 cm $H_2O$.[66] Electromyographic diaphragm action potentials elicited by the phrenic nerve stimuli can be detected with surface or esophageal electrodes to provide further information regarding the integrity of the phrenic nerve and neuromuscular junction. The normal value for phrenic nerve latency has been determined for percutaneous electrical stimulation and cutaneous chest wall action potential recording to be between 6 and 9 msec. In the event that Pdi cannot be measured, one can measure PImax. Although not as specific for diaphragmatic weakness, PImax is reduced in parallel with Pdi in the presence of diaphragmatic paralysis.

Magnetic stimulation is better tolerated than is electrical stimulation, but because both the phrenic and other nerves are stimulated, it is not as specific for the diaphragm.[66] The usual stimulation is a single electrical or magnetic impulse, which produces a twitch contraction of the diaphragm. Pdi measured during a twitch is much lower than maximal Pdi, but patients with neuromuscular diseases that involve the phrenic nerve or diaphragm have distinctly subnormal values.

## Tests of Ventilatory Drive

Ventilatory drive can be assessed by measuring minute ventilation when the subject is inhaling a gas mixture that contains a low concentration of carbon dioxide (hypercapnic response) or one that contains a subnormal concentration of oxygen (hypoxic response). The problem with these tests is that there is a wide range of normal responses, and in the presence of muscle weakness, the ventilatory responses to hypercapnic and hypoxic stimuli may be abnormally low even though neural drive is normal or increased. To circumvent this difficulty, the mouth occlusion pressure can be measured when the mouthpiece is occluded shortly after the beginning of inspiration. The pressure measured in the first 0.1 second after the occlusion ($P_{0.1}$) is not influenced by reflex or voluntary effort, or by airflow. The $P_{0.1}$ can be recorded during quiet breathing or during the administration of a hypercapnic or hypoxic challenge. Tests for control of breathing are described in detail in Chapter 8.

### Sleep Studies

Patients with neuromuscular diseases may have a variety of sleep-related breathing abnormalities, and clinicians should be alert to the possibility. Patients may be screened by recording arterial $So_2$ during sleep by means of a pulse oximeter. If there is any reason to suspect that a patient with neuromuscular disease has abnormal breathing during sleep, the optimal test is a full polysomnographic study to identify sleep stages and presence or absence of respiratory airflow as well as the frequency and duration of desaturation. When possible, it is also useful to record the movements of the chest and abdomen by using the respiratory inductive plethysmograph and to measure esophageal pressures by using a balloon catheter. Sleep studies are described in detail in Chapter 81

## DIAPHRAGMATIC PARALYSIS

### Etiology

Paralysis of one or both hemidiaphragms, often called *eventration of the diaphragm,* is a common clinical finding. A leading cause of unilateral phrenic palsy is open heart surgery; injury to a phrenic nerve occurs in 2% to 20% of such patients.[67, 68] Left-sided involvement is most frequently seen, but right-sided phrenic palsy and bilateral phrenic palsy are not uncommon. In most cases, it is thought that the portion of the phrenic nerve that courses along the pericardium is injured by the effects of the cold cardioplegia solution. In other cases, intraoperative stretching of the phrenic nerves may be at fault. Thoracotomy, pleurectomy, and even pneumonectomy are generally not accompanied by the risk for phrenic nerve injury,[69] but mediastinal and esophageal procedures do carry that risk. Attempts have been made to evaluate the incidence of phrenic nerve injury after lung transplantation. A retrospective review of 185 transplantations detected only 6 confirmed cases of phrenic injury,[70] but many subclinical or undiagnosed cases may have been missed. In two smaller prospective series, the risk was assessed as 7.4%[71] and 29.6%,[72] respectively.

Other traumatic causes of partial or complete paralysis of phrenic nerves or their roots include manipulation of the cervical spine,[73] penetrating injuries or surgery of the neck or thorax,[74] jugular or subclavian venous catheterization,[75] and birth trauma.[76] The phrenic nerves or their roots can also be injured by compression or by destruction by space-occupying lesions.[77] Examples include cervical osteoarthritis, aortic aneurysm, substernal thyroid, and bronchogenic or mediastinal tumors. Although intrathoracic malignancy is the most feared diagnosis when unilateral diaphragmatic paresis is detected, in a series of 142 cases, it accounted for only 5%.[77]

Local inflammatory conditions, such as pleurisy and pneumonia, and specific inflammations of the phrenic nerves, as in herpes zoster infection or vasculitis,[78] can also injure one or both phrenic nerves. Phrenic neuropathy has been reported 7 months[79] and 30 years[80] after mediastinal radiotherapy. The phrenic nerves are often involved in peripheral neuropathy, which appears to be particularly common in diabetes.[81] Neuralgic amyotrophy, a relatively common but poorly understood peripheral nerve disorder that usually affects the brachial plexus, may also cause unilateral or bilateral paralysis of the diaphragm.[82] Bilateral diaphragmatic paralysis may be the initial manifestation of neuromuscular diseases that are usually generalized, such as multiple sclerosis,[83] anterior horn cell disease,[84] and myopathies, particularly acid maltase deficiency.[45] In many cases of diaphragmatic paralysis, no definite cause can be established.[77]

### Clinical Features

The clinical manifestations of diaphragmatic paresis depend on the severity of the weakness, whether it is unilateral or bilateral, the rapidity of its onset, and the presence or absence of other respiratory illness. The features are also markedly different in infants as compared with older children and adults.

#### Unilateral Paralysis

More than half of adult patients with unilateral hemidiaphragmatic paralysis are entirely symptom free,[77] and another quarter experience only mild exertional dyspnea. Others experience generalized muscle fatigue, chest wall pain, cough, or dyspnea at rest. A few have severe exertional dyspnea, often associated with chest pain, and a few experience dyspnea at rest, especially if they lie with the paralyzed side down. Occasionally, a transient episode of dyspnea identifies the onset of phrenic palsy. Not surprisingly, symptoms are more common in patients with preexisting lung disease.[85]

The prognosis of adult patients with unilateral diaphragmatic paralysis is generally good, primarily because of the relatively mild pulmonary function impairment, but also because of the development of compensatory mechanisms and, in many patients, partial or full recovery by the injured phrenic nerve. Two series of patients have been studied after deliberate ablation of one phrenic nerve by local anesthesia[86] or by surgical transection.[87] The pulmonary function deficit was severe in normal subjects immediately after the phrenic nerve was anesthetized[86] but less severe over a 6- to 12-month interval after phrenic section.[87] Studies of one patient before, immediately after, and 7 weeks after right phrenic crush demonstrated an adaptive increase in the contraction characteristics of the remaining, nonparalyzed inspiratory muscles.[88]

When lung disease coexists with unilateral diaphragmatic paralysis, the prognosis is not so favorable. Lisboa and coworkers[85] reported that pulmonary function was far worse among a group of patients with unilateral diaphragmatic paralysis and concomitant lung disease than in a group with unilateral paralysis alone. We calculated from their data that two of the seven patients with lung disease had excessively high diaphragm pressure–time indices at rest and would therefore be at risk for diaphragmatic fatigue.

Regional ventilation and perfusion are mildly abnormal when one side of the diaphragm is paralyzed,[87, 88] primarily adjacent to the paralyzed hemidiaphragm. In the supine position, arterial $Po_2$ generally decreases significantly, and regional lung function is more abnormal than in the upright position. In the lateral decubitus position, perfusion of the involved side decreases when that side is uppermost and increases when it is lowermost. Exercise capacity is mildly to moderately reduced, and arterial $Po_2$ tends to increase with exercise.

### Bilateral Paralysis

Unlike unilateral phrenic palsy, bilateral paralysis of the diaphragm almost always causes severe symptoms, abnormalities of pulmonary function, and morbidity in adults and children as well as in infants. Typically, there is severe exertional dyspnea, and patients experience marked orthopnea. Many patients develop ventilatory failure, cor pulmonale, atelectasis, or pneumonia. The manifestations of bilateral diaphragmatic paralysis are much worse in the supine position, in which the beneficial gravitational effect of the weight of the abdominal contents to prevent paradoxical motion of the diaphragm is lost. As a result of the exaggerated respiratory dysfunction in the supine position, sleep disturbances are common. Furthermore, during REM sleep, activity of respiratory muscles other than the diaphragm is markedly reduced.[33, 35] Consequently, when the diaphragm is paralyzed, REM sleep is associated with particularly severe ventilatory dysfunction. Nocturnal hypoxia and worsening hypercapnia are common in patients with bilateral diaphragmatic paralysis, leading to anxiety, daytime somnolence, and morning headaches. In severe cases, confusion, memory loss, and motor impairment may occur.

The prognosis of bilateral diaphragmatic paralysis depends on the nature of the underlying disease. Enhanced use of neck and rib cage inspiratory muscles allows for better pulmonary function in the upright position, but as long as the diaphragm is weak, patients still have severe symptoms when lying down. If the nerve injury is not due to a progressive, generalized neuropathic process, phrenic nerve and diaphragm function often recover, albeit slowly, often only after 2 years.[68]

### Diaphragmatic Paralysis in Infants

Infants are much more severely affected by either unilateral or bilateral diaphragmatic paralysis than are older children and adults. Because their chest walls are relatively compliant, chest wall inspiratory muscles are needed to stabilize the chest. The inability of infants to sit up accentuates the postural problems of diaphragmatic paralysis, and the relative predominance of REM sleep reduces the ability of the other inspiratory muscles to compensate for the loss of one and especially both hemidiaphragms. Infants are particularly susceptible to atelectasis, pneumonia, and ventilatory failure even in unilateral paralysis, and they virtually always suffer ventilatory failure when the paralysis is bilateral.[76]

## Diagnosis

Physical examination of patients with *unilateral paralysis* of the diaphragm reveals dullness to percussion and absent breath sounds over the lower chest on the involved side. Frequently, the compressed lung gives rise to crackles on auscultation just above the area of dullness. On deep palpation, it may be appreciated that the inspiratory excursions of the abdomen are less on the paralyzed side than the healthy side. Paradoxically, the excursions of the lower rib cage may be greater on the side of the paralyzed hemidiaphragm (M. H. Williams, Jr., personal communication). When the normal hemidiaphragm contracts, the resultant positive abdominal pressure exerts an inspiratory effect on the lower rib cage through the zone of apposition. In unilateral diaphragmatic paralysis, this effect is greater on the paralyzed side because the zone of apposition is larger under the elevated paralyzed hemidiaphragm. The diagnosis of unilateral paralysis of the diaphragm is often suggested by the finding of an elevated hemidiaphragm on the chest radiograph, but that is a nonspecific finding. The sniff test, optimally monitored by ultrasonography,[47, 48] is usually diagnostic.

The detection of *bilateral paralysis* is much easier than of unilateral paralysis on physical examination when the condition is suspected, but it is much harder by imaging techniques because a comparison of the behavior of one side with the other does not help. The hallmark finding on physical examination is paradoxic, inward movement of the abdomen with inspiration[45]; that is, instead of the normal pattern of synchronized outward inspiratory movement of both chest and abdomen, the abdomen moves inward when the upper chest moves outward. In some cases, recruitment of the abdominal expiratory muscles masks diaphragmatic paralysis by restoring the inward movement of the abdomen on expiration and by permitting a passive outward movement of the abdomen in early inspiration, when the expiratory muscles relax. The chest radiograph shows a totally nonspecific elevation of both hemidiaphragms. Comparisons of inspiratory and expiratory chest radiographs, and even the sniff test, are often equivocal because the observer cannot rely on a comparison of the two sides, and must accurately identify both the inspiratory phase of respiration and the diaphragm's motion in that phase. Moreover, if the abdominal muscles actively contract during the expiratory phase, the diaphragm is forced upward, and its subsequent passive descent during the inspiratory phase may lead to a falsely normal examination. Thus, unless careful observations are made of inspiratory and expiratory timing and the presence or absence of abdominal muscle activity, the sniff test and its modifications are often misleading.

### Pulmonary and Ventilatory Function

Pulmonary function tests usually show a mild restrictive process in unilateral paralysis (Table 89.3). In bilateral paralysis, severe restriction is the rule, with reductions in VC and MVV averaging 55% and 45%, respectively, owing to inspiratory muscle weakness. In contrast to the findings in unilateral paralysis, the FRC and RV are decreased by 35% to 40%, respectively, because of pulmonary atelectasis. A striking finding is the difference in VC measured in the supine as compared with the upright position; supine VC is usually less than 75% of the upright value in severe bilateral diaphragmatic weakness.[89]

### Phrenic Nerve Stimulation

The most specific tests for diaphragmatic weakness or paralysis are electrophysiologic assessments of phrenic nerve competence and measurements of transdiaphragmatic pressure, described previously. If there is a neuropathic cause of diaphragm paralysis, twitch pressures are reduced or absent, and the phrenic nerve latency is prolonged, or action potentials may be absent after stimulation of the involved nerve. In myopathy, the latency and action potentials may be normal, but the mechanical responses (twitch pressures and fluoroscopically visible movements) are reduced or absent. The sensitivity and specificity of these tests are not established. Although not as specific for diaphragmatic weakness as is Pdi, PImax is reduced in parallel with Pdi in the presence of diaphragmatic paralysis.

## Differential Diagnosis

### Pleural and Pulmonary Disease

Pleural effusions, especially when subpulmonic, may produce radiographic images resembling either unilateral or bilateral diaphragmatic paralysis; lateral decubitus chest radiograms, ultrasonographic examination of the chest, or both can resolve this question. Intrapulmonary processes that reduce the compliance of the lung mimic diaphragmatic paralysis because they reduce the inspiratory excursion of the diaphragm. Atelectasis, pneumonia, edema, and fibrosis may be unilateral or bilateral. Usually, such conditions are readily apparent on chest radiographs. In most cases, the diagnosis can be established by careful physical examination, coupled with inspiratory and expiratory radiograms or fluoroscopic examination to image the diaphragm.

**Table 89.3 COMPARISON OF PULMONARY AND RESPIRATORY MUSCLE FUNCTION IN UNILATERAL AND BILATERAL PARALYSIS OF THE DIAPHRAGM***

| Variable | Unilateral | Bilateral |
|---|---|---|
| VC | 75 | 45 |
| TLC | 85 | 55 |
| FRC | 100 | 60 |
| RV | 100 | 55 |
| $FEV_1$ | 70 | 50 |
| PImax (cm $H_2O$) | −70 | −10 to −20 |
| Pdimax (cm $H_2O$) | 70 | 0 to −10 |

*Values expressed as percentage of predicted normal value unless otherwise specified.

VC = vital capacity; TLC = total lung capacity; FRC = functional residual capacity; RV = residual volume; $FEV_1$ = forced expiratory volume in 1 second; PImax and Pdimax = maximal inspiratory and transdiaphragmatic pressures, respectively.

### Other Neuromuscular Disease

Neuromuscular diseases that may be confused with diaphragmatic paralysis include alveolar hypoventilation caused by brain-stem or high cervical spinal disease, and diffuse respiratory muscle weakness consequent to anterior horn cell, neuromuscular junction, or muscle disorders.

Patients with central alveolar hypoventilation frequently have normal respiratory muscle strength, lung volumes, and maximal ventilatory capacity; that is, they are capable of normal voluntary ventilatory efforts, but automatic control is absent, as demonstrated by lack of ventilatory response to hypercapnia or hypoxia (Chapter 80).

The most reliable diagnostic methods for bilateral diaphragmatic paralysis are the observation of inward inspiratory movement of the abdomen in the supine position, fluoroscopic determination of upward movement of the diaphragm while the patient makes a full inspiration to TLC, and measurement of Pdi during the same maneuver.

## Treatment

### Unilateral Paralysis

When unilateral diaphragm paralysis is detected, a primary goal in management is to exclude serious intrathoracic pathology, such as an infection or a malignant tumor in or adjacent to the mediastinum. In most cases, no such disease is found, and no practical therapy for the diaphragmatic palsy is available. Fortunately, the relatively mild symptoms and favorable prognoses of such cases do not require aggressive treatment.

In some instances, surgical treatment is indicated. Infants with unilateral paralysis are much more severely compromised than are similarly affected adults, and surgical plication of the paralyzed hemidiaphragm can often ameliorate ventilatory failure by improving ipsilateral lung expansion and preventing excessive inefficient flailing of the paralyzed hemidiaphragm.[76] A few cases of plication of unilaterally paralyzed hemidiaphragms have been reported in adults.[90] Surgical repair of injured phrenic nerves has been accomplished in two cases.[91,92] Autologous nerve transplantation restored phrenic nerve function in a child with phrenic nerve palsy[93] and made diaphragm pacing possible in a patient with phrenic motoneuron damage.[94]

### Bilateral Paralysis

In bilateral phrenic paralysis, some form of treatment is almost always required. Plication of both hemidiaphragms or of the more severely affected hemidiaphragm is often recommended for infants.[95] The benefits are improved expansion of the lower lobes and prevention of the paradoxical motion, with resulting improved efficiency of the remaining innervated inspiratory muscles. Because many cases of phrenic nerve injury are reversible, especially those induced by trauma, and because it is likely that plication may interfere with the subsequent function of a reinnervated hemidiaphragm, bilateral plication should be reserved for cases of irreversible denervation with substantial paradoxical motion documented by fluoroscopy.

Many patients with bilateral diaphragmatic paralysis require mechanical support of ventilation. Often, this can be provided without tracheostomy by a rocking bed,[96] a negative-pressure body respirator such as the cuirass respirator,[76] nasal continuous positive airway pressure (CPAP),[95] or intermittent positive-pressure ventilation by nasal[97] or oral mask.[98] These devices are most useful when carbon dioxide retention occurs only at night. Electrophrenic respiration is not an option because this form of therapy depends on intact phrenic nerves and diaphragm muscle. A nerve that is stimulated below the site of transection may respond to pacing for a short period, but it eventually atrophies, and the threshold for activation of the muscle itself by direct stimulation is too high for pacing to be effective.

## Postoperative Diaphragmatic Dysfunction

### Clinical Features

A relatively mild and temporary form of isolated diaphragmatic dysfunction occurs in patients who undergo upper abdominal surgery[99, 100] or thoracotomy.[101] After upper abdominal surgery, the TLC, VC, $FEV_1$, tidal volume, and tidal and maximal Pdi values decrease, and respiratory rate increases. Recovery occurs over 2 to 7 days. Postoperative diaphragmatic dysfunction undoubtedly contributes to atelectasis, hypoxemia, and increased risk for surgical morbidity. Thus, measures designed to inflate the lungs and to improve inspiratory effort, such as incentive spirometry, and, in severe cases, CPAP, are indicated.

### Pathophysiology

Postoperative diaphragmatic dysfunction does not appear to be mediated by pain because it has been shown not to be abolished by opiate epidural anesthesia.[100] Animal studies show that anesthesia and lower abdominal surgery do not cause postoperative diaphragmatic dysfunction, whereas thoracotomy and upper abdominal surgery do.[102, 103] It is possible that local irritation of the diaphragm evokes afferent inhibitory neural activity. Certainly, the phrenic nerves contain plentiful afferent fibers,[104] and stimulation of these fibers, at least under some circumstances, has an inhibitory effect on ventilation.[104] Furthermore, phrenic afferents may be highly selective in their inhibitory effects, reducing only ipsilateral phrenic nerve activity.[104] Thus, local inflammation or pressure may activate free nerve endings in the diaphragm, with resulting suppression of diaphragmatic activity, while ventilatory drive to the other inspiratory muscles remains intact.

# SPINAL CORD INJURY

## General Aspects

Serious impairment of spinal cord function can result from any of a number of causes, but about three quarters of the injuries are traumatic, from motor vehicle, industrial accidents, sports accidents, or gunshot wounds. Other causes include diabetes mellitus, epidural abscesses, tumors, especially metastatic neoplasms, vascular accidents, transverse myelitis, and syringomyelia. Obviously, the onset of the disability is sudden in the case of injury, whereas it may be subacute or chronic in some of the other conditions. Nonetheless, the ultimate outcome is similar, and we focus here on spinal cord traumatic injury as the primary example of this type of neuromuscular disease.

Spinal cord injury is a catastrophic event with multiple severe consequences. Many manifestations that do not primarily involve the respiratory system nevertheless exert indirect effects on respiration. Major nonrespiratory problems include the shattering psychological impact of the disease, with severe depression; immobility; loss of bowel, bladder, and sexual functions; decubitus ulcers; and infections of the skin and urinary tract. These conditions, and sometimes the measures used to treat them, predispose to malnutrition, wasting of nonparalyzed muscles, and pulmonary infection, especially pneumonia, which is the most common cause of death.[3, 105]

Because the effects of high cervical spinal cord injury differ substantially from injuries at lower levels, we consider them separately.

## High Cervical Spinal Cord Injury

### Clinical Features

Injuries above the C-3 level produce nearly complete respiratory muscle paralysis. These patients are virtually unable to breathe or talk, and they cannot cough. Lesions that disrupt the reticulospinal pathways in the ventral aspect of the upper cervical cord eliminate automatic control of breathing, except to the limited extent that the sternomastoid and trapezius muscles receive innervation from the spinal accessory (XI) nerve. Such injuries, therefore, produce a syndrome that resembles central alveolar hypoventilation. Lesions that disrupt the more lateral cortical spinal pathways make it impossible to execute voluntary respiratory movements, but automatic control is preserved.[106] In traumatic injury, both sets of pathways are apt to be involved, so that voluntary and involuntary respiratory functions are minimal or absent.

The symptoms are dominated by asphyxia, dyspnea that may be aggravated in the sitting position, and difficulty with secretions. The physical examination during brief suspension of mechanical ventilation reveals either apnea or marked inspiratory contraction of the sternomastoid and trapezius muscles, which hypertrophy as other muscles become atrophic. Breath sounds are faint, and there may be basilar crackles. There is no diaphragmatic excursion with respiration, but the diaphragm does descend on changing from the supine to the sitting posture. The abdominal muscles are flaccid, and the patient is unable to cough.

### Pulmonary Function

Pulmonary function data are sparse for patients with high spinal cord injury. Spontaneous tidal volume varies from 60 to 500 mL.[6] The VC is 20% normal at best, and expiratory reserve volume is nearly zero. FRC is reduced, probably primarily because of an underlying atelectasis but also because the absent tone of the chest wall muscles reduces the recoil pressure.

Patients with high spinal cord injury recruit the trapezius, platysma, mylohyoid, and sternohyoid muscles to assist the sternomastoid muscles with inspiration.[107] Their synchronous contraction pulls the sternum cranially, expanding the upper rib cage, and the abdominal and lateral rib cage diameters decrease.

### Ventilatory Support

Before the advent of phrenic nerve pacing, most patients who survived high spinal cord injuries required permanent mechanical ventilatory support. Some highly motivated patients learn to perform glossopharyngeal breathing[108]; that is, they use tongue, cheek, pharyngeal, and laryngeal muscles in a coordinated way to inject successive small boluses of air into the trachea, sometimes achieving enough tidal volume to talk and to breathe without support for brief periods. Glossopharyngeal breathing also enables patients to inhale deeply from time to time, to prevent atelectasis and to improve the effectiveness of coughing.

Spinal cord injuries above C-3 denervate but do not destroy the cell bodies of the phrenic motoneuron pool. These neurons lie at levels C-3, C-4, and C-5 in humans, with the highest concentration at C-4. Because the phrenic nerves and their cell bodies in the anterior horn of the spinal cord are intact, they can be stimulated electrically. Details of the procedure for electrophrenic respiration have been summarized by Glenn and associates[109] and are reviewed later (see later section on treatment of ventilatory failure).

## Middle and Lower Cervical Spinal Cord Injury

### Clinical Features

One of the remarkable features of middle to lower cervical spinal cord injury is the extent to which the inspiratory and expiratory deficits fail to correlate with the level of injury, as assessed from peripheral sensory and motor examination. We hypothesize that several factors account for this discrepancy, not the least of which is the fact that trauma produces anatomically irregular rather than surgically precise lesions of the spinal cord. It would appear that some injuries are complete, whereas others produce only partial interruptions of spinal neural pathways.[110] Other mechanisms include recruitment of muscles not normally having phasic respiratory function, progression or partial recovery from the original injury,[111] variability in the functional status of the nonparalyzed musculature, and injury-induced, or coexistent, pulmonary mechanical abnormalities.[111]

### Respiratory Muscle Function

Both PEmax and PImax tend to be more severely impaired in mid-cervical injuries, as opposed to lower cervical or thoracic injuries, but the range of values at each injury level is so large that no statistically significant differences have been shown as a function of the level of injury. At all levels of injury, PEmax is more severely impaired than is PImax. Consequently, although the cough reflex appears to be intact,[36a] coughing is severely hampered; peak expiratory flow during cough is weakly, but significantly, correlated with the level of injury.[112]

One would expect that quadriplegic patients could not exhale below the resting, end-expiratory position (FRC) because their expiratory muscles are paralyzed. Expiratory reserve volume (ERV), however, is actually moderately well preserved, averaging 0.5 L in the 14 cases described by De Troyer and associates.[113] The mechanism of expiration is contraction of the clavicular portion of the pectoralis major muscle, with some additional help from the cranial portion of the serratus anterior muscle.[113] The latissimus dorsi and teres major muscles assist by fixating the position of the humerus. The abdominal muscles are electrically silent, but the diaphragm contracts during the early expiratory phase of cough, much as in normal subjects.[114] The expiratory action of the clavicular portion of the pectoralis major is approximately halved when the shoulders are abducted because this maneuver lessens the downward pull of the pectoralis on the manubrium. These observations help to explain why cough is partially preserved in patients with C-6 level injury.[114]

### Pulmonary Function

Patients with C-3 to C-8 lesions are usually not dependent on mechanical ventilation, and they have normal levels of arterial $P_{CO_2}$ when awake. Typical values for pulmonary and respiratory muscle function are summarized in Table 89.4; these have been compiled from data reported by many laboratories.[7] The overall pattern is that of a restrictive defect, with a normal $FEV_1$/FVC ratio and with relatively more severe reduction in ERV than in inspiratory capacity. Patients with cervical spine injuries often have hyperreactive bronchi; eight of eight chronic quadriplegics without history of asthma or cigarette smoking were found to be hyperresponsive to methacholine,[115] and eight were hyperresponsive to inhaled nebulized distilled water.[115a] Although asthma has not been reported as a common complication of spinal cord injury,

**Table 89.4 PULMONARY AND RESPIRATORY MUSCLE FUNCTION IN QUADRIPLEGIC PATIENTS WITH MIDDLE TO LOWER CERVICAL SPINAL CORD INJURY***

| Variable | C-4 to C-7 Injury | T-3 to T-12 Injury |
|---|---|---|
| FVC | 52 | 69 |
| $FEV_1$/FVC (%) | 85 | 82 |
| IC | 71 | — |
| ERV | 21 | 64 |
| TLC | 70 | 82 |
| FRC | 86 | 86 |
| RV | 141 | 91 |
| MVV | 49 | 61 |
| PImax (cm $H_2O$) | 64 | 79 |
| PEmax (cm $H_2O$) | 41 | 98 |

*Values expressed as percentage of predicted normal unless otherwise specified.

FVC = forced vital capacity; IC = inspiratory capacity; ERV = expiratory reserve volume; MVV = maximal voluntary ventilation. Other abbreviations as in Table 89.3.

this finding suggests a susceptibility, probably because of unopposed cholinergic influences.

Lung volumes in quadriplegic patients are more sensitive to changes of posture than in normal subjects. When a quadriplegic patient is upright, gravity causes the abdominal contents to pull the diaphragm down and bulge out the flaccid abdominal wall. In the supine position, gravity causes the abdominal contents to push the diaphragm craniad. Thus, RV and FRC decrease, whereas PImax and VC increase.[116] The increase in VC is usually not enough to counterbalance the reduction in RV, so that TLC is slightly smaller in the supine than in the upright position.[116]

Because of the loss of intercostal muscle function, the upper rib cage moves paradoxically inward with inspiration in quadriplegic patients, and the relative contribution of the rib cage to the tidal volume is reduced.[113, 117] The extent to which upper rib cage paradoxic motion occurs depends largely on whether scalene muscle function is preserved.[117] Upper rib cage distortion has also been shown to result in part from paralysis of the abdominal muscles, and the degree of distention can be minimized by abdominal compression.[118] Because contraction of the well-preserved diaphragm expands the lower rib cage through its action on the area of apposition,[119] lower rib cage motion is relatively normal.[118] Lung compliance is reduced, especially among patients with impaired parasternal inspiratory intercostal muscles,[110] but specific compliance, compliance corrected for lung volume, is normal.[110]

Quadriplegic patients usually have mild hypoxemia and an increase in the (A − a)$PO_2$, due to abnormally low ventilation-perfusion ratios in collapsed or partially collapsed areas of lung. There is a mild reduction of ventilation to basilar regions, even though the abdominal contribution to tidal volume that results from diaphragmatic contraction is higher than normal.

### Control of Breathing

The control of breathing may or may not be altered. In one series, the ventilatory response to carbon dioxide was normal,[120] but it was half normal in another study.[121] Axen and Bergofsky[122] found that quadriplegic patients show varying responses to added elastic loads; some did and others with equally severe levels of injury did not allow their tidal volumes to fall. The former stiffened their chest walls when presented with the elastic load and maintained inspiratory efforts for longer periods. The ability to stiffen the chest wall and preserve tidal volume is thought to be due to the influence of preserved thoracic sensory receptor on the control of the inspiratory muscles.

DiMarco and colleagues[123] reported that quadriplegic patients are able to sense the size of an inspired breath in normal fashion during passive, voluntary, and loaded breathing, even after local anesthesia of the upper airways, suggesting that this form of respiratory sensation depends on tension developed by the diaphragm or on the level of central nervous system motor command.

### Prognosis

Spontaneous partial recovery of ventilatory function usually occurs in the first few months after the initial injury.[6] For example, in patients with C-5 to C-6 injuries, VC averaged 31% of predicted initially, 51% at 3 months, and 58% at 5 months. PImax and maximal Pdi improve in parallel with VC, whereas FRC does not change, suggesting that the improved ventilatory function is due to improved inspiratory muscle strength. Wicks and Menter[124] showed that most quadriplegic patients who initially required mechanical ventilation could be weaned as their pulmonary function improved.

Quadriplegic patients are extremely vulnerable to any insult that worsens pulmonary function. Although there has been vast improvement in prognosis since the early 1980s, the rate of mortality from lower cervical spinal cord injury is still 15% to 40% in the first year, mostly from respiratory failure. After the first year, pulmonary complications, especially pneumonia, continue to take a toll, and the risk for fatal pneumonia remains several-fold higher for spinal cord–injured patients than for matched controls.[2, 105] Specific treatments to prevent pneumonia include frequent changes in the patient's position in bed, the regular use of deep-breathing exercises and incentive spirometry, and assisted coughing. When secretions are retained, chest percussion and bronchodilator and possibly mucolytic therapy are recommended, followed by therapeutic bronchoscopy in stubborn cases.

## Thoracic Spinal Cord Injury

The respiratory problems of paraplegic patients whose injuries are in the thoracic region are usually less prominent than those in quadriplegic patients. The major problem is poor cough. Expiratory muscle weakness is just as severe in midthoracic lesions as in lower cervical injuries but is significantly less in lower thoracic and upper lumbar injuries. Typical values for pulmonary function tests are summarized in Table 89.4. In general, function is better the lower the level of injury, but the mean values obscure a wide range.

## OTHER FOCAL RESPIRATORY MUSCLE PARALYSES

After isolated diaphragmatic paralysis and spinal cord injury, hemiplegia and poliomyelitis are the most common causes of focal respiratory muscle weakness or paralysis. The major respiratory complications of stroke are due to the effects on level of consciousness and ability to swallow. Hemiplegia is not usually associated with significant ventilatory impairment unless the lesion lies in the brain stem.

Large epidemics of acute poliomyelitis no longer occur in developed countries, but sporadic cases still appear in patients who have not been vaccinated. Therefore, one must think of the diagnosis and inquire into the vaccination history when one encounters a patient with an acute syndrome of fever, myalgia, and weakness. The degree of impairment in poliomyelitis varies from mild to severe, but the ventilatory deficit often worsens late in life, as one manifestation of the postpolio syndrome.

### Hemiplegia

#### Neural Pathways

The paralysis of hemiplegia results from damage to upper motor neurons. Lower motor neurons in the spinal cord remain viable and are subject to stimulation by spinal cord sensorimotor reflex arcs. As a result, the affected muscles do not respond to voluntary motor control, but they are often spastic. The respiratory muscles receive their upper motor neuronal innervation from two anatomically and functionally discrete pathways: the corticospinal tracts, which compose the pyramidal system, and the reticulospinal tracts, which course from the respiratory centers to the anterior horns of the spinal cord. The corticospinal tracts mediate voluntary respiratory motions, whereas the reticulospinal tracts mediate automatic breathing patterns. Patients with stroke usually have corticospinal tract damage but not reticulospinal tract damage unless the brain stem is infarcted.

#### Clinical Features

In hemiplegic patients, the position of the diaphragm as seen on ordinary supine chest radiographs, although usually within normal limits, can be shown to be subtly affected by hemiparesis.[125] The motion of the diaphragm, assessed by fluoroscopy with the patient supine, is mildly limited on the side of the paralysis,[126] an abnormality that is only apparent when breathing is augmented, either voluntarily or by carbon dioxide inhalation.

The motions of the chest in the anteroposterior diameter have been tested by means of calipers.[127] On the paralyzed side, the excursion of the upper chest is about 9% less than on the nonparalyzed side during quiet breathing and about 17% less during voluntary deep breathing. The motion of the lower chest is normal during quiet breathing, and lower chest excursion during deep breathing is about 10% lower on the side of the hemiplegia. De Troyer and associates[128] studied the electrical activity of the parasternal intercostal muscles and diaphragm in 20 patients with hemiplegia who were in the early stage of flaccid paralysis. In 19 patients, parasternal intercostal activity was lower on the paralyzed side, and in 15 patients, diaphragmatic electrical activity was lower on the paralyzed side. There were no obvious clinical differences between these 15 patients and the 5 whose diaphragms showed equal activity bilaterally. The investigators concluded that the upper motor innervation of the respiratory muscles was largely mediated by decussating fibers.[128]

### Poliomyelitis

#### General Considerations

Poliovirus destroys motor neurons in the anterior horns of the spinal cord. The distribution of muscle paralysis, which involves limb, truncal, and respiratory muscles, depends on the site of anterior horn cell damage. Muscle weakness and paralysis are most severe in the early, febrile stage of the illness. During convalescence, partial recovery is common; it may depend on recovery of some anterior horn cells or on improved function of the nonparalyzed muscles. The mechanism of late deterioration, which is referred to as the *postpolio syndrome*, appears to be denervation of previously reinnervated muscles. Although their number is diminishing, former victims of poliomyelitis constitute an important group of patients receiving long-term ventilatory support.[129]

#### Clinical Features and Ventilatory Function

In one large series studied after the 1953 polio epidemic, significant respiratory paresis occurred in about 15% of patients.[130] The distribution and severity of respiratory muscle involvement is variable.[6] Averaged data from two series show the relationships among dependence on mechanical ventilation, pulmonary function, and respiratory muscle strength (Table 89.5). The mean values in Table 89.5 do not reflect the wide range of values in individual patients. Moreover, because of the variable distribution of paresis, there are patients whose inspiratory and expiratory muscle weaknesses are roughly equal, others in whom expiratory muscle weakness predominates, and still others in whom inspiratory muscle weakness predominates. The general tendency is for inspiratory weakness to exceed expiratory weakness.

As in other forms of neuromuscular disease, the VC is lower than would be predicted from muscle weakness alone. This reduction is largely due to the reduction of respiratory system compliance. Compliance of the lungs is reduced to a greater extent than chest wall compliance, but both contribute to the reduction in total respiratory system compliance.

Patients with poliomyelitis often have a low ventilatory response to carbon dioxide inhalation.[130] This appears to depend more on the extent of reduction in VC or MVV than on whether the virus involved the medullary respiratory center. For example, Plum and Swanson[131] found that

Table 89.5 VITAL CAPACITY AND ITS SUBDIVISIONS, MAXIMAL VOLUNTARY VENTILATION, AND MAXIMAL RESPIRATORY PRESSURES IN THREE CATEGORIES OF PATIENTS WITH POLIOMYELITIS

| VARIABLE | GROUP 1 | GROUP 2 | GROUP 3 |
|---|---|---|---|
| VC | 15 | 34 | 56 |
| IC | 10 | 25 | 43 |
| ERV | 1 | 6 | 26 |
| MVV | 20 | 35 | 75 |
| PImax | 25 | 35 | 47 |
| PEmax | 26 | 41 | 55 |

*All values are expressed as percentage of predicted normal. Group 1 = dependent on mechanical ventilation >12 hr/day; group 2 = dependent on mechanical ventilation <12 hr/day; group 3 = not dependent on ventilatory support. Abbreviations as in Tables 89.3 and 89.4.

patients with bulbar poliomyelitis without severe muscle weakness had normal ventilatory responses, whereas the responses were less than half normal in patients who also had spinal cord and respiratory muscle involvement, irrespective of bulbar disease. The ventilatory response to hypoxia was relatively unimpaired.[130]

### Treatment

Treatment of the ventilatory complications of poliomyelitis is the same as that of other neuromuscular diseases that cause severe respiratory muscle weakness. Some lessons from the past are still relevant. Mechanical ventilatory support has been shown to correct blood gas composition and the polycythemia of chronic respiratory failure[132] but does not improve lung compliance, the work of breathing, or MVV. Glossopharyngeal breathing is a valuable technique that can increase TLC and peak expiratory flow rates.[108] Periodic hyperinflation by means of glossopharyngeal breathing should be effective in increasing lung compliance, reducing ventilation-perfusion imbalances, facilitating speech, and relieving dyspnea.

### Late Complications

Other prominent aspects of poliomyelitis are its late complications. Fischer[133] described 114 patients who have been followed since 1958 or before. By 1985, 98 (86%) required some form of ventilatory assistance, and 52 had undergone late tracheostomies, half for worsening ventilatory failure. In general, postpolio syndrome affects the same muscle groups that were affected during the original onset of the disease; thus, if respiratory insufficiency was not a feature of the initial presentation of polio, it is relatively unlikely to become manifest during the postpolio syndrome. Sleep-disordered breathing (obstructive sleep apnea, hypoventilation, or a mixed syndrome) is common in postpolio syndrome.[134]

## DIFFUSE NEUROMUSCULAR DISEASE

The disorders considered in this section have widely diverse etiologies (see Table 89.1), but their common features are that the entire respiratory musculature is involved and that respiratory muscle weakness is relatively symmetric. It is convenient to subdivide these disorders into those that have an acute onset and those with a more gradual onset. Detailed descriptions of the general clinical and neurologic characteristics of these disorders are available in several reviews[4, 5, 7, 8]; we focus here on respiratory system involvement.

### Diseases of Acute Onset

Disorders of acute onset fall into two etiologic groups. Three of the diseases are immunologic in origin: acute inflammatory polyneuropathy: Landry-Guillain-Barré-Strohl syndrome, myasthenia gravis, and Lambert-Eaton syndrome. The other three represent one or another form of toxicity, including botulism, organophosphate poisoning, and toxicity from aminoglycoside or polymyxin antibiotics. Acute inflammatory polyneuropathy affects transmission of impulses along the nerve, whereas all the other conditions affect transmission across the neuromuscular junction. Botulism, organophosphate poisoning, and antibiotic toxicity typically have acute onset. Acute inflammatory polyneuropathy may present acutely or subacutely. The symptoms of myasthenia gravis and Lambert-Eaton syndrome may be acute but often are of more gradual onset.

#### Acute Inflammatory Polyneuropathy

Acute inflammatory polyneuropathy is an acquired demyelinating neuropathy. Potential risk factors include influenza-like infection, some viral exanthems, and other viral or mycoplasmal infections. Although nerve conduction studies are usually abnormal at the time of maximal weakness, early in the clinical course, the nerve conduction studies may be normal.

Acute inflammatory polyneuropathy is an excellent model of the effects of acute respiratory muscle weakness because the ascending nature of the paralysis involves the chest wall and abdominal muscles before the laryngeal and pharyngeal muscles, and because other complications characteristic of botulism and organophosphate poisoning are absent. The clinical picture of acute ventilatory failure consequent to muscle weakness is dominated by symptoms of progressive weakness and dyspnea, difficulty in coughing, and, later on, dysphagia and difficulty with speech. Physical examination reveals limb and truncal muscle weakness, but examination of the respiratory system initially reveals only tachypnea. Later, the voice and gag reflex may fail.

The most useful parameters with which to follow the progressive ventilatory deficit are the VC and measurement of PImax and PEmax. Arterial blood gas analysis early on shows hypoxemia with an increased $(A - a)P_{O_2}$ and a low arterial $P_{CO_2}$. The $P_{CO_2}$ values rise back toward and then above normal only when VC has fallen to very low levels, usually less than one third of normal. It must be emphasized that the combination of dyspnea, tachypnea, falling VC, and low arterial $P_{CO_2}$ is a harbinger of ventilatory failure; patients should receive appropriate treatment before overt hypercapnia ensues.

At the Mayo Clinic, 21 of 79 patients with acute inflammatory polyneuropathy required admission to an intensive care unit, and 13 required mechanical ventilation.[135] The average duration of mechanical ventilation was 58 days (range: 10 to 104 days), and the average duration of weaning from mechanical ventilation was 37 days (range: 7 to 93 days). The major complications of treatment were related to tracheostomy, with one death. Two other deaths were from pulmonary embolism (in patients who had received no prophylactic therapy) and cerebellar hemorrhage (possibly related to anticoagulation). Other respiratory complications were aspiration, atelectasis, and pneumonia; nonrespiratory complications include decubitus ulcers and impaired nutrition. The prolonged course of acute inflammatory polyneuropathy in most afflicted patients is an argument for early tracheostomy.

## Myasthenia Gravis

Myasthenia gravis is a disease of the motor end plate. It produces muscle weakness that is aggravated by muscular contraction. The disease may be limited to ocular or bulbar muscles, but it often affects limb and respiratory muscles, and ventilatory failure is one of its most severe complications. In untreated states, the weakness can be severe; however, it improves when anticholinesterase therapy with drugs such as prostigmine or pyridostigmine is instituted.[136]

In mild disease, there is mild respiratory muscle weakness, with expiratory muscles affected more than inspiratory muscles.[137] Pulmonary function changes in proportion to respiratory muscle strength, but RV is relatively well preserved. A retrospective review of pulmonary function laboratory records disclosed a flow-volume pattern suggestive of variable extrathoracic upper airway obstruction in 7 of 12 myasthenia gravis patients,[42] probably as a result of weakness of upper airway abductors, such that they were unable to oppose the airway vacuum generated by relatively strong contraction of the inspiratory muscles. Respiratory muscles are sometimes more severely affected than other skeletal muscles.[138] Indeed, ventilatory failure may occasionally be the sole clinically apparent manifestation of the disease.[138]

The effects of anticholinesterase treatment are improvements in respiratory muscle strength, lung volumes, and inspiratory and expiratory flow rates,[21, 138] with no effect on the pattern of breathing.[21] The resting lung volume and the transpulmonary pressure at that volume increase, suggesting that with improved respiratory muscle tonic activity, there is an increase in the outward recoil of the chest wall.[138] Prostigmine therapy increases respiratory muscle strength but has relatively little effect on endurance, and a prolonged static effort or a maximal voluntary ventilation effort reverses the gain produced by prostigmine.[139]

Myasthenia gravis is caused by an immunoglobulin G (IgG) autoantibody that attacks the acetylcholine receptor of skeletal muscle. Treatment with anticholinesterase drugs merely increases the available acetylcholine concentration. Corticosteroids are sometimes effective, but therapy with these agents often fails. In this event, plasmapheresis to remove the IgG autoantibody may be indicated. Three to five exchanges may be required because less than half the IgG antibody is in the intravascular compartment at any one time, and a 70% reduction in concentration of the antibody at the acetylcholine receptor is needed for remission.[139]

The major problems in managing myasthenia gravis are complications of surgery, especially thymectomy, myasthenic crisis, and cholinergic crisis, each of which can result in ventilatory failure, sometimes for prolonged periods.

## Lambert-Eaton Syndrome

Lambert-Eaton syndrome, like myasthenia gravis, is an autoimmune disorder of neuromuscular transmission. Unlike in myasthenia gravis, however, muscle strength tends to improve with repeated testing.[140] About half of cases of Lambert-Eaton syndrome occur in association with small cell carcinoma of the lung (see Chapter 46), and the muscle disorder is caused by IgG antibodies to presynaptic calcium channels. Diaphragmatic weakness is common and is occasionally severe enough to produce ventilatory failure. The syndrome often improves with treatment of the underlying carcinoma. Treatment with intravenous immunoglobulin[141] or with aminopyridine derivatives[137] may be of short-term benefit.

## Botulism

Botulism is a serious, potentially fatal disease that is caused by neurotoxin from the anaerobic gram-negative bacterium *Clostridium botulinum*. The neurotoxin causes presynaptic blockade of the neuromuscular junction, thus inhibiting acetylcholine release. The classic symptoms include visual impairment, slurred speech, dysphagia, dry mouth, nausea, vomiting or diarrhea, weakness, dyspnea, and dizziness. Physical signs include ptosis, extraocular muscle paresis, pupillary abnormality, dysarthria, and extreme muscle weakness.

Ventilatory failure is common.[142] Patients who need mechanical ventilation have more dyspnea and gastrointestinal symptoms and are much more apt to have tachypnea, ptosis, and extreme muscle weakness on physical examination. The onset of ventilatory failure may be insidious, unless the physician pays careful attention to the severity and progression of dyspnea, tachypnea, reduction in VC, and reduction in maximal respiratory pressures. As with other forms of neuromuscular disease, overt hypercapnia occurs rapidly once respiratory muscle weakness has progressed far enough.

The course of botulism may be prolonged, and late residual symptoms of exertional fatigue and dyspnea are common. The mortality rate has been reduced to about 5% by aggressive therapy. Guanidine has been proposed as adjunctive therapy for muscle weakness in botulism, but it is far more effective for the ocular than for the respiratory muscles.[143]

Symptoms of dyspnea and fatigue persist for several years after recovery from botulism, even when pulmonary function tests have returned to normal.[144] Exercise intolerance in patients recovered from botulism is characterized by dyspnea, rapid shallow breathing, and reduced maximal oxygen consumption and appears to be related to low level of cardiovascular fitness, leg fatigue, or poor motivation. In a few cases, inspiratory muscle weakness also contributes.

### Organophospate Poisoning

Highly toxic organophosphates and carbonates, such as parathion, malathion, and carbaryl, are used in agricultural insecticides; similar quaternary organophosphates are used in nerve gases. These compounds cause muscle paralysis and other side effects because, like the antimyasthenic therapeutic agents edrophonium, physostigmine, prostigmine, and pyridostigmine, they inhibit acetylcholinesterase and lead to excessive concentrations of acetylcholine at the neuromuscular junction and other cholinergic synaptic sites.

Symptoms of acute intoxication reflect muscarinic and nicotinic effects. The former include sweating, excessive salivation, nausea, vomiting, abdominal cramps and diarrhea, bradycardia, and hypotension. Nicotinic effects include weakness, muscle fasciculation, and paralysis. Central nervous system effects include confusion, ataxia, loss of reflexes, convulsions, and coma. Specific respiratory manifestations include laryngospasm, excessive tracheobronchial secretions, bronchoconstriction, respiratory muscle weakness, and central depression of ventilation.

Treatment of organophosphate poisoning requires large doses of atropine to reverse the muscarinic effects and pralidoxime to reverse the neuromuscular junction paralysis. The initial dose of atropine should be 2 to 4 mg, given intravenously if possible and repeated every 5 to 10 minutes until the muscarinic symptoms disappear. Pralidoxime is given to adults in doses of 1 to 2 g intravenously, as soon as possible.

A large number of other drugs, including calcium-channel blockers, beta-blockers, antirheumatics, and diuretics, have the potential to impair respiratory muscle function.[145] For most of these, any muscle dysfunction is usually subclinical. It is likely, however, that patients with other causes of mild or subclinical respiratory muscle dysfunction may be more susceptible than healthy people to the neuropathic or myopathic effects of drugs.

### Antibiotic Toxicity

Ventilatory failure may occur after administration of aminoglycoside and polymyxin antibiotics.[145] Again, this is mediated by interference with neuromuscular transmission, and the risk is particularly high in patients with myasthenia gravis and those with renal failure. Symptoms resemble those of botulism, with diplopia, dysphagia, slurred speech, and dyspnea. Spontaneous recovery can occur within a few hours or days of stopping the antibiotic. Anticholinesterase therapy has been used effectively in reversing the effects of aminoglycoside neuromuscular blockade, but it is ineffective against blockade produced by polymyxin B and sodium colistimethate.

## Diseases of Gradual Onset

### Etiology

Although their onset may be abrupt, in most cases, the symptoms and signs of diffuse neuromuscular diseases are subacute or chronic. The major categories of diffuse neuromuscular disease are *amyotrophic lateral sclerosis,* various types of *muscular dystrophy,* and many kinds of *myopathy.* The myopathies that involve the respiratory muscles are highly diverse: they may be congenital; related to infection or diabetes mellitus; induced by steroids, alcohol, or impaired nutritional status; or related to inflammatory autoimmune disease. Many of the last type are associated with collagen-vascular diseases. Note also that the inflammatory myopathy of trichinosis has a predilection for respiratory muscles.

### Clinical Features

The clinical course varies according to the nature of the underlying disease. Patients with amyotrophic lateral sclerosis have an average life expectancy of 3 to 4 years after the onset of symptoms, and death is usually due to pneumonia or ventilatory failure. Life expectancy in muscular dystrophies is often longer, but, again, death is usually due to respiratory failure.[1] Some congenital myopathies may progress rapidly, but most cases in adults are slowly progressive. Acquired myopathies may progress rapidly or slowly, and patients may stabilize or recover, depending on removal of the inciting cause or other treatment.

Patients are usually aware of limb muscle weakness before they have respiratory symptoms, but the respiratory symptoms may appear first. Limb muscle weakness may be proximal, distal, or both. Muscle cramps and fasciculations occur in some of the disorders. In the absence of associated lung disease, the predominant respiratory symptoms are dyspnea on exertion and fatigue. As the disease progresses, dyspnea is present at rest, and difficulty in coughing, speaking, or swallowing becomes more prominent. Some patients have morning headache, disturbed sleep, and daytime somnolence, and others may develop symptoms of heart failure.

### Diagnosis

The diagnostic workup of patients suspected of having neuromuscular diseases should include tests of the neuromuscular apparatus. The pattern of muscle weakness, the presence or absence of fasciculations, and the presence or absence of hyperreflexia are important aspects of the physical examination. Electrophysiologic techniques, such as nerve conduction and electromyographic studies, are useful to differentiate among denervation, dystrophies, and myopathic processes. Biopsy of affected muscles helps to identify dystrophies and myopathies. Serum creatine kinase and aldolase levels are often elevated in dystrophies and myopathies. Improvement in strength with edrophonium indicates a neuromuscular junction defect.

### Pulmonary and Respiratory Muscle Function

Respiratory muscle weakness and impaired pulmonary function are readily detectable by objective testing well in advance of overt respiratory symptoms.[13] Because patients with neuromuscular diseases may have coincident obstructive or interstitial lung disease,[13] it is necessary to measure maximal respiratory pressures in addition to performing spirometric and lung volume measurements. In diffuse neuromuscular diseases, the inspiratory and expiratory muscles are usually weakened to the same degree.[13] On occasion, the primary manifestation of these diseases is severe diaphragmatic weakness, out of proportion to limb or other respiratory muscle involvement.[35, 45]

Pulmonary function testing of patients with respiratory muscle weakness uncomplicated by coexisting pulmonary disease reveals a typical restrictive pattern, with reductions in VC, a normal $FEV_1/FVC$ ratio, and an elevated RV.[13] The forced expiratory flow–volume curve is often truncated near RV when expiratory muscle weakness is severe.[146] MVV is almost always below normal.[1, 14] The diffusing capacity is usually normal, especially if it is corrected for the reduction in TLC.[1] All of the pulmonary function abnormalities worsen as the disease progresses, and they are usually directly related to the degree of respiratory muscle weakness.[1, 13, 146]

Again, the reduction in VC in patients with respiratory muscle weakness is out of proportion to what would be expected from muscle weakness alone.[14] The most likely reason is decrease in the distensibility of the lungs as a result of microatelectasis, coupled with a decrease in the outward pull of the chest wall. The reduction in lung compliance is not affected by intermittent positive-pressure breathing.[14] In addition, the relaxed chest wall is on average almost twice as stiff in patients with neuromuscular disease as it is in normal subjects.[15]

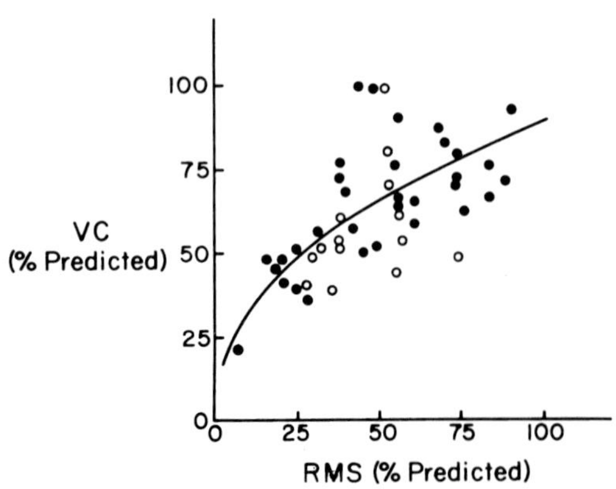


**Figure 89.1** Relationship between vital capacity (VC) and respiratory muscle strength (RMS) in patients with proximal myopathies. *Closed circles* denote patients without, and *open circles* denote patients with, coexisting lung disease. The regression lines in this and subsequent figures are calculated from data of patients with myopathy uncomplicated by lung disease. (From Braun NMT, Arora NS, Rochester DF: Respiratory muscle and pulmonary function in polymyositis and other proximal myopathies. Thorax 38:616–623, 1983.)

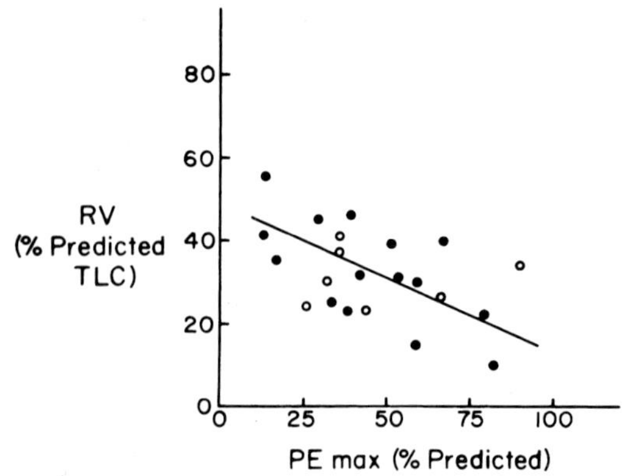


**Figure 89.2** Relationship between residual volume (RV) and maximal expiratory pressure (PE max) in patients with proximal myopathies. TLC = total lung capacity. *Closed circles* denote patients without, and *open circles* denote patients with, coexisting lung disease. (From Braun NMT, Arora NS, Rochester DF: Respiratory muscle and pulmonary function in polymyositis and other proximal myopathies. Thorax 38:616–623, 1983.)

In the early stages of neuromuscular disease, the spirometric tests may be near normal, despite considerably reduced PImax and PEmax.[1, 13] The data obtained by Braun and colleagues[13] in patients with myopathy are typical for all of the diffuse neuromuscular diseases and are consistent with data of other investigators. VC is relatively well maintained when PImax is above 40% to 50% of predicted value, but falls sharply when respiratory muscle strength is below 40% of predicted value (Fig. 89.1). The increase in RV is inversely related to PEmax (Fig. 89.2), and MVV is directly related to respiratory muscle strength (Fig. 89.3). The regression lines in Figures 89.1 to 89.3 are calculated only from patients without coexistent lung disease. It can be seen that patients with associated lung disease cannot be distinguished from those without lung disease on the VC and RV graphs (see Figs. 89.1 and 89.2), but most patients with associated lung disease have a lower MVV than could be predicted on the basis of respiratory muscle strength alone (see Fig. 89.3).

In myotonic dystrophy, there is a form of respiratory muscle dyskinesia characterized by better performance during rhythmic efforts than with static efforts, abnormal expiratory muscle activity, and prolongation of diaphragmatic activity during expiration elicited by expiratory resistive loads.[147] This may represent a form of abnormal control of breathing but more likely is a manifestation of myotonia of the respiratory muscles.[18, 148]

### Ventilatory Failure

***Respiratory Muscle Weakness.*** Most patients with neuromuscular disease who develop ventilatory failure do so because of the respiratory muscle weakness per se. The onset of ventilatory failure is likely to be abrupt, even when it has taken a long time to develop a critical degree of respiratory muscle weakness. Ventilatory failure is often precipitated by a respiratory infection, not only because of the additional respiratory loads associated with consolidation, airway mucus, reactive bronchospasm, edema, or fever-associated tachypnea, but also because of probable cytokine-mediated respiratory muscle weakness.[149] The clinical signs that indicate that ventilatory failure is imminent or in progress are increasing weakness and fatigue, dyspnea at rest, tachypnea, coughing and difficulty clearing secretions, sleep disturbances, and daytime somnolence. Most studies of patients with respiratory muscle weakness show that respiratory rate increases and arterial $P_{CO_2}$ decreases early in the course of the disease and that $P_{CO_2}$ rises to abnormally high levels only when respiratory muscle weakness is severe.[13]

***Pattern of Breathing.*** The cause of the respiratory failure is muscle weakness, but the mechanism is a progressive reduction in tidal volume, leading to an increased dead space–to–tidal volume ratio. Rapid, shallow breathing is characteristic of neuromuscular disease, despite the fact that ventilatory drive is normal or increased.[19, 21] Patients with severe respiratory muscle weakness recruit their neck inspiratory and abdominal expiratory muscles in a fashion highly reminiscent of normal subjects breathing at 50% MVV or higher.[88]

***Weakness Versus Fatigue.*** The relative magnitude of the ventilatory load in neuromuscular disease can be quantified by the intrathoracic pressure–time index, the integral over time of the intrathoracic vacuum required for tidal breathing, divided by PImax. Whenever the respiratory muscles are weak, the pressure–time index is much higher than normal, both because the load is increased and because PImax is reduced. Thus, inspiratory muscle weakness certainly predisposes to fatigue. In patients with myotonic dystrophies, the diaphragm becomes fatigued

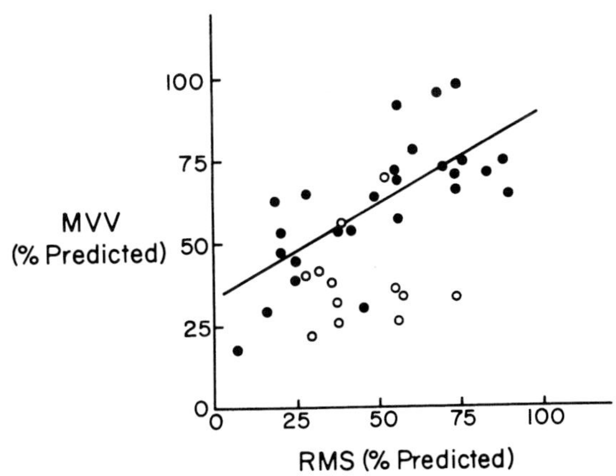


**Figure 89.3** Relationship between maximal voluntary ventilation (MVV) and respiratory muscle strength (RMS) in patients with proximal myopathies. *Closed circles* denote patients without, and *open circles* denote patients with, coexisting lung disease. (From Braun NMT, Arora NS, Rochester DF: Respiratory muscle and pulmonary function in polymyositis and other proximal myopathies. Thorax 38:616–623, 1983.)

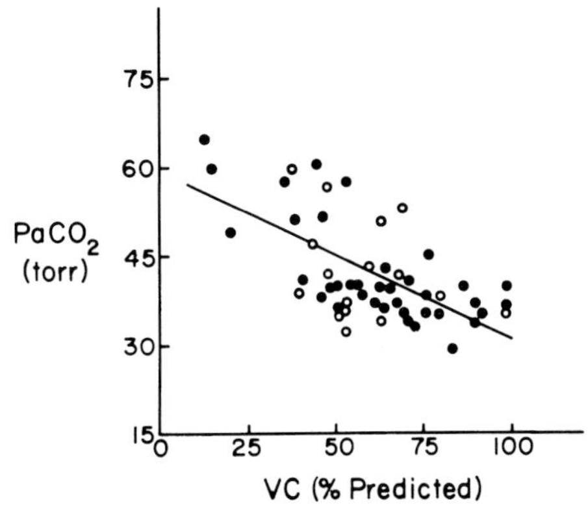


**Figure 89.4** Relationship between arterial $P_{CO_2}$ ($PaCO_2$) and vital capacity (VC) in patients with proximal myopathies. *Closed circles* denote patients without, and *open circles* denote patients with, coexisting lung disease. (From Braun NMT, Arora NS, Rochester DF: Respiratory muscle and pulmonary function in polymyositis and other proximal myopathies. Thorax 38:616–623, 1983.)

more rapidly than in normal subjects for the same relative load.[18] It is not yet known whether the diaphragm is more susceptible to fatigue in the other neuromuscular diseases. Observations in patients recovering from acute ventilatory failure caused by myasthenia gravis or acute inflammatory polyneuropathy (Landry-Guillain-Barré-Strohl syndrome) suggest that overt fatigue of the respiratory muscles is uncommon.[150] Despite considerable residual diaphragmatic and inspiratory muscle weakness, the diaphragmatic pressure–time index rarely exceeds the fatigue threshold, even in patients who cannot sustain adequate levels of ventilation, because the patients inspire very small tidal volumes.[19, 151]

***Harbingers of Ventilatory Failure.*** Overt ventilatory failure occurs abruptly; thus, measurement of arterial blood gas composition is not a reliable indicator of impending respiratory acidosis. We stress the importance of heeding the clinical observations of increasing dyspnea and tachypnea as well as sleep disturbance, morning headache, and daytime somnolence. We urge physicians to make serial measurements of VC and respiratory muscle strength in patients shown to be at risk by their symptoms. As VC decreases, there is a progressive increase in arterial $P_{CO_2}$ (Fig. 89.4), such that $P_{CO_2}$ values reach respiratory failure levels when VC is less than half normal. As respiratory muscle strength decreases from normal to half normal, arterial $P_{CO_2}$ remains normal or somewhat low (Fig. 89.5). Thereafter, $P_{CO_2}$ values rise progressively, reaching respiratory failure levels when respiratory muscle strength is less than 25% to 30% normal in patients with muscle weakness uncomplicated by lung disease.

## TREATMENT OF VENTILATORY FAILURE

### Treatment of Underlying Disease

Treatment of respiratory muscle weakness is specific in some cases and supportive in others. Examples of myopa-

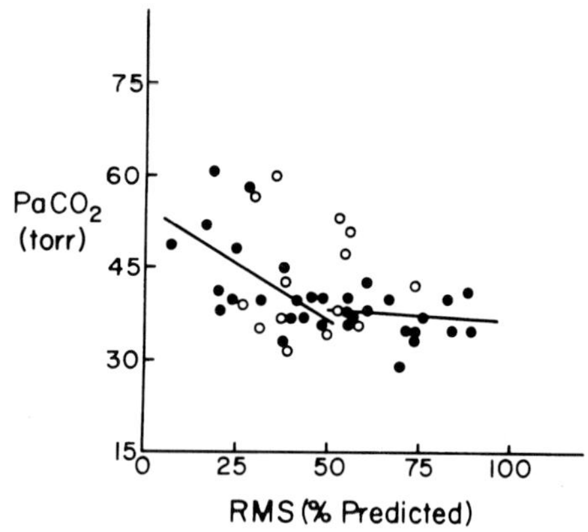


**Figure 89.5** Relationship between arterial $P_{CO_2}$ ($PaCO_2$) and respiratory muscle strength (RMS) in patients with proximal myopathies. *Closed circles* denote patients without, and *open circles* denote patients with, coexisting lung disease. (From Braun NMT, Arora NS, Rochester DF: Respiratory muscle and pulmonary function in polymyositis and other proximal myopathies. Thorax 38:616–623, 1983.)

thies that respond to specific therapy include polymyositis and dermatomyositis, hyperthyroidism and hypothyroidism, malnutrition, and alcoholic and steroid myopathies. By and large, the anterior horn cell diseases, dystrophies, and congenital myopathies are relentlessly progressive, and specific treatments are not available. Two trials of calcium-channel blocking agents in amyotrophic lateral sclerosis demonstrated no benefit.[152, 153] However, advances in neurotrophic factors, neurotransmitters, and proteases provide hope for the future.[154] Similarly, although there is currently no definitive therapy for the muscular dystrophies, preliminary animal experiments demonstrating that the gene coding for dystrophin can be delivered to the diaphragm by means of an adenoviral vector[155] suggest that specific therapy may be achievable.

## Supportive Therapy

### Oxygen, Ventilatory Stimulants, and Anabolic Agents

Several forms of supportive therapy are able to improve ventilatory and respiratory muscle function, even when the underlying disease process is progressive, as discussed in Chapters 91 to 94. Supplemental oxygen is indicated in patients with documented hypoxemia at rest, on exercise, or during sleep. Adequate oxygenation can prevent or improve cor pulmonale, polycythemia, hypoxia-related intellectual and cognitive dysfunction,[156] and possibly respiratory muscle fatigue.[157]

Ventilatory stimulants have not met with much success in the treatment or prevention of ventilatory failure in neuromuscular disease. In general, ventilatory drive is more than adequate in neuromuscular diseases, but the presence of denervation, neuropathy, or myopathy prevents an adequate response of the muscle. Thus, use of ventilatory stimulation may lead to overuse of weakened ventilatory muscles, potentially leading to further impairment of muscle function.[158] In the few cases of congenital myopathy or endocrinopathy in which control of breathing is compromised out of proportion to the degree of respiratory muscle weakness, a cautious trial of acetazolamide, doxapram, or progesterone may be warranted.[159]

### Cough, Secretions

Measures designed to assist coughing and clearance of secretions are often helpful in patients with neuromuscular diseases. A few techniques have been developed to enhance cough capacity in the presence of severe respiratory muscle weakness. For example, the effectiveness of coughing can be augmented by synchronizing coughing attempts with manual compression of the abdomen by an assistant.[108] Patients may also use an insufflator/exsufflator, or "cough machine," an instrument that provides a deep insufflation by mask, followed by rapid decompression.[160]

In patients with cervical cord injuries, the abdominal expiratory muscles, which remain innervated by intact lower motor neurons that cannot be voluntarily activated, can be stimulated electrically[161, 162] or magnetically[163] to enhance cough effectiveness. Stimulation is unlikely to be of benefit for victims of neuropathy or myopathy because the neuromuscular apparatus is not intact.

Certain types of training can improve the efficiency of coughing. With glossopharyngeal breathing, patients who otherwise would be incapable of deep inspiratory efforts can learn to augment their VC by up to 1 L. With the larger inspiration, there is more passive recoil, which promotes a more effective cough.[164] Estenne and colleagues[165] have shown that isometric exercise of the pectoralis muscle, designed to strengthen its clavicular portion, increases the expiratory capacity and thereby cough effectiveness of quadriplegic patients.

Beta-adrenergic agonists can improve clearance of secretions even in the absence of bronchial obstruction. When secretions are particularly tenacious, mucolytics, such as nebulized acetylcysteine, may help; however, nebulized acetylcysteine can precipitate severe bronchoconstriction in patients with asthma or hyperreactive airways. Nasotracheal suctioning, percussion, postural drainage, and even bronchoscopy are occasionally necessary to remove secretions from large airways.

Although tracheostomy facilitates access to large airways for clearance of secretions by suction catheter, it also virtually destroys the patient's ability to generate the strongly positive expiratory pressures and the narrow glottic orifice that are necessary for effective clearance of secretions from smaller airways by coughing.[37, 38] Thus, when possible, avoidance of tracheostomy yields important benefits.

### Inspiratory Muscle Training

Inspiratory muscle training (IMT) has been used with some success in selected patients with neuromuscular disease. In lower cervical spinal cord injury, a 6-week regimen of daily forced inspiration and expiration through resistances, coupled with manual insufflation of air to increase TLC above the spontaneously achieved value, approximately doubled the PImax, PEmax, and VC, increased TLC by about 10%, and lowered RV by about 25%.[166] Three additional studies, of 4,[162, 6,][166a] 8,[167] and 16[168] weeks of IMT demonstrated smaller, but potentially meaningful, increases in inspiratory muscle strength,[167, 168] inspiratory muscle endurance,[166a] and VC.[162, 167, 168] Both VC and PImax tended to return toward baseline after termination of the study,[167] suggesting not only that some level of continuing challenge is required for maintenance of the beneficial effect but also that the observed IMT-associated improvements were actually due to improved function, not simply improved ability to perform the tests.

The results of IMT are more variable in patients with muscular dystrophy. DiMarco and colleagues[169] reported that respiratory muscle endurance could be significantly improved by 6 to 12 weeks of IMT. The results were best in patients whose baseline PImax was at least 60% normal or higher. Wanke and coworkers[170] showed similar results after 1 to 6 months of IMT, with small improvements in inspiratory muscle strength and endurance but no improvement in VC and no improvement in strength among the most severely affected patients (VC more than 25% of predicted value). In two additional studies, IMT was not found to be of benefit.[171, 172]

IMT has shown some promise in a single case of adult-onset acid maltase deficiency[173] and in a mixed group of patients with neuromuscular disease.[174]

Results of several studies involving small numbers of patients suggest that IMT by voluntary effort[175, 176] or with phrenic nerve stimulation[177] may help to improve the strength and endurance of mechanically ventilated patients with spinal cord injury,[175–177] muscular dystrophy,[175] or neuropathies,[175] improving their chances to become independent of mechanical ventilation. These favorable results suggest that the reason that severely affected, but spontaneously breathing, patients have been found to be relatively unlikely to respond to IMT[169, 170] is that it is relatively easy for such patients to breathe around the resistor, thereby failing to achieve the inspiratory muscle overload necessary for a training effect; in patients on mechanical ventilation, the closed ventilatory circuit, and perhaps the close attention paid by therapists throughout the training sessions, makes it more likely that strong inspiratory efforts will continue throughout the sessions.[175]

## Ventilatory Assistance

When neuromuscular disease is far advanced and ventilatory failure is impending or already established, ventilatory support is necessary if patients are to survive. Many such patients do not choose to accept ventilatory support, whether delivered by traditional means, including tracheostomy and volume-cycled ventilators, or by "noninvasive" means.[178] Indeed, it has become almost a truism that the quality of life on chronic mechanical ventilation is unacceptable. There is no doubt that the cumbersome nature of ventilatory support equipment, the ever-present risk of death from disconnection or power failure, the problems of maintaining communication, and the expense of equipment and caregivers present major challenges to patients and their families. Advances in respiratory care, however, have made it possible for highly motivated patients with access to financial support and to creative and resourceful rehabilitation specialists to live long periods of acceptable quality on mechanical ventilation, with or without tracheostomy.[179]

**Techniques for Noninvasive Mechanical Ventilatory Support.** The principal categories of noninvasive mechanical ventilation are based on use of gravity (rocking bed), application of positive pressure to the body (abdominal belt), application of negative pressure to the body (iron lung, cuirass, body wrap), and application of positive pressure to the airway (nose mask or mouthpiece).

***Rocking Bed.*** The rocking bed is a conventional bed mounted on an apparatus that allows it to cycle from 30 degrees head up to 15 degrees head down several times each minute. The resulting shifting of the abdominal organs assists diaphragmatic excursion. The rocking bed is useful for patients who cannot sustain their own ventilatory support indefinitely but who have relatively good ventilatory function when sitting upright. It is particularly useful for patients with diaphragmatic paralysis or quadriplegia.

***Abdominal Pneumatic Belt.*** Similar assistance in diaphragmatic excursion can be provided by an abdominal positive-pressure belt ventilator. This consists of a pneumatic belt that is connected to a cyclic positive-pressure source. As the bladder in the belt is inflated, the abdomen is compressed. This pushes the diaphragm upward and assists expiratory airflow. When the bladder is deflated, the descent of the diaphragm and the passive recoil of the rib cage back to FRC provide the force for inspiration. Unlike the rocking bed, the abdominal ventilators function best when the patient is in a sitting position. Bach and Alba[180] have shown that selected patients can be maintained on abdominal positive-pressure breathing for long periods.

***Negative-Pressure Body Ventilators.*** Negative-pressure ventilators have been extensively used in the support of patients with a variety of neuromuscular diseases.[181] Such ventilators have the advantage that they leave the upper airway free, allowing unimpeded speech. The early versions of negative-pressure ventilators, the iron lungs, are too cumbersome for practical use by most patients at home. The smaller cuirass and body-wrap ventilators are more acceptable to most patients, although they still require considerable skill for successful operation.

A major problem with the use of negative-pressure mechanical ventilation is upper airway obstruction, occurring when the upper airway abductors fail to contract vigorously enough to oppose the intratracheal vacuum generated by the inspiratory cycle of the negative-pressure ventilator.[182] This is a particularly severe problem during sleep in patients with prominent weakness of bulbar muscles. In most cases, the solution to this problem is to switch to positive-pressure ventilation.

***Noninvasive Positive-Pressure Ventilation.*** Noninvasive intermittent positive-pressure ventilation has been used with great success in patients with neuromuscular diseases.[97, 108, 183] In most cases, positive-pressure ventilation has been delivered by a nasal mask, but in some cases, oral masks or mouthpieces are used. Patients may use a portable volume-cycled ventilator or a modified CPAP device. The tidal volume is adjusted to compensate for small leaks occurring through the mouth; if excessive leakage occurs, the mouth can be loosely held closed with a strap.

Complications of nasal positive-pressure ventilation are common and often troublesome. They include leaks at the mouth or the infraorbital area,[97] chronic nasal congestion, sinusitis, and skin breakdown at sites of contact with the mask.[183] Nevertheless, most patients who start on nasal positive-pressure ventilation are able to tolerate it,[183] and its use often prevents the need for tracheostomy.

***Continuous Positive Airway Pressure.*** In normal subjects, CPAP increases tidal volume by 25% and lowers respiratory rate by more than 30%.[184] In patients with neuromuscular and chest wall diseases, nasal CPAP prevents atelectasis.[185] Nasal CPAP also prevents the upper airway collapse and consequent functional inspiratory upper airway obstruction that occasionally complicate neuromuscular diseases. CPAP can prevent the flail action of a paralyzed hemidiaphragm as well,[95] thereby improving the efficiency of the remaining, functioning inspiratory muscles. On the other hand, CPAP often increases FRC and shortens inspiratory muscles, placing them at a mechanical disadvantage. Thus, CPAP has the potential to worsen inspiratory muscle weakness. We think that CPAP is most beneficial in patients with upper airway obstruction due to paresis of the upper airway musculature and in patients with isolated diaphragmatic paralysis. CPAP alone should be used only with caution and close monitoring in other neuromuscular diseases.

***Ventilatory Regimen.*** In patients with chronic ventilatory failure, nocturnal mechanical ventilatory support supplied by either negative-pressure or positive-pressure respirators provides at least several hours per day of adequate oxygenation, which in turn often prevents or reverses cor pulmonale, improves intellectual and cognitive function, and provides a margin of safety during the patient's most vulnerable period. A number of studies have also suggested that, perhaps by relieving fatigue, nocturnal ventilation can improve the function of the ventilatory muscles during the remaining hours, during which the patient breathes spontaneously.[183]

**Electrophrenic Respiration.** Electrophrenic respiration is indicated for patients in whom the neuromuscular apparatus is intact from the nerve to the muscle but in whom ventilatory drive fails or cannot be translated normally into neural impulses. Thus, patients with central alveolar hypoventilation or high cervical spinal cord injuries, in which the phrenic motor neurons remain intact, are appropriate candidates for phrenic pacing. In patients with ventilatory failure due to anterior horn diseases, neuropathies, or myopathies, the muscles are no more likely to respond to electrical stimulation than to voluntary or automatic respiratory effort.

Details of the procedure for electrophrenic respiration have been summarized by Glenn and associates.[109] First, the phrenic nerve must be tested for viability. This involves percutaneous stimulation of the cervical portion of the nerve and recording the diaphragmatic action potentials by using surface electrodes over the anterolateral rib cage. It is sometimes necessary to expose the phrenic nerve surgically to ensure its response to stimulation. Pacemaker electrodes are usually implanted on both phrenic nerves, so that an alternating pacing schedule can be employed. Cervical implantation is easier and carries lower risk, but it may not fully stimulate the diaphragm. Therefore, in cases in which maximal diaphragmatic response is required, for example, in patients with underlying lung disease, the thoracic implantation procedure is preferred. After implantation, the performance of each hemidiaphragm is tested fluoroscopically and spirometrically.

The electrical stimulation parameters have been selected to minimize nerve and muscle damage. The pulse waveform is bipolar. The current per pulse is adjusted to the point beyond which further increases in current no longer increase tidal volume. The stimulation frequency is usually 10 to 15 impulses/sec. Higher frequencies, 25 to 35 impulses/sec, may be required initially, when the diaphragm is deconditioned. However, animal experiments show that prolonged use of higher frequencies causes myopathic changes and weakness of the diaphragm, whereas lower frequencies of stimulation do not.[186] The duration of each train of impulses is selected to be about one fourth of the whole breath duration. At a typical stimulated respiratory rate of 12 breaths/min, the duration of each train of stimuli is 1.3 seconds, and the inspiration-to-expiration ratio is 1:3.

Various pacing patterns have been employed. If the diaphragm has atrophied before the initiation of pacing, it will rapidly fatigue when stimulated.[186] Therefore, one must start by stimulating the phrenic nerves for only a few minutes per hour, and then progress each day by a few minutes per hour until diaphragmatic endurance time is at least 30 minutes. Thereafter, pacing can be carried out on a schedule of 30 minutes of pacing alternating with 30 minutes of rest, for several hours at a time. The length of the pacing periods is increased until a single hemidiaphragm can be paced continuously for 6 to 12 hours. Note that the process of retraining an atrophied diaphragm is analogous to weaning patients with weak respiratory muscles from mechanical ventilation. The process will succeed provided that nutritional status is adequate and that complications, especially infections, are absent.

When the full pacing schedule has been achieved, additional variables must be considered. Some patients are more comfortable when both hemidiaphragms are paced simultaneously,[109] but these patients may need rest periods, during which they use a mechanical ventilator. To sustain patients without ventilators, it is often better to pace one hemidiaphragm for 6 to 12 hours, then switch to the other side. Tidal volumes and transdiaphragmatic pressures are about 50% higher when both hemidiaphragms are paced. Diaphragmatic pacing increases the inspiratory excursions of the abdomen and lower rib cage, but the upper rib cage moves paradoxically inward.[187] Diaphragmatic pacing is much more effective when the patient is supine than upright,[187] but the effectiveness of pacing in the sitting position can be enhanced by abdominal compression.[187]

The complications of electrophrenic respiration include nerve damage,[109] infection, and upper airway occlusion due to failure of the pharyngeal and laryngeal muscles to open the upper airway.[188] Tracheostomy circumvents this problem. Alternatively, because voluntary inspiratory efforts activate the upper airway abductors, another solution is to trigger the phrenic pacemaker from the electromyogram of the sternomastoid muscles.[188]

## SYNDROMES OF INAPPROPRIATE RESPIRATORY MUSCLE CONTRACTION

In this section, we discuss a number of disorders that we term *syndromes of inappropriate respiratory muscle contraction.* They share some common features in that either the timing of contraction is inappropriate, the synchronization between inspiratory and expiratory muscles is lacking or abnormal, or the intensity of the contraction is excessive (Table 89.6). As a group, these syndromes cause dyspnea and chest discomfort and interfere with speech and swallowing. Unlike other neuromuscular diseases, muscle weakness is generally not prominent, and only in extreme cases does inappropriate contraction of the respiratory muscles cause ventilatory failure.

**Table 89.6** SYNDROMES OF INAPPROPRIATE RESPIRATORY MUSCLE CONTRACTION

| SYNDROME | TYPE OF RESPIRATORY MUSCLE INVOLVEMENT |
|---|---|
| Hiccups (singultus) | Spasmodic contraction of diaphragm, other inspiratory muscles |
| | Upper airway closure |
| Respiratory myoclonus (tic, flutter of diaphragm) | Spasmodic contraction of diaphragm (most cases) or of abdominal muscles (one case) |
| Respiratory dyskinesia | Abnormal asynchronous pattern of breathing, involving all respiratory muscle groups, associated with neurocirculatory asthenia |
| | Associated facial and limb muscle dyskinesia (four cases); limited to respiratory muscles (one case) |
| Convulsive disorders | Status epilepticus, tetanus, strychnine poisoning |
| | Severe spasmodic contraction of all respiratory muscle groups causes hypoventilation |

### Hiccups

#### Etiology

Hiccup is a common phenomenon that is usually innocuous but that sometimes produces significant morbidity. Hiccups are associated with many conditions that involve the central nervous system, the vagus and phrenic nerves, the mediastinum, the diaphragm, and the gastrointestinal and genitourinary tracts.[189] In some cases, no obvious organic disease is present, and the hiccup phenomenon may be psychogenic. Examples of central nervous system conditions associated with hiccups include multiple sclerosis, toxic states such as uremia and alcohol intoxication, dexamethasone therapy, meningitis and encephalitis, vascular lesions and brain tumor, and surgery. Peripheral nerve causes include herpes zoster and irritation of branches of the vagus or phrenic nerves. Visceral causes include stimulation of the gastrointestinal tract by heat, cold, spasm, dilation, or distention and inflammatory, neoplastic, or surgical lesions of the mediastinum, diaphragm, or upper gastrointestinal tract.[189]

Hiccups are usually only a nuisance. Prolonged hiccups, however, cause discomfort and interfere with speech, eating, and sleep. Hiccups during or after surgery pose particular problems.

#### Pathophysiology

The spasm of hiccup is not limited to the diaphragm. There are short, sharp contractions of the diaphragm and inspiratory intercostal muscles, coupled with transient closure to the glottis.[190] These events occur from 10 to 30 times/min.[191] In infants, the upper airway closure involves pharyngeal muscles, and it may persist after diaphragmatic spasms have stopped.[192] Thus, in infants, the upper airway closure mechanism bears some resemblance to that occurring in obstructive sleep apnea. The pathogenesis of hiccup is unclear but appears to be related to supraspinal mechanisms as well as reflex arcs.

#### Treatment

Numerous treatments for hiccups have been described; many derive from folklore, many are ineffective, and few have been investigated systematically.[189] In one study, swallowing a teaspoonful of dry granulated sugar rapidly stopped hiccups in 19 of 20 patients, 12 of whom had the hiccups for only a few hours and 8 of whom had suffered for 1 day to several weeks.[193] In another study, stimulation of the pharynx with a catheter introduced through the nose stopped hiccups in 84 of 85 patients[194]; in our experience, however, relief is often transient. Electrical stimulation of the phrenic nerves, by means of needle electrodes in the neck or a phrenic pacemaker, has been completely or partially successful.[195] Treatment of the underlying irritative or metabolic cause is sometimes helpful; in one case, hiccups stopped when a hair in contact with the ear drum was removed from the external auditory canal.[189] Isolated successes have occurred with anesthetic or surgical block of phrenic or vagus nerves.[189] Other maneuvers have included hyperventilation, breath-holding, rebreathing or inhaling carbon dioxide, rapidly swallowing water or ice chips, induction of vomiting, carotid massage, and pressure on the eyes.

Many drug treatments have been proposed, generally involving tranquilizers, muscle relaxants, anticonvulsives, and narcotics. Chlorpromazine, carbamazepine, metoclopramide, haloperidol, amitriptyline, ketamine, nifedipine, quinidine, phenytoin, and baclofen have been used, with variable success.[189] Frequently, the doses must be increased to toxic levels. Valproic acid at levels well within the usual therapeutic range was successful in stopping hiccups in four of five patients and substantially reducing them in the fifth.[191]

On the basis of the preceding observations, we recommend the following: First, have the patient swallow 1 teaspoonful of dry granulated sugar. Next, if need be, proceed to pharyngeal stimulation with a nasogastric tube, and use the tube to decompress the stomach. Also, check for and remove foreign bodies in the external auditory canal.

If mechanical measures fail, and the hiccups persist for more than several hours, pharmacologic therapy is indicated. If immediate relief is required, intravenous chlorpromazine, 50 mg, can be used, followed by oral chlorpromazine for a few days if necessary. Haloperidol in doses up to 5 mg every 8 hours is another option, but both chlorpromazine and haloperidol should be used with caution because they may cause permanent dyskinesia. Baclofen, a centrally acting muscle relaxant, often works well[196]; the initial dose is 5 mg three times a day, increasing slowly to a maximum of 20 mg three to four times a day if necessary. Lorazepam may be a useful supplement. Additional or alternative drugs are amitriptyline and nifedipine. Metoclopramide as a treatment for hiccups should probably be reserved for patients who have gastrointestinal disease; the dose is 10 mg every 6 hours. Carbamazepine and valproic acid are potentially very toxic drugs and should be used only as a last resort. Other centrally acting drugs, such as baclofen or chlorpromazine, should be discontinued if either carbamazepine or valproic acid is given. Because phrenic stimulation and nerve block procedures require special skills, we would reserve those interventions for patients in whom all other measures fail.

## Respiratory Myoclonus

Myoclonus of the diaphragm and other respiratory muscles, often referred to as "tic," "flutter," or Leeuwenhoek's disease, is a rhythmic repetitive contraction of respiratory muscles, at a frequency of 30 to 300 per minute.[197] Myoclonus may be limited to the diaphragm or another respiratory muscle group. The duration and intensity of the contractions are less than with hiccup, and upper airway closure does not occur with myoclonus. A single episode of respiratory myoclonus may last for only a few seconds, or it may persist for hours. Repetitive bouts are common in afflicted patients.

The pathogenesis of respiratory myoclonus is unknown but may involve central nervous system dysfunction at the level of the brain or spinal cord. Respiratory myoclonus has been likened to palatal myoclonus, and the two may occur together.[197] The list of conditions that are associated with respiratory myoclonus is similar to that for hiccup.

The symptoms of respiratory myoclonus vary to some extent, according to which respiratory muscle groups are involved. In general, there is dyspnea, a sensation of muscular fatigue, and a sense of choking. Speech may be of a staccato nature. Physical examination reveals repetitive abdominal movements. Spirometric testing and quantitative examination of rib cage and abdominal motions by means of magnetometers or inductance plethysmographs show a flutter pattern on inspiration or expiration. Electromyography of the affected muscles demonstrates rhythmic bursts of activity synchronous with the waveforms on the spirogram; sometimes, these bursts are apparent on the electrocardiogram. In one patient, the ventilatory response to inhaled carbon dioxide was normal, but the patient had posthyperventilation apnea, which indicates central nervous system dysfunction.[197] Because respiratory myoclonus is a rare disorder, there are no systematic evaluations of therapy.

## Respiratory Dyskinesias

### Unclassified Dyskinesia

Respiratory dyskinesia refers to irregular breathing patterns produced by asynchronous and inappropriate respiratory muscle contractions that are variable in timing.[198, 199] In general, the contractions are not as rhythmic as in respiratory myoclonus, and the frequency is lower. Although these patients are dissimilar in many ways, they all have dyspnea in the absence of primary pulmonary disease, and they all have some abnormality of respiratory muscle motion.

In one series of 33 patients, abnormally large contractions of the diaphragm occurred at intervals of every few breaths, causing irregular variations in respiratory rate and tidal volume.[198] These patients had the syndrome of neurocirculatory asthenia, characterized by dyspnea, fatigue, faintness, dizziness, anxiety, and hyperventilation. In another group of four patients, similar symptoms and signs occurred in association with choreiform movement disorders involving facial and limb muscles.[199] Treatment of neurocirculatory asthenia is generally unsatisfactory. Patients with choreiform motion disorders due to extrapyramidal dysfunction may respond to reserpine and to reduction in doses of dopaminergic drugs.[199]

### Parkinson's Disease

Parkinson's disease is another form of extrapyramidal disorder that can affect the respiratory muscles. Its respiratory manifestations were described in a well-studied group of 23 patients.[200] The predominant respiratory symptom was dyspnea. Physical examination reveals the typical neurologic findings of rigidity, tremor, and poor performance of alternating movements of limb muscles. Excess salivation is common. Defective coordination of coughing has also been described.[201] Pulmonary function testing reveals mild tachypnea and near-normal VC, but inspiratory and expiratory flow rates are reduced by 35%

and 25%, respectively. RV is twice normal, and FRC is about 140% normal. Maximal respiratory pressures are about half normal. Lung compliance is slightly reduced, but lung resistance is twice normal. Thus, unlike most neuromuscular diseases, Parkinsons' disease produces an obstructive pulmonary function defect, attributable to abnormally high parasympathetic activity. Part of the airway obstruction may be explained by abnormal contraction of the upper airway musculature,[202] but abnormal contraction of the scalene and parasternal intercostal muscles may also contribute to abnormal oscillations of airflow. Treatment is that for Parkinson's disease.

### Myotonia Congenita

Respiratory dyskinesia of a different sort occurs in myotonia congenita (Thomsen's disease), a condition characterized by increased muscle excitability and impaired relaxation. One patient was shown to have respiratory as well as limb muscle involvement.[203] Electromyographic testing of the scalene muscles and diaphragm showed abnormal myotonic discharges in the absence of voluntary contraction and greatly prolonged afterdischarges with voluntary contraction. Abdominal pressure tracings reflected impaired diaphragmatic relaxation, and pleural pressure tracings made during sustained static inspiratory contraction showed rapid decline in strength. This patient had a normal chest radiograph and normal pulmonary function tests. He experienced dyspnea and chest tightness at the onset of exercise, but these symptoms cleared after a warm-up period, and he could then run for several miles. Rhythmic contraction of the muscles produced much less weakness than sustained static contractions.

## Convulsive Disorders

### Epilepsy

Grand mal seizures, even status epilepticus, do not usually pose a serious threat to ventilation; they are often associated with acidosis, usually due to increased blood lactate concentration rather than hypercapnia.[204] In rare cases, especially when there is underlying respiratory disease or neuromuscular weakness, alveolar hypoventilation may occur.

### Strychnine Poisoning

Strychnine, which is a common diluent of street drugs and an ingredient of many legitimate compounds, blocks inhibitory neurons in the spinal cord.[204] Consequently, motor neuron discharge can be precipitated by even trivial sensory stimuli, resulting in global muscle spasm that is somewhat difficult to differentiate clinically from a grand mal seizure. The pattern of the seizure is dominated by the more powerful extensor muscles, so that tonic and clonic activity is absent. The symptoms of strychnine poisoning begin within minutes of ingestion and progress over several hours. Patients are usually highly alert, with no postictal mental depression.

Treatment is supportive and includes measures to minimize muscle spasms. Milder spasms can be controlled with phenobarbital or diazepam, but in severe cases, it is necessary to paralyze the patient with pancuronium or d-tubocurarine, along with heavy sedation. Detoxification and excretion of strychnine occur within 72 hours, and cumulative toxicity does not occur. Therefore, one can anticipate that paralysis and mechanical ventilatory support need to be maintained for less than 24 hours in the absence of other complications. When the muscle spasms are stopped, temperature, lactic acid concentration, and blood gas composition rapidly return to normal.[204] Severe muscle damage and renal failure are the major complications. The most important aspect of the clinical management of strychnine poisoning is to think of the diagnosis in the first place. The sooner effective treatment is started, the less likelihood there is of complications.

### Tetanus

The general mechanism of action of picrotoxin and tetanus toxin is similar to the action of strychnine, although the precise nature of inhibitory transmitter blockade differs among the three substances. Tetanus produces muscle spasms virtually identical to those of strychnine poisoning, but recovery is delayed. Again, inhibitory neurotransmitter blockade is a prominent effect of tetanus toxin, although by no means the only one. Unlike the abrupt onset of symptoms in strychnine poisoning, the symptoms of tetanus progress more slowly, often over days; consequently, cases that initially appear to be mild may turn out to be extremely severe. The prevalence, underlying causes, and pathophysiology of tetanus have been reviewed by Alfery and Rauscher[205]; these authors also describe the various complicating factors and multiple aspects of treatment. Here, we wish to emphasize the life-threatening asphyxia consequent to severe and prolonged spasms of all muscles, including the respiratory muscles.

As with strychnine poisoning, mild cases of tetanus can be managed conservatively with sedation and muscle relaxants. However, severe cases require aggressive treatment with paralytic agents and mechanical ventilation.[206] The ventilatory component of management consists of sedation, muscle relaxants, tracheal intubation, and mechanical ventilation. Because the course of severe tetanus is prolonged, many physicians opt for tracheostomy early on. Patients with tetanus often experience a level of muscle spasm that produces rigidity without an overt convulsive episode. When this occurs, the ventilator pressure gauge shows high peak inspiratory pressures, not because of abnormal lung compliance or airway resistance, but because of chest wall stiffness. If severe, this is an indication for muscle paralysis, in part to facilitate ventilation and in part to minimize lactic acidosis and muscle necrosis. The principal agents for muscle paralysis are pancuronium and *d*-tubocurarine. Pancuronium is the agent of choice, despite its mild sympathomimetic side effects. *d*-Tubocurarine can cause hypotension, and its effects are to some extent cumulative. The principal pulmonary complications of tetanus and its treatment are related to intubation or tracheostomy, atelectasis, aspiration, and pneumonia. Patients with tetanus frequently have excessive sympathetic nervous system activity, which may be treated with beta-adrenergic blocking agents.

## SUMMARY

Different types of neuromuscular disease produce essentially similar ventilatory dysfunction. Pulmonary function tests typically show a restrictive pattern, with decreases in vital capacity and total lung capacity. Residual volume is often increased. There is sometimes variable extrathoracic upper airway obstruction. Tachypnea is a common feature of almost all neuromuscular diseases, and tidal volume tends to fall. Other symptoms and signs depend on the specific condition and its severity.

Respiratory complications are common in neuromuscular diseases. The most serious is ventilatory failure; carbon dioxide retention generally occurs when inspiratory muscle strength is less than half normal. The magnitude of hypercapnia is proportional to the severity of the respiratory muscle weakness. Pneumonia is a constant threat because of impaired cough, microatelectasis consequent to shallow breathing, and, in many patients, recurrent aspiration. Some patients with neuromuscular disease are also particularly susceptible to deep vein thrombosis and pulmonary embolism.

Few specific treatments are available for ventilatory insufficiency in neuromuscular disease. Nevertheless, supportive care based on administration of oxygen, assisted coughing, and attention to nutritional status can often prevent or delay the progression to ventilatory failure. Furthermore, advances in the noninvasive management of ventilatory failure have greatly improved the quality of life for such patients.

## References

1. Inkley SR, Oldenburg FC, Vignos PJ Jr: Pulmonary function in Duchenne muscular dystrophy related to stage of disease. Am J Med 56:297–306, 1974.
2. Frankel HL, Coll JR, Charlifue SW, et al: Long-term survival in spinal cord injury: A fifty year investigation. Spinal Cord 36:266–274, 1998.
3. Papastamelos C, Panitch HB, Allen JL: Chest wall compliance in infants and children with neuromuscular disease. Am J Respir Crit Care Med 154:1045–1048, 1996.
4. Lieberman SL, Young RR, Shefner JM: Neurological disorders affecting respiration. *In* Roussos C (ed): Lung Biology in Health and Disease (2nd ed). Vol 85: The Thorax. New York: Marcel Dekker, 1995, pp 2135–2175.
5. De Troyer A, Estenne M: The respiratory system in neuromuscular disorders. *In* Roussos C (ed): Lung Biology in Health and Disease (2nd ed). Vol 85: The Thorax. New York: Marcel Dekker, 1995, pp 2177–2212.
6. Aldrich TK, Rochester DF: The lungs and neuromuscular disease. *In* Murray JF, Nadel JA (eds): Textbook of Respiratory Medicine (2nd ed). Philadelphia: WB Saunders, 1994, pp 2524–2544.
7. Bennett DA, Bleck TP: Diagnosis and treatment of neuromuscular causes of acute respiratory failure. Clin Neuropharmacol 11:303–347, 1988.
8. Rochester DF, Findley LJ: Neuromuscular and skeletal diseases. *In* Murray JF (ed): Lung Biology in Health and Disease. Pulmonary Manifestations of Systemic Disease (vol 59). New York: Marcel Dekker, 1992.
9. Cohen MI, Sicca AL, Donnelly DF, et al: Differences between thoracic and airway motoneuron discharge patterns and their significance. *In* Sieck GC, Gandevia SC, Cameron WE (eds): Respiratory Muscles and Their Neuromotor Control: Proceedings of an IUPS Satellite Symposium Held in Los Angeles, California, July 22–24, 1986. New York: Alan R Liss, 1987, pp 175–184.
10. Campbell EJM, Agostoni E, Newsom-Davis J: The Respiratory Muscles: Mechanics and Neural Control. Philadelphia: WB Saunders, 1970.
11. Osmond DG: Functional anatomy of the chest wall. *In* Roussos C (ed): Lung Biology in Health and Disease (2nd ed). Vol 85: The Thorax. New York: Marcel Dekker, 1995, pp 413–444.
12. De Troyer A, Loring SH: Actions of the respiratory muscles. *In* Roussos C (ed): Lung Biology in Health and Disease (2nd ed). Vol 85: The Thorax. New York: Marcel Dekker, 1995, pp 535–563.
13. Braun NMT, Arora NS, Rochester DF: Respiratory muscle and pulmonary function in polymyositis and other proximal myopathies. Thorax 38:616–623, 1983.
14. De Troyer A, Deisser P: The effects of intermittent positive pressure breathing on patients with respiratory muscle weakness. Am Rev Respir Dis 124:132–137, 1981.
15. Estenne M, Heilporn A, Delhez L, et al: Chest wall stiffness in patients with chronic respiratory muscle weakness. Am Rev Respir Dis 128:1002–1007, 1983.
16. Gal TJ, Arora NS: Respiratory mechanics in supine subjects during progressive partial curarization. J Appl Physiol 52:57–63, 1982.
17. Begin R, Bureau MA, Lupien L, et al: Control of breathing in Duchenne's muscular dystrophy. Am J Med 69:227–234, 1980.
18. Begin P, Mathieu J, Almirall J, et al: Relationship between chronic hypercapnia and inspiratory muscle weakness in myotonic dystrophy. Am J Respir Crit Care Med 156:133–139, 1997.
19. Baydur A: Respiratory muscle strength and control of ventilation in patients with neuromuscular disease. Chest 99:330–338, 1991.
20. Holle RHO, Schoene RB, Pavlin EJ: Effect on $P_{0.1}$ of respiratory muscle weakness induced by partial curarization. J Appl Physiol 57:1150–1157, 1984.
21. Spinelli A, Marconi G, Gorini M, et al: Control of breathing in patients with myasthenia gravis. Am Rev Respir Dis 145:1359–1366, 1992.
22. Manning HL, Brown R, Scharf SM, et al: Ventilatory and $P_{0.1}$ response to hypercapnia in quadriplegia. Respir Physiol 89:97–112, 1992.
23. Weng TR, Schultz GE, Chang CH, et al: Pulmonary function and ventilatory response to chemical stimuli in familial myopathy. Chest 88:488–495, 1985.
24. Wilson DO, Saunders MH, Dauber JH: Abnormal ventilatory chemosensitivity and congenital myopathy. Arch Intern Med 147:1773–1777, 1987.
25. Carroll JE, Zwillich CW, Weil JV: Ventilatory response in myotonic dystrophy. Neurology 27:1125–1128, 1977.
26. Labanowski J, Schmidt-Nowara W, Guilleminault C: Sleep and neuromuscular disease: Frequency of sleep-disordered breathing in a neuromuscular disease clinic population. Neurology 47:1173–1180, 1996.
27. McEvoy RD, Mykytun I, Sajkov D, et al: Sleep apnoea in patients with quadriplegia. Thorax 50:613–619, 1995.
28. Thorpy MJ, Schmidt-Nowara WW, Pollack CP, et al: Sleep-induced non-obstructive hypoventilation associated with diaphragmatic paralysis. Ann Neurol 12:308–311, 1982.
29. Steljes DG, Kryger MH, Kirk BW, et al: Sleep in postpolio syndrome. Chest 98:133–140, 1990.
30. Ferguson KA, Strong MJ, Ahmad D: Sleep-disordered breathing in amyotrophic lateral sclerosis. Chest 110:664–669, 1996.
31. Hansotia P, Frens D: Hypersomnolence associated with alveolar hypoventilation in myotonic dystrophy. Neurology 31:1336–1337, 1981.
32. Marcus CL, Loughlin GM: Obstructive sleep apnea in children. Semin Pediatr Neurol 3:23–38, 1996.
33. Smith PEM, Edwards RHT, Galverley PMA: Ventilation and breathing pattern during sleep in Duchenne muscular dystrophy. Chest 96:1346–1351, 1989.
34. Khan Y, Heckmatt JZ: Obstructive apnoeas in Duchenne muscular dystrophy. Thorax 49:157–161, 1994.
35. Skatrud J, Iber C, McHugh W, et al: Determinants of hypoventilation during wakefulness and sleep in diaphragmatic paralysis. Am Rev Respir Dis 121:587–593, 1980.

36. Sajkov D, Marshall R, Walker P, et al: Sleep apnoea related hypoxia is associated with cognitive disturbances in patients with tetraplegia. Spinal Cord 36:231–239, 1998.
36a. Dicpinigaitis PV, Grimm DR, Lesser M: Cough reflex sensitivity in subjects with cervical spinal cord injury. Am J Respir Crit Care Med 159:1660–1662, 1999.
37. VanLunteren E, Daniels R, Deal EC Jr, et al: Role of costal and crural diaphragm and parasternal intercostals during coughing in cats. J Appl Physiol 66:135–141, 1989.
38. Knudson RJ, Mead J, Knudson DE: Contribution of airway collapse to supramaximal expiratory flows. J Appl Physiol 36:653–667, 1974.
39. Arora NS, Gal TJ: Cough dynamics during progressive expiratory muscle weakness in healthy curarized subjects. J Appl Physiol 51:494–498, 1981.
40. Szeinberg A, Tabachnik E, Rashed N, et al: Cough capacity in patients with muscular dystrophy. Chest 94:1232–1235, 1988.
41. Aldrich TK, Shapiro SM, Sherman MS, et al: Alveolar pressure and airway resistance during maximal and submaximal respiratory efforts. Am Rev Respir Dis 140:899–906, 1989.
42. Putman M, Wise RA: Myasthenia gravis and upper airway obstruction. Chest 109:400–404, 1996.
43. Myllynen P, Kammonen M, Rokkanen P, et al: Deep venous thrombosis and pulmonary embolism in patients with acute spinal cord injury: A comparison with nonparalyzed patients immobilized due to spinal fractures. Trauma 25:541–543, 1985.
44. Hamilton MG, Hull RD, Pineo GF: Venous thromboembolism in neurosurgery and neurology patients: A review. Neurosurgery 34:280–296, 1994.
45. Newsom-Davis J, Goldman M, Loh L, et al: Diaphragm function and alveolar hypoventilation. Q J Med 177:87–100, 1976.
46. Roussos C, Fixley M, Gross D, et al: Fatigue of inspiratory muscles and their synergistic behavior. J Appl Physiol 46:897–904, 1979.
47. Houston JG, Fleet M, Cowan MD, et al: Comparison of ultrasound with fluoroscopy in the assessment of suspected hemidiaphragm movement abnormality. Clin Radiol 50:95–98, 1995.
48. Gottesman E, McCool FD: Ultrasound evaluation of the paralyzed diaphragm. Am J Respir Crit Care Med 155:1570–1574, 1997.
49. Rochester DF, Esau SA: Assessment of ventilatory function in patients with neuromuscular disease. Clin Chest Med 15:751–763, 1994.
50. Allen SM, Hunt B, Green M: Fall in vital capacity with posture. Br J Dis Chest 79:267–271, 1985.
51. Fallat RJ, Jewitt B, Bass M, et al: Spirometry in amyotrophic lateral sclerosis. Arch Neurol 36:74–80, 1979.
52. Griggs RC, Donohoe KM, Utell MJ, et al: Evaluation of pulmonary function in neuromuscular disease. Arch Neurol 38:9–12, 1981.
53. Laroche CM, Carroll N, Moxham J, et al: Clinical significance of severe isolated diaphragm weakness. Am Rev Respir Dis 138:862–866, 1988.
54. Perez A, Mulot R, Vardon G, et al: Thoracoabdominal pattern of breathing in neuromuscular disorders. Chest 110:454–461, 1996.
55. Clanton TL, Diaz PT: Clinical assessment of the respiratory muscles. Phys Ther 75:983–95, 1995.
56. Rubinstein I, Slutsky AS, Rebuck AS, et al: Assessment of maximal expiratory pressure in healthy adults. J Appl Physiol 64:2215–2219, 1988.
57. Braun NMT, Arora NS, Rochester DF: Force-length relationship of the normal human diaphragm. J Appl Physiol 53:405–412, 1982.
58. Aldrich TK, Spiro P: Maximal inspiratory pressure: Does reproducibility indicate full effort? Thorax 50:40–43, 1995.
59. Mier-Jedrzejowicz AK, Brophy C, Moxhain J, et al: Assessment of diaphragm weakness. Am Rev Respir Dis 137:877–883, 1988.
60. Arora NS, Gal TJ: Cough dynamics during progressive expiratory muscle weakness in healthy curarized subjects. J Appl Physiol 51:494–498, 1981.
61. Iberti TJ, Lieber CE, Benjamin E: Determination of intra-abdominal pressure using a transurethral bladder catheter: Clinical validation of the technique. Anesthesiology 70:47–50, 1989.
62. Ostrander LE, Schneider AJL, Burma G, et al: A comparison of central venous and pleural pressure in supine dogs. Respir Physiol 31:63–70, 1977.
63. McCauley RGK, Labib KB: Diaphragmatic paralysis evaluated by phrenic nerve stimulation during fluoroscopy or real-time ultrasound. Radiology 153:33–36, 1984.
64. Mier A, Brophy C, Moxham J, et al: Phrenic nerve stimulation in normal subjects and in patients with diaphragmatic weakness. Thorax 42:885–888, 1987.
65. Mills GH, Kyroussis D, Hamnegard CH, et al: Cervical magnetic stimulation of the phrenic nerves in bilateral diaphragm paralysis. Am J Respir Crit Care Med 155:1565–1569, 1997.
66. Laghi F, Harrison MJ, Tobin MJ: Comparison of magnetic and electrical phrenic nerve stimulation in assessment of diaphragmatic contractility. J Appl Physiol 80:1731–1742, 1996.
67. Dimopoulou I, Daganou M, Dafni U, et al: Phrenic nerve dysfunction after cardiac operations: Electrophysiologic evaluation of risk factors. Chest 113:8–14, 1998.
68. Olopade CO, Staats BA: Time course of recovery from frostbitten phrenics after coronary artery bypass graft surgery. Chest 99:1112–1115, 1991.
69. De Troyer A, Vanderhoeft P: Phrenic nerve function after pneumonectomy. Chest 81:212–214, 1982.
70. Maziak DE, Maurer JR, Kesten S: Diaphragmatic paralysis: A complication of lung transplantation. Ann Thorac Surg 61:170–173, 1996.
71. Dorffner R, Eibenberger K, Youssefzadeh S: Diaphragmatic dysfunction after heart or lung transplantation. J Heart Lung Transplant 16:566–569, 1997.
72. Sheridan PH, Cheriyan A, Doud J, et al: Incidence of phrenic neuropathy after isolated lung transplantation. The Loyola University Lung Transplant Group. J Heart Lung Transplant 14:684–691, 1995.
73. Heffner JE: Diaphragmatic paralysis following chiropractic manipulation of the cervical spine. Arch Intern Med 145:562–563, 1985.
74. DeJong AA, Manni JJ: Phrenic nerve paralysis following neck dissection. Eur Arch Otorhinolaryngol 248:132–134, 1991.
75. Vest JV, Pereira M, Senior RM: Phrenic nerve injury associated with venipuncture of the internal jugular vein. Chest 78:777–779, 1980.
76. Aldrich TK, Herman JH, Rochester DF: Bilateral diaphragmatic paralysis in the newborn infant. J Pediatr 97:988–991, 1980.
77. Piehler JM, Pairolero PC, Gracey DR, et al: Unexplained diaphragmatic paralysis: A harbinger of malignant disease? J Thorac Cardiovasc Surg 84:861–864, 1982.
78. Stowasser M, Cameron J, Oliver WA: Diaphragmatic paralysis following cervical herpes zoster. Med J Aust 153:555–556, 1990.
79. De Vito EL, Quadrelli SA, Montiel GC, et al: Bilateral diaphragmatic paralysis after mediastinal radiotherapy. Respiration 63:187–190, 1996.
80. Brander PE, Jarvinen V, Lohela P, et al: Bilateral diaphragmatic weakness: A late complication of radiotherapy. Thorax 52:829–831, 1997.
81. Chan CK, Loke J, Virgulto JA, et al: Bilateral diaphragmatic paralysis: Clinical spectrum, prognosis, and diagnostic approach. Arch Phys Med Rehabil 67:161–165, 1988.
82. Mulvey DA, Aquilina RJ, Elliott MW, et al: Diaphragmatic dysfunction in neuralgic amyotrophy: An electrophysiologic evaluation of 16 patients presenting with dyspnea. Am Rev Respir Dis. 147:66–71, 1993.
83. Balbierz JM, Ellenberg M, Honet JC: Complete hemidiaphragmatic paralysis in a patient with multiple sclerosis. Am J Phys Med Rehabil 67:161–165, 1988.
84. Haas H, Johnson LR, Gill TH, et al: Diaphragm paralysis and ventilatory failure in proximal spinal muscular atrophy. Am Rev Respir Dis 123:465–467, 1981.
85. Lisboa C, Pare PD, Pertuze J, et al: Inspiratory muscle function in unilateral diaphragmatic paralysis. Am Rev Respir Dis 134:488–492, 1986.
86. Gould L, Kaplan S, McElhinney AJ, et al: A method for the production of hemidiaphragmatic paralysis. Am Rev Respir Dis 96:812–814, 1967.
87. Fackler CD, Perret GE, Bedell GN: Effect of unilateral phrenic nerve section on lung function. J Appl Physiol 23:923–926, 1967.
88. Easton PA, Fleetham JA, De La Rocha A, et al: Respiratory function after paralysis of the right hemidiaphragm. Am Rev Respir Dis 127:125–128, 1983.

89. Allen SM, Hunt B, Green M: Fall in vital capacity with posture. Br J Dis Chest 79:267–271, 1985.
90. Graham DR, Kaplan D, Evans CC, et al: Diaphragmatic plication for unilateral diaphragmatic paralysis: A 10-year experience. Ann Thorac Surg 49:248–252, 1990.
91. Merav AD, Attai LA, Condit DD: Successful repair of a transected phrenic nerve with restoration of diaphragmatic function. Chest 84:642–644, 1983.
92. Brouillette RT, Hahn YS, Noah ZL, et al: Successful reinnervation of the diaphragm after phrenic nerve transection. J Pediatr Surg 21:63–65, 1986.
93. Zifko U, Hartmann M, Girsch W, et al: Diaphragmatic paresis in newborns due to phrenic nerve injury. Neuropediatrics 26:281–284, 1995.
94. Kreiger AJ, Gropper MR, Adler RJ: Electrophrenic respiration after intercostal to phrenic nerve anastomosis in a patient with anterior spinal artery syndrome: Technical case report. Neurosurgery 35:760–763, 1994.
95. Haller JA, Pickard LR, Trepas JJ, et al: Management of diaphragmatic paralysis in infants with special emphasis on selection of patients for operative plication. J Pediatr Surg 14:779–785, 1979.
96. Abd AG, Braun NMT, Baskin MI, et al: Diaphragmatic dysfunction after open heart surgery: Treatment with a rocking bed. Ann Intern Med 111:881–886, 1989.
97. Bach JR, Alba AS: Management of chronic alveolar hypoventilation by nasal ventilation. Chest 97:52–57, 1990.
98. Bach JR, McDermott IG: Strapless oral-nasal interface for positive-pressure ventilation. Arch Phys Med Rehabil 71:910–913, 1990.
99. Ford GT, Whitelaw WA, Rosenal TW, et al: Diaphragm function after upper abdominal surgery in humans. Am Rev Respir Dis 127:431–436, 1983.
100. Simonneau E, Vivien A, Sartene R, et al: Diaphragm dysfunction induced by upper abdominal surgery. Am Rev Respir Dis 128:899–903, 1983.
101. Melendez JA, Alagesan R, Reinsel R, et al: Postthoracotomy respiratory muscle mechanics during incentive spirometry using respiratory inductance plethysmography. Chest 101:432–436, 1992.
102. Road JD, Burgess KR, Whitelaw WA, et al: Diaphragm function and respiratory response after upper abdominal surgery in dogs. J Appl Physiol 57:576–582, 1984.
103. Torres A, Kimball WR, Qvist J, et al: Sonomicrometric regional diaphragmatic shortening in awake sheep after thoracic surgery. J Appl Physiol 67:2357–2368, 1989.
104. Road J, Vahi R, Del Rio P, et al: In vivo contractile properties of fatigued diaphragm. J Appl Physiol 63:471–478, 1987.
105. Hartkopp A, Bronnum-Hansen H, Seidenschnur A-M, et al: Survival and cause of death after traumatic spinal cord injury: A long-term epidemiological survey from Denmark. Spinal Cord 35:76–85, 1997.
106. Newsom-Davis J: Autonomous breathing. Arch Neurol 30:480–483, 1974.
107. De Troyer A, Estenne M, Vincken W: Rib cage motion and muscle use in high tetraplegics. Am Rev Respir Dis 133:1115–1119, 1986.
108. Bach JR, Alba AS: Noninvasive options for ventilatory support of the traumatic high level quadriplegic patient. Chest 98:613–619, 1990.
109. Glenn WWL, Hogan JF, Phelps ML: Ventilatory support of the quadriplegic patient with respiratory paralysis by diaphragm pacing. Surg Clin North Am 60:1055–1078, 1980.
110. De Troyer A, Heilporn A: Respiratory mechanics in quadriplegia: The respiratory function of the intercostal muscles. Am Rev Respir Dis 122:591–600, 1980.
111. Haas F, Axen K, Pineda H, et al: Temporal pulmonary function changes in cervical cord injury. Arch Phys Med Rehabil 66:139–144, 1985.
112. Wang AY, Jaeger RJ, Yarkony GM, et al: Cough in spinal cord injured patients: The relationship between motor level and peak expiratory flow. 35:299–302, 1997.
113. De Troyer A, Estenne M, Heilporn A: Mechanism of active expiration in tetraplegic subjects. N Engl J Med 314:740–744, 1986.
114. Estenne M, Gorini M: Action of the diaphragm during cough in tetraplegic subjects. J Appl Physiol 72:1074–1080, 1992.
115. Dicpinigaitis PV, Spungen AM, Bauman WA, et al: Bronchial hyperresponsiveness after cervical spinal cord injury. Chest 105:1073–1076, 1994.
115a. Grimm DR, Arias E, Lesser M, et al: Airway hyperresponsiveness to ultrasonically nebulized distilled water in subjects with tetraplegia. J Appl Physiol 86:1165–1169, 1999.
116. Estenne M, De Troyer A: Mechanism of the postural dependence of vital capacity in tetraplegic subjects. Am Rev Respir Dis 135:367–371, 1987.
117. Estenne M, De Troyer A: Relationship between respiratory muscle electromyogram and rib cage motion in tetraplegia. Am Rev Respir Dis 132:53–59, 1985.
118. Urmey W, Loring S, Mead J, et al: Upper and lower rib cage deformation during breathing in quadriplegia. J Appl Physiol 60:618–622, 1986.
119. Macklem PT, Macklem DM, De Troyer A: A model of inspiratory muscle mechanics. J Appl Physiol 55:547–557, 1983.
120. Stone DJ, Keltz H: The effect of respiratory muscle dysfunction on pulmonary function. Am Rev Respir Dis 88:621–629, 1963.
121. Schwartzstein R, Leight D, Scharf S, et al: $CO_2$ response in chronic quadriplegics. Am Rev Respir Dis 131:A337, 1985.
122. Axen K, Bergofsky EH: Thoracic reflexes stabilizing loaded ventilation in normal and cord-injured man. J Appl Physiol 43:339–346, 1977.
123. DiMarco AF, Wolfson DA, Gottfried SB, et al: Sensation of inspired volume in normal subjects and quadriplegic patients. J Appl Physiol 53:1481–1486, 1982.
124. Wicks AB, Menter RR: Long-term outlook in quadriplegic patients with initial ventilator dependency. Chest 90:406–410, 1986.
124a. Oo T, Watt JW, Soni BM, Sett PK: Delayed diaphragm recovery in 12 patients after high cervical spine cord injury. A retrospective review of the diaphragm status of 107 patients ventilated after acute spinal cord injury. Spinal Cord 37:117–122, 1999.
125. Santamaria J, Ruiz C: Diaphragm elevation in stroke. Eur Neurol 28:81–83, 1988.
126. Korczyn AD, Leibowitz U, Bruderman I: Involvement of the diaphragm in hemiplegia. Neurology 19:97–100, 1969.
127. Fluck DC: Chest movements in hemiplegia. Clin Sci 31:383–388, 1966.
128. De Troyer A, De Beyl DZ, Thirion M: Function of the respiratory muscles in acute hemiplegia. Am Rev Respir Dis 123:631–632, 1981.
129. Adams AB, Whitman J, Marcy T: Surveys of long-term ventilatory support in Minnesota: 1986 and 1992. Chest 103:1463–1469, 1993.
130. Linderholm H, Werneman H: On respiratory regulation in poliomyelitis convalescents. Acta Med Scand Suppl 316:135–157, 1956.
131. Plum F, Swanson AG: Abnormalities in central regulation of respiration in acute and convalescent poliomyelitis. Arch Neurol Psychiatr 80:267–285, 1958.
132. Cherniack RM, Ewart WB, Hildes JA: Polycythemia secondary to respiratory disturbances in poliomyelitis. Ann Intern Med 46:720–727, 1957.
133. Fischer DA: Poliomyelitis: Late pulmonary complications and management. *In* Halstead LS, Wiechers DO (eds): Late Effects of Poliomyelitis. Miami: Symposium Foundation, 1985, pp 185–192.
134. Hsu AA, Staats BA: "Postpolio" sequelae and sleep-related disordered breathing. Mayo Clinic Proc 73:216–224, 1998.
135. Gracey DR, McMichan JC, Divertie MB, et al: Respiratory failure in Guillain-Barré syndrome. Mayo Clin Proc 57:742–746, 1982.
136. De Troyer A, Borenstein S: Acute changes in respiratory mechanics after pyridostigmine injection in patients with myasthenia gravis. Am Rev Respir Dis 121:629–638, 1980.
137. Smith AG, Wald J: Acute ventilatory failure in Lambert-Eaton myasthenic syndrome and its response to 3,4-diaminopyridine. Neurology 46:1143–1145, 1996.
138. Mier A, Laroche C, Green M: Unsuspected myasthenia gravis presenting as respiratory failure. Thorax 45:422–423, 1990.
139. Renzi G, Cournoyer G, Laporta D, et al: The effect of anticholinesterases on the respiratory muscle function in myasthenia gravis. Am Rev Respir Dis 131:A331, 1985.
140. Wilcox PG, Morrison NJ, Anzarut ARA, et al: Lambert-Eaton

myasthenic syndrome involving the diaphragm. Chest 93:604–607, 1988.
141. Bain PG, Motomura M, Newsom-Davis J: Effects of intravenous immunoglobulin on muscle weakness and calcium-channel autoantibodies in the Lambert-Eaton myasthenic syndrome. Neurology 47:678–683, 1996.
142. Schmidt-Nowara WW, Samet JM, Rosario PA: Early and late pulmonary complications of botulism. Arch Intern Med 143:451–456, 1983.
143. Puggiari M, Cherington M: Botulism and guanidine. JAMA 240:2276–2277, 1978.
144. Wilcox P, Andolfatto G, Fairbairn MS, et al: Long-term follow up of symptoms, pulmonary function, respiratory muscle strength, and exercise performance after botulism. Am Rev Respir Dis 139:157–163, 1989.
145. Aldrich TK, Prezant DJ: Adverse effects of drugs on the respiratory muscles. Clin Chest Med 11:177–189, 1990.
146. Kreitzer SM, Saunders NA, Tyler HR, et al: Respiratory muscle function in amyotrophic lateral sclerosis. Am Rev Respir Dis 117:437–447, 1978.
147. Jammes Y, Pouget J, Grimaud C, et al: Pulmonary function and electromyographic study of respiratory muscles in myotonic dystrophy. Muscle Nerve 8:586–594, 1985.
148. Rimmer KP, Golar SD, Lee MA, et al: Myotonia of the respiratory muscles in myotonic dystrophy. Am Rev Respir Dis 148:1018–1022, 1993.
149. Poponick J, Jacobs I, Supinski G, et al: Effect of upper respiratory tract infection in patients with neuromuscular disease. Am J Respir Crit Care Med 156:659–664, 1997.
150. Borel CO, Tilford C, Nichols DG, et al: Diaphragmatic performance during recovery from acute ventilatory failure in Guillain-Barré syndrome and myasthenia gravis. Chest 99:444–451, 1991.
151. Jabour ER, Rabil DM, Truwit JD, et al.: Evaluation of a new weaning index, based on ventilatory endurance and the efficiency of gas exchange. Am Rev Respir Dis 144:531–537, 1991.
152. Miller RG, Shepherd R, Dao H, et al: Controlled trial of nimodipine in amyotrophic lateral sclerosis. Neuromuscul Disord 6:101–104, 1996.
153. Miller RG, Smith SA, Murphy JR, et al: A clinical trial of verapamil in amyotrophic lateral sclerosis. Muscle Nerve 19:511–515, 1996.
154. Festoff BW: Amyotrophic lateral sclerosis: Current and future treatment strategies. Drugs 51:28–44, 1996.
155. Petroff BJ: Respiratory muscles as a target for adenovirus-mediated gene therapy. Eur Respir J 11:492–497, 1998.
156. Grant I, Prigatano GP, Heaton RK, et al: Progressive neuropsychologic impairment and hypoxemia. Arch Gen Psychiatr 44:999–1006, 1987.
157. Jardim J, Farkas G, Prefaut C, et al: The failing inspiratory muscles under normoxic and hypoxic conditions. Am Rev Respir Dis 124:274–279, 1981.
158. Braun NMT, Faulkner J: When should respiratory muscles be exercised? Chest 84:76–84, 1983.
159. Haake RE, Saxon LA, Bander SJ, et al: Depressed central respiratory drive causing weaning failure: Its reversal with doxapram. Chest 95:695–697, 1989.
159a. Schols AM, Soeters PB, Mostert R, et al: Physiologic effects of nutritional support and anabolic steroids in patients with chronic obstructive pulmonary disease. A placebo-controlled randomized trial. Am J Respir Crit Care Med 152:1268–1274, 1995.
159b. Ferreira IM, Verrewschi IT, Nery LE, et al: The influence of 6 months of oral anabolic steroids on body mass and respiratory muscles in undernourished COPD patients. Chest 114:19–28, 1998.
159c. Grinspoon S, Corcoran C, Askari H, et al: Effects of androgen administration in men with the AIDS wasting syndrome. A randomized, double-blind, placebo-controlled trial. Ann Intern Med 129:18–26, 1998.
159d. Johansen KL, Mulligan K, Schambelan M: Anabolic effects of nandrolone decanoate in patients receiving dialysis: A randomized controlled trial. JAMA 281:1275–1281, 1999.
159e. Demling RH: Comparison of the anabolic effects and complications of human growth hormone and the testosterone analog, oxandrolone, after severe burn injury. Burns 25:215–221, 1999.
159f. Spungen AM, Grimm DR, Strakhan M, et al: Treatment with an anabolic agent is associated with improvement in respiratory function in persons with tetraplegia: A pilot study. Mt Sinai J Med 66:201–205, 1999.
159g. Schambelan M, Mulligan K, Grunfeld C, et al: Recombinant human growth hormone in patients with HIV-associated wasting. A randomized, placebo-controlled trial. Ann Intern Med 125:873–882, 1996.
159h. Burdet L, deMuralt B, Schutz Y, et al: Administration of growth hormone to underweight patients with chronic obstructive pulmonary disease. A prospective, randomized, controlled study. Am J Respir Crit Care Med 156:1800–1806, 1997.
160. Bach JR, Smith WH, Michaels J, et al: Airway secretion clearance by mechanical exsufflation for post-poliomyelitis ventilator-assisted individuals. Arch Phys Med Rehabil 74:170–177, 1993.
161. Jaeger RJ, Turba RM, Yarkony GM, et al: Cough in spinal cord injured patients: Comparison of three methods to produce cough. Arch Phys Med Rehabil 74:1358–1361, 1993.
162. Zupan A, Savrin R, Erjavec T, et al: Effects of respiratory muscle training and electrical stimulation of abdominal muscles on respiratory capabilities in tetraplegic patients. Spinal Cord 35:540–545, 1997.
163. Lin VW, Singh H, Chitkara RK, et al: Functional magnetic stimulation for restoring cough in patients with tetraplegia. Arch Phys Med Rehabil 79:517–522, 1998.
164. Mazza FG, DiMarco AF, Altose MD, et al: The flow-volume loop during glossopharyngeal breathing. Chest 85:638–640, 1984.
165. Estenne M, Knoop C, Vanvaerenbergh J, et al: The effect of pectoralis muscle training in tetraplegic subjects. Am Rev Respir Dis 139:1218–1222, 1989.
166. Huldtgren AC, Fugl-Meyer AR, Jonasson E, et al: Ventilatory dysfunction and respiratory rehabilitation in post-traumatic quadriplegia. Eur J Respir Dis 61:347–356, 1980.
166a. Uijl SG, Houtman S, Folgering HT, Hepman MT: Training of the respiratory muscles in individuals with tetraplegia. Spinal Cord 37:575–579, 1999.
167. Rutchik A, Issman AR, Almenoff PL, et al: Resistive inspiratory muscle training in subjects with chronic cervical spinal cord injury. Arch Phys Med Rehabil 79:293–297, 1998.
168. Gross D, Ladd HW, Riley EJ, et al: The effect of training on strength and endurance of the diaphragm in quadriplegia. Am J Med 68:27–35, 1980.
169. DiMarco AF, Kelling JS, DiMarco MS, et al: The effects of inspiratory resistive training on respiratory muscle function in patients with muscular dystrophy. Muscle Nerve 8:284–290, 1985.
170. Wanke T, Toifl K, Merkle M, et al: Inspiratory muscle training in patients with Duchenne muscular dystrophy. Chest 105:475–482, 1994.
171. Martin AJ, Stern L, Yeates J, et al: Respiratory muscle training in Duchenne muscular dystrophy. Dev Med Child Neurol 28:314–318, 1986.
172. Smith PEM, Coakley JH, Edwards RHT: Respiratory muscle training in Duchenne muscular dystrophy. Muscle Nerve 11:784, 1988.
173. Martin RJ, Sufit RL, Ringel SP, et al: Respiratory improvement by muscle training in adult-onset acid maltase deficiency. Muscle Nerve 6:201–203, 1983.
174. Estrup C, Lyager S, Noeraa N, et al: Effect of respiratory muscle training in patients with neuromuscular diseases. Respiration 50:36–43, 1986.
175. Aldrich TK, Karpel JP, Uhrlass RM, et al: Weaning from mechanical ventilation: Adjunctive use of inspiratory muscle resistive training. Crit Care Med 17:143–147, 1989.
176. Lerman RM, Weiss MS: Progressive resistive exercises in weaning high quadriplegics from the ventilator. Paraplegia 25:130–135, 1987.
177. Nochomovitz ML, Hopkins M, Brodkey J, et al: Conditioning of the diaphragm with phrenic nerve stimulation after prolonged disuse. Am Rev Respir Dis 130:685–688, 1984.
178. Sherman MS, Paz HL: Review of respiratory care of the patient with amyotrophic lateral sclerosis. Respiration 61:61–67, 1994.
179. Bach JR, Rajaraman R, Ballanger F, et al: Neuromuscular ventilatory insufficiency: Effect of home mechanical ventilator use v oxygen therapy on pneumonia and hospitalization rates. Am J Phys Med Rehabil 77:8–19, 1998.
180. Bach JR, Alba AS: Intermittent abdominal pressure ventilator in

a regimen of noninvasive ventilatory support. Chest 99:630–636, 1991.
181. Braun SR, Sufit RL, Giovannoni R, et al: Intermittent negative pressure ventilation in the treatment of respiratory failure in progressive neuromuscular disease. Neurology 37:1874–1875, 1987.
182. Bach JR, Penek J: Obstructive sleep apnea complicating negative-pressure ventilatory support in patients with chronic paralytic/restrictive ventilatory dysfunction. Chest 99:1386–1393, 1991.
183. Gay PC, Patel AM, Viggiano RW, et al: Nocturnal nasal ventilation for treatment of patients with hypercapnic respiratory failure. Mayo Clin Proc 66:695–703, 1991.
184. Kesten S, Rebuck AS: Ventilatory effects of nasal continuous positive airway pressure. Eur Respir J 3:498–501, 1990.
185. Duncan SR, Negrin RS, Mihm FG, et al: Nasal continuous positive airway pressure in atelectasis. Chest 92:621–624, 1987.
186. Ciesielski TE, Fukuda Y, Glenn WWL, et al: Response of the diaphragm muscle to electrical stimulation of the phrenic nerve. J Neurosurg 58:92–100, 1983.
187. Mead J, Banzett RB, Lehr J, et al: Effect of posture on upper and lower rib cage motion and tidal volume during diaphragm pacing. Am Rev Respir Dis 130:320–321, 1984.
188. Scharf SM, Feldman NT, Goldman MD, et al: Vocal cord closure: A cause of upper airway obstruction during controlled ventilation. Am Rev Respir Dis 117:391–397, 1978.
189. Lewis JH: Hiccups: Causes and cures. J Clin Gastroenterol 7:539–552, 1985.
190. Newsom-Davis J: An experimental study of hiccup. Brain 93:851–872, 1970.
191. Jacobson PL, Messenheimer JA, Farmer TW: Treatment of intractable hiccups with valproic acid. Neurology 31:1458–1460, 1981.
192. Brouillette RT, Thach BT, Abu-Osba YK, et al: Hiccups in infants: Characteristics and effects on ventilation. J Pediatr 96:219–225, 1980.
193. Engleman EG, Lankton J, Lankton B: Granulated sugar as treatment for hiccups in conscious patients (letter). N Engl J Med 285:1489, 1971.
194. Salem RM, Baraka A, Rattenborg CC, et al: Treatment of hiccups by pharyngeal stimulation in anesthetized and conscious subjects. JAMA 202:126–130, 1967.
195. Fodstad H, Blom S: Phrenic nerve stimulation (diaphragm pacing) in chronic singultus. Neurochirurgia 27:115–116, 1984.
196. Guelaud C, Similowski T, Bizec JL, et al: Baclofen therapy for chronic hiccup. Eur Respir J 8:235–237, 1995.
197. Phillips JR, Eldridge FL: Respiratory myoclonus (Leeuwenhoek's disease). N Engl J Med 289:1390–1395, 1973.
198. Kimura E, Ichikawa A, Takahashi K, et al: Abnormal respiration and unusual movements of the diaphragm in patients with neurocirculatory asthenia. Am J Med Sci 265:205–214, 1973.
199. Weiner WJ, Goetz CG, Nausieda PA, et al: Respiratory dyskinesias: Extrapyramidal dysfunction and dyspnea. Ann Intern Med 88:327–331, 1978.
200. Neu HC, Connolly JJ Jr, Schwertley FW, et al: Obstructive respiratory dysfunction in parkinsonian patients. Am Rev Respir Dis 95:33–47, 1967.
201. Fontana GA, Pantaleo T, Lavorini F, et al: Defective motor control of coughing in Parkinson's disease. Am J Respir Crit Care Med 158:458–464, 1998.
202. Vincken WG, Gauthier SG, Dollfus RE, et al: Involvement of upper airway muscles in extrapyramidal disorders: A cause of airflow limitation. N Engl J Med 311:438–442, 1984.
203. Estenne M, Borenstein S, De Troyer A: Respiratory muscle dysfunction in myotonia congenita. Am Rev Respir Dis 130:691–684, 1984.
204. Boyd RE, Brennan PT, Deng JF, et al: Strychnine poisoning. Am J Med 74:507–512, 1983.
205. Alfery DD, Rauscher LA: Tetanus: A review. Crit Care Med 7:176–181, 1979.
206. Trujillo MJ, Castillo A, Espana JV, et al: Tetanus in the adult: Intensive care and management experience with 233 cases. Crit Care Med 8:419–423, 1980.

# 90 The Lungs and Chest Wall Diseases

F. Dennis McCool, M.D. • Dudley F. Rochester, M.D.

Kyphoscoliosis
- Diagnosis and Etiology
- Pathophysiology
- Clinical Course
- Treatment

Thoracoplasty
- Diagnosis and Etiology
- Pathophysiology
- Treatment

Pectus Excavatum
- Diagnosis and Etiology
- Pathophysiology
- Treatment

Flail Chest
- Diagnosis and Etiology
- Pathophysiology
- Treatment

Ankylosing Spondylitis
- Diagnosis and Etiology
- Pathophysiology
- Treatment

Obesity
- Diagnosis and Etiology
- Pathophysiology
- Treatment

Summary

This chapter focuses on diseases involving the bony structure of the rib cage, the spine, and the spine's articulations. These disorders may by themselves or in combination with other diseases interfere with inspiratory pump function and lead to respiratory failure. The diseases of the chest wall that most profoundly embarrass ventilatory function are kyphoscoliosis and restrictive disease resulting from previous thoracoplasty. Flail chest may result in respiratory failure, especially when there is associated pulmonary contusion. Other diseases that involve the bones of the rib cage or the spinal column, such as pectus excavatum, pectus carinatum, and ankylosing spondylitis, have much less effect on ventilatory capacity. Obesity is included in this section because of its profound effects on the mechanical properties of the chest wall. Diseases directly involving the respiratory muscles also depress ventilatory function and are discussed in Chapter 89.

## KYPHOSCOLIOSIS

### Diagnosis and Etiology

Kyphoscoliosis is a disease of the spine and its articulations that causes mild spinal deformities in as many as 1 in 1000 people and severe spinal deformity in as many as 1 in 10,000 people in the United States. The deformation of the spine in this disorder characteristically consists of an anteroposterior (AP) angulation (kyphosis), a lateral displacement or curvature (scoliosis), or both (Fig. 90.1). Scoliosis is almost always associated with kyphosis and the rotation of the spine around its long axis. The lateral and rotatory movement of the spine may create severe distortion of the ribs, consisting of wide separation of the interspaces posteriorly and crowding of the interspaces anteriorly.[1] Kyphosis may exist as an isolated deformity (e.g., in elderly patients with osteoporosis).

Hereditary factors may play a role in the development of kyphoscoliosis,[2] but the cause is usually unknown. Primary or idiopathic kyphoscoliosis may be related to defects in the vertebrae themselves or in the vertebral connective tissue. Idiopathic kyphoscoliosis often begins in childhood and may account for as many as 80% of cases of kyphoscoliosis. Less frequently, kyphoscoliosis is a sequela of other disease processes. Secondary kyphoscoliosis is due to diseases that affect either the vertebrae, the vertebral connective tissue, or the neuromuscular system supporting the spinal column (Table 90.1). The most common causes of secondary kyphoscoliosis are neuromuscular diseases, such as polio or muscular dystrophy. Other forms of secondary kyphoscoliosis, such as Marfan's syndrome, osteomalacia, postthoracoplasty, and Charcot-Marie-Tooth disease, are much less common.[3]

Severe kyphoscoliosis is easily recognizable on physical examination. In children and adolescents, however, the changes in spinal curvature may be subtle, and the spine should be carefully inspected for signs of mild scoliosis. Because of the rotation of the vertebrae in

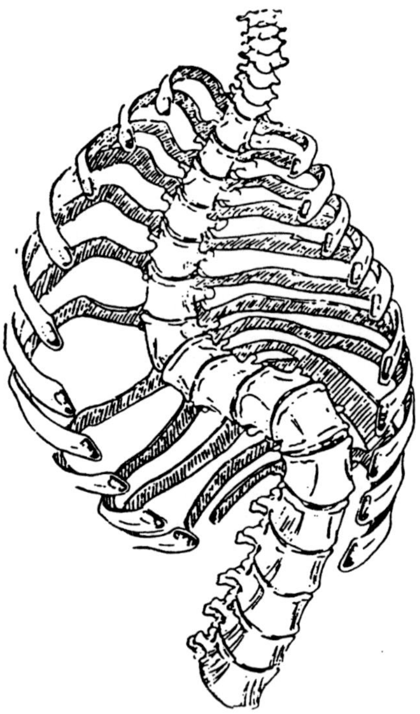

**Figure 90.1** Schema showing the rotation of the spine and rib cage in kyphoscoliosis. (From Bergofsky EH, Turino GM, Fishman AP: Cardiorespiratory failure in kyphoscoliosis. Medicine 38:263, 1959.)

scoliosis, the curvature of the vertebral column is much greater than that of the palpable spinous processes, and only radiographs can reveal the true severity. The dorsal hump seen on examination is due to the angulated ribs rather than to the spine. With severe degrees of kyphoscoliosis, chronic hypoxemia may lead to right heart failure and associated findings, including cyanosis, distended neck veins, peripheral edema, and hepatomegaly.

**Table 90.1** CAUSES OF KYPHOSCOLIOSIS

| |
|---|
| Idiopathic |
| Neuromuscular disease |
| Muscular dystrophy |
| Poliomyelitis |
| Cerebral palsy |
| Friedreich's ataxia |
| Charcot-Marie-Tooth disease |
| Vertebral disease |
| Osteoporosis |
| Osteomalacia |
| Vitamin D–resistant rickets |
| Tuberculous spondylitis |
| Neurofibromatosis |
| Disorders of connective tissue |
| Marfan's syndrome |
| Ehlers-Danlos syndrome |
| Morquio's syndrome |
| Thoracic cage abnormality |
| Thoracoplasty |
| Empyema |

The severity of the deformity can be quantified using chest radiographs to measure the acute angles formed by both limbs of the convex primary curvature of the spine (Fig. 90.2). This angle is referred to as the *Cobb angle*. It has been used to determine prognosis and to predict the effects of disease on lung function and the risk for respiratory failure. An angle greater than 100 degrees is considered a severe deformity and is more likely to be associated with respiratory failure. Although chest radiographs are useful when evaluating the degree of spinal deformity, their utility is limited when evaluating the mediastinum. In these instances, a computed tomography (CT) scan of the chest is more informative.

## Pathophysiology

### Pulmonary Function

Among the chest wall diseases, kyphoscoliosis produces the most severe reduction in total lung capacity (TLC) and vital capacity (VC).[1, 4] In adults with idiopathic kyphoscoliosis, the severity of the restrictive process is proportional to the severity of spinal deformity. The relationship between these two factors has been described as follows[5]:

$$\text{VC (\% predicted)} = 87.6 - 0.338 \times (\text{Cobb angle}).$$

Accordingly, VC is often reduced to less than 50% of the predicted value in patients with a Cobb angle of greater than 100 degrees. Those who have mild to moderate kyphoscoliosis with a Cobb angle between 60 and 90 degrees have lesser reductions of VC to 50% to 65% of predicted. Such predictive equations based on the Cobb angle are useful in differentiating the effects of spinal deformity on lung volume from other restrictive processes in adults with idiopathic kyphoscoliosis. By contrast, there is less correlation between VC and the degree of spinal deformity in patients with secondary kyphoscoliosis. In these patients, confounding factors, such as neuromuscular weakness, may have a more profound effect on VC. Similarly, in adolescents with idiopathic scoliosis,

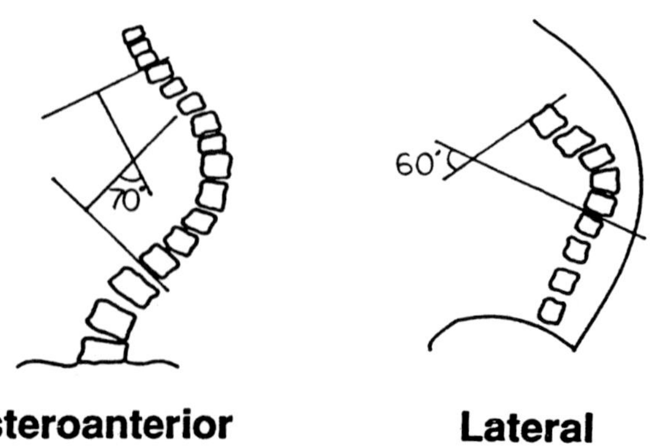


**Figure 90.2** Schematized examples of a posteroanterior chest radiograph depicting the lines constructed to measure the Cobb angle of scoliosis and of a lateral chest radiograph depicting lines drawn to measure the Cobb angle of kyphosis.

**Table 90.2 PULMONARY FUNCTION IN CHEST WALL DISEASES**

| Variable | Units | Kyphoscoliosis | Ankylosing Spondylitis | Pectus Excavatum | Postthoracoplasty |
|---|---|---|---|---|---|
| TLC | % Predicted | 44 | 85 | 90 | 64 |
| VC | % Predicted | 30 | 79 | 90 | 49 |
| RV | % Predicted | 94 | 97 | 100 | 91 |
| $FEV_1$ | % Predicted | 40 | 81 | 93 | 41 |
| $FEV_1$/FVC | — | 80 | 74 | 81 | 57 |

TLC = total lung capacity; VC = vital capacity; RV = residual volume; $FEV_1$ = forced expiratory volume in 1 second; FVC = forced vital capacity.

the presence of respiratory muscle weakness correlates more closely with mild reductions in VC than with the degree of spinal curvature.[6]

The reduction in expiratory flow rates that are seen in kyphoscoliosis reflect the overall restrictive process and are usually not related to intrinsic airway disease. Because TLC may be markedly reduced with relative preservation of residual volume (RV) (Table 90.2), the RV/TLC ratio may be elevated. The combination of reduced expiratory flow rates and an increased RV/TLC ratio may at times be mistakenly attributed to a superimposed obstructive process. Specific airway conductance, however, is usually normal or even increased despite the reduction in flow rates.[7] The increase in airway conductance may be partly explained by increased radial tension on the airways as a result of the increased elastic recoil of the lung. In rare cases, airway obstruction may occur as a consequence of torsion of the central airways or impingement of a mediastinal structure, such as the aorta, on the tracheal wall.[8]

## Respiratory Mechanics

The restrictive process in kyphoscoliosis can be partly attributed to altered volume–pressure relationships of the respiratory system (Table 90.3). Respiratory system compliance (CRS) is reduced primarily because of the stiff chest wall. In adults, when the Cobb angle is greater than 100 degrees, chest wall compliance (Ccw ) may be reduced to only 20% to 30% of predicted.[1, 5] The stiffened chest wall also places the resting position of the respiratory system (functional residual capacity [FRC]) at lower lung volumes. This further reduces respiratory system compliance by shifting tidal breathing to a flatter portion of the volume–pressure curve (Fig. 90.3). In contrast to that in adults, chest wall compliance is normal in children, even in those with severe spinal deformity.[9]

Lung compliance (CL) is also reduced in kyphoscoliosis but not to the same extent as chest wall compliance. During acute episodes of respiratory decompensation due to pneumonia or other infiltrative processes, however, lung compliance may be as severely reduced as chest wall compliance.[10] The diminished lung compliance contributes to the reduction in respiratory system compliance. The altered lung compliance is attributed to microatelectasis due to the relatively immobile chest wall and not to intrinsic lung disease.[9, 11]

The reductions in lung and chest wall compliance increase the elastic load on the respiratory muscles, thereby increasing the pressure needed to inhale (Pbreath) and the work of breathing. Because the work of breathing is positively correlated with the oxygen cost of breathing, it is not surprising that the oxygen cost of breathing in patients with kyphoscoliosis may be increased three to five times that seen in healthy subjects.[1] Such an increase in the oxygen cost of breathing may place these patients at risk for respiratory muscle fatigue.[12] Intercurrent illnesses, such as pneumonia or sepsis, may pose additional elastic loads, further increasing Pbreath and the oxygen cost of breathing.

## Respiratory Muscle Function

Inspiratory muscle weakness may also contribute to the restrictive process; however, its prevalence in kyphoscoli-

**Table 90.3 RESPIRATORY MECHANICS IN CHEST WALL DISEASES**

| Variable | Units | Kyphoscoliosis | Ankylosing Spondylitis | Pectus Excavatum | Postthoracoplasty |
|---|---|---|---|---|---|
| CRS | % Predicted | 50 | 70 | — | 50 |
| Ccw | % Predicted | 30 | 60 | — | 40 |
| CL | % Predicted | 60 | 80 | 80 | 50 |
| PImax | cm $H_2O$ | 37 | 56 | 90 | 50 |
| MVV | L/min | 37 | 80 | 107 | 37 |

CRS = compliance of respiratory system; Ccw = compliance of chest wall; CL = compliance of lungs; PImax = maximum inspiratory pressure; MVV = maximum voluntary ventilation.

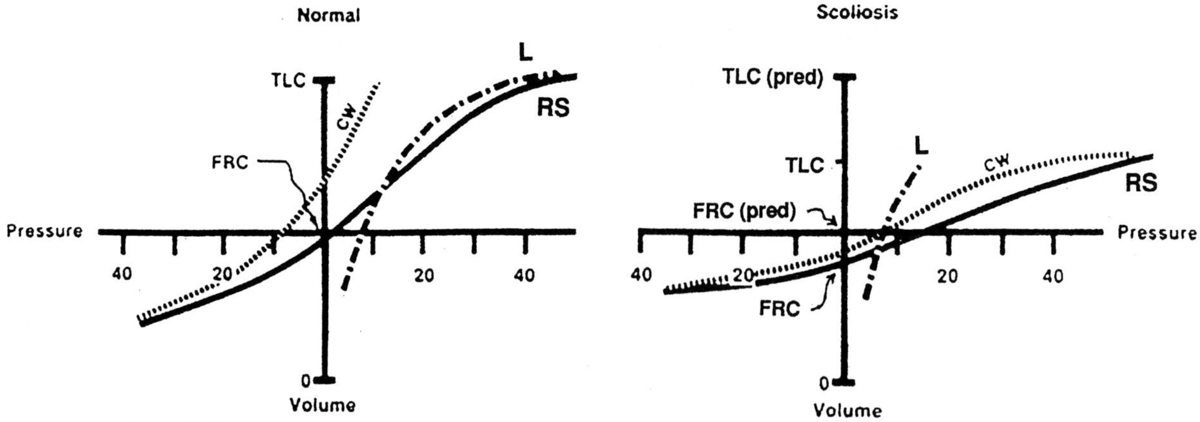


**Figure 90.3** Schema showing alterations in volume-pressure relationships of the lung (L), chest wall (CW), and respiratory system (RS) in kyphoscoliosis. The chest wall is less compliant, leading to a reduction in functional residual capacity (FRC) and tidal breathing on a flatter portion of the respiratory system volume-pressure curve. TLC = total lung capacity.

osis is unknown. Global inspiratory muscle strength can be assessed by measuring maximal voluntary static inspiratory and expiratory pressures (PImax and PEmax, respectively). In young patients with mean scoliosis Cobb angles of about 50 degrees, both PImax and PEmax are mildly decreased to 70% and 80% of control values, respectively.[6, 9] In older patients with somewhat more scoliosis, PImax is about 50% of predicted in eucapnic patients and 25% of predicted in hypercapnic patients (see Table 90.3).[4] In contrast, other investigators have found that the reduction of respiratory muscle function is not a regular feature of scoliosis in adults.[13] If present, inspiratory and expiratory muscle weakness may not be due to intrinsic muscle disease but to changes in geometry of the chest wall affecting the mechanical advantage of the inspiratory muscles. The finding that inspiratory muscle weakness is independent of the degree of spinal curvature, however, argues against this assertion.[9]

## Control and Pattern of Breathing

To compensate for the increased load on the inspiratory muscles, patients with scoliosis recruit the inspiratory muscles of the rib cage[14] and may adopt a rapid shallow breathing pattern. This decreases the work of breathing. Another advantage of breathing at low tidal volumes is reducing the ratio of Pbreath to PImax, thereby lowering the risk for inspiratory muscle fatigue and reducing the sense of respiratory effort. Disadvantages of adopting this breathing pattern include the potential for developing microatelectasis, increased dead space ventilation, and increased oxygen cost of breathing. Alternatively these patients may compensate for the increased elastic load by increasing central neural drive to the muscles.[15] Increasing ventilatory drive, as measured by mouth occlusion pressure ($P_{0.1}$), is a strategy demonstrated in young scoliotic patients without ventilatory failure.[16]

Patients with kyphoscoliosis may have either a normal or reduced ventilatory response to carbon dioxide. If the response is reduced, the magnitude of reduction is proportional to the degree of mechanical limitation imposed by the chest wall.[5] Thus, the decrement in the ventilatory response to carbon dioxide resembles that of external resistive loading and can be attributed to the restricted respiratory system rather than to an inherent problem with respiratory control. Moreover, ventilatory drive as assessed by $P_{0.1}$ is increased in young scoliotic patients.[16] These findings suggest that the drive to breathe in these patients is normal. The effects of aging and its influence on central ventilatory control, however, requires further clarification in this population.

## Gas Exchange

Hypoxemia may be attributed to ventilation-perfusion mismatch, underlying atelectasis, or shunt. The degree of ventilation-perfusion mismatching is worse in patients with Cobb angles greater than 65 degrees.[17] The maldistribution of ventilation appears to be independent of whether the hemithorax is concave or convex. Hypoventilation, if present, worsens hypoxemia.[1, 18] Persistent hypoxemia leads to pulmonary vasoconstriction, right ventricular hypertrophy, and cor pulmonale. Proliferation of pulmonary artery smooth muscle or compression of the pulmonary vascular bed by deflated lung may further increase pulmonary artery pressure at rest or during exercise. Patients with severe kyphoscoliosis may have oxyhemoglobin desaturation with minimal activity.[19]

## Exercise Capacity

Exercise capacity is most impaired in patients with severe kyphoscoliosis. Maximum oxygen consumption ($\dot{V}O_{2max}$) may be reduced to about 60% to 80% of predicted, with the lower values seen in patients with the lowest forced vital capacity (FVC), forced expiratory volume in 1 second ($FEV_1$), and maximum voluntary ventilation (MVV) (Table 90.4).[20] However, the breathing pattern response to exercise in patients with mild to moderate kyphoscoliosis (Cobb angle between 25 and 70 degrees) is similar to that

**Table 90.4** EXERCISE CAPACITY IN NORMAL SUBJECTS AND IN PATIENTS WITH THORACIC CAGE DISORDERS

| Condition | No. of Patients | Age (yr) | $\dot{V}O_{2max}$ (mL/kg/min) | $\dot{V}E$ (L/min) |
|---|---|---|---|---|
| Normal | 14 | 24 | 45.9 | 93 |
| Kyphoscoliosis | 15 | 32 | 31.6 | 66 |
| Ankylosing spondylitis | 33 | 47 | 23.4 | — |
| Thoracoplasty | 29 | 64 | 14.3 | 25 |
| Pectus excavatum | 12 | 14 | 38.5 | 73 |
| Obesity | 13 | 23 | 27.7 | 82 |

$\dot{V}O_{2max}$ = maximum oxygen consumption; $\dot{V}E$ = expired volume (minute ventilation).

seen in normal subjects. The ratio of tidal volume to vital capacity (VT/VC) is roughly 0.5, and the ratio of maximum exercise ventilation to maximal voluntary ventilation ($\dot{V}E_{max}$/MVV) reaches 70%.[20] In adolescent scoliotic patients whose respiratory muscle strength, exercise, and ventilatory capacities were on average 80% to 85% of normal, exercise capacity was related to muscle mass and strength as well as to the degree of ventilatory impairment.[21] Deconditioning and lack of regular aerobic exercise may also contribute to poor exercise performance in adolescents and adults with moderate scoliosis.

## Sleep-Disordered Breathing

When awake, patients with kyphoscoliosis may recruit the intercostal and accessory muscles to assist the diaphragm in displacing the stiff chest wall. When sleeping, these patients may hypoventilate due to hypotonia of the intercostal and accessory muscles, particularly during rapid-eye-movement (REM) sleep.[22–25] Decreased neural drive to the diaphragm during REM sleep and decreased chest wall compliance may also contribute to nocturnal hypoventilation. The degree of oxyhemoglobin desaturation during sleep in these patients appears to be more severe than that seen during sleep in patients with chronic obstructive pulmonary disease or interstitial lung disease. In addition, these patients may have recurrent episodes of obstructive sleep apnea. Distortion of the upper airway anatomy in kyphoscoliosis may predispose these patients to intermittent airway obstruction during REM-induced hypotonia of the pharyngeal muscles; however, the incidence of obstructive sleep apnea in patients with kyphoscoliosis is not increased over that seen in the general population.[23] Regardless of mechanism, recurrent hypercarbia and hypoxemia during sleep may potentiate the daytime development of hypercarbia, cor pulmonale, and respiratory muscle dysfunction.[24] Because sleep-related disorders represent a potentially treatable or reversible cause of respiratory failure, they should be evaluated in patients with kyphoscoliosis who develop carbon dioxide retention.

## Clinical Course

In general, patients with mild to moderate kyphoscoliosis have an excellent prognosis with little impairment of breathing or overall lifestyle.[18] These patients do not require special treatment to prevent ventilatory failure and are not significantly different from a control population with regard to symptoms[9] or the loss of lung volume with aging.[26] Similarly, patients with severe idiopathic kyphoscoliosis who are younger than 35 years of age also tend not to have symptoms.[18] In contrast, middle-aged patients with severe idiopathic kyphoscoliosis tend to develop dyspnea and decreased exercise tolerance, they tend to have repeated acute respiratory infections, and they are at risk for respiratory failure.[27] The onset of respiratory failure is often insidious, and its incidence is variable, accounting for less than 5% of chronic ventilatory failure in adults. After cor pulmonale develops, the prognosis is poor; without treatment, death generally occurs within a year.[1] The prognosis is worsened by any associated obstructive lung process.[28] Pregnancy usually poses no added risk for respiratory complications.[29] With severe degrees of kyphoscoliosis and reductions in VC to less than 1 L, the risk for respiratory complications during pregnancy may be increased.

Kyphoscoliosis is an easily recognizable cause of respiratory failure; the degree of spinal deformity has been associated with the development of respiratory failure. Patients with kyphosis and a Cobb angle of more than 100 degrees are at significant risk for respiratory failure. When both kyphosis and scoliosis are present, the effects are additive. Alternatively, severe scoliosis (Cobb angle of more than 100 degrees) in the absence of significant kyphosis (Cobb angle of less than 20 degrees) usually does not bring about ventilatory failure. However, the notion that the extent of the spinal deformity is the key predictor of respiratory failure has been challenged. Patients may survive into their seventh decade with minimal or mild cardiorespiratory impairment despite a Cobb angle of greater than 105 degrees.[30] Other investigators have found no correlation between the severity of hypercapnia and the degree of thoracic deformity.[4] Despite these findings, the role of reduced chest wall compliance in the evolution of respiratory dysfunction and its strong relationship to the chest wall deformity implies that the degree of spinal deformity is a key factor in the development of respiratory failure (Fig. 90.4). When respiratory failure occurs and the Cobb angle is less than 100 degrees, the etiology of respiratory failure should not be attributed solely to the skeletal deformity.

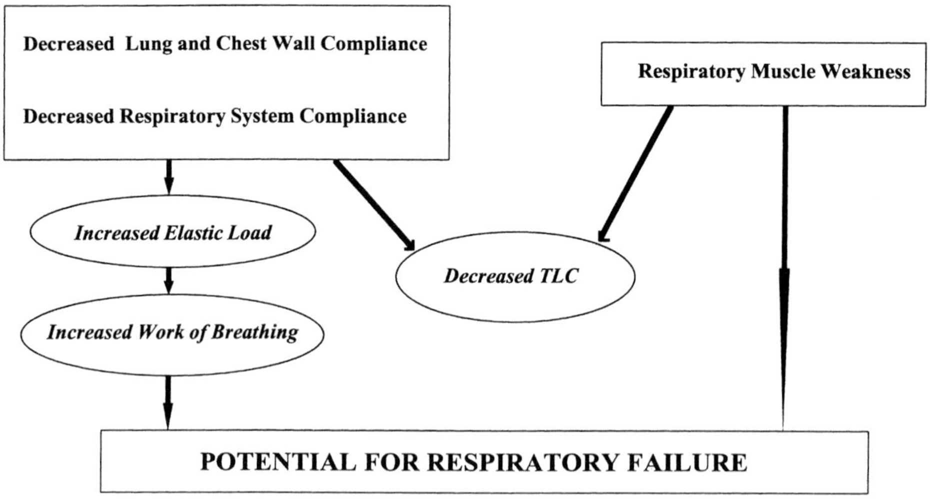


**Figure 90.4** Changes in respiratory mechanics in kyphoscoliosis and their consequences. TLC = total lung capacity.

Other factors that contribute to the development of respiratory failure (Table 90.5) include the age of onset of kyphoscoliosis and its etiology. When the onset of the spinal deformity is during childhood or adolescence, respiratory failure is more likely to occur later in life.[27] The etiology of kyphoscoliosis may also be a predictor of respiratory failure. Paralytic kyphoscoliosis and its associated inspiratory muscle weakness may result in a more rapid deterioration of pulmonary function. Other studies, however, found no such association between etiology and respiratory failure.[4, 27] The presence of hypercapnia itself may weaken the respiratory muscles and aggravate respiratory failure. Other coincident factors, such as advanced age and underlying cardiac disease, may also predispose these patients to respiratory failure.

## Treatment

### General Measures

Medical therapy for adults with kyphoscoliosis is both preventive and supportive. Immunization, adequate hydration, prompt care of respiratory infections, avoidance of sedatives, and carefully monitored supplemental oxygen are the mainstays of therapy. Physical training can improve exercise tolerance in inactive patients. If hypercapnia and cor pulmonale develop, chronic respiratory failure may be treated conservatively with chest physiotherapy, bronchodilators, oxygen therapy, and diuretics if needed. Oxyhemoglobin saturation should be routinely assessed during exercise in patients with moderate to severe kyphoscoliosis. Oxygen administered at rest or with exercise can minimize dyspnea and exercise-induced desaturation in patients with moderately severe kyphoscoliosis and chronic ventilatory failure.[31]

**Table 90.5** FACTORS PREDISPOSING TO VENTILATORY FAILURE IN KYPHOSCOLIOSIS

| |
|---|
| Spinal deformity of more than 100 degrees |
| Inspiratory muscle weakness |
| Etiology |
| Age of onset |
| Sleep-related abnormalities |

### Mechanical Ventilation

Noninvasive nocturnal ventilation is frequently used to treat chronic respiratory failure in patients with severe kyphoscoliosis. Nocturnal negative-pressure ventilation has been administered with devices such as cuirass and body-wrap ventilators and has been shown to reduce morbidity and mortality. The benefits of using these devices include improvement of blood gases, pulmonary hypertension, and right ventricular failure as well as relief of dyspnea and a marked reduction in the need for hospitalization (Table 90.6).[32–34] Disadvantages of using negative-pressure devices include the induction of upper airway obstruction during sleep and the need to custom fit a cuirass to the deformed chest wall.[32, 33]

The benefits of nocturnal positive-pressure ventilation are similar to those listed for negative-pressure ventilation. Initially, nocturnal positive-pressure ventilation was delivered through a tracheostomy. With proper care, patients could be maintained with a tracheostomy on a portable ventilator for decades. To avoid the complications of tracheostomy, however, positive-pressure ventilation is now more commonly delivered by means of nasal or face masks. Benefits reported with noninvasive positive-pressure ventilation include increased tidal volume, improved alveolar ventilation, normalization of blood gases, reduced work of breathing, improved respiratory muscle strength, better quality of life, reduced mortality, and normalized sleep patterns.[25, 35, 36] Nocturnal assisted positive-pressure ventilation may also benefit these patients by resting the respiratory muscles and alleviating inspiratory muscle fatigue. Support for this mechanism includes the observations that diaphragmatic electromyogram (EMG) activity decreases, swings in esophageal pressure become less negative during inspiration, and the rib cage and abdomen become more synchronized when breathing is assisted by positive-pressure ventilation.[36] The advantages of positive-pressure ventilation over neg-

**Table 90.6 BENEFITS OF NONINVASIVE VENTILATION IN CHEST WALL DISEASES**

| | | |
|---|---|---|
| Gas exchange | Increased $P_{O_2}$ | Decreased $P_{CO_2}$ |
| Hemodynamics | Increased pulmonary artery pressure | Increased right ventricular function |
| Mechanics | Reduced work of breathing | Increased PImax |
| Sleep hygiene | Normalized sleep patterns | Reduced apneic episodes |
| Outcomes | Reduced hospitalizations | Improved quality of life, relief of dyspnea |

PImax = maximal inspiratory pressure.

ative-pressure ventilation include the compact and portable features of the equipment and its relative ease of use. In addition, nocturnal positive-pressure ventilation may benefit these patients by reducing both obstructive and nonobstructive sleep-related events whereby negative-pressure ventilation may induce upper airway obstruction.[36] Nasal proportional assist ventilation has also been used to a limited extent in these patients.[37] In cases of acute respiratory failure refractory to the measures described previously, positive-pressure ventilation with a volume cycle ventilator delivered by an endotracheal tube may be needed to treat hypoventilation and hypoxemia.[18, 30]

The improvements noted after short-term ventilation have also been seen with long-term nocturnal ventilation. When instituted for months or years, noninvasive ventilation has resulted in improved gas exchange, ventilation, and cardiac function. In addition, long-term nocturnal noninvasive positive-pressure ventilation decreases mortality and hospitalizations for respiratory illnesses and improves quality of life, and sleep quality.[38, 39] Noninvasive positive-pressure ventilation has also been used to correct nocturnal hypoventilation that may accompany pregnancy.

Factors contributing to the improvement in pulmonary function with nocturnal positive-pressure ventilation may include reversing microatelectasis and increasing lung compliance. These benefits have been noted following brief periods (20 minutes) of intermittent positive-pressure breathing (IPPB). Improvements in lung mechanics, resting arterial $P_{CO_2}$, and oxygenation may last up to 4 hours after a single treatment of IPPB.[10] With prolonged IPPB therapy, the improvement in VC may persist for up to 9 months.[40] IPPB, however, has not been shown to be as efficacious in other diseases associated with diminished respiratory system compliance and has little effect on improving chest wall compliance.[41]

### Surgical Treatment

Attempts to avoid respiratory failure later in life by surgically stabilizing the spine have met with varied success. Procedures such as placement of Harrington rods or spinal fusion may be performed in adolescent patients. Immediately after surgery, pulmonary function may deteriorate,[42] with reductions of chest wall and respiratory system compliance of 20% to 129%.[43] This deterioration in respiratory mechanics is thought to be due to rib cage trauma and changes in chest wall caliper.[43] Despite several years of observation, the long-term benefits of spinal surgery on pulmonary function remain controversial. In adults, it is generally accepted that surgical procedures do not improve pulmonary function. Spinal fusion and Harrington rod placement did not significantly improve the FVC, $FEV_1$, or resting arterial $P_{O_2}$ in patients over the age of 20 and these procedures had associated complications.[44] In children and adolescents, there may be a role for corrective surgery. After Harrington rod instrumentation and spinal fusion, lung function was improved in children and adolescents 18 months and 3 years after surgery.[13, 42, 45] In women with an average curvature of 58 degrees, VC was improved by 12% after 3 years. In patients with kyphoscoliosis associated with neurologic disorders, early stabilization may help prevent progressive myelopathy.[46]

To summarize, patients with severe kyphoscoliosis have impaired lung function characterized by a reduction in respiratory system compliance, an increased elastic load on the respiratory muscles, and an increase in the work of breathing. As they age, adults with severe spinal deformities are at risk for respiratory failure. Although the degree of spinal distortion certainly plays a significant role in the pathogenesis of respiratory failure, other factors, such as inspiratory muscle weakness and sleep-related dysfunction, should be evaluated in patients with symptoms. After cardiorespiratory failure develops, conservative measures, coupled with nocturnal positive-pressure ventilation, improve symptoms, reduce hospitalization, and improve prognosis.

## THORACOPLASTY

### Diagnosis and Etiology

Before the advent of effective chemotherapy, thoracic surgery was a mainstay of antituberculous therapy. Thoracoplasty was one of the most common surgical procedures used to treat tuberculous empyema and cavitary pulmonary tuberculosis. It entailed removal of a number of ribs and intercostal muscles. Some of the patients who had this procedure performed in the 1940s and 1950s are still alive and often have restrictive disease as a result of distortion of the chest wall, pleural thickening, and secondary scoliosis.[47] In more recent years, thoracoplasty has been used to a limited extent to treat postpneumonic and postresectional empyema.[48, 49]

If these patients survived the initial surgery, they would typically remain symptom free for a number of years. Eventually, they would develop dyspnea on exertion, and in as many as half of the long-term survivors, the condition would deteriorate to acute or chronic respiratory failure. Of 171 patients who were operated on between 1951 and 1953, over one third had died by 1987.[50] Risk factors associated with developing respiratory failure include preoperative tuberculous cavitary disease, advanced age at the time of operation, a previous surgically induced pneumothorax on the opposite side, and male gender. The risk was greater in patients who underwent thoracoplasty than in those who underwent pneumonectomy alone.

## Pathophysiology

### Pulmonary Function

Of the chest wall disorders, thoracoplasty is second only to kyphoscoliosis in producing a severe restrictive pattern (see Table 90.2). The restrictive pattern is due to a number of factors, including a reduction in respiratory system compliance, progressive lung fibrosis related to underlying granulomatous disease, fibrothorax, phrenic nerve damage, previous lung resection, and scoliosis (Table 90.7). VC and TLC may be reduced to 40% and 70% of predicted, respectively. RV and FRC are reduced to the range of 70% and 90% of predicted, respectively.[51] Progressive scoliosis[47] and the effects of aging on respiratory system compliance worsen the restrictive process. The degree of restriction, however, does not correlate with the extent of thoracoplasty.[51]

Unlike other restrictive diseases of the chest wall, coincident airflow obstruction is common, with a prevalence ranging from 34% to 51%.[51, 52] When airflow obstruction is present, the $FEV_1$ and the $FEV_1/FVC$ ratio are reduced, and the RV/TLC ratio is increased (see Table 90.2). Airway obstruction may be due to chronic bronchitis from cigarette smoking or other factors, such as previous tuberculous bronchitis or bronchiectasis.[51] Airway obstruction becomes more prevalent with aging and is more severe in patients with carbon dioxide retention, hypoxemia, or complaints of dyspnea.[52] Although the obstructive process usually is not reversible, determining its presence and severity may help identify those at greater risk for developing respiratory failure.

**Table 90.7 FACTORS CONTRIBUTING TO PULMONARY RESTRICTION IN THORACOPLASTY**

| |
|---|
| Reduced respiratory system compliance |
| Inspiratory muscle weakness |
| Fibrothorax |
| Pulmonary fibrosis due to granulomatous disease |
| Previous lung resection |
| Phrenic nerve injury |
| Progressive scoliosis |

### Respiratory Mechanics

The long-term sequelae of thoracoplasty include a lowering of respiratory system, chest wall, and lung compliance values (see Table 90.3). As with kyphoscoliosis, respiratory system compliance may be reduced to 50% of predicted, thus imposing a substantial elastic load on the respiratory muscles. This elastic load, in combination with the resistive load due to airway obstruction, increases the work of breathing. That the oxygen cost of breathing is three to four times higher in these patients than in controls[53] reflects this added work of breathing and may predispose these patients to respiratory failure.

### Gas Exchange and Exercise Tolerance

Patients who have undergone thoracoplasty may have hypoxemia and complain of exercise intolerance. The maximal work rate and oxygen consumption are reduced, and there is a ventilatory limit to exercise. The diminished $\dot{V}O_{2max}$ has been correlated with reductions in $FEV_1$.[52] Postthoracoplasty patients may develop severe hypoxemia and hypercarbia during exercise or at rest. Diffusion capacity is moderately reduced, but when corrected for lung volume, it is within the normal range.[51] During exercise, the diffusion capacity fails to increase appropriately, indicating an irreversibly restricted pulmonary vascular bed. Cor pulmonale may develop as a result of hypoxemia or medial hypertrophy of the pulmonary arteries.

## Treatment

Treatment is supportive with the use of domiciliary oxygen, antibiotics when appropriate, and noninvasive nocturnal ventilation. In addition, any obstructive component should be vigorously treated. Positive-pressure ventilation delivered by means of an endotracheal tube or tracheostomy has been used to treat acute respiratory failure. Management of chronic respiratory failure often entails the use of positive- or negative-pressure noninvasive ventilation. Noninvasive ventilation reduces the work of breathing, alleviates respiratory muscle fatigue, relieves dyspnea, lessens sleep-induced desaturation, and improves overall prognosis.[54, 55] Improvements in VC, maximal inspiratory pressure, maximal expiratory pressure, and arterial blood gases occur soon after initiation of noninvasive ventilation and can be maintained over the long term. Even with nocturnal ventilatory assistance, however, mortality is still high, with a 55% survival rate 7 years after initiating treatment.[55]

# PECTUS EXCAVATUM

## Diagnosis and Etiology

Pectus excavatum is a chest wall deformity characterized by excessive depression of the sternum. The sternal depression may be minimal or extreme and diffuse or local; it is most often symmetric. Pectus excavatum is usually diagnosed soon after birth, affects between 0.5% and 2% of the population, and is the most common chest wall deformity seen by pediatricians and primary care providers.[56] Boys are affected about three times more often than girls.[57] The natural history of the pectus deformity is variable. It usually remains unchanged with time but may progress.

The etiology of pectus excavatum is unknown. However, the association of pectus excavatum with connective tissue disorders such as Marfan's syndrome suggests that there may be a defect in the connective tissue surrounding the sternum. There may also be a genetic predisposition to acquiring the pectus deformity. In one large series, a family history of pectus deformity was present in 41% of the family members.[58] Another series, however, noted that only 5 of 315 patients had a positive family history of pectus.[59] Scoliosis, congenital heart disease, and functional heart murmurs can be associated with pectus excavatum and were noted in 15%, 4%, and 31% of patients in one large series.[58] Pectus carinatum, a disorder in which the sternum is protuberant, is less common than pectus excavatum. It is of unknown etiology and may be associated with congenital heart disease, severe childhood asthma, and rickets.[60]

The most frequent complaints of patients with pectus deformity are cosmetic in nature. These complaints are not trivial; they may be associated with psychologic problems in as many as 85% of patients. These issues most commonly arise in patients between the ages of 15 and 20 years.[59] Another frequent complaint is dyspnea on exertion, which may occur in 30% to 70% of patients. Other symptoms include chest pain, palpitations, and frequent respiratory infections.[58, 61]

The degree of chest wall deformity with pectus excavatum can be assessed by physical examination or by using radiographic techniques. If the distance between the surface of the anterior chest wall and the deepest sternal depression is greater than 3 cm, it is considered significant for pectus. Another bedside determination, which is of historical interest, is the hollow index. This is the ratio between the amount of water contained in the chest depression and the body surface area. An index of greater than 50 mL/m$^2$ indicates the presence of pectus deformity. Currently, radiographic techniques are used to assess the degree of pectus deformity. The lateral chest radiograph can be used to measure the minimal distance between the posterior border of the sternum and the anterior border of the thoracic vertebra. A sternovertebral distance of less than 10 cm is considered significant for pectus. This measure, however, does not account for differences in body size. To address this, the ratio of the AP to transverse diameters of the rib cage (as seen on the posteroanterior and lateral chest radiograph) is calculated. A ratio of less than 0.4 indicates the presence of pectus and one less than 0.3 indicates a severe deformity. However, better anatomic definition can be obtained with CT scans. Measurements of transverse and AP chest wall diameters are taken at the level of the deepest sternal depression (Fig. 90.5).[57, 62, 63] Unlike chest radiographs, the ratio of the transverse to AP diameter of the inner chest wall is calculated. A ratio of greater than 3.25 is considered significant for pectus. In some centers, this ratio has been used to select patients for surgical correction.

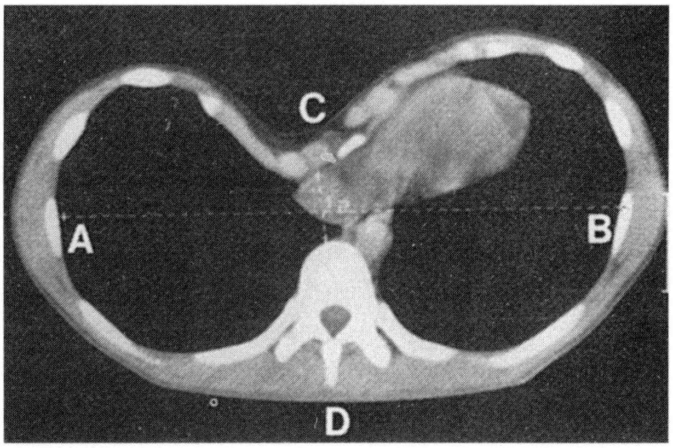


**Figure 90.5** Chest computed tomography scan of a patient with pectus excavatum, demonstrating the transverse rib cage diameter (A-B) and the reduced anteroposterior diameter (C-D). (Modified from Haller JA, Scherer LR, Turner CS, et al: Evolving management of pectus excavatum based on a single institutional experience of 664 patients. Ann Surg 209:578–582, 1989.)

## Pathophysiology

### Pulmonary Function and Respiratory Mechanics

Lung volumes are usually at the lower limits of normal or mildly reduced (see Table 90.2).[64–69] If a restrictive impairment is present, it is positively associated with the degree of sternal depression and is more severe if there is associated scoliosis.[64, 65, 69, 70] RV may be normal[69] or slightly elevated.[65, 70] Any increase in RV is unlikely to be related to an obstructive process because the $FEV_1$/FVC ratio is typically within normal limits.[70] FRC is usually within the normal range.[65, 69] Although deformed, the mobility of the rib cage is not impaired during quiet breathing or exercise.[67] Unlike kyphoscoliosis, in which lung compliance is reduced because of limited chest wall mobility, lung compliance in pectus excavatum is within normal limits unless these patients develop intrinsic lung disease (see Table 90.3).[66]

### Exercise Capacity

Despite the high prevalence of subjective complaints of exercise intolerance, cardiopulmonary exercise testing is often normal.[70] In particular, the maximal work rate, oxygen consumption, and heart rate, as well as the oxygen pulse, are similar among patients with pectus excavatum and controls. In patients with more severe deformities, however, there may be a mild reduction in the maximal work rate[68] or an increase in the oxygen consumption for a given work rate (see Table 90.4).[66]

Despite several studies evaluating cardiac function in patients with pectus excavatum, the degree of right ventricular dysfunction produced by this deformity remains unclear. The posterior displacement of the sternum may compress the right atrium, reduce cardiac output, and limit exercise. In support of this speculation, cardiac anomalies, such as compression of the right ventricle, narrowing of the right ventricular outflow tract, and sacculations of the right ventricular wall, have been observed using two-dimensional cross-sectional echocardiography.[71] In contrast, left ventricular morphology is generally normal.

## Treatment

### Surgical Approaches

Patients selected for surgical repair often have a transverse-to-AP diameter ratio of greater than 3.25 as determined by CT of the chest[72]; however, patients with lesser degrees of deformity have also undergone repair. Several surgical approaches have been used to correct the pectus deformity. The assertion that the pectus deformity is caused by an overgrowth of cartilage favors a surgical approach that removes it. Resection of costal cartilage and sternal osteotomy with or without fixation of the sternum with external or internal supports has been one of the more invasive surgical approaches.[56] A drawback of this approach is recurrence of the deformity, especially in younger children when no sternal supports are used. In procedures in which the sternum is resected and repositioned, morbidity also includes sternal necrosis and infection. Less invasive approaches in which resection of sternal cartilage is more limited and temporary struts are used to stabilize the sternum for 6 to 12 months have less associated morbidity.[59] Even less invasive techniques include placing a steel bar under the sternum with no cartilage resection or using silicone implants.[73, 74] The latter have been used to correct milder deformities in adolescents and younger adults. Problems with this approach include accurate fabrication and fit of the implant, patient discomfort, infection, and implant extrusion.

### Surgical Outcomes

Surgical repair provides cosmetic benefits, but the pathophysiologic benefits of the repair remain controversial. Subjective improvement in exercise tolerance and of dyspnea are often noted after surgery.[57, 69] Less frequently, pulmonary function improves.[75] Alternatively, others have shown a reduction in pulmonary function either within the first year[65, 68] or several years after surgical repair. The greatest reduction in lung function may occur in those patients with the mildest restrictive deficit.[64, 69] Conversely, patients with the greatest degree of pulmonary impairment (VC more than 75% of predicted) may be the most likely to have improved pulmonary function after surgery.[76] Impairment of lung function after surgery has been attributed to abnormal chest wall mechanics as a result of articular changes in the sternal and parasternal areas.[77]

The effects of surgery on exercise tolerance are also controversial. Some investigators report an improvement in exercise tolerance and an increase in $\dot{V}O_{2max}$ after surgical correction,[75] whereas others have shown no change in these parameters.[68] One small controlled study found no differences in $\dot{V}O_{2max}$, minute ventilation at maximal exercise, and cardiac output after surgery.[68] Similarly, other studies found no postoperative improvements in cardiac index or left ventricular ejection fraction when using radionuclide imaging during exercise.[61] However, a controlled study of 36 adolescents found no significant changes in VC 8 months after surgery but did report increased exercise tolerance and oxygen pulse. In addition, the resting left ventricular end-diastolic volume was increased after surgery, suggesting some relief of cardiac compression due to the depressed sternum. The latter findings are consistent with improved cardiac but not pulmonary function after surgery.[70] Discrepancies among studies regarding the benefits of surgery on pulmonary function and exercise tolerance may be related to differences in patient selection, surgical techniques, the period of time after the operation, and the effects of growth on pulmonary function.

Surgical morbidity includes sternal necrosis, infection, and worsening of pulmonary function. The most pronounced adverse effects of surgery on pulmonary function have been reported in patients younger than the age of 4 years who have had extensive repairs.[78, 79] When they grew older, these children developed severe symptoms even with minimal exercise. These changes were likely due to retardation of chest wall growth resulting in severe restrictive lung disease. This complication may be avoided by delaying repair until 6 to 8 years of age and by limiting the amount of cartilage resected. In older children, the reduction in VC after surgery is minimized when major reconstruction of the lower chest wall is avoided.[70, 76]

To summarize, pectus deformities are often accompanied by complaints of exercise intolerance but are associated with only mild reductions in TLC and VC. Radiographic techniques used to measure the transverse and AP diameters of the chest wall are used to assist in selecting patients for surgery. After surgery, there is often symptomatic improvement and cosmetic benefit but no change in pulmonary function or aerobic capacity. Most studies have evaluated postoperative changes in pulmonary function in either young adolescents or adults. Whether younger patients may benefit from minimally invasive surgical correction because of the continued growth of the thorax during adolescence is unknown.

# FLAIL CHEST

## Diagnosis and Etiology

Flail chest is a condition in which multiple rib fractures produce a segment of the rib cage that is disconnected from the rest of the chest wall and deforms markedly with breathing.[80] Usually, double fractures of three or more contiguous ribs or combined sternal and rib fractures are needed to create the flail segment.[81, 82] Flail chest occurs in as many as 25% of patients with blunt chest wall trauma. The most common causes of flail chest include falls and motor vehicle accidents. However, flail chest may also be seen after overaggressive chest compression during cardiopulmonary resuscitation, after total

**Table 90.8** PULMONARY FUNCTION IN FLAIL CHEST

| Variable | Units | Flail Chest | | Flail Chest with Pulmonary Contusion | |
|---|---|---|---|---|---|
| | | **Initial** | **6 Months** | **Initial** | **6 Months** |
| VC | % Predicted | 60 | 100 | 50 | 88 |
| FRC | % Predicted | 60 | 75 | 45 | 50 |
| $FEV_1/FVC$ | % | 78 | 81 | 83 | 83 |

VC = vital capacity; FRC = functional residual capacity; $FEV_1$ = forced expired volume in 1 second; FVC = forced vital capacity.

sternectomy, and, occasionally, with pathologic fractures such as those due to multiple myeloma. Flail chest can be diagnosed by inspection of the chest wall and subsequent documentation of rib or sternal fractures.

The mortality rate from chest wall trauma alone is high, ranging from 7% to 14%.[83] When chest wall trauma is complicated by flail chest, the mortality rate further increases.[80, 81] In a series of 1026 multiple-trauma patients, the mortality rate for those with flail chest was 68%, compared with a 27% mortality rate for the entire group.[81] This high mortality is in part attributed to other associated injuries, such as fractures of long bones or vertebra, head trauma, rupture of the aortic arch or other arteries, and laceration of the liver or spleen. If the patient survives the initial injury, long-term disability after flail chest is relatively common. Symptoms consist of chest tightness, chest pain, or dyspnea in as many as half of patients.[84]

The lung may also be injured in patients who sustain chest wall trauma. Pulmonary complications, such as pulmonary contusion, hemothorax, and pneumothorax, can occur in up to 60% of patients with flail chest.[84] Lung contusion alone has just as high a mortality rate (56%) as flail chest in multiple trauma patients.[81] Pulmonary contusion is best detected by chest CT scan. If the contusion is seen on chest radiograph, however, it may be more clinically significant.[85]

## Pathophysiology

### Pulmonary Function

Flail chest can severely impair pulmonary function. TLC, VC, and FRC can be reduced to 50% of predicted (Table 90.8). The initial reductions in FRC and VC after flail chest can be attributed to disordered chest wall motion. VC either returns to its baseline value within 6 months[86] or remains mildly reduced.[84] In contrast, patients with pulmonary contusion complicating flail chest may have persistent reductions in FRC for up to 4 years,[86] which may be due to fibrous changes in the contused area. Thus, flail chest without pulmonary contusion may cause less long-term respiratory dysfunction.

### Respiratory Mechanics

Flail chest alters the mechanics of breathing. Normally, pleural pressure is reduced during inspiration. This subatmospheric pressure is inflationary to the lung but deflationary to the rib cage. Unlike the changes in pleural pressure, it is the passive outward recoil of the rib cage, the insertional actions of the diaphragm and intercostal muscles, and the rise of abdominal pressure during inspiration that promotes rib cage expansion during inspiration. With flail chest, the multiple rib fractures uncouple the flail segment from the remainder of the chest wall. The usual factors that promote rib cage expansion, therefore, are not operant on the flail segment. Consequently, during inspiration, the subatmospheric pleural pressure is unopposed, and the uncoupled segment of chest wall moves paradoxically inward during inspiration. During expiration, pleural pressure becomes less negative, and the flail segment can be seen moving outward. A reduction in lung compliance due to pulmonary contusion or microatelectasis or an increase in airway resistance further lowers pleural pressure during inspiration and worsens the flail.

Different patterns of chest wall distortion can be seen in patients with flail chest[87] (Fig. 90.6). Paradoxical motion may occur between the rib cage and abdomen or within the rib cage itself. Abnormal patterns that have been described include (1) inward displacement of the transverse rib cage as the lower anterior rib cage and abdomen are expanding, (2) inward displacement of the anterior lower rib cage and abdomen as the transverse rib cage is expanding, and (3) inward displacement of the lower rib cage as the transverse rib cage and abdomen are expanding. These different patterns of flail may reflect differences in location of the rib cage fractures or differences in respiratory muscle recruitment patterns. Support for the latter mechanism comes from the observation that

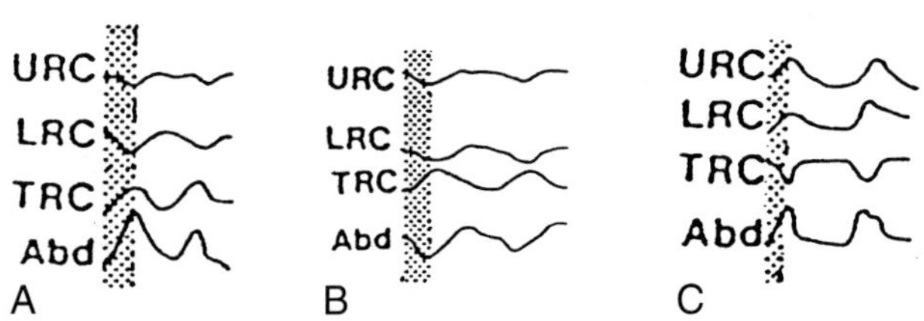


**Figure 90.6** Representative tracings of chest wall dimensions versus time, depicting three different patterns of chest wall distortion (*A* to *C*) with flail chest. The shaded area represents inspiration. URC = upper rib cage; LRC = lower rib cage; TRC = transverse lower rib cage; Abd = abdomen.

external intercostal EMG activity is increased by more than threefold in the involved area.[88, 89]

These alterations of chest wall mechanics heighten the work of breathing in patients with flail chest. The paradoxical motion of the flail segment increases the degree of muscle shortening during inspiration. This excess muscle shortening represents "internal work" that is not measured using standard techniques yet has an energetic cost. In addition to the added muscle shortening during inspiration, any associated process, such as pulmonary contusion or pleural restriction, further adds to the work of breathing by increasing the pressure needed to inhale. Because the inspiratory muscles become inefficient when operating over shorter lengths,[90] the paradoxical motion of the flail segment may result in diaphragm inefficiency. The added work of breathing, along with respiratory muscle inefficiency, increases the oxygen cost of breathing and predisposes these muscles to fatigue (Fig. 90.7).

### Gas Exchange

Hypoxemia can be pronounced in patients with flail chest and pulmonary contusion. The hypoxemia is primarily attributed to the contused lung or to microatelectasis secondary to splinting from chest wall pain.[91, 92] Hypoxemia due to either process would further contribute to respiratory muscle dysfunction by reducing energy supplies to the muscles. Flail chest in the absence of pulmonary contusion can in itself cause hypoxemia and result in respiratory failure.

## Treatment

### General Measures

Therapy for flail chest includes measures to provide adequate pulmonary toilet and pain control. Chest wall pain may cause patients to adopt a rapid shallow breathing pattern, which can lead to alveolar collapse, arteriovenous shunting, and hypoxemia. Adequate pain relief, therefore, is imperative not only for patient comfort but also because it reduces splinting, improves tidal volume, and facilitates cough. Pain control can be accomplished by direct intercostal nerve blocks or by use of epidural anesthesia.

### Mechanical Ventilation

The advent of positive-pressure ventilation provided a nonsurgical means of stabilizing the flail segment. Such "pneumatic splinting" consisted of tracheostomy with a prolonged 3- to 5-week period of mechanical ventilation. This approach had been the mainstay of therapy for nearly two decades; however, the morbidity and mortality associated with prolonged mechanical ventilation is high.[92, 93] In contrast, morbidity and mortality are significantly lower when there is either no mechanical ventilation or when the intermittent mandatory ventilation (IMV) mode is used to ventilate the patient. Consequently, continuous prolonged mechanical ventilation is no longer recommended as a primary means of stabilizing the chest wall; rather, it is recommended only when respiratory failure accompanies flail chest.

When mechanical ventilation is needed to treat respiratory failure, the mode of ventilation chosen should minimize the resistive and elastic loads imposed by the ventilator. Although IMV has been frequently used as a mode of ventilating patients with flail chest,[94] spontaneous breaths through the added resistance of the IMV circuit may aggravate chest wall distortion. In contrast, low impedance modes, such as high-flow continuous positive airway pressure (CPAP), are accompanied by less chest wall distortion during inspiration.[87] Low impedance modes of ventilation may therefore reduce the risk for inspiratory muscle fatigue and may be preferred for weaning. This speculation is supported by the observation that patients treated with CPAP alone have fewer complications, fewer hospital and intensive care unit days, and less ventilator time than patients with similar degrees of blunt thoracic trauma treated with assist control ventilation.[95] Pressure support ventilation may be an alternate means of reducing the ventilator-imposed loads, but the effects of this mode on chest wall distortion have not been evaluated.

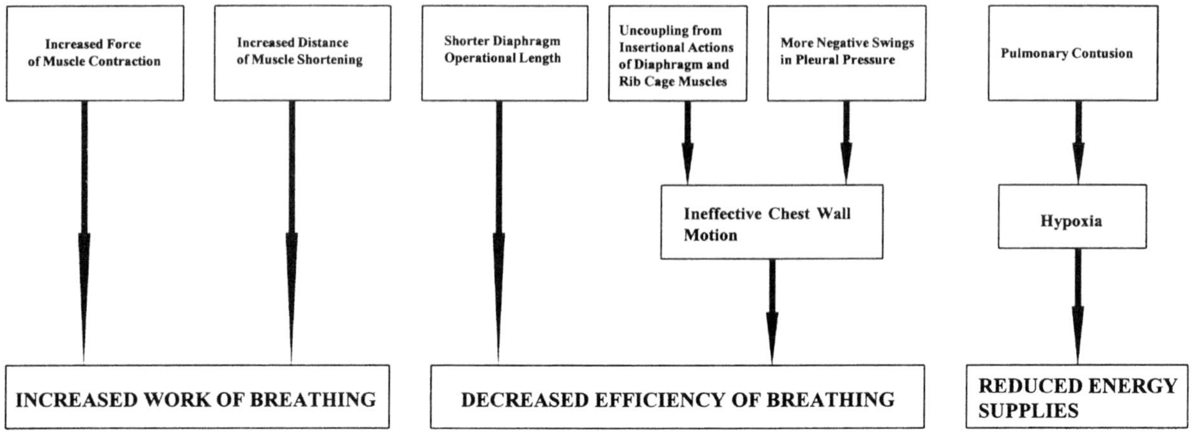


**Figure 90.7** Factors involved in the pathophysiology of flail chest.

### Surgical Management

Attempts to stabilize the flail segment surgically have been made for decades. Initial attempts consisted of applying tape, strappings, and external devices to the chest wall. These attempts met with limited success. However, the role of more invasive surgical techniques to fixate the flail segment externally has been reevaluated. Surgical techniques incorporate the use of wires, steel plates, and staples to approximate the fractured ribs. By externally stabilizing the chest wall, inward displacement of the ribs during the healing phase can be avoided, and chest wall contour can be restored to normal. Possible candidates for external fixation include patients not responding to analgesia and those who have no concurrent problems for which they need prolonged mechanical ventilation. In addition, young patients with severe chest wall deformation and patients with large, unstable segments and borderline pulmonary function may be candidates for external fixation. Chest wall external fixation in such patients improves respiratory mechanics, reduces the duration of mechanical ventilation, reduces hospital stay, and decreases the incidence of chest infection and barotrauma.[82, 96, 97]

External fixation of the flail segment has also been accomplished noninvasively using devices such as a chest cuirass to deliver constant negative extrathoracic pressure[98] or an acrylic frame. These devices have been used postoperatively for external fixation of the flail segment in a limited number of patients and were noted to reduce symptoms of pain, improve ventilatory function, and facilitate weaning from mechanical ventilation.[98] Thus, in selected patients with major chest wall resection, temporary external chest wall stabilization may enable patients to be sustained without mechanical ventilatory assistance; however, this assertion needs to be tested in larger numbers of patients.

To summarize, flail chest carries a high risk for acute respiratory failure and is associated with a high mortality rate. Complications that accompany chest trauma, such as adult respiratory distress syndrome, tracheal injury, and pneumonia, may further increase the mortality in this patient population. Adverse effects of flail chest on the respiratory system include (1) a reduction in VC as a result of inward displacement of the rib cage, (2) an increase in the work of breathing and energy demands of the inspiratory muscles, and (3) hypoxemia due to underlying pulmonary contusion or microatelectasis. The essential components of treatment include pain control and mechanical ventilation for respiratory failure. Surgical fixation of the flail segment may be indicated in some patients and may reduce the duration of mechanical ventilation. When mechanical ventilation is needed to treat respiratory failure, modes of ventilation should be chosen that reduce the elastic and resistive loads on the respiratory system.

## ANKYLOSING SPONDYLITIS

### Diagnosis and Etiology

Ankylosing spondylitis is a rheumatic disease of unknown origin that involves the axial skeleton. It is a chronic inflammatory disease that commonly afflicts men. It has a genetic predisposition: 95% of whites with primary ankylosing spondylitis have the HLA-B27 antigen, and about 20% of whites with the HLA-B27 antigen manifest some features of ankylosing spondylitis. With this disease, inflammation of the ligamentous structures of the spine, sacroiliac joint, and rib cage results in fibrosis and ossification of these structures. These processes result in rigidity of the spine and limitation of rib cage mobility as a result of bony ankylosis of the costovertebral and sternoclavicular joints.

Ankylosing spondylitis is characterized by chronic low back pain with limitation of spinal flexion and extension as well as rib cage expansion. Respiratory complaints, such as dyspnea and chest wall pain, are uncommon. If present, they may be related to chest wall restriction, kyphosis, upper lobe fibrobullous disease, or interstitial lung disease. Occasionally, patients may experience mild exercise intolerance. Respiratory failure is uncommon unless the patient has underlying lung disease, diaphragm dysfunction, or cardiac disease. Systemic manifestations occur in as many as 10% to 20% of patients and include iritis, aortic insufficiency, heart block, diastolic dysfunction, and peripheral arthritis. Upper airway obstruction is an infrequent complication of ankylosing spondylitis and is due to involvement of the cricoarytenoid cartilage. When it occurs, patients may present with hoarseness or stridor.

### Pathophysiology

#### Pulmonary Function and Mechanics

Rib cage mobility is often severely limited in patients with ankylosing spondylitis. During a VC maneuver, the rib cage may expand by only 2.5 cm, less than half of what is expected.[99] Despite this severe restriction of rib cage mobility, VC is only mildly reduced to 70% of predicted and TLC to 80% of predicted (see Table 90.2).[100–103] The reduction in lung volume, if present, is proportional to the radiographic severity of the spinal ankylosis, the degree of spinal immobility, and the degree of rib cage immobility.[102, 103] The reduced lung volume is also positively correlated with disease activity and duration.[101] Because the rib cage is often fixed in an inspiratory position, both FRC and RV may be increased above the predicted levels. Reduced rib cage mobility may also lead to a reduction in chest wall and respiratory system compliance values and to an increase in chest wall resistance.[100] Lung compliance is generally normal unless there is concomitant fibrobullous or interstitial lung disease.

The mild restrictive process seen in ankylosing spondylitis is worsened by concomitant kyphosis.[104] However, there is no correlation between the kyphosis angle and VC in ankylosing spondylitis. This lack of correlation may be due to the posterior fusion of the ribs playing a greater role in limiting VC than the degree of kyphosis.[103] Nonetheless, surgical correction of kyphosis in these patients may improve respiratory function.[105]

### Respiratory Muscle Function

Inspiratory muscle weakness may also contribute to the mild restrictive process. Modest reductions in PImax and PEmax of 56% and 76% of predicted, respectively, have been reported with ankylosing spondylitis (see Table 90.3).[102] The reduction in PImax may reflect intercostal muscle weakness rather than diaphragm dysfunction. The severe limitation of rib cage expansion with ankylosing spondylitis may promote intercostal muscle atrophy and increase the diaphragm's contribution to the inhaled volume.[106] The diaphragm appears to be strong enough to compensate for the impaired rib cage excursion because these patients have only a mild reduction in VC.

### Exercise Capacity

Exercise capacity may be reduced in patients with ankylosing spondylitis[103] and may be limited by ventilation. However, the lack of correlation between the degree of chest wall expansion and $\dot{V}O_{2max}$ or maximal work rate suggests that deconditioning also contributes to exercise intolerance in these patients (see Table 90.4).[103]

### Gas Exchange

The arterial $PO_2$ is either normal or slightly decreased in patients with ankylosing spondylitis. Reductions in diffusion capacity usually can be attributed to reductions in lung volume.[102] However, gas exchange may be severely compromised in those patients who have associated interstitial lung disease. With the exception of apical fibrobullous disease, regional ventilation is normal despite restriction of the rib cage.[107]

### Interstitial Lung Disease

About 1% to 4% of patients with ankylosing spondylitis develop fibrobullous upper lobe disease due to chronic inflammation and fibrosis of the alveolar walls.[108, 109] This complication occurs predominantly in men with longstanding disease. The spectrum of fibrobullous disease ranges from minimal upper lobe interstitial infiltrates to marked fibrosis, honeycombing, and cavity formation that may mimic tuberculosis. These patients usually do not have symptoms but are at risk for spontaneous pneumothorax and aspergillosis or mycobacteria infection. Corticosteroids have been used to treat symptoms, but they do not prevent the progression of the disease.[108] Because thoracic surgery for fibrobullous disease is complicated by bronchopleural fistula in 50% to 60% of patients, it is recommended only for the treatment of major hemoptysis.[108] Another 10% to 20% of patients with ankylosing spondylitis develop nonapical interstitial lung disease, which can be detected by high-resolution CT scan of the chest.[109]

## Treatment

Medical therapy for adult patients with ankylosing spondylitis is both preventive and supportive. Tobacco use should be avoided and baseline chest radiographs and spirometry obtained. Cardiorespiratory fitness and spinal mobility may be enhanced by instituting exercise and physiotherapy programs, but there may be little or no change in pulmonary function despite improved chest wall and spinal mobility. Similarly, specific pulmonary rehabilitation has been tried with varied success. These patients are usually managed by a clinician skillful in the treatment of rheumatic disease but are often referred to a pulmonologist for evaluation of abnormal chest radiographs, deteriorating pulmonary function, hypoxemia, or hypercapnia. If intubation is required, it should be performed with caution because these patients are at increased risk for spinal cord injury because of involvement of the cricoarytenoid joint.[110]

To summarize, ankylosing spondylitis is a chronic inflammatory disease that may limit spinal flexion and rib cage expansion and is sometimes associated with interstitial lung disease. The reduced rib cage mobility leads to only mild reductions in VC and TLC and possibly to atrophy of the inspiratory muscles of the rib cage. This mild restrictive disease may contribute to exercise intolerance in these patients.

# OBESITY

## Diagnosis and Etiology

This section focuses mainly on the respiratory effects of obesity uncomplicated by coexistent obstructive airway disease or restrictive disease of the lungs. Even uncomplicated obesity exerts substantial effects on pulmonary gas exchange, oxygenation of the blood, and the work of breathing, and it has modest effects on ventilatory drive and the pattern of breathing. Obese patients often complain of exercise intolerance and dyspnea during exertion. In addition, they are at increased risk for complications such as pneumonia, hypoxemia, atelectasis, and pulmonary embolism. Patients with uncomplicated obesity do not have ventilatory failure, but some manifestations of the obesity hypoventilation syndrome (OHS) are presented for the sake of comparison. The OHS and its relation to obstructive sleep apnea are covered in Chapters 80 and 81.

As many as one third of the adults living in the United States are overweight. The severity of obesity can be assessed from several indices that relate weight to height. In addition to calculating percentage of ideal body weight for sex and height, one can calculate the ratio of body weight to height (BW/Ht) and the body mass index (BMI), which is the ratio $BW/Ht^2$. The advantage of using the BW/Ht ratio or BMI is that no tables of height and weight are needed. The ideal BMI is 19 to 22 $kg/m^2$, but the health risks of obesity are small until the BMI exceeds 28 $kg/m^2$.[111] Obesity is mild when adipose accumulates to the extent that body weight lies between 120% and 150% of ideal body weight, the BW/Ht ratio is between 0.4 to 0.6, or the BMI lies between 28 and 40 $kg/m^2$. Obesity is severe when body weight is greater than 150% of ideal, the BW/Ht ratio is greater than 0.6, or the BMI is greater than 40 $kg/m^2$.

Table 90.9 BODY COMPOSITION IN OBESITY

| Variable | Normal | Mild Obesity | Severe Obesity |
|---|---|---|---|
| Body mass index (kg/m²) | 23 | 34 | 50 |
| Body fat (%) | 22 | 35 | 45 |
| Body weight (kg) | 65 | 96 | 132 |
| Fat-free mass (kg) | 51 | 63 | 72 |
| Body cell mass (kg) | 27 | 32 | 36 |
| Total body water (L) | 38 | 44 | 49 |
| Resting energy expenditure (watts) | 68 | 86 | 96 |

Body fat usually constitutes 15% to 20% of the body mass in healthy men and 25% to 30% in healthy women. In obesity, the body fat content may increase by as much as 500% in women and 800% in men, and body fat mass is proportional to BMI.[112, 113] Fat-free mass (FFM) increases along with fat mass, so that 15% to 30% of the weight gain in obesity results from increased FFM.[113, 114] Resting energy expenditure (REE) is proportional to FFM, and the ratio of REE to FFM is the same in patients with mild and severe obesity as it is in normal-weight subjects (Table 90.9).[113]

The distribution of obesity also has an effect on ventilatory function, independent of the body fat content per se. Methods to assess the distribution of body fat include measurement of the ratio of waist to hip circumference, the ratio of abdominal girth to hip breadth, and the thickness of skin folds in multiple sites as well as the use of CT or magnetic resonance imaging to assess the ratio of cross-sectional area of visceral fat to subcutaneous fat.

## Pathophysiology

### Pulmonary Function

Pulmonary function of obese patients is reviewed in detail in Chapter 28.

Spirometry is generally normal in uncomplicated obesity except for a modest reduction in VC or FVC when the BMI exceeds 45 kg/m².[115–120] The FVC is slightly lower in the supine position, but this is of little clinical significance.[121] Men with more central obesity have lower FVC and $FEV_1$ than women for a given BMI.[122, 123] The $FEV_1$/FVC ratio is usually normal. MVV and peak inspiratory flow rate are also normal, provided that respiratory muscle strength is normal.[119]

The effects of uncomplicated obesity on lung volume include large reductions in expiratory reserve volume (ERV) and lesser reductions in TLC and FRC (Table 90.10).[115–119] The ERV is reduced on average to 60% of predicted normal value and is inversely proportional to BMI. TLC and FRC tend to remain normal until BMI exceeds 45 kg/m².

Spirometry in OHS usually reveals a more severe restrictive pattern, with low VC, MVV, and peak inspiratory flow rate.[119, 120] This appears to be related to modest weakness of the respiratory muscles.[119] The changes in lung volumes are also more pronounced; ERV is reduced to 35% of predicted, TLC to 80% of predicted, and FVC to 60% of predicted.[120] It appears that the adverse effects of obesity on pulmonary function cannot be entirely explained by the absolute load of adipose on the chest wall because similar degrees of obesity in uncomplicated

Table 90.10 RESPIRATORY PATHOPHYSIOLOGY OF SIMPLE OBESITY AND OBESITY HYPOVENTILATION SYNDROME

| Variable | Units | Normal | Simple Obesity | Obesity Hypoventilation Syndrome |
|---|---|---|---|---|
| BW | % Ideal | 105 | 195 | 201 |
| BW/Ht | kg/cm | 0.42 | 0.75 | 0.78 |
| BMI | kg/m² | 24 | 45 | 46 |
| TLC | % Predicted | 100 | 95 | 83 |
| $C_{RS}$ | L/cm $H_2O^{-1}$ | 0.11 | 0.05 | 0.06 |
| $R_{RS}$ | cm $H_2O$ $L^{-1}$ $sec^{-1}$ | 1.2 | 4.0 | 7.8 |
| Work | J/L | 0.43 | 0.74 | 1.64 |
| MVV | L/min | 159 | 129 | 89 |
| Pimax | cm $H_2O$ | 100 | 95 | 60 |

BW = body weight; BMI = body mass index; TLC = total lung capacity; $C_{RS}$ = compliance of the respiratory system; $R_{RS}$ = respiratory system resistance; Pimax = maximal inspiratory pressure; MVV = maximum ventilatory volume.

obesity and OHS result in different patterns of lung volume changes.

## Respiratory Mechanics

Obesity generally lowers compliance of the lung, chest wall, and total respiratory system, and, as with lung volume, compliance is more severely affected in OHS.[117, 120, 124, 125] In uncomplicated obesity, chest wall and total respiratory system compliance values are generally 80% and 90% of values obtained in normal subjects; even when the BW/Ht ratio and BMI are as high as 1.2 kg/cm and 80 $kg/m^2$, respectively.[120] In OHS, the chest wall and total respiratory system compliance values are generally less than 45% of normal. The changes in compliance are thought to be due to weight pressing on the thorax and abdomen, thereby imposing an elastic load. In addition, the excess weight may also impose a threshold-type load on the chest wall; pleural pressure must be lowered to a sufficient degree before inspiratory flow can ensue.

Obesity is associated with increases in airway and respiratory system resistance, in part because of the reduction in lung volume.[115, 117, 126] After correcting for lung volume, specific airway conductance may be reduced to 50% to 70% of normal.[115, 117, 120, 125, 126] Because the $FEV_1$/FVC ratio is normal, the source of the increased airway resistance in obesity appears to lie in lung tissue and small airways rather than in the large airways. Chest wall and total respiratory system resistances are increased more in OHS than in uncomplicated obesity.[120] Total respiratory system reactance is lower in patients with simple obesity than in normal-weight subjects, and respiratory resistance rises and reactance falls when obese subjects shift from upright to supine.[126] Part of the impediment to breathing in obesity results from a two- to threefold increase in intra-abdominal pressure.[127]

The increased elastic and resistive loads imposed by the lung and chest wall, along with the threshold load imposed by the abdominal fat mass, increase the work of breathing in both uncomplicated obesity and OHS. When compared with normal, the work of breathing is 60% higher in uncomplicated obesity and may be as much as 250% higher in OHS. The increased work is accompanied by an increase in the energy cost of breathing; the oxygen cost of breathing in simple obesity is four times normal, and that in OHS is nearly 10 times normal.[120, 125]

## Gas Exchange

Hypoxemia may be mild or absent in uncomplicated obesity.[124, 128] However, gas exchange is usually impaired, and severely obese patients tend to have a widened alveolar-arterial oxygen tension gradient.[129, 130] The arterial $Po_2$ is even lower in OHS.[129–131] In both uncomplicated obesity and OHS, hypoxemia becomes more pronounced when assuming the supine position. The single-breath diffusion capacity is usually normal or increased in uncomplicated obesity[120, 132, 133] and slightly reduced in OHS.[120] The physiologic dead space ($V_D$) and the ratio of dead space to tidal volume ($V_D/V_T$) are normal.[120]

Mechanisms leading to hypoxemia include ventilation-perfusion mismatching, venous admixture, and hypoventilation in OHS. With obesity, the lung bases are well perfused but poorly ventilated because of airway closure and alveolar collapse.[134] The practical consequence of this and the increased metabolic rate in obesity is that the rate at which arterial $So_2$ falls during apnea is three times faster in obese subjects than in normal-weight subjects.[124, 135–137]

## Control of Breathing

Respiratory drive may be increased in uncomplicated obesity, even though the ventilatory response to carbon dioxide is generally reduced by about 40%.[120, 124] In contrast, the resting $P_{0.1}$ and $V_T/T_I$ ratio may be normal or higher than normal in uncomplicated obesity, and $P_{0.1}$ increases normally with carbon dioxide inhalation.[120, 124] The diaphragm electrical (EMG) response to inhalation of carbon dioxide, another index of central ventilatory drive, is also elevated in uncomplicated obesity.[120] Because the work of breathing is increased in obesity, the increase in ventilatory drive is an appropriate load compensatory response.

Ventilatory drive appears to be inappropriately low in OHS. The ventilatory response to carbon dioxide is reduced by about 65%, but arterial $Pco_2$ can be lowered to a normal level by voluntary hyperventilation in OHS.[138] Values for $P_{0.1}$ in overt OHS are unavailable; however, the respiratory muscle EMG response to carbon dioxide, which should be elevated, is inappropriately low, lying in the normal range.[120] The finding that $P_{0.1}$ in former OHS patients is the same as in uncomplicated obesity indicates that these changes are in part reversible. Because the work of breathing is excessive in OHS, the appropriate load compensatory response is an increase in ventilatory drive, rather than a normal drive.

## Pattern of Breathing

Obese patients may also alter their breathing pattern to compensate for the increased load placed on the respiratory system. During quiet breathing, the respiratory rate in subjects with uncomplicated obesity is about 40% higher than in normal-weight subjects. The increased rate is accomplished by shortening both inspiratory and expiratory time, and the ratio of inspiratory to total breath time is normal. In contrast to the increase in breathing frequency, $V_T$ is normal in uncomplicated obesity both at rest and during maximal exercise.[120, 124] In OHS, breathing frequency is 25% higher, and $V_T$ is 25% lower as compared with simple obesity, and the rapid shallow breathing pattern in OHS contributes to carbon dioxide retention.[120]

## Respiratory Muscle Function

Inspiratory and expiratory muscle strength is generally normal in uncomplicated obesity.[139–141] In severely obese subjects, there may be a mild degree of inspiratory muscle weakness, perhaps related to overstretching of the diaphragm.[142] The inspiratory muscles of subjects with uncomplicated obesity are strong enough to overcome the reduction in lung and chest wall compliance such that TLC is not reduced. Dyspnea in uncomplicated obesity is associated with greater BMI, peripheral airway disease, and mild expiratory muscle weakness.[143] In OHS, inspiratory muscle strength may be reduced by 40%,[120] perhaps because of deconditioning or other factors related to chronic disease.

### Exercise Capacity

In uncomplicated obesity, exercise capacity is near normal.[137] Minute ventilation, respiratory rate, heart rate, and oxygen consumption during treadmill exercise are higher in obese subjects than in normal-weight subjects,[144] but $\dot{V}O_2$ at anaerobic threshold is lower than in normal-weight subjects.[145, 146] With weight loss, the metabolic demands are reduced, and carbon dioxide production and alveolar ventilation during exercise fall by 12% to 22%.[120]

## Treatment

### Weight Reduction

The optimal treatment for obesity is weight loss, but it is difficult for patients to lose weight and even harder to remain at the lower weight. The problem is that losing weight decreases total energy expenditure in both normal and obese subjects, whereas the opposite is true with weight gain.[114] With weight loss, the percentage reduction in REE exceeds the percentage reduction in FFM.[137] In other words, the body has a tendency to resist changes in weight in either direction.

The effects of weight loss, induced by diet or surgery, on pulmonary function in uncomplicated obesity have been well documented.[118, 120, 128, 131, 132, 147–150] With a weight loss of 40 kg, there is either no change or a small increase in VC, TLC, or compliance. However, there is a 75% increase in ERV and lesser increases in FRC and RV. These are associated with better ventilation to the lung bases, and arterial $P_{O_2}$ may be increased by about 4 to 8 mm Hg.[120, 128] In OHS, the effects of weight loss on ERV and FRC are even more pronounced, and VC increases as well. The increases in VC and arterial $P_{O_2}$ and the fall in arterial $P_{CO_2}$ are positively correlated with weight loss.[120, 151]

Small reductions in FFM and $P_{Emax}$ may occur in uncomplicated obesity along with a small increase in MVV.[149] Alternatively, respiratory muscle strength and especially endurance may improve, with the improvement in endurance correlated with weight loss.[141] There is a significant reduction in the oxygen consumption needed for a given exercise power output.[148] Respiratory control remains essentially unaltered after weight loss.[120]

### Mechanical Ventilation

Bilevel positive airway pressure has been used successfully to treat atelectasis after gastroplasty.[152] Obese patients who experience nocturnal or nocturnal and daytime hypercapnia generally require some form of mechanical ventilation. Negative-pressure ventilation can improve nocturnal oxygenation, but it often aggravates upper airway obstruction during sleep.[153] Positive-pressure ventilation delivered by nose mask improves sleep quality, corrects hypercapnia, and improves daytime oxygenation.[154, 155]

## SUMMARY

Chest wall diseases, including obesity, exert important effects on the respiratory system. Initially, the lungs may be normal, but when the primary problem is severe, there can be multiple pulmonary complications, including atelectasis, pneumonia, hypoxemia, and hypercapnia. Among the diseases discussed in this chapter, flail chest is the most likely to precipitate acute respiratory failure. Kyphoscoliosis, restrictive disease due to previous thoracoplasty, and severe obesity are the diseases most likely to lead to chronic ventilatory failure, pulmonary hypertension, and cor pulmonale. In these patients, the stiff chest wall imposes a large elastic load on the respiratory muscles, which increases the work of breathing and impairs lung function. Coincident inspiratory muscle weakness in any of these disorders and sleep-related dysfunction also contribute to daytime hypercapnia, cor pulmonale, and pulmonary hypertension. Acute respiratory failure is treated with positive-pressure ventilation. In some patients with flail chest, surgical fixation of the flail segment may reduce the duration of mechanical ventilation. Chronic respiratory failure, which can be seen in kyphoscoliosis, after thoracoplasty, or with severe obesity, can be successfully managed with nocturnal positive-pressure ventilation. This therapy reduces morbidity and mortality from respiratory failure and improves prognosis.

Other diseases of the chest wall, such as ankylosing spondylitis, pectus excavatum, and simple obesity, impair respiratory function only mildly. These patients often have complaints of exercise intolerance but have only mild reductions in lung volumes and in exercise capacity. Surgical repair of pectus is performed in older children or adolescents. After repair of the pectus deformity, there is often symptomatic improvement but no change in aerobic capacity.

More discussion about the pathophysiology and management of pulmonary hypertension and cor pulmonale can be found in Chapter 55. Further information about the pathophysiology and treatment of respiratory failure is provided in Chapters 91 to 94. The role of rehabilitation in management is considered in Chapter 96. The interested reader should consult these chapters for further details about the diagnosis, treatment, and prevention of the pulmonary complications of chest wall disorders.

## References

1. Bergofsky EH, Turino GM, Fishman AP: Cardiorespiratory failure in kyphoscoliosis. Medicine (Baltimore) 38:263–317, 1959.
2. Litwin SD: Genetic Determinants of Pulmonary Disease. New York: Marcel Dekker, 1978, pp 182–188.
3. Walker JL, Nelson KR, Stevens DB, et al: Spinal deformity in Charcot-Marie-Tooth disease. Spine 19:1044–1047, 1994.
4. Lisboa C, Moreno R, Fava M, et al: Inspiratory muscle function in patients with severe kyphoscoliosis. Am Rev Respir Dis 132:48–52, 1985.
5. Kafer ER: Idiopathic scoliosis: Mechanical properties of the respiratory system and the ventilatory response to carbon dioxide. J Clin Invest 55:1153–1163, 1975.
6. Smyth RJ, Chapman KR, Wright TA, et al: Pulmonary function

in adolescents with mild idiopathic scoliosis. Thorax 39:901–904, 1984.
7. Baydur A, Milic-Emili J: Respiratory mechanics in kyphoscoliosis. Monaldi Arch Chest Dis 48:69–79, 1993.
8. Al-Kattan K, Simonds A, Chung KF, et al: Kyphoscoliosis and bronchial torsion. Chest 111:1134–1137, 1997.
9. Jones RS, Kennedy JD, Hasam F, et al: Mechanical inefficiency of the thoracic cage in scoliosis. Thorax 36:456–461, 1981.
10. Sinha R, Bergofsky EH: Prolonged alteration of lung mechanics in kyphoscoliosis by positive-pressure hyperinflation. Am Rev Respir Dis 106:47–57, 1972.
11. Conti G, Rocco M, Antonelli M, et al: Respiratory system mechanics in the early phase of acute respiratory failure due to severe kyphoscoliosis. Intensive Care Med 23:539–544, 1997.
12. McCool FD, Tzelepis, GE, Leith DE, et al: Oxygen cost of breathing during fatiguing inspiratory resistive loads. J Appl Physiol 66:2045–2055, 1989.
13. Szeinberg A, Canny GJ, Rashed N, et al: Forced vital capacity and maximal respiratory pressures in patients with mild and moderate scolioses. Pediatr Pulmonol 4:8–12, 1988.
14. Estenne M, Derom E, De Troyer A: Neck and abdominal muscle activity in patients with severe thoracic scoliosis. Am J Respir Crit Care Med 158:452–457, 1998.
15. Tardif C, Sohier B, Derenne JP: Control of breathing in chest wall disease. Monaldi Arch Chest Dis 48:83–86, 1993.
16. Ramonatxo M, Milic-Emili J, Prefaut C: Breathing pattern and load compensatory responses in young scoliotic patients. Eur Respir J 1:421–427, 1988.
17. Bake B, Bjure J, Kasalichy J, et al: Regional pulmonary ventilation and perfusion distribution in patients with untreated idiopathic scoliosis. Thorax 27:703–712, 1972.
18. Libby DM, Briscoe WA, Boyce B, et al: Acute respiratory failure in scoliosis or kyphosis. Am J Med 73:532–538, 1982.
19. Jones DJ, Paul EA, Bell JH, et al: Ambulatory oxygen therapy in stable kyphoscoliosis. Eur Respir J 8:819–823, 1995.
20. Kesten S, Garfinkel SK, Wright T, et al: Impaired exercise capacity in adults with moderate scoliosis. Chest 99:663–666, 1991.
21. Kearon C, Viviani GR, Killian KJ: Factors influencing work capacity in adolescent idiopathic thoracic scoliosis. Am Rev Respir Dis 148:295–303, 1993.
22. Midgren B, Petersson K, Hansson L, et al: Nocturnal hypoxemia in severe scoliosis. Br J Dis Chest 82:226–236, 1988.
23. Guilleminault C, Kurlan G, Wirkle R: Severe kyphoscoliosis, breathing, and sleep. Chest 79:626–630, 1981.
24. Sawicka EH, Branthwaite MA: Respiration during sleep in kyphoscoliosis. Thorax 42:801–808, 1987.
25. McNicholas WT: Impact of sleep in respiratory failure. Eur Respir J 10:920–933, 1997.
26. Pehrsson K, Bake JB, Larsson S, et al: Lung function in adult idiopathic scoliosis: A 20-year follow-up. Thorax 46:474–478, 1991.
27. Branthwaite MR: Cardiorespiratory consequences of unfused idiopathic scoliosis. Br J Dis Chest 80:360–369, 1986.
28. Chailleux E, Fauroux B, Binet F, et al: Predictors of survival in patients receiving domiciliary oxygen therapy or mechanical ventilation: A 10-year analysis of ANTADIR observatory. Chest 109:741–749, 1996.
29. To WW, Wong MN: Kyphoscoliosis complicating pregnancy. Int J Gynaecol Obstet 55:123–128, 1996.
30. Rom WN, Miller A: Unexpected longevity in patients with severe kyphoscoliosis. Thorax 33:106–110, 1978.
31. Strom K, Pehrsson K, Boe J, et al: Survival of patients with severe thoracic spine deformities receiving domiciliary oxygen therapy. Chest 102:164–168, 1992.
32. Wiers PWJ, Le Coultre R, Dallinga OT, et al: Cuirass respirator treatment of chronic respiratory failure in scoliotic patients. Thorax 32:221–228, 1977.
33. Fulkerson WJ, Wilkins JK, Esbenshade AM, et al: Life threatening hypoventilation in kyphoscoliosis: Successful treatment with a molded body brace-ventilator. Am Rev Respir Dis 129:185–187, 1984.
34. Kinnear W, Hockley S, Harvey J, et al: The effects of one year of nocturnal cuirass-assisted ventilation in chest wall disease. Eur Respir J 1:204–208, 1988.
35. Kerby GR, Mayer LS, Pingleton SK: Nocturnal positive pressure ventilation via nasal mask. Am Rev Respir Dis 135:738–740, 1987.
36. Carrey Z, Gottfried SG, Levy RD: Ventilatory muscle support in respiratory failure with nasal positive-pressure ventilation. Chest 97:150–158, 1990.
37. Ambrosino N, Vitacca M, Polease G, et al: Short-term effects of nasal proportional assist ventilation in patients with chronic hypercapnic respiratory insufficiency. Eur Respir J 10:2829–2834, 1997.
38. Leger P, Bedicam JM, Cornette A, et al: Nasal intermittent positive pressure ventilation: Long-term follow-up in patients with severe chronic respiratory insufficiency. Chest 105:100–105, 1994.
39. Bach JR, Robert D, Leger P, et al: Sleep fragmentation in kyphoscoliotic individuals with alveolar hypoventilation treated by NIPPV. Chest 107:1552–1558, 1995.
40. Simonds AK, Parker RA, Branthwaite MA: The effect of intermittent positive-pressure hyperinflation in restrictive chest wall disease. Respir 55:136–143, 1989.
41. McCool FD, Mayewski RJ, Shayne DS, et al: Intermittent positive pressure breathing in patients with respiratory muscle weakness: Alterations in total respiratory system compliance. Chest 90:546–552, 1986.
42. Lenke LG, Bridwell KH, Blanke K, et al: Analysis of pulmonary function and chest cage dimension changes after thoracoplasty in idiopathic scoliosis. Spine 20:1343–1350, 1995.
43. Baydur A, Swank SM, Stiles CM, et al: Respiratory mechanics in anesthetized young patients with kyphoscoliosis: Immediate and delayed effects of corrective spinal surgery. Chest 97:1157–1164, 1990.
44. Swank S, Lonstein J, Moe J, et al: Surgical treatment of adult scoliosis. J Bone J Surg 63:268–287, 1981.
45. Gagnon S, Jodoin A, Martin R: Pulmonary function test study before and after spinal fusion in young idiopathic scoliosis. Spine 14:486–490, 1989.
46. Vandenbroucke J, van Ooy A, Gfeukers C, et al: Dystrophic kyphoscoliosis in neurofibromatosis type I: A report of two cases and review of the literature. Eur Spine J 6:273–277, 1997.
47. Loynes RD: Scoliosis after thoracoplasty. J Bone Joint Surg 54B:484–498, 1972.
48. Peppas G, Molnar TF, Jeyasingham K, et al: Thoracoplasty in the context of current surgical practice. Ann Thorac Surg 56:903–909, 1993.
49. Somers J, Faber LP: Historical developments in the management of empyema. Chest Surg Clin North Am 6:403–418, 1996.
50. Phillips MS, Kinnear WJM, Shneerson JM: Late sequelae of pulmonary tuberculosis treated by thoracoplasty. Thorax 42:445–451, 1987.
51. Bredin CP: Pulmonary function in long-term survivors of thoracoplasty. Chest 95:18–20, 1989.
52. Phillips MS, Miller MR, Kinnear WJM, et al: Importance of airflow obstruction after thoracoplasty. Thorax 42:348–352, 1987.
53. Sridhar MK, Carter R, Lean ME, et al: Resting energy expenditure and nutritional state of patients with increased oxygen cost of breathing due to emphysema, scoliosis and thoracoplasty. Thorax 49:781–785, 1994.
54. Sawicka EH, Branthwaite MA, Spencer GT: Respiratory failure after thoracoplasty: Treatment by intermittent negative pressure ventilation. Thorax 38:433–435, 1983.
55. Jackson M, Smith I, King M, et al: Long term non-invasive domiciliary assisted ventilation for respiratory failure following thoracoplasty. Thorax 49:915–919, 1994.
56. Ravitch MM: Congenital Deformities of the Chest Wall and Their Operative Correction. Philadelphia: WB Saunders, 1977.
57. Haller JA, Scherer LR, Turner CS, et al: Evolving management of pectus excavatum based on a single institutional experience of 664 patients. Ann Surg 209:578–582, 1989.
58. Fonkalsrud EW, Salmon T, Guo W et al: Repair of pectus deformities with sternal support. J Thorac Cardiovasc Surg 107:37–42, 1994.
59. Dato GMA, DePaulis R, Dato AA, et al: Correction of pectus excavatum with a self-retaining seagull wing prosthesis. Chest 107:303–306, 1995.
60. Chidambaram B, Mehta AV: Currarino-Silverman syndrome (pectus carinatum type 2 deformity) and mitral valve disease. Chest 102:780–782, 1992.

61. Peterson RJ, Young WG Jr, Godwin JD, et al: Noninvasive assessment of exercise cardiac function before and after pectus excavatum repair. J Thorac Cardiovasc Surg 90:251–260, 1985.
62. Nakahara K, Kiyoshi O, Shinichiro M, et al: An evaluation of operative outcome in patients with funnel chest diagnosed by means of the computed tomogram. J Thorac Cardiovasc Surg 93:577–582, 1987.
63. Chuang J-H, Wan Y-L: Evaluation of pectus excavatum with repeated CT scans. Pediatr Radiol 25:654–656, 1995
64. Derveaux L, Ivanoff I, Rochette F, et al: Mechanism of pulmonary function changes after surgical correction for funnel chest. Eur Respir J 1:823–825, 1988.
65. Kaguraoka H, Ohnuki T, Itaoka T, et al: Degree of severity of pectus excavatum and pulmonary function in preoperative and postoperative periods. J Thorac Cardiovasc Surg 104:1483–1488, 1992.
66. Castile R, Staats B, Westbrook P: Symptomatic pectus deformities of the chest. Am Rev Respir Dis 126:564–568, 1982.
67. Mead J, Sly P, Lesouef P, et al: Rib cage mobility in pectus excavatum. Am Rev Respir Dis 130:1223–1228, 1985.
68. Wynn S, Driscol D, Ostrom N, et al: Exercise cardiorespiratory function in adolescents with pectus excavatum. J Thorac Cardiovasc Surg 99:41–47, 1990.
69. Morshuis W, Folgering H, Barentsz J, et al: Pulmonary function before surgery for pectus excavatum and at long-term follow-up. Chest 105:1646–1652, 1994.
70. Quigley PM, Haller JA, Jelus KL, et al: Cardiorespiratory function before and after corrective surgery in pectus excavatum. J Pediatr 128:638–643, 1996.
71. Mocchegiani R, Badano L, Lestuzzi C, et al: Relation of right ventricular morphology and function in pectus excavatum to the severity of the chest wall deformity. Am J Cardiol 76:941–946, 1995.
72. Haller JA Jr, Kramer SS, Lietman SA: Use of CT scans in selection of patients for pectus excavatum surgery: A preliminary report. J Pediatr Surg 22:615–622, 1988.
73. Nuss D, Kelly RE, Croitoru DP, et al: A 10 year review of a minimally invasive technique for the correction of pectus excavatum. J Pediatr Surg 33:545–552, 1998.
74. Johnson PE: Refining silicone implant correction of pectus excavatum through computed tomography. Plast Reconstr Surg 97:445–449, 1996.
75. Cahill JJ, Lees GM, Roberston HT: A summary of pre-operative and post-operative cardiorespiratory performance in patients undergoing pectus excavatum and carinatum repair. J Pediatr Surg 19:430–433, 1984.
76. Kowalewski J, Barcikowksi S, Brocki M: Cardiorespiratory function before and after operation for pectus excavatum: Medium-term results. Eur J Cardiothorac Surg 13:275–279, 1998.
77. Derveaux L, Clarysse I, Ivanoff I, et al: Preoperative and postoperative abnormalities in chest x-ray indices and in lung function in pectus deformities. Chest 95:850–856, 1989.
78. Haller JA, Colombani PM, Humphries CT, et al: Chest wall constriction after too extensive and too early operations for pectus excavatum. Ann Thorac Surg 61:1618–1625, 1996.
79. Pretorius ES, Haller JA, Fishman EK: Spiral CT with 3D reconstruction in children requiring reoperation for failure of chest wall growth after pectus excavatum surgery: Preliminary observations. Clin Imaging 22:108–116, 1998.
80. Todd TRJ, Shamji F: Pathophysiology of chest wall trauma. *In* Roussos C, Macklem PT (eds): The Thorax. Part B. New York: Marcel Dekker, 1985, pp 979–997.
81. Gaillard M, Herve C, Mandin L, et al: Mortality prognostic factors in chest injury. J Trauma 30:93–96, 1990.
82. Ahmed Z, Mohyuddin Z: Managment of flail chest injury: Internal fixation versus endotracheal intubation and ventilation. J Thorac Cardiovasc Surg 110:1676–1680, 1995.
83. Moore P, James O, Byth P, et al: Factors affecting outcome after chest injury. Anaesth Intens Care 13:362–369, 1985.
84. Landercasper J, Cogbill TH, Lindesmith LA: Long-term disability after flail chest injury. Trauma 24:410–414, 1984.
85. Smejkal R, O'Malley KF, David E, et al: Routine initial computed tomography of the chest in blunt torso trauma. Chest 100:667–669, 1991.
86. Kishikawa M, Yoshioka T, Shimazu T, et al: Pulmonary contusion causes long-term respiratory dysfunction with decreased functional residual capacity (with discussion). J Trauma 31:1203–1210, 1991.
87. Tzelepis GE, McCool FD, Hoppin FG Jr: Chest wall distortion in patients with flail chest. Am Rev Respir Dis 140:31–37, 1989.
88. Cappelo M, Yuehua C, DeTroyer A: Rib cage distortion in a canine model of flail chest. Am J Respir Crit Care Med 151:1481–1485, 1995.
89. Cappelo M, Yuehua C, DeTroyer A: Respiratory muscle response to flail chest. Am J Respir Crit Care Med 153:1897–1901, 1996.
90. Tzelepis GE, McCool FD, Leith DE, et al: Influence of lung volume on inspiratory muscle endurance. J Appl Phys 64:1796–1802, 1988.
91. Craven KD, Oppenheimer L, Wood LDH: Effects of contusion and flail chest on pulmonary perfusion and oxygen exchange. J Appl Physiol 47:729–737, 1979.
92. Trinkle JK, Richardson JD, Franz JL, et al: Management of flail chest without mechanical ventilation. Ann Thorac Surg 19:355–363, 1975.
93. Shackford SR, Smith DE, Zarins CD, et al: The management of flail chest: A comparison of ventilatory and nonventilatory treatment. Am J Surg 132:759–762, 1976.
94. Cullen P, Modell JH, Dirby RR, et al: Treatment of flail chest: Use of intermittent mandatory ventilation and positive end-expiratory pressure. Arch Surg 110:1099–1103, 1985.
95. Bolliger CT, Van Eeden SF: Treatment of multiple rib fractures: Randomized control trial comparing ventilatory and nonventilatory management. Chest 97:943–948, 1990.
96. Mouton W, Lardinois D, Furrer M, et al: Long-term follow-up of patients with operative stabilisation of a flail chest. Thorac Cardiovasc Surg 45:242–244, 1997.
97. Voggenreiter G, Neudect F, Aufmkolk M, et al: Operative chest wall stabilization in flail chest: Outcomes of patients with or without pulmonary contusion. J Am Coll Surg 187:130–138, 1998.
98. Hartke RH Jr, Block AJ: External stabilization of flail chest using continuous negative extrathoracic pressure. Chest 102:1283–1285, 1992.
99. Calin A: Ankylosing spondylitis. Clin Rheum Dis 11:41–60, 1985.
100. VanNoord JA, Caubergs M, Van de Woestigne KP, et al: Total respiratory system resistance and reactance in ankylosing spondylitis and kyphoscoliosis. Eur Respir J 4:945–951, 1991.
101. Feltelius N, Hedenstrom H, Hillerdal G, et al: Pulmonary involvement in ankylosing spondylitis. Ann Rheum Dis 45:736–740, 1986.
102. Vanderschueren D, Decramer M, Van Den Dael P, et al: Pulmonary function and maximal transrespiratory pressure in ankylosing spondylitis. Ann Rheum Dis 48:632–635, 1989.
103. Fisher LR, Cawley MI, Holgate S: Relation between chest expansion, pulmonary function, and exercise tolerance in patients with ankylosing spondylitis. Ann Rheum Dis 49:921–925, 1990.
104. Culham EG, Jimenez HA, King CE: Thoracic kyphosis, rib mobility, and lung volumes in normal women and women with osteoporosis. Spine 19:1250–1255, 1994.
105. Thiranont N, Netrawichien P: Transpedicular decancellation closed wedge vertebral osteotomy for treatment of fixed flexion deformity of spine in ankylosing spondylitis. Spine 18:2517–2522, 1993.
106. Grimby G, Fugl-Meyer AR, Blomstrand A: Partitioning of the contributions of rib cage and abdomen to ventilation in ankylosing spondylitis. Thorax 29:179–184, 1974.
107. Parkin A, Robinson PJ, Hickling P: Regional lung ventilation in ankylosing spondylitis. Br J Radiol 55:833–836, 1982.
108. Rosenow E, Strimlan C, Muhm J, et al: Pleuropulmonary manifestations of ankylosing spondylitis. Mayo Clin Proc 52:641–649, 1977.
109. Fenlon HM, Casserly I, Sant SM, et al: Plain radiographs and thoracic high-resolution CT in patients with ankylosing spondylitis. Am J Roentgenol 168:1067–1072, 1997.
110. Sinclair JR, Mason RA: Ankylosing spondylitis: The case for awake intubation. Anaesthesia 39:3–11, 1984.
111. Stevens J, Cai J, Pamuk ER, et al: The effect of age on the association between body-mass index and mortality. N Engl J Med 338:1–7, 1998.

112. Strain GW, Zumoff B: The relationship of weight-height indices of obesity to body fat content. J Am Coll Nutr 6:715–718, 1992.
113. Verga S, Buscemi C, Caimi G: Resting energy expenditure and body composition in morbidly obese, obese and control subjects. Acta Diabetol 31:47–51, 1994.
114. Leibel RL, Rosenbaum M, Hirsch J: Changes in energy expenditure resulting from altered body weight. N Engl J Med 332:621–628, 1995.
115. Rubinstein I, Zamel N, DuBarry RPT, et al: Airflow limitation in morbidly obese, nonsmoking men. Ann Intern Med 112:828–832, 1990.
116. Jenkins SC, Moxham J: The effects of mild obesity on lung function. Respir Med 85:309–311, 1991.
117. Zerah F, Harf A, Perlemuter L, et al: Effects of obesity on respiratory resistance. Chest 103:1470–1476, 1993.
118. Hakala K, Mustajoki P, Aittomaki J, et al: Effect of weight loss and body position on pulmonary function and gas exchange abnormalities in morbid obesity. Int J Obes Relat Metab Disord 19:343–346, 1995.
119. Sahebjami H, Gartside PS: Pulmonary function in obese subjects with a normal $FEV_1$/FVC ratio. Chest 110:1425–1429, 1996.
120. Rochester DF: Obesity and pulmonary function. *In* Alpert MA, Alexander JK (eds): The Heart and Lung in Obesity (1st ed). Armonk, NY: Futura, 1998, pp 109–131.
121. Gudmundsson G, Cerveny M, Shasby DM: Spirometric values in obese individuals: Effects of body position. Am J Respir Crit Care Med 156:998–999, 1997.
122. Collins LC, Hoberty PD, Walker JF, et al: The effect of body fat distribution on pulmonary function tests. Chest 107:1298–1302, 1995.
123. Lazarus R, Sparrow D, Weiss ST: Effects of obesity and fat distribution on ventilatory function. Chest 111:891–898, 1997.
124. Burki NK, Baker RW: Ventilatory regulation in eucapnic morbid obesity. Am Rev Respir Dis 129:538–543, 1984.
125. Pelosi P, Croci M, Ravagnan I, et al: Total respiratory system, lung, and chest wall mechanics in sedated-paralyzed postoperative morbidly obese patients. Chest 109:144–151, 1996.
126. Yap JCH, Watson RA, Gilbey S, et al: Effects of posture on respiratory mechanics in obesity. J Appl Physiol 79:1199–1205, 1995.
127. Sugerman H, Windsor A, Bessos M, et al: Intra-abdominal pressure, sagittal abdominal diameter and obesity comorbidity. J Intern Med 241:71–79, 1997.
128. Thomas PS, Cowen ERT, Hulands G, et al: Respiratory function in the morbidly obese before and after weight loss. Thorax 44:382–386, 1989.
129. Bradley TD, Rutherford R, Lue F, et al: Role of diffuse airway obstruction in the hypercapnia of obstructive sleep apnea. Am Rev Respir Dis 134:920–924, 1986.
130. Leech J, Onal E, Baer P, et al: Determinants of hypercapnia in occlusive sleep apnea syndrome. Chest 92:807–813, 1987.
131. Sugerman HJ, Fairman RP, Baron PL, et al: Gastric surgery for respiratory insufficiency of obesity. Chest 90:81–86, 1986.
132. Chapman KR, Himal HS, Rebuck AS: Ventilatory responses to hypercapnia and hypoxia in patients with eucapnic morbid obesity before and after weight loss. Clin Sci 78:541–545, 1990.
133. Collard P, Wilputte J-Y, Aubert G, et al: The single-breath diffusing capacity for carbon monoxide in obstructive sleep apnea and obesity. Chest 110:1189–1193, 1996.
134. Hurewitz AN, Susskind H, Harold WH: Obesity alters regional ventilation in lateral decubitus position. J Appl Physiol 59:774–783, 1985.
135. Hurewitz A, Sampson MG: Voluntary breath holding in the obese. J Appl Physiol 62:2371–2376, 1987.
136. Jense HG, Dubin SA, Silverstein PI, et al: Effect of obesity on safe duration of apnea in anesthetized patients. Anesth Analg 72:89–93, 1991.
137. Salvadori A, Fanari P, Mazza P, et al: Work capacity and cardiopulmonary adaptation of the obese subject during exercise testing. Chest 101:674–679, 1992.
138. Leech J, Onal E, Aronson R, et al: Voluntary hyperventilation in obesity hypoventilation. Chest 100:1334–1338, 1991.
139. Kelly TM, Jensen RL, Elliott CG, et al: Maximum respiratory pressures in morbidly obese subjects. Respiration 54:73–77, 1988.
140. Fiz JA, Aguilar A, Carreres A, et al: Postural variation of the maximum inspiratory and expiratory pressures in obese patients. Int J Obes Relat Metab Disord 15:655–659, 1991.
141. Weiner P, Waizman J, Weiner M, et al: Influence of excessive weight loss after gastroplasty for morbid obesity on respiratory muscle performance. Thorax 53:39–42, 1998.
142. Sharp JT, Druz WS, Kondragunta VR: Diaphragmatic responses to body position changes in obese patients with obstructive sleep apnea. Am Rev Respir Dis 133:32–37, 1986.
143. Sahebjami H: Dyspnea in obese healthy men. Chest 114:1373–1377, 1998.
144. Babb TG, Korzick D, Meador M, et al: Ventilatory response of moderately obese women to submaximal exercise. Int J Obes Relat Metab Disord 15:59–65, 1991.
145. Sakamoto S, Ishikawa K, Senda S, et al: The effect of obesity on ventilatory response and anaerobic threshold during exercise. J Med Syst 17:227–231, 1993.
146. Salvadori A, Fanari P, Mazza P, et al: Breathing pattern during and after maximal exercise testing in young untrained subjects and obese patients. Respiration 60:162–169, 1993.
147. Valtuena S, Blanch S, Barenys M, et al: Changes in body composition and resting energy expenditure after rapid weight loss: Is there an energy-metabolism adaptation in obese patients? Int J Obes Relat Metab Disord 19:119–125, 1995.
148. Refsum HE, Holter PH, Lovig T, et al: Pulmonary function and energy expenditure after marked weight loss in obese women: Observations before and one year after gastric banding. Int J Obes Relat Metab Disord 14:175–183, 1990.
149. Wadstrom C, Muller-Suur R, Backman L: Influence of excessive weight loss on respiratory function: A study of obese patients following gastroplasty. Eur J Surg 157:341–346, 1991.
150. Charuzi I, Lavie P, Peiser J, et al: Bariatric surgery in morbidly obese sleep-apnea patients: Short- and long-term follow-up. Am J Clin Nutr 55:594S–596S, 1992.
151. Sugerman HJ, Fairman RP, Sood RK, et al: Long-term effects of gastric surgery for treating respiratory insufficiency of obesity. Am J Clin Nutr 55:597S–601S, 1992.
152. Joris JL, Sottiaux TM, Chiche JD, et al: Effect of bi-level positive airway pressure (BiPAP) nasal ventilation on the postoperative pulmonary restrictive syndrome in obese patients undergoing gastroplasty. Chest 111:665–670, 1997.
153. Bach JR, Penek J: Obstructive sleep apnea complicating negative-pressure ventilatory support in patients with chronic paralytic/restrictive ventilatory dysfunction. Chest 99:1386–1393, 1991.
154. Waldhorn RE: Nocturnal nasal intermittent positive pressure ventilation with bi-level positive airway pressure (BiPAP) in respiratory failure. Chest 101:516–521, 1992.
155. Masa JF, Celli BR, Riesco JA, et al: Noninvasive positive pressure ventilation and not oxygen may prevent overt ventilatory failure in patients with chest wall diseases. Chest 112:207–213, 1997.

SECTION R

# Respiratory Failure

# 91 Principles of Critical Care of Respiratory Failure

LAWRENCE D. H. WOOD, M.D., PH.D.
GREGORY A. SCHMIDT, M.D. • JESSE B. HALL, M.D.

Introduction
A Mechanistic Approach to Respiratory Failure
- Hypoxemic vs. Ventilatory Failure
- Perioperative Respiratory Failure
- Hypoperfusion States Causing Type IV Respiratory Failure
- Respiratory Muscle Exercise and Fatigue in Respiratory Failure

Interactions Between Respiration and Circulation in Respiratory Failure
- Control of Venous Return by the Systemic Vessels
- Ventricular Dysfunction in Respiratory Failure
- Pulmonary Circulation
- Diagnosis and Management of Shock
- Approach to Inadequate Blood Transport of Oxygen

Summary

## INTRODUCTION

Respiratory failure is diagnosed when the patient loses the ability to ventilate adequately or to provide sufficient oxygen to the blood and systemic organs. Resuscitation of the patient requires urgent airway control, ventilator management, and stabilization of the circulation, whereas effective ongoing care for the patient with respiratory failure necessitates a differential diagnosis and therapeutic plan derived from an informed clinical and laboratory examination supplemented by the results of special intensive care unit (ICU) interventions. Advances in ICU management and monitoring technology facilitate early detection of pathophysiologic abnormalities of vital functions, with the potential for prevention and early treatment for the patient's continual improvement. However, this greater volume of diagnostic data and possible therapeutic interventions occasionally creates "information overload" for the physician-nurse team, confounding rather than complementing clinical skills.

The purpose of this chapter is to provide an informed, practical approach to integrating established concepts of pathophysiology with conventional clinical skills. This chapter does not provide a course in pulmonary physiology (see Chapters 4 to 9) or a comprehensive review of how to treat respiratory failure (see Chapters 92 and 93). Rather, it attempts to provide a conceptual framework of principles of critical care that have proved useful in managing the patient with respiratory failure. We begin by describing the mechanisms causing four types of respiratory failure and show how correcting each derangement enables the patient to resume spontaneous breathing effected by respiratory muscles that are not fatigued. We then review the essential pathophysiology of the pulmonary and systemic circulations as a basis for understanding the mechanical interactions between respiration and circulation and for approaching hypoperfusion states in respiratory failure.

By its very nature, critical care of patients with respiratory failure is exciting and attracts physicians who have an inclination to action. Despite its obvious utility in urgent circumstances, this inclination can replace effective clinical discipline with excessive, unfocused ICU procedures. We believe that this common approach inverts the stable pyramid of bedside skills, placing most attention on the least informative source of data while losing the rational foundation for diagnosis and treatment. An associated problem is that ICU procedures become an end in themselves rather than a means to answer thoughtful clinical questions. Thus, this chapter emphasizes up front a mechanistic approach to respiratory failure and the interpretation of ICU procedures. Beyond enhancing the clinical scholarship of critical care for respiratory failure, we contend that this approach maximizes another hallowed principle of patient care: "First, do no harm." Despite excited opinions to the contrary, we believe that effective care for respiratory failure is rarely based on brilliant, incisive, dramatic, and innovative interventions; rather, it most often derives from meticulously identifying and managing each of the patient's multiple problems toward improvement at an urgent but continuous pace. This conservative approach breeds skepticism toward innovative strategies; novel treatments require objective clinical trials before they are broadly implemented. Moreover, before traditional therapies can be used, goals must be clarified for each patient, and the least amount of intervention needed to achieve the goals must be determined; this will optimize the outcome and minimize the risk of adverse effects.[1]

We intend these principles of critical care to provide an intellectual foundation from which physicians can approach the diagnosis and management of type I respiratory failure (Chapter 92) and type II respiratory failure (Chapter 93), as well as type III respiratory failure during the perioperative period and type IV respiratory failure due to shock, both of which are described in this chapter. Through the organization of these three chapters, we hope to provide a complete educational package, allowing the reader to review the basis for detailed diagnosis and management of four types of respiratory failure. Chapter 94 then provides further details about the principles of ventilator management.

## A MECHANISTIC APPROACH TO RESPIRATORY FAILURE

### Hypoxemic vs. Ventilatory Failure

A descriptive survey of patients requiring mechanical ventilation for respiratory failure revealed four patterns of pathophysiology, each of which has a predominant mechanism[2] (Table 91.1). Intrapulmonary shunt ($\dot{Q}_S/\dot{Q}_T$) causes hypoxemia refractory to oxygen therapy despite

**Table 91.1 ACUTE RESPIRATORY FAILURE**

| | Type I: Acute Hypoxemic | Type II: Hypo-ventilatory | Type III: Peri-operative | Type IV: Shock |
|---|---|---|---|---|
| Mechanism | ↑ $\dot{Q}_S/\dot{Q}_T$ | ↓ $V_A$ | Atelectasis | Hypoperfusion |
| Etiology | Air space flooding | ↓ CNS drive<br>↓ N-M coupling<br>↑ Work/dead space | ↓ FRC<br>↑ Closing volume | Cardiogenic<br>Hypovolemic<br>Septic |
| Clinical description | Pulmonary edema<br>Cardiogenic<br>ARDS<br>Pneumonia<br>Lung hemorrhage<br>Chest trauma | Overdose/injury<br>Myasthenia gravis; polyradiculitis/ ALS; botulism/ curare<br>Asthma/COPD; pulmonary fibrosis; kyphoscoliosis | Supine/obese; ascites/ peritonitis; upper abdominal incision; anesthesia<br>Age/smoking; fluid overload; bronchospasm; airway secretions | Myocardial infarction; pulmonary hypertension<br>Hemorrhage; dehydration; tamponade<br>Endotoxemia; bacteremia |

From Hall JB, Schmidt GA, Wood LDH (eds): Principles of Critical Care. New York; McGraw-Hill, 1998, p 502.

ALS = amyotrophic lateral sclerosis; ARDS = acute respiratory distress syndrome; CNS = central nervous system; COPD = chronic obstructive pulmonary disease; FRC = functional residual capacity; $V_A$ = alveolar ventilation.

hyperventilation and reduced arterial $P_{CO_2}$ in type I failure, also called *acute hypoxemic respiratory failure* (AHRF).[2, 3] Primary failure of alveolar ventilation ($\dot{V}_A$) leads to carbon dioxide retention and arterial hypercapnia associated with reduced arterial $P_{O_2}$; this hypoxemia is easily corrected with oxygen therapy in type II failure, also called *ventilatory failure*.[2, 4] Figure 91.1 illustrates the different mechanisms for these two common abnormalities in pulmonary oxygen exchange.[4]

## Abnormalities in Pulmonary Gas Exchange

It is helpful to recall that the cause of hypercapnia (decreased $\dot{V}_A$) is often independent from the cause of

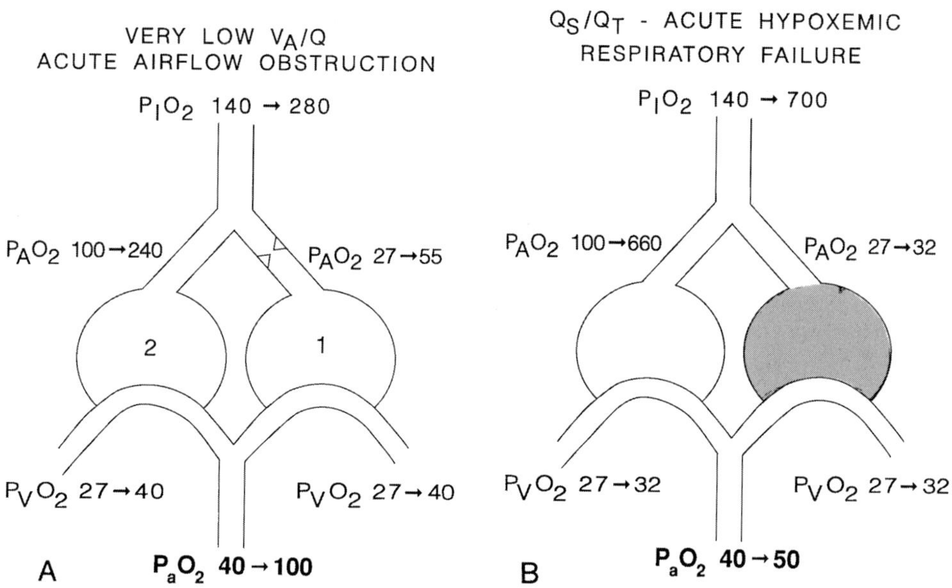


**Figure 91.1** Schematic illustration showing the effects of oxygen therapy on arterial $P_{O_2}$ ($P_aO_2$ in figure) in two conditions: acute airflow obstruction *(A)* and air space flooding with acute hypoxemic respiratory failure (AHRF) *(B)*. Each panel depicts a two-compartment lung in which each air space is perfused by half the mixed venous blood with a $P_{O_2}$ ($P_VO_2$ in figure) of 27 mm Hg while the person is breathing room air, which has a fractional concentration of oxygen in the inspired gas ($F_{I_{O_2}}$) of 0.21. Acute airflow obstruction causes severe hypoxemia that is corrected relatively easily by breathing supplementary oxygen, but hypoxemia in AHRF is much more refractory to oxygen administration and so necessitates adjunctive therapies. *A,* Because the air space distal to the obstruction is so poorly ventilated, all its inspired oxygen is absorbed and alveolar $P_{O_2}$ values ($P_AO_2$ in figure) approach mixed venous $P_{O_2}$ values (27 mm Hg). By contrast, because alveolar $P_{O_2}$ in the well-ventilated alveolus is considerably higher (100 mm Hg), its effluent blood becomes fully saturated ($S_{O_2}$ = 100%); when this blood mixes with an equal amount of effluent blood from the obstructed unit ($S_{O_2}$ = 50%), the resulting arterial blood ($Sa_{O_2}$ = 75%) has a very low $P_{O_2}$ (40 mm Hg). Raising $F_{I_{O_2}}$ to 0.4 (pressure of inspired oxygen ($P_IO_2$ in figure) = 280 mm Hg) increases both the amount of oxygen ventilating the obstructed unit and the alveolar $P_{O_2}$ (55 mm Hg). Accordingly, effluent blood from the obstructed air space ($S_{O_2}$ = 90%) mixes with fully saturated blood from the well-ventilated alveolus, which also contains more dissolved oxygen, causing arterial $S_{O_2}$ to approach 100% and arterial $P_{O_2}$ to approach 100 mm Hg. Note that this increased arterial oxygen transport is associated with increased mixed venous $P_{O_2}$ (27 to 40 mm Hg). *B,* During room air breathing, the oxygen exchange is as described in part *A,* because half the mixed venous blood traverses the flooded air space, from which no oxygen can be absorbed; accordingly, arterial $P_{O_2}$ is 40 mm Hg and mixed venous $P_{O_2}$ is 27 mm Hg. Raising $F_{I_{O_2}}$ to 1.0 increases the dissolved oxygen content in the fully saturated blood exiting the well-ventilated alveolus by about 2 mL/dL (because alveolar $P_{O_2}$ increases from 100 to 660 mm Hg), but oxygen is still not absorbed from the flooded air space. Accordingly, arterial $P_{O_2}$ increases slightly (from 40 to 50 mm Hg), and the increased $O_2$ delivery allows mixed venous $P_{O_2}$ to increase slightly (from 27 to 32 mm Hg). $Q_S/Q_T$ = intrapulmonary shunt; $V_A/Q$ = alveolar ventilation/perfusion. (From Hall JB, Schmidt GA, Wood LDH (eds): Principles of Critical Care. New York: McGraw-Hill, 1998, p 503.)

hypoxemia[2]; therefore, the treatment of hypercapnia (increased $\dot{V}_A$) is different from the treatment of hypoxemia (increased fractional concentration of inspired oxygen [$F_{IO_2}$], positive end-expiratory pressure [PEEP]). When central nervous system depression of the drive to breathe or loss of neuromuscular coupling reduces minute ventilation ($\dot{V}_E$), the carbon dioxide produced at rest each minute ($\dot{V}CO_2$ = 250 mL/min) is added to the reduced $\dot{V}_A$ (normally about 4 L/min), raising the alveolar and arterial partial pressures (P) of carbon dioxide ($P_{A_{CO_2}} = Pa_{CO_2} = k\ \dot{V}CO_2/\dot{V}_A$); recall from Chapter 4 that the P of a gas in the lungs is the product of the gas fraction (Fg) and the dry barometric pressure (Pbar $-$ $P_{H_2O}$), so $Pa_{CO_2}$ = (250/4000) $\times$ 713 $\times$ 0.86 or about 40 mm Hg. Mild alveolar hypoxia develops as the required oxygen uptake ($\dot{V}O_2$) is absorbed from the reduced $\dot{V}_A$ ($P_{A_{O_2}} = P_{I_{O_2}} - Pa_{CO_2}/R$, where $R = \dot{V}CO_2/\dot{V}O_2$), so the consequent arterial hypoxemia is corrected with small increments in inspired oxygen fraction ($F_{IO_2}$). In diseases characterized by airflow obstruction[4–7] or lung restriction,[8] $\dot{V}_A$ is reduced despite normal or increased $\dot{V}_E$ because the ratio of dead space to tidal volume ($V_D/V_T = [Pa_{CO_2} - P_{E_{CO_2}}]/Pa_{CO_2}$) is increased when large numbers of poorly perfused alveoli are excessively ventilated (high $\dot{V}_A/\dot{Q}$ units). Accordingly, when a patient requires an abnormally large $\dot{V}_E$ to maintain a normal arterial $PCO_2$, the causes are an abnormally increased $\dot{V}CO_2$, an abnormally increased $V_D/V_T$, or both. Hypoxemia develops with airflow obstruction or lung restriction when other alveoli are poorly ventilated in relation to their perfusion (low $\dot{V}_A/\dot{Q}$ units), and the hypoxemia is made worse by low mixed venous oxygen content[4–8]; again, modest increments in $F_{I_{O_2}}$ correct this hypoxemia (see Fig. 91.1*A*). In contrast, even an $F_{I_{O_2}}$ of 1.0 cannot correct the hypoxemia created by increases in $\dot{Q}_S/\dot{Q}_T$ (see Fig. 91.1*B*), and this refractory hypoxemia of acute hypoxic respiratory failure is often associated with increased $\dot{V}_E$ and $\dot{V}_A$ and, therefore, decreased arterial $PCO_2$.[2, 3]

## Abnormalities in Respiratory Mechanics

The two classical types of respiratory failure have distinctly different abnormalities in the mechanics of breathing (Fig. 91.2), while sharing mechanisms that lead to respiratory muscle dysfunction and fatigue.[9] The schematic illustration of the normal respiratory system (see Fig. 91.2*A*) indicates that spontaneous respiration is effected by the pressure ($\Delta P$) generated by inspiratory muscle to expand the lung and chest wall ($\Delta V$) against their elastance and to cause inspiratory gas flow ($\dot{V}_I$) past the airway resistance (R). When R is increased in acute-on-chronic respiratory failure (ACRF) or in status asthmaticus,[10] the $\Delta P$ necessary to breathe often exceeds the strength of the respiratory muscles, resulting in fatigue of the muscles.[9] When such a patient is mechanically ventilated, the peak pressure (Ppeak) generated at the airway opening increases well above the normal value (about 20 cm $H_2O$ in Fig. 91.2*B*, upper left) to 60 cm $H_2O$ (see Fig. 91.2*B*, lower right); however, end-inspiratory occlusion allows the airway pressure to return to the normal elastic pressure (Pel = 10 cm $H_2O$ in the same panel in Fig. 91.2*B*), which confirms that the resistive pressure (Pr = Ppeak $-$ Pel) has increased fivefold from the normal Pr value of 10 cm $H_2O$. In contrast, when air spaces become flooded with edema, pus, or blood in acute hypoxic respiratory failure, the tidal volume is delivered to a smaller number of aerated alveoli, overdistending them to increase Pel and Ppeak.[11, 12] In Figure 91.2*B*, lower left, Ppeak is increased to 60 cm $H_2O$ because end-inspiratory occlusion pressure has increased to 50 cm $H_2O$; in this instance of increased elastance, Pr (Ppeak $-$ Pel) is normal. This large increase in the ventilator pressure mirrors the increased load on the respiratory muscles during spontaneous breathing; when combined with tachypnea, oxygen desaturation, and acidosis in acute hypoxic respiratory failure, this leads to respiratory muscle fatigue.

## Clinical Presentation and Treatment Goals

These mechanical and lung gas exchange distinctions between acute hypoxic respiratory failure and ventilatory failure are paralleled by substantial differences in the clinical description and presentation of patients with type I and type II respiratory failure (see Table 91.1). In the second type, decreased $\dot{V}_A$ is caused by reduced drive to breathe (drug overdoses, head injuries) or by reduced coupling of the adequate or increased drive to breathe to the respiratory muscles (as in myasthenia gravis, Guillain-Barré syndrome, amyotrophic lateral sclerosis, or botulism, and as a reaction to muscle-relaxing drugs); often, the clinical and radiologic examinations of the chest yield normal findings in these patients. Alveolar hypoventilation also occurs commonly in respiratory diseases characterized by airflow obstruction and increased wasted ventilation; arterial $PCO_2$ increases despite increased central nervous system drive to breathe, adequate neuromuscular coupling, and increased total ventilation (status asthmaticus,[13] ACRF,[14] or restrictive disease of the respiratory system).[15] Wheezing, accessory muscle use, and hyperinflated lungs are common clinical and radiologic features in ACRF and asthma,[13, 14] whereas crackles and typical interstitial shadows without consolidated air spaces are observed in patients with respiratory failure due to pulmonary fibrosis.[8, 15] The clinical presentation of each of these categories of hypoventilating patients contrasts markedly with that of patients presenting with type I acute hypoxic respiratory failure, in whom cyanosis, tachypnea, and refractory hypoxemia lead to early identification of air space flooding by physical and radiologic examination.[16] The differential diagnosis of the air space flooding leading to $\dot{Q}_S/\dot{Q}_T$ includes cardiogenic or permeability pulmonary edema, pneumonia, or lung hemorrhage, each of which has specific etiologies and is alleviated by specific therapy (see Chapter 92).

While specific diagnostic and treatment plans are being implemented, goals of supportive therapy for types I and II respiratory failure are quite different. Therapy for patients with acute hypoxemic respiratory failure includes four objectives: (1) stabilization of the patient on the ventilator with minimal respiratory work; (2) ventilation with the least tidal volume providing adequate carbon dioxide elimination[17, 18]; (3) addition of the least amount of PEEP to prevent expiratory collapse of recruited alve-

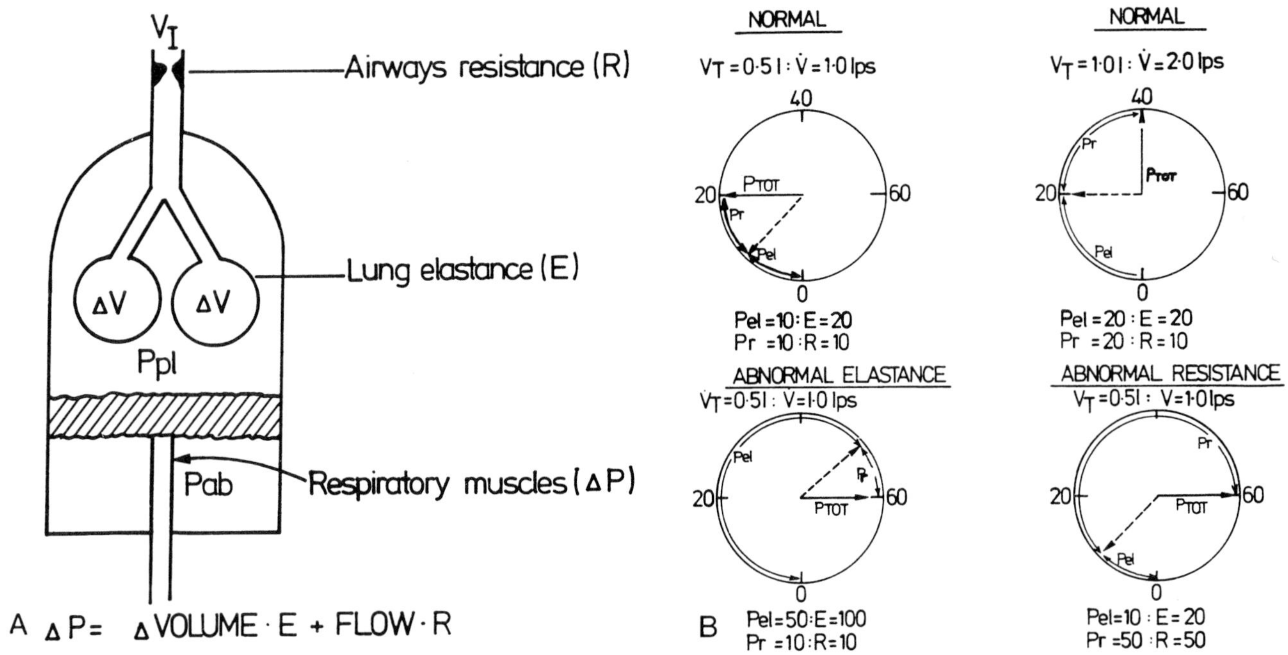


**Figure 91.2** *A,* Schematic depicts the mechanical characteristics of the respiratory system. Inspiratory flow ($V_I$ in figure) is delivered through an airway with resistance (R) to a two-compartment lung model, the units of which have elastance (E) and are distended by the delivered volume (ΔV). During positive-pressure ventilation, lung distention raises the pressure between the lungs and chest wall (Ppl) to increase the volume of the chest wall, in part by pushing the diaphragm downward (see piston at the floor of the thorax) to raise the abdominal pressure (Pab); during a spontaneous breath, the respiratory muscles (ΔP) pull the piston down to lower Ppl and inspire $\dot{V}$ across R. In either case, ΔP = the elastic pressure (Pel = ΔV × E) + the resistive pressure (Pr = $V_I$ × R). *B,* Schematic of the pressure dial on a mechanical ventilator illustrating the measurement of respiratory elastic pressures (Pel) and resistive pressures (Pr), and a calculation of E and R. The upper panels illustrate normal respiratory mechanics for a normal tidal volume and flow rate (left), and for a large tidal volume and flow rate (right panel). The lower panels illustrate abnormal elastance (left) and abnormal resistance (right panel). For discussion, see text. PTOT = total pressure; $\dot{V}$ = volume of gas; $V_T$ = tidal volume. (From Hall JB, Schmidt GA, Wood LDH (eds): Principles of Critical Care. New York: McGraw-Hill, 1998, p 504.)

oli while effecting 90% saturation of an adequate circulating hemoglobin on a nontoxic $FI_{O_2}$[11, 19, 20]; and (4) cardiovascular management to reduce air space edema by seeking the lowest pulmonary vascular pressures compatible with an adequate cardiac output and oxygen transport to the peripheral tissues[16, 21, 22] (see Chapter 92 for further discussion). Each of these goals of management of type I acute hypoxemic respiratory failure differs from the goals of management of type II ventilatory respiratory failure: patients with depressed central nervous system drive or reduced neuromuscular coupling must receive adequate ventilation and minimal oxygen supplementation with careful attention to preventing atelectasis and correcting hypoperfusion until the abnormal neurologic condition resolves; patients who require ventilation for airflow obstruction are supported with bronchodilator therapy and ventilator settings that minimize intrinsic PEEP until the airway resistance is reduced sufficiently for the respiratory muscles to achieve adequate ventilation independent from the ventilator (see Chapter 93 for further discussion).

One reason for identifying the causes of increased respiratory load is to view liberation from mechanical ventilation for patients with type I or type II respiratory failure as the mirror image of the cause of respiratory failure: that is, a systematic approach to reverse factors increasing the respiratory load and decreasing the respiratory muscle strength (Table 91.2).

## Perioperative Respiratory Failure

Physicians frequently encounter patients in the perioperative period who are unusually susceptible to atelectasis as a primary mechanism causing type III or perioperative respiratory failure.[23, 24] In general, abnormal abdominal mechanics reduce the end-expired lung volume (FRC) below the increased closing volume in these patients, which leads to progressive collapse of dependent lung units (see Table 91.1). The end result can be type I acute hypoxemic respiratory failure, type II hypoventilation, or both. However, identification of atelectasis as a distinct

**Table 91.2 LIBERATION OF THE PATIENT FROM MECHANICAL VENTILATION**

| Correctable Factors Decreasing Respiratory Muscle Load | Correctable Factors Increasing Respiratory Muscle Strength |
|---|---|
| **Type I: AHRF** | **Type IV: Shock** |
| Reduce edema production | Hypoperfusion |
| Enhance edema clearance | Hypotension |
| Treat pneumonia | Anemia |
| Drain pleural effusions | Hypoxemia |
| Stabilize chest wall | Sepsis |
| "Least" PEEP | Fever |
| Minimize dead space | Acidosis |
| **Type II: Airflow Obstruction** | Electrolytes ($K^+$, $Ca^{2+}$, $Mg^{2+}$, $PO_4^{3-}$) |
| Hypoxemia: give $O_2$ | Protein-calorie nutrition |
| Reverse sedation | Aminophylline |
| Bronchodilation | **Common Confounding Condition** |
| Clear bronchial secretions | Neuromuscular disease |
| Treat bronchial infection | Muscle-relaxing drugs |
| Pneumothorax: chest tube | Coma, sedation |
| Fractured ribs: nerve block | Cerebrovascular accident |
| Decrease intrinsic PEEP | Subclinical status epilepticus |
| Allow $HCO_3$ accumulation | Hypothyroidism |
| Reduce $CO_2$ production | Phrenic nerve paralysis |
| **Type III: Perioperative RF** | **Respiratory Muscle Fatigue** |
| Posturize and pummel | **Respiratory Muscle Exercise Program** |
| Ventilate 45 degrees upright | Tone |
| Incisional/abdominal pain | Power |
| Drain ascites | Coordination |
| Re-expand atelectasis early | Animation |
| Stop smoking | |
| Avoid overhydration | |

From Hall JB, Schmidt GA, Wood LDH (eds): Principles of Critical Care. New York: McGraw-Hill, 1998, p 505.

AHRF = acute hypoxic respiratory failure; PEEP = postiive end-expiratory pressure; RF = respiratory failure.

mechanism leading to this third type of respiratory failure can be used to prevent lung collapse by reducing the adverse effects of common clinical circumstances promoting reduction in FRC and of the conditions that promote abnormal airway closure at increased lung volume. Because many of these mechanisms are shared by patients with type I or type II respiratory failure, implementation of approaches to minimize atelectasis should be a part of the management of all patients with respiratory failure.

The principles of preventing or reversing type III perioperative respiratory failure are listed in Table 91.2.[24] Bedside nurses in the ICU turn the patient from the supine position to the left or right lateral decubitus position every 1 to 2 hours; during this time, they provide vigorous chest physiotherapy with pummeling, chest vibration, and endotracheal suction. In patients vulnerable to atelectasis, a fourth position, 30 to 45 degrees upright, helps by reducing the load imposed by the abdomen; also, the addition of sighs, continuous positive airway pressure, or PEEP returns the end-expired lung volume to a position above the patient's closing volume. Special attention to treating incisional or abdominal pain (epidural anesthesia, transcutaneous nerve stimulation) and to minimizing the intra-abdominal pressure (e.g., from ascites or tight bandages) helps prevent atelectasis. These factors cause a vertical gradient of alveolar flooding in acute respiratory distress syndrome (ARDS), in which edema tends to develop in dependent lung regions and abdominal distention and the weight of the heart aggravate dependent alveolar derecruitment.[25, 26] Ventilating the patient with ARDS in the prone position improves lung gas exchange.[27, 28]

When lobe or lung collapse is detected by physical or radiologic examination, an early aggressive approach to re-expansion includes placing the patient in the lateral decubitus position, with the collapsed lobe uppermost for vigorous pummeling and suctioning, and then increasing the tidal volume progressively to a pressure limit of 40 cm $H_2O$ with end-inspiratory pauses. Re-expansion often occurs within 10 minutes and is signaled by a fall in the $\Delta$Pel associated with the normal tidal volume at the end of the re-expansion maneuver; if this re-expansion is not confirmed radiologically, repeating these maneuvers after bronchoscopy to clear endobronchial obstruction is indicated. Once re-expansion has occurred, the implementation of increased levels of PEEP and/or sighs often prevents further episodes of atelectasis. Stopping smoking at least 6 weeks before elective operations reduces bronchorrhea and atelectasis, and avoiding overhydration in perioperative patients especially vulnerable to atelectasis is also helpful.

## Hypoperfusion States Causing Type IV Respiratory Failure

A significant number of ventilated patients do not fit in the categories of type I, II, or III respiratory failure. These are the patients who have been intubated and stabilized with ventilatory support during a hypoperfusion state, so type IV respiratory failure is most commonly due to cardiogenic, hypovolemic, or septic shock without associated pulmonary problems.[29] The appropriate rationale for ventilator therapy in these patients, who are frequently tachypneic with erratic respiratory patterns, is to stabilize gas exchange and minimize the steal of limited cardiac output by the working respiratory muscles until the mechanism for the hypoperfusion state is identified and corrected.[29, 30] Liberation from the ventilator of the patient with type IV respiratory failure is simple: when shock is corrected, the patient resumes spontaneous breathing and is extubated. Furthermore, when patients with type I, II, or III respiratory failure suffer a concurrent hypoperfusion state, the causes of reduced blood flow, hypotension, anemia, acidosis, and sepsis must be identified and corrected as part of the liberation process (see Table 91.2). Accordingly, physicians who manage respiratory failure frequently employ the principles of diagnosis and management of hypoperfusion states.

## Respiratory Muscle Exercise and Fatigue in Respiratory Failure

The respiratory muscles share with other major muscle groups of the body the characteristic that excessive work leads to fatigue.[9, 30, 31] This concept seems to explain why patients with severe airflow obstruction or air space flooding ultimately stop breathing, and why patients requiring mechanical ventilation for these and other causes of respiratory failure are unable to breathe independently from the ventilator until the load on their respiratory muscles is reduced, the respiratory muscles become stronger, or both. However, although this is a useful paradigm with which to manage patients with respiratory failure, it is exceedingly difficult to identify fatigue under clinical conditions. Nonetheless, as a rough guide, spontaneous ventilation can be sustained indefinitely when the effort of each spontaneous breath is less than one third of the maximal respiratory effort achievable.[32–34] In normal patients, the maximum negative inspiratory pressure (MIP) measured at FRC exceeds 100 cm $H_2O$, whereas the work of spontaneous breathing is less than 10 cm $H_2O$, providing considerable respiratory muscle reserve before the conditions of fatigue are approached. In contrast, patients with acute respiratory failure frequently have MIP values of less than 30 cm $H_2O$, whereas the load on the respiratory muscles, as measured by the pressure generated by the ventilator during each breath, exceeds 30 cm $H_2O$. Such values predict that the patient's respiratory muscles would fatigue quickly if spontaneous ventilation were required, a hypothesis easily confirmed in such patients who breathe rapidly and insufficiently when taken off the ventilator.[35]

Another measure of maximum respiratory effort in the conscious patient is vital capacity (VC). As a rough guideline, when VC is three times the tidal volume ($V_T$) required to maintain eucapnia and normal pH, respiratory muscle fatigue is unlikely. A corresponding alternative measure of respiratory load is the minute ventilation required to maintain normal arterial $P_{CO_2}$ and pH. Factors that increase carbon dioxide production, dead space, or metabolic acidosis necessarily increase this ventilation and thus promote respiratory muscle fatigue. Such fatigue is often signaled by increased respiratory rate ($f > 35$/min), by paradoxic respiratory motion (the abdomen moves in with inspiration as the fatigued diaphragm is pulled craniad by the negative pleural pressure), and by the patient's unexplained somnolence or decreased responsiveness. Accordingly, evaluation of the patient's ability to resume spontaneous ventilation includes measurements of MIP, VC, $V_T$, f, and $\dot{V}_E$, as well as direct observation of the respiratory motions during a period of spontaneous breathing.[36–38]

### Resting Fatigued Respiratory Muscles

Current evidence and common sense suggest that the treatment for respiratory muscle fatigue is respiratory muscle rest, a strategy that must be balanced in nearly all patients with a well-planned respiratory exercise program. Until recently, the timing of the move from respiratory muscle rest to an exercise program was not guided by objective criteria identifying fatigue.[38] Accordingly, many physicians developed empirical guidelines as to the likely presence of respiratory muscle fatigue integrated with the type of early ventilator management necessary for the patient's overall condition. For example, the cardiovascular stability and optimal ventilator management of patients with type I acute hypoxemic respiratory failure are frequently enhanced by respiratory muscle rest during the first 6 hours after elective intubation for severe hypoxemia. During this time, the acutely depleted glycogen stores of the resting respiratory muscles are replenished, and the accumulated lactic acid or other metabolites associated with fatigue are washed out[39, 40]; the patient is then ready to move to a respiratory exercise program. In contrast, the patient with ACRF who has developed respiratory muscle fatigue over a longer period of time may require up to 72 hours of respiratory muscle rest before resuming an exercise program without fatigue.

Yet these broad guidelines may cause the initiation of spontaneous breathing too soon, accompanied by failure, or too late, associated with unnecessary prolongation of ventilator support with its complications. Observation of the patient's unassisted respiratory rate (R in breaths/min) and tidal volume ($V_T$ in liters) allows calculation of the ratio (RVR) as $R/V_T$. When the RVR is less than 125, it is likely that the patient can resume spontaneous breathing, and an RVR greater than 125 signals the need for continued respiratory rest (Fig. 91.3). During the resting period, attention is directed at identifying and correcting factors to reduce the respiratory muscle load and increase respiratory muscle strength (see Table 91.2). Many patients being managed for respiratory muscle rest by me-

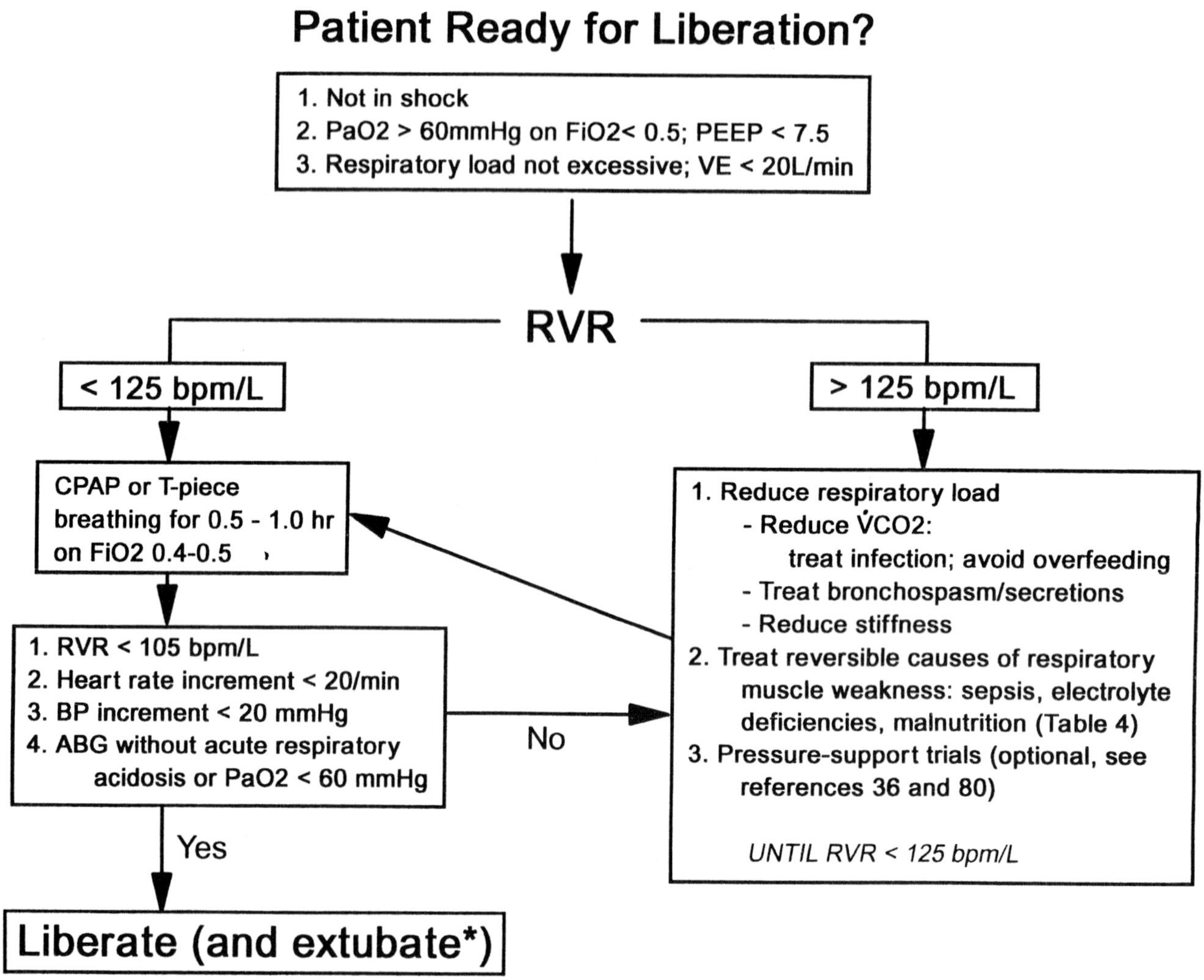


**Figure 91.3** A simple bedside algorithm for liberating patients with respiratory failure from mechanical ventilation. Note that previous studies suggest that the ratio of respiratory rate to tidal volume (RVR) threshold value of 105 breaths/min/L optimally predicts weaning outcomes and, when used in a weaning protocol, reduces duration of mechanical ventilation. Performing a trial of unassisted breathing when the RVR is < 125 breaths/min/L reduces the likelihood of a false-negative result because some patients with RVRs between 105 and 125 breaths/min/L are successful. Regardless of the threshold value used, successful liberation depends on successful completion of a trial of spontaneous, unassisted breathing; such trials are generally safe if carefully observed.

The decision to extubate depends on the patient's level of consciousness, ability to protect the airway (cough, gag reflex), and the amount of endotracheal secretion. This algorithm should be individualized; when other parameters are favorable, no single unfavorable parameter should prevent a trial of liberation. Occasionally, patients satisfy the physiologic criteria for liberation but appear distressed and uncomfortable; clinicians should exercise caution in immediately extubating such patients. Caution is also indicated for patients with evolving myocardial infarction; attempts at weaning should be initiated only when it is clear that the infarction is completed. ABG = arterial blood gas; BP = blood pressure; CPAP = continuous positive airway pressure; FiO2 = fractional inspired oxygen; PaO2 = arterial $P_{O_2}$; PEEP = positive end-expiratory pressure; $\dot{V}CO_2$ = carbon dioxide output; VE = expired volume. (From Manthous CA, Schmidt GA, Hall JB: Liberation from mechanical ventilation: A decade of progress. Chest 114:898, 1998.)

chanical ventilation are actually working as hard as or harder than they do during spontaneous ventilation by breathing actively against the ventilator.[30] This can be detected by clinical examination coupled with observation of the airway pressure, which should rise at the start of each ventilated breath. In many patients, the airway pressure stays at or below zero during inspiration, indicating active inspiration by the patient; the amount and duration of inspiratory effort can often be assessed by the fall in central venous or pulmonary artery pressure with each inspiration. When respiratory rest is indicated, it can be achieved in these circumstances by increasing the inspiratory flow rate, by increasing the minute ventilation, or, if these measures of eliminating the patient's respiratory effort are inadequate, by sedating and, sometimes, paralyzing the patient to ensure respiratory rest.

## Exercising Rested Respiratory Muscles

As soon as the patient with respiratory failure is stabilized on the ventilator, the physician should make a decision whether to rest the patient's fatigued respiratory muscles or to institute a program of respiratory muscle exercise if fatigue is neither evident nor expected. The objective of the respiratory exercise program is to increase the tone, power, and coordination of the respiratory muscles.[38] The efficacy of each program in increasing tone and power is evaluated by the daily MIP and VC measurements. Coordination is evaluated by bedside observation to determine whether the patient's respiratory efforts interact with the ventilator in a manner comfortable to the patient. Here, the goal is to adjust the ventilator so that the patient receives a breath on demand at a volume and frequency within the ranges expected for that patient off the ventilator. Several different modes of ventilation seek to achieve these goals of increased tone, power, and coordination during the liberation process.

## Liberating the Patient from Mechanical Ventilation

The aggressive approach discussed here attempts to liberate patients as soon as possible from mechanical ventilation by using the ventilator mode as an exercise program. The ventilator mode becomes a well-planned part of a larger program addressing about 50 correctable factors constraining the patient's freedom to breathe (see Table 91.2). This effective approach to liberating patients from the ventilator measures and attempts to increase the values of MIP and VC while simultaneously measuring and reducing the respiratory load.[38] The left column of Table 91.2 lists correctable factors to reduce the respiratory muscle load. As a general rule, these are the abnormal respiratory mechanics associated with the several types of acute respiratory failure, and they are discussed in detail in Chapters 92 and 93. The right column of Table 91.2 lists correctable factors to increase respiratory muscle strength, first in the context of the many disturbances of the circulation or internal environment most common to patients with type IV respiratory failure. Attempting to liberate patients with hypoperfusion states or hypotension is not successful. Correction of these hemodynamic variables complements the correction of anemia, hypoxemia, and acidosis to provide dramatic increases in the objectively measured respiratory muscle strength by MIP and VC.[41, 42] Similarly, attempting to liberate patients who are septic or have body temperatures greater than 38.5°C is often unsuccessful.

While these systemic abnormalities are being corrected, it is also helpful to initiate adequate daily protein-calorie nutrition, using protein (0.8 g/kg) and nonprotein calories (about 30 kcal/g protein), of which 20% to 50% should be supplied as lipid.[43] Elemental malnutrition is best prevented but corrected when necessary by adjustments of serum potassium, calcium, magnesium, and phosphate levels. Because severe abnormalities in the levels of each of these electrolytes are sufficient to cause respiratory muscle fatigue,[44, 45] modest abnormalities in the patient already weakened by critical illness may converge to make the patient weaker than necessary. There is some evidence that when each of these abnormalities has been corrected, respiratory muscles may be strengthened by the infusion of aminophylline in doses that achieve serum concentrations associated with effective bronchodilation.[46] When all other factors are corrected but the patient remains weak, it is helpful to assess for the presence of clinical conditions that occasionally cause reduced respiratory muscle strength. Neuromuscular disease, muscle-relaxing drugs,[47] steroids,[48] sedatives, coma, and intercurrent cerebral vascular accidents cause obscure reductions in respiratory muscle strength. Often overlooked causes of inadequate respiratory muscle function are subclinical status epilepticus, hypothyroidism, and paralysis of the phrenic nerve on one or both sides after cardiac surgery with cold cardioplegia or after other thoracic trauma.

When the patient's respiratory strength is increased and the respiratory load is reduced, several strategies are effective in completing the return to spontaneous breathing.[49–51] Each is aided when physician-patient rapport enables the patient to feel supported in the transition off the ventilator. In preparation, the patient is informed that the tidal volume will be reduced toward the patient's spontaneous volume or to the volume that the physician anticipates will be the spontaneous volume. Of course, respiratory rate on the ventilator will be increased by the patient to maintain $CO_2$ elimination, and the patient's comfort or air hunger is reevaluated. Once the patient is made comfortable with a ventilated pattern approaching his or her own, the patient is informed that the respiratory weakness or lung disease necessitating mechanical ventilation has been reversed, so a short period (1 hour) of spontaneous breathing is warranted as a prelude to liberation from the ventilator. The patient is assured that a member of the physician–nurse–respiratory therapist team will be present during this time, that a few measurements will be made toward the end of the hour (blood gas values, MIP, forced VC), and that the patient will be ventilated again while the results are interpreted. Favorable results are communicated to the patient with a plan for complete liberation as indicated. This communication minimizes the anxiety of the patient, precluding many failures to "wean."

## INTERACTIONS BETWEEN RESPIRATION AND CIRCULATION IN RESPIRATORY FAILURE

A primary role of the cardiovascular system is to deliver energy sources from the gut and liver and oxygen from the lungs via the bloodstream to all systemic organ systems for their aerobic metabolism; effluent blood flow from these tissues removes the waste products of metabolism, delivering them to the lungs, kidney, and liver for excretion. This process is facilitated by return of the whole circulation through the lungs, where carbon dioxide is eliminated and oxygen is taken up to arterialize the blood. As depicted in Figure 91.4, this central circulation is located within the thoracic cavity; movement of gas between the atmosphere surrounding the body and the alveolar space within the lungs is caused by the respiratory muscles, especially the diaphragm, depicted as a piston at the floor of the thoracic cavity. Beyond effecting ventilation to permit pulmonary gas exchange, spontaneous movement of the piston lowers the pleural pressure (Ppl), which approximates the pressure on the outside of extra-alveolar vessels, including the right and left sides of the heart (depicted as chambers labeled Pra and Pla); changes in alveolar pressure (labeled $P_A$) affect pressures within alveolar vessels. Once the blood leaves the lung and enters the left side of the heart, the ventricular pumping function ejects blood into the stiff, high-resistance arterial circulation to perfuse the systemic capillary beds, where oxygen is consumed and carbon dioxide is added, before the venous blood returns to the right side of the heart through the large-volume, very compliant, low-resistance venous circuit.[44] This section reviews the physiology of this circuit as a basis for understanding the many disturbances in circulation that are associated with respiratory failure. It begins with a discussion of the mechanisms whereby the cardiac output is controlled by the systemic vessels, followed by a description of left ventricular pumping function and then by a description of the pulmonary circulation as seen through the pulmonary artery catheter, and concludes with an approach to hypoperfusion states. Throughout this discussion, common mechanical interactions between respiration and circulation are highlighted as a basis for diagnosis and therapy of respiratory failure.

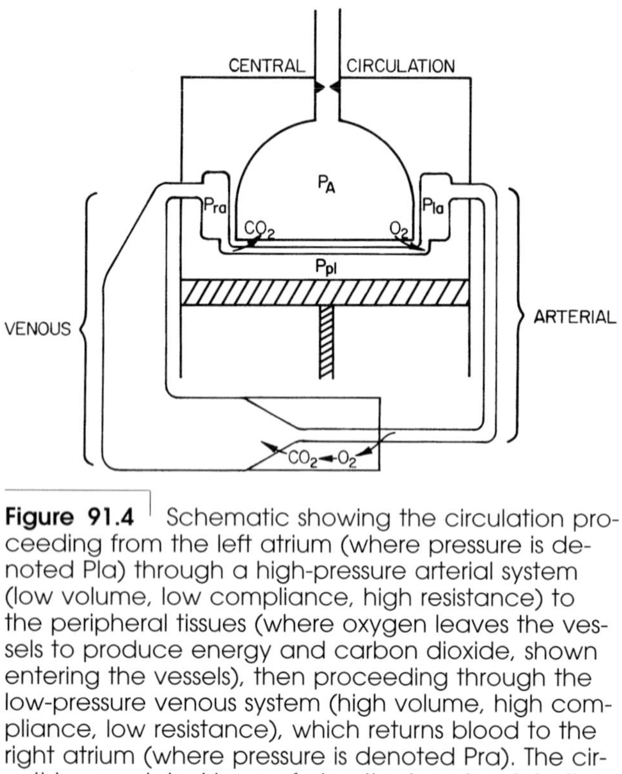


**Figure 91.4** Schematic showing the circulation proceeding from the left atrium (where pressure is denoted Pla) through a high-pressure arterial system (low volume, low compliance, high resistance) to the peripheral tissues (where oxygen leaves the vessels to produce energy and carbon dioxide, shown entering the vessels), then proceeding through the low-pressure venous system (high volume, high compliance, low resistance), which returns blood to the right atrium (where pressure is denoted Pra). The circuit is completed by perfusing the lung back to the left atrium; the pulmonary vessels are shown in close apposition with the alveoli (where pressure is denoted $P_A$), facilitating gas exchange. This central circulation is enclosed in the thorax, the floor of which is the diaphragm (indicated by the piston). Between the lungs and the thorax is the pleural space (where pressure is denoted Ppl). Ppl approximates the pressure on the outside of all extra-alveolar vessels within the central circulation, including the heart, whereas $P_A$ is the pressure outside the alveolar vessels. The anatomic arrangement accounts for the many mechanical interactions between respiration and circulation in critical illness described throughout this chapter. (From Hall JB, Schmidt GA, Wood LDH (eds): Principles of Critical Care. New York: McGraw-Hill, 1998, p 260.)

### Control of Venous Return by the Systemic Vessels

#### Mean Systemic Pressure

When the heart stops beating (see Fig. 91.4), the pressure equalizes throughout the entire vascular system, and its new value is the mean systemic pressure (Pms = 10 to 15 mm Hg). This pressure is much lower than the arterial pressure and is close to the mean right atrial pressure (PRA). When flow stops, blood drains from the high-pressure, low-volume arterial system into the large-volume, low-pressure venous system, which accommodates the displaced volume with little change in pressure. When the heart begins to beat again, the left ventricle pumps blood from the central circulation into the systemic circuit, raising the pressure there. At the same time, the right ventricle pumps blood into the lungs, thereby lowering its pressure (PRA) with regard to Pms, so blood flows from the venous reservoir to the right atrium. The pressure on the venous side falls slightly below Pms, whereas the pressure on the arterial side rises considerably above Pms with succeeding beats of the heart. This continues until a steady state is reached in which arterial pressure has risen enough to drive the whole stroke volume of each succeeding heartbeat through the high arterial resistance into the venous reservoir. Pms does not change between the state of no flow and the new state of steady flow because neither the vascular volume nor the compliance of the vessels has changed. What has changed is the distribution of the vascular volume from the compliant veins to the stiff arteries; this volume shift creates the pressure difference driving flow through the circuit.[52, 53]

Pms is the driving pressure for venous return to the right atrium when circulation resumes. It can be increased in order to increase venous return by increasing the vascular volume or by decreasing the unstressed volume and the compliance of the vessels.[52] The latter two mechanisms are mediated by vascular reflexes stimulated by hypotension or hypoxemia and so respond to the need for increased venous return and cardiac output; these usually occur together.[54, 55] The unstressed volume may also be reduced by raising the legs of a supine patient or applying military antishock trousers (MAST); both return a portion of the unstressed vascular volume from the large veins in the legs to the stressed volume, thereby increasing Pms and venous return. When the heart has either an improvement in inotropic state or a reduction in afterload, blood is shifted from the central compartment to the stressed volume of the systemic circuit, raising Pms and venous return[56]; improved ventricular pumping function also lowers PRA to increase venous return further (discussed next).

## Venous Return and Cardiac Function Curves

In the previous discussion, after the heart was stopped and before it was started, right atrial pressure was equal to the pressure throughout the vascular system (Pms). With each succeeding heartbeat, right atrial pressure decreases below Pms and venous return increases. This sequence was repeated in a more controlled steady state by replacing the heart with a pump set to keep PRA at a given value while venous return is measured.[54–56] Typical data are plotted in Figure 91.5. As PRA is reduced from 12 to 0 (indicated by the thin continuous line), venous return (VR) increases progressively with the driving pressure (Pms − PRA). The slope of the relationship between venous return and Pms − PRA is the resistance to venous return (RVR = Δ[Pms − PRA]/ΔVR). When right atrial pressure falls below zero, venous return does not increase further because blood flow becomes limited as it enters the thorax. This occurs when the pressure in these collapsible great veins falls below the atmospheric pressure outside the veins. Then further reductions in PRA and central venous pressure are associated with progressive collapse of the veins rather than increase in venous return.

For a given stressed vascular volume and compliance, Pms is set and RVR is relatively constant. In the absence of pulmonary hypertension or right ventricular dysfunction, left ventricular function determines PRA and thus determines venous return to the right side of the heart, which must equal the cardiac output from the left side of the heart. Output from the heart is described by the cardiac function curve, drawn as the thick continuous line relating PRA (abscissa) and cardiac output (ordinate) in Figure 91.5. The heart is able to eject a larger stroke volume and cardiac output when the end-diastolic pressure rises because more distended ventricles eject to about the same end-systolic volume as do less distended ventricles. Accordingly, as PRA decreases, cardiac output falls along the cardiac function curve. Yet venous return increases as PRA falls until venous return equals cardiac output at a unique value of PRA, indicated by the intersection of the cardiac function and venous return curves in Figure 91.5 (see point A in panels *A* and *B*).

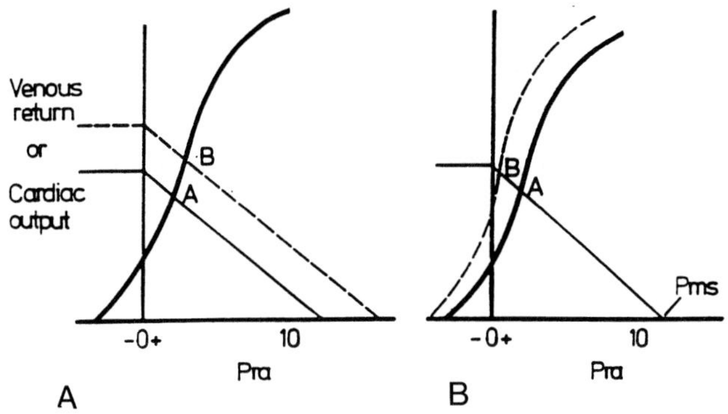


**Figure 91.5** Schematic showing mechanisms affecting venous return (VR). VR and cardiac output ($\dot{Q}T$) are plotted on the ordinate, and right atrial pressure (Pra (in figure), in mm Hg) is plotted on the abscissa. In both *A* and *B*, the thin continuous VR curve shows that VR increases as Pra decreases below the mean systemic pressure (Pms = Pra at VR = 0); therefore the inverse of the slope of this VR curve (Δ(Pms − Pra)/ΔVR) is the resistance to VR (RVR). The thick continuous cardiac function curves show that $\dot{Q}T$ increases as Pra increases because ventricular end-diastolic volume increases. The intersection of these two curves marks the unique value of Pra at which VR equals $\dot{Q}T$ in both panels *A* and *B*. When this value of $\dot{Q}T$ is insufficient, VR can be increased by increasing Pms without changing RVR, indicated by the interrupted VR curve intersecting the unchanged $\dot{Q}T$ curve at a higher $\dot{Q}T$ and Pra (see B in panel *A*). In panel *B*, VR is increased from A to B by increased cardiac function (see interrupted cardiac function curve intersecting the original VR curve at B). Accordingly, inotropic agents that increase contractility (dobutamine) can produce modest increases in VR by lowering Pra, but further increasesare limited by compression of the great veins at lower values of Pra (see *B*); note that such enhanced cardiac function displaces central blood volume into the peripheral circulation, tending to increase Pms and so promote further increases in VR, as depicted in *A*. Other inotropic agents (dopamine, epinephrine) also raise Pms by venoconstriction. (From Hall JB, Schmidt GA, Wood LDH (eds): Principles of Critical Care. New York: McGraw-Hill, 1998, p 265.)

When cardiac output is insufficient, venous return can be increased in several ways. A new steady state of increased venous return is achieved by increasing Pms with no change in RVR, indicated by the interrupted venous return curve in Figure 91.5*A*. This new venous return curve intersects the same cardiac function curve at a higher value of cardiac output at point B. This method of increasing venous return is associated with a rise in right atrial pressure. Because of the steep slope of the cardiac function curve in normal hearts, large increases in venous return occur with only small increases of right atrial pressure. Alternatively, venous return can be increased by enhanced cardiac function by increasing contractility or decreasing afterload of the heart. This is depicted as an upward shift of the cardiac function curve

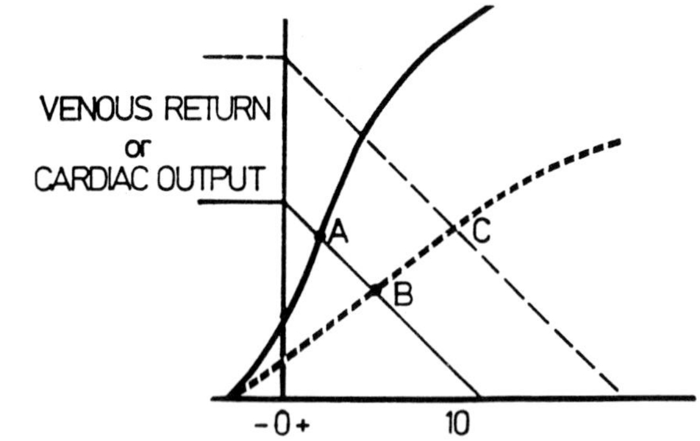


**Figure 91.6** Reduced cardiac function (*interrupted curve* from point B to point C) reduces the steady-state venous return (VR) from point A to point B, because right atrial pressure (PRA) increases along the normal VR curve (*continuous line* from point A to point B). In response, baroreceptor reflexes, vascular volume retention, or both increase mean systemic pressure (Pms) so that the new interrupted VR curve intersects the depressed cardiac function curve at C, whereby cardiac output ($\dot{Q}T$) has returned to normal at increased PRA. Note that the new steady state can be produced by systolic or diastolic dysfunction of either the left or right ventricle (for further discussion, see text). (From Hall JB, Schmidt GA, Wood LDH (eds): Principles of Critical Care. New York: McGraw-Hill, 1998, p 266.)

as in Figure 91.5*B* so that greater cardiac output occurs at each PRA. The increase on each venous return curve by this mechanism is associated with a reduction in PRA. Furthermore, in the normal heart, only a small change in venous return is possible (from point A to point B in Fig. 91.5*B*), and greater reductions in PRA do not increase cardiac output further because venous return becomes flow limited as right atrial pressure falls below zero. This explains why inotropic agents that enhance contractility are ineffective in hypovolemic shock.

When cardiac pumping function is depressed as depicted by the interrupted line in Figure 91.6, venous return is reduced from point A to point B for the same value of Pms as PRA increases. Then the patient must retain fluid or initiate cardiac reflexes to increase Pms toward the new value necessary to maintain adequate cardiac output, as in chronic congestive heart failure. This response is associated with a large increase in PRA from point B to point C, which in turn causes jugular venous distention, hepatomegaly, and peripheral edema. Diuretic reduction of vascular volumes corrects these cosmetic abnormalities at the expense of reducing Pms and venous return. In contrast, inotropic and vasodilator drugs, which improve the depressed cardiac function by shifting the interrupted cardiac function curve upward, increase cardiac output and lower PRA more effectively than in patients with normal cardiac function.[53]

### Effects of Pressure Outside the Heart on Cardiac Output

In the preceding illustrations and discussions, values of Pms and PRA were expressed in relation to atmospheric pressure. However, the transmural pressure of the right atrium exceeds PRA by the subatmospheric value (about −4 mm Hg) of the pleural pressure (Ppl) surrounding the heart. Consider the effect of opening the thorax, which raises Ppl from −4 mm Hg to 0; venous return then decreases from point A to point B in Figure 91.7 because PRA increases.[57] This is indicated by the interrupted cardiac function curve shifted to the right by the increase in pressure outside the heart but parallel to the normal cardiac function curve (continuous line through point A). Normal venous return can be restored (point B to point C) by increasing Pms by an amount equal to the rise in Ppl and PRA induced by opening the thorax. Then transmural PRA will be the same as in condition A, and PRA will have increased from point A to point C at the same cardiac output.

This mechanism for the fall in cardiac output with thoracotomy also explains the fall in cardiac output with PEEP. Pleural pressure within an intact thorax rises with

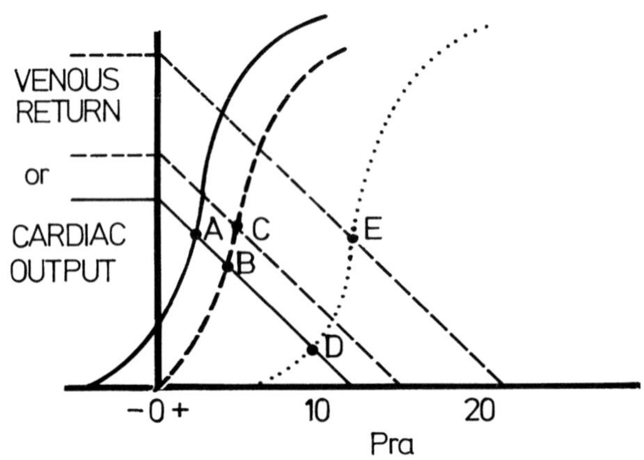


**Figure 91.7** Schematic showing effects of increased pleural pressure (Ppl) on venous return (VR) and cardiac output ($\dot{Q}T$). Compared with the normal steady state (continuous VR and cardiac function curves), increasing Ppl and right atrial pressure (Pra in figure) by 4 mm Hg shifts the normal cardiac function curves to the right (*interrupted cardiac function curve* from point B to point C), so that VR decreases from point A to point B. This accounts for the fall in $\dot{Q}T$ when thoracotomy exposes the right atrium to atmospheric pressure; similarly, the increase in Ppl and Pra when PEEP is applied to a patient with an intact thorax decreases $\dot{Q}T$. In both cases, baroreceptor reflexes or iatrogenic expansion of vascular volume increases Pms to allow the new interrupted VR curve to intersect the displaced cardiac function curve at point C, returning $\dot{Q}T$ to normal. A much larger increase in PEEP raises Ppl and Pra even more, so that the displaced normal cardiac function curve (*dotted curve* from point D to point E) intersects the normal VR curves at a very low value of $\dot{Q}T$ (point D). In this circumstance, returning $\dot{Q}T$ to a normal value (point E) requires a larger increase in Pms to allow the new interrupted VR curve to intersect the dotted cardiac function curve at point E (for further discussion, see text). (From Hall JB, Schmidt GA, Wood LDH (eds): Principles of Critical Care. New York: McGraw-Hill, 1998, p 266.)

positive-pressure ventilation, raising PRA and reducing venous return.[58–61] When 8 mm Hg PEEP (10 cm $H_2O$) is added to the ventilator, the end-expiratory value of Ppl rises by about half that amount (e.g., from −4 mm Hg to 0). Accordingly, venous return decreases with PEEP from point A to point B in Figure 91.7, with no change in cardiac function or Pms. Cardiac output is returned to normal by volume infusion or vascular reflexes, which raise Pms by an amount equal to the increase in Ppl and PRA. Of course, greater PEEP (20 cm $H_2O$ as in dotted line, Fig. 91.7) reduces venous return further (from point A to point D) and requires larger increases in Pms to return cardiac output to normal (point D to point E).

The cardiac output is much less susceptible to the deleterious effects of PEEP when Pms is high. In patients with reduced circulatory volume, vascular reflexes are already operating to maintain venous return and Pms by reducing unstressed volume, vascular compliance, or both. Such patients have little vascular reflex reserve and poorly tolerate intubation and positive-pressure ventilation without considerable intravenous infusion to increase vascular stressed volume. In contrast, well-hydrated or overhydrated patients may tolerate even large amounts of PEEP with no reduction in cardiac output, for their previously inactive vascular reflexes can increase Pms in well-filled systemic vessels by the amount that Ppl increases with PEEP. These considerations allow the physician to anticipate and treat the hypotension induced by ventilator therapy; the concept should not be interpreted as an indication for maintaining high circulatory volume in critically ill patients on ventilators, because this often increases lung edema while providing even more cardiac output than was already deemed sufficient. Furthermore, the pressure outside the heart can be increased by a variety of other concomitant conditions and complications of respiratory failure; all of these increase the pressures measured in the heart chambers while decreasing the heart volume and are thus often interpreted as diastolic dysfunction (Table 91.3).

How much is pressure surrounding the heart increased with PEEP, and is there a practical approach to relating transmural atrial pressure to stroke volume and cardiac output? When PEEP increases end-expired lung volume, the inflated lungs push the thorax to an increased volume through a greater pleural pressure, and this ΔPpl with PEEP is approximately equal to the change in pressure outside the right and left ventricles.[62] During mechanical ventilation, the ratio of ΔPpl to the change in static elastic pressure across the lung and chest wall (ΔPel) for each breath is given by the ratio of respiratory system compliance (CRS) to the compliance of the chest wall (CW); that is, ΔPpl/ΔPel = CRS/CW. When lung compliance (CL) is normal, CL = CW, so ΔPpl/ΔPel = 0.5. When the lungs' compliance decreases in acute hypoxic respiratory failure, ΔPel increases because CRS falls, but ΔPpl changes little because CW is unaffected by the lung disease,[59] and ΔPpl becomes much less than half of ΔPel. To the extent that the increase in lung volume (ΔVL) with PEEP is determined by CRS, ΔPpl/PEEP = CRS/CW, and a fall in CRS with acute hypoxic respiratory failure would decrease the ΔPpl for a given amount of PEEP well below the normal value of 0.5. Yet ΔVL with PEEP is much greater than that predicted by CRS in acute hypoxic respiratory failure because PEEP recruits many previously flooded air spaces[63, 64]; therefore, ΔPpl/PEEP is as great after acute lung injury as before[59] (Fig. 91.8). Accordingly, the ΔPpl with PEEP is difficult to measure and hard to predict; therefore, many approaches have been tested to estimate the transmural pressure of heart chambers on PEEP.[65] Because accurate knowledge of left atrial transmural pressure reveals that the value associated with an adequate cardiac output can vary among patients by as much as 20 mm Hg, a better approach is to seek the lowest pulmonary wedge pressure (PPW) that provides adequate output on each level of PEEP; in this way, therapy is not confounded by erroneous estimates of the transmural PPW.

**Table 91.3 COMMON CAUSES OF DIASTOLIC DYSFUNCTION IN CRITICALLY ILL PATIENTS SIGNALED BY HIGH LEFT ATRIAL PRESSURE AND LOW LEFT VENTRICULAR END-DIASTOLIC VOLUME**

| |
|---|
| **External Compression** |
| Pericardial effusion or constriction |
| Positive-pressure ventilation with PEEP |
| Tension pneumothorax, massive pleural effusions |
| Greatly increased abdominal pressure |
| **Myocardial Stiffness** |
| LV hypertrophy: aortic stenosis, systemic hypertension |
| Infiltrative diseases: amyloidosis |
| Ischemic heart disease |
| **Ventricular Interdependence and Right-to-Left Septal Shift** |
| Pulmonary hypertension |
| RV infarction |
| High levels of PEEP |
| **Intraventricle Filling Defects** |
| Tumor |
| Clot |
| **Rhythm or Valvular Impediments to Filling** |
| Tachycardia |
| Heart block |
| Atrial fibrillation, flutter |
| Mitral stenosis |

From Wood LDH: The pathophysiology of the circulation in critical illness. *In* Hall JB, Schmidt GA, Wood LDH (eds): Principles of Critical Care. New York: McGraw-Hill, 1998, p 263.
LV = left ventricular; PEEP = positive end-expiratory pressure; RV = right ventricular.

## Ventricular Dysfunction in Respiratory Failure

Figure 91.9*A* presents several Starling relationships of the heart.[53, 66] On the abscissa is plotted left atrial pressure (PLA), which approximates the filling pressure of the left ventricle. On the ordinate is plotted stroke volume (SV, in milliliters), or the volume ejected per beat of the heart, which is one measure of ventricular output. Another

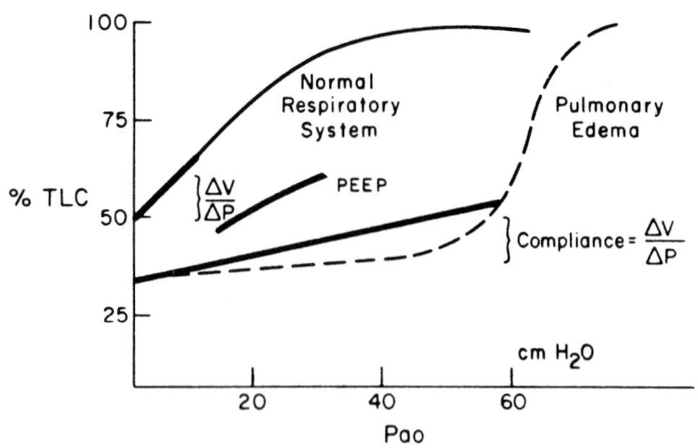


| | Before edema | After edema |
|---|---|---|
| ΔV(litres) with PEEP (20 cm $H_2O$) | 1.42±0.38 | 1.39±0.22 |
| ΔPpl (cm $H_2O$) with PEEP | 10.1±2.2 | 9.7±0.7 |
| Lung Compliance (ml/cm $H_2O$) | 102±28 | 47±17 |

**Figure 91.8** Relationships between lung volume (ordinate, percentage of total lung capacity (TLC)) and pressure across the respiratory system (abscissa, Pao in cm $H_2O$). The *thin continuous line* represents the inflation pressure-volume relationship of the normal respiratory system, showing an end-expired lung volume (Pao = 0) of 50% TLC and an inflation compliance (ΔV/ΔP) during a tidal volume breath *(thick part of thin line)*. In contrast, the *interrupted line* shows the inflation PV curve after pulmonary edema floods many lung units, reducing the end-expired lung volume to about 30% TLC; then a tidal inflation of the same ΔV causes a much larger increase in ΔPao because there are many fewer air spaces to accommodate the tidal volume. Adding 15 cm of positive end-expiratory pressure (PEEP) might be expected to produce a much smaller change in an expired lung volume in edematous lungs than in a normal respiratory system; yet when PEEP is effective in reducing shunt fraction ($\dot{Q}s/\dot{Q}_T$) by redistributing alveolar edema, the increase in end-expired lung volume (and so in pleural pressure (Ppl in figure)) is as large after pulmonary edema as in the normal respiratory system. (See table at right of graph assembled from reference 59.) (From Hall JB, Schmidt GA, Wood LDH (eds): Principles of Critical Care. New York: McGraw-Hill, 1998, p 267.)

measure of output can be expressed by multiplying by the mean arterial blood pressure (Part) developed during each beat to obtain stroke work (SW = SV × [Part − PLA]). As filling pressure of the heart increases, the ejected volume and the work done by the heart increase in a curvilinear manner; at higher filling pressures, there is less increase in stroke volume per increase in PLA than at lower values of PLA. On the continuous Starling curve in Figure 91.9*A*, the normal PLA (10 mm Hg) is associated with a normal stroke volume (75 mL) calculated from cardiac output (6.0 L/min) divided by heart rate (80 beats/min). When hypovolemia lowers PLA to 5 mm Hg, stroke volume falls to 40 mL, lowering cardiac output; if therapeutic expansion of the circulating volume raises PLA to 20 mm Hg, stroke volume increases to 100 mL, raising cardiac output above normal.

These relationships provide a common framework for understanding ventricular function in critical illness. A shift up and to the left of the Starling curve generally indicates enhanced ventricular function, with greater stroke volume for a given filling pressure (see interrupted curve). Conversely, a shift down and to the right with reduced stroke volume at a given filling pressure (see dotted Starling curve through points A and B) indicates depressed ventricular function. The lower stroke volume for PLA of 10 mm Hg at point A could be due to (1) reduced contractility; (2) increased arterial blood pressure, which causes the same stroke work to eject a smaller stroke volume at point A; or (3) a stiffer ventricle, which causes a smaller left ventricular end-diastolic volume (LVEDV) at PLA = 10. This variety of mechanisms to explain the same data is a limitation of the analysis of hemodynamics by the Starling curve; therefore, a more complete description of ventricular function is helpful.

The ventricular function revealed by the Starling relationship is based on the mechanical properties of the relaxed (diastolic) or the contracting (systolic) volume-pressure relationships of the ventricle. This section reviews the factors that influence the diastolic and systolic mechanics in health and in respiratory failure and relates these mechanics to the corresponding Starling function curves of the heart. In Figure 91.9*B*, left ventricular end-diastolic pressure (LVEDP) and end-systolic pressure (LVESP) are plotted against the corresponding volumes (LVEDV, LVESV). The continuous end-diastolic volume-pressure curve is marked with a dot at LVEDP of 10 mm Hg where the normal LVEDV is 120 mL. When the ventricle contracts, pressure rises at the same volume until the aortic valve is opened and blood is ejected until the valve closes again, at LVESV = 45 mL. The stroke volume (LVEDV − LVESV) is 75 mL as plotted on the continuous Starling curve in Figure 91.9*A*. When hypovolemia reduces LVEDV (marked 1 in Fig. 91.9*B*), both LVEDP and stroke volume decrease along the Starling curve above; if volume expansion increases LVEDV to 2 (see Fig. 91.9*B*), both stroke volume and LVEDP increase along the Starling curve.

The intracardiac pressures such as PLA are measured with regard to atmospheric pressure; therefore, they do not represent true transmural, or filling, pressures of the heart chamber when the pressure on the outside of the heart is not atmospheric. Pericardial pressure is most often equal to pleural pressure (Ppl), which is subatmospheric during spontaneous breathing (−3 to −10 mm Hg) and can become very negative in airflow obstruction or very positive with mechanical ventilation, PEEP, and pericardial disease.[62, 67] For convenience, the following discussion refers to the intravascular pressures as transmural or filling pressures, and any cause for altered pericardial or pleural pressure is noted.

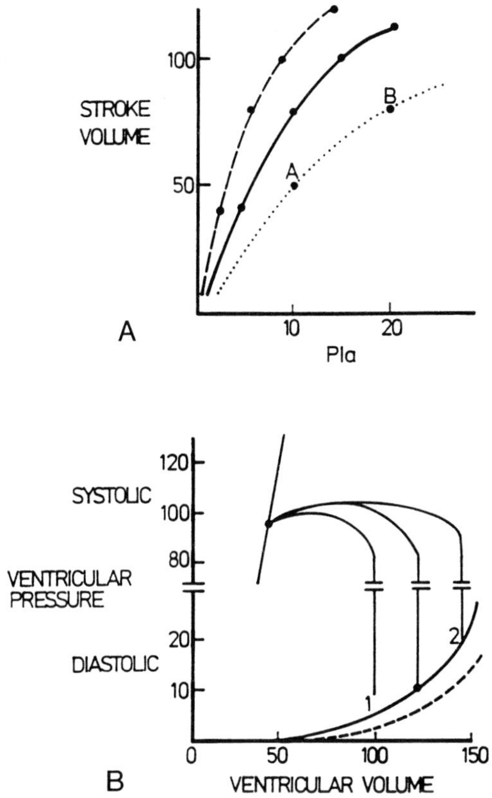


**Figure 91.9** *A,* Several Starling function curves are shown: stroke volume (SV; ordinate, in milliliters) is plotted against left atrial pressure (Pla in figure; in millimeters of mercury) on the abscissa. The middle continuous line depicts a normal Starling function curve for comparison with a depressed curve *(dotted line from point A to point B)* and with a curve depicting enhanced ventricular function *(interrupted curve);* note that all three curves may have the same systolic function (contractility) if diastolic volume-pressure (V-P) relations or afterloads differ from each other. *B,* The corresponding left ventricular volume (abscissa, in milliliters)–pressure (ordinate, in millimeters of mercury) relationships; note the break in the ordinate scale to emphasize the normal diastolic V-P curve *(continuous lines 1 and 2)* and the end-systolic V-P relationship *(continuous line up and to the left).* For discussion of the three V-P loops originating from the diastolic curve, see text. The interrupted diastolic V-P curve depicts a more compliant chamber such as the right ventricle, in which there is less diastolic pressure for each volume. (From Hall JB, Schmidt GA, Wood LDH (eds): Principles of Critical Care. New York: McGraw-Hill, 1998, p 262.)

## The Diastolic Volume-Pressure Curve and Ventricular Filling Disorders

Figure 91.9*B* plots left ventricular diastolic volume against left ventricular diastolic pressure. As ventricular volume increases from zero, the transmural pressure of the ventricle does not exceed zero until about 50 mL (the unstressed volume) is added. Then LVEDP increases in a curvilinear manner with ventricular volume (the stressed volume): first, a large change in volume occurs with a small change in pressure; then, a small change in volume occurs with a large change in pressure. If the pericardium is removed, these volume-pressure characteristics are more linear, so that the large change in LVEDP at higher values of LVEDV is no longer evident. Thus, the pericardium acts like a membrane with a large unstressed volume surrounding the heart loosely up to a given ventricular volume, but at greater LVEDV it becomes very stiff. At higher heart volumes, most of the pressure across the heart is across the pericardium, accounting for the very steep rise in the diastolic volume-pressure relationship. In the presence of pericardial effusion, the volume at which the pericardium becomes a limiting membrane is reduced by the volume of the effusion. When the effusion is large enough, reduced end-diastolic volumes are associated with extremely large end-diastolic pressures.[67] In turn, these pericardial pressures reduce venous return by raising PRA, keeping both end-diastolic volume and cardiac output abnormally low. Tension pneumothorax, massive pleural effusions, high levels of PEEP, and greatly increased abdominal pressures can all act to raise pressure outside the heart (Ppl) and thus reduce LVEDV and stroke volume despite high values of LVEDP (see Table 91.3). Intercurrent left ventricular hypertrophy or infiltrative diseases of the myocardium (e.g., amyloidosis) occasionally stiffen the relaxed ventricle so that high filling pressures are needed to maintain an adequate stroke volume, and inadequate filling time or poorly coordinated atrial contraction impairs ventricular filling as well.[68, 69]

A right-to-left shift of the interventricular septum also can restrict diastolic filling. Presumably, distention of the right ventricle causes the interventricular septum to bulge from right to left, thereby reducing the unstressed volume and compliance of the left ventricle.[70, 71] This effect of ventricular interdependence is much less marked when the pericardium is removed, perhaps because the limiting membrane of the pericardium restricts freedom of motion of the left ventricle, making it more vulnerable to displacements of the septum. Accordingly, conditions in which the right ventricle is abnormally loaded (acute pulmonary embolism; ACRF due to obstructive or restrictive lung disease) may impede the emptying of the right ventricle, causing it to work at a higher end-diastolic volume. Then left ventricular filling pressures are higher than expected for the end-diastolic volume. This provides

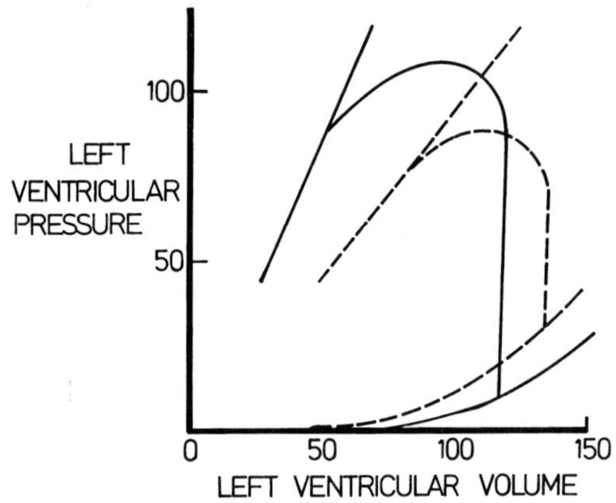


**Figure 91.10** Schematic showing left ventricular (LV) end-diastolic (ED) and end-systolic (ES) volume-pressure (V-P) relations before *(continuous curves)* and after *(interrupted curves)* acute myocardial infarction. The myocardial injury depresses the contractility to increase left ventricular end-systolic volume (LVESV) despite the fall in pressure afterload (LVESP); accordingly, left ventricular end-diastolic volume (LVEDV) increases to accommodate venous return, whereas LVEDP increases even more on account of the diastolic dysfunction due to the myocardial injury. Accordingly, left ventricular dysfunction is signaled by reduced stroke volume and cardiac output despite a large elevation in LVEDP; therapy aims to reduce preload, enhance contractility, and reduce afterload (for further discussion, see text). (From Hall JB, Schmidt GA, Wood LDH (eds): Principles of Critical Care. New York: McGraw-Hill, 1998, p 263.)

one possible explanation why PEEP is often associated with increased filling pressure to maintain a normal stroke volume even when LVEDP is corrected to the true filling pressure by subtracting the increase in Ppl (ΔPpl) measured when PEEP is applied.[59–61] Acute myocardial ischemia also displaces the diastolic volume-pressure curve of the left ventricle up and to the left (Fig. 91.10). Conceivably, the myocardial injury alters the elastic properties of the relaxed ventricle.[68] A higher ventricular filling pressure is then required at each end-diastolic volume. This accounts in part for the often noted observation that patients with acute myocardial injury need values of LVEDP as high as 30 mm Hg to maintain adequate cardiac output, whereas normal patients need filling pressures of less than 10 mm Hg.

## End-Systolic Volume-Pressure Curve and Contractility

The normal diastolic volume-pressure relationship is drawn as the continuous line in the lower right-hand portion of Figure 91.10. Consider the effects when the ventricle contracts during systole without ejecting any blood, as if the aortic valve could not open. A very large pressure is generated during this isovolumic contraction from a normal LVEDV, but when LVEDV is reduced, the pressure generated during a similar isovolumic contraction is much less as a manifestation of the force-length characteristics of the myocardium.[53] In other words, the less the muscle is stretched to begin with, the less force it can generate due to length-dependent activation of actin-myosin cross-bridges. The units of force in the hollow sphere of myocardium are the units of pressure, or force per unit area. A line connecting the end-systolic pressure volume points is linear and extrapolates toward the origin (see the continuous end-systolic volume-pressure line in Fig. 91.10, upper left).

Of course, the aortic valve does open in early systole when the isovolumic intraventricular pressure exceeds the aortic diastolic pressure; then left ventricular volume decreases as the stroke volume is ejected (see Fig. 91.10). The contracting ventricle shortens against the aortic afterload pressure until its volume reaches the end-systolic volume; at that lower volume, the maximum pressure that can be generated is equal to the afterload pressure, so the aortic valve closes and ejection is over. If the afterload pressure were reduced, the ventricle could empty more completely to a lower end-systolic volume, at which the maximum generated pressure equals the reduced afterload, and so stroke volume would increase.[53]

The line connecting all end-systolic volume-pressure points is an indicator of the pumping function or contractility of the heart, for this line defines the volume to which the ventricle can shorten against each afterload for a given contractile state.[72] Agents that enhance contractility (epinephrine, calcium, dobutamine, dopamine) shift the end-systolic volume-pressure relationship up and to the left; then the ventricle can shorten to a smaller end-systolic volume for each afterload, thereby increasing stroke volume at a given LVEDV. Conversely, negative inotropic agents, such as propranolol or myocardial ischemia, depress the end-systolic volume-pressure relationship down and to the right, as indicated by the interrupted end-systolic volume-pressure line in Figure 91.10.[73–75] Then end-systolic volume is increased for a given afterload pressure, thereby reducing the stroke volume at a given filling pressure. Such a reduction in contractility is another cause for the depressed Starling curve from point A to point B in Figure 91.9*A*.

## An Approach to Acute Ventricular Dysfunction

These concepts provide a framework for understanding the pathophysiology and therapy of acute myocardial infarction.[76, 77] Figure 91.10 depicts normal diastolic and systolic volume-pressure relationships and indicates a normal systolic ejection (continuous lines). From LVEDV = 120 mL and LVEDP = 10 mm Hg, the ventricle contracts isovolumically until the aortic valve opens at an intraventricular pressure of 80 mm Hg. Blood is then ejected as systolic pressure rises to 110 mm Hg and falls again toward LVESP = 90 mm Hg and LVESV = 50 mL, when the aortic valve closes to generate the dicrotic notch on the arterial pressure trace. Accordingly, stroke volume is 70 mL at $P_{LA}$ = 10 mm Hg and cardiac output is 5.6 L/min when heart rate = 80 beats/min. Acute myocardial infarction depresses the end-systolic volume-pressure relationship in such a way that the end-systolic volume is increased to 90 mL at a reduced LVESP (75 mm Hg) (interrupted line). At the same time, the end-diastolic volume is increased to 130 mL to accommodate the venous return, and end-diastolic pressure is increased even more than expected (LVEDP = 30 mm Hg) as a result of the shift up and to the left of the end-diastolic volume-pressure relationship (interrupted line). Thus, stroke volume (40 mL) and cardiac output (4.4 L/min) are reduced despite reflex tachycardia (heart rate = 110 beats/min) at an increased left ventricular filling pressure, and arterial blood pressure is reduced (90/70 mm Hg) despite reflex increase in systemic vascular resistance.

Conventional therapy consists of preload reduction, inotropic agents, and afterload reduction.[76, 77] Interventions such as morphine, furosemide, nitroglycerin, and rotating tourniquets reduce venous return by dilating venous capacitance beds to increase the unstressed volume and reduce mean systemic pressure (Pms; see previous discussion). In turn, this reduces LVEDV and LVEDP. The reduction in end-diastolic volume tends to reduce stroke volume along the steep diastolic volume-pressure curve so that there is a large reduction in LVEDP in response to a small reduction in LVEDV and stroke volume. Furthermore, the potential adverse effect of reduced stroke volume is often offset by increased contractility and reduced afterload when myocardial wall stress is reduced by the reduction in LVEDV and LVEDP. Reduced afterload and reduced myocardial oxygen consumption improve ventricular pumping function by shifting the end-systolic volume-pressure relationship up and to the left, so LVESV decreases and stroke volume increases. Moreover, the reduced end-diastolic pressure reduces the likelihood of complicating cardiogenic pulmonary edema. Positive inotropic agents such as dopamine and dobutamine act directly on the myocardium to reduce end-systolic volume at a given end-systolic pressure, thereby increasing stroke volume.[76–78] Afterload-reducing agents such as nitroprusside and enalapril dilate peripheral arteries to lower end-systolic pressure and afterload; in turn, end-systolic volume decreases along the depressed end-systolic volume-pressure relationship to increase stroke volume.[79] The associated reduction in LVEDV and LVEDP reduces the tendency to form pulmonary edema and may also reduce the myocardial oxygen demand by reducing ventricular wall stress.

Other concomitant effects of respiratory failure cause ventricular dysfunction characterized by reduced stroke volume at increased $P_{LA}$ (Table 91.4). Both arterial hypoxemia[73] and acidemia[74] depress the end-systolic volume-pressure curve as shown by the interrupted curve in Figure 91.10. Acute arterial hypertension raises the pressure afterload, so stroke volume decreases as end-systolic volume increases along the continuous end-systolic volume-pressure curve in Figure 91.10. Then LVEDV increases to accommodate venous return, so LVEDP increases, often more than expected, as a result of diastolic stiffness, which in turn is due to chronic left ventricular hypertrophy. Accordingly, pulmonary edema is a common complication, and it responds to vasodilator therapy when arterial blood pressure is reduced. In some or all of these conditions, diastolic dysfunction merits special management.[80] Where acute or acute-on-chronic congestive heart failure is present, reducing LVEDP and LVEDV, maintaining atrial contraction, increasing the duration of diastole, and minimizing myocardial ischemia are helpful. Each of these therapeutic measures is also helpful in managing hypoperfusion states associated with diastolic dysfunction.

**Table 91.4 ACUTE REVERSIBLE CONTRIBUTORS TO DECREASED CONTRACTILITY**

| |
|---|
| Ischemia |
| Hypoxemia |
| Respiratory acidosis |
| Metabolic acidosis |
| Hypocalcemia |
| Hypophosphatemia |
| Possibly other electrolyte abnormalities ($Mg^{2+}$, $K^+$) |
| Exogenous substances (alcohol, beta-blockers, calcium channel blockers, antiarrhythmics) |
| Endogenous substances (endotoxin, histamine, TNF, IL-1, PAF) |
| Hypothermia and hyperthermia |

From Walley KR, Wood LDH: Ventricular dysfunction in critical illness. *In* Hall JB, Schmidt GA, Wood LDH (eds): Principles of Critical Care. New York: McGraw-Hill, 1998, p 309.
IL-1 = interleukin-1; PAF = platelet-activating factor; TNF = tumor necrosis factor.

Valvular dysfunction mimics systolic and diastolic dysfunction, in such a way that LVEDV is greatly increased and the forward stroke volume is reduced.[81] With aortic regurgitation, after a vigorous systolic ejection, aortic blood flows both forward and backward in diastole so that LVEDP rises and arterial diastolic pressure falls toward equal values at a lower than normal pressure (in this instance, 40 mm Hg). The large LVEDV then ejects a large stroke volume to raise systolic pressure to 120 mm Hg, causing a bounding pulse pressure of 80 mm Hg, but the aortic regurgitation reduces forward stroke volume and cardiac output to low values. Consider also mitral valve incompetence. During systole, a large fraction of the blood ejected from the ventricle regurgitates into the left atrium, reducing forward stroke volume and cardiac output but raising LVEDV and LVEDP when the capacious left atrium fills the ventricle. In this circumstance, pulse pressure and arterial blood pressure are reduced. In both cases, the ventricular mechanics resemble the interrupted curves in Figure 91.10 and improve toward the normal continuous curves when forward flow is increased by vasodilator therapy, which lowers systemic vascular resistance to promote more peripheral runoff and less regurgitant flow.

## Pulmonary Circulation

### Pressures, Flow, and Resistance in Pulmonary Vessels

Cardiac output from the left side of the heart is equal to venous return to the right side of the heart, so all the cardiac output traverses the pulmonary circulation in a pulsatile manner (Fig. 91.11). The right ventricle ejects blood into the pulmonary artery, raising its pressure ($P_{PA}$)

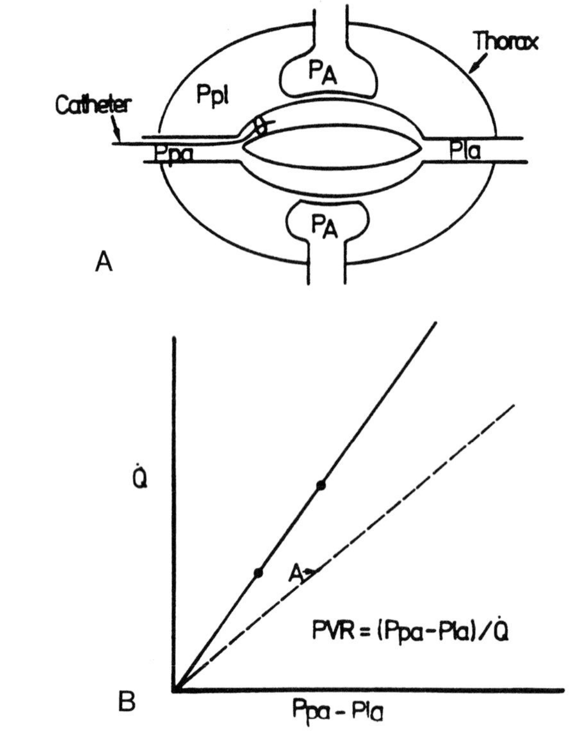


**Figure 91.11** Schematic of the pulmonary circulation *(A)* illustrating a simple view of pulmonary vascular resistance (PVR, *B*). Pulmonary blood flows from the pulmonary arteries (Ppa in figure) through branching vessels to the left atrium (Pla in figure). This central circulation is enclosed by the thorax, which contains air spaces ($P_A$ in figure) that abut alveolar vessels. Between the air spaces and thorax is the pleural (pl) space, so pleural pressure (Ppl in figure) approximates the pressure outside extra-alveolar vessels, including the heart. A balloon-tipped catheter is occluding the upper branch of the pulmonary artery so that the catheter tip sits in a stagnant column of blood, continuous with Pla, to provide an estimate of pulmonary wedge pressure (PPW)—unless $P_A$ exceeds Pla, when the occlusion pressure exceeds Pla because $P_A$ closes the alveolar vessels; in either case, when the balloon is deflated, the catheter tip measures Ppa, and a thermistor near the tip can measure pulmonary blood flow ($\dot{Q}$) by thermodilution technique. *B,* $\dot{Q}$ (ordinate) is plotted against Ppa − Pla (abscissa); the inverse of the slope of the continuous line drawn through the two P$\dot{Q}$ points is PVR; for a given $\dot{Q}$ at the lower point, Ppa − Pla increases to A on the interrupted P$\dot{Q}$ line, indicating increased PVR. (From Hall JB, Schmidt GA, Wood LDH (eds): Principles of Critical Care. New York: McGraw-Hill, 1998, p 272.)

to drive flow through a branching arteriolar system into the lung parenchyma, where a network of very small alveolar septal vessels and capillaries passes between the air spaces of the lung to effect pulmonary gas exchange. These septal vessels converge into pulmonary veins that empty into the left atrium, where the PLA is often regarded as the outflow pressure of the pulmonary circulation. When this pressure gradient across the pulmonary circulation (PPA − PLA) is divided by the pulmonary blood flow, or cardiac output ($\dot{Q}$), the pulmonary vascular resistance (PVR) is calculated (mm Hg/L per minute) and sometimes converted to metric units (dyne-sec · $cm^{-5}$) by multiplying by 80. By this analysis, increasing blood flow from one level to another is associated with increasing pressure drop across the pulmonary circulation (PPA − PLA) along a unique pressure-flow relationship depicted by the continuous line in the lower panel of Figure 91.11.[53] Resistance to pulmonary blood flow may be increased (1) by smooth muscle constriction within the pulmonary arterioles by alveolar hypoxia; (2) by compression of the alveolar septal vessels by elevated alveolar pressure; (3) by obstruction of larger pulmonary vessels by thromboembolism; or (4) by obliteration of many of the parallel vascular channels as they traverse the lung, so that the same blood flow must flow through fewer channels.[53, 71] Such an increase in pulmonary vascular resistance would be calculated as at point A on the interrupted line in Figure 91.11, where the pressure difference across the lung (PPA − PLA) has increased for the same amount of pulmonary blood flow. Pulmonary hypertension is a frequent abnormality in respiratory failure, which can lead to the acute right heart syndrome (Table 91.5).[71]

Figure 91.11 also depicts a common way to make these measurements with a pulmonary artery catheter that has been passed via systemic veins into the central circulation.[82] When the small balloon near the catheter's tip is inflated, the balloon passes with the venous blood flow through the right atrium, right ventricle, and pulmonary artery until it wedges in a pulmonary artery branch, obstructing the flow there (Fig. 91.12). Because there is no flow, the hole in the catheter tip is open to a stagnant column of blood extending through the pulmonary vessels to the pulmonary veins. Accordingly, this PPW approximates PLA, providing an estimate of LVEDP to evaluate ventricular function as discussed earlier, as well as an estimate of pulmonary microvascular (or capillary) pressure to help manage pulmonary edema (see later discussion). When the balloon is deflated and flow resumes through that vessel, the pressure there is equal to the pulmonary artery pressure. Blood drawn from the pulmonary artery provides a measure of mixed venous oxygen content ($C\bar{v}_{O_2}$); when related to the simultaneous measurement of arterial oxygen content ($Ca_{O_2}$) and cardiac output ($\dot{Q}$), the patient's oxygen consumption ($\dot{V}O_2 = \dot{Q}[Ca_{O_2} - C\bar{v}_{O_2}]$) can be calculated and interpreted in the context of the patient's oxygen transport ($\dot{Q}O_2 = \dot{Q} \times$

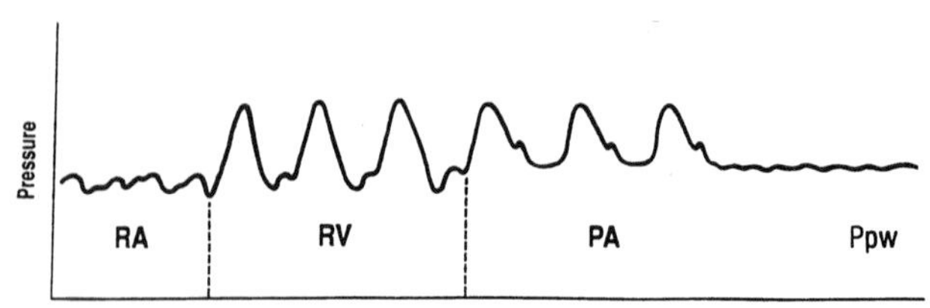


**Figure 91.12** Waveform transition as catheter is advanced from right atrial (RA) to wedge position (Ppw in figure). PA = pulmonary artery; RV = right ventricle. (From Hall JB, Schmidt GA, Wood LDH (eds): Principles of Critical Care. New York: McGraw-Hill, 1992, p 327.)

**Table 91.5 CAUSES OF THE ACUTE RIGHT HEART SYNDROME**

| |
|---|
| **ACUTE PRESSURE OVERLOAD** |
| Pulmonary embolism |
| ARDS |
| Excessive PEEP, tidal volume, and alveolar pressure |
| Air, amniotic, fat, and tumor microembolism |
| Sepsis (rarely) |
| Pulmonary leukostasis, leukoagglutination |
| Extensive lung resection |
| Drugs (e.g., heparin-protamine reaction) |
| Hypoxia |
| **ACUTE-ON-CHRONIC PA HYPERTENSION** |
| Chronic lung diseases |
| Emphysema, chronic bronchitis, bronchiectasis, cystic fibrosis |
| Restrictive diseases of the lung |
| Collagen vascular diseases of the lung |
| Thoracic cage deformities |
| Kyphoscoliosis, thoracopolasty |
| Cardiovascular disorders |
| Chronic thromboembolism |
| Primary pulmonary hypertension |
| Congenital heart diseases |
| Pulmonary veno-occlusive disease |
| Miscellaneous disorders |
| Sleep-disordered breathing |
| Hyperviscosity syndromes |
| Toxins and drugs |
| Parasites |
| End-stage liver disease |
| HIV infection |
| **RIGHT VENTRICULAR SYSTOLIC DYSFUNCTION** |
| RV infarction |
| Sepsis |
| Toxins |

From Schmidt GA, Wood LDH: Acute right heart syndromes. *In* Hall JB, Schmidt GA, Wood LDH (eds): Principles of Critical Care. New York: McGraw-Hill, 1998, p 419.
ARDS = acute respiratory distress syndrome; HIV = human immunodeficiency syndrome; PA = pulmonary artery; PEEP = positive end-expiratory pressure; RV = right ventricle.

$Ca_{O_2}$). A sensitive thermistor at the tip of the catheter may be used to detect temperature changes after the injection of a cold saline bolus into the right atrium, allowing the estimation of cardiac output from the resulting thermodilution curve.[82]

The pulmonary artery and the left atrium are surrounded by Ppl, so that the absolute values of PPA and PLA change with respiration (Fig. 91.13). When spontaneous active inspiration lowers pleural pressure, both pulmonary artery and left atrial pressure decrease, but the driving pressure of blood flow across the lung stays the same (PPA − PLA); when positive-pressure inflation raises Ppl, both PPA and PLA increase.[82] Accordingly, it is helpful to record pulmonary vascular measurements at end-expiration when the mode of ventilation has minimally different effects; even this approach can be confounded when the patient exerts vigorous respiratory activity[82] (Fig. 91.14). When alveolar pressure (PA) exceeds PLA, the true driving pressure for pulmonary blood flow is PPA − PA (see Chapter 4). One often overlooked adverse effect of positive-pressure ventilation with high PEEP or high tidal volume is the large increase in dead space (VD/VT) when pulmonary blood flow is interrupted by the high PA; not infrequently, alveolar ventilation can actually increase when tidal volume is reduced in these conditions, causing a paradoxic fall in arterial $Pco_2$. A second consequence of PA > PLA is an overestimation of PPW; this can be detected when the respiratory fluctuation of PPA is much less than that of PPW,[83] and there is considerable interobserver variability in the measurement of PPW[84a]; there are also differences in the accuracy of the various algorithms that have been proposed for estimating pulmonary capillary pressure.[84b] In view of these effects of respiration on measurements of PPA and PPW, it is not surprising that many physicians err in their interpretation of pulmonary arterial catheter data.[84] The complications of pulmonary arterial catheters abound, and it has been argued that the hemodynamic data obtained can be deduced by clinical examination or are not helpful in clinical decision making.[85, 86] On the other hand, studies have demonstrated that physicians do err in their clinical evaluations, so it seems reasonable to encourage the informed use of a pulmonary arterial catheter to obtain hemodynamic data when there is serious clinical uncertainty and when those data will be used to address important aspects of the patient's management.[82]

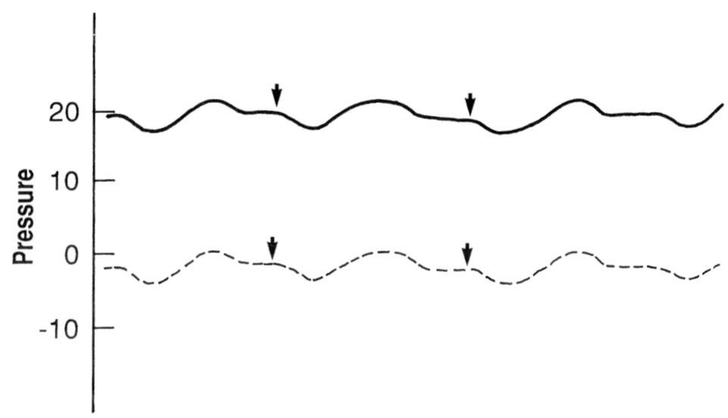


**Figure 91.13** Effect of varying intrathoracic pressure on the pulmonary vascular pressures. *Top,* Pulmonary wedge pressure (PPW) tracing; *bottom,* pleural pressure (Ppl) tracing. In this example the patient is receiving assisted mechanical ventilation. *Arrows* indicate end-expiratory pressures. Negative deflections in intrapleural pressure and PPW result from inspiratory muscle activity, and subsequent positive deflections represent lung inflation by the ventilator. At end-expiration *(arrows)* the respiratory system has returned to its relaxed state and Ppl is back to baseline (−2 cm $H_2O$). Transmural PPW remains approximately constant throughout the ventilating cycle. Because Ppl is not usually measured simultaneously with PPW, however, it is necessary that the PPW be recorded at a point where Ppl can be reliably estimated (i.e., end-exhalation, assuming no active expiratory muscle activity). A digital scan may underestimate or overestimate transmural pressure, depending on whether the pressure is sampled during a period of negative or positive change in Ppl. (From Hall JB, Schmidt GA, Wood LDH (eds): Principles of Critical Care. New York: McGraw-Hill, 1998, p 166.)

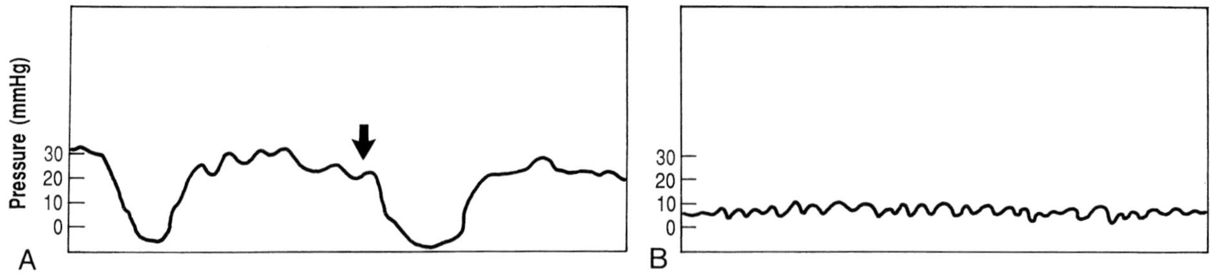


**Figure 91.14** Effect of vigorous respiratory muscle activity on end-expiratory pulmonary wedge pressure (PPW). *A,* Patient on mechanical ventilation is observed at the bedside to be making vigorous inspiratory and expiratory efforts. The PPW measured at end-exhalation *(arrow)* is 25 mm Hg. *B,* To obtain a reliable PPW, respiratory muscle activity is temporarily eliminated with a short-acting paralyzing agent. The PPW is now measured at 8 mm Hg. (From Hall JB, Schmidt GA, Wood LDH (eds): Principles of Critical Care. New York: McGraw-Hill, 1998, p 168.)

## Pulmonary Edema

Figure 91.15 is a schematic diagram depicting the circulatory factors governing the filtration of liquid ($\dot{Q}_E$) between the pulmonary vessels and the lung interstitial tissues; the Starling equation that describes lung liquid flux is written beneath the figure and is discussed in detail in Chapter 6. The hydrostatic pressure in the microvessels of the lung (Pmv; 12 mm Hg) is about halfway between PPA (normally about 15 mm Hg) and LVEDP (normally about 10 mm Hg). Hydrostatic pressure in the septal interstitial space (Pis; −4 mm Hg) is subatmospheric, in part because it drains into the peribronchovascular interstitium, which has a more negative pressure, and in part because lymph vessels, valved like veins for unidirectional flow, actively remove liquid from the interstitial spaces, which have intrinsic structural stability to resist collapse.[87] Accordingly, there is a positive hydrostatic pressure (Pmv − Pis = 16 mm Hg) driving fluid across the microvascular endothelium to the lung septal interstitium. This hydrostatic pressure difference is partially offset by the protein oncotic pressure difference that exists between plasma in the microvessels of the lung (πmv; 25 mm Hg) and liquid in the interstitial spaces (πis; 19 mm Hg). The vascular wall presents a barrier to this bulk flow of liquid characterized by its permeability to water (Kf; mL fluid flux/min per mm Hg); Kf includes surface area (S), and thus is heavily weighted by the characteristics of the alveolar vessels where so much surface resides.[87] The microvascular membrane is also characterized by its permeability to circulating proteins, dominated by albumin and globulin. If these plasma proteins were completely reflected (reflection coefficient [σ] = 1), no protein would pass from lung blood to interstitium; in contrast, if the microvascular membrane were freely permeable (σ = 0), interstitial protein concentration (CL), as measured in lung lymph, would equal that of plasma proteins (CP). Under normal steady-state conditions of liquid filtration, the ratio of CL to CP is about 0.6 in most mammals; however, when liquid filtration is progressively increased by elevating Pmv, CL/CP falls to a plateau value of about 0.3. This plateau value indicates the microvascular protein reflection coefficient (σ = 1 − CL/CP = 0.7) measured in conditions of high liquid filtration; at lower values of filtration, water diffuses from the interstitium into the blood along the concentration gradient for water established by CP > CL.[87]

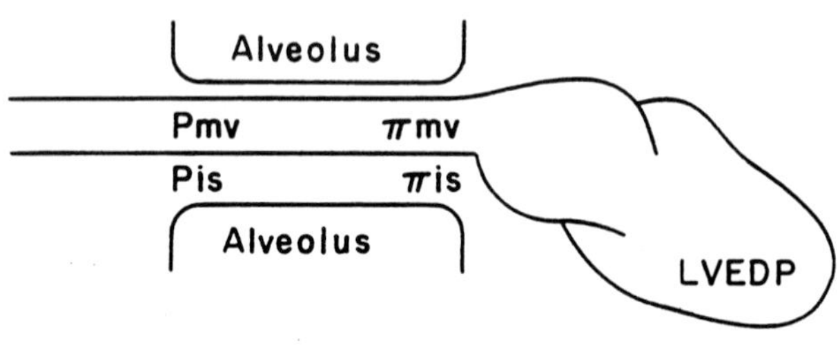


**Edema Flow = [(Pmv-Pis) - (πmv-πis) σ] Kf**

**Figure 91.15** Schematic representation of Starling forces governing the flux of lung liquid from intravascular to extravascular space (for discussion, see text). is = interstitial space; Kf = permeability to water; LVEDP = left ventricular end-diastolic pressure; mv = microvessels of the lung; P = pressure; π = colloid osmotic pressure; σ = reflection coefficient. (From Hall JB, Wood LDH: Acute hypoxemic respiratory failure. Med Grand Rounds 3:184, 1984.)

In cardiogenic pulmonary edema (see also Chapter 54), liquid filtration is increased because Pmv is greatly elevated. Several factors act to keep the lungs from accumulating excess liquid; lymphatic flow increases, CL/CP is reduced, and Pis increases. The increased septal Pis drives edema through tissue planes toward intraparenchymal peribronchovascular interstitium, where Pis becomes even more subatmospheric (−10 mm Hg) by the outward pull of alveolar walls on the adventitia surrounding the relatively stiff bronchi and vessels.[87] This adventitial pull renders Pis even more negative with each inspiration, creating a cyclic suction to move edema from the alveolar septa toward the hilum of the lung, where peribronchovascular interstitial pressures are most negative, where the tissues have the largest capacity to accommodate excess fluid, and where the most dense accumulation of lymphatics is arranged to clear the fluid to the systemic veins. This anatomic arrangement accounts for the Kerley lines, the bronchial cuffing, and the perihilar "butterfly" distribution of interstitial cardiogenic pulmonary edema seen on chest radiographs. When ongoing edema formation continues to fill these interstitial reservoirs, Pis rises at the alveolar septa, presumably disrupting tight junctions between alveolar type I epithelial cells to flood the air spaces.[88] Histologic morphometry of edematous lungs reveals that flooded alveoli have about one eighth the volume of unflooded alveoli, which indicates that a relatively small volume of alveolar edema floods eight times that volume of air space; for example, in a patient with an end-expired lung gas volume of 4 L, 250 mL of alveolar edema fills half the air spaces ($8 \times 250 = 2$ L), accounting for a large intrapulmonary shunt and for a large reduction in lung compliance because only half the lung is ventilated.[63]

In the exudative phase of ARDS, a greater proportion of increased permeability edema accumulates in air spaces, so there is a much greater shunt per volume of edema than in cardiogenic edema. Presumably, this different distribution of edema occurs because the lung injury that increases microvascular Kf and decreases $\sigma$ also damages the alveolar epithelial barrier; therefore, the increased extravascular liquid has access through a low-resistance pathway to a very large reservoir for edema: the air spaces of the lung.[89] Often, the transmural hydrostatic pressure driving edema from vessels to air space is normal or reduced; as liquid filtration increases at normal Pmv after an acute lung injury, CL/CP does not decrease as in cardiogenic edema but rather increases slightly to a value of about 0.8 (or up to 1.0 in severe injuries), so the reflection coefficient decreases ($\sigma = 1 - C_L/C_P = 0.2$). Accordingly, the protein concentration in alveolar edema from patients with ARDS is much higher than that from patients with cardiogenic edema and approaches the protein concentration in plasma.[90] When the vascular membrane is repaired, alveolar edema is cleared very slowly from the lungs by active transport of sodium; water follows the osmotic gradient through an intact alveolar membrane, and this clearance raises the concentration of protein in the remaining alveolar edema above the concentration of protein in the plasma; this concentration phenomenon has been used as a clinical marker of recovery from ARDS.[90]

Positive end-expiratory pressure increases end-expired lung volume to lower Pis and increase capacity in the peribronchovascular interstitium; in turn, this redistributes much of the alveolar edema into the expanded interstitial reservoir, in association with the aeration of flooded air spaces at a much increased alveolar volume to reduce shunt and to increase lung compliance without altering the total amount of edema.[11, 25, 63, 64] Because lung volume increases greatly when PEEP is applied, pleural pressure must increase to push the chest wall to an equivalently higher volume (see Fig. 91.8). This raises PRA to reduce venous return and arterial blood pressure[49–51] unless the patient's baroreceptor reflexes or infusions of fluid or administration of vasoactive drugs maintains mean systemic pressure (Pms; see later discussion) and cardiac output.[58, 59, 62] Because the aim of PEEP therapy is to maintain arterial saturation (>90%) of an adequate circulating hemoglobin (>10 g/dL) while breathing a nontoxic concentration of inspired oxygen (<0.6)—all to effect adequate delivery of oxygen without aggravating the lung injury with oxygen toxicity—it is helpful to use the least PEEP to achieve these goals so as to maintain adequate cardiac output.[91, 92]

Also, because PEEP already increases end-expired lung volume, superimposed large tidal volumes may cause pulmonary barotrauma and further reduce venous return; using the least tidal volume effecting adequate carbon dioxide elimination minimizes these complications.[17, 93] It is remarkable how rapidly PEEP redistributes edema to reduce hypoxemia (minutes) and how rapidly the shunt returns when PEEP is removed. Accordingly, the informed physician can implement an effective, tolerable estimate of least PEEP in less than 5 minutes in ventilated patients in whom blood pressure and pulse oximetry are being monitored continuously.[92] When PEEP is effective, plans to prevent its inadvertent removal, as during routine bedside suctioning, can prevent sudden hypoxemic cardiovascular catastrophe. Once least PEEP and least tidal volume are established, examination of the pressure-volume relationship of the respiratory system during a quasi-static tidal inflation should exclude a lower inflection point (LIP), which would signal expiratory collapse and inspiratory reopening of flooded air spaces[19]; evidence of a LIP should be countered by an increase in PEEP until the LIP goes away. Similarly, an upper inflection point should be excluded or created by decreasing the tidal volume.[17, 19] In this way, the benefits of the "open-lung" approach can be sought without the excessive values of PEEP indicated by the LIP determined from a slow inflation from zero end-expired pressure[94]; this LIP value overestimates the PEEP necessary to prevent expiratory collapse by ignoring the progressive alveolar recruitment that occurs at lower values of PEEP within the pressure-volume hysteresis of the respiratory system.[20]

Smaller tidal volumes than conventionally used are also beneficial when ventilating patients with ARDS; this was shown by the results of a recently completed National Heart, Lung, and Blood Institute (NHLBI) clinical trial of 861 patients. In this study, outcomes using traditional (12 mL/kg; "high") tidal volumes were compared with considerably diminished (6 mL/kg; "low") tidal volumes; mortality in the low tidal volume group (31%) was significantly lower than mortality in the high tidal volume group (39%).[94a] In addition to decreasing mortality in patients with ARDS, the small tidal volume approach was associated with a lower incidence of nonpulmonary organ failure. Interestingly, results from a recent Italian study showed that a low tidal volume strategy in ARDS patients attenuated the inflammatory response in both the lungs and bloodstream, as measured by a reduction in neutrophil and cytokine concentrations in bronchoalveolar lavage and a reduction in cytokines in circulating blood.[94b]

Cardiovascular management of both cardiogenic and increased permeability edema aims to reduce edema formation and accumulation and thereby to reduce the duration and complications of intensive care.[91, 92] Cardiogenic edema is caused by high Pmv, often related to acute or acute-on-chronic left ventricular dysfunction, which increases LVEDP.[77] Reducing the central blood volume by venodilating agents (morphine, furosemide, nitroglyc-

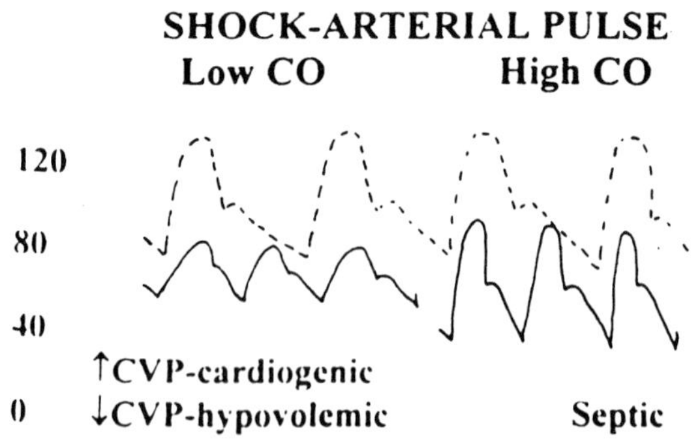


**Figure 91.17** Schematic illustrations of the normal arterial pressure wave form (interrupted pulse pressure); the continuous pressure waves in low-cardiac-output (CO) hypotension *(left)* and in high-CO hypotension *(right)* illustrate key differences from the normal pulse. The ordinate is arterial pressure (in millimeters of mercury); the abscissa is time (in seconds). As indicated below the waveforms, the difference between cardiogenic shock and hypovolemic shock is that in cardiogenic shock, central venous pressure (CVP) is increased (to 20 mm Hg); in hypovolemic shock, CVP is decreased (to 0 mm Hg). For discussion, see text. (From Hall JB, Schmidt GA, Wood LDH (eds): Principles of Critical Care. New York: McGraw-Hill, 1998, p 261.)

associated hypovolemia (Table 91.7). The end point of volume infusion is obscure because cardiac output is already increased, and although cardiac output usually increases further with intravenous infusions, the blood pressure rarely increases much with increased cardiac output. Furthermore, the need for even greater cardiac output to increase oxygen delivery is questionable because the lactic acidosis of septic shock may not be due to anaerobic metabolism.[100–102] On the one hand, there is conflicting evidence as to whether septic patients in whom oxygen transport is maximized have improved survival[103, 104] or worse survival.[105] On the other hand, pulmonary vascular pressures always rise with volume infusion, increasing the pulmonary edema when the septic process increases the permeability of lung vessels.[21, 22, 92] The frequent coincidence of ARDS and septic shock causes uncertainty concerning fluid and vasoactive drug therapy.

Our approach is to ensure resuscitation from septic shock as the first priority by aggressive volume infusion to a Ppw of 15 mm Hg and by administering dobutamine and dopamine at 5 to 10 μg/kg per minute; if ARDS does develop, we seek the lowest Ppw that preserves adequate cardiac output and systemic pressure.[92] Much evidence suggests that the septic myocardium does not function normally.[106, 107] Accordingly, infusions of positive inotropic agents such as dobutamine maintain cardiac output at a lower LVEDP to reduce lung edema. Even when cardiac output and oxygen delivery are made adequate with fluid and dobutamine infusions, the perfusion pressure for vital organs such as the brain and heart may still be too low in some septic patients. In this circumstance, norepinephrine infusion increases blood pressure and splanchnic blood flow[108, 109] without compromising renal function.[110] In contrast, dopamine and epinephrine infusions cause splanchnic hypoperfusion in septic shock.[108, 109, 111] Tachypnea and respiratory distress may be severe, so initial supportive therapy includes early intubation and mechanical ventilation as well as correction of hyperthermia with antipyretics, paralysis, and cooling (Table 91.8). This prevents catastrophic respiratory muscle fatigue, respiratory acidosis, and the complications of emergency intubation and may improve tissue oxygenation by reducing metabolic rate and oxygen requirements in patients with limited oxygen delivery.[30, 112]

## Cardiogenic Shock

In contrast to septic shock, a low cardiac output is signaled by a low pulse pressure (indicating a low stroke volume), signs of increased systemic vascular resistance (cold, cyanotic, damp extremities; poor nail-bed vascular return), and a history or presentation that includes features suggestive of cardiogenic or hypovolemic etiology of hypotension. If cardiac output is reduced, a second question is asked regarding the hypotensive patient: Is the heart too full (see Table 91.6)?

A positive answer is often signaled by symptoms of ischemic heart disease or arrhythmia, signs of cardiomegaly, the third and fourth heart sounds, gallop rhythm of heart failure, new murmurs of valvular dysfunction, increased jugular or central venous pressure, and laboratory test results suggesting ischemia (electrocardiogram [ECG], troponin, or creatine kinase) or ventricular dysfunction (chest roentgenogram suggesting cardiomegaly, venous distention, or cardiogenic edema; echocardiogram showing regional or global systolic dyskinesia). The most common cause of hypotension associated with a circulation that is too full on initial evaluation is cardiogenic shock due to myocardial ischemia.[76, 113] Initial therapy for this presumptive diagnosis is with positive inotropic drugs (dobutamine, 3 to 10 μg/kg per minute) to increase the ejection fraction of the ischemic heart. Such therapy does not directly address the coronary insufficiency and may increase the myocardial oxygen demand. Concurrent sublingual, dermal, or intravenous nitroglycerin ameliorates elements of coronary vasospasm to increase blood flow and reduces preload to reduce myocardial oxygen consumption. Morphine also reduces pain, anxiety, and preload.[76]

In this situation, even a cautious volume challenge (250 mL NaCl over 20 minutes) is relatively contraindicated before right-sided heart catheterization, because ventricular function and cardiac output are reduced as often as they are improved by this intervention and because the risk of pulmonary edema is increased. Indeed, when signs of pulmonary edema are present on clinical and radiologic examination of the thorax, diuretics, morphine, and nitroglycerin often reduce preload by relaxing the capacitance veins, in association with an increase in left ventricular systolic performance. On the other hand, about 10% of patients with myocardial ischemia present with significant hypovolemia. Accordingly, the clinical assessment of hemodynamics should be supplemented as early as possible with right-sided heart catheterization to confirm the hemo-

**Table-91.7 URGENT RESUSCITATION OF THE PATIENT WITH SHOCK: INTRAVENOUS VOLUME AND VASOACTIVE DRUG THERAPY**

| Hemorrhagic Shock, Including Trauma, Ruptured Aneurysms | Nonhemorrhagic Hypovolemia, Including Septic Shock | Cardiogenic Shock, Due to Myocardial Ischemia |
|---|---|---|
| | **Volume Therapy** | |
| Elevate legs, MAST<br>Access/infuse emergency blood<br>Group/match/administer warmed blood/components<br>>3 L/20 min warmed saline<br>Equal volumes of colloid or substitutes (albumin, dextran, hetastarch)<br>Continue aggressive volume infusion until blood pressure normal<br>Consider early surgical hemostasis | Elevate legs<br>3 L/20 min warmed saline<br>Group/match packed RBCs and plasma *re* dilutionalo anemia<br>Continue aggressive volume infusion until blood pressure normal or heart "too full"<br>Detect and treat tamponade with pericardiocentesis, thoracostomy, peritoneal drainage, or reduced PEEP | When heart is "too full," ↓ blood volume (rotating tourniquets, phlebotomy, nitroglycerin, morphine, diuretics)<br>If the heart is not "too full," or blood pressure falls with above interventions, 0.9% NaCl 250 mL/20 min<br>Repeat if blood pressure rises until heart too full |
| | **Vasoactive Drug Therapy** | |
| Awaiting adequate volume repletion, institute multipurpose agent (dopamine or *epinephrine*) and increase dose from 1 to 10 (μg/kg/min for dopamine; μg/min for epinephrine) as needed to maintain blood pressure<br>If higher doses are needed, add norepinephrine (2–20 μg/min)<br>Discontinue these drugs as urgently as volume repletion and hemostasis allow (see middle column) | Avoid vasoactive drugs until heart "too full"<br>Except dopamine (2–5 μg/kg/min) for renal perfusion early<br>Nitroglycerin and nitroprusside are contraindicated<br>Vasoconstrictors delay repletion (see left column)<br>In right heart overload with shock, norepinephrine (2–20 μg/min) may help by maintaining RV perfusion; in septic shock, vasoconstrictors may help when adequate volume replacement provides inadequate perfusion pressure (see text) | Dobutamine (5–15 μg/kg/min) to enhance contractility without excess tachycardia, arrhythmia, or vasoconstriction; higher doses dilate skeletal vascular bed<br>Dopamine (2–5 μg/kg/min) to preserve renal cortical blood flow; at higher doses (4–12 μg/kg/min), increases heart rate, contractilitiy, venous tone, and preload, like *epinephrine*<br>Nitroglycerin (25–250 μg/min) for venodilation with minimal arterial dilation except for the coronary circulation<br>Sodium nitroprusside (0.1–5 μg/kg/min) for arterial dilation to reduce afterload and allow greater output from a depressed left ventricle or regurgitant aortic/mitral valve |

From Walley KR, Wood LDH: Shock. *In* Hall JB, Schmidt GA, Wood LDH (eds): Principles of Critical Care. New York: McGraw-Hill, 1998, p 280.
MAST = military antishock trousers; PEEP = positive end-expiratory pressure; RBCs = red blood cells; RV = right ventricular.

dynamic diagnosis and the response to vasoactive agents (i.e., an increase in cardiac output and blood pressure without excessively high or low PPW); then appropriate volume infusion or reduction can be titrated according to the measured responses of PPW and cardiac output. When these measures are addressed adequately but the hypoperfusion state persists, early treatment with arteriolar vasodilator therapy or a balloon-assist device (intra-aortic balloon pump) is indicated (Fig. 91.18). These latter interventions are not relegated to a "last resort" category but, rather, are considered early in the initial stabilization of cardiogenic shock.[76, 113]

## Hypovolemic Shock

Beyond the absence of clinical features suggesting that the heart is too full, hypovolemic shock is distinguished from cardiogenic shock by several positive clinical features.[29] Often, there is an obvious source of external bleeding (multiple trauma, hemoptysis, hematemesis, hematochezia, or melena); internal bleeding is often signaled by blood aspirated from the nasal gastric tube or on stool examination, by increasing abdominal girth, or by clinical and radiologic examination of the thoracic cavity for pleural, alveolar, or periaortic blood. Each of these is often associated with a new reduction in the hematocrit. Nonhemorrhagic hypovolemia often presents with recognizable excess gastrointestinal fluid losses (vomiting, diarrhea, suctioning, and stomas), excess renal losses (osmotic or drug diuresis, diabetes insipidus), or third space losses (as in extensive burns). Physical examination reveals dry mucous membranes with decreased tissue turgor, and the routine laboratory tests often reveal increased blood urea nitrogen out of proportion to a relatively normal creatinine level, and increased hematocrit as a result of hemoconcentration.

The initial management of patients with presumed hypovolemic shock necessitates early intravenous access

**Table 91.8** OXYGEN COST ($\dot{V}O_2$) OF BREATHING AND FEVER IN 20 CRITICALLY ILL PATIENTS*

| Breathing (Mean ± SD)[30] | | Fever (Mean ± SD)[112] | |
|---|---|---|---|
| **Mode** | $\dot{V}O_2$ | **Body Temperature** | $\dot{V}O_2$ |
| CPAP | 255 ± 92 | 39.4 ± 0.8°C | 359 ± 65 |
| AC/MR | 209 ± 79 | 37.0 ± 0.5°C | 295 ± 57 |
| $\dot{V}O_2$ resp | 46 ± 21 | $\dot{V}O_2$/°C | 27.5 ± 8.1 |

From Wood LDH: The pathophysiology and differential diagnosis of acute respiratory failure. *In* Hall JB, Schmidt GA, Wood LDH (eds): Principles of Critical Care. New York: McGraw-Hill, 1998, p 501.

AC/MR = assist-control mode with muscle relaxation (full mechanical ventilation); CPAP = continuous positive airway pressure (spontaneous breathing); $\dot{V}O_2$ = oxygen consumption (mL/min) by spirometer (Deltratrac); $\dot{V}O_2$/°C = the change in $\dot{V}O_2$ per degree centigrade change in body temperature; $\dot{V}O_2$ resp = $O_2$ cost of breathing, which equals CPAP − AC/MR.

with two large-bore (No. 14 gauge) catheters for rapid infusion of warmed blood, colloid, and crystalloid solutions for hemorrhagic shock and the appropriate crystalloid solution for dehydration. Central venous access ensures adequate volume resuscitation and allows early measurement of central venous pressure. An immediate response of increased blood pressure and pulse volume supports the presumed diagnosis, whereas no improvement in these hemodynamics necessitates emergency repair of the site of the blood loss or a reevaluation of the working diagnosis. Achieving hemostasis in hemorrhagic shock is a prerequisite for adequate volume resuscitation, but delaying fluid resuscitation until hemostasis is achieved can expose the patient to more end-organ failure, so urgent simultaneous pursuit of hemostasis and volume resuscitation is appropriate.[114] Vasoconstricting drugs such as norepinephrine should be used only as short-term (<2 hours) measures to achieve adequate perfusion pressure for vital organs (brain, heart) until adequate circulating volume is restored. Prolonged use of vasoconstricting drugs confounds the physician's assessment of the end point of volume resuscitation by providing an adequate blood pressure while inadequate cardiac output and organ perfusion persist. Accordingly, we recommend early, rapid reduction to half the norepinephrine dose as soon as the physician decides that cardiac output is adequate; a consequent fall in blood pressure indicates the urgent need for more volume, but sustained blood pressure allows a subsequent halving of the vasoconstrictor dose until it is discontinued. Early endotracheal intubation and mechanical ventilation reduce the patient's work in breathing and allow respiratory compensation for lactic acidosis; warming the fluids and covering the patient with warm, dry blankets prevent the complication of hypothermia, including cold coagulopathy and further bleeding (Table 91.9).

## Other Common Causes of Shock

The purpose of this initial schema is to formulate a working diagnosis among the most common presentations

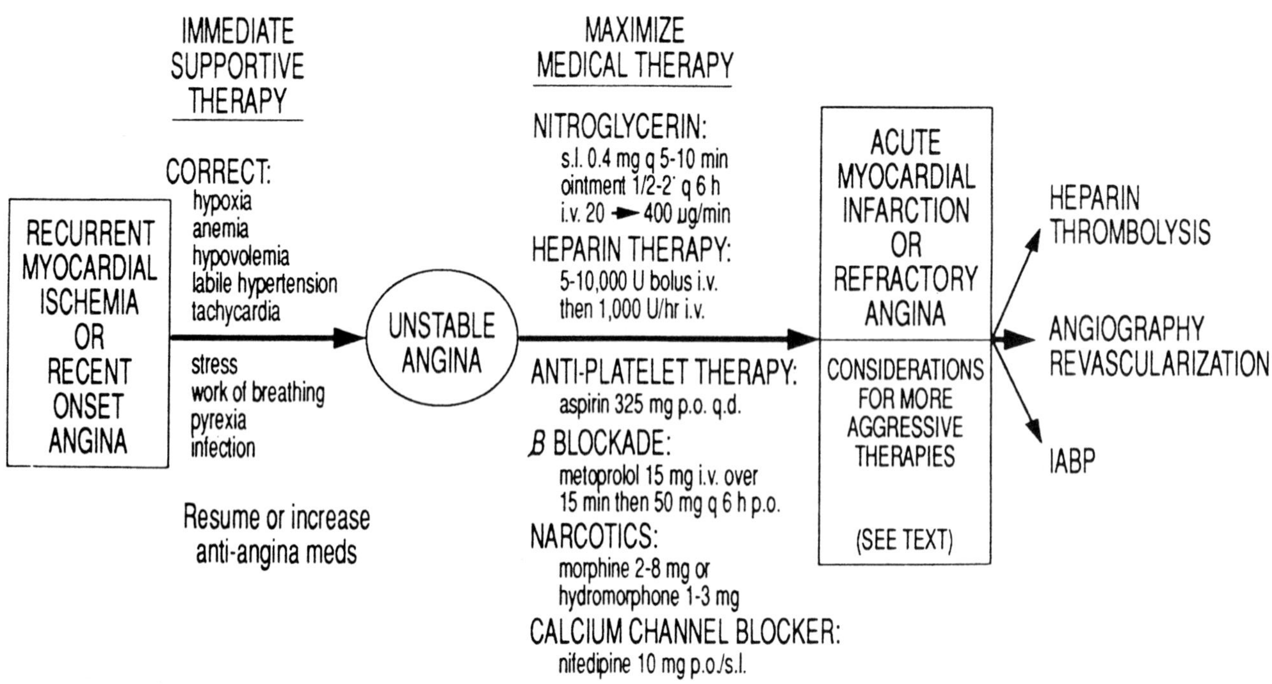


**Figure 91.18** Timeline of therapeutic modalities for myocardial ischemic syndromes. i.v. = intravenously; p.o. = orally; s.l. = sublingually. (From Hall JB, Schmidt GA, Wood LDH (eds): Principles of Critical Care. New York: McGraw-Hill, 1998, p 402.)

Table 91.9 URGENT RESUSCITATION OF THE PATIENT WITH SHOCK: MANAGING FACTORS AGGRAVATING THE HYPOPERFUSION STATE

| |
|---|
| **RESPIRATORY THERAPY** |
| Protect the airway: consider early elective intubation |
| Prevent excess respiratory work: ventilate with small volumes |
| Avoid respiratory acidosis: keep $PaCO_2$ low |
| Maintain oxygen delivery: $FI_{O_2}$, PEEP, hemoglobin |
| **INTRAVENOUS ANTIBIOSIS FOR PRESUMED SEPTIC SHOCK (EXCLUDE ALLERGIES)** |
| Empirical antimicrobial therapy for all likely microorganisms |
| Search, incise, and drain abscesses (consider laparotomy) |
| **ARRHYTHMIAS AGGRAVATING SHOCK** |
| Bradycardia (rate < 80/min in shock) |
| Correct hypoxemia: $FI_{O_2} = 1.0$ |
| Atropine 0.6 mg; repeat two times for effect |
| Increase dopamine to 10 μg/kg/min |
| Add isoproterenol, 1–4 μg/kg/min |
| Consider transvenous pacer |
| **VENTRICULAR ECTOPY, TACHYCARDIA, OR FIBRILLATION** |
| Lidocaine 1–4 mg/min |
| Detect and correct $K^+$, $Ca^{2+}$, $Mg^{3+}$ abnormalities |
| Detect and treat myocardial ischemia |
| **SUPRAVENTRICULAR TACHYCARDIA** |
| Consider defibrillation early |
| Digoxin for rate control of atrial fibrillation |
| **SINUS TACHYCARDIA >140/min** |
| Detect and treat pain and anxiety |
| Midazolam/fentanyl drip |
| Morphine |
| Detect and treat hypovolemia |
| **METABOLIC (LACTIC) ACIDOSIS** |
| Characterize to confirm anion gap without osmolal gap |
| Rule out or treat ketoacidosis, aspirin intoxication |
| Hyperventilate to keep $PaCO_2$ about 25 mm Hg |
| Calculate bicarbonate deficit and replace half if pH < 7.0 |
| Correct ionized hypocalcemia |
| Consider early dialysis |
| **HYPOTHERMIA** |
| Maintain skin dry and covered with warmed blankets |
| Warm vascular volume expanders |
| Aggressive rewarming if T < 35°C |

From Walley KR, Wood LDH: Shock. *In* Hall JB, Schmidt GA, Wood LDH (eds): Principles of Critical Care. New York: McGraw-Hill, 1998, p 284.)
PEEP, positive end-expiratory pressure; T, temperature.

of shock so that early and rapid therapy may be initiated. Then the response to the initial therapy either confirms or questions the working diagnosis. When features of the initial clinical presentation or the response of the patient to appropriate management raise questions about the working diagnosis, early acquisition of more objective hemodynamic data is encouraged to help answer the third question: What does not fit? The answer to this question often arises in other features of the clinical presentation that suggest an etiology of shock from a slightly larger differential diagnosis or from coexisting septic, cardiogenic, or hypovolemic shock (see Table 91.6). This section reviews briefly several important differential diagnostic conditions.

### Cardiac Tamponade

Although left ventricular ischemia is the most common cause of cardiogenic shock, conditions that restrict diastolic filling can produce hypoperfusion despite an apparently large heart with high diastolic pressures. Pericardial effusion is often suggested early by the clinical setting (renal failure, malignancy, chest pain), by physical examination (engorged neck veins, systolic blood pressure that falls more than 10 mm Hg on inspiration, distant heart sounds), and/or by routine investigations (chest radiograph with "water bottle" heart, low voltage on the ECG, electrical alternans). Such a constellation of clinical data requires early echocardiographic confirmation of pericardial effusion; tamponade is signaled by right ventricular and right atrial collapse, worse on inspiration, with a relatively small left ventricle.[67] Tamponade necessitates urgent pericardiocentesis or operative drainage via a pericardial window. While the definitive treatment is awaited, intravenous expansion of the circulating volume may produce small increases in blood pressure, whereas reductions in circulating volume (diuretics, nitroglycerin, morphine, intercurrent hemodialysis) are often associated with a catastrophic decrease in the cardiac output by reducing the venous tone and volume necessary to maintain the Pms required to drive venous return back against the high right atrial pressure.

Right-sided heart catheterization typically reveals a right atrial pressure increased to about 16 to 20 mm Hg and equal to both the pulmonary artery diastolic pressure and the pulmonary artery wedge pressure; cardiac output and stroke volume are much reduced.[67] This hemodynamic subset resembles that of cardiogenic shock (high PPW, low stroke volume). However, in the case of pericardial tamponade, PPW is increased because pericardial pressure is increased, so the transmural pressure of the left ventricle approaches zero, a value consistent with the very low LVEDV that accounts for the low stroke volume. Other etiologies of hypotension associated with high cardiac pressures and small ventricular volumes include constrictive pericarditis, tension pneumothorax, massive pleural effusion, positive-pressure ventilation with high PEEP, and very high intra-abdominal pressure. Up to one third of patients presenting with cardiac tamponade have increased blood pressure despite low cardiac output; this subset of patients has a high incidence of hypertension preceding the onset of tamponade.[115]

### Right Ventricular Overload and Infarction

Another clinical presentation that may simulate cardiogenic shock is the hypotension associated with acute or acute-on-chronic pulmonary hypertension (see Table 91.5). Shock that follows acute pulmonary embolism is often signaled by the clinical setting, including risk factors (recent surgery, immobilization, hypercoagulable state, prior thromboembolic events); symptoms of acute dyspnea, chest pain, or hemoptysis; physical examination revealing a loud P2 with a widened and fixed split of the second heart sound; new hypoxemia without obvious radiologic explanation; and acute right-sided heart strain on the ECG.[71] Noninvasive Doppler studies of the veins in the lower extremities, ventilation-perfusion scans, and spinal computed tomographic scans, or pulmonary angiograms confirm the diagnosis (see also Chapter 51). Heparin or placement of a filter in the inferior vena cava reduces the incidence of subsequent emboli, and some success occurs with thrombolytic therapy (or, rarely, surgical removal of the embolus) in patients with shock due to pulmonary embolism.[116] Right-sided heart catheterization reveals a unique hemodynamic profile: a very high mean pulmonary artery pressure, a pulmonary artery diastolic pressure considerably greater than the wedge pressure, and reduced cardiac output and stroke volume. Not uncommonly, the pulmonary artery wedge pressure is normal or increased despite a small LVEDV on echocardiographic examination, which also reveals right-to-left shift of the interventricular septum; presumably, this causes flattening of the diastolic volume-pressure curve of the left ventricle.

Therapy for shock due to pulmonary embolism begins with dobutamine, which increases cardiac output, blood pressure, and mixed venous $O_2$ saturation in patients.[71, 117, 118] Studies of experimental pulmonary embolism in dogs suggest that norepinephrine can increase cardiac output further by improving the perfusion pressure and oxygenation of the loaded right ventricle.[119] Potential salutary effects of intravenous vasodilators (hydralazine, nitroprusside, prostaglandin $E_1$, prostacyclin) on pulmonary hypertension are often confounded by worse systemic hypotension and right ventricular ischemia; it is conceivable that inhaled nitric oxide[120] or prostacyclin[121] may cause pulmonary vasodilation in patients with pulmonary embolism, as has been demonstrated in some patients with chronic pulmonary hypertension. Fluid therapy has deleterious effects in animal models of pulmonary embolism[119] and in patients with right ventricular infarction.[122, 123] However, some patients with shock due to pulmonary embolism or right ventricular infarction may be relatively hypovolemic, so a discrete volume challenge (250 mL of isotonic saline in 10 minutes) can be a diagnostic trial; an immediate increase in blood pressure, pulse pressure, cardiac output, and urine output confirms relative hypovolemia and suggests a further cautious fluid challenge, whereas no benefit suggests no further fluid challenge. Right ventricular infarction causes low pulmonary artery pressures in the presence of normal left ventricular filling pressures as the dilated, injured right ventricle is unable to maintain adequate flow to the left side of the heart. Engorgement of neck veins and PRA tend to decrease with dobutamine infusion, perhaps because the enhanced contractility of the left ventricle improves systolic function of the mechanically interdependent right ventricle.[122, 123]

Acute-on-chronic pulmonary hypertension causes shock in the setting of prior primary pulmonary hypertension, recurrent pulmonary emboli, progression of collagen vascular disease, or chronic respiratory failure (chronic obstructive pulmonary disease, pulmonary fibrosis) aggravated in part by hypoxic pulmonary vasoconstriction. In these circumstances, oxygen therapy and pulmonary vasodilator therapy (sodium nitroprusside, prostacyclin) combine to reduce pulmonary hypertension and increase cardiac output in a significant number of patients.[71, 116, 117] The adverse effects of systemic hypotension have been prevented by inhaled prostacyclin.[121] In ARDS, inhaled nitric oxide decreases pulmonary vascular resistance and increases cardiac output, arterial oxygenation, and oxygen delivery.[120, 124] The effect of inhaled nitric oxide on oxygenation is enhanced by the concomitant administration of almitrine bismesylate (a specific pulmonary vasoconstrictor).[124a] However, these modest effects on oxygenation last less than 72 hours[125] and do not indicate favorable outcomes regarding mortality or the number of days alive and off mechanical ventilation.[126] Accordingly, we administer inhaled nitric oxide as experimental therapy for right heart syndromes, acknowledging that it may do more harm than good.[127]

## Anaphylactic, Neurogenic, and Adrenal Shock

Other etiologies of shock have unique clinical presentations that distinguish those forms of shock from hypovolemic shock. Beyond identifying the etiology early through their association with triggering agents and trauma, the physician should note that the pathophysiology of anaphylaxis and neurogenic shock, respectively, is a dilated venous bed with greatly increased unstressed volume of the circulation leading to hypovolemic shock. Accordingly, the mainstay of therapy for both conditions is adequate volume infusion; adjunctive therapy for anaphylaxis includes antihistamines, steroids, and epinephrine to antagonize the mediators released in the anaphylactic reaction,[128] whereas a careful search for sources of blood loss and hemorrhagic shock is part of the early resuscitation of spinal shock in the traumatized patient.[29]

Not uncommonly, the presentation of patients with nonhemorrhagic hypovolemic shock raises the question of acute adrenal cortical insufficiency. When that possibility is not obviously excluded, it is appropriate to draw a serum cortisol level, provide adequate circulating steroids with dexamethasone, and, later, conduct an adrenocorticotropic hormone stimulation test to confirm or refute the diagnosis. Characteristically, the hypotension and hypoperfusion in such patients do not respond to adequate vascular volume expansion until the dexamethasone is administered.

## Multiple Etiologies of Shock

With this differential diagnosis and management evaluation in mind, the initial approach to patients with hypoperfusion states should be completed in less time than it takes to read about it. The target is to distinguish among septic shock, cardiogenic shock, and hypovolemic shock and to initiate an appropriate therapeutic challenge: antibiotics, inotropic agents, a volume challenge within 30 minutes of presentation, or all of these. From judging the response, the diagnosis is confirmed or questioned, with special regard to equivocal responses to therapy or to several other diagnostic categories of shock. The next stage of diagnosis and management may be aided by right-sided heart catheterization to confirm objectively the relationship between wedge pressure and cardiac output or to exclude errors in the initial diagnosis and management. For example, a 70-year-old woman becomes hypotensive in the immediate postoperative period after internal fixation of a recent fracture of the femur. Vague chest discomfort and ischemic changes on the ECG suggest cardiogenic shock, so dobutamine and dopamine are initiated, but they produce no improvement in the hemodynamic status. A right-sided heart catheter is inserted and reveals a cardiac output of 2.5 L/min with a wedge pressure of 3 mm Hg. An intravenous infusion of 1 L saline raises the blood pressure 10 mm Hg without raising the wedge pressure much, and the patient responds to continued transfusions of 6 units whole blood while an unusually large hemorrhage at the operative site is drained and packed.

This clinical vignette is characteristic of the overlapping clinical presentations between the major diagnostic categories of shock. Sorting out the primary etiology of the hypoperfusion state often requires considerable additional data. Indeed, this process is rendered more complex by concurrent etiologies contributing to the shock (e.g., as in the patient with septic shock who, because of intercurrent myocardial dysfunction, is unable to increase cardiac output; the patient with acute myocardial infarction who is hypovolemic; or the patient with hemorrhagic shock who becomes septic). Other combinations of these major categories overlap with confounding effects of tamponade, positive-pressure ventilation, pneumothorax, and pulmonary hypertension, all of which challenge the ongoing diagnostic and management approaches. Nonetheless, complete interpretation of data from right-sided heart catheterization and echocardiography complements the changing physical examination to provide an early move toward the correct diagnosis and management of shock. Management of associated conditions aggravating the hypoperfusion state is summarized in Table 91.9.[29]

## Approach to Inadequate Blood Transport of Oxygen

Patients with respiratory failure are susceptible to anaerobic metabolism because of the delivery of inadequate oxygen to meet the metabolic needs of their systemic organs.[130] During air breathing, arterialized blood leaves normal alveoli with an arterial $P_{O_2}$ of about 100 mm Hg. When the hemoglobin concentration is 15 g/dL, arterial oxygen content ($Ca_{O_2}$) is about 20 mL/dL of blood, 19.7 mL/dL carried by the nearly completely saturated hemoglobin (98%), and about 0.3 mL/dL in physical solution. Accordingly, a cardiac output of 5.0 L/min transports 1000 mL/min of oxygen to the tissues ($\dot{Q}_{O_2}$). There, tissue metabolism ($\dot{V}_{O_2}$) extracts 250 mL/min, so the 5.0 L/min of mixed venous blood flow to the lungs returns with 750 mL/min of oxygen, or a mixed venous oxygen content ($C\bar{v}_{O_2}$) of 15 mL/dL blood; accordingly, the normal extraction fraction (which is equal to $\dot{V}_{O_2}/\dot{Q}_{O_2} = [Ca_{O_2} - C\bar{v}_{O_2}]/Ca_{O_2}$) is 0.25. Because this oxygen content corresponds to 75% oxygen saturation (15 mL/dL ÷ 20 mL/dL × 100), mixed venous $P_{O_2}$ is 40 mm Hg, as determined by the oxyhemoglobin dissociation curve for mixed venous pH, $P_{CO_2}$, and temperature. Figure 91.19 plots the relationships between oxygen consumption ($\dot{V}_{O_2}$, left ordinate) and extraction fraction (right ordinate) with oxygen delivery ($\dot{Q}_{O_2}$, abscissa); when these values are normalized to a body size of about 65 kg, $\dot{V}_{O_2}$ is 4 mL/kg per minute and $\dot{Q}_{O_2}$ is 16 mL/kg per minute, as plotted on the continuous lines.

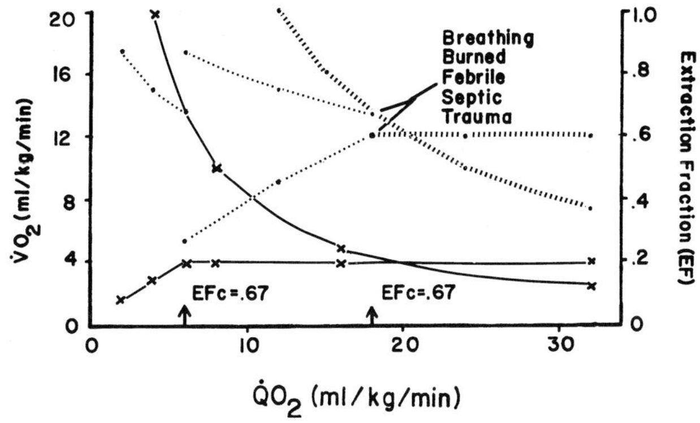


**Figure 91.19** Oxygen consumption ($\dot{V}O_2$ in figure, left ordinate) and oxygen extraction fraction (EF, right ordinate) are plotted against oxygen delivery ($\dot{Q}O_2$) (abscissa). In patients with normal metabolism *(continuous lines through Xs)*, $\dot{V}O_2$ (4 mL/kg/min) is maintained as $\dot{Q}O_2$ is decreased from 16 to 6 mL/kg/min because EF increases from 0.25 to 0.67. At lower $\dot{Q}O_2$, $\dot{V}O_2$ decreases as a result of anaerobic metabolism that leads to lactic acidemia, because EF can no longer increase sufficiently, as indicated by the dotted line departing from the continuous hyperbolic EF-$\dot{Q}O_2$ line at the critical extraction fraction (EFc) (EFc = 0.67). When $\dot{V}O_2$ is tripled *(interrupted lines through closed circles)* by one of several common manifestations of critical illness (work of breathing, burns, fever, sepsis, and trauma), EF is tripled at every value of $\dot{Q}O_2$, and supply dependence of oxygen consumption begins at a value of $\dot{Q}O_2$ three times greater than for the patient with normal $\dot{V}O_2$ despite a normal EFc of 0.67. Accordingly, $\dot{Q}O_2$ must increase with $\dot{V}O_2$ to maintain aerobic metabolism, or $\dot{V}O_2$ must be reduced. For further discussion, see text. (From Hall JB, Schmidt GA, Wood LDH (eds): Principles of Critical Care. New York: McGraw-Hill, 1998, p 500.)

In many patients with respiratory failure, the oxygen transport to the tissues is reduced by abnormally low cardiac output, hemoglobin, or oxygen saturation. Consider the effects of acute myocardial injury, which reduces cardiac output to 2.5 L/min and oxygen delivery to 8 mL/kg per min. To maintain the oxygen uptake necessary for aerobic metabolism under these conditions, the tissues must extract 250 mL/min from half the blood flow, so $C\bar{v}_{O_2}$ decreases to 10 mL/dL blood and extraction fraction increases to 0.50. Because this value corresponds to 50% saturation of the normal hemoglobin concentration, mixed venous $P_{O_2}$ decreases to 27 mm Hg. When cardiac output returns toward normal with vasoactive drug therapy, extent that pathologic supply dependence does not occur in patients[102, 135] and that the lactic acidosis of sepsis is not anaerobic,[100, 101] the common critical care practice of maximizing cardiac output and oxygen delivery confers no benefit on oxygen use.[104, 105] Even in the apparent absence of sepsis, the value of mixed venous $Po_2$ at the onset of anaerobic metabolism varies widely.[132, 133] Accordingly, measuring and monitoring changes in mixed venous $Po_2$ and venous saturation in conjunction with acid-base status and lactic acid measurements allow deductions concerning the effects of altered oxygen delivery on oxygen consumption and aerobic metabolism, but these are nonspecific and subject to errors and uncertainties. More definitive assessment is needed and may come from new, innovative, organ-specific indices of inadequate perfusion and oxygenation.[136]

## SUMMARY

The appropriate management of respiratory failure rests on identification and reversal of the underlying pathophysiologic factors eventuating in critical illness. Accordingly, we have outlined in this chapter the four major types of respiratory failure, describing how each may result in failure of respiratory gas exchange. We have specifically included hypoperfusion states that can cause respiratory failure, because mechanical ventilatory support in this setting may be viewed as adjunctive to the patient's underlying shock. Indeed, this form of respiratory failure highlights the need to understand the interactions between respiration and circulation. This understanding is crucial for the critical care physician to resuscitate the unstable patient, to treat various forms of shock, to stabilize the circulation once positive-pressure ventilation is undertaken, to treat effectively pulmonary edema and the consequent hypoxemic respiratory failure, and to provide a rational approach to inadequate blood transport of oxygen. The general schema outlined in this chapter is discussed at length in Chapters 92 and 93.

## References


1. Hall JB, Schmidt GA, Wood LDH: An approach to critical care. *In* Hall JB, Schmidt GA, Wood LDH (eds): Principles of Critical Care. New York: McGraw-Hill, 1998, pp 3–9.
2. Wood LDH: The pathophysiology and differential diagnosis of acute respiratory failure. *In* Hall JB, Schmidt GA, Wood LDH (eds): Principles of Critical Care. New York: McGraw-Hill, 1998, pp 499–508.
3. Dantzker RM: Gas exchange in the adult respiratory distress syndrome. Clin Chest Med 3:57–67, 1982.
4. Wagner P, Dantzker D, Dueck D, et al: Ventilation-perfusion inequality in chronic obstructive pulmonary disease. J Clin Invest 59:203–216, 1977.
5. Torres A, Reyes A, Roca J, et al: Ventilation-perfusion mismatching in chronic obstructive pulmonary disease during ventilator weaning. Am Rev Respir Dis 140:1246–1250, 1989.
6. Rodriquez-Roisin R, Ballester E, Roca J, et al: Mechanisms of hypoxemia in patients with status asthmaticus requiring mechanical ventilation. Am Rev Respir Dis 139:732–739, 1989.
7. Ferrer A, Roca J, Wagner PD, et al: Airway obstruction and ventilation-perfusion relationships in acute severe asthma. Am Rev Respir Dis 147:579–584, 1993.
8. Agusti AGN, Roca J, Gea J, et al: Mechanisms of gas exchange impairment in idiopathic pulmonary fibrosis. Am Rev Respir Dis 143:219–225, 1991.
9. Roussos C: Respiratory muscle fatigue and ventilatory failure. *In* Hall JB, Schmidt GA, Wood LDH (eds): Principles of Critical Care. New York: McGraw-Hill, 1992, pp 1701–1709.
10. Polese G, Rossi A, Appendini L, et al: Partitioning of respiratory mechanics in mechanically ventilated patients. J Appl Physiol 71:2435–2443, 1991.
11. Gattinoni L, Pelosi P, Crotti S, et al: Effects of positive end-expiratory pressure on regional distribution of tidal volume and recruitment in adult respiratory distress syndrome. Am J Respir Crit Care Med 151:1807–1814, 1995.
12. Marini JJ: Evolving concepts in the ventilatory management of acute respiratory distress syndrome. Clin Chest Med 17:555–556, 1996.
13. Corbridge TE, Hall JB: The assessment and management of adults with status asthmaticus. Am J Respir Crit Care Med 151:1296–1316, 1995.
14. Schmidt GA, Hall JB: Acute on chronic respiratory failure: Assessment and management of patients with COPD in the emergent setting. JAMA 261:3444–3453, 1989.
15. Corbridge T, Wood LDH: Restrictive disease of the respiratory system. *In* Hall JB, Schmidt GA, Wood LDH (eds): Principles of Critical Care. New York: McGraw-Hill, 1998, pp 595–608.
16. O'Connor MF, Hall JB, Schmidt GA, et al: Acute hypoxemic respiratory failure. *In* Hall JB, Schmidt GA, Wood LDH (eds): Principles of Critical Care. New York: McGraw-Hill, 1998, pp 537–564.
17. Hickling KG, Walsh J, Handerson S, et al: Low mortality rate in adult respiratory distress syndrome using low volume, pressure limited ventilation with permissive hypercapnia: A prospective study. Crit Care Med 22:1568–1578, 1994.
18. Thorens JB, Jolliet P, Ritz M, et al: Effects of rapid permissive hypercapnia on hemodynamics, gas exchange, and oxygen transport and consumption during mechanical ventilation for the acute respiratory distress syndrome. Intensive Care Med 22:182–191, 1996.
19. Amato MRP, Barbases V, Medeiros DM, et al: Effect of a protective-ventilation strategy on mortality in the acute respiratory distress syndrome. N Engl J Med 338:347–354, 1998.
20. Sznajder JI, Nahum A, Hansen DE, et al: Volume recruitment and oxygenation in pulmonary edema. J Crit Care 13:126–135, 1998.
21. Humphrey H, Hall J, Sznajder JI, et al: Improved survival in ARDS patients associated with a reduction in pulmonary capillary wedge pressure. Chest 97:1176–1180, 1990.
22. Mitchel JP, Schuller D, Callandrino FS, et al: Improved outcome based on fluid management in critically ill patients requiring pulmonary artery catheterization. Am J Respir Crit Care Med 145:990–998, 1992.
23. Hedenstierna G: Mechanisms of postoperative pulmonary dysfunction. Acta Chir Scand Suppl 550:152–158, 1989.
24. Ali J: Special considerations in the surgical patient. *In* Hall JB, Schmidt GA, Wood LDH (eds): Principles of Critical Care. New York: McGraw-Hill, 1998, pp 1289–1299.
25. Pelosi P, D'Andrea L, Vitale G, et al: Vertical gradient of regional lung inflation in adult respiratory distress syndrome. Am J Respir Crit Care Med 149:8–13, 1994.
26. Ranieri VM, Brienza N, Santostasi S, et al: Impairment of lung and chest wall mechanics in patients with acute respiratory distress syndrome: Role of abdominal distention. Am J Respir Crit Care Med 156:1082–1091, 1997.
27. Pelosi P, Croci M, Colappi E, et al: Prone positioning during general anesthesia minimally affects respiratory mechanics while improving functional residual capacity and increasing oxygen tension. Anesth Analg 80:955–960, 1995.
28. Albert RK: The prone position in acute respiratory distress syndrome: Where we are, and where do we go from here? Crit Care Med 25:1453–1454, 1997.
29. Walley KR, Wood LDH: Shock. *In* Hall JB, Schmidt GA, Wood LDH (eds): Principles of Critical Care. New York: McGraw-Hill, 1998, pp 277–301.
30. Manthous CA, Hall JB, Kushner R, et al: The effect of mechanical ventilation on oxygen consumption in critically ill patients. Am J Respir Crit Care Med 151:210–214, 1995.
31. Ward ME, Magder SA, Hussain SNA: Oxygen delivery–independent effect of blood flow on diaphragm fatigue. Am Rev Respir Dis 145:1058–1063, 1992.

32. Roussos CS, Macklem PT: Diaphragmatic fatigue in man. J Appl Physiol 43:189–197, 1977.
33. Respiratory Muscle Fatigue Workshop Group: NHLBI Workshop Summary: Respiratory muscle fatigue. Am Rev Respir Dis 142:474–480, 1990.
34. Zocchi L, Fitting JW, Majani U, et al: Effect of pressure and timing contraction on human rib cage muscle fatigue. Am Rev Respir Dis 147:857–864, 1993.
35. Mador MJ: Respiratory muscle fatigue and breathing pattern. Chest 100:1430–1435, 1991.
36. Yang KL, Tobin MJ: A prospective study of indexes predicting the outcome of trials of weaning from mechanical ventilation. N Engl J Med 324:1445–1450, 1991.
37. Chatila W, Jacob B, Guanglione L, et al: The unassisted respiratory rate/tidal volume ratio accurately predicts weaning outcome. Am J Med 101:61–67, 1996.
38. Manthous CA, Schmidt GA, Hall JB: Liberation from mechanical ventilation: A decade of progress. Chest 114:886–901, 1998.
39. Viires N, Sillie G, Aubier A, et al: Regional blood flow distribution in dogs during induced hypotension and low cardiac output: Spontaneous breathing versus artificial ventilation. J Clin Invest 72:935–947, 1983.
40. Jubran A, Tobin MJ: Pathophysiologic basis of acute respiratory distress in patients who fail a trial of weaning from mechanical ventilation. Am J Respir Crit Care Med 155:906–915, 1997.
41. Yanos J, Keamy MF, Leisk L, et al: The mechanisms of respiratory arrest in inspiratory loading and hypoxemia. Am Rev Respir Dis 141:933–937, 1990.
42. Yanos J, Wood LDH, Davis K, et al: The effects of respiratory and lactic acidosis on diaphragm function. Am Rev Respir Dis 147:616–619, 1993.
43. Talpers SS, Romberger DJ, Bunce SB, et al: Nutritionally associated increased carbon dioxide production. Chest 102:551–555, 1992.
44. Aubier M, Murciano D, Lecocguic Y, et al: Hypophosphatemia-associated respiratory muscle weakness in a general inpatient population. Am J Med 84:870–876, 1988.
45. Dhingra S, Solven F, Wilson A, et al. Hypomagnesemia and respiratory muscle power. Am Rev Respir Dis 129:497–498, 1984.
46. Murciano D, Aubier M, Lecocquic Y, et al: Effects of theophylline on diaphragmatic strength and fatigue in patients with chronic obstructive pulmonary disease. N Engl J Med 311:349–353, 1984.
47. Kupfer Y, Namba T, Kaldawi E, et al: Prolonged weakness after a long-term infusion of vecuronium bromide. Ann Intern Med 117:484–486, 1992.
48. Williams TJ, O'Hehir RE, Czarny D, et al: Acute myopathy in severe asthma treated with intravenously administered corticosteroids. Am Rev Respir Dis 137:460–463, 1988.
49. Esteban A, Frutos F, Tobin MJ, et al: A comparison of four methods of weaning patients from mechanical ventilation. N Engl J Med 332:345–350, 1995.
50. Brochard L, Rauss A, Benito S, et al: Comparison of three methods of gradual withdrawal from ventilatory support during weaning from mechanical ventilation. Am J Respir Crit Care Med 150:896–903, 1994.
51. Nava S, Ambrosino N, Clini E, et al: Noninvasive mechanical ventilation in the weaning of patients with respiratory failure due to chronic obstructive pulmonary disease. A randomized controlled trial. Ann Intern Med 128:721–728, 1998.
52. Goldberg HS, Rabson J: Control of cardiac output by systemic vessels. Am J Cardiol 47:696–702, 1981.
53. Wood LDH: The pathophysiology of the circulation in critical illness. *In* Hall JB, Schmidt GA, Wood LDH (eds): Principles of Critical Care. New York: McGraw-Hill, 1998, pp 259–276.
54. Mitzner W, Goldberg HS: Effects of epinephrine on resistive and compliant properties of the canine vasculature. J Appl Physiol 39:272–280, 1975.
55. Malo J, Goldberg HS, Graham R, et al: Effect of hypoxic hypoxia on systemic vasculature. J Appl Physiol 54:1403–1410, 1984.
56. Mitzner W, Goldberg HS, Lichtenstein S: Effect of thoracic blood volume changes on steady state cardiac output. Circ Res 38:255–261, 1976.
57. Fermoso JD, Richardson QT, Guyton AC: Mechanism of decrease in cardiac output caused by opening the chest. Am J Physiol 207:1112–1116, 1964.
58. Fessler HE, Brower RG, Wise RA, et al: Effects of positive end-expiratory pressure on the gradient for venous return. Am Rev Respir Dis 143:19–24, 1991.
59. Prewitt RM, Wood LDH: The effect of positive end-expiratory pressure on ventricular function in dogs. Am J Physiol 45:H534–H544, 1979.
60. Prewitt RM, Oppenheimer L, Sutherland JB, et al: The effects of positive end-expiratory pressure on left ventricular mechanics in patients with hypoxemic respiratory failure. Anesthesiology 55:409–415, 1981.
61. Pinsky MR, Desmet J-M, Vincent J: Effect of positive end-expiratory pressure on right ventricular function in humans. Am Rev Respir Dis 146:681–687, 1992.
62. Craven KD, Wood LDH: Extrapericardial and esophageal pressures with positive end expiratory pressure in dogs. J Appl Physiol 51:798–805, 1981.
63. Malo J, Ali J, Wood LDH: How does positive end-expiratory pressure reduce intrapulmonary shunt in canine pulmonary edema? J Appl Physiol 57:1002–1010, 1984.
64. Pare PD, Warriner E, Baile M, et al: Redistribution of pulmonary extravascular lung water with positive end-expiratory pressure in canine pulmonary edema. Am Rev Respir Dis 127:590–593, 1983.
65. Pinsky M, Vincent J-L, Desmet J-M: Estimating left ventricular filling pressure during positive end-expiratory pressure in humans. Am Rev Respir Dis 143:25–31, 1991.
66. Sarnoff SJ: Myocardial contractility as described by ventricular function curves: Observations on Starling's law of the heart. Physiol Rev 35:107–122, 1955.
67. Teplinsky K: Pericardial disease. *In* Hall JB, Schmidt GA, Wood LDH (eds): Principles of Critical Care. New York: McGraw-Hill, 1998, pp 451–466.
68. Spencer KT, Lang RM: Diastolic heart failure. Postgrad Med 101:63–73, 1997.
69. Lenihan DJ, Gerhson MC, Hoit BD, et al: Mechanisms, diagnosis and treatment of diastolic heart failure. Am Heart J 130:153–166, 1995.
70. Taylor RRR, Coveld JW, Sonnenblick EH, et al: Dependence of ventricular distensibility on filling of the opposite ventricle. Am J Physiol 213:711–718, 1967.
71. Schmidt GA, Wood LDH: Acute right heart syndromes. *In* Hall JB, Schmidt GA, Wood LDH (eds): Principles of Critical Care. New York: McGraw-Hill, 1998, pp 417–425.
72. Sagawa K: End-systolic pressure-volume relationship in retrospect and prospect. Fed Proc 43:2399–2401, 1984.
73. Walley KR, Becker CJ, Hogan RA, et al: Progressive hypoxemia limits left ventricular oxygen consumption and contractility. Circ Res 63:849–859, 1988.
74. Walley KR, Lewis TH, Wood LDH: Acute respiratory acidosis decreases left ventricular contractility but increases cardiac output. Circ Res 67:628–635, 1990.
75. Walley KR, Ford LE, Wood LDH: Effects of hypoxia and hypercapnia on the force-velocity relationship of rabbit myocardial muscle. Circ Res 69:1616–1625, 1991.
76. Barron JT, Parrillo JE: Myocardial ischemia. *In* Hall JB, Schmidt GA, Wood LDH (eds): Principles of Critical Care. New York: McGraw-Hill, 1998, pp 397–416.
77. Walley KR, Wood LDH: Ventricular dysfunction in critical illness. *In* Hall JB, Schmidt GA, Wood LDH (eds): Principles of Critical Care. New York: McGraw-Hill, 1998, pp 303–321.
78. Sasayoma S: Inotropic agents in the treatment of heart failure. Cardiovasc Drugs Ther 10:703–709, 1997.
79. Annane D, Bellisant E, Pussard E, et al: Placebo-controlled randomized, double-blind study of intravenous enalaprilat: Efficacy and safety in acute cardiogenic pulmonary edema. Circulation 94:1316–1324, 1996.
80. Carroll JD, Lang RM, Neuman AL, et al: The differential effects of positive inotropic and vasodilator therapy on diastolic properties in patients with congestive cardiomyopathy. Circulation 74:815–825, 1985.
81. Sorrentino MJ: Valvular heart disease. *In* Hall JB, Schmidt GA, Wood LDH (eds): Principles of Critical Care. New York: McGraw-Hill, 1998, pp 467–481.

# 92 Acute Hypoxemic Respiratory Failure

JESSE B. HALL, M.D. • GREGORY A. SCHMIDT, M.D.
LAWRENCE D. H. WOOD, M.D., PH.D.

Introduction
Classification
Diffuse AHRF: Pulmonary Edema
Diffuse AHRF: Alveolar Hemorrhage
Focal AHRF
Overlap of Diffuse and Focal AHRF
Clinical Presentation
Determining the Cause Pulmonary Edema
Defining and Scoring ARDS
Treatment of AHRF
Management of Cardiogenic Pulmonary Edema
Treatment of ARDS
Summary

## INTRODUCTION

Type I or acute hypoxemic respiratory failure (AHRF) arises from diseases causing collapse or filling of alveoli (or both) with the result that a substantial fraction of mixed venous blood traverses nonventilated air spaces, effecting a right-to-left intrapulmonary shunt[1] (Fig. 92.1; see Chapters 4 and 91). In addition to the adverse consequences on gas exchange, interstitial and alveolar fluid accumulation causes an increase in lung stiffness, imposing a mechanical load with a resulting increase in the work of breathing.[2] Uncorrected, the gas exchange and lung mechanical abnormalities may eventuate in tissue hypoxia, respiratory arrest, and death.[3]

The goals of this chapter are to classify the disorders that typically cause this pathophysiologic sequence of events; to describe the clinical presentation of this form of respiratory failure, including methods to assess the severity of underlying disease and the cause of pulmonary edema; and to explain in detail the principles of management that seek the end points of (1) correction of inadequate oxygen delivery and tissue hypoxia, (2) appropriate manipulation of the ventilator to reduce intrapulmonary shunt while avoiding the adverse consequences of ventilator-associated lung injury, barotrauma, oxygen toxicity, and diminished venous return, and (3) reduction and clearance of air space liquid without adverse consequences on oxygen delivery.

## CLASSIFICATION

As a first approximation, the disorders causing AHRF may be divided into diffuse lesions, such as pulmonary edema, and focal lung lesions, such as lobar pneumonia (Table 92.1). Because the distribution of air space involvement can have implications for the response to interventions such as positive end-expiratory pressure (PEEP),[4–6] this nosology is of both therapeutic and didactic value.

### Diffuse AHRF: Pulmonary Edema

As discussed elsewhere (see Chapters 4, 6, and 54), lung liquid flux is determined by the conductance of the pulmonary microcirculation and the accompanying driving pressure. Accordingly, excessive lung liquid accumulation may arise from hydrostatic pressure increases, leading to *cardiogenic* or *increased-pressure* edema, or from lung injury that causes an increase in conductance and a failure of the microcirculation to maintain an oncotic pressure gradient between the intravascular and interstitial spaces, which causes *increased-permeability edema* or the *acute* (formerly *adult*) *respiratory distress syndrome* (ARDS).

Cardiogenic edema most commonly arises when left ventricular end-diastolic pressure increases, as in left ventricular failure or with myocardial ischemia.[7] Less common causes of increased-pressure edema are mechanical obstruction at the level of the mitral orifice (e.g., mitral stenosis, ball-valve obstruction), which causes left atrial pressure elevation, and mitral valve incompetence with transmission of ventricular pressures to the lung circulation during systole. In the setting of critical illness, often with multiple factors contributing to impaired ventricular function or impaired renal water excretion, volume "overload" with increased hydrostatic pressure may occur. This may be encountered even without exogenous fluid administration, as when a veno-constricting drug or the Trendelenburg position results in translocation of intravascular volume from the peripheral circulation to the central compartment.

Increased-permeability pulmonary edema, also termed pulmonary capillary leak or ARDS when the condition is encountered clinically, results from injury to the lung microcirculation sustained via direct lung insults (e.g., aspiration, inhalation, infectious agents) or indirectly via systemic processes (e.g., sepsis, traumatic shock with large-volume blood product resuscitation).[8, 9] Regardless of the initiating event, the result is extravasation of fluid and protein into the interstitium (and eventually into the alveolar spaces) despite normal microvascular hydrostatic and oncotic pressures.

In cases of ARDS, it is useful to distinguish between the early phases of acute lung injury and the events that occur later[10, 11] (Fig. 92.2; see Chapter 54). By light microscopy, the early appearance is of flooding of the lung interstitium and alveoli with proteinaceous fluid with minimal evidence of cellular injury. By electron microscopy, changes of endothelial cell swelling, widening of intercellular junctions, increased numbers of pinocytotic vesicles, and disruption and denudation of the basement membrane are prominent. Some inflammatory cell infiltration of the lung interstitium may be seen (particularly in ARDS complicating sepsis or trauma), but it is often a subtle finding. This early phase of diffuse alveolar damage has been termed *exudative,* and it is a period during which pulmonary edema and its effects are most pronounced and manipulations to affect the rate of edemagenesis are most likely to have impact (see later discussion).

Over the ensuing days, hyaline membrane formation in the alveolar spaces is prominent, attributed to precipitation of serum proteins. Inflammatory cells become more numerous within the lung interstitium. As the process of alveolar damage progresses, there is extensive necrosis of type I alveolar epithelial cells. The latter phase of diffuse parenchymal injury is dominated by disordered healing. This can occur as early as 7 to 10 days after initial injury and may result in extensive pulmonary fibrosis. This has been termed the *proliferative* phase of diffuse alveolar damage, and it appears to involve abnormal collagen

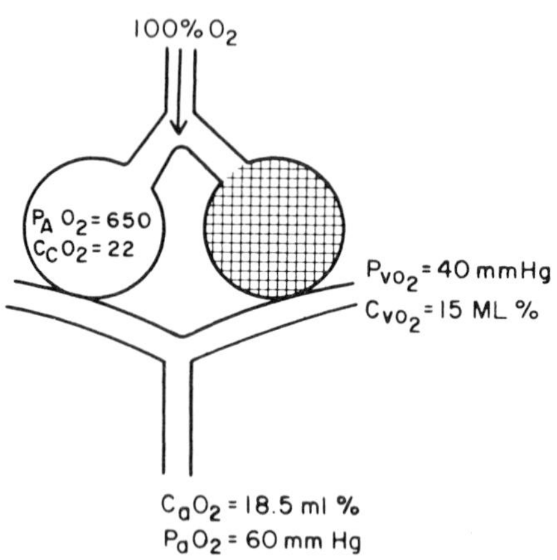


**Figure 92.1** Cartoon of a two-compartment model of lung perfusion and ventilation demonstrating the basis for gas exchange failure in acute hypoxemic respiratory failure. When large portions of the lung are nonventilated because of alveolar collapse or flooding (hatched area), blood flow to these units with a mixed venous $Po_2$ of 40 mm Hg and content of 15% by volume is effectively "shunted" through the lungs without the occurrence of resaturation. Therefore, despite a high concentration of supplemental oxygen (100% in this example) and a high alveolar $Po_2$ ($P_AO_2$ in figure) in ventilated units, these blood flows mix in accord with their contents. In this example of a 50% shunt, the result is systemic arterial hypoxemia with an arterial $Po_2$ ($P_aO_2$ in figure) of 60 mm Hg. $C_aO_2$ = arterial content of oxygen; $C_cO_2$ = content of end-capillary blood; $Cvo_2$ = content of mixed venous blood.

**Table 92.1 CAUSES OF ACUTE HYPOXEMIC RESPIRATORY FAILURE**

| |
|---|
| **Homogenous Lung Lesions (Producing Pulmonary Edema)** |
| Cardiogenic or increased-pressure edema |
| Left-ventricular (LV) failure |
| Acute LV ischemia |
| Accelerated or malignant hypertension |
| Mitral regurgitation |
| Mitral stenosis |
| Ball-valve thrombus |
| Volume overload, particularly with coexisting renal and cardiac disease |
| Increased permeability or low-pressure edema (ARDS) |
| More common |
| Sepsis and sepsis syndrome |
| Acid aspiration |
| Multiple transfusions for hypovolemic shock |
| Less common |
| Near-drowning |
| Pancreatitis |
| Air or fat emboli |
| Cardiopulmonary bypass |
| Pneumonia |
| Drug reaction or overdose |
| Leukoagglutination |
| Inhalation injury |
| Infusion of biologics (e.g., interleukin 2) |
| Ischemia-reperfusion (e.g., postthrombectomy, posttransplantation) |
| Edema of unclear or "mixed" origin |
| Reexpansion |
| Neurogenic |
| Postictal |
| Tocolysis-associated |
| Diffuse alveolar hemorrhage |
| Microscopic angiitis |
| Collagen vascular diseases |
| Goodpasture's syndrome |
| Severe coagulopathy and bone marrow transplantation |
| Retinoic acid syndrome |
| **Focal Lung Lesions** |
| Lobar pneumonia |
| Lung contusion |
| Lobar atelectasis (acutely) |

ARDS = acute respiratory distress syndrome.

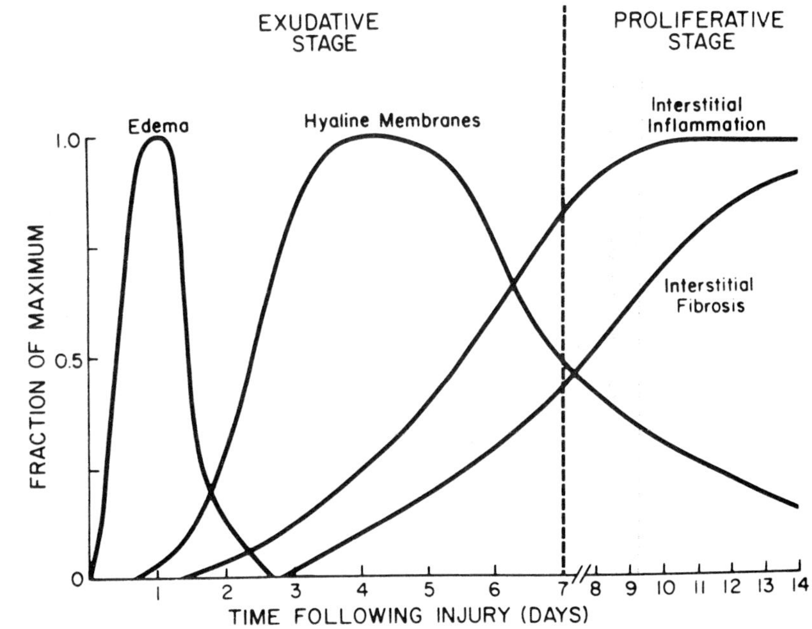


**Figure 92.2** A schematic representation of the time course of evolution of the adult respiratory distress syndrome. During the early or exudative phase, the lesion is characterized by a pulmonary capillary leak with edema and then, shortly thereafter, by hyaline membrane formation. Within as short a period as 7 to 10 days, a proliferative phase may appear, with marked interstitial inflammation, fibrosis, and disordered healing (see text for discussion). (From Katzenstein AA, Askin FB: Surgical Pathology of Non-neoplastic Lung Disease. Philadelphia: WB Saunders, 1982.)

deposition. Type II alveolar cells proliferate along alveolar septa, and within the alveolar wall fibroblasts and myofibroblasts become more prominent. Lung flooding may be minimal at this point, and the clinical picture is often dominated by a large dead-space fraction and high minute ventilation requirements, progressive pulmonary hypertension, slightly improved intrapulmonary shunt that is less responsive to PEEP, further reduction in lung compliance, and a tendency toward creation of zone I conditions within the lung if hypovolemia develops.

A number of differences between increased-permeability and increased-pressure pulmonary edema are likely to have clinical relevance. Alveolar flooding is greater with increased-permeability edema for a given increase in lung water, presumably owing to direct access through the injured alveolar epithelium, whereas in hydrostatic leak the alveolar-capillary membrane is normal and fluid tracks to the peribronchiolar interstitium.[12] In addition, active transport processes may be important in clearance of fluid from the alveolar space, and these transport mechanisms may be disrupted by acute lung injury.[13] Also, some of the mechanisms limiting edemagenesis in high-pressure pulmonary edema may not be operative in low-pressure pulmonary edema. Specifically, there is no dilution or "washout" of interstitial protein concentration in ARDS, and thus no tendency for a widened oncotic pressure gradient to oppose the hydrostatic pressures driving liquid flux. Also, the interstitial back-pressure to edemagenesis may be less because of the primary disruption of the alveolar barrier.

Some forms of pulmonary edema, although well described clinically, remain obscure as to their cause, at least in terms of basic Starling mechanisms (see Table 92.1). Neurogenic pulmonary edema, most commonly seen after catastrophic central nervous system injury, has been ascribed to both high- and low-pressure mechanisms.[14] Reexpansion pulmonary edema, relatively common unilaterally after inflation of a collapsed lung by tube thoracostomy, has been held by many to result from a sudden decrease in lung interstitial pressures that results in a widened hydrostatic pressure gradient.[15] Some evidence in animal models and from clinical cases, however, has suggested that reperfusion after reexpansion may result in lung injury (analogous to reperfusion injury after organ transplantation) with a pulmonary capillary leak.[16] Pulmonary edema can complicate tocolytic therapy, although the frequency of use of these agents is declining.[17] The cause of this form of edema remains obscure. It has also been noted under experimental conditions that transient high pulmonary microvascular pressures can result in endothelial cell injury, with a resulting low-pressure leak as a sequela.[17a] Therefore, it is at least conceivable that increased-pressure pulmonary edema may be complicated by acute lung injury in clinical settings.

## Diffuse AHRF: Alveolar Hemorrhage

The disease processes capable of producing diffuse alveolar hemorrhage (see Table 92.1) may on rare occasions cause AHRF. Diffuse alveolar hemorrhage is most often encountered in the context of collagen vascular disease,[18, 19] lung-renal syndromes, severely immunocompromised state, or cancer treatment.[20, 20a] On occasion it can be difficult to determine whether the lesion arose diffusely or was the result of focal hemorrhage with aspiration and diffuse flooding. When AHRF is accompanied by significant hemoptysis, the serologic, renal histologic, and other diagnostic clues must be pursued for specific diagnosis outlined elsewhere in this text (see Chapter 60). Supportive management remains similar to that for ARDS.

## Focal AHRF

The prototype of focal AHRF is acute lobar bacterial pneumonia. With this lung infection, calculated shunt fractions may reach 40% despite consolidation involving only a single lobe that normally receives 20% of pulmonary ventilation and perfusion. This implies a large increase in blood flow to the infected lung segment and a failure of alveolar hypoxic vasoconstriction to reduce pulmonary arterial flow. This augmentation of flow to the infected and hypoxic lobe may be mediated by local elaboration of prostaglandins, because inhibitors of these metabolic pathways allow the expected reduction in flow in animal models.[6] Another contribution to the large shunt fractions encountered in pneumonia is the consumption of oxygen by the aerobically active leukocytes and bacteria within the consolidated lobe, which causes the venous effluent from the infected region of the lung to have an oxygen saturation even lower than that of mixed venous blood.[6] Yet shunt is not the only cause of hypoxemia in pneumonia, because adjacent lung regions become hypoventilated as a result of their mechanical interaction with the consolidated lobe. Consequently, about half of the hypoxemia during air breathing is caused by low ventilation-perfusion ratios ($\dot{V}/\dot{Q}$), a situation that is very responsive to oxygen therapy.[6] When the inflammatory response is reduced by antibiotic therapy, alveolar hypoxic vasoconstriction reduces lobar blood flow and shunt, and the residual hypoxemia is much more responsive to supplemental oxygen.[20b]

Another focal lung lesion that can result in significant hypoxemia is lung contusion.[21] This lesion results from direct mechanical injury to the lung and its blood supply and emerges within minutes to hours after blunt chest trauma. The degree of lung flooding tends to be increased by fluid resuscitation and PEEP.[22] The central region of the contused lung often manifests significant hemorrhage and interruption of the pulmonary arterial circulation, so intrapulmonary shunt is minimal. Yet in the peripheral regions of the contusion and in adjacent segments and lobes mechanically interdependent with the poorly ventilated contusion, hypoventilation leads to low $\dot{V}/\dot{Q}$ and hypoxemia that is responsive to oxygen therapy. Accordingly, measures to improve ventilation (nerve blocks, analgesics, chest physiotherapy with deep breathing) and oxygen by face mask often correct the hypoxemia and are preferred to positive-pressure ventilation with PEEP, which tends to increase the injury without ameliorating the hypoxemia.[23]

## Overlap of Diffuse and Focal AHRF

Although it is useful didactically to make a distinction between focal and diffuse causes of AHRF, this classification has arisen largely from chest radiograph assessment, a relatively insensitive measure of fluid distribution.[24] When chest computed tomography scans were obtained from patients with ARDS, marked inhomogeneity of alveolar flooding was noted[4, 5, 25–27] (Fig. 92.3). Consolidation is frequently most pronounced in dependent lung regions, and if the patient is switched to the prone position, lung consolidation redistributes to the newly dependent lung regions (see Fig. 92.3). Such findings support the notion of ARDS as a disease with small or "baby" lungs of relatively preserved function. It has been hypothesized that ventilator strategies that avoid overdistention and hence injury of normal lung regions yet still achieve recruitment of flooded and collapsed lung regions optimize outcome in these patients, a perspective to be discussed at length later.

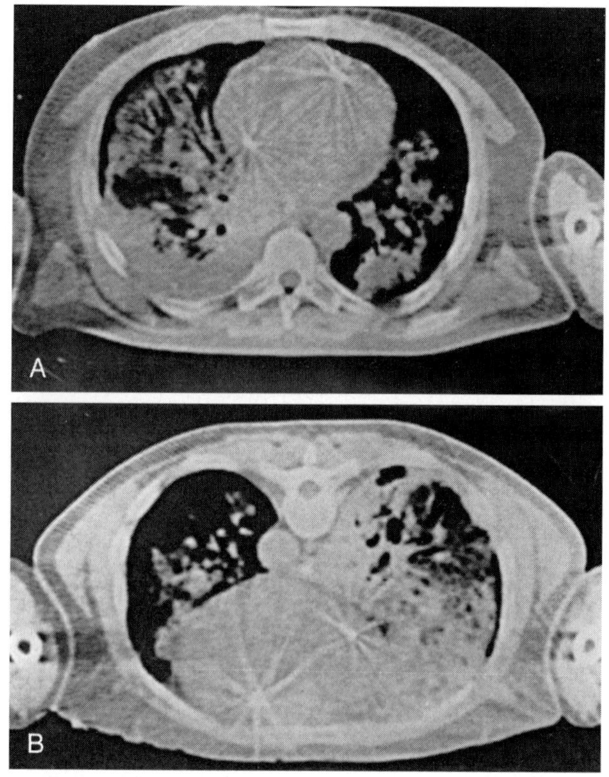


**Figure 92.3** Representative computed tomographic images of a patient with the adult respiratory distress syndrome. *A*, Supine position. *B*, Prone position. Note the focality of lung densities and their redistribution after the positioning maneuver. (From Gattinoni L, Pelosi P, Vitale G, et al: Body position changes redistribute lung computed tomographic density in patients with acute respiratory failure. Anesthesiology 42:391–407, 1991.)

By contrast, when positron emission tomography was performed in patients with lobar pneumonia, marked capillary leak of a large tracer molecule was noted in the contralateral lung.[27] The investigators speculated that this was the result of activation of inflammatory mediators during the course of the lung infection. This finding explains the propensity of patients with sepsis syndrome secondary to pneumonia to demonstrate worsened lung infiltrates during the course of fluid resuscitation. Therefore, patients with prototypical diffuse lung lesions may harbor marked regional inhomogeneities in lung flooding, and patients with focal lesions may be predisposed to develop more generalized disease.

## CLINICAL PRESENTATION

If drive to breathe is intact, the bedside appearance of patients with the various forms of AHRF is remarkably similar. Marked tachypnea (respiratory rate greater than 30 breaths/min) and dyspnea are invariably present. Physical examination reveals diffuse crackles in pulmonary edema and focal findings of consolidation in lobar pneumonia. It is not unusual to encounter a patient with pneumonia early during its evolution who has marked dyspnea but minimal physical findings and radiologic abnormalities; over ensuing hours, however, these become more pronounced as intravenous fluids are administered. This is particularly true of pneumonia complicating diabetic ketoacidosis or other conditions accompanied by dehydration. This finding probably relates to the propensity for lung regions not involved in the primary infectious process to leak fluid, as just described,[27, 28] coupled to the initially low pulmonary vascular pressures that protects against inflammatory edema. Cardiogenic pulmonary edema may be accompanied by evidence of airflow obstruction, including wheezing,[29] and on occasion it may be difficult to determine whether the primary process is asthma, chronic obstructive pulmonary disease, or cardiogenic edema. The presence of crackles, a radiologic appearance of increased-pressure edema (see later discussion), and hypoxemia refractory to oxygen therapy all suggest pulmonary edema as a primary process. Cough and purulent sputum are hallmarks of infectious processes, whereas fulminant pulmonary edema often results in copious airway secretions that produce rhonchous sounds and abundant expectoration.

Initial room-air arterial blood gas analysis or pulse oximetry in the distressed patient with severe AHRF typically reveals an arterial $Po_2$ of 30 to 50 mm Hg or saturation less than 85%. If arterial hemoglobin saturation can readily be raised to more than 95% with supplemental oxygen by mask or cannula, a large intrapulmonary shunt is unlikely. Other causes of respiratory distress should then be considered, including airway disease, pulmonary embolus, and severe metabolic acidosis. Failure to achieve more than 95% saturation of arterial blood with supplemental oxygen is consistent with AHRF and a large intrapulmonary shunt, and the presence of an alveolar filling process should be obvious by physical examination and chest radiography. In the rare instance that the chest radiograph is entirely clear of alveolar infiltrates, one should consider that the blood gas data are incorrect or that there is a right-to-left shunt at another site (e.g., pulmonary arteriovenous malformation, intracardiac shunt).

## Determining the Cause of Pulmonary Edema

The existence of pulmonary edema is often clear from the examination of the distressed patient, yet the specific cause of pulmonary edema is frequently obscure. Clinical and laboratory data should be collated to facilitate the clinical judgment of distinguishing between increased-pressure and increased-permeability types of edema.

### Clinical Setting

The most useful information derives from the setting in which the pulmonary edema develops. Cardiogenic edema is most often accompanied by systolic left ventricular or valvular dysfunction, and the abnormal heart sounds and murmurs associated with each should be sought. Electrocardiographic and serum enzyme evidence of ischemia should be reviewed in search of an obvious cause for cardiogenic edema. Review of volume administration often supplies information suggesting the explanation for pulmonary edema in patients with left ventricular or renal dysfunction.

ARDS too arises in a typical clinical context (see Table 92.1). Sepsis, blood product resuscitation after trauma, and acid aspiration account for the majority of cases of AHRF secondary to pulmonary capillary leak in most series.[8, 9] Less common causes include pancreatitis, near-drowning, leukoagglutination reactions, lung infections with viral agents or pneumocystis, fat embolism syndrome, and drug toxicities. (See Table 54.4 in Chapter 54 for complete list of clinical disorders associated with acute lung injury and ARDS.)

### Chest Radiograph

The chest radiograph is a simple and widely available test used to assess patients with pulmonary edema. However, the accuracy of the routine radiograph in distinguishing increased-pressure from increased-permeability edema is not high.[30, 31] Criteria that have been suggested to support a diagnosis of cardiogenic edema include increased heart size, increased width of the vascular pedicle, vascular redistribution toward upper lobes, septal lines, and a centrifugal pattern of spread with perihilar "bat's wing" distribution of the edema (Fig. 92.4). The lack of these findings and the presence of patchy peripheral infiltrates that extend to the lateral lung margins suggest ARDS. All of these signs overlap, however, and in the best of hands this test is unlikely to yield better than a 60% to 80% accuracy of diagnosis when applied by itself.[31]

### Edema Fluid Analysis

The protein content of edema fluid in ARDS is 70% to 90% of the plasma protein concentration.[13, 32] By contrast, cardiogenic edema is transudative in nature, with a protein content less than 50% of that in the patient's plasma.[32] This simple test is extremely useful and generally underutilized. If the patient is intubated and the cause of edema is obscure, determination of the protein content of fluid obtained by airway aspiration should be routine. This analysis loses its diagnostic value if it is not performed early in the course of edemagenesis, because there is active clearance of water from alveolar liquid across the healed alveolar membrane, so that the ratio of protein content in edema fluid to that in plasma increases as the patient recovers. Failure to concentrate alveolar protein signals persistent leak and a poorer prognosis.[13]

### Echocardiography

Echocardiography is a useful noninvasive source of information regarding cardiovascular function. Left ventricular dilation, regional or global wall motion abnormalities, and substantial mitral regurgitation on Doppler imaging are findings supporting causes for cardiogenic edema.[33] A

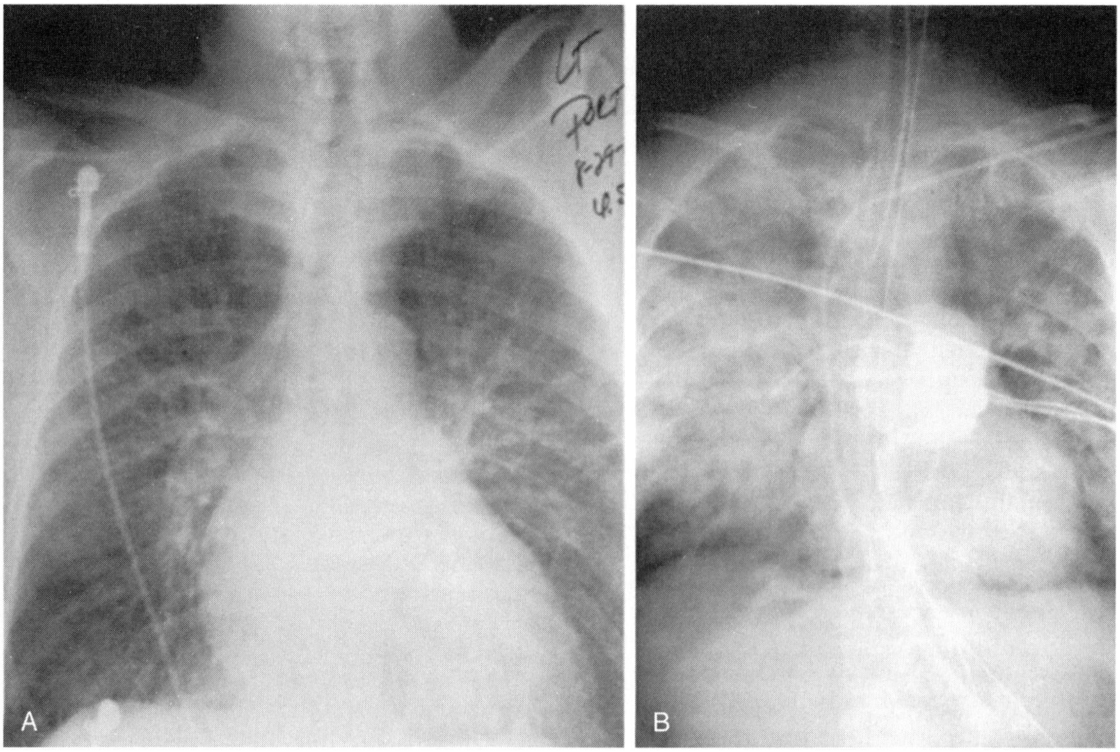


**Figure 92.4** Radiologic examples of hydrostatic (cardiogenic) and permeability (ARDS) pulmonary edema. *A,* The radiograph on the left is remarkable for a large cardiac silhouette, a hilar ``bat's wing'' appearance, and Kerley B lines, all characteristic of cardiogenic pulmonary edema. *B,* The film on the right is remarkable for infiltrates extending to the lung periphery and a very dense appearance of the edema, characteristics of ARDS. However, these signs do not have a very high accuracy in determining the cause of pulmonary edema.

small, well-contracting ventricle imaged echocardiographically in a patient with pulmonary edema suggests pulmonary vascular leak, although prior ventricular or valvular dysfunction with intercurrent resolution of the high pulmonary vascular pressures predisposing to cardiogenic edema must be kept in mind.

## Invasive Hemodynamic Monitoring

Pulmonary artery catherization with a flotation catheter is often performed for patients with pulmonary edema; the benefits of this invasive procedure continue to be debated,[34, 35] because the results of several studies suggest that the technology itself contributes to a poor patient outcome.[36] In addition, several investigations have demonstrated that physician understanding and facility with the information generated by a flotation catheter is remarkably poor.[37, 38] Safe performance of the procedure and a full understanding of the interpretation of the information generated are prerequisites for the use of such technology.

Nonetheless, it is not advisable that invasive monitoring be performed routinely in patients with AHRF. A better approach is one in which the clinician formulates specific questions regarding ventricular function, the adequacy of volume resuscitation, the degree of intrapulmonary shunt, and the adequacy of perfusion and oxygen delivery. If all other sources of information are then exhausted in pursuit of the answers to these questions and these issues remain unresolved, pulmonary artery catheterization is warranted.

The specific pulmonary capillary wedge pressure (PPW) that is selected as a determinant of high-pressure vs. low-pressure pulmonary edema is necessarily arbitrary under clinical conditions, because various degrees of lung injury, hypoalbuminemia, volume overload, and ventricular dysfunction may all promote lung flooding. In the mechanically ventilated patient with normal lung function and serum oncotic pressure, cardiogenic edema is typically associated with a PPW of 25 to 35 mm Hg or higher and ARDS, with a PPW of 0 to 18 mm Hg.

## Defining and Scoring ARDS

Because patients with ARDS have a large number of underlying medical and surgical conditions that differ in the extent and magnitude of their associated lung damage, there has long been recognition of a need for definition and assessment of severity that can help standardize patient groups for comparison. One such attempt was made by a joint American-European Consensus Conference that published its deliberations in 1994.[38] These investigators emphasized the acute nature of the syndrome and recommended that it be termed ``acute'' rather than ``adult''

Table 92.2 AMERICAN-EUROPEAN CONSENSUS CONFERENCE ON ARDS: RECOMMENDED CRITERIA FOR ACUTE LUNG INJURY (ALI) AND ACUTE RESPIRATORY DISTRESS SYNDROME (ARDS)

| Criteria | Timing | Oxygenation | Chest Radiograph | Pwedge |
|---|---|---|---|---|
| ALI | Acute onset | $Pa_{O_2}/FI_{O_2}$ < 300 mm Hg (regardless of PEEP level) | Bilateral infiltrates | <18 mm Hg or no clinical evidence left atrial hypertension |
| ARDS | Acute onset | $Pa_{O_2}/FI_{O_2}$ < 200 mm Hg (regardless of PEEP level) | Bilateral infiltrates | <18 mm Hg or no clinical evidence left atrial hypertension |

Pwedge = pulmonary capillary wedge pressure; $FI_{O_2}$ = fraction of inspired oxygen; PEEP = positive end-expiratory pressure.
From Bernard GR, Artigas A, Brigham KL, et al: The American-European Consensus Conference on ARDS: Definitions, mechanisms, relevant outcomes, and clinical trial coordination. Am J Respir Crit Care Med 149:818–824, 1994.

respiratory distress syndrome. In recognition of its range of severity, they recommended using the term *acute lung injury* (ALI) to describe the milder manifestations of evolving diffuse lung damage, and ARDS to describe the more severe end of the spectrum. Both ALI and ARDS were defined by relatively simple timing, oxygenation, chest radiographic, and hemodynamic criteria, which are given in Table 92.2.

Although these criteria carry the virtue of simplicity and constitute a "broad net" to identify patients with even mild lung injury, they are highly nonspecific and provide only a two-tier schema for the range of lung injury, with little ability to describe gradations of severity of injury. This latter goal has been sought by a number of scoring systems, of which the most widely employed is the Murray score (Table 92.3).[39]

Although these definitions and scores do not particularly illuminate individual case management, they are useful for purposes of patient recruitment to studies, and they are necessary to interpret published results of diagnostic or therapeutic trials. As mechanisms of lung injury are further elaborated, it is possible that various biochemical markers, obtained from either serum or alveolar fluid analysis, may provide further refinement of these rudimentary attempts to stage and quantify the magnitude of lung injury.[40, 40a]

## TREATMENT OF AHRF

Although the attention of the critical care physician is often focused on the details of supportive therapy for patients with AHRF, the importance of a simultaneous search for and treatment of the underlying cause of the lung failure cannot be overemphasized. Without a diagnosis and specific treatment of the underlying process or processes causing the lung injury, supportive therapy alone is likely to result ultimately in mounting complications and irreversible organ failures. ARDS represents a syndrome defined by bedside, radiologic, and physiologic criteria; it is not a specific diagnosis. The management principles detailed here are intended to stabilize the patient and to provide a window of opportunity during which the diagnostic and therapeutic interventions necessary to treat underlying diseases can be performed.

### Management of Cardiogenic Pulmonary Edema

The management of cardiogenic pulmonary edema overlaps considerably with management of left ventricular systolic and diastolic dysfunction. Most patients respond dramatically to pharmacologic interventions, and mechanical ventilatory support typically is not required. Nonetheless, on presentation hypoxemia may be severe and, as with other causes of AHRF, is minimally responsive to oxygen therapy. In contrast to other forms of AHRF, as many as one third of patients with cardiogenic pulmonary edema exhibit modest elevations of arterial $P_{CO_2}$, despite obvious increased drive to breathe and before receiving narcotics.[41] The reasons for this finding are obscure but may relate to intrapulmonary shunting of mixed venous blood with a high carbon dioxide content, or to excessive dead space caused by "cardiac asthma," which induces gas trapping and dynamic hyperinflation.

#### Pharmacologic Therapy

The primary goal of pharmacologic therapy is to reduce the left atrial and pulmonary vascular pressures that are responsible for the cardiogenic edema, which ultimately improves oxygenation and reduces the work of breathing (Table 92.4). Reduction in left ventricular preload is achieved with drugs that either translocate central blood volume to a peripheral compartment or achieve net diuresis, or both. Because ventricular systolic function is often impaired in cardiogenic pulmonary edema, inotropic support and afterload reduction are usually required as well.[42, 43] In addition, reduction of preload often reduces chamber size and, by decreasing ventricular wall tension, acts to decrease afterload.[43]

**Table 92.3 SCORING SYSTEM FOR ARDS**

| | |
|---|---|
| Chest roentgenogram score | |
| No alveolar consolidation | 0 |
| 1 quadrant consolidation | 1 |
| 2 quadrant consolidation | 2 |
| 3 quadrant consolidation | 3 |
| 4 quadrant consolidation | 4 |
| Hypoxemia score ($PaO_2/FIO_2$) | |
| ≥300 | 0 |
| 225–299 | 1 |
| 175–224 | 2 |
| 100–174 | 3 |
| ≤100 | 4 |
| Compliance (when ventilated) (mL/cm $H_2O$) | |
| ≥80 | 0 |
| 60–79 | 1 |
| 40–59 | 2 |
| 20–39 | 3 |
| ≤19 | 4 |
| PEEP required (when ventilated) (cm $H_2O$) | |
| ≤5 | 0 |
| 6–8 | 1 |
| 9–11 | 2 |
| 12–14 | 3 |
| ≥15 | 4 |
| Final score is obtained by dividing the aggregate sum by the number of components used: | |
| No injury | 0 |
| Mild to moderate injury | 0.1–2.5 |
| Severe injury (ARDS) | >2.5 |

ARDS = acute respiratory distress syndrome; $FIO_2$ = fraction of inspired oxygen; PEEP = positive end-expiratory pressure.
From Murray JF, Matthay MA, Luce J, et al: An expanded definition of the adult respiratory distress syndrome. Am Rev Respir Dis 138:720–723, 1988.

Therapy should begin with oxygen by nasal cannula or mask, titrated against oximetry or arterial blood gas measurements. Even small increases in arterial $PO_2$ increase arterial oxygen content significantly, because these increases occur on a relatively steep portion of the oxyhemoglobin dissociation curve and therefore result in relatively large increases in arterial hemoglobin saturation. Patients invariably prefer the upright position, which should be facilitated if the blood pressure permits. This positioning favors sequestration of blood volume in the peripheral venous compartment and should be maintained even after intubation and positive-pressure ventilation.

Preload reduction can be achieved by administration of morphine sulfate, 2 to 4 mg intravenously as an initial dose, followed by 2- to 4-mg doses every 5 to 10 minutes, as ascertained by the patient's level of anxiety, level of consciousness, and angina, if any.[44] Morphine is a potent anxiolytic, and the resulting reduction in sympathetic tone, coupled with its direct vascular actions, tends to reduce hypertension and tachycardia and thus myocardial oxygen demand. Further preload reduction can be accomplished with furosemide. Like morphine, furosemide has a venodilating action and results in pooling of blood volume in the venous capacitance vessels; it is also a potent loop diuretic.[45] Furosemide may also have pulmonary vascular effects that reduce intrapulmonary shunt directly.[46] An initial dose of 20 to 40 mg given intravenously is appropriate, although substantially larger doses may be required for patients with diminished renal function. The initial dose may be doubled if a response is not noted within 30 to 90 minutes. Alternative regimens to achieve diuresis include bumetanide (initial dose, 1 to 2 mg intravenously) or the combination of furosemide and metolazone (initial dose, 2.5 to 10 mg by mouth), particularly if glomerular filtration rate is reduced.[47]

Alternative rapid preload reduction is effected by rotating tourniquets or phlebotomy, or both, and may be used in conjunction with the venous dilating effects of nitroglycerin therapy, particularly if renal function is extremely compromised and there is a substantial delay in instituting hemodialysis or ultrafiltration.[48] When renal function is acceptable, longer-term diuresis may be enhanced by intravenous administration of dopamine at a dose of 1 to 4 μg/kg/min.[49]

After an initial 12-lead electrocardiogram is obtained, continuous monitoring of the electrocardiogram should

**Table 92.4 TREATMENT OF CARDIOGENIC PULMONARY EDEMA***

- Correction of hypoxemia
  - Supplemental oxygen by mask or cannula
  - Consider noninvasive positive-pressure ventilation
  - Intubation and mechanical ventilation for unstable patients
- Preload reduction
  - Upright position
  - Morphine sulfate (2–5 mg intravenously)
  - Furosemide (20–40 mg intravenously)
  - Alternative diuretic regimens
    - Bumetanide
    - Metolazone and furosemide
    - Low dose dopamine (1–4 μg/kg/min)
  - Topical or sublingual nitrates
  - If coexistent ischemia is evident, use intravenous nitroglycerin
  - Consider phlebotomy or rotating tourniquets to temporize when renal function is poor
  - Emergency renal dialysis/ultrafiltration if diuresis cannot be achieved
  - Positive end-expiratory pressure (PEEP)
- Afterload reduction
  - Treatment of anxiety to lower systemic blood pressure (e.g., morphine sulfate)
  - Specific antihypertensive therapy
    - Angiotensin-converting enzyme inhibitors
    - Nifedipine (10–20 mg by mouth or sublingually)
    - Sodium nitroprusside for accelerated hypertension
  - Intra-aortic balloon pump for refractory ventricular failure
  - PEEP
- Inotropic support
  - Dobutamine, 5–10 μg/kg/min

*Most patients improve with correction of hypoxemia and the initial therapies listed for reduction of preload and afterload; the more extensive and invasive interventions listed are required when ischemia, severe ventricular dysfunction, or renal failure complicates cardiogenic pulmonary edema.

be routine, because bradyarrhythmias and tachyarrhythmias are common among patients with cardiogenic pulmonary edema. Bradyarrhythmias may contribute significantly to cardiogenic pulmonary edema by virtue of the increase in preload and diastolic wall tension, and these disturbances should be treated early and aggressively.

If blood pressure does not fall substantially with morphine administration, a component of accelerated or malignant hypertension contributing to ventricular decompensation should be considered.[50] For moderate persistent elevations of blood pressure, an angiotensin-converting enzyme inhibitor such as lisinopril or enalapril may given either intravenously or by mouth.[51] If this class of agents is contraindicated, a calcium channel blocker such as nifedipine may be used, given as 10 or 20 mg sublingually.[52] More substantial elevations of blood pressure in the setting of cardiogenic pulmonary edema are best treated with sodium nitroprusside, started at a dose of 10 μg/min total dose and then doubled every 3 to 5 minutes until the blood pressure is reduced to the range of 140 to 160 mm Hg systolic and 90 to 100 mm Hg diastolic.[50, 53]

This relatively simple approach result in rapid, dramatic improvement in the majority of patients with mild and uncomplicated cardiogenic pulmonary edema (see Table 92.4). Predisposing causes of ventricular dysfunction should be sought, and serial enzyme and electrocardiographic studies to exclude myocardial infarction should be routine. Echocardiography is often useful to identify regional wall motion abnormalities, global left ventricular function, and valvular abnormalities. Intravenous nitroglycerin is useful if there is evidence of ongoing myocardial ischemia; it reduces preload by its effects on the venous circulation, can have a favorable effect on the distribution of myocardial blood flow, and is a mild afterload-reducing agent.[54, 55] It should be started at 10 μg/min *total* dose and then doubled every 3 to 5 minutes, titrated until pain has resolved or blood pressure begins to fall. If pain control is not achieved with nitroglycerin, intra-aortic balloon pump assistance should be considered. Anticoagulation, thrombolytic therapy, or surgical intervention should be considered in all patients with transmural infarction or unstable angina.[56] In these instances of severe ischemic injury or risk thereof, mechanical ventilatory support is likely be required and should be instituted electively.

Systolic dysfunction is signaled by hypotension or evidence of hypoperfusion, such as oliguria despite diuretic use or persistent lactic acidosis. Although diastolic dysfunction is often difficult to assess with echocardiography, systolic dysfunction is usually readily apparent in a technically adequate study. Dobutamine is the preferred catecholamine to try to correct systolic dysfunction, because it has afterload-reducing effects as well as positive inotropy.[57] It should be administered initially at a dose of 5 to 15 μg/kg/min, titrated against measured cardiac output and clinical parameters of perfusion. Tachyphylaxis to its action is not unusual, and often the dose must be increased to yield the same effect over several days.[58] Once stabilized, many patients can be switched to afterload-reducing agents such as the angiotensin-converting enzyme inhibitors for long-term management.[59, 60]

Acute mitral regurgitation should be considered as a cause of cardiogenic pulmonary edema if there is an associated systolic murmur, the cardiac silhouette is small, or the clinical setting is consistent with endocarditis.[61] Valvular incompetence can be confirmed by demonstration of a large v-wave at the time of right-sided heart catheterization (Fig. 92.5) or by echocardiography. Administration of inotropic agents may worsen the regurgitant fraction and is generally contraindicated. Therapy should begin with a rapid-acting afterload-reducing agent such as nitroprusside. Right-sided heart catheterization with continuous measurement of mixed venous oxygen saturation is a useful way to adjust therapy.

## Positive-Pressure Ventilation

Most patients respond sufficiently rapidly to pharmacologic agents to avoid mechanical ventilatory support. If improvement is noted but the patient remains in significant respiratory distress with or without hypoxemia, early consideration should be given to positive-pressure ventilation delivered noninvasively by face mask (noninvasive positive-pressure ventilation [NIPPV]).[62] NIPPV has been demonstrated to improve gas exchange,[62] reduce the work of breathing,[63] relieve dyspnea, reduce ventricular afterload,[64] and improve outcome[65–67] in patients with ventricular dysfunction and cardiogenic pulmonary edema. Two recent articles reported the results of studies of NIPPV in a total of 55 patients with "severe" cardiogenic pulmonary edema, most of whom were also hypercapnic.[67a, 67b] Only 6 patients required endotracheal intubation, and of these, 4 died from acute myocardial infarction; noninvasive ventilation worked well in most patients but

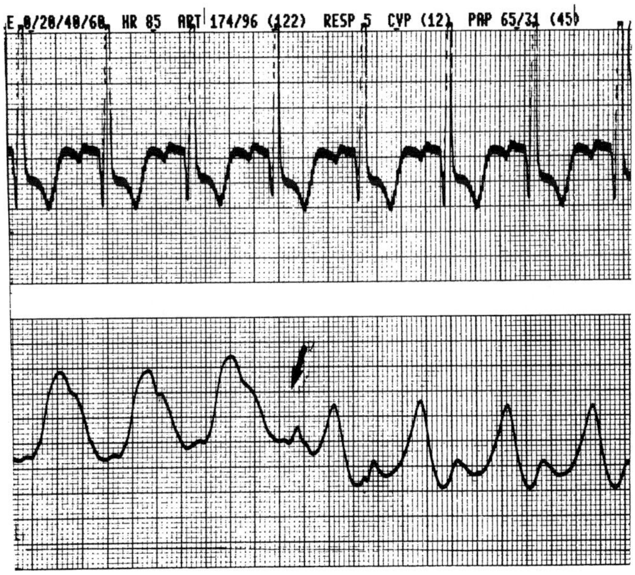


**Figure 92.5** Demonstration of a giant v-wave indicating mitral regurgitation in a patient with papillary muscle ischemia. Note that after catheter balloon inflation *(arrow)*, the pulmonary arterial waveform (identified by the dicrotic notch) converts to a three-component wedge tracing, with a v-wave greater than 30 mm Hg.

probably should not be used in patients with new infarcts as a cause of their edema. It is likely that the benefits of NIPPV also derive from avoidance of endotracheal intubation and all of its associated complications.

Effective application of NIPPV requires a coordinated team of physicians, nurses, and respiratory therapists familiar with this therapy[68] (see Chapter 93). A well-fitted nasal or face mask should be used, and the procedure should be explained to the patient, with encouragement and emphasis on the subjective improvements in dyspnea that are likely to occur. NIPPV should begin at low levels of inspiratory and expiratory pressures (e.g., 5 cm $H_2O$). Some systems provide a single continuous positive airway pressure (CPAP) throughout the respiratory cycle, whereas others permit selection of independent inspiratory and expiratory pressure levels (e.g., BiPAP). Increasing expiratory pressure benefits gas exchange primarily, whereas increasing inspiratory pressure increases the delivered tidal volume for any given patient effort. Continuous pulse oximetry should be employed to assess oxygenation, and patient respiratory rate and tidal volume should be monitored to assess the benefit on ventilation. Most patients benefitting from NIPPV do so promptly, reporting diminished dyspnea and adopting a slower, deeper breathing pattern. Inspiratory and expiratory pressures can be increased as high as 20 to 25 cm $H_2O$, but levels greater than 15 cm $H_2O$ are often associated with discomfort because of the need for an extremely tight-fitting mask. The least level of inspiratory and expiratory pressure that ensures adequate oxygenation, ventilation, and patient comfort should be sought.

Patients who present with shock, who develop significant hypotension during the course of therapy, or who fail to tolerate NIPPV should be considered for elective intubation and mechanical ventilation. At the time of intubation and immediately thereafter, the patient should be sedated; morphine sulfate can be used if blood pressure is adequate, or a short-acting benzodiazepine may be used if hypotension is present.

The institution of mechanical ventilation via an endotracheal tube confers benefits similar to NIPPV (e.g., reduced work of breathing, diminished oxygen consumption, reduction of left ventricular afterload), albeit with the risks of intubation. Initial ventilator settings should include a fraction of inspired oxygen ($F_{IO_2}$) of 1.0, a tidal volume of 6 to 8 mL/kg, and a respiratory rate of 25 breaths/min. The patient may initiate breaths in an assist-control (AC), synchronized intermittent mandatory ventilation (SIMV), pressure-support, or proportional-assist mode (see Chapter 94) with the sensitivity set at a minimal level of $-2$ cm $H_2O$. PEEP may then be titrated against arterial saturation to permit a reduction in the $F_{IO_2}$ to 0.6 or less. PEEP has fewer adverse effects on venous return when the circulatory volume is increased, as in cardiogenic edema, and PEEP tends to reduce both left ventricular preload and afterload.[64, 69]

The ongoing requirement for ventilatory support is in most instances dictated by the pace of correction of the underlying ventricular dysfunction and valvular or ischemic disease, if any. If new complications do not arise and cardiovascular function is stabilized, the patient may be returned to spontaneous breathing modes after preload is reduced and gas exchange improves, signaled by a diminishing requirement for PEEP.

## Treatment of ARDS: Pharmacologic Therapy

As already noted, the supportive management of ARDS is fruitless if it is not accompanied by aggressive diagnosis and treatment of the predisposing condition or conditions (see Table 92.1). It is also important to observe that some causes of ARDS tend to have a generally benign course. These include tocolytic- or heroin-associated pulmonary edema, postictal pulmonary edema, and pulmonary edema associated with air emboli. These forms of increased-permeability edema often respond to supplemental oxygen and diuresis alone. When mechanical ventilation is required, it is usually for a brief period, and many of the monitoring and circulatory manipulations described in this section are not indicated.

As the sequence of cellular and biochemical events resulting in acute lung injury has been described in increasing detail, a number of pharmacologic interventions to interrupt these pathways have been contemplated.[9, 70, 71] Early support for many such agents was anecdotal, but controlled trials have provided more informed guidance concerning the absence of effective specific prevention and treatment. Unfortunately, none has proved beneficial.[71a] This discussion is restricted to those therapies that have been assessed to some extent in human subjects.

**Corticosteroids.** Because neutrophil-mediated injury is probably important in many forms of acute lung injury, corticosteroids have been used, both in animal models and in uncontrolled human studies.[72] However, when evaluated prospectively in patients with sepsis syndrome, high-dose methylprednisolone did not prevent the development of ARDS, nor reduce the mortality rate, compared with an identical placebo-treated control group.[73, 74] In another prospective, randomized trial of steroids begun after ARDS was well established, no beneficial effect on gas exchange or lung mechanics could be demonstrated, nor was outcome improved.[75] In the latter study a number of conditions predisposing to ARDS were present, including sepsis, aspiration, and pancreatitis.

On the basis of these well-conducted clinical trials, use of corticosteroids cannot be supported for sepsis syndrome or established ARDS in the exudative phase. An exception to this generalization would be ARDS that is caused by an inflammatory disease that is associated with lung injury and is known to respond to corticosteroids, such as acute eosinophilic pneumonia.[76] This emphasizes the point that ARDS is not a disease-specific entity and that all patients with this syndrome require other diagnostic considerations. A separate question persists concerning the benefit of corticosteroids for treatment of the disordered healing and fibrosis that occurs during the proliferative phase of ARDS (see later discussion). Finally, some clinicians still advocate the prophylactic use of corticosteroids for specific disorders that may progress to ARDS, such as witnessed aspiration, or soon after long bone fracture to prevent fat embolization syndrome.[77, 78] However, data to support these recommendations are scant.

**Eicosanoid Administration or Inhibition.** Available data support a role for prostaglandin pathways, both in mediation of acute lung injury and in amelioration of the effects of this injury.[70, 71] Accordingly, interventions have been designed that involve both prostaglandin administration and inhibition of prostaglandin synthesis with nonsteroidal anti-inflammatory drugs. Because prostaglandin $E_1$ ($PGE_1$) inhibits platelet aggregation and neutrophil chemotaxis and is a pulmonary arterial vasodilator, it has been used to treat ARDS associated with both medical and surgical predispositions, but with negative results.[79] In the same study, a trend toward increased survival was present in the placebo-treated group, and many complications were noted in the treatment group, including hypotension, diarrhea, and fever. A second study has confirmed this negative result.[80] One pilot investigation using liposomal $PGE_1$ did demonstrate improvements in gas exchange and lung mechanics, but long-term benefits have not been adequately assessed.[80a] Two clinical trials that evaluated the nonsteroidal anti-inflammatory drug ibuprofen, a prostaglandin-blocking agent, in sepsis and included data on the incidence of lung injury failed to demonstrate benefit.[81, 82] Therefore, at the present time neither administration nor blockade of eicosanoids can be recommended for the treatment of ARDS.

**Ketoconazole.** The azole antifungal ketoconazole is a potent inhibitor of leukotriene biosynthesis. Two trials, in patients at risk of acute lung injury from sepsis and trauma, suggested a significant protective effect of this agent.[83, 84] The results of a recent multicenter trial of ketoconazole, however, showed no improvement in mortality, and the study was stopped.[84a]

**Surfactant.** The vital role played by pulmonary surfactant in normal lung function is discussed in Chapter 13. It has long been known from both animal models and human studies that surfactant levels are decreased, or the ratios of the surfactants are abnormal, in subjects with ARDS.[85, 86] Intensivists caring for adults have been encouraged by the results of surfactant therapy in premature infants who are at risk of or who have already developed the neonatal respiratory distress syndrome (NRDS); the results of several controlled trials have demonstrated better survival in surfactant-treated infants that was associated with improved gas exchange and lung mechanics, decreased requirement for CPAP, and less barotrauma.[87–89] Anzueto and colleagues[90] reported the largest prospective study of surfactant in ARDS. Their results were disappointing: There was no benefit associated with the therapy. Although concerns were raised in analysis of this study about the dose, mode, and timing of delivery and the precise surfactant formulation studied, at present surfactant therapy for ARDS should remain experimental.

## Treatment of ARDS: Supportive Therapy

In summary of the clinical trials described previously, state-of-the-art management of ARDS does not include any pharmacologic interventions that are of proven benefit to limit acute lung injury or restore physiologic function. Although it is possible that further explication of the mechanisms of lung injury will provide new avenues for intervention, these approaches must be considered experimental and the goal of ongoing trials such as those now being conducted by a National Institutes of Health–sponsored network of clinical centers for the study of ARDS.[71] At present, management of these patients relies on meticulous supportive therapy, while underlying diseases are diagnosed and treated. Even if new pharmacologic agents become available, the same supportive therapy will be necessary to maintain viability so that the patient can benefit from treatment.

### Circulatory Management

If edemagenesis could be diminished early after the lung injury, the duration of potentially dangerous ventilator, PEEP, and oxygen therapy could be reduced and outcome could conceivably be improved. Most patients with ARDS do not die during the early phase of disease as a consequence of severe hypoxemia, but rather days to weeks later, frequently with evidence of hypermetabolism, nosocomial infection, and multiple organ systems failure.[91] Some have argued that maximizing oxygen delivery to peripheral tissues is a necessary strategy in patients with ARDS and advocate approaches such as volume loading to achieve this goal.[92] This position is largely untenable, because the oxygen extraction defect purported to exist in patients with sepsis and ARDS now seems to have been artifactual or, at least, not clinically relevant.[93] The consequence of maximizing oxygen delivery with volume administration could be escalating requirements for mechanical ventilation, oxygen, and PEEP; accordingly, to the extent that intensity and duration of supportive therapy are greater determinants of complications and organ dysfunctions, the result could be detrimental. Our approach is to explore an aggressive reduction in ventricular preload without decreasing cardiac output early in the course of ARDS as a strategy to minimize edemagenesis and lessen its adverse effects. The justification for this approach derives from both animal models and clinical data.[94–98]

One clinical study reported that extravascular lung water measured by single-pass multiple-tracer technique did not correlate with the level of intrapulmonary shunt or survival in patients with ARDS.[99] This correlation did not address the specific question of whether reduction in lung water in a given patient could be accomplished safely and would have a salutary effect on outcome. Several retrospective or noninterventional studies reported data showing a correlation between survival and net diuresis or reduction in pulmonary capillary wedge pressure.[100–102] Prospective data collection has also demonstrated that titration of therapy to minimize extravascular lung water in patients with ARDS results in decreased ventilator days and decreased days in the intensive care unit.[103] Because a prospective, randomized trial of this therapy did not demonstrate improved survival, circulatory management in these cases has been described as a therapeutic dilemma.[104, 105] On the one hand, judicious volume reduction may improve lung function; in the extreme, however, hypoperfusion and other organ failure could occur. Our own experience is that PPW can safely be reduced in patients with ARDS,[102] and indeed this focuses the clinician's attention on precisely the parameters of organ function that should be followed in all critically ill patients (e.g., mental status, urine output and concentration, circulatory adequacy, metabolic evidence of anaerobic metabolism). Pressure reduction never should be misinterpreted as trading reduced pulmonary edema for a state of inadequate perfusion. Rather, seeking the lowest pulmonary vascular pressures compatible with an *adequate* cardiac output and oxygen delivery should be emphasized. Preload can be reduced, in part, by meticulous attention to limit all extraneous fluid administration. Furosemide is usually given to achieve diuresis, but this may confound interpretation of renal function as an indicator of the adequacy of perfusion. In selected patients, particularly those with manifest systolic dysfunction, dobutamine may be used to maintain perfusion at a reduced PPW. If preload is reduced excessively, our practice is to first give back packed red blood cells rather than crystalloid. Although this approach is both safe and successful anecdotally, it clearly requires confirmation by an appropriate clinical trial.

The interpretation of right-sided heart catheterization data during mechanical ventilation with PEEP can be challenging. Some have suggested utility to determining the left ventricular filling pressure, defined as the transmural pressure or left atrial pressure minus pericardial pressure.[106] Of course, the usual measurement made at right-sided heart catheterization is the PPW. Measurements of PPW may fail to reflect left ventricular filling pressure for a number of reasons. If alveolar pressure is greater than left atrial pressure at the site of measurement (West zone 1 or 2), then the downstream intravascular pressure is not measured and the heart catheter measurement reflects alveolar pressure. Existence of zone 1 or 2 conditions can be inferred from the excursion of the pulmonary arterial and wedge pressure waveforms during positive-pressure ventilation,[107] and this possibility must be considered if one attempts preload reduction in patients with ARDS requiring high PEEP levels (Fig. 92.6). However, even under zone 3 lung conditions, PPW may not reflect ventricular transmural pressure if PEEP increases pericardial pressure. To circumvent this possibility, some have suggested that the right atrial pressure be used to index pericardial pressure,[108] although this approach does not appear valid under conditions of changing PEEP, at least in postoperative cardiac patients.[109] Others have suggested that the nadir in PPW after opening the airway to atmospheric pressure[109–111] might better reflect left ventricular filling pressure. However, this approach is objectionable because even relatively short discontinuation of PEEP can have adverse effects on gas exchange. Moreover, the notion that any particular intravascular pressure measurement or extravascular lung water measurement defines the appropriate point to which therapy should be directed is an illusion and distraction. These data should contribute to the trends in many measurements (e.g., blood pressure, fluid balance, urine output, cardiac output, PPW) that guide the clinician in seeking the lowest pulmonary wedge pressures consistent with an adequate cardiac output.

## Ventilatory Management

### Lung Mechanics, Ventilator-Induced Lung Injury, and Ventilator-Associated Lung Injury

A body of knowledge has accrued from both bench and clinical investigations that has motivated intensivists to reconsider how they ventilate patients with ARDS. Much of this work was based on early observations that mechanical ventilation using large tidal volumes and high inflation pressures could cause a fatal lung injury in animals with otherwise normal lungs.[112–114] The term *ventilator-induced lung injury* (VILI) has been applied to acute lung injury that is directly induced by mechanical ventilation in animal models. VILI is indistinguishable morphologically, physiologically, and radiologically from diffuse alveolar damage resulting from other causes of acute lung injury. VILI is unique because mechanical ventilation can be identified as the cause of lung injury. *Ventilator-associated lung injury* (VALI) is defined as lung injury that resembles ARDS and that occurs in patients receiving mechanical ventilation. VALI is invariably associated with preexisting lung pathology such as ARDS. Although the experimental data are overwhelming in demonstrating the existence of VILI, one cannot be sure in any particular case whether and to what extent VALI is caused by a particular ventilator strategy.[114a]

A very large number of animal experiments have been reported since the early studies, further exploring the precise mechanisms of VILI in a variety of species, with both open- and closed-chest models, and with a variety of initial lung injuries simulating the conditions of mechanical ventilation of the patient with preexisting ARDS; these have been analyzed in an excellent review.[115] These investigations demonstrated that lung injury during mechanical ventilatory support appears to be related to the distending volume to which the lung is subjected, rather than to the distending pressure. For instance, in experimental animals with bands placed around the chest, lung injury does not occur despite ventilation with high airway pressures, because excessive lung inflation cannot occur; without the bands, lung damage is severe.[116] Such observations have created a term, *volutrauma,* to define the resulting form of microstructural injury. Volutrauma differs from the older and more familiar term, barotrauma, which is applied to the grosser forms of extra-alveolar air collections that are sought on routine radiographs obtained in patients undergoing mechanical ventilation.

In addition to the detrimental effects of overdistention, numerous investigations have suggested a protective or ameliorating effect of PEEP on VILI.[115, 117] For example, in a canine model of oleic acid injury, Corbridge and colleagues[118] reported that mechanical ventilation with large tidal volumes and low PEEP was associated with a worsening of intrapulmonary shunt, compared with ventilation with high PEEP and small tidal volumes adjusted to the same maximal transpulmonary pressure (Fig. 92.7). Morphologic studies have suggested that the beneficial effect of PEEP in this context may be related to its ability to maintain recruitment of collapsed and flooded alveoli, thereby avoiding cyclic recruitment-derecruitment with each delivered breath, a mechanical event thought to lead to shear injuries to terminal airways and alveoli.[115, 119, 120]

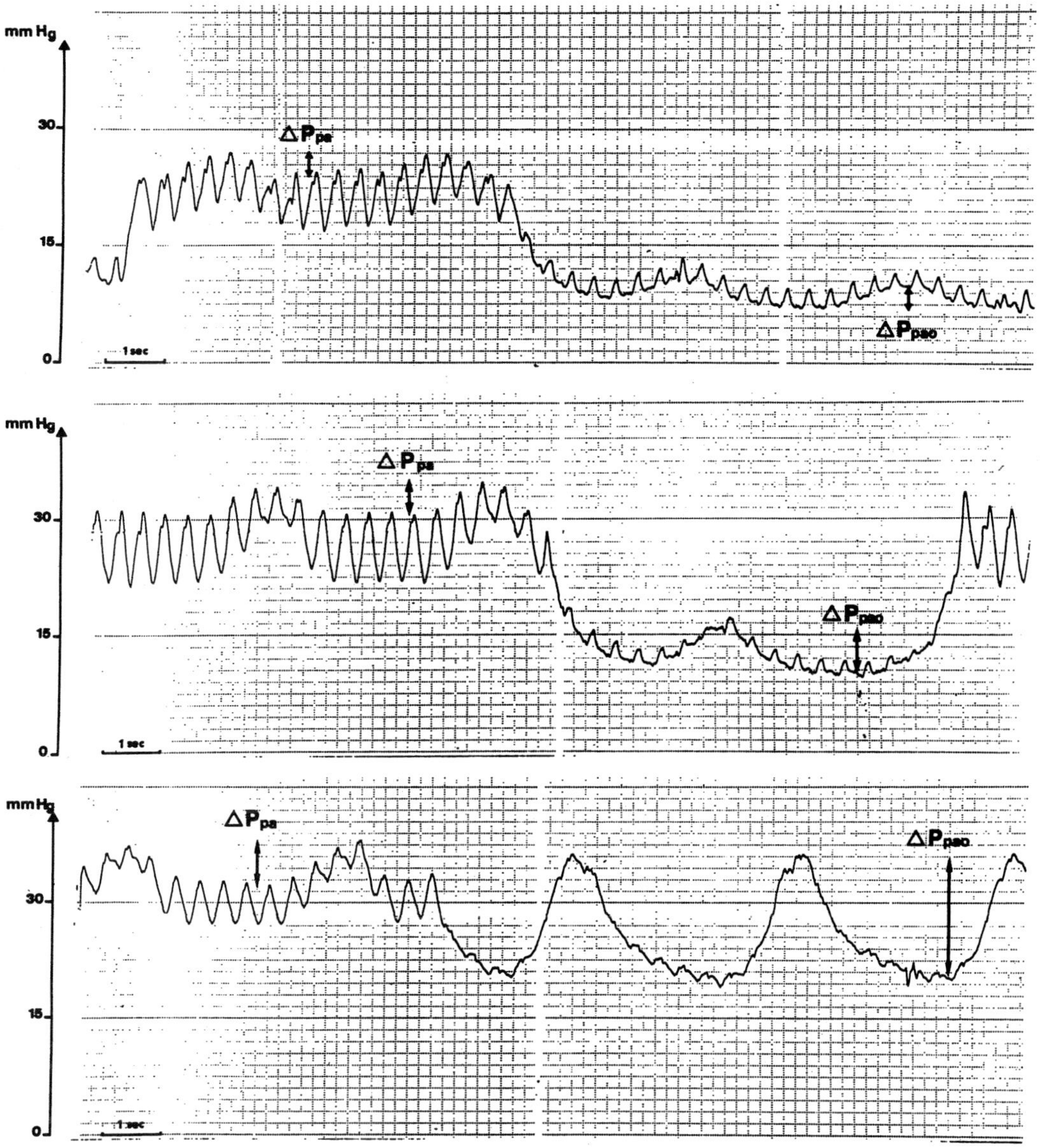


**Figure 92.6** Pressure tracings recorded in the same patient at different levels of end-expiratory pressure: zero end-expiratory pressure (ZEEP) *(top)*, positive end-expiratory pressure (PEEP) at 15 mm Hg (PEEP-15) *(center)*, and PEEP at 20 mm Hg (PEEP-20) *(bottom)*. The ratio of the change in pulmonary artery occlusion pressure to that in pulmonary arterial pressure is approximately 1 during ZEEP and PEEP-15 conditions, but increases to 2.3 during PEEP-20, suggesting a shift from West zone 3 to non–zone 3 conditions at the balloon-occluded pulmonary artery catheter tip. Also note that the end-expiratory Ppao value during PEEP-20 is markedly higher than during PEEP-15 (18 vs. 10 mm Hg), a change that cannot be explained by the PEEP increment alone. Failure to recognize this phenomenon could result in overestimation of the filling pressure of the left ventricule and failure to recognize hypovolemia. (From Teboul JL, Besbes M, Andrivet P, et al: A bedside index assessing the reliability of pulmonary artery occlusion pressure measurements during mechanical ventilation with positive end-expiratory pressure. J Crit Care 7:26, 1992.)

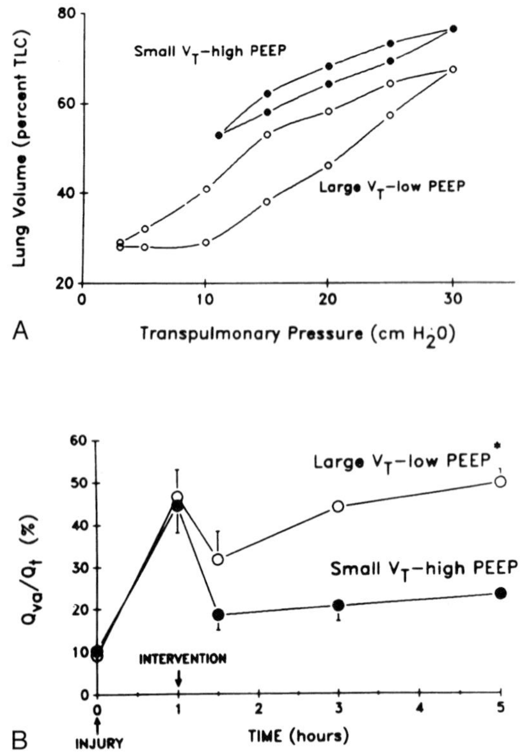


**Figure 92.7** *A,* Pulmonary pressure-volume relationships during canine acid aspiration are compared between two groups: *open circles* denote conditions of large tidal volume (VT) and low positive end-expiratory pressure (PEEP) (3 cm $H_2O$); *closed circles* denote small VT with high PEEP (13 cm $H_2O$). Note that an increase in PEEP of 10 cm $H_2O$ caused a large increase in end-expiratory lung volume such that VT was halved to maintain similar end-expiratory lung volume and transpulmonary pressure. *B,* The use of a low VT–high PEEP ventilatory pattern reduced the intrapulmonary shunt (Qva/Qt) more effectively than did the large VT–low PEEP pattern, and this improvement was maintained over the 5-hour period of observation. In the animals ventilated with lower PEEP and higher VT, the intrapulmonary shunt climbed to the earlier levels. (Adapted from Corbridge TC, Wood LDH, Crawford GP, et al: Adverse effects of large tidal volume and low PEEP in canine acid aspiration. Am Rev Respir Dis 142:311–315, 1990.)

The events of alveolar recruitment and alveolar overdistention have been related to the pressure-volume relationships of the respiratory system during inflation, as demonstrated in Fig. 92.8. Both in animal models of lung injury and in patients with ARDS (Fig. 92.9), the respiratory system inflation pressure-volume curve exhibits a sigmoidal shape, with a lower inflection point (LIP) and an upper inflection point (UIP).[121, 122] As shown in Figure 92.9, marked hysteresis is often noted when the inflation and deflation limbs are compared. The presence of the LIP is consistent with the edematous lung's behaving as a two-compartment structure, with one population of alveoli exhibiting near-normal compliance and another recruitable only at higher transpulmonary pressures.[123] As transpulmonary pressure is raised to the LIP, effecting alveolar recruitment, lung compliance improves, as reflected by the increase in the slope of the pressure-volume curve. Volume tends to increase in an almost linear fashion as pressure is increased, until the UIP is reached; the subsequent flattening of the curve is taken to represent alveolar overdistention with its attendant risks of alveolar injury.

These mechanical events—cyclic alveolar recruitment-derecruitment and overdistention—not only may carry the potential for direct lung injury but also may initiate a series of inflammatory events with widespread consequences. Several investigations have demonstrated that the serum and bronchoalveolar lavage profile of cytokines and other mediators of inflammation may be altered by ventilator strategies that result in alveolar overdistention or recruitment-derecruitment. The clinical significance of the emergence of such biochemical markers of inflammation remains to be determined, but the linkage of mechanical events during ventilatory support to inflammation could provide a mechanistic explanation for the evolution of multisystem organ failure so commonly observed during the care of patients with ARDS.[124–128a]

The pressure-volume relationships of the respiratory system described earlier have been taken by many as a

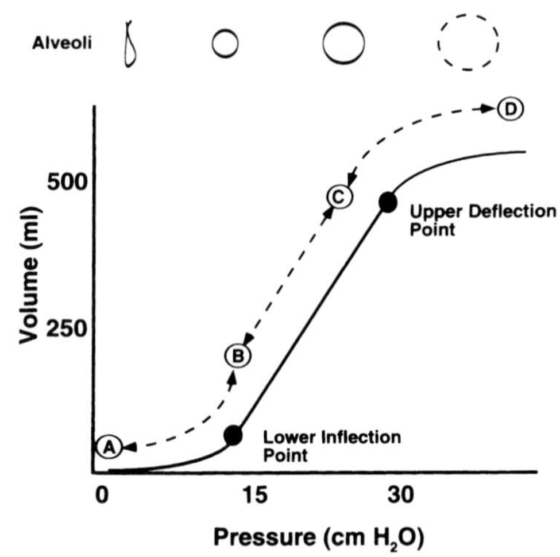


**Figure 92.8** A schematized sigmoidal pressure-volume curve of the respiratory system in a patient with the acute respiratory distress syndrome. The outlines across the top of the graph indicate the relative state of inflation of alveoli. At airway pressures greater than the upper inflection point C (30 cm $H_2O$), the curve flattens as the limits of lung compliance are reached, and there is progressive overdistention of alveoli. Airway pressures below the lower inflection point B are also associated with lower compliance and result in alveolar collapse. Cyclic recruitment-derecruitment may lead to injury as well. Some have advocated ventilator strategies that couple positive end-expiratory pressure and low tidal volumes to maintain ventilation between points B and C. (From Granton JT, Slutsky AR: Ventilator induced lung injury. *In* Hall JB, Schmidt G, Wood LDH (eds): Principles of Critical Care. New York: McGraw-Hill, 1998, p 125.)

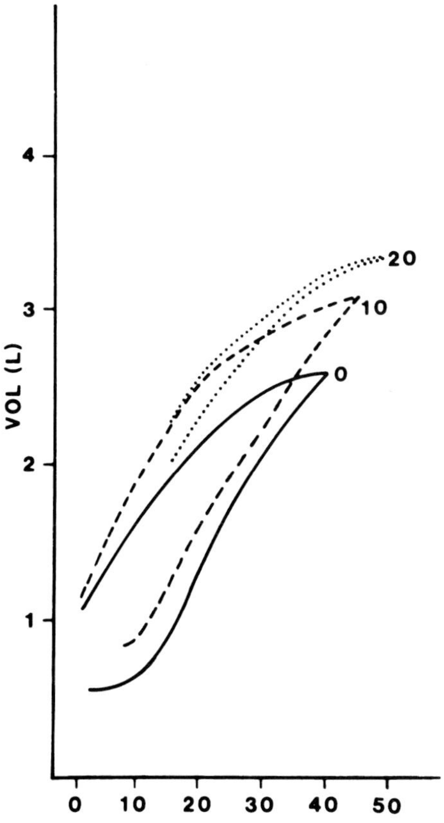


**Figure 92.9** A static pressure-volume curve is shown for a patient with early acute respiratory distress syndrome (ARDS) at various levels of positive end-expiratory pressure (PEEP). Without PEEP, the curve demonstrates marked hysteresis and an inflection point on the inflation limb. At 20 cm $H_2O$ PEEP, the inflection point is lost and the inflation-deflation curves are more nearly superimposable with an increased slope, indicating improved compliance associated with alveolar recruitment. (From Benito S, LeMaire F: Pulmonary pressure-volume relationship in acute respiratory distress syndrome in adults: Role of positive end expiratory pressure. J Crit Care 5:27–34, 1990.)

surrogate measure of lung inflation events, a perhaps naive notion that disregards the separate and potentially different contributions of lung and chest wall components (see later discussion). Nonetheless, on the basis of the accumulating information from animal studies of VILI, recommendations have been made to select PEEP and tidal volume levels that maintain the respiratory system within the bounds of LIP and UIP: that is, a PEEP level sufficiently large to maintain lung inflation above the LIP at the initiation of each breath and a tidal volume sufficiently low to maintain inflation below the UIP at the end of each breath. This strategy has been termed *open-lung ventilation,* and it has been recommended that these end points of ventilation be sought even at the cost of resulting hypercapnia *(permissive hypercapnia).*

### Clinical Studies of Ventilator Strategies for ARDS

To what extent do clinical data support the abundant evidence for VILI derived from animal investigations? As mentioned previously respiratory system pressure-volume curves in patients with ARDS often exhibit an LIP and a UIP (see Fig. 92.9), analogous to the findings in animal models. In one study of severe ARDS, when patients were initially ventilated at a tidal volume of 10 mL/kg, the plateau airway pressure rose above the UIP in 80% of cases, necessitating a reduction in mean tidal volume to 7 to 8 mL/kg.[129] These and other findings suggest that overdistention, to the extent that it is represented by the UIP, can be avoided by low tidal volume ventilation.

There is far less consensus about whether manipulation of PEEP at the bedside can minimize VALI and, if so, what level of PEEP should be used. For one thing, the LIP is really an inflection zone, across which there is progressive recruitment with progressively higher PEEP. When the pressure-volume relationship is measured in ARDS, the LIP is often in the range of 8 to 18 cm $H_2O$.[122, 129, 130] In a computed tomographic study of patients with ARDS,[130] the amount of reopening-collapsing tissue became insignificant only when PEEP reached 20 cm $H_2O$ (although the greatest reduction was seen between 10 and 15 cm $H_2O$ PEEP). Such an attempt to prevent ventilation across the LIP in dependent alveoli requires that nondependent alveoli become overdistended due to the substantial gradient of pleural pressure in edematous lungs.[131]

A second point is that the LIP determined from the inflation limb of the pressure-volume curve may bear little relation to the level of PEEP required to prevent end-expiratory derecruitment, owing to the significant hysteresis of edematous lungs. To prevent shear stress induced by recruitment-derecruitment, the necessary PEEP is that required to keep the lung above an inflection point on the *deflation* pressure-volume curve, a point that is likely to be lower than the inflation LIP, as shown in Figure 92.9. Lacking definitive clinical data, intensivists are not in agreement about the approach to PEEP, some selecting PEEP on the basis of the inflation-limb LIP (the open-lung approach) and others choosing "least PEEP," the lowest value of PEEP necessary to maintain an acceptable arterial oxygen saturation (arterial $SO_2$) with an $FI_{O_2}$ lower than 0.6.[1]

Of greatest importance have been clinical trials to determine the impact of these strategies on patient outcome. Hickling and colleagues[132, 133] reported a favorable impact on survival of tidal volume reduction and permissive hypercapnia in patients with ARDS, comparing outcome with historical controls. These studies were limited by the lack of a randomized, prospective controlled design, a crucial weakness in light of findings that the survival of patients with ARDS in the same time frame appears to have improved apart from the details of mechanical ventilatory support.[134]

The results of the first clinical trial to compare the open-lung approach with conventional ventilation (Fig. 92.10 and Fig. 92.11) were reported in 1995 by Amato and colleagues.[135] Subsequently, the same authors published the results of an even larger study using the same methods.[136] They randomly assigned patients with ARDS to one of two treatments: (1) the conventional approach, consisting of AC ventilation with tidal volumes of 12 mL/kg, PEEP sufficient to maintain an adequate arterial $S_{O_2}$ with $F_{I_{O_2}}$ lower than 0.6, and respiratory rates sufficient to maintain arterial carbon dioxide levels of 25 to 38 mm Hg, with no efforts made to control peak inspiratory or plateau airway pressures; or (2) the open-lung approach, consisting of pressure-controlled inverse ratio ventilation (PC-IRV), pressure-support ventilation, or volume-assured pressure-support ventilation with tidal volumes less than 6 mL/kg, recruitment maneuver, peak pressures less than 40 cm $H_2O$, and PEEP titrated to maintain lung inflation above the LIP, as illustrated in Figure 92.10. Patients managed with the open-lung approach demonstrated a more rapid recovery of pulmonary compliance, a decreased requirement for high $F_{I_{O_2}}$, a lower rate of barotrauma, a higher rate of liberation from the ventilator, a decreased rate of death associated with respiratory failure, and a decreased mortality rate at 28 days (although not at hospital discharge).

Although these results are striking, a number of concerns regarding this study deserve consideration. The number of patients included in the study was small (only 53). Furthermore, there were multiple treatment differences between the two groups, including PEEP strategy, tidal volume, $P_{CO_2}$, minute ventilation, lung recruitment maneuvers, and mode of ventilation. Of importance is that mortality was extremely high in the group given conventional ventilation (71%), and the early differences in mortality between the groups did not seem to be consistent with a difference between the two ventilator strategies in the accrual of progressive lung injury. Finally, patients with severe metabolic acidosis, a common feature of patients with overwhelming sepsis and ARDS, were excluded from study. Even if the results of this study are accepted, the benefit may have resulted simply from tidal volume reduction, not the PEEP strategy. Even if the PEEP strategy prevented VILI, the PEEP value selected from the LIP seen on inflation of edematous lungs from zero end-expiratory pressure is considerably larger than the PEEP value required to maintain alveolar recruitment during tidal ventilation on PEEP.[136a]

Other trials exploring the benefits of low tidal volume ventilation have yielded less encouraging results. Stewart

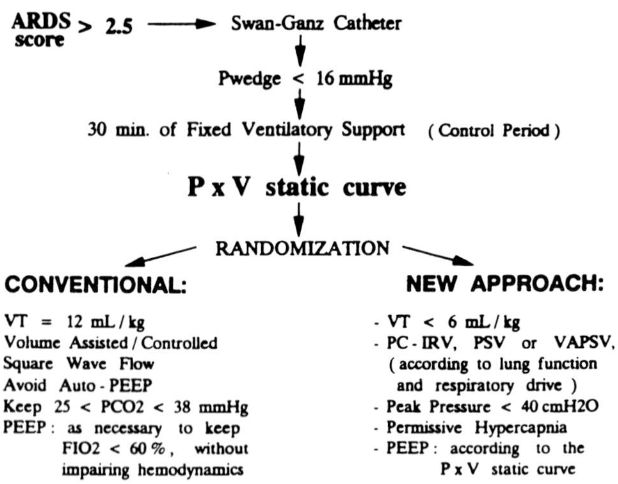


**Figure 92.10** A diagram illustrating the selection of patients and the initial evaluation procedures in a comparison of conventional ventilation with "open-lung" ventilation. ARDS = acute respiratory distress syndrome; $F_{I_{O_2}}$ = fractional concentration of oxygen in inspired gas; P = pressure; PC-IRV = pressure-controlled inverse ratio ventilation; PEEP = positive end-expiratory pressure; PSV = pressure-supported ventilation; Pwedge = pulmonary wedge pressure; V = volume of gas; VAPSV = volume-assured pressure-supported ventilation; VT = tidal volume. (Adapted from Amato MBP, Barbas CSV, Medeiros DM, et al: Beneficial effects of the "open lung approach" with low distending pressures in acute respiratory distress syndrome: A prospective randomized study on mechanical ventilation. Am J Respir Crit Care Med 152:1835, 1995.)

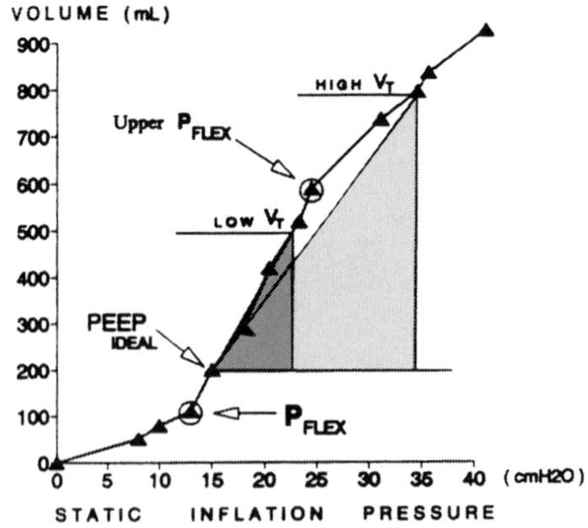


**Figure 92.11** An inspiratory static pressure-volume curve of the respiratory system obtained from a patient entered in a study of "open-lung" ventilation in ARDS. At an inflation pressure between 10 and 15 cm $H_2O$, a lower inflection point is noted (PFLEX). This describes a lung inflation point below which alveolar closure is hypothesized to occur, and selection a positive end-expiratory pressure (PEEP) level below this point causes alveolar recruitment-derecruitment with each respiratory cycle. It is speculated that such inflation-deflation, with its associated shear forces, can cause lung injury. Therefore, a PEEP level greater than this lower inflection point is shown as "PEEPIDEAL." As volume increases along the inflation curve, a second or upper inflection point (Upper PFLEX) is encountered. This is believed to reflect a point at which overdistention of alveolar units occurs, risking volutrauma. Use of high tidal volumes, as shown, can result in lung inflation exceeding this inflection point, risking alveolar overdistention and injury. The goal of "open-lung" ventilation is to maintain inflation-deflation between the two inflection points during the entire respiratory cycle. (Adapted from Amato MBP, Barbas CSV, Medeiros DM, et al: Beneficial effects of the "open lung approach" with low distending pressures in acute respiratory distress syndrome: A prospective randomized study on mechanical ventilation. Am J Respir Crit Care Med 152:1835, 1995.)

and colleagues[137] randomly assigned 120 patients either to pressure- or volume-limited ventilation (peak-inspiratory pressure maintained at 30 cm $H_2O$ or less and tidal volume at 8 mL/kg or less) or to conventional ventilation (with the peak-inspiratory pressure allowed to rise as high as 50 cm $H_2O$ and the tidal volume to 10 mL/kg). No differences in mortality rate, incidence of barotrauma, or degree of multiple-organ dysfunction were seen between the groups. Two other prospective, randomized trials of low vs. high tidal volume strategies yielded similar results.[138, 139] Also, an analysis of data from a large (N = 725) group of patients with ARDS enrolled in a trial of aerosolized synthetic surfactant failed to demonstrate any significant correlations between higher ventilatory pressures and volumes with the development of pneumothorax, air leaks, or mortality.[140] However, the incidence of barotrauma in this study was low (7%), perhaps related to current ventilator approaches, which emphasize limiting airway pressures in patients with acute lung injury. Historically, high incidences of barotrauma (greater than 40%) are often associated with mechanical ventilation with high tidal volumes that cause inspiratory airway pressures higher than 35 to 40 cm $H_2O$.

Are these results consistent with the Amato study? Sufficiently large differences exist between these studies to make direct comparisons difficult, if not impossible. The two groups in the Amato study differed greatly by both PEEP level (16 vs. 7 cm $H_2O$ in the open-lung and conventional limbs, respectively) and tidal volume (362 vs. 763 mL, respectively). The other trials comparing low and high tidal volumes did not explore differences in PEEP, and the results of studies comparing only different tidal volume strategies are not entirely consistent internally. Also, the patients in all arms of the low tidal volume studies[137–139] and the open-lung arm of the Amato study shared similar survival curves, whereas the "conventional" arm of the Amato study, in which no restriction of airway pressure was applied, exhibited an inordinately high mortality rate (71%). Therefore, the currently available clinical data support efforts to minimize VALI at the bedside and suggest that limitation of excessive distending pressures may be the most important factor in this regard. The low tidal volume trials also suggest that patients with milder forms of acute lung injury may not benefit further from reduction of distending pressures much below a level of 35 cm $H_2O$.

The debate over which tidal volume is best in ARDS may have been settled with the recent report on NIH's web site of the preliminary results from an NHLBI-supported multicenter trial of 861 patients with acute lung injury who were randomly assigned to be ventilated with either high (12-mL/kg) or low (6-mL/kg) tidal volumes; PEEP strategies were the same in the two groups. At interim analysis, the mortality rates were significantly different in the two groups: 39% of patients ventilated with high tidal volumes, in comparison with 31% of those receiving low tidal volumes. A full report is in press.[140a]

Other clinical series have elaborated other factors that may be significant in interpreting prior studies and fashioning future ones.[141] Gattinoni and colleagues[142] studied respiratory system mechanics, partitioned between lung and chest wall components, in two groups of patients with ARDS. They prospectively classified patients as having either ARDS resulting from pulmonary disease ($ARDS_p$), primarily pneumonia, or ARDS caused by extrapulmonary disease ($ARDS_{exp}$), primarily trauma and intra-abdominal sepsis. The differences between the two groups were notable. At PEEP levels of 0 cm $H_2O$, both groups had similar respiratory system (lungs plus chest wall) compliance and similar end-expiratory lung volume. However, patients with $ARDS_p$ had much stiffer lungs than patients with $ARDS_{exp}$. When patients with $ARDS_p$ had their PEEP levels increased to 15 cm $H_2O$, the respiratory system became stiffer yet, with minimal recruitment of lung volume. Patients with $ARDS_{exp}$ exhibited a much greater chest wall stiffness than patients with $ARDS_p$, and this correlated with an increased intra-abdominal pressure. Increasing the PEEP in $ARDS_{exp}$ patients from 0 to 15 cm $H_2O$ increased respiratory system compliance and resulted in a significant lung recruitment of approximately 0.3 L. The difference in lung and chest wall mechanics between the two patient groups suggested fundamental differences in lung pathophysiology to the authors. They proposed that patients with $ARDS_p$ had substantial lung consolidation and minimal recruitment with PEEP, whereas patients with $ARDS_{exp}$ had alveolar flooding and collapse, which was more amenable to recruitment with PEEP.

Ranieri and coworkers[143] compared patients with ARDS consequent to major abdominal surgery ("surgical" ARDS) to patients with "medical" ARDS. In surgical ARDS, the static inspiratory volume-pressure curve of the respiratory system and lung showed a downward concavity, indicating that compliance decreased with inflation and suggesting alveolar overdistention. Patients with ARDS consequent to medical conditions had an upward concavity on the static inspiratory volume-pressure curves of the respiratory system and lung, indicating an increase in compliance and alveolar recruitment during inflation. PEEP effects were not examined. Surgical ARDS patients who underwent operative abdominal decompression for bleeding exhibited an upward and leftward shift of the lung, chest wall, and respiratory system volume-pressure curves.

Mergoni and colleagues[144] studied patients with acute respiratory failure, partitioning respiratory system mechanics and describing PEEP effects on mechanics and gas exchange. These investigators showed that in a subset of patients with ARDS, the LIP of the static volume-pressure curve of the respiratory system was caused by the shape of the volume-pressure curve of the chest wall and not that of the lung. When this was true, PEEP was not as effective in improving arterial $Po_2$, which suggests that in these patients the LIP is not a measure of alveolar recruitment.

How do these investigations inform our understanding of trials of lung-protective ventilator strategies? Post hoc comparisons of patient groups in these outcome studies with the detailed results of studies of mechanics is difficult, if not impossible. How best may this information be used for current clinical practice or future clinical studies? Several lessons can be drawn from this group of investigations of respiratory system, lung, and chest wall mechanics in patients with ARDS: First, lung mechanics in patients with ARDS cannot be confidently inferred from measurement of respiratory system mechanics at the mouth, and partitioning of separate lung and chest wall effects is advisable. Second, the UIP and the LIP on the volume-pressure curve must be interpreted in light of contributions of deranged chest wall (including abdominal) mechanics and hence may not simply reflect properties of the injured lung. Third, overdistention of the lung cannot be predicted simply by the end-inspiratory pressure, particularly when chest wall/abdominal elastance is markedly increased. Finally, lung recruitability may be influenced by the nature of the lung insult itself, with lung consolidation perhaps somewhat refractory to the addition of PEEP.

It is certainly premature to recommend routine measurements at the bedside to partition lung mechanics in individual patients, although clinicians who are actively employing ventilator strategies to limit alveolar distention should be aware that simple measurement of the plateau pressure at end inspiration is likely to overestimate the true transpulmonary pressure when abdominal distention and other causes of chest wall stiffness are present. Of most importance is that as future studies are designed to further elucidate the clinical significance of VILI and its prevention, these principles should be extremely helpful for protocol design to more precisely define patient groups to be enrolled and to inform interpretation of results.

### Bedside Management of Ventilator Therapy: Practical Guidelines

The principles that guide our ventilatory management of ARDS are as follows: (1) avoid alveolar overdistention; (2) maintain an $F_{I_{O_2}}$ of less than 0.6; (3) use sufficient PEEP to prevent significant tidal recruitment-derecruitment; (4) consider that the mode of ventilation is usually less important than attending to goals 1 through 3; and (5) tolerate hypercapnia, if necessary, to achieve goals 1 through 3. A bedside approach to rapid adjustment of the ventilator is delineated in the following paragraphs. These goals can be achieved in more than 90% of newly ventilated ARDS patients; occasionally, the salvage therapies discussed later in this chapter may be required.

On presentation, the patient should receive oxygen provided by a high-flow or rebreather mask, although these devices rarely achieve a tracheal $F_{I_{O_2}}$ much above 0.6 in dyspneic, tachypneic patients.[145] The administration of supplemental oxygen is a diagnostic as well as therapeutic maneuver. Patients whose oxygenation improves dramatically with supplemental oxygen usually have a small shunt and a larger component of ventilation-perfusion mismatch (or hypoventilation). Even when the arterial $P_{O_2}$ improves only slightly, indicating a large shunt, oxygen delivery may rise significantly, owing to the steep nature of the oxyhemoglobin saturation relationship at low arterial $P_{O_2}$ (Fig. 92.12). The role of NIPPV has not been established in ARDS. Although NIPPV has been used successfully in this setting, it is generally not a good choice and patients must be carefully selected. Because the course of ARDS is usually longer than patients will tolerate NIPPV, and because ARDS is so often associated with hemodynamic instability, coma, and multiorgan system failure (including ileus), all but exceptional patients should be endotracheally intubated.

Intubation should be performed early and electively when it is clear that mechanical ventilation will be required, rather than waiting for severe respiratory failure. If hypoperfusion is present, as in the patient with hypotension, cardiovascular instability, or the hyperdynamic circulation of sepsis, oxygen delivery may be compromised not only by hypoxemia but also by an inadequate cardiac output. In this circumstance, sedation and muscle relaxation should be considered as a means to diminish the oxygen requirement of the skeletal muscles. Patients with extreme hypoxemia despite ventilator management, as described later, may also benefit from sedation or paralysis. Finally, muscle relaxation allows cooling of the febrile patient without causing shivering, an important consideration in this group of patients with borderline oxygen delivery.[146, 147]

***Initial Ventilator Settings.*** The initial ventilator settings include an $F_{I_{O_2}}$ of 1.0, a respiratory rate of 20 to 30 breaths/min, and a tidal volume of 6 to 8 mL/kg when AC or SIMV mode is used, or an inspiratory pressure equal to 30 to 35 cm $H_2O$ when pressure-control ventilation (PCV) is used. An expected consequence of these low tidal volumes or inflation pressures is respiratory acidosis. The benefits and risks of accepting an elevated $P_{CO_2}$ are discussed later (see section on permissive hypercapnia). Using a low triggered sensitivity ($-2$ cm $H_2O$ or flow-by) with the AC mode or providing pressure-support breaths between SIMV breaths allows patients to increase their minute ventilation should they have the drive to do so. Most patients require substantial sedation (especially with PCV) which, in addition to aiding patient-ventilator synchrony, reduces oxygen consumption and carbon dioxide production.[146]

One of the first goals of ventilator management is to reduce the $F_{I_{O_2}}$ to less than 0.6 to minimize further lung injury. Although it is clinically difficult to distinguish the sequelae of acute lung injury from the complications of the therapy it requires, including potential injury due to oxygen, it is generally agreed that an $F_{I_{O_2}}$ greater than 0.6 is toxic.[148–153] At the same time, there are limits to the degree of hypoxemia that patients tolerate; an arterial $S_{O_2}$ approaching 75% can cause global myocardial hypoxia, anaerobic metabolism, acute dilated cardiomyopathy, and bradycardic arrest.[154] Accordingly, PEEP is used to recruit alveoli, diminish intrapulmonary shunt, and permit a decrease in the $F_{I_{O_2}}$. PEEP exploits the hysteresis of the inflation and deflation limbs of each breath to recruit alveoli on inspiration, by expanding collapsed units and translocating fluid from flooded units to the interstitial space,[121, 155] then prevent derecruitment at end-expiration. The result is increased respiratory system compliance due to increased FRC and improved gas exchange due to oxygenation of perfused recruited air spaces. When severely hypoxemic patients fail to respond to PEEP, a focal lung process (e.g., lobar pneumonia, atelectasis) should be suspected (see later discussion).[156–158]

Reducing PEEP, even for short periods, is often associated with alveolar derecruitment and rapid arterial hemoglobin desaturation. Therefore, once endotracheal tube

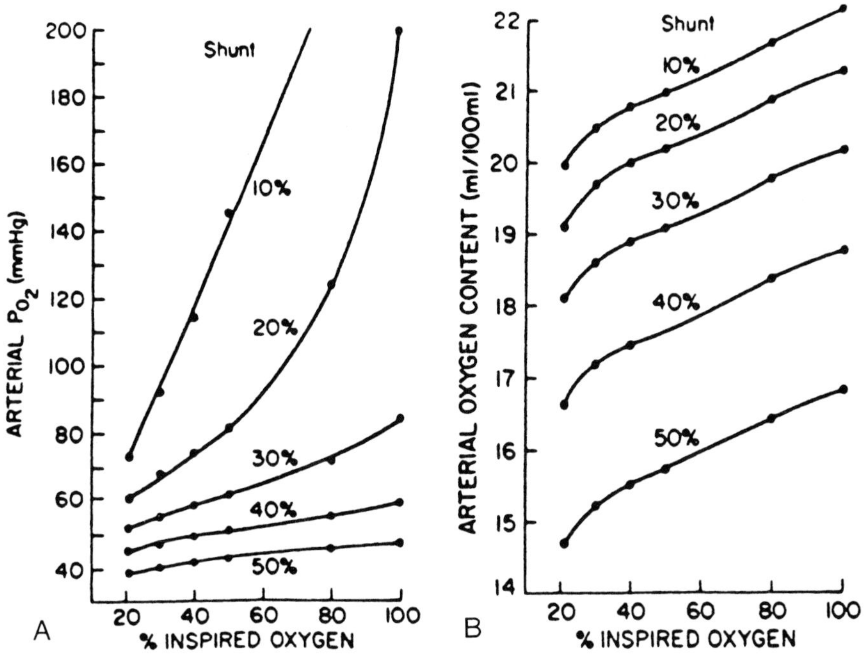


**Figure 92.12** Arterial $P_{O_2}$ is shown as a function of the percentage of inspired oxygen at various degrees of shunt *(A)*, and an increase in arterial oxygen content is shown with increased percentage of inspired oxygen at various degrees of shunt *(B)*. Even at large shunt fractions, the relative increase in content and hence oxygen delivery is great, because the small change in arterial $P_{O_2}$ occurs on the steep portion of the oxygen-hemoglobin dissociation curve. (From Dantzker RM: Gas exchange in the adult respiratory distress syndrome. Clin Chest Med 3:57, 1982.)

suctioning has been accomplished for diagnostic purposes, nursing and respiratory therapy staff should be instructed to keep airway disconnections to a minimum or to use an in-line suctioning system that maintains sterility and positive pressure, usually one in which the suctioning catheter resides in a sterile sheath and enters the endotracheal tube via a tight-sealing diaphragm. These suctioning systems usually are effective for lesser levels of PEEP (less than 15 cm $H_2O$), but they often leak if higher levels are attempted.

Because the approach to PEEP in patients with ARDS is evolving, intensivists must currently manage patients without the benefit of solid clinical data. Guidelines are provided here for both the least-PEEP and the open-lung strategies.

In the least-PEEP approach, PEEP is initially increased to 15 to 20 cm $H_2O$ in a single step as a recruitment maneuver, while pulse oximetry is used to monitor the arterial oxyhemoglobin saturation. With this high initial level of PEEP and tidal volumes of 6 to 8 mL/kg, a plateau airway pressure as high as 45 to 50 cm $H_2O$ may be encountered, a level perhaps necessary for alveolar recruitment but undesirable for application beyond the early minutes of ventilation. Consideration should be given to the possibility that certain disease processes (e.g., ARDS secondary to primary pneumonia) may result in less alveolar recruitment than others (e.g., ARDS secondary to a nonpulmonary source of sepsis), as discussed previously.

Hypotension, attributed both to a rise in pleural (and, therefore, right atrial) pressure and to increased resistance to venous return,[156] is uncommon, perhaps because the pleural pressure increment is slight, being proportional to chest wall compliance and the volume of lung recruited by the PEEP, not to the PEEP per se. Significant hypotension can be treated by reducing the PEEP temporarily, then infusing fluids or vasoactive drugs to restore cardiac output. Once the oximeter-monitored arterial $S_{O_2}$ rises to 90%, the $F_{I_{O_2}}$ is reduced to 0.6. Just as shunt lesions are poorly responsive to increased $F_{I_{O_2}}$, so are they to reduced $F_{I_{O_2}}$, and it usually is possible to achieve the target of 0.6 $F_{I_{O_2}}$ within 10 minutes of raising the PEEP. Once the $F_{I_{O_2}}$ is lowered to 0.6, PEEP is decreased in steps of 2.5 cm $H_2O$, allowing at least 15 minutes between steps, seeking the least PEEP that gives an arterial $S_{O_2}$ greater than 90% with an $F_{I_{O_2}}$ of 0.6. Finally, adequate oximeter-measured saturation is confirmed with arterial blood gas analysis. Note that the volume-pressure curve during tidal inflation from this least-PEEP value can be measured to determine the presence or absence of a LIP. When the LIP is not evident, the least-PEEP value also protects the lung from excess shear stress at a lower PEEP than does the open-lung approach. When a LIP is evident at least PEEP, it can be abolished by small increments in PEEP (2.5 to 5 cm $H_2O$) above the least PEEP.

In some patients, PEEP must be raised higher than 15 to 20 cm $H_2O$ to get the $F_{I_{O_2}}$ below 0.6. In such patients ancillary strategies, such as transfusion of packed red blood cells, augmentation of cardiac output (usually with dobutamine), or reduction of oxygen consumption (through sedation, therapeutic paralysis, and cooling) may be used to improve oxygenation, or salvage methods may be resorted to (see later discussion).

The open-lung approach uses PEEP not just to avoid oxygen toxicity but also as a lung-protective strategy. As described by Amato and colleagues,[135] the volume-pressure curve is constructed by increasing the tidal volume from 100 to 1000 mL, noting the pressures after an inspiratory pause (all with zero PEEP). The LIP of the inflation limb is determined, and PEEP is set 2 cm $H_2O$ higher. Practitioners who are uncomfortable subjecting a patient with ARDS to mechanical ventilation without PEEP for the time required to construct a volume-pressure curve, typically about 30 minutes, simply determine the curve on a PEEP of 10 to 15 cm $H_2O$. PEEP is then adjusted upward until there is no LIP. Those who find it impractical to determine volume-pressure curves on a daily basis may set the PEEP on the basis of typical values required to exceed the LIP, such as the average PEEP of 17 used in the Amato trial. This average value is often higher than the least PEEP, because the Amato method did not account for alveolar recruitment within the volume-pressure hysteresis at PEEP levels much less than the LIP observed during inflation of edematous lungs from zero end-expiratory pressure. As oxygenation improves over the first few days, the PEEP is adjusted downward and the mode is changed from pressure-control to pressure-support. Because the open-lung approach provides no guide to reducing PEEP, the least-PEEP method may be used to guide PEEP reduction as the lung edema clears.

***Ventilator Adjustment After Stabilization.*** Once the PEEP is adjusted and the $F_{I_{O_2}}$ is lowered to 0.6, the mode, tidal volume (or pressure), and rate should be reevaluated. With AC or SIMV, a 0.3-second end-inspiratory pause should be used to determine the plateau airway pressure. If it exceeds 35 cm $H_2O$, the tidal volume should be reduced progressively until this target value is achieved.[157, 158] In the use of PCV, the inspiratory pressure should be set at 30 to 35 cm $H_2O$. The use of these pressure targets assumes that they correlate with alveolar overdistention,[121, 122] an assumption that is less likely to be true under conditions of significant chest wall (including abdominal) restriction (see previous discussion).

Although the technique varies with the specific ventilator, PCV involves setting the inspiratory pressure-assist at a level such that PEEP plus the pressure-assist is 30 to 35 cm $H_2O$. The inspiratory:expiratory (I:E) ratio is typically 1:1. (A word of caution: the pressure-control mode of ventilation is an upgrade to many of the ventilators commonly used in the intensive care unit and may not be incorporated into the main controls of the ventilator. It can be difficult to ascertain exactly what state these ventilators are in without careful inspection of the waveforms on a pressure and flow monitor.) There is no clear benefit to one mode or another. Although it is simpler to use PCV (which does not require repeated determinations of plateau airway pressure in the face of changing respiratory system mechanics to avoid alveolar overdistention), equivalent ventilation can be provided with the use of AC or IMV and a decelerating flow waveform.[159] Inverse-ratio ventilation, described in more detail later, can be included with any of these modes. With PCV, the I:E ratio can usually be set directly. With AC or IMV, either the inspiratory flow rate can be set to a low value (e.g., 30 L/min or lower) or a decelerating profile, or an end-inspiratory pause can be dialed in.

The initial respiratory rate of 20 to 30 breaths/min may also need adjustment. The expiratory flow waveform should be inspected (when available) for the presence of end-expiratory flow. Alternatively, auto-PEEP (also called intrinsic PEEP; see Chapter 93) should be determined. When either of these measures of dynamic hyperinflation is encountered, the rate should generally be lowered (and consideration should be given to treating bronchospasm, if indicated). Alternatively, if there is no end-expiratory flow on the initially chosen rate, it can be raised to ameliorate the respiratory acidosis that is expected when small tidal volumes are used.

***Permissive Hypercapnia.*** Historically, physicians have attempted to ventilate patients to a normal arterial $P_{CO_2}$. In patients with severe lung disease, this arbitrary goal has a mechanical cost: the probable amplification of lung injury, as described earlier. Increasing evidence points to the safety and efficacy of allowing the arterial $P_{CO_2}$ to rise well above 40 mm Hg. When patients with severe ARDS are ventilated with volume- or pressure-limited ventilation as described previously, the arterial $P_{CO_2}$ rises typically to 60 to 70 mm Hg, but in some patients it is much higher (more than 150 mm Hg).[132, 133] The arterial pH falls to roughly 7.2, but at times below 7.0. Respiratory acidosis has many deleterious physiologic effects, including cellular metabolic dysfunction, depression of myocardial contractility, coronary vasodilation, systemic vasodilation, pulmonary vasoconstriction, enhanced hypoxic pulmonary vasoconstriction, cerebral vasodilation, increased intracranial pressure, and renal vasoconstriction. Yet even very high levels of arterial $P_{CO_2}$ seem remarkably well tolerated by adequately sedated patients.[160, 161] Perhaps this is related to highly efficient and rapidly acting cellular compensatory mechanisms,[160] which tend to defend intracellular pH. Because respiratory acidosis raises intracranial pressure, permissive hypercapnia should not be used in patients with cerebral edema, trauma, or space-occupying lesions. This and other contraindications are listed in Table 92.5. Some researchers have speculated that hypercapnia could worsen cardiac ischemia in patients with coronary artery disease through a coronary vasodilation-induced "steal" syndrome, but the significance of this effect is not known. There is also concern that permissive hypercapnia may cause deterioration in patients with left ventricular systolic dysfunction or right-sided heart syndromes.

The question for the clinician is not whether a normal arterial $P_{CO_2}$ is desirable, but which is riskier for the patient: a high arterial $P_{CO_2}$ or alveolar overdistention. Although conclusive evidence from controlled patient trials is lacking, the preponderance of evidence from animal studies and limited human data favor the use of permissive hypercapnia. For example, healthy human volunteers have been reported to tolerate levels of arterial $P_{CO_2}$ as high as 250 mm Hg (and pH levels as low as 6.72) without serious consequences.[162] Arterial $P_{CO_2}$ values greater 100 mm Hg are sometimes encountered in patients with severe asthma and do not appear to be associated

**Table 92.5 CONTRAINDICATIONS FOR PERMISSIVE HYPERCAPNEA**

| |
|---|
| Increased intracranial pressure |
| Active myocardial ischemia |
| Hypotension and/or severe left-ventricular failure with catecholamine dependence |
| Pulmonary hypertension with acute right-sided heart failure |
| Severe metabolic acidosis (?) |

with any deleterious systemic effects.[160] When a group of severe ARDS patients (lung injury score, 2.5 or greater) were ventilated to keep the peak pressure (Ppeak) no higher than 30 to 40 cm $H_2O$ (total volume, 4 to 7 mL/kg), mortality was only 26%, compared with a rate of 53% predicted from their Acute Physiology and Chronic Health Evaluation (APACHE II) scores.[132, 133] Others have reported similar results.[129, 135] The effect of respiratory acidosis superimposed on an underlying metabolic acidosis is unknown and could be much more deleterious.

How permissive hypercapnic ventilation is best done (magnitude of acidemia, rapidity of changes, use of alkalinizing agents) has not been defined. A common approach is to allow the arterial $P_{CO_2}$ to rise gradually (e.g., 10 mm Hg/hr) to allow time for cellular compensation. Some have advocated the infusion of sodium bicarbonate to raise the blood pH, but this generally has not been done in ARDS patients, and no advantage has been shown over simply allowing the pH to fall. Sodium bicarbonate delivers a substantial carbon dioxide load to a patient who is already marginally able to excrete what is produced endogenously, and such treatment further risks volume overload and potassium depletion. Given the questions regarding safety and usefulness, the role of sodium bicarbonate requires validation before it can be advocated clinically.

### Innovative Therapies for ARDS

***Prone Positioning.*** Many studies have shown that a substantial fraction of patients with ARDS exhibit improved oxygenation with prone positioning and this is not necessarily innovative therapy.[163–165] Nonetheless, it is a remarkably underutilized technique, most likely because of the difficulty providing nursing and others forms of care to patients in this position.

Hypotheses offered to explain the improvement in oxygenation include increased FRC, change in regional diaphragm motion, redistribution of perfusion, and better clearance of secretions.[166] FRC has been shown to be increased with prone positioning in intubated, mechanically ventilated patients without lung injury who are undergoing general anesthesia for surgery.[167] Animal models of $\dot{V}/\dot{Q}$ distribution have suggested that gravity has far less influence on the distribution of perfusion in the prone position and that the distribution of blood flow to regions of the lung is relatively unaffected by the change from the supine to the prone position.[168] This, coupled with the observation that turning to the prone position is associated with a migration of the edema fluid to the dependent portions of the lung (as demonstrated by computer tomography), has suggested to some investigators that $\dot{V}/\dot{Q}$ relationships might be favorably altered by prone positioning.[169] Studies in dogs with oleic acid–induced lung injury have verified that oxygenation is improved, shunt is decreased, and the distribution of flow in the acutely injured lung in the prone position is relatively uninfluenced by gravity.[170, 171] More recent animal studies suggested that there are greater variations in pleural pressure gradient than previously believed and that the prone position is associated with alveolar recruitment as a consequence of high transpulmonary pressures in regions of the lung that have high flow regardless of position.[172] Another possible explanation for the improvement in oxygenation associated with ventilation in the prone position is improved lymphatic flow. Almost all animals in nature, except humans, lie prone when they are recumbent, so it is reasonable to assume that lung lymphatics evolved to drain the lung best in this position.

In patients receiving prone ventilation, special attention is necessary to prevent pressure necrosis of the nose, face, and ears and to ensure maintenance and patency of the endotracheal tube. Pressure on the eye could lead to retinal ischemia, especially in hypotensive patients. Some patients experience cardiac arrhythmias or hemodynamic instability on being turned. Nevertheless, because it is efficacious, relatively safe, and devoid of harmful side effects when done carefully, prone ventilation is worth attempting in patients with severe ARDS and may grow to become a common strategy for ventilation in these patients.

***Tracheal Gas Insufflation.*** A potentially useful adjunctive technique, termed tracheal gas insufflation (TGI), involves the introduction of fresh gas near the carina through a modified endotracheal tube. This added flow washes carbon dioxide–rich gas out of the trachea (and, through turbulence, out of smaller airways as well), reducing anatomic dead space. The arterial $P_{CO_2}$ reducing effect of TGI is lessened by acute lung injury, but this is partially counterbalanced by the higher arterial $P_{CO_2}$ tolerated during permissive hypercapnia.[173] In patients with ARDS, TGI with 100% humidified oxygen, delivered throughout the respiratory cycle at a flow of 4 L/min, successfully lowered arterial $P_{CO_2}$ from 108 to 84 mm Hg.[174] Potential risks of TGI include tracheal erosion, oxygen toxicity related to the unknown $F_{IO_2}$, and hemodynamic compromise or barotrauma due to the occult presence of auto-PEEP.

***High-Frequency Ventilation.*** If excessive lung excursion is associated with injury to the lung, then it seems reasonable that ventilation with very small tidal volumes at high frequencies would be associated with the least possible ventilator-induced lung injury and with improved outcome. High-frequency jet ventilation (HFV) typically employs tidal volumes of 1 to 5 mL (or higher) and respiratory rates of 60 to 300 breaths/min. Gas exchange is poorly understood under these conditions, but it is thought to occur as much through augmented axial diffusion as through bulk flow.[175, 176] Current models of gas exchange during HFV cannot explain how gas exchange occurs in the normal lung, let alone under conditions that may exist in the diseased lung.[177, 178] Multiple trials of HFV have failed to demonstrate any benefit over mechanical ventilation.[179–181] HFV has never been associated with improved oxygenation, reduced barotrauma, or decreased days of mechanical ventilation, all of which are outcomes that would reasonably be expected as an extension of the physiology and concerns driving open-lung ventilation. That they have not been observed suggests that all previous investigations of HFV were conducted with the use of the wrong guidelines for ventilation (i.e., striving to maintain normocarbia), or that some other effect not yet understood precludes benefit from this technique. Future studies of HFV should compare this technique with open-lung ventilation or with the least-PEEP approach coupled with permissive hypercapnia, and must demonstrate superior benefit to gain acceptance. Until further studies are done, HFV is best viewed as a salvage therapy for patients with ARDS refractory to conventional ventilator management.

***Inverse Ratio Ventilation***. Inverse ratio ventilation (IRV) entails the use of prolonged inspiratory times (I:E ratio greater than 1) with either volume-cycled or pressure-cycled modes of mechanical ventilation. A subset of patients with hypoxemia refractory to conventional modes of mechanical ventilation respond to IRV.[182, 183] However, there is no way to prospectively identify these patients. The exact mechanisms by which IRV improves gas exchange in some patients with ARDS remain obscure but are believed to involve both alveolar recruitment at lower airway pressures and more optimal distribution of ventilation.[184, 185] Although it is tempting to attribute the beneficial effect of IRV to intrinsic PEEP, anecdotal reports have excluded intrinsic PEEP or gas trapping as the mechanism by which gas exchange improves in at least some patients.[186] An important caution for using this mode is that both auto-PEEP and the higher mean alveolar pressure typical of IRV tend to reduce cardiac output. In one study of PCV with or without IRV, cardiac output fell with IRV so that systemic oxygen delivery actually worsened.[187] Some investigators have noted a very gradual (over several hours) but progressive tendency for oxygenation to improve after a change to IRV.[188] This phenomenon has led some to suggest that a subset of lung units may be recruitable only through a prolonged inspiratory time. Further studies are needed on this aspect of IRV. Inverse ratio pressure-controlled ventilation has been used as part of the open-lung strategy for ventilation of patients with severe ARDS. Its role remains poorly defined, and it is best regarded as a salvage therapy for patients with hypoxemia refractory to more conventional approaches. Whichever approach is used, the intensivist should monitor auto-PEEP regularly, because the shortened expiratory times of IRV predispose to this effect.

***Extracorporeal Gas Exchange and Intravenous Oxygenator.*** The use of extracorporeal gas exchange (ECMO) to adequately oxygenate and ventilate the blood while allowing the lung to rest remains an attractive strategy for the management of acute lung injury, but its value has not been supported by clinical outcome studies. The earliest large-scale attempt to use ECMO in patients with severe ARDS did not demonstrate any benefit to its use, although it did generate a large database and a great deal of insight into patients with this problem.[189] However, the enrollment criteria in this study were so strict that the mortality rate among all patients entered into it was certain to be high, and consequently it was unlikely that any difference would be demonstrated between groups. Many intensivists believe that more careful patient selection, earlier randomization of patients, and better technology might have demonstrated a benefit to ECMO. A second wave of studies using ECMO was reported throughout the 1980s.[190, 191] A variety of techniques were described, including veno-venous ECMO to assist in the elimination of carbon dioxide. However, a 1994 report of ECMO in adult patients with ARDS failed to demonstrate any benefit.[192] There is little apparent future for this technique in adult patients with ARDS. ECMO is best regarded at this time as heroic salvage therapy for patients with isolated respiratory failure in whom all other supportive measures have failed.

The use of an intravenous oxygenator (IVOX) in patients with severe ARDS has been described in several reports.[193] This technology consists of a very small membrane lung that is actually inserted into the inferior vena cava. This device is capable of only limited gas exchange and, consequently, is unlikely to be developed for widespread use. Advances in technology that result in increased capacity for gas exchange would allow a smaller device to exchange more gas and would make revisiting this technology very interesting.

***Partial Liquid Ventilation.*** The literature has described the use of partial liquid ventilation via perflurocarbons instilled into the trachea of adults and children with RDS.[194–197] The preliminary results from adult use and the more extensive experience in pediatric patients suggest that this mode of therapy is both safe and efficacious in improving gas exchange. Partial liquid ventilation clearly allows oxygenation in patients who might otherwise be quite difficult to oxygenate with conventional modes of ventilation, in part because the perfluorocarbon is able to recruit dependent alveoli (by virtue of the hydraulic column), which PEEP is not. Several issues remain to be addressed before the role of perfluorocarbons can be determined, such as their impact on outcome and whether there are adverse effects associated with their use in the adult population. A practical problem is that perflurocarbons are radiodense, making the lungs appear white, so it is impossible to use chest radiographs to detect infection or to follow the progress of healing. Even if partial liquid ventilation with perfluorocarbons proves to be both safe and beneficial, its role probably will be as salvage therapy, limited to patients who cannot be adequately oxygenated with more conventional modes of mechanical ventilation.

***Inhaled Nitric Oxide.*** Since Roissant and colleagues[198] published their initial experience with the use of inhaled nitric oxide (iNO) as a therapy for ARDS, there has been a rapid expansion of interest and literature in this field.[199–202] Nitric oxide is a potent endogenous vasodilator that, when given by inhalation, selectively vasodilates the pulmonary circulation. iNO has several potentially salutary effects in ARDS. It selectively vasodilates pulmonary vessels that subserve *ventilated* alveoli, diverting blood flow to these alveoli (and away from areas of shunt). The first effect, the lowering of pulmonary vascular resistance, accompanied by a lowering of pulmonary artery pressure, appears maximal at very low concentrations (approximately 0.1 ppm) in patients with ARDS.[202] The beneficial effects on oxygenation take place at somewhat higher concentrations (1 to 10 ppm).[202] The rapid inactivation of iNO via hemoglobin binding prevents unwanted systemic hemodynamic side effects but also mandates continuous delivery of gas to the ventilator circuit. In the numerous studies evaluating the acute response to iNO, there has been a consistent finding that approximately 50% to 70% of patients show improved oxygenation.

Two prospective trials failed to demonstrate improved long-term outcome from iNO administration in ARDS. Michael and colleagues[203] randomly assigned patients to receive or not receive iNO; after 72 hours, both groups had the same degree of oxygenation perturbation, suggesting that the early effects of this therapy are not sustained for a clinically relevant period. Dellinger and associates[204] reported that a multicenter North American trial of iNO in patients with ARDS found no differences in mortality or number of days alive and off mechanical ventilation, although some subsets of patients appeared to benefit in post hoc analysis.

These trials have resulted in some controversy concerning ongoing assessment of iNO.[204a, 204b] At the present time in this country, iNO may be administered only under the auspices of protocols sanctioned by the US Food and Drug Administration. Further trials will probably be required before any use for this agent is identified to treat AHRF. These evaluations may include combining iNO with other inhaled vasodilators such as prostacyclin[205, 206] or with agents such as almitrine that enhance hypoxic vasoconstriction of the pulmonary circulation.[207, 208] One important risk of iNO therapy should be noted. If continuous delivery of iNO is interrupted (e.g., during patient transport, supply exhaustion), precipitous and life-threatening hypoxemia and right-sided heart failure can occur.[209]

### Monitoring the Patient with ARDS

Patients with ARDS, by virtue of their serious gas exchange (and sometimes hemodynamic) impairment, combined with the effects of powerful therapy (sedation, therapeutic paralysis, PEEP), are at risk for sudden and life-threatening deterioration. Changes in intrapulmonary shunt, oxygen consumption, and systemic perfusion are frequent, making arterial saturation and oxygen delivery volatile. Accordingly, careful monitoring for hypoxemia and adequacy of oxygen delivery is advisable. Continuous pulse oximetry is generally reliable (barring gross hypoperfusion) and should be used routinely, when available. Alternatively, frequent sampling of arterial blood gases is advisable throughout the first day of management and after major interventions or changes in clinical appearance of the patient.

The debate concerning use of right-sided heart catheterization has intensified. Physicians have been justly criticized for overuse, poor judgment, and inadequate interpretive skills. Although right-sided heart catheters should not be placed routinely in ARDS patients, invasive monitoring may be useful when there is a clinically relevant question that cannot be answered noninvasively. For example, there often arises the question "Is this ARDS alone or is the patient volume overloaded?" Although this determination may be made by analysis of edema fluid, empiric diuresis of the patient, or examination of the neck veins, intercurrent septic hypotension, renal failure, and ventricular dysfunction an compromise the judgment of the best clinician. Knowledge of how far to push diuresis or ultrafiltration (or even whether to give back fluid to these often hypotensive patients) may be helped by invasive hemodynamic monitoring. Positive-pressure ventilation, PEEP, and vasoactive drug infusions all have dual-edged effects on oxygen transport that are difficult to discern simply from the vital signs and arterial blood gas determinations; invasive monitoring is particularly useful in this setting. The greatest uncertainty exists early in the course of management, so a low threshold for early invasive monitoring should be accompanied by an aggressive withdrawal as soon as the questions are answered.

### Management During Recovery from the Exudative Phase of ARDS

Some patients rapidly recover from ARDS (within 2 to 3 days); the pace is likely to be determined by resolution of the predisposing cause and, arguably, by appropriate cardiovascular interventions. Such recovery is heralded by increased lung compliance and diminishing oxygen requirements. When the $FI_{O_2}$ can be reduced to 0.4 to 0.5, PEEP should cautiously be reduced. On occasion, however, even small decrements in PEEP are associated with sudden arterial desaturation, perhaps related to alveolar flooding or collapse associated with surfactant deficiency or dysfunction. When this occurs, PEEP often must be increased to higher than the former level for alveolar recruitment. Accordingly, reduction via small decrements (2 to 3 cm $H_2O$) of PEEP, with several hours of observation between adjustments, is recommended.

When an $FI_{O_2}$ of 0.4 and PEEP of less than 7.5 cm $H_2O$ have been achieved, the patient should be evaluated for spontaneous ventilation. If central nervous system depression, muscle weakness, or new lung insults have not occurred during the course of acute illness, rapid progression to a T-piece or CPAP trial is appropriate, with prompt extubation (see Chapter 93). In anticipation of these events, sedatives and muscle relaxants should be discontinued as soon as the edema resolves.

### Management of Proliferative-Phase ARDS

A subset of patients with ARDS progress over the first week of mechanical ventilation to disordered healing and severe lung fibrosis. This is usually characterized by increasing airway pressures or a falling tidal volume on PCV, a further fall in lung compliance, less response to PEEP, a "honeycomb" appearance on the chest radiograph, progressive pulmonary hypertension, and rising minute ventilation requirements (more than 20 L/min). Barotrauma is a prominent feature, and multiple organ failures often supervene. A number of observations regarding supportive therapy in this setting should be made. Increased vascular permeability at this point in the course may be minimal, and strategies to reduce preload and edema are fraught with complications. Patients are prone to increases in zone I lung conditions, and attempts to reduce the PPW may result in increased dead space and hypoperfusion. Therefore, it is no longer appropriate to seek the lowest PPW that provides adequate cardiac output; instead, liberalization of fluid intake to provide a circulating volume in excess of that just adequate is a better strategy in this later phase of ARDS.

Interventions to directly influence the course of lung fibrosis are not well established, but high-dose corticosteroid therapy has its advocates.[210–211] One prospective trial showed improved survival with the use of corticosteroids in late ARDS,[212] but routine use in such patients remains controversial; their potential benefit is being examined in a multicenter clinical trial. If corticosteroids are used in this setting, aggressive measures to monitor for ventilator-associated pneumonia are warranted. This complication of mechanical ventilation has a high incidence and a high mortality rate in patients with ARDS.[213, 214] In view of the abnormal chest radiograph findings, abnormal gas exchange, multiple causes of fever and leukocytosis, and high incidence of colonization of the airway, diagnosis is difficult and maybe aided by various techniques to obtain protected specimens from the lower respiratory tract.[212]

If there has been no substantial improvement by 10 to 14 days but recovery is still possible, tracheostomy is reasonable for patient comfort and ongoing ventilator management. Nutritional support is crucial and should be instituted if recovery is not likely to be complete within the first several days of management. Subsequent management of these patients is often protracted and difficult, with constant attention to the details of various organ failures and complications that inevitably arise over time.

#### Pulmonary Sequelae of ARDS

Although there are a limited number of long-term follow-up studies of patients with ARDS, it appears that the range of outcomes is rather wide: Patients may recover with minimal or no abnormalities by routine lung function testing shortly after acute lung insult, or they may remain substantially impaired for a year or longer, if not permanently.[215] In most studies, approximately one fourth of patients show no impairment at 1 year, one fourth have moderate impairment, roughly half have only mild impairment, and a very small fraction have severe impairment. Exertional dyspnea is the most commonly reported symptom, although cough and wheezing also are common. A reduced single-breath carbon monoxide diffusing capacity is the most common pulmonary function abnormality. Spirometry and lung volumes tend to reveal mixed restrictive-obstructive abnormalities. Determining the prognosis after ARDS may be aided by performing complete lung function studies at the time of discharge. Those patients with substantial abnormalities should be referred for appropriate follow-up.

### Management of Focal Lesions Producing AHRF

**Lobar Pneumonia.** Inflammatory pneumonias, even those involving only a modest fraction of the lung volume, can produce significant lung shunt because of the increase in pulmonary blood flow and aerobic metabolism of the consolidated region.[6] Accordingly, supplemental oxygen often has only a modest effect in resolving the associated hypoxemia, but it may correct arterial desaturation caused by hypoventilation of lung regions mechanically interdependent with the pneumonic consolidation. Many otherwise healthy patients can be stabilized with supplemental oxygen and appropriate antibiotics until inflammation subsides over the first days of therapy.

Patients with concurrent problems (e.g., old age, debilitated state, sepsis) and those with extreme hypoxemia require mechanical ventilation, in part to stabilize the cardiovascular collapse associated with pyrexia and excess work of breathing, but also to guarantee a high $F_{I_{O_2}}$. Indications for intubation are similar to those in other forms of AHRF and include tachypnea (respiratory rate greater than 35 breaths/min) and inability to achieve adequate arterial saturation. Once intubation has been performed, samples of airway secretions should be obtained for Gram staining and culture.

The guidelines for ventilator management are similar to those for patients with ARDS. However, PEEP therapy should be added cautiously and should be guided by pulse oximetry. This is particularly true in these patients with focal disease because PEEP may not recruit the consolidated lung but rather hyperinflate normal lung, redistributing blood flow to the area of consolidation and worsening intrapulmonary shunt. Nonetheless, a trial of PEEP is warranted in most patients, because varying degrees of lung edema may be present in regions distant from the radiologically apparent pneumonia. If the patient cannot be adequately oxygenated with PEEP, positioning with the healthier lung downward may help.[216] This maneuver favors blood flow to normally ventilated lung regions and improves gas exchange. In those patients with substantial airway secretions, such positioning carries the risk of soiling the normal lung.

Interventions to decrease blood flow to the infected lobe could conceivably improve gas exchange, and inhibition of prostaglandin synthesis with indomethacin was demonstrated to reduce lung shunt in a canine model of pneumonia.[217] There is little experience with such approaches in humans, however, and other effects of such agents may make their use inadvisable. iNO is potentially beneficial in this setting, as is simultaneous infusion of a pulmonary vasoconstrictor combined with iNO.[207, 208]

As in other patients with AHRF and severe hypoxemia, every attempt should be made to reduce oxygen consumption. In patients with pneumonia, adequate sedation with controlled ventilation, correction of hyperthermia, avoidance of shivering, and muscle relaxation are all simple measures that can achieve this goal.

**Lung Contusion.** Blunt chest trauma, particularly when it is sufficient to cause rib fracture, often contuses the underlying lung. As discussed earlier, the contusion essentially stops blood flow to the consolidated hemorrhagic region, probably by mechanical distortion or obliteration of the vessels. As a result, the shunt in pulmonary contusion is very small but the hypoxia can be quite profound due to mechanical interdependence of the contused regions with the surrounding lung, which leads to large numbers of low $\dot{V}/\dot{Q}$ units there.[22] This situation is important to oxygen therapy, because hypoxemic patients with large lung contusions often become well oxygenated with modest amounts of supplemental oxygen delivered via nasal prongs or mask in clinical circumstances in which the associated pain or other injuries might suggest that intubation and stabilization on a ventilator is imperative for the presumed shunt lung disease. The not infrequent concurrence of flail chest with lung contusion has little impact on the already small shunt but adds to the hypoventilation of associated regions with very low $\dot{V}/\dot{Q}$, leading to severe hypoxemia. Measures that enhance ventilation, such as adequate pain control, often allow simple oxygen supplementation to correct the hypoxemia and spare the patient intubation and positive-pressure ventilation.[218] This has a special advantage in cases of lung contusion, in which positive-pressure ventilation, especially with PEEP, is associated with an increase in the underlying lung contusion.

## SUMMARY

Since 1990, basic science research and parallel clinical investigations have brought about a renaissance in the management of ARDS. The evolution of volutrauma from an interesting laboratory finding to a major consideration in the mechanical ventilation of patients with ARDS represents one of the smoothest and most timely translations of basic science findings into clinical practice in modern medicine. Permissive hypercapnia, open-lung ventilation, and prone ventilation are all increasingly accepted as state-of-the-art strategies for the management of patients with ARDS. Finally, as success in treating patients with ARDS improves, the focus of laboratory and clinical research is shifting to prevention, treatment, and support of patients through the proliferative phase of this syndrome. It is in this area that the next important advances in treatment of this syndrome are anticipated.

## References


1. O'Connor M, Hall JB, Schmidt GA, et al: Acute hypoxemic respiratory failure. *In* Hall JB, Schmidt GA, Wood LDH (eds): Principles of Critical Care. New York: McGraw-Hill Publishers, 1998, pp 537–559.
2. Polese G, Rossi A, Appendini L, et al: Partitioning of respiratory mechanics in mechanically ventilated patients. J Appl Physiol 71:2433–2435, 1991.
3. Suchyta M, Clemmer T, Elliott C, et al: The adult respiratory distress syndrome: A report of survival and modifying factors. Chest 101:1074–1079, 1992.
4. Maunder RJ, Shuman WP, McHugh JW, et al: Preservation of normal lung regions in the adult respiratory distress syndrome. JAMA 255:2463–2465, 1986.
5. Gattinoni L, Pesenti A, Bombino M: Relationships between lung computed tomographic density, gas exchange and PEEP in acute respiratory failure. Anesthesiology 69:824–832, 1988.
6. Light RB, Mink S, Wood LDH: Pathophysiology of gas exchange and pulmonary perfusion in pneumococcal lobar pneumonia in dogs. J Appl Physiol 50:524–530, 1981.
7. Liez PL, Jacobson E, Shubin H, et al: Pulmonary edema related to changes in colloid osmotic and pulmonary artery wedge pressure in patients after acute myocardial infarction. Circulation 51:350, 1975.
8. Rinaldo JE, Christman JW: Mechanisms and mediators of the adult respiratory distress syndrome. Clin Chest Med 11:621–632, 1990.
9. Kollef MH, Schuster DP: The acute respiratory distress syndrome. N Engl J Med 332:27–37, 1995.
10. Katzenstein A, Askin FB: Surgical pathology of non-neoplastic lung disease (2nd ed). Philadelphia: WB Saunders, 1990, pp 9–36.
11. Tomashefski JF: Pulmonary pathology of the adult distress syndrome. Clin Chest Med 11:621–632, 1990.
12. Montaver JSG, Tsang J, Evans KG, et al: Alveolar epithelial damage: A critical difference between high pressure and oleic acid induced low pressure edema. J Clin Invest 77:1786–1796, 1986.
13. Matthay MA, Wiener-Kronish JP: Intact epithelial barrier function is critical for the resolution of alveolar edema in humans. Am Rev Respir Dis 142:1250–1257, 1990.
14. Colice GL, Matthay MA, Bass E, et al: Neurogenic pulmonary edema. Am Rev Respir Dis 130:941–948, 1984.
15. Shaw TJ, Caterine JM: Recurrent re-expansion pulmonary edema. Chest 86:784–786, 1984.
16. Suzuki S, Tanita T, Koike K, et al: Evidence of acute inflammatory response in reexpansion pulmonary. Chest 101:275–276, 1992.
17. Pisani RJ, Rosenow EC: Pulmonary edema associated with tocolytic therapy. Ann Intern Med 110:714, 1989.
17a. West JB, Mathieu-Costello O: Structure, strength failure and remodeling of the pulmonary capillary blood-gas barrier. Annu Rev Physiol 16:543–572, 1999.
18. Dweik RA, Arroliga AC, Cash JM: Alveolar hemorrhage in patients with rheumatic disease. Rheum Dis Clin North Am 23:395–410, 1997.
19. Jennings CA, King TE Jr, Tuder R, et al: Diffuse alveolar hemorrhage with underlying isolated pauci-immune pulmonary capillaritis. Am J Respir Crit Care Med. 155:1101–1109, 1997.
20. De Lassance A, Fleury-Feith J, Escudier E, et al: Alveolar hemorrhage: Diagnostics criteria and results in 194 immunocompromised patients. Am J Respir Crit Care Med 151:157–163, 1995.
20a. Nichols MR, Terada LS, Tuder RM, et al: Diffuse alveolar hemorrhage with underlying pulmonary capillaritis in the retinoic acid syndrome. Am J Respir Crit Care Med 158:1302–1305, 1998.
20b. Light RB, Mink SN, Cooligan TG, et al: The physiology of recovery in experimental pneumococcal pneumonia. Clin Invest Med 6:147–151, 1983.
21. Richardson JD, Adams L, Flint LM: Selective management of flail chest and pulmonary contusion. Ann Surg 196:481, 1982.
22. Oppenheimer L, Craven KD, Forkert L, et al: Pathophysiology of pulmonary contusion in dogs. J Appl Physiol 47:718–728, 1979.
23. Mackersie RC, Shackford SR, Hoyt DB, et al: Continuous epidural fentanyl analgesia: Ventilatory function improvement with routine use in treatment of blunt chest injury. J Trauma 27:1207–1212, 1987.
24. Baudendistel LJ, Shields JB, Kaminski DL: Comparison of double indicator thermodilution measurements of extravascular lung water (EVLW) with radiographic estimation of lung water in trauma patients. J Trauma 22:983–988, 1982.
25. Gattinoni L, Pesenti A, Baglioni S, et al: Inflammatory pulmonary edema and positive end-expiratory pressure: Correlations between imaging and physiologic studies. J Thorac Imag 3:59–64, 1988.
25a. Gattinoni L, Pisenti A, Terresin A, et al: Adult respiratory distress syndrome profiles by compute tomography. J Thorac Imaging 42:391–402, 1987.
26. Gattinoni L, Pelosi P, Vitale G, et al: Body position changes redistribute lung computed tomographic density in patients with acute respiratory failure. Anesthesiology 74:15–23, 1991.
27. Kaplan JD, Calandrino FS, Schuster DP: A positron emission tomographic comparison of pulmonary vascular permeability during the adult respiratory distress syndrome and pneumonia. Am Rev Respir Dis 143:150–154, 1991.
28. Cooligan T, Light RB, Wood LDH, et al: Plasma volume expansion in canine pneumococcal pneumonia. Am Rev Respir Dis 126:86–91, 1982.
29. Cabanes LR, Wever SN, Matran R, et al: Bronchial hyperresponsiveness to methacholine in patients with impaired left ventricular function. N Engl J Med 320:1317–1322, 1989.
30. Aberle DR, Wiener-Kronish JP, Webb WR, et al: Hydrostatic versus increased permeability pulmonary edema: Diagnosis based on radiographic criteria in critically ill patients. Radiology 168:73–79, 1988.
31. Aberle DR, Brown K: Radiologic considerations in the adult respiratory distress syndrome. Clin Chest Med 11:737–754, 1990.
32. Fein A, Grossman RF, Jones JG, et al: The value of edema fluid protein measurement in patients with pulmonary edema. Am J Med 67:32–38, 1979.

33. Spirito D, Maron BJ: Doppler echocardiography for assessing left ventricular diastolic function. Ann Intern Med 109:122, 1988.
34. Fein AM, Goldberg SK, Walkenstein MD, et al: Is pulmonary artery catheterization necessary for the diagnosis of pulmonary edema? Am Rev Respir Dis 129:1006–1009, 1984.
35. Dalen JE, Bone RC: Is it time to pull the pulmonary artery catheter? JAMA 276:916–917, 1996.
36. Connors AF, Speroff T, Dawson NV, et al: The effectiveness of right heart catheterization in the initial care of critically ill patients. JAMA 276:889–894, 1996.
37. Iberti TJ, Fischer EP, Leibowitz AB, et al: A multicenter study of physicians' knowledge of the pulmonary artery catheter. JAMA 264:2928–2932, 1990.
38. Bernard GR, Artigas A, Brigham KL, et al: The American-European Consensus Conference on ARDS: Definitions, mechanisms, relevant outcomes, and clinical trial coordination. Am J Respir Crit Care Med 149:818–824, 1994.
39. Murray JF, Matthay MA, Luce J, et al: An expanded definition of the adult respiratory distress syndrome. Am Rev Respir Dis 138:720–723, 1988.
40. Pittet JF, Mackersie RC, Martin TR, et al: Biological markers of acute lung injury: Prognostic and pathogenetic significance. Am J Respir Crit Care Med 155:1187–1205, 1997.
40a. Donnelly SC, Strieter RM, Reid PT, et al: The association between mortality rates and decreased concentrations of interleukin-10 and interleukin-1 receptor antagonist in the lung fluids of patients with the adult respiratory distress syndrome. Ann Intern Med 125:191–196, 1996.
41. Aberman A, Fulop M: The metabolic and respiratory acidosis of acute pulmonary edema. Ann Intern Med 76:173–184, 1972.
42. Goldberg IF, Cohn JN: New inotropic drugs for heart failure. JAMA 258:493, 1987.
43. Carroll JD, Lang RM, Neumann AL, et al: The differential effects of positive inotropic and vasodilator therapy on diastolic properties in patients with congestive cardiomyopathy. Circulation 74:815–825, 1986.
44. Vasko JS, Henney RP, Oldham HN, et al: Mechanisms of action of morphine in the treatment of experimental pulmonary edema. Am J Cardiol 18:876–883, 1966.
45. Dikshit K, Vyden JK, Forrester JS, et al: Renal and extra-renal hemodynamic effects of furosemide in congestive heart failure after acute myocardial infarction. N Engl J Med 288:1087–1090, 1973.
46. Ali J, Wood LDH: Pulmonary vascular effects of furosemide on gas exchange in pulmonary edema. J Appl Physiol 57:160–167, 1984.
47. Wollam GL, Tarazi RC, Bravo EL, et al: Diuretic potency of combined hydrochlorothiazide and furosemide therapy in patients with azotemia. Am J Med 72: 929–938, 1982.
48. Forni LG, Hilton PJ: Continuous hemofiltration in the treatment of acute renal failure. N Engl J Med 336:1303–1309, 1997.
49. Richard C, Ricome JL, Rimaiho A, et al: Combined hemodynamic effects of dopamine and dobutamine in cardiogenic shock. Circulation 67:620–626, 1983.
50. Calhoun DA, Oparil S: Current concepts: Treatment of hypertensive crisis. N Engl J Med 323:1177, 1990.
51. Hennekens CH, Albert CM, Godfried SL, et al: Adjunctive drug therapy of acute myocardial infarction: Evidence from clinical trials. N Engl J Med 335:1660–1667, 1996.
52. Polese A, Fiorentini C, Olivari MT, et al: Clinical use of a calcium antagonist (nifedipine) in acute pulmonary edema. Am J Med 66:825–830, 1979.
53. Cohn JN, Burke LP: Nitroprusside. Ann Intern Med 91:752, 1979.
54. Hill NS, Antman EM, Green LH, et al: Intravenous nitroglycerin: A review of pharmacology, indications, therapeutic effects and complications. Chest 79:69–76, 1981.
55. Gagnon RM, Fortin L, Bouches R, et al: Combined hemodynamic effects of dobutamine and IV nitroglycerin in congestive heart failure. Chest 78:694–698, 1980.
56. Hurst JW: The recognition and treatment of specific subsets of patients with atherosclerotic coronary heart disease. *In* Rackley CE, Sonnenblick EH, Wenger NK (eds): The Heart: Arteries and Veins. New York: McGraw-Hill, 1990, pp 1045–1054.
57. Leier CV, Unverferth DV: Drugs five years later: Dobutamine. Ann Intern Med 99:490–496, 1983.
58. Unverferth DV, Blanford M, Kates RE, et al: Tolerance to dobutamine after a 72-hour continuous infusion. Am J Med 69:262–266, 1980.
59. Ader R, Chatterjee K, Ports T, et al: Immediate and sustained hemodynamic and clinical improvement in chronic heart failure by an oral angiotensin-converting enzyme inhibitor. Circulation 61:931, 1980.
60. Captopril Multicenter Study Group: A placebo trial of captopril in refractory chronic congestive heart failure. J Am Coll Cardiol 2:755, 1983.
61. Sorrentino MJ: Valvular heart disease. *In* Hall JB, Schmidt GA, Wood LDH (eds): Principles of Critical Care. New York: McGraw-Hill, 1998, pp 467–481.
62. Bersten AD, Holt AW, Vedig AE, et al: Treatment of severe cardiogenic pulmonary edema with continuous positive airway pressure delivered by face mask. N Engl J Med 325:1825–1830, 1991.
63. Katz JA, Marks JD: Inspiratory work with and without continuous positive airway pressure in patients with acute respiratory failure. Anesthesiology 63:598–607, 1985.
64. Buda AJ, Pinsky MR, Ingels NB Jr, et al: Effect of intrathoracic pressure on left ventricular performance. N Engl J Med 301:453–459, 1979.
65. Patrick W, Webster K, Ludwig L, et al: Noninvasive positive-pressure ventilation in acute respiratory distress without prior chronic respiratory failure. Am J Respir Crit Care Med 153:1005–1011, 1996.
66. Abou-Shala N, Meduri U: Noninvasive ventilation in patients with acute respiratory failure. Crit Care Med 24:705–715, 1996.
67. Meduri GU, Turner RE, Abou-Shala N, et al: Noninvasive positive pressure ventilation via face mask: First-line intervention in patients with acute hypercapnic and hypoxic respiratory failure. Chest 109:179–193, 1996.
67a. Hoffmann B, Welte T: The use of noninvasive pressure support ventilation for severe respiratory insufficiency due to pulmonary edema. Intensive Care Med 25:15–20, 1999.
67b. Rusterholtz T, Kempf J, Berton C, et al: Noninvasive pressure support ventilation (NIPSV) with face mask in patients with acute cardiogenic pulmonary edema. Intensive Care Med 25:21–28, 1999.
68. Brochard L: Noninvasive ventilation. *In* Hall JB, Schmidt GA, Wood LDH (eds): Principles of Critical Care. New York: McGraw-Hill, 1998, pp 509–515.
69. Calvein JE, Driedger AA, Sibbald WJ: Positive end-expiratory pressure (PEEP) does not depress left ventricular function in patients with pulmonary edema. Am Rev Respir Dis 124:121–128, 1981.
70. Luce JM: Acute lung injury and the acute respiratory distress syndrome. Crit Care Med 26:369–376, 1998.
71. Artigas A, Bernard GR, Carlet J, et al: The American-European Consensus Conference on ARDS, part 2: Ventilatory, pharmacologic, supportive therapy, study design strategies, and issues related to recovery and remodeling. Am J Respir Crit Care Med 157:1332–1347, 1998.
71a. Ware LB, Matthay MA: The acute respiratory distress syndrome. N Engl J Med, in press.
72. Metz C, Sibbald WJ: Anti-inflammatory therapy for acute lung injury: A review of animal and clinical studies. Chest 100:1110–1119, 1991.
73. Luce JM, Montgomery B, Marks JD, et al: Ineffectiveness of high-dose methylprednisolone in preventing parenchymal lung injury and improving mortality in patients with septic shock. Am Rev Respir Dis 138:62–68, 1988.
74. Bone RC, Fisher CJ Jr, Clemmer TP, et al: Ineffectiveness of high-dose methylprednisolone in preventing parenchymal lung injury and improving mortality in patients with septic shock. Chest 92:1032–1036, 1987.
75. Bernard GR, Luce JM, Sprung CL, et al: High-dose corticosteroids in patients with adult respiratory distress syndrome. N Engl J Med 317:1565–1570, 1987.
76. Allen JN, Pacht ER, Gadek JE, et al: Acute eosinophilic pneumonia as a reversible cause of noninfectious respiratory failure. N Engl J Med 321:569–574, 1989.

77. Kallenbach J, Lewis M, Zaltzman M, et al: "Low-dose" corticosteroid prophylaxis against fat embolism. J Trauma 27:1173, 1987.
78. Schonfeld SA, Ploysonsang Y, Dilisio R, et al: Fat embolism prophylaxis with corticosteroids. Ann Intern Med 99:438, 1983.
79. Bone RC, Slotman G, Maunder R, et al: Randomized double-blind, multicenter study of prostaglandin $E_1$ in patients with the adult respiratory distress syndrome. Chest 96:114–119, 1989.
80. Melot C, Lejeune P, Leeman M, et al: Prostaglandin $E_1$ in patients with the adult respiratory distress syndrome. Chest 96:114–119, 1989.
80a. Abraham E, Park YC, Covington P, et al: Liposomal prostaglandin E1 in acute respiratory distress syndrome: A placebo-controlled, randomized, double-blind, multicenter trial. Crit Care Med 24:10–15, 1996.
81. Bernard GR, Reines HD, Halushka PV, et al: Prostacyclin and thromboxane A2 formation is increased in human sepsis: Effects of cyclo-oxygenase inhibition. Am Rev Respir Dis 144:1095–1101, 1991.
82. Haupt MT, Jastemski MS, Clemmer TP, et al: Effect of ibuprofen in patients with severe sepsis: A randomized double-blind multicenter study. Crit Care Med 19:1339–1347, 1991.
83. Slotman GJ, Burchard KW, D'Arezzo A, et al: Ketoconazole prevents acute respiratory failure in critically ill surgical patients. J Trauma 28:648–654, 1988.
84. Yu M, Thomasa G: A double-blind prospective randomized trial of ketoconazole, a thromboxane synthetase inhibitor, in the prophylaxis of the adult respiratory distress syndrome. Crit Care Med 21:1635–1642, 1993.
84a. NIH ARDS Network: Ketoconazole does not reduce mortality in patients with the acute respiratory distress syndrome. JAMA, in press.
85. Hallman M, Spragg R, Harrell JH, et al: Evidence of lung surfactant abnormality in respiratory failure. J Clin Invest 70:673–683, 1982.
86. Jobe AH, Ikegami M: Surfactant for acute respiratory distress syndrome. Adv Intern Med 42:203–230, 1997.
87. Jobe A, Ikegami M: Surfactant for the treatment of respiratory distress syndrome. Am Rev Respir Dis 136:1256–1275, 1987.
88. Merritt TA, Hallman M, Bloom BT, et al: Prophylactic treatment of very premature infants with human surfactant. N Engl J Med 315:785–790, 1986.
89. Horbar JD, Soll RF, Sutherland JM, et al: A multicenter, randomized, placebo-controlled trial of surfactant therapy for respiratory distress syndrome. N Engl J Med 320:959–965, 1989.
90. Anzueto A, Baughman RP, Guntupalli KK, et al: Aerosolized surfactant in adults with sepsis induced acute respiratory distress syndrome. N Engl J Med 334:1417–1421, 1996.
91. Bone RC, Balk R, Slotman G, et al: Adult respiratory distress syndrome: Sequence and importance of development of multiple organ failure. Chest 101:320–326, 1992.
92. Schmacker PT, Cain SM: The concept of a critical oxygen delivery. Intensive Care Med 123:223–229, 1987.
93. Ronco JJ, Phang PT, Walley KR, et al: Oxygen consumption is independent of changes in oxygen delivery in severe adult respiratory distress syndrome. Am Rev Respir Dis 143:1267–1273, 1991.
94. Prewitt RM, McCarthy J, Wood LDH: Treatment of acute low pressure edema in dogs: Relative effects of hydrostatic and oncotic pressure, nitroprusside, and positive end expiratory pressure. J Clin Invest 67:409–418, 1981.
95. Long GR, Breen PH, Mayers I, et al: Treatment of canine aspiration pneumonitis: Fluid volume reduction vs. fluid volume expansion. J Appl Physiol 65:1736–1744, 1988.
96. Sznajder JI, Zucker AR, Wood LDH, et al: Effects of plasmapheresis and hemofiltration on acid aspiration pulmonary edema. Am Rev Respir Dis 134:222–228, 1986.
97. Gottlieb SS, Wood LDH, Hansen DE, et al: The effect of nitroprusside on pulmonary edema, oxygen exchange, and blood flow in hydrochloric acid aspiration. Anesthesiology 67:47–54, 1987.
98. Zucker AR, Becker CJ, Berger S, et al: Pathophysiology of treatment of canine kerosene pulmonary injury: The effects of plasmapheresis and positive end-expiratory pressure on canine kerosene pulmonary injury. J Crit Care 4:184–193, 1989.
99. Brigham KL, Kariman K, Harris TR, et al: Correlation of oxygenation with vascular permeability-surface area but not with lung water in humans with acute respiratory failure and pulmonary edema. J Clin Invest 72:339–349, 1983.
100. Eisenberg PR, Hansrough JR, Anderson D, et al: A prospective study of lung water measurements during patient management in an intensive care unit. Am Rev Respir Dis 136:662–668, 1987.
101. Simons RS, Berdine GG, Seidenfeld JJ, et al: Fluid balance and the adult respiratory distress syndrome. Am Rev Respir Dis 135:924–929, 1987.
102. Humphrey H, Hall J, Sznajder I, et al: Improved survival in ARDS patients associated with a reduction in pulmonary capillary wedge pressure. Chest 97:1176–1180, 1990.
103. Mitchel JP, Schuller D, Calandrino FS, et al: Improved outcome based on fluid management in critically ill patients requiring pulmonary artery catheterization. Am Rev Respir Dis 145:990–998, 1992.
104. Hyers TM: ARDS: The therapeutic dilemma. Chest 97:1025, 1990.
105. Hudson LD: Fluid management strategy in acute lung injury. Am Rev Respir Dis 145:988–989, 1992.
106. O'Quinn R, Marini JJ: Pulmonary artery occlusion pressure: Clinical physiology, measurement, and interpretation. Am Rev Respir Dis 128:319–326, 1983.
107. Teboul JL, Besbes, M, Andrivet P, et al: A bedside index assessing the reliability of pulmonary artery occlusion pressure measurements during mechanical ventilation with positive end-expiratory pressure. J Crit Care 7:22–29, 1992.
108. Smiseth OA, Refsum H, Tyberg JV: Pericardial pressure assessed by right atrial pressure: A basis for calculation of left ventricular transmural pressure. Am Heart J 108:603–605, 1984.
109. Pinsky M, Vincent JL, De Smet JM: Estimating left ventricular filling pressure during positive end-expiratory pressure in humans. Am Rev Respir Dis 143:25–31, 1991.
110. Carter RS, Snyder JV, Pinsky MR: LV filling pressure during PEEP measured by nadir wedge pressure after airway disconnection. Am J Physiol 249:H770–H776, 1985.
111. Abraham E, Yoshihara G: Cardiorespiratory effects of pressure controlled inverse ratio ventilation in severe respiratory failure. Chest 96:1356–1359, 1989.
112. Webb HH, Tierney DF: Experimental pulmonary edema due to intermittent positive pressure ventilation with high inflation pressures: Protection by positive end-expiratory pressure. Am J Respir Crit Care Med 110:556–565, 1974.
113. Dreyfuss D, Basset G, Soler R, et al: Intermittent positive pressure hyperventilation with high inflation pressures produces pulmonary microvascular injury in rats. Am J Respir Crit Care Med 132:880–884, 1985.
114. Dreyfuss D, Soler P, Basset G, et al: High inflation pressure pulmonary edema. Am J Respir Crit Care Med 137:1159–1164, 1988.
114a. International Consensus Conferences in Intensive Care Medicine: Ventilator-associated lung injury in ARDS. Am J Respir Crit Care Med, in press.
115. Dreyfuss D, Saumon G: Ventilator-induced lung injury: Lessons from experimental studies. Am J Respir Crit Care Med 157:294–323, 1998.
116. Hernandez LA, Peevy KJ, Moise AA, et al: Chest wall restrictions limit high airway pressure induced lung injury in young rabbits. J Appl Physiol 66:2364–2368, 1989.
117. Muscedere JG, Mullen JBM, Gan K, et al: Tidal ventilation at low airway pressures can augment lung injury. Am J Respir Crit Care Med 149:1327–1334, 1994.
118. Corbridge TC, Wood LDH, Crawford GP, et al: Adverse effects of large tidal volume and low PEEP in canine acid aspiration. Am J Respir Crit Care Med 142:311–315, 1990.
119. Mead JT, Takishima T, Leith D: Stress distribution in lungs: A model of pulmonary elasticity. J Appl Physiol 28:596–608, 1970.
120. West JB, Tsukimoto K, Mathieu-Costello O, et al: Stress failure in pulmonary capillaries. J Appl Physiol 70:1731–1742, 1991.
121. Marini JJ: Lung mechanics in the adult respiratory distress syndrome: Recent conceptual advances and implications for management. Chest 11:673–679, 1990.
122. Benito S, LeMaire F: Pulmonary pressure-volume relationship in acute respiratory distress syndrome in adults: Role of positive end-expiratory pressure. Crit Care 5:27–34, 1990.

123. Hickling KG: The pressure-volume curve is greatly modified by recruitment: A mathematical model of ARDS lungs. Am J Respir Crit Care Med 158:194–199, 1998.
124. Slutsky AR, Tremblay LN: Multiple system organ failure: Is mechanical ventilation a contributing factor? Am J Respir Crit Care Med 157:1721–1725, 1998.
125. Imai Y, Kawano K, Tanaka H, et al: Inflammatory chemical mediators during conventional ventilation and during high frequency ventilation. Crit Care Med 150:1550–1554, 1994.
126. Tremblay LN, Valenza SP, Ribeiro J, et al: Injurious ventilatory strategies increase cytokines and c-fos m-RNA expression in an isolated rat lung model. J Clin Invest 99:944–952, 1997.
127. Douzinas EE, Tsidemiadou PD, Pitaridis MT, et al: The regional production of cytokines and lactate in sepsis-related multiple organ failure. Am J Respir Crit Care Med 155:53–59, 1997.
128. Nahum A, Hoyt J, Schmitz L, et al: Effect of mechanical ventilation strategy on dissemination of intratracheally instilled *Escherichia coli* in dogs. Crit Care Med 25:1733–1743, 1997.
128a. Ranieri VM, Suter PM, Tortorella C, et al: Effect of mechanical ventilation on inflammatory mediators in patients with acute respiratory distress syndrome. JAMA 282:54–61, 1999.
129. Roupie E, Dambrosio M, Servillo G, et al: Titration of tidal volume and induced hypercapnia in acute respiratory distress syndrome. Am J Respir Crit Care Med 152:121–129, 1995.
130. Gattinoni L, Pelosi P, Crotti S, et al: Effects of positive end-expiratory pressure on regional distribution of tidal volume and recruitment in adult respiratory distress syndrome. Am J Respir Crit Care Med 151:1807–1814, 1995.
131. Pelosi P, D'Andrea L, Vitale G, et al: Vertical gradient of regional lung inflation in adult respiratory distress syndrome. Am J Respir Crit Care Med 149:8–13, 1994.
132. Hickling KG, Henderson SJ, Jackson R: Low mortality associated with low volume pressure limited ventilation with permissive hypercapnia in severe adult respiratory distress syndrome. Intensive Care Med 16:372–377, 1990.
133. Hickling KG, Walsh J, Henderson S, et al: Low mortality rate in adult respiratory distress syndrome using low-volume, pressure-limited ventilation with permissive hypercapnia: A prospective study. Crit Care Med 22:1568–1578, 1994.
134. Milbert JA, Davis DR, Steinberg KP, et al: Improved survival of patients with acute respiratory distress syndrome (ARDS): 1983–1993. JAMA 273:306–309, 1995.
135. Amato MRP, Barbas CSV, Medeiros DM, et al: Beneficial effects of the "open lung approach" with low distending pressures in acute respiratory distress syndrome. Am J Respir Crit Care Med 152:1835–1846, 1995.
136. Amato MRP, Barbas CSV, Medeiros DM, et al: Effect of a protective ventilation strategy on mortality in the acute respiratory distress syndrome. N Engl J Med 338:347–354, 1998.
136a. Sznadjer JI, Nahum A, Hansen DE, et al: Volume recruitment and oxygenation in pulmonary edema. J Crit Care 13:126–135, 1998.
137. Stewart TE, Medade MO, Cook DJ, et al: Evaluation of a ventilation strategy to prevent barotrauma in patients at high risk for acute respiratory distress syndrome. N Engl J Med 338:355–361, 1998.
138. Brochard L, Roudot-Thoraval, Collaborative Group on VT Reduction: Tidal volume reduction in acute respiratory distress syndrome (ARDS): A multicenter randomized study. Am J Respir Crit Care Med, in press.
139. Brower R, Shanholtz C, Shade D, et al: Randomized controlled trial of small tidal volume ventilation (STV) in ARDS. Crit Care Med, in press.
140. Weg JG, Anzueto A, Balk RA, et al: The relation of pneumothorax and other air leaks to mortality in the acute respiratory distress syndrome. N Engl J Med 338:341–346, 1998.
140a. NIH ARDS Network: A trial of traditional versus a lower tidal volume strategy in acute lung injury and the acute respiratory distress syndrome. N Engl J Med, in press.
141. Hall JB: Respiratory system mechanics in adult respiratory distress syndrome: Stretching our understanding. Am J Respir Crit Care Med 158:1–2, 1998.
142. Gattinoni L, Pelosi P, Suter PM, et al: Acute respiratory distress syndrome due to pulmonary and extra-pulmonary disease: Different syndromes? Am J Respir Crit Care Med 158:3–11, 1998.
143. Ranieri VM, Brienza N, Santostasi S, et al: Impairment of lung and chest wall mechanics in patients with acute respiratory distress syndrome: Role of abdominal distension. Am J Respir Crit Care Med 156:1082–1091, 1997.
144. Mergoni M, Martelli A, Volpi A, et al: Impact of positive end-expiratory pressure on chest wall and lung pressure-volume curve in acute respiratory failure. Am J Respir Crit Care Med 156:846–854, 1997.
145. Gibson RL, Comer PB, Beckham RW, et al: Actual tracheal oxygen concentrations with commonly used oxygen equipment. Anesthesiology 44:71, 1976.
146. Manthous CA, Hall JB, Schmidt GA, et al: The effect of mechanical ventilation on oxygen consumption in critically ill patients. Am J Respir Crit Care Med 151:210–214, 1995.
147. Manthous CA, Hall JB, Wood LDH: The effect of cooling on oxygen consumption in febrile critically ill patients. Am J Respir Crit Care Med 151:10–14, 1995.
148. De Los Santos R, Seidenfeld JJ, Anzueto A, et al: One hundred percent oxygen lung injury in adult baboons. Am Rev Respir Dis 136:657–661, 1987.
149. Tierney DF, Ayers L, Kasuyama RS: Altered sensitivity to oxygen toxicity. Am J Respir Crit Care Med 115(Suppl):59–65, 1977.
150. Smith G, Winter PM, Wheelis RF: Increased normobaric oxygen tolerance of rabbits following oleic acid–induced lung damage. J Appl Physiol 35:395–400, 1973.
151. Singer MM, Wright F, Stanley L, et al: Oxygen toxicity in man: A prospective study in patients after open-heart surgery. N Engl J Med 283:1473–1478, 1970.
152. Barber RE, Lee J, Hamilton WK, et al: Oxygen toxicity in man: A prospective study in patients with irreversible brain damage. N Engl J Med 283:1478–1484, 1970.
153. Witschi HR, Hascek WM, Klein-Szanto AJ, et al: Potentiation of diffuse lung damage by oxygen: Determining variables. Am J Respir Crit Care Med 123:98–103, 1981.
154. Walley KR, Becker CJ, Hogan RA, et al: Progressive hypoxemia limits left ventricular oxygen consumption and contractility. Circ Res 63:849–859, 1988.
155. Pare PD, Warriner E, Baile M, et al: Redistribution of pulmonary extravascular water with positive end-expiratory pressure in canine pulmonary edema. Am J Respir Crit Care Med 127:590–593, 1983.
156. Fessler HE, Brower RG, Wise RA, et al: Effects of positive end-expiratory pressure on the gradient for venous return. Am J Respir Crit Care Med 143:19–24, 1991.
157. Slutsky AS: Consensus conference on mechanical ventilation, part 1. Intensive Care Med 20:64–79, 1994.
158. Slutsky AS: Consensus conference on mechanical ventilation, part 2. Intensive Care Med 20:150–162, 1994.
159. Ravenscraft SA, Burke WC, Marini JJ: Volume cycled decelerating flow. Chest 101:1342–1351, 1992.
160. Feihl F, Perret C: Permissive hypercapnia: How permissive should we be? Am J Respir Crit Care Med 150:1722–1737, 1994.
161. Tuxen DV: Permissive hypercapnic ventilation. Am J Respir Crit Care Med 150:870–874, 1994.
162. Frumin MJ, Epstein RM, Cohen G: Apneic oxygenation in man. Anesthesiology 20:789–798, 1959.
163. Douglas W, Rehder K, Beynen RM, et al: Improved oxygenation in patients with acute respiratory failure: The prone position. Am J Respir Crit Care Med 115:559–566, 1977.
164. Albert RK: The prone position in acute respiratory distress syndrome: Where we are, and where do we go from here? Crit Care Med 25:1453–1454, 1997.
165. Chatte G, Sab JM, Dubois JM, et al: Prone position in mechanically ventilated patients with severe acute respiratory failure. Am J Respir Crit Care Med 155:473–478, 1997.
166. Lamm WJ, Graham MM, Albert RK: Mechanism by which the prone position improves oxygenation in acute lung injury. Am J Respir Crit Care Med 150:184–193, 1994.
167. Pelosi P, Croci M, Calappi E, et al: The prone positioning during general anesthesia minimally affects respiratory mechanics while improving functional residual capacity and increasing oxygen tension. Anesth Analg 80:955–960, 1995.
168. Glenny RW, Lamm WJ, Albert RK, et al: Gravity is a minor de-

terminant of pulmonary blood flow distribution. J Appl Physiol 71:620–629, 1991.
169. Gattinoni L, Pelosi P, Vitale G, et al: Body position changes redistribute lung computed-tomography density in patients with acute respiratory failure. Anesthesiology 74:15–23, 1991.
170. Weiner CM, Kirk W, Albert RK: Prone position reverses gravitational distribution of perfusion in dog lungs with oleic acid induced injury. J Appl Physiol 1990; 68:1386–1392.
171. Albert RK, Leasa D, Sanderson M, et al: The prone position improves arterial oxygenation and reduces shunt in oleic acid induced acute lung injury. Am J Respir Crit Care Med 135:628–633, 1987.
172. Servillo G, Roupie E, De Robertis E, et al: Effects of ventilation in ventral decubitus position on respiratory mechanics in adult respiratory distress syndrome. Intensive Care Med 23:1219–1224, 1997.
173. Nahum A, Shapiro RS, Ravenscraft SA, et al: Efficacy of expiratory tracheal gas insufflation in a canine model of lung injury. Am J Respir Crit Care Med 152:489–495, 1995.
174. Belghith M, Fierobe L, Brunet F, et al: Is tracheal gas insufflation an alternative to extrapulmonary gas exchangers in severe ARDS? Chest 107:1416–1419, 1995.
175. Fredberg JJ: Augmented diffusion in the airways can support pulmonary gas exchange. J Appl Physiol 49:232–238, 1980.
176. Klocke RA, Saltzman AR, Grant BJB, et al: Role of molecular diffusion in conventional and high frequency ventilation. Am J Respir Crit Care Med 142:802–806, 1990.
177. Pedley TJ, Corieri P, Kamm RD, et al: Gas flow and mixing in the airways. Crit Care Med 22:s29–s36, 1994.
178. Froese AB, Bryan AC: High frequency jet ventilation. Am J Respir Crit Care Med 135:1363–1374, 1987.
179. Schuster DP, Klain M, Snyder JV: Comparison of high frequency jet ventilation to conventional ventilation during severe acute respiratory failure in humans. Crit Care Med 10:625–630, 1982.
180. Holzapfel L, Robert D, Perrin F, et al: Comparison of high frequency jet ventilation to conventional ventilation in adults with respiratory distress syndrome. Intensive Care Med 13:100–105, 1987.
181. Carlon GC, Howland WS, Ray C, et al: High frequency jet ventilation: A prospective randomized evaluation. Chest 84:551–559, 1983.
182. Tharratt RS, Allen RP, Albertson TE: Pressure controlled inverse ratio ventilation in severe adult respiratory failure. Chest 94:755–762, 1988.
183. Cole AGH, Weller SF, Sykes MK: Inverse ratio ventilation compared with PEEP in adult respiratory failure. Intensive Care Med 10:227–232, 1984.
184. Abraham E, Yoshihara G: Cardiorespiratory effects of pressure controlled inverse ratio ventilation in severe respiratory failure. Chest 96:1356–1359, 1989.
185. Gurevitch MJ, Van Dyke J, Young ES, et al: Improved oxygenation and lower peak airway pressure in severe adult respiratory distress syndrome: Treatment with inverse ratio ventilation. Chest 89:211–213, 1986.
186. Manthous CA, Schmidt GA: IRV in ARDS: Improved oxygenation without autoPEEP. Chest 103:953–954, 19 92.
187. Mercat A, Graini L, Teboul JL, et al: Cardiorespiratory effects of pressure-controlled ventilation with and without inverse ratio in the adult respiratory distress syndrome. Chest 104:871–875, 1993.
188. Sydow M, Burchardi H, Ephraim E, et al: Long term effects of two different ventilatory modes on oxygenation in acute lung injury: Comparison of airway pressure release ventilation and volume-controlled inverse ratio ventilation. Am J Respir Crit Care Med 149:1550–1556, 1994.
189. Zapol WM, Snider MT, Hill JD, et al: Extracorporeal membrane oxygenation in severe acute respiratory failure: A randomized prospective study. JAMA 242:2193–2196, 1979.
190. Egan TM, Duffin J, Glynn MFX, et al: Ten-year experience with extracorporeal membrane oxygenation for severe respiratory failure. Chest 94:681–687, 1988.
191. Snider MT, Campbell DB, Kofke WA, et al: Venovenous perfusion of adults and children with severe acute respiratory distress syndrome. ASAIO Trans 34:1014–1020, 1988.
192. Morris AH, Wallace CJ, Menlove RL, et al: Randomized clinical trial of pressure controlled inverse ratio ventilation and extracorporeal $CO_2$ removal for adult respiratory distress syndrome. Am J Respir Crit Care Med 149:295–305, 1994.
193. High KM, Snider MT Richard R, et al: Clinical trials of an intravenous oxygenator in patients with adult respiratory distress syndrome. Anesthesiology 77:856–863, 1992.
194. Hirschl RB, Pranikoff T, Wise C, et al: Initial experience with partial liquid ventilation in adult patients with the acute respiratory distress syndrome. JAMA 275:383–389, 1996.
195. Spitzer AR, Lipsky CL: Partial liquid ventilation with perflubron in premature infants with severe respiratory distress syndrome. Clin Pediatr (Phila) 36:181–182, 1997.
196. Pranikoff T, Gauger PG, Hirschl RB: Partial liquid ventilation in newborn patients with congenital diaphragmatic hernia. J Pediatr Surg 31:613–618, 1996.
197. Leach CL, Greenspan JS, Rubenstein SD, et al: Partial liquid ventilation with perflubron in premature infants with severe respiratory distress syndrome. The LiquiVent Study Group. N Engl J Med 335:761–767, 1996.
198. Roissant R, Falke KJ, Lopez F, et al: Inhaled nitric oxide for the adult respiratory distress syndrome. N Engl J Med 328:399–405, 1993.
199. Bigatello LM, Hurford WE, Kacmarek RM, et al: Prolonged inhalation of low concentrations of nitric oxide in patients with severe adult respiratory distress syndrome. Anesthesiology 80:761–770, 1994.
200. Puybasset L, Stewart T, Rouby J, et al: Inhaled nitric oxide reverses the increase in pulmonary vascular resistance induced by permissive hypercapnia in patients with adult respiratory distress syndrome. Anesthesiology 80:1254–1267, 1994.
201. Roissant R, Gerlach H, Schmidt-Ruhnke H, et al: Efficacy of inhaled nitric oxide in patients with severe ARDS. Chest 107:1107–1115, 1995.
202. Lowson SM, Rich GF, McArdle PA, et al: The response to varying concentrations of inhaled nitric oxide in patients with acute respiratory distress syndrome. Anesth Analg 82:574–581, 1996.
203. Michael JR, Barton RG, Saffle JR, et al: Inhaled nitric oxide versus conventional therapy: Effect on oxygenation in ARDS. Am J Respir Crit Care Med 157:1372–1380, 1998.
204. Dellinger RP, Zimmerman JL, Taylor RW, et al: Effects of inhaled nitric oxide in patients with acute respiratory distress syndrome: Results of a randomized phase II trial. Crit Care Med 26:15–23, 1998.
204a. Matthay MA, Pittet JF, Jayr C: Just say no to inhaled nitric oxide for the acute respiratory distress syndrome Crit Care Med 26:1–2, 1998.
204b. Zapol WM: Nitric oxide inhalation in acute respiratory distress syndrome: It works, but can we prove it? Crit Care Med 26:2–3, 1998.
205. Walmrath D, Schneider T, Schermuly R, et al: Direct comparison of inhaled nitric oxide and aerosolized prostacyclin in acute respiratory distress syndrome. Am J Respir Crit Care Med 153:991–996, 1996.
206. Meyer J, Theilmeier G, Van Aken H, et al: Inhaled prostaglandin E1 for treatment of acute lung injury in severe multiple organ failure. Anesth Analg 86:753–758, 1998.
207. Lu Q, Mourgeorn E, Law-Koune JD, et al: Dose-response curves of inhaled nitric oxide with and without intravenous almitrine in nitric oxide-responding patients with acute respiratory distress syndrome. Anesthesiology 83:929–943, 1995.
208. Jolliet P, Bulpa P, Ritz M, et al: Additive beneficial effects of the prone position, nitric oxide, and almitrine bismesylate on gas exchange and oxygen transport in acute respiratory distress syndrome. Crit Care Med 25:786–94, 1997.
209. Lavoie A, Hall JB, Olson DM, et al: Life-threatening effects of discontinuing inhaled nitric oxide in severe respiratory failure. Am J Respir Crit Care Med 153:1985–1987, 1996.
210. Hooper RG, Kearl RA: Established ARDS treated with a sustained course of adrenocortical steroids. Chest 97:138–143, 1990.
211. Meduri GU, Chinn AJ, Leeper KV, et al: Corticosteroid rescue treatment of progressive fibroproliferation in late ARDS: Patterns of response and predictors of outcome. Chest 105:1516–1527, 1994.
212. Meduri GU, Headley AS, Golden E, et al: Effect of prolonged

methylprednisolone therapy in unresolving acute respiratory distress syndrome: A randomized controlled trial. JAMA 280:159–165, 1998.
213. Wimer-Muram HT, Steiner RM, Gurney JW, et al: Ventilator-associated pneumonia in patients with adult respiratory distress syndrome: CT evaluation. Radiology 208:193–199, 1998.
214. Chastre J, Trouillet JL, Vuagnat A, et al: Nosocomial pneumonia in patients with acute respiratory distress syndrome. Am J Respir Crit Care Med 157:1165–1172, 1998.
215. Elliott CG: Pulmonary sequelae in survivors of the adult respiratory distress syndrome. Clin Chest Med 11:789–800, 1990.
216. Remolina C, Khan AU, Santiago TV, et al: Positional hypoxemia in unilateral lung disease. N Engl J Med 304:523–525, 1981.
217. Light RB: Indomethacin and acetylsalicylic acid reduce intrapulmonary shunt in experimental pneumococcal pneumonia. Am Rev Respir Dis 134:520–525, 1986.
218. Barone JE, Pizzi WF, Nealon TF: Indications for intubation in blunt chest trauma. J Trauma 26:334–338, 1986.

# 93 Ventilatory Failure

GREGORY A. SCHMIDT, M.D. • JESSE B. HALL, M.D. • LAWRENCE D.H. WOOD, M.D., PH.D.

Introduction
Consequences of Hypercapnia
- Hypoxemia
- Acidemia
- Mechanical Abnormalities
- Compensation for Metabolic Alkalosis

Type II Respiratory Failure
- Pathophysiology
- Multifactorial Respiratory Failure

Monitoring Respiratory System Mechanics
- Determination of Intrinsic Positive End-Expiratory Pressure
- Inspiratory Pressure at the Airway Opening
- Effect of Patient Effort
- Expiratory Pressure
- Respiratory Muscle Strength and Endurance

Recognizing Impending Respiratory Failure
Hemodynamic Consequences of Airflow Obstruction
- Pulsus Paradoxus
- Depressed Cardiac Output

Status Asthmaticus
- Clinical Presentation
- Management
- Liberation from Mechanical Ventilation

Acute-on-Chronic Respiratory Failure
- Clinical Presentation
- Management
- Prognosis

Summary

## INTRODUCTION

Since 1990, the approach to ventilatory failure has evolved importantly, most notably with a shift to noninvasive ventilation for a large number of selected patients and to less emphasis on normalizing the arterial partial pressure of carbon dioxide (arterial $P_{CO_2}$) in intubated patients, preferring to minimize barotrauma risk instead (permissive hypercapnia). Newer mechanical ventilators facilitate the use of flow and pressure waveforms to aid rational ventilation strategies. These and other new trends in the management of ventilatory failure are emphasized in this chapter.

In health, the arterial $P_{CO_2}$ is maintained within a narrow range (36 to 44 mm Hg) by adjusting alveolar ventilation ($\dot{V}_A$) to match the fluctuating rate of $CO_2$ production ($\dot{V}_{CO_2}$) as depicted in the alveolar equation for $CO_2$:

$$Pa_{CO_2} = (\dot{V}_{CO_2} \times k)/\dot{V}_A \qquad (1)$$

Primary failure of alveolar ventilation leads to a rising arterial $P_{CO_2}$ (and a falling arterial $P_{O_2}$), termed *ventilatory failure* or *type II respiratory failure*. In this chapter, we describe a pathophysiologic approach in which ventilatory failure is viewed as depressed central nervous system (CNS) respiratory drive, inadequate neuromuscular competence, or excessive respiratory system load. Such an approach is broadly applicable to the entire range of patients for whom mechanical ventilation is considered. Acute deterioration superimposed on chronic obstructive pulmonary disease (COPD), so-called *acute-on-chronic respiratory failure* (ACRF), and status asthmaticus are discussed in detail. More complete descriptions of less common subsets of patients in whom arterial $P_{CO_2}$ is elevated can be found in Chapters 80, 81, 89, and 90.

## CONSEQUENCES OF HYPERCAPNIA

Failure of $CO_2$ elimination is clinically important primarily because arterial pH and arterial $P_{O_2}$ fall. Although it may appear self-evident that hypercapnia is undesirable, it is worth examining its effects because treatment (increased ventilation) may have consequences as profoundly detrimental as the elevated arterial $P_{CO_2}$. For example, the greatest threat to life of the mechanically ventilated patient with status asthmaticus is barotrauma. Arterial $P_{CO_2}$ and barotrauma risk are coupled such that lowering one through a ventilatory adjustment typically raises the other.[1] Conventional ventilatory strategy has attempted to normalize the easily measured variable (arterial $P_{CO_2}$) rather than the less easily quantified risk of pneumothorax. Recent experience with intentional hypoventilation (permissive hypercapnia), however, supports the idea that it is more important to reduce alveolar pressures than the arterial $P_{CO_2}$, because this approach improves outcome with no demonstrated adverse effects of hypercapnia.[2, 3] This example points out the risk of titration of therapy against arbitrarily chosen values. Clearly, therapeutic interventions should be applied only when their expected benefits outweigh the anticipated costs, based on relevant end points. The most important effects of alveolar hypoventilation are on oxygenation, acid-base balance, and respiratory system mechanics.

## Hypoxemia

Hypoventilation causes a proportional fall in the alveolar $Po_2$ ($PA_{O_2}$):

$$PA_{O_2} = FI_{O_2} \times (PB - 47) - Pa_{CO_2}/RQ \qquad (2)$$

where $FI_{O_2}$ is the inspired oxygen fraction, PB the barometric pressure, and RQ the respiratory quotient. While breathing room air, a rise in the arterial $Pco_2$ from 40 to 80 mm Hg causes a fall in alveolar $Po_2$ to about 50 mm Hg, sufficient to cause significant hypoxemia. In the same example, however, simply raising the $FI_{O_2}$ from 0.21 to 0.28 boosts the alveolar $Po_2$ to 100 mm Hg. Because hypoxemia due to hypoventilation is easily corrected with supplemental oxygen, this consequence of hypoventilation is clinically unimportant in the hospital setting.

## Acidemia

Arterial pH is inversely proportional to arterial $Pco_2$. When the serum bicarbonate concentration ($HCO_3^-$) is 24 mEq/L, elevation of the arterial $Pco_2$ by 10 mm Hg results in a fall in the pH of 0.08 pH units. Any detrimental effects of respiratory acidemia are remarkably hard to discern because most such patients have concomitant hypoxemia, heart disease, or drug toxicity, and the results of animal experiments are often conflicting. Direct effects of acidemia include depression of cardiac contractility,[4–6] decreased respiratory muscle contractility and endurance time,[7] arterial vasodilation,[8] increased cerebral blood flow, and loss of conciousness. The seizure threshold is raised. The sympathetic response to respiratory acidemia can mask or even overwhelm these direct effects, however, with increased vascular tone, enhanced myocardial contractility, and CNS arousal. Serious arrhythmias are apparently uncommon,[9, 10] probably because of depressant effects on excitable tissues. Resuscitability from ventricular fibrillation is impaired in some models,[11] but not in others,[12, 13] and the range of arterial $Pco_2$ in which this can be demonstrated is far out of the range encountered in clinical respiratory failure.

The importance of these detrimental effects is not clearly known, but has probably been exaggerated, especially in patients in whom the arterial $Pco_2$ rises over hours to days rather than over minutes. Certainly many patients with COPD in whom the arterial $Pco_2$ has slowly risen to levels above 100 mm Hg exhibit no apparent adverse effects. Similarly benign results have been seen in children who have been markedly hypoventilated.[14] The increasing experience with permissive hypercapnia for patients with acute respiratory distress syndrome (ARDS) or status asthmaticus, in whom hypercapnia and acidemia are tolerated in order to avoid alveolar overdistention, has changed many clinicians' perspective about the adverse impact of acidemia. In sedated and ventilated patients with ARDS, rapid intentional hypoventilation (pH falling from 7.40 to 7.26 in 30 to 60 minutes) lowered systemic vascular resistance while cardiac output rose. Mean systemic arterial pressure and pulmonary vascular resistance were unchanged.[15] Furthermore, in many studies of patients undergoing permissive hypercapnia, a pH of well below 7.2 was tolerated well.[15–22] The feared consequences of acidemia, projected from the experience with patients having lactic acidosis (and, usually, concomitant sepsis), failed to materialize. With data now available from many patients permissively hypoventilated, the systemic hemodynamic effects are quite small even as the pH falls to 7.15, with the typical patient experiencing no change or small increases in cardiac output and blood pressure. Patients whose pH falls far below 7.0 are fewer in number, so firm conclusions cannot be drawn, but they similarly appear to tolerate their acidemia. The current practice of permissive hypercapnia does not generally include an attempt to alkalinize the blood to compensate for respiratory acidosis.

The encephalopathy of respiratory failure is multifactorial in etiology, possibly including elements of intracellular acidosis, hypoxia. impaired cardiac output, endogenous neuropeptide secretion, and sleep deprivation. Although acute $CO_2$ administration can cause obtundation and electroencephalographic depression[23]—probably through intracellular acidosis—the term *$CO_2$ narcosis* as applied to patients with ACRF, implying a direct effect of $CO_2$, is likely a misnomer. Hypercapnia may have more serious consequences in patients with increased intracranial pressure, acute right heart failure, or myocardial ischemia.

## Mechanical Abnormalities

When arterial $Pco_2$ rises to 80 mm Hg in a spontaneously breathing patient, the required alveolar ventilation falls to half (all else being equal), thereby roughly halving the work of breathing. Indeed, in the severely obstructed patient who is likely to have intrinsic positive end-expiratory pressure (PEEPi), hypoventilation additionally reduces the degree of PEEPi, further reducing the work of breathing (discussed subsequently).

In the mechanically ventilated patient, hypoventilation reduces mean alveolar pressure and, if present, PEEPi. Therefore, allowing the arterial $Pco_2$ to remain above normal may beneficially reduce the risk of barotrauma and lessen the hemodynamic consequences of mechanical ventilation (see Chapters 91 and 92). These potentially beneficial mechanical consequences of hypercapnia may outweigh the consequences of acidemia in an individual patient.

## Compensation for Metabolic Alkalosis

An elevated arterial $Pco_2$ level does not always indicate respiratory failure, but may be a consequence of metabolic alkalosis. Although early studies failed to demonstrate a predictable compensatory respiratory acidosis in patients with metabolic alkalosis, it is now clear that alkalemic patients will hypoventilate in an attempt to normalize arterial pH, even when such hypoventilation causes a significant fall in $Po_2$.[24] This compensatory hypoventilation is predictably related to the degree of alkalemia, similar to the expected compensations for other acid-base disorders. It is often stated that alkalosis prolongs the need for mechanical ventilation by reducing the drive to breathe. The reduced work of breathing allowed by metabolic alkalosis could, however, facilitate liberation from the ventilator. Although alkalemia has its own negative consequences and may be a clue to another underlying disorder (e.g., hypovolemia), it is likely that, when mechanical ventilation is prolonged in an alkalemic patient, the physician is responsible, not the alkalosis.

## TYPE II RESPIRATORY FAILURE

### Pathophysiology

Alveolar ventilation is maintained by the CNS, acting through nerves and the respiratory muscles, to drive the respiratory pump. The three subsets of ventilatory failure include loss of adequate drive, impaired neuromuscular competence, and excessive respiratory load. This concept is developed in Figure 93.1. The CNS drives the inspiratory muscles via the spinal cord and phrenic and intercostal nerves. Inspiratory muscle contraction lowers pleural pressure, thereby inflating the lungs. The pressure generated by the inspiratory muscles (neuromuscular competence) must be sufficient to overcome the elastance of the lungs and chest wall (elastic load), as well as the flow resistance of the airways (resistive load). Spontaneous ventilation can be sustained only as long as the inspiratory muscles are able to maintain adequate pressure generation.[25]

Relatively few patients develop ventilatory failure due to loss of drive. Most often this occurs in the setting of drug overdose or physician-directed sedation. Typically these patients present little challenge, requiring only supportive care until the drug can be metabolized or its action reversed. One exception is the group of patients with undiagnosed sleep apnea, who typically have a significant component of central apnea and who may require specific therapy directed at relief of obstructive apneas.

Far more common and difficult are patients who have adequate drive, but inadequate neuromuscular function or excessive load (or both). The pathophysiology of ventilatory failure is unknown and controversial, but the approach taken in this chapter is that a primary determinant of ventilatory failure is inspiratory muscle fatigue.[26] A muscle is fatigued when it can no longer develop the degree of tension possible before fatigue, no matter what the degree of stimulation, yet recovers with rest. Skeletal muscles fatigue when their rate of energy consumption exceeds the energy supplied by blood flow.[27] Similarly for the respiratory muscles, endurance time during inspiratory resistive loading is closely tied to the oxygen cost of breathing ($\dot{V}O_{2\,resp}$).[28] The primary determinants of $\dot{V}O_{2\,resp}$ are the time-tension index, work rate, and lung volume.[29] Several experiments in humans indicate that the intensity required of the contracting respiratory muscles, as well as their strength, are crucial factors determining fatigue.[30] Once fatigue of the respiratory muscles is established, neuromuscular competence is unable to sustain the mechanical load imposed on the respiratory system, and ventilatory failure ensues. It has been proposed that central depression of drive contributes to the terminal stages of respiratory failure,[31] irrespective of the precipitating cause. According to this hypothesis, overworked respiratory muscles generate inhibitory signals that feed back to the CNS to reduce drive, thereby protecting the muscles from fatigue.[32, 33] The relevance of this mechanism to respiratory failure remains to be demonstrated. Although the importance of muscle fatigue in human respiratory failure has not been conclusively established and central fatigue may be more important, our approach provides a useful conceptual framework for the treatment of patients with ventilatory failure.

In health, neuromuscular function far exceeds that nec-

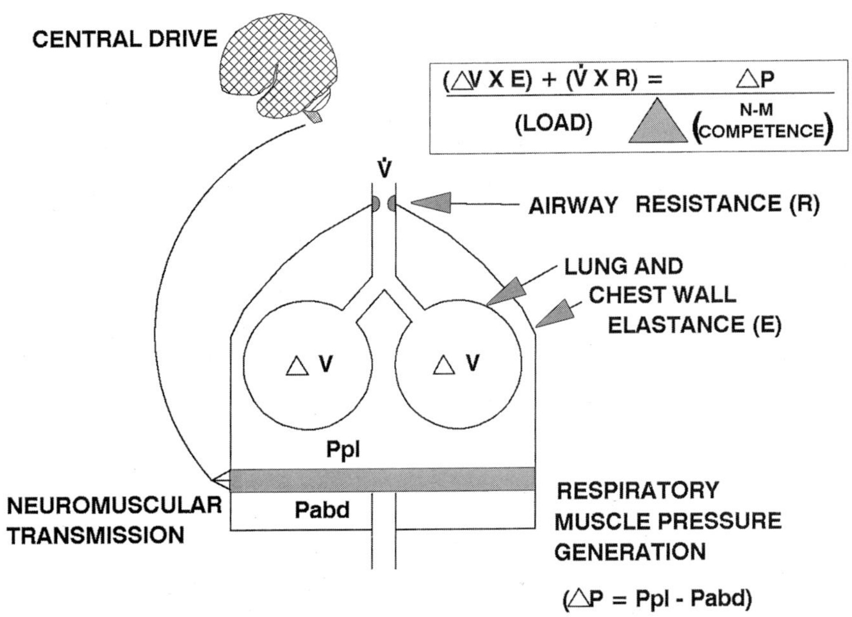


**Figure 93.1** The key elements of the ventilatory system. The central nervous system drives the respiratory muscles through neural afferents. The respiratory muscles contract (neuromuscular (N-M) competence), opposed by the abdominal pressure (Pabd), to generate a pleural pressure (Ppl). The resulting Ppl must be sufficient to overcome the combined respiratory system loads of flow resistance (R) and elastance (E) in order to maintain a given minute ventilation ($\dot{V}$).

essary to sustain ventilation against the normally small load. Dramatic increments in load (as in status asthmaticus) or decrements in strength (as in the Guillain-Barré syndrome) are required to cause hypoventilation. In patients with COPD, however, the respiratory system load, as judged by the $\dot{V}O_{2\ resp}$, is elevated to 17% to 46% of the total body $\dot{V}O_2$, due to abnormal airway resistance and increased elastance.[34] Only small increments in load or decrements in neuromuscular competence are needed to precipitate frank ventilatory failure. The many potential contributors to ventilatory failure are enumerated in Figure 93.2.

## Impaired Drive

In the usual patient who is dyspneic, tachypneic, diaphoretic, and using accessory muscles of respiration, impairment of drive is clearly not the cause of ventilatory failure. When drive has been assessed in the setting of ACRF, it is greatly elevated,[35] as it is in most patients who fail to "wean" from mechanical ventilation.[36] Nevertheless, there are patients in whom new CNS insults or drug effects contribute to respiratory failure. Even small doses of sedatives or narcotics may cause respiratory failure when superimposed on chronic ventilatory insufficiency; a careful history is essential to exclude this possibility. Occult hypothyroidism is not rare in the elderly, particularly in women. Thyroid function testing should be part of the routine screening of patients with ventilatory failure attributed to decreased drive.

**Oxygen and Drive to Breathe.** One of the most pervasive myths surrounding the treatment of ACRF is that these patients rely on hypoxic drive to breathe. Physicians are often hesitant to supply oxygen, fearing that patients will stop breathing, necessitating intubation. Because these patients are typically hypoxemic on presentation (arterial $Po_2$ usually about 30 to 40 mm Hg), failure to supply adequate oxygen is a potentially devastating treatment error. Unrelieved hypoxemia in the face of acidemia, fatiguing respiratory muscles, and an often failing right ventricle risks arrhythmia, myocardial infarction, cerebral injury, renal failure, and respiratory arrest.

In several studies performed in the 1980s, patients with COPD have been convincingly shown to nearly maintain $\dot{V}E$ despite treatment with even 100% oxygen[37, 38] and to augment their drive in response to hypercapnia.[39] When oxygen is given, the arterial $Pco_2$ typically rises, but this is attributed largely to worsened matching of ventilation and perfusion and to the Haldane effect, not to hypoventi-

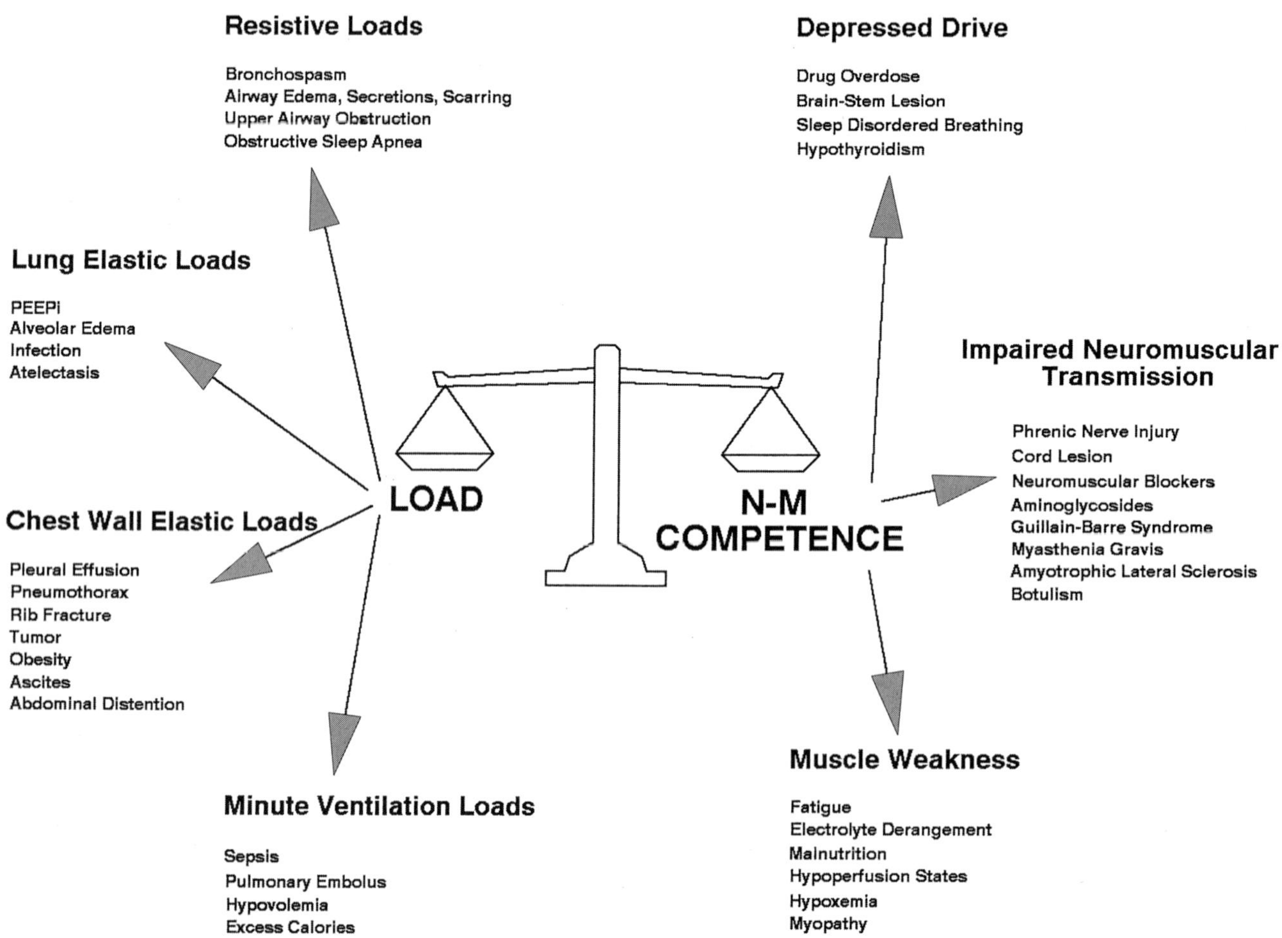


**Figure 93.2** The balance between load (resistive, elastic, and minute ventilation) and neuromuscular (N-M) competence (drive, transmission, and muscle strength) determines the ability to sustain alveolar ventilation.

lation. In one series, patients with ACRF had a mean initial arterial $P_{O_2}$ level of 38 mm Hg and an arterial $P_{CO_2}$ level of 65 mm Hg.[27] They were then placed on 100% oxygen, which raised the mean arterial $P_{O_2}$ level to 225 mm Hg, while the mean arterial $P_{CO_2}$ level plateaued at 88 mm Hg. $\dot{V}_E$ fell by a small amount (7%), and drive remained supranormal. Our point is not to claim that hypoxic drive in patients with ACRF does not exist—it clearly does[40]—but to emphasize that oxygen should be given nevertheless. High concentrations of inspired oxygen are not usually necessary in ACRF unless pneumonia or pulmonary edema is present, because hypoxemia is largely due to $\dot{V}/\dot{Q}$ mismatching, not shunt. Nevertheless, we believe that the risks of oxygen therapy have been greatly overstated,[41] often leading physicians to withhold a potentially lifesaving therapy. The goal of oxygen therapy is to maintain 90% saturation of an adequate circulating hemoglobin. This can usually be attained with a facemask at 28% to 35% or nasal cannula at 2 to 5 L/min. A rise in arterial $P_{CO_2}$ is likely, but this in itself is of little importance. Patients may progress to respiratory failure *despite* oxygen therapy, but usually not because of it. For this reason, careful serial assessments by the ICU team of physician-nurse-respiratory therapist are essential.

**Sleep-Disordered Breathing.** Sleep-disordered breathing may present as cardiopulmonary failure or be superimposed on preexisting chronic lung disease. These patients have a blunted response to respiratory acidosis and seem particularly prone to hypoventilate when given oxygen. Most patients exhibit the characteristic obese habitus and have a history of snoring, but occasionally these clues are absent. A high index of suspicion is required to detect this underrecognized condition. In particular, an untoward increase in arterial $P_{CO_2}$ with oxygen, associated with hypersomnolence, is an indication for elective intubation and mechanical ventilation for 72 hours, followed by a diagnostic search for sleep-disordered breathing when the patient awakens.

## Inadequate Neuromuscular Competence

**Failed Neuromuscular Transmission.** To effect adequate ventilation, the brain must transmit drive to the working muscles via the spinal cord and peripheral nerves. Thus causes of neuromuscular failure, such as spinal cord lesions, primary neurologic diseases, and neuromuscular blocking drugs, may produce ACRF. Aminoglycosides[42] and procainamide[43] act as mild neuromuscular blockers, a feature unimportant in most patients but relevant in those with neuromuscular diseases, such as myasthenia gravis. The clinical setting may be a clue to one of the unusual causes, such as phrenic nerve injury following cardiopulmonary bypass. This occult lesion may be induced by direct trauma to the nerve or more indirectly by cold cardioplegia.

**Muscle Weakness.** The most important causes of decreased neuromuscular competence fall into the category of muscle weakness. Especially prominent are electrolyte disturbances such as hypokalemia, hypophosphatemia,[44] and hypomagnesemia.[45] Hypophosphatemia may be exacerbated by many of the drugs used to treat ventilatory failure, such as methylxanthines, beta-agonists, corticosteroids, and diuretics, accounting for its striking prevalence in COPD patients (about 20%).[46] Malnutrition, present in 40% to 50% of hospitalized patients with emphysema,[47] can cause respiratory muscle weakness,[48] and even short-term fasting has been shown to depress diaphragm strength and endurance in experimental animals,[49] whereas short-term refeeding can improve indicies of respiratory muscle function[50] and immune response. In patients with emphysema, at the same time that the respiratory system load is elevated, the inspiratory muscles are poorly able to tolerate it because hyperexpansion forces the inspiratory muscles to operate on a disadvantageous portion of their force-length relationship. In addition, a flattened diaphragm generates less transmural pressure for a given tension than the normally curved one. In one study comparing diaphragm strength between normal persons and patients with severe, but stable, COPD (mean $FEV_1$ of 0.6 L), the patients had a maximal drop in intrathoracic pressure (sniff Pes) of only two-thirds that of the normal persons.[51] Virtually all of this difference was ascribable to the diaphragm position rather than to inherent muscle weakness. Postparalytic myopathy may contribute, especially in patients recovering from status asthmaticus.[52–54] Rarely, other myopathies, such as an adult variant of acid maltase deficiency or mitochondrial myopathy, may cause cryptic respiratory failure due to muscle weakness.

Muscle fatigue is the reversible loss of ability to develop force and is itself a cause of muscle weakness. To the extent that fatigue is central to the development of respiratory failure, it may be caused by inadequate supply of nutrients, excess generation of metabolites such as lactate or hydrogen ion, or depletion of muscle glycogen. Evidence to support the importance of blood supply in the genesis of fatigue comes from studies of respiratory failure in animals with hemorrhagic, cardiogenic, or septic shock.[55, 56] In these animals, fatigue is hastened by circulatory insufficiency. The magnitude of blood flow to respiratory muscles seems important beyond aerobic needs as demonstrated in experiments in which flow was manipulated independently of oxygen delivery.[57] Hypoperfusion states, hypoxemia, and severe anemia have the potential to contribute to muscle fatigue and thereby to hasten respiratory failure.

## Increased Respiratory System Load

**Increased Resistive Load.** In patients with COPD, the respiratory system load is chronically elevated due to abnormal airway resistance and increased elastance. The increment in airway resistance is accounted for by bronchospasm, airway inflammation, and physical obstruction by mucus and scarring. One common cause of increased flow resistance, and the most amenable to pharmacologic intervention, is bronchospasm. The disease course in most patients with COPD includes an asthmatic component. Exacerbations of bronchospasm increase resistive workload and may precipitate ACRF. Superimposed heart failure may also cause increased airway resistance, mimicking asthma ("cardiac asthma"). Upper airway obstruction is much less common, but because these patients frequently have a history of prior intubation, tracheal stenosis should be considered. Finally, sleep apnea, which commonly coexists with COPD, may need to be excluded. Especially once the patient is intubated, clues to this underlying cause of dynamic upper airway obstruction (e.g., snoring) may be impossible to discern. In the proper setting (an obese, hypersomnolent patient), this possibility should be vigorously pursued. The endotracheal tube itself presents a significant resistive workload, especially when a small size (<7.5 mm inner diameter) is chosen.[58] Tube angulation, length, and presence of secretions also affect flow resistance.

**The Role of Intrinsic Positive End-Expiratory Pressure.** The most significant contributor to the elastic load is dynamic hyperinflation.[59] Airflow obstruction, compounded by decreased elastic recoil in patients with emphysema, leads to prolongation of expiration. When the rate of alveolar emptying is slowed, expiration cannot be completed before the ensuing inspiration. Rather than reaching the normal static equilibrium of lung and chest wall recoil at functional residual capacity at the end of each breath, the respiratory system empties incompletely.

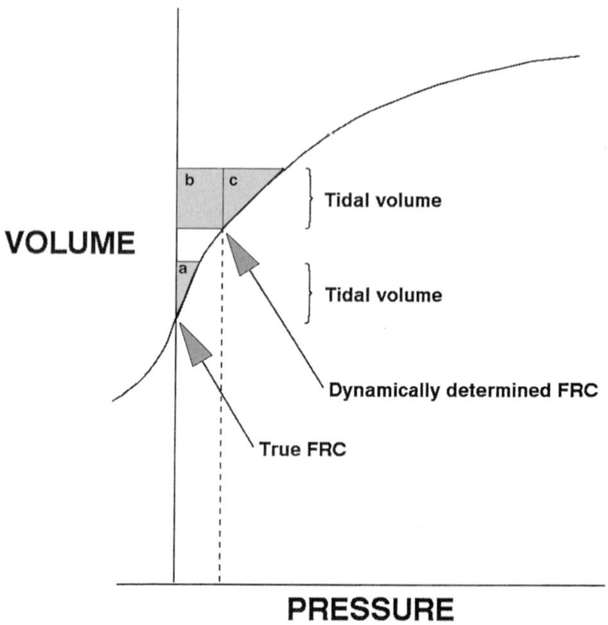


**Figure 93.3** The impact of intrinsic PEEP on work of breathing. A volume-pressure curve of the respiratory system is illustrated. Without intrinsic PEEP, inspiration begins from "true" functional residual capacity (FRC), and the external work (pressure-volume product) required to produce a tidal volume is shown in shaded area *a*. When intrinsic PEEP is present, inspiration begins from the higher, dynamically determined FRC, and the external work to produce the same tidal volume is shown in shaded areas *b* and *c*. The work represented by area *b* must be performed simply to initiate gas flow (e.g., to trigger a ventilator). Adding continuous positive airway pressure in an amount equal to intrinsic PEEP (shown as the dashed line) reduces the work of each breath to area *c*.

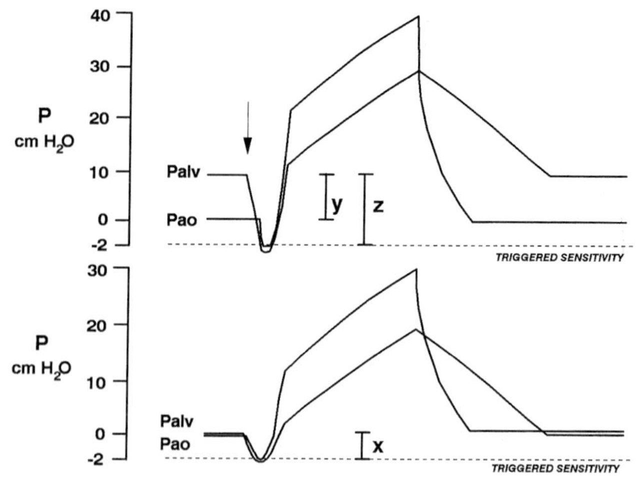


**Figure 93.4** Effect of intrinsic PEEP (PEEPi) on triggering. The lower tracings of airway opening pressure (Pao) and alveolar pressure (Palv) represent a patient who is triggering volume-cycled ventilator breaths and who does not have PEEPi. The upper tracing shows a patient similarly ventilated and with the same triggered sensitivity (− 2 cm $H_2O$), but who has 4 cm $H_2O$ PEEPi. The patient without PEEPi must lower his or her Palv by *x* (~2 cm $H_2O$) in order to lower the Pao by the same amount, triggering a breath. In contrast, the patient with PEEPi must lower his or her Palv by *y* (~4 cm $H_2O$) before having any impact on Pao, then by a further 2 cm $H_2O$ to trigger the ventilator. In the patient with PEEPi, the total reduction in Palv *(z)* required to trigger the ventilator rises as PEEPi rises and is occult. In the extreme, PEEPi may be so elevated that a weak patient is unable to trigger the ventilator despite great effort.

Expiration terminates at this higher, dynamically determined functional residual capacity. At end expiration, there remains a positive elastic recoil pressure, called *intrinsic positive end-expiratory pressure* (PEEPi). Accordingly, alveolar pressure remains positive with respect to end-expiratory pressure at the airway opening such that a greater effort must be generated by the inspiratory muscles on the subsequent breath. This adds a threshold load to spontaneous inspiration and, in mechanically ventilated patients, makes triggering of assisted breaths more difficult (Figs. 93.3 and 93.4).[60] Determinants of the magnitude of PEEPi include the degree of expiratory obstruction (including both patient and ventilator components), elastic recoil, minute ventilation, and expiratory time (therefore, respiratory rate, inspiratory flow rate, inspiratory flow profile). Methods for detecting and quantitating PEEPi are described later in this chapter. Intrinsic PEEP of about 10 cm $H_2O$ is present in most, if not all, COPD patients with acute ventilatory failure[61, 62] and can be measured in many ambulatory outpatients as well.[63] Counterbalancing this PEEPi with external PEEP provides a means by which to lower the work of breathing (or the work of triggering). When continuous positive airway pressure (CPAP) is applied by face mask in an amount less than or equal to PEEPi, the work of breathing is reduced in spontaneously breathing patients with impending respiratory failure.[64] In intubated patients with ACRF, CPAP has been demonstrated to reduce the work of breathing by nearly 50%[65] and to lessen the work of triggering the ventilator (see Fig. 93.4).[60] In addition, patients feel less dyspneic.

**Increased Lung Elastic Load.** Contributors to lung stiffness include pulmonary edema (hydrostatic and increased permeability), pneumonia, interstitial fibrosis or inflammation, tumor, and atelectasis. As noted above, at the same time that bronchospasm causes increased flow resistance, it simultaneously worsens elastic load by augmenting PEEPi.

**Increased Chest Wall Elastic Load.** The chest wall includes the thorax, diaphragm, and abdomen. Therefore, obesity, rib fracture, pneumothorax, pleural effusion, ascites, chest wall abnormalities, and abdominal distention contribute to the work of breathing. These factors are particularly relevant in the postoperative setting.

**Minute Ventilation Loads.** Dividing the work of breathing into resistive and static components is a useful way of analyzing the effort of each breath. Even if the work of each breath remains constant, however, an increase in respiratory rate increases the load. Increased minute ventilation ($\dot{V}_E$) requirements can be divided into those due to excess carbon dioxide production ($\dot{V}CO_2$) and those from worsened dead space. The first category includes excessive caloric intake, fever, agitation, muscular exertion (including shivering and respiratory distress), and hypermetabolism due to injury or infection. New dead space may be caused by pulmonary embolism, hypovolemia, PEEP (including PEEPi), or shallower breathing, which raises the dead space fraction ($V_D/V_T$).

## Multifactorial Respiratory Failure

To analyze respiratory failure in a way that facilitates management, it is important to dissect the very complex real-life patient into simple components of deranged neuromuscular competence and load. However, the patient with ACRF due to isolated rib fracture or hypokalemia is uncommon. More often, numerous contributors to both decreased strength and increased load are implicated. For example, a patient admitted with pneumonia and worsening bronchospasm may additionally have hypophosphatemia, heart failure, and malnutrition. Aspiration at the time of intubation, abdominal distention related to attempts to feed enterally, and overzealous parenteral nutrition complete the picture of multifactorial ACRF. Although such a patient may seem overwhelmingly complex, a systematic approach to each component of respiratory failure leads logically to a plan for treatment.

# MONITORING RESPIRATORY SYSTEM MECHANICS

Because most adult patients are ventilated, at least initially, with a volume-cycled mode (i.e., assist-control or intermittent mandatory ventilation), and because monitoring respiratory system mechanics in most intensive care units is practical only during volume-cycled ventilation, the following discussion is limited largely to this setting. Determination of respiratory system mechanics is an integral part of ventilator management and is a routine part of the examination of the critically ill patient.

Often the cause of ventilatory failure has not been determined by the time of endotracheal intubation. If the peak airway opening pressure (Ppeak) is not increased in a passive, ventilated patient, the physician should suspect impaired drive, neuromuscular weakness, or a transient, now resolved, problem (e.g., upper airway obstruction bypassed by the endotracheal tube) as the cause for ventilatory failure. When the Ppeak is high, partitioning its components into the resistive pressure (Presist), the static pressure (Pstat), and PEEP can aid the physician to narrow the differential diagnosis. In addition, such analysis may allow therapy to be tailored specifically to the cause of ventilatory failure. For example, for a patient with COPD and congestive heart failure who fails extubation following colon resection, bronchodilators are not helpful if Presist is normal and PEEPi is 0. Similarly, if PEEPi is elevated, measures to decompress the abdomen are not likely to get the patient off of the ventilator.

## Determination of Intrinsic Positive End-Expiratory Pressure

Dynamic hyperinflation, also called intrinsic PEEP (PEEPi) or the auto-PEEP effect, occurs when there is insufficient time for the respiratory system to return to functional residual capacity during expiration. Short expiratory times, high minute volumes, and increased expiratory resistance contribute to PEEPi, but all of these need not be present. PEEPi is present in most ventilated patients with asthma and COPD (and in many during spontaneous breathing) but is also seen in ARDS and other settings with high minute ventilations. In many regards PEEPi acts like PEEP to impede venous return, heighten the risk of barotrauma, and improve oxygenation. It has been proposed that PEEPi is the major contributor to improved oxygenation during inverse ratio ventilation and high-frequency ventilation. In addition, PEEPi increases the work of breathing and impairs the patient's ability to trigger the ventilator as described earlier in this chapter. For these reasons, it is imperative to monitor routinely the presence and amount of PEEPi in mechanically ventilated patients.

PEEPi should be suspected when, during expiration, the chest fails to come to rest before the onset of the subsequent breath or wheezes persist until inspiration.[66] These findings can be confirmed if the ventilator is made to display expiratory flow (Fig. 93.5). Several methods for quantifying PEEPi are available, but the one typically used clinically is the end-expiratory port occlusion method (Fig. 93.6).[67] Several ventilators facilitate this determination by providing an expiratory pause switch. This method does not provide accurate estimation of PEEPi if there is a leak in the tubing or around the endotracheal tube cuff, there is gas flow into the circuit during expiration (as during continuous nebulization of bronchodilators), or the patient is not fully passive during the maneuver. In one survey of ventilated patients, quanti-

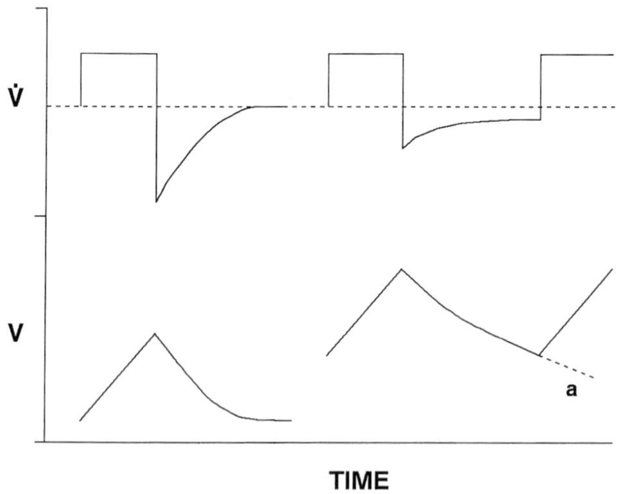


**Figure 93.5** On the left side of the figure, volume (V) and flow ($\dot{V}$) are shown during conventional volume-cycled ventilation with a square wave flow profile and no airflow obstruction. (Inspiratory flow is above the dashed, horizontal line.) On the right are V and $\dot{V}$ when significant expiratory obstruction and intrinsic PEEP are present. Note the lower peak expiratory flow, the prolongation of expiration, and the presence of persistent expiratory flow at the onset of the subsequent breath. This persistent end-expiratory flow indicates the presence of intrinsic PEEP, shown on the volume plot as a raised functional residual capacity (FRC). Dashed curve *a* represents the continued fall in lung volume toward static FRC, which would occur if the subsequent breath were not given (or came later).

tation of PEEPi was possible by the end-expiratory port occlusion technique in only one-third because patient effort confounded the airway pressure.[66] Serial measurement of PEEPi may give information regarding the obstructed patient's response to bronchodilator therapy (if $\dot{V}_E$ is constant) and is essential to safe management during inverse ratio ventilation.

## Inspiratory Pressure at the Airway Opening

Gas is driven to and from the lung by a pressure difference between alveolus and airway opening. When a muscle-relaxed patient is mechanically ventilated, the inspiratory pressure at the airway opening (Pao) consists of three components: one to drive gas across the inspiratory resistance, the second to expand the alveoli against the elastic recoil of the lungs and chest wall, and the third equal to the alveolar pressure present before inspiratory flow begins (PEEP or PEEPi) (Fig. 93.7).

$$\text{Pao} = \text{Presist} + \text{Pstat} + \text{PEEP} \qquad (3)$$

$$\text{Pao} = \dot{V}_I \times R_{AW} + \Delta V \times E_{RS} + \text{PEEP} \qquad (4)$$

where Presist is the resistive pressure component, Pstat is the static elastic pressure term, $\dot{V}_I$ is inspiratory flow, $R_{AW}$ is inspiratory resistance, ΔV is the increment in lung volume, $E_{RS}$ is elastance of the respiratory system, and PEEP is applied PEEP or intrinsic PEEP (PEEPi). Diagnostic and therapeutic information can be gleaned by distinguishing the individual components of Pao, as follows. First, PEEPi is found by the method described above, whereas PEEP is set by the ventilator. The remainder of the Pao (ΔP = Ppeak − PEEP) can be apportioned between its two components, Presist and Pstat, by stopping flow and allowing the Presist term to fall to 0. When flow is 0, Pao drops to a lower Pplateau (Fig. 93.7). Then,

$$\text{Presist} = \text{Ppeak} - \text{Pplateau} \qquad (5)$$

$$\text{Pstat} = \text{Pplateau} - \text{PEEP (or PEEPi)} \qquad (6)$$

At normal inspiratory flow rates in the range of 1 L/sec, Presist is typically between 4 and 10 cm $H_2O$. Elevated Presist is found with high inspiratory flow or increased inspiratory resistance. At constant flow, a rise in Presist may indicate, for example, increased bronchospasm or endotracheal tube obstruction. Conversely, falling Presist may correspond to a response to bronchodilators.

Because Pstat = ΔV × $E_{RS}$, elevated Pstat indicates excessive tidal volume or increased elastic recoil of the lungs or chest wall, as in pulmonary fibrosis, acute lung

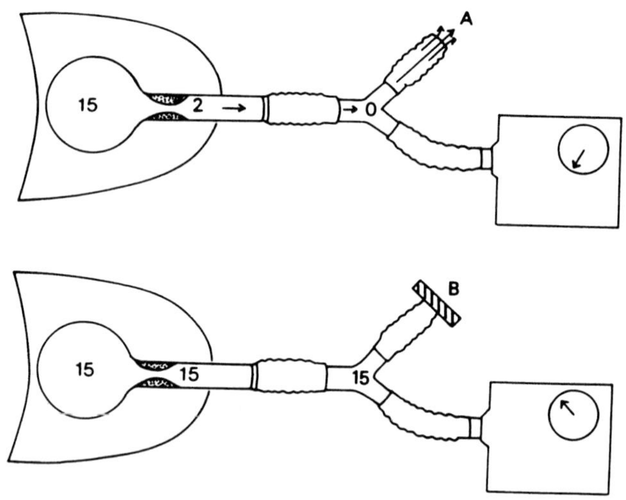


**Figure 93.6** The auto-PEEP effect and its measurement by the end-expiratory port occlusion maneuver. Just before the next ventilator inflation cycle, alveolar pressure remains markedly positive (15 cm $H_2O$) as flow continues through critically narrowed airways *(A)*. The ventilator manometer approximates auto-PEEP only when pressures equilibrate following occlusion of the expiratory port at end exhalation *(B)*. (Reproduced with permission from Pepe PE, Marini JJ: Occult positive end-expiratory pressure in mechanically ventilated patients with airflow obstruction: The auto-PEEP effect. Am Rev Respir Dis 126:166, 1982.)

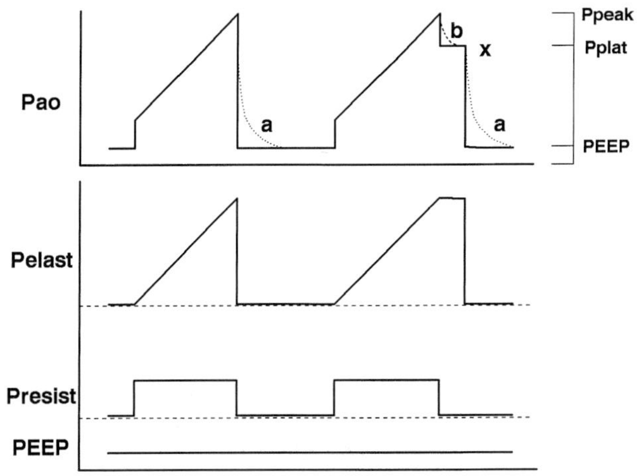


**Figure 93.7** Components of the airway opening pressure (Pao) during volume-cycled ventilation of a passive patient (assist control or intermittent mandatory ventilation breaths). The bottom tracing shows PEEP (applied PEEP or intrinsic PEEP); the second tracing from the bottom shows the pressure required to drive flow across the inspiratory resistance (Presist); the second tracing from the top shows the elastic recoil pressure of the respiratory system (Pelast); and the top tracing shows the Pao. The Pao during inspiration equals the sum of the three lower tracings. The contribution of PEEP, Presist, and Pelast to the Pao can be determined in a passive patient by (1) noting the PEEP (or measuring intrinsic PEEP); (2) stopping flow briefly at end inspiration, during which the Pao falls to a lower plateau *(x)*; (3) subtracting the plateau pressure (Pplat) from the peak pressure (Ppeak) to give the Presist; and (4) subtracting the PEEP (or intrinsic PEEP) from Pplat to give Pelast. The Pao during expiration does not fall immediately *(a)* to the PEEP level because of finite resistance in the expiratory limb of the ventilator. The expiratory pressure reflects characteristics of the ventilator circuit and the expiratory flow and does not indicate alveolar pressure. Similarly, the Ppeak does not fall immediately *(b)* to Pplat because of time required for redistribution of proximal gas.

injury, or abdominal distention. Respiratory system static compliance (CRS) is the inverse of ERS:

$$C_{RS} = \Delta V/P_{stat} \quad (7)$$

and is normally about 70 mL/cm $H_2O$.

## Effect of Patient Effort

Typically the patient performs inspiratory work during an assist-control breath.[68] This may not be obvious despite careful examination of the patient unless measures of intrathoracic pressure (esophageal pressure, central venous pressure) are available. Effort at the end of the breath will affect the Ppeak and Pplateau, making determination of respiratory system mechanics unreliable. Clues to patient effort are also often available from the airway pressure tracing, such as concavity of the rise in Pao, variability of Ppeak, and a dip in Pao before inspiration, indicating a triggering effort (Fig. 93.8).

## Expiratory Pressure

Analyzing the expiratory pressure [PAW(ex)] is substantially less useful than the inspiratory pressure because PAW(ex) is largely determined by characteristics of the mechanical ventilator, not the patient.

$$P_{AW}(ex) = PEEP + \dot{V}exp \times Rexlimb \quad (8)$$

where PEEP is the applied PEEP (not PEEPi), $\dot{V}$exp is expiratory flow rate, and Rexlimb is the resistance of the expiratory limb of the ventilator. It is important to realize that PAW(ex) does not reflect expiratory alveolar pressure or PEEPi and relates to the patient's respiratory system only indirectly through the expiratory flow. Although some ventilators display inspiratory and expiratory pressure-volume plots, only the inspiratory segment gives useful information about the patient.

## Respiratory Muscle Strength and Endurance

The patient's ability to sustain spontaneous breathing depends not only on the work of ventilation but also on

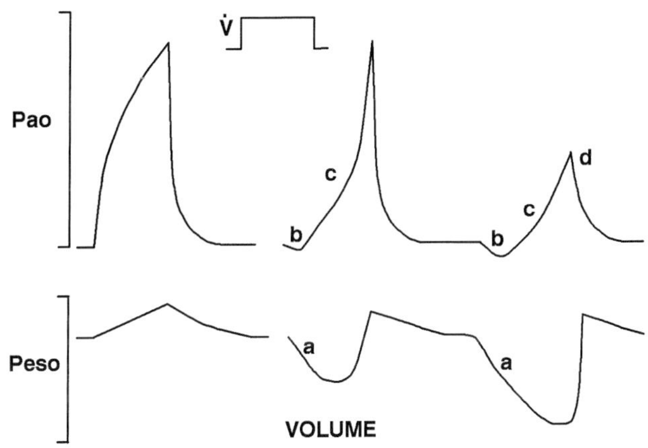


**Figure 93.8** Signs of patient effort during volume-cycled ventilation (assist-control (A/C) or intermittent mandatory ventilation (IMV) breaths). In the three breaths of equal tidal volume shown, the leftmost tracing represents a muscle-relaxed patient, whereas the other two breaths show a patient making variable inspiratory efforts. The fall in esophageal pressure (Peso) due to inspiratory muscle activity *(a)* is shown in the bottom tracings. When an esophageal balloon is not in place, similar information may be gleaned from the central venous or pulmonary artery pressure. Signs of patient effort in the airway pressure tracing include a fall in pressure at the airway opening (Pao) just before the A/C or synchronized IMV breath (triggering, *b*, a concave upward rise in Pao) during inspiration *(c)*, and a variable peak airway pressure (Ppeak; *d*). Note that the value of Pao throughout inspiration, including the Ppeak of the third breath, is reduced in proportion to the inspiratory fall in pleural pressure.

his or her respiratory muscle strength and endurance. Therefore, estimates of respiratory muscle competence go hand in hand with determinations of lung and chest wall mechanics in judging the patient's ability to maintain all or part of the effort of breathing. The maximal inspiratory pressure (MIP) generated on a voluntary (or involuntary) inspiratory effort from functional residual capacity is commonly used to test respiratory muscle strength. Normal subjects can breathe indefinitely without fatiguing when subjected to an inspiratory threshold load as long as the inspiratory pressure does not exceed 30% to 40% of MIP.[69] Whether the findings from short-term inspiratory threshhold loading in normal subjects can be extrapolated to critically ill patients, who may have less ventilatory endurance, however, is unknown. Measurement of the voluntary MIP requires patient effort and coordination and is difficult to perform reproducibly in many intubated critically ill patients. Accordingly, in clinical practice, the measured pressure is not necessarily the *maximal* inspiratory pressure. In 100 medical patients recovering from respiratory failure, the predictive value of this single test was low.[70] Thus the MIP cannot be used by itself to reliably predict weaning outcomes but, if measured correctly, it can help to identify patients with potentially treatable respiratory muscle weakness.

The vital capacity is used in many hospitals to assess single-breath respiratory muscle performance. A value greater than 10 mL/kg has been suggested to predict weaning success, but this has not been proven to be clinically useful.

## RECOGNIZING IMPENDING RESPIRATORY FAILURE

Despite aggressive attempts to find and reverse the causes of ventilatory failure, some patients will progress nonetheless to frank respiratory failure. The decision to intubate requires clinical judgment and should be assessed by a physician present at the bedside (Table 93.1). Assessment of respiratory failure based solely on results of arterial blood-gas studies is fraught with error. Certainly, a rising arterial $P_{CO_2}$ level in a patient with progressively worsening symptoms and signs of distress should be interpreted to herald impending respiratory arrest. The absolute level of the arterial $P_{CO_2}$ isolated from other clinical data, however, may be less useful. We have taken care of a small number of patients in whom the arterial $P_{CO_2}$ rose to more than 150 mm Hg while the patients were alert and conversant, and mechanical ventilation did not become necessary. On the other hand, many patients with status asthmaticus or ACRF do progress to respiratory arrest long before progressive hypercapnia is clearly documented. Respiratory arrest may be complicated by aspiration or cardiovascular instability, compromising future efforts to return the patient to spontaneous breathing. Indeed, the survival of patients who are allowed to progress to respiratory arrest is significantly lower than that of patients ventilated for acute deterioration of COPD who are electively intubated before arrest. If noninvasive ventilation (NIV) fails to stabilize the patient, the goal at this stage of management is to intubate the patient *electively* once invasive mechanical ventilation becomes unavoidable.

**Table 93.1 ASSESSMENT OF THE NEED FOR INTUBATION IN VENTILATORY FAILURE**

1. Noninvasive ventilation (NIV) should be tried in appropriate patients before intubation
2. This judgment must be made by the physician at the bedside
3. Predictors of frank ventilatory failure include
   - Respiratory rates that remain >36 breaths/min despite NIV
   - Worsening tachycardia
   - Continued use of all accessory muscles
   - Mental status deterioration
   - Patient's subjective sense of exhaustion
4. Arterial blood gas studies are of limited use in making this judgment, usually merely confirming clinical assessment
5. Concomitant hemodynamic instability or inability to protect the airway may mandate intubation

Useful bedside parameters of impending respiratory arrest include respiratory rate, mentation, rapid and shallow pattern of breathing, and the patient's own assessment. Patients may be able to tell the physician whether they are improving or not; their degree of dyspnea over time is a useful guide to likelihood of success without intubation. A breathing rate that remains above 35 to 40 breaths/min, or a rising rate despite therapy and NIV, is predictive of respiratory failure. Deterioration of mentation commonly precedes respiratory arrest. Patients become confused, less conversant, and then poorly rousable. Thoracoabdominal paradox and respiratory alternans are rarely seen and are probably not useful.

Better methods of assessing ventilatory reserve are needed, particularly to identify patients who are failing despite NIV. As the role of respiratory muscle fatigue in ventilatory failure is clarified, and as methods for assessing fatigue in spontaneously breathing patients are developed, our ability to intubate patients expeditiously, but not excessively, may improve.

## HEMODYNAMIC CONSEQUENCES OF AIRFLOW OBSTRUCTION

### Pulsus Paradoxus

During active inspiration against obstructed airways, pleural pressure falls far lower than during unloaded breathing, in extreme cases to less than $-100$ cm $H_2O$. A consequence of this is that venous return is augmented, raising right ventricular end-diastolic volume. This shifts the interventricular septum to the left, reducing the compliance of the left ventricle, decreasing left ventricular end-diastolic volume, stroke volume, and, therefore, pulse pressure. A second effect of the tremendous fall in pleural pressure comes from the dramatic increase in transmural left ventricular pressure (cavitary left ventricular pressure minus pleural pressure) during systole, which represents a sizable increment in afterload, further depressing stroke volume. The combined effects of reduced pleural pressure are clinically recognized as a fall in systolic blood pressure of greater than 10 mm Hg during inspiration (pulsus paradoxus). The degree of pulsus paradoxus has been used to gauge the course of status asthmaticus and its treatment,[71] falling as obstruction improves (and less commonly in the minutes preceeding respiratory arrest as muscle function and pressure generation decline).

### Depressed Cardiac Output

Most patients with ventilatory failure have significant airflow obstruction and consequently have PEEPi. PEEPi acts similarly to PEEP in raising pleural and, consequently, right atrial pressure, reducing the gradient for venous return, thereby causing hypotension or tachycardia. At the time of endotracheal intubation, peri-intubation drug effects, the conversion to positive pressure ventilation, and escalating PEEPi may combine to precipitate frank shock. The key to avoiding this pitfall is to prevent excessive ventilation. When hypotension occurs, the circulation can usually be restored promptly by simply ceasing ventilation for 30 seconds, then re-instituting ventilation along with measures to reduce PEEPi. A fluid bolus of 500 to 1000 mL will increase the mean systemic pressure, reestablish the gradient for venous return, and raise the cardiac output.

## STATUS ASTHMATICUS

Status asthmaticus is an attack of asthma that is severe at onset or progresses rapidly despite routine therapy and may result in ventilatory failure and death. In a subset of asthmatic patients, very rapid onset and progression of symptoms suggests a predominant role for bronchospasm.[72] In most patients with status asthmaticus, however, symptoms evolve over several days, consistent with significant airway inflammation and edema. Mucous plugging of both large and small airways is a striking finding post mortem in patients who have died of status asthmaticus.[73, 74] Further discussion of the diagnosis and treatment of asthma of varying severity is presented in Chapter 39.

### Clinical Presentation

A history is often difficult to obtain from patients with acute airflow limitation, but duration of symptoms, loss of sleep, and the patient's subjective sense of distress may be useful clues to the severity of the attack (Table 93.2). Clinical signs include tachycardia, tachypnea, hyperinflation, wheezing, accessory muscle use, pulsus paradoxus, and diaphoresis. The absence of wheezing does not exclude a diagnosis of asthma, and in the period immediately preceding respiratory arrest the chest may be completely silent.

Arterial blood gases typically show moderate hypoxemia; however, even patients requiring mechanical ventilation can usually be adequately saturated on an $FI_{O_2}$ of 0.3 to 0.5 because true intrapulmonary shunt is trivial.[75] During acute treatment with bronchodilators hypoxemia

**Table 93.2 INDICATORS OF SEVERE ASTHMA**

| |
|---|
| Long duration of symptoms |
| Progression despite optimal outpatient therapy |
| Sleep deprivation |
| Dyspnea precluding speech |
| Accessory muscle use |
| Tachycardia >120 beats/min |
| Respiratory rate >35 breaths/min |
| Pulsus paradoxus >15 mm Hg |
| $FEV_1$ <1 L |
| PEFR <120 L/min |
| Rising or elevated $Pa_{CO_2}$ |

PEFR = peak expiratory flow rate.

may worsen due to deterioration in matching of ventilation and perfusion.[76] Dead space increases substantially in asthma, presumably due to hypoperfusion of regions of hyperinflated lung.[75, 77] Despite this, most patients with asthma present with a low arterial $P_{CO_2}$ level. An elevated arterial $P_{CO_2}$ level on presentation appears to correlate with the degree of obstruction and with the propensity to frank respiratory failure,[78] but this continues to be debated.[79]

Acute electrocardiographic changes accompanying asthma include sinus tachycardia, right axis deviation, clockwise rotation, and signs of right ventricular hypertrophy. Electrocardiographic changes caused by asthma resolve within hours of response to therapy.

Lactic acidosis, which has been demonstrated in several investigations of status asthmaticus, is likely caused by increased muscle lactate production, the action of catecholamines, and, perhaps, diminished hepatic clearance.[80, 81] Its presence may predict an increased risk of progression to ventilatory failure.[78, 80]

Barotrauma is common in status asthmaticus, and both pneumomediastinum and pneumothorax predict progression to ventilatory failure. Chest pain, suddenly worsened dyspnea, tracheal deviation, subcutaneous emphysema, asymmetric breath sounds, and a mediastinal "crunch" on auscultation all should prompt a search for barotrauma with chest radiography.

### Management

#### Pharmacologic Interventions

**Oxygen.** Humidified oxygen should be given to achieve full arterial saturation. Resolution of hypoxemia improves oxygen delivery to the respiratory muscles, relieves any component of hypoxia-induced pulmonary hypertension, and protects against a paradoxical worsening of gas exchange with bronchodilator therapy. Furthermore, oxygen itself has bronchodilating properties.

**Beta-Agonists.** Inhaled beta-agonists should be initiated immediately to treat smooth muscle-mediated bronchospasm (Table 93.3). These drugs have a rapid onset of action and are generally well tolerated, even in high dose in the acute setting. Recent data are available that demonstrate that albuterol delivered by a metered-dose

**Table 93.3 BRONCHODILATOR THERAPY FOR STATUS ASTHMATICUS**

**Beta-Agonists**

- Give by inhalation, titrated to undesirable side effects (e.g., albuterol 6–12 puffs by MDI or 0.5 mL/2.5 mL saline every 20 min)
- In mechanically ventilated patients, tidal volume should be raised above 500 mL, inspiratory flow rate should be lowered to 40 L/min, actuation of the MDI should be timed to coincide with inspiration, and the breath should be followed by a brief (3 sec) pause. The effect on airway resistance should be monitored.
- If inhaled beta-agonists are not tolerated, consider parenteral epinephrine (0.3 mL 1 : 1000 SC) or terbutaline (0.25 mg SC) every 20 min.

**Corticosteroids**

- High-dose corticosteroids for the first 24–48 hr (e.g., methylprednisolone 125–250 mg IV every 6 hours)

**Methylxanthines**

- Theophylline titrated to a serum level of approximately 15 μg/mL

**Ipratropium**

- Ipratropium bromide may be of benefit in some patients (e.g., 6–10 puffs every 20 min).

IV = intravenously; MDI = metered-dose inhaler; SC = subcutaneously.

inhaler (MDI) with a spacer, to a total dose of 1600 μg over 90 minutes, does not increase cardiovascular morbidity in well-oxygenated patients with status asthmaticus.[82] Large and frequent drug doses are needed in severe asthma because the dose-response curve and duration of action are adversely affected by airway narrowing. In North America, albuterol is slightly preferred over metaproterenol because of its greater $beta_2$ selectivity and longer duration of action.[83, 84] Some clinicians prefer metaproterenol or isoetharine for initial therapy, despite the tendency of these drugs to increase side effects, because of their faster onset of action.[85] Long-acting beta-agonists are not indicated in the initial treatment of status asthmaticus because of their slow onset of action.

In most situations, beta-agonists should be administered by inhalation. There is no advantage to delivering these drugs initially by the subcutaneous route unless the patient is unable to cooperate with inhaled therapy (such as those with an impaired sensorium or those in cardiopulmonary arrest).[86–88] Subcutaneous epinephrine may, however, benefit patients not responding adequately to several hours of inhaled beta-agonists.[89] Known cardiac disease and age greater than 40 years are relative contraindications to parenteral therapy,[90] although older patients without a history of recent myocardial infarction or angina tolerate subcutaneous epinephrine reasonably well. Inhaled beta-agonists may be delivered equally well by an MDI with a spacer or by a hand-held nebulizer.[91] Even for severely obstructed patients, four puffs of albuterol (0.36 mg) delivered by an MDI with an InspirEase has been shown to be as effective as 2.5 mg of albuterol by nebulization.[92] MDIs with spacers carry the advantage of lesser cost and faster drug delivery times, whereas hand-held nebulizers require fewer instructions, less supervision, and less coordination. Patients should be treated continuously until an adequate clinical response has been achieved or toxic side effects limit further drug administration. Prior use of inhaled beta-agonists at home should not limit their use in the emergency room unless adverse effects are identified.[93] Intravenous infusion of beta-agonists is not recommended, with the possible exception of patients in cardiac arrest. Several studies have demonstrated that inhaled drug results in greater improvement in airflow and less toxicity than does intravenous administration.[94–97]

Many questions remain regarding the optimal administration of inhaled bronchodilators during mechanical ventilation.[98] There is a consensus, however, that whether MDIs or nebulizers are used, higher drug dosages are required to achieve a physiologic effect in intubated patients. In one study, only 2.9% of a radioactive aerosol delivered by nebulizer was deposited in the lungs of mechanically ventilated patients.[99] Manthous and colleagues[100] compared the efficacy of albuterol delivered by MDI via a simple inspiratory adapter (no spacer) to nebulized albuterol in mechanically ventilated patients. Using the peak-to-pause pressure gradient at a constant inspiratory flow as a measure of airway resistance, they found no effect (and no side effects) from the administration of 100 puffs (9.0 mg) of albuterol, whereas albuterol delivered by nebulizer to a total dose of 2.5 mg reduced the inspiratory flow-resistive pressure 18%. Increasing the nebulized dose to a total of 7.5 mg led to further reductions in airway resistance in 8 of 10 patients but to the development of toxic side effects in half of patients.

If MDIs are used to deliver beta-agonists during mechanical ventilation, use of a spacing device on the inspiratory limb of the ventilator is useful to optimize drug delivery.[91, 101, 101a] The minimum dose via MDI should be 4 puffs, and for some patients 10 to 20 puffs is safe and more effective.[102] Patient-ventilator synchrony is crucial to optimize drug delivery. Drug delivery may be facilitated by inserting an inspiratory pause to coincide with the dose of medication. When a nebulizer is used, the added gas flow used to drive it (typically 8 L/min) may add to adverse consequences (increased PEEPi) if not compensated for by a reduction in delivered minute ventilation. Further potential complications of nebulized drug delivery in ventilated patients include fouling of the internal filters of the ventilator, interference with the measurement of respiratory system mechanics and PEEPi (the nebulizer must be stopped to make these determinations), and inadvertent delivery of toxic fractions of oxygen (because oxygen is typically used to drive the nebulizer). In ventilated patients, MDIs require less time, have fewer complications, are less costly, and their drug delivery is more predictable, making them the preferred method of treatment.[91, 103, 104] In general, nebulizers should be placed close to the ventilator (no data are yet available for MDIs), and the tidal volume should be raised above 500 mL. Stopping the in-line humidifier improves drug deposition, but, alternatively, one can increase the dose. Inspiratory flow should be reduced to approximately 40

L/min during treatments to minimize turbulence, although this strategy has the potential to worsen lung hyperinflation (see below) and must be short lived. Heliox may improve delivery of aerosols.

Whether the drug is delivered by nebulizer or by an MDI with a spacer, dosage should be titrated to a fall in the peak-to-pause airway pressure gradient or the development of toxic side effects. When no measurable drop in airway resistance occurs, it is important to exclude other causes of elevated airway resistance such as a kinked or plugged endotracheal tube. The optimal dose interval is not known, but in the acute setting we have used both MDI and hand-held nebulizer at 20 minute intervals until there is a response or undesirable side effects occur. In ventilated patients, beta-agonists may be given continuously by inhalation.

**Corticosteroids.** Because most patients with status asthmaticus have a significant component of airway wall inflammation, corticosteroids should be administered as early as possible. In a meta-analysis, it was concluded that corticosteroids given in the emergency room significantly reduce admission rates and the number of future relapses during the first 7 to 10 days,[105] and additional evidence exists that failure to treat episodes of acute severe asthma with corticosteroids contributes to asthma deaths.[106] Both oral and intravenous routes are effective, although oral drug should be avoided in patients with gastrointestinal upset and in patients at risk for intubation. The minimum dose should be 40 mg of methylprednisolone (or its equivalent) every 6 hours.[107] The available data suggest that lower corticosteroid doses are less effective and that doses higher than 60 mg methylprednisolone intravenously every 6 hours are not significantly better.[108] The common approach of giving 60 to 125 mg methylprednisolone intravenously every 6 hours during the initial 24 hours of treatment is reasonable. Many clinicians prefer higher initial doses for patients already taking systemic corticosteroids and for patients at great risk for intubation.

**Ipratropium Bromide.** All other medications must be considered auxiliary in the treatment of status asthmaticus. Still, if use of a second-line agent produces even a marginal effect, clinical outcome may be altered. With regard to ipratropium bromide, sufficient data are available to support its use in patients with severe asthma[108–111]; however, this drug produces less bronchodilation at peak effect than beta-agonists and achieves a more variable clinical response, indicating the variable role of cholinergic mechanisms in acute asthma. In one study, 384 emergency room patients were randomized to receive nebulized albuterol 2.5 mg or albuterol 2.5 mg mixed with ipratropium 0.5 mg at entry and at 45 minutes.[112] At 45 minutes, there were significantly more responders in the group receiving both albuterol and ipratropium compared with albuterol alone; however, the median change of $FEV_1$ from baseline did not differ between groups, and by 90 minutes there was no difference in the percentage of responders and median change in $FEV_1$ between groups. In addition, there were no significant differences in the number of patients requiring additional emergency room or hospital treatment.

**Theophylline.** Several studies have demonstrated that theophylline does not add to the clinical effect of maximal doses of beta-agonists during the first few hours of treatment and that theophylline increases the incidence of tremor, nausea, anxiety, and tachyarrhythmias.[108, 113] These short-term studies are reasonably convincing; however, they were not designed to look at a possible delayed effect from the early use of theophylline. Indeed, data are available demonstrating that theophylline benefits patients after 24 hours of treatment.[114] Interestingly, nonbronchodilating properties of theophylline may warrant its use in status asthmaticus. Anti-inflammatory properties and effects on diaphragm function may help explain data that emergency room administration of theophylline possibly results in fewer hospitalizations, even when airflow is no different from that in patients receiving placebo.[115] We often use theophylline when patients fail to respond initially to beta-agonists and corticosteroids. For patients already taking theophylline, we continue its use after confirming a nontoxic serum concentration. This approach is safe if attention is paid to serum drug levels and to factors that increase serum levels, such as congestive heart failure, and coadministration of ciprofloxacin, macrolide antibiotics, or cimetidine, and if the drug is discontinued in the presence of significant tachyarrhythmias.[108]

**Magnesium.** In the late 1980s and early 1990s, magnesium sulfate was used extensively in the emergency room treatment of status asthmaticus. This practice was based on several reports demonstrating benefit; however, these studies suffered from small patient numbers, and many were anecdotal. Since then, three prospective trials have failed to confirm a benefit to administering magnesium sulfate in status asthmaticus.[116–118] In the most recent study, 135 persons with asthma were randomized to 2 g magnesium sulfate intravenously or placebo after 30 minutes in the emergency room and studied for 4 hours.[119] Hospital admission rates and $FEV_1$ values were no different between magnesium-treated patients and controls. On subgroup analysis, however, magnesium sulfate was shown to decrease admission rates and improve $FEV_1$ in patients with severe asthma ($FEV_1 < 25\%$ of predicted). Additional evidence supporting a possible benefit in severe disease comes from an uncontrolled study of five mechanically ventilated asthmatic patients given magnesium.[120] In this study, patients were given high doses of magnesium sulfate (10 to 20 g) over 1 hour, after which there was a significant decrease in peak airway pressure (from 43 cm $H_2O$ to 32 cm $H_2O$) and in inspiratory flow resistance. Other investigators have suggested the possibility that gender may also play a role in magnesium responsiveness because estrogen may augment the bronchodilator effect of magnesium.[121] Clearly, additional data are needed to determine whether there are subgroups of patients with severe asthma who might benefit from the administration of magnesium sulfate. For now, the routine use of this agent cannot be justified, with the possible exception for patients with disease severe enough to require mechanical ventilatory support. Magnesium should not be given to patients with renal insufficiency.

**Leukotriene Modifiers.** Leukotriene modifiers are mildly effective bronchodilators. We are unaware of studies with critically ill patients, but intravenous administration of one of these agents to otherwise healthy persons with asthma caused bronchodilation that was additive to that of albuterol.[122] Whether there is any role for leukotriene modifiers in patients with status asthmaticus remains to be shown.

## Noninvasive Ventilation

Noninvasive positive pressure ventilation (NIV) by facemask is a potentially useful option for patients with status asthmaticus who do not need immediate control of the airway. NIV can be delivered with either a ventilator or a continuous positive-pressure airway device.[122a] Advantages of NIV over intubation and mechanical ventilation include decreased need for sedation and paralysis, decreased incidence of nosocomial pneumonia, decreased incidence of otitis and sinusitis, and improved patient comfort.[123] Potential disadvantages include a small increased risk of aspiration of gastric contents when there is gastric insufflation, skin necrosis, and diminished control of a patient's ventilatory status compared with invasive ventilation. Data regarding the efficacy of NIV in status asthmaticus are sparse. In one study of 21 acute asthmatic patients with a mean peak expiratory flow rate of 144 L/min, nasal continuous-positive airway pressure (CPAP) of 5 or 7.5 cm $H_2O$ significantly decreased respiratory rate and dyspnea compared with placebo.[124] Presumably, applying CPAP to the mouth helps overcome the adverse effects of PEEPi (discussed previously).[125] In another study, Meduri and colleagues[126] reported their observational experience with NIV during 17 episodes of acute severe asthma. NIV was achieved with a loose-fitting full facemask with initial settings of 0 cm $H_2O$ CPAP and 10 cm $H_2O$ pressure support ventilation. Subsequently, CPAP was increased to 3 to 5 cm $H_2O$ and pressure support ventilation was increased to achieve an exhaled tidal volume of 7 mL/kg or more and a respiratory rate of less than 25 breaths/min. Initially delivered minute ventilation averaged 16 L/min, and peak inspiratory pressure was less than 25 cm $H_2O$. The average duration of NIV was approximately 16 hours. In all but one patient (who subsequently required intubation), NIV improved the sense of dyspnea. Heart rate and respiratory rate decreased over 12 to 24 hours. Arterial $P_{CO_2}$ and pH improved significantly after 2 hours of treatment in all but one patient. Two NIV-treated patients required intubation for worsening arterial $P_{CO_2}$, and there were no NIV complications. The results of this study are promising but need to be confirmed in randomized trials.

## Ventilator Management and Permissive Hypercapnia

Mechanical ventilation in status asthmaticus is particularly challenging because airway pressures are typically high and interventions to achieve normocapnia often result in more dynamic hyperinflation and greater risk of barotrauma. The goals of therapy are to achieve adequate alveolar ventilation, low levels of PEEPi, minimal circulatory compromise, and low risk of barotrauma. Often, innovative approaches are required.

Lung hyperinflation is directly proportional to minute ventilation ($\dot{V}_E$)[18, 127] and to the degree of airflow obstruction. In the postintubation period, dangerous levels of hyperinflation develop when patients are ventilated excessively. The positive intrathoracic pressure associated with positive pressure ventilation and rising PEEPi act to increase right atrial pressure. This decreases venous return to the right heart, resulting in systemic hypotension and tachycardia. This pathophysiology is demonstrated by ventilating the patient slowly (2 to 3 breaths/min) to prolong expiratory time and allow lung deflation. Restoration of blood pressure generally occurs within 60 seconds of initiating this maneuver. Tension pneumothorax, which may occur bilaterally, should be considered in patients who remain hypotensive despite a trial of hypoventilation. Chest tubes should not be placed until a trial of hypoventilation has failed unless there is clear-cut evidence of pneumothorax.

After intubation, patients should be deeply sedated and, according to some experts, therapeutically paralyzed. These minimize airway pressures; allow determination of PEEPi, Ppeak, and Pplateau; and lower $CO_2$ production.[128] Sedation can be achieved with short-acting benzodiazepines, ketamine, or droperidol.[128–130] Ideally, one would like to ventilate the patient with status asthmaticus to a normal arterial $P_{CO_2}$ level while keeping the Ppeak and PEEPi low enough to avoid barotrauma. When patients with severe asthma are ventilated to eucapnia, however, severe dynamic hyperinflation usually occurs. End-inspired volume can be as large as 3 to 4 L above apneic functional residual capacity, a feature that risks barotrauma and cardiovascular compromise. Various combinations of tidal volume and respiratory rate (at constant minute ventilation; Fig. 93.9*B*) show that at higher rates and lower tidal volumes, Ppeak and Pplateau fall, owing to the lower end-inspired lung volume, whereas there is a small increase in end-expired volume and corresponding intrinsic PEEP owing to slightly greater air trapping caused by the reduced time for expiration.[127] Figure 93.9*A* demonstrates that varying inspiratory flow from 40 to 100 L/min while maintaining tidal volume and respiratory rate reduces end-expired lung volume, end-inspired lung volume, and Pplateau by allowing more time for expiration.

Because the determinants of arterial $P_{CO_2}$ are as follows:

$$Pa_{CO_2} = \dot{V}_{CO_2} \times k/[\dot{V}_E \times (1 - V_D/V_T)] \quad (9)$$

where $V_D/V_T$ is the dead space fraction, $\dot{V}_E$ can be reduced or respiratory acidosis can be ameliorated by reducing $\dot{V}_{CO_2}$ (sedate, relax muscles, treat fever or infection) or by minimizing dead space. Manipulations of $V_T$ and respiratory rate (RR) are more complex because raising each will increase PEEPi, thereby likely raising the $V_D/V_T$. When $V_T$ or RR is augmented in an attempt to lower arterial $P_{CO_2}$, occasionally the increment in $V_D/V_T$ outweighs the increase in $\dot{V}_E$, and arterial $P_{CO_2}$ "paradoxically" rises. It is crucial to recognize this early because continued increases in $V_T$ or RR will further raise

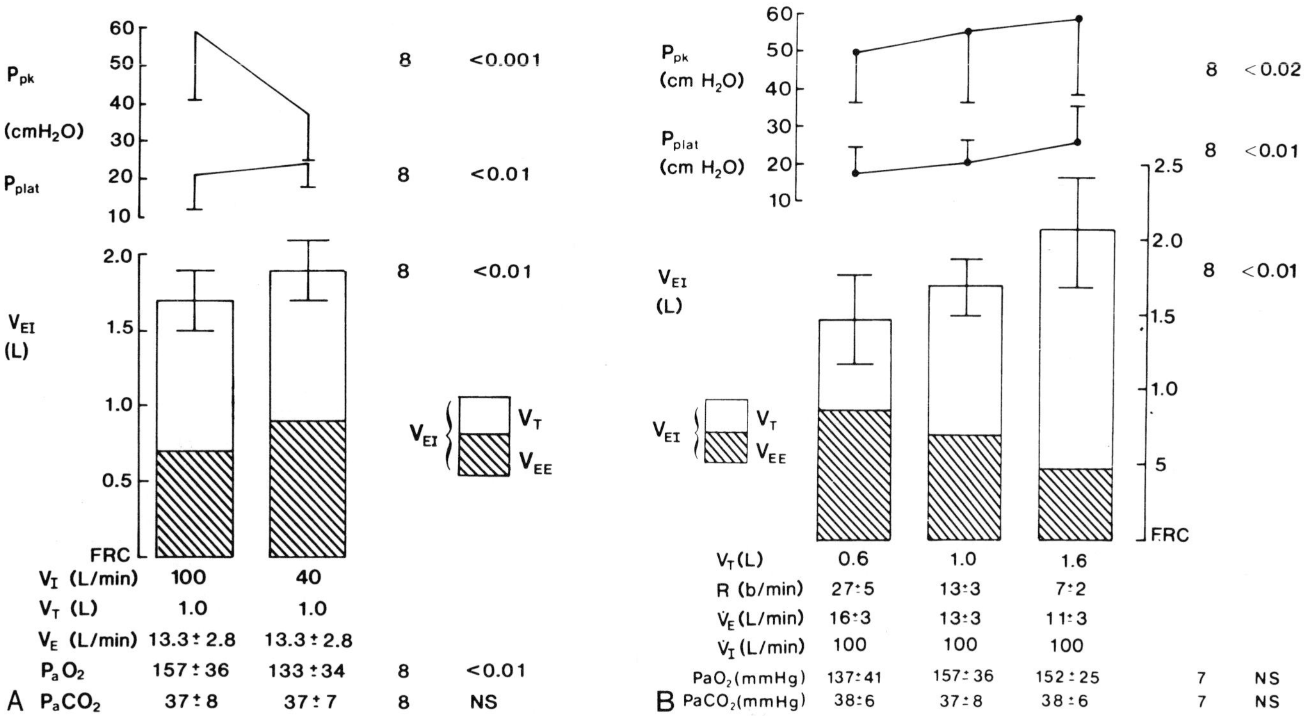


**Figure 93.9** Effects of various ventilator settings on airway pressures and dynamic hyperinflation during normocapnic ventilation of eight muscle-relaxed asthmatic patients. VEE = lung volume at end expiration; VEI = lung volume at end inspiration; Ppk = peak airway pressure; Pplat = end-inspiratory plateau pressure; $\dot{V}E$ = minute ventilation; VI = inspiratory flow.

Note that as inspiratory flow is lowered from 100 to 40 L/min at the same minute ventilation, peak airway pressures fall but dynamic gas trapping increases significantly.

Dynamic hyperinflation can be reduced by low respiratory rates with high tidal volumes, but Ppk and Pplat increase. (Reproduced with permission from Tuxen DV, Lane S: The effects of ventilatory pattern on hyperinflation, airway pressures, and circulation in mechanical ventilation of patients with severe air-flow obstruction. Am Rev Respir Dis 136:872–879, 1987.)

VD/VT, arterial $PCO_2$, and PEEPi, potentially culminating in barotrauma or shock. If initial ventilator settings fail to give acceptable Ppeak, Pplateau, and arterial $PCO_2$, VT and RR can be adjusted in graded fashion (either up or down), but should only be increased if this change leads to a clearly defined improvement in gas exchange.

To avoid significant lung hyperinflation, the ventilator should be set to allow sufficient exhalation time while continuing to optimize bronchodilator and anti-inflammatory therapy. The most important means to achieve this is to reduce the $\dot{V}E$, although increasing the $\dot{V}I$ may also be useful. For example, assume that a patient is ventilated with VT 500 mL, rate 15 breaths/min, and $\dot{V}I$ 60 L/min with a square wave. Increasing the $\dot{V}I$ dramatically, to 120 L/min, lengthens the expiratory time (TE) from 3.5 seconds to 3.75 seconds (a 7% increase). By comparison, simply decreasing the rate from 15 breaths/min to 14 lengthens TE to 3.8 seconds (an 8% increase). Although the inspiratory to expiratory ratio appears less favorable with the rate reduction (1:7 vs. 1:15), the time for exhalation is actually greater.

A strategy aimed at reducing inspiratory time (with fast inspiratory flow rates and the square inspiratory flow wave form) carries a cost of higher peak inspiratory pressures. Recent data fail to show a relationship, however, between Ppeak and complications of mechanical ventilation.[131] The reasons may be that Ppeak does not predict alveolar pressure or the degree of overdistension of alveolar structures and that the high pressures are encountered largely by robust proximal airways. In general, therefore, we accept high peak pressures for the greater good of reducing PEEPi.

Clinical studies demonstrate that an initial $\dot{V}E$ between 8 and 10 L/min (achieved by a VT between 8 and 10 mL/kg and an RR between 11 and 14 breaths/min), combined with an inspiratory flow rate of 80 to 100 L/min, is unlikely to result in a dangerous degree of lung hyperinflation as measured by end-inspired volume.[131] This volume is determined by collecting the total exhaled volume of gas during 20 to 60 seconds of apnea in a paralyzed patient. Only a end-inspired volume above 20 mL/kg (1.4 L in an average-sized adult) has been shown to predict complications of hypotension and barotrauma. Limiting the use of end-inspired volume as a routine clinical tool, however, is the need for paralysis. End-inspired volume (VEI) may be estimated from other ventilator parameters if one assumes linear compliance of the respiratory system, although this assumption has not been rigorously demonstrated in clinical studies. Specifically,

$$C = V_T/(P_{plateau} - PEEP_i) = V_{EI}/P_{plateau} \quad (10)$$

hence

$$V_{EI} = (V_T \times P_{plateau})/(P_{plateau} - PEEP_i) \quad (11)$$

Reasonable surrogate measures of lung hyperinflation, therefore, are Pplateau and PEEPi, although their reliability is subject to patient effort. In our experience (and that of others), complications are rare when Pplateau is less than 30 cm $H_2O$ and PEEPi is less than 15 cm $H_2O$.[132] In one study comparing Pplateau, PEEPi, and end-inspired volume as predictors of barotrauma and hypotension in mechanically ventilated patients with status asthmaticus, however, only end-inspired volume had a high predictive value.[131]

These data support an approach to mechanical ventilation in the patient with status asthmaticus using low minute volumes and high inspiratory flow rates to minimize dynamic hyperinflation. Typical initial ventilator settings include a tidal volume of about 8 to 10 mL/kg and an RR of 11 to 14 breaths/min, with inspiratory flows of around 80 L/min. These settings will usually lead to an arterial $P_{CO_2}$ level well above the normal range, an approach that trades the risks of barotrauma for the presumably lower risks of hypercapnia (permissive hypercapnia). Several series of asthmatic patients have been treated successfully with this approach.[2, 3] Low values of arterial pH are generally well tolerated: alkali therapy is not used. Hypercapneic acidosis does cause cerebral vasodilation, decreased myocardial contractility, vasodilation with a hyperdynamic circulation, and pulmonary vasoconstriction.[133] Accordingly, permissive hypercapnia should be avoided in patients with raised intracranial pressure (as might occur in the setting of anoxic brain injury from cardiopulmonary arrest) and in patients with severe myocardial dysfunction. Indirect evidence suggests that permissive hypercapneic ventilation in asthma decreases mortality. Although the lack of common methodology precludes fair comparison of mortality rates among studies, it can generally be stated that reported death rates are higher in series not employing permissive hypercapnia.[108]

One of the downsides of permissive hypercapneic ventilation is that patients must be fully sedated and, generally, therapeutically paralyzed. An increasing number of patients are being reported with severe neuromuscular weakness following mechanical ventilation for asthma.[134–141] Both myopathy and neuropathy[134] have been described. Various factors could contribute to neuromuscular weakness, including high-dose corticosteroids, paralytic agents,[142] disuse atrophy associated with muscle paralysis, or the polyneuropathy of critical illness.[143, 144] Neurophysiologic findings (motor axonal degeneration) in one series of three patients were not consistent with disuse atrophy.[134] Each of the three patients with neuropathy fully recovered over 2 to 12 months. Respiratory muscle strength (negative inspiratory pressure or vital capacity) should be assessed routinely following reversal of sedation and paralysis.

**Effect of Inspiratory Flow Profile.** On most ventilators the physician can choose one of several inspiratory wave forms, most commonly square or decelerating. The rationale for the use of decelerating flow is to minimize peak Pao, an effect that occurs predictably because maximal flow (and, therefore, flow-related pressure) occurs early in the breath when lung volume (and elastic recoil pressure) is minimal, whereas near the end of the breath lung volume is maximal, but flow is minimal. However, an inescapable consequence of the overall lower $V_I$ is a shorter $T_E$. Thus in patients who are obstructed or have high minute ventilations (those in whom a decelerating flow pattern will most reduce Ppeak) PEEPi is increased (Fig. 93.10). Although the relative contributions of Ppeak and PEEP (or PEEPi) to barotrauma risk are not clearly defined, it seems likely that, in most patients, barotrauma risk will be worsened with a decelerating profile, rather than improved. A sine waveform similarly lowers Ppeak while shortening expiratory time. Because the ventilator may "look better" (lower Ppeak, fewer alarms) on either

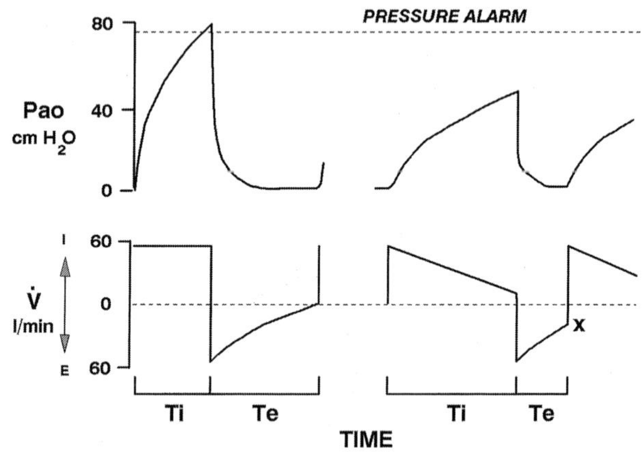


**Figure 93.10** Effect of flow profile on airway opening pressure (Pao) and inspiratory to expiratory (I:E) ratio in a patient with status asthmaticus during assist-control or intermittent mandatory ventilation breaths. The left-hand tracings show the typical high peak pressure (Ppeak) and slow explratory flow of a patient with severe obstruction ventilated with a square wave inspiratory flow profile. Note that expiratory flow just reaches zero before the next breath is delivered. The Ppeak can be dramatically reduced by changing to a decelerating flow profile (right-hand tracing) because much of the high Pao is flow related (i.e., the Presist, which is proportional to flow, is elevated). However, in order to deliver the same $V_T$ at the now lower mean inspiratory flow, the inspiratory time (Ti) must increase. If the respiratory rate is not lowered, the expiratory time (Te) falls, increasing the I:E ratio. With the now shortened Te, there is insufficient time for the respiratory system to reach functional residual capacity, expiratory flow is still detected at the onset of inspiratory flow (*x*), and intrinsic PEEP (PEEPi) is present. Therefore, the lower (improved?) Pao comes at the cost of new (or higher) PEEPi and a higher mean alveolar pressure.

of these alternate modes, while PEEPi is typically occult, such flow patterns can be insidiously threatening.

We believe that there is little reason to use anything other than the conventional square wave inspiratory flow profile, except in the rare situation when inverse ratio ventilation is desired. PEEPi should be diligently measured and the hidden complexities of this mode made clear to all caring for the patient.

**Use of PEEP.** Ventilator-applied PEEP generally should be avoided in mechanically ventilated patients with status asthmaticus who are not triggering the ventilator, because it may increase lung volume.[145] Low levels of ventilator-applied PEEP such as 5 to 10 cm $H_2O$ will, however, decrease inspiratory work of breathing in patients triggering the ventilator, and are unlikely to increase lung volume. This strategy may be useful early in the process of returning the patient to spontaneous breathing.

### Helium-Oxygen (Heliox)

It has been recognized for some time that breathing heliox, a gas consisting of 20% oxygen and 80% helium (hence a density approximately one-third that of air), results in prompt improvement in dyspnea, work of breathing, and arterial blood gas abnormalities in patients with upper airway obstruction.[146] This benefit stems from the density dependence of the flow-related pressure drop across the upper airway in cases of severe upper airway obstruction, disorders typically producing highly turbulent flow across the narrowed airway. In the normal bronchial tree, gas velocities decrease rapidly beyond third-generation airways because of the exponential increase in cross-sectional area and flow is laminar. As a result, the resistive pressure drop in peripheral airways is independent of gas density,[147] and most predicted that heliox would be ineffective in status asthmaticus. There are both animal and human data, however, that support its efficacy.[1, 148, 149] When there is narrowing of the bronchial tree, as in asthma, airway resistance increases, as does gas velocity. Perhaps flow is turbulent even in very distal airways.

When heliox was given by mask to spontaneously breathing patients with acute attacks in an emergency room, peak expiratory flow rate (PEFR) increased significantly and pulsus paradoxus decreased.[1] To the extent that the pulsus paradoxus reflects the inspiratory fall in pleural pressure and $V_I$ and $V_T$ did not fall, it follows that heliox reduced inspiratory airway resistance. The increase in PEFR is indirect evidence that expiratory airway resistance was decreased as well. Taken together, these effects should decrease work of breathing and delay inspiratory muscle fatigue, "buying time" for concurrent bronchodilator and anti-inflammatory therapy to take hold.

One interesting report describes improved gas exchange and airway pressures in seven asthmatic patients ventilated with heliox.[148] In each of the seven patients given helium (60% to 80%) and oxygen (40% to 20%), the peak airway pressure fell in minutes (mean fall 33 cm $H_2O$), and arterial $P_{CO_2}$ dropped within a half hour (mean drop 36 mm Hg).[148] It is not clear from this study whether tidal volume was truly held constant because the ventilator was changed to administer the heliox. Moreover, much, if not all, of the fall in Ppeak could be explained by reduced flow resistance through the endotracheal tube, and data sufficient to exclude this hypothesis (peak tracheal pressure, Pplateau, PEEPi) were not included in the published report. Heliox delivered through the ventilator circuit probably does decrease Ppeak and arterial $P_{CO_2}$,[148] but it is extremely important to recalibrate ventilator flow meters (from which tidal volume is derived). These meters are often gas-density dependent and inaccurately measure tidal volume during heliox administration unless they are recalibrated. If the ventilator used employs a hot-wire pneumotachometer, very large errors in measurement of flow and hence calculation of tidal volume may be seen. Careful planning, including a trial of heliox use in a lung model, is mandatory before patient use. A spirometer should be placed on the expiratory port of the ventilator during heliox administration to confirm tidal volume changes. The limited number of patients treated and the difficulty of measuring flow and volume when using helium make this approach still experimental.

### General Anesthesia

In rare cases, the aforementioned strategies are not sufficient to stabilize the patient on the ventilator, and consideration should be given to the use of other therapies. Halothane and enflurane are general anesthetic bronchodilators that can acutely reduce Ppeak and arterial $P_{CO_2}$,[150, 151] although they are associated with myocardial depression, arterial vasodilation, and arrhythmias, and benefit does not last long after discontinuation of the drug. Because virtually all patients can be successfully managed with the ventilator strategies described earlier, we believe that inhalational anesthesia should be used rarely, if at all.

### Ancillary Approaches

Strategies to mobilize mucus such as chest physiotherapy or treatment with mucolytics or expectorants have not proved efficacious in controlled trials.[108] Bronchoalveolar lavage, in contrast, with either saline or acetylcysteine may be useful in nonintubated patients to remove mucus and improve airflow.[152–154] In intubated asthmatic patients, this procedure is theoretically more risky because the presence of the bronchoscope within the lumen of the endotracheal tube and large airways increases expiratory airway resistance and may lead to dangerous levels of lung hyperinflation if minute ventilation is not decreased during the procedure. Convincing data demonstrating benefit and safety of bronchial lavage in intubated patients are needed before this practice can be advocated.

## Liberation from Mechanical Ventilation

For patients with asthma severe enough to require a paralyzing agent, the drug should be discontinued briefly every several hours to prevent accumulation. The mechanical derangements seen in the ventilated asthmatic provide a reliable measure of the degree of ongoing asthma. As airway pressures fall, sedatives and muscle relaxants can be reduced to prepare the patient for a brief period of spontaneous ventilation and then extubation. When Ppeak and PEEPi fall sufficiently, patients can usually be extubated promptly, provided that pneumonia, CNS injury, or postparalytic weakness has not supervened. Although some patients with very labile asthma respond to therapy within hours, more typically patients require 24 to 48 hours of aggressive bronchodilator and anti-inflammatory therapy until airway pressures fall. Once this occurs and arterial $P_{CO_2}$ normalizes, paralytic agents and sedatives should be withheld and the patient allowed to breathe. We favor a quick return to spontaneous breathing and extubation, without prolonged trials of spontaneous or partially assisted breathing, because the endotracheal tube itself may perpetuate bronchospasm. After extubation, close observation in the intensive care unit is recommended for an additional 12 to 24 hours during which time clinicians can focus on safe transfer to the general medical ward and on maximizing outpatient management. This time should be used to initiate an important aspect of ongoing asthma care—patient education—in an attempt to prevent future episodes of status asthmaticus.

## ACUTE-ON-CHRONIC RESPIRATORY FAILURE

In patients with severe, stable, chronic respiratory failure, the $\dot{V}O_{2\,resp}$ is twofold to fivefold higher than normal.[155] At all times, this increased load is precariously balanced by diminished and barely adequate neuromuscular competence (see Fig. 93.2). Minor additional decrements in strength or increments in load are sufficient to precipitate acute ventilatory failure. Admissions to intensive care units for exacerbations of COPD account for a substantial portion of bed days because these patients often require prolonged ventilatory support. In surgical intensive care units COPD is an important problem as well because it is one of the more common reasons for a prolonged postoperative recovery.

### Clinical Presentation

Patients usually present with dyspnea that has been worsening over days, often with increased cough and sputum production. Physical examination typically demonstrates respiratory distress, accessory muscle use, a prolonged expiratory time, recruitment of expiratory muscles, and wheezing. The chest radiograph is usually abnormal, reflecting the chronic lung disease, but only occasionally reveals a cause for the patient's acute deterioration (e.g., pneumonia or pneumothorax). Sometimes there are indicators of acute infection such as purulent sputum, fever, leukocytosis, and a new radiographic infiltrate.

Typical initial arterial blood gases while the patient is breathing room air show a $P_{O_2}$ level of 35 to 45 mm Hg and a $P_{CO_2}$ level of 60 to 70 mm Hg. Electrocardiography may show signs of right atrial enlargement or right ventricular hypertrophy and is additionally useful to exclude acute myocardial ischemia.

### Management

The patient with ACRF presents a challenge to the physician at each of three phases of management: before intubation, following institution of mechanical ventilation, and at the point of liberation from the ventilator. These three phases are discussed sequentially.

#### Management Before Intubation

The goals of management in the patient not yet intubated are to forestall invasive mechanical ventilation when this is possible and recognize progressive respiratory failure when it is not. The proven efficacy of NIV (discussed subsequently), which can avert mechanical ventilation in about 75% of patients with ACRF, is one of the most important developments in the management of these patients; NIV works because it buys time for the physician to treat precipitants of ACRF and for the patient to improve.

It is important to remember that NIV is generally only a temporizing measure, not a definitive treatment for ACRF. Avoiding intubation and conventional mechanical ventilation nearly always depends on discerning the cause of ACRF and reversing it. Thus, while NIV is initiated, each of the potential causes enumerated in Figure 93.2 should be reviewed in light of the clinical presentation. On occasion, impending respiratory failure can be averted by a specific intervention targeted to one precipitant, such as rib fracture (intercostal nerve block) or pulmonary edema (diuresis, afterload reduction). More often several contributors are identified, such as worsened bronchospasm, electrolyte derangement, and infection, and treatment must be broad based. The treatments of many of these precipitants are discussed throughout this text.

**Pharmacotherapy.** Bronchodilators are an essential part of the early management of these patients (Table 93.4). Although much of the airflow obstruction of COPD is irreversible, most patients will have some reversible component.[156–158] There is now convincing evidence, at least in stable COPD, that the combination of beta-agonist and ipratropium is superior to either drug alone, and we recommend that these drugs be given in combination.[159, 160] We administer combined therapy with beta-agonists, ipratropium, and corticosteroids to our patients with ACRF, occasionally with the addition of aminophylline, and each of these is discussed below. Respiratory stimulants would be predicted not to work in this setting because drive is already supranormal. Indeed, doxapram and similar drugs are now rarely used because their toxicity is substantial and their efficacy minimal.[161, 162] We believe there is no role for these drugs.

***Beta-Agonists.*** Inhaled, $beta_2$-selective agents (albuterol, bitolterol, terbutaline, metaproterenol) should be given by an MDI, unless patient distress makes this impractical, because these routes seem to be equally efficacious in nonventilated patients[163] and in ventilated ones[91, 164] as long as a spacer device is used and care is taken with regard to technique. Higher doses than usual can be given, such as 4 to 10 (or more) puffs every 20 to

**Table 93.4 BRONCHODILATOR THERAPY IN ACUTE-ON-CHRONIC RESPIRATORY FAILURE**

**Beta-Agonists**

Albuterol or metaproterenol by metered-dose inhaler (MDI) (3–6 puffs every 30–60 min)
or
Albuterol or metaproterenol by nebulizer (0.5 mL albuterol or 0.3 mL metaproterenol in 2.5 mL normal saline solution every 2 hr)
In mechanically ventilated patients, tidal volume should be raised above 500 mL, inspiratory flow rate should be lowered to 40 L/min, actuation of the MDI should be timed to coincide with inspiration, and the breath should be followed by a brief (3 sec) pause. The effect on airway resistance should be monitored.

**Corticosteroids**

Methylprednisolone, 0.5–1 mg/kg every 6 hr
Assess ongoing need after 72 hr

**Methylxanthines**

Loading dose is 5 mg/kg
Maintenance dose is approximately 0.5 mg/kg/hr
Must be titrated against serum levels

**Ipratropium**

3–10 puffs every 2–6 hr by MDI
Consider high doses (400 μg every 2–6 hr) in the intubated patient

60 minutes, although there is no clear benefit from very high or frequent doses. In one study of stable, ventilated COPD patients, 4 puffs of albuterol via MDI was as effective as a cumulative dose of 12 or 16 puffs.[164] Furthermore, bronchodilation was sustained for 60 minutes. A hand-held nebulizer (0.5 mL albuterol or 0.3 mL metaproterenol mixed with 2.5 mL saline solution) may be useful for patients who cannot use an MDI reliably, but otherwise this route confers no additional efficacy. Parenteral agents (e.g., epinephrine 0.3 mL subcutaneously), and their concomitant toxicity, can nearly always be avoided.

***Ipratropium.*** The anticholinergic agent ipratropium bromide is as effective as metaproterenol in the treatment of ACRF,[165] may even be better in stable COPD, and is effective when given to mechanically ventilated COPD patients.[119] An additional advantage of this drug is that, compared with metaproterenol, its use is associated with a small rise in arterial $Po_2$ rather than the small decline usually seen with beta-agonists. The addition of ipratropium to a regimen containing inhaled beta-agonists yields incremental benefit for patients with COPD.[159] The usual dose of ipratropium in ACRF is 3 puffs every 30 to 60 minutes. Much higher doses (400 μg) have been shown to be optimal for stable patients with COPD, but this has not been extheed in ACRF.[166]

***Theophylline.*** Theophylline is a mildly effective bronchodilator in patients with COPD. In addition to its actions as a bronchodilator, theophylline has salutary effects on the diaphragm in experimental settings. These include inotropy and resistance to fatigue in patients, although the clinical relevance of these findings is yet to be demonstrated, and some studies have challenged the underpinning of these clinical trials.[167] Whether theophylline should be given to patients with ACRF is controversial, and recent trends show it to be out of favor. A controlled trial in patients hospitalized for an acute exacerbation of COPD failed to show any benefit of theophylline when added to a standard regimen of beta-agonists and corticosteroids.[168] On the other hand, theophylline causes demonstrable (although generally mild) physiologic improvement in stable COPD patients, even when superimposed on a regimen of beta-agonist[156] or on a combination of high-dose inhaled beta-agonist plus ipratropium.[169]

The toxicity of these drugs is substantial, including arrhythmogenesis and CNS effects. Daily serum level measurements are necessary for safe use, especially in light of the significant interactions with other drugs. Even in therapeutic doses, theophylline may have important toxicity. In a multivariate analysis of 100 patients taking theophylline, drug level was the most important predictor of arrhythmia,[170] ahead of age and gender. Both atrial and ventricular arrhythmias were seen and correlated with theophylline level. In the group with therapeutic levels, 48% had arrhythmias. Particularly worrisome was the finding of multifocal atrial tachycardia in patients on theophylline, including those with nontoxic levels. Two of six patients with this rhythm disturbance died suddenly during hospitalization, without antecedent ventricular ectopy.

We find it difficult to give firm advice regarding the use of theophylline in ACRF but generally no longer prescribe it ourselves. It is a reasonable choice for patients who have used it with benefit in the outpatient setting, and we occasionally add it when more standard bronchodilator regimens have failed. Theophylline is initiated as a loading dose of 5 mg/kg infused over 30 minutes, then continued as an intravenous infusion at a rate of 0.5 mg/kg/hr. In patients who are already taking an oral methylxanthine, intravenous loading and maintenance dosing should be guided by serum levels. Given the mild efficacy of the drug and the substantial toxicity, it is difficult to justify empirical partial loading doses.

***Corticosteroids.*** Patients with ACRF given methylprednisolone, 0.5 mg/kg every 6 hours, in addition to standard bronchodilators show greater improvement in spirometric values than do patients who are not.[171] This benefit is demonstrable at least as early as 12 hours and, in some studies of patients with asthma, possibly after 1 hour. In another study of patients with ACRF, 0.8 mg/kg of prednisolone given intravenously reduced the inspiratory resistance and PEEPi when measured at 90 minutes.[172] Therefore, any patient with ACRF should be given methylprednisolone, 0.5 to 1 mg/kg every 6 hours. The benefit of corticosteroids beyond the first few days is not known. Because these drugs have important detrimental effects on metabolic, muscular, and immune function, their continued use should be reevaluated after the first 72 hours. Although no effect of corticosteroids on respiratory muscle function can be shown in the short term (<2 weeks[173]), they do contribute to muscle weakness in the long term.[52]

***Antibiotics.*** Bronchitis is a common precipitant of ACRF. Nevertheless, the efficacy of antibiotics is controversial. Because benefit has been demonstrated in several studies and a trend toward benefit in some others,[174] we give an inexpensive, oral, broad-spectrum antibiotic (e.g., ampicillin, doxycycline, or cotrimoxazole) empirically. For patients likely to harbor resistant organisms, such as those with serious cardiopulmonary comorbidity, frequent purulent exacerbations of COPD, or taking oral corticosteroids chronically, a quinolone may be a better choice.[175]

***Anabolic Steroids.*** A combination of anabolic steroids (nandrolone decanoate, 25 to 50 mg intramuscularly every 2 weeks) and caloric supplementation (420 kcal/day supplement) raised the mouth pressure during a maximal static inspiratory maneuver in patients with clinically stable COPD.[176] We are aware of no trials showing clinically important benefits in patients with ACRF.

***Mucolytic Therapy.*** Mucokinetic agents, including iodides and acetylcysteine, have not been found effective in ACRF.[177] Preliminary studies indicate that DNAse may be useful. Systemic hydration is also unproven.

**Noninvasive Ventilation.** Most medical centers use a facemask or nasal mask and pressure-support ventilation, although poncho wraps and other ventilator modes can support NIV. A tight-fitting mask allows substantial ventilatory assistance, yet provides for brief periods off of the ventilator during which patients can speak, inhale nebulized medications, expectorate, and swallow liquids. This form of ventilatory assistance has been used for prolonged periods (more than 1 week) and has been shown to relieve symptoms, reduce respiratory rate, increase tidal volume, improve gas exchange,[178] lessen the amplitude of the diaphragmatic electromyogram as well as the transdiaphragmatic pressure,[179] reduce the hospital length of stay, and lower in-hospital mortality.[180, 181] The overall success rate has ranged from 56% to 92%.[123, 179, 189] Complications of the mask have been minor and few; local skin breakdown has been attributed to the tight-fitting mask, but can be avoided by applying a patch of wound care dressing. Only a few patients cannot tolerate facemasks or nasal masks, and some of these respond to judicious and carefully monitored anxiolytics. Aspiration of gastric contents has only rarely been noted in these patients, even when a nasogastric tube is not routinely placed; however, impaired mentation probably increases this risk. The hemodynamic impact of NIV is generally negligible.[183]

We typically begin therapy with a facemask and an expiratory positive pressure of 5 cm $H_2O$ and inspiratory positive pressure of 15 cm $H_2O$ (equivalently, 5 cm $H_2O$ PEEP with 10 cm $H_2O$ pressure support). Higher pressures can sometimes be used, but tend to be limited by air leak or mask discomfort. The PEEP component of NIV is important[184] and does not usually cause incremental hyperinflation.[185] Indeed, CPAP alone (without ventilatory assistance) reduces the work of breathing, improves gas exchange, leads to subjective benefit, and sometimes can avert intubation when applied to patients with ACRF.[185–187] When PEEP was added to pressure-support ventilation in ventilated patients with COPD, inspiratory effort fell another 17%, and patient-ventilator synchrony improved.[184] Some patients adapt better to NIV if lower starting pressures are used (e.g., 2 cm $H_2O$ PEEP and 8 cm $H_2O$ pressure support), with escalation of pressures after the first 5 to 10 minutes until the patient's respiratory rate falls into the low twenties. A salutary response is typically evident within 10 minutes of beginning NIV, as indicated by a falling RR and heart rate, as well as by the patient's subjective assessment. Occasional patients feel claustrophobic and may objectively worsen with NIV. Although we have occasionally used pharmacologic anxiolytic therapy with success, this has obvious attendant risks and should only be undertaken with appropriate safeguards.

Early on, NIV methods were considered most appropriate in patients who refused endotracheal intubation or whose prognosis due to age or underlying disease made recovery unlikely. However, data accumulated in the past 5 years make it clear that NIV, rather than intubation, should be considered the therapy of choice for most patients with ACRF. Furthermore, we believe that intensivists should not wait with NIV until progressive ventilatory failure brings the patient to the precipice. Because this approach is quite safe, unloads the respiratory muscles, and contributes to patient comfort, we believe that any patient with ACRF who is ill enough to be admitted to an intensive care unit should be considered a candidate for NIV at the time of admission, not just if deterioration continues. By waiting until some form of ventilation is necessary to prevent respiratory arrest, patients will be less likely to tolerate NIV and less likely to be spared intubation.

A risk of NIV that is not often discussed is its potential to lull the physician-nurse team into a sense of comfort at the same time that the patient continues to worsen. NIV is unsuccessful in one fourth or more of patients with ACRF, even when these patients are carefully chosen. Time spent trying NIV will, in these patients, potentially lead to a later, more urgent intubation in a more exhausted patient.

**Arrhythmia Management.** Arrhythmias are common in the setting of respiratory failure. Fortunately, they are rarely serious, but they can serve to distract the physician from more important issues, may limit the dose of bronchodilating drugs,[188] and sometimes are significant in and of themselves. The most common rhythms are sinus tachycardia, atrial fibrillation, atrial flutter, multifocal atrial tachycardia, and ventricular premature beats. It can be difficult to judge the contributions of hypoxemia, cor pulmonale, metabolic derangements, underlying coronary artery disease, and drug toxicity. Treatment should focus on rectifying the underlying respiratory failure, because this usually has a beneficial impact on arrhythmias. Hypoxemia and electrolyte abnormalities should be corrected as a first priority. Monitoring should be initiated, and, if arrhythmias continue despite correction of apparent exacerbating factors, myocardial ischemia should be excluded. Atrial fibrillation can be controlled with a calcium channel blocker or digoxin. Beta-blockers generally should be avoided for fear of worsening lung function, although short-acting, selective drugs have occasionally been used with success. Multifocal atrial tachycardia often responds to verapamil, sometimes with restoration of sinus rhythm,[189] and there appears to be a role for parenteral magnesium as well.

## Management Immediately Following Intubation

This phase consists of the immediate peri-intubation management and the first few days of mechanical ventilation. In many respects, treatment begun in the preintubation phase (bronchodilators, in particular) is continued, but several additional concerns become relevant. Care consists of stabilizing the patient on the ventilator, ensuring rest of the patient and respiratory muscles, improving neuromuscular competence, reducing load, and giving prophylaxis against complications. Optimal treatment at this time is likely to facilitate eventual liberation from mechanical ventilation.

**Peri-intubation Risks.** There are two common pitfalls in the post-intubation period, life-threatening alkalosis and hypotension, both related to overzealous ventilation and both avoidable by considering the patient's own ventilatory pattern preceeding intubation. Most patients with ACRF have a minute ventilation of 10 L/min or less and breathe at tidal volumes of about 300 mL. Physicians commonly choose ventilator settings with higher tidal volumes and correspondingly lower deadspace to tidal volume fractions. In addition, higher minute ventilations than 10 L/min are often employed, particularly during the first few minutes of manual-assisted ventilation. Finally, as the work of breathing is assumed by the ventilator, $\dot{V}CO_2$ drops by as much as 20%. All of these factors join to dramatically lower the patient's arterial $PCO_2$ once assisted ventilation begins. Because preexisting compensatory metabolic alkalosis is the rule, life-threatening alkalemia (pH > 7.7) can be achieved easily. This scenario can be avoided by simply aiming for a more reasonable minute ventilation, approximating the patient's own pattern of breathing. Typical initial ventilator settings are described below. There is no need to attempt to normalize pH, a manuever that merely serves to waste the bicarbonate that has been so vigorously conserved during the evolution of respiratory failure.

Hypotension is a consequence of escalating PEEPi following intubation, compounded by the effect of sedative drugs and sympathetic lysis. The degree of dynamic hyperinflation is proportional to $V_E$. PEEPi has the same deleterious consequences on venous return as externally applied PEEP and can cause serious hypoperfusion. Again, the key to avoiding this pitfall is to prevent excessive ventilation. When hypotension occurs, the circulation can usually be promptly restored by simply ceasing ventilation for 30 seconds and then reinstituting ventilation along with measures to reduce PEEPi and restore circulating volume.

**Ventilator Settings.** We generally initiate ventilation using the assist-control mode because one of the goals in this phase is to ensure respiratory muscle rest. Tidal volumes of about 5 to 7 mL/kg are used (about 350 to 500 mL) with a respiratory rate of 20 to 24 breaths/min. As discussed previously, PEEPi presents an inspiratory threshold load to the patient with ACRF. The patient must generate sufficient force to counterbalance PEEPi before his efforts result in any inspiratory flow and before he can trigger the ventilator. This difficulty cannot be sidestepped by lowering the triggered sensitivity on the ventilator or by using flow triggering. Applying external PEEP, roughly equal to the PEEPi, does reduce the work of breathing (and triggering) by significant amounts, as depicted in Figure 93.4.[65, 184] In some patients, externally applied PEEP causes additional hyperinflation with detrimental hemodynamic effects and potentially increased barotrauma risk.[145, 190] However, most patients with ACRF demonstrate flow limitation so that external PEEP (in amounts up to about 85% of the PEEPi) has no significant impact on the expiratory flow-volume relationship, lung volume, or hemodynamics.[191, 192]

**Ensuring Rest and Recovery.** Following intubation, most patients are exhausted and will sleep for the first day. Typically, little sedation is necessary. The respiratory muscles require 48 to 72 hours for full recovery, so resumption of breathing efforts before that is counterproductive and likely to lead to recurrence of respiratory muscle fatigue.[193] We continue to encourage rest by maintaining ventilation, adding sedation when necessary. Rest can be achieved with any mode of ventilation as long as settings are chosen that minimize patient effort. It is important to emphasize that having the patient connected to a ventilator is no guarantee that the patient is relieved of the work of breathing. Even when the ventilator is set at a very sensitive trigger, the presence of PEEPi causes the patient to have to make a substantial inspiratory effort to get a breath, even on assist-control mode. For example, with a triggered sensitivity of $-1$ cm $H_2O$ and a PEEPi of 10 cm $H_2O$, the patient must lower the airway pressure by 11 cm $H_2O$ to trigger a breath. It is incumbent on the physician to ensure that the patient is, in fact, rested. When this is achieved, respiratory muscle strength usually improves demonstrably over the first few days.

**Improving Neuromuscular Competence.** Each of the factors discussed in phase 1 (and in Fig. 93.2) that contribute to depressed neuromuscular competence should be reviewed daily in the ventilated patient. In this phase, the signal importance of nutrition must be recognized. Malnutrition is a common partner of advanced COPD and contributes to respiratory muscle dysfunction as well as immune depression. In a randomized trial of standard feeding vs. supplementation (1000 kcal above usual), malnourished inpatients with COPD were shown to develop greater respiratory muscle endurance and strength in only 16 days when given extra calories.[50] Excessive refeeding should be avoided, however, because unnecessarily high levels of carbon dioxide production ($\dot{V}CO_2$) may result. On occasion, detailed nutritional information including indirect calorimetry may be helpful to guide nutritional management. When calorie requirements have been assessed, it is usually advisable to supply a large fraction (50% or more) of total calories in the form of lipids to minimize the respiratory quotient and hence the $\dot{V}CO_2$. Especially with refeeding, hypophosphatemia commonly develops while the patient is in the intensive care unit, and serum phosphate content should be assessed on a daily basis.

Once the respiratory muscles are rested, a program of exercise should be initiated. The goal is to encourage muscle power, tone, and coordination by allowing the patient to assume nonfatiguing breaths. This can be achieved with any ventilator mode, for example, progressively lowering the triggered sensitivity on assist-control, reducing the backup rate on intermittent mandatory ventilation, lowering the inspiratory pressure on pressure support, or through graded T-piece sprints. After a period of work, the patient is returned to full rest to facilitate sleep at night. As strength improves, the amount of exercise can be increased in step until full spontaneous breathing can be sustained.

**Decreasing Load.** Efforts to decrease respiratory load should continue. Once the patient is ventilated, it becomes possible to apportion the load into resistive and elastic components as described earlier in this chapter. These determinations may provide insight into the precipitants of respiratory failure and serve to guide therapy.

It is important to continue treatment with bronchodilators, but whether MDIs and nebulizers are equally effective in ventilated patients is controversial.[194] On the one hand, in a study of drug deposition in ventilated patients, an MDI (plus holding chamber) was more efficient than a nebulizer.[195] On the other hand, in another trial of ventilated patients, MDIs were completely ineffective despite a cumulative dose in 1 hour of 100 puffs.[100] There may be substantial differences related to method of administration or to the specific equipment used to deliver drug. We recommend that these drugs be given to effect, whether by MDI or nebulizer. If MDIs are used, the usual number of puffs should be doubled to compensate for the reduced delivery of drug to the patient as a starting point and the dose increased, as needed, until bronchodilation is achieved (assessed by determining respiratory mechanics).

Other contributors to increased load, such as congestive heart failure, pulmonary embolization, or respiratory infection, may be easier to discern once the patient is mechanically ventilated and should be sought during this phase. Congestive heart failure can usually be excluded by the physical examination and chest radiograph. Only occasionally is the additional information from pulmonary artery catheterization useful. Pulmonary embolism is much more difficult to exclude. The incidence of embolism as a precipitant of ACRF is unknown. The reported frequency of deep venous thrombosis ranges from 9% to 45%,[27] and pulmonary emboli are probably an order of magnitude less common. Nevertheless, pulmonary emboli are commonly found at autopsy. As a treatable condition, it is worth finding, but currently available methods make diagnosis difficult. Perfusion lung scanning is nearly always abnormal, and the addition of lung scanning is only occasionally useful. Noninvasive leg studies have been challenged in this setting as well. Capnography has been suggested as a method for excluding pulmonary emboli in patients with ACRF,[196] and spiral CT scans are helpful in making the diagnosis.

## Liberation from the Ventilator

The fundamental principle that guides management in this third phase is that successful liberation from the ventilator requires that the premorbid, compensated relationship between neuromuscular competence and load must be reestablished. Therefore, a strategy for successfully discontinuing mechanical ventilation emphasizes increasing the strength and decreasing the load. Therapy may be highly focused, such as repleting inorganic phosphate or relieving a pneumothorax. More often, a broad assault on many potential precipitants, namely bronchospasm, infection, electrolyte derangement, and fatigue, is used. In either case, when load has been reduced and neuromuscular competence promoted, the patient will be able to breathe free of assistance. On the other hand, if a compensated balance of strength and load cannot be restored, attempts at spontaneous breathing will be futile. A corollary principle is that the specifics of ventilator management, such as the mode chosen or the device used, are largely irrelevant details.[197] Only the patient's improving physiology determines the ability to maintain ventilation. This point has been confirmed by recent trials of weaning methods, which have shown that frequent T-piece trials are superior to intermittent mandatory ventilation (and, variably, pressure support as well), probably by more readily demonstrating to the physician that the ventilator is no longer necessary.[198–200]

The progress of the patient can be followed by measuring respiratory parameters (MIP, Ppeak, Pplateau, and PEEPi) on a daily basis. The impact of therapeutic maneuvers can be assessed in this way as well. Finally, these parameters provide clues to the ability of the patient to sustain independent ventilation. For example, while PEEPi remains at 10 cm $H_2O$, there is little point in trying to make the patient breathe. Indeed, in such a circumstance efforts should be directed at attempting to reduce the work of breathing.[201] On the other hand, when PEEPi has resolved and strength is adequate (usually when the MIP is $>$ 30 cm $H_2O$), mechanical ventilation is no longer necessary.

When discontinuation of mechanical ventilation is imminent, it is useful to anticipate the respiratory pattern that the patient will soon assume. We have been impressed that patients ventilated at a supraphysiologic $V_T$, such as 1000 mL, experience respiratory distress and agitation when resuming their usual pattern of 30 breaths/min at a $V_T$ of 300 mL. By choosing a pattern of mechanical ventilation that more closely approximates spontaneous respiration (e.g., A/C mode, $V_T$ 450 mL, rate 18 breaths/min), the transition from the ventilator is smoothed.

There may be a role for NIV in the phase of liberation as well as in the period before intubation by serving as a bridge to spontaneous breathing.[201a] We have begun to extubate carefully chosen patients somewhat earlier than in the past, knowing that we have NIV in reserve if patients do not tolerate extubation. This is particularly attractive for patients who are steadily improving, but perhaps not quite ready to take on full spontaneous breathing. In other words, a trend toward improvement in a borderline candidate for extubation makes us more eager to attempt extubation because, even if ventilatory failure reasserts itself, NIV is likely to tide the patient over the additional days until the balance of neuromuscular competence and respiratory system load is reestablished. This approach has been validated recently.[201a, 202]

Even with appropriate institution of rest while still on the ventilator, rapid application of the algorithms given above to correct abnormalities of neuromuscular competence and load, and progressive exercise, some patients require protracted periods of ventilator support. Indeed, with the wider use of NIV and the avoidance of intubation in all but the most severely impaired patients, it may be the case that in the future, truly "difficult to wean" patients will be encountered in the intensive care unit. The principles elaborated above still apply to this group, with a few additional comments. After approximately 1 to 2 weeks of ventilator dependence, we typically assess the patient for tracheostomy. If it appears that liberation from mechanical ventilation may succeed within the week, tracheostomy is usually not performed, and efforts continue to extubate the patient. If we judge the course to be protracted, we prefer tracheostomy for purposes of patient comfort, communication, and avoidance of complications associated with translaryngeal intubation. If progress to liberation is likely to be very slow after the first couple of weeks, many intensive care unit personnel will consider transfer of the stable patient to a transitional ventilator unit, given the often superior rehabilitation and physical therapy departments in these institutions.

Following extubation, careful serial assessments are in order. Deterioration in the hours just following extubation suggests upper airway edema. In the uncomplicated patient, the respiratory rate falls slightly through the first day, most often into the mid-20s to low 30s. Efforts to build strength and reduce load should continue in order to protect the gains that have already been made. Once the patient is stable off of the ventilator, a prompt transfer to the more benign setting of the general ward should be encouraged. There has been a resurgence of interest in the use of NIV to treat patients with chronic respiratory failure from COPD and other lung diseases, but the indications are controversial and in most instances clear-cut benefit has not been shown.[202a]

## Prognosis

Despite severe underlying pulmonary impairment, the prognosis for patients with ACRF is not uniformly poor. One year survival following acute respiratory failure ranges from 28% to 72%.[203, 204] The prognosis is best for patients with kyphoscoliosis or neuromuscular disease and worst for those with pneumoconiosis and pulmonary fibrosis.[205] In men with COPD who come to mechanical ventilation for ACRF, 1 year survival is about 40% to 50%.[20, 207] Some patients will return to an acceptable quality of life and even go back to work. In a cohort of 1016 patients admitted with a COPD exacerbation and $P_{CO_2}$ higher than 50 mm Hg, 1 year survival was 47%, but only 26% rated their quality of life as good or better when surveyed at 6 months.[207] Other than the underlying cause of chronic respiratory failure, predictors of survival include premorbid functional status, baseline dyspnea, serum albumin level,[208] and presence of cor pulmonale,[207] but these indicators are not refined enough to allow accurate prognostication for an individual patient. Ideally, patients studied in the clinic with known, severe COPD are encouraged to discuss their wishes regarding intensive care with their physicians before acute deterioration. Unfortunately, this is only occasionally accomplished. It is our approach to fully support patients with ACRF who believe their quality of life is acceptable, especially because the majority can be successfully managed with NIV, and most of those intubated will eventually be successfully liberated from the ventilator. On the other hand, when mechanical ventilation seems excessive in the patient's or physician's judgement, comfort-only measures may be appropriate.

## SUMMARY

Type II respiratory failure, or ventilatory failure, is due to alveolar hypoventilation resulting in a rising arterial $P_{CO_2}$ and respiratory acidosis. Adequate ventilation requires central drive, a competent neurologic system to transmit drive to the respiratory muscles, and adequate muscular strength and endurance to move the lungs and chest wall against the prevailing respiratory load. Loss of drive, inadequate neuromuscular competence, and excessive respiratory system load, alone or together, cause ventilatory failure.

Impaired drive is typically the result of drug effects, neurologic dysfunction, or sleep-disordered breathing. Neuromuscular failure is commonly due to primary neurologic diseases, electrolyte derangements, or muscle fatigue. Respiratory system loads can be divided into resistive loads, such as bronchospasm, elastic loads of the lung (e.g., pulmonary edema) or chest wall (e.g., pleural effusion), and minute ventilation loads such as acidemia or carbohydrate loading.

When the cause of ventilatory failure cannot be identified and treated, mechanical ventilation may become necessary to sustain life. The two most common syndromes of ventilatory failure are status asthmaticus and ACRF, the latter most commonly seen in patients with COPD. In all such patients the goals of management are to restore drive, improve neuromuscular function, and reduce respiratory system load in order to liberate the patient from mechanical ventilation while preventing or minimizing complications.

## References

1. Marini JJ: Paying the piper—the linkage of alveolar ventilation to alveolar pressure. Intensive Care Med 16:73–74, 1990.
2. Menitove SM, Goldring RM: Combined ventilator and bicarbonate strategy in the management of status asthmaticus. Am J Med 74:898–901, 1983.
3. Darioli R, Perret C: Mechanical controlled hypoventilation in status asthmaticus. Am Rev Respir Dis 129:385–387, 1984.
4. Walley KR, Lewis TH, Wood LDH: Acute respiratory acidosis

decreases left ventricular contractility but increases cardiac output in dogs. Circ Res 67:628–635, 1990.
5. Cingolani HE, Faulkner SL, Mattiazzi AR, et al: Depression of human myocardial contractility with "respiratory" and "metabolic" acidosis. Surgery 77:427–432, 1975.
6. Downing SE, Talner NS, Gardner TH: Cardiovascular responses to metabolic acidosis. Am J Physiol 208:237–242, 1965.
7. Juan G, Calverley P, Talamo C, et al: Effect of carbon dioxide on diaphragmatic function in human beings. N Engl J Med 310:874–879, 1984.
8. Kontos HA, Richardson DW, Patterson JL: Vasodilator effect of hypercapnic acidosis on human forearm blood vessels. Am J Physiol 215:1403–1405, 1968.
9. Molfino NA, Nannini LJ, Martelli AN, et al: Respiratory arrest in near-fatal asthma. N Engl J Med 324:285–288, 1991.
10. Rogers RM, Spear JF, Moore EN, et al: Vulnerability of canine ventricle to fibrillation during hypoxia and respiratory acidosis. Chest 63:986–994, 1973.
11. von Planta I, Weil MH, von Planta M, et al: Hypercarbic acidosis reduces cardiac resuscitability. Crit Care Med 19:1177–1182, 1991.
12. Kette F, Weil MH, von Planta M, et al: Buffer agents do not reverse intramyocardial acidosis during cardiac resuscitation. Circulation 81:1660–1666, 1990.
13. Kerber RE, Pandian NG, Hoyt R, et al: Effect of ischemia, hypertrophy, hypoxia, acidosis, and alkalosis on canine defibrillation. Am J Physiol 244:H825–H831, 1983.
14. Goldstein B, Shnnon DC, Todres ID: Supercarbia in children: Clinical course and outcome. Crit Care Med 18:166–168, 1990.
15. Thorens J-B, Jolliet P, Ritz M, et al: Effects of rapid permissive hypercapnia on hemodynamics, gas exchange, and oxygen transport and consumption during mechanical ventilation for the acute respiratory distress syndrome. Intensive Care Med 22:182–191, 1996.
16. Feihl F, Perret C: Permissive hypercapnia: How permissive should we be? Am J Respir Crit Care Med 150:1722–1737, 1994.
17. Potkin RT, Swenson ER: Resuscitation from severe acute hypercapnia: Determinants of tolerance and survival. Chest 102:1742–1745, 1992.
18. Tuxen DV, Williams TJ, Scheinkestel CD, et al: Use of a measurement of pulmonary hyperinflation to control the level of mechanical ventilation in patients with acute severe asthma. Am Rev Respir Dis 146:1136–1142, 1992.
19. Hickling KG, Walsh J, Henderson S, et al: Low mortality rate in adult respiratory distress syndrome using low-volume, pressure-limited ventilation with permissive hypercapnia: A prospective study. Crit Care Med 22:1568–1578, 1994.
20. Bidani A, Tzouanakis AE, Cardenas VJ, et al: Permissive hypercapnia in acute respiratory failure. JAMA 272:957–962, 1994.
21. Kiely DG, Cargill RI, Lipworth BJ: Effects of hypercapnia on hemodynamic, inotropic, lusitropic and electrophysiologic indices in humans. Chest 109:1215–1221, 1996.
22. Roupie E, Dambrosio M, Servillo G, et al: Titration of tidal volume and induced hypercapnia in acute respiratory distress syndrome. Am J Respir Crit Care Med 152:121–128, 1995.
23. Forslid A, Ingvar M, Rosen I, et al: Carbon dioxide narcosis: Influence of short-term high concentration carbon dioxide inhalation on EEG and cortical evoked responses in the rat. Acta Physiol Scand 127:281–287, 1986.
24. Javaheri S, Kazemi H: Metabolic alkalosis and hypoventilation in humans. Am Rev Respir Dis 136:1011–1016, 1987.
25. Grassino A, Macklem PT: Respiratory muscle fatigue and ventilatory failure. Ann Rev Med 35:625–647, 1984.
26. Zakynthinos SG, Vassilakopoulos T, Roussos C: The load of inspiratory muscles in patients needing mechanical ventilation. Am J Respir Crit Care Med 152:1248–1255, 1995.
27. Derenne JP, Fleury B, Pariente R: Acute respiratory failure of chronic obstructive pulmonary disease. Am Rev Respir Dis 138:1006–1033, 1988.
28. McCool FD, Tzelepis GE, Leith DE, et al: Oxygen cost of breathing during fatiguing inspiratory resistive loads. J Appl Physiol 66:2045–2055, 1989.
29. Mador MJ: Respiratory muscle fatigue and breathing pattern. Chest 100:1430–1435, 1991.
30. Roussos C, Fixley M, Gross D, et al: Fatigue of inspiratory muscles and their synergic behavior. J Appl Physiol 46:897–904, 1979.
31. Sassoon CS, Gruer SE, Sieck GC: Temporal relationships of ventilatory failure, pump failure, and diaphragm fatigue. J Appl Physiol 81:238–245, 1996.
32. Yanos J, Keamy MF, Leisk L, et al: The mechanism of respiratory arrest in inspiratory loading and hypoxemia. Am Rev Respir Dis 141:933–937, 1990.
33. Respiratory Muscle Fatigue Workshop Group: NHLBI workshop summary: Respiratory muscle fatigue. Am Rev Respir Dis 142:474–480, 1990.
34. Jounieaux V, Mayeux I: Oxygen cost of breathing in patients with emphysema or chronic bronchitis in acute respiratory failure. Am J Respir Crit Care Med 152:2181–2184, 1995.
35. Aubier M, Murciano D, Fournier M, et al: Central respiratory drive in acute respiratory failure of patients with chronic obstructive pulmonary disease. Am Rev Respir Dis 122:191–199, 1980.
36. Montgomery AB, Holle RHO, Neagley SR, et al: Prediction of successful ventilator weaning using airway occlusion pressure and hypercapnic challenge. Chest 91:496–499, 1987.
37. Aubier M, Murciano D, Milic-Emili J, et al: Effects of the administration of $O_2$ on ventilation and blood gases in patients with chronic obstructive pulmonary disease during acute respiratory failure. Am Rev Respir Dis 122:747–754, 1980.
38. Sassoon CSH, Hassell KT, Mahutte CK: Hyperoxic-induced hypercapnia in stable chronic obstructive pulmonary disease. Am Rev Respir Dis 135:907–911, 1987.
39. Erbland ML, Ebert RV, Snow SL: Interaction of hypoxia and hypercapnia on respiratory drive in patients with COPD. Chest 97:1289–1294, 1990.
40. Dunn WF, Nelson SB, Hubmayr RD: Oxygen-induced hypercarbia in obstructive pulmonary disease. Am Rev Respir Dis 144:526–530, 1990.
41. Schmidt GA, Hall JB: Oxygen therapy and hypoxic drive to breathe: Is there danger in the patient with COPD? Intensive Crit Care Dig 8:124–125, 1989.
42. Pittinger C, Adamson R: Antibiotic blockade of neuromuscular function. Ann Rev Pharmacol 12:169–184, 1972.
43. Miller B, Skupin A, Rubenfire M, et al: Respiratory failure produced by severe procainamide intoxication in a patient with preexisting peripheral neuropathy caused by amiodarone. Chest 94:663–665, 1988.
44. Aubier M, Murciano D, Lecocguic Y, et al: Effect of hypophosphatemia on diaphragmatic contractility in patients with acute respiratory failure. N Engl J Med 313:420–424, 1985.
45. Dhingra S, Solven F, Wilson A, et al: Hypomagnesemia and respiratory muscle power. Am Rev Respir Dis 129:497–498, 1984.
46. Fiaccadori E, Coffrini E, Ronda N, et al: Hypophosphatemia in course of chronic obstructive pulmonary disease: Prevalence, mechanisms, and relationships with skeletal muscle phosphorus content. Chest 97:857–868, 1990.
47. Openbrier D, Irwin M, Rogers RM, et al: Nutritional status and lung function in patients with emphysema and chronic bronchitis. Chest 83:17–22, 1983.
48. Arora NS, Rochester DF: Respiratory muscle strength and maximal voluntary ventilation in undernourished patients. Am Rev Respir Dis 126:5–8, 1982.
49. Shindoh C, Dimarco A, Supinski G: Effect of acute fasting on diaphragm strength and endurance. Am Rev Respir Dis 144:488–493, 1991.
50. Whittaker JS, Ryan CF, Buckley PA, et al: The effects of refeeding on peripheral and respiratory muscle function in malnourished chronic obstructive pulmonary disease patients. Am Rev Respir Dis 142:283–288, 1990.
51. Polkey MI, Kyroussis D, Hamnegard CH, et al: Diaphragm strength in chronic obstructive pulmonary disease. Am J Respir Crit Care Med 154:1310–1317, 1996.
52. Decramer M, Lacquet LM, Fagard R, et al: Corticosteroids contribute to muscle weakness in chronic airflow obstruction. Am J Respir Crit Care Med 150:11–16, 1994.
53. Decramer M, de Bock V, Dom R: Functional and histologic picture of steroid-induced myopathy in chronic obstructive pulmonary disease. Am J Respir Crit Care Med 153:1958–1964, 1996.
54. Leatherman JW, Fluegel WL, David WS, et al: Muscle weakness

in mechanically ventilated patients with severe asthma: Am J Respir Crit Care Med 153:1686–1690, 1996.
55. Aubier M, Trippenbach T, Roussos C: Respiratory muscle fatigue during cardiogenic shock. J Appl Physiol 51:499–508, 1981.
56. Hussain SNA, Graham R, Ruthledge F, et al: Respiratory muscle energetics during endotoxic shock in dogs. J Appl Physiol 60:486–493, 1986.
57. Ward ME, Magder SA, Huasain SNA: Oxygen delivery-independent effect of blood flow on diaphragm fatigue. Am Rev Respir Dis 145:1058–1063, 1992.
58. Wright PE, Marini JJ, Bernard GR, et al: In vitro versus in vivo comparison of endotracheal tube airflow resistance. Am Rev Respir Dis 140:10–16, 1989.
59. Coussa ML, Guérin C, Eissa NT, et al: Partitioning of work of breathing in mechanically ventilated COPD patients. J Appl Physiol 75:1711–1719, 1993.
60. Smith TC, Marini JJ: Impact of PEEP on lung mechanics and work of breathing in severe airflow obstruction. J Appl Physiol 65:1488–1499, 1988.
61. Broseghini C, Brandolese R, Poggi R, et al: Respiratory mechanics during the first day of mechanical ventilation in patients with pulmonary edema and chronic airway obstruction. Am Rev Respir Dis 138:355–361, 1988.
62. Murciano D, Aubier M, Bussi S, et al: Comparison of esophageal, tracheal, and mouth occlusion pressure in patients with chronic obstructive pulmonary disease during acute respiratory failure. Am Rev Respir Dis 126:837–841, 1982.
63. Aldrich TK, Hendler JM, Vizioli LD, et al: Intrinsic positive end-expiratory pressure in ambulatory patients with airways obstruction. Am Res Respir Dis 147:845–849, 1993.
64. Smith TC, Marini JJ, Lamb VJ: The inspiratory threshold load resulting from airtrapping during mechanical ventilation (abstract). Am Rev Respir Dis 135:A52, 1987.
65. Petrof BJ, Legaré M, Goldberg P, et al: Continuous positive airway pressure reduces work of breathing and dyspnea during weaning from mechanical ventilation in severe chronic obstructive pulmonary disease. Am Rev Respir Dis 141:281–289, 1990.
66. Kress JP, O'Connor MC, Schmidt GA: Clinical examination reliably detects intrinsic positive end-expiratory pressure in critically ill, mechanically ventilated patients. Am J Respir Crit Care Med 159:290–294, 1999.
67. Pepe PE, Marini JJ: Occult positive end-expiratory pressure in mechanically ventilated patients with airflow obstruction. Am Rev Respir Dis 126:166–170, 1982.
68. Marini JJ, Rodriguez RM, Lamb V: The inspiratory workload of patient-initiated mechanical ventilation. Am Rev Respir Dis 134:902–909, 1986.
69. Roussos CS, Macklem PT: Diaphragmatic fatigue in man. J Appl Physiol 43:189–197, 1977.
70. Yang KL, Tobin MJ: A prospective study of indexes predicting the outcome of trials of weaning from mechanical ventilation. N Engl J Med 324:1445–1450, 1991.
71. Knowles G, Clark T: Pulsus paradoxus as a valuable sign indicating severity of asthma. Lancet II:1356–1359, 1973.
72. Arnald A, Lane D, Zapata E, et al: The speed of onset and severity of acute severe asthma. Br J Dis Chest 76:157–163, 1982.
73. Hogg JC: The pathology of asthma. Clin Chest Med 5:567–571, 1984.
74. Aikawa T, Shimura S, Sasaki H, et al: Marked goblet cell hyperplasia with mucus accumulation in the airways of patients who died of severe acute asthma attack. Chest 101:916–921, 1992.
75. Rodriguez-Roisin R, Ballester E, Roca J, et al: Mechanisms of hypoxemia in patients with status asthmaticus requiring mechanical ventilation. Am Rev Respir Dis 139:732–739, 1989.
76. Douglas J, Rafferty P, Fergusson R: Nebulised salbutamol without oxygen in severe acute asthma: How effective and how safe? Thorax 40:180–183, 1985.
77. Roca J, Ramis L, Rodriguez-Roisin R, et al: Serial relationships between ventilation perfusion inequality and spirometry in acute severe asthma requiring hospitalization. Am Rev Respir Dis 137:1055–1061, 1988.
78. Raimondi AC, Lombardi D, Schottlender J, et al: Acid base disturbances as therapeutical and clinical predictors in 325 admissions with acute severe asthma. Am Rev Respir Dis 145:A494, 1992.
79. Mountain RD, Sahn SA: Clinical features and outcome in patients with acute asthma presenting with hypercapnia. Am Rev Respir Dis 138:535–539, 1988.
80. Appel D, Rubenstein R, Shrager K, et al: Lactic acidosis in severe asthma. Am J Med 75:580–584, 1983.
81. Jederlinic PJ, Irwin RS: Status asthmaticus. J Intensive Care Med 4:166–184, 1989.
82. Newhouse M, Chapman KR, McCallum AL, et al: Cardiovascular safety of high doses of inhaled fenoterol and albuterol in acute severe asthma. Chest 110:595–603, 1996.
83. Gern J, Lemanske R: Beta adrenergic agonist therapy. Immunol Allergy North Am 13:839, 1993.
84. Paterson J, Evans R, Prime F: Selectivity of bronchodilator action of salbutamol in asthmatic patients. Br J Dis Chest 65:21–38, 1971.
85. Shrestha M, Gourlay S, Robertson S, et al: Isoetharine versus albuterol for acute asthma. Am J Med 100:323–327, 1996.
86. Fanta CH, Rossing TH, McFadden ER: Treatment of acute asthma. Am J Med 80:5–10, 1986.
87. Uden D, Goetz D, Kohen D, et al: Comparison of nebulized terbutaline and subcutaneous epinephrine in the treatment of acute asthma. Ann Emerg Med 14:229–232, 1985.
88. Becker AB, Nelson NA, Simons FE, et al: Inhaled salbutamol (albuterol) vs injected epinephrine in the treatment of acute asthma in children. J Pediatr 102:465–469, 1989.
89. Appel D, Karpel JP, Sherman M: Epinephrine improves expiratory airflow rates in patients with asthma who do not respond to inhaled metaproterenol sulfate. J Allergy Clin Immunol 84:90–98, 1989.
90. Cydulka R, Davison R, Grammer L, et al: The use of epinephrine in the treatment of older adult asthmaticus. Ann Emerg Med 17:322–323, 1990.
91. Dhand R, Tobin MJ: Inhaled bronchodilator therapy in mechanically ventilated patients. Am J Respir Crit Care Med 156:3–10, 1997.
92. Idris AH, McDermott MF, Raucci JC, et al: Emergency department treatment of severe asthma: Metered-dose inhaler plus holding chamber is equivalent in effectiveness to nebulizer. Chest 103:665–672, 1993.
93. Rossing TH, Fanta CH, et al: Effect of outpatient treatment of asthma with beta agonists on the response to sympathomimetics in an emergency room. Am J Med 75:781–784, 1983.
94. Lawford P, Jones B, Milledge J: Comparison of intravenous and nebulised salbutamol in initial treatment of severe asthma. BMJ 1:84, 1978.
95. Williams S, Winner S, Clark T: Comparison of inhaled and intravenous terbutaline in acute severe asthma. Thorax 36:629–632, 1981.
96. Pierce RJ, Payne CR, Williams SJ, et al: Comparison of intravenous and inhaled terbutaline in the treatment of asthma. Chest 79:506–511, 1981.
97. Salmeron S, Brochard L, Mal H, et al: Nebulized versus intravenous albuterol in hypercapnic acute asthma: A multicenter, double-blind, randomized study. Am J Respir Crit Care Med 149:1466–1470, 1994.
98. Manthous CA, Hall J: Administration of therapeutic aerosols to mechanically ventilated patients. Chest 106:560–571, 1994.
99. Macintyre NR, Silver R, Miller C, et al: Aerosol delivery in intubated, mechanically ventilated patients. Crit Care Med 13:81–84, 1985.
100. Manthous CA, Hall JB, Schmidt GA, et al: Metered-dose inhaler versus nebulized albuterol in mechanically ventilated patients. Am Rev Respir Dis 148:1567–1570, 1993.
101. Manthous CA, Hall JB: Update on using therapeutic aerosols in mechanically ventilated patients. J Crit Illness 11:457–468, 1996.
101a. Marik P, Hogan J, Krikorian J: A comparison of bronchodilator therapy delivered by nebulization and metered-dose inhaler in mechanically ventilated patients. Chest 115:1653–1657, 1999.
102. British Thoracic Society: Guidelines for management of asthma in adults: Acute severe asthma. BMJ 301:797–800, 1990.
103. Bowton DL: Metered-dose inhalers versus hand-held nebulizers: Some answers and new questions. Chest 101:298–299, 1992.
104. Hess D: Aerosol bronchodilator delivery during mechanical ventilation: Nebulizer or inhaler. Chest 100:1103–1104, 1991.
105. Rowe B, Keller J, Oxman A: Effectiveness of steroid therapy in

acute exacerbations of asthma: A meta analysis. Am J Emerg Med 10:801–810, 1992.
106. Benatar SR: Fatal asthma. N Engl J Med 314:423–429, 1986.
107. McFadden ER: Dosages of corticosteroids in asthma. Am Rev Respir Dis 147:1306–1310, 1993.
108. Corbridge TC, Hall JB: The assessment and management of adults with status asthmaticus. Am J Respir Crit Care Med 151:1296–1316, 1995.
109. Bryant DH: Nebulised ipratropium bromide in the treatment of acute asthma. Chest 88:24–29, 1992.
110. Bryant DH, Rogers P: Effects of ipratropium bromide nebulizer solution with and without preservatives in the treatment of acute and stable asthma. Chest 102:742–747, 1992.
111. Lanes SF, Garrett JE, Wentworth III CE, et al: The effect of adding ipratropium bromide to salbutamol in the treatment of acute asthma: A pooled analysis of three trials. Chest 114:365–372, 1998.
112. Karpel JP, Kotch A, Zinny M, et al: A comparison of inhaled ipratropium, oral theophylline plus inhaled beta-agonist, and the combination of all three in patients with COPD. Chest 105:1089–1094, 1994.
113. Rodrigo C, Rodrigo G: Treatment of acute asthma: Lack of therapeutic benefit and increase of the toxicity from aminophylline given in addition to high doses of salbutamol delivered by metered-dose inhaler with a spacer. Chest 106:1071–1076, 1994.
114. Evans W, Monie R, Crimmins J, et al: Aminophylline, salbutamol and combined intravenous infusions in acute severe asthma. Br J Dis Chest 74:385–386, 1980.
115. Wrenn K, Slovis CM, Murphy F, et al: Aminophylline therapy for acute bronchospastic disease in the emergency room. Ann Intern Med 115:241–247, 1991.
116. Tiffany BR, Berk WA, Todd IK, et al: Magnesium bolus or infusion fails to improve expiratory flow in acute asthma exacerbations. Chest 104:831–834, 1993.
117. Green S, Rothrock S: Intravenous magnesium for acute asthma: Failure to decrease emergency treatment duration of need for hospitalization. Ann Emerg Med 21:260–265, 1992.
118. Bloch H, Silverman R, Mancuso L: Intravenous magnesium sulfate as an adjunct in the treatment of acute asthma. Chest 107:1576–1581, 1995.
119. Fernandez A, Lazaro A, Garcia A, et al: Bronchodilators in patients with chronic obstructive pulmonary disease on mechanical ventilation: Utilization of metered-dose inhalers. Am Rev Respir Dis 141:164–168, 1990.
120. Sydow M, Crozier TA, Zielmann S, et al: High-close intravenous magnesium sulfate in the management of life-threatening status asthmaticus. Intensive Care Med 19:467–471, 1993.
121. Skobeloff EM, Spivey WH, McNamara RM: Estrogen alters the response of bronchial smooth muscle (abstract). Ann Emerg Med 21:647, 1992.
122. Gaddy JN, Margolskee DJ, Bush RK, et al: Bronchodilation with a potent and selective leukotriene (LTD4) receptor antagonist (MK-571) in patients with asthma. Am Rev Respir Dis 146:358–363, 1992.
122a. Rabain JT, Gay PC: Noninvasive ventilation. Mayo Clin Proc 74:817–820, 1999.
123. Meduri GU, Abou-Shala N, Fox RC, et al: Noninvasive face mask mechanical ventilation in patients with acute hypercapnic respiratory failure. Chest 100:445–454, 1991.
124. Shivaram U, Miro AM, Cash ME, et al: Cardiopulmonary responses to continuous positive airway pressure in acute asthma. J Crit Care 8:87–92, 1993.
125. Martin JG, Shore S, Engel LA: Effect of continuous positive airway pressure on respiratory mechanics and pattern of breathing in induced asthma. Am Rev Respir Dis 126:812–817, 1982.
126. Meduri GU, Cook TR, Turner RE, et al: Noninvasive positive pressure ventilation in status asthmaticus. Chest 110:767–774, 1996.
127. Tuxen DV, Lane S: The effects of ventilatory pattern on hyperinflation, airway pressures, and circulation in mechanical ventilation of patients with severe air-flow obstruction. Am Rev Respir Dis 136:872–879, 1987.
128. Hall JB, Wood LDH: Management of the critically ill asthmatic patient. Med Clin North Am 74:779–796, 1990.
129. Strube P, Hallam P: Ketamine by continuous infusion in status asthmaticus. Anaesthesia 41:1017–1019, 1986.
130. Prezant DJ, Aldrich TK: Intravenous droperidol for the treatment of status asthmaticus. Crit Care Med 16:96–97, 1988.
131. Williams TJ, Tuxen DV, Scheinkestel CD, et al: Risk factors for morbidity in mechanically ventilated patients with acute severe asthma. Am Rev Respir Dis 146:607–615, 1992.
132. Leatherman J: Life-threatening asthma. Clin Chest Med 15:453, 1994.
133. Tuxen DV: Permissive hypercapnic ventilation. Am J Respir Crit Care Med 150:870–874, 1994.
134. Coakley JH, Nagendran K, Ormerod IEC, et al: Prolonged neurogenic weakness in patients requiring mechanical ventilation for acute airflow limitation. Chest 101:1413–1416, 1992.
135. Kuper Y, Okrent D, Twersky R, et al: Disuse atrophy in a ventilated patient with status asthmaticus receiving neuromuscular blockade. Crit Care Med 15:795–796, 1987.
136. Bachmann P, Gaussorgues P, Piperno D, et al: Hydrocortisone and pancuronium bromide: Acute myopathy during status asthmaticus. Crit Care Med 16:731–733, 1988.
137. Knox AJ, Mascie-Taylor BH, Muers M: Acute hydrocortisone myopathy in acute severe asthma. Thorax 41:411–412, 1986.
138. MacFarlane I, Rosenthal F: Severe myopathy after status asthmaticus. Lancet 2:615, 1977.
139. van Marlen W, Woods KL: Acute hydrocortisone myopathy. BMJ 281:271–272, 1980.
140. Williams TJ, O'Hehir R, Czarny D, et al: Acute myopathy in severe asthma treated with intravenously administered corticosteroids. Am Rev Respir Dis 137:460–463, 1999.
141. Brun-Buisson C, Gherardi R: Hydrocortisone and pancuronium bromide: Acute myopathy during status asthmaticus. Crit Care Med 16:731–732, 1988.
142. Gooch JL, Suchyta MR, Balbierz JM, et al: Prolonged paralysis after treatment with neuromuscular junction blocking agents. Crit Care Med 19:1125–1131, 1991.
143. Zochodne DW, Bolton CF, Wells GA: Critical illness polyneuropathy: A complication of sepsis and multiple organ failure. Brain 110:819–842, 1987.
144. Lopez-Messa JB, Garcia A: Acute polyneuropathy in critically ill patients. Intensive Care Med 16:159–162, 1990.
145. Tuxen DV: Detrimental effects of positive end-expiratory pressure during controlled mechanical ventilation of patients with severe airflow obstruction. Am Rev Respir Dis. 140:5–9, 1989.
146. Curtis JL, Mahlmeister M, Fink JB, et al: Helium-oxygen gas therapy: Use and availability for the emergency treatment of inoperable airway obstruction. Chest 90:455–457, 1986.
147. Wood LDH, Engel P, et al: Effect of gas physical properties and flow on lower pulmonary resistance. J Appl Physiol 41:234, 1976.
148. Gluck EH, Onorato DJ, Castriotta R: Helium-oxygen mixtures in intubated patients with status asthmaticus and respiratory acidosis. Chest 98:693–698, 1990.
149. Kass JE, Castriotta RJ: Heliox therapy in acute severe asthma. Chest 107:757–760, 1995.
150. Saulnier FF, Durocher AV, Deturck RA, et al: Respiratory and hemodynamic effects of halothane in status asthmaticus. Intensive Care Med 16:104–107, 1990.
151. Echeverria M, Gelb AW, Wexler HR, et al: Enflurane and halothane in status asthmaticus. Chest 89:153, 1986.
152. Smith DL, Deshazo RD: Bronchoalveolar lavage in asthma: State of the art. Am Rev Respir Dis 148:523–532, 1993.
153. Millman M, Millman FM, Goldstein IM, et al: Use of acetylcysteine in bronchial asthma: Another look. Ann Allergy 54:294, 1985.
154. Lang DM, Simon RA, Mathison DA, et al: Safety and possible efficacy of fiberoptic bronchoscopy with lavage in the management of refractory asthma with mucous impaction. Ann Allergy 67:324, 1991.
155. Donahoe M, Rogers RM, Wilson DO, et al: Oxygen consumption of the respiratory muscles in normal and in malnourished patients with chronic obstructive pulmonary disease. Am Rev Respir Dis 140:385–391, 1989.
156. Thomas P, Pugsley JA, Stewart JH: Theophylline and salbutamol improve pulmonary function in patients with irreversible chronic obstructive pulmonary disease. Chest 101:160–165, 1992.
157. Dhand R, Jubran A, Tobin MJ: Bronchodilator delivery by metered-dose inhaler in ventilator-supported patients. Am J Respir Crit Care Med 151:1827–1833, 1995.

158. Manthous CA, Chatila W, Schmidt GA, et al: Treatment of bronchospasm by metered-dose inhaler albuterol in mechanically ventilated patients. Chest 107:210–213, 1995.
159. Petty TL: The combination of ipratropium and albuterol is more effective than either agent alone. Chest 107:183S–186S, 1995.
160. Fernandez A, Muños J, de la Calle B, et al: Comparison of one versus two bronchodilators in ventilated COPD patients. Intensive Care Med 20:199–202, 1994.
161. Pourriat JL, Baud M, Lamberto C, et al: Effects of doxapram on hypercapnic response during weaning from mechanical ventilation in COPD patients. Chest 101:1639–1643, 1992.
162. Angus RM, Ahmed AA, Fenwick LJ, et al: Comparison of the acute effects on gas exchange of nasal ventilation and doxapram in exacerbations of chronic obstructive pulmonary disease. Thorax 51:1048–1050, 1996.
163. Berry RB, Shinto RA, Wong FH, et al: Nebulizer vs spacer for bronchodilator delivery in patients hospitalized for acute exacerbations of COPD. Chest 96:1241–1246, 1989.
164. Dhand R, Duarte AG, Jubran A, et al: Dose-response to bronchodilator delivered by metered-dose inhaler in ventilator-supported patients. Am J Respir Crit Care Med 154:388–393, 1996.
165. Karpel JP, Pesin J, Greenberg D, et al: A comparison of the effects of ipratropium bromide and metaproterenol sulfate in acute exacerbations of COPD. Chest 98:835–839, 1990.
166. Gross NJ, Petty TL, Friedman M, et al: Dose response to ipratropium as a nebulized solution in patients with chronic obstructive pulmonary disease. Am Rev Respir Dis 139:1188–1191, 1989.
167. Levy RD, Nava S, Gibbons L, et al: Aminophylline and human diaphragm strength in vivo. J Appl Physiol 68:2591–2596, 1990.
168. Rice KL, Leatherman JW, Duane PG, et al: Aminophylline for acute exacerbations of chronic obstructive pulmonary disease: A controlled trial. Ann Intern Med 107:305–309, 1987.
169. Nishimura K, Koyama H, Ikeda A, et al: The additive effect of theophylline on a high-dose combination of inhaled salbutamol and ipratropium bromide in stable COPD. Chest 107:718–723, 1995.
170. Bittar G, Friedman HS: The arrhythmogenicity of theophylline: A multivariate analysis of clinical determinants. Chest 99:1415–1420, 1991.
171. Albert RK, Martin TR, Lewis SW: Controlled clinical trial of methylprednisolone in patients with chronic bronchitis and acute respiratory insufficiency. Ann Intern Med 92:753–756, 1980.
172. Rubini F, Rampulla C, Nava S: Acute effect of corticosteroids on respiratory mechanics in mechanically ventilated patients with chronic airflow obstruction and acute respiratory failure. Am J Respir Crit Care Med 149:306–310, 1994.
173. Wang Y, Zintel T, Vasquez A, et al: Corticosteroid therapy and respiratory muscle function in humans. Am Rev Respir Dis 144:108–112, 1991.
174. Murphy TF, Sethi S: Bacterial infection in chronic obstructive pulmonary disease. Am Rev Respir Dis 146:1067–1083, 1992.
175. Grossman RF: The value of antibiotics and the outcomes of antibiotic therapy in exacerbations of COPD. Chest 113:249S–255S, 1998.
176. Schols AMW, Soeters PB, Mostert R, et al: Physiologic effects of nutritional support and anabolic steroids in patients with chronic obstructive pulmonary disease: A placebo-controlled randomized trial. Am J Respir Crit Care Med 152:1268–1274, 1995.
177. American Thoracic Society: Inpatient management of COPD. Am J Respir Crit Care Med 152:S97–S106, 1995.
178. Kramer N, Meyer TJ, Meharg J, et al: Randomized, prospective trial of noninvasive positive pressure ventilation in acute respiratory failure. Am J Respir Crit Care Med 151:1799–1806, 1995.
179. Brochard L, Isabey D, Piquet J, et al: Reversal of acute exacerbations of chronic obstructive lung disease by inspiratory assistance with a face mask. N Engl J Med 323:1523–1530, 1990.
180. Brochard L, Mancebo J, Wysocki M, et al: Noninvasive ventilation for acute exacerbations of chronic obstructive pulmonary disease. N Engl J Med 333:817–822, 1995.
181. Bott J, Carroll MP, Conway JH, et al: Randomized controlled trial of nasal ventilation in acute ventilatory failure due to chronic obstructive airways disease. Lancet 341:1555–1557, 1993.
182. Meduri GU, Conoscenti CC, Menashe P, et al: Noninvasive face mask ventilation in patients with acute respiratory failure. Chest 95:865–870, 1989.
183. Confalonieri M, Gazzaniga P, Gandola L, at al: Haemodynamic response during initiation of non-invasive positive pressure ventilation in COPD patients with acute ventilatory failure. Respir Med 92:331–337, 1998.
184. Appendini L, Purro A, Patessio A, et al: Partitioning of inspiratory muscle workload and pressure assistance in ventilator-dependent COPD patients. Am J Respir Crit Care Med 154:1301–1309, 1996.
185. Appendini L, Patessio A, Zanaboni S, et al: Physiologic effects of positive end-expiratory pressure and mask pressure support during exacerbations of chronic obstructive pulmonary disease. Am J Respir Crit Care Med 149:1069–1076, 1994.
186. de Lucas P, Tarancón C, Puente L, et al: Nasal continuous positive airway pressure in patients with COPD in acute respiratory failure: A study of the immediate effects. Chest 104:1694–1697, 1993.
187. Miro AM, Shivaram U, Hertig I: Continuous positive airway pressure in COPD patients in acute hypercapnic respiratory failure. Chest 103:266–268, 1993.
188. Cazzola M, Imperatore F, Salzillo A, et al: Cardiac effects of formoterol and salmeterol in patients suffering from COPD with preexisting cardiac arrhythmias and hypoxemia. Chest 114:411–415, 1998.
189. Salerno DM, Anderson B, Sharkey PJ, et al: Intravenous verapamil for treatment of multifocal atrial tachycardia with and without calcium pretreatment. Ann Intern Med 107:623–628, 1987.
190. Gay PC, Rodarte JR, Hubmayr RD: The effects of positive expiratory pressure on isovolume flow and dynamic hyperinflation in patients receiving mechanical ventilation. Am Rev Respir Dis 139:621–626, 1989.
191. Ranieri VM, Giuliani R, Cinnella G, et al: Physiologic effects of positive end-expiratory pressure in patients with chronic obstructive pulmonary disease during acute ventilatory failure and controlled mechanical ventilation. Am Rev Respir Dis 147:5–13, 1993.
192. Baigorri F, De Monte A, Blanch L, et al: Hemodynamic responses to external counterbalancing of autopositive end-expiratory pressure in mechanically ventilated patients with chronic obstructive pulmonary disease. Crit Care Med 22:1782–1791, 1994.
193. Braun NMT, Faulkner J, Hughes RL, et al: When should respiratory muscles be exercised? Chest 84:76–84, 1983.
194. Newhouse MT, Fuller HD: Rose is a rose is a rose?: Aerosol therapy in ventilated patients: Nebulizers versus metered dose inhalers—a continuing controversy. Am Rev Respir Dis 148:1444–1446, 1993.
195. Fuller HD, Dolovich MB, Posmituck G, et al: Pressurized aerosol versus jet aerosol delivery to mechanically ventilated patients: Comparison of dose to the lungs. Am Rev Respir Dis 141:440–444, 1990.
196. Chopin C, Fesard P, Mangalaboyi J, et al: Use of capnography in diagnosis of pulmonary embolism during acute respiratory failure of chronic obstructive pulmonary disease. Crit Care Med 18:353–357, 1990.
197. Schmidt GA, Hall JB: Acute on chronic respiratory failure: Assessment and management of patients with COPD in the emergent setting. JAMA 261:3444–3453, 1989.
198. Esteban A, Frutos F, Tobin MJ, et al: A comparison of four methods of weaning patients from mechanical ventilation. N Engl J Med 332:345–350, 1995.
199. Brochard L, Rauss A, Benito S, et al: Comparison of three methods of gradual withdrawal from ventilatory support during weaning from mechanical ventilation. Am J Respir Crit Care Med 150:896–903, 1994.
200. Ely EW, Baker AM, Dunagan DP, et al: Effect on the duration of mechanical ventilation of identifying patients capable of breathing spontaneously. N Engl J Med 335:1864–1869, 1996.
201. Marini JJ: Strategies to minimize breathing effort during mechanical ventilation. Crit Care Clin 6:635–636, 1990.
201a. Girault C, Daudenthun I, Chevron V, et al: Noninvasive ventilation as a systematic extubation and weaning technique in acute-

on-chronic respiratory failure. Am J Respir Crit Care Med 160:86–92, 1999.
202. Nava S, Ambrosino N, Clini E, et al: Noninvasive mechanical ventilation in the weaning of patients with respiratory failure due to chronic obstructive pulmonary disease. A randomized controlled trial. Ann Intern Med 128:721–728, 1998.
202a. Clinical indications for noninvasive positive pressure ventilation in chronic respiratory failure due to restrictive lung disease, COPD, and nocturnal hypoventilation—a consensus conference report. Chest 116:521–534, 1999.
203. Sukumalchantra Y, Dinakara P, Williams MH: Prognosis of patients with chronic obstructive pulmonary disease after hospitalization for acute ventilatory failure: A three year follow-up study. Am Rev Respir Dis 93:215–222, 1966.
204. Hudson LD: Survival data in patients with acute and chronic lung disease requiring mechanical ventilation. Am Rev Respir Dis 140:S19–S24, 1989.
205. Chailleux E, Fauroux B, Binet F, et al: Predictors of survival in patients receiving domiciliary oxygen therapy or mechanical ventilation: A 10 year analysis of ANTADIR observatory. Chest 109:741–749, 1996.
206. Stauffer JL, Fayter NA, Graves B, et al: Survival following mechanical ventilation for acute respiratory failure in adult men. Chest 104:1222–1229, 1993.
207. Connors AF, Dawson NV, Thomas C, et al: Outcomes following acute exacerbation of severe chronic obstructive lung disease. Am J Respir Crit Care Med 154:959–967, 1996.
208. Menzies R, Gibbons W, Goldberg P: Determinants of weaning and survival among patients with COPD who require mechanical ventilation for acute respiratory failure. Chest 95:398–405, 1989.

# 94 Principles of Mechanical Ventilation

NEIL R. MACINTYRE, M.D.

Introduction
Design Features of Mechanical Ventilators
Gas Delivery Systems
Subsystems
Physiologic Effects of Mechanical Ventilation
Ventilatory Pattern and Respiratory System Mechanics
Alveolar Recruitment and Gas Exchange
Lung Stretch and Stretch Injury
Mechanical Loads
Patient-Ventilator Interactions
Hemodynamic Effects
Pressure-Unrelated Complications
Oxygen Toxicity
Patient-Ventilator Interface Events
Pulmonary Infections
Summary

## INTRODUCTION

Mechanical ventilation is the process of using devices to either totally or partially provide $O_2$ and $CO_2$ transport between the environment and the alveolar spaces of the lungs. The desired result of mechanical ventilation is to maintain appropriate levels of $PO_2$ and $PCO_2$ in arterial blood while also unloading the respiratory muscles. Although negative-pressure chambers or wraps and extracorporeal circuits might fulfill this definition, this discussion focuses on the use of positive airway pressure to effect mechanical ventilatory support.

The use of positive-pressure mechanical ventilation is widespread. Each year in the United States, an estimated 1 to 3 million patients require mechanical ventilatory support outside the operating room.[1] This support is supplied by an installed base of approximately 50,000 positive-pressure ventilators in the United States. Traditionally, this support has been provided in intensive care unit settings, but there are clear trends toward expanding the venues to subacute facilities, long-term care facilities, and the home. As the American population ages and as more aggressive surgical and medical therapies are developed, the need for mechanical ventilation in all of these venues is likely to expand.[1]

## DESIGN FEATURES OF MECHANICAL VENTILATORS

### Gas Delivery Systems

**Positive-Pressure Breath Controller.** Most modern ventilators use piston/bellows systems or controllers of high-pressure sources to drive gas flow.[2, 3] Tidal breaths are generated by this gas flow and can either be controlled entirely by the ventilator or be interactive with patient efforts. In general, pneumatic, electronic, or microprocessor systems provide for various types of breaths. These can be classified by what initiates the breath (trigger variable), what controls gas delivery during the breath (target or limit variable), and what terminates the breath (cycle variable).[4, 5] The trigger variable is either patient effort (detected by the ventilator as a pressure or flow change; see later discussion) or a set machine timer. The target or limit variable is generally either a set flow or a set inspiratory pressure. The cycle variable is generally a set volume, a set inspiratory time, or a flow rate. In Figure 94.1, this classification scheme is used to depict the five most common breath types available on the current generation of mechanical ventilators.

**Mode Controller.** The availability and delivery logic of different breath types define the *mode* of mechanical ventilatory support.[4, 5] The mode controller is an electronic, pneumatic, or microprocessor-based system that is designed to provide the proper combination of breaths according to set algorithms and feedback data (conditional variables) (Table 94.1). Newer designs can incorporate advanced monitoring and feedback functions into these controllers to allow for continuous adjustments in mode algorithms as a patient's condition changes.[6]

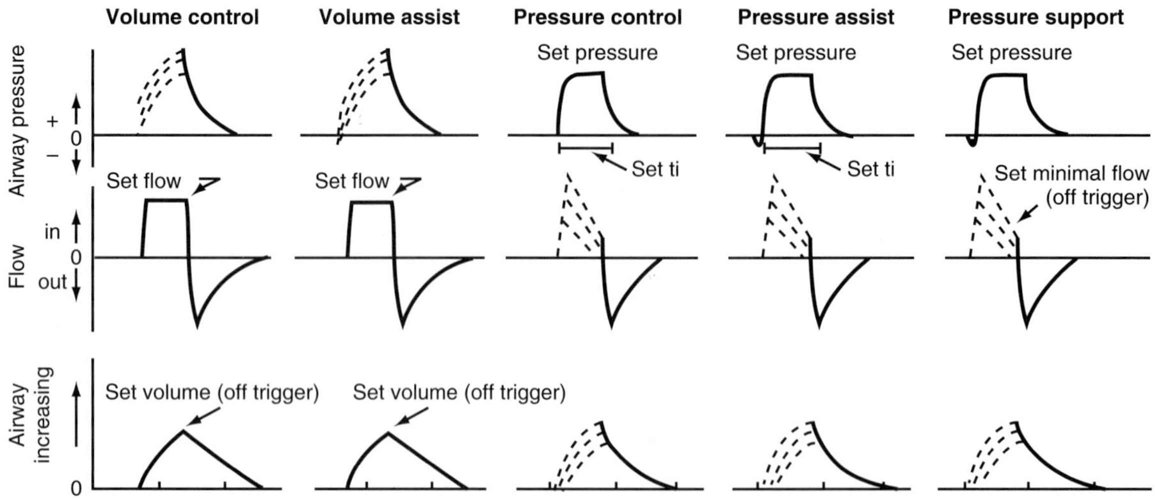


**Figure 94.1** Airway pressure, flow, and volume tracings over time, depicting the five basic breaths available on most modern mechanical ventilators. Breaths are classified by their trigger, target/limit, and cycle variables. ti = inspiratory time.

## Subsystems

**Effort (Demand) Sensors.** Current ventilators allow for a number of patient-ventilator interactions.[7] Examples include patient-triggered breaths (ventilator initiates flow in response to patient demand) and pressure-targeted/limited breaths (ventilator adjusts flow in response to patient demand) (see "Interactions" section later). Patient effort sensors are needed to allow the ventilator to deliver these interactive breaths properly. These sensors are usually either pressure or flow transducers in the ventilatory circuitry and are characterized by their sensitivity (how much of a circuit pressure or flow change must be generated to initiate a ventilator response) and their responsiveness (the delay in providing this response).[8]

**Gas Blenders.** Gas blenders mix air and $O_2$ to produce a delivered fraction of inspired oxygen ($FI_{O_2}$) that can be adjusted from 0.21 to 1.0. Some ventilators have the capacity of administering special gas mixtures (e.g., heliox).

**Humidifiers.** With the upper airway bypassed by tracheal intubation, sufficient heat and moisture must be added to the inspired gas mixtures to prevent mucosal desiccation. "Active" humidifiers use external water sources and electrical power to adjust blended gas mixtures to near body conditions (intratracheal temperature of >35°C, water content of >40 mg/L).[9] "Passive" humidifiers use simple heat-moisture exchange devices in the ventilator circuit that reutilize heat and moisture trapped from expired gas. These disposable units can usually supply adequate heat and moisture (i.e., warmer than 30°C to 33°C and higher than 28 to 32 mg $H_2O$/L) for many patients, particularly those receiving mechanical ventilation for only short periods of time.[9]

**Expiratory Pressure Generator.** Positive airway pressure can be sustained throughout expiration (positive end-expiratory pressure [PEEP]) to help maintain alveolar patency and improve ventilation/perfusion ($\dot{V}/\dot{Q}$) matching (see "Physiologic Effects" section later). PEEP is usually applied by regulating pressure in the expiratory valve of the ventilator system, but a continuous flow of source gas during the expiratory phase can provide a similar effect. Some expiratory valves, even when fully open, have measurable resistance that may result in some inadvertent applied PEEP.[10] As discussed in more detail later, PEEP can also be generated in alveoli if expiratory time is inadequate for the lung to return to its "rest volume" or significant flow limitation exists; this is called intrinsic PEEP.[11]

**Gas Delivery Circuit.** This usually consists of flexible tubing that often includes pressure or flow sensors and exhalation valve. It is important to remember that this tubing has measurable compliance (4 mL/cm $H_2O$ is a representative value), and significant amounts of delivered gas may serve only to distend this circuitry rather than enter the patient's lungs when high airway pressures are encountered.

**Patient-Ventilator Circuit Interface.** Positive-pressure ventilation is generally supplied through a tube inserted into the patient's airway (orotracheal or nasotracheal tube or tracheostomy). These tubes generally have air-filled balloons to provide a proper seal in the airway. An alternative to the tracheal tube is a mask system. Both full-face and nasal masks have been used with a variety of ventilatory support systems and modes.[12–14] Mask leakage, however, can be significant, and thus support modes involving the use of masks must be able to provide adequate volumes and proper inspiratory timing. To this end, special nasal-mask ventilators with pressure-targeted and either time-cycled or leak-compensated flow-cycled capabilities have been developed.[14]

**Aerosol Generators.** Therapeutic aerosols (e.g., bronchodilators, steroids, antibiotics) can be delivered through

Table 94.1 CURRENTLY AVAILABLE MODES OF MECHANICAL VENTILATION

| Mode (Common Names) | Breath Type: Mandatory | | | Assisted | | | Supported | | | Spontaneous | | | Conditional Variable |
|---|---|---|---|---|---|---|---|---|---|---|---|---|---|
| | *Trigger* | *Limit* | *Cycle* | *Trigger* | *Limit* | *Cycle* | *Trigger* | *Limit* | *Cycle* | *Trigger* | *Limit* | *Cycle* | |
| CMV/VCV | Time | Flow | Volume* | — | — | — | — | — | — | — | — | — | — |
| ACV | Time | Flow | Volume* | Patient† | Flow | Volume* | — | — | — | — | — | — | Patient effort/time |
| IMV | Time | Flow | Volume* | — | — | — | — | — | — | Patient† | Pressure‡ | Pressure‡ | — |
| SIMV | Time | Flow | Volume* | Patient† | Flow | Volume* | — | — | — | Patient† | Pressure | Pressure | Patient effort/time |
| PCV | Time | Pressure | Time | — | — | — | — | — | — | — | — | — | — |
| PACV | Time | Pressure | Time | Patient† | Pressure | Time | — | — | — | — | — | — | Patient effort/time |
| PIMV | Time | Pressure | Time | — | — | — | — | — | — | Patient† | Pressure | Pressure | — |
| PSIMV | Time | Pressure | Time | Patient† | Pressure | Time | — | — | — | Patient† | Pressure | Pressure | Patient effort/time |
| APRV | Time | Pressure | Time | — | — | — | — | — | — | Patient†§ | Pressure | Pressure | — |
| Assist APRV | Time | Pressure | Time | Patient† | Pressure | Time | — | — | — | Patient†§ | Pressure | Pressure | Patient effort/time |
| PSV | — | — | — | — | — | — | Patient | Pressure | Flow‖ | — | — | — | — |
| MMV | Time | Flow | Volume* | Patient† | Flow | Volume* | — | — | — | Patient† | Pressure | Pressure | Minute volume |

ACV = assist-control ventilation; APRV = airway pressure-release ventilation; CMV/VCV = controlled mechanical ventilation/volume-controlled ventilation; IMV = intermittent mandatory ventilation; MMV = mandatory minute ventilation; PACV = pressure ACV; PCV = pressure-controlled ventilation; PIMV = pressure IMV; PSIMV = pressure SIMV; PSV = pressure support ventilation; SIMV = synchronized IMV.

*Cycling can also be due to set inspiratory time in the setting of a fixed flow, with or without a pause.

†May be patient-generated pressure or flow in the circuit.

‡Pressure-limited only on demand-valve systems in which the ventilator limits and cycles to maintain constant airway pressure (thus, this applies to all modes in this column).

§Allows spontaneous breathing during both the mandatory inspiratory and expiratory time.

‖Flow reflects interaction of patient effort respiratory system impedance, and ventilator flow rate.

From the American Association for Respiratory Care: Consensus statement on the essentials of mechanical ventilators. Respir Care 37:1000–1008, 1992.

the ventilator circuitry.[15] This can be accomplished by either in-line nebulizers or by special chambers designed for metered-dose inhalers. Lung deposition is generally less than in a nonintubated patient because the endotracheal tube serves as a significant barrier to aerosol delivery. Higher dosing is thus advisable.

**Monitors and Graphic Displays.** Although electronic and microprocessor-based systems have considerable internal monitoring of electronic and pneumatic function, the three variables generally displayed for clinical use are circuit pressures, flows, and volumes (see Fig. 94.1).[16] Alarms can be utilized on all of these monitors.[5, 17] Most modern positive-pressure ventilators also have oxygen sensors in the circuitry to ensure that the desired $F_{IO_2}$ is being delivered. In addition, some ventilators may also have analyzers for exhaled $CO_2$ and inhaled therapeutic gases such as nitric oxide or heliox.

## PHYSIOLOGIC EFFECTS OF MECHANICAL VENTILATION

### Ventilatory Pattern and Respiratory System Mechanics

**Equation of Motion.** Lung inflation during mechanical ventilation occurs when pressure and flow are applied at the airway opening. These applied forces interact with respiratory system compliance (both lung and chest wall components), airway resistance, and, to a lesser extent, respiratory system inertance and lung tissue resistance to effect gas flow.[18, 19] For simplicity, because inertance and tissue resistance are relatively small, they can be ignored, so that the interactions of pressure, flow, and volume with respiratory system mechanics can be expressed by the simplified equation of motion:

$$\text{Driving pressure} = (\text{flow} \times \text{resistance}) + (\text{volume/system compliance}) \quad (1)$$

In the mechanically ventilated patient, this relationship is expressed as

$$\Delta P_{AO} = (\dot{V} \times R) + (V_T/C_{RS}) \quad (2)$$

where $\Delta P_{AO}$ is the change in pressure above baseline at the airway opening; $\dot{V}$ is the flow into the patient's lungs; R is the resistance of circuit, artificial airway, and natural airways; $V_T$ is the tidal volume; and $C_{RS}$ is the respiratory system compliance.

By performing an inspiratory hold at end-inspiration (i.e., no-flow conditions: $\dot{V} = 0$), the components of $\Delta P_{AO}$ required for flow and for alveolar distention can be separated. Specifically, when $\dot{V} = 0$ at end-inspiration, $\Delta P_{AO}$ is referred to as a "plateau" pressure and reflects the static system compliance ($C_{RS} = V_T/\Delta P_{AO_{plateau}}$). Calculating the difference in $\Delta P_{AO}$ during flow and during no-flow (the "peak to plateau difference") allows for a calculation of inspiratory airway resistance ($R = \Delta P_{AO_{peak-plateau}}/\dot{V}$).

Separating chest wall and lung compliance ($C_{CW}$ and $C_L$, respectively) during a passive machine-controlled positive-pressure breath requires an esophageal pressure measurement (Pes) in order to approximate pleural pressure. With this measurement, the inspiratory change in Pes ($\Delta$Pes) can be used in the following calculations: $C_{CW} = V_T/\Delta Pes$ and $C_L = V_T/(\Delta P_{AO} - \Delta Pes)$.

**Pressure-Targeted vs. Flow/Volume-Targeted Breaths.** In Figure 94.1 and Table 94.1, it can be seen that there are two basic approaches to delivering positive-pressure breaths: pressure targeting and flow/volume targeting.[4–6] With pressure targeting (breaths 3 to 5 in Fig. 94.1), the clinician sets an inspiratory pressure target (with either time or flow as the cycling criteria) so that flow and volume are dependent variables (i.e., varying with lung mechanics and the patient's effort to maintain the flow and volume targets). With flow/volume targeting (breaths 1 and 2 in Fig. 94.1), the clinician sets an inspiratory flow and cycling volume so that airway pressure is the dependent variable. Changes in compliance or resistance causes a change of tidal volume (but not $P_{AO}$) with the pressure-targeted breath. In contrast, similar changes in compliance or resistance change $P_{AO}$ (but not flow or volume) with a volume-targeted breath. These design characteristics need to be considered in choosing a pressure or a flow/volume-targeted breath for a given patient. Specifically, if $CO_2$ clearance is more important than limiting lung distention (e.g., mild lung injury in a patient with a head injury), volume guarantee with volume-cycled breaths would be the best choice. In contrast, if regional overdistention is more of a concern than $CO_2$ clearance (e.g., severe lung injury with high ventilatory pressures), ensuring a maximal distending pressure limit with a pressure-targeted breath would be the best choice (see "Lung Stretch Injury" section later). In addition, if a patient's spontaneous flow demand is high during patient-triggered breaths, the variable flow of the pressure-targeted breath may be more synchronous than the fixed flow of the flow/volume-targeted breath (see "Interactions" section later).

There are several ventilator modes that offer types of breath that have both pressure-targeting and volume-cycling features.[6] Although these breaths offer the variable decelerating flow pattern of pressure-targeted breaths, the volume guarantee means that pressure must increase if lung mechanics worsen. Thus, although these breaths have pressure-targeting features, they are not pressure limiting.[6]

**Intrinsic PEEP and the Ventilatory Pattern.** Measured $P_{AO}$ during breath delivery depends on both the $\Delta P_{AO}$ and the baseline pressure (both applied and intrinsic PEEP). Intrinsic PEEP is determined by three factors: minute ventilation, the expiratory time fraction, and the respiratory system's expiratory time constant (the product of resistance and compliance).[20] As minute ventilation increases, expiratory time fraction decreases, and the time constant lengthens (i.e., higher R or C values), the potential for intrinsic PEEP to develop increases.

The development of intrinsic PEEP has different effects on pressure-targeted vs. flow/volume-targeted ventilation (Fig. 94.2). In flow/volume-targeted ventilation, the constant delivered volume in the setting of a rising intrinsic

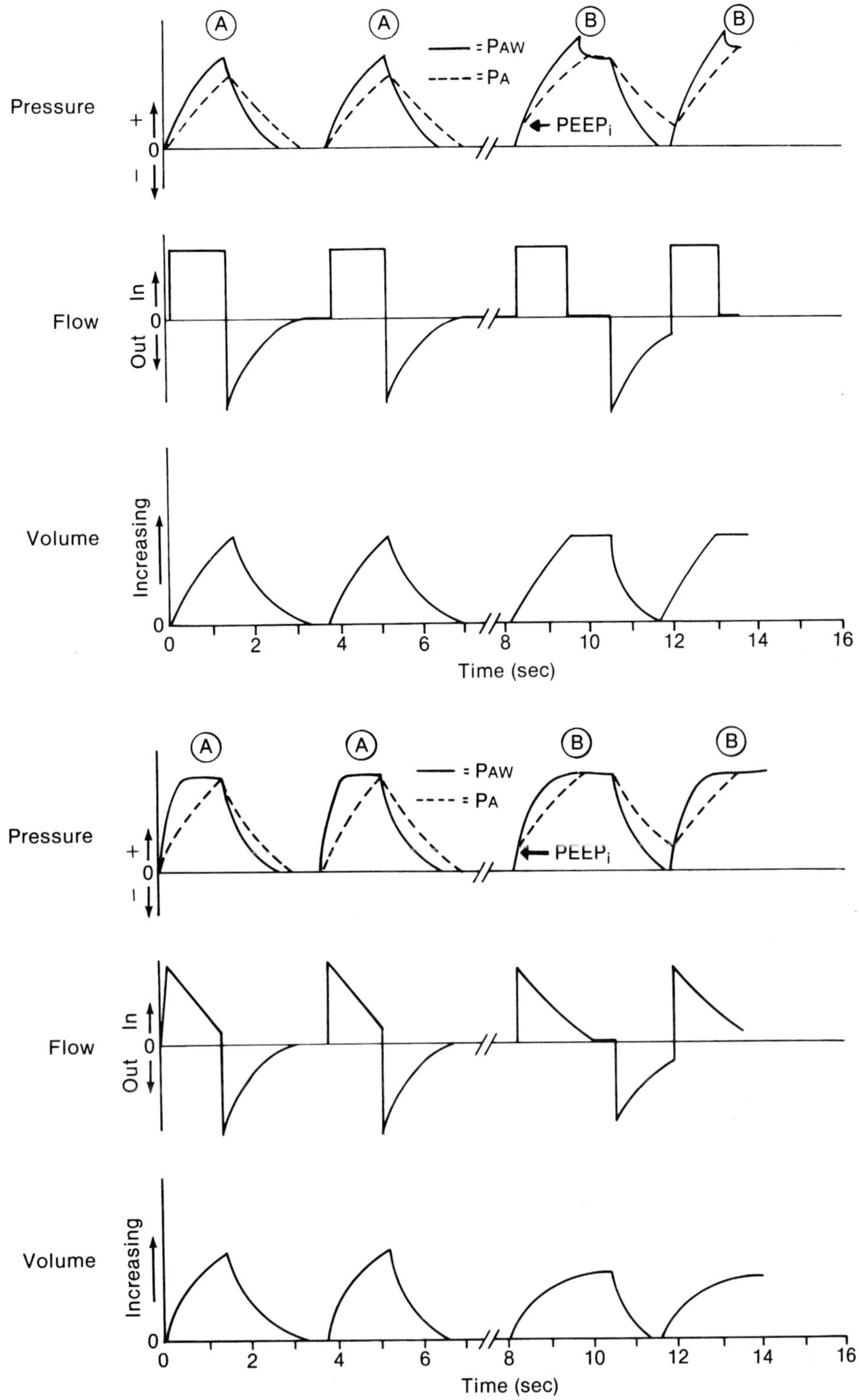


**Figure 94.2** The effects of intrinsic positive end-expiratory pressure (PEEPi, shown as PEEP$_i$ in the illustration) on flow/volume-targeted breaths *(upper panels)* and pressure-targeted breaths *(lower panels)*. In each set of panels, airway and alveolar pressures (Paw and Palv, respectively, shown as PAW and PA), flow, and volume are plotted. The first two breaths (labeled A) have sufficient expiratory time, so that expiratory flow returns to zero and alveolar pressure returns to the set baseline airway pressure. In contrast, the second two breaths (labeled B) have an inadequate expiratory time, so that expiratory flow is interrupted by the next delivered breath and alveolar pressure remains above the set baseline airway pressure (PEEPi). In flow/volume-targeted breaths, PEEPi forces the end-inspiratory alveolar pressure up in order to guarantee the tidal volume. In pressure-targeted breaths, the set pressure limit in the setting of PEEPi reduces the inspiratory driving pressure and tidal volume falls. (From MacIntyre NR: Intrinsic positive end-expiratory pressure. Prob Respir Care 4:48, 1991.)

PEEP increases the peak and plateau PAO to maintain a constant ΔPAO (see Fig. 94.2, upper panels). In contrast, in pressure-targeted ventilation, the set PAO limit coupled with a rising intrinsic PEEP level decreases ΔPAO and thus the delivered tidal volume (and minute ventilation) (see Fig. 94.2, lower panels).

In the passive patient, intrinsic PEEP can be assessed in two additional ways. First, when inadequate expiratory time is producing intrinsic PEEP, analysis of the flow graphic reveals that expiratory flow has not returned to zero before the next breath is initiated (compare expiratory flow patterns in breaths A vs. B in Fig. 94.2). Second, intrinsic PEEP in alveolar units that have patent airways can be quantified during a prolonged expiratory hold maneuver that permits equilibration of the intrinsic PEEP throughout the ventilator circuitry.[11]

**Distribution of Ventilation.** A positive-pressure tidal breath must distribute itself among the millions of alveolar units in the lung.[21, 22] Factors affecting this distribution include regional resistances, compliances, functional residual capacities, and the delivered flow pattern (including inspiratory pause). In general, delivered ventilation tends to distribute more to units with high compliance and low resistance (Fig. 94.3). This creates the potential for regional overdistention of healthier lung units, even in the presence of "normal"-sized tidal volumes (see "Lung Stretch Injury" section later).

Flow pattern may also affect ventilation distribution. Specifically, slower flows tend to distribute more evenly when there are obstructive inhomogeneities (although consequent shorter expiratory times may worsen air trapping), whereas faster flows (especially decelerating flows) tend to distribute more evenly in the presence of compliance inhomogeneities.[21] In addition, rapid initial flows (a consequence of set decelerating flow profiles or pressure-targeted breaths) pressurize the lung most rapidly and thus produce the highest mean inspiratory alveolar pressure for a given end-inflation pressure.[23] Finally, inspiratory pauses can also allow pendelluft action to fill slowly filling alveoli (see Fig. 94.3, resistance abnormality model).

More uniform ventilation distribution does not necessarily mean better ventilation-perfusion ($\dot{V}/\dot{Q}$) matching (i.e., more even ventilation distribution may actually worsen $\dot{V}/\dot{Q}$ matching in a lung with perfusion inhomogeneities). Because of all these considerations, predicting which flow pattern will optimize ventilation-perfusion matching is difficult and often an empirical trial-and-error exercise.

## Alveolar Recruitment and Gas Exchange

Infiltrative lung disease produces severe $\dot{V}/\dot{Q}$ mismatching through alveolar flooding and collapse.[24] In many (but not all) of these disease processes, these collapsed alveoli can be recruited during a positive-pressure ventilatory cycle.[25–29] Two specific techniques to maintain this recruitment are the application of PEEP and manipulations of the inspiratory:expiratory time relationships.

**Positive End-Expiratory Pressure.** PEEP is defined as an elevation of transpulmonary pressures at the end of expiration.[25, 26] As noted earlier, PEEP can be produced either by expiratory circuit valves (applied PEEP) or as a consequence of the interaction of ventilator settings with respiratory system mechanics (intrinsic PEEP). Expiratory muscle contraction can also raise intrathoracic pressures at end-expiration, but this should not be considered PEEP, because it is not a transpulmonary pressure (i.e., alveolar-pleural pressure).

Alveoli prevented from "derecruiting" by PEEP provide several patient benefits. First, recruited alveoli improve $\dot{V}/\dot{Q}$ matching and gas exchange.[25, 26] Second, as discussed in more detail later, patent alveoli throughout the ventilatory cycle are not exposed to the risk of injury from the shear stress of repeated opening and closing.[30–32] Third, PEEP prevents surfactant breakdown in collapsing alveoli and thus improves lung compliance.[33] PEEP, however, can also be detrimental. Because the tidal breath is delivered on top of the baseline PEEP, end-inspiratory pressures are raised by PEEP application. This must be considered if the lung is at risk for stretch injury (see "Lung Stretch Injury" section later). Moreover, because alveolar injury is often quite heterogeneous, PEEP that is appropriate in one region may be suboptimal in another and excessive in yet another.[27–29] Optimizing PEEP is thus a balance between recruiting the recruitable alveoli in diseased regions without overdistending already recruited alveoli in healthier regions. Another potential detrimental effect of PEEP is that it also raises mean intrathoracic pressure. This can compromise cardiac filling in susceptible patients (see "Hemodynamic Effects" section later).[34]

Criteria for determining the appropriate PEEP setting can be based on either gas exchange or mechanical goals:

Gas exchange goals are the traditional approach to setting PEEP.[25, 26] When gas exchange goals are defined, the idea is to use $F_{I_{O_2}}$ requirements, arterial $P_{O_2}$, or the calculated shunt fraction as the target. An example would be to apply whatever PEEP is necessary to attain a minimally acceptable arterial $P_{O_2}$ at the lowest possible $F_{I_{O_2}}$. A more aggressive gas exchange goal would be to normalize (or at least minimize) shunt fraction.[26, 35] This approach, however, may require very high levels of PEEP (i.e., sometimes in excess of normal maximal transpulmonary pressure). This approach is not commonly used to-

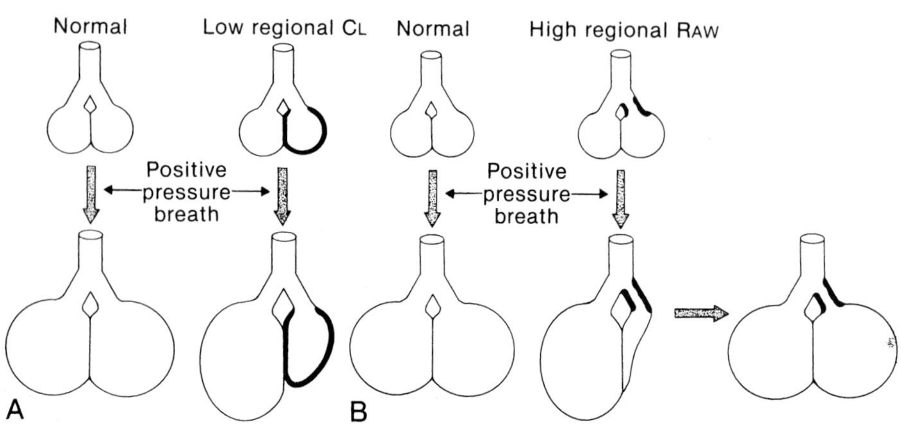


**Figure 94.3** Schematic effects of the distribution of ventilation in two-unit lung models with homogeneous mechanical properties (left breath), with abnormal compliance distribution (middle breath), and with abnormal resistance distribution (right breath). (From MacIntyre NR: Mechanical ventilatory support. *In* Dantzker DR, MacIntyre NR, Bakow ED (eds): Comprehensive Respiratory Care. Philadelphia: WB Saunders, 1995, p 453.)

day out of concern that overdistending healthier lung regions is probably an unacceptable tradeoff for aggressive shunt reduction.[25, 36] Moreover, some of the apparent shunt reduction that occurs with high PEEP levels may be a consequence of reduced cardiac output from the high intrathoracic pressures.[37]

Mechanical goals for PEEP applications have the appeal of setting ventilator pressures in accordance with the mechanical behavior of the respiratory system. This approach actually dates back several decades when "best compliance" was proposed as a reasonable way to set proper PEEP.[38] Today, the goal is similar but is often more specifically focused on static pressure-volume (P-V) relationships[39–42] (Fig. 94.4). One approach is to use the lower inflection point on a static P-V curve (see Fig. 94.4, point A) as the marker for an optimal pressure that prevents derecruitment. A variation on this approach would be to use the lower inflection point on the deflation limb of the static pressure-volume curve. Because of respiratory system compliance hysteresis,[43] this deflation limb value is generally several centimeters of water lower than the corresponding value on the inflation limb and may be a better representation of the true critical derecruitment pressure. A corollary to both of these approaches is that it may be beneficial to first perform a "volume recruitment" maneuver (e.g., a 1-minute period of 35- to 40–cm $H_2O$ inflation hold) before returning to the desired PEEP level.[36, 39]

**Inspiratory Flow Pattern and Inspiratory-Expiratory Time Manipulations.** Inspiration from a positive-pressure breath consists of a flow magnitude and a flow profile that, as noted earlier, can affect ventilation distribution (and thus $\dot{V}/\dot{Q}$). Inspiratory time (and the relationship of inspiratory to expiratory time) can be particularly important. Prolonging inspiratory time, generally by adding a pause and often used in conjunction with a rapid decelerating flow (i.e., pressure-targeted) breath, can substantially increase mean inflation pressure and lengthens gas mixing time in the lung. Moreover, if the resultant expiratory time is inadequate for the lung to return to its relaxed volume (i.e., functional residual capacity), intrinsic PEEP develops (see Fig. 94.2).

There are several physiologic effects of prolonging inspiratory time. First, the increased gas mixing time may improve $\dot{V}/\dot{Q}$ matching in infiltrative lung disease.[44–46] Second, the development of intrinsic PEEP can have effects similar to those of applied PEEP (see previous discussion). Indeed, much of the improvement in gas exchange associated with long inspiratory time strategies may be merely a PEEP phenomenon.[47] However, the distribution of intrinsic PEEP (most pronounced in lung units with long time constants) may be different from that of applied PEEP, and thus $\dot{V}/\dot{Q}$ effects may also be different. Third, because these long inspiratory times significantly increase total intrathoracic pressures, cardiac output may be affected (see "Hemodynamic Effects" section later). Finally, inspiratory:expiratory time ratios that exceed 1:1 (so-called inverse ratio ventilation) are uncomfortable, and sedation or paralysis of the patient is often required.[48]

In general, inspiratory time prolongation is reserved for patients in whom the plateau pressure from the PEEP/tidal volume combination has approached 35 cm $H_2O$ and potentially toxic concentrations of $FI_{O_2}$ are being employed without meeting arterial oxygen saturation or oxygen delivery goals.[25]

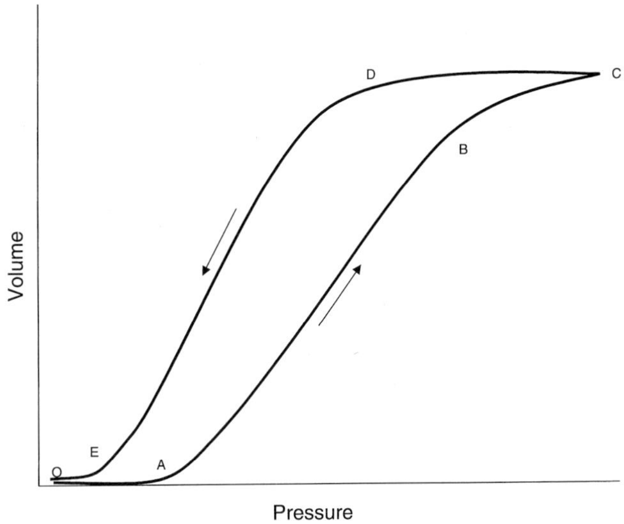


**Figure 94.4** Schematic pressure-volume plot in a patient with infiltrative lung disease and alveolar collapse at end-expiration (point 0). On the vertical axis is delivered volume and on the horizontal axis is distending pressure: ideally the alveolar–pleural pressure under static conditions. Both inflation *(upward arrow)* and deflation *(downward arrow)* phases of the breath are illustrated. Point A is the lower inflection point during inflation and represents the point when the bulk of recruitable alveoli have been opened so that inflation compliance is maximal. Point B is the upper inflection point during inflation and represents the point when recruitable alveoli begin to be overdistended and compliance falls. Point C is the maximal pressure and volume during the maneuver. Point D is the upper inflection point during deflation when alveoli begin to empty. Point E is the lower inflection point during deflation when alveoli begin to collapse or derecruit. In accordance with the concept that positive end-expiratory pressure (PEEP) should be used to prevent derecruitment and that the PEEP-tidal volume combination should not overdistend, there are two conceptual approaches to setting the PEEP-tidal volume combination by using this plot: (1) to set the PEEP just above point A and keep the PEEP-tidal volume combination below point B (inflation curve settings) and (2) to perform a volume recruitment maneuver to point C and set the PEEP-tidal volume combination between points D and E (deflation curve settings).

## Lung Stretch and Stretch Injury

The lung can be injured when it is stretched excessively by positive-pressure ventilation. The most well-recognized injury is that of alveolar rupture presenting as extra-alveolar air in the mediastinum (pneumomediastinum), pericardium (pneumopericardium), subcutaneous tissue (subcutaneous emphysema), pleura (pneumothorax), or vasculature (air emboli).[49] The risk for extra-alveolar air increases as a function of the magnitude and duration of alveolar overdistention. Thus, interactions of respiratory system mechanics (see Fig. 94.3) and mechanical ventilation strategies (high regional tidal volume and PEEP, both applied and intrinsic) that produce regions of excessive alveolar stretch (i.e., transpulmonary distending pressures in excess of 40 cm $H_2O$) for prolonged periods greatly increase the risk of rupture of alveolar units.[49]

In experimental animals, a parenchymal lung injury not associated with extra-alveolar air can also be produced by mechanical ventilation strategies that stretch the lungs beyond the normal maximum (i.e., transpulmonary distending pressures of 30 to 35 cm $H_2O$). Pathologically, this is manifested as diffuse alveolar damage[36, 50] and is associated with cytokine release[51] and bacterial translocation.[52] It also appears that this injury is potentiated by a shear stress phenomenon that occurs when injured alveoli are repetitively opened and collapsed during the ventilatory cycle.[30–32, 36] Cytokine release has also been linked to mechanical ventilation in patients with the acute respiratory distress syndrome,[52a] and ventilator settings that create overdistention and shear stress, which are known to cause lung damage in experimental animals, are also believed to worsen lung injury in these patients.[52b]

This injury may occur clinically when low resistance–high compliance units receive a disproportionately high regional tidal volume in the setting of high alveolar distending pressures (see Fig. 94.3) and appears to be potentiated in atelectatic units that do not receive levels of PEEP sufficient to prevent collapse. Concern about this injury is the rationale for using mechanical measurements of the lung to guide ventilator management in a "lung-protective" approach. The simplest guide to limiting overdistention is to manage patients below the normal maximal transpulmonary pressure of 35 cm $H_2O$ (in a patient with near-normal chest wall compliance, end-inspiratory transpulmonary pressure is approximated by the airway plateau pressure[25]). As described earlier, however, the most direct way to assess mechanical behavior fully is to construct the static P-V curve (see Fig. 94.4). The idea is to use the lower inflection point as a guide to a PEEP level that prevents collapse (see earlier discussion of alveolar recruitment strategies) and the upper inflection point as a guide to the maximal distention that would be allowed with the PEEP/tidal volume combination. When coupled with a volume recruitment maneuver, this "open-lung" approach to ventilatory support in patients with severe lung injury has been shown to improve outcome over conventional strategies in preliminary studies.[39]

Because constructing static pressure-volume curves is time-consuming and often requires heavy sedation and/or paralysis of the patient, simpler ways of determining inflection points are being investigated. Potential approaches include delivering a very slow flow (i.e., 10 L/min), constant-flow breath while recording a single dynamic pressure-volume curve.[53] Because flow is so slow, flow-resistive pressure is minimized and the curve approximates a static curve. Either corrections for endotracheal tube resistive pressure can be subtracted mathematically or pressures can be recorded from the distal end of the endotracheal tube. The addition of an esophageal pressure tracing to account for chest wall effects, which are often ignored, might also be important in patients with abnormal chest wall compliance (e.g., obese or heavily bandaged patients).

Of importance is that reducing the risk of stretch injury may necessitate the use of small tidal volumes and lower minute ventilations to keep maximal transpulmonary pressures less than 35 cm $H_2O$.[25] This may cause $P_{CO_2}$ to increase with consequent respiratory acidosis. Willingness to tolerate respiratory acidosis to prevent lung overstretch is sometimes referred to as *permissive hypercapnia*.[54, 55] Increases in $CO_2$ levels seem to be tolerated in increments of about 10 mm Hg/hr,[55] and most patients can tolerate pH values in the range of 7.1 to 7.2.[55] However, allowing acidosis should probably be avoided in patients with central nervous system mass lesions (or mass effect) and in patients with unstable hemodynamics (pressor dependence or dysrhythmias).[55]

Preliminary results (see Web site address: www.hedwig.mgh.harvard.edu) from a large multicenter trial supported by the National Heart, Lung, and Blood Institute have upheld the value of protecting the lungs by using smaller than ordinary tidal volumes. In this study of 861 patients with acute lung injury, subjects were randomized to be ventilated with either conventional (12 mL/kg, high) or small (6 mL/kg, low) tidal volumes: PEEP strategies were the same in the two groups. At interim analysis, mortality was significantly different in the two groups: 39% in patients ventilated with high tidal volumes compared with 31% in those receiving low tidal volumes; a full report is in press.[55a]

An interesting ventilatory strategy focused on lung protection involves the use of high-frequency ventilation (HFV). HFV uses much higher than normal breathing frequencies (i.e., 60 to 500 breaths/minute in the adult).[56] With this breathing pattern, tidal volumes are often smaller than anatomic dead space and thus gas transport mechanisms other than convective flow must be invoked (e.g., augmented diffusion, asymmetric flow profiles, Taylor dispersion, and pendelluft).[57] Conventional ventilators are usually incapable of responding this quickly, and thus either jet devices or high-frequency oscillators must be used to deliver this breathing pattern. The putative advantage to HFV in infiltrative lung disease is that the high delivered minute ventilation and short expiratory time produce substantial intrinsic PEEP, whereas the small tidal volumes limit maximal pressures and distending volume. Conceptually, this means that the lung is recruited and ventilated in the optimal portion of the pressure-volume curve (see Fig. 94.4, between points C and D). In infants at high risk for barotrauma, HFV has been proven safe and effective in reducing long-term lung injury.[58] Experience in adults is less extensive, and the results of clinical trials so far have not been encouraging.[59]

## Mechanical Loads

Mechanical loads describe the mechanical aspects of ventilation with a single number: an expression either of a pressure-time product (PTP) or work (W)[18, 19, 60] (Fig. 94.5 and Fig. 94.6). Because mechanical loads correlate with

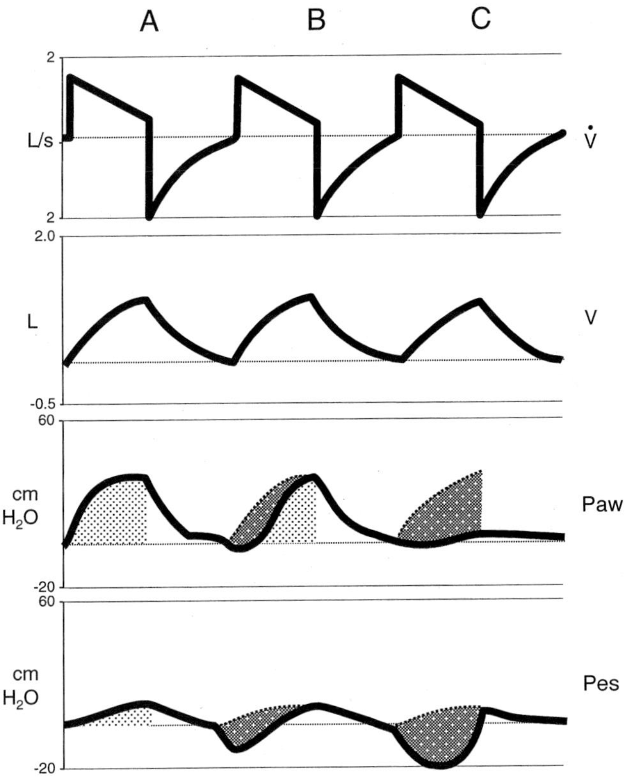


**Figure 94.5** Loads expressed as pressure time products (PTP) *(shaded areas)*. The figure depicts airway pressure (Paw) and esophageal pressure (Pes), flow ($\dot{V}$), and volume (V) tracings of a fully controlled mechanical breath (breath A), an interactive patient-ventilator breath (breath B) and a spontaneous (unassisted/unsupported) breath (breath C), with the same tidal volume and inspiratory flow profile. The lighter shaded area equals machine load, and the darker shaded area equals patient load. Note that in the machine-controlled breath, the esophageal pressure reflects loads related to chest wall expansion by the positive airway pressure; in the spontaneous breath, the esophageal pressure reflects loads related to lung and chest wall expansion by actively contracting ventilatory muscles. Note also that, given the same volume and flow profile, the total PTP for the lungs and chest wall is the same in all three breaths, regardless of machine or patient contribution.

ventilatory muscle oxygen demands,[61–63] the concept of load is useful in considering inspiratory muscle energy requirements during spontaneous or interactive partial ventilatory support (see "Interactions" section later). Moreover, when referenced to muscle strength or endurance properties, load tolerance is a useful guide to setting levels of partial ventilatory support or predicting the spontaneous breathing capabilities.[64, 65]

The pressure-time product expresses load as the integral of pressure over time (PTP = ∫Pdt) (see Fig. 94.5). Compliance, resistance, and the size of the breath all contribute to the magnitude of the PTP per breath. During spontaneous breathing, integrating Pes over time (referenced to the passive inflation pressure) quantifies the load borne by the inspiratory muscles to inflate the lungs (see Fig. 94.5, breath C). During a controlled breath, integrating PAO over time quantifies the load borne by the ventilator to inflate the entire respiratory system (lungs and chest wall; see Fig. 94.5, breath A), and integrating Pes over time describes the loads imposed only by the chest wall. For a given tidal volume, flow profile, and set of respiratory system mechanics, the PTPs related to the lungs and chest wall should be identical regardless of whether measured during a spontaneous breath (patient PTP) or a controlled breath (ventilator PTP). Moreover, during interactive, partially supported breaths in which load is shared between patient and ventilator, the sum contributions of patient and ventilator PTP should be the same as during a controlled or spontaneous breath of the same volume and flow profile[66] (see Fig. 94.5, breath B).

Work expresses load as the integral of pressure over volume (W = ∫PdV) (see Fig. 94.6). Depending on whether the measured breath is spontaneous, ventilator controlled, or interactive, work (as in the preceding PTP discussion) can reflect properties of the lung, the chest wall, or the entire respiratory system and whether the load is borne by the patient or ventilator or is shared (see Fig. 94.6, breaths C, A, and B, respectively).

Under heavy impedance loading conditions (e.g., the patient with abnormal lung mechanics and thus high pressure requirements), duration of pressure (i.e., the PTP) correlates better with muscle energetics and fatigue potential than does volume moved with pressure (i.e., work).[63, 64, 67] Indeed, during ventilation that requires high pressures, multiplying PTP by the inspiratory time fraction and referencing this to the maximal pressure that the inspiratory muscles can generate results in the pressure-time index. Muscle fatigue can be expected if the pressure-time index value exceeds 0.15.[61, 62] This concern with high pressure loads in patients receiving partial ventilatory support is one of the rationales for providing ventilator-pressure assistance with every spontaneous effort (i.e., pressure-assisted or pressure-supported breaths), as opposed to alternating fully supported breaths with unsupported breaths (i.e., intermittent mandatory ventilation; see "Interactions" section later).[68]

## Patient-Ventilator Interactions

Mechanical ventilation modes that permit spontaneous ventilatory activity are termed *interactive* modes because patients can affect various aspects of the mechanical ventilator's functions. These interactions can range from simple triggering of mechanical breaths to more complex processes affecting delivered flow patterns and breath timing. Interactive modes allow for muscle "exercise" that, when done at nonfatiguing or physiologic levels, may prevent muscle atrophy and facilitate recovery of strength.[69] In addition, permitting spontaneous patient ventilatory activity and using comfortable interactive modes may reduce the need for the sedation and neuromuscular blockers that are often required to prevent patients from fighting machine-controlled ventilation.[7, 48, 70]

Interactive modes can be either synchronous or dyssynchronous with patient efforts. Synchronous interactions mean that the ventilator is sensitive to the initiation,

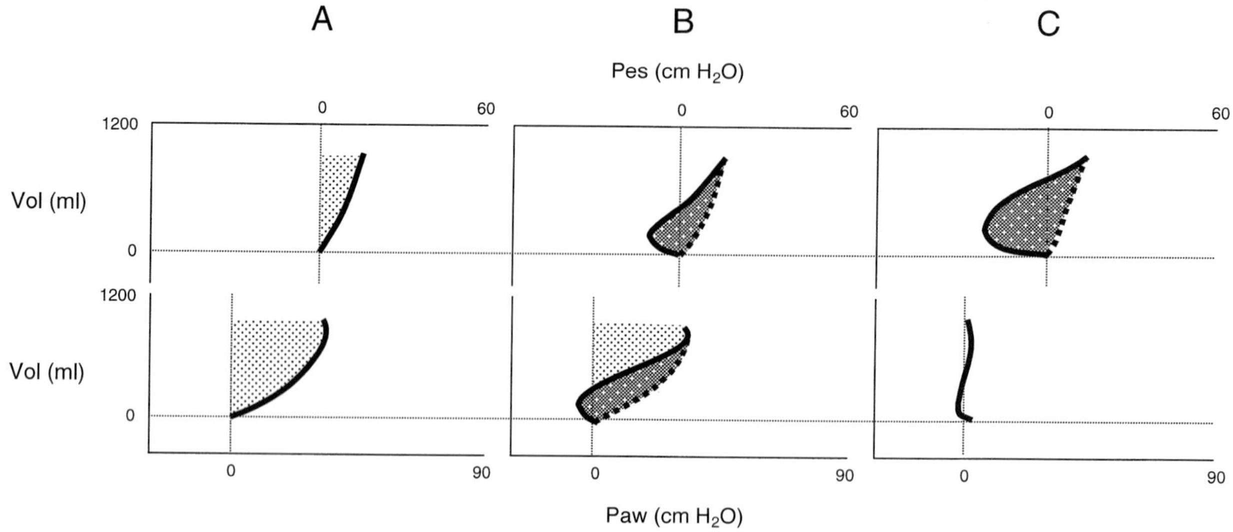


**Figure 94.6** Loads expressed as work (W) *(shaded areas).* The same machine-controlled breath (breath A), spontaneous (unassisted/unsupported) breath (breath C), and interactive breath (breath B) depicted in Figure 94.5 are now plotted as pressure (both airway (Paw) and esophageal (Pes)) versus volume (Vol). This allows for the same loads expressed as PTP in Figure 94.5 to be expressed here as ∫PdVol or W.

modulation, and termination of a patient's ventilatory effort.[70] In the ensuing discussion, synchrony is considered during the three phases of interactive breath delivery: breath triggering, ventilator flow delivery, and breath cycling:

**Ventilator Breath Triggering.** Interactive mechanical ventilation needs to sense a spontaneous effort (either an airway-pressure drop or airway-flow change; see earlier discussion of sensors) in order to trigger a mechanical response.[8] Even with modern sensors, however, there is unavoidable dyssynchrony in the triggering process.[71] First, a certain level of insensitivity must be put in the sensor to prevent artifacts from triggering the ventilator (i.e., autocycling). Second, even when the patient effort has been sensed, demand valve systems have a certain inherent delay (up to 100 milliseconds or more) before they physically open and achieve target flow into the airway (system responsiveness). Both of these factors can result in significant isometric-like pressure loads on the ventilatory muscles during the triggering process.[71] In addition, in the setting of air trapping and positive end-expiratory pressure (intrinsic PEEP), the elevated alveolar pressure at end-expiration can serve as a significant triggering threshold load on the ventilatory muscles (Fig. 94.7).[72, 73]

Several strategies can be used to minimize the magnitude of the dyssynchrony induced during breath triggering. First, ventilators with microprocessor flow controls have significantly better valve characteristics than do older generation ventilators. Second, continuous-flow systems superimposed on the demand systems can improve demand-system responsiveness in patients with high ventilatory drives (although such flows can reduce sensitivity in patients with very weak ventilatory drives).[74, 75] Third, flow-based triggers have been shown to produce a more sensitive and responsive breath-triggering process.[76] Fourth, a small amount of applied inspiratory pressure support usually increases the ventilator's initial flow delivery and can thereby improve response characteristics of the demand valve system.[76] Fifth, in patients with obstructive disease and an inspiratory threshold load induced by intrinsic PEEP, setting applied PEEP below the intrinsic PEEP level can help equilibrate the end-expiratory alveolar and circuit pressures and improve triggering (see Fig. 94.7).[72, 73, 77, 78] Finally, sensors in the pleural space or on the phrenic nerve may improve trigger performance on future systems.[79]

**Ventilator-Delivered Flow Pattern.** During an interactive breath, ventilatory muscles are contracting,[80–82] and the ventilator flow delivery should be adequate for meeting one of three goals: (1) fully unloading the contracting ventilatory muscles in patients with severely overloaded and fatigued muscles; (2) partially unloading the contracting ventilatory muscles in patients recovering from muscle fatigue; or (3) not affecting the loads (i.e., adding no imposed loads) on contracting ventilatory muscle in patients during spontaneous breathing trials. Synchronous flow interactions can be defined accordingly (Fig. 94.8):

***Breaths Designed to Fully Unload Ventilatory Muscles.*** For an interactive breath to fully unload respiratory muscles, the patient should be required only to trigger the ventilator, so that the ventilator supplies all the work of the breath.[80] The goal of synchrony during a fully unloaded breath is thus to deliver adequate flow over the entire inspiratory effort in order to totally unload the contracting muscles. Achieving this goal can be assessed by comparing the pressure pattern of the patient-triggered

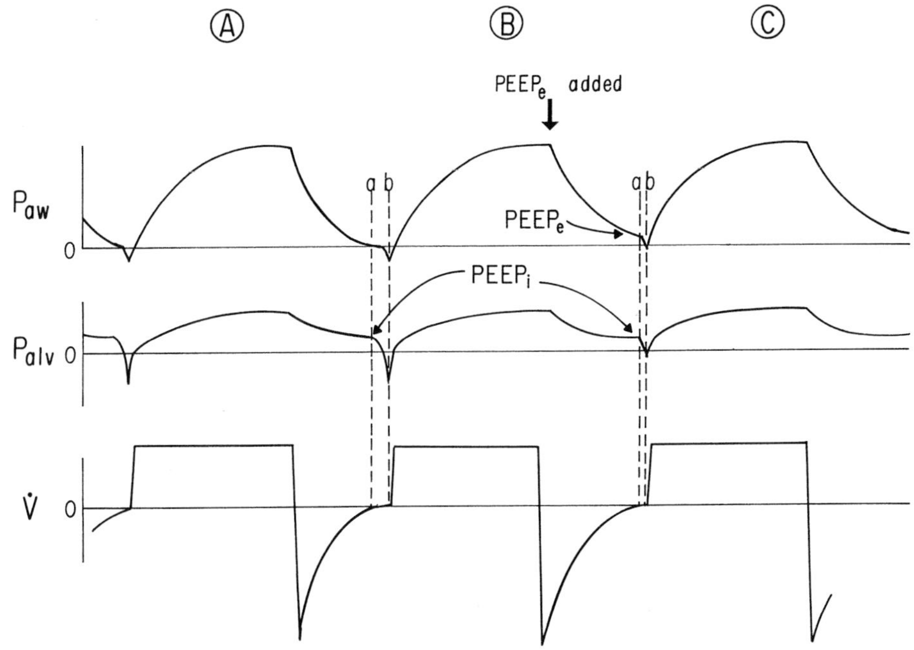


**Figure 94.7** Schematic tracings of airway pressure (Paw, shown as $P_{aw}$ on the illustration), alveolar pressure (Palv, shown as $P_{alv}$), and flow ($\dot{V}$) during patient-triggered breaths in the setting of dynamic airway collapse and consequent intrinsic positive end-expiratory pressure (PEEPi, shown as $PEEP_i$). In breath A, PEEPi is evident in the Palv tracing at end-expiration. Note that this PEEPi must be overcome by muscle contraction to lower Palv and Paw enough to trigger the assisted breath (point a to point b). In breaths B and C, a small amount of applied PEEP (PEEPe, shown as $PEEP_e$) has been added; this is less than PEEPi. This serves to partially equilibrate expiratory pressures in the lung and ventilator circuitry, thus reducing the Palv drop that must occur to lower Paw. The inspiratory threshold load imposed by PEEPi is consequently reduced. (From MacIntyre NR: Intrinsic positive end-expiratory pressure. Prob Respir Care 4:49, 1991.)

breath with a machine-triggered breath (i.e., a breath occurring without patient activity). Synchronous flow delivery should produce nearly identical airway pressure waveforms and evidence of triggering only in the pleural/esophageal pressure waveforms (see Fig. 94.8, breaths C and D). Synchrony is usually accompanied by a near-normal spontaneous respiratory frequency. In general, a pressure-targeted breath with its variable flow feature is easier to synchronize with an active patient demand than is a fixed flow breath.[83, 84]

***Breaths Designed to Partially Unload Ventilatory Muscles.*** For an interactive breath to partially unload ventilatory muscles, the patient and the ventilator need to share the work of the breath. Synchrony is then defined as having the ventilator provide a constant pressure bias on the ventilatory muscles such that their pressure-volume configuration normalizes and "unphysiologic" high-pressure–low-volume breaths are avoided (see Fig. 94.8: the abnormal load pattern in breath B is normalized in breath E but not in breath F).[68, 70] Synchronous partially unloaded breaths thus have an airway pressure waveform shape similar to (though of less magnitude than) that of a controlled breath, whereas the pleural/esophageal pressure waveforms resemble a normal loading pattern[82, 83] (Fig. 94.8, breath E). In addition, flow synchrony is usually associated with a near-normal spontaneous breathing frequency. On current systems, variable-flow, pressure-targeted breaths are better designed for partial unloading than are fixed-flow breaths. In the future, better sensors (e.g., tracheal[85] or pleural[79] sensors) or different flow control algorithms (e.g., proportional assist ventilation that governs flow by gain settings on patient flow-volume demands[86]) may further improve flow synchrony during partially unloaded breaths.

***Breaths Designed Not to Affect Ventilatory Muscle Loads.*** For an interactive breath not to affect loads on the ventilatory muscles (and not to impose loads), the ventilator must supply flow sufficient only to keep the airway pressure constant (continuous positive airway pressure). Under these conditions, flow synchrony is defined as flow that maintains a pleural/esophageal pressure waveform that would mimic that of an extubated patient. In practice, an unchanging airway pressure waveform during inspiration is often interpreted as reflecting flow synchrony during unsupported/unassisted breaths. However, because airway pressure is monitored proximal to the resistance imposed by the endotracheal tube, a better indicator of true flow synchrony under these conditions would probably be an unchanging tracheal pressure.[85] This is the rationale for arbitrarily adding small amounts

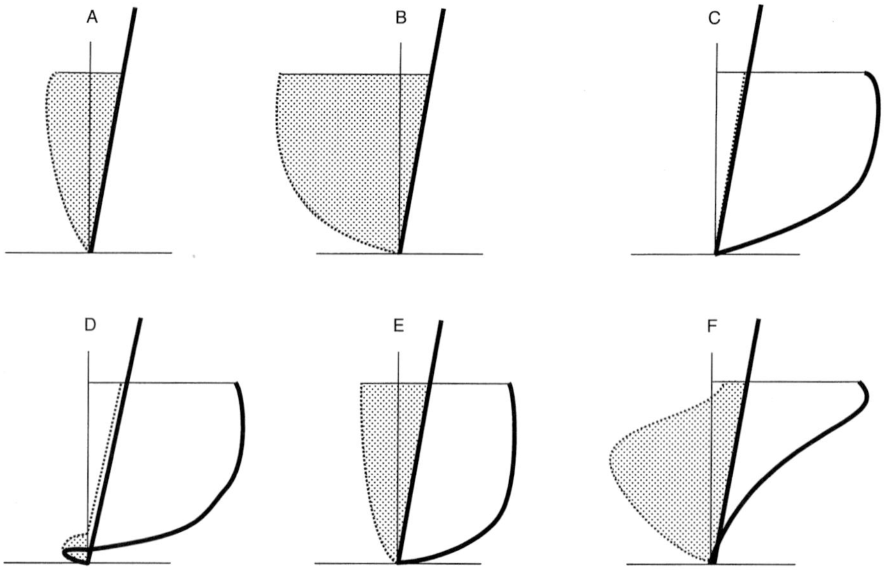


**Figure 94.8** Pressure-volume plots depicting various patient-ventilator interactions for a constant tidal volume. In each plot, volume is on the vertical axis and pressure is on the horizontal axis. Machine pressures are depicted by *solid lines;* esophageal pressures are depicted by *dashed lines.* The *solid angled line* directed upward and to the right from the origin reflects passive inflation esophageal pressure (chest wall compliance). The *shaded area* reflects patient work. Breath A depicts a normally loaded spontaneous (unsupported/unassisted) breath. Breath B depicts an abnormally loaded spontaneous breath. Breath C depicts a machine-controlled breath in the abnormal patient. Breath D depicts a synchronous-assisted breath designed to virtually unload the abnormal patient (only triggering load is evident). Breath E depicts a synchronous-assisted breath designed to partially unload the abnormal patient. Under these circumstances, synchrony is defined as a smooth airway pressure bias that converts the patient's loading pattern to a more normal configuration (i.e., resembling breath A). Breath F depicts a dyssynchronous-assisted breath in the abnormal patient. High-pressure patient loads exist through much of this breath because of inappropriate ventilator flow delivery.

of pressure support to spontaneous breaths[87] or using tracheal pressure sensors to control flow delivery from the ventilator.[85]

**Breath Cycling.** Cycling dyssynchrony can occur in one of two ways. First, if the breath lasts beyond the patient's effort, an inadequate expiratory time may develop (along with air trapping) and/or the patient's expiratory efforts may be necessary to terminate the breath.[88] Second, if the breath terminates before the patient's effort is finished, the patient may be left in need of additional flow without its being delivered. Significant imposed loading and/or double breath triggering may result. With either type of cycle dyssynchrony, it is important that the clinician recognize it and make appropriate adjustments to the cycling criteria.

## Hemodynamic Effects

In addition to affecting ventilation and the distribution of ventilation, intrathoracic pressure applications from positive-pressure ventilation can also affect cardiovascular function.[34, 89, 90] In general, as mean intrathoracic pressure is increased, right ventricular filling is decreased and cardiac output/pulmonary perfusion consequently decreases. This is the rationale for using fluid volume repletion to maintain cardiac output in the setting of high intrathoracic pressure. Of note is that the effect of reduced cardiac filling on cardiac output may be partially counteracted by better left ventricular function as a result of elevated intrathoracic pressures serving to reduce left ventricular afterload.[91]

Intrathoracic pressures can also influence distribution of perfusion. The relationship of alveolar pressures to perfusion pressures in the three-zone lung model (described fully in Chapter 4) helps explain distribution.[92] Specifically, the supine human lung is generally in a zone 3 (distention) state. As intra-alveolar pressures rise, however, zone 2 and zone 1 regions can appear, creating high $\dot{V}/\dot{Q}$ units. Indeed, increases in dead space (i.e., zone 1 lung) can be a consequence of ventilatory strategies that employ high ventilatory pressures.

Positive-pressure mechanical ventilation can affect other aspects of cardiovascular function. Specifically, dyspnea, anxiety, and discomfort with inadequate ventilatory support can lead to stress-related catechol release with subsequent increases in myocardial oxygen demands and in risk of dysrhythmias.[93] In addition, coronary blood vessel oxygen delivery can be compromised by inadequate gas exchange from the lung injury coupled with low mixed venous $P_{O_2}$ due to high oxygen consumption demands by the ventilatory muscles.

## PRESSURE-UNRELATED COMPLICATIONS

### Oxygen Toxicity

Oxygen concentrations approaching 100% are known to cause oxidant injuries in airways and lung parenchyma.[94] Much of the data supporting this concept, however, have come from animals that often have tolerances to oxygen that are quite different from those in humans. It is thus not clear what the safe oxygen concentration or duration of exposure is in sick humans. Most consensus groups have argued that $F_{I_{O_2}}$ values less than 0.4 are safe for prolonged periods and that $F_{I_{O_2}}$ values greater than 0.8 should be avoided if at all possible. As noted earlier, this means that tradeoffs among high PEEP-plateau pressures, high inspired oxygen concentrations, and arterial oxygen content goals must occur in the management of patients with severe gas exchange abnormalities.[25]

### Patient-Ventilator Interface Events

The patient-ventilator interface includes the ventilator circuitry and the artificial airway. The most important complications associated with this apparatus are ventilator disconnections (including artificial airway dislodgment), which have been reported to occur in up to 8% to 13% of ventilated patients[95] and, if left uncorrected, can be fatal. Because circuit pressure and flow can still occur when the ventilator is disconnected from the patient (e.g., the airway is in the esophagus or the disconnected circuit could be only partially occluded as it lies on the patient's chest), it is critical that carefully set, redundant (i.e., pressure *and* flow) alarms are present.[5] Other complications of the patient-ventilator interface include obstructions from secretions, circuit leaks, airway injury from inadequate heat/humidity, tracheal injury from the artificial airway, and loss of delivered tidal volume in a compliant circuit.

### Pulmonary Infections

Mechanically ventilated patients are at risk for pulmonary infections for several reasons.[96–98] First, the natural protective mechanism of glottic closure is compromised by an endotracheal tube. This permits continuous seepage of oropharyngeal material into the airways. Second, the endotracheal tube itself impairs the cough reflex and serves as an additional potential portal for pathogens to enter the lungs. This is particularly important if the circuit is contaminated. Nasotracheal tubes are also associated with a high incidence of maxillary sinusitis, which may serve as a source of ventilator-associated pneumonia.[98a] Third, airway and parenchymal injury from the underlying disease, as well as management complications noted previously, makes the lung prone to infections. Fourth, the intensive care unit environment, with its heavy use of antibiotics and presence of sick patients in proximity to each other, is itself a risk factor for a variety of infections.

Preventing ventilator-associated pneumonias is critical, as length of stay and mortality are heavily influenced by their development.[96–98, 98b] Handwashing and carefully chosen antibiotic regimens for other infections can have important beneficial effects. Management strategies that avoid breaking the integrity of the circuit (i.e., circuit changes only when visibly contaminated) also appear to be helpful.[99] Finally, continuous drainage of subglottic secretions may be a simple way of reducing lung contamination with oropharyngeal material.[100] Further information on the pathogenesis, diagnosis, treatment, and prevention of ventilator-associated pneumonia is provided in Chapter 31.

## SUMMARY

Modern medical technology has considerably improved the safety and efficacy of positive-pressure mechanical ventilators. These machines are capable of doing all or part of the work of breathing and can be programmed to interact more comfortably and effectively with patients than before. The goals of machine-assisted breathing can be focused on optimizing gas exchange or on improving respiratory system mechanics; recent emphasis has been on avoiding overdistention of the lungs, thereby preventing stretch injury, particularly in patients whose lungs are already damaged. It is important to understand the principles of mechanical ventilation, as described in this chapter, in order to take maximum advantage of its benefits, while avoiding inherent ventilator-related complications as much as possible.

## References


1. MacIntyre NR: Mechanical ventilation: The next 50 years. Respir Care 43:490–493, 1998.
2. Mushin M, Rendell-Baker W, Thompson PW, et al: Automatic ventilation of the lungs. Oxford, UK: Blackwell, 1980, pp 62–166.
3. American Society for Testing and Materials: Standard specifications for ventilators intended for use in critical care. Vol 36. Philadelphia: American Society for Testing and Materials, 1991, pp 1123–1155.
4. Chatburn RL: Classification of mechanical ventilators. Respir Care 37:1009–1025, 1992.
5. American Association for Respiratory Care Consensus Group: Essentials of mechanical ventilators. Respir Care 37:1000–1008, 1992.
6. Branson RD, MacIntyre NR: Dual control modes of mechanical ventilation. Respir Care 41:294–305, 1996.
7. MacIntyre NR: Patient ventilator interactions: Dys-synchrony and imposed loads. *In* Marini J, Slutsky A (eds): Physiologic Basis of Ventilatory Support. New York: Marcel Dekker, 1997, pp 420–435.
8. Sassoon CSH: Mechanical ventilator design and function: The trigger variable. Respir Care 37:1056–1069, 1992.
9. Branson RD, Peterson BD, Carson KD (eds): Humidification: Current therapy and controversy. Respir Care Clin North Am 4:189–341, 1998.
10. Pinsky MR, Hrehocik D, Culpepper JA, et al: Flow resistance of expiratory positive-pressure systems. Chest 94:788–791, 1988.
11. Pepe PE, Marini JJ: Occult positive end-expiratory pressure in mechanically ventilated patients with airflow obstruction. Am Rev Respir Dis 126:166–170, 1982.
12. Mehta S, Hill NS: Non-invasive ventilation in acute respiratory failure. Respir Care Clin North Am 2:267–292, 1996.
13. American Association for Respiratory Care Consensus Group:

Non-invasive positive pressure ventilation. Respir Care 42:364–369, 1997.
14. Drinkwine J, Kacmarck R: Non-invasive positive pressure ventilation: Equipment and techniques. Respir Care Clin North Am 2:183–194, 1996.
15. Hess D: Aerosol therapy. Respir Care Clin North Am 1:235–263, 1995.
16. Marini JJ: What derived variables should be monitored during mechanical ventilation? Respir Care 37:1097–1107, 1992.
17. Day S, MacIntyre NR: Ventilator alarm systems. Prob Respir Care 4:118–126, 1991.
18. Truwit JD, Marini JJ: Evaluation of thoracic mechanics in the ventilated patient: Part I. Primary measurements. J Crit Care 3:133–150, 1988.
19. Truwit JD, Marini JJ: Evaluation of thoracic mechanics in the ventilated patient: Part II. Applied mechanics. J Crit Care 3:192–213, 1988.
20. Marini JJ, Crooke PS: A general mathematical model for respiratory dynamics relevant to the clinical setting. Am Rev Respir Dis 147:14–24, 1993.
21. Macklen PT: Relationship between lung mechanics and ventilation distribution. Physiology 16:580–588, 1973.
22. Milic-Emili J, Henderson JAN, Dolovich MB, et al: Regional distribution of inhaled gas in the lung. J Appl Physiol 21:749–759, 1966.
23. Abraham E, Yoshihara G: Cardiorespiratory effects of pressure controlled ventilation in severe respiratory failure. Chest 98:1445–1449, 1990.
24. Pratt PC: Pathology of the adult respiratory distress syndrome. *In* Thurlbeck WM, Ael MR (eds): The Lung: Structure, Function and Disease. Baltimore: Williams & Wilkins, 1978, pp 43–57.
25. Slutsky AS: ACCP Consensus Conference: Mechanical ventilation. Chest 104:1833–1859, 1993.
26. Kacmarek RM, Pierson DJ (eds): AARC Conference on Positive End Expiratory Pressure. Respir Care 33:419–527, 1988.
27. Gattinoni L, Pesenti A, Baglioni S, et al: Inflammatory pulmonary edema and PEEP: Correlation between imaging and physiologic studies. J Thorac Imaging 3:59–64, 1988.
28. Gattinoni L, Pelosi P, Crotti S, et al: Effects of positive end expiratory pressure on regional distribution of tidal volume and recruitment in adult respiratory distress syndrome. Am J Respir Crit Care Med 151:1807–1814, 1995.
29. Gattinoni L, Pelosi P, Suter P, et al: ARDS caused by pulmonary and extra pulmonary disease: Different syndromes? Am J Respir Crit Care Med 158:3–11, 1998.
30. Webb HJH, Tierney DF: Experimental pulmonary edema due to intermittent positive pressure ventilation with high inflation pressures: Protection by positive end-expiratory pressure. Am Rev Respir Dis 110:556–565, 1974.
31. Dreyfus D, Soler P, Bassett G, et al: High inflation pressure pulmonary edema. Am Rev Respir Dis 137:1159–1164, 1988.
32. Muscedere JG, Mullen JB, Gan K, et al: Tidal ventilation at low airway pressures can augment lung injury. Am J Respir Crit Care Med 149:1327–1334, 1994.
33. Wyszogrodski I, Kyei-Aboagye K, Taeusch HW Jr, et al: Surfactant inactivation by hyperventilation: Conservation by end-expiratory pressure. J Appl Physiol 38:461–466, 1975.
34. Pinsky MR, Guimond JG: The effects of positive end-expiratory pressure on heart-lung interactions. J Crit Care 6:1–15, 1991.
35. DiRusso SM, Nelson LD, Safesak K, et al: Survival in patients with severe ARDS treated with high level positive end expiratory pressure. Crit Care Med 23:1485–1496, 1995.
36. Dreyfus D, Savmon G: Ventilator induced lung injury: Lessons from experimental studies. Am J Respir Crit Care Med 157:294–323, 1998.
37. Lynch JP, Mhyre JG, Dantzker DR: Influence of cardiac output on intrapulmonary shunt. J Appl Physiol 46:315–321, 1979.
38. Suter PM, Fairley HB, Isenberg MD: Optimum end-expiratory pressure in patients with acute pulmonary failure. N Engl J Med 292:284–289, 1975.
39. Amato MB, Barbas CSV, Medeivos DM, et al: Effect of a protective-ventilation strategy on mortality in the acute respiratory distress syndrome. N Engl J Med 338:347–354, 1998.
40. Salmon RB, Primiano FP, Saidel GM, et al: Human pressure-volume relationships: Alveolar collapse and airway closure. J Appl Physiol 51:353–362, 1981.
41. Servillo G, Svantesson C, Beydon L, et al: Pressure volume curves in acute respiratory failure. Am J Respir Crit Care Med 155:1629–1636, 1997.
42. Benito S, Lemaire F: Pulmonary pressure-volume relationship in acute respiratory distress syndrome in adults: Role of positive and expiratory pressure. J Crit Care 5:27–34, 1990.
43. Sharp JT, Johnson FN, Goldbert NB, et al: Hysteresis and stress adaptation in the human respiratory system. J Appl Physiol 23:487–497, 1967.
44. Cole AGH, Weller SF, Sykes MD: Inverse ratio ventilation compared with PEEP in adult respiratory failure. Intensive Care Med 10:227–232, 1984.
45. Armstrong BW, MacIntyre NR: Pressure controlled inverse ratio ventilation that avoids air trapping in ARDS. Crit Care Med 23:279–285, 1995.
46. Tharratt RS, Allen RP, Albertson TE: Pressure controlled inverse ratio ventilation in severe adult respiratory failure. Chest 94:755–762, 1988.
47. Shanholtz C, Brower R: Should inverse ratio ventilation be used in ARDS? Am J Respir Crit Care Med 149:1354–1358, 1994.
48. Hansen-Flaschen J, Brazinsky S, Bassles C, et al: Use of sedating drugs and neuromuscular blockade in patients requiring mechanical ventilation for respiratory failure. JAMA 266:2870–2875, 1991.
49. Samuelson WN, Fulkerson WJ: Barotrauma in mechanical ventilation. Prob Respir Care 4:52–67, 1991.
50. Kolobow T, Morentti MP, Fumagalli R, et al: Severe impairment in lung function induced by high peak airway pressure during mechanical ventilation. Am Rev Respir Dis 135:312–315, 1987.
51. Tremblay L, Valenza F, Ribiero SP, et al: Injurious ventilatory strategies increase cytokines and c-*fos* m-RNA expression in an isolated rat lung model. J Clin Invest 99:944–952, 1997.
52. Nahum A, Hoyt J, Schmitz L, et al: Effect of mechanical ventilation strategy on dissemination of intratracheally instilled *E. coli* in dogs. Crit Care Med 25:1733–1743, 1997.
52a. Ranieri VM, Suter PM, Tortorella C, et al: Effect of mechanical ventilation on inflammatory mediators in patients with acute respiratory distress syndrome. JAMA 282:54–61, 1999.
52b. International Consensus Conferences in Intensive Care Medicine: Ventilator-associated lung injury in ARDS. Am J Respir Crit Care Med (in press).
53. Servillo G, Svantesson C, Beydon L, et al: Pressure volume curves in acute respiratory failure: Automated low flow inflation versus occlusion. Am J Respir Crit Care Med 155:1629–1636, 1997.
54. Hickling KG, Walsh J, Henderson S, et al: Low mortality rate in adult respiratory distress syndrome using low-volume, pressure-limited ventilation with permissive hypercapnia: A prospective study. Crit Care Med 22:1568–1578, 1994.
55. Fiehl F, Perret C: Permissive hypercapnia—How permissive should we be? Am J Respir Crit Care Med 150:1722–1737, 1994.
55a. NIH ARDS Network: A trial of traditional versus a lower tidal volume strategy in acute lung injury and the acute respiratory distress syndrome. N Engl J Med (in press).
56. Froese AB, Bryan C: High frequency ventilation. Am Rev Respir Dis 135:1363–1374, 1987.
57. Chang HK: Mechanisms of gas transport during high frequency ventilation. J Appl Physiol 56:553–563, 1984.
58. Keszler M, Donn SM, Bucciarelli RL, et al: Multicenter controlled trial comparing HFJV and conventional mechanical ventilation in newborns with PIE. J Pediatr 119:85–93, 1991.
59. Froese AB: High frequency oscillatory ventilation for ARDS: Let's get it right this time. Crit Care Med 25:906–908, 1998.
60. Agostoni E, Campbell EJM, Freedman S: Energetics. *In* Campbell EJM, Agostoni E, Newsome-Davis J (eds): The respiratory muscles. Philadelphia: WB Saunders, 1970, pp 115–137.
61. Field S, Sanci S, Grassino A: Respiratory muscle oxygen consumption estimated by the diaphragm pressure-time index. J Appl Physiol 57:44–51, 1984.
62. Collett PW, Perry C, Engel LA: Pressure time product, flow, and oxygen cost of resistive breathing in humans. J Appl Physiol 58:1263–1272, 1985.
63. MacIntyre NR, Leatherman NE: Mechanical loads on the ventilatory muscles. Am Rev Respir Dis 144:968–973, 1989.

64. Bellemare F, Grassino A: Effect of pressure and timing of contraction on human diaphragm fatigue. J Appl Physiol 53:1190–1195, 1982.
65. Marini JJ: Exertion during ventilator support: How much and how important? Respir Care 31:385–387, 1986.
66. Banner MJ, Kirby RR, MacIntyre NR: Patient and ventilator work of breathing and ventilatory muscle loads at different levels of pressure support ventilation. Chest 100:531–533, 1991.
67. McGregor M, Bechlake MR: The relationship of oxygen cost of breathing to mechanical work and respiratory force. J Clin Invest 40:971–980, 1961.
68. MacIntyre NR: Weaning from mechanical ventilatory support: Volume-assisting intermittent breaths versus pressure-assisting every breath. Respir Care 33:121–125, 1988.
69. Anzueto A, Peters JI, Tobin MJ, et al: Effects of prolonged controlled mechanical ventilation on diaphragmatic function in healthy adult baboons. Crit Care Med 25:1187–1190, 1997.
70. MacIntyre NR: Patient-ventilator interactions. *In* Grenvik A (ed): Textbook of Critical Care Medicine (4th ed). Philadelphia: WB Saunders, 1999.
71. Katz J, Kraemer R, Gjerde GE: Inspiratory work and airway pressure with continuous positive airway pressure delivery systems. Chest 88:519–516–526, 1985.
72. Smith TC, Marini JJ: Impact of PEEP on lung mechanics and work of breathing in severe airflow obstruction. J Appl Physiol 65:1488–1499, 1988.
73. Gay PC, Rodarte JR, Hubmayr RD: The effects of positive expiratory pressure on isovolume flow and dynamic hyperinflation in patients receiving mechanical ventilation. Am Rev Respir Dis 139:621–626, 1989.
74. Gurevitch MJ, Gelmont D: Importance of trigger sensitivity to ventilator delay in advanced COPD. Crit Care Med 17:354–359, 1989.
75. MacIntyre NR: Importance of trigger sensitivity to ventilator response delay in advanced COPD (letter). Crit Care Med 18:581–582, 1990.
76. Sassoon CSH, Giron AE, Ely E, et al: Inspiratory work of breathing on flow-by and demand-flow continuous positive airway pressure. Crit Care Med 17:1108–1114, 1989.
77. Petrof BJ, Legare M, Goldberg P, et al: Continuous positive airway pressure reduces work of breathing and dyspnea during weaning from mechanical ventilation in severe chronic obstructive pulmonary disease. Am Rev Respir Dis 141:281–289, 1990.
78. MacIntyre NR, McConnell R, Cheng KC: Applied PEEP reduces the inspiratory load of intrinsic PEEP during pressure support. Chest 111:188–193, 1997.
79. Takahashi T, Takezawa J, Kimura T, et al: Comparison of inspiratory work of breathing in T-piece breathing, PSV, and pleural pressure support ventilation (PPSV). Chest 100:1030–1034, 1991.
80. Marini JJ: Strategies to minimize breathing effort during mechanical ventilation. Crit Care Clin 6:635–661, 1990.
81. Flick GR, Belamy PE, Simmons DH: Diaphragmatic contraction during assisted mechanical ventilation. Chest 96:130–135, 1989.
82. Marini JJ, Smith TC, Lamb VJ: External work output and force generation during synchronized intermittent mechanical ventilation. Am Rev Respir Dis 138:1169–1179, 1988.
83. MacIntyre NR, McConnell R, Cheng KC, et al: Pressure limited breaths improve flow dys-synchrony during assisted ventilation. Crit Care Med 25:16761–16767, 1997.
84. Ho L, MacIntyre NR: Effects of initial flow rate and breath termination criteria on pressure support ventilation: Chest 99:134–138, 1991.
85. Banner MJ, Blanch PB, Kirby RR: Imposed work of breathing and methods of triggering a demand-flow, continuous positive airway pressure system. Crit Care Med 21:1183–1190, 1993.
86. Younes M: Proportional assist ventilation, a new approach to ventilatory support. Am Rev Respir Dis 145:114–120, 1992.
87. Kacmarek RM: The role of pressure support ventilation in reducing imposed work of breathing. Respir Care 33:99–120, 1988.
88. Jubran A, Van de Graaf WB, Tobin MJ: Variability of patient ventilator interactions with pressure support ventilation in patients with chronic obstructive pulmonary disease. Am J Respir Crit Care Med 152:129–136, 1995.
89. Marini JJ, Culver BH, Butler J: Mechanical effect of lung inflation with positive pressure on cardiac function. Am Rev Respir Dis 124:382–386, 1979.
90. Scharf SM, Caldini P, Ingram RH Jr: Cardiovascular effects of increasing airway pressure in the dog. Am J Physiol 232:1135–1143, 1977.
91. Pinsky MR, Summer WR, Wise RA, et al: Augmentation of cardiac function by elevation of intrathoracic pressure. J Appl Physiol 54:450–455, 1983.
92. Hughes JM, Glazier JB, Maloney JE, et al: Effect of lung volume on the distribution of pulmonary blood flow in man. Respir Physiol 4:58–72, 1968.
93. Lemaire F, Teboul JL, Cinotti L, et al: Acute left ventricular dysfunction during unsuccessful weaning from mechanical ventilation. Anesthesiology 69:171–179, 1988.
94. Jenkinson SG: Oxygen toxicity. New Horiz 1:504–511, 1993.
95. Betbese AJ, Perez M, Bak E, et al: A prospective study of unplanned endotracheal extubation in ICU patients. Crit Care Med 26:1180–1186, 1998.
96. Craven DE, Kunches LM, Kilinsky V, et al: Risk factors for pneumonia and fatality in patients receiving continuous mechanical ventilation. Am Rev Respir Dis 133:792–796, 1986.
97. Langer M, Mosconi P, Cigada M, et al: Long-term respiratory support and risk of pneumonia in critically ill patients. Am Rev Respir Dis 140:302–305, 1989.
98. Fagon J, Chastre J, Domart Y, et al: Nosocomial pneumonia in patients receiving continuous mechanical ventilation. Am Rev Respir Dis 139:877–884, 1989.

98a. Holzapfel L, Chastang C, Demingeon G, et al: A randomized study assessing the systematic search for maxillary sinusitis in nasotracheally mechanically ventilated patients. Influence of nosocomial maxillary sinusitis on the occurrence of ventilator-associated pneumonia. Am J Respir Crit Care Med 159:695–701, 1999.

98b. Kollef MH: The prevention of ventilator-associated pneumonia. N Engl J Med 340:627–634, 1999.

99. Kollef MH, Shapiro SD, Fraser VG, et al: Mechanical ventilation with or without 7 day circuit change. Ann Intern Med 123:168–174, 1995.
100. Mahjul P, Auboyer C, Jospe R, et al: Prevention of nosocomial pneumonia in intubated patients: Respective role of mechanical subglottic secretion drainage and stress ulcer prophylaxis. Intensive Care Med 18:20–25, 1992.

# 95

# Ethics and Withdrawal of Life Support

THOMAS A. RAFFIN, M.D.

Introduction
Goals of Critical Care Medicine
ICU Mortality Rates
Patient and Physician Preferences in the ICU
Fundamental Principles of Biomedical Ethics
- Beneficence
- Nonmaleficence
- Autonomy
- Justice

Physician Virtues
Legal Precedents in Ethical Decision Making
Government Legislation and Regulations in Ethical Decision Making
Key Practical Principles in Ethical Decision Making
- Source of Authority
- Effective Communication
- Quality-of-Life Values
- Patients' Rights

Brain Death and Organ Transplantation
Withholding Basic Life Support
Withholding Advanced Life Support
Withdrawing Advanced Life Support
Withdrawing Basic Life Support
Euthanasia
Summary

## INTRODUCTION

Critically ill patients, especially those in respiratory failure, require management in intensive care units (ICUs). ICUs evolved from postoperative recovery rooms and specialized care units devoted to patients with severe injuries, burns, trauma, and poliomyelitis.[1] In the early 1960s, only 10% to 20% of hospitals in the United States had ICUs. However, in the 1990s, almost all of the 6000 acute care hospitals in the United States had ICUs, and many large medical centers have numerous specialty critical care units, including cardiac, cardiovascular surgical, medical, neurosurgical, surgical, trauma, and burn units.[1]

It is estimated that there are approximately 78,000 ICU beds in acute care hospitals in the United States.[2] The overall average daily charge for critical care ranges from $2000 to $10,000/day. From these charges, it is estimated that critical care costs more than $80 billion/year. Because total health care expenditures in 1998 were estimated to be more than $1 trillion, critical care expenditures now account for almost 10% of all national health care expenditures.[3] The gross domestic product (GDP) of the United States is approximately $6 trillion, and total health care expenditures are more than 14% of the GDP. Thus, the cost of intensive care accounts for almost 1% of the GDP.[2]

As ICUs were growing in number and critical care medicine was becoming a discipline, complex dilemmas arose in ethical decision making, often dealing with withholding or withdrawing life support.[1, 4] One of the key legal cases that began the national debate on this issue was the 1976 case of Karen Ann Quinlan in New Jersey. This case is discussed in the section on legal precedents in ethical decision making. Since this first major court case dealing with withdrawing life support, there have been numerous cases dealing with both withholding and withdrawing life support, and one of them, the case of Nancy Cruzan case, was heard by the US Supreme Court.

This chapter focuses on the goals of critical care medicine; the fundamental principles of biomedical ethics; the virtues of a physician; the legal precedents, government legislation, and regulations; and key practical principles in ethical decision making and in brain death and organ transplantation. It concludes with sections on withholding basic life support, withholding advanced life support, withdrawing advanced life support, withdrawing basic life support, and euthanasia.

## GOALS OF CRITICAL CARE MEDICINE

Physicians, nurses, respiratory therapists, and other members of the ICU health care team have two major goals when caring for critically ill patients. The first goal is to save the salvageable. Initially, a medical judgment must be made whether or not a patient is salvageable. Then, if the patient appears to be salvageable, the health care team does all in its power to save the patient as long as this follows the patient's wishes. Fundamentally, the critical care team is following two age-old tenets of medicine: to restore health and to relieve suffering. These two key tenets of medicine have been written about since the times of Hippocrates, Galen, and Maimonides.[5] Physicians in emergency rooms and ICUs stop patients from dying by instituting life support measures such as mechanical ventilation or massive fluid resuscitation with inotropic support. Usually, the patient is stabilized over the course of several hours to many days, and then the critical care team must wait for the patient to heal and regain strength. Essentially, it is the wisdom of the body that dictates which organ systems will heal and recover and which patients will live. Critical care team members can do only so much. The rest is in the wise hands of nature.

The second goal of physicians caring for critically ill patients is to help the dying have a peaceful and dignified death. This is an extremely important goal because many patients admitted to ICUs are admitted there to die. This can easily be understood by reviewing mortality rates of specific subpopulations of patients admitted to ICUs. Because many patients admitted to ICUs will die there, it is important for ICU health care team members to understand that death is both an enemy and a colleague. In other words, it is entirely appropriate and oftentimes a thoughtful and sensitive act to assist a hopelessly ill patient to die with peace and dignity. This should not be perceived as a failure. It takes a great deal of skill and sensitivity to work closely with patients, their families or surrogates, and other health care team members in supporting a sensitive and compassionate death. Close attention to the needs of family members who will be left behind can result in a more effective and shortened grieving process and a healthier return to functional life. Because of these complex and delicate issues, research studies on critically ill patients in the ICU pose special problems.[5a]

## ICU MORTALITY RATES

The overall death rate for all patients admitted to ICUs is approximately 15% to 20%.[6] However, this low mortality rate includes large numbers of patients in subpopulations with extremely low mortality rates. For example, patients who have coronary artery bypass graft surgery are admitted to ICUs postoperatively, usually for only 2 to 3 days. Of the more than 350,000 patients in the United States who underwent coronary artery bypass graft procedures in 1998, the mortality rate was approximately 4% to 6%, and the overall cost was $5 to $6 billion. Similar low mortality rates are also seen in other surgical subpopulations who require intensive care, such as patients who have undergone neurosurgery or major vascular surgery. Of the hundreds of thousands of Americans who take drug overdoses every year in an attempt to commit suicide, only 5% to 10% needed to be admitted to ICUs because they developed respiratory failure; the mortality rate in this subpopulation admitted to ICUs is only 5% to 6%.[6] If postoperative patients and overdose patients with low mortality rates are excluded in estimating the overall mortality rates of patients in ICUs in the United States, a truer overall value is 30% to 40%.

Investigators have been publishing mortality statistics from individual ICUs since the mid-1970s.[6] For example, in 1984, Cullen and coworkers[7] updated an earlier study published in 1976 on the outcome of critically ill patients in a surgical ICU. The overall mortality rate was 69%, in comparison with a 73% mortality rate in 1976. One difference in the two studies is that in 1984, it appeared that the survivors' quality of life improved significantly after their stay in the ICU. A study by LeGall and coworkers[8] in France revealed that 66% of patients were discharged from the ICU alive, but the survival rate fell to 50% at 6 months and was 49% at 1 year.

During the 1980s, a number of research groups attempted to develop classification systems to standardize data describing critically ill patients. One of the best-known classification systems is the Acute Physiologic Assessment and Chronic Health Evaluation (APACHE) system developed by Knaus and coworkers.[9] The original APACHE study gave rise to the APACHE II severity of disease classification system for acutely ill patients.[10] The APACHE II system uses a point score based on values of 12 routine physiologic measurements, on age, and on previous health status to provide a measure of severity of disease. Research revealed that an increasing score was closely correlated with the subsequent risk of hospital death for 5815 admissions at 13 hospitals.

APACHE II data published in 1985 shed important light on prognosis of ICU patients with organ system failures.[11] Knaus and coworkers developed objective criteria for five organ system failures (cardiovascular, respiratory, renal, hematologic, and neurologic) and then monitored ICU admissions. The number and duration of organ system failures were linked to outcome at hospital discharge for 2719 ICU patients (48%) who developed them. The data demonstrated that for all medical and most surgical admissions, a single organ system failure lasting more than a day resulted in a mortality rate approaching 40%. Two organ system failures lasting for more than a day increased the death rate to 60%. Three or more organ system failures persisting after 3 days resulted in a mortality rate of 98%. Advanced chronologic age increased both the probabilities of developing organ system failure and of death once organ system failure occurred. The APACHE II classification system has been extremely important in helping us understand the link between organ system failure and mortality in critically ill patients. Furthermore, it has given rise to larger and more widespread research and patient care tools such as APACHE III.

Numerous subpopulations of critically ill patients in the ICU have death rates from 80% to 100%. Patients with acute respiratory distress syndrome (ARDS) have death rates ranging from 40% to 100%. The prognosis is significantly worse in ARDS when it is due to bacterial sepsis.[12]

A US and international, multicenter, prospective survey was conducted to determine the hospital survival rates of patients with acute respiratory failure (ARF) managed in sophisticated ICUs.[13] A total of 1426 patients with ARF were studied. Of the survey patients, 793 (55.6%) survived their hospitalization, whereas 633 (44.4%) died in the hospital. Survival rates were higher in patients with ARF caused by pneumonia (63%) or postshock lung injury (67%) and lower in patients with ARF caused by sepsis (46%). Severity of lung injury at the time of entry into the survey was a major prognostic factor. In addition, patients with ARF and with multiorgan failure had lower survival rates (10%) than those with pulmonary dysfunction alone (45%). Patients who required more than 14 days of mechanical ventilation and were transferred to a long-term acute care hospital had a particularly bad prognosis; a 1-year follow-up study showed that 77% had died, typically after spending most of their days in a medical facility.[13a]

The development of renal failure markedly increases the risk of death in critically ill patients in ICUs.[6] Liver failure has also been demonstrated to produce a high mortality rate in ICU patients.[6] A classic study published in 1991 concerned the decision-making autonomy of burn patients when it was clear from their presentation that survival was improbable.[13b] The authors, Imbus and Zawacki, took the stance that when burns are so severe, survival is improbable, and thus an aggressive approach to decision making should be invoked to preserve patient autonomy. While patients were still lucid, and after having been told of their prognosis, they were asked whether they wanted to choose between a full therapeutic regimen or ordinary care. Because survival was improbable, it was quite reasonable for patients to consider choosing ordinary care.

The longer a patient is in the ICU, the greater is the chance for severe morbidity or death. This statement may seem paradoxical because a critically ill patient can ordinarily be saved only in an ICU. However, the reason for this statement is to emphasize the fact that a stay in the ICU carries many risks. The leading cause of death in critically ill patients in the ICU is infection. In 1985, Montgomery and colleagues[12] evaluated the causes of mortality in patients with ARDS. Among 47 patients with ARDS, the mortality rate was 68%. However, only 16% of these patients died because of respiratory failure. Seventy-three percent of the patients died from sepsis and multisystem organ failure. It is uncommon for patients in respiratory failure on mechanical ventilation to die because of difficulty in managing the ventilator. The leading infections in critically ill patients in ICUs are sepsis, nosocomial pneumonia, and other nosocomial infections such as catheter-related urinary tract infections.[14] For example, it is estimated that patients with ARDS have a 60% incidence of nosocomial pneumonia.[15] Nosocomial pneumonia, often with sepsis, can lead to multisystem organ failure and a grim prognosis. Other key factors leading to death in critically ill patients in ICUs include severe arrhythmias and cardiac arrest, acute airway problems, abdominal catastrophes, pneumothorax, catastrophic gastrointestinal bleeding, and pulmonary embolism.[16]

## PATIENT AND PHYSICIAN PREFERENCES IN THE ICU

The ICU is a foreign, frightening, and bewildering place for patients, families, and surrogates. Odd noises assault their ears: high-pitched regular beeps, alarms, buzzers, and the deep rhythmic swooshing sounds of machines that aid breathing. Intravenous bottles with tubes dangle from the ceiling like mysterious vines. Patients and family members feel a complete loss of control and believe that they are treated as if they were once again children. They are surrounded by desperately ill patients who are the center of attention in a massive struggle between sophisticated and well-trained health care providers, remarkable machinery and technology, and the unrelenting power of nature.

Since the mid-1980s, a number of investigators have attempted to define patient, family, and physician preferences regarding the delivery of critical care. In 1988, medical ICU patients who were at least 55 years old and had been in an ICU during a 1-year period were interviewed[17]; family members were interviewed if the patient had died. Of note, 70% of patients and families were 100% willing for the patient to undergo intensive care again to achieve even 1-month survival. Only 8% were completely unwilling to undergo intensive care to achieve any prolonged survival. For 82% of the respondents, patient or family preferences were not well correlated with functional status or quality of life. Severity of critical illness, length of stay, age, and charges for intensive care did not influence willingness to undergo critical care management in an ICU. In 1986, a report of the preferences of homosexual men with acquired immunodeficiency syndrome (AIDS) for life-sustaining treatment documented that many were willing to forgo life-sustaining treatment if the prognosis was extremely poor.[18]

A report published in 1991 compared physician attitudes toward decision making in the care of critically ill patients as documented in a survey conducted in 1981 and repeated in 1988.[19] In the 1988 survey, physicians were more comfortable discussing do-not-resuscitate orders with patients and were more likely to allow a critically ill patient to die if that was the patient's wish. In both the 1981 and the 1988 surveys, most physicians believed that treatment costs should not play a significant role in medical decision making. Of interest was that physicians in 1988 felt that malpractice concerns were a more important determinant in their decision-making process than did physicians in 1981.

In 1992, the Society of Critical Care Medicine Ethics Committee presented an article that evaluated the attitudes of critical care professionals concerning forgoing life-sustaining treatments in critically ill patients.[20] At the Society's 1988 meeting, 600 questionnaires were returned from registrants. Fifty-six percent of the respondents were not disturbed by withholding or withdrawing treatment, whereas 26% were more disturbed by withdrawing than by withholding treatment. Of the 600 respondents, 89% had withheld and 87% had withdrawn life-prolonging treatments. Respondents felt that a physician's foremost professional duty to his or her patient is to preserve life but that it was important to evaluate and ensure quality of life carefully.

Some individuals who have never been admitted to an ICU are concerned and hesitant about being placed on life support in an effort to save their lives, even when there might be a good chance that they could be saved.

Furthermore, many health care professionals who work in ICUs understand that the struggle of some critically ill patients can be hopeless and torturous with no chance for recovery. However, in agreement with the results from the studies just cited, it seems clear that "substituted judgments" for incompetent patients concerning whether to provide or continue critical care must be made with objectivity and great thoughtfulness to ensure reflecting the values of the patient.

Physicians have significant difficulty in determining whether critically ill patients have a hopeless prognosis. The Study to Understand Prognoses and Preferences for Outcomes and Risk of Treatments (SUPPORT) enrolled over 9000 patients with one of nine serious illnesses over 4 years at five hospitals. This carefully performed multicenter study revealed that the level of communication between physicians, patients, and families was not optimal and that the intervention used by SUPPORT to improve communication was not effective.[21]

Another study utilized the SUPPORT and APACHE III data to determine how accurately physicians used the term "terminally ill."[22] This study revealed that statistical estimates of prognosis to define a category of "terminally ill" patients for public policy purposes are unavoidably arbitrary. Patients with predicted poor prognoses in the SUPPORT and APACHE populations often had numerical predictive values that supported hopefulness just days before death. One interesting suggestion from the study is that the common teaching that one can find a time to shift from aggressive to death-accepting care may be misleading. In both situations, both approaches may have to exist at the same time. Finally, there is no satisfactory definition of terminal illness. Thus, although predictive values from prognostic systems such as APACHE III may provide prognostic insight into large populations of patients, they are not that helpful for considering a specific individual patient.

Many people would like to believe there is great similarity among physicians in their judgement and approaches to decision-making concerning when to withhold or withdraw life support. The lack of credibility of this concept was nicely demonstrated by a Canadian study published in 1995.[23] A survey instrument developed for the study consisted of 12 clinical scenarios, and the responses were analyzed from 149 ICU attending physicians, 142 ICU residents, and 1070 ICU nurses. The respondents consistently identified as important the following factors in making their decisions: likelihood of long-term survival, premorbid cognitive function, and age of the patient. In choosing the appropriate level of care for the various patient scenarios, the same option was chosen by more than 50% of the respondents in only 1 of 12 scenarios. Of interest, opposite extremes of care were chosen by more than 10% of the respondents in 8 of 12 scenarios. Thus, although ICU health care workers identified common patient factors important to decision-making in withdrawing care, there was marked variability in the level of care they chose.[24]

## FUNDAMENTAL PRINCIPLES OF BIOMEDICAL ETHICS

Biomedical ethics as a discipline flowered in the 1980s. In 1976, the case of Karen Ann Quinlan in New Jersey established that extraordinary life support could be withdrawn from patients with, in essence, no chance to regain any reasonable quality of life.[25] In 1983, the President's Commission for the Study of Ethical Problems in Medicine and Biomedical and Behavioral Research published its extensive and ground-breaking report to the nation.[26] During this period, physicians, philosophers, scholars, lawyers, ethicists, and ethics committees began to study biomedical ethics and the ethical dilemmas that confront medicine.[1, 27–33] Because of the exponential growth in technology and the remarkable capabilities of modern medicine, we are confronted with new and complex ethical quandaries wherever we turn: the use of human fetal tissue, genetic alteration of nonhuman species, gene therapy in humans, and newer approaches to in vitro fertilization. As we attempt to grapple with these advances in medicine and science, we remain conflicted over older and unresolved biomedical ethical problems: relieving suffering in irreversibly impaired patients with powerful analgesics that might hasten their deaths; withdrawing food and water from patients in chronic, persistent vegetative states; use of animals in education and research; and the role of abortion.

"Ethics" is a generic term for a variety of ways of investigating and attempting to define a moral life. Two major ethical theories, consequentialist and deontologic, provide a basis for analyzing biomedical ethical issues.[30–33] The consequentialist theory supports actions as right or wrong according to their consequences rather than any intrinsic features they may have. A key consequentialist theory is utilitarianism, whose origins are found in the writings of David Hume, Jeremy Bentham, and John Stuart Mill. Deontologic ethical theory puts forth the premise that certain acts or situations are inherently right or wrong. Both ethical theories have strengths and weaknesses. To understand, analyze thoughtfully, and make judgments about biomedical ethical dilemmas that we must deal with when caring for critically ill patients in ICUs, it is important to be well versed in the four fundamental principles of biomedical ethics (Table 95.1). These help to make ethical decision making more pragmatic and available to nonphilosophers (e.g., to health care professionals) confronting biomedical ethical questions.

### Beneficence

Beneficence means to do good or, in medicine, to restore health and relieve suffering. It is the fundamental duty of the physician to benefit the patient. This means that the health care provider attempts to preserve the patient's life.

**Table 95.1** FOUR FUNDAMENTAL BIOMEDICAL ETHICAL PRINCIPLES

| |
|---|
| Beneficence |
| Nonmaleficence |
| Autonomy |
| Justice |

The concepts of preserving life and appreciation for the sanctity of life have their roots in most religious traditions.

## Nonmaleficence

Nonmaleficence means to do no harm *(primum non nocere)*. Most health care providers believe that they do not often violate this principle. However, there are many times when health care providers order unnecessary diagnostic tests or new therapeutic drugs or techniques that result in significant morbidity or mortality. In the ICU, an example of this might be placing a nonindicated intravascular catheter, which results in a pneumothorax or sepsis. Such an act is in direct violation of the principle of nonmaleficence. Unfortunately, it is quite common for health care professionals to violate this principle because of the great numbers of available diagnostic and therapeutic modalities, many of which are not especially helpful to patients and can frankly harm them.

For example, a violation of nonmaleficence could occur when a patient asks a physician for an antibiotic to treat an ordinary (viral) cold. The physician, although knowing that the patient will not benefit from an antibiotic, nonetheless complies with the patient's request and prescribes a commonly used antibiotic such as tetracycline. Six days later the patient has a severe hypersensitivity reaction to the antibiotic, develops acute necrotizing epidermolysis, becomes critically ill, and dies. This example gives us insight into how easily the principle of nonmaleficence can be violated.

Extreme violation of the principle of nonmaleficence regularly occurs in the ICU. When health care practitioners are caring for patients on life support who have, in essence, no chance to regain a reasonable quality of life and are simply languishing and suffering, the principle of nonmaleficence or "first do no harm" is being violated. The purpose of critical care in an ICU is to save the patient's life and return the patient to a reasonable quality of life (as determined by the patient). The goal is not to prolong dying. The Hippocratic oath expresses a duty of nonmaleficence together with beneficence: "I will use treatment to help the sick according to my ability and judgment, but I will never use it to injure or wrong them."[32]

One possible violation of the ethical principle of nonmaleficence has been occurring in the United States since the rapid growth in health care costs during the past several decades: the attempt by some health care providers to accumulate great wealth by exploiting the practice of medicine. This violation is especially grave in consideration of the fact that we are rationing health care dollars. There are many examples of corporations and individuals who have attempted to accumulate inappropriate levels of wealth and to profit from their patients or society's ability to pay for health care. In the US health care system, this has been a destructive force. Actions such as these clearly wrong our patients and society. Examples include inappropriately large profits by corporations producing medical supplies, equipment, and drugs; overutilization of diagnostic and therapeutic modalities, including endoscopy and surgery; and unnecessarily high charges that allow some health care professionals to have salaries significantly greater than many hundreds of thousands of dollars per year. The great American entrepreneurial spirit has made commerce in the United States strong, but our troubled health care system must be reorganized with appropriate regulation in order to function effectively with reasonable cost.

## Autonomy

Autonomy means respecting the individuality and personhood of others. This allows patients to be self-determining agents. Patients are to be treated not as children in a paternalistic physician-patient relationship but rather as partners in adult-adult interactions. In actuality, patients are much more than equal partners in arriving at decisions affecting their own lives and should be encouraged to assume the responsibility of this partnership. The term "autonomy" is derived from the Greek word meaning self-rule or self-governance in Greek city-states. Greek citizens made their own laws, as opposed to having them imposed on them. A legally competent adult in the United States who is not trying to commit suicide is in charge of his or her own health care. The legal basis that supports the right of a patient to refuse treatment is the common-law right of self-determination and the constitutionally derived "right of privacy." The legal right of autonomy was recognized by the US Supreme Court (not specifically dealing with health care matters) as long ago as 1891, when it stated,

> "No right is held more sacred or is more carefully guarded by the common law than the right of every individual to the possession and control of his own person, free from all restraints or interference by others, unless by clear and unquestionable authority of law."[34]

It is vital in the practice of modern medicine to obtain informed consent from patients after ensuring that they understand the risks and benefits of a diagnostic or therapeutic procedure. It is extremely important when caring for critically ill patients to be honest and make sure that communication has been truthful.[35] If an adult patient is not legally competent to give informed consent, then a close relative or a surrogate decision maker should be involved in the decision making. This concept is further discussed in the section on legal precedents in ethical decision making.

In the United States, minors do not have autonomy under law to make health care decisions for themselves. In addition, US courts believe that they have more responsibility than parents in making sure appropriate health care decisions have been made for minors. For example, if parents discover that their child has acute lymphoblastic leukemia and they want to take the child to be treated with amygdalin (Laetrile) or multivitamin therapy instead of clinically proven therapy, courts will intercede and take the child away from the parents to ensure that the child receives standard-of-practice care. In contrast, if a critically ill, definitely salvageable adult who is legally competent and is clearly not trying to commit suicide elects not to be admitted to an ICU where available therapies could save the patient's life, it is the right of the patient through his or her ethical and legal autonomy to decide not to receive indicated critical care treatment. As will be emphasized again in this chapter, in almost all cases, decision-making capacity lies in the hands of the patient, not in the hands of health care providers.

### Justice

Justice is the support of the fair allocation of medical resources to citizens. Currently in the United States, we do not have just allocation of medical resources. Economically disadvantaged Americans suffer greater morbidity and mortality from illness and die younger in most disease-specific categories than do middle-class citizens. In addition, federal and state governments pass regulations and statutes that provide unjust care for the poor and disadvantaged. For example, not to allow the poor to have abortions or receive transplants while allowing the middle class to receive these treatments is not consonant with a just system of health care. This remains true even if an individual state such as Oregon decides it must ration health care to the uninsured and underinsured. It is the responsibility of the entire country to provide just health care.

The four fundamental principles of biomedical ethics can be used to analyze complex biomedical ethical issues. They help place in perspective the ethical dilemmas that confront us and lead to a more thoughtful and ethical practice of medicine. It is important to remember that these four key ethical principles are based on many complex and, at times, antagonistic ethical theories from a variety of scholars and that have evolved through history.

Depending on one's point of view, an individual can use one or more of the four principles to support an argument even though another person may use a different one of the same principles to support the opposite position. One example of how these four ethical principles can come into conflict can be seen in some of the current discussions concerning the management of human immunodeficiency virus (HIV) infections: preventing infections in persons unknowingly exposed to a patient with possible HIV infection conflicts with respecting the autonomy of that patient and the confidentiality of his or her HIV test result.

## PHYSICIAN VIRTUES

Besides using the four biomedical ethical principles in decision making, health care providers need to nurture within themselves the personal virtues paramount to medical practice.[36] The virtues addressed here are moral virtues. Key moral virtues that are often identified as important to the provision of health care include benevolence and compassion, truthfulness and trustworthiness, respect for persons, justice, piety (not relating to any specific creed or form of worship), hope, and prudence. Virtue ethics are important to all persons, but they are essential to health care providers. They identify a way of life for the physician. Furthermore, health care professionals can obtain these virtues by practicing them.

It is important to remember that medicine is a moral enterprise grounded in a covenant of trust.[37, 38] For physicians to optimize their care of patients, they must focus on ways to optimize communication. Unfortunately, the current state of physician-patient communication leaves much to be desired. Numerous studies demonstrate persistent patient dissatisfaction with the amount and type of information received from physicians.[39]

Cultural differences also play an important role in physician-patient communication. In the United States and in many other countries, it is increasingly common for health professional to find themselves in cross-cultural situations; confronted with the cultural considerations of ethical decision-making. There have been articles focusing on ethical decision-making in critical care in other countries containing unique cultural dimensions.[40]

## LEGAL PRECEDENTS IN ETHICAL DECISION MAKING

Numerous decisions by state courts and legislatures have helped build a legal framework in the approach to biomedical ethical issues in the United States. It is important to remember that a court decision or legislative action in one particular state is not accepted as law by other states. Furthermore, just as individual positions and insights into morality and ethics differ, so do the arbitrary judgments of state and federal courts and legislatures. There can be no question that the background, experiences, morality, and politics of jurors and legislators play a vital role in forming their decisions. Thus, there is always an arbitrary component in judicial and legislative action.

The case of Karen Ann Quinlan in 1976 concerned a 22-year-old woman who became comatose after the probable ingestion of alcohol and drugs.[25] She was supported on mechanical ventilation, was not brain dead, but was in a persistent vegetative state with a very poor prognosis. Her father, believing that his daughter would not want to live under such circumstances, had himself appointed her legal guardian and asked her physicians to remove her from the ventilator and allow her to die. The physicians refused, and the clinical case went to court.

The New Jersey Supreme Court evaluated "the reasonable possibility of return to cognitive and sapient life as distinguished from . . . biological vegetative existence."[25] The court believed that a benefit would exist when life-sustaining treatment would result in "at very least, a remission of symptoms enabling a return toward a normal functioning, integrated existence."[25] In addition, the court believed that such ethical decisions should be made by the physician and family.

The New Jersey Supreme Court ruled that Quinlan had a constitutional "right to privacy" to be removed from the ventilator if the family, physicians, and hospital ethics committee agreed. The court ruled that, in the absence of information from the patient or self, the physicians and family had the right to make the decision to withdraw life support. In addition, the court indicated that the family's wishes could overrule the physicians' concerns. In other words, "substituted judgments" could be made for incompetent adults. Because Quinlan was in a persistent vegetative state, she was able to breathe and remained alive after the ventilator was discontinued. She lived for 10 more years with no cognitive function.

In the case of *Saikewicz v. Superintendent of Belcher State School*, the Supreme Court of the State of Massachusetts in 1977 decided that without information from the patient and his family, only the court, not the physician and family, could make "substituted judgments" and therefore decisions to withhold life support.[41] With the advent of this decision, health care professionals in Massachusetts became frightened about making decisions concerning withholding and withdrawing life support without the assistance of the courts. In 1978, the Massachusetts Court of Appeals in the Dinnerstein case decided that family and physician could, indeed, make a thoughtful judgment concerning withholding life support without having to bring the case to the courts.[42]

In 1981, Clarence Herbert, a 55-year-old Californian, suffered postoperative cardiac arrest that left him with severe brain damage. Two days later, his family agreed with his physicians that advanced life support should be withdrawn owing to the grim prognosis and the patient's earlier comments that he did not wish to be kept alive artificially. Herbert did not die when the ventilator was discontinued. Two days later, the family agreed that basic routine life support, which included intravenous fluids and nutrition, should be stopped. One week later, Herbert died. The two physicians who cared for Herbert were prosecuted for murder by the Los Angeles District Attorney in 1983 in *Barber v. Superior Court*.[43] The court referred to the Quinlan decision when defining such terms as benefits and burdens. The Barber decision stated that nutrition and hydration were medical procedures and should be evaluated by health care providers:

> "Medical procedures to provide nutrition and hydration are more similar to other medical procedures than to typical human ways of providing nutrition and hydration. Their benefits and burdens ought to be evaluated in the same manner as any other medical procedure."[43]

Another key element from the Barber decision was the identification of who can appropriately decide for incompetent patients. The court noted that the physicians must identify a surrogate to make a "substituted judgment" on the patient's behalf. The California court stated that it was not necessary to have formal conservatorship proceedings.

The right of competent adult patients with fatal diseases to refuse treatment over the objection of physicians in hospitals was affirmed in the California case *Bartling v. Superior Court*.[44] Mr. Bartling had severe lung disease, was chronically attached to a ventilator, and also had lung cancer. He was legally competent, and he and his family wanted him removed from the ventilator because of his poor quality of life and grim prognosis. Mr. and Mrs. Bartling knew this would mean that Mr. Bartling would die. The physicians and hospital refused, and thus the case was brought to court. The California State Court of Appeals ruled in favor of Bartling after his death. They stated,

> "If the right of the patient to self-termination as to his own medical treatment is to have any meaning at all, it must be paramount to the interests of the patient's hospital and doctors. The right of a competent ill patient to refuse medical treatment is a constitutionally guaranteed right which must not be abridged."[44]

In 1986, the California case *Bouvia v. Superior Court* established the right of a patient to refuse both nourishment and hydration.[45] Ms. Bouvia was an intelligent young quadriplegic woman with cerebral palsy who had unrelenting pain and demanded that the hospital halt her food and water so that she could die. The California State Court of Appeals, in April 1986, overturned a lower court's decision and held that state policy did not require "all and every life must be preserved against the will of the sufferer." Bouvia was allowed to leave the hospital. At this writing, she remains alive.

In 1986, the Massachusetts case *Brophy v. New England Sinai Hospital* supported the withholding of nutrition and hydration from a fireman in a chronic, persistent vegetative state.[46] The Massachusetts court ruled in this manner because the evidence showed that the patient would never regain cognitive abilities, communication skills, or the capability of interacting purposefully with his environment.

In 1988, the State of California in the case of Drabick ruled that mentally incapacitated patients have the right to have appropriate decisions made on their behalf by surrogate decision makers.[47] The family wanted nutrition and hydration withdrawn from Drabick, who was in a chronic, persistent vegetative state. The court supported the Drabick family, and life support was withdrawn. In 1983, the President's Commission urged adoption of the "proportionate treatment test" in situations in which an individual did not make his or her wishes known in a legally acceptable manner by writing or leaving a living will. In the 1983 *Barber v. Superior Court* decision, the court relied on a proportionate treatment analysis. In the Drabick case, the court also focused on the question of whether the benefits of the treatment outweighed the detriments. Specifically, it stated:

> "Proportionate treatment is that which, in the view of the patient, has at least a reasonable chance of providing benefits to the patient, which benefits outweigh the burdens attendant to the treatment. Thus, even if a proposed course of treatment might be extremely painful or intrusive, it would still be proportionate treatment if the prognosis was for complete cure or significant improvement in the patient's condition. On the other hand, a treatment course which is only minimally painful or intrusive may nonetheless be considered disproportionate to the potential benefits if the prognosis is virtually hopeless for any significant condition."[47]

Although California courts delivered the progressive Drabick decision in 1988, the state courts in New York and Missouri made it more difficult to withhold or withdraw life-sustaining treatment from incompetent patients.[39, 40] In the O'Connor case in New York, the court ruled that treatment must be given unless there is unequivocal evidence that the patient would have chosen to refuse it.[48] This decision was extremely rigid and set a standard of proof that few patients were likely to fulfill. In the case of Nancy Cruzan, the Missouri court declared that the state had an "unqualified" interest in prolonging and preserving life.[49] The Missouri court markedly limited the right of families to make decisions on behalf of incompetent patients. The court wanted "the most rigid of formalities" to be used to make decisions when treatment should be stopped. The court desired a written document, a living will, or absolutely clear and convincing evidence of a patient's refusal to be treated. Then, the Missouri court went on to undermine the legality of all advance directives (living wills): "It is definitionally impossible for a person to make an informed decision—either to consent or refuse—under hypothetical circumstances."[49] Missouri's living will law did not permit the refusal of artificial feedings. The court specifically ruled that continued tube feedings were "not heroically invasive" because the "invasion took place when the gastrostomy tube was inserted."[49]

In June 1990, the US Supreme Court made its landmark ruling on the Cruzan case, which was appealed by the State of Missouri.[49–52] This was the first case the Supreme Court had ever ruled on concerning the ethics of withholding and withdrawing life support. As expected, the Supreme Court upheld the State of Missouri in its position that a state can prohibit families from withdrawing life support from an incompetent loved one if there is not clearly convincing evidence that the loved one wanted life support to be withheld or withdrawn. The Supreme Court voted 5 to 4 in support of the Missouri law. This ruling was narrow, without sweeping implications, because it upheld the rights of states to decide what type of evidence they require when allowing families and physicians to withhold or withdraw life support. It was fundamentally a states' rights issue. Chief Justice William Rehnquist wrote, "There is no automatic assurance that the view of close family members will be necessarily the same as the patient's would have been had she been confronted with her situation while competent." The chief justice implied that had Cruzan filled out a legal living will in the state of Missouri, the Supreme Court might have honored such a signed petition. Thus, the Cruzan decision both supported the right of states to decide how to handle withholding and withdrawing life support and upheld the importance of advance directives. Chief Justice Rehnquist wrote, "For purposes of this case, we assume that the United States Constitution would grant a competent person a constitutionally protected right to refuse life saving hydration and nutrition."

New evidence was brought to bear by friends of Cruzan, and the Attorney General of Missouri decided that they would not have to go back to court to allow nutrition and hydration to be withdrawn. Thus, they were withdrawn in late 1990, and Cruzan died.

## GOVERNMENT LEGISLATION AND REGULATIONS IN ETHICAL DECISION MAKING

In the 1980s, state legislatures began to pass living will legislation that allowed state citizens the right of dictating what type of health care they would receive if they became legally incompetent.[53] Three types of legislation have been passed by individual states. First, some states have passed living will legislation. Second, some states have passed statutes called natural death act directives or declarations. Third, a number of states have passed legislation to support durable powers of attorney for health care.[54] Generic living wills not passed by specific state legislatures are available. However, it is important to remember that if a living will has not been approved by a specific state legislature, then it is not legally binding. Thus, if a person has a durable power of attorney for health care from the State of California but becomes critically ill and loses legal competence in the State of Missouri, the California living will document does not have validity in Missouri. However, living will documents are still of much value to families, loved ones, friends, and health care providers in determining what the patient would have wanted. Now, virtually all states have passed some form of living will legislation.

One of the most effective types of advance directives is a durable power of attorney for health care. The first durable power of attorney for health care law was passed in the State of Pennsylvania in 1982. In 1984, the California state legislature passed the California Durable Power of Attorney for Health Care Act, which allows individuals to identify treatment preferences in various clinical situations and to designate an "attorney in fact" who is empowered to make medical decisions should the patient become legally incompetent.[54]

In the same way that a will is of great importance to citizens because it guarantees that a person's wishes are carried out after death, a living will is a document that all adult Americans should have. Extensive court precedents and legislative action strongly support the view that life-sustaining treatment can be withheld if it can be determined that the incompetent patient would not have wanted it.[1, 26, 27, 43, 47] It is not necessary for a living will to identify all specific management approaches if different illnesses or catastrophes occur. It is best to complete advanced directives with generic statements such as "If I have, in essence, no chance to regain a reasonable quality of life, please withhold and withdraw life support (including nutrition and hydration) from me so that I can die with peace and dignity."

In 1990, the federal act dealing with advance directives, known as the Patient Self-Determination Act (PSDA), was passed.[55] The PSDA requires health care providers (hospitals, nursing homes, and health maintenance organizations) to (1) provide written information to all patients at the time of admission about advance directives; (2) document whether advance directives have been executed; and (3) educate their staff and the community about these documents, or risk having their federal Medicare and Medicaid reimbursements withheld.

Because a living will filled out by an individual patient is somewhat different from a durable power of attorney for health care, which enables an "attorney in fact" to make medical decisions when the patient is legally incompetent, some authors have proposed that patients fill out both a living will and a durable power of attorney for health care.[55] In all likelihood, by writing what is desired for care either in a living will or through a durable power of attorney for health care, the necessity of filling out both types of forms should be alleviated.

## KEY PRACTICAL PRINCIPLES IN ETHICAL DECISION MAKING

Four key practical principles should be followed in caring for patients and dealing with biomedical ethical issues (Table 95.2): (1) establish the source of authority for decision making; (2) achieve effective communication with patients and families; (3) make early determination and ongoing review of patient quality-of-life values and desires; and (4) recognize patients' rights.[1, 27]

### Source of Authority

The most important practical principle in ethical decision making is the understanding that the patient is the true source of authority. The actual authority over the patient does not reside with the physician. Patients have the ethical and legal autonomy to determine the health care that they will receive. If the patient is legally incompetent, appropriately identified family members or other surrogates (e.g., "attorney-in-fact") can decide what course of treatment to choose.[56] Many of the problems in ethical decision making are a result of not following this key principle. In effect, physicians are guides and consultants engaged to evaluate their patient's problems, present reasonable options for diagnosis and management in clear and understandable language, and facilitate thoughtful decision making. Except in emergencies or when further care is clearly futile, physicians should not proceed with management plans until those with true authority have made their decisions.

### Effective Communication

The second key practical principle in ethical decision making in patient care, especially in ICUs, is the necessity of health care providers to be able to communicate effectively with patients and families. Communication skills vary considerably among health care providers. Unfortunately, in ICUs, stress, fear, intimidation, and unfamiliarity with the setting can overwhelm even sophisticated patients and families. Health care professionals are responsible not only for attempting to communicate but also for making sure that effective communication has taken place. The solution to difficult problems involving withholding and withdrawing life support is determined through effective communication with patients, families, or surrogates. There is no more important skill.

**Table 95.2 FOUR KEY PRACTICAL PRINCIPLES FOR PATIENT CARE AND ETHICAL DECISION MAKING**

| |
|---|
| Establish the source of authority for decision making |
| Achieve effective communication with patients and families |
| Make early determination and ongoing review of patient quality of life values and desires |
| Recognize patients' rights |

Obviously, some health care providers communicate better than others. When physicians are made aware of difficulties with communication, they should promptly enlist a proven facilitator: a social worker, chaplain, rabbi, minister, ethicist, or psychotherapist, for example. There are a number of reasons why communication in ICUs is difficult for physicians. First, each patient problem is stressful and emotionally wrenching, which takes a significant physical and emotional toll on physicians. Second, the accumulation of many cases exacts a high price from physicians in terms of fatigue and distance, personal fear of death, guilt, insecurity, and anxiety. Third, effective communication in emergency situations requires time, an asset that is often unavailable to physicians working in ICUs. It is important to emphasize again that outside facilitators can be extremely valuable members of a health care team because they have both the communication skills and the time to work with patients, families, or surrogates. Unfortunately, physicians and other health care providers often do not enlist facilitators, possibly because they feel a loss of control over the care of the patient. It should be a rule rather than an exception to bring a facilitator in early whenever it appears that the ethical decision making will be difficult.

To optimize communication, it is important to ensure that the environment is not rushed or chaotic. Communication should be kept simple and honest and in as much detail as is needed. Patients, families, or surrogates should be encouraged to ask questions and to repeat in their own words what they have heard from health care providers.

Information should be presented in the language and at the level of detail that enables patients, families, or surrogates to make thoughtful decisions. Esoteric medical vocabulary will cause a patient or family to feel alienated or confused. Patients, families, or surrogates should always be asked to summarize what has been said, to ensure that communication has been accurate and to provide an opportunity to correct misunderstandings. Health care providers should ask colleagues to assist in determining whether their communication skills are optimal.

One example of inadequate communication is when a physician tells a family that their critically ill loved one is "stable," without providing much in the way of further explanation. Perhaps a more truthful report to the family would be "Your wife is as sick as any person could be, and the odds are overwhelming that she will not survive. She has not improved in 24 hours, and if she does not improve over the next several days, we might have to begin to discuss decreasing her level of critical care support."

Another example of inadequate communication is when a health care provider tells a family that their critically ill son has improved after 3 days, whereas in fact his overall status still carries a dismal prognosis and only one small, relatively unimportant physiologic measurement has mildly improved. This type of inappropriate good news, although making the health care provider feel better, puts the patient's family and loved ones on an unrealistic roller coaster and inappropriately alters their expectations. It is important to tell the truth and to provide accurate prognostic information.

## Quality-of-Life Values

The third key practical principle in ethical decision making is the need for early determination and regular review of the quality-of-life values and desires of individual patients. Physicians need to learn, whenever possible, the views of each patient or surrogate on the balance between quality and mere prolongation of life. This is the concept of proportionality discussed in the section on legal precedents. Health care professionals should avoid making assumptions in this area, especially with patients of different religious, cultural, or ethnic backgrounds. The balance between the possible extension of life and the reduction in quality of life resulting from any treatment course must be clearly described and discussed with each patient, family members, or surrogates.

Health care providers should not withhold difficult information, such as the diagnosis of a terminal condition, from patients, family, or surrogates. It is a physician's duty to be honest and straightforward. Specific treatment options for probable complications should be explored as early as possible to avoid unnecessary guilt in surrogates who are forced to decide for incompetent patients. For example, having a patient agree with a do-not-resuscitate order without informing the family might result in a situation in which the patient becomes legally incompetent and the family decides not to follow the wishes of the patient even though the patient's desires were stated in front of several health care providers. The relationship between the patient's surrogates and the health care team can become complex, highly emotional, and adversarial.

When an illness progresses, patients, family, or surrogates will reassess the relative costs and benefits of treatments as they gain insight into potential therapies and prognosis. Thus, it is important to evaluate patients' thoughts concerning proportionality when their disease status changes significantly.

## Patients' Rights

The fourth key practical principle in ethical decision making is the recognition that patients have significant rights. Most physicians do not know that the American Hospital Association developed a code of patients' rights and that this code has been enacted into law in many states.[57] Health care providers need to practice in the spirit of these rights. Some of the most important patients' rights are (1) to receive considerate and respectful care; (2) to receive information about the illness, the course of treatment, and the prospects for recovery in terms that the patient can understand; (3) to receive as much information about any proposed treatment or procedure as the patient may need in order to give informed consent or to refuse this course of treatment (except in emergencies, this information should include a description of the procedure or treatment, the medically important risks involved in this treatment, alternative courses of treatment or nontreatment and the risks involved in each, and the name of the person who will carry out the treatment or procedure); (4) to participate actively in decisions regarding the medical care (to the extent permitted by law, this includes the right to refuse treatment); and (5) to have patients' rights applied to the person who may have legal responsibility to make decisions about medical care on behalf of the patient.[27]

# BRAIN DEATH AND ORGAN TRANSPLANTATION

The development and expansion of organ transplantation has been a remarkable story in modern scientific medicine. Transplantation of kidneys, hearts, and bone marrow is commonplace. As discussed in Chapter 97, heart-lung, bilateral lung, and single lung transplantations are becoming established as effective therapy for selected patients.[58] During the development of organ transplantation, the definition of death was redefined because physicians were removing organs from patients who were on life support and whose hearts were still beating. In the early to mid-1960s, there was no widely accepted definition of brain death. State legislatures and courts brought in physicians to provide expert testimony to define death. The traditional definition of death at this time was the cessation of function of both the heart and the lungs.

The Ad Hoc Committee of the Harvard Medical School in 1968 wrote their report "To Define Irreversible Coma as a New Criterion for Death."[59] This gave rise to the current definition of death, which is total and irreversible loss of brain function.[26] To make the diagnosis of brain death, one must demonstrate irreversible loss of cerebral and brain-stem function, including ventilatory reflexes. Patients who have been taking drugs that suppress the central nervous system or who are hypothermic cannot be declared brain dead until these conditions have been reversed. It is not mandatory to perform electroencephalography or cerebral blood flow studies in patients to confirm brain death. Family or surrogate approval is not mandatory before brain death is determined, because the clinical diagnosis is a medical issue. However, it is mandatory to obtain family or surrogate approval before retrieving organs for transplantation from a brain-dead patient.

Infrequently, families give instructions not to withdraw life support from their brain-dead loved ones. This is a result of their emotional turmoil. With honest and sensitive communication, this issue can be resolved in the first 1 to 2 days.

One of the major limitations of widespread transplantation in the United States is the scarcity of donor organs. Therefore, it is vital that health care providers or other facilitators discuss this issue with family members or surrogates of patients who are brain dead or near brain death, because these patients might be ideal organ donors.[60] These issues must be discussed in a truthful and compassionate manner. Some states have developed legislation that requires discussion of potential transplant donor status with the surrogates of patients who are brain dead.

# WITHHOLDING BASIC LIFE SUPPORT

It is difficult to forgo providing basic life support such as food, water, and supplementary oxygen in medical practice. Often, basic life support is provided automatically, without fully considering whether this is always a truly caring act.

In critically ill patients, health care providers should consider four important points when deciding whether to provide basic life support. First, any medical intervention should deliver what patients consider to be in their best interests. This should be determined in an active and truthful dialogue with their families and physicians. Second, it is wise to include close family members and loved ones in the decision-making process whenever possible. This will enlist the family and loved ones on the side of the eventual treatment course, minimizing the possibility of conflict. Third, health care providers should anticipate the various likely medical courses and obtain as far in advance as possible reasonable choices the patient wishes to make for each major alternative. Fourth, once any medical intervention has begun in a critically ill patient, withdrawing it to end a prolonged dying process requires a direct action that will usually result in death.

Those forced to make such decisions and those who carry them out are inevitably left with disturbing feelings. Patients who are terminally ill, suffering, and awaiting death are better served by not having infections treated with antibiotics or cerebral edema treated with steroids. It is distressing to observe comatose, hopelessly ill patients being pulled back needlessly from a painless death to live out an extra few days or weeks in pain and indignity in a hospital. Sometimes, when this situation occurs, it is due to health care providers who are frustrated by impossible-to-treat illnesses and are attempting to gain some control by treating conditions and not the patient. If family members or legal surrogates for the patient want every possible measure taken to try to keep the patient alive, professionals usually should comply with this request. However, if the desire to persist in treatment seems inappropriate to the health care providers, a direct, logical challenge will often fail, whereas a sensitive and compassionate exploration of underlying feelings can result in thoughtful ethical decision making.[27] In addition, if continued care is medically futile, physicians have the right, but not without legal liability, to make the decision independently to stop treatment. This will be further analyzed in the discussion on futility in the section on withholding advanced life support.

For dying patients, physicians need to have a reason for placing intravenous lines. Once an intravenous line is in place, it becomes difficult to stop treating infections and chemical imbalances that might provide a humane death. The same reasoning applies to ordering laboratory tests or assessing vital signs. Once a treatment problem is identified, it becomes difficult not to act, especially because of the fear of legal action. Obviously, thinking before placing intravenous lines also applies to the placement of feeding tubes, especially in patients in chronic, persistent vegetative states.

## WITHHOLDING ADVANCED LIFE SUPPORT

Withholding advanced life support usually refers to not providing cardiopulmonary resuscitation (CPR) or intubation to critically ill patients. A number of important position papers have addressed the practicalities and ethics of withholding advanced life support.[1, 26, 27, 55, 61–68] A patient in cardiac or pulmonary arrest presents health care professionals with an emergency that produces a set of automatic responses if the patient is to be saved. Unless health care professionals are aware of the patient's previously expressed desires against resuscitation, they must act first and evaluate later.

A study published in 1983 of all the resuscitations at a major medical center in 1 year revealed that only 14% of patients who received CPR left the hospital alive.[69] Only 19% of patients discussed the procedure with their physicians, and in only one third of cases was the family consulted about resuscitation, even though more than 95% of physicians believed that such consultations were appropriate.

In a 1986 study, 22% of patients and 86% of families were involved in decisions not to resuscitate.[70] Families identified the attending physician as a source of help with decision making. A 1989 study reported on the success rate of CPR in 503 patients aged 70 and over in five Boston health care institutions.[71] Initially, 111 (22%) of all patients survived, but only 19 (3.8%) left the hospital alive. Only 2 of 244 patients (0.8%) with out-of-hospital cardiopulmonary arrest left the hospital alive. Only 17 of 259 patients (6.6%) with in-hospital arrest survived to discharge. Most survivors had ventricular arrhythmias and were resuscitated within minutes. Poor outcomes were found in patients with unwitnessed arrests, terminal arrhythmias such as asystole and electromechanical dissociation, and patients in whom CPR lasted more than 15 minutes.

The above studies point out the ethical dilemma presented by CPR. Because CPR is quite invasive and often brutal, it is hard to reconcile the small chance of a successful outcome with the loss of a dignified death. This is especially so in the setting of chronic, severe, or terminal disease. In attempting to minimize the occurrence of this type of deplorable situation, the health care provider should consider four important points. First, because a cardiopulmonary arrest could easily occur in an elderly, chronically ill, or terminally ill hospitalized patient, there is little ethical justification for not discussing CPR in advance. In addition, this point applies to similar patients who remain at home or in nursing homes. Second, decisions whether or not to resuscitate patients should be made early and conveyed to patients, families, and all health care providers. Third, prominent notations identifying resuscitation status should be placed on medical charts. Fourth, attending physicians should take the lead in bringing up the matter of whether to perform CPR. Physicians who do not believe they can participate in such decision making should probably not be caring for critically ill patients. All pulmonary and critical care medicine training programs must devote a component of their educational program to this area.

Some physicians have difficulty asking patients whether they want a do-not-resuscitate (DNR) order written in the chart. The reasons for this include stress, time limitations, and the emotional difficulty of having such a discussion with a patient, especially a long-term patient. Another reason why some physicians do not regularly ask patients about DNR orders is that most severely ill patients, when asked whether they want a DNR order, elect not to have one written in the chart. The main reason for this is the human desire to do everything possible to stay alive. Looking into the jaws of death is a terrifying proposition and something that normal people attempt to avoid at all costs. However, physicians should not be dissuaded from asking patients about DNR orders. In fact, physicians should always ask the following two questions (the second question should be asked only if the patient does not want a DNR order): (1) "Would you like us to write a DNR order in your medical chart? This means that if you have a cardiopulmonary arrest, you will not be resuscitated and that you will probably die." (2) "Let's presume you are successfully resuscitated and placed on life support in an ICU. If your health care providers determine after 72 hours of doing everything possible to save your life that you have, in essence, no chance to regain a reasonable quality of life, would you agree to let us withdraw life support and let you die with peace and dignity?"

The majority of patients who do not agree to a DNR order will agree to the second question. If a patient agrees with the second question, then it should be documented in the medical chart in front of witnesses, and the family or legal surrogates should be notified immediately to make sure that they are aware of the patient's plan and will not take a different position if the patient becomes legally incompetent. Thus, talking with patients about whether they want CPR is vitally important and, in almost all cases, will assist health care providers in determining how best to care for their patients.

In the late 1980s, biomedical ethicists began to define the obligations of the physician when care was medically futile. In 1988, Tomlinson and Brody[72] stated that "the right of self-determination, as well as the patient's preferences, is irrelevant to the determination that resuscitation would be of *no* [emphasis added] medical benefit. When this is the rationale for a DNR decision, the physician has no duty to ascertain the patient's preferences." The physician should always communicate effectively with patients and learn their preferences; however, if a management option is medically futile, the health care providers are not obligated to pursue this option. Some hospitals in the United States have CPR policies that state that CPR does not have to be administered if it is deemed medically futile by the physician or physicians of record.

The key problem in all of this is: what is the definition of medical futility? Many authorities believe three strict criteria need to be met to establish medical futility. First, the disease must be terminal. Second, the disease must be irreversible. Third, death must be imminent; however, the definition of imminent is somewhat arbitrary. Most health care providers would agree that imminent death could easily be defined as that expected in 24 to 48 hours. However, does imminent also mean within 7 days, 2 weeks, or 2 months? There have not been enough significant court cases in this area to help define medical futility. Therefore, to claim care is medically futile should not be used as an excuse to avoid effective communication with the patient, family, or legal surrogates. Thoughtful decision making is a product of effective communication.

Lantos and colleagues[73] in 1989 discussed the illusion of futility in clinical practice. They pointed out that physicians are under no obligation to offer, or even discuss, futile therapies. They demonstrated how this was supported by moral reasoning in ancient and modern medical ethics, by public policy, and by case law. Furthermore, they pointed out there are no strict criteria for defining futility. They underscored the importance of health care providers' using both clinical judgment and a clear consideration of the patient's goals for therapy. They concluded that claims of medical futility should not be used to avoid difficult discussions with patients, their families, or surrogates.

Schneiderman and colleagues[74] attempted to identify a practical way of identifying medical futility. They proposed that "when physicians conclude (either through personal experience, experiences shared with colleagues, or consideration of published empiric data) that, in the last 100 cases a medical treatment has been useless, they should regard that treatment as futile. If a treatment merely preserves permanent unconsciousness or cannot end dependence on intensive medical care, the treatment should be considered futile." This is a thoughtful proposal, but is still quite complicated to use. It is not clear what medical futility means beyond its strict definition of terminal illness, irreversibility, and imminent death. In 1992, an article discussing futility made the important point that "...the problem with futility is that its promise of objectivity can rarely be fulfilled. The rapid advance of the language of futility into the jargon of bioethics should be followed by an equally rapid retreat."[75] The issue of medical futility will prove to be one of the most important biomedical ethical topics in the 21st century, especially with increased pressure for health care rationing.

## WITHDRAWING ADVANCED LIFE SUPPORT

Withdrawing advanced life support can be one of the most difficult decisions for health care providers, patients, family members, and surrogates.[1, 26, 27, 54, 61–68] There are no absolute guidelines for deciding when to withdraw advanced life support. Each specific patient and clinical situation must be analyzed in its own context and with its independent complexities. In the following paragraphs, recommendations that will be of significant assistance when deciding whether to withdraw advanced life support are identified. It is always important to provide to patients, families, or legal surrogates the most current data concerning prognosis and medical benefits. Published data from studies such as APACHE II are extremely valuable.[3]

One must first assess whether a patient is legally competent.[56] Psychiatric consultation should be obtained when the state of competence cannot be clearly identified. It must be remembered that patients on mechanical ventilators can definitely be legally competent. This has been supported by the Bartling decision in California.[44] Unanimity of decision making must be sought among members of the health care team. Difficulties arise when health care providers feel excluded from the decision-making process. Because nurses provide the great majority of critical care in intensive care units, they often have unique information and insights about patients and families that are available only to those who spend long hours at the bedside.

It is mandatory to work diligently to determine the patient's judgment regarding withdrawal of life support. Although most persons on life support are legally incompetent, a significant number have decision-making capacity. Legally competent patients on mechanical ventilators who request that life support be discontinued must be evaluated carefully. Such patients have a legal right to control their health care, and professionals who do not comply may be committing battery. On the other hand, it is quite common for critically ill patients to have severe reactive depression, and when they survive a critical illness, they repudiate their earlier claims to have life support discontinued. Thus, it is extremely difficult to assess patients who desire to have their advanced life support withdrawn.

Decision making by families and legal surrogates cannot be rushed. These are delicate processes that have their own timing, and often a resolution is not achieved for many days. Non–health care provider facilitators such as representatives from organized religion or social workers are often invaluable. Enlisting facilitators to join the health care team early rather than later is a wise choice. The goal of the health care team when working with families or legal surrogates should be toward making a unanimous decision concerning life support in incompetent patients.

In dealing with difficult cases, it is extremely valuable to establish time-limited goals based on clinical judgment and data from prognostic studies. When families or legal surrogates are advised that life support should be withdrawn, they are often overwhelmed with confusion and guilt, are in a state of emotional shock, and may resist the advice. Decision making can be significantly aided if concrete, temporal milestones that herald improvement or failure can be identified. The physician might say to the adult children of a man who has been on a ventilator with respiratory and renal failure for 2 weeks, "If we see no signs your father has improved over the next 72 hours, we believe life support should be withdrawn. In our opinion your father is suffering and has essentially no chance to regain a reasonable quality of life. To withdraw life support would allow him a peaceful and dignified death."[27]

In proposing time-limited goals for decision making, the length of time can be from several to many days. The most important thing is that if the physician attempts to make decisions only on a day-by-day basis, it is extremely difficult to step back and gain a broader perspective. Day-to-day decision making often results in prolonged and sometimes inappropriate utilization of life support. The interlude provided by time-limited goals is a period during which the family can begin to accept the tragedy of the situation. Confident and sensitive facilitation of this process is paramount. Sometimes, before patients, families, or legal surrogates can reach a thoughtful decision, they may need to overtly express anger and mistrust often generated by less-than-adequate communication with health care providers. Health care providers must be able to tolerate expressions of hostility from patients, families, or legal surrogates without becoming defensive. This is part of the practice of medicine. Anger usually subsides once it is understood that health care team members are understanding, sensitive, and supportive. Even if patients, families, or legal surrogates do not express anger, it is wise to attempt to give them the opportunity to express it. Statements such as "This is a very sad situation and I am sure it is overwhelming" and "If I were in your position I probably would be angry" can open the way to the expression and resolution of feelings.

Communication is the key in discussing extremely complex ethical issues such as withholding and withdrawing advanced life support. An effective way of telling patients or families that the physician believes life support should be withdrawn is to say, "It is my best judgment, and that of the other members of the health care team, that your relative essentially has no chance to regain a reasonable quality of life. I am saying this on the basis of what I understand to be your relative's desires for quality of life. We believe life support should be withdrawn, which means your relative will probably die." There are two important components to the above statement. First, the statement is carefully qualified in a way that implies a decision must be shared. Second, it makes clear that death is the probable result of the recommended action. Without this knowledge, there is no true informed consent, and potential emotional and legal liability looms.

It is quite common for grief-stricken or guilt-ridden family members to attempt to relieve their stress at their loved one's expense by pressing for disproportionate treatment. A good example of this would be a son returning home to visit his critically ill father who has, in essence, no chance to regain a reasonable quality of life. Because the son has not written or communicated with his father for 10 years, he is overwhelmed by guilt. It is common in such a situation for the son to be totally against withdrawing life support. Such insistence usually dissolves once the underlying feelings are acknowledged and understood. Basically, a family therapy process is begun, and after a few to many days, the son will gain the insight and understanding to support the withdrawal of advanced life support.

As a general principle, health care professionals should not involve themselves with patient cases that are inconsistent with their ethical principles. Resentment and emotional turmoil arising under such circumstances may compromise clinical judgment. If the physician desires, the care of the patient can be transferred in an orderly and appropriate manner to another physician. This is an unusual event. If involvement with a particular patient cannot be avoided by the physician, frequent venting of feelings with understanding colleagues or a professional counselor will make optimal care more likely.

When patients on advanced life support are legally incompetent and no documented written or oral communication about withdrawal treatment exists, the problem is more complex. This was true in the 1988 Supreme Court decision in the Cruzan case and the New York ruling on the O'Connor case the same year.[48, 49] However, in these two cases, the key issue was withdrawing basic life support, which in most cases is hydration and nutrition, as opposed to withdrawing advanced life support such as mechanical ventilators, inotropic agents for blood pressure support, or dialysis. It is vital for health care providers to be knowledgeable about their own state's laws when attempting to care for incompetent patients with no written or oral communication about withdrawal of treatment. Overall, the most satisfactory resolution of such cases occurs when professionals and families review and carefully explore the quality-of-life values previously held by the patient. Once family members or legal surrogates have agreed that the patient would not have wanted to have continued life support, consent to withdraw treatment usually follows. If no one knows the patient well enough to provide information about his or her quality-of-life values, an interdisciplinary group composed of physicians, nurses, family members or friends, and two to three patient advocates (at least two of whom represent an organized religion, preferably that of the patient) can be established. This group can then identify what it believes to be the most thoughtful "substituted judgment" for the patient. Decisions should be made by family, friends, health care providers, and facilitators. Legal assistance is rarely necessary. In addition, it must be remembered that physicians are attempting to identify what is in the best interests of their patients. Hospital lawyers attempt to identify what is in the best interests of the hospital's well-being and how to minimize potential hospital liability. Often, the goals of physicians and lawyers in the intensive care unit are markedly different.

## WITHDRAWING BASIC LIFE SUPPORT

The withdrawal of basic life support such as hydration or nutrition by intravenous lines or feeding tubes is legally controversial and has resulted in a number of important legal precedents. Guidelines on determining when it is permissible to withdraw basic life support are now a states' rights issue. As noted previously, Missouri and New York require clear instructions made out by patients before the fact. In California, family members or legal surrogates can identify what the patient would have wanted.

The key to resolving ethical problems in this area lies in clarifying the patient's interests. When effective informed consent has been achieved along with sensitive decision making, most difficult ambiguities can be resolved. As always, communication is the key. It is best to have the patient's wishes regarding withdrawal of treatment in writing. If possible, conflicts between the patient's wishes and those of the family should be mediated toward a consensus, although the patient's wishes must be controlling. It is vital to provide families, or legal surrogates with assurances that comfort and caring will be maintained and that health care providers will not abandon the patient.

## EUTHANASIA

There is a remarkable amount of debate and experimentation regarding euthanasia throughout the world today.[1, 27, 76, 77] From the practice of euthanasia in Holland to reports from physicians about providing enough medication to assist patients committing suicide, and the efforts of citizens who are attempting to legalize euthanasia through referendums, we are confronted with controversies surrounding euthanasia on a daily basis. One of the key difficulties in discussing euthanasia is in determining what we are talking about. What is the definition of euthanasia? Dictionaries state that euthanasia is the act of putting to death without pain a person suffering from an incurable and painful disease or condition. "Euthanasia" is derived from Greek, and its direct translation is "an easy death." However, how does withdrawing life support from a hopelessly ill patient differ from euthanasia?

People often speak of passive euthanasia, of which forgoing life support is a prime example. Active euthanasia would be the direct putting to death in a painless manner of a person who is hopelessly ill and in pain. Because of the vagueness surrounding the definition of euthanasia, and the fact that it is an emotionally loaded term, it is probably best to use this term only when describing the direct and active putting to death of a patient by a physician. An example of this would be a lethal injection. Therefore, when using the term "euthanasia" (or "active euthanasia"), one should not be describing such acts as withholding or withdrawing life support from hopelessly ill patients.

According to the results of a 1988 survey, 85% to 90% of ICU physicians have stated that they are withholding and withdrawing life-sustaining treatments from patients who are dying from terminal and irreversible diseases.[20] A study published in 1992 concerned the attitudes of medical students, housestaff, and faculty physicians toward euthanasia and termination of life-sustaining treatment.[78] The majority of respondents (76%) considered withholding and withdrawing life-support therapy consistent with passive euthanasia. Only 16% of the respondents said they would help a patient who requested assistance in dying. The majority of respondents (68%) agreed that there was a moral justification for assisting patients to die and felt "understanding" for a physician who assists a patient in dying, but only 6% of individuals surveyed were willing to terminate the life of a patient deliberately by administering medication to cause respiratory arrest, and only 1.1% of those surveyed were willing to do so to cause cardiac arrest.

Attitudes, however, are changing. A survey of physicians published in 1998 documented that physician-assisted death does occur, although in limited numbers, despite legal constraints, and it would increase substantially if the constraints were removed.[78a] Currently, under certain circumstances, 11% of physicians acknowledge that they are willing to assist suicide, 7% are willing to administer a lethal injection, and 6% of physicians have already assisted death at least once. Furthermore, the number of physicians who would be willing to comply with requests for assisted suicide and euthanasia increases severalfold, to 36% and 24%, respectively, if these practices become legal.

Many leading physicians, philosophers, and biomedical ethicists, including this author, are opposed to physicians' direct participation (e.g., administering lethal injections) in active euthanasia in the United States. There is a long and impressive history of opposition to euthanasia in the practice of medicine. The Hippocratic oath declares the opposition to the practice of euthanasia.[79, 80] In 1988, the Council on Ethical and Judicial Affairs of the American Medical Association reaffirmed its opposition to euthanasia.[81] In 1988, the Journal of the American Medical Association published an anonymous first-person account of euthanasia.[82] This resulted in a strong call to have doctors not participate in euthanasia.[81, 83]

Most health care providers are opposed to participating in euthanasia. There are a number of strong and important criticisms against physicians' practice of active euthanasia. There is grave concern that active euthanasia could evolve from a practice that is desired by a legally competent patient to a practice that is used by surrogates of legally incompetent patients and eventually to a practice that is used to terminate life at an earlier stage in patients who are in disadvantaged or vulnerable groups. In addition, active euthanasia is not consistent with the role of the physician as a healer who is committed to the sanctity of life. If a US citizen is intent on dying, it is not necessary for a physician to "pull the trigger." However, in certain carefully analyzed individual cases, it is reasonable for physicians to provide medication to assist in ending the lives of terminally ill patients who have irreversible disease and are having a lingering and painful death. This type of physician-assisted suicide was eloquently discussed in a 1991 article by Quill.[83] On the other hand, the notorious Dr. Jack Kevorkian, with his variety of "suicide machines," has assisted numerous men and woman to commit suicide, none of whom had been terminally ill.[84] Dr. Kevorkian was convicted in 1999 of second degree murder for killing a patient by intravenous injection, an event that was recorded and then televised; Dr. Kevorkian is now in prison in Michigan.

Although it seems that active euthanasia will not be widespread in the United States because of ample opposition, this is clearly not the case everywhere.[85, 86] There are strong supporters of euthanasia, and there is a large program of euthanasia in Holland, although it is not legally supported.[87] The technique in Holland for performing euthanasia is to administer an hypnotic-like barbiturate, followed by a lethal injection of a paralytic agent. It is estimated that 5000 to 10,000 Dutch citizens are euthanized each year.[87] More recently, it appeared that a significant percentage of these patients did not necessarily provide informed consent to be euthanized. Possibly, these are patients who were not legally competent but were either in a health care facility or at home with family members.

The state of Washington in 1991 attempted to pass a bill legalizing euthanasia and physician-assisted suicide. Weeks before the vote, it appeared that the referendum would pass. However, at the last minute, along with a flurry of negative advertising, the bill was defeated. In November 1992, the state of California also had a referendum on the ballot that had the potential to legalize active euthanasia and physician-assisted suicide. The bill did not pass, although it had been reported in public opinion polls that up to 70% of California citizens favored the initiative. The US Supreme Court has weighed in on the issue by decreeing that terminally ill patients do not have a constitutional right to physician-assisted suicide but added that the Court's verdict "permits this debate to continue as it should in a democratic society."

And the debate has continued. In 1994, voters in Oregon passed the Death with Dignity Act, which subsequently survived two bitterly contested referendums, and physician-assisted suicide was legalized on October 27, 1997. It is of interest that the first referendum to enact the bill was only narrowly approved, but the second to repeal it was rejected by 60% of the voters, many authorities saying because the electorate had become better informed about the issues by the intervening court battle and extensive public debate over the measure. The Act does not permit euthanasia, but it does allows state residents to receive prescriptions for self-administered lethal medications from their physicians.[88] The chief requirements for participation spelled out in the Oregon Death with Dignity Act are as follows: (1) The patient must be an adult with a terminal illness and a life expectancy of less than 6 months; (2) the request must be made by the patient and must be voluntary; (3) the initial request must be repeated after 15 days, with an opportunity to rescind it; and (4) the physician must obtain a second opinion to confirm the diagnosis of a terminal condition and the prognosis, and there must be referral for psychiatric evaluation if the patient's judgment is possibly impaired.

An evaluation after 1 year of implementation revealed that only 23 Oregonians had received prescriptions for lethal medications; of these, 15 died after taking them, 6 died from their underlying illness, and 2 were still alive.[88] The authors determined that the decision to request and carry out physician-assisted suicide was associated with concern about loss of autonomy or control of bodily functions but not with fear of intractable pain or concern about financial loss; neither the level of education nor extent of health coverage was an important factor. There was no evidence to support the fears that physician-assisted suicide, once legalized, would be forced on terminally ill patients who were poor, uneducated, uninsured, or concerned about the financial burdens of their illness. Passage of the Act may also have had an unforeseen consequence by improving palliative treatment of dying patients in the state; Oregon is third nationally in the rate of hospice admissions and among the top five in the per capita use of morphine for medical purposes.

## SUMMARY

The two major goals of health care providers when dealing with critically ill patients are to save the salvageable and to help the dying have a peaceful and dignified death. These concepts have evolved from the basis of the practice of medicine, which is to restore health and relieve suffering. Many patients who go into respiratory failure and are managed in ICUs go on to die. Thus, dealing with issues concerning withholding and withdrawing life support is extremely common and important.

There are four fundamental principles of biomedical ethics. By discussing beneficence, nonmaleficence, autonomy, and justice, one can analyze the different ethical issues in specific cases. Numerous legal precedents are of great assistance in ethical decision making, from the 1976 Quinlan case to the 1980 Cruzan case. There also are state court precedents and two US Supreme Court precedents. Fundamentally, most state courts have supported passive euthanasia: that is, withholding and withdrawing life support from patients who will not regain a reasonable quality of life. Some states, such as New York and Missouri, have made it inordinately difficult to withdraw life support without clear and convincing evidence from patients before they become legally incompetent. Advance directives are extremely important in helping patients state their desires. The new Patient Self-Determination Act has put more pressure on health care facilities to encourage patients to fill out advance directives. Physicians should recommend to all their patients that they complete advance directives and that such directives be on file in medical charts. In addition, physicians and their family members should fill out advance directives, to set an example.

There are four key practical principles in ethical decision making. First, the patient is the key source of authority. Second, the most important approach to solving ethical problems in a critical care setting is effective communication. Third, because the patient must make a decision or have his or her surrogates make the decision, it is vital to ascertain what the patient thinks (or thought) about quality-of-life values. Fourth, patients have important rights, and these must be well understood by health care providers.

Finally, there are several approaches to dealing with withholding basic life support, withholding advanced life support, withdrawing advanced life support, and withdrawing basic life support. How to communicate with patients, families, and surrogates and what words to use are probably the most important factors. Essentially, withholding and withdrawing life support constitutes passive euthanasia. Active euthanasia, for example, by administering a lethal injection, should not be performed by physicians.

## References


1. Raffin TA, Shurkin J, Sinkler WS: Intensive Care: Facing the Critical Choices. New York: WH Freeman, 1988.
2. Snider GL: Allocation of intensive care: The physician's role. Am J Respir Crit Care Med 150:575–580, 1994.
3. Angus DC, Sirio CA, Clermont G, Bien J: International comparisons of critical care outcome and resource consumption. Crit Care Clin 13:389–407, 1997.
4. Krishna G, Raffin TA: The dying thoracic patient. Chest Surg Clin North Am 8:723–739, 1998.
5. Cowley LT, Young E, Raffin TA: Care of the dying: An ethical and historical perspective. Crit Care Med 20:1473–1482, 1992.

5a. Ruberfeld GD, Angus DC, Pinsky MR, et al: Outcomes research in critical care. Results of the American Thoracic Society Critical Care Assembly Workshop on outcomes research. Am J Respir Crit Care Med 159:358–367, 1999.

6. Raffin TA: ICU survival of patients with systemic illness. Am Rev Respir Dis 140:974–980, 1989.
7. Cullen DJ, Keene R, Waternaux C, et al: Results, charges and benefits of intensive care for critically ill patients: Update 1983. Crit Care Med 12:102–106, 1984.
8. LeGall J-R, Brun-Buisson C, Trunet P, et al: Influence of age, previous health status and severity of acute illness on outcome from intensive care. Crit Care Med 10:575–577, 1982.
9. Knaus WA, Zimmerman JE, Wagner DP, et al: APACHE—Acute physiology and chronic health evaluation: A physiologically based classification system. Crit Care Med 9:951–957, 1980.
10. Knaus WA, Draper EA, Wagner DP, Zimmerman JE: APACHE II: A severity of disease classification system for acutely ill patients. Crit Care Med 13:818–829, 1985.
11. Knaus WA, Draper EA, Wagner DP, et al: Prognosis in acute organ-system failure. Ann Surg 202:685–693, 1985.
12. Montgomery AB, Stager MA, Carrico CJ, et al: Causes of mortality in patients with ARDS. Am Rev Respir Dis 132:485–489, 1985.
13. Vasilyev S, Schaap RN, Mortensen JD: Hospital survival rates of patients with acute respiratory failure in modern respiratory intensive care units. An international, multicenter, prospective survey. Chest 107:1083–1088, 1995.

13a. Carson SS, Bach PB, Brzozowski L, et al: Outcomes after long-term acute care. An analysis of 133 mechanically ventilated patients. Am J Respir Crit Care Med 159:1568–1573, 1999.

13b. Imbus SH, Zawacki BE: Autonomy for burn patients when survival is unprecedented. N Engl J Med 297:308–311, 1977.

14. Pinilla JC, Ross DF, Martin T, et al: Study of the incidence of intravascular catheter infection in associated septicemia in critically ill patients. Crit Care Med 11:21–25, 1983.
15. Tobin MJ, Grenvik A: Nosocomial lung infection and its diagnosis. Crit Care Med 12:191–199, 1984.
16. Girard K, Raffin TA: The chronically critically ill: To save or let die? Respir Care 30:339–343, 1985.
17. Danis M, Patrick DL, Sutherland LI, et al: Patients' and families' preferences for medical intensive care. JAMA 260:797–802, 1988.
18. Steinbrook R, Lo B, Moulton J, et al: Preferences of homosexual men with AIDS for life sustaining treatment. N Engl J Med 314:457–460, 1986.
19. Goetzler R, Moskowitz M: Changes in physician attitudes toward limiting care of critically ill patients. Arc Intern Med 151:1537–1540, 1991.
20. Society of Critical Care Medicine Ethics Committee: Attitudes of critical care medicine professionals concerning forgoing life-sustaining treatments. Crit Care Med 20:320–326, 1992.
21. The SUPPORT Investigators: A controlled trial to improve care for seriously ill hospitalized patients: The study to understand prognoses and preferences for outcomes and treatments (SUPPORT). JAMA 274:1591–1598, 1995.
22. Lynn J, Harrell F, Cohn F, et al: Prognoses of seriously ill hospitalized patients on the days before death: Implications for patient care and public policy. New Horizons 5:56–61, 1997.
23. Cook DJ, Guyatt GH, Jaeschke R: Determinants in Canadian health care workers of the decision to withdraw like support. JAMA 273:703–708, 1995.
24. Raffin TA: Withdrawing life support: How is the decision made? JAMA 273:738–739, 1995.
25. In re Quinlan, 70 N.J. 10, 355 A.2d 647 (1976).
26. President's Commission for the Study of Ethical Problems in Medicine and Biomedical and Behavioral Research: Deciding to forego life-sustaining treatment. Washington, DC: US Government Printing Office, 1983.
27. Ruark JE, Raffin TA: Stanford University Medical Center Committee on Ethics: Initiating and withdrawing life support: Principles and practices in adult medicine. N Engl J Med 318:25–30, 1988.
28. Thomas JA, Hamm TE Jr, Perkins PL, Raffin TA: Stanford University Medical Center Committee on Ethics. Special report: Animal research at Stanford University: Principles, policies, and practices. N Engl J Med 318:1630–1632, 1988.
29. Greely HT, Hamm T, Johnson R, Raffin TA: Stanford University Medical Center Committee on Ethics: The ethical use of human fetal tissue in medicine. N Engl J Med 320:1093–1096, 1989.
30. Brody H: Ethical Decisions in Medicine. Boston: Little, Brown, 1976.
31. Young EWD: Alpha and Omega: Ethics at the Frontiers of Life and Death. Palo Alto, CA: Addison-Wesley, 1988.
32. Beauchamp TL, Childress JF: Principles of Biomedical Ethics, 2nd ed. New York: Oxford University Press, 1983.
33. Jonsen AR, Siegler M, Winslade WJ: Clinical Ethics, 3rd ed. New York: Macmillan, 1992.
34. Society for the Right to Die: The Physician and the Hopelessly Ill Patient. New York: Society for the Right to Die, 1985.
35. Bok S: Lying: Moral Choice in Public and Private Life. New York: Pantheon, 1978.
36. Gilligan T, Raffin TA: Physician virtues and communicating with patients. New Horizons 5:6–14, 1997.

37. Crawshaw R, Rogers DE, Pelligino D, et al: Patient-physician covenant. JAMA 273:1553, 1995.
38. Cassel CK: The patient-physician covenant: An affirmation of Asklepios. Ann Intern Med 124:604–606, 1996.
39. Ong LM, deHayes JC, Hoos AM, et al: Doctor-patient communication: A review of the literature. Soc Sci Med 49:903–918, 1995.
40. Ip M, Gilligan T, Koenig B, Raffin TA: Ethical decision-making in critical care in Hong Kong. Crit Care Med 26:447–451, 1998.
41. Saikewicz v. Superintendent of Belcher State School, 373 Mass. 728, 370 N.E.2d 417 (1977).
42. In re Dinnerstein, 380 N.E. 2d 134 (1978).
43. Barber v. Superior Court of Los Angeles, 147 Cal. App. 3d 1006, 195 Cal. Rptr. 484 (1983).
44. Bartling v. Superior Court, 163 Cal. App. ed 196, 209 Cal. Rptr. 220 (1984).
45. Bouvia v. Superior Court, 179 Cal. App. 3d 1127, 225 Cal. Rptr. 297 (1986).
46. Brophy v. New England Sinai Hospital, Inc., 390 Mass. 417; 497 N.E. 2d 626 (1986).
47. In re Drabick, 200 Cal. App.3d 185, 245 Cal. Rptr. 840 (Cal. Ct. App. 1988), reviewed denied (Cal., July 28, 1988), cert. denied, 109 S.Ct. 399 (1988).
48. In re O'Connor, 72 N.Y.2d 517, 531 N.E.2d 607, 534 N.Y.S.2d 886 (1988).
49. Cruzan v. Harmon, 760 S.W.2d 408 (1988).
50. Lo B, Rouse F, Dornbrand L: Family decision making on trial: Who decides for incompetent patients? N Engl J Med 322:1228–1232, 1990.
51. Angell M: Prisoners of technology: The case of Nancy Cruzan. N Engl J Med 322:1226–1228, 1990.
52. Snyder L: Life, death, and the American College of Physicians: The Cruzan case. Ann Intern Med 112:802–804, 1990.
53. Raffin TA: Value of the living will. Chest 90:444–446, 1986.
54. Gilfix M, Raffin TA: Withholding or withdrawing extraordinary life support: Optimizing rights and limiting liability. West J Med 141:387–394, 1984.
55. Silverman HJ, Vinicky JK, Gasner MR: Advance directives: Implications for critical care. Crit Care Med 20:1027–1031, 1992.
56. Kutner JS, Ruark JE, Raffin TA: Defining patient competence for medical decision making. Chest 100:1104–1109, 1991.
57. Title 22, Section 70707, California Administrative Code.
58. Stevens JH, Raffin TA, Baldwin JC: The current status of lung transplantation. Surg Gynecol Obstet 169:179–185, 1989.
59. Guidelines for Determination of Death: Report of the medical consultants on the diagnosis of death to the President's Commission for the Study of Ethical Problems in Medicine and Biomedical and Behavioral Research. JAMA 246:2184, 1981.
60. Sanders LM, Devney P, Young E, Raffin TA: The organ donation committee: An ethically responsible approach to increase the organ donation. Chest 102:1572–1577, 1992.
61. Luce JM, Raffin TA: Withholding and withdrawal of life support from critically ill patients. Chest 94:621–626, 1988.
62. Luce JM: Ethical principles in critical care. JAMA 263:696–700, 1990.
63. Smedira NG, Evans BH, Grais LS, et al: Withholding and withdrawal of life support from the critically ill. N Engl J Med 322:309–315, 1990.
64. American College of Chest Physicians–Society of Critical Care Medicine (ACCP-SCCM) Consensus Panel: Ethical and moral guidelines for the initiation, continuation, and withdrawal of intensive care. Chest 97:949–958, 1990.
65. Raffin TA: Withholding and withdrawing life support. Hosp Pract 26:133–155, 1991.
66. Raffin TA: Biomedical ethics in the 1990s. Chest 100:4–5, 1991.
67. American Thoracic Society Bioethics Task Force: American Thoracic Society statement on withholding and withdrawing life-sustaining therapy. Ann Intern Med 155:478–485, 1991.
68. Sanders LM, Raffin TA: The ethics of withholding and withdrawing critical care. Cambr Quart Health Ethics 2:175–184, 1993.
69. Bedell SE, Delbanco TL, Cook EF, et al: Survival after cardiopulmonary resuscitation in the hospital. N Engl J Med 309:569–576, 1983.
70. Bedell SE, Pelle D, Maher PL, et al: Do-not-resuscitate orders for critically ill patients in the hospital: How are they used and what is their impact? JAMA 256:233–237, 1986.
71. Murphy DJ, Murray AM, Robinson BE, Campion EW: Outcomes of cardiopulmonary resuscitation in the elderly. Ann Intern Med 111:199–205, 1989.
72. Tomlinson T, Brody H: Ethics and communication in do-not-resuscitate orders. N Engl J Med 318:43–46, 1988.
73. Lantos JD, Singer PA, Walker RM, et el: The illusion of futility in clinical practice. Am J Med 87:81–84, 1989.
74. Schneiderman LJ, Jecker NS, Jonsen AR: Medical futility: Its meaning and ethical implications. Ann Intern Med 112:949–954, 1990.
75. Truog RD, Brett AS, Frader J: Sounding board: The problem with futility. N Engl J Med 327:125–127, 1992.
76. Singer PA, Siegler M: Euthanasia—a critique. N Engl J Med 322:1881–1883, 1990.
77. Young ED, Drought T, Mendiola M, et al: Report of the northern California conference for guidelines on aid-in-dying: Definitions, differences, convergences, conclusions. West J Med 166:381–388, 1997.
78. Caralis PV, Hammond JS: Attitudes of medical students, housestaff, and faculty physicians toward euthanasia and termination of life-sustaining treatment. Crit Care Med 20:683–690, 1992.
78a. Meier DE, Emmons CA, Wallenstein S, et al: A national survey of physician-assisted suicide and euthanasia in the United States. N Engl J Med 338:1193–1201, 1998.
79. Angell M: Euthanasia. N Engl J Med 319:1348–1350, 1988.
80. Wanser SH, Federman DD, Adelstein SJ, et al: The physician's responsibility toward hopelessly ill patients: A second look. N Engl J Med 320:844–849, 1989.
81. Council on Ethical and Judicial Affairs of the American Medical Association: Euthanasia. Report: C (A-88). AMA Council Report. Chicago, American Medical Association, 1988, p. 1.
82. Anonymous: It's over, Debbie. JAMA 259:272, 1988.
83. Quill TE: Sounding board: Death and dignity: A case of individualized decision making. N Engl J Med 324:691–694, 1991.
84. Cassel CK, Meier DE: Sounding board: Morals and moralism in the debate over euthanasia and assisted suicide. N Engl J Med 323:750–752, 1990.
85. Risley RL: A Humane and Dignified Death: A New Law Permitting Physician Aid-in-Dying. Glendale, CA: Americans Against Human Suffering, 1987.
86. Humphry D, Wickett A: The Right to Die: Understanding Euthanasia. New York: Harper & Row, 1986.
87. de Wachter MAM: Active euthanasia in the Netherlands. JAMA 262:3316–3319, 1989.
88. Chin AE, Hedberg K, Higginson GK, et al.: Legalized physician-assisted suicide in Oregon—the first year's experience. N Engl J Med 340:577–583, 1999.

# 96 Pulmonary Rehabilitation

Bartolome R. Celli, M.D. • Thomas L. Petty, M.D.

Introduction
Historical Roots
Essentials of Pulmonary Rehabilitation
- Patient Education
- Medical Management
- Breathing Training, Breathing Exercises, Coughing, Chest Physical Therapy
- Systemic Exercise
- Upper Extremity and Special Exercise
- Nutritional and Metabolic Considerations
- Oxygen

Organization of a Pulmonary Rehabilitation Program
- Individual Pulmonary Rehabilitation Programs
- Pulmonary Rehabilitation in Conjunction with Lung Volume Reduction Surgery

Outcomes of Pulmonary Rehabilitation
Importance of Early Identification and Intervention: New Directions
Summary

## INTRODUCTION

Pulmonary rehabilitation has become the standard of care for patients who are motivated to participate in a comprehensive multidisciplinary approach to improve their quality of life and perhaps also to postpone premature morbidity and mortality. Although pulmonary rehabilitation, as defined in this chapter and applied today, is designed primarily for patients who suffer from dyspnea and reduced activities of daily living due to the physiologic burdens of advancing chronic obstructive pulmonary disease (COPD), the origins of pulmonary rehabilitation techniques can be traced to the tuberculosis era.[1] Moreover, in the present period, the same fundamental principles of pulmonary rehabilitation appear applicable to other disease states with chronic airflow obstruction, including cystic fibrosis and bronchiectasis, as well as to the interstitial-infiltrative group of lung diseases.[1a] As discussed later in this chapter, pulmonary rehabilitation has also become the standard by which other treatments such as lung volume reduction surgery are judged.

In this chapter we review the state of the art of pulmonary rehabilitation, beginning with its historical roots and tracing the emergence of new concepts and evolution of technologies and their applications, up to the present time. We conclude with a look to the future, when the principles of pulmonary rehabilitation may receive even wider practice than is the case today.

## HISTORICAL ROOTS

One of the first documented examples of pulmonary rehabilitation can be found in a monograph written by Dr. Charles Denison in 1895 (Fig. 96.1). In this remarkable little book, Denison, who had left Hartford, Connecticut, for Colorado when he was debilitated from tuberculosis and suffering from hemoptysis, describes finding the "cure" in the sunshine and altitude of the Rockies. After his condition stabilized, he realized that walking each day gave him a feeling of well-being. He also learned that his exercise tolerance increased remarkably. He further observed that his pulse rate and respiratory rate became gradually reduced as he exercised more and more. Improved appetite and sleep were corollary benefits.

Denison was also interested in breathing exercises and in breathing retraining, as indicated by Figure 96.2. Obviously, the patient was taught to breathe against increasing resistances, as further described in his monograph.

Two other pioneers deserve special mention for their work in the 1950s and 1960s. The late Alvan L. Barach championed oxygen, including ambulatory oxygen using a portable compressed gas cylinder (Fig. 96.3).[2] He was keenly interested in pursed lips breathing, abdominal diaphragmatic breathing, and the leaning forward posture to relieve stress on the diaphragm.[3, 4] He also dealt with many of the psychosocial issues that plague patients with chronic respiratory insufficiency. One of us (TLP) spent many exciting hours visiting with Al, as he preferred to be called, discussing his theories on the nature of dyspnea and his philosophy of enjoying life and living prospectively.

Another giant in the field in the mid-20th century was Albert Haas, who reported on the first organized rehabilitation program that he developed at the Rusk

Institute in New York City. Many of Haas' patients had neuromuscular disorders, as well as pulmonary fibrosis, often from healed tuberculosis. A growing number of patients referred for pulmonary rehabilitation suffered from COPD. Haas and Cardon[5] were the first to show documented benefits of rehabilitation compared with a cohort of patients receiving ordinary care.

It is interesting that Haas had also suffered from tuberculosis, which he first contracted in 1932 while a medical student in Budapest, Hungary. Following a period of convalescence, which also included fresh air and good diet, Haas became bored with inactivity. He insisted on returning to his medical studies. He resumed full activities and carried his heavy books to and from class each day. During this time, he also noticed weight gain and a feeling of well-being. He hypothesized that, at least in his case, exercise was good for the recovering tuberculosis patient and not harmful, which was the dogma of the day. After Haas recovered and immigrated to the United States, he designed a program for breathing exercises to deal with the pain and physical limitations that often followed thoracoplasty, which was one of the chief surgical therapies for tuberculosis beginning in the mid-1930s. Later on, Haas realized that breathing exercises were helpful for other tuberculosis patients, not just those who were recovering from surgery.

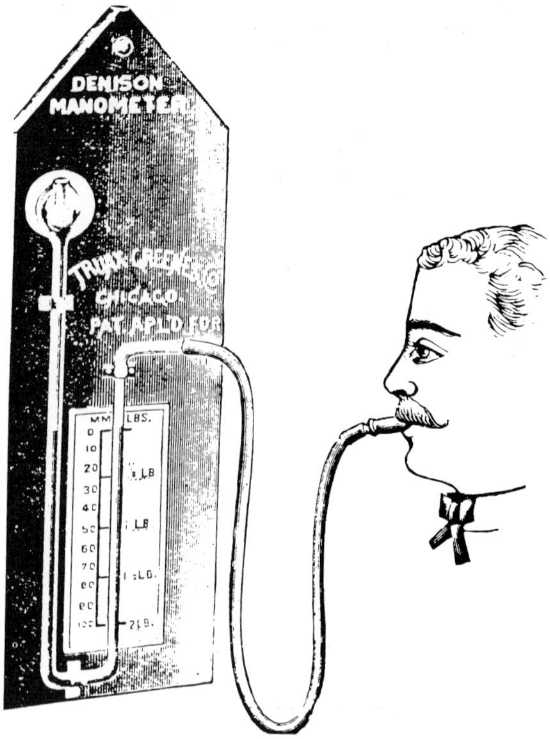


**Figure 96.2** An illustration of a crude approach to breathing exercises appearing in Dr. Denison's book.

Dr. William Miller, who still is in practice in Dallas, Texas, applied many of Barach's and Haas' techniques, as well as his own innovations such as the use of oxygen to assist with exercise training.[6] He was an early contributor to several studies that established the use of exercise as the cornerstone of pulmonary rehabilitation in patients with advanced COPD.[7]

The eighth Aspen Emphysema Conference was the first and only of the many conferences in this series (now known as the Thomas L. Petty Aspen Lung Conference) to deal with the application of the evolving methods of treatment for advanced stages of COPD. The earlier conferences had dealt with the scientific basis for emphysema and related disorders.[8] The first of these conferences was held in 1958.[9] By the mid-1960s, there was interest in improving the outcome of patients with COPD, with the various therapeutic interventions, both physical and pharmacologic. Oxygen was just emerging in the embryonic studies of the Denver Group (described subsequently).[10] Many leaders in the field participated, including William F. Miller of Dallas; Benjamin V. Brascomb of Birmingham, Alabama; Reuben M. Cherniack, at that time in Winnipeg, Canada; and Theodore Noehren, the summarizer of the 1965 Conference. The consensus reached was that COPD was not a hopeless and inexorably progressive disorder but one amenable to emerging therapies.[8]

An early study by the Denver Group reported on a comprehensive approach for patients with advanced COPD.[11] This was a demonstration project then funded through a contract from the Public Health Service, under a program known as the Chronic Respiratory Disease Control Program. Between 1966 and 1968, the Denver Group enrolled 182 consecutive patients with advanced states of COPD, all believed to be due to emphysema

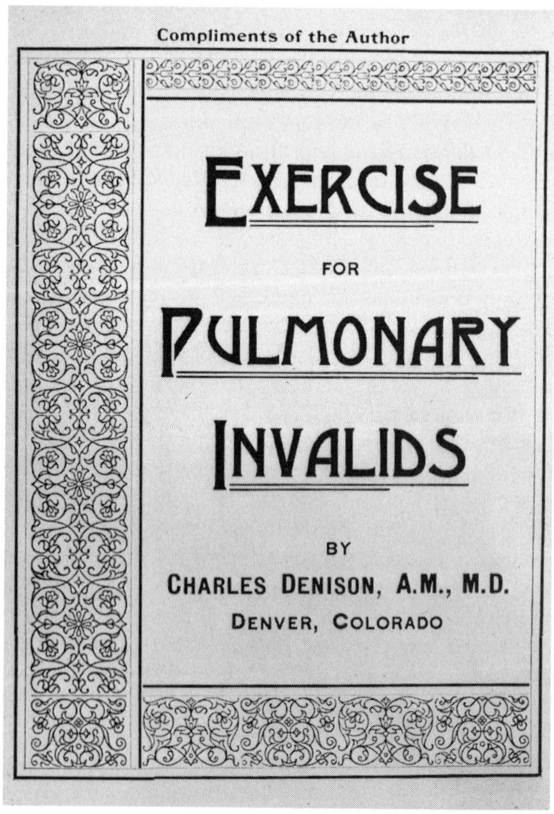
Compliments of the Author

EXERCISE

FOR

PULMONARY

INVALIDS

BY

CHARLES DENISON, A.M., M.D.

DENVER, COLORADO

**Figure 96.1** A monograph entitled *Exercise for Pulmonary Invalids,* authored and published by Dr. Charles Denison in 1895.

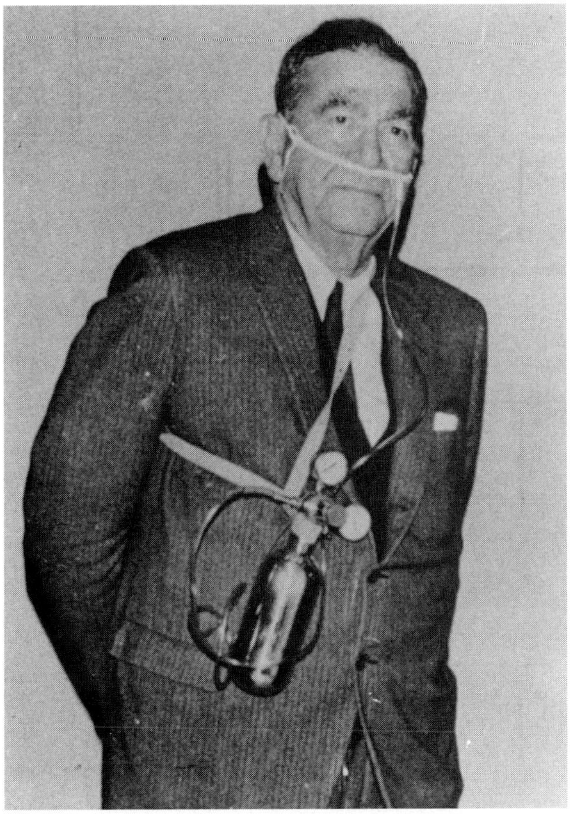

**Figure 96.3** Dr. Alvan L. Barach modeling his small portable oxygen system. (Reproduced with permission from Petty TL: Prescribing Home Oxygen for COPD. New York: Thieme-Stratton, Inc, 1982.)

and chronic bronchitis and thus irreversible. Many of the patients in this original rehabilitation program were also candidates for home oxygen, which was also under expanded study by the Denver Group, beginning in 1965.[11, 12] These early oxygen studies, which were carried out in a highly selected series of six patients who were observed in the hospital's clinical research unit, demonstrated a remarkable reduction in pulmonary vascular pressures and pulmonary vascular resistance and in the control of erythrocytosis. The most dramatic outcomes, however, were the improved exercise tolerance, weight gain, and feeling of well-being, which allowed the patients to live at home and spend considerably less time than before in the hospital.[11, 12] In fact, reduction in hospital needs was shown during the development of this rehabilitation program in an era when hospitalization was liberally offered to patients with intractable dyspnea from COPD.[13]

In 1974, a new committee of the American College of Chest Physicians, known as the Pulmonary Rehabilitation Committee, following many deliberations, arrived at the following definition of pulmonary rehabilitation:

> An art of medical practice wherein an individually tailored multidisciplinary program is formulated, which through accurate diagnosis, therapy, emotional support and education stabilizes or reverses both the physio and psychopathology of pulmonary diseases in attempts to return the patient to the highest possible functional capacity allowed by his pulmonary handicap and overall life situation.

Later, a committee of the Interagency Council on Heart Disease Resources recognized the value of pulmonary rehabilitation as a method of treatment that could help prevent or forestall the complications of cor pulmonale. The necessary community resources for the implementation of pulmonary rehabilitation principles was published.[14]

One of the most important stimuli for the expanded development and dissemination of knowledge about comprehensive care for respiratory patients came from the Human Interaction Research Institute, then directed by the late Edward Glaser of Los Angeles, California. In 1967, Glaser organized a conference, co-chaired by the late Oscar Balchum, of Los Angeles, and Albert Haas. Many who had attended the eighth Aspen Lung Conference were also in attendance. The full list of participations has been published elsewhere.[15, 16] This conference resulted in the development of a consensus statement, ultimately published by the *Journal of the American Medical Association* in 1974, in a manuscript nicely synthesized and integrated by John E. Hodgkin, an important leader in the pulmonary rehabilitation movement in the modern era.[16] That landmark article requested further consensus building by all who read it. This ultimately led to the publication of a full-length monograph on pulmonary rehabilitation, published and distributed in 1979 by the American College of Chest Physicians.[17]

The Sugarloaf Conference on the scientific basis for outpatient respiratory therapy considered the role of oxygen, physical therapy, nebulization therapy, and intermittent positive-pressure breathing (IPPB) in COPD.[18] This Conference resulted in the offering of research contracts that led to the Nocturnal Oxygen Therapy Trial (NOTT)[19] and the IPPB Trial.[20] A second conference on the scientific basis for inpatient therapy was held in Atlanta, Georgia, in November 1979. Pulmonary rehabilitation was specifically addressed at this conference.[21] On this occasion, data were presented that suggested an improvement in survival in patients who received pulmonary rehabilitation compared with a matched cohort group, which included historical controls.[21]

The most powerful scientific impetus behind the movement of pulmonary rehabilitation was the NOTT, which was published nearly two decades ago.[19] This study was proposed at the original Sugarloaf Conference. It was intended to compare the outcome of nocturnal oxygen (i.e., 12 to 15 hours per day) with continuous oxygen administration, using ambulatory sources. In the NOTT study, 12 hours of oxygen was arbitrarily chosen, including the hours of sleep, to compare with what was intended to be continuous oxygen. In fact, the continuous oxygen patients actually received oxygen only, on average, 17.9 hours per day.

Almost simultaneously, the British Medical Research Council (MRC) was conducting another study in the United Kingdom, which compared nocturnal oxygen for up to 15 hours per day with no oxygen. This conference was coordinated by the late David Flenley.[22] Because the demographic background factors and the disease severity in these two closely related studies were so similar, it was possible to compare outcomes. In brief, the results of the MRC and NOTT trials, in which pulmonary rehabilitation was also given to all enrolled patients who had chronic, stable hypoxemia, showed that survival without oxygen was poor. It was somewhat better with oxygen delivered by stationary sources for 12 or 15 hours per day. The best survival was in patients who had received oxygen even longer, nearly 18 hours per day, including from an ambulatory source.[19, 23, 24] Brain function was improved in both study groups, but this increase in mental acuity was sustained and of greater magnitude in the "continuous" oxygen patients compared with the nocturnal oxygen therapy group.[24]

Whether the improved survival was a result of the duration of oxygen therapy or the method of its administration has never been answered. It is possible that the ability to ambulate and to participate in the activities of daily living, which have a beneficial psychosocial influence and also stimulate appetite and improve sleep, could explain, in part, why those who breathed oxygen longer, including while ambulatory, did better than those who received oxygen only from stationary sources. In the NOTT study, brain function was improved more in ambulatory oxygen patients than in those allocated randomly to receive stationary oxygen at night for either 12 or 15 hours.

Now, the efficacy and scientific foundation of pulmonary rehabilitation have been firmly established and the evidence continues to mount.[24a] Rehabilitation programs are (or should be) an integral part of the continuum of therapeutic strategies available for patients with "chronic respiratory disease who remain symptomatic or continue to have decreased function despite standard medical management."[1a]

## ESSENTIALS OF PULMONARY REHABILITATION

### Patient Education

Patient education is fundamental to the solution of any chronic disease state. This is certainly true for insulin-dependent diabetes mellitus, chronic renal insufficiency, chronic congestive heart failure, obesity states, and many other chronic conditions that plague humankind. Many educational approaches to pulmonary rehabilitation have been developed, which include individual instruction periods, lectures, tapes, and brief monographs.[25] Group sessions with a professional or lay leader who has been a former patient are particularly valuable. A formalized curriculum in patient education has been organized in some centers, with 1- to 2-hour sessions daily for 5 to 10 days, to cover all of the details that a patient must know about anatomy and physiology of the lungs, body mechanics, nutrition, diet, sleep, sexuality, adaptation to dyspnea, and all the other issues that impact on patients with chronic respiratory insufficiency. Patient education has been shown to improve the health-related quality of life (assessed by a standardized questionnaire), but it seems to work better for patients with asthma than patients with COPD.[25a]

### Medical Management

Obviously, individual patients should continue with their prescribed therapeutic regimens during and after undertaking pulmonary rehabilitation. The standard treatment of patients with COPD is described in detail in Chapter 38; the principles of management of other forms of chronic lung disease are presented in the chapters that bear their names. Only two special elements that pertain to pulmonary rehabilitation are considered here.

#### Smoking Cessation

Cigarette smoking is the cause of COPD in 85% to 90% of afflicted patients. Furthermore, there is no doubt that smoking cessation is the single most important therapy that can retard the otherwise inexorable worsening of expiratory airflow obstruction, no matter when it is diagnosed; the immense value of stopping smoking by persons with early airflow obstruction is discussed and illustrated later in this chapter. The various pharmacologic and behavior-modification techniques that are available to assist persons to stop smoking are reviewed in Chapter 98. Suffice it to say here, if a patient who is still smoking enrolls in a rehabilitation program, all the educational resources of the program should be brought to bear to emphasize the vital importance of smoking cessation. Frequent contact provides the opportunity for lengthy discussions about the perils of cigarettes, the benefits of quitting, and how to succeed in stopping; this message along with the necessary counseling and reassurance should be reinforced at each visit. Continued smoking will largely offset the benefits of rehabilitation.

#### Vaccination

The causes of exacerbations of COPD are poorly understood and are probably multifactorial; both influenza virus and *Streptococcus pneumoniae* may play a role, and there is no doubt that when either of these infections occurs, patients with chronic lung disease have an increased incidence of serious complications, including death. One of the national health objectives in the United States for the year 2000 is to increase influenza and pneumococcal vaccination levels to higher than 60% among persons at high risk for complications and everyone 65 years of age or older.[25b] As just stated, this includes *all* patients with COPD and other forms of chronic lung disease, regardless of age. Because the influenza vaccine is type specific and serotypes are constantly changing, vaccination must be repeated every year, preferably at the beginning of the "flu" season in October; in contrast, the pneumococcal vaccine is polyvalent, and its benefits should last a lifetime. One of the responsibilities of a rehabilitation program is to educate enrollees about the importance of vaccination against influenza and pneumococcal infections and to ensure that it is carried out and (for influenza) repeated annually.

### Breathing Training, Breathing Exercises, Coughing, Chest Physical Therapy

As cited earlier, the original pioneers in pulmonary rehabilitation recognized that establishment of a slow, controlled breathing pattern, often with exhalation against pursed lips, is beneficial in reducing dyspnea, particularly in patients with advanced COPD with hyperinflation. One carefully controlled clinical trial showed an improvement in the oxygen ventilation equivalent, a reduction in respiratory rate, and an increasing tidal volume with pursed lips breathing compared with no pursed lips breathing.[26] The exact mechanism by which this breathing maneuver decreases dyspnea is unknown. It does not seem to change functional residual capacity or oxygen uptake (which has been shown to actually increase), but it does decrease respiratory frequency and increase tidal volume.[24] The bending forward posture has been shown to result in an improvement in dyspnea in some patients with severe COPD both at rest and during exercise. These changes can also be seen in the supine or Trendelenburg position. The best explanation for the change is that of improved diaphragmatic function as the increased abdominal pressure lengthens the diaphragm to a better contracting position.

Diaphragmatic breathing is a technique aimed at changing the breathing pattern from one where the rib cage and accessory muscles are the predominant ventilatory pressure generators to a more normal one in which inspiratory pressures are generated with the diaphragm. It is usually practiced for at least 20 minutes two or three times daily.[27] Similar to pursed lips breathing, there is usually a fall in respiratory rate and minute ventilation and an increase in tidal volume. Although it results in increased work of breathing, it may offer relief to the dyspneic patient by shifting work from the accessory muscles to the diaphragm.

Chest physical therapy aims to remove airway secretions, thereby decreasing airflow resistance and the possibility of bronchopulmonary infection. These techniques include postural drainage, chest percussion, vibration, and directed cough. Postural drainage uses gravity to help drain individual lung segments. Chest percussion should be performed with care in patients with osteoporosis or bone problems.

Cough is also an effective technique for removing excess mucus from the larger airways. Unfortunately, patients with COPD have impaired cough efficiency, maximum expiratory flow is reduced, ciliary beat is impaired, and the mucus itself has altered viscoelastic properties. Because spasms of coughing may lead to dyspnea, fatigue, and worsened airflow obstruction, directed cough may be helpful by modulating the beneficial effect and preventing the untoward ones. With controlled coughs, patients are instructed to inhale deeply, hold their breath for a few seconds, and then cough two or three times with their mouth open. They are also instructed to compress their upper abdomen to assist in the cough. It seems clear that pulmonary function tests do not improve with any of these techniques. On the other hand, programs that include a combination of postural drainage, percussion, vibration, and cough training do increase the rate of clearance of inhaled radiotracers and increase sputum volume and weight. The single most important criteria for chest physical therapy is the presence of sputum production. Many other breathing exercise techniques, including use of a variety of mechanical devices to improve respiratory muscle strength and to help clear secretions, have shown promise but lack the necessary definitive studies to be routinely recommended.[27]

With ventilatory muscle training, respiratory muscles can be specifically trained to improve their strength or their endurance. Because reduced inspiratory muscle strength is evident in patients with COPD, considerable efforts have been made to define the role of respiratory muscle training in these patients. Strength training has limited clinical significance. Controlled trials of endurance training have shown an increase in the endurance time that the ventilatory muscles could tolerate a known load. Some have shown a significant increase in strength and a decrease in dyspnea during inspiratory loading and during exercise. In the studies in which systemic exercise performance was evaluated, there was a minimal increase in walking distance. In summary, the extensive data available indicate that ventilatory muscle training with resistive breathing results in improved ventilatory muscle strength and endurance and has marginal effects on overall exercise performance. It is not clear whether this effort results in decreased morbidity or mortality or offers any other clinical advantage.[28] The conclusion of recently published evidence-based guidelines suggests that selected patients who manifest dyspnea and decreased respiratory muscle strength could undergo a trial of ventilatory muscle training. Perhaps, as more data become available and criteria for patient selection more clear, ventilatory muscle endurance training will find its true indications.

## Systemic Exercise

It is also true that the original pioneers of pulmonary rehabilitation recognized the value of systemic exercise. Maintaining a state of physical fitness is important in general health. Many investigators have pursued the methods and mechanisms of exercise training for patients with advanced COPD.[27, 29–33] High-intensity systemic exercise has been shown to improve exercise tolerance, reduce dyspnea, and reduce lactic acid production for a given level of exercise intensity.[34] The relevance of this method of heavy exercise used in research studies to daily life is debatable, because exercise training is largely task specific. Thus, normal brisk walking on the level or upstairs seems most appropriate. Patients should exercise at least 20 minutes, twice daily or more, to maintain a level of physical fitness. Although a high level of exercise performance may be achieved by high-intensity training, using treadmills and professionals to assist the patient in coping with the demands of exercise on a treadmill, this requires skills above and beyond normal walking.

Many controlled clinical trials (Table 96.1) have shown the value of systemic exercise training, which most practically includes walking on the level, such as in halls and corridors. Use of 12- or 6-minute walk tests have been one of the yardsticks of success in a pulmonary rehabilitation program.[35–37] All of these studies report in common an increase in exercise endurance, a modest but significant improvement in work or oxygen uptake, and a decrease in the perception of dyspnea.[38–41] Perhaps the most complete of these reports is the one by Ries and coworkers.[40] They randomized 119 patients to education (n = 62)

**Table 96.1 OUTCOMES OF PULMONARY REHABILITATION IN PATIENTS WITH ADVANCED COPD**

| Outcome | Effect | Grade of Evidence* |
|---|---|---|
| Exercise endurance | Large and significant increase | A |
| Exercise work capacity (watts or $\dot{V}O_2$) | Modest increase | A |
| Dyspnea | Large and significant improvement | A |
| Quality of life | Improvement | A |
| Biochemical muscle enzyme changes | Controversial | B |
| Health-related cost survival | Improvement | C |

*Evidence is graded according to these guidelines: Grade A = evidence obtained from well-controlled randomized studies. Grade B = evidence obtained from well-designed controlled trials, small numbers. Grade C = evidence obtained from multiple time series or expert opinion.

From Kravetz HM: How the office-based pulmonary rehabilitation program works. *In* Casaburi R, Petty TL (eds): Principles and Practice of Pulmonary Rehabilitation. Philadelphia: WB Saunders, 1993, pp 483–486.

and education with exercise training (n = 57). After 6 months, the trained patients significantly increased their exercise endurance time and peak oxygen uptake and reported an improvement in perception of dyspnea and self-efficacy for walking when compared with controls. A recent metaanalysis of articles published during the last 45 years on the effects of pulmonary rehabilitation in patients with asthma or COPD confirmed the improvements in physical performance (6-minute walking test) and symptoms (questionnaire).[24a] The results of 14 controlled trials were recently reviewed using graded evidence.[28] Careful analysis of these trials in over 550 patients proved that training using different forms of exercise (walking, cycle ergometry, treadmill, or a combination thereof) was equally effective in producing a beneficial effect. Therefore, it seems appropriate for most patients to train with the easiest form of exercise, including (and perhaps most important) walking, without the use of any external device. Not surprisingly, once patients improve exercise performance, usually in an organized outpatient rehabilitation program, it is vital to preserve the gain by exercising on a regular maintenance schedule.[41a]

## Upper Extremity and Special Exercises

Most of our knowledge about exercise conditioning is derived from programs emphasizing leg training. This is unfortunate because the performance of many everyday tasks requires not only the hands but also the concerted action of other muscle groups that are used in upper torso and arm positioning. Some of these muscles serve a dual function (respiratory and postural), and arm exercise increases their capacity to participate in ventilation.[42] These observations suggest that when the arms are trained to perform more work, or when the ventilatory requirement for the same work is decreased, as has been shown, the capacity to perform activities of daily living improves.[43]

Arm training results in improved performance, which is for the most part task specific. Ries and coworkers[44] studied the effects of two forms of arm exercise, gravity-resistance and modified proprioceptive neuromuscular facilitation, and compared the results with those from no arm exercise in 45 patients with COPD. The 20 patients who completed the program showed improved performance on the tests that were specific for the training. The patients also reported a decrease in fatigue for all tests performed. Martinez and coworkers[45] showed that unsupported arm training (against gravity) decreases oxygen uptake at the same workload when compared with arm cranking training. They concluded that unsupported arm exercise may be a more effective way to train patients in activities that resemble those of daily living. Therefore, upper extremity exercise is recommended as an important component in the training of patients undergoing pulmonary rehabilitation.

## Nutritional and Metabolic Considerations

A growing body of knowledge indicates a high level of energy expenditure in some patients who have advanced COPD and associated weight loss.[46–48] The reason for weight loss is probably multifactorial and may include depression, poor appetite due to chronic illness or to the use of drugs, dyspnea during eating, hypoxemia during the act of eating, or lack of interest in food.[49, 50] An intriguing interrelationship between weight loss from high energy expenditure and the presence of inflammatory cytokines suggests complex underlying metabolic disorders in weight loss and muscle weakness in COPD.[51] Weight loss and muscle wasting contributes to a reduced efficiency of the skeletal muscles.[52–54] To counteract this, emerging studies are beginning to show a positive effect of anabolic agents on increasing lean body mass in such patients.[55] How weight loss and associated muscle weakness and dysfunction may be mitigated by diet, exercise, and possible anabolic agents is a subject of current intense study. These metabolic nutritional and muscle dysfunction phenomena suggest an underlying systemic defect in at least some patients with advanced stages of COPD. (See subsequent discussion about early stages of disease.) Several studies have shown that weight gain is possible, simply with the encouragement of additional calories. Much of this weight gain is, however, in the form of fat and not lean body mass.

## Oxygen

As described earlier in the context of historical roots, two landmark studies clearly showed improved survival in selected patients with COPD who breathed supplementary oxygen at night compared with those who received no oxygen and even better survival in those who breathed oxygen for longer periods through the aid of ambulatory delivery systems.[19, 22] Contemporary guidelines for prescribing home oxygen for patients with COPD, based in part on the NOTT, are shown in Table 96.2. The chief criterion is a significant level of hypoxemia, defined as an arterial $Po_2$ of 55 mm Hg or less for 3 weeks or more when the patient is in a clinically stable state (i.e., has been free from exacerbation of bronchitis, heart failure, and other intercurrent complications). Additional criteria were also used in the North American multicenter trial to enroll stable patients with COPD whose arterial $Po_2$ values were between 55 and 59 mm Hg. These included evidence of pulmonary hypertension as judged by roentgenographic abnormalities (an enlarged pulmonary outflow tract); electrocardiographic findings of elevated right-sided intracardiac pressures (P waves in standard leads 2, 3, and aVF $>$ 2 mm); clinical evidence of cor pulmonale with heart failure; or secondary polycythemia from chronic oxygen insufficiency. Now, patients with COPD who have echocardiographic evidence of right ventricular hypertrophy and/or pulmonary hypertension also qualify.

### Dosage

The therapeutic goal of administering supplementary oxygen is to raise arterial $Po_2$ to the range of 60 to 65 mm Hg or, alternatively, to reach an oxygen saturation of 90% to 94%. The results of the NOTT established the fact that the great majority of patients with advanced COPD and hypoxemia, as defined in the previous paragraph, can achieve this goal with oxygen delivered by nasal cannulae at 1 to 2 L/min. Less than 10% of the patients required 3 L/min or more while at rest. Additional results obtained during the conduct of the trial indicated that additional oxygen, 1 L/min, was required during the stress of exercise and while sleeping; these extra needs are undoubtedly caused by the increased metabolic demands of exercise and the modest degree of hypoventilation and/or worsening of gas exchange that occurs during sleep. Thus, if the baseline flow of oxygen is 2 L/min with patients at rest, the flow rate should be turned up to 3 L/min while they are exercising or sleeping. Periodic monitoring of oxygenation is essential to determine who should receive supplementary oxygen in the first place and, in those who are being treated, to evaluate if therapeutic goals are being met or exceeded. Two techniques are available: either arterial puncture with direct measurement of $Po_2$ or pulse oximetry to quantify oxygen saturation; the latter is being increasingly used given the convenience and improved accuracy of newer oximeters.

**Table 96.2 GUIDELINES FOR PRESCRIBING HOME OXYGEN FOR ADVANCED COPD**

| |
|---|
| **Patient Selection Criteria** |
| Stable course of disease on optimum medical therapy (e.g., bronchodilators, antibiotics, and corticosteroids when indicated) |
| At least two arterial blood gas determinations while breathing room air at rest a minimum of 20 minutes |
| Resting $Pao_2$ consistently 55 mm Hg or less, or consistently 55 to 59 mm Hg, plus cor pulmonale clinically diagnosed and/or hematocrit >55% |
| Patients with substantial nocturnal hypoxemia (i.e., $Pao_2$ <55 mm Hg on multiple occasions, or patients with hematocrit >55% or clinical evidence of pulmonary hypertension) |
| Normoxic patients in whom less dyspnea and substantially increased exercise capability is demonstrated with oxygen |
| **Oxygen Dose** |
| Continuous flow by double or single nasal cannulae (see text) or by demand system with demonstration of adequate oxygen saturation |
| Lowest liter flow to raise $Po_2$ to 60–65 mm Hg or oxygen saturation to 90%–94% |
| Increase baseline liter flow by 1 L/min during exercise and sleep |

### Delivery Systems

In historical order, the systems available for home use by a physician's prescription are as follows: compressed gas in high-pressure cylinders, liquid gas in lightweight canisters, and stationary oxygen concentrators. The advantages and disadvantages of each are listed in Table 96.3. Large compressed gas cylinders are fixed in place, but patients can move short distances while using long (50 ft) tubing; smaller cylinders can be attached to wheel chairs or installed in automobiles to allow journeys out of the home. Ambulatory patients are best served with a liquid system, which is the only truly practicable way to deliver oxygen to someone who is working. New generation lightweight cylinders (2.1 kg) are available, and oxygen concentrators are being developed that can be used to fill portable cylinders at home.[55a]

## ORGANIZATION OF A PULMONARY REHABILITATION PROGRAM

There have been many organizational approaches to a pulmonary rehabilitation program. Historically, at the beginning, inpatient care was the norm. This had the advantage of a captive audience and a controlled environment that ensured a good diet. The disadvantages, of course, were economic, which became overwhelming for most patients. The inpatient experience also fostered an undesirable dependency on many patients.

Today, most pulmonary rehabilitation programs are conducted on an outpatient basis, often employing a conference room or clinic that is otherwise not in use. An outpatient rehabilitation program requires some space for exercising and socializing. The only equipment required is a movie projector, video tape player or slide projector, a blackboard, and treadmills, exercycles, spirometers, and pulse oximeters.[56–59]

### Individual Pulmonary Rehabilitation Programs

All of the principles embodied in the concept of a pulmonary rehabilitation program could be accomplished by

Table 96.3 ADVANTAGES AND DISADVANTAGES OF AVAILABLE HOME OXYGEN SYSTEMS

| | Liquid Portable | Concentrators | Compressed Gas |
|---|---|---|---|
| Advantages | Light weight | Lower cost | Lower cost in general (cost may equal liquid in continuous-use situations) |
| | Long-range portable canister | Convenient | Widespread availability |
| | Most practical ambulatory system | Attractive equipment | |
| | | Widespread availability | |
| Disadvantages | More expensive than concentrators used alone | Electricity required | Multiple tanks necessary for ambulation unless transfilling can be done at home |
| | Not available in small or rural communities | May need back-up tank system | Frequent deliveries needed |
| | | Not portable | Heavy and unsightly tanks |

individual patients, provided that they have suitable motivation and instruction. One foundation, the Pulmonary Research and Education Foundation, has published three individual instruction booklets, now bound together in a single volume, that have achieved some success.[60] This volume has also been translated into Spanish. A recent study compared the effects of an individually tailored exercise program with a standard one for patients with COPD. After 8 weeks of training, there was a significant difference in favor of the patients treated individually.[61] This report underscores the need to tailor the program to the individual's need to realize maximal benefit.

## Pulmonary Rehabilitation in Conjunction with Lung Volume Reduction Surgery

In the middle of the 1990s, Dr. Joel Cooper in St. Louis revived a surgical procedure first proposed by Otto Brantigan and coworkers[62] in 1959. This procedure, properly called *lung pneumectomy* but commonly referred to as *lung volume reduction*, involves resection of poorly functioning portions of emphysematous lung in patients with severe symptomatic COPD.[63] A recent comprehensive review reported that after lung volume reduction surgery, most patients have significant short-term physiologic improvement that is matched by functional gain in exercise capacity and subjective improvement in dyspnea and quality of life.[63a] Because of his experience with patients undergoing lung transplantation, Cooper and his group have long advocated the benefit of pulmonary rehabilitation as an important component of the perioperative treatment of patients scheduled for other surgical procedures on the lungs. Inasmuch as rehabilitation includes aspects such as patient education about the nature of the disease and the proper use of medications, and also instruction about breathing exercises and directed cough, rehabilitation has become routine in the management of patients undergoing lung volume reduction surgery. To reinforce this concept, it has recently been shown that patients who could not walk 200 m within 6 minutes before lung volume reduction had significantly higher morbidity and mortality rates than patients able to cover that timed distance.[64] Whether improvement of the walked distance by preoperative rehabilitation results in improved surgical outcome remains to be determined, but most experts familiar with the surgery have the impression that a well-prepared patient will more likely return to full mobilization, cooperate with physiotherapy, and withstand the rigors of the difficult surgical experience.[65] The conviction that rehabilitation is important is such that the two national trials (one Canadian and one in the United States) and the regional Massachusetts trial include pulmonary rehabilitation in both arms of the protocols.

Practically, the preoperative rehabilitation program for lung volume reduction and other major surgical procedures consists of the same components outlined in this chapter. Unique to surgical patients is early mobilization and exercise (even with air leaks and thoracostomy tube drainage) during the postoperative period. Throughout the recovery, emphasis is placed on breathing and systemic exercises until the patient is able to assume a normal life. The postoperative rehabilitation period varies depending on the course of the patient.

## OUTCOMES OF PULMONARY REHABILITATION STUDIES

Outcome analysis can be defined as the assessment of the "consequences" of an intervention. On the one hand, pulmonary rehabilitation does not affect the degree of respiratory impairment as measured by tests of pulmonary physiologic function. On the other hand, it has been shown that patients with COPD who complete exercise training increase the concentration of oxidative enzymes in the trained muscles and that this is accompanied by a beneficial delay in the early generation of lactate (a marker of dysfunctional muscle performance).[66] This physiologic change does prove an ameliorating effect on exercise impairment and has caused extraordinary excitement in the field.

Pulmonary rehabilitation also profoundly impacts on a patient's disability and handicap, as there are clinically significant improvements in walking distance, perception of dyspnea, and health-related quality of life after training. Very few studies have addressed the effect of pulmonary rehabilitation on other outcomes such as health care utilization or survival. Early studies suggested a decrease in the total days of hospitalization after patients underwent pulmonary rehabilitation[13]; unfortunately these studies were uncontrolled, and the findings could represent changes in overall health care practice. One recent large controlled trial did find survival to increase and the number of hospitalization days to decrease—but insignificantly—in patients undergoing rehabilitation with exercise compared with controls.[40]

Because of the documented and experienced benefits of pulmonary rehabilitation on exercise capacity and quality of life, this therapeutic concept has become a standard treatment for patients with COPD and other chronic respiratory ailments.

## THE IMPORTANCE OF EARLY IDENTIFICATION AND INTERVENTION: NEW DIRECTIONS

One of the most interesting recent developments in the field of pulmonary rehabilitation focuses on recent observations that patients with only mild degrees of expiratory airflow obstruction have poor exercise tolerance.[67] In these studies, men were not able to reach the predicted target heart rate or maximum oxygen consumption, even though their limitation did not seem to be the abnormalities of pulmonary mechanics. This raises the question of the basic nature of physiologic impairment in patients with early stages of COPD. The easiest explanation for poor athletic performance is physical unfitness. But why patients with only mild degrees of airflow obstruction become unfit was not explained by this study. Whatever the explanation, a recent report of the effects of exercise rehabilitation showed that even patients with mild COPD (i.e., similar to those just described) benefited from a 12-week program with improvement in exercise capacity.[67a]

It is also an interesting fact that patients who smoke, as they evolve into states of chronic airflow obstruction, choose a diet low in antioxidants, high in fat, and low in fiber. This is the worst possible diet for a patient who may be suffering from oxidative lung injury as a consequence of tobacco smoking. The interrelation between nutrition and lung health is just beginning to receive systematic inquiry.[68] The possibility of using antioxidants to combat the oxidant burden on the lung in COPD is being investigated.[68] Many smokers also suffer from associated affective disorders incident in COPD, which are anxiety and depression, along with a degree of somatic preoccupation. It is highly likely that tobacco smoking is used by these individuals to combat anxiety and depression and to help deal with unpleasant somatic sensations. There is no doubt that patients who take to smoking rather than to exercise for symptomatic relief could improve their state of physical conditioning. Thus, if we are to believe these early studies, it seems that pulmonary rehabilitation, at least in terms of the education and exercise component, should be initiated early. Of course, smoking cessation would be the first critical step in such an early rehabilitation program. Perhaps we should also begin to look at COPD as a systemic disease with pulmonary, cardiovascular, musculoskeletal, nutritional, and psychologic components, which are all intertwined with tobacco abuse.[69]

The evidence then suggests that early intervention may be of use. It should not be forgotten, though, that patients with symptomatic lung disease are candidates for pulmonary rehabilitation irrespective of the severity of their disease.[70] Indeed, some studies have shown that those patients with the most severe disease will improve more than those patients with lesser involvement.[71] Currently, it is believed that any patient with symptoms who is willing and capable to enroll in a pulmonary rehabilitation program should be provided with the opportunity to do so.

The 1994 Lung Health Study showed that patients with only a mild degree of airflow obstruction had accelerated losses of lung function if they continued to smoke. In contrast, those patients who were successful in stopping smoking, most of whom received specialized care for this purpose, had a slight improvement in airflow, followed by a minuscule decline at the end of 5 years (Fig. 96.4).[72] The obvious conclusion from this landmark study was that smoking cessation can alter the early course and prognosis of COPD. Another interesting finding in the Lung Health Study was the cause of death, which most commonly was lung cancer followed by heart attack, stroke, and all other causes (Table 96.4). During the course of the 5-year study, no patient died of COPD. The reason for this is that they had not reached a degree of sufficient respiratory insufficiency to increase the risk of death from exacerbations of COPD. Thus, it turns out that early states of airflow obstruction are an indicator of high risk of death from other causes, most notably lung and other cancers, heart attack, and stroke. This is all the more reason why patients with mild impairment of $FEV_1$ must be identified by simple spirometry so that they may be enrolled in aggressive programs designed to assist

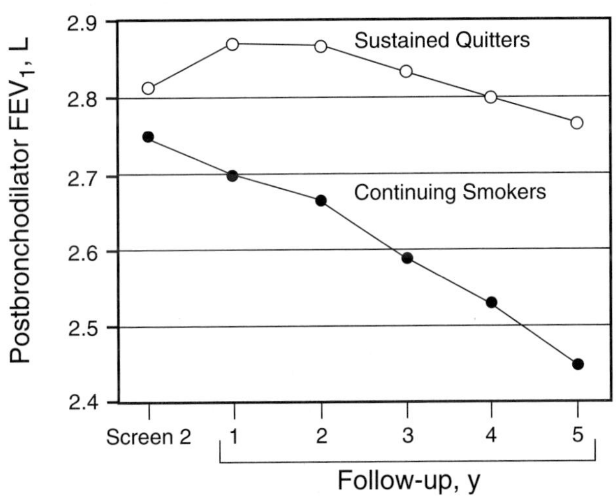


**Figure 96.4** Mean postbronchodilator forced expiratory volume at 1 second ($FEV_1$) for participants in the smoking intervention and placebo group who were sustained quitters (open circles) and continuing smokers (closed circles). The two curves diverge sharply after baseline. (From Anthonisen NR, Connett JE, Kiley JP, et al: Effects of smoking intervention and the use of an inhaled anticholinergic bronchodilator on the rate of decline of $FEV_1$. The Lung Health Study. JAMA 272:1497–1505, 1994.)

**Table 96.4 THE LUNG HEALTH STUDY: CAUSES OF DEATH WITHIN 5 YEARS**

| Cause | SIA | SIP | UC | Total |
|---|---|---|---|---|
| Lung cancer | 18 | 20 | 19 | 57 |
| Cardiovascular disease | 18 | 7 | 12 | 37 |
| Other | 18 | 17 | 20 | 55 |
| **Total** | **54** | **44** | **51** | **149** |

SIA = smoking intervention and ipratroprium; SIP = smoking intervention and placebo; UC = usual care.

From Anthonisen NR, Connett JE, Kiley JP, et al: Effects of smoking intervention and the use of an inhaled anticholinergic bronchodilator on the rate of decline of $FEV_1$. The Lung Health Study. JAMA 272:1497–1505, 1994.

smoking cessation and to improve the physical status of the patient.

At this writing, a new health care initiative for COPD is emerging. This is known as the National Lung Health Education Program (NLHEP).[73] NLHEP aims to identify COPD patients in early incipient stages of disease at which smoking cessation and other strategies can have a major impact in reducing the premature morbidity and mortality of COPD. NLHEP is aimed at all primary care physicians and the patients they see on a daily basis. Approximately 70% of all smokers see a physician once a year for some medical problem. Here is when COPD can be identified by simple spirometry. It is highly important that simple hand-held spirometers, which are accurate and easy to use, be widely employed by all primary care providers as a first step in identifying patients who are just beginning on a pathway that leads to symptomatic COPD and the need for pulmonary rehabilitation.

## SUMMARY

Patients with advanced COPD and severe physical disability profit from pulmonary rehabilitation, whether offered as part of an organized program or individually. Patient education, smoking cessation, breathing retraining, physical conditioning by daily exercise, and bronchial hygiene techniques suitable for home use can be provided in an inexpensive outpatient setting. Home oxygen is highly beneficial for selected patients. Pulmonary rehabilitation clearly improves the quality of life by reducing the symptoms and social burden of illness. Exercise tolerance is improved, and the need for hospitalization may be reduced.

Although COPD is a progressive disease, the socioeconomic gain from pulmonary rehabilitation is well documented. There is growing evidence that detecting smokers with early expiratory airflow obstruction and instituting rehabilitation, with an emphasis on smoking cessation, greatly attenuates the otherwise inexorable worsening of COPD. Widespread use of simple spirometric testing by primary care physicians is the first step in the development of programs designed to halt or forestall the progression of COPD and provides the opportunity to reduce the incidence of other smoking-related complications such as bronchogenic cancer and cardiovascular diseases.

## References


1. Petty TL: Pulmonary Rehabilitation: A Personal Historical Perspective. *In* Casaburi R, Petty TL (eds): Principles and Practice of Pulmonary Rehabilitation. Philadelphia, WB Saunders, 1993, pp 1–8.

1a. American Thoracic Society: Pulmonary rehabilitation—1999. Am J Respir Crit Care Med 159:1666–1682, 1999.

2. Barach AL: Ambulatory oxygen therapy: Oxygen inhalation at home and out of doors. Dis Chest 35:229–241, 1957.
3. Barach AL: Physiologic Therapy in Respiratory Diseases. Philadelphia: JB Lippincott, 1958.
4. Barach AL: Breathing exercises in pulmonary emphysema and allied chronic respiratory disease. Arch Phys Med Rehabil 36:379–390, 1955.
5. Haas A, Cardon H: Rehabilitation in chronic obstructive pulmonary disease: A 5-year study of 252 male patients. Med Clin North Am 53:593–606, 1969.
6. Pierce AK, Paez PN, Miller WF: Exercise training with the aid of a portable oxygen supply in patients with emphysema. Am Rev Respir Dis 91:653–659, 1965.
7. Miller WF: Rehabilitation of patients with chronic obstructive lung disease. Med Clin North Am 51:349–361, 1967.
8. Petty TL (ed): Principles of Management of Chronic Obstructive Lung Disease. Proceedings of the Eighth Aspen Emphysema Conference. Washington, DC: U.S. Department of Health, Education, and Welfare publication (PHS) 1,457, 1966.
9. Mitchell RS (ed): Symposium on emphysema and the "chronic bronchiolitis" syndrome. Am Rev Respir Dis 50(Part 2):1–213, 1959.
10. Levine BE, Bigelow DB, Hamstra RD, et al: The role of long-term continuous oxygen administration in patients with chronic airway obstruction with hypoxemia. Ann Intern Med 66:639–650, 1967.
11. Petty TL, Nett LM, Finigan MM, et al: A comprehensive care program for chronic airway obstruction: Methods and preliminary evaluation of symptomatic and functional improvement. Ann Intern Med 70:1109–1120, 1969.
12. Petty TL, Finigan MM: Clinical evaluation of prolonged ambulatory oxygen therapy in chronic airway obstruction. Am J Med 45:242–252, 1968.
13. Hudson LD, Tyler ML, Petty TL: Hospitalization needs during an outpatient rehabilitation program for severe chronic airway obstruction. Chest 70:606–610, 1976.
14. Intersociety Commission on Heart Disease. Petty TL (Chairman), Branscomb BV, Farrington JF, Kettel LJ: Pulmonary Rehabilitation Study Group. Community resources for rehabilitation of patients with chronic obstructive pulmonary disease and cor pulmonale. Circulation 49(Suppl 1):A1–A20, 1974.
15. Glaser EM: A pilot study to determine the feasibility of promoting the use of a systematized care program for patients with chronic obstructive pulmonary disease. Final Report. Los Angeles Human Interaction Research Institute. Social and Rehabilitation Service, Department of Health, Education, and Welfare. Project RD-2571-6-67, 1968.
16. Hodgkin JE, Balchum OJ, Kass I, et al: Chronic obstructive airway diseases. Current concepts in diagnosis and comprehensive care. JAMA 232:1243–1260, 1975.
17. Hodgkin JE (ed): Chronic Obstructive Pulmonary Disease: Current Concepts in Diagnosis and Comprehensive Care. Park Ridge, IL: American College of Chest Physicians, 1979.
18. Proceedings of the Conference on the Scientific Basis of Respiratory Therapy. Am Rev Respir Dis 110(Suppl):1–202, 1974.
19. Nocturnal Oxygen Therapy Trial Group: Continuous or nocturnal oxygen therapy in hypoxemic chronic obstructive lung disease. A clinical trial. Ann Intern Med 93:391–398, 1980.
20. Intermittent Positive Pressure Breathing Trial Group: Intermittent positive pressure breathing therapy of chronic obstructive pulmonary disease. A clinical trial. Ann Intern Med 99:612–620, 1983.
21. Petty TL: Pulmonary rehabilitation. *In* the Proceedings of the Conference on the Scientific Basis on In-Hospital Respiratory Therapy. Am Rev Respir Dis 122:1–161, 1980.
22. Report of the Medical Research Council Working Party: Long term domiciliary oxygen therapy in chronic hypoxic cor pulmonale complicating chronic bronchitis and emphysema. Lancet 1:681–686, 1981.

23. Cooper CB: Long-term Oxygen Therapy. *In* Casaburi R, Petty TL (eds): Principles and Practice of Pulmonary Rehabilitation. Philadelphia: WB Saunders, 1989, pp 183–203.
24. Heaton RK, Grant I, McSweeny AJ, et al: Psychologic effects of continuous and nocturnal oxygen therapy in hypoxemic chronic obstructive pulmonary disease. Arch Intern Med 143:1941–1947, 1983.
24a. Cambach W, Wagenaar RC, Koelman TW, et al: The long-term effects of pulmonary rehabilitation in patients with asthma and COPD: A research synthesis. Arch Phys Med Rehabil 80:103–111, 1999.
25. Petty TL, Nett LM: Enjoying Life with COPD, 3rd ed. Cedar Grove, NJ: Laennec Publishing, 1995, p 199.
25a. Gallefoss F, Bakke PS, Kjaersgaard P: Quality of life assessment after patient education in a randomized controlled study on asthma and chronic obstructive pulmonary disease. Am J Respir Crit Care Med 159:812–817, 1999.
25b. CDC Centers for Disease Control and Prevention: Influenza and pneumococcal vaccination levels among adults aged <65 years. MMWR 46:797–802, 1998.
26. Mueller RE, Petty TL, Filley GF: Ventilation and arterial blood gas changes induced by pursed lips breathing. J Appl Physiol 28:784–789, 1970.
27. Faling LJ: Controlled breathing techniques and chest physical therapy in chronic obstructive pulmonary disease and allied conditions. *In* Casaburi R, Petty TL (eds): Principles and Practice of Pulmonary Rehabilitation. Philadelphia: WB Saunders, 1993, pp 167–182.
28. ACCP/AACVPR Pulmonary Rehabilitation Guideline Panel. Pulmonary Rehabilitation. Joint ACCP/AACVPR Evidence-Based Guidelines. Chest 112:1363–1396, 1997.
29. Christie D: Physical training in chronic obstructive lung disease. BMJ 2:150–151, 1968.
30. Nicholas JJ, Gilbert R, Gabe R, et al: Evaluation of an exercise therapy program for patients with chronic obstructive pulmonary disease. Am Rev Respir Dis 102:1–9, 1970.
31. Brundin A: Physical training in severe chronic obstructive lung disease: I. Clinical course, physical working capacity and ventilation. Scand J Respir Dis 55:25–36, 1974.
32. Casaburi R, Wasserman K: Exercise training in pulmonary rehabilitation. N Engl J Med 314:1509–1511, 1986.
33. Ries AL, Archibald CJ: Endurance exercise training at maximal targets in patients with chronic obstructive pulmonary disease. J Cardiopulmon Rehabil 7:594–601, 1987.
34. Casaburi R, Patessio A, Ioli F, et al: Reduction in exercise lactic acidosis and ventilation as a result of exercise training in patients with obstructive lung disease. Am Rev Respir Dis 143:9–18, 1991.
35. McGavin CR, Gupta SP, McHardy GJ: Twelve-minute walking test for assessing disability in chronic bronchitis. BMJ 1:822–823, 1976.
36. Wijkstra PJ, TenVergert EM, van der Mark TW, et al: Relation of lung function, maximal inspiratory pressure, dyspnea, and quality of life with exercise capacity in patients with chronic obstructive pulmonary disease. Thorax 49:468–472, 1994.
37. Cahalin L, Pappagianopoulos P, Prevost S, et al: The relationship of the 6-min walk test to maximal oxygen consumption in transplant candidates with end-stage lung disease. Chest 108:452–459, 1995.
38. O'Donnell DE, Webb KA, McGuire MA: Older patients with COPD: Benefits of exercise training. Geriatrics 48:59–62, 65–66, 1993.
39. Reardon J, Awad E, Normandin E, et al: The effect of comprehensive outpatient pulmonary rehabilitation on dyspnea. Chest 105:1046–1052, 1994.
40. Ries AL, Kaplan RM, Linberg TM, et al: Effects of pulmonary rehabilitation on physiologic and psychosocial outcomes in patients with chronic obstructive pulmonary disease. Ann Intern Med 122:823–832, 1995.
41. Goldstein RS, Gort EH, Stubbing D, et al: Randomised controlled trial of respiratory rehabilitation. Lancet 344:1394–1397, 1994.
41a. Grosbois JM, Lamblin C, Lemaire B, et al: Long-term benefits of exercise maintenance after outpatient rehabilitation program in patients with chronic obstructive pulmonary disease. J Cardiopulm Rehabil 19:216–225, 1999.
42. Celli BR: The clinical use of upper extremity exercise. Clin Chest Med 15:339–349, 1994.
43. Couser JI, Martinez FJ, Celli BR: Pulmonary rehabilitation that includes arm exercise reduces metabolic and ventilatory requirements for simple arm elevation. Chest 103:37–41, 1993.
44. Ries AL, Ellis B, Hawkins RW: Upper extremity exercise training in chronic obstructive pulmonary disease. Chest 93:688–692, 1988.
45. Martinez FJ, Vogel PD, Dupont DN, et al: Supported arm exercise vs unsupported arm exercise in the rehabilitation of patients with severe chronic airflow obstruction. Chest 103:1397–1402, 1993.
46. Schols AM, Soeters PB, Mostert R, et al: Energy balance in chronic obstructive pulmonary disease. Am Rev Respir Dis 143:1248–1252, 1991.
47. Schols AM, Fredrix EW, Soeters PB, et al: Resting energy expenditure in patients with chronic obstructive pulmonary disease. Am J Clin Nutr 54:983–987, 1991.
48. Baarends EM, Schols AM, Pannemans DL, et al: Total free living energy expenditure in patients with severe chronic obstructive pulmonary disease. Am J Respir Crit Care Med 155:549–554, 1997.
49. Schols AM, Mostert R, Cobben N, et al: Transcutaneous oxygen saturation and carbon dioxide tension during meals in patients with chronic obstructive pulmonary disease. Chest 100:1287–1292, 1991.
50. Schols AM, Soeters PB, Dingemans AM, et al: Prevalence and characteristics of nutritional depletion in patients with stable COPD eligible for pulmonary rehabilitation. Am Rev Respir Dis 147:151–156, 1993.
51. Schols AM, Buurman WA, Staal van den Brekel AJ, et al: Evidence for a relation between metabolic derrangements and increased levels of inflammatory mediators in a subgroup of patients with chronic obstructive pulmonary disease. Thorax 51:819–824, 1996.
52. Schols AM, Mostert R, Soeters PB, et al: Body composition and exercise performance in patients with chronic obstructive pulmonary disease. Thorax 46:695–699, 1991.
53. Baarends EM, Schols AM, Akkersmans MA, Wouters EF: Decreased mechanical efficiency in clinically stable patients with COPD. Thorax 52:981–986, 1997.
54. Schols AM, Soeters PB, Mostert R, et al: Physiologic effects of nutritional support and anabolic steroids in patients with chronic obstructive pulmonary disease. A placebo-controlled randomized trial. Am J Respir Crit Care Med 152:1268–1274, 1995.
55. Lacasse Y, Guyatt GH, Goldstein RS: The components of a respiratory rehabilitation program: A systematic overview. Chest 111:1077–1088, 1997.
55a. Keller RR: Long-term oxygen therapy: Advances and perspectives in technical devices. Monaldi Arch Chest Dis 54:75–78, 1999.
56. Tietsort JA: A storefront program for pulmonary rehabilitation. *In* Casaburi R, Petty TL (eds): Principles and Practice of Pulmonary Rehabilitation. Philadelphia: WB Saunders, 1993, pp 474–477.
57. Sutton FD: The proprietary pulmonary rehabilitation program. *In* Casaburi R, Petty TL (eds): Principles and Practice of Pulmonary Rehabilitation. Philadelphia: WB Saunders, 1993, pp 478–482.
58. Kravetz HM: How the office-based pulmonary rehabilitation program works. *In* Casaburi R, Petty TL (eds): Principles and Practice of Pulmonary Rehabilitation. Philadelphia: WB Saunders, 1993, pp 483–486.
59. Mall RW, Mederios M: Reimbursement for a Community Hospital-based Program. *In* Casaburi R, Petty TL (eds): Principles and Practice of Pulmonary Rehabilitation. Philadelphia: WB Saunders, 1993, pp 487–494.
60. Petty TL, Tiep BL, Burns MR: Essentials of Pulmonary Rehabilitation: A "Do it Yourself" Program. Lomita, CA: Pulmonary Education and Research Foundation, 1991, pp 1–52.
61. Vallet G, Ahmaidi S, Serres I, et al: Comparisons of two training programs in chronic airways limitation patients: Standardized versus individual protocols. Eur Respir J 10:114–122, 1997.
62. Brantigan OC, Mueller E, Kress MB: A surgical approach to pulmonary emphysema. Am Rev Respir Dis 80:194–202, 1959.
63. Cooper JD, Trulock EP, Triantafillou AN, et al: Bilateral pneumectomy (volume reduction) for chronic obstructive pulmonary disease. J Thorac Cardiovasc Surg 109:106–119, 1995.
63a. Young J, Fry-Smith A, Hyde C: Lung volume reduction surgery

(LVRS) for chronic obstructive pulmonary disease (COPD) with underlying severe emphysema. Thorax 54:779–789, 1999.
64. Szekely LA, Oelberg DA, Wright C, et al: Preoperative predictors of operative morbidity and mortality in COPD patients undergoing bilateral lung volume reduction surgery. Chest 111:550–558, 1997.
65. Martinez FJ, de Oca MM, Whyte RI, et al: Lung-volume reduction improves dyspnea, dynamic hyperinflation, and respiratory muscle function. Am J Respir Crit Care Med 155:1984–1990, 1997.
66. Maltais F, LeBlanc P, Simard C, et al: Skeletal muscle adaptation to endurance training in patients with chronic obstructive pulmonary disease. Am J Respir Crit Care Med 154:442–447, 1996.
67. Carter R, Nicotra B, Blevins W, et al: Altered exercise gas exchange and cardiac function in patients with mild chronic obstructive pulmonary disease. Chest 103:745–750, 1993.
67a. Berry MJ, Rejeski J, Adair NE, et al: Exercise rehabilitation and chronic obstructive pulmonary disease stage. Am J Respir Crit Care Med 160:1248–1253, 1999.
68. Skidhar MK (ed): Nutrition and lung health. Should people at risk of chronic obstructive lung disease eat more fruits and vegetables? BMJ 310:75–76, 1995.
69. Petty TL: Pulmonary rehabilitation of early COPD. COPD as a systemic disease. Chest 105:1636–1637, 1994.
70. Celli BR: Pulmonary rehabilitation in patients with COPD. Am J Respir Crit Care Med 152:861–864, 1995.
71. ZuWallack RL, Patel K, Reardon JZ, et al: Predictors of improvement in the 12-minute walking distance following a six-week outpatient pulmonary rehabilitation program. Chest 99:805–808, 1991.
72. Anthonisen NR, Connett JE, Kiley JP, et al: Effects of smoking intervention and the use of an inhaled anticholinergic bronchodilator on the rate of decline of $FEV_1$. The Lung Health Study. JAMA 272:1497–1505, 1994.
73. Petty TL, Weinmann GG: Building a national strategy for the prevention and management of and research in chronic obstructive pulmonary disease. JAMA 277:246–253, 1997.

# 97 Lung Transplantation

JANET R. MAURER, M.D., F.C.C.P.
NOE ZAMEL, M.D., F.R.C.P.C., F.C.C.P.

Introduction
Clinical Lung Transplantation
- Survival Data
- Types of Lung Transplantations

Selection and Evaluation of Candidates
- Cystic Fibrosis
- Non–Cystic Fibrosis Bronchiectasis
- Nonbronchiectatic Chronic Obstructive Lung Disease
- Idiopathic Pulmonary Fibrosis
- Pulmonary Hypertension
- Pediatric Lung Transplantation

Preoperative and Perioperative Management
- Preoperative Management
- Immunosuppression

Postoperative Prophylaxis
Infectious Complications
- Bacterial Infections
- Viral Infections
- Fungal Infections
- *Pneumocystis carinii* Infections

Rejection
- Acute Rejection
- Bronchiolitis Obliterans
- Functional Outcomes
- Medical Complications of Long-Term Survivors
- Recurrent Disease

Summary and Future Issues

## INTRODUCTION

Successful lung transplantation dates to the early 1980s, although attempts at human lung transplantation had been made since 1963, when Hardy and coworkers[1] first reported a unilateral lung graft. The recipient lived only 18 days, but that report was the stimulus for more than 40 attempts at lung transplantation over the next 20 years. The longest survival during those two decades, however, was less than a year, largely because of technical issues and the lack of adequate immunosuppressive drugs.[2]

The first long-term survivor was reported in 1982. With the aid of the new and revolutionary immunosuppressive drug cyclosporine, the Stanford group, who had been pioneers in both heart and lung transplantation, reported a successful heart-lung transplantation in a patient with primary pulmonary hypertension. This patient ultimately survived more than 5 years.[3] Within 4 years of the Stanford report, both isolated unilateral and bilateral lung transplantation were successfully performed at the University of Toronto and subsequently at many other medical centers internationally.[4, 5]

A registry of the numbers and types of lung transplantations performed internationally is kept by the International Society of Heart and Lung Transplant in conjunction with the United Network for Organ Sharing. Each year an update of the Registry is published in the *Journal of Heart and Lung Transplant.* In 1998 the Registry had recorded a total of 2428 heart-lung transplantations from 122 transplantation centers and 4777 unilateral and 3278 bilateral lung transplantations from 150 transplantation centers.[6] The number of heart-lung transplantations per year rose rapidly in the late 1980s to a peak of about 240 and then fell as the numbers of isolated lung transplantations increased and competition for donor organs increased. In the late 1990s the number of isolated lung transplantations performed per year had leveled off at approximately 1200 and the number of heart-lung transplantations at approximately 150. Unilateral lung transplantations account for slightly more than half of the isolated lung transplantations performed. The limiting factor in the number of transplantations performed is donor availability. Despite the use of older donors, living donors, and so-called marginal donors, the demand for transplantable lungs still far exceeds the supply.

## CLINICAL LUNG TRANSPLANTATION

### Survival Data

Bilateral and unilateral lung transplants have nearly identical early courses with approximately 70% 1-year and 62% 2-year survivals.[6] This is considerably better than that of the heart-lung recipients of whom 60% are alive at 1 year and about 50% at 2 years. Despite the isolated transplant recipients' early similar survivals, Registry data suggest that after 3 years the survival curves begin to splay, and the bilateral transplants do somewhat better than the unilateral ones. The respective half-lives for bilateral, unilateral, and heart-lung recipients are 4.5, 3.6,

**Table 97.2 DISEASE-SPECIFIC SELECTION GUIDELINES FOR VARIOUS END-STAGE LUNG DISEASE**

| |
|---|
| NONBRONCHIECTATIC CHRONIC OBSTRUCTIVE PULMONARY DISEASE |
| $FEV_1 < 25\%$ predicted (without reversibility) |
| And/or arterial $PCO_2 \geq 55$ mm Hg |
| And/or ↑ pulmonary artery pressures (PAP) |
| CYSTIC FIBROSIS/BRONCHIECTASIS |
| $FEV_1 \leq 30\%$ predicted or |
| $FEV_1 > 30\%$ predicted *and* any of |
| Rapid fall in $FEV_1$ |
| Massive hemoptysis |
| Increase in cachexia |
| Increase in hospitalizations |
| Accessory criteria |
| Arterial $PCO_2 \geq 50$ mm Hg |
| Arterial $PO_2 \leq 55$ mm Hg |
| IDIOPATHIC PULMONARY FIBROSIS |
| Symptomatic, progressive disease despite drug therapy: reassess every 3 months |
| Rest or exercise desaturation |
| "Symptomatic" often correlates to |
| $VC < 60\%–70\%$ predicted |
| $DL_{CO} < 50\%–60\%$ predicted |
| PULMONARY HYPERTENSION |
| Symptomatic, progressive disease despite optimal medical treatment; usually NYHA III–IV; gold standard medical treatment considered to be prostacyclin |
| Useful hemodynamic predictors |
| Cardiac index < 2 L/min/m² |
| Right atrial pressure > 15 mm Hg |
| PAP mean > 55 mm Hg |

angiogram in patients at high risk for coronary artery disease; a 24-hour creatinine clearance; and liver function studies. Other investigations in selected patients may include, for example, bone densitometry or preventive screening studies such as mammography and sigmoidoscopy. Investigations often done at the transplantation center include cytomegaloviral and other serologies, tissue typing, and psychosocial evaluation. Disease-specific criteria are summarized in Table 97.2. Several issues of note in specific diseases are discussed in the following sections.

## Cystic Fibrosis

Criteria for referral of patients with cystic fibrosis are based primarily on the longitudinal study of Kerem and coworkers,[32] who evaluated predictors for mortality in a large, but single-center population of cystic fibrosis patients. These are the best available data. Concerns about the management of resistant organisms in cystic fibrosis patients remain. Recent data suggest that patients colonized with fungal or atypical mycobacterial organisms or with multiply resistant bacterial organisms may have survival rates comparable with those who are colonized with more sensitive organisms.[33] Even panresistance is now considered only a relative contraindication because in vitro sensitivities do not necessarily correspond to in vivo sensitivities. Probably the only absolute contraindication in most medical centers to transplantation in the cystic fibrosis patient that remains is resistant *Burkholderia cepacia* or similar organisms.[34] It is recommended that microbiologic review of sputum be done on a periodic basis, usually at 3-month intervals during the pretransplantation waiting period.

## Non–Cystic Fibrosis Bronchiectasis

Patients with bronchiectasis from other causes, including immunodeficiency syndromes, immotile or dysfunctional cilia syndromes, postinfectious syndromes, or unknown etiologies, are assessed according to the same guidelines as cystic fibrosis patients, as no good literature exists to determine prognosis in these patients.

## Nonbronchiectatic Chronic Obstructive Lung Disease

In patients with nonbronchiectatic chronic obstructive lung disease, those with elevated $PCO_2$ or elevated pulmonary artery pressure or both, and with progressive deterioration (especially cor pulmonale), have the poorest prognosis. This subgroup of patients probably derives a survival benefit from lung transplantation. Candidates who do not fit into this category may, however, experience an improved functional capacity without necessarily an increased survival[35] because in many cases it is inherently difficult to predict survival in patients with advanced obstructive lung disease.

## Idiopathic Pulmonary Fibrosis

Idiopathic pulmonary fibrosis patients have by far the highest death rate while waiting for transplantation; in most medical centers more than 50% of these patients die while waiting.[35, 36] It is likely that death occurs both because the disease progresses rapidly and because patients are often referred for transplantation only when they are extremely ill. In addition, because most patients with idiopathic pulmonary fibrosis are in the sixth and seventh decades, they may have comorbid conditions that influence survival or may have significant side effects from extensive steroid or cytotoxic treatment. The Guidelines reflect the need for transplantation centers to access these patients as soon as they are symptomatic or are not improving with medical therapy, or both.

## Pulmonary Hypertension

The widespread use of continuous intravenous epoprostenol to treat patients with advanced primary pulmonary hypertension has led to some cautious optimism about the prognosis of this disease.[37, 38] It has also made it more difficult to determine when such patients should be listed as transplant candidates. The Guidelines state that patients who are functionally NYHA class III or NYHA class IV despite optimal medical therapy (including epoprostenol) are potential lung transplantation candidates. Additional useful hemodynamic parameters in the assessment of failure of medical therapy include a cardiac index of less than 2 $L/min/m^2$, right atrial pressure more than 15 mm Hg, and mean pulmonary artery pressure more than 55 mm Hg.[39] Such parameters are not well defined for patients with pulmonary hypertension secondary to congenital heart disease. That group of patients appears to have better survival with similar hemodynamic parameters.[40] Nevertheless, in the absence of good data, the criteria used are severe, progressive symptoms with function at NYHA class III or IV level.

### Pediatric Lung Transplantation

Most pediatric patients presenting with advanced lung disease have either cystic fibrosis or primary or secondary pulmonary hypertension. Guidelines for pediatric cystic fibrosis patients are generally adapted from the guidelines for their adult counterparts. In cases of pulmonary hypertension, the underlying diagnoses tend to be diverse and prognostic indicators are difficult to develop. In general, the following criteria are used: the disease is no longer responding to maximal medical and surgical treatment; the patient is functioning in NYHA class III or IV; and the patient has clinical right ventricular failure, severe cyanosis and low cardiac output.[41]

## PREOPERATIVE AND PERIOPERATIVE MANAGEMENT

### Preoperative Management

Patients listed for transplantation have progressive diseases and require careful medical management during the waiting period. Any comorbid issues such as osteoporosis, systemic hypertension, or obesity should be managed aggressively to ensure that the patient remains the best possible candidate for transplantation. Maintaining good functional capacity with pulmonary rehabilitation programs for those patients without severe pulmonary hypertension and frequently measuring and adjusting supplemental oxygen therapy to ensure adequate saturations at rest and exercise are important aspects of preoperative care.

### Immunosuppression

Induction immunosuppression is now quite variable from center to center. This variability has resulted from the introduction of several new immunosuppressive agents. Most patients continue to receive intraoperative and perioperative steroid preparations with oral prednisone continued for variable periods (at least several months postoperative). The remainder of the immunosuppressive protocol can, however, include tacrolimus instead of cyclosporine preparations and mycophenolate mofetil instead of azathioprine in a number of centers. Very specific antilymphocyte activation preparations are also now available. Two new anti-interleukin-2 receptor antibodies, dacliximab and basiliximab, which are easy to administer and which have negligible toxicity, are available and may replace the cytolytic preparations in those medical centers that have depended on this type of induction. No prospective studies have, however, been done with these preparations. Within the next few years several other agents will also be approved by the Food and Drug Administration, and increasingly the immunosuppressive protocol for individual patients will be tailored to individual needs. Maintenance regimens may include low doses of prednisone, tacrolimus, or cyclosporine preparations and mycophenolate mofetil or azathioprine.

## POSTOPERATIVE PROPHYLAXIS

Early reports of infection in lung transplant recipients emphasized the high rate of bacterial postoperative infections, along with the usual opportunistic agents.[42, 43] These observations have resulted in many programs using a broad-based prophylaxis regimen directed against not only bacterial but also viral and fungal organisms. Prophylactic regimens are most intense in the first weeks after transplantation, but are often continued for months. Because prophylactic regimens are both expensive and potentially toxic, some groups are using close prospective monitoring with preemptive treatment as an alternative approach. Monitoring for cytomegalovirus antigenemia or DNA in peripheral blood, for example, is gaining increased acceptance.[44, 45]

## INFECTIOUS COMPLICATIONS

Infections and chronic rejection (bronchiolitis obliterans) remain the two major causes of death.[6] In the first year post-transplantation, infections account for about one third of all deaths; after the first year, bronchiolitis obliterans accounts for one third of deaths and the two etiologies together for about half of all deaths.[6]

### Bacterial Infections

Routine postoperative prophylaxis appears to have decreased the frequency of early postoperative bacterial infections. Typically broad-spectrum antibiotics are used initially and modified when the results of donor and recipient airway cultures are known. In recipients with preoperative diagnoses of bronchiectasis (primarily cystic fibrosis patients) who often harbor one or more species of gram-negative organisms in their airways, the prophylaxis is usually more complex. Typically, the most recently effective antibiotics or those that have shown good activity against the organism are used. Because of this approach, it is important to keep abreast of the sensitivities of the organisms in these patients. For this reason, the International Guidelines detailed above recommend that patients with known colonizing organisms have sputum cultures and antibiotic sensitivity studies repeated every 3 months during the preoperative period.[28–31]

Bacterial pneumonias represent the bulk of the severe bacterial infections. Gram-negative organisms, especially *Pseudomonas* species, account for about 75% of these.[46] Other reported bacteria run the gamut of nosocomial organisms. Legionellosis is rarely reported.[47] Bacterial bronchitis, mediastinitis, empyema, and less often sepsis account for most of the remaining bacterial processes. Bronchiectasis commonly occurs in patients who have developed bronchiolitis obliterans.[48] These patients often develop recurrent episodes of bacterial bronchitis and occasionally pneumonia. Pseudomonal species again are the predominant infecting organisms.

## Viral Infections

Viral infections are common and often cause more morbidity and mortality than do bacterial infections. Viral infections can be divided into two basic groups: those caused by members of the herpesvirus family and those caused by common respiratory viruses. The second group has only recently been recognized as important.

In the herpesvirus group, cytomegalovirus (CMV) is the most important. In patients who have not had prophylaxis, the peak incidence of CMV infection, which can be either reactivated infection (already present in recipient) or primary infection (from donor), occurs between 30 and 100 days after the transplantation.[49] Infection rates with this organism vary depending on the serologic status of the donor and recipient but can approach 100% in particularly susceptible groups.[50] All donor-recipient serologic combinations with the exception of donor-negative, recipient-negative are at significant risk of developing symptomatic infection. In lung transplant recipients, the organism appears to target the graft, and in patients who have received no or only short-term prophylaxis, the incidence of pneumonia is very high.[51]

Early detection of CMV infection and prompt institution of antiviral therapy has significantly reduced the morbidity and mortality from this disease. Fortunately, both antiviral and immunoglobulin therapies are now available to treat CMV infections. Most lung transplantation programs routinely provide prophylactic therapy for the most at-risk patients, with ganciclovir or ganciclovir plus CMV immunoglobulin for varying periods postoperatively. Although these drugs may not prevent infection, the course of the infection is modified, resulting in less morbidity.[52] Because of the expense and toxicity of pharmacologic prophylaxis, a growing number of institutions are using an alternative approach to the CMV problem. With polymerase chain reaction and other modern technology, the patient's blood is monitored for CMV activity as measured by DNA or antigenemia. When the activity levels rise appreciably, therapy is instituted preemptively before a clinical syndrome appears.[44] CMV infection (primarily when pneumonitis has been histologically diagnosed) has been identified by several authors as a risk factor for bronchiolitis obliterans.[53, 53a] This relationship, however, remains controversial.[54]

Herpes simplex and herpes zoster also occur commonly in lung transplant recipients. Acyclovir is effective prophylaxis against these infections in patients not already receiving ganciclovir prophylaxis. With proper prophylaxis, the morbidity from these viruses can be reduced to a minor problem.

Infection with another herpesvirus, Epstein-Barr virus, is intimately related to the development of post-transplant lymphoproliferative disorders (PTLD). These usually appear within the first year post-transplant in 4% to 10% of lung transplant recipients and often occur initially in the transplanted lung. Pediatric recipients who have never had Epstein-Barr virus have been known to be at high risk of developing this process, and it has also recently been shown that adult graft recipients who have never had Epstein-Barr virus have a similar risk of developing PTLD. Serology-negative recipients who receive serology-positive organs have at least an 80% chance of primary infection, and those who develop infection may have a 50% chance of developing PTLD.[55] Because this is a fatal disease in at least half of the recipients who develop it, strategies to reduce the risk should be devised. Currently, there is no specific treatment for the process; reduction of immunosuppression, administration of ganciclovir and alpha-interferon, and occasionally chemotherapeutic agents have all been used with varied success.

A second group that is emerging as important pathogens in lung transplant recipients are the common respiratory viruses. Since 1995, several reports of infections with paramyxoviruses (respiratory syncytial virus and parainfluenza virus), adenovirus, and influenza A virus have highlighted this problem.[56–60] Respiratory syncytial virus, usually of minor importance in adults, presents most frequently in the winter with a broad spectrum of respiratory signs and symptoms. Pneumonia is common. Adenoviral infections have been reported mostly in pediatric recipients and appear to have a significant impact on survival.[60] Influenza A also appears frequently as pneumonia and in conjunction with other types of infection.[61] Overall, the death rate in these series is about 20%, with the adenoviral infections reported as having the worst outcomes.[60] It is unclear whether antiviral therapy is of benefit because the data on treatment are scant.

## Fungal Infections

The most lethal infections are invasive fungal infections, particularly those caused by *Aspergillus* species. The increasing recognition of the severe morbidity caused by these organisms has led to widespread use of antifungal prophylaxis at least within the first few months postoperatively. Invasive disease is varied and includes ulcerative tracheitis, empyemas, bronchitis, localized parenchymal infection, and disseminated disease.[62–65] *Aspergillus* colonization in these reports varied between 22% and nearly 50% of patients. In one medical center, patients with single-lung transplants were prone to more invasive infections, particularly in the native lung.[63] The relationship between colonization and invasive disease has not been clearly established, although a recent case series suggests that rising antibody titers to *Aspergillus* may be an important marker.[66] Allergic bronchopulmonary aspergillosis has also been noted in a few patients.[67] In patients with complicated courses post-transplantation, fungal infection is a common terminal event. The severity of this disease and its often progressive course in immunosuppressed patients despite aggressive antifungal therapy has led increasingly to surgical approaches to management when disease is localized.[68–70] Important questions as to the best prophylactic regimen—various combinations of intravenous and aerosolized amphotericin B as well as oral drugs have been tried—remain unanswered.

Occasional cases of deep fungal infections (e.g., histoplasmosis) have been reported from areas where the fungi are indigenous. It is important to remember that, when considering the possibility of such an infection, one must take into account the geographic areas from which both the donor and recipient originate or have traveled.

### *Pneumocystis carinii* Infections

*Pneumocystis carinii* is now rarely seen as a serious pathogen in lung transplant recipients primarily because of universal prophylaxis with trimethoprim-sulfamethoxazole (or an alternative). If no prophylaxis is used, however, this disease occurs in nearly all lung recipients.[71] Most programs continue this prophylaxis indefinitely, although there are no specific data supporting this practice.

## REJECTION

### Acute Rejection

#### Clinical Signs

Acute rejection is common in the first weeks after lung transplantation. Clinically, it is often difficult to separate acute rejection from infection.[72] Symptoms include a general feeling of malaise, dyspnea, and low-grade fever. Signs are also confusing and can include a falling $FEV_1$, clear chest radiograph to radiograph with ill-defined infiltrates, pleural effusion, elevated white blood cell count, and hypoxemia.[72] Because of these nonspecific findings, a "shotgun" approach to treatment has often been used.[4] Histologic diagnosis, however, is reliably obtained by transbronchial biopsy.[73–78]

#### Histologic Diagnosis

Transbronchial biopsy is the gold standard for diagnosis of acute rejection (see Fig. 18.37). It is recommended that at least five pieces of tissue be obtained to give the most reliable information.[79] Animal studies have documented the histologic spectrum of rejection and the high sensitivity of detecting this process by transbronchial biopsy.[73, 80] It has also been shown in humans that, with adequate tissue, the sensitivity of detecting acute rejection is at least 80%, and the specificity approaches 100% in the absence of complicating infections.[81] Acute rejection is graded universally by a scheme initially set up in 1990 by a study group supported by the International Society for Heart and Lung Transplantation.[79] The group revised this scheme in 1995 to reflect increasing experience with the spectrum of pathologic changes after lung transplantation, and it remains the worldwide standard classification of acute rejection.[82]

Multiple groups have attempted to distinguish between acute rejection and infection based on cytokine milieu, cellular components in bronchoalveolar lavage fluid or other local factors.[83–85] In general, however, changes in these parameters overlap sufficiently so that clear distinctions cannot be made without histologic diagnosis. This is a continuing area of intense research as a noninvasive means of detecting acute rejection or a propensity to develop acute rejection could allow preemptive measures or tailored immunosuppressive regimens.

#### Treatment

Acute rejection is usually treated by bolus intravenous steroid therapy with or without temporary increases in the maintenance immunosuppression. In at least 80% of cases, the acute rejection is adequately treated. In 15% to 20% of acute rejection episodes, however, the process is either persistent or recurrent and presents a particularly difficult problem for the clinician.[86, 87] Intensified immunosuppression with one or more agents is usually tried, but it has been shown that persistent or recurrent or late (at least 3 months postoperative) acute rejection episodes greatly increase the risk of chronic rejection.[88, 89]

#### Surveillance Bronchoscopy

The role of surveillance bronchoscopy—bronchoscopy performed in clinically stable patients post-transplantation—to detect asymptomatic rejection or infection remains controversial. Probably more than one half of active lung transplantation centers perform at least one surveillance bronchoscopy with transbronchial biopsies in the post-transplantation period, and several studies have shown that at least 20% of asymptomatic patients had grade II or greater rejection.[90, 91] Although most centers treat patients with grade II or higher histology, no one has shown that this results in better survivals or lower rates of bronchiolitis obliterans.

### Bronchiolitis Obliterans

Bronchiolitis obliterans, or chronic rejection, is the most feared complication after lung transplantation. It is manifested by a pathologic process centered predominantly in the small airways with the resulting development of varying degrees of obstructive airway disease. It occurs in at least 50% of survivors by 5 years post-transplantation.[92] Described as early as 2 months after transplantation, the onset is more often 6 months or more after surgery, with a mean onset from 1 to 2 years.[93]

#### Clinical Signs

In most cases, the onset of bronchiolitis obliterans is insidious with the patient complaining of malaise and a vague, nonspecific ill feeling.[94] Initially, this may or may not be accompanied by mild shortness of breath and intermittent nonproductive cough, although eventually the dyspnea becomes a dominant complaint. Even before the onset of vague symptoms, a fall in the $FEF_{25-75}$ may herald the onset of this disease, as may a variety of less commonly available pulmonary function studies.[95–97] Eventually, the $FEV_1$ falls, and ultimately so does the vital capacity.[95] Chest radiographs are typically normal until very late in the disease when bronchiectasis may develop, but CT scans may show a mottled appearance with peripheral lucency, especially during expiration.[98]

**Table 97.3 CLINICAL CLASSIFICATION OF BRONCHIOLITIS OBLITERANS SYNDROME**

| |
|---|
| Grade 0: $FEV_1$ > 80% of baseline* |
| Grade 1: $FEV_1$ 66%–79% of baseline |
| Grade 2: $FEV_1$ 51%–65% of baseline |
| Grade 3: $FEV_1$ ≤ 50% of baseline |

*Baseline $FEV_1$ is the average of the two highest consecutive measurements post-transplant. Each grade is classified either a, with histologic confirmation; or b, no histologic confirmation.

Adapted from Cooper J, Billingham M, Egan T, et al: A working formulation for the standardization of nomenclature and for clinical staging of chronic dysfunction in lung allografts: International Society for Heart and Lung Transplantation. J Heart Lung Transplant 12:713–716, 1993.

### Diagnosis

As with acute rejection, the gold standard for diagnosis of bronchiolitis obliterans is transbronchial biopsy. Diagnosis by transbronchial biopsy is not, however, a sensitive means of detection. For this reason, in 1994 a clinical description (Table 97.3) was set up to characterize the development of this process in lung transplant recipients.[99] This clinical classification, now widely used in transplantation centers, describes bronchiolitis obliterans by the degree of obstructive airway disease present. When defined, according to these criteria, the process is called *bronchiolitis obliterans syndrome.* Thus, the criteria recognize, but do not require, histologic diagnosis to identify chronic rejection. Although histologic diagnosis is difficult, bronchoscopy is often performed at least once in patients suspected of having developed bronchiolitis obliterans because it is necessary to eliminate infections as a potential cause of the functional loss in these patients.

### Treatment

Treatment of bronchiolitis obliterans is largely unrewarding. A number of immunosuppressive protocols have been reported in the literature to slow or stabilize the process.[100–103] Reversal of functional loss, however, is rare. Even without treatment, the syndrome appears to have a variable course, with some patients experiencing rapid loss of function resulting in death within a few months and others having a slow loss of function over several years.[104] Many patients who develop advanced disease also develop bronchiectasis or bronchomalacia complicated by infection with *Pseudomonas* or other gram-negative organisms.[105]

### Etiology

Precipitating factors for bronchiolitis obliterans and the events that occur in its pathogenesis have been the subject of much research and debate in the lung transplantation community. Predisposing factors that have most consistently been identified include number and severity of acute rejection episodes and CMV pneumonitis.[106–107] A number of other factors that have also been identified as important by individual centers include human leukocyte antigen (HLA) mismatches,[108–110] viral infections,[111] and the development of anti-HLA antibodies.[112] Small animal models of heterotopic tracheal transplantation and some larger animal models of orthotopic whole lung transplants have been developed to study the process by which transplantation bronchiolitis obliterans occurs.[113–115] These models may help to better define the process that initiates this complication and hopefully will provide some help in dealing with this complication in human transplant recipients.

## Functional Outcomes

### Pulmonary Function

Despite the many complications that can plague lung transplant recipients, most experience a dramatic improvement in lung function that greatly improves their quality of life.[5, 116] Reports from several medical centers suggest that lung volumes in bilateral lung transplant recipients approach normal values,[116–118] whereas the lung function in unilateral recipients depends on the underlying disease.[119] Heart-lung transplant recipients tend to have restrictive pulmonary physiology, which has been attributed to a variety of factors[120] but likely is most influenced by the relationship of donor and recipient size. Diffusing capacity has been reported as remaining slightly below normal in most patients.[121] Chacon and coworkers[122] studied the factors determining respiratory mechanics after heart-lung transplantation and bilateral lung transplantation. They compared the lung volumes post-transplantation with the size of the recipient's lung pre-transplantation and the predicted size of the donor lungs. In addition, they measured pressure-volume curves and maximum respiratory pressures post-transplantation. The results suggest that at high volumes the chest wall adapts to the size of the transplanted lungs, whereas at lower volumes the transplanted lungs adapt to the recipient's chest wall.[122]

### Airway Function

The remarkable improvements in pulmonary function after transplantation are accompanied by interesting findings possibly related to the loss of innervation, relative airway ischemia, or loss of lymphatics after the surgery. Increased airway responsiveness to methacholine and histamine has been found after both heart-lung and isolated lung transplantation.[123, 124] This is not usually clinically evident, however. Patients with heart-lung grafts do not exhibit airway constriction following exercise challenge as is the case with asthmatic patients,[125] yet they respond with airway dilation to inhaled albuterol and ipratropium bromide.[126] Glanville and coworkers[126] used these findings, along with the observations that the hyperresponsiveness to methacholine was stable over 1 to 4 years and that the maximal airway narrowing to methacholine was limited (plateau of dose response), to suggest that the post-transplant changes were related to denervation hypersensitivity of muscarinic receptors. Using bronchial rings of lungs undergoing retransplantation, however, Stretton and associates[127] could not confirm this. Ward

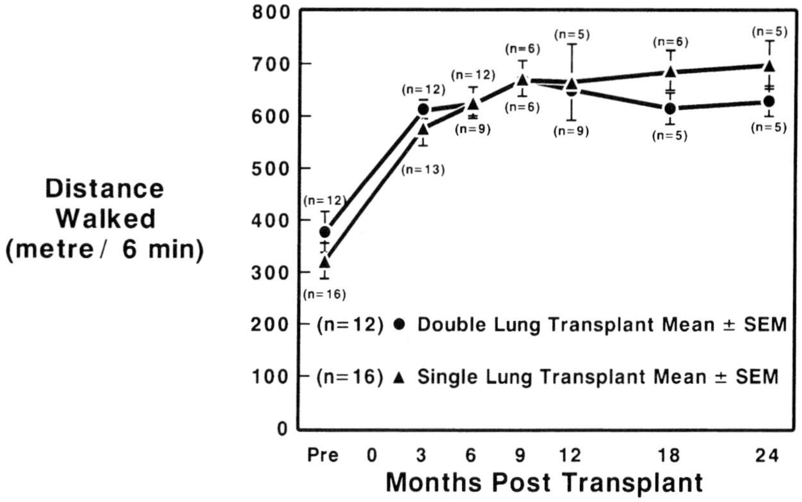


**Figure 97.1** The 6-minute walk test in single-lung and double-lung transplant recipients. The total distance walked in 6 minutes is measured. Pretransplant, the test is performed with supplemental oxygen; post-transplant, without supplemental oxygen. (Reproduced with permission from Williams TJ, Grossman RF, Maurer JR: Long-term functional follow-up of lung transplant recipients. Clin Chest Med 11:347–358, 1990.)

and coworkers[128] compared the results of methacholine and hypertonic saline challenges to amounts of inflammation in airway biopsies and found very little correlation. Snell and colleagues[129] have shown that even healthy, stable lung recipients have evidence of ongoing inflammation as demonstrated by increased numbers of CD68-positive cells on endobronchial biopsy but again were unable to correlate this with hyperresponsiveness. Thus, the mechanism of post-transplantation hyperresponsiveness remains unclear. Healthy individuals have airway dilation following a deep breath while their airways are constricted, but heart-lung transplant recipients fail to show such dilation.[130] This absence of dilation following lung inflation is similar to the findings in asthmatic patients.[131]

## Exercise Capacity

Exercise capacity increases significantly following any type of lung transplantation.[132, 133] Maximal exercise testing, as well as 6-minute walk tests, have been used to measure exercise capacity of lung transplant recipients before and after transplantation. Figure 97.1 shows that double-lung and single-lung recipients can expect to approximately double the distance covered in 6-minute walk tests after transplantation and that this improvement is maintained over time.[133] Maximal exercise capacity also increases dramatically after transplantation. Various authors have shown, however, that neither single-lung nor double-lung transplants achieve greater than about 60% of predicted maximum oxygen uptakes. Levy and colleagues[119] compared maximal, symptom-limited cycle ergometer exercise performance in 11 heart-lung, 6 double-lung, and 16 single-lung recipients and found that in all cases oxygen uptakes were in the 40% to 60% ranges, and no significant difference was apparent depending on type of transplant. Furthermore, subjects were not limited by cardiac or ventilatory capacity, but rather exercise responses were characterized by reduced aerobic capacity (Fig. 97.2).[119] Subsequent studies to further delineate the defect have suggested a role for muscle deconditioning, but of more importance may be abnormalities in systemic oxygen extraction related to skeletal muscle oxidative capacity.[134, 135] It has been suggested that immunosuppressive drugs, which have been shown in animal models to impair mitochondrial function,[136] are the cause. Other recent studies evaluating exercise performance in pretransplant patients with advanced disease have also, however, shown impairment of systemic oxygen uptake, the mechanism of which remains unclear.[137]

## Control of Breathing

Sanders and associates[138] examined the responses to hypercapnia and hypoxia in patients with heart-lung transplants and found that, while hypoxia had no effect, pulmonary denervation was associated with a reduction of the overall ventilatory response to progressive hypercapnia. Using patients with heart-lung transplants who had normal spirometry, Duncan and colleagues[139] found that

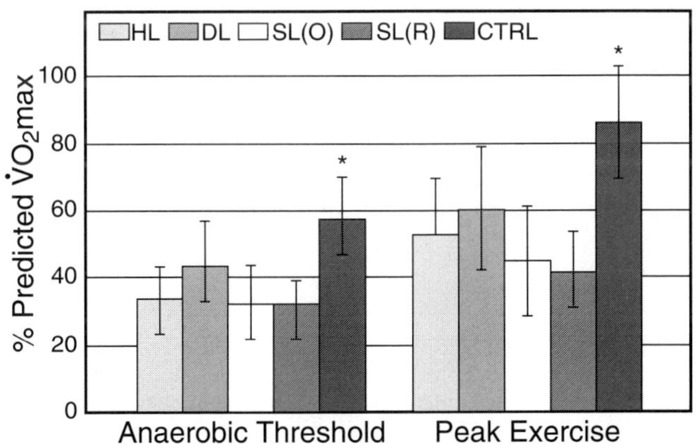


**Figure 97.2** Mean values for oxygen uptake ($\dot{V}O_2$) were similar among the different groups of lung transplant recipients at the anaerobic threshold and at peak exercise; however, these values were significantly lower than those observed in the control subjects. CTRL = control; DL = double lung; HL = heart-lung; SL(O) = single lung obstructive; SL(R) = single lung restrictive: $*P < .05$. (From Levy RD, Ernst P, Shennib H, et al: Exercise performance after lung transplantation. J Heart Lung Transplant 12:23–33, 1993.)

the ventilatory response to hypercapnia was normal but the mouth occlusion pressure was increased, and the pattern of breathing during progressive hypercapnia was consistent with the absence of vagal-mediated inflation inhibition. In a double-lung transplant population with tracheal anastomoses, Frost and coworkers[140] found that hypercapneic ventilatory responses were low or low normal, and the responses did not correlate with preoperative or postoperative $P_{CO_2}$ or muscle strength.

### Psychosocial Factors

Despite the many concerns and potential complications faced by recipients after lung transplantation, these patients generally report an improved quality of life.[141, 142] It is important to recognize, however, that many patients with advanced lung disease have significant anxiety, depression and other psychologic diagnoses, and failure to address these issues pretransplantation may result in a less than optimal post-transplantation adjustment.

## Medical Complications of Long-Term Survivors

As more recipients of lung grafts have achieved long-term survival, the impact of medical complications (Table 97.4) related to immunosuppressive therapy, to the patient's underlying illness, or to the usual diseases of aging have become of increasing concern to the transplantation pulmonologist. Nearly 10% of lung transplant recipients will die of these complications, and many more will experience significant morbidity.[143, 144] Recognition of the severity of these complications has led to more stringent selection criteria (see earlier discussion) and to aggressive preventative approaches in the hope that the impacts of these complications can be lessened.

### Nephrotoxicity

Nearly all patients receiving cyclosporine or tacrolimus immunosuppression experience a reduction in renal function. A significant fall in creatinine clearance occurs in the first few months after transplant.[145] Although only a small percentage of patients will ultimately develop renal failure requiring dialysis, care should be taken to minimize the use of concomitant nephrotoxic antibiotics and other medications.

**Table 97.4 COMMON MEDICAL COMPLICATIONS IN LUNG TRANSPLANT RECIPIENTS**

| | |
|---|---|
| Nephrotoxicity | Myopathy |
| Hypertension | Hemolytic-uremic syndrome |
| Osteoporosis | Menstrual irregularities |
| Hyperlipidemia | Lymphoproliferative disorders |
| Diabetes mellitus | Other malignancies |
| Neurotoxicity | Gastroparesis |
| Anemia | Esophagitis/gastritis |
| Hypercoaguability | Perforated bowel |
| Pancreatitis | |

### Hypertension

Almost universal after solid organ transplantation is the occurrence of systemic hypertension. The hypertension requires aggressive management to protect renal function.

### Neurotoxicity

A high rate of neurologic complications occurs in patients receiving cyclosporine or tacrolimus. One report notes an incidence of about 25% in a post–lung transplantation population.[146] The complications include seizures, severe headaches, confusion, and strokes, as well as varying levels of delirium, and they do not appear to be reliably related to immunosuppressive levels. In many cases, typical white matter changes can be seen with CT or magnetic resonance imaging techniques.

### Osteoporosis

Between 30% and 50% of patients coming to lung transplantation have osteoporosis by the World Health Organization's definition (−2.5 standard deviations from peak bone mass).[147] More importantly, post-transplantation patients have been found to have a rapid bone loss in the first 6 months after surgery,[148] and the fracture rates are excessive,[149] a problem that greatly impairs quality of life. Particularly distressing are vertebral compression fractures, which can impair cough and pulmonary function. Preventative therapy is of paramount importance.

### Other

Table 97.4 shows a myriad of other medical issues. Special note should be made of those that are potentially preventable. Thromboembolic phenomena can be minimized by use of low-dose warfarin in the presence of indwelling catheters. Gastric complications, particularly gastroparesis, as well as hyperlipidemia and hyperglycemia (often seen with tacrolimus), can be prevented or managed pharmacologically. Finally, regular preventative medicine screening should not be forgotten, because there is a significantly increased incidence of several types of malignancy, particularly skin malignancies, besides the Epstein-Barr–related lymphocytic disorders noted above (Table 97.5).

## Recurrent Disease

A number of diseases have been reported to recur in the allograft. Recurrent sarcoidosis has been reported by several authors, although it is usually subclinical.[150, 151] Other diagnoses with case reports of recurring disease include lymphangioleiomyomatosis,[152] giant cell interstitial pneumonia,[153] panbronchiolitis,[154] eosinophilic granuloma,[155] bronchoalveolar cell carcinoma,[156] and desquamative interstitial pneumonia.[157]

**Table 97.5 PREVENTIVE CARE MONITORING OF LUNG TRANSPLANT RECIPIENTS**

| |
|---|
| Provide preoperative and postoperative patient instruction regarding risks of immunosuppression, high-risk activities (e.g., sun exposure), and worrisome symptoms |
| Identify individual patient risks that predispose to postoperative problems—history of smoking, osteoporosis, family history of disease, hypercoagulability |
| Perform routine preventive medicine screens (mammograms, sigmoidoscopy, complete skin inspection) yearly for all patients and every 6 months for high-risk patients |
| When possible, institute preoperative or preemptive therapy and education to prevent postoperative problems |

Reproduced with permission from Maurer JR, Tewari S: Nonpulmonary medical complications in the intermediate and long-term survivor. Clin Chest Med 18:367–378, 1997.

## SUMMARY AND FUTURE ISSUES

Donor scarcity remains an important limitation to lung transplantation. Despite the use of living related donors, non–heart beating donors, and marginal donors, a significant discrepancy between supply and demand exists. Whether this gap will be filled by genetically engineered xenografts remains to be seen. Other major issues that continue to impair the outcomes of lung transplant recipients are organ preservation, management of acute and chronic rejection, and the many medical complications including infections. Most of these problems will be addressed as we enter the twenty-first century. We look forward to more selective immunosuppressive agents and to methods of developing allograft tolerance to enhance the quality of life of these patients.

## References


1. Hardy JD, Webb WR, Dalton ML, et al: Lung homotransplantation in man. JAMA 186:1065–1074, 1963.
2. Derom F, Barbier F, Ringoir S, et al: Ten month survival after lung homotransplantation in man. J Thorac Cardiovasc Surg 61:835–846, 1971.
3. Reitz BA, Wallwork JL, Hunt SA, et al: Heart-lung transplantation: Successful therapy for patients with pulmonary vascular disease. N Engl J Med 306:557–564, 1982.
4. Toronto Lung Transplant Group: Unilateral lung transplantation for pulmonary fibrosis. N Engl J Med 314:1140–1145, 1986.
5. Cooper JD, Patterson GA, Grossman R, et al: Double-lung transplant for advanced chronic obstructive lung disease. Am Rev Respir Dis 139:303–307, 1989.
6. Hosenpud JD, Bennett LE, Keck BM, et al: The Registry of the International Society for Heart and Lung Transplantation: Fifteenth Official Report—1998. J Heart Lung Transplant 17:656–661, 1998.
7. Lillihei CW, in discussion of Wildevuur CRH, Benfield JRA: A review of 23 human lung transplantations by 20 surgeons. Ann Thorac Surg 9:489–515, 1970.
8. Mills NL, Boyd AD, Gheranpong C: The significance of the bronchial circulation in lung transplantation. J Thorac Cardiovasc Surg 60:866–878, 1970.
9. Lima O, Cooper JD, Peters WJ, et al: Effects of methylprednisolone and azathioprine on bronchial healing following lung autotransplantation. J Thorac Cardiovasc Surg 82:211–215, 1981.
10. Morgan WE, Lima O, Goldberg M, et al: Improved bronchial healing in canine left lung reimplantation using omental pedicle wrap. J Thorac Cardiovasc Surg 85:134–139, 1983.
11. Miller JD, deHoyos A, Patterson GA, et al: An evaluation of the role of omentopexy and of early corticosteroid administration in clinical lung transplantation. J Thorac Cardiovasc Surg 105:247–252, 1993.
12. Schafers H-J, Haverich A, Wagner TOF, et al: Decreased incidence of bronchial complications following lung transplantation. Eur J Cardiovasc Surg 6:174–179, 1992.
13. Miller JD, deHoyos A: An evaluation of the role of omentopexy and of early perioperative corticosteroid administration in clinical transplantation. The University of Toronto and Washington University lung transplant programs. J Thorac Cardiovasc Surg 105:247–252, 1993.
14. Calhoon JH, Grover FL, Gibbons WJ, et al: Single lung transplantation: Alternative indications and technique. J Thorac Cardiovasc Surg 101:816–825, 1991.
15. Novick RJ, Menkis AH, Sandler D, et al: Contralateral pneumectomy after single lung transplantation for emphysema. Ann Thorac Surg 52:1317–1319, 1991.
16. Kroshus TJ, Bolman RM, Kshettry VR: Unilateral volume reduction after single-lung transplantation for emphysema. Ann Thorac Surg 62:363–368, 1996.
17. Anderson MB, Kriet JM, Kapelanski DP, et al: Volume reduction surgery in the native lung after single lung transplantation for emphysema. J Heart Lung Transplant 16:752–757, 1997.
18. Schulman LL, O'Hair DP, Cantu E, et al: Salvage by volume reduction of chronic allograft rejection in emphysema. J Heart Lung Transplant 18:107–112, 1999.
19. Horvath J, Dummer S, Loyd J, et al: Infection in the transplanted and native lung after single lung transplant. Chest 104:681–685, 1993.
20. Frost AE, Keller CA, Noon GP, et al: Outcome of the native lung after single lung transplantation. Multiorgan Transplant Group. Chest 107:981–984, 1995.
21. Westney GE, Kesten S, de Hoyos A, et al: *Aspergillus* infection in single and double lung transplant recipients. Transplantation 61:915–919, 1996.
22. Dark JH, Patterson GA, Al-Jilaihawi AN, et al: Experimental en bloc double-lung transplantation. Ann Thorac Surg 42:394–398, 1986.
23. Pasque MK, Cooper JD, Kaiser LR, et al: Improved technique for bilateral lung transplantation: Rationale and initial clinical experience. Ann Thorac Surg 49:785–791, 1990.
24. Gammie JS, Keenan RJ, Pham SM, et al: Single versus double-lung transplantation for pulmonary hypertension. J Thorac Cardiovasc Surg 115:397–402, 1998.
25. Spray TL, Mallory GB, Cantor CB, et al: Pediatric lung transplantation. Indications, techniques and early results. J Thorac Cardiovasc Surg 107:990–1000, 1994.
26. Shaw LR, Miller JD, Slutsky AS, et al: Ethics of lung transplantation with live donors. Lancet 338:678–681, 1991.
27. Starnes VA, Barr ML, Cohen RG, et al: Living-donor lobar lung transplantation experience: Intermediate results. J Thorac Cardiovasc Surg 112:1284–1290, 1996.
28. International guidelines for the selection of lung transplant candidates: Joint statement of the American Society for Transplant Physicians (ASTP)/American Thoracic Society (ATS)/European Respiratory Society (ERS)/International Society for Heart and Lung Transplantation (ISHLT). Am J Respir Crit Care Med 158:335–339, 1998.
29. Maurer JR, Frost AE, Estenne M, et al (Coordinating Committee): International guidelines for the selection of lung transplant candidates. J Heart Lung Transplant 17:703–709, 1998.
30. Maurer JR, Frost AE, Estenne M, et al: International guidelines for the selection of lung transplant candidates. The International Society for Heart and Lung Transplantation, the American Thoracic Society, the American Society of Transplant Physicians, the European Respiratory Society. Heart Lung 27:223–229, 1998.
31. Maurer JR, Frost AE, Estenne M, et al: International guidelines for the selection of lung transplant candidates. Transplantation 66:951–956, 1998.

32. Kerem H, Reisman J, Corey M, et al: Prediction of mortality in patients with cystic fibrosis. N Engl J Med 326:1187–1191, 1992.
33. Aris RM, Gilligan PH, Neuringer IP, et al: The effects of panresistant bacteria in cystic fibrosis patients on lung transplant outcome. Am J Respir Crit Care Med 155:1699–1704, 1997.
34. LiPuma JJ: *Burkholderia cepacia:* Management issues and new insights. Clin Chest Med 19:473–486, 1998.
35. Hosenpud JD, Bennett LE, Keck BM, et al: Effect of diagnosis on survival benefit of lung transplantation for end-stage lung disease. Lancet 351(9095):24–27, 1998.
36. Hayden AM, Robert RC, Kriett JM, et al: Primary diagnosis predicts prognosis of lung transplant candidates. Transplantation 55:1048–1050, 1993.
37. McLaughlin VV, Genthner DE, Panella MM, et al: Reduction in pulmonary vascular resistance with long-term epoprostenol (prostacyclin) therapy in primary pulmonary hypertension. N Engl J Med 338:273–277, 1998.
38. Rosenzweig EB, Kerstein D, Barst RJ: Long-term prostacyclin for pulmonary hypertension with associated congenital heart defects. Circulation 99:1858–1865, 1999.
39. D'Alonzo GE, Barst RJ, Ayres SM, et al: Survival in patients with primary pulmonary hypertension. Results from a national prospective registry. Ann Intern Med 115:343–349, 1991.
40. Hopkins WE, Ochoa LL, Richardson GW, et al: Comparison of the hemodynamics and survival of adults with severe primary pulmonary hypertension or Eisenmenger syndrome. J Heart Lung Transplant 15:100–105, 1996.
41. Bridges ND, Clark BJ, Gaynor JW, et al: Outcome of children with pulmonary hypertension referred for lung or heart and lung transplantation. Transplantation 62:1824–1828, 1996.
42. Brooks RG, Hofflin JM, Jamieson SW, et al: Infectious complications in heart-lung transplant recipients. Am J Med 79:412–422, 1985.
43. Maurer JR, Tullis E, Grossman RF, et al: Infectious complications following isolated lung transplantation. Chest 101:1056–1059, 1992.
44. Egan JJ, Lomax J, Barber L, et al: Preemptive treatment for the prevention of cytomegalovirus disease: In lung and heart transplant recipients. Transplantation 65:747–752, 1998.
45. Stephan F, Fajac A, Grenet D, et al: Predictive value of cytomegalovirus DNA detection by polymerase chain reaction in blood and bronchoalveolar lavage in lung transplant patients. Transplantation 63:1430–1435, 1997.
46. Kramer MR, Marshal SE, Starnes VA, et al: Infectious complications in heart-lung transplantation. Analysis of 200 episodes. Arch Intern Med 153:2010–2016, 1993.
47. Bangsborg JM, Uldum S, Jensen JS, et al: Nosocomial legionnellosis in three heart-lung transplant patients: Case reports and environmental observations. Eur J Clin Microbiol Infect Dis 14:99–104, 1995.
48. Loubeye P, Revel D, Delignette A, et al: Bronchiectasis detected with thin-section CT as a predictor of chronic lung allograft rejection. Radiology 194:213–216, 1995.
49. Smyth RL, Scott JP, Borysiewicz LK, et al: Cytomegalovirus infection in heart-lung transplant recipients: Risk factors, clinical associations, and response to treatment. J Infect Dis 164:1045–1050, 1991.
50. Ettinger NA, Bailey TC, Trulock EP, et al: Cytomegalovirus infection and pneumonitis. Impact after isolated lung transplantation. Washington University Lung Transplant Group. Am Rev Respir Dis 147:1017–1023, 1993.
51. Dauber JH, Paradis IL, Dummer JS: Infectious complications in pulmonary allograft recipients. Clin Chest Med 11:291–308, 1990.
52. Gutierrez CA, Chaparro C, Krajden M, et al: Cytomegalovirus viremia in lung transplant recipients receiving ganciclovir and immune globulin. Chest 113:924–932, 1998.
53. Kroshus TJ, Kshettry VR, Savik K, et al: Risk factors for the development of bronchiolitis obliterans syndrome after lung transplantation. J Thorac Cardiovasc Surg 114:195–202, 1997.
53a. Ettinger NA, Bailey TC, Trulock EP, et al: Cytomegalovirus infection and pneumonitis. Impact after isolated lung transplantation. Washington University Lung Transplant Group. Am Rev Respir Dis 147:1017–1023, 1993.
54. Sharples LD, Tamm M, McNeil K, et al: Development of bronchiolitis obliterans syndrome in recipients of heart-lung transplantation—early risk factors. Transplantation 61:560–566, 1996.
55. Aris RM, Maia DM, Neuringer IP, et al: Posttransplantation lymphoproliferative disorder in the Epstein-Barr virus–naïve lung transplant recipient. Am J Respir Crit Care Med 154:1712–1717, 1996.
56. Ohori NP, Michaels MG, Jaffe R, et al: Adenovirus pneumonia in lung transplant recipients. Hum Pathol 26:1073–1079, 1995.
57. Wendt C, Fox J, Hertz M: Paramyxovirus infection in lung transplant recipients. J Heart Lung Transplant 14:479–485, 1995.
58. Palmer SM, Henshaw NG, Howell DN, et al: Community respiratory viral infection in adult lung transplant recipients. Chest 113:944–950, 1998.
59. Krinzman S, Basgoz N, Kradin R, et al: Respiratory syncytial virus-associated infections in adult recipients of solid organ transplants. J Heart Lung Transplant 17:202–210, 1998.
60. Bridges ND, Spray TL, Collins MH, et al: Adenovirus infection in the lung results in graft failure after lung transplantation. J Thorac Cardiovasc Surg 116:617–623, 1998.
61. Umeh F, Sarodia BD, Haug MT, et al: Influenza A infection in patients after lung transplantation. Chest 114:399S, 1998.
62. Kramer MR, Denning DW, Marshall SE, et al: Ulcerative tracheobronchitis after lung transplantation: A new form of invasive aspergillosis. Am Rev Respir Dis 144:552–556, 1991.
63. Westney G, Kesten S, DeHoyos A, et al: *Aspergillus* infection in single and double lung transplant recipients. Transplantation 61:915–919, 1996.
64. Nunley DR, Ohori P, Grgurich WF, et al: Pulmonary aspergillosis in cystic fibrosis lung transplant recipients. Chest 114:1321–1329, 1998.
65. Cahill BC, Hibbs JR, Savik K, et al: *Aspergillus* airway colonization and invasive disease after lung transplantation. Chest 112:1160–1164, 1997.
66. Tomee JF, Mannes GP, van der Bij W, et al: Serodiagnosis and monitoring of *Aspergillus* infections after lung transplantation. Ann Intern Med 125:197–201, 1996.
67. Egan JJ, Yonan N, Carroll KB, et al: Allergic bronchopulmonary aspergillosis in a lung allograft recipients. Eur Respir J 9:169–171, 1996.
68. Salerno CT, Ouyang DW, Pederson TS, et al: Surgical therapy for pulmonary aspergillosis in immunocompromised patients. Ann Thorac Surg 65:1415–1419, 1998.
69. Caillot D, Casasnovas O, Bernard A, et al: Improved management of invasive pulmonary aspergillosis in neutropenic patients using early thoracic computed tomographic scan and surgery. J Clin Oncol 15:139–147, 1997.
70. Baron O, Guillaume B, Moreau P, et al: Aggressive surgical management in localized pulmonary mycotic and nonmycotic infections for neutropenic patients with acute leukemia: Report of eighteen cases. J Thorac Cardiovasc Surg 115:63–68, 1998.
71. Gryzan S, Paradis IL, Zeevi A, et al: Unexpectedly high incidence of *Pneumocystis carini* infection after heart-lung transplantation. Am Rev Respir Dis 137:268–274, 1988.
72. Lawrence EC: Diagnosis and management of lung allograft rejection. Clin Chest Med 11:269–278, 1990.
73. Prop J, Nieuwenhuis P, Wildevuur CRH: Lung allograft rejection in the rat. Transplantation 40:25–29, 1985.
74. Veith FJ, Sinha SBP, Blumcke S, et al: Nature and evolution of lung allograft rejection with and without immunosuppression. J Thorac Cardiovasc Surg 63:509–520, 1972.
75. Koerner SK, Hagstrom JWC, Veith FJ: Transbronchial biopsy for the diagnosis of lung transplant rejection: Comparison with needle and open-lung biopsy techniques in canine lung allografts. Am Rev Respir Dis 114:575–579, 1976.
76. Hutter J, Stewart S, Higenbottam TW, et al: Histological changes in heart-lung transplant recipients during rejection episodes and at routine biopsy. J Heart Transplant 7:440–444, 1988.
77. Higenbottam T, Stewart S, Penketh A, et al: Transbronchial lung biopsy for the diagnosis of rejection in heart-lung transplant patients. Transplantation 46:532–539, 1988.
78. Starnes VA, Theodore J, Oyer PE, et al: Evaluation of heart-lung transplant recipients with prospective serial transbronchial biopsies and pulmonary function studies. J Thorac Cardiovasc Surg 98:683–690, 1989.

79. The International Society for Heart Transplantation, Yousem SA, Berry GJ, Brunt EM, et al: A working formulation for the standardization of nomenclature in the diagnosis of heart and lung rejection: Lung rejection study group. J Heart Transplant 9:593–601, 1990.
80. Tazelaar HD, Nilsson FN, Rinaldi M, et al: The sensitivity of transbronchial biopsy for the diagnosis of acute lung rejection. J Thorac Cardiovasc Surg 105:674–678, 1993.
81. Higenbottam T, Stewart S, Penketh A, et al: Transbronchial lung biopsy for the diagnosis of rejection in heart-lung transplant patients. Transplantation 46:532–536, 1988.
82. Yousem SA, Berry GJ, Cagle PT, et al: Revision of the 1990 working formulation for the classification of pulmonary allograft rejection: Lung Rejection Study Group. J Heart Lung Transplant 15:1–15, 1996.
83. Sundaresan S, Alevy YG, Steward N, et al: Cytokine gene transcripts for tumor necrosis factor α, interleukin-2, and interferon γ in human pulmonary allografts. J Heart Lung Transplant 14:512–518, 1995.
84. Whitehead BF, Stoehr C, Wu CJ, et al: Cytokine gene expression in human lung transplant recipients. Transplantation 56:956–961, 1993.
85. Schersten H, Aarnio P, Burnett JC Jr, et al: Endothelin-1 in bronchoalveolar lavage during acute rejection of allotransplanted lungs. Transplantation 57:159–161, 1994.
86. Shennib H, Mercado M, Nguyen D, et al: Successful treatment of steroid-resistant double-lung allograft rejection with orthoclone OKT3. Am Rev Respir Dis 144:224–226, 1991.
87. Keenan RJ, Iacono A, Dauber JH, et al: Treatment of refractory acute allograft rejection with aerosolized cyclosporine in lung transplant recipients. J Thorac Cardiovasc Surg 113:335–340, 1997.
88. Cahill B, O'Rourke MK, Strasburg KA, et al: Methotrexate for lung transplant recipients with steroid resistant acute rejection. J Heart Lung Transplant 15:1130–1137, 1996.
89. Valentine VG, Robbins RC, Wehner JH, et al: Total lymphoid irradiation for refractory acute rejection in heart-lung and lung allografts. Chest 109:1184–1189, 1996.
90. deHoyos A, Chamberlain D, Schvartzman R, et al: Prospective assessment of a standardized pathological grading system for acute rejection in lung transplantation. Chest 103:1813–1818, 1993.
91. Trulock EP, Ettinger NA, Brunt EM, et al: The role of transbronchial lung biopsy in the treatment of lung transplant recipients. An analysis of 200 consecutive procedures. Chest 102:1049–1054, 1992.
92. Boehler A, Kesten S, Weder W, et al: Bronchiolitis obliterans after lung transplantation: A review. Chest 114:1411–1426, 1998.
93. McCarthy P, Starnes VA, Theordore J, et al: Improved survival following heart-lung transplant. J Thorac Cardiovasc Surg 99:54–60, 1990.
94. Burke CM, Theodore J, Baldwin JC, et al: Twenty-eight cases of human heart-lung transplantation. Lancet 1:517–519, 1986.
95. Patterson GM, Wilson S, Whang JL, et al: Physiologic definitions of obliterative bronchiolitis in heart-lung and double lung transplantation: A comparison of the forced expiratory flow between 25% and 75% of the forced vital capacity and forced expiratory volume in one second. J Heart Lung Transplant 15:175–181, 1996.
96. Bassiri AG, Girgis RE, Doyle RL, et al: Detection of small airway dysfunction using specific airway conductance. Chest 111:1533–1535, 1997.
97. Ikonen T, Harjula AL, Kinnula VL, et al: Assessment of forced expiratory volume in one second-fraction of the engrafted lung with $^{133}$-Xe radiospirometry improves the diagnosis of bronchiolitis obliterans syndrome in single lung transplant recipients. J Heart Lung Transplant 14:244–250, 1995.
98. Leung AN, Fisher KL, Valentine V, et al: Bronchiolitis obliterans after lung transplantation: Detection using expiratory HRCT. Chest 113:365–370, 1998.
99. Cooper J, Billingham M, Egan T, et al: A working formulation for the standardization of nomenclature and for clinical staging of chronic dysfunction in lung allografts: International Society for Heart and Lung Transplantation. J Heart Lung Transplant 12:713–716, 1993.
100. Kesten S, Chaparro C, Scavuzzo M, et al: Tacrolimus as rescue therapy for bronchiolitis obliterans syndrome. J Heart Lung Transplant 16:905–912, 1997.
101. Dusmet M, Maurer J, Winton T, et al: Methotrexate can halt the progression of bronchiolitis obliterans syndrome in lung transplant recipients. J Heart Lung Transplant 15:948–954, 1996.
102. Snell GI, Esmore DS, Williams TJ: Cytolytic therapy for the bronchiolitis obliterans syndrome complicating lung transplantation. Chest 109:874–878, 1996.
103. Afolabi OA, Parry G, Healy MD, et al: The role of total lymphoid irradiation (TLI) in the treatment of obliterative bronchiolitis.(abstract). J Heart Lung Transplant 15:S102, 1996.
104. Nathan SD, Ross DJ, Belman MJ, et al: Bronchiolitis obliterans in single-lung transplant recipients. Chest 107:967–972, 1995.
105. Yousem SA, Burke CM, Billingham ME: Pathologic pulmonary alterations in long-term human heart-lung transplantation. Hum Pathol 16:911–923, 1985.
106. Clellano C, Higenbottam T, Otulana B, et al: Histologic prognostic indicators for the lung allografts of heart-lung transplants. J Heart Lung Transplant 9:177–186, 1990.
107. Keenan RJ, Lega ME, Dummer JS, et al: Cytomegalovirus serologic status and postoperative infection correlated with risk of developing chronic rejection after pulmonary transplantation. Transplantation 51:433–438, 1991.
108. Schulman LL, Weinberg AD, McGregor C, et al: Mismatches at the HLA-DR and HLA-B loci are risk factors for acute rejection after transplantation. Am J Respir Crit Care Med 157:1833–1837, 1998.
109. Bando K, Paradis IL, Similo S, et al: Obliterative bronchiolitis after lung and heart-lung transplantation: An analysis of risk factors and management. J Thorac Cardiovasc Surg 110:4–13, 1995.
110. Itescu S, Weinberg AD, Burke EM, et al: Risk factors for early onset obliterative bronchiolitis after lung transplantation: Influence of donor HLA-DR4 type (abstract). J Heart Lung Transplant 16:A69, 1997.
111. Hohlfeld J, Niedermeyer J, Hamm H, et al: Seasonal onset of bronchiolitis obliterans syndrome in lung transplant recipients. J Heart Lung Transplant 15:888–894, 1996.
112. Jaramillo A, Smith MA, Phelan D, et al: Development of ELISA-detected anti-HLA antibodies precedes the development of bronchiolitis obliterans syndrome and correlates with progressive decline in pulmonary function after lung transplantation. Transplantation 67:1155–1161, 1999.
113. Hertz MI, Jessurun J, King MB, et al: Reproduction of the obliterative bronchiolitis lesion after heterotopic transplantation of mouse airways. Am J Pathol 142:1945–1951, 1993.
114. Koskinen PK, Kallio EA, Krebs R, et al: A dose-dependent inhibitory effect of cyclosporine A on obliterative bronchiolitis of rat tracheal allografts. Am J Respir Crit Care Med 155:303–312, 1997.
115. Boehler A, Chamberlain D, Kesten S, et al: Lymphocytic airway infiltration as a precursor to fibrous obliteration in a rat model of bronchiolitis obliterans. Transplantation 64:311–317, 1997.
116. Toronto Lung Transplant group: Experience with single lung transplantation for pulmonary fibrosis. JAMA 259:2258–2262, 1988.
117. Williams TJ, Grossman RF, Maurer JR: Long-term functional follow-up of lung transplant recipients. Clin Chest Med 11:347–358, 1990.
118. Gaissert HA, Trulock EP, Cooper JD, et al: Comparison of early functional results after lung volume reduction or lung transplantation for COPD. J Thorac Cardiovasc Surg 111:296–307, 1996.
119. Levy RD, Ernst P, Shennib H, et al: Exercise performance after lung transplantation. J Heart Lung Transplant 12:23–33, 1993.
120. Madden BP, Hodgson ME, Tsang V, et al: Intermediate results of heart-lung transplantation for cystic fibrosis. Lancet 339:1583–1587, 1992.
121. Williams TJ, Johns DP, Side E, et al: $D_LCO$ reduction is not associated with altered $DM/V_C$ in heart-lung transplant recipients (abstract). Am Rev Respir Dis 145:A703, 1992.
122. Chacon RA, Corris PA, Dark JH, et al: Respiratory mechanics after heart-lung and bilateral lung transplantation. Thorax 52:718–722, 1997.
123. Glanville AR, Burke CM, Theodore J, et al: Bronchial hyper-responsiveness after human cardiopulmonary transplantation. Clin Sci 73:299–303, 1987.

124. Maurer JR, McClean PA, Cooper JD, et al: Airway hyper-reactivity in patients undergoing lung and heart-lung transplantation. Am Rev Respir Dis 139:1038–1041, 1989.
125. Glanville AR, Gabb GM, Theodore J, et al: Bronchial responsiveness to exercise after human cardiopulmonary transplantation. Chest 96:281–286, 1989.
126. Glanville AR, Theodore J, Baldwin JC, et al: Bronchial responsiveness after human heart-lung transplantation. Chest 97:1360–1366, 1990.
127. Stretton CD, Mak JC, Belvisi MG, et al: Cholinergic control of human airways in vitro following extrinsic denervation of human respiratory tract by heart-lung transplantation. Am Rev Respir Dis 142:1030–1033, 1990.
128. Ward C, Snell GI, Orsida B, et al: Airway versus transbronchial biopsy and BAL in lung transplant recipients: Different but complementary. Eur Respir J 10:2876–2880, 1997.
129. Snell GI, Ward C, Wilson JW, et al: Immunopathological changes in the airways of stable lung transplant recipients. Thorax 52:322–328, 1997.
130. Glanville AR, Yeend RA, Theodore J, et al: Effect of single respiratory manoeuvres on specific airway conductance in heart-lung transplant recipients. Clin Sci 74:311–317, 1988.
131. Fish JE, Ankin MG, Kelly JF, et al: Regulation of bronchomotor tone by lung inflation in asthmatic and non-asthmatic subjects. J Appl Physiol 50:1079–1086, 1981.
132. Miyoshi S, Trulock EP, Schaefers HJ, et al: Cardio-pulmonary exercise testing after single and double lung transplantation. Chest 97:1130–1136, 1990.
133. Williams TJ, Grossman RF, Maurer JR: Long-term functional follow-up of lung transplant recipients. Clin Chest Med 11:347–358, 1990.
134. Morton JM, McKenna MJ, Carey MF, et al: Reductions in type I fibre proportions and oxidative enzyme activity in skeletal muscle exist pre and post lung transplantation. J Heart Lung Transplant 18:A66, 1999.
135. Evans AB, Al-Himyary AJ, Hrovat MI, et al: Abnormal skeletal muscle oxidative capacity after lung transplantation by $^{31}$P-MRS. Am J Respir Crit Care Med 155:615–622, 1997.
136. Mercier JG, Hokanson JF, Brooks GA: Effects of cyclosporine A on skeletal muscle mitochondrial respiration and endurance time in rats. Am J Respir Crit Care Med 151:1532–1536, 1995.
137. Oelberg DA, Medoff BD, Markowitz DH, et al: Systemic oxygen extraction during incremental exercise in patients with severe chronic obstructive pulmonary disease. Eur J Appl Physiol 78:201–207, 1998.
138. Sanders MH, Owens GR, Sciurba FC, et al: Ventilation and breathing pattern during progressive hypercapnia and hypoxia after human heart-lung transplantation. Am Rev Respir Dis 140:38–44, 1989.
139. Duncan SR, Kagawa FT, Starnes VA, et al: Hypercarbic ventilatory responses of human heart-lung transplant recipients. Am Rev Respir Dis 144:126–130, 1991.
140. Frost AE, Zamel N, McClean P, et al: Hypercapnic ventilatory response in recipients of double-lung transplants. Am Rev Respir Dis 146:1610–1612, 1992.
141. Cohen L, Littlefield C, Kelly P, et al: Predictors of quality of life and adjustment after lung transplantation. Chest 113:633–644, 1998.
142. Gross CR, Savik K, Bolman RM III, et al: Long-term health status and quality of life outcomes of lung transplant recipients. Chest 108:1587–1593, 1995.
143. Chaparro C, Kesten S, Chamberlain D, et al: Causes of death in lung transplant recipients. J Heart Lung Transplant 13:758–767, 1994.
144. Maurer JR: Medical complications following lung transplantation. Semin Respir Crit Care Med 17(2):173–185, 1996.
145. Zaltzman JS, Pei Y, Maurer J, et al: Cyclosporine nephrotoxicity in lung transplant recipients. Transplantation 54:875–878, 1992.
146. Goldstein LS, Haug MT, Perl J, et al: Central nervous system complications after lung transplantation. J Heart Lung Transplant 17:185–191, 1998.
147. Kanis JA and the World Health Organization (WHO) Study Group: Assessment of fracture risk and its application to screening for postmenopausal osteoporosis: Synopsis of a WHO report. Osteoporos Int 4:368–381, 1994.
148. Ferrari SL, Nicod LP, Hamacher J, et al: Osteoporosis in patients undergoing lung transplantation. Eur Respir J 9:2378–2382, 1996.
149. Aris RM, Neuringer IP, Weiner MA, et al: Severe osteoporosis before and after lung transplantation. Chest 109:1176–1183, 1996.
150. Johnson BA, Duncan SR, Ohori NP, et al: Recurrence of sarcoidosis in pulmonary allograft recipients. Am Rev Respir Dis 148:1373–1377, 1993.
151. Muller C, Briegel J, Haller M, et al: Sarcoidosis recurrence following lung transplantation. Transplantation 61:1117–1119, 1996.
152. Nine JS, Yousem SA, Paradis IL, et al: Lymphangioleiomyomatosis: Recurrence after lung transplantation. J Heart Lung Transplant 13:714–719, 1994.
153. Frost AE, Keller CA, Brown RW, et al: Giant cell interstitial pneumonitis. Disease recurrence in the transplanted lung. Am Rev Respir Dis 148:1401–1404, 1993.
154. Baz MA, Kussin PS, Van Trigt P, et al: Recurrence of diffuse panbronchiolitis after lung transplantation. Am J Respir Crit Care Med 151:895–898, 1995.
155. Gabbay E, Dark JH, Ashcroft T, et al: Recurrence of Langerhan's cell granulomatosis following lung transplantation. Thorax 53:326–327, 1998.
156. Garver RI, Zorn GL, Wu X, et al: Recurrence of bronchoalveolar cell carcinoma in transplanted lungs. N Engl J Med 340:1071–1074, 1999.
157. King MB, Jessurun J, Hertz MI: Recurrence of desquamative interstitial pneumonia after lung transplantation. Am J Respir Crit Care Med 157:1349–1350, 1998.

# Prevention and Control

SECTION S

# 98 Individual Measures: Social and Behavioral Aspects

NOREEN M. CLARK, PH.D.
SUSAN JANSON, R.N., A.N.P., D.N.SC.

Introduction
Smoking Interventions for Primary Prevention
- Smoking Avoidance
- Public Pressure and Policy
- Smoking Cessation

Secondary Prevention: Asthma Self-Management
- Asthma Education Programs
- Asthma Self-Management Programs
- Patient Adherence to Therapy
- Role of the Clinician in Asthma Self-Management

Gaps in Knowledge and Needed Research
- Smoking
- Asthma

Clinician-Patient Relationships

## INTRODUCTION

This chapter focuses on social and behavioral aspects of preventing and treating lung disease through interventions designed to help patients and clinicians change their behavior. Three questions are addressed. First, can the behavior of large numbers of people (i.e., a population) be changed to help reduce the prevalence of lung disease? Smoking cessation is the example for exploring this primary prevention question. Smoking is a pervasive cause or contributor to lung disease, and quitting can significantly alter prospects for lung health. Some success has been realized in getting significant numbers of people to quit smoking, but many challenges remain.

The second question addressed focuses on secondary prevention. Can patients learn to minimize the impact of disease once they have it? In considering this question, asthma self-management serves as the example. Research conducted over the 1980s and 1990s has shown that patients can be taught to manage their asthma with resulting improvements in health status and health care utilization. The lessons from these studies may suggest how interventions could be developed to foster self-management.

The advice and education given by clinicians is central to enable patients to manage disease. This precept leads to the third question to be considered: What can clinicians do to foster the goals of primary and secondary prevention in patients? Studies have defined the elements of communication between clinician and patient that lead to differences in health status.

In addressing each of these questions, attention is given to the criteria by which the success of behavioral interventions can be judged.

## SMOKING INTERVENTIONS FOR PRIMARY PREVENTION

Smoking is the leading preventable cause of death and disability in the United States,[1] and it has been the target of major educational, clinical, and legal actions since the first Surgeon General's Report.[2] In the ensuing years, the rate of smoking by American adults has declined from 42% in 1964 to 24.7% in 1997.[3, 4]

An important and relatively recent advance is the widespread recognition of the addictive property of tobacco; that is, that smoking cessation initiates both behavioral and physiologic consequences.[5] Differences in prevalence of smoking have been shown to be associated with personal and social characteristics including sex, race, education, income, employment, occupation, and habits of eating, drinking, and socializing.[3, 6–9]

Two types of interventions have been tested through evaluation research. The first type comprises programs targeted at nonsmokers with the intention of keeping them from developing the habit in the first place. Other programs have focused on getting smokers to quit, anticipating that cessation will reduce the risk of acquiring disease or reduce the impact of disease already present.

### Smoking Avoidance

Few programs aimed at helping people avoid smoking in the first place have been reported. Only six smoking prevention studies conducted in the 1990s could be located that presented statistical results of evaluation, used a randomized controlled design, and enrolled a sample size large enough for sufficient power. Three of these studies reported a significant effect of an intervention on preventing habitual smoking ($P < .05$) (Table 98.1).[10–12] These programs targeted school children in junior high or middle school and were offered as part of the school curriculum.[13] Many of the smoking prevention studies found in the literature analyzed the effects of an intervention on an outcome thought to predict adoption of smoking: for example, the feeling of self-efficacy to avoid smoking or the ability to resist peer pressure to smoke. These studies did not report actual smoking behavior. They anticipated long-term results (i.e., not smoking) based on achievement of a near-term objective (e.g., developing confidence to resist). As yet, the long-term results of these investigations have not been reported.

### Public Pressure and Policy

The denormalization of smoking through laws, local regulations restricting smoking in public places, price increases, and limitation of advertising may be the most effective current method of reducing smoking. Fierce antismoking campaigns launched and widely supported by health agencies and organizations have influenced public attitudes toward smoking and smoking prevalence. In California, public control of smoking began in 1989, and the prevalence of smoking had dropped from 26% to 16% by 1995.[14] Other states that instituted vigorous antismoking campaigns reported similar or greater declines in smoking prevalence. However, smoking continues to be a serious problem among adolescents, and the prevalence is this population is increasing. Cigarette advertising is thought to be a major contributor to this trend.

Although public policy interventions are thought to be a means of affecting the smoking behavior of large numbers of Americans, they have not received rigorous evaluation. At the local level, some attention has been paid to the effectiveness of policies aimed at decreasing the access of young people to cigarettes. There is evidence, for example, that banning of cigarette vending machines is more effective and less problematic than installation of locking devices on vending machines for deterring access of minors to cigarettes.[15] Other studies have assessed the effectiveness of community education programs for support of existing policies prohibiting sales of tobacco to school-age smokers.[16–19] Active enforcement of laws forbidding the sale of tobacco products to minors appears to be successful in the short term, but tobacco sellers appear unlikely to continue compliance with such policies in the absence of continuous enforcement. The influence

**Table 98.1** SUCCESSFUL SMOKING AVOIDANCE INTERVENTIONS*

| Study | N | Target | Methods | Outcomes |
|---|---|---|---|---|
| Telch et al[10] | 540 | Seventh grade students in southern California junior high school | A: videotape instruction; B: videotape plus peer leader; C: survey only (2 controls) | Less smoking in B (3.7%) vs. A (28.6%) or controls (18.9% and 30.4%) ($P < .05$) |
| Botvin et al[11] | 3153 | Predominantly Hispanic seventh graders | Fifteen-session prevention program vs. no intervention control | Less smoking in intervention group ($P < .05$), less new smoking in intervention group ($P < .03$) |
| Botvin et al[12] | 608 | Students in predominantly black urban junior high schools | Twelve-session smoking prevention program that taught resistance skills and life skills (treatment) vs. control | Reduced smoking in treatment group 56% ($P < .05$) |

*Successful interventions were those that showed a statistically significant ($P < .05$) treatment effect at follow-up.

of policy interventions on smoking prevention and cessation is an area that deserves study.

## Smoking Cessation

Many cessation programs have selected target populations of smokers based on both research findings and assumptions regarding disease risk. For example, programs for pregnant women have been implemented because this subgroup is identifiable and reachable, and because smoking is a threat not only to the women but also to their unborn children. Further, pregnant women may be more amenable to cessation strategies. This idea is supported by the work of Secker-Walker and associates,[20] who showed that individualized "relapse reduction" counseling of pregnant women who were smoking in early pregnancy resulted in more abstinent days during pregnancy, although the ultimate relapse rate did not differ between experimental and control groups.

Persons with lung disease, particularly chronic obstructive pulmonary disease (COPD), have been targeted for intervention, based on the idea that people with evidence of harm from smoking might be more strongly motivated to quit. Research has suggested that smokers with COPD may have greater difficulty quitting than do most smokers.[21] The high risk of harm from continued smoking in persons with early signs of COPD led the Lung Health Study to combine behavioral, social, and pharmacologic approaches to smoking cessation.[22] The Smoking Cessation Group Program used was a 12-week, 13-session intervention designed to teach smokers the skills necessary to avoid relapse and sustain nonsmoking. These behavioral activities were combined with use of nicotine gum (nicotine polacrilex) to help the participants cope with nicotine withdrawal and cravings while they acquired new behavioral skills. The need for social support was also recognized. Participants were encouraged to bring a spouse or other support person with them to the intervention program. Family members, friends, and even coworkers were invited to quit smoking along with the participant and/or instructed on how to best assist the participant's efforts at smoking cessation.[22]

One year after the intervention, 40% of the program participants were not smoking, compared with 11% of the control subjects.[23] The number of participants with sustained nonsmoking (i.e., quitting during the initial cessation program and maintaining nonsmoking status at each subsequent annual visit) declined over 5 years. By the end of the study approximately 22% of program participants were still not smoking, compared with 5% of the control participants.

In the Lung Health Study, the rate of decline in pulmonary function was dramatically slowed by sustained nonsmoking but continued without abatement in those who continued to smoke. The average decline over 5 years in $FEV_1$ was 301 mL in smokers and 72 mL in sustained nonsmokers.[24] The Lung Health Study demonstrated that, in smokers identified as having early pulmonary impairment, an intensive smoking cessation intervention can result in sustained smoking cessation and can significantly slow or even reverse the obstructive lung damage caused by smoking.

Members of minority groups also have been identified as an important audience for smoking cessation interventions, because the burdens of chronic lung disease disproportionately affect low income people in minority communities.[25] One study showed that an intervention for urban African-Americans based in community churches reached the target population but found no sustained smoking cessation from the program provided.[26]

At least two reasons account for the particular interest in providing interventions in the clinical setting. The first is related to access to smokers. The majority of Americans have contact with clinicians, some on a regular basis. Put simply, clinicians have access to patients and have opportunities to address smoking behavior. Second, clinicians are regarded by patients as a credible source of medical information; for some patients, the physician is the most trusted clinical informant.[27] Some interventions in which physicians or nurses provide direct cessation counseling to patients have demonstrated success in achieving smoking cessation.[28–31]

Most people who quit smoking do so by themselves through a variety of means often known only to them.[32] Nonetheless, interest remains high in finding ways to assist smokers to kick their habit. Since 1990, approximately 40 studies of cessation programs conducted in the United States have used randomized controlled study designs and adequate sample sizes to test the hypothesis. By the criterion of smoking cessation maintained for at least 1 year after intervention (at a significance level of $P < .05$), ten of these programs were successful (in Table 98.2).[28–31, 33–38] These successful programs were not characterized by any one specific approach. They reflect ranges of target audiences, settings for program delivery, types of educators, materials, and pharmacologic supports for quitting.

Although this review of smoking intervention articles was not intended to be exhaustive, it was reasonably thorough for the years 1989 to 1999. Slightly more than one fourth of the interventions reviewed showed success in prolonging quitting beyond 1 year. The low rate of success may indicate that many of the programs tested were not very powerful, or that the addictive nature of smoking makes cessation via behavioral interventions exceedingly difficult, or, more likely, that both factors are influential. Nonetheless, given the great benefits to be gained from cessation in terms of preserving lung function and delaying or avoiding the onset of disease, and given the relatively low cost of most programs, wider application of the interventions that proved successful seems warranted. In particular, studies of the impact of physician or nurse advice indicate a reasonably good payoff from a minimal intervention, especially when nicotine replacement is also available. Behavioral approaches to cessation, coupled with pharmacologic approaches, seem promising and worth the costs, considering the clinical benefits to be derived.

## SECONDARY PREVENTION: ASTHMA SELF-MANAGEMENT

Asthma provides a good example of a disease in which the involvement of patients in their own care produces

**Table 98.2 SUCCESSFUL SMOKING CESSATION INTERVENTIONS***

| STUDY | N | TARGET | METHODS | OUTCOMES |
|---|---|---|---|---|
| Miller et al[28] | 2024 | Hospital inpatients | Nurse-led inpatient counseling, one phone call | Higher self-reported quit rate at 1 yr in treatment group ($P < .01$) |
| Tonneson et al[29] | 507 | Smokers (<10 cigarettes/day and >10 cigarettes/day) who refused nicotine patch intervention | Nurse-conducted consultation, brochures, quitting advice, letter (motivational group) | Light and heavy smokers had double quit rate in treatment group vs. control at 1 yr ($P = .012, .20$) |
| Ockene et al[30] | 1261 | Primary care patients | Physician-delivered interventions: advice only, counseling, counseling + nicotine gum | Maintained cessation at 1 yr in more intensive treatment groups ($P = .02$) |
| Hurt et al[31] | 240 | Volunteers who smoked >20 cigarettes/day | Physician cessation advice, nurse follow-up and relapse prevention, nicotine patch/placebo | Higher smoking cessation in nicotine patch at 8 wk ($P < .001$) and 1 yr ($P = .011$) |
| Taylor et al[33] | 660 | Hospitalized patients who were motivated to quit | Nurse-managed program: meeting with nurse-case manager, videotape, workbook, relaxation audio tape, nicotine replacement therapy and two follow-up telephone calls vs. usual care | Cotinine-validated quit rate at 12 mo: 31% in intervention group vs. 21% in control ($P = .006$) |
| Simon et al[34] | 324 | Adults older than 25 yr, 98% men | Video, self-help literature, nicotine patch, 3-mo telephone follow-up | Higher quit rate at 12 mo in treatment ($P < .01$) |
| Lando et al[35] | 1083 | Hard-core smokers who completed a smoking cessation clinic | Additional telephone support vs. no further treatment | Abstinence rates higher in the telephone follow-up groups at 6, 12, and 24 mo ($P = .09$), no longer significant at 34 mo |
| Russell et al[36] | 600 | Dependent heavy smokers motivated to quit in 30 English general practices | Brief physician advice, booklet, 16 hr of nicotine patch per day (or placebo) with brief support and follow-up at 1, 3, 6, 12, 26, and 52 wk | Higher abstinence in nicotine patch group at 1 yr (36% vs. 16.5%, $P < .05$) |
| Salina et al[37] | 34 companies | Smokers in Chicago area companies | Media campaign, self-help materials (nongroup), or same plus social support (group) | 30% abstinence in group vs. 19.5% in nongroup at 24 mo ($P < .001$) |
| Zhu et al[38] | 3030 | General population | A: self-help kit; B: kit plus one telephone counseling session; C: kit plus six telephone sessions | 12-mo abstinence rates: A, 7.2%; B, 9.0%; C, 13.4%; significant difference ($P < .05$) between minimal intervention (A, B) and prolonged intervention (C) |

*Successful intervention was defined as cessation maintained at a statistically significant level ($P < .05$) for 1 yr or longer.

positive outcomes. The benefits of educating patients about asthma and of instructing them in the skills of self-assessment, use of medicine, and other strategies for disease control have been shown both in adults (Table 98.3)[39–56] and in children (Table 98.4).[46, 57–73] These benefits include a reduction in asthma-related costs.[41, 72, 74] Indeed, studies of asthma education and self-management training are so consistent in showing benefit that they are explicitly recommended in the 1997 revision of the National Guidelines for the Diagnosis and Management of Asthma.[75]

The guidelines specify the essential information that should be provided to all people with asthma. In brief, patients and families need to understand the basic pathophysiology of the disease and the actions of the medications on the airway. They need to know how to use the recommended pharmacotherapy appropriately, control exposure to exacerbating factors, monitor their own dis-

**Table 98.3 OUTCOMES OF EVALUATED ADULT ASTHMA EDUCATION PROGRAMS**

| Study | N | Evaluation Design | Follow-Up Design | Outcomes |
|---|---|---|---|---|
| Allen et al[39] | 116 | RCT | 3, 6, 9, and 12 mo | Increased knowledge ($P < .0001$)<br>Increased compliance ($P < .02$)<br>No difference in morbidity |
| Bailey et al[40] | 225 | RCT | 1 yr | Better adherence to treatment regimens ($P = .0001$)<br>Decreased ED visits and hospitalizations, but difference from control group not significant |
| Bolton et al[41] | 241 | RCT | 4, 8, and 12 mo | Fewer ED visits (most significant at 4 mo, $P = .003$, but still at 12 mo, $P = .005$)<br>Reduction in ED charges by $628 |
| Charlton et al[42] | 115 (69 adults, 46 children) | Pre/Post | Every 8 wk for 1 yr | Reduced number of MD visits (median number reduced from 8.0 to 2.0 in peak-flow educated group and 4.5 to 1.0 in symptoms only educated group)<br>Reduced use of oral steroids |
| Garrett et al[43] | 500 adults and children | RCT | 9 mo | Increased ownership of peak flow meters ($P = .0001$) and improved technique (children $P < .05$, adults $P < .005$)<br>Increased usage of preventive medication (adults $P < .05$)<br>Increased self-management plans (adults $P < .01$)<br>Increased knowledge of action plan when symptoms worsened (children $P > .05$, adults $P < .005$)<br>No difference in compliance, hospital admissions, ED use, or days lost from school or work |
| Hilton et al[44] | 339 | RCT | 1 yr | Increased knowledge in maximum intervention group ($P < .05$)<br>No difference in self-management ability or asthma morbidity |
| Huss et al[45] | 52 | Pre/Post | 3 mo | Greater adherence scores for avoidance measures ($P < .05$) |
| Jenkinson et al[46] | 177 | RCT | 3 and 12 mo | Increased knowledge of drugs (after 3 mo, $P = .002$; after 12 mo, $P = .007$)<br>More significant increase in knowledge of intervention groups given tape than given only book ($P = .007$)<br>Reduction in perception of disability |
| Kotses et al[47] | 76 | RCT | 2–12 mo | Reduced asthma attack frequency ($P < .05$)<br>Decreased use of medication (cromolyn sodium, $P < .01$; $\beta_2$-agonists, $P < .05$)<br>Fewer asthma related problems ($P < .01$) |
| Maiman et al[48] | 289 | Factorial | 6 mo | Fewer ED visits ($P = .05$ with intervention from asthmatic nurse, self-identified or not)<br>No significant results from booklet or non-asthmatic nurse plus booklet intervention |
| Mayo et al[49] | 104 | RCT | 32 mo | Threefold reduction in readmission rate ($P < .004$) in treated vs. untreated patients<br>Twofold reduction in hospital day use rate ($P < .05$) in treated vs. untreated patients<br>Threefold reduction in readmission rate and hospital day use ($P = .003$) in patients serving as their own control |
| Moldofsky et al[50] | 62 | RCT | 16 mo | No significant retention of knowledge<br>No change in medical status |
| Osman et al[51] | 801 | Factorial | 1 yr | Fewer hospital admissions than control (by 54%, $P < .05$, in those retained in clinic care and by 49%, 31% to 78%, in total intervention group)<br>Less sleep disturbance by 80%<br>No significant difference in days of restricted activity, prescription of bronchodilators, inhaled steroids, use of oral steroids, number of MD consultants, or significant interaction between having a peak flow meter and education |
| Ringsberg et al[52] | 38 | RCT | 5 and 12 mo | Decreased number of hospital days ($P = .0001$)<br>Reduced acute visits to a hospital by 44%<br>Increased knowledge<br>No change in spirometric variables |

*Table continued on following page*

**Table 98.3 OUTCOMES OF EVALUATED ADULT ASTHMA EDUCATION PROGRAMS** *Continued*

| Study | N | Evaluation Design | Follow-Up Design | Outcomes |
|---|---|---|---|---|
| Snyder et al[53] | 79 | RCT | 1, 2, and 3 mo | Increased knowledge (interaction effect, $P < .05$)<br>Decreased number of attacks (1.93 weekly compared to 2.87 weekly, $P < .05$) |
| Yoon et al[54] | 76 | RCT | 5 and 10 mo | Fewer readmissions (educated group one-seventh that of control, $P < .001$) decrease in ED visits ($P < .001$)<br>No difference in spirometric results, average PEF, or mean daily variability of PEF |
| Wilson et al[55] | 323 | RCT | 5 and 12 mo | Reduced "bother" due to asthma ($P < .05$)<br>Increased physical activity ($P < .05$)<br>Improved asthma, judged by MD ($P < .05$)<br>Better environment control ($P < .0001$)<br>Improved MDI technique ($P < .05$) |
| Windsor et al[55] | 267 | Pre/Post | 12 mo | Improvement in inhaler skills use (CI = .29, .61), inhaler adherence (CI = .24, .50), medication adherence (CI = .31, .57), and total adherence (CI = .28, .56)<br>Costs were $32.03/patient<br>Cost effectiveness was $96.09 for intervention group and $243.68 for control group |

CI = confidence interval; MDI = Metered dose inhaler; ED = emergency department; RCT = randomized clinical trial.

ease status, and take appropriate rescue actions when asthma worsens. The key educational messages to be given to patients and families about managing asthma are brief and specific:

- Asthma is a chronic inflammatory disease of the airway that waxes and wanes with periods of asthma control and occasional flares.
- Treatment is aimed at controlling airway inflammation with antiinflammatory medication and reduction or avoidance of exacerbating factors.
- Acute flares of asthma must be treated at the earliest sign to control the disease.

## Asthma Education Programs

Many researchers have explored the methods for imparting knowledge and skills to patients and their families. An important and consistent finding is that focusing on imparting knowledge without teaching skills may increase patients' knowledge of facts about asthma but is unlikely to change their ability to manage their disease.[76–78] Education programs seem to achieve best results when they use a combination of methods, adapting them to the developmental needs of patients in different age groups. Videos and interactive programs are effective in teaching parents to assess and respond to signs of wheezing in very young children.[79] Using a multidisciplinary protocol adapted to children's health beliefs, others have shown that young children can be instructed and can make important daily decisions to manage their illness.[65, 80] Well-designed, validated, and evaluated programs have been published and are available for dissemination and use in school settings.[59, 72, 81] Newsletters, learning games, and support groups designed for teenagers are being tested for effectiveness in helping adolescents assume responsibility for managing their own asthma.[82] An increasing number of programs for adults have been developed that use a variety of learning techniques, including workbooks, group teaching, and problem-solving exercises, as supplements to individualized instruction from the patient's personal clinician.[40, 47, 54, 55, 83] Recognizing that asthma is not only a disease of the young, specific strategies have been developed for teaching older patients about asthma. Large-print materials, simplified action plans, medication devices, and reminder kits are some of the effective approaches that have been tested.[66]

The setting in which asthma education is imparted may be important. Some studies suggest that in adults,[49, 84–86] and in children recently hospitalized for acute asthma,[87] individualized educational approaches are more powerful in changing self-management behavior. However, at least one study showed no difference in the effects of group and individual education programs for adults.[55]

Two important limitations of almost all asthma education programs are their reliance on written materials, handouts, and worksheets and their reliance on the English language. One survey of 273 patients visiting an emergency department for an acute asthma exacerbation showed that only 27% read at the high school level and only 33% read at the seventh to eighth grade level.[88] Poor metered-dose inhaler technique was found to correlate with low reading levels. Clearly, literacy is an important factor in patients' ability to comprehend and apply information and skills required for asthma self-management and can become a significant barrier to achieving asthma control.

## Asthma Self-Management Programs

Asthma self-management may be defined as the direct involvement of patients in strategies to control their disease. Structured self-management education programs have been shown to increase knowledge about asthma; increase confidence; improve school and work attendance;

Table 98.4 OUTCOMES OF EVALUATED PEDIATRIC ASTHMA EDUCATION PROGRAMS

| Study | N | Evaluation Design | Follow-Up Period | Outcomes |
|---|---|---|---|---|
| Jenkinson et al[46] | 177 | RCT | 3 and 12 mo | Significant knowledge increases ($P$ = .002)<br>No other significant change |
| Staudenmayer et al[57] | 40 | Pre/Post | 6 mo | Change in direction of fewer school absences ($P$ = .09)<br>Reduced number of emergency physician visits for those with baseline use ($P$ = .03)<br>Reduced hospitalizations ($P$ = .03) |
| Fireman et al[58] | 26 | RCT | 8–16 mo | Decreased school absences ($P$ < .05)<br>Reduced ED use (no statistical analysis)<br>Reduced hospitalization time (no statistical analysis) |
| Lewis et al[59] | 76 | RCT | 1 yr | Reduced ED visits ($P$ < .001)<br>Reduced number of hospital days ($P$ < .01) |
| Hindi-Alexander and Cropp[60] | 92 | Pre/Post | 1 yr | Reduced school absences ($P$ < .005)<br>Reduced ED use but not statistically significant<br>No difference in hospitalizations |
| McNabb et al[61] | 14 | Pre/Post | 1 yr | Reduced ED use (no statistical analysis) |
| LeBaron et al[62] | 31 | RCT | 4 mo | Increased knowledge about cromolyn (no statistical analysis)<br>No change in pulmonary function or systems |
| Rubin et al[63] | 54 | RCT | 1 yr | No difference in school absences<br>Improvement in ED use but not statistically significant |
| Clark et al[64] | 310 | RCT | 1 yr | Improved academic performance ($P$ < .05)<br>Increased self-management behavior: parent ($P$ = .0001); child ($P$ = .05)<br>No difference in school absences<br>Reduced ED use among those with baseline use ($P$ = .05)<br>Reduced hospitalizations among those with baseline use ($P$ = .05) |
| Mesters et al[65] | 67 | RCT | 1 yr | Higher level of asthma self-efficacy ($P$ < .02)<br>Increased self-management behavior ($P$ < .01)<br>Decreased MD visits ($P$ < .01) |
| Wilson and Starr-Schneidkraut[66] | 80 | RCT | 1 yr | Increased symptom-free days ($P$ = .004)<br>Fewer nights of parental sleep interruption |
| Rakos et al[67] | 43 | RCT | 1 yr | No significant difference in school absences<br>No significant differences in ED use or emergency MD visits |
| Mitchell et al[68] | 368 | RCT | 6 mo | Differences according to ethnicity of child<br>No differences in hospital days |
| Hughes et al[69] | 95 | RCT | 1 yr | Reduced school absences ($P$ = .04) |
| McIntosh et al[70] | 92 | RCT | 4–6 mo | More treatment (35%) than control (17%) subjects reported more smoking outside their homes at post-test (and their children's continine levels were lower) but not statistically significant |
| Parcel et al[71] | 104 | Comparison group | 1 yr | Improved ED use but not significantly significant<br>Higher levels of self-efficacy regarding asthma ($P$ = .018) |
| Evans et al[72] | 239 | RCT | 1 yr | Increased self-management ($P$ = .05)<br>Increased communication with parent ($P$ = .002)<br>Better academic grades ($P$ = .05)<br>Fewer days with symptoms ($P$ = .004) |
| Robinson[73] | 74 | Pre/Post | 3 yr | Reduced school absences (no statistical analysis)<br>Better MDI technique ($P$ = .0005)<br>Fewer hospital days ($P$ = .02) |

and reduce rescue medication use, urgent care visits, and hospitalizations in both children and adults.[40, 49, 55, 84, 89–93] There is some evidence that self-management skills develop slowly over time,[55, 94, 95] and the duration of improvement in symptoms and health care use has been variable, ranging from 4 to 18 months.[41, 81, 96] Both group and individual educational formats for teaching asthma skills have been tried. Regardless of mode of delivery, the most effective programs are those that focus on teaching self-management skills as well as imparting information about asthma.[84, 91]

Some asthma self-management programs include peak flow monitoring[84, 90–92] and suggest that it may be a useful adjunct to an overall treatment plan. In fact, the *National Guidelines*[75] recommend peak flow monitoring as a useful adjunct in patients with moderate persistent or severe persistent asthma. When patients are trained in the correct exhalation technique and checked repeatedly to ensure maintenance of the skill, peak flow monitoring is useful for detecting the effects of exposures, for assessing responses to changes in therapy, and for alerting the patient and the clinician to periods of clinical instability.[83] For these reasons, peak flow monitoring has been incorporated into action plans as an objective guide to the need to adjust therapy.

Six studies, four of which were randomized controlled trials, compared the use of daily peak flow monitoring to symptom monitoring as the basis for written self-management plans (Table 98.5).[42, 97–101] Four of these studies showed no significant differences in lung function, symptom frequency, quality of life, hospitalizations, medication use, or need for medical visits, although all of these parameters improved.[42, 98, 99, 101] Two studies showed a marked decrease in number of emergency room visits in the group using peak flow monitoring,[92, 100] and two showed no effect of peak flow monitoring on asthma morbidity.[98, 102]

The conflicting findings of these investigations probably result from differences in selection of patients, research design, and quality of the therapy provided before randomization. Two studies showed that when medical therapy was made optimum before patients were randomly assigned to educational/monitoring treatment groups, short-term compliance and knowledge of asthma improved and morbidity decreased in all groups, but there were no differences between groups in outcomes achieved.[99, 101]

In contrast, one study showed that symptoms were reduced and health care utilization was decreased after an education intervention, independent of the use of inhaled antiinflammatory medication.[103] The important implication of studies of asthma self-management programs is that educating patients to be involved directly in their care improves asthma control and clinical outcomes. The role and impact of self-monitoring is less well understood, but it may have a significant impact on some selected outcomes. Defining how optimal therapy, patient education, self-management strategies, and self-monitoring interact to affect morbidity requires further exploration.

## Patient Adherence to Therapy

One of the ways in which asthma education may most strongly improve asthma control is by fostering better adherence to the treatment plan. Studies have shown that fewer than 50% of asthma medications are taken as prescribed,[104] and nonadherence to regular use of long-term controller therapies, especially inhaled corticosteroids, results in treatment failure. Conversely, improved adherence to an effective regimen can markedly reduce asthma morbidity,[105] emergency department visits,[106] and airway inflammation.[86]

Adherence requires behavior change, not simply knowledge. Ignorance about the purposes of treatment is only one determinant of nonadherence to therapy. Other, possibly even more important causes are lack of confidence in the treatment plan[107] and lack of practice in adjusting therapy. In one study, subjects who were shown scenarios of acute asthma situations were not able to select the correct actions despite having suitable scores on an asthma knowledge test.[108] A survey of 603 people with asthma revealed that more than 46% of patients with uncontrolled asthma and bothersome symptoms were reluctant to take inhaled corticosteroids on a regular basis; this reluctance was associated with fears and concerns that most had not discussed with their doctors.[109] Nonadherence is also a problem in peak flow monitoring. Several researchers have documented the problems of missing, false, and inaccurate recording of peak flow data over time in both children[110] and adults.[111, 112] When patients are taught to use peak flow monitoring as part of an educational intervention, however, increases in adherence with therapies and improved outcomes have been noted.[84]

## Role of the Clinician in Asthma Self-Management

The importance of a patient's beliefs in the necessity, efficacy, and safety of a treatment plan as determinants

**Table 98.5** OUTCOMES OF STUDIES USING PEAK FLOW OR SYMPTOM MONITORING AS A BASIS FOR SELF-MANAGEMENT

| Study | N | Evaluation Design | Follow-Up Period | Outcomes |
|---|---|---|---|---|
| Charlton et al[42] | 69 | Group comparison | 2 yr | Decreased MD visits ($P < .05$)<br>No differences between group |
| Ignacio-Garcia and Gonzales-Santos[84] | 70 | RCT | 6 mo | Decreased ER visits and lost work days<br>Decreased exacerbation in peak flow group |
| Lahdensuo et al[91] | 115 | RCT | Every 4 mo for 1 yr | Decreased urgent care visits ($P$ = .04)<br>Missed work days ($P$ = .02)<br>Courses of steroids ($P < .006$)<br>Increased quality of life ($P$ = .009) in peak flow group |
| GRASSIC[102] | 712 | RCT | 1 yr | No differences among groups |
| Jones et al[98] | 72 | RCT | 1 yr | No effects of PEF monitoring |
| Cote et al[99] | 188 | RCT | 6 mo | Decreased morbidity in all groups ($P$ = .00)<br>No differences between groups |
| Cowie et al[100] | 150 | RCT | 6 mo | Decreased ER visits in peak flow group ($P$ = .006) |
| Turner et al[101] | 92 | RCT | 6 mo | No differences among groups<br>Significant increase in $FEV_1$, $PEF_1$, and quality of life and decrease in symptoms ($P < .0001$ for all variables) |

MD = physician; ER = emergency room; PEF = peak expiratory flow.

of adherence to the plan calls attention to the role of the clinician in patient teaching and counseling. The quality of the doctor-patient relationship appears to be one of the strongest influences on patient compliance with a treatment regimen.[104, 113]

Patient-provider relationships have been studied extensively,[114] but the particular means by which influence is exerted have not been well delineated. A subtle shift in conceptions of how clinicians should approach patient education and communication has led to less direct emphasis on adherence to medical regimens and greater emphasis on developing the capacity of patients to manage the range of factors necessary for disease control. Further, increasing attention is being given to quality of life as a desired outcome of clinical care, an idea that broadens even further the scope of clinician counseling.

Becker[114] and his colleagues suggested a conceptual model for approaching patients that went beyond focusing strictly on medicine use. Focusing instead on factors important in patients' decisions to follow therapeutic advice, the elements of this model include the beliefs that one is susceptible to a health problem, that the consequences of disease could be severe, and that the benefits of therapy outweigh the costs. Inui and colleagues[115] used this model as the basis for training physicians seeing hypertensive patients. Their randomized controlled study of 62 physicians showed that a single session of instruction in this conceptual model led physicians to allocate a greater percentage of clinic-visit time to patient teaching. The patients of the trained physicians showed greater knowledge and more appropriate patient beliefs regarding hypertension and its therapy. Patients of tutored physicians also complied more reliably with drug treatment and had better control of their blood pressure. A similar study showed that educating physicians in this model enhanced material compliance with antibiotic treatment of pediatric otitis media.[116]

Based on their review of the patient-provider literature, Clark and colleagues[27] identified ten specific techniques[117] that are central to effective communication and education (Table 98.6). An educational program[96] for general practice pediatricians seeing children with asthma was then developed and comprised three elements: information on clinical treatment of asthma, the ten communication techniques, and the educational messages and skills most needed by patients with asthma. This physician training was evaluated in a randomized study of 79 physicians and 637 of their asthmatic patients. Physicians in the program group were found to be more likely to address patients' fears about medicines, provide a sequence of educational messages, and write down how to adjust the medicines when symptoms change. The physicians in the intervention group spent no more time with their patients than did the control group of physicians. Parents of the children treated by program physicians were significantly more likely to report that the physician had been reassuring, had stated as a goal that the child be fully active, and had given information to relieve specific worries. These parents were also more likely to report that they knew how to make management decisions at home. After the intervention, the patients of physicians in the program group were more likely to have received a prescription for inhaled antiinflammatory medicine and to have been asked by the physician to demonstrate how to use a metered-dose inhaler. Two years after the intervention, the children being seen by program physicians exhibited no difference in number of nonemergency office visits or number of visits for follow-up of symptom episodes but required fewer urgent visits and hospitalizations.

**Table 98.6** TEACHING AND COMMUNICATION BEHAVIORS FOR CLINICIANS

| |
|---|
| Show nonverbal attentiveness |
| Give nonverbal encouragement |
| Give verbal praise for things done well |
| Maintain interactive conversation |
| Find out underlying worries/concerns |
| Give specific reassuring information |
| Tailor medication schedule to family's routine |
| Reach agreement on a short-term goal |
| Review the long-term therapeutic plan |
| Help patient to use criteria for making decisions about asthma management |

## GAPS IN KNOWLEDGE AND NEEDED RESEARCH

### Smoking

Although behavioral interventions have been shown to be of some value in smoking cessation or avoidance, issues regarding their utility remain:

- If clinician counseling regarding smoking cessation is effective, efficient, and can reach large numbers of people at risk, how can it be integrated routinely into practice, and what are the relative benefits of different configurations of counseling and pharmacotherapy provide by different types of clinicians?
- How effective are programs targeted at those with early signs of lung disease as a routine element of clinical care?
- What are the connections between avoidance programs that target an intermediate behavior (e.g., refusal skills in teenagers) and ultimate smoking behavior?
- Would interventions that target changes in the social environment enable smokers to quit more easily?
- What are the relative benefits of policy interventions (e.g., prohibitions, insurance requirements) vis-à-vis behavioral intervention?

### Asthma

Although much has been learned about successful educational interventions for asthma, important questions need to be addressed:

- Which components of an educational program are essential or most important in general, and for specific subgroups of patients?

- Which learning approaches are most effective for which patient groups (e.g., elderly patients, women, patients with more severe disease)?
- What is the trajectory of persistence of effects of programs over time?
- Which strategies for control of the indoor air environment produce desired effects, and how can these best be taught to patients?
- What are the key educational messages that are most critical for patients who demonstrate certain clinical, demographic, or cultural characteristics?
- What are the effective means for reaching people with low literacy skills?
- Which subgroups of patients with asthma benefit from specific monitoring techniques such as peak flow monitoring?
- What are the links between education, optimal treatment regimens, patient-clinician relationships, adherence, and outcomes?

## CLINICIAN-PATIENT RELATIONSHIPS

As the role of social and behavioral determinants in disease management and prevention becomes clearer, the need for integrating attention to these factors into clinical care becomes more salient. Important dimensions of this integration deserve study:

- What balance should be struck in the clinical visit between therapeutics and patient education to enhance outcome?
- What modes of intervention best prepare clinicians to communicate effectively with patients?
- What are the most appropriate roles of various clinical staff in educating patients?
- Can clinical settings be shaped to become optimal educational entities in which, from entering to departure, patients are routinely and systematically helped to develop their knowledge and skills?

## References

1. US Department of Health and Human Services: Reducing the Health Consequences of Smoking: 25 Years of Progress: A Report of the Surgeon General. Public Health Service, Centers for Disease Control, Center for Chronic Disease Prevention and Health Promotion, Office on Smoking and Health. DHHS Publication No. CDC 89–8411. Rockville, MD: US Government Printing Office, 1989.
2. US Department of Health, Education, and Welfare: Smoking and Health: A Report of the Advisory Committee to the Surgeon General of the Public Health Service. Public Health Service Publication No. 1103. Washington, DC: US Department of Health, Education, and Welfare, 1964.
3. Centers for Disease Control: Cigarette smoking among adults—United States, 1992, and changes in the definition of current smoking. MMWR Morb Mortal Wkly Rep 43:342–346, 1994.
4. Centers for Disease Control: Cigarette Smoking Among Adults—United States, 1997. MMWR 48:994–999, 1999.
5. Brandon SL, Tiffany ST, Baker TB: The process of smoking relapse. *In* Tims F, Leukfeld C: Relapse and Recovery in Drug Abuse. Rockville, MD: National Institute on Drug Abuse, 1986.
6. Eisenger RA: Psychosocial predictors of smoking recidivism. J Health Soc Behav 12:355–362, 1983.
7. Kabat JC, Wynder EL: Determinants of quitting smoking. Am J Public Health 77:1301–1305, 1987.
8. DuNah RE, Ahn H, Ahn DK: Demographics and cigarette smoking among women. Prev Med 20:262–270, 1991.
9. Hahn LP, Folsom AR, Sprafka JM, et al: Cigarette smoking and cessation behaviors among urban blacks and whites. Pub Health Rep 105:290–295, 1990.
10. Telch MJ, Miller LM, Killen JD, et al: Social influences approach to smoking prevention: The effects of videotape delivery with and without same-age peer leader participation. Addict Behav 15:21–28, 1990.
11. Botvin GJ, Dusenbury L, Baker E, et al: Smoking prevention among urban minority youth: Assessing effects on outcome and mediating variables. Health Psychol 11:290–295, 1992.
12. Botvin GJ, Batson HW, Witts-Vitale S, et al: A psychosocial approach to smoking prevention for urban black youth. Pub Health Rep 104:573–582, 1989.
13. Hovell MF, Russos S, Beckhelm MK, et al: Compliance with primary prevention in private practice: Creating a tobacco-free environment. Am J Prev Med 11:288–293, 1995.
14. Centers for Disease Control: Cigarette smoking among adults—United States, 1995. MMWR Morb Mortal Wkly Rep 46:1217–1220, 1997.
15. Forster JL, Hourigan ME, Kelder S: Locking devices on cigarette vending machines: Evaluation of a city ordinance. Am J Public Health 82:1217–1219, 1992.
16. Pierce JP, Mills SL, Shopland DR, et al: Accessibility of cigarettes to youths aged 12–17 years—United States, 1989. MMWR Morb Mortal Wkly Rep 41:485–488, 1992.
17. Jason LA, Ji PY, Anes MD, et al: Active enforcement of cigarette control laws in the prevention of cigarette sales to minors. JAMA 266:3159–3161, 1991.
18. DiFranza JR, Carlson RR, Caisse RE: Reducing youth access to tobacco. Tob Control 1:57–58, 1992.
19. DiFranza JR, Norwood BD, Garnder DW, et al: Legislative efforts to protect children from tobacco. JAMA 257:3387–3389, 1987.
20. Secker-Walker RH, Solomon LJ, Flynn BS, et al: Individualized smoking cessation counseling during prenatal and early postnatal care. Am J Obstet Gynecol 171:134–155, 1994.
21. Duncan CL, Cumming CR, Hudes ES, et al: Quitting smoking: Reason for quitting and predictors of cessation among medical patients. J Intern Med 7:398–404, 1992.
22. Clark NM, Bailey WC, Rand C: Advances in prevention and education in lung disease. Am J Respir Crit Care Med 157:S155–S167, 1998.
23. O'Hara P, Grill J, Rigdon MA, et al: Design and result of the initial intervention program for the Lung Health Study. Prev Med 22:304–315, 1993.
24. The Lung Health Study Research Group: Effects of smoking intervention and the use of an inhaled anticholinergic bronchodilator on the rate of decline if $FEV_1$. JAMA 272:1497–1505, 1994.
25. Kochane KD, Maurer JD, Rosenberg HM: Why did black life expectancy decline from 1984 through 1989 in the United States? Am J Public Health 84:938–944, 1994.
26. Voorhees CC, Stillman FA, Swank RT, et al: Heart, body, and soul: Impact of church-based smoking cessation interventions on readiness to quit. Prev Med 25:277–285, 1996.
27. Clark NM, Nothwehr F, Gong M, et al: Physician-patient partnership in managing chronic illness. Acad Med 70:957–959, 1995.
28. Miller NH, Smith PM, DeBusk RF, et al: Smoking cessation in hospitalized patients: Results of a randomized trial. Arch Intern Med 157:409–415, 1997.
29. Tonneson P, Mikkelsen K, Markholst C, et al: Nurse-conducted smoking cessation with minimal intervention in a lung clinic: A randomized controlled study. Eur Respir J 9:2351–2355, 1996.
30. Ockene JK, Kristeller J, Pbert L, et al: The physician-delivered smoking intervention project: Can short-term interventions produce long-term effects for a general outpatient population? Health Psychol 13:278–281, 1994.
31. Hurt RD, Dale LC, Fredrickson PA, et al: Nicotine patch therapy for smoking cessation combined with physician advice and nurse follow-up: One-year outcome and percentage of nicotine replacement. JAMA 271:595–600, 1994.
32. US Department of Health and Human Services: The Health Bene-

fits of Smoking Cessation: A Report of the Surgeon General. Public Health Service, Centers for Disease Control, Center for Chronic Disease Prevention, and Health Promotion, Office on Smoking and Health. DHHS Publication No. CDC 90–8416. Washington, DC: Government Printing Office, 1990.
33. Taylor CB, Miller NH, Herman S, et al: A nurse-managed smoking cessation program for hospitalized workers. Am J Public Health 86:1557–1560, 1996.
34. Simon JA, Solkowitz SN, Carmody TP, et al: Smoking cessation after surgery: A randomized trial. Arch Intern Med 157:1371–1376, 1997.
35. Lando HA, Pirie PL, Roski J, et al: Promoting abstinence among relapsed chronic smokers: The effect of telephone support. Am J Public Health 86:1557–1560, 1996.
36. Russell MA, Stapleton JA, Feyerabend C, et al: Targeting heavy smokers in general practice: Randomised controlled trial of transdermal nicotine patches. BMJ 306:1308–1312, 1993.
37. Salina D, Jason LA, Hedeker D, et al: A follow-up of a media-based, worksite smoking cessation program. Am J Community Psychol 22:257–271, 1994.
38. Zhu SH, Stretch V, Balabanis M, et al: Telephone counseling for smoking cessation: Effects of single-session and multiple-session interventions. J Consult Clin Psychol 64:202–211, 1996.
39. Allen RM, Jones MP, Oldenburg B: Randomized trial of asthma self-management programme for adults. Thorax 50:731–738, 1995.
40. Bailey W, Richards JJ, Brooks C, et al: A randomized trial to improve self-management practices of adults with asthma. Arch Intern Med 150:1664–1668, 1990.
41. Bolton MB, Tilley BC, Kuder J, et al: The cost and effectiveness of an education program for adults who have asthma. J Gen Intern Med 6:401–407, 1991.
42. Charlton I, Charlton G, Broomfield J, et al: Clinical trial, randomized controlled trial: Evaluation of peak flow and symptoms only self-management plans for control of asthma in general practice. BMJ 301:1355–1359, 1990.
43. Garrett J, Fenwich JM, Taylor G, et al: Prospective controlled evaluation of the effect of a community-based asthma education centre in a multiracial working class neighbourhood. Thorax 49:976–983, 1994.
44. Hilton S, Anderson H, Sibbald B, et al: Survey: Controlled evaluation of the effects of patient education on asthma morbidity in general practice. Lancet 1:26–29, 1986.
45. Huss K, Salerno M, Huss RW: Computer-assisted reinforcement of instruction: Effects on adherence in adult atopic asthmatics. Res Nurs Health 14:259–267, 1991.
46. Jenkinson D, Davidson J, Jones S, et al: Comparison of effects of a self-management booklet and audiocassette for patients with asthma. BMJ 297:267–270, 1988.
47. Kotses H, Bernstein I, Bernstein D, et al: A self-management program for adult asthma. Part I: Development and evaluation. J Allergy Clin Immunol 95:529–540, 1995.
48. Maiman LA, Green LW, Gibson G, et al: Education for self-treatment by adult asthmatics. JAMA 241:1919–1922, 1979.
49. Mayo PH, Richman J, Harris HW: Results of a program to reduce admissions for adult asthma. Ann Intern Med 112:864–871, 1990.
50. Moldofsky H, Broder I, Davies G, et al: Videotape educational program for people with asthma. Can Med Educ J 120:669–672, 1979.
51. Osman LM, Abdalla MI, Beattie JA, et al: Reducing hospital admission through computer supported education for asthma patients. Grampian Asthma Study of Integrated Cate (GRASSIC). BMJ 308:568–571, 1994.
52. Ringsberg KC, Wiflund I, Wilhelmsen L: Education of adult patients at an "asthma school": Effects on quality of life, knowledge and need for nursing. Eur Respir J 3:33–37, 1990.
53. Snyder SE, Winder JA, Creer TJ: Development and evaluation of an adult asthma self-management program: Wheezers Anonymous. J Asthma 24:153–158, 1987.
54. Yoon R, McKenzie D, Bauman A, Miles D: Controlled trial evaluation of an asthma education programme for adults. Thorax 48:1110–1116, 1993.
55. Wilson SR, Scamagas P, German DF, et al: A controlled trial of two forms of self-management education for adults with asthma. Am J Med 94:564–576, 1993.
56. Windsor RA, Bailey WC, Richards JM Jr, et al: Evaluation of the efficacy and cost effectiveness of health education methods to increase medication adherence among adults with asthma. Am J Public Health 80:1519–1521, 1990.
57. Staudenmayer H, Harris PS, Selner JC: Evaluation of a self-help education-exercise program for asthmatic children and their parents: Six-month follow-up. J Asthma 18:1–5, 1981.
58. Fireman P, Friday GA, Gira C, et al: Teaching self-management skills to asthmatic children and their parents in an ambulatory care setting. Pediatrics 68:341–348, 1981.
59. Lewis CE, Rachelsfsky G, Lewis MA, et al: A randomized trial of A.C.T. (asthma care training) for kids. Pediatrics 74:478–486, 1984.
60. Hindi-Alexander MC, Cropp GJA: Evaluation of a family asthma program. J Allergy Clin Immunol 74:505–510, 1984.
61. McNabb WL, Wilson-Pessano SR, Hughes GW, et al: Self-management education of children with asthma: AIR WISE. Am J Public Health 75:1219–1220, 1985.
62. LeBaron S, Zeltzer LK, Ratner P, et al: A controlled study of education for improving compliance with cromolyn sodium (Intal): The importance of physician-patient communication. Ann Allergy 55:811–818, 1985.
63. Rubin DH, Leventhal JM, Sadock RT, et al: Educational intervention by computer in childhood asthma: A randomized clinical trial testing the use of a new teaching intervention in childhood asthma. Pediatrics 77:1–10, 1986.
64. Clark NM, Feldman CH, Evans D, et al: Managing better: Children, parents and asthma. Patient Educ Couns 8:27–38, 1986.
65. Mesters I, Meertens R, Kok G, et al: Effectiveness of a multidisciplinary education protocol in children with asthma (0–4 years) in primary health care. J Asthma 31:347–359, 1994.
66. Wilson SR, Starr-Schneidkraut N: State of the art in asthma education: The US experience. Chest 106:197S–205S, 1994.
67. Rakos RF, Grodek MV, Mack KK: The impact of a self-administered behavioral intervention program on pediatric asthma. J Psychosomatic Res 29:101–108, 1985.
68. Mitchell EA, Ferguson V, Norwood M: Asthma education by community child health nurses. Arch Dis Child 61:1184–1189, 1986.
69. Hughes DM, McLeod M, Garner B, et al: Controlled trial of a home and ambulatory program for asthmatic children. Pediatrics 87:54–61, 1991.
70. McIntosh N, Clark NM, Howatt WF: Reducing tobacco smoke in the environment of the child with asthma: Assisted minimal contact intervention. J Asthma 6:453–462, 1994.
71. Parcel GS, Nader PR, Tiernan K: A health education program for children with asthma. J Dev Behav Pediatr 1:128–132, 1980.
72. Evans D, Clark NM, Feldman CH, et al: A school health education program for children with asthma aged 8–11 years. Health Educ Q 14:367–279, 1987.
73. Robinson LD: Evaluation of an asthma summer camp program. Chest 87:105s, 1985.
74. Trautner C, Richter B, Berger M: Cost-effectiveness of a structured treatment and teaching programme on asthma. Eur Respir J 6:1485–1491, 1993.
75. National Guidelines for the Diagnosis and Management of Asthma. Expert Panel Report 2, Publication No. 97–4051. Bethesda, MD: National Institutes of Health, National Heart, Lung, and Blood Institute, 1997.
76. Boulet LP, Chapman KR, Green LW, et al: Asthma education. Chest 106:184S–196S, 1994.
77. Clark NM: Asthma self-management education. Research and implications for clnical practice. Chest 95:1110–1113, 1989.
78. Rachelefsky GS: Review of asthma self-management programs. J Allergy Clin Immunol 80:506–511, 1987.
79. Wilson SR, Austin DM, Starr-Schneidkraut N, et al: Early intervention with parents of very young children with asthma: A developmental evaluation of the Wee Wheezers program. J Asthma 33:239–254, 1996.
80. Bush PJ, Iannotti RJ: A childrens' health belief model. Med Care 28:69–86, 1990.
81. Clark NM, Feldman CH, Evans D, et al: The impact of health education on frequency and cost of health care use by low-income children with asthma. J Allergy Clin Immunol 78:108–115, 1986.
82. Asthma and Allergy Foundation of America: Power Breathing—Asthma Education for Adolescents. New York, 1998.

83. Janson S: Value of home peak flow monitoring for asthma control. West J Med 163:370–371, 1995.
84. Ignacio-Garcia JM, Gonzales-Santos P: Asthma self-management education program by home monitoring of peak expiratory flow. Am J Respir Crit Care Med 151:353–359, 1995.
85. Kotses H, Stout C, McConnaughy K, et al: Evaluation of individualized asthma self-management programs. J Asthma 33:113–118, 1996.
86. Sont JK: How do we monitor asthma control? Allergy 54(Suppl 49):68–73, 1999.
87. Madge P, McColl J, Paton J: Impact of a nurse-led home management training programme in children admitted to hospital with acute asthma: A randomised controlled study. Thorax 2:223–228, 1997.
88. Williams MV, Baker DW, Honig EG, et al: Inadequate literacy is a barrier to asthma knowledge and self-care. Chest 114:1008–1015, 1998.
89. Clark NM, Gotsch A, Rosenstock IR: Patient, professional, and public education on behavioral aspects of asthma: A review of strategies for change and needed research. J Asthma 30:241–255, 1993.
90. Woolcock AJ, Yan K, Salome CM: Effect of therapy on bronchial hyper responsiveness in the long-term management of asthma. Clin Allergy 18:165–176, 1988.
91. Lahdensuo A, Haahtela T, Herrala J, et al: Randomised comparison of guided self management and traditional treatment of asthma over one year. BMJ 312:748–752, 1996.
92. Ghosh CS, Ravindran P, Joshi M, et al: Reductions in hospital use from self management training for chronic asthmatics. Soc Sci Med 46:1087–1093, 1998.
93. Beasley R, Cushley M, Holgate ST: A self management plan in the treatment of adult asthma. Thorax 44:200–204, 1989.
94. Balter MS, Rebuck AS: Treatment of the recalcitrant asthmatic. Ann Allergy 63:297–300, 1989.
95. Toelle BG, Peat JK, Salome CM, et al: Evaluation of a community-based asthma management program in a population sample of schoolchildren. Med J Aust 158:742–746, 1993.
96. Clark NM, Gong M, Schork MA, et al: Impact of education for physicians on patient outcomes. Pediatrics 101:831–836, 1998.
97. D'Souza W, Crane J, Burgess C, et al: Community-based asthma care: Trial of a "credit card" asthma self-management plan. Eur Respir J 7:1260–1265, 1994.
98. Jones KP, Mullee MA, Middleton M, et al: Peak flow based asthma self-management: A randomized controlled study in general practice. Thorax 50:851–857, 1995.
99. Cote J, Cartier A, Robichaud P, et al: Influence on asthma morbidity of asthma education programs based on self-management plans following treatment optimization. Am J Respir Care Crit Care Med 155:1509–1514, 1997.
100. Cowie RL, Revitt SG, Underwood MF, et al: The effect of a peak flow-based action plan in the prevention of exacerbations of asthma. Chest 112:1534–1538, 1997.
101. Turner MO, Taylor D, Bennett R, et al: A randomized trial comparing peak expiratory flow and symptom self-management plans for patients with asthma attending a primary care clinic. Am J Respir Crit Care Med 157:540–546, 1998.
102. Grampian Asthma Study of Integrated Care (GRASSIC). Integrated care for asthma: A clinical, social, and economic evaluation. BMJ 308:559–564, 1994.
103. Clark NM, Gong M, Schork MA, et al: Long-term effects of asthma education for MDs on patient satisfaction and use of health services. Eur Respir J (in press).
104. Bender B, Milgrom H, Rand C: Nonadherence in asthmatic patients: Is there a solution to the problem? Ann Allergy Asthma Immunol 79:177–184, 1997.
105. Mannino DM, Homa DM, Pertowski CA, et al: Surveillance for asthma: United States, 1960–1995. MMWR Morb Mortal Wkly Rep CDC Surveillance Summaries 47:1–27, 1998.
106. Greineder D, Loane K, Parks P: Reduction in resource utilization by an asthma outreach program. Arch Pediatr Adolesc Med 149:415–420, 1995.
107. Bender B, Milgrom H, Rand C, et al: Psychological factors associated with medication nonadherence in asthmatic children. J Asthma 35:347–353, 1998.
108. Kolbe J, Vamos M, Fergusson W, et al: Differential influences on asthma self-management knowledge and self-management behavior in acute severe asthma. Chest 110:1463–1468, 1996.
109. Boulet LP: Perception of the role of potential side effects of inhaled corticosteroids among asthmatic patients. Chest 113:587–592, 1998.
110. Redline S, Wright EC, Kattan M, et al: Short-term compliance with peak flow monitoring: Results from a study of inner city children with asthma. Pediatr Pulmonol 21:203–210, 1996.
111. Verschelden P, Cartier A, L'Archevque J, et al: Compliance with and accuracy of daily self-assessment of peak expiratory flow (PEF) in asthmatics over a 3 month period. Eur Respir J 9:880–885, 1996.
112. Cote J, Cartier A, Malo JL, et al: Compliance with peak expiratory flow monitoring in home management of asthma. Chest 113:968–972, 1998.
113. Cromer BA: Behavioral strategies to increase compliance in adolescents. *In* Cramer JA, Spilker B: Patient Compliance in Medical Practice and Clinical Trials. New York: Raven Press, 1991, pp 89–105.
114. Becker MH: Theoretical models of adherence and strategies for improving adherence. *In* Schumaker SA, Schron EG, Ockene JK (eds): The Handbook of Health Behavior Change. New York: Springer Publishing, 1990, pp 5–43.
115. Inui TS, Yourtee EL, Williamson JW: Improved outcomes in hypertension after physician tutorials: A controlled trail. Ann Intern Med 84:646–651, 1976.
116. Maiman LA, Becker MH, Liptak GS, et al: Improving pediatricians' compliance-enhancing practices: A randomized trial. Am J Dis Child 142:773–779, 1988.
117. Clark NM, Gong M, Schork MA et al: A scale for assessing clinician's teaching and communication behavior regarding asthma. Health Educ Behav 24:245–256, 1997.

# 99 Community Measures: Public Policy and Education

Virginia S. Taggart, M.P.H. • Robinson Fulwood, M.S.P.H.
Michele Hindi-Alexander, Ph.D. • Claude Lenfant, M.D.

Introduction
Role of Government in Secondary Prevention: Asthma
Assessing the Growing Public Health Problem
Developing Policy to Address the Problem
Ensuring Implementation Through the NAEPP
Evaluating Government Programs and Effects
Role of Government in Primary Prevention: Air Quality and Smoking
Assessing Air Quality
Ensuring Air Quality: The Clean Air Act
Assessing Health Effects of Environmental Tobacco Smoke
Developing Policies and Intervention Strategies to Ensure Reduced ETS
Assessing the Prevalence of Smoking Among Youth
Developing Policies and Intervention Strategies to Prevent Young People From Smoking
Summary

## INTRODUCTION

The role of the government in setting policy and educating the public about the prevention and control of lung disease has its basis in the established goal of the Constitution's framers to promote the general welfare of the population. The earliest health activities to reach this goal included quarantines in the 1700s and early 1800s to contain contagious diseases and demands in the 1800s and early 1900s for concerted community, and government, action to improve sanitation for the control and prevention of communicable, infectious diseases such as smallpox, diphtheria, and typhus. The role of government expanded as scientific research defined the causes of disease and as scientific discoveries identified the means for preventing their progression or onset.



Government statistics on the nation's health, which began to be collected in the late 1800s, indicate that much progress was made. For example, the scourges of smallpox, cholera, diphtheria, typhus, and polio were eventually eliminated. National statistics also, however, revealed much physical disability and premature death from chronic illnesses. These data fostered public recognition of the importance of personal attention to health and fitness as well as of governmental action to promote health and to prevent and control disease. The convergence of advances in science and of growth in the national commitment to reduce suffering and enhance the quality of life underlies the capacity of modern governments—both local and national—to fulfill their historic role of promoting general welfare.

In 1988, the Institute of Medicine[1] summarized the role of government in preventing and controlling disease as the identification of problems, mobilization of necessary effort and resources, and assurance of conditions in which people can be healthy. Thus, the role of the government includes

- Assessment: Collecting information systematically on the health of the nation and supporting scientific research on the causes, treatment, and prevention of disease.
- Policy development: Defining goals and priorities based on scientific knowledge and proposing measures to achieve them.
- Assurance: Taking action through public education advocacy, negotiation, mobilization of resources or, if necessary, mandating action or directly providing services.
- Evaluation: Determining whether policy goals and priorities are achieved. This evaluation can then lead into a further cycle of assessment, policy development, and assurance.

Governments at all levels share these functions. The national government has primary roles in assessment through conducting and promoting research and in overall health policy development and implementation. These roles include nationwide efforts to focus attention on major public health problems and to encourage action on the part of other levels of government as well as private groups. Local governments have primary roles in assuring that local needs are met by implementing and coordinating services based on community-specific knowledge and values. Local governments further evaluate the effects of programs on local needs and convey this information back to the national level for further research and policy development.

This chapter first illustrates government roles in secondary prevention—treatment and prevention of disease progression—with asthma as an example of a growing public health problem. This chapter then illustrates government roles in primary prevention, using as example the efforts to improve ambient air quality, reduce exposure to environmental tobacco smoke, and prevent young people from smoking.

## ROLE OF GOVERNMENT IN SECONDARY PREVENTION: ASTHMA

### Assessing the Growing Public Health Problem

#### Surveillance: The Scope of the Asthma Burden

A key role of government is monitoring the health of the nation through collection and analysis of statistics, as on the rates of hospital discharge and ambulatory care visits for different diseases. This is partly accomplished through the annual National Health and Nutrition Examination Survey of a representational sample of the American population. These surveys show clearly that asthma is a growing health problem with significant impact on the nation. It ranks among the most common chronic conditions in the United States, affecting an estimated 14.9 million persons in 1995. Asthma's prevalence increased 75% over 14 years, from 30.7 per 1000 population in 1980 to 53.8 per 1000 population in 1994; prevalence is slightly higher among African Americans[2, 3] and is increasing more rapidly among children than among adults.

National statistics further show that asthma accounts for more than 1.5 million emergency department visits, 500,000 hospitalizations, 5500 deaths, and more than 100 million days of restricted activity a year. Among diseases commonly seen in outpatient departments, asthma was the sixth most frequent in 1992. These figures do not appear to be an artifact of a change in how asthma is labeled or diagnosed but instead appear to reflect a real change in the prevalence of the disease.[4, 5]

The burden of asthma disproportionately affects minorities and the poor. For example, asthma prevalence is only slightly higher among nonwhites than among whites, yet asthma hospitalization and morbidity rates for nonwhites are more than twice larger.[3] Why this is so is not clearly understood, but it is likely due to an interaction of factors such as high levels of exposure to environmental allergens and irritants, lack of access to quality medical care, and lack of financial resources and social support to manage the disease effectively on a long-term basis.

The estimated direct and indirect costs for asthma totaled $11.3 billion in 1998,[6] with disproportionate share of costs being attributable to nonscheduled acute or emergency care.[7] One study revealed that people with severe asthma, who make up only 10% of the asthmatic population, account for roughly 51% of all direct medical care expenditures and 54% of total asthma costs.[8]

The full burden of disease, however, is not measured by the more extreme events alone. Children with asthma miss an average of twice as many school days as other children, with 21% of children with asthma missing more than 2 weeks of school a year.[9] Twenty-one per cent of people of all ages with asthma restricted their daily activities due to asthma.[10] Asthma symptoms not severe enough to require a visit to a physician can still substantially restrict activities and impair quality of life.

#### Research: Advances in Understanding and Treating Asthma

The US Congress created the National Institutes of Health (NIH) to be the "steward of biomedical and behavioral research for the nation. Its mission is science in pursuit of fundamental knowledge about the nature and behavior of living systems and the application of that knowledge to extend healthy life and reduce the burdens of illness and disability."[11] More specifically, the NIH were designed to improve the health of the nation through the conduct of research on the causes, prevention, and methods of diagnosis and treatment of disease; to assist and foster research by public and private agencies; to promote the coordination and application of research; to provide training; and to assist states and other agencies in the prevention, diagnosis, and treatment of diseases. The continuous growth and success of these efforts have led to the NIH's reputation as the world's major medical research organization.

Decisions regarding which research should be supported are the result of a deliberative assessment of the impact of a disease on public health (e.g., the number of people affected, the degree of disability or deaths caused, the effects on quality of life, and risk of spreading in the population), and the potential for scientific progress (e.g., the emergence of promising scientific discoveries and the availability of qualified investigators). In determining research priorities, the NIH seek input from a variety of sources, including formal conferences and advisory panels, individual researchers, professional societies, patient and voluntary organizations, and Congress itself.[12]

Increasing concern about the public health burden imposed by pulmonary diseases, such as chronic obstructive pulmonary disease and asthma, and scientific breakthroughs from studies of their pathogenesis and treatment led to an expansion of the National Heart Institute in 1969, when it become the National Heart and Lung Institute. The commitment continues today as one fourth of the total National Heart, Lung, and Blood Institute (NHLBI) budget is dedicated to lung diseases, a significant portion of which is spent on asthma.[13] The National Heart, Lung, and Blood Institute and the National Institute of Allergy and Infectious Diseases have the major responsibility for conducting and supporting asthma research; the National Institute of Environmental Health Sciences, the National Institute of Child Health and Human Development, and the National Institute of Nursing Research also support research on asthma. The NIH collaborate for with other federal agencies involved in different aspects of asthma research or management, such as the Centers for Disease Control and Prevention, the Environmental Protection Agency, and the Agency for Health Care Policy and Research.

The NIH support a comprehensive spectrum of research on asthma's pathogenesis, management, and prevention. This program encompasses basic research on the disease's pathogenesis, epidemiologic research on its genetic and environmental determinants, and clinical research on its therapies. The NIH also sponsors demonstration and education programs to promote the translation of scientific findings into patient care. These research programs are supported through a variety of mechanisms, including investigator-initiated grants, Institute-initiated grants and contracts to stimulate targeted research areas, and research training and career development grants to promote careers in asthma research. This variety in mechanisms of support ensures breadth in the scope of research and in the participation by researchers with different skills across the nation.

It is through the interplay of research in various scientific disciplines that advances in asthma care have been made possible. Different disciplines have made unique contributions to understanding asthma and have generated results that informed the findings of other types of asthma research.

**Basic Research.** A major focus of basic research has been the role of specific inflammatory cells and the mechanisms of their interaction with each other and with resident airway cells.[14] Research has also been directed at examining the mechanisms of neural control of airway function and defining their contribution to airway hyperresponsiveness. Genetically engineered murine models have enabled exploration of the immune and inflammatory responses of the lungs to antigen sensitization and challenge. Basic research is now beginning to clarify the mechanisms responsible for the cycle of injury, repair, and remodeling that contributes to the persistence and severity of asthma.

**Epidemiologic Research.** Longitudinal studies are focusing on identifying risk factors associated with the onset of asthma as well as with severe asthma and asthma-related death. Epidemiologic studies in the late 1990s have identified different patterns of wheezing in young children with viral illness[15] and have prompted an exciting new area of investigation into the mechanisms by which infections and other early life exposures influence development of the immune system and regulation of airway inflammation, airway hyperresponsiveness, and airway remodeling that underlie the onset and persistence of asthma.

**Genetic Research.** A genome-wide search is underway to identify genes that confer susceptibility to asthma. Early findings confirm that multiple genes may be involved in asthma and that they may vary among ethnic and racial groups.[16] Studies of known candidate genes suggest that genetically determined changes in inflammatory pathways and T-cell signaling are involved in the pathophysiology of asthma. Moreover, because the genetic background of the population has not changed significantly over the past 20 years, the rapid increase in asthma prevalence most reflects the interaction between environmental factors and genetic susceptibility. Applying recently developed techniques in cellular and molecular biology and genetics to define how this interaction predisposes certain individuals to asthma is a priority for research. Genetic studies also provide insights into clinical studies. For example, clinical and epidemiologic studies have revealed that a subset of patients may respond poorly to regular use of $beta_2$-agonist medications; genetic analyses have identified specific polymorphisms of genes for the beta receptor.[17] Future research in pharmacogenetics has the potential for defining an approach to asthma treatment that will enable physicians to target therapy based on a patient's specific genotype.

**Clinical Research.** A number of NIH programs investigate new drug therapies and evaluate the effectiveness of existing therapies in asthma management. Clinical trials in children are also exploring the effects of therapies on the course of the disease and on lung growth and development, but much research is needed to identify optimal therapeutic strategies for children at different developmental stages. Studies are underway to elucidate the interaction of pregnancy, asthma, and the potential impact of therapy on pregnancy outcomes. Little research has been done on asthma in the elderly,[18] and yet the highest number of deaths from asthma occur in people over age 55 years, and concern is increasing about the multiple therapies taken by older people with asthma and other health conditions. Clinical research provides the essential link between advances in basic scientific understanding of asthma and the ultimate improvement in health outcomes for people with the disease.

**Demonstration and Education Research.** Documentation of the value and cost-effectiveness of teaching patients self-management has prompted a dramatic shift in patient-physician relationships, with a new emphasis on encouraging partnership. Current research is focused on identifying methods to promote clinicians' adoption of practice guidelines and to foster more effective and efficient patient teaching and counseling.[19] Research is needed to identify the most essential elements of patient education. Research is also needed to develop models to extend effective asthma management into populations that have been traditionally harder to reach, such as minorities and the poor.[20] Several institutes have initiated research programs to stimulate innovative models for reaching children with asthma in their home and school environments, as through nurse case managers, peer educators visiting homes, and programs aimed at making schools "asthma friendly" by reducing exposure to environmental triggers and ensuring appropriate school policies and procedures for helping children manage their asthma at school. More recently, there has been an upsurge in local community coalitions that organize disparate groups to join in coordinating citywide or countrywide asthma medical service and education programs. Evaluation research is essential to determine their effectiveness and to encourage dissemination of appropriate models.

## Developing Policy to Address the Problem

The significant federal role in supporting and stimulating scientific investigations through a wide spectrum of basic, epidemiologic, clinical, and education/behavioral research has led to the striking advances in treatment that have made asthma a controllable disease. It is now possible for most asthma patients to expect a level of symptom control and quality of life that was unimaginable just 15 years ago.

Paradoxically, these advances have occurred at the same time that the disease has affected people at increasing rates, and evidence mounted that at least in "hot spots" of high rates of hospitalization and mortality around the country the standards of managing the disease were poor. It is apparent, then, that additional measures are necessary to ensure that the benefits of publicly supported research are widely available to fulfill the congressional mandate that the NIH translate research and provide credible, science-based information to improve the health of the public. These measures include federal policies to stimulate programs at the national and community levels that promote adequate management of disease and associated disabilities. Three examples in the area of asthma include the National Asthma Education and Prevention Program (NAEPP), the Healthy People reports, and the President's Task Force on Environmental Health Risks and Safety Risks to Children.

### National Asthma Education and Prevention Program

The National Heart, Lung, and Blood Institute established the National Asthma Education and Prevention Program in March 1989 to address the growing problem of asthma in the United States.

**Goals and Organization.** NAEPP's goals are to:

- Raise awareness of patients, health professionals and the public that asthma is a serious chronic disease.
- Ensure the recognition of the symptoms of asthma by patients, families, and the public and the appropriate diagnosis by health professionals.
- Ensure effective control of asthma by encouraging a partnership among patients, physicians, and other health professionals through modern treatment and education programs.

The NAEPP Coordinating Committee is composed of representatives from more than 30 medical professions, voluntary health organizations, patient groups, and government agencies (Table 99.1) and provides overall direction to the NAEPP programs. NAEPP activities include assessing biomedical and behavioral research findings and their relevance for wide-scale application in clinical and public health practice, clinical practice guidelines, and educational programs and materials for health professional and patient groups.

**Table 99.1 NATIONAL ASTHMA EDUCATION AND PREVENTION PROGRAM COORDINATING COMMITTEE MEMBER ORGANIZATIONS**

| |
|---|
| **Public Organizations** |
| Allergy and Asthma Network/Mothers of Asthmatics |
| American Academy of Allergy, Asthma, and Immunology |
| American Academy of Family Physicians |
| American Academy of Pediatrics |
| American Academy of Physician Assistants |
| American Association for Respiratory Care |
| American Association of Occupational Health Nurses |
| American College of Allergy, Asthma, and Immunology |
| American College of Chest Physicians |
| American College of Emergency Physicians |
| American Lung Association |
| American Medical Association |
| American Nurses' Association |
| American Pharmaceutical Association |
| American Public Health Association |
| American School Health Association |
| American Society of Health-System Pharmacists |
| American Thoracic Society |
| Association of State and Territorial Directors of Public Health Education |
| Asthma and Allergy Foundation of America |
| National Association of School Nurses |
| National Black Nurses' Association |
| National Heart, Lung, and Blood Institute Ad Hoc Committee on Minority Populations |
| National Medical Association |
| Society for Public Health Education |
| **Federal Agencies** |
| Agency for Health Care Policy and Research |
| Centers for Disease Control and Prevention |
| National Center for Environmental Health |
| National Center for Health Statistics |
| National Heart, Lung, and Blood Institute |
| National Institute for Occupational Safety and Health |
| National Institute of Allergy and Infectious Diseases |
| National Institute of Environmental Health Sciences |
| US Department of Education |
| US Environmental Protection Agency |
| US Food and Drug Administration |
| US Public Health Service |
| **Additional Representatives to the NAEPP School Asthma Education Subcommittee** |
| American Alliance for Health, Physical Education, Recreation, and Dance |
| National Association of Elementary School Principals |
| National Education Association Health Information Network |
| National School Boards Association |

**Clinical Practice Guidelines.** Increases in the complexity of medical care and in the volume of medical literature make it increasingly difficult for clinicians to keep abreast of findings relevant to numerous medical conditions. Clinical practice guidelines, which are systematically developed statements to assist practitioners in making decisions about appropriate health care for specific conditions,[21] are a major mechanism for translating scientific advances into medical practice and for ensuring that the benefits of research are extended to patient care. Guidelines review the literature and make recommendations for care based on evidence or, when evidence is controversial or lacking, on a consensus of expert opinion. As such, guidelines offer health care professionals and patients a synthesis of state-of-the-art management strategies and a common reference point for communicating with each other and for making individual treatment decisions. The objective for clinical practice guidelines are to help reduce wide variations in medical practice, improve clinical decision-making by promoting practices proven to be effective ("evidence-based practice"), eliminate inappropriate procedures, and control expenditures.

The federal government provides the research expertise and resources, impartiality, independence (from any single medical specialty or pharmaceutical interest), and capacity for consensus building that increase the likelihood of effective guidelines.[21] The NIH have successfully used guidelines as the foundation for several national-level research translation and education programs aimed at preventing and reducing illness from diseases with a high impact on public health. For example, the National High Blood Pressure Program and the National Cholesterol Education Program have contributed to significant reductions in heart disease over the last 20 years.[1]

The NAEPP developed asthma clinical practice guidelines in 1991[22] to improve asthma care and to serve as the foundation for all NAEPP education activities for health professionals, patients, and the general public. A NAEPP subcommittee continually monitors the literature in order to alert the coordinating committee when the recommendations should be updated, as was done with publication of the 1997 revision of the guidelines.[23]

The NAEPP strives to ensure the scientific validity, credibility, and practical utility of its guidelines by including a wide range of groups in both the development and the review processes. Thus the expert panels charged with evaluating the literature and drafting the guidelines have included pulmonologists, allergists, nurses, family physicians, pediatricians, emergency medicine specialists, behavioral scientists, and health educators. Furthermore, each organization represented on the NAEPP Coordinating Committee has provided input as a part of the guidelines' review cycle. For example, review of the 1997 NAEPP guidelines involved over 140 individuals from 40 public and private organizations. The broad representation not only extended the breadth of scientific review but also enhanced the usefulness of the guidelines. For example, the review process prompted the development of summary charts geared to busy primary care physicians and of sample patient education materials as integral parts of the guidelines.

## Healthy People

The Healthy People national initiative identifies opportunities to improve the health of all Americans. Since its inception in 1979, Healthy People has reflected a consensus among scientists and the public health community that the nation's health strategy must emphasize prevention. For two decades, the US Public Health Service has used Healthy People reports to set specific objectives for health promotion and disease prevention in targeted populations, to organize concerted action among the public health and private sectors to meet these objectives, and to provide indicators for monitoring progress. Implementation of Healthy People objectives is far reaching and includes providing mandates for federal programs, stimulating and prioritizing research, providing a framework for the clinical services and health education campaigns of state and county health departments, organizing school health education curricula, and mobilizing cooperative programs among private voluntary organizations and businesses to improve their community's health.

Led by the federal government, Healthy People provides an opportunity for all sectors of the nation to participate in developing national health objectives and in shaping public health programs to achieve them. Healthy People objectives are developed with input from 22 expert working panels and over 2000 individuals through regional meetings, open review (e.g., through the Internet) and from a consortium of over 300 national organizations, state and local public health agencies, voluntary organizations, health service organizations, congressional representatives, and private citizens.

Building on the successful achievement of most of the objectives outlined in the 1979 Surgeon General's Healthy People Report,[24] the Healthy People 2000 objectives[25] emphasized disease prevention and reduction of health disparities among Americans. Healthy People 2000 had three objectives specifically relevant to asthma: to reduce hospitalizations due to asthma, to reduce activity restrictions due to asthma, and to increase the proportion of people with asthma who receive formal patient education.

Healthy People 2010 objectives[26] are currently being developed, and it builds on a broader science base, improved surveillance systems, and heightened public demand for preventive health services and quality health care. Healthy People 2010 focuses on the theme that prevention is the single most important factor in maintaining good health. Thus Healthy People 2010 outlines objectives for prevention, improving quality of life, and reducing disparities. Healthy People 2010 also takes advantage of the advances in asthma care defined in the NAEPP's guidelines and has added objectives on asthma, as noted in Table 99.2.

Collaborative efforts to incorporate Healthy People 2010 objectives into asthma programs at all levels—national, state, and local, in both the public health and private sectors—will significantly increase the likelihood of success in promoting the health and well-being of all people with asthma. Use of Healthy People objectives and performance indicators will help public health planners and researchers evaluate their programs' impact compared with national goals.

**Table 99.2 HEALTHY PEOPLE OBJECTIVES FOR ASTHMA**

**Healthy People 2000**

1. Reduce asthma morbidity, as measured by a reduction in asthma hospitalizations, to no more than 160 per 100,000 people.
2. Reduce to no more than 10% the proportion of people with asthma who experience activity limitation.
3. Increase to at least 50% the proportion of people with asthma who receive formal patient education, including information about community and self-help resources, as an integral part of the management of their condition.

**Healthy People 2010**

1. Reduce asthma death rate to no more than 14 per million population.
2. Reduce the overall asthma morbidity, as measured by a reduction in asthma hospitalization rate, to 10 per 10,000 people.
3. Reduce morbidity as measured by reduction in annual rate of emergency department visits to no more than 46 per 10,000 people.
4. Reduce to no more than 10% the proportion of people with asthma who experience activity limitation.
5. (Developmental) Reduce disruption of life for people with asthma, as measured by school work days lost.
6. Increase to at least 40% the proportion of people with asthma who receive formal patient education, including information about community and self-help resources, as an integral part of the management of their condition.
7. (Developmental) Increase to ___ % the proportion of primary care physicians who have participated in continuing medical education on asthma.
8. (Developmental) Increase to ___ % the proportion of people with asthma who receive written asthma management plans from their physicians.
9. (Developmental) Increase to ___ % the proportion of patients who receive counseling form health care providers on how to recognize the early signs of worsening asthma and how to respond appropriately.
10. (Developmental) Increase to ___ % the proportion of asthma patients using daily therapy who have received instruction on peak expiratory flow monitoring to assess the course of their disease and response to treatment.
11. (Developmental) Reduce to ___ % the proportion of people with asthma who use more than one canister or equivalent a month of short-acting inhaled beta-agonists for relief of symptoms.
12. (Developmental) Increase to ___ % the proportion of people hospitalized for asthma who have received follow-up medical care for long-term management of their condition.
13. Establish in at least 15 states a surveillance system for tracking asthma mortality, morbidity, access to medical care, and asthma management.

### President's Task Force on Environmental Health Risks and Safety Risks to Children

Executive Order 13945 of April 21, 1997, Protection of Children From Environmental Health Risks and Safety Risks, directs each federal agency to make it a high priority to identify, assess, and address the illness and injury that American children suffer from environmental health and safety risks. A Task Force was also created, co-chaired by the Secretary of the Department of Health and Human Resources and the Administrator of the Environmental Protection Agency, to recommend promising strategies for protecting children's environmental health and safety. Four priority areas were identified for immediate attention: childhood asthma, unintentional injuries, developmental disorders, and childhood cancer. A 1998 Task Force report focuses on the particular contribution of environmental factors to childhood asthma and emphasizes the needs to strengthen and accelerate research into the environmental factors that cause or worsen childhood asthma, to implement public health programs that reduce environmental exposures that worsen asthma (including environmental tobacco smoke), and to establish a coordinated nationwide asthma surveillance system. The report outlines opportunities for coordination and collaboration among federal agencies.

A significant feature of the Executive Order is its mandate to review and foster public access to federal government–sponsored research related to environmental health and safety risks affecting children. Thus the Task Force is developing a computer-based inventory that will be available to the public through the Internet and will encourage sharing of information on academic and private research.

## Ensuring Implementation Through the NAEPP

The role of the government in preventing illness and promoting health, as noted earlier, is threefold: assessment (conducting research into the causes, treatment, and prevention of disease), policy development (setting goals and priorities based on that research), and assurance (taking action to ensure implementation of programs to reach those goals). The action to assure implementation can take a variety of forms. Federal or local governments may provide public information and education, mobilize resources and negotiate partnerships among private and public sector organizations, or, if necessary, require action through regulatory mechanisms or direct provision of services.

### NAEPP Partnerships and Activities

For implementing effective asthma management programs, and thus for preventing asthma-related illness and deaths, the major examples of governmental action are the programs generated by the NAEPP. In these programs, the NAEPP Coordinating Committee members work collaboratively to facilitate asthma research translation and information dissemination in a manner that engages partnerships among government agencies, voluntary organizations, and community groups. The multilevel partnerships built through the NAEPP maximize resources, minimize duplication of effort, and allow each member organization to focus on projects that can best benefit from their unique contribution to the field. For example, the NAEPP

- Leads and coordinates educational efforts of professional and voluntary organizations, civic groups, and federal and state agencies to provide for the rapid transfer of asthma research results to professional, patient, and public audiences
- Fosters and maintains collaborative partnerships to strengthen the resources available for improving the quality of life for patients with asthma
- Develops and implements culturally sensitive asthma education strategies to meet the needs of diverse populations, including the underserved, minorities, and those outside the traditional health care system

The multifaceted nature of the government's role in disease prevention programs and the integral importance of public involvement through partnership activities are demonstrated in the NAEPP's partnership activities with health care professionals, public and private groups, schools, and local asthma coalitions.

**Health Care Professionals.** Through its membership, the NAEPP has a network of physicians and other clinicians who work to increase the dissemination, adoption, and implementation of NAEPP clinical practice guidelines throughout the country. Interventions target a variety of populations and settings, including managed care and the inner city as well as other locations where asthma morbidity and mortality rates are especially high. Each professional society—for physicians, nurses, nurse practitioners and physician assistants, health educators, pharmacists, and respiratory therapists—has offered its members numerous continuing education programs devoted to the guidelines through journal articles, workshops, seminars at regional and national meetings, and innovative video and computer-assisted learning programs. The National Medical Association and American College of Chest Physicians, worked with the NAEPP to develop synopses of the guidelines in easy-to-use pocket-card formats that encouraged more widespread distribution among primary care clinicians and medical students. The NAEPP also worked with the American Academy of Allergy, Asthma, and Immunology to develop a summary guide and interactive conferences targeted specifically to primary care clinicians who care for children.

In the managed care setting, the NAEPP has worked with several groups to promote opportunities for providing quality asthma care. For example, the NAEPP and the American College of Chest Physicians organized a national conference on asthma management for managed care organizations, including those serving Medicaid populations. Another example is the NAEPP's work with the National Commission on Quality Assurance and the Institute for Health Care Improvement to implement regional seminar series on asthma and to develop general parameters for health care performance indicators based on the clinical practice guidelines.

A major goal for all of these efforts to promote adoption of NAEPP guidelines is to help different clinical disciplines appreciate how the guidelines can be appropriately adapted to the circumstances of local practice settings.

**Patient and Public Groups.** Patient and public advocacy groups work both individually and collectively with the NAEPP to increase public awareness about asthma as a serious public health problem, improve patient adherence to medical advice, and stimulate community action. The American Lung Association, for example, has an extensive network of chapters around the country that offer family education programs on asthma and has been a strong advocate for legislation to protect asthma patients from environmental tobacco smoke. The Asthma and Allergy Foundation of America is a leader in promoting support groups for asthma patients, including innovative programs for teenagers. The Allergy and Asthma Network/Mothers of Asthmatics prepares a patient-oriented and family-oriented newsletter. All these organizations continue to develop educational and advocacy materials that promote key messages from the NAEPP guidelines.

The NAEPP has a vibrant public education campaign to increase awareness of warning signs and symptoms of undiagnosed or inadequately controlled asthma. The campaign's key message focuses on encouraging those who experience signs and symptoms of asthma to see their doctor or health care provider for treatment. The campaign uses radio public service announcements that present a variety of specific messages about asthma to increase public awareness. The announcements have been distributed to more than 600 radio stations in African-American and Hispanic markets across the nation. More recently, the NAEPP's public education efforts have focused on collaborating with community-based coalitions that deal directly with asthma problems at the local level.

**Schools.** Recognizing that asthma is a particularly significant public health problem for school-age children, the NAEPP partners with organizations like the Association of Elementary School Principals, the American School Health Association, the National School Nurses Association, and the National Education Association to promote strategies that help children with asthma be healthy and ready to learn. The NAEPP has disseminated asthma education information written specifically for the school setting to more than 100,000 schools across the country.

Furthermore, the NAEPP works to mobilize activities. The NAEPP Resolution: Asthma Management in Schools, developed in collaboration with the National Association of School Board Administrators, is a policy statement emphasizing the need for prompt and reliable access to medications in the school. The NAEPP also developed a checklist, "How Asthma Friendly Is Your School?", that outlines the major components of school programs and procedures that would enable a child with asthma to participate fully in school activities. Teachers, administrators, and parents are encouraged to use the checklist as an assessment tool and NAEPP school materials as educational tools to strengthen their school's support of children with asthma. The American Lung Association, in partnership with the Environmental Protection Agency and the NAEPP, teaches asthma management skills to school children through a program conducted in elementary schools around the country.

**Local Asthma Coalitions.** A new NAEPP public education effort focuses on developing networks of community-based groups—many call themselves asthma coalitions—involved in asthma education and outreach. The coalitions are composed of members from local public health departments, hospitals and medical centers, community clinics, schools, community recreation centers, pharmacies, concerned parents groups, lung associations and other nonprofit groups, and local media. The diverse representation enhances a sense of local ownership and collaboration. This, in turn, increases participation in educational activities that improve the clinical practice skills of health care providers, the self-management skills of patients and families, and the responsiveness of community organizations (e.g., changing pharmacy hours or school policies on medication use, arranging financial assistance for families in need).

One of the earliest coalitions, the Fresno Asthma Project, demonstrates a successful community intervention model. A small federal grant initiated the project; 3 years later, the group was self-sustaining through the enthusiastic support of local foundations, pharmaceutical companies, and private organizations.[27] Coalitions have since proliferated. Representatives from 43 coalitions attended a 1998 NAEPP national meeting designed to promote exchange of information among coalitions, coordination with NAEPP, and stimulation of development of additional community asthma coalitions. Table 99.3 lists 1998 conference participants and illustrates the wide-reaching impact of a national-level program in spawning local action.

**Table 99.3 ASTHMA COALITIONS: NATIONAL ASTHMA EDUCATION AND PREVENTION PROGRAM ASTHMA COALITION CONFERENCE PARTICIPANTS, 1998**

| |
|---|
| Allina Pediatric Asthma Clinical Action Group (Minneapolis, MN) |
| American Lung Association of Oregon (Portland, OR) |
| Arizona Asthma Coalition (Phoenix, AZ) |
| Asthma Care Alliance of Southern Arizona (Tucson, AZ) |
| Asthma Coalition of Northern Virginia (Falls Church, VA) |
| Asthma Community Development Program (Indianapolis, IN) |
| Asthma Summit (Tulsa, OK) |
| Asthma Task Force: Southeast Pennsylvania (Plymouth Meeting, PA) |
| Buffalo Schools Asthma Alliance (Buffalo, NY) |
| Case Western University and Cleveland, Ohio—Partners in Asthma Education (Cleveland, OH) |
| Central California Asthma Project (Fresno, CA) |
| Chicago Asthma Consortium (Chicago, IL) |
| Childhood Asthma Task Force (Flint, MI) |
| Cuyahoga County Coalition on Indoor Urban Environmental Triggers of Asthma (Cleveland, OH) |
| Dallas Asthma Consortium (Dallas, TX) |
| Detroit Asthma Coalition (Detroit, MI) |
| East Harlem Pediatric Asthma Working Group (New York, NY) |
| Fight Asthma Milwaukee (Milwaukee, WI) |
| Fresno/Madera County Asthma Coalition (Fresno, CA) |
| Greater Baltimore Asthma Coalition (Baltimore, MD) |
| Kansas Coalition for Quality Asthma Care (Topeka, KS) |
| Kent County Pediatric Asthma Network (Grand Rapids, MI) |
| Kings County Asthma Coalition (Lemoore, CA) |
| Maine Asthma Initiative (Augusta, ME) |
| Merced/Mariposa County Asthma Coalition Merced, CA) |
| Montgomery County AIR (Rockville, MD) |
| New York City (CUES) Asthma Working Group (New York, NY) |
| New York City Childhood Asthma Initiative (New York, NY) |
| North Carolina Childhood Asthma Initiative (Raleigh, NC) |
| Pediatric Asthma Program (Greenville, NC) |
| Rochester Community Asthma Network (R-CAN) (Rochester, NY) |
| School Attendance and Asthma Management Initiative (SAAMI) (Minneapolis, MN) |
| School Initiated Good Health (SIGH) (Norfolk, VA) |
| Urban Asthma Coalition (Boston, MA) |
| Virginia Asthma Coalition (Richmond, VA) |
| Washington State Asthma Project (Seattle, WA) |
| Washtenaw County Asthma Surveillance Team (AST) (Ypsilanti, MI) |
| Zap Atlanta (Atlanta, GA) |

## Other Government Activities

In addition to the NAEPP coordinating activities, a number of federal, state, and local government agencies conduct other asthma programs related specifically to their respective agency missions. For example, several institutes of the NIH support research on asthma; the Environmental Protection Agency's environmental justice programs and its campaigns to improve the indoor air quality of schools will benefit children with asthma; the Administration for Children and Families incorporates asthma education into training for Head Start program workers; the Health Research and Services Administration and Indian Health Services provide medical care that strives to incorporate asthma clinical practice guidelines; and several state health departments have committed resources to developing surveillance systems to gather local community information about asthma prevalence and morbidity. Although conducted independently, many of these activities were influenced by the policies of the NAEPP and Healthy People, demonstrating the "multiplier" effect of nationally coordinated policy development and program implementation.

## Evaluating Government Programs and Effects

The rationale underlying government's role in preventing disease is that only the mobilization of a nation's collec-

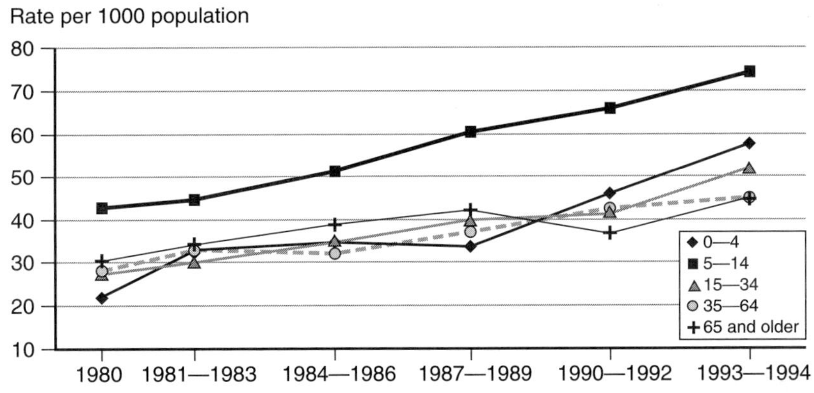


**Figure 99.1** Trends in asthma prevalence are shown by age. (Data from National Health Interview Survey, National Center for Health Statistics, CDC, Atlanta.)

tive resources can eliminate significant threats to public and individual health and improve the health of the nation. Continued support for government activity depends on its success in reducing illness and disability due to a disease and, ultimately, in preventing the disease. Evaluation of the specific impact of federal programs is complicated by the simultaneous institution of multiple interventions at the national, state, and local levels as well as in the private sector. Monitoring and evaluation are nonetheless essential to guide future efforts. Evaluating the success of government programs includes assessment of both process and outcome. Are scientific discoveries improving asthma care, fostering new therapies, and providing clues for prevention? Are policies and clinical practice guidelines implemented? Are the intended effects of these policies achieved—that is, do patients with asthma have fewer hospitalizations, fewer restrictions on activities, and an improved quality of life?

## National Survey Data

The NAEPP uses national survey data to assess program progress. Data on the trends in asthma prevalence, morbidity, and mortality are collected by the Centers for Disease Control and Prevention. Although affected by secular trends, these data provide excellent information to inform program planning and development at the federal, state, and local levels. For example, Figure 99.1 shows that the prevalence of asthma has been increasing since the early 1980s for all age, sex, and racial groups. Although some of the increase represents a true increase in disease, some reflects improved recognition and diagnosis,[5] as promulgated by NAEPP physician education programs and public media campaigns.

Figure 99.2 shows that the age-adjusted rates of asthma hospitalizations have declined in recent years, providing some reassurance about the more widespread use of improved medical treatments. The trends also, however, reveal areas of concern. The decline started about 10 years earlier for whites (1981 to 1983) than it did for African Americans (1990 to 1992), and the rate among African Americans is three and a half times that among whites. African Americans have also had consistently higher rates of emergency room visits. This disparity underscores the need for directed educational and health service programs. Furthermore, analysis of hospitalizations by age reveals that rates have risen dramatically for young children: Between 1980 and 1992, the rate for children under age 1 year increased by 81% and for children age 1 to 4 years it rose by 57%.[2] Further analyses indicate that this increase can only partially be explained by changes in diagnostic practices.[3, 5] Reviews of national trend data thus demonstrate that further research is urgently needed to understand more about the disease's expression in children and why this sharp increase is occurring only in young children.

Trends in mortality data also provide direction for public health program planning. The steady increase in asthma mortality rates over the last 15 years, following a previous 10 year decline,[3] calls for study of what changes—whether in the environment or in pharmacologic treatments—might be responsible. Furthermore, the

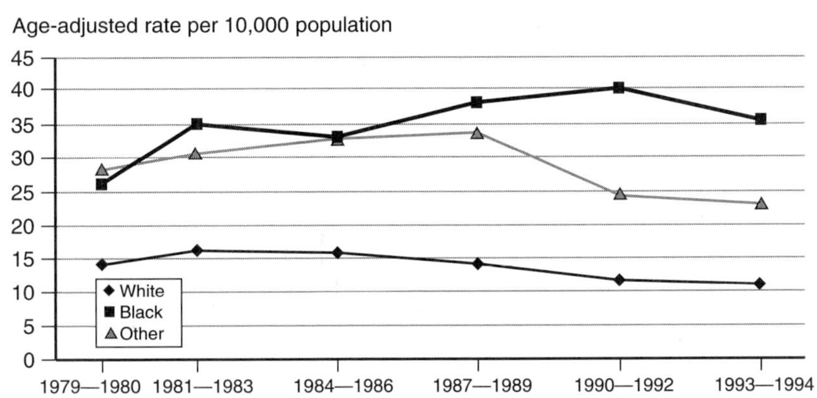


**Figure 99.2** Trends in asthma hospitalizations are shown by race. Data are age adjusted to the 1970 U.S. resident population. (Data from National Hospital Discharge Survey, National Center for Health Statistics, CDC, Atlanta.)

consistently higher death rates among African Americans require asthma management intervention programs targeted to patients at highest risk. It is encouraging, however, to note that the increase in death rates has not been commensurate with the steep rise in asthma prevalence (e.g., between 1981 and 1995 the death rates rose 37% whereas between 1980 and 1995 the prevalence rates for asthma rose 85%).[3] This may well suggest that asthma management has improved overall.

## National Commission on Quality Assurance/Health Employee Data Information Set

The NAEPP has recently begun to work with the National Commission on Quality Assurance in the development of their Health Employee Data Information Set on asthma. This effort focuses attention on the quality of asthma care delivered by managed care organizations. Their inclusion of measures on asthma will stimulate managed care organizations to implement asthma management strategies that are both evidence based and cost effective. The challenge is to balance the desire to promote a general approach to medical care known to be effective against the need to maintain flexibility in tailoring general recommendations to individual patient circumstances. Nonetheless, performance measures based on guidelines at least provide a framework for designing quality assurance programs at the local level.

To improve care for the underserved patients who carry a disproportionate burden of asthma, the NAEPP also works with government agencies that purchase health care services for Medicaid populations. Through these combined efforts, the NAEPP works to negotiate and influence changes in health care to patients with asthma.

## Healthy People Progress Reports

The Assistant Secretary of Health, Department of Health and Human Services, conducts periodic reviews of progress in meeting Healthy People objectives. A midcourse review of objectives relating to asthma revealed some progress in the population as a whole (e.g., hospitalizations were reduced overall) but not in all areas (e.g., activity restrictions increased slightly) and also revealed continued and substantial disparities among lower socioeconomic groups and minority populations. The review highlighted the need for further research and for more aggressive implementation of the guidelines. These highlights helped establish the directions for the programs of the several different federal agencies involved in asthma.

## Evidence of the Impact of Clinical Practice Guidelines

Ironically, clear evidence on the value of guidelines in changing clinician behavior and improving patient outcomes emerged only after the push for evidence based guidelines had gathered strength. A review of 59 rigorous evaluations of clinical practice guidelines for a variety of medical conditions concluded that guidelines improve clinical practice and achieve health gains when introduced in the context of rigorous evaluation.[28] The review noted that guidelines can achieve gain only if they are scientifically valid and are disseminated with specific educational and implementation strategies. That is, written guidelines alone are not sufficient to effect change. Research is needed on the relative effectiveness of different implementation strategies, but those that prompt clinician adherence to guidelines during the patient visit appear to be the most successful. Example of prompts include computer-generated reminders in the patient chart and medical records (history and physical assessment forms, treatment records, discharge instructions) designed to ensure compliance with stipulations in the guidelines. Interactive workshops, audits, chart reviews, and feedback between the medical and educational opinion leaders and the clinicians expected to implement the guidelines also provide strong impetus for adopting guidelines.[29, 30] Computer-based audits and feedback comparing patient care practices with national guidelines is also effective.[31]

The adoption of guidelines into clinical practice varies widely, especially among primary care clinicians—the group that the guidelines are most designed to reach. A review of studies evaluating use of guidelines in primary care (general medicine or family practice settings, health maintenance organizations) revealed that there were statistically significant improvements in just 5 of 13 studies, and the changes in patient outcomes were not considered "clinically dramatic" even in those 5 studies.[32] Possible explanations for these unimpressive results are that the studies examined the impact of older, non–evidence-based guidelines and used methods that were flawed or insensitive to the changes being measured.

The modesty of the demonstrable effects of guidelines among primary care clinicians may have also been due to poor dissemination rather than to deficiencies in the guidelines themselves.[33] A survey of pediatricians revealed that the most common limitation to finding guidelines helpful was a perception that they promoted "cookbook medicine" and constrained individual physician judgment.[34] Yet all good guidelines repeatedly emphasize the need to tailor the general recommendations in the guidelines to the particular needs and circumstances of individual patients. They define aims of management and show more than one route by which the aim can be reached.[35] Dissemination efforts, then, should include methods to predispose clinicians to try the guidelines. Perhaps it is noteworthy that recent medical school graduates and non–university-affiliated physicians were the most likely to find guidelines helpful and more likely to change their behavior because of them.[34]

## Evidence of the Impact of Asthma Clinical Practice Guidelines

To assess the impact of asthma guidelines in the United States, a review of the literature from February 1991 to August 1998 was conducted. A MEDLINE and HealthSTAR search used such key words as "asthma," "clinical guidelines," "NAEPP guidelines," "treatment outcomes," and "physician practices patterns." Studies were then selected if they were based on national clinical practice guidelines, focused on health care professional practices, and used a study design that included comparison groups. An initial search was limited to studies of the NAEPP guidelines, but the search was broadened due to a small yield. Surveys or audits of medical staff practices were also reviewed. Studies evaluating patient education programs were not within the scope of this review. Of 127 citations, 22 publications met the criteria for selection.

**Impact on Changing Clinician Behavior.** Eight articles reported on surveys of clinicians' asthma management practices compared with the recommendations in the NAEPP Expert Panel Reports (EPR1 and EPR2). Although there are obvious limitations to survey methodology, the results offer interesting cross-sectional observations of clinical practice in the years following publication and distribution of the guidelines. The results were mixed. One survey of emergency room physicians replicated a similar survey conducted 3 years before the guidelines and found significant and clinically meaningful changes in the use of pulmonary function testing (74% vs. 47% in 1998), inhaled beta-agonists as first-line treatment (98% vs. 17%), and early steroid use (82% vs. 21%). Fifty per cent of the respondents directly attributed changes in their own behavior to the guidelines.[36] Another study based on a mail survey of emergency department physicians showed reasonably high concordance with guidelines in the medications used but not in the use of peak flow measurements.[37] In contrast, a survey of prescription patterns in one city[38] and another study of claims data in a large health maintenance organization[39] showed asthma care that differed substantially from recommendations in the guidelines, particularly with respect to use of anti-inflammatory therapy. One of the studies revealed particular deficiencies in geographic areas serving low-income patients.[38] Three surveys of patients—two of managed care enrollees (though hampered by low response rates) and one of predominantly low-income patients hospitalized for asthma–revealed patterns of care that did not follow recommendations made in the guidelines.[40–42]

These survey studies may simply confirm the finding in other studies evaluating guidelines for other diseases that making guidelines available is a necessary but not sufficient ingredient for effecting behavior change. The NAEPP's distribution of more than 300,000 copies of its NAEPP EPR1 and the projected distribution of more than 200,000 copies of its EPR2 will certainly increase awareness of guidelines and will provide a reference point for changing asthma care practices. Targeted implementation programs are, however, also necessary to promote adoption.

Just five studies were available in the published literature that compared asthma care practices between clinicians who received an intervention that promoted use of asthma clinical practice guidelines and clinicians in a control group (Table 99.4).[43–47] The quality of the evaluation methods varied. For example, only one of the studies had a randomized control group, and sample sizes may not have been sufficient in several studies. The conclusions were similar, however, and they confirmed previous studies of guideline implementation in other diseases: Guidelines influence behavior among clinicians, but only with targeted, and fairly intensive, implementation programs.

Two studies demonstrated the importance of including the group ultimately responsible for implementing the guidelines in the adoption process. For example, in one of the emergency department studies, the local clinicians developed a critical pathway protocol based on a national guideline, but they adapted it slightly to fit the local practice setting.[45] The study in primary health care clinics was particularly noteworthy for its inclusion of all clinic staff—physicians, nurses, health assistants, laboratory technicians, and clerical staff—in interactive sessions, which increased ownership of the program, confidence in implementing it, and ability to reinforce each other for adopting practices recommended in the guidelines.[43]

All studies indicated the need for repetition and reinforcement: One noted that asthma practice behaviors in an emergency department declined after the intervention program was discontinued.[47] Another concluded that concise messages repeated in multiple formats were most likely to effect change.[46] Computer strategies were the least favored by participants in this last study, perhaps because the study was conducted in 1992 to 1993, before widespread use of computers in clinical practice.

**Impact on Patient Outcomes.** The ultimate test of guidelines is whether they improve health outcomes and quality of life. Research on whether guidelines achieve this goal is spare. Only nine studies have been published, and the quality of the methods used was uneven (Table 99.5).[48–52] The five studies with comparison groups were conducted in the comparison groups emergency department or hospital setting. All reported greater reductions in either readmission rates or emergency department visits and greater improvements in asthma management skills. One study also reported significant improvements in quality of life even 2 years after the intervention.[51] Cautions in interpreting these studies are their reliance on historical comparison groups and the potentially selective enrollment of patients in intervention groups, but it is noteworthy that the results suggest a positive impact of clinical practice guidelines on treatment of a high-risk population, that is, patients who frequently rely on the emergency department or hospital for asthma care.

**The Need for More Research.** Overall, the studies show a promising potential for clinical practice guidelines to influence medical practice and improve patient outcomes. The most striking conclusion from the studies evaluating the impact of asthma guidelines, though, may well be that much research still needs to be done in a wider variety of clinical settings and with more rigorous techniques. Although we understand how to produce evidence-based, scientifically valid guidelines that are credible to potential users, we have much to learn about how to foster their adoption and how to assure their intended effects on patient health. Perhaps focusing resources on improving and evaluating the implementation of guidelines will be more useful than creating more guidelines.[33]

The research that has been conducted confirms the value of a research continuum: Basic research in asthma led to discoveries for improved clinical treatment; clinical

**Table 99.4** IMPACT OF ASTHMA GUIDELINES ON CLINICIAN BEHAVIOR

| Authors | Design (n) | Target | Methods | Outcome |
|---|---|---|---|---|
| Evans et al., 1997[43] | 2 Year controlled trial (22 clinics), comparing treatment group to standard care | Public health clinic staff in New York City (physicians, nurses, health assistants, laboratory technicians, clerical) serving African-American and Latino children <12 years old | 15 hours of training in 6 months, based on NAEPP guidelines; 6 more hours over next year | Treatment group: greater positive changes: higher rate of new patients ($P < .01$); higher return for follow-up treatment 2 years in a row ($P < .001$); higher use of anti-inflammatory medication ($P < .001$); higher patient education ($P < .01$) |
| Feder et al., 1995[44] | Randomized controlled trial (24 practices involving 39 general practitioners); assignment to either diabetes or asthma guideline intervention | General practitioners in inner-city London, nonteaching practices | These educational outreach visits (academic detailing) over 6 months; a structured prompt for patient review in the medical record; feedback on audit of patient notes | Treatment group: improvement in prescribing preventive medicine ($P < .03$); use of prompt; improved recording of asthma review outcome variables |
| Goldberg et al., 1998[45] | Emergency department staff treatment group patients (149) compared with historical comparison group patients (97) | Emergency department clinicians in community hospital | Nurse-initiated critical pathway, based on NAEPP guidelines | Treatment group: increased use of MDIs with spacer ($P < .001$) and oral steroids ($P < .03$); decreased use of saline locks, IV steroids, and oxygen (all $P < .03$) with no difference in hospital admissions |
| Gorton et al., 1995[46] | Controlled comparison with 4-month follow-up of 3 interventions (average 16 physicians per treatment group) and standard care (22); assignment to groups was not randomized | Primary care physicians (family and general practitioners, internists, pediatricians); half in rural settings | Mailed guidelines and either (1) telephone academic detailing and CME conference; (2) computer summaries and e-mail access to expert; or (3) multimedia—CME conference, video and audio cassettes, fax and poster reminders. Note: multiple strategies were available at some practice sites | All groups increased office peak flow monitoring: group 3 increased home peak flow monitoring ($P < .01$) and improved medical plan for mild asthma ($P < .03$)<br>Use of interventions: 79% used written materials, 50% attended conference, 27% listened to cassettes. Concise messages got higher usefulness scores; computer strategies got lowest |
| Stell, 1996[47] | Emergency department treatment group audit (79 patients) compared with historical comparison (93) | Emergency department staff in city hospital, London | All members of staff involved in four audit cycles, which included feedback relative to national guidelines; asthma assessment prompt in treatment record. Note: staff audited and staff participating in feedback not always the same | Treatment group improved use of some assessment criteria, initial medication, and use of arterial blood gas (all $P < .05$), but improvements declined when audit stopped. No improvement in discharge plan (follow-up appointment, use of steroid or PEF) |

CME = Continuing medical education; MDI = metered dose inhaler.

**Table 99.5** FURTHER STUDIES ON THE IMPACT OF ASTHMA GUIDELINES ON PATIENT OUTCOMES

| Author | Design (n) | Target | Methods | Outcome |
|---|---|---|---|---|
| Bailey et al., 1998[48] | Treatment group (19) compared with standard care (23) and historical control (38) | Adults hospitalized for asthma | Medical management by clinical pathway based on NAEPP guidelines | Treatment group had greater conversion to use of MDI rather than nebulizer ($P < .05$), resulting in cost savings. No differences between groups in readmission rates |
| Gibson and Wilson, 1996[49] | 2-Year follow-up by chart audit of treatment group (135) compared with standard care (not reported); enrollment at discretion of hospital attending doctor | Adults hospitalized for asthma | Education and medical management by Australian guidelines, hospital visit plus three clinic visits<br>Continuous quality improvement used to adopt, implement, and evaluate impact of program | Treatment group: lower readmission rates ($P < .01$)<br>Treatment group pre-post: improved inhaler technique and use of written asthma action plan ($P < .01$) |
| Kelso et al., 1995[50] | 1-Year follow-up and 2 year baseline for treatment group (30) compared with historical control (27) | African-American adults in ED with history of multiple ED or hospital visits | Medical management by NAEPP guidelines plus 1-hour education, telephone follow-up, referral to clinic | Treatment group: 41% reduction in ED, control group none ($P < .01$). Both groups reduced hospitalizations<br>Treatment group: before treatment, none used inhaler correctly, used peak flow meters or inhaled steroids; all used after |
| Kelso et al., 1996[51] | 2-Year follow-up chart review and interview of treatment group (21) compared with chart review controls from local hospital seen at same time (18); enrollment from community | African-American adults with frequent ED or hospital visits | Medical management by NAEPP guidelines plus education (1 hour at enrollment and integrated in all follow-up clinic visits and telephone calls); frequency of visits varied by patient needs | Treatment group: greater reduction in ED visits ($P < .01$) (62% of treatment group had no ED in 2 years; 0.0% control had no ED); greater reduction in hospital visits ($P < .05$)<br>Treatment group pre/post: quality of life improved: less activity limits, bother with asthma at home and work, and sleep disturbance |
| Webb et al., 1992[52] | Treatment group (59) compared with historical control (67) | Children (1–6 years) hospitalized for asthma; staff model HMO | Medical management and education by protocol based on NAEPP guidelines<br>Protocol used as quality assurance tool to link hospital, ED, and clinic care | Protocol adopted by physicians (increased use of inhaled medication, oxygen; pulse oximetry; and nursing staff; decreased epinephrine); high steroid use in both groups<br>Treatment group patients: earlier treatment of severe episodes ($P < .001$) and improved compliance at follow-up ($P <$ 05); no difference in length of stay or readmission |

ED = Emergency department; HMO = health maintenance organization; MDI = metered dose inhaler; NAEPP = National Asthma Education and Prevention Program.

and demonstration research validated the importance of both pharmacologic and educational strategies; clinical guidelines translated research findings into practical recommendations for management; and clinicians' experience with implementation in different settings has now identified gaps that require additional research to be filled. Research on the effectiveness of this entire process is needed not only to improve the strategies for dissemination and implementation, but also to develop therapies that are either easier to use or more potent in achieving the desired patient outcomes. Broad government support of such research is an essential part of its mission to prevent morbidity and mortality due to asthma.

## ROLE OF GOVERNMENT IN PRIMARY PREVENTION: AIR QUALITY AND SMOKING

One government responsibility is to protect the public's health by preventing disease. Government must therefore be attentive to emerging health issues, sensitive to their potential consequences, and responsive to public needs. Within this framework, government assesses risk factors for the development of disease and stimulates the formulation and implementation of policies, rules, and regulations designed to reduce risk and, at a minimum, protect the health of its most sensitive populations. The two main areas of concern for respiratory diseases are air quality, both indoors and out, and tobacco smoke, both actively and passively inhaled. This section reviews the US government's role in preventing lung disease by improving air quality, reducing exposure to environmental tobacco smoke, and preventing youth from smoking.

### Assessing Air Quality

#### Effects of Air Pollution on Respiratory Health

Some direct effects of specific components of air pollution on respiratory health have been documented. For example

- Nitrogen dioxide ($NO_2$) has been shown to irritate the lungs and to lower resistance to respiratory infection (e.g., influenza). Although short-term effects are unclear, long-term exposure is associated with increased incidence of acute respiratory disease in children.[53]
- Sulfur dioxide ($SO_2$) has been shown to alter lung defense mechanisms, activate airway sensory nerves, aggravate respiratory and cardiovascular disease, and increase mortality. The most sensitive subgroups are those with asthma, chronic lung or cardiovascular disease, the very young, and the elderly. Persons with asthma can develop wheezing and bronchoconstriction after exercising for 1 to 3 minutes in air containing as little $SO_2$ as 0.2 ppm.[53]
- Irritant pollutant gas (such as nitrogen dioxide, acrolein, and ammonia) and particulate mixtures appear to be risk factors for the development of either emphysema or bronchitis (or both). High concentrations of sulfur combustion particulates predispose to the development of chronic bronchitis. Pre-exposure to air pollutants has also been shown to have an adjuvant effect on subsequent exposure to $SO_2$ and to allergens, resulting in IgE production.[54]

#### Exposure Research

The area of injury within the airways varies according to the agent of exposure. Oxidants cause epithelial damage; particulates often alter epithelial permeability: Because ozone ($O_3$) seems to damage the distal regions of the lungs, not the large airways, the forced expiratory flow at 25% to 75% of forced vital capacity ($FEF_{25-75}$) may be a more sensitive measure of injury than the $FEV_1$. This may explain why some earlier investigators using $FEV_1$ could not find evidence of ozone exposure effects on the lungs. Also, a lag from 1 day to 2 weeks has been documented between some exposures (to $O_3$ and to particulates) and their measurable respiratory effects, which suggests the possibility that the response is inflammatory in nature rather than an acute reflex reaction. Future field research needs to consider this lag period between exposure and observable effects, an omission in earlier studies. In addition, exposure to pollutants can modify immune function and result in sensitization or increased airway allergic responses. Whatever the exposure, persons with asthma are found to be more susceptible than people without asthma.[55, 56]

Another source of data on the effects of exposure to ambient pollutant are histopathologic studies of the lungs from young victims of traumatic death.[57] These studies have provided strong evidence of damage from air pollution, implying an association between high air pollution (mean annual concentration of inhalable particulates ranging from 80 to 100 $\mu g/m^3$) and lung inflammation and wall thickness. These associations remain after controlling for occupational exposure, passive smoking, age, and gender. The effect of smoking (additive or synergistic) is small but still measurable.[58]

### Ensuring Air Quality: The Clean Air Act

#### National Ambient Air Quality Standards

In 1970, the US Congress established the Clean Air Act (CAA), mandating the protection of the respiratory health of susceptible populations, with a margin of safety, with regard to six criteria pollutants: sulfur dioxide ($SO_2$), particulate matter ($PM_{10}$), nitrogen dioxide ($NO_2$), carbon monoxide (CO), ozone ($O_3$), and lead (Pb). To reduce the public's involuntary exposure to pollutants, enforceable standards were needed. Therefore, the act's National Ambient Air Quality Standards (NAAQS) set values based on available data for those criteria pollutants. A margin of safety was included to protect the entire population, including those thought to be most susceptible. CAA susceptible or "at-risk" populations are defined as those persons with asthma or emphysema, those with coronary artery disease, the elderly, infants, and children with cystic fibrosis or bronchopulmonary dysplasia.[53, 55, 56]

The government has an ongoing mandate to set standards, monitor implementation, promote research, and update the standards accordingly. The following discussions of ozone and particulate matter standards illustrate how the mandate is implemented.

**Ozone Standards.** The NAAQS for $O_3$ was set at 0.12 ppm as a 1 hour average concentration not to be exceeded more than once a year. Although emissions of $O_3$ decreased 18% between 1988 and 1996, the Environmental Protection Agency (EPA) designated 98 US cities as nonattainment areas for $O_3$ in October 1991. Recent data have shown a link between short-term (1 to 3 hours) increases in ambient ozone levels and increases in hospital admissions and emergency room visits for respiratory causes. Other data have shown that prolonged exposure (6 to 8 hours) to low $O_3$ concentrations (0.08 ppm) while performing intermittent moderate exercise results in chest pain, coughing, nausea, pulmonary congestion, and significant reductions in lung function in healthy people. After each $O_3$ exposure, the return to baseline takes longer and, depending on individual sensitivity, reaches a point where damage may be permanent. Given these newer data, the new standard for ozone will be revised downward to 0.08 ppm for a 3 year averaging of 8 hour daily maximum concentrations.[58]

Several current research projects are aimed at estimating past exposures and long-term (lifetime) ozone exposure, and relating them to health outcomes, particularly to changes in the small airways.[59] As more sensitive and reliable instruments to measure emissions and exposures to ambient pollution are developed, the scientific database increasingly shows that the original NAAQS set for the six criteria pollutants no longer appear as protective as originally intended and thus require regular revisions.

**Particulate Matter Standards.** The NAAQS for particulate matter (PM) have also undergone revisions as more precise data have emerged. The original standard for total suspended particulates, established in 1971, was replaced in 1987 by the $PM_{10}$ standard. This newer standard focused on smaller sized particles, because they had been shown to penetrate deeper into the lung. However, emerging data show health effects associated with even smaller particles. These particles often mix with $SO_2$, become more potent, and cause alterations in lung tissue, in lung structure, and in respiratory tract defense mechanisms. This mixture has also been linked to carcinogenesis, increased hospital admissions and emergency department visits, and even to premature mortality in sensitive individuals.[58, 60]

In 1997, the EPA completed its periodic review of the NAAQS as mandated by the Clean Air Act. Newer data showed significant increases in respiratory symptoms and acute decreases in lung function in children and adults with asthma, and in people without asthma, after exposure to $PM_{10}$ at concentrations well below the current standard.[54, 60] As a result, the Revised Ozone and Particulate Matter Standards Implementation Act of 1998 proposed two new standards for particulate matter: one for $PM_{2.5}$ (set at 15 $\mu g/m^3$ annually and at 65 $\mu g/m^3$ for 24 hours); the other, for $PM_{10}$, remains at the current level. The 1998 Act also directed the EPA to collaborate with other federal agencies to develop a coordinated interagency PM research program addressing health effects, biologic mechanisms, monitoring, speciation, and regional transport of PM and to establish a nationally consistent monitoring network to measure and analyze fine particles ($PM_{2.5}$). The National Academy of Sciences was also asked to review the $PM_{2.5}$ standards and to make recommendations by June 30, 2002.[55, 60]

## Research Questions

Each round of research answers some questions but inevitably raises new ones. The role of government is to support this continuous research process. Questions currently needing attention include the following: Does exposure to the combination of low levels of air pollutants and environmental tobacco smoke during childhood increase the risks for chronic obstructive pulmonary disease or asthma? Are some populations genetically more vulnerable to injury from specific exposures or combinations of exposures? What is the relationship between the responses to a single acute exposure and to long-term low-dose exposure to any of the criteria pollutants? Do multiple exposures exert cumulative effects? What is the best marker of exposure to use in each case?

## Need for Indoor Air Standards

The results of some two dozen human exposure studies initiated in 1980 showed that indoor air pollution also needs to be recognized as a hazard, especially because Americans spend 95% of their time, or 23 hours per day, indoors. If the same substances found outdoors were also found in indoor air, the legal machinery of the Clean Air Act of 1990 would apply, but the substances are quite different.[61] Of the hundreds of air pollutants covered by existing US laws, only ozone and sulfur dioxide remain more prevalent outdoors.[61] Small, light, monitoring instruments were used in human exposure studies to record the prevalence of volatile organic compounds (representing some 30 different chemicals), carbon monoxide, pesticides, and dangerous particles. Over 3000 people, a representative sample of the North American population, carried these instruments as they went about their daily lives. Detailed analyses showed that exposures to particles smaller than 10 μm were about 60% greater than expected during the day. Because recent epidemiologic data have shown an association between elevated concentrations of fine particles and premature death, finding this level of pollutants in indoor air is of concern. Other results have indicated that "each day the average urban infant will ingest 110 nanograms of benzo(a)pyrene, one of the most toxic polycyclic aromatic hydrocarbons (equivalent to smoking three cigarettes)."[60]

As data on the effects of pollutants on respiratory health accrue, the legislative burden increases. Ideally, the most desirable response would be for the industries involved to voluntarily accept accountability for the potential toxic chemical emissions from such products as house paints, carpets, cabinetry, and cleaning products and to take responsible remedial action. However, past experience has demonstrated that both legislation and enforcement are essential. This triggers the need to create an infrastructure to measure and monitor emissions both indoors and outdoors.

## Assessing Health Effects of Environmental Tobacco Smoke

Environmental tobacco smoke (ETS), both mainstream (secondhand smoke exhaled by individuals) and sidestream (from burning cigarettes, cigars, and pipes), is an irritant for sensitive individuals, children, and infants. Since the early 1970s, population-based epidemiologic studies have consistently shown that ETS affects the respiratory health of children, especially during the first years of life. An EPA review corroborated that ETS is a risk factor not only for lung cancer but also for lower respiratory tract infections (bronchitis and pneumonia) and middle ear effusion in infants and young children. The report estimated that between 150,000 and 300,000 of these cases are attributable to ETS annually for infants up to 18 months and that exacerbations of symptoms in children with preexisting asthma reach 200,000 to 1,000,000 annually. Furthermore, ETS is strongly associated with the onset of asthma in children, although asthma causality cannot be definitely ascribed to ETS.[62–67]

Tobacco use is the leading cause of preventable death in the United States. In 1994 alone, it was responsible for estimated direct and indirect health costs reaching $68 billion. A review of more than 30 epidemiologic studies assessing the relationship between ETS and lung cancer in never-smokers led the EPA to classify ETS as the only known human carcinogen for which typical environmental levels of exposure are associated with a demonstrated increase in the risk for cancer.[64] Up to 38% of US children aged 2 months to 5 years are exposed to ETS. Twenty-four per cent are exposed to maternal smoking during pregnancy. Maternal smoking is associated with low birth weight, increased rates of sudden infant death syndrome, and increased rates of wheeze-associated lower respiratory illness.[62, 63] Among children under 2 years exposed to prenatal smoke or to ETS of 20 or more cigarettes per day, were 2.5 times as likely to develop chronic bronchitis and twice as apt to develop asthma.[62] A 1998 study has additionally shown a link between exposure to secondhand smoke and airway complications in children receiving general anesthesia.[68]

## Developing Policies and Intervention Strategies To Ensure Reduced ETS

The government continues to have a leadership role in protecting the public from involuntary exposure to tobacco smoke. One strategy is to ban smoking in certain settings; the other is to encourage a reduction in general consumption of tobacco products by enacting further restrictions and by increasing taxes on tobacco products.

### Acts and Bans

The success of the first strategy may be appreciated most by travelers outside the United States, where involuntary exposure to ETS smoke is nearly ubiquitous. A concerted collaborative effort among individuals, voluntary agencies such as the American Lung Association, professional societies such as the American Public Health Association, and local and federal governments has reversed attitudes and perceptions, changed the culture and made smoking an unacceptable (even offensive) behavior, and led to the successful banning of smoking in many public places. Since publication of the first Surgeon General's report linking smoking to disease in 1964, 1238 state laws addressing tobacco control–related issues have been passed.[69, 70] The Pro-Children Act of 1994, which prohibits smoking in federally funded facilities where children's services are provided, gave impetus to 46 states and the District of Columbia to require smoke-free indoor air in a wide variety of public buildings. This act also forms the basis for federal rules and regulations regarding the right to work and play in a smoke-free environment.[71]

### Restrictions and Taxes

Although all states prohibit the sale and distribution of tobacco products to minors and all states tax cigarettes, only 42 states also tax chewing tobacco and snuff, and only 9 states restrict advertising of tobacco products. Most federal policies, acts, and bans are designed to cover specific aspects of tobacco use (such as advertising to minors, availability and access by minors, smoke-free indoor areas). The restrictions aimed at protecting youth have a spillover effect in reducing advertising's reach to people of all ages. The Federal Cigarette Labeling and Advertising Act of 1965 uniformly requires health warnings on cigarette packs.

In individual states, however, there is great variability in both enactment and enforcement of various acts and bans.[72] For example, the California Tobacco Control Program, enacted in 1989, is highly restrictive and prohibits smoking in all public indoor areas, including bars and taverns. This comprehensive multipronged program also imposes an additional tax and uses the proceeds to fund community intervention and education programs. As a result, California has nearly met the Year 2000 objective of reducing the prevalence of smokers to no more than 15%. For a contrasting example, Kentucky has no smoking restrictions or bans in any indoor area (private work sites, restaurants, grocery stores), and 27.8% of Kentuckians are current cigarette smokers.

The FDA declaration in 1996 that cigarettes and smokeless tobacco were devices delivering the addictive drug nicotine was a major step toward reducing involuntary exposure to ETS and preventing smoking. Through this action, the FDA asserted jurisdiction over cigarettes (but not cigars because of insufficient evidence).[73] As a result, state attorneys general and state health departments continue to be involved in ongoing legal proceedings against the tobacco industry.

### Multimedia and Multilevel Community Campaigns

A multiprong approach that delivers messages from several sources is more effective than a single effort to reduce tobacco consumption. Health behavior research has demonstrated that receiving anti-tobacco information from a variety of sources—including family, friends, physicians, clinical programs, mass media, and policies—is more likely to lead to successful cessation.[74] For example, Massachusetts instituted a state cigarette tax hike between 1992 and 1996, the proceeds of which were earmarked for a statewide media campaign that included billboards, radio, TV spots, pamphlets, and communitywide education efforts. Results showed that the per capita rate of tobacco consumption fell more than three times as fast as in the 48 states not having such a campaign.[75]

When federal and state government agencies collaborate with professional and voluntary associations to develop multilevel efforts, the combined effectiveness often exceeds the sum of its parts. For example, the American Lung Association has historically had a pioneering role in bringing air-quality issues to the fore, in initiating legal action on behalf of nonsmokers and air pollution–sensitive individuals,[75] and in developing ongoing community programs. Among these are smoking cessation and prevention programs, which are also critical for reducing smoking consumption (Chapter 98).

## Assessing the Prevalence of Smoking Among Youth

Compelling epidemiologic data have shown that 18% of those who try a cigarette do so before age 12 years, that most smokers (82%) start smoking daily before age 18 years, and that 3000 young persons start smoking each day in the United States. At least 4.5 million adolescents (ages 12 to 17 years) in the United States smoke cigarettes. Recent trends in daily cigarette smoking by high school seniors are discouraging: After a steady decline during the 1980s, rates are increasing in the 1990s.[76]

Data have also consistently shown that only minor results are achieved by even costly and effort-intensive campaigns to help smokers achieve and sustain smoking cessation. As a result, the focus of public health programs has changed. Most public health organizations now recommend that tobacco prevention activities should focus on school-age children and adolescents. Smoking prevention, especially targeted to young people, rather than smoking cessation, is considered the key approach to reducing tobacco use.[76] In addition, prevention activities should include cigars as well as cigarettes. Cigars contain up to 70 times the nicotine in cigarettes,[73] and a recent California survey found that 7.6% of males aged 12 to 13 years reported having smoked cigars.[73]

## Developing Policies and Intervention Strategies to Prevent Young People From Smoking

Government has a legitimate, possibly essential role in protecting minors from assuming risks that will lead to illness later in their lives.

### Restricted Access to Tobacco Products

The Federal Alcohol, Drug Abuse, and Mental Health Act (amended in 1992) established the age of 18 years as the minimum legal age to purchase tobacco products. Then, to ensure reduced access to all tobacco products for persons under this age, the Public Health Services Act of 1992 mandated the creation of the Tobacco Outlet Inspection Program. Cigars, previously exempt from many of the tobacco regulations, are included in this act. Local enforcement, however, remains highly variable. Research has shown that young people are often able to obtain both products from various outlets.[72]

### Anti-Tobacco Use Education

In addition to using the legal process already described, the government has strongly promoted anti–tobacco use education programs for youth. For example, the Centers for Disease Control and Prevention (CDC) issued guidelines for anti–tobacco use school programs for kindergarten through 12th grade in 1994. These guidelines were based on the report of the National Cancer Institute's Expert Panel on School-Based Smoking Prevention Programs as well as on the Surgeon General's Report on Preventing Tobacco Use Among Young People that included eight school-based program objectives for Healthy People 2000 (see Table 99.6). Implementation of the CDC guidelines would bring the United States closer to reaching the National Education Goal of having every school in America free of drugs and violence by the Year 2000.[70, 75]

The American Lung Association has also emphasized anti-tobacco use education programs by developing the Smoke Free Class of 2000 program. The program includes Teens Against Tobacco Use, a curriculum for ninth graders that is currently used in 39 states. The multitiered program first trains adults, who then train teens, who in turn teach children 9 to 12 years of age about the importance of remaining tobacco free. It is the program's goal

**Table 99.6 HEALTHY PEOPLE 2000 OBJECTIVES FOR YOUTH AND SCHOOL SMOKING PREVENTION PROGRAMS**

- Reduce the initiation of cigarette smoking by children and youth so that no more than 15% have become regular cigarette smokers by age 20. (Baseline: 30% in 1987)
- Establish tobacco-free environments and include tobacco use prevention in the curricula of all elementary, middle, and secondary schools, preferably as part of quality (comprehensive) school health education. (Baseline: 17% of school districts were smoke free, and 75% to 81% of school districts offered antismoking education in 1988)
- Increase to at least 75% the proportion of worksites (such as schools) with a formal smoking policy that prohibits or severely restricts smoking at the workplace. (Baseline: 54% of medium and large companies in 1987)
- Enact in 50 states comprehensive laws on clean indoor air that prohibit or strictly limit smoking in the workplace and enclosed public places (such as schools). (Baseline: 13 states in 1988)

to reach 30,000 teens and 450,000 children with an anti-tobacco use message by the millennium.[77,78] (See Chapter 98 for more on the effectiveness of school-based smoking prevention programs.)

Community involvement in the form of state coalitions to develop anti–tobacco use prevention programs can help amplify state resources—and thus help achieve a smoke-free society—by involving community groups, volunteer organizations, advocacy groups, educators, and representatives of target populations. Leadership from physicians and other health officials has helped to ensure the success of the programs of these coalitions, which numbered 47 in 1989.[74]

How good are these programs? Few studies have as yet evaluated smoking prevention in youth, although some have reported promising results. For example, a study of two Vermont communities revealed the powerful impact of mass media in promoting positive messages about not smoking. One of the communities received an intervention that combined school-based and mass media tobacco education programs; the other received only a school-based smoking prevention curriculum. The high-risk adolescents who received both the school curriculum and the media's explicit smoking prevention messages (on both radio and television) still had lower smoking rates 2 years later.[75] For another example, the Teenage Attitudes and Practices Surveys (TAPS I and TAPS II), an ongoing large-scale research project, have made it clear that the period just before adolescents begin to use tobacco is critical and that parental involvement, peer influence, and the introduction and practice of refusal skills in this period are crucial. These surveys also found that health professionals only counseled their patients about tobacco use 25% of the time (TAPS I and II) and that, although illegal, the sale of tobacco products to minors was extensive. The surveys further found that more than half (58.8%) of all states had recommended that schools develop tobacco-use policies that create a smoke-free environment but that less than half (46.9%) of all school districts had such policies.[76–78]

### Future Smoking Prevention Program Needs

In summary, future prevention programs need to address the following points:

- Clearly needed are greater monitoring and enforcement of existing laws and regulations. The government's role in primary prevention of tobacco use could be boosted by more effectively limiting advertising, access, and availability to underage youth.
- Consistent, ongoing anti–tobacco use guidance and advice offered by physicians (including obstetricians and pediatricians), dentists (including hygienists), and other health care providers are both effective and cost beneficial.[74]
- Schools have a captive audience for 12 years and a mandate to educate. Their role is even more important than that of government and voluntary agencies. The school setting is ideal for focusing on anti–tobacco use education and for using novel, creative approaches, such as interactive technologies, as well as approaches proven effective in developing the refusal skills necessary to prevent the onset of habitual smoking.
- The American Academy of Pediatrics has recommended a complete, across-the-board ban on all advertising of tobacco products in all media.[77] The media (including movies, videos, television, and the Wide World Web) should be strongly encouraged to recognize their accountability in this area. A requirement for equal time for presentations of scientific, medical, and clinical data on the effects of tobacco products on health would promote more responsible programming, including portrayals of role models conveying realistic verbal and nonverbal messages regarding nonsmoking behavior.
- Prospective longitudinal studies are needed to clarify the determinants of the initiation and maintenance of smoking behavior. Better knowledge of these determinants will contribute to the design of effective anti-tobacco use interventions.

The government's role in preventing young people from smoking is twofold: to promote and support research to identify effective smoking prevention strategies and to enact and enforce bans and laws to prevent involuntary exposure to tobacco smoke.

## SUMMARY

This chapter has illustrated the role of the government in the prevention and control of lung diseases—both in secondary prevention programs to reduce morbidity and halt the progression of disease and in primary prevention programs to prevent the onset of disease. The roles of government include assessment of the nation's health, research into the causes and treatment of disease; development of policies for collaborative public and private programs based on scientific knowledge, and initiation of the actions necessary to ensure that all citizens benefit from scientific advances. As illustrated by its asthma programs, the government's fulfillment of these roles has been critical in making serious and life-threatening diseases controllable and in minimizing their impact on the quality of life of those affected. Similarly, the collective action enabled through government policies and regulations on air quality and environmental tobacco smoke has been essential for preserving air quality to protect the public's health. Unfortunately, programs to prevent young people from smoking have been less successful but may have succeeded in keeping smoking rates from rising even higher: More aggressive and uniform enforcement of national regulations is needed at the local level, and more innovative and effective educational strategies are urgently needed.

Certainly, numerous lung diseases and a large array of programs could be discussed. It is, for example, difficult to leave aside the notable efforts in curbing the terrible impact of influenza and tuberculosis and the emerging urgency of rising rates of chronic obstructive lung disease among a growing number of older Americans. Nonetheless, the governmental role discussed within the parameters of this chapter apply widely to other lung diseases.

This chapter has explained the government resources available to promote lung health and prevent lung disease. Perhaps more importantly, the chapter has also demonstrated that the success of government effort is directly proportional to the involvement of its citizens. Enthusiastic congressional support has made possible the remarkable advances of government-supported research. Yet government policies and program activities, especially at the national level, can only provide a foundation for the local translation of these findings into improvements in health for all citizens. In illustrating the process, we hope to encourage the reader's participation.

## References


1. Institute of Medicine, Committee for the Study of the Future of Public Health: The Future of Public Health. Washington, DC: National Academy Press, 1988.
2. Centers for Disease Control and Prevention (CDC): Asthma Mortality and Hospitalization Among Children and Young Adults—United States, 1980–1993. MMWR 45:350–353, 1996.
3. Centers for Disease Control and Prevention (CDC), National Center for Health Statistics: National Health Interview Survey. Atlanta: CDC, 1996.
4. Gergen PJ, Weiss KB: Changing patterns of asthma hospitalization among children: 1979 to 1987. JAMA 264:1688–1692, 1990.
5. Weiss K, Gergen P, Wagener D: Breathing better or wheezing worse? The changing epidemiology of asthma morbidity and mortality. Annu Rev Public Health 14:491–513, 1993.
6. National Heart, Lung, and Blood Institute (NHLBI), National Institutes of Health: Data Fact Sheet: Asthma Statistics. Bethesda, MD: NHLBI, January 1999.
7. Weiss K, Gergen P, Hodgson TA: An economic evaluation of asthma in the United States. N Engl J Med 326:862–866, 1992.
8. Sullivan S, Ellxhauser A, Bulst AS, et al: National Asthma Education and Prevention Program working group report on the cost effectiveness of asthma care. Am J Respir Crit Care Med 154:584–595, 1996.
9. Fowler MG, Davenport MG, Garg R: School functioning of US children with asthma. Pediatrics 90:939–944, 1992.
10. Centers for Disease Control and Prevention (CDC): Surveillance Summaries: April 24, 1998. MMWR 47(SS-1), 1998.
11. National Institutes of Health: Section 1125, NIH Organization and Functions. *In* NIH Manual. Bethesda, MD: National Institutes of Health, revised October 1, 1994.
12. Institute of Medicine, Committee on the NIH Research Priority-Setting Process: Scientific Opportunities and Public Needs. Washington, DC: National Academy Press, 1998.
13. Hurd S, Lenfant C: NHLBI: Fifty years of achievement in pulmonary biology and medicine. Am J Respir Crit Care Med 157:168–171, 1998.
14. Nadel J, Busse W: Asthma. Am J Respir Crit Care Med 157:130–138, 1998.
15. Martinez FD, Wright AL, Taussig LM, et al: Asthma and wheezing in the first six years of life. N Engl J Med 332:133–138, 1995.
16. Collaborative Study of the Genetics of Asthma (CSGA): A genome wide search for asthma susceptibility loci in ethnically diverse populations. Nat Genet 15:389–392, 1997.
17. Martinez FD, Graves PE, Baldini M, et al: Association between genetic polymorphisms of the $beta_2$-adrenoceptor and response to albuterol in children with and without a history of wheezing. J Clin Invest 15:3184–3188, 1997.
18. National Heart, Lung, and Blood Institute, National Asthma Education and Prevention Program Working Group Report: Considerations for Diagnosing and Managing Asthma in the Elderly (National Institutes of Health Pub. No. 96-3662). Bethesda, MD: National Institutes of Health, 1996.
19. Clark N, Gong M, Schork M, et al: Impact of education for physicians on clinical behavior, patient outcomes, and satisfaction with care. Pediatrics 101:831–836, 1998.
20. National Heart, Lung and Blood Institute, National Asthma Education and Prevention Program—Asthma Management in Minority Children: Practical Insights for Clinicians, Researchers, and Public Health Planners (National Institutes of Health Pub. No. 95-3675). Bethesda, MD: National Institutes of Health, 1995.
21. Institute of Medicine. Field M, Lohr K (eds): Clinical Practice Guidelines: Directions for a New Program. Washington, DC: National Academy Press, 1990, pp 33–78.
22. National Heart, Lung, and Blood Institute, National Asthma Education and Prevention Program, Expert Panel Report: Guidelines for the Diagnosis and Management of Asthma (National Institutes of Health Pub. No. 91-3642). Bethesda, MD: National Institutes of Health, 1991.
23. National Heart, Lung, and Blood Institute, National Asthma Education and Prevention Program: Expert Panel Report 2: Guidelines for the Diagnosis and Management of Asthma (National Institutes of Health Pub. No. 97-4051). Bethesda, MD: National Institutes of Health, 1997.
24. Healthy People: The Surgeon General's Report on Health Promotion and Disease Prevention (DHEW Pub. No. PHS 79-55071). Washington, DC: US Government Printing Office, 1979.
25. Healthy People 2000: National Health Promotion and Disease Prevention Objectives. (DHEW Pub. No. PHS 91-50212). Washington, DC: US Government Printing Office, 1991.
26. Healthy People 2010 Objectives: Draft for Public Comment. Washington, DC: US Department of Health and Human Services, 1998.
27. Wilson S, Scamagas P, Grado J, et al: The Fresno Asthma Project: A model intervention to control asthma in multiethnic, low-income, inner-city communities. Health Educ Behav 25:79–98, 1998.
28. Grimshaw J, Russell I: Effect of clinical guidelines on medical practice: A systematic review of rigorous evaluations. Lancet 342:1317–1322, 1993.
29. Grimshaw J, Russell I: Achieving health gain through clinical guidelines II. Ensuring guidelines change medical practice. Qual Health Care 3:45–52, 1994.
30. Davis D, Thomson M, Oxman A, et al: Evidence for the effectiveness of CME: A review of 50 randomized controlled trials. JAMA 268:1111–1117, 1992.
31. Neville R, Hoskins G, Smith B, et al: Observations on the structure, process and clinical outcomes of asthma care in general practice. Br J Gen Pract 46:583–587, 1996.
32. Worrall G, Chaulk P, Freake D: The effects of clinical practice guidelines on patient outcomes in primary care: A systematic review. Can Med Assoc J 156:1705–1712, 1997.
33. Worrall G, Chaulk P: Hope or experience? Clinical practice guidelines in family practice. J Fam Pract 42:353–356, 1996.
34. Christakis D, Rivara FP: Pediatricians' awareness of and attitudes about four clinical practice guidelines. Pediatrics 101:825–830, 1998.
35. Partridge M: The impact of asthma guidelines on clinical practice. Monaldi Arch Chest Dis 48:367–368, 1993.
36. Lantner R, Ros S: Emergency management of asthma in children: Impact of NIH guidelines. Ann Allergy Asthma Immunol 74:188–190, 1995.
37. Emerman C, Cydulka R, Skobeloff E: Survey of asthma practice among emergency physicians. Chest 109:708–712, 1996.
38. Lang D, Sherman M, Polansky M: Guidelines and realities of asthma management. Arch Intern Med 157:1193–1200, 1997.
39. Buchner D, Carlson A, Stempel D: Patterns of anti-inflammatory therapy in the post-guidelines era: A retrospective claims analysis of managed care members. Am J Manag Care 3:87–93, 1997.
40. Jatulis D, Meng Y, Elashoff R: Preventive pharmacologic therapy among asthmatics: Five years after publication of guidelines. Ann Allergy Asthma Immunol 81:82–88, 1998.
41. Legorreta A, Christian-Herman J, O'Connor R, et al: Compliance with national asthma management guidelines and specialty care. Arch Intern Med 158:457–464, 1998.
42. Hartert T, Windom H, Peebles R, et al: Inadequate outpatient medical therapy for patients with asthma admitted to two urban hospitals. Am J Med 100:386–394, 1996.
43. Evans D, Mellins R, Lobach K, et al: Improving care for minority children with asthma: Professional education in public health clinics. Pediatrics 99:157–166, 1997.
44. Feder G, Griffiths C, Highton C, et al: Do clinical guidelines introduced with practice based education improve care of asthmatic and diabetic patients? A randomised controlled trial in general practices in east London. BMJ 311:1473–1478, 1995.

45. Goldberg R, Chan L, Haley P, et al: Critical pathway for the emergency department management of acute asthma: Effect on resource utilization. Ann Emerg Med 31:562–567, 1998.
46. Gorton T, Cranford C, Golden W, et al: Primary care physicians response to dissemination of practice guidelines. Arch Fam Med 4:135–142, 1995.
47. Stell I: Asthma management in accident and emergency and the BTS guidelines—A study of the impact of clinical audit. Accid Emerg Med 13:392–394, 1996.
48. Bailey R, Weingarten S, Lewis M, et al: Impact of clinical pathways and practice guidelines on the management of acute exacerbations of bronchial asthma. Chest 113:28–33, 1998.
49. Gibson PG, Wilson AJ: The use of continuous quality improvement methods to implement practice guidelines in asthma. Practice 16:87–102, 1996.
50. Kelso T, Self T, Rumbak M: Educational and long-term therapeutic intervention in the ED: Effect on outcomes in adult indigent minority asthmatics. Am J Emerg Med 13:632–637, 1995.
51. Kelso T, Abou-Shala N, Heilker G: Comprehensive long-term management program for asthma: Effect on outcomes in adult African-Americans. Am J Med Sci 311:272–280, 1996.
52. Webb L, Kuykendall D, Zeiger R: The impact of status asthmaticus practice guidelines on patient outcome and physician behavior. QRB Quality Rev Bull 18:417–476, 1992.
53. Health Effects of Ambient Air Pollution. Bethesda, MD: American Lung Association, February 1992.
54. Abbey DE, Burchette RJ, Knutsen SF, et al: Long-term particulate and other air pollutants and lung function in nonsmokers. Am J Respir Crit Care Med 158:289–298, 1998.
55. Gambling with Public Health: Who Loses Under the New Health Standards for Ozone. Bethesda, MD: American Lung Association, September 1996.
56. Health Effects Institute: Acute Effects of Ambient Ozone on Asthmatic, Wheezy, and Healthy Children. Research Report Number 82. Cambridge, MA: Health Effects Institute, May 1998.
57. Sherman CB: The health consequences of cigarette smoking: Pulmonary diseases. Med Clin North Am 76:355–357, 1992.
58. Souza MB, Saldiva PHN, Pope CA III, et al: Respiratory changes due to long-term exposure to urban levels of air pollution. Chest 113:1312–1318, 1998.
59. Health Effects Institute: Methods Development for Epidemiologic Investigations of the Health Effects of Prolonged Ozone Exposure. Research Report Number 81. Cambridge, MA: Health Effects Institute, March 1998.
60. Vedal S, Petkau J, White R, Blair J: Acute effects of ambient inhalable particles in asthmatic and nonasthmatic children. Am J Respir Crit Care Med 157:1034–1043, 1998.
61. Ott WR, Roberts JW: Everyday Exposure to Toxic Pollutants. Sci Am Feb 1988, pp 86–91.
62. Morgan WJ, Martinez FD: Maternal smoking and infant lung function. Am J Resp Crit Care Med 158:689–690, 1998.
63. Meltzer EO, Meltzer SB: Passive smoking: An underrated problem in children? J Respir Dis 14, 1993.
64. Respiratory Health Effects of Passive Smoking: Lung Cancer and Other Disorders. The US EPA, U.S. DHHS Monograph 4. NIH Publication No. 93-3605. Bethesda, MD: NIH, August 1993.
65. Eisner MD, Yelin EH, Smith S, et al: Impact of environmental tobacco smoke on asthma severity. J Invest Med 46:97A, 1998.
66. Eisner MD, Yelin EH, Henke J, et al: Environmental tobacco smoke and adult asthma: The impact of changing exposure status on health outcomes. Am J Respir Crit Care Med 158:170–175, 1998.
67. Eisner MD, Alexander KS, Blanc PD: Bartenders' respiratory health after establishment of smoke-free bars and Taverns. JAMA 280:1909–1914, 1998.
68. Voelker R: Quick Updates: Smoke, anesthesia don't mix. JAMA 279:1939, 1998.
69. Policies Restricting Smoking in Public Places and the Workplace in the Health Consequences of Involuntary Smoking: A report of the Surgeon General (Chapter 6). U.S. DHHS, PHS, CDC, 1986.
70. Centers for Disease Control and Prevention (CDC): State Tobacco Control Highlights, 1996. Atlanta: CDC, National Center for Chronic Disease Prevention and Promotion, Office of Smoking and Health. Publication No. 099-4895, 1996.
71. Centers for Disease Control and Prevention (CDC): TIPS: Pro-children Act of 1994. Atlanta: CDC, 1994.
72. Implementing the Synar Regulation: Tobacco Outlet Inspection. US Department of Health and Human Services. Publication No. (SMA) 98-3184, 1998.
73. National Cancer Institutes of Health: Cigars: Health Effects and Trends. Monograph 9. NIH Publication No. 98-4302. Bethesda, MD: NIH, 1998.
74. Health-care provider advice on tobacco use to persons aged 10–22 years—United States, 1993. US Department of Health and Human Services. MMWR 44:826–830, 1995.
75. Flynn BS, Worden JK, Secker-Walker RH, et al: Long-term responses of higher and lower risk youths to smoking prevention interventions. Prev Med 26:389–394, 1997.
76. Preventing Tobacco Use Among Young People: A Report of the Surgeon General. Chapter 3. US Department of Health and Human Services, Public Health Service, CDC, 1994.
77. American Lung Association: Lung Disease Data 1997. New York: American Lung Association, August 1997.
78. Chronic Diseases and Health Promotion. US Department of Health and Human Services. Adapted from the MMWR: Tobacco Topics 1990–1993. Atlanta: CDC.

# APPENDIX

# Glossary of Terms and Standard Symbols

## I. PRIMARY AND QUALIFYING SYMBOLS

### General

| | |
|---|---|
| P | *Pressure.* Includes also *partial pressure* of a gas in a mixture of gases or in blood |
| L | Lung |
| W | Chest Wall |
| RS | Respiratory System |
| Pl | Pleura |

### Ventilation

| | |
|---|---|
| V | Volume of Gas |
| $\dot{V}$ | Flow of Gas |
| I | Inspired |
| E | Expired |
| A | Aleolar |
| T | Tidal |
| ET | End-Tidal |
| D | Dead Space |
| STPD | Standard Conditions: *s*tandard *t*emperature 0°C, barometric *p*ressure 760 mm Hg, and *d*ry. |
| BTPS | Body Conditions: *b*ody *t*emperature and ambient *p*ressure, *s*aturated with water vapor at these conditions. |
| ATPS | Ambient Conditions: *a*mbient *t*emperature and *p*ressure, *s*aturated with water vapor at these conditions. |

### Gas Exchange—Blood Flow

| | |
|---|---|
| Q | Volume of Blood |
| $\dot{Q}$ | Flow of Blood |
| F | Fractional Concentration of Gas |
| C | Concentration in Blood |
| S | Saturation in Blood |
| b | Blood, in General |
| a | Arterial Blood |
| v | Venous Blood |
| $\bar{v}$ | Mixed Venous Blood |
| c | Capillary Blood |
| c′ | Pulmonary End-Capillary Blood |

## II. VENTILATION AND LUNG MECHANICS

### Static Lung Volumes

| | |
|---|---|
| VC | *Vital Capacity.* The maximum volume of gas that can be exhaled after fully inflating the lungs. |
| FRC | *Functional Residual Capacity.* The volume of gas remaining in the lungs at the end of quiet expiration. |
| TLC | *Total Lung Capacity.* The volume of gas in the lungs after a maximum inspiration. |
| RV | *Residual Volume.* The volume of gas remaining in the lungs after a maximum exhalation. |
| IC | *Inspiratory Capacity.* The volume of gas that can be inhaled from resting end-expiration (FRC) to full inflation (TLC). |
| ERV | *Expiratory Reserve Volume.* The volume of gas that can be exhaled from resting end-expiration (FRC) to full exhalation (RV). |
| IRV | *Inspiratory Reserve Volume.* The volume of gas that can be inhaled from resting end-inspiration to full inflation (TLC). |

### Descriptors of Forced Breathing Maneuvers

| | |
|---|---|
| FVC | *Forced Vital Capacity.* The volume of gas that can be forcibly exhaled after fully inflating the lungs. |
| $FEV_t$ | *Timed Forced Expiratory Volume.* The volume of gas exhaled at a specified time after beginning the forced vital capacity maneuver. For example, $FEV_1$ = forced expiratory volume in 1 second. |
| $FEV_t$/FVC | *Ratio of Timed Expiratory Volume to Forced Vital Capacity.* For example, $FEV_1$/FVC, usually expressed as a percentage. |
| $FEF_x$ | *Specified Forced Expiratory Flow.* The forced expiratory flow rate during a specified portion of the forced vital capacity. For example, $FEF_{200-1200mL}$ = forced expiratory flow rate between 200 and 1200 mL of the forced vital capacity; $FEF_{25-75\%}$ = forced expiratory flow rate between 25% and 75% of the forced vital capacity. |
| $\dot{V}max_{x\%}$ | *Specified Maximum Expiratory Flow.* The instantaneous expiratory flow rate when x per cent of the forced vital capacity has been exhaled. For example, $\dot{V}max_{50\%}$ = maximum expiratory flow rate at 50% of the forced vital capacity. |
| MVV | *Maximum Voluntary Ventilation.* Volume of gas exhaled while making maximum breathing efforts during a certain time interval (often 12 seconds). |
| VR | *Ventilatory Reserve.* The difference between ventilatory capacity during maximum exercise (estimated as MVV or calculated from $FEV_1$) and minute ventilation at peak exercise; VR, which is also known as *breathing reserve,* represents the potential for further increase in ventilation during maximum (or peak) exercise. |
| PImax | *Maximum Inspiratory Pressure.* The maximum pressure generated by the respiratory muscles during an attempted inspiration. |
| PEmax | *Maximum Expiratory Pressure.* The maximum pressure generated by the respiratory muscles during an attempted exhalation. |

### Descriptors of Ventilation

f — *Respiratory Frequency.* The number of breaths during 1 minute.

$V_T$ — *Tidal Volume.* The volume of gas inspired or expired during each breath.

$\dot{V}_E$ — *Expired Volume.* The volume of gas (BTPS), usually measured at the mouth, exhaled during 1 minute.

$\dot{V}_I$ — *Inspired Volume.* The volume of gas (BTPS), measured or calculated, inhaled during 1 minute.

$\dot{V}_A$ — *Alveolar Ventilation.* The volume of gas (BTPS), exhaled from the lungs during 1 minute, that contributed to gas exchange. (Calculated as expired volume minus dead space ventilation.)

$\dot{V}_D$ — *Dead Space Ventilation.* The volume of gas (BTPS), exhaled from the lungs during 1 minute, that did not contribute to gas exchange; also known as *wasted ventilation.* (Calculated from the equation:

$$\dot{V}_D = \dot{V}_E \frac{Pa_{CO_2} - PE_{CO_2}}{Pa_{CO_2} - PI_{CO_2}}$$

where $Pa_{CO_2}$, $PE_{CO_2}$, and $PI_{CO_2}$ are the partial pressures of $CO_2$ in arterial blood, mixed expired gas, and inspired gas, respectively.)

$V_D$ — *Dead Space Volume.* The volume of the physiologic dead space. (Calculated as $\dot{V}_D$/f.)

$V_D/V_T$ — *Ratio of Dead Space to Tidal Volume.* The proportion, usually expressed as a percentage, of each breath that does not contribute to $CO_2$ removal (i.e., the proportion of each breath that is wasted).

### Volume-Pressure Relationships

C — *Compliance.* General symbol for compliance, or the ratio of volume change of the structure per unit change in applied pressure across the structure.

$C_L$ — *Lung Compliance.* The volume change divided by the difference between alveolar pressure (Palv) and pleural pressure (Ppl), which is also known as the transpulmonary pressure (Pl).

$C_W$ — *Chest Wall Compliance.* The volume change divided by the difference between pleural pressure (Ppl) and body surface pressure (Pbs), which is also known as the transthoracic pressure.

$C_{RS}$ — *Respiratory System Compliance.* The volume change divided by the difference between alveolar pressure (Palv) and body surface pressure (Pbs), or transpulmonary pressure (Pl) plus transthoracic pressure (Pw).

$C_{DYN}$ — *Dynamic Compliance.* Value for compliance based on measurements made during uninterrupted breathing.

$C_{ST}$ — *Static Compliance.* Value for compliance based on measurements made during periods of no airflow.

$C/V_L$ — *Specific Compliance.* Value for compliance divided by the lung volume at which it was measured, usually FRC.

### Flow-Pressure Relationships

R — *Resistance.* General symbol for frictional resistance, or the pressure difference divided by flow.

$R_{AW}$ — *Airway Resistance.* Resistance calculated from pressure difference between airway opening (Pao) and alveoli (Palv) divided by the airflow.

$R_L$ — *Total Pulmonary Resistance.* Resistance calculated by dividing flow-dependent transpulmonary pressure by airflow at the mouth.

$G_{AW}$ — *Airway Conductance.* The reciprocal of $R_{AW}$.

$G_{AW}/V_L$ — *Specific Conductance.* Value for airway conductance divided by the lung volume at which it was measured.

## III. GAS EXCHANGE

### Blood

Examples shown are for $O_2$; other gases (e.g., $CO_2$, $N_2$, CO) or other sites (e.g., $\bar{v}$, c′) can be substituted when appropriate.

$P_{O_2}$ — *Partial Pressure of $O_2$.* General designation in mm Hg; source usually specified (e.g., arterial $P_{O_2}$ or $Pa_{O_2}$).

$S_{O_2}$ — *Blood Saturation.* General designation expressed as a percentage; source usually specified (e.g., arterial $S_{O_2}$ or $Sa_{O_2}$).

$C_{O_2}$ — *Oxygen content.* General designation expressed in mL/dL; source usually specified (e.g., arterial $C_{O_2}$).

$\dot{V}_{O_2}$ — *Oxygen Consumption.* The volume of $O_2$ (STPD) utilized by the body during 1 minute. (Usually calculated as the amount of $O_2$ extracted from inspired gas.)

$\dot{V}_{O_{2max}}$ — *Maximum Oxygen Consumption.* The maximal volume of $O_2$ (STPD) that can be utilized by the body during 1 minute of maximally attainable exercise.

$\dot{V}_{CO_2}$ — *Carbon Dioxide Output.* The volume of $CO_2$ (STPD) produced by the body during 1 minute. (Usually calculated as the amount of $CO_2$ added to exhaled gas.)

RQ — *Respiratory Quotient.* The ratio of $\dot{V}_{CO_2}$ to $\dot{V}_{O_2}$ during steady-state metabolic activity.

RER — *Respiratory Exchange Ratio.* The ratio of $\dot{V}_{CO_2}$ to $\dot{V}_{O_2}$, as in RQ, but also including the influence of transient changes in body stores of respiratory gases.

### Gas to Blood

$(A - a)P_{O_2}$ — *Alveolar-Arterial $P_{O_2}$ Difference.* The difference in $P_{O_2}$ between mean alveolar gas and arterial blood, expressed in mm Hg.

*Alveolar Air Equation.* Often used to calculate mean alveolar $P_{O_2}$ ($PA_{O_2}$):

$$PA_{O_2} = PI_{O_2} - PA_{CO_2}\left[FI_{O_2} + \frac{1 - FI_{O_2}}{R}\right]$$

where $PI_{O_2}$ = $P_{O_2}$ of inspired gas; $PA_{CO_2}$ = alveolar $P_{CO_2}$ (usually assumed to equal arterial $P_{CO_2}$); $FI_{O_2}$ = fractional concentration of $O_2$ in inspired gas; and R = respiratory exchange ratio.

**DL** *Diffusing Capacity of the Lung.* Expressed as the volume of gas transferred per minute per unit of alveolar-capillary pressure difference for the gas used, which is usually specified (e.g., $DL_{CO}$ or $DL_{O_2}$).

**DM** *Diffusing Capacity of the Alveolocapillary Membrane.*

**1/DL** *Total Resistance to Diffusion.* The sum of the resistance to diffusion of the test gas across the alveolocapillary membrane (1/DM) and the resistance to diffusion within the red blood cells attributable to the chemical reaction between the test gas and hemoglobin (1/θVC). These relationships are expressed by the Roughton-Forster equation:

$$\frac{1}{DL} = \frac{1}{DM} + \frac{1}{\theta VC}$$

**DL/VA** *Diffusion per Unit of Alveolar Volume.* The value of DL (STPD) divided by VA (BTPS), both measured in the same breathing maneuver.

## IV. HEMODYNAMIC DESCRIPTORS

**$\dot{Q}T$** *Cardiac Output.* The total output of the left ventricle.

**$\dot{Q}S$** *Pulmonary Shunt.* The total amount of blood perfusing completely nonventilated gas exchange units; hence, blood that does not come in contact with inspired gas and contribute to oxygen uptake. Often called the *right-to-left shunt,* but this term also includes intracardiac shunts.

**$\dot{Q}S/\dot{Q}T$** *Pulmonary Shunt Flow.* The total pulmonary shunt ($\dot{Q}S$), or venous admixture, expressed as a percentage of total cardiac output ($\dot{Q}T$) according to the equation

$$\frac{\dot{Q}S}{\dot{Q}T} = \frac{Cc'_{O_2} - Ca_{O_2}}{Cc'_{O_2} - C\bar{v}_{O_2}} \times 100$$

where $Cc'_{O_2}$ = $O_2$ content of end-capillary blood, $Ca_{O_2}$ = $O_2$ content of arterial blood, and $C\bar{v}_{O_2}$ = $O_2$ content of mixed venous blood. When determined from specimens obtained while breathing 100% $O_2$, $\dot{Q}S/\dot{Q}T$ is a measure of right-to-left shunting of blood.

**PPA** *Pulmonary Artery Pressure.* The pressure, systolic, diastolic, or mean, measured in the pulmonary artery.

**PLA** *Left Atrial Pressure.* The pressure, usually mean, measured in the left atrium.

**Pcap** *Pulmonary Capillary Pressure.* The mean pressure in the pulmonary capillaries, which cannot be measured directly in humans but is frequently estimated by the equation

$$Pcap = PLA + 0.4\ (PPA - PLA)$$

**PPW** *Pulmonary Wedge Pressure.* The mean pressure measured by the pulmonary artery occlusion technique, which provides an estimate of the postcapillary, or pulmonary venous, pressure.

**PVR** *Pulmonary Vascular Resistance.* The resistance to blood flow through the lungs. A calculated value from the equation

$$PVR = \frac{PPA - PLA}{\dot{Q}T},$$

in which PPW is often used to approximate PLA.

## V. OTHER USEFUL TERMS

**PEEP** *Positive End-Expiratory Pressure.* The condition in which the pressure in the airways at the end of expiration is positive (i.e., higher than atmospheric). Usually *applied* during mechanical ventilation, but may be *intrinsic.*

**$P_{0.1}$** *Mouth Occlusion Pressure.* The pressure measured in the mouth during the first 0.1 second of attempted inspiration after the airway is temporarily occluded while the subject is breathing. An estimate of the central drive to breathe.

**TI/TTOT** *Duty Cycle.* The ratio of the duration of inspiration (TI) to the duration of inspiration and expiration (TTOT), a reflection of respiratory timing.

*Henderson-Hasselbalch Equation:* Useful for calculating any one of three variables, pH, $HCO_3^-$, or $H_2CO_3$, when two of them are known:

$$pH = pK + \log\frac{[HCO_3^-]}{[H_2CO_3]}$$

where pK, the dissociation constant, is 6.10 for plasma at 37°C; $[HCO_3^-]$ is the concentration of bicarbonate in plasma; and $[H_2CO_3]$ is the concentration of carbonic acid in plasma (both in mol/L). The equation can be rearranged by using $PCO_2$ (mm Hg) and its solubility in plasma so that

$$pH = pK + \log\frac{[HCO_3^-]}{[PCO_2 \times 0.0301]}$$

# INDEX

Note: Page numbers in *italics* refer to illustrations; page numbers followed by t refer to tables.

## A


(A–a)$PO_2$. See *Oxygen, partial pressure of, alveolar-to-arterial difference in.*
A fibers, of visceral sensory neurons, 573
Abbreviations, in respiratory medicine, 2563–2565
Abdomen, disorders of. See also specific organs and systems, e.g., *Esophagus*; *Gastrointestinal system*; *Kidney*; *Liver*; *Pancreas.*
chest pain in, 580
pleural effusion in, 2027–2031, *2027*, *2029*
movement of, in diaphragmatic paralysis, 2335
in flail chest, 2367, *2367*
lung volume changes in, 105–106, *105*
muscles of, 108, 859, 2330–2331, 2330t
pneumatic belt for, in neuromuscular disorders, 2347
pressure in, in obesity, 2372
spinal rigidity in, 108
surgery on, pleural effusion after, 2030
preoperative evaluation for, 885–886
tightening of, diaphragm motion in, 106–107
tuberculosis of, 1084–1085
Abscess(es), abdominal, pleural effusion in, 2029–2030
brain, in arteriovenous malformations, 1561
in sinusitis, 916
in toxoplasmosis, 2203
disseminated, in nocardiosis, 1023
liver, amebic, lung involvement in, 1144–1146, *1145*
pleural effusion in, 2025
lung, 1030–1031
amebic, 1144–1146, *1145*
anaerobic, 1017–1018, *1018*, 1020, 1031
aortography in, *659*
bronchoscopy in, 749
computed tomography of, 688, 2007
diagnosis of, 1031
drainage of, 749
in bronchiectasis, 1328
in cancer, 1431–1432
in emphysema, 1195
in hydatid disease, 1158
liquefaction necrosis in, *448*
microbiology of, 1030–1031
pleural effusion in, 2016–2021, 2018t, *2021*
*Pseudomonas aeruginosa*, 1011, *1012*
specimen collection from, 611, *612*
*Staphylococcus aureus*, 1003–1004
*Strongyloides stercoralis*, 1152
treatment of, 727, 749, 1031
pancreatic, pleural effusion in, 2030
peritonsillar, 918
retropharyngeal, 918, 2096–2097
skin, in coccidioidomycosis, 1124
subphrenic, pleural effusion in, 2029–2030
*Absidia* infections, 1108, 1134–1135, *1135*
Absorption, of drugs, 247–248
Abuse, drug. See *Drug(s), abuse of*; specific drugs, e.g., *Cocaine.*
Acadesine, preoperative, in cardiac risk reduction, 884
Acanthosis nigricans, in lung cancer, 1421
Accelerated fractionation, in radiation therapy, 1433
Accelerated silicosis, 1818, 1818t
Acceleration, pulmonary circulation effects of, 66
Acepifylline, 272
Acetaldehyde, in smoke, 1909
Acetazolamide, in asthma, 290
in chronic obstructive pulmonary disease, 1228
in hypoventilation, 2144
in metabolic alkalosis, 173
in mountain sickness, 1932, 1939
in sleep apnea, 2165
Acetic anhydride, exposure to, 1910
Acetoacetate accumulation, in diabetic ketoacidosis, 166–167, *167*
Acetone, in multiple inert gas elimination technique, 80–81, *81*, *82*
Acetylcholine, action of, 250, *250*, *251*
excess of, in Lambert-Eaton syndrome, 1379
in mucus secretion regulation, 332, 333
in pulmonary vascular resistance control, 131
of epithelial cells, 361
release of, 252–253, *253*
Acetylcholinesterase inhibitors, respiratory effects of, 2343
*N*-Acetylcysteine, in chronic obstructive pulmonary disease, 1224
in mucus reduction, 289
in pulmonary edema, 1610
in secretion clearance, in neuromuscular disorders, 2346
in specimen processing, 613t
*N*-Acetylglucosaminyltransferase I, in lung development, 42
N-Acetyltransferase, as biomarker, for lung cancer, 1406
*Achaete-scute* homologue–1, in lung development, 42
Acid(s), nonvolatile, excretion of, 162
titratable, in urine, 162
Acid fast staining, of *Mycobacterium*, 1043, *1044*, 1046
Acid rain, 1886
Acid-base balance and imbalance, 155–178. See also *Metabolic acidosis; Metabolic alkalosis; Respiratory acidosis; Respiratory alkalosis.*
anion gap concept in, 163–164, *164*, 170
bicarbonate/carbon dioxide relationships in, 157–158, *157*, *159*
buffers in, 156, 157, 158
in exercise, 200, *200*, 205–206, *206*
in kidney, 162–163
intracellular, 163
classification of, 158–160, 160t
compensation in, 161, 161t
Acid-base balance and imbalance *(Continued)*
bicarbonate-carbon dioxide relationships in, *159*, 160t
failure of, in heavy exercise, 211
in exercise, 208–209, *209*, 211
kidney in, 162–163
laboratory definitions of, 160
respiratory, 161, 161t
Henderson-Hasselbalch equation for, 155–156, 831, 2565
in hypoxia, 130
metabolic parameters in, 157–158, *157*, 160t
mixed, 158–159, 160t
parameter selection in, 155–160, *157*, *159*, 160t
physiology of, 155–163, *157*, *159*, 160t
respiratory parameters in, 157–158, *157*, 160t
temperature effects in, 163
terminology of, 155–163, *157*, *159*, 160t
triple disorders of, 159
ventilatory response and, 192–193, *193*
Acidemia, in hypercapnia, 2444
in respiratory failure, 2444
versus acidosis, 156
Acid-fast stains, for *Mycobacterium*, 1043, *1044*, 1046
Acidosis. See also *Metabolic acidosis; Respiratory acidosis.*
anion gap. See *Anion gap acidosis.*
diabetic ketoacidosis as, 166–167, 166t, *167*, 1134
dilutional, 163, *164*, 170
gastrointestinal causes of, 169–170
hyperchloremic. See *Hyperchloremic acidosis.*
lactic. See *Lactic acidosis.*
renal tubular, 168–169, 169t
toxic, 168
uremic, 167–168
ventilatory response in, 192–193, *193*
versus acidemia, 156
Aciduria, paradoxical, in metabolic alkalosis, 162
Acinar rosette, on interstitial lung disease radiographs, 1656–1657, *1658*, 1658t
*Acinetobacter* pneumonia, 998t, 1013–1014, *1013*
Acinus(i). See also *Alveolus(i).*
definition of, 56, 1204, *1204*
Acquired immunodeficiency syndrome. See *Human immunodeficiency virus infection.*
Acramin textile dyes, exposure to, 1910
Acrolein, in smoke, 1909
Acromegaly, respiratory manifestations of, 2313
Acrosclerosis, in mixed connective tissue disease, 1708
ACTH (adrenocorticotropic hormone), in lung cancer, 1379, 1422
Actin, in fluid and solute exchange, *134–135*
in permeability regulation, 141–142
Actinin, in fluid and solute exchange, *134–135*
*Actinomadura* pneumonia, culture in, 620–621

*Actinomyces* infections, pleural effusion in, 2023
pneumonia due to, 620–621, 1019t, 1020–1022, *1021*
Actinomycetes, thermophilic, inhalation of, hypersensitivity pneumonitis in, 1868
Activated partial thromboplastin time, measurement of, in heparin therapy, 1516
Activating transcription factor, in signal transduction, 239–240, *239*
Activator protein–1, 259–260
in receptor gene regulation, 246
Activinlike kinase, defects of, in hereditary hemorrhagic telangiectasia, 1560
Acute chest syndrome, in sickle cell disease, 2287–2289
Acute hypoxemic respiratory failure. See also *Acute/adult respiratory distress syndrome.*
breathing mechanics in, 2380, *2381*
causes of, 2378t
classification of, 2413–2416, *2414–2416*, 2414t
clinical manifestations of, 2378t, 2380–2381, 2416–2419, *2418*, 2419t, 2420t
definition of, 2378t, 2379, *2379*
pathogenesis of, 2378t, 2379, *2379*, 2413, *2414*
pathophysiology of, 2379–2380, *2379*, *2381*
treatment of, 2380–2381, 2419–2437. See also *Acute/adult respiratory distress syndrome, treatment of.*
in cardiogenic pulmonary edema, 2419–2422, 2420t, *2421*
mechanical ventilation in, 2380–2381, 2382t
pharmacologic, 2422–2423
supportive, 2423–2437, *2425–2428*, *2431*, 2432t
Acute Physiologic Assessment and Chronic Health Evaluation (APACHE) system, 2488, 2490
Acute respiratory disease, in military recruits, 937–940, *939*
Acute right heart syndrome, in respiratory failure, 2395, 2395t
Acute/adult respiratory distress syndrome, 318–319, 2413–2442
amiodarone-induced, 1983
causes of, 1498, 2417
chest radiography of, 1584, *1584*, 2417, *2418*, 2420t
clinical manifestations of, 2416–2419, *2418*, 2419t, 2420t
computed tomography of, 2416, *2416*
definition of, 1576, 1592–1593, 1592t, 1593t, 2418–2419, 2419t, 2420t
diagnosis of, 1591–1600
barrier function measurement in, 1597–1598
blood gas analysis in, 1594–1595
bronchoscopy in, 756
chest radiography in, 1594
criteria for, 1591–1594, 1592t, 1593t
edema fluid analysis in, 2417
fluid protein measurement in, 1595
hemodynamic measurements in, 1595–1596
lung injury detection in, 1598–1600
lung water measurement in, 1596–1597
pulmonary function tests in, 1595
symptoms and signs in, 1591
diffuse, 2413–2415, 2414t, *2415*
diffuse alveolar damage in, 1743–1744, 1743t
drug-induced, 1990, 1990t
echocardiography in, 2417–2418
Acute/adult respiratory distress syndrome *(Continued)*
epidemiology of, 1613
evaluation of, 2417–2418, *2418*
extrapulmonary versus pulmonary, 1500
exudative phase of, pathogenesis of, 2414, *2414*, *2415*
pathophysiology of, 2397
treatment of, 2435
focal, 2415–2416, *2416*
hemodynamic monitoring in, 2418
herpes simplex virus infections in, 948
idiopathic, versus acute interstitial pneumonia, 1686
in alveolar hemorrhage, 2415
in amniotic fluid embolism, 2323
in bronchiolitis, 1362, *1362*
in focal lesions, 2414t, 2415–2416
in infection, 1587, 1588t, 1589
in inflammation, 1589–1590, 1590t
in malaria, 1147
in oxygen toxicity, 1987
in pancreatitis, 2276, 2277
in pregnancy, 2324
in sepsis, 147
in strongyloidiasis, 1152
in toxic exposures, 1362, *1362*, 1588t, 1590–1591, 1904
in transfusions, 2292
lung mechanics in, 1585
mechanisms of, 1587–1591, 1588t–1590t
mitomycin-induced, 1976–1977
mortality in, 1613, 2488, 2489
pathogenesis of, coagulation disorders in, 520
interleukin-1 family in, 499
neutrophils in, 528
platelet-activating factor in, 498
tumor necrosis factor-α in, 502
pathophysiology of, 318–319, 1584–1586, 2397–2398
permissive hypercapnia in, 2444
pressure-volume relationships in, 2426, *2426*, *2427*
prevention of, 1577
postoperative, 2382, 2382t
proliferative phase of, pathogenesis of, 2414–2415, *2415*
treatment of, 2435–2436
pulmonary edema in, 1498, 1500, 2413–2415, *2415*
causes of, 2417–2418, *2418*
treatment of, 2419–2422, 2420t, *2421*
scoring system for, 2418–2419, 2419t, 2420t
septic shock with, 2399–2400
sequelae of, in toxic exposures, 1904–1905
severity of, 2418–2419, 2419t, 2420t
stages of, 1586
surfactant alterations in, 93, 318–319
treatment of, 1600–1611, 1613–1614, *1614*
antioxidants in, 1610
cardiac catheterization in, 1600–1601
circulatory management in, 2423–2424, *2425*
corticosteroids in, 1608–1609, 2422
diuretics in, 1602–1603
extracorporeal gas exchange in, 2434
immediate, 1600
in exudative phase, 2435
in pancreatitis, 2277
in proliferative phase, 2435–2436
in pulmonary edema, 2419–2422, 2420t, *2421*
in toxic exposures, 1904–1905
innovative, 2433–2435
inotropic agents in, 1603–1604
Acute/adult respiratory distress syndrome *(Continued)*
ketoconazole in, 2423
mechanical ventilation in, 2421–2422, 2424–2436, *2426–2428*, *2431*, 2432t
monitoring of, 2435
monoclonal antibodies in, 1610–1611
options for, 1600–1604
outcome of, 1611–1614, *1614*
oxygen therapy in, 2430, *2431*
pentoxifylline in, 1610
pharmacologic, 2419–2423, 2420t, *2421*
prostaglandin inhibitors in, 2423
sequelae of, 2436
specific, 1608–1611
strategies for, 1604–1611, 1606t
surfactant in, 320–321, 1609–1610, 2423
vasodilators in, 1601–1602, 1611
versus acute lung injury, 2419, 2419t
versus high-altitude pulmonary edema, 1935
versus neonatal respiratory distress syndrome, 318
Acyclovir, in cytomegalovirus infections, 945, 2302
prophylactic, 2231
in herpes simplex virus infections, 949, 2303
in varicella-zoster virus infections, 968, 2303
Acyl coenzyme A, formation of, in ketoacidosis, 167, *167*
Addison's disease, respiratory manifestations of, 2313
Adenitis, mediastinal. See *Mediastinitis, granulomatous (chronic).*
Adenocarcinoma(s), of lung. See *Lung cancer, adenocarcinoma as.*
versus mesothelioma, 2069
Adenoids, enlarged, pharyngeal obstruction in, 1351
Adenoma(s), of bronchi, 1478
of lung, pathology of, 483t
of mucous glands, 1478
of parathyroid glands, 2128
of pituitary gland, 2313
of salivary glands, in lung, 1462–1463, 1462t
Adenosine, as inflammatory mediator, 258
in provocation testing, in asthma, 1266
receptor for, theophylline inhibition of, 273
release of, 232, *233*
Adenosine deaminase, deficiency of, in severe combined immunodeficiency, 2239
in pleural fluid, 2005–2006, 2022
Adenosine triphosphate, as energy source, 201
generation of, in exercise, 198–201, *199*, *200*, 205–206, *206*
in pyruvate metabolism, 164–165, *165*
Adenovirus infections, 931t, 937–940
bronchitis after, 934
clinical manifestations of, 938–939, *939*
diagnosis of, 625, 939–940
epidemiology of, 938
in immunodeficiency, 939, 940t
in lung transplantation, 2522
pathogenesis of, 938, *938*
pneumonia due to, in transplantation, 2232, 2302
pathology of, 470
prevention of, 940
receptors in, 938
transmission of, 938
treatment of, 940
viral characteristics in, 937–938, *938*
Adenovirus respiratory disease, definition of, 938–939
Adenylyl cyclase, in beta-adrenergic agonist action, 268, *269*

Adenylyl cyclase *(Continued)*
in signal transduction, 236, *236*
receptor cross-talk effects on, 242, *242*
Adhesion molecules, blockers of, in asthma, 287
in chronic obstructive pulmonary disease, 287
in asthma, 1261
in granulocyte movement, 527–528
in neutrophil movement, 524–525, *525*
Adhesion properties, of mucus, 365
Adhesions, pleural, 2007, *2007*
Adkins tumor, 2132
Adrenal gland, disorders of, respiratory manifestations of, 2312–2313
metastasis to, treatment of, 1431
suppression of, corticosteroid-induced, 282
Adrenal shock, 2404
Adrenergic nerves, 22
in pulmonary circulation control, 131
of airways, *250*
of pulmonary circulation, 297
Adrenergic receptor(s). See also *Alpha-adrenergic receptors; Beta-adrenergic receptor(s).*
in bronchodilation, 255–256
Adrenocorticotropic hormone, in lung cancer, 1379, 1422
Adult respiratory distress syndrome. See *Acute/adult respiratory distress syndrome.*
Advance directives, 2494
Advanced Multiple Beam Equalization Radiography (AMBER) system, 641, *641–643*
Aerodynamic diameter, of aerosols, 350
Aerosol(s), 349–360
aerodynamic diameter of, 350
antibiotics in, 359–360, 1310
clearance of, 354–355, *354*. See also *Alveolus(i), clearance from; Mucociliary transport.*
measurement of, 357, *358*
delivery of, 355–356. See also *Nebulizers.*
deposition of, diffusion in, 351, *351*
electrostatic precipitation in, 351, *351*
from metered-dose inhalers, 355–356
from powder devices, 356
in bronchioles, 57
in lower respiratory tract, 352–354, *352, 353*
in nose, 1345
in upper respiratory tract, 352
inertial impaction in, 351, *351*
interception in, 351, *351*
measurement of, 365–366, *366*
mechanisms of, 350–351, *351*
sedimentation in, 351, *351*
diagnostic use of, 356–357, *358*, 365, *366*
environmental. See *Occupational and environmental disorder(s).*
generation of, 355–356. See also *Nebulizers.*
in mechanical ventilation, 2472, 2474
hygroscopic, deposition of, 354
in alveolar diseases, 359
in asthma, 357, 359
in chronic obstructive pulmonary disease, 357, 359
in emphysema, 359
in gene therapy, 360
in immunization, 359–360
in interstitial lung disease, 359
in mucociliary transport abnormalities, 359
in pneumonia, 359–360
liquid, behavior of, 351–352
lung injury due to, agents causing, 1905t
pathogenesis of, 1903–1904
Aerosol(s) *(Continued)*
sequelae of, 1904–1905
treatment of, 1904
occupational. See *Occupational and environmental disorder(s).*
particle size distribution of, 350, 352–354, *352, 353*
phagocytosis of, 372–373, 373t
propellants for, 355–356
properties of, 350
radiolabeled, in diagnostic studies, 356–357, *358*
in ventilation-perfusion scanning, 699–700
systemic drug delivery by, 360
tonicity of, deposition and, 354
tuberculosis transmission in, 1053
water, contaminated with microbial agents, hypersensitivity pneumonitis due to, 1868
Affected relative pair methods, in genetic disease, 49–50
Afferent nerves, of autonomic nervous system, 250–252, *251*
Affinity, of drug, 243
Agammaglobulinemia, X-linked, 2233t, 2234–2235
Age, versus alveolar-arterial oxygen difference, 824
versus chronic obstructive pulmonary disease progression, 1202, *1202*
versus decompression sickness susceptibility, 1960
versus diffusing capacity, 814
versus lung cancer survival, 1397, 1397t
versus pneumonia risk factors, 987–988
versus pulmonary function, 857
Agonists, drug, 243–244, *244*
beta-adrenergic. See *Beta$_2$-adrenergic agonists.*
receptor, 242–243, *242*
AIDS. See *Human immunodeficiency virus infection.*
Air, compression of, in chest, 102
dry, water homeostasis in, 362–363
embolism of, 465, 1526
after pneumomediastinum, 2098, *2098*, 2102
in diving, 1954–1956, *1956*, 1962
in mechanical ventilation, 2478
in pregnancy, 2324
humidification of, in nasal breathing, 362
in mediastinum. See *Pneumomediastinum.*
in pleural space. See *Pneumothorax.*
reabsorption of, in pneumothorax, 2046–2047
trapping of, in expiration radiographs, 646, *647, 650*
in ventilation-perfusion scanning, 699
volume of, versus depth, in diving, 1954–1955, *1955*
warming of, in nose, 1346
Air block, in mechanical ventilation, 2102
Air flow. See *Airflow.*
Air gap, in radiography, 636, *636*
Air pollution, acid aerosols in, 1906
adverse effects of, acute, 374
animal studies of, 1215, 1891
asthma as, 1250, 1892, 1894–1895
carcinogenesis as, 1887–1888
chronic obstructive pulmonary disease as, 1215, 1893
clinical studies of, 1890–1891
defense mechanisms against, 1888–1889
definition of, 1886
epidemiologic studies of, 1890, 1891–1892
Air pollution *(Continued)*
from nitrogen dioxide, 1215, 1894–1896
from ozone, 1215, 1893–1896
from particulates, 1891–1893
from sulfur dioxide, 1215, 1891–1893
goblet cell metaplasia and hyperplasia as, 1262
lung cancer as, 1403
lung injury as, 1903–1905
mortality as, 1885, 1891, 1895
study methods for, 1890–1891
"welfare," 1885
air quality standards and, 1885, 1886t
chlorine and chlorine compounds in, 1905–1906
defense mechanisms against, 1888–1889
extreme, examples of, 1805, 1885, 1891
from large-scale conflagrations, 1909
historical aspects of, 1885, 1891
indoor, 1887t, 1888, 1894
environmental tobacco smoke in, 1399–1400, 2558–2560, 2559t
standards for, 2557–2558
nitrogen oxides in. See *Nitrogen dioxide; Nitrogen oxides.*
ozone in. See *Ozone.*
pollutants causing, 1885–1888
criteria, 1885, 1886t
definition of, 1885–1886
distribution of, 1886–1888
properties of, 1886–1888
sources of, 1886–1888
types of, 1886, 1887t
pulmonary function test effects of, 803
reduction of, government involvement in, 2556–2557
sulfur oxides in. See *Sulfur oxides (including sulfur dioxide).*
Air quality, improvement of, government role in, 2556–2558
Air surface liquid, composition of, 339–340, 340t
volume of, regulation of, 339
Air travel, after diving, 1952
oxygen therapy during, 1226–1227
pulmonary function tests for, 859–860
with lung disease, 1941
Airflow, dynamics of, 1343–1345, *1343–1345*
in cough, 369, 555–557, *555, 557*
in pharynx, 1350
in quiet breathing, determinants of, 782
in upper airway, 1343–1345, *1343–1345*
inspiratory, 1344–1345, *1345*
laminar, 97
limitation of, in chronic obstructive pulmonary disease, 1206–1207
in highly fit athletes, 218
maximal expiratory. See *Maximal expiratory flow.*
measurement of. See *Spirometry;* specific tests, e.g., *Vital capacity.*
mechanical aspects of, 95, *96*
obstruction of. See *Airway obstruction.*
resistance to. See *Airway resistance.*
turbulent, 97
velocity of, versus pressure, 97–98
versus airway generation number, 56–57, *56*, 94
maximal expiratory flow and, 98, *100*, 101
versus lung volume, during vital capacity maneuvers, 98, *99, 100*, 101
versus lung volume history, 101–103
versus pressure, 97–98, 2564
versus volume, 787–790, *787–790*
in cough, 577, *577*

Airflow *(Continued)*
normal values for, 804, 875
Airflow-pressure relationships, terminology of, 2564
Air-space consolidation. See *Consolidation*.
Air-space enlargement. See also *Emphysema (pulmonary)*.
fibrosis with, 1188–1189, 1188t, 1205
in lung injury, 1214, *1214*
simple, definition of, 1188, 1188t
pathology of, 1203–1204
Airway, glands of. See also *Bronchus(i), glands of*.
Airway(s). See also specific components, e.g., *Bronchioles; Bronchus(i); Trachea*.
aerosol deposition in. See *Aerosol(s), deposition of*.
airflow in. See *Airflow*.
anatomy of, 55–56, *56*, 1343–1344, *1343*, 1361–1362
cellular, 7, *8–12*, 9–10
circulatory, 10–11
muscular, 10
resistance and, 6–7
artificial, esophageal perforation from, 2107
autonomic innervation of, 249–256, 570
afferent nerves in, 250–252, *251*
bronchodilator nerves in, 255–256
cholinergic nerves in, *250*, 252–254, *253*
dysfunction of, 256
in mucus secretion regulation, 332–333
neurogenic inflammation and, 254–255, *254*
overview of, 249–250, *250*, *251*
burns of, bronchoscopy in, 754
cancer of, intrabronchial dissemination of, 1470–1471
clearance of, in cystic fibrosis, 1308–1309
closure of, versus lung volume, 59–60, *59*
collapse of, 783
airflow and, 1344–1345, *1344*
in sleep apnea, 1351
computed tomography of, 679, *679–681*
conducting. See also specific components, e.g., *Bronchus(i)*.
definition of, 55
cross sections of, 56–57, *56*, 94
maximal expiratory flow and, 98, *99*, 101
defense reflexes in, 252
definition of, 5–6
dehydration of, 362–363
dimensions of, aerosol studies of, 356
disorders of, hypoventilation in, 2140t, 2142, *2142*
in inflammatory bowel disease, 2270–2271, 2270t
in mediastinitis, 2113
drug delivery routes for, 248–249
edema of, in inhalation injury, 754
epithelium of. See *Epithelium and epithelial cells, airway*.
function of, after lung transplantation, 2524–2525
generations of, 56, *56*, 94
maximal expiratory flow and, 98, *100*, 101
geometry of, 94
glands of, 9, *10*
ion transport defects of, in cystic fibrosis, 1299–1300
hyperresponsiveness of, in asthma. See *Asthma*.
in byssinosis, 1861–1862
in cystic fibrosis, 1304
in spinal cord injury, 2338–2339
nonspecific, chronic obstructive pulmonary disease and, 1200
Airway(s) *(Continued)*
infection of, in cystic fibrosis, 1300–1302
inflammation of, chronic bronchitis in, 1215–1216
in asthma, 1855
in cystic fibrosis, 1301
inflammatory cells of, 232, *233*
innervation of, 570. See also *Airway(s), autonomic innervation of*.
intrapulmonary. See *Bronchioles; Bronchus(i)*.
irritation of, pain mechanisms in, 574–575
lung sequestration from. See *Sequestration(s), bronchopulmonary*.
macrophages of. See *Macrophage(s), alveolar*.
mechanical properties of, 94–95, *96*
morphology of, Weibel model of, 56, *56*
mucociliary transport in. See *Mucociliary transport*.
mucosa of, cystic fibrosis effects on, 1295–1297, 1296t, *1297*
function of, 360–361
mucus in. See *Mucus*.
muscles of, mechanical properties of, 108–109
muscles surrounding, 1346t, 1351, *1352*, *1353*
narrowing of, 1174. See also *Bronchoconstriction*.
airflow dynamics in, 1344–1345, *1344*, *1345*
at larynx, 1353
in acromegaly, 2313
in asthma, 1254, 1263–1265, *1263*, *1264*, 1274
measurement of, 1267–1268
in chronic obstructive pulmonary disease, 1216
in relapsing polychondritis, 1709, *1709*
lung function and, 1362
muscles in, 1346t
sleep apnea in, 2155–2157, *2157*
obstruction of. See *Airway obstruction*.
pain mechanisms in, 569
parenchymal interdependence with, 94
patency of, surfactant maintenance of, 309
peripheral. See *Bronchioles; Bronchus(i)*.
pharmacology of. See *Pharmacology, airway*.
physiology of, 1361–1362
plasmacytomas of, 2293
pressure losses in, 97–98
pressure-area curve of, 94
remodeling of, in asthma, 1263, *1263*, 1264t
in ozone exposure, 1896
resistance in. See *Airway resistance*.
small. See *Bronchioles; Bronchus(i)*.
smooth muscle of, 10, *12*
beta-adrenergic receptor dysfunction in, 245
of potassium channels in, 247
second messenger action in, 236, *236*
sounds generated in. See *Lung sounds*.
stimulation of, 232, *233*
types of, 6, *7*, *8*
upper. See also specific structures, e.g., *Larynx; Nose; Pharynx*.
airflow dynamics in, 1343–1345, *1343–1345*
receptors in, 181–182
Airway management. See *Airway obstruction, treatment of; Pharmacology, airway*.
Airway obstruction, after thoracoplasty, 2364
blunted perception of, 1270
cardiac output in, 2453
Airway obstruction *(Continued)*
differential diagnosis of, 1269, 1269t
flow-volume curves in, 789, *790*
functional residual capacity in, 112
hemodynamic consequences of, 2452–2453
hypercapnic response in, 820
in acromegaly, 2313
in amyloidosis, 2296
in bone marrow transplantation, 2298, 2300–2301
in cancer, bronchoscopic treatment of, 742
in carcinoid tumor, 1461
in chronic obstructive pulmonary disease, 1187–1188, *1188*
in cystic fibrosis, 1293–1294, *1294*, 1304–1305, 1304t
in inflammatory bowel disease, 2270–2271, 2270t
in kyphoscoliosis, 2361
in laryngotracheitis, 918
in lung cancer, metastatic, 1471
in lymphangio(leio)myomatosis, 1779
in mechanical ventilation, 2483
in neuromuscular disorders, 2332
in sarcoidosis, 1368, 1718
in Sjögren's syndrome, 366
in toxic exposures, 1904
laryngeal, 1351–1354, 1354t
lung injury in, 1589t
oxygen partial pressure in, versus altitude, 860
pharyngeal, 1350–1351
pulmonary edema in, 1582, 1589t
pulmonary function tests in, 789, *790*, 850–854, 851t, *852*
pulsus paradoxus in, 2452–2453
respiratory failure in, mechanical ventilation in, 2382t
pathophysiology of, *2379*
reversibility of, pulmonary function testing in, 851–852, *852*
sleep apnea in. See *Sleep apnea, obstructive*.
treatment of. See also *Pharmacology, airway*.
bronchoscopy in, 726–727, 753
stents in, 742–743, *743*
variation of, with breathing cycle, 1174
ventilation distribution in, 805, *806*, 808
Airway opening pressure, 2450–2451, *2451*
in status asthmaticus, 2458–2459, *2458*
Airway resistance, airflow and, 798, 1344, *1344*
anatomic aspects of, 6–7
at high altitude, 1918
beta-adrenergic antagonist–induced, 1983–1984
bronchiole contribution to, 1361–1362
definition of, 97
elastic recoil and, 798
high, nonrespiratory muscle recruitment in, 108
in asthma, 1856, *1856*
in chronic obstructive pulmonary disease, in exercise, 212, *213*
in heart disease, 2254–2255
in interstitial lung disease, 1662–1663, *1665*
in narrowing, 1344, *1344*
in nose, 1346
in obesity, 2372
in pregnancy, 2318
in pulmonary edema, 1579
in pulmonary venous hypertension, 2254–2255
in sleep, 2153
in thoracic mechanical time constant calculation, 215

Airway resistance *(Continued)*
inspiratory, in mechanical ventilation, 2474
lung volume and, 798
measurement of, 798–799, *799*
mechanics of, 95, *96*
normal values for, 782
pathogenesis of, in heart disease, 2255
respiratory failure in, 2447–2448
smooth muscle tone and, 798–799
ventilation-perfusion scanning in, 698
versus lung volume, 95
Albendazole, in ascariasis, 1150
in echinococcosis, 1160
in filariasis, 1155
in hookworm infections, 1151
in strongyloidiasis, 1152–1153
Albumin, binding proteins of, 140–141
electrical charge on, anion gap and, 164
endothelial cell interactions with, 144
endothelial permeability of, 139–142, 140t
safety factors and, 146, *146*
in interstitium, 137
in mucus, 329
in pulmonary edema fluid, 1500
receptors for, 140–141
technetium-99m labeled, in ventilation-perfusion scanning, 698, 828
transcytosis of, 134, *134–135*, 140–141
Albumin concentration gradient, 133
Albuterol, as bronchodilator, 270
chemical structure of, 268, *268*
in asthma, 1275, 2454, 2454t
in chronic obstructive pulmonary disease, 1221
in respiratory failure, acute-on-chronic, 2461, 2461t
in status asthmaticus, 2454, 2454t
*R*-enantiomer of, 272
Alcohol use and abuse, diving accidents in, 1964
pneumonia in, microbiology of, 988t
Aldehydes, in smoke, 1908–1909
Aldosterone, deficiency of, renal tubular acidosis in, 169
excess of, metabolic alkalosis in, 171t, 172–173
Alkalemia, versus alkalosis, 156
Alkalosis. See also *Metabolic alkalosis; Respiratory alkalosis.*
concentration, 170
ventilatory response in, 192–193, *193*
versus alkalemia, 156
Alkylating agents, pulmonary disease due to, 1974t, 1975–1976
Alleles, 46
diseases associated with, 49
exclusion of, in immunoglobulin expression, 418
in T-cell receptors, 423
Allen and Davis classification, of eosinophilic lung diseases, 1761, 1761t
Allen test, for wrist artery patency, 834
Allergen(s), asthma due to, 374–375, 1255, 1854
in airway responsiveness testing, 853
indoor, 1347
inflammatory cell response to, 232, *233*
mucosal priming by, 1348
outdoor, 1347
Allergic bronchopulmonary aspergillosis, 1131–1132, 1271–1272, 1763–1766
bronchiectasis with, 1327, 1333–1334
bronchocentric granulomatosis in, 1368
chest radiography in, 1763, 1765–1766, *1765–1767*
cystic fibrosis with, 1305, 1312
Allergic bronchopulmonary aspergillosis *(Continued)*
diagnosis of, 1763, 1763t, 1765
epidemiology of, 1763
immune response in, 1763
in asthma, 1763, 1765
in cystic fibrosis, 1763
in HIV infection, 2200
pathology of, 1763, *1764*
treatment of, 1765–1766
versus other bronchopulmonary fungoses, 1763
Allergic disease(s), asthma as, 437, 1255, 1270
epidemiology of, versus asthma prevalence, 1249–1250, *1250*
immune response in, 437
Allergic granulomatosis and angiitis (Churg-Strauss syndrome), 1538, 1769–1771, *1770*, 1770t
pleural effusion in, 2033
Allergic rhinitis, 1347–1350
classification of, 1347–1348
pathophysiology of, 1347–1348
treatment of, 1348–1349, 1348t
Allergic (leukocytoclastic) vasculitis, 1534, 1539
Allescheriosis, 1136
Almitrine, in asthma, 290
in chronic obstructive pulmonary disease, 1228
in respiratory acidosis, 174
Alpha-adrenergic blockers, as vasodilators, 300
Alpha-adrenergic receptors, functions of, *250*
in bronchodilation, 256
in mucus secretion regulation, 333
in pulmonary circulation, 131
Alpha$_1$-antitrypsin, action of, 1178
aerosolized, in emphysema, 359
augmentation therapy with, 1210
deficiency of, air pollution and, 1889
bronchiectasis with, 1334
diagnosis of, 1209–1210
disease phenotypes in, 1208–1209, *1209*
emphysema in, 1178, 1207–1210, 2276
diagnosis of, 1209–1210
elastase-antielastase hypothesis and, 1210–1214, *1210–1211*, *1214*
liver disease with, 1209
phenotypes of, 1208–1209, *1209*
treatment of, 1210
genetics of, 482, 1208–1210
liver disease in, 1209
pathology of, 480t, 482
treatment of, 1210
gene of, 1208
in mucus, 329
M alleles of, 1208
normal levels of, 1208
physiology of, 1208
Pi MM phenotype of, 1208
Pi MZ phenotype of, 1208, 1209
Pi SS phenotype of, 1208
Pi SZ phenotype of, 1208
Pi ZZ phenotype (homozygous) of, 1208–1210, 1212
structure of, 1208
Alpha-tocopherol, in lung cancer prevention, 1405
*Alternaria*, hypersensitivity pneumonitis due to, 1869
surfactant protein D binding to, 315–316
Alternobaric vertigo, 1956–1957
Altitude, high, 1915–1950
adaptation to, 1916–1929
acute, 1917–1918
biochemical, 1923
Altitude *(Continued)*
cardiovascular, 1919–1921, 1927–1928
central nervous system, 1923–1925, *1924*, *1925*
chronic, 1918
diffusing capacity increase in, 1919
fluid homeostasis in, 1925
gas exchange alterations in, 1919, *1920*, *1921*, 1926–1927, *1927*
genetic factors in, 1918, 1921
hematologic, 1921–1922, *1922*
hemodynamic, 1920–1921, *1921*
in athletic training, 1928–1929
in exercise, 1925–1929, *1925–1927*
in high-altitude residents, 1918, 1919, 1926
in mountain sickness prevention, 1932
in sleep, 1924–1925, *1924*, *1925*
morphologic, 1923
on descent, 1918
prediction of, 859–860
pulmonary function changes in, 1918–1919
tissue, 1922–1923, 1928
ventilation response in, 1916–1919, *1916*, *1917*, 1925–1926, *1926*
diffusing capacity at, 814
diving at, 1951t, 1952
dyspnea in, 220–221
exercise testing at, hematocrit in, 1922
habitable limits of, 1915
historical perspective of, 1915–1916, 1916t
maladaptation to, 1929–1942. See also specific disorders.
acute mountain sickness in, 175, 1929–1932, *1931*
cerebral edema in, 1932–1933
chronic mountain sickness in, 1938–1939, *1939*
coagulopathy in, 1937–1938
hypoxic pulmonary vasoconstriction and, 68, 130, 1634
in asthma, 1941
in congestive heart failure, 1941
in coronary artery disease, 1940
in high-altitude residents, 1938–1939, *1939*
in hypertension, 1940
in illness, 1939–1942
in lowlanders ascending to high altitude, 1929–1938
in lung disease, 1941
in pregnancy, 1942
in pulmonary hypertension, 1551
in sleep apnea, 1941, *2161*, 2162
lung injury in, 475
pulmonary edema in, 147, 1581, 1933–1937, *1934*, *1935*, 1939
retinopathy in, 1937, *1937*
subacute mountain sickness in, 1938
pulmonary function test effects of, 803
ventricular septal defects and, 298
Aluminum carbide, in hard metal products, lung disease from, 1844–1845
Aluminum industry, lung cancer in, 1400
Aluminum oxide, in pneumoconiosis, 1831t, 1842
Alveolar air equation, 58, 71–72, *72*, 180, *180*, 822, 824
Alveolar clearance. See *Alveolus(i), clearance from.*
Alveolar hemorrhage, diffuse, 1733–1748
causes of, 1653t, 1733, 1734t
chest radiography in, *1658*
clinical manifestations of, 1734, *1735*, 1736, *1736*

Alveolar hemorrhage *(Continued)*
damage in, 1743–1744, 1743t
definition of, 1733
glomerulonephritis with, *1736*, 1740–1741
in acute allograft rejection, 1741
in Behçet's syndrome, 1740
in bone marrow transplantation, 2300
in connective tissue disease, 1727t, 1739–1740, *1739*
in Goodpasture's syndrome, 1737t, 1742–1743, *1742*
in hemangiomatosis, 1746, *1746*
in hemosiderosis, 1737t, 1741–1742, *1741*
in Henoch-Schönlein purpura, 1737t, 1740
in lymphangioleiomyomatosis, 1746–1748, *1747*
in microscopic polyangiitis, *1736*, 1737t, 1739
in mitral stenosis, 1744
in mixed cryoglobulinemia, 1740
in pulmonary edema, 1579
in systemic lupus erythematosus, 1704
in tuberous sclerosis, 1748
in veno-occlusive disease, 1744, *1745*, 1746
in Wegener's granulomatosis, 1737t, 1738–1739
isolated pulmonary, 1737t, 1738
laboratory tests in, 1736, 1737t, 1738
pathogenesis of, 1738
pathology of, 1654, 1733–1734, *1734*, *1735*
penicillamine-induced, 1744
physiology of, 1736
respiratory failure in, 2415
trimellitic anhydride-induced, 1744
with capillaritis, 1734t, 1738–1741, *1739*
without capillaritis, 1734t, 1741–1748, *1741*, *1742*, 1743t, *1745–1747*
Alveolar hyperventilation. See *Hyperventilation, alveolar.*
Alveolar hypoventilation. See *Hypoventilation, alveolar.*
Alveolar macrophages. See *Macrophage(s), alveolar.*
Alveolar pressure, 60–62, *61*
blood flow distribution and, 128–129, *129*
distribution of, 128–129, *129*
elastic recoil pressure and, 799
in body plethysmography, 798–799, *799*
in pulmonary circulation three-zone model, 66, *66*
perfusion distribution and, 128–129, *129*
pulmonary vascular resistance and, 64
versus lung interstitial pressure, *137*
vessel compression and, 126
Alveolar proteinosis, pulmonary, 1789–1801
alveolar macrophage defects in, 1793
bronchoalveolar lavage in, 753, 1790, 1796–1800, *1799*
bronchoscopy in, 752
busulfan-induced, 1975
chest radiography in, 1795, *1795*
clinical features of, 1794–1796, *1795–1797*
conditions associated with, 1791, 1792t
congenital (hereditary surfactant deficiency), 318
definition of, 1789
diagnosis of, 1796
dust exposure in, 1794
etiology of, 1653t, 1793–1794
genetic defects in, 1793
in HIV infection, 1792, 1794, 2210
in immunodeficiency, 1794
in infections, 1794
Alveolar proteinosis *(Continued)*
in pulmonary edema, high-altitude, 1934–1935, *1935*
in silicosis, 1818, 1818t, 1824
natural history of, 1791–1793, 1792t
pathogenesis of, 1793–1794
pathology of, 1654, 1789–1790, *1790*, *1791*
pathophysiology of, 320
prognosis for, *1799*, 1800
pulmonary function tests in, 1795, *1796*, *1797*
secondary, 1792, 1793
surfactant excess in, 1793–1794
treatment of, 1796–1800, *1799*
Alveolar ventilation, 58. See also *Hyperventilation, alveolar; Hypoventilation, alveolar.*
at high altitude, 1919
calculation of, 824–825
carbon dioxide production rate in, 156, *157*
definition of, 58
equation for, 58, 71, 180, *180*, 822, 824
failure of, hypercapnia in, 2443
in asthma, 1265
in carbon dioxide regulation, 2443
in pneumothorax, 2045
in ventilation-perfusion ratio calculation, 77
low (hypoventilation), 71–72, *72*
versus diaphragmatic paralysis, 2336
measurement of, 58
oxygen sensitivity and, 192, *192*
versus carbon dioxide exchange rate, in exercise, 208, *209*, 210
versus carbon dioxide partial pressure, 71–72, *72*, 180–181, *180*
versus pulmonary blood flow, 825
Alveolar vessels, pressures in, 60–62, *61*
pulmonary vascular resistance and, 64
versus lung volume, 126, *127*
recruitment of, 128
Alveolar-arterial oxygen gradient (A–a)$PO_2$. See *Oxygen, partial pressure of, alveolar-to-arterial difference in.*
Alveolar-capillary block, in diffusion, 809
Alveoli. See *Alveolus(i).*
Alveolitis, cryptogenic fibrosing. See *Fibrosis, idiopathic pulmonary.*
extrinsic allergic. See *Hypersensitivity pneumonitis.*
fibrosis in, 459, 462, *463*
in asbestosis, 1833–1834
in berylliosis, 1843
in filariasis, 1153–1155, *1154*, 1761–1762, *1762*
in hard metal disease, 1845
in paracoccidioidomycosis, 1128–1129
in sarcoidosis, 752
in systemic sclerosis, 1696–1697
in usual interstitial pneumonia, 1677
lymphocytic, in inflammatory bowel disease, 2270–2271
in sarcoidosis, 1726
Alveolus(i), aerosol clearance in, 354–355, *354*
aerosol deposition in, 352–354, *352*, *353*
anatomy of, 15–21, *16–18*
asbestosis of, 1833–1834
*Ascaris lumbricoides* in, 1149–1150, 1761
barrier function of, in pulmonary edema, 1583–1584, 1597–1598
blood vessels of, 126
C fibers of, 21–22, *21*, 60–62, *61*, 64, 126, *127*
calcification in, 450
capillaries of, 16, 60–62, *61*
carbon monoxide concentration in, for diffusing capacity calculation, 811
Alveolus(i) *(Continued)*
cells of, epithelial. See *Epithelium and epithelial cells, alveolar.*
cells surrounding, 1650, *1650*
clearance from, 371–374
alveolar wall in, 371
cells in, 371–372
kinetics of, 373–374
lymphatic system in, 371
macrophages in, 371–372
measurement of, 357
mechanisms of, 372–373, 373t
collagen in, 137
concretion accumulation in, 1749–1750, *1749*, *1750*
defects of, 40–42
diffuse damage of, 1650, *1651*, 1653t
drug-induced, 479t
in HIV infection, 2210
pathology of, 456, *459*, *460*
diffusion path length in, 808–809
dimensions of, aerosol studies of, 356
edema of, barrier function in, 1582–1584
blood gas analysis in, 1594–1595
chest radiography of, 1594
in heart disease, 2247–2248, 2248t
in near drowning, 1584
in oxygen toxicity, 1987
pathology of, 1579
pathophysiology of, 1578–1579, 1578t
resolution of, 1611–1613
treatment of. See *Pulmonary edema, treatment of.*
enlargement of, in chronic obstructive pulmonary disease, 1178
epithelium of. See *Epithelium and epithelial cells, alveolar.*
ferruginous bodies in, *453*
fibrosis of, in lung injury, 1586
filling of, on interstitial lung disease radiographs, 1656, *1658*, 1658t
fluid movement into, 145
gas exchange in. See *Gas exchange.*
hemorrhage into. See *Alveolar hemorrhage.*
hemosiderosis of, 1741–1742, *1741*
hypoxia of, pulmonary vasoconstriction in, 67–68, *68*, 1633–1634
immune complex deposition in, 520
increased numbers of, 483t
inflammation of. See *Alveolitis.*
injury of, in bronchiectasis, 1326
in mechanical ventilation, 2477–2478
in ozone exposure, 1895–1896
in pulmonary edema, 1586, 2248
in transfusions, 1987
leakage into, in pulmonary capillaritis, 1733, *1735*
leukemic cells in, 2291–2292
lymphangio(leio)myomatosis of, 1776
macrophages between (interstitial), *388*, 394–396
macrophages of. See *Macrophage(s), alveolar.*
mechanical properties of, 91–93, *92*
membrane of, structure of, 91–92
microlithiasis of, 1749–1750, *1749*, *1750*
oxygen toxicity to, pulmonary edema in, 147
permeability of, in adult respiratory distress syndrome, 318–319
recruitment of, in mechanical ventilation, 2476–2477, *2477*
rupture of, pneumomediastinum in. See *Pneumomediastinum.*
septa of, anatomy of, 122
defects of, 40–42

Alveolus(i) *(Continued)*
fluid and solute exchange at, 136
structure of, 126, 136
shape of, 15–16, *17*
stability of, 16
structure of, versus ventilation inequality, 60
surface area of, diffusing capacity and, 809, *809*
surface tension in, 92–93
versus terminal respiratory unit(s), 15
volume of, during breathing, 15–16, *17*
Amantadine, in influenza, 956–957, 2320–2321
AMBER (Advanced Multiple Beam Equalization Radiography) system, 641, *641–643*
Amebae, inhalation of, hypersensitivity pneumonitis in, 1869
Amebiasis, 1144–1146, *1145*
pleural effusion in, 2026
American College of Chest Physicians, fiberoptic bronchoscopy performance guidelines of, 730
American College of Radiology, chest radiography standards of, 637
for portable equipment, 640
American Conference of Government and Industrial Hygienists, threshold limit values of, 1813
American Hospital Association, patients' rights code of, 2496
American Medical Association, impairment and disability guidelines of, 898–900, 899t, 900t
American Thoracic Society, asthma impairment rating scheme of, 900, 900t
bronchoscopy guidelines of, 729t
impairment and disability evaluation guidelines of, 900, 900t
mediastinal lymphadenopathy classification of, 2129–2130, *2130*
pulmonary function normal values of, 802, 872–881
American-European Consensus Conference Definition, of acute lung injury and ARDS, 1592–1594, 1593t
Amikacin, in cystic fibrosis, 1309t
in mycobacterial infections, 1096
in *Pseudomonas aeruginosa* pneumonia, 1012
in tuberculosis, 1070
Amiloride, in cystic fibrosis, 368
Amines, metabolism of, in lung, 720
Aminoglycosides, in cystic fibrosis, 1309t, 1311–1312
in pneumonia, 998t
Enterobacteriaceae, 1011
*Klebsiella pneumoniae*, 1009
pulmonary disease due to, 1979
Aminophylline, chemistry of, 272
in asthma, 274–275
Aminorex, pulmonary disease due to, 1336, 1988–1989
pulmonary hypertension due to, 1546
Amiodarone, pleural disease due to, 2036
pulmonary disease due to, *455*, 1973, 1981–1983, *1982*, 1982t
Amitrole, exposure to, 1910
Ammonia, inhalation of, 1909
Ammonium chloride, in metabolic alkalosis, 173
Ammonium ion, excretion of, in compensation for acid-base imbalance, 161
in urine, 162
Amniocentesis, in neonatal respiratory distress syndrome diagnosis, 317
Amniotic fluid embolism, 465, 1526–1527, 2323–2324, *2324*
Amosite, 1831t
diseases due to, 1401, 2067
Amoxicillin, in cystic fibrosis, 1309t
in endocarditis prophylaxis, 731t
in pneumonia, 995t, 998t, 1001
Amoxicillin/clavulanate, in cystic fibrosis, 1309t
in pneumonia, 922t, 995t
in tuberculosis, 1070
Amphibole asbestos, 1831t
Amphotericin B, in aspergillosis, 1133, 1134, 2198t, 2201
aerosol delivery of, 359
in blastomycosis, 1120–1121, 2198t, 2201
in coccidioidomycosis, 1127–1128, 2198t, 2200
in cryptococcosis, 1130–1131, 2197, 2198t
in fungal infections, in bone marrow transplantation, 2303
in histoplasmosis, 1116–1117, 2198t, 2199
in mucormycosis, 1134
in paracoccidioidomycosis, 1129
in penicilliosis, 2198t, 2201
in sporotrichosis, 1136
Ampicillin, in endocarditis prophylaxis, 731t
in pneumonia, *Actinomyces*, 1022
*Propionibacterium*, 1022
Ampicillin/sulbactam, in pneumonia, 998t
Amrinone, as vasodilator, 302
in pulmonary edema, 1604
Amylase, in pleural fluid, 2003, 2028
in pancreatic disease, 2029
Amyloidosis, 2295–2296
in Waldenström's macroglobulinemia, 2294
of bronchi, 1368, 1481, 1481t, 2296
of lung, nodular, 1481, 1481t
parenchymal, 2296
pathology of, 450, 454, *454*, 1653t, 1654–1655, *1655*
pathogenesis of, 2295
pleural effusions in, 2016
systemic, 2296
tracheobronchial, 1481, 1481t, 2296
Amyotrophic lateral sclerosis, 2343–2345
Anabolic agents, in chronic obstructive pulmonary disease, 2462, 2510
in respiratory failure, 2346, 2462
Anaerobic infection(s), empyema as, 1032, 2017
lung abscess as, 1031
pneumonia as, 1017–1020
clinical course of, 1020
clinical manifestations of, 1017–1018, *1018*
epidemiology of, 1017
microbiologic diagnosis of, 609, 610t, 1018–1019, *1019*, 1019t
necrotizing, 1017, *1018*
prevention of, 1020
prognosis for, 1020
treatment of, 998t, 1020
sinusitis as, 916
Anaerobic metabolism, ATP production in, 165
in exercise, 199–200, *200*, 839–840
carbon dioxide production in, 205–206, *206*
in respiratory failure, 2405–2407, *2405*, 2406t
Anaerobic pneumonitis, 1017
Anaerobic threshold. See *Lactic acid (anaerobic) threshold.*
Analeptic agents, in chronic obstructive pulmonary disease, 1228
Analgesia, pulmonary function effects of, 884–885
Anaphylactic shock, 2404
Anaphylactoid purpura (Henoch-Schönlein syndrome), 1539, 1737t, 1740
Anaphylactoid syndrome of pregnancy, 2323
Anaphylaxis, in asthma, mucociliary transport and, 367–368
in immunotherapy, for allergic rhinitis, 1349
pathology of, 465–466, *466*
recurrent, versus asthma, 1269
Anastomoses, bronchopulmonary arterial, 122, *122*
Anatomic dead space. See under *Dead space.*
Anatomy, of lung. See under *Lung.*
ANCAs (antineutrophil cytoplasmic antibodies), in Wegener's granulomatosis, 1536
Anchovy paste, in pleural fluid, in amebiasis, 2025
*Ancylostoma duodenale* (hookworm) infections, 1150–1151
Andes virus (hantavirus), 946
Anemia, dyspnea in, 220
extramedullary hematopoiesis in, pleural effusion in, 2035
hemolytic, mitomycin-induced, 1976–1977
in angioimmunoblastic lymphadenopathy, 1459
in diffuse alveolar hemorrhage, 1734, 1737t
in Goodpasture's syndrome, 1743
in hemosiderosis, 1742
in penicilliosis, 2201
sickle cell, 85, 2286–2290
Anergy, in HIV infection, 1062
T-cell, 430
Anesthesia, breathing patterns in, 181
for bronchoscopy, 726, 731–732, 732t
complications of, 755–756, 756t
for labor and delivery, in asthma, 2320
for thoracoscopy, 761
in asthma treatment, 888–889, 2320, 2459
local, contraindicated in asthma, 291
pulmonary function effects of, 884–885
vasodilation in, 302
Aneurysm(s), aortic, aortography of, *657*
pulmonary artery, 1569–1570, *1570*
in Hughes-Stovin syndrome, 1542
Rasmussen's, 1569–1570
Angiitis, allergic granulomatosis with (Churg-Strauss syndrome), 1538, 1769–1771, *1770*, 1770t
pleural effusion in, 2033
in lymphomatoid granulomatosis, 1458
in microscopic polyangiitis, diffuse alveolar hemorrhage in, *1735*, 1737t, 1739
Angina pectoris, 578, 590
at high altitude, 1940
diagnosis of, 580, 581t
in pulmonary embolism, 1507
lung compliance in, 2254, 2254t
pain mechanisms in, 570
treatment of, 2400, 2401t, *2402*
versus esophageal pain, 579
Angiofollicular lymph node hyperplasia (Castleman's disease), 1460
Angiogenesis (neovascularization), chemokines in, 508, 508t, 513–514, *513–515*
in lung cancer, 1387
in repair, 496, *496*
pulmonary circulation–systemic circulation communications in, 1565
transforming growth factor-β in, 506
Angiography, bronchial, 658, *659*
computed tomography, in pulmonary embolism, 2008
digital subtraction, 658, *660*
pulmonary, 654–657, *654–656*
balloon occlusion, 655, *656*

Angiography *(Continued)*
complications of, 656–657
contrast in, 655
interpretation of, 1513
magnification, 655, *656*
normal appearance of, 1486, *1487*
of arteriovenous malformations, 1496, 1562
of bronchiolitis obliterans, 1198
of pulmonary embolism, 702, 1512–1513, *1513*, 2008
of pulmonary hypertension, 1521, *1522*, 1549, *1550*
of sequestrations, 1568, *1568*
of vasospasm, *647*
technique for, 654–657
versus ventilation-perfusion scanning, in pulmonary embolism, 702
Angioimmunoblastic lymphadenopathy, 1459–1460
Angiomata, spider, in hepatopulmonary syndrome, 2272
Angiomyolipomas, of kidney, 1784
Angioneurotic edema, angiotensin-converting enzyme inhibitor-induced, 1981
Angioscopy, pulmonary, in thromboembolic pulmonary hypertension, 1522, *1523*
Angiostatin, in angiogenesis, in lung cancer, 1387
Angiotensin I, activation of, in pulmonary circulation, 69
Angiotensin II, excess of, in cor pulmonale, 1636–1637
in pulmonary vascular resistance control, 131
Angiotensin II receptor blockers, in pulmonary hypertension, 1645
Angiotensin-converting enzyme, elevated, in sarcoidosis, 1726
Angiotensin-converting enzyme inhibitors, as vasodilators, 302
contraindicated in asthma, 291
cough due to, *559*, 560, 564
in acute respiratory distress syndrome, 2421
in cor pulmonale, 1644–1645
in pulmonary edema, 1602, 2421
in pulmonary hypertension, 1644–1645
pulmonary disease due to, 1981
Angular cells, in fetal lung, 398
Anhydrides, in plastic manufacture, asthma due to, 1857, 1858t, 1859
Aniline, ingestion of, pulmonary hypertension due to, 1546
Animal proteins, inhalation of, asthma in, 1858t
hypersensitivity pneumonitis in, 1869
Anion gap, 163–164
calculation of, 163, *164*
urine, 170
normal, 163
profiles of, in various conditions, *164*
Anion gap acidosis, 163–164, *164*
causes of, 166t
ketoacidosis as, 166–167, 166t, *167*
lactic, 164–166, *165*, 166t, 171
toxic forms of, 168
uremic, 166t, 167–168
Ankylosing spondylitis, 1710
chest pain in, 577
diagnosis of, 2369
etiology of, 2369
exercise capacity in, 2361t
pathophysiology of, 2369–2370
pulmonary function tests in, 2359t
respiratory mechanics in, 2359t
treatment of, 2370
Anode-heel effect, in radiography, 646
Anorexia, in mediastinal mass, 2083
Anoxia, lung injury in, 465, *465*
Antagonists, drug, 243–244, *244*, 268–269
Anthophyllite, 1831t
diseases due to, 1401
Anthrax, mediastinitis in, 2109
pneumonia in, 1029
Anti–basement membrane antibody disease. See *Goodpasture's syndrome.*
Antibiotics. See also specific antibiotics and diseases.
aerosol delivery of, 359
chemotherapeutic, pulmonary disease due to, 1972–1973, 1974t, 1976–1977, *1976*
in acute chest syndrome, 2288–2289
in bronchiectasis, 1331
in chronic obstructive pulmonary disease, 1225, 2462
in cough, in bronchiectasis, 564
in cystic fibrosis, ambulatory, 1309–1310, 1309t
in hospital, 1311–1312
in pneumonia, 993–999
community-acquired, 922, 922t, 993–995, 994t, 995t, 998t
intravenous-to-oral switch in, 997
nosocomial, 995–996, 996t, 998t
in respiratory failure, 2462
in shock, 2399, 2403t
in sickle cell disease, 2288–2289
in sinusitis, 563
prophylactic, for endocarditis, in bronchoscopy, 730, 731t
in lung transplantation, 2521
resistance to, in *Acinetobacter*, 1013–1014
in anaerobic bacteria, 1020
in *Burkholderia cepacia*, 1013
in Enterobacteriaceae, 1010–1011
in *Haemophilus influenzae*, 1008
in *Moraxella catarrhalis*, 1006
in *Pseudomonas aeruginosa*, 1012
in *Staphylococcus aureus*, 1004
in *Stenotrophomonas maltophilia*, 1012–1013
in *Streptococcus pneumoniae*, 1001
in tuberculosis, 619, 2184. See also *Tuberculosis, multidrug-resistant.*
susceptibility testing of, for mycobacteria, 619–620, 1045t, 1048
for pneumococci, 1001
for tuberculosis, 619
polymerase chain reaction in, 626
toxicity of, respiratory effects of, 2343
Antibody(ies). See also *Immunoglobulin(s).*
antineutrophil cytoplasmic, in diffuse alveolar hemorrhage, 1737t, 1738
antinuclear. See *Antinuclear antibodies.*
basement membrane. See *Goodpasture's syndrome.*
*Entamoeba histolytica*, 1144
function of, 2225–2226, *2225*
in alveolar injury, in transfusions, 1987
in angioimmunoblastic lymphadenopathy, 1459
in connective tissue diseases, 1695t
in dermatomyositis, 1708
in diffuse alveolar hemorrhage, 1737t, 1738
in filariasis, 1153, 1155
in human immunodeficiency virus infection, 436–437, *436*, 2173
in influenza, 949–950, 953, 955, 956
in measles, 959
in mixed connective tissue disease, 1695t
in parainfluenza virus infections, 960
in polymyositis-dermatomyositis, 1695t, 1708
Antibody(ies) *(Continued)*
in relapsing polychondritis, 1695t
in respiratory syncytial virus infections, 962
in rheumatoid arthritis, 1695t
in rhinovirus infections, 964–965
in Sjögren's syndrome, 1695t
in systemic lupus erythematosus, 1695t
in systemic sclerosis, 1695t, 1697
lectin, in amebiasis, 1144
monoclonal. See *Monoclonal antibodies.*
p53 protein, in lung cancer, 1382–1383
precipitating, in hypersensitivity pneumonitis, 1874
Antibody-dependent cytotoxic hypersensitivity, lung injury in, 466, *467*
Anticholinergic drugs, aerosol delivery of, 357, 359
as bronchodilators, 275–277, *276*
clinical uses of, 276, *276*
future trends in, 277
in asthma, 357
in chronic obstructive pulmonary disease, 357, 359, 1221–1222
mechanisms of action of, 276
selection of, 276
side effects of, 276–277
Anticoagulants. See also specific agents, e.g., *Heparin*; *Warfarin.*
hemothorax due to, 2062
in pulmonary hypertension, 1551
International Normalized Ratio in, 1519
Anti-cytokines, in pulmonary disease, 286–287, *288*
Antidiuretic hormone (vasopressin), excess of, in cor pulmonale, 1636
in lung cancer, 1379, 1421–1422
Antigen(s), antibody interactions with, 420
cluster of differentiation system for, 413, 414t, 415t
definition of, 422
*Histoplasma capsulatum*, testing for, 1116
immunoglobulin interactions with, 422
inhalation of, hypersensitivity pneumonitis in. See *Hypersensitivity pneumonitis.*
tolerance to, dendritic cells in, 397
occupational, lung injury from, 478t
superantigens as, 428
T-lymphocyte recognition of, 426–428, 427t, *428*
tolerance to, alveolar macrophages in, 393–394, *395*
Antigenic determinant, definition of, 422
Antigenic drift, of influenza virus, 950
Antigenic shift, of influenza virus, 950
Antigen-presenting cells, 431–432, *431*
dendritic cells as, 396–397
functions of, 424–428, *425*, *426*, 427t, *428*
in asthma, 1257, *1257–1259*
interstitial macrophages as, 395
Antihistamines, in allergic rhinitis, 1349
in asthma, 284
in common cold, 933
in cough, 563
Anti-inflammatory drugs. See also specific drugs, e.g., *Aspirin*; *Corticosteroid(s)*; *Nonsteroidal anti-inflammatory drugs.*
beta-adrenergic agonists as, 269
in bronchiectasis, 1331
pulmonary disease due to, 1984–1985
Antileukoprotease, in mucus, 329
Antileukotrienes, in asthma, 284–286, *284*, 498, 2456
Antimetabolites, pulmonary disease due to, 1974t, 1977, *1977*
Antimicrobial peptides, in mucus, 332
Antimicrobials. See *Antibiotics.*

Antineutrophil cytoplasmic antibodies, in diffuse alveolar hemorrhage, 1737t, 1738
in Wegener's granulomatosis, 1536
Antinuclear antibodies, drug-induced, 1974, 1986
in systemic sclerosis, 1695t, 1697
pleural effusions in, 2005
Antioxidants, in lung cancer prevention, 1404–1405
in pulmonary edema, 1610
Antiretroviral drugs, in HIV infection, antituberculosis drug interactions with, 2184
in Kaposi's sarcoma, 2206
Antitussive agents, 289, 562–564
Antiviral drugs. See also specific drugs, e.g., *Acyclovir*; *Amantadine*.
aerosol delivery of, 359
Anxiety, exercise testing in, 849
pulmonary function tests in, 849
respiratory alkalosis in, 175
smoking and, 2513
Aorta. See also *Aortography.*
aneurysm of, aortography of, *657*
coarctation of, imaging of, 683
cystic medial necrosis of, pulmonary artery aneurysms in, 1569
disorders of, as mediastinal masses, 2130
pain in, 579
dissection of, imaging of, 683, *684*, *685*
pain in, 579, 581t
pseudoaneurysms of, imaging of, 683, *686*
rupture of, imaging of, 683, *686*
Aortic bodies, function of, 189
Aortic valve, disorders of, pain in, 579
pulmonary edema in, in pregnancy, 2321
Aortitis, pain in, 579
Aortography, in aortic dissection, 683, *684*
in catheter position detection, *638*
indications for, 658
technique for, 657–658, *657–659*
AP-1 (activator protein-1), 246, 259–260
APACHE (Acute Physiologic Assessment and Chronic Health Evaluation) system, 2488, 2490
in lung injury, 1593
Apical membrane, of airway epithelia, 335
chloride channels of, 337
sodium channels of, 336–337
Apnea, C-fiber activity in, 184
in breath-hold diving, 1952
in pontine respiratory group lesions, 187
in respiratory syncytial virus infections, 963
in spinal cord injury, 2338
sleep. See *Sleep apnea.*
Apneic threshold, breathing response at, 191
Apoptosis, defects of, in lung cancer, 1386
in lymphangio(leio)myomatosis, 1779
definition of, 444
inhibition of, in asthma, 1263
microscopic appearance of, 444, *446*
of eosinophils, 528–529, *529*, *530*
of granulocytes, 528–529, *529*, *530*
of neutrophils, 524, 528–529, *529*, *530*
of T lymphocytes, 429, *430*
steps of, 444, *445*
Appetite suppressants, pulmonary disease due to, 1988–1989
pulmonary hypertension due to, 1546
Apportionment, in impairment evaluation, 904, 910
Aquaporin-1, secretion of, in alveoli, 19
Aquaporin-5, secretion of, in alveoli, 21
Arachidonic acid metabolites. See also specific substances, e.g., *Prostaglandin(s).*
as vasodilators, 300–301
Arachidonic acid metabolites *(Continued)*
biologic effects of, 497–499, 497t
in electrolyte transport, in airway epithelium, 338
in mucus hypersecretion, 333–334
in pulmonary vascular resistance control, 297
of cyclooxygenase pathway, biologic effects of, 497–499, 497t
in mucus hypersecretion, 334
of lipoxygenase pathway, endothelial permeability and, 142, *143*
ARDS. See *Acute/adult respiratory distress syndrome.*
Ardystil syndrome, 1910
Arginine hydrochloride, in metabolic alkalosis, 173
Arginine vasopressin. See *Antidiuretic hormone (vasopressin).*
Argon, characteristics of, 1958t
Arm exercise, in pulmonary rehabilitation, 2510
β-Arrestin, action of, 245, *245*
Arrhythmias, cardiac. See *Cardiac arrhythmias.*
Arsenic exposure, lung cancer in, 1400
Arterial blood gases. See *Acid-base balance and imbalance; Blood gas(es); Carbon dioxide, partial pressure of, arterial; Oxygen, partial pressure of, arterial.*
Arterialized blood, for blood gas analysis, 834
Arteriography. See *Angiography.*
Arterioles, bronchial, 1488
pulmonary, 1631–1632
anatomy of, 120
constriction of, at high altitude, 1921
obstruction of, 1642
pressure in, 1498t
technetium-99m labeled albumin studies of, 698
Arteriolitis, pulmonary, in schistosomiasis, 1164
Arteriovenous malformations, pulmonary, 1491–1494, 1557–1565
acquired, 1495
angiography in, 654, *655*
asymptomatic, 1562
causes of, 1495, 1558
chest radiography of, 1496, 1561–1562
classification of, 1557–1558, 1558t, *1559*
clinical manifestations of, 1495–1496, 1560–1561, 1560t
congenital, 1495
diagnosis of, 1561–1563
differential diagnosis of, 1496–1497
exercise in, 1563
fistula development in, 1558, *1559*
gas exchange in, 1563
guidelines for, 1565t
hemodynamics of, 1563
idiopathic, 1565
in amyloidosis, 2296
in hereditary hemorrhagic telangiectasia, 1558–1561, 1560t
in pregnancy, 1561
left-to-right shunts in, 1495
macroscopic, 1558, 1558t
microscopic, 1558, 1558t
paradoxical embolism in, 1561
pathogenesis of, 1559–1560
pathology of, 1558, *1559*
pathophysiology of, 1495, 1563–1564
pulmonary function tests in, 1496, 1563–1564
right-to-left shunt in, 1495, 1557–1558, 1562, 1563, 1565
Arteriovenous malformations *(Continued)*
screening for, 1562–1563
treatment of, 1564–1565, *1564*, 1565t
versus systemic-pulmonary communications, 1495, 1496–1497
Arteritis, giant cell (temporal), 1541
Takayasu's, 1541
Artery(ies). See *Bronchial artery(ies); Pulmonary artery(ies); specific arteries.*
Arthralgia, in *Chlamydia psittaci* pneumonia, 1026
in histoplasmosis, 1111
in sarcoidosis, 1718
Arthritis. See also *Rheumatoid arthritis.*
in relapsing polychondritis, 1695t, 1708–1710, *1709*
infectious, pain in, 577
Arthroconidia, of *Coccidioides immitis*, 1122
Aryl hydrocarbon hydroxylase, as biomarker, for lung cancer, 1406
Asbestos, biologic potency of, 1830, 1833
deposits of, 1831t
exposure to, asbestosis in. See *Asbestosis.*
benign pleural effusions in, 1839–1840
bystander, 1832
dose-response relationships in, 1401, 1833, *1833*
lung cancer in, 1400–1401, 1836–1837, 1840
mesothelioma in. See *Mesothelioma(s).*
pleural effusion in, 2033
pleural fibrosis in, 1837, *1838*, 1839
pleural plaques in, 1837
pleural to parenchymal ratio in, 1834
sources of, 1832
fibers of, definition of, 1830
inhaled, fate of, 1832–1833
types of, 1400–1401, 2067
talc contaminated with, 1841
tissue response to, 1832–1833
uses of, 1830
Asbestos bodies, *1814*, 1832–1833, *1834*
Asbestosis, 1833–1837
causation attribution in, 910
chest radiography of, 1835
clinical features of, 1834–1835
complications of, 1836
crackles in, *595*
diagnosis of, 1835–1836
epidemiology of, 1834
ferruginous body formation in, 450, *453*
historical aspects of, 1830
latency period of, 1834
legal issues in, 1835–1836
lung cancer risk in, 1401, 1836–1837, 1840
mesothelioma risk in, 1836–1837
monitoring of, 1840
natural history of, 1834
pathogenesis of, 1833–1834
pathology of, *1814*, 1833–1834, *1834*
pleural, fibrothorax in, 2063
prevention of, 1840
pulmonary function tests in, 1835
treatment of, 1840
Ascariasis, 1149–1150, 1761
Ascites, chylous, 2057
in endometriosis, 2034
in lymphangio(leio)myomatosis, 1780
in Meigs' syndrome, 2034
in tuberculosis, 1085
pancreatic, 2029
pleural effusion with, 2015, 2271
treatment of, 2015
ultrasonography of, 660, *660*
Ascorbic acid (vitamin C), in lung cancer prevention, 1405

Aspergilloma, 1132–1133, *1132*
in tuberculosis, 1063, *1063*
Aspergillosis, 1131–1134
allergic bronchopulmonary. See *Allergic bronchopulmonary aspergillosis.*
aspergilloma as, 1063, *1063*, 1132–1133, *1132*
bronchoscopy in, 745–746
chronic necrotizing, 1133
clinical features of, 2200–2201
culture in, 621–622
diagnosis of, 610t, 2201
epidemiology of, 1131
geographic distribution of, 1108, 2200
in diabetes mellitus, 2310
in HIV infection, 1134, 2198t, 2200–2201
in lung transplantation, 2522
in sarcoidosis, 1722
in transplantation, 2229–2230, *2229*
invasive, 1133–1134, *1134*, 2200–2201
microbiologic diagnosis of, 610t
organisms causing, 1131
pathology of, 474, *475*
pleural effusion in, 2023
prevention of, 2201
skin tests for, in allergic bronchopulmonary aspergillosis, 1765
spectrum of, 1131
treatment of, 359, 2201
*Aspergillus fumigatus*, colonization by, in cystic fibrosis, 1303
surfactant protein A binding to, 312
surfactant protein D binding to, 315
*Aspergillus* spores, hypersensitivity pneumonitis due to, 1869
Asphyxia, in hemoptysis, 751
in sleep apnea, 2156
in spinal cord injury, 2337
Aspiration (during breathing), bronchiectasis in, 1336
defense mechanisms against, 986
in bone marrow transplantation, 2299
in gastroesophageal reflux, 2267–2269, *2268*
in heroin use, 1980
in near drowning, 1964–1965
in neuromuscular disorders, 2331–2332
lipid accumulation in, 454–455
lung injury in, 1588t, 1591
of baby powder, 1908
of foreign bodies. See *Foreign body(ies).*
of hydrocarbons, 1908
pneumonia in, *Actinomyces*, 1020–1021
anaerobic bacterial, 1017
diagnosis of, 920
gram-negative, 1008
in polymyositis, 1708
in pregnancy, 2324
microbiology of, 988t
*Staphylococcus aureus*, 1003
prevention of, reflux reflex in, 254
Aspiration (technique), bronchoscopic, in pneumonia, 991–992
in pneumothorax, 2047, 2055
in transbronchial biopsy, 736–737, 738t, 741t
needle. See *Needle aspiration biopsy.*
transthoracic, in pneumonia, 992–993
pneumothorax in, 2051
transtracheal, in pneumonia, 609, 992, 993t
Aspiration reflex, 181
Aspirin, anion gap acidosis due to, 168
asthma due to, 1267
contraindicated in asthma, 290–291
in amphotericin reactions, 1116
in mountain sickness, 1932
in myocardial ischemia, *2401*
Aspirin *(Continued)*
pulmonary disease due to, 1984
Association studies, in asthma, 1253, 1254t
in genetic disease, 49–50, 51t
Asthma, 1247–1289
acute, chest radiography of, 666
treatment of, 280, 281
acute severe, treatment of, 1274–1276
airflow in, versus lung volume, 102
airway resistance measurement in, 798
allergic, 1270
immune response in, 437
pathology of, 1255
anaphylaxis in, mucociliary transport and, 367–368
antigen challenge in, 1175–1176
aspirin sensitivity in, 1984
atopic, pathology of, 466, *466*
beta-adrenergic receptor function in, 256
breathing in, nasal air conditioning in, 1347
brittle, 1270
bronchial responsiveness tests in, 356, 1266
bronchitis in, 1271
bronchoalveolar lavage in, 755
bronchoscopy in, 730, 755, 757
burden of, 2544
cardiac, 2447–2448
cell abnormalities in, 1175, 1175t
chest radiography of, 666
chronic, treatment of, 1276, 1277t–1278t
chronic obstructive pulmonary disease and, 1188, *1188*, 1199–1200
chronic severe, 1276, 1277t
classification of, 1176, 1176t, 1270–1272, 1271t
clinical features of, 1181, 1266–1272, 1269t, 1271t
occupational, 1856–1857, *1856*
severe, 2453, 2453t
versus severity, 1270, 1271t
cough in, 289, 559, *559*, 563, 588
cough-variant, 1266
definition of, 1175, 1188, *1188*, 1247–1248, 1853–1854
diagnosis of, 1859, *1860*
differential diagnosis of, 1267, 1268–1269, 1269t
difficult, 1270
diving and, 1955, 1963
drug-induced, 1271
dyspnea in, 541, 543
education on, 2546–2550, 2546t, 2550t
electrocardiography in, 2453
environmental factors in, 1854–1855
epidemiology of, 1176, 1248–1252, *1250*, *1251*, 2544
national survey data on, 2551–2552, *2551*
occupational, 1854
etiology of, 1176–1178, 1175t, 1176t, *1177*
air pollution as, 1892, 1894–1895
occupational, 1853, 1853t, 1857, 1858t, 1859
exacerbation of, work-related, 1854
exercise-induced, 218, 843, 1271
extrinsic, 1176, 1176t, 1270
fatal, pathology of, 1255
fatality-prone, 1267
genetics of, 288, 1248, 1252–1253, 1254t, 2545
high altitude effects on, 1941
history in, 1266–1267
hospitalization in, 1249, 1272–1273, 1275
immediate response in, 1260, *1260*
impairment in, 900, 900t, 902, 903t
evaluation of, 907–908
in allergic bronchopulmonary aspergillosis, 1538, 1763, 1765
Asthma *(Continued)*
in allergic granulomatosis and angiitis, 1769–1770
in Churg-Strauss syndrome, 1538, 1769–1770
in elderly persons, 1269–1270
in eosinophilic pneumonia, 1767
in gastroesophageal reflux, 2267–2269, *2268*
in hard metal disease, 1845
in HIV infection, 2209
in hypersensitivity pneumonitis, 1878
in hyperthyroidism, 2310
in hyperventilation, 1270
in infections, 1251–1252, *1251*
in influenza, 953–954
in "poor perceivers," 1270
in pregnancy, 2319–2320
in rhinovirus infections, 966
inflammation in, 1175–1177, *1177*
intrinsic, 1176, 1176t, 1270
irritant-induced, 1853, 1854, 1904
laboratory studies in, 1267–1268
late response in, 1260–1261, *1260*, 1856, *1856*
lung injury in, 482
mild, treatment of, 1277t–1278t
morbidity in, 272, 1272–1273
mortality in, 1248–1249, 1272
due to beta-adrenergic agonists, 272
pathology of, 1255
mucociliary transport abnormalities in, 367–368
natural history of, 1272–1274
nocturnal, 270, 275, 1271
objectives for, in Healthy People national initiative, 2547, 2548t
occupational, 374–375, 908, 1853–1860
causes of, 1853, 1853t
definition of, 1853–1854
irritant-induced, 1853, 1854
new-onset, 1854–1860
clinical features of, 1856–1857, *1856*
diagnosis of, 1859, *1860*
epidemiology of, 1854
etiology of, 1857, 1858t, 1859
pathophysiology of, 1854–1856
treatment of, 1859–1860
sensitizer-induced, 1853
terminology of, 1853–1854
work-aggravated, 1853, 1854
pathogenesis of, 1175–1178, 1175t, 1176t, *1177*
pathology of, 480t, 482, 1175, 1175t, 1253–1256
airway mucus changes in, 1254–1255
allergic versus nonallergic, 1255
fatal, 1255
large versus small airway, 1255
structural airway changes in, 1253–1254, *1255*
versus severity, 1255
pathophysiology of, 1256–1263
airway epithelium in, 1258, 1259t
airway remodeling in, 1263, *1263*, 1264t
antigen presentation in, 1257
B lymphocytes in, *1259*, 1260
basophils in, *1259*, 1260
cytokines in, 1257–1258
dendritic cells in, 1257, *1257–1259*
eosinophils in, 1260–1261
evolution in, 1256, *1256*
immunoglobulin E in, *1259*, 1260
inflammation in, 1175–1177, *1177*, 1262–1263, *1263*, 1264t
inflammatory mediators in, 256, *257*
leukocyte accumulation in, 1261

Asthma *(Continued)*
macrophages in, 1261
mast cells in, *1259*, 1260
mucus hypersecretion in, 1262
muscarinic receptors in, 253
neural mechanisms in, 256
neurogenic mechanisms in, 1262–1263
neutrophils in, 1261
occupational, 1854–1856
overview of, 1256–1257, *1257–1259*
smooth muscle cells in, 1262
T lymphocytes in, 1257
patient education on, 2533, 2535–2540, 2535t–2539t
physical examination in, 599t, 1267
physiology of, 1263–1266, *1264*
pneumomediastinum in, 2100
precipitation of attacks in, 1274
preoperative evaluation in, 888–889
prevention of, cromones in, 283–284
government in. See *Government role, in asthma secondary prevention.*
progression of, 1273
provocation testing in, 852–853, 1266, 1268
pulmonary function tests in, 786–787, 851–853, 1265–1268
occupational, 1859, *1860*
recurrence risk of, in relatives, 48
refractory. See *Status asthmaticus.*
remission of, 1272
ventilation-perfusion ratios in, 83, *84*
research on, 2544–2546
risk factors for, 1249–1252, *1250, 1251*
seasonal, 1270
sensitizer-induced, 1853, 1853t
severe. See also *Status asthmaticus.*
chronic, 1276, 1277t
severity of, 1270, 1271t
versus pathology, 1255
smooth muscle in, hyperresponsiveness of, 1176–1177, *1177*
steroid-dependent, 1270
steroid-resistant, 280, 281, 1270
terminology of, 1853–1854
treatment of, 1274–1276. See also *Pharmacology, airway.*
acute, 280, 281
acute severe, 1274–1276
adhesion molecular blockers in, 287
aerosolized drugs in, 357, 359
aminophylline in, 274–275
anticholinergic drugs in, 275–277, *276*
anti-cytokines in, 286–287, *288*
antihistamines in, 284
antileukotrienes in, 284–286, *284*, 498, 2456
antitussives in, 289
atrial natriuretic peptide in, 278
avoidance of allergens in, 1276
beta$_2$-adrenergic agonists in, 268–272, *268–272*, 269t, 271t, 2453–2455, 2454t
chronic, 1276, 1277t–1278t
clinical practice guidelines for, 2552–2556, 2554t, 2555t
compliance with, 2538
controller drugs in, 278–284, *279–281*, 279t, 282t
corticosteroids in, 278–283, *279–281*, 279t, 282t, 286, 2454t, 2455
cough control in, 289
cromones in, 283–284
drugs contraindicated in, 290–291
enzyme inhibitors in, 288
for breathlessness, 289
furosemide in, 288

Asthma *(Continued)*
genetic aspects of, 288–289
hydrocortisone in, 280
immunomodulators in, 287–288
immunosuppressive therapy in, 286
immunotherapy in, 286
in pregnancy, 2319–2320
inflammatory mediator antagonists in, 284–286, *284*, 287t
ipratropium bromide in, 2454t, 2455
lipoxygenase inhibitors in, 284–286, *284*
magnesium in, 2455
mechanical ventilation in, 2456–2460, *2457, 2458*
mild, 1277t–1278t
mucoregulators in, 289
natural history and, 1273–1274
nedocromil in, 283–284
neuromodulators in, 288
new drugs for, 286–289, 287t, *288*
nocturnal, 270, 275
occupational, 1859–1860
outcomes of, 2553, 2555t
oxygen in, 2453
pharmacologic, 1274, 2453–2456, 2454t
phosphodiesterase inhibitors in, 287
research on, 2544–2546
self-management program for, 2533, 2535–2540, 2535t–2539t
severe, mechanical ventilation in, 2456–2460, *2457, 2458*
pharmacologic, 2453–2456, 2454t
spirometric evaluation of, 784
surfactant in, 320
theophylline in, 272–275, *273, 274*, 273t–275t, 2454t, 2455
transcription factor blockers in, 288
ventilatory stimulants in, 289–290
ventilation-perfusion ratios in, 83, *84*, 697–698
versus allergic bronchopulmonary aspergillosis, 1131–1132
wheezing in, 596
work-aggravated, 1853, 1854
Astronauts, pulmonary circulation in, 66
Asymmetric film-screen radiography systems, 640, *640*
Ataxia-telangiectasia, immunodeficiency in, 2233t, 2239–2240
Atelectasis, after cardiac surgery, 886
bronchoscopy in, 753
in cystic fibrosis, 1305, 1312
in pulmonary embolism, 1510, *1510*
in sarcoidosis, 1721–1722
in sickle cell disease, 2288
mechanical aspects of, 113
physical findings in, 599t
postoperative, 886, 2381–2383, 2382t
prevention of, 2382–2383, 2382t
round, as pseudotumor, 1481
computed tomography of, 666, *667*
in asbestos exposure, 1837, *1838*, 1839
treatment of, in cystic fibrosis, 1312
versus emphysema, 1198
Atenolol, preoperative, in cardiac risk reduction, 883
pulmonary disease due to, 1983
Atherosclerosis, high altitude effects on, 1940
Athletes. See also *Exercise.*
highly fit, ventilation response to exercise in, 218–220
pulmonary hemorrhage in, 69
training of, at high altitudes, 1928–1929
Atmosphere, barometric pressure in, versus altitude, 1915, 1916t
oxygen partial pressure in, versus altitude, 1915, 1916t

Atopy, chronic obstructive pulmonary disease in, 1199–1200
versus asthma prevalence, 1249–1250, *1250*, 1251
Atovaquone, in *Pneumocystis carinii* pneumonia, 2191t, 2192–2195, 2195t
ATP. See *Adenosine triphosphate.*
Atrial natriuretic peptide, as bronchodilator, 278
in cor pulmonale pathogenesis, 1637
Atrophy, cellular, 446
Atropine, as bronchodilator, 275, 277
in bronchoscopy, 730
in cardiac arrhythmias, in shock, 2403t
in organophosphate poisoning, 2343
side effects of, 277
Attenuation, of X-rays, in computed tomography, 661
Attorney, durable powers of, 2494
Attribution, in impairment evaluation, 910
Auramine O, for *Mycobacterium*, 1043, *1044*, 1046
Auscultation, of chest, 597–599, 599t
Authority, source of, in ethical decision making, 2495
Autoimmune disorder(s). See also *Connective tissue disease(s);* specific disorders.
angioimmunoblastic lymphadenopathy as, 1459
lymphocytic interstitial pneumonia in, 1687t
pathogenesis of, 436–437, 501
prevention of, T-lymphocyte tolerance in, 429–430
primary biliary cirrhosis as, 2275–2276
Autolysis, of cells, in necrosis, 444
Autonomic nervous system, 249–256
adrenergic receptors in, *250*, 255–256
afferent nerves in, 250–252, *251*
bronchodilator nerves in, 255–256
C fibers of, 21–22, *21*, 252
in respiratory control, 182t, 183–184
calcitonin gene-related peptide in, 250, *250*, 255
catecholamines in, 255
cholinergic nerves and reflexes in, *250*, 252–254, *253*
cotransmission in, 250, *251*
defense reflexes in, 252
dysfunction of, in asthma, 256
in chronic obstructive pulmonary disease, 256
in carotid body innervation, 189
in mucus secretion regulation, 332–333
in neurogenic inflammation, 254–255, *254*
in pulmonary circulation control, 121, 131
in visceral pain, 568
inhibitory nonadrenergic noncholinergic nerves in, *250*, 256
interactions among components of, 250
muscarinic receptors in, *240*, 242, 253, *253*
of airways. See *Airway(s), autonomic innervation of.*
of lung, 21–22
overview of, 249–250, *250, 251*
pulmonary vascular resistance effects of, 64
receptors in, 251
sympathetic nerves in, 255
tachykinins in, 254–255
Autonomy, as ethical principle, 2491–2492
Auto-PEEP effect. See *Positive end-expiratory pressure, intrinsic.*
Autosomal inheritance, 45
Avoidance, in allergic rhinitis, 1348–1349
in asthma, in pregnancy, 2319
occupational, 1859–1860
in byssinosis, 1862

Avoidance *(Continued)*
in hypersensitivity pneumonitis, 1878–1879
Azathioprine, in bronchiolitis obliterans, 1366
in drug-induced lung disease, 1693t
in microscopic polyangiitis, 1739
in pulmonary fibrosis, 1681t, 1682
pulmonary disease due to, 1977, *1977*
Azithromycin, in cystic fibrosis, 1309t
in endocarditis prophylaxis, 731t
in *Mycobacterium avium* complex infections, 1091, 2185, 2186
in pneumonia, 922t, 995t, 998t
*Legionella*, 1016
*Pneumocystis carinii*, 2195
in tuberculosis, in HIV infection, 2184
Aztreonam, in pneumonia, 998t

## B

B lymphocytes, 416–422
alternative RNA splicing in, 420
antigen interactions with, 422
cluster of differentiation system for, 413–414, 414t
defects of, common variable immunodeficiency in, 2233t, 2235
hypogammaglobulinemia with hyperimmunoglobulin M in, 2236
in severe combined immunodeficiency, 2233t, 2239
development of, 415, 421, *421*, *422*
epitopes of, 422
functions of, 421–422, 2225–2226, *2225*
immunoglobulin formation in. See *Immunoglobulin(s).*
in asthma, 1260, *1260*
in HIV infection, 2173
in lymphoma, 1456, 1456t
in sarcoidosis, 1725
intercalation of, in airway epithelium, 10, *11*
receptor editing of, 422
receptors for, 416, *417–419*, 418
receptors on, 414, 414t
self-tolerance of, 422
T lymphocyte interactions with, 414, 432–434, *433*
trafficking of, 435–436
B7-1 (CD80) molecule, in T-lymphocyte activation, 431–432, *431*
B7-2 (CD86) molecule, in T-lymphocyte activation, 431–432, *431*
Baby powder aspiration, 1908
Bacille Calmette-Guérin, in tuberculosis immunization, 1089–1090, 2185
*Bacillus anthracis* infection, mediastinitis as, 2109
pneumonia as, 1029
*Bacillus* infection, pneumonia as, 1030
Baclofen, in hiccups, 2350
BACTEC culture method, for fungi, 621
Bacteremia, *Haemophilus influenzae*, 2179
in bronchoscopy, 756
in lymphoproliferative disorders, 925
lung injury in, 1587, 1588t, 1589
*Mycobacterium tuberculosis*, 1056
pneumococcal, 1000, 2179
*Pseudomonas aeruginosa*, 1011
*Staphylococcus aureus*, 1004
Bacteria. See also specific bacteria and diseases.
alveolar macrophage protection against, 390, *391*, 392
immune response to, extracellular, 2224–2226, *2226*
intracellular, 2226, *2227*
Bacteria *(Continued)*
inhalation of, hypersensitivity pneumonitis in, 1868
pneumonia due to. See *Pneumonia, pyogenic.*
resident, virus effects on, 931–932
surfactant protein A binding to, 312
surfactant protein D binding to, 315
virulence factors of, pneumonia and, 986
*Bacterium anitratum* (*Acinetobacter*) pneumonia, 1013–1014
*Bacteroides fragilis* pneumonia, 1019, 1019t, 1020
Bagassosis, 375, 1868
BAL. See *Bronchoalveolar lavage.*
Balloons, in angiography, 655, *656*
in arteriovenous malformation embolization, 1564
in esophageal pressure measurement, 800, *800*
BALT (bronchus-associated lymphoid tissue), lymphocytes in, 435
Baritosis, 1842
Barodontalgia, 1957
Barotrauma, 1955–1957
arterial gas embolism in, 1955
clinical manifestations of, 1955–1956, *1956*
cutaneous, 1957
definition of, 1954
dental, 1957
facial, 1957
gastrointestinal, 1957
in asthma, 2453
in mechanical ventilation, in pulmonary edema, 1607
in status asthmaticus, 2456–2457, *2457*
versus hypercapnia, 2443
inner ear, 1957
lung injury in, 475
middle ear, 1956
pathophysiology of, 475, 1955
pneumomediastinum in, 475, 2099–2102, 2101t
pulmonary, 475, 1955–1956, *1956*
sinus, 1957
squeeze in, 1955
vertigo in, 1956–1957
Barrier(s), blood-gas. See *Blood-gas barrier.*
endothelial, 139
epithelial, in airway, 335
Bartter's disease, metabolic alkalosis in, 172
Basal cells, of airway epithelium, *9*, 10
of mucosa, 360
Baseline Dyspnea Index, 544
Baseline function, spirometry in, 784–785, *785*
Basement membrane, antibodies to. See *Goodpasture's syndrome.*
of endothelium, 143–144
Basidiospores, hypersensitivity pneumonitis due to, 1869
Basolateral membrane, of airway epithelium, 335
chloride channels of, 337–338
potassium channels of, 337
sodium-potassium ATPase of, 337
sodium-potassium-chloride cotransporter of, 338
Basophils, in asthma, 1260, *1260*
Bayou virus (hantavirus) infections, 945–947
B-cell–attracting chemokine, receptor for, 511–512, 511t
*BCL2* genes and products, in lung cancer, 1386
in lymphangio(leio)myomatosis, 1779
Beam equalization radiography, 640–642, *641–643*
Beclomethasone, chemical structure of, *278*
Beclomethasone *(Continued)*
in chronic obstructive pulmonary disease, 1224
pharmacokinetics of, 282
Bed, rocking, in diaphragmatic paralysis, 2337
in neuromuscular disorders, 2347
Beer's law, in oximetry, 835
Behavioral disorders, at high altitude, 1924
Behçet's syndrome, 1710, 1710t
diffuse alveolar hemorrhage in, 1740
pulmonary manifestations of, 1541–1542
Belt, pneumatic, in neuromuscular disorders, 2347
Bends. See *Decompression sickness.*
Beneficence, as ethical principle, 2490–2491
Benign metastasizing leiomyoma, 1480
Benzo(*a*)pyrene exposure, lung cancer in, 1401–1402, 1416
Bernoulli equation, for pressure drop, 97–98, *100*, 101
Beryllium lung disease, 1842–1844
cancer in, 1402–1403
pathology of, *469*
Beta$_2$-adrenergic agonists, 268–272. See also specific drugs.
anti-inflammatory effects of, 269
chemistry of, 268, *268*
clinical uses of, 269–270
corticosteroids with, 270
desensitization to, 271
future trends in, 272
in asthma, 1274–1276, 1277t–1278t, 2453–2455, 2454t
aerosol delivery of, 357
in pregnancy, 2319–2320
mortality from, 1248–1249
theophylline with, 275
in bronchiectasis, 564
in bronchiolitis obliterans, 1366
in chronic obstructive pulmonary disease, 357, 2460–2461, 2461t
in cystic fibrosis, 1310
in respiratory failure, 2460–2461, 2461t
in secretion clearance, in neuromuscular disorders, 2346
in status asthmaticus, 2453–2455, 2454t
inhaled, 268–270
long-acting, 270
mechanisms of action of, 268–269, *269*, *270*, 270t
oral, 270
safety of, 271–272
selection of, 270
side effects of, 271, 271t
vasodilating effects of, 300
Beta$_2$-adrenergic antagonists, pulmonary disease due to, 1983–1984
Beta-adrenergic receptor(s), agonist action on, 268–269, *269*, *270*, 270t
corticosteroid effects on, 245, 280
cross-talk with, 242–243, *242*
desensitization of, 244–245, *245*
distribution of, 268–269
desensitization and, 271
dysfunction of, in airway smooth muscle, 245
functions of, *250*
in bronchodilation, 255–256
in mucus secretion regulation, 333
in pulmonary circulation, 131
ontogeny of, 245
reserve numbers of, 271
structure of, 234, *235*
subtypes of, 241–242
Beta-adrenergic receptor-specific kinase, action of, 244–245, *245*

Beta-blockers, contraindicated in asthma, 290
  preoperative, in cardiac risk reduction, 883–884
Beta-carotene, lung cancer and, 1385, 1404–1405
Beta-hydroxybutyrate accumulation, in diabetic ketoacidosis, 166–167, *167*
Bicarbonate, acid-base disorder classification by, 160t
  carbon dioxide formation from, 155, 205–206, *206*
  excessive intake of, metabolic alkalosis in, 172
  formation of, 86
    from carbon dioxide, 155
    in kidney, 162
  in anion gap calculation, 163–164
  in high altitude acclimatization, *1917*
  in hypercapnia, 161
  in hypocapnia, 161
  in lactate buffering, 839–840
  in metabolic acidosis therapy, 171, 1966
  in urine, 162
  loss of, in diarrhea, 169–170
    in renal tubular acidosis, 168–169
  measurement of, 156
  normal concentration of, 156
  resorption of, 162
  standard, 156
  transport of, 86, *87*
  versus carbon dioxide, 156–160, *157*, *159*
Bile, in pleural space, 2030–2031
  pigments of, in cell injury, 450
Biliary tract, cirrhosis of, in cystic fibrosis, 1306–1307, 1312–1313
    primary, 2275–2276
  pleural fistulas with, 2030–2031
Biologic markers, for lung cancer, 1405–1406
  for smoking, 1405–1406
Biologic warfare agents, 1906–1907
Biomedical ethics. See *Ethics.*
Biopsy, bone marrow, in histoplasmosis, 1115
  brush, technique for, 733
  carinal, 741
  forceps, in bronchoscopy, 733–734
  in vasculitis, 1535
  lung, bronchoscopy in, 733–734, 741, 741t
    in allergic granulomatosis and angiitis, 1770, *1770*
    in allograft rejection, 2523, 2524
    in amyloidosis, 2296
    in ascariasis, 1150
    in aspergillosis, 1133
    in cancer, 1422, 1427
      for staging, 741
      metastatic, 1472–1473
      open, 763
      percutaneous, 760–761
      techniques for, 739t
      transbronchial, 736–737, 738t
    in carcinoid tumor, 1461
    in filariasis, *1154*
    in hepatopulmonary syndrome, 2272
    in HIV infection, 2177–2178
    in Hodgkin's disease, 1454
    in hypersensitivity pneumonitis, 1876
    in infections, 743t
    in interstitial disease, 1666, 1697
    in Kaposi's sarcoma, 2205
    in lymphangio(leio)myomatosis, 1783
    in lymphocytic interstitial pneumonia, 1687
    in lymphoma, 2207
    in metastasis, 1472–1473
    in pneumonia, 611, *612*, 993
      cytomegalovirus, 943
Biopsy *(Continued)*
      eosinophilic, 1767
      herpes simplex virus, 949
    in pulmonary edema, 1591
    in pulmonary fibrosis, 1678
    in pulmonary hypertension, 1550
    in pulmonary veno-occlusive disease, 1550
    in sarcoidosis, 1725
    in silicosis, 1823–1824
    in strongyloidiasis, 1152, *1152*
    in systemic sclerosis, 1697
    in toxoplasmosis, 1148–1149
    in tuberculosis, 1065
    in Wegener's granulomatosis, 1536, *1537*
    mediastinotomy in, 762–763
    microscopy of, 616–617
    of benign tumors, 1477
    of nodule, computed tomography guidance in, 663, *663*
    open, 763
    percutaneous, 760–761
    pneumothorax in, 2051
    radiographic guidance of, computed tomography in, 679
    specimen processing in, 611–613, *612*, 612t
    transbronchial, 734, 2177–2178
    transthoracic needle, 760–761
  lymph node, bronchoscopy in, 741, 741t
    in lung cancer, 1427
    mediastinal, 762
    scalene, 763
  mediastinal, 2087–2090
    anterior mediastinotomy in, 2089–2090
    mediastinoscopy in, 2089–2090
    mediastinotomy in, 762–763
    needle aspiration, 2088–2089, *2089*
    thoracoscopy in, 2090
  pleural, 2008–2010
    in mesothelioma, 2069
    in metastatic disease, 2074
  radiographic guidance of, computed tomography in, 663, *663*, 679
    ultrasonography in, 661
  transbronchial, in allograft rejection, 2523, 2524
    in pneumonia, 993
    of mediastinum, 2087–2090, *2089*
Biot's breathing, inspection of, 597
Bird breeder's lung. See *Hypersensitivity pneumonitis.*
Bird fever (psittacosis), 624, 998t, 1026
  genetic tests for, 626
Bischloroethyl nitrosourea, pulmonary disease due to, 1977, *1977*
Bis(chloromethyl) ether exposure, lung cancer in, 1401
Bistable oscillator model, of respiratory rhythm generation, 188–189
Bithionol, in paragonimiasis, 1162
Black Creek Canal virus (hantavirus) infections, 945–947
Black lung. See *Coal-workers' pneumoconiosis.*
Black Lung Benefits Act, impairment and disability evaluation for, 902
Blastoma(s), of lung, 1463
Blastomycosis, 1117–1121
  chest radiography of, 1119, *1121*
  clinical manifestations of, 1119–1120, *1119*, 2201
  culture in, 622–623, 1120
  diagnosis of, 626, 1120, *1120*
  dimorphism in, 1107
  epidemiology of, 1117–1118
Blastomycosis *(Continued)*
  extrapulmonary manifestations of, 1119–1120
  geographic distribution of, 2201
  histopathology of, 1119
  history of, 1117
  immune response to, 1118–1119
  in dog population, 1118
  in HIV infection, 1120, 1121, 2198t, 2201
  incubation period for, 1119
  microbiologic diagnosis of, 610t
  pathogenesis of, 1118–1119
  pleural effusion in, 2023–2024
  self-limited, 1121, *1121*
  skin tests in, 1117–1118, 1120
  treatment of, 1120–1121, *1121*, *1122*, 2201
Bleaches, chlorine exposure due to, 1905–1906
Blebs, in emphysema, 1205
  subpleural, rupture of, pneumothorax in, 2045
Bleeding. See *Hemorrhage.*
Bleomycin, in pleurodesis, in metastatic disease, 2075
  pulmonary disease due to, 1972–1973, 1976, *1976*
Blood, cancer metastasis through, 1469, *1471*, *1472*
  changes of, at high altitude, 1921–1922
  clotting of, in hemothorax, 2061
  culture of. See *Culture(s), blood.*
  dilution of, acidosis in, 163, *164*, 170
  expectoration of. See *Hemoptysis.*
  in pleural space. See *Hemothorax.*
  viscosity of, versus pulmonary vascular resistance, 126–127, *128*
  volume of, at high altitude, 1921
    distribution of, during water immersion, 1952
    in pregnancy, 2318
Blood and bone marrow transplantation, 2296–2304
  airflow obstruction in, 2300–2301
  aspiration in, 2299
  bronchiolitis obliterans in, 1364, 1366, 2300–2301
  complications of, 2297–2298, 2297t
  cytomegalovirus infections in, 942, 943, 945
  diffuse infiltrates in, 2298–2299
  graft-versus-host disease in, 2297–2298, 2300–2301
  idiopathic pneumonia syndrome in, 2299–2300
  in chronic granulomatous disease, 2237
  indications for, 2297
  mucositis in, 2299
  parenchymal lesions in, 2299
  pleural effusion in, 2033, 2299
  pneumonia in, 925
    bacterial, 2303–2304
    fungal, 2303
    mycobacterial, 2304
    *Pneumocystis carinii*, 2304
    viral, 2301–2303
  preparation for, 2297
  pulmonary function tests in, 2298, 2301
  pulmonary hemorrhage in, 2300
  pulmonary veno-occlusive disease in, 2301
  respiratory failure in, 2298
  technique for, 2297
  toxoplasmosis in, 2304
Blood flow, at high altitude, in brain, 1923
    in exercise, 1927
  in bronchial circulation, 121
  in carotid bodies, 189
  in exercise, at high altitude, 1927
  in pulmonary circulation. See *Pulmonary circulation.*

Blood flow *(Continued)*
magnetic resonance imaging appearance of, 664
symbols for, 2565
terminology of, 2563
Blood gas(es), 829–837. See also *Acid-base balance and imbalance; Carbon dioxide; Oxygen.*
criteria for, in gas exchange impairment, 901t
in acute inflammatory polyneuropathy, 2341–2342
in chronic obstructive pulmonary disease, 1192, 1194
in cystic fibrosis, 1304, 1304t
in exercise, 839, *839*, 840
in HIV infection, 2176
in near drowning, 1965, 1965t
in neuromuscular disorders, 2332
in obstructive diseases, 1182
in portopulmonary hypertension, 2275
in pulmonary edema, 1594–1595
in pulmonary embolism, 1510
in pulmonary hypertension, 1548
in sleep, 1194, 2153
measurement of, 156, 830–837
carbon dioxide as, 156, 831–832, *832*, 836–837, *836*, *837*
in impairment and disability evaluation, 899, 906
invasive, 830–834, *831*, *832*
noninvasive, 834–837, *835–837*
oxygen as, 830, 832–836, *832*, *835*, 906. See also *Oximetry.*
pH, 830–831, *831*. See also *pH, blood.*
sample collection for, 834
theoretical aspects of, 829–830
Blood pressure. See also *Hypertension; Hypotension.*
at high altitude, 1920, 1940
in exercise testing, 842
sleep apnea effects on, 2158–2159, *2158*
systemic, in venous return, 2386–2387
versus pulmonary circulation, 60
Blood-gas barrier, blood contact time with, 119
diffusion properties of, 75
dimensions of, 72
heart disease effects on, 2248–2249
oxygen diffusion through, hemoglobin reactions with, 73–74, *74*
pulmonary venous hypertension effects on, 2248–2249
stress on, 68–69
structure of, 70
structures surrounding (blood-gas interface), anatomy of, 122
thickened, oxygen diffusion through, 73, *73*
Blood-gas membrane, mechanical properties of, 91–93, *92*
Blood-gas partition coefficient, of inert gases, *81*
Blue bloaters, in chronic obstructive pulmonary disease, 1634
Bochdalek's hernia, mediastinal protrusion of, 2130–2131
Body mass index, 2370–2371, 2371t
Body plethysmography, in airway resistance measurement, 798–799, *799*
in chest wall motion measurement, 105–106
in functional residual capacity measurement, 57–58
in lung volume measurement, 793–798
pressure (closed-type), 793–794, *794*
pressure-volume, 794–795, *795*
problems with, 797–798
thoracic gas volume in, 795–797, *796*
Body plethysmography *(Continued)*
volume (open-type), 794, *794*
Body size. See also *Obesity.*
pulmonary function test effects of, 803
versus diffusing capacity, 814
Body-wrap ventilators, in neuromuscular disorders, 2347
Boerhaave's syndrome, mediastinitis in, 2106–2107, *2107*
pneumomediastinum in, 2099
Bohr effect, in oxygen dissociation curve, 86
Bohr equation, for alveolar ventilation, 58
for physiologic dead space, 58, 80, 823–824
for respiratory dead space, 822
Bohr integration, 73
Bombesin, in mucus secretion, 333
Bone(s), coccidioidomycosis of, 1124–1125
hypertrophy of, in lung disease. See *Hypertrophic pulmonary osteoarthropathy.*
infarction of, in sickle cell disease, 2288
loss of, in metabolic acidosis, 168–171
lung cancer effects on, 1421, 1421t
metastasis to, treatment of, 1435
myeloma of, 1464, 2292–2294, 2293t
pain in, in sickle cell disease, 2287
sarcoidosis of, 1723, *1723*
tuberculosis of, 1081–1083, *1082*
tumors of, metastasis of, to lung, 1474
Bone marrow, B lymphocyte development in, 421–422, *421*
biopsy of, in histoplasmosis, 1115
monocyte development in, 399, *400*
myeloma of, 1464, 2292–2294, 2293t
transplantation of. See *Blood and bone marrow transplantation.*
Bone morphogenetic protein-4, in lung development, 39
BOOP. See *Bronchiolitis obliterans organizing pneumonia.*
*Bordetella pertussis* infections, cough in, 560
Borg scale, of breathlessness, 544, 545t
in exercise, in pulmonary disease, *214*
Botulism, 2342–2343
Bötzinger complex, of medulla, 185–186, *185*
Boyle's law, 102
in diving, 1954–1955, *1955*
in functional residual capacity measurement, 58
Brachial plexopathy, computed tomography in, 671–672
in Pancoast tumor, 1430
magnetic resonance imaging in, 671–672
Brachytherapy, in lung cancer, endobronchial, 742, 1433–1434
Bradycardia, in legionellosis, 1014
Bradykinin, as inflammatory mediator, 258
in electrolyte transport, in airway epithelium, 338
in pharyngitis pathogenesis, 933
in pulmonary vascular resistance control, 131
metabolism of, in pulmonary circulation, 69
Brain, abscess of, in arteriovenous malformations, 1561
in sinusitis, 916
in toxoplasmosis, 2203
acid-base status of, ventilatory response and, 192–193, *193*
arterial air embolism in, 1955–1956
blood flow in, at high altitude, 1923
chemoreceptors of, 190, *190*
function of, at high altitude, 1917–1918
cortex of, in breathing control, 187
edema of, high-altitude, 1930t, 1932–1933
in mountain sickness, 1930
function of, at high altitude, 1923–1924
Brain *(Continued)*
hypoxia of, in hyperventilation, 2148
injury of, hyperventilation in, 2147
metastasis to, treatment of, 1431, 1435–1436
respiratory complex of, 542–543, *542*
tuberculosis of, 1083–1084, *1084*
vasoconstriction in, in hyperventilation, 2148
Waldenström's macroglobulinemia effects on, 2294
Brain death, ethical decision making in, 2496
Brain natriuretic peptide, in cor pulmonale pathogenesis, 1637
Brain stem disorders, hypoventilation in, 2140–2144, 2140t
Branches, of bronchi, development of, 35–36, *36*, *37*
of bronchial arteries, 121
of pulmonary arteries, 120, 1486, 1488, 1631–1632, *1632*
*Branhamella (Moraxella) catarrhalis* infections. See *Moraxella (Branhamella) catarrhalis infections.*
Breast carcinoma, metastasis from, to lung, *1471*, *1473*, 1474
to pleura, 2073
Breastfeeding, tuberculosis in, treatment of, 1074
Breath sounds. See *Lung sounds.*
Breath-holding time, in breathing control assessment, 818
Breathing. See also *Expiration; Inhalation; Inspiration; Ventilation.*
active cycle of, in chest physical therapy, 370
after apnea, 184
airflow in, mechanics of, *42*, 95
airway obstruction variation with, 1174
Biot's, 597
breath-holding time in, 180
cessation of. See *Apnea; Sleep apnea.*
Cheyne-Stokes, 179, 597, 2161
control of, 179–196, 2140, 2445–2446, *2445*, *2446*
after lung transplantation, 2525–2526
assessment of, 816–829
breath-holding time in, 818
factors affecting, 818
hypercapnic response in, 818–820, *819*, 877
hypoxic response in, 818–821, *820*, 878
inspiratory occlusion pressure in, 819–820, *820*
preparation for, 818
theoretical aspects of, 816–818
at high altitudes, 1916–1918, *1916*, *1917*
behavioral, 179–180
carbon dioxide levels in, 190–191, *191*
central nervous system in, 184–188, *185*, *187*
chemical, 189–193, *190–193*
chest wall receptors in, 184
constraints on, 179
disorders of. See *Hyperventilation; Hypoventilation; Sleep, disorders of; Sleep apnea.*
feedback in, 179
hydrogen ion concentration in, 192–193, *193*
hypoxia and, 191–192, *192*
in airway obstruction, 112
in chronic obstructive pulmonary disease, 1227
in kyphoscoliosis, 2360
in obesity, 2372
in pregnancy, 2318, *2318*

Breathing *(Continued)*
in sleep, 180, 2153–2154
at high altitude, 1924–1925, *1924*, *1925*
disorders of. See *Sleep apnea; Sleep, disorders of.*
in spinal cord injury, 2339
involuntary versus voluntary, 180
medulla in, 185–186, *185*, 188–189
neural, 180–189
objectives of, 179
oxygen levels in, 191–192, *192*
patterns in, 180–181, *180*, *181*
physiology of, 816–818
pons in, *185*, 186–187
receptors in, 181–184, 182t, *183*
reflexes in, 181–184, 182t, *183*
respiratory center in, 179
rhythm generation in, 188–189
sensory mechanisms in, 189–190, *190*
spinal cord in, *185*, 187–188, *187*
state-dependent, 179–180
suprapontine structures in, 187
timing in, 180–181, *180*, *181*
tracheobronchial receptors in, 182–184, 182t, *183*
upper airway receptors in, 181–182
volitional, 179–180
volume in, 180–181, *180*, *181*
diaphragmatic, in pulmonary rehabilitation, 2509
drive for. See *Ventilatory drive.*
exercises for, after abdominal surgery, 886, 886t
historical background of, 2505–2508, *2506*, *2507*
in chronic obstructive pulmonary disease, 216–217, 1227, 2464
in dyspnea, 547–548, *547*
in pulmonary rehabilitation, 2509
in ventilator liberation, 2385
frequency of, in minute ventilation calculation, 180, *181*
versus ventilation inequality, 60
glossopharyngeal, in neuromuscular disorders, 2346
in spinal cord injury, 2338
in exercise, respiratory muscle function in, 108–109
in panting mode, airway resistance measurement in, 799
in paralysis, nonrespiratory muscle recruitment for, 108
inefficient, in flail chest, 2368, *2368*
Kussmaul's, in metabolic acidosis, 161, 170
inspection of, 597
laryngeal function in, 1351
mechanics of. See *Mechanical properties.*
mouth, of dry air, water homeostasis in, 362
muscles for. See *Respiratory muscle(s).*
nasal airflow in, 1345
neuromuscular disorders affecting. See *Neuromuscular disorder(s).*
normal pattern of, 180
oxygen cost of, 2445
patient efforts at, in mechanical ventilation, 2451, *2451*, 2472, 2479–2482, *2481*, *2482*
patterns of, control of, 180–181, *180*, *181*
in asthma, 1248
in dyskinesias, 2349t, 2350–2351
in heart disease, 2261
in hemiplegia, 2340
in kyphoscoliosis, 2360
in neuromuscular disorders, 2345
in obesity, 2372
inspection of, 597

Breathing *(Continued)*
normal, 180
particulate inhalation and, 1889
pendulum, respiratory acidosis in, 174
periodic, 2147, 2161–2165
at high altitude, 1924–1925, *1924*, *1925*
clinical features of, 2162–2163
definition of, 2161
diagnosis of, 2163–2164, *2164*, *2165*
in heart disease, 2261
pathogenesis of, 2161–2162, *2163*
treatment of, 2164–2165
physiology of, 2445–2446, *2445*
pleuritic pain in, 576
pursed-lip, in chronic obstructive pulmonary disease, 1227
in dyspnea, 547
in pulmonary rehabilitation, 2509
quiet, air flow during, 782
mechanics of, 105–106, *105*
pattern of, 180
respiratory system mechanical properties and. See *Mechanical properties.*
rhythm of, generation of, 188–189
stimulation of, in hypoventilation, 2144, 2144t
in respiratory acidosis, 174
support of. See *Mechanical ventilation.*
techniques for, in chest physical therapy, 370
terminal respiratory unit changes during, 15–16
timing of, control of, 180–181, *180*, *181*
versus sleep stage, 2153–2154
volume of, control of, 180–181, *180*, *181*
voluntary pressure, pneumomediastinum in, 2099–2100
with airway resistance, 1346
work of, in asthma, 1265
in critical illness, 2407
in flail chest, 2368, *2368*
in hypercapnia, 2444
in kyphoscoliosis, 2359
in obesity, 2371t, 2372
positive end-expiratory pressure and, 2448–2449, *2448*
surfactant and, 307
Breathing reserve, in exercise, in chronic obstructive pulmonary disease, 212–213, *213*, *214*
in emphysema, 223
in interstitial pulmonary disease, 225
Breathlessness, sensation of. See *Dyspnea.*
Breuer-Hering deflation reflex, 184
Breuer-Hering inflation reflex, 21, 180–182
in heart failure, 2261
P cells and, 185
Brevotoxin, exposure to, 1909
Brisket disease, in cattle, 1634, 1638, 1938
Bromine, inhalation of, 1909
Bromocriptine, pleural disease due to, 2035
pulmonary disease due to, 1988
Bronchi. See *Bronchus(i).*
Bronchial aerosol challenge, 356
Bronchial artery(ies), anatomy of, 121–122, *122*, 1488, *1489*
angiography of, 658, *659*
branches of, 121
embolization of, in hemoptysis, 1566
in pleural blood supply, 1996–1997, *1997*
systemic circulation communications with, 1565–1566
variations in, 121
Bronchial breath sounds, 593, *593*
Bronchial circulation. See also *Bronchial artery(ies).*

Bronchial circulation *(Continued)*
anastomoses of, in bronchiectasis, 1326
anatomy of, 10–11, 121–122, *122*, 1488, *1489*
brachytherapy within, in lung cancer, 1433–1434
enlargement of, in cystic fibrosis, 1294
fetal, 121
physiology of, 1488
pressures in, pulmonary circulation pressure changes with, 1489
vessel proliferation of, in asthma, 1254
Bronchial inhibitor, low-molecular-weight, in mucus, 329
Bronchial veins, anatomy of, 121–122, *120*, 1488
Bronchiectasis, 1325–1341
angiography in, *659*
chest radiography of, 1328, *1329–1332*
classification of, 1325–1326
complications of, 1328
computed tomography of, 679, *680*, *681*, 1328–1329, *1332*
conditions associated with, 1333–1337, 1333t
cough in, *559*, 560, 564
cylindrical, 1325, 1328, *1329–1330*
cystic, 1326, 1328, *1330*, *1331*, 1722
cystic fibrosis with, 1326, 1331, 1333, 1335
definition of, 1325
diagnosis of, 1328–1331, *1329–1332*
distribution of, in lung segments, 1326
dry, 1328
epidemiology of, 1327
etiology of, 1179
focal nature of, 1325
hemoptysis in, 589, 589t
heroin-induced, 1980
impairment in, 902, 903t
in allergic bronchopulmonary aspergillosis, 1327, 1333–1334, 1763, 1765
in alpha$_1$-antitrypsin deficiency, 1334
in ankylosing spondylitis, 1710
in bronchial obstruction, 1334
in bronchopulmonary sequestration, 1334
in ciliary dyskinesia, 1336
in common variable immunodeficiency, 2235
in congenital cartilage deficiency, 1334–1335
in cystic fibrosis, 1294, *1294*, 1303
in HIV infection, 1335, 2209
in immunodeficiency, 1335–1336
in immunoglobulin A deficiency, 2235
in infections, 1336
in inflammation, 1336
in inflammatory bowel disease, 2270
in Kartagener's syndrome, 366
in rheumatoid arthritis, 1336–1337, 1701, *1701*
in sarcoidosis, 1722
in tracheobronchomegaly, 1337
laboratory tests in, 1330–1331
lung transplantation in, 2520, 2520t
mortality in, 1332, 1333
mucociliary transport abnormalities in, 366–367
pathogenesis of, 1179, 1326–1327
pathogens present in, 1328
pathology of, 1326–1327
physical signs in, 1328
postinfectious, 1327, 1328, 1336
prevention of, 1333
prognosis for, 1333
pulmonary circulation–systemic circulation communications in, 1566
pulmonary function abnormalities in, 1327

Bronchiectasis *(Continued)*
saccular, 1326
symptoms of, 1327–1328
temporary, 1325
treatment of, 1331–1333
unilateral hyperlucent lung with, 1337
varicose, 1325–1326, 1328, *1330*
ventilation-perfusion scanning in, 697–698
versus bronchitis, 1325
wet, 1328
yellow nail syndrome with, 1337
Bronchiolectasis, in cystic fibrosis, 1294, *1294*
Bronchioles. See also *Bronchiolitis.*
anatomy of, 1204, *1204*
asbestosis of, 1833
dead space in, 6
epithelium of, 16
membranous, anatomy of, 6
obstructive diseases of, 1180–1181, 1204–1205, *1204*, *1205*
pathology of, in bronchitis, 1203
terminal, anatomy of, 56, *56*
versus bronchi, 1361
Bronchiolitis, 1180, 1362–1363, *1362*
beryllium-related, 1843
chronic bronchitis in, 1215
epidemiology of, 1362
fibrosis in, 459, 462, *463*, 752
follicular, in rheumatoid arthritis, 1701
in children, 1362–1363
in chronic obstructive pulmonary disease, 1206–1207
in hypersensitivity pneumonitis, 1872, *1872*
in inflammatory bowel disease, 2270
in interstitial lung disease, 1672t
in measles, 958
in Sjögren's syndrome, 1706
infectious, 1362
obliterative. See *Bronchiolitis obliterans.*
panbronchiolitis as, 1366
respiratory, in interstitial lung disease, 1684–1686, *1685*
respiratory syncytial virus, 962–964
viral, 935–937, *936*
Bronchiolitis obliterans, 936, 1363–1366
after influenza, 953
after transplantation, bone marrow, 1364, 2300–2301
heart-lung, 1364–1365, *1365*
lung, 1364–1365, *1365*
chest radiography of, 1198, 1363
classic/proliferative, 1363
classification of, 1363, 1363t
clinical features of, 1363, 2523–2524
constrictive, 1363
diagnosis of, 2524, 2524t
drug-induced, 479t
etiology of, 1363, 2524
histology of, 1363
historical view of, 1363
in allograft rejection, 2523–2524, 2524t
in connective tissue diseases, 1364
in rheumatoid arthritis, 1700–1701, *1700*, 1703
in toxic exposures, 1362, *1362*, 1905
pathology of, 1363
penicillamine-induced, 1985
prognosis for, 1363t
proliferative, in toxic exposures, 1905
treatment of, 1363t, 1366, 2524
unilateral, with hyperinflation, 1197–1198
Bronchiolitis obliterans organizing pneumonia, 1363, 1363t, 1650–1651, *1651*, 1653t, 1686–1687
bleomycin-induced, 1976, *1976*
chest radiography of, 1365, *1658*, 1686
Bronchiolitis obliterans organizing pneumonia *(Continued)*
clinical features of, 1672t, 1686
computed tomography of, 1686
discovery of, 1365–1366
drug-induced, 479t, 1990, 1990t
etiology of, 1365, 1365t
histology of, 1365–1366
idiopathic (cryptogenic organizing pneumonitis), 1365
in bone marrow transplantation, 2300
in dermatomyositis, 1707–1708
in HIV infection, 2210
in inflammatory bowel disease, 2270–2271
in rheumatoid arthritis, 1699–1700, *1699*
in Sjögren's syndrome, 1706
in toxic exposures, 1905
pathology of, 456, 459, 462, *462*, *463*, 1672t, 1686
prognosis for, 1686–1687
pulmonary function tests in, 1686
sulfasalazine-induced, 1979
treatment of, 1366, 1686–1687
Bronchiolization, in ozone exposure, 1896
Bronchitis, acute, diagnosis of, 919
differential diagnosis of, 934
treatment of, 919
asthmatic, 1199–1200, 1271
bronchoscopic appearance of, 733
chronic, clinical features of, 1189–1195, *1190*, *1191*, *1195*, *1196*
cor pulmonale in, 1193–1194
cough in, *559*, 560, 564
crackles in, *595*
definition of, 1174, 1188
differential diagnosis of, 1195, 1197–1198
epidemiology of, 1198–1201, *1200*, *1201*
erythrocytosis in, 1192
etiology of, 1178–1179
historical background of, 1189
history in, 1189
impairment in, 903t, 907
in byssinosis, 1862
in coal working, 1825, 1828
in HIV infection, 2209
in inflammatory bowel disease, 2270
in Sjögren's syndrome, 1706
laboratory findings in, 1190–1192, *1190*, *1191*
mortality in, 1198–1199
mucociliary transport in, 364–365
abnormalities of, 366–367
natural history of, 1201–1202, *1201*, *1202*
pathogenesis of, 1178–1179, 1214–1217
airway inflammation in, 1215–1216
bronchiolitis in, 1215
chemical mediators in, 1216
epithelial cell injury and repair in, 1216
infection in, 1216–1217
secretory apparatus alterations in, 1214–1215, *1215*
pathology of, 1203, *1203*
physical examination in, 1189
pneumonia in, 1194
pneumothorax in, 1192–1193
prognosis for, 1202–1203
pulmonary function tests in, 1190–1192, 1206–1207
pulmonary rehabilitation in. See *Pulmonary rehabilitation.*
risk factors for, 1199–1202, *1200*, *1201*
silicosis with, 1819
sleep disorders in, 1194
smoking and, cessation of, 2513–2514, *2513*, 2514t
sputum examination in, 1192
Bronchitis *(Continued)*
squamous metaplasia in, *452*
structure-function correlations in, 1206–1207
treatment of. See also *Chronic obstructive pulmonary disease, treatment of; Pulmonary rehabilitation.*
antibiotics in, 1225
ventilation-perfusion scanning in, 697–698
versus asthma, 1268
eosinophilic, 289, 559
epidemiology of, 1362
hemoptysis in, 589, 589t
herpes simplex virus, 948
in cystic fibrosis, 1302
in measles, 958
in paragonimiasis, 1161
necrotizing, heroin-induced, 1980
pain in, 576
recurrent, versus asthma, 1267
rhinovirus, 966
Bronchoalveolar carcinoma, 1419
Bronchoalveolar lavage, blind, in pneumonia, 748
bronchoscopy in, 751–753, 751t
complications of, 757
culture of specimens in, 746–747, 746t, *747*
dilution markers for, 736
guidelines for, 735–736, 735t
in acute respiratory distress syndrome, 318
in alveolar proteinosis, 320, 752, 753
diagnostic, 1790, 1796
therapeutic, 1796–1800, *1799*
in asbestosis, 1835
in asthma, 755
in chemotherapy-induced disease, 1975
in cryptococcosis, 2197
in high-altitude illness, 1934–1935, *1935*
in HIV infection, 2177–2178
in hypersensitivity pneumonitis, 1871–1872, 1876
in infections, 743t
in inflammation assessment, 530
in interstitial lung disease, 319–320, 1665–1666, 1696–1697
in lung cancer, 739t, 740
in lung transplantation monitoring, 1364
in mechanical ventilation, 747, *748*
in nitrogen dioxide exposure, 1895
in ozone exposure, 1895
in pneumonia, 319, 611
cytomegalovirus, 943
nosocomial, 747, *748*
*Pneumocystis carinii*, 743–744, *744*, 2190
specimen processing after, 612
in pulmonary edema, 1595
high-altitude, 1581
in pulmonary fibrosis, 1679–1680
in sarcoidosis, 1726
in silicosis, 1824
in systemic sclerosis, 1696–1697
lymphocytes in, 752
monoclonal markers in, 742
nonbronchoscopic, in pneumonia, 748
solution characteristics in, 735–736
technique for, 734–736, 735t
therapeutic, 753–754
whole-lung, in alveolar proteinosis, 1796–1800, *1799*
Bronchoalveolar space, lymphocytes in, 435
Bronchocentric granulomatosis, 1334, 1368, 1481, 1538–1539
in allergic bronchopulmonary aspergillosis, 1765
Bronchoconstriction. See also *Bronchospasm.*
autonomic control of, *250*

Bronchoconstriction *(Continued)*
cholinergic mechanisms in, 252–253, *253*
cough and, 556
drugs inducing, 290–291
exercise-induced, 218
in asthma, 1266, 1855
in byssinosis, 1860–1862
in cholinergic reflex activation, 253–254
in lung injury, 1586
inflammatory mediators in, 256–258, *257*, *258*
inhibition of, anti-leukotrienes in, 284–286
cromones in, 283–284
limitation of, slowly adapting receptors in, 251
muscarinic receptors in, 253, *253*
paradoxical, due to ipratropium bromide, 277
pathophysiology of, 232, *233*
sulfur dioxide in, 1854, 1888–1889, 1892–1893
Bronchodilation, adrenergic receptors in, 255–256
autonomic control of, *250*, 255–256
calcitonin gene-related peptide in, 255
catecholamines in, 255
inflammatory mediators in, 256–258, *257*, *258*
nonadrenergic noncholinergic nerves in, 256
sympathetic nerves in, 255
Bronchodilator(s), 267–278. See also specific drugs.
anticholinergic drugs as, 275–277, *276*, 1221–1222
beta$_2$-adrenergic agonists as, 268–272, *268–270*, 269t, 271t, 1220–1222, 1220t
classes of, 267
delivery mechanisms for, 355–356
gastroesophageal reflux due to, 2269
in airway obstruction reversibility evaluation, 851–852, *852*
in asthma, 1276, 1277t, 2453–2455, 2454t
ventilation-perfusion ratio changes due to, 83, *84*
in chronic obstructive pulmonary disease, 1220–1223, 1220t, 1223t
in cystic fibrosis, 1304, 1310
in emphysema, 1220–1223, 1220t, 1223t
in obstructive disease evaluation, 1182
in respiratory failure, 2460–2461, 2461t
in respiratory syncytial virus infections, 963
mechanism of action of, 267
new, 277–278, 278t
phosphodiesterase inhibitors as, 277–278
potassium channel openers as, 277
response to, criteria for, 874
theophylline as. See *Theophylline*.
Bronchogenic carcinoma. See *Carcinoma(s), bronchogenic*.
Bronchogenic cysts, 483t, 2130
Bronchography, in bronchiectasis, 1328
in bronchiolitis obliterans, 1198
indications for, 654
Broncholithiasis, 727, 1368
Bronchomalacia, 1368
Bronchophony, 598
Bronchopleural fistula, bronchoscopy in, 754–755
empyema with, 2020, *2021*
in ankylosing spondylitis, 2370
Bronchopulmonary arterial anastomoses, 122, *122*
Bronchopulmonary dysplasia, 1180–1181, 1366–1367
in adrenal insufficiency, 2313
Bronchopulmonary veins, anatomy of, 121–122, 1488
Bronchorrhea, 368–369, 560
in chronic obstructive pulmonary disease, 1224
mucociliary transport in, 364–365
Bronchoscopy (flexible fiberoptic or unspecified), 727–759
anesthesia for, 731–732, 732t
complications of, 755–756, 756t
competence evaluation in, 730
complications of, 755–757, 755t, 756t
contraindications to, 728, 729t
endoscopic view in, 732–733
equipment for, 727–728
care of, 757–759
cleaning of, 758–759
damage of, 757–758
fluorescence, 728
fluoroscopic, 734, 1422–1423
guidelines for, 729t
historical development of, 727
in abscess, 1031
in acute respiratory distress syndrome, 756
in airway management, 753
in allograft rejection, 2523
in asthma, 730, 755, 757
in atelectasis, 753–754
in benign tumors, 1477
in biopsy, brush, 733
forceps, 733–734
transbronchial needle aspiration, 736–737, 738t
in brachytherapy, 742
in bronchial obstruction, 1369
in bronchiectasis, 1329
in bronchitis, 732
in bronchoalveolar lavage. See *Bronchoalveolar lavage*.
in bronchopleural fistula, 754–755
in burn injury, 754
in cough, 562
in foreign body removal, 754
in hemoptysis, 750–751, 750t, 1566
in HIV infection, 2177–2178
in infection, 743–750, 743t
abscess as, 749
bacterial, 746–749, 746t, *747*, *748*
cytomegalovirus, 749
eosinophilic, 752
fungal, 745–746
herpesvirus, 749–750
*Legionella*, 749
nosocomial, 923
*Pneumocystis carinii*, 743–744, *744*, 745t
tuberculous, 744–745, 1065
in interstitial lung diseases, 751–753, 751t
in Kaposi's sarcoma, 2205, *2206*
in laser therapy, 742
in lung cancer, 732, 733, 737, 738t, 739t, 739–743, 1422
endoscopically visible, 739–740, *739*, *740*
fluoroscopic, 1422–1423
for staging, 741
in palliative therapy, 742
in stent placement, 742–743, *743*
metastatic, 741, 741t
new modalities in, 741–742
nonendoscopically visible, 740
radiologically occult, 741
with extrinsic compression, 740
in lung transplantation monitoring, 1364
in mediastinal biopsy, 2088–2089, *2089*
in mucoepithelial malignancies, 1462
in near drowning, 1966
in pediatric patients, 753
in pleural effusion, 2009
in pneumonia. See subheading *in infection*.
Bronchoscopy (flexible fiberoptic or unspecified) *(Continued)*
in pulmonary edema, 1591
in specimen collection, 610–611
in suctioning, 753–754
in tuberculosis, 744–745, 1065
indications for, 728, 729t, 730t
insertion techniques for, 732
lavage in. See *Bronchoalveolar lavage*.
light sources for, 728
mediastinitis in, 2107–2108
mortality, 755, 755t
of larynx, 732
patient preparation for, 730–731, 731t
pneumomediastinum in, 2097
postinfectious, 1329–1330
protected sheath brush in, 991–992
for culture, 612
in infections, 743t
in specimen collection, 609, 611
technique for, 733
research uses of, 759
risks of, 728, 729t
sampling techniques in, 733–737, 735t, 738t
sizes of insertion ends in, 728
specimen handling in, 737
training for, 729–730
two bronchoscopes used for, in pneumonia, 747–748
ultrathin equipment for, 741–742, 753
versus rigid bronchoscopy, 726, 726t
video, 728
with aspiration, in pneumonia, 991–992
Bronchoscopy (rigid), 725–727
disadvantages of, 727
equipment for, 726
historical development of, 725
in cancer palliative treatment, 742
indications for, 726–727, 726t, 754
technique for, 726
versus flexible bronchoscopy, 726, 726t
Bronchospasm. See also *Asthma*.
aspirin-induced, 1984
drug-induced, 1989–1990, 1989t
exercise-induced, 1271
in gastroesophageal reflux, 2269
respiratory failure in, 2447–2448
Bronchospirometry, before pneumonectomy, 714
Bronchovascular sheath, alveolar rupture into, 2097–2098, *2097*, *2098*
Bronchovesicular breath sounds, 593, *593*
Bronchus(i), adenoma of, 1478
aerosol deposition in, 352–354, *352*, *353*
amyloidosis of, 1368, 1481, 1481t, 2296
anastomosis of, in lung transplantation, 2518
anatomy of, 1361–1362
blood supply of. See *Bronchial circulation*.
branches of, development of, 35–36, *36*
C fibers of, 252
calcified fragment in, 1368
carcinoid tumors of, 1419, 1460–1462
carcinoma of. See *Carcinoma(s), bronchogenic*.
cartilage deficiency in, 1334–1335
compression of, 1367
computed tomography of, 679, *679*
congenital malformations of, 482
constriction of. See *Bronchoconstriction*.
cough reflex receptors in, 554, *555*
dilation of. See *Bronchodilation; Bronchodilator(s)*.
abnormal. See *Bronchiectasis*.
disorders of, clinical features of, 1368–1369
diagnosis of, 1369
in mediastinitis, 2113

Bronchus(i) *(Continued)*
stents in, 1369
treatment of, 1369
edema in, prevention of, beta-adrenergic agonists in, 269
extreme enlargement of, 1337
fistulas of, bronchoscopy in, 754–755
empyema with, 2020, *2021*
in ankylosing spondylitis, 2370
foreign bodies in, *649*, 1367
glands of, 9, *10*
adenomas of, 1478
chronic obstructive pulmonary disease and, 1206
hyperplasia of, 1203, *1203*
hypertrophy of, 450, *450*
metaplasia of, 1214–1215, *1215*
mucus hypersecretion from, in asthma, 1262
tumors of, 1419
granulomatous disease of, 1367–1368
hyperreactivity of, in heart disease, 2255
inflammation of. See *Bronchitis.*
injury of, 1368
lithiasis of, 727, 1368
liver fistula with, in amebiasis, 1144–1146
lymphangio(leio)myomatosis infiltration of, 1776
medium-sized, dilation of. See *Bronchiectasis.*
metastasis to, 1367
mucoid impaction of, 1334
obstruction of, 1180–1181, 1367–1369
bronchiectasis with, 1334
in cancer, treatment of, 1431–1432
treatment of, rigid bronchoscopy in, 727
physiology of, 1361–1362
receptors in, for breathing control, 182–184, 182t, *183*
responsiveness of, segregation analysis of, 1252
tests for, 1266, 1268
rupture of, pneumothorax in, 2052–2053
sarcoidosis of, 1721–1722
sequestration of. See *Sequestration(s), bronchopulmonary.*
softening of, 1368
spasm of. See *Asthma; Bronchospasm.*
stenosis of, in tuberculosis, 745
stents in, 742–743, *743*, 1369
tumors of, 1367
benign, 1477, 1478
pleural effusion in, 2072
versus bronchioles, 1361
Bronchus-associated lymphoid tissue, lymphocytes in, 435
Brownian diffusion, inertial, 351, *351*
Brucellosis, 1030
*Brugia malayi* infections, 1153–1155, *1154*
*Bruit de moulin* (mill-wheel murmur), in pneumomediastinum, 2102
Bruits, in lung fields, in thromboembolic pulmonary hypertension, 1520
Brush, in bronchoscopy. See *Bronchoscopy, protected sheath brush in.*
Bruton's agammaglobulinemia, 2233t, 2234–2235
Bubbles, in decompression sickness, 1959–1961
Bubonic plague, 1029
Budding, in branching morphogenesis, 36, *36*, *37*
Budesonide, chemical structure of, *278*
dosage of, 281
in asthma, 1273
in croup, 935
Budesonide *(Continued)*
pharmacokinetics of, 280, 282
Buffering, isocapnic, 205–206
in exercise, 211
Buffers, in carbon dioxide-bicarbonate system, 156, 157, 158
in exercise metabolism, 200, *200*, 205–206, *206*
in kidney, 162–163
intracellular, 163
Bulk modulus, of lung, 93
Bullae, lung, impairment in, 909
in cancer, 1195
in chronic obstructive pulmonary disease, 1194–1195, *1195*, *1196*, 1205, 1219–1220, 2049
pulmonary function testing in, 853
Bumetanide, in acute respiratory distress syndrome, 2420
in pulmonary edema, 2420
Bupivacaine, contraindicated in asthma, 291
Bupropion, in smoking cessation, 1217
*Burkholderia cepacia* infections, in cystic fibrosis, 1303
pneumonia due to, 1012–1013
Burns, airway damage in, bronchoscopy in, 754
lung injury in, pathology of, 475
Busulfan, pulmonary disease due to, 1975
Byssinosis, 1860–1862
clinical features of, 1862
pathophysiology of, 1861–1862
prevention of, 1862

## C

C fibers, activation of, inflammation in, 254, *254*
function of, 252
in respiratory control, 182t, 183–184
of terminal respiratory units, 21–22, *21*
of visceral sensory neurons, 573
receptors for, 575
in cough, 554, *555*
in respiratory control, 182t, 183–184
Cabergoline, pulmonary disease due to, 1988
Cadherins, defects of, metastasis in, 1387
in fluid and solute exchange, *134–135*
Cadmium exposure, acute lung injury in, 1907
emphysema in, 1213
lung cancer in, 1403
Caisson disease. See *Decompression sickness.*
Calabar swellings, in loiasis, 1154
Calcification, fragment of, in bronchi, 1368
of lung, dystrophic, 450, *453*
in hamartoma, 1479
in hyperparathyroidism, 2312, *2312*
in kidney failure, 2279
in multiple myeloma, 2294
in silicosis, 1823
in tuberculosis, 1064
metastatic, 450, *453*
popcorn, 667
solitary nodule, 667, *668*
of lymph nodes, in sarcoidosis, 1721
of mediastinum, in histoplasmosis, 2111, *2112*
of metastases, 1471, *1473*
of pleura, *2062*, 2063
in interstitial lung disease, 1658–1659, 1660t
Calcitonin gene–related peptide, actions of, 250, *250*, 255
in mucus secretion regulation, 332, 333
Calcium, imbalance of. See also *Hypercalcemia.*
Calcium, imbalance of *(Continued)*
in renal tubular acidosis, 168–169
in respiratory alkalosis, 174
in carotid body function, 189
in chloride transport, in cystic fibrosis, 1298–1299, *1298*
in epithelial electrolyte transport regulation, 338
in vasoconstriction, 131
intracellular, endothelial permeability and, 142, *143*
receptor coupling to, 238
second messenger function of, 236, 237, *237*
in beta-adrenergic agonist action, 268, *269*
Calcium channel blockers, as vasodilators, 300
Calcium channels, 246, *246*
Calcium-calmodulin–dependent kinase, endothelial permeability and, 142
Calmodulin, in vasoconstriction, 131
cAMP. See *Cyclic adenosine monophosphate.*
Cancer, bone marrow transplantation in, 2297
bronchial, 1367
chemotherapy for. See *Chemotherapy.*
embolism from, 1527
granulocytopenia in, pneumonia in, 924–925, 925t
hemoptysis in, 589, 589t
immunodeficiency in, adenovirus infections in, 939, 940t
in common variable immunodeficiency, 2235
in transplantation, 2232
lung. See *Carcinoma(s), bronchogenic; Lung cancer.*
metastatic. See *Metastasis(es) (malignancy).*
neurogenic, of mediastinum, 2131
ovarian, Meigs' syndrome in, 2034
paraneoplastic syndromes in. See *Paraneoplastic syndrome(s).*
pleural. See *Pleura, tumors of; Pleural effusion(s), malignant.*
pneumonia in, microbiology of, 920
screening for, after transplantation, 2526
Candidate gene analysis, 49
in asthma, 1253, 1254t
Candidiasis, 1108, 1135–1136
clinical manifestations of, 1135–1136
culture in, 621–622
diagnosis of, 1136
genetic tests for, 626
geographic distribution of, 1108
in bone marrow transplantation, 2303
in HIV infection, 1135, 2202
microbiologic diagnosis of, 610t
pathogenesis of, 1135
surfactant protein D binding in, 315
treatment of, 1136
$CaO_2$. See *Oxygen concentration, arterial.*
Capillaritis, pulmonary, 1534
clinical manifestations of, 1734, *1735*, 1736, *1736*
glomerulonephritis with, *1736*, 1737t, 1740–1741
in Behçet's syndrome, 1740
in Henoch-Schönlein purpura, 1737t, 1740
in lung allograft rejection, 1741
in microscopic polyangiitis, *1735*, 1737t, 1739
in mixed cryoglobulinemia, 1740
in Wegener's granulomatosis, 1536, 1737t, 1738–1739
isolated, 1737t, 1738
laboratory tests in, 1736, 1737t, 1738
pathology of, 1733–1734, *1734*, *1735*
Capillary(ies), alveolar, 60–62, *61*
blood flow in, at high altitude, 1927

Capillary(ies) *(Continued)*
capacitance to conductance ratio of, 219
muscle, tortuosity of, at high altitude, 1923
pulmonary. See *Pulmonary capillary(ies).*
Caplan's syndrome, 1702, 1826–1830
Capnography, 836, *836*
Capreomycin, in tuberculosis, 1069t, 1070
Capsaicin, C-fiber ending stimulation by, 184
inhalation of, 1909
Captopril, as vasodilator, 302
in pulmonary hypertension, 1644–1645
Carbamino compounds, transport of, 86, *87*
Carbapenem(s), in pneumonia, 922t, 996t, 998t
anaerobic, 1019t, 1020
Enterobacteriaceae, 1011
*Klebsiella pneumoniae*, 1009
Carbohydrates, metabolism of, in exercise, 198–201, *199*, *200*
receptors for, on macrophages, 390, *391*
Carbon dioxide, absorbents for, in diving equipment, 1953, *1954*
bicarbonate formation from, 155
breathing of, in breathing control assessment, 818–820, *819*, 877
content of, measurement of, 156
diffusion of, rate of, 72
dissolved, normal concentration of, 156
transport of, 86, *87*
exchange of. See *Gas exchange.*
exhaled in unit time. See *Carbon dioxide, production of.*
hemoglobin binding to, 86
in bicarbonate form. See *Bicarbonate.*
partial pressure of, air-to-tissue gradients in, 71
alveolar, calculation of, 77
distribution of, in normal lung, 78, *78*
in alveolar ventilation equation, 58, 824–825
in exercise, heavy, 205, *206*
in physiologic dead space calculation, 58
in ventilation-perfusion ratio calculation, 77–78, *77*, *78*
measurement of, 836–837, *836*, *837*
normal, 190
ventilatory response to, 190–193, *191*, *193*
versus altitude, 1916–1917, *1916*
versus alveolar ventilation, 71–72, *72*, 180–181, *180*
versus arterial carbon dioxide, 830
versus diffusing capacity, 815
versus ventilation-perfusion ratio, 77–78, *77*, *78*
arterial. See also *Hypercapnia/hypercarbia; Hypocapnia/hypocarbia.*
acid-base disorder classification by, 160t
chemoreceptor sensing of, 189–190, *190*
criteria for, in gas exchange impairment, 901t
equation for, 2456
hydrogen ion excretion and, 162
in acute inflammatory polyneuropathy, 2341–2342
in alveolar oxygen calculation, 824
in alveolar proteinosis, 1795
in alveolar ventilation calculation, 208–209, *209*
in brain, at high altitude, 1923
in breathing control, 179
in cystic fibrosis, 1304, 1304t
in dead space calculation, 823–824
in diffusing capacity measurement, 812

Carbon dioxide *(Continued)*
in exercise, 840
heavy, 205, *206*
in pulmonary disease, 211–212, 212t
in high altitude acclimatization, 1917, *1917*
in hyperventilation, 2148
in hypoventilation, 2140–2143, *2141*
in hypoxia, 821t
in interstitial lung disease, 1663–1664
in lactic acidosis, 166
in near drowning, 1965t
in physiologic dead space calculation, 58
in portopulmonary hypertension, 2275
in pulmonary edema, 1594–1595
in pulmonary hypertension, 1548
in respiratory acidosis, 173–174
in sarcoidosis, 1723
in sleep, 2153, 2154–2155, *2155*, *2156*
in sleep apnea, 2161–2162, *2161*, *2163–2165*, 2164–2165
in total ventilation calculation, 209
in ventilatory failure, 2345, *2345*, *2346*
measurement of, 156, 831–832, *832*, 836–837, *836*, *837*
theoretical aspects of, 830
transcutaneous, 837
oxygen-hemoglobin affinity and, 1922, *1922*
respiratory responses to, 190–191, *191*
versus alveolar carbon dioxide, 830
versus alveolar ventilation, 71–72, *72*
versus bicarbonate concentration, 156–160, *157*, *159*
versus dead space/tidal volume ratio, in exercise, 209–210, *209*
arteriovenous difference of, 825
capillary, 2047
mixed venous, in exercise testing, 842
pleural fluid, 2005
urinary, in renal tubular acidosis, 168
production of, definition of, 2564
factors affecting, 156–157, *157*
from bicarbonate, 155, 205–206, *206*
from lactic acid, 205–206, *206*
in alveolar ventilation equation, 58, 208–210, *209*
in exercise, 199–200, *199*, *200*, 839, *839*, 840
heavy, 211, *211*
in emphysema, *222*, 223
in pulmonary disease, 211–212, 212t
moderate, 203–204, *204*, 210
in highly fit athletes, 218
in interstitial pulmonary disease, *223*, 225
in obesity, 220
in pregnancy, 2318
metabolic, 205
sources of, 205–206, *206*
versus oxygen consumed. See *Respiratory quotient.*
protein compounds with, transport of, 86, *87*
removal of, in hemodialysis, 2280
retention of, hypoxic response in, 821
in asthma, 1275
in chronic lung disease, 71
in hypoventilation, 71–72, *72*
ventilation-perfusion inequality and, 83, 85
versus hypoventilation, 71
transport of, 86, *87*
Carbon dioxide dissociation curve, 86, *87*
Carbon dioxide narcosis, 1265, 2444
Carbon dioxide–combining power or capacity, 156

Carbon graphite, in pneumoconiosis, 1831t, 1842
Carbon monoxide, as air pollutant, standards for, 2556
hemoglobin interactions with, 2290
in diffusing capacity, 810, *810*
in smoking, 814
in diffusing capacity measurement, 74–76, *74*, 811–814. See also *Diffusing capacity.*
oxygen binding to, 86
in smoking, 887
transfer of, diffusion-limited, 73
Carbonic acid, carbon dioxide equilibrium with, 86
dissociation of, in kidney, 162
formation of, in renal tubular acidosis, 168
in carbon dioxide–bicarbonate balance, 155
Carbonic acid–bicarbonate buffer system, in exercise metabolism, 200, *200*
Carbonic anhydrase, action of, 86, 155, 162
Carboplatin, in lung cancer, 1437, 1437t
Carborundum pneumoconiosis, 1845
Carboxyhemoglobin, formation of, 2290
in smoking, 814, 887
Carcinogen(s) and carcinogenesis, asbestos as, 1836
beryllium as, 1843
biomarkers for, 1406
in lung cancer, 1377–1378
silica as, 1822–1823
tobacco smoke as. See *Smoking.*
Carcinoid syndrome, versus asthma, 1269
Carcinoid tumor(s), of bronchi, 1460–1462
of lung, 484t, 1419, 1460–1462
of thymus, 2127
of trachea, 1461
Carcinoma(s), adenocarcinoma as. See also *Lung cancer, adenocarcinoma as.*
versus mesothelioma, 2069
bronchogenic, 1415–1451
abscess with, 749
advanced, chemotherapy for, 1437–1438, 1437t, 1438t
biopsy of, mediastinoscopy in, 2089–2090
transbronchial, 736–737, 738t
bronchoscopy in, 733
classification of, 1417, 1418t, 1419
clinical features of, 1420–1422, 1420t, 1421t
in HIV infection, 2207–2208
clubbing in, 601, 603
cough in, *559*, 560–561
diagnosis of, 1422–1423, 1422t
in HIV infection, 2208
molecular methods in, 1426, 1426t
screening, 1419–1420, 1420t
epidemiology of, 1415–1416, 1416t, 1417t, 2207
in HIV infection, 2207–2208
in pulmonary fibrosis, 1684t
mediastinal involvement in, 2083–2085
metastasis from, to pleura, 2072, *2073*
treatment of, 1435–1436
molecular biology of, 1416–1417, 1425–1426, 1426t
mortality in, 1425–1426, *1425*
natural history of, 1417, 1418t, 1419
non–small cell lung. See *Lung cancer, non–small cell.*
pain in, 577
Pancoast's syndrome in, 577, 1430
paraneoplastic syndromes in, 1421–1422
prognosis for, 1425–1426, *1425*
screening for, 1419–1420, 1420t
spinal cord compression in, 1435

Carcinoma(s) *(Continued)*
staging of, 1423–1425, 1423t–1425t, 2090–2091, *2091*
superior vena cava obstruction in, 1435
survival in, 1425–1426, *1425*
treatment of, chemotherapy for. See *Chemotherapy, for lung cancer.*
combined modalities in, 1436–1437
economic issues in, 1439, 1444
guidelines for, 1439, *1440–1444*
in HIV infection, 2208
palliative, 1431–1432, 1435–1436
radiation therapy in, 1432–1436
surgical, 1426–1432
with solitary nodule, 1439
carcinosarcomas as, 1462
embryonal cell, of mediastinum, 2128
neuroendocrine, 1460–1462
of breast, metastasis from, to pleura, 2073
of mediastinum, 2132
of parathyroid, 2128–2129
of salivary glands, in lung, 1462–1463, 1462t
of thymus, 2127
squamous cell, of lung, 1418t, 1419
bronchoscopy of, 739, *740*
pathology of, 482, 484t, *485*
smoking and, 1398–1399
Carcinoma *in situ*, of lung, 1377–1378
Carcinosarcoma(s), of lung, 1462, 1463
Cardiac. See also *Heart.*
Cardiac arrest, in near drowning, 1964–1967
in neonatal pneumothorax, 2053
Cardiac arrhythmias, in bronchoscopy, 756
in chronic obstructive pulmonary disease, 884
in hypereosinophilic syndrome, 1769
in hyperventilation, 2148
in respiratory failure, 2462–2463
in shock, 2403t
in sleep apnea, 2163
theophylline-induced, 1222
Cardiac asthma, 2447–2448
Cardiac output, after pneumonectomy, 889
at high altitude, 1920
in exercise, 1927
definition of, 2565
distribution of, in highly fit athletes, 219
estimation of, in exercise testing, 842
in airway obstruction, 2453
in arteriovenous malformations, 1563
in exercise, 838
at high altitude, 1927
in pulmonary hypertension, 1491, *1491*
in hepatopulmonary syndrome, 2273
in pneumothorax, 2054
in portopulmonary hypertension, 2275
in positive end-expiratory pressure, 2388–2389, *2388*
in pregnancy, 2318, *2318*
in pulmonary vascular resistance calculation, 123–124, 1490
in septic shock, 2399
in shunt calculation, 76
low, anaerobic metabolism in, 2405–2406, *2405*
mechanical ventilation effects on, 2482
versus gas exchange, in exercise, 202
in ventilation-perfusion inequality, 85
Cardiac silhouette, in pulmonary hypertension, 1520, *1521*
Cardiac tamponade, shock in, 2402–2403
Cardiodynamic gas exchange, 202
Cardiogenic pulmonary edema. See *Pulmonary edema, increased pressure.*
Cardiogenic shock, 2400, 2401t, *2402*
Cardiomegaly, ventilation distribution in, 2257, *2258*
Cardiomyopathy, hypertrophic, pain in, 578
peripartum, 2321
Cardiopulmonary resuscitation, in near drowning, 1965
ventilation during, pneumomediastinum in, 2101
withholding of, 2497–2498
Cardiovascular disorders, pain in, 570t, 577–579
Carina, biopsy of, 741
Carlens tube, in whole-lung lavage, 1797–1798
Carney's triad, 1480, *1481*
Carotenoids, lung cancer and, 1385, 1404–1405
Carotid bodies, chemoreceptors in, dysfunction of, respiratory acidosis in, 173
function of, 189–190
at high altitude, 1917, 1918
in heavy exercise, 211, *211*
resection of, in dyspnea, in chronic obstructive pulmonary disease, 1228
Cartilage, bronchial, deficiency of, 1334–1335
Caseation necrosis, 446, *449*
Caspases, in apoptosis, *445*
Castleman's disease, 1460
Catamenial hemoptysis, 1480
Catamenial pneumothorax, 2053–2054, *2054*, 2324
Catecholamines. See also *Epinephrine; Norepinephrine.*
beta$_2$-adrenergic agonists derived from, 268, *268*
chemical structures of, 268, *268*
in bronchodilation, 255
in cor pulmonale, 1636
in pulmonary edema, 1603–1604
metabolism of, 268
Cathepsins, in emphysema, 1212
in mucus hypersecretion, 334
Catheter(ization) (cardiac), in acute respiratory distress syndrome, 2424, *2425*
in pulmonary edema, 1600–1601, 2424, *2425*
in pulmonary hypertension, 1549
Catheter(ization) (pleural space), in malignant effusions, 2075
Catheter(ization) (tracheal), for oxygen therapy, 1226
Catheter(ization) (vascular), air embolism due to, 1526
central venous, problems with, mediastinitis in, 2108, *2108*
pain in, 576
pleural effusion in, 2036
pneumothorax in, 2051
position of, radiography in, 637, *637–639*, 639–640
pulmonary artery, aneurysms due to, 1569
in pulmonary edema, 2418
septic embolism due to, 1527
Cavalieri method, for lung volume measurement, 24, *24*
Caveolae, of alveolar epithelial cells, 19–20
Caveolin-1 secretion, in alveoli, 20
Cavernous sinus thrombosis, in sinusitis, 916–917
Cavitation, in ankylosing spondylitis, 1710
in aspergillosis, 1132–1133, *1132*
in coccidioidomycosis, 1123, *1124*, 2024
in histoplasmosis, 1111, *1112*, *1113*, 1116
in lymphomatoid granulomatosis, 1458
in pneumonia, etiologic pathogens and, 920
in tuberculosis, 1064, 2182, *2183*
CC (closing capacity), of lung volume, 111
CCAAT enhancer-binding protein family, in lung development, 40
in monocyte-macrophage development, 406–407
Ccw. See *Compliance, chest wall.*
CD (cluster of differentiation) system, for lymphocytes, 413, 414t, 415t. See also subjects starting with *CD; T lymphocytes.*
CD3 complex, T lymphocytes and, 428–429
CD2 molecule, in T-lymphocyte activation, 431–432, *431*
CD4 molecule. See *T lymphocytes, CD4+.*
CD28 molecule, in T-lymphocyte activation, 431–432, *431*
CD44 molecule, metastasis and, 1387–1388
CD80 (B7-1) molecule, in T-lymphocyte activation, 431–432, *431*
CD86 (B7-2) molecule, in T-lymphocyte activation, 431–432, *431*
CD95 (FAS) molecule, in lung cancer, 1386–1387
CD117 molecule, in lung cancer growth, 1381
*CDK* genes and products, in lung cancer, 1383–1384
CDYN (dynamic lung compliance), 800, 2564
C/EBP transcription factors, in lung development, 40
in monocyte-macrophage development, 406–407
Cefadroxil, in endocarditis prophylaxis, 731t
Cefazolin, in endocarditis prophylaxis, 731t
Cefoxitin, in anaerobic pneumonia, 1019t, 1020
in mycobacterial infections, 1096
Ceftazidime, in melioidosis, 1028
in pneumonia, in granulocytopenia, 924–925, 925t
Ceftriaxone, in *Neisseria meningitidis* pneumonia, 1006
Cell(s). See also specific types, e.g., *Epithelium and epithelial cells.*
adaptation of, to environmental changes, 446, 450, *450–452*
atrophy of, 446
death of. See *Apoptosis; Cell(s), injury and death of; Necrosis.*
dysplasia of, 450
hyperplasia of, 446, 450, *451*
hypertrophy of, 446, *450*
inflammatory, 232, *233*
injury and death of, adaptation to, 446, 450, *450–452*
calcification in, 450, *453*
causes of, 443, 444t
in amyloidosis, 450, 454, *454*
lipid accumulation in, 454–455, *455*
pathology of, 444, 444t, *445–455*, 446, 450, 454–455
recurrent, pathology of, 450, *452*, *453*
reversibility of, 444
types of, 444, *445–449*, 446
interactions among, 232, *233*
metaplasia of, 450, *452*
neoplasia of, 450
Cell culture, adenovirus, 939–940
*Chlamydia*, 624, 1027
coronavirus, 625, 940–941
cytomegalovirus, 625, 943
cytopathic effects in, 625
hantavirus, 945
influenza virus, 625, 955
parainfluenza virus, 625, 961
respiratory syncytial virus, 963
rhinovirus, 625, 966
sputum specimens for, 609
varicella-zoster virus, 968

Cell cycle, insulin-like growth factor effects on, 504–505
Cell-mediated immune response. See *Immune response, cell-mediated.*
Cellulitis, periorbital, in sinusitis, 916
Central nervous system. See also *Brain; Spinal cord.*
chemoreceptors of, 190, *190*
in breathing control, 184–188
medulla in, 185–186, *185*, 188–189
pons in, *185*, 186–187
rhythm generation and, 188–189
spinal cord in, *185*, 187–188, *187*
suprapontine structures in, 187
tuberculosis of, 1083–1084, *1084*
Central sleep apnea. See under *Sleep apnea.*
Centrilobular nodule(s), 675
Cepacia syndrome, in cystic fibrosis, 1303
Cephalexin, in endocarditis prophylaxis, 731t
Cephalosporins, in cystic fibrosis, 1309, 1309t
in pneumonia, 922t, 995t, 996t, 998t
*Haemophilus influenzae*, 1008
*Klebsiella pneumoniae*, 1009
*Moraxella catarrhalis*, 1006
pneumococcal, 1001
*Staphylococcus aureus*, 1004
resistance to, in Enterobacteriaceae, 1010–1011
Ceramic fibers, in pneumoconiosis, 1831t, 1842
Cerebral edema, high-altitude, 1930t, 1932–1933
in mountain sickness, 1930
Cerebrospinal fluid, alkalinity of, at high altitude, 1917
analysis of, in cryptococcosis, 1130
in tuberculosis, 1083–1084
culture of, in pneumonia, 989
pH of, in metabolic acidosis, 171
ventilatory response and, 193
Ceroid accumulation, in Hermansky-Pudlak syndrome, 1749
Cervical magnetic stimulation, in respiratory muscle evaluation, 858–859
Cetirizine, in allergic rhinitis, 1349
Cetylpyridinium chloride, in specimen processing, 613t
CF. See *Cystic fibrosis.*
CFTR. See *Cystic fibrosis transmembrane regulator.*
Challenge testing. See *Provocation testing.*
Channels, ion. See *Ion channels*; specific channels.
Charcot-Leyden crystals, formation of, 1763, *1764*
CHART (continuous hyperfractionated accelerated radiation therapy), in lung cancer, 1433
Chastre method, for nosocomial pneumonia diagnosis, 747, *748*
Chédiak-Higashi syndrome, 2233t, 2237–2238
Chemical(s). See also specific chemicals.
as warfare agents, 1906–1907
asthma due to. See *Asthma, occupational.*
inhalation of, hypersensitivity pneumonitis in, 1869–1870
irritant. See *Irritant gases.*
lung injury due to, 477, *477*, 478t, 479t, 1588t, 1590–1591, 1903–1914
agents causing, 1905t
pathogenesis of, 1903–1904
sequelae of, 1904–1905
treatment of, 1904
occupational exposure to. See *Occupational and environmental disorder(s).*
Chemical mediators. See *Inflammatory mediator(s);* specific substances.
Chemical pleurodesis, in metastatic disease, 2074–2075
Chemoattractants, in asthma, 1261
Chemodectoma(s), of lung, 1481
of mediastinum, 2131–2132
Chemokines, 506–507
C type, 507, 507t
CC type, 507, 507t, 516–517
in pulmonary fibrosis, 518–519
receptors for, 517–518, 517t
CXC type, 507–511, 507t, 508t
angiogenic, 508, 508t
angiostatic, 508, 508t
in pulmonary fibrosis, 512–526, *513–515*
receptors for, 511–512, 511t
CXXXC type, 507, 507t
epithelial-derived, 1259t
in allergic rhinitis, 1347–1348
in angiogenesis, 513–514, *513–515*, 1387
in asthma, 1261
in granulomatous disease, 437–438
receptors for, 238, 511–512, 511t, 517–518, 517t
Chemoreceptors. See also *Carotid bodies.*
abnormalities of, hypercapnic response in, 820
central, 190, *190*
function of, at high altitude, 1917–1918
C-fiber endings as, 184
disorders of, hyperventilation in, 2146
hypoventilation in, 2140t, 2141–2143
in acid-base balance, 173
of lung, 570
peripheral, 189–190
Chemotactic factors, for eosinophils, 1759–1760
in smoking, 1212
Chemotherapy, for angioimmunoblastic lymphadenopathy, 1460
for carcinoid tumors, 1461–1462
for erythrocytosis, 2286
for Hodgkin's disease, 1454
for Kaposi's sarcoma, 2206
for lung cancer, agents for, 1437, 1437t
dose for, 1439
economic issues in, 1444
in advanced disease, 1437–1438, 1437t, 1438t
maintenance, 1439
postoperative, 1436–1437
preoperative, 1436
radiation therapy with, 1434
radiotherapy with, 1436–1437
second-line, 1439
small cell, 1434–1435, 1438–1439
versus stage, 1429–1432
for lymphoma, 1457, 2207
for mesothelioma, 2070
granulocytopenia in, pneumonia in, 924–925, 925t
pulmonary disease due to, 1972–1978
alkylating agents in, 1974t, 1975–1976
antibiotic agents in, 1972–1973, 1974t, 1976–1977, *1976*
antimetabolites in, 1974t, 1977, *1977*
diffuse alveolar hemorrhage as, 1744
nitrosoureas in, 1974t, 1977
pathogenesis of, 1972–1974, 1974t, *1975*
tuberculosis risk in, 1059
Chest. See also *Thorax.*
barrel-shaped, in chronic obstructive pulmonary disease, 1189
clapping of, for bronchiectasis, 1331
pain in. See *Chest pain.*
percussion of, in cystic fibrosis, 1308–1309
physical examination of, 592–599
Chest *(Continued)*
auscultation in, 597–599, 599t
inspection in, 596–597, 599t
lung sounds in, adventitious, 593–596, *594–596*, 594t, 598
continuous, 595–596
discontinuous, 595, *595*, *596*
generation of, 592–593, *592*
in disorders. See under *Lung sounds.*
normal, 593, *593*
perception of, 592–593, *592*
palpation in, 597, 599t
percussion in, 597, 599t
results interpretation in, 599, 599t
radiography of. See *Chest radiography.*
size of, at high altitude, 1918–1919
tightness of, in asthma, 1266
trauma to. See *Trauma, chest.*
wall of. See *Chest wall.*
Chest pain, 567–584. See also *Angina pectoris.*
assessment of, 567–568
causes of, 575, 575t
clinical features of, 590
differential diagnosis of, 580–581, 581t
drug-induced, 2035
epidemiology of, 567–568, *578*
importance of, 567
in acute chest syndrome, 2287
in amebiasis, 1145
in ankylosing spondylitis, 577
in aortic disorders, 579
in asbestosis, 1835
in aspergillosis, 1133
in beryllium lung disease, 1843
in cardiovascular disorders, 575t, 577–579
in chest wall disorders, 576–577
in cocaine toxicity, 579
in coccidioidomycosis, 1123
in costochondritis, 577
in cryptococcosis, 1130
in decompression sickness, 1961
in diaphragmatic paralysis, 2334
in diffuse alveolar hemorrhage, 1734
in endometriosis, 2325
in esophageal disorders, 571, 579–580, 581t, 2028
in exercise testing, 842
in fibrositis, 577
in flail chest, 2368
in gastrointestinal disorders, 575t, 579–580
in histoplasmosis, 1110
in HIV infection, 2175
in infectious arthritis, 577
in interstitial lung disease, 1655–1656
in Kaposi's sarcoma, 2205
in lung cancer, 1420
in lymphangio(leio)myomatosis, 1780
in mediastinal mass, 2081
in mediastinitis, 2106, 2112
in medical history, 590
in mesothelioma, benign fibrous, 2071
malignant, 2068
treatment of, 2070
in musculoskeletal disorders, 575t, 576–577
in myocardial ischemia, 578, 590
in neuritis, 577, 590
in nitrofurantoin-induced pulmonary disease, 1978
in Pancoast's syndrome, 577
in pancreatitis, 2028, 2029
in pericarditis, 578–579
in pleural effusion, 2000, 2026, 2021
in pleural fibrosis, 1839
in pleural tumors, 2072
in pleurisy, 575–576
in pleuropulmonary disorders, 575–576

Chest pain, 567–584 *(Continued)*
in pneumomediastinum, 2083, 2102
in pneumonia, *Acinetobacter*, 1013
anaerobic, 1017
beta-hemolytic streptococcal, 1004
*Chlamydia psittaci*, 1026
*Klebsiella pneumoniae*, 1008
*Legionella*, 1014
*Nocardia*, 1022
pneumococcal, 999
in pneumothorax, 2045, 2049
in postcardiac injury syndrome, 2032
in psychiatric disorders, 575t, 580
in pulmonary artery stenosis, 576
in pulmonary embolism, 576, 1507, 2026
in pulmonary hypertension, 576, 590, 1520, 1546–1547
in radiculitis, 577, 590
in rheumatoid arthritis, 1702, 2031
in shoulder-arm and shoulder-hand syndromes, 577
in sickle cell disease, 2288
in systemic lupus erythematosus, 1705, 2031
in systemic sclerosis, 1694
in tracheobronchitis, 576
in trauma, 577, 590
in tuberculosis, 1063, 2021
neuritic, 577
neurobiology of, 568–575
hyperalgesia and, 570–573, *571*, *572*
modulation and, 574–575
peripheral mechanisms in, 569–570
sensory neurons and, 573
somatic versus visceral pain in, 568–569, 572–574
spinal mechanisms in, 573–574, *574*
noncardiac, 579–580
overlap in, 575
pleuritic, 575–576
prevalence of, 568, *568*
radicular, 577
radiography in, 580, 581t
treatment of, 581, 2070
Chest physical therapy, 370–371, 370t
assessment of, 370
for bronchiectasis, 1331
for chronic obstructive pulmonary disease, 1224–1225
for cystic fibrosis, 368, 1308–1309
for pneumonia, 997
goals of, 370
in pulmonary rehabilitation, 2509
indications for, 370
techniques for, 370–371, 370t
Chest radiography. See also *Computed tomography; Magnetic resonance imaging; Ultrasonography.*
accuracy of, versus high-resolution computed tomography, 677–678, 678t
air gap in, 636, *636*
asymmetric film-screen, 640, *640*
contrast in, 634, *635*, *636*
digital (computed), 642, 644, *644*
focal spot in, 636
geometry of, 636, *636*
goals of, 634
grid ratio in, *635*, 636
history of, 634
in impairment and disability evaluation, 905
in intensive care unit, utility of, 665
in lung volume measurement, 793
in medical history, 591
inadequate, 634
indications for, 634
methods for, 633
moving slit and beam equalization, 640–642, *641–643*
Chest radiography *(Continued)*
noise in, 636–637
normal lung in, 1–2, *2*
of acute chest syndrome, in sickle cell disease, 2288
of acute lung disease, utility of, 665–666
of acute respiratory distress syndrome, 1594, 2417, *2418*, 2420t
of allergic bronchopulmonary aspergillosis, 1334, 1763, 1765–1766, *1765–1767*
of alveolar microlithiasis, 1749, *1750*
of alveolar proteinosis, 1795, *1795*
of amebiasis, 1145, *1145*
of amiodarone-induced pulmonary disease, 1981, *1982*
of ankylosing spondylitis, 1710
of arterial gas embolism, 1956, *1956*
of arteriovenous malformations, 1496, 1561–1562
of asbestosis, 1835
of aspergillosis, 1131–1133, *1132*, *1134*
of asthma, 666
of benign tumors, 1477
of beryllium lung disease, 1843
of blastomycosis, 1119, *1121*
of bronchial obstruction, 1369
of bronchiectasis, 1328, *1329–1332*
of bronchiolitis, 936, *936*
of bronchiolitis obliterans, 1198, 1363
of bronchiolitis obliterans organizing pneumonia, 1365, *1658*, 1686
of carcinoid tumor, 1461
of chest pain, 580, 581t
of chronic obstructive pulmonary disease, 666, *706*, *707*, 1190, *1190*, 1194–1195, *1195*, *1196*, 1209, *1209*
of coal-workers' pneumoconiosis, 1829
of coccidioidomycosis, 1123, 1124, *1124*, *1126*
of cor pulmonale, 1193, 1638–1639, *1639*
of cough, 561
of croup, 935, *936*
of cryptococcosis, 1130, 2196–2197, *2197*
of cystic fibrosis, 1303–1304
of decompression sickness, 1962
of dermatomyositis, 1708
of diffuse alveolar hemorrhage, *1658*, 1734, *1735*
of dyspnea, 665–666
of emphysema, 1190, *1190*, 1194–1195, *1195*, *1196*, 1209, *1209*
of empyema, 1018, *1018*, 1032
of esophageal perforation, 2107
of filariasis, 1154, *1154*, 1761–1762, *1762*
of germ cell tumor, 2127, *2127*
of hemothorax, 2060, *2061*
of hereditary hemorrhagic telangiectasia, *1559*
of histoplasmosis, 1110, *1110*, *1112–1114*, 1114, 2199, *2199*
of Hodgkin's disease, *1454*, 1455, *1455*
of human immunodeficiency virus infection, 2176
of hydatid disease, 1159, *1159*
of hypersensitivity pneumonitis, 1874–1875, *1875*
of influenza, 954, *954*
of interstitial lung disease, 1656–1659, *1658–1661*
of Kaposi's sarcoma, 2205, *2205*
of kyphoscoliosis, 2358, *2358*
of lung abscess, 1018, *1018*, 1031
of lung cancer, 1422
for screening, 1419–1420, 1420t
metastatic, 1471–1472, *1471–1473*, 1472t
utility of, 665
Chest radiography *(Continued)*
of lung injury, 1594
of lymphangio(leio)myomatosis, 1746–1747, *1747*, 1780t, 1781–1782, 2059, *2059*
of lymphoma, 2207, *2207*
of lymphomatoid granulomatosis, 1458, *1459*
of measles, 959
of mediastinal mass, 2125
of mediastinitis, 2114
of mediastinum, 2080, *2080*, 2081, 2083
of mesothelioma, benign fibrous, 2071, *2071*
malignant, 2068–2069, *2068*
of *Mycobacterium avium* complex infections, 1091, 1092t, 1093
of *Mycobacterium kansasii* infections, 2186
of neuromuscular disorders, 2332
of normal lung, 1–2, *2*
of paragonimiasis, 1161, *1162*
of pectus excavatum, 2365, *2365*
of pleural effusion, 2006–2007, *2006*, *2007*, 2014, *2014*
of pleural fibrosis, *1838*, 1839
of pleural tumors, metastatic, 2073, *2073*
of pneumoconiosis, 1813, 1815
of pneumomediastinum, 2103–2104, *2103*, *2104*
of pneumonia, 920–921, 988–989
*Acinetobacter*, 1013, *1013*
anaerobic, 1017, *1018*
cytomegalovirus, 943, *944*, 2202
eosinophilic, 1767, *1768*, 1768
*Haemophilus influenzae*, 1007, *1007*, 2179
in granulocytopenia, 924–925
*Klebsiella pneumoniae*, 1009, *1009*
*Legionella*, 1015, *1015*
*Mycoplasma pneumoniae*, 1024, *1024*
*Nocardia*, 1022, *1023*
pneumococcal, 999–1000, *1000*, 2179
*Pneumocystis carinii*, 926, 2188–2189, *2189*
*Pseudomonas aeruginosa*, 1012, *1012*, 2180
*Staphylococcus aureus*, 1003, *1003*
varicella-zoster virus, 967, *968*
of pneumonitis, lymphocytic interstitial, 2208, *2208*
of pneumothorax, 646, *648*, *652*, 2051, *2052*
primary spontaneous, 2046, *2046*
secondary, 2049
traumatic, 2052
of pulmonary edema, 1499, 1499t, 1500, 1594, 2417, *2418*
high-altitude, 1934, *1934*
of pulmonary embolism, *708*, *709*, 1510, *1510*
of pulmonary fibrosis, idiopathic, 1673, *1674*, *1675*, 1679
of pulmonary hypertension, 1494, 1547–1548, *1548*, 1638-1639, *1639*, 1520, *1521*
of relapsing polychondritis, 1709, *1709*
of respiratory bronchiolitis-associated interstitial lung disease, 1685
of rheumatoid arthritis, 1702–1703
of sarcoidosis, 1719–1723, *1720–1723*, 1722t
of sequestrations, 1568, *1568*
of silicosis, *1661*, 1823
of solitary nodule, 665
of systemic sclerosis, 1694, *1696*
of thymoma, 2126, *2126*
of toxoplasmosis, 1148, *1148*, 2203–2204
of tuberculosis, 1063–1065, *1063–1065*
disseminated (miliary), 1078

Chest radiography *(Continued)*
in HIV infection, 2182–2183, *2183*
of Wegener's granulomatosis, 1536
peak kilovoltage in, 634, *635*, 636, *636*
portable, 637, *637–639*, 639–640, 665
problems with, 633–634
quantum mottle in, 636–637
resolution in, 636
routine, utility of, 665
screening, utility of, 665
standards for, 637
techniques for, 634–640
angiographic. See *Angiography.*
aortographic. See *Aortography.*
bronchial angiographic, 658, *658–660*
bronchographic. See *Bronchography.*
cross-sectional. See *Computed tomography; Magnetic resonance imaging.*
fluoroscopic, 654
portable, 637, *637–639*, 639–640
pulmonary angiographic. See *Angiography.*
standard film-screen, 634–637, *635*, *636*
standards for, 637
tomographic, 654
views for, 644–654
decubitus, 646, *651–653*
expiration, 644, 646, *646–650*
lateral, 644, *645*
lordotic, 654
oblique, 654
posteroanterior, 644, *645*
routine, 655, *644*
Chest tube. See *Tube thoracostomy.*
Chest wall. See also *Rib(s).*
abnormalities of, radiography of, 646, *649*
ankylosing spondylitis effects on. See *Ankylosing spondylitis.*
cancer invasion of, magnetic resonance imaging in, 670–671, *672*
compliance of, definition of, 2564
in kyphoscoliosis, 2359, 2359t, *2360*
in pulmonary edema, 1585
components of, 103
configuration of, in pregnancy, 2317
disorders of, hypoventilation in, 2140t, 2142, *2142*
pain in, 576–577, 590
elastance of, increased, 1500, 2449
flail, in multiple rib fractures, 2366–2369, *2367*, 2367t, *2368*
kyphoscoliosis effects on. See *Kyphoscoliosis.*
mechanical properties of, 103–106, *103*, *105*
movement of, dyspnea and, 543
in flail chest, 2367–2368, *2367*, *2368*
in spinal cord injury, 2339
pressure-volume relationships in, 103–105, *103*
neurofibromatosis of, 1748, 1748t
obesity effects on. See *Obesity.*
paradoxical motion of, 106, 2339
receptors of, 184
disorders of, 2146
resection of, in lung cancer, 1429–1430
restriction of, in ankylosing spondylitis, 1710
sinus tract through, in actinomycosis, 1021–1022, *1021*
sounds of, 599
sternal depression in (pectus excavatum), 2359t, 2361t, 2364–2366, *2365*
thoracoplasty of, 2359t, 2361t, 2363–2364, 2364t
trauma to, flail chest in, 2366–2369, *2367*, 2367t, *2368*
Chest wall *(Continued)*
two-compartment model of, 105–106, *105*
Cheyne-Stokes breathing, 179, 2161
in heart disease, 2261
inspection of, 597
Chicken pox, 931t, 967–968, *968*
Chief complaint, in medical history, 587
Chills, amphotericin B-induced, 1116
in blastomycosis, 1119
in bronchial disorders, 1368
in histoplasmosis, 1110
in mediastinitis, 2106
in pneumonia, beta-hemolytic streptococcal, 1004
*Chlamydia psittaci*, 1026
Enterobacteriaceae, 1010
*Klebsiella pneumoniae*, 1008
*Legionella*, 1014
*Mycoplasma pneumoniae*, 1024
pneumococcal, 999
*Pseudomonas aeruginosa*, 1011
*Chlamydia pecorum* pneumonia, 473
*Chlamydia* pneumonia, culture in, 624
genetic tests for, 626
microbiologic diagnosis of, 610t
pathology of, 473
*Chlamydia pneumoniae* pneumonia, 473, 624, 998t, 1026–1027
as asthma risk factor, 1251–1252
in sickle cell disease, 2287
*Chlamydia psittaci* pneumonia, 473, 624, 998t, 1026
genetic tests for, 626
*Chlamydia trachomatis* pneumonia, 473, 624, 1027
Chlorambucil, pulmonary disease due to, 1976
Chloramine, exposure to, 1905–1906
Chloramphenicol, in pneumonia, 998t
Chloride, in air surface liquid, 339–340, 340t
in anion gap calculation, 163–164
loss of, in cystic fibrosis, 1180, 1292, 1307
metabolic alkalosis in, 162–163, 171–173, 171t
transport of. See also *Epithelium and epithelial cells, airway, electrolyte transport across.*
in cystic fibrosis, 1292, 1296–1300, 1296t, *1297*, *1298*
water transport with, 362
Chloride channels, apical membrane, 337
apical membrane epithelial, 337
basolateral membrane, 337–338
in cystic fibrosis, 1295, *1296*, 1299
in electrolyte transport, function of, 336–338, *336*
regulation of, 338–339
Chlorine, exposure to, 1905–1906
Chlorofluorocarbons, as aerosol propellants, 355–356
Chloropicrin, 1906
Chlorpromazine, in hiccups, 2350
Choke points, in expiratory flow, 101
Chokes, in decompression sickness, 1961
Cholangitis, sclerosing, 2276
Cholesterol, embolism of, 465
in pseudochylothorax, 2057, 2059–2060
Cholinergic nerves, 22
anticholinergic drug effects on, 276
beta-adrenergic agonists effects on, 269
of airway, *250*, 252–254, *253*
of pulmonary vessels, 121, 131
Cholinergic receptors, in mucus secretion regulation, 333
Chondritis, in relapsing polychondritis, 1695t, 1708–1710, *1709*
Chondroma(s), of lung, 1478
Chondroma(s) *(Continued)*
in Carney's triad, 1480, *1481*
Choriocarcinoma, of mediastinum, 2128
Choroidal tubercle, in tuberculosis, 1077
Chromium compound exposure, lung cancer in, 1401
Chromosomes, abnormalities of, mapping of, 45–47, *46*
alleles on, 46
recombination of, 46–47, *46*
Chronic granulomatous disease, 2233t, 2237
Chronic necrotizing aspergillosis, 1133
Chronic obstructive pulmonary disease, 1187–1245
after pneumomediastinum, 2098, *2098*
air travel in, 859–860
airflow in, limitation of, 1206–1207
versus lung volume, 102
airway resistance in, respiratory failure in, 2447–2448
asthma and, 1188, *1188*, 1199–1200
blue bloaters in, 1634
breathing in, oxygen requirements for, 2446
bullae in, 1194–1195, *1195*, *1196*, 1205
surgical treatment of, 1219–1220
versus pneumothorax, 2049
centriacinar, 462, *464*
chest radiography of, 666, *706*, *707*, 1190, *1190*
classification of, 462
clinical features of, 1189–1195, *1190*, *1191*, *1195*, *1196*
compliance in, 1207
complications of, 1192–1195
computed tomography of, 676, *676*, 1190, *1191*
cor pulmonale in, 1193–1194
angiotensin II in, 1636–1637
chest radiography of, 1638–1639, *1639*
echocardiography in, 1639–1641, *1640*
electrocardiography in, 1639
hemodynamics of, 1641
left ventricular failure in, 1636
pathophysiology of, 1632, 1633–1634, *1633*
right ventricular failure in, 1635–1636, *1635*, *1636*
treatment of, 1643–1646
cough in, *559*, 560, 564
crackles in, *595*
dead space/tidal volume in, during exercise, 211–212
definitions of, 1174, 1178, 1187–1189, *1188*, 1188t
diagnosis of, 1189–1192, *1190*, *1191*
differential diagnosis of, 1195, 1197–1198, 1197t
diffusing capacity in, 1207
disability in, 901, 901t
distal acinar, 462, *464*, 465
dyspnea in, 548
epidemiology of, 1198–1201, *1200*, *1201*
erythrocytosis in, 1192
etiology of, 1178–1179
exacerbation of, 1189
chest radiography of, 666
treatment of, 1222
exercise in, 1227
for training, 216–217, *217*
oxygen during, 1225–1226
ventilation requirements for, 209–210, *209*
ventilation response limitations in, 212–217, *213–215*, *217*
exercise testing in, 848
functional residual capacity in, 104–105
heterogeneity of, 1206

Chronic obstructive pulmonary disease *(Continued)*
high altitude effects on, 1941
historical background of, 1189
hypoxic pulmonary vasoconstriction in, 68
immunization in, 1217, 2508
impairment in, 897, 907, 903t
in alpha$_1$-antitrypsin deficiency, 2276
in ankylosing spondylitis, 1710
in byssinosis, 1862
in coal working, 1825–1828, *1826*
in HIV infection, 2209
in hypersensitivity pneumonitis, 1878
in inflammatory bowel disease, 2270
in influenza, 953–954
in Marfan's syndrome, 1711
in pneumomediastinum, 2103
in Sjögren's syndrome, 1706
interlobular, 2098
irregular, 462, *464*, 465
lung volume in, 802
maximal expiratory flow in, volume history and, 102–103
mortality in, 1198–1199, 1203, 1646
mucociliary transport in, 364–367
mucous gland function in, 1206
natural history of, 1201–1202, *1201*, *1202*
cor pulmonale and, 1646–1647
pulmonary circulation changes in, 1633
occupational factors in, 1200–1201
panacinar, 462, *464*
panlobar, computed tomography in, 676, *676*
pathogenesis of, 1178–1179, 1207–1217
airway inflammation in, 1215–1216
alpha$_1$-protease inhibitor deficiency in, 1208–1210, *1209*
elastase-antielastase hypothesis of, 1210 1214, *1210–1211*, *1214*
epithelial cell injury and repair in, 1216
infection in, 1216–1217
lung injury response in, 1214
secretory apparatus alterations in, 1214–1215, *1215*
pathology of, 462, *464*, 465, 1203–1206, *1203–1205*
pathophysiology of, neural mechanisms in, 256
pulmonary circulation changes in, 1633–1634, *1633*
perinatal factors in, 1201
physical examination in, 1189
pink puffers in, 1634
pneumonia in, 988t, 1194
pneumothorax in, 1192–1193, 2049, 2050
preoperative evaluation in, 887–888, 887t, *888*
pressure-volume curve for, *103*, 104–105
prognosis for, 1202–1203
cor pulmonale and, 1646–1647
pulmonary embolism in, 1512
pulmonary function tests in, 802, 1190–1192, 1206–1207
pulmonary hypertension in, 1193
angiotensin II in, 1636–1637
hemodynamics of, 1641
left ventricular failure in, 1636
natural history of, 1646–1647
pathophysiology of, 1632–1634, *1633*
right ventricular failure in, 1635–1636, *1635*, *1636*
pulmonary rehabilitation in. See *Pulmonary rehabilitation.*
quality of life in, after lung volume reduction surgery, 1218
reduced cardiovascular function in, exercise testing in, 222–225, 224t

Chronic obstructive pulmonary disease *(Continued)*
respiratory acidosis in, 174
respiratory failure in, 2447–2448, 2460–2465
clinical features of, 2460
prognosis for, 2465
treatment of, 1228–1229, 2460–2465
after intubation, 2463–2464
before intubation, 2460–2463, 2461t
liberation from ventilator in, 2464–2465
respiratory muscle fatigue in, 109
risk factors for, 1199–1201, *1200*, *1201*, 1893
silicosis with, 1819
simple air-space enlargement in, 1203–1204
sleep disorders in, 1194
smoking and, 1178, 1199, *1200*, *1201*
animal models of, 1213–1214
bullae formation and, 1195, *1196*
cessation of, 1217, 2513–2514, *2513*, 2514t, 2533
inflammatory cells and, 1212
natural history and, 1201–1202, *1201*, *1202*
pathogenic aspects of, 1207–1209, *1209*
sputum examination in, 1192
squamous metaplasia in, *452*
structure-function correlations in, 1206–1207
surgical risks in, 883–884
synonyms for, 1188
total lung capacity in, 104–105
total vital capacity changes in, 112
treatment of, 1217–1230. See also *Pulmonary rehabilitation.*
adhesion molecular blockers in, 287
aerosolized drugs in, 357, 359
angiotensin-converting enzyme inhibitors in, 1644–1645
antibiotics in, 1225
anticholinergic drugs in, 276–277, *276*
anti-cytokines in, 286–287, *288*
antitussives in, 289
bronchodilators in, 1220–1223, 1223t
corticosteroids in, 281, 1223–1224
cromolyn in, 1224
digoxin in, 1643
drugs contraindicated in, 290–291
enzyme inhibitors in, 288
for breathlessness, 289
furosemide in, 288
genetic aspects of, 288–289
immunomodulators in, 287–288
in cor pulmonale, 1643–1646
in dyspnea, 1228
in exacerbation, 1222
in tracheal stenosis, 1229
in ventilatory failure, 1228–1229
inflammatory mediator antagonists in, 286, 287t
lung volume reduction surgery in, 715
mechanical ventilation in, 1229
mucoregulators in, 289
neuromodulators in, 288
new, 286–289, 287t, *288*, 1217–1218
nitric oxide in, 1645
nutrition in, 1227–1228
overall strategy for, 1230, *1230*
oxygen in, 299, 1225–1226, 1225t, 1229, 1643–1644, 1646–1647
phosphodiesterase inhibitors in, 287
pulmonary rehabilitation in. See *Pulmonary rehabilitation.*
secondary, 1225–1229, 1225t
secretion mobilization in, 1224–1225
smoking cessation in, 1217

Chronic obstructive pulmonary disease *(Continued)*
surfactant in, 320
surgical, 1218–1220
symptomatic, 1220–1225, 1220t, 1223t
theophylline in, 275
transcription factor blockers in, 288
vasodilators in, 1644
ventilatory stimulants in, 289–290
ventilation-perfusion scanning in, 82–83, *82*, 697–700, *706*, *707*
versus asthma, 1268
weakness in, 2447
Chronic Respiratory Disease Questionnaire, in dyspnea, 544
Chrysotile, 1831t
diseases due to, 2067
microscopic appearance of, *1814*
Churg-Strauss syndrome, 1538, 1769–1771, *1770*, 1770t
pleural effusion in, 2033
Chvostek's sign, in metabolic alkalosis, 172
in respiratory alkalosis, 175
Chyle, composition of, 2056
Chyliform pleural fluid, 2057, 2059–2060
Chylothorax, 2056–2059
clinical manifestations of, 2057
congenital, 2059
definition of, 2056
diagnosis of, 2057–2058
etiology of, 2056–2057, 2055t
iatrogenic, 2056
idiopathic, 2057
in lymphangiomyomatosis, 2059, *2059*
in neoplastic disease, 2072
neonatal, 2057
pathophysiology of, 2056
pleural fluid examination in, 2003
traumatic, 2056–2058
treatment of, 2058–2059
versus chyliform pleural fluid, 2057, 2059–2060
versus pseudochylothorax, 2057, 2059–2060
Chylous fluid collections, in lymphangio(leio)myomatosis, 1784
Chymase, in mucus hypersecretion, 334
Cidex solutions, for bronchoscope disinfection, 758
Cidofovir, in cytomegalovirus infections, 944, 2202–2203
Cigar smoking, lung cancer risk with, 1400
Cigarette smoking. See *Smoking.*
Cilia. See also *Mucociliary transport.*
of airway epithelial cells, 7, *8*, *9*
beat frequency of, 365
fluid surrounding, 362–363
function of, 360–361
immotile, 482
in cystic fibrosis, 1180, *1180*
ozone injury of, 1895–1896
primary dyskinesia of, 366, 480t, 482, 1336
regulation of, 361–362
Cimetidine, in gastroesophageal reflux, 2269–2270
Ciprofloxacin, in cystic fibrosis, 1309–1310, 1309t
in pneumonia, 995t, 1006
Circadian rhythms, pulmonary function test effects of, 803
Circulation, bronchial, anatomy of, 10–11
circuit for, 2386, *2386*
in respiratory failure. See under *Respiratory failure.*
pulmonary. See *Pulmonary circulation.*
Circulatory collapse, in pulmonary embolism, 1507, 2026

Cirrhosis, arteriovenous malformations in, 1496
biliary, in cystic fibrosis, 1306–1307, 1312–1313
primary, 2275–2276
hepatic hydrothorax in, 2015–2016
hepatopulmonary syndrome in. See *Hepatopulmonary syndrome.*
pleural effusion in, 2015–2016, 2271
portopulmonary hypertension in, 2275
Cisplatin, in lung cancer, 1437–1438, 1437t
radiation therapy with, 1434
Citric acid, as cough stimulant, 252
*Citrobacter* infections, pneumonia due to, 1010–1011
CL. See *Lung compliance.*
*Cladosporum* spores, hypersensitivity pneumonitis due to, 1869
Clapping, chest, for bronchiectasis, 1331
Clara cells, function of, 360
in airway epithelium, 10, *11*
surfactant protein A in, 310
Clarithromycin, in *Mycobacterium avium* complex infections, 1091–1092, 2185, 2186
in *Mycobacterium kansasii* infections, 2186
in pneumonia, 995t
in tuberculosis, in HIV infection, 2184
Clark oxygen electrode, 832–833, *832*
Clean Air Act of 1970, 2556–2557
Cleaning, of bronchoscopy equipment, 758
Clear cell tumors, benign, of lung, 1479–1480
Clearance, alveolar. See *Alveolus(i), clearance from.*
mucociliary. See *Mucociliary transport.*
of aerosols, 354–355, *354*
of airway, in cystic fibrosis, 1308–1309
of cough, 365, 556
of drugs, 248
of pulmonary embolism, 14
of surfactant, granulocyte-macrophage colony-stimulating factor in, 404
Clearance time, in ventilation-perfusion scanning, 698, 700
Clindamycin, in cystic fibrosis, 1309t
in endocarditis prophylaxis, 731t
in malaria, 1147
in pneumonia, 922t, 998t
anaerobic, 1019t, 1020
pneumococcal, 1001
*Pneumocystis carinii*, 2191t, 2192
in toxoplasmosis, 1149, 2204
Clodronate, alveolar macrophage depletion due to, 394
Cloning, of mucins, 328, 330t
positional, in asthma studies, 1252–1253
Closed-circuit helium method, for lung volume measurement, 791–793, *792*, 793t
Closing capacity, of lung volume, 111
Closing volume, in ventilation distribution evaluation, 806–807
of airways, 59–60, *59*
*Clostridium botulinum* toxin, respiratory effects of, 2342–2343
*Clostridium* pneumonia, 1019t
*Clostridium tetani* infections, respiratory effects of, 2351–2352
Clotting factor deficiencies, 2294–2295
Clubbing, digital, clinical features of, 600, *600–602*, 601
in cystic fibrosis, 1305
in hepatopulmonary syndrome, 2272, 2273
in interstitial lung disease, 1656
in lung abscess, 1018
in lung cancer, 1421
Clubbing *(Continued)*
in pulmonary fibrosis, 1678
pathogenesis of, 600, 601t
Cluster of differentiation system, for lymphocytes, 413, 414t, 415t. See also subjects starting with *CD*; *T lymphocytes.*
$Co_2$ (oxygen content), measurement of, 833–834
mixed venous, in moderate exercise, 202, 210
Coagulation disorder(s). See also *Thrombosis.*
at high altitude, 1937–1938
bronchoscopic complications in, 757
diffuse alveolar hemorrhage in, 1744
disseminated intravascular, 1191, 2295, 2323
evaluation for, before bronchoscopy, 730
in acute respiratory distress syndrome, 520
in amniotic fluid embolism, 1526–1527
in clotting factor deficiencies, 2294–2295
in leukemia, 2291
in lung cancer, 1421, 1421t
in lung injury, 1586
pulmonary embolism in, 1504, 1505t
venous thromboembolism in, 1504, 1505t
Coagulation necrosis, 444, 446, *447*
Coal macule, 1825–1827, *1826*
Coal-workers' pneumoconiosis, 1824–1830
chest radiography of, 1829
clinical features of, 1829
coal quality and, 1827
complications of, 1830
definition of, 1824–1825
diagnosis of, 1830
epidemiology of, 1827–1829
natural history of, 1827–1829
pathogenesis of, 1827
pathology of, 1826–1827, *1827*
pulmonary function tests in, 1828–1830
risk factors for, 1825–1826
silicosis with, 1828
surveillance for, 1815
tissue reactions to, 1824–1825, *1825*
treatment of, 1830
Coarctation, aortic, imaging of, 683
Cobalt, in hard metal products, lung disease from, 1844–1845
Cobb angle, in kyphoscoliosis, 2358, *2358*, 2359, 2361
Cocaine, in bronchoscopy, 732
pulmonary disease due to, 1980, 1980t
toxicity of, chest pain in, 579
Coccidioidin test, for coccidioidomycosis, 1126
Coccidioidomycosis, 1121–1128
asymptomatic, 1123
cavity rupture in, 2024
chest radiography of, 1123, 1124, *1124*, *1126*, 2200
clinical manifestations of, 1123–1125, *1124*, *1126*, 2200
complications of, 1123–1124, *1124*
culture in, 622–623, 1125
diagnosis of, 626, 1125–1126, 2200
dimorphism in, 1107
disseminated, 1124–1125, 1127–1128
epidemiology of, 1122
extrapulmonary, 1124–1125
genitourinary, 1125
geographic distribution of, 1107, 2100
history of, 1121–1122
immune response in, 1108, 1122–1123
in HIV infection, 1124–1125, *1126*, 1127, 2198t, 2199–2200
in immunodeficiency, 1124
in pregnancy, 2321
mediastinitis in, 2111
meningitis in, 1125, 1127–1128
Coccidioidomycosis *(Continued)*
microbiologic diagnosis of, 610t
mycologic studies in, 1125
osseous, 1124–1125
pathogenesis of, 1122–1123, *1123*, 2200
pathology of, *469*
persistent primary, 1124
pleural effusion in, 2024
prevention of, 2200
primary, 2024
self-limited, 1122
serologic studies in, 1125
skin lesions in, 1123, 1124
skin tests in, 1123, 1126
spectrum of, 1121
treatment of, 1127–1128, 2200
Codeine, in cough control, 289
Coexisting symptoms, definition of, 896
Cognitive dysfunction, at high altitude, 1923–1924
in sleep apnea, 2158
Coil embolization, of arteriovenous malformations, 1564–1565, *1564*
Coin lesions, in coccidioidomycosis, 1123
Coke oven emissions, exposure to, lung cancer in, 1401–1402
Colchicine, in amyloidosis, 2296
in pulmonary fibrosis, 1681t, 1682–1683
Cold, common. See *Common cold.*
Cold agglutinin test, for *Mycoplasma pneumoniae*, 990–991
Cold stress, in diving, 1952–1953
Colfosceril, in acute respiratory distress syndrome, 320–321
in pulmonary edema, 1609
Colitis, ulcerative, pulmonary complications of, 2270–2271, 2270t
Collagen(s), deposition of, in asthma, 1254, *1255*
in pulmonary fibrosis, 1677, 1678
in repair, 496
in lung, 93, 137
endothelial permeability and, 143–144
interstitial macrophages proximity to, 388–389, *388*
macrophage degradation of, 392–393
overgrowth of, in systemic sclerosis, 1692, 1694
type IV, metastasis effects on, 1388
Collagen vascular disease(s). See *Connective tissue disease(s).*
Collagenases, in metastasis, 1388
of alveolar macrophages, 392–393
Colloid osmotic pressure, in pulmonary circulation, 132–133, *132*, 1497, 1498t
Colon, cancer of, metastasis from, to lung, *1472*
cystic fibrosis of, pathology of, 1295
distention of, pain in, 571–573, *571*, *572*
inflammatory disease of, pulmonary complications of, 2270–2271, 2270t
tuberculosis of, 1084–1085
Colonization, *Aspergillus*, in lung transplantation, 2522
Enterobacteriaceae, 1011
gram-negative bacteria, versus superinfection, 615–616
in cystic fibrosis, 1302–1303, *1303*
*Klebsiella pneumoniae*, 1008
*Neisseria meningitidis*, 1005
nosocomial pneumonia development from, 922
pneumonia diagnosis and, 607, *607*, 608t
*Staphylococcus aureus*, 1002–1003
*Streptococcus pneumoniae*, 999
Colony-forming units, in monocyte-macrophage development, 400, *400*

Colony-stimulating factors, epithelial-derived, 1259t
Colorimetric method, for carbon dioxide measurement, 837
Coma, aspiration pneumonia in, 1017
  in respiratory acidosis, 174
Common cold, 916, 932–933, *932*
  bronchitis after, 934
  clinical manifestations of, 965–966
  coronavirus, 941
  cough in, 558
  diagnosis of, 966
  epidemiology of, 965
  pathogenesis of, 965
  pharyngitis in, 933–934, 933t, *934*
  prevention of, 966–967
  rhinovirus, 931t, 964–967, *965*
  transmission of, 965
  treatment of, 966–967
  viruses causing, 932t
Common variable immunodeficiency, 2233t, 2235
Communication, cultural factors in, 2492
  importance of, 2492
  in ethical decision making, 2495, 2499
  in physician-patient relationship, 586
Community-acquired pneumonia. See *Pneumonia, community-acquired.*
Compensation, in acid-base status. See under *Acid-base balance and imbalance.*
  workers', evaluation for, 895, 898, 902
Complement, 519–520, *519*
  action of, *2225*
  activation of, 519–520, *519*
    contrast agent-induced, 1988
    in hemodialysis, 2280
    in hypersensitivity reaction, 466, *467*
    in smoking, 1212
    in vasculitis, 1534
  deficiency of, 2233t, 2234t, 2236
Complement fixation test, for *Chlamydia*, 624
  for *Coccidioides immitis*, 1125
  for fungi, 623
  for *Histoplasma capsulatum*, 1115–1116
  for *Mycoplasma*, 624
  for *Mycoplasma pneumoniae*, 991, 1025
  for *Paracoccidioides brasiliensis*, 1129
Complex regional pain syndrome, 577
Compliance, bronchiolar, 1361–1362
  chest wall, in kyphoscoliosis, 2359, 2359t, *2360*
    in pulmonary edema, 1585
  definition of, 2564
  dynamic, definition of, 2564
  lung. See *Lung compliance.*
  pulmonary vascular, 127–128, *128*
  respiratory system, in kyphoscoliosis, 2359, 2359t
    in obesity, 2371t, 2372
  specific, definition of, 2564
  static, 2564
  thoracic, in exercise, in chronic obstructive pulmonary disease, 215
  with asthma self-management program, 2533, 2535–2540, 2535t–2539t
Compression, pneumatic, in thromboembolic disease prevention, 1514–1515
Compromised host. See *Immunodeficiency.*
Computed (digital) radiography, 642, 644, *644*
Computed tomography, 661–663
  advantages of, 661
  contrast enhancement in, 662–663
  high-resolution, 661
    accuracy of, 677–678, 678t
    in disease activity assessment, 678
    sensitivity and specificity of, 677
Computed tomography *(Continued)*
    slice parameters in, 662
    versus chest radiography, 677–678, 678t
  image display in, 661
  in percutaneous needle biopsy, 761
  interventional, 663, *663*
  of acute respiratory distress syndrome, 2416, *2416*
  of airways, 679, *679–681*
  of alveolar proteinosis, 1795
  of amiodarone-induced pulmonary disease, 1982, *1982*
  of aortic dissection, 683, *684*, *685*
  of aortic pseudoaneurysm, 683, *686*
  of arteriovenous malformations, 1562
  of asbestosis, 1835
  of benign tumors, 1477
  of brachial plexopathy, 671–672
  of brain, in lung cancer, 1423
  of bronchi, 679, *679*
  of bronchiectasis, 679, *680*, *681*, 1328–1329, *1332*
  of bronchiolitis obliterans, in rheumatoid arthritis, 1700–1701, *1700*
  of bronchiolitis obliterans organizing pneumonia, 1686
  of calcification, 2312, *2312*
  of chronic obstructive pulmonary disease, 676, *676*, 1190, *1191*
  of coal-workers' pneumoconiosis, 1829
  of congenital great vessel anomalies, 683, *687*
  of cystic fibrosis, 1303–1304
  of dermatomyositis, 1708
  of diffuse lung disease, 673–679
    parenchymal, 673–678, *674–677*, 678t
    utility of, 677–679, 678t
    with cystic lesions, 676, *676*, *677*
    with decreased opacity, 676, *676*, *677*
    with increased opacity, 675–676, *676*
    with nodules, 675, *675*
    with reticular opacities, 674–675, *674*, *675*
  of dyspnea, 547
  of emphysema, 1190, *1191*
  of empyema, 688, 1032, 2007
    with bronchopleural fistula, 2020, *2021*
  of eosinophilic granuloma, *1662*
  of hamartoma, 1479, *1479*
  of hemothorax, 688, 2060
  of HIV infection, 2176–2177
  of hydatid disease, 1159, *1159*
  of hypersensitivity pneumonitis, 1661, *1661*, 1874–1875, *1875*
  of idiopathic pulmonary fibrosis, *1662*
  of interstitial lung disease, 674, *674*, *675*, 1659–1661, *1661–1663*, 1694
  of lung abscess, 688, 2007
  of lung cancer, 750
    for screening, 1420
    for staging, 1423
    metastatic, 1472
  of lymphangio(leio)myomatosis, *1663*, 1747, *1747*, 1782–1783, *1782*
  of mediastinum, 2083–2085, *2085*, 2086
    in mass detection, 672–673, *673*, 2125
    in mediastinitis, 2110
  of mesothelioma, 2007, 2068–2069
  of nodule(s), 716
    multiple, 668–669, *669*
    solitary, 666–668, *667–669*
  of pleura, 686, *687*, 688, *688*
    in asbestos-related disease, *1838*
    in effusion, 688, 2007, 2009, 2027
    in thickening, 688, *688*
  of pneumoconiosis, 1815
Computed tomography *(Continued)*
  of pneumomediastinum, 2104
  of pneumonia, *Pneumocystis carinii*, 2189
  of pneumothorax, 688
  of pulmonary embolism, 679–681, 680t, *682*, 1512, *1512*
  of pulmonary fibrosis, 1673, 1679
  of relapsing polychondritis, 1709, *1709*
  of respiratory bronchiolitis-associated interstitial lung disease, 1685
  of rheumatoid arthritis, 1703
  of sarcoidosis, 1720, 1722
  of sequestrations, 1568
  of solitary nodule, 1439
  of systemic sclerosis, 1694
  of trachea, 679
  of tuberculosis, *687*
  patient position for, 662
  principles of, 661
  protocols for, 662–663
  scanning range for, 662
  slice parameters in, 662
  spiral/helical, 661
    contrast agents in, 663
    slice parameters in, 662
    versus conventional, 661–662
  versus magnetic resonance imaging, of mediastinum, 2085–2086
Computed tomography angiography, in pulmonary embolism, 2008
Concentration, drug, equation for, 248
Concentration alkalosis, 170
Conditional pacemaker, in respiratory rhythm generation, 188
Conductance, in airflow, 95, *96*, 787
  measurement of, 798, 799
Conducting airways. See also specific components, e.g., *Bronchus(i).*
  definition of, 55
  structure of, 56, *56*
Congenital disorder(s), chylothorax as, 2059
  in vitamin A deficiency, 38–39
  Kartagener's triad as, 1336
  of bronchi, cartilage deficiency as, 1334–1335
  of heart, imaging of, 683, 686, *687*
  of lung, 35, 482
    alveolar proteinosis as, 318
    bronchopulmonary sequestration as. See *Sequestration(s), bronchopulmonary.*
    hypoplasia as, 1198
    in Gli transcription factor defects, 39
    in retinoic acid receptor defects, 39
    in sonic hedgehog molecule defects, 38
  pulmonary artery aneurysms with, 1569
  toxoplasmosis as, 1147
  tracheobronchial, 482, 1337
Congestion, nasal, in rhinitis, 1347
Congestive heart failure. See under *Heart failure.*
Conjunctivitis, in adenovirus infections, 939, *939*
  in measles, 958
  occupational, 1859
Connective tissue, of lung, 4, *5*, 5t, *6*, 93
    alveolar septa as, 126
  of pleura, 1996, *1997*
Connective tissue activating protein-III, 508, 508t
Connective tissue disease(s). See also specific diseases, e.g., *Rheumatoid arthritis; Systemic lupus erythematosus.*
  bronchiolitis obliterans with, 1364
  diffuse alveolar hemorrhage in, 1737t, 1739–1740, *1739*
  fibrosis in, bronchoscopy in, 753

Connective tissue disease(s) *(Continued)*
interstitial lung disease in, *1650*, 1652t
kyphoscoliosis in, 2357, 2358t
overlap syndromes in, 1708
pleural effusions in, 2005
primary biliary cirrhosis with, 2275
pulmonary hypertension with, 1545
silicosis with, 1819, 1822
treatment of, lung toxicity in, 1691, 1692t, 1693t
Consciousness, alterations of, in diving, as contraindications to diving, 1963
in decompression sickness, 1961
in gas embolism, 1955–1956
in near drowning, 1964, 1965
breathing control and, 180
Consequentionalist ethical theory, 2490
Consolidation, breath sounds in, 598
computed tomography of, 675–676, *676*
in lymphoma, 1457
in pneumonia, in HIV infection, 2179
*Legionella*, 1014
in pulmonary edema, 1499
physical findings in, 599t
ventilation-perfusion scanning in, 697
Continuous diaphragm sign, in pneumomediastinum, 2103, *2103*
Continuous hyperfractionated accelerated radiation therapy (CHART), in lung cancer, 1433
Continuous positive airway pressure, in asthma, 2456
in flail chest, 2368
in neuromuscular disorders, 2348
in respiratory failure, 2462
in sleep apnea, 2160, 2165
in status asthmaticus, 2456
work of breathing and, 2448–2449
Contrast, in chest radiography, 634, *635*, 636
in computed tomography, enhancement of, 662–663
Contrast agents, in computed tomography, 662–663, 667
in mediastinal radiography, 2083
in venography, 1508, *1508*
leukostasis due to, 1988
Controller drugs, in asthma, corticosteroids as, 278–283, *279–281*, 279t, 282t
cromones as, 283–284
Contusion, lung, hypoxemia in, 2416
treatment of, 2436–2437
Cor pulmonale, 1631–1648
angiotensin in, 1636–1637
chest radiography of, 1638–1639, *1639*
clinical manifestations of, 1637–1638
definition of, 1193, 1493, 1631
diagnosis of, 1193
differential diagnosis of, 1641–1642, 1641t
echocardiography in, 1639–1641, *1640*
electrocardiography in, 1639, *1640*
hemodynamics of, 1641
in bronchiectasis, 1328, 1331
in chronic obstructive pulmonary disease, 1193–1194
in emphysema, 1193–1194
in kyphoscoliosis, 2361
in rheumatoid arthritis, 1699
in sarcoidosis, 1719
in schistosomiasis, 1163, 1164, 1525–1526
left ventricular failure in, 1636
natriuretic peptides in, 1637
natural history of, 1646–1647
neurohormones in, 1636
pathophysiology of, 1193, 1493
pulmonary circulation and, anatomy of, 1631–1633, *1632*, *1633*
Cor pulmonale *(Continued)*
pathophysiology of, 1633–1634
pulmonary hypertension in, 1493
anatomic considerations in, 1631–1632, *1632*
classification of, 1641–1643, 1641t
clinical manifestations of, 1637–1638
definition of, 1632
evaluation of, 1638–1641, *1639*, *1640*
high altitude and, 1634
pathophysiology of, 1633–1634
treatment of, 1643–1646
vasoconstrictive, 1633–1634, 1642
right ventricular failure in, 1634–1636, *1635*, *1636*
treatment of, 1193–1194, 1643–1646
Cord blood, transplantation of. See *Blood and bone marrow transplantation.*
Corner vessels, function of, 126
Coronary artery disease. See also *Angina pectoris.*
bypass surgery in, pleural effusion in, 2032
pulmonary function after, 886
high altitude effects on, 1940
in diving candidates, 1963–1964
in polyarteritis nodosa, 1541
pain in, 578
Coronavirus infections, 625, 931t, 940–941
Corticospinal tracts, in breathing control, 187, *187*
Corticosteroid(s), administration routes for, 280–281
beta-adrenergic agonist tolerance and, 271
chemistry of, 278, *278*
clinical uses of, 281
dissociated, 283
dosage for, 280–281
future trends in, 283
in acute respiratory distress syndrome, 2422
in allergic bronchopulmonary aspergillosis, 1132, 1766
in allergic granulomatosis and angiitis, 1770
in allergic rhinitis, 1349
in allograft rejection, 2523
in asthma, 278–283, *279–281*, 279t, 282t, 1270, 1273–1276, 1277t, 2454t, 2455
aerosol delivery of, 357, 359
in pregnancy, 2319–2320
steroid-sparing therapy with, 286
with beta-adrenergic agonists, 270
in bronchiolitis obliterans, 1366
in bronchiolitis obliterans organizing pneumonia, 1365–1366, 1686–1687
in chronic obstructive pulmonary disease, 1223–1224, 2461–2462, 2461t
aerosol delivery of, 357, 359
in cough, postinfectious, 564
in cystic fibrosis, 1310
in diffuse alveolar hemorrhage, in bone marrow transplantation, 2300
in emphysema, 1223–1224
in Goodpasture's syndrome, 1743
in hypereosinophilic syndrome, 1769
in hypersensitivity pneumonitis, 1879
in idiopathic pneumonia syndrome, 2300
in inflammatory bowel disease, 2271
in interstitial lung disease, 1672
in isolated pulmonary capillaritis, 1738
in microscopic polyangiitis, 1739
in nitrofurantoin-induced pulmonary disease, 1979
in nonallergic rhinitis, 1350
in pleural effusion, in systemic lupus erythematosus, 2032
in pneumonia, eosinophilic, 1767, 1769
*Pneumocystis carinii*, 2193–2194
Corticosteroid(s) *(Continued)*
in pulmonary edema, 1608–1609, 2422
in pulmonary fibrosis, 1681–1682, 1681t
in relapsing polychondritis, 1710
in respiratory failure, 2461–2462, 2461t
in respiratory syncytial virus infections, 963
in sarcoidosis, 1727
in sickle cell disease, 2289
in status asthmaticus, 2454t, 2455
in systemic lupus erythematosus, 2032
in toxic exposures, 1904
in tuberculosis, 1075
central nervous system, 1084
lymphatic, 1079
pericardial, 1086
in vasculitis, 1536
in Wegener's granulomatosis, 1738
inhaled, 248–249
advantages of, 280–281
chemical structures of, 278, *278*
clinical uses of, 281
future of, 283
in asthma, 357, 359
in chronic obstructive pulmonary disease, 357, 359, 1223
in croup, 935
mechanisms of action of, 279, *280*
pharmacokinetics of, 280, *281*
selection of, 282
side effects of, 282, 282t
intravenous administration of, 280
mechanisms of action of, 278–280, *279*, 279t, *280*
new, 283
oral, 280, 281
pharmacokinetics of, 280, *281*
pulmonary disease due to, 1985, *1986*
receptors for, 241, 245
resistance to, in asthma, 280, 281
selection of, 282
side effects of, 282, 282t, 1223, 1682
withdrawal from, 282
Corticotropin. See *Adrenocorticotropic hormone.*
Corticotropin-releasing hormone, in lung development, 41
Cortisol, excess of, respiratory manifestations of, 2312–2313
*Corynebacterium diphtheriae* infections, diagnosis of, 917
*Corynebacterium* infections. See also *Rhodococcus (Corynebacterium) equi pneumonia.*
pneumonia due to, 1030
Coryza. See *Common cold.*
Costochondritis, pain in, 577, 581t
Costophrenic angle, lateral, in pleural effusion, 2006
Cotton dust, byssinosis due to, 1860–1862
Cough, 553–566
absence of, in spinal cord injury, 2337–2338
acute, causes of, 588
definition of, 557
differential diagnosis of, 558
evaluation of, 562
afferent nerves in, 252
air volume in, 557, *557*
airflow velocity in, 369
anatomy of, 553–556, *554*
angiotensin-converting enzyme inhibitor–induced, 291, *559*, 560, 564, 1981
as particulate defense, 1889
assistance with, in neuromuscular disorders, 2346
barking, 935
brassy, 588

Cough *(Continued)*
causes of, 553, 588
central nervous system control of, 554–555, *555*
character of, 588–589
chronic, causes of, 588, *589*
definition of, 557
differential diagnosis of, 558–561, *559*
evaluation of, 561–562, 563t
clinical features of, 588–589
complications of, 370, 557, 558t
compressive phase of, *555*, 556
controlled, in chronic obstructive pulmonary disease, 1224
corticosteroid-induced, 282
croupy, 588
differential diagnosis of, 557–561, *559*, 1268, 1269t, 1877
drug-induced, 2035
dry, 556
effectiveness of, 369–370, 556
assessment of, 557, *557*
facilitation of, 1224, 2346, 2509
evaluation of, 561–562, 563t
flow-volume relationships in, 788, *790*
forced expiration technique for, 369, 1224
functions of, 369–370, 556
habit, 561
honking, 561
in acute chest syndrome, 2287
in alveolar proteinosis, 1794
in amebiasis, 1145
in asbestosis, 1835
in aspergillosis, 1133
in asthma, 559, *559*, 563, 1266, 1268
occupational, 1856, 1859
in beryllium lung disease, 1843
in blastomycosis, 1119
in bone marrow transplantation, 2299
in bronchial disorders, 1368
in bronchiectasis, *559*, 560, 564, 1327
in bronchiolitis, 1362
in bronchiolitis obliterans, 1363, 1364
in bronchiolitis obliterans organizing pneumonia, 1365
in bronchitis, *559*, 560, 564, 919, 1189
acute, 934
chronic, 367
in cancer, 560–561
in candidiasis, 1135
in carcinoid tumor, 1461
in chemotherapy-induced disease, 1974
in chronic obstructive pulmonary disease, 1189
in ciliary dyskinesia, 366
in coal-workers' pneumoconiosis, 1829
in coccidioidomycosis, 1123, 2200
in common cold, 558, *932*, 933
in cor pulmonale, 1637–1638
in croup, 935
in cryptococcosis, 1130, 2196
in cystic fibrosis, 1296–1297, 1302, 1310
in decompression sickness, 1961
in diaphragmatic paralysis, 2334
in diffuse alveolar hemorrhage, 1734
in emphysema, 1189
in filariasis, 1154
in gastroesophageal reflux disease, 559, *559*, 561–563, 2269
in Goodpasture's syndrome, 1743
in hantavirus infections, 946
in histoplasmosis, 1110, 2198
spontaneous resolution of, 1111, *1112*
in HIV infection, 2175
in hydatid disease, 1158
in hypereosinophilic syndrome, 1769

Cough *(Continued)*
in hypersensitivity pneumonitis, 1873–1874
in inflammatory bowel disease, 2270
in influenza, 951, 953
in influenza-like illness, 935
in interstitial lung disease, 561, 1655
in Kaposi's sarcoma, 2205
in laryngotracheitis, 918
in lung abscess, 1017
in lung cancer, 1420, 1471
in lymphangio(leio)myomatosis, 1780, 1780t
in malaria, 1147
in mediastinal mass, 2081
in mediastinitis, 2112
in medical history, 588–589
in mesothelioma, 2071
in neuromuscular disorders, 2331–2332
in obstructive diseases, 1174–1175
in oxygen toxicity, 1987
in ozone exposure, 1894
in paragonimiasis, 1161
in pleural effusion, 2000, 2021
in pneumonia, *Acinetobacter*, 1013
*Actinomyces*, 1021
anaerobic, 1017
beta-hemolytic streptococcal, 1004
*Chlamydia pneumoniae*, 1027
*Chlamydia psittaci*, 1026
*Chlamydia trachomatis*, 1027
*Coxiella burnetii*, 1025
Enterobacteriaceae, 1010
eosinophilic, 1767
*Haemophilus influenzae*, 1007
in elderly persons, 558
in immunodeficiency, 924
*Klebsiella pneumoniae*, 1008
*Legionella*, 1014
*Moraxella catarrhalis*, 1006
*Mycoplasma pneumoniae*, 1024
*Nocardia*, 1022
pneumococcal, 999
*Pneumocystis carinii*, 926, 2188
*Pseudomonas aeruginosa*, 1011
*Staphylococcus aureus*, 1003
in postnasal drip, 558–559, *559*, 563
in pulmonary edema, 1591
high-altitude, 1933
re-expansion, 2055
in pulmonary embolism, 558
in pulmonary fibrosis, 1672
in pulmonary hypertension, 1637–1638
in sarcoidosis, 1718
in silicosis, 1823
in Sjögren's syndrome, 366, 1705, 1706
in smoking, 560
in strongyloidiasis, 1151–1152
in systemic sclerosis, 1694
in talc granulomatosis, 1981
in toxocariasis, 1157
in tuberculosis, 1063, 2021
ineffective, 556–557, *557*
in neuromuscular disorders, 2331–2332
protussive therapy for, 564–565
inhibition of, involuntary, 554, *555*
voluntary, 553
laryngeal function in, 1351
machine for, 2346
mechanisms of, 369, 556, 2331–2332
motor outputs in, 555–556, *555*
mucociliary clearance and, 365, 369–370, 556
nonproductive, 588
pathogenesis of, in viral infections, 934
pathophysiology of, 556–557, *557*
physiology of, 553–556, *554*, *555*
pleuritic pain in, 576

Cough *(Continued)*
pneumomediastinum in, 2100
postinfectious, *559*, 560, 564
productive, 588
psychogenic, 561
receptors for, 575
respiratory muscle function in, 555–556, *555*
secretions produced in, 589. See also *Sputum.*
significance of, 553
stimulation of, agents for, 252
suppression of, for bronchoscopy, 730
syncope in, impairment in, 909
technique for, in chronic obstructive pulmonary disease, 1224
training for, 2346
treatment of, 562–565
antitussive agents for, 289
cromones in, 283–284
diagnostic information from, 561
in cystic fibrosis, 1310
nonspecific antitussive, 564
protussive, 564–565
specific antitussive, 562–564
tuberculosis transmission in, 1053
whooping (pertussis), 560
"Cough center," 554–555, *554*
Cough reflex, C fibers in, 252
hyperreactive, 556
receptors for, 553–554, *555*
Court cases, involving care decisions, 2492–2494
Cowdry type A inclusion bodies, in cytomegalovirus infections, 2302
*Coxiella burnetii* pneumonia, 473, 998t, 1025–1026
Coxsackie virus infections, 931t
pneumonia due to, 470
Coxsackie-Adeno receptor, 938
CPAP. See *Continuous positive airway pressure.*
CPR. See *Cardiopulmonary resuscitation.*
Crackles, 594, *594*, 595, *595*, *596*
in asbestosis, 1835
in beryllium lung disease, 1843
in bronchiolitis obliterans organizing pneumonia, 1365
in chronic obstructive pulmonary disease, 1189
in interstitial lung disease, 1656
in pulmonary edema, 1499
in pulmonary embolism, 1507
in pulmonary fibrosis, 1672
Cranial nerve palsy, in sarcoidosis, 1718–1719
Creatine, formation of, in exercise, 201
Creatine phosphate, hydrolysis of, in exercise, 201
CREB (cyclic adenosine monophosphate response element binding protein), as transcription factor, 261–262, *262*
Creola bodies, in asthma, 1255
CREST syndrome, 1697–1698
vasculitis in, 1539–1540, *1540*
Cricothyroid muscles, function of, 1351–1352, *1352*, 1354t
Criteria air pollutants, 1885, 1886t
Critical care unit. See *Intensive care unit.*
Critical pressure, in airway, 1344, *1344*, 1351
Crocidolite, 1831t
diseases due to, 1401, 2067
Crohn's disease, pulmonary complications of, 2270–2271, 2270t
Cromakalim, action of, on potassium channels, 247
as bronchodilator, 277
Cromolyn, 283–284

Cromolyn *(Continued)*
in allergic rhinitis, 1349
in asthma, 359, 1276, 1277t
in chronic obstructive pulmonary disease, 359
Cromones, 283–284. See also *Cromolyn; Nedocromil.*
*Crotalaria*, ingestion of, pulmonary hypertension related to, 1546
Croup, 918, 935, *936*
clinical manifestations of, 960–961
diagnosis of, 961
in measles, 958
in parainfluenza virus infections, 960–961
treatment of, 961
Crowd control agents, exposures to, 1906–1907
CRS. See *Compliance, respiratory system.*
Cryoglobulinemia, mixed, 1539, 1740
Cryotherapy, for airway obstruction, in cancer, 742
Cryptococcal antigen test, 2197
Cryptococcoma, 1130
Cryptococcosis, 1107–1108, 1129–1131
bronchoscopy in, 745
chest radiography of, 1130, 2196–2197, *2197*
clinical manifestations of, 1129–1130, 2196
culture in, 621–622, 2197
diagnosis of, 1130, 2197
epidemiology of, 1129, 2196
immune response to, 1108
in HIV infection, 1129–1131, 2196–2197
microbiologic diagnosis of, 610t
pathogenesis of, 1129
pleural effusion in, 2024
prevention of, 2197
treatment of, 1130–1131, 2197, 2198t
Cryptogenic fibrosing alveolitis. See *Fibrosis, idiopathic pulmonary.*
Cryptogenic organizing pneumonitis (idiopathic bronchiolitis obliterans organizing pneumonia), 1365
Cryptosporidiosis, in HIV infection, 2204
CST (static compliance), 2564
CT number, in computed tomography, 661
CTLA-4, in T-lymphocyte activation, 432
C-type natriuretic peptide, in cor pulmonale pathogenesis, 1637
Cuirass ventilators, in chronic obstructive pulmonary disease, 1228
in flail chest stabilization, 2369
in neuromuscular disorders, 2347
Cultural factors, in communication, 2492
Culture(s), 617–625
*Actinomadura*, 620–621
actinomycete, 618t, 620–621
*Aspergillus*, 621–622, 2201
*Blastomyces dermatitidis*, 622–623
blood, fungal, 621, 623
in histoplasmosis, 1115
in mycobacterial infections, 619
in pneumonia, 609, 617, 989
bronchial specimen, 746–747, 746t
bronchoalveolar lavage specimen, 611, 746–747, 746t, *747*
bronchoscope brush, 612
*Candida*, 621–622
cell. See *Cell culture.*
cerebrospinal fluid, in pneumonia, 989
*Chlamydia*, 618t, 624
*Coccidioides immitis*, 622–623, 2200
*Cryptococcus neoformans*, 621–622
epithelial cell, 336
fungal, 618t, 621–624. See also specific diseases and organisms.
Culture(s) *(Continued)*
*Histoplasma capsulatum*, 621–623, 1115, 2199
in pneumonia, 610t, 618t. See also *Culture(s), sputum.*
blood, 609, 617, 989
bronchoalveolar lavage specimens for, 611
bronchoscope brush, 612
cerebrospinal fluid, 989
fungal, 618t, 621–624
pleural fluid, 609, 989–990
procedures for, 618t
respiratory secretions, 991–992
throat, 609
tracheal aspirate, 609
*Micromonospora*, 620–621
*Micropolyspora*, 620–621
*Mycobacterium*, 618t, 619–620, 620t, 1044, 1045t, 1046–1047
*Mycobacterium avium* complex, 2185
*Mycobacterium kansasii*, 2186
*Mycoplasma*, 618t, 624–625
nasopharyngeal secretion, 609
*Nocardia*, 620–621
*Paracoccidioides brasiliensis*, 622–623
*Penicillium*, 2201
pleural fluid, 2005
in pneumonia, 609, 989–990
in tuberculosis, 2022
pleural tissue, in tuberculosis, 2008–2009
procedures for, 618t
respiratory secretions, in pneumonia, 991–992
*Rhodococcus equi*, 620–621
*Saccharomonospora*, 620–621
specimens for, in bacterial studies, 617, 618t
processing for, 611–613, *612*
*Sporothrix schenckii*, 622–623
sputum, for actinomycetes, 618t, 620–621
for bacteria, 617, 618t, 619, 619t
for fungi, 618t, 621–622
for mycobacteria, 618t, 619–620, 620t, 1043, *1044*, 1046
for *Mycobacterium tuberculosis*, 759–760
for *Mycoplasma*, 618t, 624–625
in chronic obstructive pulmonary disease, 1192
in HIV infection, 2183
in pneumonia, 921, 989–990. See also specific pneumonia organisms.
microscopic screening for, 614, *614*, *615*
*Streptococcus pneumoniae*, 617
*Streptomyces*, 620–621
subcultures in, for fungi, 621
*Thermoactinomyces*, 620–621
throat, in pharyngitis, 917–918
in pneumonia, 609
tracheal aspirate, 609
versus genetic testing, 626
zygomycetes, 622
Cummington-grunerite, 1831t
Currant jelly sputum, in *Klebsiella pneumoniae* pneumonia, 1008
Curschmann's spirals, in asthma, 1255
Cushing's disease, respiratory manifestations of, 2312–2313
Cushing's syndrome, in lung cancer, 1422
paraneoplastic, in lung cancer, 1379
respiratory manifestations of, 2312–2313
Cutis laxa, secondary lung injury in, 480t
$C\bar{V}O_2$. See *Oxygen concentration, mixed venous blood.*
Cw. See *Chest wall, compliance of.*
Cyanmethemoglobin method, for oxygen content, 833
Cyanosis, hemoglobin desaturation in, 86
Cyanosis *(Continued)*
in bronchiolitis, toxic, 1362
in hepatopulmonary syndrome, 2272
in hypoventilation, 2143
in pneumothorax, tension, 2054
in pulmonary fibrosis, idiopathic, 1678
in pulmonary hypertension, 1547
Cycle ergometry, in exercise testing, 841, 844–845
Cycle variable, in mechanical ventilation, 2471, *2472*, 2473t
Cyclic adenosine monophosphate, as second messenger, 236, *236*
hydrolysis of, 236, *236*
in beta-adrenergic agonist action, 268, *269*
in endothelial permeability regulation, 142, *143*, 144
in epithelial electrolyte transport regulation, 338
Cyclic adenosine monophosphate response element binding protein, as transcription factor, 261–262, *262*
Cyclic 3′,5′-guanosine monophosphate, in signal transduction, 238
Cyclin D1, in lung cancer, 1383–1384
Cyclin-dependent kinase inhibitors, in lung development, 41
Cyclohexylamine, exposure to, 1910
Cyclooxygenase pathway, products of, biologic effects of, 497–499, 497t
in mucus hypersecretion, 334
Cyclophosphamide, in allergic granulomatosis and angiitis, 1770
in drug-induced lung disease, 1693t
in interstitial fibrosis, 1697
in isolated pulmonary capillaritis, 1738
in lung cancer, 1438–1439
in lymphomatoid granulomatosis, 1459
in microscopic polyangiitis, 1739
in pulmonary fibrosis, 1681t, 1682
in systemic sclerosis, 1697
in vasculitis, 1536
in Wegener's granulomatosis, 1537, 1692t, 1738
pulmonary manifestations of, 1975–1976
Cyclopropane, in multiple inert gas elimination technique, 80–81, *81*, *82*
Cycloserine, in tuberculosis, 1069t, 1070
Cyclosporine, in asthma, 286
in drug-induced lung disease, 1693t
in lung transplantation, toxicity of, 2526
Cyst(s), bronchogenic, 483t, 2130
dermoid, of mediastinum, 2127
developmental, 2130
enteric, of mediastinum, 2130
foregut duplication, 2130
hydatid, mediastinal extension of, 2132
pleural effusion in, 2025–2026
lung, computed tomography of, 676, *677*
congenital, 482, 483t
in emphysema, 1205
in lymphangio(leio)myomatosis, 1776, *1777*, 1782
in sarcoidosis, 1722
in sequestration, 1567, *1567*
mediastinal, 2126, 2127, 2130, 2132
parasitic, *Entamoeba histolytica*, 1144
hydatid, 1157–1160, *1159*
mediastinal extension of, 2132
*Paragonimus*, 1160–1163, *1162*
*Toxocara canis*, 1157
*Toxoplasma gondii*, 1147–1148
*Trichinella spiralis*, 1156–1157
parathyroid, 2128
pericardial, 2130
pleural, in cystic fibrosis, 1294

Cysteinyl-leukotrienes, inhibitors of, in asthma, 284–286, *284*
Cystic adenomatoid malformations, pathology of, 483t
Cystic fibrosis, 1291–1323
age distribution of, 1313–1314, *1313*
allergic bronchopulmonary aspergillosis with, 1305, 1312, 1763
bronchiectasis with, 1303, 1326, 1331, 1333, 1335
CFTR protein in. See *Cystic fibrosis transmembrane regulator.*
chest radiography of, 666, 1303–1304
chloride transport abnormalities in, 1297–1299, *1298*
clinical manifestations of, 1181, 1302–1307, 1302t
complications of, 1305–1306
gastrointestinal, 1302t, 1306
genitourinary, 1307
hepatobiliary, 1306–1307
pancreatic, 1302t, 1306
respiratory, 1302–1306, 1302t, *1303*, 1304t
sweat gland dysfunction as, 1307
unusual, 1302, 1302t
colonization in, 1302–1303, *1303*
complications of, 1305–1306
computed tomography in, 1303–1304
course of, 1313–1314, *1313*, *1314*, 1314t
diagnosis of, 1181, 1307–1308, 1307t, 1308t
epidemiology of, 1292
ethnic factors in, 1292
etiology of, 1179–1180
exercise in, 1304–1305, 1310–1311
foundation for, 1291
gastrointestinal manifestations of, clinical features of, 1302t, 1306
pathology of, 1294–1295
pathophysiology of, 1302t, 1306
treatment of, 1312–1313
genetics of, 477, 1292–1293, *1293*, 1293t
genitourinary manifestations of, clinical features of, 1307
pathology of, 1295
pathophysiology of, 1307
genotypes of, 1292–1293
glandular epithelial dysfunction in, 1299–1300
hepatobiliary manifestations of, 1306–1307
historical perspectives of, 1291–1292
immunization in, 1311
in neonates, 1292, 1306, 1308, 1312
infection in, 1300–1302
ion transport defects in, 1297–1300, *1298*
lung transplantation in, 2520, 2520t
macromolecular secretion defects in, 1300
metabolic alkalosis in, 172
mortality in, 1313–1314, *1314*
mucin abnormalities in, 328
mucociliary transport in, 364–365, 368
nasal pathology in, 1294
nutrition in, 1311
pancreatic manifestations of, clinical features of, 1302t, 1306
pathology of, 1179, 1294–1295
treatment of, 1311
pathogenesis of, 1179–1180
versus chronic bronchitis pathogenesis, 1214
pathology of, 477, 480t, 1293–1295, *1294*
lung, 1293–1294, *1294*
nasal, 1294
nonrespiratory, 1294–1295
pathophysiology of, 1295–1302
airway mucosal, 1295–1297, 1296t, *1297*
Cystic fibrosis *(Continued)*
CFTR protein in, 1295, *1296*
chloride transport abnormalities in, 1297–1299
glandular epithelial, 1299–1300
in infection, 1300–1302
ion transport in, 1297–1300, *1298*
macromolecular secretion defects in, 1300
sodium transport abnormalities in, 1299
phenotypes of, 1292–1293
pneumonia in, 988t
pneumothorax in, 2049
pregnancy in, 2320
prenatal diagnosis of, 1293
prognosis for, 1313–1314, *1313*, *1314*, 1314t
*Pseudomonas aeruginosa* infections in, mucus secretion mechanisms in, 334
psychosocial aspects of, 1311, 1314
referral centers for, 1291
respiratory manifestations of, clinical features of, 1302–1306, 1302t, *1303*, 1304t
treatment of, 1312
significance of, 1291
sinus pathology in, 1294
sodium transport abnormalities in, *1298*, 1299
sweat gland dysfunction in, 1307
treatment of, 1308–1314
aerosol therapy in, 1310
airway clearance in, 1308–1309
ambulatory, 1308–1311, 1309t
antibiotics in, 1309–1312, 1309t
anti-inflammatory drugs in, 1310
bronchodilators in, 1310
corticosteroids in, 1310
DNase in, 1310
exercise in, 1310–1311
gene therapy in, 1311
hospital-based, 1311–1313
immunization program for, 1311
in gastrointestinal complications, 1312–1313
in lung complications, 1312
mucolytic drugs in, 1310
nutritional, 1311
objectives of, 1308
psychosocial support in, 1311
surgical, 1313
transplantation in, 1313
triphosphate nucleotides in, 1299
Cystic fibrosis transmembrane regulator, 1291
dysfunction of, 368
laboratory tests for, 1307
functions of, 336–338, 1295, *1296*, 1298–1300, *1298*
gene of, 1179
discovery of, 1292
in gene therapy, 1311
mutations of, 1292–1293, *1293*, 1293t, 1295
structure of, 1292–1293, *1293*
metabolism of, 1295
structure of, 337, 1295
Cystic medial necrosis, of aorta, pulmonary artery aneurysms in, 1569
Cystotomy, in echinococcosis, 1160
Cytocentrifugation, in specimen processing, 612
Cytochrome P-450, as biomarker, for lung cancer, 1406
Cytokine(s). See also specific cytokines, e.g., *Interferon(s); Interleukin(s).*
actions of, 2226, *2227*
aerosolized, 360
as inflammatory mediators, 258, *258*
chemokines as. See *Chemokines.*
Cytokine(s) *(Continued)*
dendritic cell response to, 396–397
eosinophil, 1759, 1759t
in allergic rhinitis, 1347–1348
in apoptosis, 528–529, *529*, *530*
in asthma, 1256–1258, *1257–1259*, 1259t
airway structural changes and, 1263, *1263*, 1264t
in bronchiectasis, 1326
in chest pain, 573
in dendritic cell action, 397
in goblet cell metaplasia and hyperplasia, 1262
in granulomatous disease, 437–438
in hypersensitivity pneumonitis, 1872
in influenza, 953
in lung injury, in mechanical ventilation, 2478
in malaria, 1146
in pulmonary edema, high-altitude, 1935
in sarcoidosis, 1724–1725
in silicosis, 1819
in systemic sclerosis, 1692
in tuberculosis, 1057
inhibitors of, corticosteroids as, 279
in asthma, 286–287, *288*
in chronic obstructive pulmonary disease, 286–287, *288*
interleukins as. See *Interleukin(s).*
neutrophil-derived, 521
of macrophages, 393
alveolar, 394, *395*
interstitial, 396
of T lymphocytes, 432–434, *433*
receptors for, 238
Cytology, pleural fluid, 2004
in metastatic disease, 2073–2074
Cytomegalovirus infection(s), 931t, 941–945
after lung transplantation, bronchiolitis obliterans in, 1365, *1365*
asymptomatic, 942
cell culture in, 625
chest radiography of, 2202
clinical manifestations of, 943, *944*, 2202
diagnosis of, 625, 943–944, 2202
epidemiology of, 942, 2230
immunization for, 945
in HIV infection, 749, 2202–2203
in transplantation, 2230–2231, 2230t
interstitial pattern of, 942, 943, *944*
miliary pattern of, 942, *942*, 943, *944*
natural history of, 2231
pathogenesis of, 942, *942*
pathophysiology of, 2231
pharyngitis as, 933
pneumonia as, 942–945, *942*, *944*
bronchoscopy in, 749
clinical features of, 2301–2302
genetic tests for, 626–627
in bone marrow transplantation, 2301–2302
in HIV infection, 2202–2203
in lung transplantation, 2522
in transplantation, 925
pathology of, 473, *473*
prevention of, 2302
treatment of, 2302
prevention of, 944–945, 2231
risk factors for, 2230, 2230t
spectrum of, 2230
superinfections with, 2231
transmission of, 942
treatment of, 944–945, 2202–2203
in transplantation, 2231
viral characteristics in, 941–942
Cytopathic effects, in cell cultures, 625

Cytotoxicity, of drugs. See *Drug(s), pulmonary disease(s) due to.*

## D

Danazol, in angioimmunoblastic lymphadenopathy, 1460
Dantrolene, pleural disease due to, 2035
pulmonary disease due to, 1989
Dapsone, in *Pneumocystis carinii* pneumonia, 2191–2192, 2191t, 2194–2195, 2195t
Darifenacin, anticholinergic properties of, 277
Data bases, for genetic diseases, 51–52, 52t
D-dimer, measurement of, in pulmonary embolism, 1511
Dead space, anatomic, 6, 7, 58
measurement of, 822–823, *823*
versus physiologic dead space, 823
calculation of, 822
definition of, 2564
in pulmonary embolism, 1505
in pulmonary hypertension, 1521
physiologic, 58
calculation of, 80
in exercise, in heart disease, 2259
in total ventilation calculation, 209
in ventilation-perfusion assessment, 80
measurement of, 823–824
versus anatomic dead space, 823
ventilation of, 2564
carbon dioxide production and, 156, *157*
in exercise testing, 844
Dead space/tidal volume ratio, in exercise, 844
in chronic obstructive pulmonary disease, 212, *213*, 223–224
in interstitial pulmonary disease, 225
in pulmonary disease, 211–212, 212t
versus arterial carbon dioxide, 209–210, *209*
Death and dying. See also *Mortality.*
brain death as, 2496
care goals in, 2488
euthanasia in, 2500–2501
life support and. See *Life support.*
predictive factors for, 2488–2490
Death with Dignity Act, in Oregon, 2501
Decision making, ethics of. See under *Ethics.*
in life support. See under *Life support.*
Decompression illness, air embolism in, 2102
definition of, 1954
Decompression sickness, 1959–1963
clinical manifestations of, 1960–1961, 1961t
definition of, 1954, 1959
diagnosis of, 1962
epidemiology of, 1960, 1961t
historical aspects of, 1959
massive, from blowup ascent, 1961
nonsystemic, 1960–1961
pathogenesis of, 1959–1960
risk factors for, 1960
systemic, 1960–1961
treatment of, 1961–1963
Decongestants, in bronchoscopy, 732
in common cold, 933
nasal, 1349
Decontamination, of sputum specimens, 613, 613t
Decortication, in fibrothorax, 2061, 2063
in pleural effusion, 2020
in rheumatoid arthritis, 2031
of trapped lung, 2036
Decubitus radiography, 646, *651–653*
Deep vein thrombosis, above-knee, 1505
calf-limited, 1505
clinical manifestations of, 1506–1507
Deep vein thrombosis *(Continued)*
computed tomography of, 680–681, *682*
diagnosis of, 1508–1509, *1508*, *1509*
approach to, 1513–1514, *1514*
in pregnancy, 2322
magnetic resonance imaging in, 680–681, *682*
natural history of, 1504–1505
prevention of, 1514–1515
pulmonary embolism development from. See *Pulmonary embolism.*
Defense mechanism(s). See also *Immune response.*
against air pollutants, 1888–1889
airway surface liquid as, 340
defects of, in pneumonia, correction of, 997
free radicals as. See *Free radicals.*
impaired. See *Immunodeficiency.*
in influenza, 953
in measles, 958
in pneumonia, 986
augmentation of, 997
nosocomial, 923
in respiratory syncytial virus infections, 962
in tuberculosis, 1055–1057, *1056*
in viral infections, 932
lymphatic system as, 22–23
mucus as. See *Mucus.*
of airway epithelium, 1177, *1177*
of alveoli, 371
of nasopharynx, 352
of nose, 1346–1347
overview of, 2224–2226, *2225*, *2227*, *2228*
phagocytosis as. See *Phagocytosis;* specific cells, e.g., *Macrophage(s).*
surfactant as. See *Surfactant.*
virus effects on, 931–932
Defense reflexes, in airways, 252
Defensins, in mucus, 332
Degranulation, inhibition of, in obstructive diseases, 1175
Dehydration, anion gap in, 164
of airways, 362–363
Delivery. See *Labor and delivery.*
Dendritic cells, 386, 396–397
development of, 403
in antigen presentation, 432–433
in asthma, 1257, *1257–1259*
morphology of, 389
Dengue hemorrhagic fever, pleural effusion in, 2025
Densitometry, of lung, in pulmonary edema, 1596
Dental problems, in diving, 1957
mediastinitis in, 2108
pneumomediastinum in, 2097
Deontologic ethical theory, 2490
Deoxyribonuclease. See *DNase (deoxyribonuclease).*
Deoxyribonucleic acid. See *DNA.*
Department of Veterans Affairs, impairment and disability evaluation for, 902, 903t
Deposition, alveolar. See *Alveolus(i), aerosol deposition in.*
of aerosols. See *Aerosol(s), deposition of.*
Dermatitis, in schistosomiasis, 1164
occupational, 1859
Dermatomyositis. See *Polymyositis and/or dermatomyositis.*
Dermoid cyst, of mediastinum, 2127
Desensitization, to drugs, 244–245, *245*, 271
Desert rheumatism. See *Coccidioidomycosis.*
Desflurane, pulmonary function effects of, 885
Desmopressin, in von Willebrand's disease, 2294–2295
Desmosine, excretion of, in emphysema, 1212–1213
Desquamative interstitial pneumonia, 1651–1652, *1651*, 1672t, 1684–1686
Dexamethasone, in high-altitude cerebral edema, 1933
in mountain sickness prevention, 1932
in spinal cord metastasis, 1435
Dextran, endothelial permeability of, 140
pulmonary disease due to, 1988
Diabetes mellitus, diving contraindicated in, 1963
ketoacidosis in, 166–167, *167*, 1134
lactic acidosis in, 166
mucormycosis in, 2310
recurrence risk of, in relatives, 48
respiratory manifestations of, 2309–2310, 2309t
tuberculosis risk in, 1059
Diacylglycerol, formation of, in signal transduction, 237, *237*
in electrolyte transport, in airway epithelium, 338
Diagnosis. See also specific disorders and procedures, e.g., *Biopsy*; *Mediastinoscopy.*
definition of, 585
Dialysis, peritoneal, pleural effusion in, 2016
respiratory function in, 2279–2280
Diaphoresis, in tension pneumothorax, 2054
Diaphragm, amebic liver abscess rupture through, 2025
amyloidosis of, 2296
defects of, ascites movement through, 2015, 2029
dysfunction of, after abdominal surgery, 885–886
dyskinesia of, 2349t, 2350–2351
fatigue of, mechanical aspects of, 109
function of, evaluation of, 859
mechanical aspects of, 106–107
hernia of, mediastinal protrusion of, 2130–2131
pleural effusion in, 2030
innervation of, 2330, 2330t
motion of, lung volume changes in, 105–106, *105*
myoclonus of, 2349t, 2350
paralysis of, 2334–2337
bilateral, 2335, 2336t, 2337
clinical features of, 2144, 2334–2337
diagnosis of, 2335–2336, 2336t
differential diagnosis of, 2336
etiology of, 2334
hypoventilation in, 2144
in infants, 2335
in spinal cord injury, 2338
nonrespiratory muscle recruitment in, 108
pathophysiology of, 2337
postoperative, 2337
prognosis for, 2334, 2335
respiratory acidosis in, 173–174
treatment of, 2336–2337
unilateral, 2334–2337, 2336t
plication of, in paralysis, 2336–2337
position of, in hemiplegia, 2340
in pregnancy, 2317–2318
positional changes in, 104
pressure across, measurement of, 2333
radiography of, 2332
receptors in, 184
shape of, in hyperinflation, 859
spasms of, in hiccups, 2349–2350, 2349t
strength of, evaluation of, 2333
structure of, 106
weakness of, in Lambert-Eaton syndrome, 2342
in systemic lupus erythematosus, 1704, *1704*

Diaphragmatic breathing, in pulmonary rehabilitation, 2509
Diarrhea, hyperchloremic acidosis in, 169–170
  in legionellosis, 1014–1015
  metabolic alkalosis in, 172
Diary, in disease monitoring, 591–592
Diazoxide, as vasodilator, 301
  in pulmonary edema, 1602
Diborane, exposure to, 1910
Dichloroacetate, in lactic acidosis, 171
Dideoxyarginine-vasopressin, in von Willebrand's disease, 2294–2295
Diencephalon, in breathing control, 187
Diesel exhaust, air pollution from, 1887–1888, 1887t, 1893
    lung cancer risk in, 1403
Diet, asthma risk and, 1250
  in chronic obstructive pulmonary disease, 2510
  in gastroesophageal reflux disease, 563
  in lung cancer prevention, 1404–1405
  in mountain sickness prevention, 1932
  in pulmonary rehabilitation, 2510
  in smoking, 2513
  paragonimiasis transmitted in, 1160–1163
  pulmonary hypertension related to, 1546, 1642
  trichinosis transmitted in, 1156–1157
Diethylaminoethanol, exposure to, 1910
Diethylcarbamazine, in filariasis, 1155, 1762
Diethylenetriaminepentaacetate, clearance of, from lung, 355, 1726
  technetium 99m–labeled, in ventilation-perfusion scanning, 699
    in epithelial permeability studies, 718–720, *719*
    in lung transplantation, 718
    in *Pneumocystis carinii* pneumonia, 711–712
    in tuberculosis, 713
Diffuse alveolar damage, 1650, *1651*, 1653t
  in HIV infection, 2210
Diffuse alveolar hemorrhage. See *Alveolar hemorrhage, diffuse.*
Diffusing capacity, 808–816
  after heart transplantation, 2253t
  after lung transplantation, 2524
  after pneumonectomy, 889
  age effects on, 814
  alveolar carbon dioxide pressure effects on, 815
  alveolar oxygen pressure effects on, 815
  alveolar-capillary block and, 809
  alveolar-capillary membrane and, 809
  at high altitude, 1919
  blood components of, *74*, 75–76
  body size effects on, 814
  calculation of, 811
  criteria for, in gas exchange impairment, 901t
  diffusion path length and, 808–809
  exercise effects on, 814–815
  hemoglobin-related component of, 810, *810*
  in alveolar proteinosis, 1795
  in arteriovenous malformations, 1496, 1563–1564
  in asthma, 1266
  in chemotherapy-induced disease, 1975
  in chronic obstructive pulmonary disease, 1191–1192, 1207, 1226
  in emphysema, 815, *816*, 1191–1192, 1207
  in exercise, 809
  in Goodpasture's syndrome, 1743
  in heart disease, 2252, 2253t
  in hemosiderosis, 1742
  in HIV infection, 2176
Diffusing capacity *(Continued)*
  in impairment and disability evaluation, 850t, 897–898, 899, 899t, 905–906
  in interstitial lung disease, 816, 1663–1664, 1696
  in liver disease, 2271
  in lung transplantation, 816
  in lymphangio(leio)myomatosis, 1781
  in neuromuscular disorders, 2333
  in obstructive diseases, 815, *816*
  in pancreatitis, 2276
  in *Pneumocystis carinii* pneumonia, 856, 2189
  in primary biliary cirrhosis, 2276
  in pulmonary fibrosis, 1675–1676, 1679
  in pulmonary hypertension, 1520
  in pulmonary vascular obstruction, 815–816, *817*
  in restrictive disease, 816
  in rheumatoid arthritis, 1702
  in sarcoidosis, 1723
  in smoking, 815
    carboxyhemoglobin adjustment in, 814
  in systemic sclerosis, 1696
  increased, 809
  interpretation of, 813–815, 877
  intrathoracic pressure effects on, 815
  lung volume effects on, 814
  measurement of, 74–76, *74*, 810–815
    altitude adjustments in, 814
    carbon monoxide methods for, 811–813
    carboxyhemoglobin adjustment for smokers in, 814
    gas dilution methods in, 793
    gases for, 810–811
    hemoglobin adjustment in, 813–814
    indications for, 813
    interpretation of, 813–815, 877
    intra-breath method in, 812–813
    oxygen method for, 813
    rebreathing method in, 812
    single-breath method in, 811–813
    steady-state method in, 812
    three-gas iteration method in, 812
  membrane component of, *74*, 75–76, 810, *810*
  normal values for, 814–815, 877
  oxygen-hemoglobin reaction rates and, 74
  position effects on, 815
  red blood cell status and, 810, *810*
  surface area and, 809, *809*
  theory of, 808–810, *809*, *810*
  versus age, 857
Diffusion, 57, 808–810, *809*. See also *Diffusing capacity.*
  at high altitude, 1919, *1920*, 1923
  equation for, 133–134
  Fick's law of, 70, 72
  impairment of, in highly fit athletes, 219
  in aerosol deposition, 351, *351*
  in solute transport, 133–134
  in terminal respiratory units, 15, *16*
  limitation of, 72–76, *73*, *74*
  myoglobin in, 1923
  of carbon monoxide, 811–813
  of oxygen, at high altitude, in exercise, 1927–1928
    uptake rate of, 72–73, *73*, *74*
  oxygen-hemoglobin reaction rates in, 73–74, *74*
  path length for, 808–809
  rate of, 72
  solubility and, 810, 1958–1959, *1959*
  surface area and, 809, *809*
  total resistance to, definition of, 2565
Diffusion-perfusion defect, in hepatopulmonary syndrome, 2274
DiGeorge's syndrome, 2233t, 2238
Digital clubbing. See *Clubbing.*
Digital (computed) radiography, 642, 644, *644*
Digital subtraction angiography, 658, *660*
Digitalis, in pulmonary edema, 1604
Digoxin, in cor pulmonale, 1643
Dilation. See also *Bronchodilation; Bronchiectasis; Vasodilation.*
  of nasal passages, 1345, 1346t
Diloxanide furoate, in amebiasis, 1146
Diltiazem, as vasodilator, 300
  in pulmonary hypertension, 1551
Dilutional acidosis, 163, *164*, 170
Dimethylsulfoxide, in amyloidosis, 2296
Dinucleotide repeats, 46–47, *46*
Dipalmitoylphosphatidylcholine, 308, 309, 309t
  deficiency of, in interstitial lung disease, 319
  function of, 310
  in surfactant secretion inhibition, 316, *317*
Diphenhydramine, in amphotericin reactions, 1116
2,3-Diphosphoglycerate, oxygen-hemoglobin affinity and, 1922, *1922*
Diphtheria, 917
Dipyridamole, as vasodilator, 301
Direct fluorescent antibody test, in legionellosis, 1016, *1016*
  in pneumonia, specimen processing for, 613
Direct immunofluorescence assay, in *Chlamydia* infections, 624
  in pneumonia, 616
Dirofilariasis, 1155–1156
Disability. See *Impairment and disability.*
Disinfection, of bronchoscopy equipment, 758
Dissection, aortic, imaging of, 683, *684*, *685*
    pain in, 579, 581t
Disseminated intravascular coagulation, 2295
  in amniotic fluid embolism, 2323
  in leukemia, 2291
Dissociation constants, of drugs, 243, *243*
Distal intestinal obstruction syndrome, in cystic fibrosis, 1306, 1312
Distention, of colon, pain in, 571–573, *571*, *572*
  of esophagus, pain in, 571
  of hollow viscera, pain in, 569
  of pulmonary vessels, 128
    pulmonary vascular resistance and, 62–63, *63*
Distribution, of drugs, 248
Dithiothreitol, in specimen processing, 613t
Dittrich's plugs, in bronchiectasis, 1328
Diuretics, in pulmonary edema, 1602–1603
  metabolic alkalosis due to, 172
Diving, 1951–1969
  altitude effects on, 1951t, 1952
  blowup ascent in, 1961
  Boyle's law and, 1954–1955, *1954*
  breath-hold, 1952
  commercial, decompression sickness in, 1961t
    equipment for, 1953–1954
    medical requirements for, 1963–1964
  decompression tables for, 1958, 1959
  depth effects in, 1951–1952, 1951t
  disorder(s) related to, alternobaric vertigo as, 1956–1957
    arterial gas embolism as, 1955–1956, *1956*, 2098
    cutaneous, 1957
    decompression sickness as, 1959–1963, 1961t
    dental, 1957
    dissolved inert gas-induced, 1957–1963, 1958t, *1959*, 1961t

Diving *(Continued)*
facial, 1957
gastrointestinal, 1957
hyperthermia as, 1952–1953
hypothermia as, 1952–1953, 1964
inert gas narcosis as, 1963
inner ear, 1957
middle ear, 1956
near drowning as, 1964–1967, 1965t
nomenclature of, 1954
pneumomediastinum as, 2097–2098, 2100
pressure-induced, 1954–1957, *1954*, *1956*
pulmonary, 1955–1956, *1956*
shallow water blackout as, 1952
sinus, 1957
squeeze as, 1955
energy needs for, 1953, *1953*, 1963
environment for, 1951–1953, 1951t
equipment for, 1953–1954, *1954*
for prolonged periods (weeks), 1958
Henry's law and, 1957–1959, *1959*
hyperventilation in, adverse effects of, 2147
immersion effects in, 1952
medical qualifications for, 1963–1964
mortality in, 1955, 1956, 1961, 1964, 1966–1967
pressure situation in, 1951–1952, 1951t
scuba, types of, 1953, *1954*
suits for, 1952
surface supplied air in, 1953–1954
thermal conditions in, 1952–1953
Diving reflex, 181
DL$_{CO}$. See *Diffusing capacity.*
DM (membrane diffusive conductance), definition of, 2565
in heart disease, 2252, 2253t
DNA, methylation of, abnormalities of, in lung cancer, 1378
polycyclic aromatic hydrocarbon interaction with, lung cancer in, 1401–1402
protection of, p53 protein in, 1382
DNA analysis, of cystic fibrosis, 1307–1308
of genetic diseases, 45. See also specific techniques.
of *Legionella*, 1016
of lung cancer, 1426
of *Mycobacterium*, 1045t, 1047
of pneumonia, 625–627
DNA gyrase, in tuberculosis, 1070
DNase (deoxyribonuclease), in bronchiectasis, 1331
in cystic fibrosis, 368, 1310
in mucus reduction, 289
DNR (do-not-resuscitate) orders, 2497–2498
Dobutamine, as vasodilator, 300
in acute respiratory distress syndrome, 2421
in pulmonary edema, 1603, 1604, 2421
in shock, 2401t
cardiogenic, 2400
in pulmonary embolism, 2404
septic, 2399–2400
Docetaxel, in lung cancer, 1437, 1437t
Documentation, of respiratory impairment and disability, 895–896, 909–910
Do-not-resuscitate orders, 2497–2498
Dopamine, in acute respiratory distress syndrome, 2420
in pulmonary edema, 1603–1604, 2420
in shock, 2401t
in cardiac arrhythmias, 2403t
septic, 2399–2400
Doppler studies, of bubbles, in decompression sickness, 1960
Dornase alfa, in mucus reduction, 289
Dorsal respiratory group, of medulla, 185–186, *185*
Dorsal root ganglia, in visceral innervation, 569
Down-regulation, of receptors, 245
Doxapram, in asthma, 290
in respiratory acidosis, 174
Doxorubicin, in lung cancer, 1438
in mesothelioma, 2070
Doxycycline, as pneumothorax sclerosing agent, 2048, 2050
in brucellosis, 1030
in malaria, 1147
in mycobacterial infections, 1096
in pleurodesis, in metastatic disease, 2075
in pneumonia, 922t, 995t, 998t
*Brucella*, 1030
*Chlamydia psittaci*, 1026
pneumococcal, 1001
in psittacosis, 1026
Drainage, chest tube in. See *Tube thoracostomy.*
in chylothorax, 2057–2059
in echinococcosis, 1160
in empyema, 1032
in lung abscess, 1031
in mediastinitis, 2110
in pleural effusion, 2019–2020
in pneumonia, 997
postural. See *Postural drainage.*
Dressler's syndrome, 578–579, 2032
Drive, ventilatory. See *Ventilatory drive.*
Drooling, in epiglottitis, 918
Drowning, 1964, 1966–1967. See also *Near drowning.*
Drug(s), absorption of, 247–248
abuse of. See also specific drugs, e.g., *Cocaine.*
HIV infection in, 2175
pneumomediastinum in, 2099
pneumonia in, 988t
pulmonary disease in, 1979–1981, 1980t
strychnine poisoning in, 2351
thromboembolism in, 1527
ventilation-perfusion scanning in, 704
administration routes for, 248–249
adverse reactions to, pulmonary. See *Drug(s), pulmonary disease(s) due to.*
affinity of, 243
agonists of, 243–244, *244*. See also *$Beta_2$-adrenergic agonists.*
antagonists of, 243–244, *244*
functional, 268–269
binding of, to receptors, 243–244, *243*, *244*
clearance of, 248
concentration of, equation for, 248
delivery of, routes for, 248–249
desensitization to, 244–245, *245*, 271
dissociation constants of, 243, *243*
distribution of, 248
efficacy of, 243
enzyme inhibition due to, 247
half-life of, 248
hyperventilation due to, 2147
in medical history, 591
inhaled route for. See *Inhalation, of drugs.*
interactions of, with theophylline, 274
ionized versus unionized equilibrium of, 247
lipid solubility of, 247–248
lupus due to, 2031–2032
mediastinitis due to, 2112
methemoglobinemia due to, 2290, 2291t
oral route for, 249
parenteral route for, 249
particle size of, for inhalation, 248
pharmacokinetics of, 248. See *Pharmacokinetics.*
pleural disease due to, 2035–2036
Drug(s) *(Continued)*
potentiation of, 244
pulmonary disease(s) due to, 1701, 1909, 1971–1994
acceptable risk and, 1972
acute injury as, 1588t, 1909
anti-inflammatory agents in, 1984–1985, *1986*
antimicrobial drugs in, 1978–1979
appetite suppressants in, 1988–1989
asthma as, 1271, 1858t
bromocriptine in, 1988
bronchospasm as, 1989–1990, 1989t
cardiovascular drugs in, 1981–1984, *1982*, 1982t
chemotherapy agents in, 1972–1978, 1973t, 1974t, *1975*, *1977*
contrast agents in, 1988
dantrolene in, 1989
dextran in, 1988
diffuse alveolar damage as, 1743–1744, 1743t
drug classification and, 1972, 1973t
edema as, 1588t
eosinophilic, 1762–1763, 1762t, 1990–1991, 1991t
epidemiology of, 1971–1972
hydantoin in, 1989
hydrochlorothiazide in, 1988
illicit drugs in, 1979–1981, 1980t
immunotherapy in, 1978
in connective tissue disease therapy, 1691, 1692t
infiltrative, 1990–1991, 1991t
inhaled agents in, 1986–1987
injury as, 1588t
interstitial, *1650*, 1652t
mechanisms of, 1972–1974
methysergide in, 1988
oxygen in, 1987
pathology of, 477, *477*, 479t
pleural effusion as, 1990, 1990t
pulmonary edema as, 1990, 1990t
pulmonary hypertension as, 1642
respiratory failure as, 2447
sclerotherapy in, 1989
systemic lupus erythematosus as, 1985–1986
tocolytic agents in, 1988
transfusion-related, 1987
treatment of, 1693t
tricyclic drugs in, 1989
types of, 1971–1972, 1972t
pulmonary vascular resistance effects of, 64
radioligand binding studies of, 243, *243*
radiopharmaceuticals as, for ventilation-perfusion scanning, 698–700, 718
receptor interactions with, 243–244, *243*, *244*
respiratory alkalosis due to, 175, 175t
stereoselectivity of, 244
synergism of, 244
systemic sclerosis-like syndromes due to, 1692
tachyphylactic, 244–245, *245*
thrombocytopenia due to, 2295
tolerance of, 244
Dry eyes, in Sjögren's syndrome, 1705
Dry mouth, in Sjögren's syndrome, 1705
Dry powder inhalers, 249, 1220
Dry trachea, in Sjögren's syndrome, 366
Duplex ultrasonography, in venous thrombosis, 1508–1509, *1509*
Duplication cysts, foregut, 2130
Durable powers of attorney, 2494
Duration, of lung sounds, 592

Dust(s), accumulation of, in lung, 1811–1813, *1812*
aerosol. See *Aerosol(s).*
alveolar macrophage protection against, 390, *391*, 392
exposure to, alveolar proteinosis in, 1791–1792, 1792t, 1794
asthma in, 1857
bronchiolitis in, 1366
byssinosis in, 1860–1862
lung disease in. See *Pneumoconiosis(es).*
Dust mites, asthma and, 1250
Dutch hypothesis, for asthmatic bronchitis, 1271
Duty cycle, definition of, 2565
Dying. See *Death and dying.*
Dysgerminomas, of mediastinum, 2127
Dysphagia, in lung cancer, 1420, 1421
in mediastinal mass, 2081
in peritonsillar abscess, 918
in sarcoidosis, 1719
Dysphonia, corticosteroid-induced, 282
Dysplasia, cellular, 450
in lung cancer, 1377–1378
Dyspnea, 541–552
afferent feedback in, 543
as ventilatory failure indicator, 2345
assessment of, 544, *545*, 545t, 546t
at rest, 220
central perception alterations in, 548
chest radiography of, 665–666
classification of, American Medical Association, 904t
clinical features of, 587–588
definition of, 220, 542, 896, 897
description of, 587
differential diagnosis of, 545, 545t, 1268, 1269t, 1877
disability in. See *Impairment and disability.*
drug-induced, 2035–2036
emotional component of, 542, 544
energy conservation in, 547–548
epidemiology of, 541, *568*
evaluation of, in impairment and disability determination. See *Impairment and disability, evaluation of.*
exercise testing in, 546–547, 546t
exercise training in, 548–549
functional, 896, 898
gender differences in, 220
grading of, 897
history in, 546
impairment in. See *Impairment and disability.*
in acute respiratory distress syndrome, 2416–2417
in amebiasis, 1145
in amniotic fluid embolism, 2323
in arteriovenous malformations, 1495, 1561
in asbestosis, 1835
in asthma, 1248, 1256, 1265, 1266, 1268–1269
in botulism, 2342–2343
in bronchial disorders, 1368
in bronchiectasis, 1327–1328
in bronchiolitis, 1362
in bronchiolitis obliterans, 1363, 1364
in bronchiolitis obliterans organizing pneumonia, 1365
in bronchitis, 1189
in byssinosis, 1862
in candidiasis, 1135
in chemotherapy-induced disease, 1974
in chronic obstructive pulmonary disease, 212–213, *214*, 1189, 1208
pulmonary rehabilitation in. See *Pulmonary rehabilitation.*
Dyspnea *(Continued)*
treatment of, 1228
in chylothorax, 2057
in coal-workers' pneumoconiosis, 1829
in cor pulmonale, 1637–1638
in cryptococcosis, 2196
in decompression sickness, 1961
in diaphragmatic paralysis, 2334–2335
in diffuse alveolar hemorrhage, 1734
in emphysema, 1189, 1208
in esophageal rupture, 2028
in exercise, 220–221, 542, 543
in alveolar proteinosis, 1794
in heart disease, 2262
in exercise testing, subjective description of, 845
in fat embolism, 1526
in filariasis, 1155
in Goodpasture's syndrome, 1743
in hantavirus infections, 946
in heart disease, 543–544, 2262
in hepatic hydrothorax, 2015
in Hermansky-Pudlak syndrome, 1749
in histoplasmosis, 2198
in HIV infection, 2175
in hydatid disease, 1158
in hypersensitivity pneumonitis, 1873–1874
in hyperthyroidism, 2310
in hyperventilation, 2147
in hypothyroidism, 2310
in interstitial lung disease, 1655, 1699
in Kaposi's sarcoma, 2205
in leukemia, 2291
in lung cancer, 1420, 1471
in lymphangio(leio)myomatosis, 1746, 1780, 1780t
in mediastinitis, 2112
in medical history, 587–588
in mesothelioma, benign fibrous, 2071
malignant, 2068
treatment of, 2070
in neurofibromatosis, 1748, 1748t
in nitrofurantoin-induced pulmonary disease, 1978
in pancreatitis, 2028, 2029
in pectus excavatum, 2365
in pleural effusion, 2000, 2026
in pleural fibrosis, 1839
in pleural tumors, 2072
in pneumomediastinum, 2102
in pneumonia, *Actinomyces*, 1021
beta-hemolytic streptococcal, 1004
*Chlamydia psittaci*, 1026
*Coxiella burnetii*, 1025
Enterobacteriaceae, 1010
eosinophilic, 1767
*Haemophilus influenzae*, 1007
*Klebsiella pneumoniae*, 1008
*Legionella*, 1014
*Moraxella catarrhalis*, 1006
pneumococcal, 999
*Pneumocystis carinii*, 926, 2188
*Staphylococcus aureus*, 1003
in pneumothorax, 2045, 2049, 2054
in portopulmonary hypertension, 2275
in pulmonary edema, 1498–1499, 1591
high-altitude, 1933
in heart disease, 2261
in pulmonary embolism, 1507, 2026
in pulmonary fibrosis, 1672, *1676*
in pulmonary hypertension, 1493–1494, 1520, 1546, 1637–1638
in respiratory acidosis, 174
in rheumatoid arthritis, 1699, 2031
in sarcoidosis, 1718
in sickle cell disease, 2289
Dyspnea *(Continued)*
in silicosis, 1823
in Sjögren's syndrome, 1705
in spinal cord injury, 2337–2338
in strongyloidiasis, 1151–1152
in systemic lupus erythematosus, 1704
in systemic sclerosis, 1694
in talc granulomatosis, 1981
in tuberculosis, 1063
in tuberous sclerosis, 1748
in vasculitis, 1535
laboratory tests in, 546
language of, 542
mechanical aspects of, 112
mechanisms of, 542–544, *542*
morbidity in, 541
organic, 896, 898
outcome measures of, 587
paroxysmal nocturnal, 588, 1155
pathophysiology of, 897, 2261–2262
physical examination in, 546
physiologic categories of, 545, 545t
physiologic correlates of, 897–898
position-dependent. See *Orthopnea.*
psychologic factors in, 544, 545t
pulmonary function tests in, 897–898
quality of life and, 544
questionnaires on, 544
respiratory drive reduction in, 548
respiratory muscle strengthening in, 547–548
scales for, 897
sensations experienced in, 541–542
subjective description of, 845
sudden, 588
treatment of, 547–549, *547*, 547t
drug, 289
exercise training in, 548–549
in chronic obstructive pulmonary disease, 1228
in mesothelioma, 2070
types of, 588
Dysproteinemia, in angioimmunoblastic lymphadenopathy, 1459
Dysrhythmias, cardiac. See *Cardiac arrhythmias.*


## E


E to A sign, in auscultation, 598
Ear, barotrauma of, 1956, 1957, 1962
middle, common cold manifestations in, 933
infection and inflammation of. See *Otitis media.*
Eaton-Lambert syndrome, in lung cancer, 1421
Ebola virus infections, 931t
E-cadherin defects, metastasis in, 1387
Echinococcosis (hydatid disease), 1157–1160, *1159*
mediastinal extension of, 2132
pleural effusion in, 2026–2027
Echo virus infections, 931t
Echocardiography, in acute respiratory distress syndrome, 2417–2418
in arteriovenous malformations, 1562
in cor pulmonale, 1193, 1639–1641, *1640*
in decompression sickness, 1960
in hepatopulmonary syndrome, 2273, *2273*
in pulmonary edema, 2417–2418
in pulmonary embolism, 1510
in pulmonary hypertension, 1521, 1548
Eclampsia, pulmonary edema in, 2322, *2323*
Economic issues, in lung cancer, 1439, 1444
Edema, airway, in inhalation injury, 754
aldosterone excess in, metabolic alkalosis in, 172

Edema *(Continued)*
alveolar. See *Alveolus(i), edema of.*
angioneurotic, angiotensin-converting enzyme inhibitor-induced, 1981
cerebral, high-altitude, 1930t, 1932–1933
in mountain sickness, 1930
glottic, in croup, 935, *936*
hand, in mixed connective tissue disease, 1708
in anthrax, 1029
in histoplasmosis, 1111
pulmonary. See *Pulmonary edema.*
Education, on asthma, 2533, 2535–2540, 2535t–2539t, 2545–2550, 2546t, 2550t
government in. See *Government role, in asthma secondary prevention.*
on smoking effects, 2558–2560, 2559t
patient, on dyspnea, 548, 549
on pulmonary rehabilitation, 2508
EELV. See *End-expiratory lung volume.*
Effective particle diameter, of aerosols, 350
Efficacy, of drugs, 243
Efficiency, in exercise, 202, *203*
Eggs, *Ascaris lumbricoides*, 1149–1150, 1761
*Echinococcus*, 1158
hookworm, 1150–1151
*Paragonimus westermani*, 1160–1163
*Schistosoma*, 1163–1165
*Strongyloides stercoralis*, 1151
*Toxocara canis*, 1157
Egophony, 598
Egr-1 transcription factors, in monocyte-macrophage development, 406
Ehler-Danlos syndrome, secondary lung injury in, 480t
*Eikenella corrodens* infection, pneumonia as, 998t, 1028
Elastance, in airflow, 95, *96*
increased, causes of, 2449
in interstitial pulmonary fibrosis, 217
in pulmonary edema, 1500
Elastase, excess of, in cystic fibrosis, 1179, 1301
in emphysema, 1178
in lung, localization of, 1213–1214
in mucus, 332
in mucus hypersecretion, 334
inhibitors of, in chronic obstructive pulmonary disease, 288
Elastase-antielastase hypothesis, of emphysema, 1210–1214
animal models of, 1210–1211, *1211*
human evidence in, 1212–1214
overview of, 1210, *1210*
Elastic recoil, 93, 102
airway resistance and, 798
compliance and, 800–801, *801*
determinants of, 783–784
in asthma, 1264–1265
in chronic obstructive pulmonary disease, 212, 1207
in emphysema, 802
in pulmonary fibrosis, 801–802
loss of, *103*, 104
measurement of, 784, 799–802
in disease states, 801–802
protocol for, 800–802, *800*, *801*
theoretical aspects of, 799–800
normal values for, 875
physiology of, 799–800
pressure of, 799–801, *801*
surfactant in, 308
transpulmonary pressure and, 2044
versus age, 857
Elastic resistance, in interstitial lung disease, 1662, *1664*
Elasticity, of mucus, 363
of pulmonary arteries, 120, *121*
Elastin, 93, 137
degradation of, emphysema in, 1212–1214
impaired cross-linking of, emphysema and, 1211
Elderly persons, asthma in, 1269–1270
pneumonia in, cough in, 558
pulmonary function tests in, 857
ventilation-perfusion ratios in, 82
Electrical properties, of endothelium, 139–140, 140t
of epithelium, 335–336
Electrical stimulation, in respiratory muscle strength evaluation, 2333
of phrenic nerve, in neuromuscular disorders, 2348–2349
Electrocardiography, before exercise testing, 842
in asthma, 2453
in chest pain, 580, 581t
in cor pulmonale, 1639, *1640*
in pneumomediastinum, 2102–2103
in pulmonary embolism, 1510
in pulmonary hypertension, 1520, 1548
pneumothorax effects on, 2046
Electrocautery, in cancer, in airway obstruction, 742
occult, 1428
Electrode(s), carbon dioxide, 831–832, *832*, 837
oxygen, 832–833, *832*, 835–836, *836*
pH, 830–831, *831*
Electroencephalography, at high altitude, 1923–1924
in sleep, 2155, *2156*
Electrolyte(s). See also specific electrolytes, e.g., *Calcium*; *Potassium*; *Sodium*.
transepithelial transport of. See *Epithelium and epithelial cells, airway, electrolyte transport across.*
Electromagnetic fields, lung cancer related to, 1403–1404
Electromyography, in respiratory muscle evaluation, 858–859, 2333
in sleep, 2155, *2156*
Electron microscopy, in mesothelioma, 2069
Electrooculography, in sleep, 2155, *2156*
Electrophrenic respiration, in neuromuscular disorders, 2348–2349
Electrostatic precipitation, in aerosol deposition, 351, *351*
Elephantiasis, 1153, 1154
ELISA. See *Enzyme-linked immunosorbent assay.*
Elk transcription factor, in signal transduction, 239–240, *239*
Eloesser's flap, in pleural effusion, 2020
Embolectomy, for pulmonary embolism, 1518–1519, 1522–1525, *1524*, *1525*
Embolism, air, 465, 1526
after pneumomediastinum, 2098, *2098*, 2102
in diving, 1954–1956, *1956*, 1962
in mechanical ventilation, 2478
in pregnancy, 2324
amniotic fluid, 465, 1526–1527, 2323–2324, *2324*
cholesterol, 465
fat, 465, 2288
foreign body, 465
gas, in diving, 1954–1956, *1956*, 1962
paradoxical, in arteriovenous malformations, 1561
pulmonary. See *Pulmonary embolism.*
septic, 1527
Embolism *(Continued)*
trophoblastic tissue, 2325
Embolization (therapeutic), in hemoptysis, 751, 1566
of arteriovenous malformations, 1564–1565, *1564*
of pulmonary artery aneurysms, 1569
Embryology, of lung. See *Lung, development of.*
Embryonal cell carcinoma, of mediastinum, 2128
Emotional factors, in dyspnea, 542, 544
Emphysema (mediastinal). See *Pneumomediastinum.*
Emphysema (pulmonary), airflow in, versus lung volume, 102
air-space enlargement in, fibrosis with, 1205
animal models of, 1210–1211, *1211*
basilar, 1209, *1209*
blebs in, 1205
bullae in. See *Lung, bullae of.*
centriacinar, 462, *464*, 1204, *1204*
centrilobular, 1204, *1204*
chest radiography of, 1190, *1190*
chronic, definition of, 1188–1189, 1188t
classification of, 462, 1204–1205, *1204*, *1205*
clinical features of, 1189–1195, *1190*, *1191*, *1195*, *1196*
computed tomography in, 676, *676*
congenital lobar, 1198
cor pulmonale in, 1193–1194
crackles in, *595*
cysts in, 1205
dead space/tidal volume in, during exercise, 211–212
definition of, 1174, 1178
differential diagnosis of, 1195, 1197–1198, 1197t
diffusing capacity in, 815, *816*
distal acinar, 462, *464*, 465, 1205
epidemiology of, 1198–1201, *1200*, *1201*
erythrocytosis in, 1192
etiology of, 1178
flow-volume relationships in, 789
focal, 1204
heterogeneity of, 1206
historical background of, 1189
history in, 1189
in ankylosing spondylitis, 1710
in coal working, 1825–1828, *1826*
in HIV infection, 2209
in hypersensitivity pneumonitis, 1878
in Marfan's syndrome, 1711
in pneumomediastinum, 2098, *2098*, 2103
interlobular, 2098
irregular, 462, *464*, 465
laboratory findings in, 1190–1192, *1190*, *1191*
liver disease with, 1208–1209
lung volume in, 802
mortality in, 1198–1199
natural history of, 1201–1202, *1201*, *1202*
panacinar, 462, *464*, 1204, *1205*
panlobar, 676, *676*, *1204*, *1205*
paraseptal (distal acinar), 1205
pathogenesis of, 1178, 1207–1214
$alpha_1$-protease inhibitor deficiency in, 1178, 1208–1210, *1209*, 2276
elastase-antielastase hypothesis of, 1210–1214, *1210–1211*, *1214*
pathology of, 462, *464*, 465, 1204–1206, *1204*, *1205*
physical examination in, 1189
pneumonia in, 1194
pneumothorax in, 1192–1193

Emphysema (pulmonary) *(Continued)*
pressure-volume curve for, *103*, 104–105
prognosis for, 1202–1203
pulmonary function tests in, 802, 804, 853–854, 1190–1192, 1206–1207
pulmonary rehabilitation in. See *Pulmonary rehabilitation.*
risk factors for, 1199–1202, *1200*, *1201*
silicosis with, 1819
sleep disorders in, 1194
smoking and, 1178, 1199, *1200*, *1201*
animal models of, 1213–1214
bullae formation and, 1195, *1196*
cessation of, 1217, 2513–2514, *2513*, 2514t
inflammatory cells and, 1212
natural history and, 1201–1202, *1201*, *1202*
pathogenic aspects of, 1207–1209, *1209*
sputum examination in, 1192
structure-function correlations in, 1206–1207
subpleural (distal acinar), 1205
total vital capacity changes in, 112
treatment of. See also *Chronic obstructive pulmonary disease, treatment of; Pulmonary rehabilitation.*
aerosolized drugs in, 359
alpha$_1$-protease inhibitor in, 1210
lung volume reduction surgery in, 715, 853–854
surfactant in, 320
unilateral, 1198
ventilation distribution in, 808
ventilation-perfusion scanning in, 697–698
versus asthma, 1268
versus unilateral hyperlucent lung, 1197, 1197t
with reduced cardiovascular function, exercise testing in, 222–225, 224t
without elastin damage, animal models of, 1213–1214
Emphysema (subcutaneous and tissue), in barotrauma, 1955, 1956
in diving, 1955, 1956
in esophageal rupture, 2028
in mechanical ventilation, 2477–2478
in pneumomediastinum, 2103–2104, *2104*
natural history of, 2104
treatment of, 2104
Employment. See *Occupation(s); Occupational and environmental disorder(s).*
Empyema, 1031–1032
*Acinetobacter*, 1013, *1013*
amebic, 1145, 1146
anaerobic, 1018, *1018*, 1020, 1032, 2017
bacteriology of, 2017
beta-hemolytic streptococcal, 1004–1005
bronchopleural fistula with, 2020, *2021*
causes of, 1032
clinical manifestations of, 1032
*Coccidioides immitis*, 1124, *1124*
computed tomography of, 688, 2007, 2020, *2021*
diagnosis of, 1032, 2017–2018
fibrothorax in, 2062–2063
in bronchiectasis, 1328
in cystic fibrosis, 1305
in hemothorax, 2061
in mediastinitis, 2106
*Pasteurella multocida*, 1028
pathogenesis of, 1031–1032
pathophysiology of, 2017
pleural effusion in, 2016–2021, 2018t, *2021*
postoperative, 1032
postpneumonectomy, 2020–2021
*Pseudomonas aeruginosa*, 1011, 1012
Empyema *(Continued)*
*Staphylococcus aureus*, 1003–1004, 1032
treatment of, 1020, 1032, 2018–2019, 2018t
tuberculous, 1080, 2021
versus chylothorax, 2057
Enalapril, in pulmonary hypertension, 1644
Enalaprilat, in pulmonary edema, 1602
Encephalitis, *Toxoplasma gondii*, 2203
tuberculous, 1083–1084
Encephalomyelitis/sensory neuropathy, in lung cancer, 1379
Encephalopathy, in respiratory failure, 2444
End-expiratory lung volume, in exercise, in chronic obstructive pulmonary disease, 213–215
in interstitial pulmonary fibrosis, 217
Endocarditis, in histoplasmosis, 1114–1115
in Q fever, 1026
in *Staphylococcus aureus* pneumonia, 1003–1004, *1003*
prophylaxis for, in bronchoscopy, 730, 731t
Endocrine disorders. See also specific disorders, e.g., *Diabetes mellitus.*
in lung cancer, 1421–1422, 1422t
in sarcoidosis, 1719
Endocytosis, in alveolar clearance, 373
Endoglin defects, in hereditary hemorrhagic telangiectasia, 1559–1560
Endometrioma(s), of lung, 1480
Endometriosis, 2324–2325
pleural effusion in, 2034
pneumothorax in, 2054, 2324
Endoscopy. See specific techniques, e.g., *Bronchoscopy*; *Thoracoscopy.*
Endostatin, in angiogenesis, in lung cancer, 1387
Endothelial permeability, 138–144
albumin transcytosis in, 140–141
alveolar, 135–136
decreased, cyclic nucleotides in, 144
electrical charge effects on, 139–140, 140t
increased, basement membrane and, 143–144
calcium intracellular shifts in, 142, *143*
characteristics of, 141
cytoskeletal alterations in, 141–142
mechanisms of, 141–144, *143*, 145–146
protein kinase C activation in, 142–143
pore theory of, 138–139, 138t, *139*, 138t
regional differences in, 140
to water, 144
Endothelin(s), actions of, 298
as inflammatory mediators, 257
excess of, in pulmonary hypertension, 1492
in hypoxic pulmonary vasoconstriction, 67, 130
in neonatal pulmonary vasculature remodeling, 131
in pulmonary circulation regulation, 1492
in pulmonary hypertension, 1645
in pulmonary vascular resistance control, 131
receptor for, 298
Endothelium and endothelial cells, 14–15, *15*, 122
electrical charge of, 139–140, 140t
function of, 232
heart disease effects on, 2248–2249
hydraulic conductivity of, 144
junctions in, for fluid and solute exchange, 134–135, *134–136*
of pulmonary capillaries, 1486, *1488*
fluid and solute exchange across, 134–135, *134–136*
neutrophil interactions with, 525–526, *525*
permeability of. See *Endothelial permeability.*
Endothelium and endothelial cells *(Continued)*
*Plasmodium falciparum* adherence to, 1146
products synthesized by, 232, *233*
properties of, transport and, 138, 138t
pulmonary venous hypertension effects on, 2248–2249
solute flux across, equation for, 133
structure of, 139
Endothelium-derived hyperpolarizing factor, in hypoxic pulmonary vasoconstrictor response, 130
Endothelium-derived relaxing factors. See also *Nitric oxide.*
in hypoxic pulmonary vasoconstrictor response, 130
Endotoxin, alveolar macrophage recognition of, 390, *391*
emphysema due to, 1211
in bronchoconstriction, in byssinosis, 1861
in pneumonia, lung injury from, 474
in pulmonary edema, neutralization of, 1610–1611
lung injury due to, 1587, 1588t, 1589
monoclonal antibodies to, in pulmonary edema, 1610–1611
platelet-activating factor and, 498
tumor necrosis factor-α and, 474
Endotracheal intubation, bronchoscopy in, 753
chest radiography for, 665
double-lumen, inspection of, 753
for bronchoscopy, 728, 732
for mechanical ventilation, 2472
in pregnancy, 2317–2318, 2324
pneumomediastinum in, 2097
pneumonia in, 747, *748*
Energy, conservation of, in dyspnea, 547
expenditure of, in chronic obstructive pulmonary disease, 2510
in pulmonary rehabilitation, 2510
requirements for, in cystic fibrosis, 1305, 1311
in diving, 1953, *1953*, 1963
in work situations, 906–907, 907t, 909
transfer of, in exercise, 201
Enkephalins, actions of, *251*
Enprofylline, 272, 273
*Entamoeba dispar* infections, 1144
*Entamoeba histolytica* infections (amebiasis), 1144–1146, *1145*, 2025
Enteric cysts, of mediastinum, 2130
Enteritis, tuberculous, 1084–1085
Enterobacteriaceae pneumonia, 998t, 1010–1011
Enterococcal pneumonia, in granulocytopenia, 924
Enterovirus infections, 931t
Entitlement programs, impairment and disability evaluation for. See *Impairment and disability, evaluation of.*
Environmental disorder(s). See *Occupational and environmental disorder(s).*
Environmental Protection Agency, air quality standards of, 1885, 1886t
Enzyme(s), drug inhibition of, 247
in receptor structure, 238
Enzyme immunoassay, for fungi, 616
Enzyme-linked immunosorbent assay, for *Echinococcus*, 1159
for HIV, 2173
for influenza virus, 955
for *Mycoplasma*, 624
for respiratory syncytial virus, 963
for *Schistosoma*, 1164
Eosinophil(s), 526–527
activation of, 1760
apoptosis of, 528–529, *529*, *530*

Eosinophil(s) *(Continued)*
biochemistry of, 1757–1760, 1758t, 1759t
chemotactic factors for, 1759–1760
counting of, in inflammation assessment, 529–530
development of, 527
distribution of, 1757–1758
excess of. See *Eosinophilia*; *Eosinophilic lung disease(s)*.
formation of, 1757–1758
functions of, 1757, 1759–1760
granules of, 527
harmful effects of, 1759–1760
in airway epithelium, in asthma, 1253–1254, *1255*
in allergic bronchopulmonary aspergillosis, 1763
in asthma, 1260–1261, *1260*, 1268
in mucus hypersecretion, 334
in pleural fluid, 2004
in pulmonary circulation, *525*
in sputum, in asthma, 1268
inhibition of, in asthma, 287, *288*
normal count of, 527
products secreted by, 526–527
protein constituents of, 1757–1758, 1758t
receptors on, 1758t, 1759
regulation of, 1757–1758
structure of, *522*, 526, 1758–1759, 1758t
trafficking of, 527
Eosinophil cationic protein, 334, 1758t, 1759, 1759t
Eosinophilia. See also *Eosinophilic lung disease(s)*.
drug-induced, 1990–1991, 1991t
in allergic bronchopulmonary aspergillosis, 1765
in allergic granulomatosis and angiitis, 1538, 1769
in aspergillosis, 1131–1132
in asthma, 1268
in fibrosis, 504
in filariasis, 1153, 1155, 1761–1762, *1762*
in hypereosinophilic syndrome, 1769, 1769t
in methotrexate-induced pulmonary disease, 1977
in nitrofurantoin-induced pulmonary disease, 1978
in nonallergic rhinitis with eosinophilia syndrome, 1347
in paragonimiasis, 1161
in pneumonia, *Chlamydia trachomatis*, 1027
eosinophilic, 1766–1767, *1767*, 1767t, *1768*
in strongyloidiasis, 1151–1152
in trichinosis, 1156
sulfasalazine-induced, 1979
tropical, 1760–1762, 1761t, *1762*
Eosinophilic granuloma, *1662*, 1725
Eosinophilic lung disease(s), 1760. See also *Allergic bronchopulmonary aspergillosis*.
allergic granulomatosis and angiitis as, 1538, 1769–1771, *1770*, 1770t, 2033
bronchitis as, 289, 559
classification of, 1760–1761, 1761t
drug-induced, 1762–1763, 1762t
eosinophilia-myalgia syndrome as, 1542, 1762–1763
eosinophilic granuloma as, *1662*, 1725
historical aspects of, 1760–1761
hypereosinophilic syndrome as, 1759, 1769t
parasitic, 1761–1762, 1761t, *1762*
pneumonia as, 1653t, 1654, 1760–1761
acute, 1767–1769, 1769t
bronchoscopy in, 752
chronic, 1766–1767, *1767*, 1767t, *1768*
Eosinophilic lung disease(s) *(Continued)*
drug-induced, 479t
tropical eosinophilia as, 1153–1155, *1154*, 1760–1762, 1761t, *1762*
Eotaxin, 507t, 516–517
in asthma, 287
in macrophage development, 404
receptors for, 517–518, 517t
Epidemiology. See also specific diseases.
concepts of, in occupational disorders, 1805
Epidermal growth factor receptor, in lung cancer growth, 1381
in lung development, 41–42
stimulation of, mucus secretion in, 1175
Epidural anesthesia, pulmonary function effects of, 885
Epiglottitis, 918
in croup, 935
viral, 934
Epilepsy, respiratory effects of, 2351
Epinephrine, chemical structure of, 268, *268*
in asthma, 2454, 2454t
in bronchodilation, 255
in croup, 935
in shock, 2401t
in status asthmaticus, 2454, 2454t
secretion of, theophylline effects on, 273
Epistaxis, in hereditary hemorrhagic telangiectasia, 1560, 1561
Epithelial growth factor, receptor for, 238–239
Epithelial neutrophil activating protein-78, 508, 508t
Epithelium and epithelial cells, airway, 232, *233*
barrier function of, 335
basal, *9*, 10
bronchiolar, 16
chloride channels of, *336*, 337–338
ciliated, 7, *8*, *9*
Clara, 10, *11*
culture of, 336
cytokines of, 1259t
defense function of, 1177, *1177*. See also *Mucus*.
desquamation of, in asthma, 1253
electrolyte transport across, 334–340
barriers to, 335
electrical properties in, 335–336
in cystic fibrosis, 1297–1300, *1298*
liquid composition and, 339–340, 340t
mechanisms of, 336–338, *336*
regulation of, 338, 339
goblet, 9, *9*
histology of, 7, *8–11*, 9–10
in asthma, 1243–1254, 1258, 1259t
injury of, chronic bronchitis in, 1216
in occupational asthma, 1855
innervation of, 360–361
junctional complexes between, 7, *9*
metaplasia of, chronic bronchitis in, 1216
paracellular pathway through, 338
pathology of, in asthma, 1253–1254
polarization of, 360
potassium channels of, *336*, 337
receptors on, 338
sentinel cells in, 1177, *1177*
sodium channels of, 336–338, *336*
tight junctions in, 335
toxic exposure to, pathogenic effects of, 1904
water permeability of, 338
alveolar, 16–21, 1486, *1488*
amiodarone effects on, 1973
basement membranes of, 122
bleomycin toxicity to, 1972
bronchiolar epithelial transition to, 16
Epithelium and epithelial cells *(Continued)*
culture of, 21
damage of, in lung injury, 1586
in ozone exposure, 1895–1896
in pulmonary edema, 1586
degeneration of, in hemosiderosis, 1741–1742, *1741*
differentiation of, 21
dysfunction of, in acute respiratory distress syndrome, 319
fluid movement through, 145
functions of, 19, 20t, 21, 21t, 371
heart disease effects on, 2248–2249
hyperplasia of, *451*
in clearance, 371
in fluid and solute exchange, 135–136
macrophage proximity to, 388, *388*
monolayer of, 122
ozone injury of, 1895–1896
permeability of, perfusion scanning for, 718–720, *719*
proliferation of, 19, 21
proteins produced by, 19–21, 20t, 21t
structure of, 16–17, *18*, 19–20, 371
surfactant protein A in, 310
surfactant protein B in, 313
surfactant protein C in, 313–314
surfactant secretion from, 316, *317*
toxic exposure to, pathogenic effects of, 1904
type I cells in, 19–20, 21t
type II cells in, 17, *18*, 19, 20t
bronchial, squamous metaplasia of, 1326
cystic fibrosis transmembrane regulator in, 1295
glandular, ion transport defects of, in cystic fibrosis, 1299–1300
in sputum, 614, *614*, *615*
mesenchymal interactions with, in lung development, 36, *36*, 37, *37*
pleural, mesothelioma of, 2068
pulmonary venous hypertension effects on, 2248–2249
Epithelium-derived relaxant factor, 232
Epitope, definition of, 422
Epoprostenol. See *Prostacyclin*.
Epstein-Barr virus infection(s), 931t
effusion lymphoma in, 2071
in HIV infection, 2203
in lung transplantation, 2522
in transplantation, 2231–2232
pharyngitis as, 917, 933
pneumonia as, 470
Equal pressure points, in expiration, 783
Equipment, for diving, 1953–1954, *1954*
respiratory, contamination of, gram-negative organism transmission from, 1008
*ERBB* genes and products, in lung cancer growth, 1380–1381
Ergometry, in exercise testing, 841, 844–845
Ergoreflex, in exercise, in heart failure, 2260
Erionite, diseases due to, 2067
*ERK* gene, in lung cancer, 1381–1382
ERV. See *Expiratory reserve volume*.
*Erwinia* pneumonia, 1010–1011
Erythema multiforme, in coccidioidomycosis, 1123
Erythema nodosum, in coccidioidomycosis, 1123
in histoplasmosis, 1111
in sarcoidosis, 1718, *1719*
Erythrocyte(s), alveolar macrophage sequestration of, 390, *391*, 392
formation of, at high altitude, 1921–1922, 1929
in pulmonary edema fluid, 1579

Erythrocyte(s) *(Continued)*
malaria affecting, 1146–1147
membrane of, diffusion across, 810, *810*
sickling of, in sickle cell disease and trait, 85, 2286–2290
Erythrocytosis, 2286
in bronchitis, chronic, 1192
in chronic obstructive pulmonary disease, 1192
in emphysema, 1192
in mountain sickness, 1938
Erythromycin, in cystic fibrosis, 1309t
in pneumonia, 922t, 995t, 998t
*Chlamydia trachomatis*, 1027
Erythropoiesis, at high altitude, 1921–1922, 1929
Erythropoietin, excess of, 2286
secretion of, at high altitude, 1921–1922
*Escherichia coli* infection, pneumonia due to, 1010–1011
surfactant protein A binding in, 312
surfactant protein D binding in, 315
Esophageal pressure, measurement of, 800, *800*
versus lung volume, 103–104, *103*
Esophagitis, herpes simplex virus, 948
Esophagography, 2083
Esophagoscopy, mediastinitis in, 2107
Esophagus, balloon catheter in, for inspiratory and expiratory pressure measurement, 2333
disorders of, chest pain in, 579–580, 581t
in mediastinitis, 2113
distention of, pain in, 571
irritation of, pain mechanisms in, 574–575
mechanosensitive fibers in, 570
pH monitoring in, for cough diagnosis, 562, 563t
radiation injury of, 1436
reflux into. See *Gastroesophageal reflux disease.*
rupture of, mediastinitis in, 2106–2107, *2107*
pleural effusion in, 2003, 2027–2028, *2027*
pneumomediastinum in, 2099
pneumothorax in, 2052–2053
varices of, sclerotherapy for, complications of, 1989, 2030
Estrogen receptors, lymphangio(leio)myomatosis and, 1778–1779
Ethambutol, in *Mycobacterium avium* complex infections, 2185
in *Mycobacterium kansasii* infections, 1095, 2186
in tuberculosis, 1066, 1068t, 1069
drug-resistant, 1073t
in HIV infection, 2184
regimen for, 1071–1073, 1071t
resistance to, 1073t
side effects of, 1068t, 1069
Ethane, in multiple inert gas elimination technique, 80–81, *81*, *82*
Ethanolamine oleate, for esophageal varices, pulmonary disease due to, 1989
Ether, in multiple inert gas elimination technique, 80–81, *81*, *82*
Ethics, 2487–2503
autonomy principle of, 2491–2492
beneficence principle of, 2490–2491
decision making in, governmental legislation and regulations for, 2494
in brain death, 2496
in euthanasia, 2500–2501
in life support withdrawing, 2498–2500
in life support withholding, 2496–2498
Ethics *(Continued)*
in organ transplantation, 2496
legal precedents for, 2492–2494
patient preferences in, 2489–2490
physician preferences in, 2489–2490
practical principles for, 2495–2496, 2495t
definition of, 2490
effective communication principle of, 2495
intensive care milieu and, 2487–2490
justice principle of, 2492
moral virtues in, 2492
nonmaleficence principle of, 2491
patient attitudes and, 2489–2490
patients' rights and, 2496
physician attitudes and, 2489–2490
principles of, for practical decision making, 2495–2496, 2495t
fundamental, 2490–2492, 2490t
quality-of-life value principle of, 2496
source of authority principle of, 2495
theories of, 2490
Ethionamide, in tuberculosis, 1069t, 1070
Ethmoid sinusitis, 916–917
Ethnic factors, in chronic obstructive pulmonary disease, 1199
in cystic fibrosis, 1292
in lung cancer, 1396, *1396*, 1398, 1417t
in pulmonary function tests, 803, 899, 905
in sarcoidosis, 1717–1718
in smoking, 1398, 2533
in tuberculosis, 1059
Ethylene glycol toxicity, anion gap acidosis due to, 168
Ethylene oxide, for bronchoscope disinfection, 758
inhalation of, 1909
Etoposide, in lung cancer, 1438
pulmonary disease due to, 1978
Ets transcription factors, in monocyte-macrophage development, 405–406
Eupnea, C-fiber activity in, 184
definition of, 180
respiratory muscle function in, 188
Eustachian tube dysfunction, diving disorders in, 1956–1957
Euthanasia, 2500–2501
Eventration, of diaphragm. See *Diaphragm, paralysis of.*
Exercise, 197–229. See also *Exercise testing; Exercise training.*
adenosine triphosphate generation in, 198–201, *199*, *200*
air pollutant inhalation during, 1888
airflow augmentation during, 1344
anaerobic metabolism in, 199–200, *200*, 839–840
arm, in pulmonary rehabilitation, 2510
asthma in, 843, 1271
at high altitude, 1925–1929
cardiovascular response in, 1927–1928
gas exchange in, 1926–1927, *1927*
maximal work in, 1925, *1925*
performance at, 1928–1929
tissue alterations in, 1928
ventilation in, 1925–1926, *1927*
breathing, after abdominal surgery, 886, 886t
historical background of, 2505–2508, *2506*, *2507*
in pulmonary rehabilitation, 2509
bronchospasm in, 1271
carbohydrate metabolism in, 198–201, *199*, *200*
carbon dioxide output in, in heavy exercise, 205–206, *206*
in moderate exercise, 203–204, *204*
in severe exercise, 205–206, *206*
Exercise *(Continued)*
sources of, 205–206, *206*
cardiac output in, 838
cardiovascular response in, at high altitude, 1927–1928
chest pain in, 577
dead space in, 2259
diffusing capacity in, 809, 814–815
dyspnea in, 220–221, 542, 543
in alveolar proteinosis, 1794
in heart disease, 2262
in lymphangio(leio)myomatosis, 1780, 1780t
efficiency in, 202, *203*
energy sources for, 838
energy transfer in, 201
fat metabolism in, 198–201, *199*, *200*
fatigue in, 221
gas exchange in, 201–206
at high altitude, 1926–1927, *1927*
in heart disease, 2259
in heavy exercise, 204–206, *206*
in moderate exercise, 201–204, *203*
in severe exercise, 204–206, *206*
glycogen utilization in, 200–201
heat produced in, 837–838, 838t
heavy, carbon dioxide output in, 205–206, *206*
definition of, 201
oxygen uptake in, 204–205
ventilation patterns in, 211, *211*
hyperventilation in, 2260
in arteriovenous malformations, gas exchange in, 1563
in asthma, 218
in chronic obstructive pulmonary disease, 212–217, *213–215*, *217*, 1227
oxygen during, 1225–1226
in cystic fibrosis, 1304–1305, 1310–1311
in diving, 1952, 1953, *1953*, 1963
in heart disease/failure, 2258–2260, 2259t, 2260t
dyspnea in, 2262
pulmonary hemodynamics in, 2249–2251, 2249t
in highly fit athletes, 218–220
in interstitial lung disease, 217–218, 1664, *1665*
in pulmonary fibrosis, 1676, *1676*
in pulmonary rehabilitation, historical background of, 2505–2508, *2506*, *2507*
systemic, 2509–2510, 2510t
techniques for, 2508–2509
upper extremity, 2510
in ventilation, in heart disease, 2258–2259, 2259t
insulin in, 201
intolerance of. See also *Exercise, tolerance of.*
definition of, 197
in arteriovenous malformations, 1495
in hyperthyroidism, 2310
in pulmonary hypertension, 1637
lactate paradox in, at high altitude, 1928
lactate threshold in. See *Lactic acid (anaerobic) threshold.*
lactic acid production in, 166
limitation of, in chronic obstructive pulmonary disease, 212–216, *213–215*, *217*
in highly fit athletes, 218–220
reasons for, 220–221
maximal work in, at high altitude, 1925, *1925*
moderate, carbon dioxide output in, 203–204, *204*
definition of, 201

Exercise *(Continued)*
oxygen uptake in, 201–203, *203*
ventilation patterns in, 210
muscle structure and, 197–198, 198t
oxygen availability limitation in, 206–208, *207*
oxygen uptake in, 838t
in moderate exercise, 201–203, *203*
pain in, 221
physiology of, 837–839, *839*
pulmonary artery pressure in, versus cardiac output, 1491, *1491*
pulmonary artery wedge pressure in, 2249t, 2250
pulmonary blood flow distribution in, 1489, 1491t
pulmonary edema in, high-altitude, 1937
pulmonary function testing in, for obstructive disease, 1182
pulmonary hemorrhage in, 69
respiratory muscle, 108–109
in chronic obstructive pulmonary disease, 2464
in pulmonary rehabilitation, 2509
in ventilator liberation, 2385
severe, carbon dioxide output in, 205–206, *206*
definition of, 201
oxygen uptake in, 204–205
ventilation patterns in, 211, *211*
substrate utilization in, 198–201, *199*, *200*
systemic, in pulmonary rehabilitation, 2509–2510, 2510t
tissue alterations in, at high altitude, 1928
tolerance of. See also *Exercise, intolerance of.*
after thoracoplasty, 2364
at high altitude, 1925, *1925*
in ankylosing spondylitis, 2370
in chest wall disorders, 2361t
in chronic obstructive pulmonary disease, 215–217
in kyphoscoliosis, 2360–2361, 2361t
in obesity, 2373
in pectus excavatum, 2365–2366
questionnaires for, in dyspnea, 544
versus age, 857
versus heart size, 840
ventilation in, 839, *839*
at high altitude, 1925–1926, *1927*
in pulmonary disease, 211–212, 212t
limitation of, in asthma, 218
in chronic obstructive pulmonary disease, 212–217, *213–215*, *217*
in highly fit athletes, 218–220
in interstitial pulmonary fibrosis, 217–218
patterns of, 210–212, *211*, 212t
requirements for, 208–210, *209*
respiratory muscle function in, 108–109
ventilation threshold in, 840
Exercise testing, 221–226, 837–849
activities versus work rate in, 837, 838t
after lung transplantation, 2525, *2525*
anaerobic threshold in, 839–840, 845–846, *846*, *847*
arterial catheterization with, 842
at high altitude, 1922
automated, 841–842
before lung transplantation, 2519–2520
calculations for, 843–844
cessation of, criteria for, 842
complex ergometery/treadmill systems in, 841
contraindications to, 842
controversial issues in, 844–846, *846*, *847*
Exercise testing *(Continued)*
cycle, oxygen uptake in, 202, *203*
efficiency in, 202, *203*, 844
electrocardiography before, 842
energy requirements for, 906–907, 907t, 909
ergometry in, 841, 844–845
gas exchange responses in, 205–206, *206*
gas pressures in, 844
gas volumes in, 843
in anxiety, 849
in asthma, exercise-induced, 843
in chronic obstructive pulmonary disease, 848
in disability evaluation, 846
in dyspnea, 544, 546–547, 546t, 899, 900
in emphysema with reduced cardiovascular function, 222–225, 224t
in heart disease, 846–847
in impairment and disability evaluation, 897–900, 906–907, 907t
in interstitial lung disease, 225–226, 225t, 848
in lymphangio(leio)myomatosis, 1781
in neuromuscular disease, 849
in obesity, 848–849
in obstructive disease, 847–848
in poor physical condition, 849
in pulmonary hypertension, 1548
in pulmonary vascular obstruction, 848
in restrictive disease, 848, 855, 855t
incremental method in, 842
indications for, 837
maximum tests in, 845
normal values for, 878–881
objectives of, 221
of ventilatory drive, 818
oxygen administration during, 843
oxygen pulse in, 844
oxygen uptake in, 204
physiology of, 837–839, *839*
poor motivation in, 849
principles of, 221
protocols for, 842–843
pulmonary function tests before, 842
ramp, 202–203, *203*, 843
rebreathing methods in, 842
reproducibility of, 844
respiratory gas ratio in, 844
steady-state, 842, 845
subjective responses in, 845
systems for, 841–842, 849
theoretical aspects of, 837–841, 838t, *839*, 878–881
treadmills in, 844–845
ventilatory equivalents in, 844
walk tests in, 841
work rate versus activities in, 837, 838t
Exercise training, at high altitudes, 1928–1929
endurance, lactic acid threshold in, 207, 208
physiology of, 840–841
in chronic obstructive pulmonary disease, 216–217, *217*
in cystic fibrosis, 1304–1305
in dyspnea, 547–548, *547*
physiology of, 840–841
Exhaust, from motor vehicles, air pollution from, 1887–1888, 1887t, 1893
Exoantigen testing, in coccidioidomycosis, 1125
in fungal infections, 623
Exocytosis, in mucus secretion, 332–334
Exotoxins, in pneumonia, lung injury from, 474
Expectorants, in asthma, 289
in chronic obstructive pulmonary disease, 1224
Expectorants *(Continued)*
in cystic fibrosis, 1310
Expectoration. See *Sputum, production of.*
Expiration, airflow in, in exercise, in chronic obstructive pulmonary disease, 213–214
chest radiography during, 644, 646, *646–650*
control of, ventral respiratory group in, 186
equal pressure points in, 783
flow-volume relationships for, 787–790, *787–790*
in highly fit athletes, 218
in cough, 555, *555*, 556
muscles of, 2330, 2330t
prolonged, in chronic obstructive pulmonary disease, 2448
time for, 108
respiratory frequency and, 181
Expiratory axons, in breathing control, 187–188, *187*
Expiratory flow. See also *Maximal expiratory flow.*
in pulmonary fibrosis, 1675
Expiratory neurons, in medulla, 186
Expiratory pressure, in mechanical ventilation, 2451
maximal. See *Maximal expiratory pressure.*
versus volume, normal values for, 875
Expiratory reserve volume, definition of, 57, *57*, *783*, 2563
in heart disease, 2251, *2251*, 2252t
in obesity, 2371
in spinal cord injury, 2338
measurement of, 790–791
Expiratory residual capacity, normal, *57*
Expired volume, definition of, 2564
Exposures, to harmful substances. See *Occupational and environmental disorder(s); Toxic exposure(s).*
External fixation, of flail chest, 2369
Extracellular matrix, of pulmonary capillaries, 135
permeability and, 143–144
Extracorporeal gas exchange, in acute respiratory distress syndrome, 2434
Extramedullary hematopoiesis, pleural effusion in, 2035
Extrinsic allergic alveolitis. See *Hypersensitivity pneumonitis.*
Extubation, from mechanical ventilation. See *Mechanical ventilation, liberation from.*
Exudates, pleural fluid. See *Pleural effusion(s), exudative.*
Eye disorders, at high altitude, 1937, *1937*
in lung disease, 603, 603t
in sarcoidosis, 1718
in tuberculosis, 1077

## F

Fabry's disease, secondary lung injury in, 480t
Face, barotrauma of, 1957
trauma to, pneumomediastinum in, 2097
Facial nerve palsy, in sarcoidosis, 1718–1719
$FA_{CO_t}$ (alveolar carbon monoxide concentration), for diffusing capacity calculation, 811
F-actin, in endothelium, in permeability regulation, 141–142
Factor V Leiden mutation, thromboembolism risk in, 1514
Factor VIII deficiency, 2294–2295
Factor IX deficiency, 2294–2295
Famciclovir, in herpes simplex virus infections, 949
Familial aggregation, of asthma, 1252–1253, 1254t

Familial aggregation *(Continued)*
of genetic disease, 48
of lung cancer, 1405, 1416
of smoking, 1405
Familial multifocal fibrosclerosis, 2111
Familial risk, of genetic disease, 48
Family history, 591
Farmer's lung. See *Hypersensitivity pneumonitis.*
Fas and Fas ligand, in apoptosis, *445*
in lung cancer, 1386–1387
Fast receptors, 240, *240*
Fat, body, loss of, in cystic fibrosis, 1306
metabolism of, in exercise, 198–201, *199*, *200*
dietary, in lung cancer, 1405
embolism of, 465, 1526
in sickle cell disease, 2288
Fatigue, definition of, 109
in alveolar proteinosis, 1794
in arteriovenous malformations, 1495
in chronic obstructive pulmonary disease, 215–217, *217*
in chylothorax, 2057
in exercise, 215–217, *217*, 220, 221
in pulmonary hypertension, 1546
in radiation therapy, 1436
of respiratory muscles, in chronic obstructive pulmonary disease, 216–217
in highly fit athletes, 219
in respiratory failure, 2385, *2386*, 2387, 2445–2447, *2445*, *2446*
mechanical aspects of, 109
threshold of, in chronic obstructive pulmonary disease, 216
versus weakness, 109
in neuromuscular disorders, 2345
Feedback, in breathing control, 179
Feeding tubes, misplacement of, pleural effusion in, 2036
Fenfluramine-dexfenfluramine, pulmonary hypertension due to, 1546
Fenoterol, as bronchodilator, 270
in asthma, 357
morbidity and mortality due to, 272, 1248–1249
in chronic obstructive pulmonary disease, 357
side effects of, 272
Ferruginous bodies, 1832–1833
in cell injury, 450, *453*
Fetus, bronchial circulation importance in, 121
cord blood from, transplantation of. See *Blood and bone marrow transplantation.*
high altitude effects on, 1942
macrophage development in, 387, 397–399
pulmonary circulation in, 68, 131
$FEV_1$. See *Forced expiratory volume in one second.*
Fever, amphotericin B-induced, 1116
hemorrhagic, Korean, 945–947
hyperventilation in, 2147
in amebiasis, 1145
in aspergillosis, 1131, 1133
in blastomycosis, 1119
in bronchial disorders, 1368
in bronchiectasis, 1327
in bronchoscopy, 756
in candidiasis, 1135
in chemotherapy-induced disease, 1974
in coccidioidomycosis, 1107
in cryptococcosis, 1130
in epiglottitis, 918
in fat embolism, 1526
in granulocytopenia, 924–925, 925t
Fever *(Continued)*
in histoplasmosis, 1110
in influenza, 953
in Kaposi's sarcoma, 2205
in lung injury, 1591
in mediastinal mass, 2083
in mediastinitis, 2106
in mesothelioma, 2071
in nitrofurantoin-induced pulmonary disease, 1978
in paragonimiasis, 1161
in pharyngitis, 917
in pneumomediastinum, 2102
in pneumonia, *Acinetobacter*, 1013
*Actinomyces*, 1021
anaerobic, 1017
beta-hemolytic streptococcal, 1004
*Chlamydia psittaci*, 1026
*Coxiella burnetii*, 1025
Enterobacteriaceae, 1010
*Haemophilus influenzae*, 1007
in immunodeficiency, 924
*Klebsiella pneumoniae*, 1008
*Legionella*, 1014
*Mycoplasma pneumoniae*, 1024
pneumococcal, 999
*Pneumocystis carinii*, 926
*Staphylococcus aureus*, 1003
in tuberculosis, 1062
Lassa, pharyngitis in, 933
pharyngoconjunctival, 937, 939
Pontiac, 1014
Q (*Coxiella burnetii* infection), 473, 998t, 1025–1026
reduction of, oxygen consumption reduction in, 2407
valley. See *Coccidioidomycosis.*
$FEV_t$ (timed forced expiratory volume), 2563
Fexofenadine, in allergic rhinitis, 1349
*FHIT* gene and product, in lung cancer, 1384
Fiberoptic bronchoscopy. See *Bronchoscopy (flexible fiberoptic or unspecified).*
Fibrin, radiopharmaceuticals seeking, 718
Fibrinogen, in disseminated intravascular coagulation, 2295
Fibrinolysis, disorders of, at high altitude, 1938
Fibroblast(s), in pulmonary fibrosis, 1677, 1678
proliferation of, interleukins in, 503–504
transforming growth factor-β effects on, 506
tumor necrosis factor-α effects on, 501
Fibroblast growth factors and receptors, 505
in lung cancer, 1387
in lung development, 39–41
Fibroma(s), of lung, 1478, 1479
Fibromyalgia, pain in, 576–577
Fibronectin, in fluid and solute exchange, *134–135*
Fibrosclerosis, familial multifocal, 2111
Fibrosis, air-space enlargement with, 1188–1189, 1188t, 1205
angiogenesis in, 513–514, *513–515*
bleomycin-induced, 1976
bronchoscopy in, 752–753
causes of, *1651*
cyclophosphamide-induced, 1975
cystic. See *Cystic fibrosis.*
diffusing capacity in, 816
dust accumulation in, versus occupation, *1812*
eosinophilia in, 504
familial idiopathic, 480t
from particulates, macrophages in, 1889
gold-induced, 1984
granulocyte-macrophage colony-stimulating factor in, 404
Fibrosis *(Continued)*
idiopathic pulmonary, 1671–1684
bronchoalveolar lavage in, 1679–1680
bronchoscopy in, 752–753
chest radiography of, 1673, *1674*, *1675*, 1679
clinical features of, 1671–1673, 1678–1679
complications of, 1683–1684, 1684t
computed tomography of, *1662*, 1673, 1679
diagnosis of, 1678
disease overlapping with, *1650*, 1652t
epidemiology of, 1671
exercise in, 1676, *1676*
familial, 1684
gallium scan in, 1673
histopathology of, 1677, 1678, *1679*
laboratory studies in, 1679
lung transplantation in, 2520, 2520t
natural history of, 1680
pathogenesis of, 1677–1678
arachidonic acid metabolites in, 498
chemokines in, 512–516, *513–515*
interleukin-1 family in, 500
neutrophils in, 512–513
platelet-derived growth factor in, 504
pathology of, 466, *468*
pressure-volume relationships in, *1664*
prognosis for, 1678, 1679, *1679*
pulmonary circulation in, 1676
pulmonary function tests in, 1662, *1664*, 1673, 1675–1676, *1675*, *1676*, 1679
sleep disorders in, 1676–1677
smoking and, 1677
staging of, 1678–1680, *1679*
treatment of, 1680–1684, 1681t, 1683t, 1684t
ventilation-perfusion scan in, 1673–1675
in acute respiratory distress syndrome, 2435–2436
in alveolar microlithiasis, 1749–1750, *1749*, *1750*
in alveolar proteinosis, 1792–1793
in ankylosing spondylitis, 2370
in asbestosis. See *Asbestosis.*
in beryllium lung disease, 1843–1844
in coal-worker's pneumoconiosis. See *Coal-workers' pneumoconiosis.*
in filariasis, 1154
in hard metal disease, 1845
in Hermansky-Pudlak syndrome, 1749
in histoplasmosis, 1111
in lung injury, 1586
in oxygen toxicity, 1987
in paraquat exposure, 1908
in pulmonary edema, 1586, 1614
in pulmonary venous hypertension, 2248
in radiation injury, 475, *476*, 477
in sarcoidosis, 1727
in silicosis. See *Silicosis.*
inflammatory mediators in. See *Inflammatory mediator(s).*
interstitial, biopsy in, 1697
bronchoalveolar lavage in, 1696–1697
chest radiography in, 1694, *1696*
clinical features of, 1694, 1695t
drug-induced, 1692t
exercise in, 209–210, *209*, 217–218
in ankylosing spondylitis, 1710
in dermatomyositis, 1707–1708, *1707*
in HIV infection, 2210
in rheumatoid arthritis, 1698–1699, 1702–1703
in Sjögren's syndrome, 1705–1706
in systemic lupus erythematosus, 1703–1704

Fibrosis *(Continued)*
in systemic sclerosis, 1692, 1694, 1695t, 1696–1697, *1696*
pathogenesis of, 1692, 1694
predisposition to, 1692
prognosis for, 1697
pulmonary function tests in, 1694, 1696
serology in, 1697
treatment of, 1697
interstitial macrophages in, 396
lung volume in, 801–802
mediastinal. See *Mediastinum, fibrosis of.*
nitrosourea-induced, 1977
pathogenesis of, chemokines in, 518–519
fibroblast growth factors in, 505
insulin-like growth factor in, 505
interferon-τ in, 503–504
interleukin-1 family in, 499–501
interleukin-4 in, 503–504
interleukin-5 in, 503–504
transforming growth factor-β in, 506
tumor necrosis factor-α in, 501–502
pathology of, 459, *461*, 462, *463*
pathophysiology of, 495–496, *496*
peribronchial, in chronic obstructive pulmonary disease, 1216
pleural. See *Pleura, fibrosis of.*
progressive massive, 1818, *1821*
in coal working, 1825–1828, *1825*, *1826*
in silicosis, 1818, *1821*, 1823
pulmonary hypertension in, 1633
radiation, 716, 1436
ventilation distribution in, 808
Fibrositis, of chest wall, pain in, 577
Fibrothorax, 2062–2063, *2062*
in hemothorax, 2061
Fibrous histiocytomas, of lung, 1480
Fick equation, for cardiac output, 838
Fick's law of diffusion, 70, 72
for diffusing capacity, 75
in exercise, 202
Field cancerization, in lung cancer, 1377–1378
Filariasis, 1153–1155, *1154*, 1761–1762, *1762*
Filley equations, for diffusing capacity, 812
Films, X-ray. See *Chest radiography.*
Filovirus infections, 931t
Filters, inferior vena cava, in pulmonary embolism prevention, 1517, *1518*
Filtration, in pulmonary circulation, 70
versus lymph flow, 136, *136*
Fingers, clubbing of. See *Clubbing.*
Fires, smoke inhalation in, bronchoscopy in, 754
lung injury in, 1908–1909
First messengers, definition of, 236
Fistula(s), arteriovenous, 1558, *1559*
bronchopleural, bronchoscopy in, 754–755
empyema with, 2020, *2021*
in ankylosing spondylitis, 2370
hepatobronchial, in amebiasis, 1144–1146
pancreaticopleural, 2029, 2277, *2278*
pleurobiliary, 2030–2031
Fixation, of lung tissue, for quantitative morphology, 23
Flail chest, 2366–2369
diagnosis of, 2366–2367
etiology of, 2366–2367
pathophysiology of, 2367–2369, *2367*, 2367t, *2368*
respiratory acidosis in, 173
treatment of, 2368–2369
Flax dust, byssinosis due to, 1860–1862
Flecainide, pulmonary disease due to, 1984
Fleischner's sign, in pulmonary embolism, 1510
Flexible fiberoptic bronchoscopy. See *Bronchoscopy (flexible fiberoptic or unspecified).*
Flow, air. See *Airflow.*
Flow cytometry, of pleural fluid, 2005, 2074
Fluconazole, in coccidioidomycosis, 1127–1128, 2198t, 2200
in cryptococcosis, 1130–1131, 2197, 2198t
in histoplasmosis, 1117
5-Flucytosine, in cryptococcosis, 1130–1131
Fluid(s), excess of, metabolic alkalosis in, 171t, 172–173
homeostasis of, at high altitude, 1925
loss of, metabolic alkalosis in, 171–173, 171t
Fluid and solute exchange, 132–147. See also *Pulmonary edema.*
at alveolar endothelium, 135–136
at alveolar-capillary septum, 136
at capillary endothelium, 134–135, *134–136*
endothelial permeability in. See *Endothelial permeability.*
factor affecting, 1497, 1498t
for barrier function evaluation, 1597–1598
in lung vascular injury, 146–147
in pulmonary edema, 144–147, 1576–1577
lung vascular injury and, 146–147
mechanisms of, 145–146, *145*, *146*
phases of, 144–145
sites of fluid accumulation in, 145
interstitium in, 136–138, *137*
lymphatic system in, 136, *136*
plasma molecules as, 138, 138t
sites of, 134–136, *134–136*
transcapillary, 132–134, *132*
diffusion in, 133–134
fluid flux equation for, 132–133, *132*
solute flux equation for, 133
Fluid therapy. See also *Life support.*
ethical decisions concerning, 2493, 2500
for decompression sickness, 1962
for metabolic alkalosis, 173
for pneumonia, 997, 999
for pulmonary edema, 1606
for shock, 2401t
cardiogenic, 2400
hypovolemic, 2401
septic, 2399
for sickle cell disease, 2289
Fluke infection. See *Platyhelminth infection(s).*
Flumazenil, in asthma, 290
Flunisolide, chemical structure of, *278*
pharmacokinetics of, 282
Fluorescence bronchoscopy, in lung cancer, 1422–1423
Fluorochrome stain, for mycobacteria, 616
Fluoro-2-deoxyglucose, in positron emission tomography, in lung cancer, 715–716, *715*, 1422, 1422t
Fluoroquinolones, in pneumonia, 995t, 996t, 998t
Enterobacteriaceae, 1011
*Legionella*, 1016
pneumococcal, 1001
in tuberculosis, 1070, 1073t
Fluoroscopy, 654
in bronchoscopy, 734
in diaphragm evaluation, 859
in percutaneous needle biopsy, 761
Fluticasone propionate, chemical structure of, *278*
pharmacokinetics of, 280, 282
Foam cells, in hypersensitivity pneumonitis, 1872
Focal spot, in radiography, 636
Folinic acid, in toxoplasmosis, 1149
Follicular bronchiolitis, in rheumatoid arthritis, 1701
Fontan's procedure, pleural effusion after, 2016
Foramen ovale, patent, decompression sickness in, 1960
in pulmonary hypertension, 1549, *1549*
Forced expiration technique, in chest physical therapy, 369, 370
Forced expiratory flow, average, measurement of, 786, *786*
definition of, 2563
Forced expiratory flow in one second, normal values for, 872t, 873t
Forced expiratory flow per volume segment, measurement of, 785t
Forced expiratory volume, definition of, 2563
theoretical aspects of, 782–783
Forced expiratory volume in one second, after heart transplantation, 2253, 2253t
after lung volume reduction surgery, 1218
impairment rating with, 901t
in asthma, 851, 1265
impairment rating with, 900, 900t
in chronic obstructive pulmonary disease, 1206–1207
in bronchial provocation testing, 852–853
in byssinosis, 1862
in chronic obstructive pulmonary disease, 1191, 1201–1202, *1201*, *1202*
after lung volume reduction surgery, 1218
impairment rating with, 901t
in cystic fibrosis, 1304, 1304t
in impairment and disability evaluation, 850t, 897–898, 899, 899t, 905–906
in interstitial lung disease, 1663
in kyphoscoliosis, 2359t
in lymphangio(leio)myomatosis, 1781
in pulmonary fibrosis, 1675, *1676*
measurement of, 785–786, 785t, *786*
postoperative, prediction of, 714
versus age, 857
versus position, 2252t
Forced expiratory volume in one second/forced vital capacity ratio, in asthma, 1265
in bronchiectasis, 1327
in chronic obstructive pulmonary disease, 1191, 1201–1202, 1206–1207
in cystic fibrosis, 1304, 1304t
in disease states, mechanical aspects of, 112
in flail chest, 2367, 2367t
in impairment and disability evaluation, 850t, 897–899, 899t
in interstitial lung disease, 1662–1663
in kyphoscoliosis, 2359t
in neuromuscular disorders, 2332
measurement of, 785–786, 785t
normal values for, 873t
Forced midexpiratory flow, measurement of, 785t
Forced vital capacity, definition of, 2563
impairment rating with, in restrictive ventilatory disorders, 901t
in airway obstruction, for reversibility evaluation, 851
in asthma, 1265
in bronchiectasis, 1327
in cystic fibrosis, 1304t
in impairment and disability evaluation, 897–899, 899t, 905–906
in restrictive ventilatory disorders, impairment rating with, 901t
measurement of, 785, 785t, *786*
postoperative, prediction of, 714
theoretical aspects of, 782–783
Forceps biopsy, in bronchoscopy, 733–734
Foreign body(ies), bronchoscopy of, 726, 754
embolism of, 465
in bronchus, *649*, 1367
Formaldehyde exposure, in smoke, 1909

Formaldehyde exposure *(Continued)*
lung cancer in, 1403
Formoterol, chemical structure of, 268, *268*
in asthma, 357
in chronic obstructive pulmonary disease, 357
*fos* gene, transcription of, 259–260
Foscarnet, in cytomegalovirus infections, 944, 945, 2202–2203
in herpes simplex virus infections, 949
Fractalkine, 507
Fracture(s), fat embolism in, 1526
rib. See *Rib(s), fractures of.*
*Francisella tularensis* pneumonia, 1028–1029
FRC. See *Functional residual capacity.*
Free radicals, absence of, in chronic granulomatous disease, 2237
as inflammatory mediators, 257–258, 334
injury from, 392, 1987
drug-induced, 1972–1973
pulmonary edema in, 147
macrophage generation of, 390, 392
scavengers for. See *Antioxidants;* specific substances.
Fremitus, 597
Frequency, of lung sounds, 592, *592*
Friction rub, pleural, 598–599, 2000
Friedlander's (*Klebsiella pneumoniae*) pneumonia, 998t, 1008–1009, *1009*
Frontal sinusitis, 916–917
Fulvine, ingestion of, pulmonary hypertension related to, 1546
Fumes. See also *Metal(s);* specific metals.
lung injury from, pathology of, 478t
polymer, 1907
Functional antagonism, of drugs, 244
Functional cloning, in lung disease, 47
Functional residual capacity, after thoracoplasty, 2364
definition of, 57, *57*, *783*, 2563
in ankylosing spondylitis, 2369
in asthma, 1264, 1266
in chronic obstructive pulmonary disease, 104–105, 1191, 1207
in cystic fibrosis, 1304t
in diaphragmatic paralysis, 2335, 2336t
in disease states, mechanical aspects of, 112
in exercise, in obstructive disease, 847–848
respiratory muscle function and, 108–109
in flail chest, 2367, 2367t
in interstitial lung disease, 1662, *1664*
in kyphoscoliosis, 2359, 2359t, *2360*
in neuromuscular disorders, 2333
in obstructive disease, in exercise, 847–848
in pregnancy, 2317–2318
in pulmonary fibrosis, 1675
in spinal cord injury, 2339, 2339t
measurement of, 57–58, *57*
chest radiography in, 793
gas dilution methods in, 791–793, *791*, *792*, 793t, 874
normal, *57*
positive end-expiratory pressure and, 2448, *2448*
versus age, 857
versus position, 2251–2252, 2252t, 2433
Functional vital capacity, normal values for, 872t, 873t
Fungal infection(s), 610t, 1107–1141
aspergillosis as. See *Aspergillosis.*
blastomycosis as. See *Blastomycosis.*
bronchoscopy in, 745–746
candidiasis as. See *Candidiasis.*
classification of, 1108, 1108t
coccidioidomycosis as. See *Coccidioidomycosis.*
Fungal infection(s) *(Continued)*
cryptococcosis as. See *Cryptococcosis.*
cultures in, 618t, 621–624
diagnosis of, bronchoscopy in, 743t
endemic regions for, 1107–1108
genetic tests in, 626
histoplasmosis as. See *Histoplasmosis.*
in bone marrow transplantation, 2303
in granulocytopenia, 924–925
in HIV infection, 2187. See also *Pneumocystis carinii pneumonia;* specific disorders.
treatment of, 2198t
in lung transplantation, 2522–2523
in transplantation, 925, 2229–2230, *2229*
microbiologic diagnosis of, 610t, 616
cultures in, 618t, 621–624
genetic tests in, 626
microorganisms causing, 608t
mucormycosis as, 610t, 1108, 1134–1135, *1135*
paracoccidioidomycosis as, 622–623, 1107, 1128–1129
pneumonia as, in pregnancy, 2321
pathology of, 474–475, *475*, *476*
pseudoallescheriosis as, 1136
sporotrichosis as, 622–623, 1108, 1136
zygomycosis as, 610t, 622, 1108, 1134–1135, *1135*
Fungi, culture of. See also specific diseases and organisms.
sputum specimen for, 609
inhalation of, 1910
hypersensitivity pneumonitis in, 1868–1869
surfactant protein A binding to, 312
surfactant protein D binding to, 315–316
Fungus ball, *Aspergillus*, 1132–1133, *1132*
*Coccidioides immitis*, 1124
*Pseudoallescheria boydii*, 1136
Furosemide, in acute respiratory distress syndrome, 2420
in airway disease, 288
in mountain sickness, 1932
in pulmonary edema, 1602, 2420
high-altitude, 1936–1937
*Fusarium* infections, 1136
Fused plasmalemmal channels, fluid and solute transport in, 138t
*Fusobacterium nucleatum* infection, pneumonia as, 1018–1020, 1019t
Futility, medical, 2498
FVC. See *Forced vital capacity.*


## G


G proteins, in beta-adrenergic agonist action, 268, *269*
receptor interactions with, 233–236, *234*, *235*
Galanin, actions of, 250, *250*, *251*
Gallbladder, cystic fibrosis of, 1295, 1306–1307
Gallium 67 scan, in Kaposi's sarcoma, 2206
in pneumoconiosis, 1815
in pulmonary fibrosis, 1673
of mediastinum, 2086
ventilation-perfusion, 700–701
in interstitial pneumonitis, 713
in lymphoma, 716
in *Pneumocystis carinii* pneumonia, 711–712, *712*, 2189–2190
in sarcoidosis, 713, *714*
in tuberculosis, 712
Galvanic cell method, for oxygen content, 833
Ganciclovir, in cytomegalovirus infections, 944, 945, 2202–2203, 2231
in bone marrow transplantation, 2302
in lung transplantation, 2522
Ganglioglomerular nerve, in carotid body innervation, 189
Ganglioneuroblastoma(s), of mediastinum, 2131
Ganglioneuroma(s), of mediastinum, 2131
Gangrene, lung, in pneumonia, 1009
Gas(es). See also specific gases, e.g., *Air; Blood gas(es); Carbon dioxide; Oxygen.*
blending of, in ventilators, 2472
clearance of, 354–355, *354*
density of, flow-volume curves and, 789–790, *790*
versus maximal flow, 101
diffusion of. See *Diffusion.*
embolism of, in diving, 1954–1956, *1956*, 1962
expired, analysis of, in exercise testing, 841
for mechanical ventilation, delivery of, 2471–2472, *2472*, 2473t
for ventilation-perfusion scanning, 699–700
in mediastinum. See *Pneumomediastinum.*
in pleural space. See *Pneumothorax.*
inert. See also specific gases.
characteristics of, 1958t
kinetics of, 1958, *1959*
narcosis from, 1958t, 1963
tissue supersaturation with, 1958–1959, *1959*
irritant. See *Irritant gases.*
solubility of, 1957–1959, 1958t, *1959*
supersaturation with, 1958–1960, *1959*
volume of, versus depth, in diving, 1954–1955, *1955*
Gas dilution methods, in lung volume measurement, 791–793, *791*, *792*, 793t, 874
Gas exchange, 70–86
after thoracoplasty, 2364
alveolar gas equation in, 71–72, *72*
anatomic aspects of, 15–16, *16*
at high altitude, 1919, *1920*
in exercise, 1926–1927, *1927*
blood flow for. See *Pulmonary circulation.*
blood-gas barrier in. See *Blood-gas barrier.*
blood-gas transport and, 85–86, *86*, *87*
cardiac output effects on, 85
cardiodynamic, 202
chronic impairment of, Social Security Administration criteria for, 901t
diffusing capacity and. See *Diffusing capacity.*
diffusion in. See *Diffusion.*
extracorporeal, in acute respiratory distress syndrome, 2434
impairment of, diffusion limitation in, 72–76, *73*, *74*
hypoventilation in, 71–72, *72*
in hepatopulmonary syndrome, 2274
shunts in, 76
ventilation-perfusion and. See *Ventilation-perfusion ratio.*
in ankylosing spondylitis, 2370
in arteriovenous malformations, 1495, 1496, 1563
in asthma, 1265
in bone marrow transplantation, 2298
in exercise, 201–206
at high altitude, 1926–1927, *1927*
heavy, 204–206, *206*
in chronic obstructive pulmonary disease, 216
in heart disease, 2259

Gas exchange *(Continued)*
in interstitial pulmonary fibrosis, 217
moderate, 201–204, *203*
severe, 204–206, *206*
in exercise testing, 205–206, *206*
in flail chest, 2368
in heart disease, 2258, *2258*, 2259
in hepatopulmonary syndrome, 2271
in hypoventilation, 71–72, *72*
in interstitial lung disease, 1663–1664
in kyphoscoliosis, 2360
in lung disease, 82–83, *84*
in mechanical ventilation, 2476–2477, *2477*
in obesity, 2372
in pulmonary edema, 1579, 1585–1586
in pulmonary venous hypertension, 2258, *2258*
in respiratory failure, 2379–2380
in single lung unit, 77–78, *77*, *78*
oxygen uptake in, 72–73, *73*, *74*
oxygen-hemoglobin reaction rates in, 73–74, *74*
partial pressures and, 70–71, *70*
pattern of, in normal lung, 78, *78*
perfusion-limited, 73
pulmonary vessels for, 13
shunt effects on, 76
terminology of, 2563–2565
transit time for, 13
ventilation for. See *Ventilation*.
ventilation-perfusion relationships in. See *Ventilation-perfusion ratio*.
Gas flow. See *Airflow*.
Gas transfer index, in dermatomyositis, 1708
Gastric acid, reflux of. See *Gastroesophageal reflux disease*.
Gastric lavage, in tuberculosis specimen collection, 1065
Gastrin-releasing peptide, in lung cancer growth, 1380
in mucus secretion, 333
Gastroesophageal reflux disease, 2267–2270
bronchoconstriction in, 254
chest pain in, 579–580
cough in, 559, *559*, 561–563, 588
definition of, 2267
diagnosis of, 2269
epidemiology of, 2267
pathogenesis of, 2268–2269, *2268*
treatment of, 2269–2270
Gastrointestinal system. See also specific organs.
barotrauma of, 1957
disorders of, chest pain in, 579–580
hyperchloremic acidosis in, 169–170
in cystic fibrosis, clinical features of, 1302t, 1306
pathology of, 1294–1295
pathophysiology of, 1302t, 1306
treatment of, 1312–1313
in sarcoidosis, 1719
metabolic alkalosis in, 171–173, 171t
parasitic infections of, amebiasis as, 1144–1146
ascariasis as, 1149–1150
hookworm disease as, 1150–1151
strongyloidiasis as, 1151–1153
pneumomediastinum originating in, 2096t, 2099
telangiectasia of, 1560
tuberculosis of, 1084–1085
Gastroplasty, in obesity, 2373
GATA-6 transcription factor, in lung development, 37–38
Gaucher's disease, 1748
secondary lung injury in, 480t
GAW. See *Conductance*.
Gelatinases, in metastasis, 1388
of monocytes, 393
Gemcitabine, in lung cancer, 1437–1438, 1437t
GEMM colony-forming unit, 400
GenBank, for genetic disease information, 51, 52t
Gender differences, in chronic obstructive pulmonary disease, 1199
in dyspnea, 220
in lung cancer, 1395–1396, *1395*, 1396t
in lymphangio(leio)myomatosis, 1780
in pulmonary function tests, 803
in smoking, lung cancer rates and, 1398
Gene(s), human leukocyte antigen, 425–426, *427*
immunoglobulin, 416, 418, *418–420*
in lung development. See *Lung, development of*.
mucin, 328–329, 330t
mutations of. See *Mutations*.
transcription of. See also *Transcription factor(s)*.
corticosteroids and, 278–279, *279*, 279t, *280*
tumor suppressor, mutations of, in lung cancer, 1382–1386, 1416, 1426t
Gene association studies, of asthma, 1252–1253, 1254t
Gene therapy, aerosol delivery of, 360
Gene transfer, in cystic fibrosis, 1311
Genetic disease(s). See also specific diseases, e.g., *Cystic fibrosis*.
alveolar proteinosis as, 1793
asthma as, 288, 480t, 1248, 1252–1253, 1254t, 2545
cancer as. See *Lung cancer, genetics of*.
candidate gene assessment in, 49, 1253, 1254t
comparative genomics in, 50–51
complex (multifactorial), approach to, 48–50, 48t, 51t
emphysema as, in alpha$_1$-antitrypsin deficiency, 1207–1210, *1209*
familial aggregation in, 48
familial risk of, 48
Human Genome Project and, 45, 47
interstitial pulmonary fibrosis as, 1692
linkage analysis in, 49–50
lung disease as, 45–53
interstitial, 1656
pathology of, 477, 480t, 481t, 482, *482*, 483t–484t, *485*, 486, *487–489*
lymphangio(leio)myomatosis as, 1778
mapping of, 45–47, *46*
Mendelian inheritance and, 45, 48–49
on-line information on, 51–52, 52t
pathology of, 477, 480t, 481t, 482, *482*, 483t–484t, *485*, 486, *487–489*
pectus excavatum as, 2365
pneumothorax as, 2045
positional cloning in, 47
primary, 477, 480t
pulmonary fibrosis as, 1684
sarcoidosis as, 1717–1718
secondary injury in, 477, 480–481t
sickle cell disease and trait as, 85, 2286–2290
systemic sclerosis as, 1692
Genetic testing, 625–627. See also specific tests, e.g., *Polymerase chain reaction*.
Genetics, of antigenic drift and antigenic shift, in influenza virus, 950
of high altitude response, 1634, 1918, 1921
Genitourinary tract, coccidioidomycosis of, 1125
Genitourinary tract *(Continued)*
cystic fibrosis of, 1295, 1307
sarcoidosis of, 1719
tuberculosis of, 1080–1081
Genome Data Base, 51–52, 52t
Genomic mismatch scanning, in genetic disease, 51
Gentamicin, in cystic fibrosis, 1309t, 1312
in pneumonia, 998t
*Geotrichum* infections, 1136
GERD. See *Gastroesophageal reflux disease*.
Germ cell tumors, metastasis from, 1473
of mediastinum, 2127–2128, *2127*
Ghon lesion, in tuberculosis, 1056
Giant cell(s), in sarcoidosis, 1725
Giant cell (temporal) arteritis, 1541
Giant cell interstitial pneumonitis, 1652
Gingivostomatitis, herpes simplex virus, 933, 947–948
Gitelman's syndrome, metabolic alkalosis in, 172
Glands, of bronchial submucosa. See *Bronchus(i), glands of*.
tracheal, innervation of, 22
Glasgow Coma Scale, in lung injury, 1593
in pulmonary edema, 1593
Glass wool, in lung cancer, 1403
in pneumoconiosis, 1831t, 1842
Glaucoma, ipratropium bromide-induced, 277
Gli transcription factors, in lung development, 39
Glomerulonephritis, diffuse alveolar hemorrhage with, *1736*, 1737t, 1740–1741
in Goodpasture's syndrome, 1742–1743
in microscopic polyangiitis, 1739
penicillamine-induced, 1744
Glomus cells, in carotid body, 189
Glomus tumors, of lung, 1478
Glossary, of terms and symbols, 2563–2565
Glossopharyngeal breathing, in neuromuscular disorders, 2346
in spinal cord injury, 2338
Glottis, edema of, in croup, 935, *936*
function of, 1351, *1352*, *1353*
in cough, 555–556, *555*
Glucocerebrosidase deficiency, in Gaucher's disease, 1748
Glucocorticoid(s). See also *Corticosteroid(s)*.
receptors for, 241
as transcription factors, 261
corticosteroid binding to, 278–279
Glucocorticoid receptor kinase (beta-adrenergic receptor-specific kinase), action of, 244–245, *245*
Glucocorticoid response elements, 241
in beta-receptors, 245
Glucose, in pleural fluid, 2003
Glutamate, actions of, *251*
in pain transmission, 574
Glutaraldehyde, for bronchoscope disinfection, 758
Glutathione-S-transferase, as biomarker, for lung cancer, 1406
Glycerol, iodinated, in chronic obstructive pulmonary disease, 1224
Glycogen, lactic acid synthesis from, 204
metabolism of, at high altitude, 1923
in exercise, 200–201
Glycoproteins, of mucus. See *Mucins*.
Glycopyrrolate, in chronic obstructive pulmonary disease, 1221
Glycosaminoglycans, in lung, 137
Glycosylation, of G protein–coupled receptors, 234
Goblet cells, function of, 360
hyperplasia of, *451*

Goblet cells *(Continued)*
in asthma, 1253, *1255*, 1263, *1263*, 1264t
hypersecretion of, in asthma, 1262
in mucus secretion, 332
metaplasia of, in asthma, 1263, *1263*, 1264t
of bronchial epithelium, 9, *9*
of nose, 1346
overactivity of, in cystic fibrosis, 1294, *1294*
physiology of, 1175, *1177*, 1361
Goiter, 2128, 2311, *2311*
Gold preparations, in asthma, 286
pulmonary disease due to, 1984–1985
in connective tissue disease therapy, 1692t
in rheumatoid arthritis therapy, 1702
Golgi tendon organs, as chest wall receptors, 184
Goodpasture's syndrome, diffuse alveolar hemorrhage in, 1737t, 1742–1743, *1742*
pathogenesis of, 437
pathology of, 466, *467*
penicillamine-induced, 1985
Gottron's tubercles, in dermatomyositis, 1706
Government role, 2543–2562
in air quality protection, 2556–2558
in asthma secondary prevention, 2544–2556
assessment of problem in, 2544–2546
policy development for, 2546–2548, 2546t, 2548t
policy implementation in, 2548–2550, 2550t
program evaluation in, 2550–2556, *2551*, 2554t, 2555t
in smoking prevention, 2558–2560, 2559t
overview of, 2543–2544
*Gp-100* gene and product, mutations of, in lymphangio(leio)myomatosis, 1778
Graft-versus-host disease, bronchiolitis obliterans in, 1364, 1366
in bone marrow transplantation, 2297–2298, 2300–2301
in severe combined immunodeficiency, 2233t, 2239
pathology of, 468, *470*
Graham Steell murmur, in cor pulmonale, 1638
in pulmonary hypertension, 1547
Graham three-gas iteration method, for diffusing capacity measurement, 812
Gram stain, of actinomycotic sulfur granule, 1021, *1021*
of anaerobic bacteria, 1019, *1019*
of beta-hemolytic streptococci, 1005
of empyema, 1032
of *Haemophilus influenzae*, 1007, *1007*
of *Klebsiella pneumoniae*, 1009, *1009*
of *Legionella*, 1015
of *Neisseria meningitidis*, 1005
of *Pseudomonas aeruginosa*, 1012
of sputum, in pneumonia, 614–617, *614*, *615*, 989–990, *990*
of *Staphylococcus aureus*, 1003, *1003*
of *Streptococcus pneumoniae*, 1000, *1000*
Gram-negative bacillary pneumonia, 1008–1014
*Acinetobacter*, 1013–1014, *1003*
*Citrobacter*, 1010–1011
*Enterobacter*, 998t, 1010–1011
Enterobacteriaceae, 998t, 1010–1011
*Erwinia*, 1010–1011
*Escherichia coli*, 1010–1011
*Hafnia*, 1010–1011
*Klebsiella pneumoniae*, 998t, 1008–1009, *1009*
*Morganella*, 1010–1011
*Proteus*, 1010–1011
*Pseudomonas aeruginosa*. See under *Pseudomonas aeruginosa infections.*
Gram-negative bacillary pneumonia *(Continued)*
*Salmonella*, 1010–1011
*Serratia*, 1010–1011
Granular cell myoblastoma, tracheobronchial, 1478
Granulation tissue, formation of, 496
Granule(s), of eosinophils, 527, 1758–1759, 1758t
of neutrophils, 521, 523, 523t
Granulocyte(s), 520–530. See also *Eosinophil(s); Neutrophil(s).*
accumulation of, contrast agent-induced, 1988
apoptosis of, 528–529, *529*, *530*
clearance of, in repair, 528–529, *529*, *530*
counting of, in inflammation assessment, 529–530
tissue injury mechanisms of, 527–528
types of, 520–521
Granulocyte chemotactic protein-2, 508, 508t
Granulocyte colony-stimulating factor, in pneumonia, in immunodeficiency, 997
Granulocyte-macrophage colony-stimulating factor, action of, in macrophage development, 398–400, *400*, 403–404
on alveolar macrophages, 394, *395*
as inflammatory mediator, 258, *258*
deficiency of, alveolar proteinosis in, 1793
animal studies of, 404
macrophage status in, 403–404
excess of, animal studies of, 404
in eosinophil development, 1757–1758
in pneumonia, in immunodeficiency, 997
receptor for, 238, *402*, 403–404
structure of, 403
Granulocytopenia. See also *Neutropenia.*
infections in, 2237
pneumonia in, 924–925, 925t, 997
Granuloma(s), eosinophilic, computed tomography of, *1662*
versus sarcoidosis, 1725
hyalinizing, 1480
immune response to, 437–438
in beryllium lung disease, 1843–1844
in chronic granulomatous disease, 2233t, 2237
in coccidioidomycosis, 1122–1123
in common variable immunodeficiency, 2235
in cryptococcosis, 1129
in filariasis, 1153
in histoplasmosis, 1111, *1115*
in hypersensitivity pneumonitis, 1872, *1872*, 1876
in pneumonitis, 1653t, 1655, *1655*
in sarcoidosis, 752, 1723–1724, *1724*
in schistosomiasis, 1163–1164
in tuberculosis, 1057
infectious, 1481
plasma cell, 1480
rheumatoid, 1481
Granulomatosis, allergic, and angiitis (Churg-Strauss syndrome), 1538, 1769–1771, *1770*, 1770t
pleural effusion in, 2033
bronchial, in tuberculosis, 1367–1368
bronchocentric, 1334, 1368, 1481, 1538–1539
in allergic bronchopulmonary aspergillosis, 1765
drug-induced, 479t
in talc pneumoconiosis, 1841
inflammation in, pathology of, 455, *457*
lymphomatoid, 1458–1459, *1459*, 1537–1538
mediastinal. See *Mediastinitis, granulomatous (chronic).*
Granulomatosis *(Continued)*
necrotizing sarcoid, 1538
pathology of, 466, *469*
talc, 1980–1981
Wegener's. See *Wegener's granulomatosis.*
Gravity, lung volume effects of, 109–111, *110*
pleural pressure effects of, 109–111, *110*
pulmonary circulation effects of, 64–66, *65*, 129
transpulmonary pressure effects of, 109–111, *110*
ventilation distribution effects of, 59, *59*, 109–111, *110*
Great vessels. See also *Aorta*; specific vessels.
congenital anomalies of, imaging of, 683, 686, *687*
Grepafloxacin, in pneumonia, 995t
Grid ratio, in radiography, *635*, 636
Ground itch, in hookworm disease, 1151
Ground-glass opacity, computed tomography of, 675–676, *676*
Growth, corticosteroid effects on, 282
retardation of, in cystic fibrosis, 1306
Growth factor(s). See also specific growth factors.
in clubbing, 601
in lung cancer, 1379–1382, *1380*
in monocyte-macrophage development, 401–404, 401t, *402*
in silicosis, 1819
receptors for, 238–239, *239*, 524
secretion of, in alveoli, 19, 20t
Growth hormone, excess of, respiratory manifestations of, 2313
Growth-related oncogenes, 508, 508t, 510
Guaifenesin, in allergic rhinitis, 1349
Guanine-nucleotide shift, 236
Guanosine triphosphatase, in G protein action, 235, *235*
Guanosine triphosphate, in signal transduction, 235, *235*
Guanylyl cyclase, in signal transduction, 238
Guillain-Barré syndrome, after influenza vaccination, 955
respiratory function in, 2341–2342
Gynecologic disorder(s), 2324–2325
catamenial hemoptysis as, 1480
catamenial pneumothorax as, 2053–2054, *2054*
endometriosis as. See *Endometriosis.*
lymphangio(leio)myomatosis as. See *Lymphangio(leio)myomatosis.*
trophoblastic embolization as, 2325

## H

HA-1A monoclonal antibody, in pulmonary edema, 1610
Habit cough, 561
HACE (high-altitude cerebral edema), 1930t, 1932–1933
*Haemophilus influenzae* infection(s), bacteremia as, 2179
bronchitis as, 934
diagnosis of, laboratory methods for, 990
epiglottitis as, 934
immunization for, in HIV infection, 2180
in cystic fibrosis, 1303, 1309, 1309t
otitis media as, 918–919
pneumonia as, 1006–1008, *1007*, 1007t
clinical features of, 2179
diagnosis of, 2179
in HIV infection, 2178–2180

*Haemophilus influenzae* infection(s) *(Continued)*
in influenza, 954
in lymphoproliferative disorders, 925
microbiologic diagnosis of, 615
risk factors for, 920
treatment of, 998t, 2179–2180
sinusitis as, 916
surfactant protein A binding in, 312
*Hafnia* pneumonia, 1010–1011
Haldane effect, 86
Half-life, of drugs, 248
Haloperidol, in hiccups, 2350
Halothane, in multiple inert gas elimination technique, 80–81, *81*, *82*
pulmonary function effects of, 884–885
Hamartoma(s), of lung, 1478–1479, *1479*
computed tomography of, 667, *669*
endobronchial, 1478
Hamman's crunch, in pneumomediastinum, 2102
Hamman's sign, in mediastinal emphysema, 1956
in mediastinitis, 2106
in pneumomediastinum, 2102
Hamman's syndrome, 2100
Hampton's hump, in pulmonary embolism, 1510
Hand, edema of, in mixed connective tissue disease, 1708
Handicap. See also *Impairment and disability.*
definition of, 896
*Hansenula* infections, 1136
Hantavirus infections, 945–947
in pregnancy, 2321
pathology of, 471
pleural effusion in, 2025
HAPE. See *Pulmonary edema, high-altitude.*
Haploinsufficiency, in hereditary hemorrhagic telangiectasia, 1559–1560
Hard metal disease, 1403, 1844–1845
Harrington rod placement, in kyphoscoliosis, 2363
Hay exposure, hypersensitivity pneumonitis in. See *Hypersensitivity pneumonitis.*
Hay fever. See *Allergic rhinitis.*
Headache, in coccidioidomycosis, 1123
in high-altitude disorders, 1932–1933
in mountain sickness, 1929–1932
in pneumonia, *Chlamydia psittaci*, 1026
*Legionella*, 1014
*Mycoplasma pneumoniae*, 1024
Healthy People national initiative, asthma objectives of, 2547, 2548t, 2552
smoking objectives of, 2559, 2559t
Hearing loss, in decompression sickness, 1961
in otitis media, 919
Heart. See also *Cardiac; Heart disease; Heart failure; Pericarditis.*
amyloidosis of, 2296
anatomy of, 1634–1635, *1635*
arrhythmias of. See *Cardiac arrhythmias.*
catheterization of, in pulmonary hypertension, 1549
changes of, in pregnancy, 2318, *2318*
congenital defects of, imaging of, 683, 686, *687*
function of, in respiratory failure. See *Respiratory failure, circulation in.*
in sleep, 2154
mechanical ventilation effects on, 2482
mechanosensitive fibers in, 570
pain originating in, 577–579
palpitations of, $beta_2$-adrenergic agonist-induced, 271
pectus excavatum effects on, 2366
Heart *(Continued)*
pericardium of. See *Pericarditis; Pericardium.*
sarcoidosis of, 1719, 1723, *1723*
size of, versus exercise tolerance, 840
sleep apnea effects on, 2155, 2158–2159, *2158*
surgery on, diaphragmatic paralysis in, 2334
mediastinitis after, 2109–2110
pleural effusion in, 2032
preoperative evaluation for, 886
transplantation of. See also *Heart-lung transplantation.*
pneumonia in, 2229
pulmonary function after, 2253, 2253t
tumors of, magnetic resonance imaging of, 673, *674*
Heart disease, 2247–2265. See also *Heart failure;* specific disease.
acute respiratory distress syndrome in, 2417
airway resistance in, 2254–2255
assessment for, preoperative, 883–884, 884t, 885t
diffusing capacity in, 2252, 2253t
dyspnea in, 220, 543–544, 2261–2262
exercise response in, 2258–2260, 2259t, 2260t
exercise testing in, 846–847
fatigue in, 221
gas exchange in, 2258, *2258*
hemodynamics in, 2249–2251, 2249t
in diving candidates, 1963–1964
in pulmonary dysfunction. See *Cor pulmonale.*
in pulmonary fibrosis, 1684t
lung compliance in, 2253–2254, 2254t, *2255*
lung volumes in, 2251–2252, *2251*, 2252t
orthopnea in, 2261–2262
pulmonary. See *Cor pulmonale.*
pulmonary circulation in, 67
pulmonary edema in, 1580, 1591, 2247–2248, 2248t
acute, 2261
in pregnancy, 2321
pulmonary venous hypertension in, 2247–2261
airway resistance in, 2254–2255
diffusing capacity in, 2252, 2253t
exercise response in, 2258–2260, 2259t, 2260t
gas exchange in, 2258, *2258*
hemodynamics of, 2249–2251, 2249t
histopathology of, 2248–2249, 2249t
lowering of, 2253, 2253t
lung compliance in, 2253–2254, 2254t, *2255*
lung volumes in, 2251–2252, *2251*, 2252t
pulmonary edema in, 2247–2248, 2248t
regional lung function in, 2256–2257, *2257*, *2258*
respiratory muscle function in, 2255–2256, 2256t
sleep disorders in, 2261
regional lung function in, 2256–2257, *2257*, *2258*
respiratory failure in, 2392–2393, 2393t
respiratory muscle function in, 2255–2256, 2256t
shock in, 2400
shunts in, gas exchange in, 76
sleep disorders in, 2261
Heart failure, acute, airway resistance in, 2254
congestive, airway resistance in, 2254–2255
diffusing capacity in, 2252, 2253t
exercise in, hyperventilation in, 2260
methoxamine in, 2260
Heart failure *(Continued)*
oxygen therapy for, 2259–2260, 2260t
pulmonary hemodynamics in, 2249–2251, 2249t
high altitude effects on, 1941
hyperventilation in, 2146, 2260
in hypoventilation, 2143
in pregnancy, 2321
in pulmonary hypertension, 1637–1638
lung volumes in, 2251, 2252t
orthopnea in, 2261–2262
oxygen therapy for, in exercise, 2259–2260, 2260t
pleural effusion in, 2013–2014, *2014*
position changes in, versus lung volume, 2251–2252, 2252t
preoperative risk assessment in, 883–884, 884t, 885t
pulmonary edema in, 1580, 1591, 2249t, 2250
treatment of, 1604, 1605
pulmonary hemodynamics in, 2249–2251, 2249t
respiratory muscle function in, 2255–2256, 2256t
sleep apnea in, 2162–2163, *2163*
treatment of, 1604, 1605, 2250–2251
ventilation distribution in, 2257, *2258*
in cor pulmonale, 1193
in diabetes mellitus, 2310
in kidney failure, pulmonary edema in, 2278–2279
in sleep apnea, 2159
oxygen partial pressure in, 2258, *2258*
pulmonary edema in, 2247–2248, 2248t
right-sided, in mountain sickness, 1938
in respiratory failure, 2395, 2395t
Heart rate, at high altitude, 1920
in acute mountain sickness, 1930
in exercise, 1927, *1927*
in exercise, at high altitude, 1927, *1927*
in emphysema, *222*, 224
in interstitial pulmonary disease, 226
in exercise testing, 842
in interstitial pulmonary disease, *223*
in pregnancy, 2318, *2318*
Heart rate reserve, in exercise, in chronic obstructive pulmonary disease, 215
Heart sounds, in cor pulmonale, 1638
in lymphangio(leio)myomatosis, 1781
in pulmonary embolism, 1507
in pulmonary hypertension, 1494, 1547, 1520
Heart-lung transplantation, 2518–2519
bronchiectasis after, 1336
bronchiolitis obliterans after, 1364–1365, *1365*, 1366
in bronchiectasis, 1333
in pulmonary hypertension, 1551
Heartworm infections, 1155–1156
Heat, as tracer, in lung water measurement, 1597
Heat stress, in diving, 1952–1953
Heath and Edwards classification, of pulmonary hypertension, 1543
Heerfordt's syndrome, 1718–1719
Height, pulmonary function test effects of, 803
Heimlich valves, for pneumothorax aspiration, 2047, 2050
Heitzman classification, of mediastinum anatomy, 2080–2081
Helical computed tomography, 661–663
Helium, in lung volume measurement, 791–793, *792*, 793t
solubility of, in diving, 1958, 1958t
Helium dilution method, for functional residual capacity, 57–58

Helium-oxygen mixtures, in asthma, 2459
Helminth infection(s). See *Nematode infection(s); Platyhelminth infection(s).*
Helodermin, actions of, *251*
Hemagglutinin, of influenza virus, 949–950
Hemangioma, sclerosing, of lung, 1479
Hemangiomatosis, pulmonary capillary, 1746, *1746*
Hematemesis, in esophageal rupture, 2028
versus hemoptysis, 590
Hematocrit, at high altitude, 1921–1922
high, in erythrocytosis, 2286
in mountain sickness, 1938–1939
versus pulmonary vascular resistance, 126–127, *128*
Hematogenous dissemination, of cancer, 1469, 1471, *1471*, *1472*
Hematologic disease(s), amyloidosis as. See *Amyloidosis.*
bone marrow transplantation in. See *Blood and bone marrow transplantation.*
coagulation disorders as. See *Coagulation disorder(s).*
erythrocytosis as. See *Erythrocytosis.*
hemoglobinopathies as, 2290
leukemia as. See *Leukemia(s).*
lung injury in, 1588t
lymphomas as. See *Lymphoma(s).*
multiple myeloma as, 1464, 2292–2294, 2293t
sickle cell disease and trait as, 85, 2286–2290
stem cell transplantation in. See *Blood and bone marrow transplantation.*
Waldenström's macroglobulinemia as, 1464, 2294
Hematologic disorder(s), pulmonary edema in, 1588t
Hematoma(s), of lung, 1481
Hematopoiesis, extramedullary, in mediastinum, 2132
pleural effusion in, 2035
overview of, 399, *400*
Hemiplegia, respiratory function in, 2340
Hemithorax, volume of, in pneumothorax, 2046
Hemodialysis, respiratory function in, 2279–2280
Hemodynamics, disorders of, lung injury in, 1588t
of mechanical ventilation, 2482–2483
of pulmonary circulation. See under *Pulmonary circulation.*
of pulmonary edema, 1595–1596
terminology of, 2565
Hemofiltration, in pulmonary edema, 1603
Hemoglobin, abnormal, 85
pulse oximetry errors in, 835
buffer action of, 157, 163
carbon dioxide binding to, 86
carbon monoxide binding to, 887, 2290
in diffusing capacity measurement, 810, *810*
in smoking, 814
chemical structure of, 85
disorder(s) of, 2290
sickle cell disease and trait as, 85, 2286–2290
fetal, 85
gas interactions with, in diffusing capacity, 810, *810*
in oxygen transport, 85–86, *86*
increase of, at high altitude, 1921–1922
measurement of, in arteriovenous malformations, 1562
oxidized (ferric) iron in (methemoglobin), 85
Hemoglobin *(Continued)*
oxygen content of, measurement of, 833–834
oxygen reactions with, 830
at high altitude, 1922, *1922*
hyperventilation effects on, 2147–2148
rates of, 73–74, *74*
Hemolytic anemia, microangiopathic, mitomycin-induced, 1976–1977
Hemophilia, 2294–2295
Hemopneumothorax, radiography of, *652*, *2061*
Hemopoietic stem cell transplantation. See *Blood and bone marrow transplantation.*
Hemoptysis, bronchial arteriography in, 658, *659*
bronchoscopy in, 750–751, 750t
catamenial, 1480
causes of, 589, 589t, 750t
chest radiography of, 666
clinical features of, 589–590
diagnosis of, 589–590, 750–751, 750t, 1566
differential diagnosis of, 1733, 1734t
in amebiasis, 1145
in amyloidosis, 2296
in ankylosing spondylitis, 1710
in aspergilloma, 1132–1133
in Behçet's syndrome, 1710, 1740
in bronchial disorders, 1368
in bronchiectasis, 1328, 1333
in bronchiolitis, 1362
in bronchitis, 1189
in cancer, treatment of, 1431–1432
in carcinoid tumor, 1461
in chronic obstructive pulmonary disease, 1189
in clotting factor deficiencies, 2294
in cystic fibrosis, 1305, 1312, 1313
in diffuse alveolar hemorrhage, 1733, 1734, 1740, 1743–1744
in emphysema, 1189
in endometriosis, 2325
in Goodpasture's syndrome, 1743
in hydatid disease, 1158
in Kaposi's sarcoma, 2205
in lung cancer, 1420, 1431–1432, 1471
in lymphangio(leio)myomatosis, 1780, 1780t
in mediastinal mass, 2081
in mediastinitis, 2112
in medical history, 589–590, 589t
in mitral stenosis, 1744
in paragonimiasis, 1161
in pleural effusion, 2026
in pneumonia, *Coxiella burnetii*, 1025
*Legionella*, 1014
in pneumothorax, 2052
in pulmonary capillary hemangiomatosis, 1746
in pulmonary circulation–systemic circulation communications, 1566
in pulmonary embolism, 1507, 2026
in pulmonary hypertension, 1547
in sarcoidosis, 1718
in systemic sclerosis, 1694
in tuberculosis, 1063, 1075
intolerance of, in arteriovenous malformations, 1495–1496
massive, 726–727, 751
treatment of, 1566
bronchoscopy in, 751
in bronchiectasis, 1333
Hemorrhage. See also *Hemoptysis.*
alveolar. See *Alveolar hemorrhage.*
hypovolemic shock in, 2400–2402
in bronchoscopy, 734, 756–757
in clotting factor deficiencies, 2294–2295
in coagulation disorders, 2294–2295
Hemorrhage *(Continued)*
in disseminated intravascular coagulation, 2295
pulmonary, drug-induced, 479t
in bone marrow transplantation, 2300
in galloping racehorses, 69
in influenza, 951, *952*
retinal, at high altitude, 1937, *1937*
Hemorrhagic fever, dengue, 2025
Korean, 945–947
Hemorrhagic shock, pulmonary edema in, 147
Hemorrhagic telangiectasia, hereditary. See *Hereditary hemorrhagic telangiectasia.*
Hemosiderosis, 1741–1742, *1741*
cell injury in, 450, *452*
diffuse alveolar hemorrhage in, 1734
Hemostasis, evaluation of, in pulmonary embolism, 1511
pulmonary circulation role in, 69–70
Hemothorax, 2060–2062
causes of, 2062
complications of, 2061
computed tomography of, 688
definition of, 2060
diagnosis of, 2060, *2061*
fibrothorax in, 2062–2063
iatrogenic, 2062
in anticoagulant therapy, 2062
in coronary artery bypass surgery, 2032
in endometriosis, 2325
in pleural biopsy, 2009
in pulmonary embolism, 2027
nontraumatic, 2062
pleural fluid examination in, 2002, 2004
traumatic, 2060–2062, *2061*
treatment of, 2060–2061
Hemp dust, byssinosis due to, 1860–1862
Henderson-Hasselbalch equation, 155–156, 831, 2565
Henoch-Schönlein purpura, 1539, 1737t, 1740
Henry's law, diving and, 1957–1959, *1959*
Heparin, complications of, 1517
hemothorax due to, 2062
in disseminated intravascular coagulation, 2295
in myocardial ischemia, *2401*
in pulmonary embolism, 1516–1517
in pregnancy, 2323
in thromboembolic disease, prophylactic, 1514–1515
low-dose, in thromboembolic disease prevention, 1514–1515
low-molecular weight, in thromboembolic disease, prophylactic, 1515
therapeutic, 1516–1517
Hepatic disease(s). See *Liver disease(s).*
Hepatic hydrothorax, 2015–2016, 2271
Hepatitis, chronic active, 2276
in Q fever, 1026
pleural effusion in, 2025
Hepatitis B, transmission of, in bronchoscopy, 758–759
Hepatocyte growth factor/scatter factor, in lung cancer growth, 1381
Hepatopulmonary syndrome, 2271–2274
arteriovenous malformations in, 1558
blood gases in, 2271
clinical features of, 2271–2272, *2272*
definition of, 2271
diagnosis of, 2273–2274, *2273*
gas exchange abnormalities in, 2274
pathogenesis of, 2272
treatment of, 2274
Hereditary hemorrhagic telangiectasia, 1558–1561
clinical features of, 1560–1561, 1560t

Hereditary hemorrhagic telangiectasia *(Continued)*
diagnosis of, 1561
epidemiology of, 1558
hemodynamics in, 1563
inheritance of, 1558–1559
lung injury in, 481t
pathogenesis of, 1559–1560
screening for, 1562–1563
Heredity. See *Genetic disease(s); Genetics.*
Hering-Breuer reflex. See *Breuer-Hering inflation reflex.*
Hermansky-Pudlak syndrome, 481t, 1749
*HER2/neu* gene and product, in lung cancer growth, 1380–1381
Hernia, diaphragmatic, mediastinal protrusion of, 2130–2131
pleural effusion in, 2030
Heroin, pulmonary disease due to, 1979–1980
Herpangina, 933
Herpes simplex virus infection(s), 931t, 947–949
clinical manifestations of, 947–948
diagnosis of, 948–949
disseminated, 947
epidemiology of, 947
genetic tests for, 626
gingivostomatitis as, 947–948
in HIV infection, 2203
in immunodeficiency, 947–949
in lung transplantation, 2522
latent, 947
pathogenesis of, 947
pharyngitis as, 933–934, *934*, 947–948
pneumonia as, bronchoscopy in, 749–750
in bone marrow transplantation, 2302–2303
in HIV infection, 2203
in transplantation, 2229
pathology of, 468, 470, *471*
prevention of, 949
surfactant protein A binding in, 312
transmission of, 947
treatment of, 949
type 1 versus type 2, 947
virus characteristics in, 947
Herpes zoster, 967–968, *968*
in lung transplantation, 2522
pain in, 577, 581t
Herpesvirus infections, 931t. See also specific infections.
Heterolysis, in necrosis, 444
Hiccups, 2349–2350, 2349t
High altitude. See *Altitude, high.*
High endothelial venules, 416
High-frequency mechanical ventilation, 2478
Hippocratic oath, on nonmaleficence, 2491
Histaminase, of eosinophils, 1758t, 1759
Histamine, as inflammatory mediator, 257
in allergic rhinitis, 1347
in endothelial permeability mediation, 141, 142
in provocation testing, 852, 1266
in pulmonary vascular resistance control, 131
inhibitors of. See *Antihistamines.*
rapidly adapting receptors response to, 251
receptors for, 257
release of, 232, *233*
Histiocytoma(s), of lung, 1480
Histiocytosis X, cell morphology in, 389, *390*
lung cysts in, 676, *677*
Histoplasma polysaccharide antigen test, 2199
Histoplasmosis, 1108–1117
antigen testing in, 1116
calcification in, 1109, 1110, *1110*
Histoplasmosis *(Continued)*
chest radiography of, 1110, *1110*, *1112–1114*, 1114, 2199, *2199*
chronic pulmonary, 1111, *1112*, *1113*
clinical manifestations of, 1109–1115, *1110*, *1112–1115*, 2197–2198
complications of, 1111
culture in, 621–623, 1115, 2199
diagnosis of, 1115–1116, 2199
enzyme immunoassay in, 616
genetic tests in, 626
dimorphism in, 1107
epidemiology of, 1109
geographic distribution of, 1107, 2197
healing of, 1109, 1110, *1110*
historical review of, 1108–1109
immune response to, 1108, 1109, 1111
in HIV infection, 1114, 1115, 2197–2199, 2198t
treatment of, 1116–1117, 2199
incubation time of, 1110
mediastinal fibrosis in, 1367
mediastinitis in, 2110–2111, *2112*
microbiologic diagnosis of, 610t
miliary pattern of, *1114*
mycologic studies in, 1115
pathogenesis of, 1109, 2197
physical examination in, 1109–1110
pleural effusion in, 2024
progressive disseminated, 1111, 1114–1115, *1114*, *1115*
serologic studies in, 1115–1116, 2199
skin tests for, 1109, 1115
spontaneous resolution of, 1111, *1112*
treatment of, 1116–1117, 2199
History, medical. See *Medical history;* specific diseases.
HIV infection. See *Human immunodeficiency virus infection.*
HNF-3β protein, in lung development, 38
Hoarseness, in *Chlamydia pneumoniae* infections, 1027
in laryngitis, 934
in laryngotracheitis, 918
in lung cancer, 1420, 1421
in sarcoidosis, 1718
Hodgkin's disease, cryptococcosis in, 1129, 1130
of bronchi, 1367
of lung, 1453–1455
differential diagnosis of, 1454
from mediastinal lymph nodes, 1454, *1454*
nodular sclerosing, 1454, *1454*
pneumonia in, 925
primary, 1453–1454
recurrent, 1455, *1455*
ventilation-perfusion scanning in, 716
of mediastinum, 2128
of pleura, metastatic, 2073
Holding chambers, for aerosol delivery, 356
Hollow index, in pectus excavatum, 2365
Homans' sign, in venous thrombosis, 1506–1507
Homocysteinemia, thromboembolism risk in, 1514
Honeycomb lung, 459, *461*, 1653, 1653t, *1654*, 1657–1658, *1660*, 1660t
computed tomography of, 674–675, *675*
in hypersensitivity pneumonitis, 1873
Hookworm disease, 1150–1151
Horder's spots, in psittacosis, 1026
Hormone(s). See also specific hormones.
Hormone response elements, in receptors, 241
Horner's syndrome, in Pancoast tumor, 1430
in pneumothorax, 2045–2046
Horse race effect, in chronic obstructive pulmonary disease, 1201–1202, *1201*, *1202*
Hospitalization, in pneumonia, 921–922
infections in. See *Nosocomial infection(s).*
Host defenses. See *Defense mechanism(s).*
Hot potato voice, in pneumomediastinum, 2102
Hot tubs, hypersensitivity pneumonitis related to, 1868
Hounsfield units, in computed tomography, 661
House dust mites, asthma and, 1250
Hoxa-5 protein, in lung development, 40, *40*
Hu antigen, antibodies to, in lung cancer, 1379
Hughes-Stovin syndrome, 1542
Human chorionic gonadotropin, in ovulation induction, pleural effusion due to, 2034–2035
Human Gene Mutation Database, 52t
Human Genome Project, 45, 47
Human herpesvirus 6 infections, 931t
pneumonia due to, 2232
in transplantation, 2302
Human herpesvirus 8 infections, in Kaposi's sarcoma, 2204–2205
Human immunodeficiency virus infection, 2171–2221
adenovirus infections in, 939, 940t
alveolar proteinosis in, 1792, 1794, 2210
amebiasis in, 1144–1145
anergy in, 1062
angioimmunoblastic lymphadenopathy in, 1459
aspergillosis in, 1134, 2198t, 2200–2201
asthma in, 2209
Bacille Calmette-Guérin infections in, 1090
blastomycosis in, 1120, 1121, 2198t, 2201
bronchial involvement in, 1367, 2209
bronchiectasis in, 1335, 2209
bronchiolitis obliterans organizing pneumonia in, 2210
cancer in, 2204. See also *Kaposi's sarcoma.*
bronchogenic carcinoma as, 2207–2208
lymphoma as, 1457, 2071
candidiasis in, 1135, 2202
Castleman's disease in, 1460
chest radiography of, 2176
chronic obstructive pulmonary disease in, 2209
coccidioidomycosis in, 1124–1125, *1126*, 1127, 2198t, 2199–2200
cryptococcosis in, 1129–1131, 2024, 2196–2197, *2197*, 2198t
cryptosporidiosis in, 2204
cytomegalovirus infections in, 749, 943, 2202–2203
diffuse alveolar damage in, 2210
emphysema in, 2209
epidemiology of, 2172–2173
Epstein-Barr virus infections in, 2203
ethical conflicts in, 2492
fungal infections in, 1108, 2187. See also *Pneumocystis carinii pneumonia;* specific disorders.
treatment of, 2198t
*Haemophilus influenzae* pneumonia in, 2178–2180
herpes simplex virus infections in, 947–949, 2203
histoplasmosis in, 1114, 1115, 2197–2199, 2198t, *2199*
treatment of, 1116–1117
immunologic abnormalities in, 1273
in hemophiliacs, 2294
infections in, ventilation-perfusion scanning in, 711–712, *712*

Human immunodeficiency virus infection *(Continued)*
influenza in, 2203
interstitial lung disease in, 2208–2210, *2208*
legionellosis in, 2180
lung transplantation contraindicated in, 2519
lymphadenopathy in, mediastinal, 2129–2130
lymphocytic interstitial pneumonitis in, 2208–2209, *2208*
lymphoma in, 1457, 2071
measles in, 958
mediastinal masses in, 2124
microsporidiosis in, 2204
mortality in, 2172–2173
mycobacterial infections in, 2186–2187. See also *Tuberculosis, in HIV infection.*
*Mycobacterium avium* complex infections in, 1091, 1092t, 1093–1094, *1094*, 2185–2186
*Mycobacterium kansasii* infections in, 1095, 2186
natural history of, tuberculosis effects on, 2182
nocardiosis in, 2181
obstructive lung disease in, 2209
parasitic infections in, 2203–2204
*Penicillium marneffei* infections in, 2198t, 2201–2202
pharyngitis in, 917, 933
pleural effusion in, 2025
pneumococcal pneumonia in, 2178–2180
*Pneumocystis carinii* pneumonia in. See *Pneumocystis carinii pneumonia.*
pneumonia in, 925–926. See also *Human immunodeficiency virus infection*, specific infections.
bronchoscopy in, 747
differential diagnosis of, 744, 745t
evaluation of, 2173–2178
microbiology of, 988t
pathology of, 470–471
versus CD4+ lymphocyte count, 2174
*Pseudomonas aeruginosa* pneumonia in, 2180
pulmonary function tests in, 856
precautions with, 860–861
pulmonary hypertension in, 2209
respiratory manifestations of, 931t. See also *Human immunodeficiency virus infection*, specific disorders.
differential diagnosis of, 2174
epidemiology of, 2174–2175
evaluation of, 2173–2178
bronchoscopy in, 2177–2178
CD4+ lymphocyte count in, 2174–2175
chest radiography in, 2176
clinical setting in, 2174
computed tomography in, 2176–2177
history in, 2175–2176
laboratory tests in, 2176
physical examination in, 2175–2176
pulmonary function tests in, 2176
radionuclide studies in, 2177
sputum examination in, 2177
spectrum of, 2172, 2172t
*Rhodococcus equi* infections in, 1030, 2180–2181
risk factors for, 2172–2173
sarcoidosis in, 2210
smoking in, respiratory disorders in, 2175
strongyloidiasis in, 1151, 1152, 2204
T lymphocyte count in. See *T lymphocytes, CD4+, in HIV infection.*
toxoplasmosis in, 1147–1148, 2203–2204
transmission of, in bronchoscopy, 756, 758–759

Human immunodeficiency virus infection *(Continued)*
treatment of, T lymphocyte count and, 2174–2175
tuberculosis in. See *Tuberculosis, in HIV infection.*
varicella-zoster virus infections in, 2203
viral infections in, 937, 2202–2203
viruses causing, 2171
Human leukocyte antigens, genetics of, 425–426, *427*
in ankylosing spondylitis, 1710
in Behçet's disease, 1710
in dermatomyositis, 1707
in Goodpasture's syndrome, 1743
in polymyositis, 1707
in pulmonary fibrosis, 1684
in rheumatoid arthritis, 1698
in sarcoidosis, 1717–1718
in Sjögren's syndrome, 1705
in systemic lupus erythematosus, 1703
in systemic sclerosis, 1692
nomenclature of, 425–426, *427*
structures of, 424–425, *425*, *426*
Human papillomavirus infections, 931t
Humidification, of air, in nasal breathing, 362, 1346
Humidifier lung, 1868
Humoral hypercalcemia of malignancy, in lung cancer, 1379
Humoral immune response, 2224. See also *Immunoglobulin(s).*
in lung, 436–437, *436*
Humoral theory, of clubbing pathogenesis, 601
Hunter's syndrome, lung injury in, 481t
Hurler's syndrome, lung injury in, 481t
Hyaline membranes, in diffuse alveolar damage, 1744
in lung injury, 459, *460*, *461*
Hyalinizing granuloma, of lung, 1480
Hydantoin, pulmonary disease due to, 1989
Hydatid disease (echinococcosis), 1157–1160, *1159*
mediastinal extension of, 2132
pleural effusion in, 2025–2026
Hydatidiform mole, emboli from, 2325
Hydralazine, as vasodilator, 301
Hydration, in sickle cell disease, 2289
Hydraulic conductivity, of endothelium, 144
of lung, 1576
Hydrocarbon pneumonitis, 1908
Hydrochloric acid, exposure to, 1905–1906
Hydrochlorothiazide, pulmonary disease due to, 1988
Hydrocortisone, in asthma, 280, 281
Hydrofluoric acid, exposure to, 1906
Hydrofluoroalkane-134a, as aerosol propellant, 355
Hydrogen, characteristics of, 1958t
Hydrogen fluoride, exposure to, 1906
Hydrogen ion, exchange of, in compensation for acid-base imbalance, 161
excretion of, in compensation for acid-base imbalance, 161
loss of, transport of, 163
oxygen-hemoglobin affinity and, 1922, *1922*
transport of, in kidney, 162
Hydrogen ion concentration, chemoreceptor sensing of, 189–190, *190*
equation for, 156
negative logarithm of. See *pH.*
respiratory responses to, 192–193, *193*
Hydrogen peroxide, as inflammatory mediator, 257–258
generation of, in macrophages, 390, 392
Hydrogen selenide, exposure to, 1910

Hydrogen sulfide, exposure to, 1909
Hydromorphone, in myocardial ischemia, *2401*
Hydropneumothorax, in coccidioidomycosis, 2024
in esophageal rupture, 2027–2028, *2027*, 2052–2053
in hydatid disease, 1158
in mediastinitis, 2106, *2107*
Hydrostatic pressure, alveolar, 61–62, 67, 1583–1584
in pulmonary capillaries, 132–133, *132*, 1576
in pulmonary edema, 145, 1497–1498, 1576–1577
decreased, 1580t, 1582–1583
increased, 1580–1582, 1580t
in Starling equation, 1497
in pulmonary circulation, 1498t
interstitial, in pulmonary edema, 1583
Hydrothorax, hepatic, 2015–2016, 2271
in hydatid disease, 1158
in peritoneal dialysis, 2016
Hydroxyeicosatetraenoic acids, in mucus hypersecretion, 334
Hydroxyl radical, generation of, in macrophages, 390, 392
Hydroxyurea, in hypereosinophilic syndrome, 1769
in sickle cell disease, 2289
Hygroscopic aerosols, deposition of, 354
Hyperalgesia, esophageal, 580
primary, 573
secondary, 573
visceral, 570–573, *571*, *572*
Hyperbaric therapy, for decompression sickness, 1961, 1962
for high-altitude pulmonary edema, 1936
for mountain sickness, 1931–1932
Hypercalcemia, calcification in, 450, *453*
in lung cancer, 1422
in multiple myeloma, 2294
in sarcoidosis, 1719
of malignancy, 1379
Hypercalciuria, in sarcoidosis, 1719
Hypercapnia/hypercarbia, acidemia in, 2444
after thoracoplasty, 2364
bicarbonate concentrations in, 161
consequences of, 2443–2445
dyspnea and, 543
hypoxemia in, 2444
in asthma, 1265
in bronchoscopy, 756
in chronic obstructive pulmonary disease, 1634
in cystic fibrosis, 1306, 1312
in hypoventilation, 2140–2143, *2141*
in near drowning, 1964
in neuromuscular disorders, 2331
in respiratory failure, 2379–2380
in sleep apnea, 2159
inspiratory occlusion pressure in, 819–820
mechanical effects of, 2444
metabolic alkalosis and, 2444–2445
permissive, 2443–2445
in mechanical ventilation, 2432–2433, 2432t, 2478
pulmonary circulation effects of, 1492
respiratory acidosis in, 173–174
respiratory muscle fatigue in, 109
response to, in breathing control assessment, 818–820, *819*, 877
right ventricular dysfunction in, 1635–1636, *1636*
treatment of, in cystic fibrosis, 1312
ventilatory response to, 190–191, *191*
Hypercarbia. See *Hypercapnia/hypercarbia.*

Hyperchloremic acidosis, 163–164, *164*, 168–170, 169t
  anion gap in, 163–164, 170
  in gastrointestinal dysfunction, 169–170
  in kidney dysfunction, 162, 168–169, 169t
  in respiratory alkalosis correction, 170
  treatment of, 171
Hypercortisolism, respiratory manifestations of, 2312–2313
Hypereosinophilic syndrome, 1769, 1769t
Hyperfractionation, in radiation therapy, 1433
Hyperglobulinemia, in angioimmunoblastic lymphadenopathy, 1459
  in chlamydial pneumonia, 1027
Hyperglycemia, in cystic fibrosis, 1313
Hyperimmunoglobulin E syndrome (Job's syndrome), 2233t, 2238
Hyperimmunoglobulin M syndrome, 2236
Hyperinfection syndrome, in strongyloidiasis, 1151
Hyperinflation, diaphragm flattening in, 859
  dynamic. See *Positive end-expiratory pressure, intrinsic.*
Hyperkalemia, in metabolic acidosis, 170
  in renal tubular acidosis, 169
Hyperkinetic pulmonary hypertension, 1492t, 1543, 1642
Hyperleukocytic syndrome, 2291
Hyperlucent lung. See *Lung, hyperlucent.*
Hypermagnesemia, in pulmonary edema, in seawater near drowning, 1591
Hypernatremia, anion gap in, *164*
Hyperoxia. See also *Oxygen, toxicity of.*
  chemoreceptor function in, 191, *191*
  emphysema due to, 1213
  gas exchange in, 73, *74*
  injury from, 1987
  lactic threshold in, 207
Hyperparathyroidism, 2128, 2312, *2312*
Hyperplasia, cellular, 446, 450, *451*
  in lung cancer, 1377–1378
Hyperplastic nonallergic rhinosinusitis, 1348
Hyperpnea. See also *Hyperventilation.*
  definition of, 588
  sleep, in heart disease, 2261
  versus hyperventilation, 2145
Hyperresonance, in percussion, 597
Hypersensitivity, delayed, in beryllium lung disease, 1843
Hypersensitivity pneumonitis, 1867–1884
  acute, 1873
  animal models of, 1871
  chest radiography of, 1874–1875, *1875*
  chronic, 1873–1874
  clinical features of, 1873–1876, 1873t, *1875*
  computed tomography of, 676, *676*, 1661, *1661*
  diagnosis of, approach to, 1876, 1876t
    criteria for, 1876–1877, 1877t
    tests for, 1873–1876, 1873t, *1875*
  differential diagnosis of, 1877, 1877t
  drug-induced, 1692t
  epidemiology of, 1870
  etiology of, 1867–1870, 1868t
    animal proteins in, 1869
    chemical sensitizers in, 1869–1870
    environmental, 1870–1871
    microbial agents in, 1867–1869
    occupational, 1870–1871
  histopathology of, *469*, 1872–1873, *1872*
  host factors in, 1871
  immunopathogenesis of, 1871–1872, 1871t
  impairment in, 899–900, 908
  in bird handling, 375
  in pediatric patients, 1871
  natural history of, 1877–1878
Hypersensitivity pneumonitis *(Continued)*
  prognosis for, 1877–1878
  pulmonary function tests in, 1877–1878
  subacute, 1873–1874
  summer type, 1870
  treatment of, 1878–1880
Hypersensitivity reactions, in strongyloidiasis, 1151
  in tuberculosis, 1057, 1080, 2021
  lung injury in, drug-induced, 477, *477*, 479t
    pathology of, 465–466, *466–470*, 468
  vasculitis in, 1534, 1539
Hypertension, intracranial, neurogenic pulmonary edema in, 147
  portal. See *Portal hypertension.*
  pulmonary. See *Pulmonary hypertension.*
  systemic, after lung transplantation, 2526
    high altitude effects on, 1940
    in sleep apnea, 2158–2159, *2158*
Hyperthermia, acid-base imbalance in, 163
  in diving, 1952–1953
Hyperthyroidism, respiratory manifestations of, 2310
Hypertonic aerosols, deposition of, 354
Hypertrophic pulmonary osteoarthropathy, 600–601, *601*, 601t, *602*
  in benign fibrous mesothelioma, 2071
  in cystic fibrosis, 1305–1306
  in lung cancer, 1421
Hypertrophy, cellular, 446, *450*
Hyperventilation, alveolar, 2145–2149
    adverse effects of, 2147
    aspirin-induced, 1984
    at high altitude, 1916–1918, *1917*, 1926, *1926*
    beneficial effects of, 2147
    blood pH in, 156
    chest pain in, 580
    clinical features of, 2147–2148
    definition of, 588
    diagnosis of, 2148
    drug-induced, 2147
    dyspnea in, 544
    hypoxemia after, 2147
    in anxiety, 175
    in cardiovascular disorders, 2146
    in diving, 1964
    in exercise, 209, 1926, *1926*
    in heart failure, 2162, 2260
    in hepatopulmonary syndrome, 2271
    in hypoxemia, 2145–2146
    in metabolic acidosis, 161
    in metabolic disorders, 2146–2147
    in neurologic disorders, 2147
    in pulmonary disorders, 2146
    in pulmonary embolism, 1506
    on descent from high altitude, 1918
    pathogenesis of, 2145–2147, *2145*, 2146t
    physiologic features of, 2147–2148
    psychogenic, 2147, 2148
    respiratory alkalosis in, 174–175, 175t
    seizures in, 1942
    terminology of, 2145
    treatment of, 175, 2148
    versus asthma, 1270
    versus hyperpnea, 2145
    versus tachypnea, 2145
  in exercise, in heart failure, 2260
  in heart failure, 2260
Hyperviscosity syndrome, in Waldenström's macroglobulinemia, 2294
Hypobaric conditions. See *Altitude, high.*
Hypocapnia/hypocarbia, after hyperventilation, 2147
  bicarbonate concentrations in, 161
  in asthma, 1265, 1275
Hypocapnia/hypocarbia *(Continued)*
  in hepatopulmonary syndrome, 2271
  in hyperventilation, 2145
  in pulmonary embolism, 1510
  in sleep apnea, 2161–2162, *2161*, *2163–2165*, 2164–2165
Hypocarbia. See *Hypocapnia/hypocarbia.*
Hypochloremia, metabolic alkalosis in, 162–163, 171–173, 171t
Hypochlorite bleach, chlorine exposure due to, 1905–1906
Hypogammaglobulinemia, bronchiectasis in, 1335–1336
  with hyperimmunoglobulin M, 2236
Hypoglycemia, in benign fibrous mesothelioma, 2071
Hypokalemia, beta$_2$-adrenergic agonist-induced, 271
  in metabolic alkalosis, 172
  in renal tubular acidosis, 168–169
  in respiratory alkalosis, 174
  respiratory failure in, 2447
Hypomagnesemia, respiratory failure in, 2447
Hyponatremia, in respiratory alkalosis, 174
  in tuberculosis, 1063
Hypoperfusion, shock in. See *Shock.*
Hypophosphatemia, in respiratory alkalosis, 174
  respiratory failure in, 2447
Hypopnea, 2331. See also *Apnea; Sleep apnea; Hypoventilation.*
  central, 2144
  in chronic obstructive pulmonary disease, 1194
  in sleep, 1350–1351
Hypotension. See also *Shock.*
  in asthma, 1275
  in hepatopulmonary syndrome, 2273
  in mechanical ventilation, in respiratory failure, 2463
  in near drowning, 1966
  in pulmonary edema, 1606
  protamine-induced, 1983
  pulmonary, in arteriovenous malformations, 1563
Hypothalamic-pituitary-adrenal axis, inhibition of, corticosteroids in, 282
Hypothalamus, injury of, hyperventilation in, 2147
Hypothermia, acid-base imbalance in, 163
  in diving, 1952–1953, 1964
  in shock, 2403t
  lung injury in, pathology of, 475
Hypothyroidism, pleural effusion in, 2016
  respiratory manifestations of, 2310–2311
Hypotonic aerosols, deposition of, 354
Hypoventilation, alveolar, 2140–2145
    alkalinization in, 300
    blood pH in, 156
    carbon dioxide retention and, 83, 85
    causes of, 71
    classification of, 2140, 2140t
    clinical features of, 2143
    consequences of, 2141, *2141*
    definition of, 157
    diagnosis of, 2143–2144
    differential diagnosis of, 2144
    exercise in, ventilation requirements for, 209–210, *209*
    gas exchange in, 71–72, *72*
    in kyphoscoliosis, 2360, 2361
    in mountain sickness, 1931, *1931*
    in obesity, 2159, 2371, 2371t, 2372
    in Pickwickian syndrome, 2159
    in pneumothorax, 2045
    laboratory tests in, 2141–2142, *2142*

Hypoventilation *(Continued)*
pathogenesis of, 2140–2141, 2140t, 2143
primary, 2142–2145
clinical features of, 2143
diagnosis of, 2143–2144
differential diagnosis of, 2144
pathogenesis of, 2143
treatment of, 2144–2145, 2144t
pulmonary vasoconstriction in, 1634
respiratory acidosis in, 173–174, 173t
treatment of, 2144–2145, 2144t
versus diaphragmatic paralysis, 2336
blood gases in, 821t
hypoxemia in, 2444
respiratory failure in, clinical features of, 2380–2381
pathophysiology of, 2378–2381, 2378t, *2379*, *2381*
treatment of, 2380–2381
Hypovolemic shock, 2400–2402, 2401t, 2403t
Hypoxia and hypoxemia, after thoracoplasty, 2364
alveolar, pulmonary vascular response to, 129–131, 1490
at high altitude. See *Altitude, high.*
carbon dioxide partial pressure in, 821t
causes of, 821t
ciliary activity in, 361
diffusing capacity and, 815
dyspnea in, 220
gas exchange in, 73, *74*
heroin-induced, 1980
hyperventilation in, 2145–2146
in acute inflammatory polyneuropathy, 2341–2342
in acute respiratory distress syndrome, 318
in air travel, 859–860, 1226–1227
in alveolar proteinosis, 1794
in arteriovenous malformations, 1495, 1563
in asthma, 1275, 2453
in exercise, 218
in bronchiectasis, 1327
in bronchiolitis, 936–937, 1362
in bronchiolitis obliterans, after lung transplantation, 1364
in graft-versus-host disease, 1364
in bronchiolitis obliterans organizing pneumonia, 1365
in bronchitis, 1192
in bronchoalveolar lavage, 748
in bronchoscopy, 728, 756
in chronic obstructive pulmonary disease, 82–83, 1192, 1193
at rest, 215–216
in exercise, 212
pulmonary artery pressure and, 1634
treatment of, 1228–1229
in croup, 935, 961
in cystic fibrosis, 1304, 1304t, 1306, 1312
in diaphragmatic paralysis, 2335
in emphysema, 224, 1192
in exercise, in emphysema, 224
in interstitial pulmonary fibrosis, 217
in flail chest, 2368
in hemodialysis, 2279–2280
in hepatopulmonary syndrome, 2271, 2273, 2274
in highly fit athletes, 219
in hypercapnia, 2444
in hypersensitivity pneumonitis, 1874
in hypoventilation, 71–72, *72*, 2141–2143, *2141*, 2444
in kidney failure, 2279–2280
in kyphoscoliosis, 2360
in lymphangio(leio)myomatosis, 1781
in near drowning, 1964–1965
Hypoxia and hypoxemia *(Continued)*
in obesity, 2372
in pancreatitis, 2276–2277
in pneumonia, 2415–2416
cytomegalovirus, 943
eosinophilic, 1768
treatment of, 999
in pneumothorax, 2054
in pregnancy, 1942
in pulmonary edema, 1594–1595
in pulmonary embolism, 1506, 1510
in pulmonary hypertension, 1547, 1548
in respiratory syncytial virus infections, 963
in sarcoidosis, 1723
in sickle cell disease, 2288, 2289
in sleep, 2159
in neuromuscular disorders, 2331
in pulmonary fibrosis, 1677
in spinal cord injury, 2339
in suctioning, 728
in ventricular septal defect management, 298
individual sensitivity to, 1634
inspiratory occlusion pressure in, 819, *820*
lactic acid production in, 207, *207*
lung injury in, 465, *465*
nitric oxide deficiency in, 1645
of brain, in hyperventilation, 2148
oxygen alveolar-to-arterial difference in, 821t
oxygen partial pressure in, 821t
pathophysiology of, in near drowning, 1964–1965
position-dependent, in arteriovenous malformations, 1563
in systemic-pulmonary communications, 1497
pulmonary artery pressure in, 1632
pulmonary vascular response to, 67–68, *68*, 129–131, 1490
pulmonary vasoconstriction in, at high altitude, 130, 1581, 1634, 1935
in chronic obstructive pulmonary disease, 1193
in hepatopulmonary syndrome, 2274
pathophysiology of, 1633–1634
right ventricular failure in, 1635–1636, *1636*
respiratory alkalosis in, 174–175
respiratory failure in. See *Acute/adult respiratory distress syndrome; Acute hypoxemic respiratory failure.*
response to, in breathing control assessment, 818–821, *820*, 878
retinopathy in, 1937, *1937*
stagnant, 2146
tissue, lactic acid formation in, 164–166, *165*
treatment of, in chronic obstructive pulmonary disease, 1228–1229
in cystic fibrosis, 1312
in pneumonia, 999
vasoconstriction in, 1490
ventilatory decline and, 1917
ventilatory response to, 191–192, *192*
at high altitude, 1924, 1926, *1926*
Hypoxia-altitude simulation test, 860
Hysteresis, in lung pressure-volume relationship, 95, *96*


## I


I-309, receptors for, 507t, 516–517
I-alpha neurons, in medulla, 186
I-beta neurons, in medulla, 186
Ibuprofen, in cystic fibrosis, 1310
Ibuprofen *(Continued)*
in mountain sickness, 1932
IC. See *Inspiratory capacity.*
Identical by descent regions, in genomic mapping, 51
Idiopathic interstitial pneumonias. See *Interstitial lung disease(s), pneumonia as.*
Idiopathic pneumonia syndrome, in bone marrow transplantation, 2299–2300
Idiopathic pulmonary fibrosis. See *Fibrosis, idiopathic pulmonary.*
Ileus, meconium, in cystic fibrosis, 1292, 1306, 1312
Illness, versus sickness, 586
Imaging. See specific techniques, e.g., *Chest radiography; Computed tomography; Magnetic resonance imaging; Ultrasonography.*
Imipenem, in pneumonia, 998t
in tuberculosis, 1070
Imipenem/cilastatin, in cystic fibrosis, 1309t
Immersion effects, in diving, 1952
Immotile cilia syndrome (primary ciliary dyskinesia), 366, 480t, 482, 1336
Immune complexes, deposition of, in alveoli, 520
in glomerulonephritis, 1740–1741
in systemic lupus erythematosus, 1739, *1739*
in vasculitis, 1534, 1535
lung injury in, pathology of, 466, *467*, *468*
Immune globulin, in asthma, 286
in cystic fibrosis, 1312
in cytomegalovirus infections, 944, 945
in bone marrow transplantation, 2302
prophylactic, 2231
in immunoglobulin deficiencies, 2233
in measles, 959
in respiratory syncytial virus infections, 964, 2303
in varicella-zoster virus infections, 968
Immune response, 416–430
adaptive, suppression of, alveolar macrophages in, 393–394, *395*
antibodies in. See *Antibody(ies).*
antigen-presenting cells in. See *Antigen-presenting cells.*
B lymphocytes in. See *B lymphocytes; Immunoglobulin(s).*
cell-mediated, 437–438, 2224. See also *T lymphocytes.*
disorders of, 2233t, 2234t, 2238–2240
lung injury in, pathology of, 466, *469*
cytotoxic T-cell reactions in, 437–438
eosinophils in, 1759–1760
generation of, 431–435
antibody production in, 434
cell-mediated, 434–435
T helper cell subsets in, 432–434, *433*
T-cell activation in, 431–432, *431*
human leukocyte antigens in. See *Human leukocyte antigens.*
humoral, 2224. See also *Immunoglobulin(s).*
in lung, 436–437, *436*
immunoglobulins in. See *Immunoglobulin(s).*
in allergic disease, 437
in amebiasis, 1144–1145
in aspergillosis, 1131, 1133
in asthma, 1256–1257, *1257–1259*, 1855
in blastomycosis, 1118–1119
in coccidioidomycosis, 1108, 1122–1123
in cryptococcosis, 1108, 1129
in cystic fibrosis, 1301
in filariasis, 1153
in granulomatous disease, 437–438

Immune response *(Continued)*
in hantavirus infections, 945–946
in histoplasmosis, 1108, 1109, 1111
in hookworm disease, 1150
in influenza, 953
in lung, antibody-mediated, 436–437, *436*
cell-mediated, 437–438
cytotoxic T-cell reactions in, 437–438
in allergic disease, 437
in cancer, 1386–1387
in granulomatous disease, 437–438
lymphocyte populations and trafficking in, 435–436
to autoantigens, 436–437
to extracellular pathogens, 436, *436*
in paracoccidioidomycosis, 1128–1129
in *Paragonimus westermani* infections, 1161
in sarcoidosis, 1724–1725
in schistosomiasis, 1163–1164
in systemic sclerosis, 1692
in toxoplasmosis, 1147–1148
in tuberculosis, 1055–1057, *1056*
innate, 2224
lung injury in, pathology of, 465–466, *466–470*, 468
lymphocyte populations and trafficking in, 435–436
overview of, 2224–2226, *2225*, *2227*, *2228*
specific, 2224
surfactant protein A in, 310
T lymphocytes in. See *T lymphocytes.*
to antigens. See *Antigen(s).*
to autoantigens, 436–437
to bacteria, 436, *436*
extracellular, 2224–2226, *2225*
intracellular, 2226, *2227*
to extracellular pathogens, 436, *436*
to viruses, 2226, *2228*
Immune system, components of, 413–416, 414t, 415t
Immunization, adenovirus, 940
aerosol delivery of, 360
bacille Calmette-Guérin in, 1089–1090, 2185
*Bacillus anthracis*, 1029
cytomegalovirus, 945
*Haemophilus influenzae*, 1008, 2180
in chronic obstructive pulmonary disease, 1217, 2508
in cystic fibrosis, 1311
in lymphangio(leio)myomatosis, 1784
in pulmonary rehabilitation, 2508
in sickle cell disease, 2289
influenza, 955–956, 956t, 2508
measles, 959
meningococcal, 1006
*Neisseria meningitidis*, 1006
pneumococcal, 1001–1002, 1002t, 2508
in HIV infection, 2180
tuberculosis, 1089–1090, 2185
varicella-zoster virus, 968
Immunodeficiency. See also *Human immunodeficiency virus infection; Immunosuppressive therapy; Transplantation.*
adenovirus infections in, 939, 940t
alveolar proteinosis in, 1794
aspergillosis in, 1133–1134, *1134*
bronchiectasis in, 1335–1336
candidiasis in, 1135–1136
common variable, 2233t, 2235
cryptococcosis in, 1129–1131
cytomegalovirus infections in, 942, 943
herpes simplex virus infections in, 947–949
histoplasmosis in, 1114
immunization in, 1002, 1002t
Immunodeficiency *(Continued)*
in plasma cell dyscrasias, 2292
lung injury in, 481t
lymphoma in, clinical course of, 1457
paracoccidioidomycosis in, 1128
pneumonia in, 923–926, 925t
microbiology of, 988t
*Nocardia*, 1022
*Pseudomonas aeruginosa*, 1011
risk of, 986
specimen collection in, 611, *612*
treatment of, 997
ventilation-perfusion scanning in, 711–712, *712*
primary, 2232–2240, 2233t
cellular immunity defects in, 2233t, 2234t, 2238–2240
complement deficiency as, 2233t, 2234t, 2236
immunoglobulin defects in, 2233–2236, 2233t, 2234t
phagocyte defects in, 2233t, 2234t, 2236–2238
pseudoallescheriosis in, 1136
respiratory syncytial virus infections in, 963
*Rhodococcus equi* infections in, 1030
screening tests for, 2234t
severe combined, 2233t, 2239
strongyloidiasis in, 1151
tuberculosis risk in, 1059
varicella-zoster virus infections in, 967, 968
viral infections in, 937
Immunodiffusion test, for coccidioidomycosis, 1125
for exoantigens, in fungal infections, 623
for histoplasmosis, 623, 1116
Immunofluorescence tests, for *Pneumocystis carinii*, 759
Immunogen, definition of, 422
Immunoglobulin(s), antigen interactions with, 422
classes of, 416, 419–421, *420*, 420t
complementarity determining regions of, 416, *417*
disorders of, 2333–2336, 2333t, 2334t
in plasma cell dyscrasias, 2292
excess of, in sarcoidosis, 1725
functions of, 420, 420t, 2224–2226, *2225*
genes of, 416, 418, *418–420*
heavy chains of, 416, *417*
hypervariable regions of, 416, *417*
idiotypes of, 417
in lung, 436–437, *436*
in mucus, 329
isotype switching of, 419–420, *420*
junctional diversification of, 418
light chains of, 416, *417*
amyloid formation from, 2295
monoclonal proliferation of. See also *Multiple myeloma.*
in Waldenström's macroglobulinemia, 1464, 2294
recombination of, 416, 418, *419*
structures of, 416, *417*
synthesis of, 416, 418, *418*, *419*
in B lymphocytes, 414
regulation of, 434
therapeutic. See *Immune globulin.*
Immunoglobulin A, 420–421, 420t
deficiency of, 2233t, 2235
secretory, 329, 420–421, 420t
Immunoglobulin E, 420t, 421
antigen reactions with, in allergic rhinitis, 1347, 1348
excess of, in Job's syndrome, 2233t, 2238
in allergic bronchopulmonary aspergillosis, 1763, 1766
Immunoglobulin E *(Continued)*
in allergic disease, 437
in asthma, 1176, 1252, 1260, *1260*
occupational, 1855
Immunoglobulin G, 420, 420t
absence of, in common variable immunodeficiency, 2233t, 2235
in X-linked agammaglobulinemia, 2233t, 2234–2235
deficiency of, 2233t, 2235–2236
structure of, 416, *417*
subclasses of, 416, 420t
deficiencies of, bronchiectasis in, 1335–1336
Immunoglobulin M, 420, 420t
deficiency of, 2236
excess of, in hypogammaglobulinemia, 2236
in Waldenström's macroglobulinemia, 2294
measurement of, in *Chlamydia* infections, 624
Immunohistochemistry, in mesothelioma, 2069
in pleural metastasis, 2074
of bronchoscopic specimens, 742
Immunosuppressive therapy. See also specific drugs, e.g., *Cyclosporine.*
for asthma, 286, 287–288
for bronchiolitis obliterans, 2301
after transplantation, 1366
for chronic obstructive pulmonary disease, 287–288
for drug-induced lung disease, 1693t
for sarcoidosis, 1727
for transplantation, 2226–2227
lung, 2521, 2526
pneumonia in, 925
with bronchiolitis obliterans, 1366
Immunotherapy, for allergic rhinitis, 1349
for asthma, 286
for mesothelioma, 2070
pulmonary disease due to, 1978
Impaction, inertial, in aerosol deposition, 351, *351*
Impairment and disability, 895–912
evaluation of, American Medical Association guidelines for, 898–900, 899t, 900t
American Thoracic Society guidelines for, 900
apportionment in, 904, 910
attribution in, 910
bias in, 896
blood gas measurement in, 906
causation apportionment in, 910
chest radiography in, 905
classification systems for, 898–900, 899t, 900t
components of, 904t
dyspnea in, 896–898
exercise testing in, 846, 897–898, 906–907, 907t
extrapulmonary conditions in, 905
for Black Lung Benefits Act, 903
for Department of Veterans Affairs, 902, 903t
for entitlement systems, 900–902, 901t, 903t
for Social Security Administration, 900–902, 901t
for workers' compensation, 898, 902
guidelines for, 903t
history in, 902–904, 904t
importance of, 895–896
in asthma, 907–908
in bullous conditions, 909
in chronic airflow obstruction, 907
in interstitial lung disease, 908

Impairment and disability *(Continued)*
in pneumoconiosis, 1815–1816
in sleep apnea, 909
in upper airway obstruction, 909
job requirement assessment in, 909
laboratory tests in, 905–907, 907t
malingering in, 898
physical examination in, 904
physician role in, 896
pulmonary function tests in, 850, 850t, 897–898, 905–906
purpose of, 895–896
report of, 909–910
spirometry in, 784
terminology for, 896
versus work energy requirements, 906–907, 907t
functional, 896, 898
organic, 896, 898
permanent, 896, 908
temporary, 896
Impedance plethysmography, in venous thrombosis, 1509
Inclusions, in cytomegalovirus infections, 942, *942*, *944*, 2302
in herpes simplex virus infections, 947
in viral infections, 471, 473, *473*
Independent medical examiner, for impairment and disability evaluation, 896
Indicator dilution techniques, in lung water measurement, 1596–1597
Indirect fluorescent antibody test, in legionellosis, 1016
Indium 111 scan, in *Pneumocystis carinii* pneumonia, 711–712, *712*
Indomethacin, hypoxic pulmonary vasoconstrictor response augmentation due to, 130
in bronchiectasis, 1331
Industry, air pollution from. See *Air pollution.*
diseases associated with. See *Occupational and environmental disorder(s).*
Inertial impaction, in aerosol deposition, 351, *351*
Infarction, lung, coagulation necrosis in, *447*
in pulmonary embolism, 1506
in sickle cell disease, 2288
pathology of, 465, *465*
versus tumor, 1481
Infection(s). See also *Pneumonia; Sepsis;* specific infections.
as asthma risk, 1251–1252, *1251*
bacterial. See specific bacteria and diseases.
childhood, chronic obstructive pulmonary disease risk in, 1201
chronic bronchitis in, 1216–1217
control of, in nosocomial pneumonia prevention, 923
in pulmonary function testing, 860–861
respiratory syncytial virus, 964
cough after, *559*, 560, 564
fungal. See *Fungal infection(s).*
granulomas in, 1481
in alveolar proteinosis, 1794
in bronchoscopy, 756
in cystic fibrosis, 1300–1302
lower respiratory tract. See *Bronchitis; Pneumonia.*
lung injury in, 1587, 1588t, 1589
nosocomial. See *Nosocomial infection(s).*
odontogenic, pneumomediastinum in, 2097
pathology of. See *Pathology, of infections.*
superantigens in, 428
susceptibility to, air pollutants and, 1896
upper respiratory tract. See *Epiglottitis; Rhinitis; Otitis media; Pharyngitis; Sinusitis.*
Infection(s) *(Continued)*
viral. See *Viral infection(s);* specific infections.
Infectiousness, of pathogen, definition of, 1052
Infectivity, of pathogen, definition of, 1052
Inferior vena cava filters, in pulmonary embolism prevention, 1517, *1518*
Infertility, in cystic fibrosis, 1307
Infiltrative lung disease(s), alveolar microlithiasis as, 1749–1750, *1749*, *1750*
amyloidosis as, 2296
aspergillosis as, 1131
diffuse alveolar hemorrhage as. See *Alveolar hemorrhage, diffuse.*
drug-induced, 1990–1991, 1991t
Gaucher's disease as, 1748
Hermansky-Pudlak syndrome as, 1749
hydrochlorothiazide-induced, 1988
in bone marrow transplantation, 2298–2299
in leukemia, 2291–2292
in lymphoma, 2292
in multiple myeloma, 2293
in pulmonary embolism, 1510, *1510*, 1527
in Waldenström's macroglobulinemia, 2294
lymphangio(leio)myomatosis as, 1776
lymphoproliferative, 1458–1460, *1459*
neurofibromatosis as, 1748, 1748t
Niemann-Pick disease as, 1748–1749
sulfasalazine-induced, 1979
Inflammation. See also *Inflammatory mediator(s).*
assessment of, 529–530
beta-adrenergic agonists effects on, 269
bronchiectasis in, 1326, 1336
bronchitis in, 1215–1216, *1215*
chronic, fibrosis in, 496
pathology of, 455, *457*
definition of, 495
granulocytes in. See *Granulocyte(s);* specific granulocytes.
granulomatous, pathology of, 455, *457*
in asthma. See *Asthma, pathophysiology of.*
in interstitial lung disease, 496
in lung injury, 1589–1590, 1590t
in necrosis, 444
in nonspecific interstitial pneumonia, 1688
in pulmonary edema, 1589–1590, 1590t
high-altitude, 1936
necrotizing, pathology of, 455, *456*
neurogenic, 254–255, *254*, 1262–1263
of airways, in cystic fibrosis, 1301
of blood vessels, in vasculitis, 1534
pathology of, 455–456, *455–458*
pseudotumors in, 1480
pulmonary fibrosis in, 1677–1678
regulation of, alveolar macrophages in, 393
repair after. See *Repair.*
resolution of, 528–529, *529*, *530*
transcription factors in, 259, *259*
ventilation-perfusion scanning in, 701, 713, *714*
Inflammatory bowel disease, pulmonary complications of, 2270–2271, 2270t
Inflammatory cells, of airway, 232, *233*
Inflammatory mediator(s), 256–258, *257*, *258*. See also specific substances, e.g., *Cytokine(s); Histamine; Nitric oxide.*
antagonists of, 284–286, *284*
in asthma, 286, 287t
beta-adrenergic agonist action against, 269
chemotactic. See *Chemokines;* specific chemokines.
cytokines as. See *Cytokine(s);* specific cytokines.
early response, 499–504. See also *Interferon-τ; Interleukins 1, 4, and 5; Tumor necrosis factor-α.*
Inflammatory mediator(s) *(Continued)*
eosinophil-derived, 1759, 1759t, 1760
fibrotic, 505–506. See also *Transforming growth factor-γ.*
growth factors as. See *Growth factor(s);* specific growth factors.
in airway epithelium, 232, *233*
in asthma, *257*
in mucus secretion, 333–334
in pancreatitis, 2276
in pulmonary edema, 1589–1590, 1590t
interferons as. See *Interferon(s).*
interleukins as. See *Interleukin(s).*
lipid. See *Arachidonic acid metabolites; Platelet-activating factor;* specific substances.
multiple, 258
peptide, 519–520, *519*. See also *Complement.*
tumor necrosis factor-α as. See *Tumor necrosis factor-α.*
Inflammatory papilloma, tracheobronchial, 1478
Inflammatory polyneuropathy, acute, respiratory function in, 2341–2342
Influenza, 931t, 949–957
antibodies in, 949–950, 953, 955, 956
antigenic variation in, 949, 950
Asian (1957), 950
avian, 950
bronchitis after, 934
cell culture in, 625
chronic lung disease in, 953–954
clinical manifestations of, 953–955, *954*
clinical syndrome of, 935
complications of, 953
diagnosis of, 625, 955
epidemiology of, 949–950
Hong Kong (1968), 950, 952t
immune response in, 953
immunization for, 955–956, 956t, 2506
in HIV infection, 2203
in lung transplantation, 2520
in pediatric patients, 951
in pregnancy, 2320–2321
mortality in, 949–951, 953, 954
mucociliary transport abnormalities in, 368, *369*
pandemics of, 949, 950
pathogenesis of, 951, *952*, 952t, 953
pneumonia in, 468, 470, 937, 951, *952*, 954–955, *954*
Port Chalmers (1973), 952t
prevention of, 955–956, 956t
Spanish (1918), 950
swine, 950, 955
transmission of, 950–951
treatment of, 359, 935, 956–957
Victoria (1975), 952t
virus causing, characteristics of, 949–950
shedding of, 953
surfactant protein A binding to, 312
surfactant protein D binding to, 315
Influenza-like illness, 935
Information resources, for genetic diseases, 51–52, 52t
Informed consent, 2491
for bronchoscopy, 730
Inhalation, of aerosols. See *Aerosol(s).*
of air pollutants. See *Air pollution.*
of anesthetics, vasodilation in, 302
of anthrax spores, 1029
of antigens, hypersensitivity pneumonitis in. See *Hypersensitivity pneumonitis.*
tolerance to, alveolar macrophages in, 393–394, *395*

Inhalation *(Continued)*
dendritic cells in, 397
of *Blastomyces dermatitidis*, 1117–1118
of *Coccidioides immitis* spores, 1122
of *Cryptococcus neoformans*, 1129
of drug(s), anticholinergic, 276–277, 1221–1222
$beta_2$-adrenergic agonist, 268, 269–270, 1220–1222, 1220t
corticosteroids as. See *Corticosteroid(s), inhaled.*
cromones as, 284
devices for. See *Nebulizers; Inhalers.*
DNAse as, in cystic fibrosis, 1310
epinephrine as, in croup, 935
in asthma, 357, 359
in chronic obstructive pulmonary disease, 357, 359
in infections, 359–360
in systemic disease, 360
nitric oxide as, 301
in acute respiratory distress syndrome, 2434–2435
in pulmonary hypertension, 1645
oily, pulmonary disease due to, 1986–1987
surfactant as, 320–321
with theophylline, 1223
zanamivir as, in influenza, 957
of dusts. See *Occupational and environmental disorder(s).*
of *Histoplasma capsulatum*, 1109
of hot gases, bronchoscopy in, 754
of infectious material, 986
of irritant gases. See *Irritant gases.*
of oxygen. See *Oxygen, inhalation of; Oxygen therapy.*
of *Paracoccidioides braziliensis*, 1128
of particulates, defense mechanisms against, 1889
of saline solution, in cystic fibrosis, 368
of smoke, bronchoscopy in, 754
lung injury in, 1908–1909
of viruses, 930
of water mist, in croup, 935
pressure for, in kyphoscoliosis, 2359
target organ of, 1903
Inhalers, dry powder, in chronic obstructive pulmonary disease, 1220
metered-dose, 248–249, 355–356
for chronic obstructive pulmonary disease, 1220–1224, 1220t
for respiratory failure, 2460–2461, 2461t
for status asthmaticus, 2454–2455
usage guidelines for, 1220–1221, 1220t
powder, 356
Inheritance. See *Genetics.*
Inherited disease(s). See *Genetic disease(s); Genetics.*
Injury. See *Lung injury; Trauma.*
Innate immune response, 2224
Innervation, of airways. See *Airway(s), autonomic innervation of.*
of cough, 553–554
of diaphragm, 2330, 2330t
of larynx, 251, 1351
of lung, 21–22, *21*, *23*, 232, 570
of pleura, 1998
of pulmonary circulation, 121, 131
of respiratory muscles, 2330, 2330t
of trachea, 22
of viscera, 569
Inotropic agents, in pulmonary edema, 1603–1604
Insecticide poisoning, respiratory function in, 1909, 2343
InSight asymmetric film-screen system, 640, *640*
Inspection, of chest, 596–597, 599t
Inspiration, chest radiography during, 646, *646–650*
control of, dorsal respiratory group in, 185–186
flow-volume curves for, 788, *788*
in cough, 555, *555*, 556
inhibition of, in disease states, mechanical aspects of, 112
muscles of, 2330, 2330t
training of, in neuromuscular disorders, 2346–2347
time of, in minute ventilation calculation, 180–181, *181*
Inspiratory airflow, 1344–1345, *1345*
at larynx, 1353
in exercise, in chronic obstructive pulmonary disease, 215
in mechanical ventilation, 2477
for asthma, 2458–2459, *2458*
Inspiratory axons, in breathing control, 187–188, *187*
Inspiratory capacity, definition of, 2563
in interstitial pulmonary disease, 225
measurement of, 790–791
Inspiratory duty cycle, in chronic obstructive pulmonary disease, 215
Inspiratory neurons, in medulla, 185–186
Inspiratory occlusion pressure, measurement of, 819–820, *820*
Inspiratory pressure, at airway opening, 2450–2451, *2451*
in status asthmaticus, 2458–2459, *2458*
maximal. See *Maximal inspiratory pressure.*
maximum negative, in respiratory muscle fatigue, 2383
versus volume, normal values for, 875
Inspiratory reserve volume, definition of, 57, *57*, *783*, 2563
Inspiratory residual capacity, normal, *57*
Inspired volume, definition of, 2564
Institute of Genomic Research, data bases of, 51, 52t
Insulation, man-made fibers in, in pneumoconiosis, 1831t, 1841–1842
Insulin, decrease of, in exercise, 201
receptor for, 238–239
Insulin-like growth factors, 504–505
in lung cancer growth, 1381
Integrins, α3β1, in lung development, 40
defects of, 2233t, 2238
down-regulation of, metastasis in, 1387
in asthma, 1261
Intensity, of lung sounds, 592
Intensive care unit, airway management in, bronchoscopy in, 753
care goals of, 2487–2488
chest radiography in, 665
communication in, 2495
economic costs of, 2487
ethical considerations in. See *Ethics.*
euthanasia in, 2500–2501
evolution of, 2487
length of stay in, versus mortality rate, 2489
life support decision making in, withdrawing, 2498–2500
withholding, 2496–2498
mortality rates in, 2488–2489
nonmaleficence principle violation in, 2491
patient preferences in, 2489–2490
pediatric, bronchoscopy in, 753
physician preferences in, 2489–2490
prognosis prediction in, 2488–2490
radiography equipment for, 637, *637–639*, 639–640
Intensive care unit *(Continued)*
respiratory failure management in, 2377–2410
circulation interactions in, 2386–2407, *2386*
oxygen transport and, 2405–2407, *2405*, 2406t
pulmonary, 2393–2398, *2394–2396*, 2395t, *2398*
shock and, 2398–2405, 2399t, *2400*, 2401t–2403t, *2402*
venous return and, 2386–2389, *2387*, *2388*, 2389t, *2390*
ventricular dysfunction and, 2389–2393, *2391*, *2392*, 2393t
hypoxemic versus ventilatory, 2378–2381, 2378t, *2379*, *2381*, 2382t
in hypoperfusion, 2383
in shock, 2383
perioperative, 2381–2383, 2382t
respiratory muscle considerations in, 2383, *2384*, 2385
Intercellular adhesion molecule, in asthma, 1261
Interception, in aerosol deposition, 351, *351*
Intercostal arteries, in pleural blood supply, 1996–1997, *1997*
Intercostal muscles, function of, 2330–2331, 2330t
mechanical properties of, 107–108
paralysis of, in spinal cord injury, 2339
receptors in, 184
Intercostal region, neuritic pain in, 577
Interferon(s), in common cold, 933
in influenza, 953
of T lymphocytes, 432–434, *433*
Interferon-α, in allergic granulomatosis and angiitis, 1770
in carcinoid tumors, 1462
in hypereosinophilic syndrome, 1769
Interferon-τ, deficiency of, asthma and, 1251
in asthma, 1257–1258, *1257–1259*
in fibrosis, 503–504
in mesothelioma, 2070
in pleural fluid, 2006, 2022
in toxoplasmosis, 1148
Interferon-gamma-inducible protein, 508, 508t
in pulmonary fibrosis, 514, *514*, 516
receptor for, 511–512, 511t
Interleukin(s), as inflammatory mediators, 258, *258*
in allergic rhinitis, 1348
in asthma, 288, 1256–1258, *1257–1259*, 1259t
in Castleman's disease, 1460
in eosinophil development, 1757–1758
in eosinophilic pneumonia, 1766–1767
in influenza, 953
in JAK-STAT activation, 260–261, *261*
in pulmonary edema, high-altitude, 1935
in systemic sclerosis, 1692
inhibitors of, in asthma, 288
of eosinophils, 1759, 1759t, 1760
of T lymphocytes, 432–434, *433*
receptors for, 238
mutations of, in severe combined immunodeficiency, 2239
Interleukin-1, 499–501
in silicosis, 1819
tumor necrosis factor-α synergism with, 502
Interleukin-1α, 499–501
Interleukin-1β, 499–501
Interleukin-1 receptor antagonist, 499–501
Interleukin-2, pulmonary disease due to, 1978
Interleukin-3, in macrophage development, 404
Interleukin-4, in fibrosis, 503–504

Interleukin-5, in asthma, 287
in fibrosis, 503–504
Interleukin-8, 508–511, 508t
in chronic obstructive pulmonary disease, 287
in pulmonary fibrosis, 512–514, *513–515*
receptor for, 511–512, 511t
Interleukin-10, secretion of, theophylline effects on, 273
Interlobar effusion, of lung, 1481
Interlobular septal thickening, computed tomography of, 674, *674*
Intermittent mandatory ventilation, in flail chest, 2368
Intermittent positive-pressure ventilation, after abdominal surgery, 886t
in chronic obstructive pulmonary disease, 1228
in kyphoscoliosis, 2363
International Labour Organization, pneumoconiosis radiography classification of, 1813, 1815
International Normalized Ratio, as anticoagulant effect unit, 1519
Internet, genetic disease resources on, 51–52, 52t
Interstitial lung disease(s), 1649–1670
alveolar clearance in, 373t
alveolar proteinosis as. See *Alveolar proteinosis.*
amyloid. See under *Amyloidosis.*
bronchiolitis with, 1672t, 1684–1686, *1685*
bronchoscopy in, 751–753, 751t
chemotherapy-induced, 1974, *1975*
chest radiography of, 1656–1659, *1658–1661*, 1658t
classification of, 1650 1655, *1650*, *1651*, 1652t, 1653t, *1654*, *1655*
clinical features of, 1672t
collagen degradation defects in, 393
computed tomography in, 674, *674*, *675*
cough in, 561
definition of, 1649–1650, *1650*
diagnosis of, 1655–1667
biopsy in, 1666
bronchoalveolar lavage in, 1665–1666
functional assessment in, 1661–1664, *1664–1666*
history in, 1656
laboratory findings in, 1664, 1667t
physical findings in, 1656, 1657t
radiography in, 1656–1661, *1658–1665*, 1658t, 1660t
symptoms in, 1655–1656
diffuse alveolar damage as, 1650, *1651*, 1653t
diffuse alveolar hemorrhage as. See *Alveolar hemorrhage, diffuse.*
diffusing capacity in, 816
drug-induced, 479t
exercise in, 1664, *1665*
exercise testing in, 225–226, 225t, 848
fibrosis as. See *Fibrosis, idiopathic pulmonary; Fibrosis, interstitial.*
genetic factors in, 1656
granulomatous. See *Granuloma(s); Granulomatosis.*
honeycomb lung as, 1653, 1653t, *1654*
hypersensitivity pneumonitis as, 1872–1873
impairment and disability evaluation in, 908
in ankylosing spondylitis, 2370
in HIV infection, 2208–2209, *2208*
in inflammatory bowel disease, 2270–2271, 2270t
in primary biliary cirrhosis, 2275
in sickle cell disease, 2289
Interstitial lung disease(s) *(Continued)*
in Sjögren's syndrome, 1705–1706
lymphangio(leio)myomatosis as. See *Lymphangio(leio)myomatosis.*
nonspecific pneumonitis as, 1652, 1653t, *1654*
organizing pneumonia as. See *Bronchiolitis obliterans organizing pneumonia.*
overlap among, *1650*
pathogenesis of, interferons in, 503
interleukin-1 family in, 500
pathology of, 1672t
pathophysiology of, 496, *496*
pneumonia as, acute, 459, *462*, 1672t, 1686
clinical features of, 1672t
desquamative, 1651–1652, 1653t, *1654*, 1672t, 1684–1686
eosinophilic, 1653t, 1654
in cystic fibrosis, 1294
lymphocytic, 1653–1654, 1653t, 1687, 1687t, 1705–1706, *1706*
nonspecific, 1672t, 1687–1688
pathology of, 1672t
types of, 1672t
usual, 1652–1653, 1653t, *1654*, 1672t, 1677
primary, 1652t
pulmonary function tests in, 848
sarcoidosis as. See *Sarcoidosis.*
smoking and, 1656
surfactant alterations in, 319–320
tissue inhibitors of metalloproteinases excess in, 393
treatment of, 359
ventilation-perfusion scanning in, 713
Interstitial macrophages, *388*, 394–396
Interstitium. See also subjects starting with *Interstitial.*
compliance of, 137–138, *137*
composition of, 137
disorders of. See *Interstitial lung disease(s).*
pressures in, 136, *137*, 138
Interview, medical, 586. See also *Medical history.*
Intestine(s), cystic fibrosis of, pathology of, 1295
Intra-breath method, for diffusing capacity measurement, 812–813
Intracellular receptors, 240–241, *241*
Intracranial pressure, increased, in mountain sickness, 1930
neurogenic pulmonary edema in, 147
Intrapleural pressure. See *Pleural pressure.*
Intrathoracic pressure, versus diffusing capacity, 815
Intravascular macrophages, 397
Intubation, endotracheal. See *Endotracheal intubation.*
Inverse agonists, drugs as, 244
Iodine, radiolabeled, in lung metabolic studies, 720
Iodoamphetamine, radiolabeled, in lung metabolic studies, 720
Ion channels, 246–247, *246*. See also *Chloride channels; Sodium channels; Potassium channels.*
as receptors, 240, *240*
ATP-sensitive, 247
calcium, 246, *246*
in signal transduction, 238
N-type, 246
receptor-coupled, 247
T-type, 246
voltage-gated, 247
voltage-sensitive (L-type), 246, *246*
Ion transport, transepithelial. See *Epithelium and epithelial cells, airway, electrolyte transport across.*
IPF. See *Fibrosis, idiopathic pulmonary.*
Ipratropium bromide, as bronchodilator, 276
in allergic rhinitis, 1349
in asthma, 357, 2454t, 2455
in chronic obstructive pulmonary disease, 277, 357, 1221–1222, 2461, 2461t
in common cold, 933
in cough, in rhinosinus conditions, 563
postinfectious, 564
in respiratory failure, 2461, 2461t
in status asthmaticus, 2454t, 2455
inhalation of, 1221
mechanism of action of, 1221
preparations for, 1221
side effects of, 277, 1221
Irinotecan, in lung cancer, 1437, 1437t
Iron, accumulation of, in hemosiderosis, 1741–1742, *1741*
cell injury in, 450, *452*
diffuse alveolar hemorrhage in, 1734
analogues of, gallium as, 700–701
pneumoconiosis from, *1814*, 1842
Iron and steel industry, lung cancer in, 1402
Irritable bowel syndrome, hyperalgesia in, 571, *571*
pain distribution in, 574, *574*
Irritant gases, asthma due to, 1854, 1855
bronchiolitis due to, 1362, *1362*
bronchitis due to, 1214–1215, *1215*
clearance of, 372–373, 373t
in cholinergic reflex activation, 254
lung cancer due to, 1402
lung injury due to, 1905t. See also specific substances.
pathogenesis of, 1903–1904
pathology of, 478t
sequelae of, 1904–1905
treatment of, 1904
Irritant receptors, 182–183, 182t, *183*, 575
for cough reflex, 553–554, *555*
IRV (inspiratory reserve volume), 57, *57*, *783*, 2563
$I_{SC}$ (short-circuit current), of epithelium, 335
Ischemia, lung injury in, 465, *465*
myocardial. See *Myocardial ischemia.*
Isocapnic buffering, 205–206
in exercise, 211
Isocyanate exposure, 1909–1910
asthma due to, 1855, 1857, 1858t
hypersensitivity pneumonitis due to, 1869–1870
Isoetharine, in asthma, 2454
Isoflurane, pulmonary function effects of, 884–885
Isofosamide, in lung cancer, 1439
Isolator method, for fungal culture, 621
Isoniazid, in *Mycobacterium kansasii* infections, 1095, 2186
in tuberculosis, 1066–1067, 1068t
central nervous system, 1084
drug-resistant, 1073t
in HIV infection, 2183–2184
latent, 1086–1088, *1087*
prophylactic, 1088–1089
regimen for, 1071–1072, 1071t
resistance to, 1067, 1073t
side effects of, 1067, 1068t
transmission risk and, 1054
Isopropyl alcohol toxicity, anion gap acidosis due to, 168
Isoprostanes, as inflammatory mediators, 257
Isoproterenol, as vasodilator, 300
chemical structure of, 268, *268*
in asthma, mortality from, 1248
ventilation-perfusion ratio changes due to, 83, *84*

Isoproterenol *(Continued)*
in cardiac arrhythmias, 2403t
in chronic obstructive pulmonary disease, 1220
in pulmonary edema, 1603
mechanisms of action of, 268
Isosorbide dinitrate, as vasodilator, 301
in pulmonary edema, 1602
Isothiocyanates, exposure to, 1909–1910
Isotype switching, of immunoglobulins, 419–420, *420*
Isovolume pressure-flow curves, 787–790, *787–790*
Itch, ground, in hookworm disease, 1151
swimmer's, in schistosomiasis, 1164
Itraconazole, in allergic bronchopulmonary aspergillosis, 1132, 1766
in aspergillosis, 1133, 1134, 2198t, 2201
in blastomycosis, 1121, 2198t, 2201
in coccidioidomycosis, 1127
in histoplasmosis, 1116, 1117, 2198t, 2199
in paracoccidioidomycosis, 1129
in penicilliosis, 2198t, 2201
Ivermectin, in filariasis, 1155
in strongyloidiasis, 1152–1153

## J

J receptors, 183, 570, 575
of lung, 570
JAK-STAT pathways, in transcription, 260–261, *261*
Janus kinases, in transcription, 260–261, *261*
Jo antigen, antibodies to, in polymyositis, 1708
Jobs. See *Occupation(s); Occupational and environmental disorder(s).*
Job's syndrome, 2233t, 2238
Joint(s), coccidioidomycosis of, 1125
decompression sickness effects on, 1961
inflammation of. See *Arthritis; Hypertrophic pulmonary osteoarthropathy.*
tuberculosis of, 1081–1083, *1082*
Jugular ganglia, in visceral innervation, 569
Jun transcription factor, in signal transduction, 239–240, *239*
Junctional complexes, of airway epithelial cells, 7, *9*
Justice, as ethical principle, 2492

## K

Kampmeier's foci, in pleura, 1998
Kanamycin, in tuberculosis, 1069t, 1070
Kaolin, in pneumoconiosis, 1841
Kaposi's sarcoma, 2204–2206
chest radiography of, 2205, *2205*
clinical features of, 2205
diagnosis of, 2205–2206, *2206*
epidemiology of, 2204
lung pathology in, 471, *472*
of bronchi, 1367
physical examination in, 2176
pleural effusion in, 2025, 2205–2206
risk factors for, 2175
treatment of, 2206
ventilation-perfusion scanning in, 712
virus causing, 512, 2204–2205
Kartagener's syndrome, ciliary dyskinesia in, 366
lung injury in, 482
Kartagener's triad, 1336
Karyotyping, 45–46
Kedem-Katchalsky equation, for solute flux, 133
Keratoconjunctivitis sicca, in Sjögren's syndrome, 1705
Kerley's B lines, in interstitial lung disease, 1657, *1659*, 1660t
Ketoacidosis, diabetic, 166–167, *167*
rhinocerebral mucormycosis in, 1134
Ketoconazole, in acute respiratory distress syndrome, 2423
in histoplasmosis, 1117
in paracoccidioidomycosis, 1129
side effects of, 1117
Ketotifen, in asthma, 284
Khellin, cromolyn derived from, 283
Kidney, angiomyolipomas of, 1784
drug excretion from, 248
dysfunction/failure of, 2278–2280. See also *Glomerulonephritis.*
calcification in, 2312, *2312*
hypoxemia in, 2279–2280
in hantavirus infections, 945–947
in immunosuppressive therapy, 2526
in sarcoidosis, 1719
in tuberculosis, 1080–1081
metabolic alkalosis in, 171t, 172–173
mortality prediction in, 2489
pleural disease in, 2279
pleural effusion in, 2016, 2034
pulmonary calcification in, 2279
pulmonary edema in, 1499t, 1603, 2278–2279
renal tubular acidosis in, 168–169, 169t
sleep apnea in, 2279
thrombocytopenia in, 2295
uremic acidosis in, 167–168
in compensation for acid-base imbalance, 162–163
transplantation of, pneumonia in, 2228–2229
*KIT* gene and product, in lung cancer growth, 1381
*Klebsiella* infections, surfactant protein A binding in, 312
*Klebsiella pneumoniae* pneumonia, 998t, 1008–1009, *1009*
Koplik's spots, in measles, 958
Korean hemorrhagic fever, 945–947
*KRAS* gene and product, in lung cancer growth, 1381
Krogh equation, for diffusing capacity, 811
Krypton 81m, in ventilation-perfusion scanning, 699
preoperative, 714–715
Kussmaul's breathing, in metabolic acidosis, 161, 170
inspection of, 597
Kveim test, in sarcoidosis, 1724–1726
Kyphoscoliosis, 2357–2363
ankylosing spondylitis with, 2369
breathing control and patterns in, 2360, 2361
clinical course of, 2361–2362, *2362*, 2362t
diagnosis of, 2357–2358, *2358*, 2358t
etiology of, 2357–2358, *2358*, 2358t
exercise capacity in, 2360–2361, 2361t
gas exchange in, 2360
idiopathic, 2357
in Marfan's syndrome, 1711
in multiple myeloma, 2293
pathophysiology of, 2358–2361, 2359t, *2360*, 2361t
physical examination in, 2357–2358
pulmonary function in, 2358–2359, 2359t
respiratory mechanics in, 2359, 2359t, *2360*
respiratory muscle function in, 2359–2360
secondary, 2357–2358, 2358t
sleep-disordered breathing in, 2361
treatment of, 2362–2363, 2363t
Kyphoscoliosis *(Continued)*
ventilatory failure in, 2332

## L

Labetalol, pulmonary disease due to, 1983
Labor and delivery, acute respiratory distress syndrome in, 2324
air embolism in, 2324
amniotic fluid embolism in, 2323–2324, *2324*
aspiration pneumonitis in, 2324
cardiomyopathy and, 2321
in asthma, 2319–2320
in cystic fibrosis, 2320
pneumonia in, 2320–2321
pulmonary embolism in, 2322–2323
Laboratory tests, clinical usefulness of, 587t
Labrador lung, 1842
Lactate dehydrogenase, in HIV infection, 2176
in pleural fluid, 2003
Lactate paradox, in exercise, at high altitude, 1928
Lactate:pyruvate ratio, calculation of, 208
Lactation, tuberculosis in, treatment of, 1074
Lactic acid, antilipolytic effect of, 201
buffering of, 200, *200*, 205–206, *206*
concentration of, versus production, 206
dissociation of, 200
measurement of, 165
production of, in exercise, 199–200, *200*, 839–840
heavy, 204
in chronic obstructive pulmonary disease, 216
in heart failure, 2260
in exercise testing, 845–846, *846*, *847*
in respiratory failure, 2405–2407, *2405*, 2406t
versus consumption, 208
Lactic acid (anaerobic) threshold, 839–840
causes of, 206–208
enzymatic rate limitation as, 208
fiber-type muscle composition as, 208
oxygen availability limitation as, 206–207, *207*
production-consumption imbalance as, 208
definition of, 201
in exercise, 206–208, *207*, 845–846, *846*, *847*
in interstitial pulmonary disease, 225
lactic acid production in, 166
ventilatory, 840
Lactic acidosis, 164–166, *165*, 166t
in asthma, 2453
in exercise, 839, *839*
in respiratory failure, 2407
treatment of, 171
Lactoferrin, gallium binding to, in ventilation-perfusion scanning, 701
in mucus, 331
Lambert-Eaton syndrome, in lung cancer, 1379
respiratory function in, 2342
Lamellar bodies, of alveolar epithelial cells, 17, *18*, 19
surfactant secretion from, 316, *317*, *389*
Laminar flow, 97
Laparoscopy, abdominal, pulmonary function effects of, 886
Laplace relationship, in alveolar function, 92
in diaphragm motion, 106
Large cell lung cancer. See *Lung cancer, non-small cell.*
Larva(e), *Ascaris lumbricoides*, 1149–1150, 1761

Larva(e) *(Continued)*
hookworm, 1150–1151
*Paragonimus westermani*, 1160–1163
*Schistosoma*, 1163–1165
*Strongyloides stercoralis*, 1151–1152, *1152*
*Toxocara canis*, 1157
*Trichinella spiralis*, 1156–1157
Larva currens, in strongyloidiasis, 1151, 1152
Larva migrans, visceral, 1157
Laryngeal nerve(s), entrapment of, in mediastinitis, 2114
Laryngitis, viral, 934, 948–949
Laryngoscopy, in epiglottitis, 918
Laryngotracheitis, 918
Laryngotracheobronchitis. See *Croup*.
Larynx, 1351–1354
airflow in, 1343–1345, *1343–1345*
anatomy of, 1343–1344, *1343*
bronchoscopy of, 732
burn injury of, 754
cough reflex receptors in, 553, 554
disorders of, 1351–1354, 1354t
function of, 1351, *1352*, *1353*
innervation of, 251, 1351
muscles surrounding, 1346t
narrowing of, muscles in, 1346t
obstruction of, 1351–1354, 1354t
papillomatosis of, 1478
receptors in, 182
spasm of, 1353–1354
structure of, 1351, *1352*, *1353*
Laser therapy, for emphysema, 1218
for lung cancer, in palliation, 742
rigid bronchoscopy with, 727
Lassa fever, pharyngitis in, 933
Lavage, bronchoalveolar. See *Bronchoalveolar lavage*.
whole-lung, in alveolar proteinosis, 1796–1800, *1799*
Lead, as air pollutant, standards for, 2556
Lecithin:sphingomyelin ratio, in neonatal respiratory distress syndrome diagnosis, 317
Lectins, albumin binding to, 141
antibodies to, in amebiasis, 1144
Leeuwenhoek's disease, 2349t, 2350
Left atrial (outflow) pressure, definition of, 2565
in pulmonary vascular resistance calculation, 123–124
versus edema formation, 145, *145*
versus pulmonary artery wedge pressure, 123
versus pulmonary vascular resistance, 126, *126*, *127*
Legal issues, in asbestosis, 1835–1836
in ethical decision making, court decisions as, 2492–2494
governmental legislation and regulations as, 2494
in pneumoconiosis, 1816
in smoking, 2532–2533
*Legionella* infections, nonpneumophila, 1014, 2302–2304
pneumonia due to, 1014–1017
bronchoscopy in, 749
clinical manifestations of, 1014–1015, *1015*, 1015t
complications of, 1016
diagnosis of, 743t, 920
epidemiology of, 1014
extrapulmonary features of, 1014, 1014t
genetic tests for, 626
in bone marrow transplantation, 2302–2304
in HIV infection, 2180
*Legionella* infections *(Continued)*
in transplantation, 2229
microbiologic diagnosis of, 609–613, 610t, 1015–1016, *1016*
culture in, 617, 618t
direct immunofluorescence assay in, 616
specimen processing for, 989–990
mortality in, 1016
prevention of, 1016–1017
prognosis for, 1016
risk factors for, 920, 1014
serologic evaluation of, 991
treatment of, 998t, 1016–1017
Pontiac fever due to, 1014
species causing, 1014
*Legionella micdadei* pneumonia, in bone marrow transplantation, 2302–2304
Leiomyoma(s), benign metastasizing, 1480
endobronchial, 1478
of lung, 1479
Leiomyosarcoma(s), gastric, in Carney's triad, 1480, *1481*
Lemierre's syndrome, 1017
Length density, in lung quantitative morphology, 25–26
Leucovorin, in *Pneumocystis carinii* pneumonia, 2191t
in toxoplasmosis, 2204
Leukapheresis, in leukemia, 2291
Leukemia(s), alveolar proteinosis in, 1793
bronchial involvement in, 1367
diffuse alveolar hemorrhage in, 1744
hyperleukocytic syndrome in, 2291
infiltrates in, 2291–2292
Leukocyte(s). See also specific cells, e.g., *Granulocyte(s); Neutrophil(s)*.
accumulation of, in asthma, 1261
count of, in HIV infection, 2176
in pleural fluid, 2003–2004
in sputum, 614, *614*
indium 111–labeled, in ventilation-perfusion scanning, 711–712, *712*
iron-binding proteins in, ventilation-perfusion scanning and, 701
recruitment of, in injury, 495–496, *496*
Leukocyte adhesion defects, 2233t, 2238
Leukocytoclastic vasculitis, 1534, 1539
Leukocytosis, 2291
in leukemia, 2291
in pneumonia, in immunodeficiency, 924
Leukopenia, 2291
in hemodialysis, 2280
in measles, 958
Leukostasis, contrast agent-induced, 1988
in leukemia, 2291
Leukotriene(s), action of, 232, *233*
antagonists of, in asthma, 2456
pulmonary disease due to, 1985
as inflammatory mediators, 257
biologic effects of, 497–499, 497t
eosinophil, 1759, 1759t, 1760
in bronchoconstriction, 257
in electrolyte transport, in airway epithelium, 338
in mucus hypersecretion, 334
in pulmonary vascular resistance control, 131
inhibitors of, in asthma, 284–286, *284*, 498
Leukotriene receptor antagonists, allergic granulomatosis and angiitis due to, 1770–1771
in asthma, 284–286, *284*
Levcromakalim, action of, 247, 277
Levofloxacin, in legionellosis, 995t
Lidocaine, contraindicated in asthma, 291
Lidocaine *(Continued)*
for bronchoscopy, 731, 732t, 733, 755–756, 756t
in shock, 2403t
mucosal absorption of, 755
Life support, decision making concerning, advance directives for, 2494
communication in, 2499
competency determination in, 2498–2499
do-not-resuscitate orders and, 2497–2498
ethical principles for, 2495–2496, 2495t
euthanasia and, 2500–2501
for incompetent persons, 2493–2494
government legislation and regulations in, 2494
in medical futility, 2498
legal precedents in, 2492–2494
physician attitudes toward, 2490
surrogates for, 2493, 2499, 2500
time-limited goals for, 2499
withdrawing of, advanced, 2498–2500
basic, 2500
before organ donation, 2496
in brain death, 2496
withholding of, advanced, 2497–2498
basic, 2496–2497
Lifeguard lung, 1868
Likelihood ratio, in linkage analysis, 49
Limit variable, in mechanical ventilation, 2471, *2472*, 2473t
Line stratification scheme, for interstitial pneumonitis, 713
Linear attenuation coefficient, in computed tomography, 661
Linkage analysis, in genetic disease, 46, 49–50, 51t, 1252–1253
Linkage disequilibrium mapping, in genetic disease, 50
Lipid(s). See also specific types, e.g., *Phospholipid(s)*.
accumulation of, in lung, 454–455, *454*, *455*
aerosol, clearance of, 354–355
alveolar macrophage recognition of, 390, *391*
deposition of, in alveolar proteinosis, 1789–1790, *1791*
drug solubility in, 247–248
in mucus, 331
in pleural fluid. See *Chylothorax*.
in surfactant, 309, 309t
Lipoid pneumonia, 1481
Lipoid proteinosis, 480t
Lipoma(s), of bronchi, 1478
of lung, 1479
of mediastinum, 2129, *2129*
Lipomatosis, mediastinal, 2129
corticosteroid-induced, 1985, *1986*
Lipopolysaccharide. See *Endotoxin*.
Lipoxygenase pathway, inhibitors of, in asthma, 284–286, *284*
products of, biologic effects of, 497–499, 497t
endothelial permeability and, 142, *143*
in mucus hypersecretion, 334
Liquefaction necrosis, 446, *448*
Liquid ventilation, partial, in acute respiratory distress syndrome, 2434
*Listeria monocytogenes*, leukocyte cell action on, 397
Liver, drug metabolism in, 248
glycogen storage in, 200–201
transplantation of, in hepatopulmonary syndrome, 2274
in portopulmonary hypertension, 2275
pleural effusion in, 2030
pneumonia in, 2229

Liver disease(s), 2271–2276. See also *Alpha$_1$-antitrypsin, deficiency of.*
abscess as, amebic, 1144–1146, *1145*, 2025
bronchial fistula as, 1144–1146
chronic active hepatitis as, 2276
cirrhosis as. See *Cirrhosis.*
cystic fibrosis as, clinical manifestations of, 1306–1307
pathology of, 1295
treatment of, 1312–1313
hepatopulmonary syndrome as, 2271–2274, *2272*, *2273*
hyperventilation in, 2146–2147
paracoccidioidomycosis as, 1128
parasitic, echinococcosis as, 1157–1160
schistosomiasis as, 1163–1165
pleural effusion in, 2271
portopulmonary hypertension in, 2274–2275
pulmonary function tests in, 2271
pulmonary hypertension in, 1546
Q fever as, 1026
sarcoidosis as, 1719
sclerosing cholangitis as, 2276
Living wills, 2494
*Loa loa* infections, 1153–1155
Lobectomy, in bronchiectasis, 1332
in cancer, 1427, 1431–1432
occult, 1428
stage IA and IB, 1428–1429
stage IIA, 1429
stage IIB, 1429–1430
in echinococcosis, 1160
mortality in, 1427
physiologic changes after, 889
"toilet," in cancer, 1431–1432
ventilation-perfusion scanning before, 714
LOD (logarithm of the odds) score, in linkage analysis, 49
Loeffler's syndrome, 1760, 1761–1762, 1761t
in ascariasis, 1150, 1761
in hookworm disease, 1150
in strongyloidiasis, 1152
Löfgren's syndrome, 1718, *1719*
Logarithm of the odds score, in linkage analysis, 49
Loratadine, in allergic rhinitis, 1349
Lorazepam, in hiccups, 2350
Lordotic view, in radiography, 654
Losartan, in pulmonary hypertension, 1645
Loss modulus, of mucus, 364
Loss of heterozygosity, in lung cancer, 1417
Lower respiratory tract. See specific structures and diseases, e.g., *Lung*; *Pneumonia.*
Low-molecular-weight bronchial inhibitor, in mucus, 329
Lucency. See *Lung, hyperlucent.*
Lung. See also subjects starting with *Pulmonary;* components, e.g., *Alveolus(i).*
abscess of. See *Abscess(es), lung.*
accessory bud formation in, sequestration development in, 1566
adenocarcinoma of. See *Lung cancer, adenocarcinoma as.*
adenomas of, pathology of, 483t
aerosol deposition in, 352–354, *352*, *353*
amyloidosis of, nodular, 1481, 1481t
pathology of, 450, 454, *454*
anatomy of, 3–33
airway, 5–11, *7–12*
circulatory, 11–15, *11*, 12t, *13–15*
gross, 3–5, *4–7*, 5t
lymphatic, 22–23
neural, 21–22, *21*, *23*
quantitative morphologic, 23–29, *24–28*
subgross, 3–5, *4–7*, 5t
terminal respiratory units, 15–21, *16–18*, 20t

Lung *(Continued)*
angioimmunoblastic lymphadenopathy of, 1459–1460
arteriolitis of, in schistosomiasis, 1164
aspiration from, transthoracic, in pneumonia, 992–993
baby, in pulmonary edema, 1586
bacterial infections of. See *Pneumonia, pyogenic;* specific diseases.
barotrauma of, 1955–1956, *1956*
biopsy of. See *Biopsy, lung.*
bird breeder's. See *Hypersensitivity pneumonitis.*
black. See *Coal-workers' pneumoconiosis.*
blastomas of, 1463
blood flow in. See *Pulmonary circulation, blood flow in.*
blood supply of. See *Bronchial circulation*; *Pulmonary circulation.*
bronchiectasis in. See *Bronchiectasis.*
bullae of, impairment in, 909
in cancer, 1195
in chronic obstructive pulmonary disease, 1194–1195, *1195*, *1196*, 1205, 2049
surgery for, 1219–1220
pulmonary function testing in, 853
calcification of. See *Calcification, of lung.*
cancer of. See *Lung cancer.*
carcinoma *in situ* of, 1377–1378
carcinosarcomas of, 1462, 1463
Castleman's disease of, 1460
cavitation of. See *Cavitation.*
cells of, 232, *233*
chemodectomas of, 1481
chemoreceptors of, 570
chondromas of, 1478, 1480, *1481*
circulation in. See *Bronchial circulation, Pulmonary circulation.*
clear cell tumors of, 1479–1480
collapse of. See also *Atelectasis.*
in pneumothorax, calculation of, 2046
re-expansion of, pulmonary edema after, 2055–2056
compliance of. See *Lung compliance.*
congenital malformations of, 482
congestion of, in kidney failure, 2279
connective tissue disease effects on. See specific diseases, e.g., *Rheumatoid arthritis; Systemic lupus erythematosus.*
connective tissue of, 4, *5*, 5t, *6*, 93. See also *Collagen(s).*
alveolar septa as, 126
consolidation of. See *Consolidation.*
contusion of, hypoxemia in, 2416
treatment of, 2436–2437
cystic fibrosis of. See *Cystic fibrosis.*
cysts of. See *Cyst(s), lung.*
dendritic cells of, 386, 389, 396–397
denervation of, after transplantation, 2525–2526
density of, 4, 1596
development of, branching morphogenesis in, 36, *36*
bronchial circulation importance in, 121
canalicular stage of, 36
defects in, 40–42
embryonic stage of, 35–36
epithelial-mesenchymal interactions in, 36, *36*, 37, *37*
genes in, for cell specification, 42
in early stages, 37–40, *37*
in later stages, 40, *40*
histologic stages of, 35–36
initiation of, 36–37, *37*
lung cancer types and, 1376
macrophages and, 397–399

Lung *(Continued)*
nutrition effects on, 486
overview of, 35
postnatal, 36
pseudoglandular stage of, 36
thyroid hormones in, 2311
Web site on, 35
drug metabolism in, 1972
dust accumulation in. See *Pneumoconiosis(es).*
edema of. See *Pulmonary edema.*
elastance of. See *Elastance.*
elastic recoil of. See *Elastic recoil.*
electron microscopy of, *1488*
embolism in. See *Pulmonary embolism.*
embryology of. See *Lung, development of.*
endometriomas of, 1480
farmer's. See *Hypersensitivity pneumonitis.*
fibromas of, 1478, 1479
fibrosis of. See *Fibrosis.*
fibrous histiocytomas of, 1480
fluid and solute exchange in. See *Fluid and solute exchange; Pulmonary edema.*
fungal infections of. See *Fungal infection(s);* specific diseases.
gangrene of, in pneumonia, 1009
gas exchange in. See *Gas exchange.*
glomus tumors of, 1478
graft-versus-host disease of, 468, *470*
granulomas of. See *Granuloma(s); Granulomatosis.*
ground-glass opacity of, 675–676, *676*, 678
growth of. See *Lung, development of.*
hamartomas of, 667, *669*, 1478–1479, *1479*
hemangiomas of, sclerosing, 1479
hematomas of, 1481
hemorrhage of. See also *Alveolar hemorrhage.*
drug-induced, 479t
in galloping racehorses, 69
in influenza, 951, *952*
hemosiderosis of, 1741–1742, *1741*
hilum of, masses of, 672–673, *673*, *674*
histiocytomas of, 1480
histology of, 93
honeycomb, 459, *461*, 1653, 1653t, *1654*, 1657–1658, *1660*, 1660t
humidifier, 1868
hyperinflation of, 2518
as defense mechanism, 1266
in bronchiolitis obliterans, 1363
in cystic fibrosis, 1303
hyperlucent, causes of, 646, *648–650*
in bronchiolitis obliterans, 936, 1363
unilateral, 1197, 1197t, 1337
hypoplasia of, 1198
immune response in. See *Immune response, in lung.*
infarction of, coagulation necrosis in, *447*
in pulmonary embolism, 1506
in sickle cell disease, 2288
pathology of, 465, *465*
versus tumor, 1481
infections of, bacterial. See *Pneumonia, pyogenic;* specific diseases.
fungal. See *Fungal infection(s);* specific diseases.
parasitic. See *Parasitic infection(s).*
viral. See *Viral infection(s);* specific diseases.
inflammatory pseudotumors of, 1478
inflation of, in mechanical ventilation, mechanics of, 2474–2476, *2475*, *2476*
injury of. See *Lung injury.*
innervation of, 570
in bronchoconstriction, 232

Lung *(Continued)*
interlobar effusion in, 1481
interstitium of, compliance of, 137–138, *137*
composition of, 137
disease of. See *Interstitial lung disease(s).*
pressures in, 136, *137*
Labrador, 1842
lavage of. See *Bronchoalveolar lavage.*
leiomyomas of, 1478–1480
lifeguard, 1868
lipomas of, 1479
lymphangiectasis of, 483t
lymphatic system of. See *Lymphatic system, of lung.*
lymphoepitheliomas of, 1462–1463, 1462t
lymphomas of, Hodgkin's, 1453–1455, *1454, 1455*
non-Hodgkin's, 1455–1458, 1456t
lymphomatoid granulomatosis of, 1458–1459, *1459*
lymphoproliferative diseases of, 1458–1460, *1459*
macrophages of. See also *Macrophage(s), alveolar.*
airway, definition of, 389–390
development of, 399–407, *400*, 401t, *402*
interstitial, *388*, 394–396
intravascular, 397
morphology of, 387–389, *388–390*
origin of, 397–399
proliferation of, 399
mechanical properties of, 2424, 2426–2427, *2426, 2427*
alveolar, 91–93, *92*
parenchymal, 93–94
pulmonary vascular resistance and, 126, *126, 127*
regional volume and regional ventilation relationships and, 109–111, *110*
meningiomas of, 1479
metabolic properties of, ventilation-perfusion studies of, 720
metastasis from. See *Metastasis(es) (malignancy), from lung.*
metastasis to. See *Metastasis(es) (malignancy), to lung.*
miller's, 1869
mucoepithelial malignancies of, 1462–1463, 1462t
multiple myeloma manifestations in, 1464
mushrooms worker's. See *Hypersensitivity pneumonitis.*
myxomas of, 1478
necrosis of. See *Necrosis.*
neuroendocrine system of, 22, *23*
neuroendocrine tumors of, multiple, 1480–1481
neurofibromas of, 1478, 1479
nodules of. See *Nodule(s).*
overinflation of, capillary stress failure in, 69
congenital, 483t
in chronic obstructive pulmonary disease, 1190, *1190*
pain perception in, 575
papillomas of, 1478
paraffinomas of, 1481
parenchyma of, benign tumors of, 1478–1481, *1479, 1481*
circulation system for, 10–11, 121–122, *122*, 125–126
disorders of, pulmonary hypertension in, 1336–1337
versus pleural disease, 688
endometriosis of, 2325
isolated from airways. See *Sequestration(s), bronchopulmonary.*

Lung *(Continued)*
mechanical properties of, 93–94
pneumomediastinum originating in, 2096t, 2097–2098, *2097, 2098*
perfusion of. See *Pulmonary circulation, blood flow in; Ventilation-perfusion ratio; Ventilation-perfusion screening.*
perfusion scanning of. See *Ventilation-perfusion scanning.*
phantom tumor of, 1481
pigeon fancier's. See *Hypersensitivity pneumonitis.*
plasma cell granulomas of, 1480
plasmacytomas of, 1464, 1480, 2293
pressure-volume curves for, 92, *92*, 93
proteinosis of. See *Alveolar proteinosis, pulmonary.*
pseudolymphomas of, 1480
pseudotumors of, 1480, 1481, 1481t
quantitative morphology of, 23–29
critical data set in, 24
design-based sampling in, 23–24, *24*
fixation in, 23
hierarchical data in, 24
stereology concept in, 23
terminology of, 25–29, *28*
test grid systems in, 24–25, *25–27*
radiography of. See *Chest radiography.*
re-aeration of, after lavage, 1798, *1799*
re-expansion of, pulmonary edema in, 1582–1583
regional variations in, of alveolar carbon dioxide partial pressure, 78, *78*
of alveolar oxygen partial pressure, 78, *78*
of blood flow, 60, *61*, 64–67, *65*, 1489–1490, *1490*, 1491t
of blood pressure, diffusing capacity and, 815–816, *817*
of fluid accumulation sites, 145
of interstitial compliance, 138
of perfusion, 128–129, *129*
of pulmonary artery pressure, 123
of pulmonary vascular resistance, 124–125, *125*
of transpulmonary pressure, 109–111, *110*
of ventilation. See *Ventilation, distribution of.*
of ventilation-perfusion ratio, 80–85, *81, 82, 84*
of volume, 109–111, *110*
remodeling of, macrophages in, 392–393
reperfusion injury of, pathophysiology of, 320
pulmonary edema in, 147, 1523–1524, *1525*, 1582, 2055
resection of. See also *Lobectomy; Pneumonectomy; Segmentectomy.*
complications of, 889
in blastoma, 1463
in bronchiectasis, 1332
in cancer, 1427
in carcinoid tumor, 1461
in carcinosarcoma, 1463
in chronic obstructive pulmonary disease, 1218–1220, 2512
in metastatic cancer, 1474–1475, 1474t
in *Mycobacterium avium* complex infections, 1093
in sarcoma, 1463
in tuberculosis, 1075
in volume reduction. See *Lung volume(s), reduction of, surgical.*
mortality in, 889
preoperative evaluation for, 889–891
with minimum incisions, 889
restriction of, in systemic lupus erythematosus, 1704, *1704*

Lung *(Continued)*
sarcoidosis of. See *Sarcoidosis.*
sarcomas of, 1463
scanning of. See *Ventilation-perfusion scanning.*
schwannomas of, 1479
scintigraphic studies of. See *Radionuclide studies; Ventilation-perfusion scanning.*
sequestrations of. See *Sequestration(s), bronchopulmonary.*
shape of, positional changes in, 93–94
sleeve resection of, in cancer, 1427
solute movement into, for barrier function evaluation, 1597–1598
support of, by pleural pressure, 111
surfactant in. See *Surfactant.*
surgery on. See *Lobectomy; Lung, resection of; Lung volume(s), reduction of, surgical; Pneumonectomy; Segmentectomy.*
telangiectasias of, 1561
teratomas of, 1480
thromboembolism in. See *Pulmonary embolism.*
tissue disposition in, 4, *5*, 5t
transplantation of. See *Lung transplantation.*
trapped, 2036
tumorlets of, 1463–1464, 1480–1481
tumors of. See also *Lung cancer.*
benign, 484t, 1477–1484
classification of, 483t–484t
vanishing, in systemic lupus erythematosus, 1704, *1704*
vanishing tumor of, 1481
ventilation of. See *Ventilation.*
viral infections of. See *Viral infection(s); specific diseases.*
volume of. See *Lung volume(s).*
volutrauma of, in mechanical ventilation, 2424
Waldenström's macroglobulinemia manifestations in, 1464
water content of, 132
measurement of, 1596–1597
weight of, 4
xanthomas of, 1480
Lung bud, 35
Lung cancer, 1415–1451
abscess with, 749, 1020
adenocarcinoma as, chest radiography of, *2087*
classification of, 1417, 1418t, 1419
computed tomography in, *2087*
pathology of, 484t, 486, *488*
smoking and, 1398–1399
adenosquamous, 1419
angiogenesis in, 1387
*BCL2* genes in, 1386
biologic markers for, 1405–1406
biopsy of, metastatic, 1472–1473
open, 763
percutaneous, 760–761
scalene node, 763
transbronchial, 736–737, 738t
blastoma as, 1463
bronchoalveolar carcinoma as, 1419
bronchoalveolar lavage in, 739t, 740
bronchogenic carcinoma as. See *Carcinoma(s), bronchogenic.*
bronchoscopy in. See *Bronchoscopy (flexible fiberoptic or unspecified), in lung cancer.*
bullae and, 1195
carcinogens causing, 1400–1403. See also *Lung cancer, smoking and.*
carcinoid as, 484t, 1419, 1460–1462
carcinoma as. See *Carcinoma(s), bronchogenic.*

Lung cancer *(Continued)*
carcinosarcoma as, 1462, 1463
carotenoids and, 1385
causes of. See also *Lung cancer, smoking and.*
air pollution as, 1888
particulates as, 1891
radon as, 1888
sulfur dioxide as, 1891
chemotherapy for, agents for, 1437, 1437t
dose for, 1439
economic issues in, 1444
in advanced disease, 1437–1438, 1437t, 1438t
maintenance, 1439
postoperative, 1436–1437
preoperative, 1436
radiation therapy with, 1434, 1436–1437
second-line, 1439
small cell, 1434–1435, 1438–1439
versus stage, 1429–1432
chest radiography of, 665
for screening, 1419–1420, 1420t
metastatic, 1471–1472, *1471–1473*, 1472t
classification of, 483t–484t, 1417, 1418t, 1419
clinical features of, 1420–1422, 1420t, 1421t
metastatic, 1471
computed tomography of, 669–670, *670*, *671*, 750
Cushing's syndrome in, 1379
cyclins in, 1383
developmental aspects of, 1376
diagnosis of, 1422–1423, 1422t
chest radiography in, 665, 1471–1472, *1471–1473*, 1472t
mediastinotomy in, 762–763
molecular methods in, 1426, 1426t
screening, 1419–1420, 1420t
differential diagnosis of, metastatic, 1472, 1472t
endoscopically visible, 739–740, *739*, *740*
environmental, 1400–1404
epidemiology of, 1375, 1395–1416, 1416t, 1417t
ethnic factors in, 1396, *1396*, 1398
incidence in, 1395–1396, *1395*, 1396t
international trends in, 1396–1397
mortality in, 1395, *1395*, 1397, 1397t
racial factors in, 1396, *1396*
risk factors in, 1397–1406
survival in, 1397, 1397t
ethnic factors in, 1396, *1396*, 1398, 1417t
evolution of, 1377–1378
extrinsic compression in, biopsy in, 740
familial, 1405, 1416
*FHIT* gene in, 1384
from direct invasion, 1470
gender differences in, 1395–1396, *1395*, 1396t
genetics of, 1405, 1416
Fas and Fas ligand in, 1386–1387
in growth, 1379–1382, *1380*
major histocompatibility complex molecules in, 1386
methylation abnormalities in, 1378
microsatellite instability in, 1378
*MYC* family in, 1382
non–small cell, 1376t, 1377
*RAS* family in, 1381–1382
small cell, 1376t, 1377
telomerase activity in, 1378
transmembrane receptors and ligands in, 1380–1381
tumor suppressor genes in, 1382–1386
growth of, 1379–1382, *1380*

Lung cancer *(Continued)*
*MYC* genes in, 1382
*RAS* genes in, 1381–1382
transmembrane receptors and ligands in, 1380–1381
hemoptysis in, bronchoscopy in, 750–751, 750t
histology of, smoking and, 1398–1399
host factors in, 1386–1387, 1405–1406
hypercalcemia in, 1379
impairment in, 900
in air pollution, 1403
in asbestos exposure, 1836–1837, 1840
in electromagnetic field exposure, 1403–1404
in hard metal disease, 1845
in HIV infection, 2207–2208
bronchogenic carcinoma as, 2207–2208
Kaposi's sarcoma as. See *Kaposi's sarcoma.*
in man-made vitreous fiber exposure, 1842
in nonsmokers with environmental exposure, 1399–1400
in silicosis, 1822–1823
invasion of, chest wall, 670–671, *672*
tracheal, 669
Kaposi's sarcoma as. See *Kaposi's sarcoma.*
large cell. See *Lung cancer, non–small cell.*
locally advanced, treatment of, 1430–1431, *1442*, *1443*
lymph node examination in, 1427
lymphoepithelioma as, 1462–1463, 1462t
lymphoma as, Hodgkin's, 1453–1455, *1454*, *1455*
non-Hodgkin's, 1455–1458, 1456t
mediastinoscopy in, 1427
melanoma as, 1464
metastases from. See *Metastasis(es) (malignancy), from lung.*
metastases to. See *Metastasis(es) (malignancy), to lung.*
methylation abnormalities in, 1378
microsatellite instability in, 1378
molecular biology of, 1416–1417, 1425–1426, 1426t
mortality in, 1395, *1395*, 1397, 1397t, 1425–1426, *1425*
screening effects on, 1419–1420, 1420t
smoking-related, 1400
mucoepithelial, 1462–1463, 1462t
natural history of, 1417, 1418t, 1419
neuroendocrine differentiation and, 1376–1377
neuromyopathy in, 1379
nodular. See *Nodule(s), malignant.*
non–small cell, angiogenesis in, 1387
biologic properties of, 1376t
classification of, 1418t, 1419
clinical features of, 1420–1421
combined treatment modalities in, 1434
early-stage, treatment of, 1427–1430, *1440*, *1441*
genetic factors in, 1377
inoperable, treatment of, 1432–1434
locally advanced, treatment of, 1430–1431, *1442*, *1443*
metastatic, surgical treatment of, 1431–1432
methylation abnormalities in, 1378
microsatellite instability in, 1378
molecular detection of, 1426, 1426t
*MYC* genes in, 1382
neuroendocrine differentiation and, 1376–1377
occult, surgical treatment of, 1428
*p53* gene mutations in, 1382

Lung cancer *(Continued)*
pathology of, 484t, 486, *489*
*p16*$^{INK4A}$ gene in, 1384
*RAS* genes in, 1381–1382
superior sulcus, treatment of, 1434
telomerase activity in, 1378
transition between small cell cancer, 1377
treatment of, radiation therapy in, 1432–1436
surgical, 1427–1432
occult, bronchoscopy of, 741
treatment of, 1428
occupational, 1400–1404
p53 tumor suppressor dysfunction in, 1382–1383
Pancoast tumor in, 1430
paraneoplastic syndromes in, 1378–1379, 1421–1422
pathogenesis of, metastatic, 1469–1471
pathology of, 482, 483t–484t, *485*, 486, *487–489*
phenotypic commitment of, 1377
*p16*$^{INK4A}$ gene in, 1383–1384
preneoplastic changes and, 1377–1378
prevention of, diet for, 1404–1405
prognosis for, 1425–1426, *1425*
*PTEN* gene in, 1384
racial factors in, 1396, *1396*
radiation therapy for, versus stage, 1428–1431
recurrence of, after resection, 1428
relapsed, treatment of, 1435
retinoblastoma gene in, 1383
retinoids and, 1385
risk factors for, 1397–1406, 1416, 1417t. See also *Lung cancer, smoking and.*
dietary, 1404–1405
host factors in, 1405–1406
occupational and environmental, 1400–1404, 1888, 1891
sarcoma as, 1463
screening for, 1419–1420, 1420t
small cell, 1419
apoptosis in, *446*
biologic properties of, 1376t
clinical features of, 1420–1421
Cushing's syndrome in, 1379
genetic factors in, 1377
microsatellite instability in, 1378
molecular detection of, 1426, 1426t
*MYC* genes in, 1382
neuroendocrine differentiation and, 1376–1377
*p53* gene mutations in, 1382
paraneoplastic syndromes in, 1379
pathology of, 484t, 486, *487*
radiation therapy for, 1434–1435
retinoblastoma gene in, 1383
staging of, 1424–1426
telomerase activity in, 1378
transition between non–small cell cancer, 1377
treatment of, chemotherapy in, 1438–1439
surgical, 1432
smoking and, 1397–1400, 2558
cessation effects on, 1399
cigarette composition and, 1399
environmental, 1399–1400
epidemiology of, 1415–1416, 1416t
ethnic factors in, 1398
gender differences in, 1398
HIV infection and, 2175
in asbestos exposure, 1836–1837
international trends in, 1396–1397
mortality in, 1400
*p53* gene mutations in, 1382

Lung cancer *(Continued)*
*RAS* gene mutations in, 1381
religious factors in, 1398
versus histologic type, 1398–1399
versus noncigarette tobacco use, 1400
soft-tissue, 1418
solitary nodule as, computed tomography of, 666–668, *667*, *668*
treatment of, 1439, *1445*
squamous cell carcinoma as, 1418t, 1419
pathology of, 482, 484t, *485*
smoking and, 1398–1399
staging of, 1423–1425, 1423t–1425t
bronchoscopy in, 741
computed tomography in, 669–670, *670*, *671*
magnetic resonance imaging in, 670–671, *672*
mediastinoscopy in, 762
positron emission tomography in, 716
superior sulcus, 1430, 1434
survival in, 1397, 1397t, 1425–1426, *1425*
syndrome of inappropriate antidiuretic hormone in, 1379
telomerase activity in, 1378
transforming growth factor-β gene in, 1385
treatment of, chemotherapy in. See *Chemotherapy, for lung cancer.*
combined modalities in, 1436–1437
early-stage, non–small cell, 1427–1430, *1440*, *1441*
economic issues in, 1439, 1444
guidelines for, 1439, *1440–1444*
metastatic, 1473–1475, 1474t
non–small cell, 1427–1432
occult, 1428
surgical treatment of, 1431–1432
palliative, 742, 1431–1432, 1435–1436, 1473–1474
radiation therapy in, 1432–1436
versus stage, 1428–1431
relapsed, 1435
small cell, 1432
surgical, 1426–1432
preoperative considerations in, 889–891
with solitary nodule, 1439
tumor suppressor gene dysfunction in, 1382–1386
tumorlets as, 1463–1464, 1480–1481
unresectable, treatment of, 1431, 1432–1434
ventilation-perfusion scanning in, 715–716, *715*
Lung compliance, at high altitude, 1918
definition of, 2564
dynamic, 800, 2564
in acute respiratory distress syndrome, 2420t
in chronic obstructive pulmonary disease, 1207
in edema protection, 1577
in emphysema, 1207
in heart disease, 2253–2254, 2254t, *2255*
in kyphoscoliosis, 2359, 2359t, *2360*
in neuromuscular disorders, 2331
in obesity, 2372
in poliomyelitis, 2340, 2341t
in pulmonary edema, 1578–1579, 1585
in pulmonary fibrosis, 801–802, 1675, *1675*
in pulmonary venous hypertension, 2253–2254, 2254t, *2255*
in sarcoidosis, 1723
in spinal cord injury, 2339
interstitial, 137–138, *137*
low, ventilation-perfusion scanning in, 698
static, measurement of, 800–801, *801*
Lung disease(s). See also specific disease.
diaphragmatic paralysis with, 2335
Lung disease(s) *(Continued)*
free radical activity in, 392
functional residual capacity in, measurement of, 58
genetics of, 45–53. See also *Lung cancer, genetics of.*
pathology of, 477, 480t, 481t, 482, *482*, 483t–484t, *485*, 486, *487–489*
high altitude effects on, 1941
hypoventilation in, 2140t, 2142, *2142*
interstitial. See *Fibrosis, interstitial; Interstitial lung disease(s).*
pathology of. See *Pathology*; specific diseases.
preoperative evaluation in. See *Preoperative evaluation.*
pulmonary circulation in, 67
Lung injury, acute, bronchoconstriction in, 1586
coagulation disorders in, 1586
definition of, 1592–1593, 1592t, 1593t, 2419
diagnosis of, 1591–1600
barrier function measurement in, 1597–1598
blood gas analysis in, 1594–1595
chest radiography in, 1594
criteria for, 1591–1594, 1592t, 1593t
fluid protein measurement in, 1595
hemodynamic measurements in, 1595–1596
lung injury detection in, 1598–1600
lung water measurement in, 1596–1597
pulmonary function tests in, 1595
symptoms and signs in, 1591
direct, 1587, 1590–1591
epidemiology of, 1613
gas exchange in, 1585–1586
in acid exposures, 1906
in air pollution, 1906
in airway obstruction, 1589t
in ammonia inhalation, 1909
in aspiration, 1588t
in baby powder aspiration, 1908
in bromine compound inhalation, 1909
in chlorine and chlorine compound exposure, 1905–1906
in complement activation, 519–520
in crowd control agent exposure, 1906–1907
in drug exposure, 1588t, 1909
in ethylene oxide exposure, 1909
in hematologic disorders, 1588t
in hemodynamic disorders, 1588t
in hydrocarbon pneumonitis, 1908
in hydrogen sulfide inhalation, 1909
in immune complex deposition, 520
in infection, 1587, 1588t, 1589
in isocyanate exposure, 1909–1910
in metal exposure, 1907
in military agent exposure, 1906–1907
in neurologic disorders, 1588t
in nitrogen oxide exposure, 1906
in obstetric/gynecologic disorders, 1588t
in organic dust toxicity, 1907
in paraquat exposure, 1908
in phosphine exposure, 1910
in sepsis, 1587, 1589
in smoke inhalation, 1908–1909
in sulfur dioxide exposure, 1906
in toxic exposures, 1588t, 1590–1591, 1903–1914, 1905t
in trauma, 1588t
indirect, 1587
inflammation in, 1589–1590, 1590t
lung mechanics in, 1585
Lung injury *(Continued)*
mechanisms of, 1587–1591, 1588t–1590t
pathogenesis of, 1903–1904
coagulation cascade in, 520
complement activation in, 519–520, *519*
fibrinolysis in, 520
in immune complex deposition, 520
pathology of, 456, 459, *459–462*, 1586
pathophysiology of, 1584–1586, *1584*
platelet-activating factor in, 498
pulmonary edema in. See *Pulmonary edema, increased permeability.*
sequelae of, 1904–1905
stages of, 1586
toxic exposure route in, 1903
treatment of, 1600–1611, 1613–1614, *1614*, 1904
antioxidants in, 1610
cardiac catheterization in, 1600–1601
corticosteroids in, 1608–1609
diuretics in, 1602–1603
immediate, 1600
inotropic agents in, 1603–1604
monoclonal antibodies in, 1610–1611
options for, 1600–1604
outcome of, 1611–1614, *1614*
pentoxifylline in, 1610
specific, 1608–1611
strategies for, 1604–1611, 1606t
surfactant in, 1609–1610
vasodilators in, 1601–1602, 1611
versus acute respiratory distress syndrome, 2419, 2419t
air-space enlargement in, 1214, *1214*
at high altitudes. See *Altitude, high, maladaptation to.*
biologic agents in, pathology of. See *Pathology, of infections.*
cellular aspects of. See *Cell(s), injury and death of.*
chemical, 477, *477*, 478t, 479t
chronic, pathology of, 459, 462, *463*, *464*, 465
detection of, 1598–1600
drug-induced. See *Drug(s), pulmonary disease(s) due to.*
fibrosis after. See *Fibrosis.*
hypoxemia in, 2416
hypoxic, pathology of, 465, *465*
immunologic, pathology of, 465–466, *466–470*, 468
in acid exposures, 1906
in air pollution, 1906
in ammonia inhalation, 1909
in anaphylaxis, pathology of, 465–466, *466*
in baby powder aspiration, 1908
in bacterial infections, 473–474
in bone marrow transplantation, 2298, 2300
in bromine compound inhalation, 1909
in chlamydial infections, 473
in chlorine and chlorine compound exposure, 1905–1906
in crowd control agent exposure, 1906–1907
in diving, 1955–1956, *1956*
in ethylene oxide exposure, 1909
in fungal infections, 474–475, *475*, *476*
in genetic diseases, 477, 480t, 481t, 482, *482*, 483t–484t, *485*, 486, *487–489*
in hydrocarbon pneumonitis, 1908
in hydrogen sulfide inhalation, 1909
in hypersensitivity, 465–466, *466–470*, 468
in immune complex deposition, 466, *467*
in inappropriate free radical generation, 392
in intravascular macrophage depletion, 397
in isocyanate exposure, 1909–1910

Lung injury *(Continued)*
in malnutrition, 486
in mechanical ventilation, 2424, 2426–2427, *2426*, *2427*, 2477–2478, 2483
in metal exposure, 1907
in military agent exposure, 1906–1907
in mycoplasmal infections, 473, *474*
in near drowning, 1965, 1966
in nitrogen oxide exposure, 1906
in organic dust toxicity, 1907
in ozone exposure, 1895–1896
in pancreatitis, 2276
in paraquat exposure, 1908
in parasitic infections, 475
in phosphine exposure, 1910
in radiation exposure, 475, *476*, 477, 1436
in rib fractures, 2367
in rickettsial infections, 473
in sickle cell disease, 2288
in smoke inhalation, 1908–1909
in sulfur dioxide exposure, 1906
in toxic exposures, 1903–1914, 1905t
in transfusions, 2292
in transplantation, 466, 468, *470*
in viral infections, 468, 470–471, *471–473*, 473
inflammatory mediators in. See *Inflammatory mediator(s);* specific mediators.
inflammatory reactions in, 455–456, *455–458*
interstitial macrophage proliferation in, 395–396
markers of, 1599–1600
metabolic changes in, 1598–1599
mortality prediction in, 2489
pathogenesis of, 1903–1904
pathology of. See *Pathology;* specific diseases.
pathophysiology of, in drug reactions, 1972–1974
responses in, 1178
pressure-induced, 475, 1955–1956, *1956*
repair of. See *Repair.*
reperfusion. See *Reperfusion injury.*
sequelae of, 1904–1905
thermal, 475
treatment of, 1904
ventilator-associated, 2424, 2426–2427, *2426*, *2427*, 2477–2478, 2483
Lung Injury Score, 1592–1594, 1592t
Lung scan. See *Ventilation-perfusion scanning.*
Lung sounds. See also specific types, e.g., *Crackles.*
adventitious, 593–596
classification of, 594, 594t
continuous, 594t, 595–596
discontinuous, 594t, 595, *595*, *596*
auscultation of, 597–598
bronchial, 593, *593*
bronchovesicular, 593, *593*
character of, 592–593, *592*
definition of, 592
generation of, 592
in chronic bronchitis, 1189
in chronic obstructive pulmonary disease, 1189
in diaphragmatic paralysis, 2335
in emphysema, 1189
in lymphangio(leio)myomatosis, 1781
in pulmonary edema, 1591
in sickle cell disease, 2288
in tuberculosis, 1063
normal, 593, *593*
perception of, 592–593, *592*
tracheal, 593, *593*
vesicular, 593, *593*, 598
Lung sounds *(Continued)*
voice-generated, 598
Lung transplantation, 2517–2530
bilateral, 2518
bronchiolitis obliterans after, 1364–1365, *1365*, 1366
candidate selection and evaluation for, 2519–2521, 2519t, 2520t
complications of, 2521–2523, 2526, 2526t, 2527t
contraindications to, 2519, 2519t
diffusing capacity in, 816
double, in bronchiectasis, 1333
dyspnea after, mechanisms of, 543
heart transplantation with. See *Heart-lung transplantation.*
heart-lung, 1552
historical background of, 2517
immunosuppressive therapy for, 2521
in bronchiectasis, 2520, 2520t
in chronic obstructive pulmonary disease, 1219, 2520, 2520t
in cystic fibrosis, 1313, 2520, 2520t
in emphysema, 1219
in idiopathic pulmonary fibrosis, 2520, 2520t
in lymphangio(leio)myomatosis, 1784–1785
in pediatric patients, 2521
in pulmonary fibrosis, 1683, 1683t
in pulmonary hypertension, 2520–2521, 2520t
living donor lobe, 2519
monitoring after, 2526, 2527t
numbers of, 2517
pleural effusion in, 2033
pleurodesis and, 2050
pneumonia after, 2521–2522
postoperative management in, 2521
preoperative management in, 2521
psychosocial factors in, 2526
pulmonary function tests in, 816, 2524
recurrent disease after, 2526
registry for, 2517
rejection in, 2523–2526
acute, 2523
chronic (bronchiolitis obliterans), 2523–2524, 2524t
diffuse alveolar hemorrhage in, 1741
diffusing capacity in, 816
outcome of, 2524–2526, *2525*
pathology of, 466, 468, *470*
reperfusion injury in, surfactant alterations in, 320
survival in, 2517–2518
types of, 2518–2519
unilateral, 2518
ventilation-perfusion scanning in, 716–718, *717*
Lung volume(s). See also specific types, e.g., *Functional residual capacity; Residual volume; Tidal volume; Vital capacity.*
abdominal motion effects on, 105–106, *105*
after lung transplantation, 2524
airway resistance and, 798
alveolar pressure and, 61
bronchiole dimensional changes with, 1361–1362
chest wall motion effects on, 105–106, *105*
definitions of, 57, *57*
determinants of, 783, *783*
distribution of, 109–111, *110*
end-expiratory, in exercise, 213–215
fluid, 137–138, *137*
history of, versus airflow, 101–103
in bone marrow transplantation, 2298
in chronic obstructive pulmonary disease, 1191, 1207
Lung volume(s) *(Continued)*
in cystic fibrosis, 1302, 1304, 1304t
in emphysema, 1191, 1207
in exercise, 213–215
in heart disease, 2251, *2251*, 2252t
in hypothyroidism, 2310
in interstitial lung disease, 1662, *1664*, *1665*
in neuromuscular disorders, 2333
in obesity, 2371, 2371t
in pectus excavatum, 2365
in pleural effusion, 2000
in pneumothorax, 2044–2045, *2044*, 2046
in pregnancy, 2317–2318
in pulmonary edema, 1578–1579, *2390*
in pulmonary fibrosis, 1675–1676, *1675*, *1676*
in pulmonary venous hypertension, 2251, *2251*, 2252t
in sarcoidosis, 1723
in spinal cord injury, 2339, 2339t
in systemic lupus erythematosus, 1704, *1704*
increased, pulmonary stretch receptor activation by, 182, 183, *183*
measurement of, 57–58, *57*, 790–799
airway resistance methods in, 798–799, *799*
body plethysmography in, 57–58, 793–798, *794–796*
gas dilution methods in, 791–793, *791*, *792*, 793t, 874
radiographic methods in, 793
normal, 4, 875
positive end-expiratory pressure and, 2448, *2448*
pulmonary blood flow distribution and, 66
quantitative morphologic method for, 23–29, *24–28*
reduction of, surgical, 715, 890–891
in dyspnea, 547
in emphysema, 853–854, 1218–1219
pulmonary rehabilitation with, 2512
regional, versus pleural pressure, 806, *807*
rib cage motion effects on, 105–106, *105*
terminology of, 2563
theoretical aspects of, 783, *783*
types of, 783, *783*
versus age, 857
versus airflow, during vital capacity maneuvers, 98, *99*, *100*, 101
in exercise, in chronic obstructive pulmonary disease, 213, *215*
versus airway caliber, in asthma, 1264, *1264*, 1265
versus diaphragm motion, 107
versus diffusing capacity, 814
versus pleural pressure, 111
versus position, 2253–2254, 2254t
versus pressure, 95, *96*
surfactant and, 308, *308*
versus pulmonary vascular resistance, 63–64, *63*, 126, *127*
versus radiographic results, 646, *646–650*
versus vascular compliance, 127–128
versus ventilation, 59, *59*
Lupus erythematosus, drug-induced, 2031–2032
systemic. See *Systemic lupus erythematosus.*
Lupus pleuritis, 2031–2032
Lupus pneumonitis, 1704
versus diffuse alveolar hemorrhage, 1740
Luteinizing hormone-releasing hormone analogues, in lymphangio(leio)myomatosis, 1783
Lycoperdonosis, 1910
Lyme disease, chest pain in, 577
Lymph, circulation of, 23

Lymph *(Continued)*
flow of, in lung, 1575–1577
solute lymph-to-plasma concentration ratio in, 134–135, *136*
solutes in, endothelial barrier and, 139
Lymph nodes, biopsy of, bronchoscopy in, 741, 741t
scalene, 763
transbronchial, 736–737, 738t
calcification of, broncholithiasis in, 1368
examination of, in lung cancer, 1427, 1430
hyperplasia of, angiofollicular (Castleman's disease), 1460
mediastinal. See *Mediastinum, lymph nodes of.*
sarcoidosis of, 1719–1721, *1720*
Lymphadenitis, in *Mycobacterium avium* complex infections, 1093
Lymphadenopathy, angioimmunoblastic, 1459–1460
bronchial compression in, 1367
in coccidioidomycosis, 1123
in filariasis, 1153–1154, 1761–1762
in histoplasmosis, 1110, *1110*, 1111
in interstitial lung disease, 1660t, *1663*
in lymphoma, 2207
in paracoccidioidomycosis, 1128
in sarcoidosis, 1719–1720, *1720*
in toxoplasmosis, 1148
in tuberculosis, 1064, *1064*, *1066*
in HIV infection, 2182, *2183*
mediastinal, 2129–2130, *2130*
in parapneumonic effusion, 2018
Lymphangiectasis, of lung, 483t
Lymphangiography, in chylothorax, 2058
Lymphangio(leio)myomatosis, 1775–1788, 2325
apoptosis in, 1779
cellular characteristics in, 1777–1779
chest radiography of, 1746–1747, *1747*, 1780t, 1781–1782
chylous fluid collections in, 1784, 2059, *2059*
clinical features of, 1746, 1780–1781, 1780t
computed tomography of, 1661, *1663*, 1782–1783, *1782*
definition of, 1746, 1775
diagnosis of, 1780–1781, 1780t, 1783
diffuse alveolar hemorrhage in, 1746–1748, *1747*
epidemiology of, 1779–1780
genetics of, 1778
historical overview of, 1775–1776
hormone receptors in, 1778–1779
lung cysts in, 676, *677*
monitoring of, 1784
pathogenesis of, 1776
pathology of, 1746–1748, *1747*, 1776–1777, *1777*
pregnancy in, 1778–1779, 1781, 1783
pulmonary function abnormalities in, 1781
support groups for, 1784
treatment of, 1748, 1783–1785
tuberous sclerosis and, 1778, 1781
Lymphatic sumps, 372
Lymphatic system. See also *Lymph nodes; Lymphadenopathy.*
angio(leio)myomatosis of. See *Lymphangio(leio)myomatosis.*
cancer metastasis through, 1469–1472, *1471*
hypoplasia of, yellow-nail syndrome in, 2035
of lung, 22–23
failure of, 136, 145, 146
in acute injury, 1585
in alveolar clearance, 371, 372
Lymphatic system *(Continued)*
in fluid and solute exchange, 132, *132*, 136, *136*
in pulmonary edema, in resolution stage, 1612
increased permeability, 1585
increased pressure, 1578
lymph flow in, 1575–1577
of pleura, 1997–1998, *1998*
dysfunction of, 2000
tuberculosis of, 1078–1079, *1079*
Lymphedema, in yellow-nail syndrome, 2035
Lymphocyte(s). See also *B lymphocytes; T lymphocytes.*
cluster of differentiation system for, 413, 414t, 415t. See also subjects starting with *CD.*
development of, 415
in bronchoalveolar fluid, in sarcoidosis, 752
infiltration of, in allergic rhinitis, 1347
trafficking of, 415–416, 435–436
types of, 413
Lymphocyte function antigen, in asthma, 1261
in T-lymphocyte activation, 432
Lymphocytic alveolitis, in inflammatory bowel disease, 2270–2271
Lymphocytic interstitial pneumonia, 1653–1654, 1653t, 1687, 1687t
in Sjögren's syndrome, 1705–1706, *1706*
Lymphocytic interstitial pneumonitis, in HIV infection, 2208–2209, *2208*
Lymphoepithelioma(s), of lung, 1462–1463, 1462t
Lymphokines, in tuberculosis, 1057
Lymphoma(s), chylothorax in, 2057, 2058
disseminated, 2206
Hodgkin's. See *Hodgkin's disease.*
in HIV infection, 2206–2207, *2207*
in lymphomatoid granulomatosis, 1537–1538
in Sjögren's syndrome, 1706
in transplantation, 2232
infiltration in, 2292
metastasis from, to pleura, 2073
of bronchi, 1367
of lung, 1455–1458
B-cell, 1456, 1456t
chest radiography of, 2207, *2207*
classification of, 1455, 1456t
clinical features of, 1456–1457
epidemiology of, 1455
Hodgkin's, 1453–1455, *1454*, *1455*
in HIV infection, 1457
lymphoproliferative disease transformation into, 1458, 1459
natural killer-cell, 1456t
non-Hodgkin's, 1455–1458, 1456t
primary, 1456–1457
prognosis for, 1455, 1456t
recurrence of, 1457–1458
T-cell, 1456t
treatment of, 1457–1458
of mediastinum, 2128
of pleura, 2071–2072
of thymus, 2127
pneumonia in, 925
ventilation-perfusion scanning in, 716
versus sarcoidosis, 1725
Lymphomatoid granulomatosis, 1458–1459, *1459*, 1537–1538
Lymphopoiesis, 415
Lymphoproliferative disease(s), 1458–1460
angioimmunoblastic lymphadenopathy as, 1459–1460
Castleman's disease as, 1460
in lung transplantation, 2522
lymphomatoid granulomatosis as, 1458–1459, *1459*
Lymphoproliferative disease(s) *(Continued)*
pneumonia in, 925
posttransplantation, 2231–2232
Lymphotactins, 507, 507t
Lysophospholase, of eosinophils, 1758–1759, 1758t
Lysozyme, in macrophages, 392
in mucus, 331

## M

Mace, exposure to, 1907
McGill Pain Questionnaire, 568
Mach bands, in pneumomediastinum, 2103
Macleod's syndrome (unilateral bronchiolitis obliterans), 1197–1198
Macroglobulinemia, Waldenström's, 1464, 2294
Macroglossia, in acromegaly, 2313
Macrophage(s), 385–412
activation of, in smoking, 1212
airway, proliferation of, 387
alveolar, 22, 387–397
activation of, in hypersensitivity pneumonitis, 1872
as air pollutant defense, 1889
bacterial resistance to, 392
development of, 397–407
from monocytes, 400–407, 401t, *402*
growth factors in, 400–404, 401t, *402*
in bone marrow, 399–400, *400*
transcription regulation in, 404–407
environment of, 390
fate of, 390
free radical generation in, 390, 392
function of, 371–372, 387, 390
heterogeneity of, 393–394
immobile, in alveolar proteinosis, 1793
in adaptive immune response suppression, 393–394, *395*
in alveolar proteinosis, 1789–1790, *1790*, *1791*, 1793
in asthma, 1261
in bronchoalveolar lavage, counting of, 736
in clearance, 371–372
in cystic fibrosis, 1301
in fibrosis pathogenesis, 1889
in infection, 1589
in inflammation regulation, 393
in inhaled particle and microorganism protection, 371–372, 390, *391*, 392
in *Mycobacterium tuberculosis* destruction, 1056, 1057
in sarcoidosis, 1724–1725
in sputum, 614, *614*
in surfactant catabolism, 316, *317*
in tissue remodeling, 392–393
morphology of, 388, *388*, *389*
movement of, 372
nitric oxide generation in, 392
origin of, 397–399
phospholipidosis of, 1973
pigmented, in respiratory bronchiolitis, 1366
products secreted by, 372
proliferation of, 387, 399
surfactant protein A binding to, 312–313
surfactant protein D binding to, 316
versus airway macrophages, 389–390
versus interstitial macrophages, 395
differentiation of, functional, 401
excess of, animal studies of, 404
foamy, in lipid accumulation, 454, *454*, *455*
function of, 415

Macrophage(s) *(Continued)*
differentiation for, 401
hemosiderin accumulation in, in cell injury, 450, *452*
heterogeneity of, 401
in apoptotic cell removal, 529, *529*, *530*
in fetus, 387
in mucus hypersecretion, 334
in pulmonary fibrosis, 1678
inflammatory. See *Monocyte(s).*
interstitial, *388*, 394–396
intravascular, 397
markers for, 387t
morphology of, 387–389, *388–390*
progenitors of, in fetus, 398
markers for, 387t
proliferation of, 399
pulmonary intravascular, 385
receptors of, 390, *391*, 392
survival factors for, 403
tissue, 386, 386t
types of, 385–387, 386t
Macrophage colony-stimulating factor, action of, 402
in macrophage development, 398–399, 401–403, *402*
deficiency of, 399, 402–403
forms of, 402
gene of, 402
receptor for, 387, 402, *402*
structure of, 402
Macrophage inflammatory proteins, 507t, 516–517
in pulmonary fibrosis, 518–519
receptors for, 517–518, 517t
Macrophage procoagulant inducing factors, 507t, 516–517
Macrophage-derived chemokine, 507t, 516–517
receptors for, 507t, 516–517
Macule(s), coal, 1825–1827, *1826*
Maduromycosis, 1136
Magnesium, imbalance of, respiratory failure in, 2447
Magnesium sulfate, in asthma, 2455
Magnetic resonance imaging, 664–665
of aortic dissection, 683, *684*, *685*
of aortic pseudoaneurysm, 683, *686*
of benign fibrous mesothelioma, 2071
of brachial plexopathy, 671–672
of congenital great vessel anomalies, 683, 686, *687*
of cystic fibrosis, 1304
of lung cancer, 670–671, *672*, 1423
of lung sequestration, 683, *687*
of mediastinum, 672–673, *674*, 2085–2086, *2086*, *2087*
of pleural effusion, 2007–2008
of pulmonary embolism, 679–681, 680t, *682*
of solitary nodule, 668
of venous thrombosis, 1509
principles of, 664
safety hazards of, 664
techniques for, 664–665
versus computed tomography, 2085–2086
Magnetic stimulation, in respiratory muscle evaluation, 858–859, 2333
Magnetometry, in motion analysis, in neuromuscular disorders, 2333
Major basic protein, of eosinophils, 1758t, 1759, 1759t
Major histocompatibility complex molecules. See also *Human leukocyte antigens.*
bronchiolitis obliterans and, 1364–1365
classes of, 424–425, *425*, *426*, 427t
haplotypes of, 425, 426
in antigen recognition, 426–428, 427t, *428*
Major histocompatibility complex molecules *(Continued)*
in lung cancer, 1386
of dendritic cells, 396–397
Malabsorption, in cystic fibrosis, 1306
Malaria, 1146–1147
Maldigestion, in cystic fibrosis, 1306
Malignancy. See *Cancer*; *Carcinoma(s)*; *Lung cancer*; specific diseases.
Malignant melanoma, of lung, 1464
Malingering, 898
Malnutrition, in chylothorax drainage, 2057, 2058
lung injury in, 486
tuberculosis in, 1059
MALT (mucosa-associated lymphoid tissue), lymphoma of, 1455–1457
Man-made vitreous fibers, in pneumoconioses, 1831t, 1841–1842
Mantoux test, 1059–1062, *1060*, 1061t, *1062*
Mapping, genomic, 45–47, *46*
Marburg virus infections, 931t
Marfan's syndrome, 481t, 1710–1711
Maroteaux-Lamy syndrome, lung injury in, 481t
Mask, for mechanical ventilation, 2472
Mask squeeze, in diving, 1957
Mass. See also *Tumor(s).*
mediastinal. See *Mediastinum, mass in.*
Mass median aerodynamic diameter, of aerosols, 350
Mast cell(s), disorders of, versus asthma, 1269
function of, 232, *233*
in airways, 10, *12*
in allergic rhinitis, 1347, 1348
in asthma, 1175–1176, *1177*, 1260, *1260*
in hypersensitivity pneumonitis, 1872
in mucus hypersecretion, 334
in silicosis, 1819
Mast cell tryptase, inhibitors of, in airway disease, 288
Mastocytosis, versus asthma, 1269
Material Safety Data Sheets, in occupational diseases, 904
Matrix metalloproteinases, in lymphangio(leio)myomatosis, 1779
in metastasis, 1388
of alveolar macrophages, 392–393
Maxillary sinusitis, 916–917
Maximal breathing capacity. See *Maximal voluntary ventilation.*
Maximal expiratory flow, 98, *99*, *100*, 101
definition of, 2563
in asthma, 1265, 1267
in chronic obstructive pulmonary disease, in exercise, 212, *212*, 214
volume history and, 102–103
in cough, 556
in cystic fibrosis, 1304t
mechanics of, 98, *99*, *100*, 101, 113
normal values for, 875
Maximal expiratory pressure, definition of, 2563
in ankylosing spondylitis, 2370
in heart disease, 2255–2256, 2256t
in kyphoscoliosis, 2360
in neuromuscular disorders, 2333
in spinal cord injury, 2338
Maximal inspiratory airflow, 1345
Maximal inspiratory pressure, definition of, 2563
in ankylosing spondylitis, 2370
in heart disease, 2255–2256, 2256t
in kyphoscoliosis, 2360
in neuromuscular disorders, 2333
Maximal inspiratory pressure *(Continued)*
in obesity, 2371t
in respiratory muscle evaluation, 858
in spinal cord injury, 2338
measurement of, in mechanical ventilation, 2452
Maximal midexpiratory flow, in asthma, 1265
measurement of, 786, *786*
Maximal minute ventilation, in lymphangio(leio)myomatosis, 1781
Maximal negative airway pressure, in respiratory muscle evaluation, 858
Maximal negative inspiratory pressure, in respiratory muscle fatigue, 2383
Maximal sustained ventilatory capacity, in chronic obstructive pulmonary disease, 216
Maximal voluntary ventilation, definition of, 2563
in chronic obstructive pulmonary disease, 212–214, *213*, 216
in diaphragmatic paralysis, 2335, 2336t
in exercise, in emphysema, *222*
in interstitial pulmonary fibrosis, 217
in highly fit athletes, 218
in impairment and disability evaluation, 897–898, 901t, 905
in kyphoscoliosis, 2360–2361, 2361t
in neuromuscular disorders, 2332–2333, 2344, *2345*
in obesity, 2371t
in poliomyelitis, 2341, 2341t
in respiratory muscle evaluation, 859
indications for, 785t, 787
measurement of, 785t, 787
normal values for, 874
*MDM2* gene and product, in lung cancer, 1383
Measles, 931t, 957–959
antibodies in, 959
atypical, 959–960
clinical manifestations of, 959–960
complications of, 958
diagnosis of, 960
epidemiology of, 957–958
immunization for, 959, 960
mortality in, 958
pathogenesis of, 959
pneumonia in, 958–959
in pregnancy, 2321
pathology of, 470, *472*
prevention of, 960
transmission of, 957–958
treatment of, 960
virus causing, 957
Mebendazole, in ascariasis, 1150, 1761
in hookworm infections, 1151
in trichinosis, 1156
Mechanical properties, 91–117
during nonuniform ventilation, 111
in maximal expiratory flow, 98, *99*, *100*, 101
in mechanical ventilation, 2474–2476, *2475*, *2476*
in pathologic conditions, 111–112
in respiratory failure, 2378–2385, 2378t, *2379*, *2381*, 2382t, *2384*
of airways, 94–95, *96*
of alveoli, 91–93, *92*
of blood, pulmonary vascular resistance and, 126–127, *128*
of chest wall, 103–106, *103*, *105*
after thoracoplasty, 2364
in ankylosing spondylitis, 2369
in diseases, 2359t
in flail chest, 2367–2368, *2367*, *2368*
in obesity, 2372
in pectus excavatum, 2365

Mechanical properties *(Continued)*
of lung, in pulmonary edema, 1585
parenchymal, 93–94
pulmonary vascular resistance and, 126, *126*, *127*
regional volume and regional ventilation relationships and, 109–111, *110*
of nonrespiratory muscles, during respiratory function, 108
of pleura and pleural fluid, 111
of respiratory muscles, abdominal, 108
diaphragm as, 106–107
during nonrespiratory function, 108–109
fatigue and, 109
in chest wall, 103–106, *103*, *105*
rib cage, 107–108
upper airway, 108
pressure-flow relationships as, 97–98
pulmonary function tests based on, 782–805
clinical applications of, 802–805, *805*
elastic recoil measurement as, 799–802, *800*, *801*, 875. See also *Elastic recoil.*
flow measurements as, 784–790, *785–790*, 785t, 872–874. See also *Spirometry;* specific tests.
in quiet breathing, 782
lung volumes as. See *Lung volume(s).*
normal values for, 802–804, 875
theoretical aspects of, 782–784, *783*
trade-offs in, 91, 112–113
volume history effects on, 101–103
Mechanical ventilation, 2471–2485
accidental disconnection of, 2483
acidemia in, 2444
aerosol generator in, 2472, 2474
after thoracoplasty, 2364
air block in, 2102
air embolism in, 2102
alveolar recruitment in, 2476–2477, *2477*
breath modes in, 2471–2472, *2472*, 2473t
bronchopulmonary dysplasia due to, 1366–1367
bronchoscopy with, 728, 734
cardiac output in, 2388–2389, *2388*, 2453
complications of, 2483
continuous positive airway pressure. See *Continuous positive airway pressure.*
cycling dyssynchrony in, 2481–2482, *2482*
definition of, 2471
effort sensors in, 2472
evaluation for, 2452, 2452t
expiratory pressure in, 2451, 2472
flow/volume-targeted breaths in, 2474, *2475*
for life support. See *Life support.*
gas blenders in, 2472
gas delivery systems for, 2471, *2472*, 2473t
gas exchange in, 2476–2477, *2477*
general anesthesia in, 2459
goals of, 2471
helium-oxygen mixture in, 2459
hemodynamic effects of, 2482–2483
high-frequency, 2478
in acute respiratory distress syndrome, 2433–2434
humidifiers for, 2472
hypercapnia in, 2443–2445
in acute respiratory distress syndrome, 2432–2433, 2432t
in asthma, 2455–2459, *2457*, *2458*
hypoxemia in, 2444
in acute inflammatory polyneuropathy, 2342
in acute respiratory distress syndrome, 2421–2422, 2424–2433
circulatory management in, 2423–2424, *2425*

Mechanical ventilation *(Continued)*
clinical trials of, 2427–2429, *2428*
guidelines for, 2430–2433, *2431*, 2432t
high-frequency, 2433–2434
in exudative phase, 2435
in lung contusion, 2436–2437
in proliferative phase, 2435–2436
initial settings for, 2430–2432
inverse ratio, 2434
lung injury in, 2424, 2426–2427, *2426*, *2427*
lung mechanics and, 2424, 2426–2427, *2426*, *2427*
monitoring during, 2435
nitric oxide inhalation with, 2434–2435
open-lung approach to, 2427–2428, *2428*, 2431–2432
outcome studies of, 2427–2429, *2428*
partial liquid, 2434
permissive hypercapnia in, 2432–2433, 2432t
prone positioning with, 2433
setting adjustment in, 2432
strategies for, 2427–2430, *2428*
tidal volume and, 319, 2428–2429
tracheal gas insufflation in, 2433
with focal lesions, 2436
in air travel, 1226–1227
in airflow obstruction, 2382t
in asthma, 2456–2460, *2457*, *2458*
drugs with, 2454–2455
general anesthesia in, 2459
helium-oxygen mixture in, 2459
inspiratory flow profile in, 2458–2459, *2458*
liberation from, 2459–2460
noninvasive, 2455
permissive hypercapnia in, 2455–2459, *2457*, *2458*
in bone marrow transplantation, 2298
in bronchiectasis, 1331
in chronic obstructive pulmonary disease, 1228–1229
in cystic fibrosis, 1312
in diaphragmatic paralysis, 2337
in flail chest, 2368
in hypoventilation, 2144–2145, 2144t
in increased load, 2448–2449, *2448*
in kyphoscoliosis, 2362–2363, 2363t
in lung contusion, 2436–2437
in lung injury, 1585; 2475–2476, 2481
in mechanical abnormalities, 2444
in near drowning, 1966
in neonatal respiratory distress syndrome, 317–318
in neuromuscular disorders, 2347–2349
in obesity, 2373
in pneumonia, 2436
in poliomyelitis, 2341
in pulmonary edema, 1600, 1607–1608, 2421–2422
high-altitude, 1936
in respiratory failure, acute-on-chronic, 2462–2465
in shock, 2383
liberation from, 2382t
perioperative, 2382
with muscle fatigue, 2383, *2384*, 2385
in respiratory muscle fatigue, 109, 2382, *2384*, 2385
in shock, 2382t, 2403t
hypovolemic, 2402
septic, 2400
in sleep, disordered, 2447
in apnea, 2164
in kyphoscoliosis, 2362–2363, 2363t

Mechanical ventilation *(Continued)*
in spinal cord injury, 2338
in status asthmaticus, 2456–2460, *2457*, *2458*
in strychnine poisoning, 2351
in tetanus, 2351
in tricyclic drug overdose, 1989
inspiratory pressure at airway opening in, 2450–2451, *2451*
intermittent mandatory, 2473t
intermittent positive-pressure, after abdominal surgery, 886t
in chronic obstructive pulmonary disease, 1228
inverse ratio, in acute respiratory distress syndrome, 2434
liberation from, 2382t, 2383
evaluation for, 2383, *2384*, 2385
impaired drive effects on, 2446
in acute-on-chronic respiratory failure, 2463–2465
in asthma, 2459–2460
in Karen Ann Quinlan case, 2492
procedure for, 2385
mechanical loads in, 2478–2479, *2479*, *2480*
metabolic alkalosis and, 172, 2444–2445
monitoring during, 2449–2452, *2450*, *2451*, 2474
negative-pressure, 2347
in kyphoscoliosis, 2362, 2363t
noninvasive, 2347–2348
in chronic obstructive pulmonary disease, 2462
in respiratory failure, 2462
oxygen toxicity in, 2483
partial liquid, in acute respiratory distress syndrome, 2434
patient breathing effort and interactions in, 2451, *2451*, 2472, 2479–2482, *2481*, *2482*
permissive hypercapnia in, 2443–2445
in acute respiratory distress syndrome, 2432–2433, 2432t
in asthma, 2455–2459, *2457*, *2458*
pneumomediastinum in, 2098, 2100–2101, 2101t
pneumonia due to, 2483
bronchoscopy in, 747, *748*, 991–992
diagnosis of, 747, *748*, 923
prevention of, 1608
pneumopericardium in, 2102
pneumothorax in, 2051
neonatal, 2053
tension, 2054–2055
positive-pressure. See also *Positive end-expiratory pressure.*
in acute respiratory distress syndrome, 2421–2422
in pulmonary edema, 2421–2422
noninvasive, 2347–2348
postoperative, 2382t
in chronic obstructive pulmonary disease, 887–888
pressure assist, *2472*, 2473t
pressure control, *2472*, 2473t
pressure support, *2472*, 2473t
pressure-targeted breaths in, 2474, *2475*
pulmonary vascular pressures in, 2395, *2395*
respiratory acidosis in, 173–174
respiratory muscle assessment in, 2451–2452
subcutaneous emphysema in, 2103–2104, *2104*
subsystems for, 2472, 2474
surfactant with, 320–321
ventilatory pattern in, 2475–2476, *2475*, *2476*

Mechanical ventilation *(Continued)*
volume assist, *2472*, 2473t
volume control, *2472*, 2473t
weaning from. See *Mechanical ventilation, liberation from.*
Mechanoreceptors, C-fiber endings as, 184
chest wall, 184
esophageal, 570
Golgi tendon organs as, 184
muscle spindles as, 184
tracheobronchial, 182–184, 182t, *183*
upper airway, 181–182
Meconium ileus, in cystic fibrosis, 1292, 1306, 1312
Mediastinal crunch, auscultation of, 599
Mediastinitis, 2083, 2105–2115
acute, 2105–2110
classification of, 2105–2106, 2106t
clinical features of, 2106
complications of, 2107
epidemiology of, 2105
etiology of, 2105–2106, 2106t
from direct infection extension, 2108–2109
in anthrax, 2109
in visceral perforation, 2106–2108, *2107*, *2108*
mortality in, 2107, 2108, 2110
postoperative, 2109–2110
primary, 2109
anatomic considerations in, 2095–2096
chronic (granulomatous), 2110, *2111*
definition of, 2095, 2105
granulomatous (chronic), 2105, 2110–2115
clinical manifestations of, 2112–2114, *2113*, *2114*
diagnosis of, 2114
pathophysiology of, 2110–2112, *2112*
spectrum of, 2110, *2111*
treatment of, 2114–2115, *2115*
in esophageal rupture, 2028
pneumomediastinum in, 2099
suppurative, 2105
Mediastinoscopy, 762
cervical, 762
complications of, 762, 2090
computed tomography studies before, 670
in biopsy, 2089–2090
in lung cancer, 1427
in mediastinitis, 2114
Mediastinotomy, anterior (parasternal), 762–763, 2089–2090
Mediastinum. See also specific structures within.
air in. See *Pneumomediastinum.*
anatomy of, 2080–2081, *2080*, 2080t, *2082*, 2095–2096
biopsy of, *11*, 2087–2090
cancer invasion of, 669–670, *670*, *671*
Castleman's disease of, 1460
compartments of, 2080–2081, *2080*, 2080t, *2082*
contents of, 2080–2081, *2080*, 2080t, *2082*
cross-sectional anatomy of, 2081, *2082*
cysts of, 2126, 2130
definition of, 2079
disorders of, diagnostic approach to, 2090–2091, *2091*
emphysema of, in barotrauma, 1955, 1956
fibrosis of, 1367, 2110–2115
clinical manifestations of, 2112–2114, *2113*, *2114*
diagnosis of, 2114
etiology of, 2110–2112, *2112*
pathophysiology of, 2110–2112, *2112*
spectrum of, 2110, *2111*
Mediastinum *(Continued)*
terminology of, 2110
treatment of, 2114–2115, *2115*
imaging of, 2083–2087, 2084t
chest radiography of, 2083
computed tomography in, 2083–2085, *2085*, 2086
magnetic resonance imaging in, 2085–2086, *2086*, *2087*
radionuclide studies in, 2086–2087, *2088*
ultrasonography in, 2086
inflammation and infection of. See *Mediastinitis.*
lipomatosis of, corticosteroid-induced, 1985, *1986*
lung cancer spread to, 1421
lymph nodes of, biopsy of, 2088–2089
computed tomography of, 670, 2084
evaluation of, in carcinoma staging, 2090–2091, *2091*
Hodgkin's disease of, 1454, *1454*
mediastinoscopy of, 762
sarcoidosis of, 1721
lymphadenopathy of, in parapneumonic effusion, 2018
mass in, 2081, 2081t, 2083, 2123–2137
asymptomatic, 2081
benign, 2125–2126
biopsy of, 2087–2090, *2089*
carcinoma as, 2132
chest radiography of, 2083
classification of, 2123–2124, 2124t
clinical manifestations of, 2081, 2083, 2124–2125, 2125t
compressive effects of, 2081, 2083
computed tomography of, 672–673, *673*, 2083–2085, *2085*, 2086
developmental cyst as, 2130
diagnosis of, 2125–2126, 2125t, 2131t
diaphragmatic hernia as, 2130–2131
endocrine aspects of, 2124, 2125, 2125t
epidemiology of, 2123–2124, 2124t
evaluation of, 2090
from other compartments, 2132, *2133*
germ cell tumor as, 2127–2128, *2127*
granulomatous, 2114
imaging of, 672–673, *673*, *674*, 2083–2087, 2084t, *2085–2088*
in anterior compartment, 2126–2129, *2126*, *2127*, *2129*
in middle compartment, 2129–2131, *2130*
in pediatric patients, 2123, 2124, 2124t
in posterior compartment, 2131–2132, *2132*, 2132t
lymphadenopathy as, 2129–2130, *2130*
lymphoma as, 2128
magnetic resonance imaging of, 672–673, *674*, 2085–2086, *2086*, *2087*
malignant, 2083
mesenchymal, 2129, *2129*
neurogenic, 2131–2132, *2132*, 2132t
parathyroid, 2128–2129
radionuclide studies in, 2086–2087, *2088*
sarcoma as, 2132
systemic syndromes with, 2124–2125, 2125t
thymic, 2126–2127, *2126*
thyroid, 2128
ultrasonography in, 2086
vascular, 2130
metastasis to, 2083
computed tomography of, 670, *671*
treatment of, 1432
neurofibromatosis of, 1748, 1748t
pancreatic pseudocyst extension into, 2029, *2029*
Mediastinum *(Continued)*
shift of, in pleural tumors, 2072–2073, 2074
tumors of. See *Mediastinum, mass in.*
Mediators, inflammatory. See *Inflammatory mediator(s);* specific substances.
Medical history, 586–592. See also specific diseases.
chief complaint in, 587
clinical usefulness of, 586–587
definition of, 586
diagnostic contributions of, 586, 587t
family history in, 591
in dyspnea, 546
in impairment and disability evaluation, 902–904, 904t
occupational history in, 591, 1806, 1807t, 1815–1816
past history in, 591
present illness in, 587
pulmonary symptom(s) in, 587–590
chest pain as, 590
cough as, 588–589
dyspnea as, 587–588
hemoptysis as, 589–590, 589t
questionnaires for, 591–592
social history in, 591
Medroxyprogesterone, in chronic obstructive pulmonary disease, 1228
in lymphangio(leio)myomatosis, 1783
in mountain sickness, 1939
in sleep apnea, 2164
Medulla, chemoreceptors of, 190, *190*
cough integration in, 554–555
dyspnea perception in, 543
in respiratory control, 185–186, *185*, 188–189
Mefloquine, in malaria, 1147
Meigs' syndrome, pleural effusion in, 2034
Meiosis, 46, *46*
*MEK* gene, in lung cancer, 1381–1382
Melanoma, of lung, 1464
Melanoptysis, in coal-workers' pneumoconiosis, 1829
Melioidosis, 1027–1028
Melphalan, pulmonary disease due to, 1976
Membrane(s), pharyngeal, differential diagnosis of, 917
Membrane attack complex, 519
Membrane diffusive conductance, definition of, 2565
Mendelian inheritance, 45
on-line data base on, 51, 52t
test for, 48–49
Meningioma(s), of lung, 1479
Meningitis, in anthrax, 1029
in coccidioidomycosis, 1125, 1127–1128
in cryptococcosis, 1129–1131, 2196–2197
in tuberculosis, 1083–1084, *1084*
Meningocele, mediastinal extension of, 2132
Meningococcal pneumonia, 1005–1006
Menkes syndrome, lung injury in, 481t
Menstrual cycle, hyperventilation and, 2147
Menstruation, hemoptysis associated with, from pulmonary endometrioma, 1480
pneumothorax associated with, 2053–2054, *2054*, 2324
Meperidine, in amphotericin reactions, 1116
Mercury, exposure to, 1907
Mesencephalon, in breathing control, 187
Mesenchyme, cystic hamartomas of, 1479
epithelial cell interactions with, in lung development, 36, *36*, 37, *37*
tumors of, mediastinal, 2129, *2129*
tracheobronchial, 1478
Mesothelial cells, anatomy of, 1996, *1997*
in pleural fluid, 2004

Mesothelial cells *(Continued)*
physiology of, 1998
Mesothelioma(s), benign fibrous, 2070–2071, *2071*
biopsy of, 760–761
computed tomography of, 2007
malignant, 2067–2070
asbestos exposure sources for, 1832
benign asbestos-related pleural effusion and, 1839–1840
clinical manifestations of, 2068–2069, *2068*
diagnosis of, 2069
etiology of, 2067–2068
incidence of, 2068
pathology of, 2068
pleural plaques and, 1837
staging of, 2069–2070
treatment of, 2069–2070
pathology of, 484t
Metabolic acidosis, 163–171
anion gap concept in, 163–164, *164*
bicarbonate–carbon dioxide relationships in, *159*
causes of, 164–168, *165*, 166t, *167*
cerebrospinal fluid pH in, 171
chronic, 170–171
urine bicarbonate in, 161
classification of, 163
clinical manifestations of, 170–171
compensation for, 161, 161t
bicarbonate-carbon dioxide relationships in, *159*, 160t
in exercise, 208–209, *209*, 211
diabetic ketoacidosis as, 166–167, 166t, *167*, 1134
dilutional, 163, *164*, 170
dyspnea in, 220
gastrointestinal causes of, 169–170
hyperchloremic, 163–164, 168–170, 169t
hyperventilation in, 2146
in adult respiratory distress syndrome, 1595
in exercise, 208–209, *209*, 839, *839*
in chronic obstructive pulmonary disease, 216
in emphysema, 224
in highly fit athletes, 218
in near drowning, 1964, 1965–1966
in pulmonary edema, 1595
in shock, 2403t
in triple disorders, 159
laboratory classification of, 160t
lactic. See *Lactic acidosis.*
pulmonary hypertension in, 1492
renal tubular, 168–169, 169t
right ventricular dysfunction in, 1635–1636, *1636*
toxic, 168
treatment of, 170
in near drowning, 1965–1966
in shock, 2403t
uremic, 167–168
Metabolic alkalosis, 171–173
anion gap in, 164, *164*
bicarbonate–carbon dioxide relationships in, *159*
causes of, 162, 171–172, 171t
chloride resistant, 171t, 172
chloride responsive, 171–172, 171t
clinical manifestations of, 172–173
compensation for, 161, 161t, 162–163
bicarbonate–carbon dioxide relationships in, *159*, 160t
hypochloremic, in cystic fibrosis, 1307
hypoventilation due to, 2140
in extracellular volume depletion, 171–172, 171t
Metabolic alkalosis *(Continued)*
in extracellular volume increase, 171t, 172
in mechanical ventilation, in respiratory failure, 2463
in triple disorders, 159
laboratory classification of, 160t
paradoxical aciduria in, 162
pathogenesis of, 162–163
respiratory failure and, 2444–2445
treatment of, 173
Metabolic hyperbola (alveolar ventilation equation), 58, 180, *180*
Metabolism, anaerobic, ATP production in, 165
in exercise, 199–200, *200*, 839–840
carbon dioxide production in, 205–206, *206*
in respiratory failure, 2405–2407, *2405*, 2406t
basal, in pregnancy, 2318, *2318*
ciliary, 361
energy production in, 838
in pulmonary circulation, 69–70
muscle, at high altitude, 1928
Metaiodobenzylguanidine, radiolabeled, in lung metabolic studies, 720
Metal(s). See also specific metals.
asthma due to, 1858t
hard, lung injury due to, 1844–1845
lung injury due to, 478t, 1907
pulmonary fibrosis due to, 1677
welding of, lung cancer in, 1403
pneumoconiosis in, *1814*
Metal fume fever, 1907
Metalloelastases, formation of, in smoking, 1212
Metalloproteinases, in lymphangio(leio)myomatosis, 1779
in metastasis, 1388
inhibitors of, in chronic obstructive pulmonary disease, 288
of alveolar macrophages, 392–393
Metaplasia, cellular, 450, *452*
in lung cancer, 1377–1378
Metaproterenol, in asthma, 2454
in chronic obstructive pulmonary disease, 1221
in respiratory failure, 2461, 2461t
in status asthmaticus, 2454
Metastasis(es) (benign tumor), from leiomyoma, 1480
Metastasis(es) (calcific), in hyperparathyroidism, 2312, *2312*
in kidney failure, 2279
in multiple myeloma, 2294
to lung, 450, *453*
Metastasis(es) (malignancy), factors affecting, 1387–1388
from breast, *1471*, *1473*, 1474
from carcinoid, 1461–1462
from colon, *1472*
from germ cell tumors, 1473
from lung, distribution of, 1420, 1423
factors affecting, 1387–1388
imaging in, 1423
treatment of, 1429–1430
curative, 1431
palliative, 1431–1432
surgical, 1431–1432
from mesothelioma, 2068
to adrenal gland, 1431
to bone, 1435
to brachial plexus, 671–672
to brain, 1431, 1435–1436
to bronchi, 1367
to lung, 1421, 1469–1476
Metastasis(es) (malignancy) *(Continued)*
bronchoscopy in, 741, 741t
chest radiography of, 1471–1472, *1471–1473*, 1472t
clinical features of, 1471
computed tomography of, 668–669, *669*
diagnosis of, 1471–1473, *1471–1473*, 1472t
differential diagnosis of, 1472, 1472t
frequency of, 1469, 1470t
hematogenous dissemination of, 1469, 1471, *1472*, *1473*
intrabronchial dissemination of, 1470–1471
lymphogenous dissemination of, 1469–1472, *1471*
pathogenesis of, 1469–1471
sources of, 1469, 1470t
tissue diagnosis in, 1472–1473
treatment of, 1473–1475, 1474t
to mediastinum. See *Mediastinum, metastasis to.*
to pleura. See *Pleura, metastasis to.*
Metered-dose inhalers, 248–249, 355–356
for chronic obstructive pulmonary disease, 1220–1224, 1220t
for respiratory failure, 2460–2461, 2461t
for status asthmaticus, 2454–2455
usage guidelines for, 1220–1221, 1220t
Methacholine, in provocation testing, 852–853
after lung transplantation, 2524–2525
in asthma, 1266
in heart disease, 2255
in pregnancy, 2319
Methadone, pulmonary disease due to, 1980
Methanol toxicity, anion gap acidosis due to, 168
Methemoglobinemia, 85, 2290, 2291t
Methicillin, resistance to, in *Staphylococcus aureus*, 1004
Methotrexate, in asthma, 286
pulmonary disease due to, 1693t, 1977, 1985
bronchiolitis obliterans as, 1364
in connective tissue disease therapy, 1692t
in rheumatoid arthritis therapy, 1702
Methoxamine, in heart failure, exercise and, 2260
Methyl bromide, inhalation of, 1909
Methyl isocyanate, exposure to, 1909–1910
Methyl isothiocyanates, exposure to, 1909–1910
Methylation, of DNA, abnormalities of, in lung cancer, 1378
*N*-Methyl-D-aspartate receptor, in pain transmission, 574
Methylphenidate, pulmonary disease due to, 1980
Methylprednisolone, in asthma, 281, 2454t, 2455
in diffuse alveolar hemorrhage, in bone marrow transplantation, 2300
in idiopathic pneumonia syndrome, 2300
in pneumonia, eosinophilic, 1769
*Pneumocystis carinii*, 2194
in pulmonary fibrosis, 1682
in respiratory failure, 2461, 2461t
in status asthmaticus, 2454t, 2455
in vaso-occlusive disease, in bone marrow transplantation, 2301
Methylxanthine(s), theophylline as. See *Theophylline.*
Methysergide, mediastinitis due to, 2112
pleural disease due to, 2035
pulmonary disease due to, 1988
Metoclopramide, in hiccups, 2350
Metolazone, in acute respiratory distress syndrome, 2420

Metolazone *(Continued)*
in pulmonary edema, 1603, 2420
Metoprolol, in myocardial ischemia, *2401*
pulmonary disease due to, 1983
Metronidazole, in amebiasis, 1146
in pneumonia, 922t, 998t, 1019t
Mgat1 (*N*-acetylglucosaminyltransferase I), in lung development, 42
Mica pneumoconiosis, 1841
Miconazole, in pseudoallescheriosis, 1136
Microangiopathic hemolytic anemia, mitomycin-induced, 1976–1977
Microbiologic diagnosis, 607–631. See also specific methods.
cultures in. See *Culture(s).*
direct examination methods in, 613–617, *614, 615*
genetic tests in, 625–627. See also specific tests, e.g., *Polymerase chain reaction.*
of *Actinomyces* infections, 1021–1022, *1021*
of *Coxiella burnetii* infections, 1025
of histoplasmosis, 1114, *1115*
of *Mycobacterium*, 610t, 1045–1048, 1045t
of nocardiosis, 1022–1023, *1023*
of pleural fluid, 2005
of pneumonia, 921, 989–990, *990*
*Acinetobacter*, 1013
beta-hemolytic streptococcal, 1005
Enterobacteriaceae, 1010
*Haemophilus influenzae*, 1007, *1007*
*Klebsiella pneumoniae*, 1009, *1009*
*Legionella*, 1015
*Moraxella catarrhalis*, 1006
*Mycoplasma pneumoniae*, 1024–1025
pneumococcal, 1000, *1000*
*Pneumocystis carinii*, 2190
*Pseudomonas aeruginosa*, 1012
of *Propionibacterium* infections, 1021–1022
problems in, 607–608, *607*, 608t, 609t
serologic testing in, 610t
in chlamydial infections, 624
in fungal infections, 622–624
in mycoplasmal infections, 624–625
in viral infections, 625
specimens for, collection of, 608–611, 610t, *612*
processing of, 611–613, 612t, 613t
selection of, 608–609, 610t
Microembolism, pulmonary, edema in, 147
Microfilariasis, 1153–1155, *1154*
Microglial cells, as tissue macrophages, 386
Microlithiasis, alveolar, 1749–1750, *1749, 1750*
*Micromonospora* pneumonia, culture in, 620–621
Micronodular pneumocyte hyperplasia, 1776
*Micropolyspora* pneumonia, culture in, 620–621
Microsatellite analysis, in lung cancer, 1378, 1426, 1426t
Microsatellite repeats, 46–47, *46*
Microscopic polyangiitis, diffuse alveolar hemorrhage in, *1735*, 1737t, 1739
Microscopy. See also *Gram stain*; specific organisms.
electron, in alveolar proteinosis, 1790, *1791*
in mesothelioma, 2069
in pneumonia diagnosis, 610t, 613–617
advantages of, 614
in immunodeficiency, 616–617
procedure for, 614–615, *614, 615*
sensitivity and specificity of, 615–616
of *Mycobacterium*, 1045t, 1046
phase-contrast, in fungal infections, 616
Microsporidiosis, in HIV infection, 2204
Microvascular osmotic reflection coefficient, 1576
Midazolam, for bronchoscopy, 730
Middle lobe syndrome, 1334, 1369
Midexpiratory forced expiratory flow rate, in airway obstruction, for reversibility evaluation, 851, *852*
Migratory thrombophlebitis, in lung cancer, 1421
Military personnel, adenovirus infections in, 937–940, *939*
toxic exposure in, 1906–1907
Milk-alkali syndrome, metabolic alkalosis in, 172
Miller's lung, 1869
Mill-wheel murmur, in pneumomediastinum, 2102
Milne method, for scoring pulmonary edema radiographs, 1499, 1499t
Milrinone, as vasodilator, 302
in pulmonary edema, 1604
*Mima-Herellea* (*Acinetobacter*) pneumonia, 1013–1014
Mineral dusts, lung disease related to. See *Pneumoconiosis(es).*
Mineral oils, inhalation of, pulmonary disease due to, 1986–1987
Mineral wool, in pneumoconiosis, 1831t, 1842
Mining, of uranium, lung cancer in, 1402
pneumoconioses in. See *Pneumoconiosis(es).*
Minors, health care decisions for, 2491
Minute ventilation. See *Ventilation, minute.*
Mismatch, ventilation-perfusion. See *Ventilation-perfusion ratio, inequality of.*
Mist, particle size of, 351–352
Mitochondria, oxygen partial pressure in, *70*, 71
oxygen supply to, at high altitude, 1922–1923, *1928*
Mitogen(s), in asthma, 1262
tolerance to, alveolar macrophages in, 393–394, *395*
Mitogen-activated protein kinases, 239–240, *239*
Mitomycin, in mesothelioma, 2070
pulmonary disease due to, 1976–1977
Mitral valve, disease of, respiratory muscle function in, 2255
surgery in, pulmonary function after, 2253, 2253t
prolapse of, pain in, 578
regurgitation of blood in, and acute respiratory distress syndrome, 2421, *2421*
stenosis of, airway resistance in, 2254
diffuse alveolar hemorrhage in, 1744
diffusing capacity in, 2252
lung compliance in, 2254, *2255*
lung volume in, 2251, *2251*, 2252t
pulmonary blood flow distribution in, 2256, *2257*
pulmonary edema in, in pregnancy, 2321
pulmonary hypertension in, 1641–1642
treatment of, pulmonary hemodynamics after, 2250–2251
Mivazerol, preoperative, in cardiac risk reduction, 884
Mixed connective tissue disease, 1708
antibodies in, 1695t
diffuse alveolar hemorrhage in, 1739
vasculitis in, 1540, *1541*
Mixed venous oxygen content, in exercise, 202, 210
Molds. See *Fungi.*
Mondor's syndrome, 577
Monge's disease (chronic mountain sickness), 1938–1939, *1939*
Monoclonal antibodies, in lung cancer screening, 1419–1420, 1420t
Monoclonal antibodies *(Continued)*
in respiratory syncytial virus infections, 964
to endotoxin, in pulmonary edema, 1610–1611
Monocrotaline, ingestion of, pulmonary hypertension related to, 1546
Monocyte(s), 386
development of, 399–400, *400*
cytokines and growth factors in, 401–404, 401t, *402*
function of, 415
gelatinase of, 393
macrophage development from, 397, 400–401
markers for, 387t
morphology of, 388, *388*, 389, *389*
progenitors of, markers for, 387t
Monocyte chemotactic proteins, 507t, 508, 516–517
receptors for, 517–518, 517t
Monokine induced by interferon-gamma, 508, 508t
receptor for, 511–512, 511t
Mononuclear phagocyte system. See also *Dendritic cells*; *Macrophage(s)*; *Monocyte(s).*
overview of, 386–387, 386t, 387t
Mononucleosis, cytomegalovirus, 943
Epstein-Barr virus, 933
Montelukast, allergic granulomatosis and angiitis due to, 1770–1771
in asthma, 285
Moral virtues, physician, 2492
*Moraxella (Branhamella) catarrhalis* infection(s), otitis media as, 918–919
pneumonia as, 1006
microbiologic diagnosis of, 615
treatment of, 998t
sinusitis as, 916
Morgagni's hernia, mediastinal protrusion of, 2130–2131
*Morganella* pneumonia, 1010–1011
Morphine, in acute respiratory distress syndrome, 2420
in dyspnea, 548, 1228
in myocardial ischemia, *2401*
in pulmonary edema, 1600, 2420
high-altitude, 1937
in shock, 2400
Morphogenesis, branching, in lung, 36, *36*
Morquio's syndrome, lung injury in, 481t
Mortality, in acute interstitial pneumonia, 1686
in acute respiratory distress syndrome, 1594, 1613, 2488, 2489
in air pollution exposure, 1885, 1891, 1895
in altitude sickness, 1930, 1930t
in amniotic fluid embolism, 1527, 2323
in asthma, 272, 1248–1249, 1255, 1272
in beta-adrenergic agonist therapy, 272
in bronchiectasis, 1332, 1333
in bronchitis, 1198–1199
in bronchoscopy, 755, 755t
in busulfan-induced pulmonary disease, 1975
in carcinoid tumors, 1462
in chronic obstructive pulmonary disease, 1198–1199, 1203, 1646
in cystic fibrosis, 1313–1314, *1314*
in diving, 1955, 1956, 1961, 1964, 1966–1967
in drowning, 1964, 1966–1967
in drug use, 1971
in embolectomy, in pulmonary hypertension, 1524–1525
in emphysema, 1198–1199
in esophageal rupture, 2027

Mortality *(Continued)*
in flail chest, 2367
in Goodpasture's syndrome, 1743
in Guillain-Barré syndrome, after influenza vaccination, 955
in hantavirus infections, 945, 946
in hemoptysis surgery, 1566
in hereditary surfactant deficiency, 318
in histoplasmosis, 1110
in HIV infection, 2172–2173
in hypereosinophilic syndrome, 1769
in idiopathic pneumonia syndrome, 2300
in influenza, 949–951, 953, 954
in intensive care unit, 2488–2489
in interstitial lung disease, 1672
in lobectomy, 1427
in lung cancer, screening effects on, 1419–1420, 1420t
in lung injury, 1594
in lung surgery, 889, 1332
in measles, 958
in mediastinitis, 2107, 2108, 2110
in metabolic alkalosis, 172
in mitomycin therapy, 1976–1977
in multisystem organ failure, prediction of, 2488–2489
in neonatal respiratory distress syndrome, 317
in organ system failure, 2488–2489
in pancreatitis, 2276
in parainfluenza virus infections, 960
in pneumomediastinum, 2104
in pneumonectomy, 1427
in pneumonia, 985–986
*Acinetobacter*, 1013
adenovirus, 939
anaerobic, 1020
*Bacillus*, 1030
community-acquired, 919
Enterobacteriaceae, 1010
*Haemophilus influenzae*, 1008
herpes simplex virus, 948
in pregnancy, 2320
*Klebsiella pneumoniae*, 1009
*Legionella*, 1016
*Nocardia*, 1023
nosocomial, 922
pneumococcal, 999–1001, 1001t
*Pseudomonas aeruginosa*, 1012
in pneumothorax, 2049, 2050
in pulmonary edema, 1594
high-altitude, 1933
re-expansion, 2055
in pulmonary embolism, 1503, 1517
in pregnancy, 2322
in pulmonary fibrosis, 1684t
in pulmonary hypertension, 1552
in respiratory failure, 2488–2489
in respiratory syncytial virus infections, 963
in sarcoidosis, 1727
in sickle cell disease, 2289
in smoking, 2558
in strongyloidiasis, 1152
in systemic lupus erythematosus, 1739
in tuberculosis, 1049, 1050, *1051*
central nervous system, 1084
disseminated (miliary), 1078
in varicella-zoster virus infections, 967
in Wegener's granulomatosis, 1738
perioperative, risk assessment for, 883–884, 884t, 885t
smoking and, 887
prediction of, 2488–2489
Mosaic perfusion, of lung, computed tomography of, 676, *677*
Moses' sign, in venous thrombosis, 1507
Motoneurons, gamma, in chest wall receptors, 184
in medulla, 186
in motor units, 197–198
respiratory, of spinal cord, *185*, 187–188, *187*
Motor nerves, of lung, 22
Motor neuron disease, hypoventilation in, 2144
Motor performance, at high altitude, 1923–1924
Motor units, in breathing control, 188
recruitment of, 198
structure of, 197
Motor vehicle accidents, pneumomediastinum in, 2097, 2101–2102
Mounier-Kuhn syndrome, 480t
bronchiectasis with, 1337
Mountain sickness, acute, 175, 1929–1932, 1930t
clinical features of, 1929–1930
natural history of, 1930
pathophysiology of, 1930–1931, *1931*
prevention of, 1932
treatment of, 1931–1932
chronic, 1938–1939, *1939*
subacute, 1938
Mouth. See *Oral cavity.*
Mouth occlusion pressure, definition of, 2565
in neuromuscular disorders, 2334
Moving slit radiography, 640–642, *641–643*
Mucins, 327–329. See also *Mucus.*
cloning of, 328, 330t
composition of, 327–328, 328t
enhancers of, 329
formation of, 327
bacterial defenses against, 334
genes of, 328–329, 330t
hypersecretion of, in asthma, 1262
in cystic fibrosis, 1300
intertwining of, 363
promoters of, 329
regulation of, 329
Mucociliary transport, 360–369. See also *Mucus.*
abnormalities of, 366–369
sequelae of, 360
treatment of, 359
as particulate defense, 1889
cilia in, 7, *8*, *9*
beat frequency of, 365
fluid surrounding, 362–363
function of, 360–361
in cystic fibrosis, 1180, *1180*
ozone injury of, 1895–1896
primary dyskinesia of, 1336
regulation of, 361–362
components of, 361
cough and, 556
facilitation of, 367
in aerosol clearance, 354
in asthma, 367–368, 1262
in bronchiectasis, 366–367, 1326
in bronchitis, 364–367
in bronchorrhea, 368–369
in cystic fibrosis, 364–365, 368, 1296, 1296t, *1297*
in environmental diseases, 374–375
in influenza, 368, *369*
in Kartagener's triad, 1336
in occupational diseases, 374–375
in primary ciliary dyskinesia, 366
in rhinitis, 368
in Sjögren's syndrome, 366
measurement of, 365–366, *366*
aerosols in, 357, *358*
mucosal structure and, 360–361
Mucociliary transport *(Continued)*
mucus transport in, 364
normal, 1296, 1296t, *1297*
periciliary fluid regulation in, 362–363
rate of, 365–366, *366*
regulation of, 365–366, *366*
tracheobronchial, 365–366, *366*
Mucoepithelial malignancies, in lower airways, 1462–1463, 1462t
Mucoid impaction, of bronchi, 1334
Mucoid pseudotumors, 1481
Mucolytics, in chronic obstructive pulmonary disease, 1224, 2462
in cystic fibrosis, 1310
in respiratory failure, 2462
in sputum specimen processing, 613
Mucopolysaccharidoses, lung injury in, 481t
Mucoregulators, in airway disease, 289
Mucormycosis, 1108, 1134–1135, *1135*
culture in, 622
geographic distribution of, 1108
in diabetes mellitus, 2310
microbiologic diagnosis of, 610t
versus hypersensitivity pneumonitis due to *Mucor* spores, 1869
Mucosa, airway, blood supply of, 361
cystic fibrosis effects on, 1295–1297, 1296t, *1297*
basal cells of, 360
glands of, bronchial. See *Bronchus(i), glands of.*
inflammation of (mucositis), in bone marrow transplantation, 2299
innervation of, mucociliary transport and, 362–363
Mucosa-associated lymphoid tissue, lymphoma of, 1455–1457
Mucoviscidosis. See *Cystic fibrosis.*
Mucus, accumulation of, in cystic fibrosis, 1293–1294, *1294*, 1300–1302
as particulate defense, 1889
bioadhesion of, 365
characteristics of, in asthma, 367–368, 1254–1255
in cystic fibrosis, 368
clearance of, augmentation of, 369–371, 370t. See also *Chest physical therapy; Cough.*
components of, 327–332
composition of, 363
in asthma, 1254–1255
in cystic fibrosis, 1296t, 1300
mucins in, 327–329, 328t, 330t
nonmucin, 329, 331–332
normal, 1296t
elasticity of, 363–364
formation of, in allergic bronchopulmonary aspergillosis, 1763, *1764*, 1765, *1765*
hypersecretion of, in inflammation, 333–334
infection of, in cystic fibrosis, 1301
obstruction by, in fatal asthma, 1255
removal of, bronchoscopic, 753
rheology of, 363–364
secretion of, 332–334
abnormal, diseases associated with, 327
anticholinergic drug effects on, 277
bacterial product effects on, 334
beta-adrenergic agonists in, 269
constitutive, 332
excessive, control of, 289
in asthma, 1262
in chronic obstructive pulmonary disease, 1224–1225
in cough, 556
in cystic fibrosis, 1300
in nose, 1346

Mucus *(Continued)*
in obstructive diseases, 1174–1175
inflammatory mediator effects on, 333–334
muscarinic receptors in, 253, *253*
nervous system in, 22
regulation of, 332–333
spinnability of, 363
surface tension of, 365
transport of. See *Mucociliary transport.*
viscosity of, 363–364
Mucus protease inhibitor, in mucus, 329
Müller's maneuver, in arteriovenous malformations, 1496
Multifocal alveolar hyperplasia, 1776
Multiple inert gas elimination technique, for ventilation-perfusion, 80–81, *81*, *82*
in hepatopulmonary syndrome, 2274
Multiple myeloma, 1464, 2292–2294, 2293t
amyloidosis in, 2295–2296
Multiple symmetric lipomatosis, of mediastinum, 2129
Multiple-breath nitrogen washout test, for ventilation distribution, 808
Multiple-indicator dilution techniques, for lung water measurement, 1596–1597
Multiple-isotope method, for lung water measurement, 1596–1597
Multisystem organ failure, mortality prediction in, 2488–2489
Multivesicular bodies, of alveolar epithelial cells, 19
Muramidase. See *Lysozyme.*
Muriatic acid, exposure to, 1905–1906
Murmurs, heart, in cor pulmonale, 1638
in pneumomediastinum, 2102
in pulmonary hypertension, 1547
Murray (lung injury) score, 1592–1594, 1592t, 2419, 2420t
Muscarinic receptors, *240*, 253, *253*
anticholinergic drug effects on, 276
in mucus secretion regulation, 333
subtypes of, 242
Muscle(s), alterations of, at high altitude, 1923, 1928
lactic acid production in, 166
respiratory. See *Respiratory muscle(s).*
smooth. See *Smooth muscle.*
structure of, 197–198, 198t
Muscle fibers, fast twitch, 188, 198, 198t
slow twitch, 188, 198, 198t
types of, 188
lactic threshold and, 208
Muscle relaxants, in oxygen consumption reduction, 2407
in tetanus, 2351
Muscle spindles, as chest wall receptors, 184
Muscular dystrophies, 2343–2345
inspiratory muscle training in, 2347
Mushroom spores, inhalation of, 1910
Mushroom worker's lung. See *Hypersensitivity pneumonitis.*
Mustard gas exposure, 1906
lung cancer in, 1402
Mutations, data base for, 52t
in hereditary hemorrhagic telangiectasia, 1559–1560
in lung cancer. See *Lung cancer, genetics of.*
of activinlike kinase gene, 1560
of cystic fibrosis transmembrane regulator gene, 1292–1293, *1293*, 1293t, 1295
of endoglin gene, 1559–1560
of protein C gene, thromboembolism risk in, 1514
of prothrombin gene, thromboembolism risk in, 1514
Mutations *(Continued)*
of retinoic acid receptors, 38–39
somatic, in immunoglobulin genes, 418–419
MVV. See *Maximal voluntary ventilation.*
Myalgia, in pneumonia, *Chlamydia psittaci*, 1026
*Legionella*, 1014
Myasthenia gravis, in thymoma, 2126–2127
maximal voluntary ventilation in, 787
respiratory function in, 2342
Myb transcription factors, in monocyte-macrophage development, 404–405
*myc* genes and products, in lung cancer, 1382
in lung development, 40
Mycetoma(s), in ankylosing spondylitis, 1710
in chronic obstructive pulmonary disease, 1195
in emphysema, 1195
in sarcoidosis, 1722
in tuberculosis, 1063, *1063*
*Mycobacterium* (general), acid-fast staining of, 1043, *1044*, 1046
characteristics of, 1043–1045, *1044*, 1044t
classification of, clades in, 1045
culture of, 618t, 619–620, 620t, 1044, 1045t, 1046–1047
drug susceptibility testing of, 1045t, 1048
microscopy of, 1045t
molecular probes of, 1047
mycobacteriology of, 610t, 1045–1048, 1045t
specimen processing for, 613, 613t
restriction fragment length polymorphisms of, 1045t, 1047–1048, *1048*
surfactant protein A binding to, 312
*Mycobacterium* (nontuberculous, atypical). See also specific organisms.
classification of, 1044–1045, 1044t
colonization by, in cystic fibrosis, 1303
culture of, 620, 620t, 1047
infections with, epidemiology of, 1090
historical aspects of, 1090
in bone marrow transplantation, 2304
in coal-workers' pneumoconiosis, 1830
in silicosis, 1819, 1824
in transplantation, 2232
nonpathogenic, 1044, 1044t
pathogenic, 1044, 1044t
rapidly growing, 1044, 1044t, 1095–1096
slowly growing, 1044, 1044t
*Mycobacterium* (tuberculosis complex), 1044t, 1048. See also *Tuberculosis, organism causing (Mycobacterium tuberculosis).*
*Mycobacterium abscessus* infections, 1095–1096
*Mycobacterium africanum* infections, 1048
*Mycobacterium avium* complex infections, 620, 620t, 1090–1094
chest radiography in, 1093
clinical features of, disseminated, 1093–1094
in HIV infection, 2185
lymphatic, 1093
pulmonary, 1091
colonization in, 1093
culture in, 1047
diagnosis of, 1091, 1092t
in HIV infection, 2185
disseminated, 1093–1094, *1094*
epidemiology of, 1090, 1093
in HIV infection, 1091, 1092t, 1093–1094, *1094*, 2185–2186
lymphatic, 1093
organism causing, 1090–1091
pathogenesis of, in HIV infection, 2185
pathology of, 456, *458*
*Mycobacterium avium* complex infections *(Continued)*
prevention of, 2186
pulmonary, 1091, 1092t, 1093
treatment of, disseminated, 1094
in HIV infection, 2185–2186
lymphatic, 1093
pulmonary, 1091
*Mycobacterium bovis* infections, 1048
*Mycobacterium chelonei* infections, 1095–1096
culture in, 1047
in HIV infection, 2187
*Mycobacterium fortuitum* infections, 1095–1096
*Mycobacterium fortuitum-chelonei* infections, 620, 620t
*Mycobacterium gastri* infections, 620
*Mycobacterium genavense* infections, 1096
culture in, 1047
genetic testing in, 626
*Mycobacterium gordonae* infections, 620t
in HIV infection, 2187
*Mycobacterium haemophilum* infections, 620t, 1047, 1096
*Mycobacterium kansasii* infections, 620, 620t, 1094–1095
culture in, 1044
epidemiology of, 1090
in HIV infection, 1095, 2186
*Mycobacterium malmoense* infections, 620t, 1096
in HIV infection, 2187
*Mycobacterium marinum* infections, 620t, 1047, 1096
*Mycobacterium microti* infections, 1048
*Mycobacterium scrofulaceum* infections, 620t, 1044, 1096
*Mycobacterium simiae* infections, 620t, 1096
*Mycobacterium smegmatis* infections, 620t
*Mycobacterium szulgai* infections, 620t, 1096
*Mycobacterium terrae* infections, 620, 620t
in HIV infection, 2187
*Mycobacterium tuberculosis.* See *Tuberculosis, organism causing (Mycobacterium tuberculosis).*
*Mycobacterium ulcerans* infections, genetic testing in, 626
*Mycobacterium xenopi* infections, 620t, 1096
in HIV infection, 2187
*Mycoplasma pneumoniae* infection(s), diagnosis of, laboratory methods for, 990–991
pharyngitis as, 1024
pneumonia as, as asthma risk factor, 1251–1252
culture in, 624–625
genetic tests for, 626
in sickle cell disease, 2287
microbiologic diagnosis of, 610t
pathology of, 473, *474*
treatment of, 998t
tracheobronchitis as, 1024
Mycosis(es). See *Fungal infection(s).*
Myelin, tubular, abnormal, 318
as surfactant reservoir, 308–309, *309*
formation of, 310, 316, *317*
surfactant protein B in, 313
Myelinated receptors, in breathing control, 182, 182t, *183*
Myelitis, tuberculous, 1083–1084
Myelography, in mediastinal disorders, 2083
Myeloma, multiple, 1464, 2292–2294, 2293t
amyloidosis in, 2295–2296
Myoblastoma, granular cell, tracheobronchial, 1478
Myocardial infarction, airway resistance in, 2254

Myocardial infarction *(Continued)*
oxygen therapy for, 2406
pain in, 578, 580, 581t
pleural effusion after, 2032
pulmonary edema in, outcome of, 1613
risk assessment for, preoperative, 883–884, 884t, 885t
treatment of, 2392–2393, 2393t, 2400, 2401t, *2402*
Myocardial ischemia, at high altitude, 1940
pain in, 570, 578, 590
shock in, 2400, 2401t, *2402*
Myocarditis, pain in, 578
Myoclonus, respiratory, 2349t, 2350
Myofibroblasts, in pulmonary fibrosis, 1677
Myoglobin, in diffusion, 1923, 1928
Myopathies, 2343–2345, *2344–2346*
Myosin, in endothelium, in permeability regulation, 141–142
Myosin-ATPase, activity of, versus muscle fiber type, 198
Myositis, in mixed connective tissue disease, 1708
Myotonia congenita, respiratory dyskinesia in, 2351
Myotonic dystrophy, respiratory muscle dyskinesia in, 2344
Myxedema, pleural effusion in, 2016
Myxoma(s), of lung, 1478

## N

Nadolol, pulmonary disease due to, 1983
Nafcillin, in pneumonia, 998t
Nail(s), deformities of, in clubbing, 600, *600*
yellow, bronchiectasis with, 1337
pleural effusion in, 2035
Naloxone, in asthma, 290
NANC (nonadrenergic noncholinergic) system, in asthma, 1262–1263
Nandrolone decanoate, in respiratory failure, 2462
Narcosis, carbon dioxide, 2444
in asthma, 1265
inert gas, 1958t, 1963
Nasal structures. See *Nose.*
Nasoenteric and nasogastric tubes, misplacement of, pleural effusion in, 2036
National Ambient Air Quality Standard, 1885, 1886t, 2556–2557
National Asthma Education and Prevention Program, 2546–2550, 2546t, 2550t
National Center for Biotechnology Information, genetic disease data base of, 52t
National Commission on Quality Assurance/ Health Employee Data Information Set, in asthma surveillance, 2552
National Heart, Lung, and Blood Institute, on asthma research, 2544–2545
National Institute of Occupational Safety and Health, beryllium lung disease register of, 1843, 1844
coal worker surveillance program of, 1815
National Institutes of Health, mission of, 2544–2545
Natriuretic peptides, as bronchodilators, 278
in cor pulmonale pathogenesis, 1637
Natural killer cells, 414
in hypersensitivity pneumonitis, 1872
in lung, 435, 438
in lymphoma, 1456t
Natural killer receptors, in asthma, 1262–1263
Near drowning, 1964–1967
clinical manifestations of, 1965, 1965t
Near drowning *(Continued)*
epidemiology of, 1964
in seawater, hypermagnesemia in, 1591
pathophysiology of, 1964–1965
prognosis for, 1966–1967
pulmonary edema in, 1584
treatment of, 1965–1966
Nebacumab, in pulmonary edema, 1610
Nebulizers, 249, 356
for beta-agonists, in asthma, 2454
for chronic obstructive pulmonary disease, 1220
for corticosteroids, 281
for morphine, in dyspnea, 548
for radiopharmaceuticals, in ventilation-perfusion scanning, 699
mist formation in, particle size of, 351–352
*Necator americanus* (hookworm) infections, 1150–1151
Neck, emphysema of, in diving, 1956
Necrobiotic nodules, in inflammatory bowel disease, 2271
Necrosis, caseation, 446, *449*
coagulation, 444, 446, *447*
definition of, 444
gross appearance of, 444, 446, *446–449*
in anaerobic pneumonia, 1017, *1018*
in aspergillosis, 474, *475*, 1133
in coccidioidomycosis, 1123
in histoplasmosis, 1109
in pulmonary capillaritis, 1733, *1735*
inflammation in, 455, *456*
liquefaction, 446, *448*
microscopic appearance of, 444, 446, *446–449*
Necrotizing mediastinitis, descending, 2108
Necrotizing sarcoid granulomatosis, 1538
Necrotizing (leukocytoclastic) vasculitis, 1534, 1539
Nedocromil, in asthma, 359, 1276, 1277t
in chronic obstructive pulmonary disease, 359
Needle aspiration biopsy, bronchoscope damage during, 757–758
lung, percutaneous, 760–761
mediastinal, 2088–2089, *2089*
pleural, 2008–2009
transbronchial, 736–737, 738t, 741
Negative effort dependence, in quiet breathing, 789
Negative expiratory pressure, in obstructive disease, 848
*Neisseria meningitidis* pneumonia, 998t, 1005–1006
Nematode infection(s), ascariasis as, 1149–1150, 1761
dirofilariasis as, 1155–1156
filariasis as, 1153–1155, *1154*, 1761–1762, *1762*
hookworm as, 1150–1151
lung injury in, 475
strongyloidiasis as, 1151–1153, *1152*
trichinosis as, 1156–1157
visceral larva migrans as, 1157
Neon, characteristics of, 1958t
Neonate(s), bronchopulmonary dysplasia in, 1180–1181, 1366–1367
chylothorax in, 2057
cystic fibrosis in, 1292, 1306, 1308, 1312
high altitude effects on, 1942
hypoxia in, pulmonary vascular response to, 131
mechanical ventilation in, pneumopericardium in, 2102
pneumonia in, adenovirus, 939
herpes simplex virus, 948–949
Neonate(s) *(Continued)*
streptococcal group B, 1004
pneumothorax in, 2053
pulmonary circulation in, 68
pulmonary hypertension in, 300
respiratory distress syndrome in, pneumomediastinum in, 2103
pneumothorax in, 2053
surfactant abnormalities and deficiencies in, 93, 317–318
versus acute respiratory distress syndrome, 318
with maternal diabetes mellitus, 2310
sequestrations in, 1567–1568
Neoplasia. See also *Tumor(s);* specific neoplasms.
cellular, 450
Neovascularization. See *Angiogenesis (neovascularization).*
Nephropathica epidemica, 945
Nephrotic syndrome, pleural effusion in, 2016
Nerve growth factor, in lung cancer growth, 1381
Nerve root(s), disorders of, chest pain in, 577
Nervous system. See also *Innervation.*
autonomic. See *Autonomic nervous system.*
central. See *Brain; Central nervous system; Spinal cord.*
in breathing control, 180–189
medulla in, 185–186, *185*, 188–189
patterns in, 180–181, *180, 181*
pons in, *185*, 186–187
reflexes and receptors in, 181–184, 182t, *183*
rhythm generation in, 188–189
spinal cord in, *185*, 187–188, *187*
suprapontine structures in, 187
of lung, 21–22, *21, 23*
of pulmonary circulation, 121, 131
Network hypothesis, of respiratory rhythm generation, 188–189
Neural tumors, of lung, 1479
Neuraminidase, of influenza virus, 949–950, 957
Neuregulins, ERBB protein interactions with, in lung cancer growth, 1380–1381
Neurenteric cyst(s), of mediastinum, 2130
Neurilemoma(s), of mediastinum, 2131, *2132*
Neuritis, pain in, 577, 590
Neuroblastoma(s), of mediastinum, 2131
Neurocirculatory asthenia, 580
Neuroendocrine carcinoma(s), 1460–1462
Neuroendocrine system, multiple tumors of, 1480–1481
of lung, 22, *23*, 1376–1377
Neuroepithelial bodies, of lung, 22, *23*
Neurofibroma(s), of lung, 1478, 1479
of mediastinum, 2131
Neurofibromatosis, 1748, 1748t
lung injury in, 481t
mediastinal involvement of, 2131
Neurogenic inflammation, 254–255, *254*
in asthma, 1262–1263
Neurogenic pulmonary edema, 147
high-altitude, 1936
pathophysiology of, 1581–1582
Neurogenic shock, 2404
Neurogenic theory, of clubbing pathogenesis, 601
Neurogenic tumor(s), of mediastinum, 2131–2132, 2131t, *2132*
Neurokinin(s), actions of, 250, *250*
in asthma, 1262–1263
in mucus secretion, 333
Neurokinin A, actions of, *251*
in mucus secretion, 333

Neurokinin A *(Continued)*
inflammation in, 254–255, *254*
Neurokinin B, in mucus secretion, 333
Neurokinin receptor, 234
Neurologic disorder(s). See also *Neuromuscular disorder(s).*
hyperventilation in, 2147
hypoventilation in, 2140t, 2142, 2144
in air embolism, 1955–1956
in arteriovenous malformations, 1561
in decompression sickness, 1960, 1961, 1962
in diving, 1955–1956
in fat embolism, 1526
in hard metal disease, 1845
in high-altitude cerebral edema, 1932–1933
in hypereosinophilic syndrome, 1769
in immunosuppressive therapy, post-transplantation, 2526
in lung cancer, 1421, 1421t
in lymphomatoid granulomatosis, 1458
in mediastinal mass, 2083
in metabolic alkalosis, 172
in near drowning, 1965
in respiratory acidosis, 174
in respiratory alkalosis, 175
in sarcoidosis, 1718–1719
lung injury in, 1588t
pulmonary edema in, 1588t
respiratory alkalosis in, 174–175, 175t
Neuromodulators, in airway disease, 288
Neuromuscular disorder(s), 2329–2356
after mechanical ventilation for asthma, 2356
airway obstruction in, 2332
amyotrophic lateral sclerosis as, 2343–2345
antibiotic toxicity as, 2343
aspiration in, 2331–2332
blood gas analysis in, 2332
botulism as, 2342–2343
classification of, 2329–2330, 2330t
convulsive, 2351–2352
cough impairment in, 2331–2332
diaphragmatic paralysis in, 2334–2337, 2336t
diffuse, 2341–2345
epilepsy as, 2351
exercise testing in, 849
hemiplegia in, 2340
hiccups as, 2349–2350
hypercapnic response in, 820
hypoventilation in, 2140t, 2142
imaging in, 2332
inappropriate muscular contraction in, 2349–2352, 2349t
inflammatory polyneuropathy as, 2341–2342
kyphoscoliosis in, 2332, 2357, 2358t
Lambert-Eaton syndrome as, 1379, 2342
muscular dystrophies as, 2343–2345
myasthenia gravis as, 787, 2126–2127, 2342
myopathies as, 2343–2345, *2344–2346*
myotonia congenita as, 2351
organophosphate poisoning as, 2343
Parkinson's disease as, 2350–2351
poliomyelitis as, 2340–2341, 2341t
pulmonary embolism in, 2332
pulmonary function tests in, 849, 2331–2333
respiratory acidosis in, 173t, 174
respiratory dyskinesias as, 2350–2351
respiratory failure in, 2445–2447, *2445*, *2446*
respiratory manifestations of, 2329
respiratory muscle function and, 2330–2331, 2330t, 2333, 2344, *2344*, *2345*
respiratory myoclonus as, 2350
sleep-related breathing disorders in, 2331, 2334
Neuromuscular disorder(s) *(Continued)*
spinal cord injury as. See *Spinal cord, injury of.*
strychnine poisoning as, 2351
tetanus as, 2351–2352
ventilatory drive in, 2331, 2333–2334, 2344–2345, *2345*, *2346*
ventilatory failure in, treatment of, 2345–2349
Neuromyopathy, paraneoplastic, in lung cancer, 1379
Neuron(s). See also *Motoneurons.*
expiratory, 186
I-alpha, 186
I-beta, 186
in chest wall receptors, 184
in medulla, 186
in pons, *185*, 186–187
nociceptive-specific, 573
pacemaker, 188
postinspiratory, 186
propriobulbar, 186
respiratory, 185–186
sensory, visceral, 573
Neuropeptide(s), actions of, 250, *250*, *251*
in chronic bronchitis, 1216
in mucus secretion, 333
Neuropeptide K, actions of, *251*
Neuropeptide Y, actions of, 250, *250*, *251*
ciliary effects of, 362
in mucus secretion regulation, 332, 333
Neurotoxins, eosinophil-derived, 1758t, 1759
in chemical warfare, 1906–1907
Neurotransmitters, in airway function, 249–250, *250*, *251*
in periciliary fluid regulation, 362–363
of epithelial cells, 361
release of, 232, *233*
Neutral endopeptidase, actions of, 255
imbalance of, in asthma, 1262–1263
Neutropenia, 2291
chronic inherited, 2237
cyclic, 2237
in bone marrow transplantation, 925
in HIV infection, 2176
infections in, 2237
pneumonia in, microbiology of, 988t
*Pseudomonas aeruginosa* infections in, 1011
Neutrophil(s), 521–526
accumulation of, in cystic fibrosis, 1179
activation of, 526
in smoking, 1212
apoptosis of, 524, 528–529, *529*, *530*
counting of, in inflammation assessment, 529–530
deficiency of. See *Neutropenia.*
development of, 524
evaluation of, in hantavirus infections, 946
excess of. See *Neutrophilia.*
granules in, 521, 523, 523t
in acute respiratory distress syndrome, 528
in asthma, *1260*, 1261
in fibrosis, 512–513
in host defense, 526
infiltration of, in pulmonary capillaritis, 1733, *1734*
injury potential of, 526
inside-out signaling of, 525
normal count of, 524
priming of, 526
products secreted by, 521, 523, 523t
properties of, 521, *522*, 523–524, *523*, 523t
receptors on, 523–524
recruitment of, in injury, 496, *496*
structure of, 521, *522*
trafficking of, 524–526, *525*
Neutrophil activating protein-2, 508, 508t
Neutrophil elastase, in mucus, 332
Neutrophilia, chronic bronchitis in, 1215–1216, *1215*
emphysema in, 1211
New York virus (hantavirus) infections, 945–947
Newborns. See *Neonate(s).*
Newton's third law, applied to respiratory system, 782
Nickel and nickel compounds, exposure to, 1907
lung cancer in, 1402
Niclofolan, in paragonimiasis, 1162
Nicotinamide adenine dinucleotide phosphate, in free radical generation, in macrophages, 390, 392
Nicotine, cardiovascular effects of, 887
C-fiber ending stimulation by, 184
in cigarettes, versus cancer risk, 1399
replacement of, in smoking cessation, 1217, 2533
Nicotinic receptors, 240, *240*
in lung cancer growth, 1381
Niemann-Pick disease, 1748–1749
lung injury in, 481t
Nifedipine, as vasodilator, 300
in acute respiratory distress syndrome, 2421
in myocardial ischemia, *2401*
in pulmonary edema, 1937, 2421
in pulmonary hypertension, 1551
Nitrates, as vasodilators, 301–302. See also specific drugs, e.g., *Nitroglycerin; Nitroprusside.*
Nitric oxide, actions of, 257, 297–298
as vasodilator, 301–302
deficiency of, in pulmonary hypertension, 1492
excess of, in hepatopulmonary syndrome, 2272
formation of, in macrophages, 392, 394
in nose, 1346
in bronchodilation, 256
in hypoxic pulmonary vasoconstriction, 67, 68, 130
in neonatal pulmonary vasculature remodeling, 131
in pulmonary circulation, 297–298
in pulmonary edema, 1936
in pulmonary hypertension, 1645
in vasoactivity evaluation, 299
in vasodilation, 257
inhalation of, 301
in acute respiratory distress syndrome, 2434–2435
in pulmonary edema, 1611
in sickle cell disease, 2289
Nitrites, as vasodilators, 301–302
Nitrofurantoin, pleural disease due to, 2035
pulmonary disease due to, 1762, 1972, 1978–1979
Nitrogen, fractional concentration of, in exercise testing, 843
in lung volume measurement, 791–792, *791*
narcosis from, in diving, 1963
solubility of, in diving, 1958–1959, 1958t, *1959*
transfer of, limitation of, 73, *74*
Nitrogen dioxide, alveolar clearance of, 372
as air pollutant, standards for, 2556
chronic bronchitis due to, 1215
elastin depletion due to, 1213
Nitrogen oxides. See also *Nitrogen dioxide.*
as air pollutants, adverse effects of, 1887t, 1893–1896
chronic exposure to, 1896

Nitrogen oxides *(Continued)*
indoor, 1888
reduction of, government role in, 2556
sources of, 1887t, 1888
high-level exposure to, 1906
Nitroglycerin, as vasodilator, 301
in acute respiratory distress syndrome, 2418, 2421
in myocardial ischemia, *2401*
in pulmonary edema, 1601–1602, 2418, 2421
in shock, 2400, 2401t
Nitroprusside, as vasodilator, 301
in acute respiratory distress syndrome, 2421
in pulmonary edema, 1601–1602, 1606, 2421
in shock, 2401t
Nitrosoureas, pulmonary disease due to, 1974t, 1977
Nkx-2.1 (thyroid transcription factors–1), in lung development, 38
NMDA (*N*-methyl-D-aspartate) receptor, in pain transmission, 574
*Nocardia* infections, pleural effusion in, 2023
pneumonia due to, 1022–1023, *1023*
in HIV infection, 2181
microbiologic diagnosis of, 610t, 618t, 620–621
treatment of, 998t
Nociception, in visceral pain, 569–570, 572, *572*, 573
modulation of, 574–575
neurons specific for, 573
Nocturnal asthma, 1271
Nodose ganglia, in visceral innervation, 569
Nodule(s), benign, 1477–1481, *1479*, *1481*
versus malignant, 1472t
biopsy of, 663, *663*, 740
bleomycin-induced, 1976, *1976*
calcification of, in hyperparathyroidism, 2312, *2312*
centrilobular, 675
computed tomography of, 675, *675*, 716
imaging of, 715–716
in amyloidosis, 2296
in aspergillosis, 1134
in coal-workers' pneumoconiosis, 1825, *1825*, 1826, *1826*
in Gaucher's disease, 1748
in interstitial lung disease, 1657, *1659*
in lymphangio(leio)myomatosis, 1776
in lymphoma, 2207
in lymphomatoid granulomatosis, 1458, *1459*
in mesothelioma, 2068
in Niemann-Pick disease, 1748–1749
in paracoccidioidomycosis, 1128
in rheumatoid arthritis, 1701–1702
in sarcoidosis, 1722, *1722*
malignant, in Hodgkin's disease, 1454, *1454*
lung resection in, 1428–1429
metastatic, 1471–1472, *1471*, 1472t
treatment of, 1439, *1445*
versus benign, 716, 1472t
multiple, computed tomography in, 668–669, *669*
necrobiotic, in inflammatory bowel disease, 2271
perilymphatic, 675, *675*
random distribution, 675, *675*
silicotic, 1818–1819, 1818t, *1820*, *1821*, 1823
solitary, as imaging artifact, 666, *667*
benign, 666–668, *667–669*, 1477–1481, *1479*
diagnosis of, imaging in, 665–668, *667–669*, 715–716
Nodule(s) *(Continued)*
hamartoma as, 1478
in dirofilariasis, 1155
malignant, computed tomography in, 666–668, *667–669*
lung resection in, 1428–1429
treatment of, 1439, *1445*
Noise, in chest radiography, 636–637
Nonadrenergic noncholinergic system, functions of, *250*, 256
in asthma, 1262–1263
Nonallergic rhinitis, pathophysiology of, 1348
treatment of, 1349–1350
Nonallergic rhinitis with eosinophilia syndrome (NARES), 1347
Non-Hodgkin's lymphoma. See *Lymphoma(s)*.
Nonmaleficence, as ethical principle, 2491
Non–small cell lung cancer. See *Lung cancer, non–small cell.*
Nonspecific interstitial pneumonia/pneumonitis, 1672t, 1687–1688
in HIV infection, 2209
Nonsteroidal anti-inflammatory drugs. See also *Aspirin.*
contraindicated in asthma, 290–291
in common cold, 933
pulmonary disease due to, 1985
Nontopographic inequality, of ventilation, 60
Norepinephrine, actions of, *250*, *251*
beta$_2$-adrenergic agonists derived from, 268, *268*
chemical structure of, 268, *268*
excess of, in sleep apnea, 2162
in mucus secretion regulation, 333
in pulmonary edema, 1603
in pulmonary vascular resistance control, 131
in shock, 2401t
hypovolemic, 2401–2402
in pulmonary embolism, 2404
septic, 2400
metabolism of, in pulmonary circulation, 69
of epithelial cells, 361
Nose, 1345–1350
aerosol clearance in, 354
aerosol deposition in, 352
airflow in, 1343–1345, *1343–1345*
anatomy of, 1343–1347, *1343*, 1346t
bleeding from, in hereditary hemorrhagic telangiectasia, 1560, 1561
breathing through, humidification in, 362
bronchoscope insertion in, 732
cannula in, for oxygen therapy, 1226
congestion of, in rhinitis, 1347
continuous positive airway pressure for, in sleep apnea, 2160, 2165
decongestants for, 1349
defense mechanisms of, 352
inflammation of. See *Rhinitis.*
muscles of, function of, 1345, 1346t
obstruction of, sleep apnea in, 2157
polyps of, in cystic fibrosis, 1294, 1305, 1313
receptors in, 181
reflexes in, 181
secretions of, 1346
Nosocomial infection(s), in bronchoscopy, 756
in intensive care unit, 2489
pneumonia as, 922–923, 922t
bronchoscopy in, 747, *748*
causes of, 987, 987t
*Legionella*, 1014
organisms causing, 922–923
respiratory syncytial virus, 964
treatment of, 995–996, 996t, 998t
NRDS. See *Neonate(s), respiratory distress syndrome in.*
Nuclear factor of activated T cells, as transcription factor, 261
Nuclear factor-kappa B, 260, *260*
inhibitors of, in airway disease, 288
receptor for, subtypes of, 241, *241*
Nuclear medicine. See *Radionuclide studies; Ventilation-perfusion scanning;* specific techniques.
Nucleic acid studies, for fungi, 626
for *Mycobacterium*, 1047
Nucleus ambiguus, in breathing control, 186
Numerical density, in lung quantitative morphology, 26, *27*, *28*, 29
Nutrition, deficient. See *Malnutrition.*
ethical decisions concerning, 2493–2494
in chronic obstructive pulmonary disease, 1227–1228, 2463–2464
in chylothorax drainage, 2058
in cystic fibrosis, 1306, 1311
in pneumonia, 999
in pulmonary edema, 1608
in pulmonary rehabilitation, 2510
in ventilator liberation, 2385
withholding or withdrawing of, decision making in, 2496–2497, 2500


## O


Obesity, 2370–2373
airway narrowing in, 2156
asthma in, 1267
breathing control and patterns in, 2372
chronic obstructive pulmonary disease with, 1228
diagnosis of, 2370–2371, 2371t
dyspnea in, 220
etiology of, 2370–2371, 2371t
exercise capacity in, 2361t, 2373
exercise testing in, 848–849
fat distribution in, 2371
gas exchange in, 2372
hypoventilation in, 174, 2159
pathophysiology of, 2371–2373, 2371t
pulmonary function tests in, 848–849, 856–857, 857t, 2371–2372, 2371t
respiratory manifestations of, 2310–2311
respiratory mechanics in, 2372
respiratory muscle function in, 2372–2373
severity of, 2370, 2371t
treatment of, 2373
Objective symptoms, definition of, 896
Oblique view, in radiography, 654
Obliterative bronchiolitis. See *Bronchiolitis obliterans.*
Obliterative pulmonary hypertension, 1492–1493, 1492t, 1543
Obstetrics. See *Labor and delivery; Pregnancy.*
Obstructive disease(s). See also specific diseases, e.g., *Asthma; Bronchiectasis; Chronic obstructive pulmonary disease; Cystic fibrosis.*
airway. See *Airway obstruction.*
beta-adrenergic antagonist effects on, 1983–1984
causes of, 851t, 1174
clinical features of, 1181
common features of, 1174
diagnosis of, 1181–1182
diffusing capacity in, 815, *816*
exercise testing in, 847–848
flow-volume relationships in, 788–789, *790*
in HIV infection, 2209
pathophysiology of, 1174
pulmonary function tests in, 788–789, *790*, 804, *805*, 848, 850–854, 851t, *852*, 1181–1182

Obstructive disease(s) *(Continued)*
terminology of, 1174
treatment of, surfactant in, 320
types of, 1173
ventilation distribution in, 808
ventilation-perfusion scanning in, 697–698
volume-flow curves for, *1665*
Obstructive pulmonary hypertension, 1492–1493, 1492t, 1543, 1642
Obturator airway, esophageal perforation from, 2107
Occupation(s), energy requirements for, 906–907, 907t, 909
history of, in hypersensitivity pneumonitis, 1873, 1873t
impairment and disability evaluation for. See *Impairment and disability.*
in medical history, 591, 1806, 1807t, 1815–1816
Occupational and environmental disorder(s), 1803–1809. See also *Pneumoconiosis(es).*
acute, 374
agents causing, 1905t
air pollution and. See *Air pollution*; *Hypersensitivity pneumonitis.*
allergic, 374–375
altitude-related. See *Altitude, high.*
alveolar clearance in, 372–373
alveolar proteinosis as, 1791–1792, 1792t, 1794
anthrax as, 1029
as disease models, 1803–1804, 1804t
as subspecialty, 1804
asthma as, 374–375, 908, 1256, *1256*, 1853–1860
exacerbations of preexisting disease, 1854
new-onset, 1854–1860
bronchiolitis as, 1362, *1362*
byssinosis as, 1860–1863
chronic obstructive pulmonary disease as, 1200–1201
diagnosis of, 1806, 1807t
diffuse alveolar hemorrhage as, 1744
drug-induced. See *Drug(s), pulmonary disease(s) due to.*
economic aspects of, 1804
emphysema as, 1213
epidemiologic studies in, 1805
from remote-in-time exposures, 1806
future directions in, 1808
historical perspective of, 1804–1805
importance of, 1803–1804, 1804t
in aluminum production, 1400
in ammonia exposure, 1909
in arsenic exposure, 1400
in asbestos exposure. See *Asbestos*; *Asbestosis.*
in barium exposure (baritosis), 1842
in beryllium exposure, 1842–1844
cancer in, 1402–1403
pathology of, *469*
in bis(chloromethyl) ether exposure, 1401
in bromine and bromine compound exposure, 1909
in cadmium exposure, 1403, 1907
in carborundum exposure, 1845
in chlorine and chlorine compound exposure, 1905–1906
in chromium exposure, 1401
in coal industry. See *Coal-workers' pneumoconiosis.*
in coke oven emission exposure, 1401–1402
in diesel exhaust exposure, 1403, 1893
in diving. See *Diving.*
in electromagnetic field exposure, 1403–1404
Occupational and environmental disorder(s) *(Continued)*
in ethylene oxide exposure, 1909
in formaldehyde exposure, 1403
in glass fiber exposure, 1403
in hard metal exposure, 1844–1845
in hydrogen sulfide exposure, 1909
in iron and steel industry, 1402
in isocyanate exposure, 1909–1910
in laboratory personnel, during culture, 626
in medical history, 591
in mercury exposure, 1907
in metal exposure, 1907
in mica exposure, 1841
in military, 1906
in mixed dust exposure, 1817, 1842
in mustard gas exposure, 1402
in nickel and nickel compound exposure, 1402
in non-asbestos mineral silicate exposure, 1830, 1831t, 1841–1842
in organic dust exposure, 1907
in paraquat exposure, 1908
in phosphine exposure, 1910
in silicon-carbide exposure, 1845
in talc exposure, *1814*, 1841
in trimellitic anhydride exposure, 1744, 1857, 1859, 1910
in vermiculite exposure, 1841
in vinyl chloride exposure, 1402
infections as, in health care workers, 758–759
interstitial lung disease as, 908, *1650*, 1652t, 1656
lung cancer as, 1400–1404
from air pollution, 1403
from diesel exhaust, 1403
from electromagnetic fields, 1403–1404
from established carcinogens, 1400–1402
from suspected carcinogens, 1402–1403
passive smoke in, 1399–1400
lung injury in, 477, 478t, 1588t, 1590–1591
Material Safety Data Sheets for, 904
metal fume fever as, 1907
mucociliary transport in, 374–375
pathogenesis of, 1903–1904
pneumonia as, etiology of, 987
polymer fume fever as, 1907
population studies in, 1805–1806
prevention of, 1806–1808
psittacosis as, 998t, 1026
public health aspects of, 1804
pulmonary fibrosis as, 1677
pulmonary manifestations of, 1692
Q fever as, 473, 998t, 1025–1026
radiation-induced, 1402
research on, 1805–1806
risk estimation in, 1805
sequelae of, 1904–1905
siderosis as, 1842
silicosis as. See *Silicosis.*
spectrum of, 1803
spirometry in, 784
stannosis as, 1842
toxicology in, 1805–1806
treatment of, 1904
war-related, 1804–1805
Occupational Safety and Health Administration, asbestos fiber definition of, 1830
permissible exposure limits of, for asbestos, 1836–1837
Octreotide, in carcinoid tumors, 1462
Odontogenic infections, mediastinitis in, 2108
pneumomediastinum in, 2097
Ofloxacin, in cystic fibrosis, 1309t
Ofloxacin *(Continued)*
in pneumonia, 995t
Ogilvie equation, for diffusing capacity correction for body size, 814
Ohm's law, for pulmonary vascular resistance calculation, 123–124
Oils, inhalation of, pulmonary disease due to, 1986–1987
Omeprazole, in gastroesophageal reflux, 2270
*Onchocerca volvulus* infections, 1153
Oncogene(s), in lung cancer, 1379–1382, *1380*
Oncotic pressure, in pulmonary capillaries, 132–133, *132*
plasma, decreased, pulmonary edema in, 145, *145*
On-line sources, of information on genetic disease, 51–52, 52t
Onset of blood lactate accumulation. See *Lactic acid (anaerobic) threshold.*
Ontogeny, of receptors, 245
Oophorectomy, in lymphangio(leio)myomatosis, 1783
Opacity, lung, computed tomography of, 675–676, *676*, *677*, 678
Open-circuit nitrogen method, for lung volume measurement, 791–792, *791*
Opioid(s), in cough control, 289
in dyspnea, 548
receptors for, in lung cancer growth, 1381
Opportunistic infections, in HIV infection. See *Human immunodeficiency virus infection*, specific disorders.
Oral cavity, appliances for, in sleep apnea, 2160
candidiasis of, 1135
colonization of, pneumonia diagnosis and, 607, *607*, 608t
herpes simplex virus infections of, 933, 947–948
Koplik's spots in, 958
muscles surrounding, 1346t
paracoccidioidomycosis of, 1128
Organic dust(s), inhalation of, 1907
byssinosis in, 1860–1862
Organic impairment, definition of, 896
Organizing pneumonia, bronchiolitis obliterans with. See *Bronchiolitis obliterans organizing pneumonia.*
Organizing pneumonitis, cryptogenic (idiopathic bronchiolitis obliterans organizing pneumonia), 1365
Organophosphate poisoning, respiratory function in, 2343
Orthochlorobenzamalonitrile, exposure to, 1907
Orthodeoxia, in arteriovenous malformations, 1563
in systemic-pulmonary communications, 1497
Orthomyxovirus infections, 931t. See also *Influenza.*
Orthopnea, definition of, 588
in diaphragmatic paralysis, 2335
in heart disease, 543–544, 2261–2262
in systemic-pulmonary communications, 1497
Osmolality, serum, in ethylene glycol toxicity, 168
urine, in hyperchloremic acidosis, 170
Osmotic pressure, in lung, in edema protection, 1577
versus hydrostatic pressure, 1576
in pulmonary edema, 1578, 1583, 1585
Osmotic reflection coefficient, 1576
Osteoarthropathy, hypertrophic pulmonary, 600–601, *601*, 601t, *602*

Osteoarthropathy *(Continued)*
in benign fibrous mesothelioma, 2071
in cystic fibrosis, 1305–1306
in lung cancer, 1421
Osteoclasts, as tissue macrophages, 386
Osteomyelitis, in coccidioidomycosis, 1124–1125
in tuberculosis, 1081–1083, *1082*
Osteoporosis, in lung transplantation, 2526
in multiple myeloma, 2293
Osteosarcoma, metastasis of, to lung, 1474
Otitis media, acute, 918–919
in adenovirus infections, 939
in influenza, 953
in respiratory syncytial virus infections, 962
with common cold, 933
with effusion (serous), 919
Ovarian hyperstimulation syndrome, pleural effusion in, 2034–2035
Ovary, ablation of, in lymphangio(leio)myomatosis, 1783
tumors of, Meigs' syndrome in, 2034
Ovulation, induction of, pleural effusion in, 2034–2035
Oxacillin, in cystic fibrosis, 1309t
in pneumonia, 998t
resistance to, in *Staphylococcus aureus*, 1004
Oxalic acid, in specimen processing, 613t
Oxidants, emphysema due to, 1213
Oximetry, 834–835, *835*
in asthma, 1275
in sleep, 2154–2155, *2155*, *2156*, 2334
pulse, 834–835, *835*
in arteriovenous malformations, 1562
Oxitropium bromide, as bronchodilator, 276
in asthma, 357
in chronic obstructive pulmonary disease, 277, 357, 1221
Oxothiazolidine, in pulmonary edema, 1610
Oxygen, breathing of, alveolar-arterial oxygen difference effects of, 826, *826*, 826t, 827t
carbon monoxide binding to, 86
cilia stimulation by, 361
delivery of, in respiratory failure, optimizing of, 2406, 2406t
diffusion of, at high altitude, 1923
discovery of, 1915–1916
dissolved, 85
drive to breathe and, 2446–2447
exchange of. See *Gas exchange*.
extraction of, per beat, in exercise testing, 844, 878
hemoglobin interactions with, at high altitude, 1922, *1922*
in diffusing capacity, 810, *810*
rates of, 73–74, *74*
in breathing test at 100% concentration, in arteriovenous malformations, 1496
in chronic obstructive pulmonary disease, 1193
in cor pulmonale, 1193
in diffusing capacity measurement, 813
in single-breath test, of ventilation distribution, 805–807, *807*
inhalation of. See also *Oxygen therapy*.
at 100%, in vasoactivity evaluation, 299
in exercise testing, 843
limitation of, lactic acid production in, 206–208, *207*
partial pressure of, air-to-tissue gradients in, 70–71, *70*
alveolar, calculation of, 824
carbon dioxide sensitivity and, 191, *191*
distribution of, in normal lung, 78, *78*
in hemodialysis, 2280
Oxygen *(Continued)*
in hypoventilation, 71–72, *72*, 2444
in ventilation-perfusion ratio calculation, 77–78, *77*, *78*
ventilatory sensitivity to, 191–192, *192*
versus altitude, 1916–1917, *1916*
versus diffusing capacity, 815
versus ventilation-perfusion ratio, 77–78, *77*, *78*
alveolar-to-arterial difference in, at high altitude, 1919, *1920*, 1926
definition of, 2564
in asthma, 1265
in exercise testing, 844
in hyperventilation, 2148
in hypoventilation, 2142, *2142*, 2143
in hypoxia, 821t
in interstitial lung disease, 217–218, 225–226, 1663
in near drowning, 1965, 1965t
in pulmonary hypertension, 1521
in ventilation-perfusion ratio calculation, 79–80, *79*
oxygen breathing effects on, 826, *826*, 826t, 827t
versus age, 824
arterial, at high altitude, 1917, *1920*
bronchodilator effects on, 83, *84*
chemoreceptor sensing of, 189–190, *190*
desaturation of, at high altitude, 1926, *1927*
in acute respiratory distress syndrome, 2417, 2419t
in airway obstruction, versus altitude, 860
in alveolar proteinosis, 1795, *1796*
in arteriovenous malformations, 1495, 1562
in cystic fibrosis, 1304, 1304t
in dry air at sea level, 70
in exercise, 224, 840, 2259
in heart disease, 2258, *2258*, 2259
in hemodialysis, 2279–2280
in high altitude acclimatization, 1917, *1917*
in hyperventilation, 2145–2146
in hypoventilation, 2141, *2141*
in hypoxia, 821t
in interstitial lung disease, 1663–1664
in near drowning, 1965t
in oxygen-hemoglobin dissociation curve, 85–86, *86*
in pneumothorax, 2045, 2054
in pulmonary edema, 1594–1595, 2258, *2258*
in pulmonary hypertension, 1494, 1521, 1548
in restrictive disorders, 855, 855t
in sarcoidosis, 1723
in sleep, 1194, 2153, 2154–2155, *2155*, *2156*
in venous-to-arterial shunt, 825–827, *826*, 826t, 827t
in ventilation-perfusion ratio calculation, 79
low. See *Hypoxia and hypoxemia*.
measurement of, 832–833, *832*
in exercise testing, 842
in impairment and disability evaluation, 906
theoretical aspects of, 830
transcutaneous, 834–836, *835*, *836*
*Mycobacterium tuberculosis* proliferation and, 1056
respiratory responses to, 191–192, *192*
Oxygen *(Continued)*
versus altitude, 860
versus hemoglobin affinity, 1922, *1922*
versus position, 855, 855t
atmospheric, versus altitude, 1915, 1916t
in water vapor, 70
mixed venous, in oxygen delivery monitoring, 2407
pulmonary capillary, 72–73, *73*, *74*, 2047
pulmonary disease due to, 1987
reactive species of. See *Free radicals*.
solubility of, 85
source of, for exercise metabolism, 838, 838t
toxicity of, 1987. See also *Hyperoxia*.
in mechanical ventilation, 2430, 2483
pulmonary edema in, 147
transport of, 85–86, *86*
in respiratory failure, 2405–2407, *2405*, 2406t
inadequate, blood gases in, 821t
uptake of. See *Oxygen uptake*.
Oxygen concentration, arterial, in shunt calculation, 76, 80
in venous-to-arterial shunt, 825–827, *826*, 826t, 827t
mixed venous blood, in shunt calculation, 80
in venous-to-arterial shunt, 825–827, 827t
Oxygen consumption. See *Oxygen uptake*.
Oxygen content, measurement of, 833–834
mixed venous, in exercise, 202, 210
Oxygen dissociation curve, 85–86, *86*
in highly fit athletes, 219
Oxygen free radicals. See *Free radicals*.
Oxygen pulse, in exercise testing, 844, 878
Oxygen saturation, in mountain sickness, 1939, *1939*
in sleep, 2154–2155, *2155*, *2156*
Oxygen therapy, administration of, modes for, 1226
ambulatory system for, 1226
bronchopulmonary dysplasia due to, 1366–1367
delivery systems for, 2406, 2406t, 2511, 2512t
dissolved oxygen concentration in, 85
evaluation of, exercise testing in, 842
for acute respiratory distress syndrome, 2420, 2430, *2431*
intravenous, 2434
for air embolism, 1526
for air travel, 1226–1227
for asthma, 1275, 2453
for bronchiectasis, 1331
for bronchoscopy, 728
for chronic obstructive pulmonary disease, 1225–1227, 1225t, 1229, 1643–1644, 1646–1647, 2510–2511, 2511t, 2512t
for cor pulmonale, 1643–1644
for cystic fibrosis, 1312
for decompression sickness, 1962
for dyspnea, 548
for erythrocytosis, 2286
for heart failure, 2259–2260, 2260t
for high-altitude pulmonary edema, 1936
for hypersensitivity pneumonitis, 1879
for hypoventilation, 2144
for lung contusion, 2436–2437
for mountain sickness, acute, 1932
chronic, 1939
for myocardial infarction, 2406
for near drowning, 1965–1966
for periodic breathing, at high altitude, 1924–1925, *1924*, *1925*
for pneumomediastinum, 2104
for pneumothorax, 2047

Oxygen therapy *(Continued)*
for pulmonary edema, 1600, 1607, 2420
high-altitude, 1936
for pulmonary hypertension, 1643–1644
for pulmonary vascular resistance, 299
for respiratory acidosis, 174
for respiratory failure, 2446–2447
hypoxemic, *2379*
in airway obstruction, *2379*
for sleep apnea, 1941, 2164
for status asthmaticus, 2453
for ventilatory failure, 2346
home use of, guidelines for, 2511, 2511t, 2512t
hyperbaric, pneumothorax in, 2054
in pulmonary rehabilitation, 2507–2508, 2510–2511, 2511t, 2512t
interactions of, in bleomycin toxicity, 1976
intravenous, for acute respiratory distress syndrome, 2434
oxygen-conserving devices for, 1226
post-thoracoplasty, 2364
transtracheal catheters for, 1226
vasodilating effects of, 299
with helium, for asthma, 2459
with 100% oxygen, in shunt detection, 76
Oxygen uptake, definition of, 2564
in arteriovenous malformations, 1563
in critical illness, 2405–2406, *2405*
in cystic fibrosis, 1304t
in diving, 1952–1953, *1953*, 1963
in exercise, 199–200, *199*, *200*, 838t, 1491t
at high altitude, 1925, *1925*
heavy, 204–205
in emphysema, 222–223, *222*
in highly fit athletes, 218
in interstitial pulmonary disease, *223*, 225
moderate, 201–203, *203*
steady-state in, 840
in exercise testing, 843
in near drowning, in cold water, 1965
in obesity, 220
in pregnancy, 2318, *2318*
maximum, after thoracoplasty, 2364
at high altitude, in exercise, 1925, *1925*, 1928–1929
definition of, 201, 2564
in exercise, 201, 1925, *1925*, 1928–1929
in impairment and disability evaluation, 899, 899t, 905–906, 906–907, 907t
in kyphoscoliosis, 2360–2361, 2361t
versus age, 857
measurement of, in occupational situations, 909
of respiratory muscles, 859, 2445
versus minute ventilation, in highly fit athletes, 219
reduction of, in respiratory failure, 2406–2407
versus ventilation, 839, *839*
Oxygen–carbon dioxide diagram, for ventilation-perfusion, 77, *77*, 79, *79*
Oxygen-derived free radicals. See *Free radicals.*
Oxygen-hemoglobin dissociation curve, 73–74, *74*, 830
at high altitude, 1922, *1922*
hyperventilation effects on, 2147
Oxyhemoglobin, 85–86, *86*, 833–834
Ozone, alveolar clearance of, 372
as air pollutant, adverse effects of, 1887t, 1889–1890, 1893–1896
chronic exposure to, 1896
reduction of, government role in, 2556
sources of, 1887t
standards for, 2557
Ozone *(Continued)*
chronic bronchitis due to, 1215
lung injury due to, 1906

## P

P (pump) cells, in medulla, in breathing control, 185
*p21* gene and product, in lung cancer, 1383
*p51* gene and product, in lung cancer, 1383
*p53* gene and product, function of, 1382
mutations of, in lung cancer, 1382–1383, 1416
*p73* gene and product, in lung cancer, 1383
*p107* gene and product, in lung cancer, 1383
*p130* gene and product, in lung cancer, 1383
Pacemakers, in breathing rhythm generation, 188–189
phrenic nerve, in neuromuscular disorders, 2348–2349
Pachydermoperiostosis, 600
Paclitaxel, in Kaposi's sarcoma, 2206
in lung cancer, 1437, 1437t
$Pa_{CO_2}$. See *Carbon dioxide, partial pressure of, arterial.*
$PA_{CO_2}$. See *Carbon dioxide, partial pressure of, alveolar.*
Pain, assessment of, 567–568
back, in ankylosing spondylitis, 2369
bone, in lung cancer metastasis, 1435
in sickle cell disease, 2287
causes of, 567
chest. See *Chest pain.*
definition of, 567
euthanasia in, 2500–2501
hyperventilation in, 2147
in clubbing, 601
in exercise, 221
in herpes zoster, 967–968
in pharyngitis, 917, 918
in sinusitis, 916
in venous thrombosis, 1506–1507
in visceral distention, 569
modulation of, 574–575
pleuritic, 575–576, 590
referred, 568–569, 574, *574*
from abdomen to chest, 580
in esophageal disorders, 579
in pleurisy, 576
somatic, versus visceral, 568–569
visceral. See *Visceral pain.*
Palliative treatment, of lung cancer, 1431–1432, 1435–1436
bronchoscopic, 742
metastatic, 1473–1474
Palmitoylation, of G protein–coupled receptors, 234
Palpation, of chest, 597, 599t
PALV. See *Alveolar pressure.*
Panbronchiolitis, 1366
Pancoast tumor, 1430
Pancoast's syndrome, 577
Pancreas, abscess of, pleural effusion in, 2030
cystic fibrosis of, clinical manifestations of, 1306
pathology of, 1179, 1294–1295
treatment of, 1311
enzymes of, in cystic fibrosis, 1311
pleural fistula with, 2029, 2277, *2278*
pseudocysts of, mediastinal extension of, 2132
pleural effusions in, 2028–2029, *2029*, 2277–2278, *2278*
Pancreatitis, 2276–2278
in cystic fibrosis, 1306
Pancreatitis *(Continued)*
mediastinal spread of, 2109
pleural effusion in, 2003, 2028–2029, *2029*
Pancuronium, in tetanus, 2351
Pancytopenia, in HIV infection, 2176
Panic disorder, chest pain in, 580
Panlukast, in asthma, 285
Panting, airway resistance measurement in, 799
$Pa_{O_2}$. See *Oxygen, partial pressure of.*
Papanicolaou smear, in coccidioidomycosis, 1125
Papilloma(s), tracheobronchial, 1478
Papillomatosis, multiple, of larynx, 1478
Para-aminosalicylic acid, in tuberculosis, 1066, 1069t, 1070
Paracellular pathway, for fluid and solute exchange, 134, *134–135*
through epithelial tight junctions, 338
Paracentesis, in hepatic hydrothorax, 2015
Paracoccidioidomycosis, 622–623, 1107, 1128–1129
Paradoxical aciduria, in metabolic alkalosis, 162
Paraffinoma(s), of lung, 1481
Paraganglioma(s), in Carney's triad, 1480, *1481*
of mediastinum, 2131–2132
Paragonimiasis, 1160–1163, *1162*, 2026
Parainfluenza virus infections, 931t, 959–961
antibodies in, 960
cell culture in, 625
clinical manifestations of, 960–961
diagnosis of, 625, 961
epidemiology of, 960
mortality in, 960
pathogenesis of, 960
pneumonia due to, 470, 961, 2302–2303
prevention of, 961
transmission of, 960
treatment of, 961
virus causing, 959–960
Paralysis, breathing in, nonrespiratory muscle recruitment for, 108
of diaphragm. See *Diaphragm, paralysis of.*
of respiratory muscles, pulmonary function in, 2331
Parametric pedigree analysis, in genetic disease, 49–50
Paramyxovirus infections, 931t. See also *Measles; Parainfluenza virus infections; Respiratory syncytial virus infections.*
Paranasal sinuses. See *Sinus(es)*; *Sinusitis.*
Paraneoplastic syndrome(s), dermatomyositis as, 1708
in benign fibrous mesothelioma, 2071
in lung cancer, 1378–1379, 1421–1422
in lymphoma, 1457
polymyositis as, 1708
Paraplegia, in spinal cord metastasis, 1435
respiratory function in, 2339–2340, 2339t
Parapneumonic effusion. See *Pleural effusion(s), in pneumonia; Pleural effusion(s), parapneumonic.*
Paraquat, toxicity of, 1908
Parasitic infection(s), 1143–1171
amebiasis as, 1144–1146, *1145*, 2026
ascariasis as, 1149–1150, 1761
dirofilariasis as, 1155–1156
echinococcosis (hydatid disease) as, 1157–1160, *1159*, 2026–2027, 2132
eosinophil action in, 1760
eosinophilic lung disease in, 1761–1762, 1761t, *1762*
filariasis as, 1153–1155, *1154*, 1761–1762, *1762*

Parasitic infection(s) *(Continued)*
hookworm as, 1150–1151
host response to, 1142, 1143
in HIV infection, 2203–2204
life cycles of, 1143. See also specific diseases.
lung injury in, pathology of, 475
malaria as, 1146–1147
paragonimiasis as, 1160–1163, *1162*, 2026
schistosomiasis as, 1142, 1163–1165, 1525–1526
strongyloidiasis as, 1151–1153, *1152*
toxoplasmosis as, 626–627, 1147–1149, *1148*
treatment of, 1143
trichinosis as, 1156–1157
visceral larva migrans as, 1157
Parasympathetic nervous system, of airway, 249–250, *251*, 332–333
of lung, 21–22
of pulmonary circulation, 131
pulmonary vascular resistance effects of, 64
Parathymic syndromes, 2126
Parathyroid glands, disorders of, respiratory manifestations of, 2312, *2312*
masses in, 2128–2129
Parathyroid hormone-related peptide/protein, excess of, in lung cancer, 1422
in hypercalcemia of malignancy, 1379
Parkinson's disease, respiratory muscle effects of, 2349t, 2350–2351
Paromomycin, in amebiasis, 1146
Parotitis, in sarcoidosis, 1718–1719
Paroxysmal nocturnal dyspnea, 588
in filariasis, 1155
Parrot fever (psittacosis), 624, 626, 998t, 1026
Partial agonists, drugs as, 243
Partial pressure, in gas exchange, 70
of carbon dioxide. See *Carbon dioxide, partial pressure of.*
of oxygen. See *Oxygen, partial pressure of.*
Particulates. See also *Aerosol(s); Dust(s); Pneumoconiosis(es).*
alveolar macrophage protection against, 390, *391*, 392
as air pollutants, adverse effects of, 1887t, 1891–1893
defense mechanisms against, 1889
deposition of, 1889
distribution of, 1886–1888
properties of, 1886–1888
sizes of, 1886–1887
sources of, 1886–1888, 1887t
standards for, 2557
aspiration of, in near drowning, 1966
clearance of, 354–355, *354*, 372–373, 373t
defense mechanisms against, 986
deposition of, 374, 1345
phagocytosis of, 372–373, 373t
tolerance to, alveolar macrophages in, 393–394, *395*
Pascal's principle, in plethysmography, 796
Passive pulmonary hypertension, 1543
Pasteur effect, in lactic acid production, 165
*Pasteurella multocida* pneumonia, 1028
Patched, as sonic hedgehog signal molecule receptor, 38
Paternalism, in health care, 2491–2492
Pathogenicity, definition of, 1052
Pathology, 443–493. See also specific disorders.
of acute injury, 456, 459, *459–462*
of barotrauma, 475
of cell injury and death, 444, 444t, *445–455*, 446, 450, 454–455
of chemical injury, 477, *477*, 478t, 479t
of chronic injury, 459, 462, *463*, *464*, 465
Pathology, 443–493 *(Continued)*
of genetic disorders, 477, 480t–481t, 482, *482*, 483t–484t, *485–489*, 486
of hypoxia, 465, *465*
of immunologic reactions, 465–466, *466–470*, 468
of infections, bacterial, 473–474
chlamydial, 473
fungal, 474–475, *475*, *476*
mycoplasmal, 473, *474*
parasitic, 475
rickettsial, 473
viral, 468, 470–471, *471–473*, 473
of inflammatory reactions, 455–456, *455–458*
of nutritional disorders, 486
of radiation injury, 475, *476*, 477
of temperature injuries, 475
Patient education. See *Education.*
Patient Self-Determination Act, 2494
Patients' rights, in ethical decision making, 2496
PAVMs. See *Arteriovenous malformations, pulmonary.*
$P_{breath}$, in kyphoscoliosis, 2361
Pcap. See *Pulmonary capillary(ies), pressure in.*
$P_{crit}$ (critical pressure), in airway, 1344, *1344*, 1351
PDImax (transdiaphragmatic pressure), in respiratory muscle evaluation, 858, *858*
Peak expiratory flow rate, in chronic obstructive pulmonary disease, 1191
measurement of, 786–787
Peak flow, in asthma, 1265, 2538–2539
Pectoriloquy, 598
Pectus carinatum, 2365
Pectus excavatum, 2364–2366
diagnosis of, 2364–2365
etiology of, 2364–2365
exercise capacity in, 2361t
in Marfan's syndrome, 1711
pathophysiology of, 2365–2366
pulmonary function tests in, 2359t
respiratory mechanics in, 2359t
treatment of, 2366
Pediatric patients. See also *Congenital disorder(s); Neonate(s).*
asthma in, education on, 2537t, 2538
baby powder aspiration in, 1908
bronchomalacia in, 1368
bronchopulmonary dysplasia in, 1179–1180, 1366–1367
bronchoscopy in, 727, 753
chylothorax in, 2057–2059
diaphragmatic paralysis in, 2335
environmental smoke effects on, 2558
foreign body aspiration by, 1367
hereditary hemorrhagic telangiectasia in, 1562
hypersensitivity pneumonitis in, 1871
lung transplantation in, 2521
mechanical ventilation in, pneumopericardium in, 2102
mediastinal masses in, 2123, 2124, 2124t
tuberculosis in, treatment of, 1073–1074
Pedigree analysis, in genetic disease, 49–50
Peel, pleural, 2017, 2036
removal of. See *Decortication.*
PEEP. See *Positive end-expiratory pressure.*
PEmax. See *Maximal expiratory pressure.*
Pendulum breathing, respiratory acidosis in, 174
Penicillamine, in pulmonary fibrosis, 1682
pulmonary disease due to, 1701, 1985
diffuse alveolar hemorrhage as, 1744
Penicillamine *(Continued)*
in connective tissue disease therapy, 1692t
Penicillin(s), in cystic fibrosis, 1309, 1309t
in pharyngitis, 918
in pneumonia, 995t, 998t
anaerobic, 1019t, 1020
pneumococcal, 1001
*Staphylococcus aureus*, 1004
in retropharyngeal abscess, 918
resistance to, in anaerobic bacteria, 1020
in *Haemophilus influenzae*, 1008
in *Streptococcus pneumoniae*, 1001
Penicillin G, in anthrax, 1029
in pneumonia, *Actinomyces*, 1022
alpha-hemolytic streptococcal, 1005
anaerobic, 1020
*Bacillus anthracis*, 1029
beta-hemolytic streptococcal, 1005
*Neisseria meningitidis*, 1006
*Pasteurella multocida*, 1028
*Propionibacterium*, 1022
*Penicillium* infections, 1136
in HIV infection, 2198t, 2201–2202
*Penicillium* spores, hypersensitivity pneumonitis due to, 1869
Pentamidine, in *Pneumocystis carinii* pneumonia, 2190–2191, 2191t, 2193–2196, 2195t
aerosol delivery of, 359
regional distribution of, 744, *744*
Pentoxifylline, as vasodilator, 302
in pulmonary edema, 1610
Peptide histidine isoleucine, in mucus secretion, 333
Peptide histidine isoleucine/methionine, actions of, 250, *250*, *251*
Peptide histidine methionine, in mucus secretion, 333
Peptide histidine valine, actions of, *251*
Peptidergic nerves, 22
*Peptostreptococcus* pneumonia, 1019, 1019t
Percussion, chest, 597, 599t. See also *Chest physical therapy.*
in cystic fibrosis, 1308–1309
Percutaneous needle aspiration biopsy, of lung, 760–761
Perfluorocarbons, in partial liquid ventilation, in acute respiratory distress syndrome, 2434
Perfusion. See *Pulmonary circulation, blood flow in; Ventilation-perfusion ratio; Ventilation-perfusion scanning.*
Pericardial cyst(s), 2130
Pericardial effusion(s), in sarcoidosis, 1719
in tuberculosis, 1085
peritoneal effusion with, 2016
shock in, 2402–2403
Pericardiocentesis, in cardiac tamponade, 2403
Pericarditis, in amebiasis, 1145
in histoplasmosis, 1111
in pneumonia, 1005
in tuberculosis, 1085–1086, *1086*
pain in, 578–579, 581t
pleural effusion in, 2014–2015
uremic, 2034
Pericardium, air in (pneumopericardium), 2102, 2105
Periciliary fluid, regulation of, 362–363
Perilymphatic nodule(s), 675, *675*
Periodic breathing. See *Breathing, periodic.*
Periodontal disease, anaerobic pneumonia in, 1017
Periorbital cellulitis, in sinusitis, 916
Peritoneal dialysis, pleural effusion in, 2016
Peritoneal effusion, pericardial effusion with, 2016

Peritonitis, tuberculous, 1084–1085
Peritonsillar abscess, 918
Perivascular pressure, on pulmonary vessels, 125–126
Permeability, in pulmonary edema. See *Pulmonary edema, increased permeability.*
Peroxidase, eosinophil, 1758–1759, 1758t, 1759t
in mucus, 331
Pertechnegas, in ventilation-perfusion scanning, 699–700
Pertussis, cough in, 560
PET. See *Positron emission tomography.*
Petechiae, in fat embolism, 1526
*Pfiesteria* toxin inhalation, 1909
pH, blood, acid-base disorder classification by, 160t
alveolar, in high altitude acclimatization, *1917*
calculation of, 156
factors affecting, 158
in hypoventilation, 72, *72*, 156
in pulmonary edema, 1594–1595
measurement of, 156, 829–831, *831*
cerebrospinal fluid, in metabolic acidosis, 171
ventilatory response and, 193
esophageal, in cough diagnosis, 562, 563t
Henderson-Hasselbalch equation for, 155–156
in exercise, 840
muscle, in exercise, 845–846, *846*
pleural fluid, 2005
in esophageal rupture, 2028
urine, in renal tubular acidosis, 168–169, 169t
Phagocytosis, 2224–2225, *2225*. See also *Dendritic cells; Macrophage(s); Monocyte(s).*
disorder(s) of, 2235, 2234t, 2236–2238
Chédiak-Higashi syndrome as, 2233t, 2237–2238
chronic granulomatous disease as, 2233t, 2237
Job's syndrome as, 2233t, 2238
leukocyte adhesion defects as, 2233t, 2238
neutropenia as. See *Neutropenia.*
of apoptotic cells, 528–529, *529*, *530*
of asbestos fibers, 1832–1833
of *Mycobacterium tuberculosis*, 1056
of particulates, 372–373, 373t
surfactant protein A in, 312–313
surfactant protein D in, 316
Phagosomes, of alveolar macrophages, 372
particulates in, 390
Phantom tumor, 1481
Pharmacokinetics, in inhalation route, 248
of corticosteroids, 280, *281*
of theophylline, 273
principles of, 247–248
Pharmacology. See also *Drug(s)*; specific drugs.
airway, 267–296
antitussives in, 289
bronchodilators in. See *Bronchodilator(s).*
contraindicated drugs in, 290–291
controller drugs in, 278–284, *279–281*, 279t, 282t
epithelial, 232, *233*
in breathlessness, 289
mediator antagonists in, 284–286, *284*
mucoregulators in, 289
new drugs in, 286–289, 287t, *288*
steroid-sparing, 286
ventilatory stimulants in, 289–290
Pharmacology *(Continued)*
autonomic. See *Autonomic nervous system.*
cell interactions in, 232
enzyme, 247
inflammatory cell, 232, *233*
inflammatory mediators in, 256–258, *257*, *258*. See also specific substances.
ion channel, 246–247, *246*
nervous system, 232
pharmacokinetics in. See *Pharmacokinetics.*
principles of, 231–265
receptors in. See *Receptor(s).*
transcription factors in, 258–262, *259–262*
corticosteroid interactions with, 278–279, *279*, 279t, *280*
inhibitors of, 259, 288
receptor gene regulation and, 245–246
signal transduction and, 239–241, *239*, *241*
vascular, 297–306
clinical applications of, 298–299
evaluation for, 299
vasodilators in. See *Vasodilator(s).*
vascular endothelial, 232
Pharyngitis, *Chlamydia pneumoniae*, 1027
*Coxiella burnetii*, 1025
cytomegalovirus, 943
diagnosis of, 917–918
herpes simplex virus, 947–948
in adenovirus infections, 939, *939*
*Mycoplasma pneumoniae*, 1024
organisms causing, 917–918
treatment of, 917–918
viral, 917, 933–934, 933t, *934*
Pharyngoconjunctival fever, 937, 939
Pharynx, abscesses of, 918
airflow in, 1343–1345, *1343–1345*
anatomy of, 1343–1344, *1343*, 1350
colonization of, with gram-negative bacteria, 607, *607*
cough reflex receptors in, 554
function of, 1350
infections of, airway obstruction in, 1351
inflammation of. See *Pharyngitis.*
injury of, airway obstruction in, 1351
membranes in, differential diagnosis of, 917
muscles surrounding, 1346t
narrowing of, muscles in, 1346t
nasopharyngeal segment of, 1350
obstruction of, in sleep apnea, 1350–1351, 2155–2157, *2157*
oropharyngeal segment of, 1350
patency of, maintenance of, 1350
receptors in, 181–182
surgery for, in sleep apnea, 2160
Phenothiazine, pulmonary edema due to, 1989
Phenotyping, of genetic disease, 48
Phenoxybenzamine, as vasodilator, 300
Phentolamine, in pulmonary hypertension, 300
Phenyl diguanide, C-fiber ending stimulation by, 184
Pheochromocytoma(s), of mediastinum, 2131
Phlebitis, septic, 1527
Phlebotomy, in acute respiratory distress syndrome, 2420
in erythrocytosis, 2286
in mountain sickness, 1939
in polycythemia, in cor pulmonale, 1643
in pulmonary edema, 1600, 2420
Pholcodine, in cough control, 289
Phonation. See also *Vocal cords.*
laryngeal function in, 1351
Phosgene, 1906
Phosphatidylcholine, in surfactant, 309, 309t
Phosphatidylcholine:sphingomyelin ratio, in neonatal respiratory distress syndrome diagnosis, 317
Phosphatidylglycerol, in surfactant, 309, 309t
Phosphatidylinositol, hydrolysis of, in signal transduction, 237, *237*
Phosphine, exposure to, 1910
Phosphodiesterases, in cyclic adenosine monophosphate degradation, 236, *236*
inhibitors of, as bronchodilators, 277–278
in asthma, 287
in chronic obstructive pulmonary disease, 287
theophylline as, 273, *274*
Phospholipase(s), of eosinophils, 1758–1759, 1758t
Phospholipase $A_2$, in pancreatitis, 2276
Phospholipase C, in phosphatidylinositol hydrolysis, 237, *237*
Phospholipid(s), absorption of, surfactant in, 307–308
surfactant protein B in, 313, *313*
binding of, to surfactant protein A, 310
in alveolar proteinosis, 1790, *1791*
in mucus, 331
in surfactant, 309, 309t
organization of, surfactant protein C in, 313–314, *313*
Phospholipid-dependent protein kinase, endothelial permeability and, 142
Phospholipidosis, of alveolar macrophages, amiodarone-induced, 1973
Phosphor storage systems, in digital radiography, 642, 644, *644*
Phosphorus imbalance, in respiratory alkalosis, 174
respiratory failure in, 2447
Phosphorylation, of receptors, in desensitization, 244–245, *245*
Photochemical oxidants, as air pollutants. See *Ozone, Nitrogen oxides.*
Phrenic nerve, dysfunction of, after abdominal surgery, 885–886
entrapment of, in mediastinitis, 2114
in breathing control, 186
injury of, 2334
nucleus of, 188
paralysis of. See *Diaphragm, paralysis of.*
repair of, in diaphragmatic paralysis, 2336–2337
stimulation of, in diaphragmatic paralysis evaluation, 2336
in neuromuscular disorders, 2348–2349
in respiratory muscle evaluation, 858–859, 2333
Phthalic anhydride, hypersensitivity pneumonitis due to, 1870
Phycomycosis. See *Mucormycosis.*
Phyllosilicates, in pneumoconiosis, 1831t, 1841
Physical agents, injury from. See specific agents and disorders, e.g., *Barotrauma; Hyperthermia; Hypothermia.*
Physical examination, 592–603. See also specific disorders.
clinical usefulness of, 587t, 592
of chest, 592–599
auscultation in, 597–599, 599t
inspection in, 596–597, 599t
lung sounds in, adventitious, 593–596, *594–596*, 594t, 598
continuous, 595–596
discontinuous, 595, *595*, *596*
normal, 593, *593*
palpation in, 597, 599t
percussion in, 597, 599t
results interpretation in, 599, 599t
sound generation and perception in, 592–593, *592*
of extrapulmonary manifestations, 600–601, *600–602*, 601t–603t, 603

Physical examination *(Continued)*
of skin, 602t, 603
Physical therapy, chest. See *Chest physical therapy.*
Physicians, communication skills of, 586
reasons for visiting, 585–586
Physiologic dead space. See under *Dead space.*
Physiology. See specific topics, e.g., *Acid-base balance and imbalance; Breathing; Gas exchange; Pulmonary circulation; Ventilation.*
Pickwickian syndrome, 2159
Picornavirus infections, 931t
PIE (pulmonary infiltrates with eosinophilia) syndrome, 1760
Pigeon fancier's lung. See *Hypersensitivity pneumonitis.*
Pigment, accumulation of, in cell injury, 450, *452, 453*
Pilocarpine test, in cystic fibrosis, 1308
Pimax. See *Maximal inspiratory pressure.*
Pindolol, pulmonary disease due to, 1983
Pink puffers, in chronic obstructive pulmonary disease, 1634
*p16*$^{INK4A}$ gene and product, in lung cancer, 1383–1384
PIOPED (Prospective Investigation of Pulmonary Embolism Diagnosis) trial, 1507, 1510–1512
ventilation-perfusion scanning and, 702–704, 705t
Pipe smoking, lung cancer risk with, 1400
Piperacillin, in pneumonia, 998t
Piperazine, in ascariasis, 1150
Pirbuterol, as bronchodilator, 270
Pirodavir, in rhinovirus infections, 966
Pistolesi method, for scoring pulmonary edema radiographs, 1499
Pittsburgh pneumonia, 1014
Pituitary adenoma, respiratory manifestations of, 2313
Pituitary adenylate cyclase activating peptide, *251*
Pixels, in computed tomography, 661
Pla. See *Left atrial (outflow) pressure.*
Plague, 1029
Planimetry, in lung volume measurement, 793
Plaques, pleural. See *Pleura, plaques on.*
Plasma, oncotic pressure of, decreased, pulmonary edema in, 145, *145*
proteins in, transport of, 138, 138t
Plasma cell(s), dyscrasias of, 1464, 2292–2294, 2293t. See also *Multiple myeloma.*
immunoglobulin secretion from, 416
in granulomas, of lung, 1480
Plasmacytoma(s), 2293
of lung, 1464, 1480
Plasmapheresis, in Goodpasture's syndrome, 1743
in microscopic polyangiitis, 1739
in myasthenia gravis, 2342
*Plasmodium* infections (malaria), 1146–1147
Plateau pressure, as hyperinflation measure, 2456–2458, *2457, 2458*
Platelet(s), deficiency of. See *Thrombocytopenia.*
disorders of, 2295
radiopharmaceuticals seeking, 718
Platelet basic protein, 508, 508t
Platelet factor 4, 508, 508t
Platelet-activating factor, as inflammatory mediator, 257
biologic effects of, 497–498
in mucus hypersecretion, 334
Platelet-activating factor *(Continued)*
in pulmonary vascular resistance control, 131
Platelet-derived growth factor and receptor, 238–239, 504
in lung cancer growth, 1381
in lung development, 41
Platyhelminth infection(s), echinococcosis (hydatid disease) as, 1157–1160, *1159*, 2026–2027, 2132
paragonimiasis as, 1160–1163, *1162*
schistosomiasis as, 1143, 1163–1165, 1525–1526
Platypnea, definition of, 588
in hepatopulmonary syndrome, 2272
in systemic-pulmonary communications, 1497
Plecaronil, in rhinovirus infections, 966
Pleomorphic adenomas, of lung, 1462
Plethysmography, body, in airway resistance measurement, 798–799, *799*
in chest wall motion measurement, 105–106
in functional residual capacity measurement, 57–58
in lung volume measurement, 57–58, 793–798, *794–796*
impedance, in venous thrombosis, 1509
respiratory inductance, in neuromuscular disorders, 2333
Pleura. See also *Pleural space.*
actinomycosis of, 2023
adhesions of, 2007, *2007*
anatomy of, 1995–1998, *1996–1998*
biopsy of, 2008–2010, 2074
blood supply of, 1488, 1996–1997, *1997*
calcification of, 1658–1659, 1660t
cancer of, effusion in. See *Pleural effusion(s), malignant.*
coal dust accumulation in, 1826
computed tomography of, 686, *687*, 688, *688*
connective tissue of, 1996, *1997*
cysts of, in cystic fibrosis, 1294
embryology of, 1996
fibrosis of, 2061, 2062–2063, *2062*
diffusing capacity in, 816
in ankylosing spondylitis, 1710
in asbestos exposure, 1837, *1838*, 1839, 2033
in kidney failure, 2279
treatment of, 1840
inflammation of. See *Pleuritis.*
innervation of, 1998
lymphatic system of, 1997–1998, *1998*
dysfunction of, 2000
lymphoma of, 2071
metastasis to, 2072–2076
clinical manifestations of, 2072–2073, *2073*
diagnosis of, 2073–2074
epidemiology of, 2072
etiology of, 2072
hemothorax in, 2062
histology of, 2072
pathogenesis of, 2072, 2072t
prognosis for, 2076
treatment of, 2074–2076
with unknown primary, 2074
parietal, anatomy of, 1996, *1997*
plaques on, clinical features of, 1837, *1838*
computed tomography of, 688
epidemiology of, 1837
in mesothelioma, 2068–2069, *2068*
in talc pneumoconiosis, 1841
pathology of, 1837
Pleura *(Continued)*
treatment of, 1840
resection of, in aspergillosis, 2023
sarcoidosis of, 1721
thickening of, computed tomography of, 688, *688*
cyclophosphamide-induced, 1975
decortication of, 2020
in chyliform pleural effusion, 2060
in mesothelioma, 2068–2069, *2069*
pleural effusion in, 2036
ultrasonography of, 659–660
tuberculosis of, 1079–1080
clinical manifestations of, 2021–2022, *2022*
computed tomography in, *687*
diagnosis of, 2022
effusion in, 2004, 2008–2009, 2021–2023, *2022*
*Mycobacterium tuberculosis* detection in, 2006
pathogenesis of, 2021
pleural fluid examination in, 2022
split pleura sign in, *687*, 688
treatment of, 2022–2023
tumors of, lymphoma as, 2071–2072
mesothelioma as, benign fibrous, 2070–2071, *2071*
malignant, 2067–2070, *2068*
metastatic. See *Pleura, metastasis to.*
ultrasonography of, 2007
visceral, anatomy of, 1996, *1997*
visceroparietal reactions of, in asbestos exposure, 1837, *1838*, 1839
Pleural effusion(s), 2013–2041
adenosine deaminase in, 2005–2006, 2022
after Fontan's procedure, 2016
amylase in, 2028, 2029
antinuclear antibodies in, 2005–2006
approach to, 2000–2010
invasive tests in, 2008–2010
pleural fluid analysis in, 2001–2006
radiography in, 2006–2008, *2006, 2007*
asbestos-related, benign, 1839–1840
bacteriology of, 2017
bilious, 2030–2031
bronchoscopy in, 2009
carbon dioxide tension of, 2005
causes of, 2000, 2000t, 2001, 2001t
chest radiography of, 2006–2007, *2006, 2007*
decubitus, 646, *651–653*
chylous, 2057, 2059–2060. See also *Chylothorax.*
in lymphangio(leio)myomatosis, 1776, 1780–1781, 1784
clinical manifestations of, 2000
in heart failure, 2013–2014, *2014*
in hepatic hydrothorax, 2015
in pulmonary embolism, 2026–2027
in rheumatoid arthritis, 2031
in systemic lupus erythematosus, 2031
parapneumonic, 2017
postcardiac injury, 2032
tuberculous, 2021–2022, *2022*
computed tomography of, 688, 2007, 2009
diagnosis of, in heart failure, 2014
in hepatic hydrothorax, 2015
in nephrotic syndrome, 2016
in pulmonary embolism, 2027
in rheumatoid arthritis, 2031
in systemic lupus erythematosus, 2031–2032
parapneumonic, 2017–2018
treatment of, 2014, 2032
tuberculous, 2022

Pleural effusion(s) *(Continued)*
differential diagnosis of, 2001–2005, 2002t
drainage of, 2000
drug-induced, 1990, 1990t, 2035–2036
empyema development in. See *Empyema*.
enzymes in, 2006
epidemiology of, 2001, 2002t, 2026
examination of, 2005–2006
exudative, 2016–2036
amylase in, 2003
bilious, 2030–2031
causes of, 2001, 2001t, 2002t
definition of, 2000, 2016
differential diagnosis of, 2002–2005
drug-induced, 2035–2036
eosinophils in, 2004
glucose in, 2003
iatrogenic, 2036
in abdominal diseases, 2027–2031, *2027*, *2029*
in actinomycosis, 2023
in amebiasis, 2025
in asbestos exposure, 2033
in aspergillosis, 2023
in blastomycosis, 2023–2024
in bone marrow transplantation, 2033
in coccidioidomycosis, 2024
in connective tissue diseases, 2033
in coronary artery bypass surgery, 2032
in cryptococcosis, 2024
in diaphragmatic hernia, 2030
in echinococcosis, 2025–2026
in empyema, 2016–2021, 2018t, *2021*
in endometriosis, 2034
in esophageal perforation, 2003, 2027–2028, *2027*
in extramedullary hematopoiesis, 2035
in histoplasmosis, 2024
in HIV infection, 2025
in liver transplantation, 2030
in lung transplantation, 2033
in lupus pleuritis, 2031–2032
in Meigs' syndrome, 2034
in nocardiosis, 2023
in ovarian hyperstimulation syndrome, 2034–2035
in pancreatitis, 2003, 2028–2029, *2029*
in paragonimiasis, 2026
in parasitic diseases, 2025–2026
in *Pneumocystis carinii* pneumonia, 2026
in pneumonia, 2024–2025
in postcardiac injury syndrome, 2032
in pulmonary embolism, 2026–2027
in rheumatoid pleuritis, 2031
in sarcoidosis, 2033–2034
in trapped lung, 2036
in tuberculosis, 2004, 2021–2023, *2022*
in uremia, 2034
in urinary tract obstruction, 2034
in variceal sclerotherapy, 2030
in viral infections, 2024–2025
in yellow-nail syndrome, 2035
invasive tests for, 2008–2010
lactate dehydrogenase in, 2003
leukocytes in, 2003–2004
parapneumonic, 2016–2021, 2018t, *2021*
postoperative, 2030
protein in, 2003
radiation-induced, 2036
versus transudative, 2001–2002
iatrogenic, 2036
in abdominal diseases, 2027–2031, *2027*, *2029*
in actinomycosis, 2023
in amebiasis, 1144–1146, *1145*, 2025
in amyloidosis, 2016, 2296

Pleural effusion(s) *(Continued)*
in asbestos exposure, 2033
in ascites, 2015
in aspergillosis, 2023
in blastomycosis, 2023–2024
in bone marrow transplantation, 2033, 2299
in bronchopulmonary fistula, 2020, *2021*
in Churg-Strauss syndrome, 2033
in cirrhosis, 2015–2016
in coccidioidomycosis, 2024
in congestive heart failure, 2013–2014, *2014*
in connective tissue diseases, 2033
in cor pulmonale, 1638, *1639*
in coronary artery bypass surgery, 2032
in cryptococcosis, 2024
in cystic fibrosis, 1305
in diabetes mellitus, 2310
in diaphragmatic hernia, 2030
in echinococcosis, 2025–2026
in empyema, 1018, *1018*, 2016–2021, 2018t, *2021*
in endometriosis, 2034, 2325
in esophageal perforation, 2003, 2027–2028, *2027*
in extramedullary hematopoiesis, 2035
in hemothorax, 2061
in hepatic hydrothorax, 2015–2016
in histoplasmosis, 2024
in HIV infection, 2025, 2178
in hypereosinophilic syndrome, 1769
in hypothyroidism, 2311, 2311t
in Kaposi's sarcoma, 2205–2206
in kidney failure, 2279
in leukemia, 2291–2292
in liver disease, 2271
in liver transplantation, 2030
in lung transplantation, 2033
in lupus pleuritis, 2031–2032
in lymphangio(leio)myomatosis, 1782, 1784
in lymphoma, 2071, 2207
in Meigs' syndrome, 2034
in mesothelioma, 2068–2070
in mica pneumoconiosis, 1841
in multiple myeloma, 1464, 2293–2294
in myxedema, 2016
in nephrotic syndrome, 2016
in nitrofurantoin-induced pulmonary disease, 1978
in nocardiosis, 2023
in ovarian hyperstimulation syndrome, 2034–2035
in pancreatitis, 2003, 2028–2029, *2029*, 2277–2278, *2278*
in paragonimiasis, 1161, 2026
in parasitic diseases, 2025–2026
in pericardial disease, 2014–2015
in peritoneal dialysis, 2016
in pneumonia, 920. See also *Pleural effusion(s), parapneumonic.*
*Bacillus*, 1030
beta-hemolytic streptococcal, 1004
glucose in, 2003
pneumococcal, 999–1000
*Pneumocystis carinii*, 2026
*Staphylococcus aureus*, 1003
viral, 2024–2025
in pneumothorax, 2046
in postcardiac injury syndrome, 2032
in pulmonary edema, 1499, 1612, 2013
in pulmonary embolism, 1510, 2008, 2016, 2026–2027
in rheumatoid arthritis, 1702, 2005, 2031
in rheumatoid pleuritis, 2031
in sarcoidosis, 1721, 2016, 2033–2034
in sclerotherapy, 1989, 2107
in spontaneous bacterial pleuritis, 2015–2016

Pleural effusion(s) *(Continued)*
in systemic lupus erythematosus, 1705, 2005, 2031–2032
in trapped lung, 2036
in tuberculosis, 2004, 2021–2023, *2022*
biopsy in, 2008–2009
chyliform, 2060
interferon-τ in, 2006
in uremia, 2034
in urinary tract obstruction, 2034
in variceal sclerotherapy, 2030
in viral infections, 2024–2025
in Waldenström's macroglobulinemia, 1464
in yellow-nail syndrome, 2035
interferon-τ in, 2006, 2022
invasive tests for, 2008–2010
loculation of, 2007, *2007*
long-standing, pseudochylothorax in, 2060
lung function and, 2000
malignant, 2072–2076
biopsy in, 2008–2009
clinical manifestations of, 2072–2073, *2073*
computed tomography of, 670
diagnosis of, 2073–2074
epidemiology of, 2072
etiology of, 2072
in multiple myeloma, 2293–2294
pathogenesis of, 2072, 2072t
pleural fluid examination in, 2004–2005
prognosis for, 2076
treatment of, 2074–2076
with unknown primary, 2074
methysergide-induced, 1988
*Mycobacterium tuberculosis* detection in, 2006
parapneumonic, 1032, 2016–2021, 2018t, *2021*. See also *Pleural effusion(s), in pneumonia.*
bacteriology of, 2017
bronchopulmonary fistula with, 2020, *2021*
clinical manifestations of, 2017
complicated, 2017
diagnosis of, 2017–2018
in HIV infection, 2025
incidence of, 2017
pathophysiology of, 2017
postpneumonectomy, 2020–2021
prognosis for, 2018, 2018t
treatment of, 2018–2020, 2018t
pathogenesis of, in rheumatoid arthritis, 2031
malignant, 2072, 2072t
tuberculous, 2021
pathophysiology of, 2000
in heart failure, 2013
in hepatic hydrothorax, 2015
in pericardial disease, 2014–2015
in pulmonary embolism, 2026
parapneumonic, 2017
pH of, 2005
physical findings in, 599t
postoperative, 2030
postpneumonectomy, 2020–2021
prognosis for, in rheumatoid arthritis, 2031
radiation-induced, 2036
radiography of, 2006–2008, *2006*, *2007*
sympathetic, in amebiasis, 2025
thoracoscopy in, 2009
transudative, 2013–2016
after Fontan's procedure, 2016
causes of, 2001, 2001t, 2002t
definition of, 2000, 2013, 2016
in amyloidosis, 2016
in bronchopulmonary fistula, 2020, *2021*

Pleural effusion(s) *(Continued)*
in congestive heart failure, 2013–2014, *2014*
in empyema, 2016–2021, 2018t, *2021*
in hepatic hydrothorax, 2015–2016
in lung abscess, 2016–2021, 2018t, *2021*
in myxedema, 2016
in nephrotic syndrome, 2016
in pericardial disease, 2014–2015
in peritoneal dialysis, 2016
in pulmonary embolism, 2016
in sarcoidosis, 2016
in spontaneous bacterial pleuritis, 2015–2016
postpneumonectomy, 2020–2021
versus exudative, 2001–2002
treatment of, in hepatic hydrothorax, 2015
in mesothelioma, 2070
in nephrotic syndrome, 2016
in pulmonary embolism, 2027
in rheumatoid arthritis, 2031
malignant, 2074–2076
parapneumonic, 2018–2020, 2018t
tuberculous, 2022–2023
tuberculous, 1079–1080, 2022–2023
ultrasonography of, 659, *660*, 2007
versus diaphragmatic paralysis, 2336
Pleural fluid, absorption of, 1999, *1999*
accumulation of. See *Pleural effusion(s).*
adenosine deaminase in, 2005–2006, 2022
amylase in, 2028, 2029
analysis of. See *Pleural fluid, examination of.*
antinuclear antibodies in, 2005–2006
blood in. See *Hemothorax.*
carbon dioxide tension of, 2005
chyliform, 2057, 2059–2060
color of, 2002–2003
composition of, exudative, 2000
protein in, 1998–1999
transudative, 2000
culture of, 2005
in pneumonia, 609, 989–990
in tuberculosis, 2022
dynamics of, 1577
enzymes in, 2006
eosinophils in, 2004
examination of, 1032, 2001–2006
amylase in, 2003
appearance in, 2002–2003
bacteriologic, 2005
culture in, 2005
cytology in, 2004, 2073–2074
for exudate-transudate separation, 2001–2002
glucose in, 2003
immunohistochemical studies in, 2005
in malignancy, 2004–2005, 2073–2074
in mesothelioma, 2069
in paragonimiasis, 2026
in parapneumonic effusion, 2018
in pulmonary embolism, 2026–2027
in tuberculosis, 1079–1080, 2022
lactate dehydrogenase in, 2003
protein in, 2003
white blood cell count in, 2003–2004
flow cytometry of, 2005
hematocrit of, 2002
interferon-τ in, 2006, 2022
lipids in. See *Chylothorax.*
*Mycobacterium tuberculosis* detection in, 2006
odor of, 2002
pH of, 2005, 2028
physiology of, 1998–2000, *1999*
turbidity of, 2003
Pleural friction rub, 598–599, 2000
Pleural peel, formation of, 2017
pleural effusion in, 2036
removal of. See *Decortication.*
Pleural pressure, airway resistance and, 95, *96*
decreases of, in airway obstruction, 2452–2453
distribution of, 109–111, *110*
during vital capacity maneuvers, 98, *99*, 101
elastic recoil and, 783–784, 799–800
generation of, *2445*
in chronic obstructive pulmonary disease, in exercise, 212
in flail chest, 2367
in pneumothorax, 2044–2045, *2044*, 2054
in sleep apnea, 2163, *2164*
measurement of, 800, *800*
mechanical aspects of, 111
negative, 2044
normal, 1999, 2044
theoretical aspects of, 783
ventilation inequality and, 59, *59*
versus cardiac output, 2388–2389, *2388*
versus extra-alveolar vessel pressure, 125
versus lung volume, 104, 111
versus regional lung volumes, 806, *807*
versus volume, 787–788, *787*
Pleural space, air in. See *Pneumothorax.*
anatomy of, 1995–1998, *1996–1998*
blood in. See *Hemothorax.*
chyle in. See *Chylothorax.*
embryology of, 1996
eradication of. See *Pleurodesis.*
fluid in. See *Pleural effusion(s)*; *Pleural fluid.*
function of, 1995–1996
pathophysiology of, 2000. See also *Pleural effusion(s).*
physiology of, 1998–2000, *1999*
Pleurectomy, in chylothorax, 2058
in pleural effusions, 2076
Pleurisy, 575–576
asbestos-related, 1839–1840
clinical features of, 590
in paragonimiasis, 1161
Pleuritic pain, clinical features of, 590
Pleuritis, asbestos-related, 2033
in kidney failure, 2279
lupus, 2005, 2031–2032
reactive eosinophilic, 2105
rheumatoid, 2031
spontaneous bacterial, 2015–2016
tuberculous, 1079–1080, 2021–2023, *2022*
clinical manifestations of, 2021–2022, *2022*
diagnosis of, 2022
effusion in, 2004, 2021–2023, *2022*
*Mycobacterium tuberculosis* detection in, 2006
needle biopsy in, 2008–2009
pathogenesis of, 2021
pleural fluid examination in, 2022
split pleura sign in, *687*, 688
treatment of, 2022–2023
uremic, 2034
Pleurobiliary fistulas, 2030–2031
Pleurodesis, in chylothorax, 2058
in metastatic disease, 2074–2075
in pleural effusion, in heart failure, 2014
in pneumothorax, 2048, *2048*, 2050
technique for, 2075
Pleuroperitoneal shunt, in chylothorax, 2058, 2059
in malignant effusions, 2075–2076
Pleuroscopy, 761
Plicatic acid, asthma due to, 1857
*Pmel 17* gene and product, mutations of, in lymphangio(leio)myomatosis, 1778
PMmax (maximally negative airway pressure), in respiratory muscle evaluation, 858
Pneumatic belt, in neuromuscular disorders, 2347
Pneumatic compression devices, in thromboembolic disease prevention, 1514–1515
Pneumatoceles, in *Pneumocystis carinii* pneumonia, 2188, *2189*
Pneumectomy. See *Lung volume(s), reduction of, surgical.*
Pneumococcal infections, bacteremia due to, 2179
immunization for, in HIV infection, 2180
Pneumococcal pneumonia, 987, 999–1002
causative organism of, 1000, *1000*
clinical course of, 1000–1001, 1001t
clinical manifestations of, 999–1000, *1000*, 2179
complications of, 1000
diagnosis of, 920, 2179
epidemiology of, 999
immune response in, 436
immunization for, 1001–1002, 1002t, 2508
in HIV infection, 926, 2178–2180
in influenza, 954
in lymphoproliferative disorders, 925
in sickle cell disease, 2287
microbiologic diagnosis of, 989–990, 1000, *1000*
culture in, 617
direct examination in, 615
pathology of, *455*
prognosis for, 1000–1001, 1001t
quelling reaction in, 921
sputum examination in, 921
treatment of, 922, 998t, 1001
in HIV infection, 2179–2180
Pneumococci. See *Pneumococcal pneumonia; Streptococcus pneumoniae.*
Pneumoconiosis(es), 1811–1851
as sentinel health event, 1816
asbestos-related. See *Asbestos*; *Asbestosis.*
baritosis as, 1842
beryllium, 1402–1403, 1842–1844
carborundum, 1845
coal-workers'. See *Coal-workers' pneumoconiosis.*
computed tomography in, 675
definitions of, 1811
epidemiology of, 1816
evaluation of, 1815
exposure-response relationships in, 1813, *1813*, *1814*
ferruginous body formation in, 450, *453*
hard metal, 1403, 1844–1845
imaging in, 1813, 1815
impairment in, 900, 902, 903t, 908, 1815–1816
kaolin, 1841
legal issues in, 1816
lung dust accumulation in, 1811–1812, *1812*
man-made vitreous fibers in, 1403, 1831t, 1841–1842
mica, 1841
mixed dust, 1817, 1842
new, 1842
non-asbestos mineral silicates in, 1830, 1831t, 1841–1842
occupational exposures in, 1815–1816
particle deposition mechanisms in, 1811–1812, *1812*
pathology of, 477, 478t
pulmonary function tests in, 1815

Pneumoconiosis(es) *(Continued)*
rheumatoid, 1826–1829
risk factors for, 1816, 1817t
siderosis as, 1842
silicon-carbide, 1845
silicosis as. See *Silicosis.*
stannosis as, 1842
talc, *1814*, 1841
tissue reactions in, 1812–1813
treatment of, 1815–1816, 1816
tuberculosis in, 1816
vermiculite, 1841
*Pneumocystis carinii*, surfactant protein A binding to, 312
surfactant protein D binding to, 316
*Pneumocystis carinii* pneumonia, 2187–2196
after lung transplantation, bronchiolitis obliterans in, 1364–1365, *1365*
CD4+ lymphocyte count in, 2188
chest radiography of, 2188–2189, *2189*
clinical features of, 2188–2189, *2189*
diagnosis of, 743–744, 743t, *744*, 2189–2190
epidemiology of, 2187–2188
genetic tests for, 626
historical background of, 2187–2188
in HIV infection, 926
in severe combined immunodeficiency, 2239
in transplantation, 925, *2229*, 2230
bone marrow, 2304
lung, 2523
infections coexisting with, 744, 745t
lactate dehydrogenase in, 2176
microbiologic diagnosis of, 610t, 611–613, 612t
pathogenesis of, 2188
pathology of, 474–475, *476*
pleural effusion in, 2026
pneumothorax in, 2049, 2050
prevention of, 2194–2196, 2195t
versus T lymphocyte count, 2175
prodrome of, 2188
pulmonary function tests in, 856, 2176
risk factors for, 2188
sputum examination in, 759
transmission of, 2187–2188
treatment of, 359, 2190–2194, 2190t
ventilation-perfusion scanning in, 711–712, *712*
Pneumocytes. See *Epithelium and epithelial cells, alveolar.*
Pneumocytoma (hemangioma), sclerosing, 1479
Pneumomediastinum, 2083, 2095–2105
air embolism with, 2102
air spread after, 2098, *2098*
alveolar rupture in, 2097–2099, *2097*, *2098*, 2101t
anatomic considerations in, 2095–2096
chest radiography of, 2103–2104, *2103*, *2104*
clinical manifestations of, 2102–2104, *2103*, *2104*
definition of, 2095, 2096
diagnosis of, 2102–2104, *2103*, *2104*
diagnostic, 2083
external origin of, 2096t, 2099
gastrointestinal origin of, 2096t, 2099
historical aspects of, 2096
idiopathic, 2100
in barotrauma, 2099, 2100–2102, 2101t
in mechanical ventilation, 2477–2478
pathophysiology of, 2098, 2100–2101, 2101t
treatment of, 2104–2105
in mediastinitis, 2106, *2107*
Pneumomediastinum *(Continued)*
intrathoracic airway origin of, 2096t, 2097
lung parenchyma origin of, 2096t, 2097–2099, *2097*, *2098*
natural history of, 2104
pathophysiology of, 2096–2099, 2096t, *2097*, *2098*
pneumopericardium with, 2102
sequelae of, 2105
spontaneous, 2096, 2099–2100, 2104
treatment of, 2104–2105
upper tract origin of, 2096–2097, 2096t
versus pneumothorax, 2103
Pneumonectomy, empyema after, 2020–2021
in bronchiectasis, 1332
in cancer, 1427
occult, 1428
stage IA and IB, 1428–1429
stage IIA, 1429
stage IIB, 1429–1430
in echinococcosis, 1160
in mesothelioma, 2070
mortality in, 1427
physiologic changes after, 889
preoperative evaluation for, 889–891
pulmonary function tests before and after, 890
ventilation-perfusion scanning before, 713–715
Pneumonia, *Acinetobacter*, 998t, 1013–1014, *1013*
*Actinomadura*, 620–621
*Actinomyces*, 620–621, 1019t, 1020–1022, *1021*
acute respiratory distress syndrome in, 2416–2417
adenovirus, 939, 940t
in bone marrow transplantation, 2302
in transplantation, 2232
pathology of, 470
after lung transplantation, 2521–2522
age factors in, 987–988
anaerobic bacteria in, 998t, 1017–1020, *1018*, *1019*, 1019t
anthrax as, 1029
*Aspergillus*. See *Aspergillosis.*
aspiration. See *Aspiration (during breathing), pneumonia in.*
atypical, 1023–1027
*Chlamydia pneumoniae*, 473, 624, 998t, 1026–1027
*Chlamydia psittaci*, 624, 626, 998t, 1026
*Chlamydia trachomatis*, 1027
*Coxiella burnetii* (Q fever), 473, 998t, 1025–1026
*Mycoplasma pneumoniae*, 990–991, 998t, 1024–1025, *1024*
pleural effusion in, 2024–2025
*Bacillus*, 1030
*Bacillus anthracis*, 1029
bacterial. See *Pneumonia, pyogenic.*
*Bacterium anitratum (Acinetobacter),* 1013–1014
*Bacteroides fragilis*, 1019, 1019t, 1020
biopsy in, 760–761
breath sounds in, 598
bronchoalveolar lavage in, 736
bronchoscopy in, 743–750, 743t, *744*, 745t, 746t, *747*, *748*
*Brucella*, 1030
*Burkholderia cepacia*, 1012–1013
chest radiography of. See *Chest radiography, of pneumonia.*
*Chlamydia*, genetic tests for, 626
microbiologic diagnosis of, 610t, 624
pathology of, 473
Pneumonia *(Continued)*
*Chlamydia pneumoniae*, 624, 998t, 1026–1027
as asthma risk factor, 1251–1252
in sickle cell disease, 2287
*Chlamydia psittaci*, 624, 626, 998t, 1026
*Chlamydia trachomatis*, 624, 1027
chronic, bronchiectasis with, 1334
*Citrobacter*, 1010–1011
clinical approach to, 987–993
clinical evaluation in, 987–988, 988t
epidemiologic evaluation in, 987, 987t
invasive diagnostic techniques in, 991–993, 993t
laboratory evaluation in, 988–989
microbiologic evaluation in, 989–990, *990*
radiography in, 988–989
serologic evaluation in, 990–991
clinical manifestations of. See also specific causative organisms.
in acute respiratory distress syndrome, 2416–2417
versus etiology, 988
*Clostridium*, 1019t
community-acquired, 919–922
causes of, 987, 987t
chest radiography of, 920–921
definition of, 919
diagnosis of, 919–921
epidemiology of, 919
hospitalization indications in, 921–922
microbiology of, 920–921
risk factors for, 919
treatment of, 922, 932t, 993–995, 994t, 995t, 998t
coronavirus, 941
*Corynebacterium*, 1030
cough in. See *Cough, in pneumonia.*
*Coxiella burnetii*, 473, 998t, 1025–1026
coxsackie B virus, 470
*Cryptococcus neoformans*, 1107–1108, 1129–1131, 2196–2197, *2197*
cytomegalovirus, 942, *942*, 943–945, *944*
bronchoscopy in, 749
genetic tests for, 626–627
in bone marrow transplantation, 2301–2302
in HIV infection, 2202
in lung transplantation, 2522
in transplantation, 925
pathology of, 473, *473*
defense mechanisms against, 986
diagnosis of, 985–986, 987–993. See also specific causative organisms.
clinical evaluation in, 987–988, 988t
community-acquired, 919–921
epidemiologic evaluation in, 987, 987t
in immunodeficiency, 924
invasive diagnostic techniques in, 991–993, 993t
laboratory evaluation in, 988–989
microbiologic evaluation in, 989–990, *990*
nosocomial, 923
percutaneous needle aspiration biopsy in, 760–761
radiography in, 988–989
serologic evaluation in, 990–991
differential diagnosis of, bronchoscopy in, 748
in immunodeficiency, 924
viral, 937
diffuse alveolar damage in, 1743–1744, 1743t
diseases underlying, 987–988, 988t
*Eikenella corrodens*, 998t, 1028
empyema development in, 1032–1033. See also *Empyema.*

Pneumonia *(Continued)*
Enterobacteriaceae, 998t, 1010–1011
enterococcal, in granulocytopenia, 924
eosinophilic, 1653t, 1654
acute, 1767–1769, 1769t
bronchoscopy in, 752
chronic, 1766–1767, *1767*, 1767t, *1768*
drug-induced, 479t
epidemiology of, 985, 987, 987t. See also specific causative organisms.
community-acquired, 919
Epstein-Barr virus, 470
*Erwinia*, 1010–1011
*Escherichia coli*, 1010–1011
etiology of. See *Pneumonia, microorganisms causing.*
*Francisella tularensis*, 1028–1029
Friedlander's (*Klebsiella pneumoniae*), 998t, 1008–1009, *1009*
fungal, in bone marrow transplantation, 2303
in pregnancy, 2321
in transplantation, 2229–2230, *2229*
pathology of, 474–475, *475*, *476*
*Fusobacterium nucleatum*, 1018–1020, 1019t
*Haemophilus influenzae*. See *Haemophilus influenzae infection(s), pneumonia as.*
*Hafnia*, 1010–1011
hantavirus. See *Hantavirus infections.*
hemoptysis in, 589, 589t
herpes simplex virus, 948–949
bronchoscopy in, 749–750
in bone marrow transplantation, 2302–2303
in HIV infection, 2203
in lung transplantation, 2522
in transplantation, 2229
pathology of, 468, 470, *471*
hospitalization indications in, 921–922
human herpesvirus 6, in transplantation, 2232, 2302
hypersensitivity, *469*
idiopathic interstitial, in bone marrow transplantation, 2300
in bone marrow transplantation, 2299–2300
fungal, 2303
pyogenic, 2303–2304
viral, 2301–2303
in bronchiectasis, 1328
in bronchitis, 1194
in bronchoscopy, 756
in chronic granulomatous disease, 2237
in chronic obstructive pulmonary disease, 1194
in diabetes mellitus, 2310
in elderly persons, 558
in emphysema, 1194
in granulocytopenia, 924–925, 925t, 997
in heroin use, 1980
in HIV infection. See also *Human immunodeficiency virus infection*, specific infections.
differential diagnosis of, 744, 745t
pathology of, 470–471, *472*
in hypercortisolism, 2312–2313
in immunodeficiency, 923–926, 925t, 937
specimen collection in, 611, *612*
treatment of, 997
in immunoglobulin G deficiency, 2235–2236
in lymphangio(leio)myomatosis, 1784
in malaria, 1147
in mechanical ventilation, 2483
prevention of, 1608
in plasma cell dyscrasias, 2292
in pulmonary fibrosis, 1684t

Pneumonia *(Continued)*
in rheumatoid arthritis, 1702
in severe combined immunodeficiency, 2233t, 2239
in sickle cell disease, 2287–2288
in spinal cord injury, 2339
in transplantation, early onset of, 2228–2229
fungal, 2229–2230, *2229*
late onset of, 2232
pyogenic, 2228–2229
viral, 2229–2232, 2230t
in Waldenström's macroglobulinemia, 2294
inclusion bodies in, 471, 473, *473*
influenza virus, 951, *952*, 954–955, *954*
pathology of, 468, 470
interstitial. See *Interstitial lung disease(s), pneumonia as.*
invasive diagnostic techniques in, 991–993, 993t
*Klebsiella pneumoniae*, 998t, 1008–1009, *1009*
laboratory evaluation in, 988–989
*Legionella*, 1014–1017, *1015*, 1015t, *1016*
life-threatening, causes of, 987
lipid, endogenous, 454, *454*
lipoid, 1481
lymphocytic interstitial, 1653–1654, 1653t
measles virus, 958–959
in pregnancy, 2321
pathology of, 470, *472*
melioidosis as, 1027–1028
meningococcal, 998t, 1005–1006
microbiologic diagnosis of, 607–631, 989–990, *990*. See also specific organisms.
cultures in. See *Culture(s).*
direct examination methods in, 613–617, *614*, *615*
genetic tests in, 625–627. See also specific tests, e.g., *Polymerase chain reaction.*
serologic testing in, 622–625
specimens for, collection of, 608–611, 610t, *612*
processing of, 611–613, 612t, 613t
selection of, 608–609, 610t
*Micromonospora*, 620–621
microorganisms causing, community-acquired, 920–921
nosocomial, 922–923
versus normal microflora, 608t
viral, 937
with gram-negative bacteria, 608t
*Micropolyspora*, 620–621
*Mima-Herellea* (*Acinetobacter*), 1013–1014
*Moraxella (Branhamella) catarrhalis*, 998t, 1006
*Morganella*, 1010–1011
mortality in. See *Mortality, in pneumonia.*
multiple organisms in, 948
mycobacterial. See also *Mycobacterium*; *Tuberculosis.*
microbiologic diagnosis of, 610t
*Mycoplasma pneumoniae*, 987
as asthma risk factor, 1251–1252
genetic tests for, 626
in sickle cell disease, 2287
laboratory detection of, 990–991
microbiologic diagnosis of, 610t
pathology of, 473, *474*
treatment of, 998t
*Neisseria meningitidis*, 998t, 1005–1006
*Nocardia*, 1022–1023, *1023*
in HIV infection, 2181
microbiologic diagnosis of, 610t, 618t, 620–621
treatment of, 998t

Pneumonia *(Continued)*
nosocomial, 922–923, 922t
bronchoscopy in, 747, *748*
causes of, 987, 987t
*Legionella*, 1014
prevention of, 923
respiratory syncytial virus, 964
treatment of, 995–996, 996t, 998t
organizing, bronchiolitis obliterans with. See *Bronchiolitis obliterans organizing pneumonia.*
pain in, 581t
*Paragonimus*, 1161
parainfluenza virus, 961
in bone marrow transplantation, 2302–2303
pathology of, 470
parasitic. See also specific organisms.
pathology of, 475
*Pasteurella multocida*, 1028
pathogenesis of, arachidonic acid metabolites in, 498–499
pathology of, 455–456, *455*, *456*
pathophysiology of, 319, 986
*Peptostreptococcus*, 1019, 1019t
physical examination in, 599, 988
Pittsburgh, 1014
plague as, 1029
pleural effusion in. See *Pleural effusion(s), in pneumonia; Pleural effusion(s), parapneumonic.*
pleuritic pain in, 576
pneumococcal. See *Pneumococcal pneumonia.*
*Pneumocystis carinii*. See *Pneumocystis carinii pneumonia.*
polymicrobial, 1017
prevention of, nosocomial, 923, 2483
*Prevotella*, 1019t, 1020
prognosis for, prediction of, 921–922
*Propionibacterium*, 1020–1022, *1021*
*Proteus*, 1010–1011
*Pseudomonas aeruginosa*, 998t, 1011–1013, *1012*
in HIV infection, 926
treatment of, 359, 998t
*Pseudomonas pseudomallei* (melioidosis), 1027–1028
pulmonary edema in, 1500
pulmonary function testing in, precautions with, 860–861
pyogenic, 985–1030. See also *Pneumonia*, specific bacteria.
causes of, 987, 987t
clinical approach to, 987–993, 987t, 988t, *990*, 993t
diagnosis of, 746–749, 746t, *747*, *748*, 985–986
epidemiology of, 985
hypoxemic respiratory failure in, 2415–2416
in bone marrow transplantation, 2303–2304
in HIV infection, 2178–2181
in pregnancy, 2320
in transplantation, 2228–2229
mortality in, 985–986
pathology of, 473–474
pathophysiology of, 986, 2415–2416
treatment of, 986, 993–999, 994t–998t, 2436
Q fever as, 473, 998t, 1025–1026
radiography in. See *Chest radiography, of pneumonia.*
reovirus, 470
respiratory syncytial virus, 962–963

Pneumonia *(Continued)*
in bone marrow transplantation, 2302–2303
in transplantation, 2232
pathology of, 470, *471*
rhinovirus, 470
*Rhodococcus (Corynebacterium) equi*, 1030
culture in, 620–621
in HIV infection, 2180–2181
rickettsial, 473
risk factors for, 986–988, 988t
nosocomial, 922–923
*Saccharomonospora*, 620–621
*Salmonella*, 1010–1011
serologic evaluation in, 610t, 990–991
*Serratia*, 1010–1011
*Staphylococcus aureus*. See *Staphylococcus aureus infection(s), pneumonia as.*
*Stenotrophomonas maltophilia*, 1012–1013
streptococcal, anaerobic, 1019, 1019t
microaerophilic, 1019, 1019t
treatment of, 998t
*Streptococcus pneumoniae*. See *Pneumococcal pneumonia.*
*Streptococcus viridans*, 924
*Streptomyces*, 620–621
*Sutterelia wadsworthensis*, 1019t
*Thermoactinomyces*, 620–621
*Toxoplasma gondii*, 1148
treatment of, 986. See also specific causative organisms.
community-acquired, 922, 932t
defense defect correction in, 997
empirical, 922, 922t, 994–995, 995t, 996t
hospitalization indications in, 993, 994t
in granulocytopenia, 924–925, 925t
in immunodeficiency, 924
outpatient, 993–994, 994t, 995t
pyogenic, 993–999, 994t–998t
supportive measures in, 997, 999
viral, 937
tularemia as, 1028–1029
unusual causes of, 1027–1030
usual interstitial, 1652–1653, 1653t, *1654*
varicella-zoster virus, 967, 968, *968*
in bone marrow transplantation, 2302–2303
in HIV infection, 2203
in pregnancy, 2321
in transplantation, 2232
ventilator-associated, 923, 991–992
viral, 937. See also specific viruses.
diagnosis of, 743t
in bone marrow transplantation, 2301–2303
in lung transplantation, 2522
in pregnancy, 2320–2321
microbiologic diagnosis of, 610t
microorganisms causing, 608t
nosocomial, 922
pathology of, 455–456, *458*, 468, 470–471, *471–473*, 473
pleural effusion in, 2024–2025
*Yersinia pestis*, 1029
Pneumonia Patient Outcomes Research Team, 921–922
Pneumonitis, anaerobic, 1017
aspiration. See *Aspiration (during breathing), pneumonia in.*
beryllium-related, 1843
cryptogenic organizing (idiopathic bronchiolitis obliterans organizing pneumonia), 1365
drug-induced, amiodarone in, 1973, 1981–1983, *1982*, 1982t
azathioprine in, 1977

Pneumonitis *(Continued)*
bleomycin in, 1976
cyclophosphamide in, 1975–1976
flecainide in, 1984
gold salts in, 1984–1985
hydantoin in, 1989
methotrexate in, 1977
mitomycin in, 1976–1977
nitrofurantoin in, 1972, 1978–1979
penicillamine in, 1985
procarbazine in, 1978
tocainide in, 1984
giant cell interstitial, 1652
granulomatous, 1653t, 1655, *1655*
hookworm, 1150–1151
hydrocarbon, 1908
hypersensitivity. See *Hypersensitivity pneumonitis.*
lupus, 1704, 1740
lymphocytic interstitial, in HIV infection, 2208–2209, *2208*
metal-related, 1907
nonspecific interstitial, 1652, 1653t, *1654*, 1672t
in HIV infection, 2209
radiation, 475, *476*, 477, 1436, 2036
versus Hodgkin's disease, 1454
*Schistosoma*, 1163–1165
talcum powder, 1908
toxic, 1907
*Toxoplasma gondii*, 1148
Pneumonocytes. See *Epithelium and epithelial cells, alveolar.*
Pneumopericardium, in mechanical ventilation, 2477–2478
pneumomediastinum with, 2102
treatment of, 2105
Pneumoperitoneum, after pneumomediastinum, *2098*, 2099
Pneumoretroperitoneum, pneumomediastinum and, *2098*, 2099
Pneumotachygraphy, in body plethysmography, 794, *794*, *795*
Pneumothorax, 2043–2055, 2105. See also *Hydropneumothorax.*
after pneumomediastinum, 2098–2099, *2098*
air reabsorption in, 2046–2047
catamenial, 2053–2054, *2053*, 2324
chest radiography of, 646, *648*, *652*
iatrogenic, 2051, *2052*
primary spontaneous, 2046, *2046*
secondary, 2049
traumatic, 2052
chyliform pleural effusion after, 2060
classification of, 2043–2044
clinical manifestations of, neonatal, 2053
primary, 2045–2046
secondary, 2049
tension, 2054
computed tomography of, 688
definition of, 2043–2044
diagnosis of, catamenial, 2054
primary, 2046, *2046*
secondary, 2049
tension, 2055
traumatic, 2052–2053
diagnostic, 2083
etiology of, 2045, 2049
iatrogenic, 2044, 2051, *2052*
in asthma, 1275
in barotrauma, 1955
in bronchiectasis, 1328
in bronchoscopy, 734, 757
in chronic obstructive pulmonary disease, 1192–1193
in coccidioidomycosis, 1124, *1124*, 1127

Pneumothorax *(Continued)*
in cystic fibrosis, 1305, 1312
in decompression sickness, 1962
in emphysema, 1192–1193
in interstitial lung disease, 1660t
in lymphangio(leio)myomatosis, 1746, 1747, *1747*, 1782
in Marfan's syndrome, 1711
in mechanical ventilation, 2456, 2477–2478
in percutaneous needle biopsy, 761
in pleural biopsy, 2009
in *Pneumocystis carinii* pneumonia, 2050
in pulmonary fibrosis, 1684t
in sarcoidosis, 1721
in transthoracic lung aspiration, 993
in tuberculosis, 1063, 2050–2051
incidence of, 2045, 2049
mechanisms of, 2052
mortality in, 2049, 2050
neonatal, 2053
occult, 2052
pain in, 581t
pathogenesis of, catamenial, 2054
neonatal, 2053
pathophysiology of, 2044–2045, *2044*, 2054
physical findings in, 599t
pyothorax-associated lymphoma after, 2071–2072
recurrence of, 2046, 2049
re-expansion pulmonary edema after, 2055–2056
spontaneous, 2043
primary, clinical manifestations of, 2045–2046
diagnosis of, 2046, *2046*
etiology of, 2045
genetic disposition to, 2045
incidence of, 2045
recurrence of, 2046
treatment of, 2046–2049, *2048*
secondary, 2049–2051
tension, 2046, 2054–2055
traumatic, 2043–2044, 2051–2053
treatment of, catamenial, 2054
in chronic obstructive pulmonary disease, 1192–1193
neonatal, 2053
primary, 2046–2049, *2048*
tension, 2055
traumatic, 2052–2053
versus bulla, in chronic obstructive pulmonary disease, 2049
versus pneumomediastinum, 2103
$Po_2$. See *Oxygen, partial pressure of.*
Poiseuille's equation, for pulmonary vascular resistance calculation, 124, 126–127, *128*
Poisoning. See *Toxic exposure(s).*
Policy, public. See *Government role.*
Poliomyelitis, respiratory function in, 2144, 2340–2341, 2341t
Pollution, air. See *Air pollution.*
Polyalveolar lobe, 483t
Polyangiitis, microscopic, diffuse alveolar hemorrhage in, *1735*, 1737t, 1739
Polyarteritis nodosa, 1540–1541
versus microscopic polyangiitis, 1739
Polychondritis, relapsing, 1695t, 1708–1710, *1709*
Polycyclic aromatic hydrocarbons, as air pollutants, 1887–1888, 1887t
exposure to, lung cancer in, 1401–1402
in cigarette smoke, 1399
Polycythemia, at high altitude, 1922
in cor pulmonale, 1643
in hypoventilation, 2143, 2144
in mountain sickness, 1938–1939

Polycythemia *(Continued)*
in pulmonary hypertension, 1547
Polycythemia vera, 2286
Polygenic pulmonary hypertension, 1543
Polymer(s), thermal degradation of, in building fires, toxic fumes from, 1908–1909
Polymer fume fever, 1907
Polymerase chain reaction, 626–627
for cytomegalovirus, 943
for influenza virus, 955
for lung cancer, 1426
for *Mycobacterium*, 1047
for *Mycobacterium tuberculosis*, 760, 2183, 2006
for *Pneumocystis carinii*, 759
for respiratory syncytial virus, 963
Polymyalgia rheumatica, vasculitis in, 1541
Polymyositis and/or dermatomyositis, 1706–1708
antibodies in, 1695t
diagnosis of, 1706, 1707t
diffuse alveolar hemorrhage in, 1739
diffuse lung disease in, 1707–1708, *1707*
epidemiology of, 1707
lung cancer in, 1421
risk factors for, 1707
vasculitis in, 1540
Polymyxin, pulmonary disease due to, 1979
Polyps, nasal, in cystic fibrosis, 1294, 1305, 1313
Polysaccharide antigen test, in fungal infections, 623
Polysomnography, 2155, *2156*
in heart failure, 2261
in sleep apnea, 2163–2164, *2163*, *2164*
Polyvinylchloride production, lung cancer in, 1402
Pons, in breathing control, *185*, 186–187
Pontiac fever, 1014, 1907
Popcorn calcification, of solitary nodule, 667
Pore(s), as ion channels. See *Ion channels.*
Pore theory, of endothelial permeability, 138–139, 138t, *139*, 138t
Portable radiography, 637, *637–639*, 639–640
Portal hypertension, hyperventilation in, 2146–2147
in cystic fibrosis, 1312–1313
in hepatopulmonary syndrome, 2272
in schistosomiasis, 1163–1164
pulmonary hypertension with, 1545–1546, 2274–2275
Portopulmonary hypertension, 2274–2275
Portosystemic shunt, in ascites, 2015
Positional changes and effects, dyspnea and. See *Orthopnea.*
on acute respiratory distress syndrome, 2433
on air embolism treatment, 1526
on arterial oxygen partial pressure, 855, 855t
on arteriovenous malformation behavior, 1563
on chest wall pressure-volume relationships, 104
on computed tomography results, 662
on diaphragm, 104
on diffusing capacity, 815
on hypoxemia, in systemic-pulmonary communications, 1497
on lung shape, 93–94
on lung volume, 109–111, *110*
in heart failure, 2251–2252, 2252t
on pleural effusions, 2006–2007, *2006*, *2007*
on pulmonary circulation, 64–65, 1489–1490
on pulmonary function tests, 803
on pulmonary perfusion, 129
on right ventricular function, 1636
on ventilation distribution, 109–111, *110*
Positional changes and effects *(Continued)*
on ventilation-perfusion scanning, 700
Positional cloning, in asthma studies, 1252–1253
in lung disease, 47
Positive end-expiratory pressure, 2476–2477, *2477*
advantages of, 2476
cardiac output in, 2388–2389, *2388*
definition of, 2476, 2565
disadvantages of, 2476
generator for, 2472
hypotension due to, 2463
in acute respiratory distress syndrome, 2424, *2425*, 2427–2432, *2428*
in asthma, 2459
in chronic obstructive pulmonary disease, 1229
in lung injury, 1585, 2477–2478
in pneumonia, 2436
in pulmonary edema, 1607, 2397
in status asthmaticus, 2459
inspiratory flow pattern for, 2477
inspiratory-expiratory time manipulations in, 2477
intrinsic, 2449–2450, *2450*, 2474–2475, *2475*, 2480–2481, *2481*
as hyperinflation measure, 2458
definition of, 2448
determination of, 2449–2450, *2450*
factors contributing to, 2449
inspiratory pressure at airway opening and, 2450–2451, *2451*
pneumomediastinum in, 2105
triggering and, 2448–2449, *2448*
work of breathing and, 2448–2449, *2448*
pneumomediastinum in, 2100–2101, 2104–2105
settings for, 2476–2477, *2477*
versus diastolic filling, 2391–2392, *2392*
Positive-pressure ventilation, complications of, 2483
design features of, 2471–2474, *2472*, 2473t
gas exchange in, 2476–2477, *2477*
hemodynamic effects of, 2482–2483
in kyphoscoliosis, 2362–2363, 2363t
in neuromuscular disorders, 2347–2348
lung injury in, 2477–2478
mechanical loads in, 2478–2479, *2479*, *2480*
noninvasive, in asthma, 2456
patient interactions with, 2479–2482, *2481*, *2482*
ventilatory pattern in, 2474–2476, *2475*, *2476*
Positron emission tomography, of acute respiratory distress syndrome, 2416
of lung cancer, 715–716, *715*, 1422, 1422t, 1423
of lung metabolism, 720
of mediastinum, 2086–2087, *2088*
of solitary nodule, 1439
Postinspiratory neurons, in breathing control, 186
Postnasal drip, cough in, 558–559, *559*, 563, 588
Postpericardiotomy syndrome, 578–579, 2032
Post-polio syndrome, 2144, 2340–2341
Postural drainage, in chest physical therapy, 370
in chronic obstructive pulmonary disease, 1224–1225
in cystic fibrosis, 1308–1309
in pulmonary rehabilitation, 2509
Posture. See also *Positional changes and effects.*
Posture *(Continued)*
maintenance of, respiratory muscles in, 108
Potassium, imbalance of. See *Hyperkalemia; Hypokalemia.*
transport of, 163. See also *Epithelium and epithelial cells, airway, electrolyte transport across.*
Potassium channels, 246–247
basolateral membrane, 337
bronchodilators acting upon, 277
function of, 336–338, *336*
in beta-adrenergic agonist action, 268, *269*
of pulmonary circulation, 298
receptor coupling to, 238
regulation of, 338–339
Potentiation, of drugs, 244
Pott's disease, 1081–1083, *1082*
Powder inhalers, 356, 1220
Power-duration curve, in chronic obstructive pulmonary disease, 216
PPA. See *Pulmonary artery pressure.*
PPALV. See *Alveolar pressure.*
PPV. See *Pulmonary venous pressure.*
PPW. See *Pulmonary artery wedge pressure.*
Pralidoxime, in organophosphate poisoning, 2343
Praziquantel, in paragonimiasis, 1162, 2026
in schistosomiasis, 1165
Prazosin, in pulmonary hypertension, 300
*pRB2* gene and product, in lung cancer, 1383
Pre-B cells, 421, *421*
Pre-Bötzinger complex, of medulla, 185, *185*, 188
Precipitation, electrostatic, in aerosol deposition, 351, *351*
Precipitin test, in aspergillosis, 622, 1132
in coccidioidomycosis, 1125
in cryptococcosis, 623
in histoplasmosis, 623
in hypersensitivity pneumonitis, 1874
Prednisolone, in asthma, 280, 281
in drug-induced lung disease, 1693t
in interstitial fibrosis, 1697
in systemic sclerosis, 1697
pharmacokinetics of, 280
side effects of, 282
Prednisone, in allergic bronchopulmonary aspergillosis, 1132, 1766
in allergic granulomatosis and angiitis, 1770
in asthma, 280, 1275
in chronic obstructive pulmonary disease, 1223
in hypersensitivity pneumonitis, 1879
in pleural effusion, in systemic lupus erythematosus, 2032
in pneumonia, eosinophilic, 1767
*Pneumocystis carinii*, 2194
in pulmonary fibrosis, 1681–1682, 1681t
in sarcoidosis, 1727
in systemic lupus erythematosus, 2032
in trichinosis, 1156
in tuberculosis, 1086
Preeclampsia, pulmonary edema in, 2322, *2323*
Preexisting symptoms, definition of, 896
Pregnancy, acute respiratory distress syndrome in, 2324
air embolism in, 2324
amniotic fluid embolism in, 1526–1527, 2323–2324, *2324*
anaphylactoid syndrome of, 2323
arteriovenous malformation enlargement in, 1561
aspiration pneumonitis in, 2324
asthma in, 2319–2320
chest wall changes in, 2317
cystic fibrosis in, 1307, 2320

Pregnancy *(Continued)*
diabetes mellitus in, 2310
hantavirus infections in, 2321
high altitude effects on, 1942
hypersensitivity pneumonitis in, 1871
hyperventilation in, 2147
kyphoscoliosis in, 2361
lung injury in, 1588t
lymphangio(leio)myomatosis in, 1778–1779, 1781, 1783
neonatal asthma origins in, 1251, *1251*
normal physiologic alterations in, 2317–2318, *2318*
pneumomediastinum in, 2096, 2100
pneumonia in, bacterial, 2320
fungal, 2321
viral, 2320–2321
pulmonary edema in, 1588t, 2321–2324
hydrostatic, 2321
in preeclampsia, 2322, *2322*
tocolysis-associated, 2321–2322, *2322*
pulmonary embolism in, 2322–2323
pulmonary function tests in, 2317–2318, *2318*
pulmonary hypertension in, 1551
rhinitis in, 2317
sarcoidosis in, 1719
smoking cessation programs in, 2533
thromboembolism risk in, 1514
thrombosis in, 2322–2323
tissue embolism in, 465, 1527
tuberculosis in, 1074, 2321
Preload, reduction of, in acute respiratory distress syndrome, 2423–2424, *2425*
Premedication, for bronchoscopy, 730
Prenatal diagnosis, of cystic fibrosis, 1293
Preneoplasia, in lung cancer, 1377–1378
Preoperative evaluation, 883–894
analgesia and anesthesia considerations in, 884–885
cardiac risk assessment in, 883–884, 884t, 885t
for abdominal surgeries, 885–886, 886t
for cardiac surgeries, 886
for lung volume reduction surgery, 890–891
for pulmonary resection, 889–891
cardiovascular evaluation in, 890
lung scan in, 889–890
postresection considerations and, 889
pulmonary artery occlusion test in, 890
of high-risk patients, 886–889
smokers as, 887
with asthma, 888–889
with chronic obstructive pulmonary disease, 887–888, 887t, *888*
spirometry in, 784
ventilation-perfusion scanning in, 713–715
Present illness, in medical history, 587
President's Task Force on Environmental Health Risks and Safety Risk to Children, 2548
Presist (resistive pressure component), of inspiratory pressure at airway opening, 2450–2451, *2451*
Pressure, alveolar. See *Alveolar pressure.*
blood. See *Blood pressure*; *Hypertension*; *Hypotension.*
critical, 1344, *1344*, 1351
for inhalation, in kyphoscoliosis, 2359
in airways, airflow dynamics and, 1344–1345, *1344*, *1345*
in diving, 1951–1969
in pulmonary circulation. See *Pulmonary circulation, pressures in.*
intrathoracic, during water immersion, 1952
partial. See also *Carbon dioxide, partial pressure of*; *Oxygen, partial pressure of.*
Pressure *(Continued)*
gas solubility and, 1958–1959, *1959*
pleural. See *Pleural pressure.*
pulmonary artery. See *Pulmonary artery pressure.*
pulmonary capillary. See *Pulmonary capillary(ies), pressure in.*
pulmonary venous. See *Pulmonary venous pressure.*
transpulmonary. See *Transpulmonary pressure.*
trauma induced by. See *Barotrauma.*
Pressure body plethysmography, in lung volume measurement, 793–794, *794*
Pressure-flow relationships, terminology of, 2564
Pressure-time products, in mechanical ventilation, 2478–2479, *2479*, *2480*
Pressure-volume body plethysmography, in lung volume measurement, 794–795, *795*
Pressure-volume relationships, alveolar, versus lung volume, 61
alveolar vessels versus lung volume, 126, *127*
Boyle's law of, 102
in diving, 1954–1955, *1955*
in functional residual capacity measurement, 58
esophageal, versus lung volume, 103–104, *103*
hysteresis in, 95, *96*
in acute respiratory distress syndrome, 2426, *2426*, *2427*
in chest wall movement, 103–105, *103*
in chronic obstructive pulmonary disease, 1191
in emphysema, *103*, 104–105, 1191, 1207
in pulmonary circulation, 127–128, *128*
lung, 92, *92*, 93, 95, *96*
at total lung capacity, 104
in pneumothorax, 2044–2045, *2044*
surfactant and, 308, *308*
Newton's third law as, 782
pleural, versus lung volume, 104, 111
terminology of, 2564
Prevention, of asthma, government in. See *Government role, in asthma secondary prevention.*
of occupational disease(s), 1806–1808
asbestos-related, 1840
berylliosis as, 1844
coal-workers' pneumoconiosis as, 1830
silicosis as, 1824
of smoking, 2532–2533, 2532t
*Prevotella* pneumonia, 1019t, 1020
Primaquine, in *Pneumocystis carinii* pneumonia, 2191t, 2192
Priming, by allergens, 1348
Prinzmetal's angina, 578
Privacy, right of, 2491–2492
Procarbazine, pleural disease due to, 2036
pulmonary disease due to, 1978
Prochlorperazine, in mountain sickness, 1932
Progesterone, in asthma pathogenesis, 2319
in hypoventilation, 2144
receptors for, lymphangio(leio)myomatosis and, 1778–1779
Progressive systemic sclerosis, vasculitis in, 1539–1540, *1540*
Proline-rich proteins, in mucus, 331
Propafenone, contraindicated in asthma, 290
Propellants, for aerosol delivery, 355–356
*Propionibacterium* pneumonia, 1020–1022, *1021*
Propoxyphene, pulmonary disease due to, 1980
Propranolol, pulmonary disease due to, 1983
Propriobulbar neurons, in breathing control, 186
Prospective Investigation of Pulmonary Embolism Diagnosis trial, 1507, 1510, 1511, 1512
ventilation-perfusion scanning and, 702–704, 705t
Prostacyclin, as vasodilator, 300
in portopulmonary hypertension, 2275
in pulmonary hypertension, 1551, 1646
Prostaglandin(s), as cough stimulants, 252
as inflammatory mediators, 257
biologic effects of, 497–499, 497t
formation of, in macrophages, 394
in acute respiratory distress syndrome, 2423
in electrolyte transport, in airway epithelium, 338
in mucus hypersecretion, 334
in pulmonary edema, 1611
in pulmonary hypertension, 1645–1646
in pulmonary vascular resistance control, 131, 297
metabolism of, in pulmonary circulation, 69
Prostanoids. See *Prostaglandin(s)*; *Thromboxane.*
Prostigmine, in myasthenia gravis, 2342
Protamine, pulmonary disease due to, 1983
Protease(s). See also *Metalloproteinases.*
neutrophil, in cystic fibrosis, 1179
Protease inhibitors, in mucus, 329
Protease-activated receptors, 234–235
Protein(s), animal, inhalation of, asthma in, 1858t
hypersensitivity pneumonitis in, 1869
dietary, metabolism of, in exercise, 198–199
in edema fluid, measurement of, 1595
in lung fluid, pressure differences and, 1576
in mucus, 331
in pleural fluid, 2003
in pulmonary edema fluid, 1500
surfactant, 308–316, *309*, 309t
Protein adducts, as biomarkers, for lung cancer, 1406
Protein C, activated, resistance to, thromboembolism risk in, 1514
Protein kinase A, in signal transduction, 236, *236*
Protein kinase C, endothelial permeability and, 142–143, *143*
in electrolyte transport, 338
in signal transduction, 237, *237*
Protein sequence data bases, 51, 52t
Protein tyrosine phosphatases, as receptors, 240
Proteinases, excess of, in cystic fibrosis, 1301
Proteinosis, alveolar. See *Alveolar proteinosis, pulmonary.*
lipoid, 480t
Proteoglycans, in lung, 137
in mucus, 331–332
*Proteus* pneumonia, 1010–1011
Prothrombin defects, thromboembolism risk in, 1514
Prothrombin time, measurement of, in pulmonary embolism anticoagulant prophylaxis, 1519
Protozoal infection(s), amebiasis as, 1144–1146, *1145*, 2026
lung injury in, 475
malaria as, 1146–1147
toxoplasmosis as, 626–627, 1147–1149, *1148*, 2203–2204
Protriptyline, in asthma, 290
Protussive therapy, 564–565
Provocation testing, after lung transplantation, 2524–2525

Provocation testing *(Continued)*
in asthma, 1266, 1268
occupational, 1859, *1860*
in heart disease, 2255
in hypersensitivity pneumonitis, 1875–1876
in pregnancy, 2319
indications for, 852–853
response to, criteria for, 874
Pseudoallescheriosis, 1136
Pseudoaneurysms, aortic, 683, *686*
pulmonary artery, 1568–1569, *1570*
Pseudochylothorax, 2003, 2057, 2059–2060
Pseudocyst(s), pancreatic, mediastinal extension of, 2132
pleural effusions in, 2028–2029, *2029*, 2277–2278, *2278*
Pseudohemoptysis, in *Serratia* pneumonia, 1010
Pseudolymphoma(s), in Sjögren's syndrome, 1706
of lung, 1480
*Pseudomonas aeruginosa* infections, in bronchiectasis, 1331
in cystic fibrosis, 334, 1179–1180, 1300–1301, 1303, *1303*
mucociliary transport and, 368
treatment of, 1309–1312, 1309t
mucus secretion mechanisms in, 334
pneumonia due to, 998t, 1011–1013, *1012*
in HIV infection, 926, 2180
treatment of, aerosol delivery of, 359
*Pseudomonas pseudomallei* (melioidosis) pneumonia, 1027–1028
Pseudotumor(s), of lung, 1481, 1481t
postinflammatory, 1480
Pseudotumor cerebri, in respiratory acidosis, 174
Psittacosis, 624, 998t, 1026
genetic tests for, 626
Pstat (static elastic pressure component), of inspiratory pressure at airway opening, 2450–2451, *2451*
PSTL (elastic recoil pressure), 799–801, *801*
Psychiatric disorders, chest pain in, 580
in sleep apnea, 2158
Psychogenic disorder(s), cough as, 561
hyperventilation as, 2147, 2148
Psychologic factors, in dyspnea, 544, 545t
Psychosocial issues, in cystic fibrosis, 1311, 1314
in lung transplantation, 2526
*PTEN* gene and product, in lung cancer, 1384
PU.1 transcription factor, in monocyte-macrophage development, 405–406
Public policy. See *Government role*.
Pulmonary alveolar microlithiasis, 450
Pulmonary alveolar proteinosis. See *Alveolar proteinosis, pulmonary*.
Pulmonary angiography. See *Angiography, pulmonary*.
Pulmonary artery(ies), anatomy of, 11, *12*, *13*, 120, *121*, 1631–1632, *1632*
aneurysms of, 1542, 1569–1570, *1570*
arteritis of, in bronchiectasis, 1326–1327
branches of, 120, 1486, 1488, 1631–1632, *1632*
catheterization of, in pulmonary edema, 1600–1601, 2418
compression of, ventilation-perfusion scanning in, 704
corner, function of, 126
cross section of, versus smooth muscle content, 120, *121*
versus transmural pressure difference, 125–126
disorders of, as mediastinal masses, 2130
Pulmonary artery(ies) *(Continued)*
elastic, anatomy of, 120, *121*
emboli in. See *Pulmonary embolism*.
endothelium of, permeability of, 140
enlargement of, in pulmonary hypertension, 1638
fibrosis of, in systemic sclerosis, 1697–1698
functional description of, 125–126
hypoxic constriction of. See *Hypoxia and hypoxemia, pulmonary vasoconstriction in*.
in cystic fibrosis, 1294
inflammation of. See *Vasculitis*.
intraluminal pressure in, 125–126
left main, anatomy of, 120
muscular, anatomy of, 120, *121*
obstruction of, in mediastinitis, 2113–2114, *2114*, 2115
perivascular pressure on, 125–126
plexogenic, in portopulmonary hypertension, 2275
pressures in. See *Pulmonary artery pressure*.
pseudoaneurysms of, 1568–1569, *1570*
right main, anatomy of, 120
smooth muscle of, 120, *121*
steal in, after embolectomy, 1523, *1524*
stenosis of, angiography in, *660*
pain in, 576
stents in, in mediastinitis, 2115, *2115*
supernumerary, anatomy of, 120
venous communications with. See *Arteriovenous malformations, pulmonary*.
Pulmonary artery pressure, at high altitude, 1920–1921, *1921*
in exercise, 1927
in pulmonary edema, 1935–1936
blood flow distribution and, 128–129, *129*
capillary reserve and, 1633
diffusing capacity and, 815–816, *817*
distribution of, 128–129, *129*
high. See *Pulmonary hypertension*.
in air embolism, 1526
in exercise, 1491, *1491*, 1927
in highly fit athletes, 219
in hypoxemia, 1632
in liver disease, 2274–2275
in pulmonary edema, 1601, 1935–1936
in pulmonary embolism, 1506
in pulmonary vascular resistance calculation, 62, 123–124, 1490
measurement of, 123, *124*, 299, 890
normal, 11, 60, 123, *123*, 1498t, 1632
perfusion distribution and, 128–129, *129*
pulmonary capillary effects of, 815–816, *817*
pulmonary venous pressure effects on, 2247–2248
reduction of, drugs for, 298–299
versus capillary recruitment and distention, 62–63, *63*
versus diameter, 125–126
versus pulmonary vascular resistance, 126, *126*
Pulmonary artery wedge pressure, definition of, 2565
in acute respiratory distress syndrome, 2424, *2425*
in chronic obstructive pulmonary disease, 1633, *1633*
in exercise, 2249t, 2250
in heart disease, 2249t, 2250
in highly fit athletes, 219
in left ventricular failure, 1636
in near drowning, 1966
in pulmonary edema, 1500
in pulmonary hypertension, 1550
Pulmonary artery wedge pressure *(Continued)*
in pulmonary veno-occlusive disease, 1550
measurement of, 123, *124*, 1632–1633, *1633*
normal, 1632
positional changes in, 1632–1633
Pulmonary capillary(ies), alveolar, 16
anatomy of, 13–14, *13*, *14*, 122, 1486, *1488*
blood gas partial pressures in, 2047
cancer cell invasion of, 1469
carbon dioxide partial pressure in, 78
corner vessels as, 126
destruction of, in chronic obstructive pulmonary disease, 1633
diffusion path length in, 808–809
distensibility of, 809
distortion of, pulmonary vascular resistance and, 63
dysgenesis of, in arteriovenous malformations, 1558
endothelium of, fluid and solute exchange across, 134–135, *134–136*
permeability of. See *Endothelial permeability*.
extracellular matrix of, 135, 143–144
filtration rate in, Starling equation and, 1497
versus lymph flow, 136, *136*
fluid and solute exchange in, 132–135, *132*, *134–136*, 1497, 1498t, 1575–1576
fluid flux equation for, 132–133, *132*
function of, 1632
gas exchange in. See *Gas exchange*.
gas permeability of, at high altitude, 1919
hemangiomatosis of, 1746, *1746*
hydrostatic pressure in, 132–133, *132*, 1576
in pulmonary edema, 145, 1497–1498, 1576–1577
decreased, 1580t, 1582–1583
increased, 1580–1582, 1580t
in Starling equation, 1497
inflammation of. See *Capillaritis, pulmonary*.
injury of, in pulmonary edema, 146–147
leakage from, in hantavirus infections, 946
in high-altitude pulmonary edema, 1935–1936
neutrophils in, 524–526, *525*
obstruction of, diffusing capacity in, 815–816, *817*
oxygen partial pressure in, at high altitude, 1919, *1920*
distribution of, 78
oxygen uptake along, 72–73, *73*, *74*
permeability of. See *Endothelial permeability*.
pressure in, 60, *61*, 1498t. See also *Pulmonary capillary wedge pressure*.
definition of, 2565
disruption from, 69
edema formation and, 145, *145*
fluid flux and, 132–133, *132*
in arteriovenous malformations, 1563
measurement of, 60, *61*
pulmonary edema and, 145, *145*
pulmonary artery pressure effects on, 815–816, *817*
recruitment of, 62–63, *63*, 128
reserve in, 1633
stress failure of, in highly fit athletes, 219
surface area of, diffusing capacity and, 809, *809*
transit time of, calculation of, 219
volume of, 13–14, 127
in highly fit athletes, 219–220
Pulmonary capillary wedge pressure, in acute respiratory distress syndrome, 2418
in portopulmonary hypertension, 2275

Pulmonary capillary wedge pressure *(Continued)*
in pulmonary edema, 1601, 2418, 2419t
Pulmonary circulation, 60–70. See also *Pulmonary artery(ies)*; specific vessels.
abnormal communications in. See *Arteriovenous malformations, pulmonary.*
alveolar, 14, 1486
anastomoses of, in bronchiectasis, 1326
anatomy of, 11, *12–15*, 12t, 13–15, 119–122, 1486, *1487*, 1488, *1488*, 1631–1633, *1632*, *1633*
blood-gas interface in, 122. See also *Blood-gas barrier.*
bronchial, 10–11, 122–123, *122*
corner vessel, 126
extra-alveolar, 125
general design of, 120–121, *121*
arterioles in, 1631–1632
anatomy of, 120
obstruction of, 1642
technetium-99m labeled albumin studies of, 698
arteriovenous malformations in. See *Arteriovenous malformations.*
autonomic nervous system effects on, 64, 121
blood flow in, abnormal, 66–67
control of, 67–68, *68*
distention and, 128
distribution of, 64–67, *65*, 1489–1490, *1490*, 1491t
in heart disease, 2256–2257, *2257*
exercise effects on, 1489, 1491t
factors affecting, 66–67
in exercise, 202
in highly fit athletes, 219–220
in pulmonary edema, 1579
in respiratory failure, 2393–2395, *2394–2396*, 2395t
in shunt calculation, 825–827, *826*, 826t, 827t
increased, hyperkinetic pulmonary hypertension in, 1642
mosaic perfusion in, 676, *677*
recruitment and, 128
regional distribution of, 128–129, *129*
resistance to. See *Pulmonary vascular resistance.*
stress from, 67–68
three-zone model of, 65–66, *65*
versus alveolar ventilation, 825
versus pressures, 62–63, *62*, *63*, 123, *123*
bronchial circulation interconnections with, 121, *122*
capillaries in. See *Pulmonary capillary(ies).*
control of, 67–68, *68*
disorders of. See also specific disorders.
classification of, 1485, 1486t
diagnosis of, 1485–1486
dyspnea in, 220
drug effects on, 64
endothelial cells of. See *Endothelial permeability; Endothelium and endothelial cells.*
extra-alveolar, 14, 61–62, *61*, 1486
blood flow distribution and, 66
function of, 125
pulmonary vascular resistance and, 64
resistance in, 126, *127*
fetal, 68, 131
filtration in, 70
fluid and solute exchange in. See *Fluid and solute exchange.*
functions of, 119, 1488–1491, *1490*, 1491t
gravity effects on, 66
Pulmonary circulation *(Continued)*
hemodynamics of. See also *Pulmonary circulation, pressures in; Pulmonary vascular resistance.*
in arteriovenous malformations, 1563
in chronic obstructive pulmonary disease, 1641
in cor pulmonale, 1641
in cough, 557
in heart disease, 2249–2251, 2249t
in hypoxia, 129–131
in pulmonary embolism, 1506
perfusion and. See *Pulmonary circulation, blood flow in; Ventilation-perfusion ratio.*
plasma transport and, 138, 138t
regulation of, 131–132
vascular compliance and, 127–128, *128*
vessel functional description and, 125–126
hemostatic activity of, 70
homeostatic function of, 14
hypertrophy of, 1978
hypoxic vasoconstriction of. See *Hypoxia and hypoxemia, pulmonary vasoconstriction in.*
in acceleration, 66
in arteriovenous malformations, 1563
in chronic obstructive pulmonary disease, 1641
in cor pulmonale, 1641
in cough, 557
in heart disease, 67, 2249–2251, 2249t
in hypoxia, 129–131
in lung disease, 66–67
in pulmonary edema, 64, 2396–2398, *2396*, *2398*
in pulmonary embolism, 1506
in pulmonary fibrosis, 1676
in respiratory failure, 2392–2398, 2396–2398, *2396*, *2398*
in weightlessness, 66
injury of, pulmonary edema in, 146–147
innervation of, 121, 131
lung volume and, 63–64, *63*, 66
macrophages of, 385
metabolic functions of, 69–70
microcirculation portion of, 1486. See also *Pulmonary capillary(ies).*
neonatal, 68
neutrophils in, 524–526, *525*
obstruction of, exercise testing in, 848
pharmacology of, 297–306
clinical applications of, 298–299
endothelin-1 in, 298
evaluation in, 299
new directions in, 297–298
nitric oxide in, 297–298
overview of, 297–298
potassium channel activity in, 298
vasodilators in, 299–302
physiology of, 119, 1488–1491, *1490*, 1491t
positional effects on, 64–65
pressures in, 60, *61*, 123, *123*, *124*, 1498t. See also specific types, e.g., *Pulmonary artery pressure; Pulmonary venous pressure.*
bronchial circulation pressure changes with, 1489
damage from, 68–69
distribution of, 60, *61*
in exercise, 1491t
in highly fit athletes, 219
in mechanical ventilation, 2395, *2395*
in pulmonary edema, 1595–1596
in respiratory failure, 2393–2395, *2394–2396*, 2395t
Pulmonary circulation *(Continued)*
normal, 11, 60
pulsatile, 60, 123, *123*
versus flow, 62–63, *62*, *63*
versus systemic pressures, 1490
versus volume, 127–128, *128*
pressures outside, 60–62, *61*
remodeling of, in heart disease, 2248, 2249t
in pulmonary venous hypertension, 2248, 2249t
reservoir function of, 70, 127–128, *128*
resistance of. See *Pulmonary vascular resistance.*
solute exchange in. See *Fluid and solute exchange.*
structures included in, 119–120, 1486
systemic circulation communications with, 1565–1566
bronchopulmonary sequestration in. See *Sequestration(s), bronchopulmonary.*
vasoactivity of, 69, 297–298
vasodilators for. See *Vasodilator(s).*
vasospasm in, angiography of, *647*
versus bronchial circulation, 1488, *1489*
volume of, versus pressure, 127–128, *128*
Pulmonary edema, 1497–1500, 1575–1629
after pneumothorax treatment, 2055–2056
aspirin-induced, 1984
barrier function measurement in, 1597–1598
blood gas analysis in, 1594–1595
blood-gas barrier failure in, 69
cardiogenic. See *Pulmonary edema, increased pressure.*
causes of, 2414t, 2415, 2417–2418, *2418*
chest radiography of, 1499, 1499t, 1500, 1594, 2417, *2418*
clinical manifestations of, 1498–1500, 1499t, 1933–1934, *1934*
connective tissue distortion in, 5, *6*
contrast agent-induced, 1988
cytosine arabinoside-induced, 1977, *1977*
definition of, 132, 1497, 1591–1594, 1592t, 1593t
dextran-induced, 1988
diagnosis of, 1591–1600
barrier function measurement in, 1597–1598
blood gas analysis in, 1594–1595
chest radiography of, 1499, 1499t, 1500, 1594, 2417, *2418*
criteria for, 1591–1594, 1592t, 1593t
fluid protein measurement in, 1595
hemodynamic measurements in, 1595–1596
lung injury detection in, 1598–1600
lung water measurement in, 1596–1597
pulmonary function tests in, 1595
symptoms and signs in, 1591
differential diagnosis of, 1500
diffuse, ventilation-perfusion scanning in, 711
drug-induced, 479t, 1588t, 1990, 1990t
dyspnea in, 220, 2261
echocardiography in, 2417–2418
exudative phase of, 1586
fibrosis after, 1586
flash, 1591
fluid in, analysis of, 1595, 2417
exchange of. See *Fluid and solute exchange.*
sites of accumulation in, 145
hemodynamic measurements in, 1595–1596
heroin-induced, 1979–1980
high-altitude, 147, 1930t, 1933–1937
clinical features of, 1933–1934, *1934*
coagulation disorders in, 1938

Pulmonary edema *(Continued)*
mortality in, 1933
pathology of, 1934–1935, *1935*
pathophysiology of, 1581, 1935–1936
prevention of, 1937
reentry, 1939
treatment of, 1936–1937
high-permeability. See *Pulmonary edema, increased permeability.*
high-pressure. See *Pulmonary edema, increased pressure.*
hydrostatic. See *Pulmonary edema, increased pressure.*
in acute respiratory distress syndrome, 2413–2415, 2414t, *2415*
in airway obstruction, 1589t
in aspiration, 1588t
in beryllium lung disease, 1843
in bone marrow transplantation, 2298–2299
in bronchiolitis, 1362, *1362*
in congestive heart failure, 1580
in diabetes mellitus, 2310
in hantavirus infections, 471
in heart disease, 2247–2248, 2248t, 2249t, 2250, 2261
in heart failure, 1604, 1605, 2013
in hematologic disorders, 1588t
in hemodynamic disorders, 1588t
in hemorrhagic shock, 147
in infection, 1587, 1588t, 1589
in inflammation, 1589–1590, 1590t
in kidney dysfunction, 1499t, 2278–2279
in leukemia, 2291
in malaria, 1147
in metabolic acidosis, 170
in microembolism, 147
in mountain sickness, 1931
in myocardial infarction, outcome of, 1613
in near drowning, 1582, 1965
in neurologic disorders, 1588t
in obstetric/gynecologic disorders, 1588t
in oxygen toxicity, 147
in preeclampsia, 2322, *2323*
in pregnancy, 2321–2323, *2322*
in pulmonary veno-occlusive disease, 1550
in pulmonary venous hypertension, 1580–1581
in reperfusion, 147
in sepsis, 147, 1587, 1589
in shock, 147
in sickle cell disease, 2288
in toxic exposures, 1588t, 1590–1591, 1904
in transfusions, 1987
in trauma, 1588t
in Waldenström's macroglobulinemia, 2294
increased permeability, 69, 1498, 1500, 1584–1591. See also *Acute/adult respiratory distress syndrome.*
chest radiography of, 1584, *1584*
definition of, 1576, 1591–1594, 1592t, 1593t
diagnosis of, barrier function measurement in, 1597–1598
blood gas analysis in, 1594–1595
chest radiography of, 1594
criteria for, 1591–1594, 1592t, 1593t
fluid protein measurement in, 1595
hemodynamic measurements in, 1595–1596
lung injury detection in, 1598–1600
lung water measurement in, 1596–1597
pulmonary function tests in, 1595
symptoms and signs in, 1591
in acute respiratory distress syndrome, 2413–2415, 2414t, *2415*
in infection, 1587, 1588t, 1589

Pulmonary edema *(Continued)*
in inflammation, 1589–1590, 1590t
in toxic exposure, 1588t, 1590–1591
mechanisms of, 1587–1591, 1588t–1590t
outcome of, 1613–1614, *1614*
pathophysiology of, 1584–1586, 2415
protection against, 1577
stages of, 1586
synonyms for, 1584
treatment of. See *Pulmonary edema, treatment of.*
increased pressure, 1497–1500, 1577–1584
after airway obstruction, 1582
after collapsed lung re-expansion, 1582–1583
alveolar barrier function in, 1580t, 1583–1584
at high altitudes, 1581
chest radiography of, 1499t, 1594
clinical manifestations of, 1499
decreased perimicrovascular hydrostatic pressure in, 1582–1583
decreased transmural osmotic pressure difference in, 1583
definition of, 1576
diagnosis of, barrier function measurement in, 1597–1598
blood gas analysis in, 1594–1595
fluid protein measurement in, 1595
hemodynamic measurements in, 1595–1596
lung injury detection in, 1598–1600
lung water measurement in, 1596–1597
pulmonary function tests in, 1595
symptoms and signs in, 1591
in congestive heart failure, 1580
in pregnancy, 2321
in pulmonary venous hypertension, 1580–1581
increased hydrostatic pressure in, 1580–1582, 1580t
mechanisms for, 1580–1584, 1580t
neurogenic, 1581–1582
outcome of, 1613
pathophysiology of, 1577–1580, 1578t, 2415
protection against, 1577
treatment of. See *Pulmonary edema, treatment of.*
interstitial, in heart disease, 2247–2248, 2248t
resolution of, 1612
lung function and mechanics in, 1578–1579, 1578t
lung injury in. See also *Lung injury, acute.*
detection of, 1598–1600
lung volumes in, *2390*
lung water measurement in, 1596–1597
lymphatic insufficiency in, 146
mechanisms of, 145–146, *145*, *146*
mortality in, 1933
neurogenic, 147
at high altitude, 1936
pathophysiology of, 1581–1582
normal barrier. See *Pulmonary edema, increased pressure.*
on reentry to lower altitudes, 1939
oxygen partial pressure in, 2258, *2258*
pathogenesis of, 144–147
fluid accumulation sites in, 145
in heart disease, 2247–2248, 2248t
mechanisms of, 145–146, *145*, *146*
phases of, 144–145
vascular injury in, 146–147
pathology of, 1579
high-altitude, 1581, 1934–1935, *1935*

Pulmonary edema *(Continued)*
pathophysiology of, 1497–1498, 1498t, 1575–1591, 2396–2398, *2396*, *2398*
alveolar barrier function in, 1580t, 1583–1584
decreased perimicrovascular hydrostatic pressure in, 1582–1583
decreased transmural osmotic pressure difference in, 1583
high-altitude, 1581, 1935–1936
in increased permeability edema, 1584–1591, *1584*, 1588t–1590t
in increased pressure edema, 1577–1584, *1577*, 1578t, 1580t
in lung re-expansion, 2055
in near drowning, 1582
increased hydrostatic pressure in, 1580–1582, 1580t
neurogenic, 1581–1582
postobstructive, 1582
re-expansion, 1582
phases of, 144–145
phenothiazine-induced, 1989
plasma oncotic pressure decrease in, 145, *145*
postobstructive, 1582
prevention of, high-altitude, 1937
homeostasis safety factors in, 145, 146, *146*
in highly fit athletes, 219
safety factors for, 1576–1577, 1576t
proliferative phase of, 1586
protamine-induced, 1983
pulmonary blood flow distribution in, 2256–2257, *2257*
pulmonary capillary pressure increase in, 145, *145*
pulmonary function tests in, 1499–1500, 1578–1579, 1578t, 1595
pulmonary vascular resistance in, 64, 126
re-expansion, pathophysiology of, 1582
reperfusion, after embolectomy, 1523–1524, *1525*
resolution of, 1611–1613
respiratory failure in, 2396–2398, *2396*, *2398*
secondary. See *Pulmonary edema, increased pressure.*
stages of, 1586
symptoms and signs of, 1591
tocolytic-induced, 1988, 2321–2322, *2322*
treatment of, 1600–1611
antioxidants in, 1610
cardiac catheterization in, 1600–1601
corticosteroids in, 1608–1609
diuretics in, 1602–1603
goals of, 1600, 1605–1606, 1606t
high-altitude, 1936–1937
immediate, 1600
in heart failure, 2250
increased permeability, 1605–1608, 1606t, 1613–1614, *1614*
increased pressure, 1605, 1613, 2419–2422, 2420t, *2421*
inotropic agents in, 1603–1604
mechanical ventilation in, 2421–2422
monoclonal antibodies in, 1610–1611
options for, 1600–1604
outcome of, 1611–1614, *1614*
pentoxifylline in, 1610
specific, 1608–1611
strategies for, 1604–1611, 1606t
surfactant in, 1609–1610
vasodilators in, 1601–1602, 1611
tricyclic-induced, 1989
types of, 1497–1498, 1576

Pulmonary edema *(Continued)*
vascular injury in, 146–147
vascular permeability increase in, 145–146
Pulmonary embolism, 1503–1531
air, 465, 1526
amniotic fluid, 465, 1526–1527, 2323–2324, *2324*
angiography in, 654–657, *654–656*, 1512–1513, *1513*
atypical, 1508
cellular, 1527
chest pain in, 576
chest radiography of, *708*, *709*, 1510, *1510*
cholesterol, 465
clearance of, 14
clinical manifestations of, 1506–1508, 2026–2027
clinical studies of, PIOPED as, 702–704, 705t, 722, 723, 724, 1507
compensatory mechanisms in, 1506
computed tomography angiography of, 2008
computed tomography of, 679–681, 680t, *682*, 1512, *1512*
controversies about, 1503–1504
cough in, 558
diagnosis of, 1509–1513, 2027
algorithm for, *1514*
angiography in, 654–657, *654–656*, 702, 1512–1513, *1513*
approach to, 1513–1514, *1514*
clinical, 1507–1508
computed tomography in, 679–681, 680t, *682*, 1512, *1512*
echocardiography in, 1510
hemostasis evaluation in, 1511
laboratory tests in, 1509–1510, *1510*
magnetic resonance imaging in, 679–681, 680t, *682*
ventilation-perfusion scanning in. See *Ventilation-perfusion scanning.*
with chronic pulmonary hypertension, 1520–1522, *1521–1523*
differential diagnosis of, 1507
echocardiography in, 1510
electrocardiography in, 1510
epidemiology of, 1503
fat, 465, 1526
foreign body, 465
hemodynamics of, 1506
hemostasis evaluation in, 1511
high-altitude, 1937–1938
in chronic obstructive pulmonary disease, 1512
in nephrotic syndrome, 2016
in neuromuscular disorders, 2332
in pregnancy, 2322–2323
in pulmonary fibrosis, 1684t
infarction in, 1506
magnetic resonance imaging in, 679–681, 680t, *682*
massive, 1507, 1517–1519
microemboli in, 147
mortality in, 1503, 1517
in pregnancy, 2322
natural history of, 1505–1506
origins of, 1504–1505. See also *Deep vein thrombosis; Venous thromboembolism.*
pain in, 581t
pathology of, 465, *465*
pathophysiology of, 1505–1506, 2026
pleural effusion in, 2002, 2008, 2016, 2026–2027
prevention of, 1514–1515, 1519
pulmonary hypertension in, 1519–1525
diagnosis of, 1520–1522, *1521–1523*
forms of, 1519
Pulmonary embolism *(Continued)*
obstructive, 1642
pathophysiology of, 1506
treatment of, 1522–1525, *1524*, *1525*
recurrent, prevention of, 1519
reperfusion after, edema in, 147
residual obstruction in, 1506
resolution of, 1506
respiratory acidosis in, 173
schistosomal, 1525–1526
septic, 1527
shock in, 2403–2404
substances causing, 465
tissue fragments as, 465
treatment of, 2027
embolectomy in, 1518–1519
in shock, 2403–2404
massive, 1517–1519
thrombolytic therapy in, 1518
with chronic pulmonary hypertension, 1522–1525, *1524*, *1525*
tumor-cell, 1527
unresolved, ventilation-perfusion scanning in, 704
ventilation-perfusion scanning in, 699, 701–709, 1511–1512, *1511*, *1512*
diagnostic criteria for, 704, 705t, *706–709*
mimics in, 704, *706–710*
perfusion component of, 702–703
PIOPED study of, 702–704, 705t
radiopharmaceuticals for, 718
stripe sign in, 710, *711*
ventilation component of, 703
versus angiography, 702
versus pulmonary hypertension, 1494
Pulmonary fibrosis. See *Fibrosis.*
Pulmonary function test(s), 781–881. See also *Spirometry;* specific values, e.g., *Diffusing capacity, Vital capacity.*
abbreviations used in, 2563–2565
advantages of, 781
aerosols in, 356
after abdominal surgery, 885–886, 886t
after acute respiratory distress syndrome, 2436
after cardiac surgery, 886
after lung resection, 890
after lung transplantation, 2524
after lung volume reduction, 890–891, 1218
after pneumonectomy, 889
after thoracoplasty, 2359t, 2364, 2364t
anesthesia and analgesia effects on, 884–885
at high altitude, 1918–1919
before exercise testing, 842
before lung resection, 890
before lung volume reduction, 890–891
blood gas analysis in. See *Acid-base balance and imbalance; Blood gas(es); Carbon dioxide; Oxygen.*
definitions of, 2563–2565
diffusing capacity as. See *Diffusing capacity.*
elastic recoil measurement in, 799–802, *800*, *801*, 875
ethnic factors in, 899, 905
in acute respiratory distress syndrome, 1500, 1595
in airline travel, 859–860
in airway obstruction, 789, *790*, 851–852, *852*
in alveolar proteinosis, 1795–1796, *1796*, *1797*
in amiodarone-induced pulmonary disease, 1982
in amyotrophic lateral sclerosis, 2343–2345
in ankylosing spondylitis, 2359t, 2369
in anxiety disorder, 849
Pulmonary function test(s) *(Continued)*
in arteriovenous malformations, 1496, 1563–1564
in asbestosis, 1835
in asthma, 851–853, 1265–1268, 1859, *1860*
in baseline evaluation, 784–785, *785*
in bone marrow transplantation, 2298, 2301
in bronchiectasis, 1327
in bronchiolitis obliterans, 1198
in bronchiolitis obliterans organizing pneumonia, 1686
in bronchitis, 1190–1192, 1206–1207
in byssinosis, 1862
in chemotherapy-induced disease, 1975
in chronic obstructive pulmonary disease, 802, 1190–1192, 1206–1207
in coal-workers' pneumoconiosis, 1828–1829
in croup, 961
in cystic fibrosis, 1304–1305, 1304t
in diabetes mellitus, 2309
in diaphragmatic paralysis, 2336, 2336t
in dyspnea, 546–547, 546t, 897–898
in elderly persons, 857
in emphysema, 802, 804, 853–854, 1190–1192, 1206–1207
in exercise. See *Exercise testing.*
in flail chest, 2367, 2367t
in HIV infection, 856, 2176
precautions with, 860–861
in hypersensitivity pneumonitis, 1874, 1877–1878
in hyperthyroidism, 2310
in hypothyroidism, 2310–2311
in hypoventilation, 2143
in idiopathic pulmonary fibrosis, 1662, *1664*
in impairment and disability evaluation, 850, 850t, 897–898, 905–906
in influenza, 951, 952t
in interstitial lung disease, 848, 1661–1664, *1664–1666*, 1691, 1696
in kyphoscoliosis, 2358–2359, 2359t
in lung cancer, 1422, 1422t
in lung injury, 1595
in lung transplantation, 816
in lymphangio(leio)myomatosis, 1781
in muscular dystrophies, 2343–2345
in myasthenia gravis, 2342
in myopathies, 2343–2345, *2344–2346*
in neuromuscular disorders, 849, 2332–2333
in obesity, 848–849, 856–857, 857t, 2371–2372, 2371t
in obstructive diseases, 788–789, *790*, 804, *805*, 815, *816*, 847–848, 850–854, 851t, *852*
in oxygen toxicity, 1987
in parainfluenza virus infections, 961
in Parkinson's disease, 2350–2351
in pectus excavatum, 2359t, 2366
in pneumoconiosis, 1815
in pneumonia, *Pneumocystis carinii*, 856, 2189
varicella-zoster virus, 967
in poliomyelitis, 2340–2341, 2341t
in pregnancy, 2317–2318, *2318*
in pulmonary edema, 1499–1500, 1578–1579, 1578t, 1595
in pulmonary fibrosis, 1673, 1675–1676, *1675*, *1676*, 1678, 1679
in pulmonary hypertension, 1494, 1520, 1548
in pulmonary vascular obstruction, 848, 854–855, 855t
in respiratory muscle disorders, 857–859, *858*, 2331
in restrictive diseases, 790, 804–805, 816, 848, 854, 854t

Pulmonary function test(s) *(Continued)*
in rheumatoid arthritis, 1702
in sarcoidosis, 1662, *1664*, 1723
in silicosis, 1823
in sleep, 2153
in spinal cord injury, 2338–2339, 2339t
in systemic sclerosis, 1694, 1696
in vascular obstruction, 815–816, *817*
indications for, 784–785, *785*
infection control during, 860–861
interindividual variation in, 803
intraindividual variation in, 802–803
lung volume measurements in, 790–799. See also *Functional residual capacity; Residual volume; Tidal volume; Vital capacity.*
airway resistance methods in, 798–799, *799*
body plethysmography in, 793–798, *794–796*
gas dilution methods in, 791–793, *791*, *792*, 793t, 874
static, 790–791
mechanical properties and. See *Mechanical properties.*
Newton's third law and, 782
normal values for. See also specific tests.
at maximal power output, 878
bronchodilator response as, 874
diffusing capacity as, 814–815, 877
expiratory pressure-volume curves as, 875
forced expiratory flow in one second as, 872t, 873t
functional vital capacity as, 872t, 873t
hypercapnic response as, 877
hypoxic response as, 878
in exercise testing, 878–881
inspiratory pressure-volume curves as, 875
maximal expiratory flow as, 875
maximum voluntary ventilation as, 874
residual volume as, 874
single-breath nitrogen test as, 876
total lung capacity as, 874
variability in, 802–804
pneumomediastinum in, 2099
precautions with, 781–782
preoperative, 714, 784, 890–891
screening, 849–850, 850t
spirometry in. See *Spirometry.*
statistical considerations in, 803–804
subject cooperation or noncooperation in, 855–856, 856t
symbols for, 2563–2565
theoretical aspects of, arterial blood gases and, 829–830
diffusion and, 808–810, *809*, *810*
exercise and, 837–841, 838t, *839*, 878–881
mechanical properties and, 782–784, *783*
Newton's third law and, 782
ventilation distribution and, 805, *806*
ventilation regulation and, 816–818
ventilation-perfusion relationships and, 821–822, 821t
ventilation distribution measurement in, 805–808
clinical applications of, 808
resident gas, single-breath test in, 805–807, *807*, 876
theory of, 805, *806*
ventilation regulation measurements in, 816–829
breath-holding time in, 818
clinical applications of, 820–821
hypercapnic response in, 818–819, *819*, 877

Pulmonary function test(s) *(Continued)*
hypoxic response in, 819–821, *820*, 878
inspiratory inclusion pressure in, 819–820, *820*
theory of, 816–818
ventilation-perfusion relationships in. See *Ventilation-perfusion ratio; Ventilation-perfusion scanning.*
ventilatory function measurements in, clinical applications of, 802–805, *805*, 875
normal values of, 802–804, 875
of elastic recoil, 799–802, *800*, *801*, 875
of flow, 784–790, *785–790*, 785t, 872–874
of lung volume, 790–799, *791*, *792*, 793t, *794–796*, *799*, 874
pathophysiologic patterns in, 804–805, *805*
theoretical aspects of, 782–784, *783*
with gases of different density, 789–790, *790*
Pulmonary hyalinizing granuloma, 1480
Pulmonary hypertension, 1491–1494
acute-on-chronic, 2404
airway resistance in, 2254–2255
anatomic considerations in, 1631–1633, *1632*
appetite suppressants causing, 1988–1989
at high altitude, 1920–1921, *1921*
chest pain in, 576
chest radiography of, 1494, 1520, *1521*, 1638–1639, *1639*
classification of, 1491–1493, *1491*, 1492t, *1493*, 1542, 1641–1643, 1641t
clinical manifestations of, 1493–1494, 1520, 1546–1547, 1637–1638
definition of, 1491, 1632
diagnosis of, 1193, 1547–1550, *1548–1550*, 1544–1546
pulmonary artery wedge pressure in, 1632–1633, *1633*
thromboembolic, 1520–1522, *1521–1523*
dietary or ingestive, 1546, 1642
differential diagnosis of, 1494, 1641–1643, 1641t
diffusing capacity in, 2252, 2253t
drug-induced, 479t
echocardiography in, 1521, 1639–1641, *1640*
electrocardiography in, 1520, 1639, *1640*
etiology of, 1641–1643, 1641t
exercise in, 1491, *1491*, 2258–2260, 2259t, 2260t
gas exchange in, 2258, *2258*
hemodynamics of, 1641, 2249–2251, 2249t
high altitude effects on, 1941
histopathology of, 2248–2249, 2249t
hyperkinetic, 1492t, 1543, 1642
hypoxic, 1633–1634
idiopathic. See *Pulmonary hypertension, primary.*
impairment in, 902
in bronchiectasis, 1326–1327
in chronic obstructive pulmonary disease. See *Chronic obstructive pulmonary disease.*
in cor pulmonale. See *Cor pulmonale.*
in cystic fibrosis, 1304
in fibrosis, 1633
in HIV infection, 2209
in lymphangio(leio)myomatosis, 1781
in mediastinitis, 2114
in mountain sickness, 1938
in pulmonary capillary hemangiomatosis, 1746, *1746*
in pulmonary edema, high-altitude, 1935–1936

Pulmonary hypertension *(Continued)*
in pulmonary embolism, 1506
in pulmonary fibrosis, 1676
in sarcoidosis, 1723
in schistosomiasis, 1163
in sickle cell disease, 2289–2290
in sleep apnea, 2159
in systemic lupus erythematosus, 1705
in systemic sclerosis, 1698
in veno-occlusive disease, 1744, *1745*, 1746
left ventricular failure in, 1636
lowering of, 2253, 2253t
lung compliance in, 2253–2254, 2254t, *2255*
lung transplantation in, 2520–2521, 2520t
lung volumes in, 2251–2252, *2251*, 2252t
obliterative, 1492–1493, 1492t, 1543, 1642–1643
obstructive, 1492–1493, 1492t, 1543, 1642
pain in, 576, 590
passive, 1492t, 1543, 1642
pathogenesis of, 1544–1546
pathology of, 1543–1544, *1544*, *1545*
pathophysiology of, 1491–1493, *1491*, 1492t, *1493*, 1633–1634, 2248–2249, 2249t
endothelin in, 298
thromboembolic, 1519–1520
physical findings in, 1547
polygenic, 1492t, 1543
portal hypertension with, 2274–2275
primary, 1542–1552, 1642
classification of, 1542
clinical manifestations of, 1546–1547, 1637
definition of, 1542
diagnosis of, 1547–1550, *1548–1550*
differential diagnosis of, 1542
epidemiology of, 1542–1543
etiology of, 1544–1546
genetic factors in, 1545
pathogenesis of, 1544–1546
pathology of, 1543–1544, *1544*, *1545*
physical findings in, 1547
prognosis for, 1552
thrombotic variant of, 1519
treatment of, 1550–1552
prognosis for, 1552
pulmonary edema in, 1581–1582, 2247–2248, 2248t
pulmonary function tests in, 1494, 1520
radionuclide studies in, 1521
regional lung function in, 2256–2257, *2257*, *2258*
respiratory failure in, 2395, 2395t
respiratory muscle function in, 2255–2256, 2256t
right ventricular failure in, 1634–1636, *1635*, *1636*
sleep disorders in, 2261
thromboembolic, 1519–1525
clinical manifestations of, 1520
diagnosis of, 1520–1522, *1521–1523*
differential diagnosis of, 1522
epidemiology of, 1519
pathophysiology of, 1519–1520
treatment of, 1522–1525, *1524*, *1525*
treatment of, 1550–1552
in cor pulmonale, 1643–1646
in shock, 2403–2404
thromboembolic, 1522–1525, *1524*, *1525*
vasodilators in, 300–302
variability of, 1632
vasoconstrictive, 1492, 1492t, 1543, 1643
venous, 2247–2261
airway resistance in, 2254–2255
diffusing capacity in, 2252, 2253t

Pulmonary hypertension *(Continued)*
exercise response in, 2258–2260, 2259t, 2260t
gas exchange in, 2258, *2258*
hemodynamics of, 2249–2251, 2249t
histopathology of, 2248–2249, 2249t
lowering of, 2253, 2253t
lung compliance in, 2253–2254, 2254t, *2255*
lung volumes in, 2251–2252, *2251*, 2252t
pulmonary edema in, 1580–1581, 2247–2248, 2248t
regional lung function in, 2256–2257, *2257*, *2258*
respiratory muscle function in, 2255–2256, 2256t
sleep disorders in, 2261
versus shock, 2403–2404
vicious circle of, 1493, *1493*
Pulmonary hypotension, in arteriovenous malformations, 1563
Pulmonary infiltrates with eosinophilia syndrome, 1760
Pulmonary lymphangiomyomatosis, chylothorax in, 2059, *2059*
Pulmonary rehabilitation, 2505–2516
chest physical therapy in, 2509
definition of, 2507
early implementation of, 2513–2514, *2513*, 2514t
exercise in, breathing, 2508–2509
systemic, 2509–2510, 2510t
upper extremity, 2510
historical background of, 2505–2508, *2506*, *2507*
in chronic obstructive pulmonary disease, 1227
in lung volume reduction surgery, 2512
individual programs for, 2511–2512
metabolic considerations in, 2510
nutrition in, 2510
outcomes of, 2512–2513
oxygen in, 2510–2511, 2511t, 2512t
patient education in, 2508
program organization for, 2511–2512
smoking cessation in, 2508
vaccination in, 2508
Pulmonary shunt. See *Shunt (circulatory), right-to-left.*
Pulmonary stretch receptors, in breathing control, 182–183, 182t, *183*
Pulmonary surfactant. See *Surfactant.*
Pulmonary thromboembolism. See *Pulmonary embolism.*
Pulmonary trunk, anatomy of, 120
Pulmonary vascular compliance, 127–128, *128*
Pulmonary vascular resistance, 123–127
active changes in, 1490
after heart disease treatment, 2250–2251
anatomic aspects of, 120
at high altitude, 1921
blood viscosity effects on, 126–127, *128*
calculation of, 123–124, 1490
definition of, 62, 2565
distribution of, 124–125, *125*
factors affecting, 63–64, *63*
in chronic obstructive pulmonary disease, 1633
in erythrocytosis, 2286
in exercise, 1491t
in hypoxia, 129–131
in pulmonary edema, 126, 1579, 1601
in pulmonary hypertension, 1522–1523
in respiratory failure, 2393–2395, *2394–2396*, 2395t
lung volume effects on, 63–64, *63*, 126, *127*
Pulmonary vascular resistance *(Continued)*
mechanical effects on, 126–127, *126–128*
passive changes in, 1490
physiology of, 297–298, 1490–1491
pressure-flow relations and, 62–63, *62*, *63*
profile of, 124–125, *125*
regulation of, 131, 1490–1491, 1632
drugs for, 298–302
transmural pressure effects on, 126, *126*, *127*
versus pulmonary arterial pressure, 126, *126*
vessels function and, 125–126
Pulmonary vasculature. See *Pulmonary circulation;* specific vessels.
Pulmonary vasculitis. See *Vasculitis.*
Pulmonary vein(s), anatomy of, 120–121, 1488
arterial communications with. See *Arteriovenous malformations, pulmonary.*
compression of, ventilation-perfusion scanning in, 704
functional description of, 125–126
occlusive disease of, 1549–1550
oxygen partial pressure in, 70–71
perivascular pressure on, 125–126
pressures in. See *Pulmonary venous pressure.*
stenosis of, in mediastinitis, 2114
Pulmonary veno-occlusive disease, 1549–1550
Pulmonary venous pressure, 1498t
blood flow distribution and, 128–129, *129*
distribution of, 128–129, *129*
in mediastinitis, 2114
in pulmonary vascular resistance calculation, 62, 1490
intraluminal, 125–126
normal, 11
perfusion distribution and, 128–129, *129*
versus blood flow, 123, *123*
versus diameter, 125–126
Pulmonary venules, pressure in, 1498t
Pulmonary wedge pressure. See *Pulmonary artery wedge pressure.*
Pulse, oxygen, in exercise testing, 844, 878
Pulse oximetry, 834–835, *835*
in arteriovenous malformations, 1562
Pulse pressure, in septic shock, 2399, *2400*
Pulsus paradoxus, in airflow obstruction, 2452–2453
Pump cells, in medulla, in breathing control, 185
Puna (mountain sickness), 1930
Purified protein derivative, in tuberculin skin test, 1059–1062, *1060*, 1061t, *1062*
Purine nucleoside phosphorylase deficiency, 2233t, 2238–2239
Purpura, anaphylactoid (Henoch-Schönlein), 1539
diffuse alveolar hemorrhage in, 1737t, 1740
Pursed-lip breathing, in chronic obstructive pulmonary disease, 1227
in dyspnea, 547
in pulmonary rehabilitation, 2509
PVR. See *Pulmonary vascular resistance.*
Pwedge. See *Pulmonary artery wedge pressure.*
Pyogenic pneumonia. See *Pneumonia, pyogenic.*
Pyopneumothorax, in coccidioidomycosis, 1124, *1124*, 1127
Pyrantel pamoate, in ascariasis, 1150
in hookworm infections, 1151
Pyrazinamide, in tuberculosis, 1066–1067, 1068t, 1070
central nervous system, 1084
drug-resistant, 1073t
Pyrazinamide *(Continued)*
in HIV infection, 2184
latent, 1088
prophylactic, 1089, 2185
regimen for, 1071–1072, 1071t
resistance to, 1070, 1073t
side effects of, 1070
Pyrimethamine, in *Pneumocystis carinii* pneumonia, 2194
in toxoplasmosis, 1149, 2204
Pyruvate metabolism, lactic acidosis and, 164–165, *165*


## Q


Q fever, 473, 998t, 1025–1026
$\dot{Q}_{PS}$. See *Shunt (circulatory), physiologic.*
$\dot{Q}_{S}$. See *Shunt (circulatory), right-to-left.*
$\dot{Q}_{T}$. See *Cardiac output.*
Quadriplegia, respiratory function in, 2337–2339, 2339t
ventilatory drive reduction in, 2331
Quality, of lung sounds, 592
Quality of life, after lung transplantation, 2526
dyspnea and, 544
in chronic obstructive pulmonary disease, after lung volume reduction surgery, 1218
in ethical decision making, 2496
Quantum mottle, in radiography, 636–637
Quartz, in pneumoconiosis. See also *Silicosis.*
coal-workers', 1827
Quellung reaction, 921, 989–990
Questionnaires, for medical history, 591–592, 1807t
for pain assessment, 568
in dyspnea, 544
Quinapril, in pulmonary hypertension, 1644
Quinine, in malaria, 1147
Quinlan, Karen Ann, 2490, 2492


## R


Rabbit fever (tularemia), 1028–1029
Racial factors. See *Ethnic factors.*
Radial artery, blood gas sample from, 834
Radiation exposure, lung cancer in, 1402
pneumonitis in, versus Hodgkin's disease, 1454
Radiation therapy, conformal, 1433
endobronchial, 742, 1433–1434
fibrosis due to, 716
for carcinoid tumors, 1461
for Hodgkin's disease, 1454
for lung cancer, 1432–1436
carcinoid, 1461
chemotherapy with, 1434, 1436–1437
complications of, 1436
dose in, 1433
endobronchial, 742, 1433–1434
in superior vena cava obstruction, 1435
interruptions in, 1433
metastatic, 1435–1436
non–small cell, 1432–1434
palliative, 1435–1436
postoperative, 1436–1437
small cell, 1434–1435
superior sulcus, 1434
versus stage, 1428–1431
for lymphoma, 1457
with chylothorax, 2058
for lymphomatoid granulomatosis, 1459
for mesothelioma, 2070
for Pancoast tumor, 1430

Radiation therapy *(Continued)*
for salivary gland tumors, of lung, 1463
fractionation in, 1433
interactions of, in bleomycin toxicity, 1976
lung injury in, 475, *476*, 477, 1436
pleural effusion in, 2036
pulmonary disease due to, 1978
Radiculitis, pain in, 577, 590
Radiography. See *Chest radiography; Computed tomography; Magnetic resonance imaging; Ultrasonography.*
Radioligand binding studies, of drugs to receptors, 243, *243*
Radiometric culture systems, for *Mycobacterium*, 1047
Radionuclide studies, 697–723. See also specific techniques, e.g., *Positron emission tomography.*
aerosols in, 356–357, *358*
of alveolar barrier function, 1597–1598
of clubbing, 601, *602*
of cor pulmonale, 1193
of hepatopulmonary syndrome, 2273
of HIV infection, 2177
of interstitial fibrosis, 1694
of Kaposi's sarcoma, 2206
of lung calcification, 2312, *2312*
of mediastinum, 2086–2087
of parathyroid disorders, 2128
of pneumoconiosis, 1815
of *Pneumocystis carinii* pneumonia, 2189–2190
of pulmonary edema, 1596–1598
of sarcoidosis, 1726
of systemic sclerosis, 1694
ventilation-perfusion. See *Ventilation-perfusion scanning.*
Radiopharmaceuticals, for ventilation-perfusion scanning, 698–700
thrombus-avid, 718
Radiospirometry, xenon, preoperative, 889–890
Radiotherapy. See *Radiation therapy.*
Radon, as air pollutant, 1887t, 1888
exposure to, lung cancer in, 1402
*RAF1* gene, in lung cancer, 1381–1382
Ragweed pollen, in airway responsiveness testing, 853
Rales, 594, *594*
in filariasis, 1154
in mountain sickness, 1930
in pulmonary edema, 1934
Ramp exercise testing, 202–203, *203*, 843
Ranke complex, in tuberculosis, 1056
RANTES (released by activated normal T cells), 507t, 516–517
in systemic sclerosis, 1692
receptors for, 238, 517–518, 517t
Rapidly adapting receptors, 251
in cough, 554, *555*
*RAS* genes and products, in lung cancer growth, 1381–1382, 1417
assays for, 1426, 1426t
Rash, in coccidioidomycosis, 1123
in measles, 958
in strongyloidiasis, 1151, 1152
in varicella-zoster virus infections, 967
Rassmussen's aneurysms, 1569–1570
RAW. See *Airway resistance.*
Raynaud's phenomenon, in mixed connective tissue disease, 1708
in systemic sclerosis, 1694
pulmonary hypertension with, 1545
Reactive airway dysfunction syndrome, 1853, 1904
Reactive conductance, in heart disease, 2252, 2253t
Reactive eosinophilic pleuritis, 2105
Reactive oxygen species. See *Free radicals.*
Read's test, for ventilatory sensitivity to carbon dioxide, 191, *191*, 818–820, *819*, 877
Rebreathing test, for diffusing capacity measurement, 812
for ventilation regulation assessment, 191, *191*
hypercapnic response in, 818–820, *819*, 877
hypoxic response in, 818–821, *820*, 878
Rebreathing treatment, in respiratory alkalosis, 175
Receptor(s), 233–246
adenosine, 273
adenovirus, 938
adenylate cyclase interactions with, 236, *236*
adrenergic. See *Adrenergic receptor(s); Alpha-adrenergic receptor; Beta-adrenergic receptor(s).*
agonists of, 242–243, *242*
airway epithelial, 338
albumin, 140–141
alpha-adrenergic, 131, *250*, 256, 333
beta-adrenergic. See *Beta-adrenergic receptor(s).*
B-lymphocyte, 414, 414t, 416, *417–419*, 418
carbohydrate, 390, *391*
cell surface, 233
C-fiber, 554, *555*, 575
chemokine, 238
CC, 517–518, 517t
CXC, 511–512, 511t
chemoreceptors as. See *Chemoreceptors.*
chest wall, 184, 2146
cholinergic, 333
ciliary, 361–362
classification of, 233
cloning of, 233
corticosteroid, 245
cough, 553–554, *555*, 575
Coxsackie-Adeno, 938
cross-hybridization of, 241–242
crosstalk among, 242–243, *242*
cytokine, 238
desensitization of, 244–245, *245*, 271
diaphragm, 184
down-regulation of, 245
drug interactions with, 243–244, *243*, *244*
endothelin, 298
enzyme-linked, 238–240, *239*
eosinophil, 1758t, 1759
epidermal growth factor, 41–42
estrogen, 1778–1779
fast, 240, *240*
fibroblast growth factor, 39–41
for apoptotic cells, 529, *529*, *530*
G protein-coupled, 233–236, *234*, *235*
genes for, regulation of, 245–246
glucocorticoid, 241, 261, 278–279
glycosylation of, 234
granulocyte-macrophage colony-stimulating factor, 238, *402*, 403–404
growth factor, 238–239, *239*, 524
guanylyl cyclase interactions with, 238
histamine-2, 257
in breathing control, 181–184, 182t, *183*
in inflammatory cascade, 258–262, *259–262*
in mitogen-activated protein kinase pathways, 239–240, *240*
in pulmonary disease pathophysiology, 245
in sensory neuron activation, 573
in signal transduction, 234–236, *234*, *235*, 239
insulin, 238–239
intercostal muscle, 184
Receptor(s) *(Continued)*
interleukin, 238
intracellular, 233, 240–241, *241*
ion channel, 238, 240, *240*, 246–247, *246*
irritant, 182–183, 182t, *183*, 575
J, 183, 570, 575
laryngeal, 182
lipid, 390, *391*
macrophage, 390, *391*, 392
macrophage colony-stimulating factor, 387, 402, *402*
mechanically activated. See *Mechanoreceptors.*
*N*-methyl-D-aspartate, 574
muscarinic. See *Muscarinic receptors.*
nasal, 181
natural killer, 1262–1263
neurokinin, 234
neutrophil, 523–524
nicotinic, 240, 1381
nuclear factor-kappa B, 241, *241*
ontogeny of, 245
opioid, 1381
orphan, 240
pharyngeal, 181–182
phosphatidylinositol hydrolysis and, 237, *237*
phosphorylation of, 244–245, *245*
platelet-derived growth factor, 41
progesterone, 1778–1779
protease-activated, 234–235
protein tyrosine phosphatases as, 240
pulmonary stretch, rapidly adapting, 182t, 183, 554, *555*
slowly adapting, 182, *183*
radioligand studies of, 243, *243*
RANTES, 238
rapidly adapting, 251, 554, *555*
rapidly adapting myelinated, 182
regulation of, 244–246, *244*, *245*
retinoic acid, 38–39, 1385
retinoid X, 1385
rhinovirus, 966
rhodopsin, 234
scavenger, 390, *391*
second messenger interactions with, 236–238, *236*
secretion of, in alveoli, 19, 20t
sequestration of, 245
serine/threonine kinases as, 240
serpentine motif in, 234–235, *235*
slow, 240, *240*
slowly adapting, 251
slowly adapting myelinated, 182
steroid, 240–241, *241*
steroid effects on, 245
stretch, chest wall, 184
in airways, 575
structure of, G-protein type of, 234–235, *234*, *235*
subtypes of, 241–242
T-cell. See *T-cell receptors.*
tracheobronchial, 182–184, 182t, *183*
transcriptional control of, 245–246
tumor necrosis factor-α, 238
tyrosine kinases as, 238–239, *239*
unmyelinated, 182, 182t, 183–184
upper airway, 181–182
Recessive inheritance, 45
Recoil, elastic. See *Elastic recoil.*
Recompression therapy, for decompression sickness, 1962
Recoverin, in lung cancer, 1379
Recruitment, of motor units, 198
of pulmonary vessels, 62–63, *63*, 128
Rectum, prolapse of, in cystic fibrosis, 1306, 1312

Rectum *(Continued)*
tuberculosis of, 1084–1085
Rectus abdominis muscles, mechanical properties of, 108
Recurrence risk, in genetic disease, 48
Red blood cell(s). See *Erythrocyte(s).*
Red blood cell volume, at high altitude, 1921
Red cedar dust, asthma due to, 1857
Reed-Sternberg cells, in Hodgkin's disease, 1453, 1454
Referred pain. See under *Pain.*
Reflex(es), aspiration, 181
Breuer-Hering, 21, 180–183, 185
cholinergic, 253–254
cough. See *Cough reflex.*
diving, 181
in breathing control, receptors and, 181–184, 182t, *183*
nasal, 181
reflux, 254
sneeze, 181
sneezing, 1346–1347
sniff, 181
Reflux, esophageal. See *Gastroesophageal reflux disease.*
Rehabilitation, pulmonary. See *Pulmonary rehabilitation.*
Reid classification, of bronchiectasis, 1325–1326
Reid index, 1203, *1203*
Rejection, in lung transplantation. See under *Lung transplantation.*
Relapsing polychondritis, 1695t, 1708–1710, *1709*
antibodies in, 1695t
Relative risk, in occupational disorders, 1805
Relaxation time, of mucus, 364
Released by activated normal T cells. See *RANTES (released by activated normal T cells).*
Religion, versus smoking incidence and lung cancer rates, 1398
Remifentanil, pulmonary function effects of, 885
Renal diseases. See *Kidney.*
Renal tubular acidosis, 168–169, 169t
Rendu-Osler-Weber syndrome. See *Hereditary hemorrhagic telangiectasia.*
Renin-angiotensin-aldosterone system, activation of, in cor pulmonale, 1636–1637
Reovirus pneumonia, pathology of, 470
Repair, 495–496, *496*
fibrosis in. See *Fibrosis.*
granulocytes in. See *Granulocyte(s).*
mediators in. See *Inflammatory mediator(s).*
Reperfusion injury, of lung, pathophysiology of, 320
pulmonary edema in, 147, 1523–1524, *1525*, 1582, 2055
RER (respiratory exchange ratio), in alveolar gas equation, 71–72
in exercise, variables affecting, 209–210, *209*
in hemodialysis, 2280
Research, on air pollution effects, 2556
on asthma, 2544–2546
Reservoir, pulmonary circulation as, 70, 127–128, *128*
Resident gas, single-breath test, of ventilation distribution, 805–807, *807*
Residual volume, after thoracoplasty, 2364
at high altitude, 1918
chest wall muscle action and, 104
definition of, 57, *57*, 783, *783*, 2563
in asthma, 1266
Residual volume *(Continued)*
in chronic obstructive pulmonary disease, 1191, 1207
in cystic fibrosis, 1304t
in interstitial lung disease, 1662, *1664*
in lymphangio(leio)myomatosis, 1781
in neuromuscular disorders, 2333, 2344, *2344*
in pectus excavatum, 2365
in pulmonary fibrosis, 1675
in spinal cord injury, 2339, 2339t
measurement of, 57–58, *57*, 791
normal values for, *57*, 874
Residual volume/total lung capacity ratio, in cystic fibrosis, 1304–1305, 1304t
in kyphoscoliosis, 2359, 2359t
Resistance, airway. See *Airway resistance.*
antibiotic. See *Antibiotics, resistance to.*
pulmonary vascular. See *Pulmonary vascular resistance.*
respiratory system, in obesity, 2371t, 2372
tissue, 95
total pulmonary, definition of, 2564
Resistive pressure component, of inspiratory pressure at airway opening, 2450–2451, *2451*
Resolution, in chest radiography, 636
Resource allocation, justice in, 2492
Respiration. See *Breathing; Gas exchange; Ventilation.*
Respirators, for occupational exposures, 1879–1880
Respiratory acidosis, 173–174
bicarbonate–carbon dioxide relationships in, *159*
causes of, 173–174, 173t
chronic, urine bicarbonate in, 161
clinical manifestations of, 174
compensation for, *159*, 160t, 163
in hypoventilation, 2140, 2143
in pneumothorax, 2045, 2054
in pulmonary edema, 1595
in respiratory failure, 2444
in triple disorders, 159
laboratory classification of, 160t
pathophysiology of, 173
permissive, in mechanical ventilation, 2478
in single ventricle, 298
treatment of, 174
Respiratory alkalosis, 174–175
at high altitude, 1917, 1922, *1922*
bicarbonate–carbon dioxide relationships in, *159*
causes of, 174–175, 175t
clinical manifestations of, 175
compensation for, bicarbonate–carbon dioxide relationships in, *159*, 160t
correction of, hyperchloremic acidosis in, 170
in asthma, 1275
in hyperventilation, 2147–2148
in malaria, 1147
in pregnancy, 2318
in pulmonary edema, 1595
in triple disorders, 159
laboratory classification of, 160t
pathophysiology of, 174
treatment of, 175
vasodilation in, 299–300
Respiratory alternans, 597
Respiratory bronchiolitis, 1366
in interstitial lung disease, 1672t, 1684–1686, *1685*
Respiratory complex, of brain, 542–543, *542*
Respiratory distress syndrome, adult. See *Acute/adult respiratory distress syndrome.*
Respiratory distress syndrome *(Continued)*
neonatal. See *Neonate(s), respiratory distress syndrome in.*
Respiratory drive. See *Ventilatory drive.*
Respiratory exchange ratio, in alveolar gas equation, 71–72
in exercise, variables affecting, 209–210, *209*
in hemodialysis, 2280
Respiratory failure. See also *Ventilatory failure.*
acidemia in, 2444
acute. See also *Acute/adult respiratory distress syndrome.*
in chronic obstructive pulmonary disease, 1228–1229
mortality in, 2488–2489
acute right heart syndrome in, 2395, 2395t
acute-on-chronic, 2460–2465
clinical features of, 2460
prognosis for, 2465
treatment of, 2460–2465
after intubation, 2463–2464
before intubation, 2460–2463, 2461t
liberation from ventilator in, 2464–2465
after thoracoplasty, 2364
anaerobic metabolism in, 2405–2407, *2405*, 2406t
assessment of, 2452, 2452t
breathing mechanics in, 2380, *2381*
cardiac output in, 2388–2389, *2388*, 2389t, *2390*, 2453
causes of, 859, 2449
circulation in, 2386–2407
overview of, 2386, *2386*
oxygen transport and, 2405–2407, *2405*, 2406t
pulmonary, 2392–2398
in pulmonary edema, 2396–2398, *2396*, *2398*
pressures in, 2393–2395, *2394–2396*, 2395t
shock and. See *Shock.*
venous return control and, 2386–2389
cardiac function curves in, 2387–2388, *2387*, *2388*
extracardiac pressure in, 2388–2389, *2388*, 2389t, *2390*
mean systemic pressure in, 2386–2387
ventricular dysfunction and, 2389–2393, *2391*, *2392*
classification of, 2378–2381, 2378t, *2379*, *2381*, 2382t
clinical features of, 2380–2381
drive to breathe and, 2446–2447
encephalopathy in, 2444
gas exchange in, 2379–2380
hemodynamic consequences of, 2452–2453
hypercapnia in, 2379–2380, 2443–2445
hypoxemic, 2444. See also *Acute/adult respiratory distress syndrome; Acute hypoxemic respiratory failure.*
clinical features of, 2380–2381
mechanical ventilation in, 2380–2381, 2382t
treatment of, 2380–2381, 2382t
versus ventilatory failure, 2378–2381, 2378t, *2379*, *2381*, 2382t
impaired drive in, 2445–2447, *2445*, *2446*
in airflow obstruction, mechanical ventilation in, 2382t
in asthma. See *Status asthmaticus.*
in bone marrow transplantation, 2298
in chronic obstructive pulmonary disease, 1228–1229, 2447–2448

Respiratory failure *(Continued)*
in cystic fibrosis, 1306, 1312
in fatigue, 109
in heart disease, 2392–2393, 2393t
in hypoventilation, clinical features of, 2380–2381
pathophysiology of, 2378–2381, 2378t, *2379*, *2381*
treatment of, 2380–2381
in increased load, 2445, *2445*, *2446*, 2447–2449, *2448*
in kyphoscoliosis, 2361–2362, *2362*, 2362t
in multiple myeloma, 2293
in neuromuscular disorders, 2445–2447, *2445*, *2446*
in pancreatitis, 2276–2277
in pulmonary fibrosis, 1684t
in pulmonary hypertension, 2395, 2395t
in shock. See *Shock.*
in tuberculosis, 1063, *1063*
mechanical abnormalities in, 2444
mechanical ventilation in, in hypoxemia, 2380–2381, 2382t
in shock, 2382t, 2383
liberation from, 2382t
perioperative, 2382
postoperative, 2382, 2382t
with muscle fatigue, 2383, *2384*, 2385
metabolic alkalosis in, 2444–2445
monitoring during, 2449–2452, *2450*, *2451*
multifactorial, 2449
oxygen transport in, 2405–2407, *2405*, 2406t
pathophysiology of, 2378–2381, 2378t, *2379*, *2381*, 2445–2449, *2445*, *2446*, *2448*
perioperative, 2378t, 2381–2383, 2382t
postoperative, mechanical ventilation in, 2382, 2382t
pulmonary edema in, 2396–2398, *2396*, *2398*
pulsus paradoxus in, 2452–2453
recognition of, 2452, 2452t
respiratory muscle fatigue in, 2383, *2384*, 2385
treatment of, hypoxemic, mechanical ventilation in, 2380–2381, 2382t
in cystic fibrosis, 1312
in hypoventilation, 2380–2381
in shock, 2382t, 2383
in status asthmaticus, 2453–2459, 2454t, *2457*, *2458*
postoperative, 2382, 2382t
type II, pathophysiology of, 2445–2449, *2445*, *2446*, *2448*
ventricular dysfunction in, 2389–2393, *2391*, *2392*, 2393t
Respiratory gas exchange ratio, in alveolar oxygen calculation, 824
in body plethysmography, 797
Respiratory gas ratio, in exercise testing, 844
Respiratory impairment and disability. See *Impairment and disability.*
Respiratory inductance plethysmography, in neuromuscular disorders, 2333
Respiratory motor units, in breathing control, 188
Respiratory muscle(s). See also specific muscles, e.g., *Diaphragm; Intercostal muscles.*
abdominal, 108, 859, 2330–2331, 2330t
convulsive disorders of, 2349t, 2351–2352
dysfunction of. See also *Neuromuscular disorder(s).*
pulmonary function tests in, 857–859, *858*
dyskinesias of, 2349t, 2350–2351
efficiency of, evaluation of, 859

Respiratory muscle(s) *(Continued)*
endurance of, evaluation of, 859
in mechanical ventilation, 2451–2452
exercise for, in chronic obstructive pulmonary disease, 216–217, 1227, 2464
in dyspnea, 547–548, *547*
in pulmonary rehabilitation, 2509
in ventilator liberation, 2385
expiratory, 2330, 2330t
fast twitch fibers in, 188, 198, 198t
fatigue of, in chronic obstructive pulmonary disease, 216–217
in highly fit athletes, 219
in respiratory failure, 2445–2447, *2445*, *2446*
mechanical aspects of, 109
tests for, 857–859, *858*
fibers in, 188, 859
function of, 2330–2331, 2330t, 2445–2446, *2445*
in ankylosing spondylitis, 2370
in chronic obstructive pulmonary disease, 215–217
in heart disease, 2255–2256, 2256t
in highly fit athletes, 219
in kyphoscoliosis, 2359–2360
in obesity, 2372–2373
structural aspects of, 197–198, 198t
tests for, 857–859, *858*
hiccups of, 2349–2350, 2349t
in cough, 555–556, *555*, 2331–2332
inappropriate contraction of, 2349–2352, 2349t
inflammatory neuropathy effects on, 2341–2342
innervation of, 2330, 2330t
inspiratory, 2330, 2330t
training of, 2346–2347
inspiratory force of, versus ventilation, in exercise, *214*
mechanical properties of, abdominal, 108
chest wall, 103–106, *103*, *105*
diaphragm as, 106–107
during nonrespiratory function, 108–109
fatigue and, 109
ordinarily nonrespiratory, in pathologic states, 108
rib cage, 107–108
upper airway, 108
mechanical ventilation interactions with, 2479–2482, *2481*, *2482*
metabolism in, function and, 859
motor units of, 188
myasthenia gravis effects on, 2342
myoclonus of, 2349t, 2350
nonrespiratory effects of, 108–109
oxygen uptake of, 859, 2445
versus minute ventilation, in highly fit athletes, 219
paralysis of. See also *Diaphragm, paralysis of.*
pulmonary function in, 2331
Parkinson's disease effects on, 2350–2351
physical examination of, 2332
poliomyelitis effects on, 2340–2341, 2341t
recruitment of, 2330–2331
rest for, 2382, *2384*, 2385, 2463
slow twitch fibers in, 188, 198, 198t
spinal cord injury effects on, 2337–2340, 2339t
strength of, evaluation of, 857–859, *858*, 2333, 2344–2345, *2344–2346*
in mechanical ventilation, 2451–2452
structure of, 197–198, 198t
testing of, 216, 857–859, *858*, 2343–2345, *2344–2346*

Respiratory muscle(s) *(Continued)*
training of. See *Respiratory muscle(s), exercise for.*
upper airway, 2330
ventilatory, 2330–2331, 2330t
weakness of, dyspnea in, 545t
hypoventilation in, 2144
in neuromuscular disorders, 2344–2345
treatment of, 2345–2349
Respiratory physiology. See specific topics, e.g., *Acid-base balance and imbalance; Breathing; Gas exchange; Pulmonary circulation; Ventilation.*
Respiratory quotient, definition of, 2564
in exercise, 199, *199*
heavy, 205
moderate, 202, 203–204
Respiratory rate/tidal volume ratio, ventilator liberation and, 2382, *2384*, 2385
Respiratory syncytial virus infections, 931t, 961–964
antibodies in, 962
antigen variation in, 961–962
cell culture in, 625
clinical manifestations of, 962–963
diagnosis of, 963
epidemiology of, 962
in lung transplantation, 2522
mortality in, 963
pathogenesis of, 962
pneumonia due to, in bone marrow transplantation, 2302–2303
in transplantation, 2232
pathology of, 470, *471*
prevention of, 964
transmission of, 962
treatment of, 963–964
virus causing, 961–962
Respiratory units, terminal. See *Alveolus(i); Terminal respiratory units.*
Respiratory zone, definition of, 56
Respirometry, at rest, 822
Rest, for respiratory muscles, 2382, *2384*, 2385, 2463
Restriction fragment length polymorphism analysis, 46, *46*
for *Mycobacterium*, 1045t, 1047–1048, *1048*
Restrictive ventilatory disorder(s), after thoracoplasty, 2363–2364, 2364t
causes of, 854t
disability in, Social Security Administration criteria for, 901t
exercise testing in, 848
hypercapnic response in, 820
in ankylosing spondylitis. See *Ankylosing spondylitis.*
in kyphoscoliosis. See *Kyphoscoliosis.*
in obesity. See *Obesity.*
in pectus excavatum, 2364–2366, *2365*
in sickle cell disease, 2289
pulmonary function tests in, 790, 804–805, 816, 848, 854, 854t
ventilation distribution in, 808
ventilation-perfusion scanning in, 698
volume-flow curves for, *1665*
Resuscitation, cardiopulmonary. See *Cardiopulmonary resuscitation.*
pneumothorax in, tension, 2054–2055
Reticulonodular infiltrates, in interstitial lung disease, 1657–1658, *1659*
Reticulonodular pattern, in sarcoidosis, 1720, *1720*
Retinitis, cytomegalovirus, 2202
Retinoblastoma gene, in lung cancer, 1383
Retinoic acid receptors, in lung cancer, 1385
in lung development, 38–39

Retinoid(s). See also *Vitamin A.*
lung cancer and, 1385, 1404–1405
Retinoid X receptors, in lung cancer, 1385
Retinopathy, high-altitude, 1937, *1937*
Retropharyngeal abscess, 918, 2096–2097
Revatropate, anticholinergic properties of, 277
Reynolds number, in airflow, 97
RFLPs (restriction fragment length polymorphisms), 46, *46*
for *Mycobacterium*, 1045t, 1047–1048, *1048*
Rhamnolipids, of *Pseudomonas aeruginosa*, in mucus secretion, 334
Rheumatoid arthritis, 1698–1703
antibodies in, 1695t
classification of, 1698, 1698t
coal-workers' pneumoconiosis with, 1826–1829
diagnosis of, 1698t
epidemiology of, 1698
pleural disease in, 1702, 2005, 2031
pulmonary manifestation(s) of, 1698t
bronchiectasis as, 1336–1337, 1701, *1701*
bronchiolitis obliterans as, 1364, 1700–1701, *1700*, 1703
bronchiolitis obliterans organizing pneumonia as, 1699–1700, *1699*
chest radiography of, 1702–1703
chyliform pleural effusion in, 2060
diffuse alveolar hemorrhage as, 1739
drug-induced, 1702
follicular bronchiolitis as, 1701
interstitial fibrosis as, 1698–1699, 1702–1703
nodules as, 1701–1702
pulmonary function tests in, 1702
silicotic nodule as, 1818–1819
treatment of, 1703
risk factors for, 1698
vasculitis in, 1539, 1701
Rheumatoid granuloma, of lung, 1481
Rheumatoid nodules, in rheumatoid arthritis, 1701–1702
Rhinitis, acute, 916
allergic, 1347–1350
classification of, 1347–1348
episodic, 1347
pathophysiology of, 1347–1348
perennial, 1347
seasonal, 1347
treatment of, 1348–1349, 1348t
cough in, treatment of, 563
in adenovirus infections, 939, *939*
in allergic granulomatosis and angiitis, 1769–1770
in pregnancy, 2317
mucociliary transport abnormalities in, 368
nonallergic, pathophysiology of, 1348
treatment of, 1349–1350
occupational, 1856, 1859
vasomotor, 1347, 1348
Rhinocerebral disease, in mucormycosis, 1134–1135, 2310
Rhinorrhea, in rhinitis, 1347
treatment of, 1349
Rhinovirus infections, 931t, 964–967
antibodies in, 964–965
asthma risk in, 1251
cell culture in, 625
clinical manifestations of, 965–966
common cold as, 932–933, *932*
diagnosis of, 625, 966
epidemiology of, 965
pathogenesis of, 965
pneumonia due to, 470
prevention of, 966–967
receptor in, 966
Rhinovirus infections *(Continued)*
transmission of, 965
treatment of, 966–967
virus causing, 964–965, *965*
*Rhizopus* infections, 1108, 1134–1135, *1135*
*Rhizopus* spores, hypersensitivity pneumonitis due to, 1869
*Rhodococcus (Corynebacterium) equi* pneumonia, 1030
culture in, 620–621
in HIV infection, 2180–2181
Rhodopsin, as G protein-coupled receptor, 234
Rhonchi, 594, *594*
definition of, 596
in chronic obstructive pulmonary disease, 1189
in filariasis, 1154
Rib(s), compression by, thoracic outlet syndrome in, 577
costochondritis of, 577
deformities of, in kyphoscoliosis. See *Kyphoscoliosis.*
in pectus excavatum, 2364–2366, *2365*
fibrositis of, pain in, 577
fractures of, in multiple myeloma, 2293
multiple, flail chest in, 2366–2369, *2367*, 2367t, *2368*
pain in, 577
pneumothorax in, 2052
repair of, 2369
motion of, lung volume changes in, 105–106, *105*
muscles of, mechanical properties of, 107–108
removal of, in thoracoplasty, 2359t, 2361t, 2363–2364, 2364t
Ribavirin, aerosolized, 359
in adenovirus infections, 940
in bronchiolitis, 937
in hantavirus infections, 946–947
in parainfluenza virus infections, 2303
in respiratory syncytial virus infections, 963 964, 2303
Rickettsial pneumonia, pathology of, 473
Rifabutin, in *Mycobacterium avium* complex infections, 1091–1092, 2185, 2186
in *Pneumocystis carinii* pneumonia, 2195
in tuberculosis, 2184
Rifampin, in brucellosis, 1030
in *Mycobacterium kansasii* infections, 1095, 2186
in pneumonia, 998t
*Brucella*, 1030
*Legionella*, 1016
*Neisseria meningitidis*, 1006
in tuberculosis, 1066–1067, 1068t
central nervous system, 1084
drug-resistant, 1073t
in HIV infection, 2184
latent, 1088
prophylactic, 1088–1089, 2185
regimen for, 1071–1073, 1071t
resistance to, 1067, 1073t, 2184
side effects of, 1067, 1068t, 1069
Right middle lobe syndrome, in mediastinitis, 2113
Rigor. See *Chills.*
Rimantadine, in influenza, 956–957
Rimiterol, as bronchodilator, 270
Risk estimation, in occupational disorders, 1805
RL (total pulmonary resistance), definition of, 2564
RNA splicing, alternative, in immunoglobulin isotype switching, 420
Rocking bed, in diaphragmatic paralysis, 2337
Rocking bed *(Continued)*
in neuromuscular disorders, 2347
Rodents, in hantavirus transmission, 945–947
Round atelectasis, as pseudotumor, 1481
in asbestos exposure, 1837, *1838*, 1839
Roundworm infection(s). See *Nematode infection(s).*
RQ. See *Respiratory quotient.*
Rubeola. See *Measles.*
Runyon classification, of mycobacteria, 1044, 1044t
RV. See *Residual volume.*

## S

*Saccharomonospora* pneumonia, culture in, 620–621
Safety factors, in pulmonary edema prevention, 145, 146, *146*
Safety hazards, of magnetic resonance imaging, 664
Salbutamol, in asthma, 357
in chronic obstructive pulmonary disease, 357
Salicylates. See also *Aspirin.*
anion gap acidosis due to, 168
pulmonary disease due to, 1984
Saline solution, in bronchoalveolar lavage, 735
in cystic fibrosis, aerosolized, 1310
hypertonic, 368
in sputum induction, 609
in whole-lung lavage, in alveolar proteinosis, 1796–1800, *1799*
Salivary glands, cystic fibrosis of, 1295
tumors of, in lower airways, 1462–1463, 1462t
Salmeterol, as bronchodilator, 270
chemical structure of, 268, *268*
in asthma, 357
in chronic obstructive pulmonary disease, 357
*Salmonella* pneumonia, 1010–1011
Salt. See *Saline solution*; *Sodium.*
Salt water, diving in. See *Diving.*
near drowning in, hypermagnesemia in, 1591
pulmonary edema in, 1584
San Joaquin Valley fever. See *Coccidioidomycosis.*
Sanfilippo's syndrome, lung injury in, 481t
Saralasin, in pulmonary hypertension, 1644
Sarcoid granulomatosis, necrotizing, 1538
Sarcoidosis, 1717–1732
activity of, 1726–1727
asymptomatic, 1718
bronchial, 1721–1722
bronchoscopy in, 752
chest radiography of, 1719–1723, *1720–1723*, 1722t
clinical features of, 1718–1719, 1718t, *1719*
course of, 1727
crackles in, *595*
diagnosis of, 1725–1726
endobronchial, 1368
epidemiology of, 1717
etiology of, 1717, 1725
genetics of, 1717–1718
immunologic features of, 1724–1725
in HIV infection, 2210
Kveim test in, 1724–1726
lung cancer risk in, 1416
miliary, 1720, *1721*
mortality in, 1727
nodular, 675, *675*, 1481
organ systems involved in, 1718–1719, 1718t, *1719*

Sarcoidosis *(Continued)*
pathogenesis of, 437–438, 500
pathology of, *457*, 1723–1724, *1724*
physiologic alterations in, 1723
pleural, 1721
pleural effusion in, 2016, 2033–2034
pressure-volume relationships in, *1664*
prognosis for, 1727
pulmonary function tests in, 1662, *1664*
radionuclide studies of, 2086
spontaneous remission of, 1727
stages of, 1720
treatment of, 1727–1728
tuberculosis and, 1724, 1725
ventilation-perfusion scanning in, 713, *714*
versus beryllium lung disease, 1843, 1844
Sarcoma(s), Kaposi's. See *Kaposi's sarcoma.*
mesothelioma resembling, 2068
of lung, 1463
of mediastinum, 2129, 2132
Scalene lymph nodes, biopsy of, 763
Scalene muscles, function of, 2330–2331, 2330t
Scanning, lung. See *Ventilation-perfusion scanning.*
Scatter, in radiography, 634, *635*, 636, *636*
Scavenger receptors, 390, *391*
Schistosomiasis, 1143, 1163–1165
pulmonary embolism in, 1525–1526
Schools, asthma management in, 2549–2550
Schwannoma(s), of lung, 1479
of mediastinum, 2131, *2132*
Scintigraphic studies. See *Radionuclide studies; Ventilation-perfusion scanning.*
Scl70 antigen, in systemic sclerosis, 1692
SCLC. See *Lung cancer, small cell.*
Scleroderma. See *Systemic sclerosis (scleroderma).*
Sclerosing cholangitis, 2276
Sclerosing hemangioma, of lung, 1479
Sclerosing mediastinitis. See *Mediastinitis, granulomatous (chronic).*
Sclerotherapy, for esophageal disorders, mediastinitis due to, 2107
pulmonary disease due to, 1989
for hepatic hydrothorax, 2015
for pleural space eradication. See *Pleurodesis.*
for pneumothorax, 2047–2048, *2048*, 2050
variceal, pleural effusion in, 2030
Scoliosis. See *Kyphoscoliosis.*
Scuba diving, equipment for, 1953, *1954*
Seawater, diving in. See *Diving.*
near drowning in, hypermagnesemia in, 1591
pulmonary edema in, 1584
Second messenger(s), 236–238, *236*
calcium as, 236, 237, *237*, 268, *269*
for cytokines, 238
formation of, adenylyl cyclase in, 236, *236*
guanylyl cyclase in, 238
ion channel-coupled signaling in, 238
phosphatidylinositol hydrolysis in, 237, *237*
Secretagogues, for mucus, 333–334
Secretions. See *Mucus; Sputum; Suctioning.*
Secretory component, in mucus, 329
Sedation, contraindicated in asthma, 290
for bronchoscopy, 730
in mechanical ventilation, in status asthmaticus, 2456
in oxygen consumption reduction, 2407
Sedimentation, in aerosol deposition, 351, *351*
of inhaled particulates, 1889
Segmental contour patterns, in ventilation-perfusion scanning, 710–711
Segmentectomy, in bronchiectasis, 1332
in cancer, 1428
in echinococcosis, 1160
Segregation analysis, in genetic disease, 48–49, 1252
Seizures, at high altitude, 1942
diving contraindicated in, 1963
lidocaine-induced, 755
respiratory effects of, 2351
theophylline-induced, 1222
Selectins, in asthma, 1261
in neutrophil movement, 524–525, *525*
in pulmonary edema, 1581
Selenium, in lung cancer prevention, 1405
Selenium detector systems, in digital radiography, 642
Self-determination (autonomy), 2491–2492
Self-tolerance, of B lymphocytes, 422
of T lymphocytes, 429–430
Seminoma(s), of mediastinum, 2127
Sensation, of dyspnea, 542–543, *542*
Sensitization, to pain, 573
Sensory nerve(s), of lung, 21–22, *21*
Sensory nerve fibers, in carotid body, 189
Sensory neuron(s), visceral, 573
Sepsis, acute respiratory distress syndrome in, 2417
embolism in, 1527
hyperventilation in, 2147
in histoplasmosis, 2198
lung injury in, 1587, 1589
mortality in, 1613
pulmonary edema in, 147
*Yersinia pestis*, 1029
Septal thickening, interlobular, computed tomography of, 674, *674*
Septic shock, 2399–2400, *2400*, 2401t, 2402t
anaerobic metabolism in, 2407
in malaria, 1147
in plague, 1029
pathogenesis of, arachidonic acid metabolites in, 498
tumor necrosis factor-α in, 502
Sequence-tagged sites, in DNA analysis, 47
Sequestration(s), bronchopulmonary, angiography in, 658, *658*
bronchiectasis with, 1334
clinical features of, 1567–1568
definition of, 1566
diagnosis of, 1568, *1568*
epidemiology of, 1566–1567
extralobar, 1566–1568, *1567*
in systemic-pulmonary communications, 1496–1497
intralobar, 1566–1568, *1567*
magnetic resonance imaging of, 683, *687*
pathogenesis of, 1566
pathology of, 483t, 1566–1567, *1567*
prognosis for, 1568
treatment of, 1568
of particulates, in alveolar macrophages, 390, *391*, 392
of receptors, 245
Series inequality, of ventilation, 60
Serine/threonine kinases, as receptors, 240
Serologic testing, 610t. See also specific tests, e.g., *Enzyme-linked immunosorbent assay* and diseases.
in chlamydial infections, 624
in fungal infections, 622–624
in mycoplasmal infections, 624–625
in viral infections, 625
Serotonin, in pulmonary vascular resistance control, 131
metabolism of, in pulmonary circulation, 69
Serpentine (mineral), 1831t
Serpentine motif, in receptors, 234–235, *235*
*Serratia* pneumonia, 1010–1011
Severe combined immunodeficiency, 2233t, 2239
Sevoflurane, pulmonary function effects of, 885
Sexually transmitted diseases, pharyngitis in, 917
Shallow water blackout, in diving, 1952
Shear modulus, of lung, 93–94
Shear stress and strain, of mucus, 363–364
Sheath (sustentacular) cells, in carotid body, 189
Shh (sonic hedgehog) molecule, in lung development, 38
Shingles. See *Herpes zoster.*
Shivering, in cold exposure, in diving, 1952
Shock, 2398–2405
adrenal, 2404
anaphylactic, 2404
cardiogenic, 2400, 2401t, *2402*
clinical features of, 2398, 2399t
diagnosis of, 2398, 2399t, 2404–2405
differential diagnosis of, 2399t, 2402, 2404–2405
hemorrhagic, pulmonary edema in, 147
hypovolemic, 2400–2402, 2401t, 2403t
in cardiac tamponade, 2402–2403
in right ventricular dysfunction, 2403–2404
lung injury in, 1587, 1588t, 1589
multiple etiologies of, 2404–2405
neurogenic, 2404
respiratory failure in, causes of, 2378t
clinical features of, 2378t
mechanical ventilation in, 2382t, 2383
treatment of, 2383
septic, 2399–2400, *2400*, 2401t, 2402t
anaerobic metabolism in, 2407
in malaria, 1147
in plague, 1029
pathogenesis of, 498, 502
treatment of, 2398, 2399t, 2401t, 2403t, 2404–2405
Short-circuit current, of epithelium, 335
Shortness of breath. See *Dyspnea.*
Shoulder-arm syndrome and shoulder-hand syndrome, 577
Shunt (circulatory), calculation of, 76
definition of, 76
in bronchiectasis, 1327
in highly fit athletes, 219
intrapulmonary, in hepatopulmonary syndrome, 2274
left-to-right, arteriovenous malformation as, 1495
in pulmonary circulation–systemic circulation communications, 1565–1566
physiologic, in ventilation-perfusion inequality assessment, 80
normal, 80
right-to-left, arteriovenous malformation as, 1495, 1557–1558, 1562, 1563, 1565
blood gases in, 821t
calculation of, 825–827, *826*, 826t, 827t
definition of, 2565
in decompression sickness, 1960
in hepatopulmonary syndrome, 2274
in pancreatitis, 2276
in pneumothorax, 2045
in pulmonary hypertension, 1494
versus ventilation-perfusion imbalance, 826–827, 827t
venous-to-arterial, calculation of, 825–827, *826*, 826t, 827t
Shunt (pleuroperitoneal), in chylothorax, 2058, 2059

Shunt (pleuroperitoneal) *(Continued)*
in malignant effusions, 2075–2076
Shunt (portosystemic), in ascites, 2015
Shunt theory, of clubbing pathogenesis, 600–601
Sickle cell disease, 2286–2290
acute chest syndrome in, 2287–2289
airway hyperreactivity in, 2290
chronic lung disease in, 2289–2290
hemoglobin S in, 85
historical aspects of, 2286
mortality in, 2289
pathophysiology of, 2286–2287
sleep apnea in, 2290
vaso-occlusion in, 2287
Sickle cell trait, 2286, 2290
Sickness, versus illness, 586
Siderophores, gallium binding to, in ventilation-perfusion scanning, 701
Siderosis, *1814*, 1842
Signal transduction, 234–236, *234*, *235*, 239
Silent nociceptors, in visceral pain, 572, *572*
Silica, in pneumoconiosis. See *Silicosis.*
Silicates, asbestos. See *Asbestos; Asbestosis.*
nonasbestos, pneumoconioses due to, 1830, 1831t, 1841–1842
Silicon carbide, in pneumoconiosis, 1831t, 1842
Silicon dioxide, in pneumoconiosis. See *Silicosis.*
Silicon-carbide pneumoconiosis, 1845
Silicosis, 1816–1824
accelerated, 1818, 1818t
acute, 1818, 1818t
chest radiography of, *1661*, 1823
chronic, 1818, 1818t, *1820*
clinical features of, 1823
coal-workers' pneumoconiosis with, 1828
complications of, 1824
conglomerate (progressive massive fibrosis), 1818, *1821*, 1823
definition of, 1816
diagnosis of, 1823–1824
dust accumulation in, versus occupation, *1812*
epidemiology of, 1817–1819, 1822–1823
exposure-response relationships in, 1813, *1813*
extrathoracic manifestations of, 1819
lung cancer risk in, 1403
natural history of, 1822
pathogenesis of, 1819
pathology of, 1818–1819, 1818t, *1820*, *1821*
pulmonary function tests in, 1823
rheumatoid, 1818–1819, 1823
risk factors for, 1813, *1813*, 1816–1818, 1817t
treatment of, 1824
tuberculosis in, 1819, 1822, 1824
unrecognized, 1842
Silo filler's disease, 1906
Sin Nombre virus infections, 945–947
Single photon emission computed tomography, in ventilation-perfusion scanning, 701, 703
of mediastinum, 2086
Single-breath test, for anatomic dead space, 822–823, *823*
for carbon dioxide, 836–837, *837*
for diffusing capacity, 75, 811–813
for ventilation distribution, 805–807, *807*, 876
Single-nucleotide polymorphisms, in genetic disease, 50–51
Singultus (hiccups), 2349–2350, 2349t
Sinus(es). See also *Sinusitis.*
Sinus(es) *(Continued)*
barotrauma of, 1957
examination of, 933
injury of, pneumomediastinum in, 2097
Sinus tract, in chest wall, in actinomycosis, 1021–1022, *1021*
Sinusitis, acute, 916–917
chronic, in Kartagener's syndrome, 366
cough in, treatment of, 563
in allergic granulomatosis and angiitis, 1769–1770
in cystic fibrosis, 1294, 1305
in Wegener's granulomatosis, 1536
postnasal drip in, cough in, 558–559, *559*, 563
rhinovirus, 966
with common cold, 932–933
Sisal dust, byssinosis due to, 1860–1862
Sister chromatid exchange, in lung cancer, 1406
Situs inversus, in Kartagener's syndrome, 366
in Kartagener's triad, 1336
Six-minute walk test, after lung transplantation, 2525, *2525*
Size principle of recruitment, 198
Sjögren's syndrome, antibodies in, 1695t
bronchiolitis obliterans and, 1701
mucociliary transport abnormalities in, 366
pathology of, *457*
pulmonary manifestations of, 1705–1706, *1706*
Skin, biopsy of, in vasculitis, 1535
physical examination of, 602t, 603
sensory receptors in, 568–569
Skin disorders, in angioimmunoblastic lymphadenopathy, 1459
in anthrax, 1029
in aspergillosis, 1134
in Behçet's disease, 1710, 1710t
in blastomycosis, 1119, *1119*, 1120
in coccidioidomycosis, 1123, 1124
in cryptococcosis, 1130
in decompression sickness, 1961
in dermatomyositis, 1706–1707
in diving, 1957
in herpes simplex virus infections, 947
in Kaposi's sarcoma, 2205
in lung cancer, 1421, 1421t
in lung disease, 602t, 603
in lymphomatoid granulomatosis, 1458
in melioidosis, 1027–1028
in mesothelioma, 2069
in mixed cryoglobulinemia, 1740
in paracoccidioidomycosis, 1128
in *Pasteurella multocida* infections, 1028
in radiation injury, 1436
in sarcoidosis, 1718
in scleroderma, 1691, 1694t
in strongyloidiasis, 1151–1152
Skin tests, for *Aspergillus*, 1765
for blastomycosis, 1117–1118, 1120
for coccidioidomycosis, 1123, 1126
for histoplasmosis, 1109, 1115
for paracoccidioidomycosis, 1129
for tuberculosis, 1059–1062, *1060*, 1061t, *1062*
in HIV infection, 2184–2185
prophylactic drugs and, 1087–1088
SLE. See *Systemic lupus erythematosus.*
Sleep, arousal from, 2154, 2154t
aspiration in, pneumonia in, anaerobic bacterial, 1017
asthma during, 1271
at high altitude, altitude illness incidence and, 1930t
breathing control in, 1924–1925, *1924*, *1925*
Sleep *(Continued)*
mountain sickness in, 1939, *1939*
breathing control in, 180, 2153–2154
at high altitude, 1924–1925, *1924*, *1925*
disorders of. See *Sleep apnea; Sleep, disorders of.*
cardiovascular function in, 2154, 2155, *2155*
disorders of. See also *Sleep apnea.*
arousal in, 2154, 2154t, 2157
asthma as, 1271
at high altitude, 1930t, 1939, *1939*
cardiovascular effects of, 2154, 2154t, 2155, *2155*
consequences of, 2154, 2154t
in chronic obstructive pulmonary disease, 1194
in diaphragmatic paralysis, 2335
in heart disease, 2261
in kyphoscoliosis, 2361
in pulmonary fibrosis, 1676–1677
laboratory tests in, 2154–2155, *2155*, *2156*
hypoventilation in, 2141–2144, *2141*, *2142*
in neuromuscular disorders, oximetry in, 2334
mechanical ventilation during, in kyphoscoliosis, 2362–2363, 2363t
non-rapid eye movement (NREM, active), 2153–2154
onset of, apnea at, 2161–2162, *2161*
periodic breathing in, 2147
rapid eye movement (REM, quiet), 2153–2154
stages of, breathing during, 2153–2154
Sleep apnea, arousal during, 2154
central, 2142, 2161–2165
clinical features of, 2162–2163
definition of, 2161
diagnosis of, 2163–2164, *2164*, *2165*
in heart failure, 2261
nonhypercapnic, 2164–2165
normal periods of, 2153
pathogenesis of, 2161–2162, *2163*
polysomnography in, 2155, *2156*
treatment of, 2164–2165
versus obstructive sleep apnea, 2155
consequences of, *2157*
diagnosis of, 2447
high altitude effects on, 1941
impairment in, 900, 902, 909
in acromegaly, 2313
in chronic obstructive pulmonary disease, 1194
in diabetes mellitus, 2310
in heart disease, 2261
in hypothyroidism, 2311
in kidney failure, 2279
in Marfan's syndrome, 1711
in neuromuscular disorders, 2331
in spinal cord injury, 188
obstructive, 2155–2161
cardiovascular complications of, 2155, 2158–2159, *2158*
clinical features of, *2157*, 2158
clinical significance of, 2155
consequences of, *2157*
definition of, 2155
diagnosis of, 2159–2160
in amyloidosis, 2296
in heart disease, 2261
in kyphoscoliosis, 2361
in sickle cell disease, 2290
natural history of, 2160
pathogenesis of, 2155–2157, *2157*
polysomnography in, 2155, *2156*
termination of, 2157

Sleep apnea *(Continued)*
treatment of, 2160–2161
versus central sleep apnea, 2155
pharyngeal obstruction in, 1350–1351
Sleeve resection, in cancer, 1427
Slow receptors, 240, *240*
Slowly adapting receptors, 251
Sluice effect, in pulmonary circulation three-zone model, 65
Sly's syndrome, lung injury in, 481t
Small cell carcinoma, of lung. See *Lung cancer, small cell.*
Small intestine, inflammatory disease of, pulmonary complications of, 2270–2271, 2270t
Smears, acid-fast, for tuberculosis, 616
preparation of, 612, *612*
Smog, formation of, 1887
Smoke inhalation, bronchoscopy in, 754
lung injury in, 1908–1909
particulates in. See *Particulates.*
Smokeless tobacco, lung cancer risk with, 1400
Smoking. See also *Nicotine.*
aerosol clearance in, 355
as air pollution, 1888
asbestos fiber interactions in, 1401, 1834, 1836
asthma risk in, 1859
asthmatic bronchitis in, 1271
attitudes toward, 2532–2533
avoidance of, 2532, 2532t
biomarkers of, 1406
bronchiectasis in, 1326
bronchiolitis in, 1366
bronchitis in, 1179, 1199, *1200*, *1201*
cadmium accumulation in, 1213
carboxyhemoglobin formation in, 814, 2290
cessation of, in chronic obstructive pulmonary disease, 1217, 2508, 2513–2514, *2513*, 2514t, 2533
in erythrocytosis, 2286
in pregnancy, 2533
in pulmonary rehabilitation, 2508, 2513–2514, *2513*, 2514t
lung cancer risk and, 1399
methods for, 2533, 2534t
preoperative, 887
research needs in, 2539
target populations for, 2533, 2534t
chronic obstructive pulmonary disease and, 1178, 1199, *1200*, *1201*
animal models of, 1213–1214
bullae formation and, 1195, *1196*
cessation of, 1217, 2513–2514, *2513*, 2514t
inflammatory cells and, 1212
natural history and, 1201–1202, *1201*, *1202*
pathogenic aspects of, 1207–1209, *1209*
cigarette composition and, 1399
coal dust interactions in, 1828, 1830
cough in, 560, 564
diet chosen in, 2513
diffusing capacity in, 815
carboxyhemoglobin adjustment in, 814
education on, 2558–2560, 2559t
emphysema in. See *Smoking, chronic obstructive pulmonary disease and.*
epidemiology of, in youth, 2559
ethnic variation in, 1398
exercise in, 2513–2514, *2513*, 2514t
familial aggregation of, 1405
Goodpasture's syndrome in, 1742
history of, 591
HIV infection in, respiratory disorders in, 2175
Smoking *(Continued)*
hypersensitivity pneumonitis and, 1871
impairment attribution and, 910
in youth, 2559
influenza severity in, 953
interstitial lung disease and, 1656, 1672
lung cancer in, 1397–1400, 2558
cessation effects on, 1399
cigarette composition and, 1399
environmental, 1399–1400
epidemiology of, 1415–1416, 1416t
ethnic factors in, 1398
gender differences in, 1398
in asbestos exposure, 1836–1837
international trends in, 1396–1397
mortality in, 1400
*p53* gene mutations in, 1382
*RAS* gene mutations in, 1381
religious factors in, 1398
versus histologic type, 1398–1399
versus noncigarette tobacco use, 1400
mortality in, 2558
mucociliary transport abnormalities in, 366–367
neuropeptide release in, 254
pack-years in, 591
passive exposure to, 1399–1400
government policies on, 2558–2560, 2559t
perioperative mortality in, 887
primary prevention of, 2532–2533, 2532t
government role in, 2558–2560, 2559t
public pressure and policy concerning, 2532–2533
pulmonary fibrosis in, 1677
pulmonary function test effects of, 803
pulmonary hypertension in, complications of, 1551
regulations on, 2558–2559
respiratory bronchiolitis-associated interstitial lung disease in, 1684–1686
silica interactions in, 1819, 1822
spirometry in, 784
subpleural bleb formation in, 2045
surgical risks in, 887
taxes related to, 2558
ventilation distribution in, 808
ventilation-perfusion scanning in, 719
Smooth muscle, arachidonic acid metabolite effects on, 497–499, 497t
cellular proliferation of, in lymphangio(leio)-myomatosis. See *Lymphangio(leio)myomatosis.*
of airways, 10, *12*
beta-adrenergic receptor dysfunction in, 245
hyperplasia of, in asthma, 1254, 1262
hyperresponsiveness of, in asthma, 1176–1177, *1177*
potassium channels in, 247
resistance and, 798–799
second messenger action in, 236, *236*
of pulmonary arteries, 120, *121*
genetic differences in, 130
hypoxic response of, 129–131, 1490
Smudge cells, in adenovirus infections, 938, *938*
Sneezing, in rhinitis, 1347
pleuritic pain in, 576
reflex for, 181, 1346–1347
Sniff reflex, 181
Sniff test, in respiratory muscle evaluation, 858, 859
Snoring, in pulmonary fibrosis, 1676–1677
in sleep apnea, 2155, 2158, 2160
$SO_2$ (oxygen saturation), in mountain sickness, 1939, *1939*
$SO_2$ (oxygen saturation) *(Continued)*
in sleep, 2154–2155, *2155*, *2156*
Social factors, in pneumonia, 987–988, 988t
Social history, 591
Social Security Administration, impairment and disability evaluation for, 900–902, 901t
Socioeconomic status, pulmonary function test effects of, 803
Sodium. See also *Saline solution.*
exchange of, in compensation for acid-base imbalance, 161
imbalance of, in tuberculosis, 1063
in air surface liquid, 339–340, 340t
in anion gap calculation, 163–164
loss of, in cystic fibrosis, 1180, 1292, 1307
retention of, metabolic alkalosis in, 171t, 172–173
transport of. See also *Epithelium and epithelial cells, airway, electrolyte transport across.*
in cystic fibrosis, 1296, 1296t, *1297*, *1298*, 1299
in metabolic alkalosis, 162–163
Sodium azide, exposure to, 1910
Sodium bicarbonate, in metabolic acidosis therapy, 171, 1966
Sodium channels, 247
apical membrane epithelial, 336–337
in air surface liquid volume regulation, 339
in cystic fibrosis, 1299
in electrolyte transport, function of, 336–338, *336*
regulation of, 338–339
Sodium chloride, in aerosols, particle size distribution and, 351–352
Sodium hydroxide, in specimen processing, 613t
Sodium morrhuate, for esophageal varices, pulmonary disease due to, 1989
Sodium tetradecyl sulfate, for esophageal varices, pulmonary disease due to, 1989
Sodium warfarin. See *Warfarin.*
Sodium-potassium ATPase, in beta-adrenergic agonist action, *269*
in calcium channel function, 246
in transepithelial electrolyte transport, 336–337, *336*
Sodium-potassium-chloride cotransporter, of airway epithelium, 338
Solitary nodule(s). See under *Nodule(s).*
Solitary tract, in breathing control, 185–186, *185*
in visceral innervation, 569
Soluble-gas technique, for lung water measurement, 1597
Solute(s). See also *Fluid and solute exchange.*
diffusion of, 133–134
disappearance of, into air spaces, 1598
endothelial selectivity for, 144
lymph-to-plasma concentration ratio of, 134–135, *136*
molecular weights of, versus endothelial permeability, 139, *139*, 139t
movement of, in alveolar barrier function testing, 1597–1598
properties of, versus transport, 138, 138t
Solute flux equation of Kedem and Katchalsky, 133
Solvents, ingestion of, pneumonitis in, 1908
Somatic mutation, in immunoglobulin genes, 418–419
Somatic pain, versus visceral pain, 568–569, 572–574
Somatomedins (insulin-like growth factors), 504–505

Somatomedins (insulin-like growth factors) *(Continued)*
in lung cancer growth, 1381
Somnolence, daytime, in hypoventilation, 2143, 2144
in sleep apnea, 2158, 2162, 2163
Sonic hedgehog molecule, in lung development, 38
Sore throat. See *Pharyngitis.*
Sounds, chest wall, 599
lung. See *Lung sounds.*
Source case, of tuberculosis, 1053–1054
Space travel, pulmonary circulation effects of, 66
Spacers, for inhalers, 249, 356, 1220–1221
Spanish toxic oil syndrome, pulmonary hypertension in, 1642
Sparfloxacin, in pneumonia, 995t
Spasm(s), in hiccups, 2349–2350, 2349t
in tetanus, 2351–2352
laryngeal, 1353–1354
Spasmodic croup, 935
Specific elastance, of lung, 93
Specific immune response, 2224
Specimens, for microbiologic diagnosis, collection of, 608–611, 610t, *612*
for bacterial culture, 617, 618t
processing of, 611–613, 612t, 613t
selection of, 608–609, 610t
from bronchoscopy, handling of, 737
Spectrophotometry, in oxyhemoglobin analysis, 833
Sphenoid sinusitis, 916–917
Spherules, of *Coccidioides immitis*, 1122–1123, *1123*, 1126
Spherulin skin test, for coccidioidomycosis, 1126
Sphingomyelinase deficiency, Niemann-Pick disease in, 1748–1749
Spi-1 (PU.1) transcription factor, in monocyte-macrophage development, 405–406
Spider angiomata, in hepatopulmonary syndrome, 2272
Spinal anesthesia, pulmonary function effects of, 885
Spinal cord, compression of, in metastasis, 1435
decompression sickness affecting, 1960, 1961
dorsal horn of, cytoarchitecture of, 573
in breathing control, *185*, 187–188, *187*
injury of, 2337–2340
causes of, 2337
clinical features of, 2337–2338
consequences of, 2337
cough assistance in, 2346
electrophrenic respiration in, 2348–2349
high cervical, 2337–2338
inspiratory muscle training in, 2347
lower cervical, 2338–2339, 2339t
middle cervical, 2338–2339, 2339t
prognosis for, 2339
pulmonary function in, 2338, 2339, 2339t
radiation, 1436
respiratory failure in, 2447
thoracic, 2339–2340, 2339t
ventilatory support in, 2338, 2347–2349
tuberculosis of, 1083–1084, *1084*
visceral pain pathways in, 569, 573–574, *574*
viscerosomatic convergence in, 574, *574*
Spine. See also *Spinal cord.*
ankylosing spondylitis of. See *Ankylosing spondylitis.*
coccidioidomycosis of, 1124–1125
deformities of. See *Kyphoscoliosis.*
Spine *(Continued)*
stabilization of, respiratory muscles in, 108
surgical stabilization of, in kyphoscoliosis, 2363
tuberculosis of, 1081–1083, *1082*
Spinnability, of mucus, 363
Spin-phase effects, in magnetic resonance imaging, 664
Spiral computed tomography, 661–663
Spirometry, 784–790
description of, 784
flow-volume relationships in, 787–790, *787–790*
in asthma, 1859, *1860*
in chronic obstructive pulmonary disease, 1191
in cystic fibrosis, 1304–1305, 1304t
in dyspnea, 897–900, 899t, 900t
in impairment and disability evaluation, 897–900, 899t, 900t, 905–906
in lung cancer, 1422, 1422t
in neuromuscular disorders, 2332–2333
in obstructive diseases, 1181–1182
in pneumoconiosis, 1815
incentive, after abdominal surgery, 886t
indications for, 784–785, *785*
maximal-effort expiratory vital capacity in, 785–787, 785t, *786*, 874
measurements derived from, 57, *57*
normal values for, 784, 872–873
terminology of, 785t
Spironolactone, in metabolic alkalosis, 173
Spleen, paracoccidioidomycosis of, 1128
sickle cell disease effects on, 2287
Split pleura sign, 2007
in empyema, 2020, *2021*
in tuberculosis, *687*, 688
Spondylitis, ankylosing. See *Ankylosing spondylitis.*
tuberculous, 1081–1083, *1082*
Spores, anthrax, 1029
fungal, hypersensitivity pneumonitis due to, 1868–1869
Sporotrichosis, 622–623, 1108, 1136
Sputum, asbestos bodies in, 1833
black, in coal-workers' pneumoconiosis, 1829
blood in. See *Hemoptysis.*
characteristics of, 589
culture of. See *Culture(s), sputum.*
currant jelly, in *Klebsiella pneumoniae* pneumonia, 1008
epithelial cells in, 614, *614*, *615*
examination of, digestion for, 1046
expectorated, 609
in *Acinetobacter* pneumonia, 1013
in anaerobic pneumonia, 1017, 1019
in ascariasis, 1150
in aspergillosis, 1132, 1133
in asthma, 1254–1255, 1268
in beta-hemolytic streptococci pneumonia, 1005
in blastomycosis, 1120, *1120*
in bronchiectasis, 1328
in bronchitis, 1192
in chronic obstructive pulmonary disease, 1192
in coccidioidomycosis, 1125
in cryptococcosis, 1130
in emphysema, 1192
in Enterobacteriaceae pneumonia, 1010
in *Haemophilus influenzae* pneumonia, 1007, *1007*
in histoplasmosis, 1115
in HIV infection, 2177
in *Klebsiella pneumoniae* pneumonia, 1009, *1009*
Sputum *(Continued)*
in legionellosis, 1015
in lung cancer, 1419–1420, 1420t, 1422
in meningococcal pneumonia, 1005
in *Moraxella catarrhalis* pneumonia, 1006
in mycobacterial infections, 1043, *1044*, 1046
in *Mycoplasma pneumoniae* pneumonia, 1025
in nocardiosis, 1022–1023, *1023*
in nosocomial pneumonia, 923
in paracoccidioidomycosis, 1129
in paragonimiasis, 1161
in pneumococcal pneumonia, 1000, *1000*
in *Pneumocystis carinii* pneumonia, 759, 926
in pneumonia, 921, 989–990, *990*
in *Pseudomonas aeruginosa* pneumonia, 1012
in psittacosis, 1026
in *Staphylococcus aureus* pneumonia, 1003, *1003*
in tuberculosis, 608, 609t, 616, 759–760, 1053–1054, 1065
specimen collection and processing for, 609–610, 610t, 612–613, 921
induction of, 609, 1065
in asthma, 1268
versus sputum expectoration, 759–760
microscopy of, 613–617
advantages of, 614
in immunodeficiency, 616–617
procedure for, 614–615, *614*, *615*
sensitivity and specificity of, 615–616
production of, in alveolar proteinosis, 1794
in aspergillosis, 1131
in asthma, 1256, 1267
in blastomycosis, 1119
in bronchiectasis, 1327
in bronchitis, 367, 919
in candidiasis, 1135
in chronic bronchitis, 1189
in chronic obstructive pulmonary disease, 1189
in coal-workers' pneumoconiosis, 1829
in cor pulmonale, 1637–1638
in cystic fibrosis, 1302
in emphysema, 1189
in Enterobacteriaceae pneumonia, 1010
in *Haemophilus influenzae* pneumonia, 1007
in lung abscess, 1031
in obstructive diseases, 1174–1175
in pneumococcal pneumonia, 999
in pneumonia, in immunodeficiency, 924
in *Pseudomonas aeruginosa* pneumonia, 1011
in pulmonary hypertension, 1637–1638
in *Staphylococcus aureus* pneumonia, 1003
in streptococcal pneumonia, 1004
in strongyloidiasis, 1151–1152
Squamous cell carcinoma. See under *Carcinoma(s).*
*Stachybotrys atra*, inhalation of, 1910
Staging, of lung cancer, 1423–1425, 1423t–1425t
bronchoscopy in, 741
computed tomography in, 669–670, *670*, *671*
magnetic resonance imaging in, 670–671, *672*
mediastinal evaluation in, 2090–2091, *2091*
mediastinoscopy in, 762
positron emission tomography in, 716

Staging *(Continued)*
of lymphoma, 1457
of mesothelioma, 2069–2070
Stannosis, 1842
*Staphylococcus aureus*, characteristics of, 1003, *1003*
colonization by, 1002–1003
surfactant protein A binding to, 312
*Staphylococcus aureus* infection(s), antibiotic-resistant, 1004
bacteremia as, 1004
in cystic fibrosis, 1300–1301, 1309, 1309t, 1311–1312
mediastinal, 2109
pneumonia as, 1002–1004, *1003*
diagnosis of, 920
in granulocytopenia, 924
in HIV infection, 926
in influenza, 954–955
risk factors for, 920
sputum examination in, 921
treatment of, 998t
sinusitis as, 916–917
*Staphylococcus epidermidis* infections, mediastinal, 2109
Starling equation, for fluid flux at microvascular barrier, 132–133, *132*, 1497, 1498t, 1576
in pulmonary edema, 2396, *2396*
in respiratory failure, 2389–2391, *2391*
Starling forces, 132–133, *132*, 1497
Starvation, emphysema in, 1213
ketoacidosis in, 167
Static elastic pressure component, of inspiratory pressure at airway opening, 2450–2451, *2451*
Status asthmaticus, 1275, 2453–2460
clinical features of, 2453, 2453t
definition of, 2453
pathology of, 1175, 1175t
treatment of, general anesthesia in, 2459
helium oxygen mixture in, 2459
mechanical ventilation in, 2456–2460, *2457*, *2458*
pharmacologic, 2453–2456, 2454t
Steady-state method, for diffusing capacity measurement, 75, 812
Steal, pulmonary artery, after embolectomy, 1523, *1524*
Stem cell(s), differentiation of, 399, *400*
in lung, 1376, 1377
transplantation of. See *Blood and bone marrow transplantation.*
Stem cell factor, in lung cancer growth, 1381
in macrophage development, 404
*Stenotrophomonas maltophilia* pneumonia, 1012–1013
Stent(s), tracheobronchial, 1369
in airway obstruction, 742–743, *743*
Stereology, of lung. See *Lung, quantitative morphology of.*
Stereoselectivity, of drugs, 244
Sterilization, of bronchoscopy equipment, 758
Sternoclavicular joint, arthritis of, 577
Sternotomy, median, mediastinitis after, 2109–2110
pulmonary function after, 2253
Sternum, depression of. See *Pectus excavatum.*
osteotomy of, in pectus excavatum, 2366
protuberance of (pectus carinatum), 2365
Steroid receptors, 240–241, *241*
Steroid-dependent asthma, 1270
Steroid-resistant asthma, 1270
Stimulants, ventilatory, 289–290, 2346
Stokes-Einstein radius, of solutes, 139t
Stomach, epithelioid leiomyosarcoma of, in Carney's triad, 1480, *1481*
Stomach *(Continued)*
rupture of, in barotrauma, 1957
Stones, alveolar, in microlithiasis, 1749–1750, *1749*, *1750*
bronchial, 727, 1368
Storage modulus, of mucus, 364
Straining, pneumomediastinum in, 2100, 2101t
Stramonium, in *Datura* plant, in asthma, 275
Streptococcal infection(s), alpha-hemolytic, 1004–1005
beta-hemolytic, pharyngitis as, 917–918
pneumonia as, 1004–1005
group A, pharyngitis as, 917–918
pneumonia as, 1004–1005
anaerobic, 1019, 1019t
microaerophilic, 1019, 1019t
treatment of, 998t
*Streptococcus pneumoniae*, carriage of, 999
characteristics of, 1000, *1000*
detection of, 990
surfactant protein A binding to, 312
surfactant protein D binding to, 315
*Streptococcus pneumoniae* infection(s), antibiotic-resistant, 1001
bacteremia as, 1000
bronchitis as, 934
otitis media as, 918–919
pneumonia as. See *Pneumococcal pneumonia.*
sinusitis as, 916
*Streptococcus pyogenes* infection, pharyngitis as, versus viral pharyngitis, 934
pneumonia as, 1004–1005
*Streptococcus viridans* pneumonia, 1004–1005
in granulocytopenia, 924
Streptokinase, in pleural effusion, 2019–2020
*Streptomyces* pneumonia, culture in, 620–621
Streptomycin, in *Mycobacterium avium* complex infections, 1091
in *Mycobacterium kansasii* infections, 1095
in plague, 1029
in tuberculosis, 1065–1066, 1068t, 1069–1070
central nervous system, 1084
side effects of, 1070
in tularemia, 1029
Streptozyme Test, for *Streptococcus pyogenes*, 1005
Stress, in exercise. See *Exercise testing.*
in lung tissue, 93
on blood-gas barrier, 68–69
on pulmonary capillaries, at high altitude, 1581
in highly fit athletes, 219
Stretch receptors, airway, 575
chest wall, 184
pulmonary, in breathing control, 182–183, 182t, *183*
Stridor, definition of, 596
in laryngeal disorders, 1353
in lung cancer, 1471
Stripe sign, in ventilation-perfusion scanning, 710, *711*
Stroke, in air embolism, in diving, 1955–1956
in arteriovenous malformations, 1561
Stromal cell-derived factor 1, 508
receptor for, 511–512, 511t
Stromelysins, in metastasis, 1388
of alveolar macrophages, 393
Strongyloidiasis, 1151–1153, *1152*
in HIV infection, 2204
Structure-function relationships. See *Mechanical properties.*
Strychnine poisoning, respiratory effects of, 2351
Subjective symptoms, definition of, 896
Subphrenic abscess, pleural effusion in, 2029–2030
Substance P, actions of, 250, *250*, *251*
in cough inhibition, 554, *555*
in mucus secretion regulation, 332, 333
in pain transmission, 574
in visceral pain, 573
inflammation in, 254–255, *254*
Suctioning, hypoxemia in, 728
in mechanical ventilation, 2431
in neuromuscular disorders, 2346
in pneumonia, 997
rigid bronchoscopy in, 727
Sudden infant death syndrome, alveolar hypoventilation in, 2143
Sugar cane, exposure to, hypersensitivity pneumonitis in, 1868
Sugar tumors, of lung, 1479–1480
Sugarbaker system, for mesothelioma staging, 2069–2070
Suicide, paraquat ingestion in, 1908
physician-assisted, 2500–2501
Sulfadiazine, in nocardiosis, 1023
in paracoccidioidomycosis, 1129
in toxoplasmosis, 1149, 2204
Sulfamethoxazole, in mycobacterial infections, 1096
Sulfasalazine, pulmonary disease due to, 1692t, 1702, 1979
Sulfate, transport of, in cystic fibrosis, 1300
Sulfisoxazole, in *Chlamydia trachomatis* pneumonia, 1027
Sulfonamides, in nocardiosis, 1023
Sulfur granules, in actinomycosis, 1021, *1021*
Sulfur hexachloride, in multiple inert gas elimination technique, 80–81, *81*, *82*
Sulfur hexafluoride, transfer of, limitation of, 73, *74*
Sulfur oxides (including sulfur dioxide), as air pollutants, acid species derived from, 1892
adverse effects of, 1887t, 1891–1893
bronchoconstrictor response to, 1888–1889, 1892–1893
defense mechanisms against, 1888–1889
distribution of, 1886–1888
indoor, 1888
mortality due to, 1891
properties of, 1886–1888
reduction of, 2556
sources of, 1886–1888, 1887t
standards for, 2556
chronic bronchitis due to, 1215
high-level exposure to, 1906
in workplace, asthma due to, 1854, 1855
lung injury due to, 1906
Sulfuric acid, in specimen processing, 613t
Sumatriptan, in mountain sickness, 1932
Sunlight, in air pollution formation, 1887, 1893–1896
Superantigens, T lymphocyte recognition of, 428
Superfamily(ies), cytokine receptor, 238
G protein–coupled receptor, 234–235, *235*
hematopoietin receptor, 238
steroid receptor, 240–241, *241*
Superinfections, gram-negative bacteria, versus colonization, 615–616
in transplantation, 2231
Superior sulcus tumors, 1430, 1434
Superior vena cava syndrome, in histoplasmosis, 1111
in lung cancer, 1435, 1439, 1471
in mediastinal mass, 2081, *2087*
in mediastinitis, 2113, *2113*
Supernumerary pulmonary arteries and veins, anatomy of, 120

Superoxide anions, absence of, in chronic granulomatous disease, 2237
as inflammatory mediators, 257–258
macrophage generation of, 390, 392
Suprapontine regions, in breathing control, 187
Surface density, in lung quantitative morphology, 25, *27*
Surface tension, lowering of, surfactant in, 307–309, *308*
of alveoli, 92–93
Surfactant, 307–325
alterations of, in acute respiratory distress syndrome, 318–319
in adenocarcinoma, 320
in alveolar proteinosis, 320
in interstitial lung diseases, 319–320
in ischemia-reperfusion injury, 320
in obstructive lung diseases, 320
in pneumonia, 319
in pulmonary fibrosis, 1678, 1680
alveolar macrophages in, 390
clearance of, granulocyte-macrophage colony-stimulating factor in, 404
composition of, 92
in acute respiratory distress syndrome, 318–319
lipids in, 309, 309t
proteins in, 308–316, 309t, *309*
surfactant proteins A to D in. See specific proteins, e.g., *Surfactant protein A*.
deficiency of, hereditary, 318
in acute lung injury, 1585
in newborns, 317–318. See also *Neonate(s), respiratory distress syndrome in*.
in pulmonary edema, 1585
in pulmonary embolism, 1506
discovery of, 308
excess of, in alveolar proteinosis, 1790, *1791*, 1793–1794
functions of, 92–93, 308–309, *308*, *309*
in alveolar clearance, 371
in lamellar bodies, *389*
in large airways, 309
large aggregates (heavy forms) of, 316, *317*, 318–319
metabolism of, 70, 316, *317*
overview of, 307–308
processing of, 316, *317*
pulmonary edema pathophysiology and, 1584
secretion of, 316, *317*
small aggregates (light forms) of, 316, *317*, 318–319
therapeutic, delivery methods for, 320
future strategies for, 321
in acute respiratory distress syndrome, 318–319, 320–321, 2423
in lung transplantation, 320
in neonatal respiratory distress syndrome, 318
in obstructive disease, 320
in pneumonia, 319
in pulmonary edema, 1609–1610
mechanical ventilation with, 320–321
preparations for, 320, 321
Surfactant protein A, 308, *309*, 309t, 310–313
concentration of, 310
deficiency of, 311–312, 319
distribution of, 310
excess of, 319–320
function of, 310–312, *311*
genes for, 310
in phagocytosis, 312–313
in pleural fluid, 320
in surfactant secretion inhibition, 316, *317*
Surfactant protein A *(Continued)*
infectious organism binding to, 312
ratio to phospholipid, in interstitial lung disease, 319
secretion of, 310
structure of, 310–312, *311*
synthesis of, 310
Surfactant protein B, 308, *309*, 309t, 313, *313*
deficiency of, 318, 1793
excess of, in alveolar proteinosis, 320
Surfactant protein C, 308, *309*, 309t, 313–314, *314*
Surfactant protein D, 309t, 314–316
distribution of, 315
excess of, 319–320
function of, 315
gene for, 314
in phagocytosis, 316
in pleural fluid, 320
infectious organism binding to, 315–316
structure of, *311*, 314–315
Surfactant-associated proteins, secretion of, in alveoli, 19, 20t
Surgery. See also specific procedures, e.g., *Pneumonectomy*.
abdominal, pleural effusion after, 2030
preoperative evaluation for, 885–886
cardiac. See *Heart, surgery on*.
chylothorax after, 2056
hemothorax in, 2062
in mesothelioma, benign fibrous, 2071
malignant, 2070
preoperative evaluation for. See *Preoperative evaluation*.
respiratory failure associated with, 2378t, 2381–2383, 2382t
ventilation-perfusion scanning before, 713–715
Susceptibility testing, of antibiotics. See *Antibiotics, susceptibility testing of*.
Sustentacular (sheath) cells, in carotid body, 189
*Sutterelia wadsworthensis* pneumonia, 1019t
Swallowing, larynx in, 1351
mechanisms of, 1344
of water, during near drowning, 1964
pharyngeal function in, 1350
respiration coordination with, 181–182
Sweat, analysis of, in cystic fibrosis, 1307–1308, 1307t, 1308t
Sweat glands, dysfunction of, in cystic fibrosis, 1180, 1292, 1307
Swimmer's itch, in schistosomiasis, 1164
Swimming, indoor, hypersensitivity pneumonitis related to, 1868
underwater. See *Diving*.
Swyer-James syndrome (unilateral bronchiolitis obliterans), 1197–1198
Symbols, in respiratory medicine, 2563–2565
Sympathetic nervous system, of airway, 249–250, *250*, *251*, 255
in mucus secretion regulation, 332–333
of lung, 21–22
of pulmonary circulation, 131
pulmonary vascular compliance and, 127–128
pulmonary vascular resistance and, 64
Sympathomimetic drugs. See *Beta$_2$-adrenergic agonists*.
Syncope, cough, 909
in pulmonary embolism, 1507
in pulmonary hypertension, 1547
Syndrome of inappropriate antidiuretic hormone secretion, in lung cancer, 1379, 1421–1422
Syndrome X, chest pain in, 578
Synergism, of drugs, 244
Syphilis, aortitis in, pain in, 579
Systemic lupus erythematosus, 1703–1705
antibodies in, 1695t
diffuse alveolar hemorrhage in, 1737t, 1739–1740, *1739*
drug-induced, 1974, 1985–1986, 1989
epidemiology of, 1703
in complement C2 deficiency, 2236
pleural disease in, 1705
pleural effusions in, 2005, 2031–2032
pulmonary hypertension in, 1705
pulmonary manifestations of, 466, *467*, 1703–1705, 1703t, *1704*
risk factors for, 1703
vasculitis in, 1539
Systemic sclerosis (scleroderma), 1691–1698
antibodies in, 1694, 1695t, 1697
classification of, 1691, 1694t
epidemiology of, 1691–1692
lung cancer risk in, 1416, 1421
pulmonary manifestations of, 1692
chest radiography of, 1694, *1696*
clinical features of, 1694, 1695t
interstitial pulmonary fibrosis as, 1692, 1694, 1695t, 1696, *1696*
prognosis for, 1697
pulmonary function tests in, 1694, 1696
treatment of, 1697
vascular, 1697–1698
risk factors for, 1691–1692
syndromes resembling, 1692
vasculitis in, 1539–1540, *1540*

## T

T1 and T2 (time constants), in magnetic resonance imaging, 664
T lymphocytes, 422–430
activation of, CD3 complex and, 428–429
co-stimulatory molecules for, 431–432, *431*
in hypersensitivity pneumonitis, 1871–1872
in sarcoidosis, 1724–1725
suppression of, alveolar macrophages in, 393–394, *395*
alpha-beta, 428
antigen interactions with, 422, 426–428, 427t, *428*
apoptosis of, 429, *430*
B lymphocyte interactions with, 414, 432–434, *433*, 434
CD4+, B lymphocyte interactions with, 434
cytokine release from, 430, 433
development of, 429, *430*
function of, 429
in antigen recognition, 427–428, *428*
in granulomatous disease, 437–438
in HIV infection, depletion of, 2173
in bacterial pneumonia, 2179
in coccidioidomycosis, 2200
in cryptococcosis, 2196
in cytomegalovirus infections, 2202
in histoplasmosis, 2198–2199
in Kaposi's sarcoma, 2205
in lymphoma, 2206–2207
in *Mycobacterium avium* complex infections, 2185
in *Mycobacterium kansasii* infections, 2186
in *Pneumocystis carinii* pneumonia, 2188
in *Pseudomonas aeruginosa* pneumonia, 2180

T lymphocytes *(Continued)*
in toxoplasmosis, 2203
in tuberculosis, 2182, 2182t
measurement of, 2174–2175
in hypersensitivity pneumonitis, 1872
in lung, 435–436
CD8+, cytokine release from, 430
cytotoxicity of, 434–435
development of, 429, *430*
function of, 429
in antigen recognition, 427
in lung, 435–436, 438
cluster of differentiation system for, 413–414, 414t
cytotoxic, 414, 434–435, 438
deficiency of, in DiGeorge's syndrome, 2238
development of, 415, 429, *430*
asthma and, 1251, *1251*
dysfunction of, in ataxia-telangiectasia, 2233t, 2239–2240
in blastomycosis, 1120
in coccidioidomycosis, 1125
in histoplasmosis, 1114
in severe combined immunodeficiency, 2233t, 2239
function of, 429, 2225–2226, *2225*, *2227*, *2228*
gamma-delta, 428, 435
helper, 414, 2226
in asthma, 1251, *1251*, 1256–1258, *1257–1259*
in fibrosis, 503–504
in systemic sclerosis, 1694
interferon-τ effects on, 503–504
subsets of, 432–434, *433*
in asthma, 1251, *1251*, 1256–1258, *1257–1259*
occupational, 1855
in cell-mediated immune response, 434–435
in influenza, 953
in lymphoma, 1456t
in *Mycobacterium tuberculosis* clearance, 1057
in viral infections, 2226, *2228*
intercalation of, in airway epithelium, 10, *11*
memory, trafficking of, 435–436
nuclear factor of activated T cells in, 261
receptors on. See *T-cell receptors*.
repertoire of, selection of, 429, *430*
self-tolerance of, 429–430
suppressor, 414
toxicity to, in purine nucleoside phosphorylase deficiency, 2238–2239
trafficking of, 435–436
tumor necrosis factor-α effects on, 501
Tachycardia, beta$_2$-adrenergic agonist-induced, 271
in pneumococcal pneumonia, 999
in pneumothorax, 2046, 2054
in pulmonary edema, 1933–1934
in septic shock, 2399
Tachykinin(s). See also specific substances, e.g., *Substance P*.
in asthma, 1262–1263
in cough inhibition, 554, *555*
in neurogenic inflammation, 254–255, *254*
Tachykinin receptor antagonists, in airway disease, 288
Tachyphylaxis, of drugs, 244–245, *245*
Tachypnea, in *Acinetobacter* pneumonia, 1013
in acute respiratory distress syndrome, 2416–2417
in bone marrow transplantation, 2299
in cor pulmonale, 1637
in dyspnea, 220
in pneumococcal pneumonia, 999
Tachypnea *(Continued)*
in pneumothorax, neonatal, 2053
in pulmonary edema, 1591
in pulmonary embolism, 1507
in pulmonary fibrosis, 1675
in pulmonary hypertension, 1637
in respiratory acidosis, 174
inspection of, 597
versus hyperventilation, 2145
Tacrolimus, toxicity of, 2526
Takayasu's vasculitis, 579, 1541
Talc, as sclerosing agent, in chylothorax, 2058
in hepatic hydrothorax, 2015
in metastatic disease, 2075
in pneumothorax, 2048, 2050
in pneumoconiosis, *1814*, 1841
pulmonary disease due to, 1980–1981
pulmonary hypertension due to, 1546
Talcum powder aspiration, 1908
Talin, in fluid and solute exchange, *134–135*
Tantalum carbide, in hard metal products, lung disease from, 1844–1845
*TAP* genes and products, in lung cancer, 1386
Tar, in cigarettes, versus cancer risk, 1399
Target variable, in mechanical ventilation, 2471, *2472*, 2473t
T-cell receptors, 414, 414t
CD3 complex and, 428–429
genes of, 423–424, *423*, *424*
in sarcoidosis, 1724
in T-lymphocyte activation, 431–432, *431*
repertoire of, 429, *430*
structure of, 422–424, *422–424*
Tear gases, 1907
Technegas, in ventilation-perfusion scanning, 699–700
Technetium 99m compounds, in ventilation-perfusion scanning, 698–700, 828
in interstitial pneumonitis, 713
in sarcoidosis, 713
of epithelial permeability, 718–720, *719*
peptide type, 718
Teeth, barotrauma of, 1957
Telangiectasia, ataxia with, immunodeficiency in, 2233t, 2239–2240
hereditary hemorrhagic. See *Hereditary hemorrhagic telangiectasia*.
Telomerase, aberrant activity of, in lung cancer, 1378
Temperature, acid-base balance and, 163
Temporal (giant cell) arteritis, 1541
Tension pneumothorax, 2046, 2054–2055
Teratocarcinoma, of mediastinum, 2127
Teratoma(s), metastasis from, 1473
of lung, 1480
of mediastinum, 2127, *2127*
Terbutaline, as bronchodilator, 270
in asthma, 357, 2454t
in chronic obstructive pulmonary disease, 357, 1221
in status asthmaticus, 2454t
Terminal illness. See *Death and dying*.
Terminal respiratory units. See also *Alveolus(i)*.
anatomy of, 15–21, *16–18*
type I cell, 19–21, 21t
type II cell, 17, *18*, 19, 20t, 21, 21t
bronchiole junction with, 16
C fibers of, 21–22, *21*
cell types in, 371
definition of, 15
epithelium of, 16–21, *18*, 20t, 21t
versus alveoli, 15
volume of, in breathing, 15–16, *17*
Testis, sarcoidosis of, 1719
Tetanus, 2351–2352
Tetany, in metabolic alkalosis, 172
Tetany *(Continued)*
in respiratory alkalosis, 175
Tetracycline(s), as pneumothorax sclerosing agent, 2048, *2048*
in bronchopleural fistula, 754–755
in cystic fibrosis, 1309t
in plague, 1029
in pleurodesis, 2075
in Q fever, 1026
Tetrandine, in silicosis, 1824
Textile workers, byssinosis in, 1860–1862
Thallium 201, in ventilation-perfusion scanning, in lung transplantation, 718
in tuberculosis, 712
Theophyllinate, 272
Theophylline, 272–275
administration routes for, 274–275
as vasodilator, 302
chemistry of, 272
clinical uses of, 275
dosage for, 275, 1223
drug interactions with, 274
in asthma, 1276, 1277t, 2454t, 2455
in pregnancy, 2320
in bronchiectasis, 564
in chronic obstructive pulmonary disease, 1222–1223, 1223t, 2461, 2461t
in cough, 564
in cystic fibrosis, 1310
in respiratory failure, 2461, 2461t
in status asthmaticus, 2454t, 2455
inhaled agents with, 1223
mechanisms of action of, 273, *273*, *274*, 1222
metabolism of, 1222, 1223t
nonbronchodilator actions of, 273
pharmacokinetics of, 273–274, 274t
preparations of, 1222–1223
side effects of, 275, 275t, 1222
therapeutic range of, 274
Thermal dye method, for lung water measurement, 1596–1597
Thermal injury, of airway, bronchoscopy in, 754
of lung, pathology of, 475
*Thermoactinomyces* pneumonia, culture in, 620–621
Thiabendazole, in strongyloidiasis, 1153
Thomsen's disease (myotonia congenita), respiratory dyskinesia in, 2351
Thoracentesis, in empyema, 1032, 2019
in hepatic hydrothorax, 2015
in HIV infection, 2178
in pleural effusions, 2000, 2001–2002, 2076
in nephrotic syndrome, 2016
parapneumonic, 2018–2019
pneumothorax in, 2051
pulmonary edema after, 2055–2056
ultrasonography for, 660–661, *661*, 2007
Thoracic compliance, in exercise, in chronic obstructive pulmonary disease, 215
Thoracic duct, anatomy of, 2056
disruption of, chylothorax in, 2056–2057
ligation of, in chylothorax, 2058, 2059
Thoracic mechanical time constant, in exercise, in chronic obstructive pulmonary disease, 214–215
Thoracic outlet syndrome, 577
Thoracoplasty, respiratory manifestations of, 2359t, 2361t, 2363–2364, 2364t
Thoracoscopy, advantages of, 761
in empyema, 2020
in HIV infection, 2178
in mediastinal biopsy, 2090
in mesothelioma, 2069
in pleural effusion, 2009, 2020

Thoracoscopy *(Continued)*
in pleural metastasis, 2074
in pneumothorax, 2048, 2050
indications for, 761
technique for, 761
Thoracostomy, tube. See *Tube thoracostomy.*
Thoracotomy, atelectasis after, 886
in chylothorax, 2058
in hemothorax, 2061
in lung biopsy, 763
in lung cancer, 1422
in nodule removal, 715–716
in pleural effusion, 2009–2010
in pneumothorax, 2048–2049
pulmonary edema after, 2055–2056
pulmonary function after, 2253
Thoravision digital chest imaging system, 642
Thorax. See also *Chest.*
gas volume of, measurement of, 795–797, *796*
pressure in, during cough, 557
during water immersion, 1952
in mechanical ventilation, 2482
in sleep apnea, 2159
volume of, in heart failure, 2251–2252, 2252t
Three-gas iteration method, for diffusing capacity measurement, 812
Three-zone model, of pulmonary circulation, 65–66, *65*
Threshold limit values, for dust exposures, 1813
Throat, culture of, in pneumonia, 609
inflammation of. See *Pharyngitis.*
Thrombin, in endothelial permeability mediation, 141, 142
Thrombocytopenia, 2295
heparin-induced, 1517
in bone marrow transplantation, 2300
in hantavirus infections, 946
Thrombocytosis, 2286
Thromboembolic disease. See *Deep vein thrombosis; Pulmonary embolism; Venous thromboembolism.*
β-Thromboglobulin, 508, 508t
Thrombolytic therapy, for pleural effusion, 2019–2020
for pulmonary embolism, 1518
intrapleural, 2019–2020
Thrombophilia, 1514
Thrombophlebitis, migratory, in lung cancer, 1421
Thrombosis, cavernous sinus, in sinusitis, 916–917
in erythrocytosis, 2286
in hypereosinophilic syndrome, 1769
in leukemia, 2291
in lung transplantation, 2526
in pregnancy, 2322–2323
in systemic lupus erythematosus, 1705
pulmonary. See *Pulmonary embolism.*
venous. See *Deep vein thrombosis; Venous thromboembolism.*
Thrombospondin-1, in angiogenesis, in lung cancer, 1387
Thromboxane(s), as inflammatory mediators, 257
as vasoconstrictor, 300–301
biologic effects of, 497–499, 497t
in mucus hypersecretion, 334
in pulmonary vascular resistance control, 131, 297
Thrombus(i). See also *Deep vein thrombosis; Thrombosis; Venous thromboembolism.*
radiopharmaceuticals seeking, 718
tumor, chest radiography of, *655*
Thrush, 1135
Thumbprint sign, in epiglottitis, 918
Thymic rebound, 2127
Thymoma, 2083, 2124, 2126–2127, *2126*
Thymus, carcinoma of, 2127
T lymphocyte development in, 429, *430*
Thymus-expressed chemokine and receptor, 507t, 516–517
Thyroid gland, disorders of, respiratory manifestations of, 2310–2311, *2311*, 2311t
ectopic, 2128
Thyroid hormone, in lung development, 42
Thyroid transcription factor-1, in lung development, 38
Thyroid-specific enhancer-binding protein, in lung development, 38
Thyrotropin-releasing hormone, in lung development, 42
Tidal volume, carbon dioxide production and, 156, *157*
definition of, 57, *57*, *783*, 2564
in alveolar ventilation calculation, 58
in exercise, in emphysema, *222*, 223
in highly fit athletes, 218
in interstitial pulmonary fibrosis, 217
in interstitial pulmonary disease, *223*, 225
in mechanical ventilation, in acute respiratory distress syndrome, 2428–2429
in status asthmaticus, 2456, *2457*
to prevent lung injury, 2478
in minute ventilation calculation, 180–181, *181*
in neuromuscular disorders, 2345
in physiologic dead space calculation, 80
normal, *57*
positive end-expiratory pressure and, 2448, *2448*
surfactant aggregates and, 319
versus inspiratory capacity, in interstitial pulmonary fibrosis, 217
Tietze's syndrome, 577, 590
Tight junctions, in airway epithelia, 335
neutrophil passage through, 526
TIGR data base, for genetic disease, 51
Time constants, ventilation and, 60
Timed forced expiratory volume, definition of, 2563
Time-of-flight effects, in magnetic resonance imaging, 664
Timolol, contraindicated in asthma, 290
pulmonary disease due to, 1983
Timpe and Runyon classification, of mycobacteria, 1044, 1044t
Tin dust exposure, stannosis in, 1842
Tinidazole, in amebiasis, 1146
Tiotropium, anticholinergic properties of, 277
in chronic obstructive pulmonary disease, 1221
Tissot spirometer, 822
Tissue factor, in angiogenesis regulation, in lung cancer, 1387
Tissue inhibitors of metalloproteinases, in lung disease, 393
Tissue resistance, 95
Titanium carbide, in hard metal products, lung disease from, 1844–1845
$TL_{CO}$. See *Diffusing capacity.*
TNM staging system, for lung cancer, 1423–1425, 1424t, 1425t
Tobacco use. See also *Smoking.*
noncigarette (cigar/pipe/smokeless), lung cancer in, 1400
Tobramycin, in cystic fibrosis, 1309t, 1310, 1312
Tocainide, pulmonary disease due to, 1984
Tocolytic agents, pulmonary disease due to, 1988, 2321–2322, *2322*
Tocopherols, in lung cancer, 1385
in lung cancer prevention, 1405
Toe(s), clubbing of. See *Clubbing.*
Tolazoline, as vasodilator, 300, 301
in vasoactivity evaluation, 299
Tolerance, of drugs, 244
to commonly inhaled antigens, alveolar macrophages in, 393–394, *395*
Toluene diisocyanate, asthma due to, 1855, 1857
hypersensitivity pneumonitis due to, 1869–1870
Tomography, computed. See *Computed tomography.*
conventional, 654
Tongue, enlargement of, in acromegaly, 2313
positioning of, appliances for, in sleep apnea, 2160
Tonsillitis, 917–918, 933
Tonsils, enlarged, pharyngeal obstruction in, 1351
Toothpaste lines, in bronchiectasis, 1328, *1330*
Topographic inequality, of ventilation, 59, *59*
Topotecan, in lung cancer, 1437, 1437t, 1439
Total lung capacity, after heart transplantation, 2253, 2253t
after thoracoplasty, 2364
decreased, causes of, 791
definition of, 57, *57*, 783, *783*, 2563
in acromegaly, 2313
in alveolar proteinosis, 1795
in ankylosing spondylitis, 2369
in chronic obstructive pulmonary disease, 104–105, 1191, 1207
in cystic fibrosis, 1304t
in heart disease, 2251, *2251*, 2252t
in impairment and disability evaluation, 850t
in interstitial lung disease, 1662, *1664*
in kyphoscoliosis, 2358–2359, 2359t, *2360*
in lymphangio(leio)myomatosis, 1781
in neuromuscular disorders, 2333
in obesity, 2371, 2371t
in pulmonary fibrosis, 1675–1676, *1675*, *1676*, 1679
in spinal cord injury, 2339, 2339t
inspiration to, tissue stretching in, 102
measurement of, 57–58, *57*, 793
normal values for, *57*, 874
pressure-volume curves at, 104
reduction of, in disease states, mechanical aspects of, 112
Total ventilation, definition of, 58
Tourniquets, alternating, in acute respiratory distress syndrome, 2420
in pulmonary edema, 1600, 2420
Toxic exposure(s). See also *Occupational and environmental disorder(s).*
acute respiratory distress syndrome in, 1588t, 1590–1591
agents involved in, 1905t. See also specific agents.
anion gap acidosis in, 168
bronchiectasis in, 1336
bronchiolitis in, 1362, *1362*
lung injury in, 1588t, 1590–1591
metabolic acidosis in, 168
pathogenic effects of, 1903–1904
polymer fume fever in, 1907
pulmonary edema in, 1588t, 1590–1591
pulmonary hypertension in, 1642
sequelae of, 1904–1905
to aluminum production, 1400
to ammonia, 1909
to arsenic, 1400
to baby powder, 1908
to beryllium, *469*, 1402–1403, 1842–1844

Toxic exposure(s) *(Continued)*
to bis(chloromethyl) ether, 1401
to bromine and bromine compounds, 1909
to cadmium, 1403, 1907
to carborundum, 1845
to chloramine, 1905–1906
to chlorine, 1905–1906
to chromium, 1401
to coke oven emissions, 1401–1402
to diesel exhaust, 1403, 1893
to drugs, 1909. See also *Drug(s), pulmonary disease(s) due to.*
respiratory effects of, 2343
theophylline as, 275, 275t
to ethylene oxide, 1909
to formaldehyde, 1403
to hydrocarbons, 1908
to hydrochloric acid, 1905–1906
to hydrogen sulfide, 1909
to insecticides, 1909
to isocyanates, 1909–1910
to mercury, 1907
to metal fumes, 1907
to metals, 1844–1845, 1907
to molds, 1910
to mustard gas, 1402
to occupational agents, 1805–1806
to organic dusts, 1907
to organophosphates, 2343
to oxygen. See *Hyperoxia; Oxygen, toxicity of.*
to paraquat, 1908
to phosphine, 1910
to smoke, 1908–1909
to vinyl chloride, 1402
treatment of, 1904
Toxic oil syndrome, pulmonary hypertension in, 1642
Toxins. See also *Endotoxin; Exotoxins.*
in chemical warfare, 1906–1907
tetanus, 2351–2352
*Toxocara canis* infections, 1157
Toxoplasmosis, 1147–1149, *1148*
genetic tests for, 626–627
in bone marrow transplantation, 2304
in HIV infection, 2203–2204
Tracer studies. See also *Radionuclide studies.*
of lung water, 1596–1597
Trachea, aerosol deposition in, 352–354, *352, 353*
amyloidosis of, 1481, 1481t, 2296
aspiration through, in pneumonia, 992, 993t
cancer invasion of, computed tomography in, 669
carcinoid tumor of, 1461
computed tomography of, 679
congenital malformations of, 482
cough reflex receptors in, 554, *555*
development of, 36–37, *37*
disorders of, in mediastinitis, 2113
dry, in Sjögren's syndrome, 366, 1706
enlargement of, bronchiectasis with, 1337
fracture of, pneumothorax in, 2052–2053
glands of, innervation of, 22
injury of, bronchoscopy in, 753
pneumomediastinum in, 2097
innervation of, 22
mucociliary transport rate in, 365–366
muscles surrounding, 1346t
narrowing of, in chronic obstructive pulmonary disease, 1229
in inflammatory bowel disease, 2270
in relapsing polychondritis, 1709, *1709*
muscles in, 1346t
obstruction of, 727
stents in, 742–743, *743*, 1369
Trachea *(Continued)*
tumors of, benign, 1477, 1478
Tracheal breath sounds, 593, *593*
Tracheal gas insufflation technique, in mechanical ventilation, 2097
Tracheitis, herpes simplex virus, 948–949
Tracheobronchial osteoplastica, 2296
Tracheobronchial receptors, 182–184, 182t, *183*
Tracheobronchial tree, cough reflex receptors in, 553
Tracheobronchitis. See also *Croup.*
adenovirus, 939, *939*
influenza virus, 951, *952*
measles virus, 958
*Mycoplasma pneumoniae*, 1024
pain in, 576
pathology of, 474
Tracheobronchomegaly, 480t, 1337
Tracheopathia osteochondroplastica, 1481
Tracheostomy, in neuromuscular disorders, 2346
in sleep apnea, 2160–2161
Tracheotomy, pneumomediastinum in, 2099
Tram tracks or lines, in bronchiectasis, 1328, *1329–1330*
Transbronchial biopsy, in allograft rejection, 2523
in HIV infection, 2177–2178
in interstitial lung disease, 751–753, 751t
of mediastinum, 2087–2090, *2089*
Transcapillary oncotic pressure gradient, 133
Transcellular pathway, for fluid and solute exchange, 134, *134–135*, 138–139, 138t
Transcription factor(s), 258–262. See also specific substances, e.g., *Activator protein-1.*
blockers of, in airway disease, 288
coactivators of, 261–262, *262*
corticosteroid interactions with, 278–279, *279*, 279t, *280*
function of, 258–259
in lung development, 37–40, *40*
in monocyte-macrophage development, 404–407
in receptor gene regulation, 245–246
in signal transduction, 239–241, *239, 241*
inhibitors of, 259
secretion of, in alveoli, 21, 21t
Transcytosis, of albumin, 140–141
Transdiaphragmatic pressure, in respiratory muscle evaluation, 858, *858*
measurement of, 2333
Transducin, rhodopsin interactions with, 234
Transepithelial potential difference, in ion transport, in cystic fibrosis, 1297–1298, *1298*
Transfer factor, as synonym for diffusing capacity, 76. See also *Diffusing capacity.*
Transferrin, gallium binding to, in ventilation-perfusion scanning, 701
Transforming growth factor-β, 505–506
action of, 240
in lung cancer, 1385
in lung development, 42
in silicosis, 1819
in systemic sclerosis, 1692, 1694
Transfusions, alveolar damage due to, 1987
cytomegalovirus transmission in, 945
granulocyte, in pneumonia, 997
in pulmonary edema, 1607
in sickle cell disease, 2289
lung injury in, 2292
packed cell, in respiratory failure, 2406
platelet, 2295
Transient ischemic attack, in arteriovenous malformations, 1561
Transillumination, of sinuses, in sinusitis, 933
Transitional and respiratory zone, definition of, 56, *56*
Transmission, of pathogen, definition of, 1052
Transmission disequilibrium tests, in genetic disease, 49–50, 51t
Transmural pressure, in pulmonary arteries, in Starling equation, 1497
versus cross section, 125–126
versus pulmonary vascular resistance, 126, *126, 127*
Transplantation, adenovirus infections in, 939, 940t
allogeneic organ, 2226–2232. See also specific organ.
adenovirus infections in, 939, 940t
cancer in, 2232
complications of, early, 2228–2229
late, 2232
time course of, 2227–2228, *2229*
up to six months, 2229–2232, 2230t
cytomegalovirus infections in, 942, 943, 2230–2231, 2230t
donor for, brain death in, 2496
Epstein-Barr virus infections in, 2231–2232
fungal infections in, 2229–2230, *2229*
lymphoproliferative disorder in, 2231–2232
mycobacterial infections in, 2232
pleural effusion in, 2030
*Pneumocystis carinii* pneumonia in, *2229*, 2230
pneumonia in, 925
early onset, 2228–2229
late onset, 2232
sarcoidosis in, 1725
viral infections in, *2229*, 2230–2232, 2230t
bone marrow. See *Blood and bone marrow transplantation.*
heart, pneumonia in, 2229
pulmonary function after, 2253, 2253t
heart-lung, bronchiectasis after, 1336
bronchiolitis obliterans after, 1364–1366, *1365*
in bronchiectasis, 1333
in pulmonary hypertension, 1551–1552
immunosuppressive therapy for. See *Immunosuppressive therapy, for transplantation;* specific drugs.
kidney, pneumonia in, 2228–2229
liver, pleural effusion in, 2030
pneumonia in, 2229
lung. See *Lung transplantation.*
rejection in. See also *Lung transplantation, rejection in.*
cytomegalovirus infection and, 2231
Transporters associated with antigen presentation, down-regulation of, in lung cancer, 1386
Transpulmonary pressure, 95, *96*
distribution of, in lung, 109–111, *110*
high, in neonates, 2053
in barotrauma, 1955
in interstitial lung disease, 1662, *1664*
in pneumothorax, 2044–2045
in pulmonary fibrosis, 1675, *1675*
normal, 2044
versus airflow, 98, *99*
Transthoracic lung aspiration, in pneumonia, 992–993
Transthoracic needle biopsy, 760–761
Transtracheal aspiration, in pneumonia, 609, 992, 993t
Transudates, pleural fluid. See *Pleural effusion(s), transudative.*

Transverse abdominis muscle, mechanical properties of, 108
Trapped lung, pleural effusion in, 2036
Trauma. See also *Fracture(s); Rib(s), fractures of.*
airway, bronchoscopy in, 753, 754
bronchial, 1368
chest, bronchial injury in, 1368
flail chest in, 2366–2369, *2367*, 2367t, *2368*
hemothorax in, 2060–2062, *19*
mediastinitis in, 2107
pain in, 577, 590
pneumothorax in, 2051–2053
chylothorax in, 2056–2058
esophageal, mediastinitis in, 2106–2107
facial, pneumomediastinum in, 2097
lung injury in, 1588t, 2416
pharyngeal, airway obstruction in, 1351
phrenic nerve, diaphragmatic paralysis in, 2334
pneumothorax in, 2051–2053
pressure-induced. See *Barotrauma.*
pulmonary artery aneurysms in, 1569
pulmonary circulation-systemic circulation communications in, 1565
spinal cord. See *Spinal cord, injury of.*
tissue embolism in, 1527
tracheal, bronchoscopy in, 753
pneumomediastinum in, 2097
Travelers' disease, pneumonia as, etiology of, 987
in HIV infection, 2175
Treadmills, in exercise testing, 841, 844–845
Treatment. See also specific disorders.
definition of, 585
Tremacamra, in rhinovirus infections, 966
Tremolite, 1831t
diseases due to, 2067
microscopic appearance of, *1814*
Tremor, $beta_2$-adrenergic agonist-induced, 271
Trepopnea, definition of, 588
Triamcinolone acetonide, chemical structure of, *278*
pharmacokinetics of, 282
Tributyltin, exposure to, 1907
Trichinosis, 1156–1157
Trichiptysis, in germ cell tumor, 2127
Tricuspid insufficiency, in cor pulmonale, 1637–1638, 1641
Tricyclic antidepressants, pulmonary disease due to, 1989
Triggers, of airway reactivity, 232, *233*
of breath, in mechanical ventilation, 2471–2472, *2472*, 2473t, 2479–2482, *2481*, *2482*
Trimellitic anhydride, 1910
asthma due to, 1857, 1859
diffuse alveolar hemorrhage due to, 1744
hypersensitivity pneumonitis due to, 1870
Trimethoprim-sulfamethoxazole, in cystic fibrosis, 1309t
in melioidosis, 1028
in *Pneumocystis carinii* pneumonia, 926, 2190–2195, 2191t, 2195t, 2304
in pneumonia, 998t
in toxoplasmosis, 2204
prophylactic, in chronic granulomatous disease, 2237
side effects of, 2190, 2191t
Trimetrexate, in *Pneumocystis carinii* pneumonia, 2191t, 2193
Trinotecan, in lung cancer, 1437, 1437t
Triphosphate nucleotides, in cystic fibrosis, 1299
Trisodium phosphate/benzalkonium chloride, in specimen processing, 613t
Trophoblastic embolization, 2325
Tropical eosinophilia, 1153–1155, *1154*, 1761–1762, 1761t, *1762*
Trousseau's sign, in metabolic alkalosis, 172
in respiratory alkalosis, 175
Trousseau's syndrome, in lung cancer, 1421
Trovafloxacin, in pneumonia, 995t
Tryptophan, impurities in, eosinophilic-myalgia syndrome due to, 1762–1763
ingestion of, pulmonary hypertension due to, 1546
Tube(s), endotracheal. See *Endotracheal intubation.*
feeding, misplacement of, pleural effusion in, 2036
Tube precipitin tests, for coccidioidomycosis, 1125
Tube thoracostomy, in empyema, 2019
in hemothorax, 2060–2061
in pleural effusion, 2019
in pleurodesis, 2075
in pneumothorax, 2047–2048, *2048*, 2050, 2052
pneumomediastinum in, 2099
pulmonary edema after, 2055–2056
Tubercles, Gottron's, in dermatomyositis, 1706
Tuberculin skin test, 1059–1062, *1060*, 1061t, *1062*
in HIV infection, 2184–2185
prophylactic drugs and, 1087–1088
Tuberculomas, of central nervous system, 1083–1084, *1084*
Tuberculosis, 1043–1090
abdominal, 1084–1085
adjunctive treatment for, 1075
adrenal gland, respiratory manifestations of, 2313
"adult," 1058
bacteriologic evaluation of, 1065
body distribution of, 1063
bronchial granulomatous inflammation in, 1367–1368
caseation necrosis in, 446, *449*
CD4+ lymphocyte count in, in HIV infection, 2182, 2182t
central nervous system, 1083–1084, *1084*
chest radiography of, 1063–1065, *1063–1065*
disseminated (miliary), 1078
in HIV infection, 2182–2183, *2183*
chyliform pleural effusion in, 2060
clinical manifestations of, disseminated (miliary), 1077
in HIV infection, 2181–2183, 2182t, *2183*
pericardial, 1086
pleural, 1079
conditions associated with, treatment in, 1074
culture in, 618t, 619–620, 620t, 1044, 1047
diagnosis of, 1063–1065, *1063–1065*
abdominal, 1085
bronchoscopy in, 743t, 744–745
central nervous system, 1083–1084, *1084*
genetic methods for, 626
genitourinary, 1080–1081
in HIV infection, 2183
pericardial, 1085–1086, *1086*
pleural, 1079–1080
skeletal, 1081–1083, *1082*
with pleural effusion, 2022
differential diagnosis of, 1064
disseminated (miliary), 1064, *1064*, 1076–1078
caseation necrosis in, *449*
computed tomography of, 675, *675*
empyema in, 2021
Tuberculosis *(Continued)*
endobronchial, 1367–1368
epidemiology of, 1043, 1048–1052, *1049–1052*, 1049t, 1050t
extrapulmonary, 1075–1076, *1076*, *1077*
in HIV infection, 1058, 2181
eradication of, problems with, 1048
ethnic factors in, 1059
exogenous versus endogenous, pathogenesis of, 1057–1058
extrapulmonary, 1075–1086
abdominal, 1084–1085
central nervous system, 1083–1084, *1084*
disseminated, 1076–1078
epidemiology of, 1075–1076, *1076*, *1077*
genitourinary, 1080–1081
in HIV infection, 1063, 1076, 1076t, 2182
lymphatic, 1078–1079, *1079*
pericardial, 1085–1086, *1086*
pleural, 1079–1080
sites of, 1076, *1076*, 1076t, *1077*
skeletal, 1081–1083, *1082*
genetic factors in, 1059
genitourinary, 1080–1081
history in, 1063
immune response to, 1057
immunization for, 1089–1090, 2185
in bone marrow transplantation, 2304
in children, treatment of, 1073–1074
in coal-workers' pneumoconiosis, 1830
in diabetes mellitus, 2310
in HIV infection, 744, 745t, 926, 1048, 2175, 2181–2185
CD4+ lymphocyte count in, 2182, 2182t
central nervous system, 1083
chest radiography in, 2182–2183, *2183*
clinical features of, 1063, 2181–2183, 2182t, *2183*
diagnosis of, 2183
differential diagnosis of, 1064, *1065*
disseminated (miliary), 1076 1077
epidemiology of, 1049–1050, *1050*, 1050t, 1058, 2181
extrapulmonary, 1063, 1076, 1076t, 2182
genitourinary tract, 1080–1081
immune response in, 1057
immunization for, 2185
latent, 1087
lymphatic, 1078–1079, *1079*
multidrug-resistant, 2181
prevention of, 2184–2185
progression of, 1058–1059
reinfection in, 1058
risk factors for, 1058
skin tests in, 1061–1062, *1062*, 2184–2185
sputum examination in, 760, 2177, 2183
transmission of, 1055
treatment of, 1069, 1072, 2183–2184
in lactation, 1074
in pneumoconiosis, 1816
in pregnancy, 1074, 2321
in silicosis, 1819, 1822, 1824
in transplantation, 2232
infectiousness of, 1053–1054
latent, treatment of, 1086–1090, *1087*
lymphatic, 1078–1079, *1079*, 2182, *2183*
mediastinal fibrosis in, 1367
mediastinitis in, 2110–2111
microbiologic diagnosis of, 616
miliary (disseminated), 1064, *1064*, 1076–1078
caseation necrosis in, *449*
computed tomography of, 675, *675*
mortality in, 1049, 1050, *1051*
central nervous system, 1084

Tuberculosis *(Continued)*
disseminated (miliary), 1078
multidrug-resistant, in HIV infection, 2181
prevention of, 1089
transmission risk and, 1054
treatment of, 1072–1073
natural history of, 1056, *1056*
organism causing *(Mycobacterium tuberculosis)*, characteristics of, 1048–1049
culture of, 618t, 619–620, 620t, 1044, 1047
exposure to, circumstances of, 1055
genome of, 1048–1049
in pleural fluid, 2006
polymerase chain reaction for, 2006
restriction fragment length polymorphism analysis of, 1047–1048, *1048*
transmission of, 1052–1055, *1053*
outbreaks of, environmental factors in, 1054–1055
pathogenesis of, 1055–1058, *1056*
disseminated (miliary), 1077
immune response to, 1057
in nonimmunized host, 1056
pericardial, 1085–1086
pleural, 1079
pericardial, 1085–1086, *1086*
physical examination in, 1063
pleural, 1079–1080
clinical manifestations of, 2021–2022, *2022*
computed tomography in, *687*
diagnosis of, 2022
effusion in, 2004, 2008–2009, 2021–2023, *2022*
*Mycobacterium tuberculosis* detection in, 2006
pathogenesis of, 2021
pleural fluid examination in, 2022
split pleura sign in, *687*, 688
treatment of, 2022–2023
pleural effusion in, 2004, 2021–2023, *2022*
biopsy in, 2008
interferon-τ in, 2006
pneumothorax in, 2050–2051
prevention of, immunization in, 1089–1090
in HIV infection, 2184–2185
multidrug-resistant, 1089
progression of, in HIV infection, 1058–1059
pulmonary, 1062–1075
bacteriologic evaluation of, 1065
chest radiography in, 1063–1065, *1063–1065*
diagnosis of, 1063–1065, *1063–1065*
history in, 1063
physical examination in, 1063
systemic effects of, 1062–1063
treatment of, 1065–1075, 1068t, 1069t, 1071t, 1073t
pulmonary circulation–systemic circulation communications in, 1566
pulmonary function testing in, precautions with, 860–861
reactivation, 1057–1058, 1064, *1064*
rehabilitation in, 2505–2506
reinfection in, 1058
resection in, 1075
resistance in. See also *Tuberculosis, multidrug-resistant.*
susceptibility testing in, 619
resurgence of, 1050
risk factors for, 1058–1059
sarcoidosis and, 1724, 1725
skeletal, 1081–1083, *1082*
skin tests for, 1059–1062, *1060*, 1061t, *1062*
in HIV infection, 2184–2185

Tuberculosis *(Continued)*
prophylactic drugs and, 1087–1088
sputum examination in, 608, 609t, 759–760, 1053–1054
in HIV infection, 2177, 2183
systemic effects of, 1062–1063
transmission of, 1052–1055, *1053*
environmental factors in, 1054–1055
exposure circumstances in, 1055
host factors in, 1055
prevention of, 1053
source case for, 1053–1054
terminology of, 1052
to household contacts, 1055, 1058
treatment of, 1065–1075
abdominal, 1085
adjunctive, 1075
central nervous system, 1084
compliance with, 1074
current drugs for, 1067, 1068t, 1069–1070, 1069t
drug-resistant, 1073, 1073t
evolution of, 1065–1067
failure of, 1072
for diagnostic purposes, 1065
genitourinary, 1081
importance of, 1074–1075
in children, 1073–1074
in HIV infection, 1072, 1087, 2183–2184
in lactation, 1074
in pregnancy, 1074
latent, 1086–1090, *1087*
lymphatic, 1079
multidrug-resistant, 1072–1073, 1073t
pericardial, 1086
prophylactic, 1088–1089
regimens for, 1070–1073, 1071t, 1073t, 1088
resection in, 1075
responsibility for, 1071
skeletal, 1083
supervision of, 1074
thoracoplasty in, 2363–2364, 2364t
transmission risk during, 1054
with associated conditions, 1074
with pleural effusion, 2022–2023
ventilation-perfusion scanning in, 712
versus histoplasmosis, 1111
versus melioidosis, 1028
Tuberous sclerosis, diffuse alveolar hemorrhage in, 1748
lung injury in, 481t
lymphangio(leio)myomatosis and, 1778, 1781
Tubular myelin. See *Myelin, tubular.*
Tularemia, 1028–1029
Tulobuterol, as bronchodilator, 270
Tumor(s). See also *Cancer;* specific tumor types and locations.
chylothorax in, 2056
embolism from, 1527
of bronchi, 1367, 1477, 1478
of heart, magnetic resonance imaging of, 673, *674*
of lung. See also *Lung cancer.*
benign, 1477–1484
classification of, 1477–1481
clear cell, 1479–1480
clinical manifestations of, 1477
etiology of, 1477
multiple parenchymal, 1478–1481, *1481*
pathology of, 484t
pseudotumors as, 1481, 1481t
solitary parenchymal, 1478–1480, *1479*
tracheobronchial, 1478

Tumor(s) *(Continued)*
sugar, 1479–1480
of mediastinum. See *Mediastinum, mass in.*
of pleura. See *Pleura, tumors of.*
of trachea, 1477, 1478
pulmonary circulation–systemic circulation communications in, 1566
thrombus from, chest radiography of, *655*
ventilation-perfusion scanning in, gallium, 701
Tumor markers, in pleural metastasis, 2074
Tumor necrosis factor-α, 501–502
action of, on alveolar macrophages, 394, *395*
as inflammatory mediator, 258, *258*
in influenza, 953
in malaria, 1146
in silicosis, 1819
in systemic sclerosis, 1692
of T lymphocytes, 432–434, *433*
pulmonary disease due to, 1978
receptor for, 238
Tumorlets, pulmonary, 1463–1464, 1480–1481
Tungsten carbide, in hard metal products, lung disease from, 1844–1845
Turbidity, of pleural fluid, 2003
Tussive agents, 252
TWAR strain of *Chlamydia*, 998t, 1026–1027
Tympanic membrane, otitis media effects on, 919
Tyrosine kinases, as receptors, 238–239, *239*
Tzanck test, in herpes simplex virus infections, 948
in varicella-zoster virus infections, 968

## U

Ulcer(s), herpetic, 947–949
in Behçet's disease, 1710, 1710t
in pharyngitis, 917
in tularemia, 1028–1029
Ulcerative colitis, pulmonary complications of, 2270–2271, 2270t
Ultrafiltration, in pulmonary edema, in heart failure, 2250
Ultrasonography, in biopsy guidance, 661, 2089
in thoracentesis, 660–661, *661*
indications for, 658–661
of aortic dissection, 683
of mediastinum, 2086, 2089
of pleural effusion, 2007
of venous thrombosis, 1508–1509, *1509*
Ultraviolet light, in *Mycobacterium tuberculosis* destruction, 1054–1055
Umbilical cord blood, transplantation of. See *Blood and bone marrow transplantation.*
Unconsciousness. See *Consciousness, alterations of.*
Unmyelinated receptors, in breathing control, 182, 182t, 183–184
Upper respiratory tract. See specific structures and diseases, e.g., *Larynx; Nose; Pharynx; Pharyngitis.*
Uranium exposure, lung cancer in, 1402
Urbach-Wiethe syndrome, 480t
Uremia, acidosis in, 167–168
pleural effusion in, 2034
thrombocytopenia in, 2295
Ureteroileostomy, hyperchloremic acidosis in, 170
Uridine triphosphate, in cystic fibrosis, 368
Urinary antigen test, for *Legionella*, 616, 1016
Urinary tract. See also *Genitourinary tract.*
obstruction of, pleural effusion in, 2034

Urination, problems with, at high altitude, 1942
Urine, analysis of, in tuberculosis, 1081
anion gap in, 170
buffers in, 162
pH of, in renal tubular acidosis, 168–169, 169t
testing of, in pneumonia, 609–610
Urinoma, pleural effusion in, 2034
U1-RNP antigen, antibodies to, in mixed connective tissue disease, 1708
Urokinase, in pleural effusion, 2019–2020
Usual interstitial pneumonia, 1652–1653, 1653t, *1654*, 1672t, 1677
Uveitis, in sarcoidosis, 1718
Uveoparotid fever, in sarcoidosis, 1718–1719
Uvulopalatopharyngoplasty, in sleep apnea, 2160
Uvulopalatoplasty, in sleep apnea, 2160

## V

$\dot{V}$. See *Ventilation, minute.*
$\dot{V}_A$. See *Alveolar ventilation.*
Vaccination. See *Immunization.*
Vagal reflex, activation of, in gastroesophageal reflux, 2268–2269
Vagus nerve, in airway regulation, *250*
in cough, 553, *554*
pulmonary stretch receptors leading to, 182–184, 182t, *183*
visceral pain pathways in, 569
Valacyclovir, in herpes simplex virus infections, 949
Valley fever. See *Coccidioidomycosis.*
Valsalva maneuver, diffusing capacity in, 815
in arteriovenous malformations, 1496
in diving, inner ear barotrauma in, 1957
Van Slyke method, for oxygen content, 833
Vanadium, exposure to, 1907
Vancomycin, in cystic fibrosis, 1309t
in pneumonia, 998t
in granulocytopenia, 924–925, 925t
pneumococcal, 1001
Vanishing lung syndrome, in systemic lupus erythematosus, 1704, *1704*
Vanishing lung tumor, 1481
Variant angina, 578
Varicella-zoster virus infections, 931t, 967–968, *968*
in transplantation, 2232
pneumonia due to, in bone marrow transplantation, 2302–2303
in HIV infection, 2203
in pregnancy, 2321
Varices, esophageal, sclerotherapy for, pleural effusion in, 2030
pulmonary disease due to, 1989
Vascular cell adhesion molecule, in asthma, 1261
Vascular endothelial growth factor, in angiogenesis, in lung cancer, 1387
Vascular occlusive disease, ventilation-perfusion scanning in, 697
Vascular pharmacology. See *Pulmonary circulation, pharmacology of.*
Vasculitis. See also *Arteritis*; *Capillaritis.*
pulmonary, 1533–1542
classification of, 1533–1534, 1536, 1536t
clinical features of, 1535
diagnosis of, 1535
epidemiology of, 1534
etiology of, 1534–1535
giant cell (temporal) arteritis as, 1541
in anaphylactoid purpura, 1539
Vasculitis *(Continued)*
in Behçet's syndrome, 1541–1542, 1710
in bronchocentric granulomatosis, 1538–1539
in Churg-Strauss syndrome, 1538
in dermatomyositis, 1540
in eosinophilia-myalgia syndrome, 1542
in essential mixed cryoglobulinemia, 1539
in fat embolism, 1526
in Hughes-Stovin syndrome, 1542
in lymphoid granulomatosis, 1537–1538
in mixed connective tissue disease, 1540, *1541*
in necrotizing sarcoid granulomatosis, 1538
in polymyositis, 1540
in progressive systemic sclerosis, 1539–1540, *1540*
in relapsing polychondritis, 1709
in rheumatoid arthritis, 1539, 1701
in systemic lupus erythematosus, 1539
in Wegener's granulomatosis, 1536–1537, *1537*
leukocytoclastic, 1534, 1539
pathogenesis of, 1534–1535
pathology of, 468, 1534
polyarteritis nodosa as, 1540–1541
Takayasu's disease as, 1541
terminology of, 1533
treatment of, 1536
ventilation-perfusion scanning in, 704, *710*
Vasoactive intestinal peptide, actions of, 250, *250*, *251*
in bronchodilation, 256
in mucus secretion regulation, 332, 333
Vasoactivity. See also *Vasoconstriction; Vasodilation.*
evaluation of, 299
of arachidonic acid metabolites, 497–499, 497t
of pulmonary circulation, 297–298
Vasoconstriction, endothelin in, 298
in brain, at high altitude, 1923
in chronic obstructive pulmonary disease, 1633
in diving, 1953
in high-altitude pulmonary edema, 1935
in hyperventilation, 2148
in hypoxia. See *Hypoxia and hypoxemia, pulmonary vasoconstriction in.*
in pulmonary embolism, 1505–1506
pulmonary hypertension in, 1492, 1492t, 1544–1546, 1643
regulation of, 131–132
reversal of. See *Vasodilation.*
ventilation-perfusion scanning in, 697
Vasoconstrictive pulmonary hypertension, 1543, 1544
Vasoconstrictors, in allergic rhinitis, 1349
in bronchoscopy, 732
Vasodilation, in asthma, 1254
in hepatopulmonary syndrome, 2272, *2272*, 2274
reversal of. See *Vasoconstriction.*
Vasodilator(s), 299–302. See also specific substances.
adrenergic antagonists and agonists as, 300
alkalinizing, 299–300
arachidonic acid metabolites as, 300–301
calcium channel blockers as, 300
directly acting, 301
in cor pulmonale, 1644
in portopulmonary hypertension, 2275
in pulmonary edema, 1601–1602, 1611
high-altitude, 1936, 1937
Vasodilator(s) *(Continued)*
in pulmonary hypertension, 1551, 1644
nitric oxide as. See *Nitric oxide.*
nitroso compounds as, 301–302
nonspecificity of, 299
oxygen as, 299
prostaglandins as, 1645–1646
Vasomotor rhinitis, 1347, 1348
Vaso-occlusive disease, diffuse alveolar hemorrhage in, 1744, *1745*, 1746
drug-induced, 479t
in bone marrow transplantation, 2301
in leukemia, 2291
in sickle cell disease, 2287
pulmonary venous, 1549–1550
ventilation-perfusion scanning in, 697
Vasopressin. See *Antidiuretic hormone.*
Vasospasm, angiography of, *647*
VC. See *Vital capacity.*
$\dot{V}CO_2$. See *Carbon dioxide, production of.*
$\dot{V}_D$ (dead space ventilation). See *Dead space.*
$\dot{V}_E$. See *Ventilation, minute.*
Vegetable dusts, byssinosis due to, 1860–1862
Vena cava, inferior, filter in, for pulmonary embolism prevention, 1517, *1518*
superior, obstruction of. See *Superior vena cava syndrome.*
Venography, in venous thrombosis, 1508, *1508*, 2322
Veno-occlusive disease, pulmonary, diffuse alveolar hemorrhage in, 1744, *1745*, 1746
drug-induced, 479t
Venous return control, in respiratory failure, 2386–2389
cardiac function curves in, 2387–2388, *2387*, *2388*
extracardiac pressure in, 2388–2389, *2388*, 2389t, *2390*
Venous thromboembolism, deep. See *Deep vein thrombosis.*
diagnosis of, 1508–1509, *1508*, *1509*, 1513–1514, *1514*
in pregnancy, 1514
natural history of, 1504–1505
pathogenesis of, 1504
prevention of, 1514–1515
pulmonary embolism as complication of, 1508. See also *Pulmonary embolism.*
risk factors for, 1504, 1505t
treatment of, 1515–1517, *1518*
Virchow's triad in, 1504
Ventilation, 55–60. See also *Breathing; Hyperventilation; Hypoventilation.*
alveolar. See *Alveolar ventilation.*
anatomic aspects of, 55–57, *56*
anesthesia and analgesia effects on, 884–885
at high altitude, in exercise, 1925–1926, *1926*
capacity for, maximum sustained, in chronic obstructive pulmonary disease, 216
control of. See *Breathing, control of.*
dead space in. See *Dead space.*
distribution of, 59, *59*, 109–111, *110*, 805–808
abnormal, 805, *806*
in airway obstruction, 805, *806*, 808
in airway resistance, 698
in heart disease, 2257, *2258*
in obstructive disorders, 808
in restrictive disorders, 808
in smoking, 808
physiology of, 805, *806*
resident gas, single-breath test for, 805–807, *807*, 876
tests for, 805–808, *806*, *807*, 876

Ventilation *(Continued)*
versus pleural pressure, 806, *807*
efficiency of, in exercise, 839
impaired, dyspnea in, 545t
respiratory acidosis in, 173–174, 173t
in asthma, 218
in chronic obstructive pulmonary disease, 212–220, *213–215*, *217*
in exercise. See *Exercise, ventilation in.*
in fibrothorax, 2063
in heart disease, in exercise, 2258–2259, 2259t
in highly fit athletes, 218–220
in interstitial pulmonary fibrosis, 217–218
in metabolic acidosis, 161
in metabolic alkalosis, 161
inequality of, 58–60, *59*. See *Ventilation-perfusion ratio, inequality of.*
inspection of, 597
inspiratory muscle force and, *214*
lung volume and. See *Lung volume(s).*
maximal voluntary. See *Maximal voluntary ventilation.*
maximum sustained capacity for, in chronic obstructive pulmonary disease, 216
mechanical. See *Mechanical ventilation.*
minute, carbon dioxide production and, 156–157, *157*, 212
equation for, 180, *181*
in alveolar proteinosis, 1795
in chronic obstructive pulmonary disease, 212
in high altitude acclimatization, 1917, *1917*
in highly fit athletes, 218–219
in kyphoscoliosis, 2361, 2361t
in pregnancy, 2318, *2318*
increased, causes of, 2449
resting, 822
versus respiratory muscle oxygen uptake, in highly fit athletes, 219
neuromuscular disorders affecting. See *Neuromuscular disorder(s).*
obstructive diseases of. See *Obstructive disease(s);* specific diseases.
paradoxical, respiratory acidosis in, 173–174
regulation of. See *Breathing, control of.*
requirements for, in exercise, 208–210, *209*
resting, measurement of, 822
restrictive disorders of. See *Restrictive ventilatory disorder(s).*
stimulation of, 289–290, 543
support of. See *Mechanical ventilation.*
terminology of, 2563–2564
threshold of, in exercise, 840
total, 58
in exercise, 209
versus carbon dioxide partial pressure, 190–191, *191*
versus oxygen partial pressure, 191–192, *192*
versus oxygen uptake, 839, *839*
wasted, definition of, 2564
dyspnea in, 545t
in exercise, 839, 844
in pulmonary hypertension, 1494
in ventilation-perfusion inequality, 83, 85
Ventilation-perfusion ratio, 76–85, 821–829
analysis of, 700
assessment of, 78–81, *79*, *81*, *82*
at high altitude, 1919
hemodynamics of, 1920–1921, *1921*
Bohr's equation and, 822
calculation of, 77
carbon dioxide retention and, 83, 85
definition of, 821

Ventilation-perfusion ratio *(Continued)*
distribution of, 80–85, *81*, *82*, *84*, 828–829, *829*
in asthma, 218
in elderly persons, 82
in mechanical ventilation, 2476, *2476*, 2482
in normal lung, 78, *78*
in pulmonary edema, 1935
in pulmonary embolism, 1511–1512, *1511*, *1512*
in pulmonary fibrosis, 1673–1675
in pulmonary hypertension, 1521
inequality of, 822
after lung transplantation, 716–718, *717*
airway closure and, 59–60
assessment of, 78–81, *79*, *81*, *82*. See also *Ventilation-perfusion scanning.*
beta$_2$-adrenergic agonist-induced, 271
blood gases in, 821t
differential diagnosis of, 704, *706–710*, 710t
historical view of, 76–77
in asthma, 1265
in bronchiectasis, 1327
in bronchoscopy, 728
in chronic obstructive pulmonary disease, *706*, *707*
in compression, 704
in consolidative state, 697
in diaphragmatic paralysis, 2335
in diffuse disease, 711
in emphysema, 223–224
in exercise, 211–212, 216
in hemodialysis, 2280
in hepatopulmonary syndrome, 2274
in highly fit athletes, 219
in HIV infection, 711–712, *712*
in interstitial pulmonary disease, 225–226, 713
in kyphoscoliosis, 2360
in lung disease, 82–84, *82*, *84*
in near drowning, 1964
in normal lung, 78, *78*, 111
in obstructive disease, 697–698
in occlusive disease, 697
in *Pneumocystis carinii* pneumonia, 711–712, *712*
in pneumonia, 712
in pulmonary embolism, 701–709, 705t, *706–710*, 710t, 1511–1512, *1511*, *1512*
in restrictive disease, 698
in sarcoidosis, 713, *714*
in sickle cell disease, 2289
in tuberculosis, 712
in tumor embolism, 710–711
large, 705t
nontopographic, 60
pathophysiology of, 697–698, 700–701
physiologic implications of, 111
reverse mismatch in, 699
segmental contour pattern in, 710–711
small, 705t
stripe sign in, 710, *711*
topographic, 59, *59*
versus cardiac output, 85
versus right-to-left shunt, 826–827, 827t
wasted ventilation in, 823–824
measurement of, 822–829
alveolar air equation in, 824
alveolar ventilation calculation in, 824–825
anatomic dead space in, 822–823, *823*
Bohr's equation and, 822
insoluble gases in, 827–829, *828*, *829*
physiologic dead space in, 823–824

Ventilation-perfusion ratio *(Continued)*
preoperative, 889–890
pulmonary blood flow in, 825
respiratory dead space in, 822
resting, 822
venous-to-arterial shunt calculation in, 825–827, *826*, 826t, 827t
normal, 81–82, *82*, 821, 1511, *1511*
regional differences in. See *Ventilation-perfusion ratio, inequality of.*
resting, 822
theoretical aspects of, 821–822, 821t
versus carbon dioxide concentration, 77–78, *77*, *78*
versus oxygen concentration, 77–78, *77*, *78*
versus position, 2433
Ventilation-perfusion scanning, 78–81, *79*, *81*, *82*, 697–723, 822, 827–829, *828*, *829*
aerosols for, 357, *358*, 699–700
after lung transplantation, 716–718, *717*
analysis of, 700
clearance time in, 698, 700
compliance and, 698
gallium 67, 700–701
in interstitial pneumonitis, 713
in lymphoma, 716
in *Pneumocystis carinii* pneumonia, 711–712, *712*
in sarcoidosis, 713, *714*
in tuberculosis, 712
in chronic obstructive pulmonary disease, 699–700
in consolidative state, 697
in differential diagnosis of lung diseases, 704, 705t, *706–710*, 710t
in epithelial permeability studies, 718–720, *719*
in HIV infection, 711–712, *712*
in Hodgkin's disease, 716
in immunodeficiency, 711–712, *712*
in interstitial pneumonitis, 713
in lung cancer, diagnostic, 715–716, *716*
for surgical planning, 713–715
in lung metabolism studies, 720
in lung volume reduction surgery, 715
in lymphoma, 716
in obstructive state, 697–698
in PIOPED study, 703–704, 705t
in *Pneumocystis carinii* pneumonia, 711–712, *712*
in pneumonia, 712
in pulmonary embolism, 699, 701–709, 705t, *706–710*, 710t, 1511–1512, *1511*, *1512*
in pulmonary hypertension, 1521, 1548–1549, *1549*
in restrictive state, 698
in sarcoidosis, 713, *714*
in shunt detection, in arteriovenous malformations, 1562
in tuberculosis, 712
in tumors, 701
in vascular occlusive state, 697
krypton 81m in, 714–715
matched defects in, 699
pathophysiologic basis for, 698
patterns in, 710–711, *711*
normal, 697, 704, 705t, *706*, 1511, *1511*
positions for, 700
preoperative, 713–715
quantitative, 700
radiopharmaceuticals for, 698–700
thrombus-avid, 718
resistance and, 698
reverse mismatch in, 699
screening, in pulmonary embolism, 701

Ventilation-perfusion scanning *(Continued)*
signs in, 710–711, *711*
technetium 99m compounds in, 698–700
in epithelial permeability studies, 718–720, *719*
in interstitial pneumonitis, 713
in sarcoidosis, 713
peptide type, 718
techniques for, 698–700
in epithelial permeability studies, 718, *719*
perfusion component, 702–703
ventilation component, 703
with gallium, 701
thallium 201, 718
ventilation component of, radiopharmaceuticals for, 699–700
views for, 698–699
xenon, 699
of pulmonary blood flow distribution, 64
of ventilation inequality, 60
quantitative, 700
Ventilators. See *Mechanical ventilation.*
Ventilatory drive, assessment of, 817–818, 2333–2334, 2344–2345, *2345*, *2346*
central nervous system in. See *Central nervous system, in breathing control.*
disorders of. See *Breathing, periodic; Sleep apnea, central.*
excessive. See *Hyperventilation.*
factors affecting, 782
in dyspnea, 545t, 548
in neuromuscular disorders, 2331, 2333–2334, 2344–2345, *2345*, *2346*
in quadriplegia, 2331
oxygen and, 2446–2447
reduced. See *Hypoventilation.*
Ventilatory equivalent(s), in exercise testing, 844
Ventilatory equivalent for carbon dioxide, in exercise, in emphysema, *222*, 223
in highly fit athletes, 218
in pulmonary disease, 211–212
moderate, 210
in interstitial pulmonary disease, *223*, 225–226
Ventilatory equivalent for oxygen, in exercise, at high altitude, 1926, *1926*
in emphysema, *222*, 223
in interstitial pulmonary disease, *223*, 225
Ventilatory failure. See also *Respiratory failure.*
acidemia in, 2444
acute-on-chronic. See *Respiratory failure, acute-on-chronic.*
assessment of, for mechanical ventilation, 2452, 2452t
clinical features of, 2345
definition of, 2443
harbingers of, 2345, *2345*, *2346*
hemodynamic consequences of, 2452–2453
hypercapnia in, 2443–2445
hypoxemia in, 2444
in asthma. See *Status asthmaticus.*
in botulism, 2342–2343
in chronic obstructive pulmonary disease, 1228–1229
in impaired respiratory drive, 2445–2447, *2445*, *2446*
in increased load, 2445, *2445*, 2447–2449, *2448*
in myasthenia gravis, 2342
in neuromuscular disorders, 2344–2345, *2345*, *2346*, 2445–2447, *2445*, *2446*
mechanical abnormalities in, 2444
metabolic alkalosis in, 2444–2445
Ventilatory failure *(Continued)*
monitoring during, 2449–2452, *2450*, *2451*
multifactorial, 2449
pathophysiology of, 2445–2449, *2445*, *2446*, *2448*
treatment of, 2345–2349
supportive, 2346–2349
underlying disease treatment in, 2345–2346
versus hypoxemic respiratory failure, 2379–2381, 2382t
Ventilatory reserve, definition of, 2563
Ventilatory support. See *Mechanical ventilation.*
Ventral respiratory group, of medulla, 185–186, *185*
Ventricle(s), left, dysfunction/failure of, in cor pulmonale, 1193, 1636
in respiratory failure, 2389–2393, *2391*, *2392*, 2393t
in sleep apnea, 2159
right, anatomy of, 1634–1635, *1635*
dysfunction/failure of, in cor pulmonale, 1635–1636, *1635*, *1636*
in pulmonary embolism, 1507
shock in, 2403–2404
hypertrophy of, in pulmonary hypertension, 1548
single, therapeutic respiratory acidosis in, 298
Ventricular septal defects, drug management of, 298
Venules, high endothelial, 416
pulmonary, pressure in, 1498t
Verapamil, as vasodilator, 300
Vermiculite pneumoconiosis, 1841
Vertigo, alternobaric, 1956–1957
Very late activation molecule, in asthma, 1261
Vesicles, fluid and solute transport in, 138t
herpes simplex virus in, 947
receptor tyrosine kinase internalization in, 239
Vesicular breath sounds, 593, *593*, 598
Vesiculoulcerative pharyngitis, 933, *934*
Vessel compression, alveolar pressure and, 126
Vestibular dysfunction, in decompression sickness, 1961
Veterans, impairment and disability evaluation of, 902, 903t
$\dot{V}_E/\dot{V}_{CO_2}$. See *Ventilatory equivalent for carbon dioxide.*
Video-thoracoscopy, in pneumothorax, 2048
Vinblastine, in lung cancer, 1438
radiation therapy with, 1434
pulmonary disease due to, 1978
Vinculin, in fluid and solute exchange, *134–135*
Vinorelbine, in lung cancer, 1437, 1437t
Vinyl chloride exposure, lung cancer in, 1402
Viral infection(s), 929–984. See also specific infections.
after lung transplantation, 2522
as asthma risk, 1251, *1251*
asthma triggering in, 1176
bronchiolitis as, 935–937, *936*
bronchitis as, 934
chronic obstructive pulmonary disease development after, 1207–1208
clinical manifestations of, 932
common cold as, 932–933, *932*
croup as, 935, *936*
host response to, 932
immune response in, 2226, *2228*
immunity to, 930
in bone marrow transplantation, 1364
in HIV infection, 2202–2203
Viral infection(s) *(Continued)*
in transplantation, 2229–2232, 2230t
influenza-like illness as, 935
laryngitis as, 934
outbreaks of, 930
pathogenesis of, 930–932
pharyngitis as, 933–934, 933t, *934*
pleural effusion in, 2024–2025
pneumonia as. See *Pneumonia, viral.*
significance of, 930
systemic, with respiratory involvement, 930
transmission of, 930
viral classification and, 930, 931t
Virchow's triad, 1504
Virtues, physician, 2492
Virulence factors, of bacteria, pneumonia and, 986
Virus(es). See also *Viral infection(s);* specific viruses and infections.
characteristics of, 930–932, 931t
chemokine receptor interactions with, 512
surfactant protein A binding to, 312
surfactant protein D binding to, 315
Viscera, innervation of, 569
Visceral larva migrans, 1157
Visceral pain, neurobiology of, 568–575
hyperalgesia and, 570–573, *571*, *572*
modulation and, 574–575
peripheral mechanisms in, 569–570
sensory neurons and, 573
somatic versus visceral pain in, 568–569, 572–574
spinal mechanisms in, 573–574, *574*
Visceroparietal reactions, in asbestos exposure, 1837, *1838*, 1839
Viscoelasticity, of respiratory system, 95
Viscosity, of blood, versus pulmonary vascular resistance, 126–127, *128*
of mucus, 363–364
Visual Analogue Scale, for chest pain, 568
for dyspnea, 544, *545*, 845
Vital capacity, after heart surgery, 2253, 2253t
after thoracoplasty, 2364
as ventilatory failure indicator, 2345
at high altitude, 1918–1919
"combined," 790
decreased, causes of, 791
definition of, 57, *57*, 783, *783*, 2563
in acromegaly, 2313
in acute inflammatory polyneuropathy, 2341–2342
in airway obstruction, for reversibility evaluation, 851
in alveolar proteinosis, 1795
in ankylosing spondylitis, 2369
in chronic obstructive pulmonary disease, 1191, 1207
in cystic fibrosis, 1304, 1304t
in diaphragmatic paralysis, 2336, 2336t
in disease states, mechanical aspects of, 112
in exercise, 217
in flail chest, 2367, 2367t
in heart disease, 2251, *2251*, 2252t, 2256, 2256t
in hyperthyroidism, 2310
in impairment and disability evaluation, 850t
in interstitial lung disease, 1662, *1664*, 1696
in isovolume pressure-flow relationships, 787–788, *787*
in kyphoscoliosis, 2358–2359, 2359t
in neuromuscular disorders, 2344, *2344*, *2345*
in pneumothorax, 2044–2045, *2044*
in poliomyelitis, 2340, 2341t
in pulmonary fibrosis, 1679
in respiratory muscle fatigue, 2383

Vital capacity *(Continued)*
in respiratory muscle weakness, 859
in spinal cord injury, 2339, 2339t
in systemic sclerosis, 1696
in ventilation distribution evaluation, 807
maximal expiratory flow and, 98, *99*, *100*, 101–102
measurement of, 785–787, 785t, *786*, 874, 790–791
normal, *57*
"slow," 791
versus position, 2252t
Vitamin(s), deficiency of, in cystic fibrosis, 1306
supplementation with, in cystic fibrosis, 1311
Vitamin A, deficiency of, congenital defects in, 38–39
lung cancer and, 1385
lung injury in, 486
in lung cancer prevention, 1404–1405
Vitamin $B_6$ deficiency, lung injury in, 486
Vitamin C, in lung cancer prevention, 1405
Vitamin D deficiency, lung injury in, 486
Vitamin E, lung cancer and, 1385, 1405
Vitronectin, in fluid and solute exchange, *134–135*
$\dot{V}_{max}$ (maximal expiratory flow), 98, *99*, *100*, 101
in chronic obstructive pulmonary disease, 102–103
$\dot{V}O_2$. See *Oxygen uptake*.
Vocal cords, bronchoscopy of, 732
burn injury of, 754
disorders of, 1353–1354
dysfunction of, versus asthma, 1269, 1353–1354
Vocal disorders, in pneumomediastinum, 2102
Voice-generated sounds, auscultation of, 598
Volume body plethysmography, in lung volume measurement, 794, *794*
Volume density, in lung quantitative morphology, 25, *28*, 29
Volume of distribution, of drugs, 248
Volume-pressure relationships. See *Pressure-volume relationships*.
Voluntary pressure breathing, pneumomediastinum in, 2099–2100
Volutrauma. See also *Barotrauma*.
in mechanical ventilation, 2424
Vomiting, Boerhaave's syndrome in, 2106–2107, *2107*
laryngeal function in, 1351
metabolic alkalosis in, 162, 171–173, 171t
pneumomediastinum in, 2100
von Recklinghausen's disease. See *Neurofibromatosis*.
von Willebrand's disease, 2294–2295
VR (ventilatory reserve), definition of, 2563
VT. See *Tidal volume*.
$V_t$ (electrical potential difference), of epithelium, 335

## W

Waldenström's macroglobulinemia, 1464, 2294
Walk tests, 841
Warfare, toxic agents used in, 1906–1907
Warfarin, hemothorax due to, 2062
in pulmonary hypertension, 1551
in thromboembolic disease prevention, 1514–1515, 1519
Wasting, in histoplasmosis, 1114
Water, aerosol, behavior of, 351–352
contamination of, hypersensitivity pneumonitis due to, 1868, 1878
Water *(Continued)*
diving in. See *Diving*.
drowning in. See *Drowning; Near drowning*.
endothelial permeability to, 144
in lung, normal content of, 132
in mucus, 327
in vapor form, oxygen partial pressure in, 70
partial pressure of, in pulmonary capillaries, 2047
*Legionella* transmitted in, 1014, 1017
transport of, mucociliary, 362
through airway epithelia, 338
Water lily sign, in hydatid cyst rupture, 1158, 1159
Waterfall effect, in pulmonary circulation three-zone model, 65
Weakness. See also *Neuromuscular disorder(s)*.
dyspnea at rest in, 220
in bronchiectasis, 1327
in carcinoid tumor, 1461
in chronic obstructive pulmonary disease, 848
in dermatomyositis, 1706–1707
in heart failure, 2255–2256, 2256t
in pulmonary hypertension, 1546
respiratory failure in, 2447
versus fatigue, 109, 2345
Wedge pressure, pulmonary. See *Pulmonary artery wedge pressure*.
Wegener's granulomatosis, 1536–1537, *1537*
diffuse alveolar hemorrhage in, 1737t, 1738–1739
pseudotumors in, 1481
versus lymphomatoid granulomatosis, 1458
Weibel model, of airway system, 56, *56*, 94
Weight, excessive. See *Obesity*.
Weight loss, in alveolar proteinosis, 1794
in bronchiectasis, 1327
in carcinoid tumor, 1461
in chronic obstructive pulmonary disease, 1227–1228, 2510
in histoplasmosis, 2198
in mediastinal mass, 2083
in obesity, 2373
in pneumonia, *Actinomyces*, 1021
eosinophilic, 1767
*Nocardia*, 1022
in tuberculosis, 1062–1063
Weightlessness, pulmonary circulation effects of, 66
Welding fumes, acute lung injury from, 1906
cadmium exposure in, 1907
lung cancer from, 1403
pneumoconiosis from, *1814*
Westermark's sign, in pulmonary embolism, 1510
Western blot test, for HIV infection, 2173
Western red cedar dust, asthma due to, 1857
Wheezing, 594, *594*
definition of, 595–596
differential diagnosis of, 1268, 1269t
generation of, 596
in acute respiratory distress syndrome, 2417
in aspergillosis, 1131
in asthma, 1248, 1250, *1250*, 1251, 1256, 1266–1269
occupational, 1856, 1859
in bronchial disorders, 1368
in cor pulmonale, 1637
in cystic fibrosis, 1302
in lung cancer, 1420
in pulmonary edema, 1591
in pulmonary hypertension, 1637
in sarcoidosis, 1718
in strongyloidiasis, 1151–1152
in toxocariasis, 1157
Whipp ramp slope method, for exercise testing, 843
White blood cells. See *Leukocyte(s)*.
Whooping cough, 560
Wide dynamic range cells, in spinal cord, 573
Williams-Campbell syndrome, 480t
Window width and window level, in computed tomography, 661
Wiskott-Aldrich syndrome, 2240
Withdrawal, from corticosteroids, 282
Wood dust, pulmonary fibrosis due to, 1677
Wood's classification, of pulmonary hypertension, 1492, 1492t
Woolsorter's disease, 1029, 2109
Work, in mechanical ventilation, 2478–2479, *2479*, *2480*
of breathing. See *Breathing, work of*.
Workers' compensation, evaluation for, 895, 898, 902
Workplace. See *Occupation(s)*; *Occupational and environmental disorder(s)*.
World Health Organization, lung cancer classification of, 483t–484t, 1417, 1418t, 1419
Worm infection(s). See *Nematode infection(s)*; *Platyhelminth infection(s)*.
Wright respirometer, 822
*Wuchereria bancrofti* infections, 1153–1155, *1154*, 1761–1762, *1762*

## X

Xanthines(s), theophylline as. See *Theophylline*.
Xanthoma(s), of lung, 1480
Xenon studies, of differential lung function, 889–890
of pulmonary blood flow distribution, 64
of ventilation inequality, 59, 699, 700, 827–829, *828*, *829*
Xerotrachea, in Sjögren's syndrome, 366, 1706
X-linked disorder(s), 45
agammaglobulinemia as, 2233t, 2234–2235
chronic granulomatous disease as, 2237
hypogammaglobulinemia with hyperimmunoglobulin M as, 2236
severe combined immunodeficiency as, 2233t, 2239
Wiskott-Aldrich syndrome as, 2240
X-rays, in computed tomography, 661
of chest. See *Chest radiography*.
Xyphodynia, 577

## Y

Yeasts. See also *Fungal infection(s);* specific fungi.
alveolar macrophage protection against, 390, *391*, 392
Yellow-nail syndrome, bronchiectasis with, 1337
lung injury in, 480t
pleural effusion in, 2035
*Yersinia pestis* infection, pneumonia due to, 1029
Young's syndrome, lung injury in, 482

## Z

Zafirlukast, allergic granulomatosis and angiitis due to, 1770–1771
in asthma, 285, 498

Zafirlukast *(Continued)*
pulmonary disease due to, 1984
Zanamivir, in influenza, 359, 957
Ziehl-Neelsen stain, for *Mycobacterium*, 1043, *1044*, 1046
Zileuton, in asthma, 285, 498
Zinc chloride, exposure to, 1907
Zinc fingers, in receptors, 241
Zinostatin, pulmonary disease due to, 1978
Zoonosis(es), anthrax as, 1029
brucellosis as, 1030
hantavirus infections as, 471, 945–947, 2025, 2321
influenza as, 950
*Pasteurella multocida* infections as, 1028
plague as, 1029
psittacosis as, 998t, 1026
Q fever as, 473, 998t, 1025–1206
Zoonosis(es) *(Continued)*
*Rhodococcus equi* infections as, 620–621, 1030, 2180–2181
tularemia as, 1028–1029
Zoster. See *Herpes zoster.*
Zygomycosis. See *Mucormycosis.*
Zygomycosis (mucormycosis), culture in, 622
microbiologic diagnosis of, 610t

ISBN 0-7216-7713-4

90038

9 780721 677132